HANDBOOK OF LABORATORY AND DIAGNOSTIC TESTS

with Nursing Implications

FOURTH EDITION

Joyce LeFever Kee, RN, MSN
Associate Professor Emerita
College of Health and Nursing Science
University of Delaware

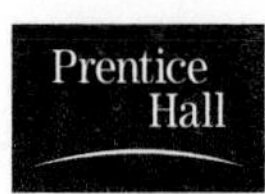
Prentice
Hall

Prentice Hall, Upper Saddle River, New Jersey 07458

Library of Congress Cataloging-in-Publication Data

Kee, Joyce LeFever.
Handbook of laboratory and diagnostic tests : with nursing implications / Joyce LeFever Kee.—4th ed.
p. cm.
Rev. ed. of: Handbook of laboratory diagnostic tests with nursing implications. 3rd ed. ©1998.
Includes bibliographical references and index.
ISBN 0-13-030517-0
1. Diagnosis, Laboratory—Handbooks, manuals, etc. 2. Diagnosis, Noninvasive—Handbooks, manuals, etc. 3. Nursing—Handbooks, manuals, etc.
I. Kee, Joyce LeFever. Handbook of laboratory diagnostic tests with nursing implications. II. Title.
[DNLM: 1. Laboratory Techniques and Procedures—Handbooks.
2. Laboratory Techniques and Procedures—Nurses' Instruction. 3. Diagnostic Tests, Routine—Handbooks. 4. Diagnostic Tests, Routine—Nurses' instruction.
QY 39 K26h 2001]
RB38.2.K44 2001
616.07'56—dc21

00-058900

Acquisitions Editor: Nancy Anselment
Executive Editor: Maura Connor
Production Editor: Marianne Hutchinson (Pine Tree Composition)
Director of Manufacturing and Production: Bruce Johnson
Managing Editor: Patrick Walsh
Manufacturing Buyer: Ilene Sanford
Project Liaison: Janet Bolton
Art Director: Marianne Frasco
Marketing Manager: Kristin Walton
Editorial Assistant: Beth Ann Romph
Cover Art: Images.com, Teofilo Olivieri
Composition: Pine Tree Composition, Inc.
Printing and Binding: R.R. Donnelley, Harrisonburg

Prentice Hall International (UK) Limited, *London*
Prentice Hall of Australia Pty. Limited, *Sydney*
Prentice Hall Canada, Inc., *Toronto*
Prentice Hall Hispanoamericana, S.A., *Mexico*
Prentice Hall of India Private Limited, *New Delhi*
Prentice Hall of Japan, Inc., *Tokyo*
Prentice Hall Singapore Pte. Ltd.
Editora Prentice Hall do Brasil Ltda., *Rio de Janeiro*

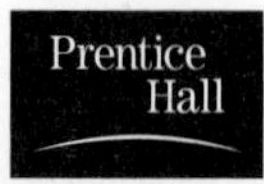
Prentice
Hall

10 9 8 7 6 5 4 3
ISBN 0-13-030517-0

I dedicate this book in loving memory of my second mother

Ruth L. LeFever

CONTENTS

Preface *ix*

Acknowledgments *xiii*

Contributors and Consultants *xv*

PART ONE

Considerations for Use of Laboratory Tests 1

List of Laboratory Tests 4

Laboratory Tests 8

PART TWO

Considerations for Use of Diagnostic Tests 315

List of Diagnostic Tests 317

Diagnostic Tests 319

APPENDIX A

Laboratory Test Values for Adults and Children 449

APPENDIX B

Clinical Problems with Laboratory and Diagnostic Tests 475

APPENDIX C

Therapeutic Drug Monitoring (TDM) 479

Bibliography *489*

Index *495*

PREFACE

Each day hundreds of thousands of laboratory and diagnostic tests are performed. Longevity and high technology promote the use of sensitive tests to monitor all clients' well-being and to make specific diagnoses.

As a health provider, you have the critical responsibility of staying current with the many facets of high-quality client care. The *Handbook of Laboratory and Diagnostic Tests with Nursing Implications,* 4th edition, gives information about the commonly ordered laboratory and diagnostic tests, along with nursing implications and client teaching. It gives quick, pertinent information about the tests, emphasizing their purposes, the procedures, the clinical problems associated with disease entities and drugs related to abnormal test results, as well as nursing implications together with client teaching. Reference values are given for children, adults, and the elderly.

Because the reference text is a handbook in pocket form, it can be easily carried to clinical settings. This text is appropriate for students in various types of nursing and non-nursing programs, including medical technology programs, baccalaureate and nursing programs, associate degree programs, diploma programs, and practical nursing programs. This book is most valuable to the nurse practitioner, registered nurse, and licensed practical nurse in hospital settings, including specialty areas such as intensive care units, emergency rooms, clinics, health care provider offices, and independent nursing practices.

THE FOURTH EDITION

The fourth edition of the handbook lists more than 400 laboratory and diagnostic tests, including 26 new tests that have been added to this edition. These are the major additions and revisions:

- New laboratory and diagnostic tests have been added, such as atrial natriuretic hormone; hemoglobin A_1c; international normalized ratio (INR); mumps antibody, rabies antibody, toxoplasmosis antibody, rotavirus antigen, and other antibody and antigen tests; opiates detection; prealbumin assay; platelet aggregation and

adhesions; glucose self-monitoring devices; glucagon; viral culture; biopsy (bone marrow, breast, endometrial tissue, kidney, and liver); bone densitometry; cervicography; colposcopy; hysteroscopy; and many more.
- Lists of all laboratory and diagnostic tests with page numbers are found at the beginning of Part One, Laboratory Tests, and Part Two, Diagnostic Tests.
- Laboratory test values have been updated, as needed, to current values. Reference values may differ among institutions. These values are guidelines; persons should check with their institutions' laboratory policies and reference values for the tests.
- Latest tests for human immunosuppressive virus-type (HIV-1 and HIV-2) have been included.
- Updated data are given for diagnostic tests: magnetic resonance imaging (MRI), gastric analysis, nuclear scans, various stress/exercise tests (treadmill exercise ECG, exercise myocardial perfusion imaging test [thallium/technetium stress test], nuclear persantine stress test, nuclear dobutamine stress test), Pap smear, positron emission tomography (PET), echocardiography, Holter monitoring, pulmonary function tests, and ultrasonography.
- Factors affecting laboratory tests and diagnostic tests have been added.
- Client teaching has been added to Nursing Implications for all laboratory and diagnostic tests.
- Appendix A has been updated with current laboratory test values and added reference values for new tests. Appendix B has also been updated with new laboratory and diagnostic tests for previous health problems and two additional health problems: pregnancy and fetal distress; and gynecologic problems.
- Updated laboratory and diagnostic tests related to clinical problems are in Appendix B.

ORGANIZATION

Each test is presented in the following sequence: name(s) of test; reference values and normal findings for adults, children, and elderly; description of the test; purpose(s); clinical problems related to the test; the effects of any medication on test results; procedure; factors affecting laboratory and diagnostic test results; and nursing implications with client teaching.

There are two parts in the text—Part I: Laboratory Tests and Part II: Diagnostic Tests—and three appendixes. Appendix A, Laboratory Test Values for Adults and Children, provides an alphabetical list of tests found in the text as well as tests that are frequently ordered. It includes the types of specimens, such as blood, plasma, serum, urine, and feces, as well as the color-top tube used for collections of venous blood. Appendix B, Clinical Problems with Laboratory and Diagnostic Tests, lists laboratory and diagnostic tests usually ordered for diagnosing common health problems. Appendix C, Therapeutic Drug Monitoring (TDM), lists over 100 drugs with their serum therapeutic range, peak time, and toxic level.

Joyce LeFever Kee, RN, MSN

ACKNOWLEDGMENTS

I would like to extend my sincere thanks and deep appreciation to the following people: Ellen Boyda, for updating Pap smears; Linda S. Farmer, for reviewing laboratory tests, giving suggestions, and making corrections; Judith Fullhart, for updating GI tests; Jane Purnell Taylor, for rewriting the human immunodeficiency virus-types (HIV-1 and HIV-2) laboratory test; David C. Sestili, for updating the pulmonary function tests; Frank DiGregorio, for updating all cardiac testing, nuclear scans, PET, and ultrasonography; Heiddy DiGregorio for updating selected nursing implications for diagnostic tests; and Ronald J. LeFever, for updating therapeutic drug monitoring (TDM) tests.

Also my appreciation goes to Don Passidomo, Head Librarian, Veterans Administration Medical Center, Wilmington, Delaware, for his assistance with researching the materials; and to Nancy Anselment, Nursing Editor, Prentice Hall Health for her helpful suggestions. To my husband, Edward, go my love and appreciation for his support.

Joyce LeFever Kee, RN, MSN

CONTRIBUTORS AND CONSULTANTS

Ellen K. Boyda, RN, MS, CRNP
Family Nurse Practitioner
Independent Practice
Boothwyn, Pennsylvania
Papanicolaou smear

Linda S. Farmer, MT, ASCP
Laboratory Manager
St. Francis Hospital
Wilmington, Delaware
Laboratory test values and procedures

Judith W. Fullhart, MS, RN, CGRN
Gastroenterology Department
Veterans Administration Hospital
Wilmington, Delaware
All GI tests

Frank DiGregorio, CNMT, RDMS
Director
Community Imaging Center
Wilmington, Delaware
Stress/Exercise tests
Echocardiography
Holter monitoring
Nuclear scans
Positron emission tomography (PET)
Ultrasonography

Heiddy M. DiGregorio, RNC
Christiana Care Health Services
Newark, Delaware
Updated selected nursing implications for diagnostic tests

Ronald J. LeFever, BS, RPh
Pharmacy Services
Medical College of Virginia
Richmond, Virginia
Therapeutic drug monitoring (TDM)

David C. Sestili, CRTT, RPFT
Manager
Pulmonary Laboratories
Christiana Care Health Services
Newark, Delaware
Pulmonary function tests

Jane Purnell Taylor, RN, MSN
Associate Professor
Neumann College
Aston, Pennsylvania
HIV tests

REVIEWERS

Cheryl Brady, RN, MSN
School of Nursing
Kent State University
East Liverpool, OH

Sheryl A. Innerarity, RN, PhD, FNP, CS
School of Nursing
University of Texas at Austin
Austin, TX

Cathy Kessenich, DSN, ARNP
School of Nursing
University of Tampa
Tampa, FL

Carolyn J. Rivard, RN, BScN, EdD
Department of Health & Human Sciences
Fanshawe College
London, Ontario
Canada

ONE

Considerations for Use of Laboratory Tests

This introductory section on laboratory tests serves a twofold orientation—to disseminate essential information and to show the basic organizational format of the individual tests.

As you know, results of laboratory tests provide the basis for diagnosis, treatment, and progress of a disease condition or health status, or both. The laboratory test is a multiphased process: identifying need for test; ordering test; generating the laboratory requisition; physical and educational preparation of the client and family; collection, labeling, and care of specimen(s); and health teaching. Naturally, the complexity of this process is dependent on many variables. For purposes of being a handy reference, general directions common to most laboratory tests related to reference values, description, purpose, clinical problems and drug effects, procedure, factors affecting laboratory results, and nursing implications with client teaching will be addressed. Only facts specific to a given test will be listed with each test. The explanations following the headings for laboratory tests help in their clarification.

Reference Values. Laboratory test values can differ among laboratories; therefore, it is important to know your institution's laboratory values. The reference values given are comparably the same in most laboratories.

Description. Information is provided about each laboratory test and its purpose(s).

Purpose(s). The purpose(s) for the laboratory tests is/are given.

Clinical Problems. The disease entities that are associated with decreased and elevated test results are listed according to decreasing frequency of occurrence. Drugs that may cause false negatives or positives could result in a misleading test report. Drugs the client is taking that could affect test results should be recorded.

Procedure. Many procedures for laboratory tests are the same. The following are helpful suggestions applicable to most tests.

1. Follow institutional policy and procedure, which may include a signed consent form.
2. Collect recommended amount of specimen (blood, urine, etc.).
3. Avoid using arm/hand with intravenous (IV) fluids for drawing venous blood specimen.
4. Clearly label specimen container with client's identifying information.
5. Note significant drug data on label or requisition, or both.
6. Avoid hemolysis; do not shake blood specimens.
7. Observe strict aseptic technique when collecting and handling each specimen.
8. Do not enforce fluid restrictions unless otherwise indicated.
9. Collect 24-hour urine specimens:
   a. Have client void prior to test, discard urine, and then save all urine for 24 hours.
   b. Refrigerate urine or keep on ice unless preservatives are added or otherwise indicated.
   c. Instruct client *not* to urinate directly into the container.
   d. Instruct client to avoid getting toilet paper and feces in urine specimens.
   e. Label the urine collection bottle/container with the client's name, date, and exact time of collection (eg, 7/12/04, 7 AM to 7/13/04, 7:01 AM).
10. List drugs and food the client is taking that could affect test results.
11. When possible, hold medications and foods that could cause false test results until after the test. Before holding drugs, check with the health care provider. This may not be practical or possible; however, if client takes medication and laboratory test is abnormal, this should be brought to the health care provider's attention.
12. Promptly send specimen to the laboratory.

Factors Affecting Laboratory Results

- Various factors that could affect test results should be identified. Drugs that affect test results are given in Clinical Problems; therefore, they are not repeated here.

Nursing Implications. Common nursing implications that may not be repeated with each laboratory test are:

1. Be knowledgeable about laboratory and diagnostic tests.
2. Provide time and be available to answer questions. Be supportive to client and family.
3. Follow procedure that is stated for each test. Label specimens with client information.
4. Relate test findings to clinical problems and drugs. Test may be repeated to confirm a suspected problem.
5. Report abnormal results to the health care provider.
6. Compare test results with other related laboratory and/or diagnostic tests.

Client Teaching

7. Explain purpose and procedure of each test to the client and family.
8. Encourage clients to keep medical appointments for follow-up.
9. Provide health teaching related to clinical problem.

List of Laboratory Tests

Acetaminophen (Serum) 8
Acid Phosphatase (ACP) (Serum) 9
Adenovirus Antibody (Serum) 11
Adrenocorticotropic Hormone (ACTH) (Plasma) 12
Alanine Aminotransferase (ALT) (Serum) 14
Albumin (Serum) 16
Alcohol (Ethyl or Ethanol) (Serum or Plasma) 17
Aldolase (ALD) (Serum) 18
Aldosterone (Serum and Urine) 20
Alkaline Phosphatase (ALP) with Isoenzyme (Serum) 22
Alpha$_1$ Antitrypsin (α_1AT) (Serum) 24
Alpha Fetoprotein (AFP) Serum 25
Aminoglycosides (Serum) 27
Ammonia (Plasma) 29
Amylase: (Serum and Urine) 31
Angiotensin-Converting Enzyme (ACE) (Serum) 33
Anion Gap 35
Antibiotic Susceptibility (Sensitivity) Test 36
Antidepressants (Tricyclics) (Serum) 37
Antidiuretic Hormone (ADH) (Plasma) 39
Antiglomerular Basement Membrane Antibody (Anti-GBM, AGBM) (Serum) 41
Antimitochondrial Antibody (AMA) (Serum) 42
Antimyocardial Antibody (Serum) 43
Antinuclear Antibodies (ANA) (Serum) 44
Antistreptolysin O (ASO) (Serum) 45
Arterial Blood Gases (ABGs) (Arterial Blood) 47
Aspartate Aminotransferase (AST) (Serum) 49
Atrial Natriuretic Hormone (ANH) (Plasma) 51
Bilirubin (Total, Direct, Indirect) (Serum) 52
Bilirubin (Urine) 55
Bleeding Time (Blood) 56
Blood Urea Nitrogen (BUN) (Serum) 58
Blood Urea Nitrogen/Creatinine Ratio (Serum) 60

Calcitonin (hCT) (Serum) 61
Calcium (Ca) (Serum and Urine) 63
Carbon Dioxide (CO_2) Combining Power (Serum or Plasma) 65
Carbon Monoxide, Carboxyhemoglogin (Blood) 67
Carcinoembryonic Antigen (CEA) (Serum or Plasma) 68
Catecholamines (Plasma and Urine) 69
Cerebrospinal Fluid (CSF) 73
Ceruloplasmin (Cp) (Serum) 74
Chlamydia Test (Serum, Tissue Smear or Culture) 76
Chloride (CI) (Serum) 78
Cholesterol (Serum) 80
Cold Agglutinins (Serum) 81
Complement: Total (Serum) 83
Complement C3 and C4 Test (Serum) 84
Coombs' Direct (Blood—RBC) 85
Coombs' Indirect (Serum) 86
Copper (Cu) (Serum and Urine) 87
Cortisol (Plasma) 89
C-Reactive Protein (CRP) (Serum) 91
Creatinine (Serum and Urine) 92
Creatinine Clearance (Urine) 93
Creatine Phosphokinase (CPK, CK), and CPK Isoenzymes (Serum) 95
Crossmatch (Blood) 97
Cryoglobulins (Serum) 98
Cultures (Blood, Sputum, Stool, Throat, Wound, Urine) 99
Cytomegalovirus (CMV) Antibody (Serum) 102
Dexamethasone Suppression Test (DST) 103
Digoxin (Serum) 106
Dilantin (Phenytoin) (Serum) 107
D-Xylose Absorption Test (Blood and Urine) 109
Encephalitis Virus Antibody (Serum) 111
Enterovirus Group (Serum) 112
Erythrocyte Sedimentation Rate (ESR) (Blood) 113
Estetrol (E_4) (Plasma and Amniotic Fluid) 115
Estradiol (E_2) (Serum) 116
Estriol (E_3) (Serum and Urine) 117
Estrogen (Serum and Urine—24 Hour) 119
Estrone (E_1) (Serum and Urine) 120
Factor Assay (Plasma) 122
Febrile Agglutinins (Serum) 125
Ferritin (Serum) 127
Fibrin (Fibrinogen) Degradation Products (FDP) (Serum) 129
Fibrinogen (Plasma) 130
Folic Acid (Folate) (Serum) 131
Follicle-Stimulating Hormone (FSH) (Serum and Urine) 132
FTA-ABS (Fluorescent Treponemal Antibody Absorption) (Serum) 134
Fungal Organisms; Fungal Antibody Test, Mycotic Infections 135
Gamma-Glutamyl Transferase (GGT) (Serum) 137
Gastrin (Serum or Plasma) 139
Glucagon (Plasma) 140
Glucose: Fasting Blood Sugar (FBS); Postprandial (Feasting) Blood Sugar (PPBS) 142
Glucose-6-Phosphate Dehydrogenase (G6PD) Blood 144
Glucose Self-Monitoring Devices (Blood and Urine) 145
Glucose Tolerance Test—Oral (OGTT) (Serum) 148

Growth Hormone (GH), Human Growth Hormone (hGH) (Serum) 150
Haptoglobin (HP) Serum 151
Helicobacter Pylori (Serum, Culture, Breath Analysis) 153
Hematocrit (Hct) (Blood) 154
Hemoglobin (Hb, Hgb) (Blood) 156
Hemoglobin A_1c (Blood) 158
Hemoglobin Electrophoresis (Blood) 160
Hepatitis Profile (Hepatitis A, B, C, D, E) 161
Hepatitis A Virus (HAV) antibody (HAV Ab, Anti-HAV) (Serum) 164
Hepatitis B Surface Antigen (HBsAG) (Serum) 166
Herpes Simplex Virus (HSV) Antibody Test (Serum) 167
Heterophile Antibody (Serum) 169
Hexosaminidase (Total, A, and A and B) (Serum and Amniotic Fluid) 170
Human Chorionic Gonadotropin (HCG) (Serum and Urine) 171
Human Immunodeficiency Virus Type 1 (HIV-1) or HIV) 173
Human Leukocyte Antigens (HLA) (Serum) 184
Human Placental Lactogen (hPL) (Plasma or Serum) 186
17-Hydroxycorticosteroids (17-OHCS) (Urine) 187
5-Hydroxyindolacetic Acid (5-HIAA) (Urine) 189
Immunoglobulins (Ig) (Serum) 190
Insulin (Serum), Insulin Antibody Test 192
International Normalized Ratio (INR) (Plasma) 194
Iron and Total Iron-Binding Capacity (TIBC) (Serum) 195
17-Ketosteroids (17-KS) (Urine) 197
Lactic Acid (Blood) 199
Lactic Dehydrogenase (LDH or LD); LDH Isoenzymes (Serum) 200
Lactose and Lactose Tolerance Test (Serum, or Plasma, Urine) 202
Lead (Blood) 203
Le Cell Test; Lupus Erythematosus Cell Test (Blood) 204
Lecithin/Sphingomyelin (L/S) Ratio (Amniotic Fluid) 206
Legionnaire's Antibody Test (Serum) 207
Leucine Aminopeptidase (LAP) (Serum) 208
Lipase (Serum) 209
Lipoproteins, Lipoprotein Electrophoresis, Lipids (Serum) 210
Lithium (Serum) 212
Luteinizing Hormone (LH) (Serum and Urine) 213
Lyme Disease Antibody Test (Serum) 215
Lymphocytes (T and B) Assay (Blood) 217
Magnesium (Mg) (Serum) 218
Mumps Antibody (Serum) 221
Myoglobin (Serum and Urine) 223
5′ Nucleotidase (5′N or 5′NT) (Serum) 224
Occult Blood (Feces) 226
Opiates (Urine and Blood) 227
Osmolality (Serum and Urine) 229
Ova and Parasites (O & P) (Feces) 231
Parathyroid Hormone (PTH) (Serum) 233

Partial Thromboplastin Time (PTT); Activated Partial Thromboplastin Time (APTT) (Plasma) 234
Phenylketonuria (PKU) (Urine); Guthrie Test for PKU (Blood) 235
Phosphorus (P) (Serum) 238
Platelet Aggregation and Adhesions (Blood) 239
Platelet Antibody Test (Blood) 241
Platelet (Thrombocyte) Count (Blood) 242
Potassium (K) (Serum and Urine) 244
Prealbumin (PA, PAB) Assay (Serum) 247
Pregnanediol (Urine) 249
Pregnanetriol (Urine) 250
Progesterone (Serum) 251
Prolactin (PRL) (Serum) 253
Prostate-Specific Antigen (PSA) (Serum) 255
Protein (Total); Protein Electrophoresis (Serum) 256
Protein (Urine) 259
Prothrombin Time (PT) (Plasma) 260
Rabies Antibody Test (Serum) 262
Rapid Plasma Reagin (RPR) (Serum) 263
RBC Indices (Red blood cell count, MCV, MCH, MCHC) Blood 264
Renin (Plasma) 267
Reticulocyte Count (Blood) 268
Rheumatoid Factor (RF); Rheumatoid Arthritis (RA) Factor (Serum) 269
RH Typing (Blood) 271
Rotavirus Antigen (Blood and Feces) 272
Rubella Antibody Detection (Serum) 274
Salicylate (Serum) 275
Semen Examination/Analysis; Antisperm Antibody Test 276
Sickle Cell (Screening) Test (Blood) 278
Sodium (Na) (Serum and Urine) 279
Testosterone (Serum or Plasma) 282
Theophylline (Serum) 283
Thyroid Antibodies (TA) (Serum) 284
Thyroid-Stimulating Hormone (TSH) (Serum) 286
Thyroxine (T_4) (Serum) 287
Torch Screen Test 289
Toxoplasmosis Antibody Test (Serum) 290
Triglycerides (Serum) 292
Triiodothyronine (T_3) (Serum) 293
Triiodothyronine Resin Uptake (T_3 Ru) (Serum) 294
Uric Acid (Serum and Urine) 296
Urinalysis (Routine) 298
Urobilinogen (Urine) 301
Viral Culture (Blood, Biopsy, CSF Pharynx, Rectum, Sputum, Stool, Urine) 302
Vitamin A (Serum) 304
Vitamin B_{12} (Serum) 305
White Blood Cells (WBC): Total (WBC) (Blood) 306
White Blood Cell Differential (Blood) 308
Zinc (Plasma) 311
Zinc Protoporphyrin (ZPP) (Blood) 313

LABORATORY TESTS

ACETAMINOPHEN (SERUM)

TYLENOL, TEMPRA, DATRIL, LIQUIPRIN, PARACETAMOL, PANADOL, ACETA

Reference Values

Adult: Therapeutic: 5–20 μg/mL, 31–124 μmol/L (SI units)
Toxic: >50 μg/mL, 305 μmol/L (SI units), >200 μg/mL, possible hepatotoxicity

Child: Same as adult

Description. Acetaminophen has antipyretic and nonnarcotic effects similar to aspirin. Acetaminophen does not inhibit platelet aggregation nor does it produce gastric distress and bleeding. It only has a weak anti-inflammatory response.

Acetaminophen is absorbed by the gastrointestinal tract and metabolized in the liver to active metabolites. Peak action time for acetaminophen occurs in 1 to 2½ hours and the half-life is 3 hours. Overdose of acetaminophen can be extremely dangerous since it may lead to hepatotoxicity. If a single dose of 10 grams or 30 tablets (325 mg each) of acetaminophen is ingested, liver damage is likely to occur. With a serum acetaminophen level >200 mg/mL in 4 hours or >50 mg/mL in 12 hours, hepatotoxicity is likely to result.

Purposes

- To determine if the therapeutic acetaminophen dose is within therapeutic range
- To check for acetaminophen toxicity

Clinical Problems

Decreased level: High-carbohydrate meal
Drugs that may decrease acetaminophen value: Anticholinergics, cholestyramine (Questran)

Elevated level: Acetaminophen overdose, liver disease
Drugs that may increase acetaminophen value: Chloramphenicol (Choromycetin), phenobarbital

Procedure

- No food or fluid restriction is required.
- Collect 3 to 5 mL of venous blood in a red-top tube.
- Record dose and time drug was taken on the laboratory requisition slip.

Nursing Implications

- Keep the acetaminophen bottle tightly closed, out of reach of children, and away from the light.
- Suggest to the health care provider to order liver function tests and serum acetaminophen periodically for clients on long-term acetaminophen therapy. Liver damage may result when taking large doses of the drug for days, weeks, or months.
- Observe for signs and symptoms of hepatotoxicity—vomiting, jaundice, clay-colored stool, itching, epigastric or abdominal pain, diarrhea, and abnormal liver function tests.

Client Teaching

- Explain to the client that the purpose of the test is to monitor therapeutic drug level and to determine if a toxic serum acetaminophen level is present.
- Instruct the client to take the prescribed dosage. Usually the drug should not be taken for more than 10 days unless prescribed by the health care provider.
- Instruct the client to keep acetaminophen products out of the reach of children. If a child ingests large amounts of the drug, call the poison control center immediately, give syrup of ipecac if indicated by the center, and take the child to the emergency room. Acetylcysteine (Mucomyst) has been used as an antidote for adults within 16 hours after drug overdose.

ACID PHOSPHATASE (ACP) SERUM

PROSTATIC ACID PHOSPHATASE (PAP)

Reference Values

Adult: <2.6 ng/mL; 0–5 U/L range; varies according to the method used; 0.2–13 IU/L (SI units)

Child: 6.4–15.2 U/L

Description. The enzyme ACP is found in the prostate gland and in semen in high concentration. It is found in lesser extent in bone marrow, red blood cells (RBCs), liver, and spleen. The highest rise in serum ACP occurs in prostatic cancer. In benign prostatic hypertrophy (BPH), the rise is also above normal level.

Purpose

- To compare ACP test with other laboratory test for diagnosing prostatic cancer, BPH

Clinical Problems

Decreased level: Down syndrome
Drugs that may decrease ACP value: Fluorides, oxalates, phosphates, alcohol

Elevated level: Carcinoma of the prostate, prostate palpation or surgery, Paget's disease, cancer of the breast and bone, multiple myeloma, osteogenesis imperfecta, benign prostatic hypertrophy, sickle cell anemia, cirrhosis, chronic renal failure, hyperparathyroidism, myocardial infarction.
Drugs that may increase ACP value: Androgens in females, clofibrate

Procedure

- No food or fluid restriction is required.
- Collect 5 to 7 mL of venous blood in a red-top tube. Avoid hemolysis. ACP is rich in blood cells.
- Take blood specimen to the laboratory *immediately.* ACP is heat- and pH-sensitive. If the specimen is exposed to air and left at room temperature, there will be a decrease in activity after 1 hour.

Nursing Implications

- Recognize clinical problems associated with an elevated serum ACP level. A high serum ACP level occurs with metastasized prostatic cancer.
- Indicate on the laboratory slip if the client had a prostate examination 24 hours before the test. Prostatic massage or extensive palpation of the prostate can elevate the serum ACP.
- Check the serum ACP following treatment for carcinoma of the prostate gland. With surgical intervention the serum level should

drop in 3 to 4 days; following successful estrogen therapy it should drop in 3 to 4 weeks. If serum ACP has not been ordered, a reminder or suggestion to the health care provider may be necessary.
- Encourage client to express concerns about prostatic problem.

ADENOVIRUS ANTIBODY (SERUM)

Reference Values

Adult and Child: Negative. Positive: fourfold titer increase in paired sera

Description: The adenovirus frequently is presented among school-aged children and military recruits; many may be asymptomatic. Adenovirus can be responsible for upper respiratory tract disease, cystitis (hemorrhagic), and keratoconjunctivitis. Transmission may be by direct or indirect contact (there are 41 different types of adenoviruses).

Purpose

- To determine the cause of upper respiratory tract disease and pharyngitis

Clinical Problems

Positive: Adenovirus infections of the upper respiratory tract, hemorrhagic cystitis, pharyngitis, keratoconjunctivitis

Procedure

- No food or fluid restriction is required.
- Collect 3 to 5 mL of venous blood in a red-top tube. Avoid hemolysis. A second blood specimen is usually obtained 2 to 3 weeks later to determine the acute and convalescent titer.
- A swab of the drainage from the infected area such as the throat, eye, or urethra may be obtained for immunofluorescence testing to determine the presence of an adenoviral infection. The swab specimen should be labeled and taken immediately to the laboratory for testing.

Nursing Implications

- Obtain a history from the client or family concerning the infected area involved. List symptoms the client may have, such as drainage and its color.

- Check with the client concerning contact with other persons who have similarly described symptoms.
- Answer the client or family's questions or refer them to an appropriate health care provider.

ADRENOCORTICOTROPIC HORMONE (ACTH) PLASMA

CORTICOTROPIN, CORTICOTROPIN-RELEASING FACTOR (CRF)

Reference Values

7 AM to 10 AM: 8–80 pg/mL; ACTH is highest in early morning
4 PM: 5–30 pg/mL
10 PM to midnight: <10 pg/mL; lowest levels occur at bedtime

Description. Adrenocorticotropic hormone (ACTH) is stored and released from the anterior pituitary gland (adenohypophysis) under the influence of corticotropin-releasing factor (CRF) from the hypothalamus and plasma cortisol from the adrenal cortex. The negative feedback mechanism controls ACTH releases: when plasma cortisol is low, ACTH is released; when plasma cortisol is high, ACTH release is inhibited. Stress caused by surgery, infections, and physical or emotional trauma increases the ACTH level. ACTH level follows a diurnal pattern, peaks in the early morning or early arising, and ebbs in the late evening or bedtime.

A plasma ACTH is performed to determine whether a decreased plasma cortisol is due to adrenal cortex hypofunction or pituitary hypofunction. Two tests, ACTH suppression and ACTH stimulation, may be ordered to identify the origin of the clinical problem, either the adrenal cortex or the pituitary.

ACTH Suppression Test. For the ACTH suppression test, a synthetic potent cortisol, dexamethasone (Decadron), is given to suppress the production of ACTH. If an extremely high dose is needed for ACTH suppression, the cause is of pituitary origin, such as pituitary tumor, producing an excess of ACTH secretion. If the plasma cortisol continues to be high with ACTH suppression, the cause could be adrenal cortex hyperfunction (Cushing's syndrome). Suppressing pituitary release of ACTH will not affect a hyperactive adrenal gland.

ACTH Stimulation. For the ACTH stimulation test, ACTH (cosyntropin) is administered, and the plasma cortisol level should double in 1 hour. If the plasma cortisol level remains the same or is lower, adrenal gland insufficiency (Addison's disease) is the cause.

To check for pituitary hypofunction, the drug *metyrapone* (*Metopirone*) is given to block the production of cortisol, thus causing an increased ACTH secretion. If the ACTH level does not increase, the problem is pituitary insufficiency.

Purposes

- To determine if a decreased plasma cortisol is due to adrenal cortex hypofunction or pituitary hypofunction
- To evaluate the ACTH suppression test results for health problem of pituitary origin
- To check for adrenal or pituitary hypofunction
- To utilize the ACTH stimulation test to determine the presence of adrenal gland insufficiency

Clinical Problems

Decreased level: Adrenocortical hyperplasia, cancer of the adrenal gland, hypopituitarism
Drugs that may decrease ACTH value: Steroids (cortisone, prednisone, dexamethasone), estrogen, amphetamines, alcohol

Elevated level: Stress (trauma, physical or emotional), Addison's disease (adrenal hypofunction), pituitary neoplasm, surgery, pyrogens, pregnancy
Drugs that may increase ACTH value: Metyrapone, vasopressin, insulin

Procedure

- Food and fluid may be restricted. A low-carbohydrate diet may be requested for 24 hours prior to the test.
- Collect 5 to 7 mL of venous blood in a lavender-top plastic tube. Pack the tube in ice immediately and send to the laboratory. Blood should not come in contact with glass. Additional testing may be needed since a single plasma value may be misleading.

- If adrenal hypofunction is suspected, blood sample is taken at the peak time (early morning). When adrenal hyperfunction is suspected, blood sample is usually taken at low time (evening).
- Note on the laboratory label the time the blood specimen was drawn. If the test is to be repeated the next morning, the blood sample should be drawn at the same time as the first specimen.
- Restrict activity and stress (if possible) for 8 to 12 hours before the test. When possible, restrict drugs such as cortisone until after the test.

Factors Affecting Laboratory Results

- Stress and physical activity

Nursing Implications

- Obtain a history of the client's clinical symptoms and drug regimen. Steroids increase the ACTH secretion.
- Relate elevated plasma ACTH levels to plasma cortisol if ordered. With an adrenal gland insufficiency or a pituitary tumor, the ACTH secretions will be increased.

Client Teaching

- Explain to the client having the ACTH suppression test with dexamethasone or ACTH stimulation with ACTH or metyrapone that drugs are used to confirm the cause of the hormonal imbalance.
- Be supportive to the client and the family. Allow time for the client to ventilate his/her fears.

ALANINE AMINOTRANSFERASE (ALT) SERUM

SERUM GLUTAMIC PYRUVIC TRANSAMINASE (SGPT)

Reference Value

Adult: 10–35 U/L; 4–36 U/L at 37°C (SI units).

Male: Levels may be slightly higher

Child: Infant: could be twice as high as adult; child: similar to adult

Elderly: Slightly higher than adult

Description. ALT/SGPT, an enzyme found primarily in the liver cells, is effective in diagnosing hepatocellular destruction. Serum ALT level could elevate before jaundice is present. With jaundice and the serum ALT >300 units, the cause is most likely due to a liver disorder and not a hemolytic disorder.

Purpose

- To detect the presence of a liver disorder

Clinical Problems

Elevated level: **Highest increase:** acute (viral) hepatitis, severe hepatotoxicity causing necrosis of liver (drug or chemical toxicity); **slight or moderate increase:** cirrhosis, cancer of the liver, congestive heart failure, acute alcohol intoxication; **marginal increase:** acute myocardial infarction (AMI)

Drugs that may increase ALT value: Antibiotics, narcotics, meth-yldopa (Aldomet), guanethidine, digitalis preparations, indomethacin (Indocin), salicylates, rifampin, flurazepam (Dalmane), propranolol (Inderal), oral contraceptives, lead, heparin

Procedure

- No food or fluid restriction is required.
- Collect 3 to 5 mL of venous blood in a red-top tube. Avoid hemolysis. RBCs have high concentration of ALT.
- Drugs that can cause false-positive levels should be listed on the laboratory slip along with the date and time last given.

Nursing Implications

Elevated levels

- Relate the client's serum ALT/SGPT to clinical problems and drugs that can cause false-positive levels.
- Check for signs of jaundice. ALT levels rise several days before jaundice begins if it is related to liver damage.
- Be supportive to the client if jaundice is present and isolation technique is enforced.

ALBUMIN (SERUM)

Reference Values

Adult: 3.5–5.0 g/dL; 52% to 68% of total protein
Child: Newborn: 2.9–5.4 g/dL; infant: 4.4–5.4 g/dL; child: 4.0–5.8 g/dL

Description. Albumin, a component of proteins, makes up more than half of plasma proteins. Albumin is synthesized by the liver. It increases osmotic pressure (oncotic pressure), which is necessary for maintaining vascular fluid (vessels). A decrease in serum albumin will cause fluid to shift from the vessels to the tissues, resulting in edema.

The *A/G ratio* is a calculation of the distribution of two major protein fractions, albumin and globulin. The reference value of A/G ratio is > 1.0, which is the albumin value divided by globulin value (albumin ÷ globulin). A high ratio value is considered insignificant; a low ratio value occurs in liver and renal diseases. Protein electrophoresis is more accurate and has replaced the A/G ratio calculation.

Purpose

- To detect an albumin deficit

Clinical Problems

Decreased level: Cirrhosis of the liver, acute liver failure, severe burns, servere malnutrition, preeclampsia, renal disorders, certain malignancies, ulcerative colitis, prolonged immobilization, protein-losing enteropathies, malabsorption
Drugs that may decrease albumin value: Penicillin, sulfonamides, aspirin, ascorbic acid

Elevated level: Dehydration, severe vomiting, severe diarrhea
Drug that may increase albumin value: Heparin

Procedure

- No food or fluid restriction is required.
- Collect 3 to 5 mL of venous blood in a red-top tube.

Nursing Implications

- Check for peripheral edema and ascites when serum albumin is low.

- Assess skin integrity if pitted edema or anasarca is present. Use measures to avoid skin breakdown.

Client Teaching

- Suggest that the client includes foods rich in protein if the serum albumin value is decreased and the client does not have cirrhosis.

ALCOHOL (ETHYL OR ETHANOL) SERUM OR PLASMA

Reference Values. 00.0%—normal, no alcohol; <0.05% or 50 mg/dL—no significant alcohol influence; 0.05–0.10% or 50–100 mg/dL—alcohol influence is present; 0.10–0.15% or 100–150 mg/dL—reaction time affected; >0.15% or 150 mg/dL—indicative of alcohol intoxication; >0.25% or 250 mg/dL—severe alcohol intoxication; >0.30% or 300 mg/dL—comatose; >0.40% or 400 mg/dL—fatal.

Description. Ethyl alcohol (ethanol) in the blood is a frequently requested laboratory test for medical and legal reasons. In most states, an alcohol level >0.1% or 100 mg/dL is considered by law to be proof of alcohol intoxication. However, some states consider 0.08% or 80 mg/dL as proof of alcohol intoxication. On an empty stomach, plasma alcohol peaks in 40 to 70 minutes.

Serum/plasma alcohol may be used as a screening test on an unconscious client. Nurses should check for any legal ramifications (state laws) in reference to drawing blood for plasma alcohol level.

Purpose

- To detect the percent of alcohol in the bloodstream and for DUI (driving under the influence)

Clinical Problems

Elevated level. Moderate to severe alcohol intoxication, chronic alcohol consumption, cirrhosis of the liver, malnutrition, folic acid deficiency, acute pancreatitis, gastritis, hypoglycemia, hyperuricemia

Procedure

- Obtain a consent form if required by law.
- Cleanse the venipuncture area with benzalkonium, and then wipe the solution off with a sterile swab. Do not use alcohol to cleanse the area.
- Collect 3 to 5 mL of venous blood in a red-top tube. A green-, lavender-, or blue-top tube can be used. Avoid hemolysis.
- Write on the specimen and laboratory slip the date and time the blood specimen was drawn. The signatures of the collector and a witness should be included on the tube.

Factors Affecting Laboratory Results

- Cleansing the venipuncture site with alcohol or tincture

Nursing Implications

Elevated level

- Follow legal ramifications in your state for drawing plasma alcohol level.
- Provide safety measures, such as side rails, to prevent physical harm to the client when the serum alcohol level is greatly increased.

Client Teaching

- Instruct the client not to consume alcoholic beverages when taking sedatives, hypnotics, narcotics, tranquilizers (Valium, Librium), anticonvulsants (Dilantin), and anticoagulants (Coumadin).
- Listen to client's concerns.

ALDOLASE (ALD) SERUM

Reference Values

Adult: <6 U/L, 22–59 mU/L at 37°C (SI units), 3–8 U/dL (Sibley-Lehninger)

Child: Infant: 12–24 U/dL; child: 6–16 U/dL

Description. Aldolase is an enzyme present in many types of cells, particularly in the skeletal and cardiac muscles. This enzyme test is used to monitor skeletal muscle disease such as muscular dystrophy, dermatomyositis, and trichinosis. Aldolase is not elevated in neural origin diseases such as multiple sclerosis and myasthenia gravis.

Serum aldolase is helpful in diagnosing early cases of Duchenne's muscular dystrophy. It is not as effective in diagnosing myocardial infarction (MI). In progressive muscular dystrophy, the serum aldolase may be ten or more times the normal value.

Purpose

- To aid in the diagnosis of skeletal muscle disease, such as muscular dystrophy

Clinical Problems

Decreased level: Late muscular dystrophy
Drugs that may decrease aldolase value: Large doses of phenothiazides

Elevated level: Early and progressive muscular dystrophy, trichinosis, dermatomyositis, acute myocardial infarction (AMI), acute hepatitis, cancer of the gastrointestinal tract, leukemia
Drugs that may increase aldolase value: Alcohol, cortisone, narcotics, aminocaproic acid, insecticides, clofibrate, and intramuscular injections

Procedure

- No food or fluid restriction is required.
- Collect 3 to 5 mL of venous blood in a red-top tube. Unhemolyzed serum must be used when measuring for aldolase.

Nursing Implications

- Check serum aldolase results, and plan the nursing care according to the symptoms present and psychologic needs.
- Assist the client with activities of daily living (ADL) as needed. Promote maximum independence.
- List on the laboratory slip any drugs the client is receiving that can elevate the serum aldolase level.
- Be supportive of the client and family regarding client's physical and psychological limitations.

ALDOSTERONE (SERUM AND URINE)

Reference Values

Adult: Serum: <16 ng/dL (fasting), 4–30 ng/dL (sitting position)
Urine: 6–25 μg/24 hours

Child: (3–11 years): 5–70 ng/dL

Pregnancy: 2 to 3 times higher than adult

Description. Aldosterone is the most potent of all mineralocorticoids produced by the adrenal cortex. The major function of aldosterone is to regulate sodium, potassium, and water balance. Aldosterone promotes sodium reabsorption from the distal tubules of the kidney, and potassium and hydrogen excretion. Twenty-five percent of this hormone secretion is influenced by the adrenocorticotropic hormone (ACTH), and 60 to 75 percent depends on the renin–angiotensin system. Renin promotes aldosterone secretion, thus causing sodium retention, which results in water retention.

A decreased renin level inhibits the conversion of angiotensinogen to angiotensin. Without angiotensin, aldosterone secretion is markedly reduced.

Serum aldosterone is not the most reliable test, because there can be fluctuations caused by various influences. A 24-hour urine test is considered more reliable than a random serum aldosterone collection. The urine and serum aldosterone levels are increased by hyponatremia, a low-salt diet, and hyperkalemia. Also, hypernatremia, a high-salt diet, and hypokalemia decrease the serum aldosterone levels.

Purposes

- To detect deficit or excess of aldosterone
- To compare serum and urine aldosterone levels with other laboratory tests for determining overhydration with elevated sodium level and adrenal hypo- or hyperfunction

Clinical Problems

Decreased level—serum and urine: Overhydration with elevated serum sodium level, severe hypernatremia, high-sodium diet, adrenal cortical hypofunction (Addison's disease), diabetes mellitus, glucose infusion, licorice

Elevated level—serum: Dehydration, hyponatremia, low-sodium diet, essential hypertension, adrenal cortical hyperfunction, cancer of the adrenal gland, cirrhosis of the liver, emphysema, severe congestive heart failure (CHF)

Drugs that may increase serum aldosterone value: Diuretics, hydralazine (Apresoline), diazoxide (Hyperstat), nitroprusside, oral contraceptives

Urine: Tumors of the adrenal cortex or primary aldosteronism, same as serum aldosterone

Drugs that may increase urine aldosterone value: Diuretics, lithium, oral contraceptives

Procedure

Serum

- Food and fluids are not restricted, but excess salt may interfere with test result. Normal salt intake is suggested.
- Collect 5 mL of venous blood in a red- or green-top tube.
- The client should be in a supine position for at least 1 hour before the blood is drawn.
- Record the date and time on the specimen. Aldosterone levels exhibit circadian rhythm, with peak levels occurring in the morning and lower levels in the afternoon.

Urine

- Collect a 24-hour urine specimen in a large container with a preservative such as a boric acid tablet.
- Have the client void and discard urine before beginning the test.
- Label the container with the exact date and time of urine collection (e.g., 7/5/02, 7 AM to 7/6/02, 7:02 AM).

Nursing Implications

- Compare the serum aldosterone and the 24-hour urine aldosterone results if both have been ordered.
- Assess the client for signs and symptoms of overhydration due to excess aldosterone secretion and water retention (e.g., constant, irritating cough, dyspnea, vein engorgement, chest rales).
- Assess the client for signs and symptoms of dehydration that may also result from elevated serum aldosterone level. Sodium reabsorption may be greater than excess water retention.

- Monitor vital signs. Report vital sign changes that may indicate dehydration or overhydration.
- Check at regular intervals to determine whether the urine collection is being properly obtained.

Client Teaching

- Instruct the client not to increase or decrease salt intake before the aldosterone tests. Normal salt intake should be encouraged for accurate test results.
- Instruct the client to remain in a supine position for at least 1 hour before blood is drawn to prevent false test results. The position of the client when blood was drawn should be noted on the laboratory slip.
- Instruct the client how to collect the 24-hour urine specimen. All urine should be saved after the initial urine specimen is discarded. Toilet paper or feces should not be in the urine.

ALKALINE PHOSPHATASE (ALP) WITH ISOENZYME (SERUM)

Reference Values

Adult: 42–136 U/L; ALP^1: 20–130 U/L; ALP^2: 20–120 U/L

Child: Infant and child (aged 0–12 years): 40–115 U/L; older child (13–18 years): 50–230 U/L

Elderly: Slightly higher than adult

Description. ALP is an enzyme produced mainly in the liver and bone and is also produced in the intestine, the kidney, and the placenta. This test is useful for determining liver and bone diseases.

To differentiate between liver and bone disorders, other enzyme tests should be performed (i.e., LAP, GGTP, and/or 5′N). ALP isoenzymes, ALP^1 (liver origin) and ALP^2 (bone origin), are helpful in distinguishing between liver and bone disease.

Purposes

- To determine the presence of a liver or a bone disorder
- To compare ALP results with other laboratory tests for confirmation of liver or bone disorder

Clinical Problems

Decreased level: Hypothyroidism, malnutrition, scurvy (vitamin C deficit), hypophosphatasia, pernicious anemia, placental insufficiency
Drugs that decrease ALP values: Fluoride, oxalate, propranolol (Inderal)

Elevated level: Obstructive biliary disease (jaundice); cancer of the liver, hepatocellular cirrhosis; hepatitis; leukemia; cancer of the bone, breast, and prostate; Paget's disease (osteitis deformans); healing fractures; multiple myeloma; osteomalacia; gastrointestinal ulcerative disease; late pregnancy; hyperthyroidism; hyperparathyroidism; rheumatoid arthritis; congestive heart failure (CHF)
Drugs that may increase ALP value: Antibiotics, colchicine, methyldopa (Aldomet), allopurinol, phenothiazines, indomethacin (Indocin), procainamide, some oral contraceptives, tolbutamine, isoniazid (INH), IV albumin

Procedure

- No food or fluid restrictions are required. For ALP isoenzymes, fasting overnight may be indicated.
- Collect 3 to 5 mL of venous blood in a red-top tube. Avoid hemolysis.
- Withhold drugs that can elevate ALP level for 8 to 24 hours with health care provider's permission.
- List client's age and drugs that may affect test results on laboratory slip.

Factors Affecting Laboratory Results

- Age of the client (youth and old age) and late pregnancy to 3 weeks postpartum can cause elevated level.

Nursing Implications

- Know factors that can elevate serum ALP levels (i.e., drugs, IV albumin [can elevate serum ALP five to ten times its normal value]); age of client (child or elderly); late pregnancy to 3 weeks postpartum; and blood drawn 2 to 4 hours after fatty meal.
- Record pertinent information from procedure on laboratory slip.

Client Teaching

- Assess for clinical signs and symptoms of liver disease or bone disease.
- Inform client that other enzyme tests may be ordered to verify diagnosis.

ALPHA$_1$ ANTITRYPSIN ($\tilde{\alpha}_1$AT) SERUM

ALPHA-1-TRYPSIN INHIBITOR

Reference Values

Adult: 78–200 mg/dL, 0.78–2.0 g/L
Child: Newborn: 145–270 mg/dL; infant: similar to adult range

Description. Antitrypsin ($\tilde{\alpha}_1$AT), a protein produced by the liver, inhibits proteolytic enzymes that are released by the lung. A deficiency of homozygous antitrypsin (heredity linked) permits proteolytic enzymes to damage lung tissue, thus causing emphysema.

An elevated serum $\tilde{\alpha}_1$AT level might be present in inflammatory conditions.

Purposes

- To determine if COPD is caused by a deficiency of alpha$_1$ antitrypsin protein
- To detect a $\tilde{\alpha}_1$AT deficiency

Clinical Problems

Decreased level: Chronic obstructive lung disease (pulmonary emphysema), severe liver damage, malnutrition, severe protein-losing disorders (eg, nephrotic syndrome)

Elevated level: Acute and chronic inflammatory conditions, infections (selected), necrosis, late pregnancy, exercise (returns to normal in 1 day)
Drugs that may increase $\tilde{\alpha}_1$AT value: Oral contraceptives

Procedure

- Restrict food and fluids, except for water, for 8 hours.
- Collect 3 to 5 mL of venous blood in red-top tube.
- Hold oral contraceptives for 24 hours before the test, with the health care provider's permission. Any oral contraceptive taken should be listed on the laboratory slip.

Factors Affecting Laboratory Results

- Oral intake of food before the test can cause an inaccurate result if the client has an elevated serum cholesterol or serum triglyceride level.

Nursing Implications. List the name of the oral contraceptive and date last taken on the lab slip.

Decreased level
Client Teaching

- Explain to the client that the test is ordered to determine an antitrypsin (protein) deficiency that can cause a lung disorder. A nonsmoker with an $\tilde{\alpha}_1$AT deficiency can have emphysema. Antitrypsin inhibits proteolytic enzymes from destroying lung tissue; with a lack of this protein, the alveoli are damaged.
- Instruct the client with an $\tilde{\alpha}_1$AT deficit to use preventive methods in protecting lungs (i.e., avoid persons with upper respiratory infection [URI], seek medical care when having a respiratory infection).
- Encourage the client to stop smoking and to avoid areas having high air pollution. Air pollution can cause respiratory inflammation and promote chronic obstructive lung disease.

Elevated level

- Check the serum $\tilde{\alpha}_1$AT level 2 to 3 days after extensive surgery. Inflammation can markedly increase the serum level. A baseline serum level may be ordered before surgery for several reasons (eg, for determining lung disease and the effects of surgery).
- Report to the health care provider if the serum $\tilde{\alpha}_1$AT remains elevated 2 weeks after surgery.
- Note that serum $\tilde{\alpha}_1$AT can be markedly elevated during late pregnancy.

ALPHA FETOPROTEIN (AFP) SERUM

Reference Values

Nonpregnancy: <15 ng/mL

Pregnancy

Serum		Amniotic Fluid	
Weeks of Gestation	*ng/mL*	*Weeks of Gestation*	*µg/mL*
8–12	0–39	14	11.0–32.0
13	6–31	15	5.5–31.0
14	7–50	16	5.7–31.5
15	7–60	17	3.8–32.5
16	10–72	18	3.6–28.0
17	11–90	19	3.7–24.5
18	14–94	20	2.2–15.0
19	24–112	21	3.8–18.0
20	31–122		
21	19–124		

Description. Serum AFP, a screening test, is usually done between 16 and 20 weeks of gestation to detect the probability of twins, infant of low birth weight, or serious birth defects, such as open neural tube defect. If a high serum AFP level occurs, the test should be repeated. Ultrasound and amniocentesis may be performed to diagnose neural tube defect in the fetus.

Purpose

- To identify the probability of neural tube defects, fetal death, or other anomalies in pregnancy (see Clinical Problems)

Clinical Problems

Elevated level

Nonpregnant: Cirrhosis of the liver (not liver metastasis), germ cell tumor of gonads, such as testicular cancer

Pregnant: Neural tube defects (spina bifida, anencephaly), fetal death, other anomalies (duodenal atresia, tetralogy of Fallot, hydrocephalus, trisomy 13, encephalocele)

Procedure

- No food or fluid restriction is required.
- Collect 5 to 7 mL of venous blood in a red-top tube. Avoid hemolysis.

Factors Affecting Laboratory Results

- Fetal blood contamination could cause an elevated amniotic AFP level.
- Inaccurate recording of gestation week could affect results.
- Multiple pregnancy or fetal death could cause false-positive test.

Nursing Implications

- Explain that the test is for screening purposes. If the test is positive, genetic counseling might be necessary.
- Be supportive to individuals and family.

AMINOGLYCOSIDES (SERUM)

AMIKACIN (AMIKIN), GENTAMICIN (GARAMYCIN), KANAMYCIN (KANTREX), NETILMICIN (NETROMYCIN), TOBRAMYCIN (NEBCIN)

Reference Values

Adult and Child

THERAPEUTIC RANGE

Drug Name	*Peak*	*Trough*	*Toxic Level*
Amikacin	15–30 μg/mL	<10 μg/mL	>35 μg/mL
Gentamicin	6–12 μg/mL	<2 μg/mL	>12 μg/mL
Kanamycin	15–30 μg/mL	1–4 μg/mL	>35 μg/mL
Netilmicin	0.5–10 μg/mL	<4 μg/mL	>16 μg/mL
Tobramycin	5–10 μg/mL	<2 μg/mL	>12 μg/mL

Description. Aminoglycosides are broad-spectrum antibiotics that are effective against gram-negative microorganisms. These agents are not well absorbed from the GI tract and so are given parenterally. Peak action after intramuscular (IM) injection is ½ to 1½ hours, and after 30 minutes IV infusion is ½ hour. Half-life is about 2 hours. Aminoglycosides cross the placental barrier but do not cross the blood-brain barrier. They are excreted mostly unchanged by the kidneys.

Ototoxicity and nephrotoxicity can result from overdose of aminoglycoside or from long-term administration. Renal function tests (i.e., creatinine, creatinine clearance, and urinalysis) should be assessed periodically (recommended creatinine levels every 2 to 3 days) while the client is receiving these agents. If clients with renal insufficiency receive any of these drugs, dosage should be adjusted (decreased). Drug half-life is usually 24 to 96 hours in clients having renal damage.

Purpose

- To assess clients receiving aminoglycosides for therapeutic effect and possible toxic effect by monitoring urinary output, BUN, and serum creatinine levels

Clinical Problems

Elevated levels: Overdose of aminoglycoside, renal insufficiency or failure
Drugs that may increase aminoglycoside value: Diuretics, cephalosporins (increase chance of nephrotoxicity)

Procedure

- No food or fluid restriction is required.
- Collect 3 to 5 mL of venous blood in a red-top tube.
- Collect specimen during steady state, usually 24 to 36 hours after drug was started.
- Record on the laboratory requisition slip drug dose, route (IM or IV), and last time the drug was administered. Specific drug levels may need to be checked concurrently with aminoglycoside levels.

Nursing Implications

- Check serum aminoglycoside (amikacin, gentamicin, kanamycin, netilmicin, tobramycin) results, and report nontherapeutic levels to the health care provider immediately.
- Assess intake and output. Notify the health care provider if urine output has greatly decreased. This could be a sign of aminoglycoside toxicity.
- Suggest renal function tests for clients receiving long-term aminoglycoside therapy, especially for those with renal insufficiency.
- Recognize that diuretics and cephalosporins co-administered with an aminoglycoside could enchance the risk of nephrotoxicity.

- Assess hearing status of the client. Any hearing impairment (e.g., loss of high tone) while the client is receiving an aminoglycoside could indicate ototoxicity.
- Observe for signs and symptoms of nephrotoxicity (i.e., proteinuria, elevated creatinine, elevated BUN, decreased creatinine clearance test).
- Observe for signs and symptoms of ototoxicity (i.e., nausea and vomiting with motion, dizziness, headache, tinnitus, decrease in ability to hear high-pitched tones).

AMMONIA (PLASMA)

Reference Values

Adult: 15–45 μg/dL, 11–35 μmol/L (SI units)
Child: Newborn: 64–107 μg/dL; child: 29–70 μg/dL; 29–70 μmol/L (SI units)

Description. Ammonia, a by-product of protein metabolism is converted in the liver to urea. The kidneys excrete urea. With severe liver disorder or when blood flow to the liver is altered, the plasma ammonia level is elevated. Although elevated plasma ammonia is correlated with hepatic failure, other conditions that interfere with liver function (CHF, acidosis) can cause a temporary ammonia elevation.

Purpose

- To detect liver disorder from the inability of the liver to convert ammonia to urea

Clinical Problems

Decreased level: Renal failure, malignant hypertension, essential hypertension
Drugs that may decrease ammonia value: Antibiotics (neomycin, kanamycin, tetracycline), monoamine oxidase inhibitors, diphenhydramine (Benadryl), potassium salts, sodium salts

Elevated level: hepatic failure, hepatic encephalopathy or coma, portacaval anastomosis, Reye's syndrome, erythroblastosis fetalis, cor pulmonale, severe congestive heart failure, high-protein diet with liver failure, acidosis, exercise, hyperalimentation

Drugs that may increase ammonia value: Ammonia chloride, diuretics (thiazides, furosemide [Lasix], ethacrynic acid [Edecrin], acetazolamide [Diamox]), ion exchange resin, isoniazid (INH)

Procedure

- No food or fluid restriction is required unless indicated by laboratory. Smoking should be avoided before the test.
- Collect 5 mL of venous blood in a green-top (heparinized) tube. Deliver blood specimen in packed ice immediately to laboratory. Ammonia levels increase rapidly after blood is drawn.
- Minimize use of tourniquet for drawing blood.
- List drugs client is taking that could affect test results.

Factors Affecting Laboratory Results

- A high- or low-protein diet can cause false test result.
- Exercise might increase the plasma ammonia level.

Nursing Implications

Elevated level

- Identify clinical problems and drugs that can increase the plasma ammonia level.
- Notify the laboratory personnel promptly when a plasma ammonia level is drawn so that it can be analyzed immediately to avoid false results.
- Recognize that exercise may be a cause of an elevated plasma ammonia level.
- Observe for signs and symptoms of hepatic failure, especially when the plasma ammonia is elevated (i.e., behavioral and personality changes, lethargy, confusion, flapping tremors of the extremities, twitching, and, later, coma).
- Know various treatments used in decreasing the plasma ammonia level, such as low-protein diet, antibiotics (neomycin) to destroy intestinal bacteria that increase ammonia production, enemas, cathartics (magnesium sulfate) to prevent ammonia formation, and sodium glutamate and L-arginine in IV dextrose solution to stimulate urea formation.

AMYLASE: (SERUM AND URINE)

Reference Values

Serum: Adult: 60–160 Somogyi U/dL, 30–170 U/L (SI units)
Pregnancy: slightly increased
Child: usually not done
Elderly: could be slightly higher than adult

Serum isoenzymes: S (salivary) type: 45–70%
P (pancreatic) type: 30–55%
Values may differ with method used

Urine: Adult: 4–37 U/L2h

Description. Amylase is an enzyme that is derived from the pancreas, salivary gland, and liver. In acute pancreatitis, serum amylase is increased to twice its normal level. Its level begins to increase 2 to 12 hours after onset, peaks in 20 to 30 hours, and returns to normal in 2 to 4 days. An increased serum amylase can occur after abdominal surgery involving the gallbladder (stones or biliary duct) and stomach (partial gastrectomy).

There are two major amylase isoenzymes, P and S types. P-type elevation may occur more frequently in acute pancreatitis. Elevated S type can be due to ovarian and bronchogenic tumors.

The urine amylase level is helpful in determining the significance of a normal or slightly elevated serum amylase, especially when the client has symptoms of pancreatitis. Urine amylase can remain elevated up to 2 weeks after acute pancreatitis.

Purpose

- To assist in the diagnosis of acute pancreatitis and other health problems (see Clinical Problems)

Clinical Problems

Decreased level: IV D_5W, advanced chronic pancreatitis, acute and subacute necrosis of the liver, chronic alcoholism, toxic hepatitis, severe burns, severe thyrotoxicosis

Drugs that may decrease amylase value: Glucose, citrates, fluorides, oxalates

Elevated level: Acute pancreatitis, chronic pancreatitis (acute onset), partial gastrectomy, peptic ulcer perforation, obstruction of pancreatic duct, acute cholecystitis, cancer of the pancreas, diabetic acidosis, diabetes mellitus, acute alcoholic intoxication, mumps, renal failure, benign prostatic hypertrophy, burns, pregnancy
Drugs that may increase amylase value: Narcotics, ethyl alcohol (large amounts), ACTH, guanethidine, thiazide diuretics, salicylates, tetracycline

Procedure

Serum

- Restrict food for 1 to 2 hours before the blood sample is drawn. If the client has eaten or has received a narcotic 2 hours before the test, the serum results could be invalid.
- Obtain 3 to 5 mL of venous blood in a red-top tube.
- List on the laboratory slip drugs that could cause false amylase levels.

Urine

- Have client void and discard urine. Collect a 2-hour urine specimen.
- Urine specimen should be refrigerated or kept on ice. No preservative is needed.

Factors Affecting Laboratory Results

- IV fluids with glucose can result in false-negative levels.

Nursing Implications

Decreased level—serum and urine

- Determine when the client has ingested food or sweetened fluids. Blood should not be drawn until 2 hours after eating, since sugar can decrease the serum amylase level.
- Know that D_5W IV can decrease the serum amylase level, causing a false-negative result.
- Check urinary output for 8 hours and 24 hours. A decreased urine output could result in a decreased urine amylase.

Client Teaching

- Encourage the client to drink water during the test unless water intake is restricted for medical reasons.

- Explain to the client the importance of collecting urine at a specified time, using a urinal or bedpan and saving all urine.

Elevated level—serum and urine

- Check serum amylase levels for several days after abdominal surgery. Surgery of the stomach or gallbladder might cause trauma to the pancreas and excess amylase to be released.
- Report symptoms of severe pain when pancreatitis is suspected. The physician may want to draw a serum amylase level before a narcotic is given. An elevated level may indicate an acute pancreatitis.
- Check the serum amylase level and compare with the urine amylase level. A low serum amylase level and an increased urine amylase level could indicate that the acute problem is no longer present.
- Report elevated serum amylase results occurring beyond 3 days. If the serum amylase levels remain elevated beyond 3 days, pancreatic cell destruction could still be occurring.

ANGIOTENSIN-CONVERTING ENZYME (ACE) SERUM

ANGIOTENSIN-1-CONVERTING ENZYME

Reference Values

Adult >20 yrs: 8–67 U/L
Child and adult <20 yrs: Not performed because they normally have elevated ACE levels

Description. Angiotensin-converting enzyme (ACE) is found primarily in the lung epithelial cells and some in blood vessels and renal cells. The purpose of ACE is to regulate arterial blood pressure by converting angiotensin I to the vasoconstrictor angiotensin II, which increases blood pressure and stimulates the adrenal cortex to release aldosterone (sodium-retaining hormone). However, this test has little value for diagnosing hypertension.

High serum ACE levels are found primarily with active pulmonary sarcoidosis. Seventy to 90% of clients with active sarcoidosis have elevated serum ACE levels. Other conditions that have elevated ACE levels include: Gaucher's disease (disorder of fat metabolism), leprosy, alcoholic cirrhosis, active histoplasmosis, tuberculosis, pulmonary embolism, hyperthyroidism, and Hodgkin's disease.

Purposes

- To assist in diagnosing various health problems such as pulmonary sarcoidosis related to elevated serum ACE level
- To compare the results of serum ACE level with other laboratory tests for diagnosing health problem

Clinical Problems

Decreased level: Therapy for sarcoidosis, diabetes mellitus, hypothyroidism, respiratory distress syndrome, severe illness, starvation
Drugs that may decrease ACE value: Steroids (prednisone, cortisone), captopril, enalapril

Elevated level: sarcoidosis, Gaucher's disease, leprosy, alcoholic cirrhosis, histoplasmosis, tuberculosis, pulmonary embolism, hyperthyroidism, Hodgkin's disease, myeloma, non-Hodgkin's lymphoma, idiopathic pulmonary fibrosis, scleroderma, diabetes mellitus, asbestosis

Procedure

- Restrict food and fluids for 12 hours prior to the test.
- Collect 7 mL of venous blood in a red-top or green-top tube. Check with the laboratory concerning which tube—for clotted blood (red-top) or heparinized (green-top). Avoid hemolysis. Deliver the blood sample immediately to the laboratory.
- Record the client's age on the laboratory slip.

Nursing Implications

- Check blood pressure. This test is not used to determine the cause of hypertension; however, ACE indirectly contributes to an increase in blood pressure.
- Report if the client is taking steroids to the health care provider and on the laboratory slip.
- Record the age of the client on the laboratory slip. Rarely is this test ordered for clients under 20 years of age as there could be a false-positive test result.

Client Teaching

- Instruct the client not to eat or drink for 12 hours prior to the test; this would most likely be NPO after dinner.
- Answer questions or concerns the client may have or refer him/her to other health care providers.

ANION GAP

Reference Values

Adult: 10–17 mEq/L (values differ from 7 to 20 mEq/L)

Description. Anion gap is the difference between the electrolytes, measured cations (sodium and potassium) and measured anions (chloride and bicarbonate [CO_2]) to determine the unmeasured cations and anions in the serum. These unmeasured ions are phosphates, sulfates, lactates, ketone bodies, and other organic acids that contribute to metabolic acid–base imbalances (metabolic acidosis or alkalosis).

The formula used to determine the anion gap is: Anion gap = (sodium + potassium) – (chloride + CO_2 [bicarbonate]).

An elevated anion gap >17 mEq/L is indicative of metabolic acidosis; a decreased anion gap <10 mEq/L is indicative of metabolic alkalosis.

Purpose

- To determine the presence of acidosis

Clinical Problems

Decreased level: High electrolyte values such as sodium, calcium, magnesium, multiple myeloma, nephrosis
Drugs that may decrease the anion gap: diuretics, lithium, chlorpropamide

Elevated level: Lactic acidosis, ketoacidosis, starvation, severe salicylate intoxication, renal failure, severe dehydration, paint thinner ingestion
Drugs that may increase the anion gap: Penicillin and carbenicillin in high doses, salicylates, diuretics (thiazides and loop diuretics), methanol ingestion, paraldehyde

Normal level occurring in metabolic acidosis: Diarrhea, renal tubular acidosis, hyperalimentation, ureterosigmoidostomy, small bowel fistula, pancreatic drainage

Procedure

- No food or fluid restriction is required.
- Obtain serum electrolyte values: sodium (Na), potassium (K), chloride (C), and CO_2 (bicarbonate determinant). If electrolytes are not available, collect 7 to 10 mL of venous blood in a red-top tube.

Nursing Implications

- Calculate anion gap from recently obtained electrolyte values of sodium, potassium, chloride, and serum CO_2. Use the formula given in "Description."
- Observe for signs and symptoms of metabolic acidosis such as rapid, vigorous breathing (Kussmaul's breathing), flushed skin, increased pulse rate.

ANTIBIOTIC SUSCEPTIBILITY (SENSITIVITY) TEST

CULTURE AND SENSITIVITY (C & S) TEST

Reference Values

Adult: Organism is sensitive, intermediate, or resistant to the antibiotic disks

Child: Same as adult

Description. It is important to identify not only the organism responsible for the infection but also the antibiotic(s) that will inhibit the growth of the bacteria. The health care provider orders a C & S test when a wound infection, urinary tract infection (UTI), or other types of infected secretions are suspected. The choice of antibiotic depends on the pathogenic organism and its susceptibility to the antibiotics.

Purpose

- To check the effectiveness of selected antibiotics to a specific bacteria from a culture

Clinical Problems

Resistant (R): Antibiotic is noneffective against the organism
Intermediate (I): Bacterial growth retardation is inconclusive
Sensitive (S): Antibiotic is effective against the organism

Procedure (See Culture Procedure)

- The specimen for C & S should be taken to the laboratory within 30 minutes of collection or refrigerated.
- It usually takes 24 hours for bacterial growth and 48 hours for the test results.

Nursing Implications

- Collect specimen for C & S before preventive antibiotic therapy is started. Antibiotic therapy started before specimen collection could cause an inaccurate result.
- Record on the laboratory slip the antibiotic(s) the client is receiving, the dosages, and how long the antibiotic(s) has (have) been taken.
- Check laboratory report for C & S result. If the client is receiving an antibiotic and the report shows the organism is resistant to that antibiotic, notify the health care provider.

Client Teaching

- Inform the client that the culture test results will be available in 48 hours.

ANTIDEPRESSANTS (TRICYCLICS) SERUM

AMITRIPTYLINE, DESIPRAMINE, DOXEPIN, IMIPRAMINE, NORTRIPTYLINE

Reference Values

Adult

DRUG NAME	THERAPEUTIC RANGE (NG/ML)	TOXIC LEVEL (NG/ML)
Amitriptyline HCl (Elavil)	75–225	>500
Desipramine HCl (Norpramin)	125–300	>500
Doxepin HCl (Sinequan)	150–300	>500
Imipramine HCl (Tofranil)	150–300	>500
Nortriptyline HCl (Aventyl)	75–150	>300

Description. Antidepressants are used primarily for unipolar or endogenous depression, which is characterized by loss of interest in work or home, inability to complete tasks, and deep depression. There are three groups of antidepressants: tricyclic antidepressants (TCAs), second-generation antidepressants (newest group), and monoamine oxidase (MAO) inhibitors. A common side effect of tricyclic antidepressants is anticholinergic symptoms. With second-generation antidepressants, extrapyramidal symptoms (EPS) are common. Clients taking MAO inhibitors, foods rich in tyramine (cheese, cream, chocolate, bananas, beer, red wines) should be avoided. Hypertensive crisis could occur when taking foods rich in tyramine and MAO inhibitors.

Purposes

- To regulate tricyclic drug level for obtaining a therapeutic drug level
- To monitor tricyclic drug dose
- To avoid toxic drug level

Clinical Problems

Decreased level: Mild, reactive, unipolar, and/or atypical depression
Drugs that may decrease antidepressant level: Barbiturates, chloral hydrate

Elevated level: Toxic tricycle antidepressant
Drugs that may increase antidepressant level: Hydrocortisone, neuroleptics, cimetidine, oral contraceptives

Procedure

- No food or fluid restriction is required.
- Collect 7 mL of venous blood in a red-top tube. Deliver blood container immediately to the laboratory.
- Obtain blood specimen 2 hours before the next drug dose.

Nursing Implications

- Assess client's history related to depression.
- Record drugs that the client presently is taking. CNS depressants and alcohol, if taken with antidepressants, could cause respiratory depression and hypotension.
- Monitor vital signs and urinary output. Report abnormal findings.

- Check serum tricyclic level of the drug client is taking. Report if the level is NOT within therapeutic range.
- Assess client's compliance to drug therapy. Report changes.

Client Teaching

- Discuss the importance of drug compliance with the client. This is important to maintain a therapeutic drug level and possibly to avoid toxic level if the drug is taken in excess.
- Discuss possible side effects, such as dry mouth, blurred vision, fatigue, urinary retention, postural hypotension, and GI disturbances, and report any of these to the health care provider.
- Discuss foods to avoid if the client is taking an MAO inhibitor (see Description).

ANTIDIURETIC HORMONE (ADH) PLASMA

VASOPRESSOR

Reference Values

Adult: 1–5 pg/mL; 1–5 ng/L

Description. Antidiuretic hormone (ADH) is produced by the hypothalamus and stored in the posterior pituitary gland (neurohypophysis). Primary function of ADH is for water reabsorption from the distal renal tubules in response to the serum osmolality. Antidiuretic means "against diuresis." There is more ADH secreted from the posterior pituitary gland when the serum osmolality is increased, >295 mOsm/kg (concentrated body fluids); thus, more water is reabsorbed, which dilutes the body fluid. When the serum osmolality is decreased, <280 mOs/kg, less ADH is secreted, and thus more water is excreted via kidneys.

Syndrome (secretion) of inappropriate ADH (SIADH) is an excess secretion of ADH that is not influenced by the serum osmolality level. SIADH causes excess water retention. Stress, surgery, pain, and certain drugs (narcotics, anesthetics) contribute to SIADH.

Purposes

- To detect a deficit or excess in ADH secretion
- To identify the presence of body fluid deficit or excess

Clinical Problems

Decreased level: Diabetes insipidus, psychogenic polydipsia, nephrotic syndrome
Drugs that may decrease ADH value: Alcohol, lithium, demeclocycline, phenytoin (Dilantin)

Elevated level: SIADH, brain tumor, cancer (ectopic ADH), pulmonary tuberculosis, pain, intermittent positive pressure breathing (IPPB), surgery, pneumonia
Drugs that may increase ADH value: Anesthetics, narcotics, estrogens, oxytocin, antineoplastic (anticancer) drugs, thiazides, antipsychotics, tricyclic antidepressants

Procedure

- Restrict food and fluids for 12 hours. Avoid strenuous exercise for 12 hours. Stress should be decreased or avoided.
- Collect 5 to 7 mL of venous blood in a lavender-top plastic tube or plastic syringe. Glass container can cause degradation of the antidiuretic hormone. If blood is drawn in glass, prechill the glass and separate immediately.
- Deliver the blood specimen immediately (within 10 minutes) to the laboratory.

Factors Affecting Laboratory Results

- Blood specimen taken at night or from a client in standing position can cause the ADH to be elevated.

Nursing Implications

- Report drugs the client is taking that can affect test results. These drugs should be withheld 12 hours prior to the test.
- Record in the client's chart and on the laboratory slip if the client is having undue stress or pain. This could increase the ADH secretion (SIADH) and plasma level.
- Take the blood specimen immediately to the laboratory. The serum should be separated from the clot within 10 minutes.
- Listen to client's concerns.

ANTIGLOMERULAR BASEMENT MEMBRANE ANTIBODY (ANTI-GBM, AGBM) SERUM

GLOMERULAR BASEMENT MEMBRANE ANTIBODY

Reference Values. Negative or none detected

Description. This test is performed to detect circulating glomerular basement membrane (GBM) antibodies that can damage the glomerular basement membranes in the glomeruli. Beta-hemolytic *Streptococcus* can cause an antibody response in the renal glomeruli.

Glomerulonephritis, caused by anti-GBM, is usually severe and rapidly progressive. Pulmonary hemorrhage often occurs due to cross-reactivity of anti-GBM with pulmonary vascular basement membrane.

Purpose. To detect GBM antibodies that could cause or is causing renal disease

Clinical Problems

Positive result: Anti-GBM nephritis, tubulointerstitial nephritis, pulmonary capillary basement membranes

Procedure

- No food or fluid restriction is required.
- Collect 5 to 7 mL of venous blood in a red-top tube. Test should be run immediately, and if not, the blood should be frozen.
- Tissue from kidney biopsy might be the specimen. Tissue should be frozen after collection.

Nursing Implications

- Obtain a history of a streptococcal throat infection.
- Monitor urine output. As the glomeruli are damaged, oliguria usually occurs.
- Assess for signs and symptoms of renal (glomerular) disease (i.e., edema of the extremities, shortness of breath, proteinuria,

hematuria, increased blood pressure, elevated serum BUN and creatinine, decreased urine output.)

Client Teaching

- Instruct the client to follow a medical regimen of diet, drugs, and rest.

ANTIMITOCHONDRIAL ANTIBODY (AMA) (SERUM)

Reference Values

Negative: At a 1:5 to 1:10 dilution
Intermediate level: 1:20 to 1:80 dilution
Strongly suggestive of primary biliary cirrhosis: >1:80
Positive for primary biliary cirrhosis: >1:160

Description. The antimitochondrial antibody (AMA) test is used to differentiate between primary biliary cirrhosis and other liver disease. Eighty percent to 90% of clients with primary biliary cirrhosis have a positive titer for AMAs. A positive test result would usually rule out extrahepatic biliary obstruction and acute infectious hepatitis. To confirm biliary cirrhosis, other liver tests should be performed, such as ALT, GGT, alkaline phosphatase, serum bilirubin.

This test is usually performed in conjunction with anti–smooth muscle antibodies (ASMA) test. ASMA titer is elevated with biliary cirrhosis and chronic active hepatitis. Like AMA, ASMA is seldom elevated with extrahepatic biliary obstruction. The antibodies may also be associated with autoimmune disease.

Purposes

- To aid in the diagnosis of biliary cirrhosis
- To determine liver function
- To differentiate between biliary cirrhosis and extrahepatic disease. Liver biopsy may be needed

Clinical Problems

Positive titer: Primary biliary cirrhosis, chronic hepatitis, autoimmune disorders (i.e., systemic erythematosus (SLE), rheumatoid arthritis, pernicious anemia)

Procedure

- NPO for 8 hours prior to the test. Food and fluids may not need to be restricted; check with the laboratory.
- Collect 2 to 5 mL of venous blood in a red-top or a gray-top tube. Avoid hemolysis. Take blood specimen immediately to the laboratory.

Nursing Implications

- Assess for the presence of jaundice.
- Check other liver tests and compare test results.
- Check with the laboratory as to whether NPO is necessary.

Client Teaching

- Listen to client's concern. Answer appropriate questions.
- Tell the client that if a hematoma occurs to apply warm wet compresses or soaks. Clients with hepatic disease have an increased bleeding tendency.

ANTIMYOCARDIAL ANTIBODY (SERUM)

Reference Values

Negative: None detected
Positive: Titer levels

Description. Antimyocardial antibody develops due to a specific antigen in the heart muscle that can cause autoimmune damage to the heart. This antibody may be detected in the blood prior to or soon after heart disease. The antibody may be present after cardiac surgery, myocardial infarction, streptococcal infection and rheumatic fever. This test may be used to monitor therapeutic response to treatment.

Purpose

- To identify the presence of antimyocardial antibody as the cause of the cardiac condition

Clinical Problems

Elevated titer: Myocardial infarction, myocarditis, pericarditis, following cardiac surgery, acute rheumatic fever, chronic rheumatic diseases, streptococcal infections, idiopathic cardiomyopathy, endomyocardial fibrosis, thoracic injury, systemic lupus erythematosus (SLE)

Procedure

- No food or fluid restriction is required.
- Collect 5 to 7 mL of venous blood in a red-top tube. Send to the laboratory immediately.

Nursing Implications

- Obtain a history of heart disease.
- Check cardiac enzyme levels, CPK, AST, LDH, and if elevated, heart disease is likely.
- Observe for signs and symptoms of heart disease, such as chest pain, dyspnea, diaphoresis, and indigestion.
- Listen to client's concerns.

ANTINUCLEAR ANTIBODIES (ANA) SERUM

Reference Values

Adult: Negative

Description. The ANA test is a screening test for diagnosing systemic lupus erythematosus (SLE) and other collagen diseases. The total ANA can also be positive in scleroderma, rheumatoid arthritis, cirrhosis, leukemia, infectious mononucleosis, and malignancy. It is normally present (95%) in lupus nephritis.

Purpose

- To compare ANA with other laboratory tests for diagnosing SLE or other collagen disease

Clinical Problems

Elevated level: (>1:20) SLE, progressive systemic sclerosis, scleroderma, rheumatoid arthritis, leukemia, cirrhosis of the liver, infectious mononucleosis, myasthenia gravis, malignancy

Drugs that may increase ANA value: Antibiotics (penicillin, tetracycline, streptomycin), antihypertensives (hydralazine [Apresoline], methyldopa [Aldomet]), isoniazid (INH), diuretics (acetazolamide [Diamox], thiazides [hydrochlorothiazide/Hydrodiuril]), phenytoin (Dilantin), oral contraceptives, antiarrhythmics (procainamide [Pronestyl], quinidine), trimethadione (Tridione), chlorpromazine (Thorazine)

Procedure

- No food or fluid restriction is required.
- Collect 3 to 5 mL of venous blood in a red-top tube. Take to the laboratory immediately, since serum needs to be separate from cells.
- Withhold drugs the client is receiving that can cause a false-positive titer before test with health care provider's permission. If given, list the drugs on the laboratory slip.

Nursing Implications

- Relate clinical problems and drugs to positive ANA results. With SLE, the ANA titer may fluctuate according to the severity of the disease.
- Compare test result with other tests for lupus.
- Assess for signs and symptoms of SLE (i.e., skin rash over the cheeks and nose, joint pain).

Client Teaching

- Promote rest during an acute phase.

ANTISTREPTOLYSIN O (ASO) SERUM

Reference Values. Upper limit of normal varies with age, season, and geographic area.
Adult: <100 IU/mL
Child: Newborn: similar to mother's; 2–5 yr: <100 IU/mL; 12–19 yr: <200 IU/mL

Description. The beta-hemolytic streptococcus secretes an enzyme known as streptolysin O that acts as an antigen and stimulates the immune system to develop antistreptolysin O (ASO) antibodies. A high serum ASO could indicate an acute rheumatic fever or acute glomerulonephritis. The ASO antibodies appear 1 to 2 weeks after an acute streptococcal infection, peak 3 to 4 weeks later, and could remain elevated for months. A fourfold increase in titer between acute and convalescent phase is suggestive of a recent group A streptococcal infection.

Purposes

- To identify clients who are susceptible to specific autoimmune disorders (i.e., collagen disease)
- To aid in determining the effect of beta-hemolytic streptococcus in secreting the enzyme streptolysin O

Clinical Problems

Drugs that may decrease ASO value: Antibiotic therapy

Elevated level: Acute rheumatic fever, acute glomerulonephritis, streptococcal upper respiratory infections, rheumatoid arthritis (mildly elevated), hyperglobulinemia with liver disease, collagen disease (mildly elevated)

Procedure

- No food or fluid restriction is required.
- Collect 3 to 5 mL of venous blood in a red-top tube. Avoid hemolysis of blood specimen.
- Repeated ASO testing (once or twice a week) is advisable to determine the highest level of increase.

Factors Affecting Laboratory Results

- An increased level may occur in healthy persons (carriers).

Nursing Implications

- Check serum ASO levels when the client is complaining of joint pain in the extremities.
- Note that antibiotic therapy could decrease antibody response.
- Check the urinary output when the serum ASO is elevated. A urinary output of less than 600 mL/24 h may be associated with acute glomerulonephritis.

ARTERIAL BLOOD GASES (ABGS) ARTERIAL BLOOD

BLOOD GASES

Reference Values

Adult: pH: 7.35–7.45; $Paco_2$: 35–45 mm Hg; $Pao_2$75–100 mg Hg; HCO_3: 24–28 mEq/L; BE: +2 to −2 (±2 mEq/L)
Child: pH: 7.36–7.44. Other measurements are same as adult

Description. Determination of ABGs is usually ordered to assess disturbances of acid–base balance caused by a respiratory disorder or a metabolic disorder, or both. A pH less than 7.35 indicates acidosis, and a pH greater than 7.45 indicates alkalosis.

To determine whether the acid–base imbalance has a respiratory cause, the $Paco_2$ should be checked. A decreased pH (<7.35) and an elevated $Paco_2$ (>45 mm Hg) indicates respiratory acidosis. An elevated pH (>7.45) and a decreased $Paco_2$ (<35 mm Hg) indicates respiratory alkalosis.

To determine whether the acid–base imbalance has a metabolic cause, the bicarbonate (HCO_3) and base excess (BE) should be checked. A decreased pH (<7.35) and a decreased HCO_3 (<24 mEq/L) indicates metabolic acidosis. An elevated pH (>7.45) and an elevated HCO_3 (>28 mEq/L) indicates metabolic alkalosis.

Acid–Base Imbalance	*pH*	*$Paco_2$*	*HCO_3*	*BE*
Respiratory acidosis	↓	↑	N	N
Respiratory alkalosis	↑	↓	N	N
Metabolic acidosis	↓	N	↓	↓
Metabolic alkalosis	↑	N	↑	↑

Purposes

- To detect metabolic acidosis or alkalosis, or respiratory acidosis or alkalosis
- To monitor blood gases during an acute illness

Clinical Problems

pH decreased level

Respiratory acidosis: (pH <7.35; $Paco_2$ >45 mm Hg) chronic obstructive lung disease (i.e., emphysema, chronic bronchitis, severe asthma),

respiratory distress syndrome (ARDS), Guillain-Barré syndrome, anesthesia, pneumonia
Metabolic acidosis: (pH <7.35; HCO_3 <24 mEq/L) diabetic ketoacidosis, severe diarrhea, starvation/malnutrition, kidney failure, burns, shock, acute myocardial infarction
Drugs that may cause a low pH: narcotics, barbiturates, acetazolamide (Diamox), ammonium chloride, paraldehyde

pH elevated level
Respiratory alkalosis: (pH >7.45; $Paco_2$ <35 mm Hg) salicylate toxicity (early phase), anxiety, hysteria, tetany, strenuous exercise (swimming, running), fever, hyperthyroidism, delirium tremens, pulmonary embolism
Metabolic alkalosis: (pH >7.45; HCO_3 > 28 mEq/L) severe vomiting, gastric suction, peptic ulcer, potassium loss (hypokalemia), excess administration of sodium bicarbonate, cystic fibrosis, hepatic failure
Drugs that may cause an elevated pH: Sodium bicarbonate, sodium oxalate, potassium oxalate

Procedure

- No food or fluid restriction is required.
- Notify the laboratory that blood gases are to be sent.
- Collect 1 to 5 mL of arterial blood in a heparinized needle and syringe, remove the needle, make sure there is no air in the syringe, and apply an airtight cap over the tip of the syringe.
- Place the syringe with arterial blood in an ice bag (to minimize the metabolic activities of the sample) and deliver it immediately to the laboratory.
- Indicate on the ABG slip whether the client is receiving oxygen and the rate of flow.
- Apply pressure to the puncture site for 2 to 5 minutes.
- Be sure the blood is not collected from the same arm used for the IV infusion.

Factors Affecting Laboratory Results

- Inaccurate results can occur as a result of suctioning, changes in O_2 therapy, ventilator use, and blood transfusion.

Nursing Implications

Respiratory acidosis

- Assess for signs and symptoms of respiratory acidosis (i.e., dyspnea, disorientation, and an increased $Paco_2$).

Client Teaching

- Perform chest clapping to break up bronchial and alveolar secretions. CO_2 can be trapped in the lungs because of excess secretions and mucous plugs.
- Check for metabolic compensatory mechanism with respiratory acidosis—HCO_3 is elevated (>28 mEq/L).
- Instruct the client in performing breathing exercises to enhance CO_2 excretion from the lungs.

Metabolic acidosis

- Assess for signs and symptoms of metabolic acidosis (i.e., rapid, vigorous breathing [Kussmaul breathing]; flushing of the skin; restlessness; and a decreased HCO_3 level, decreased BE, and decreased serum CO_2).
- Check for respiratory compensatory mechanism with metabolic acidosis—$Paco_2$ is decreased (<35 mm Hg).

Respiratory alkalosis

- Assess for signs and symptoms of respiratory alkalosis (i.e., tachypnea, dizziness, tetany spasms, and decreased CO_2).

Metabolic alkalosis

- Assess for signs and symptoms of metabolic alkalosis (i.e., shallow breathing, vomiting, increased HCO_3, increased BE, and increased serum CO_2).

ASPARTATE AMINOTRANSFERASE (AST) SERUM

SERUM GLUTAMIC OXALOACETIC TRANSAMINASE (SGOT)

Reference Values

Adult: *Average range:* 8–38 U/L; (Frankel), 4–36 IU/L, 16–60 U/mL at 30°C (Karmen), 8–33 U/L at 37°C (SI units). Female values may be slightly lower than those in men. Exercise tends to increase serum levels

Child: Newborns: four times the normal level; child: similar to adults

Elderly: Slightly higher than adults

Description. AST/SGOT is an enzyme found mainly in the heart muscle and liver; it is found in moderate amounts in the skeletal muscle, the kidneys, and the pancreas. High levels of serum AST are found following an acute myocardial infarction (AMI) and liver damage. After severe chest pain due to AMI, serum AST level rises in 6 to 10 hours and peaks in 24 to 48 hours. If there is no additional infarction, the AST level returns to normal in 4 to 6 days. Other cardiac enzyme tests are used in diagnosing an AMI (i.e., CPK, LDH).

In liver disease the serum level increases by ten times or more and remains elevated for a longer period of time. Serum levels of AST and ALT are frequently compared.

Purposes

- To detect an elevation of serum AST, an enzyme that is mainly in the heart muscle and liver that increases during an acute myocardial infarction and liver damage
- To compare AST results with CPK and LDH for diagnosing an acute myocardial infarction

Clinical Problems

Decreased level: Pregnancy, diabetic ketoacidosis, beriberi

Elevated level: Acute myocardial infarction (AMI), encephalitis, liver necrosis, musculoskeletal disease and trauma, acute pancreatitis, cancer of the liver, severe angina pectoris, strenuous exercise, acute pulmonary embolism, eclampsia, CHF
Drugs that may increase AST value: Antibiotics, narcotics, vitamins (folic acid, pyridoxine, vitamin A), antihypertensives (methyldopa [Aldomet], guanethidine), theophylline, digitalis preparations, cortisone, flurazepam (Dalmane), indomethacin (Indocin), isoniazid (INH), rifampin, oral contraceptives, salicylates, intramuscular (IM) injections

Procedure

- No food or fluid restriction is required.
- Collect 3 to 5 mL of venous blood in a red-top tube. Avoid hemolysis of blood specimen. Draw blood before drugs are given.
- List on the laboratory slip drugs that can cause false-positive levels with date and time last given.

Factors Affecting Laboratory Results

- IM injections could cause increase serum AST levels.

Nursing Implications

- Alleviate anxiety by explaining purpose of the test. Be supportive to the client and family.
- Hold drugs causing an elevated serum AST for 24 hours prior to the blood test, with the health care provider's permission.
- Do not administer IM injections before the blood test. IM injections can increase the serum AST level. A few medications (e.g., morphine) can be given IV without affecting the serum level.
- Assess the client for signs and symptoms of AMI (i.e., chest and arm pain, dyspnea, diaphoresis).
- Compare serum AST and serum ALT levels to determine if liver damage could be responsible for the abnormal values.

Client Teaching

- Instruct the client to report symptoms of chest and/or arm pain, nausea, and/or diaphoresis immediately—day or night.

ATRIAL NATRIURETIC HORMONE (ANH) (PLASMA)

ATRIAL NATRIURETIC FACTOR (ANF), ATRIAL NATRIURETIC PEPTIDES (ANP)

Reference Values. 20–77 pg/mL; 20–77 ng/L (SI units)

Description. Atrial natriuretic hormone (ANH) is secreted from the atria of the heart. It is released during expansion of the atrium, produces vasodilation, and increases glomerular filtration rate. ANH reduces renal reabsorption of sodium, blocks renin release by the kidney, and blocks aldosterone secretion from the adrenal glands; thus, it has an antihypertensive effect. With the physiologic effects of ANH, preload, afterload, and blood volume are reduced. An elevated ANH level can be used to detect cardiovascular disease, early asymptomatic left ventricular disorder, and congestive heart failure (CHF). However, with chronic level CHF, the ANH is decreased, while with acute congestive heart failure, the ANH level is elevated.

Purposes

- To detect cardiovascular disease, particularly CHF
- To detect asymptomatic fluid volume (cardiac) overload

Clinical Problems

Decreased level: Chronic CHF
Drugs that may decrease plasma ANH: Prazosin, urapidil

Elevated level: Acute CHF, paroxysmal atrial tachycardia, early cardiovascular disease, subarachnoid hemorrhage

Procedure

- NPO for 8 to 12 hours prior to test.
- Withhold cardiac drugs (i.e., beta blockers, calcium blockers, diuretics vasodilators, and digoxin) until after test.
- Collect 5 mL of venous blood in a lavender-top tube. Ice the tube and take it immediately to the laboratory.

Factors Affecting Laboratory Results

- Cardiac drugs (see Procedure)

Nursing Implications

- Obtain a health and drug history from the client.
- Take vital signs. Compare findings to baseline readings.
- Answer the client's questions. Be supportive of the client.

Client Teaching

- Inform the client that medications that were withheld may be taken following the test.
- Instruct the client to notify his/her health care provider of difficulty in breathing, shortness of breath, chest pain, and/or indigestion.

BILIRUBIN (TOTAL, DIRECT, INDIRECT) SERUM

Reference Values

Adult: Total: 0.1–1.2 mg/dL, 1.7–20.5 μmol/L (SI units)
Direct (conjugated): 0.0–0.3 mg/dL, 1.7–5.1 μmol/L (SI units)

Indirect (unconjugated): 0.1–1.0 mg/dL, 1.7–17.1 μmol/L (SI units)

Child: Total: newborn: 1–12 mg/dL, 17.1–205 μmol/L (SI units); child: 0.2–0.8 mg/dL

Description. Bilirubin is formed from the breakdown of hemoglobin by the reticuloendothelial system and is carried in the plasma to the liver, where it is conjugated (directly) and excreted in the bile. There are two forms of bilirubin in the body: the conjugated, or direct reacting (soluble); and the unconjugated, or indirect reacting (protein bound). If the total bilirubin is within normal range, direct and indirect bilirubin levels do not need to be analyzed. If one value of bilirubin is reported, it represents the total bilirubin. Jaundice is frequently present when serum bilirubin (total) is greater than 3 mg/dL. Total serum bilirubin in newborns can be as high as 12 mg/dL; the panic level is >15 mg/dL.

Increased direct or conjugated bilirubin is usually the result of obstructive jaundice, either extrahepatic (from stones or tumor) or intrahepatic (damaged liver cells). Indirect or unconjugated bilirubin is associated with increased destruction of RBCs (hemolysis).

Purposes

- To monitor bilirubin levels associated with jaundice
- To suggest the occurrence of liver disorder

Clinical Problems

Decreased level

Direct: Iron deficiency anemia

Drugs that may decrease bilirubin value: Barbiturates, aspirin (large amounts), penicillin, caffeine

Elevated level

Direct: Obstructive jaundice caused by stones or neoplasms, hepatitis, cirrhosis of the liver, infectious mononucleosis, liver cancer, Wilson's disease

Indirect: Erythroblastosis fetalis, sickle cell anemia, transfusion reaction, hemolytic anemias, pernicious anemia, malaria, septicemia, CHF, decompensated cirrhosis

Drugs that may increase bilirubin value: Antibiotics, sulfonamides; diuretics; isoniazid (INH); diazepam (Valium); narcotics; barbiturates; flurazepam (Dalmane); indomethacin (Indocin); methyldopa (Aldomet); procainamide (Pronestyl); steroids; oral contraceptives; tolbutamide (Orinase); vitamins A, C, and K

Procedure

- Restrict food and fluids, except for water.
- Collect 3 to 5 mL of venous blood in a red-top tube. Avoid hemolysis.
- List drugs client is taking that may affect test results.
- Protect the blood specimen from sunlight and artificial light, as light will reduce the bilirubin content. Blood should be sent to the laboratory immediately so that separation of serum from the cells can be performed.
- There is no laboratory test for indirect bilirubin. Indirect bilirubin is calculated by subtracting direct bilirubin from total bilirubin: Total bilirubin – direct bilirubin = indirect bilirubin

Factors Affecting Laboratory Results

- A high-fat dinner prior to the test may affect bilirubin levels.
- Carrots and yams may increase the serum bilirubin level.

Nursing Implications

- Check the serum bilirubin (total), and if it is elevated, check the direct bilirubin level. To obtain the indirect bilirubin level, subtract the direct bilirubin from the total bilirubin. An elevated direct bilirubin level is usually due to a liver problem, and an elevated indirect bilirubin level is most likely due to a hemolytic problem.
- Check the sclera of the eyes and the inner aspects of the arm for jaundice.
- Be supportive to client and family. Answer questions and refer unknown answers to other professionals.

Client Teaching

- Instruct the client not to eat carrots, yams, or foods high in fat the night before.

BILIRUBIN (URINE)

Reference Values

Adult: Negative, 0.02 mg/dL

Description. Bilirubin is not normally present in urine; however, a very small quantity may be present without being detected by routine test methods. Bilirubin is formed from the breakdown of hemoglobin; it is conjugated in the liver and is excreted as bile. Conjugated, or direct, bilirubin is water soluble and is excreted in the urine when there is an increased serum level.

Bilirubinuria (bilirubin in urine) has a characteristic color of dark amber. It is an indicator of liver damage or biliary obstruction such as stones. Bilirubinuria can be tested by the floor nurse using a dipstick such as bili-Labstix or tablet (Ictotest-Ames). The more accurate testing is Ictotest (tablet). Values of serum bilirubin should be compared with urine bilirubin to diagnose the cause of the jaundice. If serum bilirubin is elevated (hyperbilirubinemia) and the urine bilirubin is negative, unconjugated (fat-soluble) hyperbilirubinemia is probable. Conjugated (water-soluble) hyperbilirubinemia is excreted in the urine.

Purpose

- To compare urine bilrubin level with serum bilirubin and other liver enzyme tests to detect liver disorder

Clinical Problems

Elevated level: Obstructive biliary disease, liver disease (hepatitis, toxic agents), CHF with jaundice, cancer of the liver (secondary)
Drugs that may increase urine bilirubin: Phenothiazines, chlorprothixene (Taractan), phenazopyridine (Pyridium), chlorzoxazone (Paraflex)

Procedure

- No food or fluid restriction is required.
- Use either bili-Labstix or Ictotest reagent tablets for the bilirubinuria test. The bili-Labstix is dipped in urine and, after 20 seconds, is compared to a color chart on the bottle.

- With the Ictotest, place 5 drops of urine on the asbestos-cellulose test mat. Place the reagent tablet on the mat and add 2 drops of water. If the test is positive for bilirubin, the mat color will turn blue or purple. Pink or red color indicates a negative test result.
- Urine bilirubin test should be performed within 1 hour. Keep urine away from ultraviolet light.

Nursing Implications

- Compare the urine bilirubin result with the serum bilirubin test (direct and total). If the serum bilirubin (direct) is elevated and the urine bilirubin is positive (bilirubinuria), the cause of the jaundice is most likely conjugated hyperbilirubinemia.
- Check the color of the urine. If it is dark amber in color, shake the urine specimen and note whether a yellow foam appears.
- Record the results of the bili-Labstix and the urine color on the client's chart.
- Notify the health care provider of amber urine with yellow foam and test results.

BLEEDING TIME (BLOOD)

Reference Values

Adult: Ivy method: 3–7 minutes; Duke method: 1–3 minutes (seldom performed)

Description. Two methods, Ivy and Duke, are used to determine whether bleeding time is normal or prolonged. Bleeding time is lengthened in thrombocytopenia (decreased platelet count [<50,000]). The test is frequently performed when there is a history of bleeding (easy bruising), familial bleeding, or preoperative screening. The Ivy technique, in which the forearm is used for the incision, is the most popular method. Aspirins and anti-inflammatory medications can prolong the bleeding time.

Purpose

- To check bleeding time for various health problems

Clinical Problems

Prolonged time: Thrombocytopenic purpura, platelet function abnormality, vascular abnormalities, severe liver disease, disseminated intravascular coagulation (DIC), aplastic anemia, factor deficiencies (V, VII, XI), Christmas disease, hemophilia, leukemia

Drugs that may increase bleeding time: Salicylates (aspirins, others), warfarin (Coumadin), dextran, streptokinase (fibrinolytic agent)

Procedure

Ivy method

- Test should NOT be performed while taking anticoagulant or aspirin. Client should withhold these medications 3 to 7 days prior to test, with health care provider's permission. Aspirin therapy will prolong bleeding time.
- Cleanse the volar surface of the forearm (below the antecubital space) with alcohol and allow it to dry. Inflate the blood pressure cuff to 40 mm Hg, and leave it inflated during the test. Puncture the skin 2.5 mm deep on the forearm; start timing with a stopwatch. Blot blood drops carefully every 30 seconds until bleeding ceases. The time required for bleeding to stop is recorded.

Duke method

- The area used is the earlobe.
- No food or fluid restriction is required.

Nursing Implications

- Explain the procedure step by step.
- Allow time for the client to ask questions.
- Obtain a drug history of the last time (date) the client took aspirin or anticoagulants. Aspirin prevents platelet aggregation, and bleeding can be prolonged by taking only one aspirin tablet (5 grains or 325 mg) 3 days prior to test. A history of taking cold medications should be recorded, since many cold remedies contain salicylates.

Client Teaching

- Instruct the client not to take aspirin and over-the-counter cold remedies for 3 days before the test. Notify the health care provider or laboratory, or both, if client has taken aspirin compounds.

BLOOD UREA NITROGEN (BUN) SERUM

Reference Values

Adult: 5–25 mg/dL
Child: Infant: 5–15 mg/dL; child: 5–20 mg/dL
Elderly: Could be slightly higher than adult
Urea nitrogen/creatinine ratio: 12:1–20:1

Description. Urea is an end product of protein metabolism. An elevated BUN level could be an indication of dehydration, prerenal failure, or renal failure or gastrointestinal bleeding, or both. Dehydration from vomiting, diarrhea, inadequate fluid intake, or all three is a common cause of an elevated BUN (up to 35 mg/dL). With dehydration, the serum creatinine level would most likely be normal or high normal. Once the client is hydrated (if dehydrated), the BUN should return to normal; if it does not, pre-renal or renal failure should be suspected. Digested blood from gastrointestinal bleeding is a source of protein and can cause the BUN to elevate. A low BUN value usually indicates overhydration (hypervolemia).

Urea nitrogen/creatinine ratio may be affected due to liver function, dietary protein intake, and muscle mass. A decreased ratio can occur from acute renal tubular necrosis, malnutrition, low-protein diet, or overhydration. The ratio may be increased due to reduced renal perfusion, obstructive uropathy, shock, GI bleeding, dehydration, and high protein intake.

Purpose

- To detect renal disorder or dehydration associated with increased BUN levels

Clinical Problems

Decreased level: Overhydration (hypervolemia); severe liver damage, low-protein diet, malnutrition (negative nitrogen balance), IV glucose fluids, pregnancy
Drugs that may decrease BUN value: Phenothiazines

Increased level: Dehydration, high protein intake, prerenal failure (low blood supply), renal insufficiency/failure, kidney diseases (glomeru-

lonephritis, pyelonephritis, acute nephritis), gastrointestinal bleeding, sepsis, AMI, diabetes mellitus, licorice (excessive ingestion)
Drugs that may increase BUN value: Diuretics, antibiotics, methyldopa (Aldomet), guanethidine (Ismelin), sulfonamides, propranolol (Inderal), morphine, lithium carbonate, salicylates

Procedure

- No food or fluid restriction is required. Test results may be more accurate if the patient is NPO for 8 hours.
- Collect 5 to 10 mL of venous blood in a red-top tube.

Factors Affecting Laboratory Results

- Hydration status of the client should be known. Dehydration or overhydration may cause false results.

Nursing Implications

- Compare serum BUN and serum creatinine results. If both BUN and creatinine levels are elevated, kidney disease should be highly suspected.
- Check vital signs every 8 hours and urinary output in 8 and 24 hours for decreased urinary output due to dehydration or renal disease.
- Assess for sign and symptoms of dehydration (i.e., poor skin turgor, increased pulse rate and respiration, dry mucous membrane, decrease in urine output [<25 mL per hour]).
- Observe for signs and symptoms of overhydration due to renal disorder (glomerulonephritis), such as dyspnea, neck vein engorgement, peripheral edema, puffy eyelids, and weight gain.
- Assess client's dietary intake.

Client Teaching

- Encourage client to increase fluid intake when BUN is 26 to 35 mg/dL, with health care provider's permission, to help correct dehydration status.

BLOOD UREA NITROGEN/CREATININE RATIO (SERUM)

UREA NITROGEN/CREATININE RATIO

Reference Values

Adult: 10:1 to 20:1 (BUN:creatinine); average: 15:1

Description. The BUN:creatinine ratio is a test primarily for determining renal function. BUN level can increase due to dehydration or a high-protein diet as well as renal dysfunction. The creatinine level does not increase with dehydration but definitely increases with renal dysfunction. This ratio test is more sensitive to the relationship of BUN to creatinine than separate tests of BUN and creatinine. However, liver function, dietary protein intake, and muscle mass may affect test result.

A decreased ratio can occur from acute renal tubular necrosis and low protein intake. The ratio may be increased due to reduced renal perfusion, glomerular disease, obstructive uropathy, or high protein intake.

Purpose

- To determine renal function

Clinical Problems

Decreased ratio: Acute renal tubular necrosis, low protein intake, malnutrition, pregnancy, liver disease, hemodialysis (urea loss), prolonged IV fluid therapy, ketosis
Drug that may decrease ratio: Phenacemide

Elevated ratio: Overproduction or lowered excretion of urea nitrogen, reduced renal perfusion (dehydration, heart failure), glomerular disease, tissue or muscle destruction, high protein intake, obstructive uropathy, azotemia, shock, hypotension, GI bleeding
Drugs that may increase ratio: Tetracycline, corticosteroids

Procedure

- No food or fluid restriction is required.
- Collect 5 to 7 mL of venous blood in a red-top tube.

Nursing Diagnoses

- Altered patterns of urinary elimination related to a decreased or elevated BUN:creatinine ratio secondary to renal disorder
- Ineffective coping related to renal impairment

Nursing Implications

- Assess the client's renal function including urine output, BUN, and serum creatinine level. Urine output should be at least 600 mL per day.
- Assess the client's dietary intake. Record increase or decrease in protein intake.
- Check his or her hydration status. Dehydration may cause increase in the BUN:creatinine ratio.

Client Teaching

- Instruct the client that urine needs to be measured and to urinate in a urinal or bedpan. Inform the health care providers after each voiding so that urine can be measured. Tell the client not to put toilet paper in the urine.

CALCITONIN (hCT) SERUM

Reference Values

Adult: Male: <40 pg/mL or ng/L; female: <25 pg/mL or ng/L
Child: <70 pg/mL; <70 ng/L (SI units)

Description. Calcitonin is a potent hormone secreted by the thyroid gland to maintain serum calcium and phosphorus levels. This hormone inhibits calcium reabsorption in the bone and promotes calcium excretion by the kidneys, thus lowering the serum calcium level. Calcitonin acts as an antagonist to the parathyroid hormone (PTH) and vitamin D.

Excess calcitonin secretion occurs in medullary carcinoma of the thyroid gland. Serum has higher values than plasma. A serum calcitonin value between 500 and 2000 pg/mL most likely indicates thyroid medullary carcinoma; a value greater than 2000 pg/mL is a definite indicator of thyroid medullary carcinoma.

When the serum calcitonin level is slightly to moderately elevated (100–500 pg/mL), a calcitonin stimulation test may be conducted to diagnose thyroid medullary carcinoma. This test consists of either a calcium infusion or a 10-second pentagastrin infusion with measurement of serum calcitonin before and after the infusion. Positive test result is a rapid rise over the baseline result.

Purpose

- To aid in the diagnosis of thyroid medullary carcinoma or parathyroid hyperplasia or adenoma

Clinical Problems

Elevated level: Thyroid medullary carcinoma, carcinoma of the lung or breast, chronic renal failure, parathyroid hyperplasma or adenoma, pernicious anemia, Zollinger–Ellison syndrome, acute or chronic thyroiditis, islet cell tumors, pheochromocytoma
Drugs that may increase calcitonin value: Calcium infusion, epinephrine, estrogens, glucagon, pentagastrin, oral contraceptives

Procedure

- Restrict food and fluids after midnight. A small amount of water may be given if needed.
- Collect 5 to 7 mL of venous blood in a green- or lavender-top tube or in a chilled red-top tube. Avoid hemolysis. Send blood specimen immediately to the laboratory for analysis or freeze to avoid deterioration.

Nursing Implication

- Obtain a health history that may suggest thyroid medullary carcinoma as indicated by a markedly elevated serum calcitonin value. If a slightly elevated serum calcitonin value is present, the nurse may collaborate with the health care provider regarding a calcitonin stimulation test.

CALCIUM (Ca) SERUM AND URINE

QUANTITATIVE (24-HOUR URINE COLLECTION)

Reference Values

Adult: Serum: 4.5–5.5 mEq/L, 9–11 mg/dL, 2.3–2.8 mmol/L (SI units). *Ionized Ca:* 4.25–5.25 mg/dL, 2.2–2.5 mEq/L, 1.1–1.24 mmol/L

Urine: 24-hour: low-calcium diet <150 mg/24 hours, <3.75 mmol/24 hours (SI units); average-calcium diet 100–250 mg/24 hours, 2.5–6.25 mmol/24 hours; high-calcium diet 250–300 mg/24 hours, 6.25–7.50 mmol/24 hours

Child: Serum: newborn: 3.7–7.0 mEq/L, 7.4–14.0 mg/dL; infant: 5.0–6.0 mEq/L, 10–12 mg/dL; child: 4.5–5.8 mEq/L, 9–11.5 mg/dL

Description. Approximately 50% of the calcium is ionized, and only ionized calcium can be used by the body; however, in most laboratories the total serum calcium level determination does not differentiate between ionized and nonionized calcium. In acidosis, more calcium is ionized, regardless of the serum level, and in alkalosis, most of the calcium is protein bound and cannot be ionized. Calcium imbalances require immediate attention, for serum calcium deficit can cause tetany symptoms, unless acidosis is present, and serum calcium excess can cause cardiac dysrhythmias.

A 24-hour urine specimen for calciuria is useful for determining parathyroid gland disorders. In hyperparathyroidism, hyperthyroidism, and osteolytic disorders, the urinary calcium excretion is usually increased; it is decreased in hypoparathyroidism.

Purposes

- To check for serum calcium excess or deficit
- To monitor calcium levels
- To detect calcium imbalance

Clinical Problems

Serum

Decreased level: Malabsorption of calcium from the gastrointestinal tract, lack of calcium and vitamin D intake, hypoparathyroidism, chronic renal failure caused by phosphorus retention, laxative abuse, extensive infections, burns, pancreatitis, alcoholism, diarrhea, pregnancy

Drugs that may decrease calcium value: Cortisone preparations, antibiotics (gentamicin, methicillin), magnesium products (antacids), excessive use of laxative, heparin, insulin, mithramycin, acetazolamide (Diamox)

Elevated level: Hyperparathyroidism; malignant neoplasm of the bone, lung, breast, bladder, or kidney; hypervitaminosis D, multiple myeloma, prolonged immobilization, multiple fractures, renal calculi, exercise, milk-alkali syndrome

Drugs that may increase calcium value: Thiazide diuretics, alkaline antacids, estrogen preparation, calcium salts, vitamin D

Procedure

Serum

- No food or fluid restriction is required, unless SMA_{12} is ordered. Many laboratories prefer that breakfast be withheld until after blood specimen is drawn.
- Collect 3 to 5 mL of venous blood in a red-top tube.

Urine

- Label the bottle for a 24-hour urine collection with the exact date and time of the urine collection. Preservatives are required by some laboratories; however, the urine specimen may be refrigerated or kept on ice.
- Indicate on the laboratory slip the client's calcium intake (limited, average, or high).

Nursing Implications

Decreased level

- Observe for signs and symptoms of tetany due to hypocalcemia (i.e., muscular twitching and tremors, spasms of the larynx, parathesia, facial spasms, and spasmodic contractions).
- Check serum calcium values and report abnormal results to the physician, especially if tetany symptoms are present.
- Assess for positive Chvostek's and Trousseau's signs of hypocalcemia.
- Observe for symptoms of tetany when the client is receiving massive transfusions of citrated blood. Citrates prevent calcium ionization. The serum calcium level may not be affected.

- Monitor the pulse regularly if the client is receiving a digitalis preparation and calcium supplements. Calcium excess enhances the action of digitalis and can cause digitalis toxicity (nausea, vomiting, anorexia, bradycardia).
- Administer IV fluids with 10% calcium gluconate slowly. Calcium should be administered in D_5W and not in a saline solution, as sodium promotes calcium loss. Calcium should not be added to solutions containing bicarbonate, since rapid precipitation will occur.

Client Teaching

- Instruct the client to avoid overuse of antacids and to prevent the chronic laxative habit, which could lower calcium level.
- Encourage the client to consume foods high in calcium and protein needed to enhance calcium absorption.

Elevated level

- Observe for signs and symptoms of hypercalcemia (i.e., lethargy, headaches, weakness, muscle flaccidity, heart block, anorexia, nausea, and vomiting).
- Promote active and passive exercises for bedridden clients. This will prevent calcium loss from the bone.
- Identify symptoms of digitalis toxicity when the client has an elevated serum calcium and is receiving a digitalis preparation.
- Notify the health care provider if the client is receiving a thiazide diuretic, for this will inhibit calcium excretion and promote hypercalcemia.

Client Teaching

- Instruct clients to avoid foods high in calcium, to be ambulatory when possible, and to increase oral fluid intake.

CARBON DIOXIDE (CO_2) COMBINING POWER (SERUM OR PLASMA)

CO_2 COMBINING POWER

Reference Values

Adult: 22–30 mEq/L, 22–30 mmol/L (SI units)
Panic Range: <15 mEq/L and >45 mEq/L
Child: 20–28 mEq/L

Description. The serum CO_2 test, usually included with the electrolyte (lyte) test, is performed to determine metabolic acid–base abnormalities. The serum CO_2 acts as a bicarbonate (HCO_3) determinant. When serum CO_2 is low, HCO_3 is lost and acidosis results (metabolic acidosis). With an elevated serum CO_2 excess, HCO_3 is conserved and alkalosis results (metabolic alkalosis).

Purpose

- To check for the presence of metabolic acidosis or alkalosis

Clinical Problems

Decreased level: Metabolic acidosis, diabetic ketoacidosis, starvation, severe diarrhea, dehydration, shock, acute renal failure, salicylate toxicity, exercise
Drugs that may decrease CO_2 value: Thiazide, diuretics, triamterene (Dyrenium), antibiotics (methicillin, tetracycline), nitrofurantoin (Furadantin), paraldehyde

Elevated level: Metabolic alkalosis, severe vomiting, gastric suction, peptic ulcer, hypothyroidism, potassium deficit
Drugs that may increase CO_2 value: Barbiturates, steroids, loop diuretics

Procedure

- No food or fluid restriction is required.
- Collect 3 to 5 mL of venous blood in a red- or green-top tube.

Nursing Implications

Decreased level

- Assess for signs and symptoms of metabolic acidosis when serum CO_2 is decreased, especially when <15 mEq/L. Symptoms include deep, vigorous breathing (Kussmaul's breathing) and flushed skin.
- Report clinical findings of metabolic acidosis to the health care provider.

Elevated level

- Assess for signs and symptoms of metabolic alkalosis with vomiting or gastric suction for several days. Signs and symptoms include shallow breathing, a serum CO_2 greater than 30 mEq/L, and a base excess greater than +2.

CARBON MONOXIDE, CARBOXYHEMOGLOBIN (BLOOD)

Reference Values

Adult: Nonsmoker: <2.5% of hemoglobin; smoker: 4–5% saturation of hemoglobin; heavy smoker: 5–12% saturation of hemoglobin. Toxic: >15% saturation of hemoglobin
Child: Similar to adult nonsmoker

Description. Carbon monoxide (CO) combines with hemoglobin to produce carboxyhemoglobin, which can occur 200 times more readily than the combination of oxygen with hemoglobin (oxyhemoglobin). When CO replaces oxygen in the hemoglobin in excess of 25%, CO toxicity occurs.

CO is formed from incomplete combustion of carbon-combining compounds, as in automobile exhaust, fumes from improperly functioning furnaces, and cigarette smoke. Continuous exposure to CO, increasing carboxyhemoglobin by more than 60%, leads to coma and death. The treatment for CO toxicity is to administer a high concentration of oxygen.

Purpose

- To determine the percentage of carbon monoxide in the hemoglobin; if high, it could be fatal

Clinical Problems

Elevated level: Smoking and exposure to smoking, automobile exhaust fumes, defective gas-burning appliances

Procedure

- No food or fluid restriction is required.
- Collect 5 to 7 mL of venous blood in a lavender-top tube.
- The most common method of analysis is performed with a CO oximeter, a direct-reading instrument.

Factors Affecting Laboratory Results

- Heavy smoking

Nursing Implications

- Determine from the client's history (obtained from the client, family, or friends) where carbon monoxide inhalation could have occurred.
- Assess for mild to severe carbon monoxide toxicity. Symptoms of mild CO toxicity are headache, weakness, malaise, dizziness, and dyspnea with exertion. Symptoms of moderate to severe toxicity are severe headache, bright red mucous membranes, and cherry-red blood. When carboxyhemoglobin exceeds 40%, the blood's residue is brick red.
- Identify individuals who might be candidates for CO poisoning. Clients who are living 24 hours a day in a house with an old heating system in the winter should have a blood CO test performed. This is especially true if those persons have continuous headaches.

CARCINOEMBRYONIC ANTIGEN (CEA) (SERUM OR PLASMA)

Reference Values

Adult: Nonsmokers: <2.5 ng/mL; smokers: <5 ng/mL
Acute inflammatory disorders: >10 ng/mL; neoplasms: >12 ng/mL

Description. CEA has been found in the gastrointestinal epithelium of embryos and has been extracted from tumors in the gastrointestinal tract. Originally, the CEA test was to detect colon cancer, especially adenocarcinoma. Elevated levels might occur during an acute inflammatory disorder. CEA should never be used as the sole criterion for diagnosis of colon and pancreatic cancer.

The primary role of the CEA test is to monitor the treatment of colon and pancreatic carcinoma. If the levels fall after treatment, the cancer is most likely under control. CEA test may also be useful for clinical staging of the carcinoma and for determining if client has had a recurrence or relapse of cancer.

Purposes

- To monitor the treatment for colon or pancreatic carcinoma
- To compare with other laboratory tests for diagnosing an inflammatory condition, or gastrointestinal or pancreatic cancer

Clinical Problems

Elevated level: Cancer: gastrointestinal tract (esophagus, stomach, small and large intestine, rectum), pancreas, liver, lung, breast, cervix, prostate, bladder, testes, kidney, leukemia; inflammatory bowel disease; chronic cigarette smoking; ulcerative colitis; cirrhosis of the liver; bacterial pneumonia; pulmonary emphysema; acute pancreatitis; acute renal failure; chronic ischemic heart disease

Procedure

- Heparin should not be administered for 2 days before the test, since it interferes with the results.
- No food or fluid restriction is required.
- Collect 10 mL of venous blood in a red- or lavender-top tube. Avoid hemolysis.

Factors Affecting Laboratory Results

- Heparin interferes with the result of the CEA test.

Nursing Implications

- Relate clinical problems to elevated CEA levels. CEA levels over 2.5 ng/mL do not always indicate cancer, nor do levels below 2.5 ng/mL indicate an absence of cancer. Usually, the CEA is used for management of cancer treatment.
- Be supportive of client and family while awaiting test results. Answer questions or, if unable to, refer the questions to health professionals.
- If heparin is given, note date and time on the laboratory slip.

CATECHOLAMINES (PLASMA AND URINE)

Reference Values

Plasma: Epinephrine: supine: <50 pg/mL; sitting: <60 pg/mL; standing: <90 pg/mL

Norepinephrine: supine: 110–410 pg/mL; sitting: 120–680 pg/mL; standing: 125–700 pg/mL

Dopamine: supine and standing: <87 pg/mL

Pheochromocytoma: Total catecholamines: >1000 pg/mL

Urine

Adult: total: <100 μg/24 h (higher with activity), <0.59 μmol/24 h (SI units), 0–14 μg/dL (random); epinephrine: <20 μg/24 h; norepinephrine: <100 μg/24 h. Values may differ with laboratories

Child: Level less than adult because of weight differences

Description. The three main catecholamines are epinephrine (adrenaline), norepinephrine, and dopamine, which are hormones secreted by the adrenal medulla. These catecholamines respond to stress, fear, hypoxia, hemorrhage, and strenuous exercise by increasing the blood pressure. Catecholamines can be measured from plasma or by a 24-hour urine collection specimen. The 24-hour urine catecholamine collection has the advantage of determining the daily secretion of hormones. A single plasma catecholamine level could be misleading due to catecholamine fluctuation, but it is considered 75% effective in diagnosing pheochromocytomas. Urinary catecholamine levels are 3 to 100 times greater than normal in cases of pheochromocytoma. In children, the urine test may be used to diagnose malignant neuroblastoma.

Fractional analysis of catecholamine levels (epinephrine, norepinephrine, dopamine) is helpful for identifying certain adrenal medullary tumors suspected in hypertensive clients. A comparison of plasma catecholamine level with a 24-hour urine catecholamine test can aid in diagnosing pheochromocytoma.

Purpose

- To assist in the diagnosis of the health problem related to the abnormal amount of catecholamines in the plasma and urine

Clinical Problems

Decreased level: Norepinephrine: anorexia nervosa, orthostatic hypotension; dopamine: parkinsonism

Elevated level: Epinephrine and norepinephrine: pheochromocytoma (continuous elevation with epinephrine); ganglioblastoma, ganglioneuroma, and neuroblastoma (higher elevations with norepinephrine); diabetic ketoacidosis; kidney disease; shock; thyrotoxicosis; acute myocardial infarction (AMI); strenuous exercise; manic-depressive disorder

Drugs that may increase plasma and urine catecholamines: Epinephrine, norepinephrine, bronchodilators, amphetamines, aminophylline, selected beta adrenergics (isoproterenol), antihypertensives, antibiotics, chlorpromazine (Thorazine)

Procedure

Plasma

- Avoid foods rich in amines 2 days prior to test, such as chocolate, cocoa, wine, beer, tea, aged cheese, nuts (especially walnuts), and bananas.
- Avoid selected drugs 2 days prior to the test, such as OTC cold medications that contain sympathomimetics, diuretics, or antihypertensives.
- Avoid strenuous exercise and smoking prior to the test.
- Restrict food and fluids 12 hours prior to the test.
- An indwelling venous catheter may be inserted for collection of blood samples. Having an IV in place helps to avoid a surge in catecholamine release when a venipuncture is performed during collection of blood sample. The test may require a blood sample while the client is in a supine position and a sample while in standing position. Blood should be collected early in the morning.
- Collect 7 to 10 mL of venous blood in a green- or lavender-top tube. Place the blood sample immediately in an ice bath and take to the laboratory. The laboratory should be notified when the specimen is obtained, because the blood should be spun down and frozen immediately. This blood sample is usually sent to another laboratory.

Urine

- Avoid drugs, coffee, chocolate, bananas, and vanilla for 3 to 7 days before the test. Check with the laboratory. No other food or fluid restriction is necessary.
- Collect urine for 24 hours in a large container with a preservative (10 to 15 mL of hydrochloric acid), and keep the bottle refrigerated. The pH of the urine collection should be below 3.0, and if not, more hydrochloric acid may be required.

- Label the large container with the client's name and the dates and exact times of the 24-hour urine collection (e.g., 4/15/03, 7:15 AM to 4/16/03, 7:15 AM).

Nursing Implications

- Monitor the client's blood pressure. Report blood pressure that remains elevated and responds poorly to drug therapy.
- Check urine output. Report abnormal decreases in urine output. This may indicate renal insufficiency as well as affect the urine catecholamine test results.
- Ascertain if the client is extremely apprehensive or has given indications of stressful situation(s). Catecholamine levels are increased during stressful conditions.
- Report to the health care provider and record any strenuous activity, severe anxiety, and rising blood pressure readings.

Plasma

- Alert the laboratory of the order for plasma catecholamine. This is necessary so that the test can be processed in the laboratory within 5 minutes after blood sample is obtained.

Client Teaching

- Explain the procedure for the plasma catecholamine test to the client. Explanations should be given at least 24 hours before the test. Writing the procedure for the client may be helpful in relieving anxiety.
- Encourage the client to relax as much as possible prior to the test and not exercise or smoke before the test.
- Listen to the client's concerns. Refer questions to other health care providers as needed.

Urine

- Withhold drugs that can cause false positives for 3 days or more, with physician's permission. Record the drugs that the client must take on the laboratory slip.

Client Teaching

- Explain that all urine should be saved in the refrigerated container. Inform the client that toilet paper and feces should not be put in the urine.
- Explain to the client that there is a strong acid as a preservative in the urine container and not to urinate directly into the container.

- Explain that fasting can increase catecholamine levels. Foods are not restricted except for those listed under Procedure.

CEREBROSPINAL FLUID (CSF)

SPINAL FLUID

Reference Values

	Color	Pressure (mm H_2O)	mm^3 WBC	Protein mg/dL	Chloride mEq/L	Glucose mg/dL
Adult	Clear, colorless	75–175	0–8	15–45	118–132	40–80
Child	Clear	50–100	0–8	14–45	120–128	35–75
Premature infant			0–20	<400		
Newborn	Clear		0–15	30–200	110–122	20–40
1–6 months				30–100		

Description. CSF/spinal fluid is obtained by a lumbar puncture (spinal tap) performed in the lumbar sac at L3–4 or at L4–5. First, CSF pressure is measured, then fluid is aspirated and placed in sterile test tubes. Data from the analysis of the spinal fluid is important for diagnosing spinal cord and brain diseases.

Purpose

- To detect color, pressure, WBC, protein, glucose, and presence of bacteria in CSF

Clinical Problems

Elevated level: Intracranial pressure (ICP) due to meningitis, subarachnoid hemorrhage, brain tumor, brain abscess, encephalitis, viral infection

Procedure

- No food or fluid restriction is required.

- Collect a sterile lumbar puncture tray, an antiseptic solution, a local anesthetic, sterile gloves, and tape.
- Place the client in a fetal position, with the back bowed, the head flexed on the chest, and the knees drawn up to the abdomen.
- Label the three test tubes 1, 2, and 3.
- The physician checks the spinal fluid pressure, using a manometer attached to the needle, and collects a total of 10 to 12 mL of spinal fluid: 3 mL in tube 1, 3 mL in tube 2, and 3 mL in tube 3. The first tube is most likely contaminated (with blood from the spinal tap) and is usually discarded; the second tube is for cell count, glucose, and protein determination; and the third tube is for microbiologic studies.
- Use aseptic technique in collecting and handling specimen.
- Label the tubes with the client's name, date, and room number. Take the test tubes immediately to the laboratory.

Nursing Implications

- Explain the procedure for the lumbar puncture to the client by giving a step-by-step explanation.
- Collect specimen in numerical order of tubes.
- Check the vital signs before the procedure and afterwards at specified times (i.e., ½, 1, 2, and 4 hours).
- Assess for changes in the neurologic status after the procedure (i.e., increased temperature, increased blood pressure, irritability, numbness and tingling in the lower extremities, and nonreactive pupils).
- Administer an analgesic as ordered to relieve a headache.
- Be supportive of client before, during, and after procedure.

Client Teaching

- Instruct the client to remain flat in bed in the prone or supine position for 4 to 8 hours following the lumbar puncture. Headaches are common because of spinal fluid leaking from the site of the lumbar puncture.

CERULOPLASMIN (Cp) SERUM

Reference Values

Adult: 18–45 mg/dL, 180–450 mg/L (SI units)

Child: Infant: <23 mg/dL; 1–5 years old: 26–55 mg/dL; >6 years old: same as adult

Description. Ceruloplasmin (Cp) is a copper-containing glycoprotein known as one of the alpha$_2$ globulins in the plasma. Ceruloplasmin is produced in the liver and binds with copper. With decreased serum ceruloplasmin levels, there is increased urinary excretion of copper and increased deposits of copper in the cornea (Kayser-Fleischer rings [green-gold rings]), brain, liver, and kidneys, thus causing damage and destruction to the organs. A deficit of ceruloplasmin or hypoceruloplasmin may result in Wilson's disease, usually seen between the ages of 7 and 15 and in early middle age.

Purpose

- To detect Wilson's disease or liver disorder

Clinical Problems

Decreased level: Wilson's disease (hepatolenticular degeneration), protein malnutrition, nephrotic syndrome, newborns and early infancy

Elevated level: Cirrhosis of the liver, hepatitis, pregnancy, Hodgkin's disease, cancer of the bone, stomach, lung, myocardial infarction, rheumatoid arthritis, infections and inflammatory process, exercise, ingestion of excess copper, estrogen therapy, lymphomas, systemic lupus erythematosus (SLE)
Drugs that may increase ceruloplasmin value: Carbamazepine, estrogen products, oral contraceptives, phenytoin, methadone, barbiturates

Procedure

- No food or fluid restriction is required.
- Withhold drugs containing estrogen for 24 hours before the blood test, with the health care provider's permission.
- Collect 5 mL of venous blood in a red-top tube.

Factors Affecting Laboratory Results

- Estrogen therapy, pregnancy exercise could cause an elevated serum ceruloplasmin level.

Nursing Implications

- Associate a decreased serum ceruloplasmin to Wilson's disease, a genetic problem in which there is excess accumulation of copper in the liver, eye, brain, and kidney.
- Assess for jaundice due to liver disorder from excess copper deposits.
- Check the cornea of the eye for a discolored (green-gold) ring from copper deposits.
- Assess for signs and symptoms of Wilson's disease, such as abnormal muscular rigidity (dystonia), tremors of the fingers, dysarthria, and mental disturbances.

CHLAMYDIA TEST (SERUM AND TISSUE SMEAR OR CULTURE)

Reference Values

Normal titer: <1:16
Positive titer: >1:64

Description. *Chlamydia* is a bacteria-like organism and has some features of a virus. There are two species of *Chlamydia: C psittaci,* which can cause psittacosis in birds and humans, and *C trachomatis,* which appears in three types (lymphogranuloma venereum [venereal disease], genital and other infections, and trachoma [eye disorder]).

The occurrence of *C psittaci* organism is more common for persons working in pet stores who may have contact with infected birds such as parakeets, and those working in the poultry industry who may come in contact with infected turkeys. A respiratory infection may result, causing chlamydial pneumonia. Serologic testing or tissue culture may be performed for diagnosis.

The strain of *C trachomatis,* lymphogranuloma venereum (LGV), venereal disease, is transmitted through sexual intercourse. It can occur in both male and female, causing enlargement of the inguinal and pelvic lymph nodes. Pregnant women can pass chlamydia infection to the newborn during birthing. This can cause trachoma ophthalmia neonatorum in the infant, which may lead to blindness later if untreated. Untreated genital infections caused by *C trachomatis* could lead to sterility.

With psittacosis and LGV, the serum titer level is greater than 1:64 (greater than fourfold of the reference value). The titer for genital infection caused by *C trachomatis* is usually between 1:16 and 1:64. Normally, the general population has a titer level less than 1:16. Tissue culture may be used to confirm test results with titer level. Tetracycline or erythromycin are usually the antibiotics used to treat chlamydia, not penicillin.

Purpose

- To identify the presence of a chlamydia infection, *C psittaci* or *C trachomatis*

Clinical Problems

Positive titer: Psittacosis; lymphogranuloma venereum (LGV); genital infections—pelvic inflammatory disease (PID), salpingitis, endometriosis; trachoma ophthalmia neonatorum; chlamydial pneumonia
Negative titer: Antibiotic therapy

Procedure

- No food or fluid restriction is required.
- Collect 3 to 5 mL of venous blood in a red-top tube. Avoid hemolysis.
- Tissue smear or culture may be obtained from the cervix or other areas.

Factors Affecting Laboratory Results

- Antibiotic therapy taken before tests could cause negative test results.

Nursing Implications

- Obtain a history from the client of any contact with birds that may be infected with *C psittaci.* Employees who work in pet shops or the poultry industry may be infected with *C psittaci* and have psittacosis.
- Check for signs and symptoms of psittacosis, which include a nonproductive or slightly productive cough, chills, fever, headache, gastrointestinal symptoms, bradycardia, and mental changes.
- Assess if the woman is pregnant and has enlargement of the pelvic or inguinal lymph nodes. Genital infection from *Chlamydia* could be passed to the infant during the vaginal birthing process. Prenatal screening of pregnant women for chlamydial infection is being

considered. Symptoms can be vague. The incidence of chlamydial infection in infants is 28 out of 1000 live births.

- Withhold antibiotic drug, with physician's approval, until after the specimen has been obtained.

Client Teaching

- Encourage the client with *C trachomatis* infection to give name(s) of sexual partner(s). Certain antibiotic therapies can eliminate the organism and prevent passing the infection to others. The sexual partner(s) may also need treatment.
- Explain to the mother with a chlamydial infection that the infant should be checked.
- Inform clients with titer less than 1:16 that an acute chlamydial infection is unlikely.
- Listen to the client's concern. Respond or refer questions to other health care providers.

CHLORIDE (Cl) SERUM

Reference Values

Adult: 95–105 mEq/L, 95–105 mmol/L (SI units)

Child: Newborn: 94–112 mEq/L; infant: 95–110 mEq/L; child: 98–105 mEq/L

Description

Chloride, an anion found mostly in the extracellular fluid, plays an important role in maintaining body water balance, osmolality of body fluids (with sodium), and acid–base balance. Most of the chloride ingested is combined with sodium (sodium chloride (NaCl), or salt).

Purpose

- To check chloride level in relation to potassium, sodium, acid–base balance

Clinical Problems

Decreased level: Vomiting, gastric suction, diarrhea, low serum potassium or sodium (or both), low-sodium diet, continuous IV D_5W, gastroenteritis, colitis, adrenal gland insufficiency, heat exhaustion, acute infections, burns, excessive diaphoresis, metabolic alkalosis, chronic respiratory acidosis, CHF

Drugs that may decrease chloride value: Thiazide and loop diuretics, bicarbonates

Elevated level: Dehydration, high serum sodium level, adrenal gland hyperfunction, multiple myeloma, head injury, eclampsia, cardiac decompensation, excessive IV saline (0.9% NaCl), kidney dysfunction, metabolic acidosis

Drugs that may increase chloride value: Ammonium chloride, cortisone preparations, ion exchange resins, prolonged use of triamterene (Dyrenium), acetazolamide (Diamox)

Procedure

- No food or fluid restriction is required.
- Collect 3 to 5 mL of venous blood in a red- or green-top tube.

Nursing Implications

Decreased level

- Assess for signs and symptoms of hypochloremia (i.e., hyperexcitability of the nervous system and muscles, tetany, slow and shallow breathing, and hypotension).
- Inform the health care provider when the client is receiving IV D_5W continuously. A chloride deficit could occur.
- Check the serum potassium and sodium levels. Chloride is frequently lost with sodium and potassium.
- Observe for symptoms of overhydration when the client is receiving several liters of normal saline for sodium and chloride replacement. Sodium holds water. Symptoms of over- hydration include a constant, irritating cough, dyspnea, neck-and-hand vein engorgement, and chest rales.

Client Teaching

- Encourage the client with deficit to drink fluids containing sodium and chloride (e.g., broth, tomato juice, *no* plain water).

Elevated level

- Assess for signs and symptoms of hyperchloremia (similar to acidosis: i.e., weakness; lethargy; and deep, rapid, vigorous breathing).
- Monitor daily weights and intake and output to determine whether fluid retention is present because of sodium and chloride excess.

- Notify the health care provider if the client is receiving IV fluids containing normal saline and has an elevated serum chloride level. Check for symptoms of overhydration.

Client Teaching

- Instruct the client to avoid drinking or eating salty foods and to use salt substitute.
- Instruct the client to read labels of salt substitutes, since many contain calcium chloride and potassium chloride.

CHOLESTEROL (SERUM)

Reference Values. (See also lipoproteins)

Adult: Desirable level: <200 mg/dL; moderate risk: 200–240 mg/dL; high risk: >240 mg/dL. Pregnancy: high risk levels but returns to prepregnancy values 1 month after delivery

Child: Infant: 90–130 mg/dL; child 2–19 yr; desirable level: 130–170 mg/dL; moderate risk: 171–184 mg/dL; high risk: >185 mg/dL

Description. Cholesterol is a blood lipid synthesized by the liver. Cholesterol is used by the body to form bile salts for fat digestion and for the formation of hormones by the adrenal glands, ovaries, and testes. Thyroid and estrogen hormones decrease the concentration of cholesterol. Approximately one third of American people have serum cholesterol levels below 200 mg/dL.

Purposes

- To check client's cholesterol level
- To monitor cholesterol levels

Clinical Problems

Decreased level: Hyperthyroidism, starvation, malabsorption

Drugs that may decrease cholesterol value: Thyroxine, estrogens, aspirin, antibiotics (tetracycline and neomycin), nicotinic acid, heparin, colchicine

Elevated level: Hypercholesterolemia; AMI; atherosclerosis; hypothyroidism; uncontrolled diabetes mellitus; biliary cirrhosis; pancreatectomy; pregnancy (third trimester); heavy stress periods; type II, III, V hyperlipoproteinemia; high-cholesterol diet; nephrotic syndrome

Drugs that may increase cholesterol value: Oral contraceptives, epinephrine, phenothiazines, vitamins A and D, sulfonamides, phenytoin (Dilantin)

Procedure

- Restrict food and fluids for 12 hours prior to test. List food and drugs taken prior to laboratory test on the laboratory slip.
- Instruct client to have a low-fat meal the night prior to the test.
- Collect 3 to 5 mL of venous blood in a red-top tube. Avoid hemolysis.

Factors Affecting Laboratory Results

- A high-cholesterol diet before the test could cause an elevated serum cholesterol level.
- Severe hypoxia could increase the serum cholesterol level.

Nursing Implications

Client Teaching

- Instruct the client with hypercholesterolemia to decrease the intake of foods rich in cholesterol (i.e., bacon, eggs, fatty meats, seafood, chocolate, and coconut).
- Encourage client to lose weight if overweight and has hypercholesterolemia. If obese, losing weight can decrease serum cholesterol level.
- Answer questions regarding cholesterol and the blood test.
- Explain to the client and family what is considered a normal serum cholesterol level and the effects of an elevated cholesterol level.

COLD AGGLUTININS (SERUM)

COLD HEMAGGLUTININ

Reference Values

Adult: Normal: 1:8 antibody titer (elderly may have higher levels); >1:16 significantly increased; >1:32 definitely positive
Child: Similar to adult

Description. Cold agglutinins (CAs) are antibodies that agglutinate RBCs at temperatures between 0°C and 10°C. Elevated titers (>1:32) are usually found in clients with primary atypical pneumonia or with other clinical problems, such as influenza and pulmonary embolism. The CAs test is often done during the acute and convalescent phases of illness.

Purposes

- To determine the presence of an increased antibody titer significant for atypical pneumonia, influenza, or leukemia
- To compare test results with other laboratory tests

Clinical Problems

Elevated level: Primary atypical pneumonia, influenza, cirrhosis, lymphatic leukemia, multiple myeloma, pulmonary embolism, acquired hemolytic anemias, malaria, infectious mononucleosis, viral infections (Epstein-Barr [EB] virus [mononucleosis] and cytomegalovirus), tuberculosis (TB)

Procedure

- No food or fluid restriction is required.
- Collect 5 to 7 mL of venous blood in a red-top tube. Keep specimen warm. Take to laboratory immediately.
- The laboratory may rewarm the blood sample for 30 minutes before the serum is separated from the cells.

Factors Affecting Laboratory Results

- Antibiotic therapy may cause inaccurate results.
- Elevated cold agglutinins may interfere with type- and cross-matching.

Nursing Implications

- Answer the client's questions concerning the significance of the test.
- Assess for signs and symptoms of viral infection (e.g., elevated temperature).
- Notify the health care provider of a recurrence of an acute inflammation. The health care provider may wish to order a serum C-reactive protein (CRP) test.
- Check the results of the serum CRP level. If the titer is decreasing, the client is responding to treatment, and/or the acute phase is declining.

- Compare CRP with erythrocyte sedimentation rate (ESR). The serum CRP level will elevate and return to normal faster than the ESR level.

COMPLEMENT: TOTAL (SERUM)

Reference Values

Adult: 75–160 U/mL; 75–160 kU/L (SI units)

Description. Total complement plays an important role in the immunologic enzyme system reacting to an antigen–antibody response. The complements make up about 10% of the serum globulins. The complement system has over twenty components, with nine major components numbered C1 to C9. C3 and C4 are the most abundant complements and are discussed separately in the text. The total complement may be referred to as total hemolytic complement or CH_{50}. CH_{50} assesses the function of the complement system. When the complement system is stimulated, it increases phagocytosis, lysis, or destruction of bacteria, and produces an inflammatory response to infection.

Most assays for CH_{50} are most senstive to changes in C2, C4, and C5. Assay should be used as a screen for overall complement function and not as a quantitiative measure of C1 activation during the course of disease states.

Purposes

- To identify the effects of the immunologic enzyme system regarding the presence of inflammatory condition(s) or tissue rejection
- To compare serum complement tests with serum immu-noglobulins to determine the cause of the health problem

Clinical Problems

Decreased level: Allograft rejection, hypogammaglobulinemia, acute poststreptococcal glomerulonephritis, acute serum sickness, systemic lupus erythematosus (SLE), lupus nephritis, hepatitis, subacute bacterial endocarditis, hemolytic anemia, rheumatic fever, multiple myeloma, advanced cirrhosis

Elevated level: Acute rheumatic fever, rheumatoid arthritis, acute myocardial infarction (AMI), ulcerative colitis, diabetes mellitus, thyroiditis, Wegener's granulomatosis, obstructive jaundice

Procedure

- No food or fluid restriction is required.
- Collect 3 to 5 mL of venous blood in a red-top tube. Avoid hemolysis. Allow to clot at room temperature. Spin at 4°C. Transfer serum and freeze immediately. This test may be sent to a large reference laboratory.

Nursing Implications

- Obtain a history from the client of an infectious process or abnormal response to infection. Complement deficiency may occur to those persons susceptible to infection and with certain autoimmune diseases.
- Assess the client's vital signs and urine output. Report abnormal findings.
- Compare total complement results with serum immunoglobulins. Complement results give information about the client's immune system.

COMPLEMENT C3 AND C4 TEST (SERUM)

C3 AND C4 COMPONENT OF THE COMPLEMENT SYSTEM

Reference Values

Adult: C3: *Male:* 80–180 mg/dL. *Female:* 76–120 mg/dL; C4: 15–45 mg/dL, 150–450 mg/L (SI units)
Elderly: Slightly higher than adult

Description. The complement system (a group of 11 proteins) is activated when the antibodies are combined with antigens. C3 is the most abundant component of the complement system and contributes about 70% of the total protein. Increased C3 levels occur in inflammatory disorders. A decrease in C3 and C4 is commonly found in diseases such as systemic lupus erythematosus (SLE), glomerulonephritis, and renal transplant rejection.

Purposes

- To assist in the detection of acute inflammatory disease (e.g., rheumatoid arthritis) and other health problems (see Clinical Problems)
- To compare test results with other laboratory tests to determine health problem

Clinical Problems

Decreased level: SLE (C4 decreased time is longer than C3), glomerulonephritis, lupus nephritis, acute renal transplant rejection, protein malnutrition, anemias (pernicious, folic acid), multiple sclerosis (slightly lower), cirrhosis of the liver

Elevated level: Acute inflammatory disease, acute rheumatic fever, rheumatoid arthritis, early SLE, AMI, ulcerative colitis, cancer

Procedure

- No food or fluid restriction is required.
- Collect 3 to 5 mL of venous blood in a red-top tube; take to the laboratory *immediately*. C3 is unstable at room temperature.

Nursing Implications

- Compare the serum C3 value with other laboratory studies that are ordered and related to the specific health problem.
- Compare the serum C3 and C4 results.
- Be supportive of client and family.

COOMBS' DIRECT (BLOOD—RBC)

DIRECT ANTIGLOBULIN TEST

Reference Values

Adult: Negative
Child: Negative

Description. The direct (antiglobulin) Coombs' test detects antibodies other than the ABO group, which attach to RBCs.

The RBCs are tested and if sensitized will agglutinate. A positive Coombs' test reveals antibodies present on RBCs, but the test does not identify the antibody responsible.

Purpose

- To detect antibodies on red blood cells

Clinical Problems

Positive (+1 to +4): Erythroblastosis fetalis, hemolytic anemia (autoimmune or drugs), transfusion hemolytic reactions (blood incompatibility), leukemias, SLE
Drugs that may increase Coomb's direct: Antibiotics (cephalosporins [Keflin], penicillin, tetracycline, streptomycin), aminopyrine (Pyradone), phenytoin (Dilantin), chlorpromazine (Thorazine), sulfonamides, antiarrhythmics (quinidine, procainamide [Pronestyl]), L-dopa, methyldopa (Aldomet), antituberculins (isoniazid [INH], rifampin)

Procedure

- No food or fluid restriction is required.
- Collect 5 to 7 mL of venous blood in a lavender-top tube. A red-top tube could be used. Avoid hemolysis. Venous blood from the umbilical cord of a newborn may be used.

Nursing Implications

- Report previous transfusion reactions.
- Observe for signs and symptoms of blood transfusion reactions (i.e., chills, fever [slight temperature elevation], and rash).

COOMBS' INDIRECT (SERUM)

ANTIBODY SCREEN TEST

Reference Values

Adult: Negative
Child: Negative

Description. The indirect Coombs' test detects free circulating antibodies in the serum. This screening test will check for antibodies in recipient's and donor's serum prior to transfusions to avoid a transfusion reaction. It does not directly identify the specific antibody. It is done as part of crossmatch blood test.

Purpose

- To check recipient's and donor's blood for antibodies prior to blood transfusion

Clinical Problems

Positive (+1 to +4): Incompatible crossmatched blood, specific antibody (previous transfusion), anti-Rh antibodies, acquired hemolytic anemia
Drugs that may increase Coombs' indirect: Same as for direct Coombs' test

Procedure

- No food or fluid restriction is required.
- Collect 5 or 7 mL of venous blood in a red-top tube.

Nursing Implications

- Obtain a history of previous transfusions, and report any previous transfusion reactions.
- Observe for transfusion reactions.
- List drugs that can cause false-positive test results on the laboratory slip.

COPPER (Cu) (SERUM AND URINE)

Reference values

Serum: Male: 70–140 μg/dL, 11–22 μmol/L (SI units); Female: 80–155 μg/dL, 12.6–24.3 μmol/L (SI units); Pregnancy: 140–300 μg/dL
Child: Newborn: 20–70 μg/dL; child: 30–190 μg/dL; adolescent: 90–240 μg/dL

Urine: Adult and child: 0–60 μg/24 h, 0.095 μmol/24 h
Wilson's disease: > 100 μg/24 h

Description. Copper (Cu) is required for hemoglobin synthesis and activation of respiratory enzymes. Approximately 90% of the copper is bound to alpha$_2$ globulin, referred to as ceruloplasmin, which is the means of copper transportation in the body. In hepatolenticular disease (Wilson's disease), the serum copper level is <20 μg/dL, and the urinary copper level is >100 μg/24 hours. There is a decrease in copper metabolism with Wilson's disease, and excess copper is deposited in the brain (basal ganglia) and liver, causing degenerative changes. Wilson's disease is more likely to be found in the Italian and Sicilian populations and in the Eastern European Jewish people.

Serum copper and serum ceruloplasmin tests are frequently ordered together and compared. Both show decreased serum levels with Wilson's disease, and the urine copper level is elevated.

Purposes

- To aid in the diagnosis of Wilson's disease (hepatolenticular disease)
- To screen infants and children with familiar history of Wilson's disease

Clinical Problems

Serum:

Decreased level: Wilson's disease, protein malnutrition, chronic ischemic heart disease

Elevated level: Cancer (bone, stomach, large intestine, liver, lung), Hodgkin's disease, leukemias, hypo/hyperthyroidism, anemias (pernicious and iron deficiency), rheumatoid arthritis, systemic lupus erythematosus, pregnancy, cirrhosis of the liver
Drug that may increase copper level: Oral contraceptives
Urine:
Elevated level: Wilson's disease, biliary cirrhosis, rheumatic arthritis, nephrotic syndromes

Procedure: A serum and a urine specimen may be requested simultaneously.
Serum:

- Collect 5 mL of venous blood in a royal blue-top tube (used for trace metal).
- No food or fluid restriction.

Urine:

- Discard the first morning urine specimen and then begin a 24-hour urine collection in a container specified for this test.

Factors Affecting Laboratory Results

- Blood sample inserted into a siliconized stopper may cause a false reading.

Nursing Implications

- Assess for signs and symptoms of Wilson's disease (i.e., rigidity, dysarthria, dysphagia, incoordination, and tremors).
- Check for a Kayser-Fleischer ring (dark ring) around the cornea. This is a copper deposit that the body has not been able to metabolize.
- Compare the serum copper level with the urine copper level and the serum ceruloplasmin level if ordered. With Wilson's disease, the serum copper and ceruloplasmin levels would be decreased and the urine copper level would be increased.

Client Teaching

- Explain to the client with Wilson's disease that foods rich in copper, such as organ meats, shellfish, mushrooms, whole-grain cereals, bran, nuts, and chocolate, should be avoided. Canned foods should be omitted. A low-copper diet and D-penicillamine promote copper excretion.

CORTISOL (PLASMA)

Reference Values

Adult: 8 AM–10 AM: 5–23 μg/dL, 138–635 nmol/L (SI units). 4 PM–6 PM: 3–13 μg/dL, 83–359 nmol/L (SI units)
Child: 8 AM–10 AM: 15–25 μg/dL; 4 PM–6 PM: 5–10 μg/dL

Description. Cortisol is a potent glucocorticoid released from the adrenal cortex in response to adrenocorticotropic hormone (ACTH) stimulation. Levels of plasma cortisol are higher in the morning and lower in the afternoon. When there is adrenal or pituitary dysfunction, the diurnal variation in cortisol function ceases.

Purposes

- To determine the occurrence of an elevated or decreased plasma cortisol level
- To associate a decreased cortisol level with an adrenocortical hypofunction

Clinical Problems

Decreased level: Adrenocortical hypofunction (Addison's disease), anterior pituitary hypofunction, respiratory distress syndrome (low-birth-weight newborns), hypothyroidism
Drugs that may decrease cortisol value: Androgens, phenytoin (Dilantin)

Elevated level: Adrenocortical hyperfunction (Cushing's syndrome), cancer of the adrenal gland, stress, pregnancy, AMI, diabetic acidosis, hyperthyroidism, pain, fever
Drugs that may increase cortisol value: Oral contraceptives, estrogens, spironolactone (Aldactone), triparanol

Procedure

- Have client rest in bed for 2 hours before blood is drawn.
- Draw blood before meals.
- Collect 5 to 7 mL of venous blood in a green-top (heparinized) tube.
- If the client has taken estrogen or oral contraceptives in the last 6 weeks, the drug(s) should be listed on the laboratory slip. Recommendation: stop medication 2 months before test.

Factors Affecting Laboratory Results

- Physical activity prior to the test might decrease the cortisol level.
- Obesity can cause an elevated serum level.

Nursing Implications

- Obtain a history of drugs taken prior to test. List drugs, especially oral contraceptives and estrogen, on the laboratory slip and inform the health care provider.

Client Teaching

- Instruct the client to rest for 2 hours prior to the test.
- Instruct client to be NPO 2 hours before test, both AM and PM.

Decreased level

- Observe for signs and symptoms of Addison's disease. Symptoms are anorexia, vomiting, abdominal pain, fatigue, dizziness, trembling, and diaphoresis.

Elevated level

- Observe for signs and symptoms of Cushing's syndrome. Symptoms are fat deposits in the face (moon face), neck, and back of chest; irritability; mood swings; bleeding (gastrointestinal or under skin); muscle wasting; weakness.

C-REACTIVE PROTEIN (CRP) SERUM

Reference Values

Adult: Not usually present; >1:2 titer, positive
Child: Not usually present

Description. CRP appears in the blood 6 to 10 hours after an acute inflammatory process or tissue destruction, or both, and it peaks within 48 to 72 hours. CRP is a nonspecific test ordered for diagnostic reasons and in monitoring the effect of therapy. CRP elevates during bacterial infections but not viral infections. It often is used as an aid in differential diagnosis: pyelonephritis vs. cystitis; and acute bronchitis vs. asthma.

Purposes

- To associate an increased CRP titer with an acute inflammatory process
- To compare test results with other laboratory tests (e.g., ASO)

Clinical Problems

Elevated level: Rheumatoid arthritis, rheumatic fever, AMI, pyelonephritis, inflammatory bowel disease, cancer with metastasis, SLE, bacterial infections, late pregnancy, Burkitt's lymphoma
Drugs that may increase CRP value: Oral contraceptives

Procedure

- Restrict food and fluids, except for water, for 8 to 12 hours before the test.
- Collect 3 to 5 mL of venous blood in a red-top tube. Avoid heat, since CRP is thermolabile.

Factors Affecting Laboratory Results

- Pregnancy (third trimester) could elevate the CRP level.

Nursing Implications

- Recognize that an elevated serum CRP level is associated with an active inflammatory process and tissue destruction (necrosis).
- Assess for signs and symptoms of an acute inflammatory process (i.e., pain and swelling in joints, heat, redness, increased body temperature).

CREATININE (SERUM AND URINE)

Reference Values

Adult: Serum: 0.5–1.5 mg/dL; 45–132.5 μmol/L (SI units). Females may have slightly lower values due to less muscle mass

Urine: 1–2 g/24 h

Child: Newborn: 0.8–1.4 mg/dL; infant: 0.7–1.7 mg/dL; 2–6 yr: 0.3–0.6 mg/dL, 27–54 μmol/L (SI units); older child: 0.4–1.2 mg/dL, 36–106 μmol/L (SI units; values increase slightly with age due to muscle mass)

Elderly: May have decreased values due to decreased muscle mass and decreased creatinine production

Description. Creatinine, a by-product of muscle catabolism, is derived from the breakdown of muscle creatine and creatine phosphate. The amount of creatinine produced is proportional to muscle mass. The kidneys excrete creatinine. When 50% or more nephrons are destroyed, serum creatinine level increases. Serum creatinine is especially useful in evaluation of glomerular function.

Serum creatinine is considered a more sensitive and specific indicator of renal disease than BUN. It rises later and is not influenced by diet or fluid intake. Normal BUN/creatinine ratio is 10:1. Values significantly higher than this suggest to be prerenal.

Purpose

- To diagnose renal dysfunction

Clinical Problems

Elevated level: Acute and chronic failure (nephritis, chronic glomerulonephritis), shock (prolonged), cancers, lupus erythematosus, diabetic nephropathy, CHF, AMI, diet (i.e., beef [high], poultry, and fish [minimal effect])
Drugs that may increase creatinine value: Antibiotics (cephalosporins, amphotericin B, aminoglycosides, kanamycin), ascorbic acid, L-dopa, methyldopa (Aldomet), lithium carbonate

Procedure

- No food or fluid restriction is required. Suggest avoiding red meats the night before the test, since these meats could increase the level.
- Collect 3 to 5 mL of venous blood in a red-top tube.
- List any drugs the client is taking that could elevate the serum level on the laboratory slip.

Nursing Implications

- Relate the elevated creatinine levels to clinical problems. Serum creatinine may be low in clients with small muscle mass, amputees, and clients with muscle disease. Older clients may have decreased muscle mass and a decreased rate of creatinine formation.
- Check the amount of urine output in 24 hours. Less than 600 mL/24 h and an elevated serum creatinine can indicate renal insufficiency.
- Compare the BUN and creatinine levels. If both are increased, the problem is most likely kidney disease.
- Limit beef and poultry if the serum creatinine level is very high.

CREATININE CLEARANCE (URINE)

Reference Values

Urine Creatinine Clearance:

Adult: 85–135 mL/min. Females may have somewhat lower values
Child: Similar to adult
Elderly: Slightly decreased values than adult due to decreased glomerular filtration rate (GFR) caused by reduced renal plasma flow
Urine creatinine: 1–2 g/24 h

Description. Creatinine clearance is considered a reliable test for estimating glomerular filtration rate (GFR). With renal dysfunction, creatinine clearance test is decreased.

The creatinine clearance test consists of a 12- or 24-hour urine collection and a blood sample. A creatinine clearance less than 40 mL/min is suggestive of moderate to severe renal impairment.

Purposes

- To detect renal dysfunction
- To monitor renal function

Clinical Problems

Decreased level: Mild to severe renal impairment, hyperthyroidism, progressive muscular dystrophy, amyotrophic lateral sclerosis (ALS)
Drugs that may decrease urine creatinine clearance: Phenacetin, steroids, thiazides

Elevated level: Hypothyroidism, hypertension (renovascular), exercise, pregnancy
Drugs that may increase urine creatinine clearance: Ascorbic acid, steroids, L-dopa, methyldopa (Aldomet), cefoxitin

Procedure

- Hydrate client well before test.
- Avoid meats, poultry, fish, tea, and coffee for 6 hours before the test and during the test, with health care provider's permission.
- List drugs on the laboratory slip that could affect test results.
- **Blood:** Collect 3 to 5 mL of venous blood in a red-top tube the morning of the test or anytime during the test, as specified.
- **Urine:** Have client void and discard the urine before the test begins. Note the time and save all urine for 24 hours in a urine container, without preservative. Refrigerate the urine collection or keep

in ice. Encourage water intake during the test to have sufficient urine output.

- Toilet paper and feces should not be in the urine.

Nursing Implications

Client Teaching

- Instruct the client not to eat meats, poultry, fish, or drink tea or coffee for 6 hours before the test. Check laboratory policy.
- Encourage water intake throughout the test.
- Instruct client not to do strenuous exercise during the test.
- Answer questions.

CREATINE PHOSPHOKINASE (CPK, CK), AND CPK ISOENZYMES (SERUM)

CREATINE KINASE (CK)

Reference Values

Adult: Male: 5–35 μg/mL, 30–180 IU/L; female: 5–25 μg/mL, 25–150 IU/L

Child: Newborn: 65–580 IU/L at 30°C. Child: male: 0–70 IU/L at 30°C; female: 0–50 IU/L at 30°C

CPK Isoenzymes

CPK-MM:	94–100% (muscle)
CPK-MB:	0–6% (heart)
CPK-BB:	0% (brain)

Description. Creatine phosphokinase (CPK) is an enzyme found in high concentration in the heart and skeletal muscles and in low concentration in the brain tissue. CPK/CK has two types of isoenzymes: M, associated with muscle; and B, associated with the brain. Electrophoresis separates the isoenzymes into three subdivisions: MM (in skeletal muscle and some in the heart), MB (in the heart), and BB (in brain tissue). When CPK/CK is elevated, a CPK electrophoresis is done to determine which group of isoenzymes is elevated. The isoenzyme CPK-MB could indicate damage to the myocardial cells.

Serum CPK/CK and CPK-MB rise within 4 to 6 hours after an acute myocardial infarction, reach a peak in 18 to 24 hours (>6 times the normal value), and then return to normal within 3 to 4 days, unless new necrosis or tissue damage occurs.

Purposes

- To suggest myocardial or skeletal muscle disease
- To compare test results with AST and LDH to determine myocardial damage

Clinical Problems

Elevated level: Acute myocardial infarction (AMI), skeletal muscle disease, cerebrovascular accident (CVA), and with elevated CPK isoenzymes
CPK-MM isoenzyme: Muscular dystrophy, delirium tremens, crush injury/trauma, surgery and postoperative state, vigorous exercise, IM injections, hypokalemia, hemophilia, hypothyroidism
CPK-MB: AMI, severe angina pectoris, cardiac surgery, cardiac ischemia, myocarditis, hypokalemia, cardiac defibrillation
CPK-BB: CVA, subarachnoid hemorrhage, cancer of the brain, acute brain injury. Reye's syndrome, pulmonary embolism and infarction, seizures
Drugs that may increase CPK value: IM injections, dexamethasone (Decadron), furosemide (Lasix), aspirin (high doses), ampicillin, carbenicillin, clofibrate

Procedure

- No food or fluid restriction is required.
- Collect 5 to 7 mL of venous blood in a red-top tube. Avoid hemolysis. Take blood specimen to the laboratory immediately.
- Note on the laboratory slip the number of times the client has received IM injections in the last 24 to 48 hours.

Nursing Implications

- Avoid IM injections; they may increase serum CPK level.
- Relate elevated serum CPK/CK and isoenzymes to clinical problems. The CPK-MB is useful in making the differential diagnosis of myocardial infarction.

- Indicate whether the client has received an IM injection in the last 24 to 48 hours on the laboratory slip, chart, Kardex.
- Assess the client's signs and symptoms of an AMI (i.e., pain; dyspnea; diaphoresis; cold, clammy skin; pallor; and cardiac dysrhythmia).
- Assess anxiety state of client and family. Be supportive.
- Provide measures for alleviating pain.
- Check the serum CPK/CK level at intervals, and notify the physician of serum level changes. High levels of CPK/CK and CPK-MB indicate the extent of myocardial damage.
- Compare serum AST/SGOT and LDH levels with CPK and CPK-MB.

CROSSMATCH (BLOOD)

BLOOD TYPING TESTS, TYPE AND CROSSMATCH

Reference Values

Adult: Compatibility: absence of agglutination (clumping) of cells
Child: Same as adult

Description. The four major blood types (A, B, AB, and O) belong to the ABO blood group system. RBCs have either antigen A, B, or AB, or none (O) on the surface of the cells. Antigens are capable of producing antibodies.

ABO blood type and Rh factor are first determined. Then the compatibility of donor and recipient blood is determined by major crossmatch. The major crossmatch is between the donor's RBC and the recipient's serum; check to determine if the recipient has any antibodies to destroy donor's RBC.

Purpose

- To determine blood type

Procedure

- No food or fluid restriction is required.
- Collect 7 to 10 mL of venous blood in a red-top tube.

Nursing Implications

- Observe for signs and symptoms of fluid volume deficit (i.e., tachycardia, tachypnea, pale color, clammy skin, and low blood pressure [late symptoms]). Crystalloid solutions (saline, lactated Ringer's) might be given rapidly to replace fluid volume until a transfusion can be prepared. Usually 15 to 45 minutes are required to type and crossmatch blood.
- Check the date of the unit of blood. Usually blood should be used within 28 days. Blood that is older than 28 days should not be given to a client having hyperkalemia.
- Monitor the recipient's vital signs before and during transfusions. Signs and symptoms of transfusion reaction can include temperature increase of 1.1°C, chills, dyspnea, etc.
- Start the blood transfusion at a slow rate for the first 15 minutes; stay with client and observe for adverse reactions.
- Flush the transfusion tubing with normal saline if other IV solutions are ordered to follow blood.

CRYOGLOBULINS (SERUM)

Reference Values

Adult: Negative to 6 mg/dL
Child: Negative

Description. Cryoglobulins are serum globulins (protein) that precipitate from the plasma at 4°C and return to a dissolved status when warmed. They are present in IgG and IgM groups and are usually found in such pathologic conditions as leukemia, multiple myeloma, rheumatoid arthritis, systemic lupus erythematosus (SLE), and hemolytic anemia.

Purposes

- To aid in the diagnose of leukemia, SLE, hemolytic anemia (see Clinical Problems)
- To compare test result with other laboratory tests

Clinical Problems

Elevated level: Lymphocytic leukemia, multiple myeloma, Hodgkin's disease, SLE, rheumatoid arthritis, polyarteritis nodosa, acquired hemolytic anemias (autoimmune), cirrhosis (biliary), Waldenström's macroglobulinemia

Procedure

- No food or fluid restriction unless indicated. Some institution protocols require food and fluid restriction for 4 to 6 hours.
- Collect 3 to 5 mL of venous blood in a red-top tube.
- The blood sample should not be refrigerated before it is taken to the laboratory.

Nursing Implications

- Recognize that elevated serum cryoglobulins may be caused by autoimmune disease, collagen diseases, or leukemia.
- Observe for signs and symptoms of rheumatoid arthritis (pain and stiffness in the joints, or swollen, red, tender joints) or SLE.
- Compare serum cryoglobulins test results with other related data.

CULTURES (BLOOD, SPUTUM, STOOL, THROAT, WOUND, URINE)

Reference Values

Adult: Negative or no pathogen
Child: Same as adult

Description. Cultures are taken to isolate the microorganism that is causing the clinical infection. The culture specimen should be taken to the laboratory immediately after collection (no longer than 30 minutes). It usually takes 24 to 36 hours to grow the organisms.

Purpose

- To isolate the microorganism in body tissue or body fluid

Clinical Problems

Specimen	*Clinical Condition or Organism*
Blood	Bacteremia, septicemia, postoperative shock, fever of unknown origin (FUO)
Sputum	Pulmonary tuberculosis, bacterial pneumonia, chronic bronchitis, bronchiectasis
Stool	*Salmonella* species, *Shigella* species, *Escherichia coli, Staphylococcus* species, *Campylobacter*
Throat	β-hemolytic streptococci, thrush (*Candida* species), tonsillar infection, *Staphyloccus aureus*
Wound	*S aureus, Pseudomonas aeruginosa, Proteus* species, *Bacteroides* species, *Klebsiella* species, *Serratia* species
Urine	*E coli, Klebsiella* species, *Pseudomonas, Serratia* species, *Shigella* species, *Candida* species, *Enterobacter, Proteus*

Procedure

- Hand washing is essential before and after collection of the specimen.
- Send specimen to the laboratory immediately.
- Obtain specimen before antibiotic therapy is started. If the client is receiving antibiotics, the drug(s) should be listed on the laboratory slip.
- Use sterile collection containers or tubes and aseptic technique during collection.
- Check with the laboratory for specific techniques used; there may be variations with procedure.

Blood: Cleanse the client's skin according to the institution's procedure. Usually, the skin is scrubbed first with povidone–iodine (Betadine). Iodine can be irritating to the skin, so it is removed and an application of benzalkonium chloride or alcohol is applied. Cleanse the top(s) of culture bottle(s) with iodine and allow to dry. The bottle(s) should contain a culture medium. Collect 5 to 10 mL of venous blood and place in the sterile bottle. Special vacuum tubes containing a culture medium for blood may be used instead of a culture bottle.

Sputum: Sterile container or cup: obtain sputum for culture early in the morning, before breakfast. Instruct the client to give several deep coughs to raise sputum. Tell the client to avoid spitting saliva secretion into the sterile container. Saliva and postnasal drip secretions can contaminate the sputum specimen. Keep a lid on the sterile container; it should not be completely filled. If a 24-hour sputum specimen is needed, then several sterile containers should be used. **Acid-Fast Bacilli (TB culture):** Follow the instructions on the container. Collect 5 to 10 mL of sputum and take the sample immediately to the laboratory or refrigerate the specimen. Three sputum specimens may be requested, one each day for 3 days. Check for proper labeling.

Stool: Collect an approximately 1-inch diameter feces sample. Use a sterile tongue blade, and place the stool specimen in a sterile container with a lid. The suspected disease or organism should be noted on the laboratory slip. The stool specimen should not contain urine. The client should not be given barium or mineral oil, which can inhibit bacteria growth.

Throat: Use a sterile cotton swab or a polyester-tipped swab. The sterile throat culture kit could be used. Swab the inflamed or ulcerated tonsillar or postpharyngeal areas of the throat. Place the applicator in a culturette tube with its culture medium. Do not give antibiotics before taking culture.

Wound: Use a culture kit containing a sterile cotton swab or a polyester-tipped swab and a tube with culture medium. Swab the exudate of the wound, and place the swab in the tube containing a culture medium. Wear sterile gloves when there is an excess amount of purulent drainage.

Urine: Clean-caught (midstream) urine specimen: Clean-caught urine collection is the most common method for collecting a urine specimen for culture. There are noncatheterization kits giving step-by-step instructions. The penis or vulva should be well cleansed. At times, two urine specimens (2 to 10 mL) are requested to verify the organism and in case of possible contamination. Collect a midstream urine specimen early in the morning, or as ordered, in a sterile container. The urine specimen should be taken immediately to the bacteriology laboratory or should be refrigerated. Label the urine specimen with the client's name, date, and exact time of collection. List any antibiotics or sulfonamides the client is taking on the laboratory slip.

Factors Affecting Laboratory Results

- Antibiotics and sulfonamides may cause false-negative results.

Nursing Implications

- Hold antibiotics or sulfonamides until after the specimen has been collected. If these drugs have been given, they should be listed on the laboratory slip.

- Deliver all specimens immediately to the laboratory, or refrigerate the specimen.
- Handle the specimen(s) using strict aseptic technique.
- Keep lids on sterile specimen containers. Sputum cups should not be uncovered by the bedside.

Client Teaching

- Explain the procedure for obtaining the culture specimen. Answer questions. If the client participates in the collection of the specimen (e.g., urine), review the procedure.
- Suggest a culture if a pathogenic organism is suspected. Check the client's temperature.

CYTOMEGALOVIRUS (CMV) ANTIBODY (SERUM)

Reference Values. (Enzyme immunoassay (EIA) for IgG and IgM)
Adult and Child: Negative to <0.30: no CMV IgM Ab detected. 0.30–0.59: weak positive for CMV IgM Ab (suggestive of a recent infection in neonates. Significance of this low level in adults is not determined). >0.60: positive for CMV IgM Ab.

Description. Cytomegalovirus (CMV) belongs to the herpes virus family; it causes congenital infection in infants. CMV can be found in most body secretions (saliva, cervical secretions, urine, breast milk, and semen). If the pregnant woman is infected with CMV, it crosses the placenta, infecting the fetus. In infants, this virus can cause cerebral tissue malformation and damage. Urine specimens for CMV bodies or throat swabs may be used to detect CMV, but they frequently are not as helpful in detection as the serology test.

Many adults have been exposed to the virus and have developed immunity to CMV. Transmission of the CMV virus to immunocompromised persons such as persons with AIDS is serious. Also, transmission of CMV can be via blood transfusions from CMV-positive donors. Serologic studies (CMV-IgM antibodies and CMV-IgG antibodies) yield results in a shorter period than by culture. Cultures may be used to confirm the findings.

Purpose

- To identify the CMV of possible infected childbearing or pregnant women, infants, or immunocompromised persons

Clinical Problems

Elevated: CMV-infected childbearing or pregnant women, infants, persons with AIDS or other immune deficiency, post-transplant organ recipients, following open heart surgery, hepatitis syndromes

Procedure

Serum

- No food or fluid restriction is required.
- Collect 5 to 7 mL of venous blood in a red-top tube. Two blood samples are usually requested; the first blood specimen is drawn during the acute phase, and 10 to 14 days later the second specimen for the convalescent phase.

Culture/Swab

- Obtain a culture of the infected area. Send the specimen immediately to the laboratory. Cultures are usually used to confirm serologic findings.

Factors Affecting Laboratory Results

- A false-positive test result may occur to those with the rheumatoid factor in the serum or those exposed to the Epstein-Barr virus.

Nursing Implications

- Obtain a history from the client of possible herpes-like viral infection.
- Assess the client for chronic respiratory infection or changes in vision. CMV retinitis can occur, which may result in blindness. Antiviral drugs may be used to treat CMV.
- Use aseptic technique when caring for clients infected with CMV.
- Listen to the client concerns about the possible effects of this virus on self or infant. Refer questions to appropriate health care provider as necessary.

DEXAMETHASONE SUPPRESSION TEST (DST)

ADRENOCORTICOTROPIC HORMONE (ACTH) SUPPRESSION TEST

Reference Values. >50% reduction of plasma cortisol and urine 17-hydroxycorticosteroids (17-OHCS)

Rapid or overnight screening test: Plasma cortisol: 8 AM: <10 μg/dL; 4 PM: <5 μg/dL. Urine 17-OHCS (5-hour specimen): <4 mg/5 h.
Increased dexamethasone dose: *Low dose:* Plasma cortisol is one half of client's baseline level. Urine 17-OHCS: <2.5 mg/24 h/second day. *High dose:* plasma cortisol and urine 17-OHCS are one half of client's baseline level.

Note: High dose is given if results do not change with low dose of dexamethasone.

Description. Dexamethasone (Decadron) is a potent glucocorticoid. The dexamethasone suppression distinguishes between adrenal hyperplasia and adrenal tumor as the cause of adrenal hyperfunction and is used to diagnose and manage depression. When given dexamethasone, there is a reduction (suppression) in ACTH secretion (negative feedback), thus causing a lower plasma and urine cortisol. Low-dose and high-dose dexamethasone are used to distinguish between adrenal hyperplasia and adrenal tumor (nonsuppress at low or high doses). Adrenal hyperplasia will suppress at high doses but not at low doses.

In psychiatry the DST is useful in diagnosing affective diseases, such as endogenous depression (melancholia). In approximately 50% of these clients, suppression of plasma cortisol does not occur.

Purpose

- To distinguish between adrenal hyperplasia and adrenal tumor as the cause of adrenal hyperfunction

Clinical Problems

Plasma cortisol or urine 17-OHCS nonsuppression: Adrenal tumor, ectopic ACTH-producing tumor, bilateral adrenal hyperplasia (except with high steroid doses), affective disorders (endogenous depression), severe stress, anorexia nervosa, trauma, pregnancy, unstable diabetes
Drugs that may cause false negatives: Synthetic steroid therapy, high doses of benzodiazepines
Drugs that may cause false positives: Phenytoin, barbiturates, meprobamate, carbamazepine

Procedure

- Avoid tea, caffeinated coffee, and chocolates. No other food or fluid restriction is required.

- Refrigerate urine for 17-OHCS levels.
- Obtain a baseline plasma cortisol and urine 17-OHCS 24 hours before the test.

Rapid or overnight screening test

- Restrict food and fluids after midnight. Check with laboratory policy.
- Give dexamethasone 1 mg or 5 μg/kg PO at 11 PM.
- Start at 7 AM, a 5-hour urine test for 17-OHCS. Draw blood at 8 AM for plasma cortisol. Obtain a urine OHCS at 12 noon.

Increased dexamethasone dose: 2 days of low or high doses of dexamethasone (Decadron)

Low Dose

- Give dexamethasone, 0.5 mg every 6 hours for 2 days (total 4 mg).
- Obtain a plasma cortisol level at 8 AM, 4 PM and 11 PM and 24-hour urine OHCS after 2-day low-dose test. If no suppression, the high-dose test may be recommended.

High Dose

- Give dexamethasone, 2 mg every 6 hours for 2 days (total 16 mg).
- Obtain a plasma cortisol level at 8 AM, 4 PM, and 11 PM and 24-hour urine OHCS after 2-day high-dose test.

Nursing Implications

- Administer dexamethasone at specified times on time. Milk or antacids may be required to decrease gastric irritation.
- Provide ample time for the client to ask questions. Refer unknown answers to appropriate health professionals.
- Report anxiety, stress, fever, or infection to the health care provider.
- Assess for side effects of dexamethasone resulting from high doses (i.e., gastric discomfort, weight gain, peripheral edema).
- Monitor electrolytes during low- and high-dose tests. Steroids cause serum potassium loss and serum sodium excess.
- Check blood glucose with Chemstrip bG for hyperglycemia while the client is taking high doses of dexamethasone. This drug is a glucocorticosteroid and can elevate blood glucose levels.
- Be supportive of client and family members during this time-consuming test procedure. Cooperation from client and family members is needed for accurate results.

DIGOXIN (SERUM)

LANOXIN

Reference Values

Adult: Therapeutic: 0.5–2 ng/mL; 0.5–2 nmol/L (SI units); infant: 1–3 ng/mL; child: same as adult

Toxic: >2 ng/mL; >2.6 nmol/L (SI units); infant: >3.5 ng/mL

Child: Same as adult

Description. Digoxin, a form of digitalis, is a cardiac glycoside given to increase the force and velocity of myocardial contraction. Serum plateau levels of digoxin occur 6 to 8 hours after an oral dose, 2 to 4 hours after IV administration, and 10 to 12 hours after IM administration.

The half-life of digoxin is 35 to 40 hours, with a shorter half-life in neonates and infants.

Purpose

- To monitor digoxin levels

Clinical Problems

Decreased level: Decreased gastrointestinal absorption or gastrointestinal motility

Drugs that may decrease digoxin level: Antacids, Kaopectate, metoclopramide (Reglan), barbiturates, cholestyramine (Questran), spironolactone (Aldactone)

Elevated level: Digoxin overdose, renal disease, liver disease

Drugs that may increase digoxin level: Diuretics, amphotericin B, quinidine, reserpine (Serpasil), succinylcholine, sympathomimetics, corticosteroids

Procedure

- No food or fluid restriction is required.
- Collect 1 to 5 mL of venous blood in a red-top tube.
- Obtain a blood sample 6 to 10 hours after administration of oral digoxin or prior to next digoxin dose or as ordered.

Factors Affecting Laboratory Results

- Administering digoxin IM might cause the absorption rate to be erratic.

Nursing Implications

- Report nontherapeutic levels to health care provider STAT.
- Obtain a blood sample for serum digoxin during predicted plateau levels for oral, IV, and IM administration or as ordered. Administering digoxin IM might cause the absorption rate to be erratic.
- Take apical pulse for 1 minute prior to administering digoxin. If the pulse rate is below 60 per minute, do not give the digoxin and notify the health care provider.
- Check serum potassium and magnesium levels. Hypokalemia and hypomagnesemia enhance the action of digoxin and could cause digitalis toxicity.
- Observe for signs and symptoms of digitalis toxicity (i.e., pulse rate <60 per minute, anorexia, nausea, vomiting, headache, visual disturbance).

Client Teaching

- Instruct the client to take pulse rate before taking digoxin and to call the health care provider if the rate is <60 beats per minute in adults and <70 in children.

DILANTIN (PHENYTOIN) SERUM

DIPHENYLHYDANTOIN

Reference Values

Adult: Therapeutic range: as an anticonvulsant: 10–20 μg/mL, 39.6–79.3 μmol/L (SI units); as antiarrhythmic agent: 10–18 μg/mL, 39.6–71.4 μmol/L (SI units); in saliva: 1–2 μg/mL, 4–9 μmol/L

Toxic range: >20 μg/mL, >79.3 μmol/L (SI units)

Child: Toxic range: >15–20 μg/mL, 56–79 μmol/L (SI units)

Description. Dilantin (phenytoin) is primarily used for inhibiting grand mal seizures. It is not effective in petit mal seizures. Dilantin is also used as an antiarrhythmic drug for decreasing force of myocardial contraction, improving atrioventricular conduction depressed by a digitalis preparation. Half-life in adults is an average of 24 hours and in children an average of 15 hours. Frequent monitoring is suggested to avoid toxic level.

Purpose

- To monitor phenytoin levels

Clinical Problems

Decreased level: Pregnancy, infectious mononucleosis
Drugs that may decrease Dilantin level: Alcohol, folate, carbamazepine (Tegretol)

Elevated level: Dilantin overdose, uremia, liver disease
Drugs that may increase Dilantin level: Aspirin, dicumarol, sulfonamides, phenylbutazone (Butazolidin), thiazide diuretics, tranquilizers, isoniazid (INH), phenobarbital, propoxyphene (Darvon)

Procedure

- No food or fluid restriction is required.
- Collect 5 to 7 mL of venous blood in a red-top tube. Avoid hemolysis.
- List on the laboratory slip drugs client is taking that could affect test results.

Nursing Implications

- Report immediately nontherapeutic and toxic levels to the health care provider.
- Record dose, route, and last time the drug was given on the requisition slip.
- Observe for signs and symptoms of Dilantin toxicity (i.e., nystagmus, slurred speech, ataxia, drowsiness, lethargy, confusion, and rash).

D-XYLOSE ABSORPTION TEST (BLOOD AND URINE)

Reference Values

Adult: 25 grams: Blood: 25–75 mg/dL/2 h (= 45 mg/dL/2 h)
Urine: >3.5 g/5 h; >5 g/24 h
5 grams: Blood: 8–28 mg/dL (= 15.7 mg/dL)
Urine: 1.2–2.4 g/5 h (= 1.8 g)
Child: Blood: 30 mg/dL/1 h

Description. The D-xylose absorption test determines the absorptive capacity of the small intestine. After ingestion of D-xylose, a pentose sugar, serum and urine D-xylose levels are measured. Usually, a low serum D-xylose level, <25 mg/dL, and a low urine D-xylose level, <3.0 g, are indicative of malabsorption syndrome. A common cause of a decreased D-xylose value is small intestinal bacterial overgrowth.

The test may cause mild diarrhea and abdominal discomfort. Both blood and urine specimens need to be obtained. Poor renal function can result in an elevated blood D-xylose levels.

Various clinical problems such as vomiting, hypomotility, dehydration, alcoholism, rheumatoid arthritis, severe congestive heart failure, ascites, and poor renal function could cause low urine D-xylose levels that are not secondary to intestinal malabsorption. To verify a positive test result, endoscopic examination and biopsy frequently are necessary.

Purpose

- To aid in the diagnosis of gastrointestinal disturbance/disorder

Clinical Problems

Decreased level: Celiac disease, small-bowel ischemia, small-bowel bacterial overgrowth, Whipple's disease, Zollinger–Ellison syndrome, multiple jejunal diverticula, radiation enteritis, massive intestinal resection, diabetic neuropathy, diarrhea, lymphoma

Procedure

- Restrict foods for 8 hours for adults and for 4 hours for children prior to the test. Foods that contain pentose, such as fruits, jams, jellies, and pastries, should be withheld for 24 hours prior to the test.
- Client ingests 25 g of D-xylose dissolved in 8 ounces (240 mL) of water. An additional 8 ounces of water should follow the mixture of D-xylose and water. Child's dose is based on weight: 0.5 g/kg but not more than 25 g. (Five g of D-xylose may be given instead of 25 g.)
- Collect 10 mL of venous blood in a gray-top tube. Blood specimens are drawn at 30, 60, and 120 minutes or at 2 hours only after D-xylose ingestion.
- Discard urine specimen before test. Keep all urine refrigerated; at the end of 5 hours, send the urine collection to the laboratory.
- Note client's age on the laboratory slip. Older adults with mild renal impairment can have a decreased 5-hour test result.
- Note on the laboratory slip if the client is taking aspirin, NSAIDs (nonsteroidal anti-inflammatory drugs), atropine. These drugs can decrease intestinal absorption.

Nursing Implications

- Explain the blood and urine test procedures to the client.
- Be supportive to the client and family members. Client compliance during the procedure is essential for accurate test results.
- Report to the health care provider if the client is having severe diarrhea, vomiting, and dehydration. These clinical problems could cause a decreased urine D-xylose level.

Client Teaching

- Closely monitor that the test procedure is correctly followed by the client during the 5 hours.
- Instruct the client that food is restricted but fluids are not. Instruct the client not to eat foods containing pentose (see Procedure).
- Instruct the client to save all urine during the 5-hour urine test. Refrigerate the urine collection.
- Instruct the client to withhold aspirin, all other NSAIDs, atropine and/or atropine products, with health care provider's approval, for 24 hours before the test.

ENCEPHALITIS VIRUS ANTIBODY (SERUM)

Reference Values

Titer: <1:10. Definite confirmation of the virus: a fourfold rise in titer level between the acute and convalescent blood specimens

Description. Encephalitis is inflammation of the brain tissue, which is frequently due to an arbovirus transmitted by a mosquito after the mosquito has been in contact with an animal host. There are several groups of arbovirus causing encephalitis. The animal host varies according to location.

Eastern equine encephalitis virus: It is mainly found in the eastern United States from New Hampshire to Texas. Transmission is by the mosquito from animal hosts: birds, ducks, fowl, and horses. Symptoms include fever, frontal headaches, drowsiness, nausea and vomiting, abnormal reflexes, rigidity, and bulging of the fontanel in infants. The mortality rate of 65% to 75% is one of the highest for viral encephalitis.

California encephalitis virus: Incidence is highest in children in the north central states of the United States. It is transmitted by infected mosquitoes and ticks. Symptoms include fever, severe headaches, stiff neck, and sore throat.

St. Louis encephalitis virus: This virus occurs most frequently in the southern, central, and western United States. It is a group B arbovirus and is transmitted by an infected mosquito. The animal host is the bird. The symptoms of headache, stiff neck, and abnormal reflexes may be mild or severe.

Venezuelan equine encephalitis virus: Incidence of this virus is most common in South America, Central America, Mexico, Texas, and Florida. It is a group A arbovirus and is transmitted by an infected mosquito. The animal hosts are the rodent and horse. Symptoms can be mild, such as flu-like symptoms, or severe, such as disorientation, paralysis, seizures, and coma.

Western equine encephalitis virus: Occurrence is primarily west of the Mississippi, particularly California, in the summer months and early fall. The virus is transmitted by infected mosquitoes infected by animal hosts: birds, squirrels, snakes, and horses. Symptoms include sore throat, stiff neck, lethargy, stupor, and coma in severe cases.

Purposes

- To detect the presence of an elevated encephalitis virus antibody titer that indicates an inflammation of the brain tissue caused by an arboviral infection
- To screen for an arbovirus

Clinical Problems

Elevated titer: Viral encephalitis (identified strain), meningoencephalitis

Procedure

- No food or fluid restriction is required.
- Collect 3 to 5 mL of venous blood in a red-top tube. Two blood specimens should be taken at least 2 to 3 weeks apart: the first during the acute phase of the viral infection, and the second during the convalescent phase.
- CSF may be tested for identifying the virus.

Nursing Implications

- Obtain a history of client's contact with mosquitoes. Ascertain when the client first became ill.
- Assess for symptoms associated with encephalitis, such as fever, frontal headaches, sore throat, stiff neck, lethargy.
- Listen to the client's concern. Answer the client's questions or refer the questions to other health care providers.

ENTEROVIRUS GROUP (SERUM)

Reference Values

Norm: Negative

Positive: Fourfold rise in titer between the acute and convalescent period

Description. The enterovirus group includes many types of viruses that are found in the alimentary tract. Examples of those serotype viruses include coxsackie A and B, echovirus, and poliomyelitis virus. Testing for the enterovirus group is usually indicated when there is an epidemic outbreak of one of these viruses. Other methods for enteroviral testing include specimens from oropharynx, stool, and CSF.

Purpose

- To identify the presence of an enterovirus associated with an epidemic outbreak such as coxsackie A and B

Clinical Problem

Positive titer: Enteroviral infections

Procedure

- No food or fluid restriction is required.
- Collect 3 to 5 mL of venous blood in a red-top tube. Usually two blood specimens are required: the first at the acute phase, and the second during the convalescent phase (2 to 3 weeks between the two phases).

Nursing Implications

- Obtain a history of an alimentary tract infection. Symptoms may vary, so the client's description of the symptoms should be recorded.
- Assess the client's vital signs. Report abnormal findings.

ERYTHROCYTE SEDIMENTATION RATE (ESR) BLOOD

SEDIMENTATION (SED) RATE

Reference Values

Adult: Westergren method: <50 yr old: male: 0–15 mm/h; female: 0–20 mm/h. >50 yr old: male: 0–20 mm/h; female: 0–30 mm/h. Wintrobe method: male: 0–9 mm/h; female: 0–15 mm/h

Child: Newborn: 0–2 mm/h; 4–14 yr old: 0–20 mm/h

Description. The ESR test measures the rate at which RBCs settle out of unclotted blood in millimeters per hour (mm/h). The ESR test is nonspecific.

The C-reactive protein (CRP) test is considered more useful than the ESR test because CRP increases more rapidly during an acute inflammatory process and returns to normal faster than ESR.

Purpose

- To compare with other laboratory tests for diagnosing inflammatory conditions (see Clinical Problems)

Clinical Problems

Decreased level: Polycythemia vera, CHF, sickle-cell anemias, infectious mononucleosis, factor V deficiency, degenerative arthritis, angina pectoris
Drugs that may decrease ESR value: Ethambutol (Myambutol), quinine, aspirin, cortisone preparations

Elevated level: Rheumatoid arthritis; rheumatic fever; acute myocardial infarction (AMI); cancer of the stomach, colon, breast, liver, and kidney; Hodgkin's disease; multiple myeloma; lymphosarcoma; bacterial infections; gout; acute pelvic inflammatory disease; systemic lupus erythematosus (SLE); erythroblastosis fetalis; pregnancy (second and third trimesters); surgery; burns
Drugs that may increase ESR value: Dextran, methyldopa (Aldomet), penicillamine (Cuprimine), theophylline, oral contraceptives, procainamide (Pronestyl), vitamin A

Procedure

- Hold medications that can cause false-positive results for 24 hours before the test with health care provider's permission.
- No food or fluid restriction is required.
- Collect 5 to 7 mL of venous blood in a lavender-top tube and keep the specimen in a vertical position.

Nursing Implications

- Answer the client's questions about the significance of an increased ESR level. An answer could be that other laboratory tests are usually performed in conjunction with the ESR test for adequate diagnosis of a clinical problem.
- Compare ESR with CRP tests results.

ESTETROL (E_4) (PLASMA AND AMNIOTIC FLUID)

Reference Values
Pregnancy

Plasma

Week of Gestation	*pg/mL*
20–26	140–210
30	>350
36	>900
40	>1050

Amniotic Fluid

Week of Gestation	*ng/mL*
32+	0.8
40+	13.0

Description. Estetrol (E_4) is an effective indicator of fetal distress during the third trimester of pregnancy. E_4 increases during gestation. One test alone should not determine fetal distress; several tests, such as estriol (E_3) and human placental lactogen, are usually performed to verify the possible diagnosis.

Purpose
- To detect the occurrence of fetal distress

Clinical Problems
Decreased level: Fetal distress, intrauterine fetal death, anencephalic fetus, fetal malformations

Procedure
- No food or fluid restriction is required.
- Collect 5 to 7 mL of venous blood in a red-top tube.

Nursing Implications
- Obtain a history of client's signs and symptoms related to the pregnancy.
- Monitor fetal heart rate.

- Compare serum E_4 with serum E_3 and human placental lactogen. Report laboratory values to the health care provider.
- Listen to the client's and family's concerns. Refer unknown answers to client's and family's questions to the appropriate health professionals.

ESTRADIOL (E_2) SERUM

Reference Values

Adult: Female: Follicular phase: 20–150 pg/mL
Midcycle phase: 100–500 pg/mL
Luteal phase: 60–260 pg/mL
Menopause: <30 pg/mL
Male: 15–50 pg/mL
Child (6 mo to 10 yr old): 3–10 pg/mL

Description. Estradiol (E_2) is a more potent estrogen than estrone (E_1) and estriol (E_3). This serum test is ordered for determining the presence of gonadal dysfunction. It is useful for evaluating menstrual and fertility problems in the female. Estradiol is produced mostly by the ovaries and also by the adrenal cortex and the testes. The serum estradiol levels are likely to be increased in males who have testicular or adrenal tumors and in females with estrogen-secreting ovarian tumors. Because serum estradiol level of prepubertal children may not be accurate, the serum test may need to be repeated.

Purposes

- To determine the presence of gonadal dysfunction
- To evaluate menstrual and fertility problems in the female

Clinical Problems

Decreased level: Primary and secondary hypogonadism, amenorrhea due to anorexia nervosa, ovarian insufficiency, pituitary insufficiency
Drugs that may decrease estradiol value: Oral contraceptives, megestrol

Elevated level: Estrogen-producing tumors, gynecomastia (male), testicular tumor, liver failure, renal failure
Drugs that may increase estradiol value: Diazepam, clomiphene

Procedure

- No food or fluid restriction is required.
- Record the phase of the menstrual cycle on the laboratory slip.
- Collect 5 to 7 mL of venous blood in a red-top tube.

Nursing Implications

- Obtain a history of signs and symptoms related to the clinical problem.
- Allow the female or male to express her/his feelings regarding symptoms and test findings. Refer client's questions to health professionals when appropriate.

ESTRIOL (E_3) SERUM AND URINE

Reference Values

Pregnancy

Serum

Weeks of Gestation	*ng/dL*
25–28	25–165
29–32	30–230
33–36	45–370
37–38	75–420
39–40	95–450

Urine

Weeks of Gestation	*mg/24 h*
25–28	6–28
29–32	6–32
33–36	10–45
37–40	15–60

Description. E_3 is a major estrogenic compound produced largely by the placenta. It increases in maternal serum and urine after 2 months of pregnancy and continues at high levels until term. If toxemia, hypertension, or diabetes is present after 30 weeks' gestation, E_3 levels are monitored. A decline in serum or urine E_3 levels suggests fetal distress caused by placental malfunction.

Purposes

- To monitor estriol levels
- To determine fetal distress after 30 weeks' gestation
- To compare test results with estetrol test results regarding fetal distress

Clinical Problems

Decreased level: Fetal distress, diabetic pregnancy, pregnancy with hypertension, impending toxemia

Elevated level: Urinary tract infection, glycosuria
Drugs that may increase estriol value: Antibiotics (ampicillin, neomycin), hydrochlorothiazide (Hydrodiuril), cortisone preparations

Procedure

- No food or fluid restriction is required.

Serum

- Collect 5 to 7 mL of venous blood in a red-top tube.

Urine

- Collect urine for 24 hours in a large container with preservative.
- Label with the client's name, the date, and the exact times of collection (e.g., 3/26/03, 8 AM to 3/27/03, 8:03 AM).
- Two 24-hour urine specimens (taken a day apart) are usually ordered for more valid results.

Nursing Implications

- Monitor the fetal heart rate, the client's blood pressure, and sugar in the urine. Hypertension and diabetes could cause placental dysfunction, leading to fetal distress.
- Report glycosuria and urinary tract infection during pregnancy; both could cause a false result.
- Be supportive of client and family.

ESTROGEN (SERUM AND URINE—24 HOUR)

Reference Values

Adult: Serum: female: early menstrual cycle: 60–200 pg/mL; mid-menstrual cycle: 120–440 pg/mL; late menstrual cycle: 150–350 pg/mL; postmenopausal: <30 pg/mL. Male: 40–115 pg/mL
Child: 1–6 yr old: 3–10 pg/mL; 8–12 yr old: <30 pg/mL
Adult: Urine: female: preovulation: 5–25 μg/24 h; follicular phase: 24–100 μg/24 h; luteal phase: 22–80 μg/24 h; postmenopausal: 0–10 μg/24 h. Male: 4–25 μg/24 h
Child: <12 yr old: 1 μg/24 h; postpuberty: same as adult

Description. There are over 30 estrogens identified in the body but only three measurable types of estrogens: estrone (E_1), estradiol (E_2), and estriol (E_3). Total serum estrogen reflects E_1, mostly E_2, and some E_3. For fetal well-being during pregnancy, serum E_3 is used.

The 24-hour urine estrogen test is useful for diagnosing ovarian dysfunction. Client's age and the phase of the menstrual cycle should be known.

Purpose

- To diagnose ovarian dysfunction and other health problems (see Clinical Problems)

Clinical Problems

Decreased level: Ovarian failure or dysfunction, infantilism, primary hypogonadism, Turner's syndrome, intrauterine death in pregnancy, menopausal and postmenopausal symptoms, pituitary insufficiency, anorexia nervosa, psychogenic stress
Drugs that may decrease estrogen value: Some phenothiazines, vitamins

Elevated level: Ovarian tumor, adrenocortical tumor, adrenocortical tumor or hyperplasia, some testicular tumors, pregnancy (gradual increase from the first trimester on)
Drugs that may increase estrogen value: Tetracycline

Procedure

- No food or fluid restriction is required.
- Note on laboratory slip the phase of client's menstrual cycle.

Serum

- Collect 5 to 10 mL of venous blood in a red-top tube.
- Indicate on the laboratory slip the phase of the menstrual cycle.

Urine

- Collect a 24-hour urine sample in a refrigerated container. The urine container should contain a preservative.
- Label with the client's name, the date, and the exact time of collection (e.g., 5/2/03, 7:02 AM to 5/3/03, 7:01 AM). No toilet paper or feces should be in the urine collection.

Nursing Implications

- Indicate on the laboratory slip if the client is taking steroids, oral contraceptives, or estrogens.
- Obtain a history of menstrual problems and the present menstrual cycle.

Client Teaching

- Encourage ventilation of feelings through provision of a private, calm environment.
- Teach the client to keep accurate records on the time of menstruation, how long each menstrual period lasts, and the amount of menstrual flow.

Urine

- Collect specimen in container with preservative.
- Follow strictly the date and times for the urine collection.

ESTRONE (E_1) SERUM AND URINE

Reference Values

Serum	Urine
Adult	
Female:	Female:
Follicular phase: 30–100 pg/mL	Follicular phase: 4–7 µg/24 h
Ovulatory phase: > 150 pg/mL	Ovulatory phase: 11–30 µg/24 h

Serum	Urine
Adult	
Female:	Female:
Luteal phase: 90–160 pg/mL	Luteal phase: 10–22 μg/24 h
Postmenopausal: 20–40 pg/mL	Postmenopausal: 1–7 μg/24 h
Male: 10–50 pg/mL	
Child (1–10 years old): <10 pg/mL	

Description. Estrone (E_1) is a potent estrogen; however, estrone and estriol (E_3) are not as potent as estradiol (E_2). E_1 is a metabolite of E_2. During the third trimester of pregnancy, the E_1 levels can increase up to tenfold the level for a nonpregnant female. E_1 is the major estrogen occurring after menopause. The serum estrone test is frequently ordered with other estrogen tests.

Purposes

- To determine ovarian failure
- To check occurrence of menopause
- To compare test results with other laboratory estrogen tests

Clinical Problems

Decreased level: Ovarian failure or dysfunction, intrauterine death in pregnancy, menopausal and postmenopausal symptoms

Procedure

Serum

- No food or fluid restriction is required.
- Note on the laboratory slip the phase of the client's menstrual cycle.
- Collect 7 to 10 mL of venous blood in a red-top tube.

Urine:

- Collect a 24-hour urine sample in a collection container that contains a boric acid preservative.
- Label the urine with the client's name, date, and exact time of collection.

Nursing Implications

- Obtain a history of signs and symptoms related to the clinical problem.

- Report laboratory value of E_1 and other estrogen factors to the health care provider. Compare serum total estrogen and serum E_1 results.
- Be supportive to the client and family. Refer client's and family's questions to health professionals when appropriate.

FACTOR ASSAY (PLASMA)

COAGULATION FACTORS, BLOOD CLOTTING FACTORS

Reference Values

Adult and Child

Factor I (fibrinogen): 200–400 mg/dL, minimal for clotting: 75–100 mg/dL

Factor II (prothrombin): Minimal hemostatic level: 10%–15% concentration

Factor III (thromboplastin): Variety of substances

Factor IV (calcium): 4.5–5.5 mEq/L or 9–11 mg/dL

Factor V (proaccelerin): 50%–150% activity; minimal hemostatic level: 5%–10% concentration

Factor VI: Not used

Factor VII (proconvertin stable factor): 65%–135% activity; minimal hemostatic level concentration

Factor VIII (antihemophilic factor [AHF], VIII-A): 55%–145% activity; minimal hemostatic level: 30%–35% concentration

Factor IX (Christmas factor, IX-B): 60%–140% activity; minimal hemostatic level: 30% concentration

Factor X (Stuart factor): 45%–150% activity; minimal hemostatic level: 7%–10% concentration

Factor XI (plasma thromboplastin antecedent [PTA] XI-C): 65%–135% activity; 20%–30% minimal hemostatic level: 20%–30% minimal hemostatic level: 20%–30% concentration

Factor XII (Hageman factor): Minimal hemostatic level: 0% concentration

Factor XIII (fibrin stabilizing factor [FSF]): Minimal hemostatic level: 1% concentration

Description. Factor assays (coagulation factors) are ordered for identification of defects in the blood coagulation mechanism due to a lack of one or more of the 12 plasma factors. A deficiency in one or more factors usually causes bleeding disorders.

Purpose

- To identify the blood factor that is causing the bleeding or blood disorder

Clinical Problems. The associated clinical problems and the causes of these problems are outlined in the following table.

COAGULATION FACTOR DEFICIENCIES

Factor	*Clinical Problems (Decreased Levels)*	*Rationale*
I	Hypofibrinogenemia Severe liver disease Disseminated intravascular coagulation (DIC) Leukemia	Deficiency of fibrinogen and fibrinolysis
II	Hypoprothrombinemia Severe liver disease Vitamin K deficiency Drugs: salicylates (excessive), anticoagulants, antibiotics (excessive), hepatotoxic drugs	Impaired liver function, vitamin K deficit
III	Thrombocytopenia	Low platelet count
IV	Hypocalcemia Malabsorption syndrome Malnutrition Hyperphosphatemia	Low calcium intake in diet
V	Parahemophilia Severe liver disease DIC	Congenital problem, impaired liver function
VI	Not used	

COAGULATION FACTOR DEFICIENCIES (*continued*)

Clinical Factor	*Problems (Decreased Levels)*	*Rationale*
VII	Hepatitis Hepatic carcinoma Hemorrhagic disease of newborn Vitamin K deficiency Drugs: antibiotics (excessive), anticoagulants	Impaired liver function, certain drugs affecting the clotting time, vitamin K deficit
VIII	Hemophilia A (classic) Von Willebrand's disease DIC Multiple myeloma Lupus erythematosus	Congenital disorder (sex linked) occurring mostly in males; circulating factor VIII inhibitors
IX	Hemophilia B (Christmas disease) Hepatic disease Vitamin K deficiency	Congenital disorder (sex linked) occurring mostly in males; circulating factor IX inhibitors
X	Severe liver disease Hemorrhage disease of newborn DIC Vitamin K deficiency	Impaired liver function; vitamin K deficit
XI	Hemophilia C Congenital heart disease Intestinal malabsorption of vitamin K Liver disease Drugs: anticoagulants	Congenital deficiency in both males and females; circulating factor XI inhibitors
XII	Liver disease	
XIII	Agammaglobulinemia Myeloma Lead poisoning Poor wound healing	Circulating factor XIII inhibitors; mild bleeding tendency

Procedure

- No food or fluid restriction is required.
- Collect 5 to 7 mL of venous blood in a blue-top tube. Apply pressure to the venipuncture. Deliver blood specimen to laboratory immediately.

Nursing Implications

- Obtain a familial history of bleeding disorders and a history of the client's bleeding tendency.
- Observe the venipuncture site for oozing of blood.
- Observe and report signs of bleeding (i.e., purpura; petechiae; or frank, continuous bleeding).

FEBRILE AGGLUTININS (SERUM)

Reference Values

Adult (febrile, titers): *Brucella:* <1:20, <1:20–1:80 (individuals working with animals); tularemia: <1:40; Widal (*Salmonella*): <1:40 (nonvaccinated; Weil-Felix (*Proteus*): <1:40
Child: Same as adult

Description. Febrile agglutination tests (febrile group) identify infectious diseases causing fever of unknown origin. Isolating the invading organism (pathogen) is not always possible, especially if the client has been on antimicrobial therapy, so indirect methods are used to detect antibodies in the serum. Detection of these antibodies is determined by the titer of the serum in highest dilution that will cause agglutination (clumping) in the presence of a specific antigen. The test should be done during the acute phase of the disease (maybe several times) and then done about 2 weeks later. A single agglutination titer is of minimal value. These tests can be used to confirm pathogens already isolated or to identify the pathogen present late in the disease (after several weeks).

Diseases commonly associated with febrile agglutination tests are brucellosis (undulant fever), salmonellosis, typhoid fever, paratyphoid fever, tularemia, and certain rickettsial infections (typhus fever).

Purpose

- To detect elevated titer caused by febrile agglutinins denoting a specific pathogen

Clinical Problems

Test	*Pathogen(s) Antigen(s)*	*Elevated Levels*
Brucella	*Brucella abortus* (cattle) *B suis* (hogs) *B melitensis* (goats)	Brucellosis titer >1:100
Pasteurella (tularemia)	*Pasteurella tularensis*	Tularemia (rabbit fever) titer: >1:80
Widal	*Salmonella* O (somatic) *Salmonella* H (flagellar) O and H portions of the organism act as antigens to stimulate antibody production	Salmonellosis Typhoid fever Paratyphoid fever titer: O antigen—>1:80 suspicious, >1:160 definite; H antigen—>1:40 suspicious, >1:80 definite
	Salmonella VI (capsular)	Nonvaccinated or vaccinated over 1 year before
Weil-Felix	*Proteus* X *Proteus* OX19	Rickettsial diseases Epidemic typhus Tick-borne typhus (Rocky Mountain spotted fever)
	Proteus OX2	Boutonneuse tick fever Queensland tick fever Siberian tick fever
	Proteus OXK	Scrub typhus titer—>1:80 significant, >1:60 definite

Procedure

- No food or fluid restriction is required.
- Collect 5 mL of venous blood in a red-top tube. Avoid hemolysis.
- Draw blood before starting antimicrobial therapy, if possible. If the client is receiving drugs for an elevated temperature, write the names of the drugs on the laboratory slip.

- The blood sample should be refrigerated if it is not tested immediately or frozen if it is to be kept 24 hours or longer.

Factors Affecting Laboratory Results

- Vaccination could increase the titer level.
- Antimicrobial therapy could decrease the titer level.

Nursing Implications

- Obtain a history of the client's occupation, geographic location prior to the fever, and recent vaccinations. Exposure to animals and ticks could be suggestive of the causative organism.
- Record on the laboratory slip and in the client's chart whether the client has been vaccinated against the pathogen within the last year. Vaccinations can increase the antibody titer.
- Be aware that leukemia, advanced carcinoma, some congenital deficiencies, and general debilitation could cause false-negative results.
- Monitor the temperature every 4 hours when elevated.
- Remind the health care provider of the need to repeat the tests when the fever persists and/or titer levels are suspicious. Titer levels could rise fourfold in 1 to 2 weeks.
- Check to determine whether the blood sample has been taken before you give antibiotics or other drugs to combat fever for a suspected organism. Antibiotic therapy could depress the titer level.

Client Teaching:

- Instruct the client to keep a record of temperatures and to notify the health care provider of changes in body temperature.

FERRITIN (SERUM)

Reference Values

Adult: Female: <40 y: 10–120 ng/mL, 10–120 µg/L (SI units); >40 y: 10–235 ng/mL, 10–235 µg/L (SI units); Postmenopausal: 10–310 ng/mL, 10–310 µg/L (SI units)

Male: 15–300 ng/mL, 15–300 µg/L

Child: Newborn: 20–200 ng/mL, 20–200 μg/L (SI units); 1 month: 200–550 ng/mL, 200–550 μg/L (SI units); Infant: 40–200 ng/mL, 40–200 μg/L (SI units); 1–16 years: 8–140 ng/mL, 8–140 μg/L (SI units)

Description. Ferritin, an iron-storage protein, is produced in the liver, spleen, and bone marrow. The ferritin levels are related to the amount of iron stored in the body tissues. It will release iron from tissue reserve as needed and will store excess iron to prevent damage from iron overload.

Serum ferritin level is useful in evaluating the total body storage of iron. It can detect early iron deficiency anemia and anemias due to chronic disease that resemble iron deficiency. Serum ferritin is not affected by hemolysis and drugs.

Purposes

- To evaluate the amount of iron stored in the body
- To detect early iron deficiency anemia

Clinical Problems

Decreased level: Iron deficiency anemia, inflamed bowel disease, gastrointestinal surgery, pregnancy

Elevated level: Anemias (hemolytic, pernicious, thalassemia, megaloblastic), metastatic carcinomas, leukemias, lymphomas, hepatic diseases (cirrhosis, hepatitis, cancer of the liver), iron overload (hemochromatosis), acute and chronic infection and inflammation, chronic renal disease, hyperthyroidism, polycythemia, rheumatoid arthritis
Drugs that may increase serum ferritin level: Oral or injectable iron drugs

Procedure

- Collect 2 to 5 mL of venous blood in a red-top tube.
- Food and fluids are not restricted.
- Note on the laboratory slip if the client is taking iron preparations.

Nursing Implications

- Compare serum ferritin level with serum iron and transferrin percent saturation. Serum ferritin levels tend to be more reliable in

determining iron deficiencies than serum iron levels. Serum ferritin levels decrease before iron stores are depleted.
- Assess if the client is taking iron preparations. They can influence test results.

Client Teaching
- Explain to the client the purpose of the test.
- Explain to the client the importance of intake of various groups of nutritional foods.

FIBRIN (FIBRINOGEN) DEGRADATION PRODUCTS (FDP) (SERUM)

FIBRIN OR FIBRINOGEN SPLIT PRODUCTS (FSP)

Reference Values

Adult: 2–10 μg/mL
Child: Not usually done

Description. The FDP test is usually done in an emergency when the client is hemorrhaging as the result of severe injury, trauma, or shock. Thrombin, which initially accelerates coagulation, promotes the conversion of plasminogen into plasmin, which in turn breaks fibrinogen and fibrin into FDP. The fibrin degradation (split) products act as anticoagulants, causing continuous bleeding from many sites. A clinical condition resulting from this fibrinolytic (clot-dissolving) activity is disseminated intravascular coagulation (DIC).

Purpose

- To aid in the diagnosis of DIC

Clinical Problems

Elevated level: DIC caused by severe injury, trauma, or shock; massive tissue damage; surgical complications; septicemia; obstetric complications (abruptio placentae, preeclampsia, intrauterine death, postcesarean birth), acute myocardial infarction (AMI), pulmonary embolism, acute necrosis of the liver, acute renal failure, burns, acute leukemia
Drugs that may increase FDP value: Streptokinase, urokinase

Procedure

- No food or fluid restriction is required.
- Collect 5 to 7 mL of venous blood in a blue-top tube. Avoid hemolysis.
- Draw blood before administering heparin.

Nursing Implications

- Monitor vital signs and report shock-like symptoms (i.e., tachycardia; hypotension; pallor; and cold, clammy skin).
- Observe and report bleeding sites (i.e., chest, nasogastric tube, incisional or injured areas, and others).
- Report progressive discoloration of the skin (i.e., petechiae, ecchymoses).
- Check urine output hourly. Report decreased urine output, <25 mL/h, and blood-colored urine.
- Provide comfort and support to the client and family.

FIBRINOGEN (PLASMA)

FACTOR I

Reference Values

Adult: 200–400 mg/dL
Child: Newborn: 150–300 mg/dL; child: same as adult

Description. Fibrinogen, a plasma protein synthesized by the liver, is split by thrombin to produce fibrin strands necessary for clot formation. A deficiency of fibrinogen results in bleeding. Low fibrinogen levels are life-threatening in *disseminated intravascular coagulation (DIC)* caused by severe trauma or obstetric complications. Markedly prolonged prothrombin time (PT) and partial thromboplastin time (PTT) and a low platelet count suggest a fibrinogen deficiency and signs of DIC. Fibrin degradation products (FDPs) are usually ordered to confirm DIC.

Purposes

- To check for a deficiency of fibrinogen as a cause of bleeding
- To compare test results with FDPs in diagnosing DIC

Clinical Problems

Decreased level: Severe liver disease, hypofibrinogenemia, DIC, leukemia, obstetric complications

Elevated level: Acute infections, collagen diseases, inflammatory diseases, hepatitis
Drugs that may increase fibrinogen value: Oral contraceptives

Procedure

- No food or fluid restriction is required.
- Collect 5 to 7 mL of venous blood in a blue-top tube. Avoid hemolysis. Take blood specimen to laboratory within 1 hour.

Factors Affecting Laboratory Results

- Postoperative surgery and third trimester of pregnancy could cause a false-positive fibrinogen elevation.

Nursing Implications

- Report if client had blood transfusion within 4 weeks.
- Monitor for signs and symptoms of DIC (i.e., petechiae and ecchymoses, hemorrhage, tachycardia, hypotension).
- Check laboratory results of PT, INR, PTT, and platelet count.
- Notify health care provider if active bleeding occurs.

FOLIC ACID (FOLATE) (SERUM)

Reference Values

Adult: 3–16 ng/mL (bioassay), >2.5 ng/mL (radioimmunoassay [RIA] serum), >200–700 ng/mL (RBC)
Child: Same as adult

Description. Folic acid, one of the B vitamins, is needed for normal RBC and WBC function. Usually, the serum folic acid or folate test is performed to detect folic acid anemia, which is a megaloblastic anemia (abnormally large RBCs). Other causes of serum folic acid deficit are pregnancy, chronic alcoholism, and old age.

Purposes

- To check for folic acid deficiency during early pregnancy
- To detect folic acid anemia

Clinical Problems

Decreased level: Folic acid anemia, vitamin B_6 deficiency anemia, malnutrition, malabsorption syndrome, pregnancy, malignancies, liver disease, celiac sprue disease
Drugs that may decrease folic acid value: Anticonvulsants, folic acid antagonists (methotrexate), oral contraceptives

Elevated level: Pernicious anemia

Procedure

- No food or fluid restriction is required. Avoid alcohol.
- Collect 7 to 10 mL of venous blood in a red-top tube. Avoid hemolysis. Send to the laboratory immediately.
- Collect 7 mL of venous blood in a lavender-top tube for RBC folic acid determination. Send it to the laboratory immediately.

Nursing Implications

- Collaborate with the dietitian and client on formulating a diet high in folic acid (i.e., liver, lean meats, milk, eggs, leafy vegetables, bananas, oranges, beans, and whole-wheat bread).
- Observe for signs and symptoms of folic acid deficiency (i.e., fatigue, pallor, nausea, anorexia, dyspnea, palpitations, and tachycardia).

Client Teaching

- Encourage the client to eat foods rich in folic acid, such as liver, lean meats, milk, eggs, leafy vegetables, bananas, oranges, beans, and whole-wheat bread.

FOLLICLE-STIMULATING HORMONE (FSH) SERUM AND URINE

Reference Values

Adult: *Serum*: female: follicular phase: 4–30 mU/mL; midcycle: 10–90 mU/mL; luteal phase: 4–30 mU/mL; menopause: 40–170 mU/mL.

Male: 4–25 mU/mL. *Urine*: female: follicular phase: 4–25 IU/24 h; midcycle: 8–60 IU/24 h; luteal phase: 4–20 IU/24 h; menopause: 50–150 IU/24 h. Male: 4–18 IU/24 h.

Child (prepubertal): *Serum:* 5–12 mU/mL; *urine:* <10 IU/mL

Description. FSH, a gonadotrophic hormone from the pituitary gland, stimulates the growth and maturation of the ovarian follicle to produce estrogen in females and to promote spermatogenesis in males. Infertility disorders can be determined by a serum and urine FSH test. Increased and decreased FSH levels can indicate gonad failure due to pituitary dysfunction.

Purposes

- To check for FSH-producing pituitary tumor
- To compare serum and urine FSH levels for determining the cause of infertility

Clinical Problems

Decreased level: Neoplasms of the ovaries, testes, adrenals; polycystic ovarian disease; hypopituitarism; anorexia nervosa

Drugs that may decrease FSH value: Estrogens, oral contraceptives, testosterone

Elevated level: Gonadal failure, such as menopause, precocious puberty, FSH-producing pituitary tumor, Turner's syndrome, Klinefelter's syndrome, orchiectomy, hysterectomy, primary testicular failure

Procedure

- No food or fluid restriction is required.
- State phase of menstrual cycle or if menopausal on the laboratory slip.
- Note on the laboratory slip if the client is taking oral contraceptives or any type of hormones.

Serum

- Rest 30 minutes to 1 hour before blood is drawn.
- Collect 5 to 7 mL of venous blood in a red-top tube. Avoid hemolysis.

Urine

- Collect a 24-hour urine specimen in a large container with a preservative. The pH of the 24-hour urine specimen should be maintained between 5 and 6.5 (glacial acetic acid or boric acid may be added).

- Label container with the client's name, the dates, and the exact times of urine collection (e.g., 5/10/03, 8 AM to 5/11/03, 8:01 AM).
- Avoid getting feces and toilet paper in the urine.

Nursing Implications

Client Teaching

- Instruct the client to rest prior to a serum test, since exercise can increase FSH release.
- Answer client questions concerning the test. Be supportive of client and family.

FTA-ABS (FLUORESCENT TREPONEMAL ANTIBODY ABSORPTION) SERUM

Reference Values

Adult: Nonreactive (negative)
Child: Nonreactive (negative)

Description. The FTA-ABS test is the treponemal antibody test, which uses the treponemal organism to produce and detect these antibodies. This test is most sensitive, specific, and reliable for diagnosing syphilis. It is more sensitive than the Venereal Disease Research Laboratory (VDRL) or rapid plasma reagin (RPR) tests. Test results can remain positive after treatment or forever, and it does not indicate the stage and activity of the disease.

Purpose

- To aid in the diagnosis of syphilis

Clinical Problems

Reactive: Primary and secondary syphilis; false positives (rare): lupus erythematosus, pregnancy, acute genital herpes

Procedure

- No food or fluid restriction is required.

- Collect 3 to 5 mL of venous blood in a red-top tube. Avoid hemolysis.
- A borderline FTA-ABS should be repeated.

Nursing Implications

- Keep information confidential except for what is required by law.
- Encourage medical care for sexual partner(s) if test is positive.
- Check the results of other serology tests for syphilis. A positive VDRL could be false positive because of acute or chronic illness.
- Recognize that a positive FTA-ABS result can occur after treatment (penicillin, erythromycin) for months or several years.
- Assess for signs and symptoms of syphilis. The primary stage begins with a small papule filled with liquid, which ruptures, enlarges, and becomes a chancre. With secondary syphilis, a generalized rash (macular and papular) develops (found on the arms, palms, face, and soles of the feet).

FUNGAL ORGANISMS; FUNGAL ANTIBODY TEST; FUNGAL DISEASE; MYCOTIC INFECTIONS (SMEAR, SERUM, CULTURE—SPUTUM, BRONCHIAL, LESION)

Reference Values

Adult: Negative, serum: <1:8
Child: Same as adult

Description. There are more than 45,000 species of fungi, but about 45 species of fungi (0.01%) are considered pathogenic to man. Fungal infections are more common today and can be classified as (1) superficial and cutaneous mycoses (tinea pedis, athlete's foot; tinea capitis, ringworm of the scalp), (2) subcutaneous mycoses, and (3) systemic mycoses (histoplasmosis, blastomycosis).

The persons most susceptible to fungal infections are those with debilitating or chronic diseases (e.g., diabetes) or those who are receiving drug therapy (i.e., steroids, prolonged antibiotics, antineoplastic agents, and oral contraceptives).

Purpose

- To assist in the diagnosis of selected fungal organisms

Clinical Problems

Positive response: Actinomycosis, histoplasmosis, blastomycosis, coccidioidomycosis, cryptococcosis meningitis, candidiasis (moniliasis, thrush), aspergillosis

Procedure

Serum

- No food or fluid restriction is required. Suggest NPO for 12 hours. Check with your laboratory.
- Collect 7 to 10 mL of venous blood in a red-top tube.
- Obtain serum antibody test 2 to 4 weeks after exposure to organism.

Culture

- Follow directions from the special laboratory on collection of the specimen.

Organism	*Disease Entity*	*Tests*
Actinomyces israelli	Actinomycosis	Smear and culture of lesion Biopsy
Histoplasma capsulatum	Histoplasmosis	Sputum Histoplasmin skin test Serum test: complement fixation or latex agglutination
Blastomyces dermatitidis	Blastomycosis	Culture Smear, wet-mount examination of the material from the lesion Biopsy, histologic examination Skin test Serum test: complement fixation
Coccidioides immitis	Coccidioidomycosis	Culture Sputum smears Skin test Serum test: complement

	Organism	Disease Entity Tests
		fixation (sensitive), latex agglutination (very sensitive)
Cryptococcus neoformans	Cryptococcosis meningitis	Culture of CSF Serum test: latex agglutination (sensitive)
Candida albicans	Candidiasis (moniliasis thrush)	Smear and culture of the skin, mucous membrane, and vagina
Aspergillus fumigatus	Aspergillosis	Sputum culture Skin test Serum IgE level and complement fixation

Nursing Implications

- Associate mycotic infections with high-risk clients having chronic illnesses or debilitating diseases.
- Obtain a history from the client as to where he or she has been living and his or her occupation.
- Monitor the client's temperature.
- Report clinical signs and symptoms of respiratory problems (i.e., cough, sputum, dyspnea, and chest pain).
- Check the color of the sputum. Certain fungi can be identified by the color of their secretions.
- Assess the neurologic status when cryptococcosis is suspected. Report headaches and changes in sensorium, pupil size and reaction, and motor function.

Client Teaching

- Inform the client to wear a mask when exposed to chicken feces. *H capsulatum* spores in the feces can be inhaled.

GAMMA-GLUTAMYL TRANSFERASE (GGT) SERUM

GAMMA-GLUTAMYL TRANSPEPTIDASE (GGTP OR GTP)

Reference Values

Adult: 0–45 IU/L (overall average); *male:* 4–23 IU/L, 9–69 U/L at 37°C (SI units); *female:* 3–13 IU/L, 4–33 U/L at 37°C (SI units)

Values may differ among institutions.

Child: Newborn: 5× higher than adult; premature: 10× higher than adult; child: similar to adult
Elderly: Slightly higher than adult

Description. The enzyme GGT is found primarily in the liver and kidney. GGT is sensitive for detecting a wide variety of hepatic diseases. The serum level will rise early and will remain elevated as long as cellular damage persists.

High levels of GGT occur after 12 to 24 hours and heavy alcohol intake. Levels may remain increased for several days to weeks after alcohol intake stops.

Purposes

- To detect the presence of a hepatic disorder
- To monitor the liver enzyme GGT during the liver disorder and treatment
- To compare with other liver enzymes for identifying liver dysfunction

Clinical Problems

Elevated level: Cirrhosis of the liver, acute and subacute necrosis of the liver, alcoholism, acute and chronic hepatitis, cancer (liver, pancreas, prostate, breast, kidney, lung, and brain), infectious mononucleosis, renal disease, acute myocardial infarction (AMI) [fourth day], acute pancreatitis, CHF
Drugs that can increase GGT value: Aminoglycosides, phenytoin (Dilantin), phenobarbital, warfarin (Coumadin)

Procedure

- No food or fluid restriction is required.
- Collect 3 to 5 mL of venous blood in a red-top tube. Avoid hemolysis.

Nursing Implications

- Compare serum GGT with serum alkaline phosphatase (ALP), leucine aminopeptidase (LAP), and alanine aminotransferase (ALT or SGPT). The GGT test tends to be more sensitive for detecting liver dysfunction than the others.

- Observe for signs and symptoms of liver damage (i.e., restlessness, jaundice, twitching, flapping tremors, spider angiomas, bleeding tendencies, purpura, ascites, and others).

Client Teaching

- Teach the client to maintain a well-balanced diet with adequate protein and carbohydrate.

GASTRIN (SERUM OR PLASMA)

Reference Values

Adult: Fasting: <100 pg/mL; nonfasting: 50–200 pg/mL
Child: not usually performed

Description. Gastrin is a hormone secreted by the G cells of the pyloric mucosa which stimulates the secretion of gastric juices, namely hydrochloric acid (HCl). A very small amount of gastrin is secreted by the islets of Langerhans in the pancreas. Gastrin values follow a circadian rhythm, with the highest values occurring during the day, especially during meals. Hypersecretion of HCl inhibits gastrin secretion.

This test is usually ordered to diagnose pernicious anemia and gastric ulcer (mildly increased serum levels), and Zollinger-Ellison syndrome (high serum levels). Zollinger-Ellison syndrome may be due to pancreatic gastrinoma.

Gastrin stimulation tests aid in differentiating between Zollinger-Ellison syndrome and hypergastrinemia due to other causes. Either calcium infusion or secretion is administered intravenously. A marked increase in serum gastrin values occurs with Zollinger-Ellison syndrome and not with other probable causes of hypergastrinemia.

Purposes

- To aid in the diagnosis of pernicious anemia
- To aid in the diagnosis of gastric ulcer
- To differentiate between Zollinger-Ellison syndrome and hypergastrinemia from other causes

Clinical Problems

Decreased level: Vagotomy, hypothyroidism
Drug that may decrease serum gastrin value: Atropine sulfate

Elevated level: Pernicious anemia, Zollinger-Ellison syndrome, malignant neoplasm of the stomach, peptic ulcer, chronic atrophic gastritis, cirrhosis of the liver, acute and chronic renal failure
Drugs that may increase serum gastrin value: Calcium products, insulin, catecholamines, caffeine

Procedure

- Food and fluids (except water) are restricted for 12 hours before the test.
- Collect 5 to 7 mL of venous blood in a red- or lavender-top tube.

Nursing Implications

- For the gastrin stimulation test, infuse calcium gluconate intravenously over a period of 3 to 4 hours. Blood sample is taken before the test and then drawn every 30 minutes to 1 hour during the infusion. For the secretin test, infuse secretin intravenously over 1 hour. Obtain a blood sample before the test and then every 15 to 30 minutes for one hour as prescribed by the health care provider.
- Check the serum gastrin value. In Zollinger-Ellison syndrome, the serum level may reach 2,800 to 300,000 pg/mL.

Client Teaching

- Instruct the client that food and beverages are restricted (with the exception of water) for 12 hours before the test. A fasting blood sample is usually ordered.

GLUCAGON (PLASMA)

Reference Values

Adult: 50–200 pg/mL, 50–200 ng/L (SI units)
Newborn: 0–1750 pg/mL, 0–1750 ng/L (I units)

Description. Glucagon is secreted by the alpha cells of the pancreas. It functions as a counterregulatory hormone to insulin in regulating glucose metabolism. In response to hypoglycemia, glucagon increases blood glucose level by converting glycogen to glucose.

Very high glucagon levels (500–1000 pg/mL) occur in glucagonoma, pancreatic alpha cell tumor.

Purposes

- To detect an increase or deficit in the serum glucagon
- To screen for glucagonoma

Clinical Problems

Decreased level: Glucose tolerance test during first hour, idiopathic glucagon deficiency, loss of pancreatic tissue

Elevated level: Glucagonoma, acute pancreatitis, severe diabetic ketoacidosis, trauma, infections, pheochromocytoma
Drugs that may increase glucagon level: Glucocorticoids, insulin, sympathomimetic amines

Procedure

- Collect 5 to 10 mL of venous blood in a lavender-top tube. Avoid hemolysis. Chill the tube with ice and take to the laboratory immediately.
- Food and fluids are restricted for 10 to 12 hours prior to the test.
- Have client relax for 30 minutes prior to the test.
- Withhold drugs such as insulin, cortisone, growth hormones, and epinephrine, with health care provider's permission, until the test is completed.

Factors Affecting Laboratory Results

- Infections, trauma, steroids, insulin, excessive exercise, uncontrolled diabetes mellitus, acute pancreatitis, and/or undue stress may elevate glucagon level.

Nursing Implications

- Compare serum glucose and insulin levels. Glucose and insulin influence plasma glucagon levels.

- Record on the laboratory slip and report if client has taken large doses of steroids in the last 24 hours.
- Observe for signs and symptoms of hyperglycemia.

Client Teaching

- Instruct the client to relax in chair or lie down for at least 30 minutes prior to the test. Stress and activity could cause false-positive test results.

GLUCOSE: FASTING BLOOD SUGAR (FBS); POSTPRANDIAL (FEASTING) BLOOD SUGAR (PPBS)

Reference Values

Fasting blood sugar (FBS)

Adult: Serum or plasma: 70–110 mg/dL; whole blood: 60–100 mg/dL; *Panic value:* <40 mg/dL and >700 mg/dL
Child: Newborn: 30–80 mg/dL; child: 60–100 mg/dL
Elderly: Serum: 70–120 mg/dL

Postprandial (feasting) blood sugar (PPBS)

Adult: Serum or plasma: <140 mg/dL/2 h; blood: <120 mg/dL/2 h
Child: <120 mg/dL/2 h
Elderly: Serum: <160 mg/dL/2 h; blood: <140 mg/dL/2 h

Description. A fasting blood sugar greater than 125 mg/dL might indicate diabetes, and to confirm the diagnosis when the blood sugar is borderline or slightly elevated, a feasting (postprandial) blood sugar or a glucose tolerance test, or both, may be ordered.

A 2-hour PPBS or feasting blood sugar is usually done to determine the client's response to a high carbohydrate intake 2 hours after a meal. This test is a screening test for diabetes, normally ordered if the fasting blood sugar was high normal or elevated.

Purposes

- To confirm a diagnosis of prediabetic state or diabetes mellitus
- To monitor blood glucose levels for diabetic clients taking an antidiabetic agent (insulin or oral hypoglycemic drug)

Clinical Problems

Decreased level: Hypoglycemic reaction (insulin shock), cancer (stomach, liver, and lung), adrenal gland hypofunction, malnutrition, alcoholism, cirrhosis of the liver, hyperinsulinism, strenuous exercise

Elevated level: Diabetes mellitus, diabetic acidosis, adrenal gland hyperfunction (Cushing's syndrome), stress, burns, exercise, infections, acute myocardial infarction (AMI), acute pancreatitis, extensive surgery, acromegaly, CHF

Drugs that may increase glucose value: Cortisone preparations, diuretics (thiazides and loop or high ceiling), ACTH, levodopa, anesthetic drugs, epinephrine, phenytoin (Dilantin)

Procedure

Fasting blood sugar (FBS)

- Restrict food and fluids 12 hours prior to test.
- Collect 3 to 5 mL of venous blood in a red- or gray-top tube. Blood is usually drawn between 7 AM and 9 AM.

Postprandial (feasting) blood sugar (PPBS)

- Collect 3 to 5 mL of venous blood in a red- or gray-top tube 2 hours after breakfast or lunch.

Nursing Implications

- Hold AM insulin and drugs until blood specimen is taken.
- Record on the laboratory slip if the client has been taking cortisone preparations, thiazides, or loop diuretics on a daily basis.

Decreased level

- Observe for signs and symptoms of hypoglycemia (i.e., nervousness, weakness, confusion, cold and clammy skin, diaphoresis, and increased pulse rate).

Client Teaching

- Instruct the client to carry sugar or candy at all times. Most diabetic persons have warnings when hypoglycemia occurs.
- Explain to the client and family that strenuous exercise can lower the blood sugar. Carbohydrate or protein intake should be increased before exercise or immediately after exercise.

- Instruct clients with a hypoglycemic problem (blood sugar <50 mg/dL) to eat food high in protein and fat and low in carbohydrates. Too much sugar stimulates insulin secretion.

Elevated level

- Observe for signs and symptoms of hyperglycemia (i.e., excessive thirst [polydipsia], excessive urination [polyuria], excessive hunger [polyphagia], and weight loss).
- Consider drugs, such as cortisone, thiazides, or loop diuretics, severe stress, or extensive surgery as a cause of slightly elevated blood sugar level.

Client Teaching

- Explain to the client that infections can increase the blood sugar level. He or she should seek medical advice.

GLUCOSE-6-PHOSPHATE DEHYDROGENASE (G6PD) BLOOD

Reference Values

Adult: Screen test: negative; quantitative test: 8–18 IU/g Hb, 125–281 U/dL packed RBC, 251–511 U/10^6 cells, 1211–2111 mIU/mL packed RBC (varies with methods used)

Child: Similar to adult

Description. G6PD is an enzyme present in the RBCs. A G6PD deficit is a sex-linked genetic defect carried by the female (X) chromosome, which will, in conjunction with infection, disease, and drugs, make a person susceptible to developing hemolytic anemia. A screen test is usually done before the quantitative test.

Purpose

- To screen for hemolytic anemia

Clinical Problems

Decreased level: Hemolytic anemia, infections (bacterial and viral), septicemia, diabetes acidosis

Drugs that may increase G6PD value: Aspirin, ascorbic acid, acetanilid, nitrofurantoin (Furadantin), phenacetin, primaquine, thiazide diuretics, probenecid (Benemid), quinidine, sulfonamides, vitamin K, tolbutamide (Orinase)

Procedure

- No food or fluid restriction is required.
- Screening test for G6PD is methemoglobin reduction (Brewer's test) or ascorbate and fluorescent spot test and others.
- Collect a small amount of capillary blood in a heparinized microhematocrit tube, or collect 5 mL of venous blood in a lavender- or green-top tube. Avoid hemolysis.

Nursing Implications

- Obtain a familial history of RBC enzyme deficiency.
- Observe for signs of hemolysis, such as jaundice of the sclera and skin.
- Check for decreased urinary output (expected to be at least 25 mL/h or 600 mL/d). Prolonged hemolysis can be toxic to the kidney cells.
- Record oxidative drugs (see drug list). Hemolysis usually occurs 3 days after taking an oxidative drug. Hemolytic symptoms will disappear 2 to 3 days after the drug has been stopped.

Client Teaching

- Instruct the susceptible person to read labels on over-the-counter (OTC) medicines and not to take drugs that contain phenacetin and aspirin. Most of these drugs, if taken continuously, can cause hemolytic anemia.

GLUCOSE SELF-MONITORING (SELF-TESTING) DEVICES

GLUCOSE FINGER-STICK, GLUCOSE CAPILLARY TEST

Reference Values

Adult: ***Blood:*** 60–110 mg/dL, 3.3–6.1 μmol/L (SI units)
Child: ***Blood:*** 50–85 mg/dL, 2.7–4.7 μmol/L (SI units)
Urine: Negative

Description. To control blood glucose levels, glucose monitoring devices are available for checking blood glucose levels. The glucose monitoring devices can be used in institutions such as hospitals, and the clients with insulin-dependent (IDDM) or type 1 diabetes mellitus and non–insulin-dependent diabetes mellitus (NIDDM) or type 2 diabetes mellitus can use it in their homes for managing diabetes mellitus. The test takes about 2 minutes, test results are reliable, and the cost is approximately 1/20th of a laboratory test.

The use of reagent strips for urine testing (e.g., Clinistix, Diastix, Tes-tape, and Clinitest tablets) are less desirable for glucose accuracy than the self-monitoring metered devices. Clients who are unable to perform a finger-stick and use the meter machine should use the urine testing method to evaluate blood glucose levels.

Purpose

- To check the blood glucose level

Clinical Problems

Decreased level: Insulin overdose

Elevated level: Diabetes mellitus, hyperalimentation, excessive stress
Drugs that may increase glucose value: Steroids, thiazide diuretics

Procedure

- NPO prior to the test unless otherwise instructed.

Blood

Finger-stick capillary method

- Check procedure on the specific glucose monitoring device.
- Cleanse the finger site with alcohol; wipe dry.
- Puncture the lateral side of the finger. Wipe off first drop of blood. Do not "milk" the finger.
- Let a large drop of blood drop onto the reagent strip. The blood should cover the pad of the strip.
- Place the reagent strip into the meter for reading. Follow directions on the meter.
- Apply pressure to the site until bleeding has stopped.

Heelstick: Use the same method for obtaining a finger-stick; however, hold the heel in a dependent position to allow the blood drop to accumulate. The use of a capillary tube to obtain the blood specimen may be necessary for blood glucose testing.

Urine

Clinitest: Dip the reagent strip into the urine specimen, remove the strip, wait 10 seconds, read by comparing strip to the color blocks.

Diastix: Dip the reagent strip in the urine specimen, remove the strip, wait 30 seconds, read by comparing strip to the color chart.

Tes-tape: Tear off 1½ inches of reagent tape, dip into the urine specimen, remove tape, wait 60 seconds, read tape by comparing the dark part of tape to color chart.

Factors Affecting Laboratory Results

Blood

- A blood drop that is insufficient for the test.
- Milking the finger can cause false-low results.

Urine

- Stale urine interferes with test results.
- Drugs that may cause a false-negative result include levodopa, aspirin, ascorbic acid, tetracycline, and methyldopa.

Nursing Implications

- Obtain a history regarding the client's glucose testing method including the past glucose testing results.

Client Teaching

- Discuss the procedure (blood and/or urine) with the client. Have the client demonstrate the procedure.
- Discuss the course of action the client should take if the test result is abnormal.
- Instruct the client to take insulin or the oral hypoglycemic agent at the prescribed time.
- Tell the client to report immediately signs and symptoms of hypoglycemia or hyperglycemia.
- Instruct the client to keep accurate records of the glucose tests.
- Encourage the client to keep all medical appointments.

GLUCOSE TOLERANCE TEST–ORAL (OGTT) SERUM

Reference Values

Adult

Time	Serum (mg/dL)	Blood (mg/dL)
Fasting	70–110	60–100
0.5 hour	<160	<150
1 hour	<170	<160
2 hours	<125	<115
3 hours	Fasting level	Fasting level

Child: Infant: lower blood sugar level than adult; <6 years: similar to adult

Description. A GTT is done to diagnose diabetes mellitus in persons having high normal or slightly elevated blood sugar values. The test may be indicated when there is a familial history of diabetes in women having babies weighing 10 pounds or more, in persons having extensive surgery or injury, and in obese persons. The test should not be performed if the fasting blood sugar (FBS) is over 200 mg/dL. The peak glucose level for the OGTT is ½ to 1 hour after the ingestion of 100 g of glucose, and the blood sugar should return to normal range in 3 hours. OGTT can be a 3- to 6-hour test.

An IV GTT may be done if the person cannot eat or tolerate the oral glucose. The blood glucose returns to the normal range in 2 hours after IV GTT.

Purpose

- To confirm the diagnosis of diabetes mellitus

Clinical Problems

Decreased level: Hyperinsulinism, adrenal gland insufficiency, malabsorption, protein malnutrition

Elevated level: Diabetes mellitus, latent diabetes, adrenal gland hyperfunction (Cushing's syndrome), stress, infections, extensive surgery or injury, acute myocardial infarction (AMI), cancer of the pancreas, insulin resistance condition
Drugs that may increase OGTT values: Steroids, oral contraceptives, estrogens, thiazide diuretics, salicylates

Procedure

- Restrict food and fluids except for water for 12 hours before the test.
- Collect 5 to 7 mL of venous blood in a red- or gray-top tube for the FBS. Collect a fasting urine specimen.
- Record on laboratory slip if client has been taking cortisone preparations, thiazide diuretics, or oral contraceptives daily.
- Give 100 g of glucose solution. Some health care providers will give glucose according to body weight (1.75 g/kg), as in pediatrics.
- Obtain blood and urine specimens ½, 1, 2, 3 hours or longer after glucose intake.
- NPO except for water during test. No coffee, tea, or smoking are allowed during test.

Nursing Implications

- Check previous FBS results before the test. A known diabetic normally does not have this test performed.
- Notify the laboratory of exact time the client drank the glucose solution.
- Minimize activities during the test.
- Identify factors affecting glucose results (i.e., emotional stress, infection, vomiting, fever, exercise, inactivity, age, drugs, and body weight). These should be reported to the health care provider.

Client Teaching

- Explain to the client that he or she may perspire or feel weak and giddy during the 2- to 3-hour test. This is frequently transitory; however, the nurse should be notified, and these symptoms should be recorded. They could be signs of hyperinsulinism.
- Explain the procedure for the test.

GLYCOSYLATED HEMOGLOBIN. *SEE* HEMOGLOBIN A_1c (BLOOD)

GROWTH HORMONE (GH), HUMAN GROWTH HORMONE (hGH) SERUM

SOMATOTROPHIC HORMONE (STH)

Reference Values

Adult: Male: <5 ng/mL; female: <10 ng/mL (norms vary with method)
Child: <10 ng/mL

Description. Human growth hormone (hGH) is secreted from the anterior pituitary gland and regulates the growth of bone and tissue. Growth hormone levels are elevated by exercise, deep sleep, protein food, and fasting. Highest levels occur during sleep. GH levels are decreased with obesity and in corticosteroid therapy.

A low serum hGH level may be a cause of dwarfism. Elevated hGH levels can cause gigantism in children and acromegaly in adults. From a single blood sample to determine the serum growth hormone level, a positive diagnosis cannot be made; therefore, growth hormone stimulation or suppression test might be suggested. A glucose loading GH suppression test should suppress hGH secretion. Failure to suppress hGH levels confirms gigantism (children) or acromegaly (adult).

Purposes

- To determine the presence of human growth hormone deficit or excess
- To aid in the diagnosis of dwarfism, gigantism, or acromegaly

Clinical Problems

Decreased level: Dwarfism in children, hypopituitarism
Drugs that may decrease hGH value: Cortisone preparations, glucose, phenothiazines

Elevated level: Gigantism (children), acromegaly (adult), major surgery, stress, exercise, uncontrolled diabetes mellitus, premature and newborn infants

Drugs that may increase hGH value: Estrogens, insulin, amphetamines, glucagon, levodopa, beta blockers, methyldopa (Aldomet), oral contraceptives

Procedure

- Restrict food and fluids except for water for 8 to 10 hours.
- Have the client rest for 30 minutes to 1 hour before taking a blood sample.
- Collect 7 to 10 mL of venous blood in a red-top tube, preferably in the early morning. Avoid hemolysis. Deliver the blood specimen immediately to the laboratory because hGH has a short half-life.

Factors Affecting Laboratory Results

- Stress, exercise, food (protein), and deep sleep could cause an elevated hGH level.

Nursing Implications

- Obtain a history of the client's activities and behavior that could affect the test results, such as stress, exercise, and food intake.

Client Teaching

- Instruct the client not to eat 8 to 10 hours before the test. Encourage the client to rest and not to exercise prior to the test.
- Encourage the client to express his/her feeling as it relates to the test and health problem. Be supportive to client and family.

HAPTOGLOBIN (HP) SERUM

Reference Values

Adult: 60–270 mg/dL, 0.6–2.7 g/L (SI units)

Child: Newborn: 0–10 mg/dL (absent in 90%); infant: 0–30 mg/dL, then gradual increase

Description. Haptoglobins are α_2 globulins in the plasma, and these globulin molecules combine with free (released) hemoglobin during hemolysis (RBC destruction). A haptoglobin–hemoglobin complex occurs, and the iron in the hemoglobin is able to be conserved. A decreased level of serum haptoglobin indicates hemolysis. After a hemolytic transfusion reaction, the serum haptoglobin level begins to fall within a few hours. It may take several days before the haptoglobin level returns to normal. A hemolytic process may be masked in persons taking steroids.

Purposes

- To identify the occurrence of hemolysis
- To assist in the diagnosis of selected health problems (see Clinical Problems)

Clinical Problems

Decreased level: Hemolysis, anemias (pernicious, vitamin B_6 deficiency, hemolytic, sickle cell), severe liver disease (hepatic failure, chronic hepatitis), thrombotic thrombocytopenic purpura, disseminated intravascular coagulation (DIC), malaria

Elevated level: Inflammation, acute infections, malignancies (lung, large intestine, stomach, breast, liver), Hodgkin's disease, ulcerative colitis, chronic pyelonephritis (active stage), rheumatic fever, acute myocardial infarction
Drugs that may increase haptoglobin value: Steroids (cortisone), estrogens, oral contraceptives, dextran

Procedure

- No food or fluid restriction is required.
- Collect 5 to 10 mL of venous blood in a red-top tube. Avoid hemolysis.

Nursing Implications

- Assess the client's vital signs. Report abnormal vital signs, especially if the client is having breathing problems related to a reduced oxygen-carrying capacity.
- Assess the client's urinary output. Excess amounts of free hemoglobin may cause renal damage.
- Check the serum haptoglobin level. The haptoglobin level may be masked by steroid therapy and inflammation. If hemolysis is suspected, the serum level may be normal instead of low due to steroids or inflammation. Notify the health care provider of the findings.

HELICOBACTER PYLORI (SERUM, CULTURE, BREATH ANALYSIS)

Reference Values: Negative findings
Positive: Elevated titer level using ELISA testing, presence of *H pylori*, urea breath test

Description. The gram-negative bacillus *Helicobacter pylori* is found in the gastric mucus layer of the epithelium in about 50% of the population by age 55. The majority of persons with the infection remain asymptomatic. *H pylori* was first identified in 1983 as a cause of peptic ulcer disease. It is recognized as a primary cause of chronic gastritis, and it may progress over years to gastric cancer or gastric lymphoma. *H pylori* is associated with 70% to 85% of clients with gastric ulcers and with 90% to 95% of clients with duodenal ulcers.

Eradication of *H pylori* for asymptomatic clients usually is not suggested or prescribed but is definitely indicated for perforated, bleeding, or refractory ulcers. Treatment to eradicate the infection includes using either a dual, triple, or quadruple drug therapy program using a variety of drug combinations. Dual drug therapy (omeprazole and amoxicillin) for 14 days has fewer side effects but is not as effective in eradicating *H pylori* as the use of triple or quadruple therapy. Quadruple therapy has a 7-day treatment course which eliminates some of the side effects. After the drug therapy program, a 6-week standard acid suppression drug (histamine-2 blocker) usually is recommended.

Purpose

- To detect the cause of the gastrointestinal disorder
- To determine the presence of *H pylori*

Clinical Problems

Elevated titer or positive culture: Presence of *H pylori* causing acute or chronic gastritis, peptic ulcer disease, gastric carcinoma, gastric lymphoma

Procedure

Serum (enzyme-linked immunosorbent assay [ELISA] serology test)

- No food or fluid restriction is required.

- Collect 7 mL of venous blood in a red-top tube.
- Use of a variety of commercial diagnostic kits.

Culture or biopsy (endoscopy)

- Obtain a culture or biopsy using endoscopy for detection of urease produced by *H pylori.*

Urea breath test

- Use the urea breath test to diagnose urease which is given off by *H pylori.* It has a sensitivity of 92% to 94%.

Nursing Implications

- Obtain a familial history of gastrointestinal disorders, such as gastritis or peptic ulcer disease.
- Record symptoms client has related to gastritis or peptic ulcer disease, such as pain, abdominal cramping, gastroesophageal reflux disease (GERD), dyspepsia (heartburn), anorexia, nausea, vomiting, GI bleeding, and tarry stools.

Client Teaching

- Encourage the client to avoid smoking (if client smokes) because smoking reduces bicarbonate content in the GI tract, allows reflux of the duodenum into the stomach, and slows the healing process.
- Listen to client's concerns. Answer client's questions or refer unknown answers to other health care providers.

HEMATOCRIT (Hct) BLOOD

Reference Values

Adult: Male: 40%–54%, 0.40–0.54 (SI units); female: 36%–46%, 0.36–0.46 (SI units)

Child: Newborn: 44%–65%; child: 1–3 years: 29%–40%; 4–10 years: 31%–43%

Description. The hematocrit (Hct) is the volume of packed RBCs in 100 mL of blood, expressed as a percentage. It is the proportion of RBCs to plasma. The test is prescribed to measure the concentration of

RBCs, also called erythrocytes, in the blood. To obtain an accurate hematocrit, the client should NOT be dehydrated.

Purposes

- To check the volume of red blood cells in the blood
- To monitor the volume of RBCs to plasma during a debilitating illness

Clinical Problems

Decreased level: Acute blood loss, anemias, leukemias, Hodgkin's disease, lymphosarcoma, multiple myeloma, chronic renal failure, cirrhosis of the liver, malnutrition, vitamin B and C deficiencies, pregnancy, systemic lupus erythematosus (SLE), rheumatoid arthritis, peptic ulcer, bone marrow failure
Drugs that may decrease Hct value: Penicillin, chloramphenicol

Elevated level: Dehydration/hypovolemia, severe diarrhea, polycythemia vera, diabetic acidosis, pulmonary emphysema (later stage), transient cerebral ischemia (TIA), eclampsia, trauma, surgery, burns

Procedure

- No food or fluid restriction is required.

Venous blood

- Collect 3 to 5 mL of venous blood in a lavender-top tube. Mix well. Tourniquet should be on for less than 2 minutes.
- Do not take blood specimen from the same arm as IV.

Capillary blood

- Collect capillary blood using the microhematocrit method. Blood is obtained from a finger-prick, using a heparinized capillary tube.

Nursing Implications

Decreased level

- Assess for signs and symptoms of anemia (i.e., fatigue, paleness, and tachycardia).
- Assess changes in vital signs for shock (i.e., tachycardia, tachypnea, and normal or decreased blood pressure).

- Recommend a repeat hematocrit several days after moderate/severe bleeding or transfusions. A hematocrit taken immediately after blood loss and after transfusions may appear normal.

Elevated level

- Assess for signs and symptoms of dehydration/hypovolemia (i.e., a history of vomiting, diarrhea, marked thirst, lack of skin turgor, and shock-like symptoms).
- Assess changes in urinary output; urine output of less than 25 mL/h or 600 mL daily could be due to dehydration.

HEMOGLOBIN (Hb, Hgb) BLOOD

Reference Values

Adult: Male: 13.5–17 g/dL; female: 12–15 g/dL
Child: Newborn: 14–24 g/dL; 6 mo to 1 yr old: 10–17 g/dL; 5–14 yr old: 11–16 g/dL

Description. Hemoglobin, a protein substance in red blood cells, is composed of iron, which is an oxygen carrier. Hemoglobin test aids in assessing the presence of anemia. Hemoglobin (erythrocyte) indices are needed to determine the type of hemoglobin disorder (see Hemoglobin Electrophoresis). Hematocrit is approximately three times the hemoglobin value if the hemoglobin is within normal level.

Abnormally high hemoglobin levels may be due to hemoconcentration resulting from dehydration. Low hemoglobin values are related to clinical problems, such as anemia.

Purposes

- To monitor the hemoglobin value in red blood cells
- To assist in diagnosing anemia
- To suggest the presence of body fluid deficit due to an elevated hemoglobin level

Clinical Problems

Decreased level: Anemias, cancers, kidney diseases, excess IV fluids, Hodgkin's disease

Drugs that may decrease hemoglobin value: Antibiotics, aspirin, antineoplastic drugs, doxapram (Dopram), indomethacin (Indocin), sulfonamides, primaquine, rifampin, trimethadione (Tridione)

Elevated level: Dehydration/hemoconcentration; polycythemia; high altitudes; chronic obstructive lung disease (COLD), such as emphysema and asthma; CHF; severe burns

Drugs that may increase hemoglobin value: Methyldopa (Aldomet), gentamicin

Procedure

- No food or fluid restriction is required.
- The tourniquet should be on less than a minute.
- Do not take the blood sample from the extremity receiving IV fluids.

Venous blood

- Collect 3 to 5 mL of venous blood in a lavender-top tube. Avoid hemolysis. Pediatric tube can also be used.

Capillary blood

- Puncture the cleansed earlobe, finger, or heel with a sterile lancet. Do not squeeze the puncture site tightly, for serous fluid and blood would thus be obtained. Wipe away the first drop of blood. Collect drops of blood in micropipettes with small rubber tops or microhematocrit tubes. Expel blood into the tubes with diluents.

Nursing Implications

Decreased level

- Recognize clinical problems and drugs that could cause a decreased hemoglobin level (i.e., anemia with Hgb <10.5 g/dL).
- Observe the client for signs and symptoms of anemia (i.e., dizziness, tachycardia, weakness, dyspnea at rest). Symptoms vary with decreased hemoglobin level.
- Check the hematocrit if the hemoglobin level is low.

Elevated level

- Observe for signs and symptoms of dehydration (i.e., marked thirst, poor skin turgor, dry mucous membranes, and shock-like symptoms [tachycardia, tachypnea, and, later, a decreased blood pressure]).

- Instruct the client to maintain an adequate fluid intake.

HEMOGLOBIN A_1c (Hgb A_1c or Hb A_1c) (BLOOD)

GLYCOSYLATED HEMOGLOBIN (Hgb A_1a, Hgb A_1b, Hgb A_1c), GLYCOHEMOGLOBIN

Reference Values

Total glycosylated hemoglobin: 5.5–9% of total Hgb (Hb)
Adult: Hgb (Hb) A_1c: Nondiabetic: 2–5%. Diabetic control: 2.5–6%; high average: 6.1–7.5%. Diabetic uncontrolled: >8.0%
Child: Hgb (Hb) A_1c: Nondiabetic: 1.5–4%

Description. Hemoglobin A (Hgb or Hb A) composes 91% to 95% of total hemoglobin. Glucose molecule is attached to Hb A_1, which is a portion of hemoglobin A. This process of attachment is called *glycosylation* or *glycosylated hemoglobin* (or *hemoglobin A_1*). There is a bond between glucose and hemoglobin. Formation of Hb A_1 occurs slowly over 120 days, the life span of red blood cells (RBCs). Hb $A_1$is composed of three hemoglobin molecules—Hb A_1a, Hb A_1b, and Hb A_1c—of which 70% Hb A_1c is 70% glycosylated (absorbs glucose). The amount of glycosylated hemoglobin depends on the amount of blood glucose available. When the blood glucose level is elevated over a prolonged period of time, the red blood cells (RBCs) become saturated with glucose; glycohemoglobin results.

A glycosylated hemoglobin represents an average blood glucose level during a 1- to 4-month period. This test is used mainly as a measurement of the effectiveness of diabetic therapy. Fasting blood sugar reflects the blood glucose level at a one-time fasting state, whereas the Hgb or Hb A_1c is a better indicator of diabetes mellitus control. However, a false decreased Hb A_1c level can be caused by a decrease in red blood cells.

An elevated Hb A_1c >p8% indicates uncontrolled diabetes mellitus, and the client is at a high risk of developing long-term complications, such as nephropathy, retinopathy, neuropathy, and/or cardiopathy. Total glycohemoglobin may be a better indicator of diabetes control for clients with anemias or blood loss.

Purposes

- To monitor and evaluate diabetes mellitus control
- To provide information regarding the presence of diabetes mellitus

Clinical Problems

Decreased level: Anemias (pernicious, hemolytic, sickle-cell), thalassemia, long-term blood loss, chronic renal failure

Elevated level: Uncontrolled diabetes mellitus, hyperglycemia, recently diagnosed diabetes mellitus, alcohol ingestion, pregnancy, hemodialysis
Drugs that may increase Hb A_1c value: Prolonged cortisone intake, ACTH

Procedure

- Schedule client 6 to 12 weeks from the last Hb A_1c test.
- Food restriction prior to the test is not required but is suggested.
- Collect 5 mL of venous blood in a lavender- or green-top tube. Avoid hemolysis; send specimen immediately to the laboratory.

Factors Affecting Laboratory Results

- Anemias may cause a low-value result.
- Hemolysis of the blood specimen can cause an inaccurate test result.
- Heparin therapy may cause a false test result.

Nursing Implications

- Monitor blood and/or urine glucose levels. Compare monthly fasting blood sugar with glycosylated hemoglobin (Hb A_1c) test result.
- Determine client's compliance to diabetic treatment regimen.
- Check the dose of daily insulin or oral hypoglycemic agent.
- Recognize clinical problems that can cause a false glycosylated hemoglobin result (see Clinical Problems).
- Observe for signs and symptoms of hyperglycemia.
- Report any complications client has due to diabetes mellitus.

Client Teaching

- Inform the client that fasting prior to the test may or may not be prescribed. The laboratory person should be told if the client has not fasted prior to the test.
- Explain the purpose of the test.
- Instruct the client to comply with the diabetic treatment regimen, such as prescribed insulin, diet, and glucose monitoring.

HEMOGLOBIN ELECTROPHORESIS (BLOOD)

HGB OR HB ELECTROPHORESIS

Reference Values

Adult: **Hb A_1:** 95%–98% total Hb; **A_2:** 1.5%–4%; **F:** <2%, **C:** 0%; **D:** 0%, **S:** 0%
Child: Newborn: **Hb F:** 50%–80% total Hb; 6 mo: **Hb F:** 8%; Child: **Hb F:** 1%–2% after 6 mo

Description. Hemoglobin electrophoresis is useful for identifying more than 150 types of normal and abnormal hemoglobin. Many abnormal hemoglobin types do not produce harmful diseases; the common hemoglobinopathies are identified through electrophoresis.
Hemoglobin S: Hb S is the most common hemoglobin variant. If both genes have Hb S, sickle-cell anemia will occur; but if only one gene has Hb S, then the person simply carries the sickle trait. Approximately 1% of the black population in the United States has sickle-cell anemia, and 8% to 10% carry the sickle-cell trait.

Purpose

- To detect abnormal hemoglobin type in the red blood cells (e.g., sickle-cell anemia, which is characterized by the S-shaped hemoglobin)

Clinical Problems

Hemoglobin Type	*Elevated Level*
Hemoglobin F	Thalassemia (after 6 months)
Hemoglobin C	Hemolytic anemia
Hemoglobin S	Sickle-cell anemia

Procedure

- No food or fluid restriction is required.
- Collect 3 to 5 mL of venous blood in a lavender-top tube. Send immediately to the laboratory. Abnormal hemoglobin is unstable.

Nursing Implications

- Observe for signs and symptoms of sickle-cell anemia. Early symptoms are fatigue and weakness. Chronic symptoms are fatigue, dyspnea on exertion, swollen joints, bones that ache, and chest pains.

Client Teaching

- Encourage genetic counseling.
- Instruct the client to take rest periods, to minimize strenuous activity, and to avoid high altitudes and extreme cold.
- Encourage client to avoid infections.
- Suggest a medical alert bracelet or card.

HEPATITIS PROFILE (HEPATITIS A, B, C, D, E)

Five major types of hepatitis virus can be identified through laboratory testing: hepatitis A virus (HAV), hepatitis B virus (HBV), hepatitis C virus (HCV), hepatitis D virus (HDV), and hepatitis E virus (HEV). These hepatitis viruses can be detected by testing serum antigens, antibodies, DNA, RNA, and/or the immunoglobins IgG and IgM. The following table differentiates between the hepatitis viruses according to method of transmission, incubation time, jaundice, acute and chronic phases of the disease, carrier status, immunity, and mortality rate.

Hepatitis A Virus (HAV). Hepatitis A virus is transmitted primarily by oral–fecal contact. Jaundice is an early sign of HAV, which can occur a few days after the viral infection and may last up to 12 weeks. The antibodies to hepatitis A, anti-HAV-IgM and anti-HAV-IgG, are used to confirm the phase of the hepatitis A infection. Anti-HAV-IgM denotes an acute phase of the infection, while anti-HAV-IgG indicates recovery, past infection, or immunity. Approximately 45% to 50% of clients having HAV may have a positive anti-HAV-IgG for life.

Hepatitis B Virus (HBV). The hepatitis B virus was once called serum hepatitis. There are numerous laboratory tests for diagnosing the acute or chronic phase of HBV. These include hepatitis B surface antigen (HBsAg), antibody to HBsAg (anti-HBs), hepatitis Be antigen (HBeAg), antibody to HBeAg (anti-HBe), and antibody to core antigen (anti-HBc-total).

HbsAg: The earliest indicator for diagnosing hepatitis B viral infection is the hepatitis B surface antigen. This serum marker can be present as early as 2 weeks after being infected, and it persists during the acute phase of the infection. If it persists after 6 months, the client could have chronic hepatitis and be a carrier. The hepatitis B vaccine will not cause a positive HBsAg. Clients who have a positive HBsAg should NEVER donate blood.

Antibody to hepatitis B surface antigen (anti-HBs): With HBV, the acute phase of viral hepatitis B usually lasts for 12 weeks; therefore, HBsAg is absent and anti-HBs (antibodies to HBsAg) develop. This serum marker indicates recovery and immunity to the hepatitis B virus. An anti-HBs-IgM would determine if the client is still infectious. An anti-HBs titer of >10 mIU/mL and without HBsAg presence, confirms that the client has recovered from HBV.

Hepatitis B e antigen (HBeAg): This serum marker occurs only with HBsAg. It usually appears one week after HBsAg and disappears before anti-HBs. If HBeAg is still present after 10 weeks, the client could be developing a chronic carrier state.

Antibody to HBeAg (anti-HBe): The presence of anti-HBe indicates the recovery phase.

Antibody to core antigen (anti-HBc): The anti-HBc occurs with a positive HBsAg approximately 4 to 10 weeks of acute HBV. An elevated anti-HBc-IgM titer indicates the acute infection process. Anti-HBc can detect clients who have been infected with HBV. This serum marker may persist for years, and clients with a positive anti-HBc should not give blood.

Hepatitis C Virus (HCV). HCV is formerly non-A, non-B hepatitis. It is transmitted parenterally. It occurs more frequently with post-transfusion hepatitis, but also should be considered with drug addicts, needle sticks, hemodialysis, and hemophilias. Approximately half of the acute cases of HCV become chronic carriers.

Antibody to hepatitis C virus (anti-HCV): HCV is confirmed by the anti-HCV test. Anti-HCV does not indicate immunity as it can with anti-HBs and anti-HBe.

Hepatitis D Virus (HDV). Hepatitis D (delta) virus is transmitted parenterally. HDV can be present only with HBV. It is coated by the HBsAg and depends upon the HBV for replication. HDV is severe and usually occurs 7 to 14 days after an acute, severe HBV infection. It has a low occurrence rate except for IV drug abusers and clients receiving multiple transfusions. Its presence is in the acute phase of HBV or as a chronic carrier of HBV. Of all the types of hepatitis, it has the greatest incidence of fulminant hepatitis and death.

COMPARISON OF THE TYPES OF VIRAL HEPATITIS

	Types of Hepatitis				
Factors Associated with Hepatitis	*HAV*	*HBV*	*HCV*	*HDV*	*HEV*
Method of transmission	Enteral (oral–fecal) Water and food	Parenteral Intravenous Sexual Perinatal	Parenteral Sexual (possible) Perinatal	Parenteral Sexual (possible) Perinatal	Enteral (oral–fecal) Water and food
Incubation time	Abrupt onset; 2–12 weeks	Insidious onset; 6–24 weeks	Insidious onset; 2–26 weeks	Abrupt onset; 3–15 weeks	Abrupt onset; 2–8 weeks
Jaundice	Adult: 70%–80% Child: 10%	20%–40%	10%–25%	Varies	25%–60%
Hepatocellular carcinoma	None	Possible	Possible	Possible	None
Acute disease: serum markers	Anti-HAV-IgM	HBsAg, HBeAg, Anti-HBc -IgM	Anti-HCV	HDAg	Anti-HEV

(continued)

Types of Hepatitis (continued)

Factors Associated with Hepatitis	*HAV*	*HBV*	*HCV*	*HDV*	*HEV*
Chronic disease: serum markers	None	HBsAg	Anti-HCV (50% of cases)	Anti-HD	None
Infective state: serum markers	None (HAV-RNA)	HBsAg, HBeAg, HBV-DNA	Anti-HCV HCV-RNA	Anti-HD HDV-RNA	None (HEV-RNA)
Fulminant hepatitis	Very low	Very low	Very low	High	Low
Chronic carrier	None	HbsAg (low incidence in adult; high incidence in children	High incidence	Anti-HDV, HDAg low incidence (10%–15%)	None
Immunity; serum markers	Anti-HAV total, Anti-HAV-IgG	Anti-HBs, Anti-HBc total	None	None	Anti-HEV
Mortality rate	<2%	<2%	<2%	≤30%	<2%

Hepatitis D antigen (HDAg): Detection of HDAg and HDV-RNA indicates the acute phase of HBV and HDV infection. When HBsAg diminishes, so does HDAg. Anti-HDV appears later and may suggest chronic hepatitis D.

Hepatitis E Virus (HEV). HEV is transmitted by oral–fecal contact and not parenterally. It can occur due to unsafe water as well as traveling in Mexico, Russia, India, or Africa. It is rare in the United States. Antibodies to hepatitis E (Anti-HEV) detect hepatitis E infection.

HEPATITIS A VIRUS (HAV) ANTIBODY (HAV ab, ANTI-HAV) (SERUM)

Reference Value

None detected

Description. Hepatitis A virus (HAV), previously called *infectious hepatitis,* usually is transmitted by oral–fecal contact. The incubation period for HAV is 2 to 6 weeks, unlike the 7 to 25 weeks for hepatitis B virus. HAV is not associated with chronic liver disease.

Antibodies to hepatitis A virus (IgM and IgG) indicate present or past infection and possible immunity. Anti-HAV IgM (Hav ab IgM) appears early after exposure and is detectable for 4 to 12 weeks. Anti-HAV IgG appears postinfection (>4 weeks) and usually remains present for life. Approximately 50% of the population in the United States have a positive anti-HAV IgG.

Purpose

- To determine the presence or past infection of HAV

Clinical Problems

Positive: Hepatitis A virus (HAV)

Procedure:

- No food or fluid restriction is required.
- Collect 3 to 5 mL of venous blood in a red-top tube.

Nursing Implications

- Obtain a history from the client of a possible contact with a person having HAV. Record if the client has eaten shellfish that may have been taken from contaminated water.

Client Teaching

- Explain to the client that HAV is normally transmitted by oral–fecal contact. Inform the client to wash hands after toileting.
- Alert the client that HAV can spread in institutions such as daycare centers, prisons, state mental institutions.

Positive test

- Rest and nutritional dietary intake are indicated for several weeks according to the severity of the HAV. Fatigue is common. Rest periods are necessary as long as jaundice is present.
- Instruct the client that effective personal hygiene is very important.

HEPATITIS B SURFACE ANTIGEN (HBsAg) SERUM

HEPATITIS-ASSOCIATED ANTIGEN (HAA), AUSTRALIAN ANTIGEN TEST

Reference Values

Adult: Negative
Child: Negative

Description. The HBsAg test is done to determine the presence of hepatitis B virus in the blood in either an active or a carrier state. It is routinely performed on donor's blood to identify the hepatitis B antigen. Approximately 5% of persons with diseases other than hepatitis B (serum hepatitis), such as leukemia, Hodgkin's disease, and hemophilia, will have a positive HBsAg test.

In hepatitis B, the antigen in the serum can be detected 2 to 24 weeks (average 4 to 8 weeks) after exposure to the virus. The positive HBsAg may be present 2 to 6 weeks after onset of the clinical disease.

HBsAg test does not diagnose hepatitis A virus. Two tests for hepatitis A are anti-HAV-IgM (indicates an acute infection) and anti-HAV-IgG (indicates a past exposure).

Purposes

- To screen for the presence of hepatitis B in the client's blood
- To detect the presence of hepatitis B in donor's blood

Clinical Problems

Elevated level (positive): Hepatitis B, chronic hepatitis B; less common: hemophilia, leukemia

Procedure

- No food or fluid restriction is required.
- Collect 5 to 7 mL of venous blood in a red-top tube.

Nursing Implications

- Obtain a history of any previous hepatitis infection and report it to the physician.

- Handle blood specimen with strict aseptic technique.
- Follow the institution's isolation procedure in discarding disposable equipment.
- Observe for signs and symptoms of hepatitis (i.e., lethargy, anorexia, nausea and vomiting, fever, dark-colored urine, and jaundice).

Client Teaching

- Instruct the client to get plenty of rest, a nutritional diet, and fluids.

HERPES SIMPLEX VIRUS (HSV) ANTIBODY TEST (SERUM)

Reference Values

Negative: <1:10

Positive: Early primary herpes simplex infection: 1:10 to 1:100. Late primary herpes simplex infection: 1:100 to 1:500. Latent herpes simplex infection: >1:500. Fourfold titer increase between the acute and convalescent period.

Description. Herpes simplex, a member of the herpesvirus group, is an infectious virus that produces antibody titers. The two types of herpes simplex are herpes simplex virus 1 (HSV-1) and herpes simplex virus 2 (HSV-2). HSV-1 infects the mouth, mostly the mucous membrane around the lip (cold sores), eyes, or upper respiratory tract. HSV-1 commonly occurs to the young as stomatitis (mouth ulcers) prior to the age of 20. HSV-2 is frequently referred to as genital herpes infecting the genitourinary tract. HSV-2 is transmitted primarily through sexual contact and can infect the newborn during vaginal delivery. Neonatal herpes may be mild, resulting in eye infection or skin rash, or it may result in a fatal systemic infection. Congenital herpes is not as common but may be acquired during early pregnancy, resulting in central nervous system disorders causing brain damage. Severe HSV infection can occur in immunosuppressed clients and neonates.

In addition to the serology blood test, a culture may be obtained for HSV-2 using the HERPCHEK test. The scrapings from suspected HSV genital vesicular lesions are obtained.

Antibodies for HSV-1 and HSV-2 begin to rise in 7 days and reach peak titers in 4 to 6 weeks after infection. HSV-IgM usually denotes acute infection, whereas HSV-IgG can indicate the convalescent phase. Those infected may have an increased titer level for 6 months after infection or it may persist throughout their life. Genital herpes (HSV-2) tends to be more severe and needs appropriate medical care, such as an antiviral drug.

Purposes

- To detect the presence of HSV
- To diagnose the convalescent phase of HSV

Clinical Problems

Positive titer: HSV-1, HSV-2, HSV-1 encephalitis, cervicitis, congenital herpes

Procedure

Serum

- No food or fluid restriction is required.
- Collect 3 to 5 mL of venous blood in a red-top tube. Avoid hemolysis. Deliver the blood sample to the laboratory within 1 hour. Gloves should be worn when obtaining a blood specimen.
- Indicate on the laboratory slip to test for HSV-1 or HSV-2, or both.
- CSF may be obtained to determine the presence of HSV if HSV-1 encephalitis is suspected.

Culture

- Swab the infected area of the throat, skin, genital area, or eye.
- Obtain respiratory or body secretions through lavage or washing.
- Deliver the specimen immediately to the microbiology lab.

Nursing Implications

- Obtain a history from the client of a possible herpes infection of the mouth (HSV-1) or the genital area (HSV-2). Ascertain when the symptoms first occurred.
- Use gloves when inspecting the area as herpes simplex can be infectious.
- Avoid giving antiviral drugs until the specimen has been obtained.

Client Teaching

- Listen to the client's concerns. If the herpes simplex is HSV-2, the client should be encouraged to have her or his sexual partner tested for HSV-2.

- Encourage the pregnant client to speak with the appropriate health care provider. This helps in alleviating the client's fears and making the client well informed. The health care provider will most likely culture the genital area near the time of birthing.

HETEROPHILE ANTIBODY (SERUM), AND MONO-SPOT

Reference Values

Adult: Normal: <1:28 titer; abnormal: >1:56 titer
Child: Same as adult
Elderly: Normal: slightly higher titer than adult

Description. This is a test primarily for infectious mononucleosis (IM). IM is thought to be caused by the Epstein-Barr virus (EBV).

Heterophiles are a group of antibodies that react to sheep and horse RBCs and, if positive (titer), an agglutination occurs. Titers of 1:56 to 1:224 are highly suspicious of infectious mononucleosis; those of 1:224 or greater are positive for infectious mononucleosis. Elevated heterophile titers occur during the first 2 weeks, peak in 3 weeks, and remain elevated for 6 weeks.

Mono-Spot: There are several commercially prepared tests: Mono-Spot by Ortho Diagnostics; Monoscreen by Smith, Kline and Beecham; and Monotest by Wapole. Mono-Spot test is usually done first and, if positive, then the titer test.

Purposes

- To check for elevated heterophile titer
- To aid in the diagnosis of infectious mononucleosis

Clinical Problems

Elevated level: Infectious mononucleosis, serum sickness, viral infections

Procedure

Heterophile antibody (HA) test: There are several HA tests: Paul–Bunnell test, Davidsohn differential test

- No food or fluid restriction is required.
- Collect 3 to 5 mL of venous blood in a red-top tube.

Mono-Spot test: Follow directions listed on the kit.

Nursing Implications

- Obtain a history of the client's contact with any person or persons recently diagnosed as having infectious mononucleosis.
- Observe for signs and symptoms of infectious mononucleosis (i.e., fever, sore throat, fatigue, swollen glands).
- Determine when the symptoms first occurred. A repeat heterophile or Mono-Spot test may be needed if the first was done too early.

Client Teaching

- Encourage the client to rest, drink fluids, and have a nutritional diet.

HEXOSAMINIDASE (TOTAL, A, AND A AND B) SERUM, AMNIOTIC FLUID

Reference Values

Adult: Total: 5–20 U/L. Hexosaminidase A: 55%–80%

Description. Hexosaminidase is a group of enzymes (isoenzymes A and B) responsible for the metabolism of gangliosides. It is found in brain tissue. Lack of the hexosaminidase A causes Tay-Sachs disease because of the accumulation of gangliosides in the brain. The total hexosaminidase may be normal or decreased. This test is used to confirm Tay-Sachs disease or to identify Tay-Sachs carriers.

Tay-Sachs disease is an autosomal-recessive disorder resulting in progressive destruction of central nervous system (CNS) cells. It is characterized by mental retardation, muscular weakness, and blindness. It affects primarily the Ashkenazic Jewish population. Death usually occurs before the age of 5 years.

Sandhoff's disease, a variant of Tay-Sachs, progresses more rapidly than Tay-Sachs disease. With this disorder, there is a deficiency of hexosaminidase A and B. It is not prevalent in any ethnic group.

Purposes

- To diagnose a deficit of hexosaminidase A (Tay-Sachs disease) or hexosaminidase A and B (Sandhoff's disease)
- To identify carriers of Tay-Sachs disease or Sandhoff's disease

Clinical Problems

Decreased level: Hexosaminidase A: Tay-Sachs disease. Hexosaminidase A and B: Sandhoff's disease

Procedure

- No food or fluid restriction is required.
- Collect 5 to 7 mL of venous blood in a red-top tube. Avoid hemolysis.
- Collect cord blood from the newborn.

Nursing Implications

Client Teaching

- Inform the Ashkenazic Jewish couple that the hexosaminidase screening test is to determine if they are Tay-Sachs carriers. Explain to the couple that it is a recessive trait and that both must carry the gene for their offspring to get Tay-Sachs disease.
- Have client communicate with health care providers such as the physician, nurse, and/or genetic counselor when both partners have a hexosaminidase A deficiency.
- Be supportive of the partners and child with Tay-Sachs disease. Answer questions or refer them to other health care providers.

HUMAN CHORIONIC GONADOTROPIN (HCG) SERUM AND URINE

PREGNANCY TEST

Reference Values. Values may be expressed as IU/mL or ng/mL. Check with your laboratory.

Adult: Serum: nonpregnant female: <0.01 IU/mL

Pregnant (Weeks)	*Values*	
1	0.01–0.04	IU/mL
2	0.03–0.10	IU/mL
4	0.10–1.0	IU/mL
5–12	10–100	IU/mL
13–25	10–30	IU/mL
26–40	5–15	IU/mL

Urine: Nonpregnant female: negative
Pregnant: 1–12 weeks: 6,000–500,000 IU/24 h
Many over-the-counter (OTC) pregnancy kits available.
Usually tested 3 days after missed menstrual period.

Description. HCG is a hormone produced by the placenta. In pregnancy, HCG appears in the blood and urine 14 to 26 days after conception, and the HCG concentration peaks in approximately 8 to 12 weeks. After the first trimester of pregnancy, HCG production declines. HCG is not found in nonpregnant females, in death of the fetus, or after 3 to 4 days postpartum.

Purposes

- To determine if the client is pregnant
- To detect a threatened abortion or dead fetus

Clinical Problems

Decreased level: Nonpregnant, dead fetus, postpartum (3 to 4 days), incomplete abortion, threatened abortion

Elevated level: Pregnancy, hydatidiform mole, chorionepithelioma, choriocarcinoma, erythyroblastosis fetalis
Drugs that may increase HCG value: Anticonvulsants, hypnotics, phenothiazines, antiparkinsonism drugs

Procedure

Serum

- Perform the pregnancy test no earlier than 5 days after the first missed menstrual period.
- Collect 3 to 5 mL of venous blood in a red-top tube. Avoid hemolysis.

Urine

- Restrict fluids for 8 to 12 hours; no food is restricted.
- Take a morning urine specimen (60 mL) with specific gravity >1.010 to the laboratory immediately. A 24-hour urine collection may be requested.
- Instruct client to follow directions when using commercial kit.
- Avoid blood in the urine, as false positives could occur.

Factors Affecting Laboratory Results

- Diluted urine (specific gravity <1.010) could cause a false-negative test result.
- Protein and blood in the urine could cause false-positive test results.

Nursing Implications

Client Teaching

- Ask the client when she had her last period. The test should be done 5 or more days after the missed period to avoid a false negative. Blood in the urine can cause false-positive result.
- Listen to client's concerns.

HUMAN IMMUNODEFICIENCY VIRUS TYPE 1 (HIV-1) OR HIV*

Note: The retrovirus designated human immunodeficiency virus type 2 (HIV-2) exhibits a pattern of transmission, and causes clinical disease features, similar to those of HIV-1. Prevalent in Africa, with equal numbers of infected men and women, HIV-2 is generally spread through heterosexual contact as a classical sexually transmitted disease, often concurrent with other genital lesions. HIV-2 cases in the United States are currently more limited. The long-term concern is that the African pattern may, in the future, be duplicated in North America.

Reference Values

Antibody screening

HIV-1/2 antibody screen (ELISA, EIA)

Adult: Seronegative for antibodies to HIV-1/2; nonreactive

---

*This test contributed by Jane Purnell Taylor, RN, MSN.

Child: Seronegative for antibodies to HIV-1/2; nonreactive

HIV-1 Western blot (confirmatory test that directly detects HIV viral gene proteins)

HIV-2 Western blot (confirmatory test that directly detects HIV viral gene proteins)

Adult: Negative

Child: Negative

Antigen screening

HIV-1 p24 Antigen

Adult: Negative for p24 antigen of HIV; nonreactive

Child: Negative for p24 antigen of HIV; nonreactive

(*Note:* There is no HIV-2 p24 antigen test; confirmatory test for the HIV-1 p24 antigen is a neutralization.)

Viral load tests: Sensitive assay that measures levels of HIV's ribonucleic acid (RNA) in plasma (to predict disease course). Uses polymerase chain reaction (PCR) to amplify HIV RNA. Used as a marker for basing treatment decisions and evaluating effectiveness of anti-HIV drug therapy (rechecked 4–8 weeks after changes in drug therapy as monitoring technique). Expressed as the number of copies of HIV RNA in a 1-mL sample of plasma

Low numbers: Represents suppressed replication

High numbers: Represents increased replication and disease progression

Description. The retrovirus HIV-1, identified as the cause of acquired immunodeficiency syndrome (AIDS), was first recognized in 1981. However, it is now believed that HIV has existed in human populations for at least 70 years, based on genetic work comparing genetic composition of many current HIV strains and extrapolation back to a common origin. The infection is expressed along a progressive continuum extending from clinically asymptomatic (although seropositive for HIV-1 antibodies) to expression of a severely damaged (suppressed) immune system due to T-helper lymphocyte (T4 lymphocyte) destruction manifested by clinical signs and symptoms, altered laboratory values, and increased susceptibility to AIDS-defining opportunistic infections (including pneumocystis carinii pneumonia; chronic cryptosporidiosis; toxoplasmosis; cryptococcosis; disseminated histoplasmosis; mycobacterial infection; disseminated cytomegalovirus infection; chronic mucocutaneous or disseminated herpes simplex virus infection; and esophageal, bronchial, or pulmonary candidiasis that rarely cause disease in an immune-competent person) and rarer forms of cancer (including Kaposi's sarcoma and lymphomas [Non-Hodgkin lymphoma and primary brain lymphoma]).

The incubation time between HIV infection and the development of HIV-1-related disease is highly individualized. Until recently, it was thought that an initial dormant phase occurred during the early and middle years of the infection. New research now shows that HIV multiplies rapidly with high viral blood levels in the first few weeks of infection. HIV viral antigen may become detectable approximately two weeks after infection and last for 3 to 5 months. Following exposure to HIV, 2 to 6 weeks later an influenza-type illness (fever, muscle aches, sweating, rash, sore throat, headache, fatigue, swollen lymph nodes) is demonstrable in up to 70% of clients. The client recovers, but over a 12-day to 5-year period (most often 6 to 12 weeks) the immune system develops antibodies to the virus (seroconversion). Depending upon individual variables, many clients next enter into a symptomless stage of infection that may last up to 8 to 12 years, during which the infection may be unknowingly transmitted. Prevention of transmission is critically important; the recent addition of the HIV-1 p24 antigen test (approved by the FDA in March 1996) may identify HIV infection in an individual within two weeks (approximately a week earlier than the anti-HIV-1/2 test), thus narrowing the vulnerable period when the virus may be passed to others while screening tests can't detect it.

In 1993, the CDC revised the system by which HIV infection and the definition of AIDS is classified to include the CD4+ T-lymphocyte count as a marker for the degree of immunosuppression related to HIV. This new definition adds to the previous operational definition of AIDS that included 23 clinical conditions. Now, the definition includes those individuals with pulmonary tuberculosis, recurrent pneumonia (within a 12-month period), and invasive cervical cancer in addition to laboratory confirmation of HIV infection with a <200 CD4+ T lymphocyte/μL or a CD4+ T lymphocyte percentage of total lymphocytes less than 14 percent. It is expected that the new working definition will promote earlier diagnosis of those at risk and that treatment modalities will be instituted with close monitoring. New treatment therapies using protease inhibitors (affecting viral reproduction) in combination, and often also including nucleoside [e.g., zidovudine] and non-nucleoside [e.g., sustiva] reverse transcriptase inhibitors, in early (rather than later) stages of the infection is leading to the hope that HIV may, in the future, be manageable as a chronic disease. Major hurdles to be overcome include development of viral strains resistant to treatment; overwhelmingly expensive drug therapies involving a complex treatment regimen (important to both individuals and the developing countries most afflicted by the AIDS epidemic); product availability; and the ability of the virus to remain hidden (non-detectable) throughout the body (in the brain, testes, lymph nodes) outside the bloodstream. Although one non-live attenuated vaccine is undergoing formal trial with volunteers considered at high risk of contracting the HIV virus, no magic-bullet vaccine is expected in the near future. The infection remains preventable, possibly chronically manageable, but not curable at the present time.

It is estimated by the Centers for Disease Control and Prevention that as many as 900,000 people in the United States manifest HIV infection, with about 40,000 new infections per year during the 1990s. Through mid-1998, 665,357 have developed AIDS and over 401,028 have died (not specifically from AIDS). In the United States, AIDS has become the second leading cause of death for all people aged 25–44 as a group (behind accidents), with AIDS the leading cause for men and the third leading cause for women. Overall, AIDS incidence decreased 18% (1996–1997) and 11% (1997–1998). Despite a continued significant decrease in the total number of reported cases, the 1997–1998 data suggest that the hoped-for continued rate of decline in the incidence of AIDS is slowing. The percentage of deaths decreased 42% (1996–1997), dropping to 20% from 1997–1998, while the percentage increase of those living with AIDS by the end of 1998 was 10%, representing 297,137 persons. These findings raise concern that the new combination drug therapies benefits in controlling viral progression may have been largely realized in combination with other factors, including untested and untreated individuals, noncompliance with treatments, and drug-resistant viral strains. As of June 1999, decreases in the number of children diagnosed with AIDS continue. Estimates are that 1 in 200 young adults in the United States is infected. Women, minorities (Black Americans, Hispanics), and young adults are among the most rapidly escalating groups of affected individuals. Overall, of the total number of people with HIV, the largest rate of increase is being observed in the heterosexual community. Current evidence suggests male-to-female transmission of HIV is more likely based upon anatomical and social factors including lack of use of barrier-type birth control methods or barrier-method failure. It has been found that in noncondom users, viral load is the greatest predictor of heterosexual HIV transmission. In addition, the baby of an untreated HIV-positive pregnant woman has a 25.5 percent chance of being infected before or during birth, or afterward, if breastfed. Child-to-child transmission of HIV-1 infection in school and day care settings is rare, as 1985 guidelines established through the CDC in regard to infected children remain effective. Risk of HIV infection in the health care setting is small (55 documented health care workers seroconverted to HIV following occupational exposure, with 25 of these having developed AIDS as of June 1999); approximately 800,000 needlesticks occur per year using conventional devices. As an outcome of this finding, a national campaign was initiated during 1996 to motivate health care settings to select newer and safer products (particularly protected or needleless equipment) in addition to use of standard precautions.

Worldwide, the World Health Organization (WHO) estimates that 40 million may exhibit HIV/AIDS by the year 2000, including 10 million HIV-infected infants and children. Approximately 90% of new cases occur in individuals who live in the developing world, including Southeast Asia and sub-Saharan Africa, with United Nations estimates of the total number currently infected at 22.6 million, with over 7.7 million who exhibit symptoms of AIDS. The global death toll due to AIDS was 2.6 million in 1998 (85% of these occurred in Africa). By the end of 2000, the number of orphaned African children under age 15 who will have lost one or both parents to AIDS is expected to be over 10 million. The pandemic will be stopped only through a reexamination of culture (including gender and sexual customs) and implementation of major prevention strategies.

Although HIV-1 has been isolated from blood, semen, saliva, vaginal secretions, breast milk, tears, cerebrospinal fluid, amniotic fluid, and urine, actual transmission occurs via infected lymphocytes carried by blood, semen, vaginal secretions, and breast milk. Those *at risk* for acquiring HIV infection include: noninfected persons who have unprotected direct sexual contact (vaginal, oral, or rectal) with an infected person of either sex; multiple partners; homosexual and bisexual men; persons with hemophilia or related clotting disorders who have received clotting factor concentrates; other recipients of infected blood or blood products (particularly prior to 1985); persons who have had, or have been treated for, syphilis or gonorrhea during the past 12 months; persons who have had a positive screening test for syphilis in the past 12 months without a negative confirmatory test; persons who have been in jail within the past 12 months; those who share infected needles with others as a component of illicit IV drug use; persons who subsequently have sexual contact with someone included in one or more of these groups; and fetuses or neonates exposed to an infected mother during the perinatal period (possibly secondary to maternal IV drug use or maternal heterosexual contact with an IV drug user).

Screening of blood products by blood banks in the United States was instituted in 1985 using the enzyme-linked immunosorbent assay (ELISA). Blood banks are required to test donors for antibodies to HIV-1 and -2. Blood banks have also implemented six additional infectious disease tests to ensure safety of the blood reaching hospitals nationally. In March 1996, the FDA-approved HIV-1 p24 antigen test was added to help identify infection earlier (because a person can be infected and have a negative antibody test). Screening of donors and public education has also been enhanced to assure the public concerning blood safety. All blood that tests positive is destroyed. Donors notified of confirmed-positive test results are included on a permanent deferral list and asked not to donate in the future. Nationally, the safety record is positive; over 37 million people have received transfusions since 1985 with only 38 documented cases of AIDS from that blood. From 1981 through 1998 (reflecting both pre- and post-1985, when screening requirements were implemented), 8,382 cases have been documented, including those who have received transfusions, organs, and donations of tissue and sperm, collectively.

Purposes

- To screen for the presence of HIV infection
- To monitor HIV during drug therapy

Clinical Problems

Seropositive test: Blood shows evidence of infection; blood test detects antibodies to HIV-1/2; or viral antigen is detected (p24 antigen of HIV).

Recall that a positive test indicative of HIV infection does not diagnose AIDS (which is defined as a clinical diagnosis with defining characteristics). HIV infection is expressed on a continuum from seropositive asymptomatic infection to disease expression. *Note:* Diagnosing HIV infection in children born to HIV-infected mothers is complicated by maternal antibodies which transplacentally affect the fetus, giving a positive HIV antibody result at birth (although only 15% to 30% are truly infected); the antibody usually becomes undetectable by 9 months of age (occasionally as long as 18 months). Thus, standard antibody tests are not reliable, and polymerase chain reaction (PCR) and virus culture are the most specific and sensitive means for detection of infection in children whose mothers are infected. These additional tests can identify 30% to 50% of infected infants at the time of birth and, by 3 to 6 months of age, close to 100%.

Procedure

- A signed consent form for the HIV-1/2 antibody screen is usually required and should include appropriate pre- and post-counseling.
- No food or fluid restriction is required.
- Collect 5 to 10 mL of venous blood in a red-top tube.

Two tests are most commonly employed for HIV-1/2 antibody screening (not for the virus itself). These include ELISA (enzyme-linked immunosorbent assay) and EIA (enzyme immunoassay). ELISA testing is reliable, specific, and highly sensitive. When a positive HIV-1 test result occurs, the test is generally repeated twice on the same sample; if two out of three of these tests are positive, an HIV-1 Western blot is done as well as an HIV-2 antibody screen. If the HIV-2 antibody screen is positive, an HIV-2 Western blot is performed. A second quickly performed confirmatory test commonly used is the immunofluorescence assay (IFA), but it is slightly less reliable than the Western blot. Collectively, when the ELISA plus Western blot show a persistently positive outcome, the specificity and sensitivity rates are both 99%, and the accuracy rate is 99%. False-positive Western blot results in low-risk populations are possible but less likely than with ELISA. False positives may be retested using an alternate laboratory; false-negative results are usually noted when testing is done prior to seroconversion.

If the client tests positive (reactive) when screening is for the HIV-1 p24 antigen, the test is repeated twice more on the same sample. A separate confirmatory test (called a neutralization) may be performed. If a client tests positive for the antigen but doesn't neutralize, both an antibody and an antigen test may be redone in approximately 4 weeks; at 8 weeks, just an antibody test may be done. It must be recalled that the HIV-1 p24 antigen generally disappears from the blood during the asymptomatic phase and is undetectable.

Nursing Implications

- Ascertain the purpose of being tested for each peson screened and assess the risk potential for HIV using information provided.
- Obtain a signed consent form from the client for HIV antibody test and/or antigen screening test.
- Provide clients being screened for HIV antibody or antigen with comprehensive pretest counseling, protection for confidential information obtained, and consistently accurate and comprehensive posttest education, support, and follow-up.
- Become knowledgeable about commercially available HIV home blood test kits in order to be able to accurately provide advice for clients who may elect self-testing and experience a variety of positive and negative issues as an outcome.
- Recognize the role of education as a highly effective preventive strategy.
- Develop a full knowledge of HIV infection and AIDS-related diseases in order to adequately address actual and potential client concerns in the role of nurse-educator.
- Be prepared to clearly explain and clarify meaning of test results for clients who may be experiencing situational crisis associated with the testing process and/or outcome.
- Monitor laboratory reports for indication of decreasing CD4+ T-lymphocyte cell counts; inform the health care provider.
- Assess for signs and symptoms related to clinical progression toward a depressed immune system, including profound involuntary weight loss, chronic diarrhea, chronic weakness, and intermittent or constant fever.

- Implement standard precautions, which combine the major features of universal (blood and body fluid) precautions (designed to reduce risk of blood-borne pathogen transmission) and body substance isolation (designed to reduce the risk of transmission of pathogens from moist body substances), and apply them to all clients regardless of diagnosis or presumed infection status; these precautions apply to blood, all body fluids, secretions, and excretions (except sweat), regardless of whether visible blood is present, nonintact skin, and mucous membranes.
- In obstetric settings, gloves should be worn whenever handling placentas; also when handling newborns who have not had initial baths; when changing diapers; obtaining urine or fecal samples; and during suctioning, heelsticks for blood glucose determination, and vitamin K administration.
- Request and use tight-fitting collection containers for all laboratory specimens involving blood and body fluids, followed by placing containers into plastic cover bags for safe handling and transport.
- Be nonjudgmental with HIV/AIDS clients and their families with regard to how the illness may have been acquired.
- Recognize that infants born to HIV/AIDS-infected mothers will exhibit and maintain a positive HIV antibody response (reflecting maternal antibodies) for up to 18 months. However, only 15% to 30% are truly infected. Those who do become infected become symptomatic more quickly than adults and may have a decreased survival period. Many children (both infected and noninfected) may be orphaned if their mothers die, necessitating interdisciplinary planning for the family.
- Recognize actual and/or at-risk clients for HIV/AIDS. HIV-infected clients should be screened for the presence of co-infection with TB. Anergy testing may be necessary.
- Become knowledgeable concerning institutional policies in compliance with CDC guidelines and the OSHA Blood-borne Pathogen Standard concerning needlestick/penetrating injurics and blood or secretion splash incidents.
- Screen women for the presence of frequent vaginal yeast infections.

- Review client records for adequate immunization status; recognize that HIV-infected clients are also high-risk for coinfection with hepatitis B virus. Screen client records for documentation of hepatitis B vaccine; inform the health care provider of findings; tetanus booster should be current within 10 years; documentation should show receipt of annual flu shot and a single dose of pneumococcal vaccine.

Client Teaching

- Provide clients with an overview about HIV and the testing available for antibodies.
- Explain to the client that if a first HIV test indicates a positive response, a repeat test and confirmatory tests will need to be made prior to reaching any conclusions.
- Explain to the client that a confirmed positive HIV antibody test indicates exposure to HIV that has stimulated an immune system response; the person is infected and able to transmit the infection. Explain that a negative test is not a guarantee that infection has not occurred; variables include the time frame in relation to exposure and when the test is done. For both outcomes, plan strategies with the client to ensure risk reduction related to HIV for both self and others; include relationship and sexual boundary setting as part of the discussion.
- Discuss the meaning of test results for the client's desired or planned life events (e.g., sexual contact, marriage, childbearing, breastfeeding, etc.). Refer the client to other health professionals as necessary. Provide the National AIDS Hotline phone number (1-800-342-AIDS) (1-800-342-2437); if needed, suggest Spanish AIDS Hotline (1-800-342-SIDA); Hearing Impaired AIDS Hotline (TDD Service; 1-800-243-7889). Provide these Internet Web sites: American Social Health Association (www.ashastd.org) and Centers for Disease Control (www.cdc.gov/HIV).
- Explain that there is no definitive cure for HIV/AIDS; however, well-being and survival are effected through early intervention strategies, including early diagnosis and the use of combination drug therapy.
- Teach awareness and prevention to at-risk clients who demonstrate knowledge deficits about HIV/AIDS, particularly in primary care settings.

- Stress elimination of substance abuse and to expose oneself to only low-risk sexual behavior as a preventive strategy; explain that sexual abstinence is 100% effective.
- Suggest that clients facing elective surgery discuss autologous transfusion with their health care providers to allay fears related to blood transfusions.
- Explain to members in the community that casual contact with a person with HIV/AIDS does not put them at high risk for contracting HIV/AIDS. However, intimate sexual contact (oral, genital, rectal) with a person with HIV/AIDS puts the individual at high risk.
- Address anxiety and fear reactions about HIV/AIDS within the public sector. Stress that HIV/AIDS is not spread by talking to, shaking hands with, sharing glasses with, embracing, sharing spoons with, or sharing a household with an HIV/AIDS-infected client. Stress that there are no known cases transmitted by kissing, as saliva is low in lymphocytes; nor spread by insect bites.
- Encourage clients with HIV/AIDS to identify persons with whom they have had sexual contact. At times, clients are more likely to tell the nurse names of partners than they are to tell the health care provider.
- Encourage childbearing-age women to voluntarily and routinely be tested for their HIV status to assist with childbearing decisions and allow for early intervention with any subsequent offspring.
- Explain to HIV-positive pregnant clients that the American College of Obstetricians and Gynecologists (ACOG) currently recommends (effective July 1999) that *all* HIV-positive pregnant women should be offered scheduled C-section deliveries at 38 weeks' gestation to decrease the risk of transmission to the newborn; also that HIV risk to the infant can be further reduced to approximately 2% when a combination of a scheduled C-section plus treatment with ZDV (Zidovudine) is employed (as compared to a 25% risk when untreated vaginal delivery is elected).
- Inform infected pregnant women who labor with an anticipated vaginal delivery that internal fetal monitoring will not be used during labor (to maintain fetal skin integrity and prevent exposure to potentially bloody amniotic fluid).
- Explain that breastfeeding is permitted if a client is initially negative and remains so at the time of delivery; breastfeeding is not initiated when the mother is untested for HIV or determined to be

positive, because breast milk contains HIV-infected lymphocytes, colostrum has high concentrations, and maternal nipples may become sore and crack, with potential HIV exposure for the neonate.

- Inform families that HIV-infected infants and children will need to receive all routine immunizations *except* oral polio vaccine. Only injectable killed polio vaccine should be given. These babies should also receive flu shots in the fall of the year. Hepatitis B vaccine should also be given.
- Discuss with clients the need to have a tetanus booster that is current within 10 years; also, clients should be instructed to receive an annual flu shot and a single dose of pneumococcal vaccine.
- Inform women clients to seek gynecologic evaluation if an infection is persistent and/or unresponsive to nonprescription treatment (e.g., Monistat-7 and/or Gyne-Lotrimin). Teach clients to wear cotton underwear and avoid douching. Tell clients to not douche prior to a gynecologic examination because PAP tests and specimen quality may be adversely affected.
- Encourage low-risk healthy individuals to donate blood because sterile needles are used and are discarded, with no risk of infection. The donor does not have contact with other blood.
- Advise clients not to use the toothbrushes or razors of high-risk or HIV/AIDS-infected individuals because of the possibility of blood contamination; women should be taught to safely dispose of menstrual blood-containing items.

HUMAN LEUKOCYTE ANTIGENS (HLA) SERUM

HLA TYPING, ORGAN-DONOR TISSUE TYPING

Reference Values. Histocompatibility match or nonmatch; no norms

Description. The human leukocyte antigens (HLA) are on the surface membranes of leukocytes, platelets, and many tissue cells. This antigenic system is very complex as it relates to tissue compatibility for transplantation and immune response. There are five different antigens that belong to the HLA system; A, B, C, D, and DR (D-related). Each of these antigens contains many groups (20 A antigens, 40 B antigens, 8 C antigens, 12 D antigens, and 10 DR antigens) that can be HLA phenotyped to determine histocompatibility.

The four main purposes for HLA testing are: (1) organ transplantation; (2) transfusion; (3) disease association, such as juvenile rheumatoid arthritis, ankylosing spondylitis, myasthenia gravis, Addison's disease, and insulin-dependent diabetes mellitus; and (4) paternity testing may be verified when the putative father has one haplotype (phenotyping) that is identical to the child. This test may be useful in genetic counseling when associated with susceptibility to certain diseases.

Purposes

- To screen for histocompatibility in tissue typing
- To determine paternity of the child

Clinical Problems

Positive histocompatibility: Tissue compatibility for grafts and organ transplants, father of the child

Procedure

- No food or fluid restriction is required.
- Collect 5 to 7 mL of venous blood in a green-top tube. Avoid hemolysis. Blood samples should be analyzed immediately.

Factors Affecting Laboratory Results

- Blood transfusion in the last 3 days could affect test results.

Nursing Implications

Client Teaching

- Encourage the client to express concerns related to the health problem.
- Listen to client's and family's concerns. Refer questions to appropriate health professionals if necessary.

HUMAN PLACENTAL LACTOGEN (hPL) PLASMA OR SERUM

CHORIONIC SOMATOMAMMOTROPIN

Reference Values

Nonpregnant female: <0.5 μg/mL

Pregnant female

Weeks of Gestation	*Reference Values*
5–7	1.0 μg/mL
8–27	<4.6 μg/mL
28–31	2.4–6.0 μg/mL
32–35	3.6–7.7 μg/mL
36–term	5.0–10.0 μg/mL

Male: <0.5 μg/mL

Description. Human placental lactogen (hPL) is a hormone secreted by the placenta and can be detected in the maternal blood after 5 weeks of gestation. During pregnancy, the hPL increases slowly. This test is useful for evaluating placental function and fetal well-being, especially from the 28th week to term. A decreased hPL level, <4.0 μg/mL, during the third trimester of pregnancy is indicative of fetal distress, retarded fetal growth, threatened abortion, toxemia, or post-fetal maturity. A serum estriol and nonstress test are frequently ordered to verify the hPL test result.

Purposes

- To evaluate placental function
- To determine fetal well-being after 28th week to term

Clinical Problems

Decreased level: Fetal distress, toxemia of pregnancy, threatened abortion, trophoblastic neoplastic disease (hydatidiform mole, choriocarcinoma)
Elevated level: Multiple pregnancy, diabetes mellitus, bronchogenic carcinoma, liver tumor, lymphoma

Procedure

- No food or fluid restriction is required.

- Collect 5 to 7 mL of venous blood in a red- or green-top tube. Avoid hemolysis.
- hPL value fluctuates; therefore, the test may need to be repeated.

Nursing Implications

- Record the gestation week on the laboratory slip.
- Correlate the serum/plasma human placental lactogen result with the serum or urine estriol level. The hPL value can fluctuate daily, so the hPL test is usually repeated. Other tests for detecting fetal distress may also be ordered.
- Be supportive of the client and family. Allow the client time to express her concerns. Be a good listener. Direct appropriate questions to other health professionals, such as the physician or midwife.

17-HYDROXYCORTICOSTEROIDS (17-OHCS) URINE

PORTER-SIBER CHROMOGENS

Reference Values

Adult: Male: 3–12 mg/24 h; female: 2–10 mg/24 h; average: 2–12 mg/24 h
Child: Infant to 1 yr: <1 mg/24 h; 2 to 4 yr: 1–2 mg/24 h; 5–12 yr: 6–8 mg/24 h
Elderly: Lower than adult

Description. 17-OHCS are metabolites of adrenocortical steroid hormones, mostly of cortisol, and are excreted in the urine. Because the excretion of the metabolites is diurnal, varying in rate of excretion, a 24-hour urine specimen is necessary for accuracy of test results. This test is useful for assessing adrenocortical hormone function.

Purposes

- To assess adrenocortical hormone function
- To detect disorders caused by deficit or excess of adrenocortical hormone

Clinical Problems

Decreased level: Addison's disease, androgenital syndrome, hypopituitarism, hypothyroidism, liver disease

Drugs that may decrease urine 17-OHCS: Calcium gluconate, dexamethasone (Decadron), phenytoin (Dilantin), promethazine (Phenergan), reserpine (Serpasil)

Elevated level: Cushing's syndrome, adrenal cancer, hyperpituitarism, hyperthyroidism, extreme stress, eclampsia
Drugs that may increase urine 17-OHCS: Antibiotics (penicillin and erythromycin), cortisone, acetazolamide (Diamox), ascorbic acid, thiazide diuretics, phenothiazides, digoxin, estrogen, colchicine, hydroxyzine (Atarax), iodides, oral contraceptives, quinidine, spironolactone (Aldactone), paraldehyde

Procedure

- Withhold drugs (with health care provider's approval) for 3 days before the test to prevent false results. Any drugs given should be listed on the laboratory slip.
- No food or fluid is restricted except for coffee and tea. Fluid intake should be encouraged.
- Collect urine in a large container/bottle, and add an acid preservative to prevent bacterial degradation of the steroids. The urine collection should be refrigerated if no preservative is added. No toilet paper or feces should be in the urine.
- Label container with client's name, date, and exact time of collection (e.g., 9/23/03, 7:30 AM to 9/24/03, 7:30 AM).

Nursing Implications

- Encourage the client to increase fluid intake, except coffee, during the 24-hour test.
- If levels are decreased, observe for signs and symptoms of hypoadrenalism (i.e., fatigue, weakness, weight loss, bronze coloration of the skin, postural hypotension, cardiac dysrhythmia, craving for salty food, and fasting hypoglycemia).
- If levels are elevated, observe for signs and symptoms of hyperadrenalism (i.e., "moon face," "buffalo hump," fluid retention, hypertension, hyperglycemia, petechiae or ecchymosis, and hirsutism).

5-HYDROXYINDOLACETIC ACID (5-HIAA) URINE

5-OH-INDOLACETIC ACID

Reference Values

Adult: Qualitative random samples: negative; quantitative 24-hour: 2–10 mg/24 h
Child: Usually not done

Description. 5-HIAA, a metabolite of serotonin, is excreted in the urine as the result of carcinoid tumors found in the appendix or in the intestinal wall. Serotonin is a vasoconstricting hormone secreted by the argentaffin cells of the gastrointestinal (GI) tract and is responsible for peristalsis. Carcinoid tumor cells, which secrete excess serotonin, are of low-grade malignancy; removal ensures an 80% to 90% cure. Some noncarcinoid tumors may produce high levels of 5-HIAA.

Purposes

- To confirm carcinoid tumor of the intestine
- To compare with other laboratory tests for confirmation of carcinoid tumor

Clinical Problems

Drugs that may decrease urine 5-HIAA: ACTH, heparin, imipramine (Tofranil), phenothiazines, methyldopa (Aldomet), MAO inhibitors, promethazine (Phenergan)

Elevated level: Carcinoid tumors of the appendix and intestine, carcinoid tumor with metastasis (>100 mg/24 h), sciatica pain, skeletal and smooth muscle spasm
Drugs that may increase urine 5-HIAA: Acetophenetidin (Phenacetin), reserpine (Serpasil), methamphetamine (Desoxyn)
Foods that may increase urine 5-HIAA: Banana, pineapple, plums, avocados, eggplant, walnuts

Procedure

- Eliminate the foods and drugs listed above for 3 days before the test. Check with health care provider.

Qualitative random urine sample (screening)

- Collect a random urine sample and take to the laboratory immediately. The random urine test is usually done first.

Quantitative 24-hour urine collection

- Collect urine for 24 hours in a large container with an acid preservative. Urine collection should have a pH <4.0.

Nursing Implications

- Check the 5-HIAA result of the random urine test. A repeat test may be needed if the client has taken drugs that can depress the 5-HIAA. If the urine test is positive, the health care provider may order the 5-HIAA 24-hour urine test.

Client Teaching

- Instruct the client not to eat food listed or to take drugs for 3 days before test without health care provider's permission. Foods and drugs taken should be listed on the laboratory slip.

IMMUNOGLOBULINS (Ig) SERUM

IgG, IgA, IgM, IgD, IgE

Reference Values. Values may differ in institutions.

	Total Ig (99%; mg/dL)	*IgG (80%; mg/dL)*	*IgA (15%; mg/dL)*	*IgM (4%; mg/dL)*	*IgD 0.2%; mg/dL)*	*IgE (0.0002; U/mL)*
Adult	900–2,200	650–1,700	70–400	40–350	0–8	<40 (IgE 0–120 mg/dL)
6–16 yr	800–1,700	700–1,650	80–230	45–260		<62
4–6 yr	700–1,700	550–1,500	50–175	22–100		<25
1–3 yr	400–1,500	300–1,400	20–150	40–230		<10
6 mo	225–1,200	200–1,100	10–90	10–80		
3 mo	325–750	275–750	5–55	15–70		
Newborn	650–1,450	700–1,480	0–12	5–30		

Description. Immunoglobulins (Ig) are classes of proteins referred to as antibodies. They are divided into five groups found in gamma globulin (IgG, IgA, IgM, IgD, IgE) and can be separated by the process of immunoelectrophoresis. As individuals are exposed to antigens, immunoglobulin (antibody) production occurs, and with further exposure to the same antigen, immunity results.

IgG: IgG results from secondary exposure to the foreign antigen and is responsible for antiviral and antibacterial activity. This antibody passes through the placental barrier and provides early immunity for the newborn.

IgA: IgA is found in secretions of the respiratory, GI, and genitourinary (GU) tracts, tears, and saliva. It protects mucous membranes from viruses and some bacteria. IgA does not pass the placental barrier. Those having congenital IgA deficiency are prone to autoimmune disease.

IgM: IgM antibodies are produced 48 to 72 hours after an antigen enters the body and are responsible for primary immunity. IgM does not pass the placental barrier. It is produced early in life, after 9 months.

IgD: Unknown

IgE: Increases during allergic reactions and anaphylaxis

Purposes

- To identify the occurrence of total or a specific elevated immunoglobulin
- To associate a specific immunoglobin elevation with a health problem (see Clinical Problems)

Clinical Problems

Ig	*Decreased Level*	*Elevated Level*
IgG	Lymphocytic leukemia	Infections (all types)
	Agammaglobulinemia	Severe malnutrition
	Preeclampsia	Chronic granulomatous infection
	Amyloidosis	Hyperimmunization
		Liver disease
		Rheumatic fever
		Sarcoidosis
IgA	Lymphocytic leukemia	Autoimmune disorders
	Agammaglobulinemia	Rheumatic fever

(continued)

Ig	*Decreased Level*	*Elevated Level*
	Malignancies	Chronic infections
		Liver disease
IgM	Lymphocytic leukemia	Lymphosarcoma
	Agammaglobulinemia	Brucellosis
	Amyloidosis	Trypanosomiasis
		Infectious mononucleosis
		Rubella virus in newborns
IgE		Allergic reactions (asthma)
		Skin sensitivity
		Drugs: tetanus toxoid and antitoxin, gamma globulin

Procedure

- No food or fluid restriction is required. Some laboratories request NPO 12 hours before the test. Check with your laboratory.
- Collect 5 to 7 mL of venous blood in a red-top tube.
- Record on the laboratory slip if client has received any vaccination or immunization (including toxoid) in the last 6 months; any blood transfusion, gamma globulin, or tetanus antitoxin in the last 6 weeks.

Factors Affecting Laboratory Results

- Immunizations and toxoids received in the last 6 months and blood transfusions received in the last 6 weeks can affect test results.

Nursing Implications

- Obtain vaccination, immunization, transfusion, and gamma globulin history.

Client Teaching

- Instruct the client to avoid infections.

INSULIN (SERUM), INSULIN ANTIBODY TEST

Reference Values

Adult: Serum insulin: 5–25 μU/mL, 10–250 μIU/mL. Panic Value: 7 μU/mL

Insulin antibody test: <4% serum binding of beef or pork

Description. Insulin, hormone from the beta cells of the pancreas, is essential in transporting glucose to the cells. Increased glucose levels stimulate insulin secretion. Serum insulin and blood glucose levels are compared to determine the glucose disorder. Serum insulin level is valuable in diagnosing insulinoma (islet cell tumor) and islet cell hyperplasia, and in evaluating insulin production in diabetes mellitus (DM). Insulin values are more helpful during an OGTT (oral glucose tolerance test) for diagnosing an early pre-hyperglycemic DM state. A normal fasting insulin level and a delayed rise in GTT curves occur frequently with a mildly diabetic individual. In insulinoma the serum insulin is high, and blood glucose is <30 mg/dL.

Insulin antibody test: This test is ordered when a diabetic, taking pork or beef insulin, requires larger and larger insulin dosages. Insulin antibodies develop as the result of impurities in animal insulins. These antibodies are of immunoglobulin types such as IgG (most common), IgM, and IgE. The IgG antibodies neutralize the insulin, thus preventing glucose metabolism. IgM antibodies can cause insulin resistance, and IgE may be responsible for allergic effects.

Purposes

- To assist in the detection of an early pre-hyperglycemic diabetes mellitus state
- To check for the presence of insulin antibody that can affect insulin absorption and dosage

Clinical Problems

Decreased level: Diabetes mellitus (insulin-dependent diabetes mellitus [IDDM] or type I), hypopituitarism
Drugs that may decrease insulin value: Beta blockers (e.g., propranolol), cimetidine, calcitonin, loop and thiazide diuretics (i.e., furosemide, hydrochlorothiazide), phenytoin, calcium channel blockers, phenobarbital

Elevated level: Insulinoma, noninsulin-dependent diabetes mellitus (NIDDM or type II), liver disease, Cushing's syndrome (hyperactive adrenal cortex), acromegaly, obesity (may double its value)
Drugs that may increase insulin value: Cortisone preparations, oral contraceptives, thyroid hormones, epinephrine, levodopa, terbutaline

(Brethine), tolazamide (Priscoline), oral antidiabetic drugs (i.e., tolbutamide [Orinase], acetohexamide [Dymelor])

Procedure

- Restrict food and fluids for 10 to 12 hours with the exception of water. Insulin secretion reaches its peak in 30 minutes to 2 hours after meals.
- Withhold medications that may affect test results, such as insulin and cortisone, until after the test.
- Collect 3 to 5 mL of venous blood in a red-top tube. Avoid hemolysis. If the test is to be conducted with OGTT, draw blood specimen for serum insulin before administering glucose.

Nursing Implications

- Obtain a history of clinical symptoms related to a glucose disorder. Report client's complaints.
- Report if the client's insulin dosage has increased over a period of time due to an increase in blood sugar. This may result from insulin antibody formation.

Client Teaching:

- Instruct the client to report signs and symptoms of insulin reaction, such as nervousness, sweating, weakness, rapid pulse rate, and/or confusion.

INTERNATIONAL NORMALIZED RATIO (INR) (PLASMA)

Reference Values

Oral anticoagulant therapy: 2.0–3.0 INR
Higher value for mechanical heart value: 3.0–4.5 INR

Description. The International Normalized Ratio (INR) was devised to monitor more correctly anticoagulant therapy for clients receiving warfarin (Coumadin) therapy. The World Health Organization (WHO) recommends the use of INR for a more consistent reporting of prothrombin time results. The INR is calculated by the use of a nomogram demonstrating the relationship between the INR and the PT ratio. Usually both PT and INR values are reported for monitoring Coumadin therapy.

Refer to Prothrombin Time (PT) for the purposes, clinical problems, procedure, factors affecting laboratory results, nursing implications, and client teaching.

IRON AND TOTAL IRON-BINDING CAPACITY (TIBC) SERUM

IRON-BINDING CAPACITY (IBC)

Reference Values

Serum iron

Adult: 50–150 μg/dL, 10–27 μmol/L (SI units); men slightly higher than women. *Elderly:* 60–80 μg/dL

Child: Newborn: 100–200 μg/dL; 6 mo–2 yr: 40–100 μg/dL

TIBC

Adult: 250–450 μg/dL (2 to 3× greater than serum iron level). *Elderly:* <250 μg/dL

Child: Newborn: 60–175 μg/dL; infant: 100–400 μg/dL; 6 mo–2 yr: 100–135 μg/dL; child over 2 yr: same as adult

Transferrin saturation percent: 20%–50% saturation

Description. Iron is coupled with plasma transferrin (protein), which is responsible for iron transportation to the bone marrow for the purpose of hemoglobin synthesis. Serum iron levels are elevated when there is excessive red blood cell destruction (hemolysis), and levels are decreased in iron deficiency anemia. Usually, serum iron and TIBC are determined together.

The TIBC measures the amount of additional iron with which transferrin is able to combine. When the serum iron is decreased, the TIBC is increased, and when serum iron is increased, the TIBC is decreased.

Purposes

- To determine a probable cause of iron excess (e.g., hemolysis) or deficit (e.g., iron deficiency anemia)

- To compare serum iron and total iron-binding capacity (TIBC) for diagnosing iron deficiency anemia

Clinical Problems

Decreased level

Serum iron: Iron deficiency anemia; cancer of the stomach, small and/or large intestines, rectum, and breast; rheumatoid arthritis; bleeding peptic ulcer; chronic renal failure; pregnancy; low-birth-weight infants; protein malnutrition; chronic blood loss (GI, uterine)
TIBC: Hemochromatosis (excess iron deposits in organs and tissues), anemias (hemolytic, pernicious, sickle cell), renal failure, cirrhosis of the liver, rheumatoid arthritis, infections, cancer of the GI tract

Elevated level

Serum iron: Hemochromatosis, anemias (hemolytic, pernicious, and folic acid deficiency), liver damage, thalassemia, lead toxicity
TIBC: Iron deficiency anemia, acute chronic blood loss, polycythemia
Drugs that may increase TIBC value: Oral contraceptives, iron preparations

Procedure

- No food or fluid restriction is required.
- Collect 5 to 7 mL of venous blood in a red-top tube. Avoid hemolysis; false elevated readings can occur.

Nursing Implications

Decreased level

- Observe for signs and symptoms of iron deficiency anemia (i.e., pallor, fatigue, headache, tachycardia, dyspnea on exertion).

Client Teaching

- Encourage the client to eat foods rich in iron (i.e., liver, shellfish, lean meat, egg yolk, dried fruits, whole grain, wines, and cereals). Milk has little or no iron.
- Recommend rest and avoidance of strenuous activity.
- Instruct how to take iron supplements. Iron should be given following meals or snacks because it irritates the gastric mucosa. Orange juice (ascorbic acid) promotes iron absorption.

- Explain that iron supplements can cause constipation and that stools will have a tarry appearance.

Elevated level

- Observe for signs and symptoms of hemochromatosis (i.e., bronze pigmentation of the skin, cardiac dysrhythmias, and heart failure).

17-KETOSTEROIDS (17-KS) URINE

Reference Values

Adult: Male: 5–25 mg/24 h; female: 5–15 mg/24 h
Child: Infant: <1 mg/24 h; 1–3 yr: <2 mg/24 h; 3–6 yr: <3 mg/24 h; 7–10 yr: 3–4 mg/24 h; 10–12 yr: 1–6 mg/24 h. Adolescent: male: 3–15 mg/24 h; female: 3–12 mg/24 h
Elderly: 4–8 mg/24 h

Description. 17-KS are metabolites of male hormones that are secreted from the testes and adrenal cortex. In men, approximately one third of the hormone metabolites come from the testes and two thirds from the adrenal cortex. In women, nearly all of the excreted hormones (androgens) are derived from the adrenal cortex. Since most of the 17-KS is from the adrenal cortex, this test is useful for diagnosing adrenal cortex dysfunction.

Purpose

- To assist in the diagnosis of adrenal cortex dysfunction

Clinical Problems

Decreased level: Adrenal cortical hypofunction (Addison's disease), hypogonadism, hypopituitarism, myxedema, nephrosis, severe debilitating diseases
Drugs that may decrease urine 17-KS: Thiazide diuretics, estrogen, oral contraceptives, reserpine, chlordiazepoxide (Librium), probenecid (Benemid), promazine, meprobamate (Miltown), quinidine, prolonged use of salicylates

Elevated level: Adrenal cortical hyperfunction (adrenocortical hyperplasia, Cushing's syndrome, adrenocortical carcinoma); testicular neoplasm; ovarian neoplasm; hyperpituitarism; severe stress or infection, or both

Drugs that may increase urine 17-KS: ACTH, antibiotics, phenothiazines, dexamethasone (Decadron), spironolactone (Aldactone)

Procedure

- No food or fluid restriction is required.
- If possible, drugs that interfere with test results should not be given for 48 hours before the test.
- Collect a 24-hour urine specimen in a large container and keep refrigerated. An acid preservative is usually added to keep the urine at a pH <4.5, thus preventing steroid decomposition by bacterial growth.
- List on the laboratory slip the client's sex and age.
- Postpone test if female has her menstrual period. Blood in urine can cause false-positive results.

Nursing Implications

- Encourage the client to increase fluid intake.

Decreased level

- Observe for signs and symptoms of adrenal gland insufficiency (i.e., weakness, weight loss, polyuria, hypotension, tachycardia).
- Record fluid intake and output. Report if client's urine output is >2,000 mL/24 h. Dilute urine can cause a false-negative test result.
- Monitor weight loss. In Addison's disease, sodium is not retained. Weight loss and dehydration usually occur.

Client Teaching

- Suggest medical alert bracelet or card.

Elevated level

- Observe for signs and symptoms of adrenal gland hyperfunction (i.e., "moon face," cervical–dorsal fat pad ["buffalo hump"], weight gain, bleeding tendency, hyperglycemia).
- Check serum potassium and blood glucose levels. Hypokalemia and hyperglycemia frequently occur; potassium supplements and insulin or a low-carbohydrate diet may be indicated.

LACTIC ACID (BLOOD)

Reference Values

Adult:

Arterial blood:	0.5–2.0 mEq/L, 11.3 mg/dL, 0.5–2.0 mmol/L (SI units).
Venous blood:	0.5–1.5 mEq/L, 8.1–15.3 mg/dL, 0.5–1.5 mmol/L (SI units)
Panic range:	>5 mEq/L, >45 mg/dL, >5 mmol/L (SI units)

Description. Increased secretion of lactic acid occurs following strenuous exercise, and acute or prolonged hypoxemia (tissue hypoxia). A major cause of metabolic acidosis is excess circulating lactic acid.

Shock and severe dehydration cause cell catabolism (cell breakdown) and an accumulation of acid metabolites, such as lactic acid. When the anion gap is >18 mEq/L, pH <7.25, and the $Paco_2$ remains within normal range (35–45 mm Hg), blood lactic acid level should be checked to determine if lactic acidosis is present.

Purpose

- To detect the presence of acidosis related to shock, trauma, or severe illness (also see Anion Gap)

Clinical Problems

Decreased level: High lactic dehydrogenases (LDH) value

Elevated level: Shock, severe dehydration, severe trauma, ketoacidosis, severe infections, neoplastic conditions, hepatic failure, renal disease, chronic alcoholism, severe salicylate toxicity

Procedure

- Collect 5 to 10 mL of blood in a green- or gray-top tube.
- Instruct the client to avoid hand clenching, which can lead to a buildup of lactic acid caused by a release of lactic acid from muscle of the clenched hand.
- Avoid using a tourniquet if possible; it could increase the blood lactic acid level.
- Deliver the blood specimen on ice to the laboratory immediately.

Factors Affecting Laboratory Results

- Use of tourniquet could elevate lactic acid value.

Nursing Implications

- Obtain a history of the clinical problem as described by the client, family, or referral report.
- Compare laboratory values that may indicate acidotic state, such as low pH, low bicarbonate, normal $Paco_2$, or low serum CO_2.
- Observe for signs and symptoms of acidosis, such as dyspnea or Kussmaul's breathing, increased pulse rate.
- Be supportive of client and family. If shock is present, anxiety and fear are common.

LACTIC DEHYDROGENASE (LDH OR LD); LDH ISOENZYMES SERUM

Reference Values

Adult: Total LDH: 100–190 IU/L, 70–250 U/L, 70–200 IU/L (differs among institutions)
LDH isoenzymes: LDH_1: 14%–26%, LDH_2: 27%–37%; LDH_3: 13%–26%; LDH_4: 8%–16%; LDH_5: 6%–16%. Differences of 2% to 4% are usually normal.

Child: Newborn: 300–1,500 IU/L; child: 50–150 IU/L

Description. LDH is an intracellular enzyme present in nearly all metabolizing cells, with the highest concentrations in the heart, skeletal muscle, RBCs, liver, kidney, lung, and brain. Two subunits, H (heart) and M (muscle), are combined in different formations to make five isoenzymes.

- LDH_1: cardiac fraction; H, H, H, H; in heart, RBCs, kidneys, brain (some)
- LDH_2: cardiac fraction; H, H, H, M; in heart, RBCs, kidneys, brain (some)
- LDH_3: pulmonary fraction; H, H, M, M; in lungs and other tissues: spleen, pancreas, adrenal, thyroid, lymphatics
- LDH_4: hepatic fraction; H, M, M, M; liver, skeletal muscle, kidneys and brain (some)

- LDH_5: hepatic fraction; M, M, M, M; liver, skeletal muscle, kidneys (some)

Serum LDH and LDH_1 are used for diagnosing acute myocardial infarction (AMI). A high serum LDH (total) occurs 12 to 24 hours after an AMI, reaches its peak in 2 to 5 days, and remains elevated for 6 to 12 days. It is a useful test for diagnosing a delayed reported myocardial infarction. A flipped LDH_1/ LDH_2 ratio, with LDH_1 higher indicates a myocardial infarction.

Purposes

- To aid in the diagnosis of myocardial or skeletal muscle damage
- To compare test results with other cardiac enzyme tests (i.e., CPK, AST)
- To check LDH isoenzyme results to determine organ involvement

Clinical Problems

Elevated level: AMI, acute pulmonary embolus and infarction, cerebral vascular accident (CVA), acute hepatitis, cancers, anemias, acute leukemias, shock, skeletal muscular diseases, heat stroke
Drugs that may increase LDH value: Narcotics

Procedure

- No food or fluid restriction is required.
- Collect 5 to 7 mL of venous blood in a red-top tube. Avoid hemolysis.
- List narcotics or IM injections given in the last 8 hours on the laboratory slip.

Nursing Implications

- Obtain a history of the client's discomfort. A complaint of severe indigestion for several days could be indicative of a myocardial infarction.
- Assess for signs and symptoms of an AMI (i.e., pale or gray color; sharp, stabbing pain or heavy pressure pain; shortness of breath [SOB], diaphoresis, nausea and vomiting; and indigestion).

Client Teaching

- Instruct the client to notify the nurse of any recurrence of chest discomfort.

LACTOSE AND LACTOSE TOLERANCE TEST (SERUM)

Reference Values

Serum/Plasma: <0.5 mg/dL, <14.5 µmol/L (SI units)
Urine: 12–40 mg/dL
Lactose test: Tolerance: fasting serum glucose plus 20–50 mg/dL
Intolerance: fasting serum glucose plus <20 mg/dL

Description. Lactose is a disaccharide sugar. Milk is rich in lactose; one glass of milk may contain 12 grams of lactose. For lactose to be absorbed, lactase (an intestinal enzyme) converts lactose to glucose and galactose. With a deficiency of the lactase enzyme, diarrhea, flatus, and abdominal cramping commonly occur due to excess lactose in the intestine.

When lactose intolerance is suspected, a lactose tolerance test is usually conducted. A large amount of lactose is ingested, and serum glucose levels are drawn at specified times. If the serum glucose level is more than 20 mg/dL, greater than the fasting glucose level, lactose is tolerated and is being converted into glucose; if the increase in the serum glucose level is less than 20 mg/dL of the fasting glucose, lactose intolerance is occurring. Milk products should be avoided to decrease lactose intolerance.

Purposes

- To compare serum and urine lactose results for determining lactose deficit
- To diagnose lactose intolerance

Clinical Problems

Decreased glucose level: Excess lactose in intestine, lactose intolerance

Elevated glucose level: Normal lactose tolerance

Procedure

Lactose tolerance test

- Restrict food and fluids for 8 to 12 hours before the test.
- Administer 50 to 100 grams of lactose in 200+ mL of water. The amount of lactose is determined by the laboratory. Fifty grams of lactose is equivalent to a quart of milk.

- Collect four venous blood specimens, 5 mL each, in gray-top tubes. The first blood specimen should be collected before the test. After oral administration of lactose solution, collect the next three blood samples ½ hour, 1 hour, and 2 hours after lactose ingestion.
- Conduct test adjacent to bathroom in the event that diarrhea due to lactose intolerance occurs.

Nursing Implications

- Explain to the client the test procedure. Instruct the client to remain NPO for 8 to 12 hours (as determined by the institution's protocol) before the test. Tell the client that he or she will have 4 blood specimens collected within 2 to 2½ hours.

Client Teaching

- Instruct the client who has a lactose intolerance to avoid milk products. Suggest lactose-free milk. Calcium supplements may be necessary.
- Instruct the client not to exercise 8 hours before the test and not to smoke during the test because smoking can increase the blood glucose level.

LEAD (BLOOD)

Reference Values

Adult: Normal: 10–20 μg/dL; acceptable: 20–40 μg/dL; excessive: 40–80 μg/dL; toxic: >80 μg/dL

Child: Normal: 10–20 μg/dL; acceptable: 20–30 μg/dL; excessive: 30–50 μg/dL; toxic: >50 μg/dL

Description. Excessive lead exposure due to occupational contact is hazardous to adults; however, most industry will accept a 40 μg/dL blood lead level as a normal value. Lead toxicity can occur in children from eating chipped lead-based paint.

Lead is usually excreted rapidly in the urine, but if excessive lead exposure persists, the lead will accumulate in the bone and soft tissues. Chronic lead poisoning is more common than acute poisoning.

Purpose

- To check for lead toxicity

Clinical Problems

Elevated level: Lead gasoline, fumes from heaters, lead-based paint, unglazed pottery, batteries, lead containers used for storage, heat stroke

Procedure

- No food or fluid restriction is required.
- Collect 5 to 7 mL of venous blood in a lavender- or green-top tube.
- Urine may be requested for a 24-hour quantitative test; a lead-free container must be used.

Nursing Implications

- Observe for signs and symptoms of lead poisoning (i.e., lead colic [crampy abdominal pain], constipation, occasional bloody diarrhea, behavioral changes [from lethargy to hyperactivity, aggression, impulsiveness], tremors, and confusion).
- Monitor the urinary output, as lead toxicity can decrease kidney function. A urine output <25 mL/h should be reported.
- Monitor medical treatment for removing lead from the body (e.g., chelation therapy).
- Provide adequate fluid intake.

Client Teaching

- Instruct those in high-risk groups to have their blood lead levels monitored.
- Instruct client(s) that paint chips from woodwork in house may contain lead and that some children have tendencies to eat paint chips.

LE CELL TEST; LUPUS ERYTHEMATOSUS CELL TEST (BLOOD)

LUPUS TEST, LE PREP, LE PREPARATION, LE SLIDE CELL TEST

Reference Values

Adult: Negative, no LE cells

Child: Negative

Description. LE cell test, a screening test for systemic lupus erythematosus (SLE), is a nonspecific test. Positive results have been reported in those having rheumatoid arthritis, scleroderma, and drug-induced lupus, such as penicillin, tetracycline, dilantin, oral contraceptives. The test is positive in 60% to 80% of those having SLE. Antinuclear antibodies (ANA) and anti-DNA are more sensitive tests for lupus and should be used to confirm SLE.

Purposes

- To aid in the diagnosis of SLE
- To compare with ANA and/or anti-DNA tests for diagnosing SLE

Clinical Problems

Elevated level: SLE, scleroderma, rheumatoid arthritis, chronic hepatitis

Drugs that may increase LE cells: Hydralazine (Apresoline), procainamide (Pronestyl), quinidine, anticonvulsants (phenytoin [Dilantin], Mesantoin, Tridione), oral contraceptives, methysergide, antibiotics (penicillin, tetracycline, streptomycin, sulfonamides), methyldopa (Aldomet), isoniazid (INH), clofibrate, reserpine, phenylbutazone

Procedure

- No food or fluid restriction is required.
- Collect 3 to 5 mL of venous blood in a red- or green-top tube. Avoid hemolysis.
- On laboratory slip, list drugs taken that might affect test results.

Nursing Implications

- Compare LE test results with serum ANA or serum anti-DNA, or both. LE test should not be the only test used to diagnose SLE.
- Observe for signs and symptoms of SLE (i.e., fatigue, fever, rash [butterfly over nose], leukopenia, thrombocytopenia).
- Be supportive of client and family. Encourage daily rest periods, which help in decreasing symptoms.

Client Teaching:

- Instruct the client to have daily rest periods, which help to decrease symptoms.

LECITHIN/SPHINGOMYELIN (L/S) RATIO (AMNIOTIC FLUID)

Reference Values

Before 35 weeks' gestation: 1:1. Lecithin (L): 6–9 mg/dL. Sphingomyelin (S): 4–6 mg/dL
After 35 weeks' gestation: 4:1. Lecithin (L): 15–21 mg/dL. Sphingomyelin (S): 4–6 mg/dL

Description. The L/S ratio can be used to predict neonatal respiratory distress syndrome (also called hyaline membrane disease) before delivery. Lecithin (L), a phospholipid, is responsible mostly for the formation of alveolar surfactant. Surfactant lubricates the alveolar lining and inhibits alveolar collapse, thus preventing atelectasis. Sphingomyelin (S) is another phospholipid, the value of which remains the same throughout the pregnancy. A marked rise in amniotic lecithin after 35 weeks (to a level three or four times higher than that of sphingomyelin) is considered normal, and so chances for having hyaline membrane disease are small. The L/S ratio is also used to determine fetal maturity in the event that the gestation period is uncertain. In this situation, the L/S ratio is determined at intervals of a period of several weeks.

Purpose

- To check for possible neonatal respiratory distress syndrome (hyaline membrane disease) to the unborn prior to delivery

Clinical Problems

Decreased ratio after 35 weeks: Respiratory distress syndrome, hyaline membrane disease

Procedure

- No food, fluid, or drug restriction is necessary.
- The physician performs an amniocentesis to obtain amniotic fluid. The specimen should be cooled immediately to prevent the destruction of lecithin by certain enzymes in the amniotic fluid. The specimen should be frozen if testing cannot be done at a specified time (check with the laboratory).

- Care should be taken to prevent puncture of the mother's bladder. If urine in the specimen is suspected, then the specimen should be tested for urea and potassium. If these two levels are higher than blood levels, the specimen could be urine and not amniotic fluid.
- Ultrasound is frequently used when obtaining amniotic fluid.

Nursing Implications

- Check the procedures for amniocentesis. Explain the procedure to the client. Assist the health care provider in obtaining amniotic fluid. Maternal vaginal secretions or a bloody tap into the amniotic fluid may cause a false, increased reading for lecithin.
- Obtain a fetal history of problems occurring during gestation. Also ask for and report information on any previous children born with respiratory distress syndrome.
- Be supportive of the mother and her family before, during, and after the test.
- Assess the newborn at delivery for respiratory complications (substernal retractions, increased respiratory rate, labored breathing, and expiratory grunts).

LEGIONNAIRE'S ANTIBODY TEST (SERUM)

Reference Value. Negative

Description. Legionnaire's disease, caused by a gram-negative bacillus, *Legionella pneumophila,* causes acute respiratory infection such as severe, consolidated pneumonia. This organism is in the soil and water (lakes, streams, reservoirs) and is passed by inhalation in aerosol form through plumbing fixtures (shower heads, whirlpool baths) and air conditioning systems (cooling towers and condensers). The bacteria can be isolated from blood, sputum, pleural fluid, and lung-tissue specimen.

A fourfold rise in antibody titer >1:128 during the acute and convalescent phase or a single titer >1:256 is evidence of the disease. Several blood samples and a tissue specimen are useful in confirming Legionnaire's disease.

Purpose

- To diagnose the presence of Legionnaire's disease

Clinical Problems

Elevated antibody titer: Legionnaire's disease

Procedure

- No food or fluid restriction is required.
- Collect 3 to 5 mL of venous blood in a red-top tube. Tissue specimen from the lung or bronchiole site may be used.

Nursing Implications

- Obtain a history from the client as to where he or she has been in the last weeks, such as a hotel or institutional site.
- Assess the client's respiratory status by inspection, palpation, percussion, and auscultation.
- Observe the signs and symptoms of Legionnaire's disease, such as malaise, high fever, chills, cough, chest pain, and tachypnea. Fever rises rapidly to 39°C to 41°C, or 102°F to 105°F.

Client Teaching

- Inform the client that Legionnaire's disease is not transmitted from person to person but through aerosol means such as exhaust vents and fans.

LEUCINE AMINOPEPTIDASE (LAP) SERUM

Reference Values

Adult: 8–22 μU/mL, 12–33 IU/L, 75–200 U/mL, 20–50 U/L at 37°C (SI units) (varies according to laboratory method)

Description. Leucine aminopeptidase (LAP) is an enzyme produced mainly by the liver. This test may be used to differentiate between liver and bone disease. LAP is normal in bone disease, whereas alkaline phosphatase (ALP) may be abnormal in liver and bone disease.

This enzyme test is not frequently ordered but is sometimes used to assist with the evaluation of hepatobiliary disease. Elevated level can indicate biliary obstruction due to liver metastases and choledocholithiasis (calculi in the common bile duct).

Purpose

- To compare with other liver enzyme tests for diagnosing liver disease

Clinical Problems

Elevated level: Cancer of the liver, extrahepatic biliary obstruction (stones), acute necrosis of the liver, viral hepatitis, severe preeclampsia, pregnancy (mild)
Drugs that may increase LAP value: Estrogens, progesterone, oral contraceptives

Procedure

- No food or fluid restriction is required.
- Collect 3 to 5 mL of venous blood in a red-top tube. Avoid hemolysis of the blood specimen that may result from rough handling.

Nursing Implications

- Obtain a history of the client's signs and symptoms of the clinical problem.
- Compare LAP with other tests for liver dysfunction, such as alkaline phosphatase (ALP), alanine aminotransferase (ALT or SGPT), gamma-glutamyl transpeptidase (GGT), and/or 5′ nucleotidase (5′N). LAP is not considered as sensitive as the other tests, but it may be ordered to verify liver dysfunction.

LIPASE (SERUM)

Reference Values

Adult: 20–180 IU/L, 14–280 mU/mL, 14–280 U/L (SI units)
Child: Infant: 9–105 IU/L at 37°C; child: 20–136 IU/L at 37°C

Description. Lipase, an enzyme secreted by the pancreas, aids in digesting fats in the duodenum. Lipase, like amylase, appears in the bloodstream following damage to the pancreas. Lipase and amylase levels increase in 2 to 12 hours in acute pancreatitis, but serum lipase can be elevated for up to 14 days after an acute episode, whereas the serum amylase returns to normal after approximately 3 days. Serum lipase is useful for a late diagnosis of acute pancreatitis.

Purpose

- To suggest acute pancreatitis or other pancreatic disorders (see Clinical Problems)

Clinical Problems

Elevated level: Acute pancreatitis, chronic pancreatitis, cancer of the pancreas, obstruction of the pancreatic duct, perforated ulcer, acute renal failure (early stage)
Drugs that may increase lipase value: Narcotics, steroids, bethanechol (Urecholine)

Procedure

- Restrict food and fluids except water for 8 to 12 hours before test.
- Narcotics should be withheld for 24 hours prior to the test. If given, note time on the laboratory slip.
- Collect 3 to 5 mL of venous blood in a red-top tube. Avoid hemolysis.

Factors Affecting Laboratory Results

- Most narcotics elevate the serum lipase level.

Nursing Implication

- Alert health care provider when abdominal pain persists for several days. A serum lipase determination may be ordered, as it is effective for diagnosing latent acute pancreatitis.

LIPOPROTEINS, LIPOPROTEIN ELECTROPHORESIS, LIPIDS (SERUM)

Reference Values

Adult: Total: 400–800 mg/dL, 4–8 g/L (SI units); cholesterol: 150–240 mg/dL (see test on cholesterol); triglycerides: 10–190 mg/dL (see test on triglycerides); phospholipids: 150–380 mg/dL

LDL: 60–160 mg/dL; risk for CHD: high: >160 mg/dL, moderate: 130–159 mg/dL, low: <130 mg/dL
HDL: 29–77 mg/dL; risk for CHD: high: <35 mg/dL, moderate: 35–45 mg/dL, low: 46–59 mg/dL, very low: >60 mg/dL
Child: See tests on cholesterol and triglycerides

Description. The three main lipoproteins are cholesterol, triglycerides, and phospholipids. The two fractions of lipoproteins—alpha (α), high-density lipoproteins (HDL) and beta (β), low-density lipoproteins (chylomicrons, VLDL, LDL)—can be separated by electrophoresis. The β groups are the largest contributors of atherosclerosis and coronary artery disease. HDL, called "friendly lipids," are composed of 50% protein and aid in decreasing plaque deposits in blood vessels.

Increased lipoproteins (hyperlipidemia or hyperlipoproteinemia) can be phenotyped into five major types (I, IIA and IIB, III, IV, V).

Purposes

- To identify clients with hyperlipoproteinemia
- To distinguish between the phenotypes of lipidemias
- To monitor lipid counts for clients with hyperlipidemia

LIPOPROTEIN PHENOTYPE: HYPERLIPIDEMIA

Type	Lipid Composition*
I	Increased chylomicrons; increased triglycerides; normal or slightly increased very low-density lipoproteins (VLDLs)
IIA	Increased low-density lipoproteins (LDL); increased cholesterol; slightly increased triglycerides or normal; normal VLDL (common pattern of hyperlipidemia)
IIB	Increased LDL, VLDL; both cholesterol and triglycerides are elevated (common pattern of hyperlipidemia)
III	Moderately increased cholesterol triglycerides; and normal VLDL. Normal or decreased LDL
IV	Increased VLDL; slightly increased cholesterol and markedly increased triglycerides; (common pattern of hyperlipidemia)
V	Increased chylomicrons, VLDL, and triglycerides; and slightly increased cholesterol

*Types II and IV are increased in atherosclerosis and coronary artery disease.

Clinical Problems

Elevated level: Hyperlipoproteinemia, acute myocardial infarction (AMI), hypothyroidism, diabetes mellitus, nephrotic syndrome, Laennec's cirrhosis, diet high in saturated fats, eclampsia
Drugs that may increase lipoprotein values: Aspirin, cortisone preparations, oral contraceptives, phenothiazines, sulfonamides

Procedure

- Restrict food and fluids except for water for 12 to 14 hours prior to the test. No alcohol intake is allowed for 24 hours, and a regular diet is maintained for 3 days before test.
- Collect 5 to 7 mL of venous blood in a red-top tube.

Nursing Implications

- Check the client's serum cholesterol and serum triglyceride levels and compare with the lipoprotein electrophoresis results.

Client Teaching

- Instruct client with hyperlipoproteinemia to avoid foods high in saturated fats and sugar (i.e., bacon, cream, butter, fatty meats, and candy). Limit excess alcohol intake
- Answer client's questions concerning risk of coronary heart disease related to high LDL and low HDL.

LITHIUM (SERUM)

Reference Values

Adult: Normal: negative; therapeutic: 0.5–1.5 mEq/L; toxic: >1.6 mEq/L; lethal: >4.0 mEq/L
Child: Not usually given to children

Description. Lithium or lithium salt is used to treat manic-depressive psychosis. This agent is used to correct the mania in manic depression and to prevent depression. Since therapeutic and toxic lithium levels are narrow ranges, serum lithium should be closely monitored.

Purposes

- To identify lithium toxicity
- To monitor lithium levels for therapeutic effect and toxicity

Clinical Problems

Elevated level: Lithium toxicity

Procedure

- No food or fluid restriction is required.
- Collect 5 to 7 mL of venous blood in a red-top tube 8 to 12 hours after last lithium dose.
- Lithium tolerance test is an alternative. A base blood specimen is obtained, and then the lithium dose is given. Blood specimens are collected 1, 3, and 6 hours after the lithium dose.

Nursing Implications

- Observe for signs and symptoms of lithium overdose (i.e., slurred speech, muscle spasm, confusion, and nystagmus). Lithium dosage should be lower in the older adult.

Client Teaching

- Instruct the patient to take prescribed lithium dosage daily, to keep medical appointments, and to have periodic blood specimens drawn to determine lithium levels.
- Encourage adequate fluid and sodium intake while the patient is on lithium. Diuretics should be avoided.
- Instruct nursing mother to consult health care provider. Breast milk can contain high levels of lithium.

LUTEINIZING HORMONE (LH) SERUM AND URINE

INTERSTITIAL CELL-STIMULATING HORMONE (ICSH)

Reference Values. Ranges vary among laboratories

Serum: Adult: female: follicular phase: 5–30 mIU/mL; midcycle: 50–150 mIU/mL; luteal phase: 2–25 mIU/mL. Postmenopausal: 40–100 mIU/mL. Male: 5–25 mIU/mL. Child: 6–12 yr: <10 mIU/mL; 13–18 yr: <20 mIU/mL

Urine: Adult: female: follicular phase: 5–25 IU/24 h; midcycle: 30–90 IU/24 h; luteal phase: 2–24 IU/24 h; postmenopausal: >40 IU/24 h. Male: 7–25 IU/mL

Description. Luteinizing hormone (LH), gonadotropic hormone secreted by the anterior pituitary gland, is needed (with follicle-stimulating hormone [FSH]) for ovulation to occur. After ovulation, LH aids in stimulating the corpus luteum in secreting progesterone. FSH values are frequently evaluated with LH values. In men, LH stimulates testosterone production, and with FSH, they influence the development and maturation of spermatozoa.

LH is usually ordered to evaluate infertility in women and men. High serum values are related to gonadal dysfunction, and low serum values are related to hypothalamus or pituitary failure. Women taking oral contraceptives have an absence of midcycle LH peak until the contraceptives are discontinued. This test might be used to evaluate hormonal therapy for inducting ovulation.

Purposes

- To evaluate the serum or urine luteinizing hormone level for determining the cause of hormonal dysfunction
- To identify the gynecological problem related to excess or deficit of LH

Clinical Problems

Decreased level: Hypogonadotropinism (defects in pituitary gland or hypothalamus), anovulation, amenorrhea (pituitary failure), hypophysectomy, testicular failure, hypothalamic dysfunction, adrenal hyperplasia or tumors

Drugs that may decrease LH value: Oral contraceptives, estrogen compounds, testosterone administration

Elevated level: Amenorrhea (ovarian failure), tumors (pituitary, testicular), precocious puberty, testicular failure, Turner's syndrome, Klinefelter's syndrome, premature menopause, Stein-Leventhal syndrome, polycystic ovary syndrome, liver disease

Procedure

Serum

- No food or fluid restriction is required.
- Withhold medications that could interfere with test results for 24 to 48 hours before the test (check with the health care provider).
- Collect 3 to 5 mL of venous blood in a red- or lavender-top tube. Avoid hemolysis. Daily blood samples must be taken at the same time each day to determine if ovulation occurs.
- Note on the laboratory slip the phase of the menstrual cycle, client's age, and if client is postmenopausal.

Urine

- Collect 24-hour urine specimen in a container with a preservative, or keep refrigerated if no preservative is added.
- Label the specimen with the client's name, date, and time.

Nursing Implications

- Obtain a menstrual history from the client. Record the menstrual phase on the laboratory slip.
- Check with the health care provider about withholding medications that could affect test results.

Client Teaching

- Encourage the client to express concerns about infertility or other health problems.
- Be supportive of client and family.

LYME DISEASE ANTIBODY TEST (SERUM)

Reference Values

Adult and Child: Titer: <1:256; indirect fluorescent antibody (IFA) titer: ELISA or Western blot: negative for Lyme disease

Description. *Borrelia burgdorferi* is the spirochete that causes Lyme disease. Several tick vectors, primarily the deer tick, carry the spirochete. The spirochete can be cultivated, with difficulty, from blood, CSF, or skin biopsies. Lyme disease is most prevalent in the northeastern states, upper midwestern states, and western states.

A reddish, macular lesion usually occurs about 1 week after the tick bite. It can affect the CNS and the peripheral nervous system (PNS), causing a neuritis or aseptic meningitis. It can also affect the heart and joints, causing transient ECG abnormalities, carditis, and problems in one or more joints, mostly the knees, leading to arthritis. It may take a few weeks to 2 years to become symptomatic.

Immunoglobulins (IgM and IgG) aid in diagnosing early, late, or remission stage of Lyme disease. IgM titers occur approximately 2 to 4 weeks after the onset of disease, peaking at 6 to 8 weeks before levels decrease. IgG titers occur 1 to 3 months after onset of Lyme disease and peak at 4 to 6 months. IgG may remain elevated for months or years. Symptoms such as fever with flu-like symptoms may begin 1 week after the spirochete infection. An erythematous, circular rash at the tick site frequently appears. The client may also suffer with malaise, headache, and muscle or joint aches and pain. Testing should be done 4 to 6 weeks after being infected. If the client has symptoms and the test is performed earlier with negative findings, a repeated test should be performed a week or two later. Antibiotic therapy is usually prescribed when symptoms are apparent even if the test result is negative.

Purpose

- To detect the occurrence of Lyme disease

Clinical Problems

Low titers: Infectious mononucleosis, hepatitis B, autoimmune disease (rheumatoid arthritis, SLE), and periodontal disease
Positive titer (fourfold increase): Lyme disease

Procedure

- No food or fluid restriction is required.
- Collect 3 to 5 mL of venous blood in a red-top tube. Avoid hemolysis.
- Repeat Lyme disease antibody test for symptomatic clients with early negative test result.

Factors Affecting Laboratory Results

- Persons with a high rheumatoid factor could have a false-positive test result.

Nursing Implications

- Obtain a history regarding a tick bite.
- Assess for a macular lesion at the site of the tick bite and elsewhere.
- Check titer level. A fourfold rise in titer is indicative of a recent infection.

Client Teaching

- Instruct the client to wear clothing that covers entirely the extremities when in the woods and areas infested by ticks and deer.
- Instruct the client to see a health care provider immediately if bitten by a tick or if a macular lesion results from a tick bite. Antibiotic therapy is frequently started.

LYMPHOCYTES (T AND B) ASSAY (BLOOD)

(T AND B LYMPHOCYTES; LYMPHOCYTE MARKER STUDIES; LYMPHOCYTE SUBSET TYPING)

Reference Values

Adult: T cells: 60%–80%, 600–2400 cells/μL. B cells: 4%–16%, 50–250 cells/μL

Description. The two categories of lymphocytes are T lymphocytes and B lymphocytes. The T lymphocytes are associated with cell-mediated immune responses (cellular immunity), such as rejection of transplant and graft, tumor immunity, and microorganism (bacterial and viral) death. If the surface of the host's tissue cell is altered, the T cells might perceive that altered cell as foreign and attack it. This might be helpful if the altered surface is of tumor development; however, this T-cell attack might give rise to autoimmune disease.

The B lymphocytes, derived from bone marrow, are responsible for humoral immunity. The B cells synthesize immunoglobulins to react to specific antigens. An interaction between T and B lymphocytes is necessary for a satisfactory immune response.

Measurement of T and B lymphocytes is valuable for diagnosing autoimmune disease (i.e., immunosuppressive diseases, such as AIDS, lymphoma, and lymphocytic leukemia). T and B cells can be used to monitor changes during the treatment of immunosuppressive diseases.

Purposes

- To detect selected autoimmune diseases, such as lymphoma and lymphocytic leukemia
- To monitor the effects of treatment for immunosuppressive diseases, such as AIDS

Clinical Problems

Decreased level: T lymphocytes: lymphoma, lupus disease (SLE), thymic hypoplasia (DiGeorge's syndrome), acute viral infections. B lymphocytes: IgG, IgA, IgM deficiency, lymphomas, nephrotic syndrome, sex-linked agammaglobulinemia. T and B lymphocytes: immunodeficiency diseases

Drugs that may decrease T lymphocytes: Immunosuppressive agents

Elevated level: T lymphocytes: Autoimmune disorders, such as Graves' disease. B lymphocytes: Acute and chronic lymphocytic leukemias, multiple myeloma, Waldenström's macroglobulinemia

Procedure

- No food or fluid restriction is required.
- Collect 10 mL of venous blood in each of two lavender-top tubes. Refrigerate blood specimens. Check with laboratory procedure in your institution.

Nursing Implications

- Observe for signs and symptoms of lymphocytic leukemias (i.e., fatigue, pallor, vesicular skin lesions, increased WBC).
- Listen to the client's concern. Respond to questions or refer the questions to other health care provider(s) if necessary.

Client Teaching

- Instruct the client to stay away from persons with colds or communicable diseases.

MAGNESIUM (Mg) SERUM

Reference Values

Adult: 1.5–2.5 mEq/L; 1.8–3.0 mg/dL

Child: Newborn: 1.4–2.9 mEq/L; child: 1.6–2.6 mEq/L

Description. Magnesium (Mg) is the second most plentiful cation (positive ion electrolyte) in the cells/intracellular fluid. One third of the magnesium ingested is absorbed through the small intestine, and the remaining unabsorbed magnesium is excreted in the stools. The absorbed magnesium is eventually excreted through the kidneys.

Magnesium influences use of potassium, calcium, and protein. With a magnesium deficit, there is frequently a potassium and calcium deficit. Magnesium, like potassium, sodium, and calcium, is needed for neuromuscular activity. This electrolyte activates many enzymes for carbohydrate and protein metabolism. A serum magnesium deficit is known as hypomagnesemia, and a serum magnesium excess is called hypermagnesemia.

Purposes

- To detect hypomagnesemia or hypermagnesemia
- To monitor magnesium levels when there is a probable magnesium loss

Clinical Problems

Decreased level: Protein malnutrition, malabsorption, cirrhosis of the liver, alcoholism, hypoparathyroidism, hyperaldosteronism, hypokalemia, IV solutions without magnesium, chronic diarrhea, bowel resection complications, dehydration

Drugs that may decrease magnesium value: Diuretics, calcium gluconate, amphotericin B, neomycin, insulin

Elevated level: Severe dehydration, renal failure, leukemia (lymphocytic and myelocytic), diabetes mellitus (early phase)

Drugs that may increase magnesium value: Antacids that contain magnesium, such as Maalox, Mylanta, Aludrox, DiGel; laxatives that control magnesium, such as milk of magnesia, magnesium citrate, epsom salts ($MgSO_4$)

Procedure

- No food or fluid restriction is required.
- Collect 3 to 5 mL of venous blood in a red-top tube. Avoid hemolysis.

Nursing Implications

Decreased level

- Check serum potassium, sodium, calcium, and magnesium levels. Electrolyte deficits may accompany a magnesium deficit. If hypokalemia and hypomagnesemia are present, potassium supplements will not totally correct the potassium deficit until the magnesium deficit is corrected.
- Observe for signs and symptoms of hypomagnesemia, such as tetany symptoms (twitching and tremors, carpopedal spasm, and generalized spasticity), restlessness, confusion, and dysrhythmias. Neuromuscular irritability can be mistakenly attributed to hypocalcemia.
- Report to the health care provider if the client has been NPO and receiving IV fluids without magnesium salts for several weeks. Hyperalimentation solutions should contain magnesium.
- Check if the client is taking a digitalis preparation, such as digoxin. A magnesium deficit enhances the action of digitalis, causing digitalis toxicity. Signs and symptoms of digitalis toxicity include anorexia, nausea, vomiting, and bradycardia.
- Assess renal function when the client is receiving magnesium supplements. Excess magnesium is excreted by the kidneys.
- Assess ECG changes. A flat or inverted T wave can be indicative of hypomagnesemia. It can also indicate hypokalemia.
- Administer IV magnesium sulfate in solution slowly to prevent a hot or flushed feeling. IV calcium gluconate should be available to reverse hypermagnesemia due to overcorrection. Calcium antagonizes the sedative effect of magnesium.

Client Teaching

- Instruct the client to eat foods rich in magnesium (fish, seafood, meats, green vegetables, whole grains, and nuts).

Elevated level

- Observe for signs and symptoms of hypermagnesemia, such as flushing, a feeling of warmth, increased perspiration (with a serum magnesium level at 3 to 4 mEq/L), muscular weakness, diminished reflex, respiratory distress, hypotension, or a sedative effect (with the magnesium level at 9 to 10 mEq/L).
- Monitor urinary output. Effective urinary output (>750 mL daily) will decrease the serum magnesium level.

- Provide adequate fluids to improve kidney function and restore body fluids. Dehydration can cause hemoconcentration and, as a result, magnesium excess.
- Assess the client's level of sensorium and muscle activity. Severe hypermagnesemia causes sedation, and decreases muscular tone and reflex activity.
- Assess ECG strip for changes. A peaked T wave and wide QRS complex can indicate hypermagnesemia and hyperkalemia. Serum potassium and magnesium levels should be checked.
- Check for digitalis toxicity if the client is taking digoxin and is receiving calcium gluconate for hypermagnesemia. Calcium excess enhances the action of digitalis, and digitalis toxicity can result.

Client Teaching

- Instruct the client to avoid constant use of laxatives and antacids containing magnesium. Suggest that the client increase dietary fiber to avoid constipation and laxative use.

MUMPS ANTIBODY (SERUM)

Reference Values

Negative: <1:8 titer

Positive or Immunization: >1:8 (recent infection or immunization undetermined)

Description. Mumps, infectious parotitis, is an acute, contagious viral infection causing an inflammation of the parotid and salivary glands. The mumps virus can be spread by droplets or by direct contact with the saliva of an infected person. Complications of mumps include (1) in adolescent or adult males, unilateral orchitis in approximately 20% of reported cases; (2) in adult women, oophoritis; and (3) in persons of all ages and genders, meningoencephalitis in 1% to 10% of infected cases.

Diagnosis may be made by blood specimen, culture of saliva, or mumps skin test. With a blood specimen two blood samples should be taken, one during the acute phase and one during the convalescent phase. For those persons who are at high risk or who have not had mumps, there is a vaccine to provide immunity.

Purpose

- To detect the presence of the mumps antibody in a person who may be at risk

Clinical Problems

Positive: Mumps virus. *Complications:* Orchitis, oophoritis, meningo-encephalitis

Procedure

- Collect a total of two 3- to 5-mL samples of venous blood in a red-top tube, 1 to 2 weeks apart. The first specimen is drawn during the acute phase, and the second is taken 1 to 2 weeks later during the convalescent phase. Place ice around specimen tube.
- Label the first specimen "acute."
- No food or fluids are restricted.

Nursing Implications

- Assess the client for symptoms of mumps, such as malaise, headache, chills, fever, pain below the ear, and swelling of the parotid glands.
- Assess if the client has been in contact with a person diagnosed as having mumps. Clients who are suspected of having mumps may be isolated up to 9 days after swelling occurs.
- Check if the client had received the mumps vaccine. Those who develop mumps normally have a lifetime immunity.

Client Teaching

- Explain to the client that he/she is to return for a second blood test 1 to 2 weeks later for the convalescent phase of the mumps infection.
- Explain to the client that mumps is contagious and that he/she will be isolated for about 9 days from other persons who have never had mumps or the vaccine. The incubation period for mumps is 16 to 18 days.
- Inform the pregnant female that if mumps occurs during the first trimester of pregnancy, the fetus may have a higher risk of developing congenital anomalies. It is suggested to many young females that if they have not had mumps, they should be tested for mumps antibody; and if the result is negative, they should receive the mumps vaccine.

MYOGLOBIN (SERUM AND URINE)

Reference Values

Serum: Adult: female: 12–75 ng/mL, 12–75 μg/L (SI units); male: 20–90 ng/mL, 20–90 μg/L (SI units)
Urine: Negative or <20 ng/mL, <20 μg/L (SI units)

Description. Myoglobin is an oxygen-binding protein, similar to hemoglobin, that is found in skeletal and cardiac muscle cells. Myoglobin is released into circulation after an injury. Increased serum myoglobin occurs about 2 to 6 hours following muscle tissue damage, and it reaches its peak following a myocardial infarction (MI) in approximately 8 to 12 hours. Elevated serum myoglobin (myoglobinemia) is short-lived; in 50% of persons having an MI, the serum level begins to return to normal range in 12 to 18 hours. Urine myoglobin may be detected for 3 to 7 days following muscle injury.

Because serum myoglobin is nonspecific concerning which muscle is damaged, myocardium or skeletal, cardiac enzymes should be ordered and checked. The serum myoglobin is not performed following cardioversion or after an angina attack.

Myoglobin passes rapidly from the blood through the glomeruli in the kidney and is excreted in the urine. Myoglobinuria can appear within 3 hours after an MI and may be present in the urine up to 72 hours or longer.

Purpose

- To detect myoglobin protein, which is released in high amount during skeletal or cardiac muscle injury

Clinical Problems

Elevated level: Acute MI, skeletal muscle injury, severe burns, trauma, surgical procedure, polymyositis, acute alcohol toxicity (delirium tremens), renal failure, metabolic stress

Procedure

- No food or fluid restriction is required.

Serum: Collect 3 to 5 mL of venous blood in a red-top tube. Avoid hemolysis. The blood sample should be drawn soon after an acute MI or following acute pain.
Urine: Collect 5 to 10 mL of random urine specimen in a sterile plastic container.

Factors Affecting Laboratory Results

- A blood sample taken for a serum myoglobin 1½ to 2 days following acute chest pain

Nursing Implications

- Obtain a history of the current muscle discomfort (skeletal or cardiac). Report findings.
- Assess the client for signs and symptoms of an MI, such as sharp, penetrating pain in the chest, radiating pain in the left arm, diaphoresis, dyspnea, nausea, and vomiting.
- Check vital signs and report abnormal findings.
- Compare elevated serum myoglobin level with positive urine myoglobin. Cardiac enzymes should be ordered.

Client Teaching

- Instruct the client to inform you when pain occurs or recurs. Have the client describe the pain (type, intensity, duration).
- Explain the procedure for urine collection to the client.
- Explain to the client that a blood sample and urine specimen may both be ordered and explain why (see Description).
- Answer client's and family's questions or refer the questions to the appropriate health care professional. Listen to their concerns.

5′ NUCLEOTIDASE (5′N OR 5′NT) SERUM

Reference Values

Adult: <17 U/L
Pregnancy: Third trimester: slightly above normal value
Child: Values lower than adults, except infants

Description. Serum 5′ nucleotidase (5′N) is a liver enzyme test used to diagnose hepatobiliary disease. 5′N is not elevated in bone disorders; alkaline phosphatase (ALP) may be elevated in bone and liver disorders. Elevated ALP and 5′N indicate liver disorder; elevated ALP and a normal 5′N indicate bone disorder. Usually, several other liver enzyme tests may be used to diagnose liver disorders such as gamma-glutamyl transferase (GGT), and leucine aminopeptidase (LAP).

Purpose

- To compare test results with other liver enzyme tests for diagnosing a liver disorder

Clinical Problems

Elevated level: Cirrhosis of the liver, biliary obstruction from calculi or tumor, and metastasis to the liver
Drugs that may increase 5′N value: Acetaminophen, aspirin, narcotics, phenothiazines, phenytoin

Procedure

- No food or fluid restriction is required.
- Collect 3 to 5 mL of venous blood in a red-top tube. Avoid hemolysis.

Nursing Implications

- Compare 5′N levels with other liver enzyme levels. Elevated ALP, GGT, LAP, and 5′N values indicate that the problem is of liver origin.

Client Teaching

- Instruct the client to maintain effective oral hygiene as bleeding of the gums commonly occurs. With liver disorder, the prothrombin time is usually prolonged.
- Encourage the client to eat well-balanced meals.

OCCULT BLOOD (FECES)

Reference Values

Adult: Negative

Child: Negative

Note: A diet rich in meats, poultry, and fish, as well as certain drugs (i.e., cortisone, aspirin, iron, and potassium preparations) could cause a false-positive occult blood test.

Description. Occult (nonvisible or hidden) blood in the feces usually indicates GI bleeding. Bright red blood from the rectum can be indicative of bleeding from the lower large intestine (e.g., hemorrhoids), and tarry black stools indicate blood loss of >50 mL from the upper GI tract.

Purpose

- To detect blood in the feces

Clinical Problems

Drugs that may cause false negatives: Large amounts of ascorbic acid

Positive results: Bleeding peptic ulcers, gastritis, gastric carcinoma, bleeding esophageal varices, colitis, intestinal carcinoma, diverticulitis
Drugs that may cause false positives: Aspirin, cortisone, iron, and potassium preparations, NSAIDs drugs (indomethacin [Indocin], ibuprofens), thiazide diuretics, colchicine, reserpine

Procedure

- A variety of blood test reagents may be used. Orthotolidine (Occultest) is considered the most sensitive test.
- Avoid meats, poultry, and fish 2 to 3 days prior to stool specimen.
- On the laboratory slip list drugs the client is taking.
- Obtain a single, random stool specimen (small amount) and send it to the laboratory, or test using a kit to detect occult blood. Stool specimen could be obtained from a rectal examination.

Nursing Implications

- Obtain a history of bleeding episodes, dental hygiene, and/or bleeding gums. Only 2 mL or more blood can cause a positive test result.
- Determine whether the client has had epigastric pain between meals, which could be indicative of a peptic ulcer.
- Be sure the stool is not contaminated with menstrual discharge.

Client Teaching

- Instruct the client not to eat meats, poultry, and fish for 2 to 3 days before the test. Excessive green, leafy vegetables could cause a false-positive result.
- Encourage the client to report abnormally colored stools (e.g., tarry stools). Oral iron preparations can cause the stool to be black.

OPIATES (URINE AND BLOOD)

Reference Values (Urine and Blood)

Negative

Toxic Values

Urine: *Codeine:* >0.005 mg/dL (0.2 μmol/L). *Hydroxmorphone:* > 0.1 mg/dL (5 μmol/L). *Meperidine:* > 0.5 mg/dL (20 μmol/L). *Methadone:* > 0.2 mg/dL (10 μmol/L). *Morphine:* >0.005 mg/dL (0.2 μmol/L). *Propoxyphene:* >0.5 mg/dL (20 μmol/L)

Blood: *Cocaine:* >1000 ng/mL (>3300 μmol/L) (SI units)

Description. Testing for opiates is primarily done to screen for drug abuse or narcotic toxicity, or to check the progress of opiate detoxification. Specific opiates, such as codeine, morphine, methadone, hydroxmorphone, and meperidine, can be individually tested. Urine is the preferred specimen for checking for these opiates; however, gastric secretions could be analyzed.

The liver detoxifies opiates, and the urine excretes 90% of the opiates in 24 hours. The peak effect of opiates in the body occurs in approximately 1 hour.

Cocaine, another narcotic that is frequently abused, is a central nervous system stimulant. It increases blood pressure, respiratory rate, and heart rate and may lead to cardiopulmonary failure. Cocaine has many street names, such as coke, crack, gold dust, stardust, and happy dust.

Purposes

- To detect the presence of opiates
- To check for opiate toxicity
- To monitor the progress of opiate detoxification

Clinical Problems

Elevated level: Specific opiate presence or toxicity
Drugs that may increase opiate levels: Use of other opiates

Procedure

- No food or fluid restriction is required.
- List drugs taken by the client in the last 24 hours on the laboratory sheet, including over-the-counter (OTC) drugs.
- A signed consent may be necessary.

Urine

- Collect a random urine specimen and send the specimen immediately to the laboratory.
- Refrigerate the urine specimen if the test cannot be done immediately.

Blood

- Collect 5 to 10 mL of venous blood in a lavender- or green-top tube. Place tube on ice and send it to the laboratory immediately.
- If the test is for a legal purpose, have a witness present when obtaining the blood specimen. A signed consent form may be needed; check with hospital or state policy.
- Used for legal evidence, special handling and labeling of the specimen is essential; that is, it should be placed in a sealed container or bag and labeled with the date and time of the drawn blood specimen and the witness's name and signature.

Factors Affecting Laboratory Results

- Blood specimen not tested within an hour after drawing and the tube not placed on ice

- Blood specimen not drawn soon after cocaine use (cocaine has a short action)

Nursing Implications

- Obtain a drug history including OTC drugs. Explain that the information will be given to the health care provider.
- Send the random urine specimen immediately to the laboratory. If the opiate test is for methadone, a 24-hour urine specimen is needed. Inform the laboratory that the urine specimen should be tested immediately or refrigerated. Delay in testing can cause false-negative test result.

Client Teaching

- Explain to the client that addictive narcotic drugs can cause withdrawal symptoms when the drug is abruptly stopped
- Inform the client of the adverse reactions to cocaine, such as lung and kidney problems, heart attacks, suicidal tendency, hallucinations, and others.

OSMOLALITY (SERUM AND URINE)

Reference Values

Adult: Serum: 280–300 mOsm/kg H_2O; urine: 50–1200 mOsm/kg H_2O
Child: Serum: 270–290 mOsm/kg H_2O; urine: child: same as adult; newborn: 100–600 mOsm/kg H_2O
Panic Value: <240 mOsm/kg and >320 mOsm/kg

Description. Serum osmolality is an indicator of serum concentration. An elevated serum osmolality indicates hemoconcentration and dehydration, and a decreased serum level indicates hemodilution or overhydration. Osmolality measures the number of dissolved particles (electrolytes, sugar, urea) in the serum. Doubling the serum sodium, which accounts for 85% to 95% of the serum osmolality, can give a rough estimate of the serum osmolality. The serum osmolality can be calculated if the sodium, glucose, and urea are known.

$$\text{Serum osmolality} = 2 \times \text{Na} + \frac{\text{BUN}}{3} + \frac{\text{glucose}}{18}$$

Urine osmolality is more accurate than the specific gravity in determining the concentration, since it is influenced by the number of particles. The state of hydration affects the urine osmolality.

Purposes

- To monitor body fluid balance
- To determine the occurrence of body fluid overload or dehydration

Clinical Problems

Decreased level: Excessive fluid intake, continuous IV D_5W, SIADH (serum only), hyponatremia, acute renal disease, and diabetes insipidus (urine only)

Elevated level: Dehydration, hyperglycemia, hypernatremia, diabetes insipidus (serum only), SIADH (urine only), ethanol

Procedure

Serum

- No food or fluid restriction is required.
- Collect 5 to 7 mL of venous blood in a red-top tube. Avoid hemolysis.

Urine

- Give a high-protein diet for 3 days prior to test. Check with your laboratory.
- Restrict fluids for 8 to 12 hours.
- Collect a random, morning urine specimen. The first urine specimen in the morning is discarded, and the second specimen, taken 2 hours later, is sent to the laboratory. Urine osmolality should be high in the morning.

Nursing Implications

Client Teaching

- Inform client that no food and fluids are restricted with serum osmolality test. Fluids are restricted with urine.

Decreased level

- Associate a decreased serum osmolality with serum dilution caused by excessive fluid intake (overhydration).

- Observe for signs and symptoms of overhydration (i.e., a constant, irritating cough; dyspnea; neck-and-hand vein engorgement; and chest rales). Instruct to decrease fluid intake.
- Determine whether the decreased urine osmolality could be caused by excessive water intake (>2 quarts daily) or continuous IV administration of D_5W. A urine osmolality <200 mOsm/kg after fluids are restricted could be indicative of early kidney impairment.
- Observe for signs and symptoms of water intoxication (i.e., headaches, confusion, irritability, weight gain).

Elevated level

- Determine the hydration status of the client. Dehydration will cause an elevated serum and urine osmolality.
- Assess for signs and symptoms of dehydration (i.e., thirst, dry mucous membranes, poor skin turgor, and shock-like symptoms). Encourage the client to increase fluid intake.
- Check for hyperglycemia and glycosuria. Both could cause an elevation of serum and urine osmolality.
- Compare the serum osmolality with the urine osmolality. If the serum is hypo-osmolar (hypo-osmolality), the problem could be due to the syndrome of inappropriate ADH (SIADH).

OVA AND PARASITES (O & P) FECES

Reference Values

Adult: Negative
Child: Negative

Description. Parasites may be present in various forms in the intestine, including the ova, larvae, cysts, and trophozoites of the protozoa. Some of the organisms identified are amoeba, flagellates, tapeworms, hookworms, and roundworms. A history of recent travel outside the United States should be reported to the laboratory to help in identifying the parasite.

Purpose

- To identify specific ova and parasites in fecal matter

Clinical Problems

Positive result: Protozoa: *Balantidium coli, Chilomastix mesnili, Entamoeba histolytica, Giardia lamblia, Trichomonas hominis;* helminths (adults): *Ascaris lumbricoides* (roundworm), *Diphyllobothrium latum* (fish tapeworm), *Enterobius vermicularis* (pinworm), *Necator americanus* (American hookworm), *Strongyloides stercoralis* (threadworm), *Taenia saginata* (beef tapeworm), *Taenia solium* (pork tapeworm)

Procedure

- Collect stool specimen daily for 3 days or every other day. Take to the laboratory immediately, within 1 hour, or refrigerate.
- Mark on the laboratory slip countries the client has visited in the last 1 to 3 years.
- A loose or liquid stool is likely to indicate trophozoites and needs to be kept warm and taken to the laboratory within 30 minutes.
- If the stool is tested for tapeworm, the entire stool should be sent to the laboratory so that the head (scolex) of the tapeworm can be identified.
- Anal swabs are used to check for pinworm eggs, and the swabbing should be done in the morning before defecation or the morning bath.
- No tissue paper or urine in the fecal collection.
- Avoid taking mineral oil, castor oil, metamucil, barium, antacids, or tetracycline for 1 week before the test.
- Laboratory results are available in 24 to 48 hours.

Nursing Implications

- Obtain a history of the client's recent travel, and notify the laboratory and health care provider.
- Handle the stool specimen with care to prevent parasitic contamination of yourself and other clients.
- Check for occult blood in stool. The worm attaches itself to the bowel's lining.

Client Teaching

- Explain that the stool specimen should be collected in the morning. Explain that a soap suds enema should not be used, as this may destroy the parasite. The stool specimen should be obtained before treatment is initiated.

PARATHYROID HORMONE (PTH) SERUM

Reference Values

Adult: Intact PTH: 11–54 pg/mL; C-terminal PTH: 50–330 pg/mL; N-terminal PTH: 8–24 pg/mL

Description. Parathyroid hormone (PTH), secreted by the parathyroid glands, regulates the concentration of calcium and phosphorus in the extracellular fluid (ECF). The main function of PTH is to promote calcium reabsorption and phosphorus excretion. A low serum calcium level stimulates the secretion of PTH and a high serum calcium level inhibits PTH secretion.

Two forms of PTH, inactive C-terminal PTH and active N-terminal PTH, are used in diagnosing parathyroid disorders. C-terminal assays (PTH-C) are an effective indicator of chronic hyperparathyroidism. N-terminal assays (PTH-N) detect acute changes in the PTH secretion, can differentiate between hypercalcemia due to malignancy or parathyroid disorder, and are useful for monitoring the client's response to PTH therapy. Both assays and serum calcium values are used in diagnosing early and borderline parathyroid disorders.

Purposes

- To identify hypo- or hyperparathyroidism (see Clinical Problems)
- To monitor the client's response to PTH therapy

Clinical Problems

Decreased level: *PTH-C levels:* hypoparathyroidism, nonparathyroid hypercalcemia. *PTH-N levels:* hypoparathyroidism, nonparathyroid hypercalcemia, certain tumors, pseudohyperparathyroidism. *PTH-serum:* hypoparathyroidism, nonparathyroid hypercalcemia, Graves' disease, sarcoidosis

Elevated level: *PTH-C levels:* secondary hyperparathyroidism, tumors, hypercalcemia, pseudohypoparathyroidism. *PTH-N levels:* primary and secondary hyperparathyroidism, pseudohypoparathyroidism. *PTH-serum:* primary and secondary hyperparathyroidism, hypercalcemia, chronic renal failure, pseudohyperparathyroidism (defect in renal tubular response)

Procedure

- Restrict food and fluids for 8 hours prior to the test.
- Collect 5 to 7 mL of venous blood in a red-top tube in AM. Morning PTH is usually at its lowest point. Avoid hemolysis. N-terminal PTH is unstable and needs to be chilled or frozen if test is not immediately done.
- N-terminal PTH levels decrease during hemodialysis; collect blood specimens before dialysis.

Factors Affecting Laboratory Results

- Food, especially milk products, might lower the PTH level.

Nursing Implications

- Recognize the relationship of serum calcium levels and PTH secretion and serum level.
- Assess for signs and symptoms of hypocalcemia (tetany symptoms), and hypercalcemia (lethargy, muscle flaccidity, weakness, headaches).

Client Teaching

- Instruct the client not to eat until after the blood sample is taken. Foods high in calcium (milk products) may lower PTH level.

PARTIAL THROMBOPLASTIN TIME (PTT); ACTIVATED PARTIAL THROMBOPLASTIN TIME (APTT) PLASMA

Reference Values

Adult: PTT: 60–70 seconds; APTT: 20–35 seconds

Anticoagulant therapy: 1.5–2.5 times the control in seconds. *Note:* Most laboratories do APTT only

Description. The PTT is a screening test used to detect deficiencies in all clotting factors except VII and XIII and to detect platelet variations. The PTT is useful for monitoring heparin therapy.

The APTT is more sensitive in detecting clotting factor defects than the PTT, because the activator added in vitro shortens the clotting time. APTT is also used to monitor heparin therapy and is useful in preoperative screening for bleeding tendencies.

Purposes

- To monitor heparin therapy
- To screen for clotting factor deficiencies

Clinical Problems

Increased (prolonged) levels: Factor deficiencies (V, VIII, IX, X, XI, XII), cirrhosis of the liver, vitamin K deficiency, leukemias, Hodgkin's disease, disseminated intravascular coagulation (DIC), hypofibrinogenemia, von Willebrand's disease (vascular hemophilia)
Drugs that may increase PTT value: Heparin, salicylates

Procedure

- No food or fluid restriction is required.
- APTT test should be drawn 1 hour before next heparin dosage.
- Collect 3 to 5 mL of venous blood in a blue-top tube. Blood specimen should be taken to the laboratory *immediately.*

Nursing Implications

- Report APTT or PTT results to the physician.
- Assess the client for signs and symptoms of bleeding (i.e., purpura, hematuria, and nosebleeds).
- Administer heparin subcutaneously (SC) or IV through a heparin lock/IV reservoir. **Do not** aspirate when giving heparin SC, as a hematoma could occur at the injection site.

PHENYLKETONURIA (PKU) URINE; GUTHRIE TEST FOR PKU (BLOOD)

Reference Values

Child: Phenylalanine: 0.5–2.0 mg/dL; PKU: negative, but positive when the phenylalanine is 12–15 mg/dL; Guthrie: negative, but positive when the serum phenylalanine is 4 mg/dL

Description. The urine PKU and Guthrie tests are two screening tests used for detecting a hepatic enzyme deficiency, phenylalanine hydroxylase, which prevents the conversion of phenylalanine (amino acid) to tyrosine in the infant. Phenylalanine from milk and other protein products accumulates in the blood and tissues and can lead to brain damage and mental retardation.

The Guthrie procedure is the test of choice because a positive test result occurs when the serum phenylalanine reaches 4 mg/dL, 3 to 5 days of life after milk ingestion. If Guthrie test is positive, a specific blood phenylalanine test should be performed. The PKU urine test is done after the infant is 3 to 4 weeks old and should be repeated a week or two later. Significant brain damage usually occurs when the serum phenylalanine level is 15 mg/dL.

Purposes

- To screen for phenylalanine hydroxylase deficiency
- To repeat phenylketonuria test as indicated

Clinical Problems

Elevated level: PKU, low-birth-weight infants, hepatic encephalopathy, septicemia, galactosemia
Drugs that may increase PKU value: Aspirins, ketone bodies

Procedure

Guthrie test (Guthrie bacterial inhibition test): Phenylalanine promotes bacterial growth (*Bacillus subtilis*) when the serum level is greater than 4 mg/dL.

- Cleanse the infant's heel, and prick it with a sterile lancet. Obtain several drops of blood on a filter paper streaked with *B subtilis*. If the bacillus grows, the test is positive.
- Test should be performed on the fourth day after 2 to 4 days of milk ingestion (either cow's milk or breast milk).
- Note on the laboratory slip the date of birth and the date of the first milk ingested.

Urine PKU: Phenylalanine is converted to phenylpyruvic acid and is excreted in the urine when the serum level is 12 to 15 mg/dL.

- Dip Phenistix (dipstick with ferric salt) in fresh urine, or press against a fresh wet diaper. If positive, the dipstick will turn green.
- Perform PKU urine test 3 to 6 weeks after birth, preferably at 4 weeks, and repeat if necessary.

Nursing Implications

- Determine if the infant has had at least 3 days of milk intake before performing the Guthrie test. Vomiting and refusing to eat are common problems of PKU infants. This may cause a normal serum phenylalanine level.
- Compare the Guthrie test with serum phenylalanine.
- Obtain history if mother was a "PKU baby." If so, the mother should be on a low phenylalanine diet before and during pregnancy.

Client Teaching

- Explain to the mother the screening tests used to detect PKU. The Guthrie test is normally done while in the hospital. Many pediatricians want the urine PKU done 4 weeks after birth as a follow-up test.
- Teach the mother how to perform a urine PKU test accurately. Fresh urine on diaper or urine specimen should be used.
- Instruct that the baby should not receive aspirin or salicylate compounds for 24 hours before testing the urine to prevent a false-positive test. Tylenol should be given instead of aspirin.
- Tell the mother which foods the baby should and should not have. The preferred milk substitute is Lofenalac (Mead Johnson) with vitamins and minerals. Other low-phenylalanine foods are fruits, fruit juices, vegetables, cereals, and breads. Avoid high-protein foods, such as milk, ice cream, and cheese.

PHENYTOIN (*SEE* DILANTIN)

PHOSPHORUS (P) SERUM

PHOSPHATE (PO_4)

Reference Values

Adult: 1.7–2.6 mEq/L, 2.5–4.5 mg/dL, 0.78–1.52 mmol/L (SI units)
Child: Newborn: 3.5–8.6 mg/dL; infant: 4.5–6.7 mg/dL; child: 4.5–5.5 mg/dL
Elderly: Slightly lower than adult

Description. Phosphorus is the principal intracellular anion, and most exists in the blood as phosphate. From 80% to 85% of the total phosphates in the body are combined with calcium in the teeth and bones. Phosphates also regulate enzymatic activity for energy transfer.

Phosphorus and calcium concentrations are controlled by the parathyroid hormone. Usually there is a reciprocal relationship between calcium and phosphorus (i.e., when serum phosphorus levels increase, serum calcium levels decrease, and vice versa).

Purposes

- To check phosphorus level
- To monitor phosphorus levels during renal insufficiency or failure
- To compare phosphorus level with other electrolytes (i.e., potassium, calcium)

Clinical Problems

Decreased level: Starvation, malabsorption syndrome, hyperparathyroidism, hypercalcemia, hypomagnesemia, chronic alcoholism, vitamin D deficiency, diabetic acidosis, myxedema, continuous IV fluids with glucose, nasogastric (NG) suctioning, and vomiting
Drugs that may decrease phosphorus value: Antacids (aluminum hydroxide [Amphojel]); epinephrine (adrenalin); insulin, mannitol

Elevated level: Renal insufficiency, renal failure, hypoparathyroidism, hypocalcemia, hypervitaminosis D, bone tumors, acromegaly, healing fractures, sarcoidosis, Cushing's syndrome
Drugs that may increase phosphorus value: Methicillin, phenytoin (Dilantin), heparin, Lipomul, laxatives with phosphate

Procedure

- Restrict food and fluids except for water 4 to 8 hours. Carbohydrate lowers serum phosphorus levels.
- Hold IV fluids with glucose for 4 to 8 hours.
- Collect 3 to 5 mL of venous blood in a red-top tube. Avoid hemolysis. Take to the laboratory *immediately*.

Nursing Implications

Decreased level: Hypophosphatemia

- Check the serum phosphorus, calcium, and magnesium levels. An elevated calcium level causes a decreased phosphorus level.
- Observe for signs and symptoms of hypophosphatemia (i.e., anorexia, pain in the muscles and bone).

Client Teaching

- Instruct the client to eat foods rich in phosphorus (i.e., meats [beef, pork, turkey], milk, whole-grain cereals, and almonds) if the decrease is caused by malnutrition. Most carbonated drinks are high in phosphates.
- Instruct *not* to take antacids that contain aluminum hydroxide (Amphojel). Phosphorus binds with aluminum hydroxide; a low serum phosphorus level results.

Elevated level: Hyperphosphatemia

- Check serum calcium level; if low, observe for tetany symptoms.
- Monitor urinary output. A decreased urine output, <25 mL/h or <600 mL/d, can increase the serum phosphorus level.

Client Teaching

- Instruct the client to eat foods that are low in phosphorus (i.e., vegetables). Avoid drinking carbonated sodas that contain phosphates.

PLATELET AGGREGATION AND ADHESIONS (BLOOD)

Reference Values

Adult: Aggregation in 3 to 5 minutes

Description. ***Platelet aggregation test*** measures the ability of platelets to adhere to each other when mixed with an aggregating agent such as collagen, ADP, or ristocetin (an antibiotic). This test is performed to detect abnormality in platelet function and to aid in diagnosing hereditary and acquired platelet deficiencies such as von Willebrand's disease. Increased bleeding tendencies result from a decrease in platelet aggregation time.

Platelet adhesion test, like platelet aggregation, evaluates platelet function and helps to confirm hereditary diseases such as von Willebrand's disease. This test is also performed on clients taking large doses of aspirin for several weeks and on persons having a prolonged bleeding time. It is not performed in many laboratories because of the difficulty in standardizing the technique.

Purposes

- To evaluate platelet function
- To detect platelet bleeding disorders

Clinical Problems

Decreased platelet aggregation: von Willebrand's disease (ristocetin test), Bernard-Soulier syndrome (ristocetin test), cirrhosis of the liver, afibrinogenemia, Glanzmann's disease (thrombasthenia) (ADP, epinephrine, or collagen test), idiopathic thrombocytopenic purpura, platelet release defects, uremia

Drugs that may decrease platelet aggregation: Aspirin and aspirin compounds, anti-inflammatory agents such as NSAIDS (ibuprofen and others), 5-fluorouracil, phenothiazines, tricyclic antidepressants, diazepam (Valium), antihistamines, dipyridamole (Persantine), cortisone preparations, theophylline, marijuana, cocaine, heparin, furosemide (Lasix), penicillins, Vitamin E, volatile general anesthetics, theophylline, propranolol, pyrimidine compounds, and others

Elevated platelet aggregation: Diabetes mellitus, hyperlipemia, hypercoagulability, polycythemia vera

Procedure

- Collect 7 to 10 mL of venous blood in a blue-top tube. Avoid hemolysis. Test of blood should be tested within 2 hours after collection. Do not refrigerate.
- NPO, including medications, after midnight, except for water.

- No aspirin or aspirin compounds for 7 to 10 days prior to the test. List drugs the client is taking on the laboratory slip.

Factors Affecting Laboratory Results

- Foods high in fat content eaten before the test (hyperlipemia increases platelet aggregation)

Nursing Implications

- Obtain a drug history from the client.
- Check for bleeding tendencies, petechiae, purpura.

Client Teaching

- Instruct the client about the importance of not taking aspirin or aspirin compounds 7 to 10 days before the test (check with the health care provider). Aspirin inhibits clotting time.
- Inform the client that medications, food, and fluids (except water) should not be taken after midnight. It may be necessary to take some medications.

PLATELET ANTIBODY TEST (BLOOD)

PLATELET ANTIBODY DETECTION TEST, ANTIPLATELET ANTIBODY DETECTION

Reference Values

Negative

Description. When client becomes sensitized to platelet antigen of transfused blood, platelet antibodies (autoantibodies or isoantibodies) develop, thus causing thrombocytopenia because of destruction to the platelets. The platelet autoantibodies are IgG immunoglobulins of autoimmune origin. With idiopathic thrombocytopenic purpura (ITP), platelet autoantibodies are present.

Drug-induced thrombocytopenia is caused by platelet-associated IgG autoantibodies because of hypersensitivity to certain drugs. Some of the drugs that may cause drug-induced immunologic thrombocytopenia include salicylates, acetaminophen, antibiotics (sulfonamides, penicillin, cephalosporins, quinidine and quinidine-like drugs, gold, cimetidine, oral hypoglycemic agents, heparin, digoxin.)

Maternal-fetal platelet antigen incompatibility can occur if the mother has ITP autoantibodies that are passed to the fetus. Neonatal thrombocytopenia may result.

Purpose

- To detect the presence of platelet antibodies

Clinical Problems

Positive test: Thrombocytopenia because of platelet autoantibodies or isoantibodies, idiopathic thrombocytopenic purpura, post-transfusion purpura, drug-induced thrombocytopenia.
Drugs that may cause drug-induced thrombocytopenia: See Description.

Procedure

- No food or fluid restriction is required.
- Collect two (2) 10 mL of venous blood in a blue-top tube. Deliver to the laboratory immediately with the time of collection written on the requisition form.

Nursing Implications

- Obtain a drug history from the client.
- Check platelet count. If thrombocytopenia is present, a platelet antibody test may be ordered.
- Check for sites of petechiae, purpura.

Client Teaching

- Instruct the client to report any abnormal bleeding.
- Listen to client's and family's concerns.

PLATELET (THROMBOCYTE) COUNT (BLOOD)

Reference Values

Adult: 150,000–400,000 μL (mean, 250,000 μL); 0.15–0.4 × 10^{12}/L (SI units)
Child: Premature: 100,000–300,000 μL; newborn: 150,000–300,000 μL; infant: 200,000–475,000 μL

Description. Platelets (thrombocytes) are basic elements in the blood that promote coagulation. A low platelet count (thrombocytopenia) is associated with bleeding, and an elevated platelet count (thrombocytosis) may cause increased clotting. With a platelet count of 100,000 μL, bleeding is likely to occur, and with a platelet count <50,000 μL, hemorrhage is apt to occur.

Purposes

- To check platelet count
- To monitor platelet count during cancer chemotherapy

Clinical Problems

Decreased level: Idiopathic thrombocytopenic purpura, cancer (bone, GI, and brain), leukemias, aplastic anemia, liver disease, kidney disease, disseminated intravascular coagulation (DIC), SLE

Drugs that can decrease platelet count: Aspirin, chloromycetin, sulfonamides, quinidine, thiazide diuretics, phenylbutazone (Butazolidin), chemotherapeutic agents, tolbutamide (Orinase)

Increased level: Infections, acute blood loss, splenectomy, polycythemia vera, myeloproliferative disorders

Procedure

- No food or fluid restriction is required.

Venous

- Collect 3 to 5 mL of venous blood in a lavender-top tube.

Capillary blood

- Discard the first few drops of blood, and collect the next drops of blood from a finger puncture. Dilute with appropriate solution.

Factors Affecting Laboratory Results

- Chemotherapy and X-ray therapy can cause a decreased platelet count.

Nursing Implications

- Check the platelet count, especially with bleeding episodes, and report abnormal levels to the health care provider.

- Observe for signs and symptoms of bleeding (i.e., purpura, petechiae, hematemesis, rectal bleeding), and report to the health care provider.
- Monitor the platelet count, especially when the client is receiving chemotherapy or radiation therapy.

Client Teaching

- Teach the client to avoid injury.

POTASSIUM (K) SERUM AND URINE

Reference Values

Serum: Adult: 3.5–5.3 mEq/L, 3.5–5.3 mmol/L (SI units).
Child: 3.5–5.5 mEq/L; infant: 3.6–5.8 mq/L

Urine: Adult: Broad range: 25–120 mEq/24 h; average range: 40–80 mEq/24 h, 40–80 mmol/24 h (SI units)

Description. Serum potassium (K) has a narrow range; therefore, potassium values should be closely monitored; death could occur if serum levels are <2.5 mEq/L or >7.0 mEq/L. Eighty to 90% of the body's potassium is excreted in the urine. When there is tissue breakdown, potassium leaves the cells and enters the extracellular fluid. With adequate kidney function, the potassium in the vascular fluid will be excreted, and if renal shutdown or insufficiency occurs, then potassium will continue to increase in the vascular fluid.

The body does not conserve potassium, and the kidneys excrete an average of 40 mEq/L daily (the range is 25 to 120 mEq/24 h), even with a low dietary potassium intake. A decrease in urinary potassium can indicate hyperkalemia (elevated serum potassium), and an increase in urinary potassium can indicate hypokalemia (low serum potassium).

Purposes

- To check potassium level
- To detect the presence of hypo- or hyperkalemia

- To monitor potassium levels during health problems (i.e., renal insufficiency, debilitating illness, cancer) and with certain drugs (e.g., thiazide diuretics)

Clinical Problems

Decreased level (Hypokalemia)

Serum: Vomiting/diarrhea, laxative abuse, dehydration, malnutrition/starvation, crash diet, stress, trauma, injury and surgery (with renal function), gastric suction, diabetic acidosis, burns, hyperaldosteronism, excessive ingestion of licorice, metabolic alkalosis

Drugs that may decrease potassium value: Diuretics (potassium wasting), cortisone, estrogen, insulin, laxatives, lithium carbonate, sodium polystyrene sulfonate (Kayexalate), and aspirin

Urine: Elevated serum potassium level, acute renal failure

Elevated level (Hyperkalemia)

Serum: Oliguria and anuria, acute renal failure, IV potassium in fluids, Addison's disease, severe tissue injury or burns (with kidney shutdown), metabolic acidosis

Drugs that may increase potassium value: Diuretics (potassium sparing–spironolactone), antibiotics (penicillin, cephalosporins, heparin, epinephrine, histamine, isoniazid)

Urine: Decreased serum potassium level, dehydration, starvation, vomiting, and diarrhea

Procedure

Serum

- No food, fluid, or drug restrictions are necessary.
- Collect 3 to 5 mL of venous blood in a red-top tube. Avoid leaving tourniquet on for >2 minutes if possible. Avoid hemolysis.

Urine

- The 24-hour urine specimen should be kept on ice or refrigerated.
- Potassium supplements given as salt replacement should be eliminated for 48 hours.

Factors Affecting Laboratory Results

- The use of a tourniquet can cause an increase in the serum potassium level.

Nursing Implications

- Compare serum potassium levels with urine potassium levels. When serum potassium level is decreased, urine potassium level is frequently increased and vice versa.

Decreased serum level

- Observe for signs and symptoms of hypokalemia (i.e., vertigo, hypotension, cardiac dysrhythmias, nausea, vomiting, diarrhea, abdominal distention, decreased peristalsis, muscle weakness, and leg cramps).
- Record intake and output. Polyuria can cause an excessive loss of potassium.
- Determine the client's hydration status when hypokalemia is present. Overhydration can dilute the serum potassium level.
- Recognize behavioral changes as a sign of hypokalemia. Low potassium levels can cause confusion, irritability, and mental depression.
- Report ECG changes. A prolonged and depressed S-T segment and a flat or inverted T-wave is indicative of hypokalemia.
- Dilute oral potassium supplements in at least 6 ounces of water or juice to reduce irritation to the gastric mucosa.
- Monitor the serum potassium level in clients receiving potassium-wasting diuretics and steroids. Cortisone steroids cause sodium retention and potassium excretion.
- Assess for signs and symptoms of digitalis toxicity when the client is receiving a digitalis preparation and a potassium-wasting diuretic or steroid. A lower serum potassium level enchances the action of digitalis. Signs and symptoms of digitalis toxicity are nausea and vomiting, anorexia, bradycardia, dysrhythmia, and visual disturbances.
- Administer IV KCl in a liter of IV fluids. *Never* give an IV or bolus push of KCl, as cardiac arrest can occur. KCl can be administered IV only when it is diluted (20 to 40 mEq/L of KCl) and should never be given SC or IM. Concentrated IV KCl is irritating to the heart muscle and to the veins, causing phlebitis.

Client Teaching

- Teach the client and family to eat foods high in potassium (i.e., fruits, fruit juices, dry fruits, vegetables, meats, nuts, coffee, tea, and cola).

Elevated serum level

- Observe for signs and symptoms of hyperkalemia (i.e., bradycardia, abdominal cramps, oliguria or anuria, tingling, and twitching or numbness of the extremities).
- Assess urine output to determine renal function; urine output should be at least 25 mL/h or 600 mL daily, and a urine output of less than 600 mL/d may cause hyperkalemia.
- Report serum potassium levels >5.0 mEq/L. Restriction of potassium intake may be necessary, and if serum level is higher, Kayexalate (ion exchange resin) may be needed. High serum potassium levels, >7.0 mEq/L, could cause cardiac arrest.
- Regulate the rate of IV fluids so that no more than 10 mEq KCl/h are administered.
- Check the age of whole blood before administering it to a client with hyperkalemia. Blood 3 to 4 weeks old or older has an elevated serum potassium level, which could be five times the normal serum potassium level.
- Monitor the ECG for QRS spread and peaked T waves, a sign of hyperkalemia. The pulse may be rapid, but if hyperkalemia persists, bradycardia can occur.
- Observe for signs and symptoms of hypokalemia when administering Kayexalate for a prolonged period (2 or more days).

PREALBUMIN (PA, PAB) ASSAY (SERUM)

TRANSTHYRETIN (TTR), TRYPTOPHAN-RICH PREALBUMIN

Reference Values

Adult: 17–40 mg/dL, 170–400 mg/L (SI units); Female (average): 18 mg/dL, 180 mg/L (SI units); Male (average): 21.6 mg/dL, 216 mg/L (SI units)

Child: Newborn: 10–11.5 mg/dL, 100–115 mg/L (SI units); 2 to 3 years: 16–28 mg/dL, 160–280 mg/L (SI units)

Description. Prealbumin, also known as thyroxin-binding protein or transthyretin, is a test used primarily for nutritional assessment.

Transthyretin, a transport protein, is a precursor of albumin. Prealbumin has a shorter half-life (2 to 4 days) than albumin (20 to 24 days); it can readily indicate any change affecting protein synthesis and catabolism. This test is more sensitive for determining nutritional status and liver dysfunction than an albumin test. It is also useful in monitoring the effectiveness of total parenteral nutrition (TPN) and evaluating the nutritional needs in critically ill clients. A prealbumin value of <5 mg/dL indicates severe protein depletion, and a value <10 mg/dL indicates severe nutritional deficiency.

Purposes

- To assess the client's nutritional status
- To evaluate the client's nutritional needs on admission to the hospital, or following a surgical procedure, or during a critical illness.

Clinical Problems

Decreased level: Protein-wasting diseases, malnutrition, malignancies, cirrhosis of the liver, zinc deficiency (zinc is required for synthesis of prealbumin), chronic illness
Drugs that decrease prealbumin value: Estrogen, oral contraceptives

Elevated level: Hodgkin's disease, chronic kidney disease, adrenal hyperfunction
Drugs that increase prealbumin value: Steroids (high doses), nonsteroidal anti-inflammatory drugs (NSAIDs) (high doses)

Procedure

- No food or fluid restriction; some institutions request NPO 8–12 hours prior to the test.
- Collect 2 to 5 mL of venous blood in a red-top tube. Avoid hemolysis.

Nursing Implications

- Obtain a history of the client's nutritional intake. Record findings.
- Check vital signs and weight.
- Listen to the client's concerns; answer questions or refer them to other health care providers.

Client Teaching

- Inform the client of ways in which nutritional status can be improved.

PREGNANEDIOL (URINE)

Reference Values

Adult: Female: 0.5–1.5 mg/24 h (proliferative phase), 2–7 mg/24 h (luteal phase), 0.1–1.0 mg/24 h (postmenopausal); male: 0.1–1.5 mg/24 h

Pregnancy: 10–19 gestation weeks: 5–25 mg/24 h; 20–28 gestation weeks: 15–42 mg/24 h; 28–32 gestation weeks: 25–49 mg/24 h

Child: 0.4–1.0 mg/24 h

Description. Pregnanediol is the major metabolite of progesterone produced by the ovary during the luteal phase of the menstrual cycle and by the placenta. Progesterone is responsible for uterine changes after ovulation and for maintaining pregnancy after fertilization. A steady rise in urine pregnanediol levels occurs during pregnancy, and a decrease in these levels indicates placental, not fetal, dysfunction and the possibility of an abortion.

Urine pregnanediol levels may be used to determine menstrual disturbances and are used to verify ovulation in those who have not been able to become pregnant.

Purposes

- To determine the occurrence of placental dysfunction
- To compare test results with other laboratory tests for determining cause of menstrual disorder

Clinical Problems

Decreased level: Menstrual disorders (amenorrhea), ovarian hypofunction, threatened abortion, fetal death, placental failure, preeclampsia, benign neoplasms of the ovary and breast

Elevated level: Pregnancy, ovarian cyst, choriocarcinoma of the ovary, adrenal cortex hyperplasia

Procedure

- No food or fluid restriction is required.
- Collect urine over a 24-hour period in a large refrigerated container with preservative.
- Label the bottle with the client's name, date, and exact times of collection (e.g., 11/7/03, 8 AM to 11/8/03, 8 AM).
- Record on the laboratory slip the date of the last menstrual period or weeks of gestation.
- Post urine collection time and procedure at appropriate places.

Nursing Implications

- Obtain a history of menstrual changes (patterns, frequency, length of period, flow, and discomfort).
- Obtain a history of pregnancy complications or problems. Record when the client had her last menstrual period.
- Give support to the client and family.
- Monitor the urine pregnanediol levels if sequential tests have been ordered. Progesterone therapy may be needed.

PREGNANETRIOL (URINE)

Reference Values

Adult: Male: 0.4–2.4 mg/24 h; female: 0.5–2.0 mg/24 h
Child: Infant: 0–0.2 mg/24 h; child: 0–1.0 mg/24 h

Description. Pregnanetriol comes from adrenal corticoid synthesis. It should not be mistaken for pregnanediol. The pregnanetriol test is useful in diagnosing congenital adrenocortical hyperplasia.

Purpose

- To detect anterior pituitary hypofunction or adrenocortical hyperfunction (see Clinical Problems)

Clinical Problems

Decreased level: Anterior pituitary hypofunction

Elevated level: Adrenogenital syndrome, congenital adrenocortical hyperplasia, adrenocortical hyperfunction, malignant neoplasm of the adrenal gland

Procedure

- No food or fluid restriction is required.
- Collect urine for 24 hours in a large, refrigerated container.
- Label the bottle with the client's name, date, and exact times of collection.

Nursing Implications

- Assess for changes in external genitalia.
- Monitor urine pregnanetriol levels with cortisone replacement.
- Be supportive of client and family.

PROGESTERONE (SERUM)

Reference Values

Adult: Female: Follicular phase: 0.1–1.5 ng/mL; 20–150 ng/dL
Luteal phase: 2–28 ng/mL; 250–2800 ng/dL
Postmenopausal: <1.0 ng/mL; <100 ng/dL
Pregnancy: First trimester: 9–50 ng/mL
Second trimester: 18–150 ng/mL
Third trimester: 60–260 ng/mL
Male: <1.0 ng/mL; <100 ng/dL

Description. Progesterone, a hormone produced primarily by the corpus luteum of the ovaries and a small amount by the adrenal cortex, peaks during the luteal phase of the menstrual cycle for 4 to 5 days and during pregnancy. It prepares the endometrium for implantation of the fertilized egg. This hormone remains elevated during early pregnancy. Higher levels of progesterone occur when there are twins or more than a single fetus. Placenta secretes about ten times the normal amount (luteal phase). Only a small amount of progesterone is detected in the blood, since most is metabolized in the liver to pregnanediol, a progesterone metabolite.

Serum progesterone is useful in evaluating infertility problems, confirming ovulation, assessing placental functions in pregnancy, and determining the risk of a possible threatened abortion. A urine pregnanediol might be ordered to verify serum progesterone results.

Purposes

- To aid in the diagnosis of ovarian or adrenal tumor
- To assist in the diagnosis of placental failure
- To evaluate infertility problems resulting from a decreased progesterone level

Clinical Problems

Decreased levels: Gonadal dysfunction, luteum deficiency, threatened abortion, toxemia of pregnancy, placental failure, fetal death
Drugs that may decrease progesterone value: Oral contraceptives

Elevated levels: Ovulation, pregnancy, ovarian cysts, tumors of the ovary or adrenal gland
Drugs that may increase progesterone value: ACTH, progesterone preparations

Procedure

- No food or fluid restriction is required.
- Collect 5 to 7 mL of venous blood in a red- (preferred) or green-top tube. Avoid hemolysis. Invert the green-top tube several times to mix with the anticoagulant in the tube.
- Note on the laboratory slip the phase of the client's menstrual cycle, or weeks of gestation if pregnant.

Nursing Implications

- Obtain a history from the client of her menstrual phase or weeks or months of gestation.
- Listen to the client's concerns and fears. Refer client's questions to health professionals when appropriate.

Client Teaching

- Inform the client that the blood test may be repeated or that a urine test may be ordered. Repeated tests may be indicated to obtain complete information concerning progesterone secretion.

PROLACTIN (PRL) SERUM

LACTOGENIC HORMONE, LACTOGEN

Reference Values

Female: Follicular phase: 0–23 ng/mL
Luteal phase: 0–40 ng/mL
Postmenopausal <12 ng/mL
Pregnancy: First trimester: <80 ng/mL
Second trimester: <160 ng/mL
Third trimester: <400 ng/mL
Male: 0.1–20 ng/mL
Pituitary adenoma: >100–300 ng/mL

Description. Prolactin is a hormone secreted by the adenohypophysis (anterior pituitary gland) and is necessary in developing the mammary glands for lactation. If breast feeding after delivery, prolactin levels remain elevated for maintaining lactation. Impotence in the male might be attributed to excess prolactin secretion that suppresses gonad function.

Serum prolactin levels greater than 100–300 ng/mL in nonpregnant females and in males may indicate a pituitary adenoma (tumor). Bromocriptine (Parlodel) decreases the serum prolactin level and tumor growth until the pituitary tumor can be removed.

Purposes

- To detect various health problems related to an increased prolactin level (see Clinical Problems)
- To check drugs that the client is taking which influence increased prolactin levels

Clinical Problems

Decreased level: Postpartum pituitary infarction

Drugs that may decrease prolactin value: Bromocriptine, levodopa, ergot derivatives, apomorphine

Elevated level: Pregnancy, breast feeding, pituitary tumor, amenorrhea, galactorrhea, ectopic prolactin-secreting tumors (such as the lung), primary hypothyroidism, hypothalamic disorder, endometriosis, chronic renal failure, polycystic ovary, Addison's disease, stress, sleep, coitus, exercise

Drugs that may increase prolactin value: Amphetamine, estrogens, antihistamines, oral contraceptives, phenothiazines, tricyclic antidepressants, monoamine oxidase inhibitors (MAO inhibitors), methyldopa (Aldomet), haloperidol (Haldol), cimetidine (Tagamet), procainamide derivatives, reserpine (Serpasil), isoniazid (INH), verapamil

Procedure

- Withhold medications that interfere with the test.
- Fasting specimen is preferred.
- Collect 3 to 5 mL of venous blood in a red- or lavender-top tube. Avoid hemolysis. Client should be awake for 1 to 2 hours before blood test; sleep elevates the serum prolactin level.

Factors Affecting Laboratory Results

- Exercise, stress, pain, surgical trauma, and sleep may affect test results.

Nursing Implications

- List drugs the client is taking that may affect test results on the laboratory slip.
- Listen to the client's concerns.

Client Teaching

- Instruct the client about the test procedure, such as blood specimen to be drawn 1 to 2 hours after awakening.
- Instruct the client to avoid stress and exercise prior to the test. Note the presence of stress or pain on the laboratory slip.

PROSTATE-SPECIFIC ANTIGEN (PSA) SERUM

Reference Values

Male: No prostatic disorder: 0–4 ng/mL
Benign prostatic hypertrophy (BPH): 4–19 ng/mL
Prostate cancer: 10–120 ng/mL (depends on the stage of prostatic cancer)

Description. Prostate-specific antigen (PSA), a glycoprotein from the prostatic tissues, is increased in both BPH and prostatic cancer; however, it is markedly increased in prostatic cancer. PSA is more sensitive than prostatic acid phosphatase (PAP), also known as acid phosphatase (ACP), in early detection of prostatic cancer. The use of PSA and PAP, along with rectal examination, assists with making an accurate diagnosis.

PSA may be used to diagnose, monitor effect of prostatic cancer treatment with chemotherapy or radiation, and determine disease process and prognosis. Repeating the PSA test may be necessary.

Purpose

- To aid in the diagnosis of prostatic cancer

Clinical Problems

Elevated level: Prostatic cancer, benign prostatic hypertrophy (BPH) (low elevation)

Procedure

- No food or fluid restriction is required.
- Collect 3 to 5 mL of venous blood in a red-top tube.

Nursing Implications

- Obtain a history regarding changes in urinary pattern such as interrupted urine flow, frequent urination (especially at night), difficulty in starting and stopping the urine flow, hematuria, and/or pain in the back or during urination.

Client Teaching

- Explain to the client that the test is painless.
- Instruct the client that a manual rectal examination is part of the test regimen to determine prostatic changes.
- Be supportive of the client. Provide an atmosphere in which the client feels comfortable expressing his concerns.

PROSTATIC ACID PHOSPHATASE (PAP) (SEE ACID PHOSPHATASE [ACP])

PROTEIN (TOTAL); PROTEIN ELECTROPHORESIS (SERUM)

Reference Values

Adult: Total protein: 6.0–8.0 g/dL

Protein Fraction	*Weight (g/dL)*	*% of Total Protein*
Albumin	3.5–5.0	52–68
Globulin	1.5–3.5	32–48
Alpha-1	0.1–0.4	2–5
Alpha-2	0.4–1.0	7–13
Beta	0.5–1.1	8–14
Gamma	0.5–1.7	12–22

Child: Total protein: premature: 4.2–7.6 g/dL; newborn: 4.6–7.4 g/dL; infant: 6.0–6.7 g/dL; child: 6.2–8.0 g/dL

	Albumin (g/dL)		*Globulins (g/dL)*		
	(g/dL)	*Alpha-1*	*Alpha-2*	*Beta*	*Gamma*
Premature	3.0–4.2	0.1–0.5	0.3–0.7	0.3–1.2	0.3–1.4
Newborn	3.5–5.4	0.1–0.3	0.3–0.5	0.2–0.6	0.2–1.2
Infant	4.4–5.4	0.2–0.4	0.5–0.8	0.5–0.9	0.3–0.8
Child	4.0–5.8	0.1–0.4	0.4–1.0	0.5–1.0	0.3–1.0

Description. The total protein is composed mostly of albumin and globulins. The use of the total serum protein test is limited unless the protein electrophoresis test is performed.

Serum protein electrophoresis is a process that separates various protein fractions into albumin and alpha-1, alpha-2, beta, and gamma globulins. Albumin plays an important role in maintaining serum colloid osmotic pressure. The gamma globulin is the body's antibodies, which contribute to immunity.

Purposes

- To associate and differentiate between albumin and globulin
- To monitor protein levels
- To identify selected health problems associated with protein deficit

Clinical Problems

Total Protein and Protein Fraction	*Decreased Level*	*Elevated Level*
Total Protein	Malnutrition, starvation Malabsorption syndrome Severe liver disease Cancer of GI tract Severe burns Hodgkin's disease Ulcerative colitis Chronic renal failure	Dehydration Vomiting, diarrhea Multiple myeloma Sarcoidosis Respiratory distress syndrome
Albumin	Chronic liver disease Malnutrition, starvation Malabsorption syndrome Leukemia, malignancies Chronic renal failure SLE Severe burns Nephrotic syndrome Toxemia of pregnancy CHF	Dehydration Exercise

Globulins	*Decreased Level*	*Elevated Level*
Alpha-1	Emphysema due to alpha-1 antitrypsin deficiency, nephrosis	Pregnancy Neoplasm Acute and chronic infection Tissue necrosis
Alpha-2	Hemolytic anemia Severe liver disease	Acute infection Injury, trauma Severe burns Extensive neoplasm Rheumatic fever Rheumatoid arthritis

Globulins	*Decreased Level*	*Elevated Level*
		AMI Nephrotic syndrome Biliary cirrhosis Obstructive jaundice
Beta	Hypocholesterolemia	Hypothyroidism Biliary cirrhosis Kidney nephrosis Nephrotic syndrome Diabetes mellitus Cushing's disease Malignant hypertension
Gamma	Nephrotic syndrome Lymphocytic leukemia Lymphosarcoma Hypogammaglobulinemia or agammaglobulinemia	Collagen disease Rheumatoid arthritis Lupus erythematosus Malignant lymphoma Hodgkin's disease Chronic lymphocytic leukemia Multiple myeloma Liver disease Chronic infections

Procedure

- Collect 5 to 7 mL of venous blood in a red-top tube. Avoid hemolysis.
- No food or fluid restriction is required. Check with your laboratory.

Factors Affecting Laboratory Results

- A high-fat diet before the test

Nursing Implications

- Assess client's dietary intake. Suggest foods high in protein (i.e., beans, eggs, meats, milk).
- Assess for peripheral edema in the lower extremities when the albumin level is decreased.
- Assess urinary output. Urinary output should be 25 mL/h or 600 mL/24 h.
- Check for albumin/protein in the urine.

PROTEIN (URINE)

Reference Values

Random specimen: Negative: 0–5 mg/dL; positive: 6–2,000 mg/dL (trace to +2)
24-hour specimen: 25–150 mg/24 h

Description. Proteinuria is usually caused by renal disease due to glomerular damage or impaired renal tubular reabsorption, or both. With a random urine specimen, protein can be detected by using a reagent strip or dipstick, such as Combstix. If a random specimen is positive for proteinuria, a 24-hour urine specimen is usually ordered for protein. The amount of protein is an indicator of severity of renal involvement. Emotions and physiologic stress may cause transient proteinuria. Newborns may have an increased proteinuria during the first 3 days of life.

Purposes

- To compare urine protein with serum protein level in relation to health problems (see Clinical Problems)
- To identify renal dysfunction with increased protein level in the urine

Clinical Problems

Elevated level: *Heavy proteinuria:* acute or chronic glomerulonephritis, nephrotic syndrome, lupus nephritis, amyloid disease; *Moderate proteinuria:* drug toxicities (aminoglycosides), cardiac disease, acute infectious disease, multiple myeloma, chemical toxicities; *Mild proteinuria:* chronic pyelonephritis, polycystic kidney disease, renal tubular disease
Drugs that may increase urine protein: Penicillin, gentamicin, sulfonamides, cephalosporins, contrast media, tolbutamide (Orinase), acetazolamide (Diamox)

Procedure

- No food or fluid restriction is required.
- List drugs client is taking that could affect test results.

Qualitative test: Random urine specimen

- Collect clean-caught or midstream urine specimen.

- Place the reagent strip/dipstick in the urine specimen. Match the dipstick with the color chart on the bottle for results.

Quantitative analysis test: 24-hour specimen

- Discard first urine specimen. Then save all urine for 24 hours in a refrigerated urine-collection bottle.
- Label the urine bottle with client's name, date, exact time of collection (e.g., 7/12/04, 8:01 AM to 7/13/04, 8:02 AM).

Nursing Implications

- Explain the test procedure to the client.
- Assess for signs and symptoms of renal dysfunction (i.e., fatigue, decreased urine output, peripheral edema, increased serum creatinine).
- Notify the health care provider if the urine output is <25 mL/h.

PROTHROMBIN TIME (PT) PLASMA

PRO-TIME, INR

Reference Values

Adult: 10–13 seconds (depending on the method and reagents used); anticoagulant therapy: PT: 1.5–2.0 times the control in seconds; *INR (international normalized ratio):* 2.0–3.0

Child: Same as adult

Description. Prothrombin, synthesized by the liver, is an inactive precursor in the clotting process. The PT test measures the clotting ability of factors I (fibrinogen), II (prothrombin), V, VII, and X. The major use of the PT test is to monitor oral anticoagulant therapy (e.g., warfarin sodium [Coumadin]). If PT is >2.5 times the control value, bleeding is likely to occur.

See International Normalized Ratio (INR) test.

Purpose

- To monitor oral anticoagulant (warfarin) therapy

Clinical Problems

Decreased level: Thrombophlebitis, myocardial infarction, pulmonary embolism

Drugs that may decrease PT time and INR: Barbiturates, oral contraceptives, diphenhydramine (Benadryl), rifampin, metaproterenol (Alupent), vitamin K, digitalis, diuretics

Increased (prolonged) level: Liver diseases; afibrinogenemia; factor deficiencies II, V, VII, X; leukemias; erythroblastosis fetalis; CHF
Drugs that may increase PT time and INR: Oral anticoagulants (Coumadin, Dicumarol), antibiotics, salicylates (aspirin), sulfonamides, phenytoin (Dilantin), chlorpromazine (Thorazine), chlordiazepoxide (Librium), methyldopa (Aldomet), mithramycin, reserpine (Serpasil)

Procedure

- No food or fluid restriction is required.
- Collect 3 to 5 mL of venous blood in a blue-top or black-top tube. The blood must be tested within 2 hours. Fill tube to capacity.
- Control values are given with the client's PT and INR values.
- List drugs on the laboratory slip that can affect test results.

Factors Affecting Laboratory Results

- A high-fat diet (decreases PT) and alcohol use (increases PT)

Nursing Implications

- Monitor the plasma PT and/or INR when the client is receiving oral anticoagulant therapy.
- Inform the health care provider of the client's PT daily or as ordered. The health care provider may want the anticoagulant held or the dose adjusted.
- Observe for signs and symptoms of bleeding (i.e., purpura, nosebleeds, hematemesis, hematuria). Report and record symptoms.
- Administer vitamin K as ordered when the PT is over 40 seconds or when bleeding is occurring.
- Assess the alcohol consumption and diet. Alcohol intake can increase PT, INR; and a high-fat diet may decrease PT, INR.

Client Teaching

- Instruct the client not to self-medicate when receiving anticoagulant therapy. Over-the-counter (OTC) drugs may either increase or decrease the effects of the anticoagulant.

- Instruct the client to take the prescribed anticoagulant as ordered by the health care provider and not to miss a dose.

RABIES ANTIBODY TEST (SERUM)

FLUORESCENT RABIES ANTIBODY (FRA)

Reference Values

Indirect fluorescent antibody (IFA) <1:16

Description. The rabies rhabdovirus affecting the central nervous system may be present in the saliva, brain, spinal cord, urine, and feces of rabid animals. The virus can be transmitted to the human by an infected dog, bat, skunk, squirrel, or other animal and is nearly 100% fatal if the person does not receive treatment before the symptoms occur.

This rabies antibody test is performed to diagnose rabies both in animals and in humans that have been bitten by a rabid animal. Also, it is useful to test the effects of rabies immunization on employees working in animal shelters. Both the rabies antibody test and the animal's brain tissue are preferred to positively diagnose rabies that was transmitted to the human. If the animal suspected of having rabies survives longer than 10 days, it is unlikely that the animal is rabid.

Purpose

- To aid in the diagnosis of rabies in animals and humans

Clinical Problems

Elevated titer count: Rabies transmission

Procedure

- Collect 5 to 7 mL of venous blood in a red-top tube. The animal brain should be sent along with the blood sample to the laboratory if possible.
- No food or fluid restriction is required.

Nursing Implications

- Obtain a history of the animal bite. Rabies immunoglobulin (RIG) may be given soon after the exposure to neutralize the virus.
- The animal responsible for the animal bite should be captured. If the animal's rabies vaccination is not current, the animal is usually destroyed in order to test the brain tissue. A wait of 10 days to determine the survival of a "wild" animal is not suggested.

Client Teaching

- Suggest to persons working with animals, such as those working in veterinary practices, in kennels, in wildlife areas, and research laboratories, that they receive a preexposure rabies vaccine such as HDVC (human diploid cell rabies vaccine) to protect them from rabies exposure.
- Instruct the person who was bitten or the family to seek medical care immediately. Encourage the family to notify the humane society concerning the animal bite. The animal should be captured.
- Inform the client and/or family that if the animal is not located, then a series of rabies vaccinations is necessary and should be taken.
- Answer the client's questions or refer the questions to appropriate health professionals.

RAPID PLASMA REAGIN (RPR) SERUM

Reference Values

Adult: Nonreactive
Child: Nonreactive

Description. The RPR test is a rapid-screening test for syphilis. A nontreponemal antibody test like VDRL, the RPR test detects reagin antibodies in the serum and is more sensitive but less specific than VDRL. Frequently it is used on donor's blood as a syphilis detection test. As with other nonspecific reagin tests, false positives can occur as the result of acute and chronic diseases. A positive RPR should be verified by VDRL and/or FTA-ABS tests.

Purpose

- To compare test results with other laboratory tests for diagnosing syphilis

Clinical Problems

Reactive (positive): Syphilis. False positives: tuberculosis, pneumonia, infectious mononucleosis, chickenpox, smallpox vaccination (recent), rheumatoid arthritis, lupus erythematosus, hepatitis, pregnancy

Procedure

- Follow the directions on the RPR kit. Positive test: Flocculation occurs on the plastic card.

Nursing Implications

- If test result is positive, explain to the client that further testing will be done to verify test results.
- If repeat result is positive, sexual contacts need to be notified for treatment.

RBC INDICES (RED BLOOD CELL COUNT, MCV, MCH, MCHC) BLOOD

ERYTHROCYTE INDICES

Reference Values

	Adult	*Newborn*	*Child*
RBC count (million)/μL or $\times 10^{12}$/L [SI units])	Male: 4.6–6.0 Female: 4.0–5.0 4.6–6.0 $\times 10^{12}$	4.8–7.2 4.8–7.2 $\times 10^{12}$	3.8–5.5 3.8–5.5 $\times 10^{12}$
MCV (cuμ [conventional] or fL [SI units])	80–98	96–108	82–92
MCH (pg [conventional and SI units])	27–31	32–34	27–31
MCHC (% or g/dL [conventional] or SI units)	32%–36% 0.32–0.36	32%–33% 0.32–0.33	32%–36% 0.32–0.36
RDW (coulter S)	11.5–14.5		

Description. RBC indices provide information about the size (MCV; mean corpuscular volume), weight (mean corpuscular hemoglobin [MCH]), and hemoglobin concentration (mean corpuscular hemoglobin concentration [MCHC]) of RBCs. A decreased MCV or microcytes, small-sized RBCs, is indicative of iron deficiency anemia and thalassemia. An increased MCV or macrocytes, large-sized RBCs, is indicative of pernicious anemia and folic acid anemia. In macrocytic anemias, the MCH is elevated, and it is decreased in hypochromic anemia. The MCHC can be calculated from MCH and MCV as follows:

$$\text{MCHC} = \frac{\text{MCH}}{\text{MCV}} \times 100 \text{ or MCHC} - \frac{\text{Hb}}{\text{Hct}} \times 100$$

Purposes

- To monitor red blood cell count
- To differentiate between the components of RBC indices for determining health problem (see Clinical Problems)

Clinical Problems

Indices	*Decreased Level*	*Elevated Level*
RBC count	Hemorrhage (blood loss)	Polycythemia vera
	Anemias Chronic infections	Hemoconcentration/ dehydration
	Leukemias	High altitude
	Multiple myeloma	Cor pulmonale
	Excessive IV fluids	Cardiovascular disease
	Chronic renal failure	
	Pregnancy	
	Overhydration	
MCV	Microcytic anemia: iron deficiency Malignancy Rheumatoid arthritis	Macrocytic anemia; aplastic, hemolytic, pernicious, folic acid deficiency
		Chronic liver disease
	Hemoglobinopathies; thalassemia, sickle cell anemia, hemoglobin C	Hypothyroidism (myxedema) Drugs affect vitamin B_{12}

(continued)

Indices	*Decreased Level*	*Elevated Level*
	Lead poisoning Radiation	anticonvulsants, antimetabolics
MCH	Microcytic, hypochromic anemia	Macrocytic anemias
MCHC	Hypochromic anemia Iron deficiency anemia Thalassemia	
RDW		Iron-deficiency anemia Folic acid deficiency Pernicious anemia Homozygous hemoglobinopathies (S, C, H)

Procedure

- No food or fluid restriction is required.
- Collect 3 to 5 mL of venous blood in a lavender-top tube. Avoid hemolysis
- Usually a particle counter is used, which will provide all CBC results along with all the indices.

Nursing Implications

- Assess for the cause(s) of a decreased RBC count. Check for blood loss, and obtain a history of anemias, renal insufficiency, chronic infection, or leukemia. Determine whether the client is overhydrated.
- Observe for signs and symptoms of advanced iron deficiency anemia (i.e., fatigue, pallor, dyspnea on exertion, tachycardia, and headache). Chronic symptoms include cracked corners of the mouth, smooth tongue, dysphagia, and numbness and tingling of the extremities.
- Assess for signs and symptoms of hemoconcentration. Dehydration, shock, and severe diarrhea can elevate the RBC level.

Client Teaching

- Instruct the client to eat foods rich in iron (i.e., liver, red meats, green vegetables, and iron-fortified bread).
- Explain to the client who is taking iron supplements that the stools usually appear dark in color (tarry). Tell the client to take iron medication with meals. Milk and antacids can interfere with iron absorption.

RENIN (PLASMA)

PLASMA RENIN ACTIVITY (PRA)

Reference Values

Adult: Thirty minutes supine: 0.2–2.3 ng/mL; upright: 1.6–4.3 ng/mL; restricted salt diet: 4.1–10.8 ng/mL

Child: 1–3 yr old: 1.7–11.0 ng/mL; 3–5 yr old: 1.0–6.5 ng/mL; 5–10 yr old: 0.5–6.0 ng/mL

Description. Renin is an enzyme secreted by the juxtaglomerular cells of the kidneys. This enzyme activates the renin-angiotensin system, which causes the release of aldosterone and causes vasoconstriction. Aldosterone promotes sodium reabsorption from the kidneys, thus sodium and water retention. Vasoconstriction and aldosterone can cause hypertension. Elevated plasma renin rarely occurs in essential hypertension, but its value is frequently elevated in renovascular and malignant hypertension.

Postural changes (from a recumbent to an upright position) and a decreased sodium (salt) intake will stimulate renin secretion. Plasma renin levels are usually higher from 8 AM to 12 noon and lower from noon to 6 PM.

Purpose

- To identify a possible cause of hypertension

Clinical Problems

Decreased level: Essential hypertension, Cushing's syndrome, diabetes mellitus, hypothyroidism, high-sodium diet

Drugs that may decrease renin value: Antihypertensives, levodopa, propranolol (Inderal)

Elevated level: Hypertension (malignant, renovascular), hyperaldosteronism, cancer of the kidney, acute renal failure, Addison's disease, cirrhosis, chronic obstructive pulmonary disease (COPD), manic-depressive disorder, pregnancy (first trimester), preeclampsia and eclampsia, hyperthyroidism, low-sodium diet, hypokalemia

Drugs that may increase renin value: Estrogens, diuretics, certain anti-hypertensives, oral contraceptives

Procedure

- Keep the syringe and collecting tube cold in an ice bath before collection.
- The tourniquet should be released before the blood is drawn.
- Collect 5 to 7 mL of venous blood in a lavender-top tube.
- Note on the laboratory slip if the client is in a supine or upright position. Note also if the client is on a normal or low-salt diet.
- Take the blood specimen (in ice) to the laboratory immediately.

Nursing Implications

- Check with the laboratory on procedural changes or modifications.
- Monitor the client's blood pressure every 4 to 6 hours or as indicated.
- Assess kidney function by recording urinary output. Urine output should be at least 600 mL per day.

RETICULOCYTE COUNT (BLOOD)

Reference Values

Adult: 0.5%–1.5% of all RBCs, 25,000–75,000 μL
Reticulocyte count = reticulocytes (%) × RBC count
Child: Newborn: 2.5%–6.5% of all RBCs; infant: 0.5%–3.5% of all RBCs; child: 0.5%–2.0% of all RBCs

Description. The reticulocyte count is an indicator of bone marrow activity and is used in diagnosing anemias. Reticulocytes are immature, non-nucleated RBCs that are formed in the bone marrow, pass into circulation, and in 1 to 2 days are matured RBCs. If the reticulocyte percent or count is abnormal, the test should be repeated, since the results can be different according to the time when the blood was tested. Both the RBC count and the reticulocyte count should be reported.

Purpose

- To aid in the diagnosis of anemias (pernicious, folic acid deficiency, hemolytic, sickle cell) (see Clinical Problems)

Clinical Problems

Decreased level: Anemias (pernicious, folic acid deficiency, aplastic), radiation therapy, x-ray irradiation, adrenocortical hypofunction, anterior pituitary hypofunction, cirrhosis of the liver (alcohol suppresses reticulocytes)

Elevated level: Anemias (hemolytic, sickle cell), treatment for anemias (iron deficiency, vitamin B_{12}, folic acid), thalassemia major, leukemias, posthemorrhage (3 to 4 days), erythroblastosis fetalis, hemoglobin C and D diseases, pregnancy

Procedure

Venous blood

- No food or fluid restriction is required.
- Collect 3 to 5 mL of venous blood in a lavender-top tube.

Capillary blood

- Cleanse the finger, and puncture the skin with a sterile lancet. Wipe the first drop of blood away.
- Collect blood by using a micropipette.

Nursing Implications

- Obtain a history regarding radiation exposure.
- Check the reticulocyte count and the RBC count. If the reticulocyte count is given as a percentage, convert the percentage to the count. See reference values.
- Monitor the reticulocyte count when the client is taking iron supplements for iron deficiency anemia or is being treated for pernicious anemia or folic acid anemia. An increased count suggests that the marrow is responding.

RHEUMATOID FACTOR (RF); RHEUMATOID ARTHRITIS (RA) FACTOR (SERUM)

RA LATEX FIXATION

Reference Values

Adult: <1:20 titer; 1:20–1:80 positive for rheumatoid and other conditions; >1:80 positive for rheumatoid arthritis

Child: Not usually done
Elderly: Slightly increased

Description. The rheumatoid factor (RF), or rheumatoid arthritis (RA) factor, test is a screening test to detect antibodies (IgM, IgG, or IgA) found in the serum of clients with rheumatoid arthritis. The RF occurs in 53% to 94% of clients with rheumatoid arthritis, and if the test is negative, it should be repeated.

Purposes

- To screen for IgM, IgG, or IgA antibodies present in clients with possible rheumatoid arthritis
- To aid in the diagnosis of rheumatoid arthritis
- To compare test results in relation to other laboratory tests for diagnosing rheumatoid arthritis

Clinical Problems

Elevated level: Rheumatoid arthritis, lupus erythematosus, dermatomyositis, scleroderma, infectious mononucleosis, tuberculosis, leukemia, sarcoidosis, cirrhosis of the liver, hepatitis, syphilis, chronic infections, myocardial infarction, renal disease

Procedure

- No food or fluid restriction is required.
- Collect 3 to 5 mL of venous blood in a red-top tube.

Factors Affecting Laboratory Results

- A positive RF test result frequently remains positive regardless of clinical improvement.
- The RF test result can be positive in various clinical problems, such as collagen diseases, cancer, and liver cirrhosis.
- The older adult may have an increased RF titer without the disease.

Nursing Implications

- Consider the age of the client when the RF is slightly increased. Elderly may have slightly increased RF titers without clinical symptoms of RA. With juvenile rheumatoid arthritis, only 10% of the children have a positive RF titer.

- Assess for pain in the small joints of the hands and feet, which could be indicative of early-stage rheumatoid arthritis.
- Compare RF test results with C-reactive protein test. With RF test it may take 6 months for a significant elevation of the RF titer.

RH TYPING (BLOOD)

Reference Values

Adult: Rh^+ (positive). Rh^- (negative)
Child: Same as adult

Description. Rh typing is performed when typing donor/recipient blood and for crossmatching blood for transfusion. Rh positive (most common Rh factor) indicates the presence of antigen on RBCs, and Rh negative indicates an absence of the antigen. An Rh-negative woman carrying a fetus with an Rh-positive blood group can cause Rh-positive antigens from the fetus to seep into the mother's blood, causing Rh antibody formation. To prevent Rh antibodies, the Rh-negative woman is given Rho(D) immune globulin, such as RhoGAM, within 3 days after delivery with the first child or after a miscarriage to neutralize any anti-Rh antibodies.

Purpose

- To identify client's Rh factor during pregnancy or for blood transfusion

Clinical Problems

Elevated anti-Rh antibodies
Infant: erythroblastosis fetalis

Procedure

- No food or fluid restriction is required.
- Collect 5 mL of venous blood in a red-top tube or 7 mL in a lavender-top tube.

Nursing Implications

- Obtain a history of previous blood transfusions. If pregnant, determine whether she has been pregnant before and whether the child was born jaundiced.
- Compare the tested Rh factor with the client's stated Rh factor.

Client Teaching

- Inform the pregnant woman with Rh-negative blood that her blood will be tested at intervals during pregnancy to determine if antibodies are produced. Rh-negative women usually receive RhoGAM after delivery to prevent anti-Rh antibody production.

ROTAVIRUS ANTIGEN (BLOOD AND FECES)

Reference Values

Blood and Stool: Negative

Description. Rotavirus is an RNA virus that frequently causes infectious diarrhea in infants and young children, usually between 2 months and 2 years old. Rotavirus is a significant cause of enteritis in infants and gastroenteritis in very young children. It is more prevalent in the winter months in the United States; it is year-round in the tropical areas. Adults can also become infected with this virus. Clinical symptoms include vomiting (usually precedes diarrhea), diarrhea, fever, and abdominal pain. This virus is frequently transmitted to infants and children in daycare centers, group homes, and preschools, and to the elderly in nursing homes. Symptoms in adults are normally mild.

The rotavirus is mainly transmitted by the fecal-oral route. It can be detected in the stool using electron microscopy or preferable ELISA screening. Kits are available for testing the stool specimen.

Purpose

- To identify the rotavirus that is causing gastroenteritis in infants and young children

Clinical Problems

Positive test result: Gastroenteritis caused by the rotavirus

Procedure

- Food and fluid are not restricted.

Blood

- Collect 5 mL of venous blood in a red-top tube. Avoid hemolysis.
- Test results are available in 24 hours.

Stool

- Obtain liquid stool and place the specimen in a closed container. The container should be placed on ice. A freshly soiled diaper may be used. Take immediately to the laboratory.
- A cotton-tip swab may be used to swab the rectum in a rotating motion. Leave the swab in the rectum for a few seconds for absorption. Place the swab in a tube or container, pack in ice, and send it immediately to the laboratory.
- No preservatives or metal container should be used. It interferes with ELISA testing.
- Test results are available in approximately 24 hours.

Nursing Implications

- Obtain a history of diarrhea, vomiting, and fever occurring in the child. Record the frequency of the symptoms and the color of the stool and vomitus.
- Take vital signs. Keep a chart of body temperatures.
- Collect stool according to the procedure. Have the specimen container iced and taken immediately to the laboratory.
- Answer the family's questions. Be supportive of the child and family members.

Client Teaching

- Demonstrate to the parent collection of the stool specimen. The stool specimen should be collected during the acute stage.
- Instruct the family member that the stool can be infectious and that the rotavirus could be transmitted to others if precautiosn are not taken. Hands should be thoroughly washed after changing soiled diapers. Diapers should be carefully placed in plastic bag and properly discarded.
- Instruct the parent to check the child's body temperature at specified intervals.
- Encourage the parent to increase the child's fluid intake, particularly electrolyte-based fluids.

- Inform the parent that the rotavirus is easily transmitted and that there is a higher risk of transmission in nurseries, day-care centers, group homes, and nursing homes.

RUBELLA ANTIBODY DETECTION (SERUM)

HEMAGGLUTINATION INHIBITION TEST (HAI OR HI) FOR RUBELLA

Reference Values

Adult: Titer <1:8. Susceptibility to rubella: titer 1:8–1:32. Past rubella exposure and immunity: titer 1:32–1:64; definite immunity: >1:64

Description. Rubella (German measles) is a mild viral disease of short duration causing a fever and a transient rash. The rubella virus produces antibodies against future rubella infections, but the exact antibody titer is unknown. Hemagglutination inhibition (HI or HAI) measures rubella antibody titers and is considered to be a sensitive and reliable test. Women should be immune to rubella or should receive the rubella vaccine before marriage and definitely before pregnancy. When women contract rubella during the first trimester of pregnancy, serious congenital deformities in the fetus could result.

Purpose

- To identify clients who are susceptible to rubella or have immunity to the rubella virus

Clinical Problems

Decreased level: <1:8: susceptible to rubella

Elevated level: >1:32: immunity; >1:64: definite immunity

Procedure

- No food or fluid restriction is required.
- Collect 5 mL of venous blood in a red-top tube.

Nursing Implications

- Obtain a history of having rubella and recent exposure to rubella virus.

Client Teaching

- Teach women the need to have their blood checked for rubella immunity before marriage and pregnancy. If the titer is <1:8, rubella vaccine should be received.
- Instruct pregnant women who are susceptible to German measles to avoid exposure to the disease. If exposed, the obstetrician should be notified immediately so that an HAI antibody titer test can be done.
- Explain to interested persons that fetal abnormalities can occur if the woman develops German measles during the first trimester of pregnancy. Professional help may be needed.
- Be supportive of individual and family.

SALICYLATE (SERUM)

Reference Values

Adult: Normal: negative; therapeutic: 5 mg/dL (headache), 10–30 mg/dL (rheumatoid arthritis); mild toxic: >30 mg/dL; severe toxic: >50 mg/dL; lethal: >60 mg/dL
Child: Toxic: >25 mg/dL
Elderly: Mild toxic: >25 mg/dL

Description. Salicylate levels are measured to check the therapeutic level, as in the treatment of rheumatic fever, and to check the levels caused by an accidental or deliberate overdose. Blood salicylate reaches its peak in 2 to 3 hours, and the blood level can be elevated for as long as 18 hours. Prolonged use of salicylates (aspirins) can cause bleeding tendencies, since it inhibits platelet aggregation.

Purposes

- To monitor salicylate level for daily therapeutic range
- To check for salicylate toxicity

Clinical Problems

Elevated level: >30 mg/dL: overdose or large, continuous doses of aspirin or drugs containing aspirin

Procedure

- No food or fluid restriction is required.
- Collect 5 to 7 mL of venous blood in a red- or green-top tube.
- A urine test may also be done as a screening test.

Nursing Implications

- Observe for signs and symptoms of early aspirin overdose (i.e., hyperventilation, flushed skin, and ringing in the ears).
- Obtain a history from the child or parent concerning the approximate number of aspirins taken. A toxic dose for a small child is 3.33 grains/kg, or 299 mg/kg. Salicylates are not the choice agent for children with virus because of the possibility of developing Reye's syndrome.

Client Teaching

- Instruct the client who takes aspirins regularly that before any surgery the surgeon should be informed of the number of aspirins taken daily.

SEMEN EXAMINATION/ANALYSIS

Reference Values

Male adult: Count: 50–150 million/mL (20 million/mL–low, low normal); volume: 1.5–5.0 mL; morphology: >75% mature spermatozoa; motility: >60% actively mobile spermatozoa
Child: Not usually done
Antisperm Antibody Test: Adult: Negative to 1:32

Description. Semen examination is one test that may determine the cause of infertility. The sperm count, volume of fluid, percent of normal mature spermatozoa (sperms), and the percent of actively mobile spermatozoa are studied when analyzing the semen content. Sexual abstinence is usually required for 3 days before the test. Masturbation is the usual method for obtaining a specimen; however, for religious reasons, intercourse with a condom is sometimes preferred.

Sperm count can be used to monitor the effectiveness of sterilization after a vasectomy. In cases of rape, a forensic or medicolegal analysis is done to detect semen in vaginal secretions or on clothes.

The *antisperm antibody test* could be ordered to identify a possible cause of infertility. Autoantibodies to sperm might result from a blocking of the efferent ducts in the testes.

Purposes

- To check the sperm count
- To determine if the decreased sperm count could be the cause of infertility

Clinical Problems

Decreased level: Infertility (0–2 million/mL), vasectomy
Drugs that may cause a low count: Antineoplastic agents, estrogen

Procedure

- Avoid alcoholic beverages for several days (at least 24 hours) before the test. No other food or fluid restrictions are required.
- Instruct client to abstain from intercourse for 3 days before collection of semen.
- Collect semen by
  - Masturbation: collect in a clean container.
  - Coitus interruptus: collect in a clean glass container.
  - Intercourse with a clean, washed condom: place the condom in a clean container.
- Keep the semen specimen from chilling, and take it to the laboratory within 30 minutes.

Factors Affecting Laboratory Results

- Recent intercourse (within 3 days) could have an effect on the sperm count.

Nursing Implications

- Be available to discuss methods of semen collection with the client and his spouse/partner.
- Be supportive of the client and his spouse/partner. Be a good listener, and give them time to express their concerns.
- Answer their questions, or refer the questions to the appropriate person (i.e., health care provider, clergy).
- Avoid giving your moral convictions about the test or the surgical procedure (vasectomy).

SICKLE CELL (SCREENING) TEST (BLOOD)

Reference Values

Adult: 0
Child: 0

Description. Hemoglobin S (sickle cell), an abnormal hemoglobin, causes RBCs to form a crescent or sickle shape when deprived of oxygen. With adequate oxygen, the red cells with hemoglobin S will maintain a normal shape.

If a sickle cell screening test is positive for hemoglobin S, hemoglobin electrophoresis should be ordered to differentiate between sickle cell anemia caused by hemoglobin S/S and sickle cell trait caused by hemoglobin A/S. If the client's hemoglobin level is less than 10 g/dL or the hematocrit is less than 30%, test results could be falsely negative.

Purpose

- To screen for sickle cell anemia

Clinical Problems

Positive results: Sickle cell anemia, sickle cell trait

Procedure

- No food or fluid restriction is required.
- Collect 3 to 7 mL of venous blood in a lavender-top tube.
- Note on the laboratory slip if blood transfusion was given 3 to 4 months before the screening test. If so, inaccurate results could result.
- If a commercial test kit (e.g., Sickledex) is used, follow the directions given on the kit.

Factors Affecting Laboratory Results

- A blood transfusion given within 3 to 4 months could cause inaccurate results.
- Hemoglobin <10 g/dL or hematocrit <30% could cause false-negative test results.

Nursing Implications

- Observe for signs nad symptoms of sickle cell anemia. Early symptoms are fatigue and weakness. Chronic symptoms are dyspnea on exertion, swollen joints, "aching bones," and chest pains

Client Teaching

- Instruct the client to avoid people with infections and colds.
- Encourage the client to seek genetic counseling if he or she has sickle cell anemia or the sickle cell trait.
- Instruct the client with sickle cell anemia to minimize strenuous activity and to avoid high altitudes and extreme cold. Encourage the client to take rest periods.

SODIUM (Na) SERUM AND URINE

Reference Values

Serum

Adult: 135–145 mEq/L; 135–145 mmol/L (SI units)
Infant: 134–150 mEq/L
Child: 135–145 mEq/L

Urine

Adult: 40–220 mEq/L/24 h
Child: Same as adult

Description. Sodium (Na) is the major cation in the extracellular fluid (ECF), and it has a water-retaining effect. Sodium has many functions: it helps to maintain body fluids, it is responsible for conduction of neuromuscular impulses via the sodium pump; and it is involved in enzyme activity.

The urine sodium level should be monitored when edema is present and the serum sodium level is low or normal. In congestive heart failure (CHF) the urine sodium level is usually low, and the serum sodium level is low-normal or normal due to hemodilution, or it is elevated.

Purposes

- To monitor sodium level
- To detect sodium imbalance (hypo- or hypernatremia)
- To compare sodium level with other electrolytes (i.e., calcium, potassium, sodium, chloride)

Clinical Problems. Serum sodium and urine sodium have many different clinical and drug problems.

Serum

Decreased level: Vomiting, diarrhea, gastric suction, syndrome of inappropriate antidiuretic hormone (SIADH), continuous IV D_5W, tissue injury, low-sodium diet, burns, salt-wasting renal disease

Drugs that may decrease sodium value: Diuretics (furosemide [Lasix], ethacrynic acid [Edecrin], thiazides, mannitol)

Elevated level: Dehydration, severe vomiting and diarrhea, CHF, adrenal hyperfunction, high-sodium diet, hepatic failure

Drugs that may increase sodium value: Cortisone preparations, antibiotics, laxatives, cough medicines

Urine

Decreased level: Adrenal hyperfunction, CHF, hepatic failure, renal failure, low-sodium diet

Drugs that may decrease urine sodium: Cortisone preparations

Elevated level: Adrenal hypofunction, dehydration, essential hypertension, anterior pituitary hypofunction, high-sodium diet

Drugs that may increase urine sodium: Loop or high-ceiling diuretics

Procedure

Serum

- No food or fluid restriction is required. If the client has eaten large quantities of foods high in salt content in the last 24 to 48 hours, this should be noted on the laboratory slip.
- Collect 3 to 5 mL of venous blood in a red- or green-top tube.

Urine

- Collect a 24-hour urine specimen, place all urine in a large container, and refrigerate. Label the container with the exact times the urine collection started and ended. First-voided specimen should be discarded.

Factors Affecting Laboratory Results

- A diet high in sodium

Nursing Implications

Decreased level: Hyponatremia

- Assess for signs and symptoms of hyponatremia (i.e., apprehension, anxiety, muscular twitching, muscular weakness, headaches, tachycardia, and hypotension).
- Recognize that hyponatremia may occur after surgery as the result of SIADH.
- Monitor the medical regimen for correcting hyponatremia (i.e., water restriction, normal saline solution to correct a serum sodium level of 120 to 130 mEq/L, and 3% saline to correct a serum sodium level of less than 115 mEq/L).
- Check the specific gravity of urine. A specific gravity of less than 1.010 could indicate hyponatremia.
- Irrigate NG tubes and wound sites with normal saline instead of sterile water.
- Compare the serum sodium level with the urine sodium level. A low or normal serum sodium and a low urine sodium could indicate sodium retention or a decrease in sodium intake.

Client Teaching

- Suggest that client drink fluids with solutes, such as broth and juices; client should avoid drinking only plain water.

Elevated level: Hypernatremia

- Observe for signs and symptoms of hypernatremia (i.e., restlessness; thirst; flushed skin; dry, sticky mucous membranes; a rough, dry tongue; and tachycardia).
- Check for body fluid loss by keeping an accurate intake and output record and weighing the client daily.
- Check the specific gravity of the urine. A specific gravity over 1.030 could indicate hypernatremia.
- Observe for edema and overhydration resulting from an elevated serum sodium level. Signs and symptoms of overhydration are a constant, irritating cough; dyspnea; neck-and-hand vein engorgement; and chest rales.

Client Teaching

- Instruct the client to avoid foods that are high in sodium (i.e., corned beef, bacon, ham, canned or smoked fish, cheese, celery, catsup, pickles, olives, potato chips, and Pepsi Cola). Also, avoid using salt when cooking or at mealtime.

TESTOSTERONE (SERUM OR PLASMA)

Reference Values

Adult: Male: 0.3–1.0 µg/dL, 300–1,000 ng/dL; female: 0.03–0.1 µg/dL, 30–100 ng/dL
Child: Male: 12–14 years: >0.1 µg/dL, >100 ng/dL

Description. Testosterone, a male sex hormone, is produced by the testes and adrenal glands in the male and by the ovaries and adrenal glands in the female. It is useful in diagnosing male sexual precocity before the age of 10 years and male infertility. The highest serum testosterone levels occur in the morning.

Purposes

- To assess testosterone value
- To detect testicular hypofunction
- To aid in the diagnosis of male sexual precocity

Clinical Problems

Decreased level: Testicular hypofunction, primary hypogonadism (Klinefelter's syndrome), alcoholism, anterior pituitary hypofunction, estrogen therapy

Elevated level: Male sexual precocity, adrenal hyperplasia, adrenogenital syndrome in women, polycystic ovaries

Procedure

- No food or fluid restriction is required.
- Collect 5 to 7 mL of venous blood in a red- or green-top tube. Avoid hemolysis.

Nursing Implications

- Be supportive of the male patient and his family concerning physical changes caused by hormonal deficiency.
- Observe for signs and symptoms of excess testosterone secretion (i.e., hirsutism, masculine voice, and increased muscle mass).

THEOPHYLLINE (SERUM)

AMINOPHYLLINE, THEO-DUR, THEOLAIRE, SLO-PHYLLIN

Reference Values

Therapeutic range: Adult: 5–20 μg/mL, 28–112 μmol/L (SI units); elderly: 5–18 μg/mL; **premature** infants: 7–14 μg/mL; **neonate:** 3–12 μg/mL; child: same as adult
Toxic level: Adult: >20 μg/mL, >112 μmol/L (SI units); elderly: same as adult; child: premature infants: >14 μg/mL; neonate: >13 μg/mL; child: same as adult

Description. Theophylline, a xanthine derivative, relaxes smooth muscle of the bronchi and pulmonary blood vessels; stimulates the CNS; stimulates myocardium; increases renal blood flow, causing diuresis; and relaxes smooth muscles of the GI tract. Usually, theophylline products are given to control asthmatic attacks and to treat acute attack. Theophylline has a shorter half-life in smokers and children, so dosage may need to be increased. It has a narrow therapeutic range, and serum levels should be monitored. If severe theophylline toxicity occurs, >30 μg/mL, cardiac dysrhythmias, seizures, respiratory arrest, and/or cardiac arrest might result.

Purpose

- To monitor theophylline levels

Clinical Problems

Decreased level: Smoking
Drugs that may decrease serum theophylline: Phenytoin (Dilantin), barbiturate

Elevated level: Theophylline overdose, CHF, liver disease, lung disease, renal disease
Drugs that may increase serum theophylline: Cimetidine (Tagamet), propranolol (Inderal), erythromycin, allopurinol

Procedure

- No food or fluid restriction is required, except no coffee, tea, colas, or chocolates 8 hours prior to test.

- Collect 3 to 5 mL of venous blood in a red-top tube. Avoid hemolysis.
- Record the name of the drug, dose, route, and last dose administered on the laboratory requisition slip.
- List drugs the client is taking that could affect test results on the laboratory slip.

Factors Affecting Laboratory Tests

- Chocolate, coffee, tea, and colas could increase serum theophylline level.

Nursing Implications

- Check theophylline level, and report nontherapeutic levels to the health care provider immediately.
- Recognize that smoking and the drug phenytoin (Dilantin) shorten half-life and promote a faster theophylline clearance.
- Observe for signs and symptoms of theophylline toxicity (i.e., anorexia, nausea, vomiting, abdominal discomfort, nervousness, jitters, irritability, tachycardia, and cardiac dysrhythmias).
- Monitor pulse rate, and report signs of tachycardia and skipped beats.
- Monitor intake and output. Report if client's output has greatly increased due to the theophylline effect.

THYROID ANTIBODIES (TA) SERUM

THYROID AUTOANTIBODIES; ANTITHYROGLOBULIN ANTIBODY AND ANTIMICROSOMAL ANTIBODY

Reference Values. Antithyroglobulin: negative to titer <1:20; antimicrosomal: negative to titer <1:100

Description. Thyroid autoimmune disease produces thyroid antibodies (antithyroglobulin antibodies and antimicrosomal antibodies). If thyroglobulin breaks away from thyroxine and enters the circulation, antithyroglobulin antibodies usually form. Antimicrosomal antibodies form if the microsomes of the thyroid epithelial cells are attacked. An increase in these thyroid antibodies damage the thyroid gland. Usually, serum titers are ordered to detect the presence of one or both of the thyroid antibodies.

With thyrotoxicosis, a positive titer of 1:1600 may occur and with Hashimoto's thyroditis, the titer may be greater than 1:5000. Antibodies to thyroglobulin may be detected in 40% to 70% of clients with chronic thyroiditis, 40% of clients with Graves' disease (thyrotoxicosis), and 70% of clients having hypothyroidism (low to moderate titer elevation). Antibodies to thyroid microsomes occur in 70% to 90% of clients with chronic thyroiditis.

Purposes

- To aid in the diagnosis of Graves' disease
- To detect the presence of thyroid antibodies which may cause a thyroid autoimmune disease

Clinical Problems

Elevated titer: Chronic thyroiditis, Hashimoto's thyroiditis, Graves' disease (thyrotoxicosis), pernicious anemia, lupus erythematosus, rheumatoid arthritis

Procedure

- No food or fluid restriction is required.
- Collect 5 mL of venous blood in a red-top tube. Avoid hemolysis.

Nursing Implications

- Obtain a family history of thyroid disease. Determine whether the client has had a viral infection in the last few weeks or months. It is believed that viral infections can trigger autoimmune disease.
- Check the serum thyroglobulin antibody and serum microsomal antibody results. An extremely high serum thyroglobulin test can indicate Hashimoto's thyroditis.
- Be supportive to the client and family.

THYROID-STIMULATING HORMONE (TSH) SERUM

Reference Values. Values differ according to laboratory method used
Adult: ***0.35–5.5*** μIU/mL, <10 μU/mL, <10^3 IU/L (SI units), <3 ng/mL
Child: Newborn: <25 μIU/mL by the third day

Description. The anterior pituitary gland secretes thyroid-stimulating hormone (TSH) in response to thyroid-releasing hormone (TRH) from the hypothalamus. TSH stimulates the secretion of thyroxine (T_4) produced in the thyroid gland. TSH and T_4 levels are frequently measured to differentiate pituitary from thyroid dysfunctions. A decreased T_4 level and a normal or elevated TSH level can indicate a thyroid disorder. A decreased T_4 level with a decreased TSH level can indicate a pituitary disorder.

Purposes

- To suggest secondary hypothyroidism due to pituitary involvement
- To compare test results with T_4 level to differentiate between pituitary and thyroid dysfunction

Clinical Problems

Decreased level: Secondary hypothyroidism (pituitary involvement), hyperthyroidism, anterior pituitary hypofunction
Drugs that may decrease TSH value: Aspirin, steroids, dopamine, and heparin

Elevated level: Primary hypothyroidism (thyroid involvement), thyroiditis (Hashimoto's autoimmune disease), antithyroid therapy for hyperthyroidism
Drugs that may increase TSH value: Lithium, potassium iodide

Procedure

- No food or fluid restriction is required. Avoid shellfish for several days prior to test.
- Collect 5 mL of venous blood in a red- or green-top tube. Avoid hemolysis.
- Neonate measurement: see Thyroxine.

Nursing Implications

- Recognize the cause of hypothyroidism by comparing the TSH level with the T_4 level. Decreased TSH and T_4 levels could be due to anterior pituitary dysfunction causing secondary hypothyroidism. A normal or elevated TSH and a decreased T_4 could be due to thyroid dysfunction.
- Observe for signs and symptoms of hypothyroidism (i.e., anorexia; fatigue; weight gain; dry and flaky skin; puffy face, hands, and feet; abdominal distention; bradycardia; infertility; and ataxia).
- Monitor vital signs before and during treatment for hypothyroidism. Report if tachycardia occurs.

THYROXINE (T_4) SERUM

Reference Values

Adult: Reported as serum thyroxine: T_4 by column: 4.5–11.5 μg/dL. T_4 RIA: 5–12 μg/dL; free T_4: 1.0–2.3 ng/dL; reported as thyroxine iodine: T_4 by column: 3.2–7.2 μg/dL

Child: Newborn: 11–23 μg/dL; 1–4 mo: 7.5–16.5 μg/dL; 4–12 mo: 5.5–14.5 μg/dL; 1–6 yr: 5.5–13.5 μg/dL; 6–10 yr: 5–12.5 μg/dL

Description. Thyroxine (T_4) is the major hormone secreted by the thyroid gland and is at least 25 times more concentrated than triiodothyronine (T_3). The serum T_4 levels are commonly used to measure thyroid hormone concentration and to determine thyroid function. Other thyroid laboratory tests should be performed to verify and confirm thyroid gland disorders.

In some institutions the T_4 test is required for all newborns to detect a decreased thyroxine secretion, which could lead to irreversible mental retardation.

Purposes

- To determine thyroid function
- To aid in the diagnosis of hypo- or hyperthyroidism
- To compare test results with other laboratory thyroid tests

Clinical Problems

Decreased level: Hypothyroidism (cretinism, myxedema), protein malnutrition, anterior pituitary hypofunction, strenuous exercise, renal failure

Drugs that may decrease T_4 value: Cortisone, chlorpromazine (Thorazine), phenytoin (Dilantin), heparin, lithium, sulfonamides, reserpine (Serpasil), testosterone, propranolol (Inderal), tolbutamide (Orinase), salicylates (high doses)

Elevated level: Hyperthyroidism, acute thyroiditis, viral hepatitis, myasthenia gravis, pregnancy, preeclampsia

Drugs that may increase T_4 value: Oral contraceptives, estrogen, clofibrate, perphenazine (Trilafon)

Procedure

- No food or fluid restriction is required.
- Collect 5 to 7 mL of venous blood in a red-top tube. Prevent hemolysis.
- List drugs that may affect test results on the laboratory slip.
- Neonate measurement: Warm or massage heel of neonate; clean area; wipe alcohol from site; wipe off first drop of blood; touch special filter paper with drops of blood. Test is usually performed after third day.

Nursing Implications

Decreased level

- Observe for signs and symptoms of hypothyroidism (i.e., fatigue, forgetfulness, weight gain, dry skin with poor turgor, dry and thin hair, bradycardia, decreased peripheral circulation, depressed libido, infertility, and constipation).

Elevated level

- Observe for signs and symptoms of hyperthyroidism (i.e., nervousness, tremors, emotional instability, increased appetite, weight loss, palpitations, tachycardia, diarrhea, decreased fertility, and exophthalmos).
- Monitor the pulse rate. Tachycardia is common and, if severe, could cause heart failure and cardiac arrest.

TORCH SCREEN TEST

TORCH BATTERY, TORCH TITER

Reference Values

Maternal: IgG titer antibodies: negative
IgM titer antibodies: negative

Infant: Same as mother; infant should be tested under 2 months of age

Description. TORCH stand for toxoplasmosis, rubella, cytomegalovirus (CMV), and herpes simplex. It is a screen test to detect the presence of these organisms in the mother and newborn infant. The two common viruses that affect the infant most are CMV and rubella. During pregnancy, TORCH infections can cross the placenta and could result in mild or severe congenital malformation, abortion, or stillbirth. The severe effect from these organisms occurs during the first trimester. If the fetus is infected, the organism remains throughout the pregnancy.

TORCH screening test is more frequently performed when congenital infection in the newborn is suspected. The IgG titers are compared with both the mother and newborn serum. If the IgG titer level is higher in the fetus than the mother, congenital TORCH infection is likely. The test may be repeated in several weeks. Individual testing may be necessary along with a clinical examination and history taking to identify the TORCH infection.

Purpose

- To detect TORCH infection in newborns and mothers

Clinical Problems

Positive IgG, IgM titers: Toxoplasmosis, rubella, CMV, herpes simplex

Procedure

- No food or fluid restriction is required.
- Collect 7 mL of venous blood in a red-top tube.
- TORCH kits: Follow directions on the kit.

Nursing Implications

- Obtain a history from the client about any previous infection.
- Be supportive to the client and family regarding their concerns and fear.

Client Teaching

- Inform the client that several tests may be necessary to confirm a diagnosis.

TOXOPLASMOSIS ANTIBODY TEST (SERUM)

Reference Values

Titer: <1:4, no previous infection from *T. gondii*
Titer: 1:4 to 1:64, past exposure, many persist for life
Titer: >1:256, recent infection
Titer: >1:424, acute infection

Description. *Toxoplasma gondii (T. gondii)* is a protozoan organism that causes the parasitic disease, toxoplasmosis. In the United States 25% to 40% of the population have antibodies to *T. gondii.* Half of these persons are asymptomatic. This organism can remain in body muscle and be dormant for years or life. This organism is transmitted in raw or poorly cooked meat or by ingesting occysts from feces of infected cats. Transmission from the latter may occur when changing the cat litter.

Congenital form of toxoplasmosis occurs to the fetus when the mother is acutely infected with the *T. gondii* during pregnancy and passed the organism via placenta to the unborn child. Congenital toxoplasmosis may cause mental retardation, hydrocephalus, microcephalus, and chronic retinitis, or could lead to fetal death. The Centers for Disease Control recommends a serological test for *T. gondii* antibody titer for all pregnant women before the 20th week. Toxoplasmosis is not communicable between individuals except for maternal-fetal transfer.

The IgM antibody titer begins to rise 1 week after infection and peaks in 1 to 3 weeks. The IgG antibody titer rises in approximately 4 to 7 days after the IgM antibody, peaks 1 to 3 weeks later, and falls slowly within 6 months. Sulfonamides may be used to treat toxoplasmosis.

Purposes

- To identify the *T. gondii* organism
- To detect the *T. gondii* organism in pregnant woman before the 20th week

Clinical Problems

Elevated titers: Toxoplasmosis. Low positive titer: Past infection of *T. gondii.* High positive titer: Current active infection of *T. gondii.*

Procedure

- No food or fluid restriction is required.
- Collect 5 to 7 mL of venous blood in a red-top tube during early weeks of pregnancy or if suggestive symptoms are present. Test may be repeated in 2 weeks to determine if there is a rise in antibody titer.

Nursing Implications

- Obtain a history of meat ingested that was raw or poorly cooked or of contact with a cat and cat litter. Ask whether the cat roams the street or is completely housebound.
- Check if the client is pregnant and has a cat. Ascertain if the pregnant woman handles the cat litter.
- Check if the client has ever been serologically tested for toxoplasmosis. Chronic toxoplasmosis has a low-positive titer.

Client Teaching

- Instruct the client to cook all meat thoroughly. Raw or poorly cooked meat may have the *T. gondii* organism.
- Inform cat owners that meticulous handwashing is essential after changing the cat litter.
- Instruct the pregnant woman not to handle the cat litter. Cats that are allowed to roam the streets may have acquired the *T. gondii* organism.
- Instruct the pregnant woman with an outdoor cat to inform her obstetrician so that a titer level could be taken and monitored.
- Answer client's questions or refer them to appropriate personnel.

TRIGLYCERIDES (SERUM)

Reference Values

Adult: 12–29 yr: 10–140 mg/dL; 30–39 yr: 20–150 mg/dL; 40–49 yr: 30–160 mg/dL; >50 yr: 40–190 mg/dL, 0.44–2.09 mmol/L (SI units)
Child: Infant: 5–40 mg/dL; 5–11 yr: 10–135 mg/dL

Description. Triglycerides are a blood lipid carried by the serum lipoproteins. Triglycerides are a major contributor to arterial diseases and are frequently compared with cholesterol with the use of lipoprotein electrophoresis. As the concentration of triglycerides increases, so will the very low density lipoproteins (VLDL) increase, leading to hyperlipoproteinemia. Alcohol intake can cause a transient elevation of serum triglyceride levels.

Purposes

- To monitor triglyceride levels
- To compare test results with lipoprotein groups (VLDL) that indicate hyperlipemia

Clinical Problems

Decreased level: Congenital β-lipoproteinemia, hyperthyroidism, protein malnutrition, exercise
Drugs that may decrease triglyceride value: Ascorbic acid, clofibrate (Atromid-S), phenformin, metformin

Elevated level: Hyperlipoproteinemia, acute myocardial infarction (AMI), hypertension, hypothyroidism, nephrotic syndrome, cerebral thrombosis, alcoholic cirrhosis, uncontrolled diabetes mellitus, Down syndrome, stress, high-carbohydrate diet, pregnancy
Drugs that may increase triglyceride value: Estrogen, oral contraceptives

Procedure

- Restrict food, fluids, and medications after 6 PM the night before the test, except for water. Hold medications until blood is drawn. Maintain a normal diet for 2 or more days before the test.

- No alcohol is allowed for 24 hours before the test.
- Collect 3 to 5 mL of venous blood in a red-top tube.
- Note on laboratory slip if client's weight has increased or decreased in the last 2 weeks.

Factors Affecting Laboratory Results

- A high-carbohydrate diet and alcohol can elevate the serum triglyceride level.

Nursing Implications

- Check to see if a lipoprotein electrophoresis has been ordered, which is frequently done when the triglycerides are elevated.

Client Teaching

- Instruct the client with a high serum triglyceride level to avoid eating excessive amounts of sugars and carbohydrates as well as dietary fats. The client should be encouraged to eat fruits.

TRIIODOTHYRONINE (T_3) SERUM

T_3 RIA

Reference Values

Adult: 80–200 ng/dL
Child: Newborn: 40–215 ng/dL; 5 to 10 yr: 95–240 ng/dL; 10 to 15 yr: 80–210 ng/dL

Description. Triiodothyronine (T_3), one of the thyroid hormones, is present in small amounts in blood and is more short acting and more potent than thyroxine (T_4). Both T_3 and T_4 have similar actions in the body. Serum T_3 radioimmunoassay (RIA) measures both bound and free T_3. It is effective for diagnosing hyperthyroidism, especially T_3 thyrotoxicosis, in which T_3 is increased and T_4 is in normal range. It is not as reliable for diagnosing hypothyroidism, for T_3 remains in normal range. T_3 RIA and T_3 update are two different tests.

Purposes

- To aid in the diagnosis of hyperthyroidism
- To compare T_3 with T_4 for determining thyroid disorder

Clinical Problems

Decreased level: Severe illness and trauma, malnutrition
Drugs that may decrease T_3 value: Propylthiouracil, methylthiouracil, methimazole (Tapazole), lithium, phenytoin (Dilantin), propranolol (Inderal), reserpine (Serpasil), aspirin (large doses), steroids, sulfonamides

Elevated level: Hyperthyroidism, T_3 thyrotoxicosis, toxic adenoma, Hashimoto's thyroiditis
Drugs that may increase T_3 value: Estrogen, progestins, oral contraceptives, liothyronine (T_3), methadone

Procedure

- No food or fluid restriction is required.
- Withhold drugs that affect test results for 24 hours with health care provider's approval.
- Collect 5 to 7 mL of venous blood in a red-top tube. Avoid hemolysis.

Nursing Implications

Elevated level

- Observe for signs and symptoms of hyperthyroidism (i.e., nervousness, tremors, emotional instability, increased appetite, weight loss, palpitations, tachycardia, diarrhea, decreased fertility, and exophthalmos).
- Monitor pulse rate. Tachycardia is common and, if severe, could cause heart failure.

TRIIODOTHYRONINE RESIN UPTAKE (T_3 RU) SERUM

T_3 UPTAKE

Reference Value

Adult: 25%–35% uptake

Description. T_3 resin uptake is an indirect measure of free thyroxine (T_4), whereas serum T_3 RIA is a direct measurement of T_3. This is an in vitro test in which the client's blood is mixed with radioactive T_3 and synthetic resin material in a test tube. The radioactive T_3 will bind at available thyroid-binding globulin (protein) sites. The unbound radioactive T_3 is added to resin for T_3 uptake. In hyperthyroidism there are few binding sites left, so more T_3 is taken up by the resin, thus causing a high T_3 resin uptake. In hypothyroidism there is less T_3 resin uptake.

This test is performed when clients receive drugs, diagnostic agents, inorganic or organic iodine. It should not be used as the only test to determine thyroid dysfunction.

Purposes

- To differentiate between hypo- or hyperthyroidism
- To compare test result with T_3 for determining thyroid disorder

Clinical Problems

Decreased level: Hypothyroidism (cretinism, myxedema), pregnancy, Hashimoto's thyroiditis, menstruation, acute hepatitis
Drugs that may decrease T_3 RU: Corticosteroids, estrogen, oral contraceptives, antithyroid agents (methimazole, propylthiouracil), thiazides, chlordiazepoxide (Librium), tolbutamide (Orinase), clofibrate

Elevated level: Hyperthyroidism, protein malnutrition, metastatic carcinoma, myasthenia gravis, nephrotic syndrome, threatened abortion, renal failure, malnutrition
Drugs that may increase T_3 RU: Corticosteroids, warfarin (Coumadin), heparin, phenytoin (Dilantin), phenylbutazone (Butazolidin), aspirin (high doses), thyroid agents, salicylates (high doses)

Procedure

- No food or fluid restriction is required.
- Collect 5 to 7 mL of venous blood in a red-top tube. Prevent hemolysis.
- List drugs that may affect test results on the laboratory slip.

Nursing Implications

Decreased level: See Thyroxine (serum)

Elevated level: See Thyroxine (serum)

URIC ACID (SERUM AND URINE)

Reference Values. Values may differ among laboratories.

Serum

Adult: Male: 3.5–8.0 mg/dL; female: 2.8–6.8 mg/dL. *Panic values:* >12 mg/dL

Child: 2.5–5.5 mg/dL

Elderly: 3.5–8.5 mg/dL

Urine

Adult: 250–500 mg/24 h (low-purine diet); 250–750 mg/dL (normal diet)

Child: Same as adult

Description. Uric acid is a by-product of purine metabolism. An elevated urine and serum uric acid (hyperuricemia) depend on renal function, purine metabolism rate, and dietary intake of purine foods. Excess quantities of uric acid are excreted in the urine. Uric acid can crystallize in the urinary tract in acidic urine; therefore, effective renal function and alkaline urine are necessary with hyperuricemia. The most common problem associated with hyperuricemia is gout. Uric acid levels frequently change day by day; thus, uric acid levels may be repeated several days or weeks.

Purposes

- To monitor serum uric acid during treatment for gout
- To aid in the diagnosis of health problems (see Clinical Problems)

Clinical Problems

Serum

Decreased level: Wilson's disease, proximal renal tubular acidosis, folic acid anemia, burns, pregnancy

Drugs that may decrease uric acid value: Allopurinol, azathioprine (Imuran), warfarin (Coumadin), probenecid (Benemid), sulfinpyrazone

Elevated level: Gout, alcoholism, leukemias, metastatic cancer, multiple myeloma, severe eclampsia, hyperlipoproteinemia, diabetes mellitus (severe), renal failure, glomerulonephritis, stress, congestive heart failure, lead poisoning, strenuous exercise, malnutrition, lymphoma, hemolytic anemia, megaloblastic anemia, infectious mononucleosis, polycythemia vera

Drugs that may increase uric acid value: Acetaminophen, ascorbic acid, diuretics (thiazides, acetazolamide [Diamox], furosemide [Lasix]), levodopa, methyldopa (Aldomet), phenothiazine, prolonged use of aspirin, theophylline, 6-mercaptopurine

Urine

Decreased level: Renal diseases (glomerulonephritis [chronic], urinary obstruction, uremia), eclampsia, lead toxicity

Elevated level: Gout, high-purine-diet leukemias, neurologic disorders, manic-depressive disease, ulcerative colitis

Procedure

Serum

- No food or fluid restriction is necessary, unless purine diet is restricted.
- Collect 3 to 5 mL of venous blood in a red-top tube.
- List drugs the client is taking that can affect test results on the laboratory slip.

Urine

- Collect a 24-hour urine specimen in a large container and refrigerate. A preservative in the container may be necessary.
- Label the container with the client's name, dates of collection, and times (e.g., 9/23/04, 7:11 AM to 9/24/04, 7:15 AM).
- Note on the laboratory slip if client is on a low, high, or normal purine diet.

Nursing Implications

- Request the dietitian to visit the client to discuss food preferences and to plan a low-purine diet.
- Observe for signs and symptoms of gout (i.e., tophi [crystallized uric acid deposits] of the ear lobe and joints, joint pain, and edema in the "big toe").
- Monitor urinary output. Poor urine output could indicate inadequate fluid intake or poor kidney function.

- Check urine pH, especially if hyperuremia is present. Uric acid stone can occur when the urine pH is low (acidic). Alkaline urine helps to prevent stones in urinary tract.
- Compare the serum uric acid level with the urine uric acid level. An elevated serum uric acid level (hyperuricemia) and a decreased urine uric acid level can indicate kidney dysfunction. Increased serum and urine uric acid levels are frequently seen in gout.

Client Teaching

- Teach the client to avoid eating foods that have moderate or high amounts of purines, such as:

  High (100–1,000 mg purine nitrogen): brains, heart, kidney, liver, sweetbreads, roe, sardines, scallops, mackerel, anchovies, broth, consommé, mincemeat

  Moderate (9–100 mg purine nitrogen): meat, poultry, fish, shellfish, asparagus, beans, mushrooms, peas, spinach
- Instruct the client to decrease alcoholic intake, since alcohol can cause renal retention of urate.

URINALYSIS (ROUTINE)

Reference Values

	Adult	*Newborn*	*Child*
Color	Light straw to dark amber		Light straw to dark yellow
Appearance	Clear	Clear	Clear
Odor	Aromatic		Aromatic
pH	4.5–8.0	5.0–7.0	4.5–8.0
Specific gravity	1.005–1.030	1.001–1.020	1.005–1.030
Protein	2–8 mg/dL; negative reagent strip test		
Glucose	Negative		Negative
Ketones	Negative		Negative
Microscopic examination	1–2 per low-power field		

(continued)

	Adult	*Newborn*	*Child*
RBC			Rare
WBC	3–4		0–4
Casts	Occas. hyaline		Rare

Description. Urinalysis is useful for diagnosing renal disease and urinary tract infection and for detecting metabolic disease not related to the kidneys. Many routine urinalyses are done in the health care provider's office.

Purposes

- To detect normal vs abnormal urine components
- To detect glycosuria
- To aid in the diagnosis of renal disorder

Clinical Problems

Color: **Colorless or pale:** large fluid intake, diabetes insipidus, chronic kidney disease, alcohol ingestion. **Red or red-brown:** hemoglobinuria, porphyrins, menstrual contamination; Drugs: sulfisoxazole–phenazopyridine (Azo Gantrisin), phenytoin (Dilantin), cascara, chlorpromazine (Thorazine), docusate calcium and phenolphthalein (Doxidan), phenolphthalein; Foods: beets, rhubarb, food color; **Orange:** restricted fluid intake, concentrated urine, urobilin, fever; Drugs: amidopyrine, nitrofurantoin, phenazopyridine (Pyridium), sulfonamides; Foods: carrots, rhubarb, food color; **Blue or green:** *Pseudomonas* toxemia; Drugs: amitriptyline (Elavil), methylene blue, methacarbanol (Robaxin), yeast concentrate; **Brown or black:** Lysol poisoning, melanin, bilirubin, methemoglobin, porphyrin; Drugs: cascara, iron injectable

Appearance: **Hazy or cloudy:** bacteria, pus, RBC, WBC, phosphates, prostatic fluid spermatozoa, urates; **Milky:** fat, pyuria

Odor: **Ammonia:** urea breakdown by bacteria; **Foul or putrid:** bacteria (urinary tract infection); **Mousey:** phenylketonuria; **Sweet or fruity:** diabetic ketoacidosis, starvation

Foam: **Yellow:** severe cirrhosis of the liver, bilirubin, or bile

pH: **<4.5:** Metabolic acidosis, respiratory acidosis, starvation diarrhea, diet high in meat protein; Drugs: ammonium chloride, mandelic acid; >8.0: bacteriuria, urinary tract infection; Drugs: antibiotics (neomycin, kanamycin), sulfonamides, sodium bicarbonate, acetazolamide (Diamox), potassium citrate

Specific gravity: **<1.005:** diabetes insipidus, excess fluid intake, overhydration, renal disease, severe potassium deficit; **>1.026:** decreased fluid intake, fever, diabetes mellitus, vomiting, diarrhea, dehydration. Contrast media

Protein: **>8 mg/dL or >80 mg/24 h:** proteinuria, exercise, severe stress, fever, acute infectious diseases, renal diseases, lupus erythematosus, leukemia, multiple myeloma, cardiac disease, toxemia of pregnancy, septicemia, lead, mercury; Drugs: barbiturates, neomycin, sulfonamides

Glucose: **>15 mg/dL or +4:** diabetes mellitus, CNS disorders (stroke), Cushing's syndrome, anesthesia, glucose infusions, severe stress, infections; Drugs: ascorbic acid, aspirin, cephalosporins, epinephrine

Ketones: **+1 to +3:** ketoacidosis, starvation, diet high in proteins

RBCs: **>2 per low-power field:** trauma to the kidneys, renal diseases, renal calculi, cystitis, lupus nephritis, excess aspirin, anticoagulants, sulfonamides, menstrual contamination

WBCs: **>4 per low-power field:** urinary tract infection, fever, strenuous exercise, lupus nephritis, renal diseases

Casts: fever, renal diseases, heart failure

Procedure

- No food or fluid restriction is required, unless NPO for an early morning specimen is ordered by the health care provider.
- Collect a freshly voided urine specimen (50 mL) in a clean, dry container and take it to the laboratory within 30 minutes. An early morning urine specimen collected before breakfast is preferred. The urine specimen could be refrigerated for 6 to 8 hours.
- A clean-caught or midstream urine specimen may be requested if bacteria or WBCs are suspected. Follow directions on the clean-caught urine container.
- Make sure there are no feces or toilet paper in the urine specimen.

Factors Affecting Laboratory Results

- A urine specimen that has been sitting for an hour or longer without refrigeration.

Nursing Implications

- Assist the client with the urine collection as needed.
- Obtain a history of any drugs the client is currently taking.
- Obtain a history of foods taken in excess amounts that could affect test results.
- Assess the fluid status of the client. Early morning urine specimen, dehydration, and decreased fluid intake usually result in concentrated urine.

Client Teaching

- Instruct client that the urine specimen should be taken to the laboratory within 30 minutes or else refrigerated.

UROBILINOGEN (URINE)

Reference Values

Adult: Random: negative or <1.0 Ehrlich units; 2-hour specimen: 0.3–1.0 Ehrlich units; 24 hour: 0.5–4.0 mg/24 h, 0.5–4.0 Ehrlich units/24 h, 0.09–4.23 μmol/24 h (SI units)
Child: Similar to adult

Description. Urobilinogen test is one of the most sensitive tests for determining liver damage, hemolytic disease, and severe infections. In early hepatitis, mild liver cell damage, or mild toxic injury, the urine urobilinogen level will increase despite an unchanged serum bilirubin level. The urobilinogen level will frequently decrease in severe liver damage, since less bile will be produced. The urobilinogen test may be one of the tests performed during urinalysis.

Purpose

- To aid in determining liver damage

Clinical Problems

Decreased level: Biliary obstruction, severe liver disease, cancer of the pancreas, severe inflammatory disease
Drugs that may decrease urine urobilinogen: Antibiotics, ammonium chloride, ascorbic acid

Elevated level: Cirrhosis of the liver (early), infectious hepatitis, toxic hepatitis, hemolytic and pernicious anemia, erythroblastosis fetalis, infectious mononucleosis
Drugs that may increase urine urobilinogen: Sulfonamides, phenothiazines, cascara, phenazopyridine (Pyridium), methenamine mandelate (Mandelamine), sodium bicarbonate

Procedure

- No food or fluid restriction is required.

2-hour urine specimen

- Collect 2-hour specimen between 1 and 3 PM or 2 and 4 PM, as urobilinogen peaks in the afternoon. Urine should be kept refrigerated or in a dark container. Urine should be tested within ½ hour, as urine urobilinogen oxidizes to urobilin (orange substance).

24-hour urine specimen

- Collect 24-hour urine specimen, place in a large container, and keep refrigerated. A preservative may be added to the container.
- Label the container with the client's name, date, and time of urine collection.
- List drugs that affect test results on the laboratory slip.

Nursing Implications

- Check for an elevated urobilinogen level in freshly voided urine with a reagent color dipstick. Record the results of the single test.
- Assess for signs and symptoms of jaundice (i.e., yellow sclera, skin on the forearm is yellow).

Client Teaching

- Explain the procedure to the client for the 2-hour or 24-hour test.

VIRAL CULTURE (BLOOD, BIOPSY, CEREBROSPINAL FLUID, PHARYNX, RECTUM, SPUTUM, STOOL, URINE)

Reference Value

Negative culture result

Description. The virus culture is performed to confirm a suspected viral infection. A blood sample, sputum, and a pharyneal swab are the most common specimens to obtain for identifying a virus. The specimen is placed on a special viral culture medium of growing cells; it will not grow on nonliving media.

Purpose

- To identify a viral infection

Clinical Problems

Positive: Pneumonia (viral), meningitis (viral), rhinovirus, sinusitus, conjunctivitis, shingles, varicella-zoster virus, herpes simplex, enteroviruses, influenza, cytomegalovirus (CMV)

Procedure

- No food or fluid restriction is required.
- Collect 5 mL of venous blood in a green-top tube. Tube should be chilled. A repeated test is suggested in 14 to 28 days as a convalescent specimen.
- A culturette swab may be used to obtain a specimen from the conjunctiva, lesion, throat, and rectum. The swab should be placed in a chilled viral transport media.
- Obtain 5 mL of cerebrospinal fluid and place in a chilled sterile vial.
- Obtain a midstream, clean-caught urine specimen in a sterile container.
- Deliver the specimen immediately to the laboratory.

Nursing Implications

- Obtain a history regarding the possibility of a viral infection. Note the severity of the infection.
- Record symptoms that the client is having in relation to the suspected virus.

Client Teaching

- Explain the procedure for collecting the specimen to the client.
- Inform the client that a second blood sample may be needed in 2 to 4 weeks. Check with the health care provider.
- Listen to the client's concerns.

VITAMIN A (SERUM)

RETINOL

Reference Values

Adult: 30–95 μg/dL, 1.05–3.0 μmol/L (SI units); 125–150 IU/dL
Child: 1–6 Years: 20–43 μg/dL, 0.7–1.5 μmol/L (SI units); 7–12 Years: 20–50 μg/dL, 0.91–1.75 μmol/L (SI units); 13–19 Years: 26–72 μg/dL, 0.91–2.5 μmol/L (SI units)

Description. Vitamin A is a fat-soluble vitamin that is absorbed from the intestine in the presence of lipase and bile. Vitamin A moves to the liver and is stored there as retinyl ester and in the body as retinol. It binds to the serum protein prealbumin.

The functions of vitamin A include the mucous membrane epithelial cell integrity of the eyes, cornea, and the respiratory, gastrointestinal, and genitourinary tracts; body growth; night vision; and skin integrity. Vitamin A has played a major role for years in treating acne; however, high doses of vitamin A can be toxic because it is a fat-soluble vitamin and accumulates in the body tissues.

Purposes

- To detect a vitamin A deficit
- To check for vitamin A toxicity

Clinical Problems

Decreased level: Night-blindness; liver, intestinal, or pancreatic diseases; chronic infections; carcinoid syndrome; cystic fibrosis; protein malnutrition; malabsorption; celiac disease
Drugs that may decrease vitamin A level: Mineral oil, neomycin, cholestyramine

Elevated level: Hypervitaminosis, chronic kidney disease
Drugs that may increase vitamin A level: Glucocorticoids, oral contraceptives

Procedure

- NPO for 8 to 12 hours before the test except for water.

- Collect 5 to 7 mL of venous blood in a red-top tube. Avoid hemolysis and protect the specimen from light. The blood specimen may be placed in a paper bag.

Nursing Implications

- Obtain a history of the client's nutrient intake and supplementary vitamin intake. Note if the client avoids foods that are rich in vitamin A, such as green leafy and yellow vegetables; yellow fruits such as apricots and canteloupe; eggs, whole milk, liver. Individuals with a well-balanced dietary intake normally do not need vitamin supplements.

Client Teaching

Decreased level

- Encourage the client to eat foods rich in vitamin A.
- Inform the client that vitamin supplements can be helpful in preventing vitamin deficiency. The client may wish to contact the health care provider concerning vitamin supplements.

Elevated level

- Instruct the client that megadoses of vitamin A for treating acne can be toxic. The health care provider should be contacted before taking megadoses of vitamin A.
- Instruct pregnant women that vitamins are usually prescribed during pregnancy; however, megadoses of vitamin A should be avoided because it may cause a birth defect in the newborn.

VITAMIN B_{12} (SERUM)

Reference Values

Adult: 200–900 pg/mL

Child: Newborn: 160–1200 pg/mL

Description. Vitamin B_{12} is essential for RBC maturation. The extrinsic factor of vitamin B_{12} is obtained from foods and is absorbed in the small intestines when the intrinsic factor is present. The intrinsic factor is produced by the gastric mucosa, and when this factor is missing, pernicious anemia, a megaloblastic anemia, develops.

Purposes

- To detect pernicious anemia as determined by a decreased vitamin B_{12}
- To suggest other health problems (see Clinical Problems)

Clinical Problems

Decreased level: Pernicious anemia, malabsorption syndrome, inadequate intake, liver diseases, hypothyroidism, sprue, pancreatic insufficiency, gastrectomy, Crohn's disease
Drugs that may decrease vitamin B_{12} value: Neomycin, metformin, ethanol, anticonvulsants

Elevated level: Acute hepatitis, acute and chronic myelocytic leukemia, polycythemia vera
Drugs that may increase vitamin B_{12} value: Oral contraceptives

Procedure

- No food or fluid restriction is required.
- Collect 3 to 5 mL of venous blood in a red-top tube. Prevent hemolysis.

Nursing Implications

- Assess for signs and symptoms of pernicious anemia (i.e., pallor, fatigue, dyspnea, sore mouth, smooth beefy-red tongue, indigestion, tingling numbness in the hands and feet, and behavioral changes).

Client Teaching

- Inform the client of foods high in vitamin B_{12}, such as milk, eggs, meat, and liver. Contact the dietitian to assist the client in meal planning. IM vitamin B_{12} may be ordered.

WHITE BLOOD CELLS (WBCs): TOTAL (WBC) BLOOD

LEUKOCYTES

Reference Values

Adult: Total WBC count: 4,500–10,000 μL
Child: Newborn: 9,000–30,000 μL; 2 yr: 6,000–17,000 μL; 10 yr: 4,500–13,500 μL

Description. (See White Blood Cell Differential.) WBCs (leukocytes) are divided into two groups, the polymorphonuclear leukocytes (neutrophils, eosinophils, and basophils) and the mononuclear leukocytes (monocytes and lymphocytes). Leukocytes are a part of the body's defense system; they respond immediately to foreign invaders by going to the site of involvement. An increase in WBCs is called leukocytosis, and a decrease in WBCs is called leukopenia.

Purposes

- To assess WBCs as a part of a complete blood count (CBC)
- To determine the presence of an infection
- To check WBC values for diagnosing health problems (see Clinical Problems)

Clinical Problems

Decreased level: Hematopoietic diseases (aplastic anemia, pernicious anemia, hypersplenism, Gaucher's disease), viral infections, malaria, agranulocytosis, alcoholism, SLE, RA

Drugs that may decrease WBC value: Antibiotics (penicillins, cephalothins, chloramphenicol), acetaminophen (Tylenol), sulfonamides, propylthiouracil, barbiturates, cancer chemotherapy agents, diazepam (Valium), diuretics (furosemide [Lasix], ethacrynic acid [Edecrin]), chlordiazepoxide (Librium), oral hypoglycemic agents, indomethacin (Indocin), methyldopa (Aldomet), rifampin, phenothiazine

Elevated level: Acute infection (pneumonia, meningitis, appendicitis, colitis, peritonitis, pancreatitis, pyelonephritis, tuberculosis, tonsillitis, diverticulitis, septicemia, rheumatic fever), tissue necrosis (myocardial infarction, cirrhosis of the liver, burns, cancer of the organs, emphysema, peptic ulcer), leukemias, collagen diseases, hemolytic and sickle cell anemia, parasitic diseases, stress (surgery, fever, emotional upset [long lasting]), histamine

Drugs that may increase WBC value: Aspirin, antibiotics (ampicillin, erythromycin, kanamycin, methicillin, tetracyclines, vancomycin, streptomycin), gold compounds, procainamide (Pronestyl), triamterene (Dyrenium), allopurinol, potassium iodide, hydantoin derivatives, sulfonamides (long acting), heparin, digitalis, epinephrine, lithium

Procedure

Venous blood

- No food or fluid restriction is required.
- Collect 7 mL of venous blood in a lavender-top tube. Avoid hemolysis.

Capillary blood

- Collect blood from a finger puncture with a micropipette. Dilute immediately with the proper reagent.

Factors Affecting Laboratory Results

- The age of the individual. Children can have a high WBC count, especially during the first 5 years of life.

Nursing Implications

- Check the vital signs and signs and symptoms of inflammation and infection.
- Notify the health care provider of changes in the client's condition (e.g., fever, increased pulse and respiration rate, and leukocytosis)

Client Teaching

- Teach the client to check the side effects of patent medicines such as cold medications, which could cause agranulocytosis or severe leukopenia.
- Instruct clients with leukopenia to avoid persons with any contagious condition. Their body resistances are reduced, and they are prime candidates for severe colds or infections.

WHITE BLOOD CELL DIFFERENTIAL (BLOOD)

DIFFERENTIAL WBC

Reference Values

DIFFERENTIAL WBC VALUES

	Adult		*Child*
WBC Type	*%*	*µL*	*Same as adult except*
Neutrophils (total)	50–70	2500–7000	Newborn: 61%; 1 year: 32%

WBC Type	Adult %	Adult µL	Child: Same as adult except
Segments	50–65	2500–6500	
Bands	0–5	0–500	
Eosinophils	1–3	100–300	
Basophils	0.4–1.0	40–100	
Monocytes	4–6	200–600	1–12 yr: 4%–9%
Lymphocytes	25–35	1700–3500	Newborn: 34%; 1 yr: 60%; 6 yr: 42%; 12 yr: 38%

Description. Differential WBC count, part of the complete blood count (CBC), is composed of five types of WBC (leukocytes): neutrophils, eosinophils, basophils, monocytes, and lymphocytes. The differential WBC count is expressed as cubic millimeters (µL) and percent of the total number of WBCs. Neutrophils and lymphocytes make up 80% to 90% of the total WBCs. Differential WBC count provides more specific information related to infections and disease process.

Neutrophils: Neutrophils are the most numerous circulating WBCs, and they respond more rapidly to the inflammatory and tissue injury sites than other types of WBC. During an *acute* infection, the body's first line of defense is the neutrophils. The segments are mature neutrophils, and the bands are immature ones that multiply quickly during an acute infection.

Eosinophils: Eosinophils increase during allergic and parasitic conditions. With an increase in steroids, either produced by the adrenal glands during stress or administered orally or by injection, eosinophils decrease in number.

Basophils: Basophils increase during the healing process. With an increase in steroids, the basophil count will decrease.

Monocytes: Monocytes are the second line of defense against bacterial infections and foreign substances. They are slower to react to infections and inflammatory diseases, but they are stronger than neutrophils and can ingest larger particles of debris.

Lymphocytes: Increased lymphocytes (lymphocytosis) occur in chronic and viral infections. Severe lymphocytosis is commonly caused by chronic lymphocytic leukemia. Lymphocytes play a major role in the immune response system with B lymphocytes and T lymphocytes.

Purpose

- To differentiate between the various types of WBCs for diagnosing health problems (see Description)

Clinical Problems

Decreased level

Neutrophils: Viral diseases, leukemias, agranulocytosis, aplastic and iron deficiency anemias
Eosinophils: Stress (burns, shock), adrenocortical hyperfunction
Basophils: Stress, hypersensitivity reaction, pregnancy
Monocytes: Lymphocytic leukemia, aplastic anemia
Lymphocytes: Cancer, leukemia, adrenocortical hyperfunction, agranulocytosis, aplastic anemia, multiple sclerosis, renal failure, nephrotic syndrome, SLE

Elevated level

Neutrophils: Acute infections, inflammatory diseases, tissue damage (AMI), Hodgkin's disease, hemolytic disease of newborns, acute appendicitis, acute pancreatitis
Eosinophils: Allergies; parasitic disease; cancer of bone, ovary, testes, brain; phlebitis and thrombophlebitis
Basophils: Inflammatory process, leukemia, healing stage of infection or inflammation
Monocytes: Viral diseases, parasitic diseases, monocytic leukemia, cancer, collagen diseases
Lymphocytes: Lymphocytic leukemia, viral infections, chronic infections, Hodgkin's disease, multiple myeloma, adrenocortical hypofunction

Procedure

- No food or fluid restriction is required.
- Collect 7 mL of venous blood in a lavender-top tube. Prevent hemolysis.

Factors Affecting Laboratory Results

- Steroids could decrease eosinophil and lymphocyte values.

Nursing Implications

- Check the WBC count and the differential WBC count. Elevated neutrophils may be indicative of an acute infection. Elevated eosinophils may be a sign of allergy. Increased basophils can be caused by the healing process. Increased monocytes occur during infection, and increased lymphocytes occur in chronic or viral infections.
- Assess the client for signs and symptoms of an infection (i.e., elevated temperature, increased pulse rate, edema, redness, and exudate [wound drainage]).
- Assess the client for signs and symptoms of allergies, such as tearing, runny nose, rash, and more severe reactions.
- Assess for signs and symptoms of healing (i.e., ability to increase movement at the injured site, decreased edema, and exudate).

ZINC (PLASMA)

Reference Values

Plasma: Adult: 60–150 μg/dL, 11–23 μmol/L (SI units)
Urine: 150–1250 μg/24 h

Description. Zinc (ZN), a heavy metal, is an element found in the body and required for body growth and metabolism. Approximately 80% of zinc is in the blood cells. About 30% of the zinc ingested is absorbed from the small intestine. Most of the body's excretion of zinc is in the stool, but a small amount is excreted in the urine.

Zinc is a component of many enzymes, such as carbonic anhydrase, DNA and RNA polymerases, lactic dehydrogenase, and alkaline phosphatase, and it plays an important role in enzyme catalytic reactions. Zinc deficiency is not apparent until it becomes severe, when it is manifested by growth retardation, delayed sexual development, severe dermatitis, alopecia, or poor wound healing. Zinc toxicity is rare but it can be related to workers' inhaling zinc oxide during industry exposure.

Purposes

- To detect a zinc deficiency

- To determine the cause of diarrhea, malnutrition, growth retardation, delayed sexual development, alopecia, and poor healing
- To detect zinc toxicity due to industry exposure (inhaling zinc oxide)

Clinical Problems

Decreased level: Malnutrition, malabsorption, diarrhea, anemia, alcoholism, myocardial infarction, hereditary deficiency, cirrhosis of the liver, chronic renal failure, gallbladder disease
Drugs that decrease zinc levels: Corticosteroids, estrogens, penicillamine, anticancer agents, antimetabolites, cisplatin, diuretics

Elevated level: Ingestion of acidic food or beverages from galvanized containers, industrial exposure

Procedure

- No food or fluid restriction is required.
- Collect 3 to 5 mL of venous blood in a metal-free, navy blue–top tube. Avoid hemolysis.
- Send the blood specimen to the laboratory immediately.

Factors Affecting Laboratory Results

- Use of a tube or needle containing metal

Nursing Implications

- Obtain a history of the client's nutritional intake. Zinc is present in many foods. Malnutrition, cirrhosis of the liver, alcoholism, or severe diarrhea contributes to a zinc deficit. Zinc is required for the synthesis of prealbumin.
- Monitor intravenous therapy including total parenteral nutrition (TPN); continuous use can cause a zinc deficit.
- Check the history for anemia. With sickle cell anemia, the zinc level is decreased because abnormal red blood cells cause excess loss of zinc.

Client Teaching

- Instruct the pregnant client that vitamins prescribed should contain zinc. An increase in zinc requirement is needed during pregnancy and for lactation.

- Instruct the client who has poor nutrition to take vitamins. Tell the client to check the label on vitamin container to determine that zinc is one of the elements.

ZINC PROTOPORPHYRIN (ZPP) (BLOOD)

FREE ERYTHROCYTE PROTOPORPHYRIN (FEP)

Reference Values

Adult and Child: 15–77 μg/dL, 0.24–1.23 μmol/L (SI units). *Average:* <35 μg/dL, <0.56 μmol/L (SI units)

Description. Zinc protoporphyrin (ZPP) is a screening test to check for lead poisoning and iron deficiency. It can be checked by drawing a blood sample or by use of a hematofluorometer using several drops of blood. With iron deficiency, the ZPP level does not become elevated until after a few weeks. After iron therapy, the ZPP level returns to normal in 2 to 2½ months.

The use of the ZPP test for screening for increased blood lead levels has more than doubled within a year. ZPP is an effective indicator of the total body of lead. After exposure to lead ceases, blood lead becomes more normal in several weeks or months. The Centers for Disease Control (Atlanta, GA) is now recommending that children suspected of lead poisoning be checked using the blood lead test.

Purpose

- To screen for lead poisoning or for iron deficiency

Clincal Problems

Elevated level: Lead poisoning, iron deficiency, anemia of chronic disease, sickle-cell disease, occupational exposure, accelerated erythropoiesis, acute inflammatory processes

Procedure

- No food or fluid restriction is required.

- Collect 3 to 5 mL of venous blood in a green- or lavender-top tube. Avoid hemolysis. A hematofluorometer with a few drops of blood may be used.

Nursing Implications

- Obtain a history from the client or family concerning the child's ingesting paint containing lead. Older houses may still have lead paint, which might be eaten by a child.
- Obtain a history from the adult client concerning excessive lead exposure due to occupational contact. Other possible contact with lead includes eating or drinking from unglazed pottery, drinking "moonshine" whiskey prepared in lead containers, breathing leaded gasoline fumes.
- Compare the blood lead level with the blood ZPP level.
- Observe for signs and symptoms of lead poisoning, such as lead colic (crampy abdominal pain), constipation, occasional bloody diarrhea, behavioral changes (from lethargy to hyperactivity, aggression, impulsiveness), tremors, and confusion.
- Obtain a history of iron deficiency. Check serum iron level and serum ferritin level. Compare the above levels with the ZPP level.
- Check that blood ZPP levels are repeated after 2 months of iron therapy.

TWO

Considerations for Use of Diagnostic Tests

Millions of diagnostic tests are performed daily throughout the world. These tests monitor client/patient well-being and assist in the diagnosis of specific conditions.

This introductory chapter to diagnostic tests has a twofold purpose. The first is to disseminate essential information related to all diagnostic tests, and the second is to describe the basic organizational format of the individual tests.

General directions common to most diagnostic tests are normal finding, description, purpose(s), clinical problems, procedure, factors affecting diagnostic results, and nursing implications with client teaching. Only facts specific to a given test are given.

Normal Finding(s). Normal size, structure, and function of the organ under examination are stated.

Description. Information about the test is briefly described.

Purpose(s). The purpose(s) is/are given for each diagnostic test.

Clinical Problems. This covers either disease entities or conditions that are associated with abnormal findings or indications for the test.

Procedure. The procedure usually differs among tests; however, common procedures for most tests are:

1. A signed consent form.
2. Food and fluid restriction.
3. Institutional policies that must be followed.

Factors Affecting Diagnostic Results. Various factors that could affect test results should be identified. Drugs that affect test results are given in Clinical Problems; therefore, they are not repeated here.

Nursing Implications

1. Be knowledgeable about test.
2. Provide time and be available to answer questions. Be supportive of client and family.
3. Obtain history of allergies to iodine, seafood. Observe for severe allergic reaction to contrast dye.
4. Obtain baseline vital signs. Monitor vital signs as indicated following test.
5. Have client void before test.
6. If sedative is used, instruct client not to drive home.

Client Teaching

7. Explain test procedure to the client or family, or both.
8. Provide teaching related to care of health problem.

List of Diagnostic Tests

Amniotic Fluid Analysis 319
Angiography (Angiogram) 320
Arthrography 323
Arthroscopy 325
Barium Enema 326
Biopsy (Bone Marrow, Breast, Endometrium, Kidney, Liver) 328
Bone Densitometry 332
Bronchography (Bronchogram) 334
Bronchoscopy 335
Cardiac Catheterization 337
Cervicography (Cervigram) 340
Cholangiography (IV), Percutaneous Cholangiography, T-Tube Cholangiography 341
Cholecystography (Oral) 343
Chorionic Villi Biopsy (CVB) 345
Colonoscopy 346
Colposcopy 348
Computed Tomography (CT) Scan, Computed Axial Tomography (CAT) 350
Cystoscopy, Cystography (Cystogram) 354
Echocardiography (Echocardiogram) 356
Electrocardiography (ECG, EKG) 361
Electroencephalography, Electroencephalogram (EEG) 364
Electromyography, Electromyogram (EMG) 365
Endoscopic Retrograde Cholangiopancreatography (ERCP) 367
Esophogeal Studies 368
Esophagogastroduodenoscopy, Esophagogastroscopy 373
Gastric Analysis 374
Gastrointestinal (GI) Series 377
Holter Monitoring 379
Hysterosalpingography (Hysterosalpingogram) 381
Hysteroscopy 383
Intravenous Pyelography (IVP) 384
Lymphangiography (Lymphangiogram) 386
Magnetic Resonance Imaging (MRI) 388
Mammography (Mammogram) 390
Multigated Acquisition (MUGA) Scan 392
Myelography (Myelogram) 393
Nuclear Scans (Bone, Brain, Brain Perfusion, Heart, Kidney, Liver and Spleen, Colon and Ovary, Gastroesophageal Reflux, GI Bleeding, Gastric Emptying, Gallbladder, Lung, and Thyroid Studies) 395

Papanicolaou Smear (PAP Smear) 405
Positron Emission Tomography (PET) 408
Proctosigmoidoscopy, Proctoscopy, Sigmoidoscopy 410
Pulmonary Function Tests 412
Radioactive Iodine (RAI) Uptake Test 420
Schilling Test 422
Sinus Endoscopy 424
Skin Tests (Tuberculin, Blastomycosis, Coccidioidomycosis, Histoplasmosis, Trichinosis, Toxoplasmosis) 426
Stress/Exercise Tests (Treadmill Exercise Electrocardiology, Exercise Myocardial Perfusion Imaging Test [Thallium/Technetium Stress Test], Nuclear Persantine (Dipyridamole) Stress Test, Nuclear Dobutamine Stress Test) 428
Ultrasonography (Abdominal Aorta, Brain, Breast, Carotid, Doppler—Arteries and Veins, Eye and Eye Orbit, Gallbladder, Heart, Kidney, Liver, Pancreas, Pelvis [Uterus, Ovaries, Pregnant Uterus], Prostate, Scrotum, Spleen, Thoracic, and Thyroid 435
Venography (Lower Limb) 442
Ventilation Scan 444
X-Ray (Chest, Heart, Flat Plate of the Abdomen, Kidney, Ureter, Bladder, Skull, Skeletal) 445

DIAGNOSTIC TESTS

AMNIOTIC FLUID ANALYSIS

Normal Findings. Clear amniotic fluid; no chromosomal or neural tube abnormalities

Description. Amniotic analysis is useful for detecting chromosomal abnormalities (Down syndrome, trisomy 21), neural tube defects (spina bifida), sex-linked disorders (hemophilia), and for determining fetal maturity. The amniotic fluid is obtained by amniocentesis, performed during the 14th to the 16th weeks of pregnancy, for chromosomal and neural tube defects.

Amnioscopy: Insertion of a fiberoptic, lighted instrument (amnioscope) into the cervical canal to visualize the amniotic fluid. Because of possible infection, the test is rarely performed.

Purposes

- To detect chromosomal abnormalities, neural tube defects, and sex-linked disorders
- To determine fetal maturity

Clinical Problems

Abnormal findings: Chromosomal disorders, neural tube defects (alpha-fetoprotein), hemolytic disease due to Rh incompatibility, X-linked disorders, fetal maturity, fetal stress (meconium), pulmonary maturity of fetus (L/S ratio)

Procedure

- Obtain a signed consent form.
- No food or fluid is restricted.
- Have client void prior to procedure to prevent puncturing the bladder and aspirating urine.
- Cleanse suprapubic area with an antiseptic. A local anesthetic is injected at needle site for the amniocentesis.

- The placenta and fetus are located by ultrasound or manually (fetus only).
- Aspirate 5 to 15 mL of amniotic fluid. Apply dressing to needle insertion site.

Foam stability test: This test determines if surfactant from mature fetal lungs is present in the amniotic fluid. When the test tube of amniotic fluid is shaken, bubbles appear around the surface if adequate amounts of surfactant are present.

Nursing Implications

- Obtain a signed consent form.
- Have the client void before the test.

Client Teaching

- Explain that the test screens only for specific abnormalities.
- Inform the client that normal results do not guarantee a normal infant. The health care provider should tell the woman of potential risks, such as premature labor, spontaneous abortion, infection, and fetal or placental bleeding. Complications are rare.
- Inform the client that the test takes about 30 minutes.
- Be supportive. Be a good listener.

Post-test

- Encourage the family to seek genetic counseling if chromosomal abnormality has been determined.
- Instruct the client to notify the health care provider immediately of any of the following: bleeding or leaking fluid from the vagina, abdominal pain or cramping, chills and fever, or lack of fetal movement.

ANGIOGRAPHY (ANGIOGRAM)

ARTERIOGRAPHY: CARDIAC (SEE CARDIAC CATHETERIZATION), CEREBRAL ANGIOGRAPHY, PULMONARY ANGIOGRAPHY, AND RENAL ANGIOGRAPHY

Normal Findings. Normal structure and patency of blood vessels

Description. The terms angiography (examination of the blood vessels) and arteriography (examination of the arteries) are used interchangeably.

A catheter is inserted into the femoral or brachial artery, and a contrast dye is injected to allow visualization of the blood vessels. Angiographies are useful for evaluating patency of blood vessels and for identifying abnormal vascularization resulting from tumors. This test may be indicated when computed tomography (CT) or radionuclide scanning suggests vascular abnormalities.

The new contrast medium has a low osmolality; examples include iopamidol, iohexol, and ioxaglate. The older media were hyperosmolar with a high content of iodine.

Cerebral angiography: The injected dye outlines the carotid and vertebral arteries, large blood vessels of the circle of Willis, and small cerebral arterial branches.

Pulmonary angiography: The catheter inserted in the brachial or femoral artery is threaded into the pulmonary artery, and dye is injected for visualizing pulmonary vessels. During the test, the client should be monitored for cardiac dysrhythmias.

Renal angiography: This test permits visualization of the renal vessels and the parenchyma. An aortogram may be performed with renal angiography to detect any vessel abnormality in the aorta and to show the relationship of the renal arteries to the aorta.

Clinical Problems

Type of Angiography	*Indications/Purposes*
Cerebral	To detect cerebrovascular aneurysm; cerebral thrombosis; hematomas; tumors from increased vascularization; cerebral plaques or spasm; cerebral fistula
	To evaluate cerebral blood flow; cause of increased intracranial pressure
Pulmonary	To detect pulmonary emboli; tumors; aneurysms; congenital defects; vascular changes associated with emphysema, blebs, and bullae; heart abnormality
	To evaluate pulmonary circulation
Renal	To detect renal artery stenosis; renal thrombus or embolus; space-occupying lesions (i.e., tumor, cyst, aneurysm)
	To determine the causative factor of hypertension; cause of renal failure
	To evaluate renal circulation

Procedure

All angiographies

- Obtain a signed consent form.
- Restrict food and fluids for 8 to 12 hours. Anticoagulants (e.g., heparin) are discontinued.
- Record vital signs. Void before test.
- Remove dentures and metallic objects before the test.
- If the client has a history of severe allergic reactions to various substances or drugs, steroids or antihistamines may be given before and after the procedure as a prophylactic measure.
- A sedative or narcotic analgesic, if ordered, is administered 1 hour before the test.
- IV fluids may be started before the procedure so that emergency drugs, if needed, can be administered.
- Client is in supine position on an x-ray table. A local anesthetic is administered to the injection/incisional site.
- The test takes 1 to 2 hours.

Renal: A laxative or cleansing enema is usually ordered the evening before the test.

Pulmonary: ECG/EKG electrodes are attached to the chest for cardiac monitoring during angiography. Pulmonary pressures are recorded, and blood samples are obtained before the contrast dye is injected.

Factors Affecting Diagnostic Results

- Feces, gas, and barium sulfate can interfere with test results.

Nursing Implications

Pre-test

- Obtain a history of hypersensitivity to iodine, seafood, or contrast dye from other x-ray procedure (e.g., intravenous pyelogram [IVP]).
- Record baseline vital signs.

Client Teaching

- Explain the purpose and procedure of the angiography.
- Inform the client that when the dye is injected there could be a warm, flushed sensation lasting a minute or two. Client must remain still so that the pictures are clear.
- Explain that the test should not cause pain, but there may be moments of discomfort.

Test

- Monitor vital signs.
- Assess for vasovagal reaction (common complication; i.e., decreased pulse rate and blood pressure, cold and clammy). Give IV fluids and atropine IV. This reaction lasts about 15 to 20 minutes.

Post-test

- Apply pressure on the injection site for 5 to 10 minutes or longer until bleeding has stopped.
- Monitor vital signs as ordered.
- Enforce bedrest for 12 to 24 hours or as ordered. Activities should be restricted for a day.
- Check peripheral pulses in the extremities (i.e., dorsalis pedis, femoral, and radial).
- Check injection site for bleeding.
- Apply cold compresses or an ice pack to the injection site for edema or pain if ordered.
- Monitor ECG tracings, urine output, and IV fluids.
- Inform client that coughing is a common occurrence following a pulmonary angiography.
- Assess for weakness or numbness in an extremity, confusion, or slurred speech following a cerebral angiography. These could be symptoms of transient ischemic attack (TIA).
- Observe for a delayed allergic reaction to the contrast dye (i.e., tachycardia, dyspnea, skin rash, urticaria, decreased BP, and decreased urine output).
- Be supportive of client and family.

ARTHROGRAPHY

Normal Findings

Knee: Normal medial meniscus

Shoulder: Bicipital tendon sheath, normal joint capsule, and intact subscapular bursa

Description. Arthrography is an x-ray examination of a joint using air or contrast media, or both, in the joint space. It can visualize abnormal joint capsule and tears to the cartilage or ligaments. This procedure is performed when clients complain of peristent knee or shoulder pain or discomfort. It is usually performed on an outpatient basis.

Arthrography is not indicated if the client is having acute arthritic attack, joint infection, or is pregnant. This procedure is usually performed prior to an arthroscopy.

Purposes

- To visualize the structures of the joint capsule
- To detect abnormalities of the cartilage and/or ligaments (tears)

Clinical Problems

Abnormal findings: Osteochondritis dissecans, osteochondral fractures, cartilage and synovial abnormalities, tears of the ligaments, and joint capsule abnormalities. *Shoulder:* adhesive capsulitis, tears of rotator cuff, bicipital tenosynovitis or tears

Procedure

- No food or fluid restriction is required.
- Prepare the knee or shoulder area using aseptic technique.
- Local anesthetic is administered to puncture site.
- A needle is inserted into the joint space (e.g., knee), and synovial fluid is aspirated for synovial fluid analysis.
- Air and/or contrast medium is injected into the joint space, and x-rays are taken.
- The knee may be bandaged.

Nursing Implications

- Obtain a history of type of pain to knee and shoulder, and possible allergies to seafood, iodine, or contrast dye.
- Check vital signs.

Client Teaching

- Explain the procedure to the client (see Procedure).
- Inform the client that changes in body positions may be requested during the procedure. At other times, the client is to remain still. The client will not be asleep.

Post-test

- Apply an Ace bandage to the leg, including the knee, if indicated, to decrease swelling and pain.

Client Teaching

- Instruct the client to rest the joint for a specified time, usually 12 hours.
- Inform the client that a crepitant noise may be heard with joint movement; if it persists, the surgeon should be notified.
- Instruct the client to apply an ice bag with a cover to the affected joint to decrease swelling. An analgesic for pain/discomfort may be ordered.

ARTHROSCOPY

Normal Findings. Normal lining of the synovial membrane; ligaments and tendons intact

Description. Arthroscopy is an endoscopic examination of the interior aspect of a joint, usually the knee, using a fiberoptic endoscope. Normally, *arthrography* (x-ray examination of a joint using air or contrast media, or both, in the joint space) is performed prior to arthroscopy.

Arthroscopy is used to perform joint surgery and diagnose meniscal, patellar, extrasynovial, and synovial diseases. Frequently, biopsy or surgery is performed during the test procedure. Arthroscopy is contraindicated if a wound or severe skin infection is present.

Purposes

- To diagnose meniscal, patellar, extrasynovial, and synovial diseases
- To perform joint surgery

Clinical Problems

Abnormal findings: Meniscal disease with torn lateral or medial meniscus, patellar disease, chondromalacia, patellar fracture, osteochondritis dissecans, osteochondromatosis, torn ligaments, Baker's cysts, synovitis, and rheumatoid and degenerative arthritis.

Procedure

- Obtain a signed consent form.
- No food or fluid is restricted for local anesthetic; NPO after midnight with spinal and general anesthesia.

- The arthrosope is inserted into the interior joint for visualization, draining fluid from the joint, biopsy, and/or surgery.
- Ace bandage or tourniquet may be applied above the joint to decrease blood volume in the leg.

Nursing Implications

- Assess the involved area for possible skin lesion or infection.
- Determine the client's anxiety level, and be available to answer questions. Be prepared to repeat information if the level of anxiety or fear is determined to be high.

Post-test

- Assess client before, during, and after procedure, including vital signs, bleeding, swelling, etc.
- Apply ice to the area as indicated.
- Administer analgesic for pain or discomfort as ordered.

Client Teaching

- Instruct client to avoid excessive use of joint for 2 to 3 days or as ordered. Limited walking is usually permitted soon after the procedure.

BARIUM ENEMA

LOWER GASTROINTESTINAL (COLON) TEST

Normal Findings. Normal filling, normal structure of the large colon

Description. The barium enema is an x-ray examination of the large intestine. Barium sulfate (single contrast) or barium sulfate and air (double contrast) is administered slowly through a rectal tube. The filling process is monitored by fluoroscopy, and then x-rays are taken. The colon must be free of fecal material so that the barium will outline the large intestine to detect any disorders. The double-contrast technique (barium and air) is useful for identifying polyps.

The test can be performed in a hospital, clinic, or at a private health facility.

Purpose

- To detect disorders of the large intestine

Clinical Problems

Abnormal findings: Tumor in the colon; inflammatory disease: ulcerative colitis, granulomatous colitis, diverticulitis; diverticula; fistulas; polyps; intussusception

Procedure. Abdominal x-rays, ultrasound studies, radionuclide scans, upper gastrointestinal (GI) series, and proctosigmoidoscopy should be done before the barium enema. It is important that the colon is fecal free.

Pre-preparation

- A clear liquid diet for 18 to 24 hours before the test (broth, ginger ale, cola, black coffee or tea with sugar only, gelatin, and syrup from canned fruit). Some institutions permit a white chicken sandwich (no butter, lettuce, or mayonnaise) or hard-boiled eggs and gelatin for lunch and dinner; then NPO after dinner.
- Encourage the client to increase water or clear liquid intake 24 hours before the test to maintain adequate hydration.
- Prescribe laxatives (castor oil or magnesium citrate), which should be taken the day before the test in the late afternoon or early evening (4 PM to 8 PM).
- A cleansing enema or laxative suppository such as bisacodyl (Dulcolax) may be ordered the evening before the test.
- Saline enemas should be given early in the morning (6 AM) until returns are clear (maximum of three enemas). Some private laboratories have clients use laxative suppositories instead of enemas in the morning.
- Black coffee or tea is permitted 1 hour before the test. Some institutions permit dry toast.

Post-preparation

- The client should expel the barium in the bathroom or bedpan immediately after the test.
- Fluid intake should be increased for hydration and to prevent constipation due to retained barium.
- A laxative such as milk of magnesia or magnesium citrate or an enema should be given to get the barium out of the colon. A laxative may need to be repeated on the next day.

Factors Affecting Diagnostic Results

- Inadequate bowel preparation with fecal material remaining in the colon

Nursing Implications

- List the procedure step by step for the client. Most private laboratories have written preparation slips.
- Notify the health care provider if the client has severe abdominal cramps and pain prior to the test. Barium enema should not be performed if the client has severe ulcerative colitis, suspected perforation, or tachycardia.
- Administer a laxative or cleansing enema after the test. Instruct the client to check the color of the stools for 2 to 3 days. Stools may be light in color because of the barium sulfate. Absence of stool should be reported.

Client Teaching

- Emphasize the importance of dietary restrictions and bowel preparation. Adequate preparation is essential, or the test may need to be repeated.
- Explain that he or she will be lying on an x-ray table.
- Inform the client that the test takes approximately ½ to 1 hour. Tell the client to take deep breaths through the mouth, which helps to decrease tension and promote relaxation.

BIOPSY (BONE MARROW, BREAST, ENDOMETRIUM, KIDNEY, LIVER)

Normal Finding. Normal cells and tissue from the bone marrow, breast, endometrium of the uterus, kidney, and liver

Description. Biopsy is the removal and examination of tissue from the body. Usually biopsies are performed to detect malignancy or to identify the presence of a disease process. Biopsies can be obtained by (1) aspiration by applying suction, (2) the brush method, using stiff bristles that scrape fragments of cells and tissue, (3) excision by surgical cutting at tissue site, (4) fine-needle aspiration at tissue site with or without the guidance of ultrasound, (5) insertion of a needle through the skin, and (6) punch biopsy, using a punch-type instrument.

Bone marrow: The bone marrow is composed of red and yellow marrow. The red marrow produces blood cells and the yellow marrow has fat cells and connective tissue. The sternum and iliac crest are the most common sites for bone marrow aspiration.

Breast: Biopsy of the breast is mainly performed to determine if a breast lesion (nodule or mass) is a cyst, benign, or cancerous. The majority of breast lumps are benign. The site of the breast lesion can be identified with the use of a fixed grid on the mammogram.

Endometrium of the uterus: Endometrial biopsy can detect polyps, cancer, inflammatory condition, and defect in ovulation. The biopsy collection using a probe (blind technique) can be performed in the health care provider's office. Complications include perforation of the uterus, excessive bleeding, and aborting an early pregnancy. This procedure should not be performed if there is purulent discharge from the vagina. An endometrial biopsy differs from a D & C (dilation and curettage) in that dilation of cervix is not needed. D & C requires general anesthesia because the entire endometrium is curettaged. With an endometrial biopsy, the affected tissue in the uterus could be missed with a sample biopsy, while with the D & C the total endometrium is obtained.

Kidney (renal): A kidney biopsy is usually done with the guidance of ultrasound or fluoroscopy. The biopsy is performed to determine the cause of renal disease, to rule out metastatic malignancy of the kidney, or to determine if rejection of a kidney transplant is occurring. The biopsy can be obtained in three ways: (1) by use of a cystocope, (2) by excision of the kidney, taking a wedge of issue, and (3) percutaneously, using a needle.

Liver: Liver biopsy is not usually done unless the liver enzymes are greatly increased. It is performed to rule out metatastic malignancy or to detect a cyst or the presence of cirrhosis. Ultrasound is used to guide the biopsy needle to the pathologic site. Prior to a liver biopsy, the following laboratory levels should be checked: prothrombin time (PT), partial thromboplastin time (PTT), and platelet count. The liver is vascular, and if these laboratory results are abnormal, bleeding could occur following the test procedure.

Purposes

- To identify abnormal tissue from various body sites
- To detect the presence of a disease process

Clinical Problems

Indications: Blood disorders, malignancies, cysts, polyps, infectious process, progressive disease entities (cirrhosis, nephrosis, lupus nephritis), ovulative defects, rejection of an organ transplant

Procedure

- A consent form should be signed.
- Baseline vital signs are taken.
- Biopsy site is anesthetized.

Bone marrow

- A local anesthetic is injected at site (sternum or iliac spine).
- A needle with a stylet is inserted through a skin slit into the bone about 3 mm deep.
- The stylet is removed, and a 10 mL syringe is attached to the needle. Bone marrow is aspirated; part is used for a blood smear, and the remaining amount is placed in a green- or lavender-top tube.

Breast

- Needle aspiration or an excision of breast tissue can be performed.
- The skin is anesthetized; general anesthesia may be used if biopsy tissue is difficult to obtain.
- A mammogram or ultrasound is usually needed to determine the placement of needle or the excision site.
- Tissue obtained from biopsy is placed in formalin and sent immediately to the laboratory. The specimen from a needle aspiration is placed on cytologic slide.

Endometrium of the uterus

- The client is placed in the lithotomy position
- A sound (probe) is inserted into the cavity of the uterus to determine its size. This is done as a precaution to prevent perforation of the uterus.
- A suction tube with curette is inserted into the cavity of the uterus, and sample specimens are obtained from the lateral, anterior, and/or posterior uterine wall.
- Specimen(s) is/are placed in formalin solution and sent to the laboratory for histologic testing.

Kidney (renal)

This test can be performed by use of a cystoscope with the brush method, excision of a wedge of renal tissue, or percutaneously with a special needle.

- The client is placed in the prone position.
- With the percutaneous method, the site is determined with the use of ultrasound or fluoroscopy.
- Anesthetic is given according to the procedure chosen.
- With needle insertion, the client is asked to take a breath and hold it. A small tissue specimen is obtained. Pressure is applied to the site for approximately 20 minutes to prevent bleeding because the kidney tissue is very vascular.

Liver

- NPO for at least 6 hours prior to the test. The liver is less congested without food intake.
- Check that PT, APTT (PTT), and platelet count have been done and documented. Abnormal findings should be reported prior to procedure to decrease/avoid excessive bleeding following the biopsy.
- A fine needle is inserted, usually with the guidance of ultrasound.
- The client is asked first to take a deep breath, then to exhale and hold breath. With expiration, the diaphragm is motionless and remains high in the thorax.
- Apply a pressure dressing.
- The tissue specimen is placed in formalin solution, or the specimen is swabbed on a slide and fixed in 95% alcohol.
- Place the client on his or her right side to decrease the chance of hemorrhage.

Factors Affecting Diagnostic Results

- Blind biopsy can result in missing the diseased tissue.
- Improper care of the tissue specimen

Nursing Implications

- Check that the consent form has been signed.
- Check that the prescribed laboratory tests have been done.
- Monitor vital signs as prescribed (i.e., every 15 minutes for the first hour, every 30 minutes for the second hour, and then hourly).
- Observe for bleeding and shortness of breath.

- Report absence or decreased bowel sounds following renal or liver biopsy test.

Client Teaching

- Explain the biopsy procedure to the client.
- Instruct the client to report excessive bleeding immediately to the health care provider.
- Instruct the client to report an elevated temperature.
- Instruct the client to take the prescribed pain medication as needed.
- Advise the client to rest for 24 hours following the test procedure.
- Instruct the client to avoid heavy lifting for at least 24 hours, or longer if indicated (i.e., following liver and renal biopsies).

Kidney

- Increase fluid intake following the biopsy.
- Check bowel sounds for several hours following the test. Abdominal intervention can cause a decrease in bowel sounds (decreased peristalsis).
- Instruct the client to report decreased urination or burning when urinating.

Liver

- Avoid heavy lifting.

BONE DENSITOMETRY

BONE DENSITY (BD), BONE MINERAL DENSITY (BMD), BONE ABSORPTIOMETRY

Normal Finding. Normal bone densitometry scan is determined according to the client's age, sex, and height.

Normal: 1 standard deviation below peak bone mass level

Osteoporosis: >2.5 standard deviations below peak bone mass level (WHO standard)

Description. A bone density test is done to detect early osteoporosis by determining the density of bone mineral content. Clients who have a loss of bone mineral are readily prone to fractures. The bones that are usually examined are the lumbar spine and the proximal hip (neck of the femur).

Another bone site, the heel bone, can be evaluated according to the client's symptoms.

The dual energy x-ray absorptiometry (DEXA) measures bone mineral density and exposes the client to only a minimal amount of radiation. Images from the detector/camera are computer analyzed to determine the bone mineral content. The computer can calculate the size and thickness of the bone.

Purposes

- To evaluate the bone mineral density
- To identify early and progressive osteoporosis

Clinical Problems

Abnormal findings: Loss of bone mineral content, early and progressive osteoporosis

Procedure

- A signed consent form may be required.
- No food or fluid restriction is required.
- Client is to remove all metal objects at the area to be scanned (i.e., keys, coins, zippers, belts, etc.).
- The client lies on an imaging table with a radiation source below and the detector above, which measures the bone's radiation absorption.
- The bone density test takes approximately 30 to 60 minutes.

Factors Affecting Diagnostic Results

- Metallic objects in the bone scanning site
- Previous fractures of the bone may increase the bone density.

Nursing Implications

- Obtain family history of osteoporosis and client's skeletal problems, such as loss of height, fractures, and others.

Client Teaching

- Explain the procedure for bone density test.
- Inform the client that the test should not cause pain and that the radiation is considered minimal.
- Instruct the client to remove all metal objects that would be within the scanning area.
- Tell the client that the test should take approximately 30 to 60 minutes.

BRONCHOGRAPHY (BRONCHOGRAM)

Normal Finding. Normal tracheobronchial structure

Description. Bronchography is an x-ray test to visualize the trachea, bronchi, and the entire bronchial tree after a radiopaque iodine contrast liquid is injected through a catheter into the tracheobronchial space. The bronchi are coated with the contrast dye, and a series of x-rays is then taken. Bronchography may be done in conjunction with bronchoscopy.

Bronchography is contraindicated during pregnancy. This test should not be done if the client is hypersensitive to anesthetics, iodine, or x-ray dyes.

Purpose

- To detect bronchial obstruction, such as foreign bodies, tumors, etc.

Clinical Problems. Foreign bodies in the bronchial tubes, tumors, cysts, bronchiectasis

Procedure

- Obtain a signed consent form.
- Restrict foods and fluids for 6 to 8 hours before the test.
- Oral hygiene should be given the night before the test and in the morning to lessen the number of bacteria introduced into the lung.
- Postural drainage may be performed for 3 days before the test.
- A sedative and atropine are usually given 1 hour before the test.
- A topical anesthetic is sprayed into the pharynx and trachea. A catheter is passed through the nose into the trachea, and a local anesthetic and iodized contrast liquid are injected through the catheter.
- The client is usually asked to change body positions so that the contrast dye can reach most areas of the bronchial tree.
- After bronchography, the client may receive nebulization and should perform postural drainage to remove contrast dye. Food and fluids are restricted until the gag (cough) reflex is present.

Factors Affecting Diagnostic Results

- Secretions in the tracheobronchial tree can prevent the contrast dye from coating the bronchial walls.

Nursing Implications

- Obtain a signed consent form.
- Obtain a history of hypersensitivity to anesthetics, iodine, and x-ray dyes.
- Record vital signs.
- Answer client's questions and concerns or refer to other health professionals, if necessary. Reassure the client that the airway will not be blocked. Inform the client that he or she may have a sore throat after the test.

Client Teaching

- Explain the procedure of the test (see Procedure).
- Encourage the client to practice good oral hygiene the night before and the morning of the test. Dentures should be removed before the test.

Post-test

- Assess for signs and symptoms of laryngeal edema (i.e., dyspnea, hoarseness, apprehension).
- Monitor vital signs. The temperature may be slightly elevated for 1 to 2 days after the test.
- Assess for allergic reaction to the anesthetic and iodized contrast dye (i.e., apprehension, flushing, rash, urticaria, dyspnea, tachycardia, and/or hypotension).
- Check the gag reflex before offering fluids and food.
- Check breath signs. Report abnormal findings.
- Have the client perform postural drainage for removal of contrast dye.
- Offer throat lozenges or an ordered medication for sore throat.
- Be supportive of the client and family.

BRONCHOSCOPY

Normal Finding. Normal structure and lining of the bronchi

Description. Bronchoscopy is the direct inspection of the larynx, trachea, and bronchi through a standard metal bronchoscope or a flexible fiberoptic bronchoscope called bronchofibroscope (preferred instrument). Through the bronchoscope, a catheter brush or biopsy forceps can be passed to obtain secretions and tissues for cytologic examination. The two main purposes of bronchoscopy are visualization and specimen collection.

Purposes

- To inspect the larynx, trachea, and bronchus for lesions
- To remove foreign bodies and secretions from the tracheobronchial area
- To improve tracheobronchial drainage

Clinical Problems

Abnormal findings: Tracheobronchial lesion (tumor), bleeding site, foreign bodies, mucous plugs

Procedure

- Obtain a signed consent form.
- Restrict food and fluids for 6 hours before the bronchoscopy, preferably for 8 to 12 hours.
- Dentures, contact lenses, and jewelry should be removed.
- Obtain a history of hypersensitivity to analgesics, anesthetics, and antibiotics.
- Check vital signs and record.
- Administer premedications.
- The client will be lying on a table in the supine or semi-Fowler's position with head hyperextended or will be seated in a chair. The throat will be sprayed with a local anesthetic. The bronchoscope can be inserted through the nose or mouth.
- Specimen containers should be labeled, and specimens should be taken immediately to the laboratory.
- The procedure takes about 1 hour.

Nursing Implications

Pre-test

- Obtain vital signs and record.

Client Teaching

- Instruct the client to relax before and during the test. Instruct the client to practice breathing in and out through the nose with the mouth opened; this breathing will be used during the insertion of the bronchoscope.

- Inform the client that there may be hoarseness or sore throat after the test.
- Encourage the client to ask questions, and give client time to express concerns.
- Tell the client the test takes about 1 hour.

Post-test

- Recognize the complications that can follow bronchoscopy (i.e., laryngeal edema, bronchospasm, pneumothorax, cardiac dysrhythmias, and bleeding).
- Check blood pressure frequently as prescribed until stable.
- Assess for signs and symptoms of respiratory difficulty (i.e., dyspnea, sneezing, apprehension, and decreased breath sounds).
- Check for hemoptysis. Inform client that blood-tinged mucus is not necessarily abnormal.
- Assess the gag reflex before giving food and liquids.
- Offer lozenges or prescribed medication for mild throat irritation after gag reflex is present.

Client Teaching

- Instruct client not to smoke for 6 to 8 hours. Smoking may cause coughing and start bleeding, especially after a biopsy.
- Be supportive of client and family. Answer questions.

CARDIAC CATHETERIZATION

CARDIAC ANGIOGRAPHY (ANGIOCARDIOGRAPHY), CORONARY ARTERIOGRAPHY

Normal Findings. Patency of coronary arteries; normal heart size, structure, valves; normal heart and pulmonary pressures

Description. Cardiac catheterization is a procedure in which a long catheter is inserted in a vein or artery of the arm or leg. This catheter is threaded to the heart chambers or coronary arteries, or both, with the guidance of fluoroscopy. Contrast dye is injected for visualizing the heart structures. During injection of the dye, cineangiography is used for filming heart activity. Complications that can occur, though rare, are myocardial infarction, cardiac dysrhythmias, cardiac tamponade, pulmonary embolism, and CVA.

With *right cardiac catheterization,* the catheter is inserted into the femoral vein or an antecubital vein and is threaded through the inferior vena cava into the right atrium to the pulmonary artery. Right atrium, right ventricle, and pulmonary artery pressures are measured, and blood samples from the right side of the heart can be obtained. While the dye is being injected, the functions of the tricuspid and pulmonary valves can be observed.

For *left cardiac catheterization,* the catheter is inserted into the brachial or femoral artery and is advanced retrograde through the aorta to the coronary arteries and/or left ventricle. Dye is injected. The patency of the coronary arteries and/or functions of the aortic and mitral valves and the left ventricle can be observed. This procedure is indicated before heart surgery.

Purposes

- To identify coronary artery disease (CAD)
- To determine cardiac valvular disease

Clinical Problems

Abnormal findings: *Right-sided cardiac catheterization:* tricuspid stenosis, pulmonary stenosis, pulmonary hypertension, septal defects; *left-sided cardiac catheterization:* coronary artery disease (partial or complete coronary occlusion), mitral stenosis, mitral regurgitation, aortic regurgitation, left ventricular hypertrophy, ventricular aneurysm, septal defect

Procedure

- Obtain a signed consent form. Check that the health care provider has discussed possible risk factors before the consent form is signed.
- No food or fluid is allowed for 6 to 8 hours before the test.
- Antihistamines (e.g., Benadryl) may be ordered the evening before and the morning of the test if an allergic reaction is suspected.
- Oral anticoagulant therapy is discontinued. Heparin may be ordered to prevent thrombi.
- Client voids before taking premedications (sedative, tranquilizer, analgesic).

- The client is positioned on a padded table that tilts. Skin anesthetic is given at the site of catheter insertion. Client lies still during insertion of the catheter and filming.
- ECG leads are applied to the chest to monitor heart activity. D_5W infusion is started at a keep-vein-open (KVO) rate for administering emergency drugs as needed.
- Vital signs and heart rhythm are monitored during the procedure.
- Coughing and deep breathing are frequently requested. Coughing can decrease nausea and dizziness and possible dysrhythmia.
- The procedure takes 1½ to 3 hours.

Nursing Implications

Pre-test

- Explain the purpose and procedure of the test.
- Obtain a history of allergies to dye, seafood, or iodine.
- Record baseline vital signs and take ECG.
- Administer premedication, if prescribed, ½ to 1 hour before the test.
- Give time for client to express feelings of concern.

Client Teaching

- Inform client that a hot, flushing sensation may be felt for a minute or two when the dye is injected. Explain that clacking noises may be heard as the film advances.
- Inform the client that there should be no pain, except for some discomfort from lying on the table and at the catheter insertion.

Post-test

- Monitor vital signs every 15 minutes for the first hour and then every 30 minutes until stable.
- Observe catheter insertion site for bleeding or hematoma. Change dressings as needed.
- Check peripheral pulses below the insertion site.
- Take ECG or check heart monitor.
- Administer narcotic or non-narcotic analgesics as ordered for discomfort.

Client Teaching

- Instruct the client to remain on bedrest for 8 to 12 hours or as ordered.
- Encourage fluid intake unless contraindicated (e.g., congestive heart failure).

CERVICOGRAPHY (CERVIGRAM)

Normal Finding. Normal cervical tissue; no abnormal cells found.

Description. Cervicography is a photographic method to record an image of the cervix. This test may be done in conjunction with a Pap smear, colposcopy, and/or routine gynecologic examination. The Pap smear detects cellular changes, whereas the cervicography is a more sensitive means for detecting cervical cancer. It can identify some cancerous lesions that were missed by the Pap smear.

Purpose

- To detect cervical cancer

Clinical Problems

Abnormal findings: Cancer of the cervix, invasive cervical cancer

Procedure

- A consent form should be signed.
- No food or fluid restriction is required.
- The client is placed in the lithotomy position.
- Acetic acid (5%) is swabbed on the cervical area.
- Pathographs are taken of the cervix.
- Aqueous iodine is then swabbed on the cervix; photos follow.
- An endocervical smear is taken; tissue obtained is applied to a slide(s).

Factors Affecting Diagnostic Results

- Cervical mucus that was not removed from the cervix before applying acetic acid and the photography

Nursing Implications

- Obtain a signed consent form.
- Obtain a history of any gynecologic health problems (i.e., discharge, abnormal bleeding).

Client Teaching

- Explain the procedure to the client.
- Inform the client that she may experience a brown vaginal discharge following the procedure for a few days. This could be due to the iodine swabbed on the cervix.
- Instruct the client to inform the health care provider if great discomfort or heavy discharge occurs.

CHOLANGIOGRAPHY (IV), PERCUTANEOUS CHOLANGIOGRAPHY, T-TUBE CHOLANGIOGRAPHY

Normal Findings. Patent biliary ducts; no stones or strictures

Description. *IV cholangiography* examines the biliary ducts (hepatic ducts within the liver, the common hepatic duct, the cystic duct, and the common bile duct) by radiographic and tomographic visualization. The contrast substance, an iodine preparation such as iodipamide meglumine (Cholografin), is injected IV, and approximately 15 minutes later x-rays are taken.

Percutaneous cholangiography is indicated when biliary obstruction is suspected. The contrast substance is directly instilled into the biliary tree. The process is visualized by fluoroscopy, and spot films are taken.

T-tube cholangiography, known as postoperative cholangiography, may be done 7 to 8 hours after a cholecystectomy to explore the common bile duct for patency and to see if any gallstones remain. During the operation, a T-shaped tube is placed in the common bile duct to promote drainage. The contrast substance is injected into the T tube.

Clinical Problems

Test	*Indications/Purposes*
IV cholangiography	To detect stricture, stones, or tumor in the biliary system
Percutaneous cholangiography	To detect obstruction of the biliary system caused from stones, cancer of the pancreas

(continued)

Test	*Indications/Purposes*
T-tube cholangiography	To detect obstruction of the common bile duct from stones or stricture; fistula

Procedure

- Obtain a signed consent form.
- Restrict food and fluids for 8 hours before test.

IV cholangiography

- A laxative may be given the night before the test and a cleansing enema in the morning.
- A contrast agent, iodipamide meglumine (Cholografin) is injected IV while the client is lying on a tilting x-ray table. X-rays are taken every 15 to 30 minutes until the common bile duct is visualized.

Percutaneous cholangiography

- A laxative the night before and cleansing enema the morning of the test may be ordered.
- Preoperative medications usually include sedatives/tranquilizers. An antibiotic may be ordered for 24 to 72 hours before the test for prophylactic purposes.
- The client is placed on a tilting x-ray table that rotates. The upper right quadrant of the abdomen is cleansed and draped. A skin anesthetic is given.
- The client should exhale and hold breath while a needle is inserted with the guidance of fluoroscopy into the biliary tree. Bile is withdrawn, and the contrast substance is then injected. Spot films are taken.
- A sterile dressing will be applied to the puncture site.

T-tube cholangiography

- A cleansing enema may be ordered in the morning before the test.
- The client lies on an x-ray table and a contrast agent, such as sodium diatrizoate (Hypaque), is injected into the T tube and an x-ray is taken. Final x-ray is taken 15 minutes later.

Factors Affecting Diagnostic Results

- Obesity, gas, and fecal material in the intestines can affect the clarity of the x-ray.

Nursing Implications

- List the procedure steps for the client to alleviate anxiety.

- Recognize that obesity, gas, or fecal material in the intestines can affect the clarity of the x-ray.
- Obtain a history of allergies to seafood, iodine, or x-ray dye.
- Permit the client to express concerns. Be supportive.
- Observe for signs and symptoms of allergic reaction to contrast agents (i.e., nausea; vomiting; flushing; rash; urticaria; hypotension; slurred, thick speech; and dyspnea).
- Check the infusion site for signs of phlebitis (i.e., pain, redness, swelling). Apply warm compresses to the infusion site if symptoms are present.
- Monitor vital signs as ordered for percutaneous cholangiography. Instruct the client to remain in bed for several hours following the test.

Client Teaching

- Inform the client having IV cholangiography that the test may take several hours.

CHOLECYSTOGRAPHY (ORAL)

GALLBLADDER RADIOGRAPHY, GALLBLADDER (GB) SERIES

Normal Findings. Normal size and structure of gallbladder; no gallstones

Description. Oral cholecystography is an x-ray test used to visualize gallstones. A contrast material (radiopaque dye) is taken orally the night before, and it takes 12 to 14 hours for the dye to be concentrated in the gallbladder. Nonfunctioning liver cells can hamper the excretion of the dye. Immediately after the oral cholecystography test, the client may be given a fat-stimulus meal. Fluoroscopic examination and x-rays are taken to observe the ability of the gallbladder to empty the dye.

When the gallbladder cannot be visualized using an oral contrast substance, the IV cholangiography may be ordered. If GI x-rays are ordered, the gallbladder x-ray should be obtained first because barium could interfere with the test results.

Purposes

- To detect stones or tumor in the gallbladder
- To check for obstruction of the cystic duct

Clinical Problems

Abnormal findings: Cholelithiasis, neoplasms of the gallbladder, cholecystitis, obstruction of the cystic duct

Procedure

- The client should have a fat-free diet 24 hours before the x-ray. Restrict food and fluids except for sips of water 12 hours before the test.
- Two hours after the dinner meal, radiopaque tablets are administered according to the directions on the folder. Various commercial contrast agents are available (i.e., iopanoic acid [Telepaque], calcium or sodium ipodate [Oragrafin], iodoalphionic acid [Priodax], and iodipamide meglumine [Cholografin]).
- No laxatives should be taken until after the x-ray tests.
- A high-fat meal may be given in the x-ray department after the fasting x-rays are taken. Post–fatty-meal films will be taken at intervals to determine how fast the gallbladder expels the dye.
- The fasting x-ray test takes 45 minutes to 1 hour, and the post–fatty-meal test takes an hour or two.

Factors Affecting Diagnostic Results

- Diarrhea or vomiting can inhibit absorption of the contrast substance.
- Liver disease

Nursing Implications

- Obtain a history of allergies to seafood, iodine, or x-ray dye, as many of these agents contain iodine.
- Observe for signs and symptoms of jaundice (i.e., yellow sclera of the eyes, yellow skin, and a serum bilirubin level >3 mg/dL). Test is not done if there is severe liver disease.
- Administer the radiopaque tablets every 5 minutes with a full glass of water 2 hours after the dinner meal. Clients may take the tablets on their own.
- Observe for signs and symptoms of allergic reaction to the radiopaque tablets (i.e., elevated temperature, rash, urticaria, hypotension, thick speech, or dyspnea).
- Report vomiting and diarrhea prior to the test. Tablets may not be absorbed because of hypermotility.

Client Teaching

- Inform the client that the evening meal before the test should be fat free.
- Inform the client that the test does not hurt.
- Inform the client that a second stage of the test may be ordered. It would include a high-fat meal and then more x-rays taken.

CHORIONIC VILLI BIOPSY (CVB)

Normal Finding. Normal fetal cells

Description. Chorionic villi sampling can detect early fetal abnormalities. Fetal cells are obtained by suction from fingerlike projections around the embryonic membrane, which eventually becomes the placenta. The test is performed between the eighth and tenth week of pregnancy. After the tenth week maternal cells begin to grow over the villi.

Advantage of CVB over amniocentesis is that CVB may be performed earlier, and results can be obtained in a few days and not weeks. Disadvantage is that CVB cannot determine neural tube defects and pulmonary maturity.

Purpose

- To detect chromosomal disorders

Clinical Problems

Abnormal findings: Chromosomal disorders; hemoglobinopathies (e.g., sickle-cell anemia); lysosomal storage disorders, such as Tay-Sachs disease.

Procedure

- Obtain a signed consent form.
- No food or fluid restriction is required.
- Place client in lithotomy position.
- Ultrasound is used to verify the placement of the catheter at the villi. Suction is applied, and tissue is removed from the villi.
- Test takes approximately 30 minutes.

Factors Affecting Diagnostic Results

- Performing the test 10 weeks after gestation

Nursing Implications

- Assess for signs of spontaneous abortion resulting from procedure (i.e., cramps, bleeding).
- Be supportive of client and family. Be a good listener.
- Assess for infection resulting from the procedure (i.e., chills, fever).

Client Teaching

- Instruct the client to report if excessive bleeding or severe cramping occurs after the procedure.

COLONOSCOPY

Normal Findings. Normal mucosa of the large intestine; absence of pathology

Description. Colonoscopy, an endoscopic procedure, is an inspection of the large intestine (colon) using a long, flexible fiberscope (colonoscope). This test is useful for evaluating suspicious lesions in the large colon (i.e., tumor mass, polyps, and inflammatory tissue). Biopsy of the tissue or polyp can be obtained. Polyps can be removed with the use of an electrocautery snare.

Colonoscopy should not be done on pregnant women near term, following an acute myocardial infarction, after recent abdominal surgery, in acute diverticulitis, in severe (active) ulcerative colitis, or in a confused/uncooperative patient. Occasionally, colon perforation is caused by the fiberscope; however, this is rare. Bleeding may be a side effect of the biopsy or polypectomy.

Purposes

- To detect the origin of lower intestinal bleeding
- To identify polyps in the large intestine
- To screen for benign or malignant lesions (tumors) in the colon

Clinical Problems

Abnormal findings: Lower intestinal bleeding, diverticular disease, benign or malignant lesions (i.e., polyps or tumors), ulcerative colitis

Procedure. Bowel preparation procedure may vary among institutions.

- Obtain a signed consent form.
- Specific laboratory tests (hemoglobin, hematocrit, PT, PTT, and platelet count) should be done within 2 days before the test.
- Iron medication should be withheld at least 4 days before the procedure.
- A sedative/tranquilizer may be ordered prior to the test to promote relaxation. A narcotic analgesic may be titrated IV during the procedure.
- Glucagon or IV anticholinergics may be given to decrease bowel spasms.
- Barium sulfate from other diagnostic studies can decrease visualization; therefore, the study should not be attempted within 10 days to 2 weeks of a barium study.
- Avoid using soapsuds enemas. These can irritate intestine.

Preparation A (use of GoLYTELY/Colyte solution)

- Instruct the client to take magnesium citrate at 4 PM two days prior to test.

Day before test

- Prepare GoLYTELY or Colyte solution according to instructions, and refrigerate solution.
- Instruct the client to have a regular lunch and a liquid dinner (i.e., broth, gelatin, etc).
- Have the client drink GoLYTELY/Colyte as instructed at 7 PM to 10 PM.

Morning of test

- Client may drink 8 ounces of clear liquid (black coffee, tea, water, clear juice) up to 1 hour before test.

Preparation B (72-hour clear liquid/enemas)

- Instruct the client to have only a clear liquid diet for 3 days before test.
- Follow 48-hour Fleet Prep Kit No. 2.

Nursing Implications

Pre-test

- Record baseline vital signs and pertinent laboratory values.
- Report anxiety and fears to the health care provider conducting the procedure.

Client Teaching

- Explain the procedure of the test. The client lies in Sims position on left side. A lubricated colonoscope is inserted. Air may be insufflated for better visualization. X-rays are taken.
- Instruct the client to bring someone to drive him or her home.
- Inform the client that the procedure takes from ½ to 1½ hours.
- Instruct client to breathe deeply and slowly through the mouth during the insertion of the colonoscope.

Post-test

- Monitor vital signs every ½ hour for 2 hours or until stable.
- Assess for anal bleeding, abdominal distention, severe pain, severe abdominal cramps, and fever, and report any of these signs or symptoms to the health care provider immediately.

Client Teaching

- Instruct the client to rest for 2 to 6 hours following the procedure.

COLPOSCOPY

Normal Finding. Normal appearance of the vagina and cervical structures

Description. Colposcopy is the examination of the vagina and cervix using a binocular instrument (colposcope) that has a magnifying lens and a light. This test can be performed in the gynecologist's office or in the hospital. After a positive Pap smear or a suspicious cervical lesion, colposcopy is indicated for examining the vagina and cervix more thoroughly. Atypical epithelium, leukoplakia vulvae, and irregular blood vessels can be identified with this procedure, and photographs and a biopsy specimen can be obtained.

Since the test has become more popular, there has been a decreased need for conization (surgical removal of a cone of tissue from the cervical os). Colposcopy is also useful for monitoring women whose mothers received diethylstilbestrol during pregnancy; these women are prone to develop precancerous and cancerous lesions of the vagina and cervix.

Purpose

- To identify precancerous lesions of the cervix

Clinical Problems

Indications: Vaginal and cervical lesions, abnormal cervical tissue after a positive Pap smear, irregular blood vessels, leukoplakia vulvae, dysplasia and cervical lesions, vaginal and cervical tissue changes for women whose mothers took diethylstilbestrol during pregnancy

Procedure

- A consent form should be signed.
- No food or fluid restriction is required.
- The client's clothes should be removed, and the client should wear a gown and be properly draped.
- The client assumes a lithotomy position (legs in stirrups).
- 3% acetic acid is applied to the vagina and cervix. This produces color changes in the cervical epithelium and helps in detecting abnormal changes.
- A biopsy specimen of suspicious tissues and photographs may be taken.
- A vaginal tampon may be worn after the procedure.
- The test takes approximately 15 to 20 minutes.

Factors Affecting Diagnostic Results

- Mucus, cervical secretions, creams, and medications can decrease visualization.

Nursing Implications

- Obtain a signed consent form.
- Be present during the test.
- Place the biopsy tissue into a bottle containing a preservative; place the cells, if obtained, on a slide; and spray them with a fixative solution.

Client Teaching

- Inform the client that she should not experience pain but that there may be some discomfort with the insertion of the speculum or when the biopsy is taken.
- Inform the client that the test takes 15 to 20 minutes

Post-test client teaching

- Inform the client that she may have some bleeding for a few hours because of the biopsy. Tell the client that she can use tampons and that if bleeding becomes heavy and it is not her menstrual period, she should call the gynecologist.
- Instruct the client not to have intercourse for a week, until the biopsy side is healed, or as ordered by the health care provider.
- Inform the client that she should be notified of the results of the test, and tell her to call if she has not heard from the office in a week.

COMPUTED TOMOGRAPHY (CT) SCAN, COMPUTED AXIAL TOMOGRAPHY (CAT)

CAT SCAN, COMPUTED TRANSAXIAL TOMOGRAPHY (CTT), EMI SCAN

Normal Findings. Normal tissue; no pathologic findings

Description. The computed tomography (CT) scan, or CAT scan, was developed in England in 1972 and was called the EMI scan. The CT scanner produces a narrow x-ray beam that examines body sections from many different angles. It produces a series of cross-sectional images in sequence that build up a three-dimensional picture of the structure.

The CT scan can be performed with or without iodine contrast media (dye). It is not an invasive test unless contrast dye is used. The contrast dye causes a greater tissue absorption and is referred to as contrast enhancement. This enhancement enables small tumors to be seen.

CT is capable of scanning the head, abdomen (stomach, small and large intestines, liver, spleen, pancreas, bile duct, kidney, and adrenals), pelvis (bladder, reproductive organs, and small and large bowel within pelvis), and chest (lung, heart, mediastinal structure). The CT scan detects most types of body tissue, but NOT nerves. This procedure does not cause pain; however, there may be some discomfort from lying still.

High-speed CT is available at most institutions. This CT uses a "slip ring" that provides continuous spiral scanning, enabling large areas to be scanned in half the time. This allows data to be reconstructed into a three-dimensional image. This type of CT is most helpful to orthopedic and plastic surgeons by showing fractures in the facial area, hip fractures, and other areas. Cine CT (ultrafast CT) measures blood flow to the brain and through the heart.

Purposes

- To screen for coronary artery disease; head, liver, and renal lesions; tumors; edema; abscess; bone destruction
- To locate foreign objects in soft tissues, such as the eye

Clinical Problems

CT Type	*Abnormal Findings*
Head	Cerebral lesions: hematomas, tumors, cysts, abscess, infarction, edema, atrophy, hydrocephalus
Internal auditory canal	Acoustic neuroma, cholesteatoma, bone erosion
Eye orbits	Bone destruction, optic nerve tumors, muscle tumor
Sinus	Bone destruction, sinusitis, polyps, tumors
Neck (soft tissue)	Tumors, abscess, stones in the salivary ducts, enlarged nodes
Abdomen:	
Liver	Hepatic lesions: cysts, abscess, tumors, hematomas, cirrhosis with ascites
Biliary	Obstruction due to calculi
Pancreatic	Acute and chronic pancreatitis; pancreatic lesions: tumor, abscess, pseudocysts
Kidney	Renal lesions: tumors, calculi, cysts, congenital anomalies; perirenal hematomas and abscesses
Adrenal	Adrenal tumors
Chest and thoracic	Chest lesions: tumors, cysts, abscesses; aortic aneurysm; enlarged lymph nodes in mediastinum; pleural effusion

(continued)

CT Type	*Abnormal Findings*
Spine	Tumors, paraspinal cysts, vascular malformation, congenital spinal anomalies (e.g., spina bifida, herniated intervertebral disk)
Bony pelvis, long bones, joints	Bone destruction, fractures, tumors
Guided needle biopsy	For lung or liver masses, adrenal mass, kidney

Procedure

General preparation for all scans

- Obtain a signed consent form.
- For AM scheduling: NPO 8 hours before test. For PM scheduling: NPO after a full liquid breakfast. Small sips of water may be taken 2 hours before test. NPO may not be necessary if contrast dye is *not* used. Check with CT supervisor for food and fluid restrictions.
- Medications can be taken until 2 hours before the test.
- With a possible allergic reaction to contrast dye, prednisone, diphenhydramine (Benadryl), and ranitidine (Zantac) may be given one hour prior to CT. With a possible severe allergic reaction, these drugs may be given 6 and 12 hours prior to CT.
- IV infusion or heparin lock inserted may be required prior to test.
- CT scanning usually takes 30 minutes to 1½ hours.

Head CT

- Remove hairpins, clips, and jewelry (earrings) before the test.
- A mild sedative or analgesic may be ordered for restless clients or for those who have aches and pains of the neck or back.
- Head is positioned in a cradle, and a wide, rubberized strap is applied snugly around the head to keep it immobilized during test.

Abdominal and pelvic CT

- Abdominal x-ray (KUB) may be requested before CT scan.
- Laboratory reports of serum creatinine and BUN should be available.
- GI tract must be free from barium. An enema may be ordered.
- For an AM abdominal/pelvic scan, give the oral contrast media (15 oz) between 8 PM and 10 PM the evening before the scan. NPO after 10 PM. One hour prior to the CT, give ½ bottle of the oral contrast. One-half hour prior to the CT, give the remaining ½ bottle of oral contrast.
- For a PM abdominal/pelvic scan, give 1 bottle (15 oz) of oral contrast media at 7 AM the morning of the scan. NPO after 7 am. One

hour prior to the CT, give ½ bottle of the oral contrast. One-half hour prior to the CT, give ½ bottle of the oral contrast.

- For abdominal scan, give the oral contrast media (15 oz) 1 hour before scan. Half of the oral solution may be given 1 hour before and the remaining solution ½ hour before scan.
- For pelvic scan, give the oral contrast media (15 oz) between 8 PM and 10 PM the evening before the scan. Additional oral contrast media is usually given the morning of the scan.

Chest CT

- A chest x-ray may be requested before a chest scan.
- IV contrast media is frequently given in left arm.

Spine CT

- NPO is not indicated, as contrast media is usually not ordered.
- Spine x-rays taken prior to scan should be available.

Neck CT

- IV contrast media is used. Check general preparation for scan for IV contrast injection studies.

Bony pelvis, long bones, and joints CT

- Nuclear medicine study to locate "hot areas" should be done before the CT scan of the bones and joints.

Factors Affecting Diagnostic Results

- Barium sulfate, flatus, and metal plates can obscure visualization.

Nursing Implications

- Obtain a history of allergies to seafood, iodine, and contrast dye from other x-ray tests. Contrast enhancement is not always done with CT, especially for head, chest, and spinal CT scanning.
- Observe for signs and symptoms of a severe allergic reaction to the dye (i.e., dyspnea, palpitations, tachycardia, hypotension, itching, and urticaria). Emergency drugs should be available.
- Observe for delayed allergic reaction to the contrast dye (i.e., skin rash, urticaria, headache, and vomiting). An oral antihistamine may be ordered for mild reactions.
- Be supportive of the client and family.

Client Teaching

- Explain the procedure to the client. The CT scanner is circular with a doughnut-like opening. The client is strapped to a special table with the scanner revolving around the body area that is to be examined. Clicking noises will be heard from the scanner. The radiologist or specialized technician is in a control room and can observe and communicate all times through an intercom system. The test is *not* painful.

- Inform the client that holding breath may be requested several times during an abdominal scan.
- Inform the client that the CT of the head takes 30 minutes without contrast media and 1 to 1½ hours with use of contrast. For body CT, the test takes 1½ hours.
- Advise the client that if contrast dye is injected IV, a warm, flushed sensation may be felt in the face or body. A salty or metallic taste may be experienced. Nausea is not uncommon. These sensations usually last for 1 or 2 minutes.
- Instruct the client to resume usual level of activity and diet, unless otherwise indicated.

CYSTOSCOPY, CYSTOGRAPHY (CYSTOGRAM)

CYSTOURETHROSCOPY

Normal Findings. Normal structure of the urethra, bladder, prostatic urethra, and ureter orifices

Description. Cystoscopy is the direct visualization of the bladder wall and urethra with the use of a cystoscope. With this procedure, small renal calculi can be removed from the ureter, bladder, or urethra, and a tissue biopsy can be obtained. A *retrograde pyelography,* injection of contrast dye through the catheter into the ureters and renal pelvis, may be performed during the cystoscopy.

Cystography is the instillation of a contrast dye into the bladder via a catheter. This procedure can detect neurogenic bladder, fistulas, tumors, and a rupture in the bladder.

Purposes

- To detect renal calculi and renal tumor
- To remove renal stones
- To determine the cause of hematuria or urinary tract infection (UTI)

Clinical Problems

Abnormal findings: Renal calculi, tumors, prostatic hyperplasia, urethral stricture, hematuria, urinary tract infection

Procedure

- Obtain a signed consent form.
- Provide a full liquid breakfast in the AM if local anesthetic is used. Several glasses of water before the test may be ordered. Restrict food and fluids for 8 hours before cystoscopy if general anesthesia is given.
- Record baseline vital signs.
- A narcotic analgesic may be ordered 1 hour before cystoscopy. The procedure is done under local or general anesthesia.
- The client is placed in the lithotomy position. A local anesthetic is injected into the urethra. Water may be instilled to enhance better visualization. A urine specimen may be obtained.
- Test procedure takes about 30 minutes to 1 hour.

Nursing Implications

- Obtain history concerning the presence of cystitis or prostatitis, which could result in sepsis following the procedure.
- Check for hypersensitivity to anesthetics.
- Assess urinary patterns—amount, color, odor, specific gravity—and take vital signs.

Client Teaching

- Explain the test procedure.
- Inform the client that there may be some pressure or burning discomfort during or following the test.

Post-test

- Recognize the complications that can occur as the result of a cystoscopy: hemorrhaging, perforation of the bladder, urinary retention, and infection.
- Monitor vital signs. Compare with baseline vital signs.
- Monitor urinary output for 48 hours following a cystoscopy.
- Report gross hematuria. Inform the client that blood-tinged urine is not uncommon.

- Observe for signs and symptoms of an infection: fever, chills, tachycardia, burning on urination, pain. Antibiotics may be given before and after the test as a prophylactic measure.
- Apply heat to the lower abdomen to relieve pain and muscle spasm as ordered. A warm sitz bath may be ordered.

Client Teaching

- Advise client to avoid alcoholic beverages for 2 days after the test.
- Inform client that a slight burning sensation when voiding might occur for a day or two.

ECHOCARDIOGRAPHY (ECHOCARDIOGRAM)*

M-MODE, TWO-DIMENSIONAL (2D), SPECTRAL DOPPLER, COLOR FLOW DOPPLER, TRANSESOPHAGEAL, CONTRAST, AND STRESS ECHOCARDIOGRAPHY

Normal Findings. Normal heart size and structure; normal movements of heart valves and heart chambers

Description. Echocardiography (echocardiogram) is a noninvasive ultrasound test used to identify abnormal heart size, structure, and function, and valvular disease. A hand-held transducer (probe) moves over the chest area of the heart and other specified surrounding areas. The transducer sends and receives high-frequency sound waves. The sound waves that are reflected (echo) from the heart back to the transducer produce pictures. These pictures appear on a television-like screen and are recorded on videotape and moving graph paper.

There are several types of echocardiographic studies, which include M-mode, two-dimensional (2D), spectral Doppler, color flow Doppler, transesophageal, contrast, and stress echocardiography. Transesophageal echocardiography (TEE) is gaining popularity for diagnosing and managing a wide range of cardiovascular diseases, such as valvular heart dys-

---

*Revised by Frank Di Gregorio, CNMT, RDMS, Director, Community Imaging Center, Wilmington, Delaware.

function and aortic pathology. Stress echocardiography is a valuable tool for assessing myocardial ischemia at half the cost of other cardiac studies.

M-mode echocardiography: M-mode echocardiography, the earliest type of echocardiography, is used to record the motion of various heart structures (M is for *motion*). This test assesses the dimension of the left ventricle and its degree of dilatation and contractility related to myocardial disease or volume overload. It is useful for measuring the thickness of the right and left ventricles (hypertrophy). M-mode echocardiography is also used for assessing the cardiac valves and valvular movements for stenosis, regurgitation, or prolapse.

Two-dimensional (2D) echocardiography: This test employs M-mode echocardiography, which records motion, and provides two-dimensional (cross-sectional) views of the heart structures. It is used to evaluate the size, shape, and movement of the chambers and valves of the heart and it is useful in detecting valvular disease and in assessing congenital heart disease.

Spectral Doppler echocardiography: Spectral Doppler measures the amount, speed, and dissection of blood passing through the heart valves and heart chambers. A swishing sound is heard as the blood flows throughout the heart. This test can detect turbulent blood flow through the heart valves and may indicate valvular disease. Septal wall defects may also be detected.

Color Doppler echocardiography: The color flow Doppler (red and blue) shows the direction of blood flowing through the heart. It can identify leaking heart valves (regurgitation) or hardened valves (stenosis), function of prosthetic valves, and the presence of shunts (holes) in the heart. The use of the color flow Doppler complements the 2-D echocardiogram and the spectral Doppler study.

Transesophageal echocardiography: With transesophageal echocardiography (TEE), a transducer (probe) is attached to an endoscope and is inserted into the esophagus to visualize adjacent cardiac and extracardiac structures with greater acuity than most echocardiography studies, including transthoracic (TTE). TEE can be used in the intensive care unit, emergency department and operating room, as well as in cardiac testing facilities. This type of echocardiography is useful for diagnosing mitral and aortic valvular pathology; determining the presence of a possible intracardiac thrombus in the left atrium; detecting suspected acute dissection of the aorta and endocarditis; monitoring left ventricular function before, during, or after surgery; and evaluating intracardiac repairs during surgery.

This test is contraindicated if esophageal pathology (e.g., strictures, varices, trauma) exists. Also, TEE should not be performed if undiagnosed active gastrointestinal bleeding is occurring or if the client is uncooperative. A light sedative is frequently given prior to testing. TEE can be performed on an unconscious client. TEE is tolerated well, with approximately 1% of clients being intolerant of the esophageal probe. The rate of complications is <0.2%.

Contrast echocardiography: This test assists in determining intracardiac communications and myocardial ischemia and perfusion defects. Microbubbles are injected into the venous circulation for the purpose of recording showers of echoes by M-mode or 2D tests. The microbubbles pass through the right atrium and ventricle, where they are absorbed in the lung; they do not pass to the left side of the heart. If the microbubbles are detected on the left side of the heart, an intracardiac communication or shunt is present. New contrast agents are under development which may allow visualization of the coronary arteries with echocardiography.

Stress echocardiography: It may be necessary to evaluate the function of the left ventricle under stress. Physical exercise hampers good imaging, so the ventricle is stressed pharmacologically using the inotropic drugs dobutamine and dipyridamole (Persantine). Dobutamine is a most effective nonexercise stressor. The object of this test is to detect myocardial ischemia caused by coronary artery disease (CAD). To determine perfusion and wall motion abnormalities, dipyridamole and a contrast agent are used. Some facilities use a combination of dipyridamole and dobutamine for stress echocardiographic testing. This combination increases the effectiveness of detecting multivessel coronary artery disease (CAD) from 72% with one pharmacologic agent to 92% using both. Arbutamine is a new inotropic agent in use in Europe and is being tested in the United States.

Purposes

- To identify abnormal heart size, structure, and function
- To detect cardiac valvular disease and septal wall defects
- To determine the function of prosthetic heart valves
- To assess the effects of congenital heart disease
- To monitor left ventricular function before, during, and after surgery
- To evaluate and rule out coronary artery disease

Clinical Problems

Abnormal findings: Abnormal heart size, structure, and function, heart valvular disease (regurgitation or stenosis of the aortic or mitral valves); congenital heart disease; heart wall damage after a myocardial infarction; cardiomyopathy mural thrombi; pericardial effusion; aortic pathology; and endocarditis

Diagnostic Tests	*Indications to Determine/Detect*
M-mode echocardiography	Dimension of the left ventricle Degree of ventricular dilatation and contractility Ventricular hypertrophy Function of cardiac valves—stenosis or regurgitation
Two-dimensional (2D) echocardiography	Cardiac valvular disease
Spectral Doppler echocardiography	Blood flow through heart chambers and valves Septal wall defects
Color Doppler echocardiography	Direction of blood flow through the heart Function of cardiac valves—stenosis or regurgitation Function of prosthetic valves Presence of shunting in the heart
Transeosphageal echocardiography	Function of left ventricle before, during, or after surgery Cardiac valvular disease Presence of intracardiac thrombus in left atrium Aortic disease (e.g., dissection of aorta) Presence of endocarditis
Contrast echocardiography	Perfusion defects Presence of shunting in the heart
Stress echocardiography	Function of left ventricle under stress Perfusion defects Wall motion abnormalities

Procedure

- Obtain a signed consent form.
- No food or fluid restriction is required.
- No medications should be omitted before the test unless indicated by the institution or health care provider.

- The client undresses from the waist up and wears a hospital gown. The client is positioned on his or her left side or in supine position.
- Vital signs are recorded. Three electrode patches are applied to the chest area to monitor heart rate and changes in cardiac rhythm.
- Water-soluble gel is applied to the skin areas that are to be scanned. The transducer, with slight pressure, moves over different areas of the chest. Some clients may require pictures to be taken under the neck.
- The 2D echo takes about 20 to 30 minutes, and the 2D echo with Doppler studies takes approximately 30 to 45 minutes.
- The cardiologist interprets the test results and sends report to the client's personal health care provider (HCP). The HCP gives test results to the client.

Transesophageal echocardiography (TEE):

- The client should be NPO for at least 4 hours prior to test.
- A light sedative is given prior to the test.
- An IV sedative (e.g., Versed) is given.
- The endoscopic transducer is inserted into the esophagus.
- The test takes 15 to 30 minutes.
- The client is monitored (Dynamap) during recovery for 1 to 2 hours.

Contrast echocardiography

- An IV line is inserted for injection of contrast media.

Stress echocardiography

- The client should be NPO for 4 hours before the test.
- The client may be placed on a treadmill or receive a pharmacologic agent.
- Images are acquired during rest (pretest) and then during stress or immediately following stress (post-test).

Factors Affecting Diagnostic Results

- Large body habitus may cause poor image quality.
- Severe respiratory disease may affect test results.

Nursing Implications

- Obtain a history of the client's physical complaints.
- Obtain vital signs and an ECG recording as indicated. These are for baseline readings.
- Check that the consent form has been signed.

Client Teaching

- Explain the procedure to the client (see Procedure).
- Inform the client that he or she will be positioned on his or her back and/or left side during the test procedure.
- Inform the client that a gel will be applied to the skin area and that the transducer (probe) moves over the gel area. The sound waves are transmitted as a picture on videotape and on graph paper.
- Inform the client that he or she will receive test results from either the cardiologist or the health care provider.
- Answer client's questions or refer questions to health care providers.

ELECTROCARDIOGRAPHY (ELECTROCARDIOGRAM—ECG OR EKG), VECTORCARDIOGRAPHY (VECTORCARDIOGRAM—VCG)

Normal Finding. Normal electrocardiogram deflections, P, PR, QRS, QT, S-T, and T

Description. An electrocardiogram (ECG) records the electrical impulses of the heart by means of electrodes and a galvanometer (ECG machine). These electrodes are placed on the legs, arms, and chest. Combinations of two electrodes are called bipolar leads (i.e., lead I is the combination of both arm electrodes, lead II is the combination of right-arm and left-leg electrodes, and lead III is the combination of the left-arm and left-leg electrodes). The unipolar leads are AVF, AVL, and AVR; the A means augmented, V is the voltage, and F is left foot, L is left arm, and R is right arm. There are at least six unipolar chest or precordial leads. A standard ECG consists of 12 leads; six limb leads (I, II, III, AVF, AVL, AVR) and six chest (precordial) leads (V_1, V_2, V_3, V_4, V_5, V_6).

The electrical activity that the ECG records is in the form of waves and complexes: P wave (atrial depolarization); QRS complex (ventricular depolarization); and ST segment, T wave, and U wave (ventricular repolarization). An abnormal ECG indicates a disturbance in the electrical activity of the myocardium. A person could have heart disease and have a normal ECG as long as the cardiac problem did not affect the transmission of electrical impulses.

P wave (atrial contraction or depolarization): The normal time is 0.12 seconds. An enlarged P-wave deflection could indicate atrial enlargement. An absent or altered P wave could suggest that the electrical impulse did not come from the SA node.

PR interval (from the P wave to the onset of the Q wave): The normal time interval is 0.12 to 0.2 seconds. An increased interval could imply a conduction delay in the AV node that could result from rheumatic fever or arteriosclerotic heart disease. A short interval could indicate Wolff-Parkinson-White syndrome.

QRS complex (ventricular contraction or depolarization): The normal time is less than 0.12 seconds. An enlarged Q wave may imply an old myocardial infarction. An enlarged R wave deflection could indicate ventricular hypertrophy. An increased time duration may indicate a bundle-branch block.

QT interval (ventricular depolarization and repolarization): The normal time interval is 0.36 to 0.44 seconds. A shortened or prolonged QT interval could imply ischemia or electrolyte imbalances.

ST segment (beginning ventricular repolarization): A depressed ST segment indicates myocardial ischemia. An elevated ST segment can indicate acute myocardial infarction (AMI) or pericarditis. A prolonged ST segment may imply hypocalcemia or hypokalemia. A short ST segment may be due to hypercalcemia.

T wave (ventricular repolarization): A flat or inverted T wave can indicate myocardial ischemia, myocardial infarction, or hypokalemia. A tall, peaked T wave, >10 mm in precordial leads, or >5 mm in limb leads, can indicate hyperkalemia.

Vectorcardiogram (VCG): The VCG records electrical impulses from the cardiac cycle, making it similar to the ECG. However, it shows a three-dimensional view (frontal, horizontal, and sagittal planes) of the heart, whereas the ECG shows a two-dimensional view (frontal and horizontal planes). The VCG is considered more sensitive than the ECG for diagnosing a myocardial infarction. It is useful for assessing ventricular hypertrophy in adults and children.

Purposes

- To detect cardiac dysrhythmias

- To identify electrolyte imbalance (e.g., hyperkalemia [peaked T wave])
- To monitor ECG changes during the stress/exercise tests and the recovery phase after a myocardial infarction

Clinical Problems

Abnormal findings: Cardiac dysrhythmias, cardiac hypertrophies, myocardial ischemia, electrolyte imbalances, myocardial infarction, pericarditis

Procedure

- No food, fluid, or medication is restricted.
- Clothing should be removed to the waist, and the female client should wear a gown.
- Nylon stockings should be removed, and trouser legs should be raised.
- The client lies in the supine position.
- The skin surface should be prepared. Excess hair should be shaved from the chest if necessary.
- Electrodes with electropaste or pads are strapped to the four extremities. Chest electrodes are applied. The lead selector is turned to record the 12 standard leads.
- The ECG takes approximately 15 minutes.

Nursing Implications

- List medications the client is taking and the last time they were taken. The health care provider may want to compare ECG results with prescribed medications.

Client Teaching

- Instruct the client to relax and to breathe normally during the ECG procedure. Tell the client to avoid tightening the muscles, grasping bed rails or other objects, and talking during the ECG tracing.
- Tell the client that the ECG does not cause pain or any discomfort.
- Instruct the client to tell you if he or she is having chest pain during the ECG tracing. Mark the ECG paper at the time the client is having chest pain.
- Allow the client time to ask questions.

ELECTROENCEPHALOGRAPHY, ELECTROENCEPHALOGRAM (EEG)

Normal Finding. Normal tracing

Description. The electroencephalogram (EEG) measures the electrical impulses produced by brain cells. Electrodes, applied to the scalp surface at predetermined measured positions, record brain-wave activity on moving paper. EEG tracings can detect patterns characteristic of some diseases (i.e., seizure disorders, neoplasms, strokes, head trauma, infections of the nervous system, and cerebral death). At times, recorded brain waves may be normal when there is pathology.

Purposes

- To detect seizure disorder
- To identify a brain tumor, abscess, intracranial hemorrhage
- To assist in the determination of cerebral death

Clinical Problems

Abnormal tracing: Seizure disorders (i.e., grand mal, petit mal, psychomotor); brain tumor; brain abscesses; head injury; intracranial hemorrhage; encephalitis; cerebral death

Procedure. The procedure may be performed while the client is (1) awake, (2) drowsy, (3) asleep, (4) undergoing stimuli (rhythmic flashes of bright light), or (5) a combination of any of these.

- Shampoo hair the night before. Instruct the client not to use oil or hair spray on the hair.
- The decision concerning withdrawal or holding of medications before the EEG is made by the health care provider.
- No food or fluid is restricted, with the exception of *no* coffee, tea, cola, and alcohol.
- The EEG tracing is usually obtained with the client lying down; however, the client could be seated in a reclining chair.
- For a sleep recording, keep the client awake 2 to 3 hours later the night before the test, and wake the client at 6 AM. A sedative such as chloral hydrate may be ordered.
- The EEG takes approximately 1½ to 2 hours.

Post-test

- Remove the collodion or paste from the client's head. Acetone may be used to remove the paste.
- Normal activity may be resumed, unless the client was sedated.

Nursing Implications

- Report medications that the client is taking that could change the EEG result.
- Report to the health care provider and EEG laboratory any apprehension, restlessness, or anxiety of client.
- Observe for seizures, and describe the seizure activity.

Client Teaching

- Inform client that getting an electric shock from the machine does not occur. Also the EEG machine does not determine intelligence and cannot read the mind. Many clients are apprehensive about the test.
- Encourage the client to eat before the test. Hypoglycemia should be prevented because it can affect normal brain activity. Coffee, tea, and any other stimulants should be avoided. Alcohol and tranquilizers are depressants that can affect test results.
- Inform client that the test does not produce pain.
- Advise the client to be calm and to relax during the test. If rest and stimuli recordings are ordered, inform the client that there will be a brief time when there are flashing lights.
- Instruct the client that normal activity can be resumed following the test.

ELECTROMYOGRAPHY, ELECTROMYOGRAM (EMG)

Normal Findings. At rest: minimal electrical activity; voluntary muscle contraction: markedly increased electrical activity

Description. Electromyography (EMG) measures electrical activity of skeletal muscles at rest and during voluntary muscle contraction. A needle electrode is inserted into the skeletal muscle to pick up electrical activity, which can be heard over a loudspeaker, viewed on an oscilloscope, and recorded on graph paper all at the same time. Normally there is no (or minimal) electrical activity at rest; however, in motor disorders, abnormal patterns occur. With voluntary muscle contraction, there is a loud popping sound and increased electrical activity (waves).

The test is useful in diagnosing neuromuscular disorders. EMG can be used to differentiate between myopathy and neuropathy.

Purposes

- To diagnose neuromuscular disorders, such as muscular dystrophy
- To differentiate between myopathy and neuropathy

Clinical Problems

Abnormal findings: Muscular dystrophy; peripheral neuropathy due to diabetes mellitus, alcoholism; myasthenia gravis, myotonia; amyotrophic lateral sclerosis (ALS), anterior poliomyelitis

Procedure

- Obtain a signed consent form.
- No food or fluid is restricted, with the exception of *no* coffee, tea, colas, or other caffeine drinks, and *no* smoking for 3 hours before the test.
- Medications such as muscle relaxants, anticholinergics, and cholinergics should be withheld until after the test with the health care provider's approval. If specific medication is needed, the time of the test should be rearranged.
- The client lies on a table or sits in a chair in a room free of noise. Needle electrodes are inserted in selected or affected muscles. If the client experiences marked pain, the needle should be removed and reinserted.
- The procedure takes approximately 1 to 2 hours.
- If serum enzyme tests are ordered (i.e., SGOT, CPK, LDH), the specimen should be drawn before the EMG or 5 to 10 days after the test.

Post-test

- If residual pain occurs, analgesic may be given.

Nursing Implications

- Withhold medications that could affect EMG results with permission.
- Draw blood for serum enzymes prior to the test if ordered.
- Administer analgesic if residual pain is present.

Client Teaching

- Inform client that the test will not cause electrocution; however, there may be a slight, temporary discomfort when the needle electrodes are inserted. If pain persists for several minutes, the technician should be told.
- Instruct the client to follow the technician's instructions (i.e., to relax specified muscle(s) and to contract the muscle(s) when requested).

ENDOSCOPIC RETROGRADE CHOLANGIOPANCREATOGRAPHY (ERCP)

Normal Findings. Normal biliary and pancreatic ducts

Description. Endoscopic retrograde cholangiopancreatography (ERCP) is an endoscopic and x-ray examination of the biliary pancreatic ducts after contrast medium is injected into the duodenal papilla. The purpose of this procedure is to identify the cause of the biliary obstruction, which could be due to stricture, cyst, stones, or tumor.

ERCP is performed following abdominal ultrasound, CT, liver scanning, or biliary tract x-ray studies to confirm or diagnose hepatobiliary or pancreatic disorder.

Purposes

- To detect biliary stones, stricture, cyst, or tumor
- To identify biliary obstruction, such as stones or stricture
- To confirm biliary or pancreatic disorder

Clinical Problems

Abnormal findings: Biliary stones, stricture, cyst, or tumor; primary cholangitis; pancreatic stones, stricture, cysts or pseudocysts, or tumor; chronic pancreatitis; pancreatic fibrosis; or duodenal papilla tumors

Procedure

- Obtain a signed consent form.
- Restrict food and fluids for 8 hours before the test.

- Obtain baseline vital signs. Have the client void.
- Premedicate with mild narcotic or sedative. Atropine may be given prior to or after insertion of the endoscope.
- Local anesthetic is sprayed in the pharynx to decrease the gag reflex prior to the insertion of the fiberoptic endoscope.
- Secretin may be given IV to paralyze the duodenum. Contrast medium is injected after the endoscope is at the duodenal papilla and the catheter is in the pancreatic duct.
- Test takes ½ to 1 hour.

Nursing Implications

- Obtain a client history of allergies to seafood, iodine, and contrast dye. Report allergic findings.
- Determine whether anxiety level may interfere with client's ability to absorb information concerning the procedure.
- Monitor the vital signs during the test and compare to baseline vital signs. Rupture within the GI tract caused by endoscope perforation could cause shock.

Client Teaching

- Inform client that the endoscope will not obstruct breathing.
- Explain that there may be a sore throat for a few days after the test.
- Be supportive of the client prior to and during the test procedure.

Post-test

- Monitor vital signs. A rise in temperature might indicate infection.
- Check skin color. Jaundice is an indicator of disease process.
- Check the gag reflex before offering food or drink.
- Check for signs and symptoms of urinary retention caused by atropine.

Client Teaching

- Suggest warm saline gargle and lozenges to decrease throat discomfort, which may persist for a few days after the test.

ESOPHAGEAL STUDIES

ESOPHAGEAL ACIDITY, ESOPHAGEAL MANOMETRY, ACID PERFUSION (BERNSTEIN TEST)

Normal Finding. Esophagus secretions of pH 5 to 6

Description. Esophageal studies are performed mainly to determine pyrosis (heartburn) and dysphagia (difficulty in swallowing). Most esophageal problems result from a reflux of gastric juices into the lower part of the esophagus because of inadequate closure of the cardioesophageal (low esophageal) sphincter.

Gastric secretions are highly acidic with a pH of 1.0 to 2.5, whereas the pH in the esophagus is 5.0 to 6.0. Backflow of gastric juices causes esophageal irritation or esophagitis. The three common esophageal studies are esophageal acidity, esophageal manometry, and acid perfusion (Bernstein test).

Esophageal acidity: A pH electrode attached to a catheter is passed into the lower esophagus to measure esophageal acidity. If there is no acid reflux, 0.1–N of HCl is instilled into the stomach. A pH <2.0 indicates acid reflux, caused mostly by an incompetent lower esophageal sphincter. The one-time measurement of esophageal acidity has largely been replaced by the 24-hour pH monitoring.

24-hour pH monitoring: A pH electrode probe is passed through the nostril into the lower esophagus to measure esophageal acidity. The probe is connected to a recording device, which is worn by the client. The client keeps a diary of all symptoms and activities as they occur and marks them by an indicator on the recorder. After 24 hours the data is analyzed and interpreted.

Esophageal manometry: This test measures esophageal sphincter pressure and records peristaltic contractions. It detects esophageal motility disorder, such as achalasia (failure to relax GI tract smooth muscles, e.g., lower esophagus when swallowing). In achalasia, the baseline cardioesophageal sphincter pressure may be as high as 50 mm Hg, with a relaxation pressure of 24 mm Hg. Food and fluid cannot pass into the stomach until the weight of the contents is increased. With spasms of the esophagus, the sphincter is normal and peristalsis has irregular motility and force.

Acid perfusion (Bernstein test): This test is useful to distinguish between gastric acid reflux causing "heartburn" or esophagitis, and cardiac involvement (i.e., angina, myocardial infarction). Saline and HCl (0.1–N) are dripped through tubing, one at a time, into the esophagus. If the client complains of symptoms of esophagitis (i.e., epigastric discomfort, heartburn) after ½ hour of IV HCl drip, the diagnosis is usually acid reflux. Additional GI studies would be needed to confirm the diagnosis.

Purposes

- To distinguish between gastric acid reflux and cardiac involvement
- To diagnose gastric acid reflux
- To determine the cause of heartburn or difficulty in swallowing

Clinical Problems

Esophageal acidity: Incompetent lower esophageal sphincter, chronic reflux esophagitis

Esophageal manometry: Achalasia, spasm of esophagus, esophageal scleroderma

Acid perfusion: Esophagitis, epigastric pain or discomfort

Procedure

- Food and fluids are restricted 8 to 12 hours prior to the test. Avoid alcohol intake 24 hours prior to the test.
- Place client in high Fowler's position.
- Monitor pulse during test procedure to detect dysrhythmias from catheter insertion.
- Withhold antacids and autonomic nervous system agents for 24 hours before the test with health care provider's approval.

Esophageal acidity: *one-time measurement*

- Catheter with pH electrode is inserted into the esophagus through the client's mouth.
- The client is asked to stimulate acid reflux by performing Valsalva's maneuver or lifting the legs.
- If there is no acid reflux, 300 mL of HCl 0.1N is administered over 3 minutes, and the Valsalva's maneuver or lifting the legs is repeated.

Esophageal acidity: *24-hour pH monitoring*

- NPO of solid foods for 8 hours prior to the test.
- The catheter with the pH probe is inserted into the esophagus through the client's nostril.
- The probe is taped securely at the nose.
- Secure the recorder to the client's belt or provide a shoulder strap.
- The client records symptoms and activities in a diary and on the recorder over a 24-hour period of time.

Esophageal manometry

- A manometric catheter with a pressure transducer is inserted through the mouth into the esophagus.
- Esophageal sphincter pressure is measured before and after swallowing.
- Peristaltic contractions are recorded.

Acid perfusion (Bernstein test)

- A catheter is passed through the nose into the esophagus.
- Saline solution is dripped (6 to 10 mL/min) through the catheter. The client is told to indicate when pain occurs.
- HC1 0.1–N is dripped through the catheter for ½ hour. The client is told to indicate when pain occurs.
- When pain or discomfort is reported, the HCl line is turned off, and saline solution is started until symptoms have subsided.

Factors Affecting Diagnostic Results

- Antacids, anticholinergics, and cimetidine-like drugs may increase the pH, thus reducing acidity and causing false test results.

Nursing Implications

- Explain the test procedure(s) to the client (see Procedure). Note the presence of anxiety and fear. Report findings.
- Monitor pulse and blood pressure during the procedure. Baseline vital signs should be recorded. Report irregularity of pulse rate immediately to the health care provider. Check for signs of respiratory distress during catheter insertion.

Client Teaching

- Instruct the client that food and fluids are restricted for 8 to 12 hours before the test. Avoid alcohol for 24 hours before test.
- Instruct the client to sit in high Fowler's position for insertion of the catheter.

Esophageal acidity

Client Teaching

- Inform the client that a catheter (with electrode) will be swallowed and the pH of the esophagus secretions are recorded.
- Tell the client to perform the Valsalva's maneuver (bear down and hold breath) or to lift legs to stimulate gastric acid reflux as directed by the health care provider.

- Instruct the client to inform the health care provider of any pain or discomfort.

Esophageal acidity: *24-hour pH monitoring*

Client Teaching

- Instruct the client to have a regular diet during the 24 hours of recording unless otherwise indicated.
- Inform the client that a catheter with electrode will be inserted through the nostril and that the pH of the esophageal secretions will be recorded for 24 hours.
- Instruct the client that a diary will be provided. Symptoms and activities should be noted in the diary at the time they occur.
- Instruct the client not to operate the microwave oven during the 24 hours.
- Inform the client that the recorder should not get wet. A sponge bath rather than a shower is suggested.
- Instruct the client to return to the department in 24 hours to have the probe removed.

Esophageal manometry

Client Teaching

- Inform the client that a manometric catheter is to be swallowed. The esophageal pressure and peristaltic contractions are recorded.
- Instruct the client that drinking water may be requested (check with the health care provider first).

Acid perfusion

Client Teaching

- Inform the client that a catheter is inserted through the nose into the esophagus.
- Tell the client there will be two IV solutions and that only one will be dripping into the catheter at a time.
- Instruct the client to inform the health care provider immediately when pain or discomfort occurs during the procedure.

ESOPHAGOGASTRODUODENOSCOPY, ESOPHAGOGASTROSCOPY

GASTROSCOPY, ESOPHAGOSCOPY, DUODENOSCOPY, ENDOSCOPY

Normal Findings. Normal mucous membranes of the esophagus, stomach, and duodenum

Description. Esophagogastroscopy includes gastroscopy and esophagoscopy. If duodenoscopy is included, the term is esophagogastroduodenoscopy. This test is performed under local anesthesia in a gastroscopic room of a hospital or clinic, usually by a gastroenterologist.

A flexible fiberoptic endoscope is used for visualization of the internal structures of the esophagus, stomach, and duodenum. Biopsy forceps or a cytology brush can be inserted through a channel of the endoscope. The major complications are perforation and hemorrhage.

Purposes

- To visualize the internal esophagus, stomach, and duodenum
- To obtain cytologic specimen
- To confirm the presence of gastrointestinal pathology

Clinical Problems

Esophageal: Esophagitis, hiatal hernia, esophageal stenoses, achalasia, esophageal neoplasms (benign or malignant), esophageal varices, Mallory-Weiss tear

Gastric: Gastritis, gastric neoplasm (benign or malignant), gastric ulcer, gastric varices

Duodenal: Duodentitis, diverticula, duodenal ulcer, neoplasm

Procedure

- Obtain a signed consent form.
- Restrict food and fluids for 8 to 12 hours before test. Client may take prescribed medications at 6 AM on the day of the test.

- A sedative/tranquilizer, a narcotic analgesic, and/or atropine are given an hour before the test or are titrated IV immediately prior to the procedure and/or during the procedure.
- The client should not drive self home following test because of sedative.
- A local anesthetic may be used.
- Dentures, jewelry, and clothing should be removed from the neck to the waist.
- Record baseline vital signs.
- Test should *not* be performed within 2 days after a GI series.
- The test takes approximately 1 hour or less.

Factors Affecting Diagnostic Results

- Barium from a recent GI imaging series can decrease visualization of the mucosa.

Nursing Implications

Client Teaching

- Explain the procedure. Inform the client that the instrument is flexible.
- Have the client void. Take vital signs.
- Explain that some pressure will be felt with the insertion of the endoscope. Fullness in the stomach when air is injected is usually noted.
- Be a good listener. Be supportive.

Post-test

- Keep the client NPO for 2 to 4 hours after the test or as ordered. Check the gag reflex before offering food and fluids.
- Monitor vital signs frequently as indicated.
- Give throat lozenges or analgesics for throat discomfort. Inform client that flatus or belching is normal.
- Observe for possible complications, such as perforation in GI tract from the endoscope. These symptoms might include epigastric or abdominal pain, dyspnea, tachycardia, fever, subcutaneous emphysema.

GASTRIC ANALYSIS

Normal Findings. Fasting: 1.0–5.0 mEq/L/h
Stimulation: 10–25 mEq/L/h
Tubeless: detectable dyes in the urine

Description. The gastric analysis test examines the acidity of the gastric secretions in the basal state (without stimulation) and the maximal secretory ability with stimulation (i.e., histamine phosphate, betazole hydrochloride [Histalog], pentagastrin). An increased amount of free hydrochloric acid could indicate a peptic ulcer, and an absence of free HCl (achlorhydria) could indicate gastric atrophy, probably caused by a malignancy or pernicious anemia. Gastric contents may be collected for cytologic examination.

Basal gastric analysis: Gastric secretions are aspirated through a nasogastric tube after a period of fasting. Specimens are obtained to evaluate the basal acidity of gastric content, and the gastric stimulation test follows.

Stimulation gastric analysis: The stimulation test is usually a continuation of the basal gastric analysis. A gastric stimulant (i.e., Histalog or pentagastrin) is administered, and gastric contents are aspirated every 15 to 20 minutes until several samples are obtained.

Tubeless gastric analysis: This test detects the presence or absence of hydrochloric acid (HCl); however, it will NOT indicate the amount of free acid in the stomach. A gastric stimulant (caffeine, Histalog) is given, and an hour later a resin dye (Azuresin, Diagnex Blue) is taken orally by the client. The free HCl releases the dye from the resin base; the dye is absorbed by the GI tract and is excreted in the urine. Absence of the dye in the urine 2 hours later is indicative of gastric achlorhydria. This test method saves the client the discomfort of being intubated with a nasogastric tube; however, it does lack accuracy.

There is controversy over the usefulness of gastric acid secretory tests; however, they are still used to document gastric acid hypersecretions (e.g., Zollinger-Ellison syndrome and hypergastrinemia).

Purposes

- To evaluate gastric secretions
- To detect an increase or decrease of free hydrochloric acid

Clinical Problems

Decreased level: Pernicious anemia, gastric malignancy, atrophic gastritis

Elevated level: Peptic ulcer (duodenal), Zollinger-Ellison syndrome

Procedure

Basal and stimulation

- Restrict food, fluids, and smoking for 8 to 12 hours prior to test.
- Anticholinergics, cholinergics, adrenergic blockers, antacids, steroids, alcohol, and coffee should be restricted for at least 24 hours before the test.
- Baseline vital signs should be recorded.
- Loose dentures should be removed.
- A lubricated nasogastric tube is inserted through the nose or mouth.
- A residual gastric specimen and four additional specimens taken 15 minutes apart should be labeled with the client's name, the time, and specimen number.

Stimulation: Continuation of the basal gastric analysis

- A gastric stimulant is administered (i.e., betazole hydrochloride [Histalog] or histamine phosphate IM; pentagastrin subcutaneously).
- Several gastric specimens are obtained over a period of 1 to 2 hours: histamine, four 15-minute specimens in 1 hour; and Histalog, eight 15-minute specimens in 2 hours. Specimens should be labeled.
- Vital signs should be monitored.
- The test usually takes 2½ hours for both basal and stimulation tests.

Tubeless gastric analysis

- Restrict food and fluids for 8 to 12 hours before the test.
- AM urine specimen is discarded.
- Certain drugs are withheld for 48 hours before the tests with health care provider's permission (i.e., antacids, electrolyte preparations [potassium], quinidine, quinine, iron, B vitamins).
- Give the client caffeine sodium benzoate 500 mg in a glass of water.
- Collect a urine specimen 1 hour later. This is the control urine specimen.
- Give the client the resin dye agent (Azuresin or Diagnex Blue) in a glass of water.
- Collect a urine specimen 2 hours later. The urine may be colored blue or blue-green for several days. Absence of color in the urine usually indicates absence of HCl in the stomach.

Factors Affecting Diagnostic Results

- Stress, smoking, and sensory stimulation can increase HCl secretion.

Nursing Implications

- Obtain a history of categories of drugs that can affect test results (i.e., antacids, antispasmodics, adrenergic blockers, cholinergics, and steroids).
- Monitor vital signs. Observe for possible side effects from use of stimulants (i.e., dizziness, flushing, tachycardia, headache, and decreased systolic blood pressure).
- Label the specimens (gastric or urine) with the client's name, date, and time.
- Be supportive of the client.

Client Teaching

- Explain the purpose and procedure of the tube or tubeless gastric analysis test to the client (see Procedures).
- Explain to the client how the nasogastric tube is inserted (through the nose or mouth) and that swallowing during its insertion will be requested.

GASTROINTESTINAL (GI) SERIES, UPPER GI AND SMALL-BOWEL SERIES, BARIUM SWALLOW, HYPOTONIC DUODENOGRAPHY

Normal Findings. Normal structure of the esophagus, stomach, and small intestine, and normal peristalsis

Description. Upper GI and small-bowel series are fluoroscopic and x-ray examinations of the esophagus, stomach, and small intestine. Oral barium meal (barium sulfate) or water-soluble contrast agent, meglumine diatrizoate (Gastrografin), is swallowed. By means of fluoroscopy, the barium is observed as it passes through the digestive tract, and spot films are taken. Inflammation, ulcerations, and tumors of the esophagus, stomach, and duodenum can be detected.

If increased peristalsis, a spastic duodenal bulb, or a space-occupying lesion is observed or suspected in the duodenal area during the GI series, a hypotonic duodenography procedure can be performed by giving glucagon, atropine, propantheline (Pro-Banthine), or like drug to slow down the action of the small intestine.

Purposes

- To detect an esophageal, gastric, or duodenal ulcer
- To identify polyps, tumor, or hiatal hernia in the GI tract
- To detect foreign bodies, esophageal varices, or esophageal or small bowel strictures

Clinical Problems

Abnormal findings: Hiatal hernia; esophageal varices; esophageal or small bowel strictures; gastric or duodenal ulcer; gastritis or gastroenteritis; gastric polyps; benign or malignant tumor of the esophagus, stomach, or duodenum; diverticula of the stomach and duodenum; pyloric stenosis; malabsorption syndrome; volvulus of the stomach; foreign bodies

Procedure

- Restrict food, fluids, medications, and smoking for 8 to 12 hours before the test. A low-residue diet may be ordered for 2 to 3 days before the test.
- Withhold medications 8 hours before the test unless otherwise indicated. Narcotics and anticholinergic drugs are withheld for 24 hours to avoid intestinal immobility.
- Laxatives may be ordered the evening before the test.
- The client swallows a chalk-flavored (chocolate, strawberry) barium meal or meglumine diatrizoate (Gastrografin) in calculated amounts (16 to 20 oz).
- Spot films are taken during the fluoroscopic examination. The procedure takes approximately 1 to 2 hours but could take 4 to 6 hours if the test is to include the small-bowel series. A 24-hour x-ray film, post-GI series, may be requested.
- A laxative is usually ordered after the completion of the test to rid the GI tract of barium.

Factors Affecting Diagnostic Results

- Excessive air in the stomach and small intestine

Nursing Implications

- Record vital signs. Note in the chart any epigastric pain or discomfort.

Client Teaching

- Inform the client that all of the chalk-flavored liquid must be swallowed. Tell client that the test should not cause pain or any discomfort.

Post-test

- Confirm with the radiology department that the upper GI series or small-bowel studies are completed before giving the late breakfast or late lunch.
- Administer the ordered laxative after the test. Inform the client that the stools should be light in color for the next several days. Barium can cause fecal impaction.

HOLTER MONITORING

AMBULATORY ELECTROCARDIOGRAPHY, DYNAMIC ELECTROCARDIOGRAPHY

Normal Finding. No abnormal or insignificant ECG findings

Description. Holter monitoring (ambulatory electrocardiography) evaluates the client's heart rate and rhythm during normal daily activities, rest, and sleep over 24 hours (occasionally 48 hours). For Holter monitoring, there is a continuous electrocardiogram (ECG) recording on a cassette tape that is boxed inside an approximately 1-pound monitor. The client is given a diary to record symptoms, such as palpitations, chest pain, shortness of breath, syncope, and vertigo, as well as the time of the symptoms. After 24 hours, the monitor with the tape and diary are returned to the cardiac center, and the tape is scanned or reviewed for abnormal findings, such as cardiac dysrhythmias.

The primary purpose for Holter monitoring is to identify suspected and unsuspected cardiac dysrhythmias which can be correlated between the recorder, event marking of symptoms, and transient symptoms marked in the diary. It is infrequently ordered for clients having Prinzmetal's variant angina, a form of myocardial ischemia, that results from spasms of the coronary arteries. Holter monitoring is more sensitive for identifying the cause of the symptoms than a routine electrocardiogram.

Purpose

- To identify cardiac dysrhythmias related to cardiac symptoms as marked on the monitor and recorded in the diary

Clinical Problems

Indications: Suspected and unsuspected cardiac dysrhythmias (supraventricular and ventricular), correlation of symptoms with the ECG tape, mitral valve prolapse causing dysrhythmia, hypertrophic obstructive cardiomyopathy causing atrial and ventricular dysrhythmias, and pacemaker dysfunction

Procedure

- No food or fluid restriction is required.
- The skin is cleansed, shaved as needed, and electrodes are placed over bony areas for eliminating artifacts that could be caused from skeletal muscle movement and insufficient attachment to the skin due to hair.
- Five to seven electrode patches are placed on the chest area.
- The client is given a diary to record the present activity when symptoms such as palpitations, chest pain, shortness of breath, and others occur.
- The client should not take a bath, shower, or swim until the electrodes are removed.

Post-test

- The client returns the Holter monitor the next day (24 hours later) with the diary.
- The tape is scanned (reviewed) by the cardiologist and the diary reviewed. A written report is submitted to the client's health care provider.

Factors Affecting Diagnostic Results

- The client does not record activities correlated with symptoms in the diary.

Nursing Implications

- Check that a consent form has been signed.
- Record the client's history of cardiac disorders and/or symptoms.

- Check that a baseline ECG has been received. A comparison of the baseline ECG with the 24-hour ECG monitoring could be requested.

Client Teaching

- Instruct the client that the monitor device will be attached either by a shoulder strap or as a belt.
- Review the procedure for Holter monitoring with the client (see Procedure).
- Emphasize the importance of pushing the event marker button on the monitor when symptoms occur and recording in the diary the time, symptoms, and activity that is present at the time of symptoms.
- Inform the client that the monitor should not get wet. Bathing, showering, and swimming should be avoided. The client should avoid using an electric razor or electric toothbrush during the 24 hours of monitoring.
- Instruct the client to return the Holter monitor and diary the next day at approximately the same time the test was started.
- Explain to the client that the cardiologist or health care provider will discuss the findings with him or her.

HYSTEROSALPINGOGRAPHY (HYSTEROSALPINGOGRAM)

Normal Findings. Normal structure of the uterus and patent fallopian tubes

Description. Hysterosalpingography is a fluoroscopic and x-ray examination of the uterus and fallopian tubes. A contrast medium, either oil-base Ethiodol or Lipiodol, or water-soluble Salpix, is injected into the cervical canal. It flows through the uterus and into the fallopian tubes and spills into the abdominal area for visualizing the uterus.

The hysterosalpingogram should be done on the seventh to the ninth day after the menstrual cycle. The client should not be pregnant, have bleeding, or have an acute infection.

Ultrasonography is replacing hysterosalpingography, except that the latter test is more effective in determining tubal patency.

Purposes

- To identify uterine fibroids, tumor, or fistula

- To identify fallopian tube occlusion
- To evaluate repeated fetal losses

Clinical Problems

Abnormal findings: Uterine masses (i.e., fibroids, tumor), uterine fistulas, bleeding (e.g., injury), fallopian tube occlusion (i.e., adhesions, stricture), extrauterine pregnancy

Procedure

- Obtain a signed consent form.
- No food or fluid is restricted.
- A mild sedative (e.g., diazepam [Valium]) may be ordered prior to the test.
- A cleansing enema and douche may be ordered prior to the test.
- The client lies on an examining table in the lithotomy position. A speculum is inserted into the vaginal canal, and the contrast medium is injected into the cervix under fluoroscopic control. X-rays are taken throughout the 15- to 30-minute procedure.

Nursing Implications

- Obtain a history of hypersensitivity to iodine, seafood, or previous use of contrast dye.
- Ask the client the date of her last menstrual period. If pregnancy is suspected, the procedure should not be done.
- Check for signs and symptoms of infection following the test, such as fever, increased pulse rate, and pain. If the client is at home, instruct her to call the health care provider to report these symptoms.

Client Teaching

- Inform client that some abdominal cramping and some dizziness may be experienced. Explain that it is normal; however, if it is continuous or if severe cramping occurs, the examiner should be notified.
- Encourage the client to ask questions and express concerns. Be a good listener.
- Inform client that there may be some bloody discharge for several days following the test. If it continues after 3 to 4 days, she should notify her health care provider.

HYSTEROSCOPY

Normal Finding

Normal uterine cavity; normal endometrial uterine tissue

Description. Hysteroscopy allows visualization of the entire endometrial cavity of the uterus. This test is considered more effective for viewing and obtaining endometrial pathology than the D & C (dilation and curettage) or hysterosalpingography. With D & C, scraping of the endometrial tissue is done without visualization, which may result in failure to obtain the pathologic tissue. With the use of the hysteroscope, a biopsy can be taken and polyp(s) removed.

Hysteroscopy is contraindicated if there is cervical or vaginal infection, pelvic inflammatory disease, or purulent vaginal discharge, or if cervical surgery had been performed previously. Risks of hysteroscopy include perforation of the uterus or infection.

Purposes

- To visualize the uterine cavity
- To obtain a biopsy of the endometrial lining of the uterus
- To remove a uterine polyp

Clinical Problems

Abnormal findings: Hyperplasia of the endometrial tissue in the uterus; endometrial cancer; polyps

Procedure

- Obtain a signed consent form.
- Food and fluids are restricted for 8 hours prior to the test.
- The client is placed in the lithotomy position.
- A hysteroscope is placed through the cervical os into the endometrial cavity of the uterus. Carbon dioxide is usually instilled to distend the uterine cavity.
- Biopsy of tissue can be obtained.
- The test takes approximately 30 minutes.

Nursing Implications

- Obtain a menstrual history. The test should be performed after menstruation and prior to ovulation.

Client Teaching

- Explain the procedure to the client.
- Inform the client that discomfort following the carbon dioxide instillation is possible. Lower abdominal distention (uterus) and bloating can result.

Post-test

- Monitor vital signs.
- Check for excessive bleeding or discharge.

Client Teaching

- Inform the client that cramping or a slight vaginal bleeding may occur following the test for one to two days. Use of a mild analgesic decreases discomfort.
- Instruct the client to report severe discomfort, signs of a fever, heavy vaginal bleeding, or shortness of breath immediately to the health care provider.
- Tell the client that sexual intercourse or douching should be avoided for 2 weeks or as instructed by the health care provider.

INTRAVENOUS PYELOGRAPHY (IVP)

INTRAVENOUS PYELOGRAM, EXCRETORY UROGRAPHY

Normal Findings. Normal size, structure, and functions of the kidneys, ureters, and bladder

Description. Intravenous pyelography (IVP) visualizes the entire urinary tract. A radiopaque substance is injected IV, and a series of x-rays is taken at specific times. IVP is useful for locating stones and tumors and for diagnosing kidney diseases.

Purposes

- To identify abnormal size, shape, and functioning of the kidneys
- To detect renal calculi, tumor, cyst

Clinical Problems

Abnormal findings: Renal calculi, tumor, cyst, hydronephrosis, pyelonephritis, renovascular hypertension

Procedure

- Obtain a signed consent form.
- Restrict food and fluids for 8 to 12 hours before the test.
- Give client a laxative the night before and a cleansing enema(s) the morning of the test. Check with radiology department for preparation.
- An antihistamine or a steroid may be given prior to the test for those who are hypersensitive to iodine, seafood, and contrast dye.
- Record baseline vital signs.
- The client lies in the supine position on an x-ray table. X-rays are taken 3, 5, 10, 15, and 20 minutes after the dye is injected.
- Emergency drugs and equipment should be available at all times.
- The test takes approximately 30 to 45 minutes.
- The client voids at the end of the test, and another x-ray is taken to visualize the residual dye in the bladder.

Nursing Implications

- Obtain a history of known allergies, especially to seafood, iodine preparations, or contrast dye.
- Check the BUN. If BUN levels are greater than 40 mg/dL, notify the health care provider.
- Report to health care provider if client had a recent barium enema or GI series, as these tests can interfere with IVP findings.

Client Teaching

- Inform client that a transient flushing or burning sensation and a salty or metallic taste may occur during or following the IV injection of contrast dye.
- Encourage the client to ask questions and to express any concerns.

Post-test

- Monitor vital signs and urinary output.
- Observe and report possible delayed reactions to the contrast dye (i.e., dyspnea, rashes, flushing, urticaria, tachycardia).
- Check the site where the dye was injected for irritation or hematoma. Apply warm or cold compresses as ordered.

LYMPHANGIOGRAPHY (LYMPHANGIOGRAM)

LYMPHOGRAPHY

Normal Findings. Normal lymphatic vessels and lymph nodes

Description. Lymphangiography is an x-ray examination of the lymphatic vessels and lymph nodes. A radiopaque iodine contrast oil substance (e.g., Ethiodol) is injected into the lymphatic vessels of each foot; the dye can also be injected into the hands to visualize axillary and supraclavicular nodes. Fluoroscopy is used with x-ray filming to check on lymphatic filling of the contrast dye and to determine when the infusion of the contrast dye should be stopped. The infusion rate is controlled by a lymphangiographic pump, and approximately 1½ hours are required for dye to reach the level of the third and fourth lumbar vertebrae.

Other tests, such as ultrasonography, computed tomography, and/or biopsy, may be used to confirm the diagnosis and to stage lymphoma involvement.

Lymphangiography is usually contraindicated if the client is hypersensitive to iodine or has severe chronic lung disease, cardiac disease, or advanced liver or kidney disease. Lipid pneumonia may occur if the contrast dye flows into the thoracic duct and sets up microemboli in the lungs.

Purposes

- To detect metastasis of the lymph nodes
- To identify malignant lymphoma
- To determine the cause of lymphedema
- To assist with the staging of malignant lymphoma

Clinical Problems

Abnormal findings: Malignant lymphoma (e.g., Hodgkin's disease), metastasis to the lymph nodes, lymphedema

Procedure

- Obtain a signed consent form.
- No food or fluid is restricted.

- Antihistamines and a sedative may be ordered prior to the test.
- Contrast dye (blue) is injected intradermally between several toes of each foot, staining the lymphatic vessels of the feet in 15 to 20 minutes. This is for visualization of the lymphatic vessels.
- A local skin anesthetic is injected, and small incisions are made on the dorsum of each foot.
- The contrast dye is slowly infused with the aid of the infusion pump. The client should remain still during the procedure. X-rays are taken of the lymphatics in the leg, pelvic, abdominal, and chest areas.
- Twenty-four hours later, a second set of films is taken to visualize the lymph nodes. X-ray filming usually takes 30 minutes. The contrast dye remains in the lymph nodes for 6 months to a year; thus, repeated x-rays can be taken to determine the disease process and the response to treatment.
- The procedure takes 2½ to 3 hours.

Nursing Implications

- Obtain a history of allergies to seafood, iodine preparations, or contrast dye used in another x-ray test.
- Record baseline vital signs.
- Have client void before test.

Client Teaching

- Inform the client that it is a prolonged procedure and that lying still during the test is essential. Give a sedative if one is ordered.
- Inform the client that the blue contrast dye discolors the urine and stool for several days and could cause the skin to have a bluish tinge for 24 to 48 hours.
- Tell the client that the test takes about 2½ to 3 hours.

Post-test

- Monitor vital signs as indicated. Observe for dyspnea, pain, and hypotension, which could be due to microemboli from the spillage of the contrast dye.
- Assess the incisional site for signs of an infection (i.e., redness, oozing, and swelling).
- Check for leg edema. Elevate lower extremities as indicated.

MAGNETIC RESONANCE IMAGING (MRI)

NUCLEAR MAGNETIC RESONANCE (NMR) IMAGING

Normal Findings. Normal tissue and structure

Description. MRI, a noninvasive test, uses a magnetic field with aid of radiofrequency waves to produce cross-sectional images of the body. The magnet for MRI is encased in a large doughnut-shaped cylinder. The client lies on a narrow table, and the body part to be scanned is placed within the cylinder-type scanner. Since MRI was first introduced in 1983 for tissue visualization, the imaging quality has greatly improved. There is no risk of radiation. The cost of MRI is approximately one third more than the cost of computed tomography (CT) scan.

MRI is sensitive in detecting edema, infarcts, hemorrhage, blood flow, tumors, infections, plaques due to multiple sclerosis, and defining internal organ structure. It can differentiate between edema and a tumor. MRI excels in diagnosing pathologic problems associated with the central nervous system (CNS), such as tumor, hemorrhage, edema, cerebral infarction, and subdural hematoma. Bone does not hamper its ability to visualize tissue. Bone artifacts do not occur, and MRI can identify tumors hidden by the bone (e.g., pituitary gland tumor).

Pacemakers, aneurysm or surgical clips, certain heart artifical valves, jewelry, watches, credit cards, and hair clips can affect the magnetic field. When an emergency situation occurs during the imaging, the client must be moved from the MRI room to use resuscitation equipment. MRI is difficult to use to study critically ill clients on life-support systems because of the magnetic effect.

MRI and CT can be used for similar tissue studies. MRI does use contrast media in certain circumstances, but the IV contrast for MRI is chemically unrelated to the iodinated contrast used in CT and conventional radiography. Presently, the only commercially available intravascular contrast for MRI is gadolinium-DTPA. Gadolinium (Magnavist) and Ferodax are frequently used to evaluate CNS problems (i.e., brain, base of skull, and spine). This contrast agent can cross the blood–brain barrier. Imaging can occur after 5 to 60 minutes of the gadolinium infusion.

Cine MRI is a fast-moving MRI procedure that can image the heart in a continuous motion. With the original MRI, a picture is imaged every 1 to 2 seconds.

Magnetic resonance angiography (MRA): MRA is a noninvasive means of displaying vessels by imaging. It maximizes the signals in structures containing blood flow and reconstructs only the structures with flow. Other structures of lesser interest are subtracted from the image by the computer.

Purpose

- To detect abnormal masses, tissue structures and tears, neurologic and vascular disorders, fluid accumulation

Clinical Problems

Abnormal findings: Tumors, blood clots, cysts, edema, hemorrhage, abscesses, infarctions, aneurysm, plaque formation, demyelinating disease (e.g., multiple sclerosis), dementia, muscular disease, skeletal abnormalities, congenital heart disease, acute renal tubular necrosis (ATN), blood flow abnormalities

Procedure

- Obtain a signed consent form.
- No food or fluid is restricted for adults; NPO for 4 hours for children.
- Remove all jewelry, including watches, glasses, hairpins, and any metal objects. Magnetic field can damage watches. Those with pacemakers are not candidates for MRI, and some with metal prosthetics (i.e., hip, knee, heart valves) may not be candidates for MRI.
- Occupational history is important. Metal in the body, such as shrapnel or flecks of ferrous metal in the eye, may cause critical injury, such as retinal hemorrhage.
- The client must lie absolutely still on a narrow table with a cylinder-type scanner around the body area being scanned.
- The procedure takes approximately 45 minutes to 1½ hours.

Blood flow: Extremities

- The limb to be examined is rested in a cradle-like support. Reference sites to be imaged are marked on the leg or arm, and the extremity is moved into a flow cylinder.
- The procedure takes approximately 15 minutes for arms and 15 minutes for legs.

Factors Affecting Diagnostic Results

- Ferrous metal in the body could cause critical injury to the client.
- Nonferrous metal may produce artifacts that degrade the images.

Nursing Implications

- Ascertain from the client the presence of a pacemaker, previous pacemaker wire left in the body, heart valve, any metal prosthetics, or shrapnel left in the body (such as in the eye) which could cause serious tissue injury as the result of the magnetic pull.
- Alert health care provider if client is on an IV controller or pump. MRI can disrupt IV flow.
- Elicit any past problems for claustrophobia. Relaxation technique may need to be tried or a sedative used.

Client Teaching

- Explain the procedure. Inform the client that various noises from the scanner will be heard. Ear plugs are available. Inform client that the MRI personnel will be in another room but can communicate via an intercom system.
- Explain that there is no exposure to radiation.
- Instruct the client to remove watches, credit cards, hairpins, and jewelry. Magnetic field can damage a watch.
- Inform the client who has metal fillings in teeth that a "tingling sensation" may be felt during imaging.

MAMMOGRAPHY (MAMMOGRAM)

Normal Findings. Normal ducts and glandular tissue; no abnormal masses

Description. Mammography is an x-ray of the breast to detect cysts or tumors. Benign cysts are seen on the mammogram as well-outlined, clear lesions that tend to be bilateral, whereas malignant tumors are irregular and poorly defined and tend to be unilateral. A mammogram can detect a breast lesion approximately 2 years before it is palpable.

There have been technical improvements in the equipment, mammographic units, and the recording system used for mammography. The use of radiographic grids has improved the imaging quality of mammograms by decreasing image density. With the use of grids, the visibility of small cancers is increased. Also, the use of magnification mammography has improved the capability to identify cancers; however, the magnification increases the client's radiation dose by prolonging exposure time.

The American Cancer Society and the American College of Radiologists have suggested that women between 35 and 40 years have a mammogram every 2 years and that women over 40 years have an annual mammogram. Radiation received is very low dose.

Purposes

- To screen for breast mass(es)
- To detect breast cyst or tumor

Clinical Problems

Abnormal finding: Breast mass (cyst or tumor)

Procedure

- Food and fluids are not restricted.
- The client removes clothes and jewelry from the neck to the waist and wears a paper or cloth gown that opens in the front. Powder and ointment on the breast should be removed to avoid false-positive result.
- The client is standing, and each breast, one at a time, rests on an x-ray cassette table. As the breast is compressed, the client will be asked to hold her breath while the x-ray is taken. Two x-rays are taken of each breast from different angles.
- The procedure takes about 15 to 30 minutes.

Nursing Implications

- Ascertain whether the client is pregnant or suspected of being pregnant. Test is contraindicated during pregnancy.
- Ask the client to identify the lump in the breast if one is present.

Client Teaching

- Instruct client not to use ointment, powder, or deodorant on the breast or under the axilla on the day of the mammogram.
- Inform the client not to be alarmed if an additional x-ray is needed.

- Be supportive of the client. Allow the client time to express her fears and concerns.
- Encourage the client to self-examine the breast every month. If premenopausal, breast examination should be done after menstrual period. Demonstrate breast examination if necessary.

MULTIGATED ACQUISITION (MUGA) SCAN

Normal Findings. Normal heart size, ventricular wall motion, and ejection fractions.

Description. MUGA scan is a rapid, safe method to evaluate the heart size, ventricular wall motion, and ejection fraction. The client's blood is tagged with a radioactive tracer, such as technetium-99m, which permits the heart and its function to be visualized. There is multiple imaging during acquisition (MUGA) scanning. Gated refers to the synchronizing of images with the client's ECG and the computer. MUGA identifies changes occurring with contraction and expansion of the ventricles of the heart. With cardiac disease, there may be reduced ability of the heart to pump blood sufficiently.

Because a radioactive substance is used with the test, the MUGA is a nuclear medicine (scan) procedure. The amount of radiation exposure used is comparable to that of a CT scan. MUGA may be performed with the stress test.

Purposes

- To evaluate the heart's size, ventricular wall motion, and ejection fraction
- To evaluate the effect of an acute myocardial infarction for prognosis
- To evaluate cardiovascular disease
- To detect ventricular aneurysm
- To evaluate pharmaceutical and chemotherapy response

Clinical Problems

Abnormal findings: Congestive heart failure (CHF), valvular disease (regurgitation), ventricular aneurysm, acute myocardial infarction, cardiac ventricular dysfunction

Procedure

- No food or fluid restriction is required.
- A pyrophosphate material which tags to the red blood cells is injected intravenously. A second IV injection of a radioactive tracer is given.
- ECG electrodes are attached and the ECG is monitored.
- Client is in a supine position with a gamma camera over the chest. The radioactive tracer (contains no dye) allows visualization of the heart and its function.

Nursing Implications

- Obtain a history of drugs the client is taking. They may interfere with the test result.
- Monitor vital signs and ECG.

Client Teaching

- Explain the MUGA test procedure (see Procedure).
- Answer client's questions and refer unknown answers to appropriate health professionals.

MYELOGRAPHY (MYELOGRAM)

Normal Findings. Normal spinal subarachnoid space; no obstructions

Description. Myelography is a fluoroscopic and radiologic examination of the spinal subarachnoid space using air or a radiopaque contrast agent (oil or water soluble). With clients who are hypersensitive to iodine and seafood, air is the contrast agent used. This procedure is performed in an x-ray department by a radiologist, a neurologist, or a neurosurgeon. After the contrast dye is injected into the lumbar area, the fluoroscopic table is tilted until the suspected problem area can be visualized, and spot films are taken. This procedure is contraindicated if increased intracranial pressure is suspected.

Purposes

- To identify herniated intervertebral disks
- To detect cysts or tumor at or within the spinal column
- To detect spinal nerve root injury

Clinical Problems

Abnormal findings: Herniated intervertebral disks, metastatic tumors, cysts, astrocytomas and ependymomas (within the spinal cord), neurofibromas and meningiomas (within the subarachnoid space), spinal nerve root injury, arachnoiditis

Procedure

- Obtain a signed consent form.
- Restrict food and fluids for 4 to 8 hours before the test. If the myelogram is scheduled in the afternoon, then the client may have a light breakfast or clear liquids in the morning.
- A cleansing enema may be ordered the night before or early on the morning of the test to remove feces and gas for improving visualization.
- Premedications may include a sedative or narcotic analgesic, or both.
- The client is placed in the prone position on a fluoroscopic table and is secured to the table. A spinal puncture is performed, and contrast dye is injected. As the dye enters the spinal canal, the table is tilted.
- The myelogram takes approximately 1 hour.

Post-test

- The radiopaque oil is removed, and the client should remain flat for 6 to 8 hours. If a water-soluble radiopaque agent was used, the client's head should be elevated at 60° for 8 hours.

Nursing Implications

- Obtain a history of allergies to iodine, seafood, and radiopaque dye used in other x-ray test.
- Record baseline vital signs.
- Recognize conditions in which myelography would be contraindicated (i.e., multiple sclerosis [could cause exacerbation] and increased ICP).
- Allow the client time to ask questions and express concerns or fear.

Client Teaching

- Inform the client that the table will be tilted as the dye circulates in the spinal canal. A transient burning sensation and/or a flushed, warm feeling may be felt as the dye is injected and may last for a short time after the test.

- Instruct the client to let the health care provider know of any discomfort (e.g., pain down the leg).

Post-test

- Monitor vital signs as indicated.
- Monitor urinary output. The client should void in 8 hours.
- Observe for signs and symptoms of chemical or bacterial meningitis (i.e., severe headache, fever, stiff neck, irritability, and convulsions).

Client Teaching

- Instruct the client to lie in the prone and/or supine position for 6 to 8 hours. If a water-soluble contrast agent was used or if not all of the contrast oil was removed, the head of the bed should be elevated at a 60° angle for 8 hours or longer.
- Encourage the client to increase fluid intake. The fluids will help restore the cerebrospinal fluid loss.

NUCLEAR SCANS (BONE, BRAIN PERFUSION, HEART, KIDNEY, LIVER AND SPLEEN, COLON AND OVARY, GASTROESOPHAGEAL REFLUX, GASTROINTESTINAL BLEEDING, GASTRIC EMPTYING, GALLBLADDER, LUNG, AND THYROID STUDIES)*

RADIONUCLIDE SCANS, RADIOISOTOPE IMAGING

Normal Finding. Normal; no observed pathology

Description. Nuclear medicine is the clinical field concerned with the diagnostic and therapeutic uses of radioactive isotopes. A radioactive isotope is an unstable isotope that decays or disintegrates, emitting radiation. Radioisotopes, known as radionuclides, concentrate in certain organs of the body and are distributed more readily in diseased tissues. Scintillation (gamma) camera detectors are used for imaging. Equal or uniform gray distribution is normal, but lighter areas, referred to as *hot*

---

*Revised by Frank Di Gregorio, CNMT, RDMS, Director, Community Imaging Center, Wilmington, Delaware.

spots, indicate hyperfunction, and darker areas, *cold spots,* indicate hypofunction.

There are two types of imaging systems: (1) planar imaging, which projects images acquired from two or three different angles, and (2) single photon emission computed tomography (SPECT), in which the scintillation camera rotates and projects images in an arc of 180° (for cardiac imaging) to 360°, acquiring 32 or more images. The advantage of SPECT over planar imaging is that with SPECT the images are not obscured by overlying organs, tissue, or bone. The camera orbits around a client lying on a special table. Nuclear medicine imaging is moving toward a new era with the use of high-speed computers.

The use of radionuclides as radiopharmaceuticals is considered safe. The radionuclide used in most studies is technetium 99m (Tc-99m), which accounts for 70% of the nuclear imaging procedures. Other radionuclides include, iodine 123 and 125 (I-123, I-125), thallium (T-201), xenon (Xe-133), indium 111 (In-111)-labeled white blood cells, and gallium (Ga-67) citrate.

Positron emission tomography (PET) is discussed separately in the text.

Clinical Problems

Test	*Indications/Purposes*
Bone	To detect early bone disease (osteomyelitis); carcinoma metastasis to the bone; bone response to therapeutic regimens (i.e., radiation therapy, chemotherapy) To determine unexplained bone pain To detect fractures and abnormal healing of fractures; degenerative bone disorders
Brain	To detect an intracranial mass and disorder: tumors, abscess, cancer metastasis to the brain, head trauma (subdural hematoma), cerebrovascular accident (stroke), aneurysm
Brain perfusion study	To diagnose Alzheimer's disease, brain death, AIDS dementia To locate seizure foci To determine the location and size of cerebral ischemia

(continued)

Test	*Indications/Purposes*
Heart (cardiac) MUGA	To identify cardiac hypertrophy (cardiomegaly) To quantify cardiac output (ejection fraction) wall motion To detect congestive heart failure (CHF) or an aneurysm
Kidney	To detect parenchymal renal disease: tumor, cysts, glomerulonephritis, urinary tract obstruction To assess the function of renal transplantation
Liver and spleen	To detect tumors, cysts, or abscesses of the liver and spleen, hepatic metastasis, splenic infarct To assess liver response to therapeutic regimens (i.e., radiation, chemotherapy) To identify hepatomegaly and splenomegaly To identify liver position and shape
Lung	To detect pulmonary emboli, tumors, pulmonary diseases with perfusion changes (i.e., emphysema, bronchitis, pneumonia) To assess arterial perfusion changes secondary to cardiac disease
Monoclonal antibodies for colon and ovarian cancer	To detect colon and ovarian cancer cells in the body
Gastrointestinal bleeding study	To detect the localization of gastrointestinal and nongastrointestinal bleeding sites
Gastric emptying study	To diagnose gastric obstruction and the cause of dysmotility
Gastrointestinal reflux	To detect esophageal reflux syndrome
Gallbladder study (CCK hepatobiliary)	To diagnose chronic cholecystitis To detect hypercholestosis conditions
Thyroid	To detect thyroid mass (tumors), diseases of thyroid gland (Graves', Hashimoto's thyroiditis) To determine the size, structure, and position of the thyroid gland To evaluate thyroid function resulting from hyperthyroidism and hypothyroidism

Procedure. The radionuclide (radioisotope) is administered orally or IV. The interval from the time the radionuclide is given to the time of imaging can differ according to the radionuclide and organ in question. Normally, masses such as tumors absorb more of the radioactive substance than does normal tissue.

For diagnostic purposes, the dose of radionuclide is low (<30 mCi) and should have little effect on visitors, other clients, and nursing and medical personnel. Usually food and fluids are not restricted except in the case of gallbladder studies.

The procedures for the organ scans are listed according to the radionuclides used, the method of administration, the waiting period after injection, the food and fluid allowed, and other instructions.

Bone

- Radionuclides: technetium (Tc)-99m-labeled phosphate compounds (Tc-99m diphosphonate, pyrophosphate, medronate sodium)
- Administration: IV
- Waiting period after injection: Can differ according to the radionuclides used (e.g., for Tc-99m the period is 2 to 3 hours [3 hours for an edematous person])
- Food and fluids: no restrictions; for Tc-99m, water is encouraged during the waiting period (six glasses)
- Other instructions: Void before imaging begins. Remove metal objects, jewelry, keys. Scanning occurs 2 to 4 hours after IV radionclicide injection and takes 1 to 2 hours. A sedative may be ordered if the client has difficulty lying quietly during imaging

Brain: Radionuclide brain scanning is very effective for identifying metastatic disease, strokes, subdural abscesses, and hematomas.

- Radionuclides: Tc-99m-glucoheptonate, Tc-99m-O_4, Tc-99m-DTPA (diethylenetriamine penta-acetic acid), Tl-201 NaCl
- Administration: IV
- Waiting period after injection: Tc-99m-O_4, 1 to 3 hours; Tc-99m-DTPA, 45 minutes to 1 hour. Frequently a few photo scans taken before the waiting period is over
- Food and fluids: No restrictions
- Other instructions: With Tc-99m-O_4, 10 drops of Lugol's solution are given the night before or at least 1 hour before the scan, or

potassium perchlorate 200 mg to 1 g given 1 to 3 hours before brain scan. These agents block the uptake of Tc-99m-O_4 in the salivary glands, thyroid, and choroid plexus. With Tc-99m-DTPA, blocking agents are not necessary

Brain perfusion study: Perfusion study to diagnose Alzheimer's disease, locate seizure foci and cerebral ischemia, Parkinson's disease

- Radionuclides: Tc-99m-hexamethylpropyleneamineoxime (Tc-99m-HM-PAO)
- Administration: IV
- Waiting period after injection: 15 to 30 minutes after Tc-99m-HM-PAO injection
- Food and fluids: No restriction
- Other instructions: Imaging room should be quiet and lights dimmed. IV line should be inserted before the test. Client lies still 15 minutes before the Tc-99m-HM-PAO injection. During imaging the client is in supine position with the head in a head holder. The entire brain, including the cerebellum, is imaged

Heart (cardiac) MUGA: *(For myocardial perfusion imaging studies with stress imaging, see Stress/Exercise Tests.)*

Multigated acquisition (MUGA) scanning is a rapid, safe method to evaluate the heart size, ventricle wall motion, and ejection fraction. The client's blood is tagged with a radioactive tracer, such as technetium-99m, which permits the heart and its function to be visualized. There is multiple imaging during MUGA scanning. MUGA identifies changes occurring with contraction and expansion of the ventricles of the heart. With cardiac disease, the heart's ability to pump blood sufficiently may be reduced. The amount of radiation exposure is comparable to that of a CT scan. MUGA may be performed with the stress test.

- Radionuclides: Tc-99m-O_4 tagged red blood cells (RBCs)
- Administration: IV
- Waiting period after injection: None
- Food and fluids: None
- Other instructions: The electrocardiogram is monitored. The client is in a supine position with a gamma camera over the chest. The radioactive tracer (containing no dye) allows visualization of the heart and its function

Heart

- Radionuclides: Tc-99m-pyrophosphate or Tc-99-m-pertechnetate. To confirm if a myocardial infarction (MI) occurred. This test is ordered 2 to 6 days after a suspected myocardial infarction. Tc-99m-labeled RBCs or albumin are used for ejection fraction studies (MUGA)
- Administration: IV
- Waiting period after injection: Tc-99m, 30 minutes to 1 hour
- Food and fluids: NPO may be required from midnight to study
- Other instructions: Client lies quietly for 15 to 30 minutes during the imaging for a myocardial infarction

Kidney: For renal blood-flow (renogram) studies and imaging. Two drugs may be used with renal imaging: furosemide (Lasix) for determining renal excretory function, and captopril for identifying renovascular hypertension.

- Radionuclides: Tc-99m-pertechnetate, Tc-99m-glucoheptonate for renal cortical and tubular disorders; Tc-99 diethylenetriamine pentaacetic acid (Tc-99m-DTPA) for evaluating renal function and perfusion disorders; Tc-99m glucoheptonate and I-131 hippuran (for renal perfusion studies); Tc-99m mercaptylacetyltriglycine (Tc-99m-MAG3) for evaluating renal clearance related to renal insufficiency
- Administration: IV
- Waiting period after injection: Renal perfusion study: Imaging is done immediately after the radiopharmaceutical is given intravenously. Renogram curves are plotted. Kidney disorders: 3 to 30 minutes after Tc-99m-DTPA is injected
- Foods and fluids: No restrictions. The client should be well hydrated. Drink 2 to 3 glasses of water 30 minutes before the scan. Dehydration could lead to false test results
- Other instructions: Void before the scan. If the client had IVP, the renogram or scan should be delayed 24 hours. Lugol's solution, 10 drops, may be ordered if I-131 hippuran is given. Client lies quietly for 30 minutes to 1 hour during imaging

Liver and spleen: Liver imaging can detect 90% of hepatic metastases and 85% of hepatocellular diseases. It is useful for screening the liver and spleen for lacerations and hematomas following trauma. SPECT improves lesion/mass detection.

- Radionuclides: Tc-99m compounds: Tc-99m-sulfur colloid
- Administration: IV
- Waiting period after injection: Tc-99m-sulfur colloid, 15 minutes. Spleen scan can be done at the same time
- Food and fluids: no restrictions. NPO after midnight may be ordered
- Other instructions: Client lies quietly for 30 minutes to 1 hour during the imaging. Client may be asked to turn from side to side and onto abdomen during imaging

Colon and ovary: The use of radiolabeled monoclonal antibodies: used to identify colon and ovarian cancer cells in areas of the body. The radiolabeled monoconal antibodies attach to cancer cells. The cancer cells can then be detected with use of a gamma camera.

- Radionuclides: Monoclonal antibodies labeled with 111 Indium (111 In)
- Administration: IV. Infusion takes 5 to 30 minutes
- Waiting period after injection: 3 to 5 days after radiolabeled monoclonal antibodies. Usually, two sets of images are taken at different times using the nuclear gamma camera
- Food and fluids: Light breakfast or lunch
- Other instructions: Regular medications can be taken. Client voids prior to the test. Allergic reaction to the monoclonal antibodies, though uncommon (less than 4%), may occur. Monoclonal antibodies are obtained from mice (human cancer cells are injected in the mice to produce antibodies)

Gastroesophageal reflux: Esophageal clearance is determined following a swallowed radioactive tracer. Numerous esophageal tests, such as endoscopy, barium esophagoscopy, and acid reflux testing may be performed to detect esophageal reflux syndrome. The radionuclide gastroesophageal reflux scan is highly sensitive (99%) for esophageal reflux.

- Radionuclides: Solution containing 150 mL of orange juice, 150 mL of 0.1 N hydrochloric acid, and 300 μCi Tc-99m sulfur colloid (Tc-99m-SC). Child: 250 μCi Tc-99m-SC in 10 mL of sterile water via a feeding tube
- Administration: Orally
- Waiting period: 30 seconds

- Food and fluids: Fasting for at least 4 hours prior to the study
- Other instructions: The client is in an upright or supine position. The procedure may require that the client perform a Valsalva maneuver

Gastrointestinal (GI) bleeding: The radionuclide GI bleeding study is more sensitive than angiography. For a positive test result the client must be actively bleeding at the time of imaging for accurate identification of the bleeding site.

- Radionuclides: Tc-99m-labeled RBCs
- Administration: Intravenously by bolus injection. For Tc-99m-labeled (tagged) RBCs, withdraw 5 to 8 mL of whole blood into a shielded syringe containing Tc-99m sodium pertechnetate. After processing the blood, Tc-99m-labeled RBCs are injected as a bolus
- Waiting period after injection: Imaging begins immediately after injection or until the site of bleeding is located. If negative after 2 hours, imaging may be repeated when client begins active bleeding or imaging at different time periods during the 24 hours after injection
- Food and fluids: NPO unless otherwise indicated
- Other instructions: Client is in supine position. Imaging is usually over the abdominal and pelvic areas. This test may be done as an emergency study, pre-surgery to locate the site of gastric bleeding, or pre-angiography

Gastric emptying: Delayed gastric emptying could be due to acute disorders, such as trauma, postoperative ileus, gastroenteritis, or chronic disorders, such as diabetes gastroparesis, peptic ulcers, pyloric stenosis, and Zollinger-Ellison syndrome.

- Radionuclides: 111 In DTPA or Tc-99m labeled juice and Tc-99m AC labeled eggs
- Administration: Client ingests scrambled egg sandwich and juice (all radiolabeled). Tc-99m-sulfur colloid-labeled instant oatmeal may be ordered instead of eggs
- Waiting period after oral meal: Immediately after ingesting the oral meal and continuously for 1 hour. A 2-hour imaging may also be requested following the oral meal
- Food and fluids: NPO for 4 hours and no smoking prior to the test

- Other instructions: Client is in a mid-Fowler's position for the meal and during imaging. The test should be performed in the morning because during the day the gastric emptying time can vary

Gallbladder (hepatobiliary scan): Hepatobiliary radioactive scanning is more sensitive for diagnosing acute cholecystitis than other standard gallbladder diagnostic tests. With hepatobiliary scanning, accurate imaging of the biliary tract can be performed even when there is marked hepatic dysfunction and jaundice.

- Radionuclides: Tc-99m disofenin, Tc-99m mebrofenin, or and other Tc-IDA derivatives
- Administration: IV. Cholecytokinin (CCK), a hormone that stimulates the gallbladder (GB) to contract and empty, may be used with normal saline solution as an infusion to promote GB emptying for imaging purposes
- Waiting period after injection: Immediate after CCK and radionuclide infusions
- Food and fluids: NPO for 4 hours before the test with use of CCK
- Other instructions: Usually CCK is given pre-radiopharmaceutical injection to stimulate the gallbladder of clients who have not eaten. CCK is short acting (20 to 30 minutes). Normal value for gallbladder ejection fraction (GBEF%) is >35%. Lower values indicate chronic cholecystitis. Higher values usually indicate hypercholestosis conditions. Nausea and abdominal discomfort may occur for a few minutes after the CCK infusion

Lung (pulmonary): Lung perfusion and ventilation scannings are sensitive for detecting pulmonary emboli (PE), obstructive pulmonary disease, and lung carcinoma. Both types of lung scans may be performed to identify the pulmonary disorder.

- Radionuclides: Perfusion study: TC-99m compounds: macroaggregated albumin (Tc-99m-MAA), Tc-99m human albumin microspheres (Tc-99m-HAM). Ventilation study: Xe-133 (more commonly used), Xe-127 (not commonly used), krypton (Kr) 81m, and Tc-99m-DTPA aerosol
- Administration: Intravenously (perfusion) or inhaled (ventilation)
- Waiting period after injection: Tc-99m compounds, 5 minutes after the injection of the radionuclide
- Food and fluids: No restrictions

- Other instructions: A chest radiograph is usually ordered for comparison with the nuclear medicine study. The client should lie quietly for 30 minutes during the imaging; however, for the inhaled test, the client is seated. Usually the camera is positioned behind the client

Thyroid: This test differentiates between primary thyroid carcinoma and metastases to the thyroid gland. Radioactive iodine is the most frequently used radionuclide because iodine is easily taken up in the thyroid gland. Iodine is a precursor in thyroid hormone synthesis.

- Radionuclides: I-131 sodium iodide, I-123, I-125, Tc-99m-pertechnetate
- Administration: I-123, I-125, I-131 (orally). I-123 has a short half-life and is the choice radionuclide. Tc-99m-pertechnetate (IV)
- Waiting period after injection: I-123, I-125, I-131—2 to 24 hours. I-123 is the radionuclide most commonly used because it has a shorter half-life. Tc-99m-pertechnetate, 30 minutes
- Food and fluids: No breakfast and NPO for 2 hours following oral iodine
- Other instructions: Three days before the scan (imaging), iodine preparations, thyroid hormones, phenothiazines, corticosteroids, aspirin, sodium nitroprusside, cough syrups containing iodides, and multivitamins are usually discontinued with health care provider's permission. Seafoods and iodized salt should be avoided. If the drugs cannot be withheld for 3 days, the drugs should be listed on the nuclear medicine request slip. The client should lie quietly for 30 minutes during the imaging procedure

Factors Affecting Diagnostic Results

- Two radionuclides administered in one day may interfere with each other.
- Too short or too long a waiting period after injection of the radionuclide could affect test results.

Nursing Implications

- Explain to the client the purpose and procedure for the ordered study. Procedures will differ according to the type of study (see Procedure).

- Check if a consent form is needed. Usually a consent form is not needed unless the radionuclide is >30 mCi.
- Obtain a brief health history in regard to recent exposure to radioisotopes, allergies that could cause an adverse reaction, being pregnant, breast feeding, and drugs.
- Adhere to the instructions from the nuclear medicine laboratory concerning the client and the procedure. The client should arrive on time.
- Report to the health care provider if the client is extremely apprehensive.
- Be supportive to the client. Advise the client to ask questions and to communicate concerns.
- List restricted drugs containing iodine that the client is taking on the request slip. This is important if the radionuclide is iodine.

Client Teaching

- Explain that the dose of radiation from radionuclide imaging is usually less than the amount of radiation received from diagnostic x-ray.
- Inform client and family that the injected radionuclide should not affect the family, visitors, other clients, or hospital staff members. The radionuclide is excreted from the body in about 6 to 24 hours.
- Explain that the detection equipment will move over a section or sections of the body. No physical discomfort should be felt.
- Inform the client that the scanning may take 30 minutes to 1 hour, depending on the organ being studied.
- Instruct the client to remove jewelry or any metal object.

PAPANICOLAOU SMEAR (PAP SMEAR)*

CYTOLOGY TEST FOR CERVICAL CANCER

Normal Finding. No abnormal or atypical cells

Description. The Papanicolaou (Pap) smear became internationally known and used in the early 1950s for detecting cervical cancer and precancerous tissue. Malignant tissue change usually takes many years, so yearly

*Updated with the assistance of Ellen K. Boyda, RN, MS, CRNP, Family Nurse Practitioner, Pennsylvania.

examination of exfoliative cervical cells (sloughed-off cells) allows detection of early precancerous conditions. It has been suggested that women from age 18 to 40 years have yearly Pap smears and that women from age 40 years on have either twice-a-year or yearly smears. How often the Pap smear test should be performed is determined by the client's health care provider.

The Pap smear (cytology) results are reported by the Bethesda system. General categories of The Bethesda System (TBS) are as follows:

I. Within normal limits.
II. Abnormal changes
   A. Benign cellular changes
      1. Differentiates reactive or inflammatory changes from true dysplastic changes.
      2. Most important features of TBS. *Management:* Repeat smears yearly.
   B. Epithelial abnormalities
      1. Atypical cells of undetermined significance (ASCUS): favoring a neoplastic process or a reactive process. *Management:* Repeat smears at closer intervals, recall for colposcopy and/or combine repeat cytology with cervicography of HPV-DNA type.
      2. Low-grade squamous intraepithelial lesion (LGSIL): shows the earliest abnormal nuclear changes; combines diagnosis of HPV and mild dysplagia. *Management:* Repeat cytology at close intervals, recall for colposcopy.
      3. High-grade squamous intraepithelial lesion (HGSIL): includes moderate and severe dysplastic changes. *Management of HGSIL:* Recall for colposcopy.
      4. Squamous cell carcinoma: changes consistent with cancer. *Management:* Recall for colposcopy.
      5. Glandular cell abnormalities
         a. Atypical cells of undetermined significance, atypical endocervical cells. *Management:* In young women, check for endocervicitis, repeat smear, refer to colposcopy; in older women; refer for colposcopy with endocervical sample.
         b. Cancer *Management:* Refer for colposcopy.

For suggestive or positive Pap smears, colposcopy and/or a cervical biopsy are frequently ordered to confirm the test results. Atypical cells can occur following cervicitis and after excessive or prolonged use of hormones.

Purposes

- To detect precancerous and cancerous cells of the cervix
- To assess the effects of sex hormonal replacement
- To identify viral, fungal, and parasitic conditions
- To evaluate the response to chemotherapy or radiation therapy to the cervix

Clinical Problems

***Abnormal findings*:** Precancerous and cancerous cells of the cervix, cervicitis; viral, fungal, and parasitic conditions

Procedure

- No food or fluid is restricted.
- The client should not douche, insert vaginal medications, or have sexual intercourse for at least 24 hours, preferably 48 hours, before the test. The test should be done between menstrual periods.
- The client is generally asked to remove all clothes, as the breasts are examined after the Pap smear is taken. A paper or cloth gown is worn.
- Instruct the client to lie on the examining table in the lithotomy position.
- A speculum, which may be lubricated with warm running water, is inserted into the vagina.
- A curved, wooden spatula (Pap stick) is used to scrape the cervix. The obtained specimen is transferred onto a slide and is immersed in a fixative solution or sprayed with a commercial fixation spray. Label the slide with the client's name and the date.
- The procedure takes approximately 10 minutes.

Factors Affecting Diagnostic Results

- Douching, use of vaginal suppositories, or sexual intercourse within 24 hours before the test

Nursing Implications

- Obtain a history regarding menstruation and any menstrual problems.

Client Teaching

- Answer client's questions if possible. Be a good listener.

at a bimanual examination of the vagina, lower ab-
m may or will follow the Pap smear.
louching, insertion of vaginal suppositories, or
ntercourse for at least 24 hours, preferably 48 hours,
aindicated before a Pap smear.
Tell client that the test results should be back in about 3 to 5 days. Reporting test results to clients differs; some institutions send cards while others call only if results are abnormal.

POSITRON EMISSION TOMOGRAPHY (PET)*

Normal Findings. Normal brain, lung, heart and gastrointestinal activities and blood flow

Description. Positron emission tomography (PET), a relatively noninvasive test, measures areas of positron-emitting isotope concentration. PET is used to study the brain, heart, lungs, and abdominal organs, and for oncologic purposes. For brain studies, PET assesses normal brain function; regional cerebral blood flow and volume; glucose, protein, and oxygen metabolism; blood–brain barrier function, neuroreceptor-neurotransmitter systems; and the pathophysiology of neurologic and psychiatric disorders. For heart studies, PET assesses cardiac perfusion or blood flow; glucose and oxygen metabolism; and receptor functions. PET perfusion imaging provides information concerning the severity of coronary artery disease (CAD). In oncology, PET has recently been approved for lung nodules and colorectal imaging.

The client receives a substance tagged with a radionuclide by gas or injectable form (e.g., radioactive glucose, rubidium-82, oxygen-15, nitrogen-13). Flurodeoxyglucose (FDG) is the most common radioisotope used in PET. Tomographic slices from cross-sections of tissue are detected and visually displayed by computer. PET is most effective in determining blood flow (brain, heart). Radiation from PET is a quarter of that received by CT.

---

*Revised by Frank Di Gregorio, CNMT, RDMS, Director, Community Imaging Center, Wilmington, Delaware.

Purposes

- To detect a decreased blood flow or perfusion with coronary artery disease
- To determine the size of infarct and myocardial viability
- To detect transient ischemia
- To detect decreased oxygen utilization and decreased blood flow with brain disorders such as cerebral vascular accident (CVA)
- To differentiate between types of dementia (i.e., Alzheimer's disease and other dementias, such as parkinsonism)
- To identify stages of cranial tumors
- To identify lung nodules
- To identify colorectal metastasis

Clinical Problems

Abnormal findings: Hypoperfusion to brain and heart, stroke, epilepsy, migraine, Parkinson's disease, dementia, Alzheimer's disease, AMI for first 72 hours

Procedure

- Obtain a signed consent form.
- Start two IVs, one for radioactive substance and the second to draw blood gas samples. A blindfold may be used to keep the client from being distracted, since alertness is necessary.
- No coffee, alcohol, or tobacco is allowed for 24 hours before the test.
- Empty bladder 1 to 2 hours before the test.
- No sedatives are given, since client needs to follow instructions.
- Test takes 1 to 1½ hours.

Nursing Implications

- Explain procedure (see Procedure).
- Obtain a signed consent form.
- Monitor vital signs.

Client Teaching

Pre-test

- Inform client that instructions given during test should be followed.
- Assess IV site.
- Listen to client's concerns.

Post-test

- Encourage fluid post-test to get rid of radioactive substance.
- Avoid postural hypotension by slowly moving the client to upright position.

PROCTOSIGMOIDOSCOPY, PROCTOSCOPY, SIGMOIDOSCOPY

Normal Findings. Normal mucosa and structure of the rectum and sigmoid colon

Description. Proctosigmoidoscopy is the term for proctoscopy, an examination of the anus and rectum, and sigmoidoscopy, an examination of the anus, rectum, and sigmoid colon. Three types of instruments are used: (1) a 7-cm rigid proctoscope or anoscope, (2) a 25- to 30-cm rigid sigmoidoscope, and (3) a 60-cm flexible sigmoidscope.

With this procedure the rectum and distal sigmoid colon can be visualized, and specimens can be obtained by a biopsy forceps or a snare, or by cytology brush or culture swab. The test is usually indicated when there are changes in bowel habits, chronic constipation, or bright blood or mucus in the stool, or it can be part of an annual physical examination for those over 40 years old. With asymptomatic clients, proctosigmoidoscopy is usually performed every 3 to 5 years.

Purposes

- To examine the anus, rectum, and sigmoid colon
- To detect blood or tumor in the sigmoid colon
- To obtain a culture of tissue or secretion for cytologic study

Clinical Problems

Abnormal findings: Hemorrhoids, rectal and sigmoid colon polyps; fistulas, fissures; rectal abscesses; neoplasms (benign or malignant); ulcerative or granulomatous colitis; infections or inflammation of the rectosigmoid area

Procedure

- Obtain a signed consent form.
- Client is allowed a light dinner the night before the test and a lighter breakfast or NPO 8 hours prior to test. Usually heavy meals, vegetables, and fruits are prohibited within 24 hours of the test.
- Client may take prescribed medications by 6 AM the morning of the test with health care provider's permission.
- No barium studies should be performed within 3 days of the test.
- A saline or warm tap water enema(s) or hypertonic salt enema(s), such as Fleet's, is given the morning of the test. If enemas are contraindicated, then a rectal suppository, such as bisacodyl (Dulcolax), could be given. Prep with GoLYTELY could be used. If so, follow those instructions. Oral cathartics are seldom used because they may increase fecal flow from the small intestine during the test.
- The client should assume either a knee-chest position or Sims' (side-lying) position.
- As the lubricated endoscope is inserted into the rectum, the patient should be instructed to breathe deeply and slowly. Sometimes air is injected into the bowel to improve visualization. Specimens can be obtained during the procedure.
- The procedure takes approximately 15 to 30 minutes.

Factors Affecting Diagnostic Results

- Barium from barium studies can decrease visualization.
- Fecal material in the lower colon can decrease visualization.

Nursing Implications

- Check the chart to determine if the client has had a barium study within 3 days before the scheduled proctosigmoidoscopy.
- Record baseline vital signs before the test.
- Allow the client time to ask questions and to express concerns. Be supportive of the client.

Client Teaching

- Explain the procedure to the client regarding body position, pre-test preparation (enema and diet), and the time required for the procedure.
- Encourage the client to breathe deeply and slowly and to relax during the test. Explain that there may be some gas pains if air is injected for better visualization.

Post-test

- Monitor vital signs as indicated.
- Observe for signs and symptoms of bowel perforation (i.e., pain, abdominal distention, and rectal bleeding). Check for shock-like symptoms (i.e., tachycardia, paleness, diaphoresis) if perforation is suspected.

Client Teaching

- Encourage the client to rest for an hour or so after the test, if possible.

PULMONARY FUNCTION TESTS*

PULMONARY DIAGNOSTIC TESTS

Normal Finding. Normal values according to client's age, sex, weight, and height; >80% of the predicted value

Description. Pulmonary function tests (PFTs) are useful in differentiating between obstructive and restrictive lung diseases and in quantifying the degree (mild, moderate, or severe) of obstructive or restrictive lung disorders. Other purposes for pulmonary tests include: to establish baseline for comparison with future pulmonary tests; to evaluate pulmonary status before surgery, pulmonary disability for insurance; to track the progress of lung disease; and to assess the response to therapy.

In pulmonary physiologic testing, the lungs are monitored by many complex devices and tests, the most basic device being the spirometer. This device is used to measure flows, volumes, and capacities.

A number of pulmonary tests are conducted, since no single measurement can evaluate pulmonary function. The tests frequently used for PFTs are the slow vital-capacity group, lung volume group, forced vital capacity, diffusion capacity study, and the flow-volume loop.

Pulmonary function tests

1. *Slow vital-capacity tests*

   Tidal volume (TV): the amount of air inhaled and exhaled during rest or quiet respiration or normal breathing

---

*This test contributed by David C. Sestili, CRTT, RPFT.

Inspiratory capacity (IC): the maximal inspired amount of air from end expiratory tidal volume in normal breathing

Expiratory reserve volume (ERV): the maximal amount of air that can be exhaled from end expiratory tidal volume in normal breathing

Inspiratory reserve volume (IRV): the maximal amount of air that can be inspired from end inspiratory tidal volume in normal breathing

Vital capacity (VC): the maximal amount of air exhaled after a maximal inhalation. VC = ERV + IC or VC = IC + ERV

2. *Lung-volume measurements*

   Residual volume (RV): the amount of air that remains in the lungs after maximal expiration

   Functional residual capacity (FRC): the amount of air left in the lungs after tidal or normal expiration. FRC = ERV + RV. In obstructive disorders, FRC is increased because of hyperinflation of the lungs due to air trapping. In restrictive disorders, FRC and RV can be normal or decreased

   Total lung capacity (TLC): the total amount of air that is in the lungs at maximal inspiration; TLC = VC + RV, FRC + IC

3. *Forced vital capacity (FVC):* Decreased in obstructive lung disease; normal or decreased in restrictive lung disease; FVC = IC + ERV

   Forced inspiratory volume (FIV): greatest amount of air inhaled after a maximal expiration

   Forced expiratory volume timed (FEV_T): greatest amount of air exhaled in FEV 0.5 second, 1 second FEV_1, 2 seconds FEV_2, 3 seconds FEV_3. See Figure 1 for graphic of lung volume and capacity. FEV_1 is most important to monitor, i.e., asthmatic, preoperative >1.5 liters is preferred

4. *Flow volume loop (FVL):* Another method to visualize forced vital capacity measurement by graphing flow vs. volume is FVL, seen in Figure 2. Abnormal FLVs in Figure 3 indicate types of pulmonary problems

   Peak expiratory flow (PEF): the highest flow rate achieved at the beginning of the FVC and reported in liters per second. *Note:* Peak flow meters measure in liters per minute.

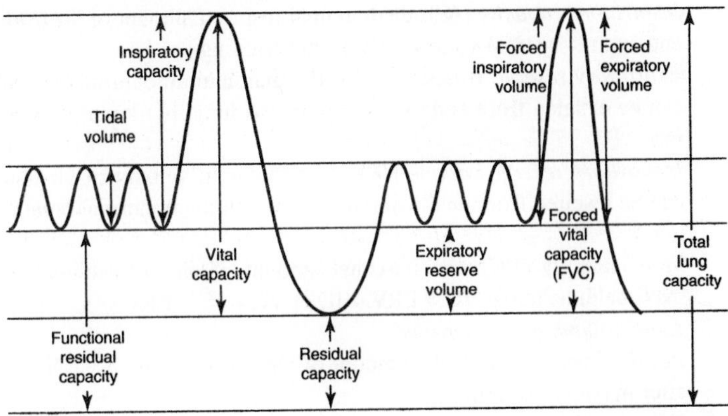
Inspiratory capacity
Tidal volume
Vital capacity
Functional residual capacity
Residual capacity
Expiratory reserve volume
Forced inspiratory volume
Forced expiratory volume
Forced vital capacity (FVC)
Total lung capacity

FIGURE 1. Graphic of lung volume and capacity. *(From Kee, JL [1999]. Laboratory and Diagnostic Tests with Nursing Implications [5th ed]. Norwalk, CT: Appleton & Lange.)*

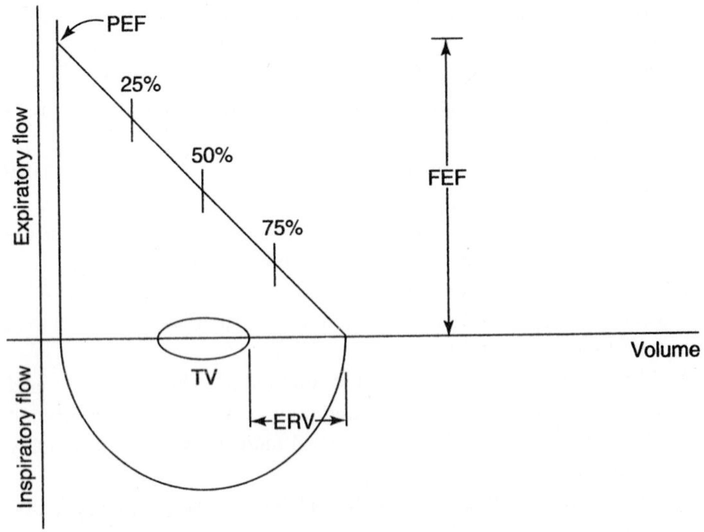
PEF
25%
50%
75%
FEF
Expiratory flow
Inspiratory flow
Volume
TV
ERV

FIGURE 2. Flow volume loop (FVL) and force expiratory flow (FEF). *(Courtesy of David C. Sestili, CRTT, RPFT.)*

Peak inspiratory flow (PIF): the highest flow rate achieved at the beginning of the forced inspiratory capacity

Forced expiratory flow (FEF): Figure 2 demonstrates the rate of flow at selected points on the flow volume loop. The FEF looks at flow at the 25%, 50%, and 75% of the FVC and evaluates flow in various size airways. It can evaluate the effectiveness of bronchodilator therapy. FEF 25% reflects flow through large airways; FEF 50% reflects flow through medium airways; and FEF 75% reflects flow through small airways. Decreased FEF 75% indicates small airway disease.

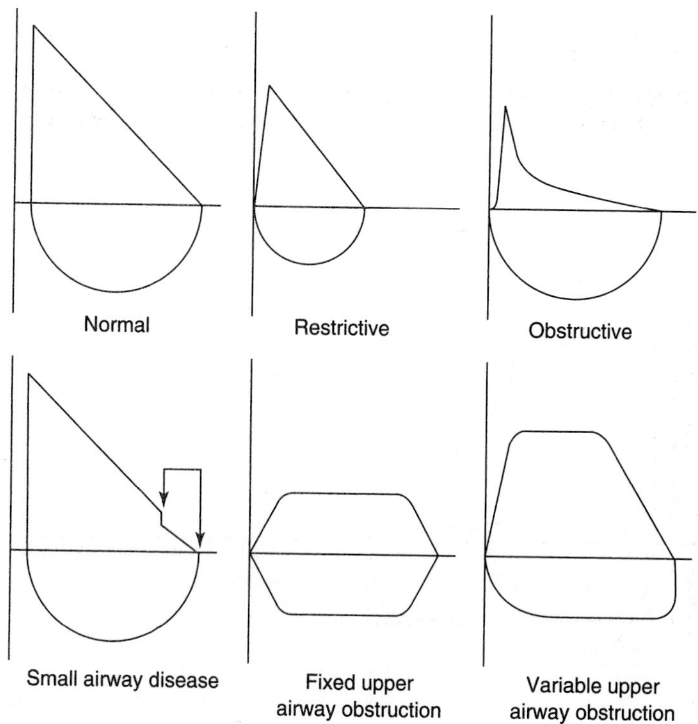
Normal
Restrictive
Obstructive
Small airway disease
Fixed upper airway obstruction
Variable upper airway obstruction

FIGURE 3. Abnormal flow volume loops (FVL). *(Courtesy of David C. Sestili, CRTT, RPFT.)*

5. *Diffusion capacity test:* Diffusion tests can be done by a number of techniques. The most commonly used one is the single breath test. This requires the client to inspire from RV to TLC. The gas inhaled is a mixture of helium 10%, carbon monoxide 0.3%, oxygen 21%, and nitrogen 68.7%. The client holds his or her breath for 10 seconds prior to expiration. After the first 750 mL is discarded to wash out dead-space gas, an alveolar sample is collected and analyzed for helium and CO concentration. Results of this reflect the state of the alveolar capillary barrier. Decreased diffusing capacity occurs in disease states such as interstitial fibrosis, interstitial edema, and emphysema. It will also decrease in persons with abnormal hemoglobin, such as anemias, smokers, HbCO. Cardiac output can effect result.
6. *Bronchial provocation studies:* Inhalation of pharmacologic and antigenic substances are used to test the sensitivity of the airways toward hyperreactivity and obstruction. Serial spirometry tests are performed to document the amount or degree of reactivity (a drop in FEV_1 greater than 20% of baseline spirometry). Indications for these tests are: (1) normal spirometric test, (2) a history of symptoms such as wheezing, or coughing without a cause, and (3) symptoms related to exposure to industrial substances.

   Methacholine chloride is usually the testing drug of choice due to its short-acting time in causing bronchoconstriction. The client inhales progressively larger doses of the drug until all levels are administered without change in FEV_1, or a drop of 20% of baseline FEV_1 is reached. The drug is then reversed by administration of a bronchodilator.
7. *Exercise studies:* Pulmonary function studies are done at a resting state. The exercise studies evaluate clients under an active state. These tests are performed by having the subject walk on a treadmill or pedal an ergometer to a set protocol to stimulate activity at progressive work loads. During the test, a 12-lead electrocardiogram is taken and expired gases are analyzed for oxygen consumption and carbon dioxide production, tidal volume, respiratory rate, blood pressure, and oxygen saturation by oximetry and/or arterial blood gases. These tests are used to determine the amount of disability and to evaluate the person with exertional dyspnea. This allows the client to have an exercise prescription for activities for pulmonary cardiac rehabilitation.

8. *Pulse oximetry:* This is a noninvasive procedure to measure oxygen saturation in the blood. The device measures the oxygen saturation via two wavelengths of infrared light. The light is passed through an extremity, such as a finger. The device then is able to measure the saturation of the blood in that area. This method is an excellent noninvasive trending device. When values vary a blood gas for PO_2 and/or CO oximetry to measure % HbO_2 and SaO_2 should be done to validate the results. A note of caution: Blood gas results normally do not measure oxygen saturation; they are calculated. Check with your blood gas laboratory for this information.

   The pulse oximeter is a very useful tool, but it has some drawbacks. It should be trusted after direct comparison to CO oximetry is done. Abnormal hemoglobins such as HbCO, MetHb, and SulfaHb could fool the device. These hemoglobins are measured around the same infrared wavelengths and may falsely be considered by the oximeter to be oxygen. Blood flow to an area may be impeded and will also affect the pulse oximeter. Correlation with the client's true pulse will assist in correcting this problem. Light sources may also affect the results; the area should be guarded against external light sources.
9. *Body plethysmograph (body box):* Body plethysmograph is a method to measure the exact amount of air in the thorax. This is accomplished by having the subject sit inside an airtight box and breathe through a flow-measuring device. A panting maneuver is done, and a shutter is closed to measure pressure at the mouth and pressure changes of the box. By knowing these measurements and applying Boyle's Law, the thoracic gas volume (TGV), which correlates to functional residual capacity (FRC) can be measured. The compliance and resistances to the lung can also be measured by this device. Advantages are that the body box measures all air in the chest. Volumes tend to be larger in box studies. Disadvantages to the body box test are that some clients have claustrophobia, and persons with perforated eardrums will tend to have readings higher than normal, which could be misleading. This test requires total client cooperation.
10. *Nutritional studies:* Indirect calorimetry is the measurement of CO_2 production and O_2 consumption. From this, respiratory quotient

(RQ) is obtained ($PO_2 + CO_2 = RQ$) which yields the type of substrate utilized in metabolism (i.e., carbohydrate, fat, protein). This noninvasive test gives useful information as energy expenditure (EE) and the amount of calories needed for minimal existence expressed in kcal per 24 hours. The RQ tells about the type of fuel being metabolized, such as RQ 1.0 is carbohydrates, RQ 0.80 indicates mixed carbohydrates and fats, and RQ 0.75 indicates lipids.

Purposes

- To assess pulmonary/respiratory function
- To detect the occurrence of pulmonary dysfunction
- To differentiate between obstructive and restrictive lung diseases
- To evaluate the response of drug therapy for decreasing lung dysfunction

Clinical Problems

Obstructive diseases: Emphysema, chronic bronchitis, bronchiectasis, bronchospasm, bronchial secretions, airway inflammation caused by bacterial or viral infections

Restrictive diseases: Pulmonary fibrosis, pneumonia, lung tumors, kyphoscoliosis, neuromuscular diseases, chest trauma, obesity, scleroderma, sarcoidosis, pulmonary edema, surgical removal of lung tissue, pregnancy

Procedure

- Eating a heavy meal before the test should be discouraged.
- Client should avoid smoking 4 to 6 hours before the tests.
- Client should wear nonrestrictive clothing.
- Record client's age, height, and weight, which may be used to predict normal range.
- Medications are not restricted unless indicated by the health care provider. Usually sedatives and narcotics are not given.
- Postpone procedure if the client has an active cold or is under the influence of alcohol.
- Dentures may be left in during testing.
- ·st can be performed in a sitting or standing position (children ınding position only). A nose clip is applied, and the client is ıcted to breathe in and out through the mouth.

- Practice sessions on fast and deep breathing are given. Normally the test is repeated twice, and the best tracing is used. The test may be repeated after using a bronchodilator.

Bronchial provocation studies

- The client must not exercise, smoke, or consume caffeine (coffee, cola, or chocolate) for a minimum of 6 hours before testing.
- Discontinue bronchodilator therapy for at least 48 hours prior to testing with health care provider's permission.

Exercise studies

- The client will be walking on a treadmill or riding a stationary bike. The heart rate and rhythm will be monitored by a 12-lead ECG.
- The client will be breathing through a mouthpiece during the test.

Nutritional studies

- The client should fast for at least 12 hours before the test.
- The test is performed approximately ½ hour after waking. There should be no activity before testing.
- The client exhales into an analyzing device.
- This test can be conducted for clients on ventilators, hyperalimentation, or tube feeding as long as there are no changes in the diet or ventilator settings until the test is completed.

Factors Affecting Diagnostic Results

- Use of bronchodilators 4 hours before the pulmonary function test may produce falsely improved pulmonary results.
- Sedatives and narcotics given before the test could decrease test results.

Nursing Implications

- List on the request slip the oral bronchodilators and steroids the client is taking. Record client's age, height, and weight.
- Record vital signs.
- Assess for signs and symptoms of respiratory distress (i.e., breathlessness, dyspnea, tachycardia, severe apprehension, and gray or cyanotic color).
- Be supportive of client and answer questions if possible.

Client Teaching

- Explain the purpose of the tests and the procedure.

- Practice breathing patterns for pulmonary function tests with the client (i.e., normal breathing, rapid breathing, forced deep inspiration, and forced deep expiration).

RADIOACTIVE IODINE (RAI) UPTAKE TEST

I-131 UPTAKE TEST, RADIOIODINE THYROID UPTAKE TEST

Normal Findings. Adult: 1%–13% (thyroid gland); 6 hours: 2%–25% (thyroid gland); 24 hours: 15%–45% (thyroid gland)

Description. The radioactive iodine uptake test is used to determine the metabolic activity of the thyroid gland by measuring the absorption of I-131 or I-123 in the thyroid. The uptake test is one of the tests used in diagnosing hypothyroidism and hyperthyroidism. It tends to be more accurate for diagnosing hyperthyroidism than for diagnosing hypothyroidism. It is also useful for differentiating between hyperthyroidism (Graves' disease) and an overactive toxic adenoma.

A calculated dose of I-131 or I-123, in liquid or capsule form, is given orally. The client's thyroid is scanned at three different times. The tracer dose has a small amount of radioactivity and is considered harmless. The client's urine may be checked for radioactive iodine excretion.

Purposes

- To determine the metabolic activity of the thyroid gland
- To diagnose hypothyroidism and hyperthyroidism
- To differentiate between hypoerthyroidism and an overactive toxic adenoma

Clinical Problems

Decreased level: Hypothyroidism (myxedema)

Drugs that may decrease RAI uptake: Lugol's solution, vitamins, expec-
ᵔnts (SSKI), antithyroid agents, cortisone preparation, ACTH, aspirin,
ᵎnes, phenylbutazone (Butazolidin), anticoagulants, thiopental
ᵎntothal)

t may cause false negatives: Seafood, cabbage, iodized salt

Elevated level: Hyperthyroidism (Graves' disease), thyroiditis, cirrhosis of the liver

Drugs that may increase RAI uptake: Barbiturates, estrogens, lithium carbonate, phenothiazines

Procedure

- Restrict food and fluids for 8 hours prior to the test. The client can eat an hour after the radioiodine capsule or liquid has been taken.
- The amount of radioactivity in the thyroid gland may be measured three times (after 2, 6, and 24 hours).
- The client should return to the nuclear medicine laboratory at specified times to measure the I-131 uptake level with the scintillation counter.

Factors Affecting Diagnostic Results

- Severe diarrhea, intestinal malabsorption, and x-ray contrast media studies may cause a decreased I-131 uptake level, even in normal thyroid glands.
- Renal failure could cause an increased iodine uptake.

Nursing Implications

- Ask client for any known allergic reaction to iodine.
- Write down the times for returning to the nuclear medicine laboratory. Emphasize the importance of being on time for each determination.
- List on the request slip the x-ray studies and drugs the client has received in the last week, which could affect test results.
- Draw blood for T_3 and/or T_4 tests, if ordered, before the client takes the radioiodine capsule or liquid.
- Observe for signs and symptoms of hyperthyroidism (i.e., nervousness, tachycardia, excessive hyperactivity, exophthalmos, mood swings, and weight loss).

Client Teaching

- Inform client that eating an hour after the radioiodine capsule or liquid has been taken is usually permitted unless otherwise indicated by the nuclear medicine laboratory.

- Inform the client that the test should not be painful and that the amount of radiation received should be harmless.
- Inform client that the radioactive substance should not harm family members, visitors, or other clients, since the dosage is low and gives off very little radiation. Women who are pregnant should not be given this test.

SCHILLING TEST (URINE)

CO-57-TAGGED VITAMIN B_{12}, (COBALT-57-TAGGED CYANOCOBALAMINE)

Normal Finding

Adult: >7% excretion of radioactive vitamin B_{12} within 24 hours. Usual range is 10%–40% of vitamin B_{12} excretion. Pernicious anemia: excretion of vitamin B_{12} is <3%. Intestinal malabsorption: excretion is 3%–5%

Description. The Schilling test is primarily ordered to diagnose pernicious anemia, a macrocytic anemia. The test determines if the client lacks the intrinsic factor in the gastric mucosa that is necessary for the absorption of vitamin B_{12} from food. With impaired absorption due to the lack of intrinsic factor or from intestinal malabsorption, little to no vitamin B_{12} is absorbed and therefore less is excreted in the urine.

A vitamin B_{12} defiency affects the bone marrow, the gastrointestinal tract, and neurologic system. The bone marrow becomes hyperplastic, having many bizarre red blood cell forms. The gastrointestinal mucosa atrophies, and there is a decrease in hydrochloric acid. Classic symptoms of pernicious anemia include a beefy, red tongue; indigestion; abdominal pain; diarrhea; and tingling and numbness of the hands and feet.

The test consists of collecting a 24-hour urine specimen after the client has taken a radioactive capsule of vitamin B_{12} administered by a technician from the nuclear medicine laboratory and an injection of in-
...uscular vitamin B_{12} given by the nurse. The intramuscular vitamin
...urate the liver and the protein-binding sites, thus permitting
...tion of the capsule cobalt-tagged vitamin B_{12} by the small in-
...nd its excretion in the urine. There are various types of radioac-

tive cobalt (Co-57, Co-56, Co-60), but Co-57 is preferred because of its shorter half-life and its low-energy gamma radiation.

Purposes

- To determine if there is a vitamin B_{12} deficiency
- To detect pernicious anemia and intestinal malabsorption syndrome

Clinical Problems

Decreased level: Pernicious anemia, intestinal malabsorption syndrome, liver diseases, hypothyroidism (myxedema), pancreatic insufficiency, sprue

Procedure

- Obtain a signed consent form.
- Restrict food and fluids for 8 to 12 hours before the test. Food and fluids are permitted after the IM vitamin B_{12} dose.
- Avoid ingestion of B vitamins for 3 days prior to the test and no laxatives for 1 day prior to test.
- A sample of urine (25–50 mL) should be collected before cobalt-tagged vitamin B_{12} is given to determine if there are radionuclide contaminants. A recent radionuclide scan within 7 days prior to the test could affect test result.
- The radioactive Co-57-tagged vitamin B_{12} capsule(s) or liquid is/are administered orally by a technician from nuclear medicine.
- Vitamin B_{12} (usually 1 mg) is given IM by the nurse 1 to 2 hours after the radioactive dose.
- Collect urine in a large container for 24 hours, according to the institution's procedure. No preservative is needed in the urine container. Check laboratory's policy.
- Label the urine container with the client's name, date, time, and room.
- Rubber gloves should be worn to handle the 24-hour urine specimen.

Nursing Implications

- Assess for signs and symptoms of pernicious anemia, such as beefy, red tongue; indigestion; abdominal pain; diarrhea; and tingling and numbness of the hands and feet.
- Assess urine output; low urine output affects test results.

- Do not administer laxatives the night before the test, as they could decrease absorption rate.
- Observe the client for at least 1 hour after the administration of the radionuclide for possible anaphylactic reaction.
- Release the breakfast tray after the nonradioactive vitamin B_{12} is given.
- Label the urine container and laboratory slip with the exact dates and times of collection. Tell client and family not to throw away the urine.

Client Teaching

- Discuss the test procedure with the client (see Procedure).
- Explain to the client that the radioactive substance should not be harmful to family members, visitors, or self unless the person is pregnant.
- Instruct the client that foods high in vitamin B_{12} are mostly animal products, such as milk, eggs, meat, and liver. Vitamin B_{12} is low in vegetables. Refer the client to the dietitian as needed.

SINUS ENDOSCOPY

Normal Finding. Normal sinuses; no infection or structural abnormalities noted

Description. Sinus endoscopy examines the anterior ethmoids and the middle meatal sinus areas. The primary purposes are to correct structural abnormalities and alleviate an infectious process. Sinus endoscopy is frequently prescribed for clients with chronic sinusitis who are nonresponsive to antibiotic therapy.

Purpose

- To diagnose the presence of a chronic sinus infection or structural abnormality

Clinical Problems. Acute or chronic sinusitis, cysts, sinus erosion, structural abnormality

Procedure

- Obtain a signed consent form.
- Restrict food and fluids after midnight or 12 hours prior to the procedure.
- Remove dentures, jewelry, and hairpins if present.
- Intravenous fluids are usually started prior to the procedure.
- Eye pads may be used to protect the eyes from injury during the procedure.
- The nostrils are sprayed with topical anesthetic. The procedure may be performed in the health care provider's office or in an outpatient department.
- CT scan may be needed during the procedure to visualize the sinus area.
- Nasal packing may be inserted into the nostril(s) post-procedure.

Factors Affecting Diagnostic Results

- Severe nasal septal defect.

Nursing Implications

- Obtain a history of the sinus problem(s) from the client.
- Check that the consent form is signed.
- Monitor vital signs.

Client Teaching

- Explain the procedure for sinus endoscopy (see Procedure). Answer questions that the client may have or if unknown, refer questions to appropriate health professionals.

Post-test

- Continue monitoring client's vital signs until stabilized.
- Check for excessive bleeding or discharge.

Client Teaching

- Instruct client to call health care provider if excessive bleeding or discharge occurs and for elevated body temperature.
- Instruct the client to take prescribed drugs (antibiotic and pain medication). Discuss post-test care as indicated by the health care provider.

SKIN TESTS (TUBERCULIN, BLASTOMYCOSIS, COCCIDIOIDOMYCOSIS, HISTOPLASMOSIS, TRICHINOSIS, AND TOXOPLASMOSIS)

Normal Finding. Negative results

Description. Skin testing is useful for determining present or past exposure to an infectious organism: bacterial (tuberculosis); mycotic (blastomycosis, coccidioidomycosis, histoplasmosis); or parasitic (trichinosis and toxoplasmosis). The types of skin tests include scratch, patch, multipuncture, and intradermal. With intradermal, the antigen of the organism is injected under the skin, and if the test is positive in 24 to 72 hours, the injection site becomes red, hard, and edematous.

Bacterial organism and disease: *Tuberculosis:* The tuberculin skin test indicates whether a person has been infected by the tubercle bacilli.

Testing methods

- *Mantoux Test:* Purified protein derivative tuberculin (PPD) is injected intradermally. PPD has several strengths, but the intermediate strength is usually used unless the client is known to be hypersensitive to skin tests. The client should not receive PPD if there was a previous positive test. The test is read in 48 to 72 hours.
- *Tine Test or Mono-Vacc Test:* These are multipuncture tests that use tines impregnated with PPD. Method is for mass screening. The tine test is read in 48 to 72 hours, and the Mono-Vacc Test is read in 48 to 96 hours.
- *Vollmer's Patch Test:* This test "patch" resembles a Band-Aid; however, the center piece is impregnated with concentrated old tuberculin (OT). The patch is removed in 48 hours, and the test result is read.

Mycotic organisms and diseases

- *Blastomycosis:* The organism *Blastomyces dermatitidis* causes blastomycosis. The antigen blastomycin is injected intradermally, and if an erythematous area greater than 5 mm in diameter occurs, the test is positive. The skin test should be read in 48 hours. Positive sputum and tissue specimens will confirm the blastomycin skin test.
- *Coccidioidomycosis:* The organism *Coccidioides immitis* causes the fungal disease coccidioidomycosis. The antigen, coccidioidin, is injected intradermally, and the skin test is read in 24 to 72 hours.

- *Histoplasmosis:* The organism *Histoplasma capsulatum* causes histoplasmosis. On chest x-ray the lung infection resembles tuberculosis. The histoplasmin test is not always reliable. The antigen is injected intradermally, and the skin test is read in 24 to 48 hours. To confirm the skin test result, sputum and tissue specimens should be obtained.

Parasites

- *Trichinosis:* The parasitic organism *Trichinella spiralis* causes trichinosis. Symptoms of nausea, diarrhea, pain, colic, fever, and swelling of the muscles occur approximately 2 weeks after ingesting the organism. The antigen is injected intradermally, and the test is read in 15 to 20 minutes. A positive test is a blanched wheal with an erythematous area surrounding it.
- *Toxoplasmosis:* The organism *Toxoplasma gondii* causes toxoplasmosis. This organism is found in the eye ground and brain tissue of man. The antigen, toxoplasmin, is injected intradermally, and the test result is read in 24 to 48 hours. A positive test is an erythematous area over 10 mm in diameter.

Purposes

- To determine the present or past exposure to an infectious organism
- To determine if the client has been infected by the tubercle bacilli using the TB skin test

Clinical Problems

Antigen Skin Test	*Organism*	*Disease*
Tuberculin	Tubercle bacilli	Tuberculosis
Blastomycin	*Blastomyces dermatitidis*	Blastomycosis
Coccidioidin	*Coccidioides immitis*	Coccidioidomycosis
Histoplasmin	*Histoplasma capsulatum*	Histoplasmosis
Trichinellin	*Trichinella spiralis*	Trichinosis
Toxoplasmin	*Toxoplasma gondii*	Toxoplasmosis

Procedure

- No food or fluid is restricted.
- Cleanse the inner aspect of the forearm with alcohol and let it dry.

- Inject intradermally 0.1 mL of the antigen into the inner aspect of forearm.
- Indicate injection site for reading of test result.

Nursing Implications

- Obtain a client history about hypersensitivity to skin tests. Ask the client if the skin test was performed before and if so, the result. The skin test should only be repeated if it was negative.
- Report if the client has taken steroids or immunosuppressant drugs in the last 4 to 6 weeks, since false test results could occur.

Client Teaching

- Inform the client that a pinprick will be felt. A small amount of solution is injected under the skin.
- Inform the client that the result of the skin test must be read during the stated time.
- Ask the client about contact with a bacterial, fungal, or parasitic organism.
- Tell the client that a positive skin test does not always indicate active infectious disease. However, the positive test does indicate that the organism is present in the body in either an active or a dormant state.

STRESS/EXERCISE TESTS: TREADMILL EXERCISE ELECTROCARDIOLOGY, EXERCISE MYOCARDIAL PERFUSION IMAGING TEST (THALLIUM/TECHNETIUM STRESS TEST), NUCLEAR PERSANTINE (DIPYRIDAMOLE) STRESS TEST, NUCLEAR DOBUTAMINE STRESS TEST*

Normal Findings. Normal ECG with little or no ST-segment depression or arrhythmia with exercise; normal myocardial perfusion.

Description. Stress testing is based on the theory that clients with coronary artery disease will have marked ST-segment depression when exer-

*Updated and revised by Frank Di Gregorio, CNMT, RDMS, Director, Community Imaging Center, Wilmington, Delaware.

cising. Depression of the ST segment and depression or inversion of the T wave indicate myocardial ischemia. ST segment depression usually occurs before the onset of pain and remains present for some time after the pain has subsided. Mild segment depression after exercise can occur without coronary artery disease (CAD).

Treadmill and Bicycle Exercise Electrocardiology: This type of stress test is frequently prescribed to determine the presence of CAD. The bicycle ergometer test may be used; however, the treadmill seems to be the choice. The body muscles do not seem to tire with the treadmill method as much as leg muscles with the bicycle ergometer. For clients who cannot walk (i.e., hemiplegics, amputees), an arm ergometer can be used. With the treadmill stress test, the work rate is changed every 3 minutes for 15 minutes by increasing the speed slightly and the degree of incline (grade) by 3% each time (3%, 6%, 9%, etc). The clients will exercise until they are fatigued, develop symptoms, or reach their maximum predicted heart rate (MPHR).

Exercise thallium perfusion test: The radioisotope thallium-201, which accumulates in the myocardial cells, is used during the stress test to determine myocardial perfusion during exercise. With severe narrowing of the coronary arteries, there is less thallium accumulation in the heart muscle. If a coronary vessel is completely occluded, no uptake of thallium will occur at the myocardial area that the vessel supplies.

Clients with coronary artery disease may have normal thallium perfusion scans at rest; however, during exercise, when the heart demands more oxygen, myocardial perfusion decreases. The client returns 2 to 3 hours later for a second scan of the heart at rest. Frequently second scans are done to differentiate between an ischemic area and an infarcted or scarred area of the myocardium.

Exercise Technetium Perfusion Test: This is a useful stress test for detecting myocardial ischemia using technetium 99m-laced (TC-99m) compounds, such as Tc-99m-sestamibi (Cardiolite). The technetium compounds are used for perfusion scanning because they are trapped in the myocardium and do not cause redistribution of the compound. Technetium compounds provide more clinical information by allowing the assessment of perfusion, wall motion, and ejection fraction in one test procedure. Other technetium agents approved by the U.S. Food and Drug Administration (FDA) are Tc-99m-tebroxime and Tc-99m-tetrofosmin. Tc-99m-furifusion is a new technetium agent whose approval by the FDA is pending.

Cardiolite imaging is perhaps the most useful noninvasive test for diagnosing and following CAD at the present time. Positive stress Cardiolite scanning usually indicates CAD; however, a more markedly abnormal scan is more likely to indicate serious CAD. It is important to correlate the scan findings with the ECG, the exercise stress test, and the client's symptoms. The use of gated single positron emission (SPECT) (gated refers to the synchronizing of images with the computer and the client's heart rhythm) greatly improves the sensitivity and specificity of the Cardiolite scan.

Nuclear Persantine (Dipyridamole) Stress Test: This is an alternative stress test usually ordered when the client is not physically able to exercise or to walk on a treadmill. Persantine is administered intravenously to dilate the coronary arteries and increase blood flow to the myocardium. Arteries that have become narrowed because of coronary artery disease (CAD) cannot expand.

Thallium-201, Cardiolite, or other Tc-based compounds, administered intravenously, detect decreased blood flow to the heart muscle (myocardium). The isotope is administered 3 minutes after the 4-minute IV Persantine infusion. The client must avoid foods, beverages, and medications containing xanthines (caffeine and theophyllines) 24 hours prior to the test, and theophylline preparations 36 hours prior to the test.

Nuclear persantine stress testing is contraindicated for clients who have severe bronchospastic lung disease, such as asthma or advanced atrioventricular heart block. Other unfavorable conditions in which this test is not indicated include acute myocardial infarction (AMI) within 48 hours of the test, severe aortic or mitral stenosis, resting systolic blood pressure less than 90 mm Hg, and allergy to dipyridamole.

Nuclear Dobutamine Stress Test: Dobutamine is an adrenergic (sympathomimetic) drug that increases myocardial contractility, heart rate, and systolic blood pressure, which increases the myocardial oxygen consumption and thus increases coronary blood flow. If the client has heart block or asthma and takes a theophylline preparation daily, this test may be ordered instead of the nuclear Persantine (dipyridamole) stress test. Dobutamine is an alternative stressor test.

Contraindications for nuclear dobutamine test include clients having acute myocardial infarction (AMI) within 10 days, acute myocarditis or pericarditis, unstable angina pectoris (prolonged episodes, episodes at rest), ventricular and atrial antidysrhythmias, severe aortic or mitral stenosis, hyperthyroidism, and acutely severe infections. Propranolol (Inderal) should be available for any possible adverse reaction to the dobutamine infusion.

Purposes

- To screen for coronary artery disease (CAD)
- To evaluate myocardial perfusion
- To differentiate between an ischemic area and an infarcted or scar area of the myocardium
- To develop a cardiac rehabilitation program
- To evaluate cardiac status for work capability
- To evaluate drug efficiency

Clinical Problems

Abnormal finding: Positive: >2 mm ST depression, coronary artery disease, myocardial hypoperfusion

Procedure

- Obtain a signed consent form.
- NPO for 2 to 3 hours before the test. Avoid alcohol, caffeine-containing drinks, and smoking for 2 to 3 hours before the test. Most medications should be taken.
- Comfortable clothes should be worn (i.e., shorts or slacks, sneakers with socks, and *no* bedroom slippers).
- The chest is shaved as needed, and the skin is cleansed with alcohol.
- Electrodes are applied to the chest according to the lead selections.
- Baseline ECG, pulse rate, and blood pressure are taken and then monitored throughout the test.
- The test is stopped if the client becomes dyspneic, suffers severe fatigue, complains of chest pain, has a rapid increase in pulse rates or blood pressure, or both, or develops life-threatening arrhythmias (i.e., ventricular tachycardia, premature ventricular contractions [PVCs] over 10 PVC in 1 minute).
- The test takes approximately 30 minutes, which includes up to 10 to 15 minutes of exercising.

Treadmill stress test: Usually, there are five stages: first the speed is 2 mph at a 3% incline for 3 minutes. In the second stage the speed is 3.3

mph at a 6% incline for another 3 minutes. The speed usually does not go beyond 3.3 mph. With each stage the incline is increased 3% and the time is increased by 3 minutes, unless fatigue or adverse reactions occur.

Bicycle ergometer test: The client is instructed to pedal the bike against an increased amount of resistance. A shower or hot bath should *not* be taken for 2 hours after testing.

Exercise thallium perfusion test: An IV line is inserted. Exercise time for the stress test is determined. The client obtains the maximal exercise level, and thallium is injected intravenously one minute before the test ends. The client continues to exercise for 1 more minute. A scan taken by a nuclear camera (scintillator) visualizes thallium perfusion of the myocardium. Client returns in 3 or more hours for a second scan.

Exercise technetium perfusion test: With the Cardiolite stress test, the client receives two injections intravenously, one at rest and one at stress. The client should be NPO for 2 to 3 hours prior to the test. Any medications that may affect the blood pressure or heart rate should be discontinued 24 to 36 hours prior to the test unless the test is used to evaluate the efficacy of cardiac medication. The total time for the test is 3 hours, a shorter time than thallium imaging.

Nuclear persantine (dipyridamole) stress test: The client remains NPO after midnight except for water. A diabetic client should check with the health care provider concerning diet. Caffeine-containing drugs, food, and beverages such as colas must be avoided 24 hours prior to the test. Decaffeinated beverages should also be avoided. Certain drugs (e.g., theophylline preparations) should be stopped 36 hours before the test.

The client is in a supine position during the test. The client receives a total of 0.56 mg/kg/dose of IV Persantine (dipyridamole) over a period of 4 minutes. Three minutes after the Persantine infusion, the isotope (thallium, Cardiolite, or other Tc-based compound) is injected intravenously. Aminophylline should be available to reverse any adverse reaction to Persantine. Imaging procedure begins 15 to 30 minutes after the isotope infusion. Heart rate, blood pressure, and ECG will be monitored before and during the test.

The test is terminated if any of the following occur: ventricular tachycardia, second degree heart block, severe ST segment depression, severe hypotension (<90 mmHg), and severe wheezing. The asthmatic client may use the beta-agonist inhaler if necessary during the procedure.

Nuclear dobutamine stress test: The client remains NPO after midnight except for water. Beta blockers, calcium channel blockers, and ACE inhibitors should be discontinued for 36 hours prior to the test. Nitrates should not be taken 6 hours before the test. Dobutamine is administered IV using an infusion pump. The dobutamine is mixed in 1 L of normal saline solution, and the dose and infusion rate is increased until the client's heart rate reaches approximately 85% of his or her maximum predicted heart rate. If the heart rate is less than 110 beats per minute, IV atropine sulfate may be given. The isotope is injected when the maximum heart rate is achieved.

The test is terminated if atrial or ventricular tachycardia, atrial flutter or fibrillation, severe ST-segment depression, progressive anginal pain, or severe hypotension or hypertension occurs. Imaging begins 5 to 10 minutes after the completion of the dobutamine infusion. Propranolol (Inderal) should be available for adverse reaction to dobutamine.

Nursing Implications

- Recognize when the stress test is contraindicated (i.e., recent myocardial infarction); severe, unstable angina; uncontrolled cardiac dysrhythmias, CHF; or recent pulmonary embolism.
- Check that the consent form has been signed.
- Review medications that may interfere with the test (e.g., beta blockers decrease heart rate).
- Recognize whether a treadmill stress test or pharmacologic stress test is appropriate.

Client Teaching—Treadmill Stress Test

- Explain the procedure to the client in regard to NPO 2 to 3 hours prior to test; not smoking, continuing with medications; the clothing and shoes that should be worn; shaving and cleansing the chest area; electrode application; continuous monitoring the ECG, pulse rate, and BP; and not leaning on the rails of the treadmill or the handlebars of the bike.
- Instruct the client to inform the cardiologist or technician if he or she experiences chest pain, difficulty in breathing, or severe fatigue. The risk of having a myocardial infarction during the stress test is less than 0.2%.
- Inform the client that after 10 to 15 minutes of testing or when the heart rate is at a desired or an elevated rate, the test is stopped. It will be terminated immediately if there are any severe ECG changes (i.e., multiple PVCs, ventricular tachycardia).

- Instruct the client to continue the walking exercise at the completion of the test for 2 to 3 minutes to prevent dizziness. The treadmill speed will be decreased. Tell the client that he or she may be perspiring and may be "out of breath." Profuse diaphoresis, cold and clammy skin, severe dyspnea, and severe tachycardia are not normal, and the test will be terminated.
- Inform the client that an ECG and vital signs are taken 5 to 10 minutes after the stress test (recovery stage).
- Encourage the client to participate in a cardiac/exercise rehabilitation program as advised by the health care provider/cardiologist. Tell the client of the health advantages—constant heart monitoring, improved collateral circulation, increased oxygen supply to the heart, and dilating coronary resistance vessels.
- Discourage the client over 35 years of age from doing strenuous exercises without having a stress/exercise test or a cardiac evaluation.
- Inform the client that he or she can resume activity as indicated.

Exercise Thallium Perfusion Test—Client Teaching

- Explain the procedure for the test (see Procedure). Explain that the difference between the routine stress test and the exercise thallium perfusion test is an injection of thallium 201 during the routine stress test followed by scans and/or x-rays. Nursing implications are the same for both tests.
- Instruct the client to return for additional pictures in 2 to 4 hours as indicated by the technician or cardiologist.

Exercise Technetium Perfusion Test—Client Teaching

- Explain the procedure.
- The client should lie quietly for approximately 30 minutes during the imaging.
- Inform the client that the test should last no more than 3 hours.
- Instruct the client taking medications that affect the blood pressure or heart rate to check with the health care provider as for discontinuing the medications for 24 to 48 hours prior to testing.

Nuclear Persantine (Dipyridamole) Stress Test—Client Teaching

- Explain the procedure for the test to the client (see Procedure). The client should be NPO after midnight except for water.
- Instruct the client to avoid food, beverages, and drugs that contain caffeine. Beverages and foods rich in caffeine include colas (Coke and Pepsi), Dr. Pepper, Mountain Dew, Tab, chocolate (syrup and

candy), tea, and coffee. Decaffeinated coffee and tea should also be avoided. Drugs containing caffeine include Anacin, Excedrin, NoDoz, Wigraine, Darvon compound, cafergot, fiorinal. Theophylline preparations should be avoided 36 hours before the test; the client should check with the health care provider in case it is not possible to discontinue the theophylline drug for that period of time.

- Explain to the client that first Persantine will be given intravenously and then an isotope. The client is positioned under a camera with his or her left arm over the head. The camera will be moving very close to the chest for taking pictures (imaging). The imaging takes approximately 20 to 30 minutes.
- Instruct the client to return for additional pictures in 2 to 4 hours as indicated by the technician or cardiologist.
- Explain to the client that a written report is submitted to the client's personal health care provider from the cardiologist.

Nuclear Dobutamine Stress Test—Client Teaching

- Explain the procedure for the test to the client (see Procedure). The client should be NPO after midnight except for water.
- Instruct the client to discontinue drugs that are beta blockers, calcium channel blockers, ACE inhibitors for 36 hours prior to the test with the health care provider's approval. Give the client the date and time for stopping the drug. Nitrates should not be taken 6 hours before the test unless necessary (check with the health care provider).

ULTRASONOGRAPHY (ABDOMINAL AORTA, BRAIN, BREAST, CAROTID, DOPPLER—ARTERIES AND VEINS, EYE AND EYE ORBIT, GALLBLADDER, HEART, KIDNEY, LIVER, PANCREAS, PELVIS [UTERUS, OVARIES, PREGNANT UTERUS], PROSTATE, SCROTUM, SPLEEN, THORACIC, AND THYROID)*

ULTRASOUND, ECHOGRAPHY (ECHOGRAM), SONOGRAM

Normal Finding. A normal pattern image of the organ or Doppler spectral analysis

---

*Revised by Frank Di Gregorio, CNMT, RDMS, Director, Community Imaging Center, Wilmington, Delaware.

Description. Ultrasonography (ultrasound or sonogram) is a diagnostic procedure used to visualize body tissue structure or wave-form analysis of Doppler studies. An ultrasound probe called a transducer is held over the skin surface or in a body cavity to produce an ultrasound beam to the tissues. The reflected sound waves or echoes from the tissues can be transformed by a computer into either scans, graphs, or audible sounds (Doppler).

Ultrasound can detect tissue abnormalities (i.e., masses, cysts, edema, stones). It cannot be used to determine bone abnormalities or for air-filled organs. In obese persons it is difficult for sound waves to pass through fat layers.

Diagnostic ultrasound examinations are relatively inexpensive and cause no known harm to the clients. Most ultrasound studies (e.g., gallstones) do not need other modalities for confirmation; however, CT, MRI, or radionuclide scanning may be used to confirm certain ultrasound results.

Abdominal aorta: The area for abdominal scanning includes the xyphoid process to the umbilicus. Ultrasound can detect aortic aneurysms with 98% accuracy.

Arteries and veins (Doppler): Doppler ultrasonography evaluates the blood flow in arteries and veins anywhere in the body. The Doppler transducer can detect decreased blood flow caused by partial arterial occlusion or by deep-vein thrombosis. It can be used in fetal monitoring during labor and delivery. A Doppler instrument is available to nurses for monitoring blood flow for those who have altered circulation. Low-frequency waves usually indicate low-velocity blood flow.

Brain: Brain echoencephalography is ultrasound of the brain. If the third ventricle, which is normally midline, is shifted to one side, then pathologic findings, such as intracranial lesion or intracranial hemorrhage, may be suspected. It is most useful to evaluate hydrocephalus and intracranial hemorrhage in newborns.

Breast: Ultrasound of the breast is helpful for (1) diagnosing breast lesions in women who have dense breasts, (2) differentiating between cystic and solid lesions, (3) follow-up of fibrocystic breast disease, and (4) evaluating women with silicone breast implants for breast lesions. The breast ultrasound may be suggested for pregnant women as well as any woman with a palpable breast mass. X-ray mammography remains the *screening* examination of choice, as ultrasound cannot detect microcalcification. Still, ultrasound serves as a valuable adjunctive tool.

Carotid artery with doppler: Blood flow in the cartoid artery can be measured by using Doppler technique to determine carotid stenosis. During a carotid sonogram, vertebral arteries can be visualized by this Doppler technique to determine antegrade or retrograde blood flow through these vessels.

Eye and eye orbit: Ultrasound of the eye and eye orbital area may be used to (1) determine abnormal tissue of the eye (vitreous adhesions, retinal detachment) when opacities within the eye are present, and (2) detect orbital lesions. With this test, orbital lesions can be distinguished from orbital inflammation.

Gallbladder and bile ducts: Ultrasonography can evaluate the size, structure, and position of the gallbladder and can determine the presence of gallstones.

Heart: Echocardiography is ultrasound of the heart. It can determine the size, shape, and position of the heart and the movement of heart valves and chambers. The methods commonly used are the M-mode and the two-dimensional. The M-mode records the motion of the intracardiac structures, such as valves, and the two-dimensional records a cross-sectional view of cardiac structures (See Echocardiography for detailed data).

Intravascular ultrasonography: An ultrasound transducer mounted on a catheter is used to obtain pathologic changes to the arterial wall and to evaluate vascular procedures such as angioplasty placement. This test is usually performed in large medical centers.

Kidneys: Ultrasound is a reliable test to identify and to differentiate renal cyst and tumor. The cyst is echo free, and the tumor and renal calculi record multiple echoes. This test is highly recommended when the client is hypersensitive to iodinated contrast dye used in x-ray tests (e.g., IVP).

Liver: The liver was one of the first organs examined by ultrasound. It is useful for distinguishing between a cyst or tumor and for determining the size, structure, and position of the liver. It is very helpful in differentiating obstructive from nonobstructive jaundice.

Pelvis: *Uterus:* Ultrasonography may be used to distinguish between cystic, solid, and complex masses as well as to localize free fluid and inflammatory processes. *Ovaries:* The dimensions of the ovaries, as well as ovarian cysts and solid lesions, can be identified by pelvic sonography. Pelvic ultrasonography is a valuable tool but should not replace a gynecologic examination. *Pregnancy:* In pregnancy the amniotic fluid enhances reflection of sound waves from the placenta and fetus, thus revealing their size, shape, and position. Echoes from the pregnancy may be seen after as few as 4 weeks of amenorrhea. For visualization of pelvic structures, a full bladder is indicated in the nongravid and first-trimester pregnancy. The uterus is sometimes evaluated with a transvaginal transducer with the bladder empty.

Pancreas: The pancreas is a more difficult organ to examine and may require distending the stomach with water to create an acoustic window. Ultrasonography does not measure pancreatic function, but it can determine overall size of the gland and detect pancreatic abnormalities, such as pancreatic tumors, pseudocysts, and pancreatitis. This test is useful for clients who are too thin for adequate CT scanning.

Prostate (transrectal): Ultrasound of the prostate gland is used to (1) evaluate palpable prostate nodules and seminal vesicles, (2) determine if urinary problems may be related perhaps to benign prostatic hypertrophy (BPH), (3) detect early small prostate tumor, and (4) identify tumor location for biopsy and/or radiation purposes. A rectal examination and the laboratory test, prostate-specific antigen (PSA), should be included for diagnosing prostatic lesions.

Scrotum/testes: Ultrasound of the scrotum sac contents is helpful in diagnosing abscess, cyst, hydrocele, spermatocele, varicocele, testicular tumors, torsion, and chronic scrotal swelling.

Spleen: Ultrasonography can be used for determining the size, structure, and position of the spleen. This procedure can identify splenic masses. In some cases it is a useful tool for evaluating the need for splenectomy, follow-up of pathologies such as hematoma or abscess.

Thoracic: Ultrasound is useful in identifying lesions, but it is not diagnostic on air-filled cavities such as the lungs unless a lesion is present adherent to the chest wall. It may be used to identify pleural fluid, malposition of the diaphragm, and the presence of an abscess. Ultrasound of the thoracic area may be used in combination with x-ray and thoracic scans.

Thyroid: Ultrasonography of the thyroid is 85% accurate in determining the size and structure of the thyroid gland. It can differentiate between a cyst and tumor and can determine the depth and dimension of thyroid nodules.

Purposes

- To evaluate the size, structure, and position of body organs
- To evaluate the blood flow in arteries and veins
- To detect cysts, tumors, and calculi

Clinical Problems

Organ	*Abnormal Findings*
Abdominal aorta	Aortic aneurysms, aortic stenosis
Arteries and veins (Doppler)	Arterial occlusion (partial or complete), deep-vein thrombosis, chronic venous insufficiency, arterial trauma
Brain	Intracranial hemorrhage, lesions (tumors, abscess), hydrocephalus
Breast	Cysts, tumors (benign or malignant), metastasis to the lymph nodes and muscle tissue
Carotid artery	Carotid plaque, thrombus, degree of stenosis
Eye and eye orbit	Vitreous opacities, detached retina, foreign bodies, orbital lesion, orbital inflammation, meningioma, glioma, neurofibroma, cyst, keratoprosthesis
Gallbladder	Acute cholecystitis, cholelithiasis, biliary obstruction
Heart (Cardiac)	Cardiomegaly, mitral stenosis, aortic stenosis and insufficiency, pericardial effusion, congenital heart disease, left ventricular hypertrophy, ischemic heart disease, septal defects
Kidney (Renal)	Renal cysts and tumors, hydronephrosis, perirenal abscess, acute pyelonephritis, acute glomerulonephritis
Liver (Hepatic)	Hepatic cysts, abscesses, tumor; hepatic metastasis; hepatocellular disease, congenital abnormalities
Pelvis	
Uterus	Uterine tumor, fibroids; hydatiform mole, endometrial changes
Ovaries	Ovarian cysts or tumor
Pregnancy	Fetal age, fetal death, placenta previa, abruptio placenta; hydrocephalus; breech fetal presentation
Pancreas	Pancreatic tumors, pseudocysts, acute pancreatitis
Prostate	Cancer of the prostate gland, benign prostatic hypertrophy (BPH), prostatitis

(continued)

Organ	Abnormal Findings
Scrotum	Hydrocele, spermatocele, varicocele, testicular tumors, torsion, acute/chronic epididymitis, cyst, abscess, chronic scrotal swelling
Spleen	Splenomegaly; splenic cysts, abscesses, tumor, congenital anomalies
Thoracic	Pleural fluid, abscess formation, malposition of the diaphragm
Thyroid	Thyroid tumors (benign or malignant), thyroid goiters or cysts

Procedure

- Obtain a signed consent form.
- Restrict food and fluids for 4 to 8 hours before test for abdomina aorta, gallbladder, liver, spleen, and pancreas ultrasound studies.
- The client should eat a fat-free meal the night prior to the test for abdominal, gallbladder, liver, pancreas, and kidney sonograms.
- Premedications are seldom given unless the client is extremely apprehensive or has nausea and vomiting.
- Mineral oil or conductive gel is applied to the skin surface at the site to be examined. The transducer is hand held and moved smoothly back and forth across the oiled or gel-skin surface.
- The client's position may vary from supine to oblique, prone, semirecumbent, and erect.
- The average time for a procedure is 30 minutes.
- The client should not smoke or chew gum prior to the examination to prevent swallowing air.

Brain

- Remove jewelry and hairpins from neck and head.

Breast

- Hand-held, real-time contact scanning over palpable mass is the most widely used method for breast imaging.
- An automated system utilizing full-breast water immersion and a reproducible, systematic survey is less widely used due to higher cost, space requirements, and lack of real-time capability.
- No lotion or powder should be applied under the arm or breast area the day of the test.

Doppler

- Blood pressure will be taken at certain limb sites.

Eye and eye orbit

- Anesthetize the eye and eye area.
- With contact method, the probe touches the corneal surface.

Heart and liver

- Ask the client to breathe slowly and to hold breath after deep inspiration.

Obstetrics (First Trimester), Pelvic and Renal

- The client should drink 24 ounces of water 1 hour prior to the examination, or three to four 8-ounce glasses of clear liquid 90 minutes prior to the test. The client should not void until the test is completed. Second and third trimester clients need not drink large amounts of water *unless* bleeding has occurred, in which case the above procedure is followed.

Prostate

- Administer an enema 1 hour prior to the test.
- The client should drink two 8-ounce glasses of clear fluid 1 hour prior to the test.
- The client should *not* void 1 hour prior to the test.
- The client lies on his left side.
- Rectal examination is usually performed before the transducer is inserted into the rectum. Lubricate the rectal probe and insert it into the rectum. The test takes approximately ½ hour.

Scrotum

- The penis is strapped back to the abdominal area.
- Gel is applied and the transducer is passed over the scrotum.

Factors Affecting Diagnostic Results

- Residual barium sulfate in the GI tract from previous x-ray studies will interfere with ultrasound results. Ultrasonography should be performed before barium studies.
- Air and gas (bowel) will not transmit the ultrasound beam.
- Excess fecal material in the colon and rectum (prostate).

Nursing Implications

- Obtain a signed consent form.
- NPO for 6 hours prior to all abdominal studies (e.g., gallbladder, aorta).
- Confirm that the client has not had any other tests that may interfere with test results (e.g., upper GI series).

Client Teaching

- Explain the procedure to the client (see Description and Procedure).
- Inform the client that this is a painless procedure, that there is no exposure to radiation, and that the ultrasound test is considered to be safe and fast.
- Instruct the client to remain still during the procedure. Inform him or her that the test usually takes 30 minutes or less, except for a few ultrasound tests (e.g., arterial, venous, and carotid ultrasonography), which could take 1 hour.
- Encourage the client to ask questions and to express any concerns. Refer questions you cannot answer to the ultrasonographer or the health care provider.
- Be supportive of the client and the family.

Eye

- Avoid rubbing the eyes until the anesthetic effect has worn off in order to avoid corneal abrasion.
- Inform the client that blurred vision may be present for a short time until the anesthetic has worn off.

VENOGRAPHY (LOWER LIMB)

PHLEBOGRAPHY

Normal Finding. Normal, patent, deep leg veins

Description. Lower-limb venography is a fluoroscopic or x-ray examination of the deep leg veins after injection of a contrast dye. This test is useful for identifying venous obstruction caused by a deep-vein thrombosis (DVT). This procedure is frequently done after Doppler ultrasonography to confirm a positive or questionable DVT. *Radionuclide venography* using I-125 fibrinogen IV with scintillation scanning may be done for clients who are too ill for venography or are hypersensitive to contrast dye. It may take 6 to 72 hours for the isotope to collect at the thrombus site, and so the scanner could be used to check the leg daily for 3 days. This type should not be used for screening purposes.

Purposes

- To detect deep-vein thrombosis (DVT)

- To identify congenital venous abnormalities
- To select a vein for arterial bypass grafting

Clinical Problems

Abnormal findings: Deep-vein thrombosis, congenital venous abnormalities

Procedure

- Obtain a signed consent form.
- Restrict food and fluids for 4 hours before the test; some permit clear liquids before the test.
- Anticoagulants may be temporarily discontinued.
- The client lies on a tilted radiographic table at a 40- to 60-degree angle. A tourniquet is applied above the ankle, a vein is located in the dorsum of the client's foot, a small amount of normal saline is administered IV into the vein, and then the contrast dye is injected slowly over a period of 2 to 4 minutes.
- Fluoroscopy may be used to monitor the flow of the contrast dye, and spot films are taken.
- Normal saline is used after the procedure to flush the contrast dye from the veins.
- A sedative may be indicated prior to the test for clients who are extremely apprehensive and for those who have a low threshold of pain.
- The test takes 30 minutes to 1 hour.

Factors Affecting Diagnostic Results

- Weight on the leg being tested can cause a decrease in the flow of the contrast dye.

Nursing Implications

- Obtain a history of allergies to iodine, iodine substance, and seafood. Antihistamines or steroids may be given for 2 to 3 days before the test.
- Record baseline vital signs. Have client void before test.

Client Teaching

- Inform the client that a slight burning sensation may be felt when the dye is injected. Instruct the client not to move the leg being tested during the injection of the dye or during x-ray filming.

Post-test

- Monitor vital signs as indicated.

- Check the pulse in the dorsalis pedis, popliteal, and femoral arteries for volume intensity and rate.
- Observe for signs and symptoms of latent allergic reaction to the contrast dye (i.e., dyspnea, skin rash, urticaria, and tachycardia).
- Observe the injection site for bleeding, hematoma, and signs and symptoms of infection (i.e., redness, edema, and pain).
- Elevate the affected leg as ordered.
- Be supportive of the client.

VENTILATION SCAN

PULMONARY VENTILATION SCAN

Normal Finding. Normal lung tissue with normal gas distribution in both lungs

Description. The ventilation scan is a nuclear scan of the lungs. The client inhales a mixture of air, oxygen, and radioactive gas (xenon [Xe-127 or Xe-133] or krypton-85 [Kr-85]). A single-breath scan is taken first. Then three phases of scanning follow: (1) the wash-in phase which is the build-up of gas distribution in the lungs; (2) the equilibrium phase in which radioactive gas reaches a steady state; and (3) the wash-out phase in which room air is breathed to remove radioactive gas from the lungs.

The pulmonary ventilation scan is usually performed with the *pulmonary perfusion scan* to differentiate between a ventilatory problem and vascular abnormalities in the lung. The pulmonary perfusion scan indirectly evaluates problems related to blood flow to the lungs (e.g., pulmonary embolism). The radioactive substance used is technetium or iodine, and images are displayed by a scintillator. A ventilation scan can reveal decreased ventilation (uptake of radioactive gas) caused by chronic obstructive pulmonary disease (COPD), atelectasis, and pneumonia; the pulmonary perfusion scan is normal. However, pulmonary embolus can cause an abnormal perfusion scan and a normal ventilation scan.

Purposes

- To differentiate between a ventilatory problem and vascular abnormalities in the lung

- To detect lung cancer, sarcoidosis, or tuberculosis
- To determine hypoventilation due to excess smoking or COPD

Clinical Problems. Parenchymal lung disease (COPD), vascular abnormalities (pulmonary emboli), tuberculosis, sarcoidosis, lung cancer, hypoventilation due to excess smoking or COPD

Procedure

- No food or fluid restriction is required.
- Remove all metal objects (jewelry) from around the neck and chest.
- The client inhales gas (radioactive xenon or krypton). The client will be asked to take a deep breath and to hold it for a short time (single breath) while the scanner takes an image of the lung. Other images will be recorded during three phases of the test: wash-in, equilibrium, and wash-out.

Factors Affecting Diagnostic Results

- Metal objects could cause inaccurate recorded images.

Nursing Implications

- Record and report any respiratory distress the client is having. Check breath sounds.
- Report if the client is having chest pain, especially if pulmonary embolism is suspected.
- Assess communications for verbal and nonverbal expressions of anxiety and fear about tests and/or potential or actual health problem.
- Be supportive of client and family.

Client Teaching

- Explain the procedure to the client (see Procedure). Explain that the radioactive gas is minimal.

X-RAY (CHEST, HEART, FLAT PLATE OF THE ABDOMEN, KIDNEY, URETER, BLADDER, SKULL, SKELETAL)

ROENTGENOGRAPHY, RADIOGRAPHY

Normal Findings

Chest: Normal bony structure and normal lung tissue

Heart: Normal size and shape of the heart and vessel

Flat plate of abdomen: Normal abdominal structures

Kidney, ureter, bladder (KUB): Normal kidney size and structure

Skull and skeletal: Normal structures

Description. In the body there are four densities—air, water, fat, and bone—that will absorb varying degrees of radiation. Air has less density, causing dark images on the film, and bone has high density, causing light images. Bone contains a large amount of calcium and will absorb more radiation, allowing less radiation to strike the x-ray film; thus, a white structure is produced.

Today, x-ray studies cause only small amounts of radiation exposure because of the high quality of x-ray film and procedure. X-ray studies are requested primarily for screening purposes and are followed by other extensive diagnostic tests.

Purposes

- To identify bone structure and tissue in the body
- To detect abnormal size, structure, and shape of bone and body tissues

Clinical Problems

Test	*Abnormal Findings*
Chest	Atelectasis, pneumonias, tuberculosis, tumors, lung abscess, pneumothorax, sarcoma, sarcoidosis, scoliosis/kyphosis
Heart	Cardiomegaly, aneurysms, anomalies of the aorta
Abdominal (flat plate)	Abdominal masses, small bowel obstruction, abdominal tissue trauma, ascites
KUB	Abnormal size and structure of KUB, renal calculi, kidney and bladder masses
Skull	Head trauma (intracranial pressure, skull fractures), congenital anomalies, bone defects
Skeletal	Fractures, arthritic conditions, osteomyelitis

Procedure

Chest

- No food or fluid is restricted.

- A posteroanterior (PA) chest film is usually ordered with the client standing. An anteroposterior (AP) chest film could be ordered. A lateral chest film may also be ordered.
- Clothing and jewelry should be removed from the neck to the waist, and a paper or cloth gown should be worn.
- The client should take a deep breath and hold it as the x-ray is taken.

Heart

- No food or fluid is restricted.
- PA and left-lateral chest films are usually indicated for evaluating the size and shape of the heart.
- Clothing and jewelry should be removed from the neck to the waist, and a paper or cloth gown should be worn.
- Client instructions include body position and when to take a deep breath and hold it.

Abdomen and KUB

- No food or fluid is restricted.
- X-rays should be taken before an IVP or GI studies.
- Clothes are removed, and a paper or cloth gown is worn.
- Client lies in a supine position with arms away from the body on a tilted x-ray table.
- Testes should be shielded as an added precaution.

Skull

- No food or fluid is restricted.
- Remove hairpins, glasses, and dentures before the test.
- Various positions may be needed so that different areas of the skull can be x-rayed.

Skeletal

- Restrict food and fluids if fracture is suspected.
- Immobilize suspected fracture site.

Factors Affecting Diagnostic Results

- Radiopaque materials for IVP and GI studies administered within 3 days of routine x-rays (chest, flat plate of the abdomen, and KUB) could distort the pictures.

Nursing Implications

Client Teaching

- Inform the client that the x-ray test usually takes 10 to 15 minutes.

- Inform the client that there may be several x-rays taken, one or two chest films, or five skull films. The client may be asked to remain in the waiting room for 10 to 15 minutes after x-rays are taken to be sure the films are readable.
- Ask the female client if she is pregnant or if pregnancy is suspected. X-rays should be avoided during the first trimester of pregnancy. A lead apron covering the abdomen and pelvic area may be used.
- Explain that today's x-ray equipment and film are of good quality and decrease the exposure to radiation.

Appendix A

Laboratory Test Values for Adults and Children

Laboratory tests and their reference values for adults and children are listed alphabetically, including types of specimens and color-top tubes. Reference values differ from laboratory to laboratory, so nurses should refer to the published laboratory values used in each hospital or private laboratory for any differences. Note: µg/mL is the same as mg/L; µg is the same as mcg (microgram).

Test	*Specimen (Color-top Tube)*	*Reference Values*
Acetaminophen	Serum (Red)	*Adult and Child:* Therapeutic: 5–20 µg/mL, 31–124 µmol/L (SI units); toxic: >50 µg/mL, >305 µmol/L (SI units); >200 µg/mL—possible hepatotoxicity
Acetone	Serum (Red) or plasma (Green)	*Adult and Child:* 0.3–2.0 mg/dL, 51.6–344 µmol/L (SI units), ketones: 2–4 mg/dL; qualitative will show negative. *Newborn:* slightly higher than adult
Acid phosphatase	Serum (Red)	*Adult:* <2.6 ng/mL; 0–5 U/L range; varies according to the method used; 0.2–13 IU/L (SI units) *Child:* 6.4–15.2 U/L
Activated partial thromboplastin time (APTT)	Plasma (Blue)	*Adult:*20–35 seconds
Adenovirus antibody	Serum (Red)	Negative

Test	*Specimen (Color-top Tube)*	*Reference Values*
Adrenocorticotropic hormone (ACTH)	Plasma (Green)	*Adult:* 7–10 AM: 8–80 pg/mL; 4 PM: 5–30 pg/mL; 10 PM–12 midnight: <10 pg/mL
Alanine aminotransferase (ALT or SGPT)	Serum (Red)	*Adult and Child:* 10–35 U/L; 4–36 U/L (SI units). *Infant:* could be twice as high *Elderly:* Slightly higher than adult
Albumin	Serum (Red)	*Adult:* 3.5–5.0 g/dL, 52%–68% of total protein *Child:* 4.0–5.8 g/dL *Newborn:* 2.9–5.4 g/dL *Infant:* 4.4–5.4 g/dL
Alcohol	Serum (Red) or plasma (Green)	*Adult or Child:* 0% alcohol influence: > 0.10%. Alcohol toxicity: > 0.25%
Aldolase (ALD)	Serum (Red)	*Adult:* < 6 U/L; 22–59 mU/L at 37°C (SI units) *Child:* 6–16 U/dL *Infant:* 12–24 U/dL
Aldosterone	Serum (Red) or plasma (Green)	*Adult:* <16 ng/dL (fasting); 4–30 ng/dL (sitting position) *Child:* (3–11 yrs): 5–70 ng/dL *Pregnancy:* 2 to 3 times higher than adult
	Urine	*Adult:* 6–25 µg/24 h
Alkaline phosphatase (ALP)	Serum (Red)	*Adult:* 42–136 U/L; ALP[1]: 20–130 U/L; ALP[2]: 20–120 U/L *Elderly:* slightly higher *Infant and child (0–12 years):* 40–115 U/L *Older child:* (13–18 yrs): 50–230 U/L
$Alpha_1$ antitrypsin	Serum (Red)	*Adult and child:* 78–200 mg/dL, 0.78–2.0 g/L *Newborn:* 145–270 mg/dL
Alpha fetoprotein (AFP)	Serum (Red)	*Nonpregnancy:* <15 ng/mL

Test	*Specimen (Color-top Tube)*	*Reference Values*	
		Pregnancy:	
		Weeks of gestation	*ng/mL*
		8–12	0–39
		13	6–31
		14	7–50
		15	7–60
		16	10–72
		17	11–90
		18	14–94
		19	24–112
		20	31–122
		21	19–124
(AFP)	Amniotic fluid	*Weeks of gestation*	*μg/mL*
		15	5.5–31
		16	5.7–31.5
		17	3.8–32.5
		18	3.6–28
		19	3.7–24.5
		20	2.2–15
		21	3.8–18
Amikacin	Serum (Red)	*Adult:* Therapeutic, peak: 15–30 mg/L; trough: <10 mg/L; toxic: >35 mg/L	
Ammonia	Plasma (Green)	*Adult:* 15–45 μg/dL, 11–35 μmol/L (SI units)	
		Child: 29–70 μg/dL; 29–70 μmol/L (SI units)	
		Newborn: 64–107 μg/dL	
Amylase	Serum (Red)	*Adult:* 60–160 Somogyi U/dL, 30–170 U/L (SI units)	
		Elderly: could be slightly high	
	Urine	*Adult:* 4–37 U/L/2 h	
Angiotensin-converting enzyme (ACE)	Serum (Red) or plasma (Green)	*Adult >20 yr:* 8–67 U/L	
		Child: usually not performed	
Anion gap	Serum (Red)	10–17 mEq/L	

Test	*Specimen (Color-top Tube)*	*Reference Values*
Antibiotic sensitivity test (C & S)	Culture	*Adult and child:* sensitive or resistant to antibiotic
Antidiuretic hormone (ADH)	Plasma (Lavender)	Adult: 1–5 pg/mL; 1–5 ng/L
Anti-DNA	Serum (Red)	*Adult:* <1:85 *Child:* <1:60–1:70
Antiglomerular basement membrane (Anti-GBM)	Serum (Red)	Negative
Antimitochondrial antibody (AMA)	Serum (Red or Gray)	*Reference Values* *Adult:* Negative: 1:5–1.10 dilution Intermediate level: 1:20–1:80 dilution Strongly suggestive of biliary cirrhosis: >1:80 Positive for biliary cirrhosis: >1:160
Antimyocardial antibody (AMA)	Serum (Red)	None detected
Antinuclear antibodies (ANA)	Serum (Red)	*Adult and child:* negative
Antistreptolysin O (ASO)	Serum (Red)	*Adult:* <100 IU/mL *Newborn:* same as mother *2–5 years:* <100 IU/mL *12–19 years:* <200 IU/mL
Arterial blood gases (ABGs)	Blood	*Adult:* pH: 7.35–7.45; $Paco_2$: 35–45 mmHg; PaO_2: 75–100 mmHg; HCO_3: 24–28 mEq/L; BE: −2 to +2 *Child:* pH: 7.36–7.44; others are same as adult
Ascorbic acid	Plasma (Gray)	*Adult and Child:* 0.6–2.0 mg/dL, 34–114 µmol/dL (SI units)
	Serum (Red)	0.2–2.0 mg/dL

Test	*Specimen (Color-top Tube)*	*Reference Values*
Aspartate aminotransferase (AST) (SGOT)	Serum (Red)	*Adult and child: average range:* 8–38; 5–40 U/L (Frankel), 4–36 IU/L, 16–60 U/mL 30°C (Karen), 8–33 U/L 37°C (SI units). Female lower than male. Exercise increases levels *Elderly:* slightly higher *Newborn:* four times the normal
Atrial natriuretic hormone (ANH)	Plasma (Lavender)	*Reference Values* *Adult:* 20–77 pg/mL; 20–77 ng/L (SI units)
Barbiturate	Serum (Red)	*Phenobarbital* *Adult and child:* therapeutic: 15–40 mg/L; toxic: >40 mg/L *Amobarbital* *Adult and child:* therapeutic: 3–12 mg/L; toxic: >12 mg/L
Bence-Jones protein	Urine	*Adult and child:* negative to trace
Bilirubin	Serum (Red)	Total: *Adult:* 0.1–1.2 mg/dL, 1.7–20.5 μmol/L (SI units) *Child:* 0.2–0.8 mg/dL *Newborn:* 1–12 mg/dL, 17.1–205 μmol/L (SI units) Direct: *Adult:* 0.0–0.3 mg/dL, 1.7–5.1 μmol/L (SI units) Indirect: *Adult:* 0.1–1.0 mg/dL, 1.7–17.1 μmol/L (SI units)
	Urine	*Adult and child:* negative to 0.02 mg/dL
Bleeding time	Blood	*Adult:* Ivy method: 3–7 minutes; Duke method: 1–3 minutes
Blood urea nitrogen (BUN)	Serum (Red)	*Adult:* 5–25 mg/dL *Elderly:* slightly higher *Child:* 5–20 mg/dL *Newborn:* 5–15 mg/dL

Test	*Specimen (Color-top Tube)*	*Reference Values*
Blood urea nitrogen/creatinine ratio	Serum (Red)	BUN: creatinine 10:1 to 20:1 Average: 15:1
Bromide	Serum (Red)	*Adult and child:* 0 Therapeutic: <80 mg/dL; toxic: >100 mg/dL
Calcitonin (hCT)	Serum (Red)	*Adult:* Male: <40 pg/mL or ng/L; female: <25 pg/mL or ng/L *Child:* <70 pg/mL; <70 ng/L (SI units)
Calcium (Ca)	Serum (Red)	*Adult:*4.5–5.5 mEq/L, 9–11 mg/dL, 2.3–2.8 mmol/L (SI units). *Ionized Ca:* 4.25–5.25 mg/dL; 2.2–2.5 mEq/L, 1.1–1.24 mmol/L *Child:* 4.5–5.8 mEq/L, 9–11.5 mg/dL *Newborn:* 3.7–7.0 mEq/L, 7.4–14.0 mg/dL *Infant:* 5.0–6.0 mEq/L, 10–12 mg/dL
	Urine	*Adult:* low calcium diet: <150 mg/24 h; average calcium diet: 100–250 mg/24 h; high calcium diet: 250–300 mg/24
Carbamazepine	Serum (Red)	*Adult:* Therapeutic: 4–12 mg/mL; toxic: >12–15 mg/mL
Carbon dioxide combining power (CO_2)	Serum (Red) or plasma (Green)	*Adult:* 22–30 mEq/L, 22–30 mmol/L (SI units) *Panic Range:* <15 mEq/L and >45 mEq/L *Child:* 20–28 mEq/L
Carbon monoxide (CO) blood carboxyhemoglobin	Blood (Lavender)	*Adult and child:* Nonsmoker: <2.5% saturation of Hb; smoker: average (1–2 pk): 4–5% saturation of Hb; heavy: 5–12% saturation of Hb; life threatening: >15% saturation of Hb

Test	*Specimen (Color-top Tube)*	*Reference Values*
Carcinoembryonic antigen (CEA)	Plasma (Lavender)	*Adult:* nonsmokers: <2.5 ng/mL; smokers: <5.0 ng/mL; neoplasm: >12 ng/mL; inflammatory: >10 ng/mL
Carotene	Serum (Red)	*Adult:* 60–200 µg/dL *Child:* 40–130 µg/dL
Catecholamines	Serum: see test Urine	*Adult:* total: <100 µg/24 h, 0–14 µg/dL (random) Epinephrine: <20 µg/24 h Norepinephrine: <100 µg/24 h *Child:* less than adult due to weight differences
Cerebrospinal	Spinal	*Adult:* pressure: 75–175 mm H_2O; WBC: 0–8 µL; protein: 15–45 mg/dL; glucose: 40–80 mg/dL *Child:* pressure: 50–100 mm H_2O; WBC: 0–8 µL; protein: 14–45 mg/dL; glucose: 35–75 mg/dL
Ceruloplasmin (Cp)	Serum (Red)	*Adult and child:* 18–45 mg/dL, 180–450 mg/L (SI units) *Infant:* <23 mg/dL
Chlamydia	Serum (Red)	*Adult: Normal titer:* <1:16 *Positive titer:* >1:64
Chloride (Cl)	Serum (Red)	*Adult:* 95–105 mEq/L, 95–105 mmol/L (SI units) *Child:* 98–105 mEq/L *Newborn:* 94–112 mEq/L *Infant:* 95–110 mEq/L
Cholesterol	Serum (Red)	*Adult:* <200 mg/dL; moderate risk: 200–240 mg/dL; high risk: >240 mg/dL *Child:* 2–19 years: 130–170 mg/dL; moderate risk: 171–184 mg/dL; high risk: >185 mg/dL *Infant:* 90–130 mg/dL

Test	*Specimen (Color-top Tube)*	*Reference Values*
Cholinesterase (pseudocholinesterase)	Blood, plasma (Green)	*Adult and child:* 0.5–1.0 mg/dL, 6–8 IU/L *Adult and child:* 3–8 units, 8–18 IU/L 37°C
Clot retraction	Blood (Red)	*Adult and child:* 1–24 hours
Cold agglutinins (CA)	Serum (Red)	*Adult and child:* 1–8 antibody titer; positive: >1:16 titer
Complement: Total	Serum (Red)	*Adult:* 75–160 kU/L (SI units)
Complement C_3	Serum (Red)	*Adult:* *Male:* 80–180 mg/dL *Female:* 76–120 mg/dL *Elderly:* slightly higher
Complement C_4	Serum (Red)	*Adult:* 15–45 mg/dL
Coombs' direct	Blood (Lavender)	*Adult and child:* negative
Coombs' indirect	Serum (Red)	*Adult and child:* negative
Copper (Cu)	Serum (Red)	*Adult:* male: 70–140 μg/dL; female: 80–155 μg/dL; pregnancy: 140–300 μg/dL *Child:* 30–190 μg/dL *Adolescent:* 90–240 μg/dL *Newborn:* 20–70 μg/dL
	Urine	*Adult:* 0–60 μg/24 h Wilson's disease: >100 μg/24 h
Corticotropin	Plasma (Green)	*Adult:* 8–10 AM: up to 80 pg/mL
Cortisol	Plasma (Green)	*Adult:* 8–10 AM: 5–23 μg/dL; 4–6 PM: 3–13 μg/dL *Child:* 8–10 AM: 15–25 μg/dL; 4–6 PM: 5–10 μg/dL
	Urine	*Adult:* 24–105 μg/24 h
C-Reactive Protein (CRP)	Serum (Red)	*Adult:* 0; positive: >1:2 titer
Creatine phosphokinase (CPK)	Serum (Red)	*Adult:* male: 5–35 μg/mL, 30–180 IU/L; female: 5–25 μg/mL, 25–150 IU/L *Child:* male: 0–70 IU/L 30°C; female: 0–50 IU/L 30°C *Newborn:* 65–580 IU/L at 30°C
CPK isoenzymes	Serum (Red)	*Adult:* CPK-MM: 94%–100% (muscle); CPK-MB: 0%–6% (heart); CPK-BB: 0% (brain)

Test	*Specimen (Color-top Tube)*	*Reference Values*
Creatinine (Cr)	Serum (Red)	*Adult:* 0.5–1.5 mg/dL, 45–132.5 umol/L (SI units) *Elderly:* slightly lower *Child:* 0.4–1.2 mg/dL *Newborn:* 0.8–1.4 mg/dL *Infant:* 0.7–1.7 mg/dL
	Urine	*Adult:* 0.9–1.9 g/24 h
Creatinine clearance	Urine	*Adult:* male: 85–135 mg/min; female: 85–120 mL/min *Elderly:* slightly lower *Child:* males slightly higher
Cross-match	Blood (Red)	*Adult and child:* compatible
Cryoglobulins	Serum (Red)	*Adult:* up to 6 mg/dL *Child:* 30 mg/dL/1 h
Cultures	Various specimens	*Adult and child:* negative or no pathogen
Cytomegalovirus (CMV) antibody	Serum (Red)	*Adult and Child:* Negative to <0.30
Dexamethasone suppression test	Plasma Urine	*Adult:* Cortisol: <5 µg/dL; 17-OHCS: <4 mg/5 h (>50% reduction of plasma cortisol and urine 17-OHCS)
Diazepam (Valium)	Serum (Red)	*Adult:* therapeutic: 0.5–2.0 mg/L, 400–600 ng/mL; toxic: >3 mg/L, >3,000 ng/mL
Digoxin	Serum (Red)	*Adult and child:* therapeutic: 0.5–2.0 ng/mL, 0.5–2 nmol/L (SI units); toxic: >2 ng/mL *Infant:* therapeutic: 1–3 ng/mL; toxic: >3.5 ng/mL
Dilantin (Phenytoin)	Serum (Red)	*Adult:* therapeutic: 10–20 µg/mL; toxic: >20 µg/mL *Child:* toxic: >15–20 µg/mL
Diltiazem (Cardizem)	Serum (Red)	*Adult:* therapeutic: 50–200 ng/mL; toxic: >200 ng/mL
Disseminated intravascular coagulation (DIC)	Plasma (Blue)	*Adult:* platelet, PT, APTT, fibrinogen, thrombin time, fibrin split products, and plasma paraprotamine

Test	*Specimen (Color-top Tube)*	*Reference Values*	
D-xylose absorption test	Blood (Gray)	25 g: 25–75 mg/dL/2 h; 5 g: 8–28 mg/dL/2 h	
	Urine	25 g: >3.5 g/5 h; >5 g/24 h; 5 g: 1.2–2.4 g/5 h	
Encephalitis virus antibody	Serum (Red)	<1:10	
Enterovirus group	Serum (Red)	Negative	
Erythrocyte sedimentation rate (ESR, sed rate)	Blood (Lavender)	*Adult:* Westergren method: <50 years, male: 0–15 mm/h; female: 0–20 mm/h; >50 years, male: 0–20 mm/h; female: 0–30 mm/h	
		Wintrobe method: male: 0–9 mm/h; female: 0–15 mm/h	
		Child: 0–20 mm/h	
		Newborn: 0–2 mm/h	
Estetrol (E_4)	Plasma (Red)	*Pregnancy:*	
		Weeks of gestation	*pg/mL*
		20–26	140–210
		30	350
		36	900
		40	>1050
	Amniotic fluid	*Weeks of Gestation*	*ng/mL*
		32+	0.8
		40+	13.0
Estradiol (E_2)	Serum (Red)	*Female:* follicular phase: 20–150 pg/mL; midcycle phase: 100–500 pg/mL; luteal phase: 60–260 pg/mL; menopause: <30 pg/mL	
		Child: <30 pg/mL; 6 mo to 10 yr: 3–10 pg/mL	
		Male: 15–50 pg/mL	
Estriol (E_3)	Serum (Red)	*Pregnancy:*	
		Weeks of gestation	*ng/dL*
		25–28	25–165
		29–32	30–230
		33–36	45–370
		37–38	75–420
		39–40	95–450

Test	Specimen (Color-top Tube)	Reference Values	
	Urine	*Weeks of gestation*	*ng/dL*
		25–28	6–28
		29–32	6–32
		33–36	10–45
		37–40	15–60
Estrogen	Serum (Red)	*Adult:* early menstrual cycle: 60–200 pg/mL; midcycle: 120–440 pg/mL; late cycle: 150–350 pg/mL; postmenopause: <30 pg/mL; male: 12–34 pg/mL *Child:* 1–6 yr: 3–10 pg/mL; 8–12 yr: <30 pg/mL	
	Urine	*Adult:* preovulation: 5–25 μg/24 h; follicular phase: 24–100 μg/24 h; luteal phase: 22–80 μg/24 h; post-menopause: 0–10 μg/24 h; male: 4–25 μg/24 h *Child:* <12 yr: 1 μg/24 h; >12 years: same as adult	
Estrone (E_1)	Serum (Red)	*Adult: Female:* follicular phase: 30–100 pg/mL; ovulatory phase: > 150 pg/mL; luteal phase: 90–160 pg/mL; postmenopausal: 20–40 pg/mL *Male:* 10–50 pg/mL *Child* (1–10 years old): < 10 pg/mL	
	Urine	*Female:* follicular phase: 4–7 μg/24 h; ovulatory phase: 11–30 μg/24 h; luteal phase: 10–22 μg/24 h; postmenopausal: 1–7 μg/24 h	
Ethosuximide	Serum (Red)	*Adult:* therapeutic: 40–100 μg/mL; toxic: >100 μg/mL *Child:* therapeutic: 2–4 mg/kg/d; toxic: same as adult or higher	
Factor assay	Plasma (Blue)	See Factor Assay in text	
Febrile agglutinins	Serum (Red)	*Adult and child:* *Brucella:* <1:20 Tularemia: <1:40	

Test	*Specimen (Color-top Tube)*	*Reference Values*
		Salmonella: <1:40 *Proteus:* <1:40
Ferritin	Serum (Red)	See Ferritin in text
Fibrin degradation products (FD)	Blood (Blue)	*Adult:* 2–10 µg/mL
Fibrinogen	Plasma (Blue)	*Adult and child:* 200–400 mg/dL *Newborn:* 150–300 mg/dL
Folic acid (Folate)	Serum (Red)	*Adult and child:* 3–16 ng/mL, >2.5 ng/mL (RIA)
	Blood (Lavender)	*Adult:* 200–700 ng/mL
Follicle-stimulating hormone (FSH)	Serum (Red)	*Adult:* follicular phase: 4–30 mU/mL; midcycle: 10–90 mU/mL; luteal phase: 4–30 mU/mL; postmenopause: 40–170 mU/mL; male: 4–25 mU/mL *Child:* prepubertal: 5–12 mU/mL
FTA-ABS	Serum (Red)	*Adult and child:* negative
Fungal organisms	Various specimens	*Adult and child:* negative
Gamma-glutamyl transferase (GGT)	Serum (Red)	*Adult and child:* average: 0–45 IU/L; male: 4–23 IU/L, 9–69 U/L at 37°C (SI units) ; female: 3–13 IU/L, 4–33 U/L at 37°C (SI units) *Elderly:* slightly higher *Newborn:* 5× higher *Premature:* 10× higher
Gastrin	Serum (Red) or plasma (Lavender)	*Adult:* fasting: <100 pg/mL; nonfasting: 50 to 200 pg/mL
Gentamicin	Serum (Red)	*Adult:* therapeutic, peak: 6–12 µg/mL; trough: <2 µg/mL; toxic: >12 µg/mL
Glucose fasting (FBS)	Serum (Red)	*Adult:* 70–110 mg/dL *Elderly:* 70–120 mg/dL *Panic value:* <40 mg/dL, >700 mg/dL *Child:* 60–100 mg/dL *Newborn:* 30–80 mg/dL

Test	*Specimen (Color-top Tube)*	*Reference Values*
Postprandial (PPBS)	Blood (Gray)	*Adult:* 60–100 mg/dL
	Serum (Red)	*Adult:* <140 mg/dL/2 h *Elderly:* <160 mg/dL/2 h *Child:* <120 mg/dL/2 h
	Blood (Gray)	*Adult:* <120 mg/dL/2 h
Glucagon	Plasma (Lavender)	*Adult:* 50–200 pg/mL, 50–200 ng/L (SI units) *Newborn:* 0–1750 pg/mL
Glucose-6-phosphate dehydrogenase (G6PD)	Blood (Green or Lavender)	*Adult and child:* quantitative test: 8–18 IU/g Hb, 125–281 U/dL packed RBC, 251–511 U/dL (cells)
Glucose tolerance test (OGTT)	Serum (Red)	*Adult:* fasting: 70–110 mg/dL; one-half hour: <160 mg/dL; 1 hour: <170 mg/dL; 2 hours: <125 mg/dL; 3 hours: same as fasting
	Blood (Gray)	*Adult:* fasting: 60–100 mg/dL; one-half hour: <150 mg/dL; 1 hour: <160 mg/dL; 2 hours: <115 mg/dL; 3 hours: same as fasting
Growth hormone (GH or hGH)	Serum (Red)	*Adult:* male: <5 ng/mL; female: <10 ng/mL *Child:* <10 ng/mL
Haptoglobin (Hp)	Serum (Red)	*Adult and child:* 60–270 mg/dL, 0.6–2.7 g/L (SI units) *Newborn:* 0–10 mg/dL *Infant:* 1–6 months: 0–30 mg/dL
Helicobacter pylori	Serum (Red)	Negative
Hematocrit (Hct)	Blood (Lavender)	*Adult:* male: 40%–54%; female: 36%–46% *Child:* 1–3 yr: 29%–40%; 4–10 yr: 31%–43% *Newborn:* 44%–65%

Test	*Specimen (Color-top Tube)*	*Reference Values*
Hemoglobin (Hb or Hgb)	Blood (Lavender)	*Adult:* male: 13.5–17 g/dL; female: 12–15 g/dL *Child:* 6 mo–1 yr; 10–17 g/dL; 5–14 yr: 11–16 g/dL *Newborn:* 14–24 g/dL
Hemoglobin A_1c	Plasma (Lavender, Green)	*Adult: Nondiabetic:* 2–5%; *diabetic control:* 2.5–6%; *diabetic uncontrol:* >8.0%; *Child: Nondiabetic:* 1.5–4%
Hemoglobin electrophoresis	Blood (Lavender)	*Adult:* Hb A_1: 95%–98% total Hb; A_2: 1.5%–4%; F: <2%; C: 0%; D: 0%; S: 0% *Child:* Hb F: 1%–2% after 6 mo *Newborn:* Hb F: 50%–80% total Hb *Infant:* Hb F: 8%
Hepatitis A virus	Serum (Red)	Negative
Hepatitis B surface antigen (HB_sAg)	Serum (Red)	*Adult and child:* negative
Herpes simplex virus antibody	Serum (Red)	Negative: <1:10 Positive: >1:10 Positive >1:10 to 1:500
Heterophile antibody	Serum (Red)	*Adult and child:* normal: <1:28 titer; abnormal: >1:56
Hexosaminidase (A and B)	Serum (Red) Aminotic fluid	Total: 5–20 U/L 55%–80% *Elderly:* slightly higher
Human chorionic gonadotropin (hCG)	Serum (Red)	*Adult:* nonpregnant: <0.01 IU/mL Pregnant:

Weeks of gestation	*Values (IU/mL)*
1	0.01–0.04
2	0.03–0.10
4	0.10–1.0
5–12	10–100
13–25	10–30
26–40	5–15

	Urine	*Adult:* Nonpregnant: negative; pregnant: 1–12 weeks: 6,000–500,000 IU/24 h

Test	*Specimen (Color-top Tube)*	*Reference Values*
Human immunodeficiency virus (HIV), AIDS virus	Serum (Red)	*Adult and child:* seronegative
Human leukocyte antigen (HLA)	Serum (Green)	Histocompatibility match or non-match
Human placental lactogen (HPL)	Serum (Red)	*Nonpregnant female:* <0.5 μg/mL *Pregnant female* *Weeks of Gestation* — *Reference values* 5–7 — 1.0 μg/mL 8–27 — <4.6 μg/mL 28–31 — 2.4–6.0 μg/mL 32–35 — 3.6–7.7 μg/mL 36–term — 5.0–10.0 μg/mL *Male:* <0.5 μg/mL
17-OHCS	Urine	*Adult:* average: 2–12 mg/24 h; male: 3–12 mg/24 h; female: 2–10 mg/24 h *Elderly:* lower than adult *Child:* 2–4 yr: 1–2 mg/24 h; 5–12 yr: 6–8 mg/24 h *Infant:* <1 mg/24 h
5-HIAA	Urine	*Adult:* random sample: negative; quantitative: 2–10 mg/24 h
Immunoglobulins (Ig)	Serum (Red)	*Adult:* total Ig: 900–2,200 mg/dL; IgG: 650–1,700 mg/dL; IgA: 70–400 mg/dL; IgM: 40–350 mg/dL; IgD: 0–8 mg/dL; IgE: 0–120 mg/dL *Child:* 6–16 yr: total Ig: 800–1,700; IgG: 700–1650 mg/dL; IgA: 80–230 mg/dL; IgM: 45–260 mg/dL; IgE: <62 U/mL
Insulin	Serum (Red)	*Adult:* 5–25 μU/mL, 10–250 μIU/mL. *Panic Value:* 7 μU/mL
Insulin antibody test	Serum (Red)	<4% serum binding of beef or pork

Test	*Specimen (Color-top Tube)*	*Reference Values*
International Normalized Ratio (INR)	Plasma (Blue)	For anticoagulant therapy: 2.0–3.0 INR
Iron	Serum (Red)	*Adult:* 50–150 μg/dL, 10–27 μmol/L (SI units) *Child:* 6 mo–2 yr: 40–100 μg/dL *Newborn:* 100–250 μg/dL *Elderly:* 60–80 μg/dL
Iron-binding capacity (IBC; TIBC)	Serum (Red)	*Adult and child:* 250–450 μg/dL *Newborn:* 60–175 μg/dL *Infant:* 100–135 μg/dL
Ketone bodies	Urine	*Adult and child:* negative
17-Ketosteroids (17-KS)	Urine	*Adult:* male: 5–25 mg/24 h; female: 5–15 mg/24 h *Elderly:* 4–8 mg/24 h *Child:* 1–3 yr: <2 mg/24 h; 3–6 yr: <3 mg/24 h; 7–10 yr: <4 mg/24 h; 10–12 yr: <5–6 mg/24 h *Adolescent:* male: 3–15 mg/24 h; female: 3–12 mg/24 h
Lactic acid	Blood (Green)	*Adult: arterial* blood: 0.5–2.0 mEq/L, 11.3 mg/dL, 0.5–2.0 mmol/L (SI units); *venous* blood: 0.5–1.5 mEq/L, 8.1–15.3 mg/dL, 0.5–1.5 mmol/L (SI units); *panic:* >5 mEq/L, >45 mg/dL, >5 mmol/L (SI units)
Lactic dehydrogenase (LD or LDH)	Serum (Red)	*Adult:* 100–190 IU/L, 70–250 U/L *Child:* 50–150 IU/L *Newborn:* 300–1500 IU/L
LDH isoenzymes	Serum (Red)	*Adult:* LDH_1: 14%–26%; LDH_2: 27%–37%; LDH_3: 13%–26%; LDH_4: 8%–16%; LDH_5: 6%–16%
Lactose	Serum/plasma (Gray)	<0.5 mg/dL
	Urine	12–40 mg/dL
Lactose	Serum/plasma (Gray)	*Adult and child:* <0.5 mg/dL, <14.5 μmol/L (SI units)
	Urine	12–40 mg/dL

Test	*Specimen (Color-top Tube)*	*Reference Values*
Lactose test tolerance	Serum/plasma (Gray)	Tolerance: FBS + 20–50 mg/dL; intolerance: <20 mg/dL
Lead	Blood (Brown)	*Adult:* 10–20 μg/dL; acceptable: 20–40 μg/dL, toxic: >80 μg/dL *Child:* <20 μg/dL, toxic: >50 μg/dL
Lecithin/sphingomyelin ratio (L/S)	Amniotic fluid	*Adult:* 1:1 before 35 weeks' gestation; L: 6–9 mg/dL; S: 4–6 mg/dL 4:1 after 35 weeks' gestation. L: 15–21 mg/dL; S: 4–6 mg/dL
Legionnaire's antibody	Serum (Red)	Negative
Leucine aminopeptidase (LAP)	Serum (Red)	*Adult:* 8–22 μU/mL, 12–33 IU/L, 20–50 U/L at 37°C (SI units)
Lidocaine	Serum (Red)	*Adult:* therapeutic: 1.5–5.0 μg/mL; toxic: >6 μg/mL
Lipase	Serum (Red)	*Adult:* 20–180 IU/L, 14–280 mU/mL, 14–280 U/L (SI units) *Child:* 20–136 IU/L *Infant:* 9–105 IU/L
Lipoproteins	Serum (Red)	*Adult:* total lipids: 400–800 mg/dL, 4–8 g/L (SI units) Cholesterol: 150–240 mg/dL Triglycerides: 10–190 mg/dL Phospholipids: 150–325 mg/dL LDL: 60–130 mg/dL; HDL: 29–77 mg/dL; low-risk HDL: >46 mg/dL
Lithium	Serum (Red)	*Adult:* therapeutic: 0.5–1.5 mEq/L; toxic: >1.5 mEq/L; lethal: >4.0 mEq/L
Lupus erythematosus (LE) cell test	Blood (Green or Red)	*Adult and child:* No LE cells
Luteinizing hormone (LH)	Serum (Red)	*Serum:* Adult: female: follicular phase: 5–30 mIU/mL; midcycle: 50–150 mIU/mL; luteal phase: 2–25 mIU/mL. Postmenopausal: 40–100 mIU/mL. Male: 5–25 mIU/mL. Child: 6–12 yr: <10 mIU/mL; 13–18 yr: <20 mIU/mL

Test	Specimen (Color-top Tube)	Reference Values
		Urine: Adult: female: follicular phase: 5–25 IU/24 h; midcycle: 30–90 IU/24 h; luteal phase: 2–24 IU/24 h; postmenopausal: >40 IU/24 h. Male: 7–25 IU/mL
Lyme disease test	Serum (Red)	<1:256
Lymphocytes (T and B) assay	Blood (Lavender)	T cells: 60%–80%; 600–2400 cells/μL B cells: 4%–16%; 50–250 cells/μL
Magnesium (Mg)	Serum (Red)	*Adult:* 1.5–2.5 mEq/L, 1.8–3.0 mg/dL *Child:* 1.6–2.6 mEq/L *Newborn:* 1.4–2.9 mEq/L
Malarial smear	Blood (Lavender)	*Adult and child:* negative
Mumps antibody	Serum (Red)	*Adult and child:* Negative: <1:8 titer; Positive: >1:8
Myoglobin	Serum (Red)	Serum: *Adult:* 12–90 ng/mL; Urine: Negative, <20 ng/mL
Nifedipine (Procardia)	Serum (Red)	*Adult:* therapeutic: 50–100 ng/mL; toxic: >100 ng/mL
5-Nucleotidase	Serum (Red)	*Adult:* < 17 U/L
Occult blood	Feces	*Adult and child:* negative
Opiates	Serum and Urine	Negative (see text)
Osmolality	Serum (Red)	*Adult:* 280–300 mOsm/kg H_2O *Child:* 270–290 mOsm/kg H_2O *Panic Value:* <240 mOsm/kg and >320 mOsm/kg
	Urine	*Adult and child:* 50–1,200 mOsm/kg H_2O *Newborn:* 100–600 mOsm/kg H_2O
Ova and parasites	Feces	*Adult and child:* negative
Parathyroid hormone (PTH)	Serum (Red)	*Adult:* C-terminal/midregion: 50–330 pg/mL; intact/midregion: 11–54 pg/mL; N-terminal: 8–24 pg/mL
Partial thromboplastin time (PTT)	Plasma (Blue)	*Adult:* 60–70 seconds; APTT: 20–35 seconds

Test	***Specimen (Color-top Tube)***	***Reference Values***
Phenylalanine	Serum (Red)	*Child:* 0.5–2.0 mg/dL
Phenylketonuria	Urine	*Child:* negative
Phospholipids	Serum (Red)	*Adult:* 150–325 mg/dL
Phosphorus (P)	Serum (Red)	*Adult:* 1.7–2.6 mEq/L, 2.5–4.5 mg/dL, 0.78–1.52 mmol/L (SI units) *Child:* 4.5–5.5 mg/dL *Infant:* 4.5–6.7 mg/dL *Elderly:* slightly lower than adult
Platelet aggregation and adhesions	Blood (Blue)	*Adult:* aggregation in 3–5 min
Platelet antibody test	Blood (Blue)	*Adult:* Negative
Platelet count	Blood (Lavender)	*Adult and child:* 150,000–400,000 μL, 0.15–0.4 × 10^{12}/L (SI units) *Premature:* 100,000–300,000 μL *Newborn:* 150,000–300,000 μL *Infant:* 200,000–475,000 μL
Porphobilinogen	Urine	*Adult and child:* random, negative quant: 0–2 mg/24 h
Porphyrins:		
Coproporphyrins	Urine	*Adult:* random: negative or 3–20 μg/dL; quantitative: 15–160 μg/24 h *Child:* 0–80 μg/24 h
Uroporphyrins	Urine	*Adult:* random: negative; quant: <30 μg/24 h *Child:* 10–30 μg/24 h
Potassium (K)	Serum (Red)	*Adult:* 3.5–5.3 mEq/L, 3.5–5.0 mmol/L (SI units) *Child:* 3.5–5.5 mEq/L *Infant:* 3.6–5.8 mEq/L
	Urine	*Adult:* 25–120 mEq/24 h
Prealbumin assay	Serum (Red)	*Adult:* 17–40 mg/dL; *Female:* 18 mg/dL; *Male:* 21.6 mg/dL *Child:* 2–3 yrs: 16–28 mg/dL *Newborn:* 10–11.5 mg/dL

Test	Specimen (Color-top Tube)	Reference Values
Pregnanediol	Urine	*Adult:* female: proliferative phase: 0.5–1.5 mg/24 h; luteal phase: 2–7 mg/24 h; postmenopause: 0.1–1.0 mg/24 h; male: 0.1–1.5 mg/24 h *Pregnancy:* *Weeks of gestation* — *mg/24 h* 10–19 — 5–25 20–28 — 15–42 28–32 wks — 25–49 mg/24 h *Child:* 0.4–1.0 mg/24 h
Pregnanetriol	Urine	*Adult:* male: 0.4–2.4 mg/24 h; female: 0.5–2.0 mg/24 h *Child:* 0–1.0 mg/24 h *Infant:* 0–0.2 mg/24 h
Primidone	Serum (Red)	*Adult:* therapeutic: 5–12 μg/mL; toxic: >12–15 μg/mL *Child:* <5 years: therapeutic: 7–10 μg/mL; toxic: >12 μg/mL
Procainamide	Serum (Red)	*Adult:* therapeutic: 4–10 μg/mL; toxic: >10 μg/mL
Progesterone	Serum (Red) or plasma (Lavender)	*Adult:* Female: follicular phase: 0.1–1.5 ng/mL; 20–150 ng/dL; luteal phase: 2–28 ng/mL; 250–2800 ng/dL; postmeno-pausal: <1.0 ng/mL; <100 ng/dL. Pregnancy: first trimester: 9–50 ng/mL; second trimester: 18–150 ng/mL; third trimester: 60–260 ng/mL. Male: <1.0 ng/mL; <100 ng/dL
Prolactin	Serum (Red) or plasma (Lavender)	*Adult:* follicular phase: 0–23 ng/mL; luteal phase 0–40 ng/mL; male: 0.1–20 ng/mL. Pituitary tumor: >100–300 ng/mL; pregnancy: trimester: 1st: <80 ng/mL; 2nd: <160 ng/mL; 3rd: <400 ng/mL
Propranolol (Inderal)	Serum (Red)	*Adult:* therapeutic: 50–100 ng/mL; toxic: >500 ng/mL

Test	*Specimen (Color-top Tube)*	*Reference Values*
Prostate-specific antigen (PSA)	Serum (Red)	Male: normal: 0–4 ng/mL BPH: 4–19 ng/mL; prostate CA: 10–120 ng/mL
Protein (total)	Serum (Red)	*Adult:* 6.0–8.0 g/dL *Child:* 6.2–8.0 g/dL *Premature:* 4.2–7.6 g/dL *Newborn:* 4.6–7.4 g/dL *Infant:* 6.0–6.7 g/dL
Protein electrophoresis	Serum (Red)	
Albumin		*Adult:* 3.5–5.0 g/dL *Child:* 4.0–5.8 g/dL
Globulin		*Adult:* 1.5–3.5 g/dL
Protein	Urine	*Adult:* random: 0–5 mg/dL; 25–150 mg/24 h
Prothrombin time	Plasma (Blue)	*Adult:* 11–13 seconds PT: 1.5–2.0 times the control in seconds
Quinidine	Serum (Red)	*Adult:* therapeutic: 2–5 μg/mL; toxic: >5 μg/mL
Rabies antibody test	Serum (Red)	*Adult:* Negative, IFA <1:16
Rapid plasma reagin (RPR)	Serum (Red)	*Adult and child:* nonreactive
Red blood cell (RBC) indices	Blood (Lavender)	*Adult:* RBC count: 4.6–6.0 × 10^{12} (million/μL) MCV: 80–98 cubic microns (cuu) or fL (SI units) MCH: 27–31 pg MCHC: 32%–36% or 0.32–0.36 g/dL *Child:* RBC: 3.8–5.5 × 10^{12} MCV: 82–92 cuμ or fL MCH: 27–31 pg MCHC: 32%–36% or 0.32–0.36 g/dL *Newborn:* RBC: 4.8–7.2 × 10^{12} MCV: 96–108 cuμ or fL MCH: 32–34 pg

Test	*Specimen (Color-top Tube)*	*Reference Values*
		MCHC: 32%–33% or 0.32–0.33 g/dL RDW (coulter S): 11.5–14.5
Renin	Plasma (Lavender)	*Adult:* 30 minutes supine: 0.2–2.3 ng/mL; upright: 1.6–4.3 ng/mL; restricted salt diet: 4.1–10.8 ng/mL
Reticulocyte count	Blood (Lavender)	*Adult:* 0.5%–1.5% of all RBCs, 25,000–75,000 μL *Child:* 0.5%–2.0% of all RBCs *Newborn:* 2.5%–6.5% of all RBCs *Infant:* 0.5%–3.5% of all RBCs
Rheumatoid factor (RF)	Serum (Red)	*Adult:* <1:20 titer, 1:20–1:80 positive for rheumatoid conditions; >1:80 for rheumatoid arthritis *Elderly:* slightly increased
Rh typing	Blood (Lavender or Red)	*Adult and child:* Rh+ and Rh–
Rubella antibody detection	Serum (Red)	*Adult:* <1:8. Rubella exposure and immunity: 1:32–1:64 titer; definite immunity: >1:64
Rotavirus antigen	Blood and Feces	Negative
Salicylate aspirin	Serum (Red or Green)	*Adult:* therapeutic: 5 mg/dL (headache), 10–30 mg/dL rheumatoid arthritis; mild toxic: >30 mg/dL; severe toxic: >50 mg/dL; lethal: >60 mg/dL *Child:* mild toxic: >25 mg/dL *Elderly:* Mild toxic: >25 mg/dL
Semen analysis	Semen	*Adult:* 50–150 million/mL
Sickle cell test	Blood (Lavender)	*Adult and child:* 0 sickle cells
Sodium (Na)	Serum (Red)	*Adult and child:* 135–145 mEq/L, 135–145 mmol/L (SI units) *Infant:* 134–150 mEq/L
	Urine	*Adult and child:* 40–220 mEq/L/24 h
T_3 (Triiodothyronine)	Serum (Red)	*Adult:* 80–200 ng/dL *Child:* 5–10 yr: 95–240 ng/dL; 10–15 yr: 80–210 ng/dL *Newborn:* 40–215 ng/dL

Test	*Specimen (Color-top Tube)*	*Reference Values*
T_4 (Thyroxine)	Serum (Red)	*Adult:* 4.5–11.5 μg/dL. T_4 RIA: 5–12 μg/dL; free T_4: 1.0–2.3 ng/dL *Child:* 1–6 yr: 5.5–13.5 μg/dL; 6–10 yr: 5–12.5 μg/dL *Newborn:* 11–23 μg/dL *Infant:* 1–4 mo: 7.5–16.5 μg/dL; 4–12 mo: 5.5–14.5 μg/dL
Testosterone	Serum or plasma (Red or Green)	*Adult:* male: 0.3–1.0 μg/dL, 300–1,000 ng/dL; female: 0.03–0.1 μg/dL, 30–100 ng/dL *Child:* male: 12–14 yr: >0.1 μg/dL, >100 ng/dL
Theophylline	Serum (Red)	*Adult and child:* therapeutic: 5–20 μg/mL, 28–112 μmol/L (SI units); toxic: >20 μg/mL *Elderly:* 5–18 μg/mL; toxic: >20 μg/mL *Newborn:* 3–12 μg/mL; Toxic: >13 μg/mL
Thyroid antibodies	Serum (Red)	*Adult:* negative or <1:20
Thyroid-binding globulin (TBG)	Serum (Red)	*Adult:* 10–36 μg/dL
Thyroid-stimulating hormone (TSH)	Serum (Red)	*Adult:* 0.35–5.5 μIU/mL, <10 μU/mL, <10^3 IU/L (SI units), <3 ng/mL *Newborn:* <25 μIU/mL (third day)
Tobramycin	Serum (Red)	*Adult:* therapeutic: peak: 5–10 μg/mL; trough: <2 μg/mL; toxic: >12 μg/mL
Torch test	Serum (Red)	*Child:* negative
Toxoplasmosis antibody test	Serum (Red)	*Adult and Child:* Negative or <1:4, past exposure: 1:4–1:64; acute infection: >1:424
T_3 resin-uptake	Serum (Red)	*Adult:* 25%–35% uptake

Test	*Specimen (Color-top Tube)*	*Reference Values*
Triglycerides	Serum (Red)	*Adult:* 12–29 yr: 10–140 mg/dL; 30–39 yr: 20–150 mg/dL; 40–49 yr: 30–160 mg/dL; >50 yr: 40–190 mg/dL *Child:* 5–11 yr: 10–135 mg/dL *Infant:* 5–40 mg/dL
Uric acid	Serum (Red)	*Adult:* male: 3.5–8.0 mg/dL; female: 2.8–6.8 mg/dL *Panic Value:* >12 mg/dL *Elderly:* 3.5–8.5 mg/dL *Child:* 2.5–5.5 mg/dL
	Urine	*Adult:* 250–750 mg/24 h (normal diet)
Urinalysis	Urine	*Adult, child, and newborn:* See urinalysis in text
Urobilinogen	Urine	*Adult and child:* Random: negative or <1.0 Ehrlich units, 2 hr: 0.3–1.0 Ehrlich units, 24 hours: 0.5–4.0 mg/24 h, 0.09–4.23 µmol/24 h (SI units)
Valproic acid	Serum (Red)	*Adult and child:* Therapeutic: 50–100 µg/mL; toxic: >100 µg/mL
Vanillylmandelic acid (VMA)	Urine	*Adult and child:* 1.5–7.5 mg/24 h *Adolescent:* 1–5 mg/24 h
VDRL	Serum (Red)	*Adult and child:* negative
Verapamil (Calan)	Serum (Red)	*Adult:* therapeutic: 100–600 µg/L; toxic: >600 µg/L
Viral culture		Negative
Vitamin A	Serum (Red)	See text
Vitamin B_{12}	Serum (Red)	*Adult:* 200–900 pg/mL
White blood cells (WBCs)	Blood (Lavender)	*Adult:* Total: 4,500–10,000 µL *Child:* 2 yr: 6,000–17,000 µL *Newborn:* 9,000–30,000 µL
WBC differential: neutrophils (total)	Blood (Lavender)	*Adult:* 50%–70%, 2,500–7,000 µL *Child:* 1 yr: 32% *Newborn:* 61%
Segments		*Adult:* 50%–65%, 2,500–6,500 µL
Bands		*Adult:* 0%–5%, 0–500 µL

Test	*Specimen (Color-top Tube)*	*Reference Values*
Eosinophils		*Adult:* 1%–3%, 100–300 μL
Basophils		*Adult:* 0.4%–1%, 40–100 μL
Monocytes		*Adult:* 4%–6%, 200–600 μL *Child:* 1–12 yr: 4–9%
Lymphocytes		*Adult:* 25%–35%, 1,700–3500 μL *Child:* 6 yr: 42%, 12 yr: 38% *Infant:* 60% *Newborn:* 61%
Zinc	Plasma (Navy blue)	*Adult:* 60–150 μg/dL, 11–23 μmol/L (SI units)
	Urine	150–1250 μg/24 h
Zinc Protoporhyrin	Plasma (Lavender, Green)	*Adult and Child:* 15–77 μg/dL, 0.24–1.23 μmol/L (SI units); Average: <35 μg/dL

Appendix B

Clinical Problems with Laboratory and Diagnostic Tests

Various laboratory and diagnostic tests are ordered for diagnosing clinical health problems. Twenty common health problems with frequently ordered laboratory and diagnostic tests are listed.

1. **Cerebrovascular accident (CVA)**
   Laboratory tests: CBC, serum cholesterol, cerebrospinal fluid
   Diagnostic tests: CT brain scan, nuclear brain scan, MRI, cerebral angiography, positron emission tomography (PET), oculoplethysmography
2. **Cholecystitis (acute)**
   Laboratory tests: CBC, direct bilirubin, serum alkaline phosphatase
   Diagnostic tests: Gallbladder and biliary ultrasound, CT gallbladder scan, cholangiogram, nuclear gallbladder scan
3. **Cirrhosis of the liver**
   Laboratory tests: Liver enzyme tests: alkaline phosphatase (ALP), gamma-glutamyl transferase (GGT), alanine aminotransferase (ALT/SGPT), 5′nucleotidase (5′N); total and direct bilirubin; serum protein; serum albumin; prealbumin assay; CBC; platelet aggregation; prothrombin time (PT); serum electrolytes; plasma ammonia; antimitochondrial antibody; zinc; zinc protoporhyrin
   Diagnostic tests: Nuclear liver scan, CT liver scan, liver biopsy, hepatic angiography, biopsy
4. **Colorectal cancer**
   Laboratory tests: Carcinoembryonic antigen (CEA), serum electrolytes, fecal analysis for occult blood
   Diagnostic tests: Barium enema, proctosigmoidoscopy, colonoscopy, biopsy

5. **Congestive heart failure (CHF)**
   Laboratory tests: CBC, serum electrolytes, serum and urine osmolality.
   Diagnostic tests: X-ray of heart and chest, ECG/EKG, CVP, pulmonary artery catheter (monitoring PCWP), echocardiography
6. **Deep-vein thrombophlebitis (DVT)**
   Laboratory tests: CBC, PT, PTT/APTT
   Diagnostic tests: Doppler ultrasonography, venography
7. **Diabetes mellitus (DM)**
   Laboratory tests: CBC, serum/blood FBS (fasting blood sugar or blood glucose) and postprandial blood sugar (PPBS or feasting blood sugar), glucose self-monitoring, hemoglobin A_1c, insulin and insulin antibody, glucagon serum electrolytes, serum acetone, arterial blood gases (ABGs), oral glucose tolerance test, serum BUN
8. **Emphysema**
   Laboratory tests: Arterial blood gases (ABGs), serum alpha-1-antitrypsin
   Diagnostic tests: Chest x-ray, pulmonary function tests, nuclear lung scan
9. **Lung cancer**
   Laboratory tests: Arterial blood gases (ABGs), sputum cytology
   Diagnostic tests: Chest x-ray, bronchoscopy, CT lung scan, lung biopsy, MRI, mediastinoscopy
10. **Multiple sclerosis (MS)**
    Laboratory tests: CSF analysis
    Diagnostic tests: MRI, CT scan, EMG
11. **Myocardial infarction—Acute (AMI)**
    Laboratory tests: Cardiac enzymes: creatinine phosphokinase (CPK) and CPK isoenzymes (CPK-MB), aspartate aminotransferase (AST/SGOT), lactic dehydrogenase (LDH) and LDH isoenzymes with LDH_1 greater than LDH_2; CBC; lipoproteins: cholesterol, triglycerides, LDL, HDL; serum electrolytes; PT, PTT/APTT; serum and urine myoglobin; serum/blood glucose; sed rate (ESR); arterial blood gases (AGBs); AMA
    Diagnostic tests: ECG/EKG 12 leads, thallium myocardial imaging, echocardiography, cardiac angiography (cardiac catheterization), x-ray of heart and chest, exercise/stress testing, positron emission tomography (PET)

12. **Osteoporosis**
    Laboratory tests: Serum calcium, serum phosphorus, serum alkaline phosphatase (ALP), protein electrophoresis
    Diagnostic tests: X-ray of bone, bone density scan
13. **Pancreatitis (acute)**
    Laboratory tests: Serum and urine amylase, serum lipase
    Diagnostic tests: CT of pancreas, ultrasound of the pancreas
14. **Peptic ulcer**
    Laboratory tests: serum electrolytes; *Helicobacter pylori*
    Diagnostic tests: Upper GI series, gastric analysis studies, gastric acid stimulation test, esophagogastroduodenoscopy
15. **Pneumonia**
    Laboratory tests: CBC, sputum culture, blood culture, arterial blood gases (ABGs)
    Diagnostic tests: Chest x-ray, pulmonary function tests, nuclear lung scan
16. **Pulmonary embolism (PE)**
    Laboratory tests: CBC, PT, PTT/APTT
    Diagnostic tests: Chest x-ray, nuclear lung (perfusion) scan, pulmonary angiography
17. **Renal failure (RF)**
    Laboratory tests: Serum BUN, serum creatinine, urinalysis, serum and urine osmolality, arterial blood gases (ABGs), anti-GBM, BUN/creatinine ratio
    Diagnostic tests: KUB x-ray, nuclear renal scan, renal angiography
18. **Rheumatoid arthritis (RA)**
    Laboratory tests: CBC, rheumatoid factor (RF), antinuclear antibodies (ANA), antimitochondrial, C-reactive protein (CRP), complements 3 and 4, erythrocyte sedimentation rate (sed rate or ESR), protein electrophoresis
    Diagnostic tests: Synovial fluid analysis, x-ray of joints, nuclear bone scan
19. **Systemic lupus erythematosus (SLE or lupus)**
    Laboratory tests: CBC, erythrocyte sedimentation rate (sed rate or ESR), antinuclear antibodies (ANA), anti-DNA, lupus erythematosus cell test (LE cell test), C-reactive protein (CRP), urinalysis, complements 3 and 4
    Diagnostic tests: Kidney biopsy

20. **Ulcerative colitis**
Laboratory tests: CBC, serum electrolytes, sed rate (ESR)
Diagnostic tests: Barium enema
21. **Pregnancy and fetal distress**
Laboratory tests: alpha fetoprotein, estrone (E_1), estriol (E_3), estetrol (E_4), ferritin, human chorionic gonadotropin, pregnanediol, progesterone
22. **Gynecologic problems**
Laboratory tests: estrone (E_1), estrogen, estradiol (E_2), prolactin
Diagnostic tests: biopsy, cervicography, colposcopy, hysteroscopy

Appendix C

Therapeutic Drug Monitoring (TDM)*

Selective drugs are monitored by serum and urine for the purposes of achieving and maintaining therapeutic drug effect and for preventing drug toxicity. Drugs with a wide therapeutic range (window), the difference between effective dose and toxic dose, are not usually monitored. Drug monitoring is important in maintaining a drug concentration-response relationship, especially when the serum drug range (window) is narrow, such as with digoxin and lithium. Therapeutic drug monitoring (TDM) is the process of following drug levels and adjusting them to maintain a therapeutic level. Not all drugs can be dosed and/or monitored by their blood levels alone.

Drug levels are obtained at peak time and trough time after a steady state of the drug has occurred in the client. Steady state is reached after four to five half-lives of a drug and can be reached sooner if the drug has a short half-life. Once steady state is achieved, serum drug level is checked at the peak level (maximum drug concentration) and/or at trough/residual level (minimum drug concentration). If the trough or residual level is at the high therapeutic point, toxicity might occur. Careful assessment is needed by both physical and laboratory means.

TDM is required for drugs with a narrow therapeutic index or range (window); when other methods for monitoring drugs are noneffective, such as blood pressure (BP) monitoring; for determining when adequate blood concentrations are reached; for evaluating client's compliance to drug therapy; for determining whether other drugs have

*Revised and updated by Ronald J. Lefever, RPh., Pharmacy Services, Medical College of Virginia, Richmond, VA.

altered serum drug levels (increased or decreased) that could result in drug toxicity or lack of therapeutic effect; and for establishing new serum-drug level when dosage is changed.

Drug groups for TDM include analgesics, antibiotics, anticonvulsants, antineoplastics, bronchodilators, cardiac drugs, hypoglycemics, sedatives, and tranquilizers. To effectively conduct TDM, the laboratory must be provided with the following information: the drug name and daily dosage, time and amount of last dose, time blood was drawn, route of administration, and client's age. Without complete information, serum drug reporting might be incorrect.

Drug	*Therapeutic Range*	*Peak Time*	*Toxic Level*
Acetaminophen (Tylenol)	10–20 μg/mL	1–2½ hours	>50 μg/mL Haptotoxicity: >200 μg/mL
Acetohexamide (Dymelor)	20–70 μg/mL (should be dosed according to blood glucose levels)	2–4 hours	>75 μg/mL
Alcohol	Negative		Mild toxic: 150 mg/dL Marked toxic: >250 mgL
Alprazolam (Xanax)	10–50 ng/mL	1–2 hours	>75 ng/mL
Amikacin (Amikin)	Peak: 20–30 μg/mL	Intravenously: ½ hour	Peak: >35 μg/mL
	Trough: ≤10 μg/mL	½–1½ hours	>10 μg/mL
Aminocaproic acid (Amicar)	100–400 μg/mL	1 hour	>400 μg/mL
Aminophylline (see Theophylline)			
Amiodarone (Cardarone)	0.5–2.5 μg/mL	2–10 hours	>2.5 μg/mL

Drug	*Therapeutic Range*	*Peak Time*	*Toxic Level*
Amitriptyline (Elavil) + nortriptyline (parent and active metabolite)	110–225 ng/mL	2–4 hours (and up to 12 hours)	>500 ng/mL
Amobarbital (Amytal)	1–5 μg/mL	2 hours	>15 μg/mL Severe toxicity: >30 μg/mL
Amoxapine (Asendin)	200–400 ng/mL	1½ hours	>500 ng/mL
Amphetamine:			
Serum	20–30 ng/mL		0.2 μg/mL
Urine		Detectable in urine after 3 hours; positive for 24–48 hours	>30 μg/mL urine
Aspirin (see Salicylates)			
Atenolol (Tenormin)	200–500 ng/mL	2–4 hours	>500 ng/mL
Beta carotene	48–200 μg/dL	Several weeks	>300 μg/dL
Bromide	20–80 mg/dL		>100 mg/dL
Butabarbital (Butisol)	1–2 μg/mL	3–4 hours	>10 μg/mL
Caffeine	Adult: 3–15 μg/mL Infant: 8–20 μg/mL	½–1 hour	>50 μg/mL
Carbamazepine (Tegretol)	4–12 μg/mL	6 hours (range 2–24 hours)	>9–15 μg/mL
Chloral hydrate (Noctec)	2–12 μg/mL	1–2 hours	>20 μg/mL
Chloramphenicol (Chloromycetin)	10–20 mg/L		>25 mg/L
Chlordiazepoxide (Librium)	1–5 μg/mL	2–3 hours	>5 μg/mL

Drug	*Therapeutic Range*	*Peak Time*	*Toxic Level*
Chlorpromazine (Thorazine)	50–300 ng/mL	2–4 hours	>750 ng/mL
Chlorpropamide (Diabinese)	75–250 µg/mL	3–6 hours	>250–750 µg/mL
Clonidine (Catapres)	0.2–2.0 ng/mL (Hypotensive effect)	2–5 hours	>2.0 ng/mL
Clorazepate (Tranxene)	0.12–1.0 µg/mL	1–2 hours	>1.0 µg/mL
Cimetidine (Tagamet)	Trough: 0.5–1.2 µg/mL	1–1½ hours	Trough: >1.5 µg/mL
Clonazepam (Klonopin)	10–60 ng/mL	2 hours	>80 ng/mL
Codeine	10–100 ng/mL	1–2 hours	>200 ng/mL
Cyclosporine	100–300 ng/mL	3–4 hours	>400 ng/mL
Dantrolene (Dantrium)	1–3 µg/mL	5 hours	>5 µg/mL
Desipramine (Norpramin)	125–300 ng/mL	4–6 hours	>500 ng/mL
Diazepam (Valium)	0.5–2 mg/L 400–600 ng/mL Therapeutic	1–2 hours	>3 mg/L >3000 ng/mL
Digitoxin (rarely administered)	10–25 ng/mL	Noticeable: 2–4 hours Peak: 12–24 hours	>30 ng/mL
Digoxin	0.5–2 ng/mL	PO: 6–8 hours IV: 1½–2 hours	2–3 ng/mL
Dilantin (see Phenytoin)			
Diltiazem (Cardizem)	50–200 ng/mL	2–3 hours	>200 ng/mL
Disopyramide (Norpace)	2–4 µg/mL	2 hours	>4 µg/mL
Doxepin (Sinequan)	150–300 ng/mL	2–4 hours	>500 ng/mL
Ethchlorvynol (Placidyl)	2–8 µg/mL	1–2 hours	>20 µg/mL

Drug	*Therapeutic Range*	*Peak Time*	*Toxic Level*
Ethosuximide (Zarontin)	40–100 μg/mL	2–4 hours	>150 μg/mL
Flecainide (Tambocor)	0.2–1.0 μg/mL	3 hours	>1.0 μg/mL
Fluoxetine	90–300 ng/mL	2–4 hours	>500 ng/mL
Flurazepam (Dalmane)	20–110 ng/mL	0.5–1 hour	>1500 ng/mL
Folate	>3.5 μg/L	1 hour	
Gentamicin (Garamycin)	Peak: 6–12 μg/mL Trough: <2 μg/mL	IV: 15–30 minutes	Peak: >12 μg/mL >2 μg/mL
Glutethimide (Doriden)	2–6 μg/mL	1–2 hours	>20 μg/mL
Gold	1.0–2.0 μg/mL	2–6 hours	>5.0 μg/mL
Haloperidol (Haldol)	5–15 ng/mL	2–6 hours	>50 ng/mL
Hydromorphone (Dilaudid)	1–30 ng/mL	½–1½ hours	>100 ng/mL
Ibuprofen (Motrin, etc)	10–50 μg/mL	1–2 hours	>100 μg/mL
Imipramine (Tofranil) + desipramine (parent and active metabolite)	200–350 ng/mL	PO: 1–2 hours IM: 30 minutes	>500 ng/mL
Isoniazid (INH, Nydrazid)	1–7 mg/mL (dose usually adjusted based on liver function tests)	1–2 hours	>20 mg/mL
Kanamycin (Kantrex)	Peak: 15–30 μg/mL	PO: 1–2 hours IM: 30 minutes–1 hour	Peak: >35 μg/mL Trough: >10 μg/mL
Lead	<20 μg/dL Urine: <80 μg/24 hours		>80 μg/dL Urine: >125 μg/24 hours

Drug	*Therapeutic Range*	*Peak Time*	*Toxic Level*
Lidocaine (Xylocaine)	1.5–5 µg/mL	IV: 10 minutes	>6 µg/mL
Lithium	0.8–1.2 mEq/L	½–4 hours	>1.5 mEq/L
Lorazepam (Ativan)	50–240 ng/mL	1–3 hours	>300 ng/mL
Maprotiline (Ludiomil)	200–300 ng/mL	12 hours	>500 ng/mL
Meperidine (Demerol)	0.4–0.7 µg/mL	2–4 hours	>1.0 µg/mL
Mephenytoin (Mesantoin)	15–40 µg/mL	2–4 hours	>50 µg/mL
Meprobamate (Equanil, Miltown)	15–25 µg/mL	2 hours	>50 µg/mL
Methadone (Dolophine)	100–400 ng/mL	½–1 hour	>2000 ng/mL or >0.2 µg/mL
Methaqualone	1–5 µg/mL		>10 µg/mL
Methyldopa (Aldomet)	1–5 µg/mL	3–6 hours	>7 µg/mL
Methyprylon (Noludar)	8–10 µg/mL	1–2 hours	>50 µg/mL
Metoprolol (Lopressor)	75–200 ng/mL	2–4 hours	>225 ng/mL
Methotrexate	<0.1 µmol/L after 48 h	1–2 hours	1.0×10^6 at 48 h
Methsuximide	<1.0 µg/mL	1–4 hours	>40 µg/mL
Mexiletine (Mexitil)	0.5–2 µg/mL	2–3 hours	>2 µg/mL
Morphine	10–80 ng/mL	IV: immediately IM: ½–1 hour SC: 1–1½ hours	>200 ng/mL
Netilmicin (Netromycin)	Peak: 0.5–10 µg/mL Trough: <4 µg/mL	IV: 30 minutes	Peak: >16 µg/mL >4 µg/mL
Nifedipine (Procardia)	50–100 ng/mL	½–2 hours	>100 ng/mL
Nortriptyline (Aventyl)	50–150 ng/mL	8 hours	>200 ng/mL

Drug	*Therapeutic Range*	*Peak Time*	*Toxic Level*
Oxazepam (Serax)	0.2–1.4 μg/mL	1–2 hours	
Oxycodone (Percodan)	10–100 ng/mL	½–1 hour	>200 ng/mL
Pentazocine (Talwin)	0.05–0.2 μg/mL	1–2 hours	>1.0 μg/mL Urine: >3.0 μg/mL
Pentobarbital (Nembutal)	1–5 μg/mL	½–1 hour	>10 μg/mL Severe toxicity: >30 μg/mL
Phenmetrazine (Preludin)	5–30 μg/mL (Urine)	2 hours	>50 μg/mL (urine)
Phenobarbital (Luminal)	15–40 μg/mL	6–18 hours	>40 μg/mL Severe toxicity: >80 μg/mL
Phenytoin (Dilantin)	10–20 μg/mL	4–8 hours	>20–30 μg/mL Severe toxicity: >40 μg/mL
Pindolol (Visken)	0.5–6.0 ng/mL	2–4 hours	>10 ng/mL
Primidone (Mysoline)	5–12 μg/mL	2–4 hours	>12–15 μg/mL
Procainamide (Pronestyl)	4–10 μg/mL	1 hour	>10 μg/mL
Procaine (Novocain)	<11 μg/mL	10–30 minutes	>20 μg/mL
Prochlorperazine (Compazine)	50–300 ng/mL	2–4 hours	>1000 ng/mL
Propoxyphene (Darvon)	0.1–0.4 μg/mL	2–3 hours	>0.5 μg/mL
Propranolol (Inderal)	>100 ng/mL	1–2 hours	>150 ng/mL
Protriptyline (Vivactil)	50–150 ng/mL	8–12 hours	>200 ng/mL
Quinidine	2–5 μg/mL	1–3 hours	>6 μg/mL
Ranitidine (Zantac)	100 ng/mL	2–3 hours	>100 ng/mL

Drug	*Therapeutic Range*	*Peak Time*	*Toxic Level*
Reserpine (Serpasil)	20 ng/mL	2–4 hours	>20 ng/mL
Salicylates (Aspirin)	10–30 mg/dL	1–2 hours	Tinnitis: 20–40 mg/mL Hyperventilation: >35 mg/dL Severe toxicity: >50 mg/dL
Secobarbital (Seconal)	2–5 µg/mL	1 hour	>15 µg/mL Severe toxicity: >30 µg/mL
Theophylline (Theodur, Aminodur)	10–20 µg/mL	PO: 2–3 hours IV: 15 minutes (depends on smoking or nonsmoking)	>20 µg/mL
Thiocyanate	4–20 µg/mL		>60 µg/mL
Thioridazine	100–600 ng/mL		>2000 ng/mL
(Mellaril)	1.0–1.5 µg/mL	2–4 hours	>10 µg/mL
Timolol (Blocadren)	3–55 ng/mL	1–2 hours	>60 ng/mL
Tobramycin (Nebcin)	Peak: 5–10 µg/mL	IV: 15–30 minutes	Peak: >12 µg/mL
	Trough: 1–1.5 µg/mL	IM: ½–1½ hours	Trough: >2 µg/mL
Tocainide (Tonocard)	4–10 µg/mL	½–3 hours	>12 µg/mL
Tolbutamide (Orinase)	80–240 µg/mL	3–5 hours	>640 µg/mL
Trazodone (Desyrel)	500–2500 ng/mL	1–2 weeks	>4000 ng/mL
Trifluoperazine (Stelazine)	50–300 ng/mL	2–4 hours	>1000 ng/mL
Valproic Acid (Depakene)	50–100 µg/mL	½–1½ hours	>100 µg/mL Severe toxicity: >150 µg/mL

Drug	*Therapeutic Range*	*Peak Time*	*Toxic Level*
Vancomycin (Vanocin)	Peak: 20–40 μg/mL Trough: 5–10 μg/mL	IV: Peak: 5 minutes IV: Trough: 12 hours	Peak: >80 μg/mL
Verapamil (Calan)	100–300 ng/mL	PO: 1–2 hours IV: 5 minutes	>500 ng/mL
Warfarin (Coumadin)	1–10 μg/mL (dose usually adjusted by 1 to 2.5 × control)	1½–3 days	>10 μg/mL

Note: HIV drugs are dosed and monitored by other laboratory tests.

Bibliography

Abrams DI, Parker-Martin J, Unger KW (1989). AIDS: Caring for the dying patient. *Patient Care,* 23:22–36.

AIDS in humans dates to 1930, researcher finds (2000, February 2). *The News Journal,* A4.

Angelidis, PA (1994). MR image compression using a wavelet transform coding algorithm. *Magnetic Resonance Imaging,* 12(7):1111–1112.

Barrick B, Vogel S (1996). Application of laboratory diagnostics in HIV testing. *Nursing Clinics of North America,* 31(1): 41–45.

Bartholet J (2000, January 17). The years. *Newsweek,* 32–37.

Black JM, Matassarin-Jacobs E (1997). *Luckmann and Sorensen's Medical–Surgical Nursing.* 5th ed. Philadelphia: WB Saunders.

Brooks DJ, Beany RP, Thomas DGT (1986). The role of positron emission tomography in the study of cerebral tumors. *Seminars in Oncology,* 13:83–93.

Brown CH (1989). *Handbook of Drug Therapy Monitoring.* Baltimore: Williams & Wilkins.

Bynum R (1999, August 31). Drop in deaths from AIDS slows. *The New Journal,* A5.

Cassetta RA (1993). AIDS: Patient care challenges nursing. *The American Nurse,* 25:1, 24.

Cassetta RA (1993). The new faces of the epidemic. *The American Nurse,* 25:16.

CDC revises AIDS definition (1993). *The American Nurse,* 25:20.

Chernecky CC, Krech RL, Berger BJ (1993). *Cholesterol Uptake in Laboratory Tests and Diagnostic Procedures.* Philadelphia: Saunders. 1: 7,8.

Chernecky CC, Berger BJ, (eds). (1997). *Laboratory Tests and Diagnostic Procedures.* 2nd ed. Philadelphia: Saunders.

Cholesterol Uptake. (1988) 1(6): 7, 8.

Corbett JV (1996). *Laboratory Tests and Diagnostic Procedures with Nursing Diagnoses.* 4th ed. Norwalk, CT: Appleton & Lange.

Cose E (2000, January 17). A cause that crosses the color line. *Newsweek,* 49.

Cowley G (2000, January 17). Fighting the disease: What can be done. *Newsweek,* 38.

Crandall BF, Kulch P, Tabsh K (1994). Risk assessment of amniocentesis between 11 and 15 weeks: Comparison to later amniocentesis controls. *Prenatal Diagnosis,* 14: 913–939.

C-Sections recommended for HIV positive pregnant women (1999, October/November). *AWHONN Lifelines,* 3(5): 17.

Curry JC (1994). Interpreting laboratory data. In: Muma RD, Lyons BA, Borucki MJ, Pollard RB, eds. *HIV Manual for Health Care Professionals.* Norwalk, CT: Appleton & Lange, pp 111–122.

DeLorenzo L (1993). The changing face of AIDS. *The Nursing Spectrum,* 2: 19.

DeVita VT Jr, Hellman S, Rosenberg SA (1992). *AIDS: Etiology, Diagnosis, Treatment and Prevention.* 3rd ed. Philadelphia: Lippincott.

Epstein JD (1998, September 19). Dupont AIDS drug gets FDA approval. *The News Journal,* A1, A8.

Fahey JL, Nishanian P (1997). Laboratory diagnosis and evaluation of HIV infection. In: Fahey JL, Flemmig DS, eds. *AIDS/HIV Reference Guide for Medical Professionals.* 4th ed. Baltimore: Wilkins and Wilkins, pp 232–242.

Fischbach FT (1996). *A Manual of Laboratory Diagnostic Tests.* 5th ed. Philadelphia: Lippincott.

Fisher M, Prichard JW, Warach S (1995). New magnetic resonance techniques for acute ischemic stroke. *Journal of the American Medical Association,* 274(11): 908–911.

Flake KJ (2000). HIV testing during pregnancy: Building the case for voluntary testing. *AWHONN Lifelines,* 4C: 13–16.

Flaskerud JH (1992). Psychosocial aspects. In: Flaskerud JH, Unguarski PJ, eds. *HIV/AIDS: A Guide to Nursing Care.* 2nd ed. Philadelphia: Saunders, pp 239–274.

Flemmig DS, Johiro AK (1997). HIV counseling and testing. In: Fahey JL, Flemmig DS, eds. *AIDS/HIV Reference Guide for Medical Professionals.* 4th ed. Baltimore: Wilkins and Wilkins, pp 57–74.

Food and Drug Administration (1995). Mammography quality deadline. *FDA Medical Bulletin,* 25(1): 3.

Froelicher, ES (1994). Usefulness of exercise testing shortly after acute myocardial infarction for predicting 10 year mortality. *American Journal of Cardiology,* 74: 318–323.

Gefter WB (1988). Chest applications of magnetic resonance imaging: An update. *Radiologic Clinics of North America,* 26: 573–586.

Gerberding JL (1992). HIV transmission to providers and their patients. In: Sande MA, Volberding PA, eds. *The Medical Management of AIDS.* 3rd ed. Philadelphia: Saunders, pp 54–64.

Goldstein RA, Mullani NA, Wong WH (1986). Positron imaging of myocardial infarction with rubidium-82. *Journal of Nuclear Medicine,* 27: 1824–1829.

Gorman C (1997, January 6; 1996, December 30). The disease detective. *Time,* 148(29): 56–62, 63.

Grady C (1992). HIV disease: Pathogens and treatment. In: Flaskerud JH, Unguarski PJ, eds. *HIV/AIDS: A Guide to Nursing Care.* 2nd ed. Philadelphia: Saunders, pp 30–53.

Guzman ER, Rosenberg JC, Houlihan C (1994). A new method using vaginal ultrasound and transfundal pressure to evaluate the asymptomatic incompetent cervix. *Obstetrics and Gynecology,* 83(2): 248–252.

Haney DQ (2000, January 31). Virus levels linked to AIDS transmission. *The News Journal,* A3.

Hardy CE, Helton GJ, Kondo C, et al (1994). Usefulness of magnetic resonance imaging for evaluating great-vessel anatomy after arterial switch operation for D-transposition of the great arteries. *American Heart Journal,* 128: 326–332.

Henry JB (1996). *Todd-Sanford-Davidsohn: Clinical Diagnosis and Management by Laboratory Methods.* 19th ed. Philadelphia: WB Saunders.

HIV/AIDS Surveillance Reports (June, 1999). Atlanta: Centers for Disease Control and Prevention. 11(1).

Hochrein MA, Sohl L (1992). Heart smart: A guide to cardiac tests. *American Journal of Nursing,* 92(12): 22–25.

Hyman RA, Gorey MT (1988). Imaging strategies for MR of the brain. *Radiologic Clinics of North America,* 26(3): 471–502.

Intermountain Thoracic Society. (1984). *Clinical Pulmonary Function Testing, a Manual of Uniform Laboratory Procedures.* 2nd ed.

Itchhaporia D, Cerqueira MD (1995). New agents and new techniques and nuclear cardiology. *Current Opinion in Cardiology,* 10(6): 650–655.

IV Persantine Thallium Imaging: Protocol (1990). Delaware: DuPont-Merck Pharmaceutical Company.

Jaffe MS (1996). *Medical–Surgical Nursing Care Plans: Nursing Diagnoses & Interventions.* 3rd ed. Stamford, CT: Appleton & Lange.

Johnson LL, Lawson MA (1996). New imaging techniques for assessing cardiac function. *Critical Care Clinics,* 12(4): 919–937.

Johnson D, Silverstein-Currier J, Sanchez-Keeland L (1999). Building barriers to HIV: Protecting women through contraception and infection prevention. *Advance for Nurse Practitioners,* 7(5): 40–44.

Kanal E, Shaibani A (1994). Firearm safety in the MR imaging environment. *Radiology,* 193: 875–876.

Kaplan A, Jack R, Opheim KE, et al. (1995). *Clinical Chemistry. Interpretation and Techniques,* 4th ed. Baltimore: Williams & Wilkins.

Kee JL (1999). *Fluids and Electrolytes with Clinical Applications,* 6th ed. New York: Delmar Publishers.

Kee JL (1999). *Laboratory and Diagnostic Tests with Nursing Implications.* 5th ed. Norwalk, CT: Appleton & Lange.

Kee JL, Hayes ER (2000). *Pharmacology: A Nursing Process Approach.* 3rd ed. Philadelphia: Saunders.

Keeys, MU (1994). Nuclear cardiology stress testing. *Nursing 94,* 24(1): 63, 64.

Knoben JE, Anderson PO (1993). *Clinical Drug Data.* 7th ed. Hamilton, IL: Drug Intelligence Publications.

Kramer DM (1984). Basic principles of magnetic resonance imaging. *Radiologic Clinics of North America,* 22(4): 765–778.

Kurytka D (1996). Advances in HIV/AIDS care. *The Nursing Spectrum,* 5(26): 6.

Locher AW (1996, July/August). Ethics, women with HIV, and procreation: Implications for nursing practice. *Journal of Obstetric, Gynecologic and Neonatal Nursing,* 25(6): 465–469.

Lopez M, Fleisher T, deShazo RD (1992). Use and interpretation of diagnostic immunologic laboratory tests. *Journal of the American Medical Association,* 268(20): 2970–2990.

Masland T, Norland R (2000, January 17). 10 Orphans. *Newsweek,* 42–45.

Maule WF (1994). Screening for colorectal cancer by nurse endoscopists. *New England Journal of Medicine,* 330(3): 183–184.

McClatchey KD ed. (1994). *Clinical Laboratory Medicine.* Baltimore: Williams & Wilkins.

Mellico KD (1993). Interpretation of abnormal laboratory values in older adults. Part I. *Journal of Gerontological Nursing,* 19(1): 39–45.

Mennemeyer ST, Winkelman JW (1993). Searching for inaccuracy in clinical laboratory testing using Medicare data: Evidence for prothrombin time. *Journal of the American Medical Association,* 269: 1030–1033.

Mettler FA (1996). *Essentials of radiology.* Philadelphia: WB Saunders.

Miller WF, Scacci R, Fast LR (1987). *Laboratory Evaluation of Pulmonary Function.* Philadelphia: Lippincott.

Moran BA (2000). Maternal infections. In: Mattson, S, Smith, JE, eds. *Core Curriculum for Maternal-Newborn Nursing.* 2nd ed. Philadelphia: WB Saunders, 419–448.

Moulton-Barrett R, Triadafilopoulos G, Michener R, et al. (1993). Serum C-bicarbonate in the assessment of gastric *Helicobacter pylori* urease activity. *American Journal of Gastroenterology,* 88(3): 369–373.

Myers MC, Page MD (1996). Caring for the laboring woman with HIV infection on AIDS. In: Martin EJ, ed. *Intrapartum Management Modules.* 2nd ed. Baltimore: Wilkins and Wilkins, pp 451–486.

National Committee for Clinical Laboratory Standards (1995). *How to define, determine, and utilize reference intervals in the clinical laboratory, approved guidelines.* NCCLS Document C-28-A. 25(4).

National Multiple Sclerosis Society. (1987). MRI—no mystique. *Inside,* 5(4): 24–27.

Noble D (1993). Controversies in the clinical chemistry laboratory. *Analytical Chemistry,* 84(6): 797–800.

Norris MKG (1993). Evaluating serum triglyceride levels. *Nursing 93,* 23(5): 31.

Nyamath A, Flemmig DS (1997). Prevention consideration for women. In: Fahey JL, Flemmig, DS, eds. *AIDS/HIV Reference Guide for Medical Professionals.* 4th ed. Baltimore: Wilkins and Wilkins, pp 232–242.

Pagana KD, Pagana TJ (1999). *Diagnostic and Laboratory Test Reference.* 4th ed. St. Louis: C. V. Mosby Co.

Pasquale MJ (1992). *Application of Radionuclide Stress Tests.* Wilmington, DE: Cardiac Diagnostic Center.

Peterson KL, Nicod P (1997). *Cardiac catheterization methods, diagnosis, and therapy.* Philadelphia: WB Saunders.

Peterson KJ, Solie CJ (1994). Interpreting laboratory values in chronic renal insufficiency. *American Journal of Nursing,* 94(5): 56B, 56E, 56H.

Porembka, DT (1996). Transesophageal echocardiography. *Critical Care Clinics,* 12(4): 875–903.

Purvis A (1997, January 6; 1996, December 30). The global epidemic. *Time,* 148(29): 76–78.

Rakel RE (1996). *Saunders' manual of medical practice.* Philadelphia: WB Saunders.

Ravel R (1995). *Clinical laboratory medicine.* 6th ed. Chicago: Year Book.

Reed JD, Soulen RL (1988). Cardiovascular MRI: Current role in patient management. *Radiologic Clinics of North America,* 26: 589–600.

Renkes, J (1993). GI endoscopy: Managing the full scope of care. *Nursing 93,* 23(6): 50–55.

Romancyzuk AN, Brown JP (1994). Folic acid will reduce risk of neural tube defects. *American Journal of Maternal Child Nursing,* 19(6): 331–334.

Rotello, LS, Radin, EJ, Jastremski, MS, et al. (1994). MRI protocol for critically ill patients. *American Journal of Critical Care,* 3(3): 187–190.

Sacher RA, McPherson RA (1991). *Widmann's Clinical Interpretation of Laboratory Tests.* 10th ed. Philadelphia: F.A. Davis.

Sayad DE, Clarke GD, Peshock RM (1995). Magnetic resonance imaging of the heart and its role in current cardiology. *Current Opinion in Cardiology.* 10(6): 640–649.

Selig PM (1996). Pearls for practice: Management of anticoagulation therapy with the international normalized ratio. *Journal of the American Academy of Nursing Practitioners,* 8(2): 77–80.

Sipes, C. (1995, January/February). Guidelines for assessing HIV in women. *MCN: The American Journal of Maternal Child Nursing,* 20(1): 29–33.

Smith S, Forman D (1994). Laboratory analysis of cerebrospinal fluid. *Clinical Laboratory Science,* 7(4): 32–38.

Strimike C (1996). Understanding intravascular ultrasound. *American Journal of Nursing,* 96(6): 40–43.

Stringer M, Librizzi R (1994). Complications following prenatal genetic procedures. *Nursing Research,* 43(2): 184–186.

Sutton D (1995). Angiography. In: Sutton D, Young JWR. *A Concise Textbook of Clinical Imaging.* 2nd ed. St. Louis: CV Mosby.

TB Facts for Health Care Workers (1993). Atlanta, GA: Department of Health and Human Services, Public Health Service, Centers for Disease Control and Prevention, National Center for Prevention Services, Division of Tuberculosis Elimination.

Thompson E, Detwiler DS, Nelson CM (1996). Dobutamine stress echocardiography: A new, noninvasive method for detecting ischemic heart disease. *Heart & Lung,* 25(2): 87–97.

Thompson L (1995). Percutaneous endoscopic gastrostomy. *Nursing 95,* 25(4): 62–63.

Thrall JH, Ziessman HA (1995). *Nuclear Medicine.* St. Louis: CV Mosby.

Tietz NW ed. (1997). *Clinical Guide to Laboratory Tests.* 3rd ed. Philadelphia: Saunders.

Topol EJ, Holmes DR, Rogers WJ (1991). Coronary angiography after thrombolytic therapy for acute myocardial infarction. *Annual of Internal Medicine,* 114(10): 877–885.

Vannier MW, Marsh JL (1996). Three-dimensional imaging surgical planning, and image-guided therapy. *Radiologic Clinics of North America,* 34(3): 545–561.

Wallach J (1998). *Handbook of Interpretation of Diagnostic Tests.* Philadelphia: Lippincott-Raven.

Washington JA (1993). Laboratory diagnosis of infectious diseases. *Infectious Disease Clinics of North America,* 7(2): 13.

Wilde P, Hartnell GC (1995). Cardiac imaging. In: Sutton D, Young JWR. *A Concise Textbook of Clinical Imaging.* 2nd ed. St. Louis: CV Mosby.

Williamson MR (1996). *Essentials of ultrasound.* Philadelphia: WB Saunders.

Wofson AB, Paris PM (1996). *Diagnostic testing in emergency medicine.* Philadelphia: WB Saunders.

Womack C, Thomas JD (1996). Easing the way through an MRI. *RN,* 59(10): 34–37.

Wong ND, Vo W, Abrahamson D, et al. (1994). Detection of coronary artery calcium by ultrafast computed tomography and its relation to clinical evidence of coronary artery disease. *American Journal of Cardiology,* 73: 223–227.

Wormser GP, Horowitz H (1992). Care of the adult patient with HIV infection. In: Wormser GP, ed. *AIDS and Other Manifestations of HIV Infection.* 2nd ed. New York: Raven, pp 173–200.

Young SW (1984). *Nuclear Magnetic Resonance Imaging.* New York: Raven Press.

Zaret BL, Wackers FJ (1993). Nuclear cardiology. *New England Journal of Medicine,* 329(12): 855–863.

Zubal IG (1996). The evolution of imaging devices: A constant challenge with combining progress. In: *Yearbook of Nuclear Medicine.* St. Louis: CV Mosby.

INDEX

ABGs, 47–49
ACE, 33–35
Acetaminophen, 8, 9
Acid-fast bacilli (TB culture), 101
Acid perfusion test, 368–372
Acid phosphatase (ACP), 9–11
ACTH stimulation test, 13
ACTH suppression test, 12, 13
ACTH, 12–14
Actinomyces israelii, 136
Activated partial thromboplastin time (APTT), 234, 235
Adenovirus antibody, 11, 12
ADH 30, 40
Adrenocorticotropic hormone, (ACTH), 12–14
Adrenocorticotropic hormone suppression, 103–105
A/G ratio, 16
Alanine aminotransferase (ALT), 14, 15
Albumin, 16, 17, 256, 257
Alcohol (ethyl), 17, 18
Aldolase (ALD), 18, 19
Aldosterone, 20–22
  serum, 20–22
  urine, 20–22
Alkaline phosphatase (ALP), 22, 23
  isoenzyme, 22
ALP, 22, 23
Alpha fetoprotein (AFP), 25–27
$Alpha_1$-trypsin inhibitor, 24, 25
$Alpha_1$-antitrypsin, 24, 25
ALT/SGPT 14, 15
Ambulatory electrocardiography, 379–381
Amikacin, 27–29
Aminoglycosides, 27–29
Aminophylline, 283–284
Amitriptyline, 37–39
Ammonia, 29, 30
Amnioscopy, 319
Amniotic fluid analysis, 319, 320
Amylase, 31–33
  isoenzymes, 31

Amylase (*cont.*)
serum, 31–33
urine, 31–33
ANA, 44, 45
Angiocardiography, 337–339
Angiography, 320–323
cerebral, 321
pulmonary, 321, 322
renal, 321, 322
Angiotensin-converting enzyme (ACE), 33–35
Anion gap, 36, 37
Antibiotic susceptibility, 36, 37
Antibiotic sensitivity test, 36, 37
Antibody screen test, 86, 87
Antidepressants, 37–39
Antidiuretic hormone (ADH), 39, 40
Antiglomerular basement membrane antibody (AntiGBM, AGBM), 41, 42
Antihemophilic factor, 122–124
Antimicrosomal antibody, 284, 285
Antimitochondrial antibody (AMA), 42, 43
Antimyocardial antibody, 43, 44
Antinuclear antibodies (ANA), 44, 45
Antisperm antibody test, 276, 277
Antistreptolin O, 45, 46
Antithyroglobulln antibody, 284, 285
APTT, 234, 235
Arterial blood gases (ABGs), 47–49
Arteriography, 320–323
Arthrography, 323–325
Arthroscopy, 325, 326
ASO, 45, 46
Aspartate aminotransferase (AST), 49–51
Aspergillus, 143
Aspirin, 275, 276
AST/SGOT, 49–51
Atrial natriuretic hormone (ANH), 51, 52

Barium swallow, 377–379
Barium enema, 326–328
Basophils, 309, 310
Bernstein test, 368–372
Bibliography, 489–497
Bilirubin, 52–56
direct, 52–54
indirect, 52—54
total, 52—54
urine, 55, 56
Biopsy, 328–332
bone marrow, 329, 330
breast, 329, 330
endometrium, 329, 330
kidney, 329–332
liver, 329–332
Blastomyces dermatitidis, 136, 426
Bleeding time, 56, 57
Ivy method, 56, 57
Duke method, 56, 57
Blood gases, 47–49
Blood urea nitrogen (BUN), 58, 59

Blood urea nitrogen/Creatinine ratio, 60, 61
Blood typing tests, 97, 98
Bone absorpiometry, 332, 333
Bone densitometry, 332, 333
Bone density, 332, 333
Bone marrow biopsy, 329, 330
Bone mineral density (BMD), 332, 333
Breast biopsy, 329, 330
Bronchogram, 334, 335
Bronchography, 334, 335
Bronchoscopy, 335–337
Brucella, 126
BUN, 58, 59

C-reactive protein (CRP), 91, 92
Calcitonin, 61, 62
Calcium (CA), 63–65
  serum, 63–65
  urine, 63–65
California encephalitis virus, 111
Candida albicans, 137
Carbon dioxide combining power, 65, 66
Carbon monoxide (CO), 67, 68
Carboxyhemoglobin, 67, 68
Carcinoembryonic antigen
(CEA), 68, 69
Cardiac angiography, 337–339
Cardiac catheterization, 337–339
CAT scan, 350–354
Catecholamines, 69–73
  plasma, 69–73
  urine, 69–73
CEA, 68, 69
Cerebral angiography, 321
Cerebrospinal fluid (CSF), 73, 74
Ceruloplasmin (Cp), 74–76
Cervical cancer test, 405–408
Cervicography, 340, 341
Chlamydia test, 76–78
  C psittaci, 76, 77
  C trachomatic, 76–77
Chloride (Cl), 78–80
Cholangiography, 341–343
  intravenous, 341, 342
  percutaneous, 341, 342
  T-tube, 341, 342
Cholecystography, 343–345
Cholesterol, 80, 81
Chorionic somatomammotropin, 185–187
Chorionic villi biopsy (CVB), 345, 346
Christmas factor, 122–124
Clinical problems with laboratory and diagnostic tests, 475–478
  cerebrovascular accident, 475
  cholecystitis, 475
  cirrhosis of the liver, 475
  colorectal cancer, 475
  congestive heart failure (CHF), 476
  deep-vein thrombophlebitis, 476

Clinical problems with laboratory and diagnostic tests *(cont.)*
- diabetes mellitus, 476
- emphysema, 476
- gynecologic problems, 478
- lung cancer, 476
- multiple sclerosis, 476
- myocardial infarction, 476
- osteoporosis, 477
- pancreatitis, 477
- peptic ulcer, 477
- pneumonia, 477
- pregnancy and fetal distress, 478
- pulmonary embolism (PE), 477
- renal failure, 477
- rheumatoid arthritis, 477
- systemic lupus erythematosus, 477
- ulcerative colitis, 478

CO_2 combining power, 65, 66
Coagulation factors, 122–125
Coccidioides immitis, 136
Coccidoidomycosis, 426, 427
Cold agglutinins, 81–83
Cold hemagglutinin, 81–83
Colonoscopy, 346–348
Color flow Doppler echocardiography, 357–359
Colposcopy, 348–350
Complement, 83–85
- C_3, 84, 85
- C_4, 84, 85
- total, 83, 84

Computed tomography scan, 350–354
- abdominal, 351–353
- bone, 353
- chest, 351, 353
- eye, 351
- head, 351, 352
- neck, 351, 352
- pelvis, 352, 353
- sinus, 352, 353
- spine, 351, 353

Computed transaxial tomography (CTT), 350–354
Considerations for use of laboratory tests, 1–3
Considerations for use of diagnostic tests, 315, 316
Coombs' test, 85–87
- direct, 85, 86
- indirect, 86, 87

Copper (Cu), 87–89
Coronary arteriography, 337–339
Corticotropin, 12–14
Corticotropin-releasing factor (CRF), 12–14
Cortisol, 89–91
CPK, 95–97
Creatine phosphokinase (CPK), 95–97
- isoenzymes, 95, 96

Creatinine (Cr), 92, 93
- serum, 92, 93
- urine, 92, 93

Crcatinine clearance, 93–93
Crossmatch, 97, 98

Cryoglobulins, 98, 99
CSF, 73, 74
CT scan, 350–354
Culture and sensitivity test (C & S), 36, 37
Cultures, 99–103
blood, 100
sputum, 100, 101
stool, 101
throat, 101
urine, 101
wound, 101
Cytomegalovirus (CMV) antibody, 102, 103
CVB, 345, 346
Cystogram, 354
Cystography, 354
Cystoscopy, 354–356
Cystourethroscopy, 354–356

D-Xylose absorption test, 109, 110
Datril, 8, 9
Desipramine HCI, 37–39
Dexamethasone suppression test (DST), 103–105
Digoxin, 106, 107
Dilantin, 107, 108
Diphenylhydantoin, 107, 108
Direct antiglobulin test, 85, 86
DST test, 103–105
Duodenoscopy, 373, 374
Dynamic electrocardiography, 379–381

E_1, 120–122
E_2, 116, 117
E_3, 117, 118
E_4 115, 116
Eastern equine encephalitis virus, 111
ECG/EKG, 361–363
Echogram, 435–442
Echography, 435–442
EEG, 364, 365
Electrocardiogram, 361–363
Electrocardiography (ECG), 356–361
color Doppler, 357, 359
contrast, 358–360
M-mode, 357, 359
spectral Doppler, 357, 359
stress, 358–360
transesophageal (TEE), 357, 358, 360
two-dimensional (2D), 357, 359
Electroencephalogram, 364, 365
Electroencephalography, 364, 365
Electromyography (EMG), 365–367
Electromyogram, 365–367
EMG, 365–367
Emission computed tomography (ECT) scan, 408–410
Encephalitis virus antibody, 111, 112
eastern equine, 111
California, 111
St. Louis, 111
Venezuelan equine, 111
Western equine, 111
Enterovirus group, 112, 113

Endometrial biopsy, 329, 330
Endoscopic retrograde cholangiopancreatography (ERCP), 367, 368
Eosinophils, 309, 310
ERCP, 367, 368
Erythrocyte sedimentation rate (ESR), 113, 114
Esophageal manometry, 368–372
Esophageal studies, 368–372
 acid perfusion, 368–372
 esophageal acidity, 368–372
 esophageal manometry, 368–372
Esophageal acidity, 368–372
Esophagogastroduodenoscopy, 373–374
Esophagogastroscopy, 373, 374
Esophagoscopy, 373–374
ESR, 113, 114
Estetrol (E_4), 115, 116
Estradiol (E_2), 116, 117
Estriol (E_3), 117, 118
Estrogen, 119, 120
 serum, 119, 120
 urine, 119, 120
Estrone (E_1), 120–122
Ethanol, 17, 18
Excretory urography, 384, 385

Factor I, 122–124, 130, 131
Factor VIII, 122–124
Factor assay, 122–125
Fasting blood sugar, 142–144
FBS, 142–144
FDP, 129, 130
Feasting blood sugar, 142–144
Febrile agglutinins, 125–127
Ferritin, 127–129
Fibrin degradation products (FDP), 129, 130
Fibrin split products (FSP), 129, 130
Fibrin stabilizing factor, 122–124
Fibrinogen, 122–124, 130, 131
Fluorescent treponemal antibody absorption, 134, 135
Foam stability test, 320
Folate, 131, 132
Folic acid, 131, 132
Follicle-stimulating hormone (FSH), 132–134
FSH, 132–134
FTA-ABS, 134, 135
Fungal antibody test, 135–137
Fungal organism test, 135–137

Gallbladder radiography, 342–345
Gallbladder series, 343–345
Gamma-glutamyl transferase (GGT), 137–139
Gamma-glutamyl transpeptidase (GGTP), 137–139
Gastric analysis, 374–377
 basal, 375, 376
 stimulation, 374–376
 tubeless, 374–376
Gastrin, 139, 140
Gastrointestinal (GI) series, 377–379

Gastrointestinal test, 326–328, 377–379
lower, 326–328
upper, 377–379
Gastroscopy, 363, 364
Gentamicin, 27–29
GGT, 137–139
G1 series, 377–379
Globulin, 256–258
Glomerular basement membrane antibody, 41, 42
Glucagon, 140–142
Glucose self-monitoring devices, 145–147
Glucose tolerance test, 148, 149
Glucose blood sugar, 142–144
Glucose-6-phosphate dehydrogenase (G6PD), 144, 145
Glycosylated hemoglobin, 158–160
Growth hormone (GH). 150, 151
Guthrie test, 235–237

Hageman factor, 122–124
HAI for rubella, 274, 275
Haptoglobin, 151, 152
HAV, 161, 163, 164
Hb A_{1c}, 158–160
HBV, 161, 163, 164
HCG, 171–173
Hct, 154–156
HCV, 162–164
HDV, 163,164
Helicobacter pylori, 153, 154
Hemagglutination inhibition test (HAI, HI), 274, 275
Hemoglobin A_{1c}, 158–160
Hematocrit (Hct), 154–156
Hemoglobin (Hb), 156–158
Hemoglobin electrophoresis, 160, 161
Hepatitis A virus, 161, 163–165
Hepatitis Bc antigen antibody (anti-HBc), 162
Hepatitis Be antigen antibody (anti-HBe), 162
Hepatitis Be antigen (HbeAg), 162
Hepatitis B surface antigen (HbsAg), 162, 166, 167
Hepatitis B surface antigen antibody (anti-HBs), 162
Hepatitis B virus, 162–164
Hepatitis C virus, 162–164
Hepatitis C virus antibody (anti-HCV), 163
Hepatitis D antigen (HDAg), 164
Hepatitis D virus, 163, 164
Hepatitis E virus, 163, 164
Hepatitis profile, 161–164
HERPCHEK, 167
Herpes simplex virus (HSV) antibody test, 167–169
Heterophile antibody, 169, 170
HEV, 163, 164
Hexosaminidase test, 170, 171
Hgb/Hb electrophoresis, 160, 161
Hgb, 156–158
5-HIAA, 189, 190

High density lipoprotein (HDL), 210, 211
Histoplasma capsulatum, 136, 147
HIV, 173–184
HLA typing, 184, 185
Holter monitoring, 379–381
HSV, 167–169
Human chorionic gonadotropin (HCG), 171–173
Human growth hormone (HGH), 150, 151
Human immunodeficiency virus (HIV), 173–184
Human leukocyte antigens (HLA), 184, 185
Human placental Iactogen (HPL), 186, 187
17-Hydroxycorticosteroids (17-OHCS), 187, 188
5-Hydroxyindolacetic acid (5-HIAA), 189, 190
Hyperkalemia, 245–247
Hyperlipidemia, 211, 212
Hypernatremia, 279–281
Hypokalemia, 244–246
Hyponatremia, 279–281
Hypotonic duodenography, 378, 379
Hysterosalpingogram, 381, 382
Hysterosalpingography. 381, 382
Hysteroscopy, 383, 384

IgA, 190, 191
IgD, 190, 191
IgE, 190–192
IgG, 190, 191
IgM, 190–192
Imipramine HCl, 37–39
Immunoglobulins (Ig), 190–192
INR, 194, 195, 260–262
Insulin test, 192–194
Insulin antibody test, 193, 194
International normalized ratio (INR), 194, 195, 260–262
Interstitial cell stimulating hormone (ICSH), 213–215
Intravenous pyelography (IVP), 384, 385
Intravenous pyelogram, 384, 385
Iron, 195–197
Iron-binding capacity (IBC), 195–197

Kanamycin, 27–29
I 7-Ketosteroids (17-KS), 197, 198
Kidney biopsy, 329–332

L/S ratio, 206, 207
Laboratory test values for adults and children, 449–473
Lactic dehydrogenase (LDH/LD), 200, 201
  isoenzymes, 200, 201
Lactic acid, 199, 200
Lactogen, 253, 254
Lactogenic hormone, 253, 254
Lactose, 202, 203

Lactose tolerance test, 202, 203
Lanoxin, 106, 107
LAP, 208, 209
LDH, 200, 201
LDH isoenzymes, 200, 201
LE cell test, 204, 205
LE prep, 204, 205
LE slide cell test, 204, 205
Lead, 203, 204
Lecithin/sphingomyelin (L/S) ratio, 206, 207
Legionnaire's antibody test, 207, 208
Leucine aminopeptidase, (LAP), 208, 209
Leukocytes, 306–308
LH, 213–215
Lipase, 209, 210
Lipid composition, 210, 211
Lipids, 210–212
Lipoprotein electrophoresis, 210–212
Lipoprotein phenotype, 211
Lipoproteins, 210–212
List of laboratory tests, 4–7
Lithium, 212, 213
Liver biopsy, 329–332
Low-density lipoproteins, 210, 211
Lower gastrointestinal, 326–328
Lupus test, 204, 205
Lupus erythematosus test, 204, 205
Luteinizing hormone (LH), 213–215
    serum, 213–215
    urine, 213–215
Lyme disease antibody test, 215–217
Lymphangiography 386, 387
Lymphocytes, 309, 310
Lymphocytes (T and B) assay, 217, 218
Lymphography, 386, 387

Magnesium (Mg), 218–221
Magnetic resonance angiography (MRA), 389
Magnetic resonance imaging (MRI), 388–390
Mammogram, 390–392
Mammography, 390–392
Mantoux test, 426
MCH, 264, 265
MCHC, 264–265
MCV, 264, 265
Mean corpuscular hemoglobin (MCH), 264, 265
Mean corpuscular hemoglobin concentration (MCHC), 264, 265
Mean corpuscular volume (MCV), 264, 265
Metabolic alkalosis, 47–49
Metabolic acidosis, 47–49
Monocytes, 309, 310
Mono-spot, 169, 170
Mono-vacc test, 426
MRI, 388–390

MUGA scan, 392, 393
Multigated aquisition (MUGA) scan, 392, 393
Mump antibody, 221, 222
Mycotic infection test, 135–137, 426, 427
Myelography, 393–395
Myelogram, 393–395
Myoglobin, 223, 224

5′N, 224, 225
Netilmicin, 27–29
Neutrophils, 308–310
NMR, 388–390
Nortriptyline, 37–39
Nuclear dobutamine stress test, 430, 431, 435
Nuclear magnetic resonance (NMR), 388–390
Nuclear Persantine stress test, 430, 432, 434, 435
5′Nucleotidase (5′N or 5′NT), 224, 225
Nuclear scans, 395–405
  bone, 396, 398
  brain, 396, 398
  brain perfusion, 396, 399
  colon and ovary, 397, 401
  gallbladder study, 397, 403
  gastric emptying study, 397, 402, 403
  gastrointestinal bleeding study, 397, 403
  heart, 397, 400
  kidney, 397, 400
  liver and spleen, 397, 400, 401
  lung, 397, 403, 404
  thyroid, 397, 404

Occult blood, 226, 227
17-OHCS, 187, 188
Opiates, 227–229
Oral glucose tolerance test, 148, 149
Organ–donor tissue typing, 184, 185
Osmolality, 229–231
  serum, 229–231
  urine, 229–231
Ova and parasites. 231, 232

Panadol, 8, 9
PAP smear, 405–408
Papanicolaou (PAP) smear, 405–408
Paracetatmol, 8, 9
Parasites, 427
Parathyroid hormone (PTH), 233, 234
Partial thromboplastin time (PTT), 234, 235
Pasteurella, 126
Percutaneous cholangiography, 341, 342
PET, 408–410
Phenylketonuria (PKU), 235–237
Phlebography, 442–444

Phospholipids, 210
Phosphorus (P), 238, 239
PKU, 235–237
Plasma renin activity (PRA), 267, 268
Plasma thromboplastin antecedent (PTA), 122–124
Platelet adhesions, 239–241
Platelet aggregation, 239–241
Platelet antibody test, 241, 242
Platelet count, 242–244
Porter-Siber chromogens, 187, 188
Positron emission tomography (PET), 408–410
Postprandial blood sugar, 142–144
Potassium (K), 244–247
PPBS, 142–144
Prealbumin assay, 247–249
Pregnanediol, 249, 250
Pregnanetriol, 250, 251
Proaccelerin, 122–124
Proconvertin stable factor, 122–124
Proctoscopy, 410–412
Proctosigmoidoscopy, 410–412
Progesterone, 251–253
Prolactin (PRL), 253, 254
Prostate-specific antigen (PSA), 255
Prostatic acid phosphatase (PAP), 9–11
Protein, 256–260
  electrophoresis, 256–258
  total, 256–258
  urine, 259, 260
Protein electrophoresis, 256–258
  albumin, 256, 257
  globulin, 256–258
Prothrombin, 122–124
Prothrombin time (PT), 260–262
PSA, 255
Psittaci, 76, 77
PT, 260–262
PTT, 234, 235
Pulmonary angiography, 321, 322
Pulmonary ventilation scan, 444, 445
Pulmonary diagnostic tests, 412–420
Pulmonary function tests, 412–420
  body plethysmograph, 417
  bronchial provocative studies, 416, 419
  diffusion capacity test, 416
  exercise studies, 416, 419
  flow volume loop, 413–415
  forced vital capacity, 413
  lung volume measurements, 413
  nutritional studies, 417–419
  pulse oximetry, 417
  slow vital capacity tests, 412, 413
Pulse oximetry, 417

RA latex fixation, 269–271
Rabies antibody test, 262, 263
Radioactive iodine (RAI) uptake test, 420–422
Radiography, 445–448
Radioiodine thyroid uptake test, 420–422

Radioisotope imaging, 395–405
Radionuclide scans, 395–405
RAI uptake test, 420–422
Rapid plasma reagin (RPR), 263, 264
RBC count, 264–266
RBC indices, 264–266
Red blood cell indices, 264–266
  MCH, 264, 265
  MCHC, 264, 265
  MCV, 264, 265
  RDW, 264, 265
Renal angiography, 321, 322
Renin, 267, 268
Respiratory alkalosis, 47–49
Respiratory acidosis, 47–49
Reticulocyte count, 268, 269
Retinol, 304, 305
Rh factor, 271, 272
Rh typing, 271, 272
Rheumatoid arthritis (RA), 270, 271
Rheumatoid factor (RF), 270, 271
Roentgenography, 445–448
Rotavirus antigen, 272–274
RPR, 263, 264
Rubella antibody detection, 274, 275

Salicylate, 275, 276
Salmonellosis, 126
Schilling test, 422–424
Sedimentation (Sed) rate, 113, 114
Semen analysis, 276, 277
Semen examination, 276, 277
Serum glutamic pyruvic transaminase (SGPT), 14, 15
Serum glutamic oxaloacetic transaminase (SGOT), 49–51
SGOT, 49–51
SGPT, 14, 15
Sickle cell screening test, 278, 279
Sickle cell test, 278, 279
Sigmoidoscopy 410–412
Sinus endoscopy, 424, 425
Skin tests, 426–428
  blastomycosis, 426, 427
  coccidioidomycosis, 426, 427
  histoplasmosis, 427
  testing methods, 426
  toxoplasmosis, 427
  trichinosis, 427
  tuberculosis, 426
Slo-Phyllin, 283, 284
Small bowel series, 377–379
Sodium (Na), 279–281
  serum, 279–281
  urine, 279, 281
Somatotrophic hormone (STH), 150, 151
Sonogram, 435–442
Spinal fluid, 73, 74
St. Louis encephalitis virus, 111
Stress/exercise testing, 428–435
  bicycle ergometer test, 432

dobutamine, 430, 431, 435
exercise perfusion test, 432
persantine, 430, 432, 434, 435
Stuart factor, 122–124

T_3, 293, 294
T_3 RIA, 293, 294
T_3 RU, 294, 295
T_3 uptake, 294, 295
T_4, 287, 288
TDM, 479–487
Tempra, 8, 9
Testosterone, 282
Theo-Dur, 283, 284
Theolaire, 283, 284
Theophylline, 283, 284
Therapeutic drug monitoring (TDM), 479–487
Thrombocyte count, 242–244
Thromboplastin, 122–124
Thyroid antibodies (TA), 284, 285.
Thyroid-stimulating hormone (TSH), 286, 287
Thyroxine (T_4), 287, 288
TIBC, 195–197
Tine test, 426
Tobramycin, 27–29
Torch battery, 289, 290
Torch screen test, 289, 290
Torch titer, 289, 290
Total iron-binding capacity, (TIBC), 195–197
Toxoplasmosis antibody test, 290, 291
Trachomatis, 76, 77
Transthyretin (TTR), 247–249
Triglycerides, 292, 293
Triiodothyronine (T_3), 293, 294
Triiodothyronine resin uptake (T_3 RU), 294, 295
Tryptophan-rich prealbumin, 247–249
T-tube cholangiography, 341, 342
Tylenol 8, 9
Type and crossmatch, 97, 98

Ultrasonography, 435–442
abdominal aorta, 436, 440
arteries and veins (doppler), 436, 440
brain, 436, 440
breast, 436, 437, 440
carotid, 437
eye and eye orbit, 437, 439–441
gallbladder, 437, 439
heart, 437, 439, 441
kidneys, 437, 439
liver, 437, 439
pancreas, 438, 439
pelvic, 437, 438, 441
prostate, 438, 439, 441
scrotum and testes, 438, 439, 441
spleen, 438, 440

Ultrasonography *(cont.)*
thoracic, 438, 440
thyroid, 438, 440
Ultrasound, 435–442
Upper GI series, 377–379
Urea nitrogen creatinine ratio, 58, 60, 61
Uric acid, 296–298
serum, 296–298
urine, 296–298
Urinalysis, 298–301
Urobilinogen, 301, 302

Vasopressor, 39, 40
Vectorcardiography, 361, 362
Vectorcardiogram, 361, 362
Venography, 442–444
Ventilation scan, 444, 445
Venezuelan equine encephalitis virus, 111
Very low-density lipoproteins, 211
Viral cultures, 302, 303
Vitamin A, 304, 305
Vitamin B_{12}, 305, 306
Vitamin B_1, deficiency test, 422–424
Vollmer's patch test, 426

WBCs, 306–308
Weil-Felix, 126
Western equine encephalitis virus, 111
White blood cells, 306–308
differential, 308–311
total, 306–308

White blood cell differential, 308–311
basophils, 309, 310
eosinophils, 309, 310
lymphocytes, 309, 310
monocytes, 309, 310
neutrophils, 308–310

Widal test, 126

Wound culture, 100, 101

X-ray, 445–448
abdominal, 446, 447
chest, 446, 447
heart, 446, 447
KUB (kidney, ureter, bladder) 446, 447
skeletal, 446, 447
skull, 446, 447

Zinc, 311–313

Zinc protoporphyrin (ZPP), 313, 314

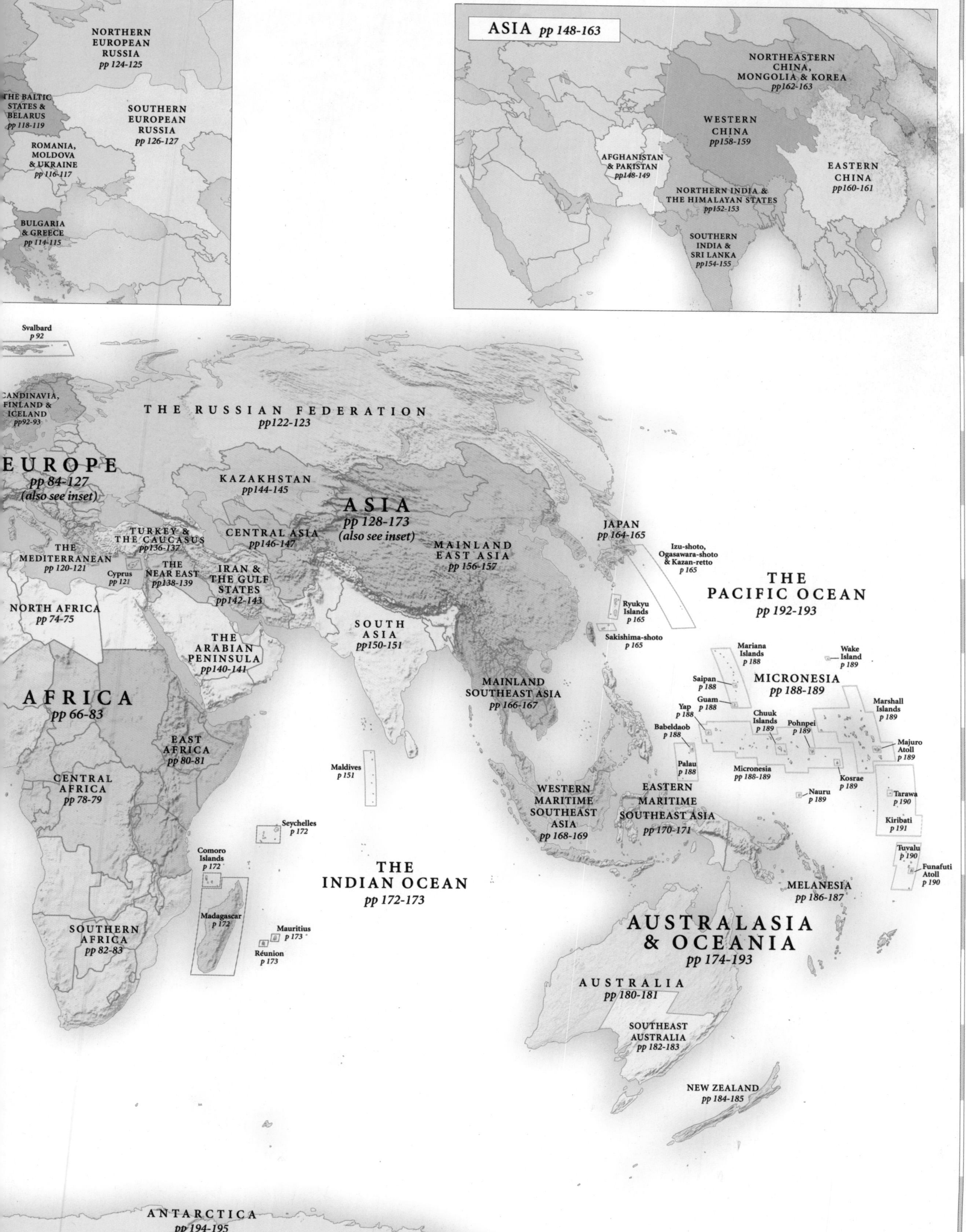

NORTHERN EUROPEAN RUSSIA pp 124-125
THE BALTIC STATES & BELARUS pp 118-119
SOUTHERN EUROPEAN RUSSIA pp 126-127
ROMANIA, MOLDOVA & UKRAINE pp 116-117
BULGARIA & GREECE pp 114-115
ASIA pp 148-163
NORTHEASTERN CHINA, MONGOLIA & KOREA pp162-163
WESTERN CHINA pp158-159
AFGHANISTAN & PAKISTAN pp148-149
EASTERN CHINA pp160-161
NORTHERN INDIA & THE HIMALAYAN STATES pp152-153
SOUTHERN INDIA & SRI LANKA pp154-155
Svalbard p 92
SCANDINAVIA, FINLAND & ICELAND pp92-93
THE RUSSIAN FEDERATION pp122-123
EUROPE pp 84-127 (also see inset)
KAZAKHSTAN pp144-145
ASIA pp 128-173 (also see inset)
TURKEY & THE CAUCASUS pp136-137
CENTRAL ASIA pp146-147
THE MEDITERRANEAN pp 120-121
Cyprus pp 121
THE NEAR EAST pp138-139
IRAN & THE GULF STATES pp142-143
MAINLAND EAST ASIA pp 156-157
JAPAN pp 164-165
Izu-shoto, Ogasawara-shoto & Kazan-retto p 165
THE PACIFIC OCEAN pp 192-193
NORTH AFRICA pp 74-75
SOUTH ASIA pp150-151
Ryukyu Islands p 165
Sakishima-shoto p 165
THE ARABIAN PENINSULA pp140-141
Mariana Islands p 188
Wake Island p 189
MICRONESIA pp 188-189
Saipan p 188
Guam p 188
Yap p 188
MAINLAND SOUTHEAST ASIA pp 166-167
AFRICA pp 66-83
Marshall Islands p 189
Chuuk Islands p 189
Pohnpei p 189
Babeldaob p 188
EAST AFRICA pp 80-81
Majuro Atoll p 189
Palau p 188
Micronesia pp 188-189
Kosrae p 189
Maldives p 151
CENTRAL AFRICA pp 78-79
WESTERN MARITIME SOUTHEAST ASIA pp 168-169
EASTERN MARITIME SOUTHEAST ASIA pp 170-171
Nauru p 189
Tarawa p 190
Kiribati p 191
Seychelles p 172
Comoro Islands p 172
THE INDIAN OCEAN pp 172-173
Tuvalu p 190
Funafuti Atoll p 190
MELANESIA pp 186-187
Madagascar p 172
Mauritius p 173
Réunion p 173
SOUTHERN AFRICA pp 82-83
AUSTRALASIA & OCEANIA pp 174-193
AUSTRALIA pp 180-181
SOUTHEAST AUSTRALIA pp 182-183
NEW ZEALAND pp 184-185
ANTARCTICA pp 194-195

DORLING KINDERSLEY

CONCISE ATLAS *of the* WORLD

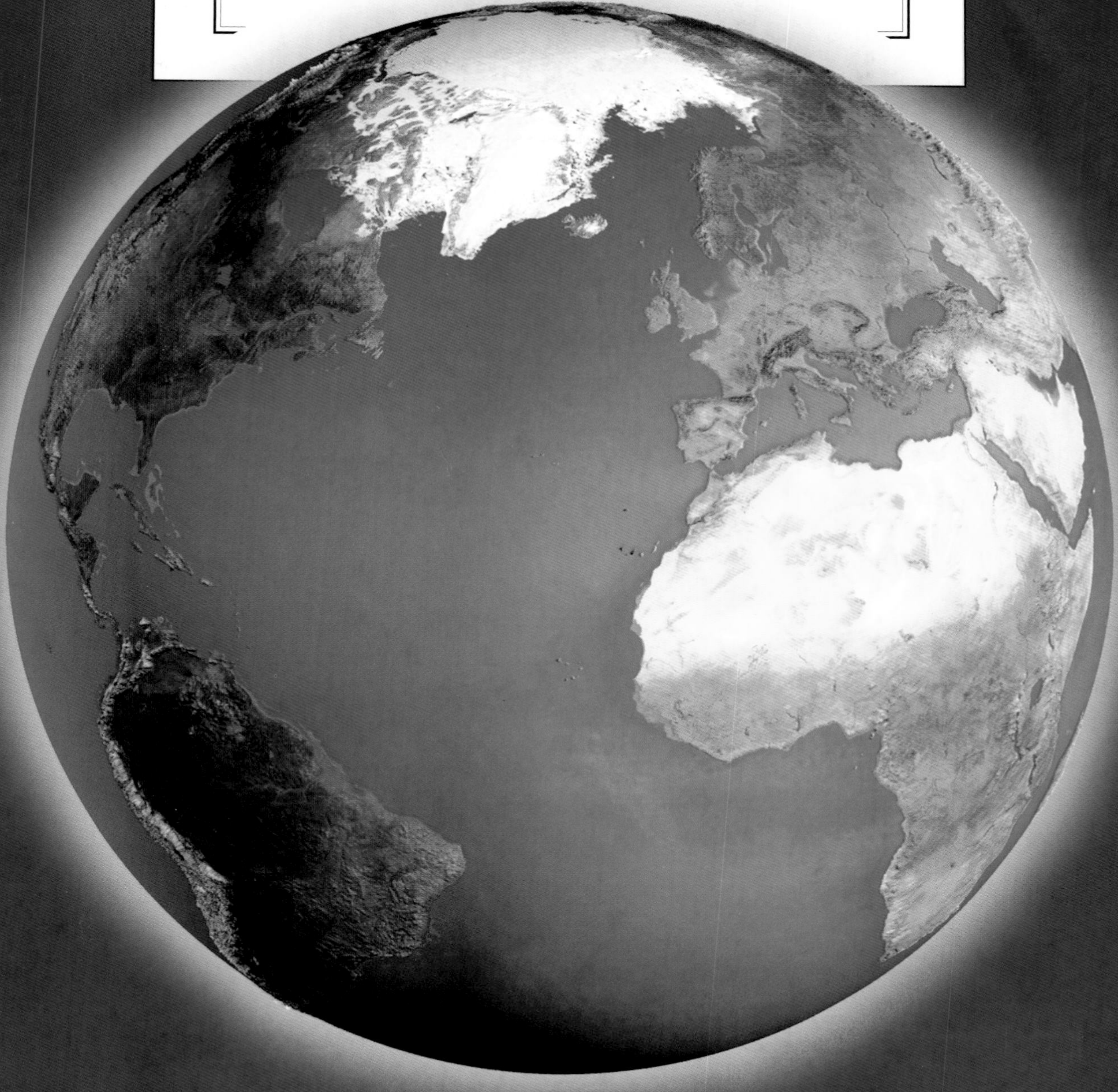

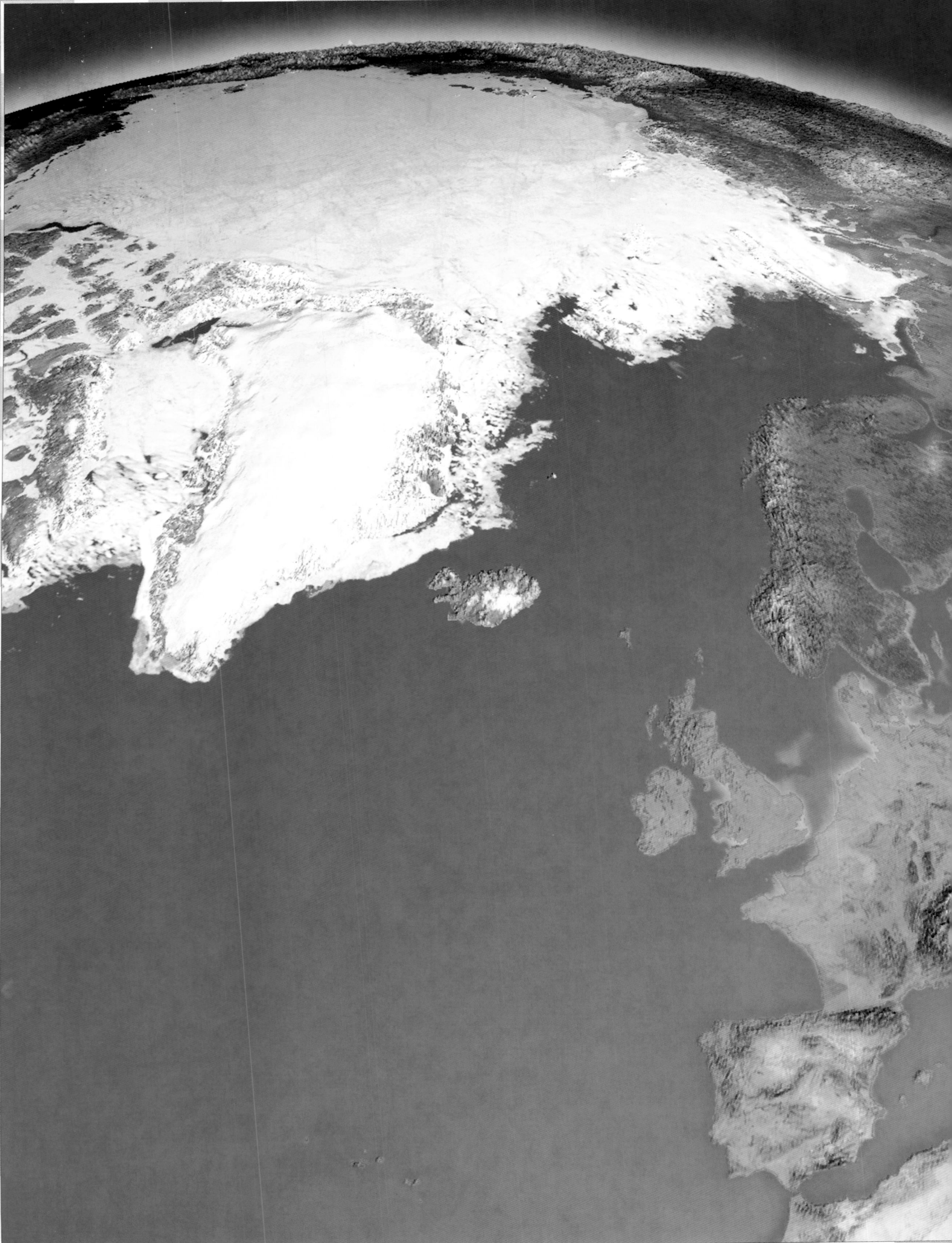

DORLING KINDERSLEY

CONCISE ATLAS *of the* WORLD

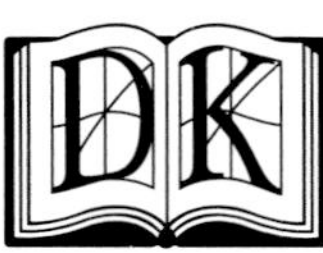

A Dorling Kindersley Book

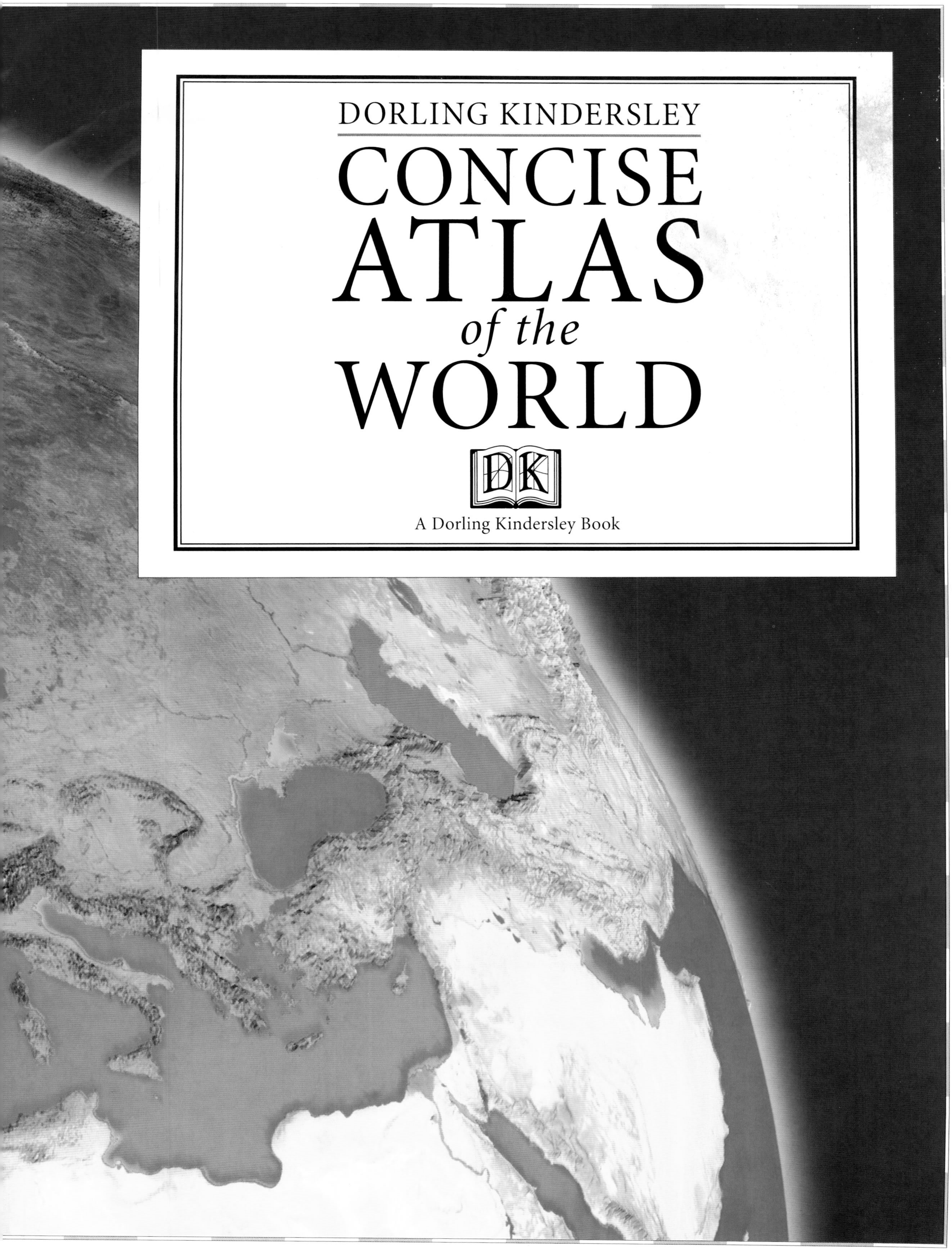

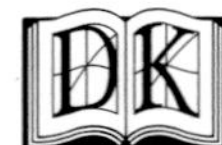

LONDON, NEW YORK, DELHI, PARIS,
MUNICH, AND JOHANNESBURG

GENERAL GEOGRAPHICAL CONSULTANTS

Physical Geography • Denys Brunsden, Emeritus Professor, Department of Geography, King's College, London

Human Geography • Professor J Malcolm Wagstaff, Department of Geography, University of Southampton

Place Names • Caroline Burgess, Permanent Committee on Geographical Names, London

Boundaries • International Boundaries Research Unit, Mountjoy Research Centre, University of Durham

DIGITAL MAPPING CONSULTANTS

DK Cartopia developed by George Galfalvi and XMap Ltd, London

Professor Jan-Peter Muller, Department of Photogrammetry and Surveying, University College, London

Cover globes, planets and information on the Solar System provided by Philip Eales and Kevin Tildsley, Planetary Visions Ltd, London

REGIONAL CONSULTANTS

North America • Dr David Green, Department of Geography, King's College, London
Jim Walsh, Head of Reference, Wessell Library, Tufts University, Medford, Massachussetts

South America • Dr David Preston, School of Geography, University of Leeds

Europe • Dr Edward M Yates, formerly of the Department of Geography, King's College, London

Africa • Dr Philip Amis, Development Administration Group, University of Birmingham
Dr Ieuan L Griffiths, Department of Geography, University of Sussex
Dr Tony Binns, Department of Geography, University of Sussex

Central Asia • Dr David Turnock, Department of Geography, University of Leicester

South and East Asia • Dr Jonathan Rigg, Department of Geography, University of Durham

Australasia and Oceania • Dr Robert Allison, Department of Geography, University of Durham

ACKNOWLEDGMENTS

Digital terrain data created by Eros Data Center, Sioux Falls, South Dakota, USA. Processed by GVS Images Inc, California, USA and Planetary Visions Ltd, London, UK • CIRCA Research and Reference Information, Cambridge, UK • Digitization by Robertson Research International, Swanley, UK • Peter Clark

---

Editor-in-Chief
Andrew Heritage

Managing Editor
Lisa Thomas

Senior Managing Art Editor
Philip Lord

Senior Cartographic Manager
David Roberts

Managing Cartographer
Roger Bullen

Senior Cartographic Editor
Simon Mumford

Database Manager
Simon Lewis

Cartographers
Pamela Alford • James Anderson • Sarah Baker-Ede • Caroline Bowie • Dale Buckton Tony Chambers • Jan Clark • Tom Coulson • Bob Croser • Martin Darlison • Claire Ellam • Sally Gable • Jeremy Hepworth • Geraldine Horner • Chris Jackson • Christine Johnston • Julia Lunn • Michael Martin • James Mills-Hicks • John Plumer • Rob Stokes • John Scott • Ann Stephenson • Julie Turner • Iorwerth Watkins • Jane Voss • Scott Wallace • Bryony Webb • Alan Whitaker • Peter Winfield

Editors
Debra Clapson • Thomas Heath • Wim Jenkins • Jane Oliver
Siobhān Ryan • Elizabeth Wyse

Editorial Research
Helen Dangerfield • Andrew Rebeiro-Hargrave

Additional Editorial Assistance
Margaret Hynes • Robert Damon • Ailsa Heritage • Constance Novis • Jayne Parsons • Chris Whitwell

Designers
Scott David • Carol Ann Davis • David Douglas
Rhonda Fisher • Karen Gregory • Nicola Liddiard • Paul Williams

Illustrations
Ciárán Hughes • Advanced Illustration, Congleton, UK

Picture Research
Melissa Albany • James Clarke • Anna Lord • Christine Rista • Sarah Moule • Louise Thomas

Editorial Direction • Louise Cavanagh

Art Direction • Chez Picthall

Systems Coordinator Phil Rowles

Production Michelle Thomas

Digital Maps Created in DK Cartopia by
Tom Coulson • Thomas Robertshaw
Philip Rowles • Rob Stokes

Placenames Database Team
Natalie Clarkson • Ruth Duxbury • Caroline Falce • John Featherstone • Dan Gardiner
Ciárán Hynes • Margaret Hynes • Helen Rudkin • Margaret Stevenson • Annie Wilson

Published in the United States by
Dorling Kindersley Publishing Inc.
95 Madison Avenue, New York, New York 10016

First American Edition, 2001
2 4 6 8 10 9 7 5 3 1

A CIP catalog record for this book is available from the Library of Congress/ ISBN: 0-7894-7437-9

Reproduction by Colourscan, Singapore. Printed and bound by Graficas Estella, Spain.

INTRODUCTION

FOR MANY, THE OUTSTANDING LEGACY OF THE TWENTIETH CENTURY was the way in which the Earth shrank. As we enter the third millennium, it is increasingly important for us to have a clear vision of the World in which we live. The human population has increased fourfold since 1900. The last scraps of *terra incognita* – the polar regions and ocean depths – have been penetrated and mapped. New regions have been colonized, and previously hostile realms claimed for habitation. The advent of aviation technology and mass tourism allows many of us to travel further, faster, and more frequently than ever before. In doing so we are given a bird's-eye view of the Earth's surface denied to our forebears.

AT THE SAME TIME, the amount of information about our World has grown enormously. Telecommunications can span the greatest distances in fractions of a second: our multimedia environment hurls uninterrupted streams of data at us, on the printed page, through the airwaves, and across our television and computer screens; events from all corners of the globe reach us instantaneously, and are witnessed as they unfold. Our sense of stability and certainty has been eroded; instead, we are aware that the World is in a constant state of flux and change. Natural disasters, manmade cataclysms, and conflicts between nations remind us daily of the enormity and fragility of our domain.

OUR CURRENT "GLOBAL" CULTURE has made the need greater than ever before for everyone to possess an atlas. This atlas has been conceived to meet this need. At its core, like all atlases, it seeks to define where places are, to describe their main characteristics, and to locate them in relation to other places. Every attempt has been made to make the information on the maps as clear and accessible as possible. In addition, each page of the atlas provides a wealth of further information, bringing the maps to life. Using photographs, diagrams, "at-a-glance" thematic maps, introductory texts, and captions, the atlas builds up a detailed portrait of those features – cultural, political, economic, and geomorphological – which make each region unique, and which are also the main agents of change.

THESE WORDS, which formed the introduction to the first edition of the *DK World Atlas* in 1997, remain as true today as they were then. This *Concise Edition* incorporates thousands of revisions and updates affecting every map and every page, and features a new typographic design for the maps. The *Concise Edition* has been created to bring all these benefits to a new audience, in a handier format and at a more affordable price.

ANDREW HERITAGE
EDITOR-IN-CHIEF

CONTENTS

INTRODUCTION v

CONTENTS .... vi–vii

HOW TO USE THIS ATLAS .... viii–ix

THE WORLD TODAY

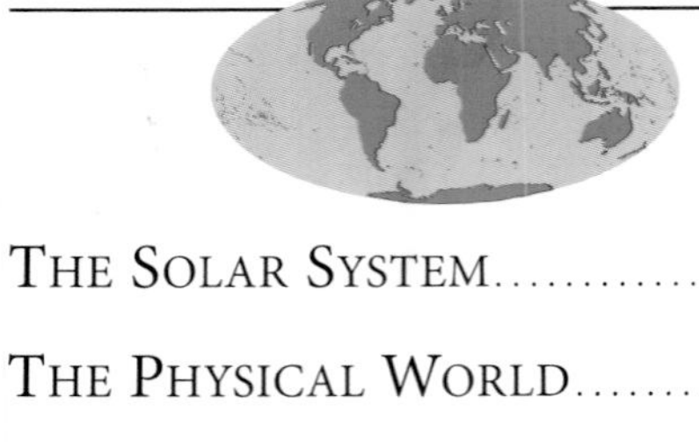

THE SOLAR SYSTEM .... x–xi

THE PHYSICAL WORLD .... xii–xiii

STRUCTURE OF THE EARTH .... xiv–xv

SHAPING THE LANDSCAPE .... xvi–xvii

THE WORLD'S OCEANS .... xviii–xix

THE GLOBAL CLIMATE .... xx–xxi

LIFE ON EARTH .... xxii–xxiii

POPULATION AND SETTLEMENT .... xxiv–xxv

THE ECONOMIC SYSTEM .... xxvi–xxvii

THE POLITICAL WORLD .... xxviii–xxix

STATES AND BOUNDARIES .... xxx–xxxi

INTERNATIONAL DISPUTES xxxii

ATLAS OF THE WORLD

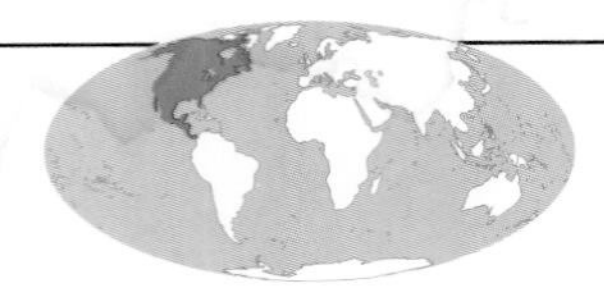

NORTH AMERICA

NORTH AMERICA 1

PHYSICAL NORTH AMERICA 2–3

POLITICAL NORTH AMERICA 4–5

NORTH AMERICAN RESOURCES 6–7

CANADA 8–9

CANADA: WESTERN PROVINCES 10–11
Alberta, British Columbia, Manitoba, Saskatchewan, Yukon

CANADA: EASTERN PROVINCES 12–13
New Brunswick, Newfoundland & Labrador, Nova Scotia, Ontario, Prince Edward Island, Québec, St Pierre & Miquelon

SOUTHEASTERN CANADA 14–15
Southern Ontario, Southern Québec

UNITED STATES OF AMERICA 16–17

USA: NORTHEASTERN STATES 18–19
Connecticut, Maine, Massachussetts, New Hampshire, New Jersey, New York, Pennsylvania, Rhode Island, Vermont

USA: MID-EASTERN STATES 20–21
Delaware, District of Columbia, Kentucky, Maryland, North Carolina, South Carolina, Tennessee, Virginia, West Virginia

USA: SOUTHERN STATES 22–23
Alabama, Florida, Georgia, Louisiana, Mississippi

USA: TEXAS 24–25

USA: SOUTH MIDWESTERN STATES 26–27
Arkansas, Kansas, Missouri, Oklahoma

USA: UPPER PLAINS STATES 28–29
Iowa, Minnesota, Nebraska, North Dakota, South Dakota

USA: GREAT LAKES STATES 30–31
Illinois, Indiana, Michigan, Ohio, Wisconsin

USA: NORTH MOUNTAIN STATES 32–33
Idaho, Montana, Oregon, Washington, Wyoming

USA: CALIFORNIA & NEVADA 34–35

USA: SOUTH MOUNTAIN STATES 36–37
Arizona, Colorado, New Mexico, Utah

USA: HAWAII & ALASKA 38–39

MEXICO 40–41

CENTRAL AMERICA 42–43
Belize, Costa Rica, El Salvador, Guatemala, Honduras, Nicaragua, Panama

THE CARIBBEAN 44–45
Anguilla, Antigua & Barbuda, Aruba, Bahamas, Barbados, British Virgin Islands, Cayman Islands, Cuba, Dominica, Dominican Republic, Grenada, Guadeloupe, Haiti, Jamaica, Martinique, Montserrat, Navassa Island, Netherlands Antilles, Puerto Rico, St. Kitts & Nevis, St. Lucia, St. Vincent & the Grenadines, Trinidad & Tobago, Turks & Caicos Islands, Virgin Islands (US)

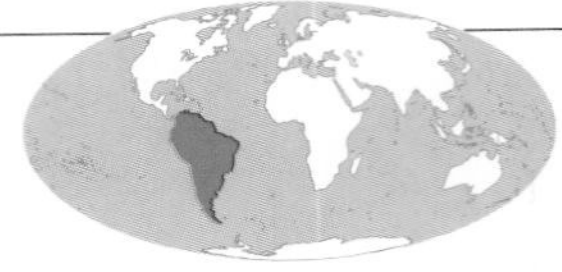

SOUTH AMERICA

SOUTH AMERICA 46–47

PHYSICAL SOUTH AMERICA 48–49

POLITICAL SOUTH AMERICA 50–51

SOUTH AMERICAN RESOURCES 52–53

NORTHERN SOUTH AMERICA 54–55
Colombia, French Guiana, Guyana, Suriname, Venezuela

WESTERN SOUTH AMERICA 56–57
Bolivia, Ecuador, Peru

BRAZIL 58–59

EASTERN SOUTH AMERICA 60–61
Southeast Brazil, Northeast Argentina, Uruguay

SOUTHERN SOUTH AMERICA 62–63
Argentina, Chile, Paraguay

THE ATLANTIC OCEAN 64–65

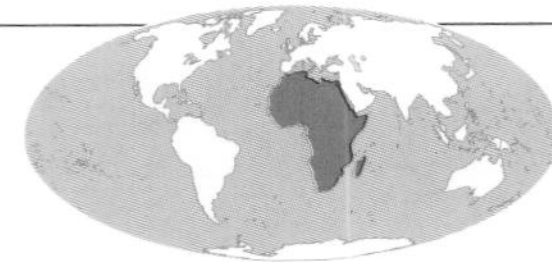

AFRICA

AFRICA 66–67

PHYSICAL AFRICA 68–69

POLITICAL AFRICA 70–71

AFRICAN RESOURCES 72–73

NORTH AFRICA 74–75
Algeria, Egypt, Libya, Morocco, Tunisia, Western Sahara

WEST AFRICA 76–77
Benin, Burkina, Cape Verde, Gambia, Ghana, Guinea, Guinea-Bissau, Ivory Coast, Liberia, Mali, Mauritania, Niger, Nigeria, Senegal, Sierra Leone, Togo

CENTRAL AFRICA 78–79
Cameroon, Central African Republic, Chad, Congo, Dem. Rep. Congo (Zaire), Equatorial Guinea, Gabon, Sao Tome & Principe

EAST AFRICA 80–81
Burundi, Djibouti, Eritrea, Ethiopia, Kenya, Rwanda, Somalia, Sudan, Tanzania, Uganda

SOUTHERN AFRICA 82–83
Angola, Botswana, Lesotho, Malawi, Mozambique, Namibia, South Africa, Swaziland, Zambia, Zimbabwe

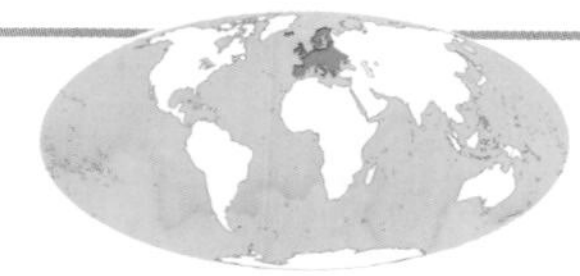

Europe

EUROPE 84–85

PHYSICAL EUROPE 86–87

POLITICAL EUROPE 88–89

EUROPEAN RESOURCES 90–91

SCANDINAVIA, FINLAND, & ICELAND . 92–93
Denmark, Finland, Iceland, Norway, Svalbard, Sweden

SOUTHERN SCANDINAVIA 94–95
Denmark, Faeroe Islands, Southern Norway, Southern Sweden

THE BRITISH ISLES 96–97
Channel Islands, Isle of Man, Republic of Ireland, United Kingdom

THE LOW COUNTRIES 98–99
Belgium, Luxembourg, Netherlands

GERMANY 100–101

FRANCE 102–103
France, Monaco

THE IBERIAN PENINSULA 104–105
Andorra, Gibraltar, Portugal, Spain

THE ITALIAN PENINSULA 106–107
Italy, San Marino, Vatican City

THE ALPINE STATES 108–109
Austria, Liechtenstein, Slovenia, Switzerland

CENTRAL EUROPE 110–111
Czech Republic, Hungary, Poland, Slovakia

SOUTHEAST EUROPE 112–113
Albania, Bosnia & Herzegovina, Croatia, Macedonia, Yugoslavia

BULGARIA & GREECE 114–115
(including European Turkey)

ROMANIA, MOLDOVA, & UKRAINE 116–117

THE BALTIC STATES & BELARUS 118–119
Belarus, Estonia, Latvia, Lithuania, Kaliningrad

THE MEDITERRANEAN 120–121

THE RUSSIAN FEDERATION 122–123

NORTHERN EUROPEAN RUSSIA 124–125

SOUTHERN EUROPEAN RUSSIA 126–127

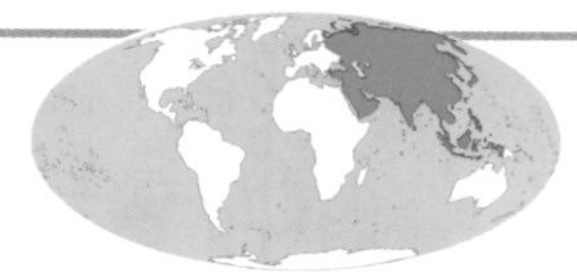

Asia

ASIA 128–129

PHYSICAL ASIA 130–131

POLITICAL ASIA 132–133

ASIAN RESOURCES 134–135

TURKEY & THE CAUCASUS 136–137
Armenia, Azerbaijan, Georgia, Turkey

THE NEAR EAST 138–139
Iraq, Israel, Jordan, Lebanon, Syria

THE ARABIAN PENINSULA 140–141
Bahrain, Kuwait, Oman, Qatar, Saudi Arabia, United Arab Emirates, Yemen

IRAN & THE GULF STATES 142–143
Bahrain, Iran, Kuwait, Qatar, United Arab Emirates

KAZAKHSTAN 144–145

CENTRAL ASIA 146–147
Kyrgyzstan, Tajikistan, Turkmenistan, Uzbekistan

AFGHANISTAN & PAKISTAN 148–149

SOUTH ASIA 150–151
Bangladesh, Bhutan, India, Maldives, Nepal, Pakistan, Sri Lanka

NORTHERN INDIA & THE HIMALAYAN STATES 152–153
Bangladesh, Bhutan, Nepal, Northern India

SOUTHERN INDIA & SRI LANKA 154–155

MAINLAND EAST ASIA 156–157
China, Mongolia, North Korea, South Korea, Taiwan

WESTERN CHINA 158–159

EASTERN CHINA 160–161
Eastern China, Taiwan

NORTHEASTERN CHINA, MONGOLIA & KOREA 162–163
Mongolia, Northeastern China, North Korea, South Korea

JAPAN 164–165

MAINLAND SOUTHEAST ASIA 166–167
Myanmar, Cambodia, Laos, Paracel Islands, Philippines, Spratly Islands, Thailand, Vietnam

WESTERN MARITIME SOUTHEAST ASIA 168–169
Brunei, Indonesia, Malaysia, Singapore

EASTERN MARITIME SOUTHEAST ASIA 170–171
East Timor, Indonesia, Philippines

THE INDIAN OCEAN 172–173

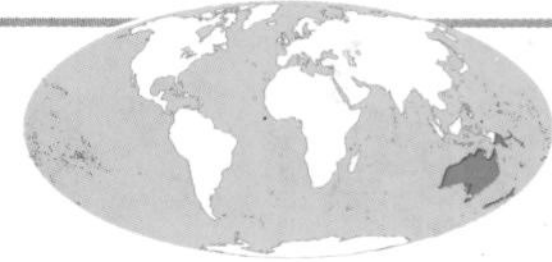

Australasia and Oceania

AUSTRALASIA & OCEANIA 174–175

POLITICAL AUSTRALASIA & OCEANIA 176–177

AUSTRALASIAN & OCEANIAN RESOURCES 178–179

AUSTRALIA 180–181

SOUTHEAST AUSTRALIA 182–183
New South Wales, South Australia, Tasmania, Victoria

NEW ZEALAND 184–185

MELANESIA 186–187
Papua New Guinea, Fiji, Solomon Islands, Vanuatu, New Caledonia

MICRONESIA 188–189
Guam, Marshall Islands, Micronesia, Nauru, Northern Mariana Islands, Palau, Wake Island

POLYNESIA 190–191
Cook Islands, Easter Island, French Polynesia, Kiribati, Niue, Pitcairn Islands, Tokelau, Tuvalu, Wallis & Futuna

THE PACIFIC OCEAN 192–193

ANTARCTICA 194–195

THE ARCTIC 196–197

INDEX-GAZETTEER

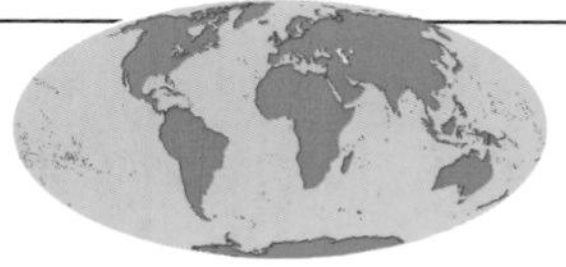

GEOGRAPHICAL COMPARISONS 198–199

COUNTRIES OF THE WORLD
including World Timezones 200–207

GEOGRAPHICAL GLOSSARY 208–210

GEOGRAPHICAL NAMES 211

INDEX 212–349

CREDITS/ACKNOWLEDGEMENTS .. 350

KEY TO REGIONAL MAPS

PHYSICAL FEATURES

elevation

6000m / 19,686ft
4000m / 13,124ft
3000m / 9843ft
2000m / 6562ft
1000m / 3281ft
500m / 1640ft
250m / 820ft
100m / 328ft
sea level
below sea level

elevation above sea level (mountain height)
volcano
pass
elevation below sea level (depression depth)

sand desert
lava flow
coastline
reef
atoll

sea depth

sea level
-250m / -820ft
-500m / -1640ft
-1000m / -3281ft
-2000m / -6562ft
-3000m / -9843ft

seamount / guyot symbol
undersea spot depth

DRAINAGE FEATURES

main river
secondary river
tertiary river
minor river
main seasonal river
secondary seasonal river
canal
waterfall
rapids
dam
perennial lake
seasonal lake
perennial salt lake
seasonal salt lake
reservoir
salt flat / salt pan
marsh / salt marsh
mangrove
wadi
spring / well / waterhole / oasis

ICE FEATURES

ice cap / sheet
ice shelf
glacier / snowfield
summer pack ice limit
winter pack ice limit

COMMUNICATIONS

highway
highway (under construction)
major road
minor road
tunnel (road)
main line
minor line
tunnel (railroad)
international airport

BORDERS

full international border
undefined international border
disputed *de facto* border
disputed territorial claim border
indication of country extent (Pacific only)
indication of dependent territory extent (Pacific only)
demarcation/ cease-fire line
autonomous / federal region border
2nd order internal administrative border
3rd order internal administrative border

SETTLEMENTS

built-up area

settlement population symbols

more than 5 million
1 million to 5 million
500,000 to 1 million
100,000 to 500,000
50,000 to 100,000
10,000 to 50,000
fewer than 10,000

country/dependent territory capital city
autonomous / federal region / 2nd order internal administrative center
3rd order internal administrative center

MISCELLANEOUS FEATURES

ancient wall
site of interest
scientific station

GRATICULE FEATURES

lines of latitude and longitude / Equator
Tropics / Polar circles
45° degrees of longitude / latitude

TYPOGRAPHIC KEY

PHYSICAL FEATURES

landscape features	*Namib Desert* *Massif Central* ***ANDES***
headland	***Nordkapp***
elevation / volcano / pass	**Mount Meru 4556 m**
drainage features	***Lake Rudolf***
rivers / canals spring / well / waterhole / oasis / waterfall / rapids / dam	***Mekong***
ice features	***Vatnajökull***
sea features	*Golfe de Lion* *Andaman Sea* ***INDIAN OCEAN***
undersea features	*Barracuda Fracture Zone*

REGIONS

country	**ARMENIA**
dependent territory with parent state	**NIUE (to NZ)**
region outside feature area	ANGOLA
autonomous / federal region	MINAS GERAIS
2nd order internal administrative region	MINSKAYA VOBLASTS'
3rd order internal administrative region	Vaucluse
cultural region	New England

SETTLEMENTS

capital city	**BEIJING**
dependent territory capital city	FORT-DE-FRANCE
other settlements	**Chicago** **Adana** **Tizi Ozou** **Yonezawa** **Farnham**

MISCELLANEOUS

sites of interest / miscellaneous	Valley of the Kings
Tropics / Polar circles	*Antarctic Circle*

HOW TO USE THIS ATLAS

THE ATLAS IS ORGANIZED BY CONTINENT, moving eastward from the International Dateline. The opening section describes the world's structure, systems, and its main features. The Atlas of the World that follows, is a continent-by-continent guide to today's world, starting with a comprehensive insight into the physical, political, and economic structure of each continent, followed by integrated mapping and descriptions of each region or country.

THE WORLD

THE INTRODUCTORY SECTION of the Atlas deals with every aspect of the planet, from physical structure to human geography, providing an overall picture of the world we live in. Complex topics such as the landscape of the Earth, climate, oceans, population, and economic patterns are clearly explained with the aid of maps and diagrams drawn from the latest information.

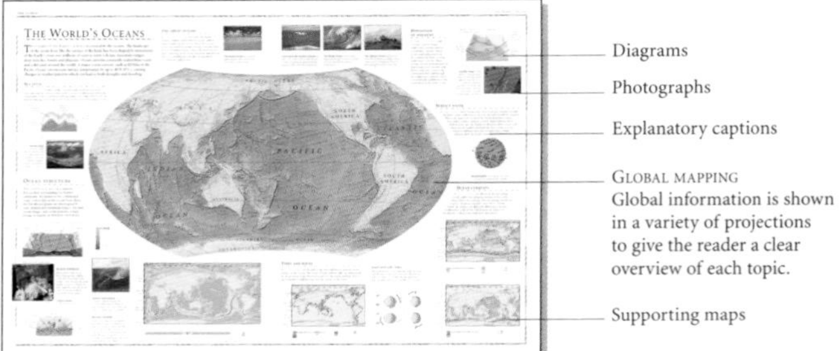
THE WORLD'S OCEANS

Diagrams
Photographs
Explanatory captions
GLOBAL MAPPING
Global information is shown in a variety of projections to give the reader a clear overview of each topic.
Supporting maps

THE POLITICAL CONTINENT

THE POLITICAL PORTRAIT of the continent is a vital reference point for every continental section, showing the position of countries relative to one another, and the relationship between human settlement and geographic location. The complex mosaic of languages spoken in each continent is mapped, as is the effect of communications networks on the pattern of settlement.

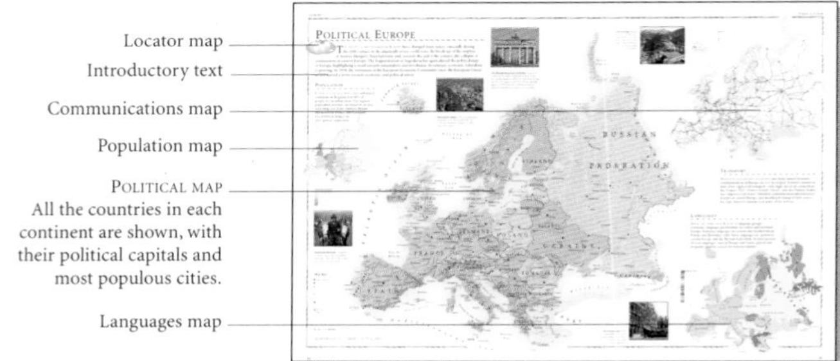
POLITICAL EUROPE

Locator map
Introductory text
Communications map
Population map
POLITICAL MAP
All the countries in each continent are shown, with their political capitals and most populous cities.
Languages map

CONTINENTAL RESOURCES

THE EARTH'S RICH NATURAL RESOURCES, including oil, gas, minerals, and fertile land, have played a key role in the development of society. These pages show the location of minerals and agricultural resources on each continent, and how they have been instrumental in dictating industrial growth and the varieties of economic activity across the continent.

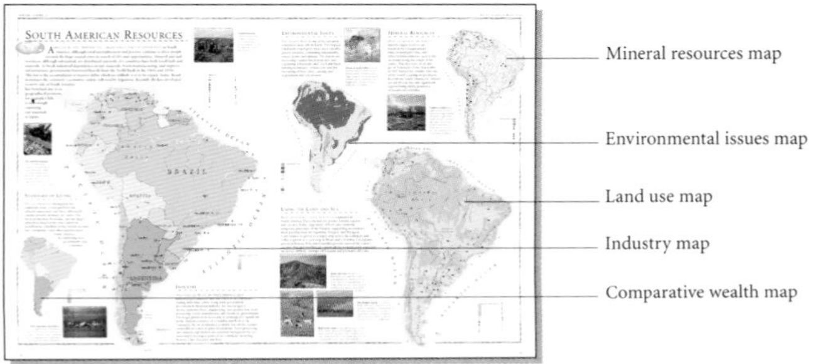
SOUTH AMERICAN RESOURCES

Mineral resources map
Environmental issues map
Land use map
Industry map
Comparative wealth map

The Physical Continent

The astonishing variety of landforms, and the dramatic forces that created and continue to shape the landscape, are explained in the continental physical spread. Cross-sections, illustrations, and terrain maps highlight the different parts of the continent, showing how nature's forces have produced the landscapes we see today.

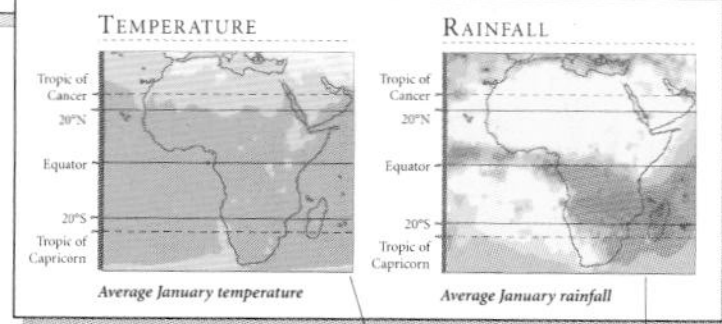

Temperature
Rainfall
Average January temperature
Average January rainfall

Climate charts
Rainfall and temperature charts clearly show the continental patterns of rainfall and temperature.

Climate map
Climatic regions vary across each continent. The map displays the differing climatic regions, as well as daily hours of sunshine at selected weather stations.

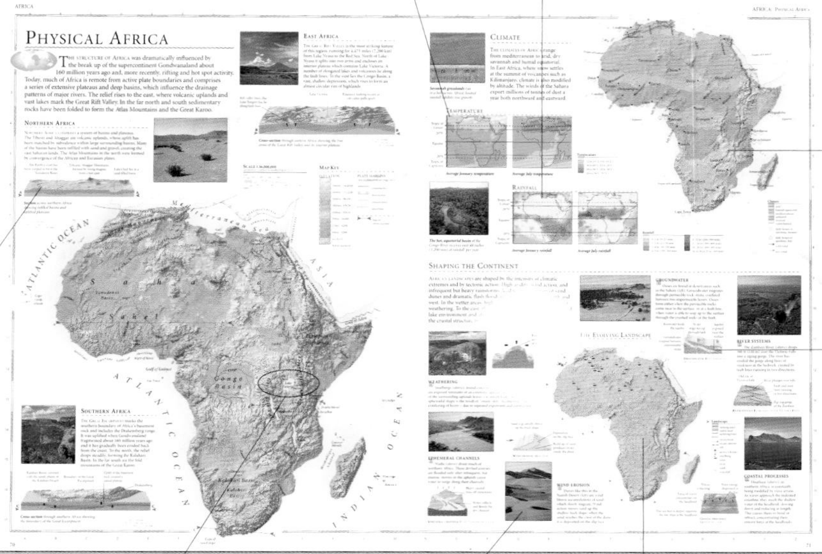

Physical Africa

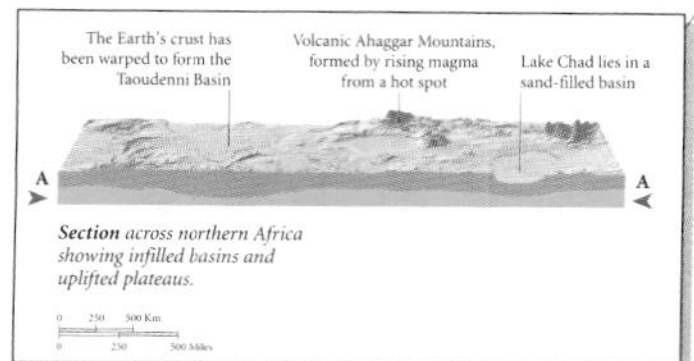

The Earth's crust has been warped to form the Taoudenni Basin
Volcanic Ahaggar Mountains, formed by rising magma from a hot spot
Lake Chad lies in a sand-filled basin
Section across northern Africa showing infilled basins and uplifted plateaus.

Cross-sections
Detailed cross-sections through selected parts of the continent show the underlying geomorphic structure.

Rainwater feeds the aquifer | Water migrates up through fault | Aquifer exposed near the surface | Groundwater trapped between impermeable strata | Groundwater: Replenishment of an oasis

Landform diagrams
The complex formation of many typical landforms is summarized in these easy-to-understand illustrations.

Main physical map
Detailed satellite data has been used to create an accurate and visually striking picture of the surface of the continent.

Photographs
A wide range of beautiful photographs bring the world's regions to life.

Landscape evolution map
The physical shape of each continent is affected by a variety of forces which continually sculpt and modify the landscape. This map shows the major processes which affect different parts of the continent.

Regional Mapping

The main body of the Atlas is a unique regional map set, with detailed information on the terrain, the human geography of the region and its infrastructure. Around the edge of the map, additional 'at-a-glance' maps, give an instant picture of regional industry, land use and agriculture. The detailed terrain map (shown in perspective), focuses on the main physical features of the region, and is enhanced by annotated illustrations, and photographs of the physical structure.

Regional Locator
This small map shows the location of each country in relation to its continent.

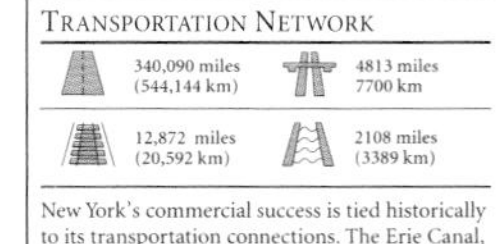

Transportation Network

340,090 miles (544,144 km)	4813 miles 7700 km
12,872 miles (20,592 km)	2108 miles (3389 km)

New York's commercial success is tied historically to its transportation connections. The Erie Canal, completed in 1825, opened up the Great Lakes and the interior to New York's markets and carried a stream of immigrants into the Midwest.

Transportation network
The differing extent of the transportation network for each region is shown here, along with key facts about the transportation system.

Key to main map
A key to the population symbols and land heights accompanies the main map.

World locator
This locates the continent in which the region is found on a small world map.

Land use map
This shows the different types of land use which characterize the region, as well as indicating the principal agricultural activities.

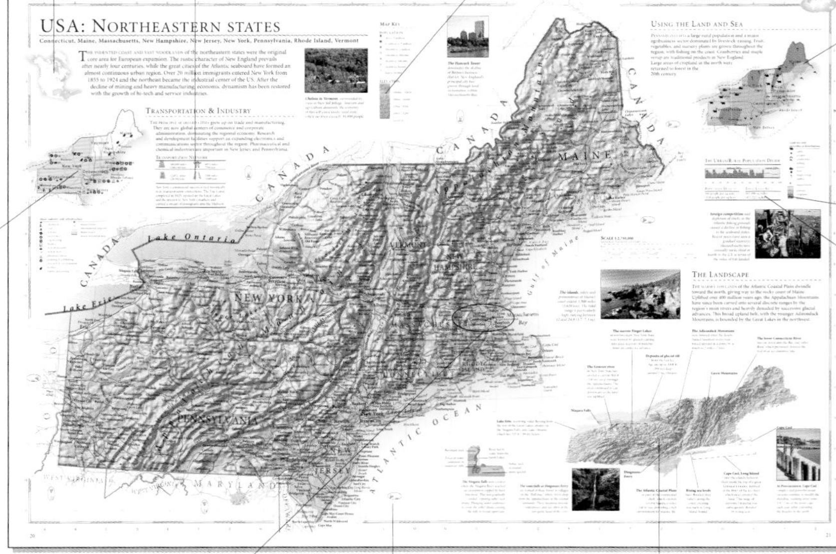

USA: Northeastern States

Grid reference
The framing grid provides a location reference for each place listed in the Index.

Map keys
Each supporting map has its own key.

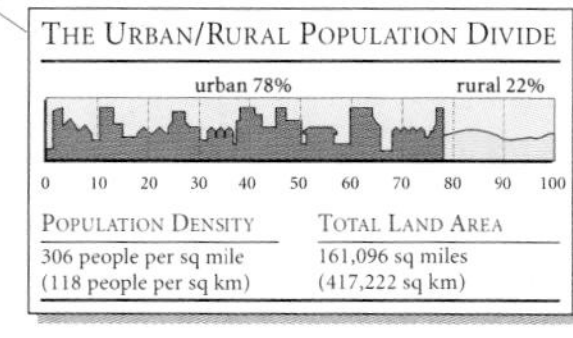

The Urban/Rural Population Divide

urban 78% | rural 22%

0 10 20 30 40 50 60 70 80 90 100

Population Density	Total Land Area
306 people per sq mile (118 people per sq km)	161,096 sq miles (417,222 sq km)

Urban/rural population divide
The proportion of people in the region who live in urban and rural areas, as well as the overall population density and land area are clearly shown in these simple graphics.

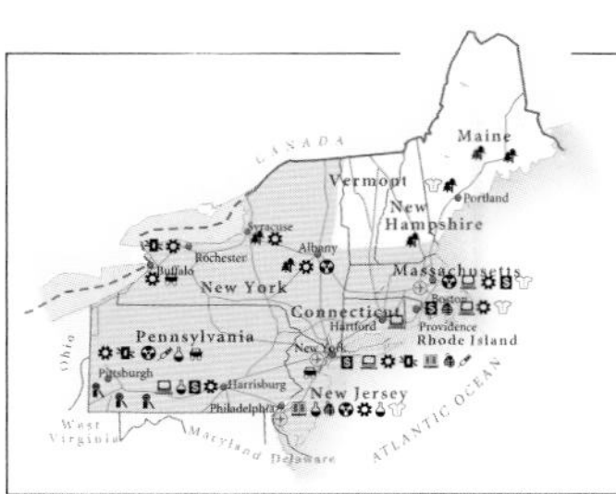

Transportation and industry map
The main industrial areas are mapped, and the most important industrial and economic activities of the region are shown.

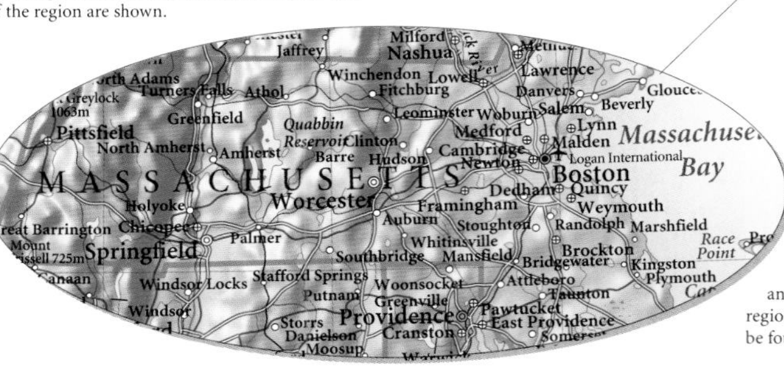

Continuation symbols
These symbols indicate where adjacent maps can be found.

Main regional map
A wealth of information is displayed on the main map, building up a rich portrait of the interaction between the physical landscape and the human and political geography of each region. The key to the regional maps can be found on page viii.

Landscape map
The computer-generated terrain model accurately portrays an oblique view of the landscape. Annotations highlight the most important geographic features of the region.

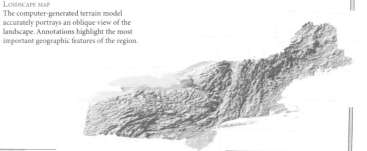

Jupiter

- **Diameter:** 88,846 miles (142,984 km)
- **Mass:** 1,900,000 million million million tons
- **Temperature:** -153°C (extremes not available)
- **Distance from Sun:** 483 million miles (778 million km)
- **Length of day:** 9.84 hours
- **Length of year:** 11.86 earth years
- **Surface gravity:** 1 kg = 2.53 kg

Mars

- **Diameter:** 4,217 miles (6,786 km)
- **Mass:** 642 million million million tons
- **Temperature:** -137 to 37°C
- **Distance from Sun:** 142 million miles (228 million km)
- **Length of day:** 24.623 hours
- **Length of year:** 1.88 earth years
- **Surface gravity:** 1 kg = 0.38 kg

Earth

- **Diameter:** 7,926 miles (12,756 km)
- **Mass:** 5,976 million million million tons
- **Temperature:** -70 to 55°C
- **Distance from Sun:** 93 million miles (150 million km)
- **Length of day:** 23.92 hours
- **Length of year:** 365.25 earth days
- **Surface gravity:** 1 kg = 1 kg

Venus

- **Diameter:** 7,520 miles (12,102 km)
- **Mass:** 4,870 million million million tons
- **Temperature:** 457°C (extremes not available)
- **Distance from Sun:** 67 million miles (108 million km)
- **Length of day:** 243.01 earth days
- **Length of year:** 224.7 earth days
- **Surface gravity:** 1 kg = 0.88 kg

Mercury

- **Diameter:** 3,031 miles (4,878 km)
- **Mass:** 330 million million million tons
- **Temperature:** -173 to 427°C
- **Distance from Sun:** 36 million miles (58 million km)
- **Length of day:** 58.65 earth days
- **Length of year:** 87.97 earth days
- **Surface gravity:** 1 kg = 0.38 kg

The Solar System

Nine major planets, their satellites, and countless minor planets (asteroids) orbit the Sun to form the Solar System. The Sun, our nearest star, creates energy from nuclear reactions deep within its interior, providing all the light and heat which make life on Earth possible. The Earth is unique in the Solar System in that it supports life: its size, gravitational pull and distance from the Sun have all created the optimum conditions for the evolution of life. The planetary images seen here are composites derived from actual spacecraft images (not shown to scale).

The Sun

- **Diameter:** 864,948 miles (1,392,000 km)
- **Mass:** 1990 million million million million tons

The Sun was formed when a swirling cloud of dust and gas contracted, pulling matter into its center. When the temperature at the center rose to 1,000,000°C, nuclear fusion – the fusing of hydrogen into helium, creating energy – occurred, releasing a constant stream of heat and light.

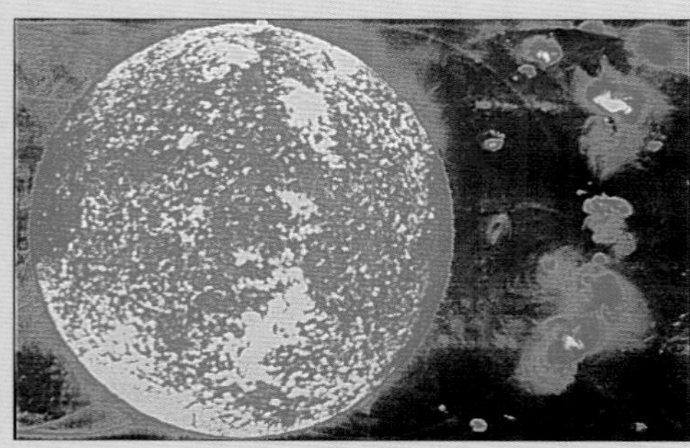

Solar flares are sudden bursts of energy from the Sun's surface. They can be 125,000 miles (200,000 km) long.

The Formation of the Solar System

The cloud of dust and gas thrown out by the Sun during its formation cooled to form the Solar System. The smaller planets nearest the Sun are formed of minerals and metals. The outer planets were formed at lower temperatures, and consist of swirling clouds of gases.

The Milankovitch Cycle

The amount of radiation from the Sun which reaches the Earth is affected by variations in the Earth's orbit and the tilt of the Earth's axis, as well as by "wobbles" in the axis. These variations cause three separate cycles, corresponding with the durations of recent ice ages.

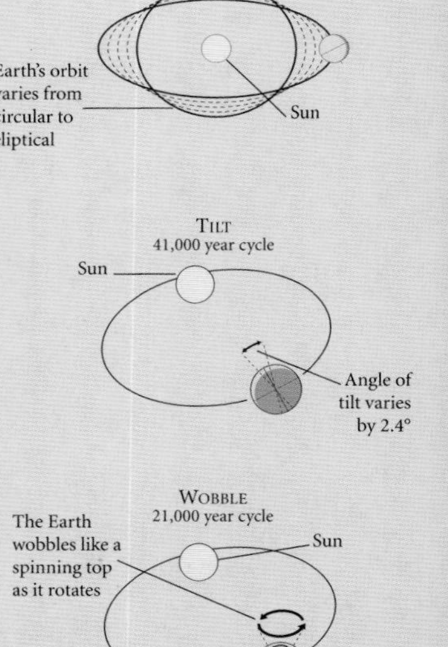
Stretch
100,000 year cycle
Earth's orbit varies from circular to eliptical
Sun
Tilt
41,000 year cycle
Sun
Angle of tilt varies by 2.4°
Wobble
21,000 year cycle
The Earth wobbles like a spinning top as it rotates
Sun

Saturn

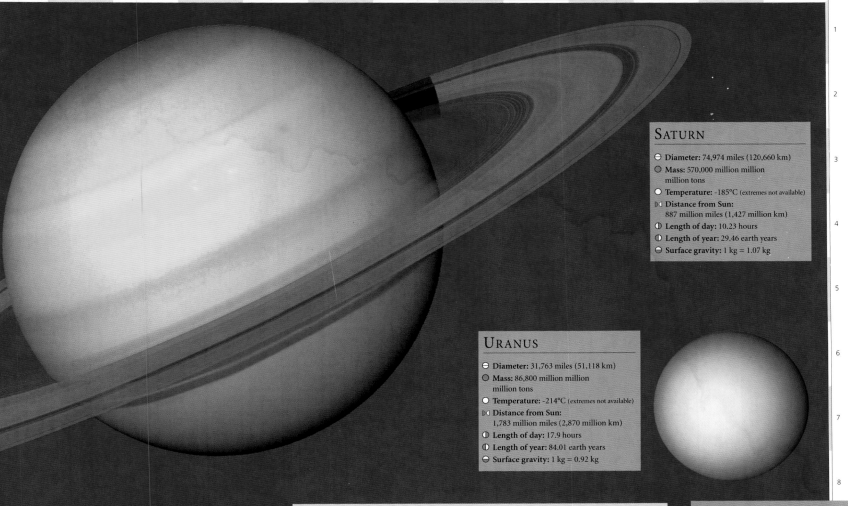

- **Diameter:** 74,974 miles (120,660 km)
- **Mass:** 570,000 million million million tons
- **Temperature:** -185°C (extremes not available)
- **Distance from Sun:** 887 million miles (1,427 million km)
- **Length of day:** 10.23 hours
- **Length of year:** 29.46 earth years
- **Surface gravity:** 1 kg = 1.07 kg

Uranus

- **Diameter:** 31,763 miles (51,118 km)
- **Mass:** 86,800 million million million tons
- **Temperature:** -214°C (extremes not available)
- **Distance from Sun:** 1,783 million miles (2,870 million km)
- **Length of day:** 17.9 hours
- **Length of year:** 84.01 earth years
- **Surface gravity:** 1 kg = 0.92 kg

Space Debris

Millions of objects, remnants of planetary formation, circle the Sun in a zone lying between Mars and Jupiter: the asteroid belt. Fragments of asteroids break off to form meteoroids, which can reach the Earth's surface. Comets, composed of ice and dust, originated outside our Solar System. Their elliptical orbit brings them close to the Sun and into the inner Solar System.

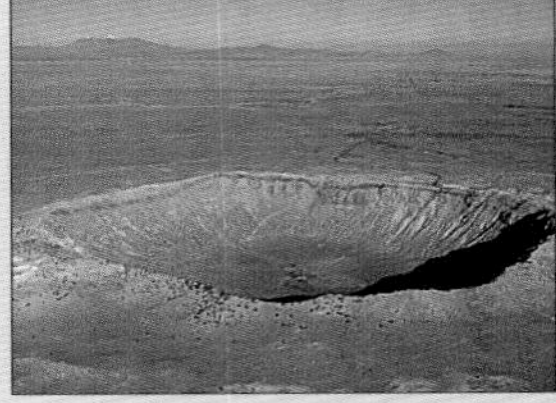

***Meteor Crater in Arizona** is 4200 ft (1300 m) wide and 660 ft (200 m) deep. It was formed over 10,000 years ago.*

Meteoroids

Meteoroids are fragments of asteroids which hurtle through space at great velocity. Although millions of meteoroids enter the Earth's atmosphere, the vast majority burn up on entry, and fall to the Earth as a meteor or shooting star. Large meteoroids traveling at speeds of 155,000 mph (250,000 kmph) can sometimes withstand the atmosphere and hit the Earth's surface with tremendous force, creating large craters on impact.

Possible and actual meteorite craters

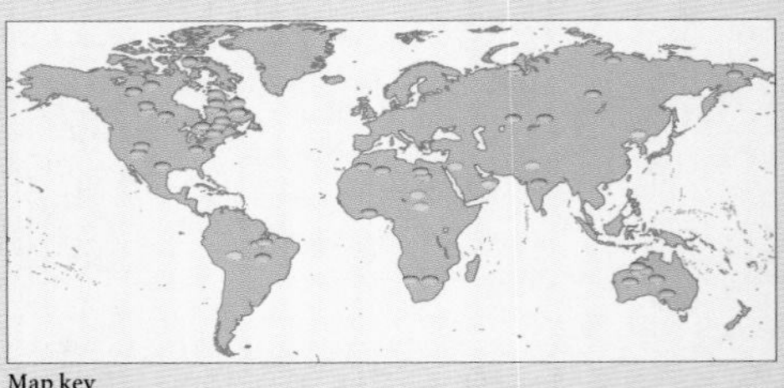

Map key
Possible impact craters — Meteorite impact craters

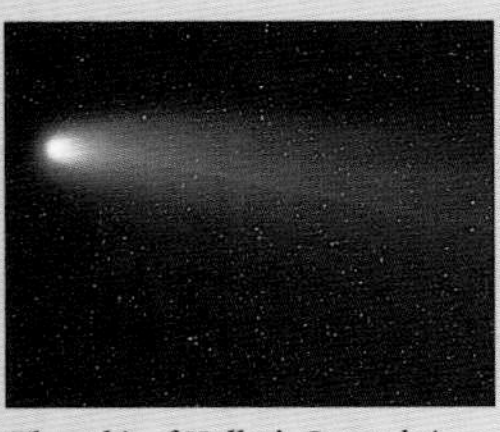

***The orbit of Halley's Comet** brings it close to the Earth every 76 years. It last visited in 1986.*

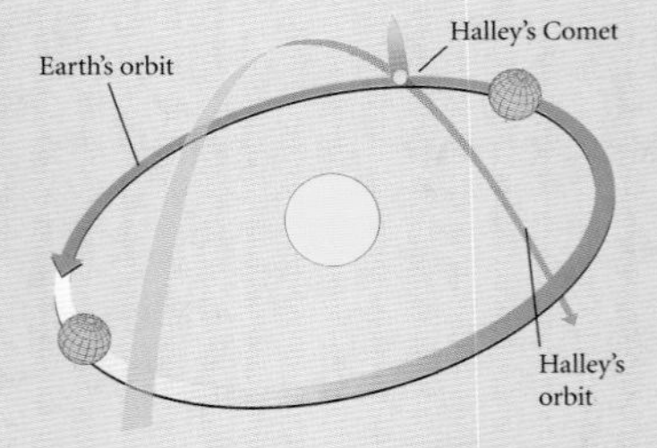
Earth's orbit
Halley's Comet
Halley's orbit

Orbit of Halley's Comet around the Sun

Neptune

- **Diameter:** 30,775 miles (49,528 km)
- **Mass:** 102,000 million million million tons
- **Temperature:** -225°C (extremes not available)
- **Distance from Sun:** 2794 million miles (4497 million km)
- **Length of day:** 19.2 hours
- **Length of year:** 164.79 earth years
- **Surface gravity:** 1 kg = 1.18 kg

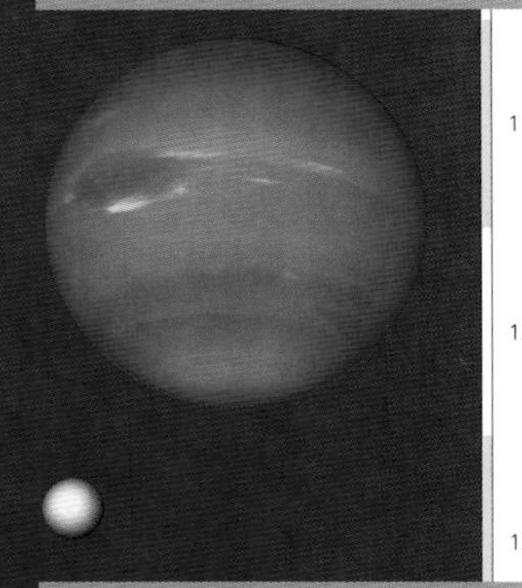

The Earth's Atmosphere

During the early stages of the Earth's formation, ash, lava, carbon dioxide, and water vapor were discharged onto the surface of the planet by constant volcanic eruptions. The water formed the oceans, while carbon dioxide entered the atmosphere or was dissolved in the oceans. Clouds, formed of water droplets, reflected some of the Sun's radiation back into space. The Earth's temperature stabilized and early life forms began to emerge, converting carbon dioxide into life-giving oxygen.

***It is thought** that the gases that make up the Earth's atmosphere originated deep within the interior, and were released many millions of years ago during intense volcanic actvity, similar to this eruption at Mount St. Helens.*

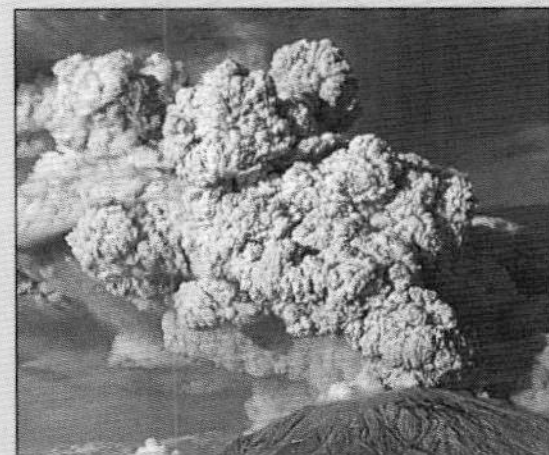

Pluto

- **Diameter:** 1,429 miles (2,300 km)
- **Mass:** 13 million million million tons
- **Temperature:** -236°C (extremes not available)
- **Distance from Sun:** 3,666 million miles (5,900 million km)
- **Length of day:** 6.39 hours
- **Length of year:** 248.54 earth years
- **Surface gravity:** 1 kg = 0.30 kg

Order and relative distance from the Sun of planets

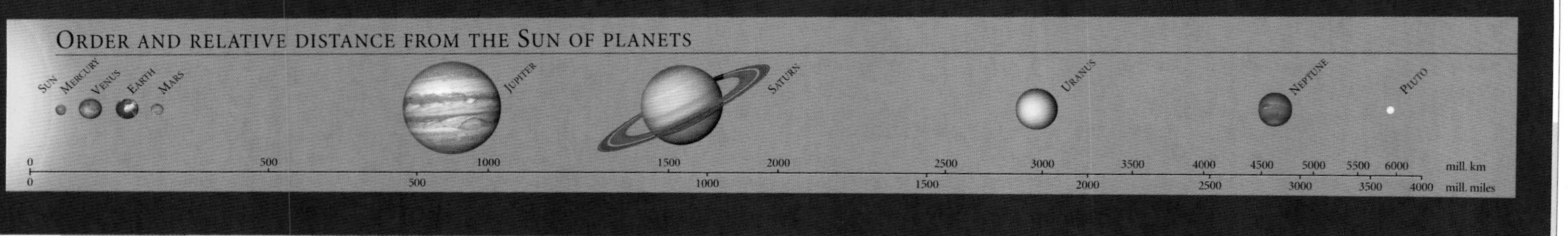
Sun
Mercury
Venus
Earth
Mars
Jupiter
Saturn
Uranus
Neptune
Pluto
0 500 1000 1500 2000 2500 3000 3500 4000 4500 5000 5500 6000 mill. km
0 500 1000 1500 2000 2500 3000 3500 4000 mill. miles

THE PHYSICAL WORLD

THE EARTH'S SURFACE is constantly being transformed: it is uplifted, folded and faulted by tectonic forces; weathered and eroded by wind, water, and ice. Sometimes change is dramatic, the spectacular results of earthquakes or floods. More often it is a slow process lasting millions of years. A physical map of the world represents a snapshot of the ever-evolving architecture of the Earth. This terrain map shows the whole surface of the Earth, both above and below the sea.

THE WORLD IN SECTION

These cross-sections around the Earth, one in the northern hemisphere; one straddling the Equator, reveal the limited areas of land above sea level in comparison with the extent of the sea floor. The greater erosive effects of weathering by wind and water limit the upward elevation of land above sea level, while the deep oceans retain their dramatic mountain and trench profiles.

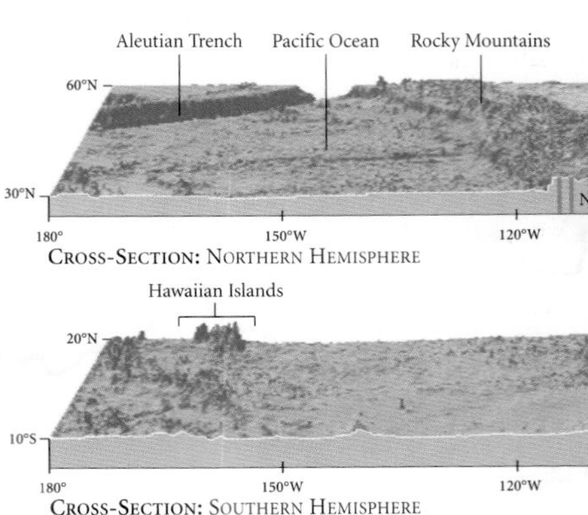

Aleutian Trench
Pacific Ocean
Rocky Mountains
60°N
30°N
180°
150°W
120°W
CROSS-SECTION: NORTHERN HEMISPHERE
Hawaiian Islands
20°N
10°S
180°
150°W
120°W
CROSS-SECTION: SOUTHERN HEMISPHERE

MAP KEY

GEOGRAPHICAL REGIONS

- ice
- tundra
- needleleaf forest
- broadleaf forest
- cultivated land
- hot desert
- cold desert
- tropical grassland
- tropical rainforest
- mountain
- submarine regions

SCALE 1:73,000,000
(projection: Wagner VII)

Km 0 250 500 1,000 1,500 2,000
Miles 0 250 500 1,000 1,500 2,000

PACIFIC OCEAN

NORTH AMERICA

SOUTH AMERICA

ATLANTIC OCEAN

SOUTHERN OCEAN

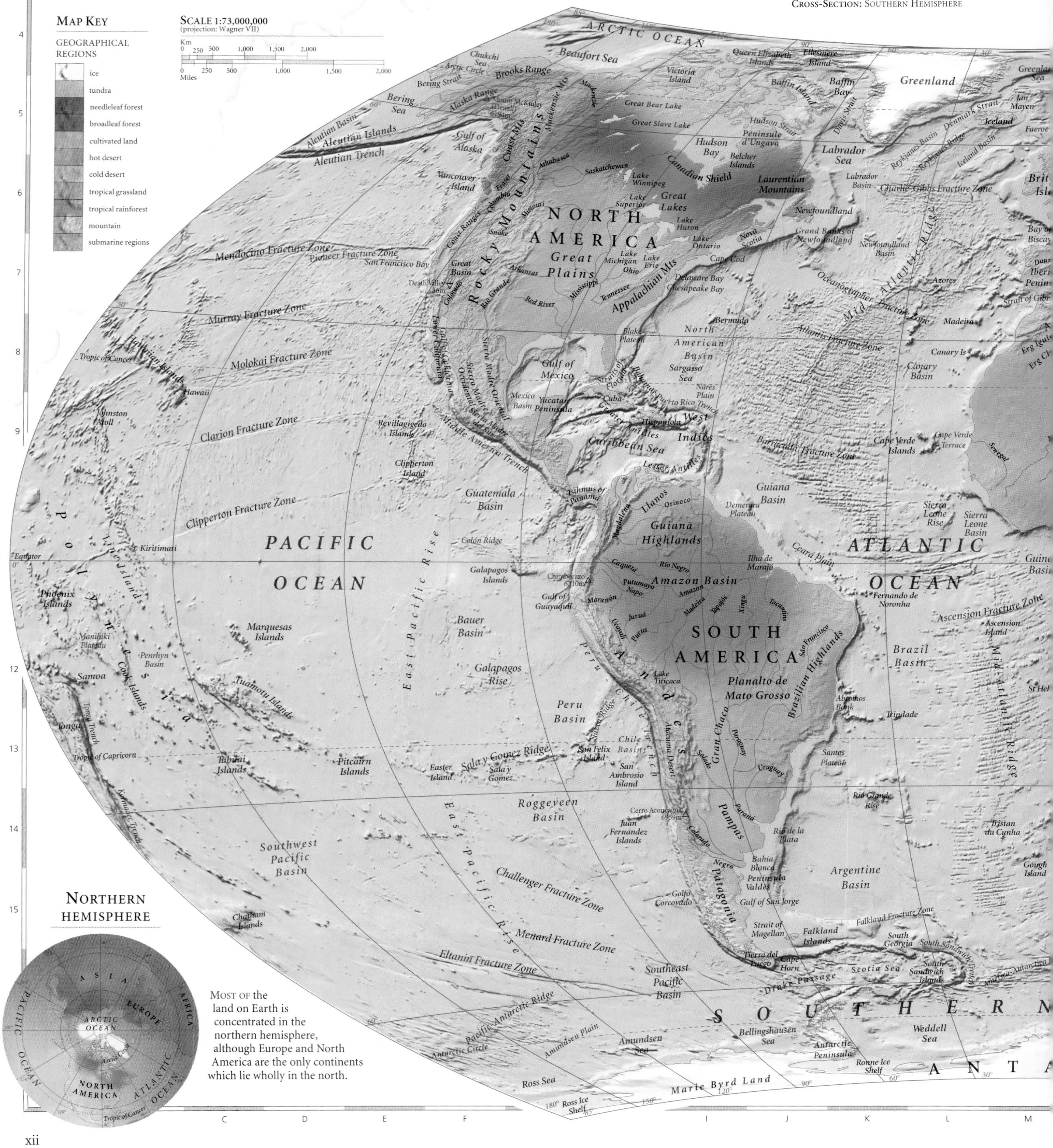

NORTHERN HEMISPHERE

MOST OF the land on Earth is concentrated in the northern hemisphere, although Europe and North America are the only continents which lie wholly in the north.

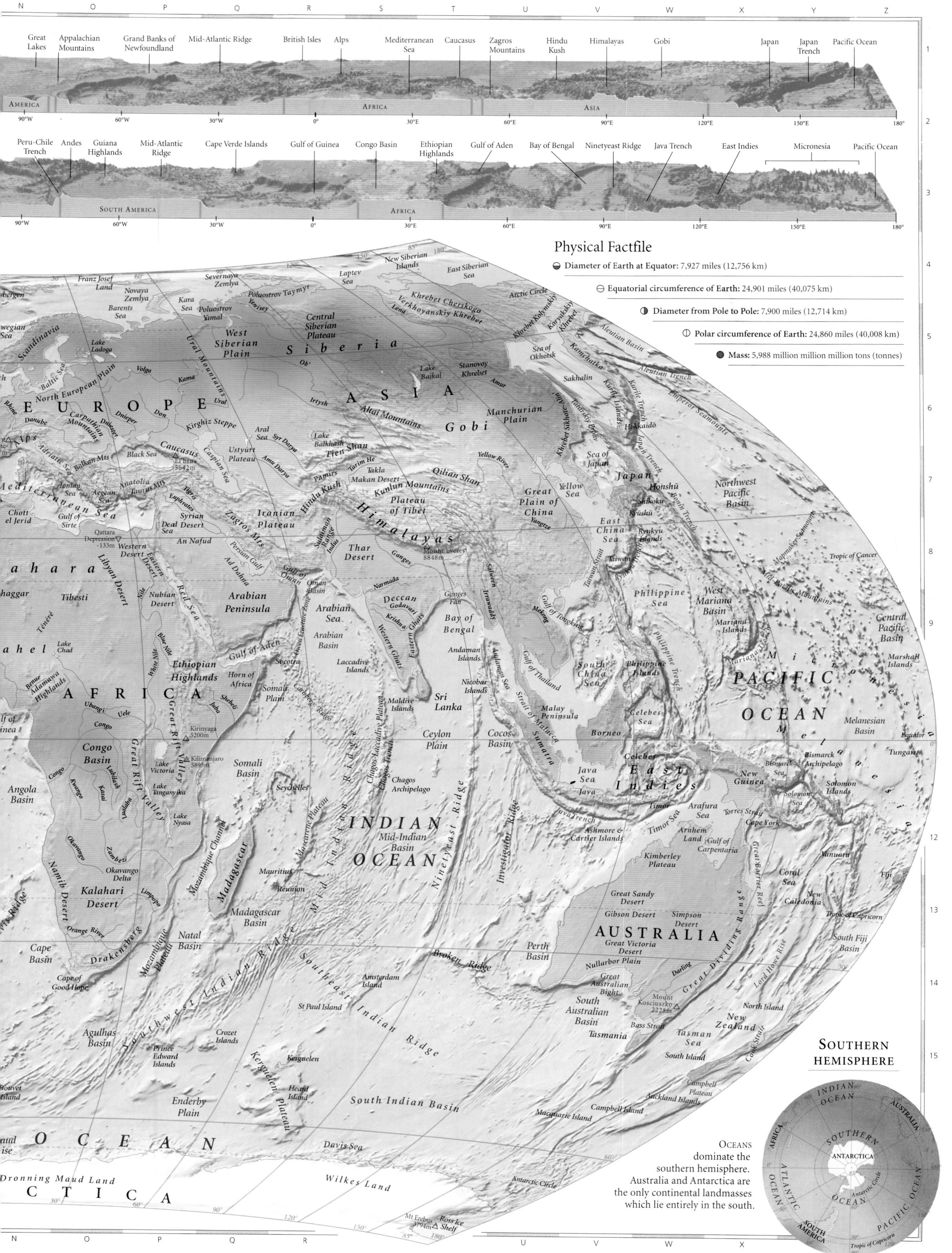

Great Lakes
Appalachian Mountains
Grand Banks of Newfoundland
Mid-Atlantic Ridge
British Isles
Alps
Mediterranean Sea
Caucasus
Zagros Mountains
Hindu Kush
Himalayas
Gobi
Japan
Japan Trench
Pacific Ocean
AMERICA
AFRICA
ASIA
Peru-Chile Trench
Andes
Guiana Highlands
Mid-Atlantic Ridge
Cape Verde Islands
Gulf of Guinea
Congo Basin
Ethiopian Highlands
Gulf of Aden
Bay of Bengal
Ninetyeast Ridge
Java Trench
East Indies
Micronesia
Pacific Ocean
SOUTH AMERICA
AFRICA
Physical Factfile
Diameter of Earth at Equator: 7,927 miles (12,756 km)
Equatorial circumference of Earth: 24,901 miles (40,075 km)
Diameter from Pole to Pole: 7,900 miles (12,714 km)
Polar circumference of Earth: 24,860 miles (40,008 km)
Mass: 5,988 million million million tons (tonnes)
EUROPE
ASIA
Siberia
West Siberian Plain
Central Siberian Plateau
Gobi
Himalayas
Plateau of Tibet
Arabian Peninsula
AFRICA
Congo Basin
Kalahari Desert
INDIAN OCEAN
Mid-Indian Basin
PACIFIC OCEAN
AUSTRALIA
Borneo
East Indies
Madagascar
Sri Lanka
Tasmania
New Zealand
South Indian Basin
Kerguelen Plateau
Southeast Indian Ridge
Southwest Indian Ridge
Ninetyeast Ridge
Wilkes Land
Dronning Maud Land
SOUTHERN HEMISPHERE
OCEANS dominate the southern hemisphere. Australia and Antarctica are the only continental landmasses which lie entirely in the south.
INDIAN OCEAN
AUSTRALIA
SOUTHERN
ANTARCTICA
ATLANTIC OCEAN
PACIFIC OCEAN
SOUTH AMERICA
AFRICA

Structure of the Earth

The Earth as it is today is just the latest phase in a constant process of evolution which has occurred over the past 4.5 billion years. The Earth's continents are neither fixed nor stable; over the course of the Earth's history, propelled by currents rising from the intense heat at its center, the great plates on which they lie have moved, collided, joined together, and separated. These processes continue to mold and transform the surface of the Earth, causing earthquakes and volcanic eruptions and creating oceans, mountain ranges, deep ocean trenches, and island chains.

Inside the Earth

The Earth's hot inner core is made up of solid iron, while the outer core is composed of liquid iron and nickel. The mantle nearest the core is viscous, whereas the rocky upper mantle is fairly rigid. The crust is the rocky outer shell of the Earth. Together, the upper mantle and the crust form the lithosphere.

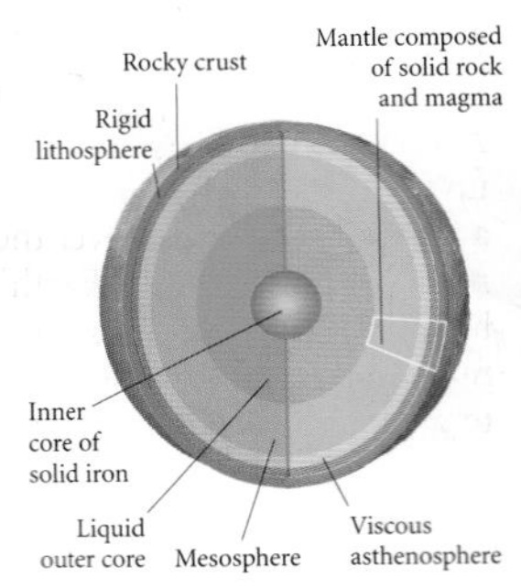
Rocky crust
Mantle composed of solid rock and magma
Rigid lithosphere
Inner core of solid iron
Liquid outer core
Mesosphere
Viscous asthenosphere

The Dynamic Earth

The Earth's crust is made up of eight major (and several minor) rigid continental and oceanic tectonic plates, which fit closely together. The positions of the plates are not static. They are constantly moving relative to one another. The type of movement between plates affects the way in which they alter the structure of the Earth. The oldest parts of the plates, known as shields, are the most stable parts of the Earth and little tectonic activity occurs here.

Continental plate
Rigid tectonic plate
Oceanic plate
Shield area in middle of plate: little tectonic activity occurs here
Plate boundary: most tectonic activity takes place here

Inner core
Outer core
Subduction zone
Ocean crust
Movement of plate
Mid-ocean ridge
Lithosphere
Asthenosphere
Mesosphere
Continental crust

Convection currents

Deep within the Earth, at its inner core, temperatures may exceed 8,100°F (4,500°C). This heat warms rocks in the mesosphere which rise through the partially molten mantle, displacing cooler rocks just below the solid crust, which sink, and are warmed again by the heat of the mantle. This process is continuous, creating convection currents which form the moving force beneath the Earth's crust.

Plate boundaries

The boundaries between the plates are the areas where most tectonic activity takes place. Three types of movement occur at plate boundaries: the plates can either move toward each other, move apart, or slide past each other. The effect this has on the Earth's structure depends on whether the margin is between two continental plates, two oceanic plates, or an oceanic and continental plate.

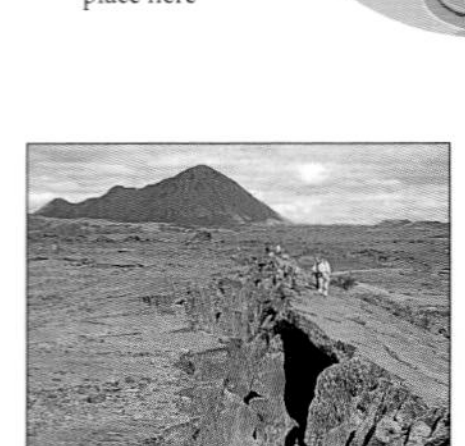

The Mid-Atlantic Ridge *rises above sea level in Iceland, producing geysers and volcanoes.*

Mid-ocean ridges

Mid-ocean ridges are formed when two adjacent oceanic plates pull apart, allowing magma to force its way up to the surface, which then cools to form solid rock. Vast amounts of volcanic material are discharged at these mid-ocean ridges which can reach heights of 10,000 ft (3,000 m).

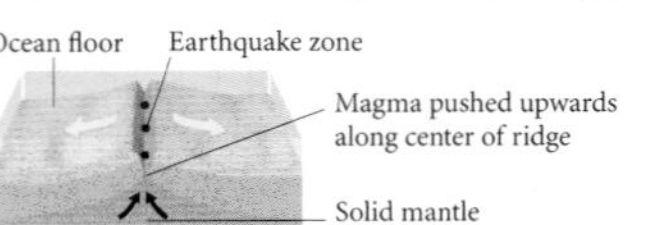
Ocean floor
Earthquake zone
Magma pushed upwards along center of ridge
Solid mantle

Formation of a mid-ocean ridge

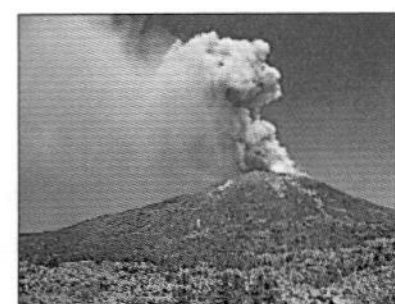

Mount Pinatubo *is an active volcano, lying on the Pacific "Ring of Fire."*

Ocean plates meeting

Oceanic crust is denser and thinner than continental crust; on average it is 3 miles (5 km) thick, while continental crust averages 18–24 miles (30–40 km). When oceanic plates of similar density meet, the crust is contorted as one plate overrides the other, forming deep sea trenches and volcanic island arcs above sea level.

Overriding plate
Chain of islands
Ocean trench
Diving plate
Volcanic activity

Ocean plates meeting to form an island arc

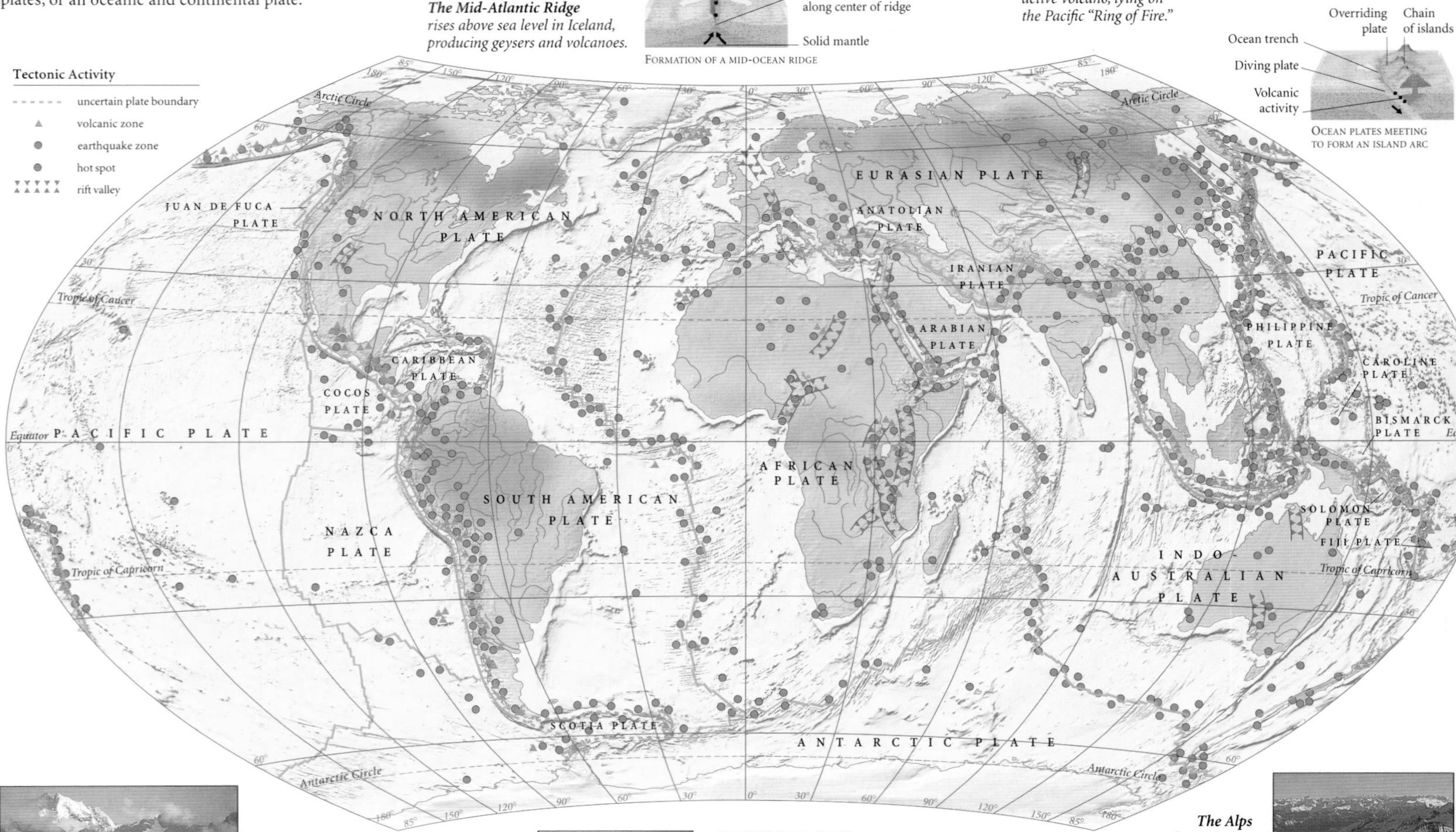
Tectonic Activity
uncertain plate boundary
volcanic zone
earthquake zone
hot spot
rift valley
Arctic Circle
Tropic of Cancer
Equator
Tropic of Capricorn
Antarctic Circle
JUAN DE FUCA PLATE
NORTH AMERICAN PLATE
EURASIAN PLATE
ANATOLIAN PLATE
IRANIAN PLATE
ARABIAN PLATE
PACIFIC PLATE
PHILIPPINE PLATE
CAROLINE PLATE
BISMARCK PLATE
CARIBBEAN PLATE
COCOS PLATE
PACIFIC PLATE
AFRICAN PLATE
SOUTH AMERICAN PLATE
NAZCA PLATE
SOLOMON PLATE
FIJI PLATE
INDO-AUSTRALIAN PLATE
SCOTIA PLATE
ANTARCTIC PLATE

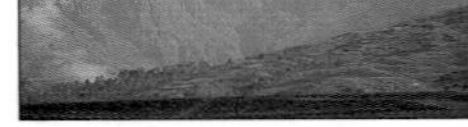

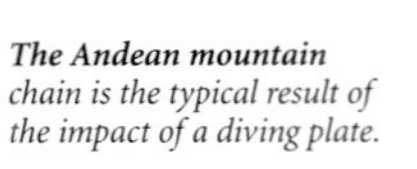

The Andean mountain *chain is the typical result of the impact of a diving plate.*

Diving plates

When an oceanic and a continental plate meet, the denser oceanic plate is driven underneath the continental plate, which is crumpled by the collision to form mountain ranges. As the ocean plate plunges downward, it heats up, and molten rock (magma) is forced up to the surface.

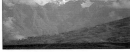

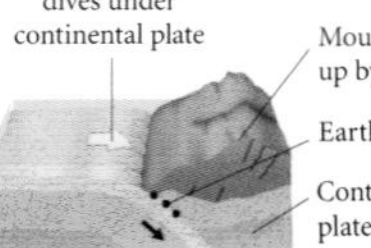
Oceanic plate dives under continental plate
Mountains thrust up by collision
Earthquake zone
Continental plate

Diving plate

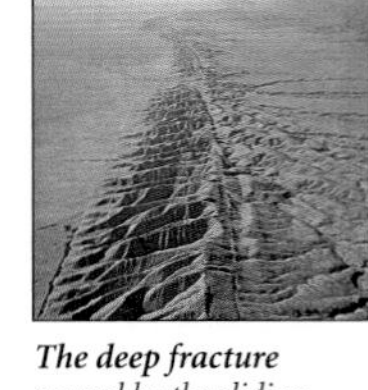

The deep fracture *caused by the sliding plates of the San Andreas Fault can be clearly seen in parts of California.*

Sliding plates

When two plates slide past each other, friction is caused along the fault line which divides them. The plates do not move smoothly, and the uneven movement causes earthquakes.

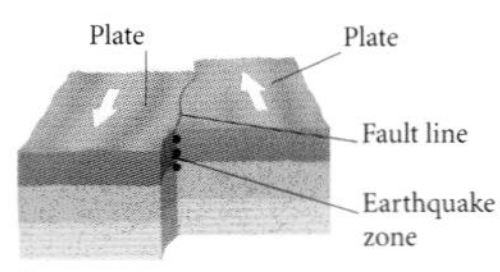
Plate
Plate
Fault line
Earthquake zone

Sliding plates

The Alps *were formed when the African plate collided with the Eurasian Plate, about 65 million years ago.*

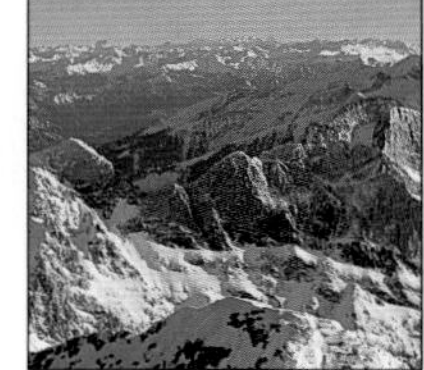

Plate buckles as it collides
Mountains thrust upwards
Earthquake zone
Crust thickens in response to the impact

Continental plates colliding to form a mountain range

Colliding plates

When two continental plates collide, great mountain chains are thrust upward as the crust buckles and folds under the force of the impact.

Continental drift

Although the plates which make up the Earth's crust move only a few inches in a year, over the millions of years of the Earth's history, its continents have moved many thousands of miles, to create new continents, oceans, and mountain chains.

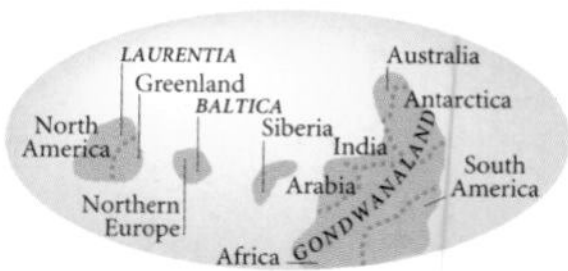
LAURENTIA
Greenland
BALTICA
Australia
Siberia
India
Antarctica
North America
South America
Arabia
Northern Europe
Africa
GONDWANALAND

1: CAMBRIAN PERIOD

570–510 million years ago. *Most continents are in tropical latitudes. The supercontinent of Gondwanaland reaches the South Pole.*

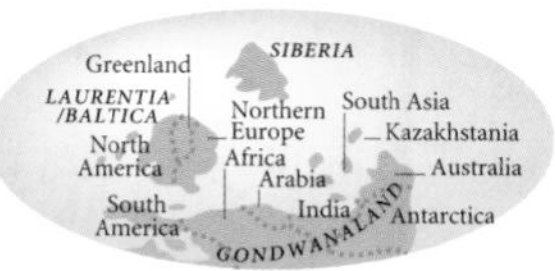
Greenland
SIBERIA
LAURENTIA /BALTICA
Northern Europe
South Asia
Kazakhstania
North America
Africa
Arabia
Australia
South America
India
Antarctica
GONDWANALAND

2: DEVONIAN PERIOD

408–362 million years ago. *The continents of Gondwanaland and Laurentia are drifting northward.*

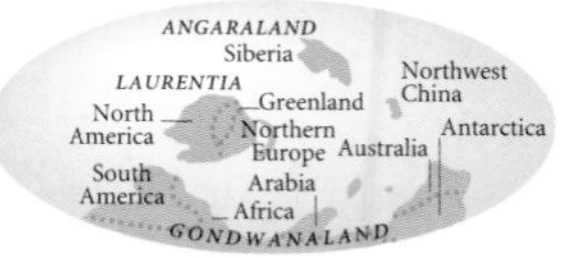
ANGARALAND
Siberia
LAURENTIA
Northwest China
North America
Greenland
Northern Europe
Antarctica
Australia
South America
Arabia
Africa
GONDWANALAND

3: CARBONIFEROUS PERIOD

362–290 million years ago. *The Earth is dominated by three continents; Laurentia, Angaraland, and Gondwanaland.*

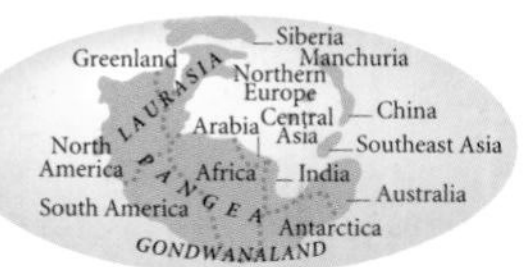
Greenland
Siberia
Manchuria
Northern Europe
China
Arabia
Central Asia
Southeast Asia
North America
Africa
India
South America
Australia
Antarctica
LAURASIA
PANGEA
GONDWANALAND

4: TRIASSIC PERIOD

245–208 million years ago. *All three major continents have joined to form the supercontinent of Pangea.*

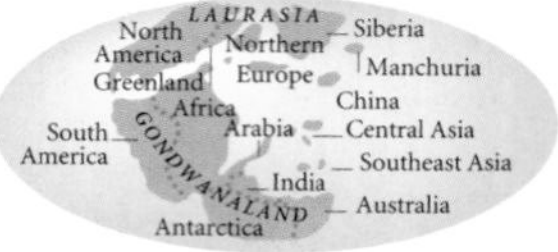
LAURASIA
North America
Siberia
Northern Europe
Greenland
Manchuria
China
Africa
South America
Arabia
Central Asia
Southeast Asia
India
Australia
Antarctica
GONDWANALAND

5: JURASSIC PERIOD

208–145 million years ago. *The supercontinent of Pangea begins to break up, causing an overall rise in sea levels.*

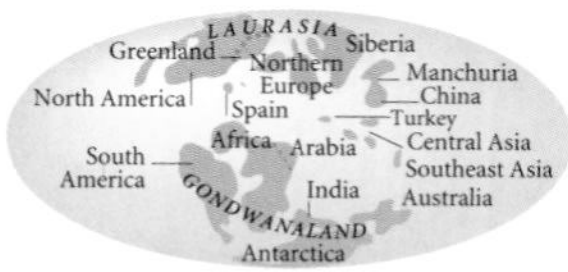
LAURASIA
Greenland
Siberia
Northern Europe
Manchuria
North America
Spain
China
Turkey
Africa
Arabia
Central Asia
South America
Southeast Asia
India
Australia
GONDWANALAND
Antarctica

6: CRETACEOUS PERIOD

145–65 million years ago. *Warm, shallow seas cover much of the land: sea levels are about 80 ft (25 m) above present levels.*

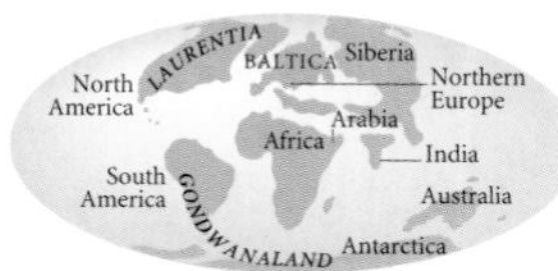
LAURENTIA
BALTICA
Siberia
North America
Northern Europe
Arabia
Africa
India
South America
Australia
GONDWANALAND
Antarctica

7: TERTIARY PERIOD

65–2 million years ago. *Although the world's geography is becoming more recognizable, major events such as the creation of the Himalayan mountain chain, are still to occur during this period.*

Continental shields

The centers of the Earth's continents, known as shields, were established between 2500 and 500 million years ago; some contain rocks over three billion years old. They were formed by a series of turbulent events: plate movements, earthquakes, and volcanic eruptions. Since the Pre-Cambrian period, over 570 million years ago, they have experienced little tectonic activity, and today, these flat, low-lying slabs of solidified molten rock form the stable centers of the continents. They are bounded or covered by successive belts of younger sedimentary rock.

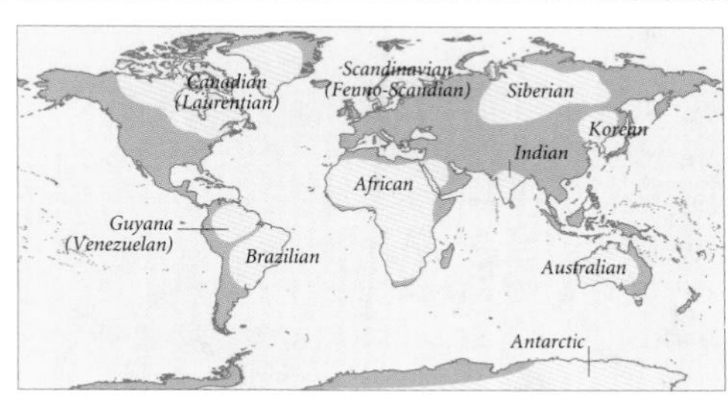
Canadian (Laurentian)
Scandinavian (Fenno-Scandian)
Siberian
Korean
Indian
African
Guyana (Venezuelan)
Brazilian
Australian
Antarctic

Creation of the Himalayas

Between 10 and 20 million years ago, the Indian subcontinent, part of the ancient continent of Gondwanaland, collided with the continent of Asia. The Indo-Australian Plate continued to move northward, displacing continental crust and uplifting the Himalayas, the world's highest mountain chain.

Movements of India

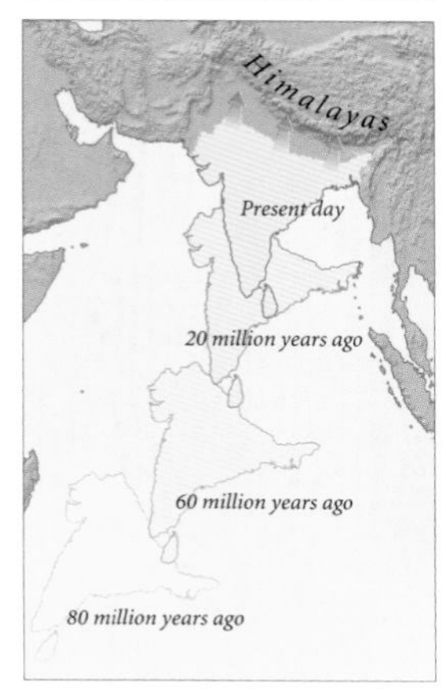
Himalayas
Present day
20 million years ago
60 million years ago
80 million years ago

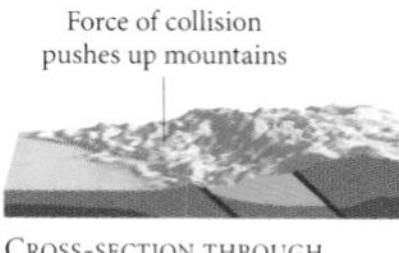
Force of collision pushes up mountains

Cross-section through the Himalayas

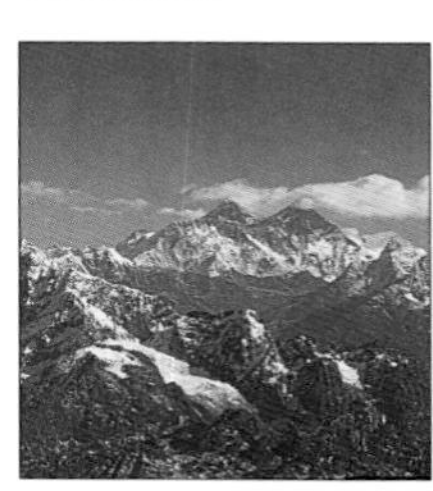

The Himalayas *were uplifted when the Indian subcontinent collided with Asia.*

The Hawaiian Island chain

A hot spot lying deep beneath the Pacific Ocean pushes a plume of magma from the Earth's mantle up through the Pacific Plate to form volcanic islands. While the hot spot remains stationary, the plate on which the islands sit is moving slowly. A long chain of islands has been created as the plate passes over the hot spot.

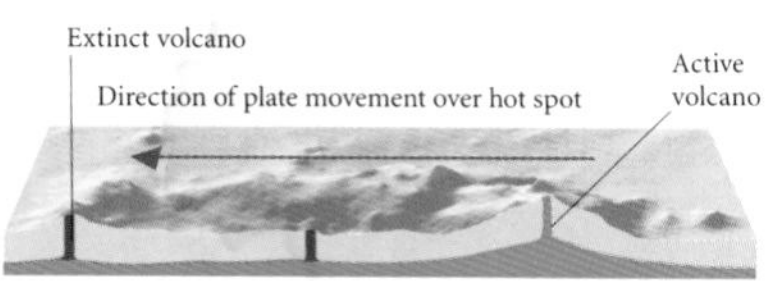
Extinct volcano
Active volcano
Direction of plate movement over hot spot

Cross-section through the Hawaiian Islands

Evolution of the Hawaiian Islands

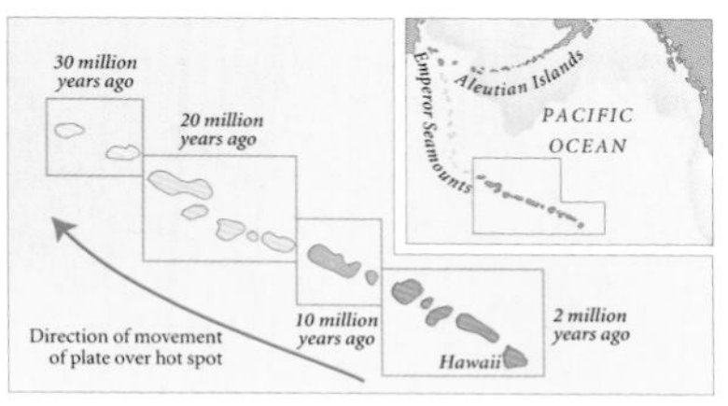
30 million years ago
20 million years ago
10 million years ago
2 million years ago
Aleutian Islands
Emperor Seamounts
PACIFIC OCEAN
Hawaii
Direction of movement of plate over hot spot

The Earth's Geology

The Earth's rocks are created in a continual cycle. Exposed rocks are weathered and eroded by wind, water and chemicals and deposited as sediments. If they pass into the Earth's crust they will be transformed by high temperatures and pressures into metamorphic rocks or they will melt and solidify as igneous rocks.

GNEISS

1 Gneiss is a metamorphic rock made at great depth during the formation of mountain chains, when intense heat and pressure transform sedimentary or igneous rocks.

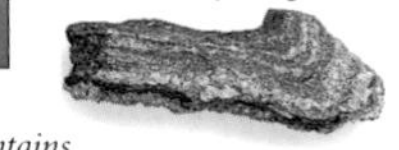

Gneiss *formations in Norway's Jotunheimen Mountains.*

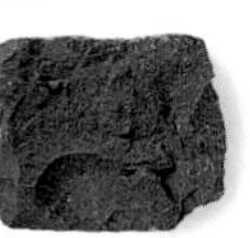

BASALT

2 Basalt is an igneous rock, formed when small quantities of magma lying close to the Earth's surface cool rapidly.

Basalt *columns at Giant's Causeway, Northern Ireland, UK.*

LIMESTONE

3 Limestone is a sedimentary rock, which is formed mainly from the calcite skeletons of marine animals which have been compressed into rock.

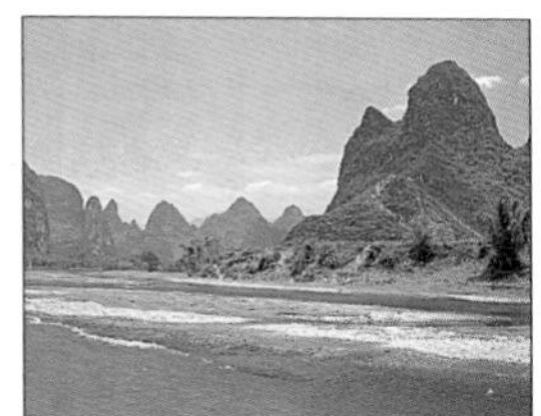

Limestone hills*, Guilin, China.*

CORAL

4 Coral reefs are formed from the skeletons of millions of individual corals.

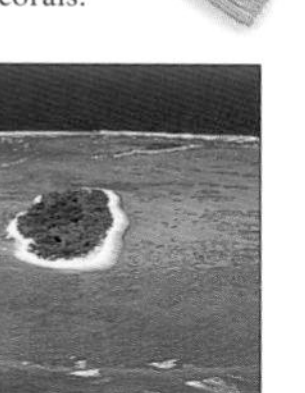

Great Barrier Reef*, Australia.*

SANDSTONE

8 Sandstones are sedimentary rocks formed mainly in deserts, beaches, and deltas. Desert sandstones are formed of grains of quartz which have been well rounded by wind erosion.

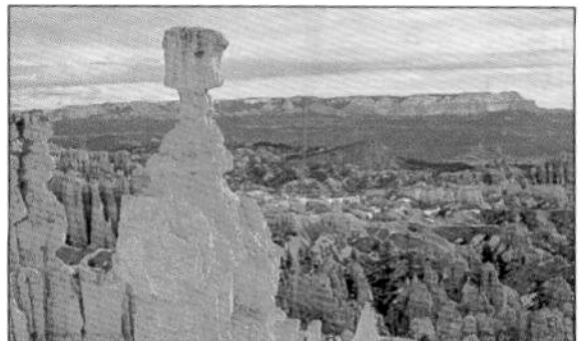

Rock stacks *of desert sandstone, at Bryce Canyon National Park, Utah.*

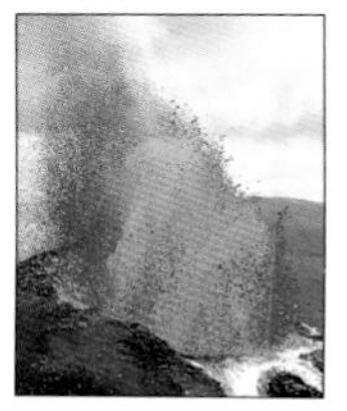

Extrusive igneous rocks *are formed during volcanic eruptions, as here in Hawaii.*

ANDESITE

7 Andesite is an extrusive igneous rock formed from magma which has solidified on the Earth's crust after a volcanic eruption.

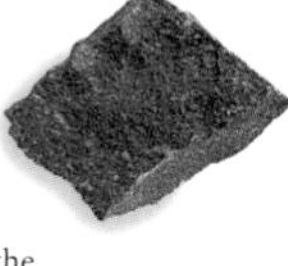

The world's major geological regions

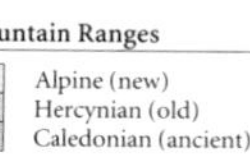
Geological Regions
continental shield
sedimentary cover
coral formation
igneous rock types
Mountain Ranges
Alpine (new)
Hercynian (old)
Caledonian (ancient)

SCHIST

6 Schist is a metamorphic rock formed during mountain building, when temperature and pressure are comparatively high. Both mudstones and shales reform into schist under these conditions.

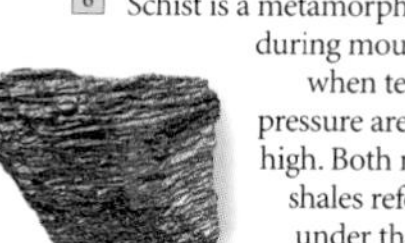

Schist formations *in the Atlas Mountains, northwestern Africa.*

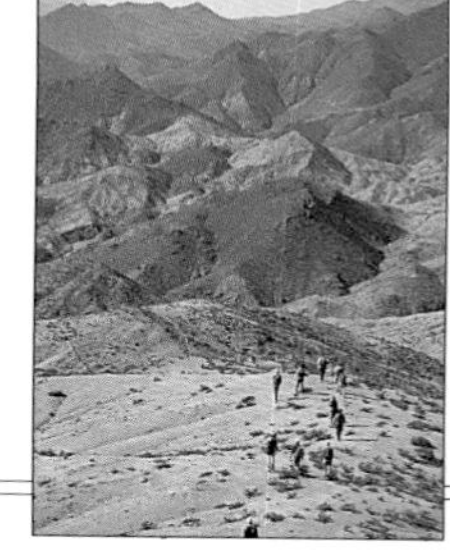

GRANITE

5 Granite is an intrusive igneous rock formed from magma which has solidified deep within the Earth's crust. The magma cools slowly, producing a coarse-grained rock.

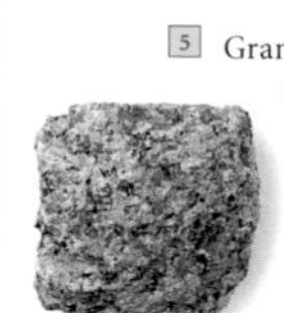

Namibia's *Namaqualand Plateau is formed of granite.*

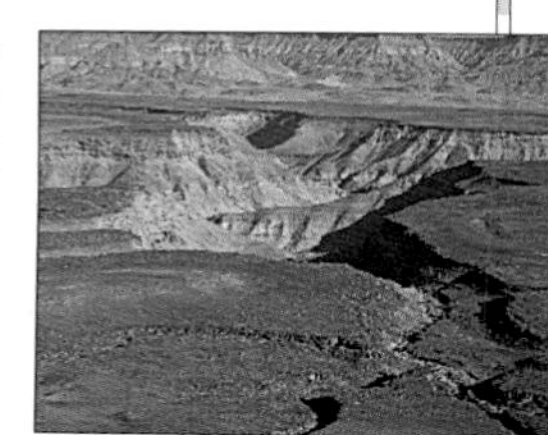

Shaping the Landscape

The basic material of the Earth's surface is solid rock: valleys, deserts, soil, and sand are all evidence of the powerful agents of weathering, erosion, and deposition which constantly shape and transform the Earth's landscapes. Water, either flowing continually in rivers or seas, or frozen and compacted into solid sheets of ice, has the most clearly visible impact on the Earth's surface. But wind can transport fragments of rock over huge distances and strip away protective layers of vegetation, exposing rock surfaces to the impact of extreme heat and cold.

Water

Less than 2% of the world's water is on the land, but it is the most powerful agent of landscape change. Water, as rainfall, groundwater, and rivers, can transform landscapes through both erosion and deposition. Eroded material carried by rivers forms the world's most fertile soils.

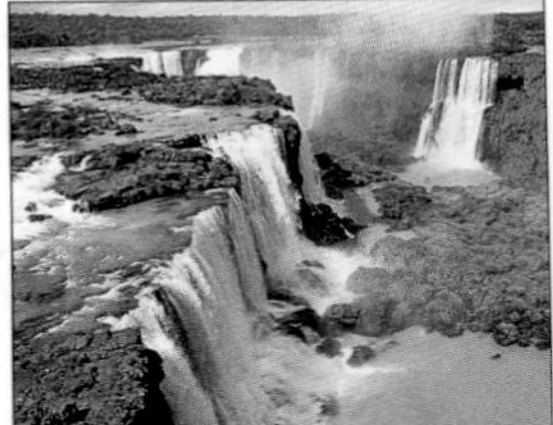

Waterfalls such as the Iguaçu Falls *on the border between Argentina and southern Brazil, erode the underlying rock, causing the falls to retreat.*

Coastal water

The world's coastlines are constantly changing; every day, tides deposit, sift and sort sand and gravel on the shoreline. Over longer periods, powerful wave action erodes cliffs and headlands and carves out bays.

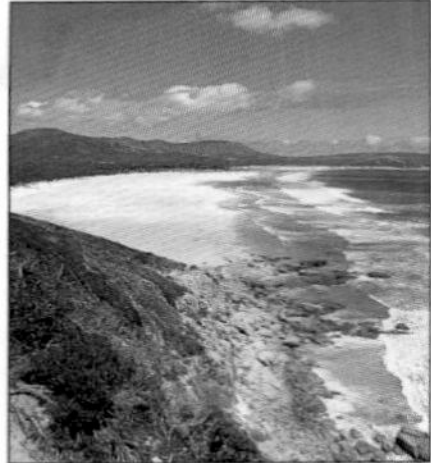

A low, wide sandy beach *on South Africa's Cape Peninsula is continually re-shaped by the action of the Atlantic waves.*

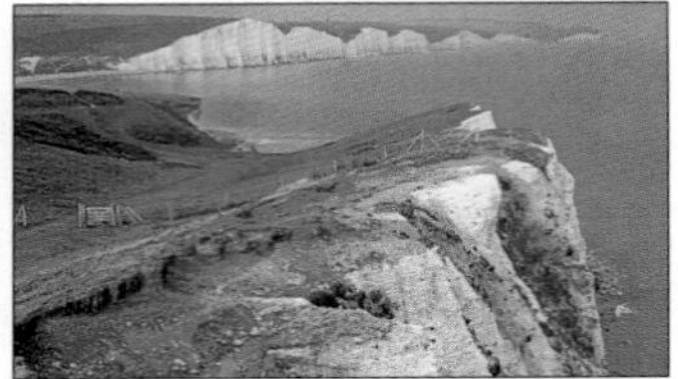

The sheer chalk cliffs *at Seven Sisters in southern England are constantly under attack from waves.*

Groundwater

In regions where there are porous rocks such as chalk, water is stored underground in large quantities; these reservoirs of water are known as aquifers. Rain percolates through topsoil into the underlying bedrock, creating an underground store of water. The limit of the saturated zone is called the water table.

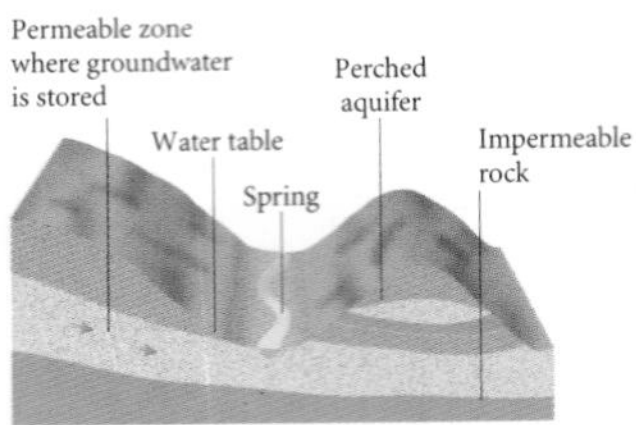
Permeable zone where groundwater is stored
Perched aquifer
Water table
Impermeable rock
Spring

Storage of groundwater in an aquifer

World river systems

drainage basin

World river systems: Sediment deposited annually per drainage basin

tons per sq mile per year: 9120, 6080, 1520, 760

tonnes per sq km per year: 2400, 1600, 400, 200 and less

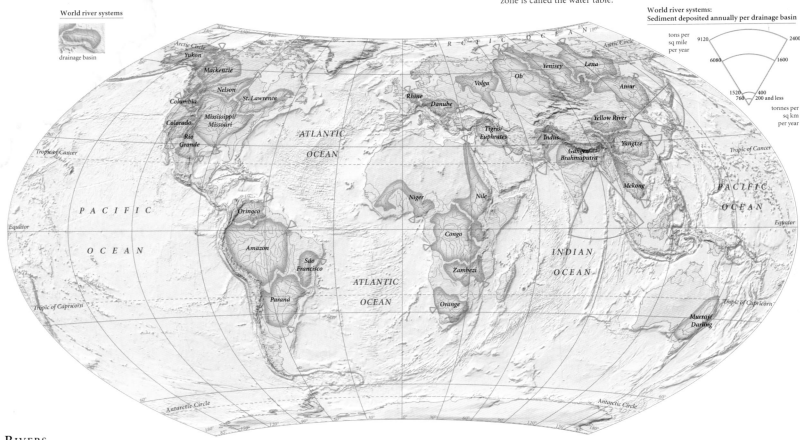

Arctic Circle, Tropic of Cancer, Equator, Tropic of Capricorn, Antarctic Circle

ARCTIC OCEAN, ATLANTIC OCEAN, PACIFIC OCEAN, INDIAN OCEAN

Yukon, Mackenzie, Nelson, St. Lawrence, Columbia, Colorado, Mississippi/Missouri, Rio Grande, Orinoco, Amazon, São Francisco, Paraná, Rhine, Danube, Volga, Ob', Yenisey, Lena, Amur, Tigris/Euphrates, Indus, Ganges/Brahmaputra, Yellow River, Yangtze, Mekong, Niger, Nile, Congo, Zambezi, Orange, Murray/Darling

Rivers

Rivers erode the land by grinding and dissolving rocks and stones. Most erosion occurs in the river's upper course as it flows through highland areas. Rock fragments are moved along the river bed by fast-flowing water and deposited in areas where the river slows down, such as flat plains, or where the river enters seas or lakes.

River valleys

Over long periods of time rivers erode uplands to form characteristic V-shaped valleys with smooth sides.

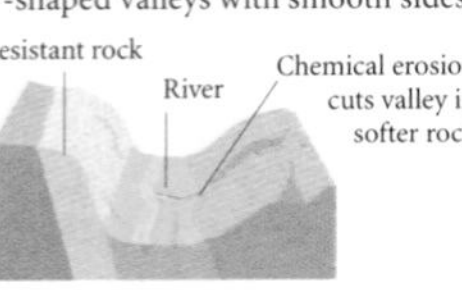
Resistant rock
River
Chemical erosion cuts valley in softer rock

River valley erosion

Deltas

When a river deposits its load of silt and sediment (alluvium) on entering the sea, it may form a delta. As this material accumulates, it chokes the mouth of the river, forcing it to create new channels to reach the sea.

The Nile *forms a broad delta as it flows into the Mediterranean.*

Drainage basins

The drainage basin is the area of land drained by a major trunk river and its smaller branch rivers or tributaries. Drainage basins are separated from one another by natural boundaries known as watersheds.

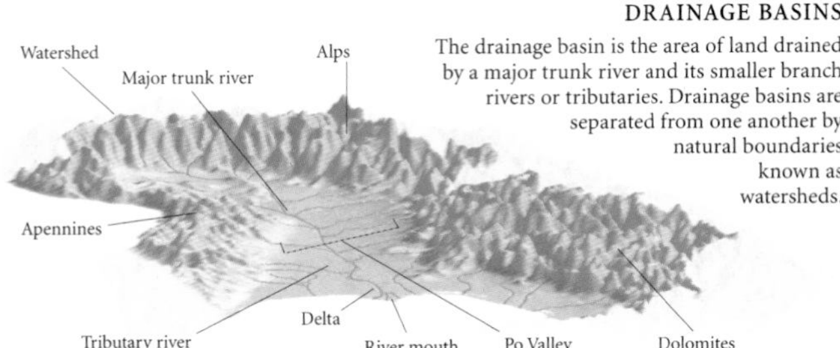
Watershed
Major trunk river
Alps
Apennines
Tributary river
Delta
River mouth
Po Valley
Dolomites

The drainage basin *of the Po River, northern Italy.*

The Mississippi River *forms meanders as it flows across the southern US.*

Meanders

In their lower courses, rivers flow slowly. As they flow across the lowlands, they form looping bends called meanders.

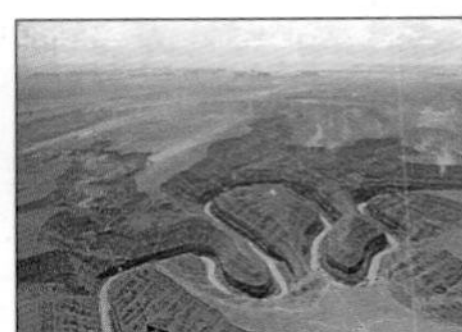

The meanders *of Utah's San Juan River have become deeply incised.*

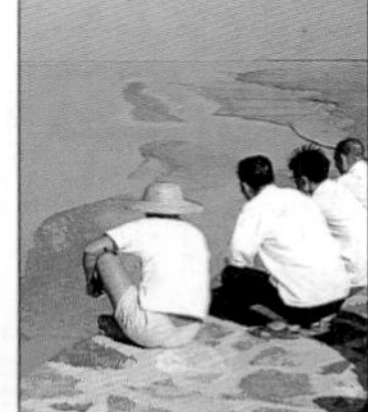

Mud is *deposited by China's Yellow River in its lower course.*

Deposition

When rivers have deposited large quantities of fertile alluvium, they are forced to find new channels through the alluvium deposits, creating braided river systems.

Landslides

Heavy rain and associated flooding on slopes can loosen underlying rocks, which crumble, causing the top layers of rock and soil to slip.

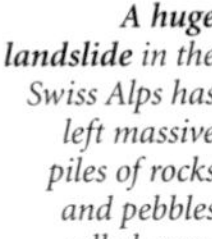

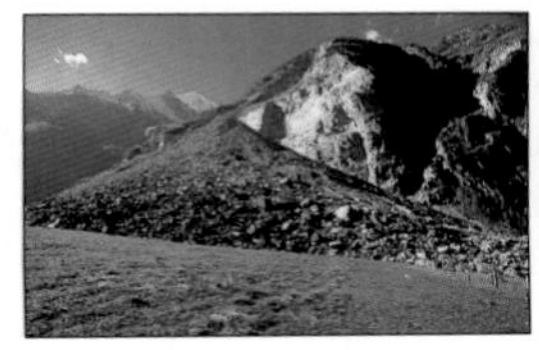

A huge landslide *in the Swiss Alps has left massive piles of rocks and pebbles called scree.*

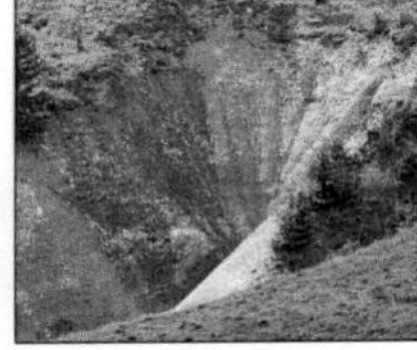

A deep gully *in the French Alps caused by the scouring of upper layers of turf.*

Gullies

In areas where soil is thin, rainwater is not effectively absorbed, and may flow overland. The water courses downhill in channels, or gullies, and may lead to rapid erosion of soil.

Ice

During its long history, the Earth has experienced a number of glacial episodes when temperatures were considerably lower than today. During the last Ice Age, 18,000 years ago, ice covered an area three times larger than it does today. Over these periods, the ice has left a remarkable legacy of transformed landscapes.

Glaciers

Glaciers are formed by the compaction of snow into "rivers" of ice. As they move over the landscape, glaciers pick up and carry a load of rocks and boulders which erode the landscape they pass over, and are eventually deposited at the end of the glacier.

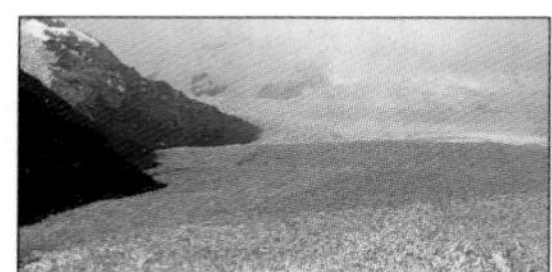

***A massive glacier** advancing down a valley in southern Argentina.*

Glacial valleys

Glaciers can erode much more powerfully than rivers. They form steep-sided, flat-bottomed valleys with a typical U-shaped profile. Valleys created by tributary glaciers, whose floors have not been eroded to the same depth as the main glacial valley floor, are called hanging valleys.

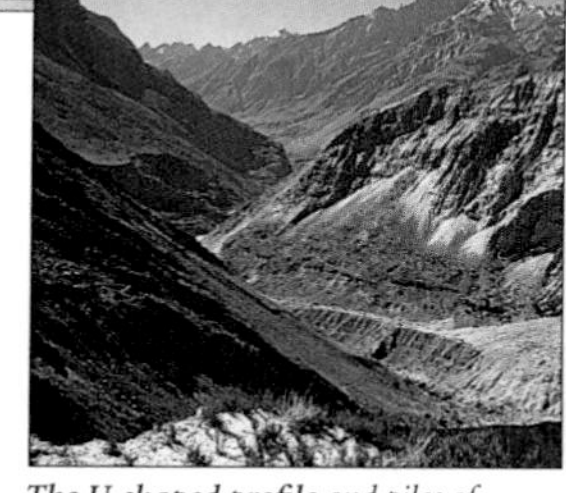

***The U-shaped profile** and piles of morainic debris are characteristic of a valley once filled by a glacier.*

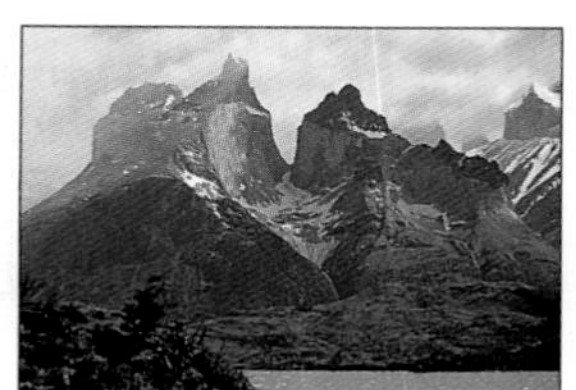

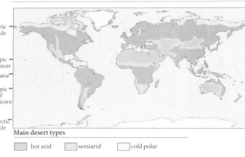

***A series of hanging valleys** high up in the Chilean Andes.*

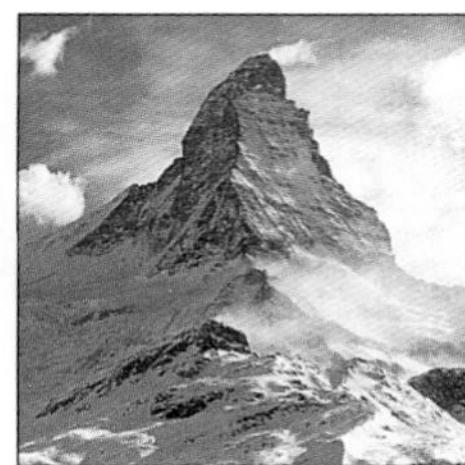

***The profile** of the Matterhorn has been formed by three cirques lying "back-to-back."*

Cirques

Cirques are basin-shaped hollows which mark the head of a glaciated valley. Where neighboring cirques meet, they are divided by sharp rock ridges called arêtes. It is these arêtes which give the Matterhorn its characteristic profile.

Fjords

Fjords are ancient glacial valleys flooded by the sea following the end of a period of glaciation. Beneath the water, the valley floor can be 4,000 ft (1,300 m) deep.

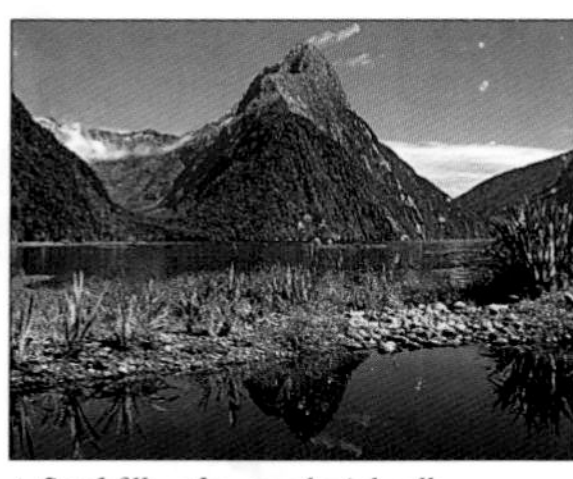

***A fjord** fills a former glacial valley in southern New Zealand.*

Past and present world ice-cover and glacial features

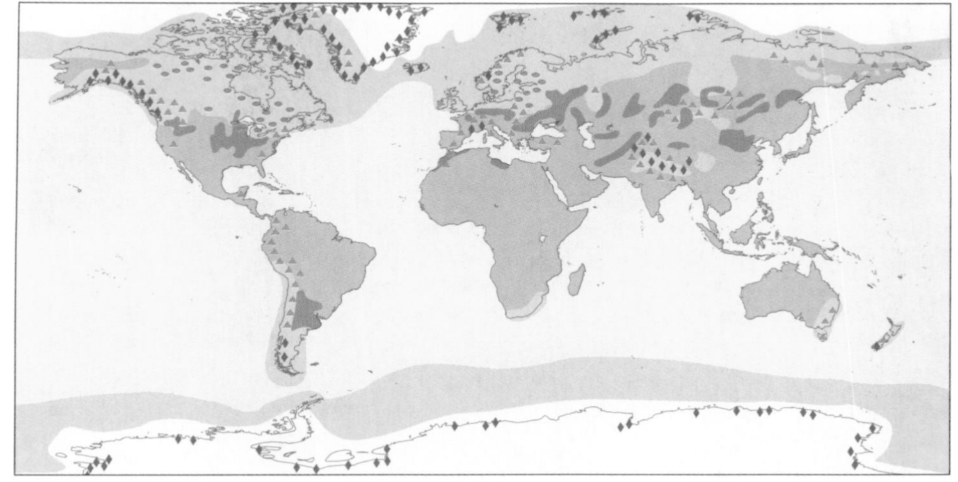

Past and present world ice cover and glacial features

- extent of last Ice Age
- loess deposits
- post-glacial feature
- glacial feature
- present day ice cover
- glacial field

Post-glacial features

When a glacial episode ends, the retreating ice leaves many features. These include depositional ridges called moraines, which may be eroded into low hills known as drumlins; sinuous ridges called eskers; kames, which are rounded hummocks; depressions known as kettle holes; and windblown loess deposits.

Kame terrace
Kettle hole
Esker
Braided river
Windblown loess
Retreating glacier
Drumlin
Terminal moraine
Glacial till
Bedrock

Post-glacial landscape features

Ice shattering

Water drips into fissures in rocks and freezes, expanding as it does so. The pressure weakens the rock, causing it to crack, and eventually to shatter into polygonal patterns.

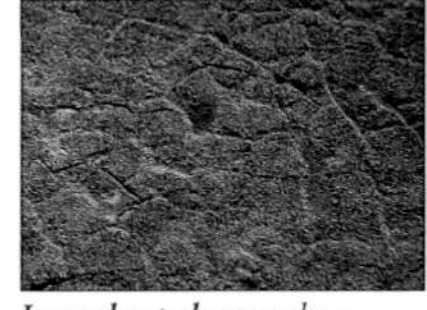

***Irregular polygons** show through the sedge-grass tundra in the Yukon, Canada.*

Periglaciation

Periglacial areas occur near to the edge of ice sheets. A layer of frozen ground lying just beneath the surface of the land is known as permafrost. When the surface melts in the summer, the water is unable to drain into the frozen ground, and so "creeps" downhill, a process known as solifluction

Wind

Strong winds can transport rock fragments great distances, especially where there is little vegetation to protect the rock. In desert areas, wind picks up loose, unprotected sand particles, carrying them over great distances. This powerfully abrasive debris is blasted at the surface by the wind, eroding the landscape into dramatic shapes.

Prevailing winds and dust trajectories

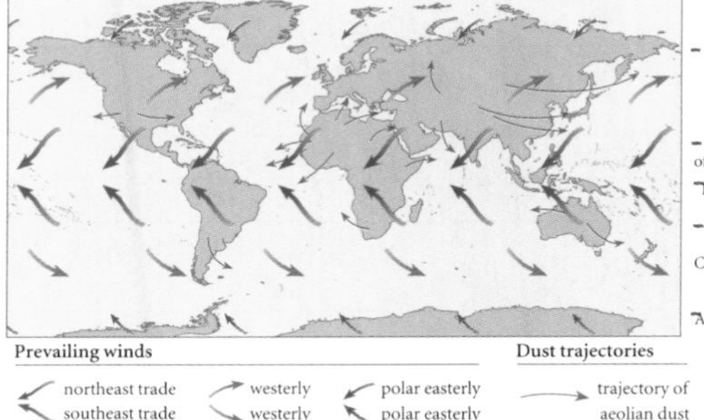

Arctic Circle
Tropic of Cancer
Equator
Tropic of Capricorn
Antarctic Circle

Prevailing winds: northeast trade, southeast trade; westerly, westerly; polar easterly, polar easterly

Dust trajectories: trajectory of aeolian dust

Deposition

The rocky, stony floors of the world's deserts are swept and scoured by strong winds. The smaller, finer particles of sand are shaped into surface ripples, dunes, or sand mountains, which rise to a height of 650 ft (200 m). Dunes usually form single lines, running perpendicular to the direction of the prevailing wind. These long, straight ridges can extend for over 100 miles (160 km).

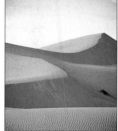

***Barchan dunes** in the Arabian Desert.*

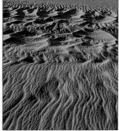

***Complex dune system** in the Sahara.*

Dunes

Dunes are shaped by wind direction and sand supply. Where sand supply is limited, crescent-shaped barchan dunes are formed.

Types of Dune

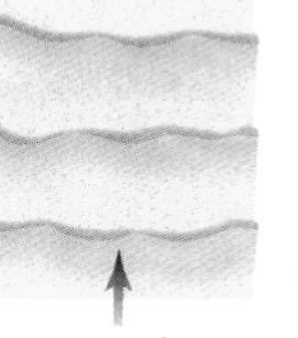

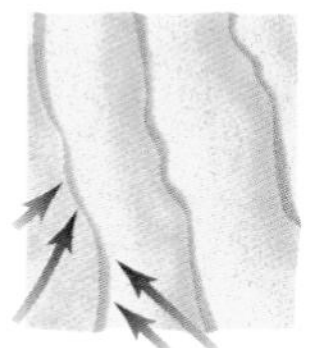

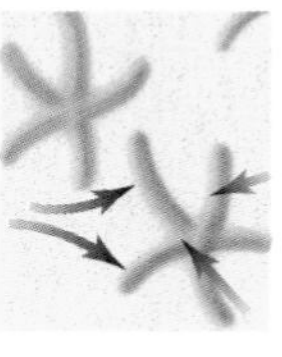

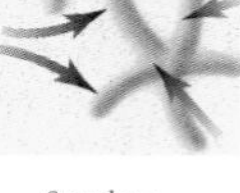

wind direction

Transverse dune · Barchan dune · Linear dune · Star dune

Temperature

Hot and cold deserts

Main desert types: hot arid; semiarid; cold polar

Most of the world's deserts are in the tropics. The cold deserts which occur elsewhere are arid because they are a long way from the rain-giving sea. Rock in deserts is exposed because of lack of vegetation and is susceptible to changes in temperature; extremes of heat and cold can cause both cracks and fissures to appear in the rock.

Heat

Fierce sun can heat the surface of rock, causing it to expand more rapidly than the cooler, underlying layers. This creates tensions which force the rock to crack or break up. In arid regions, the evaporation of water from rock surfaces dissolves certain minerals within the water, causing salt crystals to form in small openings in the rock. The hard crystals force the openings to widen into cracks and fissures.

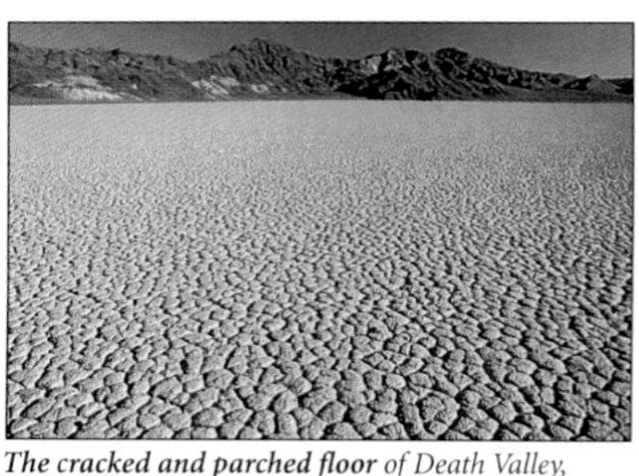

***The cracked and parched floor** of Death Valley, California. This is one of the hottest deserts on Earth.*

Desert abrasion

Abrasion creates a wide range of desert landforms from faceted pebbles and wind ripples in the sand, to large-scale features such as yardangs (low, streamlined ridges), and scoured desert pavements.

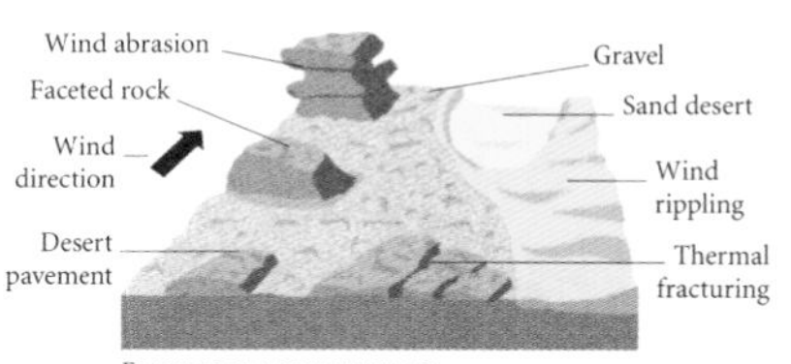

Wind abrasion
Faceted rock
Wind direction
Desert pavement
Gravel
Sand desert
Wind rippling
Thermal fracturing

Features of a desert surface

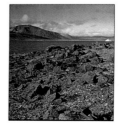

***This dry valley at Ellesmere Island** in the Canadian Arctic is an example of a cold desert. The cracked floor and scoured slopes are features also found in hot deserts.*

The World's Oceans

TWO-THIRDS OF THE EARTH'S SURFACE is covered by the oceans. The landscape of the ocean floor, like the surface of the land, has been shaped by movements of the Earth's crust over millions of years to form volcanic mountain ranges, deep trenches, basins, and plateaus. Ocean currents constantly redistribute warm and cold water around the world. A major warm current, such as El Niño in the Pacific Ocean, can increase surface temperature by up to 46°F (8°C), causing changes in weather patterns which can lead to both droughts and flooding.

The great oceans

THERE ARE FIVE OCEANS on Earth: the Pacific, Atlantic, Indian, and Southern oceans, and the much smaller Arctic Ocean. These five ocean basins are relatively young, having evolved within the last 80 million years. One of the most recent plate collisions, between the Eurasian and African plates, created the present-day arrangement of continents and oceans.

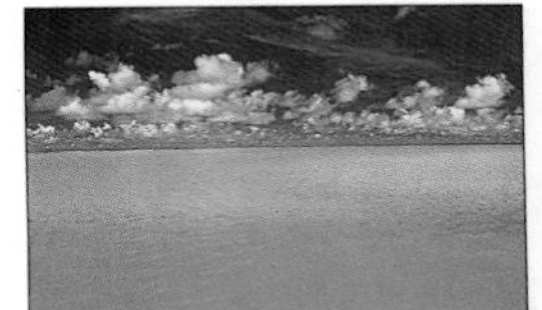

***The Indian Ocean** accounts for approximately 20% of the total area of the world's oceans.*

Sea level

IF THE INFLUENCE of tides, winds, currents, and variations in gravity were ignored, the surface of the Earth's oceans would closely follow the topography of the ocean floor, with an underwater ridge 3,000 ft (915 m) high producing a rise of up to 3 ft (1 m) in the level of the surface water.

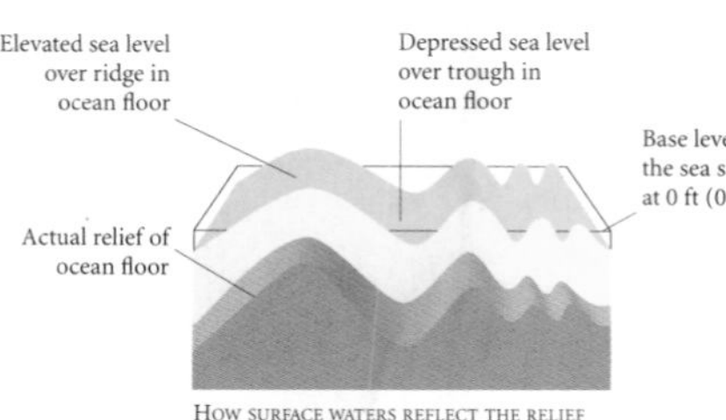
Elevated sea level over ridge in ocean floor
Depressed sea level over trough in ocean floor
Base level of the sea surface at 0 ft (0 m)
Actual relief of ocean floor

HOW SURFACE WATERS REFLECT THE RELIEF OF THE OCEAN FLOOR

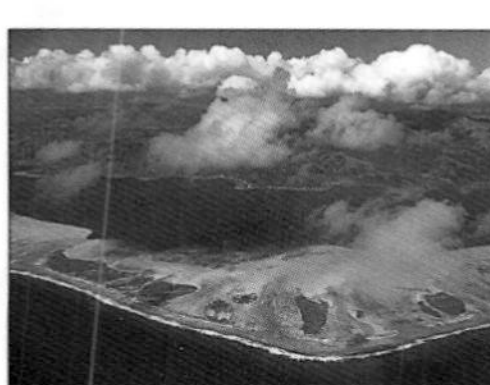

***The low relief** of many small Pacific islands such as these atolls at Huahine in French Polynesia makes them vulnerable to changes in sea level.*

Ocean structure

THE CONTINENTAL SHELF is a shallow, flat seabed surrounding the Earth's continents. It extends to the continental slope, which falls to the ocean floor. Here, the flat abyssal plains are interrupted by vast, underwater mountain ranges, the mid-ocean ridges, and ocean trenches which plunge to depths of 35,828 ft (10,920 m).

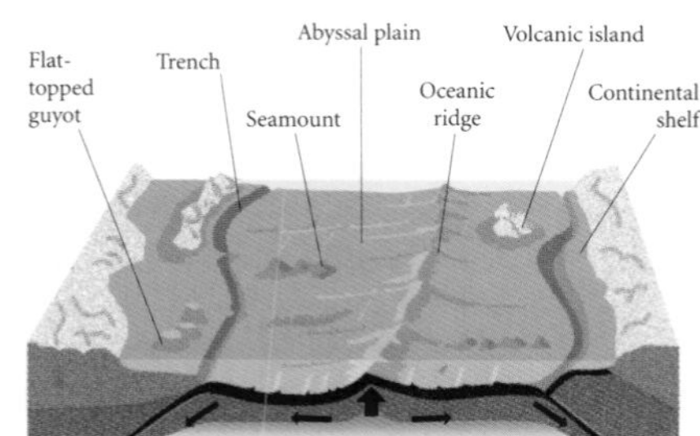
Flat-topped guyot
Trench
Seamount
Abyssal plain
Oceanic ridge
Volcanic island
Continental shelf

TYPICAL SEA-FLOOR FEATURES

Ocean depth
Sea level
200m / 656ft
1000m / 3281ft
2000m / 6562ft
3000m / 9843ft
4000m / 13,124ft
5000m / 16,400ft
6000m / 19,686ft

EUROPE
ASIA
AFRICA
AUSTRALIA
ANTARCTICA
ARCTIC
INDIAN OCEAN
SOUTHERN
Arctic Circle
Barents Sea
Kara Sea
Laptev Sea
East Siberian Sea
North Sea
Baltic Sea
Sea of Okhotsk
Black Sea
Caspian Sea
Adriatic Sea
Mediterranean Sea
Sea of Japan
Kurile Trench
Emperor Seamounts
Northwest Pacific Basin
Japan Trench
Yellow Sea
East China Sea
Taiwan Strait
Persian Gulf
Tropic of Cancer
Red Sea
Arabian Sea
Mid-Pacific Mountains
Bay of Bengal
Philippine Sea
Mariana Trench
Gulf of Thailand
South China Sea
Sunda Shelf
Strait of Malacca
Celebes Sea
Carlsberg Ridge
Chagos-Laccadive Plateau
Gulf of Guinea
Equator
Somali Basin
Mid-Indian Ridge
Mid-Indian Basin
Ninetyeast Ridge
Bismarck Sea
Solomon Sea
Melanesian Basin
Angola Basin
Mozambique Channel
Mascarene Plateau
Arafura Sea
Timor Sea
Coral Sea
Great Barrier Reef
Tropic of Capricorn
Walvis Ridge
Madagascar Basin
Perth Basin
South Fiji Basin
Cape Basin
Mozambique Plateau
Southwest Indian Ridge
South Australian Basin
Bass Strait
Tasman Sea
Agulhas Basin
Southeast Indian Ridge
Kerguelen Plateau
Campbell Plateau
South Indian Basin
Enderby Plain
Antarctic Circle

Black smokers

These vents in the ocean floor disgorge hot, sulfur-rich water from deep in the Earth's crust. Despite the great depths, a variety of lifeforms have adapted to the chemical-rich environment which surrounds black smokers.

***A black smoker** in the Atlantic Ocean.*

***Surtsey, near Iceland**, is a volcanic island lying directly over the Mid-Atlantic Ridge. It was formed in the 1960s following intense volcanic activity nearby.*

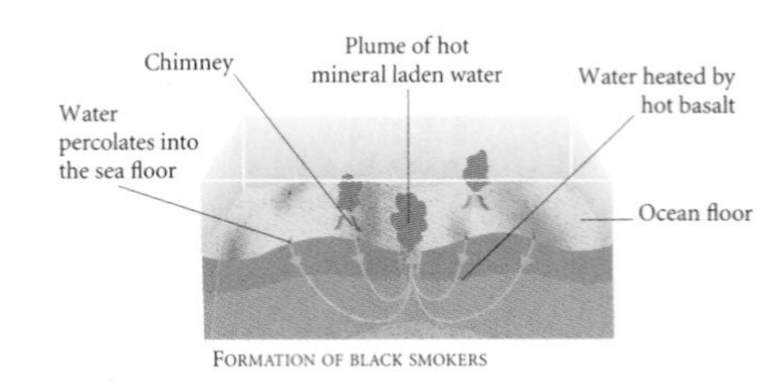
Chimney
Plume of hot mineral laden water
Water heated by hot basalt
Water percolates into the sea floor
Ocean floor

FORMATION OF BLACK SMOKERS

Ocean floors

Mid-ocean ridges are formed by lava which erupts beneath the sea and cools to form solid rock. This process mirrors the creation of volcanoes from cooled lava on the land. The ages of sea floor rocks increase in parallel bands outward from central ocean ridges.

Ages of the ocean floor

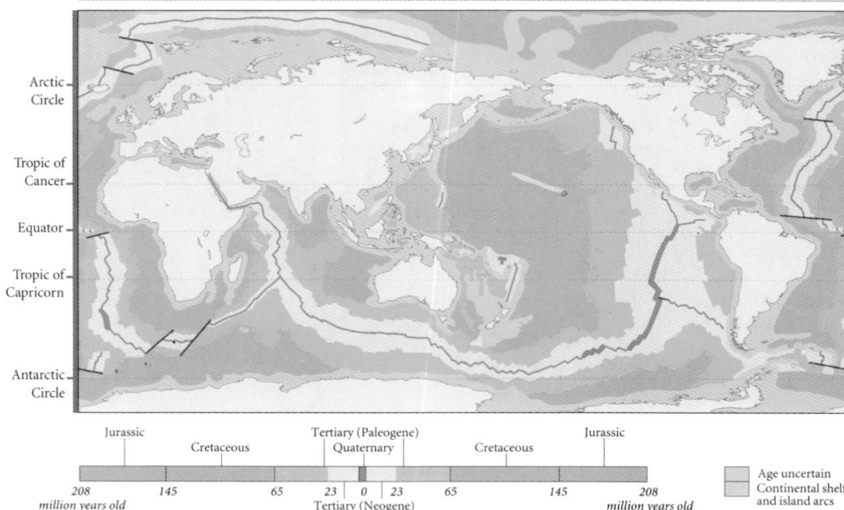
Arctic Circle
Tropic of Cancer
Equator
Tropic of Capricorn
Antarctic Circle
Jurassic
Cretaceous
Tertiary (Paleogene)
Quaternary
Cretaceous
Jurassic
208 million years old
145
65
23
0
23
65
145
208 million years old
Tertiary (Neogene)
Age uncertain
Continental shelf and island arcs

Currents in the Southern Ocean *are driven by some of the world's fiercest winds, including the Roaring Forties, Furious Fifties, and Shrieking Sixties.*

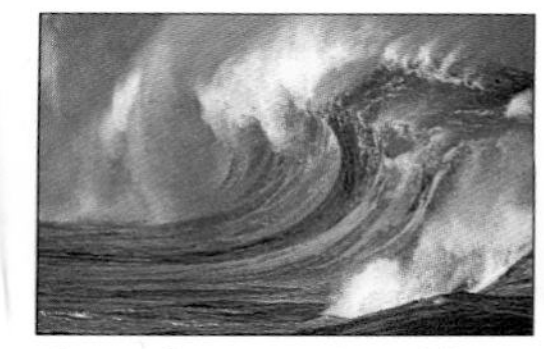

The Pacific Ocean *is the world's largest and deepest ocean, covering over one-third of the surface of the Earth.*

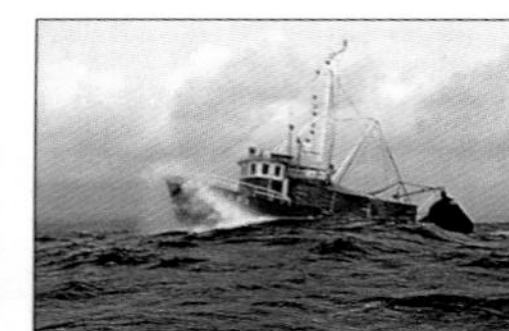

The Atlantic Ocean *was formed when the landmasses of the eastern and western hemispheres began to drift apart 180 million years ago.*

DEPOSITION OF SEDIMENT

STORMS, EARTHQUAKES, and volcanic activity trigger underwater currents known as turbidity currents which scour sand and gravel from the continental shelf, creating underwater canyons. These strong currents pick up material deposited at river mouths and deltas, and carry it across the continental shelf and through the underwater canyons, where it is eventually laid down on the ocean floor in the form of fans.

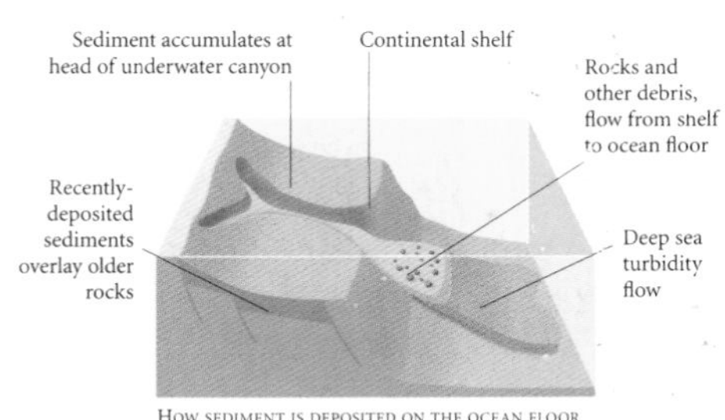
Sediment accumulates at head of underwater canyon
Continental shelf
Rocks and other debris, flow from shelf to ocean floor
Recently-deposited sediments overlay older rocks
Deep sea turbidity flow

HOW SEDIMENT IS DEPOSITED ON THE OCEAN FLOOR

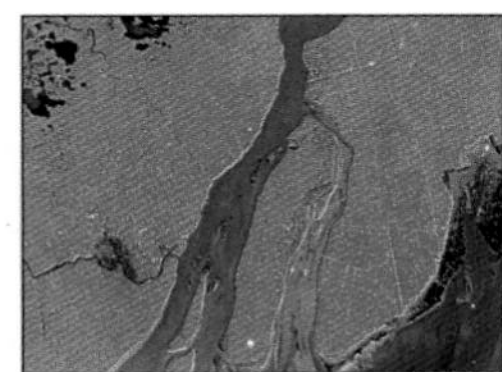

Satellite image *of the Yangtze (Chang Jiang) Delta, in which the land appears red. The river deposits immense quantities of silt into the East China Sea, much of which will eventually reach the deep ocean floor.*

SURFACE WATER

OCEAN CURRENTS move warm water away from the Equator toward the poles, while cold water is, in turn, moved towards the Equator. This is the main way in which the Earth distributes surface heat and is a major climatic control. Approximately 4,000 million years ago, the Earth was dominated by oceans and there was no land to interrupt the flow of the currents, which would have flowed as straight lines, simply influenced by the Earth's rotation.

Idealized globe *showing the movement of water around a landless Earth.*

OCEAN CURRENTS

SURFACE CURRENTS are driven by the prevailing winds and by the spinning motion of the Earth, which drives the currents into circulating whirlpools, or gyres. Deep sea currents, over 330 ft (100 m) below the surface, are driven by differences in water temperature and salinity, which have an impact on the density of deep water and on its movement.

SURFACE TEMPERATURE AND CURRENTS

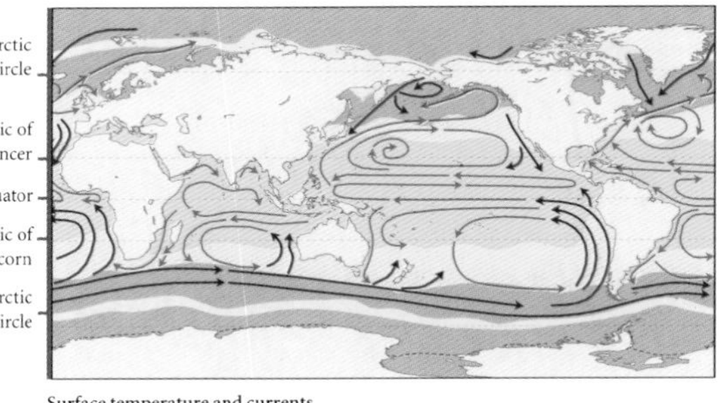
Arctic Circle
Tropic of Cancer
Equator
Tropic of Capricorn
Antarctic Circle

Surface temperature and currents

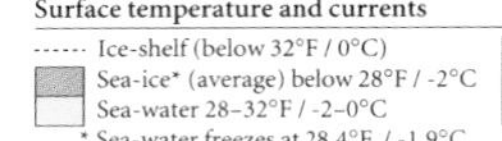
Ice-shelf (below 32°F / 0°C)
Sea-ice* (average) below 28°F / -2°C
Sea-water 28–32°F / -2–0°C
* Sea-water freezes at 28.4°F / -1.9°C

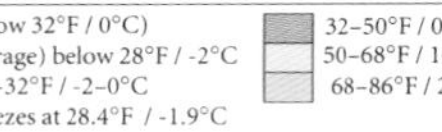
32–50°F / 0–10°C
50–68°F / 10–20°C
68–86°F / 20–30°C
warm current
cold current

TIDES AND WAVES

TIDES ARE CREATED by the pull of the Sun and Moon's gravity on the surface of the oceans. The levels of high and low tides are influenced by the position of the Moon in relation to the Earth and Sun. Waves are formed by wind blowing over the surface of the water.

TIDAL RANGE AND WAVE ENVIRONMENTS

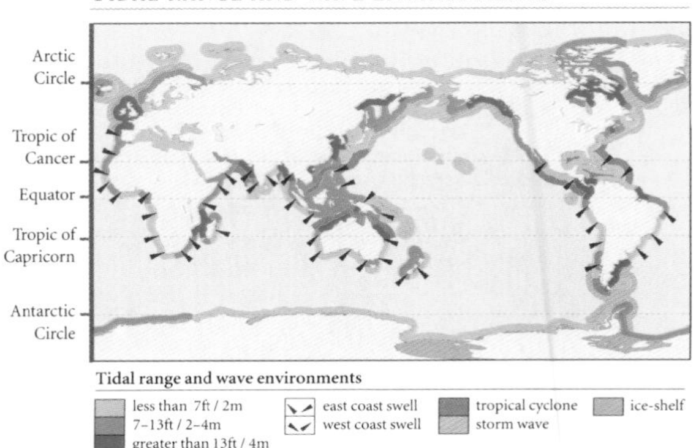
Arctic Circle
Tropic of Cancer
Equator
Tropic of Capricorn
Antarctic Circle
Tidal range and wave environments
less than 7ft / 2m
7–13ft / 2–4m
greater than 13ft / 4m
east coast swell
west coast swell
tropical cyclone storm wave
ice-shelf

HIGH AND LOW TIDES

The highest tides occur when the Earth, the Moon and the Sun are aligned *(below left)*. The lowest tides are experienced when the Sun and Moon align at right angles to one another *(below right)*.

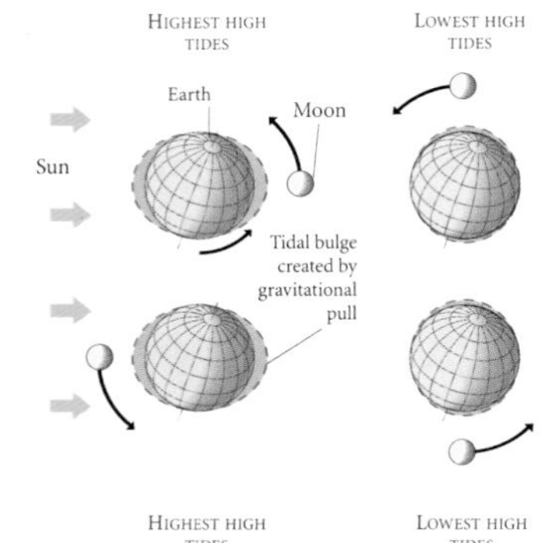
HIGHEST HIGH TIDES
LOWEST HIGH TIDES
Earth
Moon
Sun
Tidal bulge created by gravitational pull
HIGHEST HIGH TIDES
LOWEST HIGH TIDES

DEEP SEA TEMPERATURE AND CURRENTS

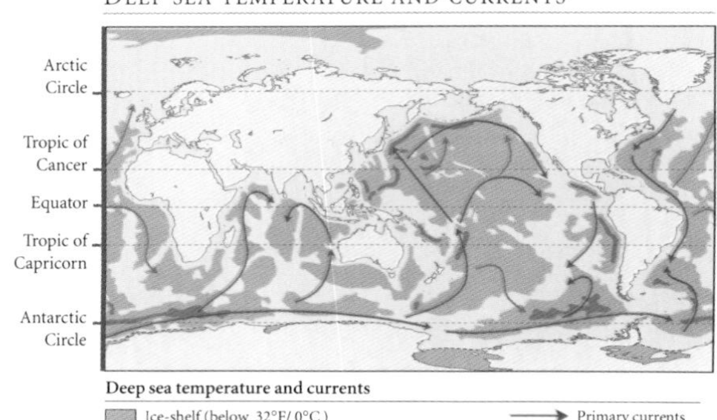
Arctic Circle
Tropic of Cancer
Equator
Tropic of Capricorn
Antarctic Circle
Deep sea temperature and currents
Ice-shelf (below 32°F/ 0°C)
Sea-water 28–32°F / -2–0°C (below 16,400ft/ 5000m)
Sea-water 32–41° F/0–5°C (below 13,120ft/4000m)
Primary currents
Secondary currents

The Global Climate

The Earth's climatic types consist of stable patterns of weather conditions averaged out over a long period of time. Different climates are categorized according to particular combinations of temperature and humidity. By contrast, weather consists of short-term fluctuations in wind, temperature, and humidity conditions. Different climates are determined by latitude, altitude, the prevailing wind, and circulation of ocean currents. Longer-term changes in climate, such as global warming or the onset of ice ages, are punctuated by shorter-term events which comprise the day-to-day weather of a region, such as frontal depressions, hurricanes, and blizzards.

Global Air circulation

Air does not simply flow from the Equator to the poles, it circulates in giant cells known as Hadley and Ferrel cells. As air warms it expands, becoming less dense and rising; this creates areas of low pressure. As the air rises it cools and condenses, causing heavy rainfall over the tropics and slight snowfall over the poles. This cool air then sinks, forming high pressure belts. At surface level in the tropics these sinking currents are deflected poleward as the westerlies and toward the Equator as the trade winds. At the poles they become the polar easterlies.

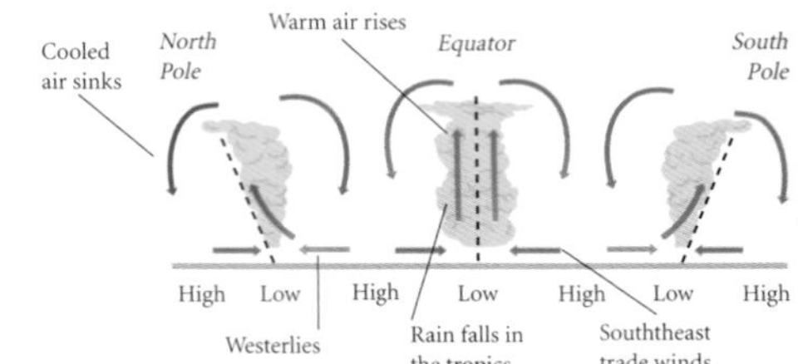
Cooled air sinks
North Pole
Warm air rises
Equator
South Pole
High
Low
High
Low
High
Low
High
Westerlies
Rain falls in the tropics
Souththeast trade winds

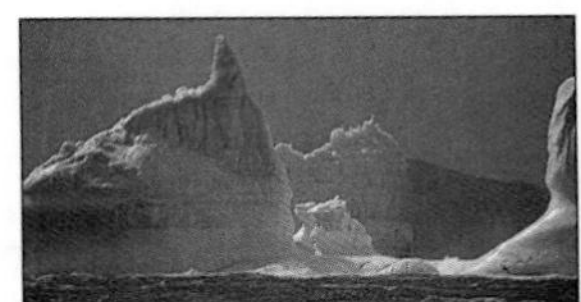

The Antarctic pack ice *expands its area by almost seven times during the winter as temperatures drop and surrounding seas freeze.*

The Atmosphere, Wind, and Weather

The Earth's atmosphere has been compared to a giant ocean of air which surrounds the planet. Its circulation patterns are similar to the currents in the oceans and are influenced by three factors; the Earth's orbit around the Sun and rotation about its axis, and variations in the amount of heat radiation received from the Sun. If both heat and moisture were not redistributed between the Equator and the poles, large areas of the Earth would be uninhabitable.

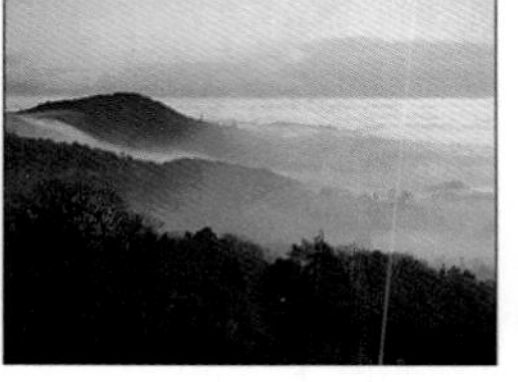

Heavy fogs, *as here in southern England, form as moisture-laden air passes over cold ground.*

Temperature

The world can be divided into three major climatic zones, stretching like large belts across the latitudes: the tropics which are warm; the cold polar regions and the temperate zones which lie between them. Temperatures across the Earth range from above 86°F (30°C) in the deserts to as low as -70°F (-55°C) at the poles. Temperature is also controlled by altitude; because air becomes cooler and less dense the higher it gets, mountainous regions are typically colder than those areas which are at, or close to, sea level.

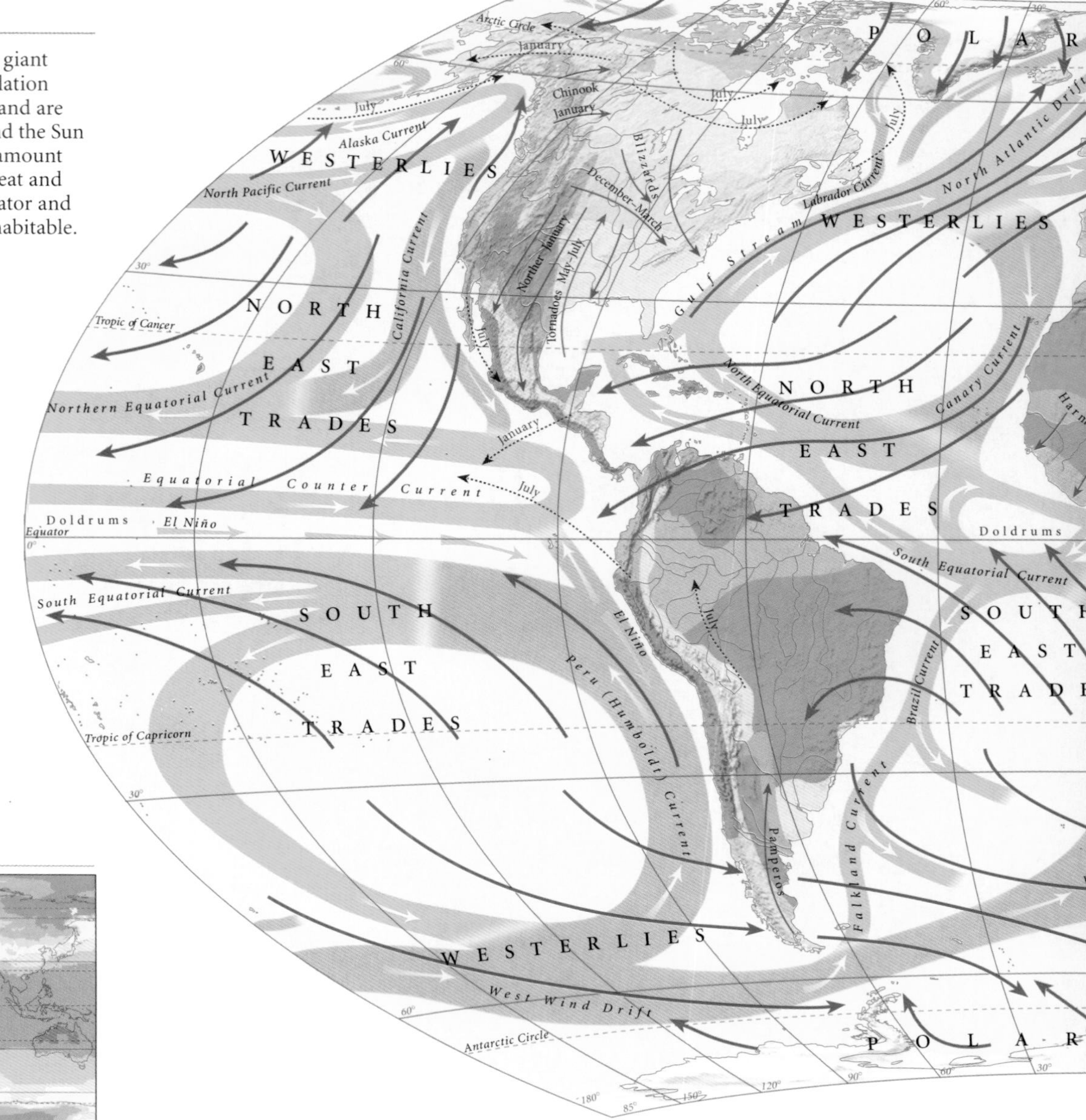
Arctic Circle
January
Chinook
July
POLAR
WESTERLIES
Alaska Current
North Pacific Current
Blizzards
December–March
Labrador Current
North Atlantic Drift
Gulf Stream
California Current
Northers January
Tornadoes May–July
Tropic of Cancer
NORTH EAST TRADES
Northern Equatorial Current
North Equatorial Current
Canary Current
Harmattan
Equatorial Counter Current
Doldrums
El Niño
Equator
South Equatorial Current
SOUTH EAST TRADES
Peru (Humboldt) Current
Brazil Current
Tropic of Capricorn
Pamperos
Falkland Current
West Wind Drift
Antarctic Circle

Average January temperatures

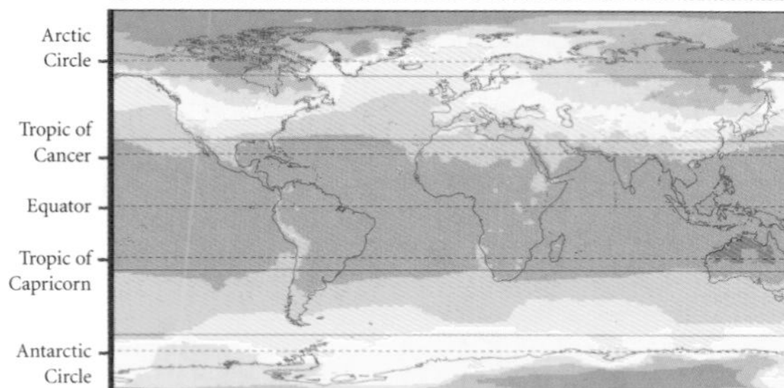
Arctic Circle
Tropic of Cancer
Equator
Tropic of Capricorn
Antarctic Circle

Average July temperatures

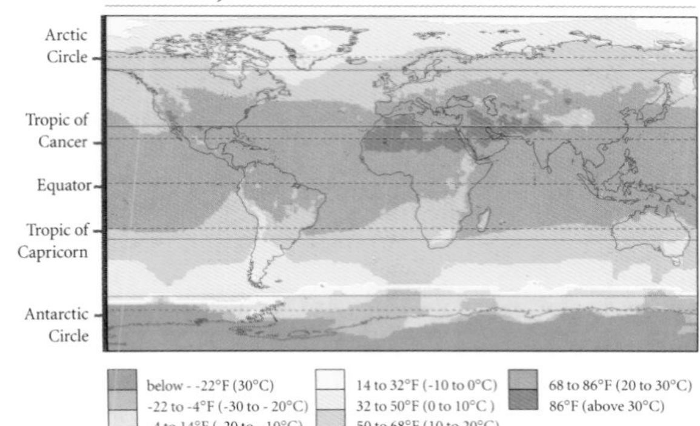
Arctic Circle
Tropic of Cancer
Equator
Tropic of Capricorn
Antarctic Circle
below - -22°F (30°C)
-22 to -4°F (-30 to - 20°C)
-4 to 14°F (-20 to - 10°C)
14 to 32°F (-10 to 0°C)
32 to 50°F (0 to 10°C)
50 to 68°F (10 to 20°C)
68 to 86°F (20 to 30°C)
86°F (above 30°C)

Climatic change

The Earth is currently in a warm phase between ice ages. Warmer temperatures result in higher sea levels as more of the polar ice caps melt. Most of the world's population lives near coasts, so any changes which might cause sea levels to rise, could have a potentially disastrous impact.

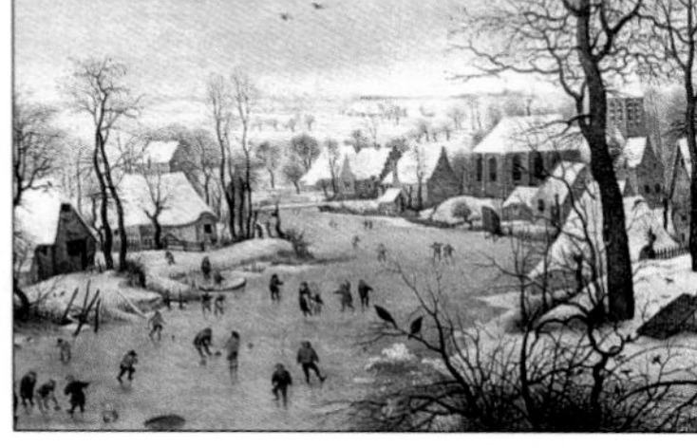

This ice fair, *painted by Pieter Brueghel the Younger in the 17th century, shows the Little Ice Age which peaked around 300 years ago.*

The greenhouse effect

Gases such as carbon dioxide are known as "greenhouse gases" because they allow shortwave solar radiation to enter the Earth's atmosphere, but help to stop longwave radiation from escaping. This traps heat, raising the Earth's temperature. An excess of these gases, such as that which results from the burning of fossil fuels, helps trap more heat and can lead to global warming.

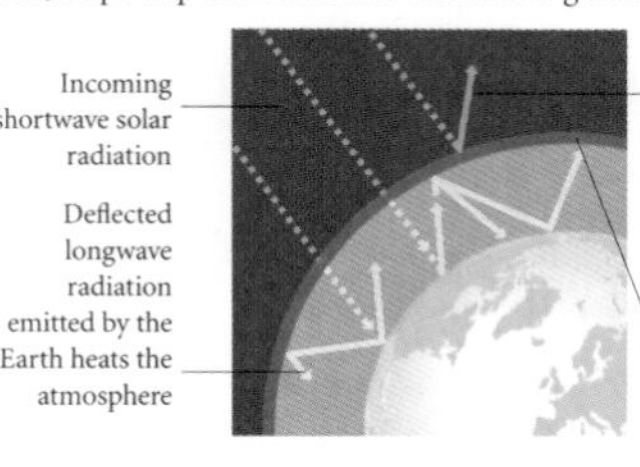
Incoming shortwave solar radiation
Deflected longwave radiation emitted by the Earth heats the atmosphere
Deflected shortwave solar radiation
Greenhouse gases prevent the escape of longwave radiation

The islands of the Caribbean, Mexico's Gulf coast and the southeastern US are often hit by hurricanes formed far out in the Atlantic.

OCEANIC WATER CIRCULATION

IN GENERAL, OCEAN CURRENTS parallel the movement of winds across the Earth's surface. Incoming solar energy is greatest at the Equator and least at the poles. So, water in the oceans heats up most at the Equator and flows poleward, cooling as it moves north or south toward the Arctic or Antarctic. The flow is eventually reversed and cold water currents move back toward the Equator. These ocean currents act as a vast system for moving heat from the Equator toward the poles and are a major influence on the distribution of the Earth's climates.

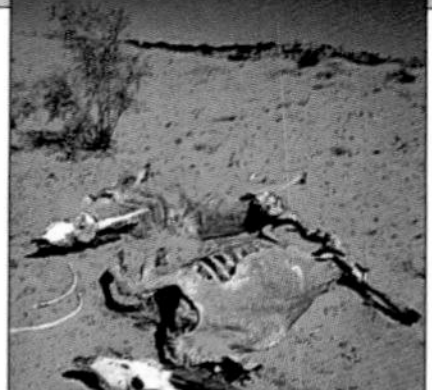

***In marginal climatic zones** years of drought can completely dry out the land and transform grassland to desert.*

TILT AND ROTATION

The tilt and rotation of the Earth during its annual orbit largely control the distribution of heat and moisture across its surface, which correspondingly controls its large-scale weather patterns. As the Earth annually rotates around the Sun, half its surface is receiving maximum radiation, creating summer and winter seasons. The angle of the Earth means that on average the tropics receive two and a half times as much heat from the Sun each day as the poles.

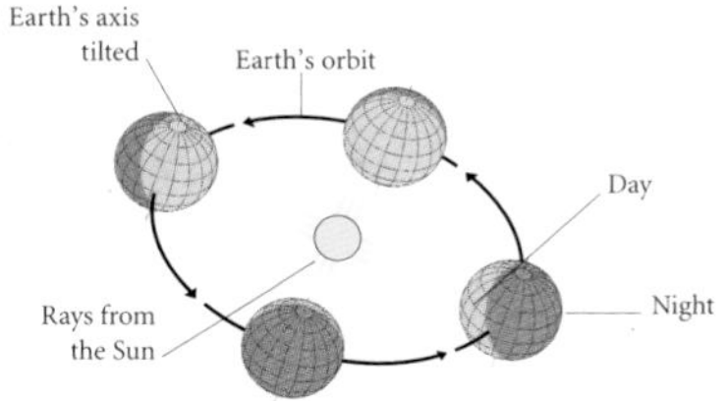

Earth's axis tilted
Earth's orbit
Day
Night
Rays from the Sun

MAP KEY

Climate zones: ice cap; subarctic; tundra; continental; temperate; warm temperate; mediterranean; semiarid; arid; hot humid; humid equatorial; tropical

Ocean currents: warm; cold

Prevailing winds: warm; cold

Local winds: warm; cold; seasonal*

* (seasonal winds which can either be warm or cold)

The wide range of environments found in the Andes is strongly related to their altitude, which modifies climatic influences. While the peaks are snow-capped, many protected interior valleys are semitropical.

THE CORIOLIS EFFECT

The rotation of the Earth influences atmospheric circulation by deflecting winds and ocean currents. Winds blowing in the northern hemisphere are deflected to the right and those in the southern hemisphere are deflected to the left, creating large-scale patterns of wind circulation, such as the northeast and southeast trade winds and the westerlies. This effect is greatest at the poles and least at the Equator.

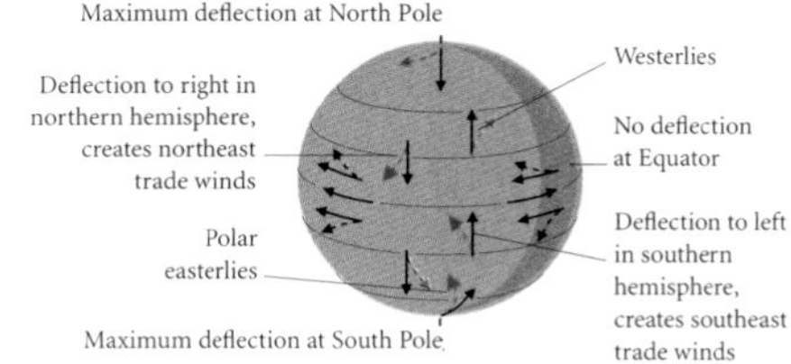

Maximum deflection at North Pole
Deflection to right in northern hemisphere, creates northeast trade winds
Polar easterlies
Maximum deflection at South Pole
Westerlies
No deflection at Equator
Deflection to left in southern hemisphere, creates southeast trade winds

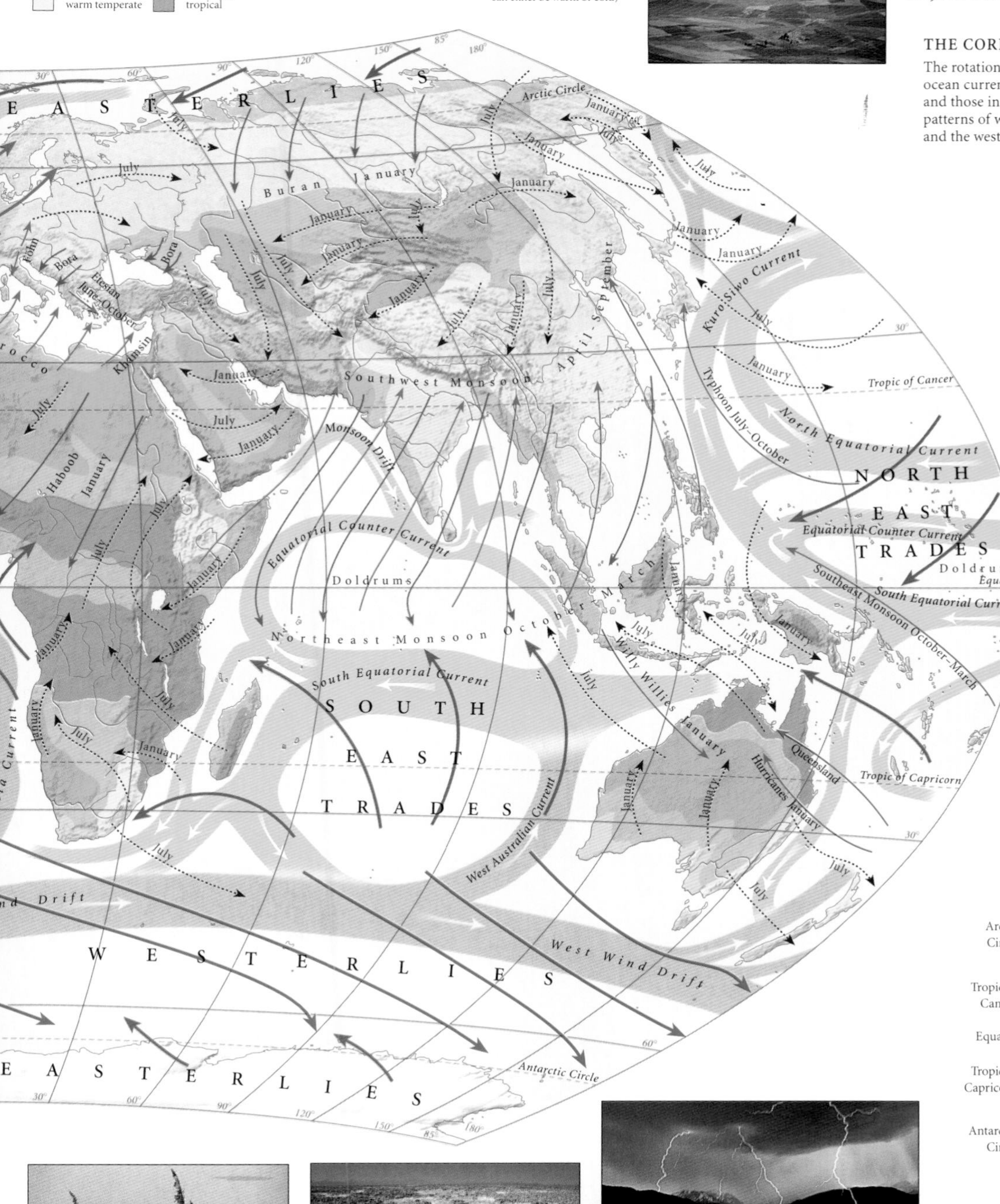

EASTERLIES
Arctic Circle
Buran
January
July
Bora
Etesian June–October
Sirocco
Khamsin
Haboob
Southwest Monsoon
Monsoon Drift
Kuro Siwo Current
Typhoon July–October
Tropic of Cancer
North Equatorial Current
NORTH EAST TRADES
Equatorial Counter Current
Doldrums
Equator
South Equatorial Current
Southeast Monsoon October–March
Northeast Monsoon October–March
South Equatorial Current
SOUTH EAST TRADES
Willy Willies
Hurricanes January
Queensland
Tropic of Capricorn
West Australian Current
West Wind Drift
WESTERLIES
Antarctic Circle
EASTERLIES

PRECIPITATION

WHEN WARM AIR EXPANDS, it rises and cools, and the water vapor it carries condenses to form clouds. Heavy, regular rainfall is characteristic of the equatorial region, while the poles are cold and receive only slight snowfall. Tropical regions have marked dry and rainy seasons, while in the temperate regions rainfall is relatively unpredictable.

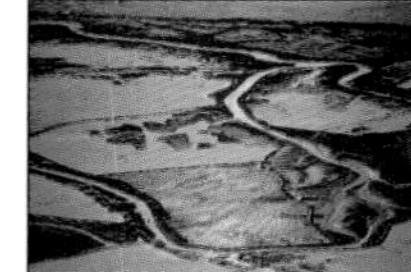

***Monsoon rains**, which affect southern Asia from May to September, are caused by sea winds blowing across the warm land.*

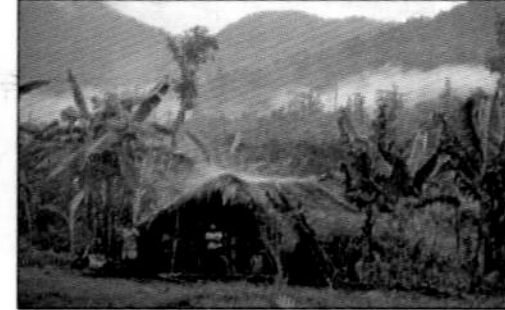

***Heavy tropical rainstorms** occur frequently in Papua New Guinea, often causing soil erosion and landslides in cultivated areas.*

AVERAGE JANUARY RAINFALL

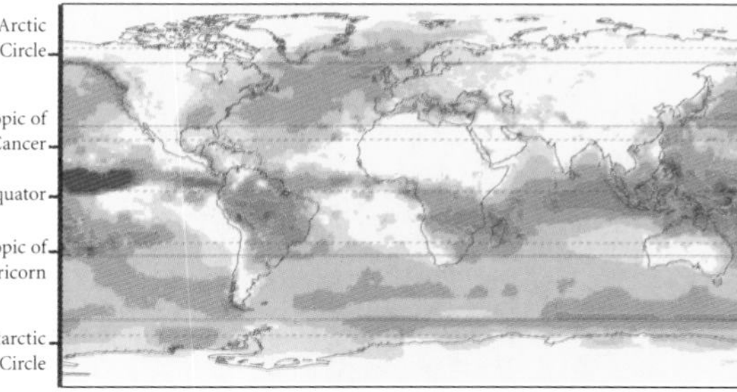

Arctic Circle
Tropic of Cancer
Equator
Tropic of Capricorn
Antarctic Circle

AVERAGE JULY RAINFALL

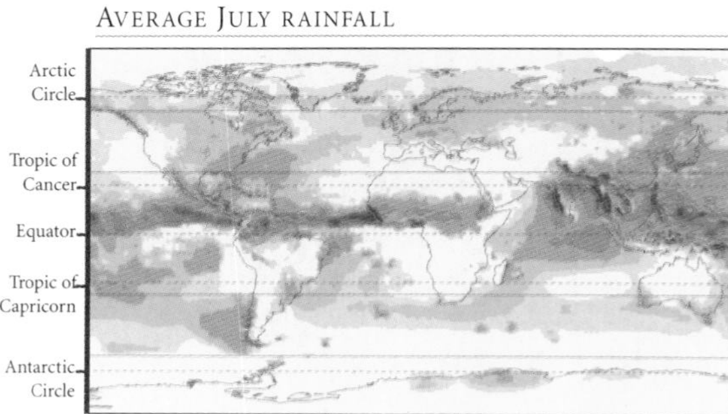

Arctic Circle
Tropic of Cancer
Equator
Tropic of Capricorn
Antarctic Circle

0–1 in (0–25 mm); 1–2 in (25–50 mm); 2–4 in (50–100 mm); 4–8 in (100–200 mm); 8–12 in (200–300 mm); 12–16 in (300–400 mm); 16–20 in (400–500 mm); 20 in (above 500 mm)

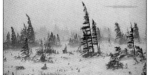

***The intensity of some blizzards** in Canada and the northern US can give rise to snowdrifts as high as 10 ft (3 m).*

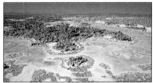

***The Atacama Desert in Chile** is one of the driest places on Earth, with an average rainfall of less than 2 inches (50 mm) per year.*

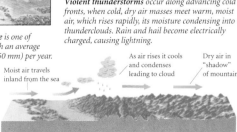

***Violent thunderstorms** occur along advancing cold fronts, when cold, dry air masses meet warm, moist air, which rises rapidly, its moisture condensing into thunderclouds. Rain and hail become electrically charged, causing lightning.*

THE RAINSHADOW EFFECT

When moist air is forced to rise by mountains, it cools and the water vapor falls as precipitation, either as rain or snow. Only the dry, cold air continues over the mountains, leaving inland areas with little or no rain. This is called the rainshadow effect and is one reason for the existence of the Mojave Desert in California, which lies east of the Coast Ranges.

Moist air travels inland from the sea

As air rises it cools and condenses leading to cloud

Dry air in "shadow" of mountain

THE RAINSHADOW EFFECT

Life on Earth

A UNIQUE COMBINATION of an oxygen-rich atmosphere and plentiful water is the key to life on Earth. Apart from the polar ice caps, there are few areas which have not been colonized by animals or plants over the course of the Earth's history. Plants process sunlight to provide them with their energy, and ultimately all the Earth's animals rely on plants for survival. Because of this reliance, plants are known as primary producers, and the availability of nutrients and temperature of an area is defined as its primary productivity, which affects the quantity and type of animals which are able to live there. This index is affected by climatic factors – cold and aridity restrict the quantity of life, whereas warmth and regular rainfall allow a greater diversity of species.

Biogeographical Regions

THE EARTH CAN BE DIVIDED into a series of biogeographical regions, or biomes, ecological communities where certain species of plant and animal coexist within particular climatic conditions. Within these broad classifications, other factors including soil richness, altitude, and human activities such as urbanization, intensive agriculture, and deforestation, affect the local distribution of living species within each biome.

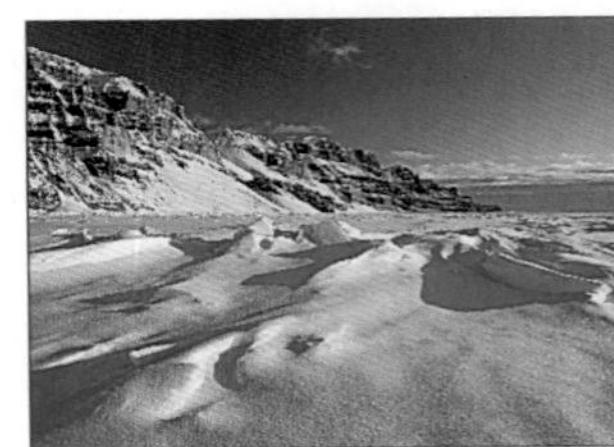

POLAR REGIONS

A layer of permanent ice at the Earth's poles covers both seas and land. Very little plant and animal life can exist in these harsh regions.

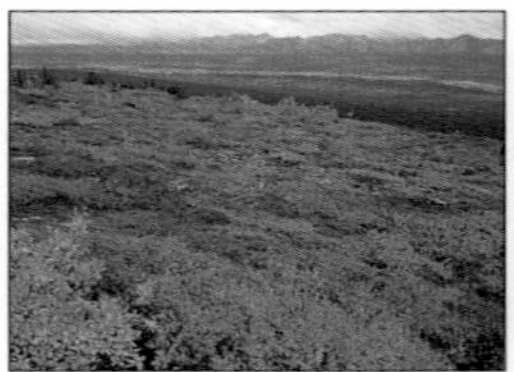

TUNDRA

A desolate region, with long, dark freezing winters and short, cold summers. With virtually no soil and large areas of permanently frozen ground known as permafrost, the tundra is largely treeless, though it is briefly clothed by small flowering plants in the summer months.

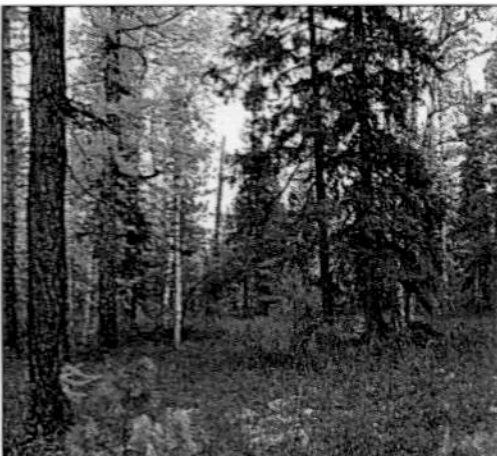

NEEDLELEAF FORESTS

With milder summers than the tundra and less wind, these areas are able to support large forests of coniferous trees.

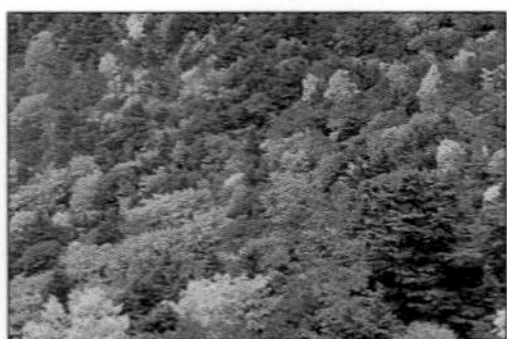

BROADLEAF FORESTS

Much of the northern hemisphere was once covered by deciduous forests, which occurred in areas with marked seasonal variations. Most deciduous forests have been cleared for human settlement.

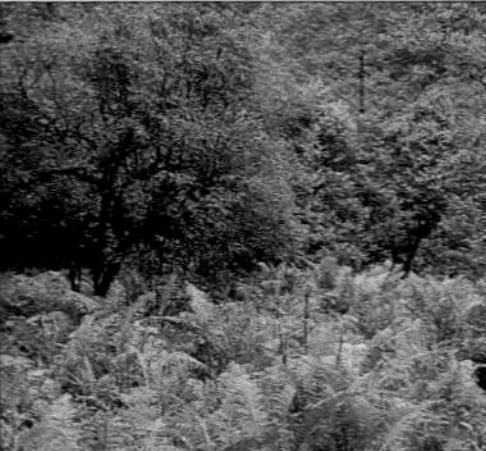

TEMPERATE RAIN FORESTS

In warmer wetter areas, such as southern China, temperate deciduous forests are replaced by evergreen forest.

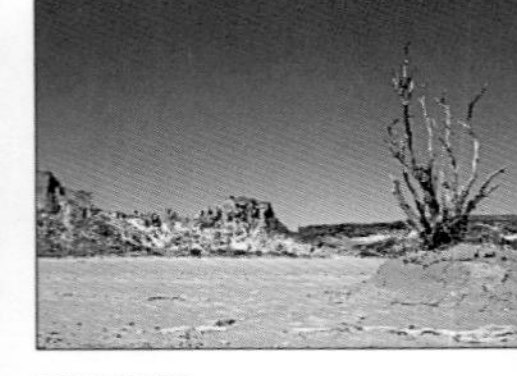

DESERTS

Deserts are areas with negligible rainfall. Most hot deserts lie within the tropics; cold deserts are dry because of their distance from the moisture-providing sea.

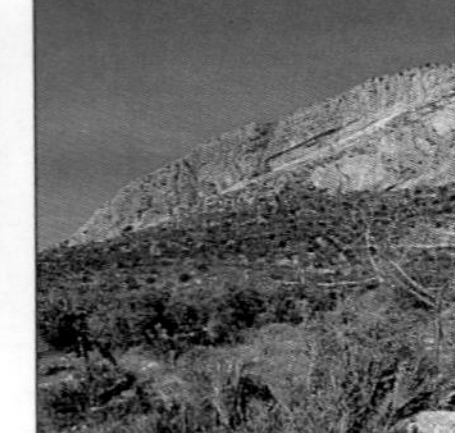

MEDITERRANEAN

Hot, dry summers and short winters typify these areas, which were once covered by evergreen shrubs and woodland, but have now been cleared by humans for agriculture.

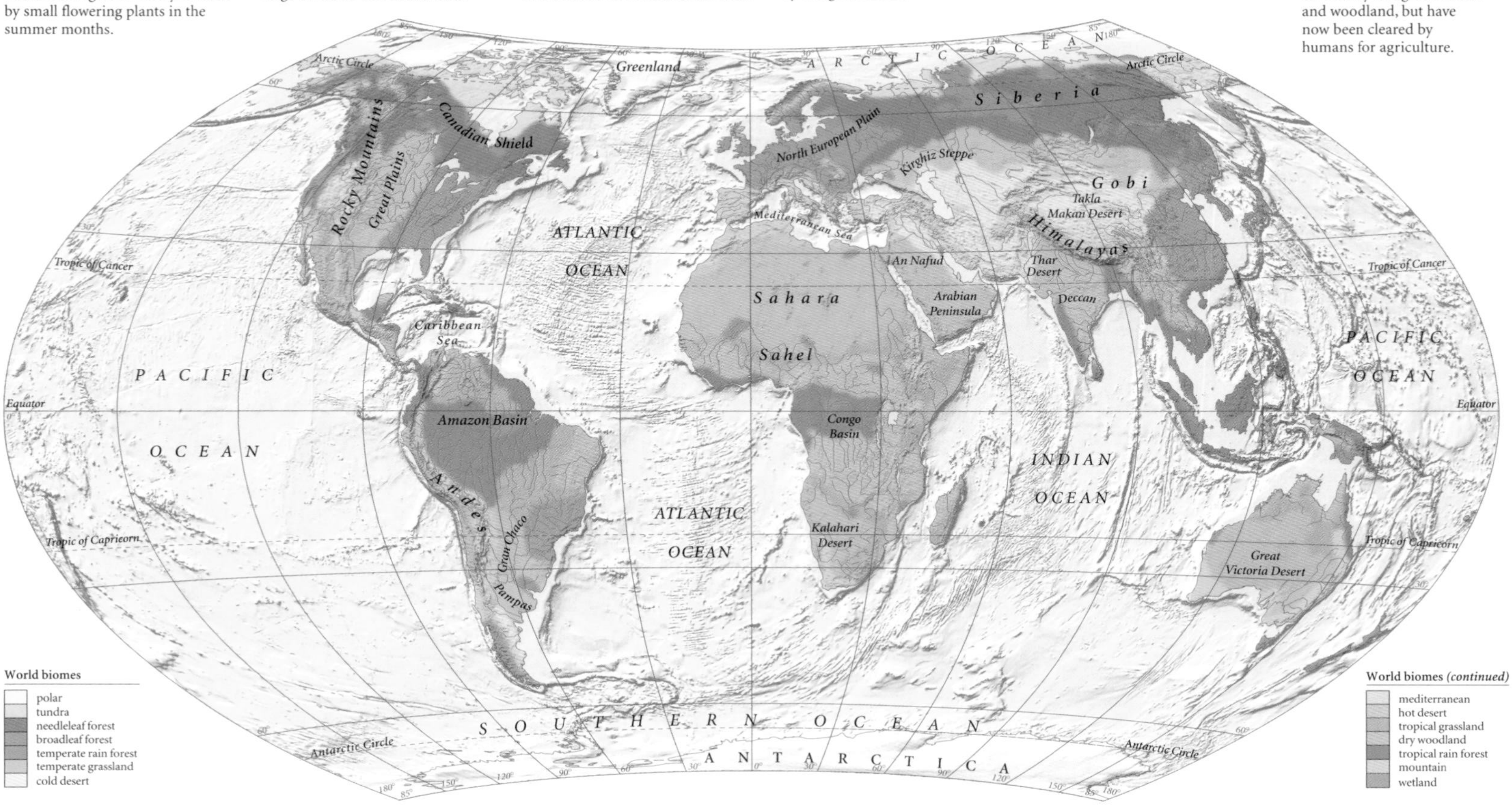

Arctic Circle
Greenland
ARCTIC OCEAN
Siberia
Canadian Shield
Rocky Mountains
Great Plains
North European Plain
Kirghiz Steppe
Gobi
Takla Makan Desert
Himalayas
Mediterranean Sea
ATLANTIC OCEAN
Tropic of Cancer
An Nafud
Thar Desert
Deccan
Arabian Peninsula
Sahara
Sahel
Caribbean Sea
PACIFIC OCEAN
Equator
Amazon Basin
Congo Basin
INDIAN OCEAN
Andes
Gran Chaco
Pampas
Kalahari Desert
Tropic of Capricorn
Great Victoria Desert
SOUTHERN OCEAN
Antarctic Circle
ANTARCTICA

World biomes

- polar
- tundra
- needleleaf forest
- broadleaf forest
- temperate rain forest
- temperate grassland
- cold desert

World biomes *(continued)*

- mediterranean
- hot desert
- tropical grassland
- dry woodland
- tropical rain forest
- mountain
- wetland

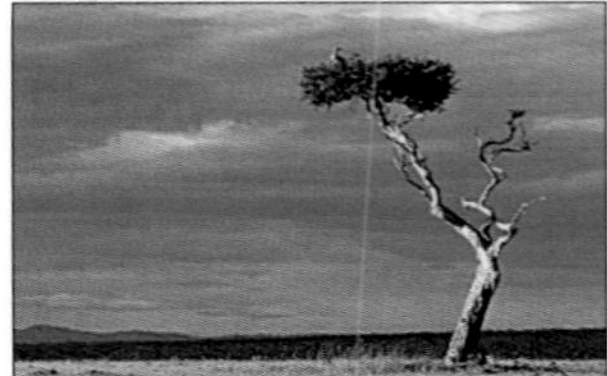

TROPICAL AND TEMPERATE GRASSLANDS

The major grassland areas are found in the centers of the larger continental landmasses. In Africa's tropical savannah regions, seasonal rainfall alternates with drought. Temperate grasslands, also known as *steppes* and *prairies* are found in the northern hemisphere, and in South America, where they are known as the *pampas*.

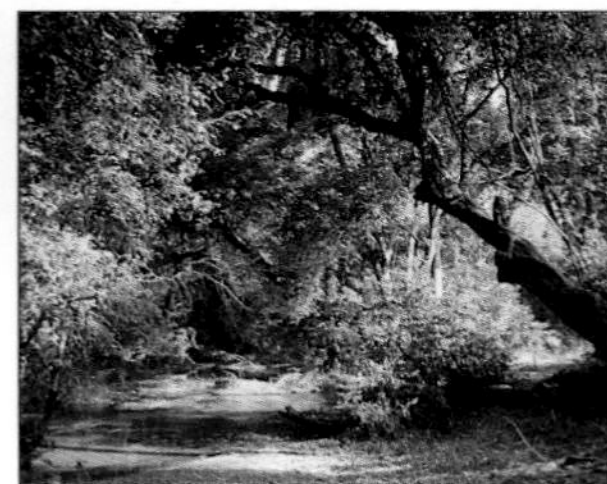

DRY WOODLANDS

Trees and shrubs, adapted to dry conditions, grow widely spaced from one another, interspersed by savannah grasslands.

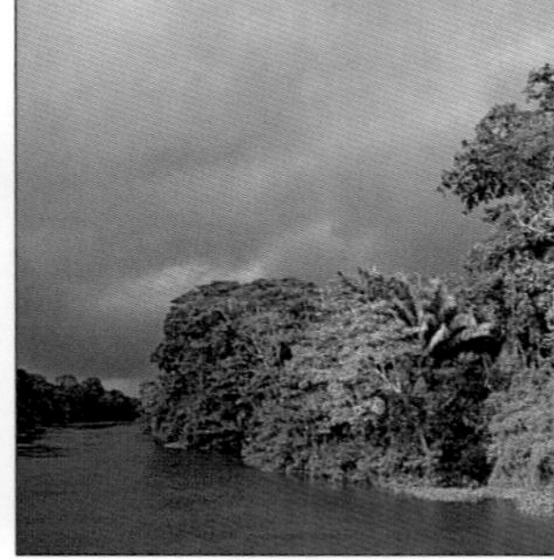

TROPICAL RAIN FORESTS

Characterized by year-round warmth and high rainfall, tropical rain forests contain the highest diversity of plant and animal species on Earth.

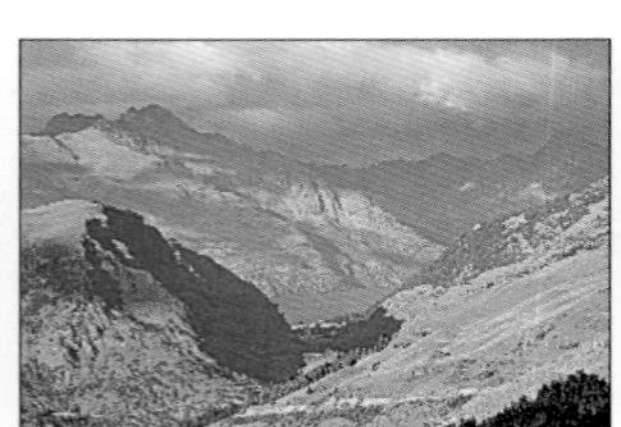

MOUNTAINS

Though the lower slopes of mountains may be thickly forested, only ground-hugging shrubs and other vegetation will grow above the tree line which varies according to both altitude and latitude.

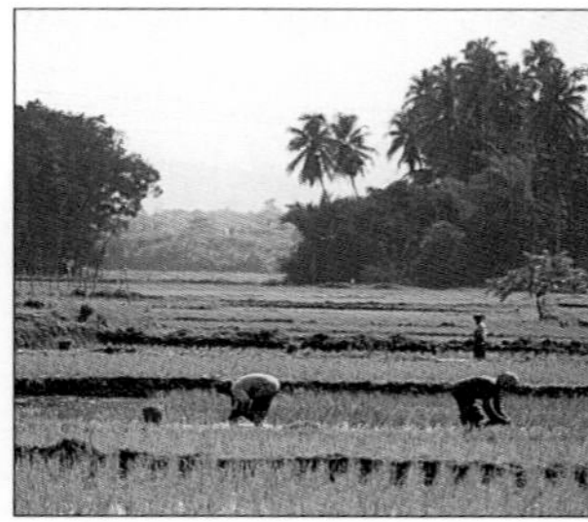

WETLANDS

Rarely lying above sea level, wetlands are marshes, swamps and tidal flats. Some, with their moist, fertile soils, are rich feeding grounds for fish and breeding grounds for birds. Others have little soil structure and are too acidic to support much plant and animal life.

BIODIVERSITY

THE NUMBER OF PLANT AND ANIMAL SPECIES, and the range of genetic diversity within the populations of each species, make up the Earth's biodiversity. The plants and animals which are endemic to a region – that is, those which are found nowhere else in the world – are also important in determining levels of biodiversity. Human settlement and intervention have encroached on many areas of the world once rich in endemic plant and animal species. Increasing international efforts are being made to monitor and conserve the biodiversity of the Earth's remaining wild places.

ANIMAL ADAPTATION

THE DEGREE OF AN ANIMAL'S ADAPTABILITY to different climates and conditions is extremely important in ensuring its success as a species. Many animals, particularly the largest mammals, are becoming restricted to ever-smaller regions as human development and modern agricultural practices reduce their natural habitats. In contrast, humans have been responsible – both deliberately and accidentally – for the spread of some of the world's most successful species. Many of these introduced species are now more numerous than the indigenous animal populations.

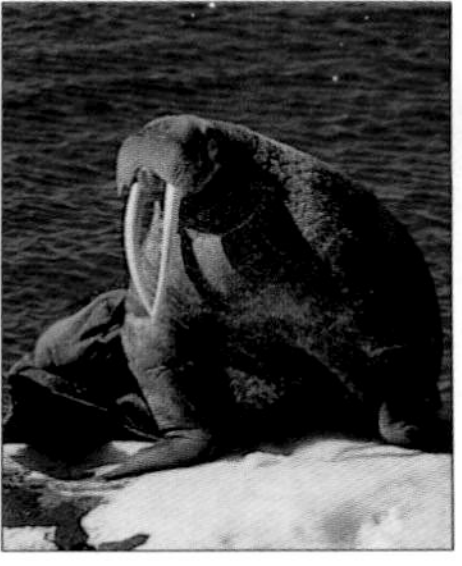

POLAR ANIMALS

The frozen wastes of the polar regions are able to support only a small range of species which derive their nutritional requirements from the sea. Animals such as the walrus *(left)* have developed insulating fat, stocky limbs, and double-layered coats to enable them to survive in the freezing conditions.

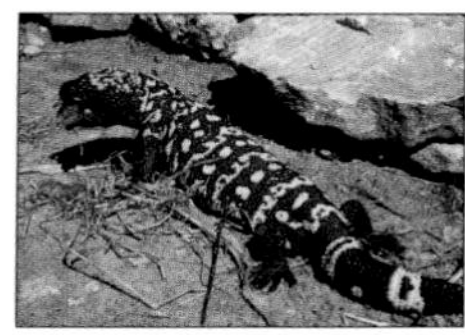

DESERT ANIMALS

Many animals which live in the extreme heat and aridity of the deserts are able to survive for days and even months with very little food or water. Their bodies are adapted to lose heat quickly and to store fat and water. The Gila monster *(above)* stores fat in its tail.

AMAZON RAINFOREST

The vast Amazon Basin is home to the world's greatest variety of animal species. Animals are adapted to live at many different levels from the treetops to the tangled undergrowth which lies beneath the canopy. The sloth *(below)* hangs upside down in the branches. Its fur grows from its stomach to its back to enable water to run off quickly.

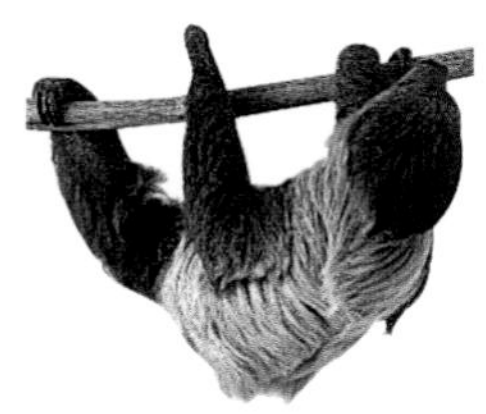

DIVERSITY OF ANIMAL SPECIES

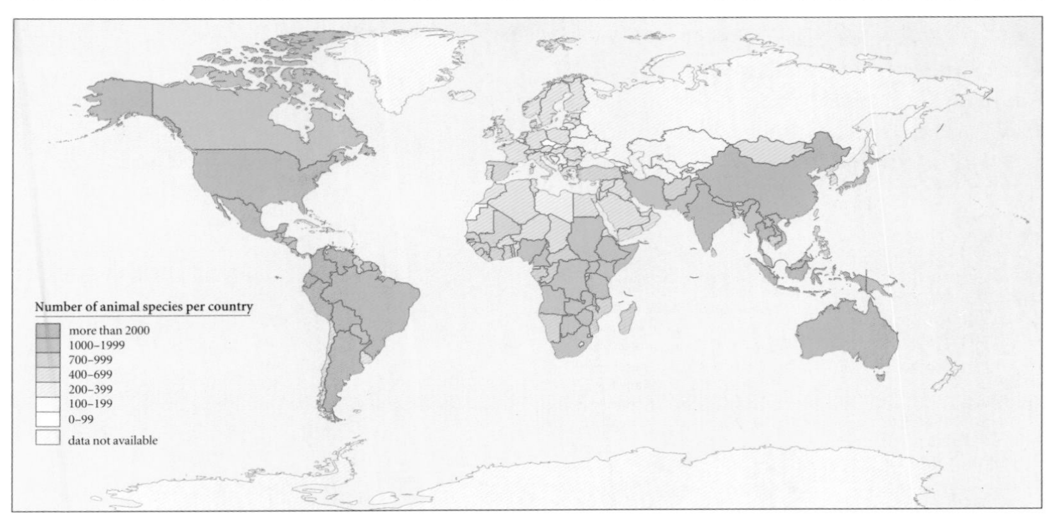
Number of animal species per country
more than 2000
1000–1999
700–999
400–699
200–399
100–199
0–99
data not available

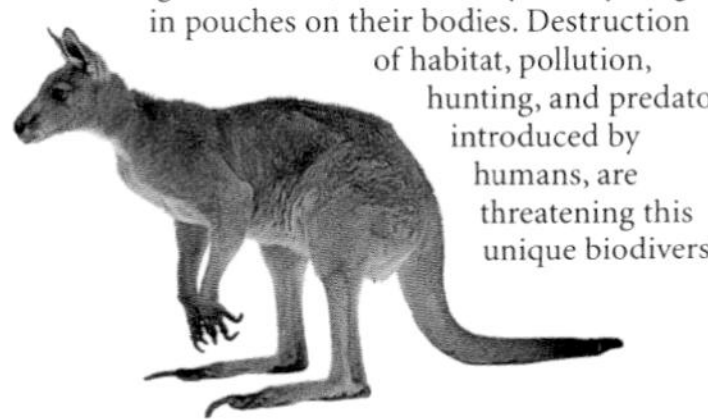

MARINE BIODIVERSITY

The oceans support a huge variety of different species, from the world's largest mammals like whales and dolphins down to the tiniest plankton. The greatest diversities occur in the warmer seas of continental shelves, where plants are easily able to photosynthesize, and around coral reefs, where complex ecosystems are found. On the ocean floor, nematodes can exist at a depth of more than 10,000 ft (3,000 m) below sea level.

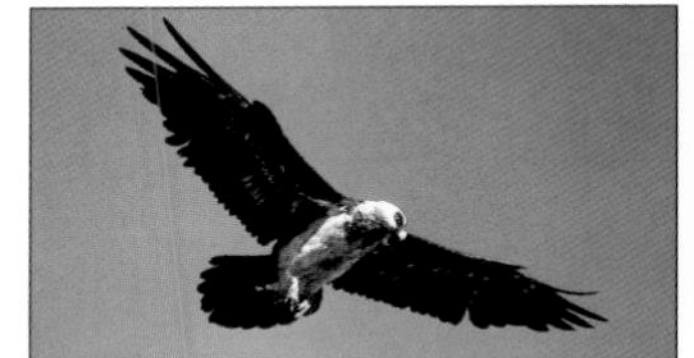

HIGH ALTITUDES

Few animals exist in the rarefied atmosphere of the highest mountains. However, birds of prey such as eagles and vultures *(above)*, with their superb eyesight can soar as high as 23,000 ft (7,000 m) to scan for prey below.

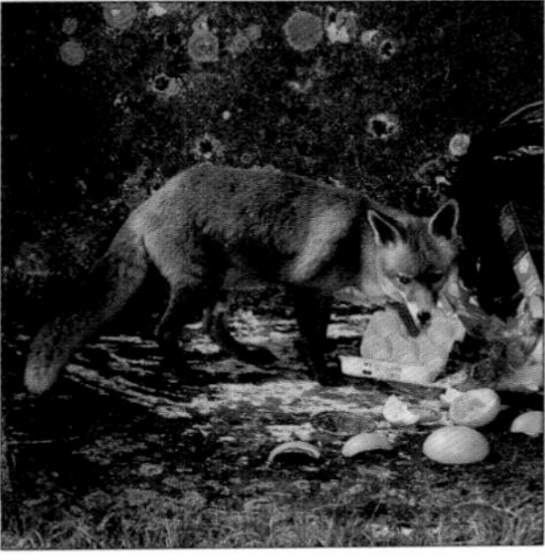

URBAN ANIMALS

The growth of cities has reduced the amount of habitat available to many species. A number of animals are now moving closer into urban areas to scavenge from the detritus of the modern city *(left)*. Rodents, particularly rats and mice, have existed in cities for thousands of years, and many insects, especially moths, quickly develop new coloring to provide them with camouflage.

ENDEMIC SPECIES

Isolated areas such as Australia and the island of Madagascar, have the greatest range of endemic species. In Australia, these include marsupials such as the kangaroo *(below)*, which carry their young in pouches on their bodies. Destruction of habitat, pollution, hunting, and predators introduced by humans, are threatening this unique biodiversity.

PLANT ADAPTATION

ENVIRONMENTAL CONDITIONS, particularly climate, soil type, and the extent of competition with other organisms, influence the development of plants into a number of distinctive forms. Similar conditions in quite different parts of the world create similar adaptations in the plants, which may then be modified by other, local, factors specific to the region.

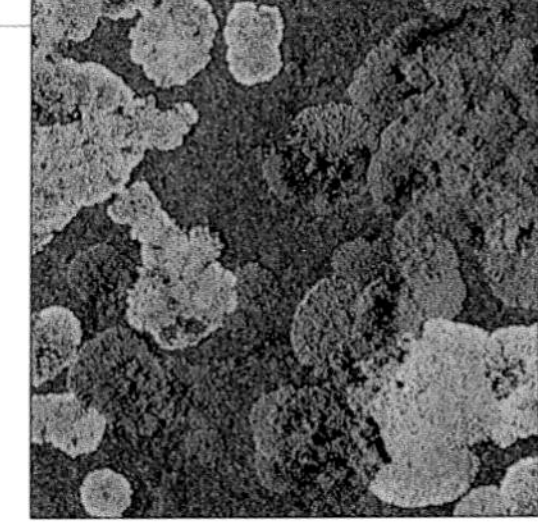

COLD CONDITIONS

In areas where temperatures rarely rise above freezing, plants such as lichens *(left)* and mosses grow densely, close to the ground.

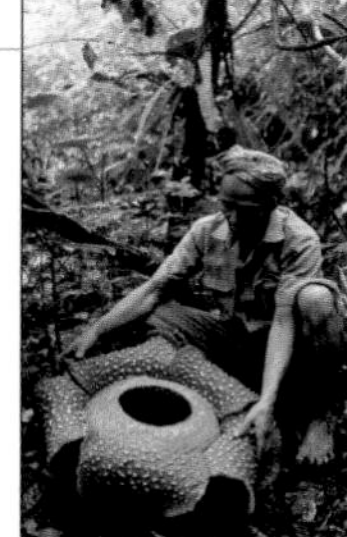

RAIN FORESTS

Most of the world's largest and oldest plants are found in rain forests; warmth and heavy rainfall provide ideal conditions for vast plants like the world's largest flower, the rafflesia *(left)*.

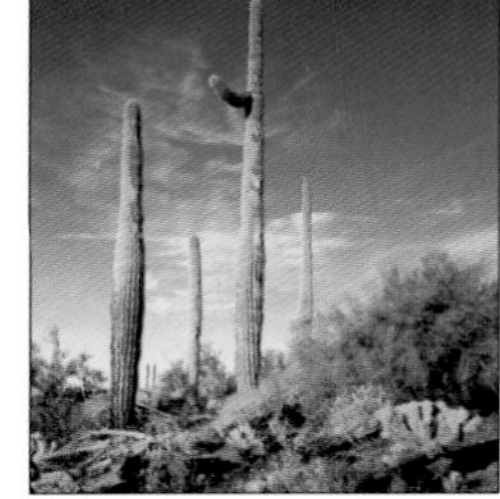

HOT, DRY CONDITIONS

Arid conditions lead to the development of plants whose surface area has been reduced to a minimum to reduce water loss. In cacti *(above)*, which can survive without water for months, leaves are minimal or not present at all.

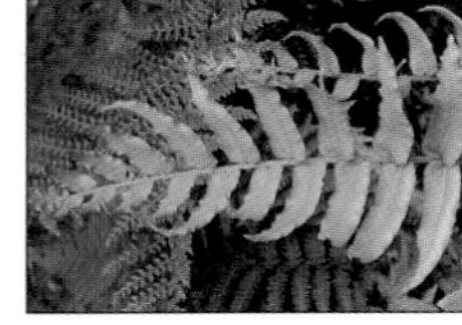

ANCIENT PLANTS

Some of the world's most primitive plants still exist today, including algae, cycads, and many ferns *(above)*, reflecting the success with which they have adapted to changing conditions.

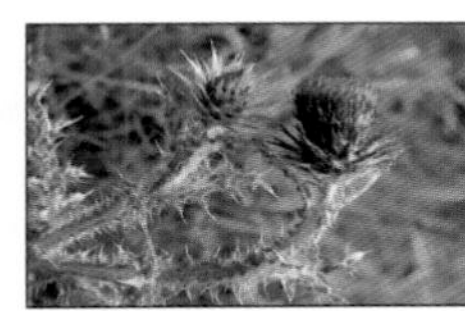

RESISTING PREDATORS

A great variety of plants have developed devices including spines *(above)*, poisons, stinging hairs, and an unpleasant taste or smell to deter animal predators.

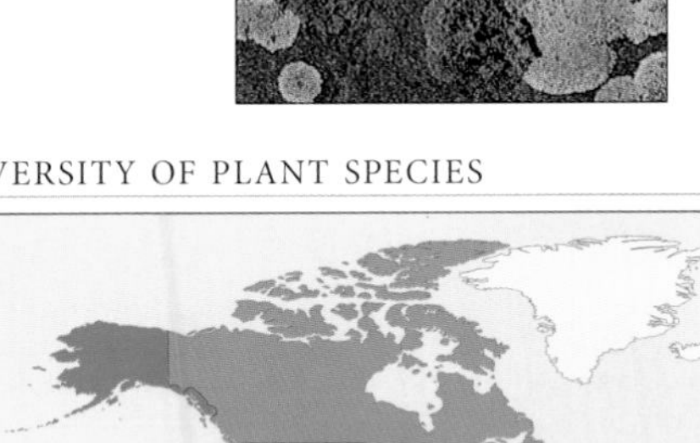

DIVERSITY OF PLANT SPECIES

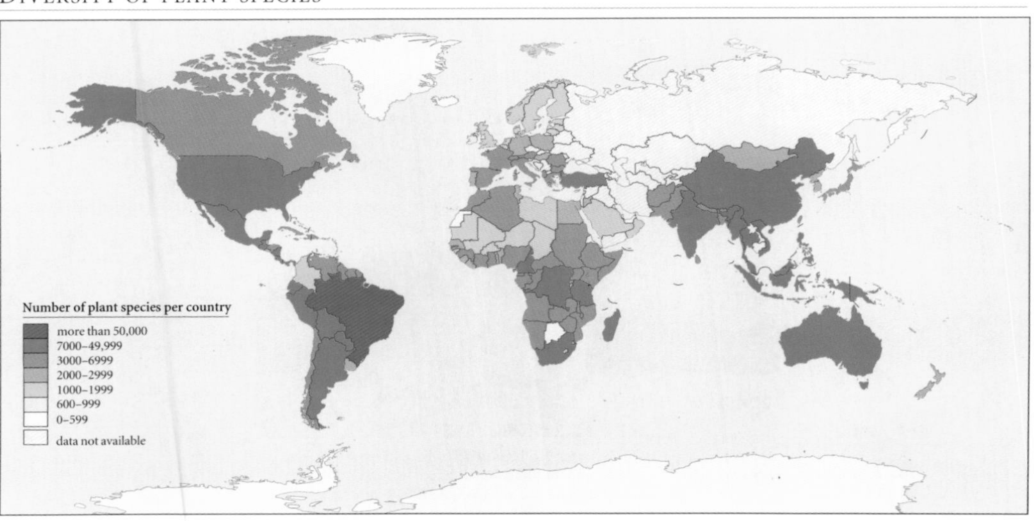
Number of plant species per country
more than 50,000
7000–49,999
3000–6999
2000–2999
1000–1999
600–999
0–599
data not available

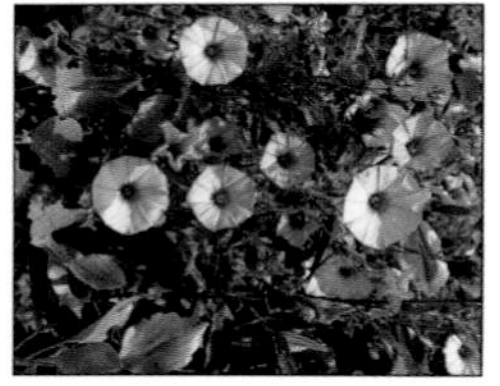

WEEDS

Weeds such as bindweed *(above)* are fast-growing, easily dispersed, and tolerant of a number of different environments, enabling them to quickly colonize suitable habitats. They are among the most adaptable of all plants.

POPULATION AND SETTLEMENT

THE EARTH'S POPULATION IS PROJECTED to rise from its current level of about 5.5 billion to reach some 10 billion by 2025. The global distribution of this rapidly growing population is very uneven, and is dictated by climate, terrain, and natural and economic resources. The great majority of the Earth's people live in coastal zones, and along river valleys. Deserts cover over 20% of the Earth's surface, but support less than 5% of the world's population. It is estimated that over half of the world's population live in cities – most of them in Asia – as a result of mass migration from rural areas in search of jobs. Many of these people live in the so-called "megacities," some with populations as great as 40 million.

NORTH AMERICA

THE EASTERN AND WESTERN SEABOARDS of the US, with huge expanses of interconnected cities, towns, and suburbs, are vast, densely-populated megalopolises. Central America and the Caribbean also have high population densities. Yet, away from the coasts and in the wildernesses of northern Canada the land is very sparsely settled.

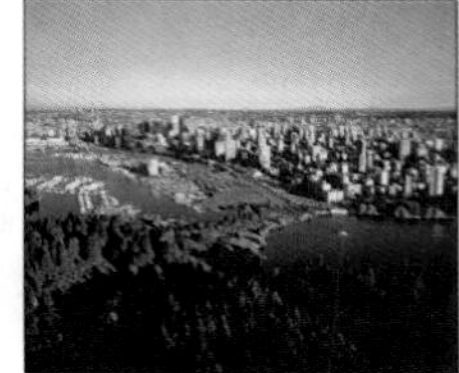

__Vancouver__ on Canada's west coast, grew up as a port city. In recent years it has attracted many Asian immigrants, particularly from the Pacific Rim.

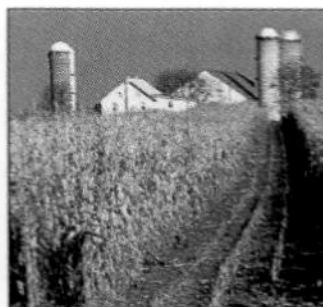

__North America's__ central plains, the continent's agricultural heartland, are thinly populated and highly productive.

EUROPE

WITH ITS TEMPERATE CLIMATE, and rich mineral and natural resources, Europe is generally very densely settled. The continent acts as a magnet for economic migrants from the developing world, and immigration is now widely restricted. Birthrates in Europe are generally low, and in some countries, such as Germany, the populations have stabilized at zero growth, with a fast-growing elderly population.

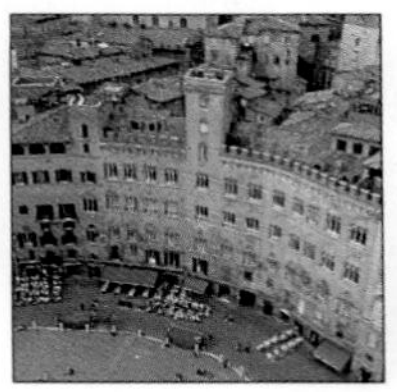

__Many European cities__, like Siena, once reflected the "ideal" size for human settlements. Modern technological advances have enabled them to grow far beyond the original walls.

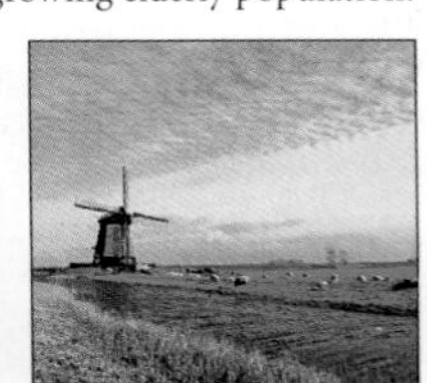

__Within__ the densely-populated Netherlands the reclamation of coastal wetlands is vital to provide much-needed land for agriculture and settlement.

PATTERNS OF SETTLEMENT

THE PAST 200 YEARS have seen the most radical shift in world population patterns in recorded history.

NOMADIC LIFE

ALL THE WORLD'S PEOPLES were hunter-gatherers 10,000 years ago. Today nomads, who live by following available food resources, account for less than 0.0001% of the world's population. They are mainly pastoral herders, moving their livestock from place to place in search of grazing land.

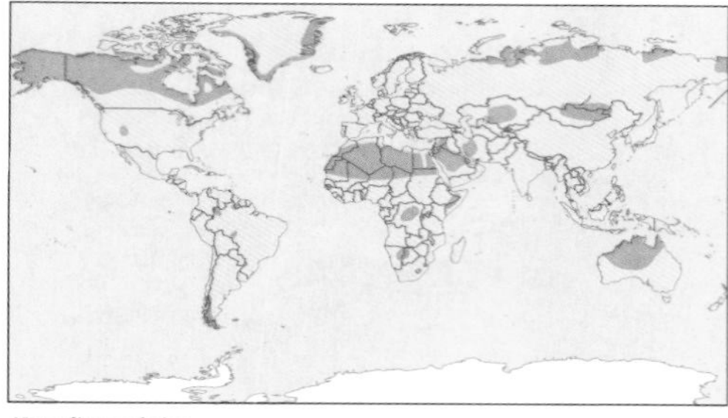

Nomadic population

Nomadic population area

THE GROWTH OF CITIES

IN 1900 there were only 14 cities in the world with populations of more than a million, mostly in the northern hemisphere. Today, as more and more people in the developing world migrate to towns and cities, there are 29 cities whose population exceeds 5 million, and around 200 "million-cities."

MILLION-CITIES IN 1900

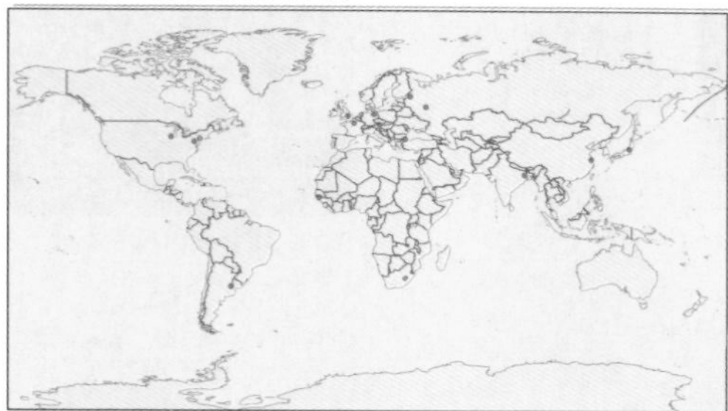

Million-cities in 1900

• Cities over 1 million population

MILLION-CITIES IN 1995

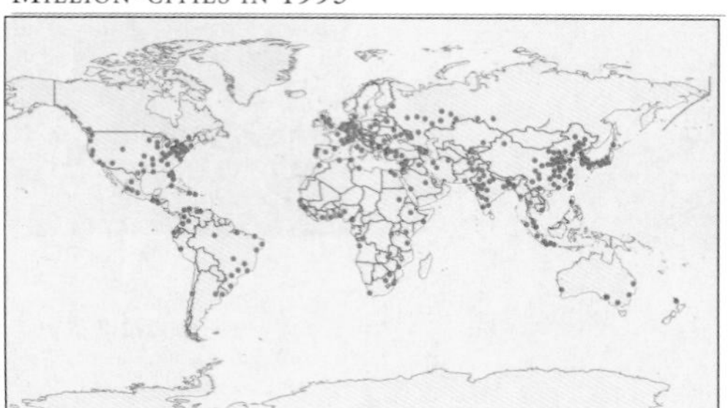

Million-cities in 1995

• Cities over 1 million population

Population density (inhabitants per sq mile)

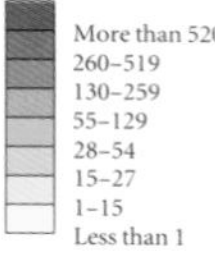
More than 520
260–519
130–259
55–129
28–54
15–27
1–15
Less than 1

NORTH AMERICA

Population 9% World land area 17%

EUROPE

Population 14% World land area 7.1%

AFRICA

Population 12% World land area 20.2%

SOUTH AMERICA

Population 5.5% World land area 11.8%

SOUTH AMERICA

MOST SETTLEMENT IN SOUTH AMERICA is clustered in a narrow belt in coastal zones and in the northern Andes. During the 20th century, cities such as São Paulo and Buenos Aires grew enormously, acting as powerful economic magnets to the rural population. Shantytowns have grown up on the outskirts of many major cities to house these immigrants, often lacking basic amenities.

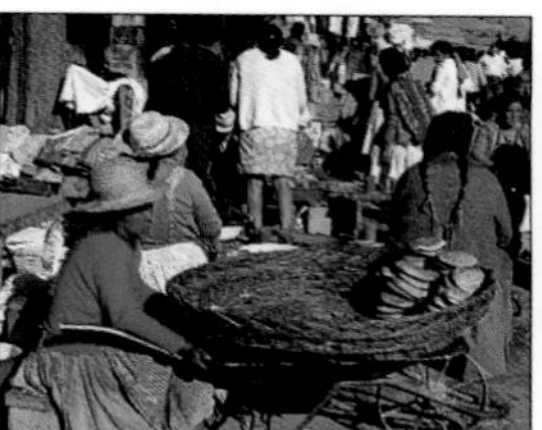

__Many people in western__ South America live at high altitudes in the Andes, both in cities and in villages such as this one in Bolivia.

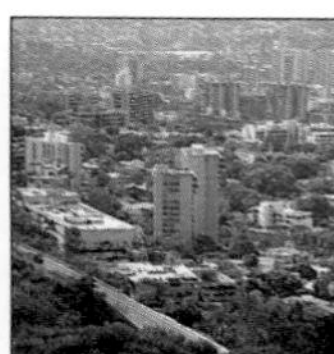

__Venezuela__ is the most highly urbanized country in South America, with more than 90% of the population living in cities such as Caracas.

AFRICA

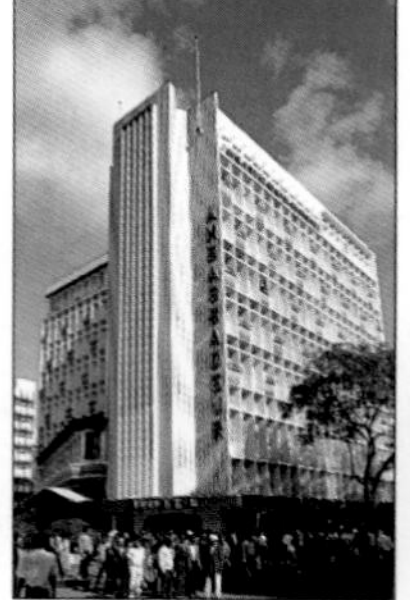

__Cities such as Nairobi__ (above), Cairo and Johannesburg have grown rapidly in recent years, although only Cairo has a significant population on a global scale.

THE ARID CLIMATE of much of Africa means that settlement of the continent is sparse, focusing in coastal areas and fertile regions such as the Nile Valley. Africa still has a high proportion of nomadic agriculturalists, although many are now becoming settled, and the population is predominantly rural.

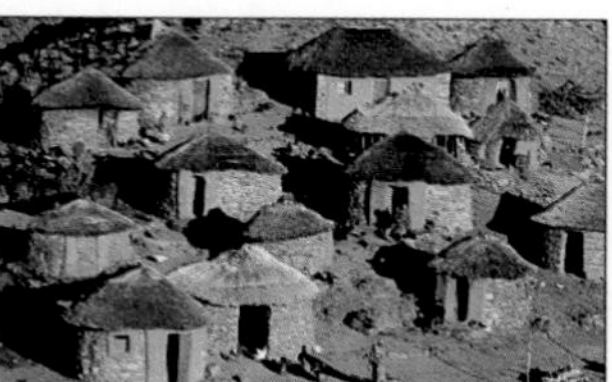

__Traditional lifestyles__ and homes persist across much of Africa, which has a higher proportion of rural or village-based population than any other continent.

ASIA

MOST ASIAN SETTLEMENT originally centered around the great river valleys such as the Indus, the Ganges, and the Yangtze. Today, almost 60% of the world's population lives in Asia, many in burgeoning cities – particularly in the economically-buoyant Pacific Rim countries. Even rural population densities are high in many countries; practices such as terracing in Southeast Asia making the most of the available land.

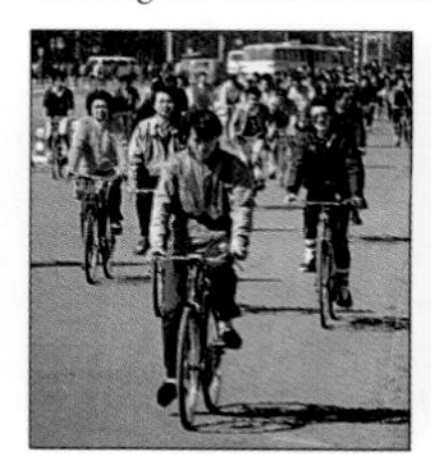

__Many of China's cities__ are now vast urban areas with populations of more than 5 million people.

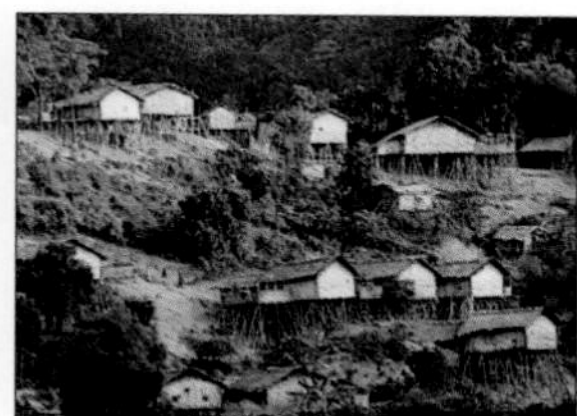

__This stilt village in Bangladesh__ is built to resist the regular flooding. Pressure on land, even in rural areas, forces many people to live in marginal areas.

POPULATION STRUCTURES

POPULATION PYRAMIDS are an effective means of showing the age structures of different countries, and highlighting changing trends in population growth and decline. The typical pyramid for a country with a growing, youthful population, is broad-based *(left)*, reflecting a high birthrate and a far larger number of young rather than elderly people. In contrast, countries with populations whose numbers are stabilizing have a more balanced distribution of people in each age band, and may even have lower numbers of people in the youngest age ranges, indicating both a high life expectancy, and that the population is now barely replacing itself *(right)*. The Russian Federation *(center)* still bears the scars of World War II, reflected in the dramatically lower numbers of men than women in the 60–80+ age range.

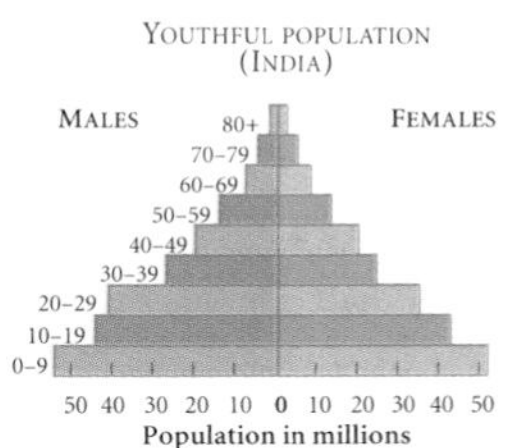
YOUTHFUL POPULATION (INDIA)
MALES
FEMALES
80+
70–79
60–69
50–59
40–49
30–39
20–29
10–19
0–9
50 40 30 20 10 0 10 20 30 40 50
Population in millions

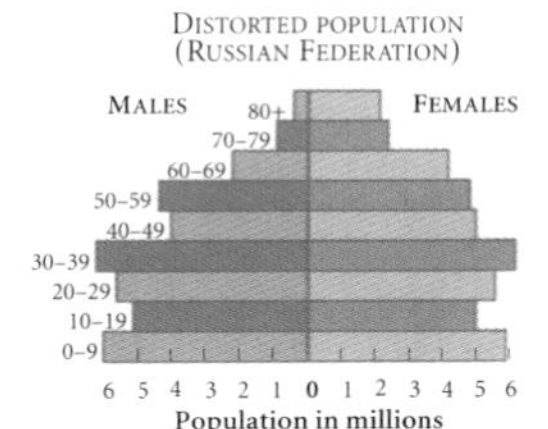
DISTORTED POPULATION (RUSSIAN FEDERATION)
MALES
FEMALES
80+
70–79
60–69
50–59
40–49
30–39
20–29
10–19
0–9
6 5 4 3 2 1 0 1 2 3 4 5 6
Population in millions

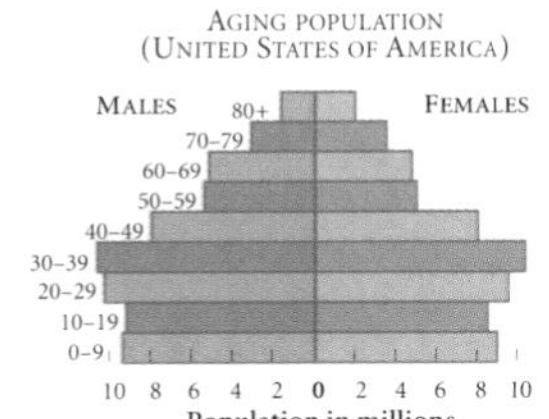
AGING POPULATION (UNITED STATES OF AMERICA)
MALES
FEMALES
80+
70–79
60–69
50–59
40–49
30–39
20–29
10–19
0–9
10 8 6 4 2 0 2 4 6 8 10
Population in millions

POPULATION GROWTH

IMPROVEMENTS IN FOOD SUPPLY and advances in medicine have both played a major role in the remarkable growth in global population, which has increased five-fold over the last 150 years. Food supplies have risen with the mechanization of agriculture and improvements in crop yields. Better nutrition, together with higher standards of public health and sanitation, have led to increased longevity and higher birthrates.

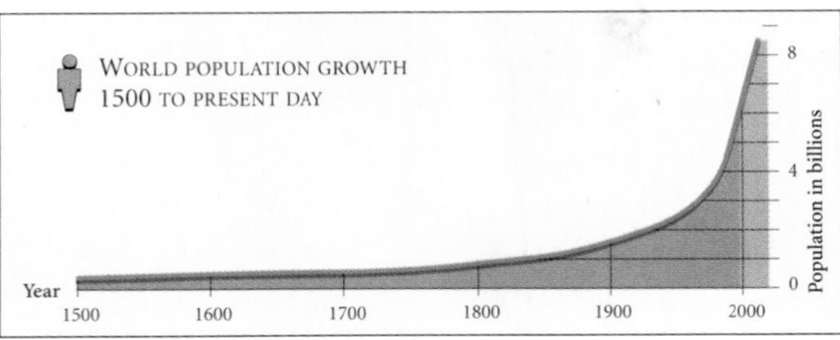
WORLD POPULATION GROWTH
1500 TO PRESENT DAY
Year
1500
1600
1700
1800
1900
2000
0
4
8
Population in billions

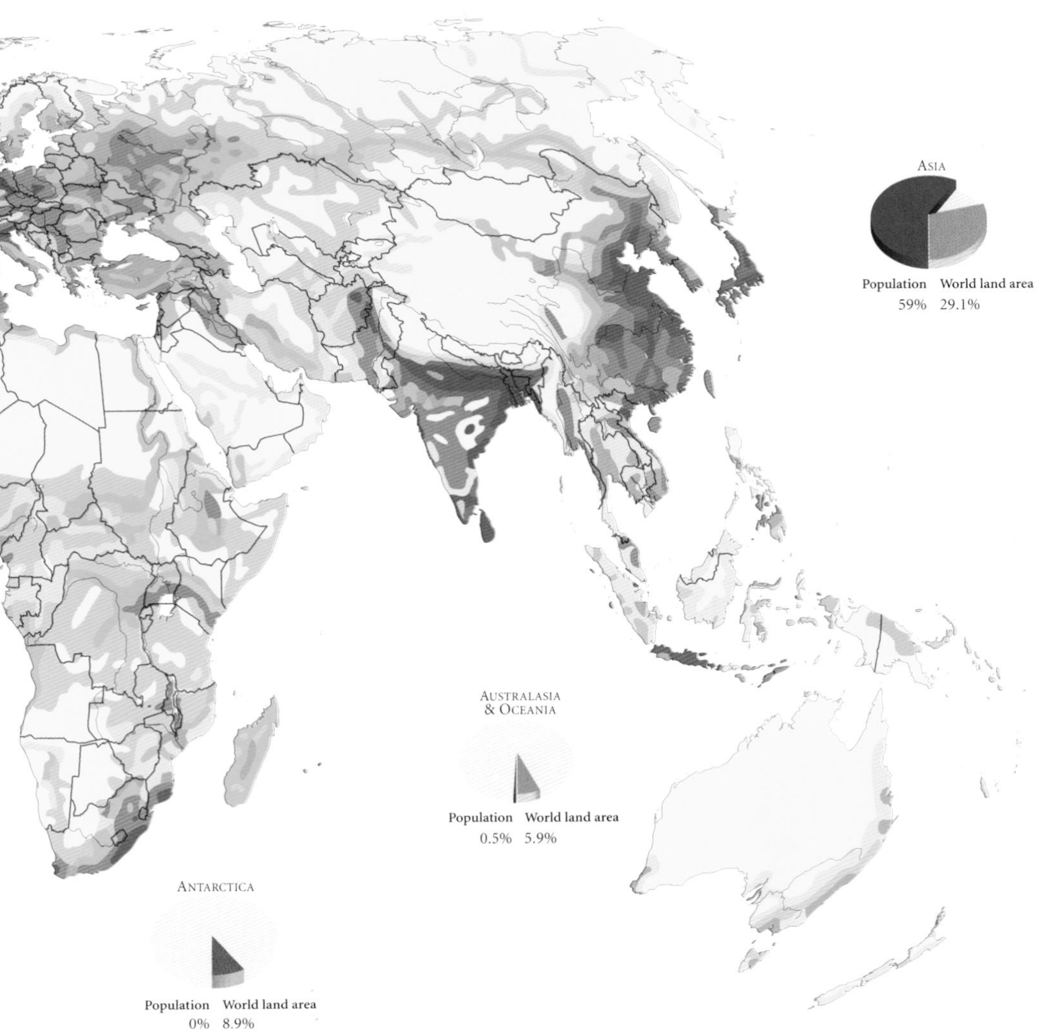
ASIA
Population 59%
World land area 29.1%
AUSTRALASIA & OCEANIA
Population 0.5%
World land area 5.9%
ANTARCTICA
Population 0%
World land area 8.9%

WORLD NUTRITION

TWO-THIRDS OF THE WORLD'S food supply is consumed by the industrialized nations, many of which have a daily calorific intake far higher than is necessary for their populations to maintain a healthy body weight. In contrast, in the developing world, about 800 million people do not have enough food to meet their basic nutritional needs.

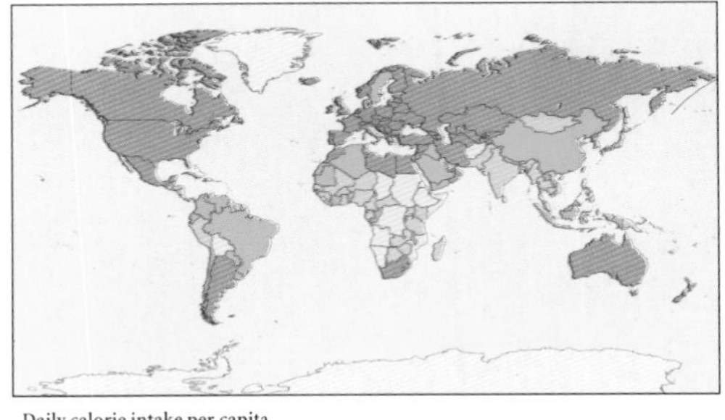

Daily calorie intake per capita
above 3,000 / 2,500–2,999 / 2,000–2,499 / below 2,000 / data not available

WORLD LIFE EXPECTANCY

IMPROVED PUBLIC HEALTH and living standards have greatly increased life expectancy in the developed world, where people can now expect to live twice as long as they did 100 years ago. In many of the world's poorest nations, inadequate nutrition and disease, means that the average life expectancy still does not exceed 45 years.

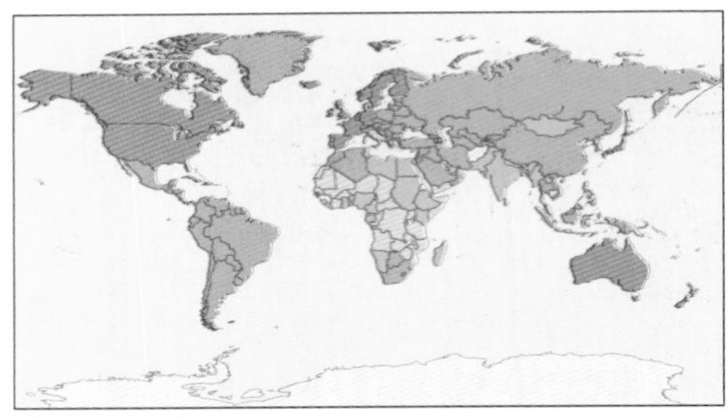

Life expectancy at birth
above 75 years / 65–74 years / 55–64 years / 45–54 years / below 44 years / data not available

AUSTRALASIA & OCEANIA

THIS IS THE WORLD'S most sparsely settled region. The peoples of Australia and New Zealand live mainly in the coastal cities, with only scattered settlements in the arid interior. The Pacific islands can only support limited populations because of their remoteness and lack of resources.

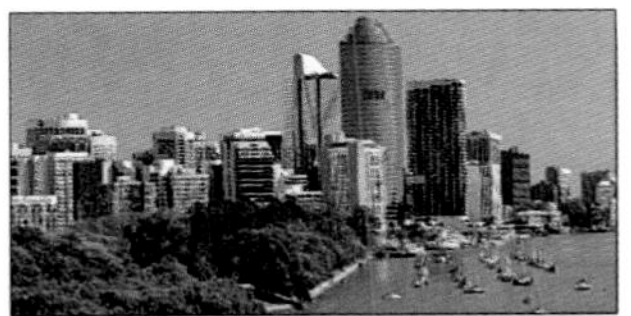

***Brisbane**, on Australia's Gold Coast is the most rapidly expanding city in the country. The great majority of Australia's population lives in cities near the coasts.*

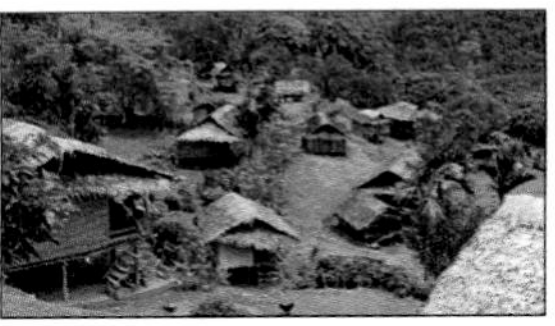

***The remote highlands** of Papua New Guinea are home to a wide variety of peoples, many of whom still subsist by traditional hunting and gathering.*

AVERAGE WORLD BIRTHRATES

BIRTHRATES ARE MUCH HIGHER in Africa, Asia, and South America than in Europe and North America. Increased affluence and easy access to contraception are both factors which can lead to a significant decline in a country's birthrate.

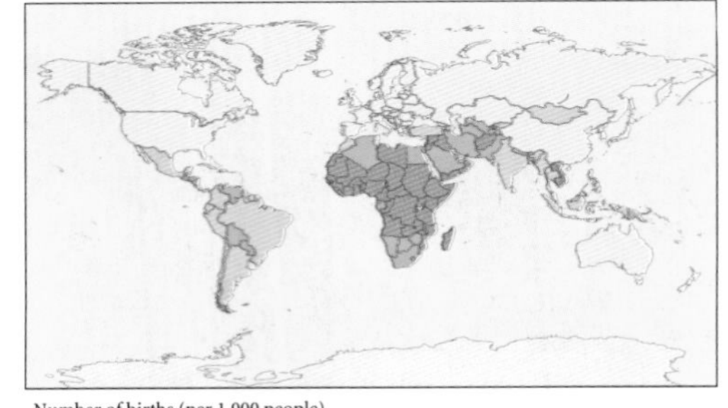

Number of births (per 1,000 people)
above 40 / 30–39 / 20–29 / below 20 / data not available

WORLD INFANT MORTALITY

IN PARTS OF THE DEVELOPING WORLD infant mortality rates are still high; access to medical services such as immunization, adequate nutrition, and the promotion of breast-feeding have been important in combating infant mortality.

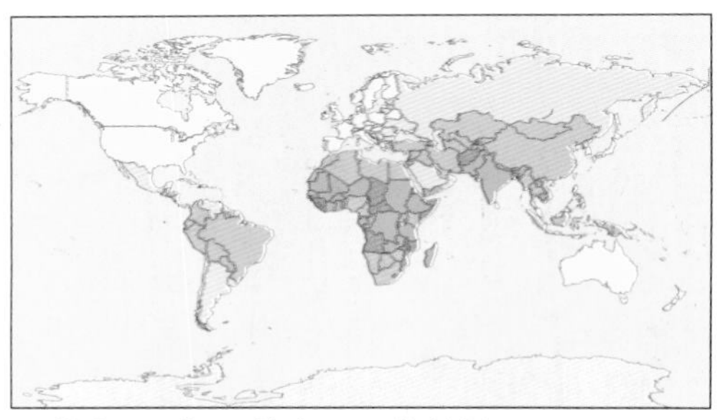

World infant mortality rates (deaths per 1,000 live births)
above 125 / 75–124 / 35–74 / 15–43 / below 15 / data not available

The Economic System

The wealthy countries of the developed world, with their aggressive, market-led economies and their access to productive new technologies and international markets, dominate the world economic system. At the other extreme, many of the countries of the developing world are locked in a cycle of national debt, rising populations, and unemployment. The state-managed economies of the former communist bloc began to be dismantled during the 1990s, and China is emerging as a major economic power following decades of isolation.

Trade blocs

EU · CACM · NAFTA · SADC · ASEAN · ECOWAS · LAIA · CEEAC

Trade blocs

International trade blocs are formed when groups of countries, often already enjoying close military and political ties, join together to offer mutually preferential terms of trade for both imports and exports. Increasingly, global trade is dominated by three main blocs: the EU, NAFTA, and ASEAN. They are supplanting older trade blocs such as the Commonwealth, a legacy of colonialism.

International Trade Flows

World trade acts as a stimulus to national economies, encouraging growth. Over the last three decades, as heavy industries have declined, services – banking, insurance, tourism, airlines, and shipping – have taken an increasingly large share of world trade. Manufactured articles now account for nearly two-thirds of world trade; raw materials and food make up less than a quarter of the total.

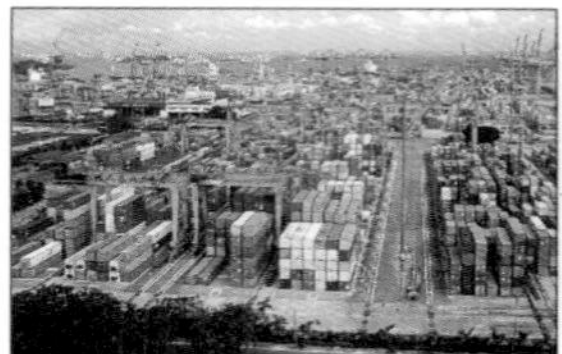

SHIPPING
Ships carry 80% of international cargo, and extensive container ports, where cargo is stored, are vital links in the international transportation network.

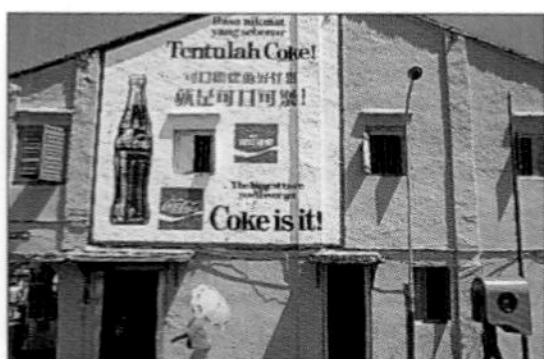

Tentulah Coke!
Coke is it!

MULTINATIONALS
Multinational companies are increasingly penetrating inaccessible markets. The reach of many American commodities is now global.

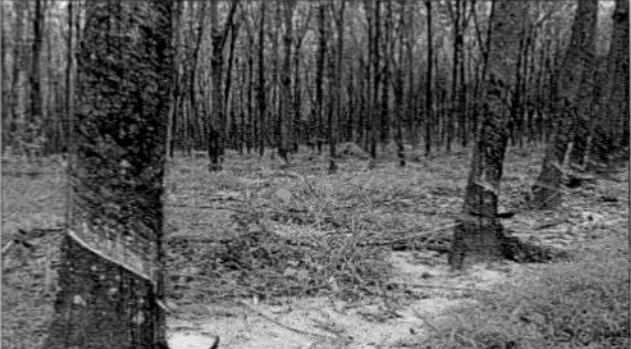

PRIMARY PRODUCTS
Many countries, particularly in the Caribbean and Africa, are still reliant on primary products such as rubber and coffee, which makes them vulnerable to fluctuating prices.

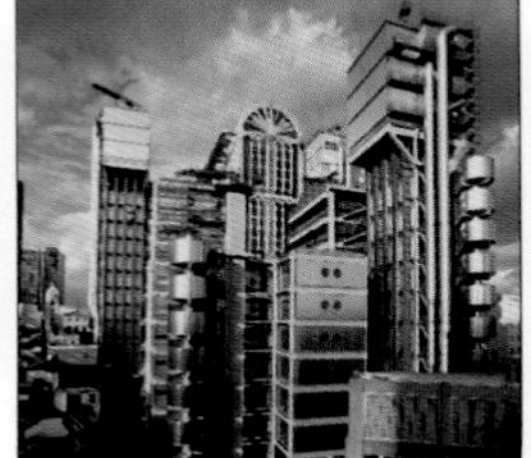

SERVICE INDUSTRIES
Service industries such as banking, tourism and insurance were the fastest-growing industrial sector in the last half of the 20th century. Lloyds of London is the center of the world insurance market.

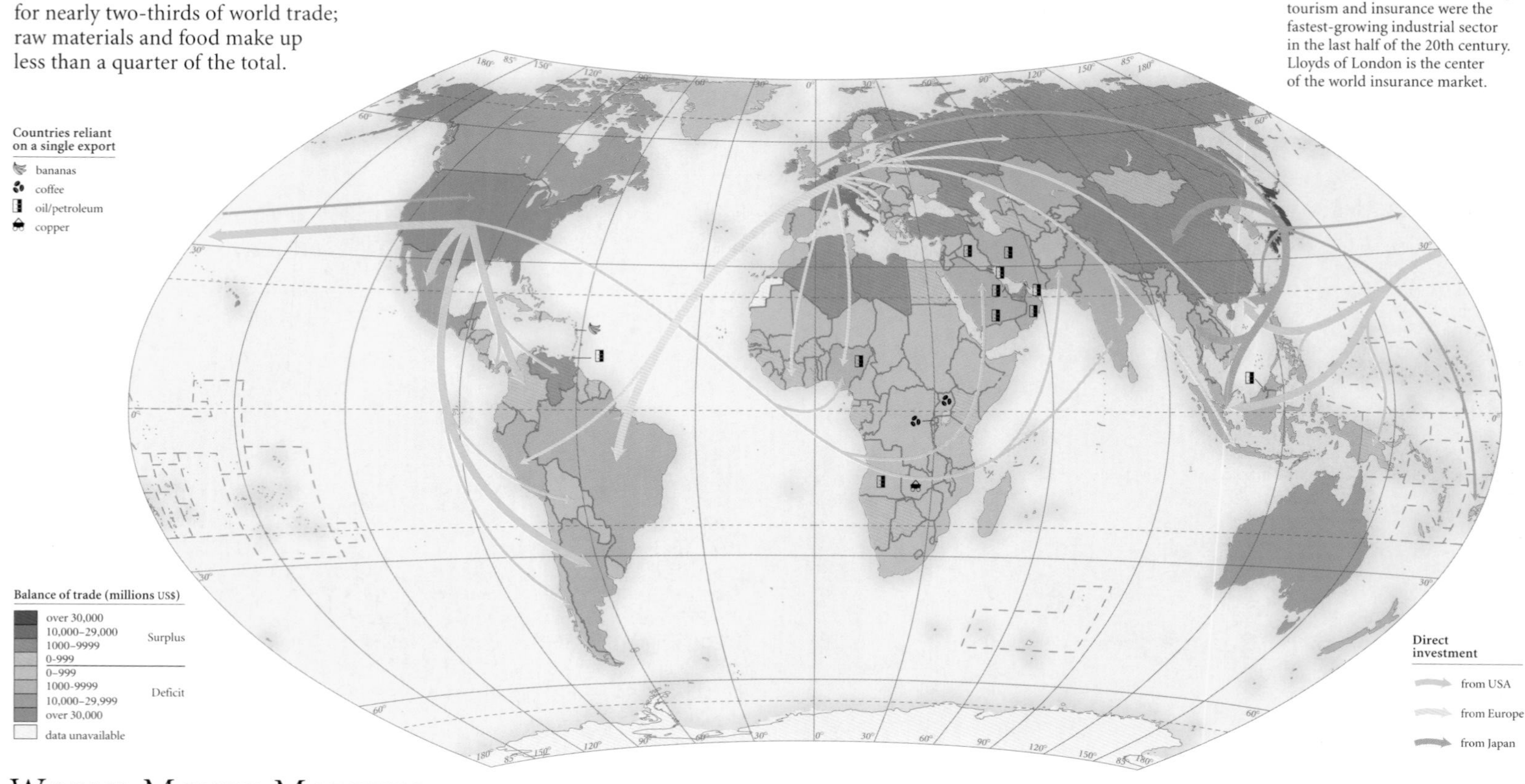

Countries reliant on a single export
bananas
coffee
oil/petroleum
copper
Balance of trade (millions US$)
Surplus
over 30,000
10,000–29,000
1000–9999
0–999
Deficit
0–999
1000–9999
10,000–29,999
over 30,000
data unavailable
Direct investment
from USA
from Europe
from Japan

World Money Markets

The financial world has traditionally been dominated by three major centers – Tokyo, New York and London, which house the headquarters of stock exchanges, multinational corporations and international banks. Their geographic location means that, at any one time in a 24-hour day, one major market is open for trading in shares, currencies, and commodities. Since the late 1980s, technological advances have enabled transactions between financial centers to occur at ever-greater speed, and new markets have sprung up throughout the world.

Major money markets

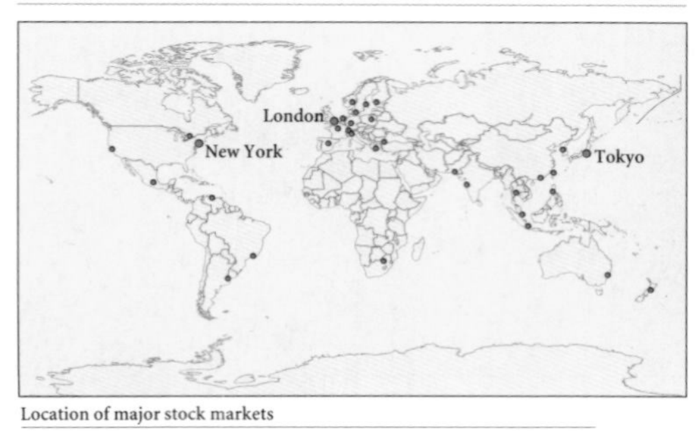

London
New York
Tokyo

Location of major stock markets

● Major stock markets

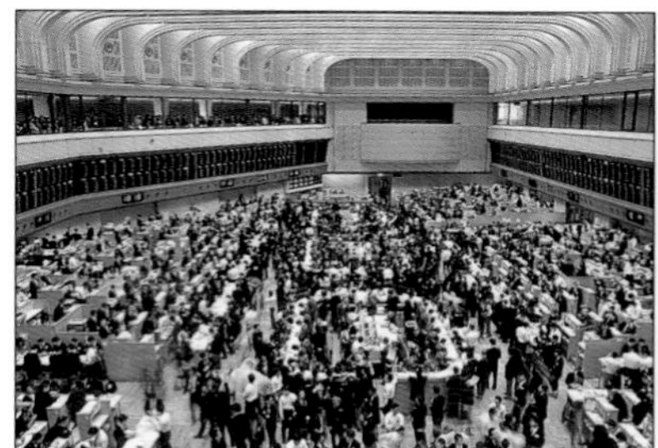

The Tokyo Stock Market crashed in 1990, leading to a slow-down in the growth of the world's most powerful economy, and a refocusing on economic policy away from export-led growth and toward the domestic market.

New stock markets

New stock markets are now opening in many parts of the world, where economies have recently emerged from state controls. In Moscow and Beijing, and several countries in eastern Europe, newly-opened stock exchanges reflect the transition to market-driven economies.

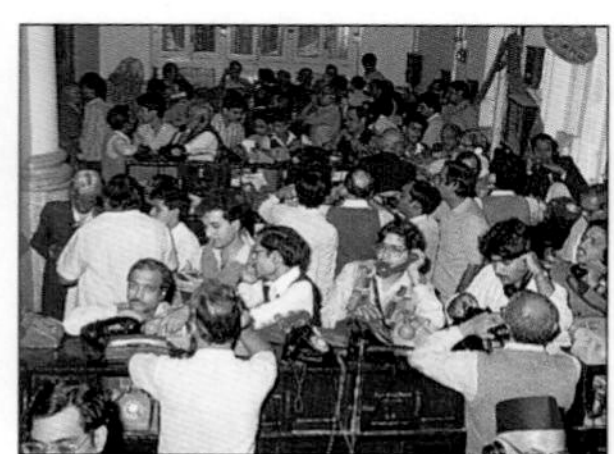

Dealers at the Calcutta Stock Market. *The Indian economy has been opened up to foreign investment and many multinationals now have bases there.*

The developing world

International trade in capital and currency is dominated by the rich nations of the northern hemisphere. In parts of Africa and Asia, where exports of any sort are extremely limited, home-produced commodities are simply sold in local markets.

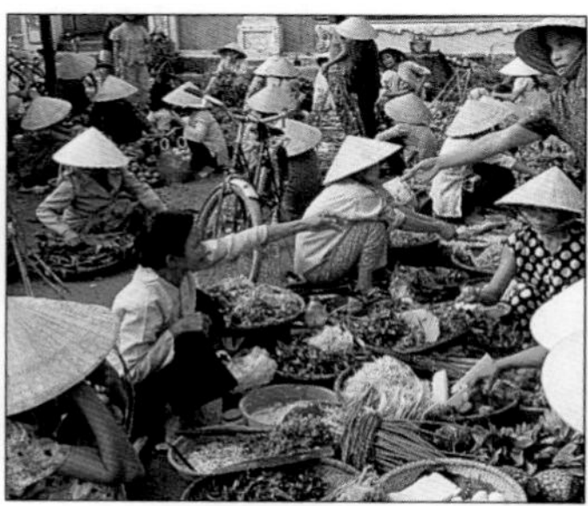

Markets have thrived *in communist Vietnam since the introduction of a liberal economic policy.*

World Wealth Disparity

A global assessment of Gross Domestic Product (GDP) by nation reveals great disparities. The developed world, with only a quarter of the world's population, has 80% of the world's manufacturing income. Civil war, conflict, and political instability further undermine the economic self-sufficiency of many of the world's poorest nations.

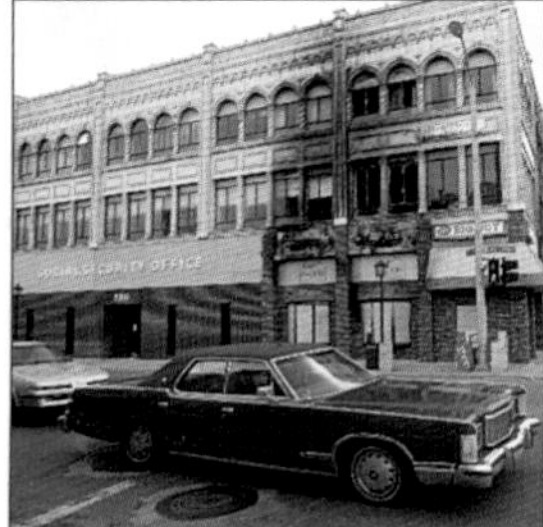

***Cities such as Detroit** have been badly hit by the decline in heavy industry.*

Urban Decay

Although the US still dominates the global economy, it faces deficits in both the federal budget and the balance of trade. Vast discrepancies in personal wealth, high levels of unemployment, and the dismantling of welfare provisions throughout the 1980s have led to severe deprivation in several of the inner cities of North America's industrial heartland.

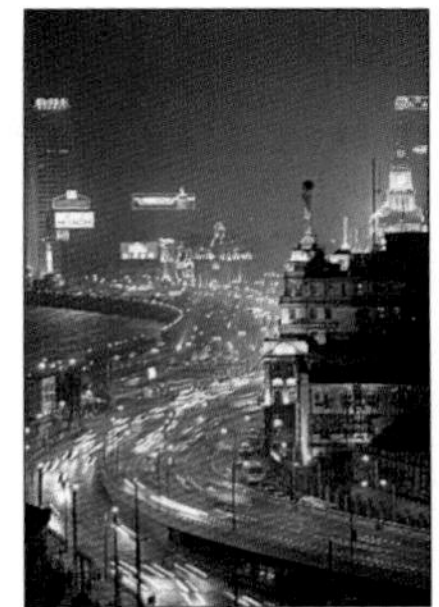

Booming Cities

Since the 1980s the Chinese government has set up special industrial zones, such as Shanghai, where foreign investment is encouraged through tax incentives. Migrants from rural China pour into these regions in search of work, creating "boomtown" economies.

***Foreign investment** has encouraged new infrastructure development in cities like Shanghai.*

Urban Sprawl

Cities are expanding all over the developing world, attracting economic migrants in search of work and opportunities. In cities such as Rio de Janeiro, housing has not kept pace with the population explosion, and squalid shanty towns *(favelas)* rub shoulders with middle-class housing.

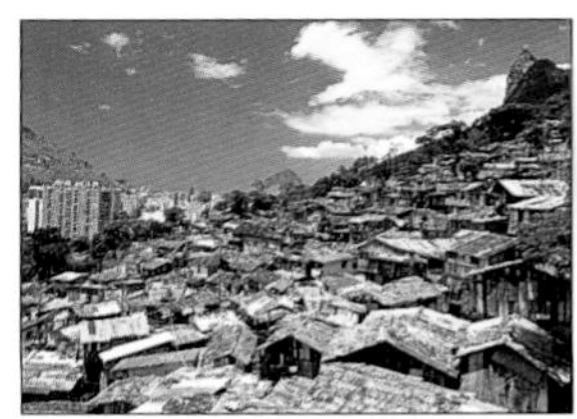

***The favelas of Rio de Janeiro** sprawl over the hills surrounding the city.*

Comparative World Wealth

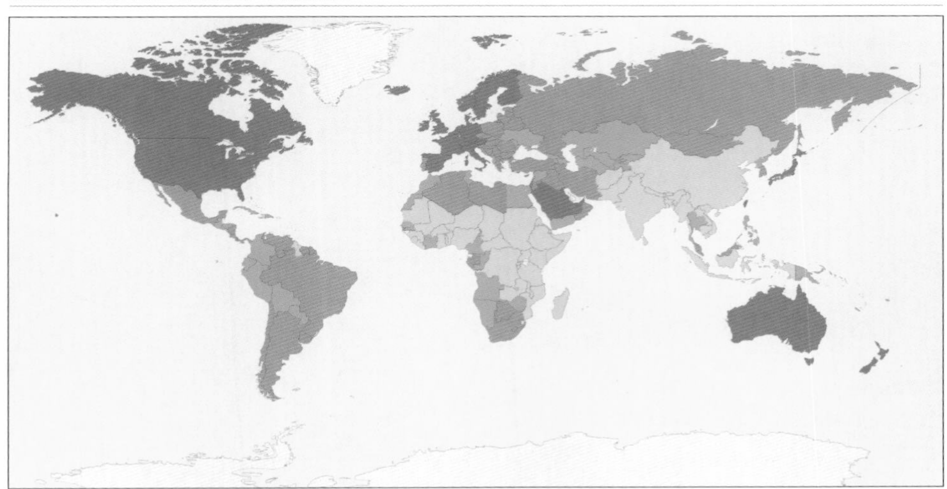

World economies
- high income
- upper-middle income
- lower-middle income
- low income
- data unavailable

Economic "Tigers"

The economic "tigers" of the Pacific Rim – Taiwan, Singapore, and South Korea – have grown faster than Europe and the US over the last decade. Their export- and service-led economies have benefited from stable government, low labor costs, and foreign investment.

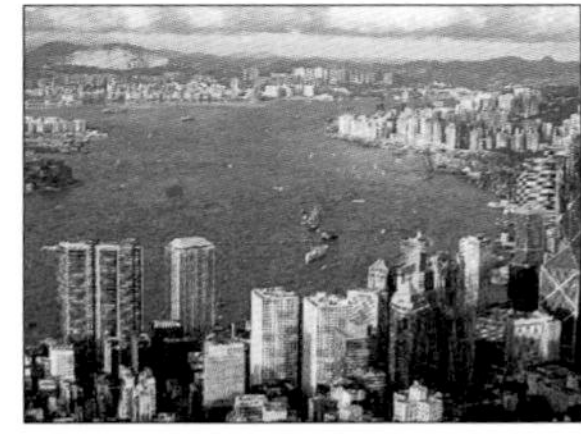

***Hong Kong**, with its fine natural harbor, is one of the most important ports in Asia.*

Agricultural Economies

In parts of the developing world, people survive by subsistence farming – only growing enough food for themselves and their families. With no surplus product, they are unable to exchange goods for currency, the only means of escaping the poverty trap. In other countries, farmers have been encouraged to concentrate on growing a single crop for the export market. This reliance on cash crops leaves farmers vulnerable to crop failure and to changes in the market price of the crop.

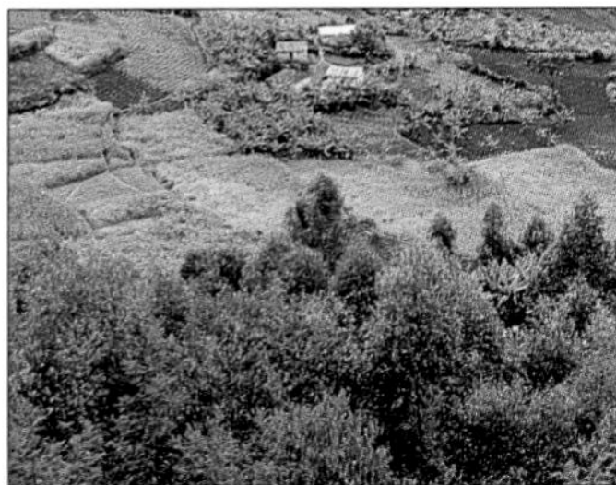

***The Ugandan uplands** are fertile, but poor infrastructure hampers the export of cash crops.*

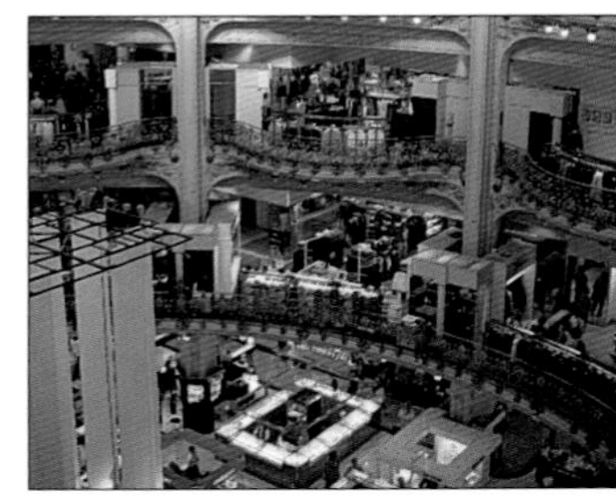

***A shopping arcade** in Paris displays a great profusion of luxury goods.*

The Affluent West

The capital cities of many countries in the developed world are showcases for consumer goods, reflecting the increasing importance of the service sector, and particularly the retail sector, in the world economy. The idea of shopping as a leisure activity is unique to the western world. Luxury goods and services attract visitors, who in turn generate tourist revenue.

Tourism

In 1995, there were 567 million tourists worldwide. Tourism is now the world's biggest single industry, employing 127 million people, though frequently in low-paid unskilled jobs. While tourists are increasingly exploring inaccessible and less-developed regions of the world, the benefits of the industry are not always felt at a local level. There are also worries about the environmental impact of tourism, as the world's last wildernesses increasingly become tourist attractions.

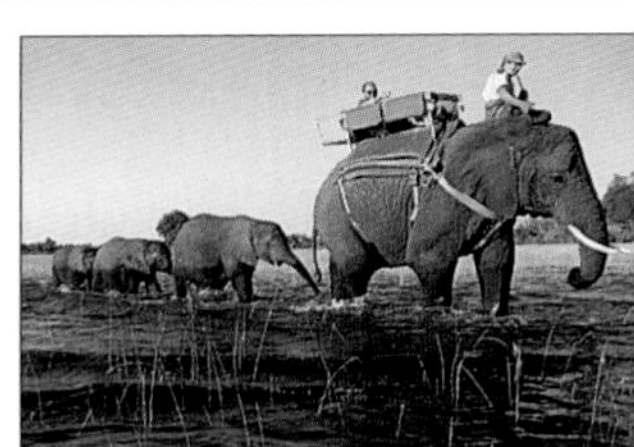

***Botswana's Okavango Delta** is an area rich in wildlife. Tourists go on safaris to the region, but the impact of tourism is controlled.*

Money Flows

Foreign investment in the developing world during the 1970s led to a global financial crisis in the 1980s, when many countries were unable to meet their debt repayments. The International Monetary Fund (IMF) was forced to reschedule the debts and, in some cases, write them off completely. Within the developing world, austerity programs have been initiated to cope with the debt, leading in turn to high unemployment and galloping inflation.
In many parts of Africa, stricken economies are now dependent on international aid.

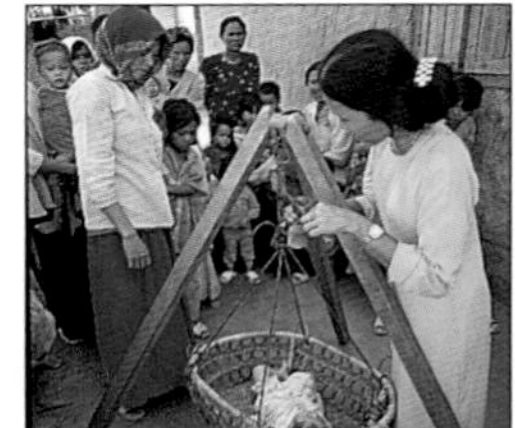

***In rural Southeast Asia**, babies are given medical checks by UNICEF as part of a global aid program sponsored by the UN.*

Tourist Arrivals

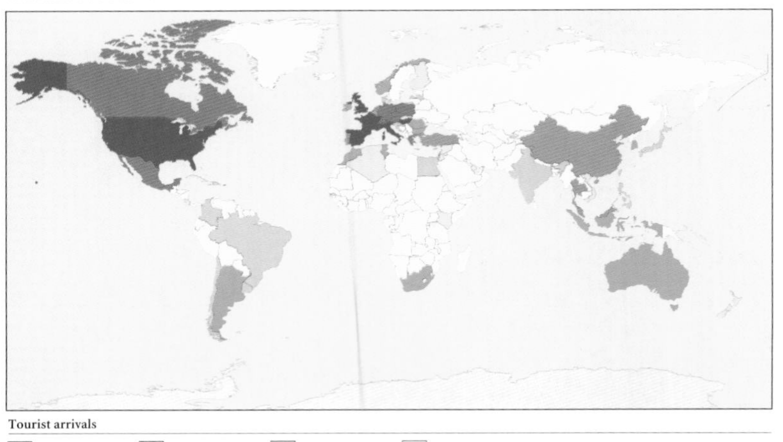

Tourist arrivals
- over 20 million
- 10–20 million
- 5–10 million
- 2.5–5 million
- 1–2.5 million
- 700,000–999,000
- under 700,000
- data unavailable

International Debt: Donors and Receivers

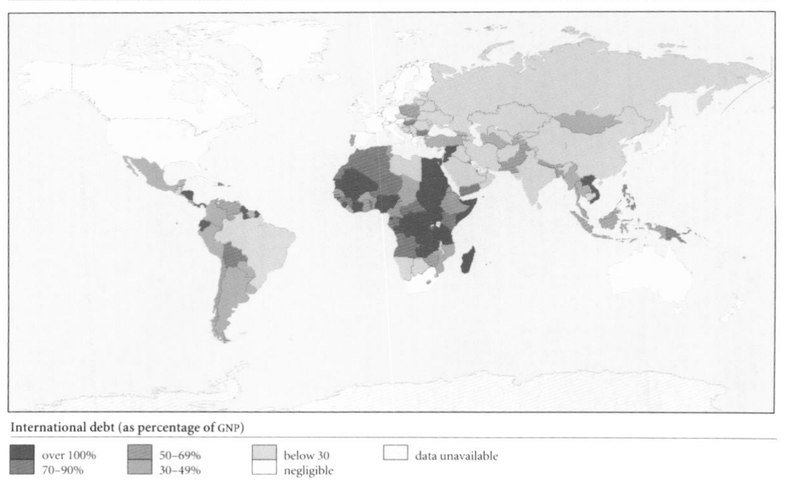

International debt (as percentage of GNP)
- over 100%
- 70–90%
- 50–69%
- 30–49%
- below 30
- negligible
- data unavailable

The Political World

There are 192 independent countries in the world today. With the exception of Antarctica, where territorial claims have been deferred by international treaty, every land area of the Earth's surface either belongs to, or is claimed by, one country or another. The largest country in the world is the Russian Federation, the smallest is Vatican City. Some 60 overseas dependent territories remain, administered variously by France, Australia, Denmark, New Zealand, Norway, Portugal, the UK, the US, and the Netherlands.

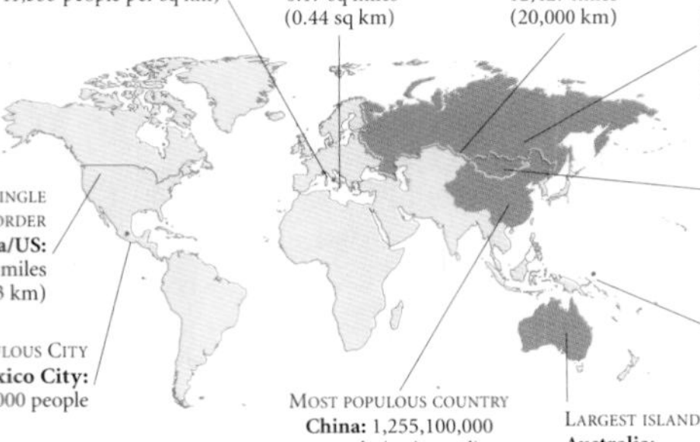

Most densely populated country
Monaco: 15,897 people per sq mile (41,333 people per sq km)

Smallest country
Vatican City: 0.17 sq miles (0.44 sq km)

Longest land borders
Russian Federation: 12,427 miles (20,000 km)

Largest country
Russian Federation: 6,592,863 sq miles (17,075,400 sq km)

Least densely populated country
Mongolia: 5 people per sq mile (2 people per sq km)

Smallest island country
Nauru: 8.2 sq miles (21 sq km)

Largest island country
Australia: 2,967,915 sq miles (7,686,850 sq km)

Most populous country
China: 1,255,100,000 people (estimated)

Most populous city
Mexico City: 16,700,000 people

Longest single land border
Canada/US: 5,526 miles (8,893 km)

International Borders

The map shows three main types of boundary between states. Full borders represent internationally agreed and recognized territorial boundaries. Undefined borders exist where no fixed boundary between states has been demarcated; the boundaries indicated in this way show approximate areas of sovereignty. A disputed border is indicated where a *de facto* territorial boundary exists, which is not agreed or is subject to arbitration.

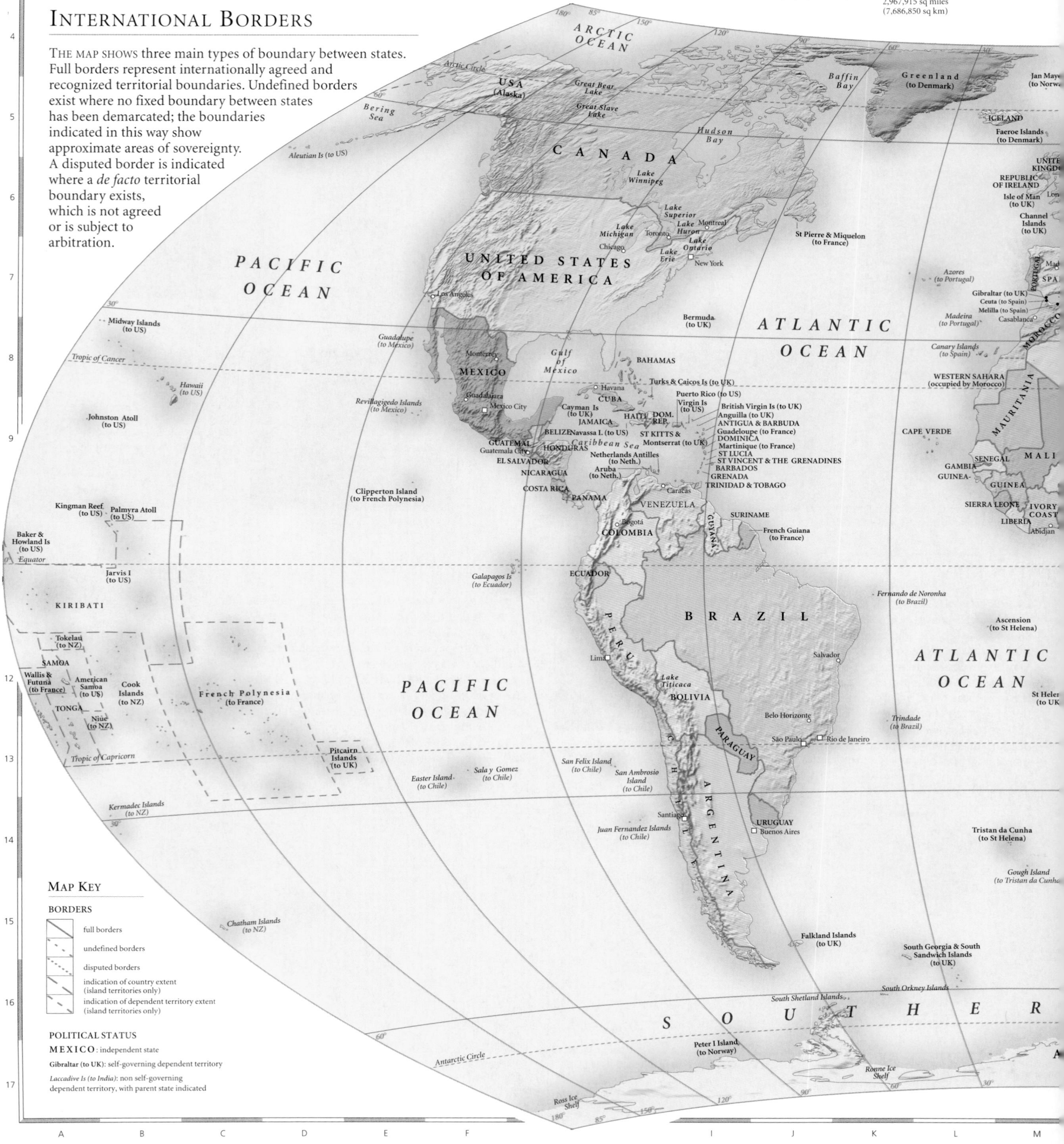

Map Key

BORDERS

- full borders
- undefined borders
- disputed borders
- indication of country extent (island territories only)
- indication of dependent territory extent (island territories only)

POLITICAL STATUS

MEXICO: independent state

Gibraltar (to UK): self-governing dependent territory

Laccadive Is (to India): non self-governing dependent territory, with parent state indicated

The World in 1914

The early years of the 20th century saw the mainly European colonial empires reaching their greatest extents by 1914. Two world wars inaugurated their disintegration, but even in 1950 there were only 82 independent countries. Since then, over 100 have gained their independence, culminating in the breakup of the Soviet Union and former Yugoslavia in the early 1990s.

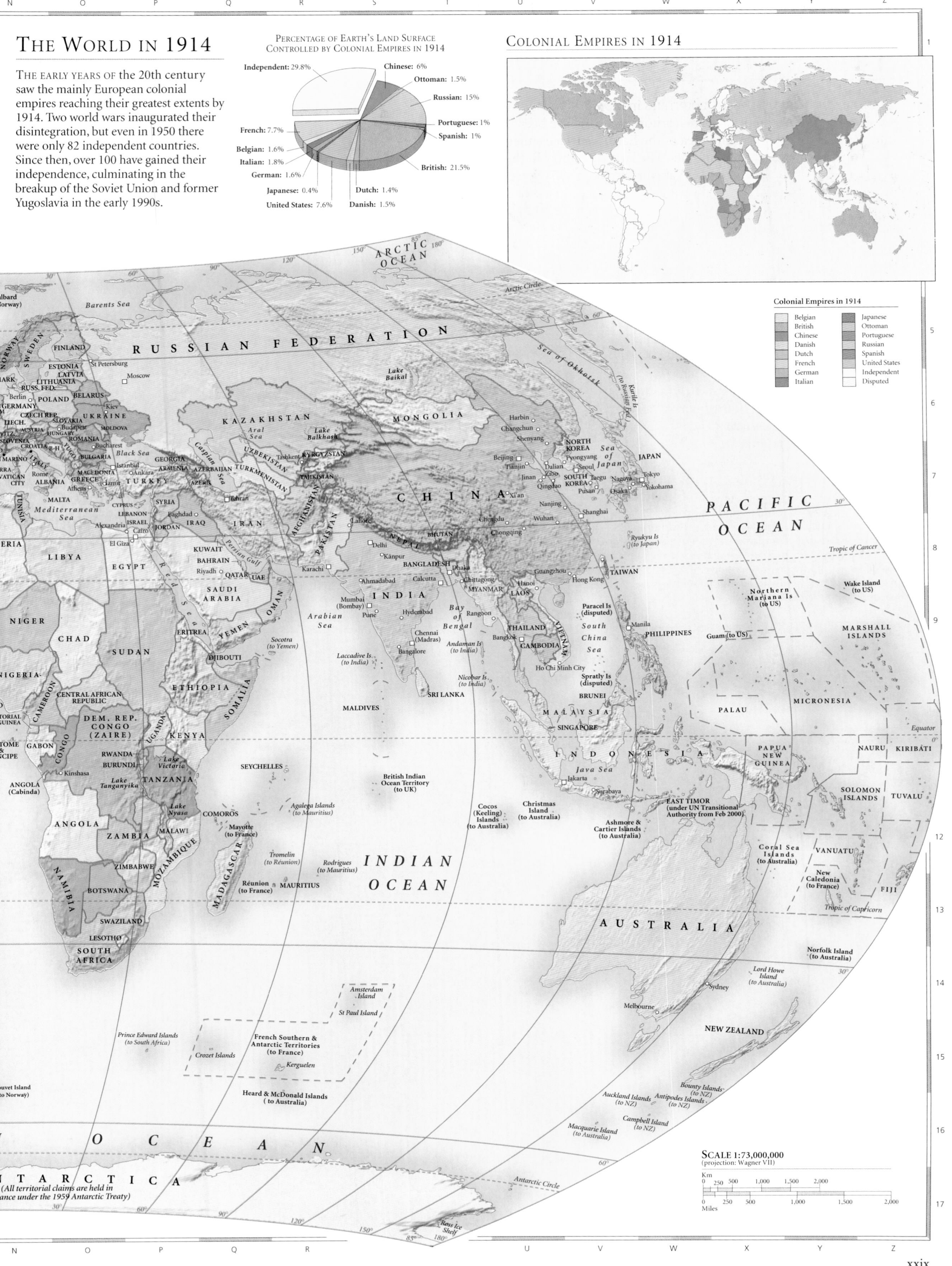

Percentage of Earth's Land Surface Controlled by Colonial Empires in 1914
Independent: 29.8%
Chinese: 6%
Ottoman: 1.5%
Russian: 15%
Portuguese: 1%
Spanish: 1%
British: 21.5%
Danish: 1.5%
Dutch: 1.4%
United States: 7.6%
Japanese: 0.4%
German: 1.6%
Italian: 1.8%
Belgian: 1.6%
French: 7.7%
Colonial Empires in 1914
Colonial Empires in 1914
Belgian
British
Chinese
Danish
Dutch
French
German
Italian
Japanese
Ottoman
Portuguese
Russian
Spanish
United States
Independent
Disputed
ARCTIC OCEAN
Barents Sea
RUSSIAN FEDERATION
Sea of Okhotsk
KAZAKHSTAN
MONGOLIA
CHINA
PACIFIC OCEAN
INDIAN OCEAN
AUSTRALIA
NEW ZEALAND
INDIA
JAPAN
PHILIPPINES
INDONESIA
MALAYSIA
Mediterranean Sea
Black Sea
Caspian Sea
Arabian Sea
Bay of Bengal
South China Sea
Java Sea
Tropic of Cancer
Tropic of Capricorn
Equator
Arctic Circle
Antarctic Circle
ANTARCTICA
(All territorial claims are held in abeyance under the 1959 Antarctic Treaty)
Scale 1:73,000,000
(projection: Wagner VII)
Km
Miles

STATES AND BOUNDARIES

THERE ARE OVER 190 SOVEREIGN STATES in the world today; in 1950 there were only 82. Over the last half-century national self-determination has been a driving force for many states with a history of colonialism and oppression. As more borders are added to the world map, the number of international border disputes increases.

In many cases, where the impetus toward independence has been religious or ethnic, disputes with minority groups have also caused violent internal conflict. While many newly-formed states have moved peacefully toward independence, successfully establishing government by multi-party democracy, dictatorship by military regime or individual despot is often the result of the internal power-struggles which characterize the early stages in the lives of new nations.

THE CHANGING WORLD MAP

DECOLONIZATION

In 1950, large areas of the world remained under the control of a handful of European countries (*page xxviii*). The process of decolonization had begun in Asia, where, following World WarII, much of southern and southeastern Asia sought and achieved self-determination. In the 1960s, a host of African states achieved independence, so that by 1965, most of the larger tracts of the European overseas empires had been substantially eroded. The final major stage in decolonization came with the breakup of the Soviet Union and the Eastern bloc after 1990. The process continues today as the last toeholds of European colonialism, often tiny island nations, press increasingly for independence.

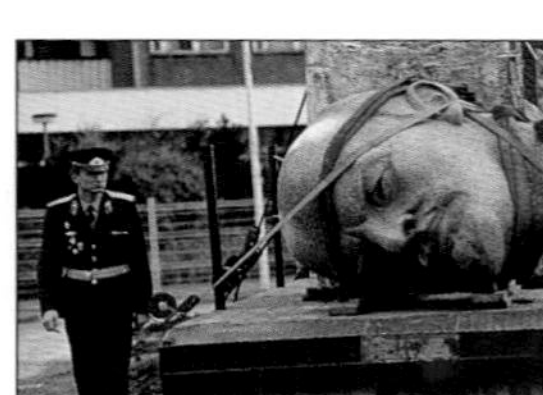

***Icons of communism**, including statues of former leaders such as Lenin and Stalin, were destroyed when the Soviet bloc was dismantled in 1989, creating several new nations.*

NEW NATIONS 1945–1965

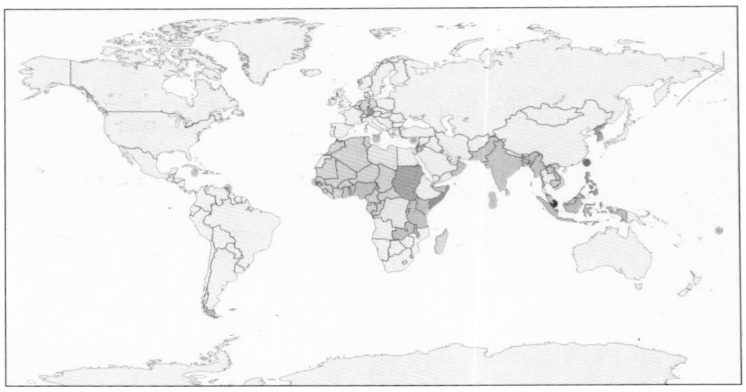

NEW NATIONS 1965–1996

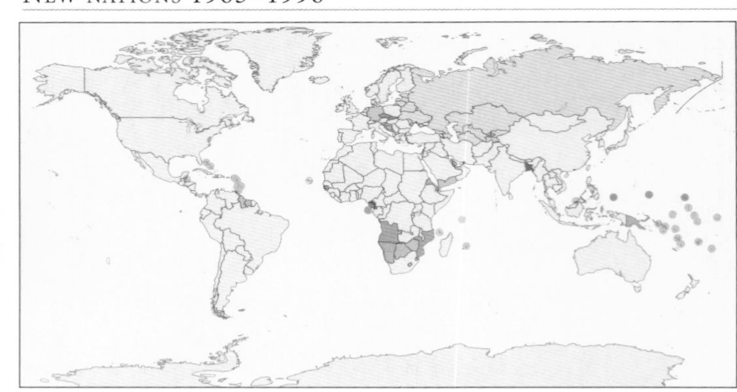

Administration at the time of independence

Australia	Netherlands
Aust/NZ/UK	New Zealand
Belgium	Pakistan
China	Portugal
Czechoslovakia	South Africa
Egypt/UK	Spain
Ethiopia	UK
France	Unified country
France/UK	USA
Italy	USSR
Japan	Yugoslavia
Malaysia	

THE NATURE OF POLITICS

Democracy is a broad term: it can range from the ideal of multiparty elections and fair representation to, in countries such as Singapore and Indonesia, a thin disguise for single-party rule. In despotic regimes, on the other hand, a single, often personal authority has total power; institutions such as parliament and the military are mere instruments of the dictator.

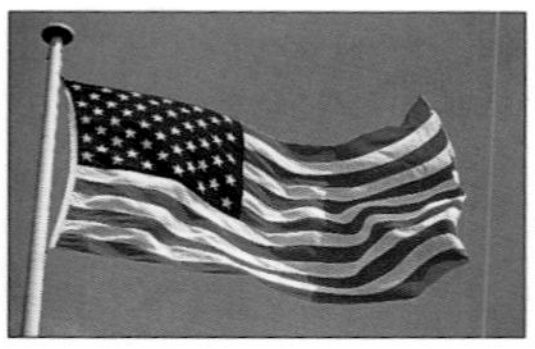

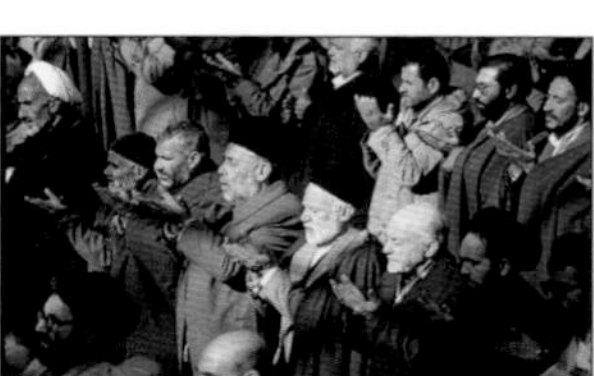

***Iran** is one of the world's true theocracies; Islam has an impact on every aspect of political life.*

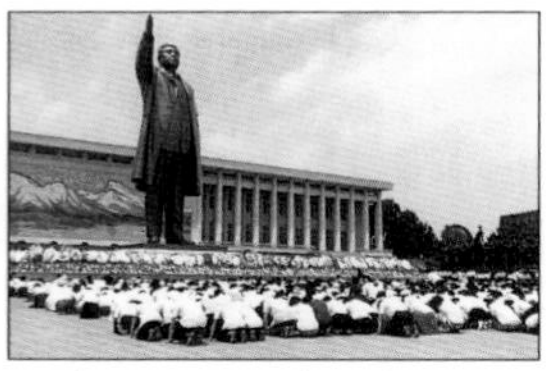

***North Korea** is an independent communist republic. Power is concentrated in the hands of Kim Jong Il.*

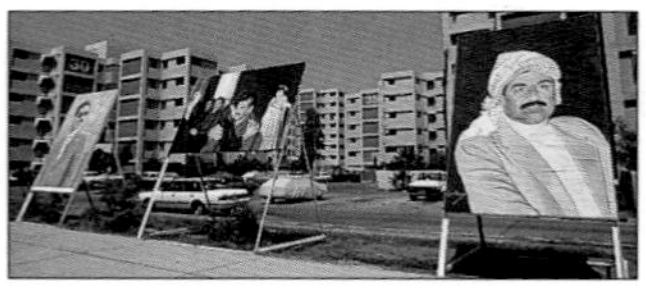

***The stars and stripes** of the US flag are a potent symbol of the country's status as a federal democracy.*

***Saddam Hussein** overthrew his predecessor in 1979. Since then he has promoted an extreme personality cult, with autocratic control over 21.8 million Iraqis.*

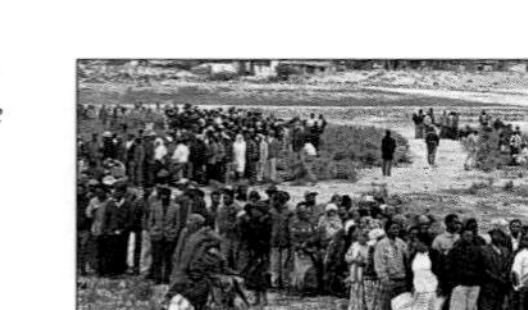

***South Africa** became a democracy in 1994, when elections ended over a century of white minority rule.*

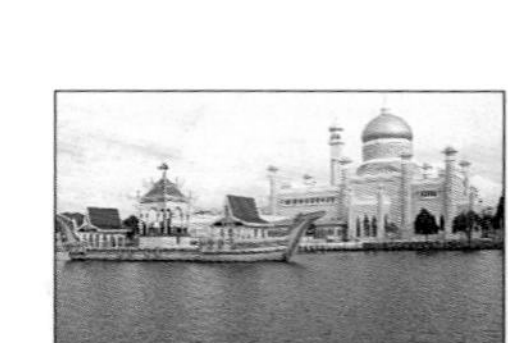

***In Brunei** the Sultan has ruled by decree since 1962; power is closely tied to the royal family. The Sultan's brothers are responsible for finance and foreign affairs.*

Types of government

- Multiparty democracy for more than 10 yrs
- Multiparty/transitional democracy within last 10 yrs
- Single-party government
- Military regime
- Theocracy
- Absolute monarchy
- Current civil unrest

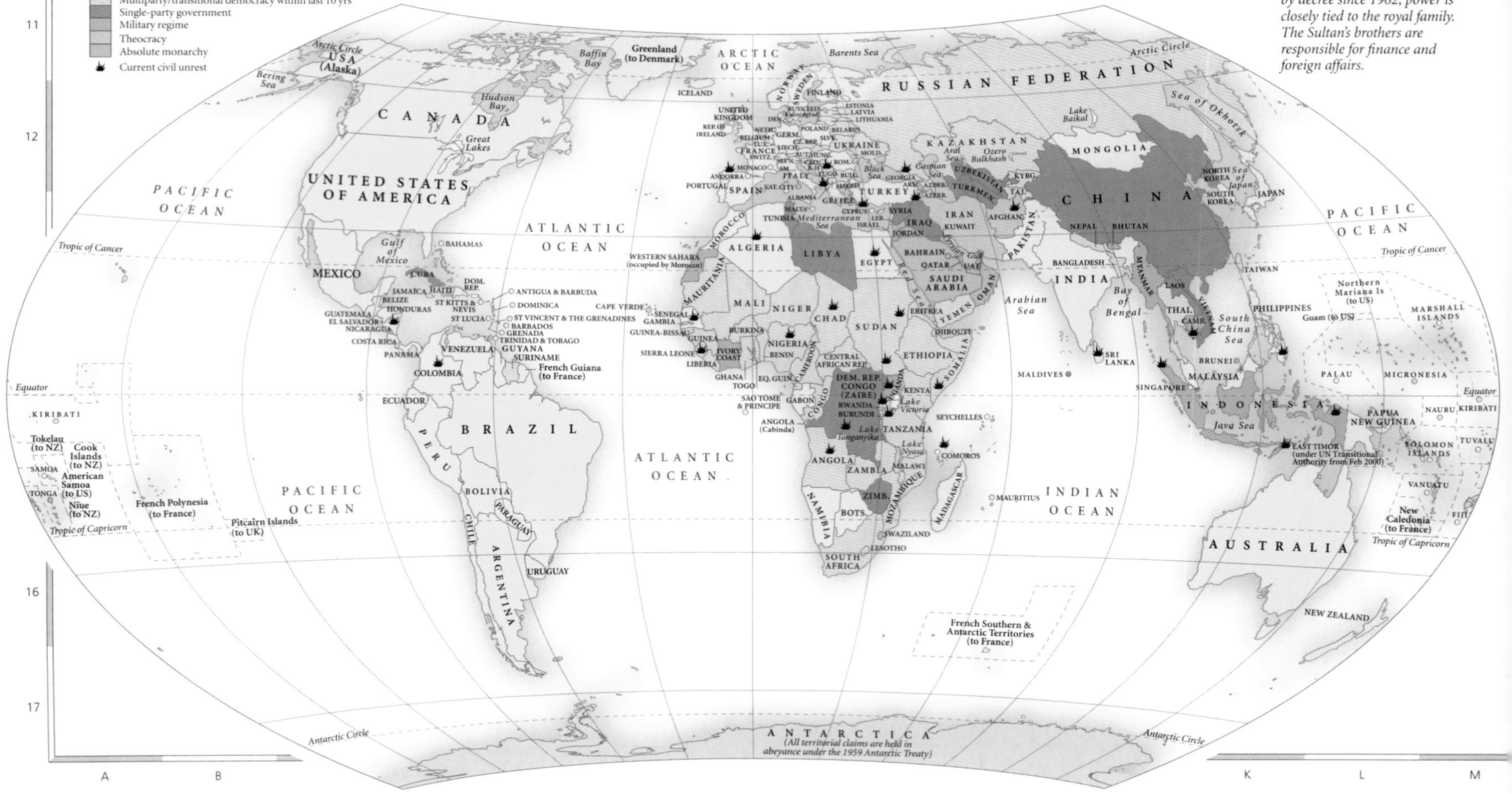

Lines on the Map

The determination of international boundaries can use a variety of criteria. Many of the borders between older states follow physical boundaries; some mirror religious and ethnic differences; others are the legacy of complex histories of conflict and colonialism, while others have been imposed by international agreements or arbitration.

Enclaves

The shifting political map over the course of history has frequently led to anomalous situations. Parts of national territories may become isolated by territorial agreement, forming an enclave. The West German part of the city of Berlin, which until 1989 lay several hundred miles within East German territory, was a famous example.

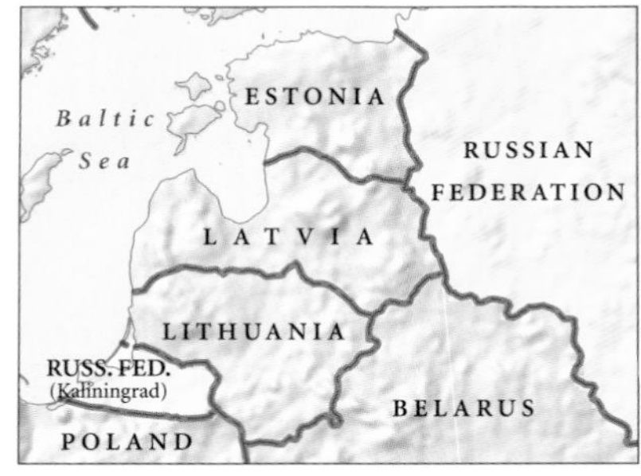
Baltic Sea
ESTONIA
RUSSIAN FEDERATION
LATVIA
LITHUANIA
RUSS. FED. (Kaliningrad)
BELARUS
POLAND

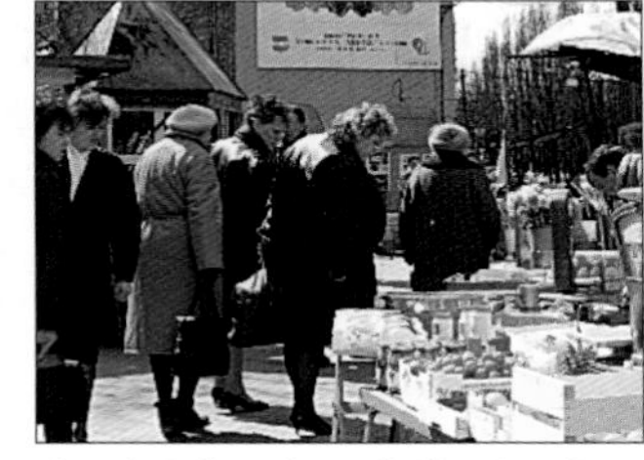

Since the independence of Lithuania and Belarus, the peoples of the Russian enclave of Kaliningrad have become physically isolated.

Post-colonial borders

When the European colonial empires in Africa were dismantled during the second half of the 20th century, the outlines of the new African states mirrored colonial boundaries. These boundaries had been drawn up by colonial administrators, often based on inadequate geographical knowledge. Such arbitrary boundaries were imposed on people of different languages, racial groups, religions, and customs. This confused legacy often led to civil and international war.

WESTERN SAHARA
ALGERIA
MAURITANIA
MALI

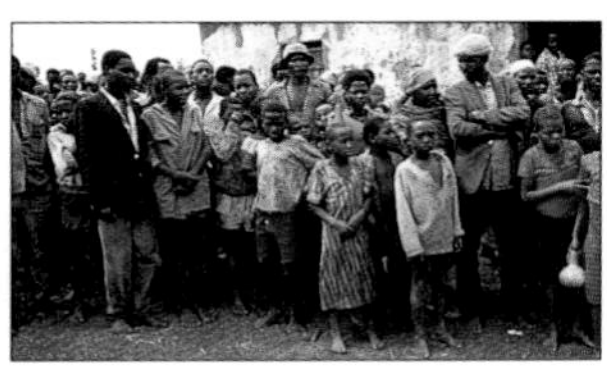

The conflict that has plagued many African countries since independence has caused millions of people to become refugees.

Antarctica

When Antarctic exploration began a century ago, seven nations, Australia, Argentina, Britain, Chile, France, New Zealand, and Norway, laid claim to the new territory. In 1961 the Antarctic Treaty, signed by 39 nations, agreed to hold all territorial claims in abeyance.

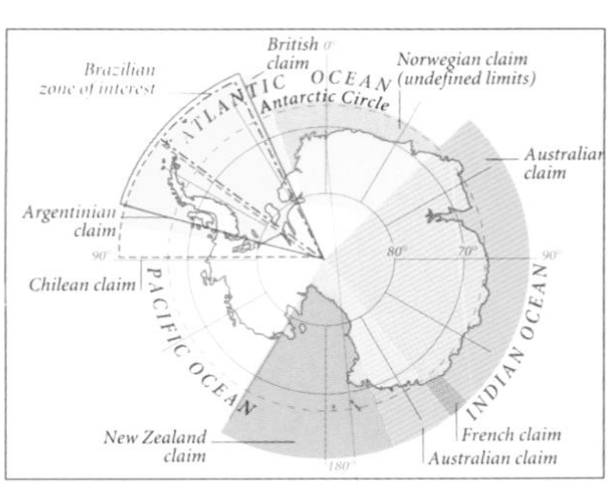
Brazilian zone of interest
British claim
Norwegian claim (undefined limits)
ATLANTIC OCEAN
Antarctic Circle
Australian claim
Argentinian claim
Chilean claim
PACIFIC OCEAN
INDIAN OCEAN
New Zealand claim
French claim
Australian claim

Geometric borders

Straight lines and lines of longitude and latitude have occasionally been used to determine international boundaries; and indeed the world's longest international boundary, between Canada and the USA follows the 49th Parallel for over one-third of its course. Many Canadian, American and Australian internal administrative boundaries are similarly determined using a geometric solution.

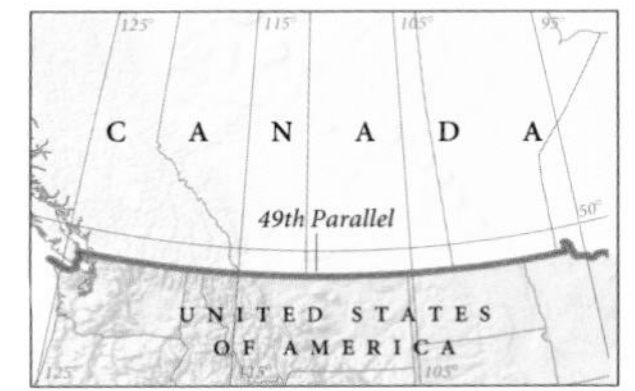
CANADA
49th Parallel
UNITED STATES OF AMERICA

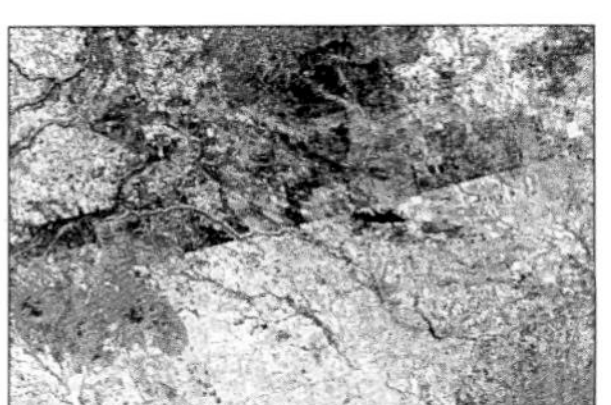

Different farming techniques in Canada and the US clearly mark the course of the international boundary in this satellite map.

World boundaries

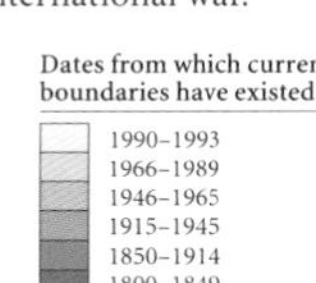
Dates from which current boundaries have existed
1990–1993
1966–1989
1946–1965
1915–1945
1850–1914
1800–1849
Pre-1800

Physical borders

Many of the world's countries are divided by physical borders: lakes, rivers, mountains. The demarcation of such boundaries can, however, lead to disputes. Control of waterways, water supplies, and fisheries are frequent causes of international friction.

Lake borders

Countries which lie next to lakes usually fix their borders in the middle of the lake. Unusually the Lake Nyasa border between Malawi and Tanzania runs along Tanzania's shore.

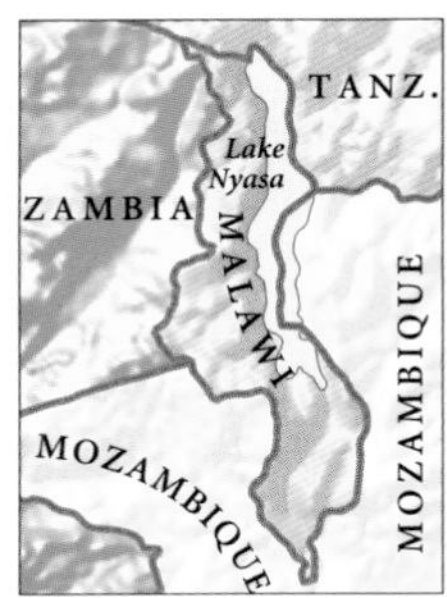
TANZ.
Lake Nyasa
ZAMBIA
MALAWI
MOZAMBIQUE
MOZAMBIQUE

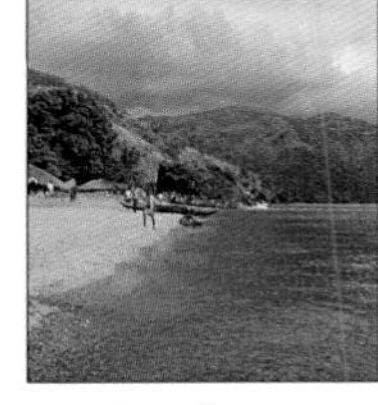

Complicated agreements between colonial powers led to the awkward division of Lake Nyasa.

River borders

Rivers alone account for one-sixth of the world's borders. Many great rivers form boundaries between a number of countries. Changes in a river's course and interruptions of its natural flow can lead to disputes, particularly in areas where water is scarce. The center of the river's course is the nominal boundary line.

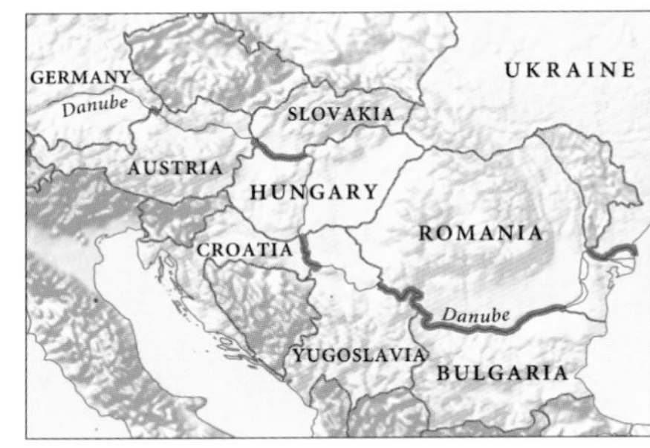
GERMANY
Danube
UKRAINE
SLOVAKIA
AUSTRIA
HUNGARY
ROMANIA
CROATIA
Danube
YUGOSLAVIA
BULGARIA

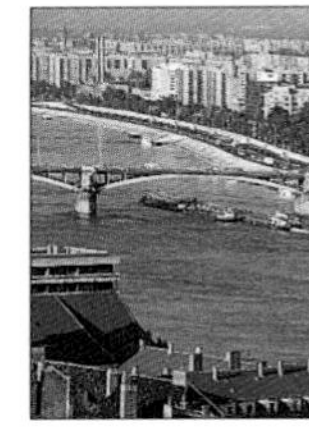

The Danube forms all or part of the border between nine European nations.

Mountain borders

Mountain ranges form natural barriers and are the basis for many major borders, particularly in Europe and Asia. The watershed is the conventional boundary demarcation line, but its accurate determination is often problematic.

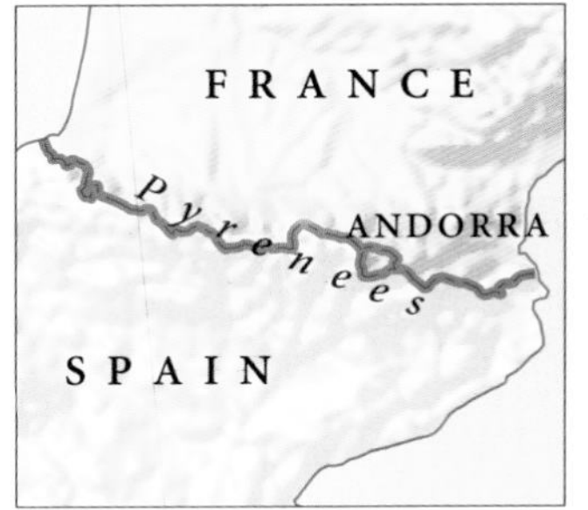
FRANCE
Pyrenees
ANDORRA
SPAIN

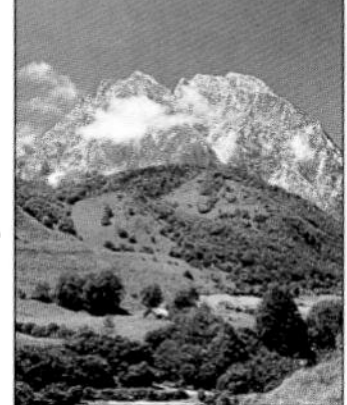

The Pyrenees form a natural mountain border between France and Spain.

Shifting boundaries – Poland

Borders between countries can change dramatically over time. The nations of eastern Europe have been particularly affected by changing boundaries. Poland is an example of a country whose boundaries have changed so significantly that it has literally moved around Europe. At the start of the 16th century, Poland was the largest nation in Europe. Between 1772 and 1795, it was absorbed into Prussia, Austria, and Russia, and it effectively ceased to exist. After World War I, Poland became an independent country once more, but its borders changed again after World War II following invasions by both Soviet Russia and Nazi Germany.

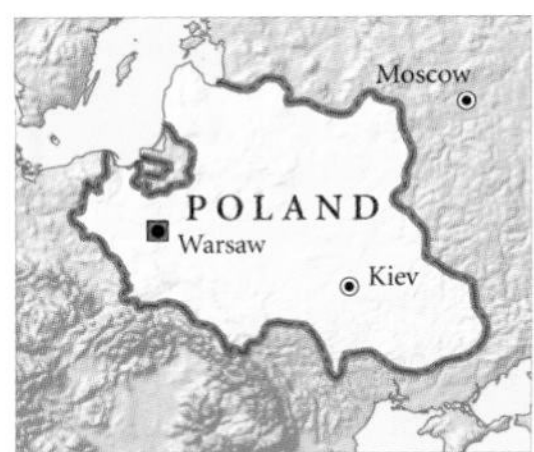
Moscow
POLAND
Warsaw
Kiev

In 1634, Poland was the largest nation in Europe, its eastern boundary reaching toward Moscow.

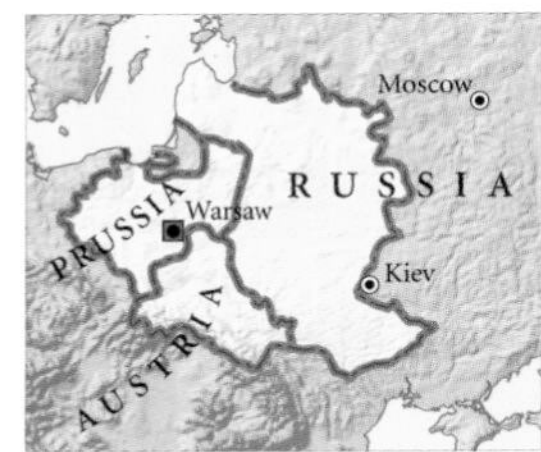
Moscow
PRUSSIA
Warsaw
RUSSIA
Kiev
AUSTRIA

From 1772–1795, Poland was gradually partitioned between Austria, Russia, and Prussia. Its eastern boundary receded by over 100 miles (160 km).

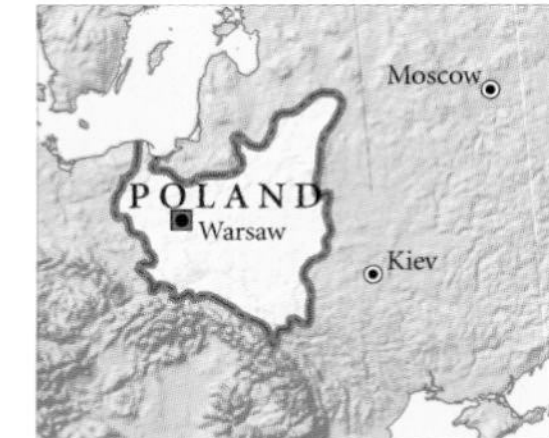
Moscow
POLAND
Warsaw
Kiev

Following World War I, Poland was reinstated as an independent state, but it was less than half the size it had been in 1634.

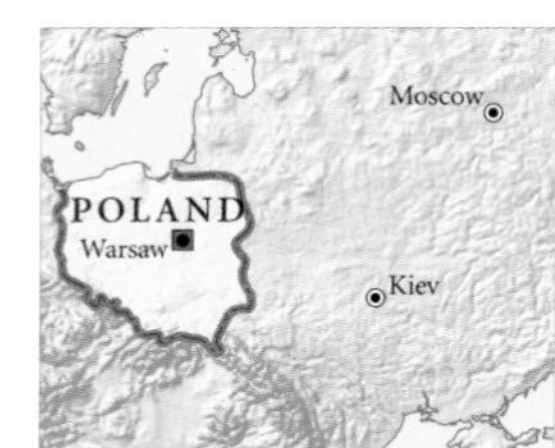
Moscow
POLAND
Warsaw
Kiev

After World War II, the Baltic Sea border was extended westward, but much of the eastern territory was annexed by Russia.

INTERNATIONAL DISPUTES

THERE ARE MORE THAN 60 DISPUTED BORDERS or territories in the world today. Although many of these disputes can be settled by peaceful negotiation, some areas have become a focus for international conflict. Ethnic tensions have been a major source of territorial disagreement throughout history, as has the ownership of, and access to, valuable natural resources. The turmoil of the postcolonial era in many parts of Africa is partly a result of the 19th century "carve-up" of the continent, which created potential for conflict by drawing often arbitrary lines through linguistic and cultural areas.

JAMMU AND KASHMIR

DISPUTES OVER JAMMU AND KASHMIR have caused three serious wars between India and Pakistan since 1947. Pakistan wishes to annex the largely Muslim territory, while India refuses to cede any territory or to hold a referendum, and also lays claim to the entire territory. Most international maps show the "line of control" agreed in 1972 as the *de facto* border. In addition, both Pakistan and India have territorial disputes with neighboring China. The situation is further complicated by a Kashmiri independence movement, active since the late 1980s.

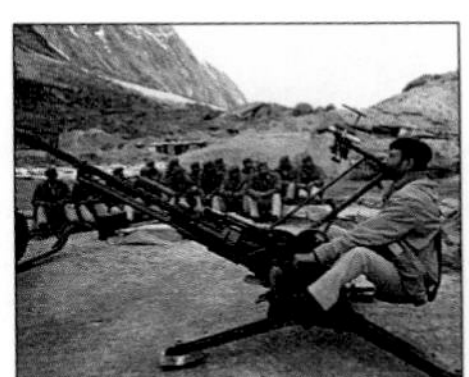

Indian army troops *maintain their positions in the mountainous terrain of northern Kashmir.*

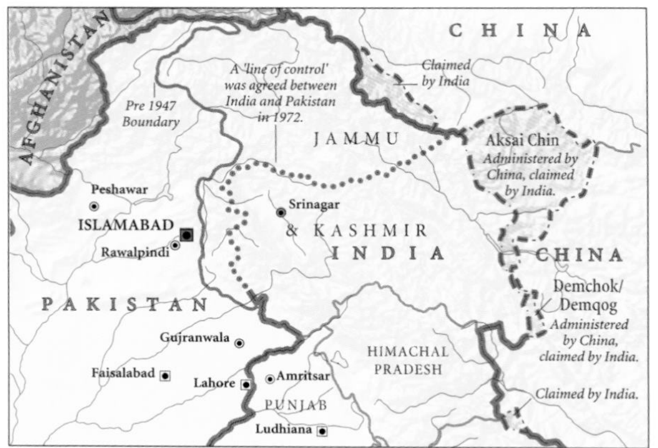
CHINA
AFGHANISTAN
A 'line of control' was agreed between India and Pakistan in 1972.
Claimed by India
Pre 1947 Boundary
JAMMU
Aksai Chin
Administered by China, claimed by India.
Peshawar
Srinagar
ISLAMABAD
& KASHMIR
Rawalpindi
INDIA
CHINA
PAKISTAN
Demchok/Demqog
Administered by China, claimed by India.
Gujranwala
HIMACHAL PRADESH
Faisalabad
Lahore
Amritsar
PUNJAB
Claimed by India.
Ludhiana

NORTH AND SOUTH KOREA

SINCE 1953, the *de facto* border between North and South Korea has been a ceasefire line which straddles the 38th Parallel and is designated as a demilitarized zone. Both countries have heavy fortifications and troop concentrations behind this zone.

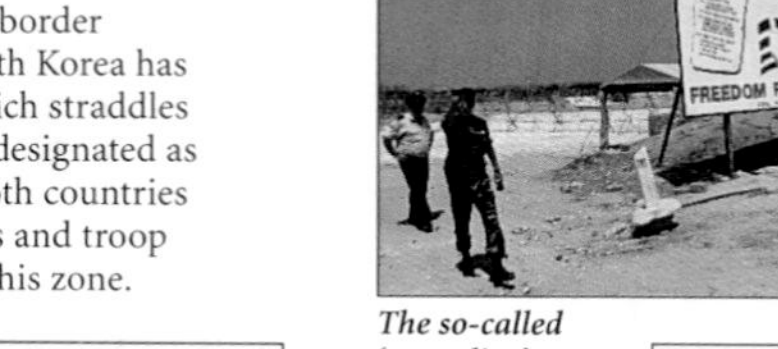

Heavy fortifications *on the border between North and South Korea.*

The so-called 'green line' *divides Cyprus into Greek and Turkish sectors.*

CYPRUS

CYPRUS WAS PARTITIONED in 1974, following an invasion by Turkish troops. The south is now the Greek Cypriot Republic of Cyprus, while the self-proclaimed Turkish Republic of Northern Cyprus is recognized only by Turkey.

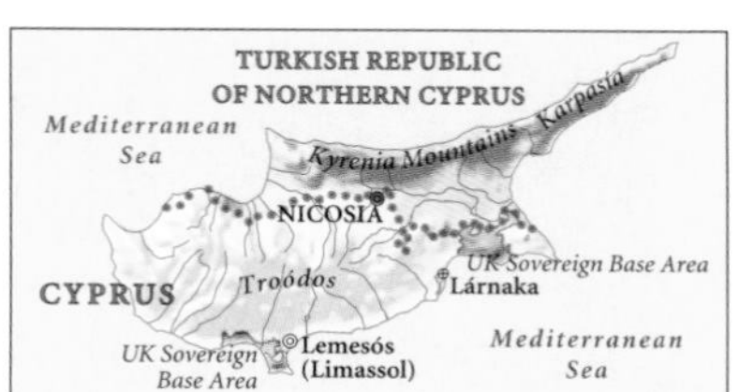
TURKISH REPUBLIC OF NORTHERN CYPRUS
Mediterranean Sea
Kyrenia Mountains
Karpasia
NICOSIA
UK Sovereign Base Area
CYPRUS
Troodos
Larnaka
UK Sovereign Base Area
Lemesós (Limassol)
Mediterranean Sea

Disputed territories and borders

- Countries involved in active territorial or border disputes
- Disputed borders
- Undefined borders
- Disputed territories

THE FALKLAND ISLANDS

THE BRITISH DEPENDENT TERRITORY of the Falkland Islands was invaded by Argentina in 1982, sparking a full-scale war with the UK. In 1995, the UK and Argentina reached an agreement on the exploitation of oil reserves around the islands.

British *warships in Falkland Sound during the 1982 war with Argentina.*

ISRAEL

ISRAEL WAS CREATED IN 1948 following the 1947 UN Resolution (147) on Palestine. Until 1979 Israel had no borders, only ceasefire lines from a series of wars in 1948, 1967 and 1973. Treaties with Egypt in 1979 and Jordan in 1994 led to these borders being defined and agreed. Negotiations over Israeli settlements in disputed territories such as the West Bank, and the issue of self-government for the Palestinians, continue.

- Israeli settlement
- Major settlement
- Palestinian settlement
- Area under Palestinian control

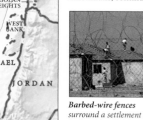

Barbed-wire fences *surround a settlement in the Golan Heights.*

YUGOSLAVIA

FOLLOWING THE DISINTEGRATION in 1991 of the communist state of Yugoslavia, the breakaway states of Croatia and Bosnia-Herzegovina came into conflict with the "parent" state (consisting of Serbia and Montenegro). Warfare focused on ethnic and territorial ambitions in Bosnia. The tenuous Dayton Accord of 1995 sought to recognize the post-1990 borders, whilst providing for ethnic partition and required international peace-keeping troops to maintain the terms of the peace.

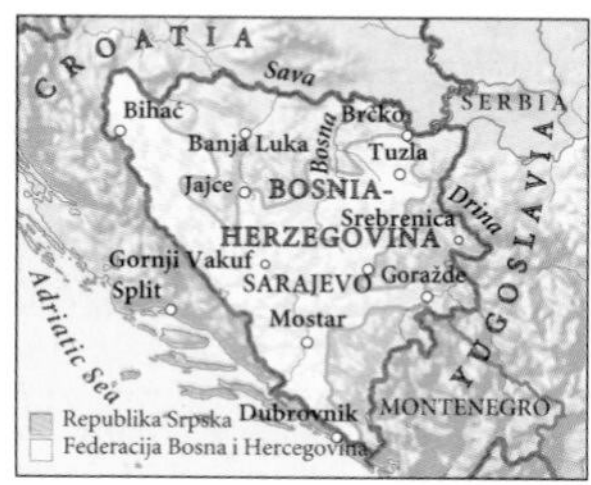
CROATIA
Sava
SERBIA
Bihać
Banja Luka
Brčko
Tuzla
Jajce
BOSNIA-
Srebrenica
HERZEGOVINA
Drina
Gornji Vakuf
SARAJEVO
Goražde
Split
Mostar
YUGOSLAVIA
Adriatic Sea
Dubrovnik
MONTENEGRO
Republika Srpska
Federacija Bosna i Hercegovina

Most claimant *states have small military garrisons on the Spratly Islands.*

THE SPRATLY ISLANDS

THE SITE OF POTENTIAL OIL and natural gas reserves, the Spratly Islands in the South China Sea have been claimed by China, Vietnam, Taiwan, Malaysia, and the Philippines since the Japanese gave up a wartime claim in 1951.

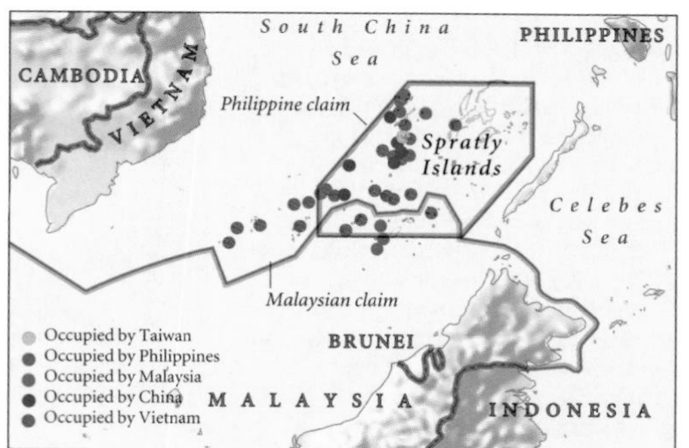
South China Sea
PHILIPPINES
CAMBODIA
VIETNAM
Philippine claim
Spratly Islands
Celebes Sea
Malaysian claim
BRUNEI
Occupied by Taiwan
Occupied by Philippines
Occupied by Malaysia
Occupied by China
Occupied by Vietnam
MALAYSIA
INDONESIA

ATLAS OF THE WORLD

THE MAPS IN THIS ATLAS ARE ARRANGED CONTINENT BY CONTINENT, STARTING FROM THE INTERNATIONAL DATE LINE, AND MOVING EASTWARD. THE MAPS PROVIDE A UNIQUE VIEW OF TODAY'S WORLD, COMBINING TRADITIONAL CARTOGRAPHIC TECHNIQUES WITH THE LATEST REMOTE-SENSED AND DIGITAL TECHNOLOGY.

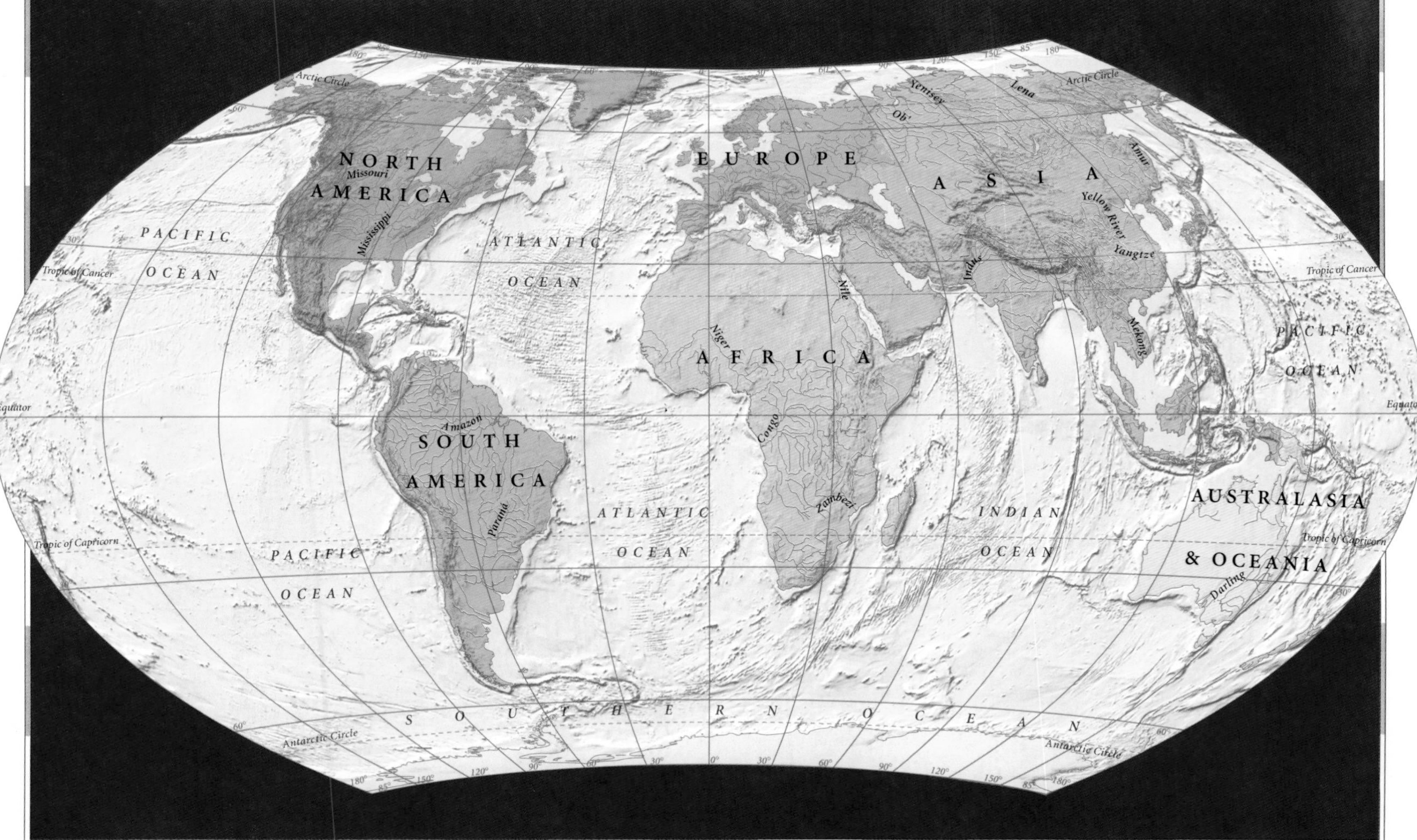
NORTH AMERICA
Missouri
Mississippi
PACIFIC OCEAN
ATLANTIC OCEAN
EUROPE
ASIA
Yenisey
Ob'
Lena
Amur
Yellow River
Yangtze
Indus
Mekong
Nile
Niger
AFRICA
Congo
Zambezi
SOUTH AMERICA
Amazon
Paraná
INDIAN OCEAN
AUSTRALASIA & OCEANIA
Darling
SOUTHERN OCEAN
Arctic Circle
Tropic of Cancer
Equator
Tropic of Capricorn
Antarctic Circle

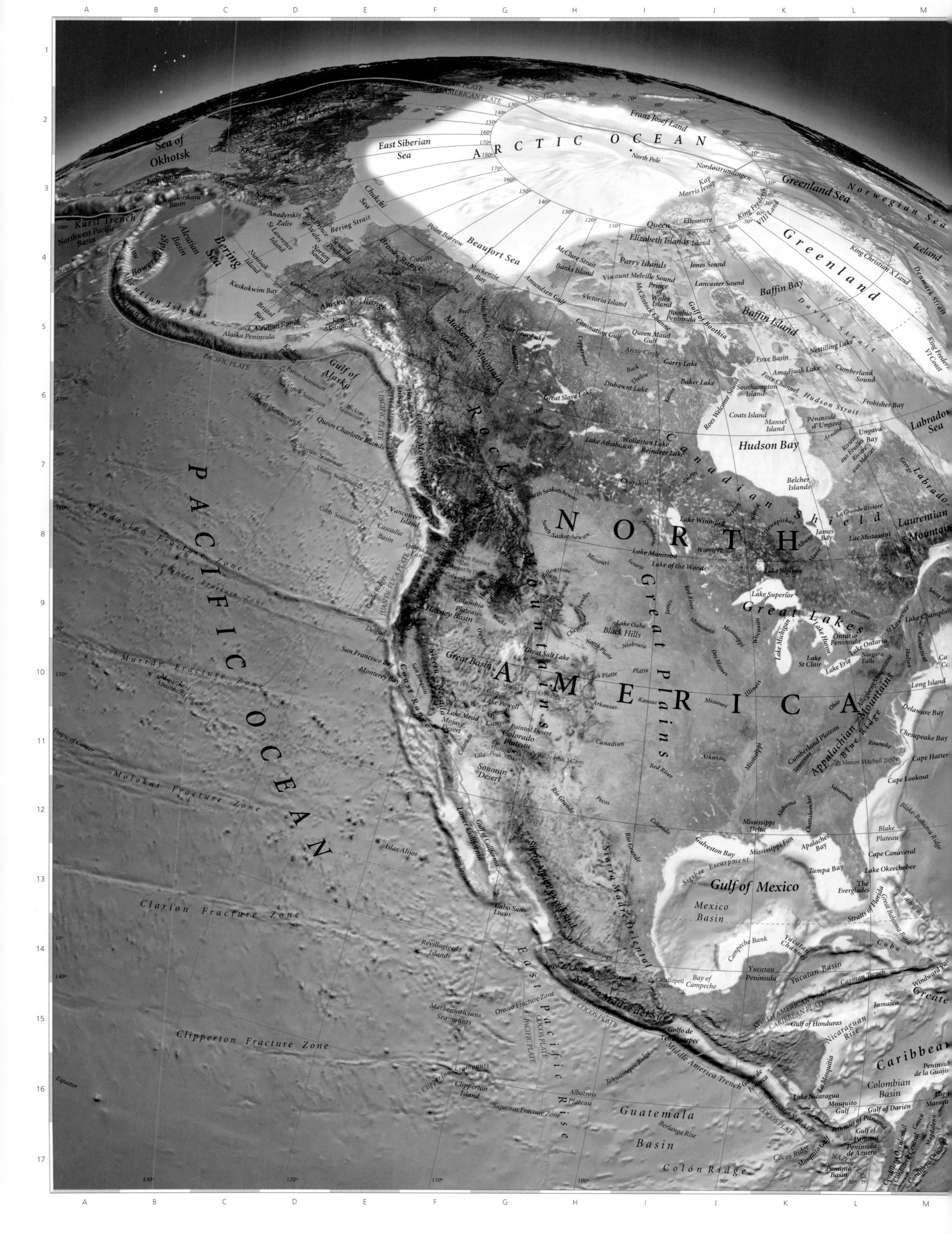

A B C D E F G H I J K L M

ARCTIC OCEAN
North Pole
East Siberian Sea
Sea of Okhotsk
Chukchi Sea
Bering Strait
Bering Sea
Beaufort Sea
Greenland Sea
Norwegian Sea
Greenland
Iceland
Baffin Bay
Baffin Island
Davis Strait
Queen Elizabeth Islands
Parry Islands
Banks Island
Victoria Island
Ellesmere Island
Jones Sound
Lancaster Sound
Prince of Wales Island
Boothia Peninsula
Gulf of Boothia
Amundsen Gulf
Coronation Gulf
Queen Maud Gulf
Mackenzie Bay
Brooks Range
Alaska Range
Alaska Peninsula
Aleutian Islands
Aleutian Trench
Aleutian Basin
Bowers Ridge
Kuril Trench
Northwest Pacific Basin
Kodiak Island
Gulf of Alaska
Mackenzie Mountains
Great Bear Lake
Great Slave Lake
Lake Athabasca
Hudson Bay
Hudson Strait
Foxe Basin
Southampton Island
Coats Island
Belcher Islands
James Bay
Labrador Sea
Ungava Bay
Canadian Shield
Laurentian Mountains
Queen Charlotte Islands
Vancouver Island
Cascadia Basin
Rocky Mountains
NORTH AMERICA
Great Plains
Lake Winnipeg
Lake Manitoba
Lake of the Woods
Lake Superior
Great Lakes
Lake Michigan
Lake Huron
Lake Erie
Lake Ontario
Black Hills
Great Salt Lake
Great Basin
Columbia Plateau
Colorado Plateau
Grand Canyon
Mojave Desert
Sonoran Desert
San Francisco Bay
Monterey Bay
Appalachian Mountains
Blue Ridge
Cape Hatteras
Chesapeake Bay
Delaware Bay
Long Island
Mississippi Delta
Mississippi Fan
Galveston Bay
Sigsbee Escarpment
Gulf of Mexico
Mexico Basin
Campeche Bank
Bay of Campeche
Yucatan Peninsula
Yucatan Channel
Yucatan Basin
Cayman Trench
Cuba
Straits of Florida
The Everglades
Lake Okeechobee
Cape Canaveral
Tampa Bay
Apalachee Bay
Blake Plateau
Lower California
Gulf of California
Cabo San Lucas
Sierra Madre Occidental
Sierra Madre Oriental
Sierra Madre del Sur
Golfo de Tehuantepec
Middle America Trench
Gulf of Honduras
Nicaraguan Rise
Lake Nicaragua
Caribbean
Colombian Basin
Isthmus of Panama
Gulf of Panama
PACIFIC OCEAN
Mendocino Fracture Zone
Pioneer Fracture Zone
Murray Fracture Zone
Molokai Fracture Zone
Clarion Fracture Zone
Clipperton Fracture Zone
East Pacific Rise
Revillagigedo Islands
Mathematicians Seamounts
Clipperton Island
Albatross Plateau
Guatemala Basin
Cocos Ridge
Colón Ridge
Tropic of Cancer
Equator

A B C D E F G H I J K L M

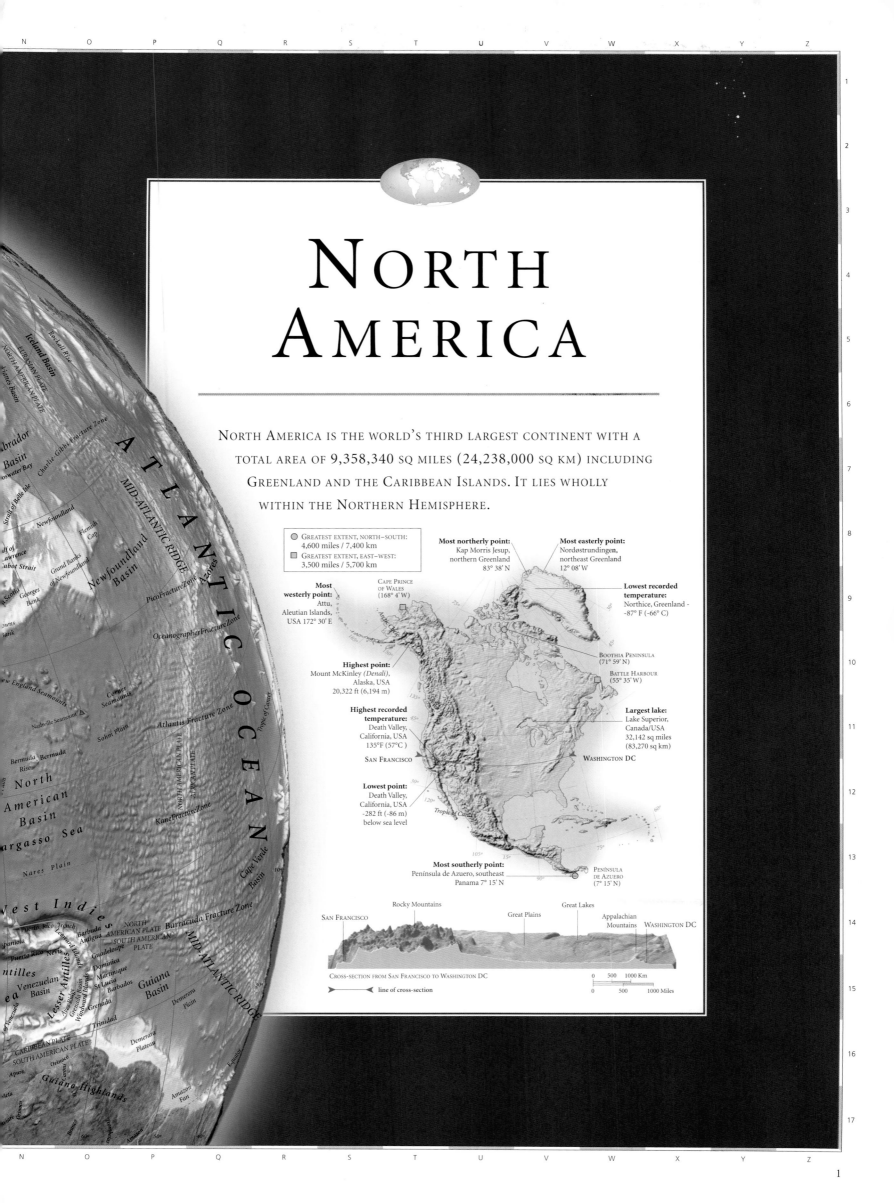

North America

North America is the world's third largest continent with a total area of 9,358,340 sq miles (24,238,000 sq km) including Greenland and the Caribbean Islands. It lies wholly within the Northern Hemisphere.

Greatest extent, north–south: 4,600 miles / 7,400 km
Greatest extent, east–west: 3,500 miles / 5,700 km
Most northerly point: Kap Morris Jesup, northern Greenland 83° 38' N
Most easterly point: Nordøstrundingen, northeast Greenland 12° 08' W
Most westerly point: Attu, Aleutian Islands, USA 172° 30' E
Cape Prince of Wales (168° 4' W)
Lowest recorded temperature: Northice, Greenland -87° F (-66° C)
Boothia Peninsula (71° 59' N)
Battle Harbour (55° 35' W)
Highest point: Mount McKinley (Denali), Alaska, USA 20,322 ft (6,194 m)
Highest recorded temperature: Death Valley, California, USA 135°F (57°C)
Largest lake: Lake Superior, Canada/USA 32,142 sq miles (83,270 sq km)
San Francisco
Washington DC
Lowest point: Death Valley, California, USA -282 ft (-86 m) below sea level
Tropic of Cancer
Most southerly point: Península de Azuero, southeast Panama 7° 15' N
Península de Azuero (7° 15' N)
Rocky Mountains
Great Plains
Great Lakes
Appalachian Mountains
Cross-section from San Francisco to Washington DC
line of cross-section
0 500 1000 Km
0 500 1000 Miles
Atlantic Ocean
Mid-Atlantic Ridge
North American Basin
Sargasso Sea
West Indies
Newfoundland Basin
Iceland Basin
Guiana Basin
Guiana Highlands

PHYSICAL NORTH AMERICA

THE NORTH AMERICAN CONTINENT can be divided into a number of major structural areas: the Western Cordillera, the Canadian Shield, the Great Plains, and Central Lowlands, and the Appalachians. Other smaller regions include the Gulf Atlantic Coastal Plain which borders the southern coast of North America from the southern Appalachians to the Great Plains. This area includes the expanding Mississippi Delta. A chain of volcanic islands, running in an arc around the margin of the Caribbean Plate, lie to the east of the Gulf of Mexico.

THE CANADIAN SHIELD

SPANNING NORTHERN CANADA and Greenland, this geologically stable plain forms the heart of the continent, containing rocks more than two billion years old. A long history of weathering and repeated glaciation has scoured the region, leaving flat plains, gentle hummocks, numerous small basins and lakes, and the bays and islands of the Arctic.

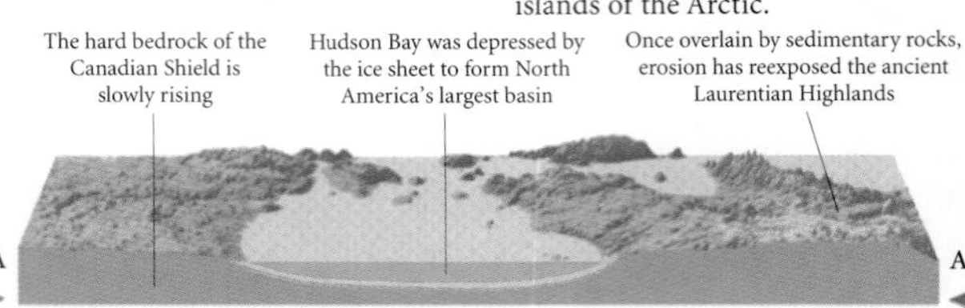
The hard bedrock of the Canadian Shield is slowly rising
Hudson Bay was depressed by the ice sheet to form North America's largest basin
Once overlain by sedimentary rocks, erosion has reexposed the ancient Laurentian Highlands
A
A

***Section** across the Canadian Shield showing where the ice sheet has depressed the underlying rock and formed bays and islands.*

0 100 200 Km
0 100 200 Miles

THE WESTERN CORDILLERA

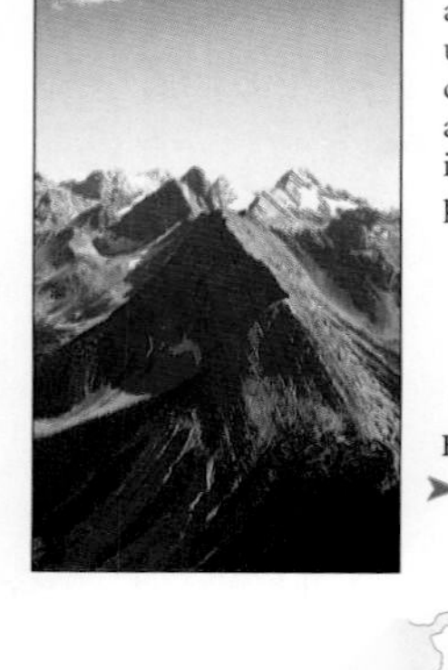

ABOUT 80 MILLION YEARS ago the Pacific and North American plates collided, uplifting the Western Cordillera. This consists of the Aleutian, Coast, Cascade and Sierra Nevada mountains, and the inland Rocky Mountains. These run parallel from the Arctic to Mexico.

Strata have been thrust eastward along fault lines

The Rocky Mountain Trench is the longest linear fault on the continent

B

B

Volcanic rock

***Cross-section** through the Western Cordillera showing direction of mountain building.*

0 50 100 Km
0 50 100 Miles

The weight of the ice sheet, 1.8 miles (3 km) thick, has depressed the land to 0.6 miles (1 km) below sea level

***This computer-generated** view shows the ice-covered island of Greenland without its ice cap.*

MAP KEY

ELEVATION

3500m / 11,484ft
3000m / 9843ft
2500m / 8203ft
2000m / 6562ft
1500m / 4922ft
1000m / 3281ft
500m / 1640ft
250m / 820ft
100m / 328ft
sea level

PLATE MARGINS (for explanation see page xiv)

constructive
destructive
conservative
uncertain
physiographic regions
line of cross-section

SCALE 1:42,000,000
(projection: Lambert Azimuthal Equal Area)

Km 0 100 200 400 600 800 1000
Miles 0 50 100 200 300 400 500 600 700 800 900 1000

THE APPALACHIANS

THE APPALACHIAN MOUNTAINS, uplifted about 400 million years ago, are some of the oldest in the world. They have been lowered and rounded by erosion and now slope gently toward the Atlantic across a broad coastal plain.

Horizontal strata

Sedimentary strata folded and faulted into ridges and valleys

Softer strata has been crumpled against the harder basement rock

Hard basement rock

C

C

***Cross-section** through the Appalachians showing the numerous folds, which have subsequently been weathered to create a rounded relief.*

0 50 100 Km
0 50 100 Miles

THE GREAT PLAINS & CENTRAL LOWLANDS

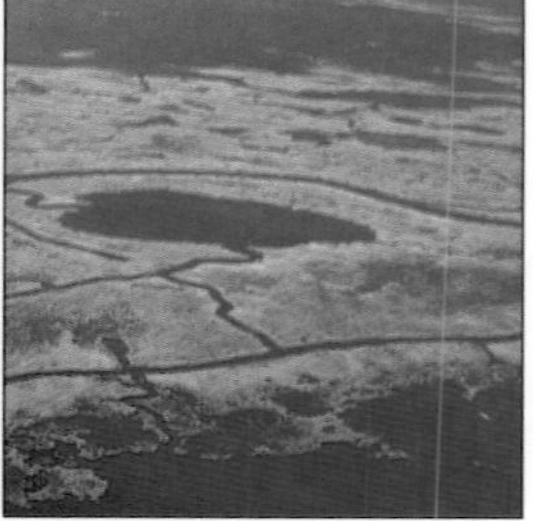

DEPOSITS LEFT by retreating glaciers and rivers have made this vast flat area very fertile. In the north this is the result of glaciation, with deposits up to one mile (1.7 km) thick, covering the basement rock. To the south and west, the massive Missouri/Mississippi river system has for centuries deposited silt across the plains, creating broad, flat floodplains and deltas.

Sedimentary layers overlay domed basement rock

Upland rivers drain south toward the Mississippi Basin

Confluence of the Missouri and Mississippi Rivers

D

D

***Section** across the Great Plains and Central Lowlands showing river systems and structure.*

0 200 400 Km
0 200 400 Miles

CLIMATE

"Tornado alley" *in the Mississippi Valley suffers frequent tornadoes.*

NORTH AMERICA'S climate includes extremes ranging from freezing Arctic conditions in Alaska and Greenland, to desert in the southwest, and tropical conditions in southeastern Florida, the Caribbean, and Central America. Central and southern regions are prone to severe storms including tornadoes and hurricanes.

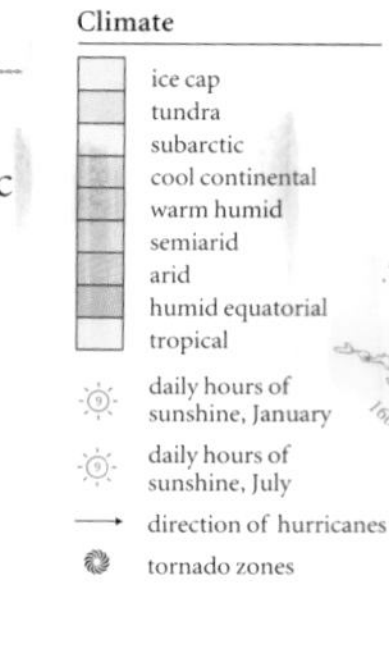
Climate
ice cap
tundra
subarctic
cool continental
warm humid
semiarid
arid
humid equatorial
tropical
daily hours of sunshine, January
daily hours of sunshine, July
direction of hurricanes
tornado zones

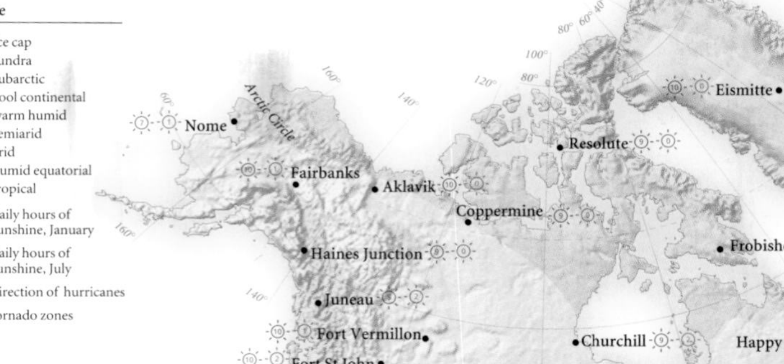
Nome
Eismitte
Arctic Circle
Resolute
Fairbanks
Aklavik
Coppermine
Frobisher Bay
Haines Junction
Juneau
Fort Vermillon
Churchill
Happy Valley - Goose Bay
Fort St John
Torbay

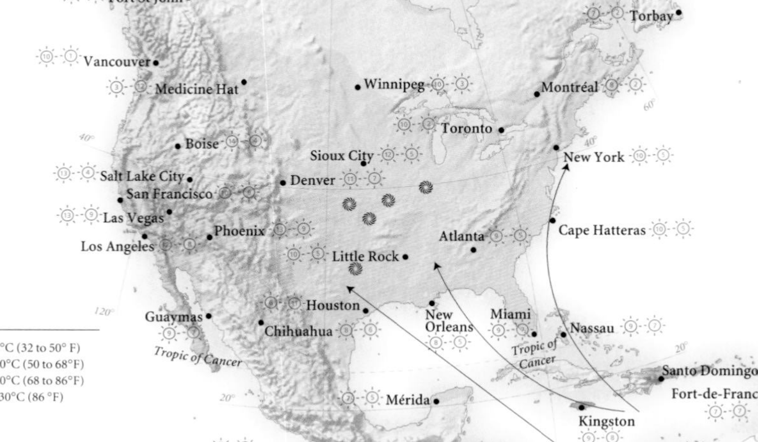
Vancouver
Medicine Hat
Winnipeg
Montréal
Toronto
Boise
Sioux City
New York
Salt Lake City
Denver
San Francisco
Las Vegas
Cape Hatteras
Phoenix
Atlanta
Los Angeles
Little Rock
Guaymas
Houston
New Orleans
Miami
Nassau
Chihuahua
Tropic of Cancer
Santo Domingo
Fort-de-France
Mérida
Kingston
Acapulco
San Salvador
San José

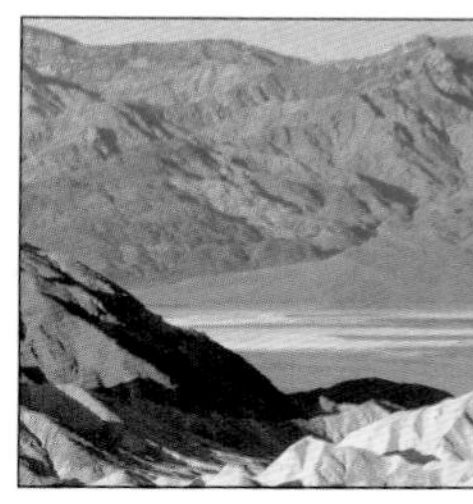

***Much of the southwest** is semi-desert; receiving less than 12 inches (300 mm) of rainfall a year.*

TEMPERATURE

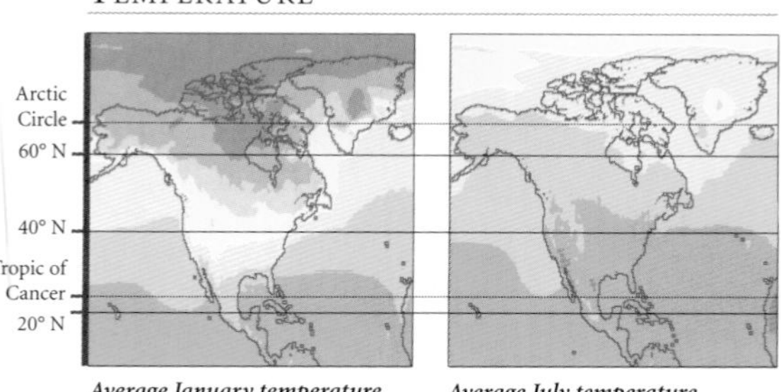
Arctic Circle
60° N
40° N
Tropic of Cancer
20° N

Average January temperature *Average July temperature*

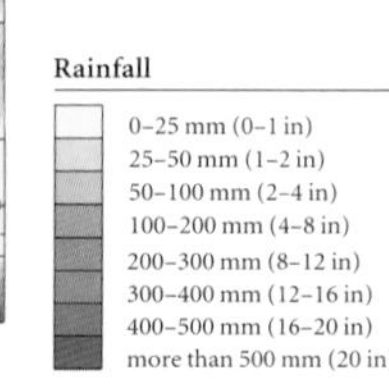
Temperature
below -30°C (-22°F)
-30 to -20°C (-22 to -4°F)
-20 to -10°C (-4 to 14°F)
-10 to 0°C (14 to 32°F)
0 to 10°C (32 to 50° F)
10 to 20°C (50 to 68°F)
20 to 30°C (68 to 86°F)
above 30°C (86 °F)

RAINFALL

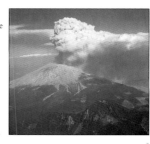

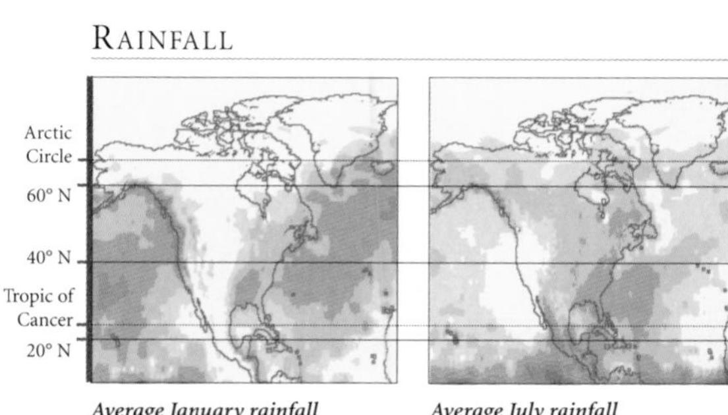
Arctic Circle
60° N
40° N
Tropic of Cancer
20° N

Average January rainfall *Average July rainfall*

Rainfall
0–25 mm (0–1 in)
25–50 mm (1–2 in)
50–100 mm (2–4 in)
100–200 mm (4–8 in)
200–300 mm (8–12 in)
300–400 mm (12–16 in)
400–500 mm (16–20 in)
more than 500 mm (20 in)

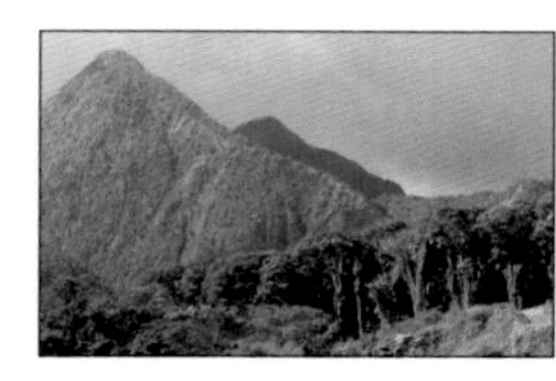

***The lush**, green mountains of the Lesser Antilles receive annual rainfalls of up to 360 inches (9,000 mm).*

SHAPING THE CONTINENT

GLACIAL PROCESSES affect much of northern Canada, Greenland and the Western Cordillera. Along the western coast of North America, Central America, and the Caribbean, underlying plates moving together lead to earthquakes and volcanic eruptions. The vast river systems, fed by mountain streams, constantly erode and deposit material along their paths.

VOLCANIC ACTIVITY

1 Mount St. Helens volcano *(right)* in the Cascade Range erupted violently in May 1980, killing 57 people and leveling large areas of forest. The lateral blast filled a valley with debris for 15 miles (25 km).

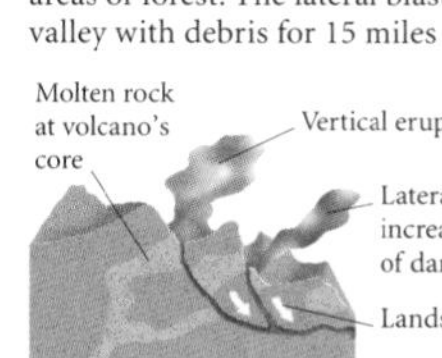
Molten rock at volcano's core
Vertical eruption
Lateral explosion increases extent of damage
Landslide fills valley

VOLCANIC ACTIVITY: ERUPTION OF MOUNT ST. HELENS

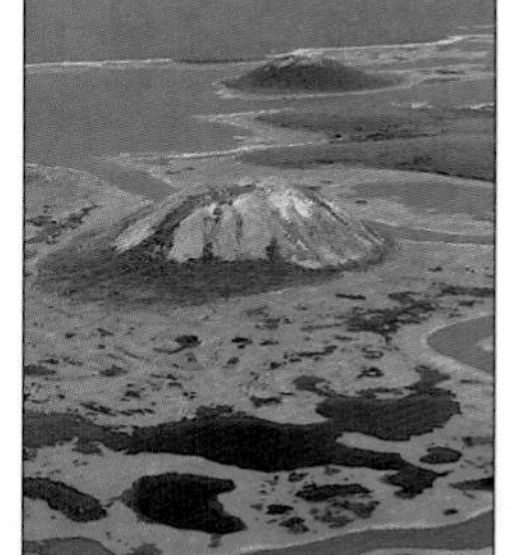

PERIGLACIATION

2 The ground in the far north is nearly always frozen: the surface thaws only in summer. This freeze-thaw process produces features such as pingos *(left)*; formed by the freezing of groundwater. With each successive winter ice accumulates producing a mound with a core of ice.

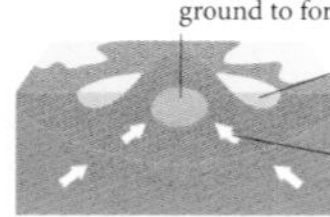
Ice core pushes up ground to form pingo
Unfrozen lake
Groundwater attracted to ice core

PERIGLACIATION: FORMATION OF A PINGO IN THE MACKENZIE DELTA

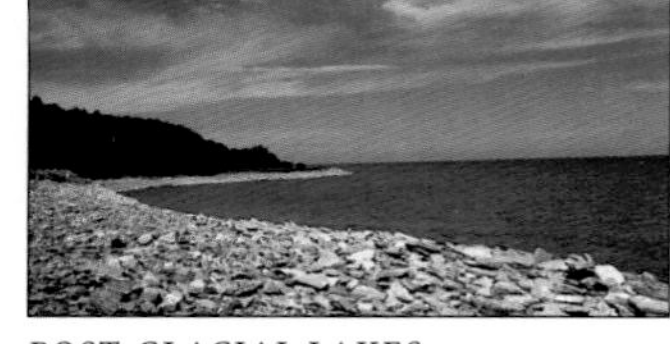

POST-GLACIAL LAKES

3 A chain of lakes from Great Bear Lake to the Great Lakes *(above)* was created as the ice retreated northward. Glaciers scoured hollows in the softer lowland rock. Glacial deposits at the lip of the hollows, and ridges of harder rock, trapped water to form lakes.

Retreating glacier
Ice-scoured hollow filled with glacial meltwater to form a lake
Harder rock creates a barrier between lakes
Softer lowland rock

POST-GLACIAL LAKES: FORMATION OF THE GREAT LAKES

THE EVOLVING LANDSCAPE

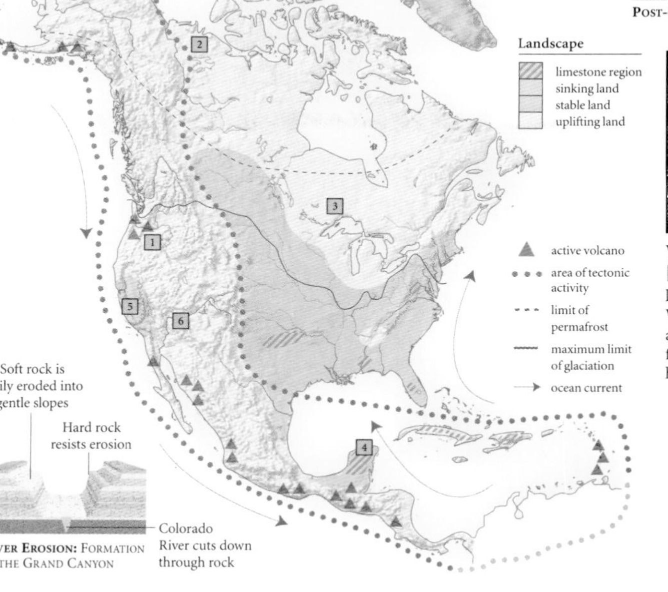
Landscape
limestone region
sinking land
stable land
uplifting land
active volcano
area of tectonic activity
limit of permafrost
maximum limit of glaciation
ocean current
Soft rock is easily eroded into gentle slopes
Hard rock resists erosion
Colorado River cuts down through rock

RIVER EROSION: FORMATION OF THE GRAND CANYON

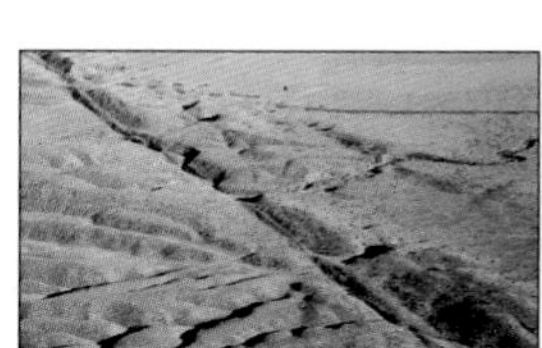

SEISMIC ACTIVITY

5 The San Andreas Fault *(above)* places much of the North America's west coast under constant threat from earthquakes. It is caused by the Pacific Plate grinding past the North American Plate at a faster rate, though in the same direction.

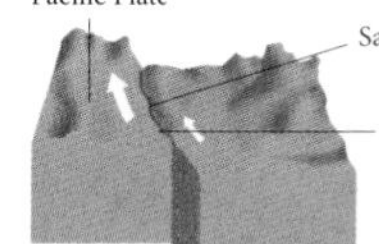
Pacific Plate
San Andreas Fault
Fault is caused by faster movement of Pacific Plate
North American Plate

SEISMIC ACTIVITY: ACTION OF THE SAN ANDREAS FAULT

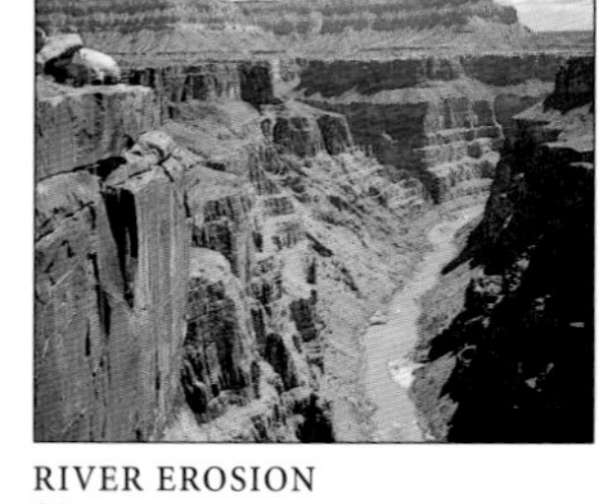

RIVER EROSION

6 The Grand Canyon *(above)* in the Colorado Plateau was created by the downward erosion of the Colorado River, combined with the gradual uplift of the plateau, over the past 30 million years. The contours of the canyon formed as the softer rock layers eroded into gentle slopes, and the hard rock layers into cliffs. The depth varies from 3,855–6,560 ft (1,175–2,000 m).

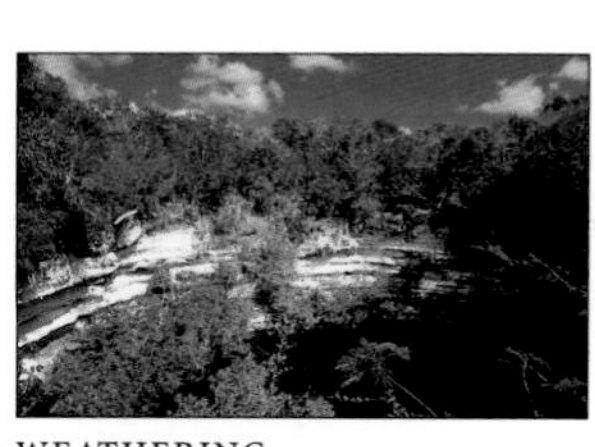

WEATHERING

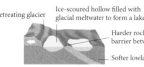

4 The Yucatan Peninsula is a vast, flat limestone plateau in southern Mexico. Weathering action from both rainwater and underground streams has enlarged fractures in the rock to form caves and hollows, called sinkholes *(above)*.

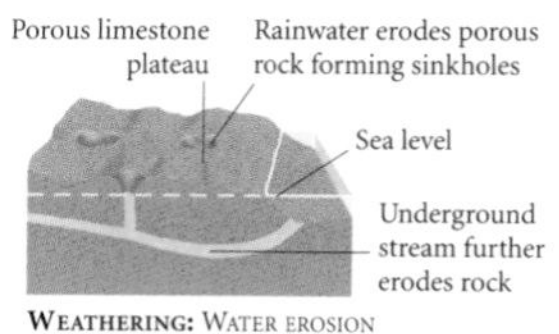
Porous limestone plateau
Rainwater erodes porous rock forming sinkholes
Sea level
Underground stream further erodes rock

WEATHERING: WATER EROSION ON THE YUCATAN PENINSULA

Political North America

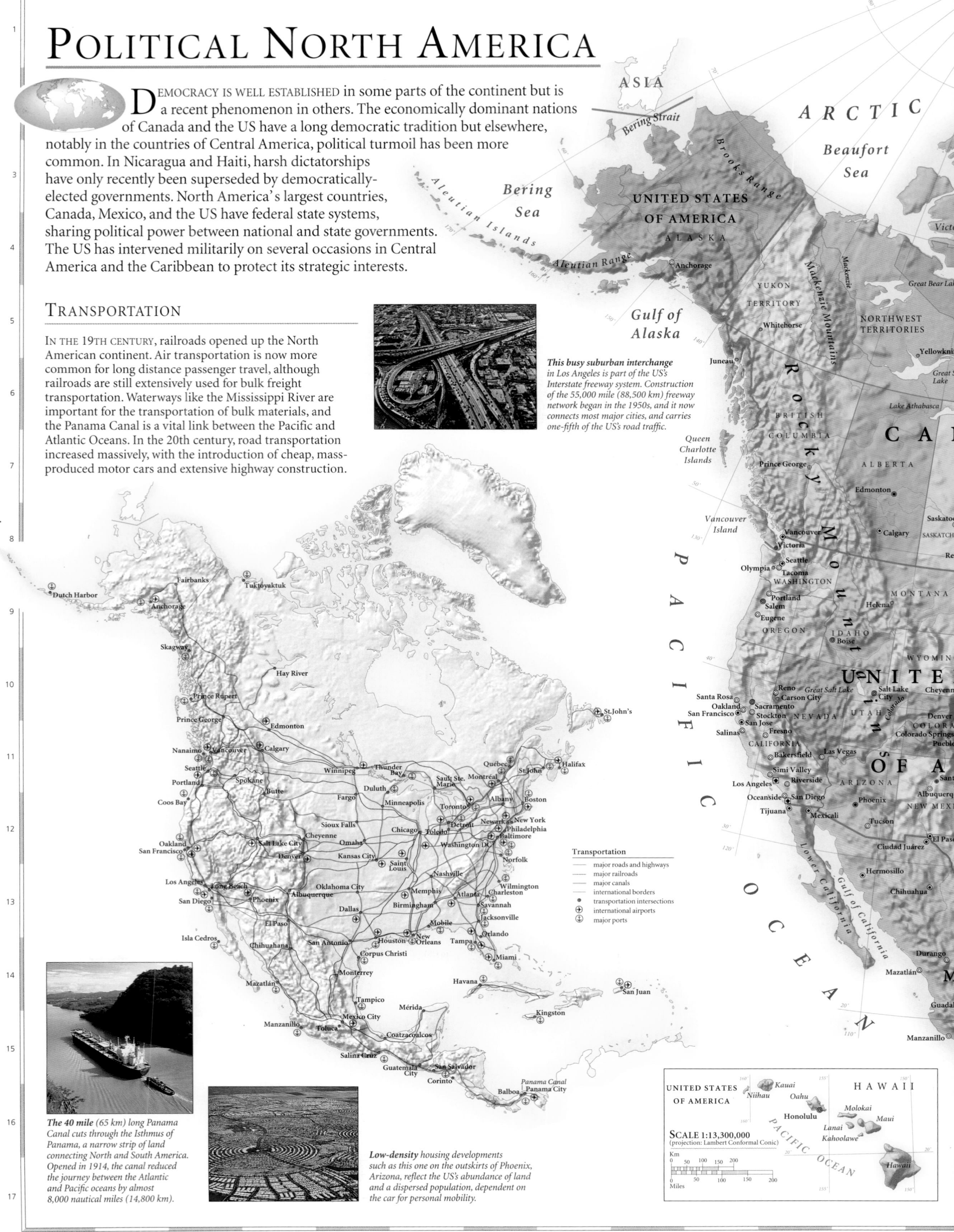

ASIA
Bering Strait
ARCTIC
Beaufort Sea
Brooks Range
Bering Sea
Aleutian Islands
UNITED STATES OF AMERICA
ALASKA
Aleutian Range
Anchorage
YUKON TERRITORY
Mackenzie Mountains
Mackenzie
Great Bear Lake
Gulf of Alaska
Whitehorse
NORTHWEST TERRITORIES
Yellowknife
Juneau
Rocky Mountains
BRITISH COLUMBIA
Lake Athabasca
Queen Charlotte Islands
Prince George
ALBERTA
Edmonton
Vancouver Island
Vancouver
Victoria
Calgary
Saskatoon
Olympia
Seattle
Tacoma
WASHINGTON
PACIFIC OCEAN
Portland
Salem
Eugene
OREGON
Helena
MONTANA
IDAHO
Boise
WYOMING
Reno
Carson City
Great Salt Lake
Salt Lake City
Cheyenne
Santa Rosa
Oakland
San Francisco
Sacramento
Stockton
San Jose
NEVADA
UTAH
Colorado
Denver
COLORADO
Colorado Springs
Pueblo
Salinas
Fresno
CALIFORNIA
Bakersfield
Las Vegas
Simi Valley
Los Angeles
Riverside
ARIZONA
Oceanside
San Diego
Tijuana
Mexicali
Phoenix
Albuquerque
NEW MEXICO
Tucson
El Paso
Ciudad Juárez
Lower California
Gulf of California
Hermosillo
Chihuahua
Durango
Mazatlán
Manzanillo
Dutch Harbor
Fairbanks
Tuktoyaktuk
Skagway
Hay River
Prince Rupert
Edmonton
St.John's
Nanaimo
Calgary
Spokane
Butte
Coos Bay
Winnipeg
Thunder Bay
Duluth
Sault Ste. Marie
Montreal
Québec
St.John
Halifax
Fargo
Minneapolis
Toronto
Albany
Boston
Sioux Falls
Detroit
Newark
New York
Philadelphia
Baltimore
Chicago
Toledo
Washington DC
Omaha
Kansas City
Saint Louis
Norfolk
Nashville
Oklahoma City
Memphis
Atlanta
Wilmington
Charleston
Long Beach
Birmingham
Savannah
Dallas
Jacksonville
Mobile
Orlando
Isla Cedros
Houston
New Orleans
Tampa
San Antonio
Corpus Christi
Miami
Monterrey
Havana
San Juan
Tampico
Mérida
Mexico City
Kingston
Toluca
Coatzacoalcos
Salina Cruz
Guatemala City
San Salvador
Corinto
Panama Canal
Panama City
Balboa
Transportation
major roads and highways
major railroads
major canals
international borders
transportation intersections
international airports
major ports
UNITED STATES OF AMERICA
HAWAII
Niihau
Kauai
Oahu
Honolulu
Molokai
Maui
Lanai
Kahoolawe
Hawaii
PACIFIC OCEAN
SCALE 1:13,300,000
(projection: Lambert Conformal Conic)
Km
Miles

Democracy is well established in some parts of the continent but is a recent phenomenon in others. The economically dominant nations of Canada and the US have a long democratic tradition but elsewhere, notably in the countries of Central America, political turmoil has been more common. In Nicaragua and Haiti, harsh dictatorships have only recently been superseded by democratically-elected governments. North America's largest countries, Canada, Mexico, and the US have federal state systems, sharing political power between national and state governments. The US has intervened militarily on several occasions in Central America and the Caribbean to protect its strategic interests.

Transportation

In the 19th century, railroads opened up the North American continent. Air transportation is now more common for long distance passenger travel, although railroads are still extensively used for bulk freight transportation. Waterways like the Mississippi River are important for the transportation of bulk materials, and the Panama Canal is a vital link between the Pacific and Atlantic Oceans. In the 20th century, road transportation increased massively, with the introduction of cheap, mass-produced motor cars and extensive highway construction.

This busy suburban interchange *in Los Angeles is part of the US's Interstate freeway system. Construction of the 55,000 mile (88,500 km) freeway network began in the 1950s, and it now connects most major cities, and carries one-fifth of the US's road traffic.*

The 40 mile *(65 km) long Panama Canal cuts through the Isthmus of Panama, a narrow strip of land connecting North and South America. Opened in 1914, the canal reduced the journey between the Atlantic and Pacific oceans by almost 8,000 nautical miles (14,800 km).*

Low-density *housing developments such as this one on the outskirts of Phoenix, Arizona, reflect the US's abundance of land and a dispersed population, dependent on the car for personal mobility.*

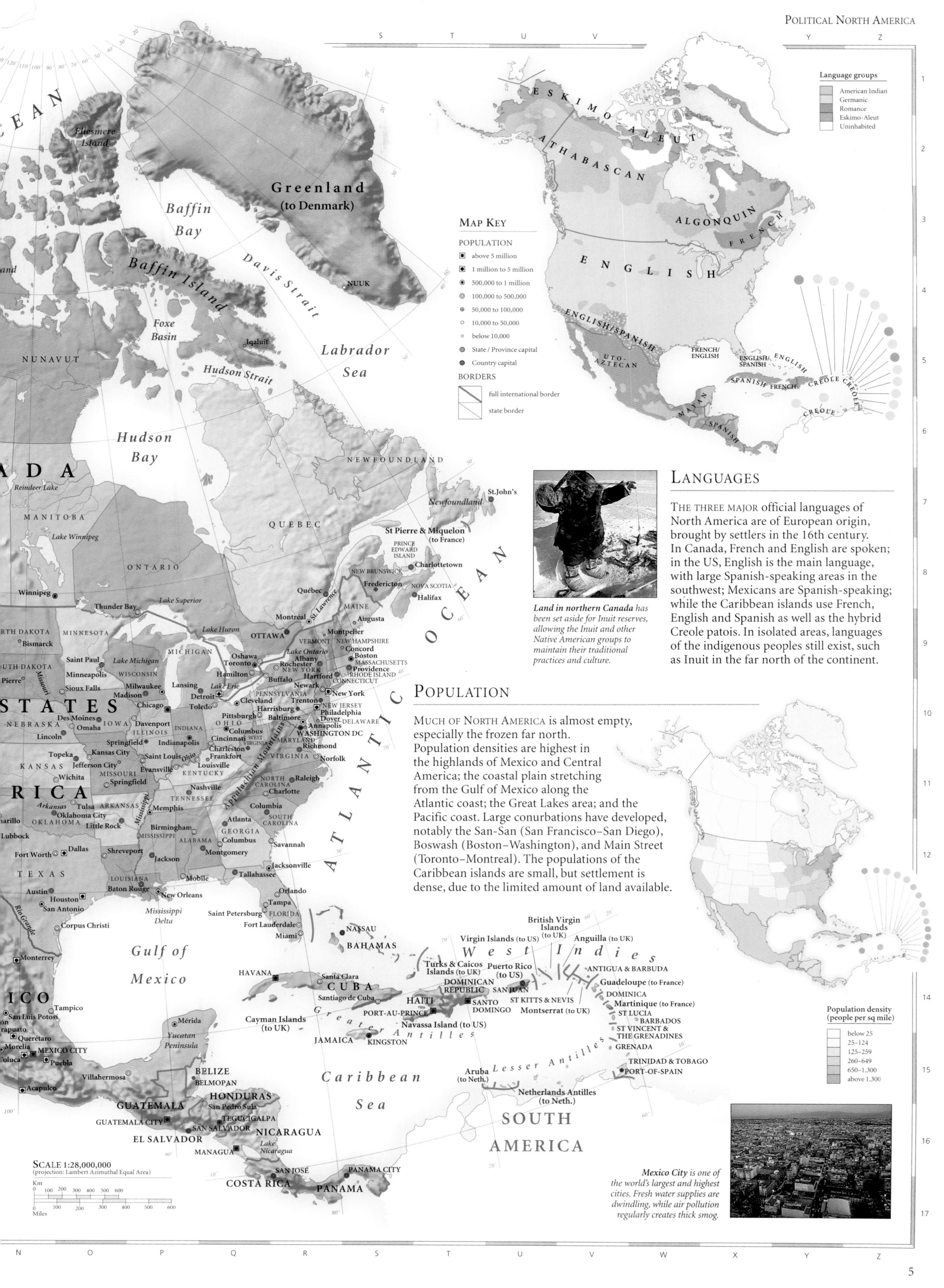
S T U V Y Z
1 2 3 4 5 6 7 8 9 10 11 12 14 15 16 17
N O P Q R S T U V W X Y Z
Language groups
American Indian
Germanic
Romance
Eskimo-Aleut
Uninhabited
ESKIMO-ALEUT
ATHABASCAN
ALGONQUIN
FRENCH
ENGLISH
ENGLISH/SPANISH
UTO-AZTECAN
FRENCH/ ENGLISH
ENGLISH/ SPANISH
ENGLISH
SPANISH
FRENCH
CREOLE
CREOLE
CREOLE
MAYAN
SPANISH
MAP KEY
POPULATION
above 5 million
1 million to 5 million
500,000 to 1 million
100,000 to 500,000
50,000 to 100,000
10,000 to 50,000
below 10,000
State / Province capital
Country capital
BORDERS
full international border
state border
Ellesmere Island
Greenland (to Denmark)
Baffin Bay
Baffin Island
Davis Strait
NUUK
Foxe Basin
Iqaluit
NUNAVUT
Labrador Sea
Hudson Strait
Hudson Bay
NEWFOUNDLAND
Newfoundland
St.John's
QUEBEC
MANITOBA
Reindeer Lake
Lake Winnipeg
ONTARIO
Winnipeg
Thunder Bay
Lake Superior
St Pierre & Miquelon (to France)
PRINCE EDWARD ISLAND
Charlottetown
NEW BRUNSWICK
Fredericton
NOVA SCOTIA
Halifax
Québec
Montréal
OTTAWA
MAINE
Augusta
Montpelier
VERMONT
NEW HAMPSHIRE
Concord
Boston
MASSACHUSETTS
Providence
RHODE ISLAND
Hartford
CONNECTICUT
NEW YORK
Albany
Lake Ontario
Rochester
Buffalo
Toronto
Oshawa
Hamilton
Lake Huron
MICHIGAN
Lake Michigan
Lake Erie
Lansing
Detroit
Toledo
Cleveland
PENNSYLVANIA
Harrisburg
Pittsburgh
Newark
Trenton
New York
NEW JERSEY
Philadelphia
Baltimore
Dover
DELAWARE
Annapolis
WASHINGTON DC
MARYLAND
Richmond
Norfolk
VIRGINIA
WEST VIRGINIA
Charleston
OHIO
Columbus
Cincinnati
INDIANA
Indianapolis
ILLINOIS
Springfield
Chicago
Milwaukee
Madison
WISCONSIN
MINNESOTA
Saint Paul
Minneapolis
NORTH DAKOTA
Bismarck
SOUTH DAKOTA
Pierre
Sioux Falls
Missouri
STATES
NEBRASKA
Lincoln
Omaha
Des Moines
IOWA
Davenport
KANSAS
Topeka
Kansas City
Jefferson City
Saint Louis
Ohio
Frankfort
Louisville
KENTUCKY
Evansville
Wichita
MISSOURI
Springfield
RICA
Arkansas
Tulsa
Oklahoma City
OKLAHOMA
ARKANSAS
Little Rock
Memphis
Mississippi
TENNESSEE
Nashville
Appalachian Mountains
NORTH CAROLINA
Raleigh
Charlotte
Columbia
SOUTH CAROLINA
Atlanta
GEORGIA
Birmingham
MISSISSIPPI
ALABAMA
Columbus
Savannah
Montgomery
Jackson
Shreveport
Dallas
Fort Worth
Lubbock
TEXAS
LOUISIANA
Baton Rouge
New Orleans
Mobile
Tallahassee
Jacksonville
Austin
Houston
San Antonio
Rio Grande
Corpus Christi
Mississippi Delta
Orlando
Tampa
Saint Petersburg
FLORIDA
Fort Lauderdale
Miami
ATLANTIC OCEAN
Gulf of Mexico
Monterrey
Tampico
San Luis Potosí
Querétaro
Morelia
MEXICO CITY
Puebla
Acapulco
Mérida
Yucatan Peninsula
Villahermosa
NASSAU
BAHAMAS
HAVANA
Santa Clara
CUBA
Santiago de Cuba
Cayman Islands (to UK)
JAMAICA
KINGSTON
Greater Antilles
PORT-AU-PRINCE
HAITI
Navassa Island (to US)
Turks & Caicos Islands (to UK)
DOMINICAN REPUBLIC
SANTO DOMINGO
Puerto Rico (to US)
SAN JUAN
Virgin Islands (to US)
British Virgin Islands (to UK)
Anguilla (to UK)
West Indies
ANTIGUA & BARBUDA
ST KITTS & NEVIS
Montserrat (to UK)
Guadeloupe (to France)
DOMINICA
Martinique (to France)
ST LUCIA
BARBADOS
ST VINCENT & THE GRENADINES
GRENADA
TRINIDAD & TOBAGO
PORT-OF-SPAIN
Lesser Antilles
Aruba (to Neth.)
Netherlands Antilles (to Neth.)
Caribbean Sea
BELIZE
BELMOPAN
HONDURAS
San Pedro Sula
TEGUCIGALPA
GUATEMALA
GUATEMALA CITY
SAN SALVADOR
EL SALVADOR
NICARAGUA
Lake Nicaragua
MANAGUA
SAN JOSÉ
COSTA RICA
PANAMA CITY
PANAMA
SOUTH AMERICA
SCALE 1:28,000,000
(projection: Lambert Azimuthal Equal Area)
Km
0 100 200 300 400 500 600
0 100 200 300 400 500 600
Miles
Population density (people per sq mile)
below 25
25–124
125–259
260–649
650–1,300
above 1,300

LANGUAGES

THE THREE MAJOR official languages of North America are of European origin, brought by settlers in the 16th century. In Canada, French and English are spoken; in the US, English is the main language, with large Spanish-speaking areas in the southwest; Mexicans are Spanish-speaking; while the Caribbean islands use French, English and Spanish as well as the hybrid Creole patois. In isolated areas, languages of the indigenous peoples still exist, such as Inuit in the far north of the continent.

***Land in northern Canada** has been set aside for Inuit reserves, allowing the Inuit and other Native American groups to maintain their traditional practices and culture.*

POPULATION

MUCH OF NORTH AMERICA is almost empty, especially the frozen far north. Population densities are highest in the highlands of Mexico and Central America; the coastal plain stretching from the Gulf of Mexico along the Atlantic coast; the Great Lakes area; and the Pacific coast. Large conurbations have developed, notably the San-San (San Francisco–San Diego), Boswash (Boston–Washington), and Main Street (Toronto–Montreal). The populations of the Caribbean islands are small, but settlement is dense, due to the limited amount of land available.

***Mexico City** is one of the world's largest and highest cities. Fresh water supplies are dwindling, while air pollution regularly creates thick smog.*

North American Resources

The two northern countries of Canada and the US are richly endowed with natural resources that have helped to fuel economic development. The US is the world's largest economy, although today it is facing stiff competition from the Far East. Mexico has relied on oil revenues but there are hopes that the North American Free Trade Agreement (NAFTA), will encourage trade growth with Canada and the US. The poorer countries of Central America and the Caribbean depend largely on cash crops and tourism.

Standard of Living

The US and Canada have one of the highest overall standards of living in the world. However, many people still live in poverty, especially in urban ghettos and some rural areas. Central America and the Caribbean are markedly poorer than their wealthier northern neighbors. Haiti is the poorest country in the western hemisphere.

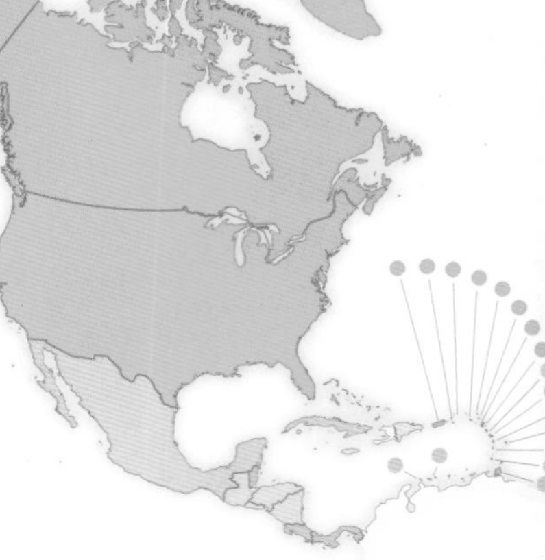

Standard of Living (UN Human Development Index)
high
low

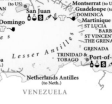

Industry

The modern, industrialized economies of the US and Canada contrast sharply with those of Mexico, Central America, and the Caribbean. Manufacturing is especially important in the US; vehicle production is concentrated around the Great Lakes, while electronic and hi-tech industries are increasingly found in the western and southern states. Mexico depends on oil exports and assembly work, taking advantage of cheap labor. Many Central American and Caribbean countries rely heavily on agricultural exports.

After its purchase *from Russia in 1867, Alaska's frozen lands were largely ignored by the US. Oil reserves similar in magnitude to those in eastern Texas were discovered in Prudhoe Bay, Alaska in 1968. Freezing temperatures and a fragile environment hamper oil extraction.*

Fish such as cod, *flounder, and plaice are caught in the Grand Banks, off the Newfoundland coast, and processed in many North Atlantic coastal settlements.*

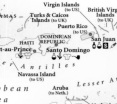

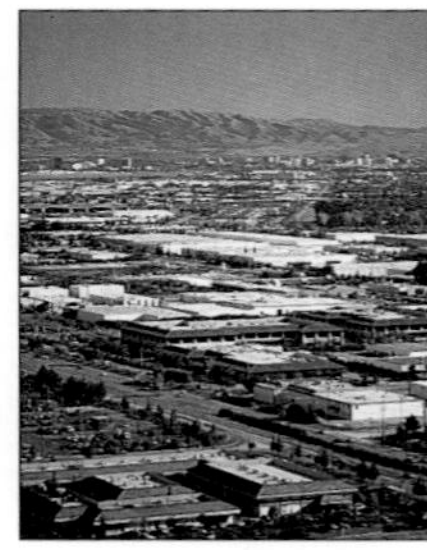

South of San Francisco, *"Silicon Valley" is both a national and international center for hi-tech industries, electronic industries, and research institutions.*

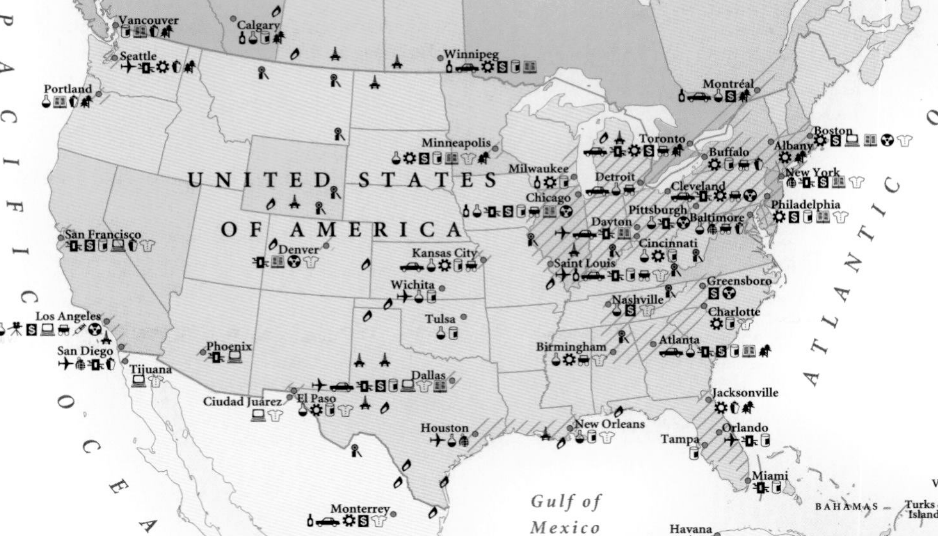
ARCTIC OCEAN
PACIFIC OCEAN
ATLANTIC OCEAN
Greenland (to Denmark)
CANADA
UNITED STATES OF AMERICA
USA
MEXICO
Bering Sea
Beaufort Sea
Baffin Bay
Labrador Sea
Hudson Bay
Gulf of Alaska
Gulf of Mexico
Caribbean Sea
Prudhoe Bay
Vancouver
Calgary
Seattle
Winnipeg
Portland
Montréal
Toronto
Minneapolis
Boston
Buffalo
Albany
Milwaukee
Detroit
New York
Chicago
Cleveland
Pittsburgh
Baltimore
Philadelphia
Dayton
Cincinnati
Denver
Kansas City
Saint Louis
San Francisco
Wichita
Greensboro
Nashville
Charlotte
Los Angeles
Tulsa
San Diego
Phoenix
Birmingham
Atlanta
Tijuana
Dallas
Ciudad Juárez
El Paso
Jacksonville
Houston
New Orleans
Orlando
Tampa
Miami
Monterrey
Guadalajara
Mexico City
West Indies
BAHAMAS
CUBA
Havana
HAITI
Port-au-Prince
DOMINICAN REPUBLIC
Santo Domingo
JAMAICA
Cayman Islands (to UK)
Greater Antilles
Lesser Antilles
Turks & Caicos Islands (to UK)
Virgin Islands (to US)
British Virgin Islands (to UK)
Puerto Rico (to US)
San Juan
Anguilla (to UK)
ST KITTS & NEVIS
ANTIGUA & BARBUDA
Montserrat (to UK)
Guadeloupe (to France)
DOMINICA
Martinique (to France)
ST LUCIA
BARBADOS
ST VINCENT & THE GRENADINES
GRENADA
TRINIDAD & TOBAGO
Port-of-Spain
Navassa Island (to US)
Aruba (to Neth.)
Netherlands Antilles (to Neth.)
VENEZUELA
COLOMBIA
BELIZE
GUATEMALA
Guatemala City
HONDURAS
Tegucigalpa
EL SALVADOR
San Salvador
NICARAGUA
Managua
COSTA RICA
San José
PANAMA
Panama City
RUSS. FED.
Bering Strait
Hudson Strait

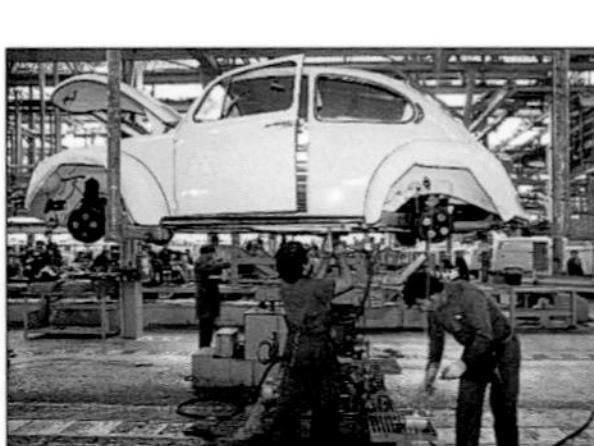

Multinational companies *rely on cheap labor and tax benefits to assemble vehicles in Mexican factories.*

The World Trade Center, *destroyed by terrorists in September 2001, was a potent symbol of New York's leading role in world trade and finance.*

Industry

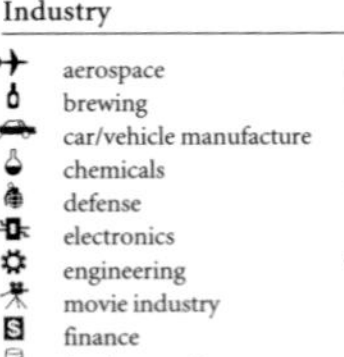
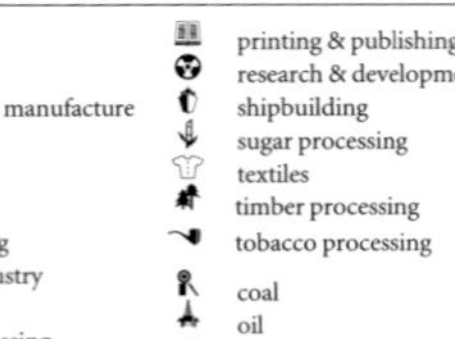
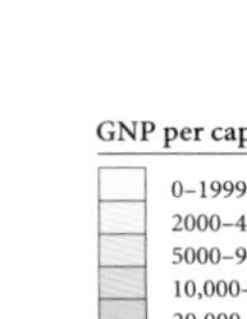
aerospace
brewing
car/vehicle manufacture
chemicals
defense
electronics
engineering
movie industry
finance
food processing
hi-tech industry
iron & steel
pharmaceuticals
printing & publishing
research & development
shipbuilding
sugar processing
textiles
timber processing
tobacco processing
coal
oil
gas
industrial cities
major industrial areas

GNP per capita (US$)
0–1999
2000–4999
5000–9999
10,000–19,999
20,000–24,999
25,000+

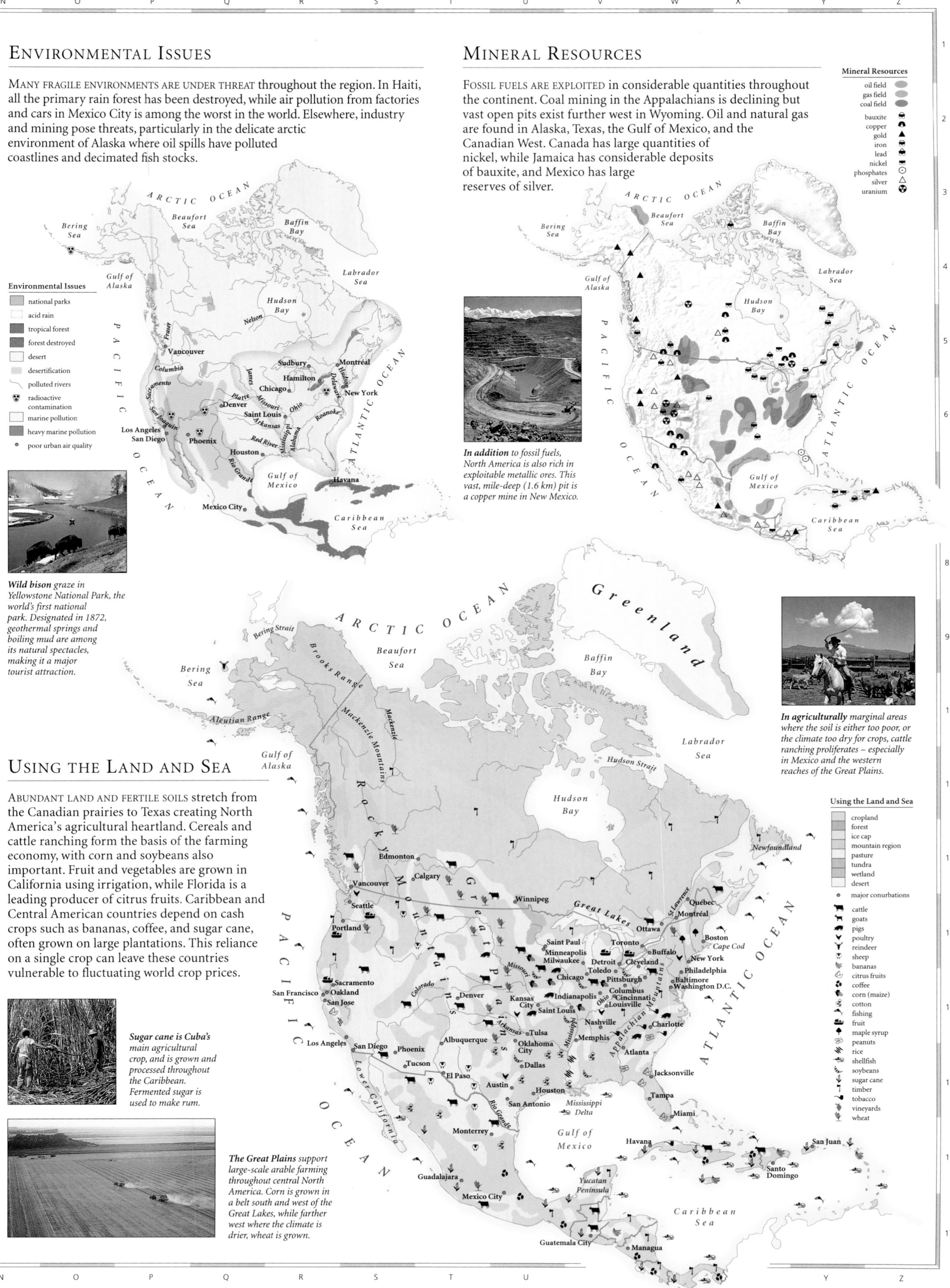
Environmental Issues
national parks
acid rain
tropical forest
forest destroyed
desert
desertification
polluted rivers
radioactive contamination
marine pollution
heavy marine pollution
poor urban air quality
Mineral Resources
oil field
gas field
coal field
bauxite
copper
gold
iron
lead
nickel
phosphates
silver
uranium
Using the Land and Sea
cropland
forest
ice cap
mountain region
pasture
tundra
wetland
desert
major conurbations
cattle
goats
pigs
poultry
reindeer
sheep
bananas
citrus fruits
coffee
corn (maize)
cotton
fishing
fruit
maple syrup
peanuts
rice
shellfish
soybeans
sugar cane
timber
tobacco
vineyards
wheat

Environmental Issues

Many fragile environments are under threat throughout the region. In Haiti, all the primary rain forest has been destroyed, while air pollution from factories and cars in Mexico City is among the worst in the world. Elsewhere, industry and mining pose threats, particularly in the delicate arctic environment of Alaska where oil spills have polluted coastlines and decimated fish stocks.

***Wild bison** graze in Yellowstone National Park, the world's first national park. Designated in 1872, geothermal springs and boiling mud are among its natural spectacles, making it a major tourist attraction.*

Mineral Resources

Fossil fuels are exploited in considerable quantities throughout the continent. Coal mining in the Appalachians is declining but vast open pits exist further west in Wyoming. Oil and natural gas are found in Alaska, Texas, the Gulf of Mexico, and the Canadian West. Canada has large quantities of nickel, while Jamaica has considerable deposits of bauxite, and Mexico has large reserves of silver.

***In addition** to fossil fuels, North America is also rich in exploitable metallic ores. This vast, mile-deep (1.6 km) pit is a copper mine in New Mexico.*

Using the Land and Sea

Abundant land and fertile soils stretch from the Canadian prairies to Texas creating North America's agricultural heartland. Cereals and cattle ranching form the basis of the farming economy, with corn and soybeans also important. Fruit and vegetables are grown in California using irrigation, while Florida is a leading producer of citrus fruits. Caribbean and Central American countries depend on cash crops such as bananas, coffee, and sugar cane, often grown on large plantations. This reliance on a single crop can leave these countries vulnerable to fluctuating world crop prices.

***In agriculturally** marginal areas where the soil is either too poor, or the climate too dry for crops, cattle ranching proliferates – especially in Mexico and the western reaches of the Great Plains.*

***Sugar cane is Cuba's** main agricultural crop, and is grown and processed throughout the Caribbean. Fermented sugar is used to make rum.*

***The Great Plains** support large-scale arable farming throughout central North America. Corn is grown in a belt south and west of the Great Lakes, while farther west where the climate is drier, wheat is grown.*

CANADA

CANADA IS THE THIRD LARGEST COUNTRY in the world, and with only about one-tenth of its land area inhabited, it is one of the most sparsely populated. Canada became a confederation in 1867, though Newfoundland did not join until 1949. As a founding member of the UN and of the Commonwealth, Canada has played an important role in international affairs. A constitutional crisis, focusing on the French-speaking Québécois, and Inuit and Native American land rights, dominated politics in the 1990s. In 1999, part of the Northwest Territories, Nunavut, became a self-governing homeland for the Inuit.

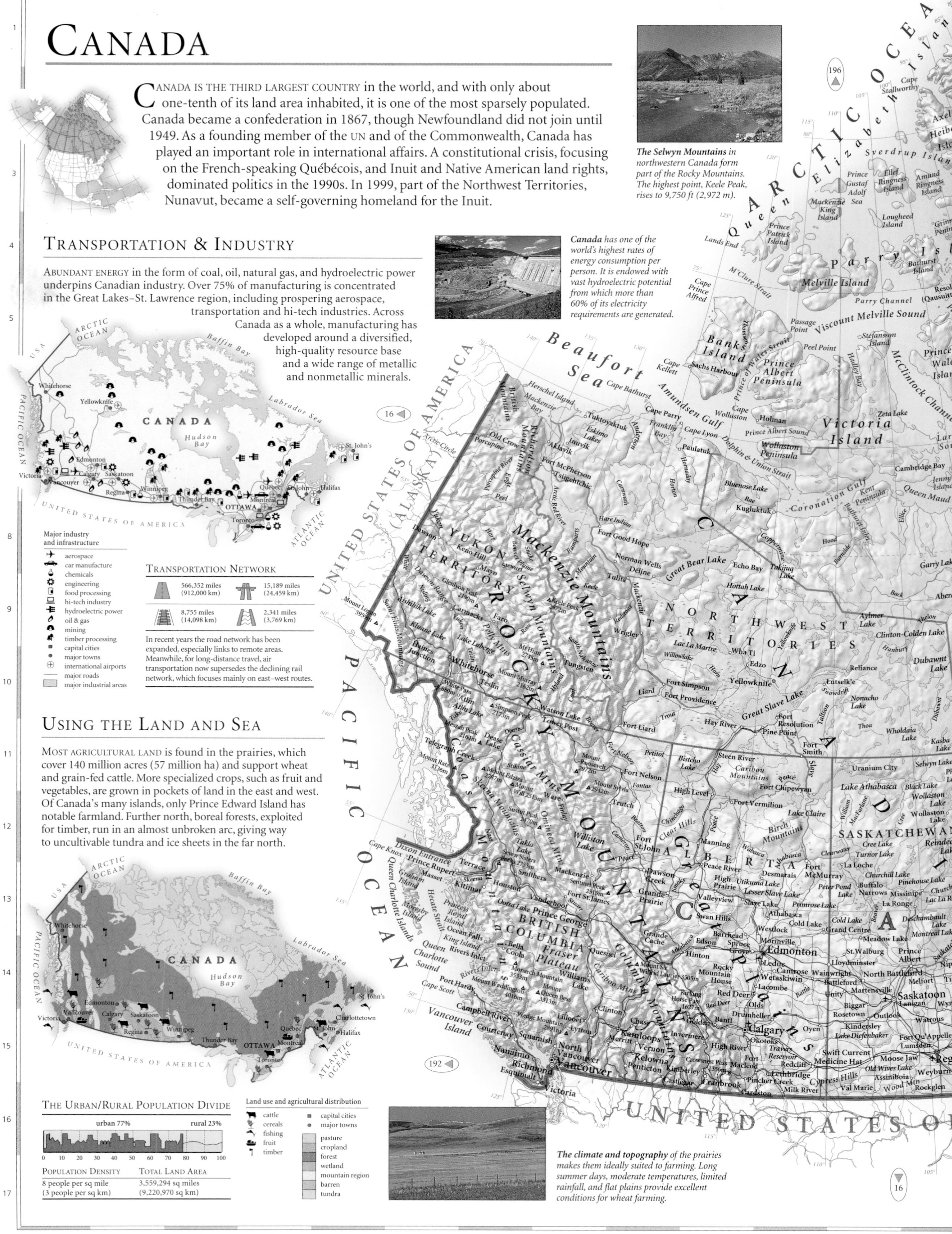

ARCTIC OCEAN
Queen Elizabeth Islands
Beaufort Sea
UNITED STATES OF AMERICA (ALASKA)
PACIFIC OCEAN
YUKON TERRITORY
NORTHWEST TERRITORIES
ROCKY MOUNTAINS
Mackenzie Mountains
BRITISH COLUMBIA
ALBERTA
SASKATCHEWAN
Victoria Island
Banks Island
Melville Island
Great Bear Lake
Great Slave Lake
Lake Athabasca
Whitehorse
Yellowknife
Edmonton
Calgary
Vancouver
Victoria
Saskatoon
UNITED STATES OF
196
16
192

The Selwyn Mountains in northwestern Canada form part of the Rocky Mountains. The highest point, Keele Peak, rises to 9,750 ft (2,972 m).

TRANSPORTATION & INDUSTRY

ABUNDANT ENERGY in the form of coal, oil, natural gas, and hydroelectric power underpins Canadian industry. Over 75% of manufacturing is concentrated in the Great Lakes–St. Lawrence region, including prospering aerospace, transportation and hi-tech industries. Across Canada as a whole, manufacturing has developed around a diversified, high-quality resource base and a wide range of metallic and nonmetallic minerals.

Canada has one of the world's highest rates of energy consumption per person. It is endowed with vast hydroelectric potential from which more than 60% of its electricity requirements are generated.

Major industry and infrastructure

- aerospace
- car manufacture
- chemicals
- engineering
- food processing
- hi-tech industry
- hydroelectric power
- oil & gas
- mining
- timber processing
- capital cities
- major towns
- international airports
- major roads
- major industrial areas

TRANSPORTATION NETWORK

566,352 miles (912,000 km)	15,189 miles (24,459 km)
8,755 miles (14,098 km)	2,341 miles (3,769 km)

In recent years the road network has been expanded, especially links to remote areas. Meanwhile, for long-distance travel, air transportation now supersedes the declining rail network, which focuses mainly on east–west routes.

USING THE LAND AND SEA

MOST AGRICULTURAL LAND is found in the prairies, which cover 140 million acres (57 million ha) and support wheat and grain-fed cattle. More specialized crops, such as fruit and vegetables, are grown in pockets of land in the east and west. Of Canada's many islands, only Prince Edward Island has notable farmland. Further north, boreal forests, exploited for timber, run in an almost unbroken arc, giving way to uncultivable tundra and ice sheets in the far north.

Land use and agricultural distribution

- cattle
- cereals
- fishing
- fruit
- timber
- capital cities
- major towns
- pasture
- cropland
- forest
- wetland
- mountain region
- barren
- tundra

THE URBAN/RURAL POPULATION DIVIDE

urban 77% — rural 23%

0 10 20 30 40 50 60 70 80 90 100

POPULATION DENSITY	TOTAL LAND AREA
8 people per sq mile (3 people per sq km)	3,559,294 sq miles (9,220,970 sq km)

The climate and topography of the prairies makes them ideally suited to farming. Long summer days, moderate temperatures, limited rainfall, and flat plains provide excellent conditions for wheat farming.

The Landscape

Glaciers on islands in the Arctic Ocean are the last remnants of the ice sheet that once covered and shaped Canada. Hudson Bay is the center of the Canadian Shield, a huge, eroded plateau marked at its southern extremity by a string of lakes running southeastward from Great Bear Lake to the Great Lakes. In contrast to the rolling relief of the Shield and the central lowland region, the Rocky Mountains rise to peaks of over 13,000 ft (4,000 m), stretching 500 miles (800 km) along the west coast.

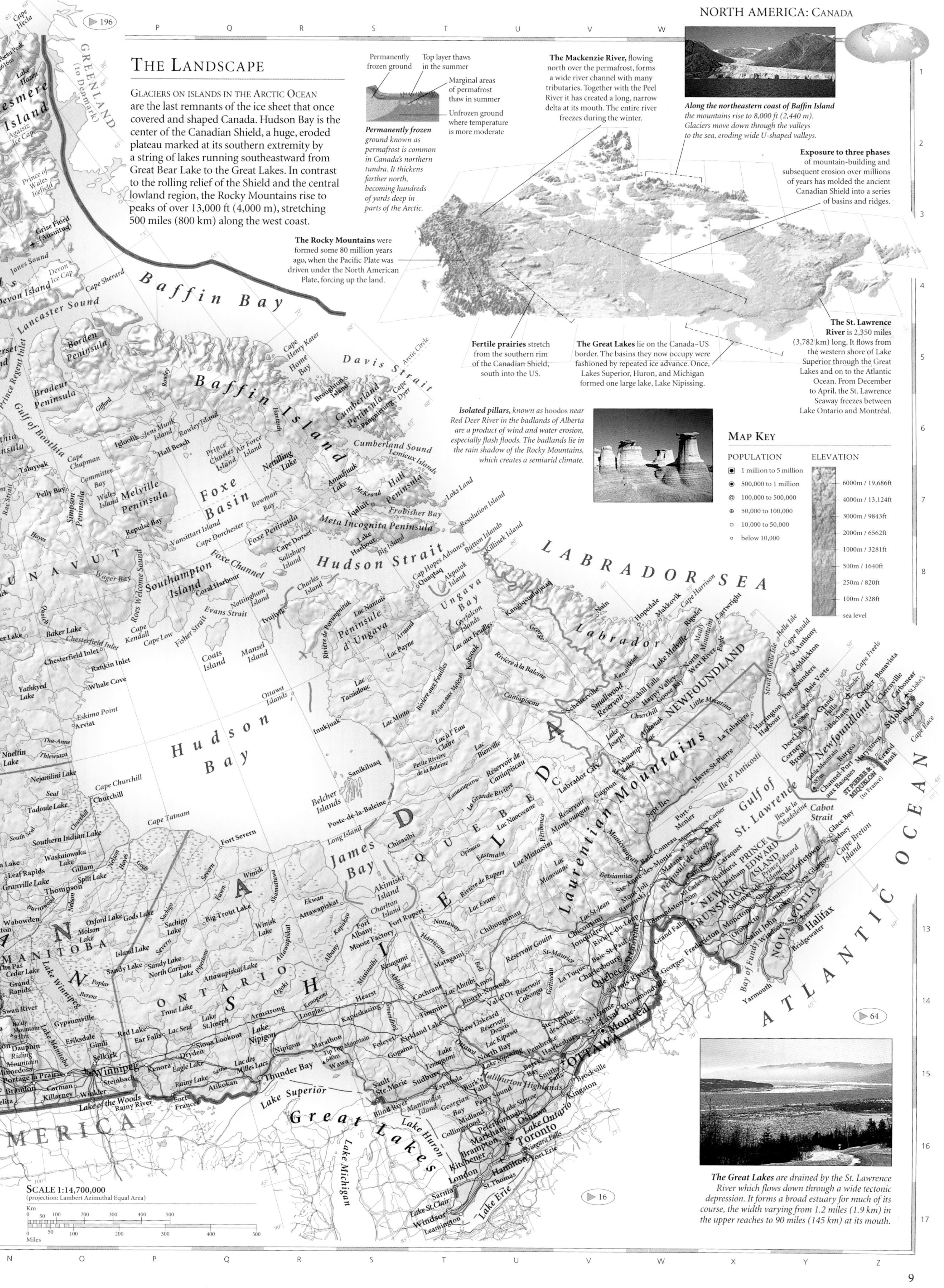

Permanently frozen ground
Top layer thaws in the summer
Marginal areas of permafrost thaw in summer
Unfrozen ground where temperature is more moderate
Permanently frozen *ground known as permafrost is common in Canada's northern tundra. It thickens farther north, becoming hundreds of yards deep in parts of the Arctic.*
The Mackenzie River, flowing north over the permafrost, forms a wide river channel with many tributaries. Together with the Peel River it has created a long, narrow delta at its mouth. The entire river freezes during the winter.
Along the northeastern coast of Baffin Island the mountains rise to 8,000 ft (2,440 m). Glaciers move down through the valleys to the sea, eroding wide U-shaped valleys.
Exposure to three phases of mountain-building and subsequent erosion over millions of years has molded the ancient Canadian Shield into a series of basins and ridges.
The Rocky Mountains were formed some 80 million years ago, when the Pacific Plate was driven under the North American Plate, forcing up the land.
Fertile prairies stretch from the southern rim of the Canadian Shield, south into the US.
The Great Lakes lie on the Canada–US border. The basins they now occupy were fashioned by repeated ice advance. Once, Lakes Superior, Huron, and Michigan formed one large lake, Lake Nipissing.
The St. Lawrence River is 2,350 miles (3,782 km) long. It flows from the western shore of Lake Superior through the Great Lakes and on to the Atlantic Ocean. From December to April, the St. Lawrence Seaway freezes between Lake Ontario and Montréal.
Isolated pillars, known as hoodos near Red Deer River in the badlands of Alberta are a product of wind and water erosion, especially flash floods. The badlands lie in the rain shadow of the Rocky Mountains, which creates a semiarid climate.
Map Key
Population
1 million to 5 million
500,000 to 1 million
100,000 to 500,000
50,000 to 100,000
10,000 to 50,000
below 10,000
Elevation
6000m / 19,686ft
4000m / 13,124ft
3000m / 9843ft
2000m / 6562ft
1000m / 3281ft
500m / 1640ft
250m / 820ft
100m / 328ft
sea level
Baffin Bay
Baffin Island
Davis Strait
Foxe Basin
Hudson Strait
Hudson Bay
James Bay
Labrador Sea
Atlantic Ocean
Great Lakes
Lake Superior
Lake Huron
Lake Michigan
Lake Erie
Lake Ontario
Laurentian Mountains
Gulf of St. Lawrence
Newfoundland
Nova Scotia
New Brunswick
Prince Edward Island
Manitoba
Ontario
Québec
Nunavut
Labrador
Greenland (to Denmark)
Ottawa
Montréal
Québec
Toronto
Winnipeg
Halifax
St. John's
Scale 1:14,700,000
(projection: Lambert Azimuthal Equal Area)

The Great Lakes are drained by the St. Lawrence River which flows down through a wide tectonic depression. It forms a broad estuary for much of its course, the width varying from 1.2 miles (1.9 km) in the upper reaches to 90 miles (145 km) at its mouth.

196 · 64 · 16

CANADA: WESTERN PROVINCES

Alberta, British Columbia, Manitoba, Saskatchewan, Yukon Territory

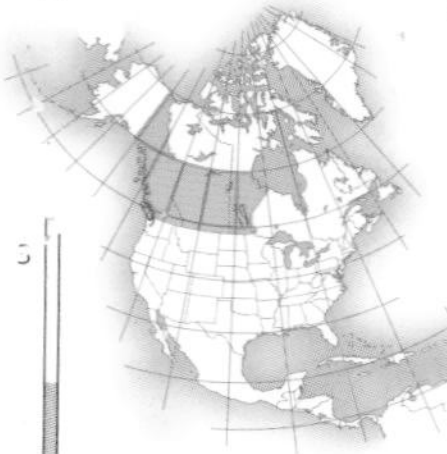

THE MOUNTAINS OF THE WEST COAST, incorporating British Columbia and the Yukon Territory, descend into the vast, flat prairies of Alberta, Saskatchewan, and Manitoba. The empty lands and fertile soils of the prairie provinces attracted migrants, and the descendants of early European immigrants still make up a large proportion of the population. The mechanization of agriculture has reduced the need for labor, and rural population densities remain low. The majority of the people live within 100 miles (160 km) of the southern Canada–US border, and in British Columbia, one of the leading Canadian provinces in terms of economic wealth. The Yukon Territory, in the far north, remains a relatively unspoiled wilderness, containing large, untapped mineral reserves. This province has a significant population of Native Americans people, many of whom maintain a traditional lifestyle.

USING THE LAND AND SEA

WHEAT FARMING IS THE ECONOMIC MAINSTAY of Alberta, Manitoba, and Saskatchewan, which contain 82% of farmland in Canada. Cattle are also raised on the prairies. Forestry and fishing are the most prominent resource-based industries in British Columbia. Despite the mountainous terrain, fruit and specialized grains can be grown in the Okanagan and Fraser valleys.

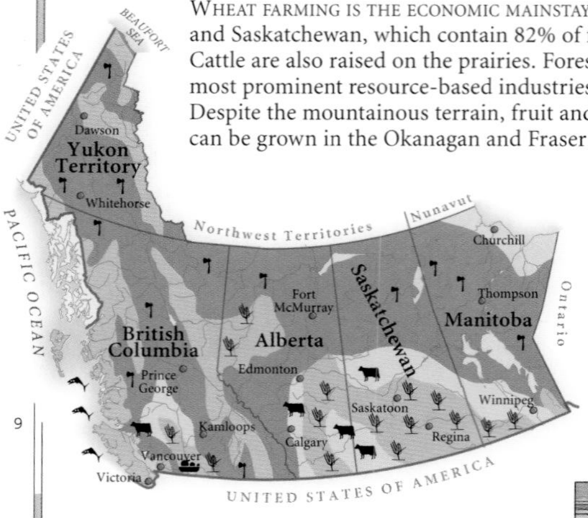

Land use and agricultural distribution: cattle, cereals, fishing, fruit, timber, major towns; pasture, cropland, forest, wetland, barren, tundra

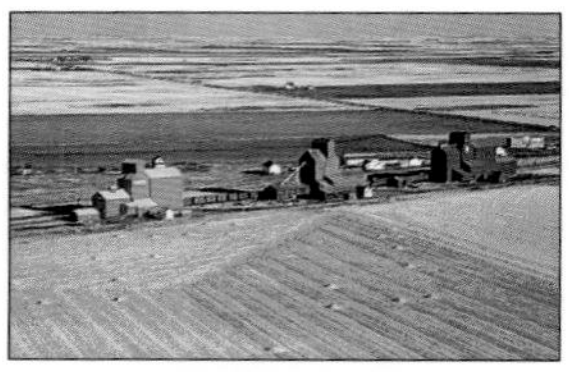

THE URBAN/RURAL POPULATION DIVIDE

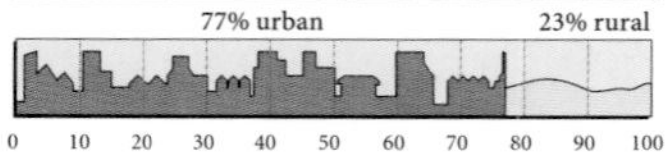

77% urban — 23% rural

POPULATION DENSITY	TOTAL LAND AREA
7 people per sq mile (3 people per sq km)	1,224,449 sq miles (3,172,150 sq km)

***Large, highly-mechanized** and often very specialized farms, requiring huge investment but little labor, characterize modern farming in the prairies.*

TRANSPORTATION & INDUSTRY

THE WESTERN PROVINCES contain a wealth of mineral resources. Alberta holds the bulk of Canada's fossil fuels; the other provinces contain reserves of metallic ores, such as zinc, lead, and silver. Isolation from markets has slowed the development of manufacturing, restricting it to the large cities like Vancouver, Winnipeg, and Calgary. Hydroelectric power is widely exploited, although there is increasing concern about potential ecological damage.

Major industry and infrastructure: aerospace, chemicals, coal, engineering, food processing, hydroelectric power, mining, oil & gas, timber processing, major towns, international airports, major roads, major industrial areas

TRANSPORTATION NETWORK

82,438 miles (135,145 km)
6,459 miles (10,401 km)
10,811 miles (17,410 km)
None

The transportation network of the western provinces is dominated by east–west routes that weave through mountain passes and spread across the plains. Access to some northern areas is restricted to air travel.

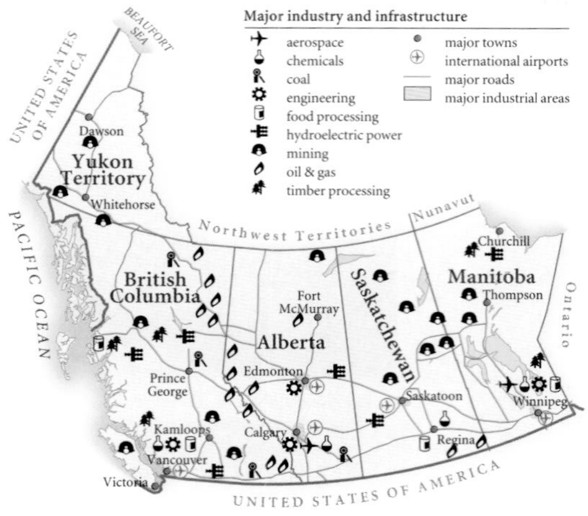

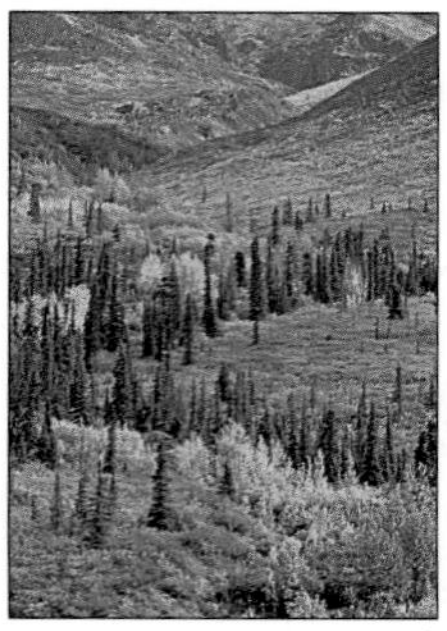

***Much of the Yukon Territory** is uninhabited tundra. Industry is based on the extraction of mineral resources, and to a lesser extent, on the scattered forests of the south.*

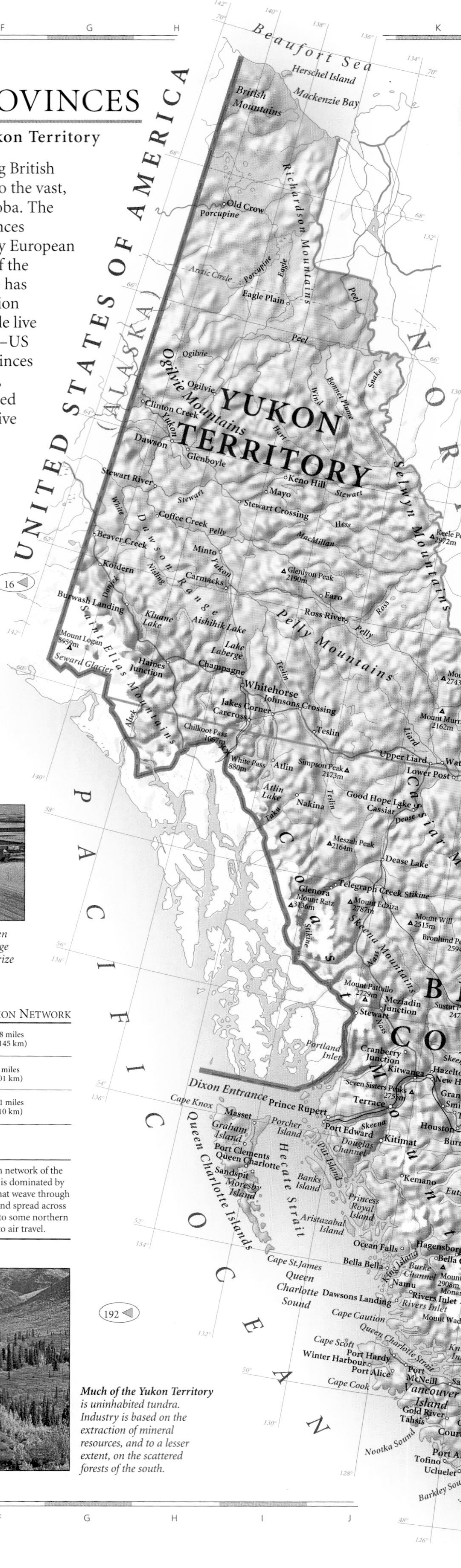

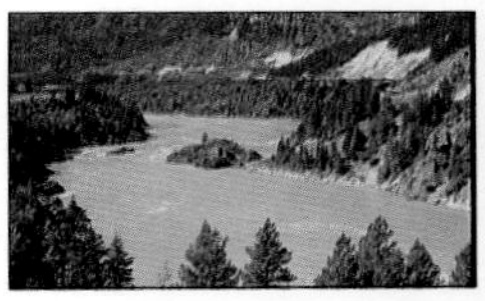

***The Fraser River valley** is a major area of settlement in British Columbia. Railraods cross the Rocky Mountains via this valley.*

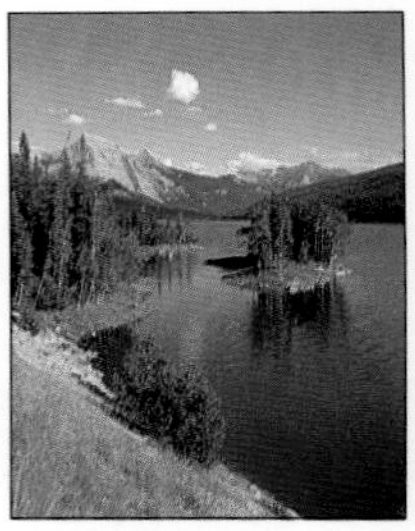

***Established in 1907,** Jasper National Park lies in the heart of the Rocky Mountains. It is noted for its spectacular alpine scenery and contains part of the large Columbia Icefield.*

16
192

The Landscape

The massive Rocky Mountains form a continental divide between rivers flowing eastward and westward. The interior plains lie east of the mountains, stretching from the Arctic Circle south into the US. Covered with glacial deposits from the last Ice Age, these are interspersed with hilly regions and long, steep escarpments.

The Columbia Icefield in the Rocky Mountains is the source of two major rivers, the Athabasca and the North Saskatchewan.

Vegetated island
River flow is diverted by deposited sediments
Bar
Sand flat

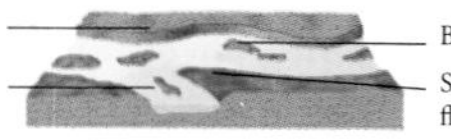

***Braided rivers** are shallow and fast-flowing. The interlaced branches are formed when excess sediments, which can no longer be transported, are deposited. The sediments collect in the river channel forming bars and sand flats. Islands form when the bars are colonized by vegetation.*

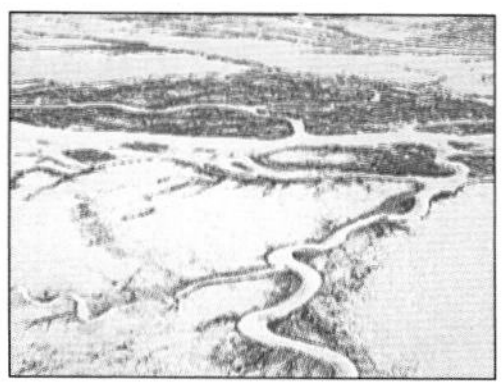

***Across the tundra** of northern Manitoba, widespread permafrost inhibits water from permeating the soil. This causes rivers like the Churchill to flow in many channels, which can be frozen for up to six months during the winter.*

The badlands of Alberta were created when east-flowing rivers, swollen by meltwater at the end of the last Ice Age, cut deep, wide canyons producing eroded, barren landscapes.

South Saskatchewan River

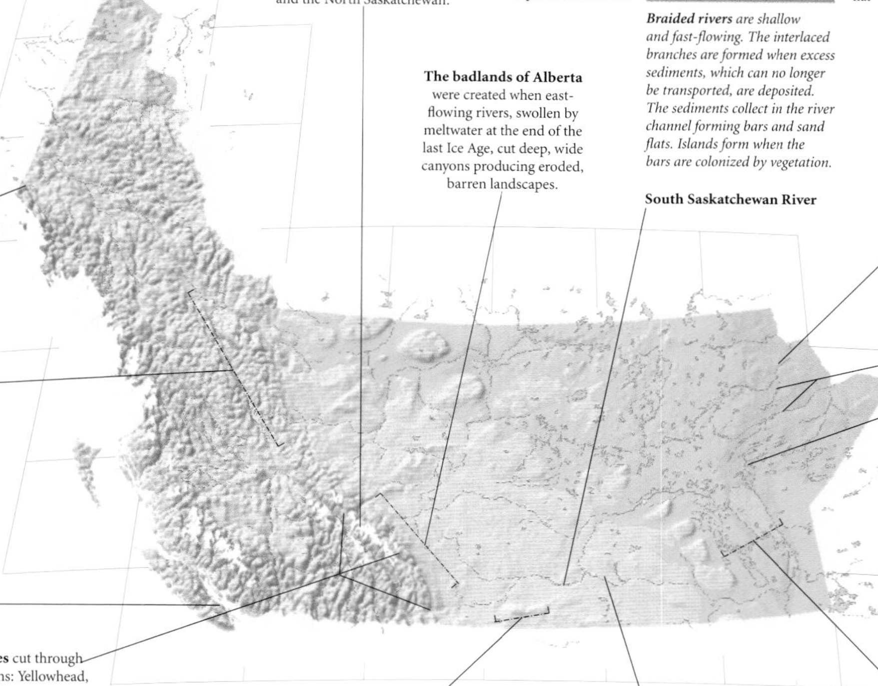

Mount Logan rises 19,551 ft (5,959 m). It is the highest peak in Canada.

The Nelson and Churchill Rivers drain northward across the Canadian Shield to Hudson Bay. The shield covers three-fifths of Saskatchewan.

Setting Lake

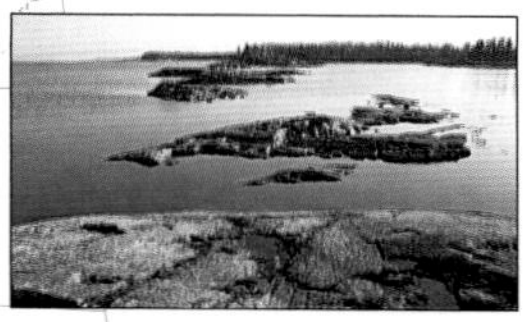

The Rocky Mountain Trench is the longest linear fault in the world. It has formed a straight, flat-bottomed valley between 2–9 miles (4–15 km) wide, and up to 3,280 ft (1,000 m) deep.

Hundreds of islands dot the fjord-indented coast of British Columbia; the largest is Vancouver Island.

***Ancient granite outcrops**, part of the Canadian Shield, rise above the surface of Setting Lake, which was initially formed by meltwater from the last Ice Age.*

Three major passes cut through the Rocky Mountains: Yellowhead, Kicking Horse, and Crowsnest. They are all used as transportation routes through the mountains.

The Cypress Hills rise to 4,806 ft (1,465 m) above the surrounding plain. Having escaped the last glaciation they contain unique plant and animal life. The silvery lupine, bunchberry, and lodgepole pine all grow in the cool, moist climate of the hills.

The Alberta and Saskatchewan plains bear strong testament to past glaciations. The Assiniboine, Saskatchewan and Qu'Appelle Rivers occupy flat-bottomed, steep-sided valleys eroded during the last Ice Age by glacial meltwater.

The lowlands of Manitoba are a basin that once held the vast post-glacial Lake Agassiz, remnants of which include Lake Winnipeg, Lake Winnipegosis, and Lake Manitoba.

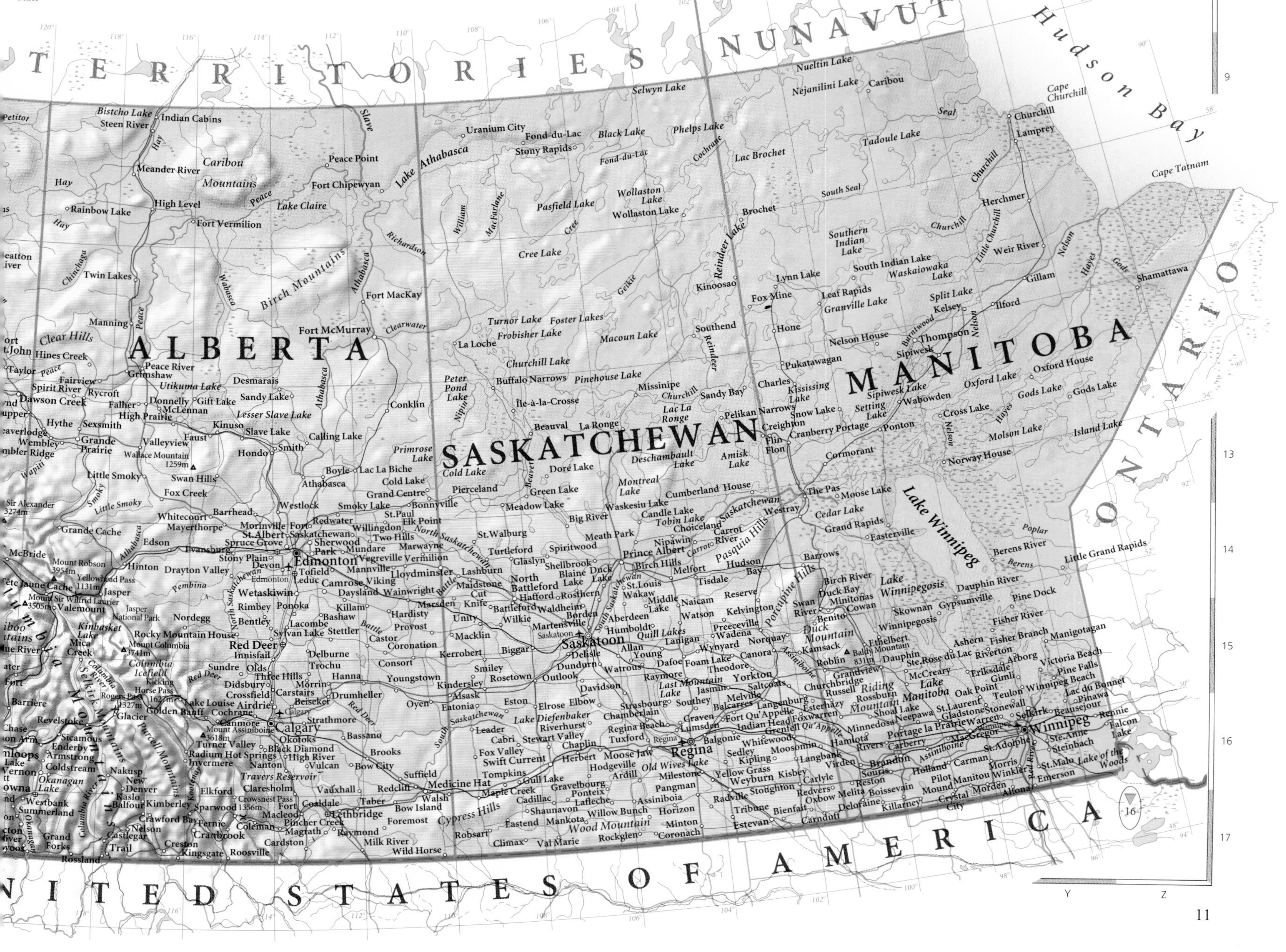

Map Key

POPULATION
- 500,000 to 1 million
- 100,000 to 500,000
- 50,000 to 100,000
- 10,000 to 50,000
- below 10,000

ELEVATION
- 6000m / 19,686ft
- 4000m / 13,124ft
- 3000m / 9843ft
- 2000m / 6562ft
- 1000m / 3281ft
- 500m / 1640ft
- 250m / 820ft
- 100m / 328ft
- sea level

Scale 1:8,250,000
(projection: Lambert Conformal Conic)

Km 0 25 50 100 150 200 250
Miles 0 25 50 100 150 200 250

CANADA: EASTERN PROVINCES

New Brunswick, Newfoundland, Nova Scotia, Ontario, Prince Edward Island, Quebec, *St. Pierre & Miquelon* (to France)

COLONIZED BY BOTH THE ENGLISH AND THE FRENCH during the 16th century, Canada's eastern provinces are still marked by their dual influences. They contain the last fragment of once-sizeable French territories, the islands of St. Pierre and Miquelon. French remains Canada's second official language and Quebec's first language. The population of the eastern provinces is highly concentrated in the south, especially along the border with the US. A recent decline in fishing in the Atlantic provinces has encouraged a steady flow of westerly migration to more properous regions. The north, around Hudson Bay, remains snow-covered for most of the year and the indigenous Inuit people make up the bulk of its sparse population.

Rocher Percé, is 290 ft (88 m) high. Lying off the southeastern coast of Quebec, it is a sanctuary for sea birds.

SCALE 1:7,750,000
(projection: Lambert Conformal Conic)

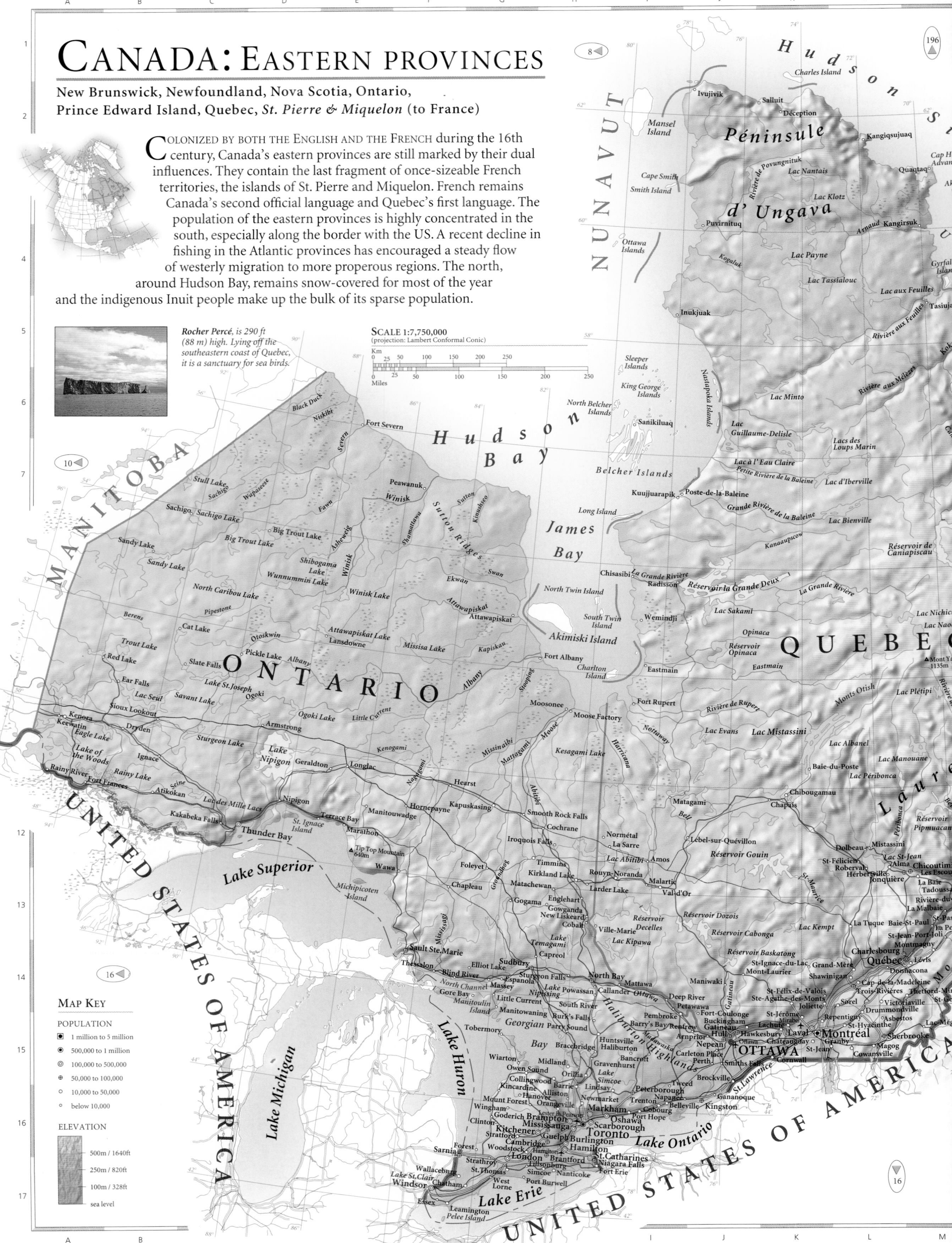

A B C D E F G H I J K L M
1 2 3 4 5 6 7 8 9 10 11 12 13 14 15 16 17
Km 0 25 50 100 150 200 250
Miles 0 25 50 100 150 200 250
MAP KEY
POPULATION
1 million to 5 million
500,000 to 1 million
100,000 to 500,000
50,000 to 100,000
10,000 to 50,000
below 10,000
ELEVATION
500m / 1640ft
250m / 820ft
100m / 328ft
sea level
NUNAVUT
MANITOBA
ONTARIO
QUEBEC
UNITED STATES OF AMERICA
Hudson Bay
Hudson Strait
James Bay
Péninsule d' Ungava
Lake Superior
Lake Michigan
Lake Huron
Lake Erie
Lake Ontario
Georgian Bay
Mansel Island
Charles Island
Ivujivik
Salluit
Déception
Kangiqsujuaq
Quaqtaq
Cape Smith
Smith Island
Lac Nantais
Lac Klotz
Puvirnituq
Kangirsuk
Lac Payne
Lac Tassialouc
Lac aux Feuilles
Tasiujaq
Ottawa Islands
Inukjuak
Sleeper Islands
King George Islands
North Belcher Islands
Sanikiluaq
Belcher Islands
Nastapoka Islands
Lac Minto
Lac Guillaume-Delisle
Lacs des Loups Marin
Lac à l' Eau Claire
Lac d'Iberville
Kuujjuarapik
Poste-de-la-Baleine
Lac Bienville
Réservoir de Caniapiscau
Long Island
Chisasibi
Radisson
Réservoir la Grande Deux
North Twin Island
South Twin Island
Wemindji
Lac Sakami
Réservoir Opinaca
Akimiski Island
Charlton Island
Eastmain
Mont Yapeitso 1135m
Fort Albany
Fort Severn
Peawanuk
Winisk
Sutton Ridges
Big Trout Lake
Sandy Lake
Sachigo Lake
Stull Lake
North Caribou Lake
Winisk Lake
Attawapiskat
Attawapiskat Lake
Lansdowne
Missisa Lake
Cat Lake
Pickle Lake
Slate Falls
Trout Lake
Red Lake
Ear Falls
Lac Seul
Savant Lake
Sioux Lookout
Kenora
Keewatin
Dryden
Eagle Lake
Lake of the Woods
Rainy River
Fort Frances
Rainy Lake
Atikokan
Ignace
Sturgeon Lake
Armstrong
Lake Nipigon
Geraldton
Longlac
Nipigon
Kakabeka Falls
Thunder Bay
Terrace Bay
Marathon
Manitouwadge
Tip Top Mountain 640m
Wawa
Michipicoten Island
Hearst
Hornepayne
Kapuskasing
Moosonee
Moose Factory
Fort Rupert
Lac Mistassini
Lac Evans
Lac Albanel
Chibougamau
Chapais
Matagami
Smooth Rock Falls
Cochrane
Iroquois Falls
Timmins
Kirkland Lake
Rouyn-Noranda
Normétal
La Sarre
Lac Abitibi
Amos
Lebel-sur-Quévillon
Réservoir Gouin
Malartic
Val-d'Or
Larder Lake
Foleyet
Chapleau
Matachewan
Gogama
Englehart
New Liskeard
Cobalt
Ville-Marie
Réservoir Decelles
Lac Kipawa
Réservoir Dozois
Réservoir Cabonga
Réservoir Baskatong
Lake Temagami
Capreol
Sudbury
Sault Ste. Marie
Thessalon
Elliot Lake
Blind River
Espanola
Sturgeon Falls
North Bay
Mattawa
Manitoulin Island
Little Current
Manitowaning
Tobermory
Parry Sound
Huntsville
Haliburton
Bracebridge
Pembroke
Petawawa
Deep River
Maniwaki
Ottawa
OTTAWA
Hull
Gatineau
Montréal
Laval
Québec
Lévis
Trois-Rivières
Sherbrooke
Granby
Drummondville
Victoriaville
Saint-Hyacinthe
Chicoutimi
Jonquière
Alma
Dolbeau
Roberval
La Tuque
Kingston
Brockville
Cornwall
Belleville
Peterborough
Oshawa
Markham
Scarborough
Toronto
Mississauga
Brampton
Burlington
Hamilton
St. Catharines
Niagara Falls
Fort Erie
Kitchener
Guelph
Cambridge
Stratford
Woodstock
London
Brantford
Sarnia
Chatham
Windsor
Lake St. Clair
Leamington
Pelee Island
Barrie
Orillia
Owen Sound
Collingwood
Wiarton
Goderich
Kincardine
Orangeville

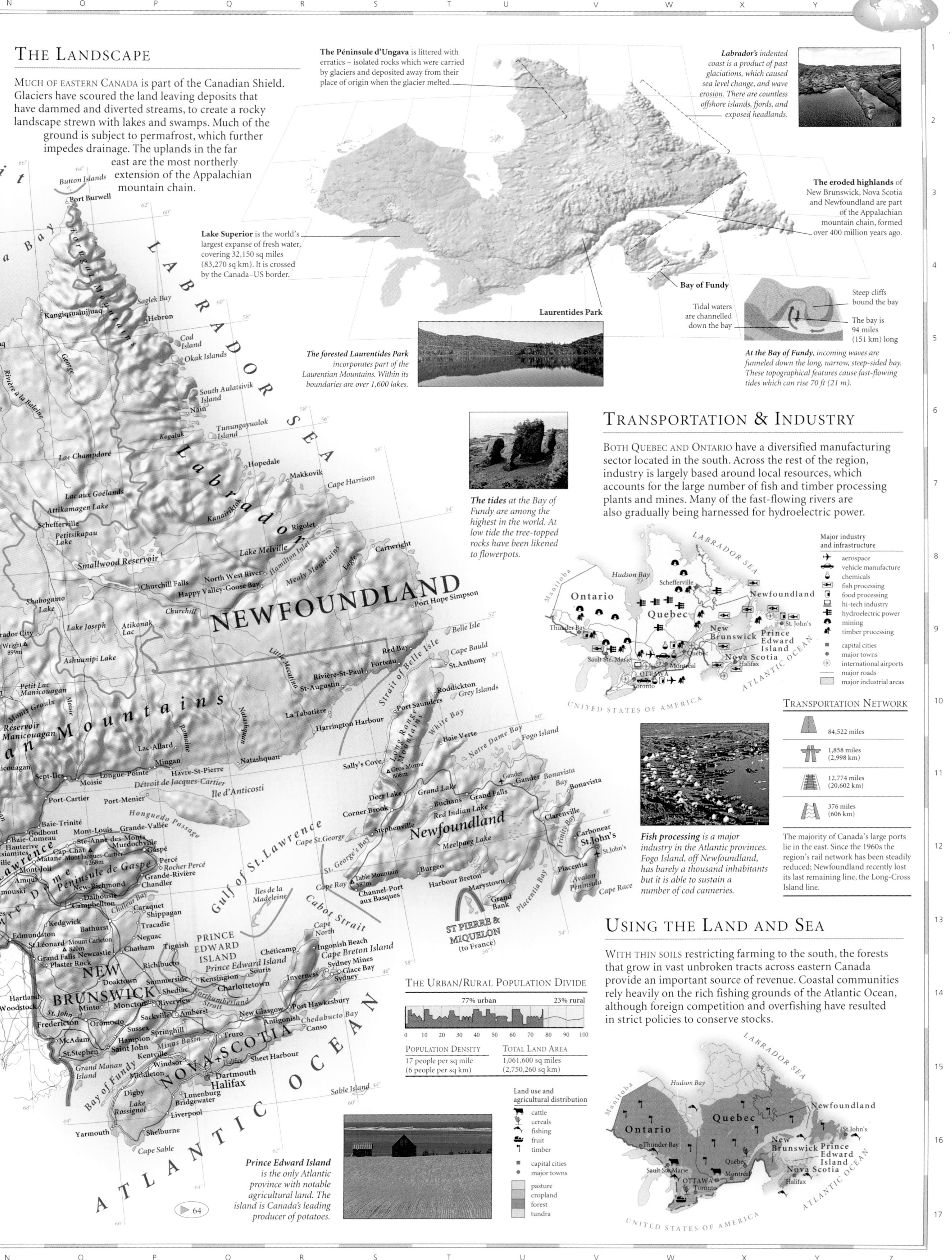
LABRADOR SEA
Labrador
NEWFOUNDLAND
Newfoundland
Gulf of St. Lawrence
Cabot Strait
Strait of Belle Isle
NEW BRUNSWICK
NOVA SCOTIA
PRINCE EDWARD ISLAND
ATLANTIC OCEAN
Bay of Fundy
Halifax
St.John's
Charlottetown
Fredericton
ST PIERRE & MIQUELON (to France)
Île d'Anticosti
Cape Breton Island
Sable Island
Smallwood Reservoir
Lake Melville
Happy Valley-Goose Bay
Schefferville
Sept-Îles
Péninsule de Gaspé
Corner Brook
Gander
Sydney
Moncton
Saint John
Yarmouth
Ontario
Quebec
Hudson Bay
Thunder Bay
Sault Ste. Marie
OTTAWA
Toronto
Montreal
UNITED STATES OF AMERICA

The Landscape

Much of eastern Canada is part of the Canadian Shield. Glaciers have scoured the land leaving deposits that have dammed and diverted streams, to create a rocky landscape strewn with lakes and swamps. Much of the ground is subject to permafrost, which further impedes drainage. The uplands in the far east are the most northerly extension of the Appalachian mountain chain.

The Péninsule d'Ungava is littered with erratics – isolated rocks which were carried by glaciers and deposited away from their place of origin when the glacier melted.

Labrador's indented coast is a product of past glaciations, which caused sea level change, and wave erosion. There are countless offshore islands, fjords, and exposed headlands.

The eroded highlands of New Brunswick, Nova Scotia and Newfoundland are part of the Appalachian mountain chain, formed over 400 million years ago.

Lake Superior is the world's largest expanse of fresh water, covering 32,150 sq miles (83,270 sq km). It is crossed by the Canada–US border.

Bay of Fundy

Laurentides Park

Tidal waters are channelled down the bay

Steep cliffs bound the bay

The bay is 94 miles (151 km) long

***At the Bay of Fundy**, incoming waves are funneled down the long, narrow, steep-sided bay. These topographical features cause fast-flowing tides which can rise 70 ft (21 m).*

***The forested Laurentides Park** incorporates part of the Laurentian Mountains. Within its boundaries are over 1,600 lakes.*

***The tides** at the Bay of Fundy are among the highest in the world. At low tide the tree-topped rocks have been likened to flowerpots.*

Transportation & Industry

Both Quebec and Ontario have a diversified manufacturing sector located in the south. Across the rest of the region, industry is largely based around local resources, which accounts for the large number of fish and timber processing plants and mines. Many of the fast-flowing rivers are also gradually being harnessed for hydroelectric power.

Major industry and infrastructure: aerospace; vehicle manufacture; chemicals; fish processing; food processing; hi-tech industry; hydroelectric power; mining; timber processing; capital cities; major towns; international airports; major roads; major industrial areas

Transportation Network

84,522 miles
1,858 miles (2,998 km)
12,774 miles (20,602 km)
376 miles (606 km)

The majority of Canada's large ports lie in the east. Since the 1960s the region's rail network has been steadily reduced; Newfoundland recently lost its last remaining line, the Long-Cross Island line.

***Fish processing** is a major industry in the Atlantic provinces. Fogo Island, off Newfoundland, has barely a thousand inhabitants but it is able to sustain a number of cod canneries.*

Using the Land and Sea

With thin soils restricting farming to the south, the forests that grow in vast unbroken tracts across eastern Canada provide an important source of revenue. Coastal communities rely heavily on the rich fishing grounds of the Atlantic Ocean, although foreign competition and overfishing have resulted in strict policies to conserve stocks.

The Urban/Rural Population Divide

77% urban | 23% rural

Population Density	Total Land Area
17 people per sq mile (6 people per sq km)	1,061,600 sq miles (2,750,260 sq km)

Land use and agricultural distribution: cattle; cereals; fishing; fruit; timber; capital cities; major towns; pasture; cropland; forest; tundra

***Prince Edward Island** is the only Atlantic province with notable agricultural land. The island is Canada's leading producer of potatoes.*

▶ 64

SOUTHEASTERN CANADA

Southern Ontario, Southern Quebec

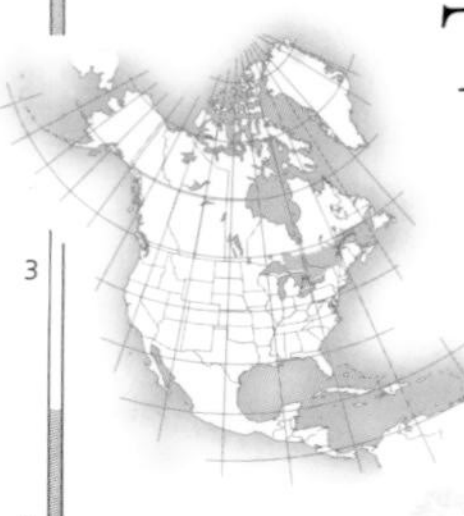

THE SOUTHERN PARTS of Quebec and Ontario form the economic heart of Canada. The two provinces are divided by their language and culture; in Quebec, French is the main language, whereas English is spoken in Ontario. Separatist sentiment in Quebec has led to a provincial referendum on the question of a sovereignty association with Canada. The region contains Canada's capital, Ottawa and its two largest cities: Toronto, the center of commerce and Montréal, the cultural and administrative heart of French Canada.

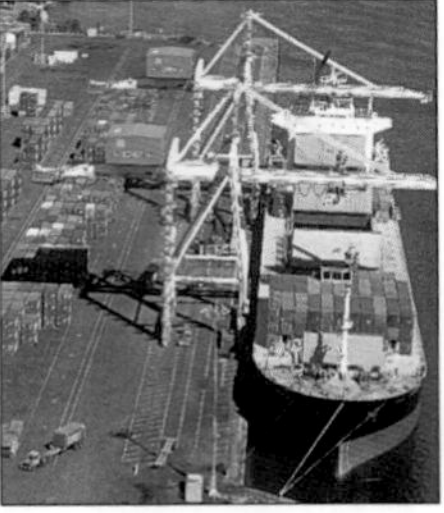

***The port at Montréal** is situated on the St. Lawrence Seaway. A network of 16 locks allows sea-going vessels access to routes once plied by fur-trappers and early settlers.*

TRANSPORTATION & INDUSTRY

THE CITIES OF SOUTHERN QUEBEC AND ONTARIO, and their hinterlands, form the heart of Canadian manufacturing industry. Toronto is Canada's leading financial center, and Ontario's motor and aerospace industries have developed around the city. A major center for nickel mining lies to the north of Toronto. Most of Quebec's industry is located in Montréal, the oldest port in North America. Chemicals, paper manufacture, and the construction of transportation equipment are leading industrial activities.

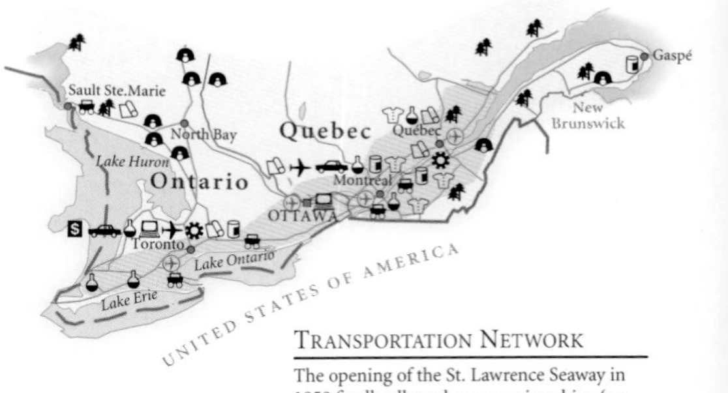

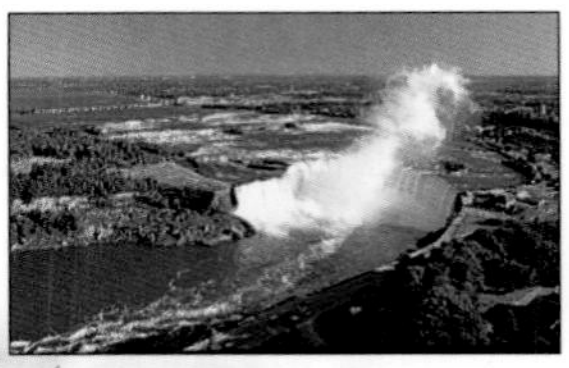

***Niagara Falls** lies on the border between Canada and the US. It comprises a system of two falls: American Falls, in New York, is separated from Horseshoe Falls, in Ontario, by Goat Island. Horseshoe Falls, seen here, plunges 184 ft (56 m) and is 2,500 ft (762 m) wide.*

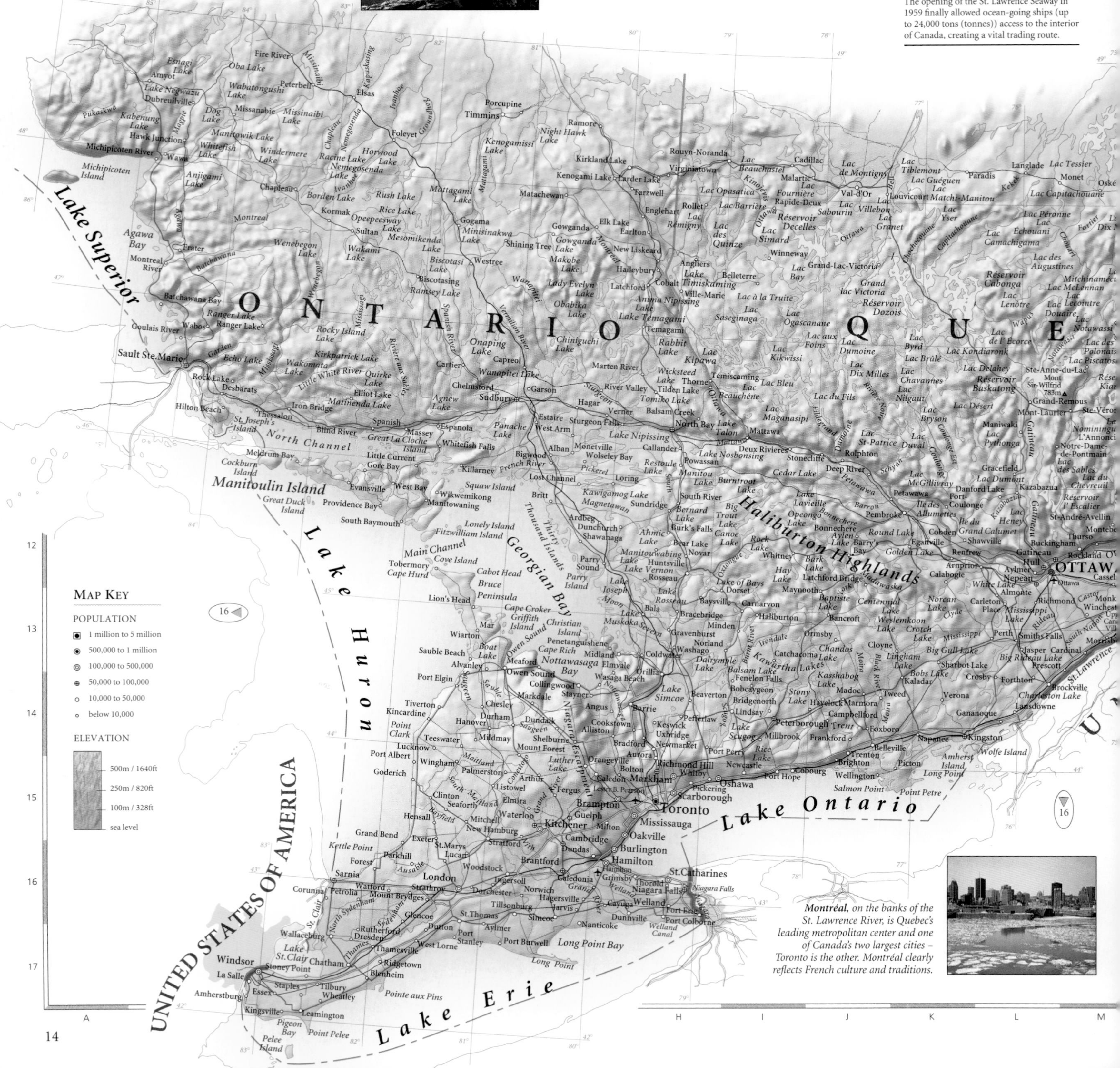

Major industry and infrastructure

car manufacture	textiles
chemicals	paper industry
engineering	timber processing
finance	capital cities
food processing	major towns
hi-tech industry	international airports
mining	major roads
iron & steel	major industrial areas

TRANSPORTATION NETWORK

The opening of the St. Lawrence Seaway in 1959 finally allowed ocean-going ships (up to 24,000 tons (tonnes)) access to the interior of Canada, creating a vital trading route.

MAP KEY

POPULATION

- 1 million to 5 million
- 500,000 to 1 million
- 100,000 to 500,000
- 50,000 to 100,000
- 10,000 to 50,000
- below 10,000

ELEVATION

- 500m / 1640ft
- 250m / 820ft
- 100m / 328ft
- sea level

***Montréal**, on the banks of the St. Lawrence River, is Quebec's leading metropolitan center and one of Canada's two largest cities – Toronto is the other. Montréal clearly reflects French culture and traditions.*

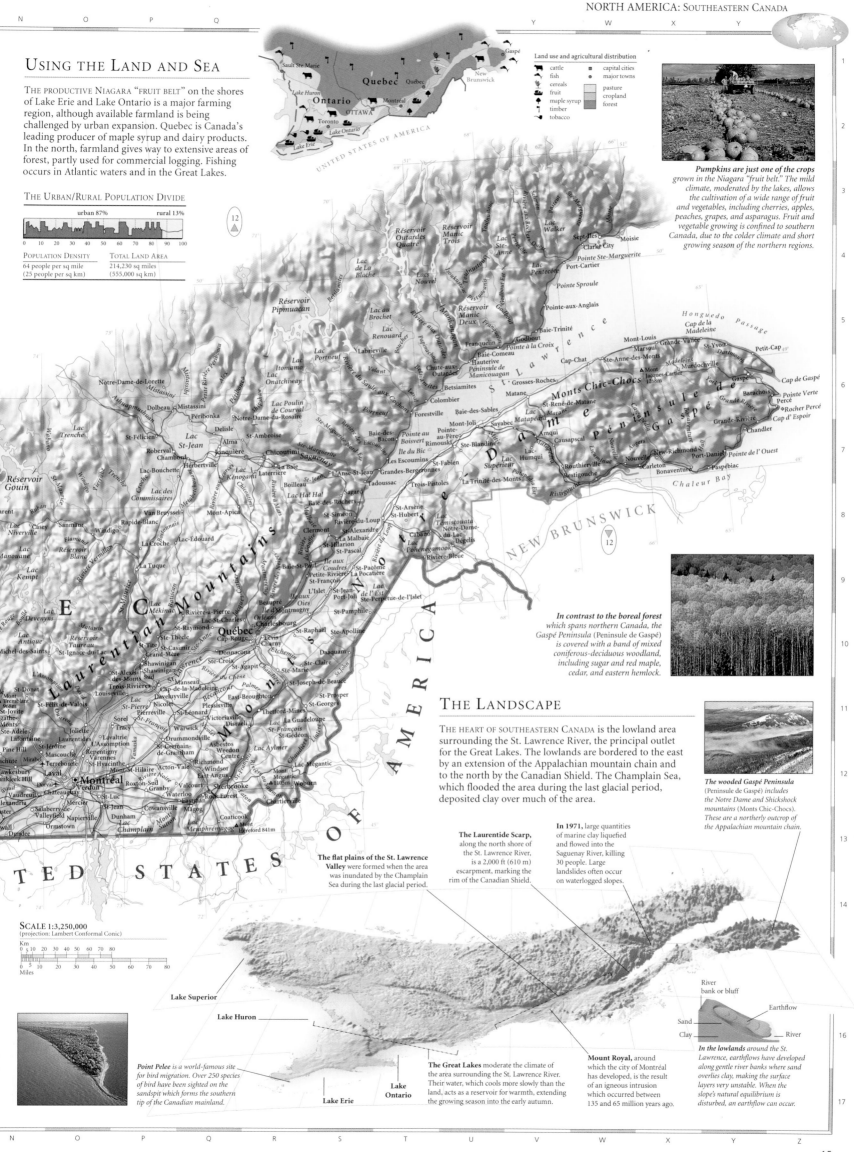

USING THE LAND AND SEA

THE PRODUCTIVE NIAGARA "FRUIT BELT" on the shores of Lake Erie and Lake Ontario is a major farming region, although available farmland is being challenged by urban expansion. Quebec is Canada's leading producer of maple syrup and dairy products. In the north, farmland gives way to extensive areas of forest, partly used for commercial logging. Fishing occurs in Atlantic waters and in the Great Lakes.

Land use and agricultural distribution

cattle
fish
cereals
fruit
maple syrup
timber
tobacco
capital cities
major towns
pasture
cropland
forest

THE URBAN/RURAL POPULATION DIVIDE

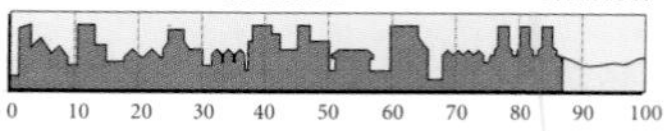

urban 87% rural 13%

0 10 20 30 40 50 60 70 80 90 100

POPULATION DENSITY	TOTAL LAND AREA
64 people per sq mile (25 people per sq km)	214,230 sq miles (555,000 sq km)

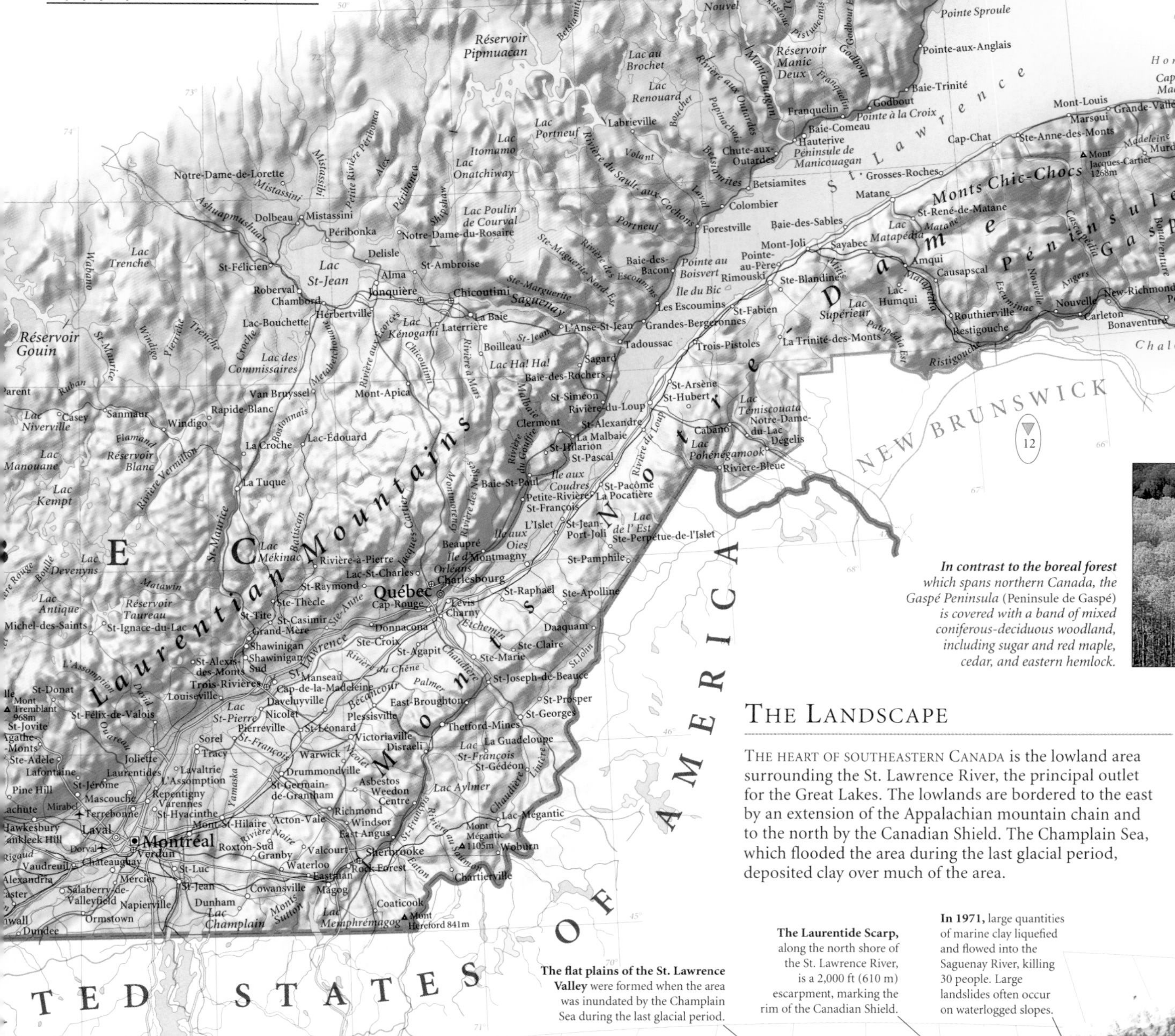

Pumpkins are just one of the crops *grown in the Niagara "fruit belt." The mild climate, moderated by the lakes, allows the cultivation of a wide range of fruit and vegetables, including cherries, apples, peaches, grapes, and asparagus. Fruit and vegetable growing is confined to southern Canada, due to the colder climate and short growing season of the northern regions.*

In contrast to the boreal forest *which spans northern Canada, the Gaspé Peninsula (Peninsule de Gaspé) is covered with a band of mixed coniferous-deciduous woodland, including sugar and red maple, cedar, and eastern hemlock.*

THE LANDSCAPE

THE HEART OF SOUTHEASTERN CANADA is the lowland area surrounding the St. Lawrence River, the principal outlet for the Great Lakes. The lowlands are bordered to the east by an extension of the Appalachian mountain chain and to the north by the Canadian Shield. The Champlain Sea, which flooded the area during the last glacial period, deposited clay over much of the area.

The wooded Gaspé Peninsula *(Peninsule de Gaspé) includes the Notre Dame and Shickshock mountains (Monts Chic-Chocs). These are a northerly outcrop of the Appalachian mountain chain.*

SCALE 1:3,250,000
(projection: Lambert Conformal Conic)

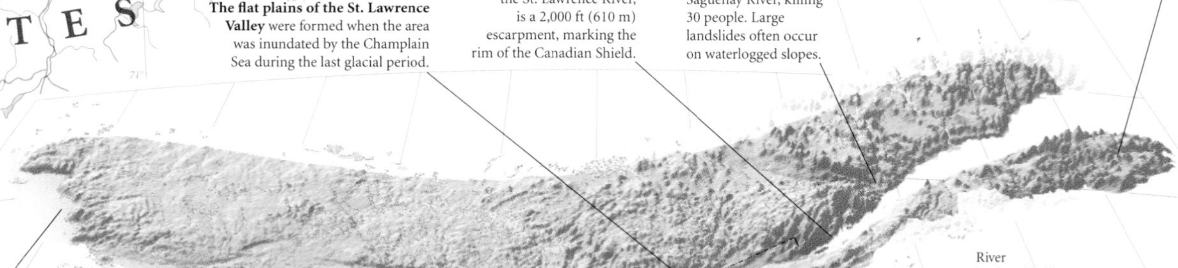

The flat plains of the St. Lawrence Valley were formed when the area was inundated by the Champlain Sea during the last glacial period.

The Laurentide Scarp, along the north shore of the St. Lawrence River, is a 2,000 ft (610 m) escarpment, marking the rim of the Canadian Shield.

In 1971, large quantities of marine clay liquefied and flowed into the Saguenay River, killing 30 people. Large landslides often occur on waterlogged slopes.

Lake Superior

Lake Huron

Lake Erie

Lake Ontario

River bank or bluff
Earthflow
Sand
Clay
River

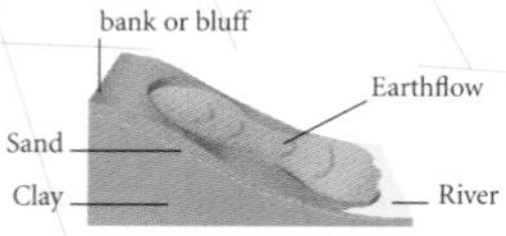

In the lowlands *around the St. Lawrence, earthflows have developed along gentle river banks where sand overlies clay, making the surface layers very unstable. When the slope's natural equilibrium is disturbed, an earthflow can occur.*

Point Pelee *is a world-famous site for bird migration. Over 250 species of bird have been sighted on the sandspit which forms the southern tip of the Canadian mainland.*

The Great Lakes moderate the climate of the area surrounding the St. Lawrence River. Their water, which cools more slowly than the land, acts as a reservoir for warmth, extending the growing season into the early autumn.

Mount Royal, around which the city of Montréal has developed, is the result of an igneous intrusion which occurred between 135 and 65 million years ago.

THE UNITED STATES OF AMERICA

CONTERMINOUS USA (FOR ALASKA AND HAWAII SEE PAGES 38–39)

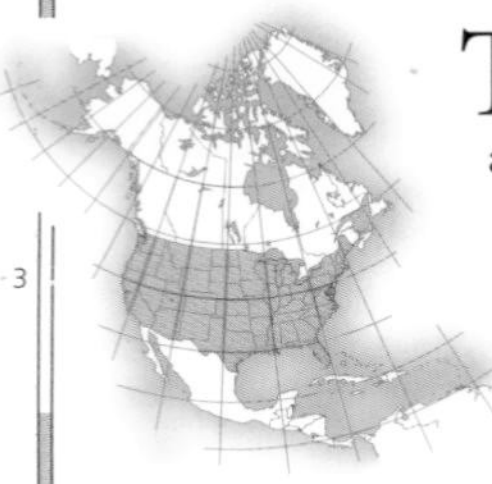

THE US'S PROGRESSION FROM FRONTIER TERRITORY to economic and political superpower has taken less than 200 years. The 48 conterminous states, along with the outlying states of Alaska and Hawaii, are part of a federal union, held together by the guiding principles of the US Constitution, which embodies the ideals of democracy and liberty for all. Abundant fertile land and a rich resource-base fueled and sustained US economic development. With the spread of agriculture and the growth of trade and industry came the need for a larger workforce, which was supplied by millions of immigrants, many seeking an escape from poverty and political or religious persecution. Immigration continues today, particularly from Central America and Asia.

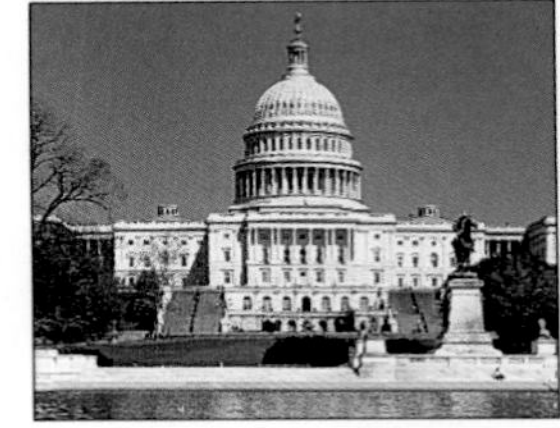

Washington D.C. was established as the nation's capital in 1790. It is home to the seat of national government, on Capitol Hill, as well as the President's official residence, the White House.

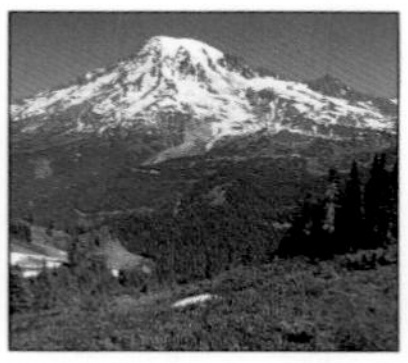

SCALE 1: 12,700,000
(projection: Lambert Azimuthal Equal Area)

***Mount Rainier** is a dormant volcano in the Cascade Range, Washington. This 14,090 ft (4392 m) peak is flanked by the most extensive glacier outside Alaska.*

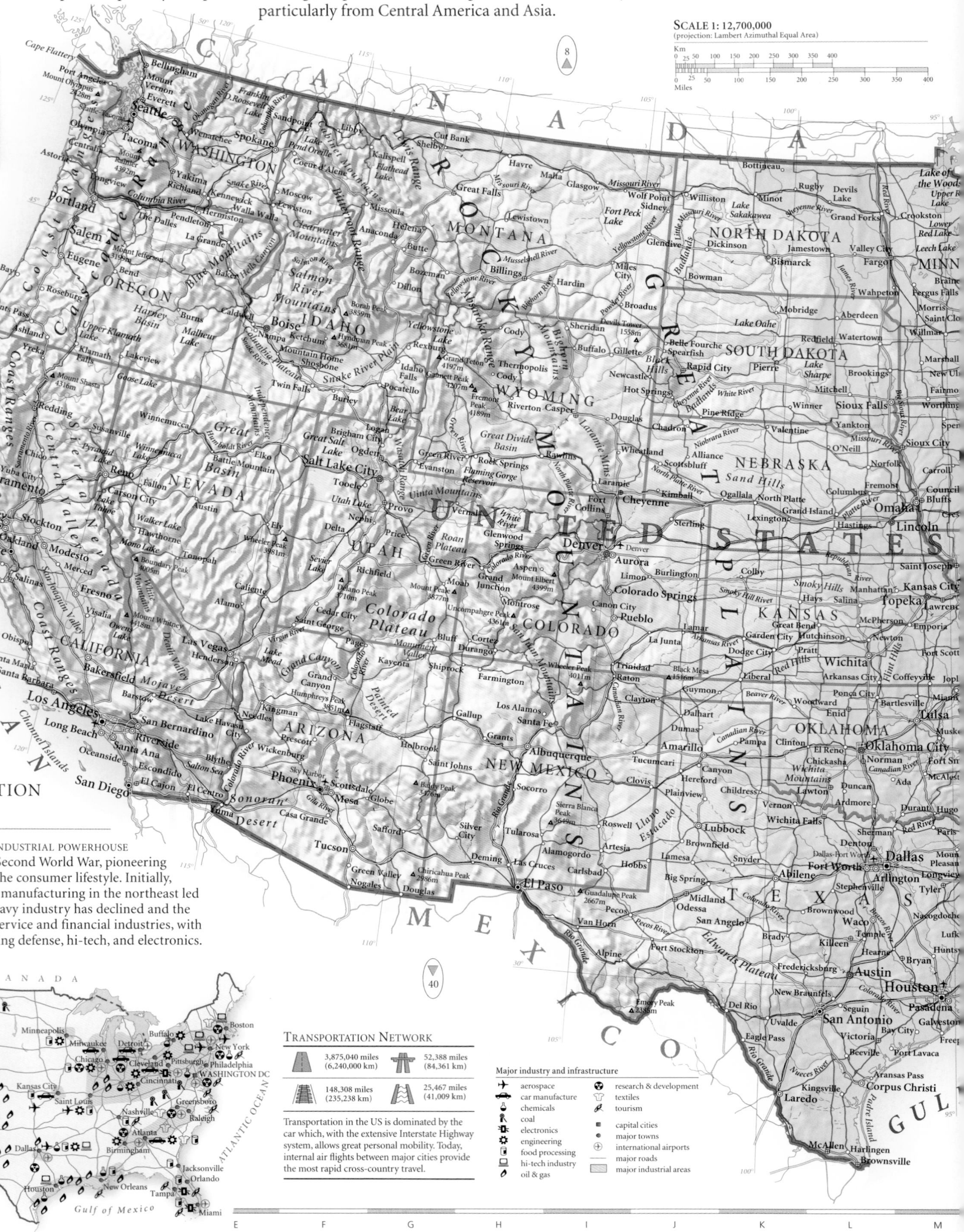

TRANSPORTATION & INDUSTRY

THE US HAS BEEN THE INDUSTRIAL POWERHOUSE of the world since the Second World War, pioneering mass-production and the consumer lifestyle. Initially, heavy engineering and manufacturing in the northeast led the economy. Today, heavy industry has declined and the economy is driven by service and financial industries, with the most important being defense, hi-tech, and electronics.

TRANSPORTATION NETWORK

3,875,040 miles (6,240,000 km)	52,388 miles (84,361 km)
148,308 miles (235,238 km)	25,467 miles (41,009 km)

Transportation in the US is dominated by the car which, with the extensive Interstate Highway system, allows great personal mobility. Today, internal air flights between major cities provide the most rapid cross-country travel.

Major industry and infrastructure

- aerospace
- car manufacture
- chemicals
- coal
- electronics
- engineering
- food processing
- hi-tech industry
- oil & gas
- research & development
- textiles
- tourism
- capital cities
- major towns
- international airports
- major roads
- major industrial areas

THE LANDSCAPE

THE HIGH, RUGGED MOUNTAIN RANGES of the west are about 80 million years old, geologically young compared to the old, eroded, Appalachian mountain chain, which dates from when North America and Europe were joined together as part of the supercontinent Pangaea, 400 million years ago. In contrast, the Great Plains and Mississippi Basin have a low relief and fertile soils.

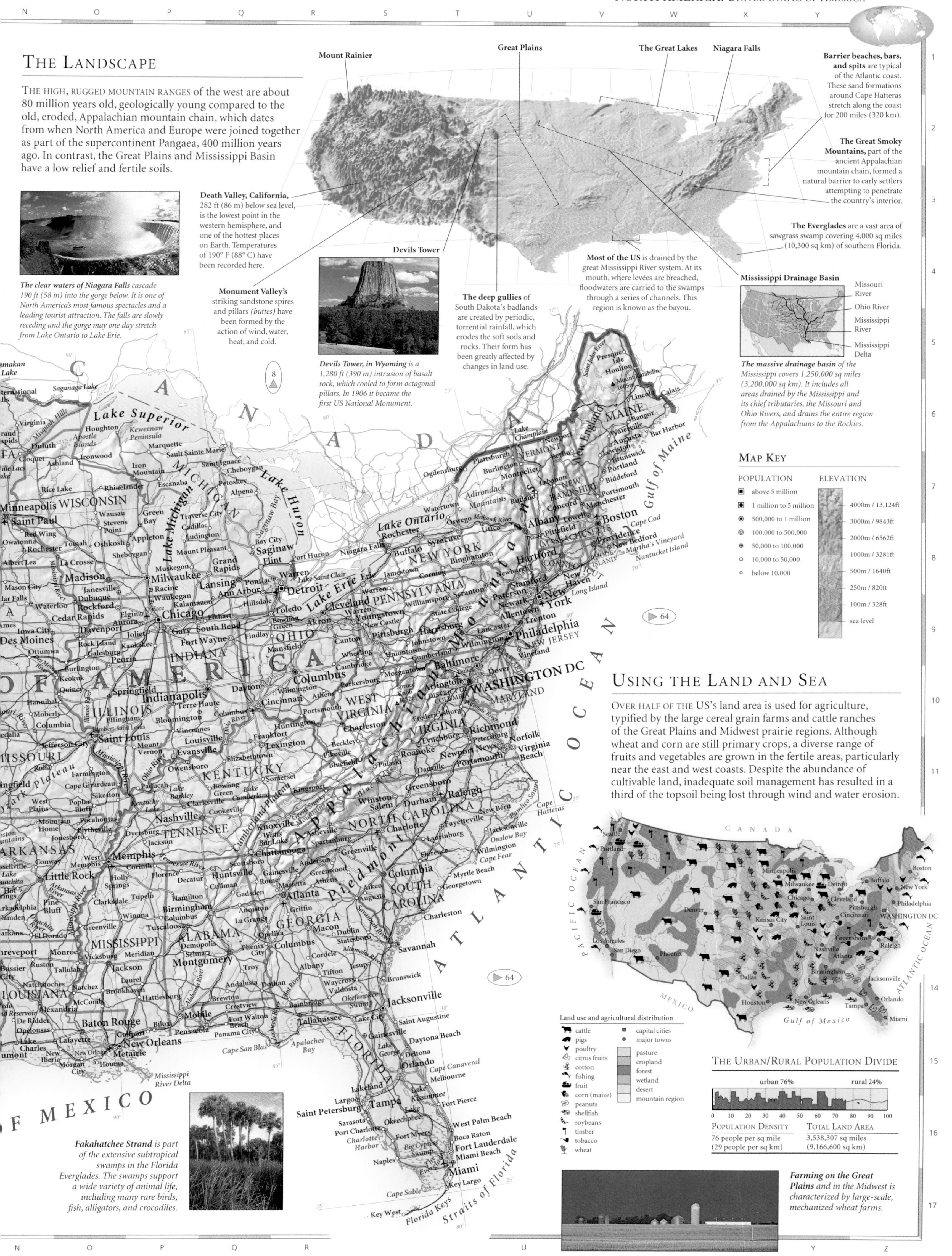

Mount Rainier
Great Plains
The Great Lakes
Niagara Falls
Barrier beaches, bars, and spits are typical of the Atlantic coast. These sand formations around Cape Hatteras stretch along the coast for 200 miles (320 km).
The Great Smoky Mountains, part of the ancient Appalachian mountain chain, formed a natural barrier to early settlers attempting to penetrate the country's interior.
The Everglades are a vast area of sawgrass swamp covering 4,000 sq miles (10,300 sq km) of southern Florida.
Death Valley, California, 282 ft (86 m) below sea level, is the lowest point in the western hemisphere, and one of the hottest places on Earth. Temperatures of 190° F (88° C) have been recorded here.
Devils Tower
Most of the US is drained by the great Mississippi River system. At its mouth, where levées are breached, floodwaters are carried to the swamps through a series of channels. This region is known as the bayou.
Monument Valley's striking sandstone spires and pillars *(buttes)* have been formed by the action of wind, water, heat, and cold.
The deep gullies of South Dakota's badlands are created by periodic, torrential rainfall, which erodes the soft soils and rocks. Their form has been greatly affected by changes in land use.
Mississippi Drainage Basin
Missouri River
Ohio River
Mississippi River
Mississippi Delta
MAP KEY
POPULATION
above 5 million
1 million to 5 million
500,000 to 1 million
100,000 to 500,000
50,000 to 100,000
10,000 to 50,000
below 10,000
ELEVATION
4000m / 13,124ft
3000m / 9843ft
2000m / 6562ft
1000m / 3281ft
500m / 1640ft
250m / 820ft
100m / 328ft
sea level
CANADA
UNITED STATES OF AMERICA
ATLANTIC OCEAN
GULF OF MEXICO
Appalachian Mountains
Lake Superior
Lake Michigan
Lake Huron
Lake Erie
Lake Ontario
Gulf of Maine
WASHINGTON DC
New York
Boston
Philadelphia
Chicago
Detroit
Atlanta
Miami
New Orleans
Land use and agricultural distribution
cattle
pigs
poultry
citrus fruits
cotton
fishing
fruit
corn (maize)
peanuts
shellfish
soybeans
timber
tobacco
wheat
capital cities
major towns
pasture
cropland
forest
wetland
desert
mountain region
THE URBAN/RURAL POPULATION DIVIDE
urban 76%
rural 24%
POPULATION DENSITY
76 people per sq mile (29 people per sq km)
TOTAL LAND AREA
3,538,307 sq miles (9,166,600 sq km)

The clear waters of Niagara Falls cascade 190 ft (58 m) into the gorge below. It is one of North America's most famous spectacles and a leading tourist attraction. The falls are slowly receding and the gorge may one day stretch from Lake Ontario to Lake Erie.

Devils Tower, in Wyoming is a 1,280 ft (390 m) intrusion of basalt rock, which cooled to form octagonal pillars. In 1906 it became the first US National Monument.

The massive drainage basin of the Mississippi covers 1,250,000 sq miles (3,200,000 sq km). It includes all areas drained by the Mississippi and its chief tributaries, the Missouri and Ohio Rivers, and drains the entire region from the Appalachians to the Rockies.

USING THE LAND AND SEA

OVER HALF OF THE US's land area is used for agriculture, typified by the large cereal grain farms and cattle ranches of the Great Plains and Midwest prairie regions. Although wheat and corn are still primary crops, a diverse range of fruits and vegetables are grown in the fertile areas, particularly near the east and west coasts. Despite the abundance of cultivable land, inadequate soil management has resulted in a third of the topsoil being lost through wind and water erosion.

***Fakahatchee Strand** is part of the extensive subtropical swamps in the Florida Everglades. The swamps support a wide variety of animal life, including many rare birds, fish, alligators, and crocodiles.*

***Farming on the Great Plains** and in the Midwest is characterized by large-scale, mechanized wheat farms.*

USA: NORTHEASTERN STATES

Connecticut, Maine, Massachusetts, New Hampshire, New Jersey, New York, Pennsylvania, Rhode Island, Vermont

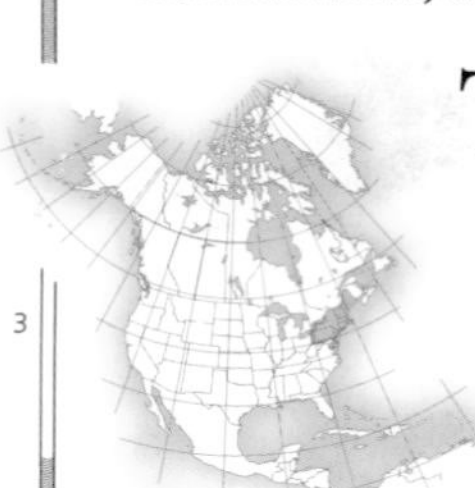

THE INDENTED COAST AND VAST WOODLANDS of the northeastern states were the original core area for European expansion. The rustic character of New England prevails after nearly four centuries, while the great cities of the Atlantic seaboard have formed an almost continuous urban region. Over 20 million immigrants entered New York from 1855 to 1924 and the northeast became the industrial center of the US. After the decline of mining and heavy manufacturing, economic dynamism has been restored with the growth of hi-tech and service industries.

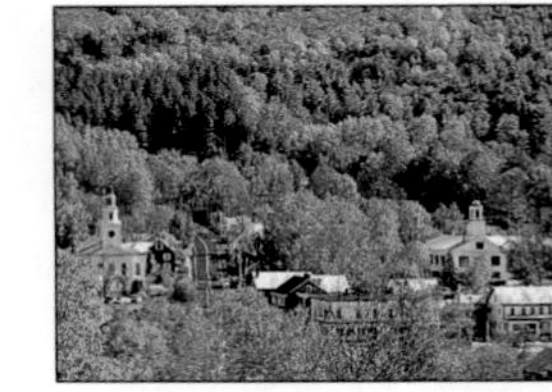

Chelsea in Vermont, surrounded by trees in their fall foliage. Tourism and agriculture dominate the economy of this self-consciously rural state, where no town exceeds 30,000 people.

MAP KEY

POPULATION

- above 5 million
- 1 million to 5 million
- 500,000 to 1 million
- 100,000 to 500,000
- 50,000 to 100,000
- 10,000 to 50,000
- below 10,000

ELEVATION

- 1000m / 3281ft
- 500m / 1640ft
- 250m / 820ft
- 100m / 328ft
- sea level

TRANSPORTATION & INDUSTRY

THE PRINCIPAL SEABOARD CITIES grew up on trade and manufacturing. They are now global centers of commerce and corporate administration, dominating the regional economy. Research and development facilities support an expanding electronics and communications sector throughout the region. Pharmaceutical and chemical industries are important in New Jersey and Pennsylvania.

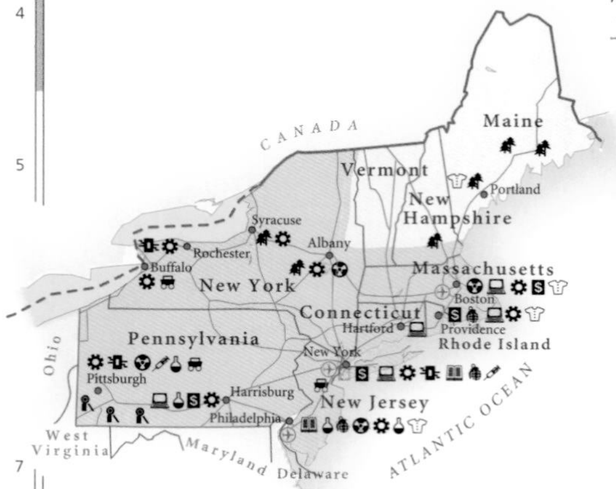

TRANSPORTATION NETWORK

340,090 miles (544,144 km)	4813 miles 7700 km
12,872 miles (20,592 km)	2108 miles (3389 km)

New York's commercial success is tied historically to its transportation connections. The Erie Canal, completed in 1825, opened up the Great Lakes and the interior to New York's markets and carried a stream of immigrants into the Midwest.

Major industry and infrastructure

- chemicals
- coal
- defense
- electronics
- engineering
- finance
- hi-tech industry
- iron & steel
- pharmaceuticals
- printing & publishing
- research & development
- textiles
- timber processing
- major towns
- international airports
- major roads
- major industrial area

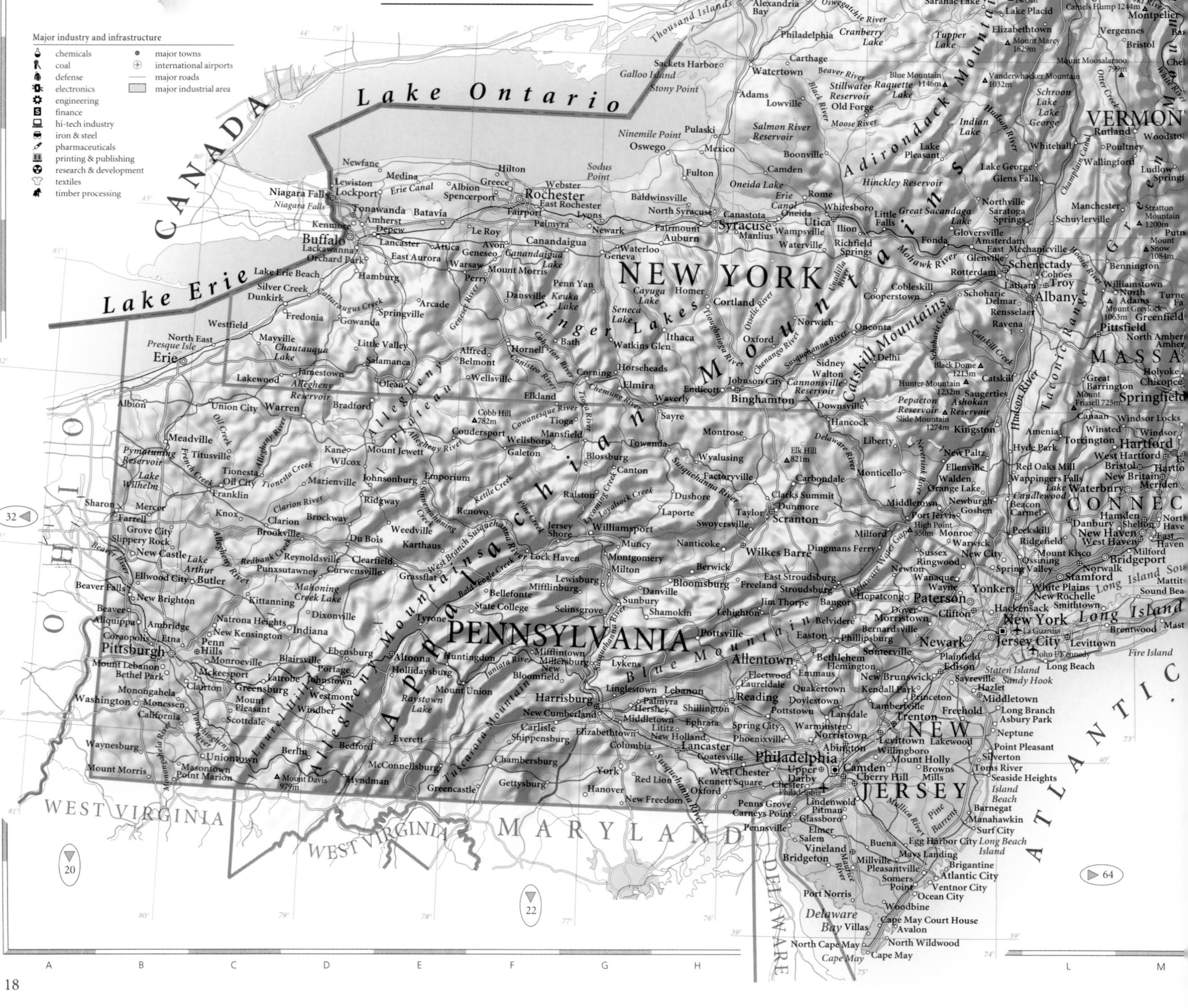

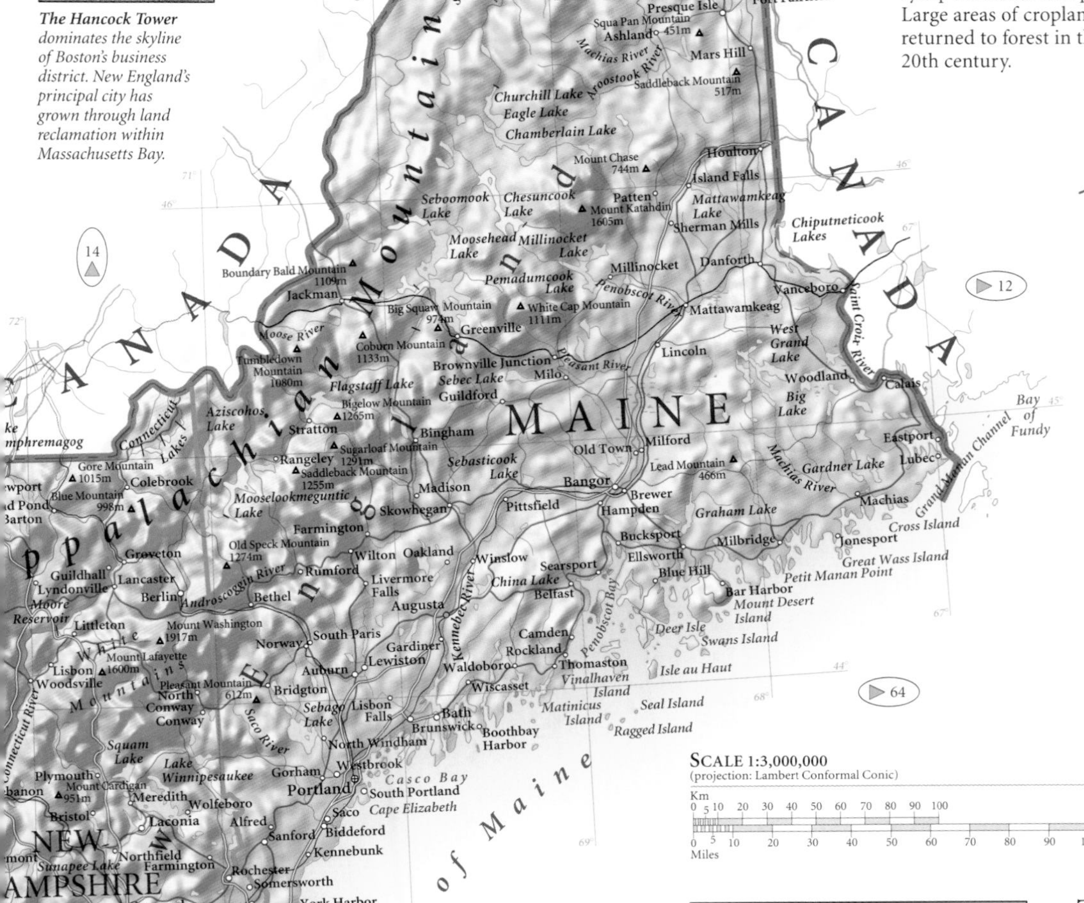

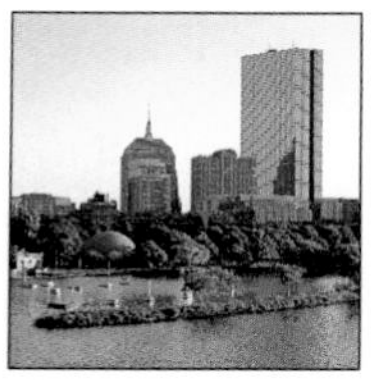

The Hancock Tower *dominates the skyline of Boston's business district. New England's principal city has grown through land reclamation within Massachusetts Bay.*

USING THE LAND AND SEA

PENNSYLVANIA HAS a large rural population and a major agribusiness sector dominated by livestock-raising. Fruit, vegetables, and nursery plants are grown throughout the region, with fishing on the coast. Cranberries and maple syrup are traditional products in New England. Large areas of cropland in the north were returned to forest in the 20th century.

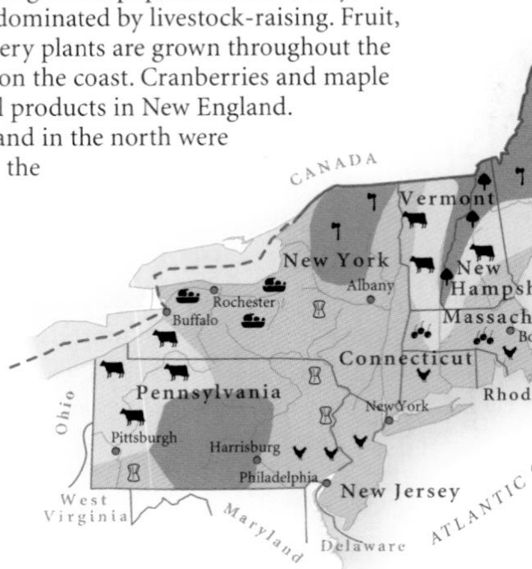

Land use and agricultural distribution

- cattle
- poultry
- cranberries
- fishing
- fodder
- fruit
- maple syrup
- timber
- major towns
- pasture
- cropland
- forest

THE URBAN/RURAL POPULATION DIVIDE

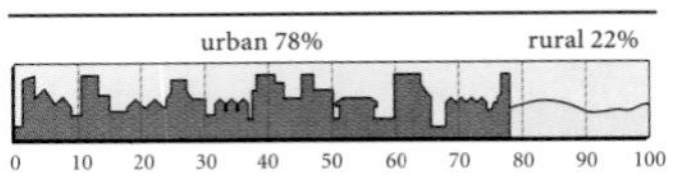

urban 78% | rural 22%

0 10 20 30 40 50 60 70 80 90 100

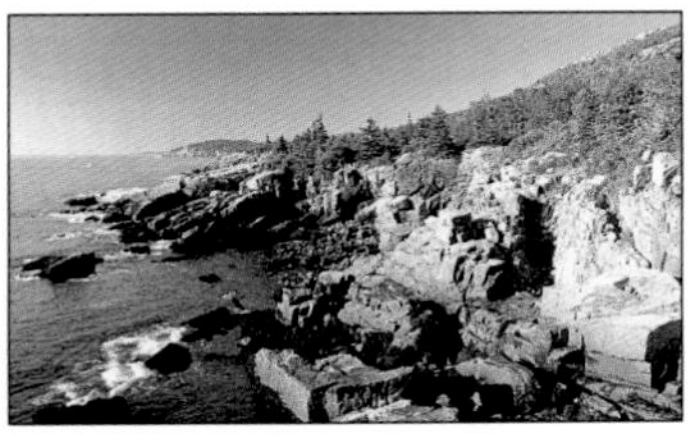

POPULATION DENSITY	TOTAL LAND AREA
306 people per sq mile (118 people per sq km)	161,096 sq miles (417,222 sq km)

Foreign competition *and depletion of stocks in the Atlantic fishing grounds caused a decline in fishing in the seaboard states. Recent years have seen a gradual recovery; Massachusetts now annually ranks third or fourth in the US in terms of the value of fish landed.*

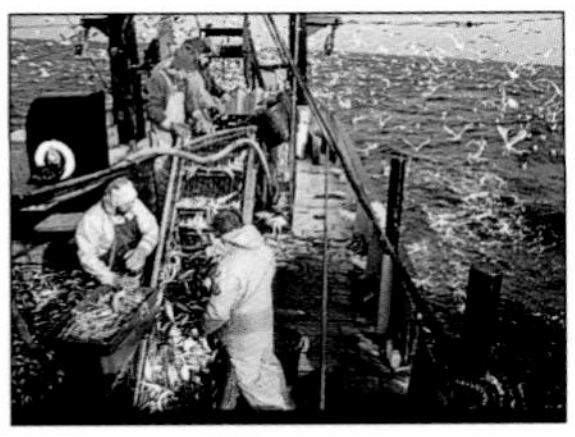

SCALE 1:3,000,000
(projection: Lambert Conformal Conic)

The islands, *inlets and promontories of Maine's coast extend 3,500 miles (5,630 km). The tidal range is particularly high, varying between 12 and 24 ft (3.7–7.3 m).*

THE LANDSCAPE

THE MARSHY LOWLANDS of the Atlantic Coastal Plain dwindle toward the north, giving way to the rocky coast of Maine. Uplifted over 400 million years ago, the Appalachian Mountains have since been carved into several discrete ranges by the region's main rivers and heavily denuded by successive glacial advances. This broad upland belt, with the younger Adirondack Mountains, is bounded by the Great Lakes in the northwest.

The narrow Finger Lakes of northwestern New York State were formed by glaciers cutting into deep deposits of material from an earlier ice advance.

The Adirondack Mountains were formed when the deeply buried basement rocks were forced upward in a dome by as much as 2 miles (3 km).

The lower Connecticut River has cut down into the flat, clay valley floor, which previously formed the bed of an ice-dammed lake.

Deposits of glacial till from the last Ice Age are up to 1000 ft (300 m) deep around Lake Ontario.

The Genesee river in New York State has eroded a canyon 800 ft (240 m) deep through the Appalachians. The river continued to cut downward as the land was uplifted.

Green Mountains

Niagara Falls

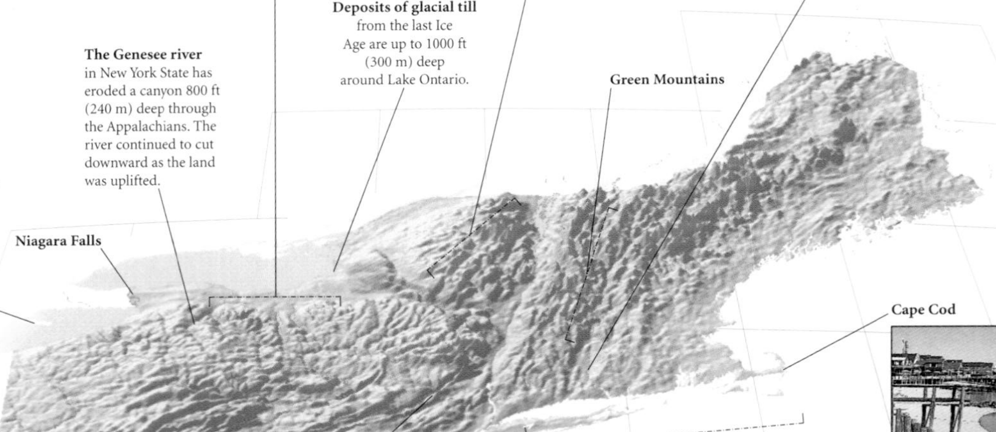

Lake Erie, receiving water flowing from the rest of the Great Lakes, drains via the Niagara Falls, into Lake Ontario, which lies 325 ft (99 m) below.

Cape Cod

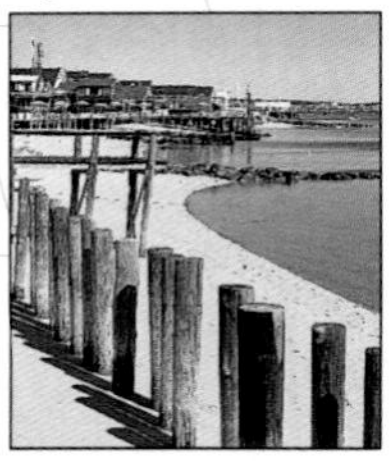

Resistant rock

River fed by water from the Great Lakes

Force of water continues to undercut cliffs

Softer rock is eroded more quickly

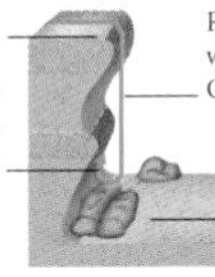

The Niagara Falls *were created where the Niagara River reached an escarpment capped by hard limestone. This was gradually eroded, exposing softer rock strata. Plunging water continues to erode the softer strata causing the falls to recede upstream.*

Dingmans Ferry

The waterfalls at Dingmans Ferry *are typical of those found in villages on the "Fall-line," where rivers drop from the Appalachians to the coastal lowlands. These locations provide waterpower and are often at the navigable head of the river.*

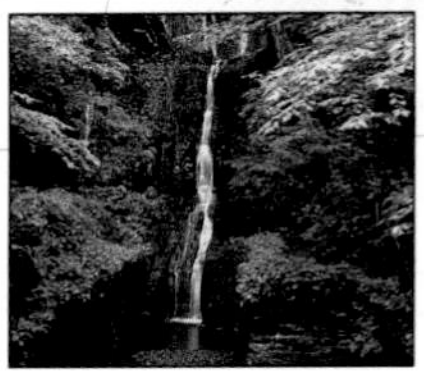

The Atlantic Coastal Plain is part of the continental shelf, which extends several hundred miles out to sea, providing a rich environment for marine life.

Rising sea levels have flooded river valleys along the coast, creating rias such as Long Island Sound.

Cape Cod, Long Island and the islands between them mark the top of a great terminal moraine, formed at the front of the ice sheet which once covered the land. This ridge of deposited material was subsequently flooded by rising seas.

At Provincetown, Cape Cod, *complex and powerful ocean currents continue to modify the shoreline, washing away some 3 ft (1 m) of the lower cape each year, while extending the beaches in the north.*

USA: MID-EASTERN STATES

Delaware, District of Columbia, Kentucky, Maryland, North Carolina, South Carolina, Tennessee, Virginia, West Virginia

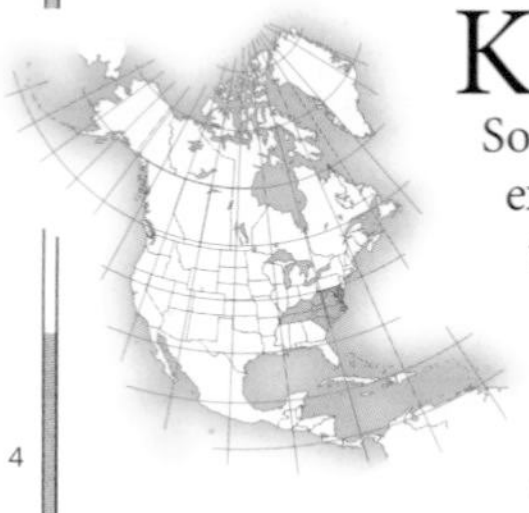

KEY EVENTS IN AMERICAN HISTORY took place in this diverse region, which became the front line between the North and the South during the Civil War of the 1860s. Strong regional contrasts exist between the fertile coastal plains, the isolated upcountry of the Appalachian Mountains, and the cotton-growing areas of the Mississippi lowlands to the west. While coal mining, a traditional industry in the Appalachians, has declined in recent years leaving much rural poverty, service industries elsewhere have increased, especially in Washington D.C, the nation's capital.

MAP KEY

POPULATION
- 500,000 to 1 million
- 100,000 to 500,000
- 50,000 to 100,000
- 10,000 to 50,000
- below 10,000

ELEVATION
- 6000m / 19,686ft
- 4000m / 13,124ft
- 3000m / 9843ft
- 2000m / 6562ft
- 1000m / 3281ft
- 500m / 1640ft
- 250m / 820ft
- 100m / 328ft
- sea level

SCALE 1:3,250,000
(projection: Lambert Conformal Conic)

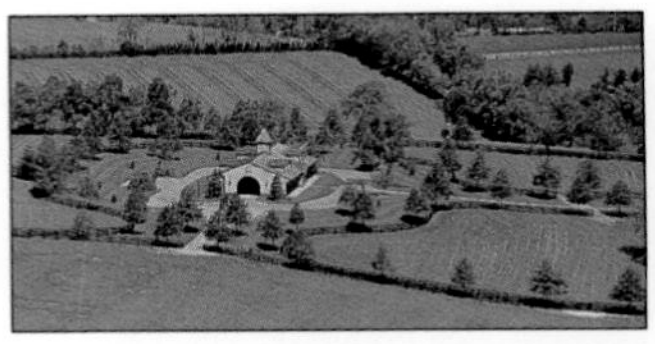

The Bluegrass region of Kentucky centers on the town of Lexington. This exceptionally fertile rolling plain is well known for its thoroughbred horse-breeding ranches.

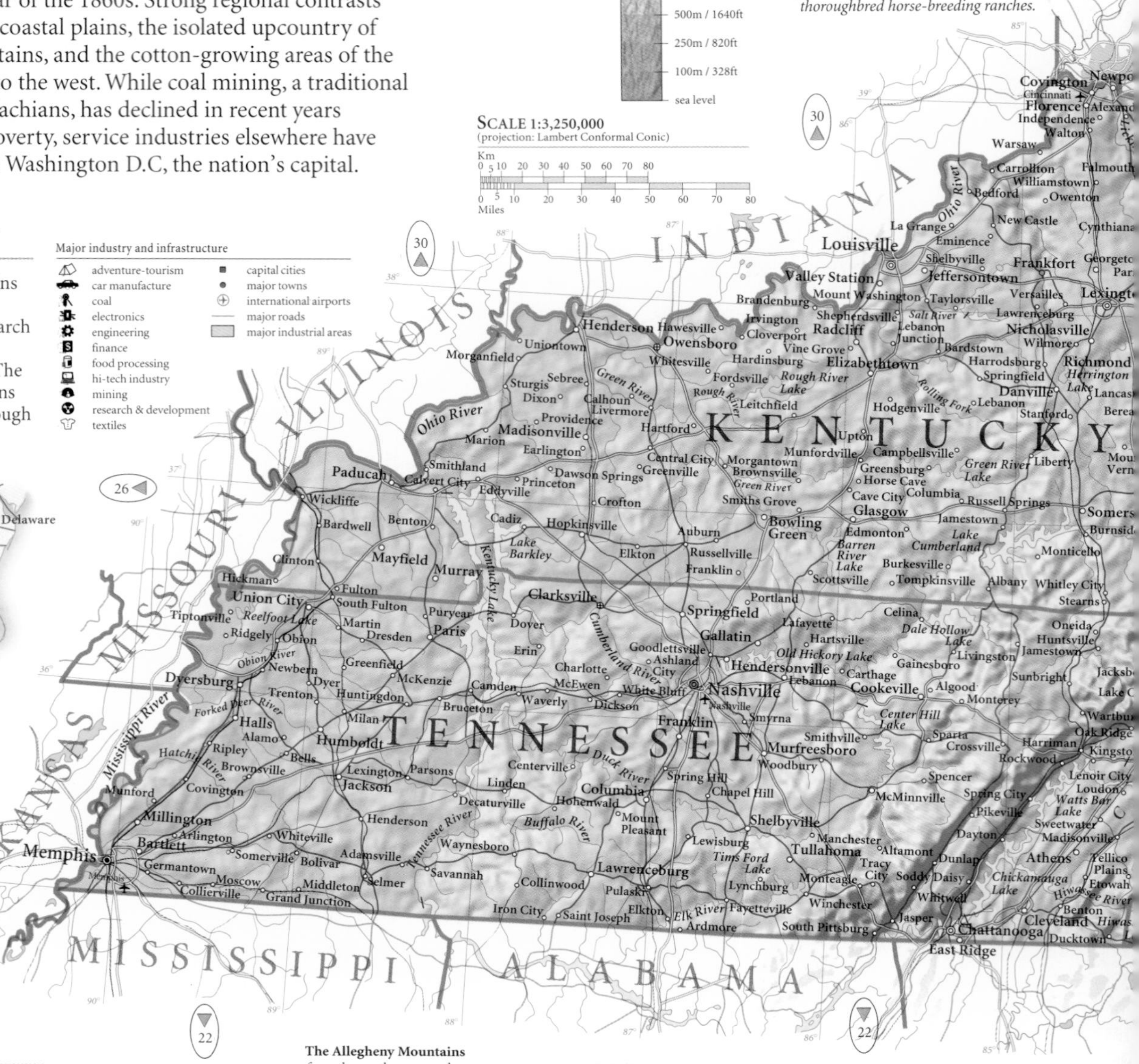

TRANSPORTATION & INDUSTRY

IN THE URBANIZED NORTHEAST, manufacturing remains important, alongside a burgeoning service sector. North Carolina is a major center for industrial research and development. Traditional industries include Tennessee whiskey and textiles in South Carolina. The decline of open-cast coal mining in the Appalachians has been hastened by environmental controls, although adventure-tourism is a flourishing new industry.

Major industry and infrastructure
- adventure-tourism
- car manufacture
- coal
- electronics
- engineering
- finance
- food processing
- hi-tech industry
- mining
- research & development
- textiles
- capital cities
- major towns
- international airports
- major roads
- major industrial areas

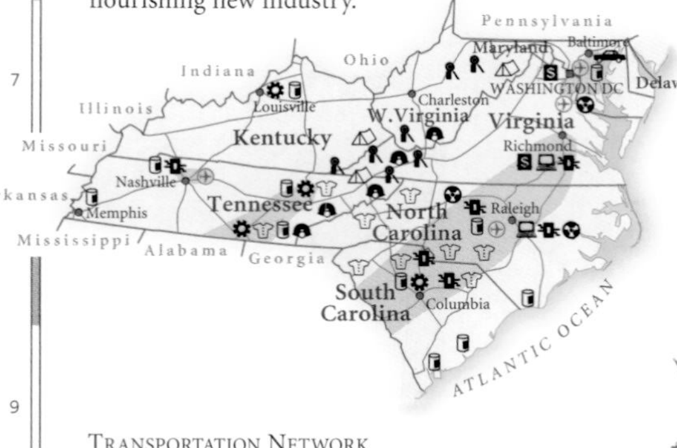

TRANSPORTATION NETWORK

452,218 miles (723,548 km)	5,737 miles (8,267 km)
18,336 miles (29,503 km)	4,404 miles (7,081 km)

Tennessee's rivers are part of an important inland bulk-transportation network. Memphis connects with New Orleans in the south, and with cities as distant as Minneapolis, Sioux City, Chicago, and Pittsburgh, via the Mississippi and its tributaries.

THE LANDSCAPE

THE EASTERN TRIBUTARIES OF THE MISSISSIPPI drain the interior lowlands. The Cumberland Plateau and the parallel ranges of the Appalachians have been successively uplifted and eroded over time, with the eastern side reduced to a series of foothills known as the Piedmont. The broad coastal plain gradually falls away into salt marshes, lagoons, and offshore bars, broken by flooded estuaries along the shores of the Atlantic.

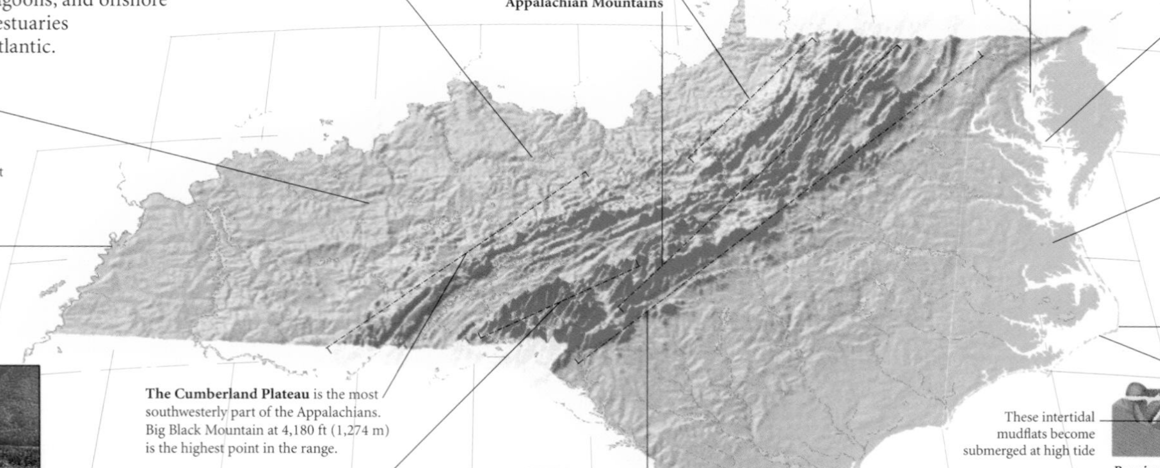

The Mammoth Cave is part of an extensive cave system in the limestone region of southwestern Kentucky. It stretches for over 300 miles (485 km) on five different levels and contains three rivers and three lakes.

The Mississippi River and its tributary the Ohio River form the western border of the region.

Natural Bridge in eastern Kentucky is an arch 78 ft (26 m) long and 65 ft (20 m) high. It has been shaped from resistant sandstone by gradual weathering processes, which removed the softer rock lying underneath.

The Allegheny Mountains form the northwestern edge of the Appalachian mountain chain. Continuous folding has formed rich seams of bituminous coal.

Appalachian Mountains

Farmland on the eastern shores of Chesapeake Bay is sustained by artificial drainage. The area also provides refuge for a variety of waterfowl.

The many inlets of Chesapeake Bay are the flooded tributaries of the main river valley, which have been inundated by rising sea levels.

Salt marshes such as Great Dismal Swamp, develop where the coast is sheltered. Vast areas of such marshland have been reclaimed for farmland and settlement.

Cape Hatteras is the easternmost point of an offshore barrier island; a wave-deposited sand-bar which has become permanent, establishing its own vegetation.

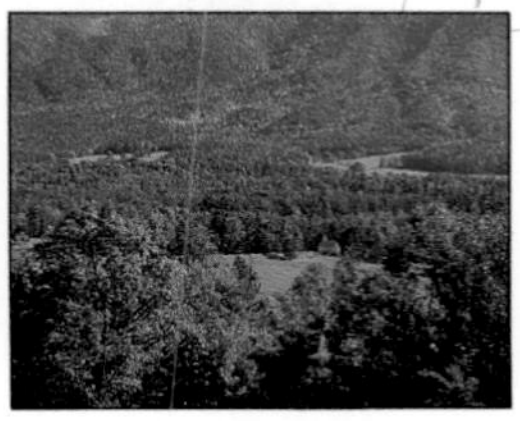

Barrier islands

Tidal inlet

Barrier island

These intertidal mudflats become submerged at high tide

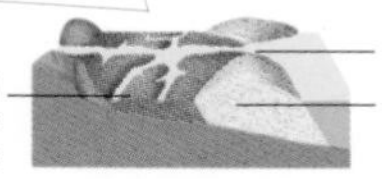

Barrier islands are common along the coasts of North and South Carolina. As sea levels rise, wave action builds up ridges of sand and pebbles parallel to the coast, separated by lagoons or intertidal mudflats, which are flooded at high tide.

The Cumberland Plateau is the most southwesterly part of the Appalachians. Big Black Mountain at 4,180 ft (1,274 m) is the highest point in the range.

The Great Smoky Mountains form the western escarpment of the Appalachians. The region is heavily forested, with over 130 species of tree.

The Blue Ridge Mountains are a steep ridge, culminating in Mount Mitchell, the highest point in the Appalachians, at 6,684 ft (2,037 m).

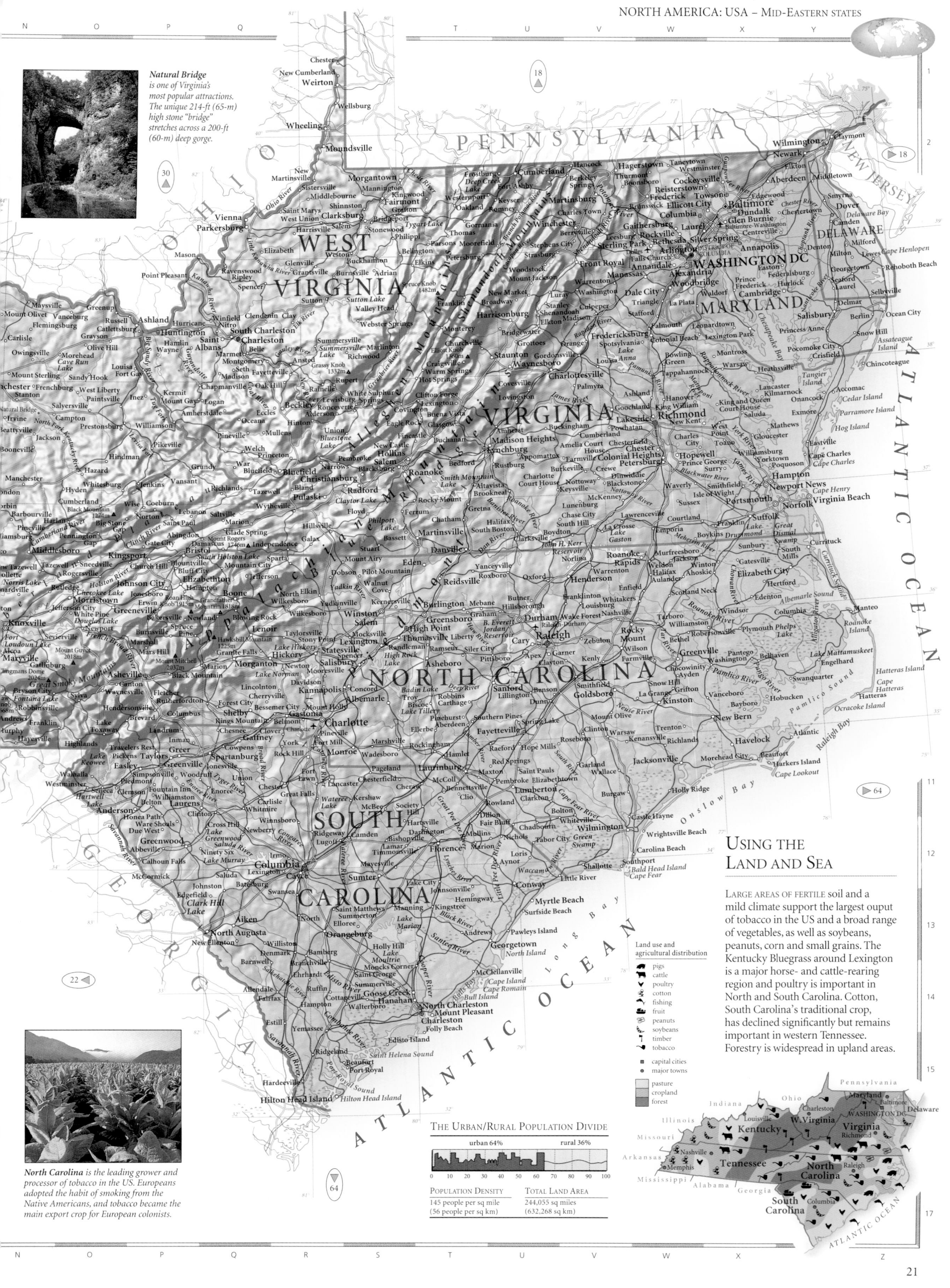
PENNSYLVANIA
OHIO
WEST VIRGINIA
VIRGINIA
MARYLAND
DELAWARE
NEW JERSEY
NORTH CAROLINA
SOUTH CAROLINA
GEORGIA
ATLANTIC OCEAN
WASHINGTON DC
Appalachian Mountains
Allegheny Mountains
Blue Ridge
Shenandoah Mountains
Chesapeake Bay
Albemarle Sound
Pamlico Sound
Onslow Bay
Long Bay
Land use and agricultural distribution
pigs
cattle
poultry
cotton
fishing
fruit
peanuts
soybeans
timber
tobacco
capital cities
major towns
pasture
cropland
forest
Pennsylvania
Ohio
Indiana
Illinois
Missouri
Arkansas
Mississippi
Alabama
Georgia
Kentucky
W.Virginia
Virginia
Tennessee
North Carolina
South Carolina
Maryland
Delaware
Louisville
Charleston
Baltimore
Richmond
Nashville
Memphis
Raleigh
Columbia
ATLANTIC OCEAN

Natural Bridge *is one of Virginia's most popular attractions. The unique 214-ft (65-m) high stone "bridge" stretches across a 200-ft (60-m) deep gorge.*

North Carolina *is the leading grower and processor of tobacco in the US. Europeans adopted the habit of smoking from the Native Americans, and tobacco became the main export crop for European colonists.*

Using the Land and Sea

Large areas of fertile soil and a mild climate support the largest ouput of tobacco in the US and a broad range of vegetables, as well as soybeans, peanuts, corn and small grains. The Kentucky Bluegrass around Lexington is a major horse- and cattle-rearing region and poultry is important in North and South Carolina. Cotton, South Carolina's traditional crop, has declined significantly but remains important in western Tennessee. Forestry is widespread in upland areas.

The Urban/Rural Population Divide

urban 64% | rural 36%

0 10 20 30 40 50 60 70 80 90 100

Population Density	Total Land Area
145 people per sq mile (56 people per sq km)	244,055 sq miles (632,268 sq km)

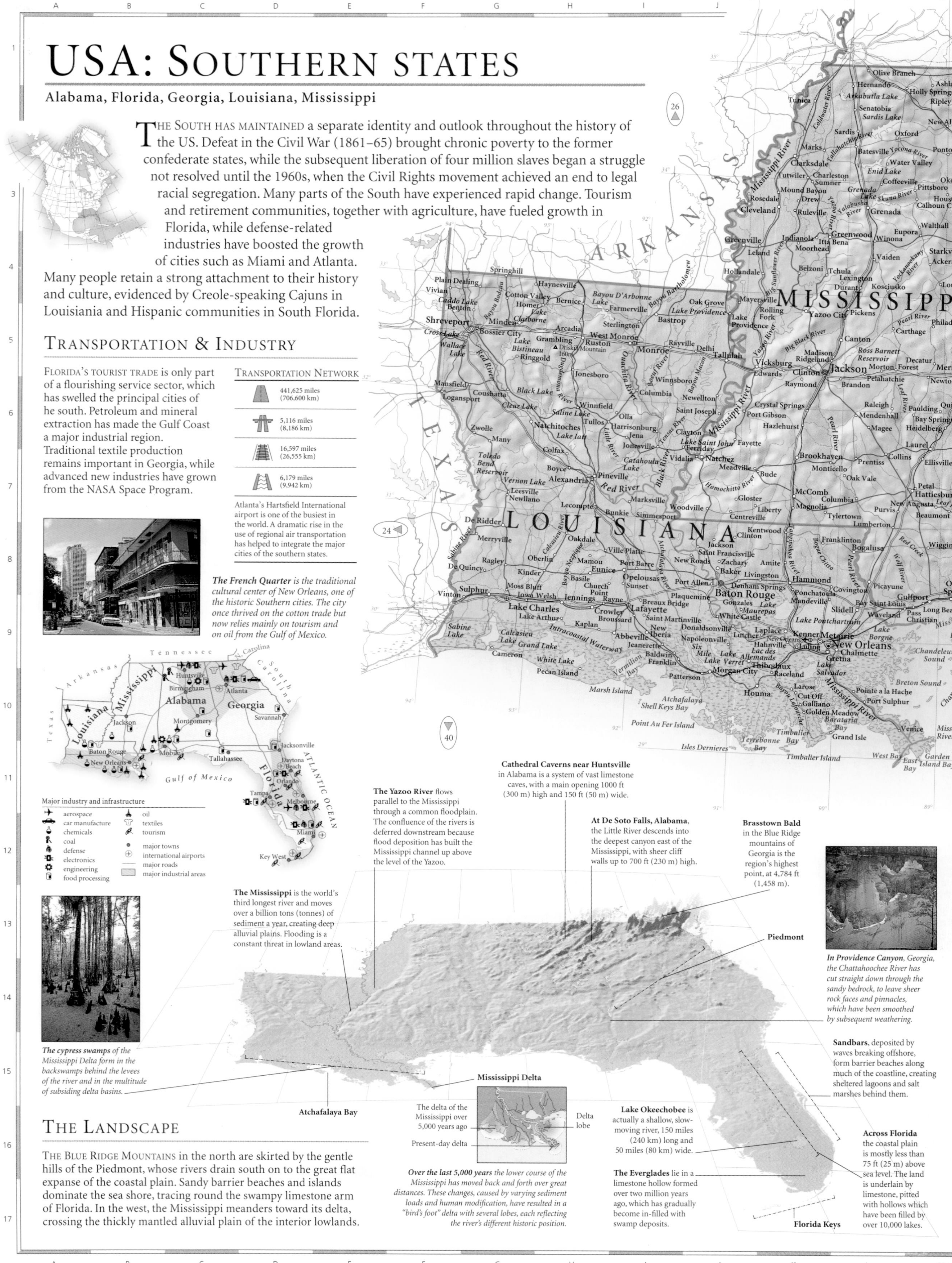

USA: Southern states

Alabama, Florida, Georgia, Louisiana, Mississippi

THE SOUTH HAS MAINTAINED a separate identity and outlook throughout the history of the US. Defeat in the Civil War (1861–65) brought chronic poverty to the former confederate states, while the subsequent liberation of four million slaves began a struggle not resolved until the 1960s, when the Civil Rights movement achieved an end to legal racial segregation. Many parts of the South have experienced rapid change. Tourism and retirement communities, together with agriculture, have fueled growth in Florida, while defense-related industries have boosted the growth of cities such as Miami and Atlanta. Many people retain a strong attachment to their history and culture, evidenced by Creole-speaking Cajuns in Louisiana and Hispanic communities in South Florida.

Transportation & Industry

FLORIDA'S TOURIST TRADE is only part of a flourishing service sector, which has swelled the principal cities of he south. Petroleum and mineral extraction has made the Gulf Coast a major industrial region. Traditional textile production remains important in Georgia, while advanced new industries have grown from the NASA Space Program.

Transportation Network

441,625 miles (706,600 km)

5,116 miles (8,186 km)

16,597 miles (26,555 km)

6,179 miles (9,942 km)

Atlanta's Hartsfield International airport is one of the busiest in the world. A dramatic rise in the use of regional air transportation has helped to integrate the major cities of the southern states.

The French Quarter is the traditional cultural center of New Orleans, one of the historic Southern cities. The city once thrived on the cotton trade but now relies mainly on tourism and on oil from the Gulf of Mexico.

Major industry and infrastructure

aerospace
car manufacture
chemicals
coal
defense
electronics
engineering
food processing
oil
textiles
tourism
major towns
international airports
major roads
major industrial areas

The cypress swamps of the Mississippi Delta form in the backswamps behind the levees of the river and in the multitude of subsiding delta basins.

Cathedral Caverns near Huntsville in Alabama is a system of vast limestone caves, with a main opening 1000 ft (300 m) high and 150 ft (50 m) wide.

The Yazoo River flows parallel to the Mississippi through a common floodplain. The confluence of the rivers is deferred downstream because flood deposition has built the Mississippi channel up above the level of the Yazoo.

At De Soto Falls, Alabama, the Little River descends into the deepest canyon east of the Mississippi, with sheer cliff walls up to 700 ft (230 m) high.

Brasstown Bald in the Blue Ridge mountains of Georgia is the region's highest point, at 4,784 ft (1,458 m).

The Mississippi is the world's third longest river and moves over a billion tons (tonnes) of sediment a year, creating deep alluvial plains. Flooding is a constant threat in lowland areas.

Piedmont

In Providence Canyon, Georgia, the Chattahoochee River has cut straight down through the sandy bedrock, to leave sheer rock faces and pinnacles, which have been smoothed by subsequent weathering.

Sandbars, deposited by waves breaking offshore, form barrier beaches along much of the coastline, creating sheltered lagoons and salt marshes behind them.

Mississippi Delta

The delta of the Mississippi over 5,000 years ago

Present-day delta

Delta lobe

Atchafalaya Bay

Over the last 5,000 years the lower course of the Mississippi has moved back and forth over great distances. These changes, caused by varying sediment loads and human modification, have resulted in a "bird's foot" delta with several lobes, each reflecting the river's different historic position.

Lake Okeechobee is actually a shallow, slow-moving river, 150 miles (240 km) long and 50 miles (80 km) wide.

The Everglades lie in a limestone hollow formed over two million years ago, which has gradually become in-filled with swamp deposits.

Florida Keys

Across Florida the coastal plain is mostly less than 75 ft (25 m) above sea level. The land is underlain by limestone, pitted with hollows which have been filled by over 10,000 lakes.

The Landscape

THE BLUE RIDGE MOUNTAINS in the north are skirted by the gentle hills of the Piedmont, whose rivers drain south on to the great flat expanse of the coastal plain. Sandy barrier beaches and islands dominate the sea shore, tracing round the swampy limestone arm of Florida. In the west, the Mississippi meanders toward its delta, crossing the thickly mantled alluvial plain of the interior lowlands.

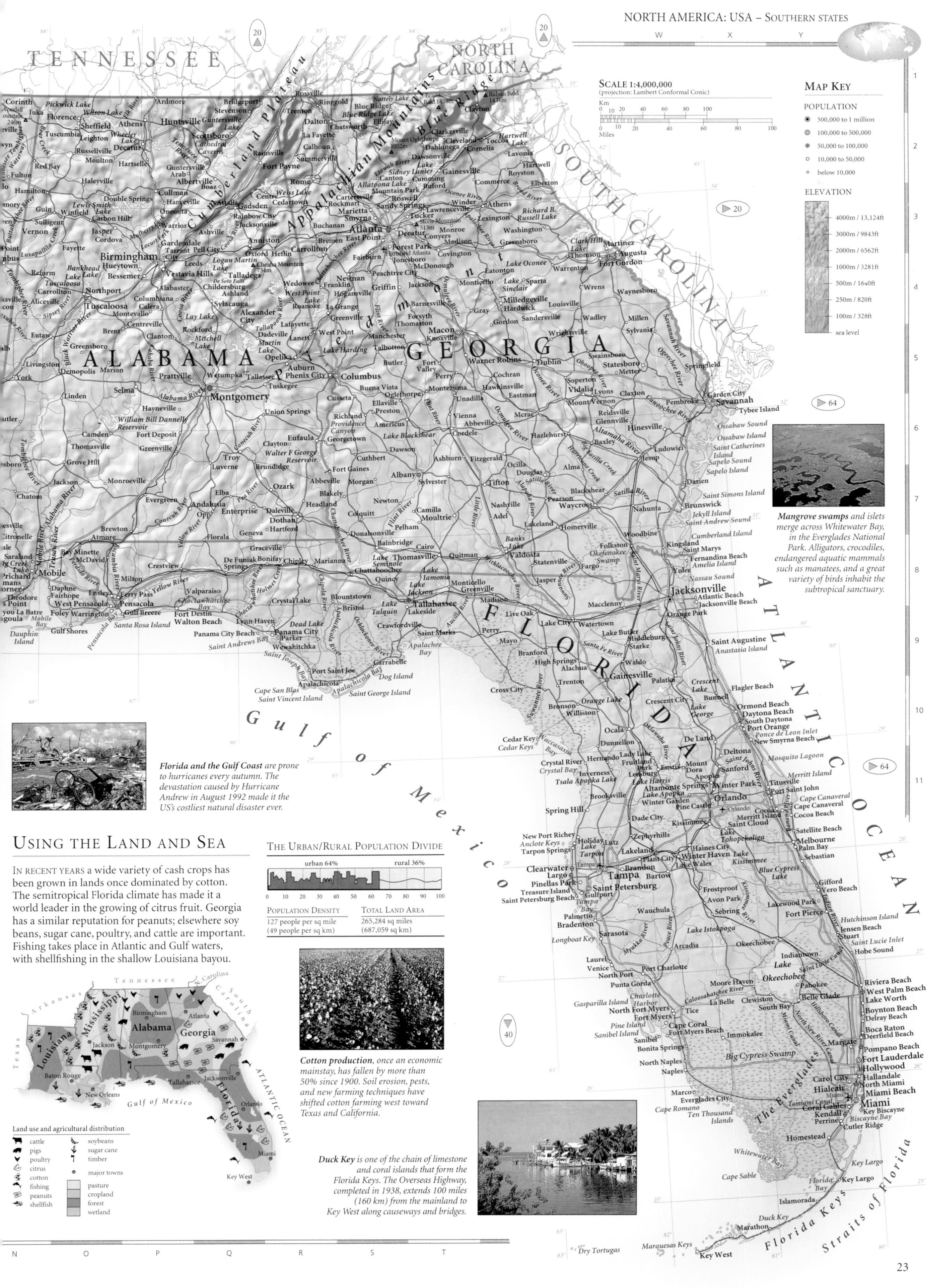
TENNESSEE
NORTH CAROLINA
SOUTH CAROLINA
ALABAMA
GEORGIA
FLORIDA
ATLANTIC OCEAN
Gulf of Mexico
Straits of Florida
Florida Keys
SCALE 1:4,000,000
(projection: Lambert Conformal Conic)
MAP KEY
POPULATION
500,000 to 1 million
100,000 to 500,000
50,000 to 100,000
10,000 to 50,000
below 10,000
ELEVATION
4000m / 13,124ft
3000m / 9843ft
2000m / 6562ft
1000m / 3281ft
500m / 1640ft
250m / 820ft
100m / 328ft
sea level
Land use and agricultural distribution
cattle
pigs
poultry
citrus
cotton
fishing
peanuts
shellfish
soybeans
sugar cane
timber
major towns
pasture
cropland
forest
wetland

Florida and the Gulf Coast are prone to hurricanes every autumn. The devastation caused by Hurricane Andrew in August 1992 made it the US's costliest natural disaster ever.

Mangrove swamps *and islets merge across Whitewater Bay, in the Everglades National Park. Alligators, crocodiles, endangered aquatic mammals such as manatees, and a great variety of birds inhabit the subtropical sanctuary.*

Using the Land and Sea

In recent years a wide variety of cash crops has been grown in lands once dominated by cotton. The semitropical Florida climate has made it a world leader in the growing of citrus fruit. Georgia has a similar reputation for peanuts; elsewhere soy beans, sugar cane, poultry, and cattle are important. Fishing takes place in Atlantic and Gulf waters, with shellfishing in the shallow Louisiana bayou.

The Urban/Rural Population Divide

urban 64% — rural 36%

Population Density	Total Land Area
127 people per sq mile (49 people per sq km)	265,284 sq miles (687,059 sq km)

Cotton production, *once an economic mainstay, has fallen by more than 50% since 1900. Soil erosion, pests, and new farming techniques have shifted cotton farming west toward Texas and California.*

Duck Key *is one of the chain of limestone and coral islands that form the Florida Keys. The Overseas Highway, completed in 1938, extends 100 miles (160 km) from the mainland to Key West along causeways and bridges.*

USA: Texas

First explored by Spaniards moving north from Mexico in search of gold, Texas was controlled by Spain and then by Mexico, before becoming an independent republic in 1836, and joining the Union of States in 1845. During the 19th century, many migrants who came to Texas raised cattle on the abundant land; in the 20th century, they were joined by prospectors attracted by the promise of oil riches. Today, although natural resources, especially oil, still form the basis of its wealth, the diversified Texan economy includes thriving hi-tech and financial industries. The major urban centers, home to 80% of the population, lie in the south and east, and include Houston, the "oil-city," and Dallas Fort Worth. Hispanic influences remain strong, especially in southern and western Texas.

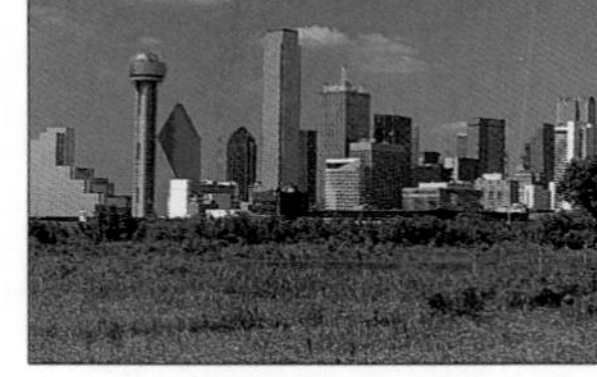

***Dallas was founded** in 1841 as a prairie trading post and its development was stimulated by the arrival of railroads. Cotton and then oil funded the town's early growth. Today, the modern, high-rise skyline of Dallas reflects the city's position as a leading center of banking, insurance, and the petroleum industry in the southwest.*

Using the Land

Cotton production and livestock-raising, particularly cattle, dominate farming, although crop failures and the demands of local markets have led to some diversification. Following the introduction of modern farming techniques, cotton production spread out from the east to the plains of western Texas. Cattle ranches are widespread, while sheep and goats are raised on the dry Edwards Plateau.

Land use and agricultural distribution

- cattle
- goats
- sheep
- cereals
- cotton
- major towns
- pasture
- cropland
- forest
- barren

The Urban/Rural Population Divide

urban 80% | rural 20%

0 10 20 30 40 50 60 70 80 90 100

Population Density	Total Land Area
73 people per sq mile (28 people per sq km)	267,338 sq miles (692,402 sq km)

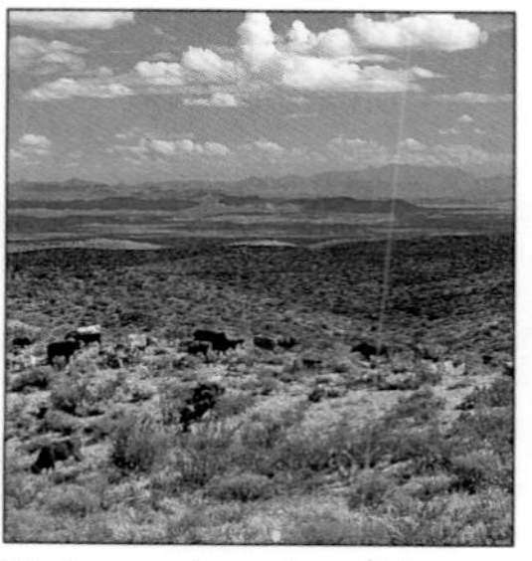

***The huge cattle ranches of Texas** developed during the 19th century when land was plentiful and could be acquired cheaply. Today, more cattle and sheep are raised in Texas than in any other state.*

Oklahoma · Arkansas · New Mexico · Louisiana · Amarillo · Dallas · El Paso · Texas · Austin · Houston · San Antonio · MEXICO

The Landscape

Texas is made up of a series of massive steps descending from the mountains and high plains of the west and northwest to the coastal lowlands in the southeast. Many of the state's borders are delineated by water. The Rio Grande flows from the Rocky Mountains to the Gulf of Mexico, marking the border with Mexico.

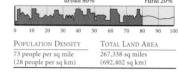

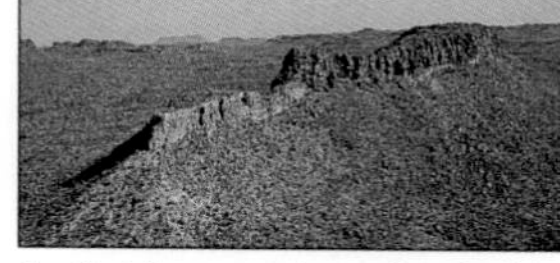

***Cap Rock Escarpment** juts out from the plains, running 200 miles (320 km) from north to south. Its height varies from 300 ft (90 m) rising to sheer cliffs up to 1,000 ft (300 m).*

40 ◀

36 ◀

The Llano Estacado or Staked Plain in northern Texas is known for its harsh environment. In the north, freezing winds carrying ice and snow sweep down from the Rocky Mountains. To the south, sandstorms frequently blow up, scouring anything in their paths. Flash floods, in the wide, flat riverbeds that remain dry for most of the year, are another hazard.

The Guadalupe Mountains lie in the southern Rocky Mountains. They incorporate Guadalupe Peak, the highest in Texas, rising 8,749 ft (2,667 m).

The Red River flows for 1300 miles (2090 km), marking most of the northern border of Texas. A dam and reservoir along its course provide vital irrigation and hydro-electric power to the surrounding area.

The Rio Grande flows from the Rocky Mountains through semi-arid land, supporting sparse vegetation. The river actually shrinks along its course, losing more water through evaporation and seepage than it gains from its tributaries and rainfall.

Sabine River

Extensive forests of pine and cypress grow in the eastern corner of the coastal lowlands where the average rainfall is 45 inches (1145 mm) a year. This is higher than the rest of the state and over twice the average in the west.

In the coastal lowlands of southeastern Texas the Earth's crust is warping, causing the land to subside and allowing the sea to invade. Around Galveston, the rate of downward tilting is 6 inches (15 cm) per year. Erosion of the coast is also exacerbated by hurricanes.

Big Bend National Park

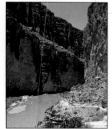

Edwards Plateau is a limestone outcrop. It is part of the Great Plains, bounded to the southeast by the Balcones Escarpment, which marks the southerly limit of the plains.

Flowing through 1,500 ft (450 m) high gorges, the shallow, muddy Rio Grande makes a 90° bend. This marks the southern border of Big Bend National Park, and gives it its name. The area is a mixture of forested mountains, deserts, and canyons.

Laguna Madre in southern Texas has been almost completely cut off from the sea by Padre Island. This sand bank was created by wave action, carrying and depositing material along the coast. The process is known as longshore drift.

Padre Island

Oil deposits

Oil trapped by fault

Oil deposits migrate through reservoir rocks such as shale

Oil accumulates beneath impermeable cap rock

Impermeable rock strata

Salt dome

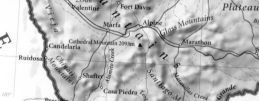

***Oil deposits** are found beneath much of Texas. They collect as oil migrates upward through porous layers of rock until it is trapped, either by a cap of rock above a salt dome, or by a fault line which exposes impermeable rock through which the oil cannot rise.*

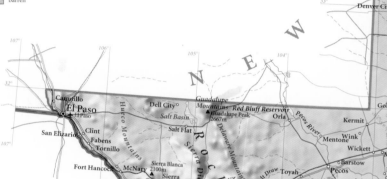

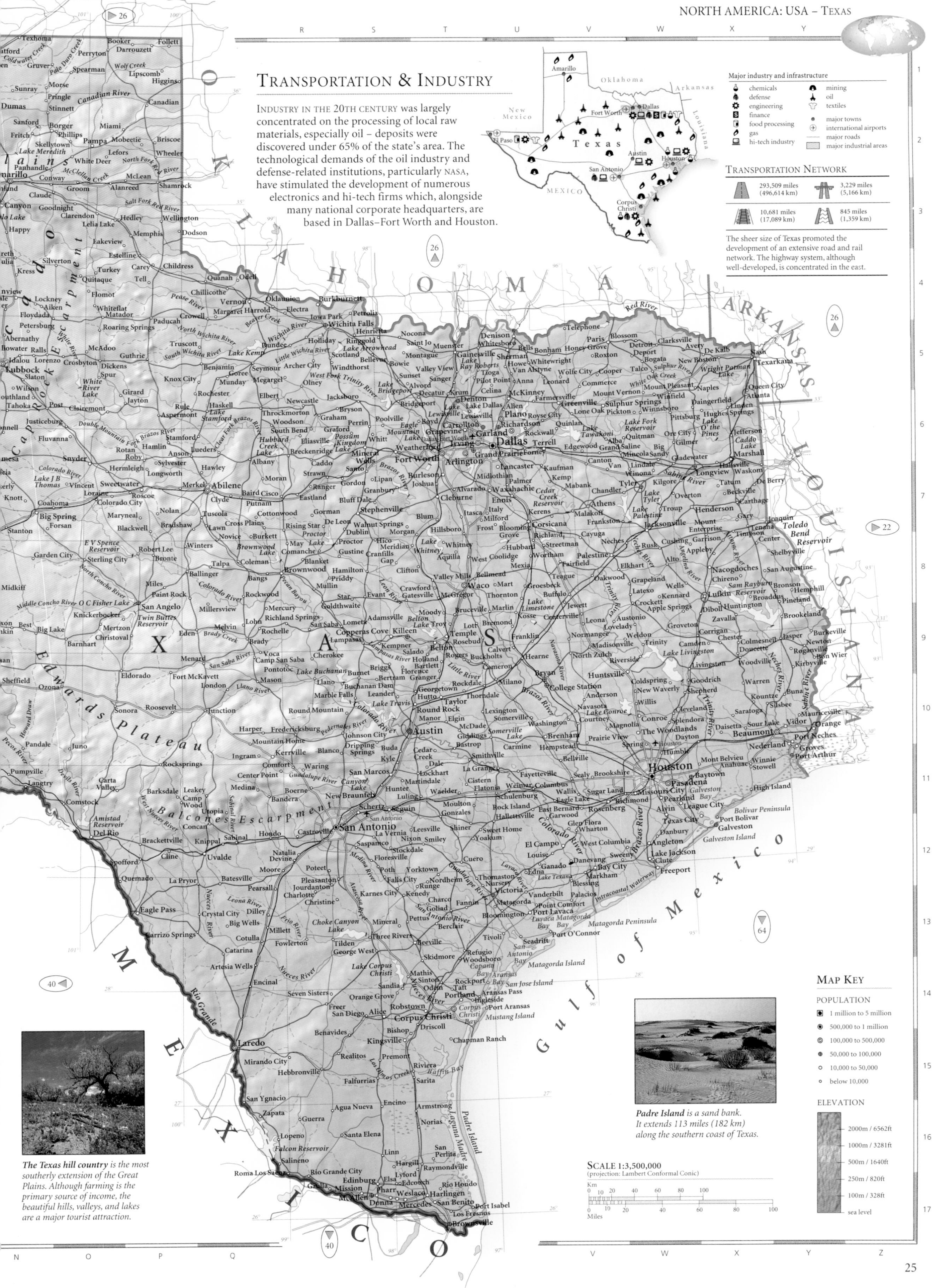
TRANSPORTATION & INDUSTRY
INDUSTRY IN THE 20TH CENTURY was largely concentrated on the processing of local raw materials, especially oil – deposits were discovered under 65% of the state's area. The technological demands of the oil industry and defense-related institutions, particularly NASA, have stimulated the development of numerous electronics and hi-tech firms which, alongside many national corporate headquarters, are based in Dallas–Fort Worth and Houston.
Major industry and infrastructure
chemicals
defense
engineering
finance
food processing
gas
hi-tech industry
mining
oil
textiles
major towns
international airports
major roads
major industrial areas
TRANSPORTATION NETWORK
293,509 miles (496,614 km)
3,229 miles (5,166 km)
10,681 miles (17,089 km)
845 miles (1,359 km)
The sheer size of Texas promoted the development of an extensive road and rail network. The highway system, although well-developed, is concentrated in the east.
OKLAHOMA
ARKANSAS
LOUISIANA
TEXAS
MEXICO
Gulf of Mexico
Edwards Plateau
Balcones Escarpment
Dallas
Fort Worth
Austin
Houston
San Antonio
Corpus Christi
El Paso
Amarillo
Lubbock
Laredo
Brownsville
MAP KEY
POPULATION
1 million to 5 million
500,000 to 1 million
100,000 to 500,000
50,000 to 100,000
10,000 to 50,000
below 10,000
ELEVATION
2000m / 6562ft
1000m / 3281ft
500m / 1640ft
250m / 820ft
100m / 328ft
sea level
SCALE 1:3,500,000
(projection: Lambert Conformal Conic)

Padre Island is a sand bank. It extends 113 miles (182 km) along the southern coast of Texas.

The Texas hill country is the most southerly extension of the Great Plains. Although farming is the primary source of income, the beautiful hills, valleys, and lakes are a major tourist attraction.

USA: South Midwestern States

Arkansas, Kansas, Missouri, Oklahoma

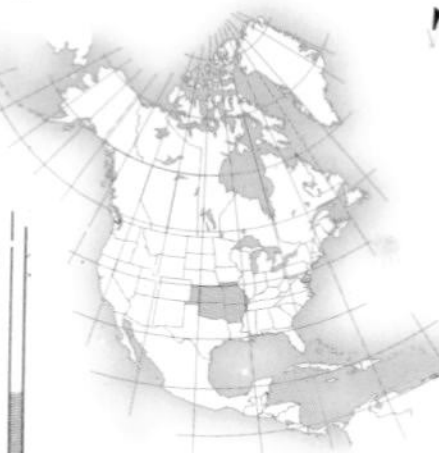

The expansion of the US focused on this region in the mid-19th century. Settlers spread from the confluence of the Missouri and Mississippi Rivers up onto the Great Plains. This treeless expanse, which early explorers had called the Great American Desert was turned into one of the world's richest agricultural regions. But periodic droughts, coupled with overintensive farming, led to the "dustbowl" soil erosion crisis of the 1930s, the abandonment of many farms, and a mass exodus to the west coast. The land has since recovered, although the mechanization of agriculture has led to a decline in the rural population. In recent years, suburban residential development has spread rapidly across the wooded Ozark Plateau in the east of the region.

Transportation & Industry

The processing of agricultural products, such as brewing and meatpacking, has been traditionally important in these states. In Kansas and Oklahoma, diversified manufacturing now supplements income from fossil fuels; Wichita has become a world center for aeronautical engineering, an industry which also employs many people in neighboring Missouri.

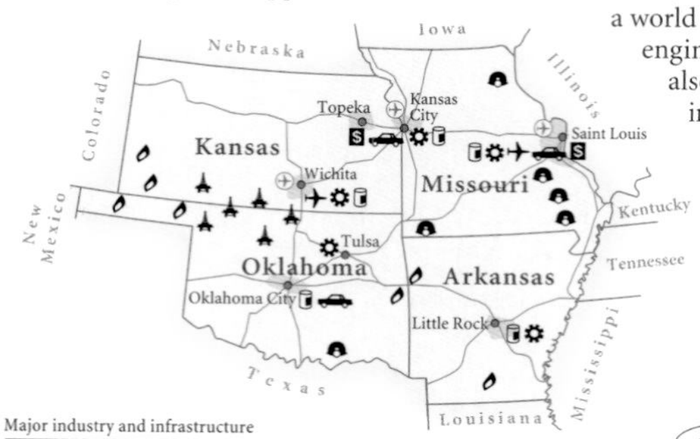

Nebraska, Iowa, Illinois, Colorado, Kansas, Topeka, Kansas City, Saint Louis, Wichita, Missouri, Kentucky, New Mexico, Tulsa, Oklahoma, Oklahoma City, Arkansas, Tennessee, Little Rock, Mississippi, Texas, Louisiana

Major industry and infrastructure

- aerospace
- engineering
- finance
- food processing
- gas
- mining
- oil
- vehicle manufacture
- major towns
- international airports
- major roads
- major industrial areas

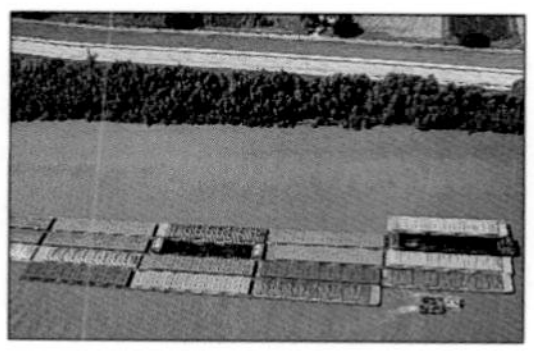

Agricultural produce from the plains is moved by barges along the Mississippi. The river now carries a far greater tonnage of freight than any other waterway system in the US.

Transportation Network

380,307 miles (608,491 km)	4068 miles (6508 km)
16,185 miles (25,896 km)	1994 miles (3208 km)

The Arkansas River and its tributaries allow access to over half of the US's navigable inland waterways. A system of locks and dams along the river provides Tulsa, in Oklahom, with a navigable water route to the Gulf of Mexico.

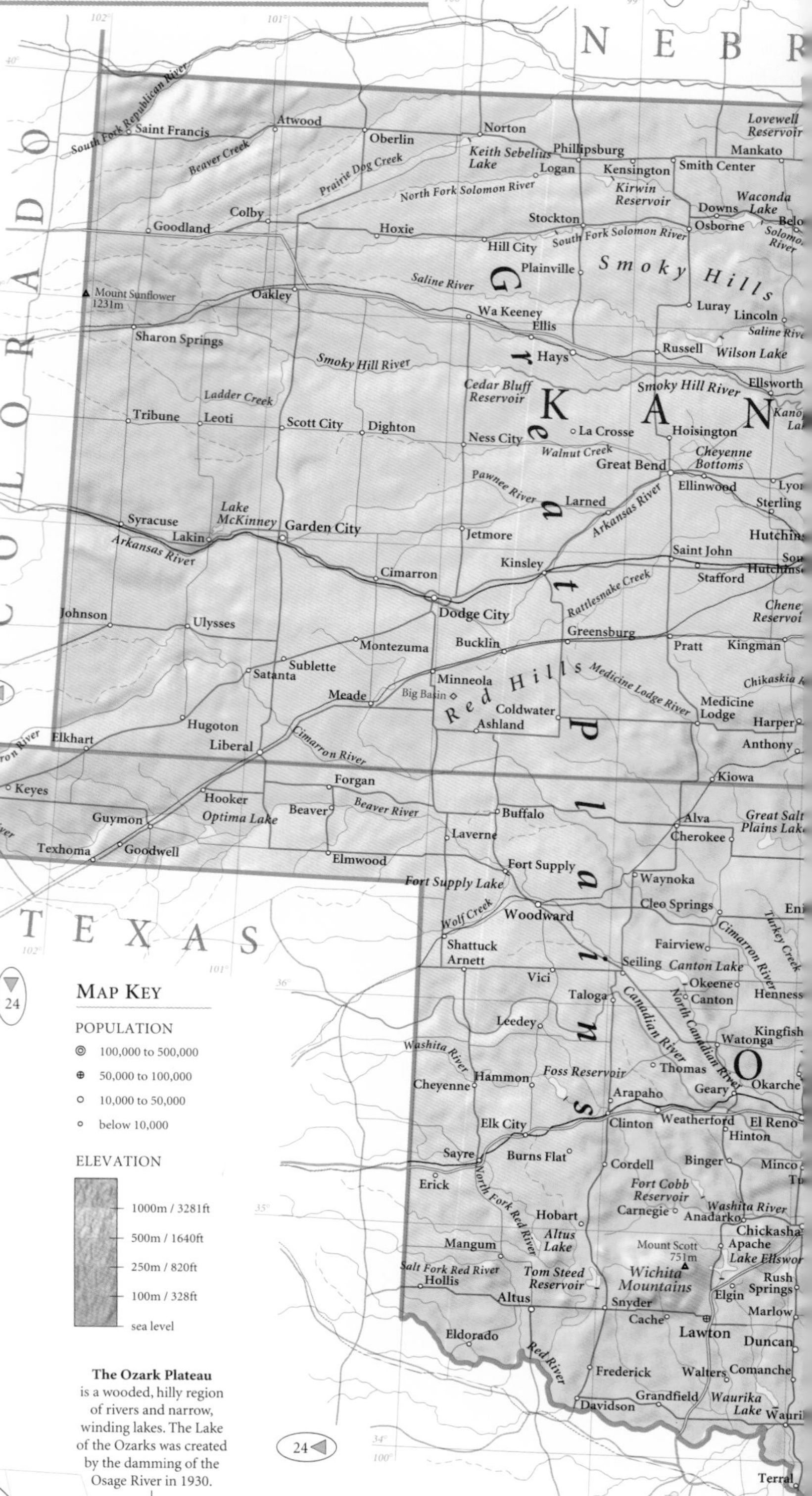

Map Key

Population

- 100,000 to 500,000
- 50,000 to 100,000
- 10,000 to 50,000
- below 10,000

Elevation

- 1000m / 3281ft
- 500m / 1640ft
- 250m / 820ft
- 100m / 328ft
- sea level

SCALE 1:3,250,000
(projection: Lambert Conformal Conic)

Km 0 5 10 20 30 40 50 60 70
Miles 0 5 10 20 30 40 50 60 70

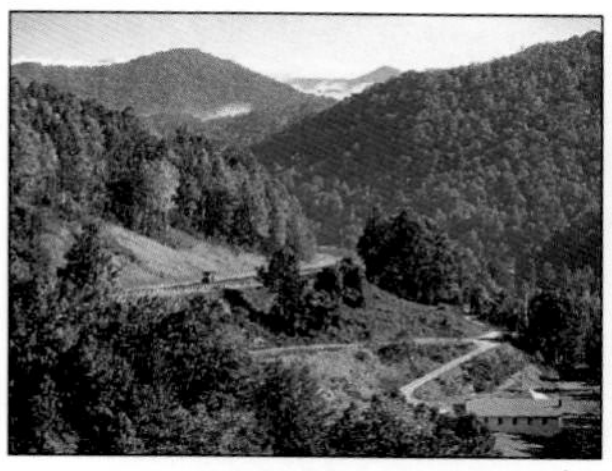

28 24 36 36 24

The Landscape

Most of the region consists of high, treeless plains, which gradually descend east from the Rocky Mountains. Drainage follows this slope, with rivers flowing toward the alluvial lowlands of the Mississippi in the southeast. Between the plains and the lowlands lie various ranges of wooded hills, including the deeply incised Ozark Plateau.

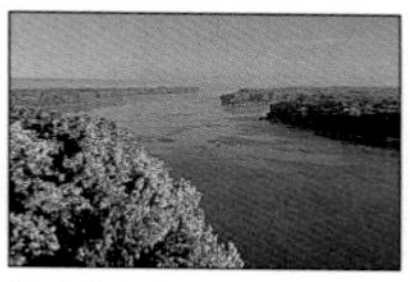

The Mississippi, North America's longest river, is joined by the Missouri, its main tributary, on a flood plain which spreads south to the Gulf of Mexico.

The Ozark Plateau is a wooded, hilly region of rivers and narrow, winding lakes. The Lake of the Ozarks was created by the damming of the Osage River in 1930.

Collapsed limestone caverns led to the formation of Big Basin in Kansas; a depression 100 ft (33 m) deep and 1 mile (1.6 km) wide.

Flint Hills is the region's easternmost major escarpment. Steep, grassy uplands are interspersed with rocky, wooded ravines and outcrops of limestone and chert.

Missouri River

The Great Salt Plains of northern Oklahoma cover 45 sq miles (116 sq km). The arid, white flats were left by the gradual evaporation of an ancient salt lake.

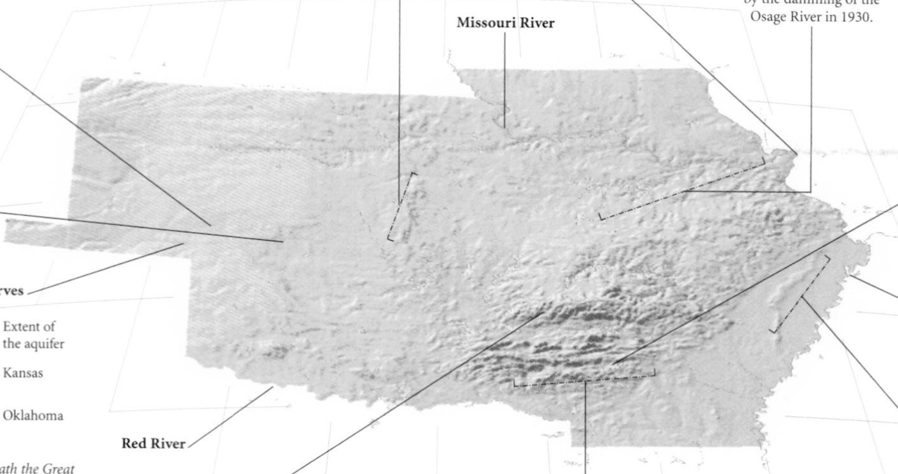

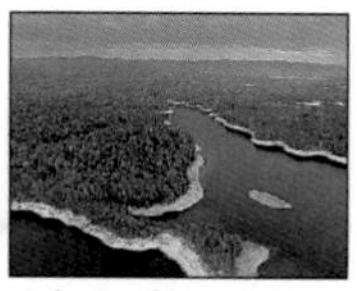

Lake Ouachita, in Arkansas is one of a number of irregularly-shaped lakes found among the ridges of the Ouachita Mountains.

Underground water reserves

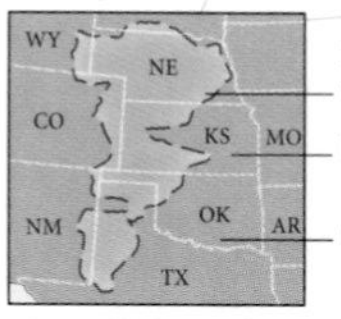

WY, NE, CO, KS, MO, NM, OK, AR, TX — Extent of the aquifer; Kansas; Oklahoma

The Ogallala Aquifer, beneath the Great Plains, is the largest known source of underground water in the world. There is concern about the rapid depletion of this finite water supply by irrigation schemes.

Mississippi River

Red River

Devil's Den is a dry badland area. The rugged landscape, strewn with large boulders, is the eroded remnant of a spur extending from the Arbuckle mountains to the west.

Ouachita Mountains

Crowleys Ridge is a long, sandy ridge, rising from the Mississippi floodplain. It was formed over thousands of years by the deposition of sand blown eastward from the Great Plains.

The landscape of northeast Kansas is interlaced by rivers which have cut broad wooded valleys through the gentle hills. All the rivers in Kansas form part of the massive Missouri/Mississippi drainage basin.

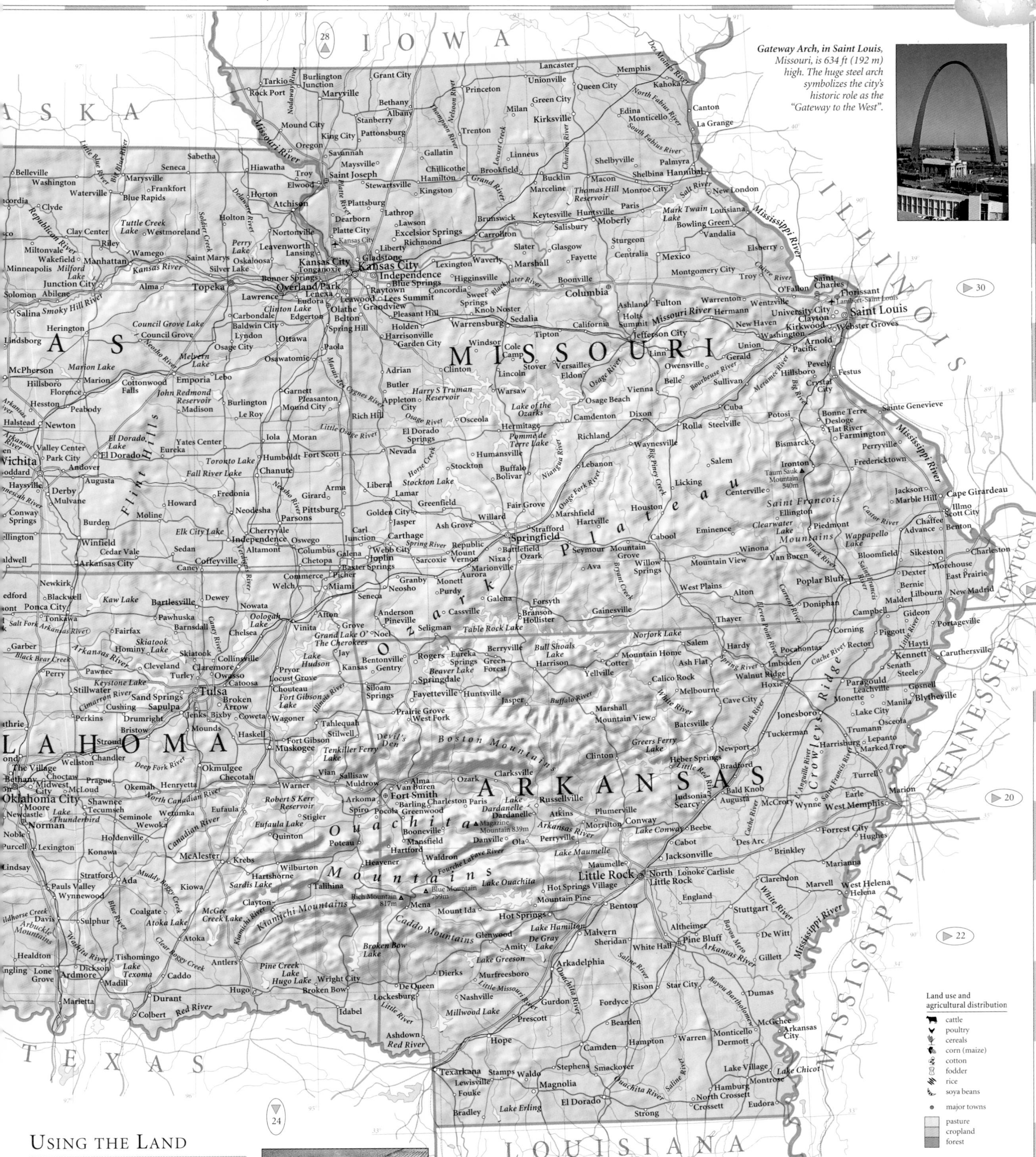

Gateway Arch, in Saint Louis, *Missouri, is 634 ft (192 m) high. The huge steel arch symbolizes the city's historic role as the "Gateway to the West".*

Land use and agricultural distribution

- cattle
- poultry
- cereals
- corn (maize)
- cotton
- fodder
- rice
- soya beans
- major towns
- pasture
- cropland
- forest

Using the Land

The problems of a harsh continental climate, with severe winters and hot, dry summers, are partially offset by the rich soils of the plains. Kansas is a major cereal crop producer, ranking first in US production of wheat and sorghum. Rainfall increases toward the east, favoring the cultivation of soybeans, cotton, and rice, with corn concentrated in Missouri. Huge herds of cattle are raised in Oklahoma, Kansas, and Missouri.

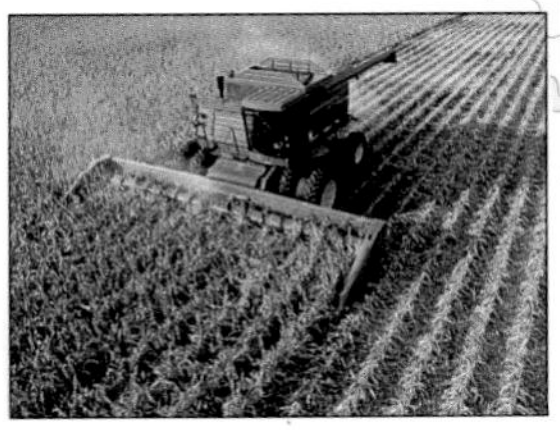

A combine harvester *works the land on the great plains. A hundred years ago this region, also known as the prairies – the French word for pasture – was covered with tall, wild grasses.*

The Urban/Rural Population Divide

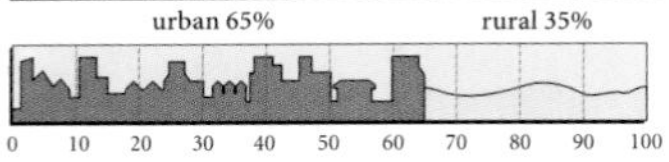

urban 65% | rural 35%

0 10 20 30 40 50 60 70 80 90 100

Population Density	Total Land Area
50 people per sq mile (19 people per sq km)	274,900 sq miles (712,177 sq km)

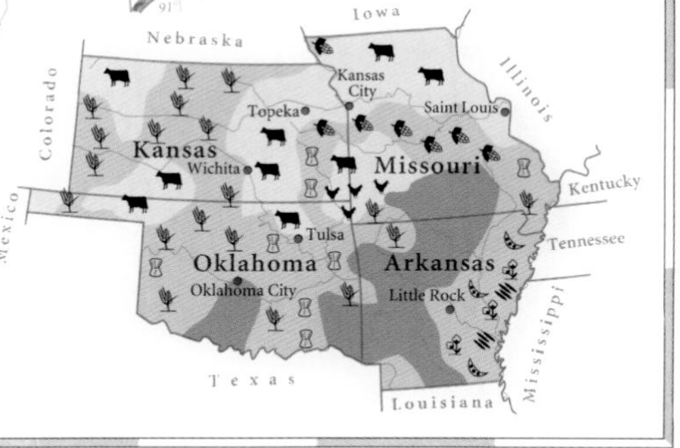

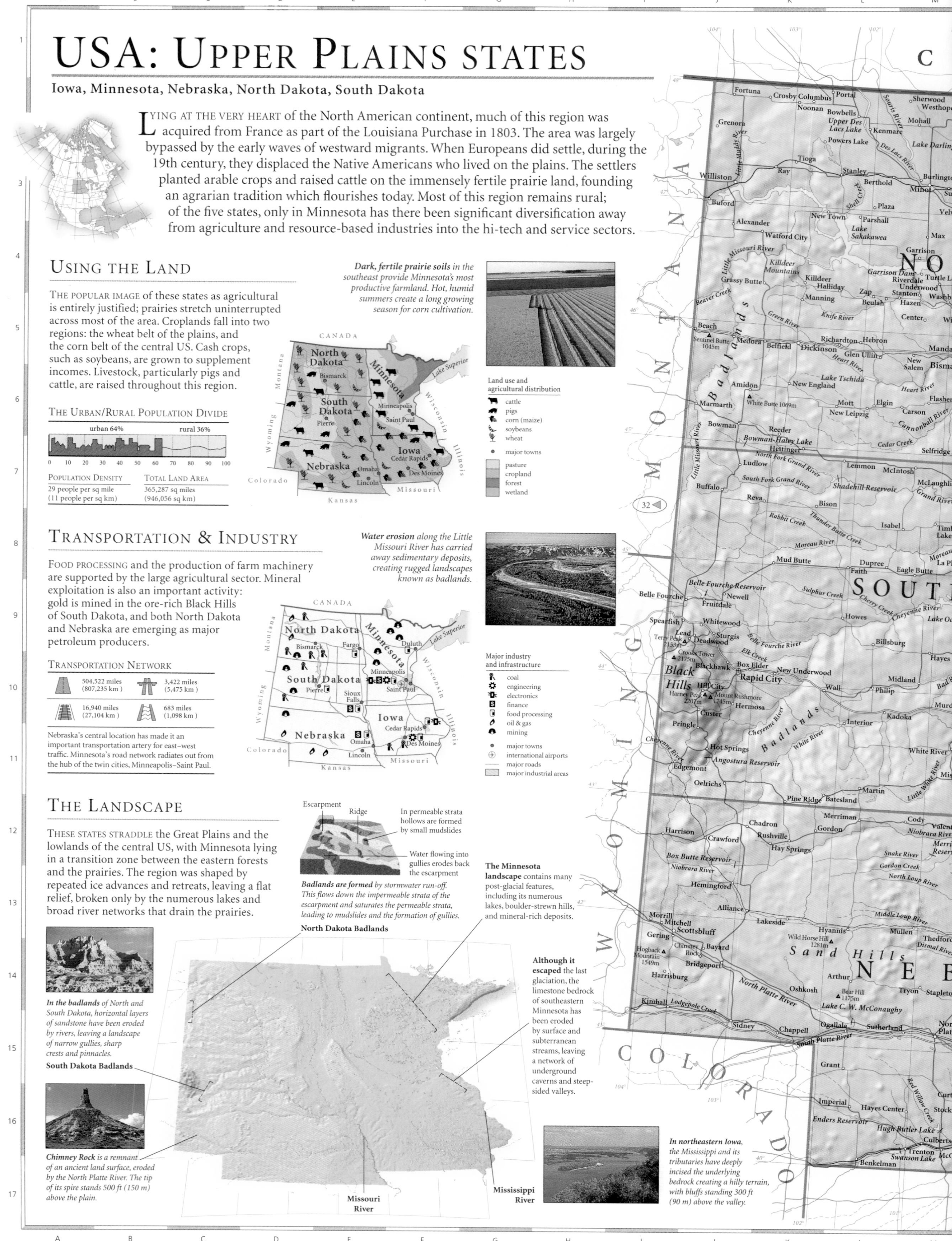

USA: Upper Plains States

Iowa, Minnesota, Nebraska, North Dakota, South Dakota

Lying at the very heart of the North American continent, much of this region was acquired from France as part of the Louisiana Purchase in 1803. The area was largely bypassed by the early waves of westward migrants. When Europeans did settle, during the 19th century, they displaced the Native Americans who lived on the plains. The settlers planted arable crops and raised cattle on the immensely fertile prairie land, founding an agrarian tradition which flourishes today. Most of this region remains rural; of the five states, only in Minnesota has there been significant diversification away from agriculture and resource-based industries into the hi-tech and service sectors.

Using the Land

The popular image of these states as agricultural is entirely justified; prairies stretch uninterrupted across most of the area. Croplands fall into two regions: the wheat belt of the plains, and the corn belt of the central US. Cash crops, such as soybeans, are grown to supplement incomes. Livestock, particularly pigs and cattle, are raised throughout this region.

The Urban/Rural Population Divide

urban 64% | rural 36%

Population Density	Total Land Area
29 people per sq mile (11 people per sq km)	365,287 sq miles (946,056 sq km)

Dark, fertile prairie soils in the southeast provide Minnesota's most productive farmland. Hot, humid summers create a long growing season for corn cultivation.

Land use and agricultural distribution: cattle; pigs; corn (maize); soybeans; wheat; major towns; pasture; cropland; forest; wetland

Transportation & Industry

Food processing and the production of farm machinery are supported by the large agricultural sector. Mineral exploitation is also an important activity: gold is mined in the ore-rich Black Hills of South Dakota, and both North Dakota and Nebraska are emerging as major petroleum producers.

Transportation Network

504,522 miles (807,235 km)	3,422 miles (5,475 km)
16,940 miles (27,104 km)	683 miles (1,098 km)

Nebraska's central location has made it an important transportation artery for east–west traffic. Minnesota's road network radiates out from the hub of the twin cities, Minneapolis–Saint Paul.

Water erosion along the Little Missouri River has carried away sedimentary deposits, creating rugged landscapes known as badlands.

Major industry and infrastructure: coal; engineering; electronics; finance; food processing; oil & gas; mining; major towns; international airports; major roads; major industrial areas

The Landscape

These states straddle the Great Plains and the lowlands of the central US, with Minnesota lying in a transition zone between the eastern forests and the prairies. The region was shaped by repeated ice advances and retreats, leaving a flat relief, broken only by the numerous lakes and broad river networks that drain the prairies.

Escarpment / Ridge / In permeable strata hollows are formed by small mudslides / Water flowing into gullies erodes back the escarpment

***Badlands are formed** by stormwater run-off. This flows down the impermeable strata of the escarpment and saturates the permeable strata, leading to mudslides and the formation of gullies.*

North Dakota Badlands

***In the badlands** of North and South Dakota, horizontal layers of sandstone have been eroded by rivers, leaving a landscape of narrow gullies, sharp crests and pinnacles.*

South Dakota Badlands

***Chimney Rock** is a remnant of an ancient land surface, eroded by the North Platte River. The tip of its spire stands 500 ft (150 m) above the plain.*

The Minnesota landscape contains many post-glacial features, including its numerous lakes, boulder-strewn hills, and mineral-rich deposits.

Although it escaped the last glaciation, the limestone bedrock of southeastern Minnesota has been eroded by surface and subterranean streams, leaving a network of underground caverns and steep-sided valleys.

Missouri River / **Mississippi River**

In northeastern Iowa, the Mississippi and its tributaries have deeply incised the underlying bedrock creating a hilly terrain, with bluffs standing 300 ft (90 m) above the valley.

32

***Along the shores** of Lake Superior in Minnesota, the average number of frost-free days can be as few as 90, and frosts may occur in any month of the year.*

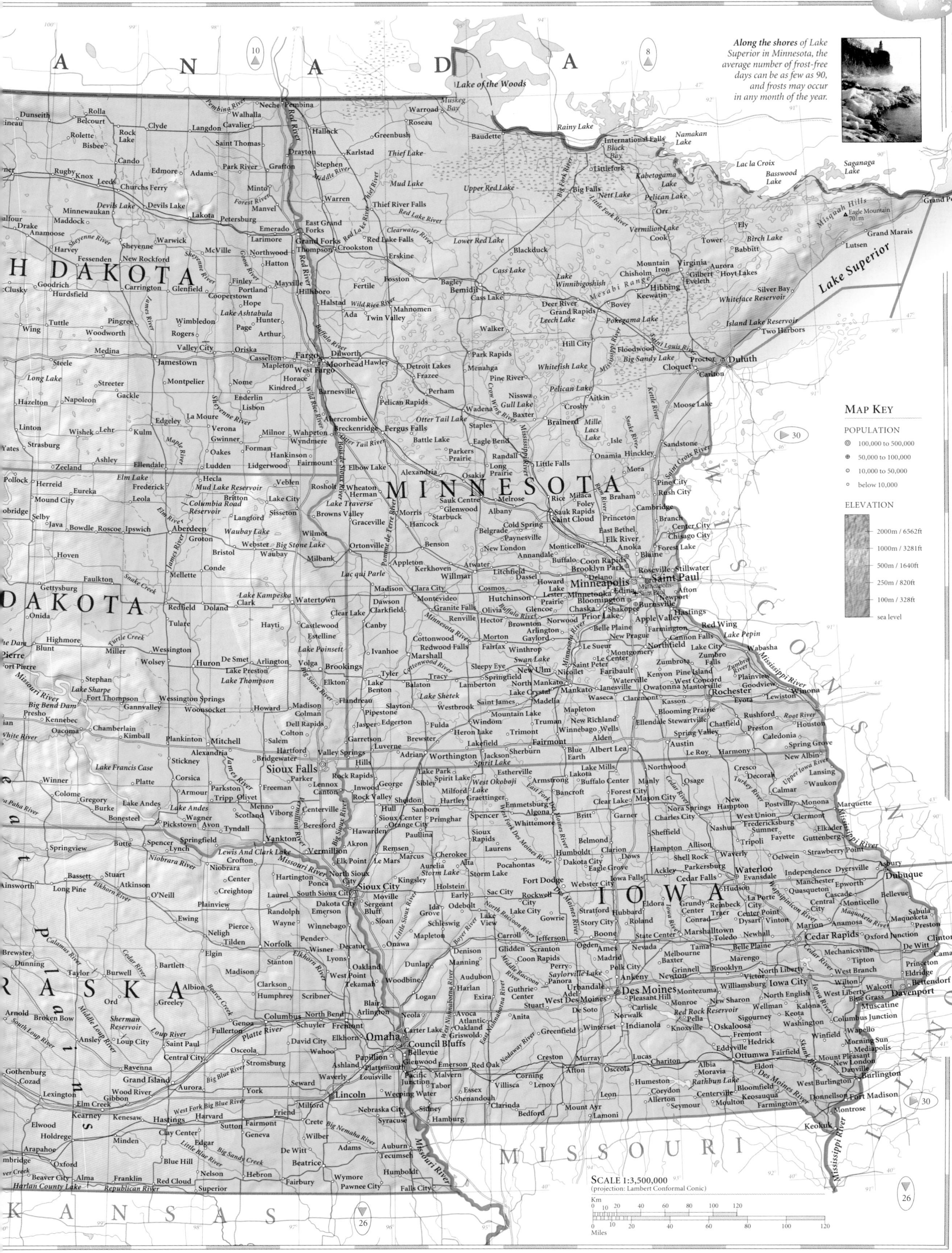

MAP KEY

POPULATION

- 100,000 to 500,000
- 50,000 to 100,000
- 10,000 to 50,000
- below 10,000

ELEVATION

- 2000m / 6562ft
- 1000m / 3281ft
- 500m / 1640ft
- 250m / 820ft
- 100m / 328ft
- sea level

SCALE 1:3,500,000
(projection: Lambert Conformal Conic)

Km 0 10 20 40 60 80 100 120

Miles 0 10 20 40 60 80 100 120

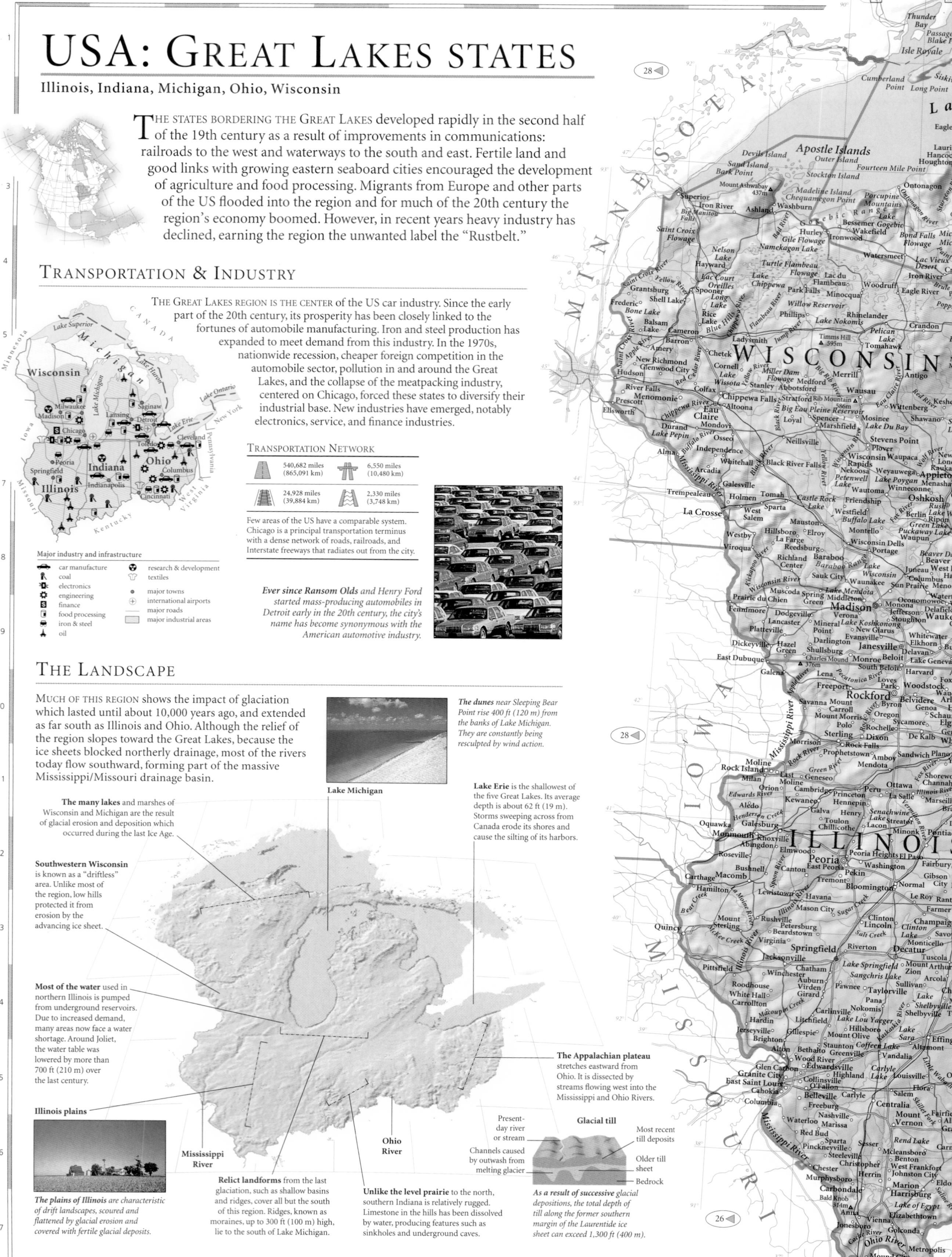
MINNESOTA
WISCONSIN
IOWA
ILLINOIS
MISSOURI
Lake Superior
Apostle Islands
Mississippi River

USA: Great Lakes states

Illinois, Indiana, Michigan, Ohio, Wisconsin

The states bordering the Great Lakes developed rapidly in the second half of the 19th century as a result of improvements in communications: railroads to the west and waterways to the south and east. Fertile land and good links with growing eastern seaboard cities encouraged the development of agriculture and food processing. Migrants from Europe and other parts of the US flooded into the region and for much of the 20th century the region's economy boomed. However, in recent years heavy industry has declined, earning the region the unwanted label the "Rustbelt."

Transportation & Industry

The Great Lakes region is the center of the US car industry. Since the early part of the 20th century, its prosperity has been closely linked to the fortunes of automobile manufacturing. Iron and steel production has expanded to meet demand from this industry. In the 1970s, nationwide recession, cheaper foreign competition in the automobile sector, pollution in and around the Great Lakes, and the collapse of the meatpacking industry, centered on Chicago, forced these states to diversify their industrial base. New industries have emerged, notably electronics, service, and finance industries.

Major industry and infrastructure: car manufacture; coal; electronics; engineering; finance; food processing; iron & steel; oil; research & development; textiles; major towns; international airports; major roads; major industrial areas

Transportation Network

540,682 miles (865,091 km)	6,550 miles (10,480 km)
24,928 miles (39,884 km)	2,330 miles (3,748 km)

Few areas of the US have a comparable system. Chicago is a principal transportation terminus with a dense network of roads, railroads, and Interstate freeways that radiates out from the city.

***Ever since Ransom Olds** and Henry Ford started mass-producing automobiles in Detroit early in the 20th century, the city's name has become synonymous with the American automotive industry.*

The Landscape

Much of this region shows the impact of glaciation which lasted until about 10,000 years ago, and extended as far south as Illinois and Ohio. Although the relief of the region slopes toward the Great Lakes, because the ice sheets blocked northerly drainage, most of the rivers today flow southward, forming part of the massive Mississippi/Missouri drainage basin.

***The dunes** near Sleeping Bear Point rise 400 ft (120 m) from the banks of Lake Michigan. They are constantly being resculpted by wind action.*

Lake Michigan

The many lakes and marshes of Wisconsin and Michigan are the result of glacial erosion and deposition which occurred during the last Ice Age.

Lake Erie is the shallowest of the five Great Lakes. Its average depth is about 62 ft (19 m). Storms sweeping across from Canada erode its shores and cause the silting of its harbors.

Southwestern Wisconsin is known as a "driftless" area. Unlike most of the region, low hills protected it from erosion by the advancing ice sheet.

Most of the water used in northern Illinois is pumped from underground reservoirs. Due to increased demand, many areas now face a water shortage. Around Joliet, the water table was lowered by more than 700 ft (210 m) over the last century.

The Appalachian plateau stretches eastward from Ohio. It is dissected by streams flowing west into the Mississippi and Ohio Rivers.

Illinois plains

Mississippi River

Ohio River

***The plains of Illinois** are characteristic of drift landscapes, scoured and flattened by glacial erosion and covered with fertile glacial deposits.*

Relict landforms from the last glaciation, such as shallow basins and ridges, cover all but the south of this region. Ridges, known as moraines, up to 300 ft (100 m) high, lie to the south of Lake Michigan.

Unlike the level prairie to the north, southern Indiana is relatively rugged. Limestone in the hills has been dissolved by water, producing features such as sinkholes and underground caves.

Glacial till

Present-day river or stream; Channels caused by outwash from melting glacier; Most recent till deposits; Older till sheet; Bedrock

***As a result of successive** glacial depositions, the total depth of till along the former southern margin of the Laurentide ice sheet can exceed 1,300 ft (400 m).*

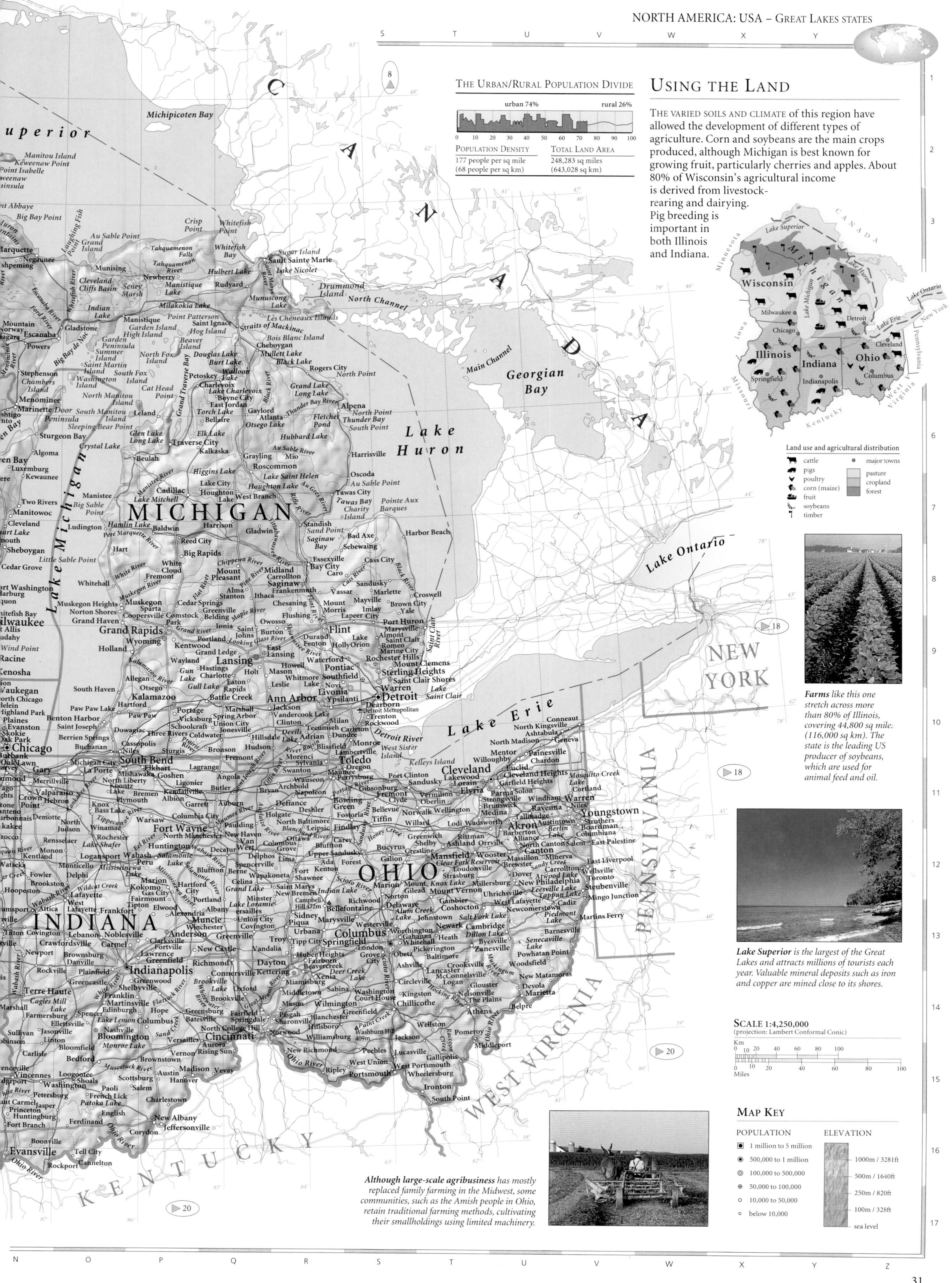
MICHIGAN
INDIANA
OHIO
CANADA
NEW YORK
PENNSYLVANIA
WEST VIRGINIA
KENTUCKY
Lake Huron
Lake Erie
Lake Ontario
Lake Michigan
Georgian Bay
Detroit
Chicago
Indianapolis
Columbus
Toledo
Cleveland
Cincinnati
Fort Wayne
Grand Rapids
Lansing
Flint
South Bend
Akron
Youngstown
Dayton
Evansville
THE URBAN/RURAL POPULATION DIVIDE
urban 74%
rural 26%
0 10 20 30 40 50 60 70 80 90 100
POPULATION DENSITY
177 people per sq mile
(68 people per sq km)
TOTAL LAND AREA
248,283 sq miles
(643,028 sq km)
Land use and agricultural distribution
cattle
pigs
poultry
corn (maize)
fruit
soybeans
timber
major towns
pasture
cropland
forest
SCALE 1:4,250,000
(projection: Lambert Conformal Conic)
MAP KEY
POPULATION
1 million to 5 million
500,000 to 1 million
100,000 to 500,000
50,000 to 100,000
10,000 to 50,000
below 10,000
ELEVATION
1000m / 3281ft
500m / 1640ft
250m / 820ft
100m / 328ft
sea level

USING THE LAND

THE VARIED SOILS AND CLIMATE of this region have allowed the development of different types of agriculture. Corn and soybeans are the main crops produced, although Michigan is best known for growing fruit, particularly cherries and apples. About 80% of Wisconsin's agricultural income is derived from livestock-rearing and dairying. Pig breeding is important in both Illinois and Indiana.

***Farms** like this one stretch across more than 80% of Illinois, covering 44,800 sq miles (116,000 sq km). The state is the leading US producer of soybeans, which are used for animal feed and oil.*

***Lake Superior** is the largest of the Great Lakes and attracts millions of tourists each year. Valuable mineral deposits such as iron and copper are mined close to its shores.*

***Although large-scale agribusiness** has mostly replaced family farming in the Midwest, some communities, such as the Amish people in Ohio, retain traditional farming methods, cultivating their smallholdings using limited machinery.*

USA: North Mountain States

Idaho, Montana, Oregon, Washington, Wyoming

THE REMOTENESS OF THE NORTHWESTERN STATES, coupled with the rugged landscape, ensured that this was one of the last areas settled by Europeans in the 19th century. Fur-trappers and gold-prospectors followed the Snake River westward as it wound its way through the Rocky Mountains. The states of the northwest have pioneered many conservationist policies, with the first US National Park opened at Yellowstone in 1872. More recently, the Cascades and Rocky Mountains have become havens for adventure tourism. The mountains still serve to isolate the western seaboard from the rest of the continent. This isolation has encouraged West Coast cities to expand their trade links with countries of the Pacific Rim.

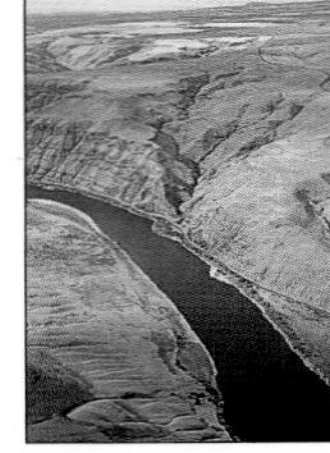

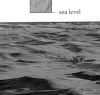

***The Snake River** has cut down into the basalt of the Columbia Basin to form Hells Canyon, the deepest in the US, with cliffs up to 7,900 ft (2,408 m) high.*

Map Key

POPULATION

- 500,000 to 1 million
- 100,000 to 500,000
- 50,000 to 100,000
- 10,000 to 50,000
- below 10,000

ELEVATION

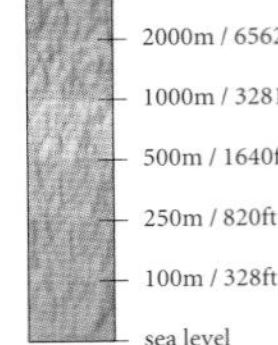

4000m / 13,124ft
3000m / 9843ft
2000m / 6562ft
1000m / 3281ft
500m / 1640ft
250m / 820ft
100m / 328ft
sea level

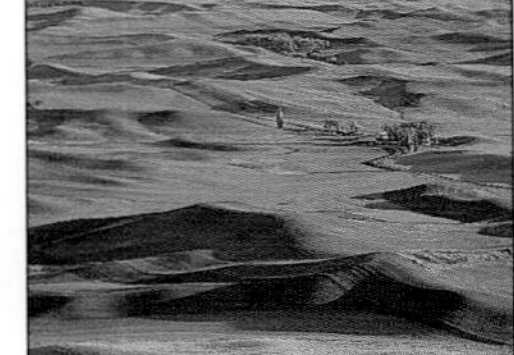

***Fine-textured, volcanic soils** in the hilly Palouse region of eastern Washington are susceptible to erosion.*

Using the Land

WHEAT FARMING IN THE EAST gives way to cattle ranching as rainfall decreases. Irrigated farming in the Snake River valley produces large yields of potatoes and other vegetables. Dairying and fruit-growing take place in the wet western lowlands between the mountain ranges.

The Urban/Rural Population Divide

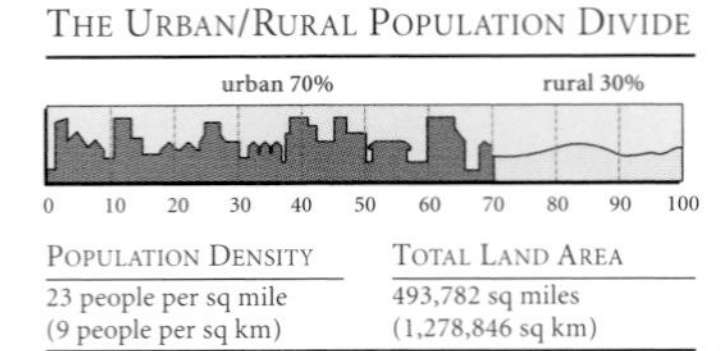

urban 70%
rural 30%
0 10 20 30 40 50 60 70 80 90 100

Population Density	Total Land Area
23 people per sq mile (9 people per sq km)	493,782 sq miles (1,278,846 sq km)

SCALE 1:4,250,000 (projection: Lambert Conformal Conic)

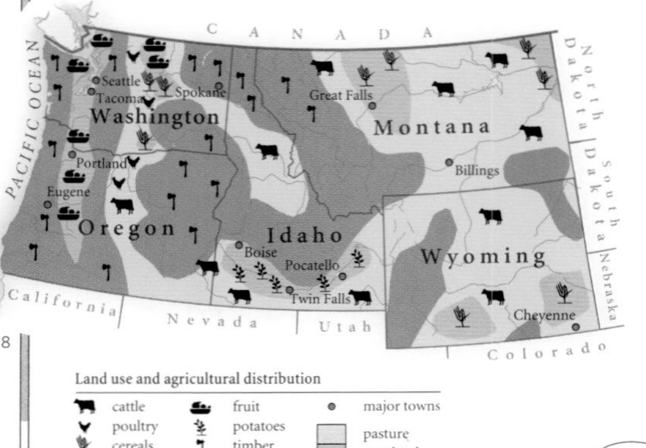

CANADA
PACIFIC OCEAN
Seattle
Tacoma
Spokane
Washington
Great Falls
Montana
Portland
Eugene
Oregon
Billings
Idaho
Boise
Pocatello
Twin Falls
Wyoming
Cheyenne
North Dakota
South Dakota
Nebraska
California
Nevada
Utah
Colorado

Land use and agricultural distribution

- cattle
- poultry
- cereals
- fruit
- potatoes
- timber
- major towns
- pasture
- cropland
- forest

192

Transportation & Industry

MINERALS AND TIMBER are extremely important in this region. Uranium, precious metals, copper, and coal are all mined, the latter in vast open-cast pits in Wyoming; oil and natural gas are extracted further north. Manufacturing, notably related to the aerospace and electronics industries, is important in western cities.

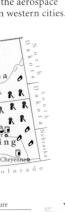

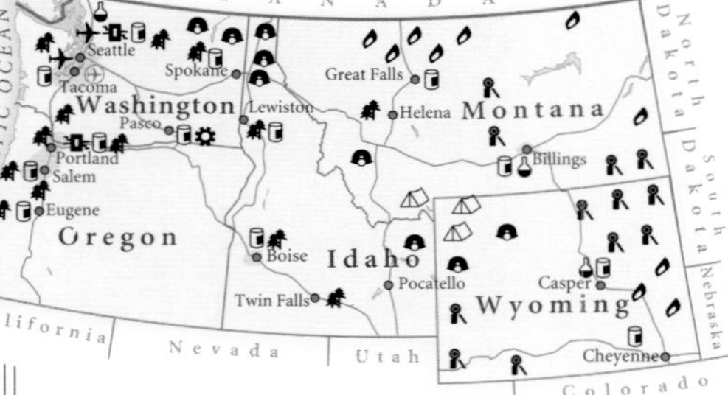

CANADA
PACIFIC OCEAN
Seattle
Tacoma
Spokane
Washington
Pasco
Lewiston
Great Falls
Helena
Montana
Portland
Salem
Billings
Eugene
Oregon
Boise
Idaho
Pocatello
Twin Falls
Casper
Wyoming
Cheyenne
North Dakota
South Dakota
Nebraska
California
Nevada
Utah
Colorado

Transportation Network

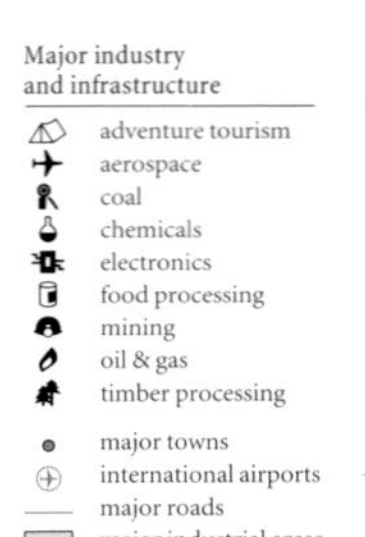

347,857 miles (556,571 km)
4,200 miles (6,720 km)
12,354 miles (19,766 km)
1,108 miles (1,782 km)

The Union Pacific Railroad has been in service across Wyoming since 1867. The route through the Rocky Mountains is now shared with the Interstate 80, a major east-west highway.

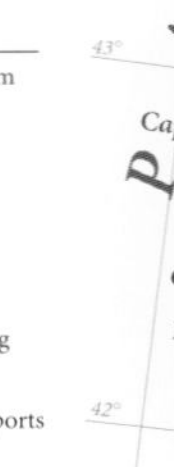

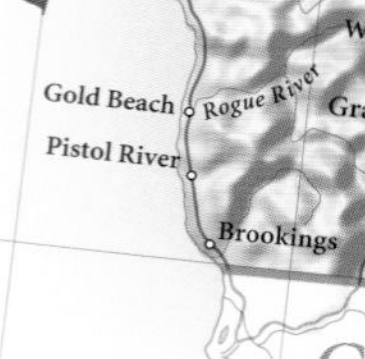

Major industry and infrastructure
adventure tourism
aerospace
coal
chemicals
electronics
food processing
mining
oil & gas
timber processing
major towns
international airports
major roads
major industrial areas

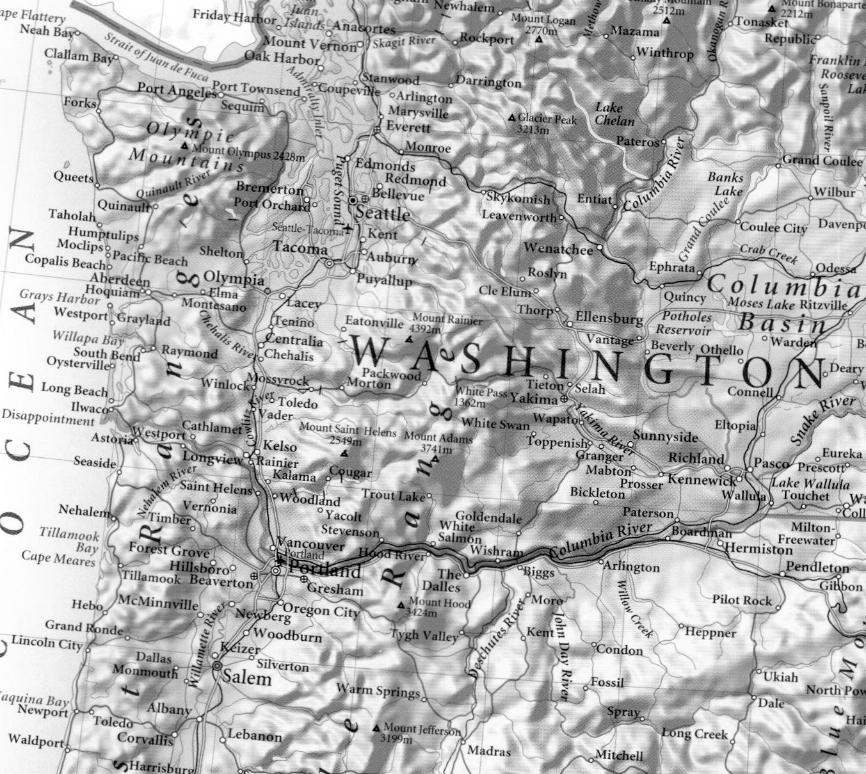

C
WASHINGTON
Columbia Basin
Olympic Mountains
Mount Olympus 2428m
Mount Baker 3254m
Glacier Peak 3213m
Mount Rainier 4392m
Mount Saint Helens 2549m
Mount Adams 3741m
Mount Hood 3424m
Mount Jefferson 3199m
Three Sisters 3157m
Matterhorn 3049m
Seattle
Tacoma
Olympia
Bellingham
Everett
Spokane
Yakima
Wenatchee
Richland
Kennewick
Pasco
Walla Walla
Vancouver
Portland
Salem
Eugene
The Dalles
Pendleton
La Grande
Columbia River
Snake River
Blue Mountains
Cascade Range
Coast Ranges
PACIFIC OCEAN
OREGON

Harney Basin

Mount Thielsen 2799m

Mount Scott 2722m

Mount McLoughlin 2894m

Crater Lake

Hart Mountain 2331m

Strawberry Mountain 2755m

CALIFORNIA

NEVADA

***Seattle lies** in one of Puget Sound's many inlets. The city receives oil and other resources from Alaska, and benefits from expanding trade across the Pacific.*

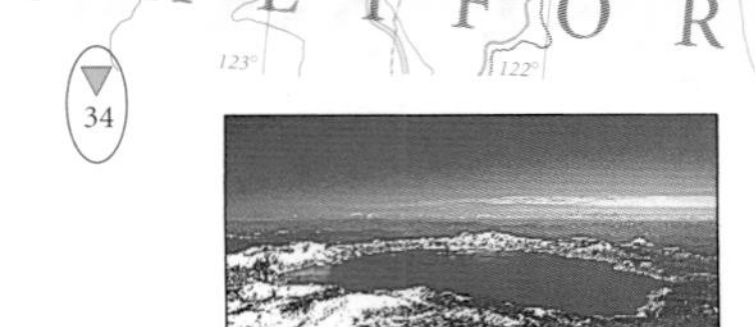
34

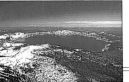

***Crater Lake, Oregon,** is 6 miles (10 km) wide and 1,800 ft (600 m) deep. It marks the site of a volcanic cone, which collapsed after an eruption within the last 7,000 years.*

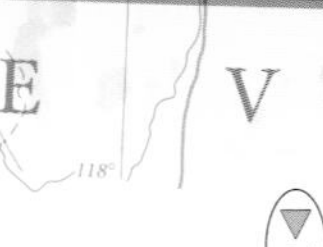
34

THE LANDSCAPE

THE ROCKY MOUNTAINS are flanked by lower parallel ranges, which spread onto the Great Plains in the east and surmount the broad lava plateau which extends westward. The Cascade Range divides the Columbia Basin from the coastlands, where the low areas around Puget Sound are broken by the steep, volcanic Olympic Mountains and the wooded hills of the Coast Ranges.

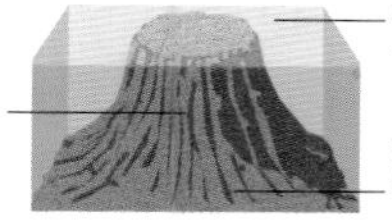

Molten rock cools, forming parallel columns

Surrounding strata eroded away

Molten rock wells up from the Earth's core

***Devil's Tower in Wyoming** is an igneous intrusion, formed below the Earth's surface. Molten rock intruded through cracks in the overlying strata and cooled. Over time, the softer rock layers have been eroded away, leaving only the tower standing.*

Glacial valleys on the seaward side of the Olympic Mountains receive about 142 inches (3,600 mm) of rain per year, supporting the only true rain forest of the northern hemisphere.

The Cascades are glacially scoured volcanic mountains, the highest of which is Mount Rainier, a dormant volcano at 14,409 ft (4,392 m).

Coast Ranges

Mount St. Helens erupted in 1980, killing 57 people and devastating a huge area.

Puget Sound

Columbia Basin

Grand Coulee and the lesser *coulées* (ravines) were cut by cataclysmic floods, from the release of an ice-dammed lake, at the end of the last ice age.

The Continental Divide, or watershed, crosses the Lewis Range. From here, rivers flow east to Hudson Bay, south to the Gulf of Mexico and west to the Pacific Ocean.

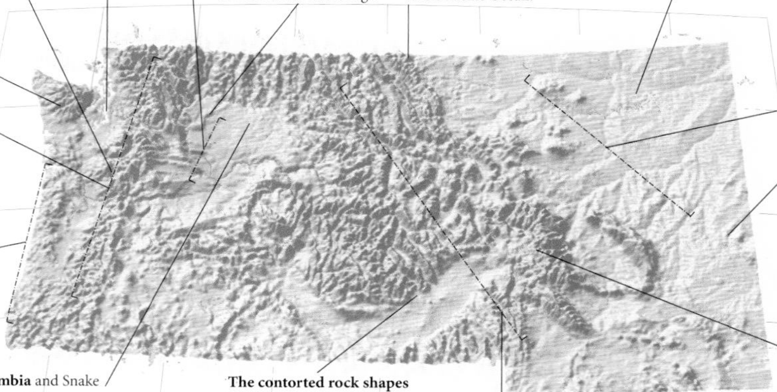

***Piney Buttes** are the remnants of an older, higher land surface gradually weathered and eroded into isolated outcrops with flat tops and steep sides.*

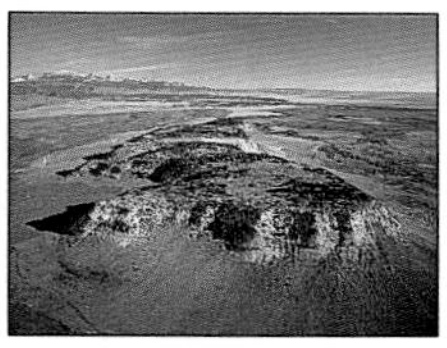

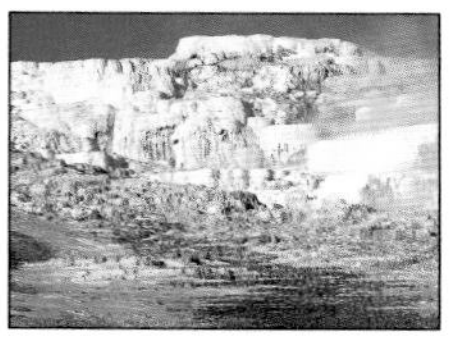

Great Plains

Devil's Tower

The plateaus of the Columbia and Snake Rivers represent one of the world's largest accumulations of lava. Over 5 million years ago, successive flows of molten basalt buried the existing land surface by up to 450 ft (150 m).

The contorted rock shapes at "Craters of the Moon" National Monument in Idaho were left 2,000 years ago by the sporadic upwelling of viscous lava from fissures in the basalt plateau.

Rocky Mountains

***Water from the hot springs** in Yellowstone National Park deposits minerals as it cools in rock pools. Long periods of deposition have created these rock terraces.*

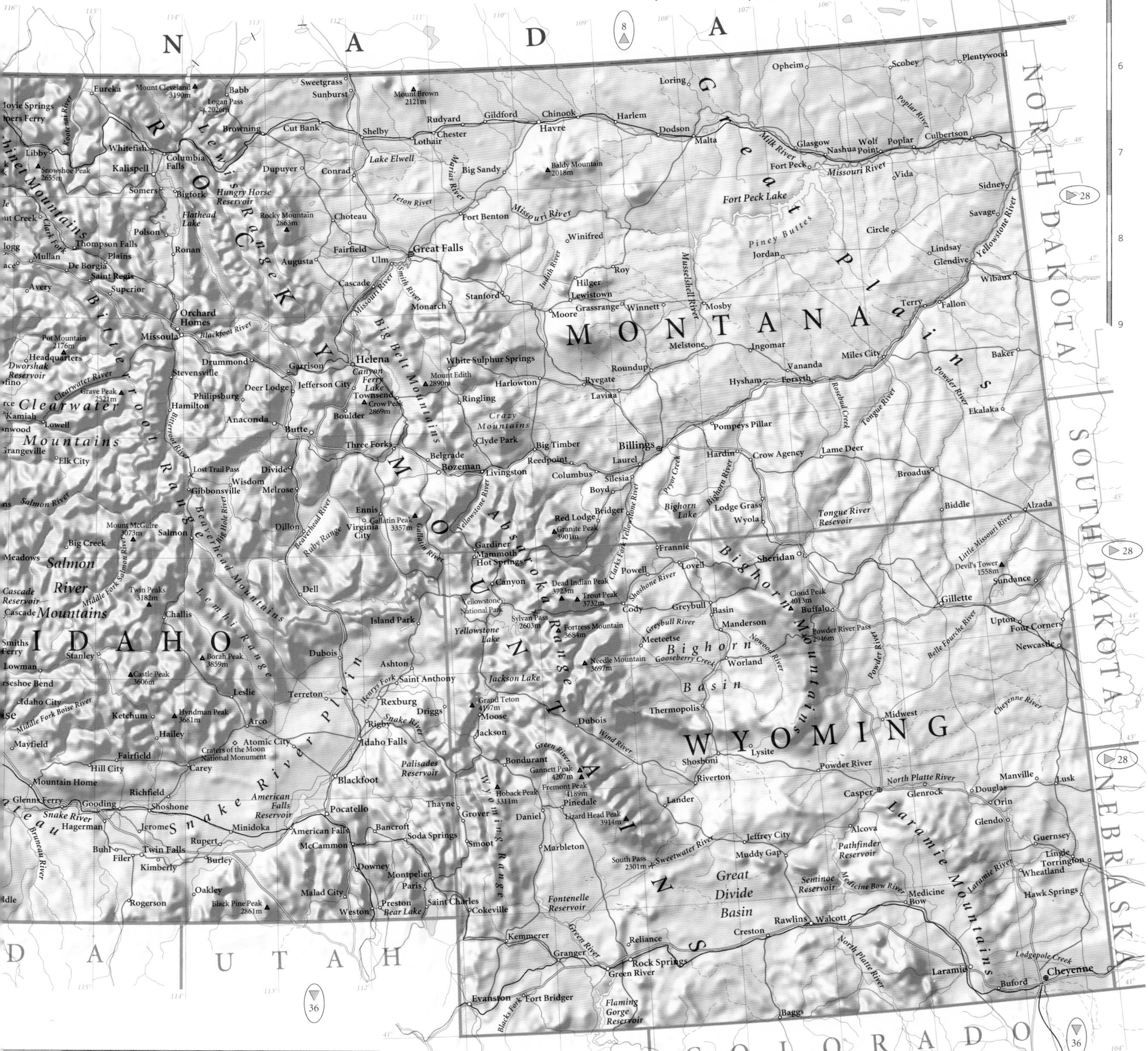

USA: CALIFORNIA & NEVADA

THE GOLD RUSH OF 1849 attracted the first major wave of European settlers to the West Coast. The pleasant climate, beautiful scenery and dynamic economy continue to attract immigrants – despite the ever-present danger of earthquakes – and California has become the US's most populous state. The overwhelmingly urban population is concentrated in the vast conurbations of Los Angeles, San Francisco, and San Diego; new immigrants include people from South Korea, the Philippines, Vietnam, and Mexico. Nevada's arid lands were initially exploited for minerals; in recent years, revenue from mining has been superseded by income from the tourist and gambling centers of Las Vegas and Reno.

MAP KEY

POPULATION
- 1 million to 5 million
- 500,000 to 1 million
- 100,000 to 500,000
- 50,000 to 100,000
- 10,000 to 50,000
- below 10,000

ELEVATION
- 4000m / 13,124ft
- 3000m / 9843ft
- 2000m / 6562ft
- 1000m / 3281ft
- 500m / 1640ft
- 250m / 820ft
- 100m / 328ft
- sea level

SCALE 1:3,250,000
(projection: Lambert Conformal Conic)

TRANSPORTATION & INDUSTRY

NEVADA'S RICH MINERAL RESERVES ushered in a period of mining wealth which has now been replaced by revenue generated from gambling. California supports a broad set of activities including defense-related industries and research and development facilities. "Silicon Valley," near San Francisco, is a world leading center for microelectronics, while tourism and the Los Angeles film industry also generate large incomes.

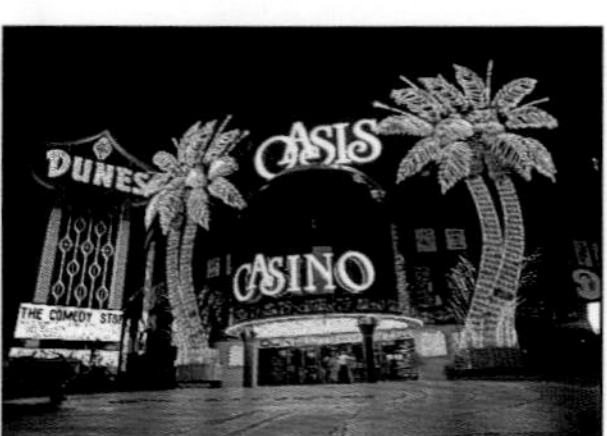

DUNES
OASIS
CASINO

Gambling was legalized in Nevada in 1931. Las Vegas has since become the center of this multimillion dollar industry.

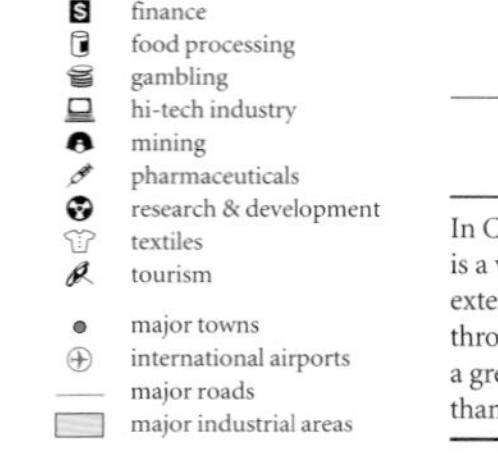

Major industry and infrastructure
- aerospace
- car manufacture
- defense
- movie industry
- finance
- food processing
- gambling
- hi-tech industry
- mining
- pharmaceuticals
- research & development
- textiles
- tourism
- major towns
- international airports
- major roads
- major industrial areas

TRANSPORTATION NETWORK

- 211,459 miles (338,334 km)
- 2,944 miles (4,710 km)
- 7,872 miles (12,595 km)
- 190 miles (306 km)

In California, the motor vehicle is a vital part of daily life, and an extensive freeway system runs throughout the state, which has a greater *per capita* car ownership than anywhere else in the world.

THE LANDSCAPE

THE BROAD CENTRAL VALLEY divides California's coastal mountains from the Sierra Nevada. The San Andreas Fault, running beneath much of the state, is the site of frequent earth tremors and sometimes more serious earthquakes. East of the Sierra Nevada, the landscape is characterized by the basin and range topography with stony deserts and many salt lakes.

Rising molten rock causes stretching of the Earth's crust

Extensive cracking (faulting) uplifted a series of ridges

As ridges are eroded they fill intervening valleys with sediments

***Molten rock** (magma) welling up to form a dome in the Earth's interior, causes the brittle surface rocks to stretch and crack. Some areas were uplifted to form mountains (ranges), while others sunk to form flat valleys (basins).*

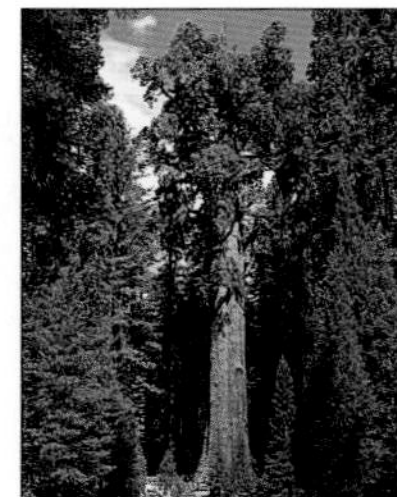

***The General Sherman** sequoia tree in Sequoia National Park is 3000 years old and at 275 ft (84 m) is one of the largest living things on earth.*

Most of California's agriculture is confined to the fertile and extensively irrigated Central Valley, running between the Coast Ranges and the Sierra Nevada. It incorporates the San Joaquin and Sacramento valleys.

The dramatic granitic rock formations of Half Dome and El Capitan, and the verdant coniferous forests, attract millions of visitors annually to Yosemite National Park in the Sierra Nevada.

The Great Basin dominates most of Nevada's topography containing large open basins, punctuated by eroded features such as *buttes* and *mesas*. River flow tends to be seasonal, dependent upon spring showers and winter snow melt.

Sierra Nevada

Wheeler Peak is home to some of the world's oldest trees, bristlecone pines, which live for up to 5,000 years.

When the Hoover Dam across the Colorado River was completed in 1936, it created Lake Mead, one of the largest artificial lakes in the world, extending for 115 miles (285 km) upstream.

The San Andreas Fault is a transverse fault which extends for 650 miles (1,050 km) through California. Major earthquakes occur when the land either side of the fault moves at different rates. San Francisco was devastated by an earthquake in 1906.

Death Valley

Named by migrating settlers in 1849, Death Valley is the driest, hottest place in North America, as well as being the lowest point on land in the western hemisphere, at 282 ft (86 m) below sea level.

The sparsely populated Mojave Desert receives less than 8 inches (200 mm) of rainfall a year. It is used extensively for testing weapons and other military purposes.

The Salton Sea was created accidentally between 1905 and 1907 when an irrigation channel from the Colorado River broke out of its banks and formed this salty 300 sq mile (777 sq km), landlocked lake.

Amargosa Desert

The Sierra Nevada create a "rainshadow," preventing rain from reaching much of Nevada. Pacific air masses, passing over the mountains, are stripped of their moisture.

USING THE LAND

CALIFORNIA is the leading agricultural producer in the US, although low rainfall makes irrigation essential. The long growing season and abundant sunshine allow many crops to be grown in the fertile Central Valley including grapes, citrus fruits, vegetables, and cotton. Almost 17 million acres (6.8 million hectares) of California's forests are used commercially. Nevada's arid climate and poor soil are largely unsuitable for agriculture; 85% of its land is state owned and large areas are used for underground testing of nuclear weapons.

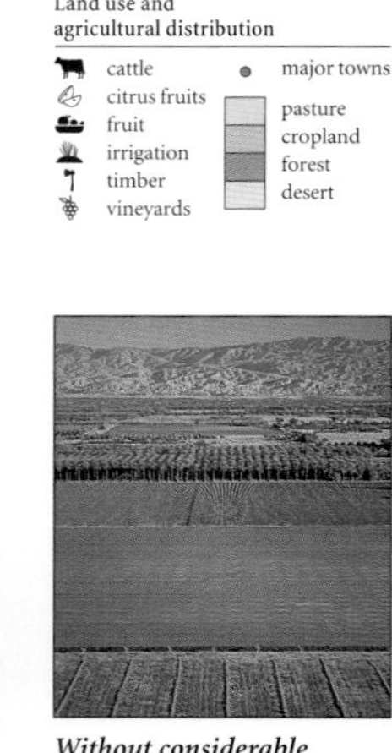

***Without considerable** irrigation, this fertile valley at Palm Springs would still be part of the Sonoran Desert. California's farmers account for about 80% of the state's total water usage.*

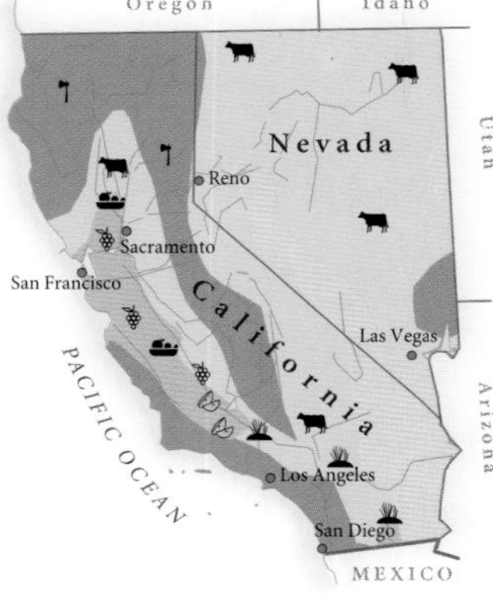

Oregon
Idaho
Nevada
Utah
Reno
Sacramento
San Francisco
California
Las Vegas
Arizona
PACIFIC OCEAN
Los Angeles
San Diego
MEXICO

Land use and agricultural distribution
- cattle
- citrus fruits
- fruit
- irrigation
- timber
- vineyards
- major towns
- pasture
- cropland
- forest
- desert

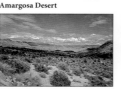

THE URBAN/RURAL POPULATION DIVIDE

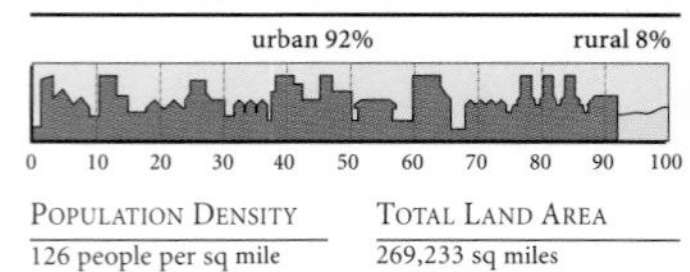

urban 92%
rural 8%
0 10 20 30 40 50 60 70 80 90 100

POPULATION DENSITY	TOTAL LAND AREA
126 people per sq mile (49 people per sq km)	269,233 sq miles (697,286 sq km)

192

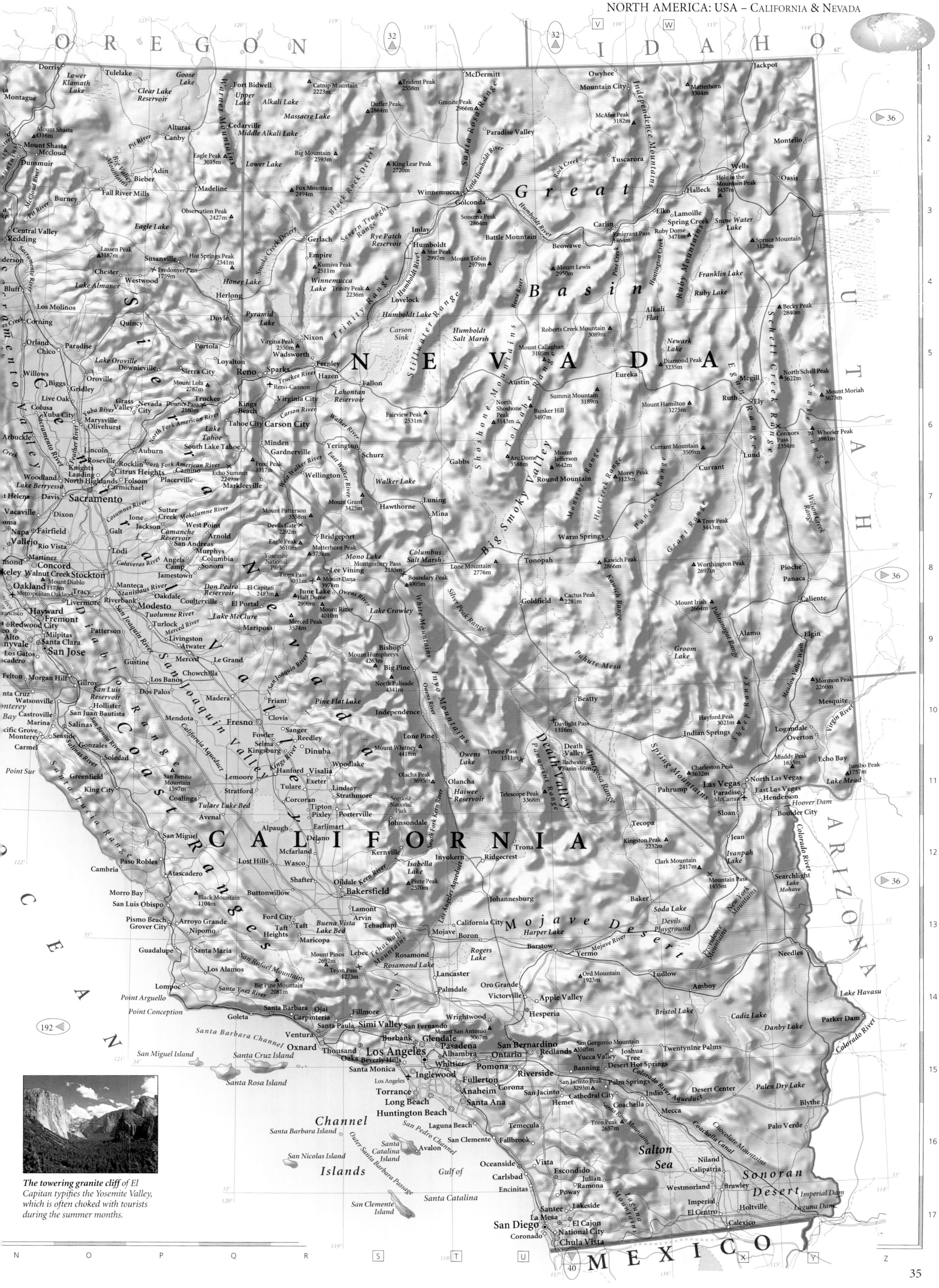

The towering granite cliff *of El Capitan typifies the Yosemite Valley, which is often choked with tourists during the summer months.*

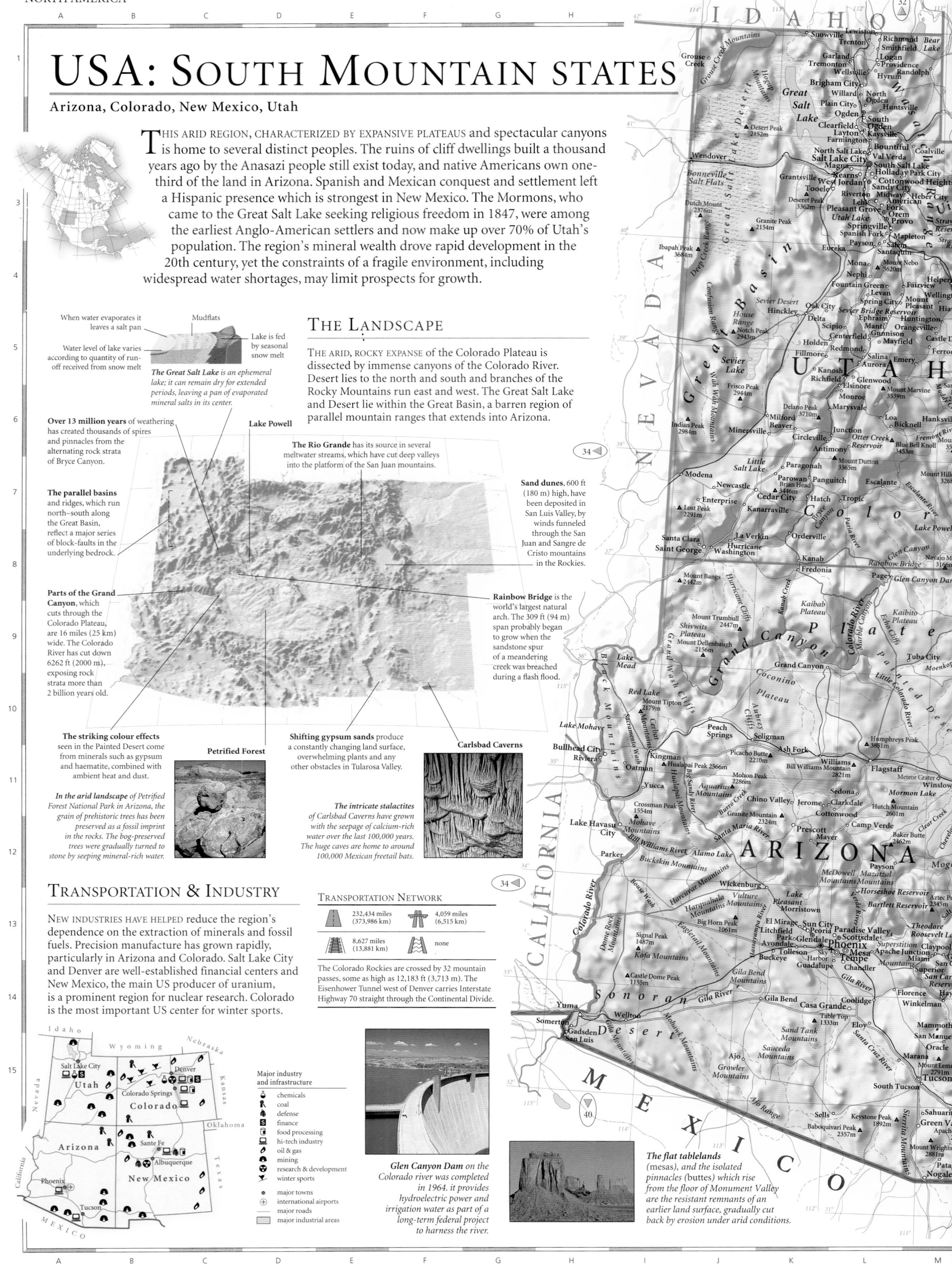

USA: South Mountain States

Arizona, Colorado, New Mexico, Utah

This arid region, characterized by expansive plateaus and spectacular canyons is home to several distinct peoples. The ruins of cliff dwellings built a thousand years ago by the Anasazi people still exist today, and native Americans own one-third of the land in Arizona. Spanish and Mexican conquest and settlement left a Hispanic presence which is strongest in New Mexico. The Mormons, who came to the Great Salt Lake seeking religious freedom in 1847, were among the earliest Anglo-American settlers and now make up over 70% of Utah's population. The region's mineral wealth drove rapid development in the 20th century, yet the constraints of a fragile environment, including widespread water shortages, may limit prospects for growth.

When water evaporates it leaves a salt pan

Mudflats

Lake is fed by seasonal snow melt

Water level of lake varies according to quantity of run-off received from snow melt

The Great Salt Lake is an ephemeral lake; it can remain dry for extended periods, leaving a pan of evaporated mineral salts in its center.

The Landscape

The arid, rocky expanse of the Colorado Plateau is dissected by immense canyons of the Colorado River. Desert lies to the north and south and branches of the Rocky Mountains run east and west. The Great Salt Lake and Desert lie within the Great Basin, a barren region of parallel mountain ranges that extends into Arizona.

Over 13 million years of weathering has created thousands of spires and pinnacles from the alternating rock strata of Bryce Canyon.

Lake Powell

The Rio Grande has its source in several meltwater streams, which have cut deep valleys into the platform of the San Juan mountains.

Sand dunes, 600 ft (180 m) high, have been deposited in San Luis Valley, by winds funneled through the San Juan and Sangre de Cristo mountains in the Rockies.

The parallel basins and ridges, which run north–south along the Great Basin, reflect a major series of block-faults in the underlying bedrock.

Parts of the Grand Canyon, which cuts through the Colorado Plateau, are 16 miles (25 km) wide. The Colorado River has cut down 6262 ft (2000 m), exposing rock strata more than 2 billion years old.

Rainbow Bridge is the world's largest natural arch. The 309 ft (94 m) span probably began to grow when the sandstone spur of a meandering creek was breached during a flash flood.

The striking colour effects seen in the Painted Desert come from minerals such as gypsum and haematite, combined with ambient heat and dust.

Petrified Forest

In the arid landscape of Petrified Forest National Park in Arizona, the grain of prehistoric trees has been preserved as a fossil imprint in the rocks. The bog-preserved trees were gradually turned to stone by seeping mineral-rich water.

Shifting gypsum sands produce a constantly changing land surface, overwhelming plants and any other obstacles in Tularosa Valley.

Carlsbad Caverns

The intricate stalactites of Carlsbad Caverns have grown with the seepage of calcium-rich water over the last 100,000 years. The huge caves are home to around 100,000 Mexican freetail bats.

Transportation & Industry

New industries have helped reduce the region's dependence on the extraction of minerals and fossil fuels. Precision manufacture has grown rapidly, particularly in Arizona and Colorado. Salt Lake City and Denver are well-established financial centers and New Mexico, the main US producer of uranium, is a prominent region for nuclear research. Colorado is the most important US center for winter sports.

Transportation Network

232,434 miles (373,986 km)	4,059 miles (6,515 km)
8,627 miles (13,881 km)	none

The Colorado Rockies are crossed by 32 mountain passes, some as high as 12,183 ft (3,713 m). The Eisenhower Tunnel west of Denver carries Interstate Highway 70 straight through the Continental Divide.

Major industry and infrastructure

- chemicals
- coal
- defense
- finance
- food processing
- hi-tech industry
- oil & gas
- mining
- research & development
- winter sports
- major towns
- international airports
- major roads
- major industrial areas

Glen Canyon Dam on the Colorado river was completed in 1964. it provides hydroelectric power and irrigation water as part of a long-term federal project to harness the river.

***The flat tablelands** (mesas), and the isolated pinnacles (buttes) which rise from the floor of Monument Valley are the resistant remnants of an earlier land surface, gradually cut back by erosion under arid conditions.*

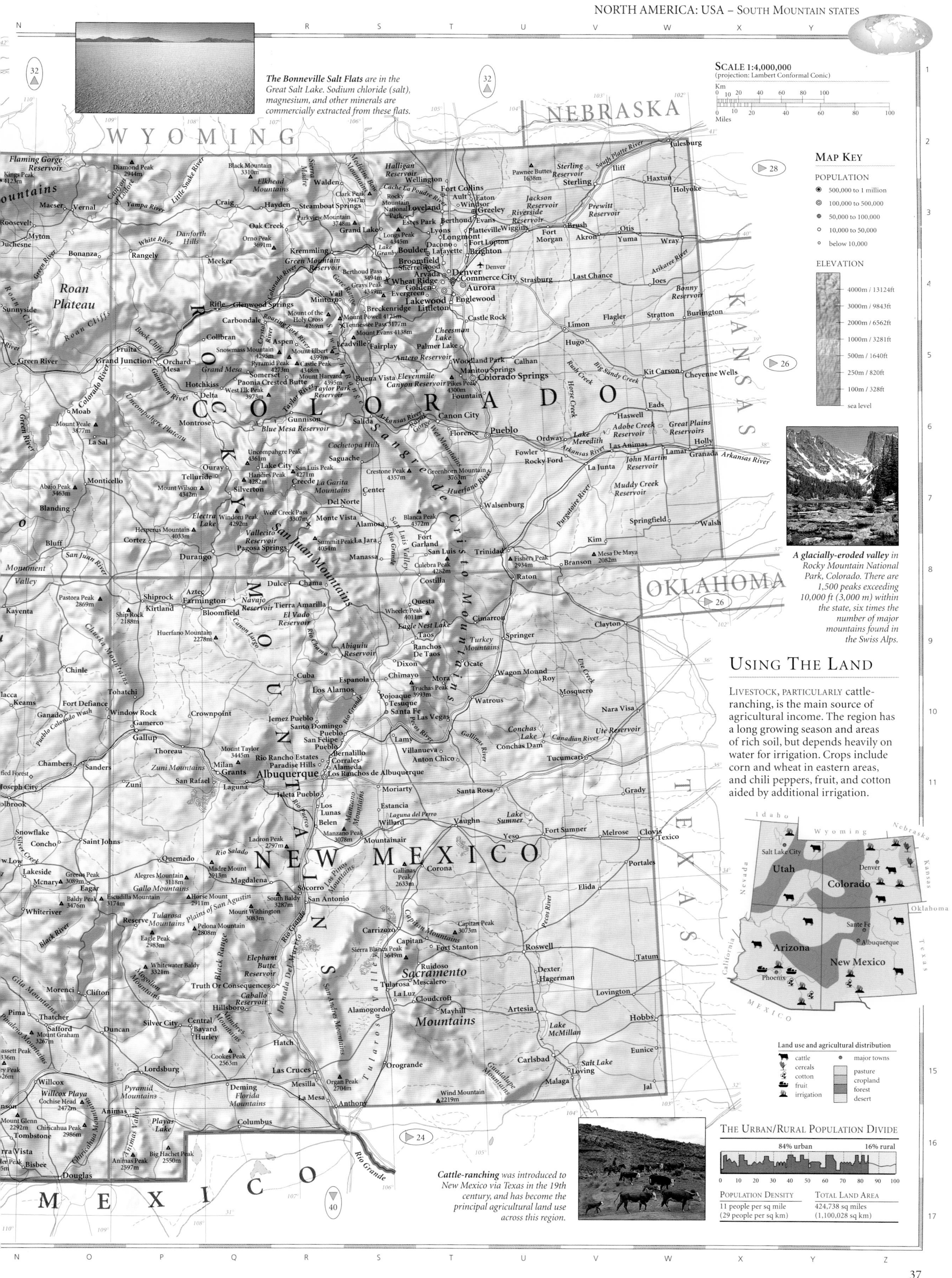
SCALE 1:4,000,000
(projection: Lambert Conformal Conic)
Km
Miles
MAP KEY
POPULATION
500,000 to 1 million
100,000 to 500,000
50,000 to 100,000
10,000 to 50,000
below 10,000
ELEVATION
4000m / 13124ft
3000m / 9843ft
2000m / 6562ft
1000m / 3281ft
500m / 1640ft
250m / 820ft
100m / 328ft
sea level
WYOMING
NEBRASKA
KANSAS
OKLAHOMA
TEXAS
COLORADO
NEW MEXICO
MEXICO
ROCKY MOUNTAINS
Sangre de Cristo Mountains
San Juan Mountains
Roan Plateau
Denver
Aurora
Colorado Springs
Pueblo
Fort Collins
Boulder
Grand Junction
Albuquerque
Santa Fe
Las Cruces
Roswell
Farmington
Rio Grande
Arkansas River
Sacramento Mountains
Land use and agricultural distribution
cattle
cereals
cotton
fruit
irrigation
major towns
pasture
cropland
forest
desert
Utah
Colorado
Arizona
New Mexico
Salt Lake City
Denver
Santa Fe
Albuquerque
Phoenix
THE URBAN/RURAL POPULATION DIVIDE
84% urban
16% rural
POPULATION DENSITY
11 people per sq mile
(29 people per sq km)
TOTAL LAND AREA
424,738 sq miles
(1,100,028 sq km)

The Bonneville Salt Flats are in the Great Salt Lake. Sodium chloride (salt), magnesium, and other minerals are commercially extracted from these flats.

A glacially-eroded valley in Rocky Mountain National Park, Colorado. There are 1,500 peaks exceeding 10,000 ft (3,000 m) within the state, six times the number of major mountains found in the Swiss Alps.

USING THE LAND

LIVESTOCK, PARTICULARLY cattle-ranching, is the main source of agricultural income. The region has a long growing season and areas of rich soil, but depends heavily on water for irrigation. Crops include corn and wheat in eastern areas, and chili peppers, fruit, and cotton aided by additional irrigation.

Cattle-ranching was introduced to New Mexico via Texas in the 19th century, and has become the principal agricultural land use across this region.

USA: HAWAII

THE 122 ISLANDS of the Hawaiian archipelago – which are part of Polynesia – are the peaks of the world's largest volcanoes. They rise approximately 6 miles (9.7 km) from the floor of the Pacific Ocean. The largest, the island of Hawaii, remains highly active. Hawaii became the US's 50th state in 1959. A tradition of receiving immigrant workers is reflected in the islands' ethnic diversity, with peoples drawn from around the rim of the Pacific. Only 2% of the current population are native Polynesians.

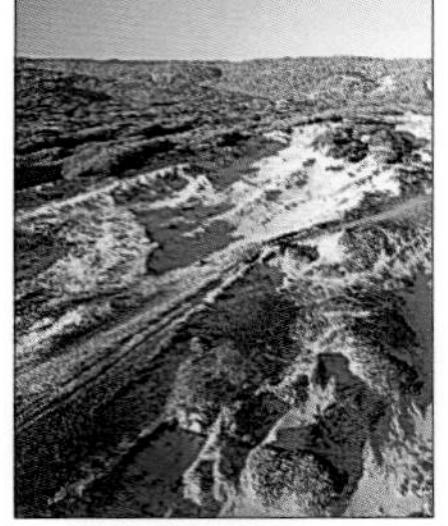
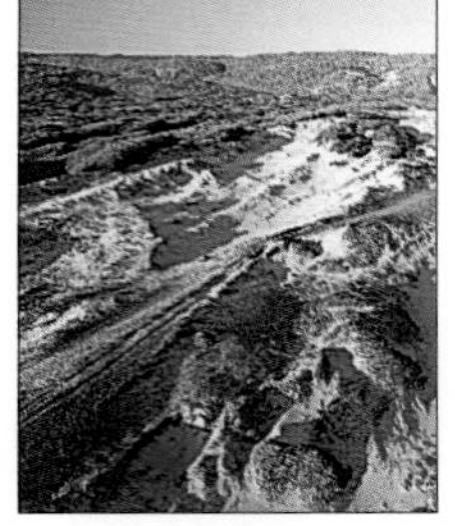

The island of Molokai *is formed from volcanic rock. Mature sand dunes cover the rocks in coastal areas.*

TRANSPORTATION & INDUSTRY

TOURISM DOMINATES the economy, with over half of the population employed in services. The naval base at Pearl Harbor is also a major source of employment. Industry is concentrated on the island of Oahu and relies mostly on imported materials, while agricultural produce is processed locally.

TRANSPORTATION NETWORK

roads	4,102 miles (6,600 km)	motorways	43 miles (69 km)
railways	none	waterways	none

Hawaii relies on ocean-surface transportation. Honolulu is the main focus of this network, bringing foreign trade and the markets of mainland US to Hawaii's outer islands.

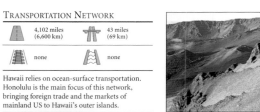

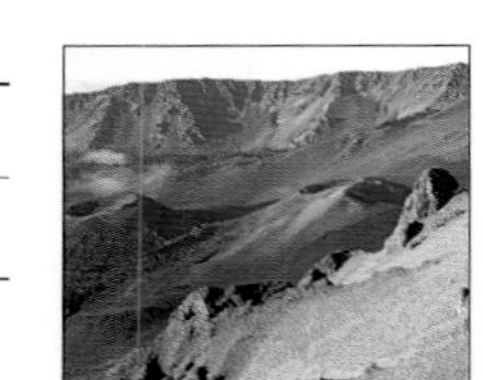

Haleakala's extinct volcanic crater is the world's largest. The giant caldera, containing many secondary cones, is 2,000 ft (600 m) deep and 20 miles (32 km) in circumference.

Major industry and infrastructure
- food processing
- military base
- textiles
- tourism
- major towns
- international airports
- major roads
- major industrial areas

Niihau Kauai Oahu Honolulu Molokai Lanai Kahoolawe Maui Hawaii Hilo
Hawaii
PACIFIC OCEAN

SCALE 1:4,000,000 (projection: Lambert Conformal Conic)

MAP KEY

POPULATION
- 100,000 to 500,000
- 50,000 to 100,000
- 10,000 to 50,000
- below 10,000

ELEVATION
- 4000m / 13,124ft
- 3000m / 9843ft
- 2000m / 6562ft
- 1000m / 3281ft
- 500m / 1640ft
- 250m / 820ft
- 100m / 328ft
- sea level

USING THE LAND AND SEA

THE VOLCANIC SOILS are extremely fertile and the climate hot and humid on the lower slopes, supporting large commercial plantations growing sugar cane, bananas, pineapples, and other tropical fruit, as well as nursery plants and flowers. Some land is given to pasture, particularly for beef and dairy cattle.

Land use and agricultural distribution
- cattle
- fishing
- fruit
- sugar cane
- major towns
- pasture
- cropland
- forest
- mountain region

The island of Kauai is one of the wettest places in the world, receiving some 450 inches (11,500 mm) of rain a year.

THE URBAN/RURAL POPULATION DIVIDE

urban 89% rural 11%

POPULATION DENSITY	TOTAL LAND AREA
183 people per sq mile (71 people per sq km)	6,423 sq miles (16,636 sq km)

USING THE LAND AND SEA

THE ICE-FREE COASTLINE of Alaska provides access to salmon fisheries and more than 5.5 million acres (2.2 million ha) of forest. Most of Alaska is uncultivable, and around 90% of food is imported. Barley, hay, and hothouse products are grown around Anchorage, where dairy farming is also concentrated.

THE URBAN/RURAL POPULATION DIVIDE

urban 68% rural 32%

POPULATION DENSITY	TOTAL LAND AREA
1 person per sq mile (0.4 people per sq km)	586,412 sq miles (1,518,800 sq km)

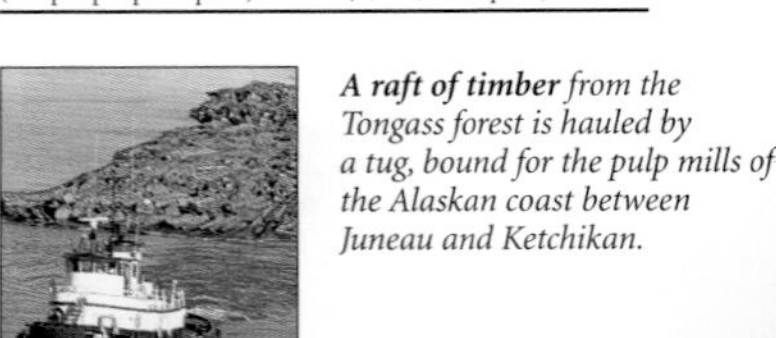

A raft of timber from the Tongass forest is hauled by a tug, bound for the pulp mills of the Alaskan coast between Juneau and Ketchikan.

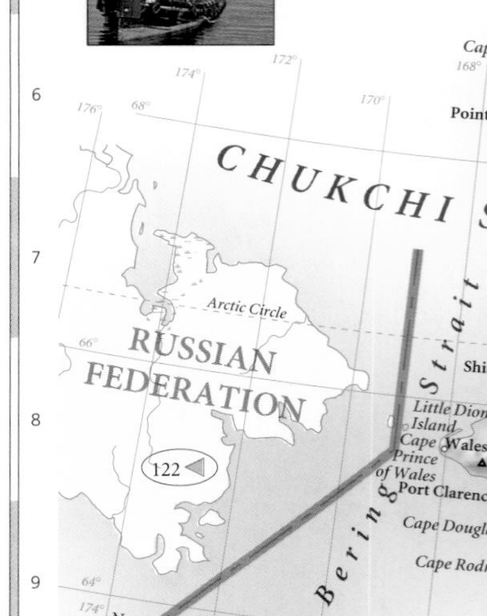

CHUKCHI SEA
RUSSIAN FEDERATION
Arctic Circle
Bering Strait
Point Hope
Cape Lisburne
Kivalina
Shishmaref
Little Diomede Island
Cape Prince of Wales
Port Clarence
Teller
Cape Douglas
Cape Rodney
Nome
Cape Nome

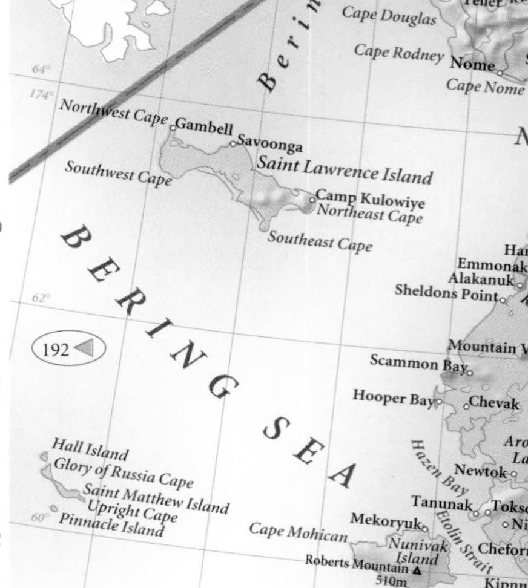

Northwest Cape
Gambell
Savoonga
Saint Lawrence Island
Southwest Cape
Southeast Cape
BERING SEA
Emmonak
Alakanuk
Sheldons Point
Mountain Village
Scammon Bay
Hooper Bay
Chevak

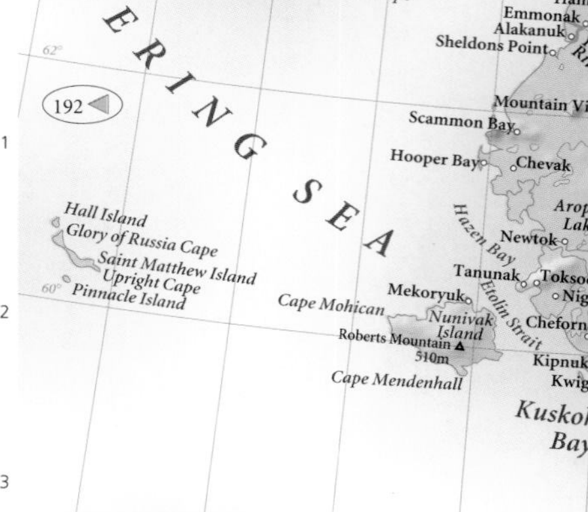

Hall Island
Glory of Russia Cape
Saint Matthew Island
Upright Cape
Pinnacle Island
Cape Mohican
Nunivak Island
Mekoryuk
Tununak
Toksook Bay
Newtok
Chefornak
Kipnuk
Kwigillingok
Cape Mendenhall
Kuskokwim Bay

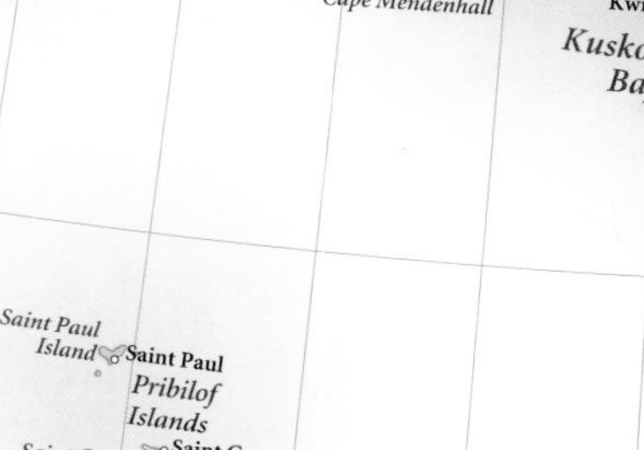

Saint Paul Island
Saint Paul
Pribilof Islands
Saint George Island
Saint George

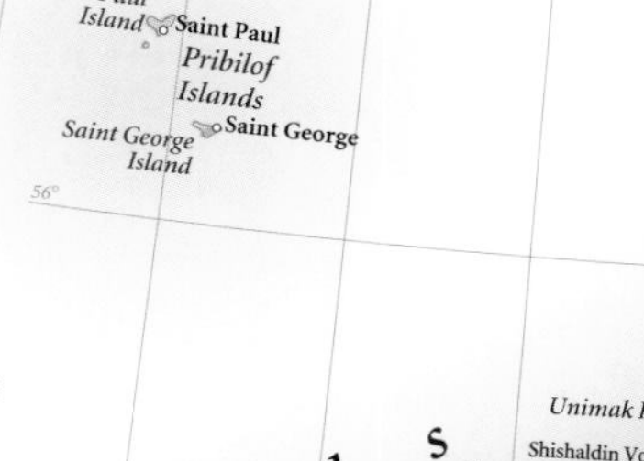

MAP KEY

POPULATION
- 100,000 to 500,000
- 50,000 to 100,000
- 10,000 to 50,000
- below 10,000

ELEVATION
- 4000m / 13,124ft
- 3000m / 9843ft
- 2000m / 6562ft
- 1000m / 3281ft
- 500m / 1640ft
- 250m / 820ft
- 100m / 328ft
- sea level

SCALE 1:9,000,000 (projection: Lambert Conformal Conic)

Aleutian Islands
Near Islands
Rat Islands
Andreanof Islands
Fox Islands
PACIFIC OCEAN

USA: ALASKA

Just over half a million people live in Alaska, a wilderness of ice, forest, mountains, and plains, purchased from Russia in 1867 and twice the size of Texas. The discovery of large oil reserves has brought prosperity to the US's "last frontier," while advancing the need to preserve natural habitats and the traditional livelihoods of indigenous peoples, such as the Aleuts and Inupiaq.

Land use and agricultural distribution
- fishing
- reindeer
- fruit
- major towns
- forest
- barren
- tundra

THE LANDSCAPE

The mountains of the Pacific coast culminate in the heavily glaciated Alaska Range and extend west, to the Alaska Peninsula and the great volcanic arc of the Aleutian Islands. The interior plains are drained by the Yukon River and bounded by the bare, jagged peaks of the Brooks Range to the north.

The Yukon Delta is a fan of alluvial material eroded by the Yukon River and its tributaries. It is approximately twice the size of the Mississippi Delta.

Brooks Range

West Fork Glacier

The ten highest mountains in the US are all in the Alaska Range, Mount McKinley *(Denali)*, at 20,321 ft (6,194 m) is the highest.

Yukon River

Alaska Range

The arc of the Aleutian Islands marks the boundary between the Eurasian and Pacific tectonic plates.

Fjords are found along the coast where valleys, deeply excavated by large glaciers, were inundated by rising seas.

***By August**, the Alaska Range is covered with autumnal tundra vegetation.*

West Fork Glacier

The surging ice mass shears along the glacier margin

Deep crevasses divide the front of the surging glacier into large ice blocks

***Surging glaciers** make rapid and dramatic advances, normally after periods of snow accumulation. West Fork Glacier in the Susitna River Basin traveled 2.5 miles (4 km) in 1987.*

TRANSPORTATION & INDUSTRY

Large areas of Alaska are undeveloped, and much of the existing infrastructure is a legacy of Cold War military investment. Mineral ores, including gold, have been mined for over a century, but the oil business now dominates the economy. Processing industries such as paper-pulp mills supply Japan and other markets on the Pacific Rim.

Major industry and infrastructure
- fish processing
- gold mining
- oil
- timber processing
- major towns
- international airports
- major roads

***The Trans-Alaska Pipeline** has carried crude oil from Prudhoe Bay since 1977. The oilfield is the US's largest and is estimated to be equal in size to the biggest oilfields of the Persian Gulf.*

TRANSPORTATION NETWORK

13,524 miles (21,760 km)	49 miles (78 km)
482 miles (772 km)	none

Nearly 80 million gallons of oil are pumped through the Trans-Alaska Pipeline every day. The oil takes six days to travel the 789 miles (1,262 km) from Prudhoe Bay to Valdez.

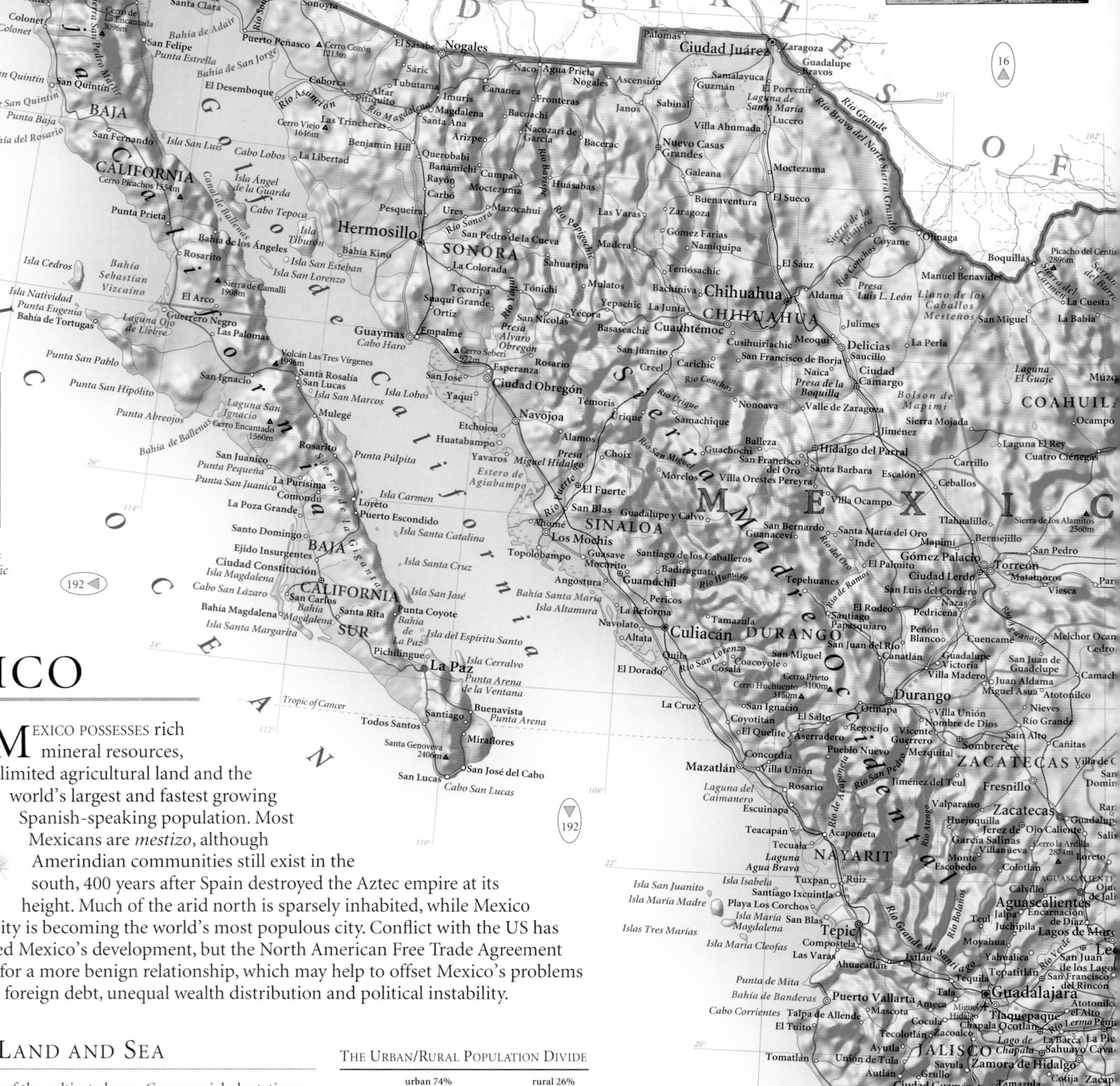

SCALE 1:7,000,000
(projection: Lambert Conformal Conic)

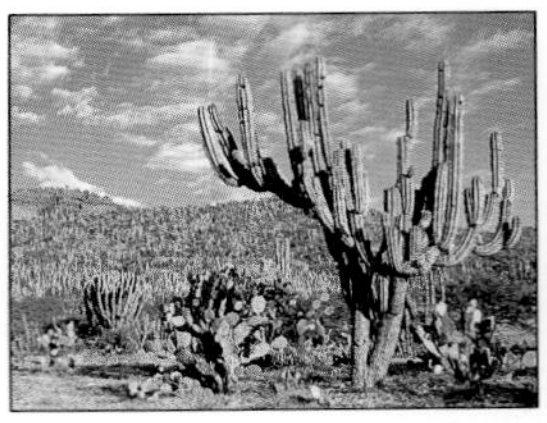

The rugged, desert landscape of the Sierra Madre del Sur is a product of complex tectonic processes, where the fold mountains in western North America, running north–south, meet the Caribbean mountain arc which runs east–west.

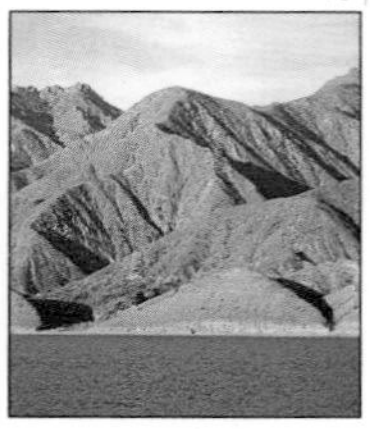

***Wave action** has cut steep cliffs into the igneous rocks of Isla Cedros, off the Pacific coast of Baja California. The island is home to sea lions, reptiles, and deer.*

MEXICO

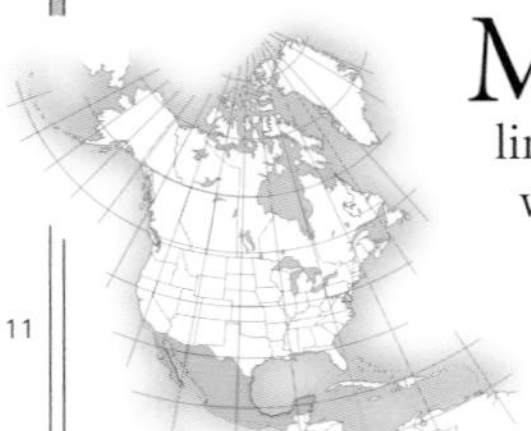

MEXICO POSSESSES rich mineral resources, limited agricultural land and the world's largest and fastest growing Spanish-speaking population. Most Mexicans are *mestizo*, although Amerindian communities still exist in the south, 400 years after Spain destroyed the Aztec empire at its height. Much of the arid north is sparsely inhabited, while Mexico City is becoming the world's most populous city. Conflict with the US has long overshadowed Mexico's development, but the North American Free Trade Agreement offers the chance for a more benign relationship, which may help to offset Mexico's problems of hyperinflation, foreign debt, unequal wealth distribution and political instability.

USING THE LAND AND SEA

CORN OCCUPIES much of the cultivated area. Commercial plantations of coffee, sugar, vanilla, and cotton are found along the Gulf coastal plain and in irrigated parts of the arid north, which is otherwise used for extensive ranching. Fishing is important, particularly shellfish for export. A soaring population has created the need for grain imports since 1980.

Land use and agricultural distribution

cattle, coffee, corn (maize), cotton, fishing, shellfish, sugar cane, timber, vanilla, capital cities, major towns, pasture, cropland, forest, desert

THE URBAN/RURAL POPULATION DIVIDE

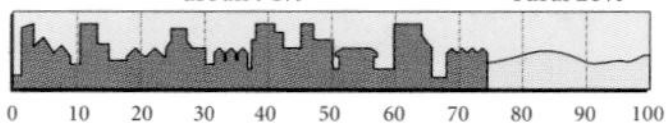

urban 74% — rural 26%

POPULATION DENSITY	TOTAL LAND AREA
130 people per sq mile (50 people per sq km)	755,865 sq miles (1,958,200 sq km)

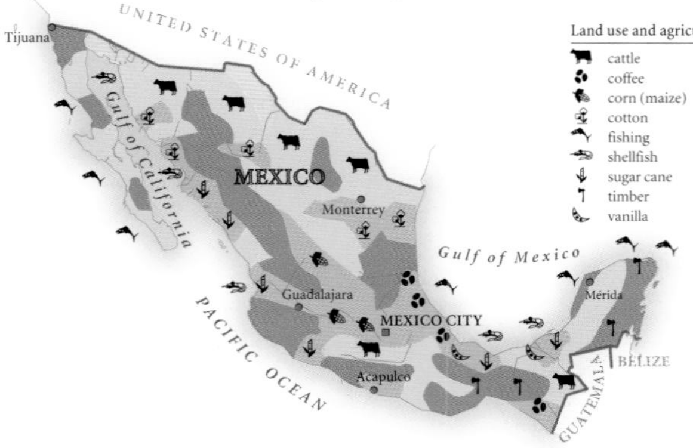

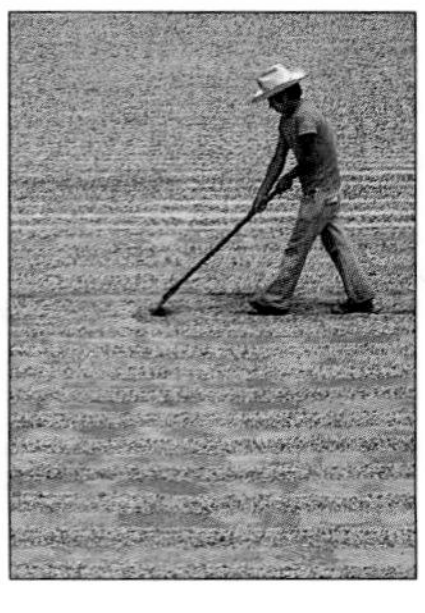

***Coffee beans** spread out to dry in the sun. Coffee, grown mainly on the Gulf coastal plain, is Mexico's most valuable export crop.*

MEXICO: ADMINISTRATIVE REGIONS

① DISTRITO FEDERAL

MAP KEY

POPULATION	ELEVATION
above 5 million	4000m / 13,124ft
1 million to 5 million	3000m / 9843ft
500,000 to 1 million	2000m / 6562ft
100,000 to 500,000	1000m / 3281ft
50,000 to 100,000	500m / 1640ft
10,000 to 50,000	250m / 820ft
below 10,000	100m / 328ft
	sea level

THE LANDSCAPE

THE GREAT CENTRAL PLATEAU rises gently southward from the Rio Grande, isolated from the coastal plains by the Sierra Madre Oriental and Occidental. The two ranges converge from east and west respectively, culminating in high volcanic peaks around Mexico City. Further ranges of the Sierra Madre rise to the south of the Balsas Basin, skirted by the low-lying Isthmus of Tehuantepec *(Istmo de Tehuantepec)* and Yucatan Peninsula.

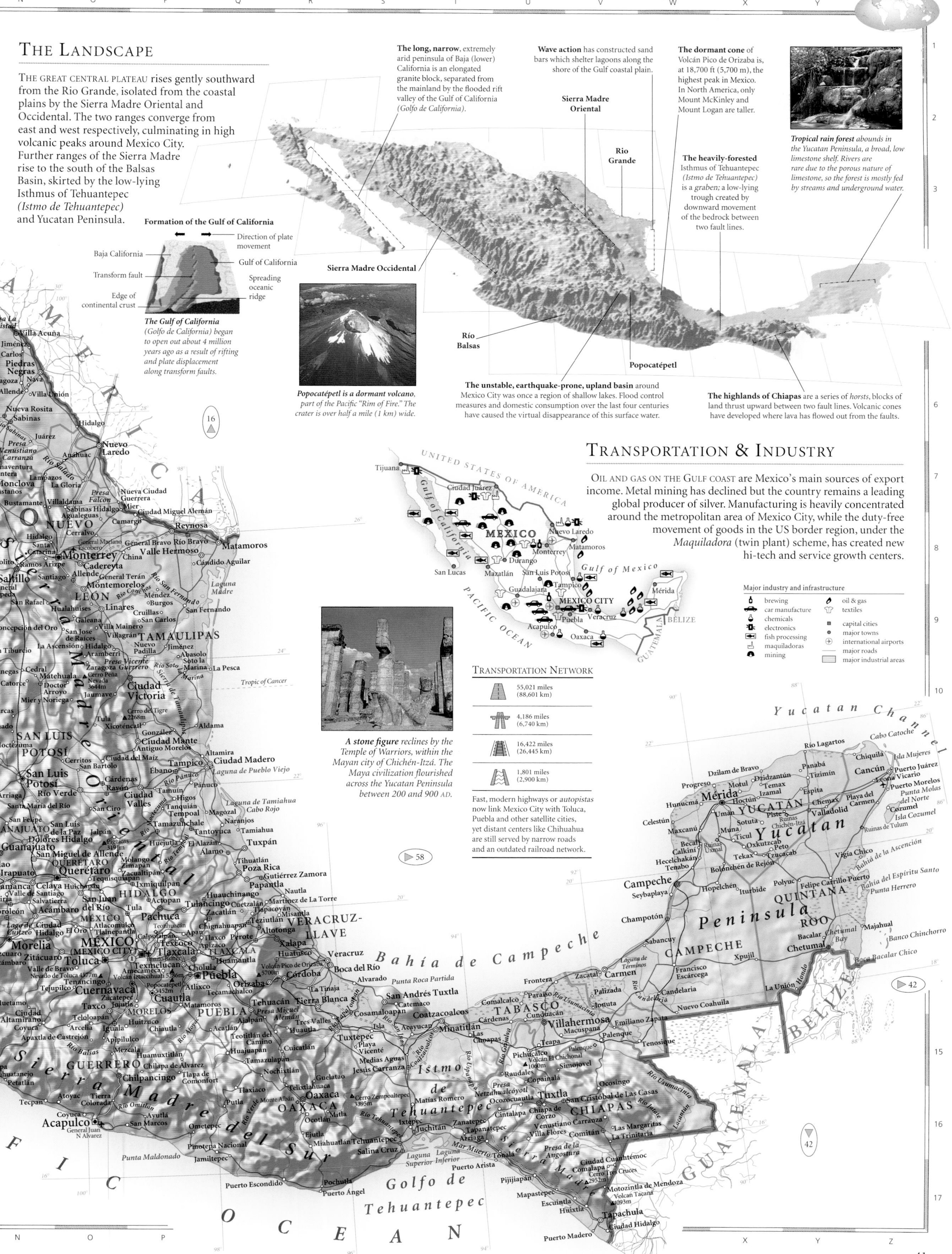

The long, narrow, extremely arid peninsula of Baja (lower) California is an elongated granite block, separated from the mainland by the flooded rift valley of the Gulf of California *(Golfo de California).*
Wave action has constructed sand bars which shelter lagoons along the shore of the Gulf coastal plain.
The dormant cone of Volcán Pico de Orizaba is, at 18,700 ft (5,700 m), the highest peak in Mexico. In North America, only Mount McKinley and Mount Logan are taller.
Sierra Madre Oriental
Rio Grande
The heavily-forested Isthmus of Tehuantepec *(Istmo de Tehuantepec)* is a *graben;* a low-lying trough created by downward movement of the bedrock between two fault lines.
Formation of the Gulf of California
Direction of plate movement
Baja California
Gulf of California
Transform fault
Spreading oceanic ridge
Edge of continental crust
Sierra Madre Occidental
Río Balsas
Popocatépetl
The unstable, earthquake-prone, upland basin around Mexico City was once a region of shallow lakes. Flood control measures and domestic consumption over the last four centuries have caused the virtual disappearance of this surface water.
The highlands of Chiapas are a series of *horsts,* blocks of land thrust upward between two fault lines. Volcanic cones have developed where lava has flowed out from the faults.
UNITED STATES OF AMERICA
Gulf of California
MEXICO
PACIFIC OCEAN
Gulf of Mexico
MEXICO CITY
BELIZE
GUATEMALA
Major industry and infrastructure
brewing
car manufacture
chemicals
electronics
fish processing
maquiladoras
mining
oil & gas
textiles
capital cities
major towns
international airports
major roads
major industrial areas
Bahía de Campeche
Golfo de Tehuantepec
Yucatan Channel
Peninsula Yucatan
Istmo de Tehuantepec
Sierra Madre Oriental
Sierra Madre del Sur
PACIFIC OCEAN

The Gulf of California *(Golfo de California) began to open out about 4 million years ago as a result of rifting and plate displacement along transform faults.*

Tropical rain forest *abounds in the Yucatan Peninsula, a broad, low limestone shelf. Rivers are rare due to the porous nature of limestone, so the forest is mostly fed by streams and underground water.*

Popocatépetl is a dormant volcano, *part of the Pacific "Rim of Fire." The crater is over half a mile (1 km) wide.*

A stone figure *reclines by the Temple of Warriors, within the Mayan city of Chichén-Itzá. The Maya civilization flourished across the Yucatan Peninsula between 200 and 900 AD.*

TRANSPORTATION & INDUSTRY

OIL AND GAS ON THE GULF COAST are Mexico's main sources of export income. Metal mining has declined but the country remains a leading global producer of silver. Manufacturing is heavily concentrated around the metropolitan area of Mexico City, while the duty-free movement of goods in the US border region, under the *Maquiladora* (twin plant) scheme, has created new hi-tech and service growth centers.

TRANSPORTATION NETWORK

55,021 miles (88,601 km)
4,186 miles (6,740 km)
16,422 miles (26,445 km)
1,801 miles (2,900 km)

Fast, modern highways or *autopistas* now link Mexico City with Toluca, Puebla and other satellite cities, yet distant centers like Chihuahua are still served by narrow roads and an outdated railroad network.

16 58 42 42

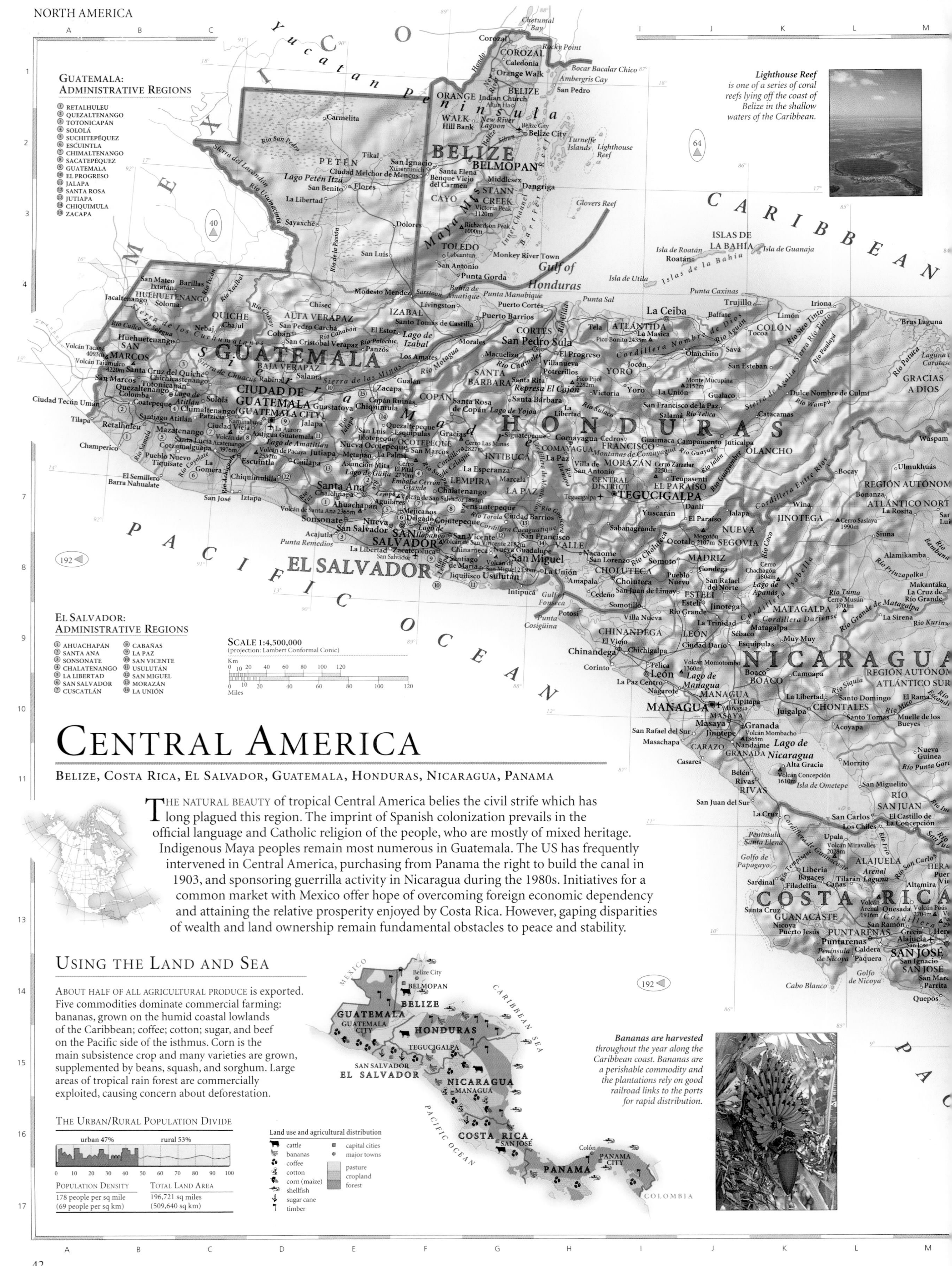

Guatemala: Administrative Regions
① RETALHULEU
② QUEZALTENANGO
③ TOTONICAPÁN
④ SOLOLÁ
⑤ SUCHITEPÉQUEZ
⑥ ESCUINTLA
⑦ CHIMALTENANGO
⑧ SACATEPÉQUEZ
⑨ GUATEMALA
⑩ EL PROGRESO
⑪ JALAPA
⑫ SANTA ROSA
⑬ JUTIAPA
⑭ CHIQUIMULA
⑮ ZACAPA
El Salvador: Administrative Regions
① AHUACHAPÁN
② SANTA ANA
③ SONSONATE
④ CHALATENANGO
⑤ LA LIBERTAD
⑥ SAN SALVADOR
⑦ CUSCATLÁN
⑧ CABAÑAS
⑨ LA PAZ
⑩ SAN VICENTE
⑪ USULUTÁN
⑫ SAN MIGUEL
⑬ MORAZÁN
⑭ LA UNIÓN
SCALE 1:4,500,000
(projection: Lambert Conformal Conic)
Km
Miles
MEXICO
Yucatan Peninsula
GUATEMALA
BELIZE
BELMOPAN
HONDURAS
TEGUCIGALPA
EL SALVADOR
SAN SALVADOR
NICARAGUA
MANAGUA
COSTA RICA
SAN JOSÉ
CARIBBEAN
PACIFIC OCEAN
Gulf of Honduras
Lago de Nicaragua

Lighthouse Reef is one of a series of coral reefs lying off the coast of Belize in the shallow waters of the Caribbean.

Central America

Belize, Costa Rica, El Salvador, Guatemala, Honduras, Nicaragua, Panama

The natural beauty of tropical Central America belies the civil strife which has long plagued this region. The imprint of Spanish colonization prevails in the official language and Catholic religion of the people, who are mostly of mixed heritage. Indigenous Maya peoples remain most numerous in Guatemala. The US has frequently intervened in Central America, purchasing from Panama the right to build the canal in 1903, and sponsoring guerrilla activity in Nicaragua during the 1980s. Initiatives for a common market with Mexico offer hope of overcoming foreign economic dependency and attaining the relative prosperity enjoyed by Costa Rica. However, gaping disparities of wealth and land ownership remain fundamental obstacles to peace and stability.

Using the Land and Sea

About half of all agricultural produce is exported. Five commodities dominate commercial farming: bananas, grown on the humid coastal lowlands of the Caribbean; coffee; cotton; sugar, and beef on the Pacific side of the isthmus. Corn is the main subsistence crop and many varieties are grown, supplemented by beans, squash, and sorghum. Large areas of tropical rain forest are commercially exploited, causing concern about deforestation.

The Urban/Rural Population Divide

urban 47% — rural 53%

0 10 20 30 40 50 60 70 80 90 100

Population Density	Total Land Area
178 people per sq mile (69 people per sq km)	196,721 sq miles (509,640 sq km)

Land use and agricultural distribution

- cattle
- bananas
- coffee
- cotton
- corn (maize)
- shellfish
- sugar cane
- timber
- capital cities
- major towns
- pasture
- cropland
- forest

Bananas are harvested throughout the year along the Caribbean coast. Bananas are a perishable commodity and the plantations rely on good railroad links to the ports for rapid distribution.

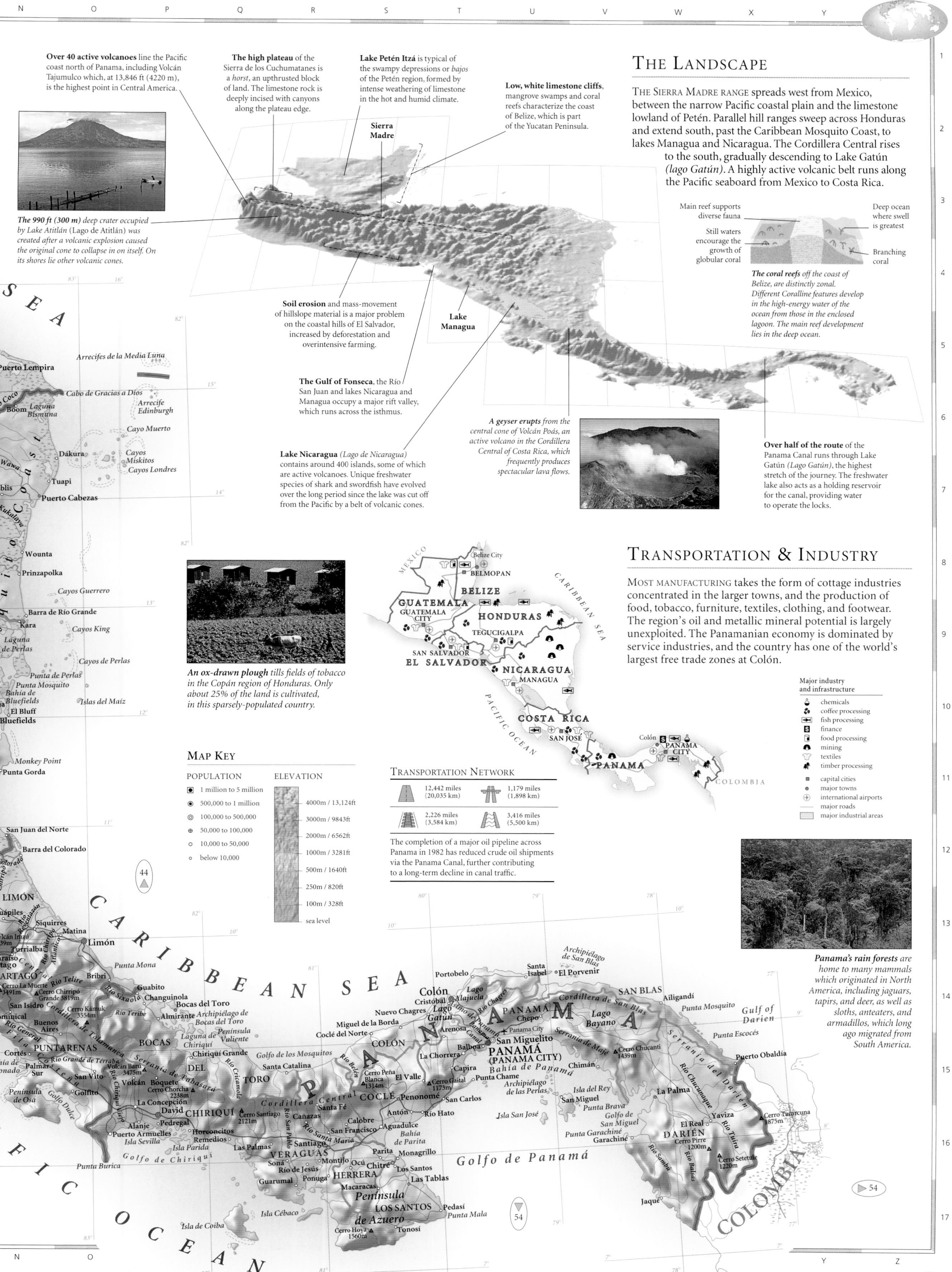
Sierra Madre
Lake Managua
Main reef supports diverse fauna
Still waters encourage the growth of globular coral
Deep ocean where swell is greatest
Branching coral
MEXICO
CARIBBEAN SEA
PACIFIC OCEAN
BELIZE
Belize City
BELMOPAN
GUATEMALA
GUATEMALA CITY
HONDURAS
TEGUCIGALPA
SAN SALVADOR
EL SALVADOR
NICARAGUA
MANAGUA
COSTA RICA
SAN JOSÉ
PANAMA
PANAMA CITY
Colón
COLOMBIA
Major industry and infrastructure
chemicals
coffee processing
fish processing
finance
food processing
mining
textiles
timber processing
capital cities
major towns
international airports
major roads
major industrial areas
MAP KEY
POPULATION
1 million to 5 million
500,000 to 1 million
100,000 to 500,000
50,000 to 100,000
10,000 to 50,000
below 10,000
ELEVATION
4000m / 13,124ft
3000m / 9843ft
2000m / 6562ft
1000m / 3281ft
500m / 1640ft
250m / 820ft
100m / 328ft
sea level
TRANSPORTATION NETWORK
12,442 miles (20,035 km)
1,179 miles (1,898 km)
2,226 miles (3,584 km)
3,416 miles (5,500 km)
CARIBBEAN SEA
PACIFIC OCEAN
Puerto Lempira
Arrecifes de la Media Luna
Cabo de Gracias a Dios
Arrecife Edinburgh
Laguna Bismuna
Cayo Muerto
Dákura
Cayos Miskitos
Cayos Londres
Tuapi
Puerto Cabezas
Wounta
Prinzapolka
Cayos Guerrero
Barra de Río Grande
Kara
Cayos King
Laguna de Perlas
Cayos de Perlas
Punta de Perlas
Punta Mosquito
Bahía de Bluefields
Islas del Maíz
El Bluff
Bluefields
Monkey Point
Punta Gorda
San Juan del Norte
Barra del Colorado
LIMÓN
Siquirres
Matina
Limón
Turrialba
CARTAGO
Punta Mona
Bribri
Guabito
Changuinola
Bocas del Toro
Archipiélago de Bocas del Toro
Almirante
Laguna de Chiriquí
Península Valiente
BOCAS
PUNTARENAS
Cortés
Palmar Sur
San Vito
Golfito
Península de Osa
Golfo Dulce
Volcán Barú 3475m
Volcán
Boquete
Cerro Chorcha 2238m
La Concepción
David
CHIRIQUÍ
Chiriquí Grande
Golfo de los Mosquitos
Santa Catalina
Cerro Santiago 2121m
Alanje
Pedregal
Horconcitos
Remedios
Puerto Armuelles
Isla Sevilla
Isla Parida
Golfo de Chiriquí
Punta Burica
Las Palmas
VERAGUAS
Santiago
Soná
Río de Jesús
Guarumal
Ponuga
Montijo
Ocú
Chitré
HERRERA
Macaracas
Península de Azuero
LOS SANTOS
Los Santos
Las Tablas
Pedasí
Punta Mala
Tonosí
Cerro Hoya 1560m
Isla Cébaco
Isla de Coiba
Portobelo
Colón
Cristóbal
Lago Gatún
Nuevo Chagres
Miguel de la Borda
Coclé del Norte
COLÓN
La Chorrera
Capira
Cerro Peña Blanca 1314m
El Valle
Cerro Gaital 1173m
Punta Chame
Penonomé
COCLÉ
San Carlos
Santa Fé
Cañazas
Calobre
San Francisco
Aguadulce
Antón
Río Hato
Bahía de Parita
Parita
Monagrillo
Golfo de Panamá
Balboa
San Miguelito
PANAMÁ (PANAMA CITY)
Bahía de Panamá
Archipiélago de las Perlas
Isla del Rey
San Miguel
Punta Brava
Golfo de San Miguel
Isla San José
Punta Garachiné
Garachiné
Chepo
Lago Bayano
Cerro Chucanti 1439m
Chimán
Serranía de Majé
Santa Isabel
El Porvenir
Archipiélago de San Blas
SAN BLAS
Cordillera de San Blas
Ailigandí
Punta Mosquito
Gulf of Darien
Punta Escocés
Puerto Obaldía
Serranía del Darién
La Palma
Yaviza
El Real
DARIÉN
Cerro Pirre 1200m
Cerro Tacarcuna 1875m
Cerro Setetule 1220m
Jaqué
COLOMBIA
Cordillera Central
PANAMÁ

THE LANDSCAPE

THE SIERRA MADRE RANGE spreads west from Mexico, between the narrow Pacific coastal plain and the limestone lowland of Petén. Parallel hill ranges sweep across Honduras and extend south, past the Caribbean Mosquito Coast, to lakes Managua and Nicaragua. The Cordillera Central rises to the south, gradually descending to Lake Gatún *(lago Gatún)*. A highly active volcanic belt runs along the Pacific seaboard from Mexico to Costa Rica.

Over 40 active volcanoes line the Pacific coast north of Panama, including Volcán Tajumulco which, at 13,846 ft (4220 m), is the highest point in Central America.

The high plateau of the Sierra de los Cuchumatanes is a *horst*, an upthrusted block of land. The limestone rock is deeply incised with canyons along the plateau edge.

Lake Petén Itzá is typical of the swampy depressions or *bajos* of the Petén region, formed by intense weathering of limestone in the hot and humid climate.

Low, white limestone cliffs, mangrove swamps and coral reefs characterize the coast of Belize, which is part of the Yucatan Peninsula.

***The 990 ft (300 m)** deep crater occupied by Lake Atitlán (Lago de Atitlán) was created after a volcanic explosion caused the original cone to collapse in on itself. On its shores lie other volcanic cones.*

***The coral reefs** off the coast of Belize, are distinctly zonal. Different Coralline features develop in the high-energy water of the ocean from those in the enclosed lagoon. The main reef development lies in the deep ocean.*

Soil erosion and mass-movement of hillslope material is a major problem on the coastal hills of El Salvador, increased by deforestation and overintensive farming.

The Gulf of Fonseca, the Río San Juan and lakes Nicaragua and Managua occupy a major rift valley, which runs across the isthmus.

***A geyser erupts** from the central cone of Volcán Poás, an active volcano in the Cordillera Central of Costa Rica, which frequently produces spectacular lava flows.*

Lake Nicaragua *(Lago de Nicaragua)* contains around 400 islands, some of which are active volcanoes. Unique freshwater species of shark and swordfish have evolved over the long period since the lake was cut off from the Pacific by a belt of volcanic cones.

Over half of the route of the Panama Canal runs through Lake Gatún *(Lago Gatún)*, the highest stretch of the journey. The freshwater lake also acts as a holding reservoir for the canal, providing water to operate the locks.

TRANSPORTATION & INDUSTRY

MOST MANUFACTURING takes the form of cottage industries concentrated in the larger towns, and the production of food, tobacco, furniture, textiles, clothing, and footwear. The region's oil and metallic mineral potential is largely unexploited. The Panamanian economy is dominated by service industries, and the country has one of the world's largest free trade zones at Colón.

***An ox-drawn plough** tills fields of tobacco in the Copán region of Honduras. Only about 25% of the land is cultivated, in this sparsely-populated country.*

The completion of a major oil pipeline across Panama in 1982 has reduced crude oil shipments via the Panama Canal, further contributing to a long-term decline in canal traffic.

***Panama's rain forests** are home to many mammals which originated in North America, including jaguars, tapirs, and deer, as well as sloths, anteaters, and armadillos, which long ago migrated from South America.*

44
54
54

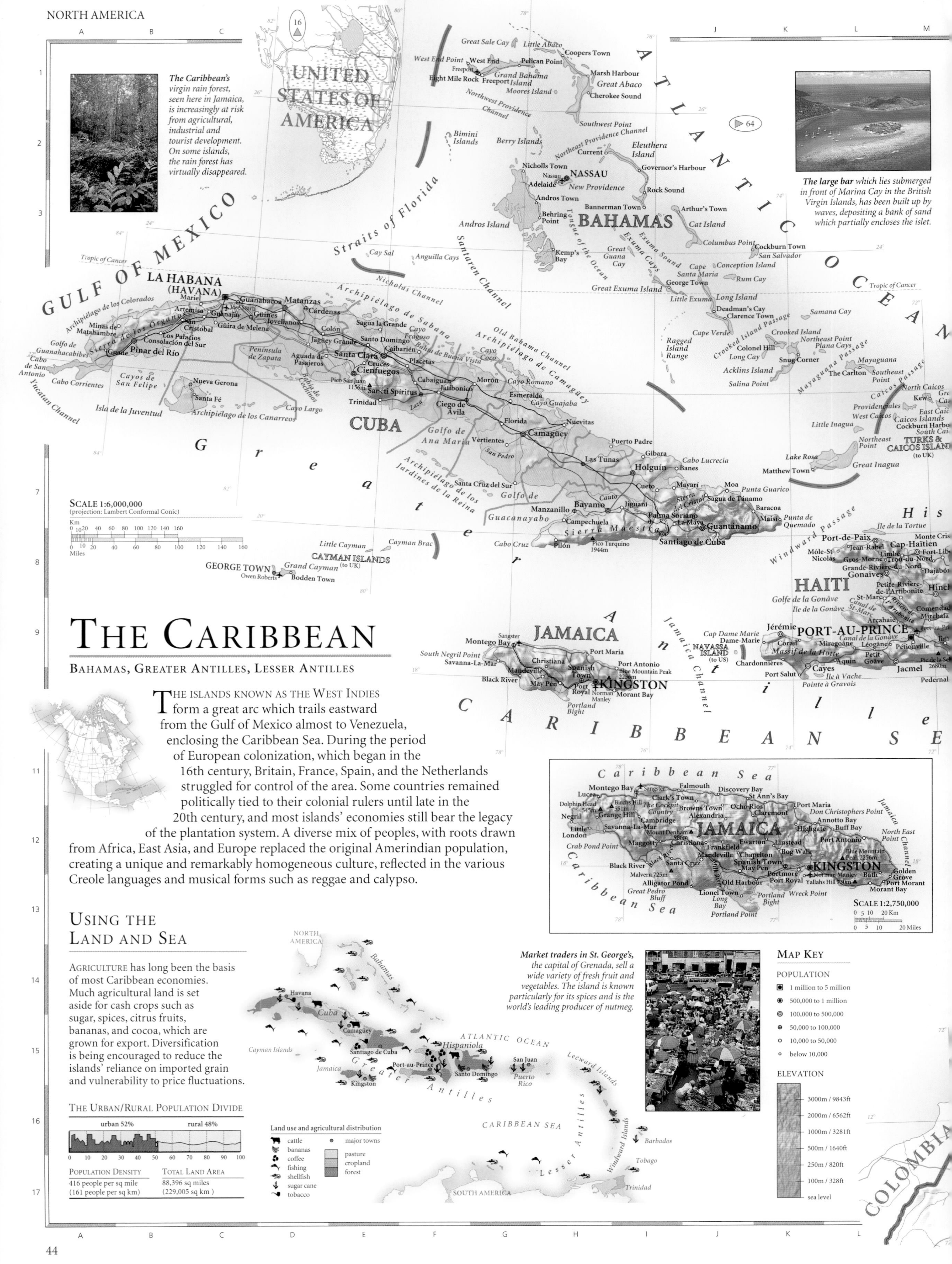

UNITED STATES OF AMERICA
GULF OF MEXICO
ATLANTIC OCEAN
BAHAMAS
NASSAU
CUBA
LA HABANA (HAVANA)
CAYMAN ISLANDS (to UK)
GEORGE TOWN
JAMAICA
KINGSTON
HAITI
PORT-AU-PRINCE
TURKS & CAICOS ISLANDS (to UK)
NAVASSA ISLAND (to US)
Greater Antilles
CARIBBEAN SEA
COLOMBIA
Straits of Florida
Tropic of Cancer
Windward Passage
Jamaica Channel
Yucatan Channel
SCALE 1:6,000,000
(projection: Lambert Conformal Conic)
SCALE 1:2,750,000

The Caribbean's virgin rain forest, seen here in Jamaica, is increasingly at risk from agricultural, industrial and tourist development. On some islands, the rain forest has virtually disappeared.

The large bar which lies submerged in front of Marina Cay in the British Virgin Islands, has been built up by waves, depositing a bank of sand which partially encloses the islet.

THE CARIBBEAN

BAHAMAS, GREATER ANTILLES, LESSER ANTILLES

THE ISLANDS KNOWN AS THE WEST INDIES form a great arc which trails eastward from the Gulf of Mexico almost to Venezuela, enclosing the Caribbean Sea. During the period of European colonization, which began in the 16th century, Britain, France, Spain, and the Netherlands struggled for control of the area. Some countries remained politically tied to their colonial rulers until late in the 20th century, and most islands' economies still bear the legacy of the plantation system. A diverse mix of peoples, with roots drawn from Africa, East Asia, and Europe replaced the original Amerindian population, creating a unique and remarkably homogeneous culture, reflected in the various Creole languages and musical forms such as reggae and calypso.

USING THE LAND AND SEA

AGRICULTURE has long been the basis of most Caribbean economies. Much agricultural land is set aside for cash crops such as sugar, spices, citrus fruits, bananas, and cocoa, which are grown for export. Diversification is being encouraged to reduce the islands' reliance on imported grain and vulnerability to price fluctuations.

THE URBAN/RURAL POPULATION DIVIDE

urban 52% | rural 48%

POPULATION DENSITY	TOTAL LAND AREA
416 people per sq mile (161 people per sq km)	88,396 sq miles (229,005 sq km)

Land use and agricultural distribution: cattle, bananas, coffee, fishing, shellfish, sugar cane, tobacco, major towns, pasture, cropland, forest

Market traders in St. George's, the capital of Grenada, sell a wide variety of fresh fruit and vegetables. The island is known particularly for its spices and is the world's leading producer of nutmeg.

MAP KEY

POPULATION
- 1 million to 5 million
- 500,000 to 1 million
- 100,000 to 500,000
- 50,000 to 100,000
- 10,000 to 50,000
- below 10,000

ELEVATION
- 3000m / 9843ft
- 2000m / 6562ft
- 1000m / 3281ft
- 500m / 1640ft
- 250m / 820ft
- 100m / 328ft
- sea level

TRANSPORTATION & INDUSTRY

CARIBBEAN INDUSTRY remains, with few exceptions, agricultural, and export-led, or service-based, supporting the flourishing tourist industry. However, several countries including Jamaica, Barbados, Trinidad and Tobago, and Puerto Rico have developed important mineral industries, and Cuba is attempting to diversify its economy by importing capital goods to start up new manufacturing businesses.

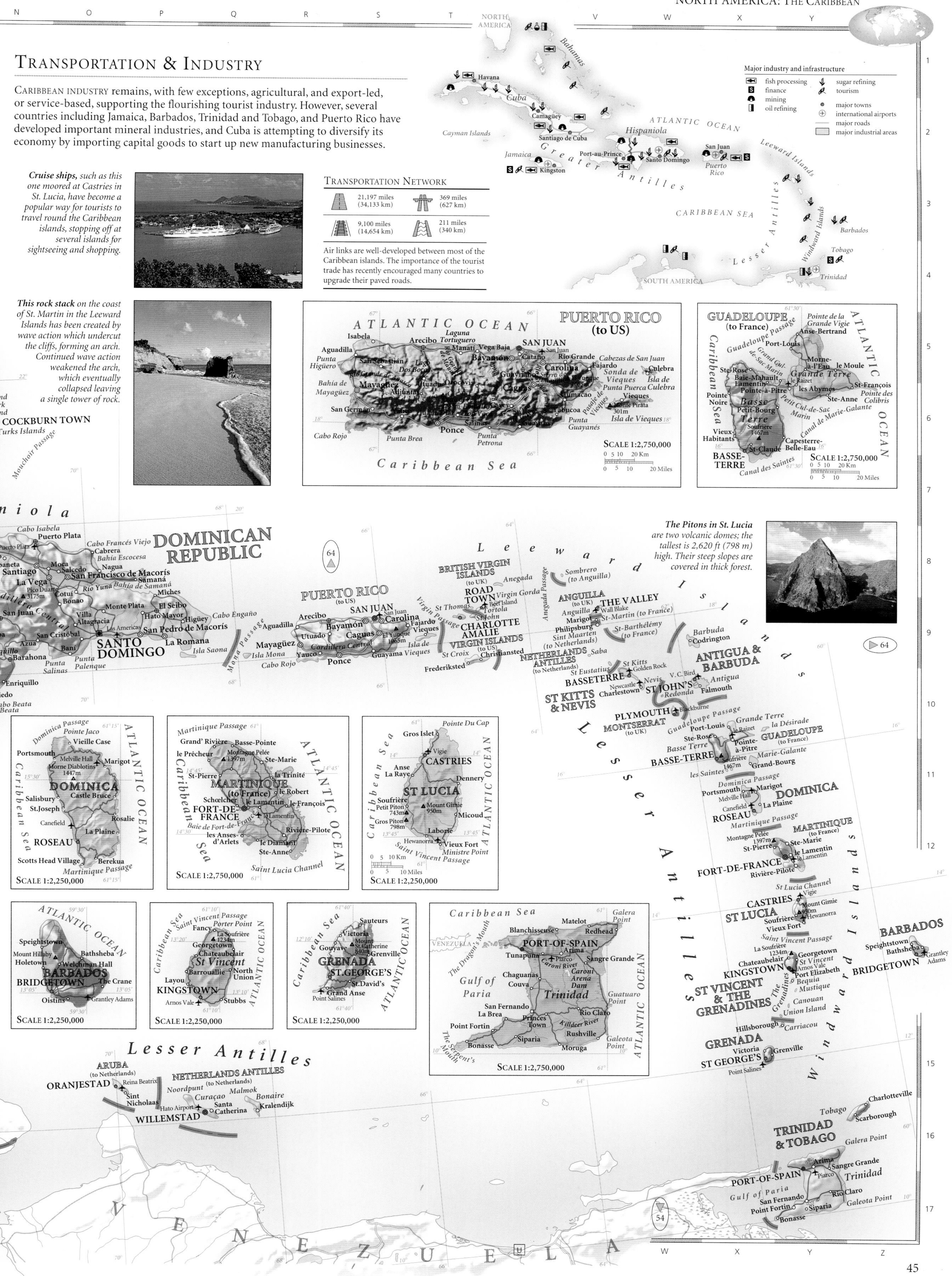

N O P Q R S T V W X Y Z
Major industry and infrastructure
fish processing
finance
mining
oil refining
sugar refining
tourism
major towns
international airports
major roads
major industrial areas
NORTH AMERICA
SOUTH AMERICA
Havana
Cuba
Camagüey
Santiago de Cuba
Cayman Islands
Jamaica
Kingston
Port-au-Prince
Hispaniola
Santo Domingo
San Juan
Puerto Rico
Bahamas
ATLANTIC OCEAN
CARIBBEAN SEA
Greater Antilles
Lesser Antilles
Leeward Islands
Windward Islands
Barbados
Tobago
Trinidad
TRANSPORTATION NETWORK
21,197 miles (34,133 km)
369 miles (627 km)
9,100 miles (14,654 km)
211 miles (340 km)
Air links are well-developed between most of the Caribbean islands. The importance of the tourist trade has recently encouraged many countries to upgrade their paved roads.
PUERTO RICO (to US)
SAN JUAN
Caribbean Sea
SCALE 1:2,750,000
GUADELOUPE (to France)
BASSE-TERRE
SCALE 1:2,750,000
DOMINICAN REPUBLIC
SANTO DOMINGO
BRITISH VIRGIN ISLANDS (to UK)
ROAD TOWN
VIRGIN ISLANDS (to US)
CHARLOTTE AMALIE
ANGUILLA (to UK)
THE VALLEY
NETHERLANDS ANTILLES (to Netherlands)
ST KITTS & NEVIS
BASSETERRE
ANTIGUA & BARBUDA
ST JOHN'S
PLYMOUTH
MONTSERRAT (to UK)
DOMINICA
ROSEAU
SCALE 1:2,250,000
MARTINIQUE (to France)
FORT-DE-FRANCE
SCALE 1:2,750,000
ST LUCIA
CASTRIES
SCALE 1:2,250,000
BARBADOS
BRIDGETOWN
SCALE 1:2,250,000
St Vincent
KINGSTOWN
SCALE 1:2,250,000
GRENADA
ST.GEORGE'S
SCALE 1:2,250,000
Trinidad
PORT-OF-SPAIN
SCALE 1:2,750,000
ST VINCENT & THE GRENADINES
GRENADA
ST GEORGE'S
TRINIDAD & TOBAGO
ARUBA (to Netherlands)
ORANJESTAD
NETHERLANDS ANTILLES (to Netherlands)
WILLEMSTAD
Lesser Antilles
VENEZUELA

Cruise ships, such as this one moored at Castries in St. Lucia, have become a popular way for tourists to travel round the Caribbean islands, stopping off at several islands for sightseeing and shopping.

This rock stack on the coast of St. Martin in the Leeward Islands has been created by wave action which undercut the cliffs, forming an arch. Continued wave action weakened the arch, which eventually collapsed leaving a single tower of rock.

The Pitons in St. Lucia are two volcanic domes; the tallest is 2,620 ft (798 m) high. Their steep slopes are covered in thick forest.

SOUTH AMERICA

REACHING FROM THE HUMID TROPICS DOWN INTO THE COLD SOUTH ATLANTIC, SOUTH AMERICA HAS AN AREA OF 6,886,000 SQ MILES (17,835,000 SQ KM). THERE ARE 12 SEPARATE COUNTRIES, WITH THE LARGEST, BRAZIL, COVERING ALMOST HALF THE CONTINENT.

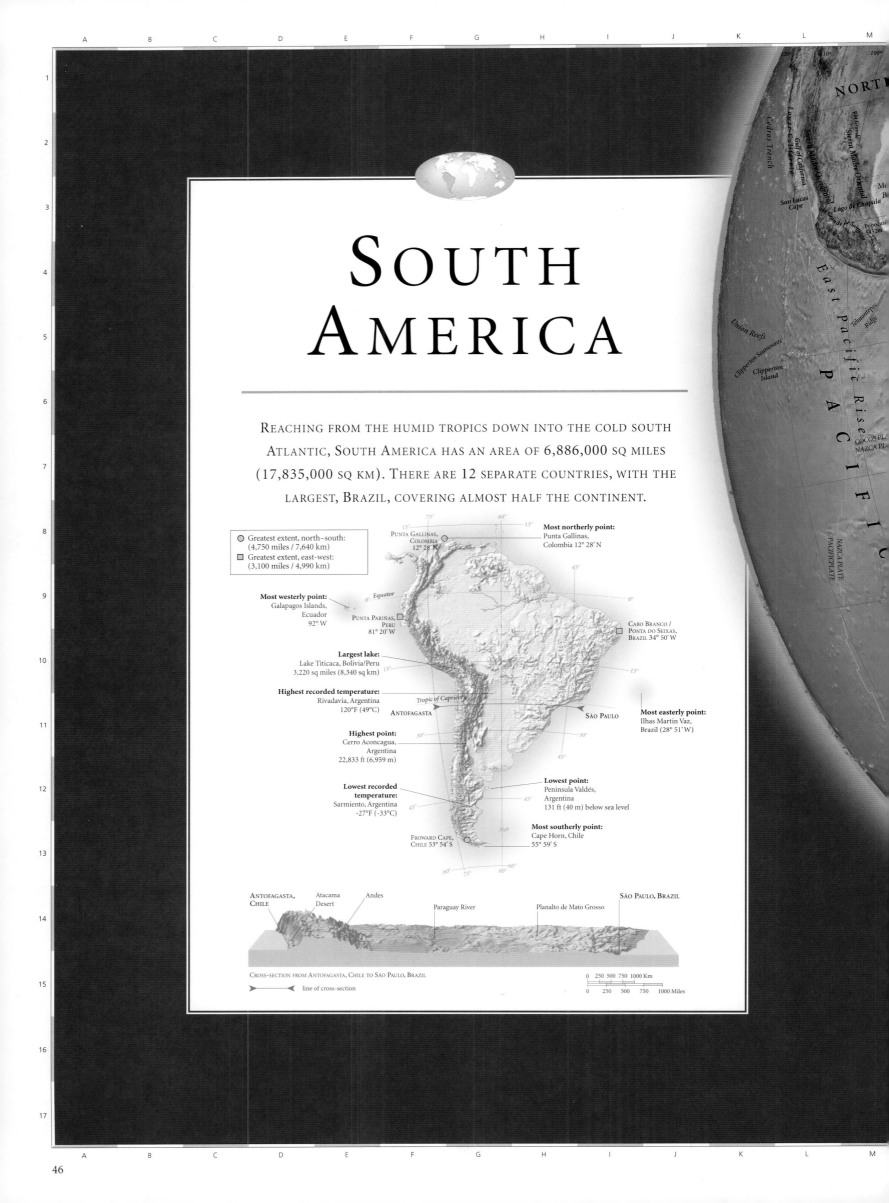

Greatest extent, north–south: (4,750 miles / 7,640 km)
Greatest extent, east-west: (3,100 miles / 4,990 km)
PUNTA GALLINAS, COLOMBIA 12° 28' N
Most northerly point: Punta Gallinas, Colombia 12° 28' N
Most westerly point: Galapagos Islands, Ecuador 92° W
Equator
PUNTA PARIÑAS, PERU 81° 20' W
CABO BRANCO / PONTA DO SEIXAS, BRAZIL 34° 50' W
Largest lake: Lake Titicaca, Bolivia/Peru 3,220 sq miles (8,340 sq km)
Highest recorded temperature: Rivadavia, Argentina 120°F (49°C)
Tropic of Capricorn
ANTOFAGASTA
SÃO PAULO
Most easterly point: Ilhas Martin Vaz, Brazil (28° 51' W)
Highest point: Cerro Aconcagua, Argentina 22,833 ft (6,959 m)
Lowest recorded temperature: Sarmiento, Argentina -27°F (-33°C)
Lowest point: Peninsula Valdés, Argentina 131 ft (40 m) below sea level
Most southerly point: Cape Horn, Chile 55° 59' S
FROWARD CAPE, CHILE 53° 54' S
ANTOFAGASTA, CHILE
Atacama Desert
Andes
Paraguay River
Planalto de Mato Grosso
SÃO PAULO, BRAZIL
CROSS-SECTION FROM ANTOFAGASTA, CHILE TO SÃO PAULO, BRAZIL
line of cross-section
0 250 500 750 1000 Km
0 250 500 750 1000 Miles
NORT
Cedros Trench
Gulf of California
Sierra Madre Occidental
Sierra Madre Oriental
San Lucas Cape
Lago de Chapala
East Pacific Rise
Union Reefs
Clipperton Seamounts
Clipperton Island
PACIFIC
COCOS PLA
NAZCA PLA
NAZCA PLATE

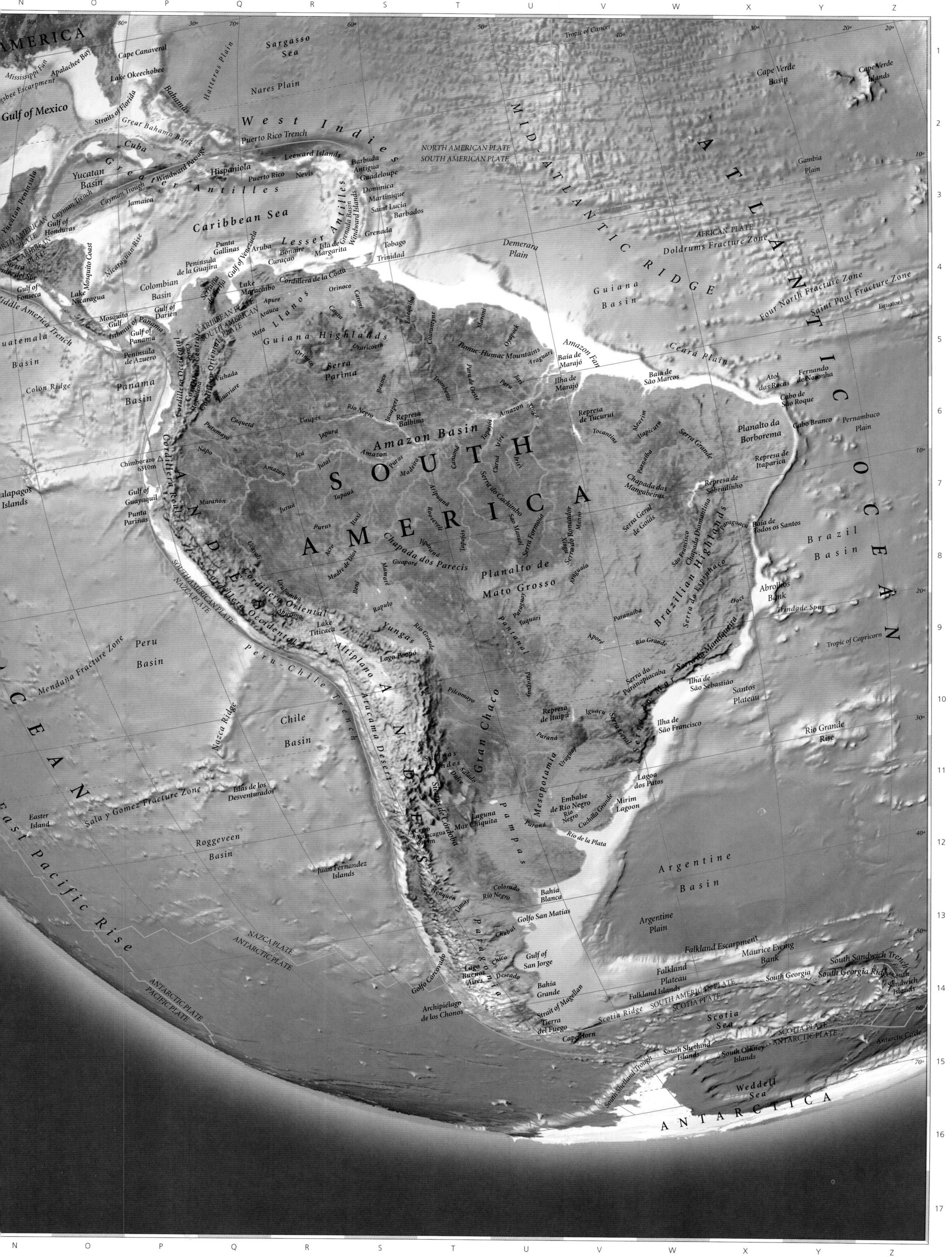

N O P Q R S T U V W X Y Z
1 2 3 4 5 6 7 8 9 10 11 12 13 14 15 16 17
AMERICA
Sargasso Sea
Tropic of Cancer
Cape Canaveral
Mississippi Fan
Apalachee Bay
Lake Okeechobee
Hatteras Plain
Cape Verde Basin
Cape Verde Islands
Nares Plain
Gulf of Mexico
Straits of Florida
Bahamas
West Indies
Great Bahama Bank
Puerto Rico Trench
Cuba
Greater Antilles
Windward Passage
Hispaniola
Leeward Islands
Barbuda
Antigua
Guadeloupe
NORTH AMERICAN PLATE
SOUTH AMERICAN PLATE
MID-ATLANTIC RIDGE
ATLANTIC OCEAN
Gambia Plain
Yucatan Peninsula
Yucatan Basin
Cayman Trench
Cayman Trough
Puerto Rico
Nevis
Dominica
Martinique
Saint Lucia
Barbados
Jamaica
Grenada Basin
Windward Islands
Caribbean Sea
Gulf of Honduras
Lesser Antilles
Grenada
Tobago
Trinidad
Nicaraguan Rise
Punta Gallinas
Aruba
Bonaire
Isla de Margarita
Curaçao
Demerara Plain
AFRICAN PLATE
Doldrums Fracture Zone
Mosquito Coast
Peninsula de la Guajira
Gulf of Venezuela
Lake Maracaibo
Cordillera de la Costa
Orinoco
Caroní
Colombian Basin
Gulf of Fonseca
Lake Nicaragua
Apure
Arauca
Guiana Basin
Four North Fracture Zone
Saint Paul Fracture Zone
Equator
Middle America Trench
Mosquito Gulf
Gulf of Darien
Isthmus of Panama
Gulf of Panama
Llanos
Guiana Highlands
Essequibo
Courantyne
Maroni
Oyapock
Tumuc-Humac Mountains
Amazon Fan
Ceara Plain
Guatemala Basin
Peninsula de Azuero
Meta
Uraricoera
Serra Parima
Araguari
Baía de Marajó
Baía de São Marcos
Atol das Rocas
Fernando de Noronha
Colón Ridge
Panama Basin
Cordillera Occidental
Cordillera Central
Cordillera Oriental
Vichada
Guaviare
Branco
Trombetas
Pará de Oeste
Jari
Pará
Ilha de Marajó
Cabo de São Roque
Caquetá
Vaupés
Rio Negro
Juauperi
Represa Balbina
Amazon
Xingu
Represa de Tucuruí
Mearim
Itapicuru
Serra Grande
Planalto da Borborema
Cabo Branco
Pernambuco Plain
Putumayo
Japurá
Amazon Basin
Tapajós
Tocantins
Parnaíba
Napo
Içá
Jutaí
Madeira
Purus
Canamã
Teles Pires
Iriri
Chimborazo 6310m
Amazon
SOUTH AMERICA
Represa de Itaparica
Chapada das Mangabeiras
Represa de Sobradinho
Galapagos Islands
Gulf of Guayaquil
Tapauá
Serra do Cachimbo
Marañón
Juruá
Aripuanã
Roosevelt
São Manuel
Serra Formosa
Serra do Roncador
Serra Geral de Goiás
Baía de Todos os Santos
Punta Pariñas
Purus
Ituxi
Brazil Basin
Acre
Chapada dos Parecis
Ucayali
Madre de Dios
Guaporé
Mamoré
Planalto de Mato Grosso
Araguaia
São Francisco
Chapada Diamantina
Brazilian Highlands
Serra do Espinhaço
Paraguaçu
SOUTH AMERICAN PLATE
NAZCA PLATE
Cordillera Oriental
Cordillera Occidental
Beni
Abrolhos Bank
Trindade Spur
Lake Titicaca
Rapulo
Paraguay
Taquari
Pantanal
Paranaíba
Doce
Peru Basin
Yungas
Rio Grande
Aporé
Rio Grande
Tropic of Capricorn
Mendaña Fracture Zone
Peru-Chile Trench
Altiplano
Lago Poopó
ANDES
Serra do Paranapiacaba
Serra do Mar
Serra da Mantiqueira
Ilha de São Sebastião
Santos Plateau
Pilcomayo
Represa de Itaipu
Iguaçu
Serra Geral
Ilha de São Francisco
Chile Basin
Atacama Desert
Nazca Ridge
Gran Chaco
Paraná
Rio Grande Rise
OCEAN
Salado
Dulce
Uruguay
Mesopotamia
Lagoa dos Patos
Sala y Gomez Fracture Zone
Islas de los Desventurados
Embalse de Río Negro
Cuchilla Grande
Mirim Lagoon
Easter Island
Pampas
Laguna Mar Chiquita
Paraná
Río de la Plata
Roggeveen Basin
Aconcagua
Juan Fernández Islands
Argentine Basin
East Pacific Rise
Colorado
Río Negro
Bahía Blanca
Neuquén
Limay
Golfo San Matías
Argentine Plain
Chubut
Patagonia
NAZCA PLATE
ANTARCTIC PLATE
Gulf of San Jorge
Falkland Escarpment
Maurice Ewing Bank
South Sandwich Trench
Chico
Lago Buenos Aires
Deseado
Falkland Plateau
South Georgia
South Georgia Ridge
South Sandwich Islands
Golfo Corcovado
ANTARCTIC PLATE
PACIFIC PLATE
Bahía Grande
Falkland Islands
SOUTH AMERICAN PLATE
SCOTIA PLATE
Archipiélago de los Chonos
Strait of Magellan
Tierra del Fuego
Scotia Ridge
Scotia Sea
Cape Horn
SCOTIA PLATE
ANTARCTIC PLATE
Antarctic Circle
South Shetland Islands
South Orkney Islands
South Shetland Trough
Weddell Sea
ANTARCTICA

PHYSICAL SOUTH AMERICA

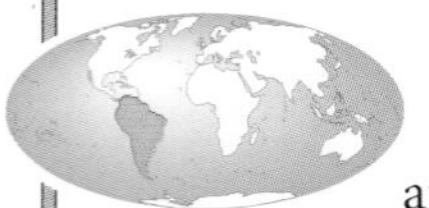

THREE MAJOR PHYSIOGRAPHIC REGIONS characterize South America. The oldest, the ancient Brazilian Shield and the smaller Guyana and Patagonian shields, form the stable core of the continent. Stretching along the entire west coast are the younger Andean fold mountains with many summits rising to 20,000 ft (6,100 m). These two diverse regions are separated by a number of sedimentary basins carrying South America's large river systems to the sea. These include the massive Amazon Basin and the basin of the Gran Chaco.

THE AMAZON BASIN AND GUYANA SHIELD

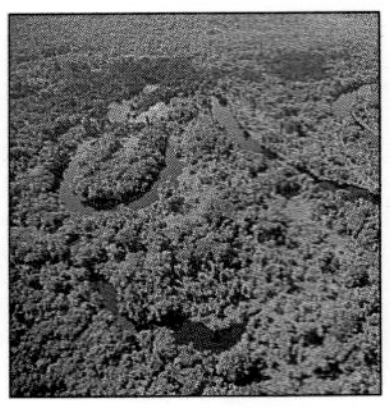

THE RIVER AMAZON occupies a large depression in the Earth's crust, formed by the uplift of the Andes. It is covered by thick volcanic deposits and layers of alluvium – these have been laid down by the Amazon's many tributaries. To the north is the smaller Guyana Shield.

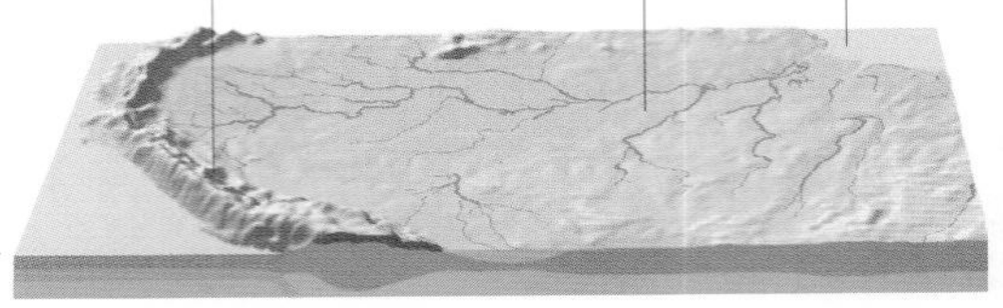

Headwaters of the Amazon rise in the Andes
Thick alluvium deposits
Mouths of the Amazon
A A

Section across northern South America showing Amazon Basin and its drainage pattern.

0 500 1000 Km
0 500 1000 Miles

SCALE 1:30,500,000 (projection: Lambert Azimuthal Equal Area)

Km 0 100 200 400 600 800
Miles 0 100 200 400 600 800

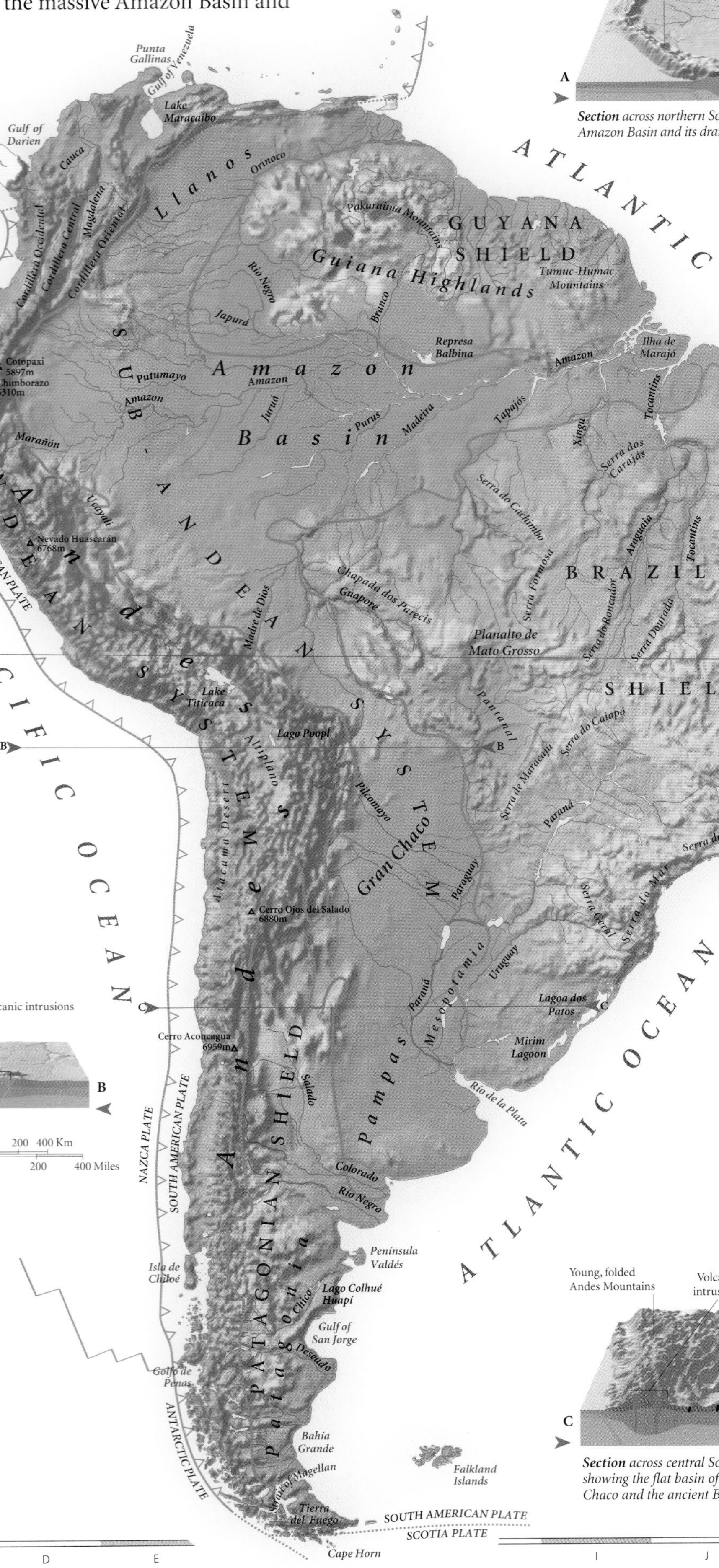

Punta Gallinas
Gulf of Venezuela
Lake Maracaibo
Gulf of Darien
Gulf of Panama
Cauca
Cordillera Occidental
Cordillera Central
Magdalena
Cordillera Oriental
Llanos
Orinoco
Pakaraima Mountains
GUYANA SHIELD
Guiana Highlands
Tumuc-Humac Mountains
Rio Negro
Branco
Japurá
Represa Balbina
Amazon
Ilha de Marajó
Putumayo
Amazon Basin
Juruá
Purus
Madeira
Tapajós
Xingu
Tocantins
Serra dos Carajás
Cotopaxi 5897m
Chimborazo 6310m
Cordillera Real
Gulf of Guayaquil
Marañón
Punta Negra
Ucayali
Nevado Huascarán 6768m
Serra do Cachimbo
Araguaia
Tocantins
Planalto da Borborema
Cabo de São Roque
Represa de Sobradinho
BRAZILIAN SHIELD
Brazilian Highlands
São Francisco
Serra do Espinhaço
Chapada dos Parecis
Guaporé
Madre de Dios
Planalto de Mato Grosso
Serra Formosa
Serra do Roncador
Serra Dourada
Pantanal
Serra do Caiapó
Serra de Maracaju
SUB-ANDEAN SYSTEM
ANDEAN SYSTEM
Andes
Lake Titicaca
Lago Poopó
Altiplano
Atacama Desert
Pilcomayo
Gran Chaco
Paraguay
Paraná
Serra da Mantiqueira
Serra Geral
Serra do Mar
Cerro Ojos del Salado 6880m
Uruguay
Mesopotamia
Lagoa dos Patos
Mirim Lagoon
Cerro Aconcagua 6959m
Salado
Pampas
Río de la Plata
PATAGONIAN SHIELD
Patagonia
Colorado
Río Negro
Península Valdés
Isla de Chiloé
Lago Colhué Huapí
Chico
Gulf of San Jorge
Deseado
Golfo de Penas
Bahía Grande
Strait of Magellan
Falkland Islands
Tierra del Fuego
Cape Horn
ATLANTIC OCEAN
PACIFIC OCEAN
ATLANTIC OCEAN
COCOS PLATE
NAZCA PLATE
SOUTH AMERICAN PLATE
NAZCA PLATE
SOUTH AMERICAN PLATE
ANTARCTIC PLATE
SOUTH AMERICAN PLATE
SCOTIA PLATE

THE ANDEAN UPLANDS

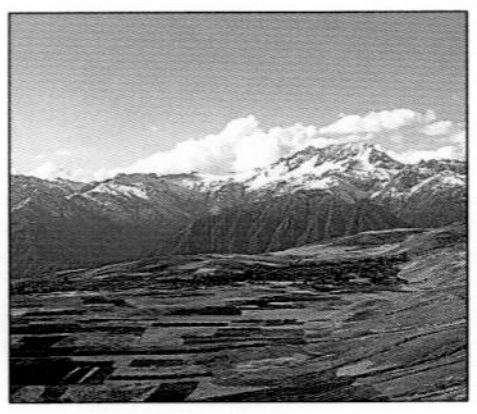

THE ANDEAN UPLANDS run along the west coast of South America. They are being uplifted as the Nazca Plate is subducted beneath the South American Plate. They contain some of the world's largest volcanoes, such as Cotopaxi, and Lake Titicaca which occupies a dormant site. The far south has many large ice-sheets and a fragmented coastline.

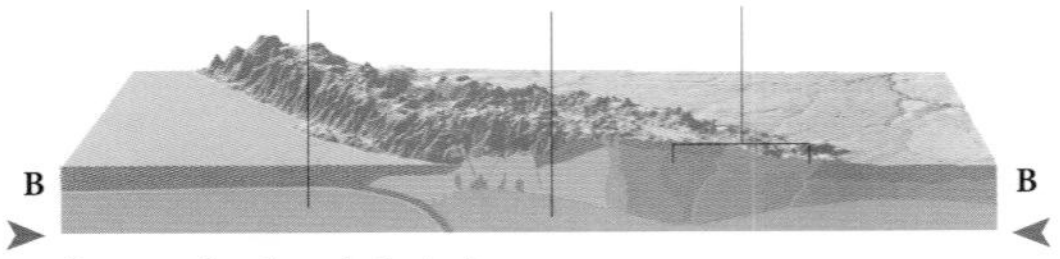

Nazca Plate
South American Plate
Volcanic intrusions
B B

Cross-section through the Andes showing the subduction of the Nazca Plate beneath the South American Plate.

0 200 400 Km
0 200 400 Miles

MAP KEY

ELEVATION

6000m / 19,686ft
4000m / 13,124ft
3000m / 9843ft
2000m / 6562ft
1500m / 4922ft
1000m / 3281ft
500m / 1640ft
250m / 820ft
100m / 328ft
sea level

PLATE MARGINS (for explanation see page xiv)

constructive
destructive
conservative
uncertain

physiographic regions
line of cross-section

THE BRAZILIAN SHIELD AND GRAN CHACO

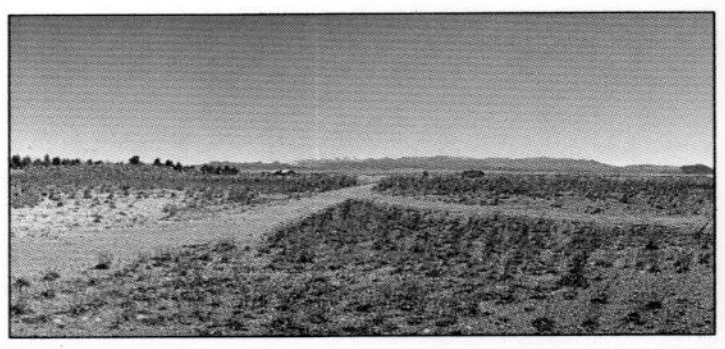

THE IMMENSE BRAZILIAN SHIELD underlies more than one-third of South America. It is pitted with numerous volcanic intrusions, and a large basaltic plateau exists between the Paraná River and the Atlantic Ocean. The flat Gran Chaco lies to the west of the shield, covered by sedimentary deposits eroded from the Andes, and transported by South America's mighty rivers.

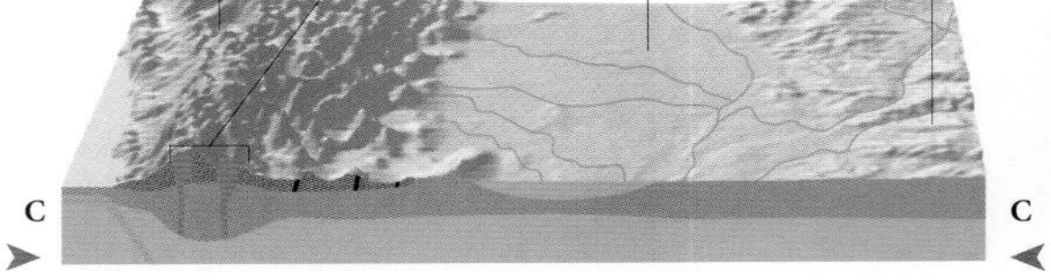

Young, folded Andes Mountains
Volcanic intrusions
Major rivers drain to the south through the Gran Chaco
Ancient resistant shield
C C

Section across central South America showing the flat basin of the Gran Chaco and the ancient Brazilian Shield.

0 200 400 Km
0 200 400 Miles

Climate

The climate of South America is influenced by three principal factors: the seasonal shift of high pressure air masses over the tropics, cold ocean currents along the western coast, affecting temperature and precipitation, and the mountain barrier produced by by the Andes, which creates a rain shadow over much of the south.

Mild winters and cool summers typify the extensive Pampas grasslands of Argentina.

Chile's hyperarid Atacama Desert is renowned as one of the driest places on Earth.

Climate
- tundra
- cool continental
- warm humid
- semiarid
- arid
- humid equatorial
- tropical
- daily hours of sunshine, January
- daily hours of sunshine, July
- cold wind

Maracaibo, Caracas, Georgetown, Cayenne, Bogotá, Quito, Equator, Belém, Manaus, Altos, Recife, Lima, Brasília, La Paz, Santa Cruz, Belo Horizonte, La Quiaca, Tropic of Capricorn, Antofagasta, Rio de Janeiro, Asunción, Cordoba, Porto Alegre, Santiago, Buenos Aires, Montevideo, Concepción, Pamperos, Stanley

Temperature

Equator, 20°, Tropic of Capricorn, 40°

Average January temperature

Average July temperature

Temperature
- below -22°F (-30°C)
- -22 to -4°F (-30 to -20°C)
- -4 to 14°F (-20 to -10°C)
- 14 to 32°F (-10 to 0°C)
- 32 to 50°F (0 to 10°C)
- 50°F (10 to 20°C)
- 68 to 86°F (20 to 30°C)
- above 86°F (30°C)

Rainfall

Equator, 20°, Tropic of Capricorn, 40°

Average January rainfall

Average July rainfall

Rainfall
- 0–1 in (0–25 mm)
- 1–2 in (25–50 mm)
- 2–4 in (50–100 mm)
- 4–8 in (100–200 mm)
- 8–12 in (200–300 mm)
- 12–16 in (300–400 mm)
- 16–20 in (400–500 mm)
- more than 20 in (500 mm)

***Tropical conditions** are found across over half of South America. When both rainfall and temperatures are high, hot humid rain forests prevail.*

Shaping the Continent

South America's active tectonic belt has been extensively folded over millions of years; landslides are still frequent in the mountains. The large river systems that erode the mountains flow across resistant shield areas, depositing sediment. Present-day glaciation affects the distinctive landscape of the far south.

Mass Movement

6 Debris slides are common in the highlands of South America *(left)*. They occur where soil on a slope is saturated by rainwater and therefore less stable. The actual slides are often triggered by earthquakes.

Scarp face left after soil has moved to the base of the slope
Failure plane
Toe of debris slide

Mass movement: A section of a debris slide

Chemical Weathering

1 Table mountains *(left)* are the eroded remnants of an ancient upland. As water percolates along cracks in these high, flat-topped mountains it forms intricate cave systems. Chemical weathering also isolates large blocks which then collapse, accumulating as rockfalls at the foot of scarp slopes.

Smooth summit dissected by deep gorges
Rainfall
Runoff surges down caverns as waterfalls

Chemical weathering: Erosion of the Guyana Shield

River Systems

2 Along the Amazon *(above)* there is a great variation in rates of erosion. As the headwaters of the Amazon flow down from the Andes, they erode and transport vast quantities of sediment, and are known as whitewaters. Across the shield areas erosion rates are very low. These rivers, carrying rotting vegetation, are called blackwaters.

Whitewater river
Blackwater river
Little erosion in shield areas
Confluence of whitewater with blackwater

River systems: Suspended sediments in the Amazon

The Evolving Landscape

Landscape
- uplifting land
- stable land
- sinking land
- glacier
- ocean current
- aluvial fan
- inselberg
- river

Folding

5 Folding occurs beneath the surface under high temperatures and pressures. Rocks become sufficiently malleable to flow and not fracture as tectonic plates collide. In the Valley of the Moon in Chile *(above)*, anticlines (or upfolds) and synclines (or troughs) have been exploited by erosion.

Fold axis
Anticline
Syncline
Fold axis

Folding: Synclines and anticlines

Deposition

4 Large alluvial fans are found extensively across South America *(above)*. Confined mountain rivers, carrying large quantities of eroded material, emerge from a mountain gorge onto the plains, where they deposit their load in huge fans.

Mountain front
Subsequent fan
Confined stream in the mountains
Fan forms as stream emerges onto the plain

Deposition: Formation of an alluvial fan

Glaciation

3 As fjord glaciers in Patagonia *(above)* retreat, they become grounded on shoals. In deeper water the base of the glacier becomes unstable, and icebergs break off (calve) until the glacier snout grounds once more.

Unstable front in deep water, where ice is fracturing
Original extent of glacier
Icebergs
Stable front
Glacier was grounded against a shoal

Glaciation: Retreating glacier in Patagonia

POLITICAL SOUTH AMERICA

MODERN SOUTH AMERICA'S POLITICAL BOUNDARIES have their origins in the territorial endeavors of explorers during the 16th century, who claimed almost the entire continent for Portugal and Spain. The Portuguese land in the east later evolved into the federal state of Brazil, while the Spanish vice-royalties eventually emerged as separate independent nation-states in the early 19th century. South America's growing population has become increasingly urbanized, with the growth of coastal cities into large conurbations like Rio de Janeiro and Buenos Aires. In Brazil, Argentina, Chile and Uruguay, a succession of military dictatorships has given way to fragile, but strengthening, democracies.

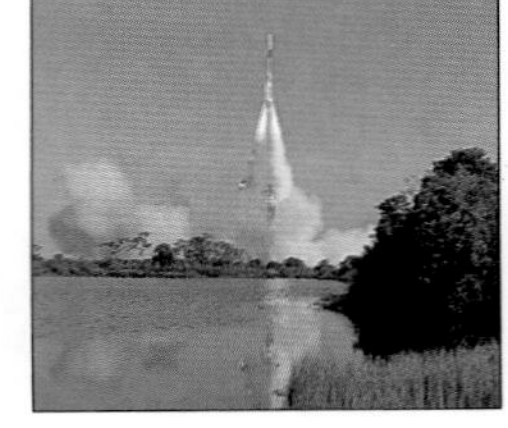

***Europe retains** a small foothold in South America. Kourou in French Guiana was the site chosen by the European Space Agency to launch the Ariane rocket. As a result of its status as a French overseas department, French Guiana is actually part of the European Union.*

SCALE 1:24,000,000
(projection: Lambert Azimuthal Equal Area)

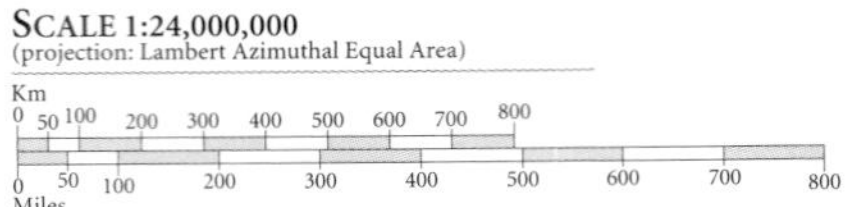
Km
0 50 100 200 300 400 500 600 700 800
0 50 100 200 300 400 500 600 700 800
Miles

TRANSPORTATION

MOST MAJOR ROAD AND RAIL ROUTES are confined to the coastal regions by the forbidding natural barriers of the Andes Mountains and the Amazon Basin. Few major cross-continental routes exist, although Buenos Aires serves as a transportation center for the main rail links to La Paz and Valparaíso, while the construction of the Trans-Amazon and Pan-American Highways have made direct road travel possible from Recife to Lima and from Puerto Montt up the coast into central America. A new waterway project is proposed to transform the River Paraguay into a major shipping route, although it involves considerable wetland destruction.

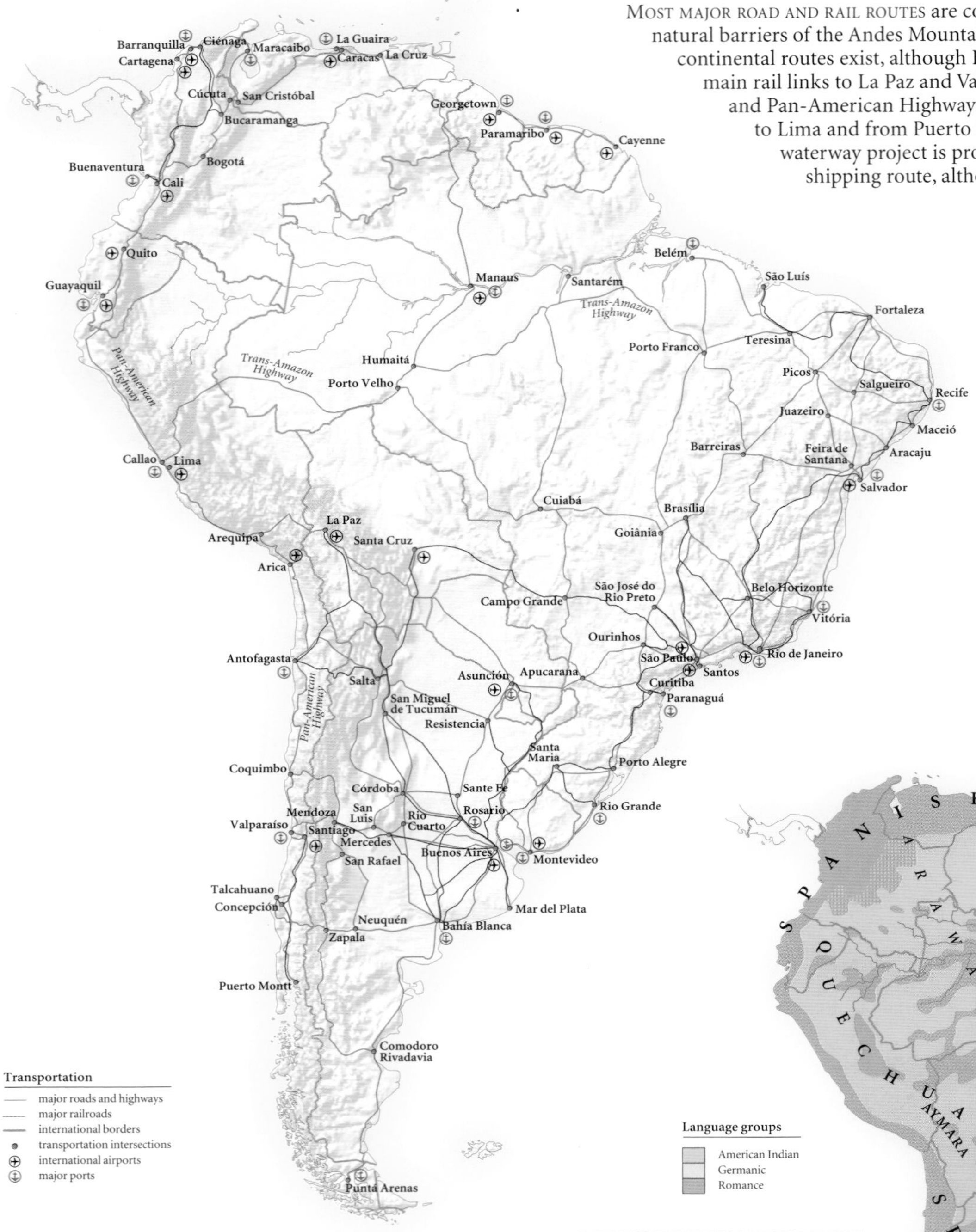

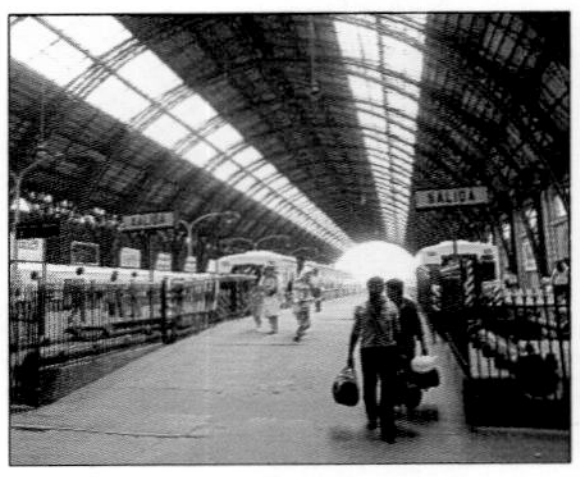

***South America's** most extensive rail network is centered on the Argentinian capital, Buenos Aires. The construction of new rail lines ouward from this important port, allowed the colonization of the Pampas lands for agriculture.*

Transportation
- major roads and highways
- major railroads
- international borders
- transportation intersections
- international airports
- major ports

LANGUAGES

PRIOR TO EUROPEAN EXPLORATION in the 16th century, a diverse range of indigenous languages were spoken across the continent. With the arrival of Iberian settlers, Spanish became the dominant language, with Portuguese spoken in Brazil, and Native American languages such as Quechua and Guaraní, becoming concentrated in the continental interior. Today this pattern persists, although successive European colonization has led to Dutch being spoken in Suriname, English in Guyana, and French in French Guiana, while in large urban areas, Japanese and Chinese are increasingly common.

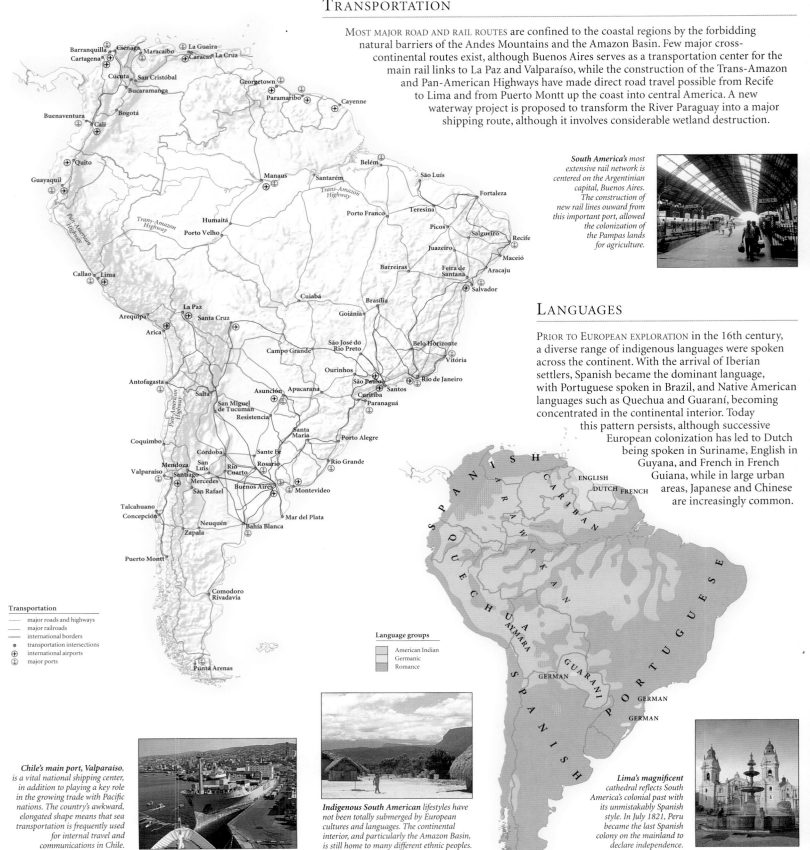

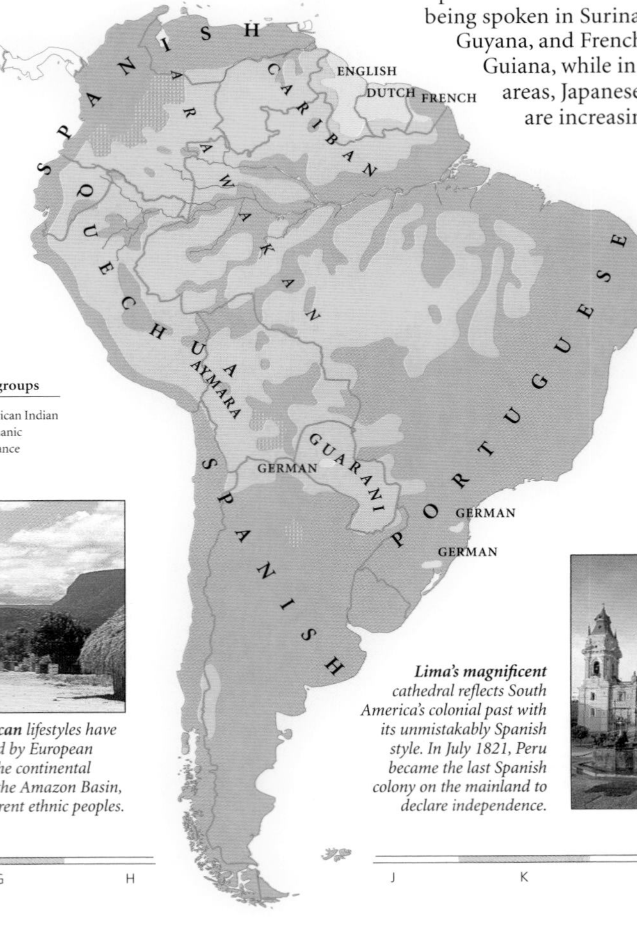

Language groups
- American Indian
- Germanic
- Romance

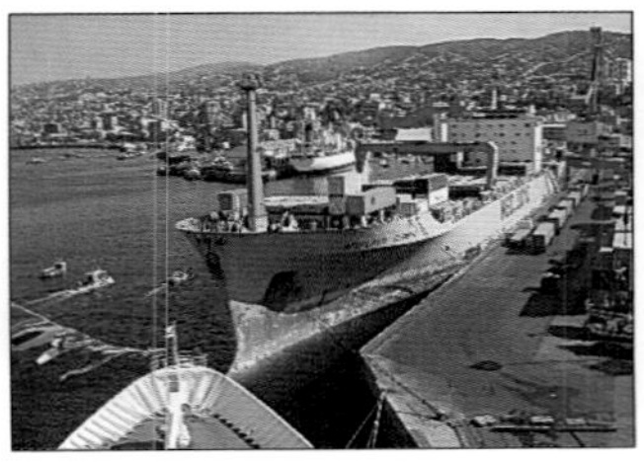

***Chile's main port, Valparaíso,** is a vital national shipping center, in addition to playing a key role in the growing trade with Pacific nations. The country's awkward, elongated shape means that sea transportation is frequently used for internal travel and communications in Chile.*

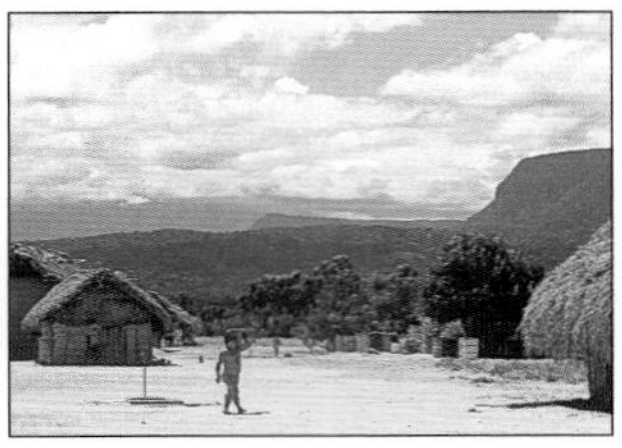

***Indigenous South American** lifestyles have not been totally submerged by European cultures and languages. The continental interior, and particularly the Amazon Basin, is still home to many different ethnic peoples.*

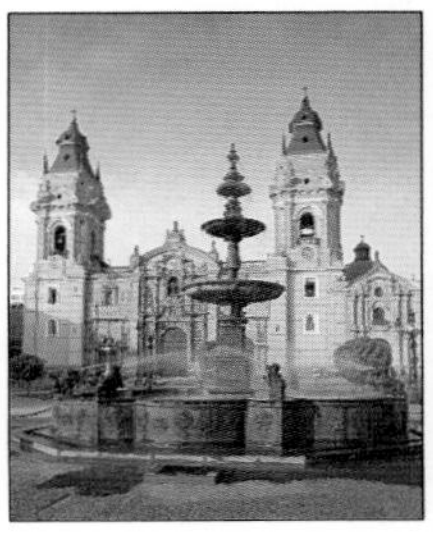

***Lima's magnificent** cathedral reflects South America's colonial past with its unmistakably Spanish style. In July 1821, Peru became the last Spanish colony on the mainland to declare independence.*

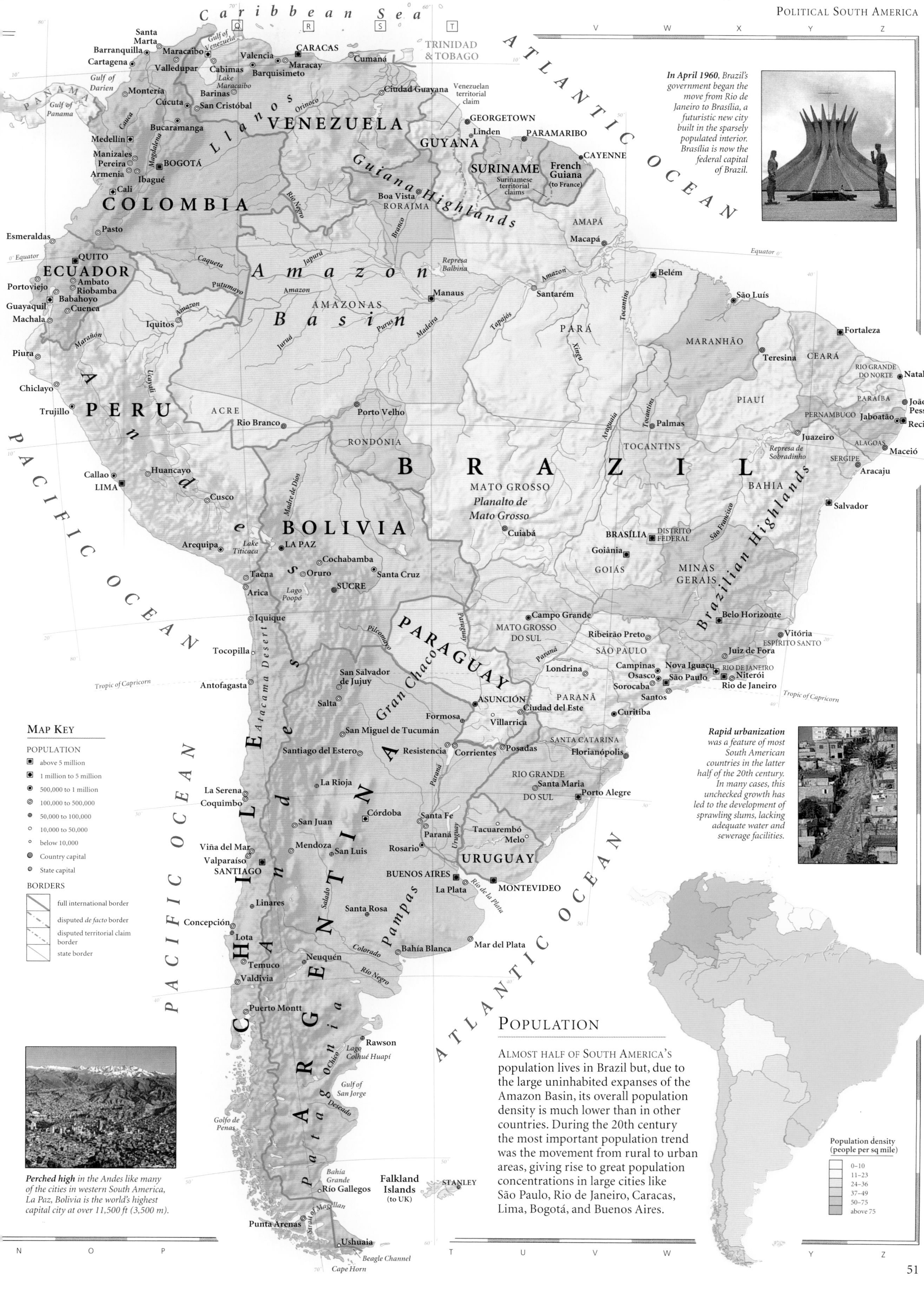

***In April 1960,** Brazil's government began the move from Rio de Janeiro to Brasília, a futuristic new city built in the sparsely populated interior. Brasília is now the federal capital of Brazil.*

***Rapid urbanization** was a feature of most South American countries in the latter half of the 20th century. In many cases, this unchecked growth has led to the development of sprawling slums, lacking adequate water and sewerage facilities.*

MAP KEY

POPULATION

- above 5 million
- 1 million to 5 million
- 500,000 to 1 million
- 100,000 to 500,000
- 50,000 to 100,000
- 10,000 to 50,000
- below 10,000
- Country capital
- State capital

BORDERS

- full international border
- disputed *de facto* border
- disputed territorial claim border
- state border

***Perched high** in the Andes like many of the cities in western South America, La Paz, Bolivia is the world's highest capital city at over 11,500 ft (3,500 m).*

POPULATION

ALMOST HALF OF SOUTH AMERICA'S population lives in Brazil but, due to the large uninhabited expanses of the Amazon Basin, its overall population density is much lower than in other countries. During the 20th century the most important population trend was the movement from rural to urban areas, giving rise to great population concentrations in large cities like São Paulo, Rio de Janeiro, Caracas, Lima, Bogotá, and Buenos Aires.

Population density (people per sq mile)

- 0–10
- 11–23
- 24–36
- 37–49
- 50–75
- above 75

South American Resources

Agriculture still provides the largest single form of employment in South America, although rural unemployment and poverty continue to drive people toward the huge coastal cities in search of jobs and opportunities. Mineral and fuel resources, although substantial, are distributed unevenly; few countries have both fossil fuels and minerals. To break industrial dependence on raw materials, boost manufacturing, and improve infrastructure, governments borrowed heavily from the World Bank in the 1960s and 1970s. This led to the accumulation of massive debts which are unlikely ever to be repaid. Today, Brazil dominates the continent's economic output, followed by Argentina. Recently, the less-developed western side of South America has benefited due to its geographical position; for example Chile is increasingly exporting raw materials to Japan.

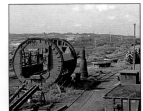

Ciudad Guayana is a planned industrial complex in eastern Venezuela, built as an iron and steel centre to exploit the nearby iron ore reserves.

Industry

aerospace, brewing, car/vehicle manufacture, chemicals, electronics, engineering, finance, fish processing, food processing, hi-tech industry, iron & steel, meat processing, metal refining, narcotics, pharmaceuticals, printing & publishing, shipbuilding, sugar processing, textiles, timber processing, tobacco processing, wine, oil, gas, industrial cities, major industrial areas

***The cold Peru Current** flows north from the Antarctic along the Pacific coast of Peru, providing rich nutrients for one of the world's largest fishing grounds. Overexploitation has severely reduced Peru's anchovy catch.*

Standard of Living

Wealth disparities throughout the continent create a wide gulf between affluent landowners and the chronically poor in inner-city slums. The illicit production of cocaine, and the hugely influential drug barons who control its distribution, contribute to the violent disorder and corruption which affect northwestern South America, de-stabilizing local governments and economies.

Standard of Living (UN Human Development Index): low – high

GNP per capita (US$): 0–499; 500–999; 1000–1499; 1500–2999; 3000–5999; 6000+

***Both Argentina and Chile** are now exploring the southernmost tip of the continent in search of oil. Here in Punta Arenas, a drilling rig is being prepared for exploratory drilling in the Strait of Magellen.*

Industry

Argentina and Brazil are South America's most industrialized countries and São Paulo is the continent's leading industrial center. Long-term government investment in Brazilian industry has encouraged a diverse industrial base; engineering, steel production, food processing, textile manufacture, and chemicals predominate. The illegal production of cocaine is economically significant in the Andean countries of Colombia and Bolivia. In Venezuela, the oil-dominated economy has left the country vulnerable to world oil price fluctuations. Food processing and mineral exploitation are common throughout the less industrially developed parts of the continent, including Bolivia, Chile, Ecuador, and Peru.

Environmental Issues

The Amazon Basin is one of the last great wilderness areas left on Earth. The tropical rain forests which grow there are a valuable genetic resource, containing innumerable unique plants and animals. The forests are increasingly under threat from new and expanding settlements and "slash and burn" farming techniques, which clear land for the raising of beef cattle, causing land degradation and soil erosion.

Clouds of smoke billow *from the burning Amazon rain forest. Over 25,000 sq miles (60,000 sq km) of virgin rain forest are being cleared annually, destroying an ancient, irreplaceable, natural resource and biodiverse habitat.*

Environmental Issues

- national parks
- tropical forest
- forest destroyed
- desert
- desertification
- polluted rivers
- marine pollution
- heavy marine pollution
- poor urban air quality

Mineral Resources

Over a quarter of the world's known copper reserves are found at the Chuquicamata mine in northern Chile, and other metallic minerals such as tin are found along the length of the Andes. The discovery of oil and gas at Venezuela's Lake Maracaibo in 1917 turned the country into one of the world's leading oil producers. In contrast, South America is virtually devoid of coal, the only significant deposit being on the peninsula of Guajira in Colombia.

Copper is Chile's *largest export, most of which is mined at Chuquicamata. Along the length of the Andes, metallic minerals like copper and tin are found in abundance, formed by the excessive pressures and heat involved in mountain-building.*

Mineral Resources

- oil field
- gas field
- coal field
- bauxite
- copper
- diamonds
- gold
- iron
- lead
- silver
- tin

Using the Land and Sea

Many foods now common worldwide originated in South America. These include the potato, tomato, squash, and cassava. Today, large herds of beef cattle roam the temperate grasslands of the Pampas, supporting an extensive meatpacking trade in Argentina, Uruguay and Paraguay. Corn (maize) is grown as a staple crop across the continent and coffee is grown as a cash crop in Brazil and Colombia. Coca plants grown in Bolivia, Peru, and Colombia provide most of the world's cocaine. Fish and shellfish are caught off the western coast, especially anchovies off Peru, shrimps off Ecuador and pilchards off Chile.

South America*, and Brazil in particular, now leads the world in coffee production, mainly growing Coffea Arabica in large plantations. Coffee beans are harvested, roasted, and brewed to produce the world's second most popular drink, after tea.*

The Pampas region *of southeast South America is characterized by extensive, flat plains, and populated by cattle and ranchers (gauchos). Argentina is a major world producer of beef, much of which is exported to the US for use in hamburgers.*

High in the Andes*, hardy alpacas graze on the barren land. Alpacas are thought to have been domesticated by the Incas, whose nobility wore robes made from their wool. Today, they are still reared and prized for their soft, warm fleeces.*

Using the Land and Sea

- barren land
- cropland
- desert
- forest
- mountain region
- pasture
- major conurbations
- cattle
- pigs
- sheep
- bananas
- corn
- citrus fruits
- cocoa
- cotton
- coffee
- fishing
- oil palms
- peanuts
- rubber
- shellfish
- soybeans
- sugar cane
- vineyards
- wheat

NORTHERN SOUTH AMERICA

COLOMBIA, GUYANA, SURINAME, VENEZUELA, *French Guiana* (to France)

FRINGED BY THE PACIFIC AND ATLANTIC OCEANS and the Caribbean Sea, South America's northern region has a rich range of natural resources, some exploited for centuries by colonial powers including the Spanish, French, Dutch, and British, others still to be fully explored. The prospects for further economic development in Colombia, Guyana and Suriname are blighted by drug-related violence and political instability. Venezuela, despite huge incomes from its oil reserves, remains less developed in other industrial sectors. French Guiana is an overseas *département* of France, now seeking greater autonomy. Most of the major population centers, such as Bogotá, have grown up in the temperate conditions of the high Andes or, like Caracas, at strategic points along the Caribbean coast.

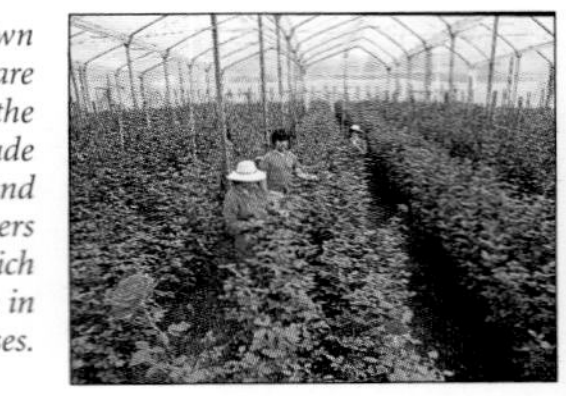

***Flowers** grown in Colombia are exported all over the world, and include fine carnations and roses. Here, workers are cutting roses which have been grown in plastic greenhouses.*

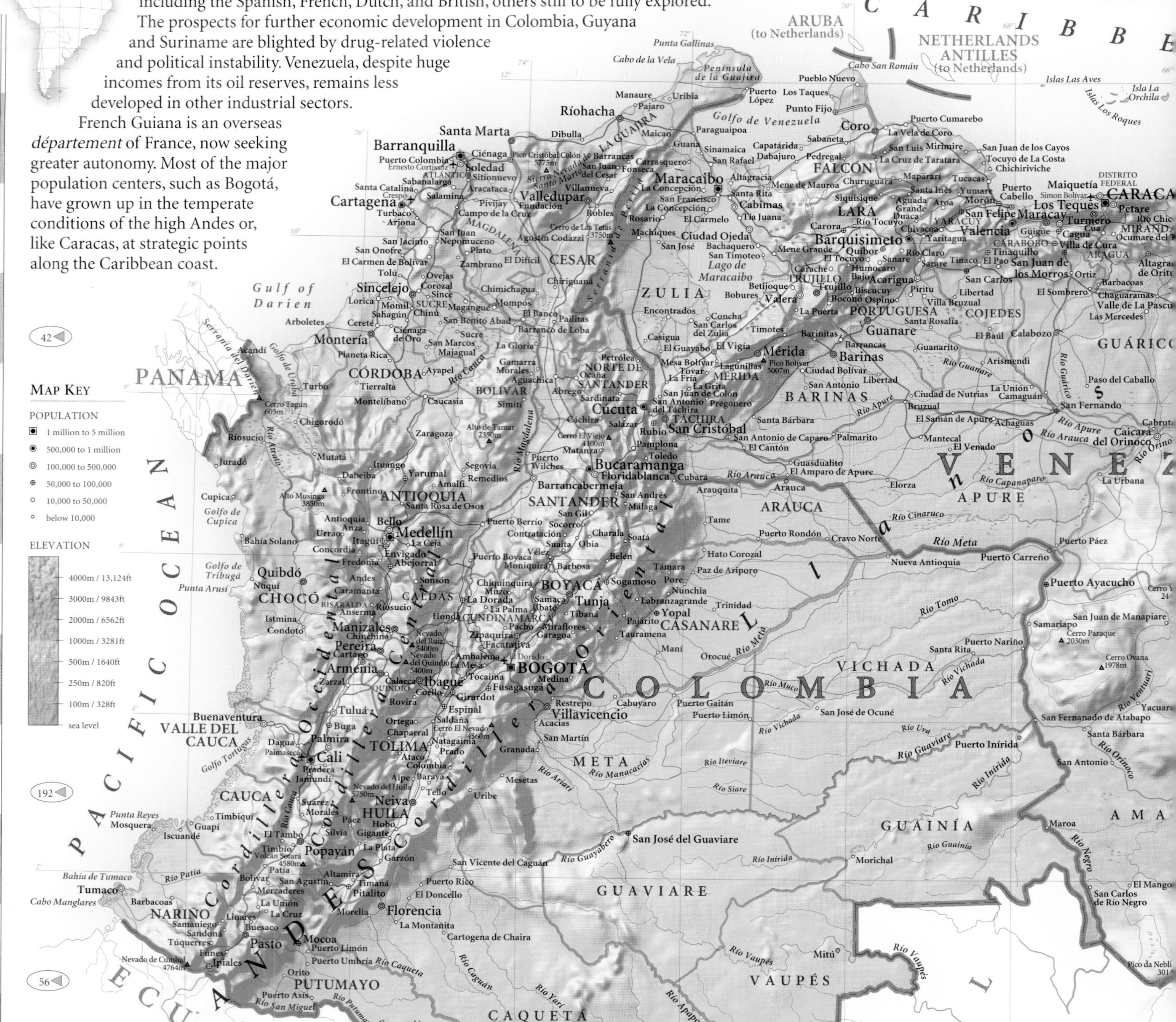

MAP KEY

POPULATION
- 1 million to 5 million
- 500,000 to 1 million
- 100,000 to 500,000
- 50,000 to 100,000
- 10,000 to 50,000
- below 10,000

ELEVATION
- 4000m / 13,124ft
- 3000m / 9843ft
- 2000m / 6562ft
- 1000m / 3281ft
- 500m / 1640ft
- 250m / 820ft
- 100m / 328ft
- sea level

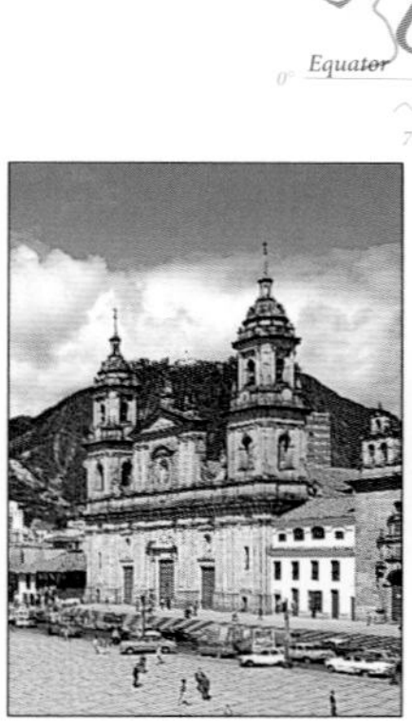

***Large open squares** like the Plaza Bolivia in Bogotá are characteristic of many cities founded by the Spanish.*

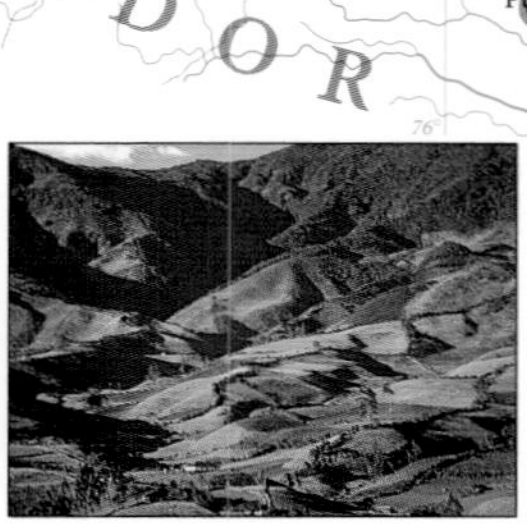

***Scattered farms** and villages have grown up on the gentle slopes of this Colombian river valley, utilizing the fertile soils for farming.*

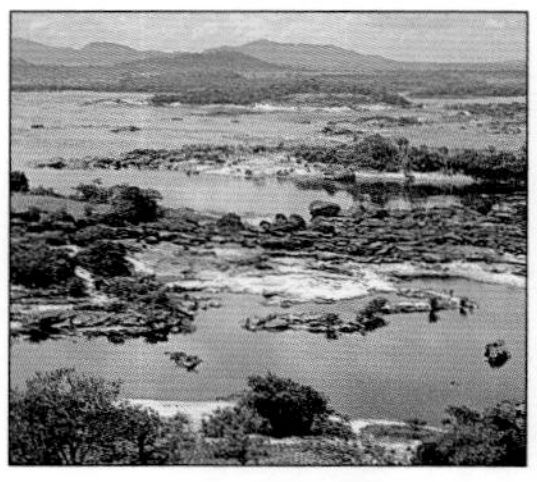

SCALE 1:7,250,000
(projection: Lambert Azimuthal Equal Area)

Km 0 25 50 100 150 200
Miles 0 25 50 100 150 200

***The River Orinoco** flows from its source in the southern Guiana Highlands to form a broad delta on Venezuela's Atlantic coast. One of its distributary channels opens into a wide bay called the Serpent's Mouth.*

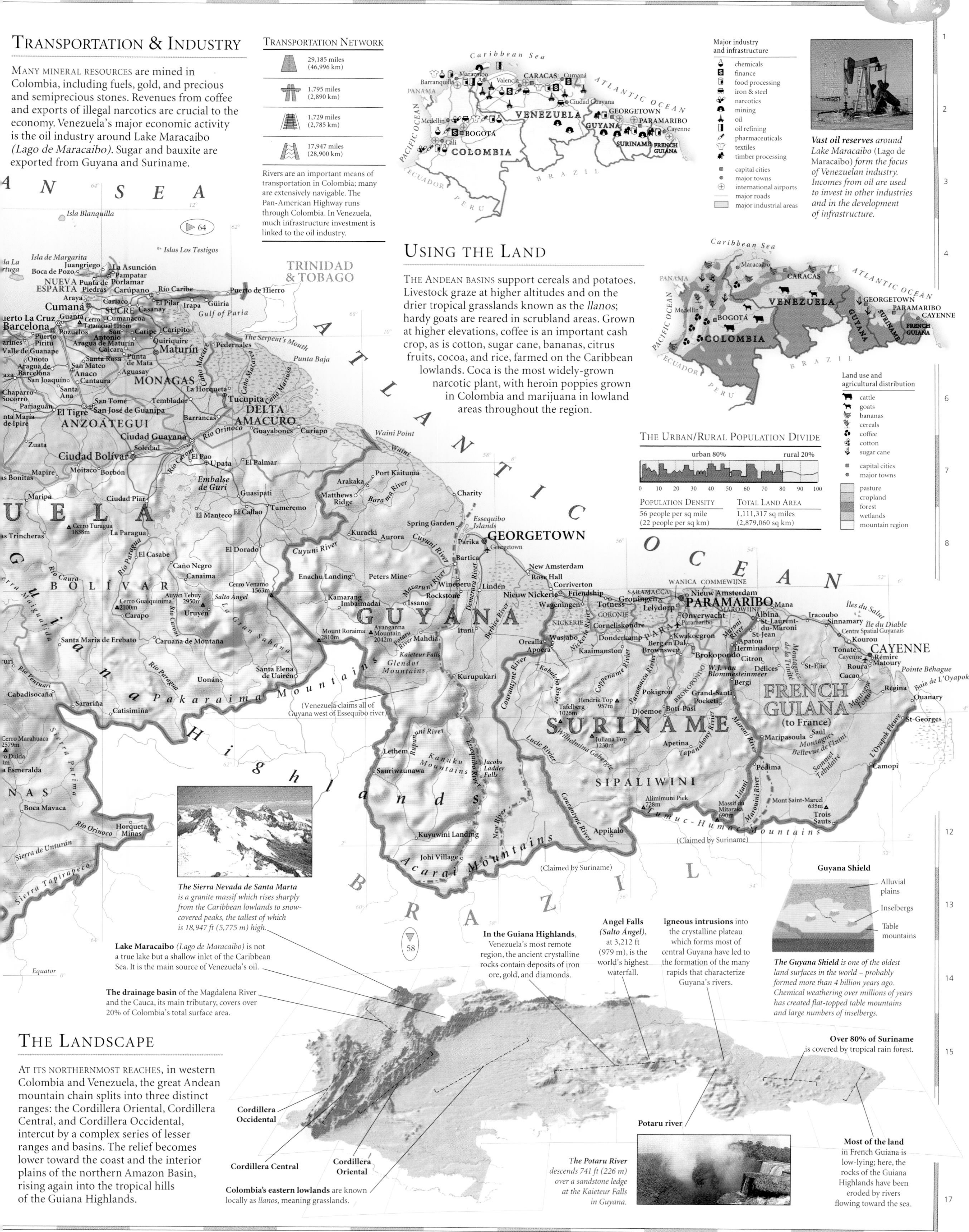

Transportation & Industry

Many mineral resources are mined in Colombia, including fuels, gold, and precious and semiprecious stones. Revenues from coffee and exports of illegal narcotics are crucial to the economy. Venezuela's major economic activity is the oil industry around Lake Maracaibo *(Lago de Maracaibo)*. Sugar and bauxite are exported from Guyana and Suriname.

Transportation Network

29,185 miles (46,996 km)

1,795 miles (2,890 km)

1,729 miles (2,785 km)

17,947 miles (28,900 km)

Rivers are an important means of transportation in Colombia; many are extensively navigable. The Pan-American Highway runs through Colombia. In Venezuela, much infrastructure investment is linked to the oil industry.

Major industry and infrastructure
chemicals
finance
food processing
iron & steel
narcotics
mining
oil
oil refining
pharmaceuticals
textiles
timber processing
capital cities
major towns
international airports
major roads
major industrial areas
Caribbean Sea
ATLANTIC OCEAN
PACIFIC OCEAN
CARACAS
VENEZUELA
COLOMBIA
BOGOTÁ
GEORGETOWN
PARAMARIBO
Cayenne
GUYANA
SURINAME
FRENCH GUIANA
BRAZIL
PERU
ECUADOR
PANAMA

***Vast oil reserves** around Lake Maracaibo (Lago de Maracaibo) form the focus of Venezuelan industry. Incomes from oil are used to invest in other industries and in the development of infrastructure.*

Using the Land

The Andean basins support cereals and potatoes. Livestock graze at higher altitudes and on the drier tropical grasslands known as the *llanos*; hardy goats are reared in scrubland areas. Grown at higher elevations, coffee is an important cash crop, as is cotton, sugar cane, bananas, citrus fruits, cocoa, and rice, farmed on the Caribbean lowlands. Coca is the most widely-grown narcotic plant, with heroin poppies grown in Colombia and marijuana in lowland areas throughout the region.

Land use and agricultural distribution
cattle
goats
bananas
cereals
coffee
cotton
sugar cane
capital cities
major towns
pasture
cropland
forest
wetlands
mountain region

The Urban/Rural Population Divide

urban 80% | rural 20%

Population Density	Total Land Area
56 people per sq mile (22 people per sq km)	1,111,317 sq miles (2,879,060 sq km)

ATLANTIC OCEAN
GUYANA
SURINAME
FRENCH GUIANA (to France)
GEORGETOWN
PARAMARIBO
CAYENNE
TRINIDAD & TOBAGO
ANZOÁTEGUI
MONAGAS
DELTA AMACURO
BOLÍVAR
SIPALIWINI
Guiana Highlands
Pakaraima Mountains
Acarai Mountains
Tumuc-Humac Mountains
Kanuku Mountains
Wilhelmina Gebergte
Gran Sabana
(Venezuela claims all of Guyana west of Essequibo river)
(Claimed by Suriname)
BRAZIL

The Sierra Nevada de Santa Marta is a granite massif which rises sharply from the Caribbean lowlands to snow-covered peaks, the tallest of which is 18,947 ft (5,775 m) high.

64

58

The Landscape

At its northernmost reaches, in western Colombia and Venezuela, the great Andean mountain chain splits into three distinct ranges: the Cordillera Oriental, Cordillera Central, and Cordillera Occidental, intercut by a complex series of lesser ranges and basins. The relief becomes lower toward the coast and the interior plains of the northern Amazon Basin, rising again into the tropical hills of the Guiana Highlands.

Lake Maracaibo *(Lago de Maracaibo)* is not a true lake but a shallow inlet of the Caribbean Sea. It is the main source of Venezuela's oil.

The drainage basin of the Magdalena River and the Cauca, its main tributary, covers over 20% of Colombia's total surface area.

In the Guiana Highlands, Venezuela's most remote region, the ancient crystalline rocks contain deposits of iron ore, gold, and diamonds.

Angel Falls *(Salto Angel)*, at 3,212 ft (979 m), is the world's highest waterfall.

Igneous intrusions into the crystalline plateau which forms most of central Guyana have led to the formation of the many rapids that characterize Guyana's rivers.

Guyana Shield

Alluvial plains
Inselbergs
Table mountains

***The Guyana Shield** is one of the oldest land surfaces in the world – probably formed more than 4 billion years ago. Chemical weathering over millions of years has created flat-topped table mountains and large numbers of inselbergs.*

Over 80% of Suriname is covered by tropical rain forest.

Cordillera Occidental
Cordillera Central
Cordillera Oriental
Potaru river

Colombia's eastern lowlands are known locally as *llanos*, meaning grasslands.

The Potaru River descends 741 ft (226 m) over a sandstone ledge at the Kaieteur Falls in Guyana.

Most of the land in French Guiana is low-lying; here, the rocks of the Guiana Highlands have been eroded by rivers flowing toward the sea.

Western South America

Bolivia, Ecuador, Peru

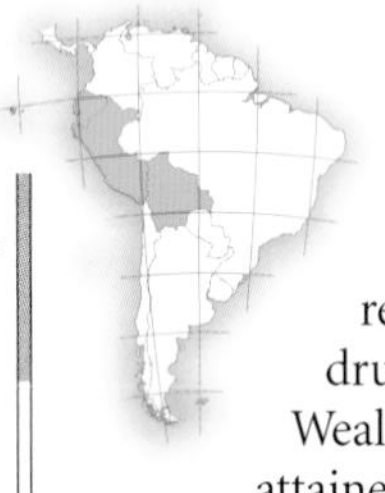

The three states of Western South America share a similar geography and recent history. Dominated by the Inca empire until Spanish conquest in the 16th century, they achieved independence from Spain in the early 19th century. The precipitous terrain of the Andes presents severe difficulties for overland transportation and continues to be a barrier to national unity and stability. Although Ecuador is now a relatively stable democracy, the military is highly influential in Peru and Bolivia, while the drug trade and associated corruption discourages external aid and economic progress. Wealth and power are still largely concentrated in the hands of a small elite of families, who attained their position during the Spanish colonial period. Land rights and political recognition for the indigenous peoples are becoming increasingly important issues, particularly in Ecuador.

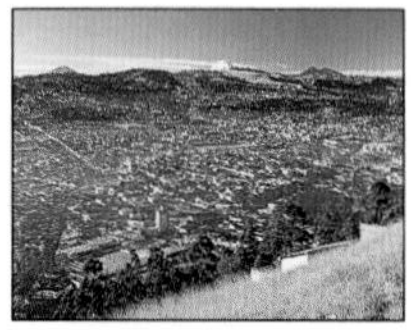

Ecuador's capital city, Quito, lies high in the Andes, nestling between snowcapped peaks. At 9,350 ft (2,850 m), Quito is the second highest capital in the world – La Paz in Bolivia is the highest.

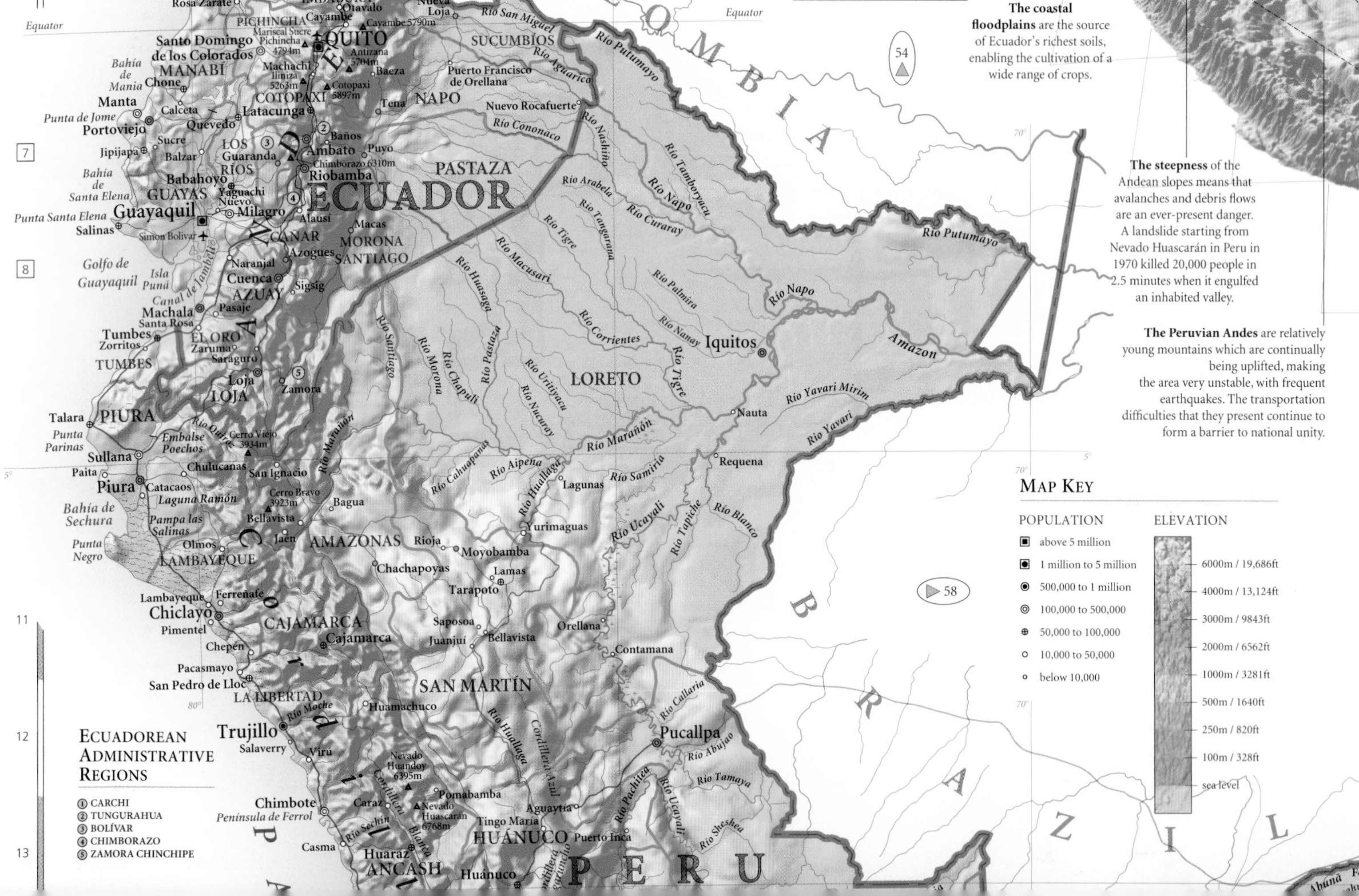

The Landscape

Bolivia, Peru, and Ecuador each possess a high Andean mountain region and an eastern region consisting of tropical lowlands and the Andean slope leading down to them. Toward the south of the region, the mountains widen to form the high plateau of the Altiplano. Peru and Ecuador also have fertile, lowland coastal plains. A wide variety of environments include *selva* (tropical rain forest), *montaña* (mountain forest), and grassland.

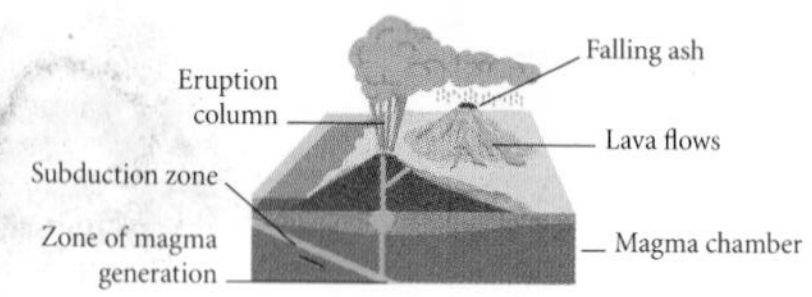

Eruption column — Falling ash — Lava flows — Subduction zone — Zone of magma generation — Magma chamber

***There are many large** and active volcanoes in the Andes. Magma generated in the heart of the volcano erupts in a huge cloud of ash. Ash-fall deposits are common throughout the Andes and the rock produced is known as andesite. This is rapidly soaked by heavy rain, causing massive debris flows.*

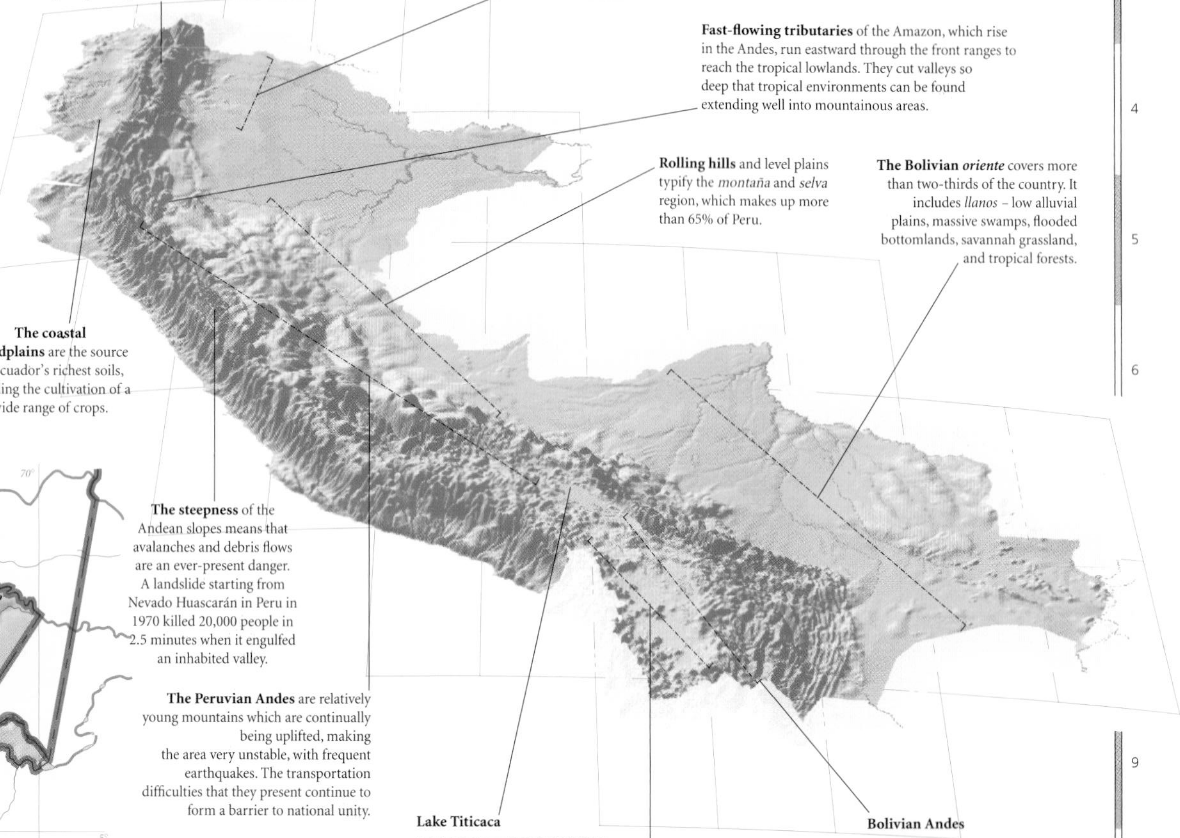

Cotopaxi is the world's highest active volcano, with a peak 19,347 ft (5,897 m) high. A massive eruption in 1877 caused a mudflow which destroyed everything in its path for 150 miles (240 km).

Much of eastern Ecuador is covered by the tropical rain forest of the Amazon Basin.

Fast-flowing tributaries of the Amazon, which rise in the Andes, run eastward through the front ranges to reach the tropical lowlands. They cut valleys so deep that tropical environments can be found extending well into mountainous areas.

Rolling hills and level plains typify the *montaña* and *selva* region, which makes up more than 65% of Peru.

The Bolivian *oriente* covers more than two-thirds of the country. It includes *llanos* – low alluvial plains, massive swamps, flooded bottomlands, savannah grassland, and tropical forests.

The coastal floodplains are the source of Ecuador's richest soils, enabling the cultivation of a wide range of crops.

The steepness of the Andean slopes means that avalanches and debris flows are an ever-present danger. A landslide starting from Nevado Huascarán in Peru in 1970 killed 20,000 people in 2.5 minutes when it engulfed an inhabited valley.

The Peruvian Andes are relatively young mountains which are continually being uplifted, making the area very unstable, with frequent earthquakes. The transportation difficulties that they present continue to form a barrier to national unity.

Lake Titicaca

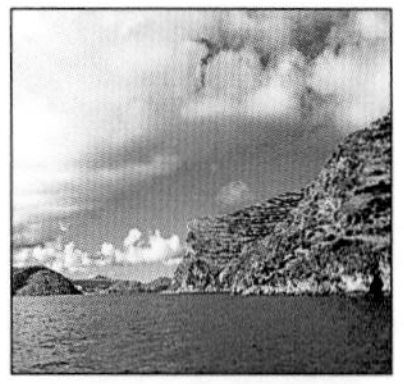

***Lake Titicaca**, which forms part of the border between Peru and Bolivia, is the largest lake in South America and the highest significant body of water in the world at an altitude of 12,507 ft (3,812 m).*

The Altiplano is a flat, high plateau lying between the Cordillera Oriental and the Cordillera Occidental at a height of up to 12,500 ft (3,800 m). At its margins lie many spurs and alluvial fans.

Bolivian Andes

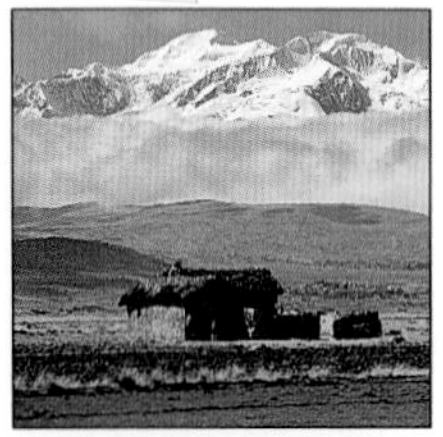

***Nevado de Illampu and Nevado de Ancohuma**, at 21,275 ft (6,485 m) and 21,490 ft (6,550 m) respectively, form Illampu, the highest mountain in the Bolivian Andes.*

Map Key

POPULATION	ELEVATION
above 5 million	6000m / 19,686ft
1 million to 5 million	4000m / 13,124ft
500,000 to 1 million	3000m / 9843ft
100,000 to 500,000	2000m / 6562ft
50,000 to 100,000	1000m / 3281ft
10,000 to 50,000	500m / 1640ft
below 10,000	250m / 820ft
	100m / 328ft
	sea level

Ecuadorean Administrative Regions

1. Carchi
2. Tungurahua
3. Bolívar
4. Chimborazo
5. Zamora Chinchipe

Scale 1:8,500,000 (projection: Lambert Azimuthal Equal Area)

Km 0 25 50 100 150 200 250 300

Miles 0 25 50 100 150 200 250 300

192 ◀ 54 ▲ ▶ 58

COLOMBIA
ECUADOR
PERU
BRAZIL
Quito
Guayaquil
Iquitos
Pucallpa
Trujillo
Chiclayo
Piura
Amazon
Río Napo
Río Putumayo
Río Marañón
Río Ucayali
Equator

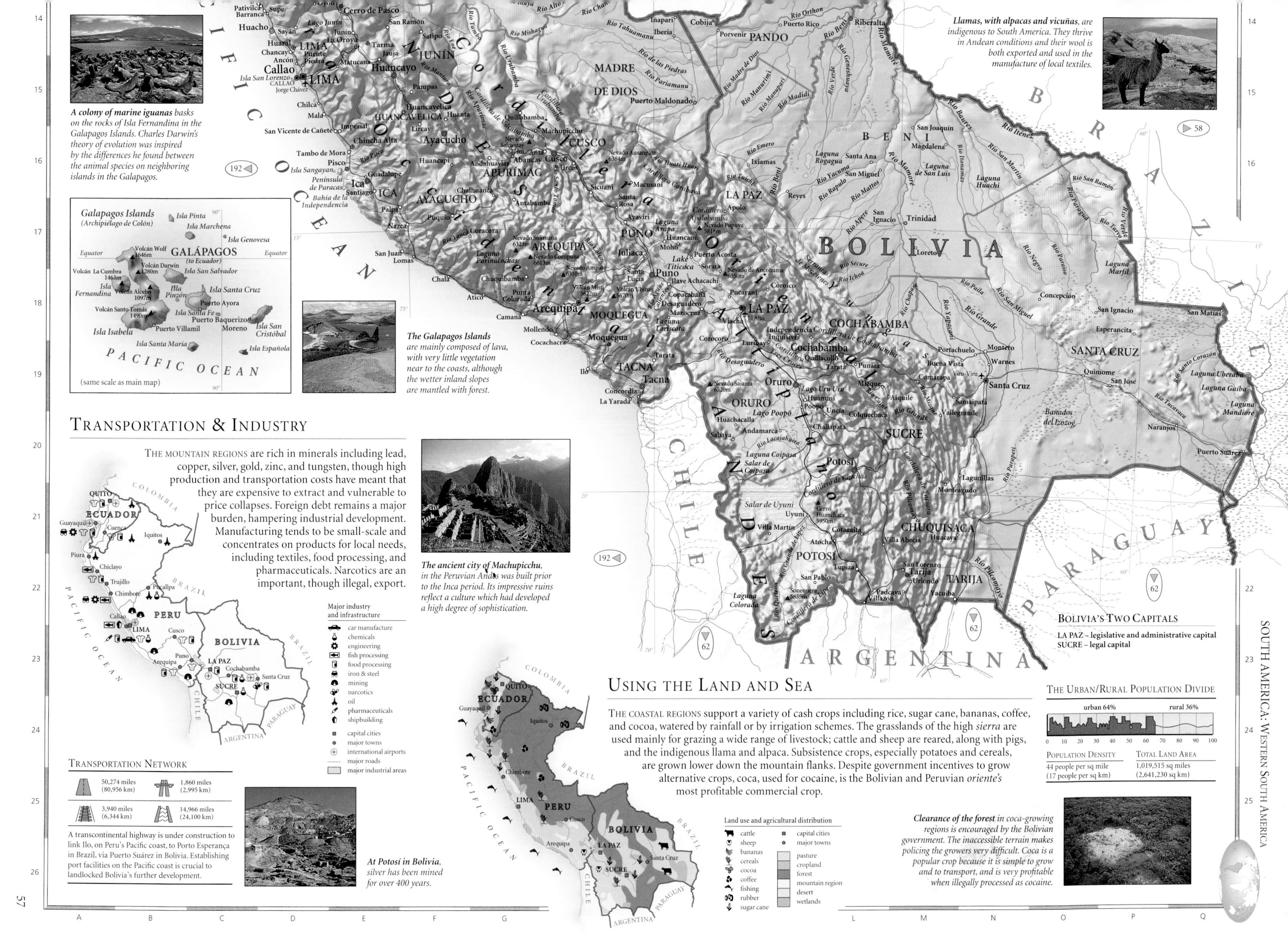
BRAZIL
BOLIVIA
PARAGUAY
ARGENTINA
CHILE
PACIFIC OCEAN
Cordillera Oriental
Cordillera Occidental
Altiplano
ANDES
PANDO
BENI
LA PAZ
COCHABAMBA
SANTA CRUZ
ORURO
POTOSÍ
CHUQUISACA
TARIJA
SUCRE
MADRE DE DIOS
CUSCO
PUNO
AREQUIPA
MOQUEGUA
TACNA
APURÍMAC
AYACUCHO
HUANCAVELICA
ICA
JUNÍN
LIMA
Lake Titicaca
Salar de Uyuni
Bañados del Izozog
Galapagos Islands
(Archipiélago de Colón)
GALÁPAGOS
(to Ecuador)
Isla Pinta
Isla Marchena
Isla Genovesa
Isla San Salvador
Isla Santa Cruz
Isla Fernandina
Isla Isabela
Isla Pinzón
Isla Santa Fe
Isla San Cristóbal
Isla Santa María
Isla Española
Puerto Ayora
Puerto Baquerizo Moreno
Puerto Villamil
Volcán Wolf 1646m
Volcán Darwin 1280m
Volcán La Cumbra 1463m
Volcán Alcedo 1097m
Volcán Santo Tomás 1490m
Equator
PACIFIC OCEAN
(same scale as main map)
192
58
62
Major industry and infrastructure
car manufacture
chemicals
engineering
fish processing
food processing
iron & steel
mining
narcotics
oil
pharmaceuticals
shipbuilding
capital cities
major towns
international airports
major roads
major industrial areas
TRANSPORTATION NETWORK
50,274 miles (80,956 km)
1,860 miles (2,995 km)
3,940 miles (6,344 km)
14,966 miles (24,100 km)
Land use and agricultural distribution
cattle
sheep
bananas
cereals
cocoa
coffee
fishing
rubber
sugar cane
capital cities
major towns
pasture
cropland
forest
mountain region
desert
wetlands
THE URBAN/RURAL POPULATION DIVIDE
urban 64%
rural 36%
0 10 20 30 40 50 60 70 80 90 100
POPULATION DENSITY
44 people per sq mile
(17 people per sq km)
TOTAL LAND AREA
1,019,515 sq miles
(2,641,230 sq km)

A colony of marine iguanas *basks on the rocks of Isla Fernandina in the Galapagos Islands. Charles Darwin's theory of evolution was inspired by the differences he found between the animal species on neighboring islands in the Galapagos.*

The Galapagos Islands *are mainly composed of lava, with very little vegetation near to the coasts, although the wetter inland slopes are mantled with forest.*

Llamas, with alpacas and vicuñas, *are indigenous to South America. They thrive in Andean conditions and their wool is both exported and used in the manufacture of local textiles.*

TRANSPORTATION & INDUSTRY

THE MOUNTAIN REGIONS are rich in minerals including lead, copper, silver, gold, zinc, and tungsten, though high production and transportation costs have meant that they are expensive to extract and vulnerable to price collapses. Foreign debt remains a major burden, hampering industrial development. Manufacturing tends to be small-scale and concentrates on products for local needs, including textiles, food processing, and pharmaceuticals. Narcotics are an important, though illegal, export.

The ancient city of Machupicchu, *in the Peruvian Andes was built prior to the Inca period. Its impressive ruins reflect a culture which had developed a high degree of sophistication.*

A transcontinental highway is under construction to link Ilo, on Peru's Pacific coast, to Porto Esperança in Brazil, via Puerto Suárez in Bolivia. Establishing port facilities on the Pacific coast is crucial to landlocked Bolivia's further development.

At Potosí in Bolivia, *silver has been mined for over 400 years.*

BOLIVIA'S TWO CAPITALS

LA PAZ – legislative and administrative capital
SUCRE – legal capital

USING THE LAND AND SEA

THE COASTAL REGIONS support a variety of cash crops including rice, sugar cane, bananas, coffee, and cocoa, watered by rainfall or by irrigation schemes. The grasslands of the high *sierra* are used mainly for grazing a wide range of livestock; cattle and sheep are reared, along with pigs, and the indigenous llama and alpaca. Subsistence crops, especially potatoes and cereals, are grown lower down the mountain flanks. Despite government incentives to grow alternative crops, coca, used for cocaine, is the Bolivian and Peruvian *oriente's* most profitable commercial crop.

Clearance of the forest *in coca-growing regions is encouraged by the Bolivian government. The inaccessible terrain makes policing the growers very difficult. Coca is a popular crop because it is simple to grow and to transport, and is very profitable when illegally processed as cocaine.*

BRAZIL

BRAZIL IS THE LARGEST COUNTRY in South America, with a population of over 165 million – greater than the combined total for the whole of the rest of the continent. The 26 states which make up the federal republic of Brazil are administered from the purpose-built capital, Brasília. Tropical rain forest, covering more than one-third of the country, contains rich natural resources, but great tracts are sacrificed to agriculture, industry and urban expansion on a daily basis. Most of Brazil's multiethnic population now live in cities, some of which are vast areas of urban sprawl; São Paulo is one of the world's biggest conurbations, with more than 17 million inhabitants. Although prosperity is a reality for some, many people still live in great poverty, and mounting foreign debts continue to damage Brazil's prospects of economic advancement.

USING THE LAND

BRAZIL HAS IMMENSE NATURAL RESOURCES, including minerals and hardwoods, many of which are found in the fragile rain forest. Brazil is the world's leading coffee grower and a major producer of livestock, sugar, and orange juice concentrate. Soybeans for animal feed, particularly for poultry feed, have become the country's most significant crop.

THE URBAN/RURAL POPULATION DIVIDE

urban 78% — rural 22%

0 10 20 30 40 50 60 70 80 90 100

POPULATION DENSITY	TOTAL LAND AREA
50 people per sq mile (19 people per sq km)	3,286,472 sq miles (8,511,970 sq km)

Land use and agricultural distribution: cattle, pigs, sheep, citrus fruits, coffee, cotton, soya beans, sugar cane, timber; capital cities, major towns; pasture, cropland, forest

The fecundity of parts of Brazil's rain forest results from exceptionally high levels of rainfall and the quantities of silt deposited by the Amazon River system.

THE LANDSCAPE

THE AMAZON BASIN, containing the largest area of tropical rain forest on Earth, covers nearly half of Brazil. It is bordered by two shield areas: in the south by the Brazilian Highlands, and in the north by the Guiana Highlands. The east coast is dominated by a great escarpment which runs for 1,600 miles (2,565 km).

The Amazon Basin is the largest river basin in the world. The Amazon River and over a thousand tributaries drain an area of 2,375,000 sq miles (6,150,000 sq km) and carry one-fifth of the world's fresh water out to sea.

Guiana Highlands

The ancient Brazilian Highlands have a varied topography. Their plateaus, hills, and deep valleys are bordered by highly-eroded mountains containing important mineral deposits. They are drained by three great river systems, the Amazon, the Paraguay–Paraná, and the São Francisco.

The São Francisco Basin has a climate unique in Brazil. Known as the "drought polygon," it has almost no rain during the dry season, leading to regular disastrous droughts.

The northeastern scrublands are known as the *caatinga*, a virtually impenetrable thorny woodland, sometimes intermixed with cacti where water is scarce.

Brazil's highest mountain is the Pico da Neblina which was only discovered in 1962. It is 9,888 ft (3,014 m) high.

The floodplains which border the Amazon River are made up of a variety of different features including shallow lakes and swamps, mangrove forests in the tidal delta area, and fertile leveés on river banks and point bars.

Pantanal swamps

*The **Pantanal region** in the south of Brazil is an extension of the Gran Chaco plain. The swamps and marshes of this area are renowned for their beauty, and abundant and unique wildlife, including wildfowl and these caimans, a type of crocodile.*

*The **Iguaçu River** surges over the spectacular Iguaçu Falls (Saltos do Iguaçu) toward the Paraná River. Falls like these are increasingly under pressure from large-scale hydroelectric projects such as that at Itaipú.*

The famous Sugar Loaf Mountain *(Pão de Açúcar)* which overlooks Rio de Janeiro is a fine example of a volcanic plug a domed core of solidified lava left after the slopes of the original volcano have eroded away.

Hillslope gullying

Rainfall; Direction of growth; Overland water flow; Water seeps through hillslope; Gully

***Large-scale** gullies are common in Brazil, particularly on hillslopes from which vegetation has been removed. Gullies grow headwards (up the slope), aided by a combination of erosion through water seepage and rainwater runoff.*

Deep natural harbors such as Baia de Guanabara were created where the steep slopes of the Serra da Mantiqueira plunge directly into the ocean.

MAP KEY

POPULATION	ELEVATION
above 5 million	3000m / 9843ft
1 million to 5 million	2000m / 6562ft
500,000 to 1 million	1000m / 3281ft
100,000 to 500,000	500m / 1640ft
50,000 to 100,000	250m / 820ft
10,000 to 50,000	100m / 328ft
below 10,000	sea level

VENEZUELA · COLOMBIA · GUYANA · SURINAME · FRENCH GUIANA (to France) · ATLANTIC OCEAN

54 · 56 · 64

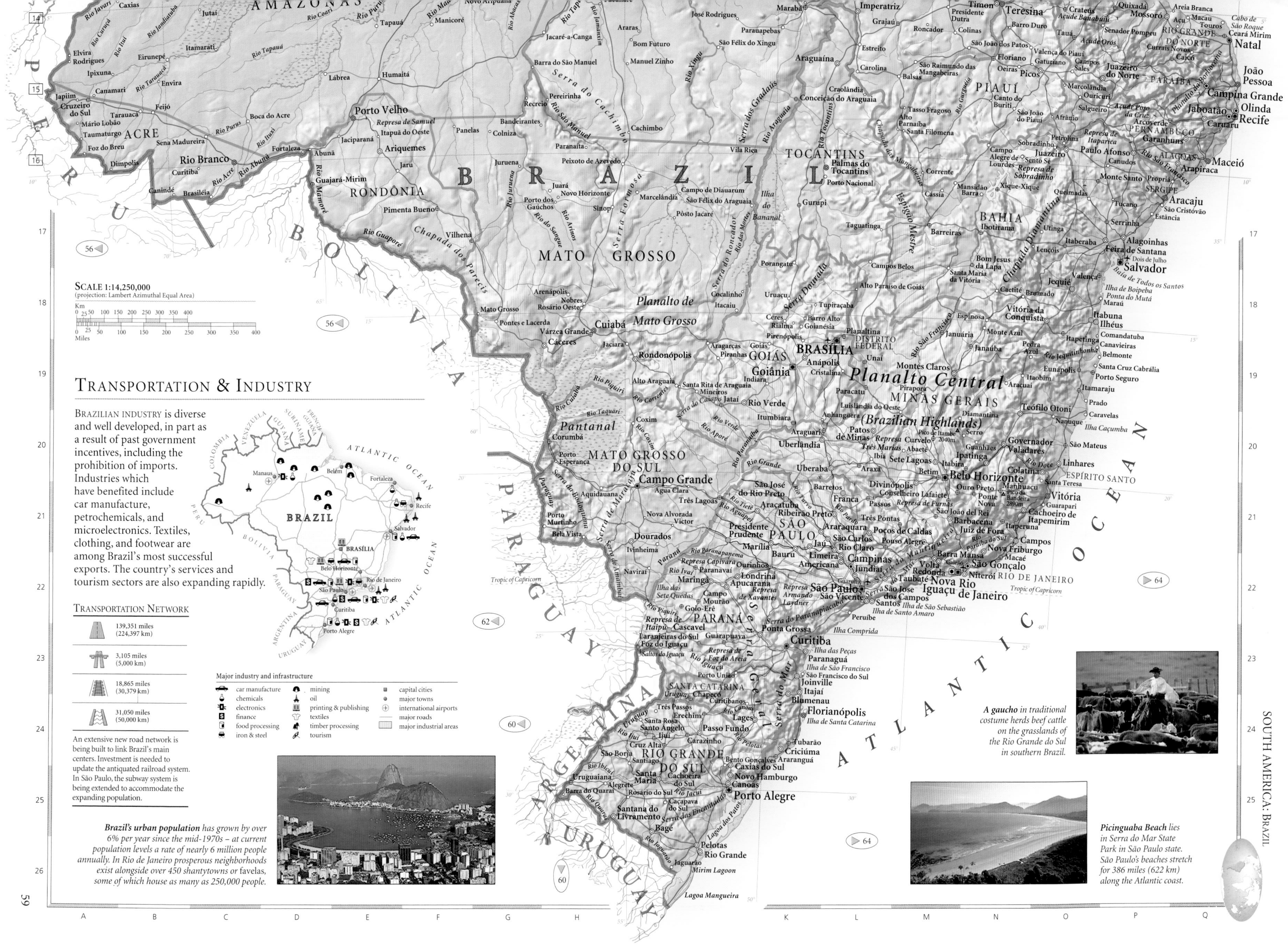
SCALE 1:14,250,000
(projection: Lambert Azimuthal Equal Area)
Km 0 25 50 100 150 200 250 300 350 400
Miles 0 25 50 100 150 200 250 300 350 400
Major industry and infrastructure
car manufacture
chemicals
electronics
finance
food processing
iron & steel
mining
oil
printing & publishing
textiles
timber processing
tourism
capital cities
major towns
international airports
major roads
major industrial areas

Transportation & Industry

Brazilian industry is diverse and well developed, in part as a result of past government incentives, including the prohibition of imports. Industries which have benefited include car manufacture, petrochemicals, and microelectronics. Textiles, clothing, and footwear are among Brazil's most successful exports. The country's services and tourism sectors are also expanding rapidly.

Transportation Network

- 139,351 miles (224,397 km)
- 3,105 miles (5,000 km)
- 18,865 miles (30,379 km)
- 31,050 miles (50,000 km)

An extensive new road network is being built to link Brazil's main centers. Investment is needed to update the antiquated railroad system. In São Paulo, the subway system is being extended to accommodate the expanding population.

Brazil's urban population *has grown by over 6% per year since the mid-1970s – at current population levels a rate of nearly 6 million people annually. In Rio de Janeiro prosperous neighborhoods exist alongside over 450 shantytowns or favelas, some of which house as many as 250,000 people.*

A gaucho *in traditional costume herds beef cattle on the grasslands of the Rio Grande do Sul in southern Brazil.*

Picinguaba Beach *lies in Serra do Mar State Park in São Paulo state. São Paulo's beaches stretch for 386 miles (622 km) along the Atlantic coast.*

Eastern South America

Uruguay, Northeast Argentina, Southeast Brazil

The vast conurbations of Rio de Janeiro, São Paulo, and Buenos Aires form the core of South America's highly-urbanized eastern region. São Paulo state, with almost 35 million inhabitants, is among the world's 20 most powerful economies, and São Paulo is the fastest growing city on the continent. Rio de Janeiro and Buenos Aires, transformed in the last hundred years from port cities to great metropolitan areas each with more than 10 million inhabitants, typify the unstructured growth and wealth disparities of South America's great cities. In Uruguay, over half of the population lives in the capital, Montevideo, which faces Buenos Aires across the Plate River *(Río de la Plata)*. Immigration from the countryside has created severe pressure on the urban infrastructure, particularly on available housing, leading to a profusion of crowded shanty settlements *(favelas or barrios)*.

Using the Land

Most of Uruguay and the Pampas of northern Argentina are devoted to the rearing of livestock, especially cattle and sheep, which are central to both countries' economies. Soybeans, first produced in Brazil's Rio Grande do Sul, are now more widely grown for large-scale export, as are cereals, sugar cane, and grapes. Subsistence crops, including potatoes, corn and sugar beets, are grown on the remaining arable land.

Land use and agricultural distribution

- cattle
- sheep
- cereals
- coffee
- fruit
- soybeans
- sugar cane
- capital cities
- major towns
- pasture
- cropland
- forest
- wetlands
- barren land

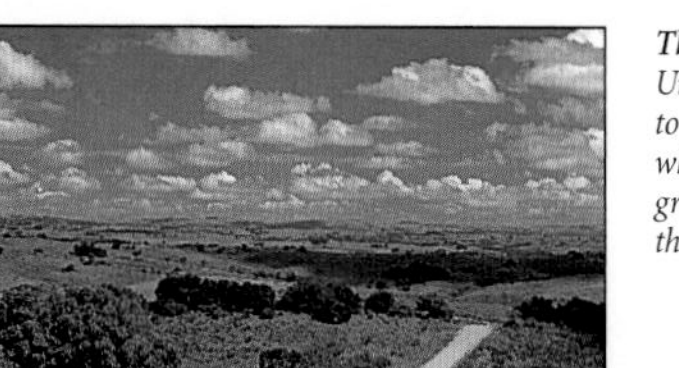

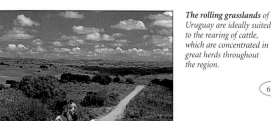

The rolling grasslands *of Uruguay are ideally suited to the rearing of cattle, which are concentrated in great herds throughout the region.*

Scale 1: 7,000,000
(projection: Lambert Azimuthal Equal Area)

Km 0 25 50 100 150 200
Miles 0 25 50 100 150 200

Soybeans are harvested*, pressed, and processed into soycake, which is used as animal feed. The cake is fed mainly to chickens on large-scale factory farms, and the growth in soy production has been an important factor in the expansion of the Brazilian poultry trade.*

Transportation & Industry

Southeast Brazil is home to much of the important motor and capital goods industry, largely based around São Paulo; iron and steel production is also concentrated in this region. Uruguay's economy continues to be based mainly on the export of livestock products including meat and leather goods. Buenos Aires is Argentina's chief port, and the region has a varied and sophisticated economic base including service-based industries such as finance and publishing, as well as primary processing.

Map Key

Population	Elevation
above 5 million	2000m / 6562ft
1 million to 5 million	1000m / 3281ft
500,000 to 1 million	500m / 1640ft
100,000 to 500,000	250m / 820ft
50,000 to 100,000	100m / 328ft
10,000 to 50,000	sea level
below 10,000	

Major industry and infrastructure

- car manufacture
- chemicals
- engineering
- finance
- food processing
- iron & steel
- meat processing
- printing & publishing
- shipbuilding
- textiles
- timber processing
- capital cities
- major towns
- international airports
- major roads
- major industrial areas

Transportation Network

Throughout the region, road networks need to be expanded to cope with urban development. Plans are underway to build a bridge over the Plate River *(Río de la Plata)* to link Colonia and Buenos Aires.

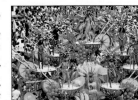

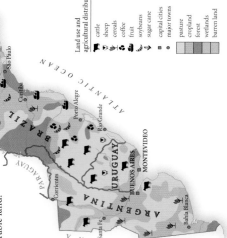

The Itaipú dam *on the Paraná River is one of the largest hydroelectric projects in the world, jointly financed by Brazil and Paraguay.*

Rio de Janeiro's *annual carnival, Mardi Gras, which ushers in the start of Lent, is an extravagant five-day parade through the city, characterized by fantastically decorated floats, exuberant dancing, and samba music.*

58 ▲
62 ◀
▶ 64

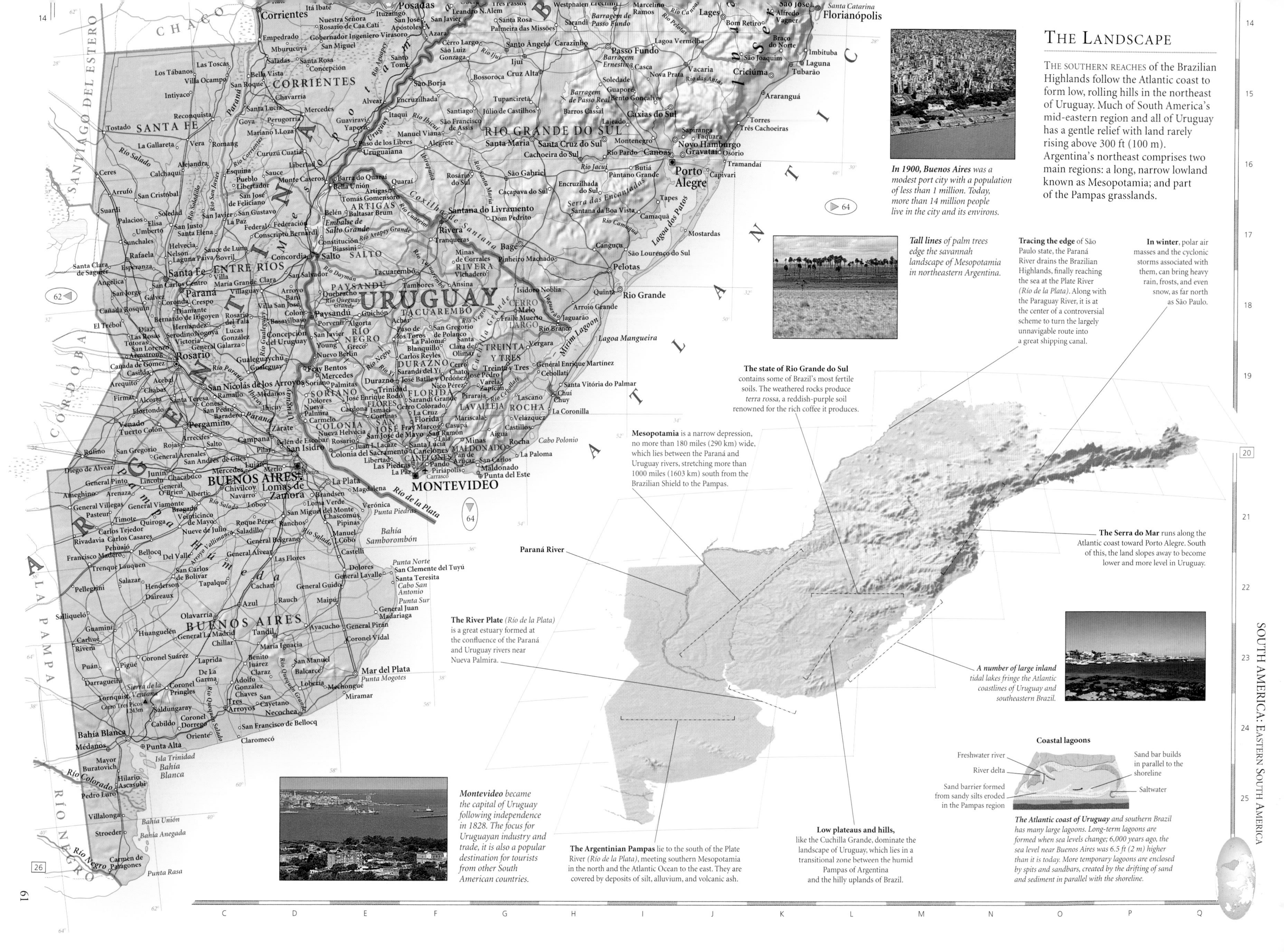

THE LANDSCAPE

THE SOUTHERN REACHES of the Brazilian Highlands follow the Atlantic coast to form low, rolling hills in the northeast of Uruguay. Much of South America's mid-eastern region and all of Uruguay has a gentle relief with land rarely rising above 300 ft (100 m). Argentina's northeast comprises two main regions: a long, narrow lowland known as Mesopotamia; and part of the Pampas grasslands.

***In 1900, Buenos Aires** was a modest port city with a population of less than 1 million. Today, more than 14 million people live in the city and its environs.*

***Tall lines** of palm trees edge the savannah landscape of Mesopotamia in northeastern Argentina.*

Tracing the edge of São Paulo state, the Paraná River drains the Brazilian Highlands, finally reaching the sea at the Plate River (*Río de la Plata*). Along with the Paraguay River, it is at the center of a controversial scheme to turn the largely unnavigable route into a great shipping canal.

In winter, polar air masses and the cyclonic storms associated with them, can bring heavy rain, frosts, and even snow, as far north as São Paulo.

The state of Rio Grande do Sul contains some of Brazil's most fertile soils. The weathered rocks produce *terra rossa*, a reddish-purple soil renowned for the rich coffee it produces.

Mesopotamia is a narrow depression, no more than 180 miles (290 km) wide, which lies between the Paraná and Uruguay rivers, stretching more than 1000 miles (1603 km) south from the Brazilian Shield to the Pampas.

The Serra do Mar runs along the Atlantic coast toward Porto Alegre. South of this, the land slopes away to become lower and more level in Uruguay.

Paraná River

The River Plate (*Río de la Plata*) is a great estuary formed at the confluence of the Paraná and Uruguay rivers near Nueva Palmira.

***A number of large inland** tidal lakes fringe the Atlantic coastlines of Uruguay and southeastern Brazil.*

Coastal lagoons

Freshwater river
River delta
Sand barrier formed from sandy silts eroded in the Pampas region
Sand bar builds in parallel to the shoreline
Saltwater

***The Atlantic coast of Uruguay** and southern Brazil has many large lagoons. Long-term lagoons are formed when sea levels change; 6,000 years ago, the sea level near Buenos Aires was 6.5 ft (2 m) higher than it is today. More temporary lagoons are enclosed by spits and sandbars, created by the drifting of sand and sediment in parallel with the shoreline.*

***Montevideo** became the capital of Uruguay following independence in 1828. The focus for Uruguayan industry and trade, it is also a popular destination for tourists from other South American countries.*

The Argentinian Pampas lie to the south of the Plate River (*Río de la Plata*), meeting southern Mesopotamia in the north and the Atlantic Ocean to the east. They are covered by deposits of silt, alluvium, and volcanic ash.

Low plateaus and hills, like the Cuchilla Grande, dominate the landscape of Uruguay, which lies in a transitional zone between the humid Pampas of Argentina and the hilly uplands of Brazil.

Southern South America

Argentina, Chile, Paraguay

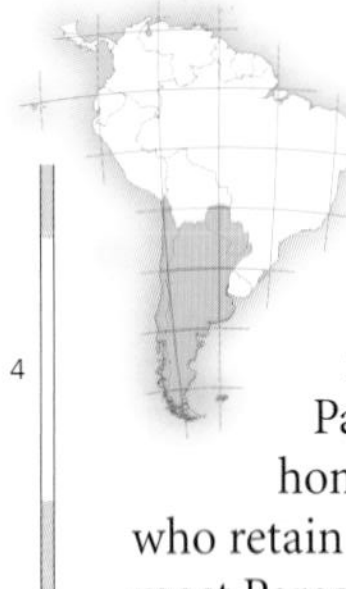

South America's cone-shaped southern region is shared by Argentina and Chile, two overwhelmingly urbanized nations whose populations live mainly in or around the capital cities, Buenos Aires and Santiago. The people are largely *mestizo* or of European origin; in the early 20th century Argentina absorbed waves of new European immigrants, many from Italy and Germany. Paraguay is far less urbanized than its neighbors, with a homogeneous population of mixed Spanish and Guaraní origin, who retain their Indian roots through the Guaraní language. Though most Paraguayans live in the southeast, near Asunción, the indigenous Indians live in the sparsely populated Gran Chaco. The Gran Chaco is also home to some of Argentina's minority indigenous peoples, who otherwise live mainly in Andean regions. Chile's estimated 800,000 Mapauche Indians live almost exclusively in the south.

Transportation & Industry

Food processing and agricultural exports remain a fundamental part of Argentina's economy. The growth of manufacturing is regularly hampered by hyper-inflation and massive foreign debts. The world's most important copper-producer and one of the top ten gold producers, Chile also has a thriving wine and grape industry. Most Paraguayan exports involve primary processing, although domestic goods are produced for home markets.

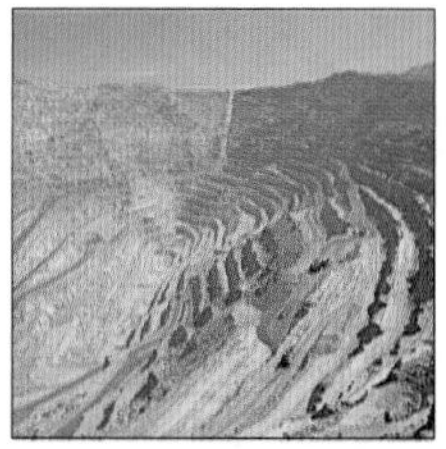

Chuquicamata copper mine, *lies on a desert plateau near Calama in the Andes of northern Chile. It is the world's largest open-pit copper mine.*

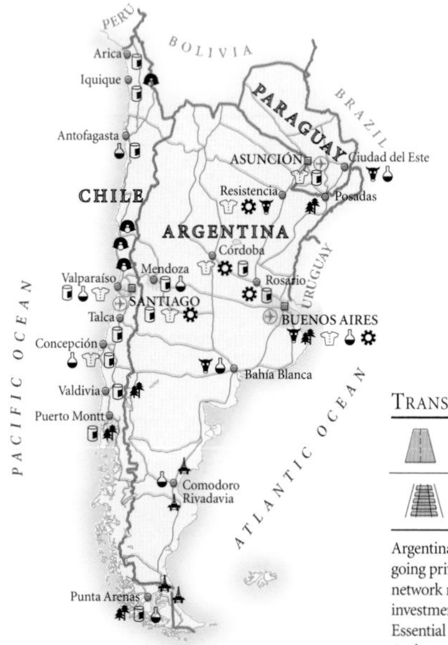

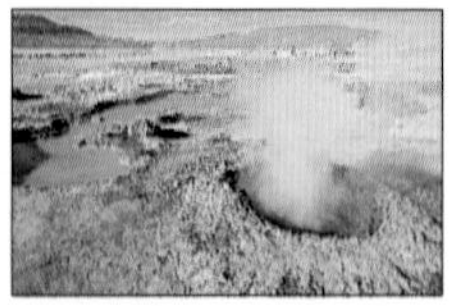

Boiling water *and steam emerge from a volcanic vent, one of the Tatio geysers which lie at the foot of Cerro de Tocorpuri near Chile's border with Bolivia.*

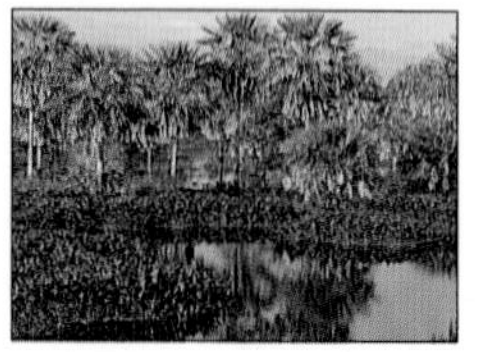

Floodwaters cover *the land in the Gran Chaco, partly submerging its vegetation of fan palms and hyacinths.*

Major industry and infrastructure

- chemicals
- engineering
- food processing
- meat processing
- mining
- oil
- textiles
- timber processing
- capital cities
- major towns
- international airports
- major roads
- major industrial areas

Transportation Network

89,104 miles (143,485 km)	2,809 miles (4,523 km)
23,107 miles (37,210 km)	9,206 miles (14,825 km)

Argentina's state transportation system is undergoing privatization, though the outmoded rail network requires updating. Paraguay requires foreign investment to upgrade its roads and railroads. Essential internal air routes, especially across the Andes, are well developed in all three countries.

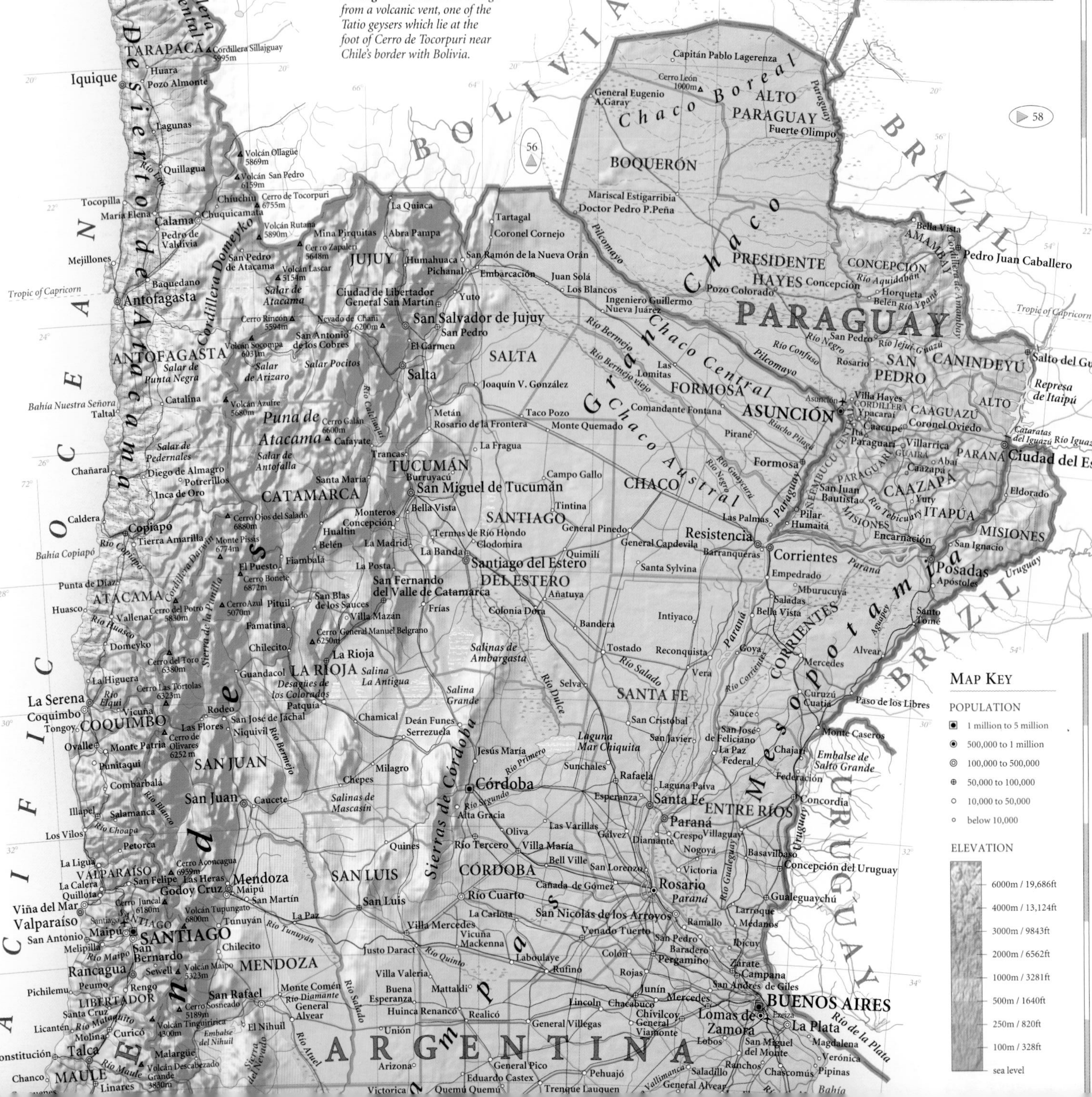

Map Key

POPULATION

- 1 million to 5 million
- 500,000 to 1 million
- 100,000 to 500,000
- 50,000 to 100,000
- 10,000 to 50,000
- below 10,000

ELEVATION

- 6000m / 19,686ft
- 4000m / 13,124ft
- 3000m / 9843ft
- 2000m / 6562ft
- 1000m / 3281ft
- 500m / 1640ft
- 250m / 820ft
- 100m / 328ft
- sea level

56

58

THE LANDSCAPE

THE ANDES RUN FROM NORTH TO SOUTH, forming a precipitous natural border between Chile and Argentina. East of the Andes are the scrublands of the Gran Chaco and the plains of the Pampas, which extend northward toward Paraguay. In the far southwest, Chile's indented Pacific coastline has many features typical of areas which have been affected by glaciation.

The Atacama Desert (Desierto de Atacama) *in Chile is one of the driest places on Earth where some areas have never recorded any rain. It contains a number of salt lakes.*

Landlocked Paraguay relies on its river system for access to the sea and to produce hydroelectric power. The most important river system is the Paraguay–Paraná which provides links into neighboring countries including Brazil, Uruguay, and Argentina.

The Gran Chaco combines poor drainage, extremely hot temperatures and thorn-infested scrub to make it one of South America's most inhospitable regions.

Most of the highest mountains in Chile's northern Andes are volcanoes like Volcán Lascar and Volcán Rutana.

Cerro Aconcagua in the central Andes is the tallest mountain in the whole chain, rising to 22,834 ft (6,959 m).

Alluvial deposits from the many rivers in central Chile have created rich soils, ideal for a wide range of agriculture.

The Pampas derive their name from an Indian word meaning flat surface. The dry western region is largely desert, whereas the east is well-watered, supporting temperate grasses.

Andes

Patagonia divides into two zones, with the Andes in the west, and the lower main plateau, extending east toward the Atlantic. It is a desolate area with climatic extremes; dark lava fields scattered with light bunchgrass give a "leopard skin" effect to the landscape.

The Andean mountain system, which forms Argentina's western border, was created by folding and faulting, following the convergence of the Nazca and South American tectonic plates.

The Patagonian ice sheet is the world's third largest ice field, covering 6,560 sq miles (17,000 sq km). Patagonia also contains many typical features from past glaciations. These include glacial lakes, U-shaped valleys, fjords, and deep-cut channels.

Cape Horn is the most southerly point of South America. The severity of the "Roaring Forties" winds makes the Horn one of the world's most treacherous shipping regions.

Argentinian Pampas

Jet stream
Rainfall
Windblown particles
Ice-capped Andes are source of loess
Thick layer of loess sediments

A thick, fertile layer of loess lies in the basin underlying the Argentinian Pampas. It has been laid down following successive periods of glaciation. The minute loess particles are transported as dust and deposited by a downward air motion, or following rainfall.

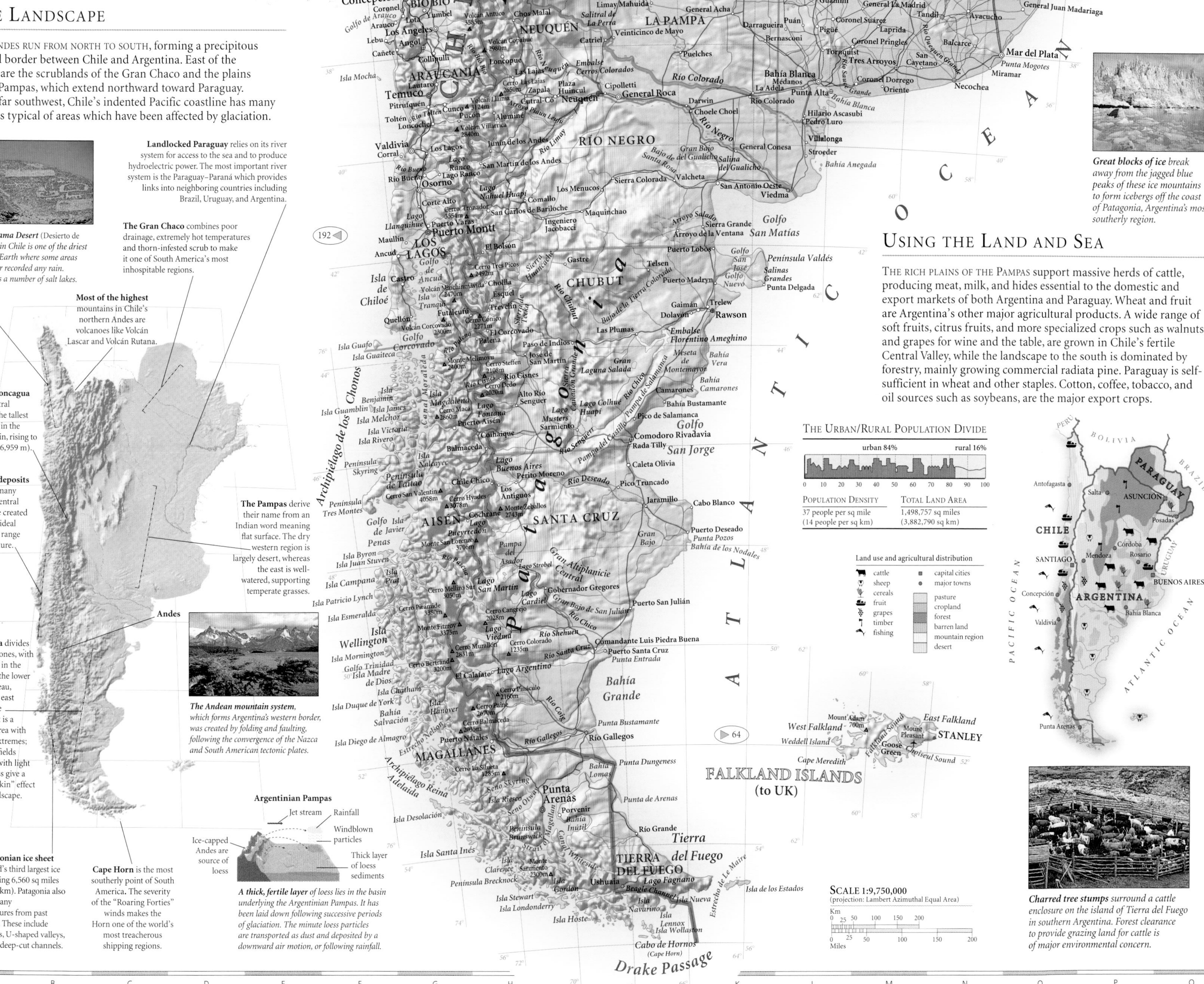

CHILE
ARGENTINA
NEUQUÉN
LA PAMPA
RÍO NEGRO
CHUBUT
SANTA CRUZ
ARAUCANÍA
BÍO BÍO
LOS LAGOS
AISÉN
MAGALLANES
TIERRA DEL FUEGO
Patagonia
ATLANTIC OCEAN
Archipiélago de los Chonos
Golfo San Matías
Golfo San Jorge
Bahía Grande
Drake Passage
Mar del Plata
Bahía Blanca
Viedma
Rawson
Comodoro Rivadavia
Puerto Montt
Punta Arenas
Ushuaia
Río Gallegos
Cabo de Hornos (Cape Horn)
FALKLAND ISLANDS (to UK)
West Falkland
East Falkland
STANLEY
192
64

Great blocks of ice break away from the jagged blue peaks of these ice mountains to form icebergs off the coast of Patagonia, Argentina's most southerly region.

USING THE LAND AND SEA

THE RICH PLAINS OF THE PAMPAS support massive herds of cattle, producing meat, milk, and hides essential to the domestic and export markets of both Argentina and Paraguay. Wheat and fruit are Argentina's other major agricultural products. A wide range of soft fruits, citrus fruits, and more specialized crops such as walnuts, and grapes for wine and the table, are grown in Chile's fertile Central Valley, while the landscape to the south is dominated by forestry, mainly growing commercial radiata pine. Paraguay is self-sufficient in wheat and other staples. Cotton, coffee, tobacco, and oil sources such as soybeans, are the major export crops.

THE URBAN/RURAL POPULATION DIVIDE

urban 84% — rural 16%

0 10 20 30 40 50 60 70 80 90 100

POPULATION DENSITY	TOTAL LAND AREA
37 people per sq mile (14 people per sq km)	1,498,757 sq miles (3,882,790 sq km)

Land use and agricultural distribution

cattle, sheep, cereals, fruit, grapes, timber, fishing

capital cities, major towns

pasture, cropland, forest, barren land, mountain region, desert

PARAGUAY, ASUNCIÓN, CHILE, SANTIAGO, ARGENTINA, BUENOS AIRES, PACIFIC OCEAN, ATLANTIC OCEAN, BOLIVIA, BRAZIL, URUGUAY, PERU

Charred tree stumps surround a cattle enclosure on the island of Tierra del Fuego in southern Argentina. Forest clearance to provide grazing land for cattle is of major environmental concern.

SCALE 1:9,750,000
(projection: Lambert Azimuthal Equal Area)

The Atlantic Ocean

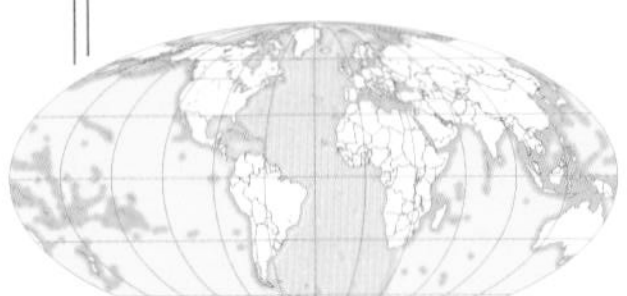

The Atlantic is the youngest of the world's oceans, formed about 180 million years ago when the landmasses of the eastern and western hemispheres separated. Its underwater topography is dominated by the Mid-Atlantic Ridge, a huge mountain system running north to south along the center of the ocean. Although most of the ridge's peaks lie below the sea, some emerge as volcanic islands, like Iceland and the Azores. The Atlantic contains a wealth of resources, including substantial oil and gas reserves and rich fishing grounds. Until the 1950s, the north Atlantic was the world's busiest shipping route; cheaper air transportation and alternative routes have shifted patterns of world trade.

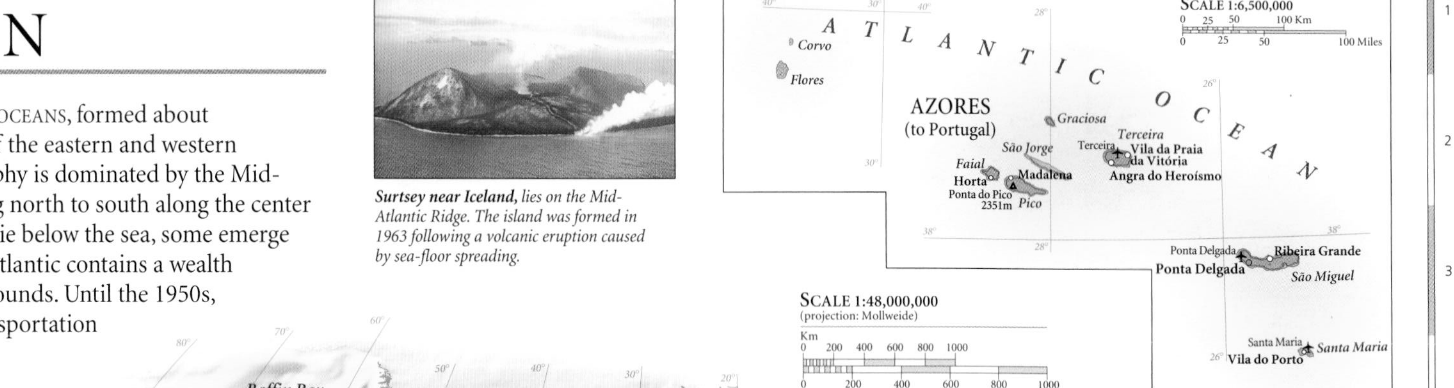
AZORES
(to Portugal)
ATLANTIC OCEAN
Corvo
Flores
Graciosa
Terceira
São Jorge
Faial
Horta
Madalena
Pico
Ponta do Pico 2351m
Vila da Praia da Vitória
Angra do Heroísmo
Ponta Delgada
Ribeira Grande
São Miguel
Santa Maria
Vila do Porto
Scale 1:6,500,000

Surtsey near Iceland, *lies on the Mid-Atlantic Ridge. The island was formed in 1963 following a volcanic eruption caused by sea-floor spreading.*

Resources

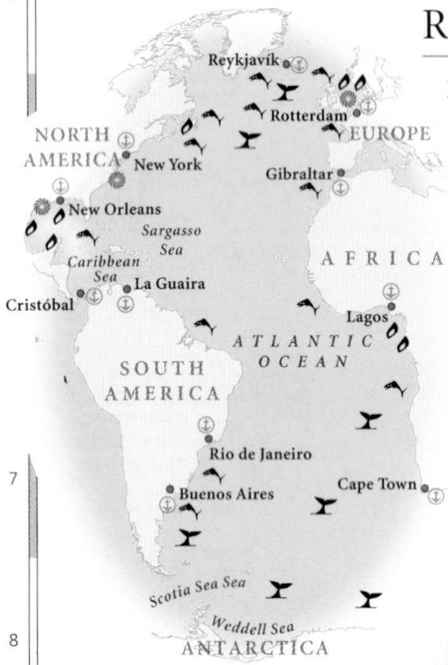

Development of the oil and gas reserves in the Atlantic began in the 1940s around the Gulf of Mexico. Since then other areas have been exploited, including the North Sea, the west coast of Africa and the area east of Newfoundland and Nova Scotia. There is also extensive mining of sand, gravel, and shell deposits by the US and UK. For centuries, the north Atlantic's fishing grounds have been utilized more heavily than other oceans, leading to a serious decline in many fish stocks.

Resources (including wildlife)
- fish
- whales
- aggregates
- oil & gas
- major towns
- major ports

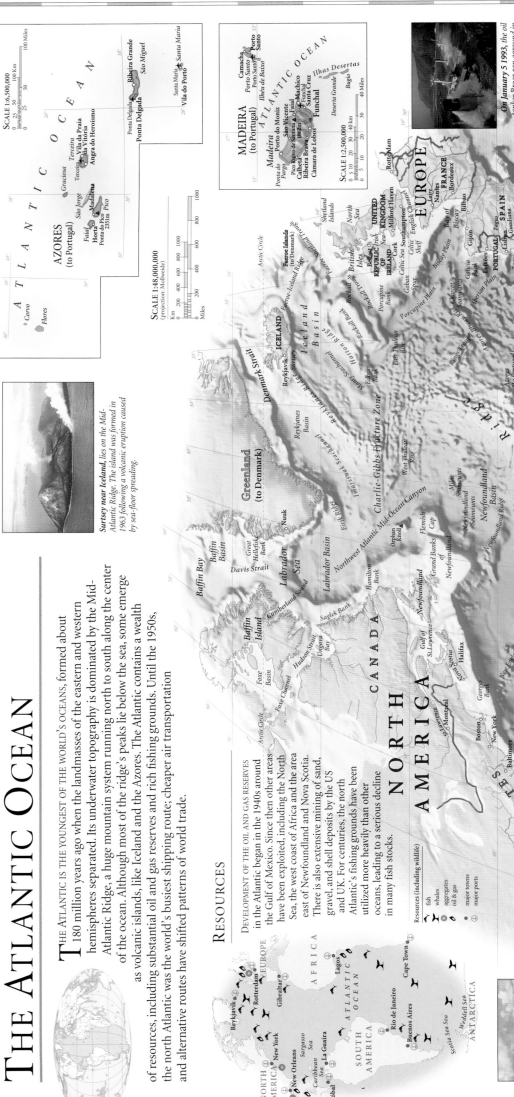

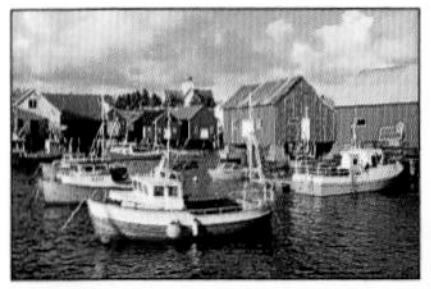

Fishing *in the seas around northwestern Europe dates back over 1,500 years. The high nutrient content of the seas makes them ideal breeding grounds for many species of fish.*

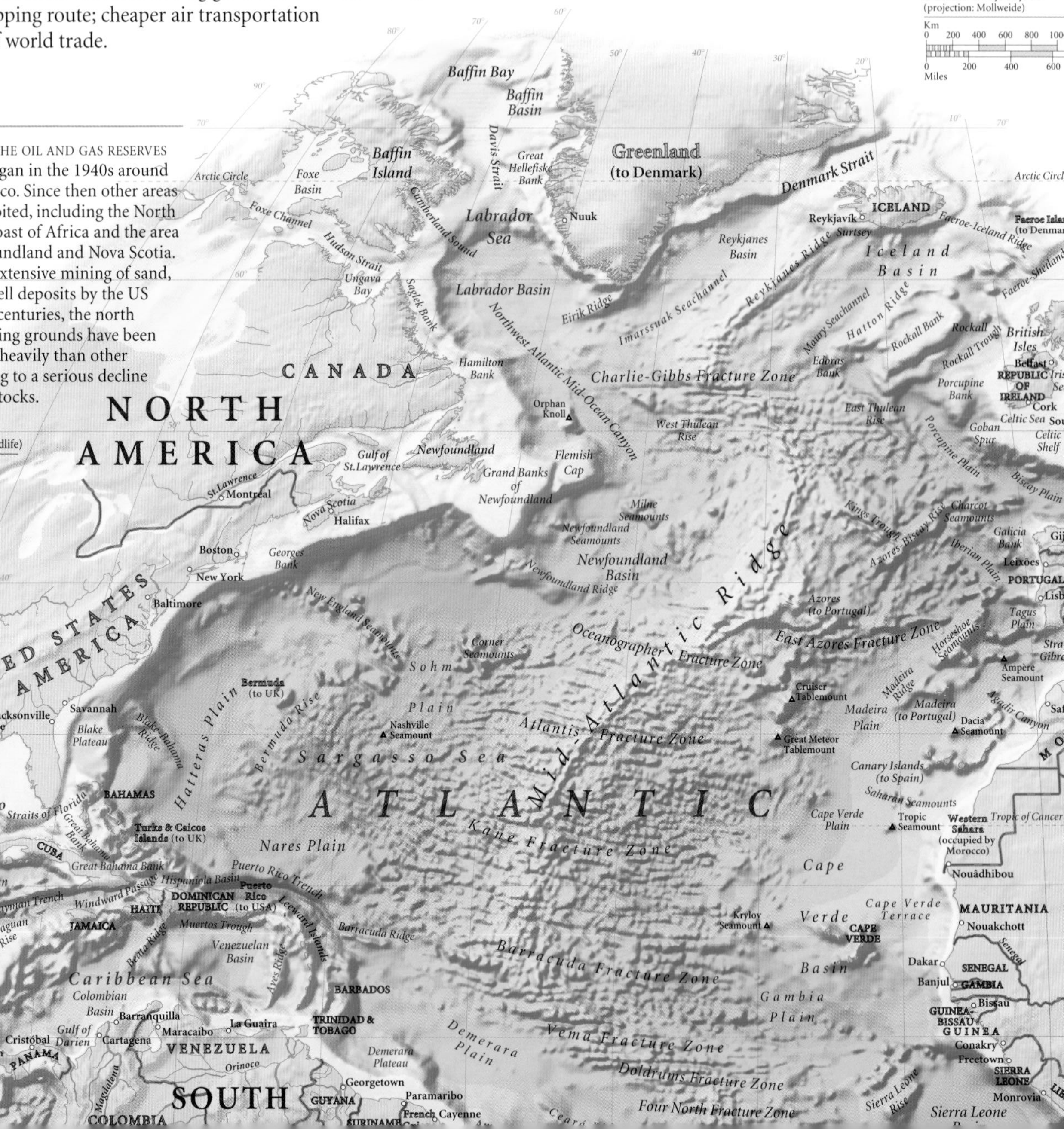

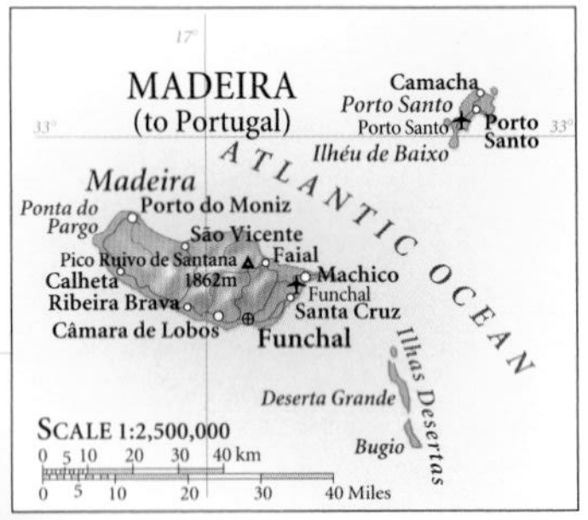

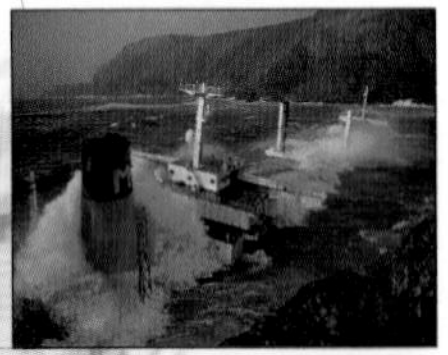

On January 5 1993, *the oil tanker Braer ran aground in the Shetland Islands, spilling 83,660 tons (85,000 tonnes) of light crude oil into the ocean, devastating the local marine ecosystem.*

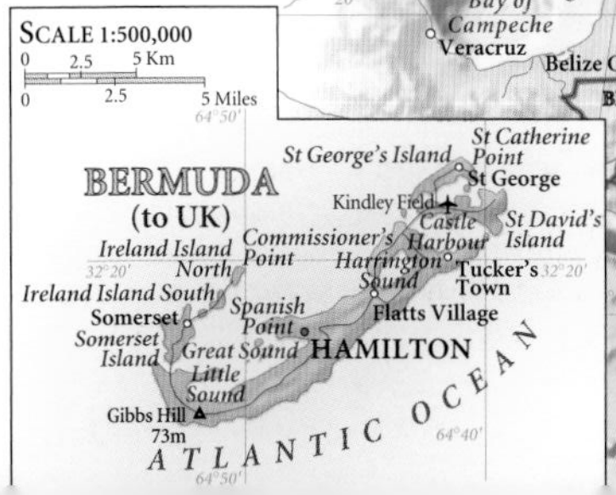

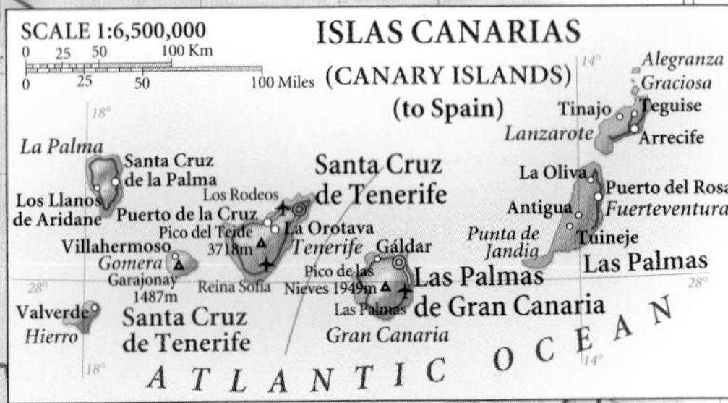

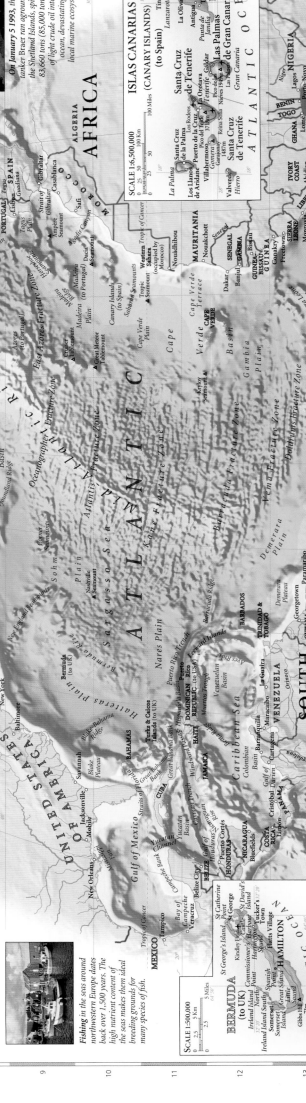

Scale 1:48,000,000 (projection: Mollweide)

The Landscape

The floor of the Atlantic is spreading by about one inch (2.5 cm) a year. The South American and African plates are moving apart drawing molten rock up from the Earth's core. The Mid-Atlantic Ridge lies along the boundary of the two plates, forming the world's longest mountain range and dividing the Atlantic floor into two parallel troughs. These troughs are subdivided into numerous smaller basins by transform faults. Most of the oceanic islands in the Atlantic are volcanic in origin; either part of the Mid-Atlantic Ridge or the Caribbean arc.

The Gulf Stream is driven by westerly winds and ocean circulation. It flows like a river of warm water along the coast of America and then across the north Atlantic where it becomes known as the North Atlantic Drift.

The Caribbean Sea only adopted its present shape 3 million years ago, when the Isthmus of Panama closed by continental drift.

Ice breaking away from the Greenland ice sheet presents a constant threat to shipping in the north Atlantic. Icebergs are carried out of the Davis Strait by sea currents.

Volcanism in the Azores *occurs because they lie over a hot spot in the oceanic crust. There are ten volcanoes clustered around the Azores. Many are still classified as active, although there has not been an eruption for over a century.*

The overall salinity of the north Atlantic is increased by highly saline water flowing out from the Mediterranean through the Strait of Gibraltar.

The Mid-Atlantic Ridge is marked along its length by numerous east–west valleys and ridges; these are caused by localized transform faulting. Some of these faults extend for 1,250 miles (2,000 km).

Silt, mud, and clay deposited at the delta of the Amazon have been carried over the continental shelf by underwater currents, forming a deep-water fan on the floor of the Atlantic Ocean.

The South Sandwich Trench is the deepest part of the Atlantic; its base lies 30,000 ft (9,144 m) below sea level. The trench is frequently subjected to earthquakes.

Icebergs in the Antarctic are larger than those in the Arctic and can be up to 50 miles (80 km) long. They can drift to latitudes of around 40°S before melting.

Floating ice shelves extend over 100 miles (160 km) into the Weddell Sea, off the coast of Antarctica.

Running the length *of the ocean, the Mid-Atlantic Ridge is a complex system of sea-floor spreading, transform faults, and volcanic islands. At its center is a large rift valley 15–30 miles (24–48 km) wide, formed by the upwelling of the ocean floor toward both Africa and South America.*

Most of the whales *in the Atlantic Ocean are found in the cooler waters of the south Atlantic, although many species migrate north to tropical waters to breed.*

Rocky breakwaters *have been built along the coast of Ghana to protect local fishing boats from being destroyed by powerful Atlantic waves.*

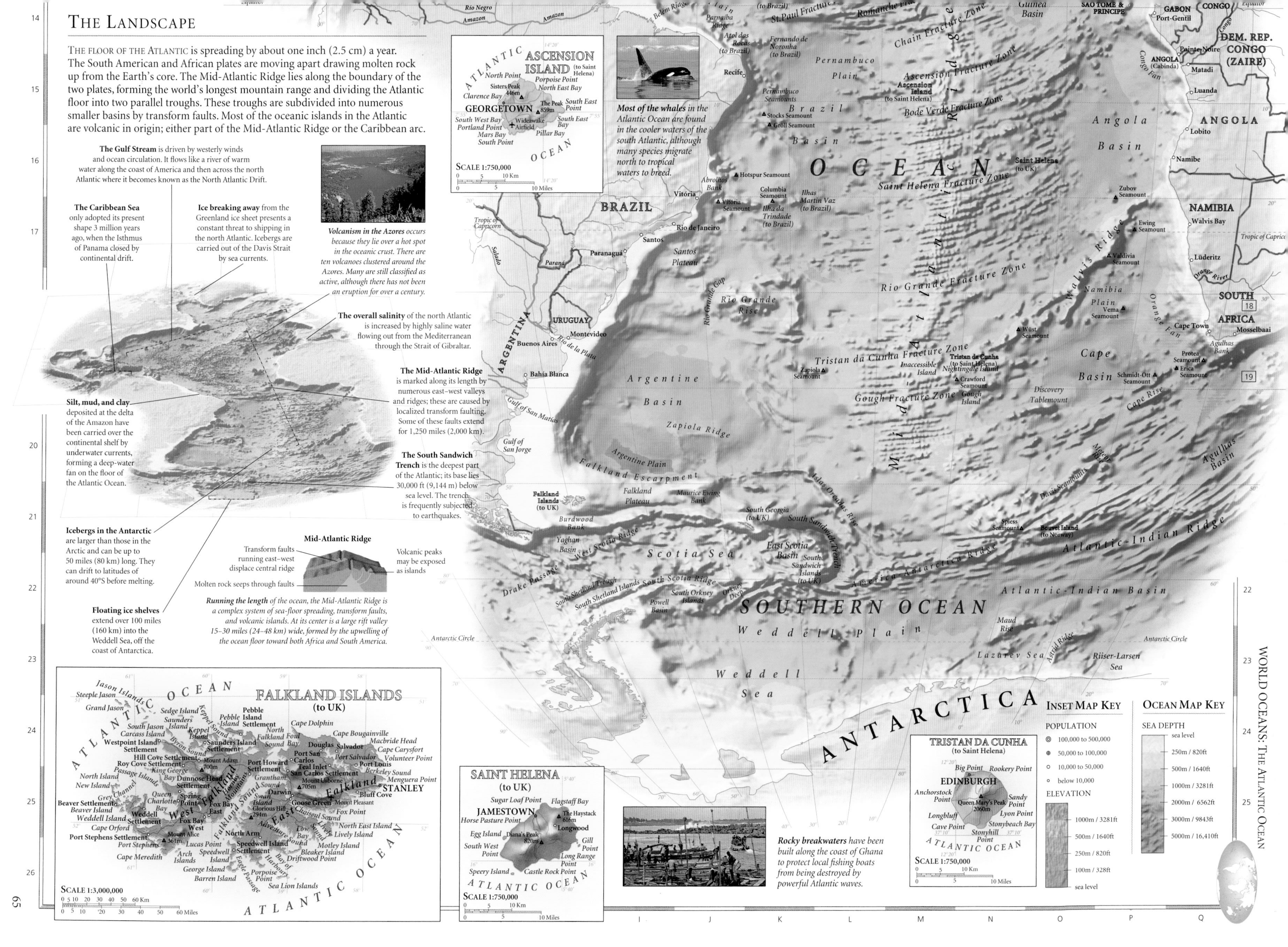
Mid-Atlantic Ridge
Transform faults running east–west displace central ridge
Volcanic peaks may be exposed as islands
Molten rock seeps through faults
ASCENSION ISLAND (to Saint Helena)
GEORGETOWN
North Point
Porpoise Point
North East Bay
Sisters Peak 446m
Clarence Bay
The Peak 859m
South East Point
South West Bay
Portland Point
Wideawake Airfield
Mars Bay
South Point
Pillar Bay
ATLANTIC OCEAN
SCALE 1:750,000
BRAZIL
URUGUAY
ARGENTINA
Rio Negro
Amazon
Recife
Vitória
Rio de Janeiro
Santos
Paranaguá
Montevideo
Buenos Aires
Río de la Plata
Bahía Blanca
Gulf of San Matías
Gulf of San Jorge
Falkland Islands (to UK)
Santos Plateau
Argentine Basin
Zapiola Ridge
Argentine Plain
Falkland Escarpment
Falkland Plateau
Maurice Ewing Bank
Burdwood Bank
Yaghan Basin
Drake Passage
Scotia Sea
South Georgia (to UK)
South Sandwich Trench
East Scotia Basin
South Sandwich Islands (to UK)
South Shetland Islands
South Orkney Islands
Powell Basin
Islas Orcadas Rise
Rio Grande Rise
Rio Grande Gap
Pernambuco Plain
Brazil Basin
St. Paul Fracture Zone
Romanche Fracture Zone
Chain Fracture Zone
Ascension Fracture Zone
Bode Verde Fracture Zone
Saint Helena Fracture Zone
Rio Grande Fracture Zone
Tristan da Cunha Fracture Zone
Gough Fracture Zone
Mid-Atlantic Ridge
OCEAN
Saint Helena (to UK)
Tristan da Cunha (to Saint Helena)
Inaccessible Island
Nightingale Island
Gough Island
Angola Basin
Guinea Basin
Walvis Ridge
Namibia Plain
Cape Basin
Cape Rise
Discovery Tablemount
Agulhas Basin
Atlantic-Indian Ridge
Atlantic-Indian Basin
America-Antarctica Ridge
Bouvet Island (to Norway)
SOUTHERN OCEAN
Weddell Plain
Weddell Sea
Lazarev Sea
Riiser-Larsen Sea
Maud Rise
ANTARCTICA
Antarctic Circle
GABON
CONGO
DEM. REP. CONGO (ZAIRE)
ANGOLA
NAMIBIA
SOUTH AFRICA
Luanda
Lobito
Namibe
Walvis Bay
Lüderitz
Cape Town
Mosselbaai
FALKLAND ISLANDS (to UK)
STANLEY
West Falkland
East Falkland
Falkland Sound
SCALE 1:3,000,000
SAINT HELENA (to UK)
JAMESTOWN
Diana's Peak 820m
SCALE 1:750,000
TRISTAN DA CUNHA (to Saint Helena)
EDINBURGH
Queen Mary's Peak 2060m
SCALE 1:750,000
INSET MAP KEY
POPULATION
100,000 to 500,000
50,000 to 100,000
10,000 to 50,000
below 10,000
ELEVATION
1000m / 3281ft
500m / 1640ft
250m / 820ft
100m / 328ft
sea level
OCEAN MAP KEY
SEA DEPTH
sea level
250m / 820ft
500m / 1640ft
1000m / 3281ft
2000m / 6562ft
3000m / 9843ft
5000m / 16,410ft

AFRICA

THE WORLD'S SECOND LARGEST CONTINENT, AFRICA COVERS AN AREA OF 11,712,434 SQ MILES (30,335,000 SQ KM). IT HAS 53 SEPARATE COUNTRIES, INCLUDING MADAGASCAR IN THE INDIAN OCEAN – THE HIGHEST NUMBER OF ANY CONTINENT.

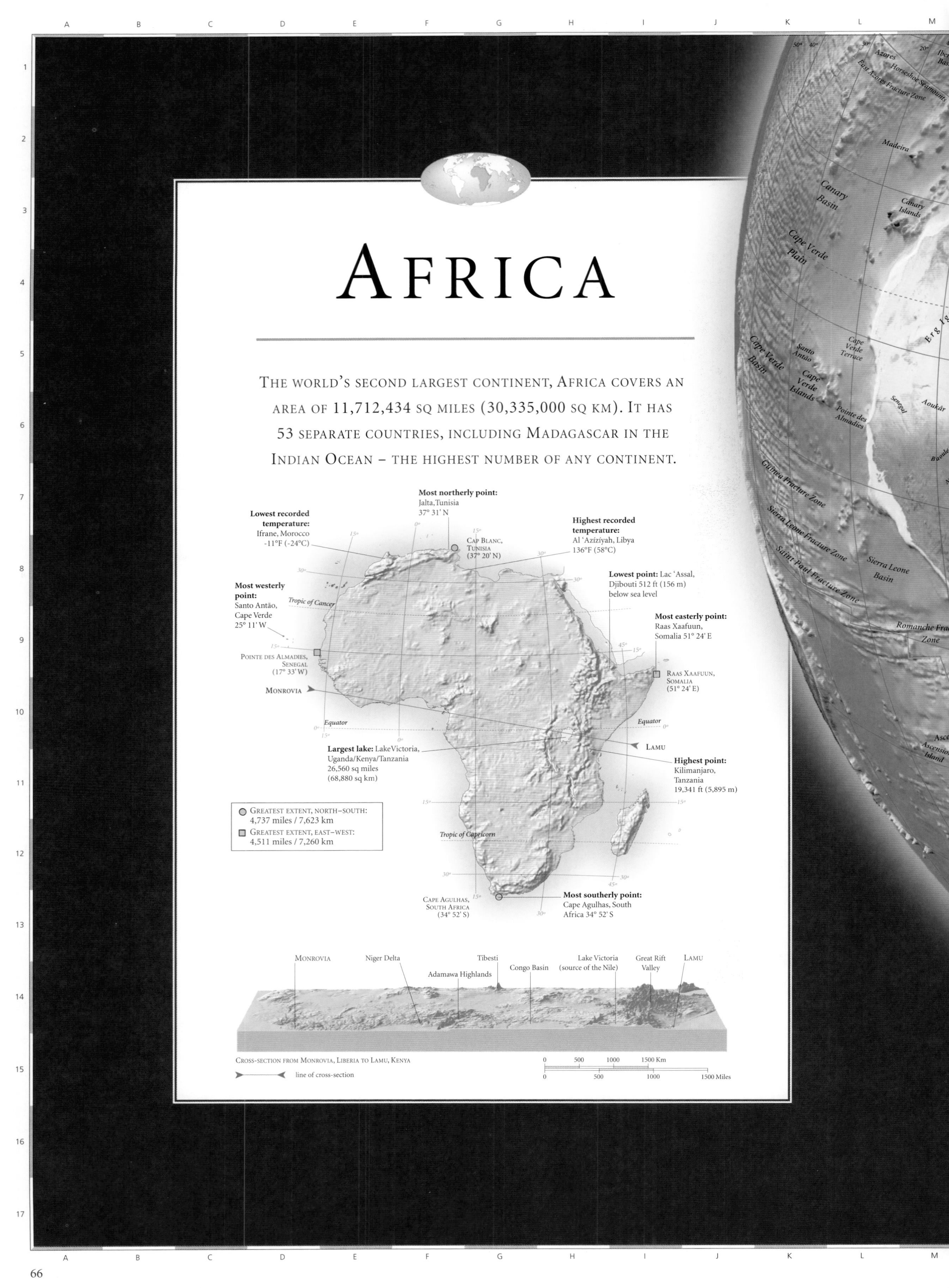

Most northerly point: Jalta, Tunisia 37° 31' N
Lowest recorded temperature: Ifrane, Morocco -11°F (-24°C)
Cap Blanc, Tunisia (37° 20' N)
Highest recorded temperature: Al 'Azízíyah, Libya 136°F (58°C)
Lowest point: Lac 'Assal, Djibouti 512 ft (156 m) below sea level
Most westerly point: Santo Antão, Cape Verde 25° 11' W
Tropic of Cancer
Most easterly point: Raas Xaafuun, Somalia 51° 24' E
Pointe des Almadies, Senegal (17° 33' W)
Raas Xaafuun, Somalia (51° 24' E)
Monrovia
Equator
Largest lake: Lake Victoria, Uganda/Kenya/Tanzania 26,560 sq miles (68,880 sq km)
Lamu
Highest point: Kilimanjaro, Tanzania 19,341 ft (5,895 m)
Greatest extent, north–south: 4,737 miles / 7,623 km
Greatest extent, east–west: 4,511 miles / 7,260 km
Tropic of Capricorn
Cape Agulhas, South Africa (34° 52' S)
Most southerly point: Cape Agulhas, South Africa 34° 52' S
Monrovia
Niger Delta
Adamawa Highlands
Tibesti
Congo Basin
Lake Victoria (source of the Nile)
Great Rift Valley
Lamu
Cross-section from Monrovia, Liberia to Lamu, Kenya
line of cross-section
0 500 1000 1500 Km
0 500 1000 1500 Miles
Azores
Horseshoe Seamounts
East Azores Fracture Zone
Madeira
Canary Basin
Canary Islands
Cape Verde Plain
Cape Verde Terrace
Santo Antão
Cape Verde Basin
Cape Verde Islands
Pointe des Almadies
Senegal
Aoukâr
Guinea Fracture Zone
Sierra Leone Fracture Zone
Saint Paul Fracture Zone
Sierra Leone Basin
Romanche Fracture Zone
Ascension Island

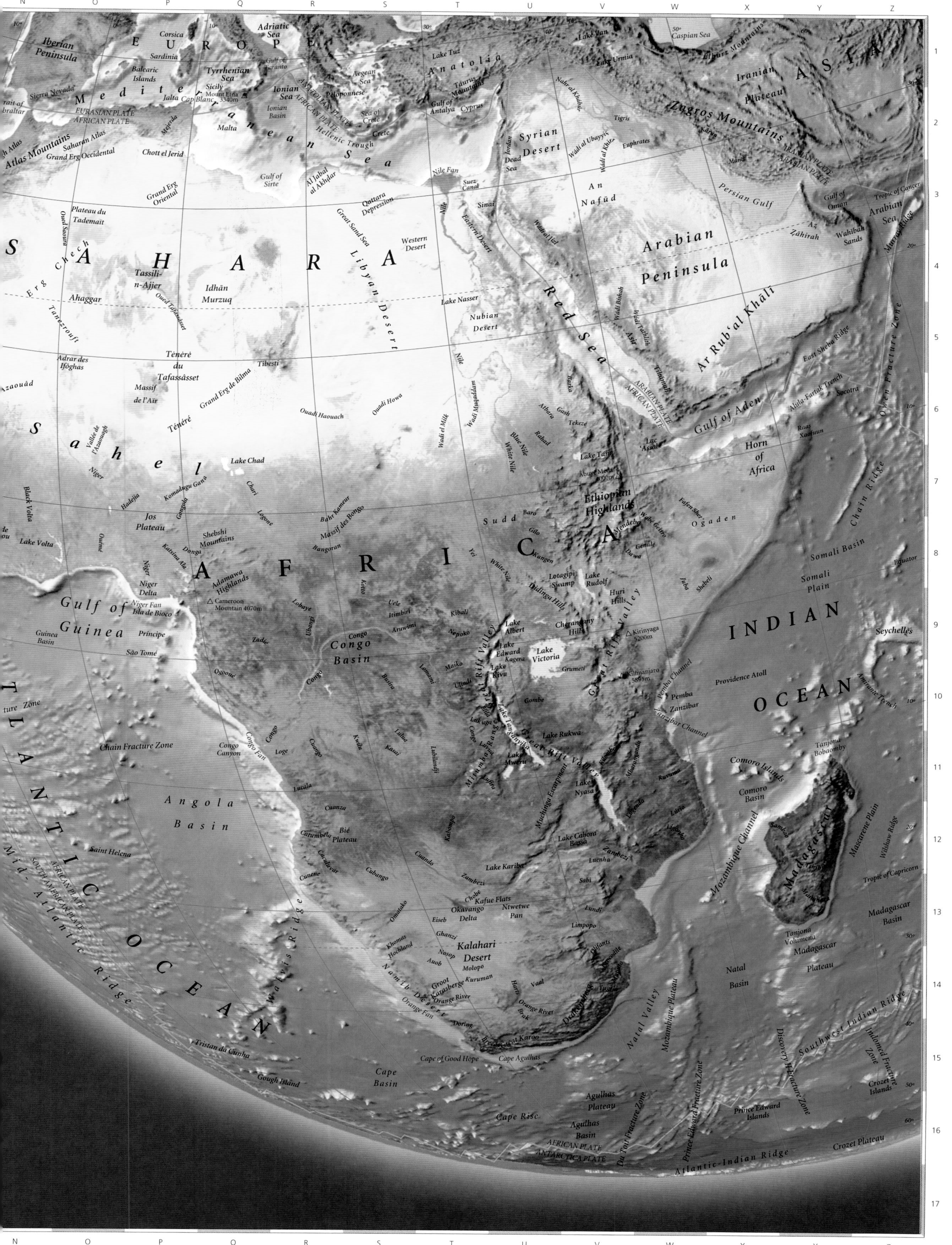
N O P Q R S T U V W X Y Z
1 2 3 4 5 6 7 8 9 10 11 12 13 14 15 16 17
EUROPE
Iberian Peninsula
Corsica
Sardinia
Balearic Islands
Adriatic Sea
Gulf of Taranto
Tyrrhenian Sea
Sicily
Mount Etna 3340m
Malta
Ionian Sea
Ionian Basin
Aegean Sea
Peloponnese
Sea of Crete
Crete
Hellenic Trough
Mediterranean Sea
EURASIAN PLATE
AFRICAN PLATE
Sierra Nevada
Atlas Mountains
Saharan Atlas
Grand Erg Occidental
Chott el Jerid
Grand Erg Oriental
Gulf of Sirte
Al Jabal al Akhdar
Qattara Depression
Great Sand Sea
Plateau du Tademaït
Oued Saoura
SAHARA
Erg Chech
Tassili-n-Ajjer
Idhān Murzuq
Ahaggar
Tanezrouft
Libyan Desert
Western Desert
Adrar des Ifôghas
Ténéré du Tafassâsset
Tibesti
Massif de l'Aïr
Grand Erg de Bilma
Ténéré
Ouadi Haouach
Ouadi Howa
Sahel
Lake Chad
Niger
Black Volta
Lake Volta
Jos Plateau
Shebshi Mountains
Adamawa Highlands
Cameroon Mountain 4070m
Niger Delta
Niger Fan
Isla de Bioco
Gulf of Guinea
Guinea Basin
Príncipe
São Tomé
AFRICA
Congo Basin
Congo
Ubangi
Lake Albert
Lake Edward
Lake Kivu
Lake Victoria
Western Rift Valley
Lake Tanganyika
Lake Rukwa
Lake Mweru
Great Rift Valley
Lake Nyasa
Lake Cabora Bassa
Lake Kariba
Zambezi
Okavango Delta
Kafue Flats
Kalahari Desert
Namib Desert
Orange River
Orange Fan
Cape of Good Hope
Cape Agulhas
Drakensberg
Limpopo
Angola Basin
Bié Plateau
Congo Canyon
Congo Fan
Chain Fracture Zone
Saint Helena
Walvis Ridge
Mid-Atlantic Ridge
SOUTH AMERICAN PLATE
AFRICAN PLATE
ATLANTIC OCEAN
Tristan da Cunha
Gough Island
Cape Basin
Cape Rise
Agulhas Plateau
Agulhas Basin
ANTARCTICA PLATE
Du Toit Fracture Zone
Prince Edward Fracture Zone
Prince Edward Islands
Discovery II Fracture Zone
Atlantic-Indian Ridge
Crozet Plateau
Crozet Islands
Southwest Indian Ridge
Natal Valley
Mozambique Plateau
Natal Basin
Madagascar Plateau
Madagascar Basin
Madagascar
Mozambique Channel
Comoro Islands
Comoro Basin
Mascarene Plain
Tropic of Capricorn
INDIAN OCEAN
Providence Atoll
Seychelles
Pemba
Zanzibar
Kilimanjaro 5895m
Kirinyaga 5200m
Lake Rudolf
Ethiopian Highlands
Lake Tana
Horn of Africa
Ogaden
Somali Basin
Somali Plain
Equator
Gulf of Aden
Socotra
Red Sea
ARABIAN PLATE
AFRICAN PLATE
Nubian Desert
Lake Nasser
Nile
Blue Nile
White Nile
Sudd
Eastern Desert
Sinai
Suez Canal
Nile Fan
Dead Sea
Syrian Desert
Cyprus
Gulf of Antalya
Taurus Mountains
Anatolia
Lake Tuz
Lake Van
Lake Urmia
Caspian Sea
Elburz Mountains
Iranian Plateau
ASIA
Zagros Mountains
Tigris
Euphrates
An Nafūd
Persian Gulf
Gulf of Oman
Tropic of Cancer
Arabian Sea
Arabian Peninsula
Ar Rub'al Khālī
East Sheba Ridge
Owen Fracture Zone
Chain Ridge

Physical Africa

The structure of Africa was dramatically influenced by the break up of the supercontinent Gondwanaland about 160 million years ago and, more recently, rifting and hot spot activity. Today, much of Africa is remote from active plate boundaries and comprises a series of extensive plateaus and deep basins, which influence the drainage patterns of major rivers. The relief rises to the east, where volcanic uplands and vast lakes mark the Great Rift Valley. In the far north and south sedimentary rocks have been folded to form the Atlas Mountains and the Great Karoo.

Northern Africa

Northern Africa comprises a system of basins and plateaus. The Tibesti and Ahaggar are volcanic uplands, whose uplift has been matched by subsidence within large surrounding basins. Many of the basins have been infilled with sand and gravel, creating the vast Saharan lands. The Atlas Mountains in the north were formed by convergence of the African and Eurasian plates.

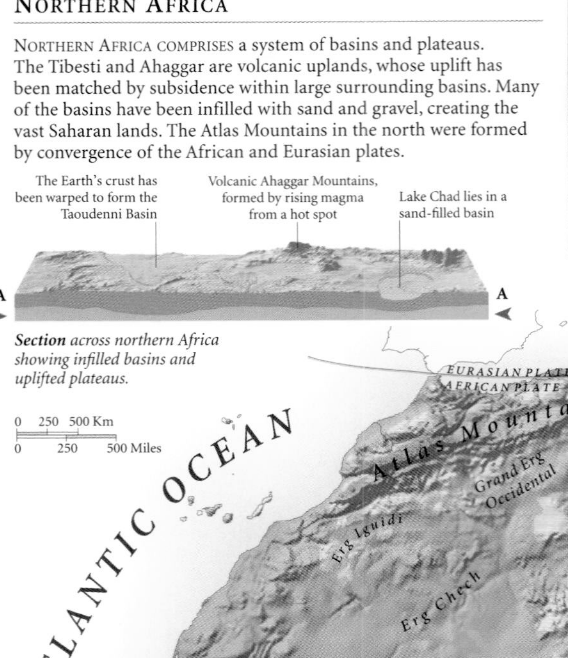

The Earth's crust has been warped to form the Taoudenni Basin
Volcanic Ahaggar Mountains, formed by rising magma from a hot spot
Lake Chad lies in a sand-filled basin
A
A

Section across northern Africa showing infilled basins and uplifted plateaus.

East Africa

The Great Rift Valley is the most striking feature of this region, running for 4,475 miles (7,200 km) from Lake Nyasa to the Red Sea. North of Lake Nyasa it splits into two arms and encloses an interior plateau which contains Lake Victoria. A number of elongated lakes and volcanoes lie along the fault lines. To the west lies the Congo Basin, a vast, shallow depression, which rises to form an almost circular rim of highlands.

Rift valley lakes, like Lake Tanganyika, lie along fault lines

Lake Victoria

Extensive faulting occurs as rift valley pulls apart

***Cross-section** through eastern Africa showing the two arms of the Great Rift Valley and its interior plateau.*

0 50 100 Km
0 50 100 Miles

Scale 1:40,000,000
(projection: Lambert Azimuthal Equal Area)

Map Key

Elevation: 5000m / 16,405ft; 4000m / 13,124ft; 3000m / 9843ft; 2000m / 6562ft; 1000m / 3281ft; 500m / 1640ft; 250m / 820ft; 100m / 328ft; sea level; below sea level

Plate margins (for explanation see page xiv): constructive; destructive; conservative; uncertain

line of cross-section

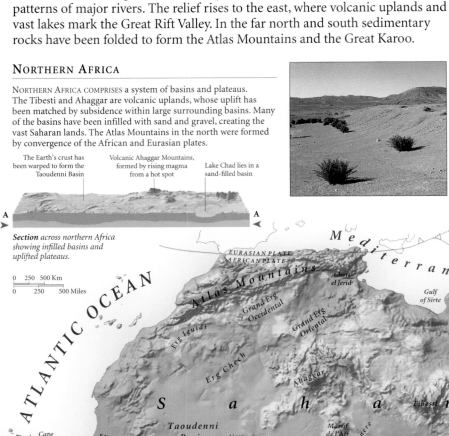

Southern Africa

The Great Escarpment marks the southern boundary of Africa's basement rock and includes the Drakensberg range. It was uplifted when Gondwanaland fragmented about 160 million years ago and it has gradually been eroded back from the coast. To the north, the relief drops steadily, forming the Kalahari Basin. In the far south are the fold mountains of the Great Karoo.

Kalahari Basin, covered with the sandy plains of the Kalahari Desert

Boundary of the Great Escarpment

Uplift of the basement rock created a raised plateau

Drakensberg

***Cross-section** through southern Africa showing the boundary of the Great Escarpment.*

0 100 200 Km
0 100 200 Miles

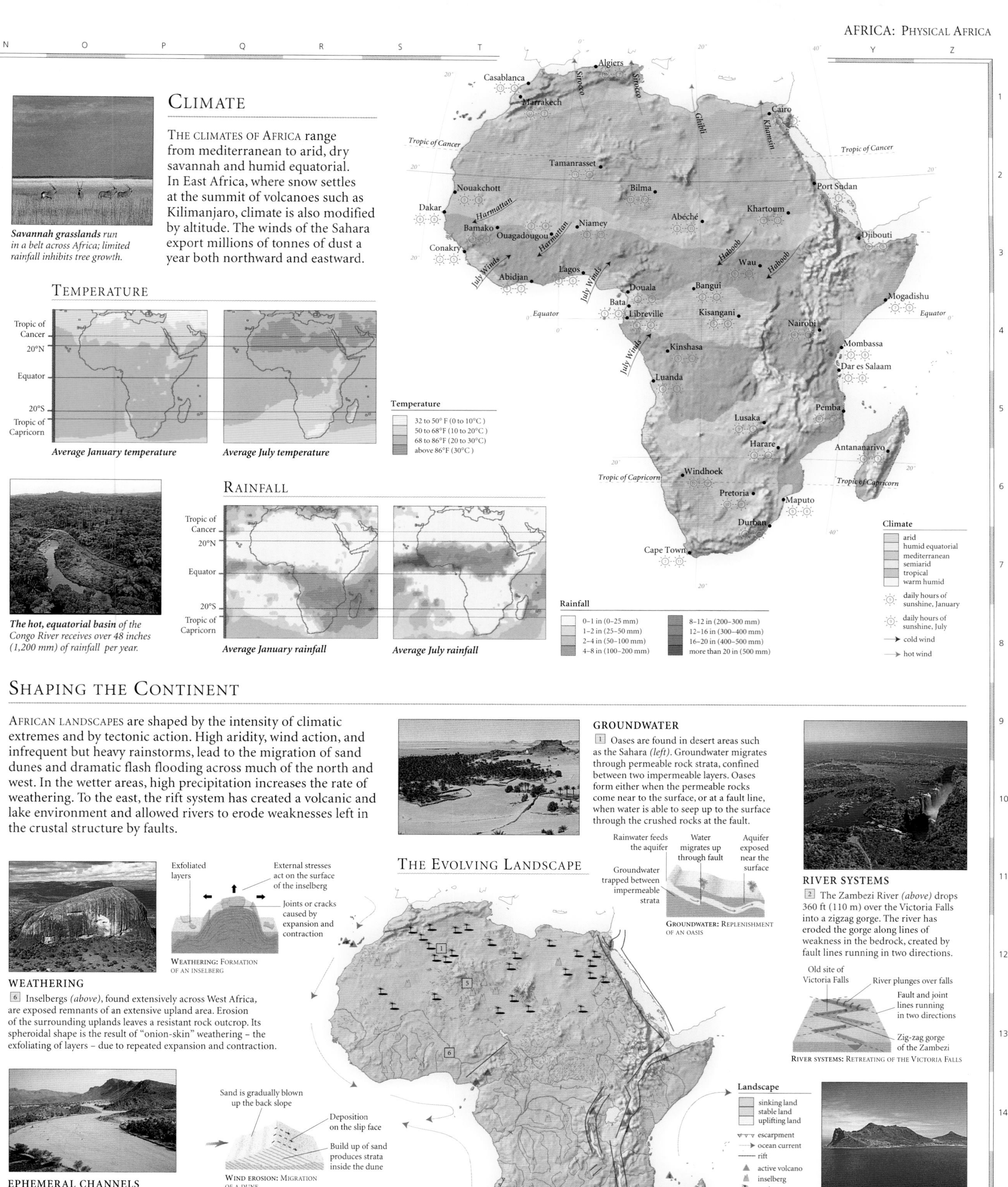

N O P Q R S T U V W X Y Z
1 2 3 4 5 6 7 8 9 10 11 12 13 14 15 16 17
Casablanca
Marrakech
Algiers
Sirocco
Ghibli
Cairo
Khamsin
Tropic of Cancer
Tamanrasset
Nouakchott
Bilma
Port Sudan
Dakar
Harmattan
Khartoum
Niamey
Abéché
Bamako
Ouagadougou
Djibouti
Conakry
Haboob
July Winds
Lagos
Wau
Abidjan
Douala
Bangui
Mogadishu
Bata
Libreville
Kisangani
Equator
Nairobi
Kinshasa
Mombassa
Dar es Salaam
Luanda
Pemba
Lusaka
Harare
Antananarivo
Tropic of Capricorn
Windhoek
Pretoria
Maputo
Durban
Cape Town
Temperature
32 to 50° F (0 to 10°C)
50 to 68°F (10 to 20°C)
68 to 86°F (20 to 30°C)
above 86°F (30°C)
Tropic of Cancer
20°N
Equator
20°S
Tropic of Capricorn
Rainfall
0–1 in (0–25 mm)
1–2 in (25–50 mm)
2–4 in (50–100 mm)
4–8 in (100–200 mm)
8–12 in (200–300 mm)
12–16 in (300–400 mm)
16–20 in (400–500 mm)
more than 20 in (500 mm)
Climate
arid
humid equatorial
mediterranean
semiarid
tropical
warm humid
daily hours of sunshine, January
daily hours of sunshine, July
cold wind
hot wind

CLIMATE

THE CLIMATES OF AFRICA range from mediterranean to arid, dry savannah and humid equatorial. In East Africa, where snow settles at the summit of volcanoes such as Kilimanjaro, climate is also modified by altitude. The winds of the Sahara export millions of tonnes of dust a year both northward and eastward.

***Savannah grasslands** run in a belt across Africa; limited rainfall inhibits tree growth.*

TEMPERATURE

Average January temperature

Average July temperature

RAINFALL

***The hot, equatorial basin** of the Congo River receives over 48 inches (1,200 mm) of rainfall per year.*

Average January rainfall

Average July rainfall

SHAPING THE CONTINENT

AFRICAN LANDSCAPES are shaped by the intensity of climatic extremes and by tectonic action. High aridity, wind action, and infrequent but heavy rainstorms, lead to the migration of sand dunes and dramatic flash flooding across much of the north and west. In the wetter areas, high precipitation increases the rate of weathering. To the east, the rift system has created a volcanic and lake environment and allowed rivers to erode weaknesses left in the crustal structure by faults.

GROUNDWATER

1 Oases are found in desert areas such as the Sahara *(left)*. Groundwater migrates through permeable rock strata, confined between two impermeable layers. Oases form either when the permeable rocks come near to the surface, or at a fault line, when water is able to seep up to the surface through the crushed rocks at the fault.

Rainwater feeds the aquifer
Water migrates up through fault
Aquifer exposed near the surface
Groundwater trapped between impermeable strata

GROUNDWATER: REPLENISHMENT OF AN OASIS

THE EVOLVING LANDSCAPE

Landscape
sinking land
stable land
uplifting land
escarpment
ocean current
rift
active volcano
inselberg
oasis
river
wadi
waterfall

RIVER SYSTEMS

2 The Zambezi River *(above)* drops 360 ft (110 m) over the Victoria Falls into a zigzag gorge. The river has eroded the gorge along lines of weakness in the bedrock, created by fault lines running in two directions.

Old site of Victoria Falls
River plunges over falls
Fault and joint lines running in two directions
Zig-zag gorge of the Zambezi

RIVER SYSTEMS: RETREATING OF THE VICTORIA FALLS

Exfoliated layers
External stresses act on the surface of the inselberg
Joints or cracks caused by expansion and contraction

WEATHERING: FORMATION OF AN INSELBERG

WEATHERING

6 Inselbergs *(above)*, found extensively across West Africa, are exposed remnants of an extensive upland area. Erosion of the surrounding uplands leaves a resistant rock outcrop. Its spheroidal shape is the result of "onion-skin" weathering – the exfoliating of layers – due to repeated expansion and contraction.

Sand is gradually blown up the back slope
Deposition on the slip face
Build up of sand produces strata inside the dune

WIND EROSION: MIGRATION OF A DUNE

EPHEMERAL CHANNELS

5 Wadis *(above)* drain much of northern Africa. These drybed courses are flooded only after infrequent, but intense, storms in the uplands cause water to surge along their channels.

Heavy rainfall runs off mountains
Water collects and floods the dry channel

EPHEMERAL CHANNELS: FLASH FLOODING OF A WADI

WIND EROSION

4 Dunes like this in the Namib Desert *(left)* are wind-blown accumulations of sand, which slowly migrate. Wind action moves sand up the shallow back slope; when the sand reaches the crest of the dune it is deposited on the slip face.

Waves refracting
Wave energy dispersed in the bay
Force of waves concentrates on the headland
The sea bed is deeper opposite the bay than at the headland

COASTAL PROCESSES: EROSION OF A BAY

COASTAL PROCESSES

3 Houtbaai *(above)*, in southern Africa, is constantly being modified by wave action. As waves approach the indented coastline, they reach the shallow water of the headland, slowing down and reducing in length. This causes them to bend or refract, concentrating their erosive force at the headlands.

POLITICAL AFRICA

THE POLITICAL MAP OF MODERN AFRICA only emerged following the end of the Second World War. Over the next half-century, all of the countries formerly controlled by European powers gained independence from their colonial rulers – only Liberia and Ethiopia were never colonized. The postcolonial era has not been an easy period for many countries, but there have been moves toward multiparty democracy in much of West Africa, and in Zambia, Tanzania, and Kenya. In South Africa, democratic elections replaced the internationally-condemned apartheid system only in 1994. Other countries have still to find political stability; corruption in government, and ethnic tensions are serious problems. National infrastructures, based on the colonial transportation systems built to exploit Africa's resources, are often inappropriate for independent economic development.

Language groups

- Afro-Asiatic (Hamito-Semitic)
- Niger-Congo
- Nilo-Saharan
- Khoisan
- Indo-European
- Austronesian

LANGUAGES

THREE MAJOR WORLD LANGUAGES act as *lingua francas* across the African continent: Arabic in North Africa; English in southern and eastern Africa and Nigeria; and French in Central and West Africa, and in Madagascar. A huge number of African languages are spoken as well – over 2,000 have been recorded, with more than 400 in Nigeria alone – reflecting the continuing importance of traditional cultures and values. In the north of the continent, the extensive use of Arabic reflects Middle Eastern influences while Bantu is widely-spoken across much of southern Africa.

OFFICIAL AFRICAN LANGUAGES

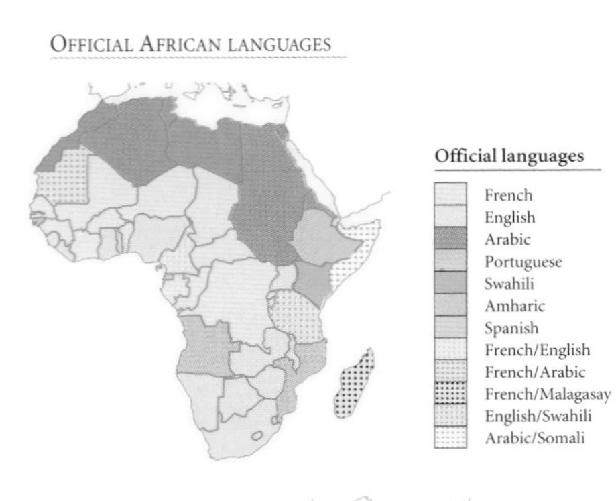
Official languages
French
English
Arabic
Portuguese
Swahili
Amharic
Spanish
French/English
French/Arabic
French/Malagasay
English/Swahili
Arabic/Somali

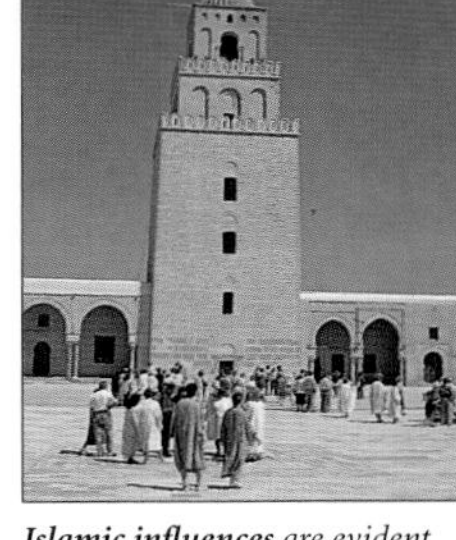

Islamic influences *are evident throughout North Africa. The Great Mosque at Kairouan, Tunisia, is Africa's holiest Islamic place.*

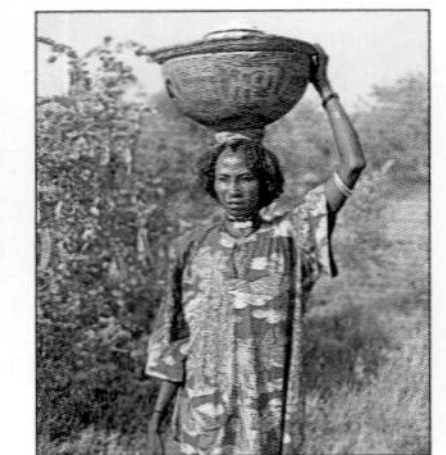

In northeastern Nigeria, *people speak Kanuri – a dialect of the Saharan language group.*

TRANSPORTATION

AFRICAN RAILROADS WERE BUILT to aid the exploitation of natural resources, and most offer passage only from the interior to the coastal cities, leaving large parts of the continent untouched – five landlocked countries have no railroads at all. The Congo, Nile, and Niger River networks offer limited access to land within the continental interior, but have a number of waterfalls and cataracts which prevent navigation from the sea. Many roads were developed in the 1960s and 1970s, but economic difficulties are making the maintenance and expansion of the networks difficult.

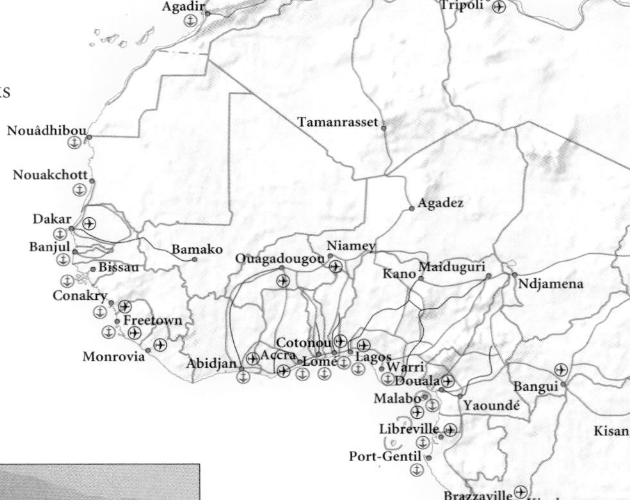

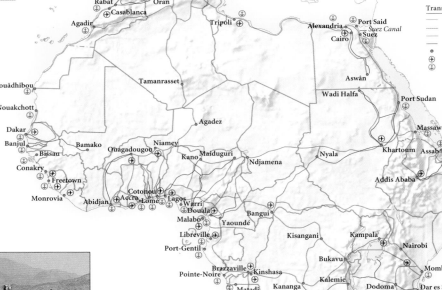

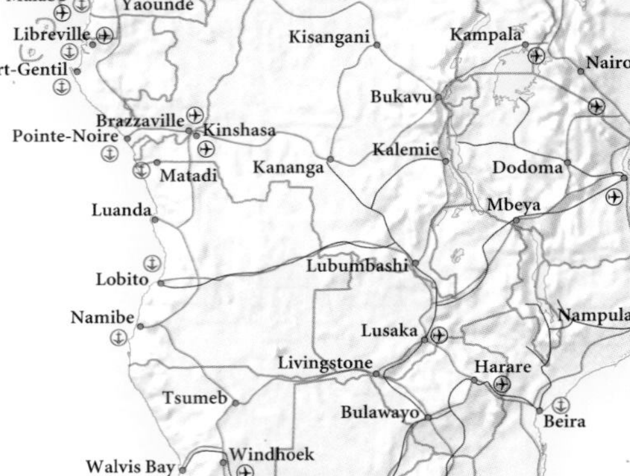
Transportation
major roads and highways
major railroads
major canal
international borders
transportation intersections
international airports
major ports

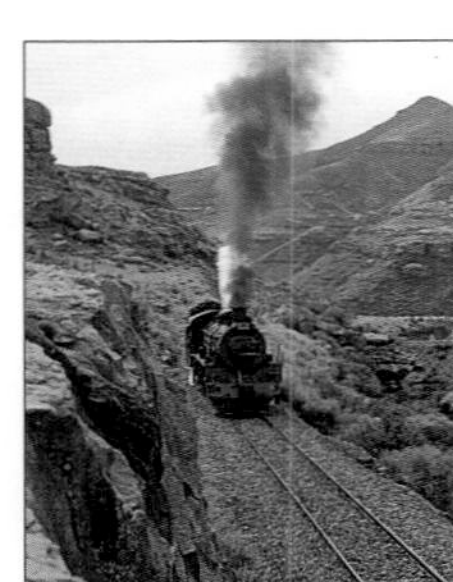

South Africa *has the largest concentration of railroads in Africa. Over 20,000 miles (32,000 km) of routes have been built since 1870.*

Traditional means of transportation, *such as the camel, are still widely used across the less accessible parts of Africa.*

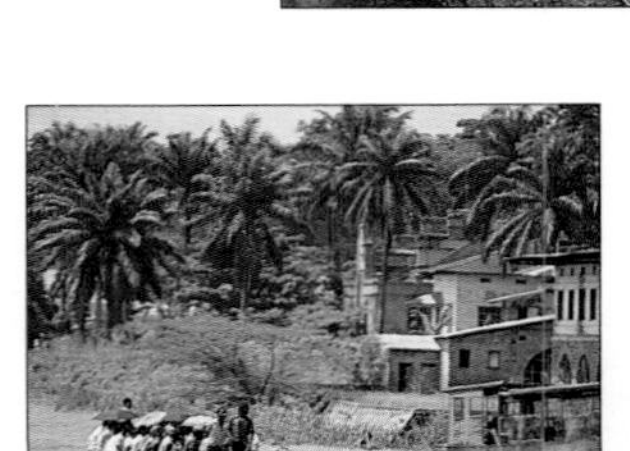

The Congo River, *though not suitable for river transportation along its entire length, forms a vital link for people and goods in its navigable inland reaches.*

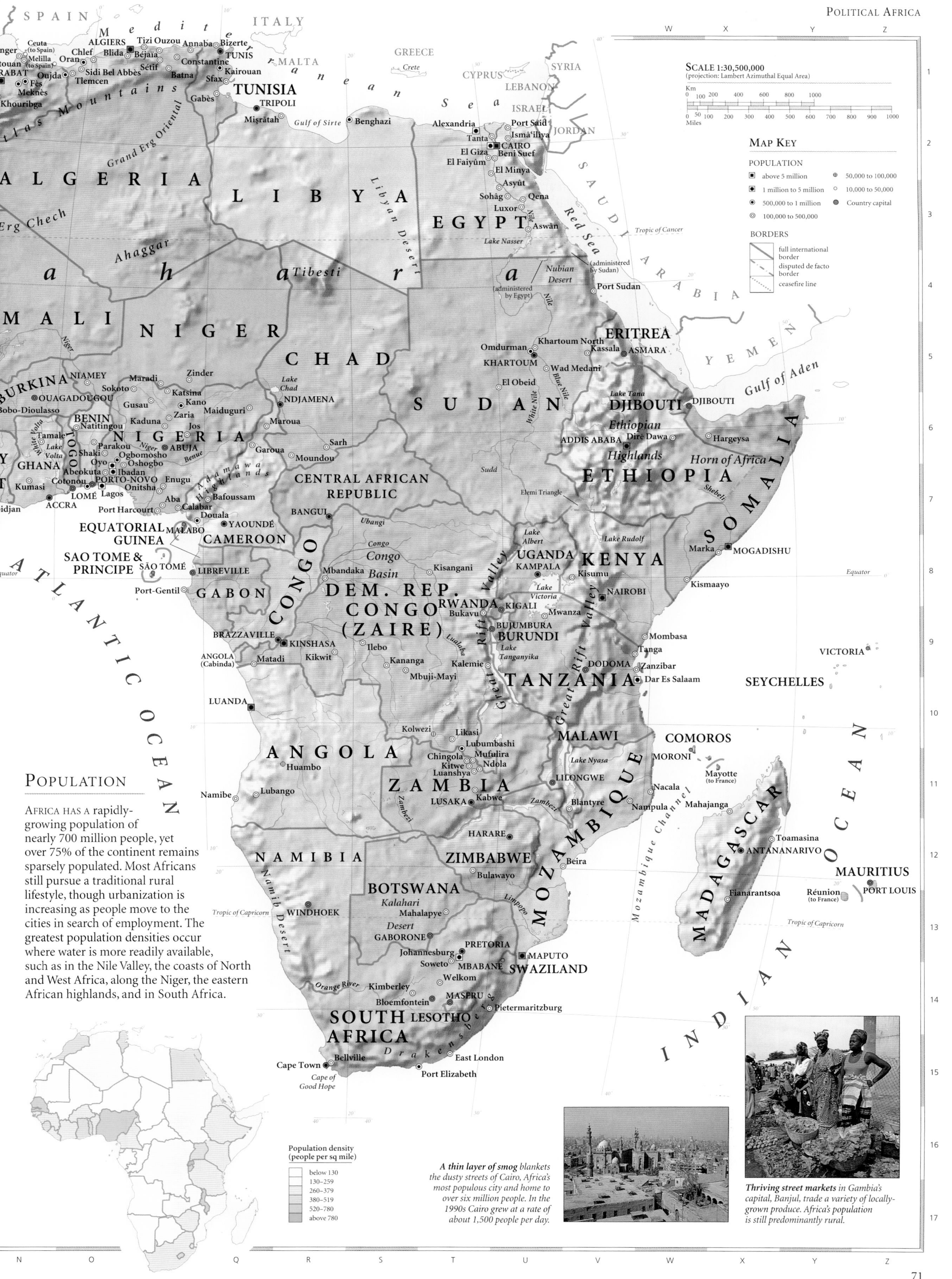
SCALE 1:30,500,000
(projection: Lambert Azimuthal Equal Area)
Km
Miles
MAP KEY
POPULATION
above 5 million
1 million to 5 million
500,000 to 1 million
100,000 to 500,000
50,000 to 100,000
10,000 to 50,000
Country capital
BORDERS
full international border
disputed de facto border
ceasefire line
ALGERIA
LIBYA
EGYPT
TUNISIA
MALI
NIGER
CHAD
SUDAN
ERITREA
DJIBOUTI
ETHIOPIA
SOMALIA
BURKINA
BENIN
TOGO
GHANA
NIGERIA
CAMEROON
CENTRAL AFRICAN REPUBLIC
EQUATORIAL GUINEA
SAO TOME & PRINCIPE
GABON
CONGO
DEM. REP. CONGO (ZAIRE)
UGANDA
KENYA
RWANDA
BURUNDI
TANZANIA
ANGOLA
ZAMBIA
MALAWI
MOZAMBIQUE
ZIMBABWE
NAMIBIA
BOTSWANA
SOUTH AFRICA
LESOTHO
SWAZILAND
MADAGASCAR
COMOROS
SEYCHELLES
MAURITIUS
ATLANTIC OCEAN
INDIAN OCEAN
Mediterranean Sea
Red Sea
Gulf of Aden
Mozambique Channel
Sahara
Population density (people per sq mile)
below 130
130–259
260–379
380–519
520–780
above 780

Population

Africa has a rapidly-growing population of nearly 700 million people, yet over 75% of the continent remains sparsely populated. Most Africans still pursue a traditional rural lifestyle, though urbanization is increasing as people move to the cities in search of employment. The greatest population densities occur where water is more readily available, such as in the Nile Valley, the coasts of North and West Africa, along the Niger, the eastern African highlands, and in South Africa.

***A thin layer of smog** blankets the dusty streets of Cairo, Africa's most populous city and home to over six million people. In the 1990s Cairo grew at a rate of about 1,500 people per day.*

***Thriving street markets** in Gambia's capital, Banjul, trade a variety of locally-grown produce. Africa's population is still predominantly rural.*

African Resources

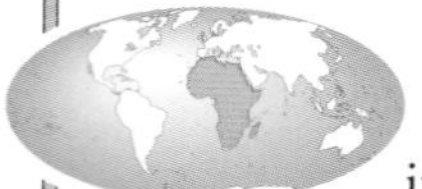

The economies of most African countries are dominated by subsistence and cash crop agriculture, with limited industrialization. Manufacturing is largely confined to South Africa. Many countries depend on a single resource, such as copper or gold, or a cash crop, such as coffee, for export income, which can leave them vulnerable to fluctuations in world commodity prices. In order to diversify their economies and develop a wider industrial base, investment from overseas is being actively sought by many African governments.

Industry

Many African industries concentrate on the extraction and processing of raw materials. These include the oil industry, food processing, mining, and textile production. South Africa accounts for over half of the continent's industrial output with much of the remainder coming from the countries along the northern coast. Over 60% of Africa's workforce is employed in agriculture.

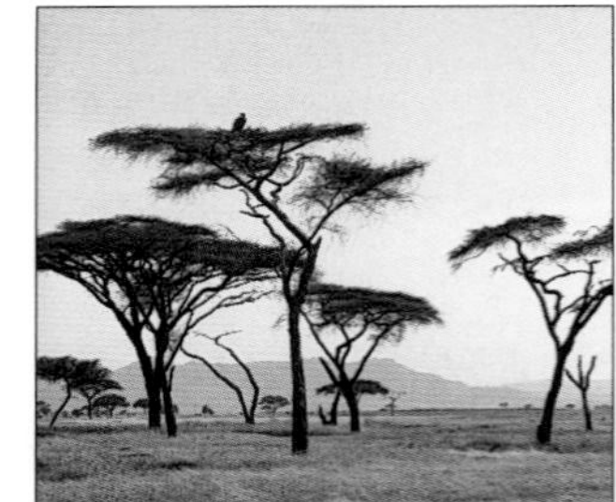

The unspoiled natural splendor *of wildlife reserves, like the Serengeti National Park in Tanzania, attract tourists to Africa from around the globe. The tourist industry in Kenya and Tanzania is particularly well developed, where it accounts for almost 10% of GNP.*

Standard of Living

Since the 1960s most countries in Africa have seen significant improvements in life expectancy, healthcare and education. However, 18 of the 20 most deprived countries in the world are African, and the continent as a whole lies well behind the rest of the world in terms of meeting many basic human needs.

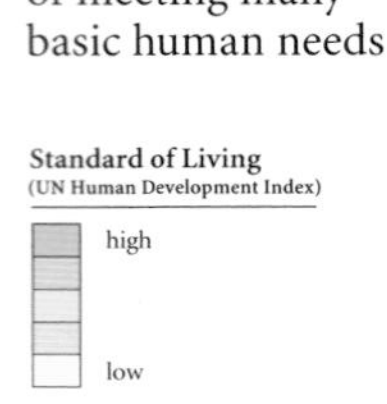
Standard of Living
(UN Human Development Index)
high
low

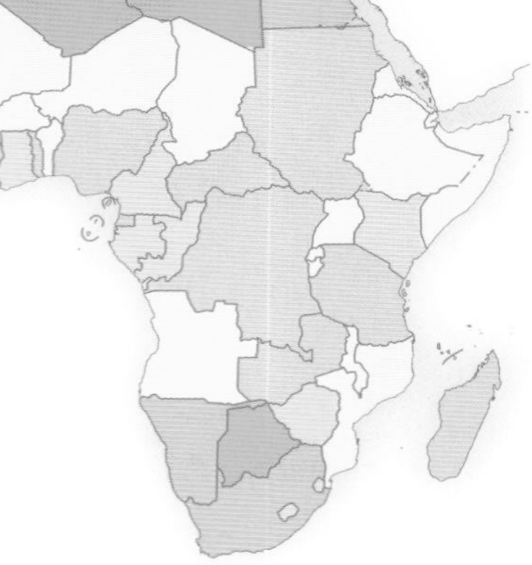

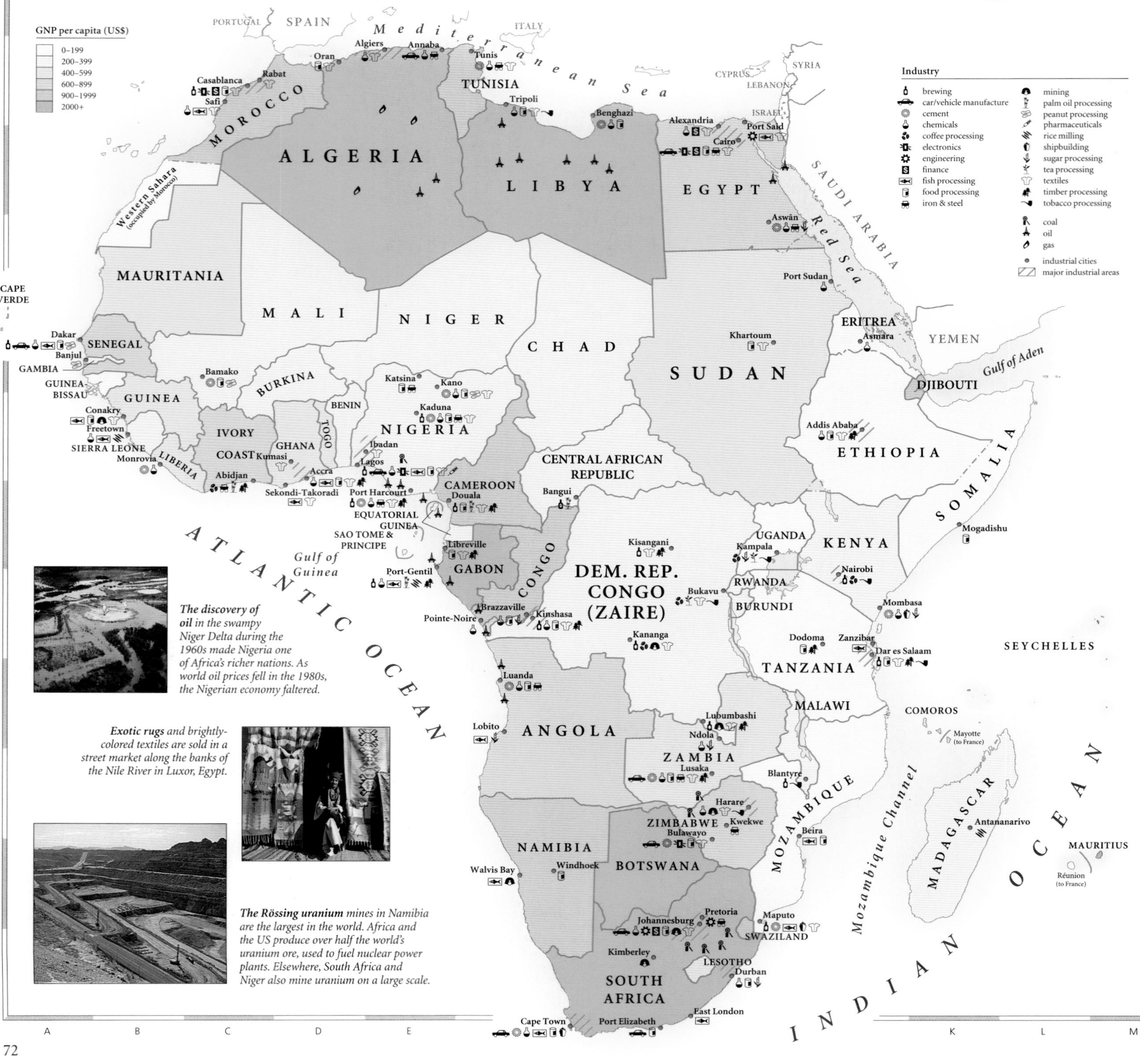

GNP per capita (US$)

- 0–199
- 200–399
- 400–599
- 600–899
- 900–1999
- 2000+

Industry

- brewing
- car/vehicle manufacture
- cement
- chemicals
- coffee processing
- electronics
- engineering
- finance
- fish processing
- food processing
- iron & steel
- mining
- palm oil processing
- peanut processing
- pharmaceuticals
- rice milling
- shipbuilding
- sugar processing
- tea processing
- textiles
- timber processing
- tobacco processing
- coal
- oil
- gas
- industrial cities
- major industrial areas

The discovery of oil *in the swampy Niger Delta during the 1960s made Nigeria one of Africa's richer nations. As world oil prices fell in the 1980s, the Nigerian economy faltered.*

Exotic rugs *and brightly-colored textiles are sold in a street market along the banks of the Nile River in Luxor, Egypt.*

The Rössing uranium *mines in Namibia are the largest in the world. Africa and the US produce over half the world's uranium ore, used to fuel nuclear power plants. Elsewhere, South Africa and Niger also mine uranium on a large scale.*

Environmental Issues

One of Africa's most serious environmental problems occurs in marginal areas such as the Sahel where scrub and forest clearance, often for cooking fuel, combined with overgrazing, are causing desertification. Game reserves in southern and eastern Africa have helped to preserve many endangered animals, although the needs of growing populations have led to conflict over land use, and poaching is a serious problem.

Environmental Issues: national parks; tropical forest; forest destroyed; desert; desertification; polluted rivers; radioactive contamination; marine pollution; heavy marine pollution; poor urban air quality

The Sahel's delicate natural equilibrium is easily destroyed by the clearing of vegetation, drought, and overgrazing. This causes the Sahara to advance south, engulfing the savannah grasslands.

Mineral Resources

Africa's ancient plateaus contain some of the world's most substantial reserves of precious stones and metals. About 30% of the world's gold is mined in South Africa; Zambia has great copper deposits; and diamonds are mined in Botswana, Dem. Rep. Congo (Zaire), and South Africa. Oil has brought great economic benefits to Algeria, Libya, and Nigeria.

Mineral Resources: oil field; gas field; coal field; bauxite; copper; diamonds; gold; iron; phosphates; tin; uranium

North and West Africa have large deposits of white phosphate minerals, which are used in making fertilizers. Morocco, Senegal, and Tunisia are the continent's leading producers.

Workers on a tea plantation gather one of Africa's most important cash crops, providing a valuable source of income. Coffee, rubber, bananas, cotton, and cocoa are also widely grown as cash crops.

Surrounded by desert, the fertile floodplains of the Nile Valley and Delta have been extensively irrigated, farmed, and settled since 3,000 BC.

Using the Land and Sea

Some of Africa's most productive agricultural land is found in the eastern volcanic uplands, where fertile soils support a wide range of valuable export crops including vegetables, tea, and coffee. The most widely-grown grain is corn and peanuts are particularly important in West Africa. Without intensive irrigation, cultivation is not possible in desert regions and unreliable rainfall in other areas limits crop production. Pastoral herding is most commonly found in these marginal lands. Substantial local fishing industries are found along coasts and in vast lakes such as Lake Nyasa and Lake Victoria.

Using the Land and Sea: cropland; desert; forest; pasture; wetland; major conurbations; cattle; goats; cereals; sheep; bananas; corn (maize); citrus fruits; cocoa; cotton; coffee; dates; fishing; fruit; oil palms; olives; peanuts; rice; rubber; shellfish; sugar cane; tea; tobacco; vineyards; wheat

North Africa

Algeria, Egypt, Libya, Morocco, Tunisia, Western Sahara

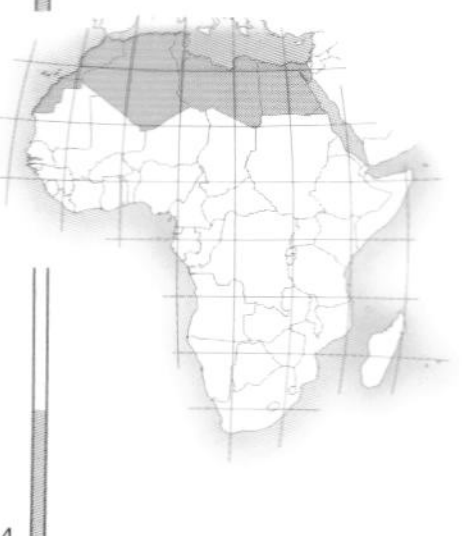

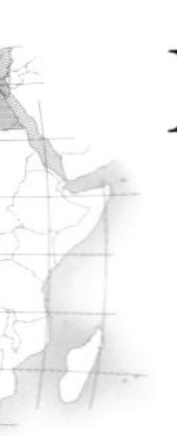

Fringed by the Mediterranean along the northern coast and by the arid Sahara in the south, North Africa reflects the influence of many invaders, both European and, most importantly, Arab, giving the region an almost universal Islamic flavor and a common Arabic language. The countries lying to the west of Egypt are often referred to as the Maghreb, an Arabic term for "west." Today, Morocco and Tunisia exploit their culture and landscape for tourism, while rich oil and gas deposits aid development in Libya and Algeria, despite political turmoil. Egypt, with its fertile, Nile-watered agricultural land and varied industrial base, is the most populous nation.

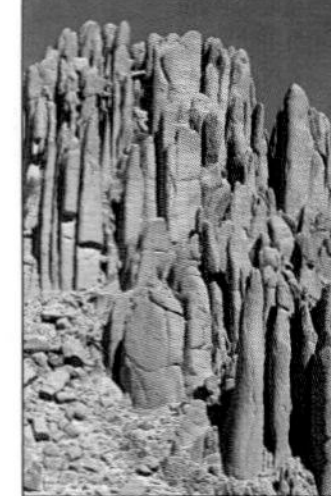

***These rock piles** in Algeria's Ahaggar Mountains are the result of weathering caused by extremes of temperature. Great cracks or joints appear in the rocks, which are then worn and smoothed by the wind.*

The Landscape

The Atlas Mountains, which extend across much of Morocco, northern Algeria, and Tunisia, are part of the fold mountain system which also runs through much of southern Europe. They recede to the south and east, becoming a steppe landscape before meeting the Sahara desert which covers more than 90% of the region. The sediments of the Sahara overlie an ancient plateau of crystalline rock, some of which is more than four billion years old.

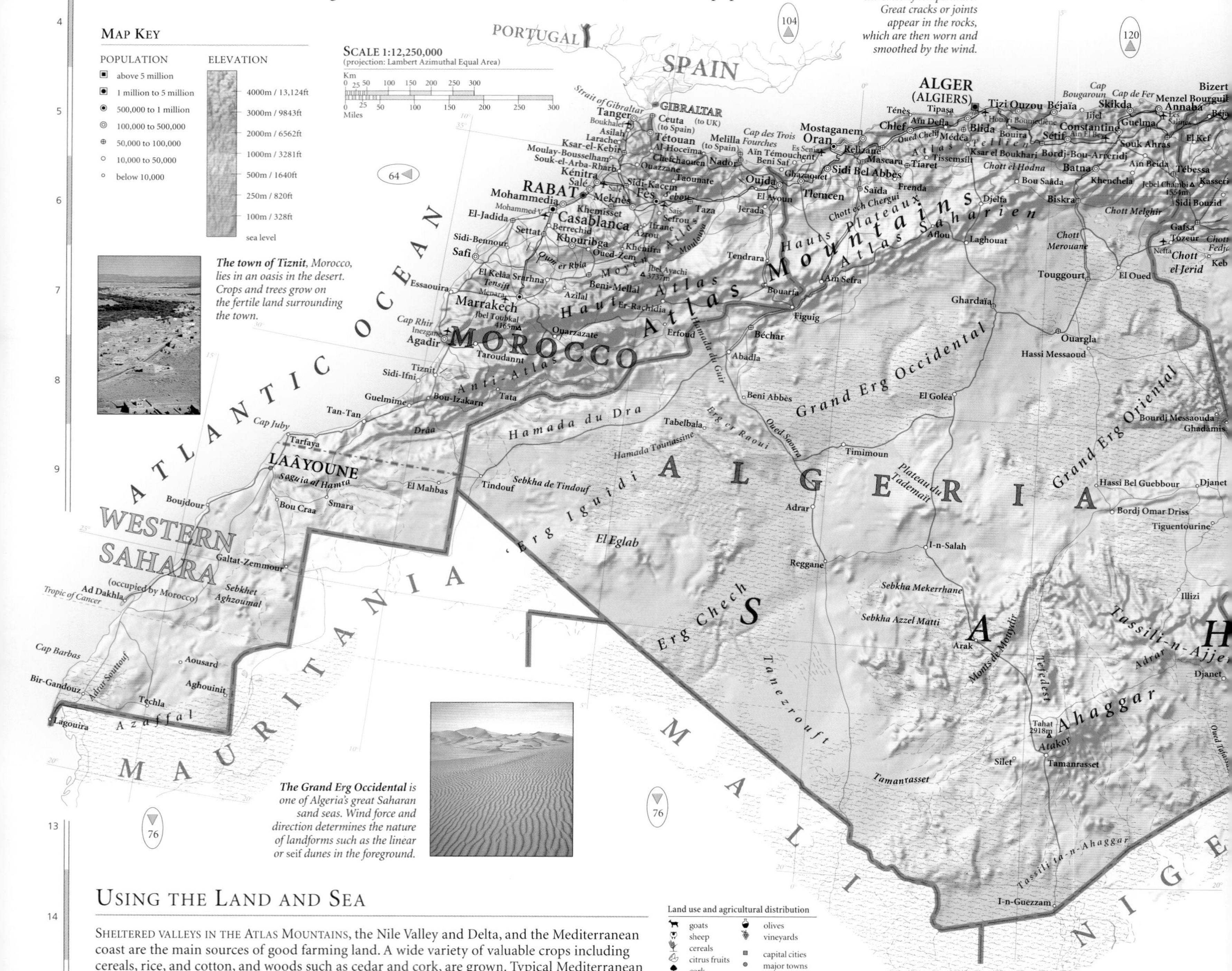

Map Key

Population	Elevation
above 5 million	4000m / 13,124ft
1 million to 5 million	3000m / 9843ft
500,000 to 1 million	2000m / 6562ft
100,000 to 500,000	1000m / 3281ft
50,000 to 100,000	500m / 1640ft
10,000 to 50,000	250m / 820ft
below 10,000	100m / 328ft
	sea level

Scale 1:12,250,000 (projection: Lambert Azimuthal Equal Area)

***The town of Tiznit**, Morocco, lies in an oasis in the desert. Crops and trees grow on the fertile land surrounding the town.*

***The Grand Erg Occidental** is one of Algeria's great Saharan sand seas. Wind force and direction determines the nature of landforms such as the linear or seif dunes in the foreground.*

Using the Land and Sea

Sheltered valleys in the Atlas Mountains, the Nile Valley and Delta, and the Mediterranean coast are the main sources of good farming land. A wide variety of valuable crops including cereals, rice, and cotton, and woods such as cedar and cork, are grown. Typical Mediterranean crops such as olives, figs, dates, and citrus fruits also thrive in these areas. The Nile Valley is particularly fertile, and most of Egypt's population lives close to the river. Elsewhere, irrigation is essential to improve crop yields on the desert margins.

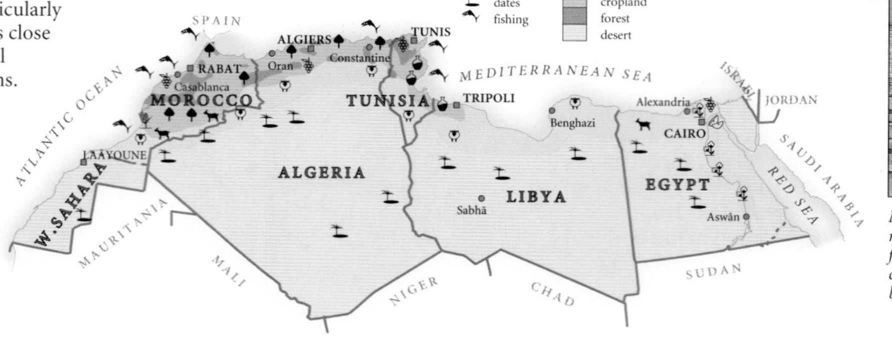

The Urban/Rural Population Divide

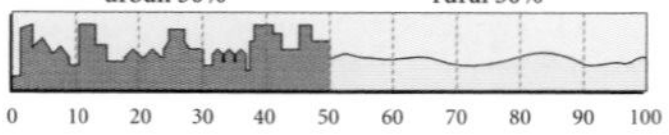

urban 50% | rural 50%

Population Density

62 people per sq mile (24 people per sq km)

Total Land Area

2,215,020 sq miles (5,738,394 sq km)

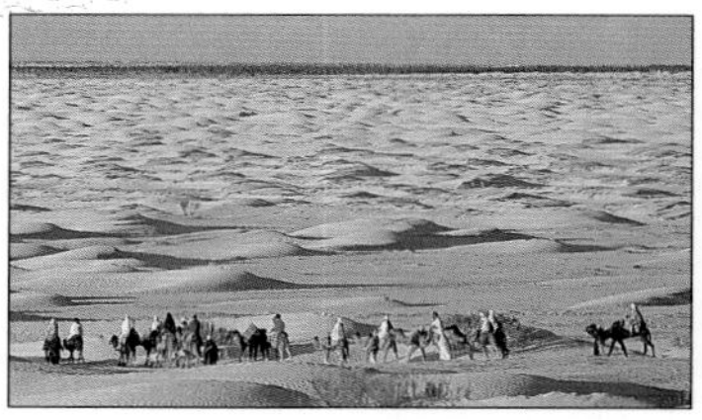

Land use and agricultural distribution: goats, sheep, cereals, citrus fruits, cork, cotton, dates, fishing, olives, vineyards, capital cities, major towns, pasture, cropland, forest, desert

***Many North African nomads**, such as the Bedouin, maintain a traditional pastoral lifestyle on the desert fringes, moving their herds of sheep, goats, and camels from place to place – crossing country borders in order to find sufficient grazing land.*

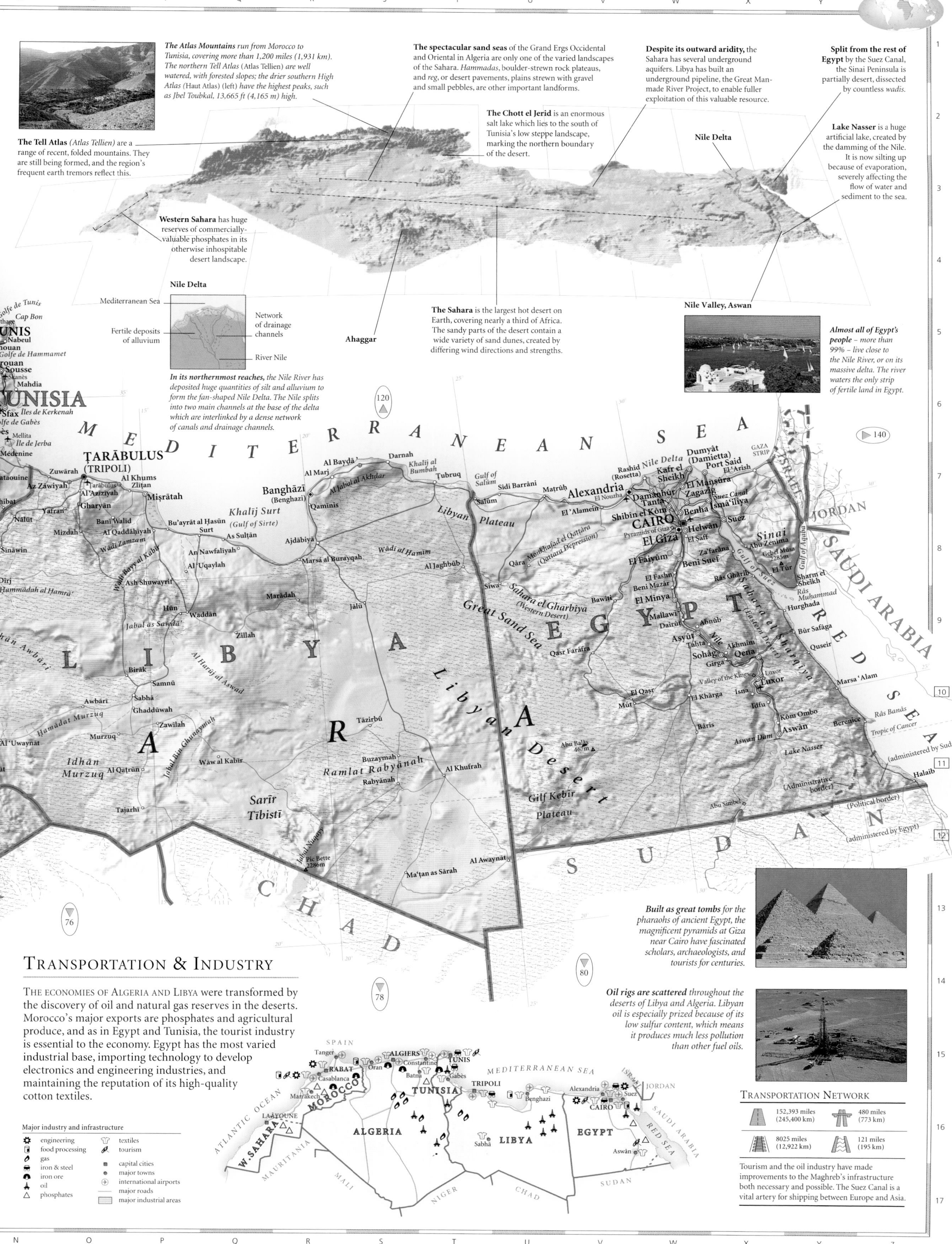

N O P Q R S T U V W X Y
Nile Delta
Mediterranean Sea
Fertile deposits of alluvium
Network of drainage channels
River Nile
Ahaggar
Nile Valley, Aswan
MEDITERRANEAN SEA
LIBYA
EGYPT
SUDAN
CHAD
SAUDI ARABIA
RED SEA
JORDAN
ISRAEL
TUNISIA
ṬARĀBULUS (TRIPOLI)
Banghāzī (Benghazi)
Khalīj Surt (Gulf of Sirte)
Alexandria
CAIRO
El Giza
Port Said
Suez
Sinai
Great Sand Sea
Libyan Desert
Libyan Plateau
Gilf Kebir Plateau
Ramlat Rabyānah
Sarīr Tibistī
Idhān Murzuq
Al Khufrah
Sabhā
Aswân
Luxor
Lake Nasser
Tropic of Cancer
Halaib
(administered by Sudan)
(administered by Egypt)
(Political border)
(Administrative border)

The Atlas Mountains *run from Morocco to Tunisia, covering more than 1,200 miles (1,931 km). The northern Tell Atlas* (Atlas Tellien) *are well watered, with forested slopes; the drier southern High Atlas* (Haut Atlas) (left) *have the highest peaks, such as Jbel Toubkal, 13,665 ft (4,165 m) high.*

The spectacular sand seas of the Grand Ergs Occidental and Oriental in Algeria are only one of the varied landscapes of the Sahara. *Hammadas*, boulder-strewn rock plateaus, and *reg*, or desert pavements, plains strewn with gravel and small pebbles, are other important landforms.

Despite its outward aridity, the Sahara has several underground aquifers. Libya has built an underground pipeline, the Great Man-made River Project, to enable fuller exploitation of this valuable resource.

Split from the rest of Egypt by the Suez Canal, the Sinai Peninsula is partially desert, dissected by countless *wadis*.

The Chott el Jerid is an enormous salt lake which lies to the south of Tunisia's low steppe landscape, marking the northern boundary of the desert.

Lake Nasser is a huge artificial lake, created by the damming of the Nile. It is now silting up because of evaporation, severely affecting the flow of water and sediment to the sea.

The Tell Atlas *(Atlas Tellien)* are a range of recent, folded mountains. They are still being formed, and the region's frequent earth tremors reflect this.

Western Sahara has huge reserves of commercially-valuable phosphates in its otherwise inhospitable desert landscape.

The Sahara is the largest hot desert on Earth, covering nearly a third of Africa. The sandy parts of the desert contain a wide variety of sand dunes, created by differing wind directions and strengths.

In its northernmost reaches, *the Nile River has deposited huge quantities of silt and alluvium to form the fan-shaped Nile Delta. The Nile splits into two main channels at the base of the delta which are interlinked by a dense network of canals and drainage channels.*

Almost all of Egypt's people *– more than 99% – live close to the Nile River, or on its massive delta. The river waters the only strip of fertile land in Egypt.*

Built as great tombs *for the pharaohs of ancient Egypt, the magnificent pyramids at Giza near Cairo have fascinated scholars, archaeologists, and tourists for centuries.*

Oil rigs are scattered *throughout the deserts of Libya and Algeria. Libyan oil is especially prized because of its low sulfur content, which means it produces much less pollution than other fuel oils.*

Transportation & Industry

The economies of Algeria and Libya were transformed by the discovery of oil and natural gas reserves in the deserts. Morocco's major exports are phosphates and agricultural produce, and as in Egypt and Tunisia, the tourist industry is essential to the economy. Egypt has the most varied industrial base, importing technology to develop electronics and engineering industries, and maintaining the reputation of its high-quality cotton textiles.

Major industry and infrastructure

- engineering
- food processing
- gas
- iron & steel
- iron ore
- oil
- phosphates
- textiles
- tourism
- capital cities
- major towns
- international airports
- major roads
- major industrial areas

Transportation Network

152,393 miles (245,400 km)	480 miles (773 km)
8025 miles (12,922 km)	121 miles (195 km)

Tourism and the oil industry have made improvements to the Maghreb's infrastructure both necessary and possible. The Suez Canal is a vital artery for shipping between Europe and Asia.

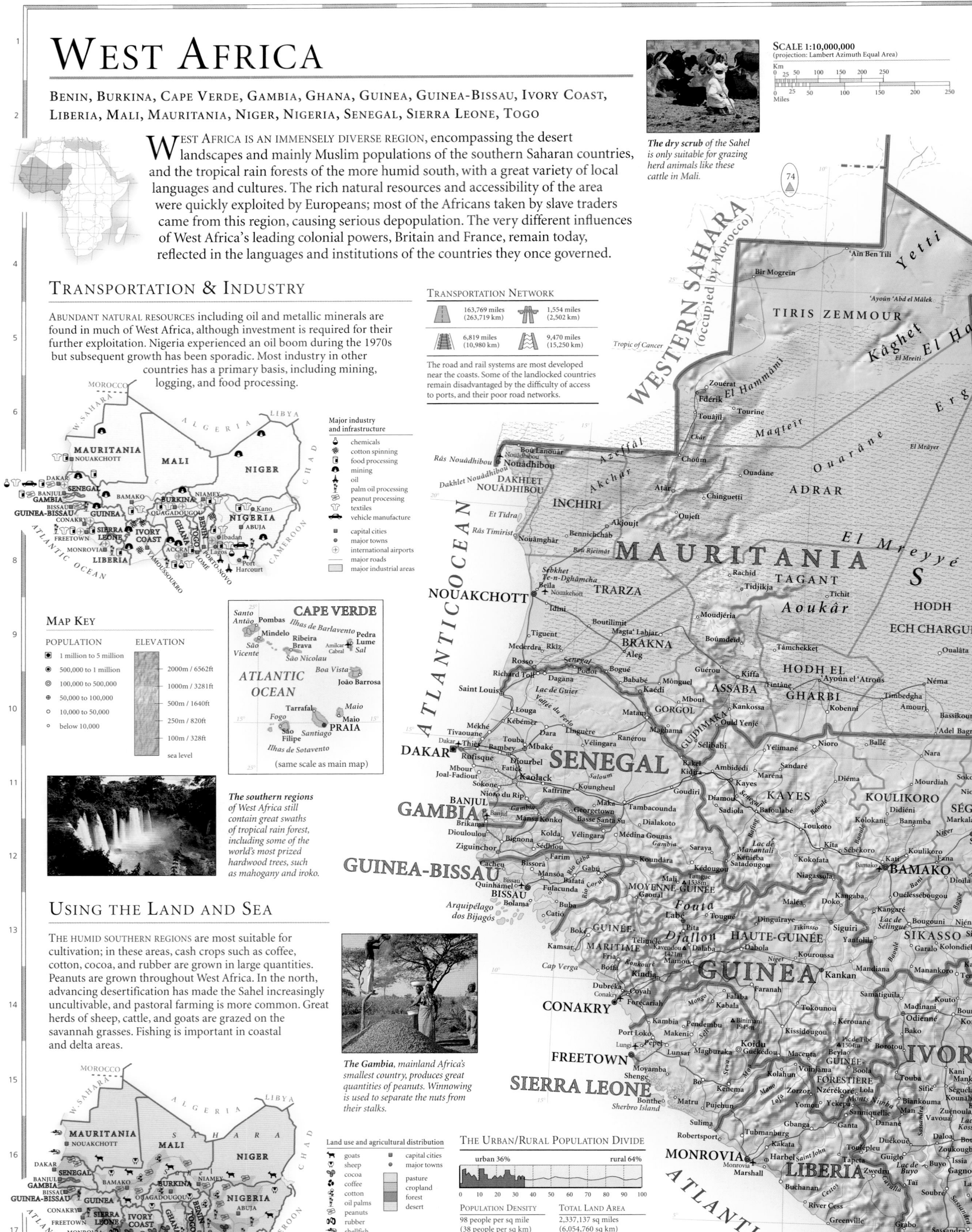
SCALE 1:10,000,000
(projection: Lambert Azimuth Equal Area)
WESTERN SAHARA (occupied by Morocco)
MAURITANIA
SENEGAL
GAMBIA
GUINEA-BISSAU
GUINEA
SIERRA LEONE
LIBERIA
ATLANTIC OCEAN
NOUAKCHOTT
DAKAR
BANJUL
BISSAU
CONAKRY
FREETOWN
MONROVIA
BAMAKO
Tropic of Cancer
TIRIS ZEMMOUR
ADRAR
INCHIRI
TRARZA
TAGANT
BRAKNA
ASSABA
GORGOL
HODH EL GHARBI
HODH ECH CHARGUI
KAYES
KOULIKORO
SIKASSO
MOYENNE-GUINÉE
HAUTE-GUINÉE
GUINÉE MARITIME
GUINÉE FORESTIÈRE
Fouta Djallon
Arquipélago dos Bijagós
Cap Verga
Sherbro Island
Cap des Palmés
CAPE VERDE
Santo Antão
São Vicente
São Nicolau
Boa Vista
Sal
Maio
Santiago
Fogo
PRAIA
Ilhas de Barlavento
Ilhas de Sotavento
(same scale as main map)

WEST AFRICA

BENIN, BURKINA, CAPE VERDE, GAMBIA, GHANA, GUINEA, GUINEA-BISSAU, IVORY COAST, LIBERIA, MALI, MAURITANIA, NIGER, NIGERIA, SENEGAL, SIERRA LEONE, TOGO

WEST AFRICA IS AN IMMENSELY DIVERSE REGION, encompassing the desert landscapes and mainly Muslim populations of the southern Saharan countries, and the tropical rain forests of the more humid south, with a great variety of local languages and cultures. The rich natural resources and accessibility of the area were quickly exploited by Europeans; most of the Africans taken by slave traders came from this region, causing serious depopulation. The very different influences of West Africa's leading colonial powers, Britain and France, remain today, reflected in the languages and institutions of the countries they once governed.

***The dry scrub** of the Sahel is only suitable for grazing herd animals like these cattle in Mali.*

TRANSPORTATION & INDUSTRY

ABUNDANT NATURAL RESOURCES including oil and metallic minerals are found in much of West Africa, although investment is required for their further exploitation. Nigeria experienced an oil boom during the 1970s but subsequent growth has been sporadic. Most industry in other countries has a primary basis, including mining, logging, and food processing.

TRANSPORTATION NETWORK

163,769 miles (263,719 km)	1,554 miles (2,502 km)
6,819 miles (10,980 km)	9,470 miles (15,250 km)

The road and rail systems are most developed near the coasts. Some of the landlocked countries remain disadvantaged by the difficulty of access to ports, and their poor road networks.

Major industry and infrastructure: chemicals; cotton spinning; food processing; mining; oil; palm oil processing; peanut processing; textiles; vehicle manufacture; capital cities; major towns; international airports; major roads; major industrial areas

MAP KEY

POPULATION
- 1 million to 5 million
- 500,000 to 1 million
- 100,000 to 500,000
- 50,000 to 100,000
- 10,000 to 50,000
- below 10,000

ELEVATION
- 2000m / 6562ft
- 1000m / 3281ft
- 500m / 1640ft
- 250m / 820ft
- 100m / 328ft
- sea level

***The southern regions** of West Africa still contain great swaths of tropical rain forest, including some of the world's most prized hardwood trees, such as mahogany and iroko.*

USING THE LAND AND SEA

THE HUMID SOUTHERN REGIONS are most suitable for cultivation; in these areas, cash crops such as coffee, cotton, cocoa, and rubber are grown in large quantities. Peanuts are grown throughout West Africa. In the north, advancing desertification has made the Sahel increasingly uncultivable, and pastoral farming is more common. Great herds of sheep, cattle, and goats are grazed on the savannah grasses. Fishing is important in coastal and delta areas.

***The Gambia**, mainland Africa's smallest country, produces great quantities of peanuts. Winnowing is used to separate the nuts from their stalks.*

Land use and agricultural distribution: goats; sheep; cocoa; coffee; cotton; oil palms; peanuts; rubber; shellfish; capital cities; major towns; pasture; cropland; forest; desert

THE URBAN/RURAL POPULATION DIVIDE

urban 36% — rural 64%

POPULATION DENSITY
98 people per sq mile (38 people per sq km)

TOTAL LAND AREA
2,337,137 sq miles (6,054,760 sq km)

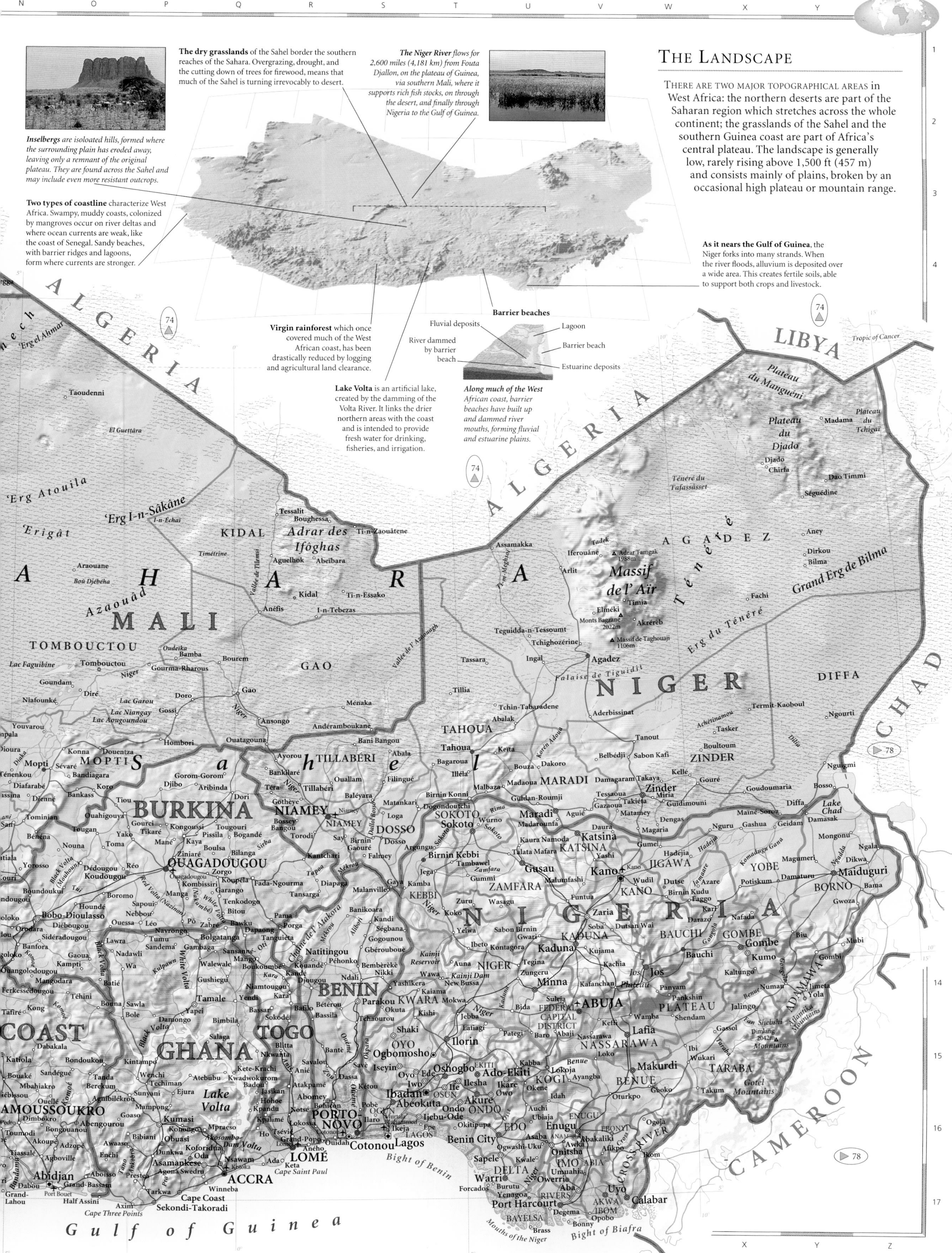

THE LANDSCAPE
THERE ARE TWO MAJOR TOPOGRAPHICAL AREAS in West Africa: the northern deserts are part of the Saharan region which stretches across the whole continent; the grasslands of the Sahel and the southern Guinea coast are part of Africa's central plateau. The landscape is generally low, rarely rising above 1,500 ft (457 m) and consists mainly of plains, broken by an occasional high plateau or mountain range.
Inselbergs are isoloated hills, formed where the surrounding plain has eroded away, leaving only a remnant of the original plateau. They are found across the Sahel and may include even more resistant outcrops.
The dry grasslands of the Sahel border the southern reaches of the Sahara. Overgrazing, drought, and the cutting down of trees for firewood, means that much of the Sahel is turning irrevocably to desert.
The Niger River flows for 2,600 miles (4,181 km) from Fouta Djallon, on the plateau of Guinea, via southern Mali, where it supports rich fish stocks, on through the desert, and finally through Nigeria to the Gulf of Guinea.
Two types of coastline characterize West Africa. Swampy, muddy coasts, colonized by mangroves occur on river deltas and where ocean currents are weak, like the coast of Senegal. Sandy beaches, with barrier ridges and lagoons, form where currents are stronger.
As it nears the Gulf of Guinea, the Niger forks into many strands. When the river floods, alluvium is deposited over a wide area. This creates fertile soils, able to support both crops and livestock.
Virgin rainforest which once covered much of the West African coast, has been drastically reduced by logging and agricultural land clearance.
Barrier beaches
Fluvial deposits
Lagoon
River dammed by barrier beach
Barrier beach
Estuarine deposits
Lake Volta is an artificial lake, created by the damming of the Volta River. It links the drier northern areas with the coast and is intended to provide fresh water for drinking, fisheries, and irrigation.
Along much of the West African coast, barrier beaches have built up and dammed river mouths, forming fluvial and estuarine plains.
N O P Q R S T U V W X Y
ALGERIA
LIBYA
MALI
NIGER
CHAD
BURKINA
GHANA
TOGO
BENIN
NIGERIA
CAMEROON
COAST
SAHARA
Sahel
Gulf of Guinea
Bight of Benin
Bight of Biafra
Tropic of Cancer
Massif de l'Aïr
Grand Erg de Bilma
Erg du Ténéré
Adrar des Ifôghas
NIAMEY
OUAGADOUGOU
ABUJA
ACCRA
LOMÉ
PORTO NOVO
Lagos
Abidjan
Kano
Lake Chad
Lake Volta
74
78
1 2 3 4 14 15 16 17
X Y Z

Central Africa

Cameroon, Central African Republic, Chad, Congo, Dem. Rep. Congo (Zaire), Equatorial Guinea, Gabon, Sao Tome & Principe

The great rain forest basin of the Congo River embraces most of remote Central Africa. The interior was largely unknown to Europeans until late in the 19th century, when its tribal kingdoms were split – principally between France and Belgium – with Sao Tome and Principe the lone Portuguese territory, and Equatorial Guinea controlled by Spain. Open democracy and regional economic integration are important goals for these nations – several of which have only recently emerged from restrictive regimes – and investment is needed to improve transportation infrastructures. Many of the small, but fast-growing and increasingly urban population, speak French, the regional *lingua franca*, along with several hundred Pygmy, Bantu, and Sudanic dialects.

The Landscape

Lake Chad lies in a desert basin bounded by the volcanic Tibesti Mountains in the north, plateaus in the east and, in the south, the broad watershed of the Congo Basin. The vast circular depression of the Congo is isolated from the coastal plain by the granite Massif du Chaillu. To the northwest, the volcanoes and fold mountains of the Cameroon Ridge *(Dorsale Camerounaise)* extend as islands into the Gulf of Guinea. The high fold mountains fringing the east of the Congo Basin fall steeply to the lakes of the Great Rift Valley.

A plug of resistant lava, at the southwestern end of the Cameroon Ridge (Dorsale Camerounaise), is all that remains of an eroded volcano.

The volcanic massif of Cameroon Mountain occupies an area which remains volcanically active.

Gulf of Guinea

Massif du Chaillu

Lake Chad is the remnant of an inland sea, which once occupied much of the surrounding basin. A series of droughts since the 1970s has reduced the area of this shallow freshwater lake to about 1,000 sq miles (2,599 sq km).

The lake-like expansion of the Congo River at Stanley Pool is the lowest point of the interior basin, although the river still descends more than 1,000 ft (300 m) to reach the sea.

Rich mineral deposits in the "Copper Belt" of Dem. Rep. Congo (Zaire) were formed under intense heat and pressure when the ancient African Shield was uplifted to form the region's mountains.

The Tibesti Mountains are the highest in the Sahara. They were pushed up by the movement of the African Plate over a hot spot, which first formed the northern Ahaggar Mountains and is now thought to lie under the Great Rift Valley.

The Congo River is second only to the Amazon in the volume of water it carries, and in the size of its drainage basin.

Lake Tanganyika, the world's second deepest lake, is the largest of a series of linear "ribbon" lakes occupying a trench within the Great Rift Valley.

Broad, shallow basin

Waterfalls and cataracts

Submarine canyon

The Congo River flows sluggishly through the rain forest of the interior basin. Toward the coast, the river drops steeply in a series of waterfalls and cataracts. At this point, the erosional power of the river becomes so great that it has formed a deep submarine canyon offshore.

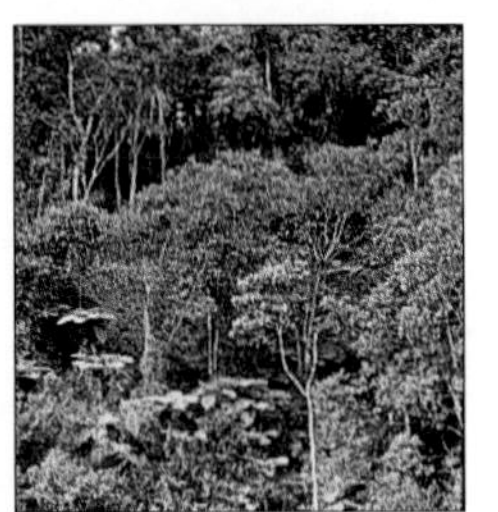

***Virgin tropical rain forest** covers the Ruwenzori range on the borders of Dem. Rep. Congo and Uganda.*

The vast sandflats surrounding Lake Chad were once covered by water. Changing climatic patterns caused the lake to shrink, and desert now covers much of its previous area.

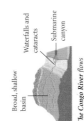

Transportation & Industry

Large reserves of valuable minerals are found in Central Africa: copper, cobalt, zinc, and tin are mined in Dem. Rep. Congo (Zaire) and Cameroon; diamonds in the Central African Republic, and manganese in Gabon. Congo, Cameroon, Gabon, and Dem. Rep. Congo (Zaire) have oil deposits and oil has also been recently discovered in Chad. Goods such as palm oil and rubber are processed for export.

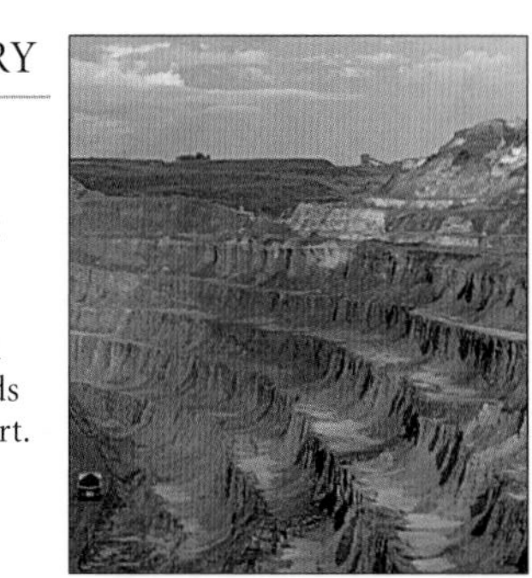

***The ancient rocks** of Dem. Rep. Congo (Zaire) hold immense and varied mineral reserves. This open pit copper mine is at Kolwezi in the far south.*

Major industry and infrastructure

- brewing
- chemicals
- cobalt
- copper
- diamonds
- food processing
- manganese
- oil
- palm oil processing
- textiles
- tin
- capital cities
- major towns
- international airports
- major roads
- major industrial areas

Transportation Network

124,349 miles (200,240 km)	342 miles (550 km)
3,830 miles (6,167 km)	15,261 miles (24,575 km)

The Trans-Gabon railroad, which began operating in 1987, has opened up new sources of timber and manganese. Elsewhere, much investment is needed to update and improve road, rail, and water transportation.

74

76

Map Key

Population

- 1 million to 5 million
- 500,000 to 1 million
- 100,000 to 500,000
- 50,000 to 100,000
- 10,000 to 50,000
- below 10,000

Elevation

- 4000m / 13,124ft
- 3000m / 9843ft
- 2000m / 6562ft
- 1000m / 3281ft
- 500m / 1640ft
- 250m / 820ft
- 100m / 328ft
- sea level

Scale 1:10,500,000
(projection: Lambert Azimuthal Equal Area)

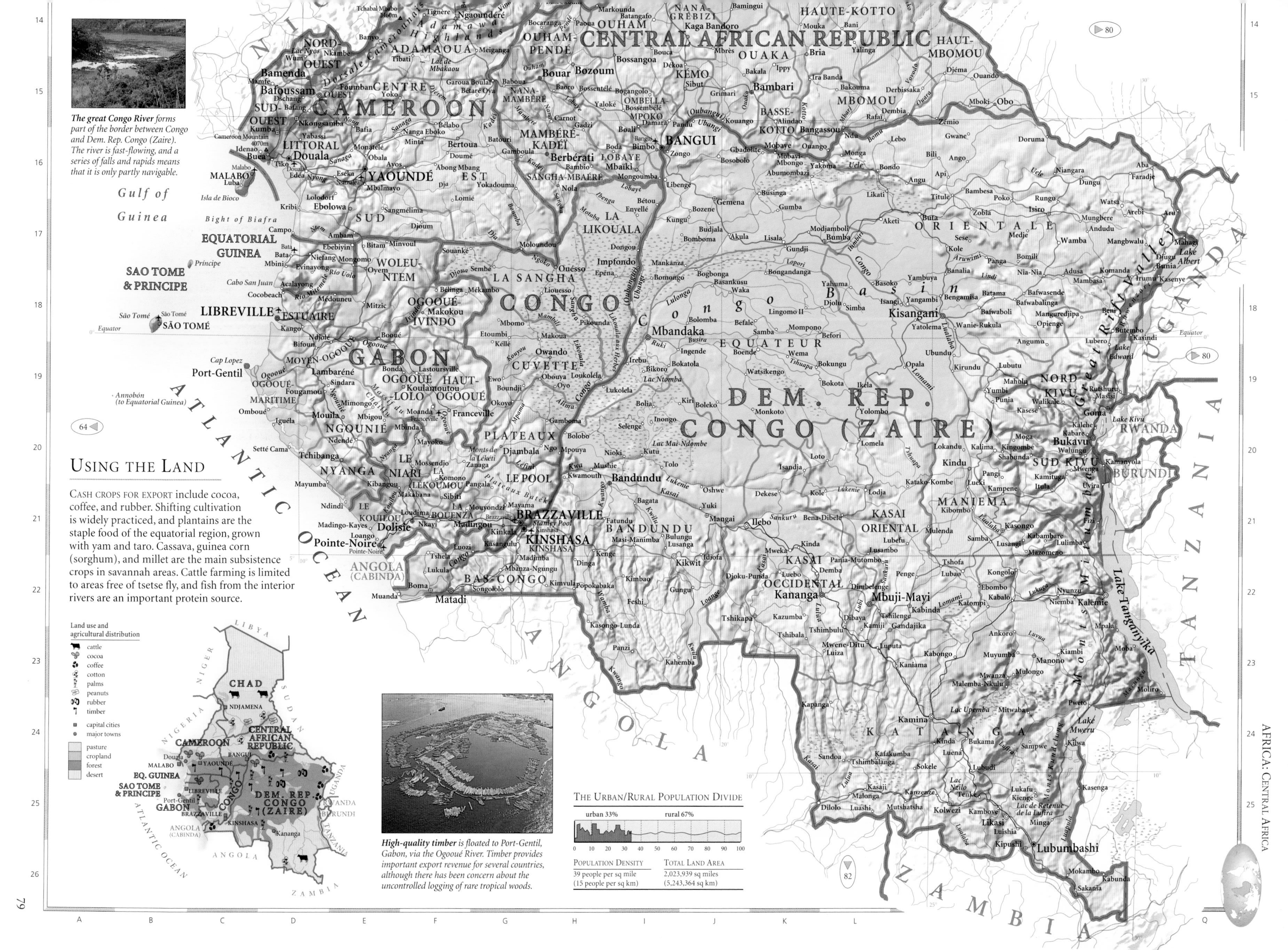
CENTRAL AFRICAN REPUBLIC
CAMEROON
EQUATORIAL GUINEA
SAO TOME & PRINCIPE
GABON
CONGO
DEM. REP. CONGO (ZAIRE)
ANGOLA
ANGOLA (CABINDA)
ZAMBIA
TANZANIA
UGANDA
RWANDA
BURUNDI
ATLANTIC OCEAN
Gulf of Guinea
Bight of Biafra
Congo Basin
Lake Tanganyika
Lake Albert
Lake Edward
Lake Kivu
Lake Mweru
Great Rift Valley
Mitumba Mountains
BANGUI
YAOUNDÉ
MALABO
LIBREVILLE
SÃO TOMÉ
BRAZZAVILLE
KINSHASA
Douala
Port-Gentil
Pointe-Noire
Matadi
Mbandaka
Kisangani
Kananga
Mbuji-Mayi
Lubumbashi
Likasi
Kolwezi
Bukavu
Goma
Bandundu
Berbérati
Bambari
Franceville
Equator
Land use and agricultural distribution
cattle
cocoa
coffee
cotton
palms
peanuts
rubber
timber
capital cities
major towns
pasture
cropland
forest
desert
THE URBAN/RURAL POPULATION DIVIDE
urban 33%
rural 67%
0 10 20 30 40 50 60 70 80 90 100
POPULATION DENSITY
39 people per sq mile
(15 people per sq km)
TOTAL LAND AREA
2,023,939 sq miles
(5,243,364 sq km)

The great Congo River *forms part of the border between Congo and Dem. Rep. Congo (Zaire). The river is fast-flowing, and a series of falls and rapids means that it is only partly navigable.*

Using the Land

CASH CROPS FOR EXPORT include cocoa, coffee, and rubber. Shifting cultivation is widely practiced, and plantains are the staple food of the equatorial region, grown with yam and taro. Cassava, guinea corn (sorghum), and millet are the main subsistence crops in savannah areas. Cattle farming is limited to areas free of tsetse fly, and fish from the interior rivers are an important protein source.

***High-quality timber** is floated to Port-Gentil, Gabon, via the Ogooué River. Timber provides important export revenue for several countries, although there has been concern about the uncontrolled logging of rare tropical woods.*

East Africa

Burundi, Djibouti, Eritrea, Ethiopia, Kenya, Rwanda, Somalia, Sudan, Tanzania, Uganda

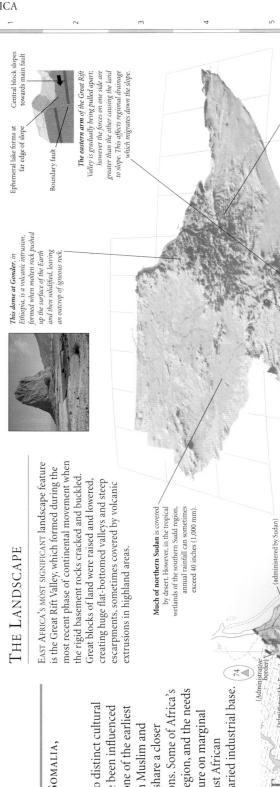

The countries of East Africa divide into two distinct cultural regions. Sudan and the "Horn" nations have been influenced by the Middle East; Ethiopia was the home of one of the earliest Christian civilizations, and Sudan reflects both Muslim and Christian influences. The southern countries share a closer cultural affinity with other sub-Saharan nations. Some of Africa's most densely populated countries lie in this region, and the needs of a growing number of people have put pressure on marginal lands and fragile environments. Although most East African economies remain strongly agricultural, Kenya has developed a varied industrial base.

The Landscape

East Africa's most significant landscape feature is the Great Rift Valley, which formed during the most recent phase of continental movement when the rigid basement rocks cracked and buckled. Great blocks of land were raised and lowered, creating huge flat-bottomed valleys and steep escarpments, sometimes covered by volcanic extrusions in highland areas.

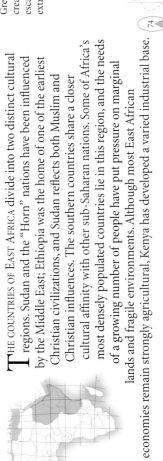

This dome at Gonder, in Ethiopia, is a volcanic intrusion, formed when molten rock pushed up the surface of the Earth and then solidified, leaving an outcrop of igneous rock.

Ephemeral lake forms at far edge of slope
Central block slopes towards main fault
Boundary fault

***The eastern arm** of the Great Rift Valley is gradually being pulled apart; however the forces on one side are greater than the other causing the land to slope. This affects regional drainage which migrates down the slope.*

Much of northern Sudan is covered by desert. However, in the tropical wetlands of the southern Sudd region, annual rainfall can sometimes exceed 40 inches (1,000 mm).

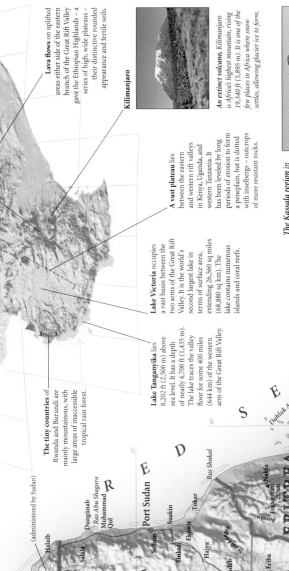

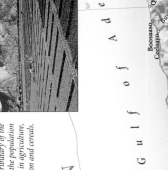

The tiny countries of Rwanda and Burundi are mainly mountainous, with large areas of inaccessible tropical rain forest.

Lava flows on uplifted areas either side of the eastern branch of the Great Rift Valley gave the Ethiopian Highlands – a series of high, wide plateaus – their distinctive rounded appearance and fertile soils.

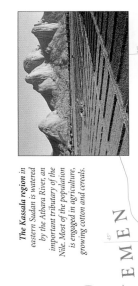

Kilimanjaro

Lake Tanganyika lies 8,202 ft (2,500 m) above sea level. It has a depth of nearly 4,700 ft (1,435 m). The lake traces the valley floor for some 400 miles (644 km) of the western arm of the Great Rift Valley.

Lake Victoria occupies a vast basin between the two arms of the Great Rift Valley. It is the world's second largest lake in terms of surface area, extending 26,560 sq miles (68,880 sq km). The lake contains numerous islands and coral reefs.

A vast plateau lies between the eastern and western rift valleys in Kenya, Uganda, and western Tanzania. It has been leveled by long periods of erosion to form a peneplain, but is dotted with inselbergs – outcrops of more resistant rocks.

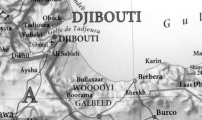

***An extinct volcano,** Kilimanjaro is Africa's highest mountain, rising 19,340 ft (5,895 m). It is one of the few places in Africa where snow settles, allowing glacier ice to form.*

***The Kassala region** in eastern Sudan is watered by the Atbara River, an important tributary of the Nile. Most of the population is engaged in agriculture, growing cotton and cereals.*

74
78
140

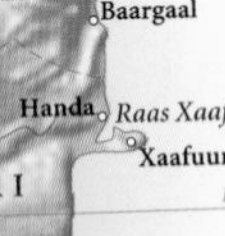

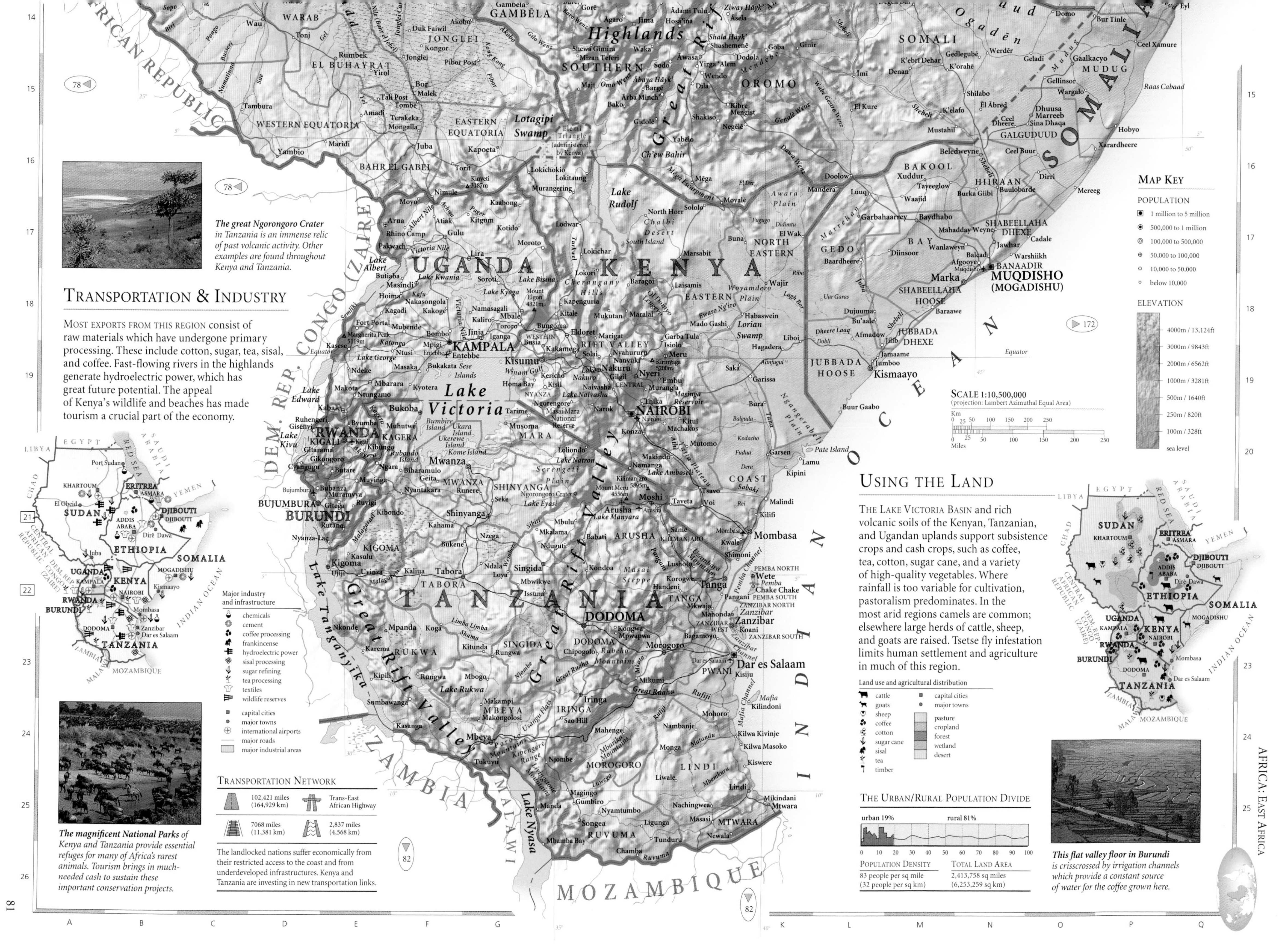
MAP KEY
POPULATION
1 million to 5 million
500,000 to 1 million
100,000 to 500,000
50,000 to 100,000
10,000 to 50,000
below 10,000
ELEVATION
4000m / 13,124ft
3000m / 9843ft
2000m / 6562ft
1000m / 3281ft
500m / 1640ft
250m / 820ft
100m / 328ft
sea level
SCALE 1:10,500,000
(projection: Lambert Azimuthal Equal Area)
UGANDA
KENYA
TANZANIA
SOMALIA
INDIAN OCEAN
Lake Victoria
NAIROBI
KAMPALA
DODOMA
MUQDISHO (MOGADISHU)
Dar es Salaam
Mombasa
Zanzibar
RWANDA
BURUNDI
DEM. REP. CONGO (ZAIRE)
ZAMBIA
MALAWI
MOZAMBIQUE
Lake Tanganyika
Lake Nyasa
Lake Rudolf
Great Rift Valley

The great Ngorongoro Crater in Tanzania is an immense relic of past volcanic activity. Other examples are found throughout Kenya and Tanzania.

TRANSPORTATION & INDUSTRY

MOST EXPORTS FROM THIS REGION consist of raw materials which have undergone primary processing. These include cotton, sugar, tea, sisal, and coffee. Fast-flowing rivers in the highlands generate hydroelectric power, which has great future potential. The appeal of Kenya's wildlife and beaches has made tourism a crucial part of the economy.

Major industry and infrastructure
chemicals
cement
coffee processing
frankincense
hydroelectric power
sisal processing
sugar refining
tea processing
textiles
wildlife reserves
capital cities
major towns
international airports
major roads
major industrial areas

TRANSPORTATION NETWORK

102,421 miles (164,929 km)		Trans-East African Highway	
7068 miles (11,381 km)		2,837 miles (4,568 km)	

The landlocked nations suffer economically from their restricted access to the coast and from underdeveloped infrastructures. Kenya and Tanzania are investing in new transportation links.

The magnificent National Parks of Kenya and Tanzania provide essential refuges for many of Africa's rarest animals. Tourism brings in much-needed cash to sustain these important conservation projects.

USING THE LAND

THE LAKE VICTORIA BASIN and rich volcanic soils of the Kenyan, Tanzanian, and Ugandan uplands support subsistence crops and cash crops, such as coffee, tea, cotton, sugar cane, and a variety of high-quality vegetables. Where rainfall is too variable for cultivation, pastoralism predominates. In the most arid regions camels are common; elsewhere large herds of cattle, sheep, and goats are raised. Tsetse fly infestation limits human settlement and agriculture in much of this region.

Land use and agricultural distribution
cattle
goats
sheep
coffee
cotton
sugar cane
sisal
tea
timber
capital cities
major towns
pasture
cropland
forest
wetland
desert

THE URBAN/RURAL POPULATION DIVIDE

urban 19% — rural 81%

POPULATION DENSITY	TOTAL LAND AREA
83 people per sq mile (32 people per sq km)	2,413,758 sq miles (6,253,259 sq km)

This flat valley floor in Burundi is crisscrossed by irrigation channels which provide a constant source of water for the coffee grown here.

SOUTHERN AFRICA

ANGOLA, BOTSWANA, LESOTHO, MALAWI, MOZAMBIQUE, NAMIBIA, SOUTH AFRICA, SWAZILAND, ZAMBIA, ZIMBABWE

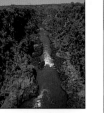

AFRICA'S VAST SOUTHERN PLATEAU has been a contested homeland for disparate peoples for many centuries. The European incursion began with the slave trade and quickened in the 19th century, when the discovery of enormous mineral wealth secured South Africa's regional economic dominance. The struggle against white minority rule led to strife in Namibia, Zimbabwe, and the former Portuguese territories of Angola and Mozambique. South Africa's notorious apartheid laws, which denied basic human rights to more than 75% of the people, led to the state being internationally ostracized until 1994, when the first fully democratic elections inaugurated a new era of racial justice.

TRANSPORTATION & INDUSTRY

SOUTH AFRICA, the world's largest exporter of gold, has a varied economy which generates about 75% of the region's income and draws migrant labor from neighboring states. Angola exports petroleum; Botswana and Namibia rely on diamond mining; and Zambia is seeking to diversify its economy to compensate for declining copper reserves.

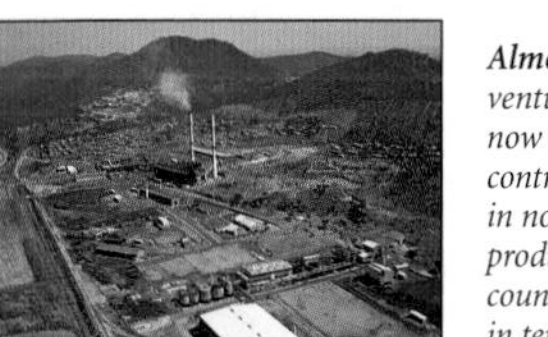

Almost all new mining ventures in Zimbabwe are now subject to government control. This mine at Bindura in northeastern Zimbabwe produces nickel, one of the country's top three minerals in terms of economic value.

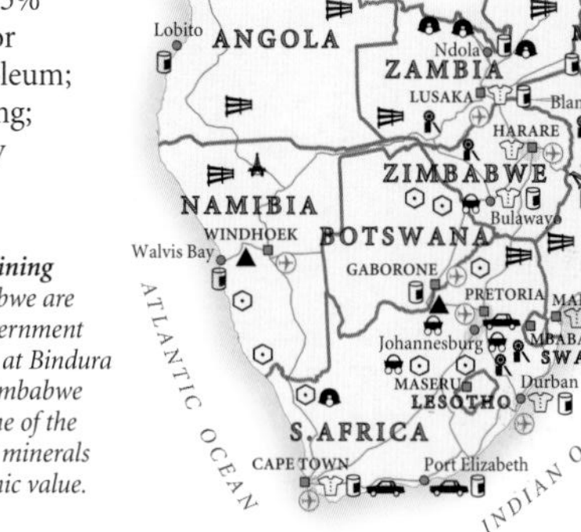
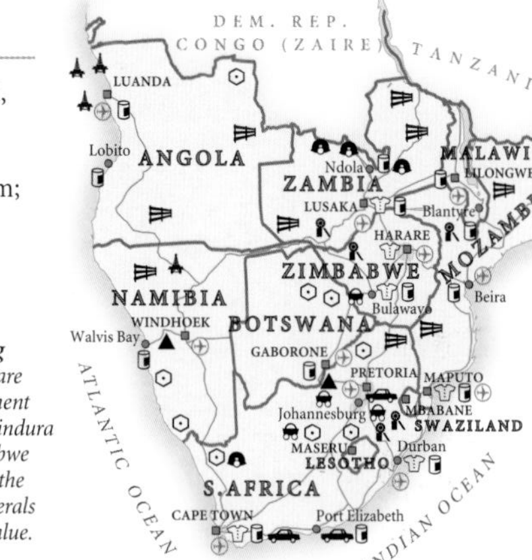

DEM. REP. CONGO (ZAIRE)
TANZANIA
LUANDA
Lobito
ANGOLA
ZAMBIA
Ndola
LUSAKA
MALAWI
LILONGWE
Blantyre
HARARE
MOZAMBIQUE
ZIMBABWE
Bulawayo
Beira
NAMIBIA
WINDHOEK
Walvis Bay
BOTSWANA
GABORONE
PRETORIA
MAPUTO
Johannesburg
MBABANE
SWAZILAND
MASERU
LESOTHO
Durban
S. AFRICA
CAPE TOWN
Port Elizabeth
ATLANTIC OCEAN
INDIAN OCEAN
Major industry and infrastructure
car manufacture
coal
copper
diamonds
food processing
gold
oil
textiles
uranium
wildlife reserves
capital cities
major towns
international airports
major roads
major industrial areas

THE LANDSCAPE

MOST OF SOUTHERN AFRICA rests on a concave plateau comprising the Kalahari basin and a mountainous fringe, skirted by a coastal plain which widens out in Mozambique. The plateau extends north, toward the Planalto de Bié in Angola, the Congo Basin and the lake-filled troughs of the Great Rift Valley. The eastern region is drained by the Zambezi and Limpopo Rivers, and the Orange is the major western river.

Thousands of years of evaporating water have produced the Etosha Pan, one of the largest salt flats in the world. Lake and river sediments in the area indicate that the region was once less arid.

Finger Rock, near Khorixas, Namibia is a remnant of a former land surface, which has been denuded by erosion over the last 5 million years. These occasional stacks of partially weathered rocks interrupt the plains of the dry southern interior.

TRANSPORTATION NETWORK

84,213 miles (135,609 km)		746 miles (1,202 km)	
23,208 miles (37,372 km)		3,815 miles (6,144 km)	

Southern Africa's Cape-gauge rail network is by far the largest in the continent. About two-thirds of the 20,000 mile (32,000 km) system lies within South Africa. Lines such as the Harare–Bulawayo route have become corridors for industrial growth.

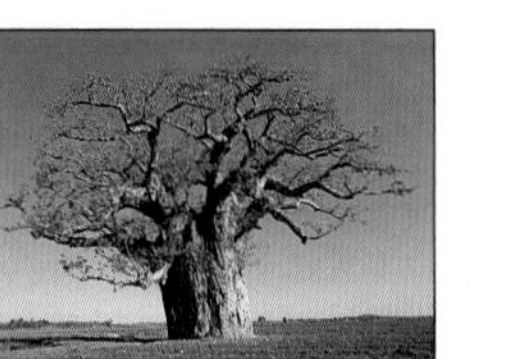

Following a series of droughts, this baobab tree in Zimbabwe now stands alone in a field once filled by sugar cane. The thick trunk and small leaves of the baobab help it to conserve water, enabling it to survive even in drought conditions.

At Victoria Falls, the Zambezi River has cut a spectacular gorge taking advantage of large joints in the basalt, which were first formed as the lava cooled and contracted.

The Okavango/Cubango River flows from the Planalto de Bié to the swamplands of the Okavango Delta, one of the world's largest inland deltas, where it divides into countless distributary channels, feeding out into the desert.

The fast-flowing Zambezi River cuts a deep, wide channel as it flows along the Zimbabwe/Zambia border.

Planalto de Bié

Khorixas, Namibia

Namib Desert

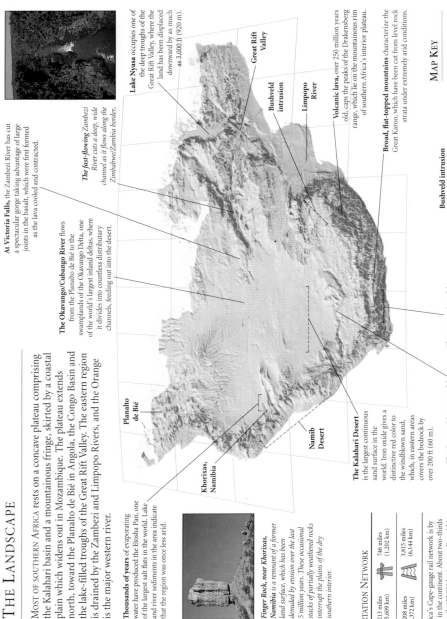

Lake Nyasa occupies one of the deep troughs of the Great Rift Valley, where the land has been displaced downward by as much as 3,000 ft (920 m).

Great Rift Valley

Bushveld intrusion

Limpopo River

Volcanic lava, over 250 million years old, caps the peaks of the Drakensberg range, which lie on the mountainous rim of southern Africa's interior plateau.

Broad, flat-topped mountains characterize the Great Karoo, which have been cut from level rock strata under extremely arid conditions.

The Kalahari Desert is the largest continuous sand surface in the world. Iron oxide gives a distinctive red color to the windblown sand, which, in eastern areas covers the bedrock by over 200 ft (60 m).

The Orange River, one of the longest in Africa, rises in Lesotho and is the only major river in the south which flows westward, rather than to the east coast.

The mountains of the Little Karoo are composed of sedimentary rocks which have been substantially folded and faulted.

Bushveld intrusion

Gabbro and peridotite · Granite · Magnetite · Chromite · Platinum minerals

The Bushveld intrusion lies on South Africa's high "veld." Molten magma intruded into the Earth's crust creating a saucer-shaped feature, more than 180 miles (300 km) across, containing regular layers of precious minerals, overlain by a dome of granite.

SCALE 1:10,500,000

(projection: Lambert Azimuthal Equal Area)

Km 0 25 50 100 150 200 250 300
Miles 0 25 50 100 150 200 250 300

SOUTH AFRICA'S THREE CAPITALS

PRETORIA – administrative capital
CAPE TOWN – legislative capital
BLOEMFONTEIN – judicial capital

MAP KEY

POPULATION
- 1 million to 5 million
- 500,000 to 1 million
- 100,000 to 500,000
- 50,000 to 100,000
- 10,000 to 50,000
- below 10,000

ELEVATION
- 3000m / 9843ft
- 2000m / 6562ft
- 1000m / 3281ft
- 500m / 1640ft
- 250m / 820ft
- 100m / 328ft
- sea level

78 · 80

CONGO · DEM. REP. CONGO (ZAIRE) · ANGOLA · TANZANIA · CABINDA (To Angola) · LUANDA · Lake Tanganyika · Lake Mweru · Lake Nyasa · Great Rift

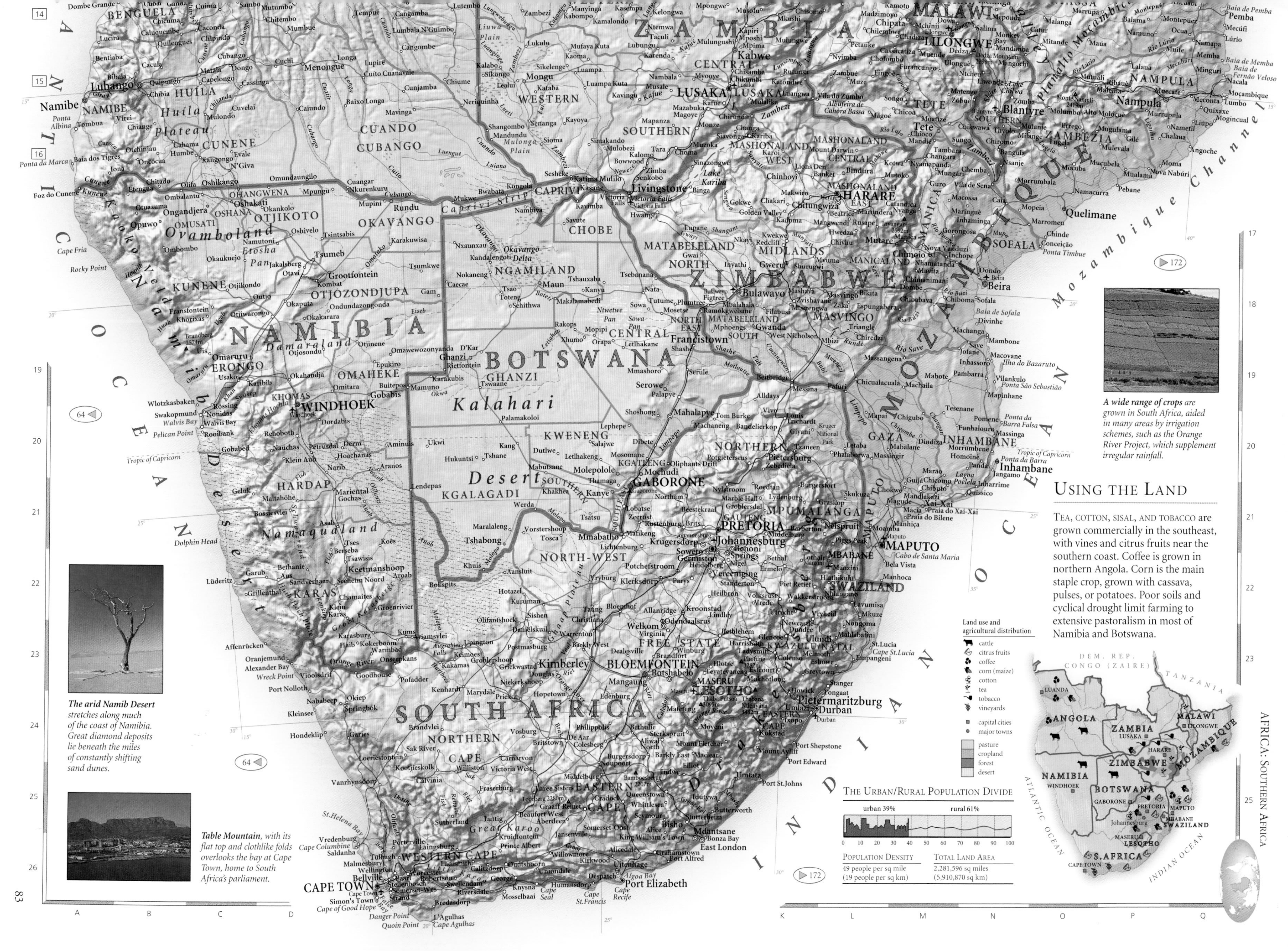

ZAMBIA
MALAWI
MOZAMBIQUE
ZIMBABWE
BOTSWANA
NAMIBIA
SOUTH AFRICA
SWAZILAND
LESOTHO
LUSAKA
LILONGWE
HARARE
WINDHOEK
GABORONE
PRETORIA
MAPUTO
MBABANE
MASERU
BLOEMFONTEIN
CAPE TOWN
Johannesburg
Durban
Port Elizabeth
East London
Kalahari
Desert
Mozambique Channel
INDIAN OCEAN
ATLANTIC OCEAN
Tropic of Capricorn
Land use and agricultural distribution
cattle
citrus fruits
coffee
corn (maize)
cotton
tea
tobacco
vineyards
capital cities
major towns
pasture
cropland
forest
desert
The Urban/Rural Population Divide
urban 39%
rural 61%
0 10 20 30 40 50 60 70 80 90 100
Population Density
49 people per sq mile
(19 people per sq km)
Total Land Area
2,281,596 sq miles
(5,910,870 sq km)
DEM. REP. CONGO (ZAIRE)
TANZANIA
ANGOLA
LUANDA

A wide range of crops are grown in South Africa, aided in many areas by irrigation schemes, such as the Orange River Project, which supplement irregular rainfall.

Using the Land

Tea, cotton, sisal, and tobacco are grown commercially in the southeast, with vines and citrus fruits near the southern coast. Coffee is grown in northern Angola. Corn is the main staple crop, grown with cassava, pulses, or potatoes. Poor soils and cyclical drought limit farming to extensive pastoralism in most of Namibia and Botswana.

The arid Namib Desert stretches along much of the coast of Namibia. Great diamond deposits lie beneath the miles of constantly shifting sand dunes.

Table Mountain, with its flat top and clothlike folds overlooks the bay at Cape Town, home to South Africa's parliament.

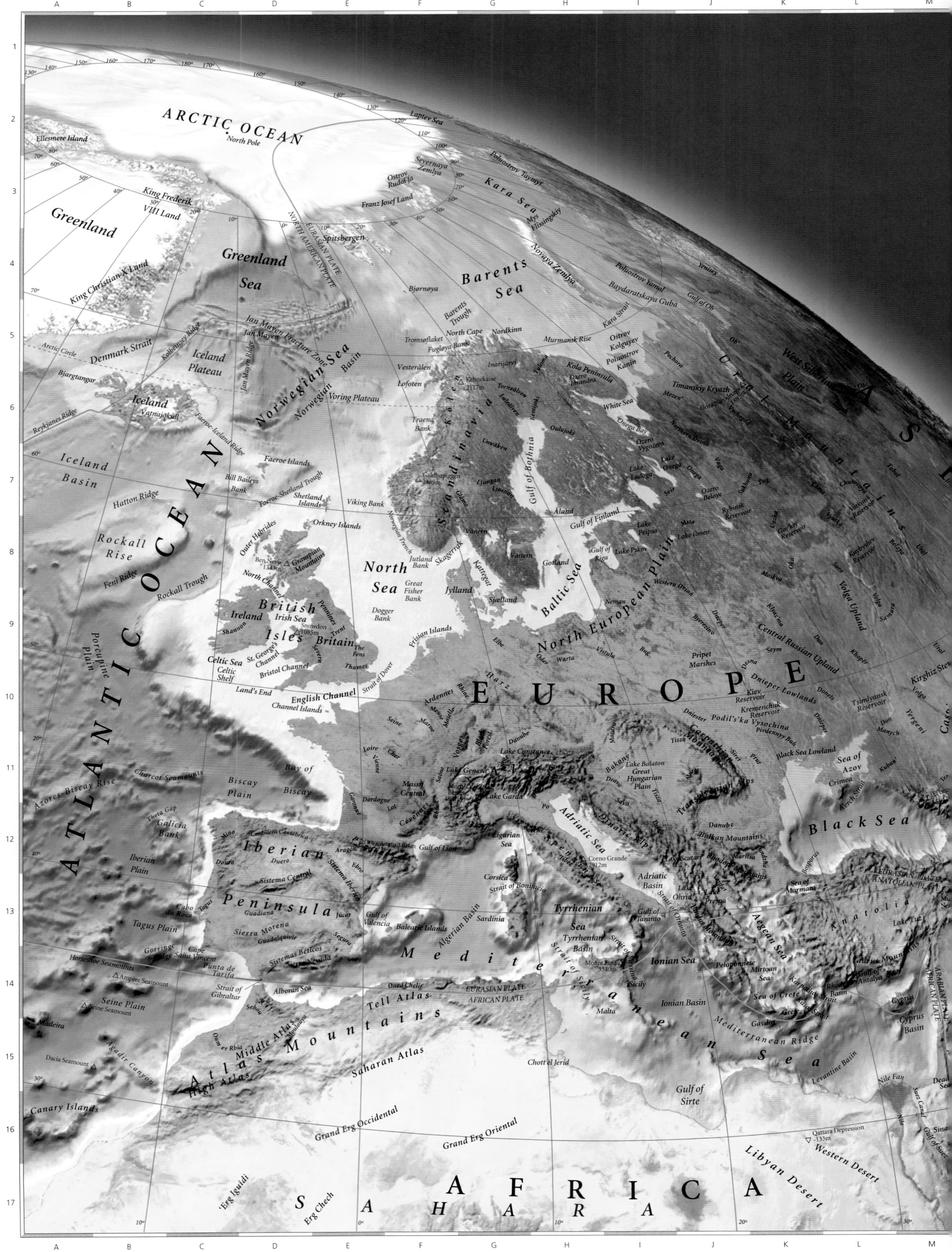
ARCTIC OCEAN
North Pole
Ellesmere Island
Greenland
King Frederik VIII Land
King Christian X Land
Greenland Sea
NORTH AMERICAN PLATE
EURASIAN PLATE
Laptev Sea
Severnaya Zemlya
Poluostrov Taymyr
Kara Sea
Ostrov Rudol'fa
Franz Josef Land
Mys Flissingskiy
Spitsbergen
Novaya Zemlya
Barents Sea
Bjørnøya
Barents Trough
Poluostrov Yamal
Baydaratskaya Guba
Gulf of Ob
Yenisey
Kara Strait
Jan Mayen Fracture Zone
Jan Mayen
Jan Mayen Ridge
Kolbeinsey Ridge
Denmark Strait
Arctic Circle
Iceland Plateau
Norwegian Sea
Norwegian Basin
Voring Plateau
North Cape
Nordkinn
Tromsøflaket
Fugløya Bank
Murmansk Rise
Ostrov Kolguyev
Poluostrov Kanin
Pechora
Ob'
West Siberian Plain
Ural Mountains
ASIA
Vesterålen
Lofoten
Kebnekaise 2117m
Inarijärvi
Kola Peninsula
Ozero Imandra
Tuloma
Timanskiy Kryazh
Mezen'
Gora Narodnaya 1895m
Vychegda
Bjargtangar
Iceland
Vatnajökull
Reykjanes Ridge
Faeroe-Iceland Ridge
Traena Bank
Kølen
Scandinavia
Torneälven
Luleälven
Kemijoki
White Sea
Onega Bay
Oulujoki
Northern Dvina
Umeälven
Gulf of Bothnia
Ozero Vygozero
Lake Onega
Lake Ladoga
Onega
Vaga
Iceland Basin
Faeroe Islands
Bill Baileys Bank
Faeroe-Shetland Trough
Shetland Islands
Galdhøpiggen 2469m
Ljungan
Ljusnan
Glåma
Åland
Svir
Ozero Beloye
Sukhona
Yug
Kama
Chusovaya
Votkinsk Reservoir
Vyatka
Hatton Ridge
Viking Bank
Norwegian Trench
Orkney Islands
Gulf of Finland
Rybinsk Reservoir
Msta
Lake Il'men
Unzha
Gor'kiy Reservoir
Kuybyshev Reservoir
Belaya
Ural
Rockall Rise
Outer Hebrides
Ben Nevis 1343m
Grampian Mountains
Vänern
Vättern
Lake Peipus
Gulf of Riga
Lake Pskov
North European Plain
Feni Ridge
Rockall Trough
North Channel
North Sea
Jutland Bank
Skagerrak
Kattegat
Gotland
Great Fisher Bank
Jylland
Moskva
Oka
Sura
Volga Upland
Volga
Samara
Sjælland
Baltic Sea
Western Dvina
Neman
British Isles
Ireland
Irish Sea
Pennines
Britain
Snowdon 1085m
Trent
Shannon
Dogger Bank
Frisian Islands
Porcupine Plain
Celtic Sea
Celtic Shelf
St. George's Channel
Severn
Bristol Channel
The Fens
Thames
Elbe
Oder
Warta
Vistula
Bug
Pripet Marshes
Berezina
Dnieper
Desna
Central Russian Upland
Don
Seym
Khoper
Harz
EUROPE
Dnieper Lowlands
Kiev Reservoir
Kremenchuk Reservoir
Donets
Tsimlyansk Reservoir
Kirghiz Steppe
Land's End
English Channel
Channel Islands
Strait of Dover
Ardennes
Rhine
Meuse
Moselle
Seine
Marne
Black Forest
Danube
Dniester
Podil's'ka Vysochina
Pivdennyy Buh
Carpathian Mountains
Tisza
Siret
Prut
Manych
Volga
Caspian
Loire
Vienne
Cher
Vosges
Lake Constance
Bakony
Lake Balaton
Great Hungarian Plain
Black Sea Lowland
Sea of Azov
Kuban'
Crimea
Kerch Strait
Charcot Seamounts
Azores-Biscay Rise
Biscay Plain
Bay of Biscay
Massif Central
Saône
Lake Geneva
Alps
Mont Blanc 4807m
Drava
Sava
Transylvanian Alps
ATLANTIC OCEAN
Theta Gap
Galicia Bank
Garonne
Dordogne
Lot
Cévennes
Rhône
Lake Garda
Po
Adriatic Sea
Dinaric Alps
Drina
Danube
Balkan Mountains
Black Sea
Miño
Cordillera Cantábrica
Iberian Peninsula
Aragon
Pyrenees
Aneto 3404m
Gulf of Lion
Ligurian Sea
Apennines
Tiber
Corno Grande 2912m
Lake Scutari
Maritsa
Rhodope Mountains
Bosporus
Sea of Marmara
EURASIAN PLATE
ANATOLIAN PLATE
Iberian Plain
Douro
Duero
Ebro
Sistema Ibérico
Sistema Central
Corsica
Strait of Bonifacio
Adriatic Basin
Lake Ohrid
Lake Prespa
Cabo da Roca
Tagus
Guadiana
Júcar
Gulf of Valencia
Balearic Islands
Algerian Basin
Sardinia
Tyrrhenian Sea
Tyrrhenian Basin
Gulf of Taranto
Strait of Otranto
Pindus Mountains
Aegean Sea
Anatolia
Lake Tuz
Tagus Plain
Sierra Morena
Guadalquivir
Segura
Gorringe Ridge
Cape Saint Vincent
Sistemas Béticos
Sierra Nevada
Mediterranean Sea
Strait of Messina
Strait of Sicily
Monte Etna 3340m
Ionian Sea
Peloponnese
Myrtoan Sea
Taurus Mountains
Gulf of Antalya
Horseshoe Seamounts
Ampère Seamount
Punta de Tarifa
Strait of Gibraltar
Alboran Sea
Oued Chelif
EURASIAN PLATE
AFRICAN PLATE
Tell Atlas
Sicily
Malta
Ionian Basin
Sea of Crete
Karpathos Strait
Rhodes Basin
Rhodes
Crete
Cyprus
Cyprus Basin
ARABIAN PLATE
AFRICAN PLATE
Seine Plain
Seine Seamount
Madeira
Sebou
Rif
Moulouya
Oum er Rbia
Middle Atlas
Atlas Mountains
Gavdos
Mediterranean Ridge
Agadir Canyon
Dacia Seamount
High Atlas
Saharan Atlas
Chott el Jerid
Levantine Basin
Nile Fan
Dead Sea
Canary Islands
Gulf of Sirte
Suez Canal
Nile
Gulf of Suez
Sinai
Grand Erg Occidental
Grand Erg Oriental
Qattara Depression -133m
Western Desert
Libyan Desert
'Erg Iguidi
Erg Chech
AFRICA
SAHARA

EUROPE

EUROPE IS THE WORLD'S SECOND SMALLEST CONTINENT, COVERING 4,053,309 SQ MILES (10,498,000 SQ KM). IT COMPRISES 44 SEPARATE COUNTRIES, INCLUDING TURKEY AND THE RUSSIAN FEDERATION, ALTHOUGH THE GREATER PARTS OF THESE NATIONS LIE IN ASIA.

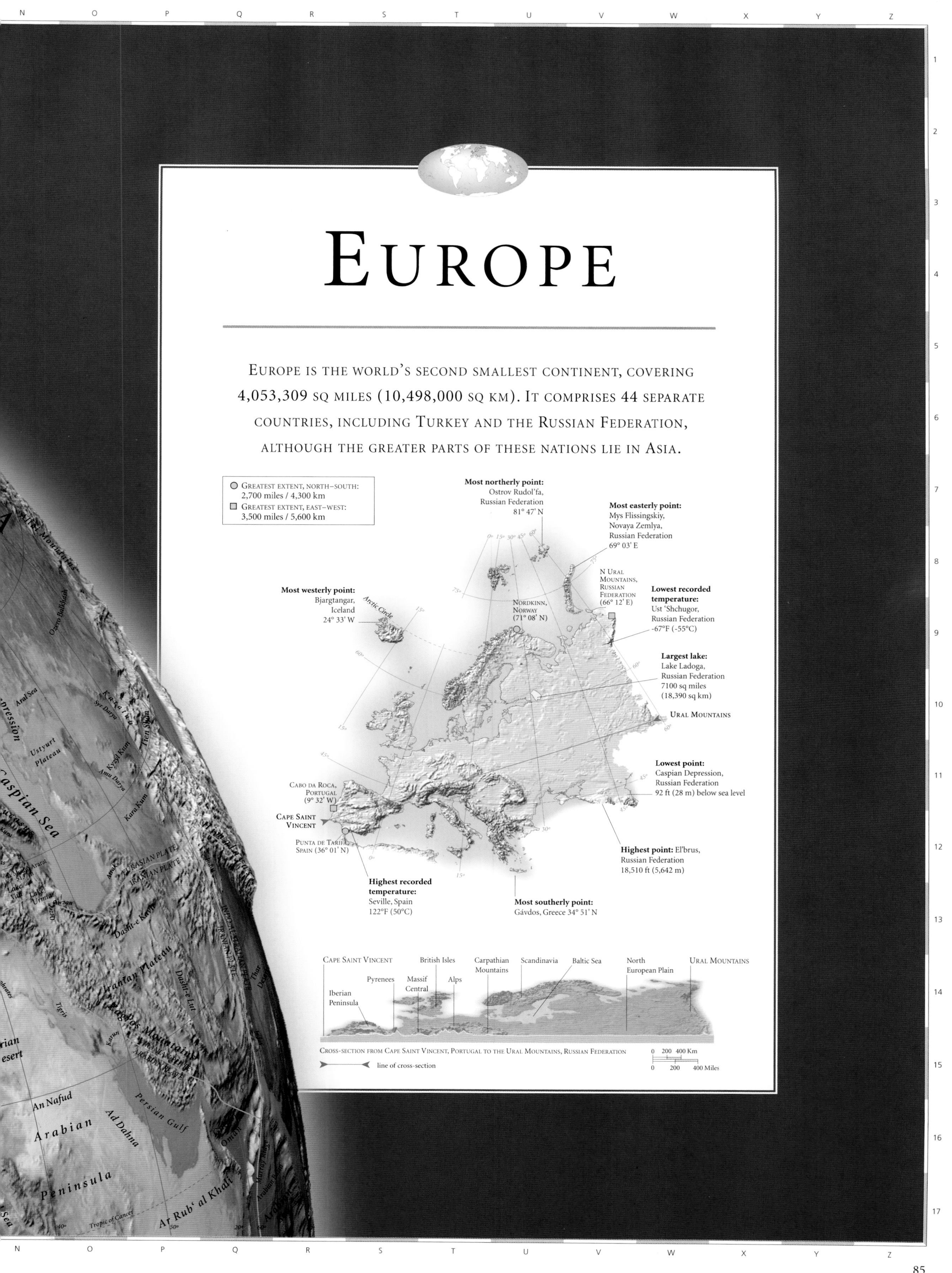

○ Greatest extent, north–south: 2,700 miles / 4,300 km
□ Greatest extent, east–west: 3,500 miles / 5,600 km
Most northerly point: Ostrov Rudol'fa, Russian Federation 81° 47' N
Most easterly point: Mys Flissingskiy, Novaya Zemlya, Russian Federation 69° 03' E
N Ural Mountains, Russian Federation (66° 12' E)
Most westerly point: Bjargtangar, Iceland 24° 33' W
Arctic Circle
Nordkinn, Norway (71° 08' N)
Lowest recorded temperature: Ust 'Shchugor, Russian Federation -67°F (-55°C)
Largest lake: Lake Ladoga, Russian Federation 7100 sq miles (18,390 sq km)
Ural Mountains
Lowest point: Caspian Depression, Russian Federation 92 ft (28 m) below sea level
Cabo da Roca, Portugal (9° 32' W)
Cape Saint Vincent
Punta de Tarifa, Spain (36° 01' N)
Highest point: El'brus, Russian Federation 18,510 ft (5,642 m)
Highest recorded temperature: Seville, Spain 122°F (50°C)
Most southerly point: Gávdos, Greece 34° 51' N
Cape Saint Vincent
Iberian Peninsula
Pyrenees
British Isles
Massif Central
Alps
Carpathian Mountains
Scandinavia
Baltic Sea
North European Plain
Ural Mountains
Cross-section from Cape Saint Vincent, Portugal to the Ural Mountains, Russian Federation
line of cross-section
0 200 400 Km
0 200 400 Miles
Aral Sea
Caspian Sea
Ustyurt Plateau
Kyzyl Kum
Kara Kum
Tien Shan
Eurasian Plate
Iranian Plate
Iranian Plateau
Zagros Mountains
Dasht-e Lut
Persian Gulf
An Nafud
Ad Dahna
Arabian Peninsula
Ar Rub' al Khali
Tropic of Cancer

Physical Europe

The physical diversity of Europe belies its relatively small size. To the northwest and south it is enclosed by mountains. The older, rounded Atlantic Highlands of Scandinavia and the British Isles lie to the north and the younger, rugged peaks of the Alpine Uplands to the south. In between lies the North European Plain, stretching 2,485 miles (4,000 km) from The Fens in England to the Ural Mountains in Russia. South of the plain lies a series of gently folded sedimentary rocks separated by ancient plateaus, known as massifs.

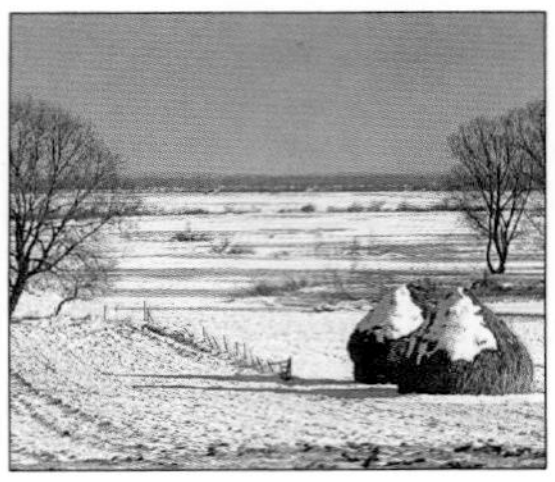

The North European Plain

Rising less than 1,000 ft (300 m)above sea level, the North European Plain strongly reflects past glaciation. Ridges of both coarse moraine and finer, wind-blown deposits have accumulated over much of the region. The ice sheet also diverted a number of river channels from their original courses.

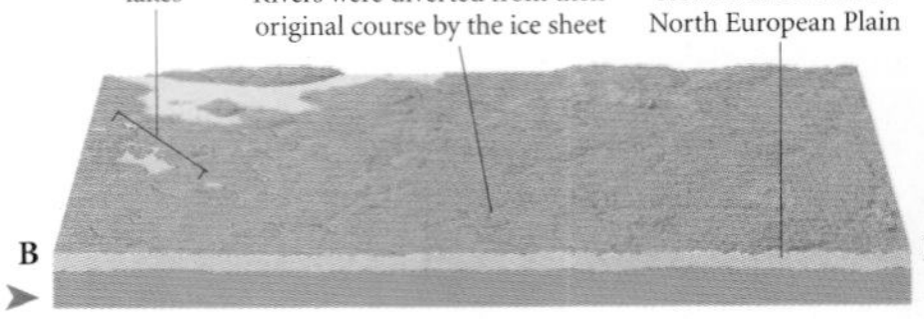

Glacial lakes

Rivers were diverted from their original course by the ice sheet

A layer of glacial sediments covers the North European Plain

Section across the North European Plain showing its low relief and drainage.

0 100 200 Km
0 100 200 Miles

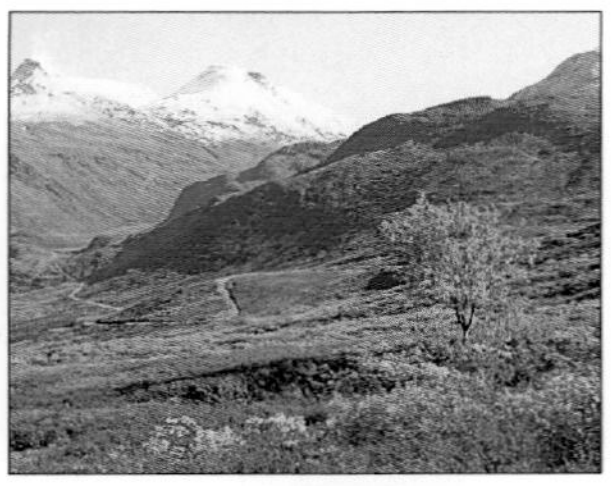

The Atlantic Highlands

The Atlantic Highlands were formed by compression against the Scandinavian Shield during the Caledonian mountain-building period over 500 million years ago. The highlands were once part of a continuous mountain chain, now divided by the North Sea and a submerged rift valley.

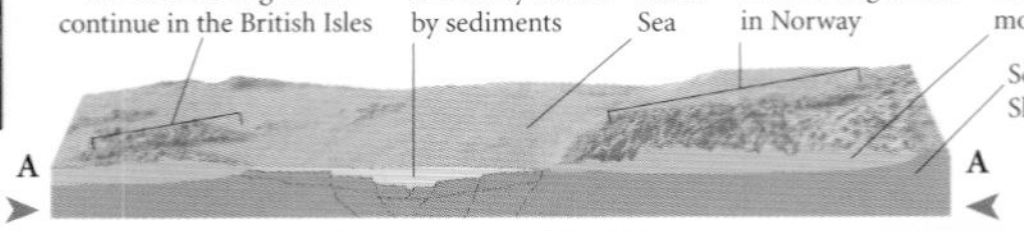

The Atlantic Highlands continue in the British Isles

Rift valley buried by sediments

North Sea

Atlantic Highlands in Norway

Rocks affected by ancient mountain-building

Scandinavian Shield

Cross-section through northeastern Europe showing the continuous mountain chain and rift valley system.

0 100 200 Km
0 100 200 Miles

SCALE 1:25,500,000
(projection: Lambert Azimuthal Equal Area)

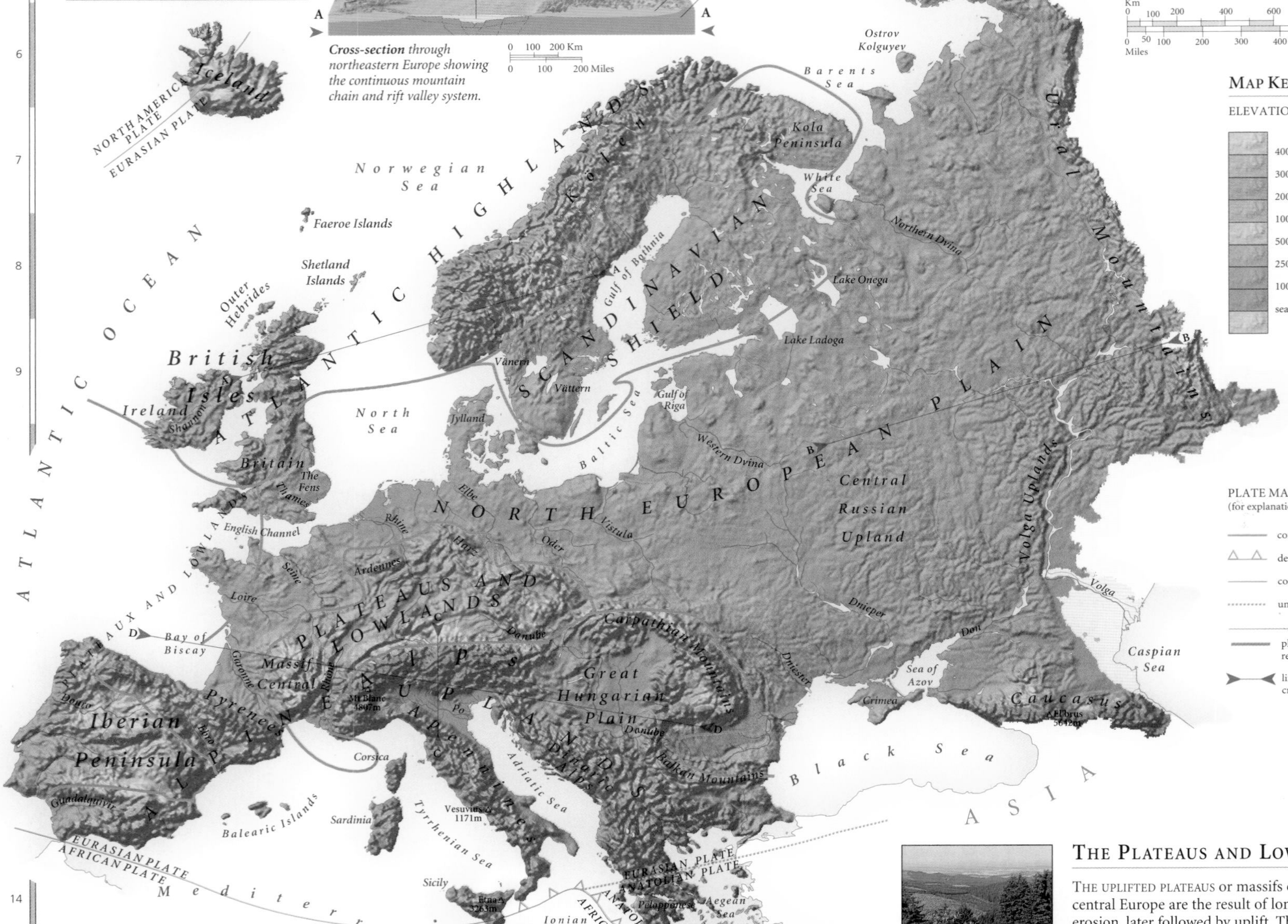

Map Key

ELEVATION

4000m / 13,124ft
3000m / 9843ft
2000m / 6562ft
1000m / 3281ft
500m / 1640ft
250m / 820ft
100m / 328ft
sea level

PLATE MARGINS
(for explanation see page xiv)

constructive
destructive
conservative
uncertain
physiographic regions
line of cross-section

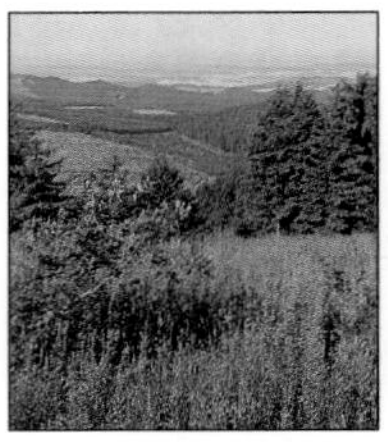

The Plateaus and Lowlands

The uplifted plateaus or massifs of southern central Europe are the result of long-term erosion, later followed by uplift. They are the source areas of many of the rivers which drain Europe's lowlands. In some of the higher reaches, fractures have enabled igneous rocks from deep in the Earth to reach the surface.

The Alpine Uplands

The collision of the African and European continents, which began about 65 million years ago, folded and then uplifted a series of mountain ranges running across southern Europe and into Asia. Two major lines of folding can be traced: one includes the Pyrenees, the Alps, and the Carpathian Mountains; the other incorporates the Apennines and the Dinaric Alps.

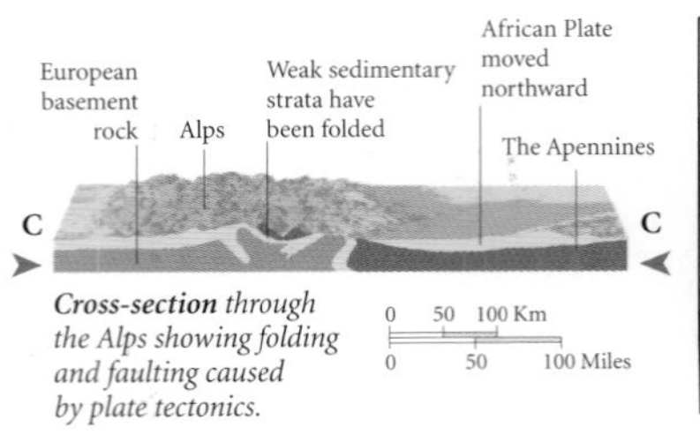
European basement rock
Alps
Weak sedimentary strata have been folded
African Plate moved northward
The Apennines
C
C

Cross-section through the Alps showing folding and faulting caused by plate tectonics.

0 50 100 Km
0 50 100 Miles

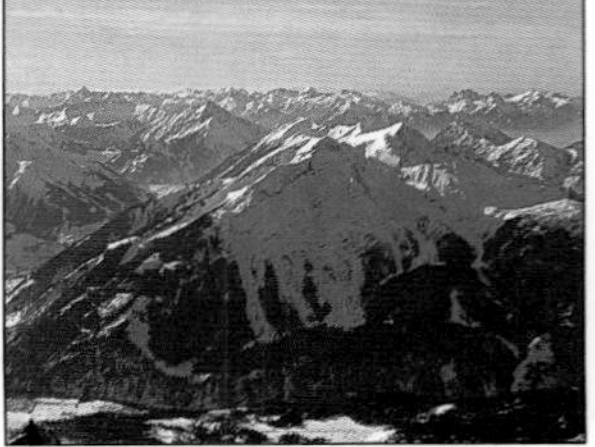

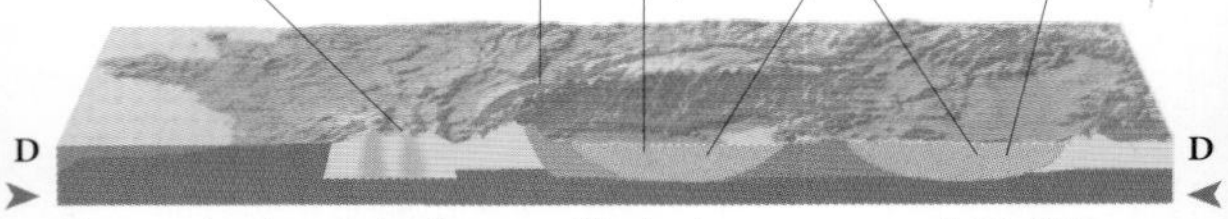

Igneous rocks have intruded into the Massif Central

Older, eroded massifs lie behind the arc of the Alps

Tectonically formed basins

Po Valley

Great Hungarian Plain

Cross-section through the plateaus and lowlands showing the lower elevation of the ancient massifs.

0 100 200 Km
0 100 200 Miles

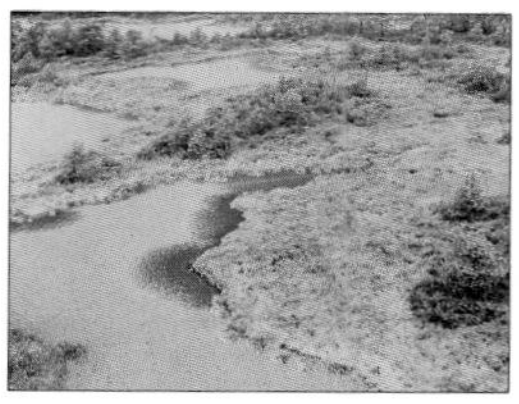

CLIMATE

Frost grips northern and eastern Europe during the long cold winters. Lakes and rivers frequently freeze.

EUROPE EXPERIENCES few extremes in either rainfall or temperature, with the exception of the far north and south. Along the west coast, the warm currents of the North Atlantic Drift moderate temperatures. Although east–west air movement is relatively unimpeded by relief, the Alpine Uplands halt the progress of north–south air masses, protecting most of the Mediterranean from cold, north winds.

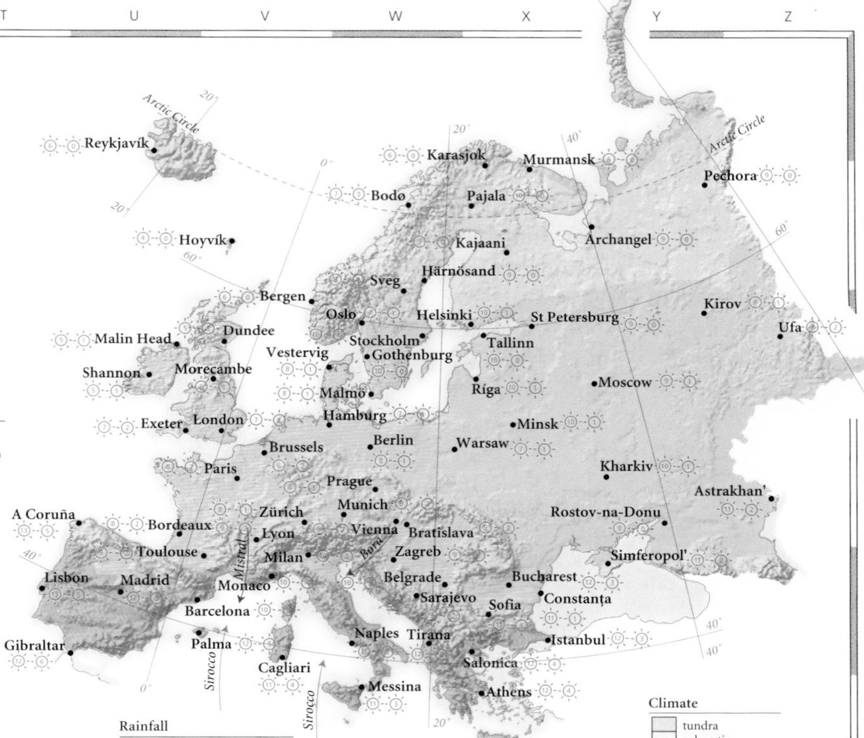

TEMPERATURE

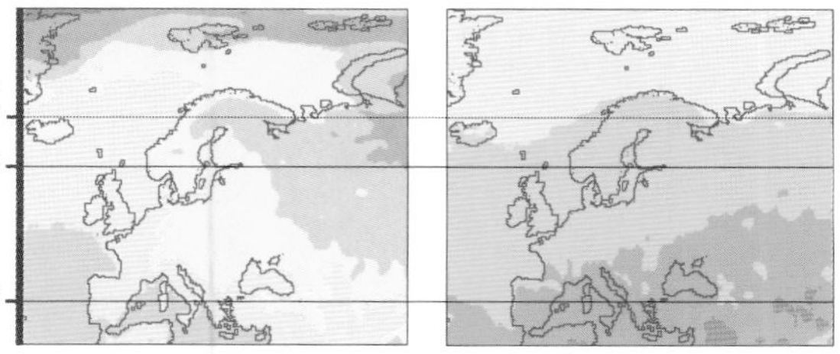

Arctic Circle — 60°N — 40°N

Average January temperature *Average July temperature*

Temperature
- below -30°C (-22°F)
- -30 to -20°C (-22 to -4°F)
- -20 to -10°C (-4 to 14°F)
- -10 to 0°C (14 to 32°F)
- 0 to 10°C (32 to 50° F)
- 10 to 20°C (50 to 60°F)
- 20 to 30°C (68 to 86°F)
- above 30°C (86°F)

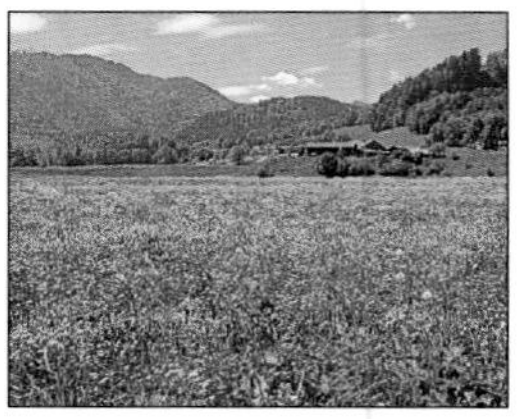

Mild temperatures and frequent rainfall contribute to the fertile farming land found over much of northwestern Europe.

RAINFALL

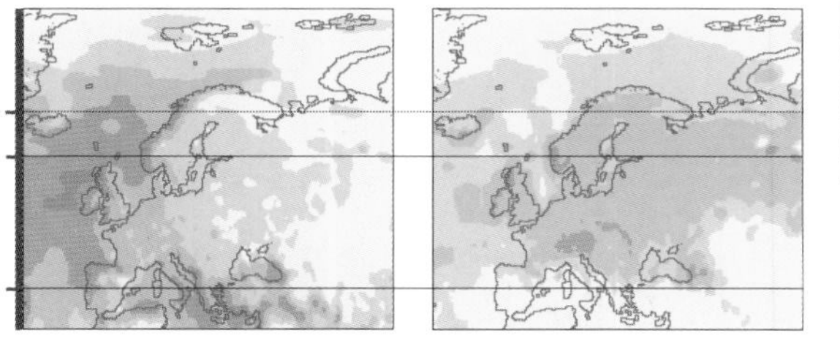

Arctic Circle — 60°N — 40°N

Average January rainfall *Average July rainfall*

Rainfall
- 0–25 mm (0–1 in)
- 25–50 mm (1–2 in)
- 50–100 mm (2–4 in)
- 100–200 mm (4–8 in)
- 200–300 mm (8–12 in)
- 300–400 mm (12–16 in)
- 400–500 mm (16–20 in)
- more than 500 mm (20 in)

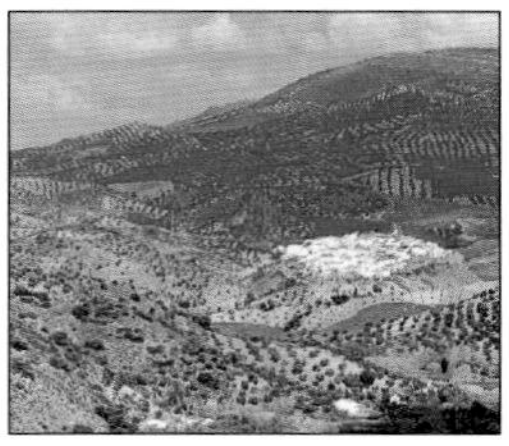

Dusty Sirocco winds from Africa help create the semiarid scrubland common across the Mediterranean coastlands of southern Europe.

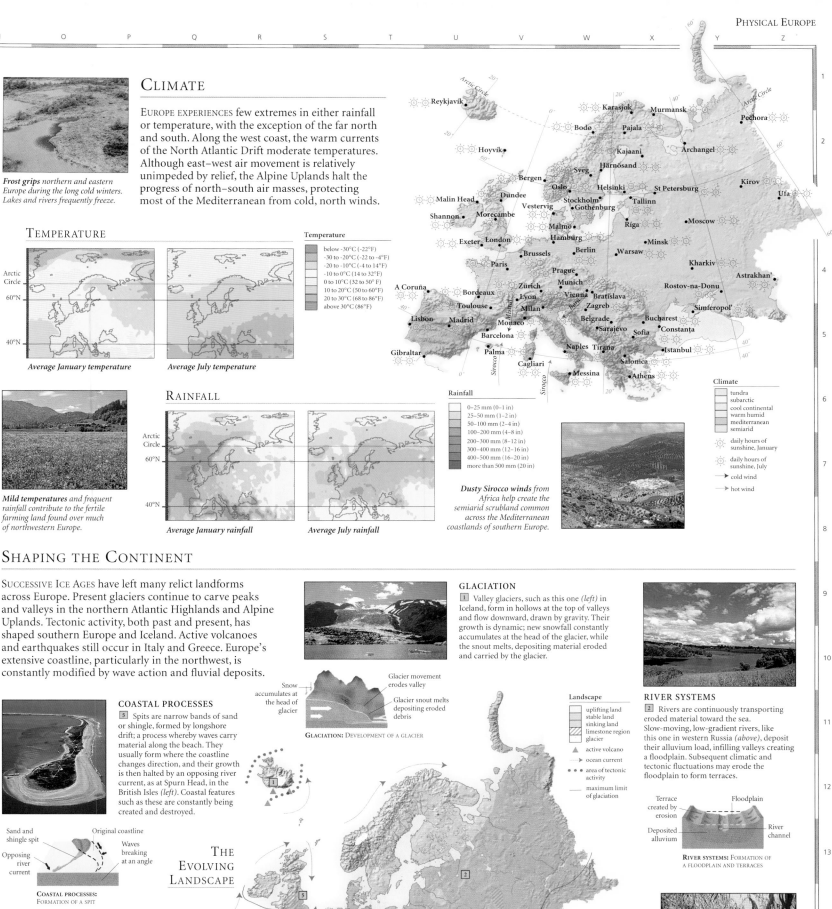

Climate
- tundra
- subarctic
- cool continental
- warm humid
- mediterranean
- semiarid
- daily hours of sunshine, January
- daily hours of sunshine, July
- cold wind
- hot wind

SHAPING THE CONTINENT

SUCCESSIVE ICE AGES have left many relict landforms across Europe. Present glaciers continue to carve peaks and valleys in the northern Atlantic Highlands and Alpine Uplands. Tectonic activity, both past and present, has shaped southern Europe and Iceland. Active volcanoes and earthquakes still occur in Italy and Greece. Europe's extensive coastline, particularly in the northwest, is constantly modified by wave action and fluvial deposits.

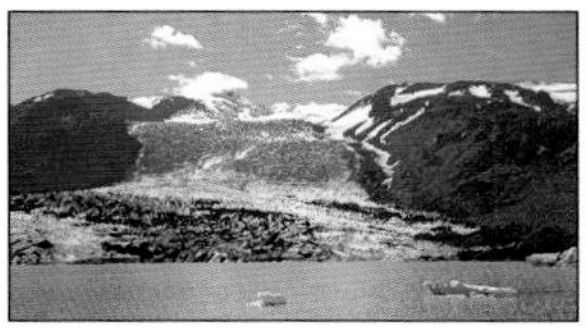

GLACIATION

1 Valley glaciers, such as this one *(left)* in Iceland, form in hollows at the top of valleys and flow downward, drawn by gravity. Their growth is dynamic; new snowfall constantly accumulates at the head of the glacier, while the snout melts, depositing material eroded and carried by the glacier.

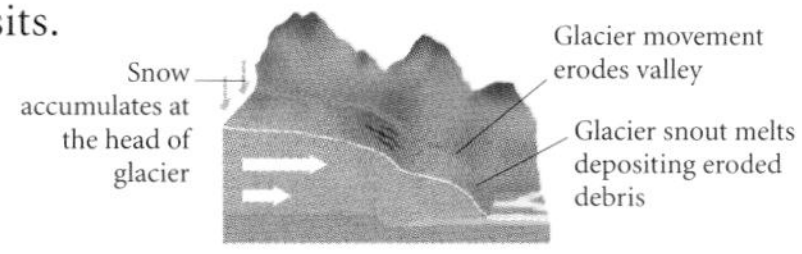

Snow accumulates at the head of glacier

Glacier movement erodes valley

Glacier snout melts depositing eroded debris

GLACIATION: DEVELOPMENT OF A GLACIER

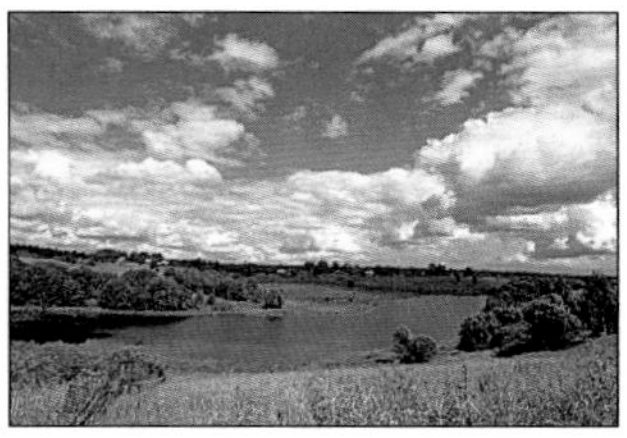

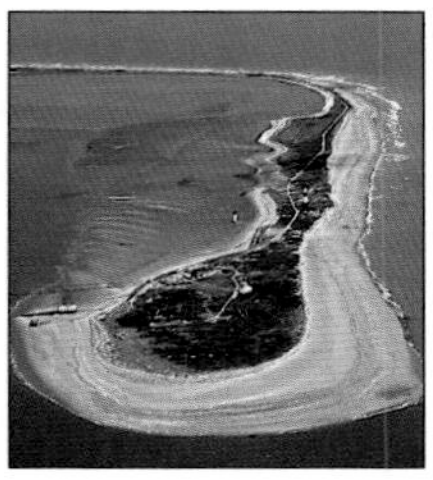

COASTAL PROCESSES

5 Spits are narrow bands of sand or shingle, formed by longshore drift; a process whereby waves carry material along the beach. They usually form where the coastline changes direction, and their growth is then halted by an opposing river current, as at Spurn Head, in the British Isles *(left)*. Coastal features such as these are constantly being created and destroyed.

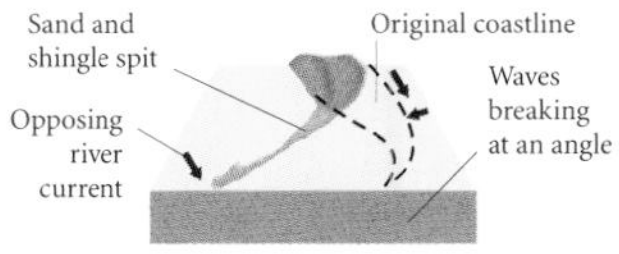

Sand and shingle spit

Original coastline

Opposing river current

Waves breaking at an angle

COASTAL PROCESSES: FORMATION OF A SPIT

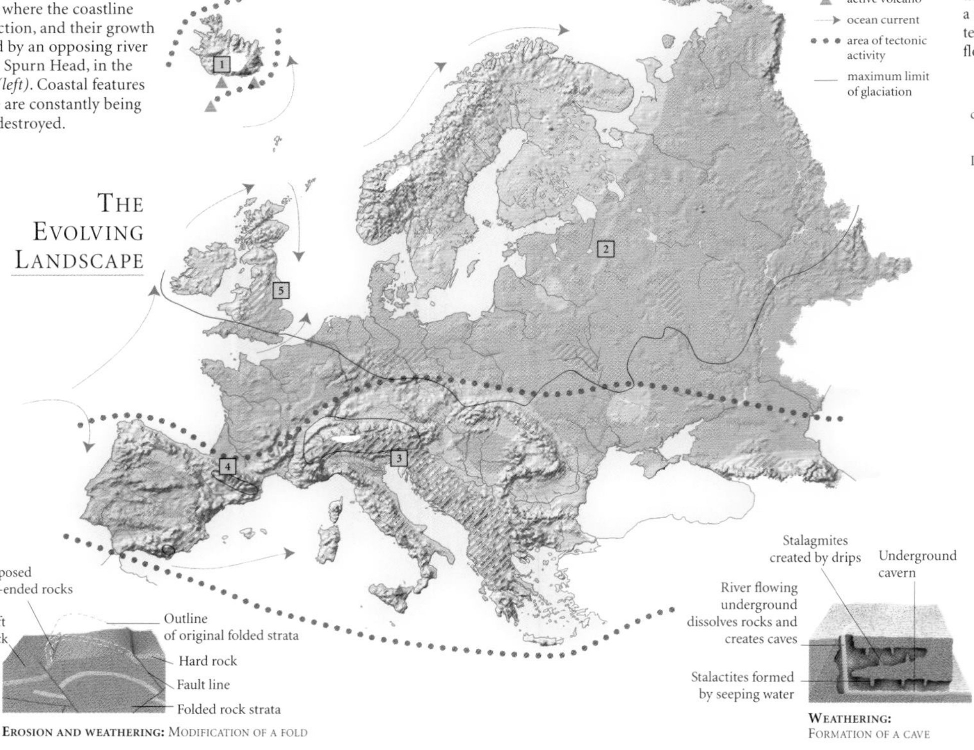
THE EVOLVING LANDSCAPE
Landscape
uplifting land
stable land
sinking land
limestone region
glacier
active volcano
ocean current
area of tectonic activity
maximum limit of glaciation

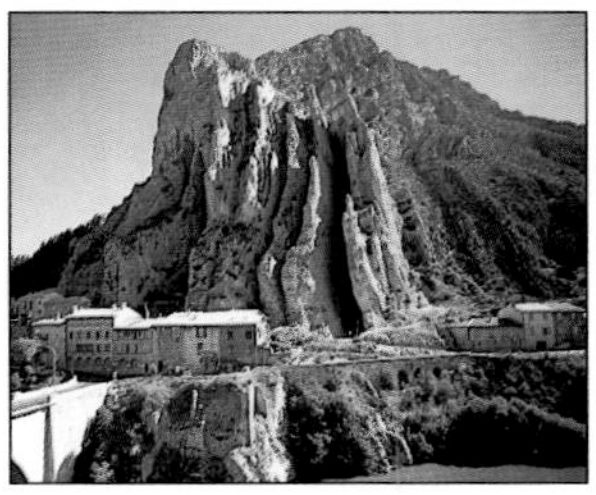

RIVER SYSTEMS

2 Rivers are continuously transporting eroded material toward the sea. Slow-moving, low-gradient rivers, like this one in western Russia *(above)*, deposit their alluvium load, infilling valleys creating a floodplain. Subsequent climatic and tectonic fluctuations may erode the floodplain to form terraces.

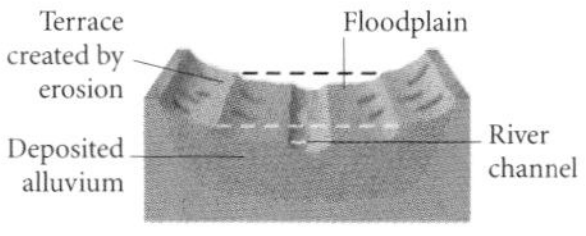

Terrace created by erosion

Floodplain

Deposited alluvium

River channel

RIVER SYSTEMS: FORMATION OF A FLOODPLAIN AND TERRACES

EROSION AND WEATHERING

4 Much of Europe was once subjected to folding and faulting, exposing hard and soft rock layers. Subsequent erosion and weathering has worn away the softer strata, leaving up-ended layers of hard rock as in the French Pyrenees *(above)*.

Exposed up-ended rocks

Soft rock

Outline of original folded strata

Hard rock

Fault line

Folded rock strata

EROSION AND WEATHERING: MODIFICATION OF A FOLD

Stalagmites created by drips

Underground cavern

River flowing underground dissolves rocks and creates caves

Stalactites formed by seeping water

WEATHERING: FORMATION OF A CAVE

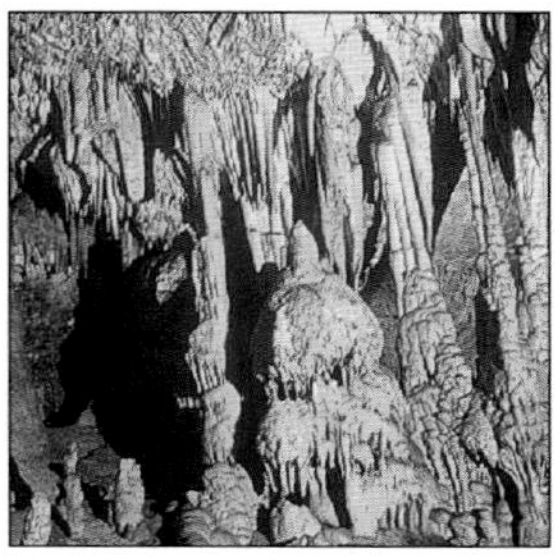

WEATHERING

3 As surface water filters through permeable limestone, the rock dissolves to form underground caves, like Postojna in the Karst region of Slovenia *(above)*. Stalactites grow downward as lime-enriched water seeps from roof fractures; stalagmites grow upward where drips splash down.

A B C D E F G H I J K L M

POLITICAL EUROPE

THE POLITICAL BOUNDARIES OF EUROPE have changed many times, especially during the 20th century in the aftermath of two world wars, the breakup of the empires of Austria-Hungary, Nazi Germany and, toward the end of the century, the collapse of communism in eastern Europe. The fragmentation of Yugoslavia has again altered the political map of Europe, highlighting a trend toward nationalism and devolution. In contrast, economic federalism is growing. In 1958, the formation of the European Economic Community (now the European Union or EU) started a move toward economic and political union.

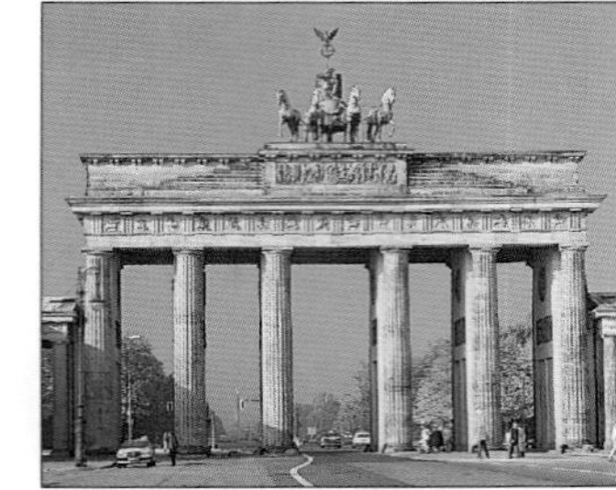

The Brandenburg Gate in Berlin is a potent symbol of German reunification. From 1961, the road beneath it ended in a wall, built to stop the flow of refugees to the West. It was opened again in 1989 when the wall was destroyed and East and West Germany were reunited.

POPULATION

EUROPE IS A DENSELY POPULATED, urbanized continent; in Belgium over 90% of people live in urban areas. The highest population densities are found in an area stretching east from southern Britain and northern France, into Germany. The northern fringes are only sparsely populated.

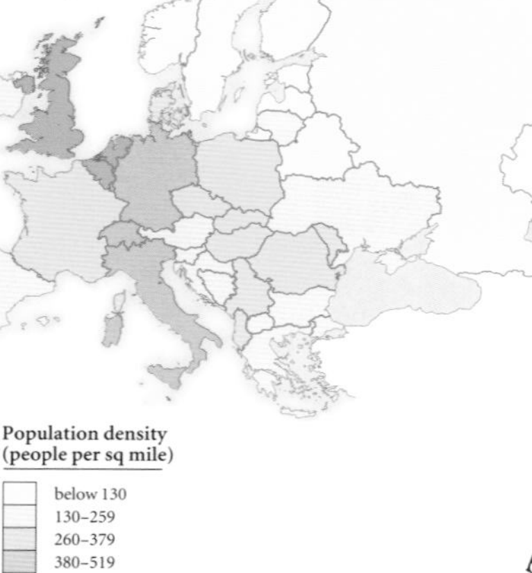

Population density (people per sq mile)

- below 130
- 130–259
- 260–379
- 380–519
- 520–780
- above 780

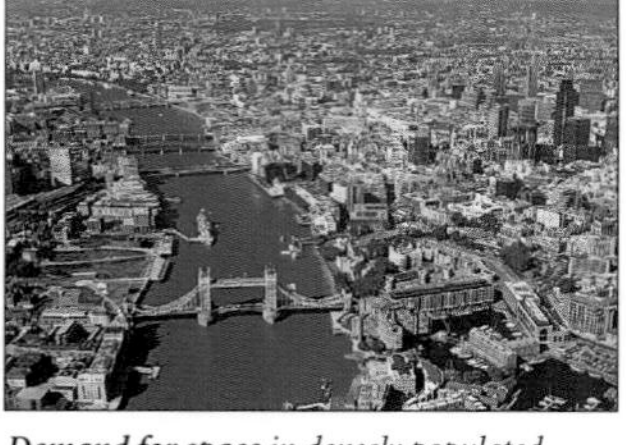

Demand for space in densely populated European cities like London has led to the development of high-rise offices and urban sprawl.

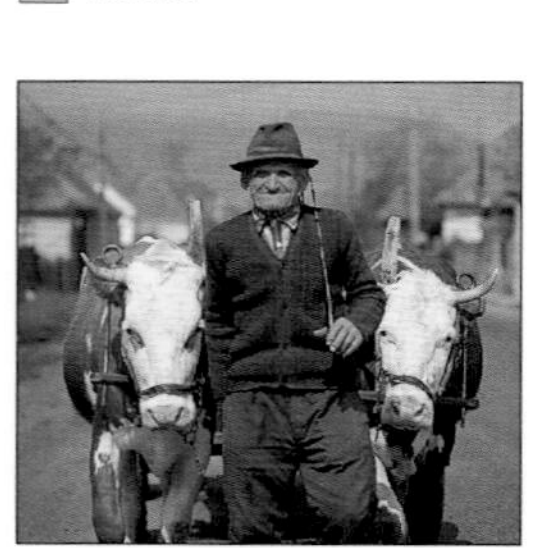
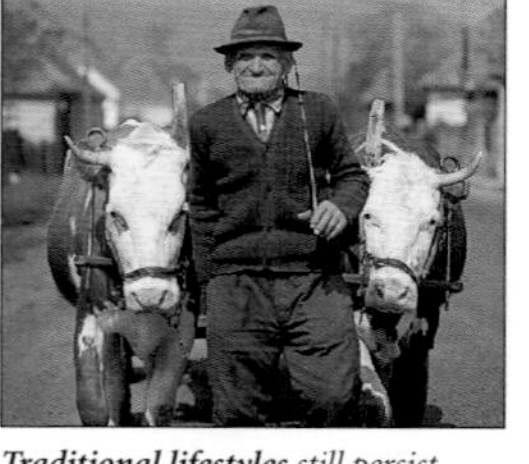

Traditional lifestyles still persist in remote and rural parts of Europe, especially in the south, east, and in the far north.

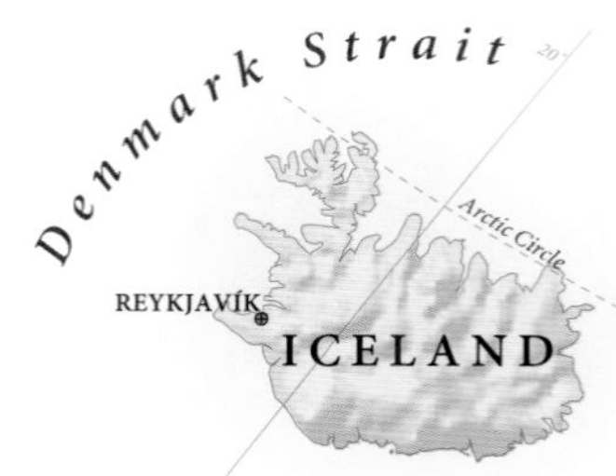
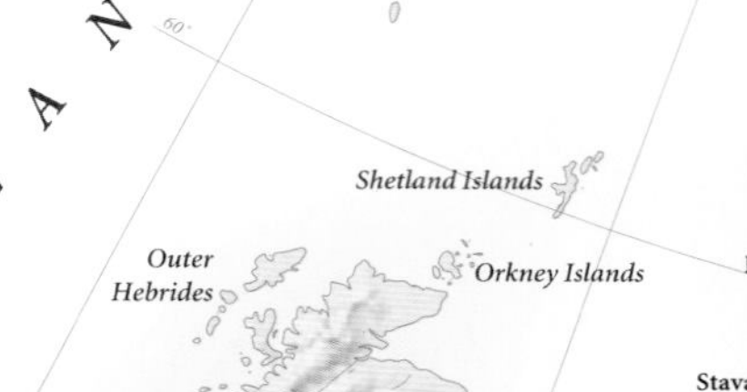
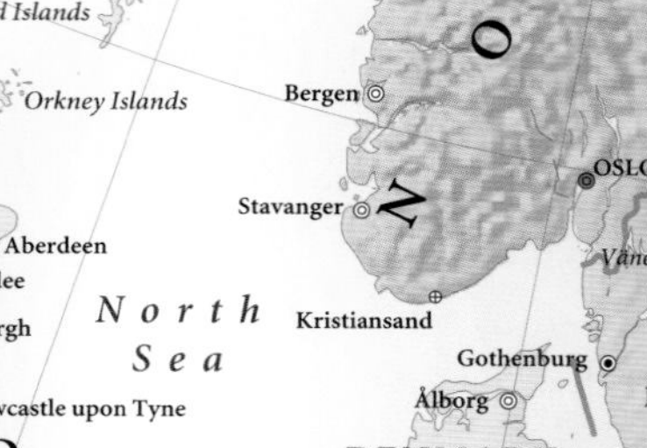
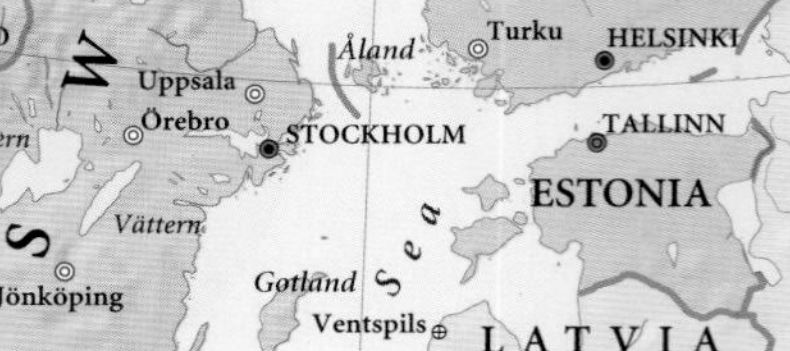
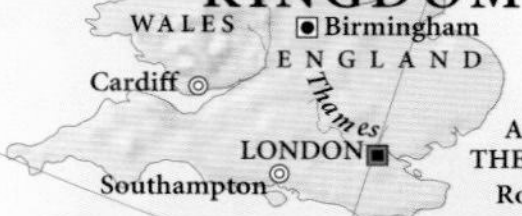
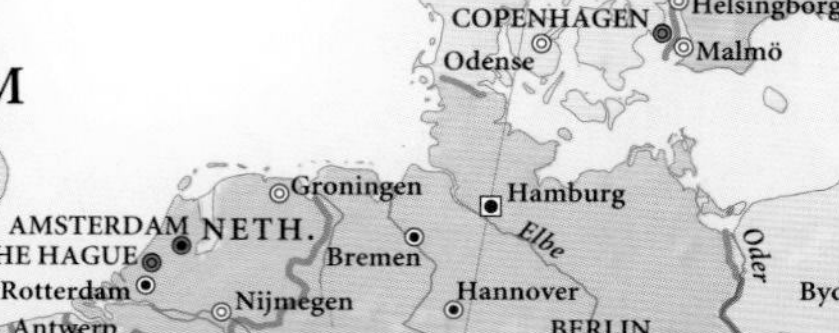
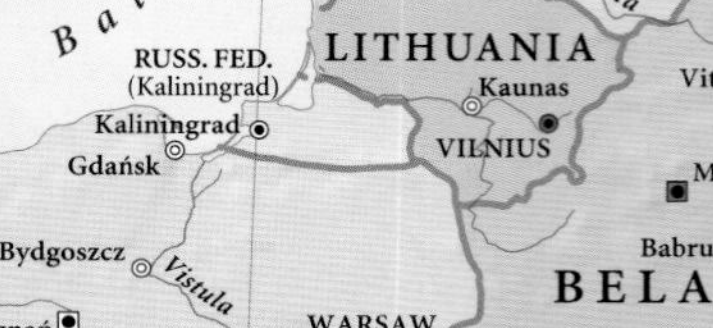
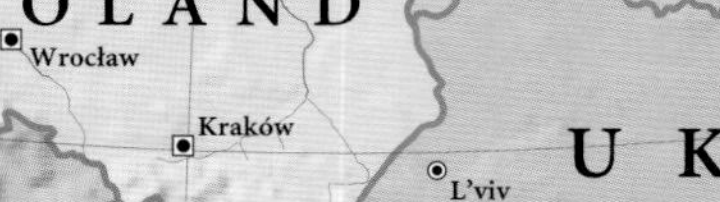
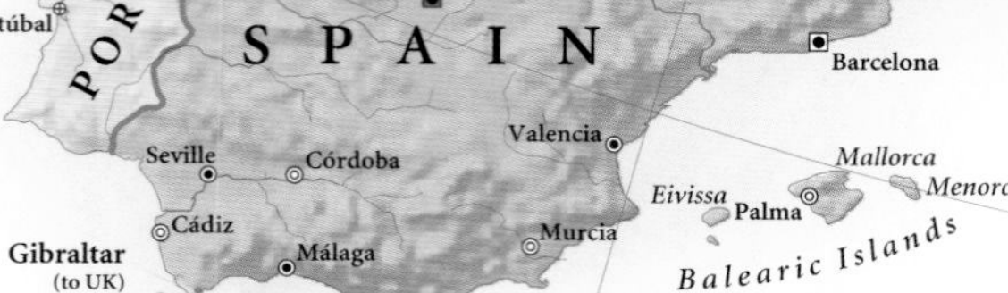
Denmark Strait
Arctic Circle
REYKJAVÍK
ICELAND
Norwegian Sea
Faeroe Islands (to Denmark)
ATLANTIC OCEAN
Shetland Islands
Orkney Islands
Outer Hebrides
SCOTLAND
Aberdeen
Dundee
Glasgow
Edinburgh
NORTHERN IRELAND
Belfast
REPUBLIC OF IRELAND
DUBLIN
Isle of Man (to UK)
Newcastle upon Tyne
UNITED KINGDOM
Leeds
Liverpool
Manchester
Sheffield
WALES
Birmingham
ENGLAND
Cardiff
Thames
LONDON
Southampton
North Sea
Channel Islands (to UK)
English Channel
NORWAY
Trondheim
Bergen
Stavanger
OSLO
Kristiansand
SWEDEN
Uppsala
Örebro
STOCKHOLM
Vänern
Vättern
Jönköping
Gothenburg
Gulf of Bothnia
FINLAND
Tampere
Turku
HELSINKI
Åland
Lake Ladoga
St Petersburg
Murmansk
TALLINN
ESTONIA
DENMARK
Ålborg
COPENHAGEN
Odense
Helsingborg
Malmö
Gotland
Ventspils
LATVIA
RIGA
Western Dvina
Liepāja
Baltic Sea
RUSS. FED. (Kaliningrad)
Kaliningrad
Gdańsk
LITHUANIA
Kaunas
VILNIUS
Vitsyebsk
MINSK
Babruysk
BELARUS
Homyel
Brest
Groningen
Hamburg
AMSTERDAM
NETH.
Bremen
THE HAGUE
Rotterdam
Nijmegen
Hannover
Elbe
Oder
Bydgoszcz
Vistula
Antwerp
BELGIUM
BERLIN
Poznań
WARSAW
Düsseldorf
BRUSSELS
Bonn
GERMANY
Łódź
Liège
Leipzig
POLAND
Rhine
Frankfurt am Main
Dresden
Wrocław
LUXEMBOURG
PRAGUE
Kraków
CZECH REPUBLIC
Nuremberg
Stuttgart
Strasbourg
Munich
Salzburg
KIEV
UKRAINE
L'viv
SLOVAKIA
Chernivtsi
Dniester
MOLDOVA
CHIŞINĂU
BRATISLAVA
VIENNA
Danube
Győr
Miskolc
AUSTRIA
BUDAPEST
Cluj-Napoca
HUNGARY
Zürich
Innsbruck
BERN
SWITZERLAND
LIECHTENSTEIN
Alps
LJUBLJANA
SLOVENIA
ROMANIA
Braşov
ZAGREB
CROATIA
Trieste
Venice
Verona
Milan
Turin
Genoa
Po
Bologna
Florence
SAN MARINO
BOS. & HERZ.
SARAJEVO
Mostar
BELGRADE
SERBIA
BUCHAREST
Constanţa
Danube
Ruse
Varna
Burgas
YUGOSLAVIA
MONTENEGRO
BULGARIA
SOFIA
Stara Zagora
Istanbul
SKOPJE
MACEDONIA
TIRANA
ALBANIA
Salonica
Adriatic Sea
le Havre
Seine
Rennes
PARIS
Nantes
St-Nazaire
Loire
Orléans
FRANCE
Bay of Biscay
Limoges
Bordeaux
Geneva
Lyon
Rhône
Toulouse
Pyrenees
Marseille
Nice
MONACO
Corsica
Pisa
ITALY
VATICAN CITY
ROME
Sardinia
Tyrrhenian Sea
Naples
Bari
Cagliari
Cosenza
Palermo
Messina
Sicily
Catania
MALTA
VALLETTA
Ionian Sea
A Coruña
Bilbao
Porto
Duero
Valladolid
Ebro
ANDORRA LA VELLA
ANDORRA
PORTUGAL
LISBON
Tagus
Setúbal
MADRID
Zaragoza
SPAIN
Barcelona
Valencia
Seville
Córdoba
Cádiz
Málaga
Murcia
Gibraltar (to UK)
Ceuta (to Spain)
Melilla (to Spain)
Eivissa
Palma
Mallorca
Menorca
Balearic Islands
Mediterranean Sea
GREECE
Larisa
Aegean Sea
ATHENS
Piraeus
Crete
Iráklion

MAP KEY

POPULATION

- above 5 million
- 1 million to 5 million
- 500,000 to 1 million
- 100,000 to 500,000
- 50,000 to 100,000
- 10,000 to 50,000
- Country capital

BORDERS

- full international border

SCALE 1:17,250,000
(projection: Lambert Azimuthal Equal Area)

Km 0 50 100 200 300 400 500 600 700 800 900 1000
Miles 0 50 100 200 300 400 500 600 700

A B C D E F G H

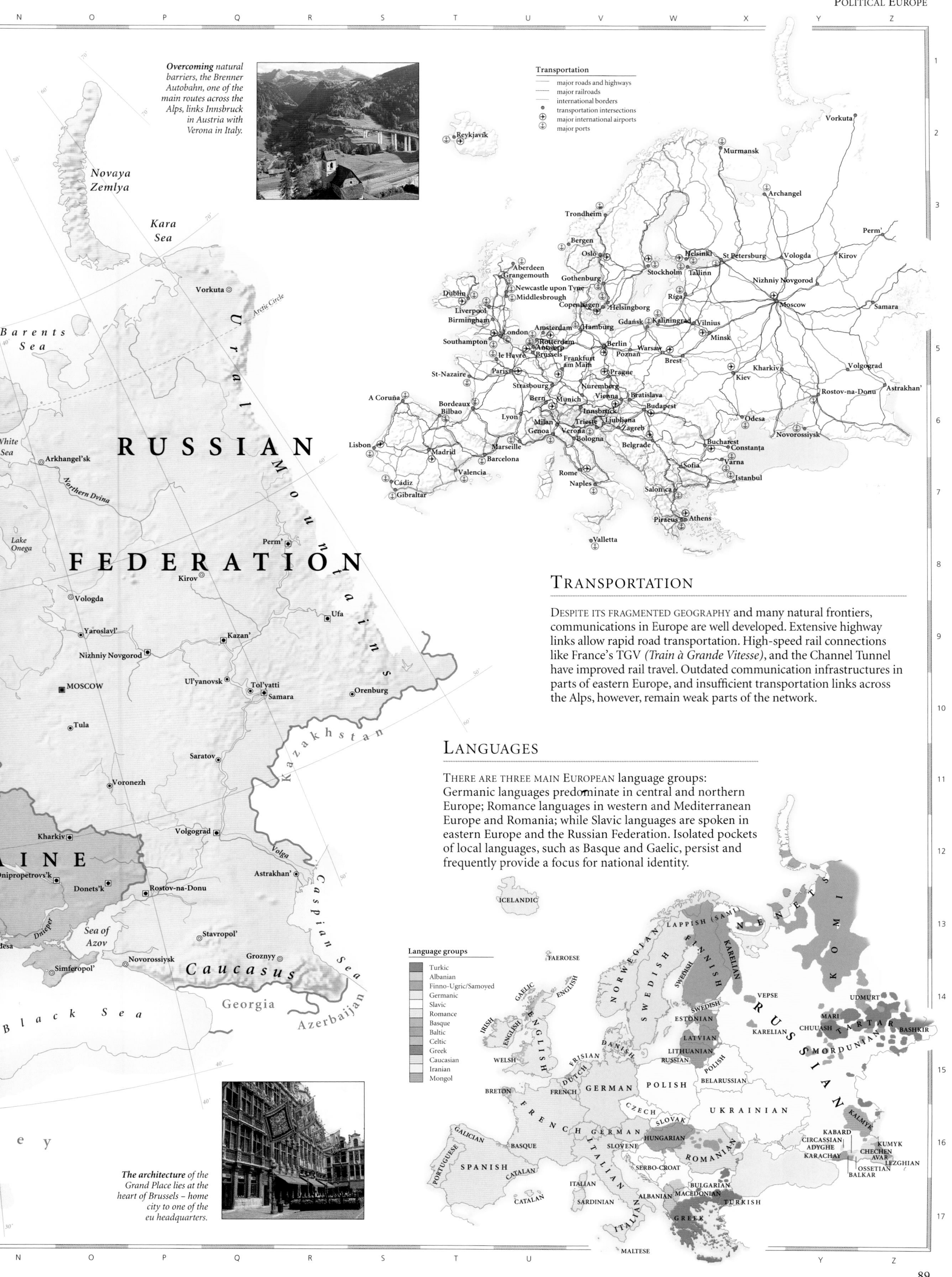
N O P Q R S T U V W X Y Z
1 2 3 4 5 6 7 8 9 10 11 12 13 14 15 16 17
Novaya Zemlya
Kara Sea
Barents Sea
White Sea
Arctic Circle
Ural Mountains
RUSSIAN FEDERATION
Vorkuta
Arkhangel'sk
Northern Dvina
Lake Onega
Perm'
Kirov
Vologda
Ufa
Yaroslavl'
Kazan'
Nizhniy Novgorod
Ul'yanovsk
Tol'yatti
Samara
MOSCOW
Orenburg
Tula
Kazakhstan
Saratov
Voronezh
Kharkiv
Volgograd
Volga
UKRAINE
Dnipropetrovs'k
Donets'k
Rostov-na-Donu
Astrakhan'
Caspian Sea
Dnieper
Sea of Azov
Stavropol'
Simferopol'
Novorossiysk
Groznyy
Caucasus
Georgia
Azerbaijan
Black Sea
Transportation
major roads and highways
major railroads
international borders
transportation intersections
major international airports
major ports
Reykjavík
Murmansk
Vorkuta
Archangel
Trondheim
Bergen
Oslo
Helsinki
St Petersburg
Vologda
Kirov
Perm'
Aberdeen
Grangemouth
Stockholm
Tallinn
Gothenburg
Nizhniy Novgorod
Newcastle upon Tyne
Middlesbrough
Dublin
Riga
Moscow
Samara
Liverpool
Birmingham
Copenhagen
Helsingborg
Gdańsk
Kaliningrad
Vilnius
Amsterdam
Hamburg
Minsk
London
Southampton
Rotterdam
Antwerp
Brussels
Berlin
Poznan
Warsaw
Brest
le Havre
Frankfurt am Main
Paris
Prague
Kharkiv
Kiev
Volgograd
St-Nazaire
Strasbourg
Nuremberg
Rostov-na-Donu
Astrakhan'
A Coruña
Bordeaux
Bilbao
Bern
Munich
Vienna
Bratislava
Budapest
Innsbruck
Lyon
Milan
Trieste
Ljubljana
Zagreb
Odesa
Genoa
Verona
Bologna
Lisbon
Madrid
Marseille
Barcelona
Belgrade
Bucharest
Constanța
Novorossiysk
Valencia
Sofia
Varna
Rome
Istanbul
Cádiz
Gibraltar
Naples
Salonica
Piraeus
Athens
Valletta
Language groups
Turkic
Albanian
Finno-Ugric/Samoyed
Germanic
Slavic
Romance
Basque
Baltic
Celtic
Greek
Caucasian
Iranian
Mongol
ICELANDIC
FAEROESE
NORWEGIAN
SWEDISH
LAPPISH (SAMI)
FINNISH
KARELIAN
NENETS
KOMI
GAELIC
ENGLISH
IRISH
WELSH
VEPSE
SWEDISH
ESTONIAN
UDMURT
MARI
CHUVASH
TARTAR
BASHKIR
KARELIAN
RUSSIAN
MORDUNIAN
LATVIAN
LITHUANIAN
DANISH
FRISIAN
DUTCH
POLISH
BELARUSSIAN
BRETON
FRENCH
GERMAN
CZECH
SLOVAK
UKRAINIAN
KALMYK
GALICIAN
BASQUE
SLOVENE
HUNGARIAN
ROMANIAN
KABARD
CIRCASSIAN
ADYGHE
KARACHAY
BALKAR
OSSETIAN
KUMYK
CHECHEN
AVAR
LEZGHIAN
PORTUGUESE
SPANISH
CATALAN
ITALIAN
SERBO-CROAT
BULGARIAN
MACEDONIAN
ALBANIAN
TURKISH
SARDINIAN
GREEK
MALTESE

Overcoming natural barriers, the Brenner Autobahn, one of the main routes across the Alps, links Innsbruck in Austria with Verona in Italy.

Transportation

Despite its fragmented geography and many natural frontiers, communications in Europe are well developed. Extensive highway links allow rapid road transportation. High-speed rail connections like France's TGV *(Train à Grande Vitesse)*, and the Channel Tunnel have improved rail travel. Outdated communication infrastructures in parts of eastern Europe, and insufficient transportation links across the Alps, however, remain weak parts of the network.

Languages

There are three main European language groups: Germanic languages predominate in central and northern Europe; Romance languages in western and Mediterranean Europe and Romania; while Slavic languages are spoken in eastern Europe and the Russian Federation. Isolated pockets of local languages, such as Basque and Gaelic, persist and frequently provide a focus for national identity.

The architecture of the Grand Place lies at the heart of Brussels – home city to one of the eu headquarters.

European Resources

Europe's large tracts of fertile, accessible land, combined with its generally temperate climate, have allowed a greater percentage of land to be used for agricultural purposes than in any other continent. Extensive coal and iron ore deposits were used to create steel and manufacturing industries during the 19th and 20th centuries. Today, although natural resources have been widely exploited, and heavy industry is of declining importance, the growth of hi-tech and service industries has enabled Europe to maintain its wealth.

Industry

Europe's wealth was generated by the rise of industry and colonial exploitation during the 19th century. The mining of abundant natural resources made Europe the industrial center of the world. Adaptation has been essential in the changing world economy, and a move to service-based industries has been widespread except in eastern Europe, where heavy industry still dominates.

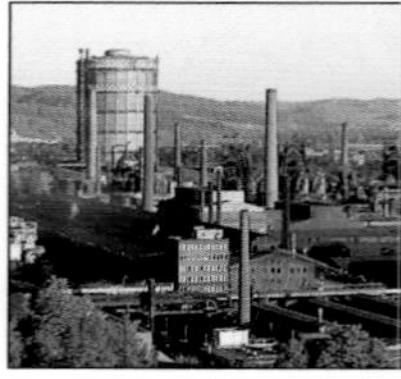

***Countries like Hungary** are still struggling to modernize inefficient factories left over from extensive, centrally-planned industrialization during the communist era.*

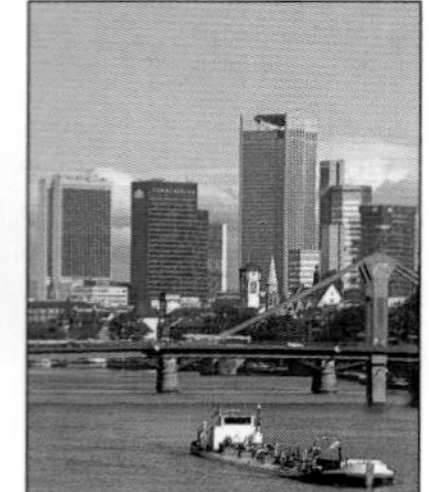

***Frankfurt am Main** is an example of a modern service-based city. The skyline is dominated by headquarters from the worlds of banking and commerce.*

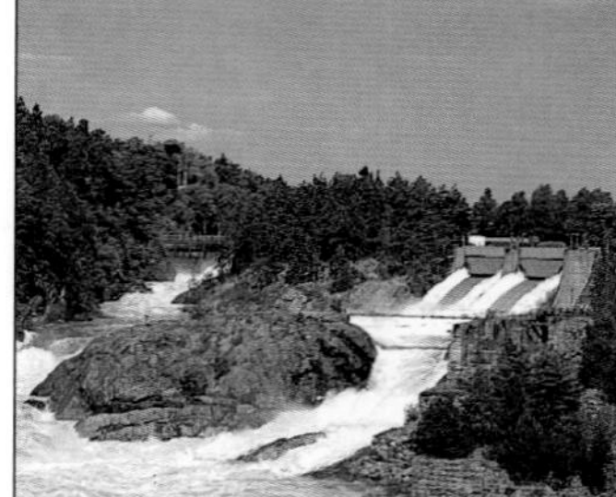

***Other power sources** are becoming more attractive as fossil fuels run out; 16% of Europe's electricity is now provided by hydroelectric power.*

Standard of Living

Living standards in western Europe are among the highest in the world, although there is a growing sector of homeless, jobless people. Eastern Europeans have lower overall standards of living – a legacy of stagnated economies.

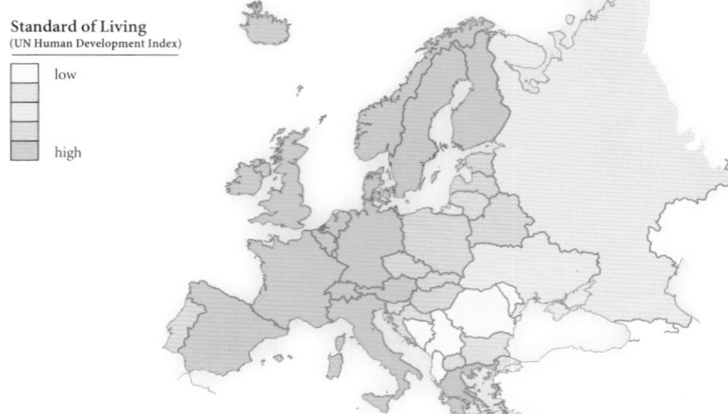
Standard of Living
(UN Human Development Index)
low
high

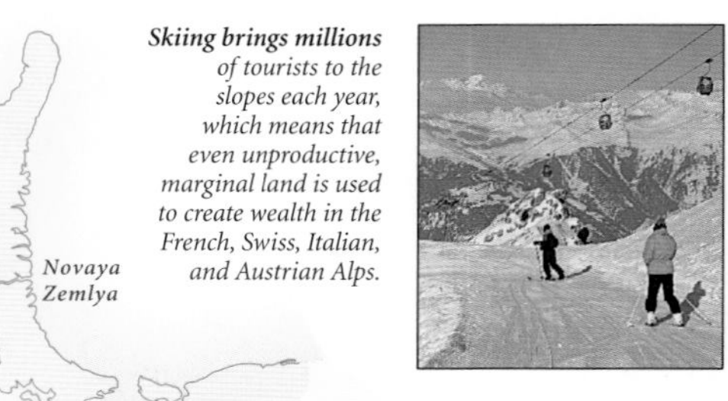

***Skiing brings millions** of tourists to the slopes each year, which means that even unproductive, marginal land is used to create wealth in the French, Swiss, Italian, and Austrian Alps.*

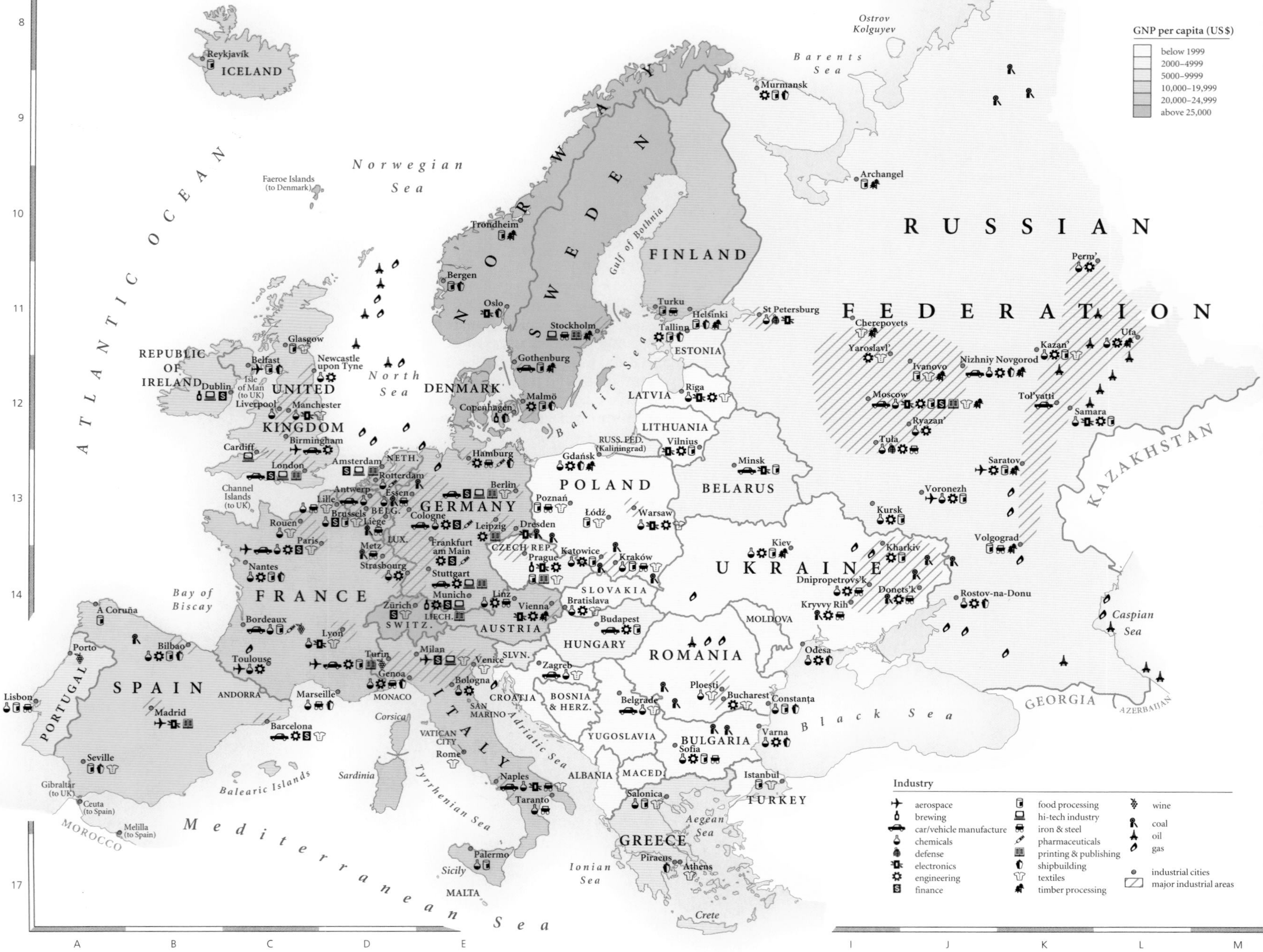

GNP per capita (US$)

- below 1999
- 2000–4999
- 5000–9999
- 10,000–19,999
- 20,000–24,999
- above 25,000

Industry

- aerospace
- brewing
- car/vehicle manufacture
- chemicals
- defense
- electronics
- engineering
- finance
- food processing
- hi-tech industry
- iron & steel
- pharmaceuticals
- printing & publishing
- shipbuilding
- textiles
- timber processing
- wine
- coal
- oil
- gas
- industrial cities
- major industrial areas

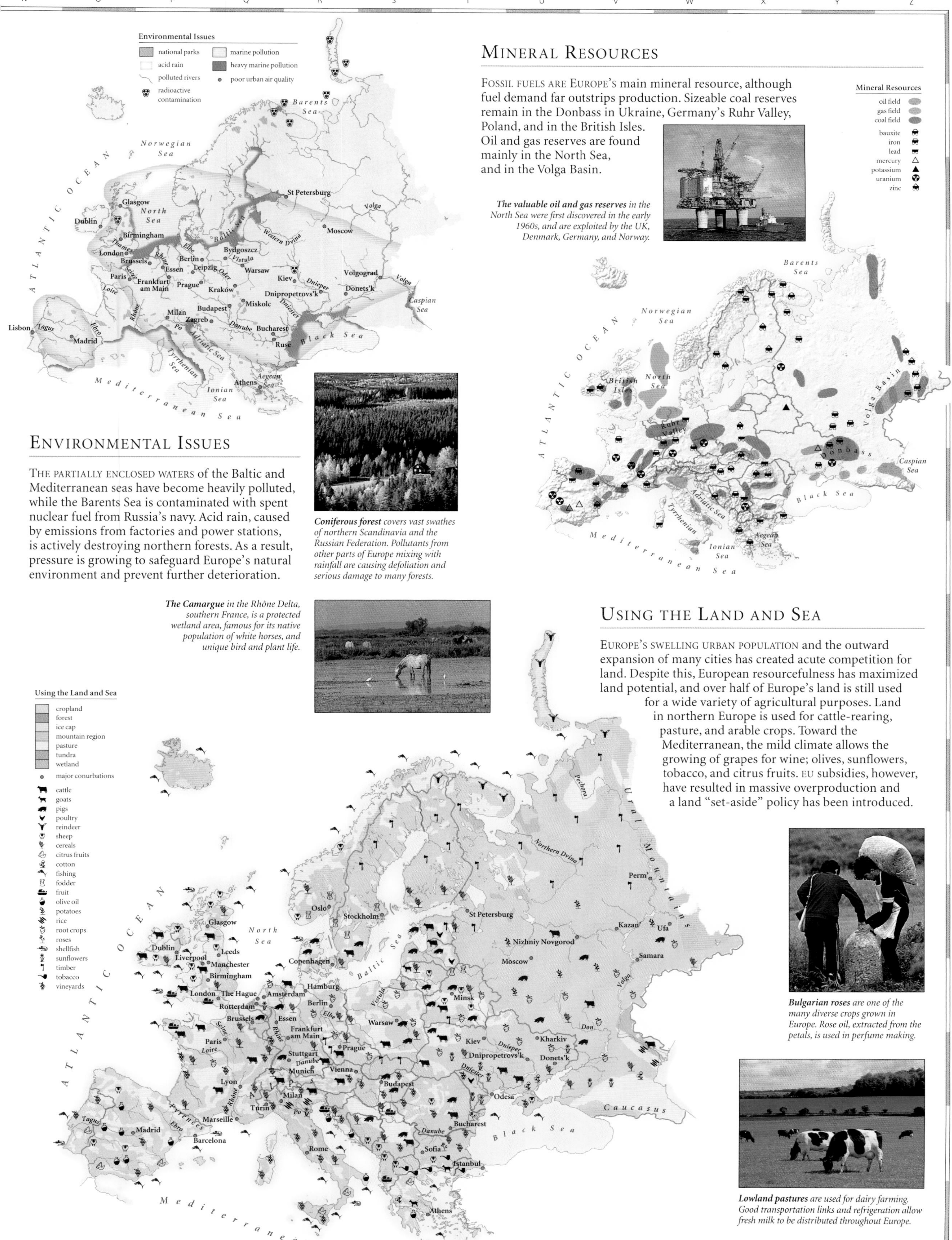
N O P Q R S T U V W X Y Z
1 2 3 4 5 6 7 8 9 10 11 12 13 14 15 16 17
Environmental Issues
national parks
acid rain
polluted rivers
radioactive contamination
marine pollution
heavy marine pollution
poor urban air quality
Barents Sea
Norwegian Sea
Atlantic Ocean
North Sea
Baltic Sea
Black Sea
Caspian Sea
Adriatic Sea
Tyrrhenian Sea
Ionian Sea
Aegean Sea
Mediterranean Sea
Glasgow
Dublin
Birmingham
London
Brussels
Paris
Frankfurt am Main
Essen
Berlin
Leipzig
Prague
Bydgoszcz
Warsaw
Kraków
Kiev
Dnipropetrovs'k
Volgograd
Donets'k
Miskolc
Budapest
Zagreb
Bucharest
Ruse
Milan
Madrid
Lisbon
Athens
St Petersburg
Moscow
Mineral Resources
oil field
gas field
coal field
bauxite
iron
lead
mercury
potassium
uranium
zinc
British Isles
Ruhr Valley
Volga Basin
Donbass
Using the Land and Sea
cropland
forest
ice cap
mountain region
pasture
tundra
wetland
major conurbations
cattle
goats
pigs
poultry
reindeer
sheep
cereals
citrus fruits
cotton
fishing
fodder
fruit
olive oil
potatoes
rice
root crops
roses
shellfish
sunflowers
timber
tobacco
vineyards
Oslo
Stockholm
Copenhagen
Liverpool
Leeds
Manchester
The Hague
Amsterdam
Rotterdam
Hamburg
Minsk
Stuttgart
Munich
Vienna
Lyon
Turin
Marseille
Barcelona
Rome
Sofia
Istanbul
Odesa
Kharkiv
Nizhniy Novgorod
Kazan'
Ufa
Samara
Perm'
Ural Mountains
Caucasus

Environmental Issues

The partially enclosed waters of the Baltic and Mediterranean seas have become heavily polluted, while the Barents Sea is contaminated with spent nuclear fuel from Russia's navy. Acid rain, caused by emissions from factories and power stations, is actively destroying northern forests. As a result, pressure is growing to safeguard Europe's natural environment and prevent further deterioration.

***Coniferous forest** covers vast swathes of northern Scandinavia and the Russian Federation. Pollutants from other parts of Europe mixing with rainfall are causing defoliation and serious damage to many forests.*

***The Camargue** in the Rhône Delta, southern France, is a protected wetland area, famous for its native population of white horses, and unique bird and plant life.*

Mineral Resources

Fossil fuels are Europe's main mineral resource, although fuel demand far outstrips production. Sizeable coal reserves remain in the Donbass in Ukraine, Germany's Ruhr Valley, Poland, and in the British Isles. Oil and gas reserves are found mainly in the North Sea, and in the Volga Basin.

***The valuable oil and gas reserves** in the North Sea were first discovered in the early 1960s, and are exploited by the UK, Denmark, Germany, and Norway.*

Using the Land and Sea

Europe's swelling urban population and the outward expansion of many cities has created acute competition for land. Despite this, European resourcefulness has maximized land potential, and over half of Europe's land is still used for a wide variety of agricultural purposes. Land in northern Europe is used for cattle-rearing, pasture, and arable crops. Toward the Mediterranean, the mild climate allows the growing of grapes for wine; olives, sunflowers, tobacco, and citrus fruits. EU subsidies, however, have resulted in massive overproduction and a land "set-aside" policy has been introduced.

***Bulgarian roses** are one of the many diverse crops grown in Europe. Rose oil, extracted from the petals, is used in perfume making.*

***Lowland pastures** are used for dairy farming. Good transportation links and refrigeration allow fresh milk to be distributed throughout Europe.*

Scandinavia, Finland & Iceland

Denmark, Norway, Sweden, Finland, Iceland

Jutting into the Arctic Circle, this northern swath of Europe has some of the continent's harshest environments, but benefits from great reserves of oil, gas, and natural evergreen forests. While most early settlers came from the south, migrants to Finland came from the east, giving it a distinct language and culture. Since the late 19th century, the Scandinavian states have developed strong egalitarian traditions. Today, their welfare benefits systems are among the most extensive in the world, and standards of living are high. The Lapps, or Sami, maintain their traditional lifestyle in the northern regions of Norway, Sweden, and Finland.

GREENLAND SEA
Denmark Strait
ICELAND
REYKJAVÍK
ATLANTIC OCEAN
Vatnajökull
(same scale as main map)

SCALE 1:9,000,000
(projection: Lambert Conformal Conic)

ARCTIC OCEAN
SVALBARD (to Norway)
Spitsbergen
Nordaustlandet
BARENTS SEA
GREENLAND SEA

The Landscape

Glaciers up to 10,000 ft (3,000 m) deep covered most of Scandinavia and Finland during the last Ice Age. The effects of glaciation mark the entire landscape, from the mountains to the lowlands, across the tundra landscape of Lapland, and the lake districts of Sweden and Finland.

Halti Mountain is Finland's highest point, at 4,356 ft (1,328 m).

Lapland, north of the Arctic Circle, is an area of undulating fells and plains known as tundra. The subsoil is permanently frozen and therefore impermeable. There are many peat bogs. Pools reappear in the summer when the surface thaws.

The Lofoten Islands were one of the first areas exposed as the ice sheet melted.

Geysers are a by-product of Iceland's volcanic activity. Geysir, Iceland's largest spring, gives them their name.

Finland's landscape was fashioned by ice action. Glaciers gouged out its distinctive shallow lake basins, such as Oulujärvi, and left debris called moraines in their wake.

Oulujärvi

Fjords

The fjords on the western coast of Norway were once gentle river valleys. Their deep floors and steep sides were carved out by glaciers during the last Ice Age, and they were later flooded by the sea.

Sjælland coast

On the coast of Sjælland, these cliffs have been eroded by the sea, exposing layers of chalk and limestone.

Area of maximum yearly uplift 0.3 in/yr (9 mm/yr)

Slower rates of uplift 0.1 in/yr (3 mm/yr)

Scandinavia is still recovering from the last Ice Age, when ice depressed the land by 2,000 ft (600 m). This gradual uplift is known as isostatic rebound.

SCALE 1:5,500,000
(projection: Lambert Conformal Conic)

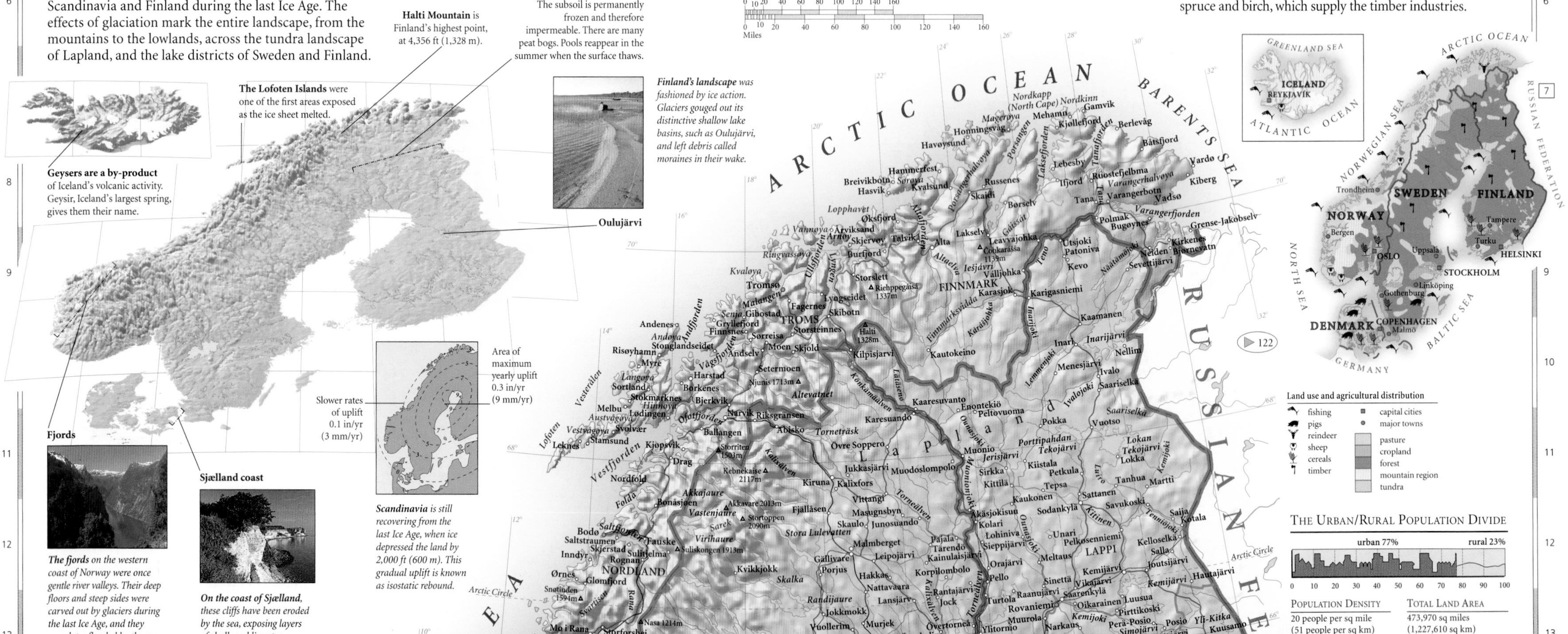

ARCTIC OCEAN
BARENTS SEA
RUSSIAN FEDERATION
FINNMARK
TROMS
NORDLAND
NORRBOTTEN
Lapland
LAPPI

122

Using the Land and Sea

The cold climate, short growing season, poorly developed soil, steep slopes, and exposure to high winds across northern regions means that most agriculture is concentrated, with the population, in the south. Most of Finland and much of Norway and Sweden are covered by dense forests of pine, spruce and birch, which supply the timber industries.

Land use and agricultural distribution: fishing, pigs, reindeer, sheep, cereals, timber; capital cities, major towns; pasture, cropland, forest, mountain region, tundra

The Urban/Rural Population Divide

urban 77% · rural 23%

Population Density	Total Land Area
20 people per sq mile (51 people per sq km)	473,970 sq miles (1,227,610 sq km)

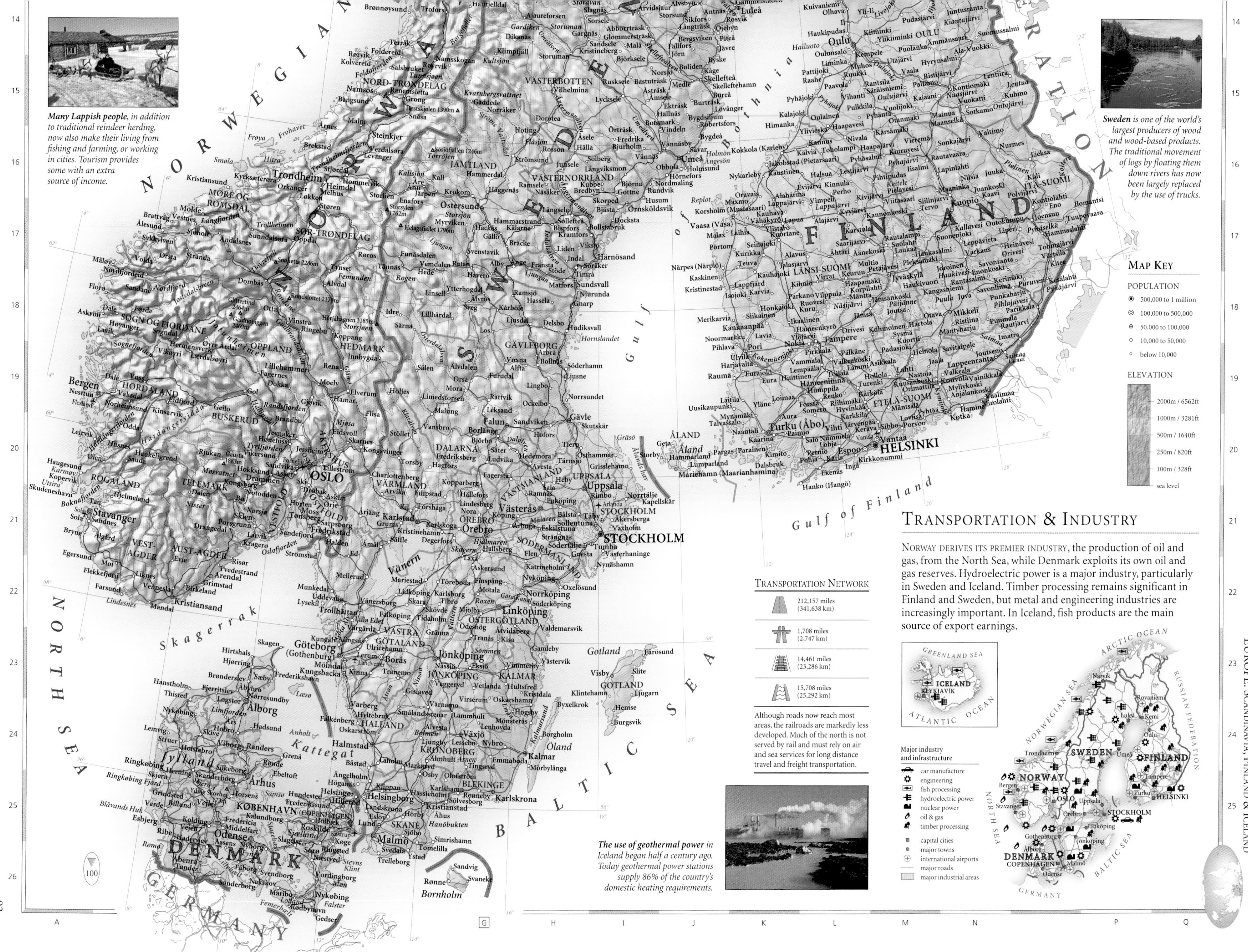

Many Lappish people, in addition to traditional reindeer herding, now also make their living from fishing and farming, or working in cities. Tourism provides some with an extra source of income.
Sweden is one of the world's largest producers of wood and wood-based products. The traditional movement of logs by floating them down rivers has now been largely replaced by the use of trucks.
MAP KEY
POPULATION
500,000 to 1 million
100,000 to 500,000
50,000 to 100,000
10,000 to 50,000
below 10,000
ELEVATION
2000m / 6562ft
1000m / 3281ft
500m / 1640ft
250m / 820ft
100m / 328ft
sea level
TRANSPORTATION & INDUSTRY
NORWAY DERIVES ITS PREMIER INDUSTRY, the production of oil and gas, from the North Sea, while Denmark exploits its own oil and gas reserves. Hydroelectric power is a major industry, particularly in Sweden and Iceland. Timber processing remains significant in Finland and Sweden, but metal and engineering industries are increasingly important. In Iceland, fish products are the main source of export earnings.
TRANSPORTATION NETWORK
212,157 miles (341,638 km)
1,708 miles (2,747 km)
14,461 miles (23,286 km)
15,708 miles (25,292 km)
Although roads now reach most areas, the railroads are markedly less developed. Much of the north is not served by rail and must rely on air and sea services for long distance travel and freight transportation.
The use of geothermal power in Iceland began half a century ago. Today geothermal power stations supply 86% of the country's domestic heating requirements.
Major industry and infrastructure
car manufacture
engineering
fish processing
hydroelectric power
nuclear power
oil & gas
timber processing
capital cities
major towns
international airports
major roads
major industrial areas
NORWEGIAN SEA
NORTH SEA
BALTIC SEA
Gulf of Bothnia
Gulf of Finland
Skagerrak
Kattegat
NORWAY
SWEDEN
FINLAND
DENMARK
GERMANY

Southern Scandinavia

Southern Norway, Southern Sweden, Denmark

Scandinavia's economic and political hub is the more habitable and accessible southern region. Many of the area's major cities are on the southern coasts, including Oslo and Stockholm, the capitals of Norway and Sweden. In Denmark, most of the population and the capital, Copenhagen, are located on its many islands. A cultural unity links the three Scandinavian countries. Their main languages, Danish, Swedish, and Norwegian, are mutually intelligible, and they all retain their monarchies, although the parliaments have legislative control.

Using the Land

Agriculture in southern Scandinavia is highly mechanized although farms are small. Denmark is the most intensively farmed country and its western pastureland is used mainly for pig farming. Cereal crops including wheat, barley, and oats, predominate in eastern Denmark and in the far south of Sweden. Southern Norway, and Sweden have large tracts of forest which are exploited for logging.

The Urban/Rural Population Divide

urban 87% — rural 13%

Population Density	Total Land Area
152 people per sq mile (61 people per sq km)	173,487 sq miles (456,564 sq km)

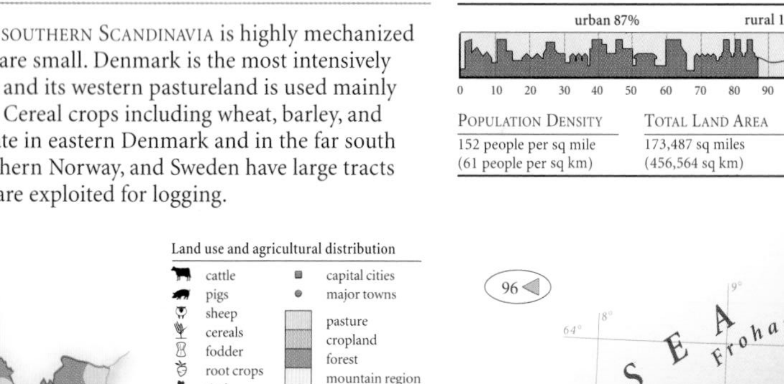

Land use and agricultural distribution
cattle
pigs
sheep
cereals
fodder
root crops
timber
capital cities
major towns
pasture
cropland
forest
mountain region
NORWEGIAN SEA
NORTH SEA
BALTIC SEA
GERMANY
NORWAY
SWEDEN
DENMARK
Trondheim
Bergen
OSLO
STOCKHOLM
Uppsala
Örebro
Linköping
Gothenburg
Ålborg
COPENHAGEN
Odense
Malmö

The Landscape

Southern Scandinavia, with the exception of Norway, has a flatter terrain than the rest of the region. Denmark and southern Sweden are both extensions of the North European Plain. In this area, because of glacial deposition rather than erosion, the soils are deeper and more fertile.

In the past, glaciers such as this one in Olden, Norway, were much larger. Today, many are retreating to yield the spectacular glacial scenery.

Olden

Distinctive low ridges, called eskers, are found across southern Sweden. They are formed from sand and gravel deposits left by retreating glaciers.

The peak of Glittertind in the Jotunheimen Mountains is 8,044 ft (2,452 m) high.

Limestone pillars eroded by the sea dot the coast of Gotland and surrounding islands.

Acid rain, caused by industrial pollution carried north from elsewhere in Europe, harms plant and animal life in Scandinavian forests and lakes. The region's surface rocks lack lime to neutralize the acid, so making the problem more serious.

The lakes of southern Sweden remain from a period when the land was completely flooded. As the ice which covered the area melted, the land rose, leaving lakes in shallow, ice-scoured depressions. Sweden has over 90,000 lakes.

Sognefjorden

Erosion by glaciers deepened existing river valleys

Sea level

When the ice retreated the valley was flooded by the sea

Old valley floor

Sognefjorden is the deepest of Norway's many fjords. It drops to 4,291 ft (1,308 m) below sea level.

Vänern in Sweden is the largest lake in Scandinavia. It covers an area of 2,080 sq miles (5,390 sq km).

Denmark's flat and fertile soils are formed on glacial deposits between 100–160 ft (30–50 m) deep.

In Norway *winters are longer and colder inland than in coastal areas, where the warm current of the North Atlantic Drift moderates the climate.*

Scale 1:3,250,000
(projection: Lambert Conformal Conic)

Map Key

Population
- 500,000 to 1 million
- 100,000 to 500,000
- 50,000 to 100,000
- 10,000 to 50,000
- below 10,000

Elevation
- 2000m / 6562ft
- 1000m / 3281ft
- 500m / 1640ft
- 250m / 820ft
- 100m / 328ft
- sea level

92
96

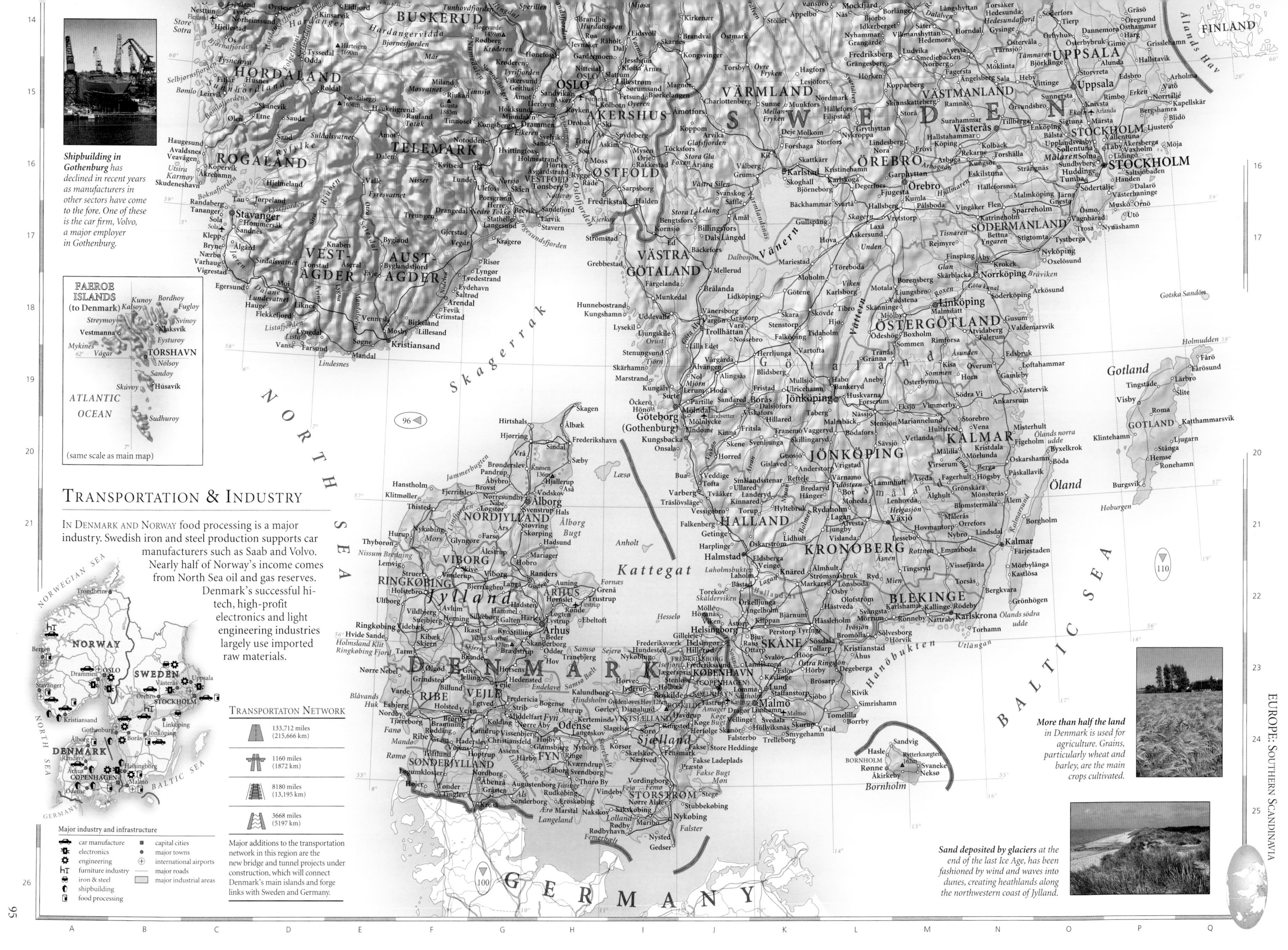
NORWAY
SWEDEN
DENMARK
FINLAND
GERMANY
NORTH SEA
BALTIC SEA
Skagerrak
Kattegat
Ålands Hav
Hanöbukten
BUSKERUD
HORDALAND
ROGALAND
TELEMARK
VEST-AGDER
AUST-AGDER
VESTFOLD
ØSTFOLD
AKERSHUS
OSLO
VÄRMLAND
VÄSTMANLAND
UPPSALA
STOCKHOLM
ÖREBRO
SÖDERMANLAND
VÄSTRA GÖTALAND
ÖSTERGÖTLAND
JÖNKÖPING
KALMAR
HALLAND
KRONOBERG
BLEKINGE
SKÅNE
Götaland
Småland
Gotland
GOTLAND
Öland
Bornholm
NORDJYLLAND
VIBORG
RINGKØBING
ÅRHUS
VEJLE
RIBE
SØNDERJYLLAND
FYN
VESTSJÆLLAND
STORSTRØM
KØBENHAVN
Jylland
Sjælland
Göteborg (Gothenburg)
Kristiansand
Stavanger
Malmö
København
Vänern
Vättern
Mälaren
96
100
110
FAEROE ISLANDS (to Denmark)
TÓRSHAVN
ATLANTIC OCEAN
(same scale as main map)

Shipbuilding in Gothenburg has declined in recent years as manufacturers in other sectors have come to the fore. One of these is the car firm, Volvo, a major employer in Gothenburg.

More than half the land in Denmark is used for agriculture. Grains, particularly wheat and barley, are the main crops cultivated.

Sand deposited by glaciers at the end of the last Ice Age, has been fashioned by wind and waves into dunes, creating heathlands along the northwestern coast of Jylland.

Transportation & Industry

In Denmark and Norway food processing is a major industry. Swedish iron and steel production supports car manufacturers such as Saab and Volvo. Nearly half of Norway's income comes from North Sea oil and gas reserves. Denmark's successful hi-tech, high-profit electronics and light engineering industries largely use imported raw materials.

NORWEGIAN SEA
NORWAY
SWEDEN
DENMARK
NORTH SEA
BALTIC SEA
GERMANY
Trondheim
Bergen
Stavanger
Drammen
OSLO
Kristiansand
Gothenburg
Västerås
Uppsala
STOCKHOLM
Örebro
Linköping
Jönköping
Borås
Helsingborg
Malmö
COPENHAGEN
Århus
Randers
Odense

Major industry and infrastructure
car manufacture
electronics
engineering
furniture industry
iron & steel
shipbuilding
food processing
capital cities
major towns
international airports
major roads
major industrial areas

Transportaton Network

133,712 miles (215,666 km)

1160 miles (1872 km)

8180 miles (13,195 km)

3668 miles (5197 km)

Major additions to the transportation network in this region are the new bridge and tunnel projects under construction, which will connect Denmark's main islands and forge links with Sweden and Germany.

THE BRITISH ISLES

UNITED KINGDOM, REPUBLIC OF IRELAND

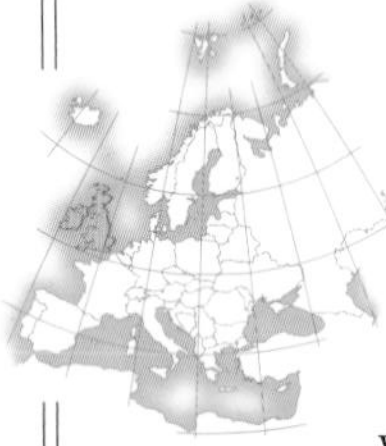

THE BRITISH ISLES have for centuries played a central role in European and world history. England, Wales, Scotland, and Northern Ireland together form the United Kingdom (UK), while the southern portion of Ireland is an independent country, self-governing since 1921. Although England has tended to be the politically and economically dominant partner in the UK, the Scots, Welsh and Irish maintain independent cultures, distinct national identities and languages. Southeastern England is the most densely populated part of this crowded region, with over nine million people living in and around the London area.

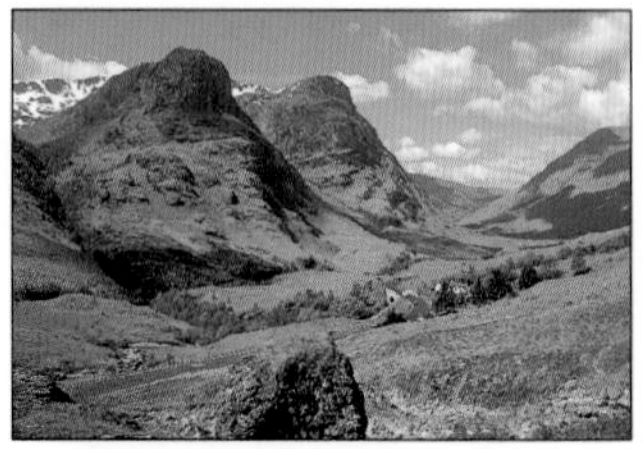

The valley of Glen Coe *in the Scottish Highlands is a U-shaped valley, typical of the north and west of the British Isles, where glaciers shaped much of the landscape.*

TRANSPORT AND INDUSTRY

THE BRITISH ISLES' INDUSTRIAL BASE was founded primarily on coal, iron and textiles, based largely in the north. Today, the most productive sectors include hi-tech industries clustered mainly in southeastern England, chemicals, finance and the service sector, particularly tourism.

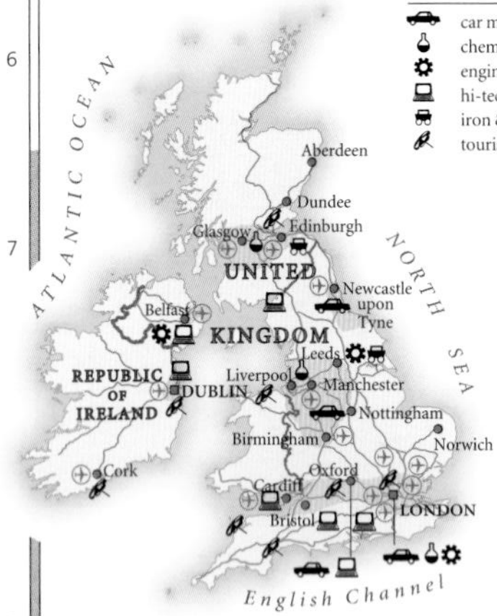

Major industry and infrastructure

car manufacture
chemicals
engineering
hi-tech industry
iron & steel
tourism
capital cities
major towns
international airports
major roads
major industrial areas

TRANSPORTATION NETWORK

288,330 miles (464,300 km)		2,046 miles (3,295 km)	
11,874 miles (19,121 km)		3,806 miles (6,129 km)	

The UK's congested roads have become a major focus of environmental concern in recent years. No longer an island, the UK was finally linked to continental Europe by the Channel Tunnel in 1994.

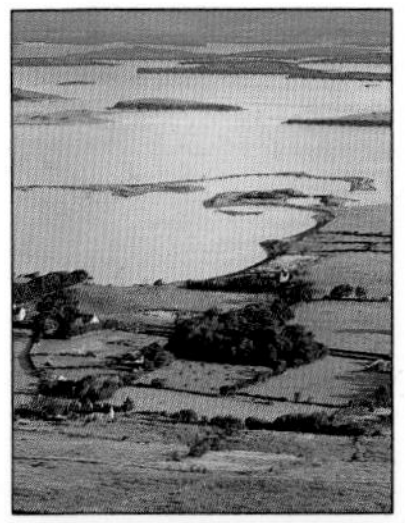

Clew Bay *in western Ireland, is characteristic of the heavily indented west coast, where deep wide-mouthed bays separate the mountains of Mayo, Donegal, and Kerry as they thrust out into the Atlantic Ocean.*

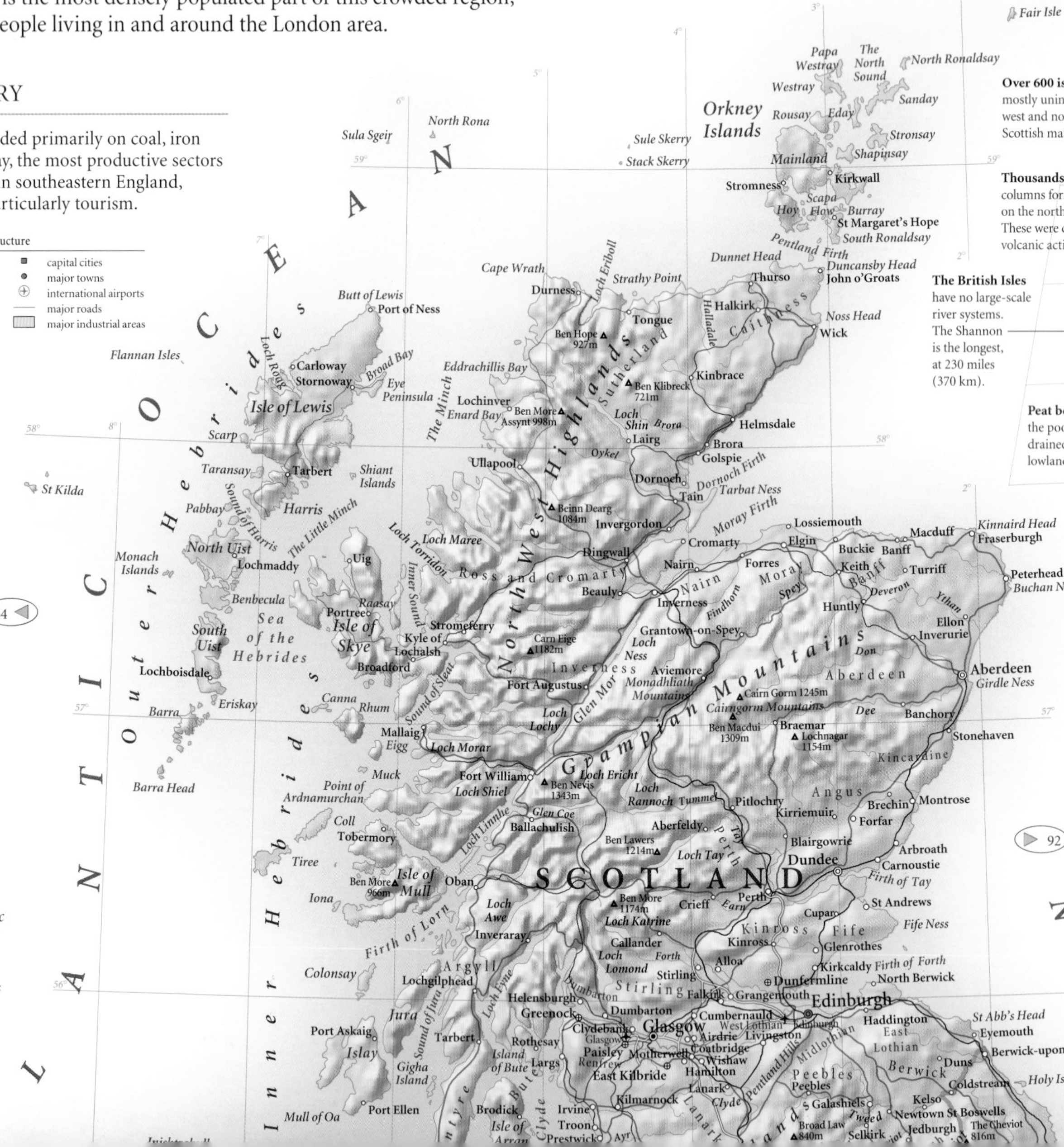

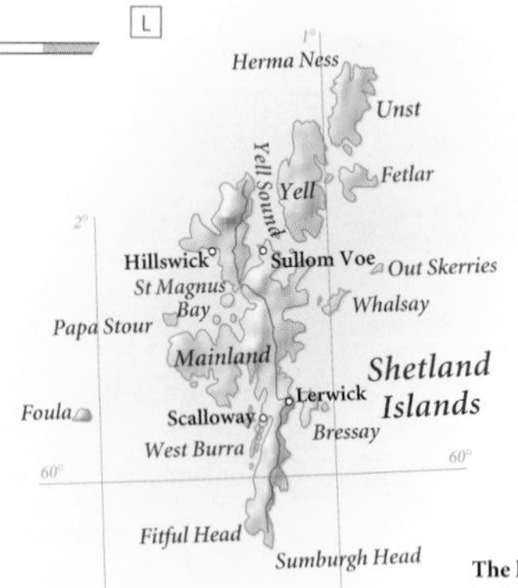

THE LANDSCAPE

RUGGED UPLANDS dominate the landscape of Scotland, Wales, and northern England. All the peaks in the British Isles over 4,000 ft (1,219 m) lie in highland Scotland. Lowland England rises into several ranges of rolling hills, including the older Mendips, and the Cotswolds and the Chilterns, which were formed at the same time as the Alps in southern Europe.

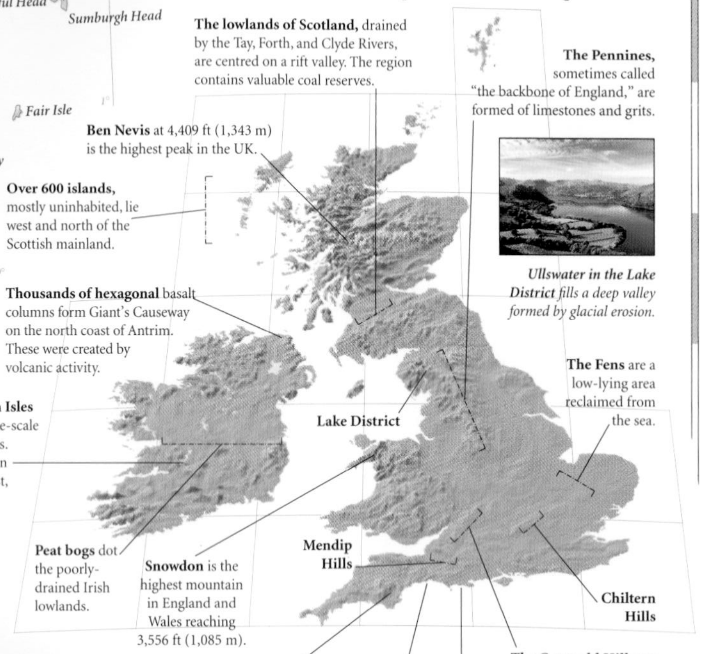

The lowlands of Scotland, drained by the Tay, Forth, and Clyde Rivers, are centred on a rift valley. The region contains valuable coal reserves.

The Pennines, sometimes called "the backbone of England," are formed of limestones and grits.

Ben Nevis at 4,409 ft (1,343 m) is the highest peak in the UK.

Over 600 islands, mostly uninhabited, lie west and north of the Scottish mainland.

Ullswater in the Lake District *fills a deep valley formed by glacial erosion.*

Thousands of hexagonal basalt columns form Giant's Causeway on the north coast of Antrim. These were created by volcanic activity.

The Fens are a low-lying area reclaimed from the sea.

Lake District

The British Isles have no large-scale river systems. The Shannon is the longest, at 230 miles (370 km).

Peat bogs dot the poorly-drained Irish lowlands.

Snowdon is the highest mountain in England and Wales reaching 3,556 ft (1,085 m).

Mendip Hills

Chiltern Hills

The Cotswold Hills are characterized by a series of limestone ridges overlooking clay vales.

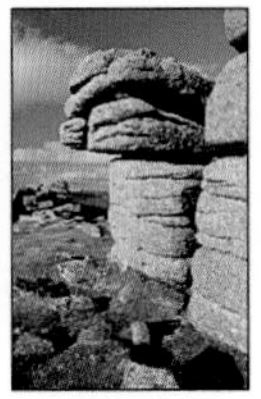

Dartmoor, *studded with tors, is an exposed part of a vast granite dome, formed when molten rock intruded into the Earth's crust.*

Durdle Door

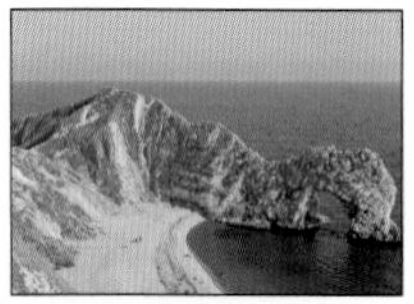

Coastal erosion *around the British Isles forms striking features such as this limestone arch, Durdle Door in Dorset.*

Black Ven, Lyme Regis

Water
Mudslide
Sea
Cracks
Sandstone
Clay
Limestone

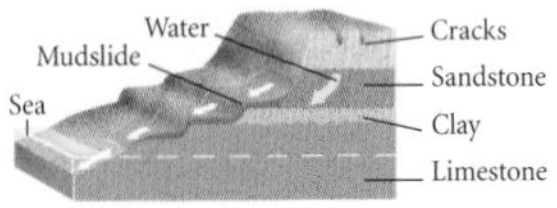

Much of the south coast *is subject to landslides. Following rain, porous sandstones feed water into the underlying, less permeable clays which then crumble and slide into the sea.*

MAP KEY

POPULATION

- above 5 million
- 1 million to 5 million
- 500,000 to 1 million
- 100,000 to 500,000
- 50,000 to 100,000
- 10,000 to 50,000
- below 10,000

ELEVATION

- 1000m / 3281ft
- 500m / 1640ft
- 250m / 820ft
- 100m / 328ft
- sea level

64

92

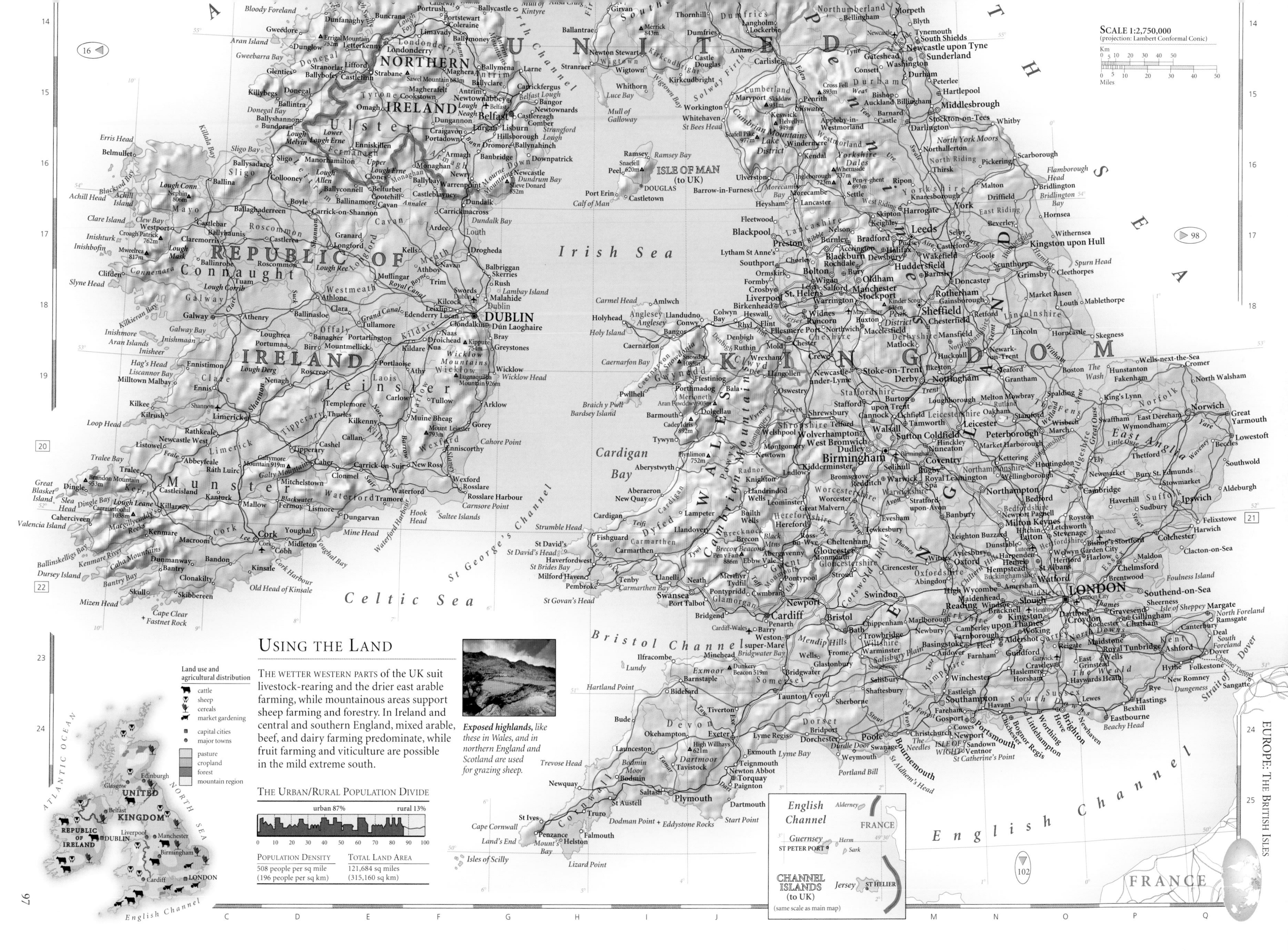
SCALE 1:2,750,000
(projection: Lambert Conformal Conic)
Km 0 5 10 20 30 40 50
Miles 0 5 10 20 30 40 50
REPUBLIC OF IRELAND
NORTHERN IRELAND
UNITED KINGDOM
ENGLAND
WALES
ISLE OF MAN (to UK)
DUBLIN
LONDON
Irish Sea
Celtic Sea
Bristol Channel
English Channel
St George's Channel
North Channel
Cardigan Bay
Ulster
Connaught
Leinster
Munster
Pennines
Cambrian Mountains
FRANCE
English Channel
CHANNEL ISLANDS (to UK)
(same scale as main map)
Alderney
Guernsey
ST PETER PORT
Herm
Sark
Jersey
ST HELIER
16
98
102
Land use and agricultural distribution
cattle
sheep
cereals
market gardening
capital cities
major towns
pasture
cropland
forest
mountain region
ATLANTIC OCEAN
NORTH SEA
English Channel
Exposed highlands, like these in Wales, and in northern England and Scotland are used for grazing sheep.
THE URBAN/RURAL POPULATION DIVIDE
urban 87%
rural 13%
0 10 20 30 40 50 60 70 80 90 100

USING THE LAND

THE WETTER WESTERN PARTS of the UK suit livestock-rearing and the drier east arable farming, while mountainous areas support sheep farming and forestry. In Ireland and central and southern England, mixed arable, beef, and dairy farming predominate, while fruit farming and viticulture are possible in the mild extreme south.

POPULATION DENSITY	TOTAL LAND AREA
508 people per sq mile	121,684 sq miles
(196 people per sq km)	(315,160 sq km)

The Low Countries

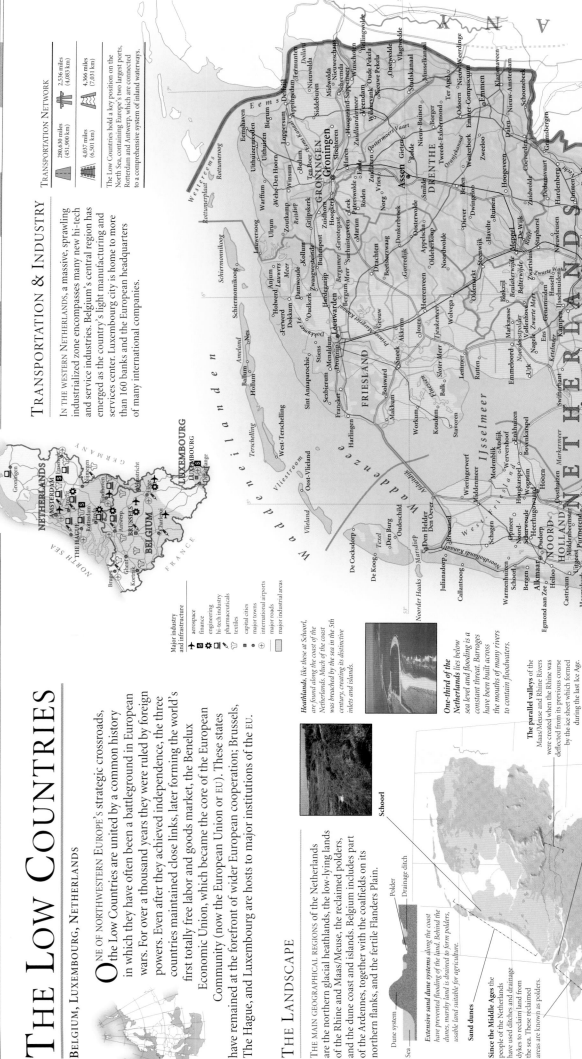

Belgium, Luxembourg, Netherlands

One of northwestern Europe's strategic crossroads, the Low Countries are united by a common history in which they have often been a battleground in European wars. For over a thousand years they were ruled by foreign powers. Even after they achieved independence, the three countries maintained close links, later forming the world's first totally free labor and goods market, the Benelux Economic Union, which became the core of the European Community (now the European Union or EU). These states have remained at the forefront of wider European cooperation; Brussels, The Hague, and Luxembourg are hosts to major institutions of the EU.

Transportation & Industry

In the western Netherlands, a massive, sprawling industrialized zone encompasses many new hi-tech and service industries. Belgium's central region has emerged as the country's light manufacturing and services center. Luxembourg city is home to more than 160 banks and the European headquarters of many international companies.

Transportation Network

280,630 miles (451,900 km)	2,536 miles (4,083 km)
4,037 miles (6,501 km)	4,366 miles (7,031 km)

The Low Countries hold a key position on the North Sea, containing Europe's two largest ports, Rotterdam and Antwerp, which are connected to a comprehensive system of inland waterways.

Major industry and infrastructure
- aerospace
- finance
- engineering
- hi-tech industry
- pharmaceuticals
- textiles
- capital cities
- major towns
- international airports
- major roads
- major industrial areas

The Landscape

The main geographical regions of the Netherlands are the northern glacial heathlands, the low-lying lands of the Rhine and Maas/Meuse, the reclaimed polders, and the dune coast and islands. Belgium includes part of the Ardennes, together with the coalfields on its northern flanks, and the fertile Flanders Plain.

Dune system — Sea — Polder — Drainage ditch

Extensive sand dune systems along the coast have prevented flooding of the land. Behind the dunes, marshy land is drained to form polders, usable land suitable for agriculture.

Heathlands, like these at Schoorl, are found along the coast of the Netherlands. Much of the coast was breached by the sea in the 5th century, creating its distinctive inlets and islands.

***One-third of the Netherlands** lies below sea level and flooding is a constant threat. Barrages have been built across the mouths of many rivers to contain floodwaters.*

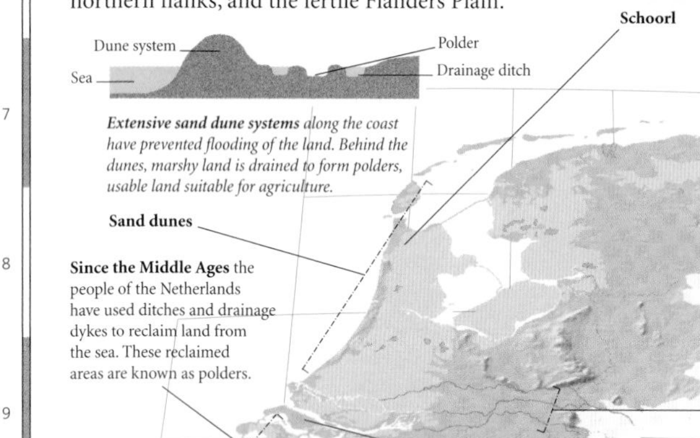

Schoorl

Sand dunes

Since the Middle Ages the people of the Netherlands have used ditches and drainage dykes to reclaim land from the sea. These reclaimed areas are known as polders.

The parallel valleys of the Maas/Meuse and Rhine Rivers were created when the Rhine was deflected from its previous course by the ice sheet which formed during the last Ice Age.

Silts and sands eroded by the Rhine throughout its course are deposited to form a delta on the west coast of the Netherlands.

The loess soils of the Flanders Plain in western Belguim provide excellent conditions for arable farming.

Ardennes

***Uplifted and folded** 220 million years ago, the Ardennes have since been reduced to relatively level plateaus, then sharply incised by rivers such as the Maas/Meuse.*

Hautes Fagnes is the highest part of Belgium. The bogs and streams in this upland region result from high rainfall and low temperatures.

▶ 100

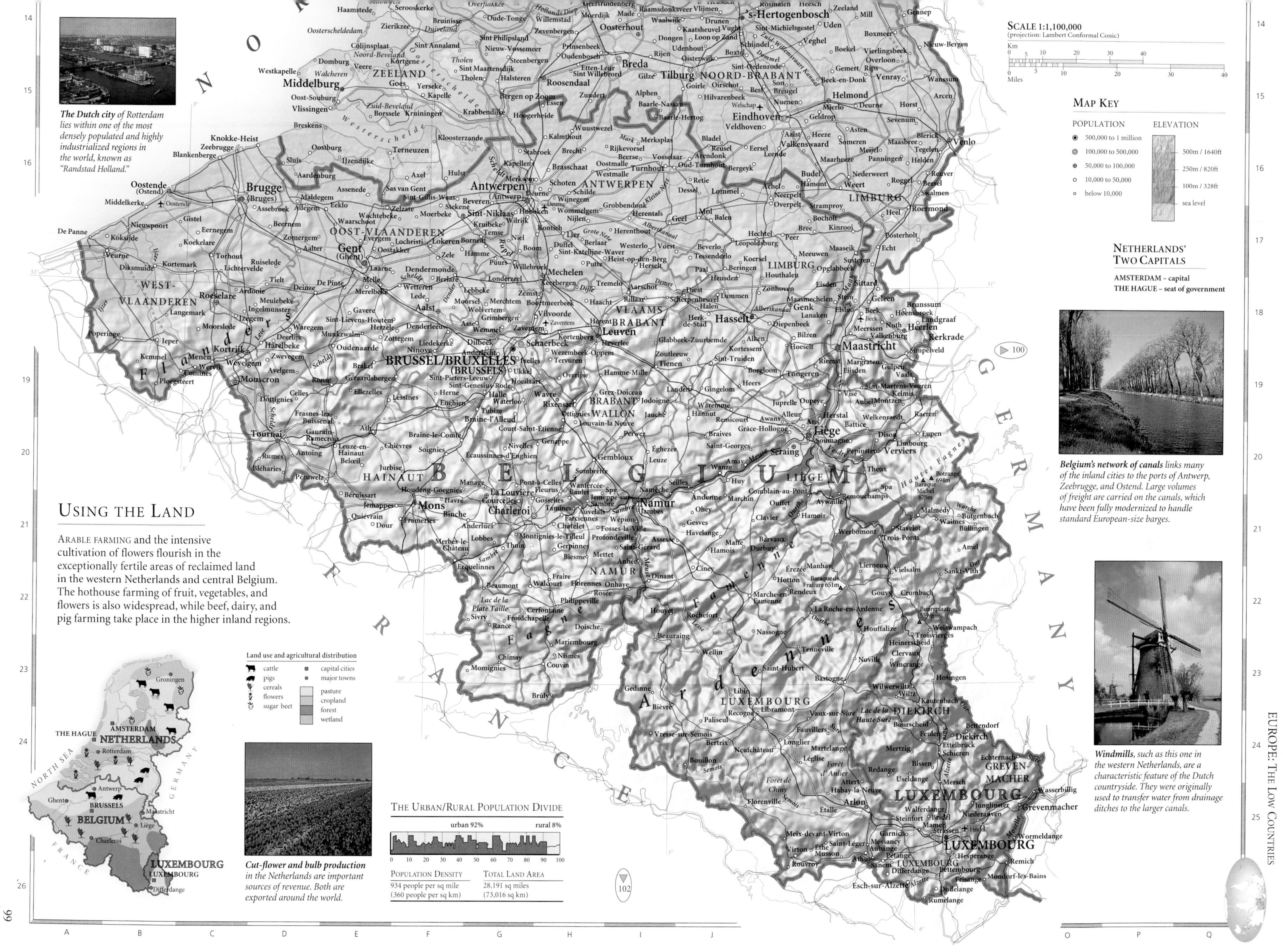

SCALE 1:1,100,000
(projection: Lambert Conformal Conic)
Km 0 5 10 20 30 40
Miles 0 5 10 20 30 40
MAP KEY
POPULATION
500,000 to 1 million
100,000 to 500,000
50,000 to 100,000
10,000 to 50,000
below 10,000
ELEVATION
500m / 1640ft
250m / 820ft
100m / 328ft
sea level
NORTH SEA
GERMANY
FRANCE
BELGIUM
LUXEMBOURG
ZEELAND
NOORD-BRABANT
LIMBURG
WEST-VLAANDEREN
OOST-VLAANDEREN
ANTWERPEN
VLAAMS BRABANT
BRABANT WALLON
HAINAUT
NAMUR
LIÈGE
DIEKIRCH
GREVENMACHER
Flanders
Famenne
Fagne
Ardennes
BRUSSEL/BRUXELLES (BRUSSELS)
Antwerpen (Antwerp)
Gent (Ghent)
Brugge (Bruges)
Oostende (Ostend)
Liège
Charleroi
Namur
Mons
Leuven
Hasselt
Maastricht
Eindhoven
Tilburg
Breda
's-Hertogenbosch
Middelburg
Kortrijk
Roeselare
Mouscron
Tournai
Sint-Niklaas
Mechelen
Aalst
Verviers
Seraing
La Louvière
Arlon
Luxembourg
100
102

The Dutch city of Rotterdam lies within one of the most densely populated and highly industrialized regions in the world, known as "Randstad Holland."

Using the Land

ARABLE FARMING and the intensive cultivation of flowers flourish in the exceptionally fertile areas of reclaimed land in the western Netherlands and central Belgium. The hothouse farming of fruit, vegetables, and flowers is also widespread, while beef, dairy, and pig farming take place in the higher inland regions.

Land use and agricultural distribution
cattle
pigs
cereals
flowers
sugar beet
capital cities
major towns
pasture
cropland
forest
wetland
NORTH SEA
GERMANY
FRANCE
THE HAGUE
AMSTERDAM
NETHERLANDS
Groningen
Rotterdam
Antwerp
Ghent
BRUSSELS
BELGIUM
Maastricht
Liège
Charleroi
LUXEMBOURG
Differdange

Cut-flower and bulb production in the Netherlands are important sources of revenue. Both are exported around the world.

The Urban/Rural Population Divide

urban 92% rural 8%

0 10 20 30 40 50 60 70 80 90 100

Population Density	Total Land Area
934 people per sq mile	28,191 sq miles
(360 people per sq km)	(73,016 sq km)

Netherlands' Two Capitals

AMSTERDAM – capital
THE HAGUE – seat of government

Belgium's network of canals links many of the inland cities to the ports of Antwerp, Zeebrugge, and Ostend. Large volumes of freight are carried on the canals, which have been fully modernized to handle standard European-size barges.

Windmills, such as this one in the western Netherlands, are a characteristic feature of the Dutch countryside. They were originally used to transfer water from drainage ditches to the larger canals.

GERMANY

DESPITE THE DEVASTATION of its industry and infrastructure during the Second World War and its separation from eastern Germany during the Cold War, West Germany made a rapid recovery in the following generation to become Europe's most formidable economic power. When the Berlin Wall was dismantled in 1989, the two halves of Germany were politically united for the first time in 40 years. Complete social and economic unity remain a longer term goal, as East German industry and society adapt to a free market. Germany has been a key player in the creation of the European Union (EU) and in moves toward a single European currency.

USING THE LAND

GERMANY has a large, efficient agricultural sector, and produces more than three-quarters of its own food. The major crops grown are cereals and sugar beet on the more fertile soils, and root crops, rye, oats, and fodder on the poorer soils of the northern plains and central uplands. Southern Germany is also a principal producer of high quality wines. Vineyards cover the slopes surrounding the Rhine and its tributaries.

Land use and agricultural distribution

- cattle
- pigs
- cereals
- sugar beet
- vineyards
- capital cities
- major towns
- pasture
- cropland
- forest

THE URBAN/RURAL POPULATION DIVIDE

urban 87% — rural 13%

POPULATION DENSITY	TOTAL LAND AREA
598 people per sq mile (231 people per sq km)	13,804 sq miles (356,910 sq km)

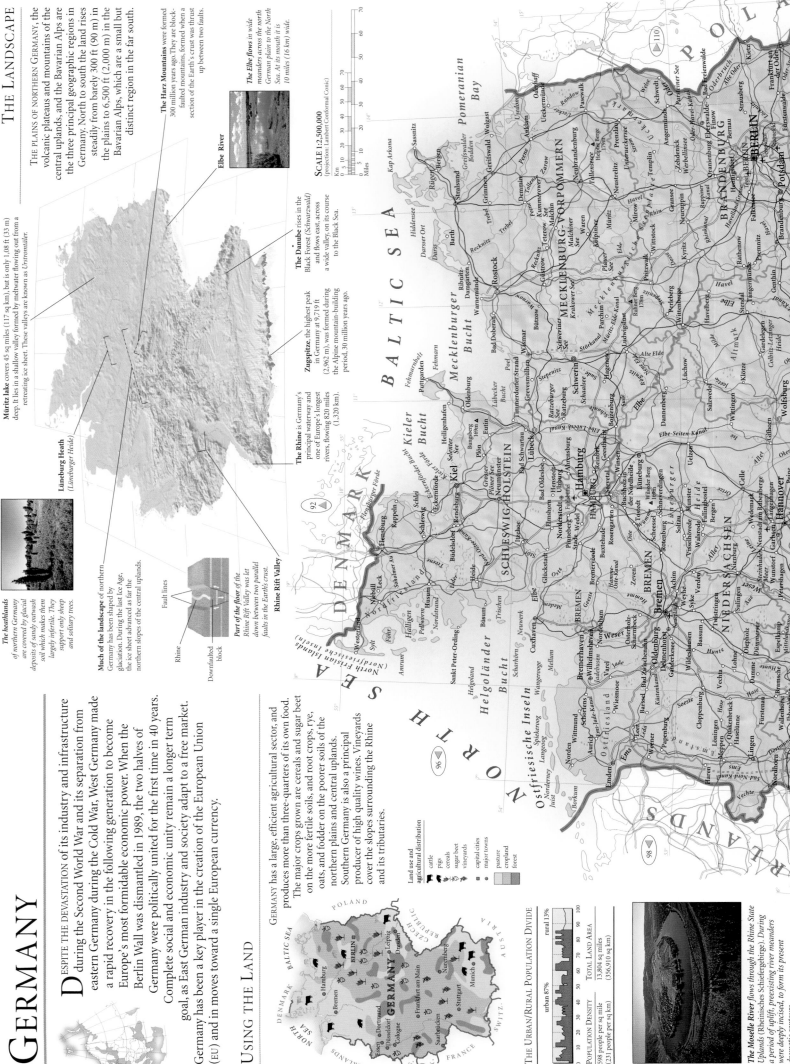

***The Moselle River** flows through the Rhine State Uplands* (Rheinisches Schiefergebirge). *During a period of uplift, preexisting river meanders were deeply incised, to form its present dramatic contours.*

THE LANDSCAPE

THE PLAINS OF NORTHERN GERMANY, the volcanic plateaus and mountains of the central uplands, and the Bavarian Alps are the three principal geographic regions in Germany. North to south the land rises steadily from barely 300 ft (90 m) in the plains to 6,500 ft (2,000 m) in the Bavarian Alps, which are a small but distinct region in the far south.

***The heathlands** of northern Germany are covered by glacial deposits of sandy outwash soil which makes them largely infertile. They support only sheep and solitary trees.*

Lüneburg Heath (*Lüneburger Heide*)

Much of the landscape of northern Germany has been shaped by glaciation. During the last Ice Age, the ice sheet advanced as far the northern slopes of the central uplands.

Müritz lake covers 45 sq miles (117 sq km), but is only 1,08 ft (33 m) deep. It lies in a shallow valley formed by meltwater flowing out from a retreating ice sheet. These valleys are known as *Urstromtäler.*

Fault lines

Rhine

Downfaulted block

***Part of the floor** of the Rhine Rift Valley was let down between two parallel faults in the Earth's crust.*

Rhine Rift Valley

The Harz Mountains were formed 300 million years ago. They are block-faulted mountains, formed when a section of the Earth's crust was thrust up between two faults.

Elbe River

***The Elbe flows** in wide meanders across the north German plain to the North Sea. At its mouth it is 10 miles (16 km) wide.*

The Rhine is Germany's principal waterway and one of Europe's longest rivers, flowing 820 miles (1,320 km).

Zugspitze, the highest peak in Germany at 9,719 ft (2,962 m), was formed during the Alpine mountain-building period, 30 million years ago.

The Danube rises in the Black Forest (*Schwarzwald*) and flows east, across a wide valley, on its course to the Black Sea.

SCALE 1:2,500,000
(projection: Lambert Conformal Conic)

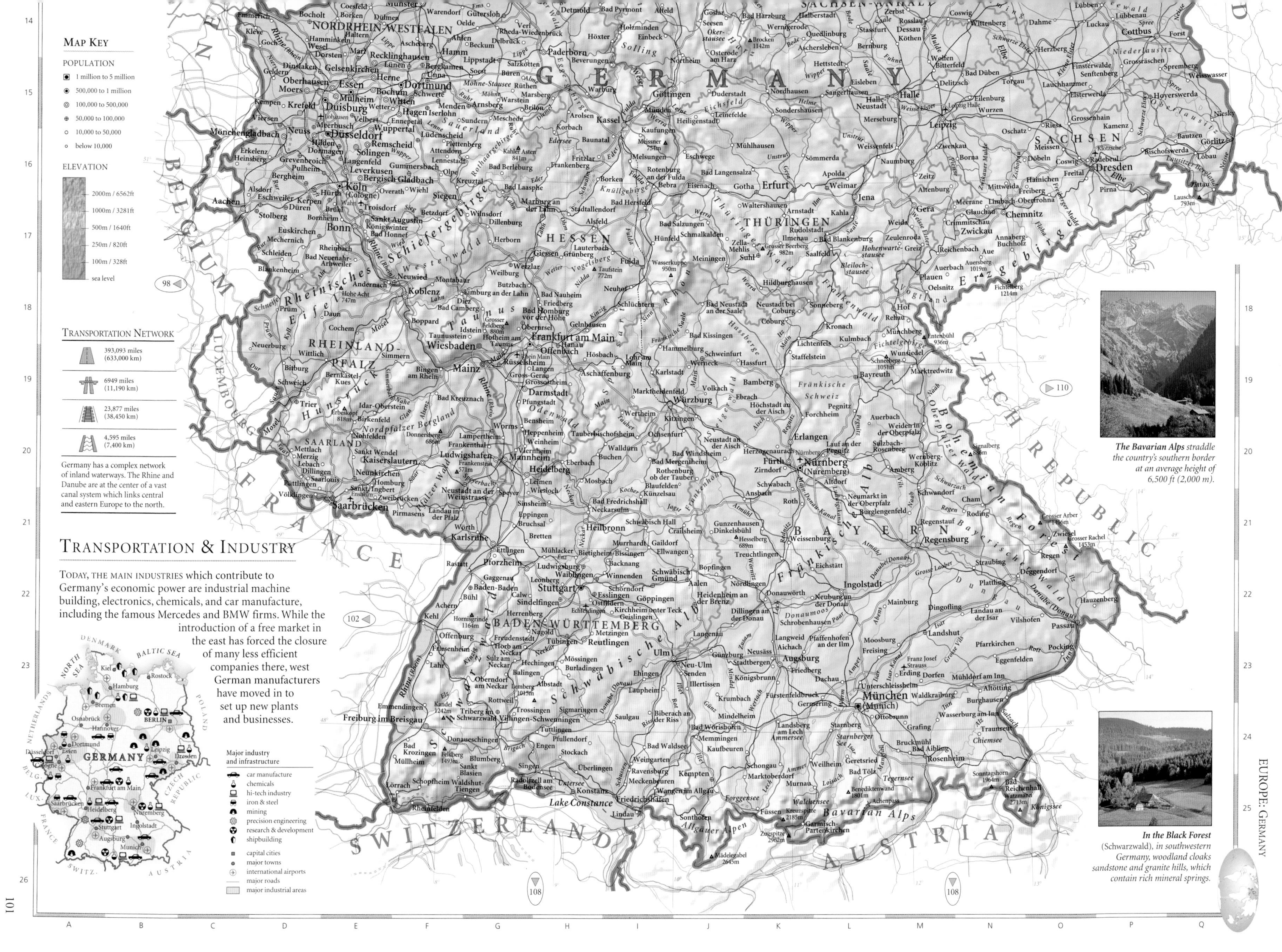
GERMANY
NORDRHEIN-WESTFALEN
HESSEN
THÜRINGEN
SACHSEN
RHEINLAND-PFALZ
SAARLAND
BADEN-WÜRTTEMBERG
BAYERN
BELGIUM
LUXEMBOURG
FRANCE
SWITZERLAND
AUSTRIA
CZECH REPUBLIC
Lake Constance
Bavarian Alps
Erzgebirge
Schwäbische Alb
Fränkische Alb
Bohemian Forest
Köln
Düsseldorf
Essen
Dortmund
Bonn
Frankfurt am Main
Wiesbaden
Mainz
Saarbrücken
Kaiserslautern
Mannheim
Heidelberg
Karlsruhe
Stuttgart
Freiburg im Breisgau
Ulm
Augsburg
München (Munich)
Nürnberg (Nuremberg)
Würzburg
Regensburg
Ingolstadt
Erfurt
Jena
Leipzig
Halle
Dresden
Chemnitz
Zwickau
Kassel
Göttingen
Cottbus
98
102
108
110

Map Key

POPULATION
- 1 million to 5 million
- 500,000 to 1 million
- 100,000 to 500,000
- 50,000 to 100,000
- 10,000 to 50,000
- below 10,000

ELEVATION
- 2000m / 6562ft
- 1000m / 3281ft
- 500m / 1640ft
- 250m / 820ft
- 100m / 328ft
- sea level

Transportation Network

- 393,093 miles (633,000 km)
- 6949 miles (11,190 km)
- 23,877 miles (38,450 km)
- 4,595 miles (7,400 km)

Germany has a complex network of inland waterways. The Rhine and Danube are at the center of a vast canal system which links central and eastern Europe to the north.

Transportation & Industry

Today, the main industries which contribute to Germany's economic power are industrial machine building, electronics, chemicals, and car manufacture, including the famous Mercedes and BMW firms. While the introduction of a free market in the east has forced the closure of many less efficient companies there, west German manufacturers have moved in to set up new plants and businesses.

DENMARK
NORTH SEA
BALTIC SEA
POLAND
NETHERLANDS
BELG.
LUX.
FRANCE
SWITZ.
AUSTRIA
CZECH REPUBLIC
GERMANY
BERLIN
Kiel
Rostock
Hamburg
Bremen
Hannover
Osnabrück
Dortmund
Essen
Düsseldorf
Cologne
Leipzig
Dresden
Frankfurt am Main
Saarbrücken
Heidelberg
Stuttgart
Nuremberg
Ingolstadt
Augsburg
Munich
Major industry and infrastructure
car manufacture
chemicals
hi-tech industry
iron & steel
mining
precision engineering
research & development
shipbuilding
capital cities
major towns
international airports
major roads
major industrial areas

The Bavarian Alps straddle the country's southern border at an average height of 6,500 ft (2,000 m).

In the Black Forest (Schwarzwald), *in southwestern Germany, woodland cloaks sandstone and granite hills, which contain rich mineral springs.*

FRANCE

FRANCE, MONACO

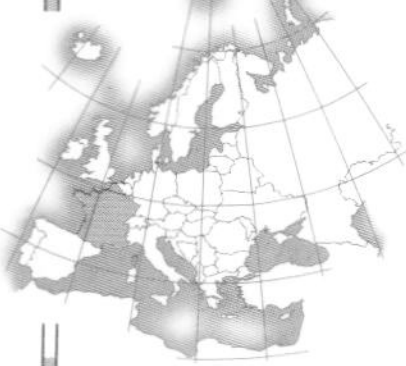

EUROPE'S SECOND LARGEST nation and the founder of modern Republican government, France is a major center of culture and fashion, and a leading producer of both agricultural and industrial goods. It has played a leading role in European events for centuries, and remains a key player in the push toward European unity. The Paris Basin is the most highly populated area; Île de France is home to over nine million people. Large parts of France remain thinly populated, particularly the mountainous Massif Central, Pyrennees, and southern Alps.

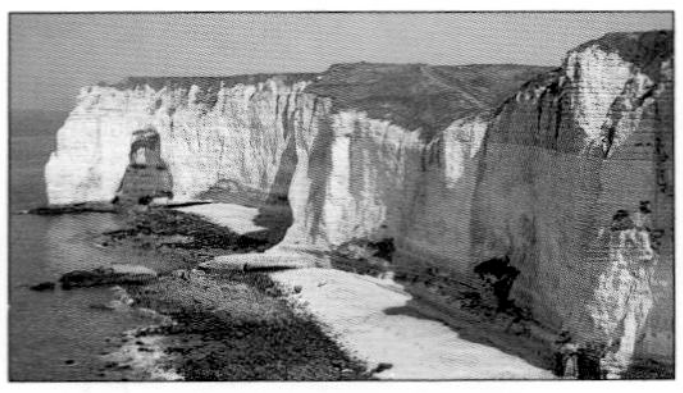

The chalk cliffs of Normandy (Normandie) *and southeastern England form part of a single geological region, now divided in two by the English Channel.*

THE LANDSCAPE

FRANCE'S LANDSCAPE was fashioned by two phases of mountain-building. The northwestern peninsula, the Massif Central, and the Vosges date from 220 million years ago. The complex folds of the Alps and Pyrenees, the gently-folded Jura, and the low-lying sedimentary areas of the Paris, Garonne, and Rhône basins started to form 65 million years ago.

The coast of Brittany *(Bretagne)* is highly indented where deep valleys in the northwestern peninsula were drowned by the sea.

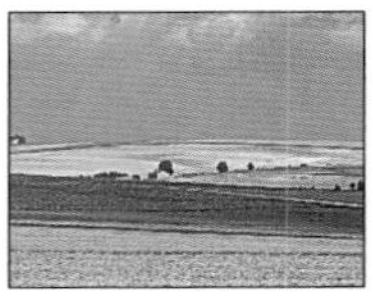

The Normandy *(Normandie)* coastline is characterized by high chalk cliffs.

The coastline of France is 2,141 miles (3,427 km) long.

The Paris Basin consists of a layered sequence of sedimentary rocks. Fertile soils over much of the area make good agricultural land.

The gently rounded summits of the Vosges are over 200 million years old.

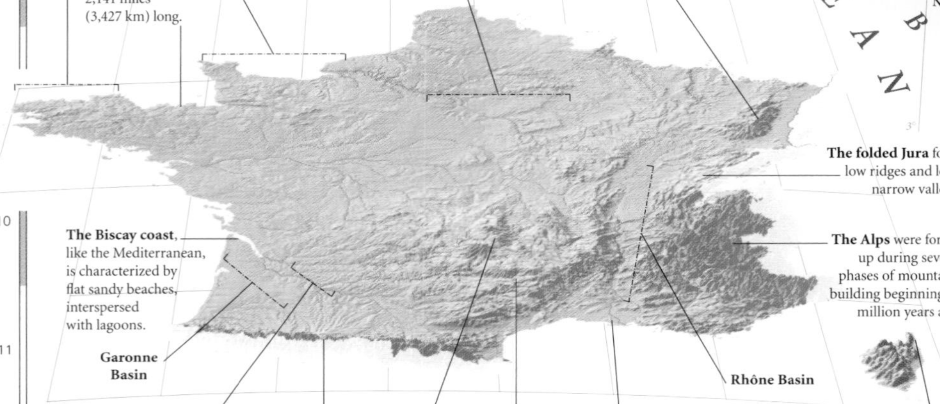

The folded Jura form low ridges and long narrow valleys.

The Alps were forced up during several phases of mountain-building beginning 65 million years ago.

The Biscay coast, like the Mediterranean, is characterized by flat sandy beaches, interspersed with lagoons.

Garonne Basin

Rhône Basin

The Dordogne region contains spectacular examples of limestone scenery including caves and gorges.

The Pyrenees form a natural border between France and Spain.

The ancient Massif Central, disturbed by the formation of the Alps, was subject to volcanism that only ceased during the last 10,000 years.

Rhône Delta

Rhône

Delta plain

The marshes of the Camargue

Corsica's northeastern peninsula has dramatic cliffs of folded limestone.

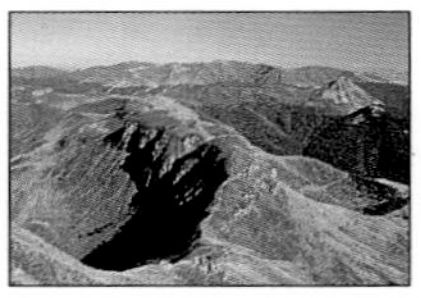

The volcanic landscape of the Auvergne where the cones of its extinct volcanoes have worn away to leave "plugs" of lava.

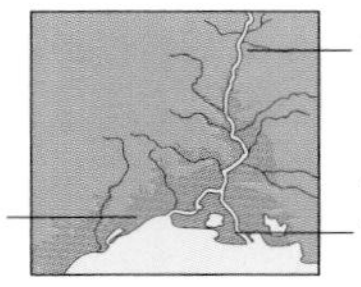

***Deposition in the Rhône Delta** is wave-dominated. Sea currents carry river sediments extending the delta plain westwards.*

TRANSPORTATION & INDUSTRY

TODAY THE MAIN FRENCH GROWTH INDUSTRIES are hi-tech, including microelectronics, telecommunications, and aerospace. Other important sectors are the nuclear industry, only rivalled in scale by that of the USA, car manufacture, dominated by the giants Renault and Peugeot and a highly diversified tourist industry.

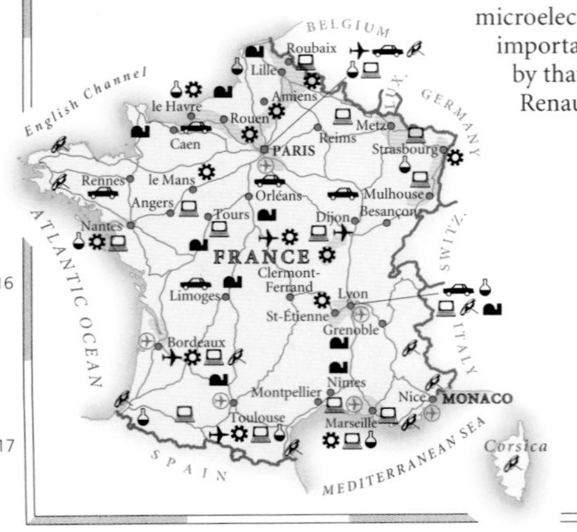

Major industry and infrastructure
- aerospace industry
- car manufacture
- chemicals
- engineering
- hi-tech industry
- nuclear power
- tourism
- capital cities
- major towns
- international airports
- major roads
- major industrial areas

TRANSPORTATION NETWORK

599,017 miles (964,600 km)	5,900 miles (9,500 km)
19,761 miles (31,821 km)	5,279 miles (8,500 km)

The French TGV (*Train à Grande Vitesse*) leads the world in high-speed train technology, and provides a service which is faster, door-to-door, than air travel.

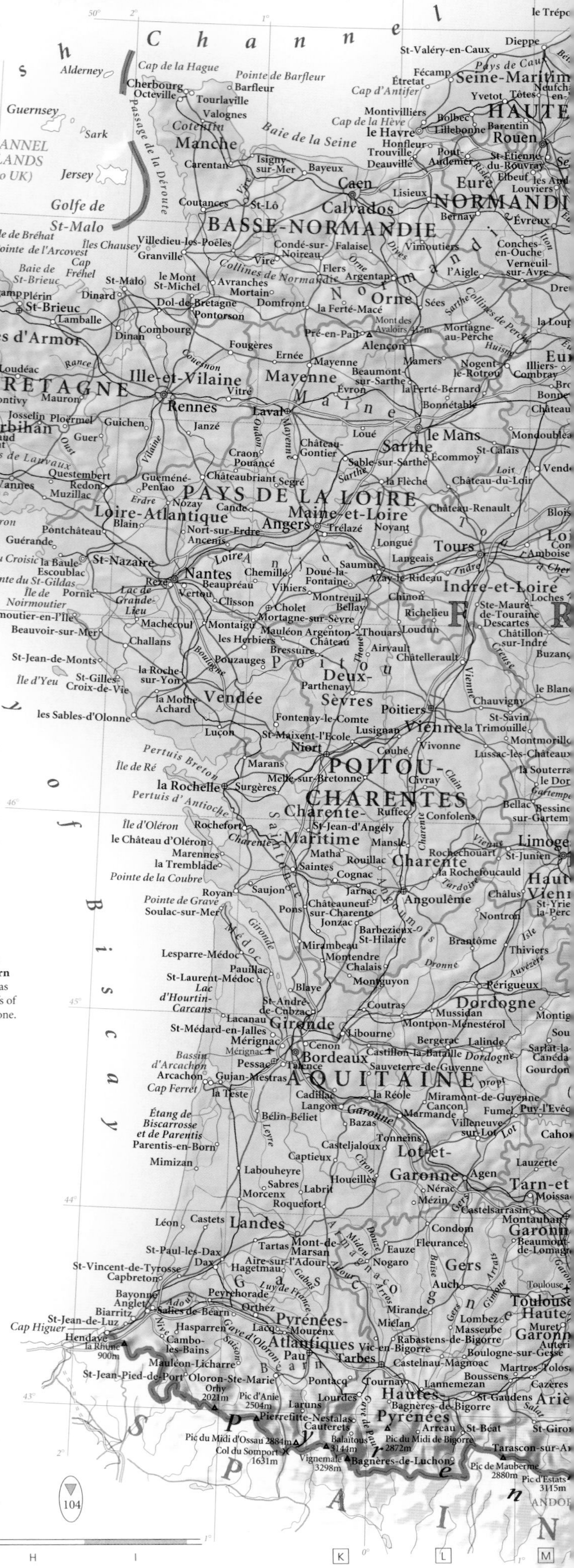

64
96
104

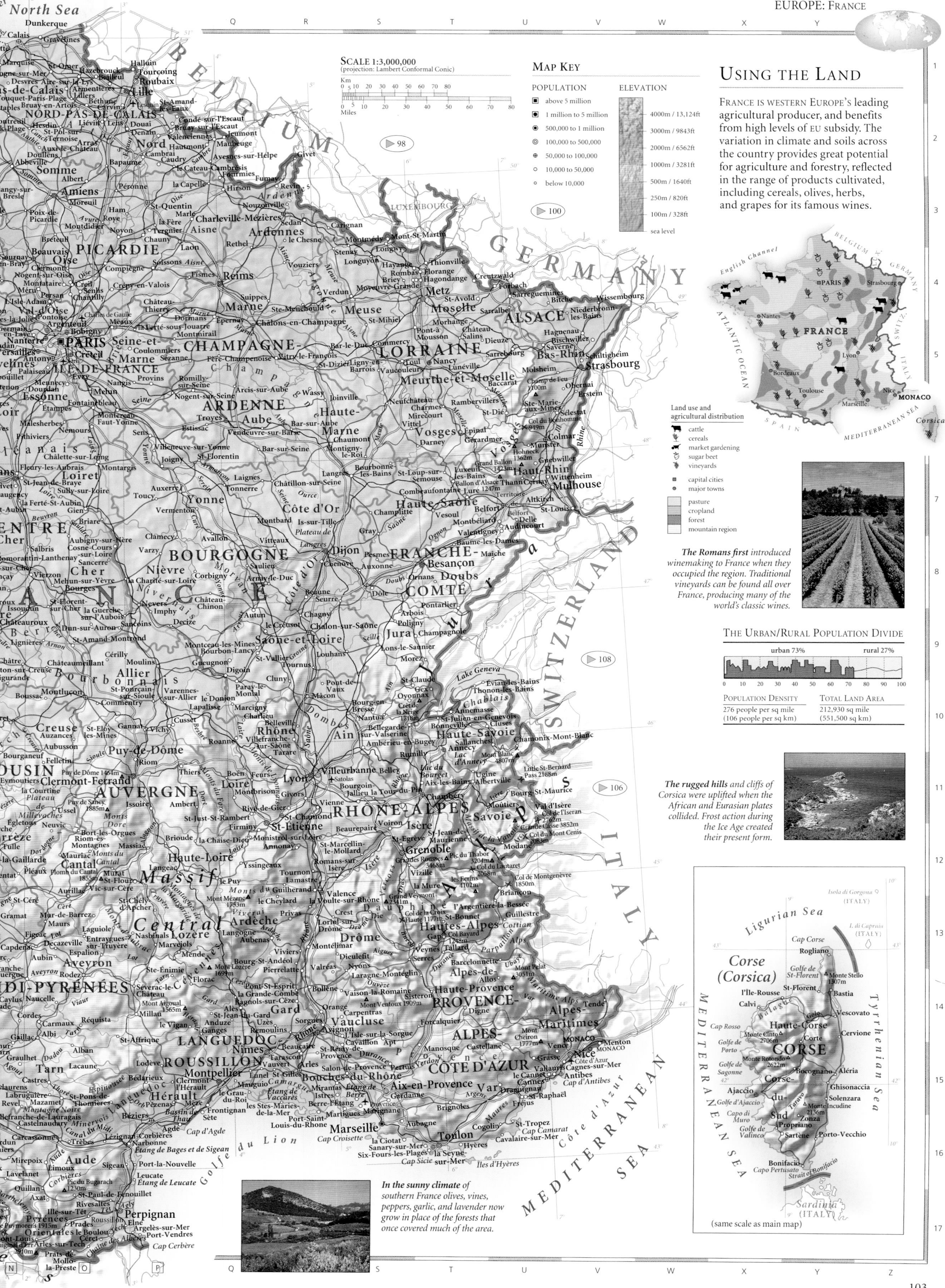
USING THE LAND
FRANCE IS WESTERN EUROPE'S leading agricultural producer, and benefits from high levels of EU subsidy. The variation in climate and soils across the country provides great potential for agriculture and forestry, reflected in the range of products cultivated, including cereals, olives, herbs, and grapes for its famous wines.
SCALE 1:3,000,000
(projection: Lambert Conformal Conic)
Km
Miles
MAP KEY
POPULATION
above 5 million
1 million to 5 million
500,000 to 1 million
100,000 to 500,000
50,000 to 100,000
10,000 to 50,000
below 10,000
ELEVATION
4000m / 13,124ft
3000m / 9843ft
2000m / 6562ft
1000m / 3281ft
500m / 1640ft
250m / 820ft
100m / 328ft
sea level
Land use and agricultural distribution
cattle
cereals
market gardening
sugar beet
vineyards
capital cities
major towns
pasture
cropland
forest
mountain region
THE URBAN/RURAL POPULATION DIVIDE
urban 73%
rural 27%
POPULATION DENSITY
276 people per sq mile
(106 people per sq km)
TOTAL LAND AREA
212,930 sq mile
(551,500 sq km)
North Sea
BELGIUM
LUXEMBOURG
GERMANY
SWITZERLAND
ITALY
MEDITERRANEAN SEA
Golfe du Lion
PARIS
Lille
Amiens
Reims
Metz
Strasbourg
Mulhouse
Dijon
Besançon
Lyon
Grenoble
Marseille
Toulon
Nice
MONACO
Montpellier
Perpignan
PICARDIE
CHAMPAGNE-ARDENNE
LORRAINE
ALSACE
ÎLE-DE-FRANCE
BOURGOGNE
FRANCHE-COMTÉ
AUVERGNE
RHÔNE-ALPES
LANGUEDOC-ROUSSILLON
PROVENCE-ALPES-CÔTE D'AZUR
MIDI-PYRÉNÉES
Massif Central
Jura
Alps
Vosges
Corse (Corsica)
Ligurian Sea
Tyrrhenian Sea
Strait of Bonifacio
(same scale as main map)

The Romans first introduced winemaking to France when they occupied the region. Traditional vineyards can be found all over France, producing many of the world's classic wines.

The rugged hills and cliffs of Corsica were uplifted when the African and Eurasian plates collided. Frost action during the Ice Age created their present form.

In the sunny climate of southern France olives, vines, peppers, garlic, and lavender now grow in place of the forests that once covered much of the area.

The Iberian Peninsula

Andorra, Gibraltar, Portugal, Spain *(Azores, Canary Islands, Madeira on p.64)*

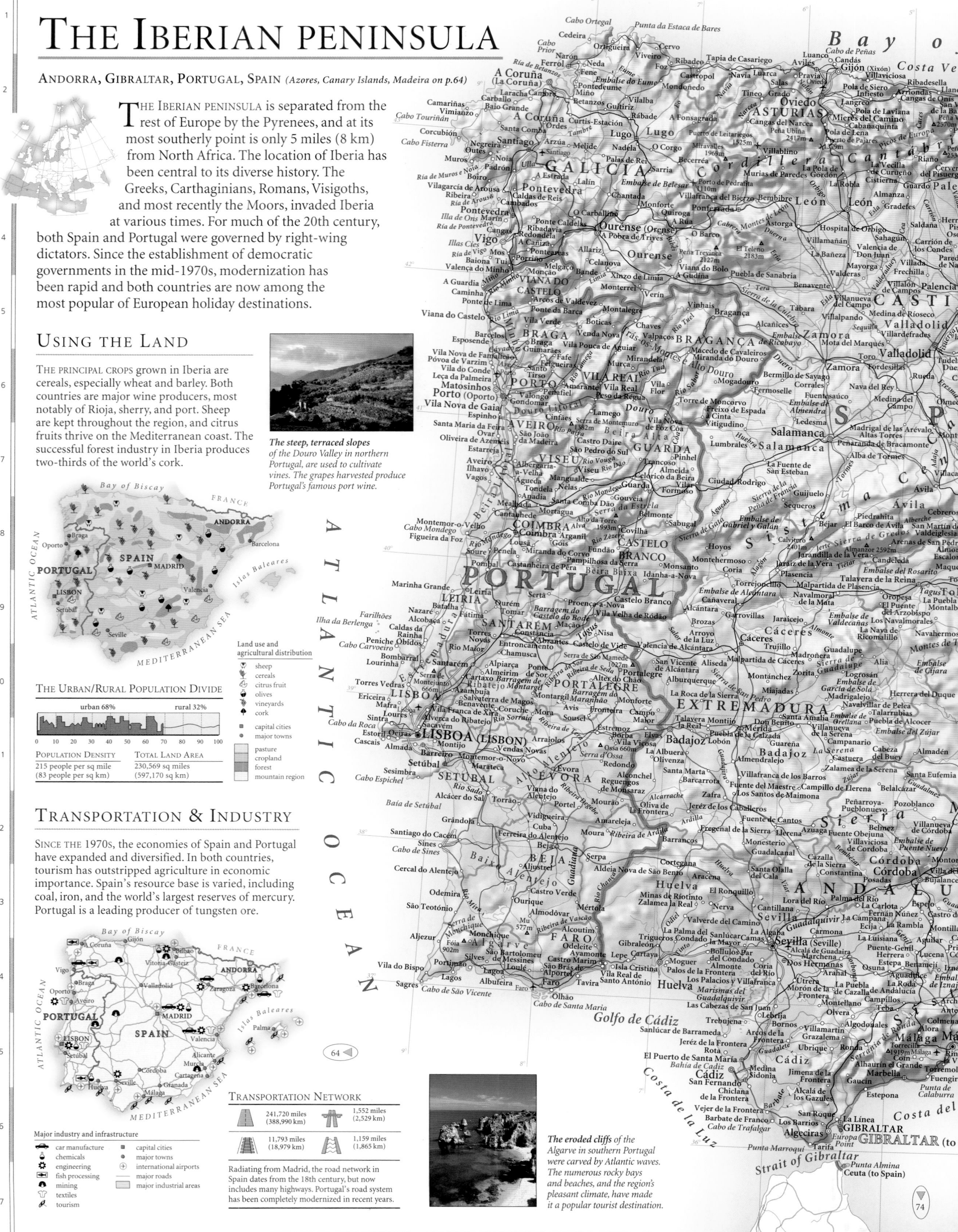
Bay of Biscay
ATLANTIC OCEAN
PORTUGAL
GALICIA
ASTURIAS
Cordillera Cantábrica
Sistema Central
EXTREMADURA
ANDALUCÍA
Golfo de Cádiz
Costa de la Luz
Strait of Gibraltar
GIBRALTAR (to UK)
MOROCCO
Lisboa (Lisbon)
Porto (Oporto)
Coimbra
Sevilla (Seville)
Salamanca
Valladolid
Badajoz
Cádiz
Huelva
Córdoba
Málaga
A Coruña (La Coruña)
Vigo
Faro
Évora
Bragança
Ceuta (to Spain)
64
74

The Iberian peninsula is separated from the rest of Europe by the Pyrenees, and at its most southerly point is only 5 miles (8 km) from North Africa. The location of Iberia has been central to its diverse history. The Greeks, Carthaginians, Romans, Visigoths, and most recently the Moors, invaded Iberia at various times. For much of the 20th century, both Spain and Portugal were governed by right-wing dictators. Since the establishment of democratic governments in the mid-1970s, modernization has been rapid and both countries are now among the most popular of European holiday destinations.

Using the Land

The principal crops grown in Iberia are cereals, especially wheat and barley. Both countries are major wine producers, most notably of Rioja, sherry, and port. Sheep are kept throughout the region, and citrus fruits thrive on the Mediterranean coast. The successful forest industry in Iberia produces two-thirds of the world's cork.

The steep, terraced slopes *of the Douro Valley in northern Portugal, are used to cultivate vines. The grapes harvested produce Portugal's famous port wine.*

Land use and agricultural distribution: sheep; cereals; citrus fruit; olives; vineyards; cork; capital cities; major towns; pasture; cropland; forest; mountain region

The Urban/Rural Population Divide

urban 68% — rural 32%

Population Density	Total Land Area
215 people per sq mile (83 people per sq km)	230,569 sq miles (597,170 sq km)

Transportation & Industry

Since the 1970s, the economies of Spain and Portugal have expanded and diversified. In both countries, tourism has outstripped agriculture in economic importance. Spain's resource base is varied, including coal, iron, and the world's largest reserves of mercury. Portugal is a leading producer of tungsten ore.

Major industry and infrastructure: car manufacture; chemicals; engineering; fish processing; mining; textiles; tourism; capital cities; major towns; international airports; major roads; major industrial areas

Transportation Network

241,720 miles (388,990 km)	1,552 miles (2,529 km)
11,793 miles (18,979 km)	1,159 miles (1,865 km)

Radiating from Madrid, the road network in Spain dates from the 18th century, but now includes many highways. Portugal's road system has been completely modernized in recent years.

The eroded cliffs *of the Algarve in southern Portugal were carved by Atlantic waves. The numerous rocky bays and beaches, and the region's pleasant climate, have made it a popular tourist destination.*

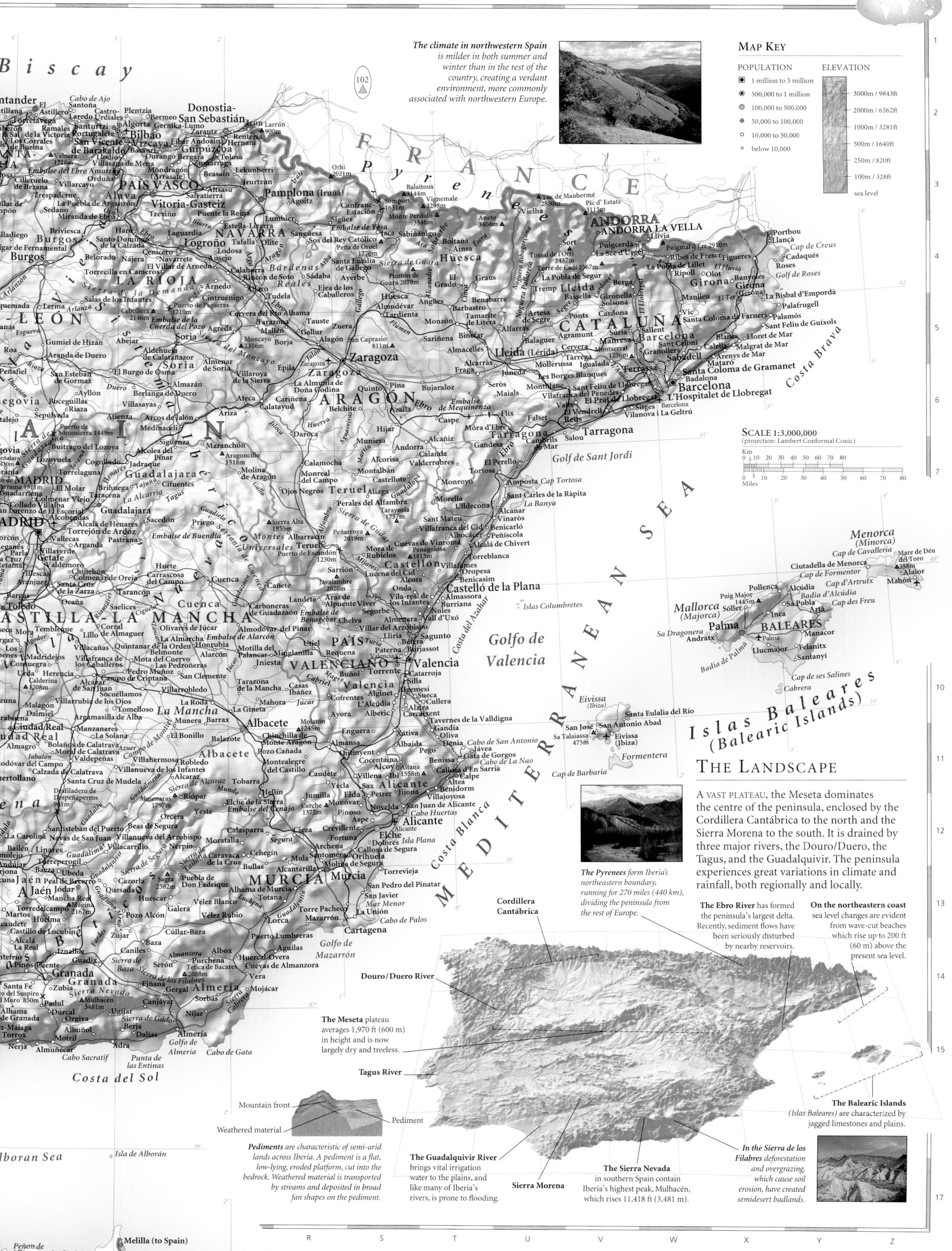

The climate in northwestern Spain is milder in both summer and winter than in the rest of the country, creating a verdant environment, more commonly associated with northwestern Europe.
MAP KEY
POPULATION
1 million to 5 million
500,000 to 1 million
100,000 to 500,000
50,000 to 100,000
10,000 to 50,000
below 10,000
ELEVATION
3000m / 9843ft
2000m / 6562ft
1000m / 3281ft
500m / 1640ft
250m / 820ft
100m / 328ft
sea level
SCALE 1:3,000,000
(projection: Lambert Conformal Conic)
FRANCE
Pyrenees
ANDORRA
MEDITERRANEAN SEA
Islas Baleares (Balearic Islands)
Golfo de Valencia
Costa Brava
Costa Blanca
Costa del Sol
Alboran Sea
Biscay
Madrid
Barcelona
Valencia
Zaragoza
Mallorca (Majorca)
Menorca (Minorca)
Eivissa (Ibiza)
Formentera

The Landscape

A vast plateau, the Meseta dominates the centre of the peninsula, enclosed by the Cordillera Cantábrica to the north and the Sierra Morena to the south. It is drained by three major rivers, the Douro/Duero, the Tagus, and the Guadalquivir. The peninsula experiences great variations in climate and rainfall, both regionally and locally.

The Pyrenees form Iberia's northeastern boundary, running for 270 miles (440 km), dividing the peninsula from the rest of Europe.

Cordillera Cantábrica
Douro/Duero River
Tagus River
Sierra Morena
Mountain front
Weathered material
Pediment

The Ebro River has formed the peninsula's largest delta. Recently, sediment flows have been seriously disturbed by nearby reservoirs.

On the northeastern coast sea level changes are evident from wave-cut beaches which rise up to 200 ft (60 m) above the present sea level.

The Meseta plateau averages 1,970 ft (600 m) in height and is now largely dry and treeless.

The Balearic Islands *(Islas Baleares)* are characterized by jagged limestones and plains.

***Pediments** are characteristic of semi-arid lands across Iberia. A pediment is a flat, low-lying, eroded platform, cut into the bedrock. Weathered material is transported by streams and deposited in broad fan shapes on the pediment.*

The Guadalquivir River brings vital irrigation water to the plains, and like many of Iberia's rivers, is prone to flooding.

The Sierra Nevada in southern Spain contain Iberia's highest peak, Mulhacén, which rises 11,418 ft (3,481 m).

***In the Sierra de los Filabres** deforestation and overgrazing, which cause soil erosion, have created semidesert badlands.*

The Italian Peninsula

Italy, San Marino, Vatican City

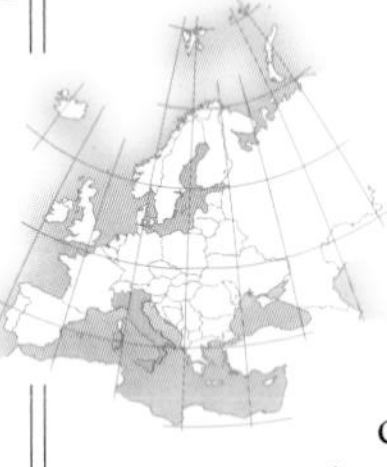

The Italian peninsula is a land of great contrasts. Until unification in 1861, Italy was a collection of independent states, whose competitiveness during the Renaissance resulted in the architectural and artistic magnificence of cities such as Rome, Florence, and Venice. The majority of Italy's population and economic activity is concentrated in the north, centered on the sophisticated industrial city of Milan. Southern Italy, the *Mezzogiorno*, has a harsh terrain, and remains far less developed than the north. Attempts to attract industry and investment in the south are frequently deterred by the entrenched network of organized crime and corruption.

The Landscape

The mainly mountainous and hilly Italian peninsula took its present form following a collision between the African and Eurasian tectonic plates. The Alps in the northwest rise to a high point of 15,772 ft (4,807 m) at Mont Blanc *(Monte Bianco)* on the French border, while the Apennines *(Appennino)* form a rugged backbone, running along the entire length of the country.

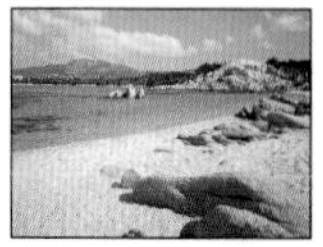

The island of Sardinia is an ancient land mass; an uplifted section of very old igneous rocks. Its rugged mountainous regions provide pasture for sheep and goats, while its valleys support some agriculture.

Costa Smeralda

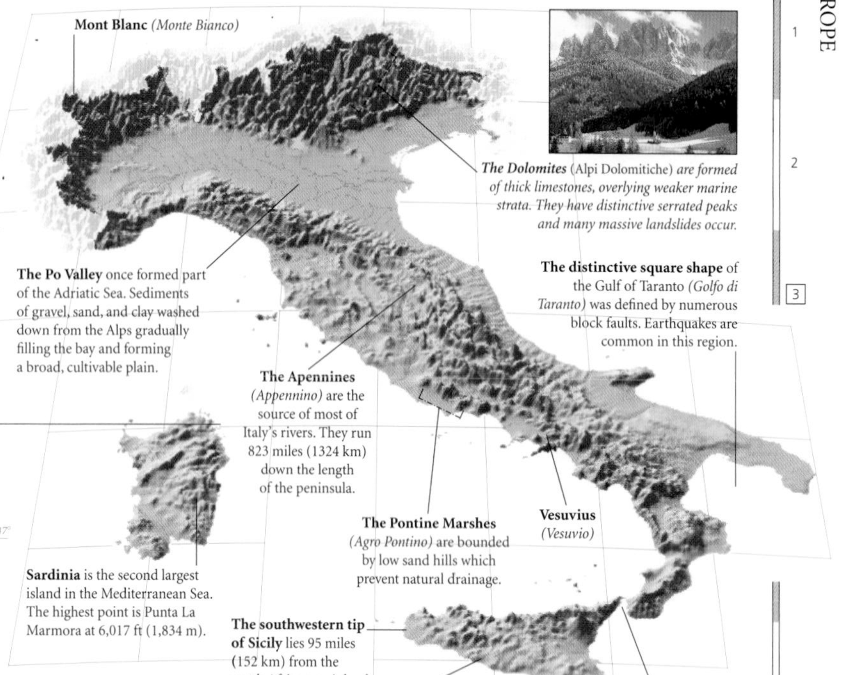

Mont Blanc *(Monte Bianco)*

***The Dolomites** (Alpi Dolomitiche) are formed of thick limestones, overlying weaker marine strata. They have distinctive serrated peaks and many massive landslides occur.*

The Po Valley once formed part of the Adriatic Sea. Sediments of gravel, sand, and clay washed down from the Alps gradually filling the bay and forming a broad, cultivable plain.

The distinctive square shape of the Gulf of Taranto *(Golfo di Taranto)* was defined by numerous block faults. Earthquakes are common in this region.

The Apennines *(Appennino)* are the source of most of Italy's rivers. They run 823 miles (1324 km) down the length of the peninsula.

Sardinia is the second largest island in the Mediterranean Sea. The highest point is Punta La Marmora at 6,017 ft (1,834 m).

The Pontine Marshes *(Agro Pontino)* are bounded by low sand hills which prevent natural drainage.

Vesuvius *(Vesuvio)*

The southwestern tip of Sicily lies 95 miles (152 km) from the north African mainland and is part of the same geological region.

Sicily is the largest island in the Mediterranean at 9,926 sq miles (25,708 sq km).

The Strait of Messina *(Stretto di Messina)* is between 2 and 12 miles (3–19 km) wide, and is a rich fishing ground.

Vesuvius *(Vesuvio)*

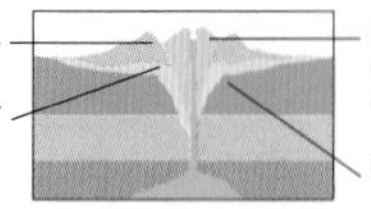

Monte Somma
Old crater
Present-day crater has developed within the old crater of Monte Somma
Old crater

***There have been four volcanoes** on the site of Vesuvius since volcanic activity began here more than 10,000 years ago.*

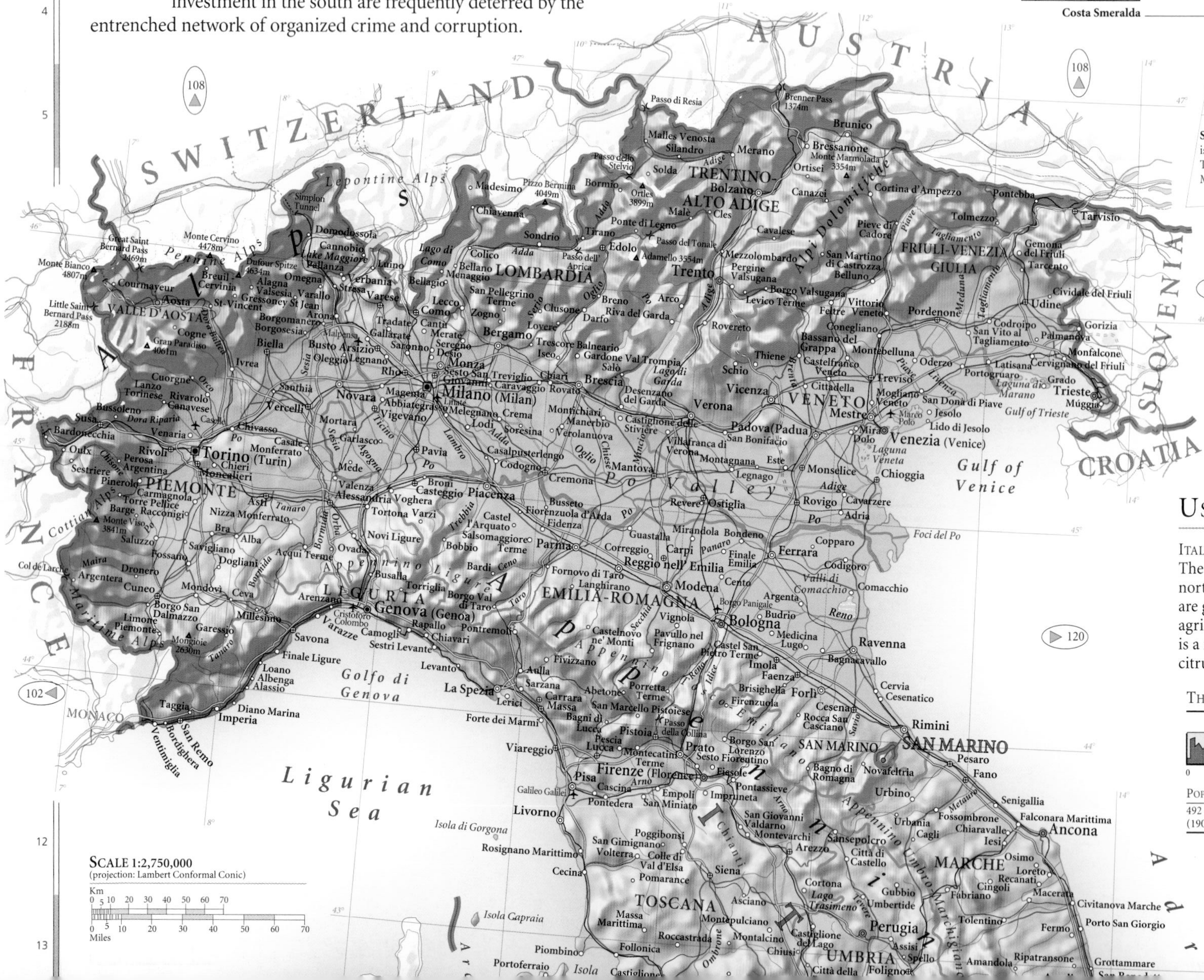

Using the Land

Italy produces 95% of its own food. The best farming land is in the Po Valley in northern Italy, where soft wheat and rice are grown. Irrigation is essential to agriculture in much of the south. Italy is a major producer and exporter of citrus fruits, olives, tomatoes, and wine.

The Urban/Rural Population Divide

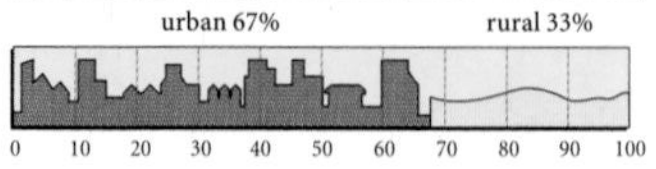

urban 67% — rural 33%

0 10 20 30 40 50 60 70 80 90 100

Population Density	Total Land Area
492 people per sq mile (190 people per sq km)	116,320 sq miles (301,270 sq km)

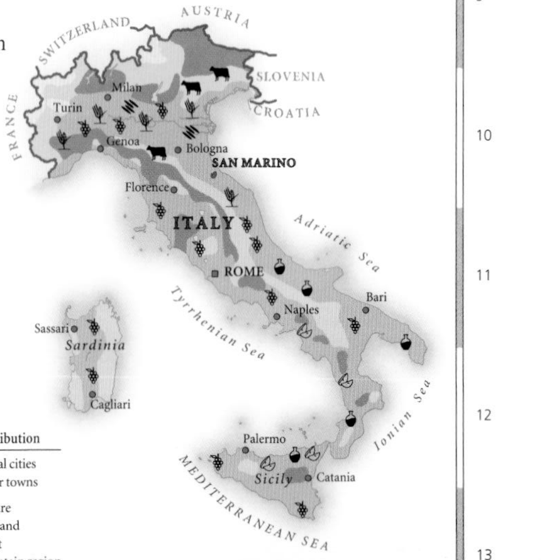

Land use and agricultural distribution

cattle, cereals, citrus fruits, olive oil, rice, vineyards; capital cities, major towns; pasture, cropland, forest, mountain region

Scale 1:2,750,000 (projection: Lambert Conformal Conic)

Km 0 5 10 20 30 40 50 60 70
Miles 0 5 10 20 30 40 50 60 70

108 · 108 · 108 · 112 · 120 · 102

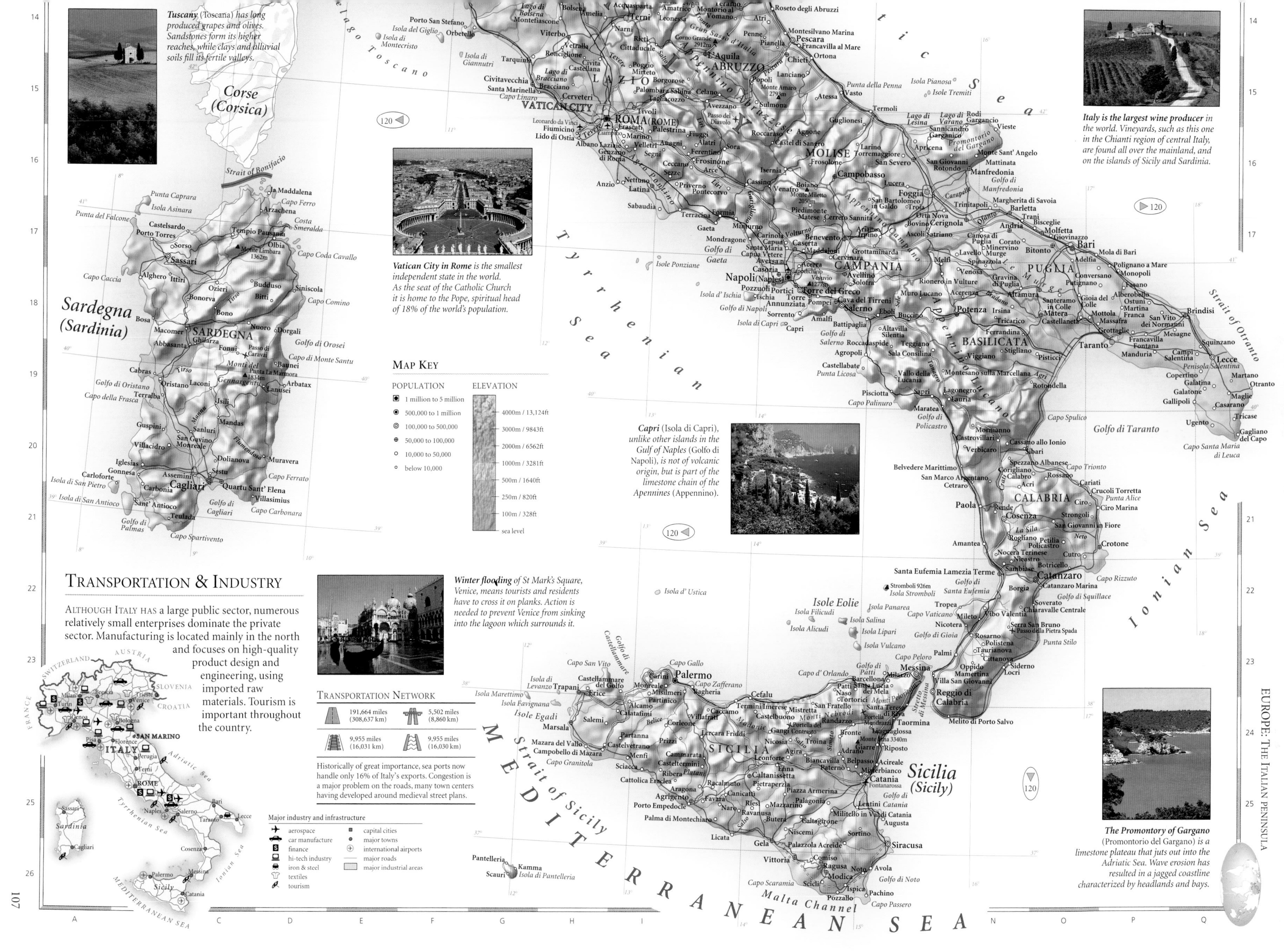
Corse
(Corsica)
Sardegna
(Sardinia)
SARDEGNA
Strait of Bonifacio
Tyrrhenian Sea
Adriatic Sea
Ionian Sea
MEDITERRANEAN SEA
Strait of Sicily
Strait of Otranto
Malta Channel
Sicilia
(Sicily)
SICILIA
Isole Eolie
Isole Egadi
LAZIO
ABRUZZO
MOLISE
CAMPANIA
PUGLIA
BASILICATA
CALABRIA
VATICAN CITY
ROMA (ROME)
Napoli (Naples)
Palermo
Cagliari
Sassari
Bari
Taranto
Brindisi
Lecce
Foggia
Pescara
Messina
Catania
Siracusa
Reggio di Calabria
Catanzaro
Golfo di Taranto
Appennino Lucano
Appennino Campano
Promontorio del Gargano

Tuscany (Toscana) has long produced grapes and olives. Sandstones form its higher reaches, while clays and alluvial soils fill its fertile valleys.

Italy is the largest wine producer in the world. Vineyards, such as this one in the Chianti region of central Italy, are found all over the mainland, and on the islands of Sicily and Sardinia.

Vatican City in Rome is the smallest independent state in the world. As the seat of the Catholic Church it is home to the Pope, spiritual head of 18% of the world's population.

Capri (Isola di Capri), unlike other islands in the Gulf of Naples (Golfo di Napoli), is not of volcanic origin, but is part of the limestone chain of the Apennines (Appennino).

Winter flooding of St Mark's Square, Venice, means tourists and residents have to cross it on planks. Action is needed to prevent Venice from sinking into the lagoon which surrounds it.

The Promontory of Gargano (Promontorio del Gargano) is a limestone plateau that juts out into the Adriatic Sea. Wave erosion has resulted in a jagged coastline characterized by headlands and bays.

Map Key

POPULATION

- 1 million to 5 million
- 500,000 to 1 million
- 100,000 to 500,000
- 50,000 to 100,000
- 10,000 to 50,000
- below 10,000

ELEVATION

- 4000m / 13,124ft
- 3000m / 9843ft
- 2000m / 6562ft
- 1000m / 3281ft
- 500m / 1640ft
- 250m / 820ft
- 100m / 328ft
- sea level

Transportation & Industry

Although Italy has a large public sector, numerous relatively small enterprises dominate the private sector. Manufacturing is located mainly in the north and focuses on high-quality product design and engineering, using imported raw materials. Tourism is important throughout the country.

Transportation Network

191,664 miles (308,637 km)	5,502 miles (8,860 km)
9,955 miles (16,031 km)	9,955 miles (16,030 km)

Historically of great importance, sea ports now handle only 16% of Italy's exports. Congestion is a major problem on the roads, many town centers having developed around medieval street plans.

Major industry and infrastructure

- aerospace
- car manufacture
- finance
- hi-tech industry
- iron & steel
- textiles
- tourism
- capital cities
- major towns
- international airports
- major roads
- major industrial areas

The Alpine States

Austria, Liechtenstein, Slovenia, Switzerland

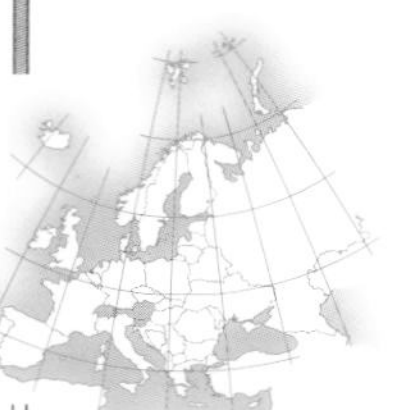

The Alpine countries of Austria, Switzerland, Liechtenstein, and Slovenia form a narrow strip across western Europe's geographical core, lying on the main north–south trading routes across the Alps. Switzerland, politically neutral since 1815, is an important international meeting place and houses one of the headquarters of the United Nations, although not itself a member. Austria, once at the heart of the great Habsburg Empire has been a fully independent nation since 1955, and maintains a deserved reputation as an international center of culture. Slovenia declared independence from the former Yugoslavia in 1991 and despite initial economic hardship, is now starting to achieve the prosperity enjoyed by its Alpine neighbors.

Using the Land

The Alpine region's mountainous terrain discourages cultivation over much of the land area. The primary agricultural activity is the raising of dairy and beef cattle on the pasture land of the lower mountain slopes. Austria is self-supporting in grains, and crops such as wheat, barley, and grapes are grown on the east Austrian lowlands. Woodlands are more prevalent in the eastern Alps; both Austria and Slovenia have large tracts of forest.

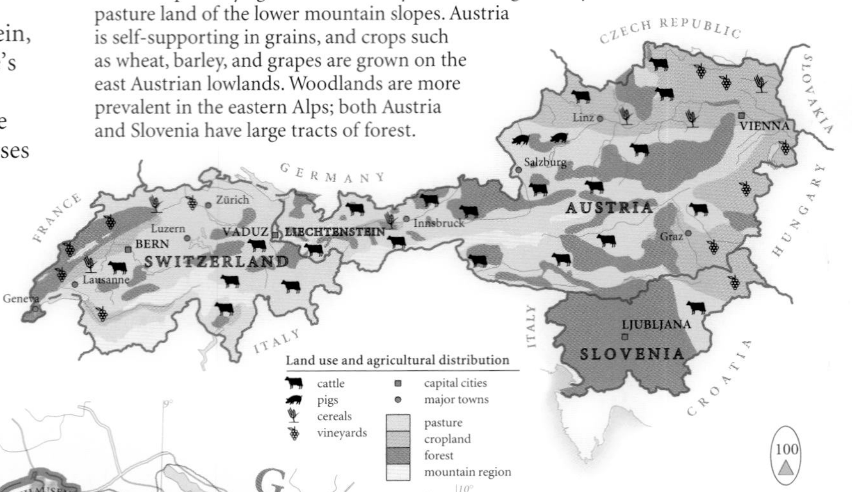

Land use and agricultural distribution

cattle
pigs
cereals
vineyards
capital cities
major towns
pasture
cropland
forest
mountain region

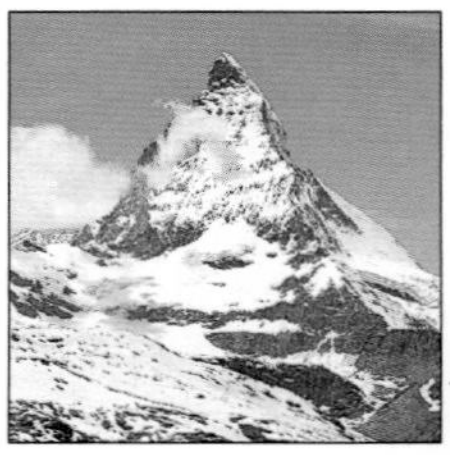

The Matterhorn, on the Swiss-Italian border, is one of the highest mountains in the Alps, at 14,692 ft (4,478 m). The term "horn" refers to its distinctive peak, formed by three glaciers eroding hollows, known as cirques, in each of its sides.

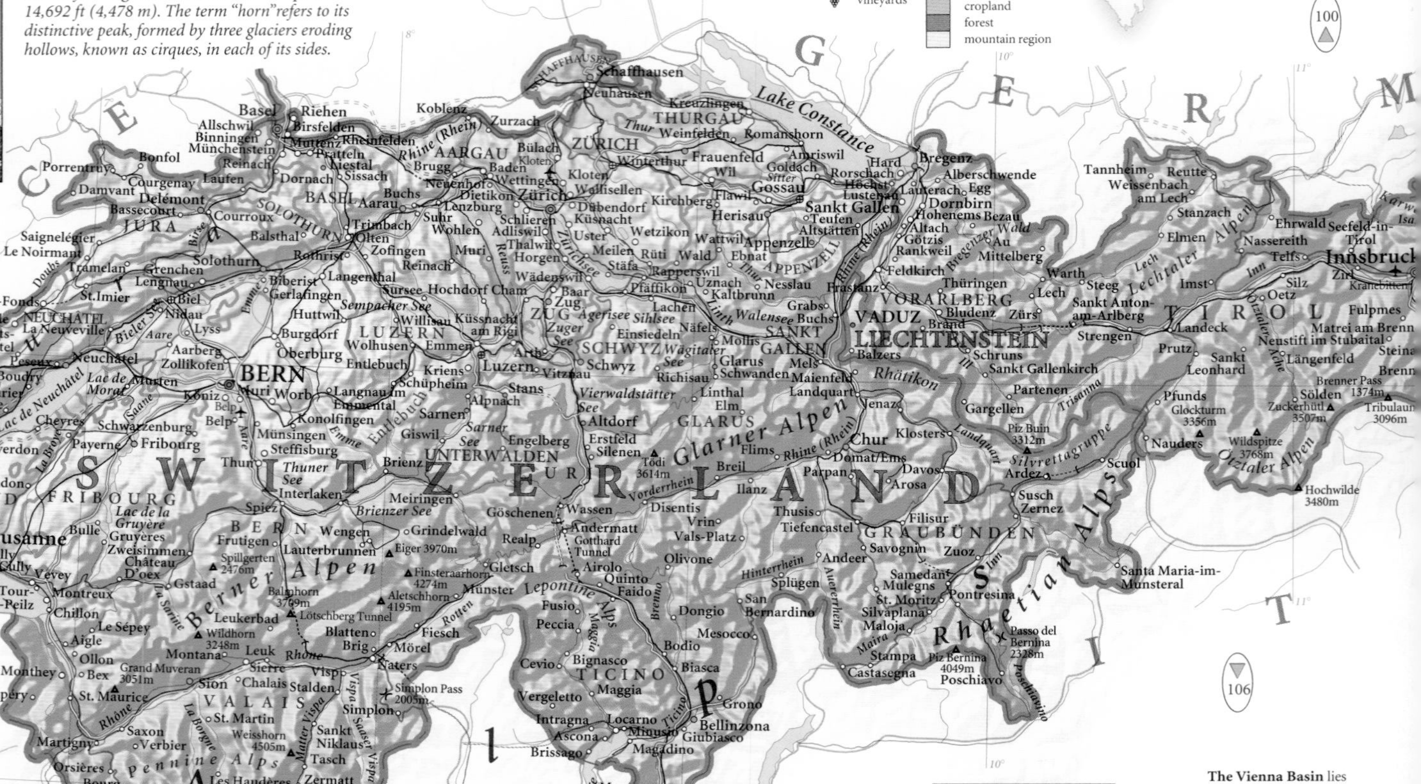

102

100

106

102

The Landscape

The Alps occupy three-fifths of Switzerland, most of southern Austria and the northwest of Slovenia. They were formed by the collision of the African and Eurasian tectonic plates, which began 65 million years ago. Their complex geology is reflected in the differing heights and rock types of the various ranges. The Rhine flows along Liechtenstein's border with Switzerland, creating a broad floodplain in the north and west of Liechtenstein. In the far northeast and east are a number of lowland regions, including the Vienna Basin, Burgenland, and the plain of the Danube. Slovenia's major rivers flow across the lower eastern regions; in the west, the rivers flow underground through the limestone Karst region.

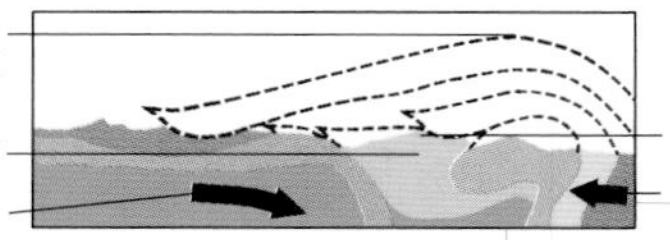

Original height after uplift and folding

Folded strata are overturned creating a *nappe*

Eurasian Plate

Present-day height of Alps

African Plate

***The convergence of the African and Eurasian plates** compressed and folded huge masses of rock strata. As the plates continued to move together, the folded strata were overturned, creating complex nappes. Much of the rock strata has since been eroded, resulting in the current topography of the Alps.*

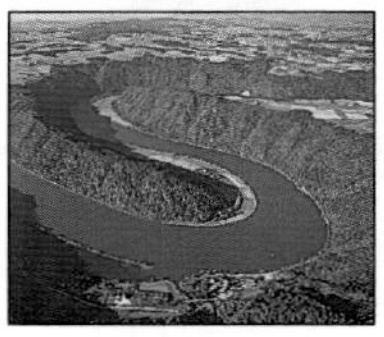

***Constricted as it cuts through** ridges in the Alps, the Danube meanders across the lowlands, where uplift combined with river erosion has deepened meanders.*

The Vienna Basin lies mainly below 390 ft (120 m). It gradually subsided and filled with sediment as the Alps were uplifted.

Neusiedler See straddles the border of Austria and Hungary; the area around it provides some of the best wine-growing land in Austria.

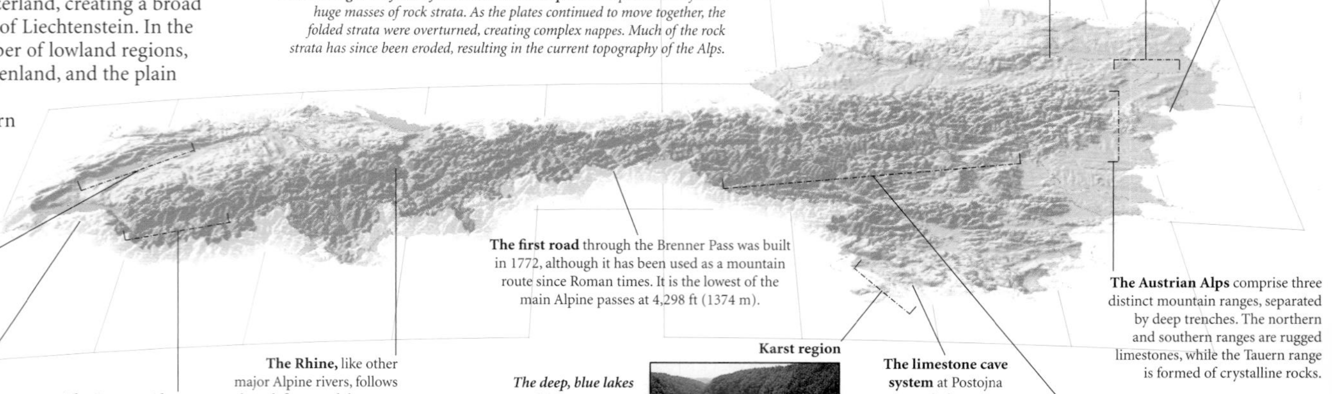

The mountains of the Jura form a natural border between Switzerland and France. Their marine limestones date from over 200 million years ago. When the Alps were formed the Jura were folded into a series of parallel ridges and troughs.

Tectonic activity has resulted in dramatic changes in land height over very short distances. Lake Geneva, lying at 1,221 ft (372 m) is only 43 miles (70 km) away from the 15,772 ft (4,807 m) peak of Mont Blanc, on the France–Italy border.

The Bernese Alps *(Berner Alpen)* contain the Aletsch, which at 15 miles (24 km) is the longest Alpine glacier.

The Rhine, like other major Alpine rivers, follows a broad, flat trough between the mountains. Along part of its course, the Rhine forms the boundary between Switzerland and Liechtenstein.

The first road through the Brenner Pass was built in 1772, although it has been used as a mountain route since Roman times. It is the lowest of the main Alpine passes at 4,298 ft (1374 m).

Karst region

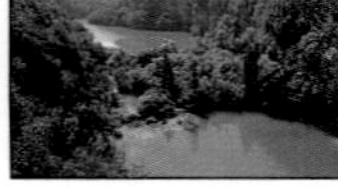

***The deep, blue lakes** of the Karst region are part of a drainage network which runs largely underground through this limestone area.*

The limestone cave system at Postojna extends for more than 10 miles (16 km) and includes caverns reaching 125 ft (40 m) in height and width.

The Austrian Alps comprise three distinct mountain ranges, separated by deep trenches. The northern and southern ranges are rugged limestones, while the Tauern range is formed of crystalline rocks.

The Tauern range in the central Austrian Alps contains the highest mountain in Austria, the towering Grossglockner, rising 12,461 ft (3,798 m).

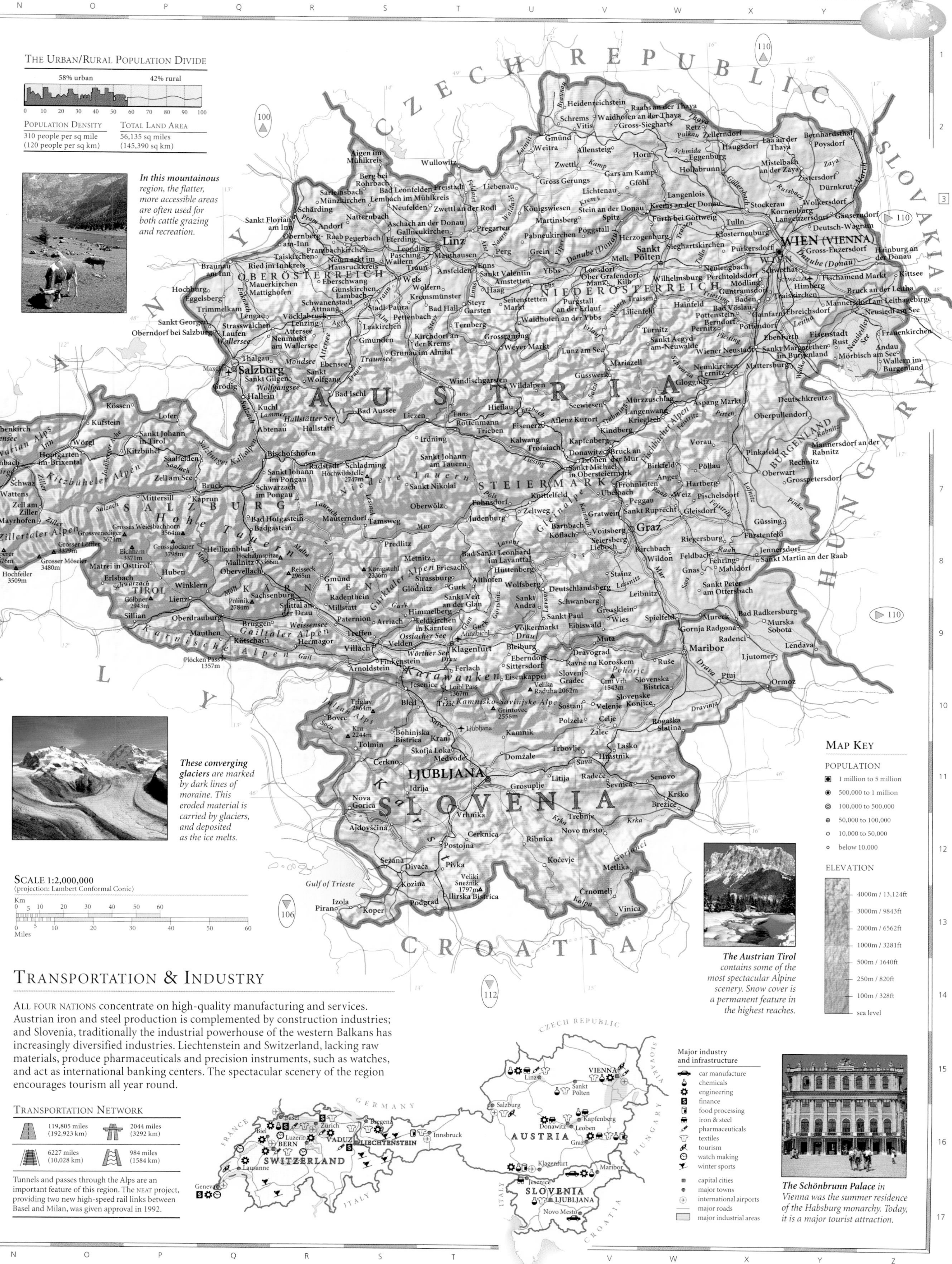
N O P Q R S T U V W X Y
CZECH REPUBLIC
SLOVAKIA
HUNGARY
GERMANY
ITALY
CROATIA
AUSTRIA
SLOVENIA
OBERÖSTERREICH
NIEDERÖSTERREICH
STEIERMARK
SALZBURG
KÄRNTEN
TIROL
BURGENLAND
WIEN (VIENNA)
Linz
Salzburg
Graz
Klagenfurt
Innsbruck
LJUBLJANA
Maribor
Sankt Pölten
Hohe Tauern
Niedere Tauern
Karawanken
Gulf of Trieste
THE URBAN/RURAL POPULATION DIVIDE
58% urban
42% rural
0 10 20 30 40 50 60 70 80 90 100
POPULATION DENSITY
310 people per sq mile
(120 people per sq km)
TOTAL LAND AREA
56,135 sq miles
(145,390 sq km)
SCALE 1:2,000,000
(projection: Lambert Conformal Conic)
MAP KEY
POPULATION
1 million to 5 million
500,000 to 1 million
100,000 to 500,000
50,000 to 100,000
10,000 to 50,000
below 10,000
ELEVATION
4000m / 13,124ft
3000m / 9843ft
2000m / 6562ft
1000m / 3281ft
500m / 1640ft
250m / 820ft
100m / 328ft
sea level
TRANSPORTATION NETWORK
119,805 miles (192,923 km)
2044 miles (3292 km)
6227 miles (10,028 km)
984 miles (1584 km)
Major industry and infrastructure
car manufacture
chemicals
engineering
finance
food processing
iron & steel
pharmaceuticals
textiles
tourism
watch making
winter sports
capital cities
major towns
international airports
major roads
major industrial areas
SWITZERLAND
LIECHTENSTEIN
VADUZ
BERN

In this mountainous region, the flatter, more accessible areas are often used for both cattle grazing and recreation.

These converging glaciers are marked by dark lines of moraine. This eroded material is carried by glaciers, and deposited as the ice melts.

The Austrian Tirol contains some of the most spectacular Alpine scenery. Snow cover is a permanent feature in the highest reaches.

TRANSPORTATION & INDUSTRY

ALL FOUR NATIONS concentrate on high-quality manufacturing and services. Austrian iron and steel production is complemented by construction industries; and Slovenia, traditionally the industrial powerhouse of the western Balkans has increasingly diversified industries. Liechtenstein and Switzerland, lacking raw materials, produce pharmaceuticals and precision instruments, such as watches, and act as international banking centers. The spectacular scenery of the region encourages tourism all year round.

Tunnels and passes through the Alps are an important feature of this region. The NEAT project, providing two new high-speed rail links between Basel and Milan, was given approval in 1992.

The Schönbrunn Palace in Vienna was the summer residence of the Habsburg monarchy. Today, it is a major tourist attraction.

Central Europe

Czech Republic, Hungary, Poland, Slovakia

When Slovakia and the Czech Republic became separate countries in 1993, they joined Hungary and Poland in a new role as independent nation states, following centuries of shifting boundaries and imperial strife. This turbulent history bequeathed the region a rich cultural heritage, shared through the works of its many great writers and composers, and celebrated in the vibrant historic capitals of Prague, Budapest, and Warsaw. Having shaken off Soviet domination in 1989, these states are facing up to the challenge of winning commercial investment to modernize outmoded industry, while bearing the severe environmental impact from forty years of large-scale industrialization.

The Landscape

The forested Carpathian Mountains, uplifted with the Alps, lie southeast of the older Bohemian massif, which contains the Sudeten and Krušné Hory *(Erzgebirge)* ranges. They divide the fertile plains of the Danube to the south and the Vistula *(Wisła)*, which flows north across vast expanses of glacial deposits into the Baltic Sea.

Hot mineral springs occur where geothermally heated water wells up through faults and fractures in the rocks of the Sudeten Mountains.

Pomerania is a sandy coastal region of glacially-formed lakes stretching west from the Vistula *(Wisła)*.

Longshore currents moving east along the Baltic coast have built a 40 mile (65 km) spit composed of material from the Vistula *(Wisła)* River.

***The Biebrza River** has left meanders and oxbow lakes as it flows across low-lying ground.*

Gerlachovský štít, in the Tatra Mountains, is Slovakia's highest mountain, at 8,711ft (2,655 m).

Carpathian Mountains

Danube River

Krušné Hory *(Erzgebirge)*

Bohemian Massif

The Berounka River cuts through the precipitous wooded landscape of the Bohemian massif, banked by a broad floodplain.

The Slovak Ore Mountains *(Slovenské Rudohorie)* are noted for their mineral resources, including high-grade iron ore.

The Great Hungarian Plain formed by the floodplain of the Danube is a mixture of steppe and cultivated land, covering nearly half of Hungary's total area.

Bluff

Slip-off slope

Direction of flow

***Meanders** form as rivers flow across plains at a low gradient. A steep cliff or bluff, forms on the outside curve, and a gentler slip-off slope on the inside bend.*

Transportation & Industry

Heavy industry has dominated postwar life in Central Europe. Poland has large coal reserves, having inherited the Silesian coalfield from Germany after the Second World War, allowing the export of large quantities of coal, along with other minerals. Hungary specializes in consumer goods and services, while Slovakia's industrial base is still relatively small. The Czech Republic's traditional glassworks and breweries bring some stability to its precarious Soviet-built manufacturing sector.

Major industry and infrastructure

- car manufacture
- chemicals
- engineering
- food processing
- mining
- shipbuilding
- tourism
- capital cities
- major towns
- international airports
- major roads
- major industrial areas

Transportation Network

213,997 miles (344,600 km)	817 miles (1,315 km)
27,479 miles (44,249 km)	3,784 miles (6,094 km)

The huge growth of tourism and business has prompted major investment in the transportation infrastructure, with new roadbuilding schemes within and between the main cities of the region.

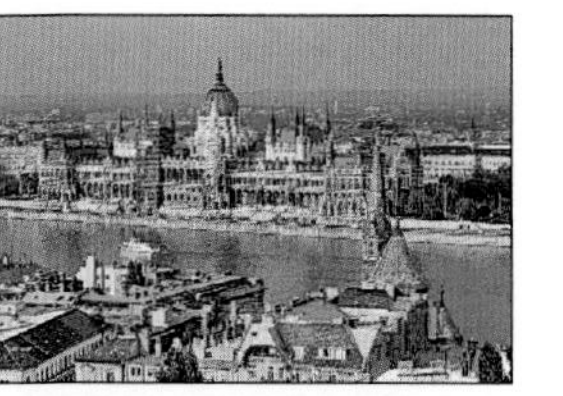

***Budapest, the capital of Hungary,** straddles the Danube. It comprises the historic towns of Buda, on the west bank, and Pest, which contains the Parliament Building, seen here on the far bank.*

▶ 118
▶ 118

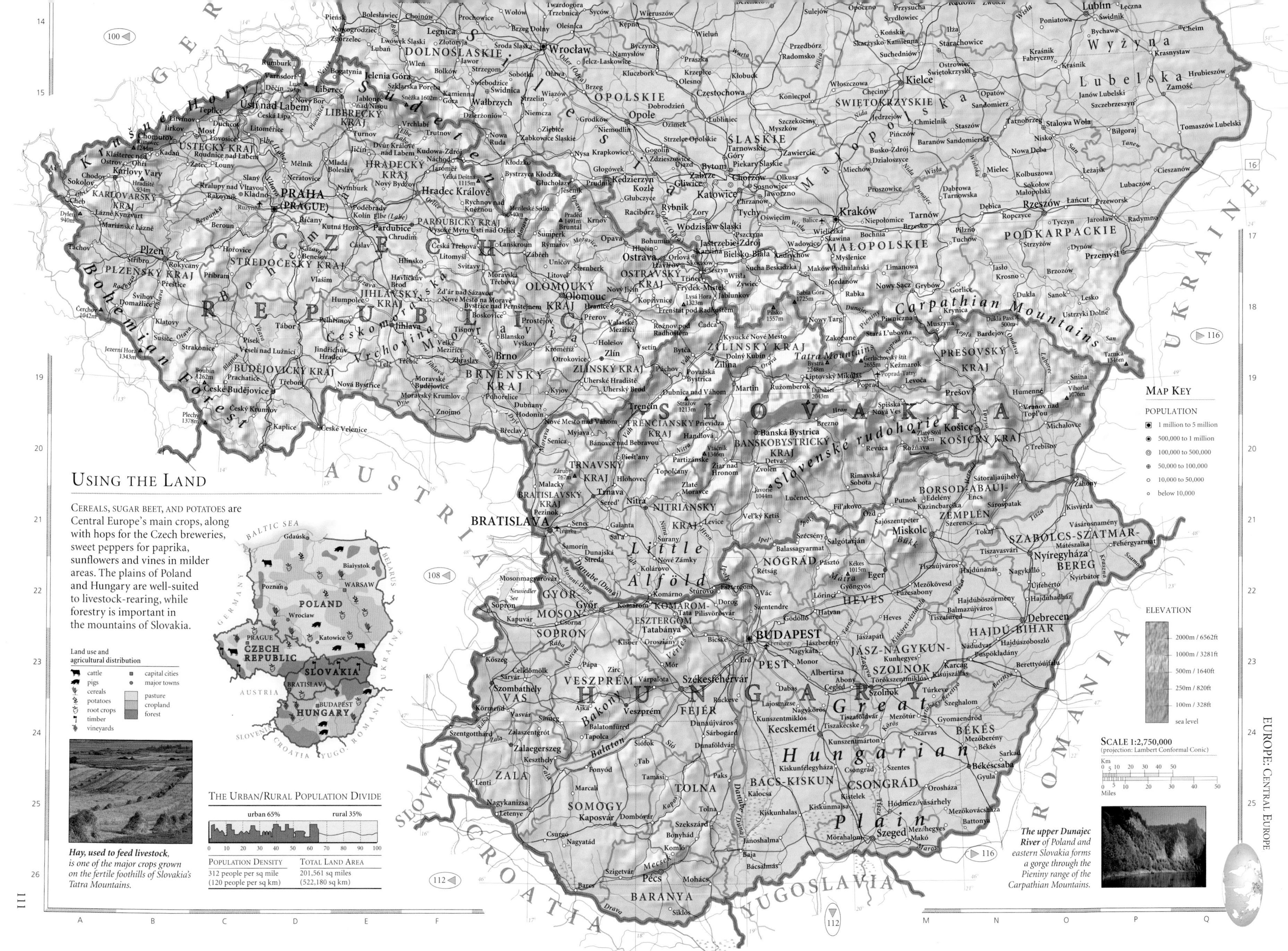
MAP KEY
POPULATION
1 million to 5 million
500,000 to 1 million
100,000 to 500,000
50,000 to 100,000
10,000 to 50,000
below 10,000
ELEVATION
2000m / 6562ft
1000m / 3281ft
500m / 1640ft
250m / 820ft
100m / 328ft
sea level
SCALE 1:2,750,000
(projection: Lambert Conformal Conic)
Land use and agricultural distribution
cattle
pigs
cereals
potatoes
root crops
timber
vineyards
capital cities
major towns
pasture
cropland
forest
THE URBAN/RURAL POPULATION DIVIDE
urban 65%
rural 35%
POPULATION DENSITY
312 people per sq mile
(120 people per sq km)
TOTAL LAND AREA
201,561 sq miles
(522,180 sq km)

USING THE LAND

CEREALS, SUGAR BEET, AND POTATOES are Central Europe's main crops, along with hops for the Czech breweries, sweet peppers for paprika, sunflowers and vines in milder areas. The plains of Poland and Hungary are well-suited to livestock-rearing, while forestry is important in the mountains of Slovakia.

Hay, used to feed livestock, *is one of the major crops grown on the fertile foothills of Slovakia's Tatra Mountains.*

The upper Dunajec River *of Poland and eastern Slovakia forms a gorge through the Pieniny range of the Carpathian Mountains.*

Southeast Europe

Albania, Bosnia & Herzegovina, Croatia, Macedonia, Yugoslavia

For 46 years the federation of Yugoslavia held together the most diverse ethnic region in Europe, along the picturesque mountain hinterland of the Dalmatian coast. Economic collapse resulted in internal tensions. In the early 1990s, civil war broke out in both Croatia and Bosnia as the ethnic populations struggled to establish their own exclusive territories. Peace was only restored by the UN after NATO launched air strikes in 1995. In the province of Kosovo, attempts to gain autonomy from Yugoslavia in 1998 were crushed by the Serbian government. The slaughter of ethnic Albanians in Kosovo provoked the West to launch NATO air strikes yet again in the region, and Yugoslav forces withdrew. The flood of refugees from Kosovo has severely strained Albania.

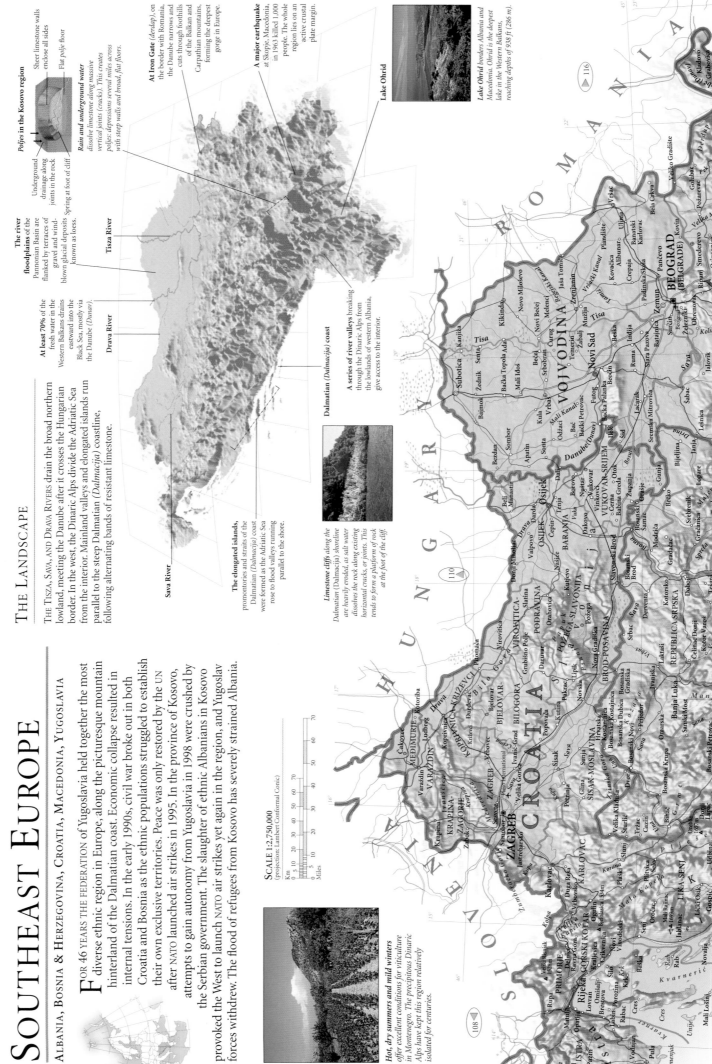

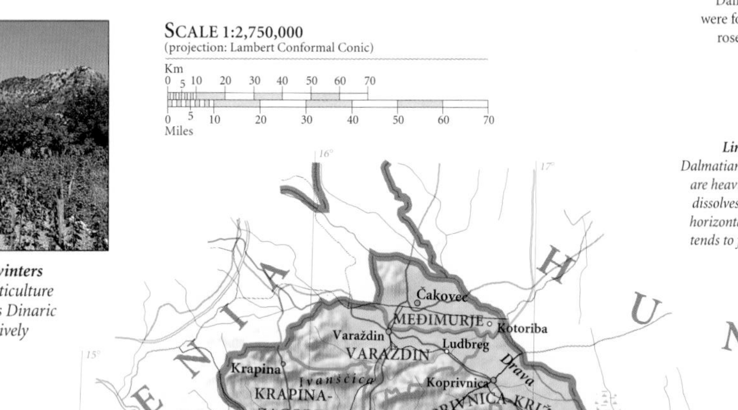

Hot, dry summers and mild winters offer excellent conditions for viticulture in Montenegro. The precipitous Dinaric Alps have kept this region relatively isolated for centuries.

Scale 1:2,750,000
(projection: Lambert Conformal Conic)
Km 0 5 10 20 30 40 50 60 70
Miles 0 5 10 20 30 40 50 60 70

The Landscape

The Tisza, Sava, and Drava Rivers drain the broad northern lowland, meeting the Danube after it crosses the Hungarian border. In the west, the Dinaric Alps divide the Adriatic Sea from the interior. Mainland valleys and elongated islands run parallel to the steep Dalmatian *(Dalmacija)* coastline, following alternating bands of resistant limestone.

At least 70% of the fresh water in the Western Balkans drains eastward into the Black Sea, mostly via the Danube *(Dunav)*.

The river floodplains of the Pannonian Basin are flanked by terraces of gravel and wind-blown glacial deposits known as loess.

Poljes in the Kosovo region

Underground drainage along joints in the rock

Spring at foot of cliff

Sheer limestone walls enclose all sides

Flat polje floor

***Rain and underground water** dissolve limestone along massive vertical joints (cracks). This creates poljes: depressions several miles across with steep walls and broad, flat floors.*

Drava River

Tisza River

Sava River

At Iron Gate *(derdap)*, on the border with Romania, the Danube narrows and cuts through foothills of the Balkan and Carpathian mountains, forming the deepest gorge in Europe.

The elongated islands, promontories and straits of the Dalmatian *(Dalmacija)* coast were formed as the Adriatic Sea rose to flood valleys running parallel to the shore.

A major earthquake at Skopje, Macedonia, in 1963 killed 1,000 people. The whole region lies on an active crustal plate margin.

Dalmatian *(Dalmacija)* **coast**

__Limestone cliffs__ along the Dalmatian (Dalmacija) shoreline are heavily eroded, as salt water dissolves the rock along existing horizontal cracks, or joints. This tends to form a platform of rock at the foot of the cliff.

A series of river valleys breaking through the Dinaric Alps from the lowlands of western Albania, give access to the interior.

Lake Ohrid

***Lake Ohrid** borders Albania and Macedonia. Ohrid is the deepest lake in the Western Balkans, reaching depths of 938 ft (286 m).*

SLOVENIA HUNGARY ROMANIA CROATIA VOJVODINA BOSNIA & HERZEGOVINA SERBIA YUGO

108 110 116 120

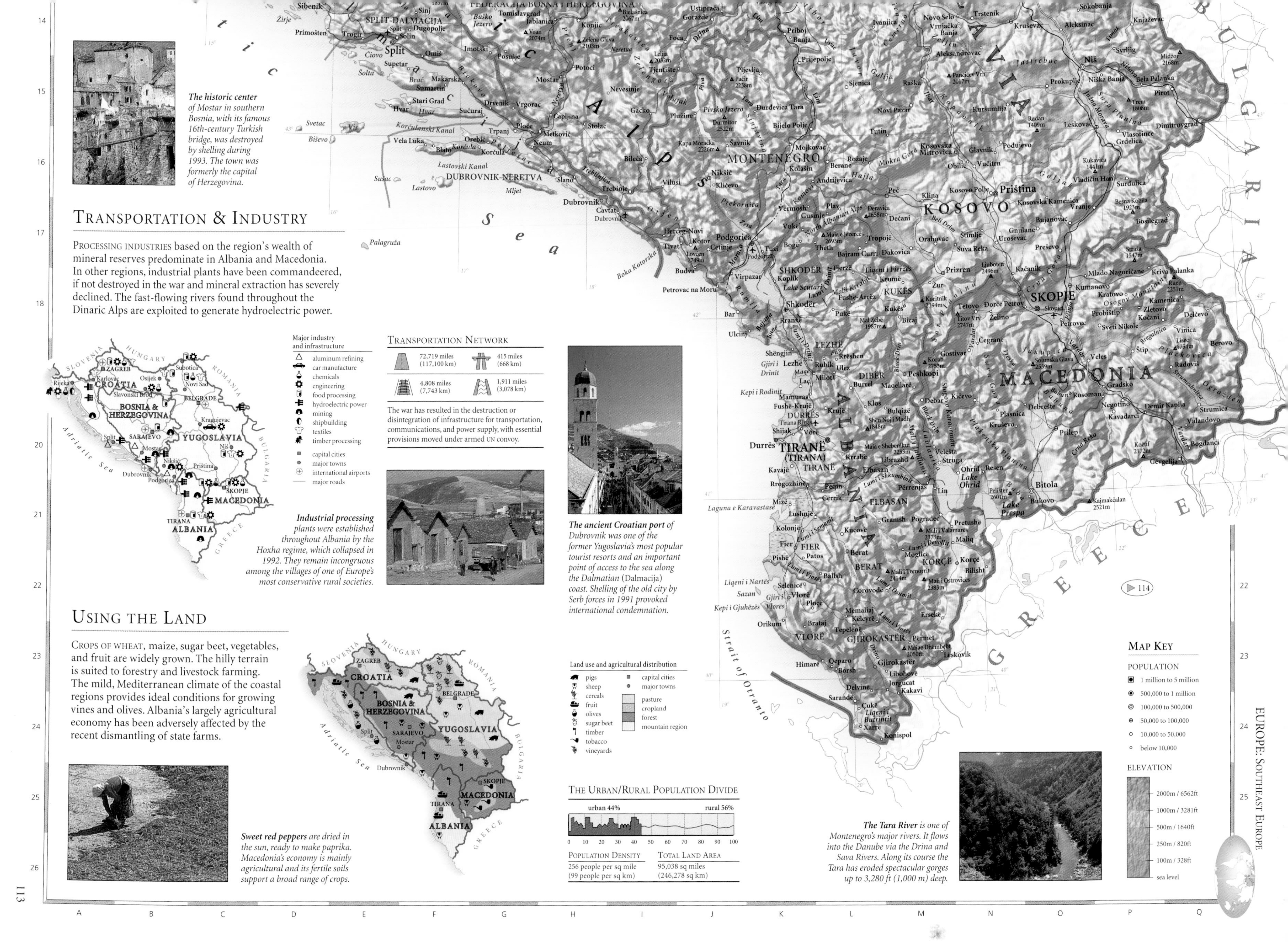
Major industry and infrastructure
aluminum refining
car manufacture
chemicals
engineering
food processing
hydroelectric power
mining
shipbuilding
textiles
timber processing
capital cities
major towns
international airports
major roads
Transportation Network
72,719 miles (117,100 km)
415 miles (668 km)
4,808 miles (7,743 km)
1,911 miles (3,078 km)
Land use and agricultural distribution
pigs
sheep
cereals
fruit
olives
sugar beet
timber
tobacco
vineyards
capital cities
major towns
pasture
cropland
forest
mountain region
The Urban/Rural Population Divide
urban 44%
rural 56%
Population Density
256 people per sq mile (99 people per sq km)
Total Land Area
95,038 sq miles (246,278 sq km)
Map Key
Population
1 million to 5 million
500,000 to 1 million
100,000 to 500,000
50,000 to 100,000
10,000 to 50,000
below 10,000
Elevation
2000m / 6562ft
1000m / 3281ft
500m / 1640ft
250m / 820ft
100m / 328ft
sea level

The historic center of Mostar in southern Bosnia, with its famous 16th-century Turkish bridge, was destroyed by shelling during 1993. The town was formerly the capital of Herzegovina.

Transportation & Industry

Processing industries based on the region's wealth of mineral reserves predominate in Albania and Macedonia. In other regions, industrial plants have been commandeered, if not destroyed in the war and mineral extraction has severely declined. The fast-flowing rivers found throughout the Dinaric Alps are exploited to generate hydroelectric power.

The war has resulted in the destruction or disintegration of infrastructure for transportation, communications, and power supply, with essential provisions moved under armed UN convoy.

***Industrial processing** plants were established throughout Albania by the Hoxha regime, which collapsed in 1992. They remain incongruous among the villages of one of Europe's most conservative rural societies.*

***The ancient Croatian port** of Dubrovnik was one of the former Yugoslavia's most popular tourist resorts and an important point of access to the sea along the Dalmatian (Dalmacija) coast. Shelling of the old city by Serb forces in 1991 provoked international condemnation.*

Using the Land

Crops of wheat, maize, sugar beet, vegetables, and fruit are widely grown. The hilly terrain is suited to forestry and livestock farming. The mild, Mediterranean climate of the coastal regions provides ideal conditions for growing vines and olives. Albania's largely agricultural economy has been adversely affected by the recent dismantling of state farms.

***Sweet red peppers** are dried in the sun, ready to make paprika. Macedonia's economy is mainly agricultural and its fertile soils support a broad range of crops.*

***The Tara River** is one of Montenegro's major rivers. It flows into the Danube via the Drina and Sava Rivers. Along its course the Tara has eroded spectacular gorges up to 3,280 ft (1,000 m) deep.*

114

BULGARIA & GREECE

Including EUROPEAN TURKEY

GREECE IS RENOWNED as the original hearth of Western civilization. The rugged terrain and numerous islands have profoundly affected its development, creating a strong agricultural and maritime tradition. In the past 50 years, this formerly rural society has rapidly urbanized, with more than half the population now living in the capital, Athens, and in the northern city of Salonica. Bulgaria, dominated for centuries by the Ottoman Turks, became part of the eastern bloc after the Second World War, only slowly emerging from Soviet influence in 1989. Moves toward democracy have led to some political instability and Bulgaria has been slow to align its economy with the rest of Europe.

TRANSPORTATION & INDUSTRY

SOVIET INVESTMENT introduced heavy industry into Bulgaria, and the processing of agricultural produce, such as tobacco, is important throughout the country. Both countries have substantial shipyards and Greece has one of the world's largest merchant fleets. Many small craft workshops, producing textiles and processed foods, are clustered around Greek cities. The service and construction sectors have profited from the successful tourist industry.

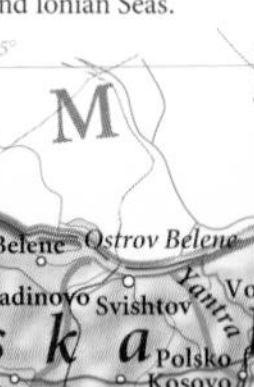
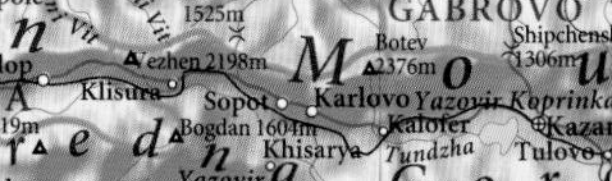
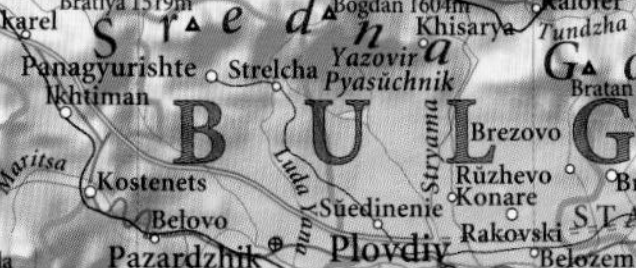
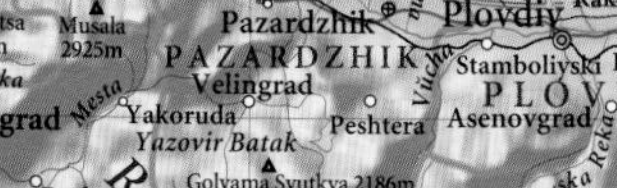
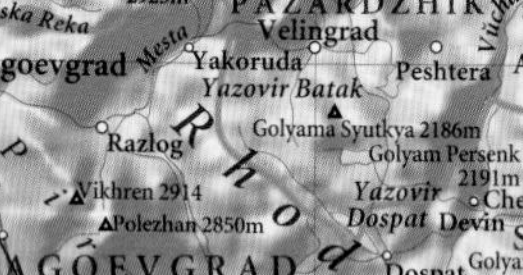
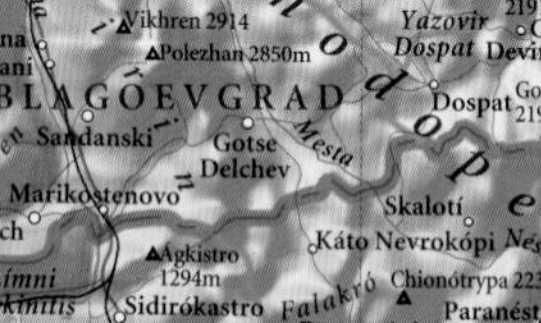

Major industry and infrastructure

- chemicals
- engineering
- food processing
- shipbuilding
- textiles
- tourism
- capital cities
- major towns
- international airports
- major roads
- major industrial areas

TRANSPORTATION NETWORK

- 103,930 miles (167,630 km)
- 345 miles (557 km)
- 4,346 miles (6,995 km)
- 294 miles (474 km)

Bulgaria's railroads require investment to revive an outdated infrastructure. In Greece, despite a developing road network, ferry-boats remain the most effective form of transportation in many areas.

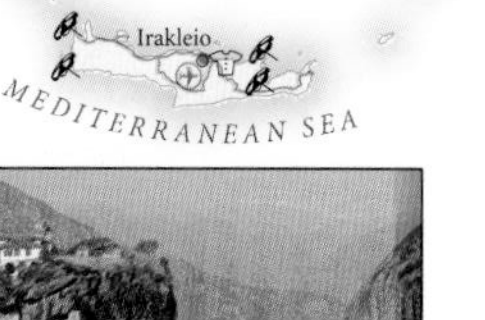

***A towering pinnacle** at Metéora in central Greece is home to the monastery of Roussanou. The 24 rock towers which dominate the plain of Thessaly (Thessalía) are remnants of an old plateau. Long-term weathering along fissures in the rock has worn away the rest of the plateau.*

THE LANDSCAPE

BULGARIA'S BALKAN MOUNTAINS divide the Danubian Plain *(Dunavska Ravnina)* and Maritsa Basin, meeting the Black Sea in the east along sandy beaches. The steep Rhodope Mountains form a natural barrier with Greece, while the younger Pindus form a rugged central spine which descends into the Aegean Sea to give a vast archipelago of over 2000 islands, the largest of which is Crete.

Mount Olympus is the mythical home of the Greek Gods and, at 9,570 ft (2,917 m), is the highest mountain in Greece.

Limestone rocks exposed by erosion of metamorphic rocks

Mount Olympus

Younger limestones created in shallow seas

Ancient metamorphic rock, formed miles below the surface

***Mount Olympus** is a composite of rocks formed by two major tectonic events. First the older metamorphic rocks were thrust over the limestones, then two million years ago regional warping and subsequent erosion, reexposed the limestone.*

The Peloponnese consist of several mountainous peninsulas, linked to the mainland by the Isthmus of Corinth. The Corinth Canal *(Dioryga Korinthou)*, built in 1893, cuts through the isthmus, linking the Aegean and Ionian Seas.

The Danube, Europe's second longest river, forms most of Bulgaria's northern border. The Danubian Plain *(Dunavska Ravnina)*, extending from the southern bank, is extremely fertile.

Balkan Mountains

Maritsa Basin

Rhodope Mountains

Pindus Mountains

Corinth Canal *(Dioryga Korinthou)*

Kythira

Crete

Karpathos

Rhodes

*The **Arda river** cuts through the Rhodope mountains in rugged, rocky gorges.*

The islands of Crete, Kythira, Karpathos, and Rhodes are part of an arc which bends southeastward from the Peloponnese, forming the southern boundary of the Aegean.

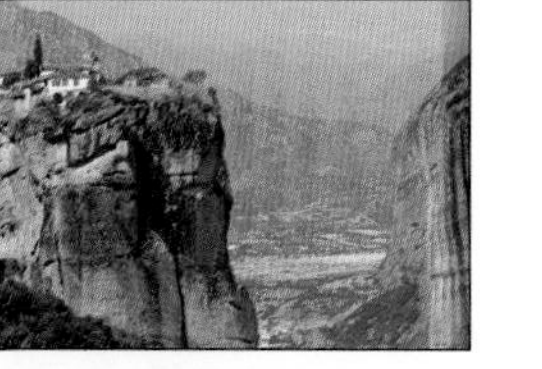

***Layers of black volcanic ash** still cover the island of Thira. This volcano last erupted 3,500 years ago, but still shows signs of volcanic activity.*

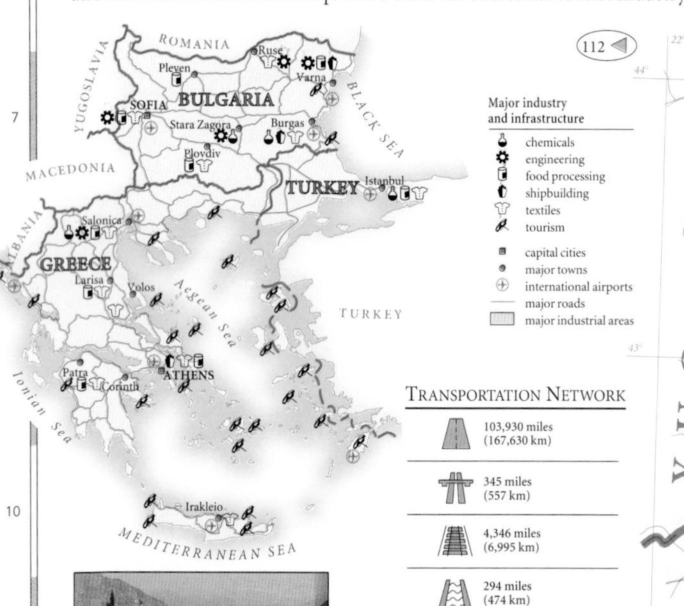

SCALE 1:2,750,000
(projection: Lambert Conformal Conic)

112
116
112

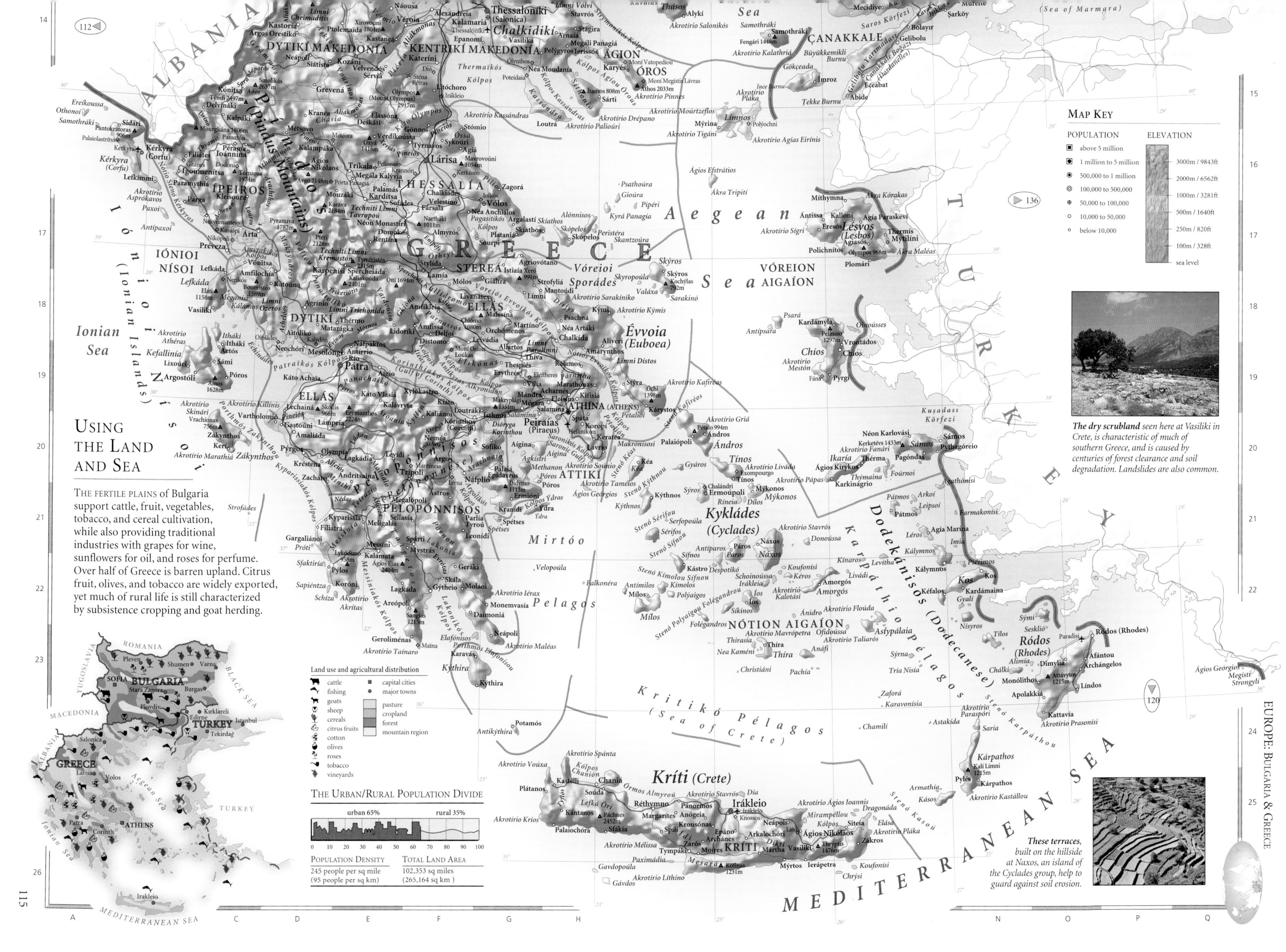

112
136
120
ALBANIA
GREECE
TURKEY
Píndos (Pindus Mountains)
DYTIKÍ MAKEDONÍA
KENTRIKÍ MAKEDONÍA
Chalkidikí
ÁGION ÓROS
ÍPEIROS
THESSALÍA
STEREÁ ELLÁS
DYTIKÍ ELLÁS
PELOPÓNNISOS
ATTIKÍ
ATHÍNA (ATHENS)
Thessaloníki (Salonica)
Lárisa
Pátra
Peiraiás (Piraeus)
IÓNIOI NÍSOI
Iónioi Nísoi (Ionian Islands)
Ionian Sea
Aegean Sea
VÓREION AIGAÍON
NÓTION AIGAÍON
Vóreioi Sporádes
Évvoia (Euboea)
Kykládes (Cyclades)
Dodekánisos (Dodecanese)
Kárpathio Pélagos
Kritikó Pélagos (Sea of Crete)
Mirtóo Pelagos
Kríti (Crete)
Irákleio
Ródos (Rhodes)
Lésvos (Lesbos)
Chíos
Sámos
ÇANAKKALE
(Sea of Marmara)
MEDITERRANEAN SEA
MAP KEY
POPULATION
above 5 million
1 million to 5 million
500,000 to 1 million
100,000 to 500,000
50,000 to 100,000
10,000 to 50,000
below 10,000
ELEVATION
3000m / 9843ft
2000m / 6562ft
1000m / 3281ft
500m / 1640ft
250m / 820ft
100m / 328ft
sea level
Land use and agricultural distribution
cattle
fishing
goats
sheep
cereals
citrus fruits
cotton
olives
roses
tobacco
vineyards
capital cities
major towns
pasture
cropland
forest
mountain region
ROMANIA
BULGARIA
SOFIA
Plovdiv
Stara Zagora
Burgas
Varna
Shumen
Pleven
BLACK SEA
YUGOSLAVIA
MACEDONIA
ALBANIA
GREECE
Salonica
Larisa
Volos
Patra
Corinth
ATHENS
Irakleio
Edirne
Kirklareli
Istanbul
Tekirdag
Aegean Sea
Ionian Sea
MEDITERRANEAN SEA

Using the Land and Sea

The fertile plains of Bulgaria support cattle, fruit, vegetables, tobacco, and cereal cultivation, while also providing traditional industries with grapes for wine, sunflowers for oil, and roses for perfume. Over half of Greece is barren upland. Citrus fruit, olives, and tobacco are widely exported, yet much of rural life is still characterized by subsistence cropping and goat herding.

The Urban/Rural Population Divide

urban 65% | rural 35%

0 10 20 30 40 50 60 70 80 90 100

Population Density
245 people per sq mile
(95 people per sq km)

Total Land Area
102,353 sq miles
(265,164 sq km)

The dry scrubland seen here at Vasiliki in Crete, is characteristic of much of southern Greece, and is caused by centuries of forest clearance and soil degradation. Landslides are also common.

These terraces, built on the hillside at Naxos, an island of the Cyclades group, help to guard against soil erosion.

Romania, Moldova & Ukraine

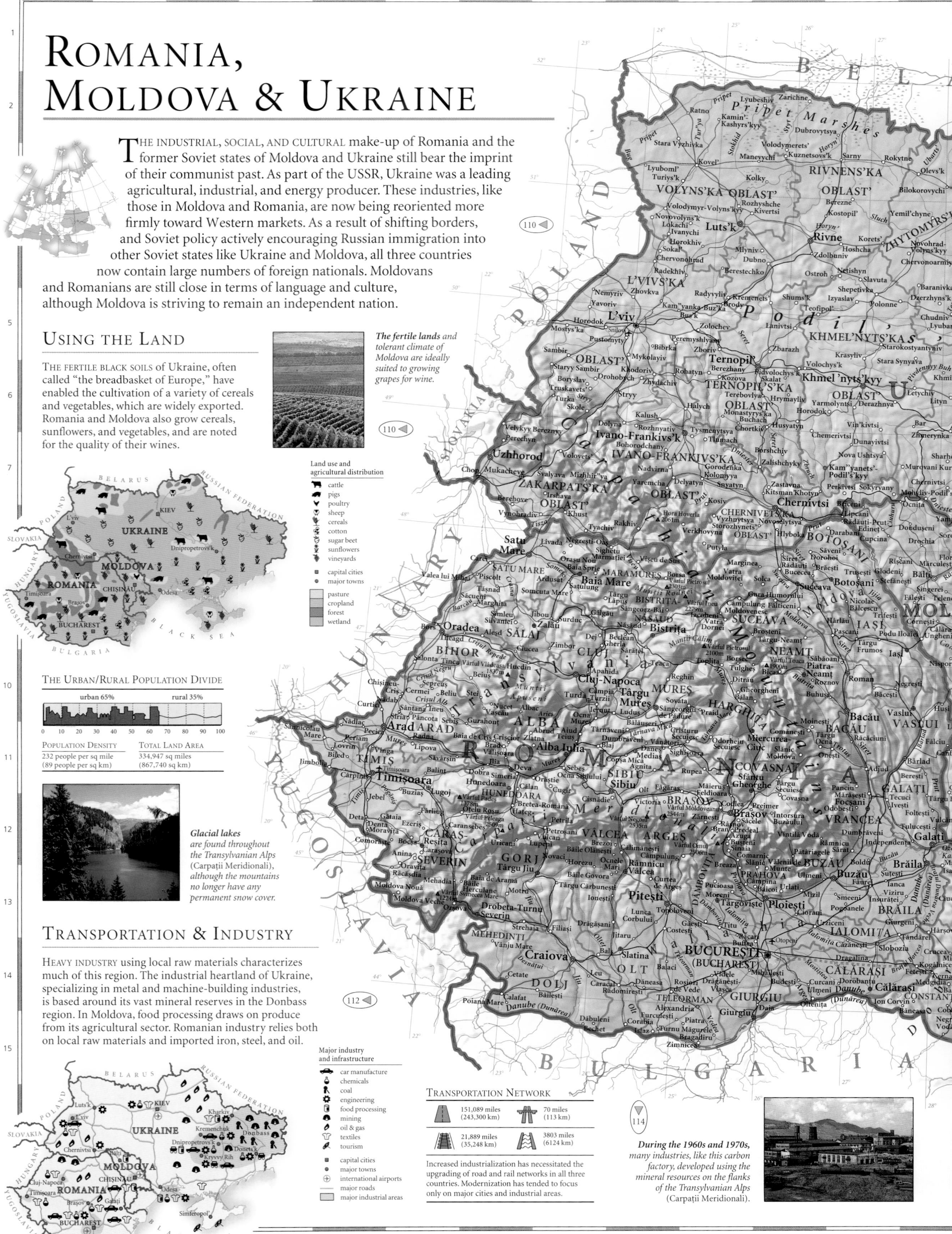

The industrial, social, and cultural make-up of Romania and the former Soviet states of Moldova and Ukraine still bear the imprint of their communist past. As part of the USSR, Ukraine was a leading agricultural, industrial, and energy producer. These industries, like those in Moldova and Romania, are now being reoriented more firmly toward Western markets. As a result of shifting borders, and Soviet policy actively encouraging Russian immigration into other Soviet states like Ukraine and Moldova, all three countries now contain large numbers of foreign nationals. Moldovans and Romanians are still close in terms of language and culture, although Moldova is striving to remain an independent nation.

Using the Land

The fertile black soils of Ukraine, often called "the breadbasket of Europe," have enabled the cultivation of a variety of cereals and vegetables, which are widely exported. Romania and Moldova also grow cereals, sunflowers, and vegetables, and are noted for the quality of their wines.

The fertile lands and tolerant climate of Moldova are ideally suited to growing grapes for wine.

Land use and agricultural distribution

- cattle
- pigs
- poultry
- sheep
- cereals
- cotton
- sugar beet
- sunflowers
- vineyards
- capital cities
- major towns
- pasture
- cropland
- forest
- wetland

The Urban/Rural Population Divide

urban 65% | rural 35%

Population Density	Total Land Area
232 people per sq mile (89 people per sq km)	334,947 sq miles (867,740 sq km)

***Glacial lakes** are found throughout the Transylvanian Alps (Carpaţii Meridionali), although the mountains no longer have any permanent snow cover.*

Transportation & Industry

Heavy industry using local raw materials characterizes much of this region. The industrial heartland of Ukraine, specializing in metal and machine-building industries, is based around its vast mineral reserves in the Donbass region. In Moldova, food processing draws on produce from its agricultural sector. Romanian industry relies both on local raw materials and imported iron, steel, and oil.

Major industry and infrastructure

- car manufacture
- chemicals
- coal
- engineering
- food processing
- mining
- oil & gas
- textiles
- tourism
- capital cities
- major towns
- international airports
- major roads
- major industrial areas

Transportation Network

151,089 miles (243,300 km)	70 miles (113 km)
21,889 miles (35,248 km)	3803 miles (6124 km)

Increased industrialization has necessitated the upgrading of road and rail networks in all three countries. Modernization has tended to focus only on major cities and industrial areas.

During the 1960s and 1970s, many industries, like this carbon factory, developed using the mineral resources on the flanks of the Transylvanian Alps (Carpaţii Meridionali).

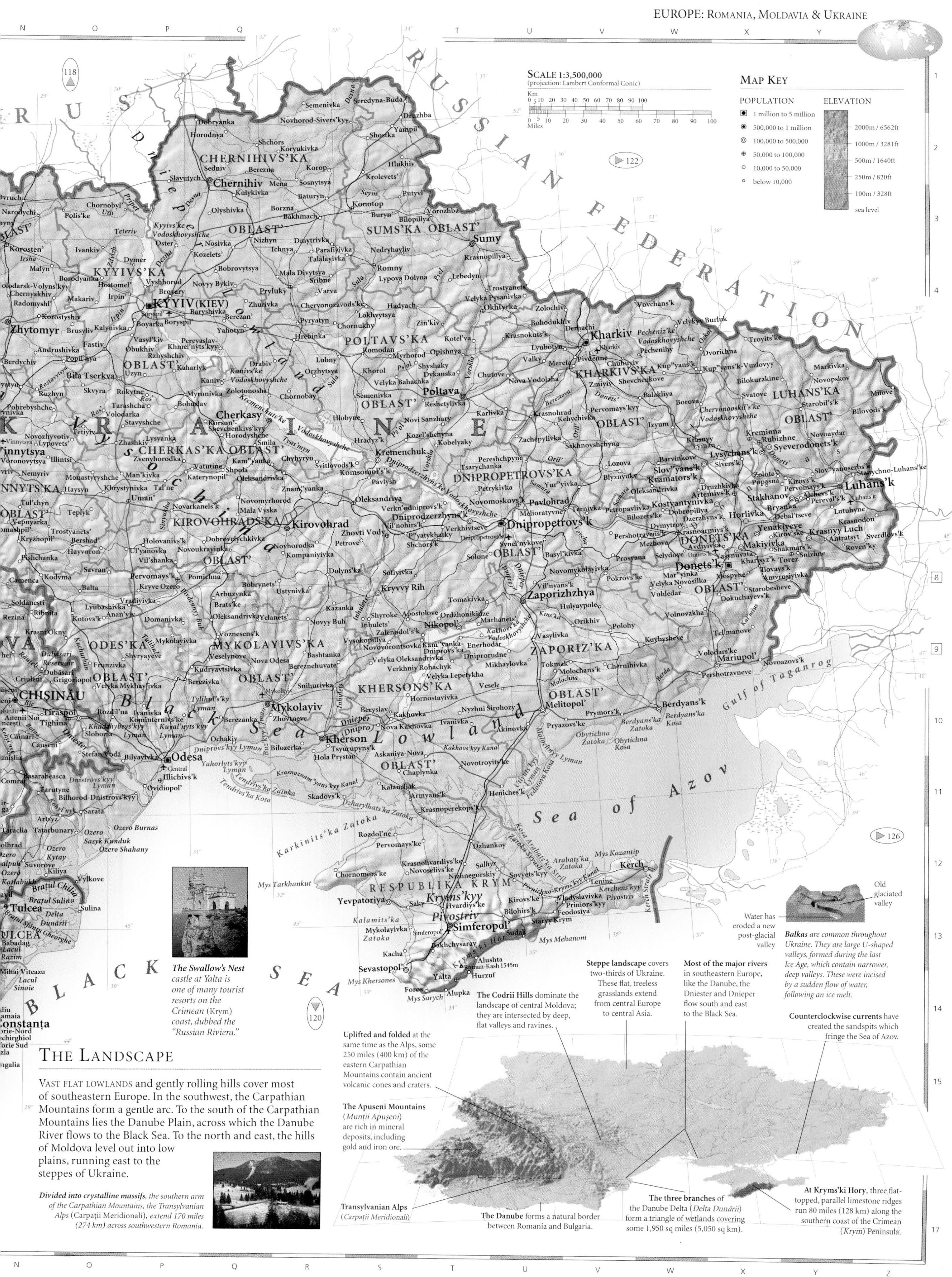
SCALE 1:3,500,000
(projection: Lambert Conformal Conic)
Km
Miles
MAP KEY
POPULATION
1 million to 5 million
500,000 to 1 million
100,000 to 500,000
50,000 to 100,000
10,000 to 50,000
below 10,000
ELEVATION
2000m / 6562ft
1000m / 3281ft
500m / 1640ft
250m / 820ft
100m / 328ft
sea level
RUSSIAN FEDERATION
UKRAINE
BLACK SEA
Sea of Azov
Gulf of Taganrog
Black Sea Lowland
Dnieper Lowland
CHERNIHIVS'KA OBLAST'
SUMS'KA OBLAST'
KYYIVS'KA OBLAST'
POLTAVS'KA OBLAST'
KHARKIVS'KA OBLAST'
LUHANS'KA OBLAST'
CHERKAS'KA OBLAST'
DNIPROPETROVS'KA OBLAST'
DONETS'KA OBLAST'
KIROVOHRADS'KA OBLAST'
ODES'KA OBLAST'
MYKOLAYIVS'KA OBLAST'
KHERSONS'KA OBLAST'
ZAPORIZ'KA OBLAST'
RESPUBLIKA KRYM
KYYIV (KIEV)
Chernihiv
Sumy
Kharkiv
Poltava
Cherkasy
Kremenchuk
Kirovohrad
Dnipropetrovs'k
Zaporizhzhya
Donets'k
Luhans'k
Mykolayiv
Kherson
Odesa
Simferopol'
Sevastopol'
Yalta
Kerch
Melitopol'
Berdyans'k
Mariupol'
Zhytomyr
Vinnytsya
CHIŞINĂU
Tulcea
Constanța
Yevpatoriya
Kryvyy Rih
Nikopol'
Kryms'kyy Pivostriv
Old glaciated valley
Water has eroded a new post-glacial valley
Balkas are common throughout Ukraine. They are large U-shaped valleys, formed during the last Ice Age, which contain narrower, deep valleys. These were incised by a sudden flow of water, following an ice melt.
The Swallow's Nest castle at Yalta is one of many tourist resorts on the Crimean (Krym) coast, dubbed the "Russian Riviera."
The Codrii Hills dominate the landscape of central Moldova; they are intersected by deep, flat valleys and ravines.
Steppe landscape covers two-thirds of Ukraine. These flat, treeless grasslands extend from central Europe to central Asia.
Most of the major rivers in southeastern Europe, like the Danube, the Dniester and Dnieper flow south and east to the Black Sea.
Counterclockwise currents have created the sandspits which fringe the Sea of Azov.
Uplifted and folded at the same time as the Alps, some 250 miles (400 km) of the eastern Carpathian Mountains contain ancient volcanic cones and craters.
The Apuseni Mountains (Munții Apuseni) are rich in mineral deposits, including gold and iron ore.
Transylvanian Alps (Carpații Meridionali)
The Danube forms a natural border between Romania and Bulgaria.
The three branches of the Danube Delta (Delta Dunării) form a triangle of wetlands covering some 1,950 sq miles (5,050 sq km).
At Kryms'ki Hory, three flat-topped, parallel limestone ridges run 80 miles (128 km) along the southern coast of the Crimean (Krym) Peninsula.

THE LANDSCAPE

VAST FLAT LOWLANDS and gently rolling hills cover most of southeastern Europe. In the southwest, the Carpathian Mountains form a gentle arc. To the south of the Carpathian Mountains lies the Danube Plain, across which the Danube River flows to the Black Sea. To the north and east, the hills of Moldova level out into low plains, running east to the steppes of Ukraine.

Divided into crystalline massifs, the southern arm of the Carpathian Mountains, the Transylvanian Alps (Carpații Meridionali), *extend 170 miles (274 km) across southwestern Romania.*

The Baltic states & Belarus

Belarus, Estonia, Latvia, Lithuania, Kaliningrad

Occupying Europe's main corridor to Russia, the four distinct cultures of Estonia, Latvia, Lithuania, and Belarus share a history of struggle for nationhood against the interests of more powerful neighbors. As the first republics to declare their independence from the Soviet Union in 1990–91, the Baltic states of Estonia, Latvia, and Lithuania have sought an economic role in the EU, while reaffirming their European cultural roots through the church and a strong musical tradition. Meanwhile, Belarus has shown economic and political allegiance to Russia by joining the Commonwealth of Independent States.

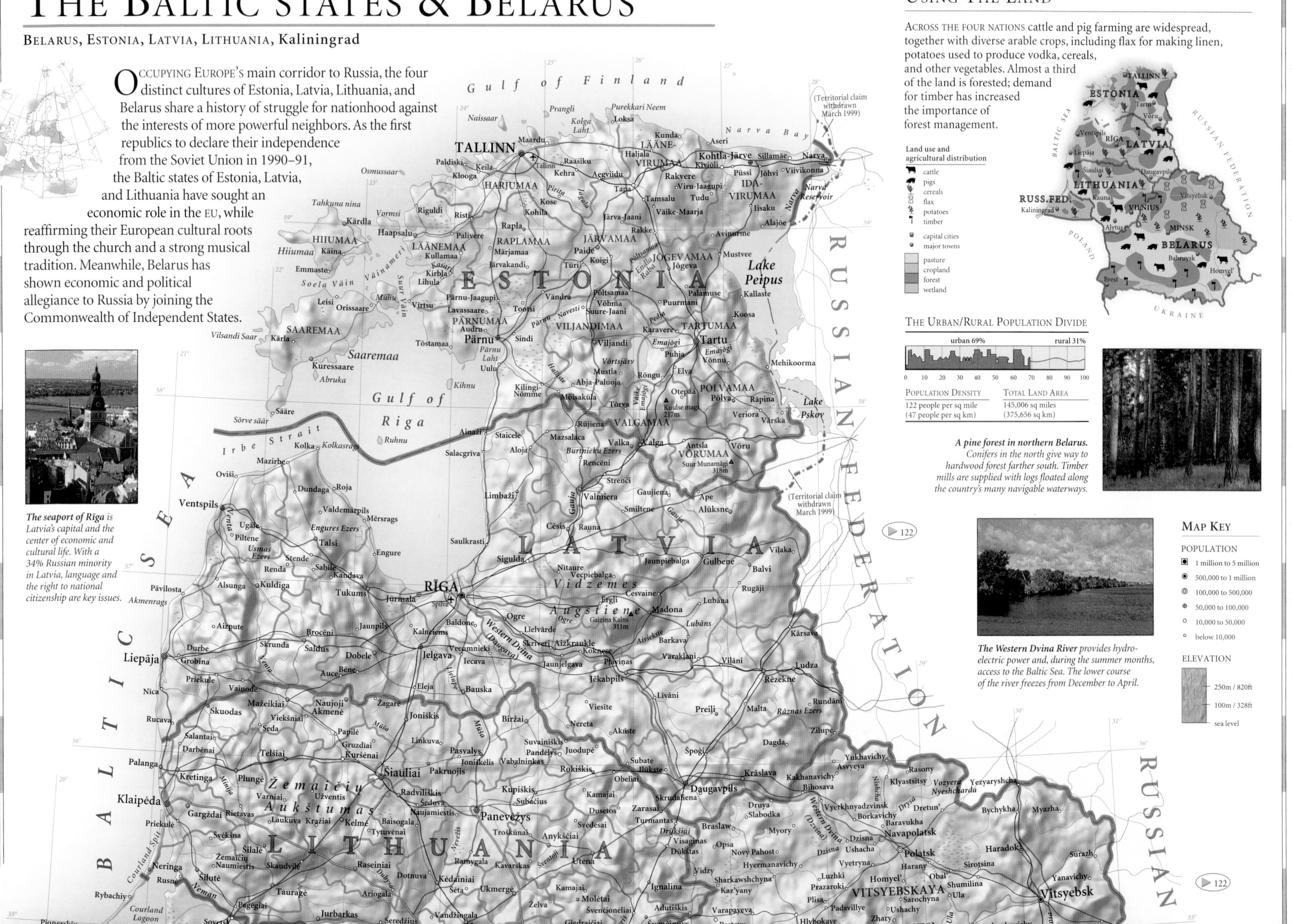

Gulf of Finland
Gulf of Riga
Irbe Strait
BALTIC SEA
RUSSIAN FEDERATION
ESTONIA
LATVIA
LITHUANIA
TALLINN
RĪGA
Tartu
Pärnu
Lake Peipus
Lake Pskov
Saaremaa
Hiiumaa
Ventspils
Liepāja
Klaipėda
Šiauliai
Panevėžys
Daugavpils
Jelgava
Vitsyebsk
Polatsk
Navapolatsk
VITSYEBSKAYA VOBLASTS'
Western Dvina (Daugava)
Courland Lagoon
(Territorial claim withdrawn March 1999)
122

The seaport of Rīga is Latvia's capital and the center of economic and cultural life. With a 34% Russian minority in Latvia, language and the right to national citizenship are key issues.

Using The Land

Across the four nations cattle and pig farming are widespread, together with diverse arable crops, including flax for making linen, potatoes used to produce vodka, cereals, and other vegetables. Almost a third of the land is forested; demand for timber has increased the importance of forest management.

Land use and agricultural distribution: cattle, pigs, cereals, flax, potatoes, timber, capital cities, major towns, pasture, cropland, forest, wetland

The Urban/Rural Population Divide

urban 69% — rural 31%

Population Density	Total Land Area
122 people per sq mile (47 people per sq km)	145,006 sq miles (375,656 sq km)

A pine forest in northern Belarus. *Conifers in the north give way to hardwood forest farther south. Timber mills are supplied with logs floated along the country's many navigable waterways.*

The Western Dvina River *provides hydro-electric power and, during the summer months, access to the Baltic Sea. The lower course of the river freezes from December to April.*

Map Key

POPULATION
- 1 million to 5 million
- 500,000 to 1 million
- 100,000 to 500,000
- 50,000 to 100,000
- 10,000 to 50,000
- below 10,000

ELEVATION
- 250m / 820ft
- 100m / 328ft
- sea level

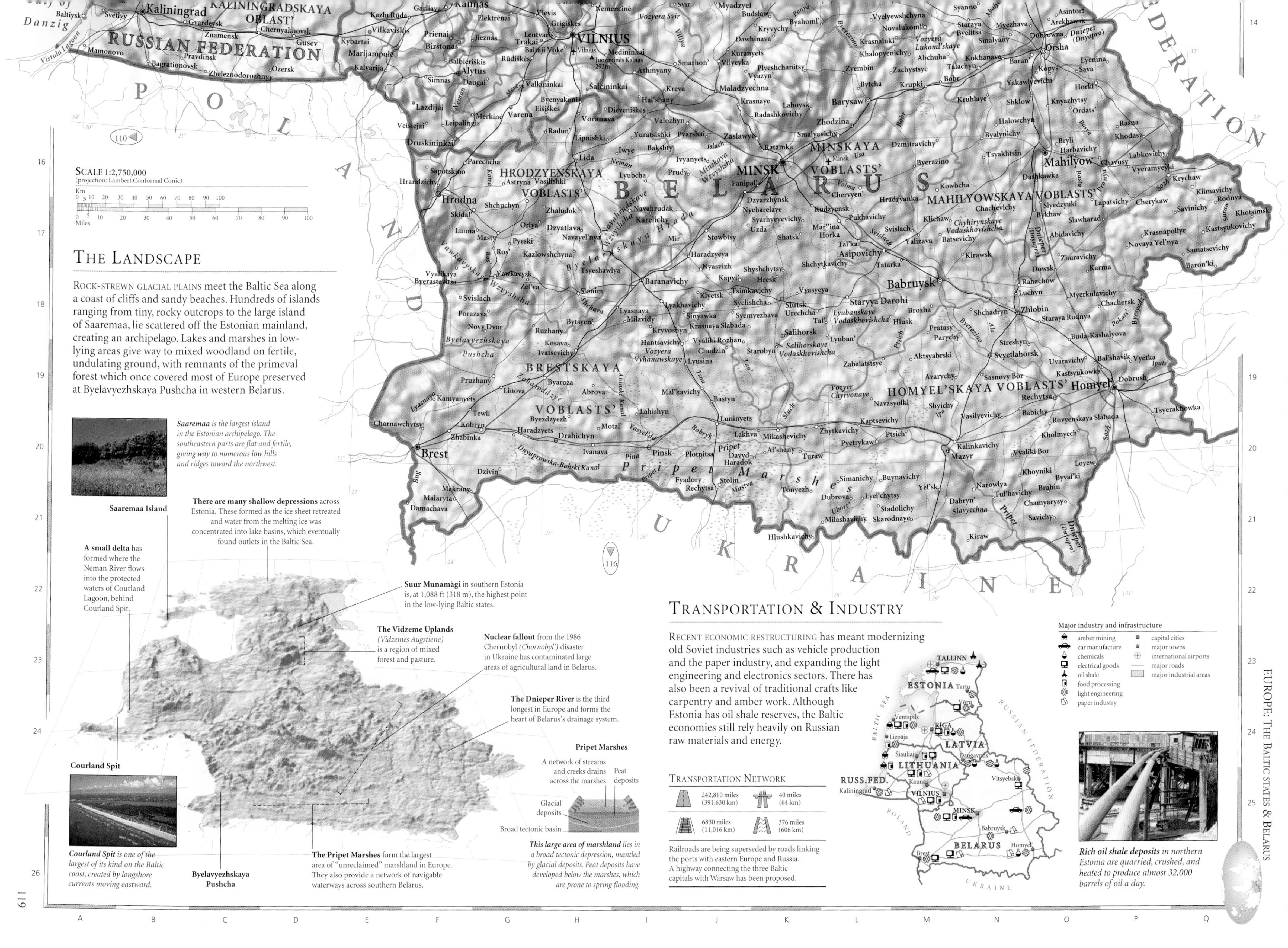

RUSSIAN FEDERATION
KALININGRADSKAYA OBLAST'
POLAND
BELARUS
UKRAINE
HRODZYENSKAYA VOBLASTS'
MINSKAYA VOBLASTS'
MAHILYOWSKAYA VOBLASTS'
BRESTSKAYA VOBLASTS'
HOMYEL'SKAYA VOBLASTS'
Kaliningrad
VILNIUS
MINSK
Hrodna
Brest
Babruysk
Mahilyow
Homyel'
Pripet Marshes
Dnieper (Dnyapro)
Pripet
Juozapinės Kalnas 292m
SCALE 1:2,750,000
(projection: Lambert Conformal Conic)
Km
Miles
Saaremaa Island
Courland Spit
Byelavyezhskaya Pushcha
Pripet Marshes
A network of streams and creeks drains across the marshes
Peat deposits
Glacial deposits
Broad tectonic basin
Major industry and infrastructure
amber mining
car manufacture
chemicals
electrical goods
oil shale
food processing
light engineering
paper industry
capital cities
major towns
international airports
major roads
major industrial areas
TALLINN
ESTONIA
RIGA
LATVIA
LITHUANIA
VILNIUS
MINSK
BELARUS
RUSS.FED.
BALTIC SEA
RUSSIAN FEDERATION
POLAND
UKRAINE

110
116

THE LANDSCAPE

ROCK-STREWN GLACIAL PLAINS meet the Baltic Sea along a coast of cliffs and sandy beaches. Hundreds of islands ranging from tiny, rocky outcrops to the large island of Saaremaa, lie scattered off the Estonian mainland, creating an archipelago. Lakes and marshes in low-lying areas give way to mixed woodland on fertile, undulating ground, with remnants of the primeval forest which once covered most of Europe preserved at Byelavyezhskaya Pushcha in western Belarus.

Saaremaa is the largest island in the Estonian archipelago. The southeastern parts are flat and fertile, giving way to numerous low hills and ridges toward the northwest.

There are many shallow depressions across Estonia. These formed as the ice sheet retreated and water from the melting ice was concentrated into lake basins, which eventually found outlets in the Baltic Sea.

A small delta has formed where the Neman River flows into the protected waters of Courland Lagoon, behind Courland Spit.

Suur Munamägi in southern Estonia is, at 1,088 ft (318 m), the highest point in the low-lying Baltic states.

The Vidzeme Uplands *(Vidzemes Augstiene)* is a region of mixed forest and pasture.

Nuclear fallout from the 1986 Chernobyl *(Chornobyl')* disaster in Ukraine has contaminated large areas of agricultural land in Belarus.

The Dnieper River is the third longest in Europe and forms the heart of Belarus's drainage system.

Courland Spit is one of the largest of its kind on the Baltic coast, created by longshore currents moving eastward.

The Pripet Marshes form the largest area of "unreclaimed" marshland in Europe. They also provide a network of navigable waterways across southern Belarus.

***This large area of marshland** lies in a broad tectonic depression, mantled by glacial deposits. Peat deposits have developed below the marshes, which are prone to spring flooding.*

TRANSPORTATION & INDUSTRY

RECENT ECONOMIC RESTRUCTURING has meant modernizing old Soviet industries such as vehicle production and the paper industry, and expanding the light engineering and electronics sectors. There has also been a revival of traditional crafts like carpentry and amber work. Although Estonia has oil shale reserves, the Baltic economies still rely heavily on Russian raw materials and energy.

TRANSPORTATION NETWORK

242,810 miles (391,630 km)	40 miles (64 km)
6830 miles (11,016 km)	376 miles (606 km)

Railroads are being superseded by roads linking the ports with eastern Europe and Russia. A highway connecting the three Baltic capitals with Warsaw has been proposed.

***Rich oil shale deposits** in northern Estonia are quarried, crushed, and heated to produce almost 32,000 barrels of oil a day.*

The Mediterranean

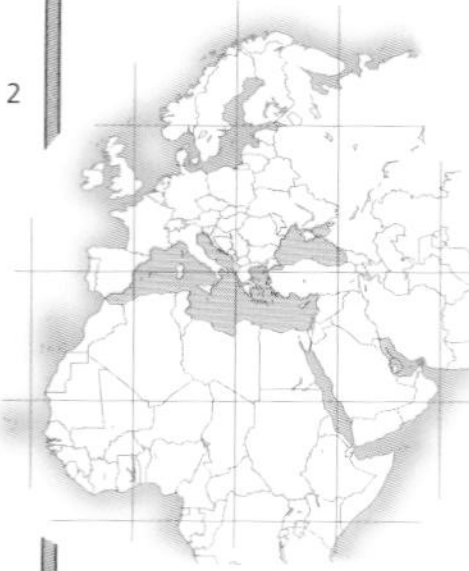

The Mediterranean Sea stretches over 2,500 miles (4,000 km) east to west, separating Europe from Africa. At its westernmost point it is connected to the Atlantic Ocean through the Strait of Gibraltar. In the east, the Suez Canal, opened in 1869, gives passage to the Indian Ocean. In the northeast, linked by the Sea of Marmara, lies the Black Sea. Throughout history the Mediterranean has been a focal area for many great empires and civilizations, reflected in the variety of cultures found in the 28 states and territories that border its shores. Since the 1960s, development along the southern coast of Europe has expanded rapidly to accommodate increasing numbers of tourists and to enable the exploitation of oil and gas reserves. This has resulted in rising levels of pollution, threatening the future of the sea.

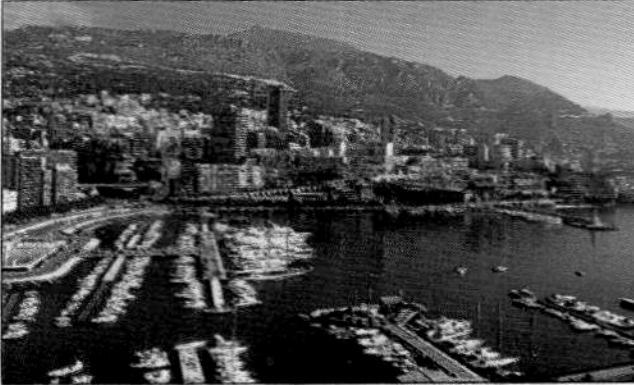

***Monte Carlo in Monaco** is just one of the luxurious resorts scattered along the Riviera, which stretches along the coast from Cannes in France to La Spezia in Italy. The region's mild winters and hot summers have attracted wealthy tourists since the early 19th century.*

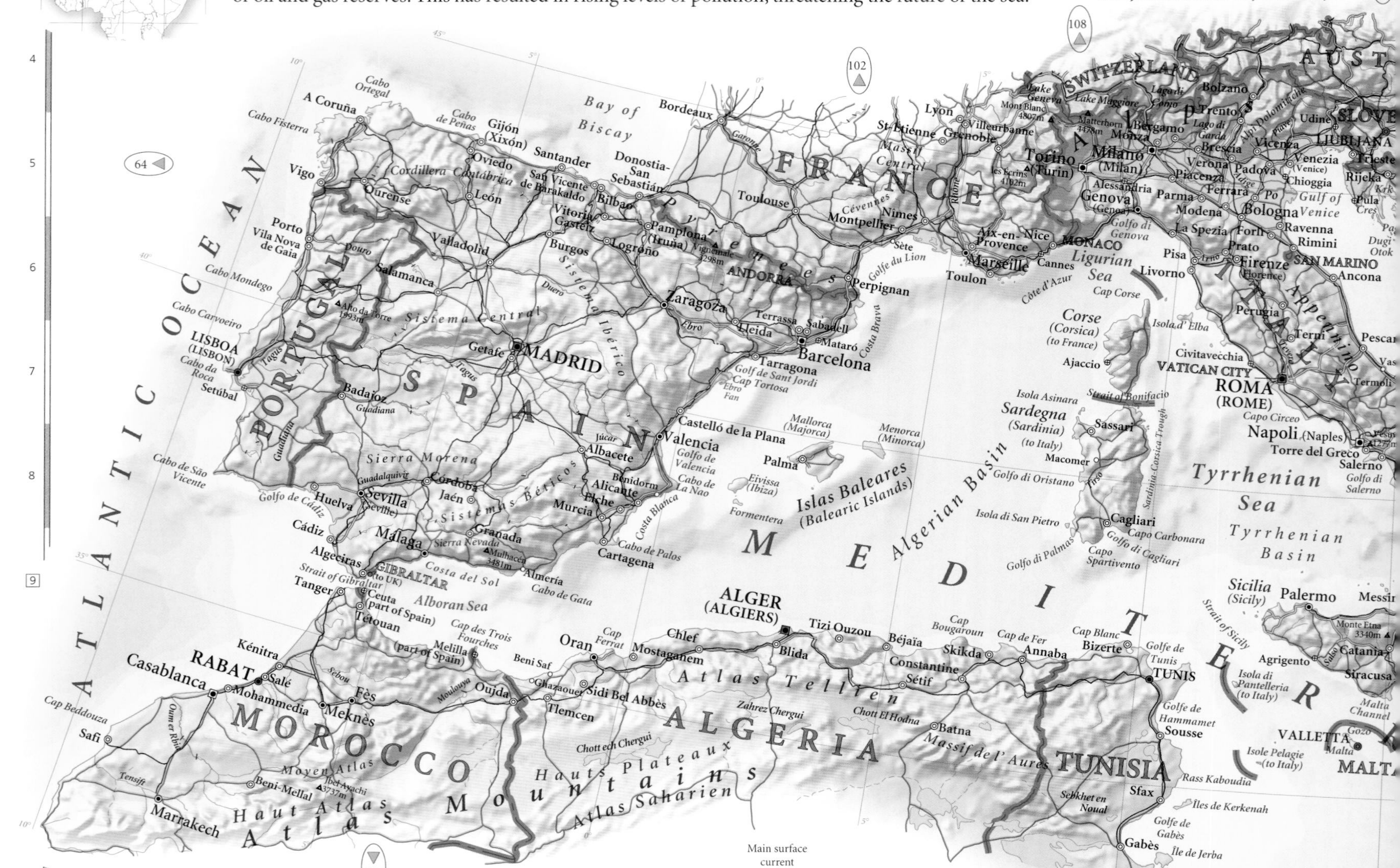

The Landscape

The Mediterranean Sea is almost totally landlocked, joined to the Atlantic Ocean through the Strait of Gibraltar, which is only 8 miles (13 km) wide. Lying on an active plate margin, sea floor movements have formed a variety of basins, troughs, and ridges. A submarine ridge running from Tunisia to Sicily divides the sea into two distinct basins. The western basin is characterized by broad, smooth abyssal (or ocean) plains. In contrast, the eastern basin is dominated by a large ridge system, running east to west.

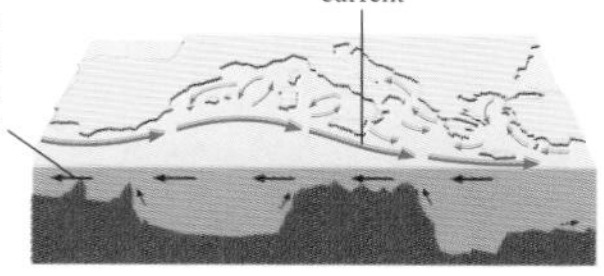

Main surface current

Denser, more saline currents flow back to Atlantic

***Atlantic surface water** enters the Mediterranean Sea via the Straits of Gibraltar and generally flows eastward, becoming progressively more saline and dense as water evaporates. This denser water sinks and at depths below 280 ft (80 m), flows back to the Atlantic Ocean.*

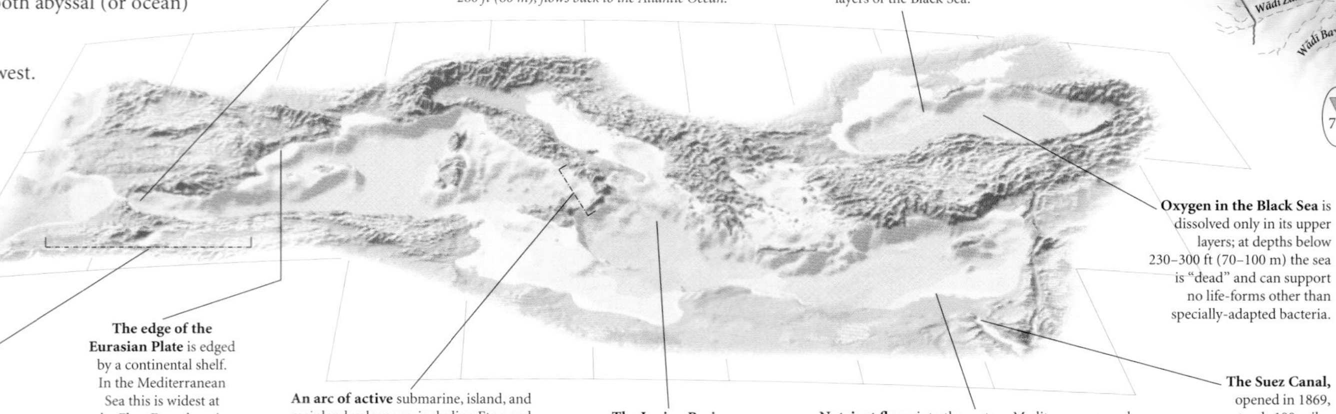

Industrial pollution flowing from the Dnieper and Danube Rivers has destroyed a large proportion of the fish population that used to inhabit the upper layers of the Black Sea.

Oxygen in the Black Sea is dissolved only in its upper layers; at depths below 230–300 ft (70–100 m) the sea is "dead" and can support no life-forms other than specially-adapted bacteria.

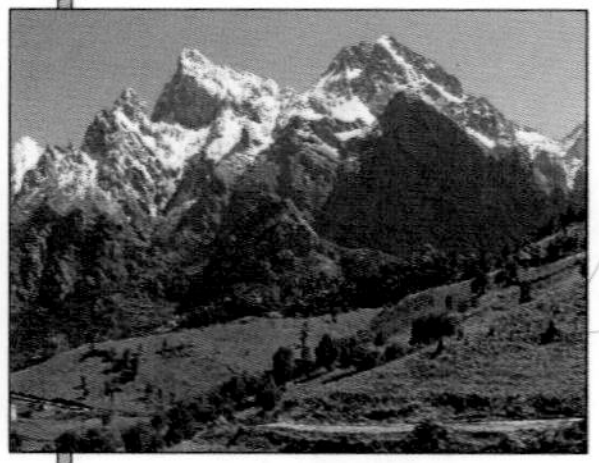

***The Atlas Mountains** are a range of fold mountains that lie in Morocco and Algeria. They run parallel to the Mediterranean, forming a topographical and climatic divide between the Mediterranean coast and the western Sahara.*

The edge of the Eurasian Plate is edged by a continental shelf. In the Mediterranean Sea this is widest at he Ebro Fan where it extends 60 miles (96 km).

An arc of active submarine, island, and mainland volcanoes, including Etna and Vesuvius, lie in and around southern Italy. The area is also susceptible to earthquakes and landslides.

The Ionian Basin is the deepest in the Mediterranean, reaching depths of 16,800 ft (5,121 m).

Nutrient flows into the eastern Mediterranean, and sediment flows to the Nile Delta have been severely lowered by the building of the Aswan Dam across the Nile in Egypt. This is causing the delta to shrink.

The Suez Canal, opened in 1869, extends 100 miles (160 km) from Port Said to the Gulf of Suez.

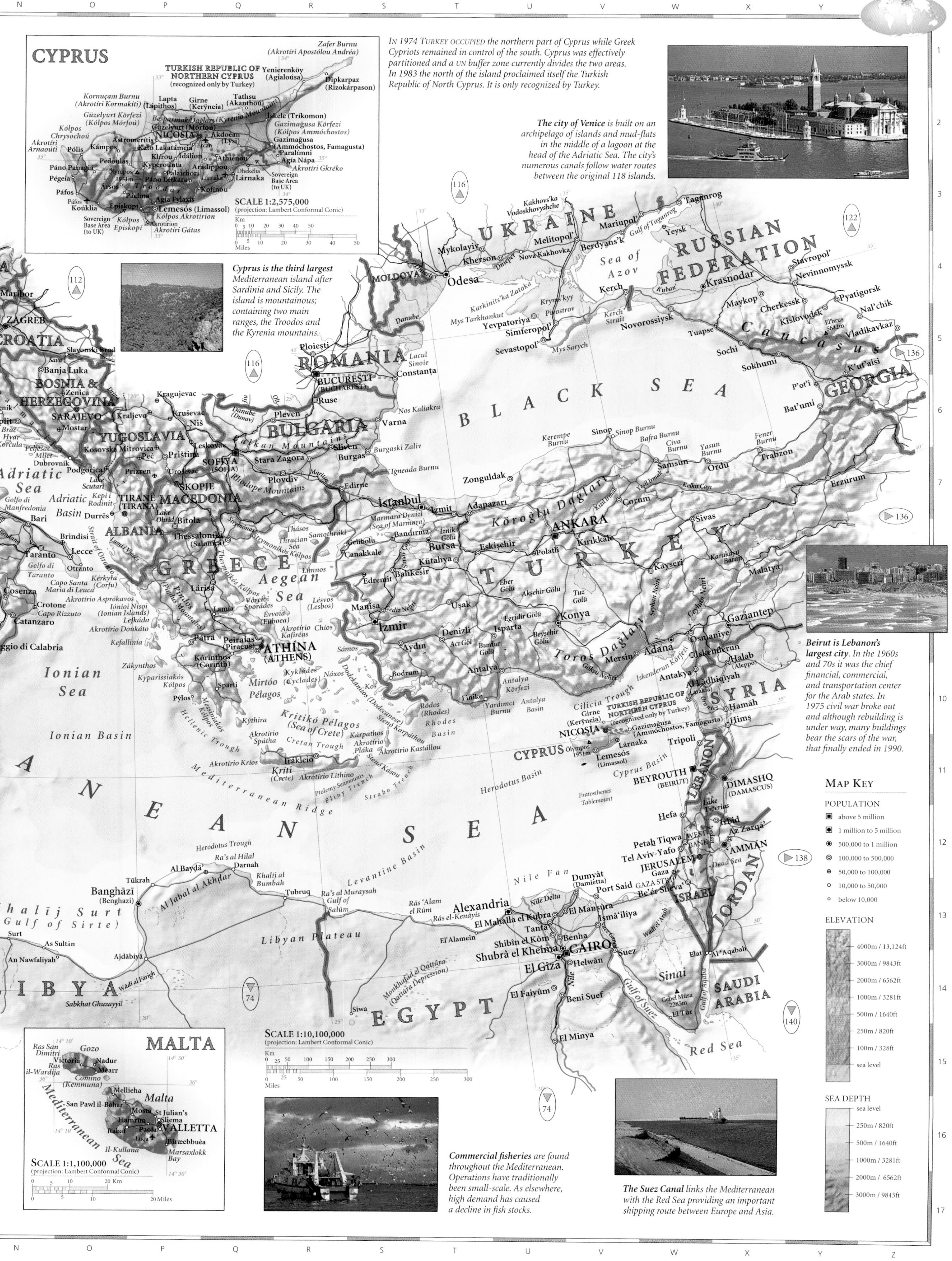
N O P Q R S T U V W X Y Z
1 2 3 4 5 6 7 8 9 10 11 12 13 14 15 16 17
CYPRUS
TURKISH REPUBLIC OF NORTHERN CYPRUS (recognized only by Turkey)
Zafer Burnu (Akrotíri Apostólou Andréa)
Yenierenköy (Agialoúsa)
Dipkarpaz (Rizokárpason)
Kornuçam Burnu (Akrotíri Kormakíti)
Lapta (Lápithos)
Girne (Kerýneia)
Tatlısu (Akanthoú)
Güzelyurt Körfezi (Kólpos Mórfou)
Kólpos Chrysochoú
Akrotíri Arnaoúti
Pólis
İskele (Tríkomon)
Gazimağusa Körfezi (Kólpos Ammóchostos)
Gazimağusa (Ammóchostos, Famagusta)
Paralimni
Agía Nápa
Akrotíri Gkréko
NICOSIA
Kámpos
Pedoulas
Páno Panagiá
Pégeia
Olympos 1951m
Páfos
Koúklia
Larnaka
Lemesós (Limassol)
Agia Fylaxis
Episkopí
Kólpos Akrotíriou
Akrotírion
Akrotíri Gátas
Kólpos Episkopí
Sovereign Base Area (to UK)
SCALE 1:2,575,000 (projection: Lambert Conformal Conic)
Km 0 5 10 20 30 40 50
Miles 0 5 10 20 30 40 50
116
112
122
136
138
140
74
UKRAINE
RUSSIAN FEDERATION
MOLDOVA
Odesa
Mykolayiv
Kherson
Melitopol'
Mariupol'
Berdyans'k
Taganrog
Yeysk
Sea of Azov
Kerch
Krasnodar
Stavropol'
Nevinnomyssk
Maykop
Cherkessk
Pyatigorsk
Kislovodsk
Nal'chik
Vladikavkaz
Novorossiysk
Tuapse
Sochi
Sokhumi
Caucasus
El'brus 5642m
Yevpatoriya
Simferopol'
Sevastopol'
Mys Sarych
Karkinits'ka Zatoka
Mys Tarkhankut
Kerch Strait
Danube
ROMANIA
Ploiești
BUCUREȘTI (BUCHAREST)
Constanța
Lacul Sinoie
Ruse
BLACK SEA
GEORGIA
K'ut'aisi
P'ot'i
Bat'umi
BULGARIA
Pleven
Varna
Burgas
Sliven
Stara Zagora
Plovdiv
SOFIYA (SOFIA)
Balkan Mountains
Rhodope Mountains
Nos Kaliakra
Burgaski Zaliv
Edirne
İğneada Burnu
Maribor
ZAGREB
CROATIA
BOSNIA & HERZEGOVINA
Banja Luka
Zenica
SARAJEVO
Mostar
YUGOSLAVIA
Kragujevac
Kraljevo
Kruševac
Niš
Leskovac
Priština
Peć
Kosovska Mitrovica
Prizren
Podgorica
Dubrovnik
SKOPJE
MACEDONIA
Bitola
Lake Ohrid
TIRANË (TIRANA)
Durrës
ALBANIA
Adriatic Sea
Adriatic Basin
Bari
Brindisi
Taranto
Lecce
Otranto
Golfo di Taranto
Crotone
Cosenza
Catanzaro
Reggio di Calabria
Ionian Sea
Ionian Basin
GREECE
Thessaloníki (Salonica)
Lárisa
Lamía
Pátra
ATHÍNA (ATHENS)
Peiraias (Piraeus)
Kórinthos (Corinth)
Spárti
Pýlos
Kérkyra (Corfu)
Kefallinía
Zákynthos
Aegean Sea
Thracian Sea
Thásos
Samothráki
Límnos
Lésvos (Lesbos)
Chíos
Sámos
Kykládes (Cyclades)
Náxos
Dodekánisos (Dodecanese)
Ródos (Rhodes)
Kárpathos
Kríti (Crete)
Irákleio
Kritikó Pélagos (Sea of Crete)
Mirtóo Pélagos
Hellenic Trough
Mediterranean Ridge
MEDITERRANEAN SEA
TURKEY
İstanbul
Marmara Denizi (Sea of Marmara)
İzmit
Adapazarı
Bursa
Bandırma
Çanakkale
Gelibolu
Balıkesir
Kütahya
Eskişehir
ANKARA
Polatlı
Kırıkkale
Çorum
Zonguldak
Sinop
Samsun
Ordu
Trabzon
Erzurum
Sivas
Kayseri
Malatya
Gaziantep
Osmaniye
Adana
Mersin
İskenderun
Antakya
Konya
Isparta
Burdur
Denizli
Uşak
Manisa
İzmir
Aydın
Bodrum
Antalya
Finike
Antalya Körfezi
Köroğlu Dağları
Toros Dağları
Tuz Gölü
CYPRUS
NICOSIA
SYRIA
Al Lādhiqīyah (Latakia)
Ḩamāh
Ḩimṣ
Ḩalab (Aleppo)
Tripoli
BEYROUTH (BEIRUT)
LEBANON
DIMASHQ (DAMASCUS)
Hefa
Irbid
Az Zarqā'
'AMMĀN
Petah Tiqwa
Tel Aviv-Yafo
JERUSALEM
WEST BANK
Gaza
GAZA STRIP
Be'ér Sheva'
ISRAEL
JORDAN
Dead Sea
Elat
Al 'Aqabah
SAUDI ARABIA
Herodotus Basin
Eratosthenes Tablemount
Levantine Basin
Nile Fan
Nile Delta
Dumyât (Damietta)
Port Said
El Manṣûra
Ismâ'îlîya
Suez
Alexandria
El Maḥalla el Kubra
Tanta
Benha
Shibîn el Kôm
Shubrâ el Kheima
CAIRO
El Gîza
Helwân
El Faiyûm
Beni Suef
El Minya
Sinai
Gebel Mûsa 2285m
El Ṭûr
Gulf of Suez
Red Sea
EGYPT
Siwa
Libyan Plateau
Monkhafad el Qattâra (Qattara Depression)
El'Alamein
Râs 'Alam el Rûm
Tubruq
Gulf of Salûm
Darnah
Al Bayḍā'
Al Jabal al Akhḑar
Tūkrah
Banghāzī (Benghazi)
Ajdābiyā
Khalīj Surt (Gulf of Sirte)
Surt
LIBYA
Sabkhat Ghuzayyil
SCALE 1:10,100,000 (projection: Lambert Conformal Conic)
Km 0 25 50 100 150 200 250 300
Miles 0 25 50 100 150 200 250 300
MALTA
Gozo
Victoria
Nadur
Mġarr
Comino (Kemmuna)
Mellieħa
San Pawl il-Baħar
Mosta
St Julian's
Sliema
VALLETTA
Rabat
Paola
Birżebbuġa
Marsaxlokk Bay
Mediterranean Sea
SCALE 1:1,100,000 (projection: Lambert Conformal Conic)
0 5 10 20 Km
0 5 10 20 Miles
MAP KEY
POPULATION
above 5 million
1 million to 5 million
500,000 to 1 million
100,000 to 500,000
50,000 to 100,000
10,000 to 50,000
below 10,000
ELEVATION
4000m / 13,124ft
3000m / 9843ft
2000m / 6562ft
1000m / 3281ft
500m / 1640ft
250m / 820ft
100m / 328ft
sea level
SEA DEPTH
sea level
250m / 820ft
500m / 1640ft
1000m / 3281ft
2000m / 6562ft
3000m / 9843ft

In 1974 Turkey occupied the northern part of Cyprus while Greek Cypriots remained in control of the south. Cyprus was effectively partitioned and a UN buffer zone currently divides the two areas. In 1983 the north of the island proclaimed itself the Turkish Republic of North Cyprus. It is only recognized by Turkey.

***The city of Venice** is built on an archipelago of islands and mud-flats in the middle of a lagoon at the head of the Adriatic Sea. The city's numerous canals follow water routes between the original 118 islands.*

***Cyprus is the third largest** Mediterranean island after Sardinia and Sicily. The island is mountainous; containing two main ranges, the Troodos and the Kyrenia mountains.*

***Beirut is Lebanon's largest city.** In the 1960s and 70s it was the chief financial, commercial, and transportation center for the Arab states. In 1975 civil war broke out and although rebuilding is under way, many buildings bear the scars of the war, that finally ended in 1990.*

***Commercial fisheries** are found throughout the Mediterranean. Operations have traditionally been small-scale. As elsewhere, high demand has caused a decline in fish stocks.*

***The Suez Canal** links the Mediterranean with the Red Sea providing an important shipping route between Europe and Asia.*

The Russian Federation

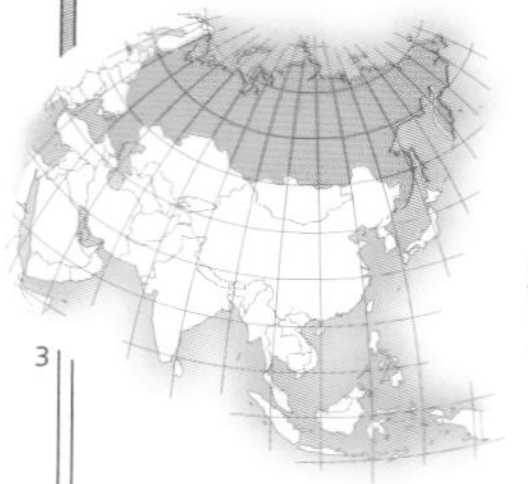

The Cold War era of global relations was concluded in 1991 with the formal dissolution of the Soviet Union. The Russian Federation declared its separate sovereignty from the foundering communist empire following independence declarations from a number of former Soviet republics. As the leading member of the Commonwealth of Independent States, the Russian Federation has a central role in the development of post-Soviet Eurasia. Crossing 11 time zones, the Russian Federation is almost twice the size of the US, and with more than 150 ethnic minorities and 21 autonomous republics, regionalist dissent within its own territory remains a danger.

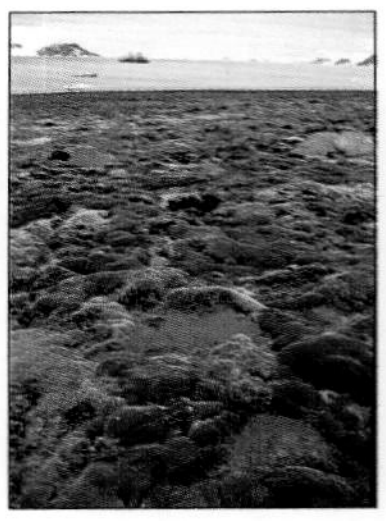

Summer beds of moss and lichen *scatter a 90% surface cover of ice across the islands of Franz Josef Land (Zemlya Frantsa-Iosifa), the northernmost land in the eastern hemisphere.*

The Russian Federation: Administrative Regions

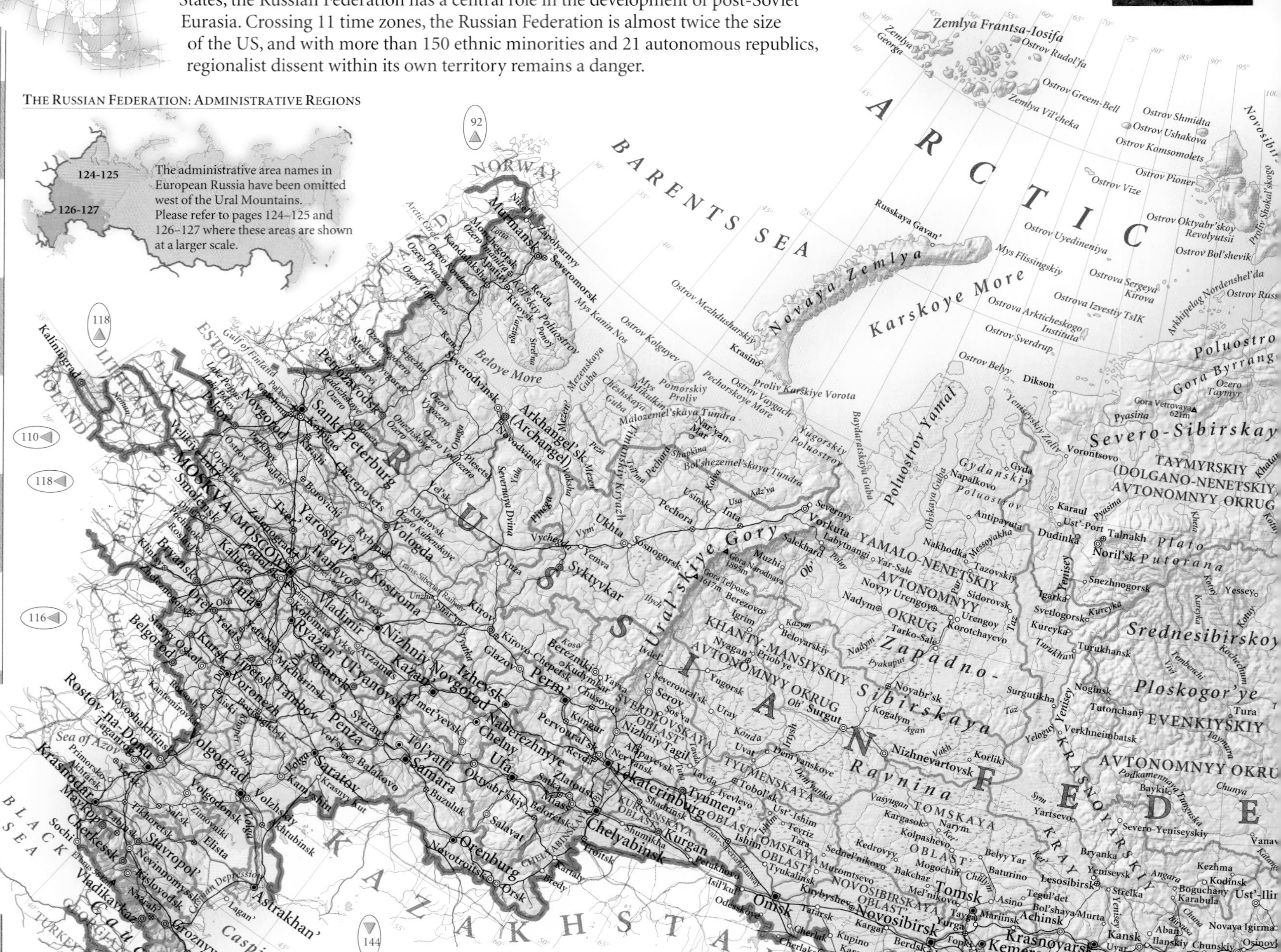

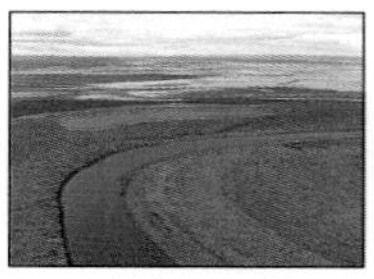

124-125

126-127

The administrative area names in European Russia have been omitted west of the Ural Mountains. Please refer to pages 124–125 and 126–127 where these areas are shown at a larger scale.

The North European Plain is marked by huge moraine ridges left by the Scandinavian Ice Sheet and by long intermoraine drainage channels, known as *Urstromtäler*.

The Khatanga River *meanders slowly across the Poluostrov Taymyr, a low-lying tundra landscape which floods in the spring thaw, until the water can escape to the sea.*

The Landscape

The Ural Mountains *(Ural'skiye Gory)* divide the fertile North European Plain from the West Siberian Plain *(Zapadno-Sibirskaya Ravnina)*, the world's largest area of flat ground, crossed by giant rivers flowing north to the Kara Sea *(Karskoye More)*. The land rises to the Central Siberian Plateau *(Srednesibirskoye Ploskogor'ye)* and becomes more mountainous to the southeast. These immense topographic regions intersect with latitudinal vegetation bands. The tundra of the extreme north gives way to a vast area of coniferous woodland, which is known as *taiga*, larger than the Amazon rain forest. This belt turns to mixed forest and then steppe grasslands towards the south.

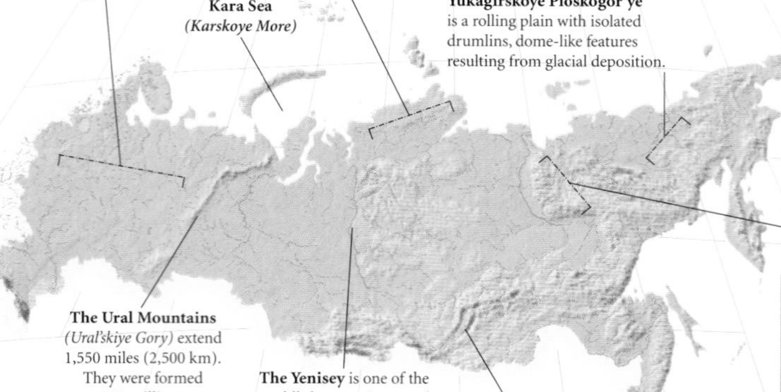

Kara Sea *(Karskoye More)*

Poluostrov Taymyr

Yukagirskoye Ploskogor'ye is a rolling plain with isolated drumlins, dome-like features resulting from glacial deposition.

The mountains of Verkhoyanskiy Khrebet were formed by movement between the Eurasian and North American plates, during the same period of folding that created the Urals.

The Ural Mountains *(Ural'skiye Gory)* extend 1,550 miles (2,500 km). They were formed over 280 million years ago, folded as the East European and Siberian plates moved closer together.

The Yenisey is one of the world's longest rivers, and also among the most languid, dropping only 500 ft (152 m) over 1,200 miles (2,000 km).

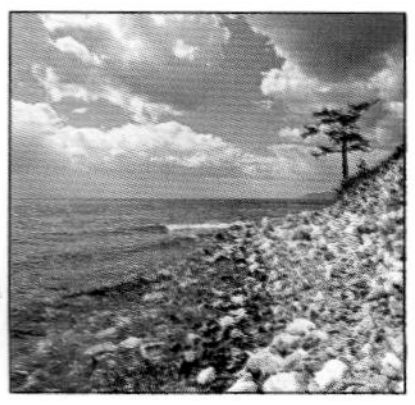

Lake Baikal (Ozero Baykal), *occupies a rift valley and is the world's deepest lake, over 1 mile (1.6 km) in depth. It is fed by over 300 rivers and drained by just one, the Angara.*

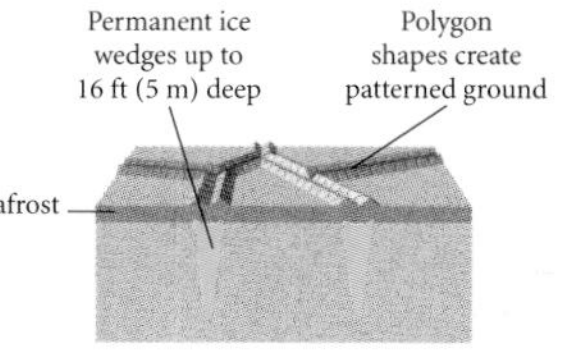

Permanent ice wedges up to 16 ft (5 m) deep

Polygon shapes create patterned ground

Permafrost

Patterned ground *is a permafrost feature found extensively across northern Russia. Seasonal contraction of the permafrost creates polygonal cracks, which are filled by ice wedges.*

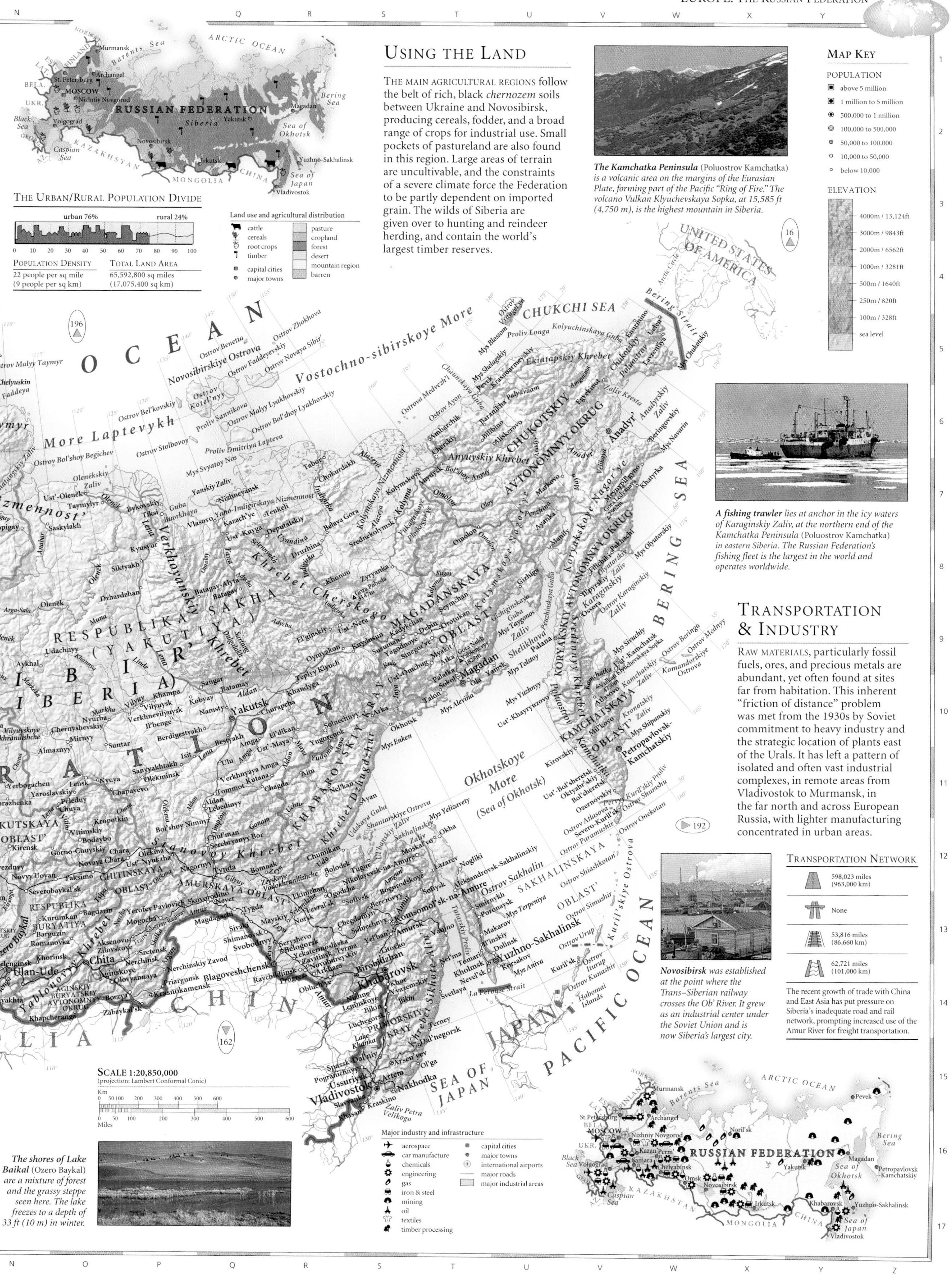

THE URBAN/RURAL POPULATION DIVIDE
urban 76%
rural 24%
POPULATION DENSITY
22 people per sq mile
(9 people per sq km)
TOTAL LAND AREA
65,592,800 sq miles
(17,075,400 sq km)
Land use and agricultural distribution
cattle
cereals
root crops
timber
capital cities
major towns
pasture
cropland
forest
desert
mountain region
barren
MAP KEY
POPULATION
above 5 million
1 million to 5 million
500,000 to 1 million
100,000 to 500,000
50,000 to 100,000
10,000 to 50,000
below 10,000
ELEVATION
4000m / 13,124ft
3000m / 9843ft
2000m / 6562ft
1000m / 3281ft
500m / 1640ft
250m / 820ft
100m / 328ft
sea level
TRANSPORTATION NETWORK
598,023 miles (963,000 km)
None
53,816 miles (86,660 km)
62,721 miles (101,000 km)
SCALE 1:20,850,000
(projection: Lambert Conformal Conic)
Major industry and infrastructure
aerospace
car manufacture
chemicals
engineering
gas
iron & steel
mining
oil
textiles
timber processing
capital cities
major towns
international airports
major roads
major industrial areas

USING THE LAND

THE MAIN AGRICULTURAL REGIONS follow the belt of rich, black *chernozem* soils between Ukraine and Novosibirsk, producing cereals, fodder, and a broad range of crops for industrial use. Small pockets of pastureland are also found in this region. Large areas of terrain are uncultivable, and the constraints of a severe climate force the Federation to be partly dependent on imported grain. The wilds of Siberia are given over to hunting and reindeer herding, and contain the world's largest timber reserves.

The Kamchatka Peninsula (Poluostrov Kamchatka) *is a volcanic area on the margins of the Eurasian Plate, forming part of the Pacific "Ring of Fire." The volcano Vulkan Klyuchevskaya Sopka, at 15,585 ft (4,750 m), is the highest mountain in Siberia.*

A fishing trawler *lies at anchor in the icy waters of Karaginskiy Zaliv, at the northern end of the Kamchatka Peninsula* (Poluostrov Kamchatka) *in eastern Siberia. The Russian Federation's fishing fleet is the largest in the world and operates worldwide.*

TRANSPORTATION & INDUSTRY

RAW MATERIALS, particularly fossil fuels, ores, and precious metals are abundant, yet often found at sites far from habitation. This inherent "friction of distance" problem was met from the 1930s by Soviet commitment to heavy industry and the strategic location of plants east of the Urals. It has left a pattern of isolated and often vast industrial complexes, in remote areas from Vladivostok to Murmansk, in the far north and across European Russia, with lighter manufacturing concentrated in urban areas.

Novosibirsk *was established at the point where the Trans-Siberian railway crosses the Ob' River. It grew as an industrial center under the Soviet Union and is now Siberia's largest city.*

The recent growth of trade with China and East Asia has put pressure on Siberia's inadequate road and rail network, prompting increased use of the Amur River for freight transportation.

The shores of Lake Baikal *(Ozero Baykal) are a mixture of forest and the grassy steppe seen here. The lake freezes to a depth of 33 ft (10 m) in winter.*

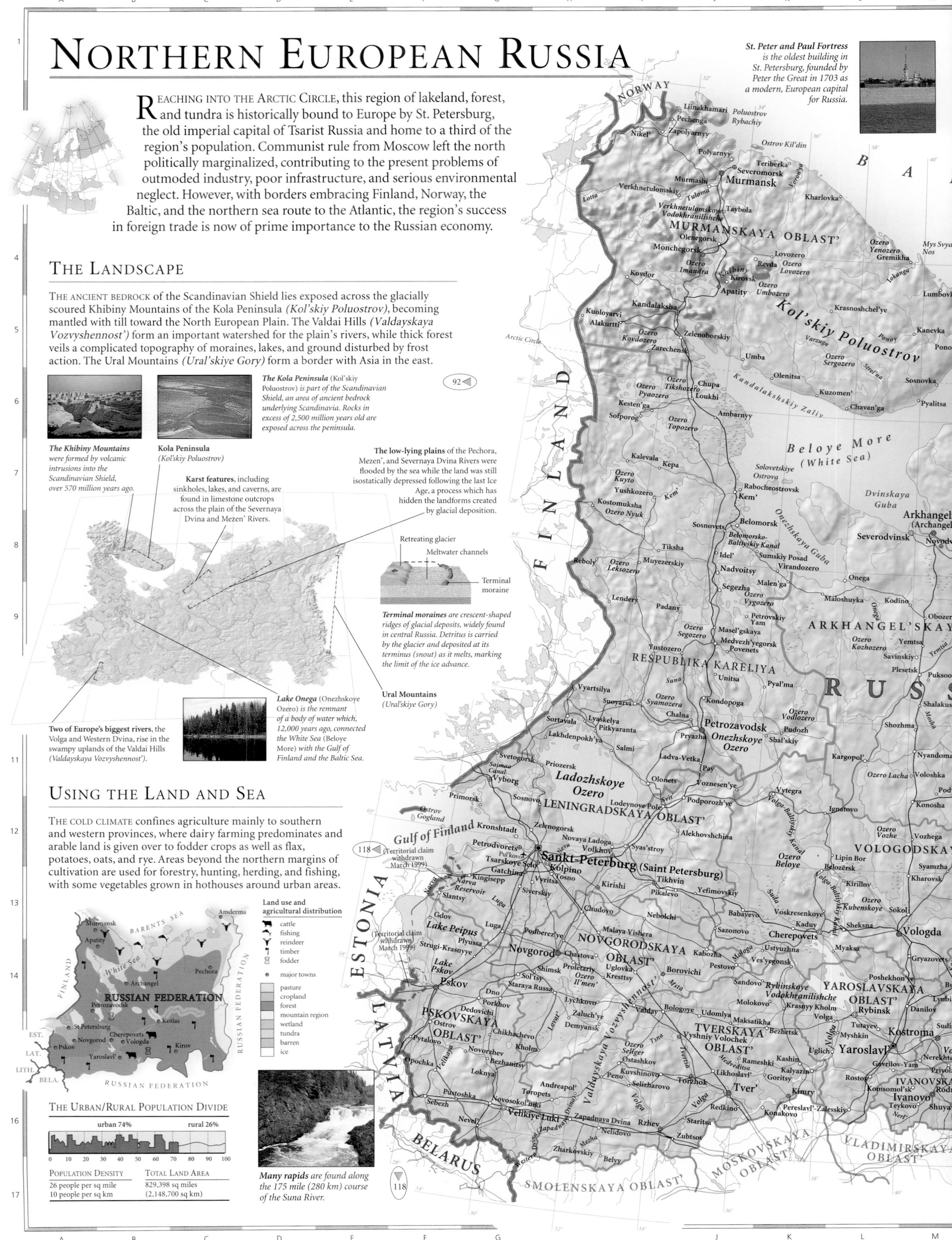

NORTHERN EUROPEAN RUSSIA

REACHING INTO THE ARCTIC CIRCLE, this region of lakeland, forest, and tundra is historically bound to Europe by St. Petersburg, the old imperial capital of Tsarist Russia and home to a third of the region's population. Communist rule from Moscow left the north politically marginalized, contributing to the present problems of outmoded industry, poor infrastructure, and serious environmental neglect. However, with borders embracing Finland, Norway, the Baltic, and the northern sea route to the Atlantic, the region's success in foreign trade is now of prime importance to the Russian economy.

St. Peter and Paul Fortress *is the oldest building in St. Petersburg, founded by Peter the Great in 1703 as a modern, European capital for Russia.*

THE LANDSCAPE

THE ANCIENT BEDROCK of the Scandinavian Shield lies exposed across the glacially scoured Khibiny Mountains of the Kola Peninsula *(Kol'skiy Poluostrov)*, becoming mantled with till toward the North European Plain. The Valdai Hills *(Valdayskaya Vozvyshennost')* form an important watershed for the plain's rivers, while thick forest veils a complicated topography of moraines, lakes, and ground disturbed by frost action. The Ural Mountains *(Ural'skiye Gory)* form a border with Asia in the east.

The Khibiny Mountains *were formed by volcanic intrusions into the Scandinavian Shield, over 570 million years ago.*

Kola Peninsula *(Kol'skiy Poluostrov)*

The Kola Peninsula (Kol'skiy Poluostrov) *is part of the Scandinavian Shield, an area of ancient bedrock underlying Scandinavia. Rocks in excess of 2,500 million years old are exposed across the peninsula.*

Karst features, including sinkholes, lakes, and caverns, are found in limestone outcrops across the plain of the Severnaya Dvina and Mezen' Rivers.

The low-lying plains of the Pechora, Mezen', and Severnaya Dvina Rivers were flooded by the sea while the land was still isostatically depressed following the last Ice Age, a process which has hidden the landforms created by glacial deposition.

Retreating glacier
Meltwater channels
Terminal moraine

Terminal moraines *are crescent-shaped ridges of glacial deposits, widely found in central Russia. Detritus is carried by the glacier and deposited at its terminus (snout) as it melts, marking the limit of the ice advance.*

Ural Mountains *(Ural'skiye Gory)*

Lake Onega (Onezhskoye Ozero) *is the remnant of a body of water which, 12,000 years ago, connected the White Sea (Beloye More) with the Gulf of Finland and the Baltic Sea.*

Two of Europe's biggest rivers, the Volga and Western Dvina, rise in the swampy uplands of the Valdai Hills (Valdayskaya Vozvyshennost').

USING THE LAND AND SEA

THE COLD CLIMATE confines agriculture mainly to southern and western provinces, where dairy farming predominates and arable land is given over to fodder crops as well as flax, potatoes, oats, and rye. Areas beyond the northern margins of cultivation are used for forestry, hunting, herding, and fishing, with some vegetables grown in hothouses around urban areas.

Land use and agricultural distribution
cattle
fishing
reindeer
timber
fodder
major towns
pasture
cropland
forest
mountain region
wetland
tundra
barren
ice

THE URBAN/RURAL POPULATION DIVIDE

urban 74% | rural 26%

0 10 20 30 40 50 60 70 80 90 100

POPULATION DENSITY	TOTAL LAND AREA
26 people per sq mile	829,398 sq miles
10 people per sq km	(2,148,700 sq km)

Many rapids *are found along the 175 mile (280 km) course of the Suna River.*

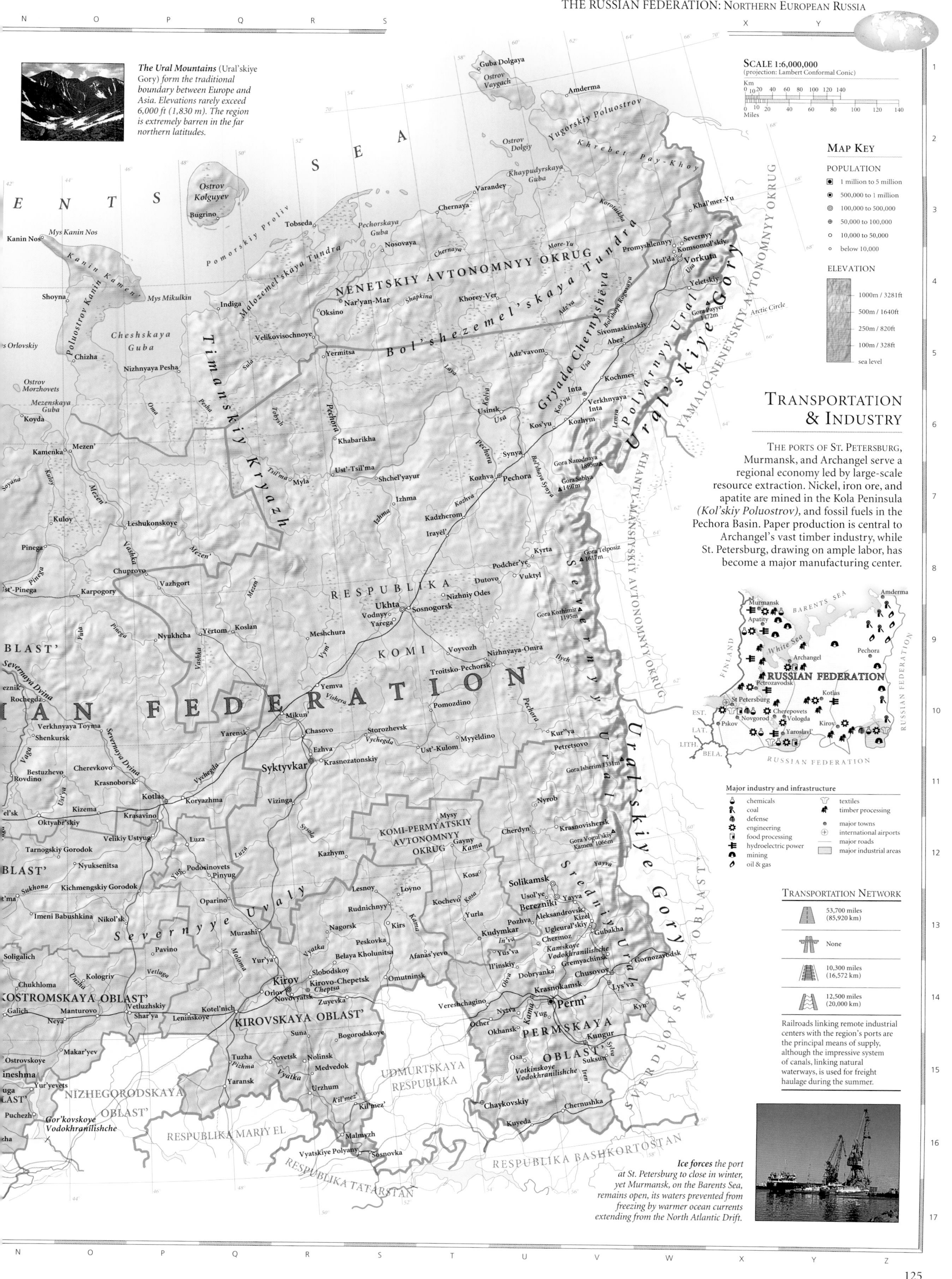
SCALE 1:6,000,000
(projection: Lambert Conformal Conic)
MAP KEY
POPULATION
1 million to 5 million
500,000 to 1 million
100,000 to 500,000
50,000 to 100,000
10,000 to 50,000
below 10,000
ELEVATION
1000m / 3281ft
500m / 1640ft
250m / 820ft
100m / 328ft
sea level
BARENTS SEA
NENETSKIY AVTONOMNYY OKRUG
RESPUBLIKA KOMI
RUSSIAN FEDERATION
KOMI-PERMYATSKIY AVTONOMNYY OKRUG
KIROVSKAYA OBLAST'
PERMSKAYA OBLAST'
KOSTROMSKAYA OBLAST'
NIZHEGORODSKAYA OBLAST'
UDMURTSKAYA RESPUBLIKA
RESPUBLIKA MARIY EL
RESPUBLIKA TATARSTAN
RESPUBLIKA BASHKORTOSTAN
SVERDLOVSKAYA OBLAST'
KHANTY-MANSIYSKIY AVTONOMNYY OKRUG
YAMALO-NENETSKIY AVTONOMNYY OKRUG
Ural'skiye Gory
Timanskiy Kryazh
Bol'shezemel'skaya Tundra
Severnyye Uvaly
Syktyvkar
Kirov
Perm'
Vorkuta
Ukhta
Pechora
Major industry and infrastructure
chemicals
coal
defense
engineering
food processing
hydroelectric power
mining
oil & gas
textiles
timber processing
major towns
international airports
major roads
major industrial areas
TRANSPORTATION NETWORK
53,700 miles (85,920 km)
None
10,300 miles (16,572 km)
12,500 miles (20,000 km)

The Ural Mountains (Ural'skiye Gory) *form the traditional boundary between Europe and Asia. Elevations rarely exceed 6,000 ft (1,830 m). The region is extremely barren in the far northern latitudes.*

Transportation & Industry

The ports of St. Petersburg, Murmansk, and Archangel serve a regional economy led by large-scale resource extraction. Nickel, iron ore, and apatite are mined in the Kola Peninsula *(Kol'skiy Poluostrov)*, and fossil fuels in the Pechora Basin. Paper production is central to Archangel's vast timber industry, while St. Petersburg, drawing on ample labor, has become a major manufacturing center.

Railroads linking remote industrial centers with the region's ports are the principal means of supply, although the impressive system of canals, linking natural waterways, is used for freight haulage during the summer.

***Ice forces** the port at St. Petersburg to close in winter, yet Murmansk, on the Barents Sea, remains open, its waters prevented from freezing by warmer ocean currents extending from the North Atlantic Drift.*

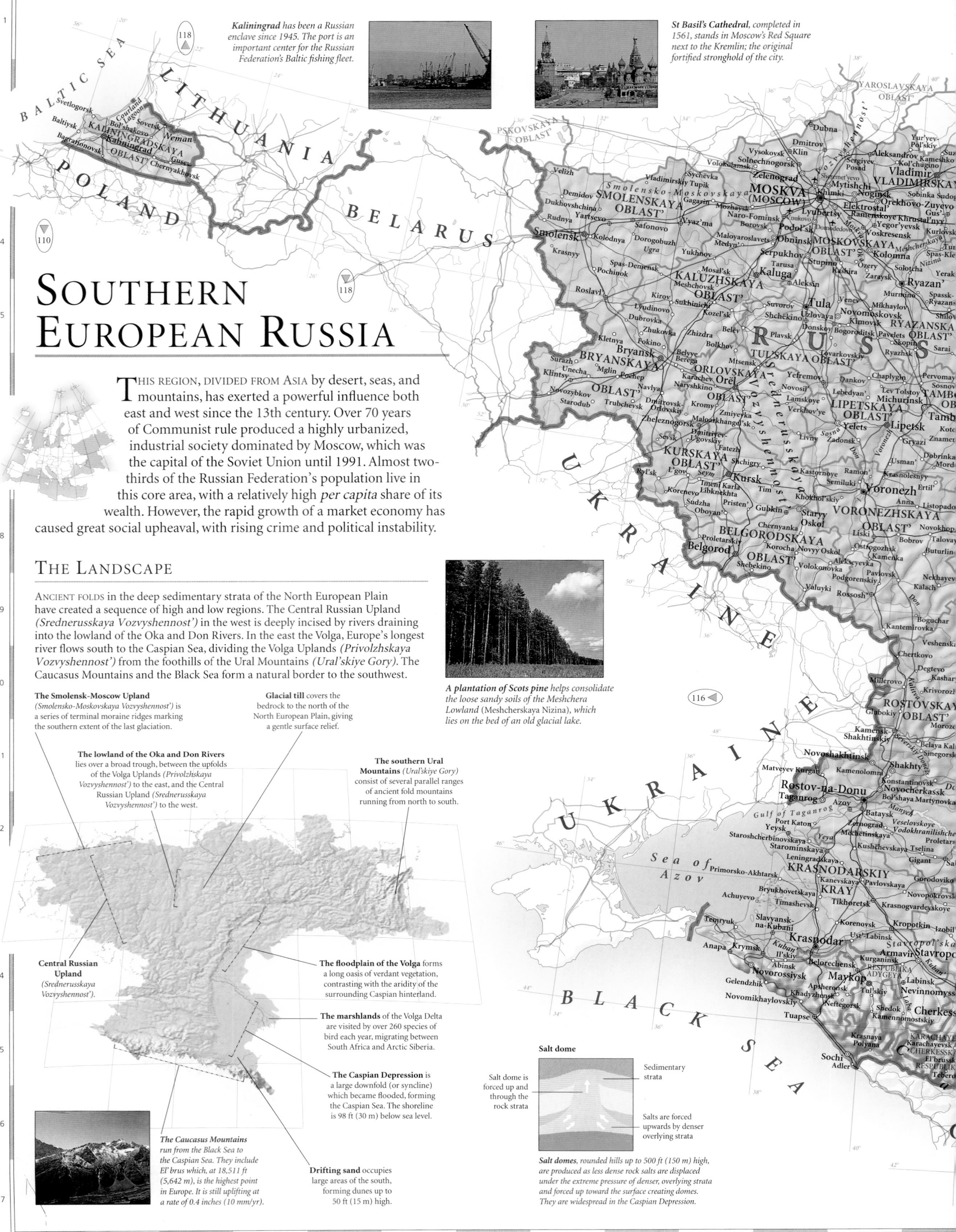
BALTIC SEA
LITHUANIA
POLAND
KALININGRADSKAYA OBLAST'
BELARUS
UKRAINE
SEA OF AZOV
BLACK SEA
MOSKVA (MOSCOW)
SMOLENSKAYA OBLAST'
KALUZHSKAYA OBLAST'
BRYANSKAYA OBLAST'
ORLOVSKAYA OBLAST'
TUL'SKAYA OBLAST'
KURSKAYA OBLAST'
BELGORODSKAYA OBLAST'
LIPETSKAYA OBLAST'
VORONEZHSKAYA OBLAST'
RYAZANSKAYA OBLAST'
MOSKOVSKAYA OBLAST'
ROSTOVSKAYA OBLAST'
KRASNODARSKIY KRAY
118
110
116

SOUTHERN EUROPEAN RUSSIA

THIS REGION, DIVIDED FROM ASIA by desert, seas, and mountains, has exerted a powerful influence both east and west since the 13th century. Over 70 years of Communist rule produced a highly urbanized, industrial society dominated by Moscow, which was the capital of the Soviet Union until 1991. Almost two-thirds of the Russian Federation's population live in this core area, with a relatively high *per capita* share of its wealth. However, the rapid growth of a market economy has caused great social upheaval, with rising crime and political instability.

Kaliningrad *has been a Russian enclave since 1945. The port is an important center for the Russian Federation's Baltic fishing fleet.*

St Basil's Cathedral, *completed in 1561, stands in Moscow's Red Square next to the Kremlin; the original fortified stronghold of the city.*

THE LANDSCAPE

ANCIENT FOLDS in the deep sedimentary strata of the North European Plain have created a sequence of high and low regions. The Central Russian Upland *(Srednerusskaya Vozvyshennost')* in the west is deeply incised by rivers draining into the lowland of the Oka and Don Rivers. In the east the Volga, Europe's longest river flows south to the Caspian Sea, dividing the Volga Uplands *(Privolzhskaya Vozvyshennost')* from the foothills of the Ural Mountains *(Ural'skiye Gory)*. The Caucasus Mountains and the Black Sea form a natural border to the southwest.

***A plantation of Scots pine** helps consolidate the loose sandy soils of the Meshchera Lowland* (Meshcherskaya Nizina), *which lies on the bed of an old glacial lake.*

The Smolensk-Moscow Upland *(Smolensko-Moskovskaya Vozvyshennost')* is a series of terminal moraine ridges marking the southern extent of the last glaciation.

Glacial till covers the bedrock to the north of the North European Plain, giving a gentle surface relief.

The lowland of the Oka and Don Rivers lies over a broad trough, between the upfolds of the Volga Uplands *(Privolzhskaya Vozvyshennost')* to the east, and the Central Russian Upland *(Srednerusskaya Vozvyshennost')* to the west.

The southern Ural Mountains *(Ural'skiye Gory)* consist of several parallel ranges of ancient fold mountains running from north to south.

Central Russian Upland *(Srednerusskaya Vozvyshennost')*.

The floodplain of the Volga forms a long oasis of verdant vegetation, contrasting with the aridity of the surrounding Caspian hinterland.

The marshlands of the Volga Delta are visited by over 260 species of bird each year, migrating between South Africa and Arctic Siberia.

The Caspian Depression is a large downfold (or syncline) which became flooded, forming the Caspian Sea. The shoreline is 98 ft (30 m) below sea level.

***The Caucasus Mountains** run from the Black Sea to the Caspian Sea. They include El' brus which, at 18,511 ft (5,642 m), is the highest point in Europe. It is still uplifting at a rate of 0.4 inches (10 mm/yr).*

Drifting sand occupies large areas of the south, forming dunes up to 50 ft (15 m) high.

Salt dome

Sedimentary strata

Salt dome is forced up and through the rock strata

Salts are forced upwards by denser overlying strata

***Salt domes**, rounded hills up to 500 ft (150 m) high, are produced as less dense rock salts are displaced under the extreme pressure of denser, overlying strata and forced up toward the surface creating domes. They are widespread in the Caspian Depression.*

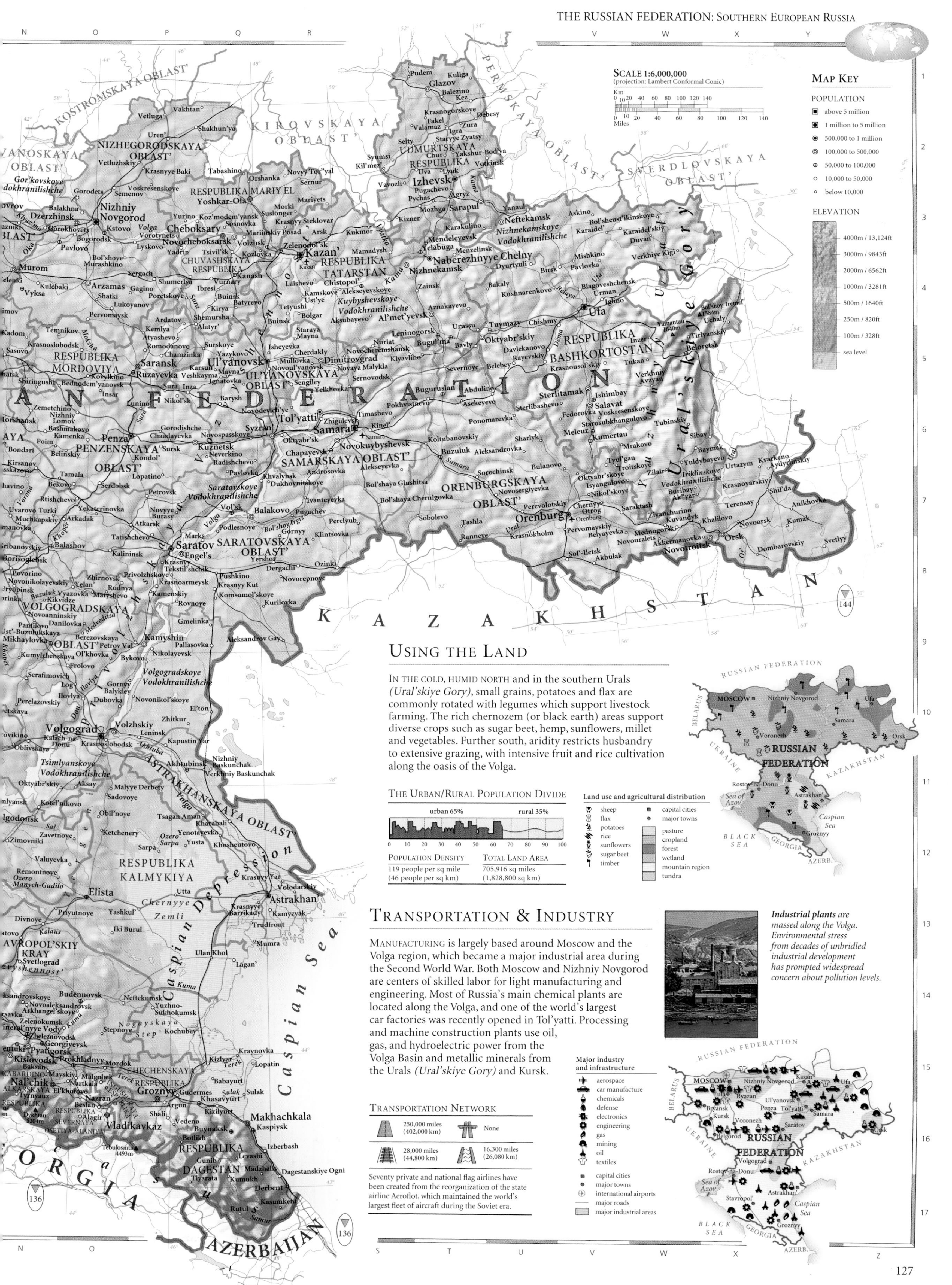

SCALE 1:6,000,000
(projection: Lambert Conformal Conic)
MAP KEY
POPULATION
above 5 million
1 million to 5 million
500,000 to 1 million
100,000 to 500,000
50,000 to 100,000
10,000 to 50,000
below 10,000
ELEVATION
4000m / 13,124ft
3000m / 9843ft
2000m / 6562ft
1000m / 3281ft
500m / 1640ft
250m / 820ft
100m / 328ft
sea level
KAZAKHSTAN
Caspian Sea
RESPUBLIKA TATARSTAN
RESPUBLIKA BASHKORTOSTAN
ORENBURGSKAYA OBLAST'
SAMARSKAYA OBLAST'
SARATOVSKAYA OBLAST'
VOLGOGRADSKAYA OBLAST'
ASTRAKHANSKAYA OBLAST'
RESPUBLIKA KALMYKIYA
RESPUBLIKA DAGESTAN
AZERBAIJAN
GEORGIA
Kazan'
Samara
Ufa
Orenburg
Saratov
Volgograd
Astrakhan'
Nizhniy Novgorod
Makhachkala

USING THE LAND

IN THE COLD, HUMID NORTH and in the southern Urals *(Ural'skiye Gory)*, small grains, potatoes and flax are commonly rotated with legumes which support livestock farming. The rich chernozem (or black earth) areas support diverse crops such as sugar beet, hemp, sunflowers, millet and vegetables. Further south, aridity restricts husbandry to extensive grazing, with intensive fruit and rice cultivation along the oasis of the Volga.

THE URBAN/RURAL POPULATION DIVIDE

urban 65% — rural 35%

POPULATION DENSITY	TOTAL LAND AREA
119 people per sq mile (46 people per sq km)	705,916 sq miles (1,828,800 sq km)

Land use and agricultural distribution: sheep, flax, potatoes, rice, sunflowers, sugar beet, timber, capital cities, major towns, pasture, cropland, forest, wetland, mountain region, tundra

TRANSPORTATION & INDUSTRY

MANUFACTURING is largely based around Moscow and the Volga region, which became a major industrial area during the Second World War. Both Moscow and Nizhniy Novgorod are centers of skilled labor for light manufacturing and engineering. Most of Russia's main chemical plants are located along the Volga, and one of the world's largest car factories was recently opened in Tol'yatti. Processing and machine construction plants use oil, gas, and hydroelectric power from the Volga Basin and metallic minerals from the Urals *(Ural'skiye Gory)* and Kursk.

***Industrial plants** are massed along the Volga. Environmental stress from decades of unbridled industrial development has prompted widespread concern about pollution levels.*

TRANSPORTATION NETWORK

250,000 miles (402,000 km)	None
28,000 miles (44,800 km)	16,300 miles (26,080 km)

Seventy private and national flag airlines have been created from the reorganization of the state airline Aeroflot, which maintained the world's largest fleet of aircraft during the Soviet era.

Major industry and infrastructure: aerospace, car manufacture, chemicals, defense, electronics, engineering, gas, mining, oil, textiles, capital cities, major towns, international airports, major roads, major industrial areas

ASIA

ASIA, THE WORLD'S LARGEST CONTINENT, COVERS 16,838,365 SQ MILES (43,608,000 SQ KM). IT COMPRISES 48 SEPARATE COUNTRIES, INCLUDING 97% OF TURKEY AND 72% OF THE RUSSIAN FEDERATION. ALMOST 60% OF THE WORLD'S POPULATION LIVES IN ASIA.

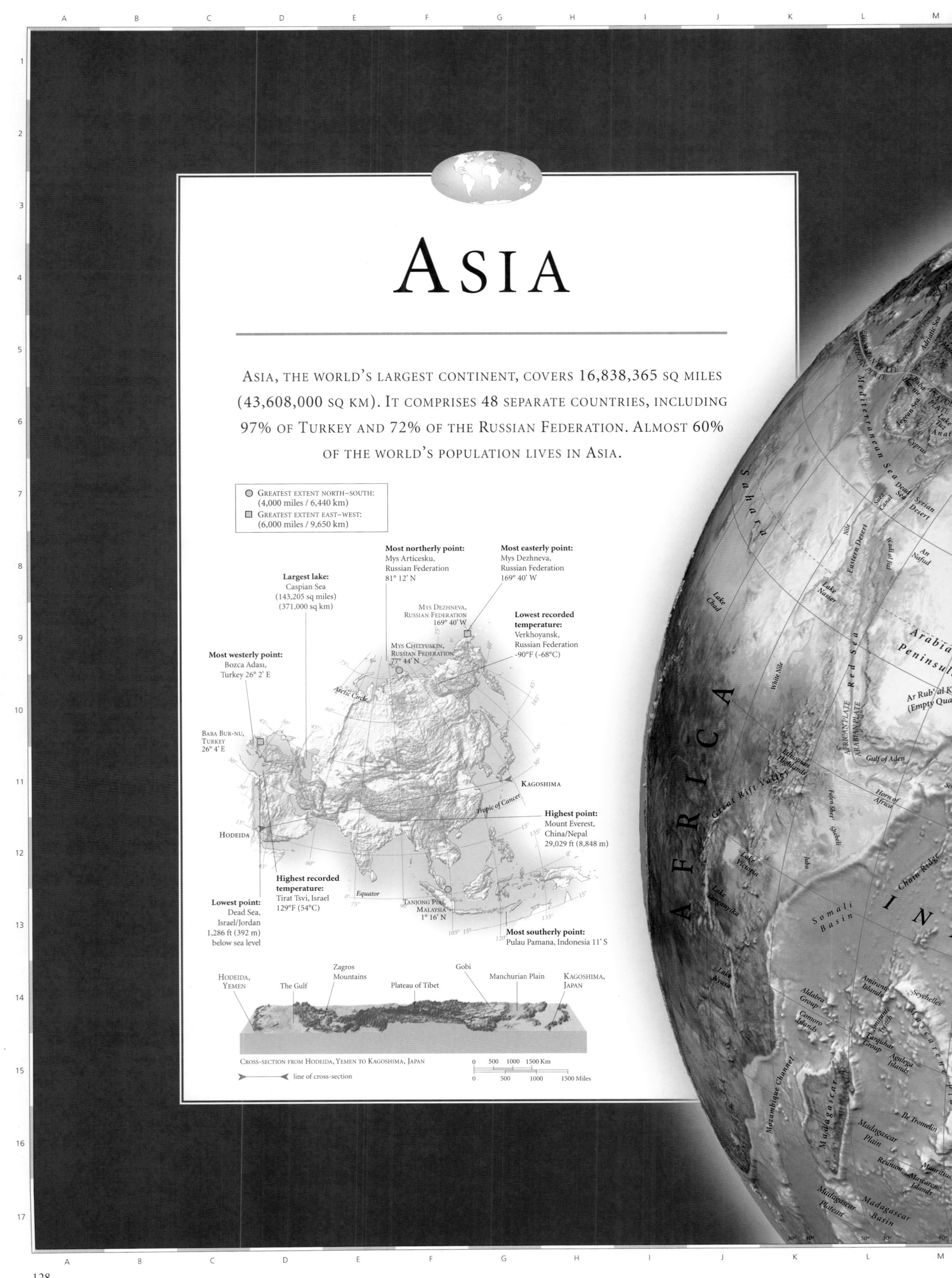

GREATEST EXTENT NORTH–SOUTH: (4,000 miles / 6,440 km)
GREATEST EXTENT EAST–WEST: (6,000 miles / 9,650 km)
Most northerly point: Mys Articesku, Russian Federation 81° 12' N
Most easterly point: Mys Dezhneva, Russian Federation 169° 40' W
Largest lake: Caspian Sea (143,205 sq miles) (371,000 sq km)
MYS DEZHNEVA, RUSSIAN FEDERATION 169° 40' W
Lowest recorded temperature: Verkhoyansk, Russian Federation -90°F (-68°C)
MYS CHELYUSKIN, RUSSIAN FEDERATION 77° 44' N
Most westerly point: Bozca Adası, Turkey 26° 2' E
Arctic Circle
BABA BUR-NU, TURKEY 26° 4' E
KAGOSHIMA
Tropic of Cancer
Highest point: Mount Everest, China/Nepal 29,029 ft (8,848 m)
HODEIDA
Highest recorded temperature: Tirat Tsvi, Israel 129°F (54°C)
Equator
TANJONG PIAI, MALAYSIA 1° 16' N
Lowest point: Dead Sea, Israel/Jordan 1,286 ft (392 m) below sea level
Most southerly point: Pulau Pamana, Indonesia 11' S
HODEIDA, YEMEN
The Gulf
Zagros Mountains
Plateau of Tibet
Gobi
Manchurian Plain
KAGOSHIMA, JAPAN
CROSS-SECTION FROM HODEIDA, YEMEN TO KAGOSHIMA, JAPAN
line of cross-section
0 500 1000 1500 Km
0 500 1000 1500 Miles
AFRICA
Sahara
Mediterranean Sea
Aegean Sea
Cyprus
Dead Sea
Syrian Desert
Suez Canal
Nile
Eastern Desert
An Nafud
Lake Nasser
Lake Chad
Red Sea
Arabian Peninsula
Ar Rub' al Khali (Empty Quarter)
White Nile
AFRICAN PLATE
ARABIAN PLATE
Ethiopian Highlands
Great Rift Valley
Gulf of Aden
Horn of Africa
Lake Victoria
Lake Tanganyika
Lake Nyasa
Somali Basin
Chain Ridge
Amirante Islands
Seychelles
Aldabra Group
Comoro Islands
Farquhar Group
Agalega Islands
Mozambique Channel
Madagascar
Madagascar Plain
Île Tromelin
Réunion
Mauritius
Mascarene Islands
Madagascar Plateau
Madagascar Basin

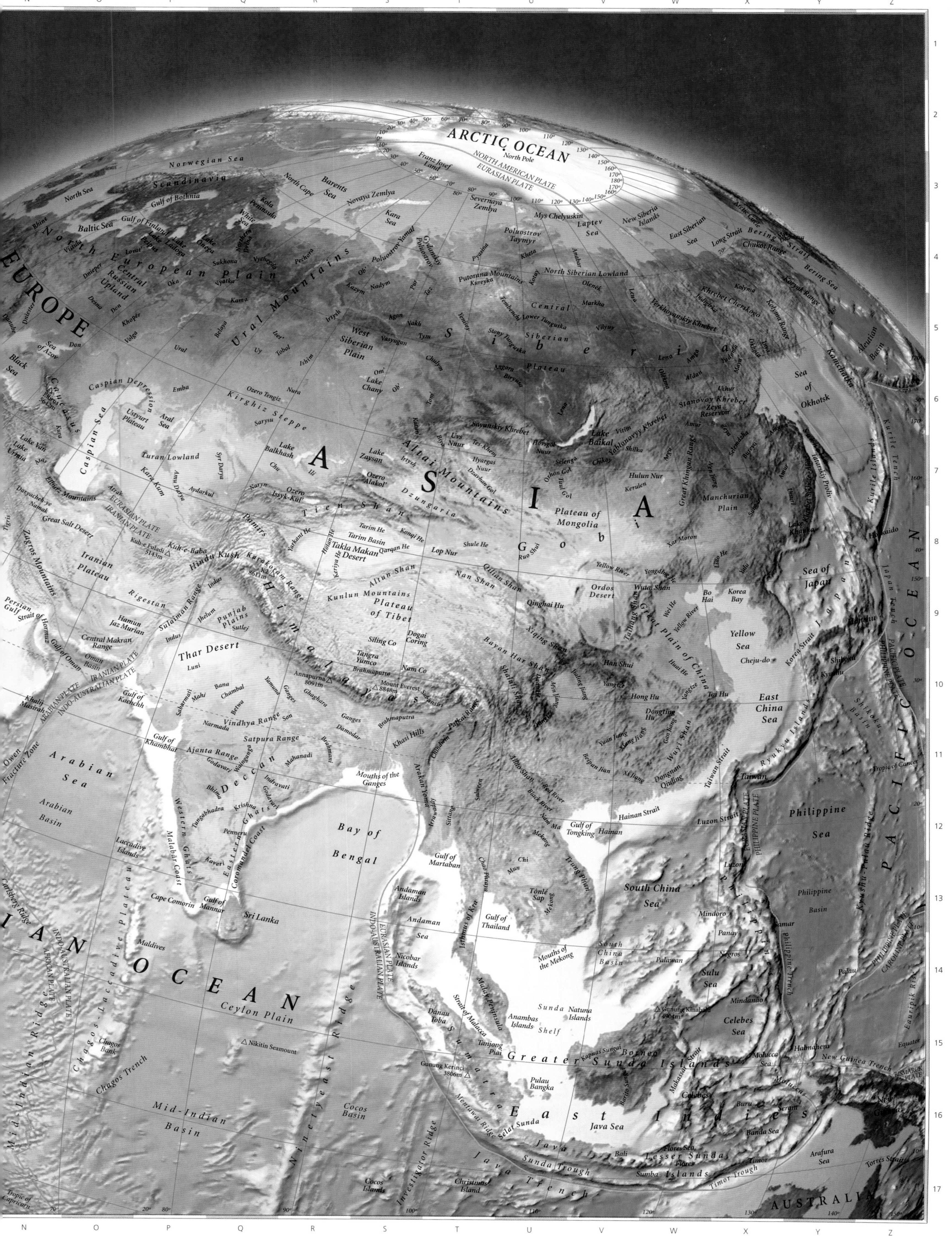

N O P Q R S T U V W X Y Z
1 2 3 4 5 6 7 8 9 10 11 12 13 14 15 16 17
ARCTIC OCEAN
North Pole
NORTH AMERICAN PLATE
EURASIAN PLATE
Franz Josef Land
Norwegian Sea
Scandinavia
North Sea
Gulf of Bothnia
North Cape
Barents Sea
Novaya Zemlya
Kara Sea
Severnaya Zemlya
Mys Chelyuskin
Laptev Sea
New Siberian Islands
East Siberian Sea
Long Strait
Bering Strait
Chukot Range
Bering Sea
Baltic Sea
Gulf of Finland
Lake Ladoga
Lake Onega
White Sea
Kola Peninsula
North European Plain
Central Russian Upland
EUROPE
Ural Mountains
Poluostrov Yamal
Poluostrov Taymyr
Putorana Mountains
North Siberian Lowland
Central Siberian Plateau
West Siberian Plain
Siberia
Khrebet Cherskogo
Verkhoyanskiy Khrebet
Sea of Okhotsk
Kamchatka
Aleutian Basin
Black Sea
Sea of Azov
Caspian Depression
Caucasus
Caspian Sea
Ustyurt Plateau
Aral Sea
Kirghiz Steppe
Lake Balkhash
Lake Zaysan
Lake Baikal
Sayanskiy Khrebet
Stanovoy Khrebet
Yablonovyy Khrebet
Turan Lowland
Kara Kum
Altai Mountains
Dzungaria
Tien Shan
ASIA
Plateau of Mongolia
Gobi
Manchurian Plain
Great Khingan Range
Elburz Mountains
Great Salt Desert
EURASIAN PLATE
IRANIAN PLATE
Zagros Mountains
Iranian Plateau
Pamirs
Hindu Kush
Karakoram Range
Tarim Basin
Takla Makan Desert
Lop Nur
Kunlun Mountains
Plateau of Tibet
Altun Shan
Qilian Shan
Nan Shan
Ordos Desert
Qinghai Hu
Great Plain of China
Bo Hai
Korea Bay
Yellow Sea
Sea of Japan
Japan
Hokkaido
Kurile Islands
Kurile Trench
Japan Trench
PACIFIC OCEAN
PACIFIC PLATE
PHILIPPINE PLATE
Persian Gulf
Strait of Hormuz
Gulf of Oman
Rigestan
Sulaiman Range
Punjab Plains
Thar Desert
Himalayas
Annapurna 8091m
Mount Everest 8848m
Bayan Har Shan
East China Sea
Shikoku Basin
Gulf of Kachchh
Gulf of Khambhat
INDO-AUSTRALIAN PLATE
ARABIAN PLATE
Vindhya Range
Satpura Range
Ajanta Range
Deccan
Khasi Hills
Mouths of the Ganges
Arabian Sea
Arabian Basin
Owen Fracture Zone
Western Ghats
Eastern Ghats
Malabar Coast
Coromandel Coast
Laccadive Islands
Bay of Bengal
Gulf of Martaban
Gulf of Tongking
Hainan
Hainan Strait
Taiwan
Taiwan Strait
Luzon Strait
Ryukyu Islands
Tropic of Cancer
Philippine Sea
Philippine Basin
Kyushu-Palau Ridge
Cape Comorin
Gulf of Mannar
Sri Lanka
Andaman Islands
Andaman Sea
Gulf of Thailand
Isthmus of Kra
South China Sea
South China Basin
Mouths of the Mekong
Nicobar Islands
Maldives
Chagos-Laccadive Plateau
INDIAN OCEAN
Ceylon Plain
Nikitin Seamount
Chagos Bank
Chagos Trench
Mid-Indian Ridge
Mid-Indian Basin
Ninetyeast Ridge
Investigator Ridge
Cocos Basin
Cocos Islands
Christmas Island
Malay Peninsula
Strait of Malacca
Sumatra
Sunda Shelf
Natuna Islands
Anambas Islands
Gunung Kinabalu 4094m
Borneo
Greater Sunda Islands
Gunung Kerinci 3806m
Pulau Bangka
Mentawai Ridge
Selat Sunda
Java
Java Sea
Java Trench
Sunda Trough
East Indies
Bali
Lesser Sunda Islands
Flores Sea
Timor Trough
Timor
Banda Sea
Arafura Sea
Torres Strait
Sulu Sea
Celebes Sea
Mindanao
Palawan
Mindoro
Luzon
Philippine Trench
Molucca Sea
Moluccas
New Guinea Trench
Equator
Palau
AUSTRALIA

Physical Asia

The natural landscape of Asia can be divided into two distinct physical regions; one covers the north, while the other spans the south. Northern Asia consists of old mountain chains like the Ural Mountains, plateaus, including the vast Plateau of Tibet, shields, and basins. In contrast, the landscapes of the south are much younger, formed by tectonic activity beginning c. 65 million years ago, leading to an almost continuous mountain chain running from Europe, across much of Asia, and culminating in the mighty Himalayan mountains. North of the mountains lies a belt of deserts. In the far south, tectonic activity has formed narrow island arcs. To the west lies the Arabian Shield, once part of the African Plate. As it was rifted apart from Africa, the Arabian Plate collided with the Eurasian Plate, uplifting the Zagros Mountains.

Coastal Lowlands and Island Arcs

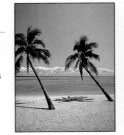

The coastal plains that fringe Southeast Asia contain many large delta systems, caused by high levels of rainfall and erosion of the Himalayas, the Plateau of Tibet, and relict loess deposits. To the south is an extensive island archipelago, lying on the drowned Sunda Shelf. Most of these islands are volcanic in origin, caused by the subduction of the Indo-Australian Plate beneath the Eurasian Plate.

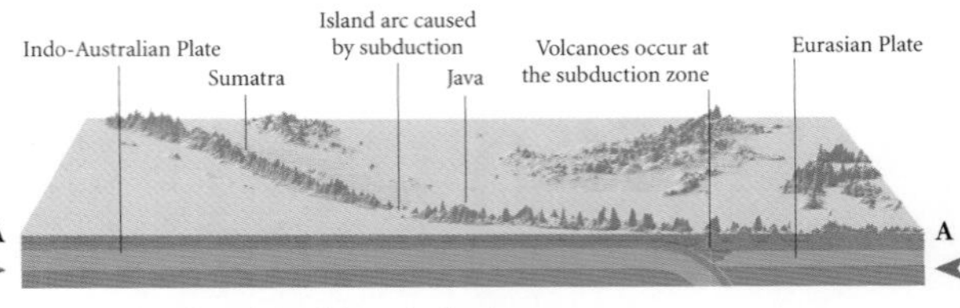
Indo-Australian Plate
Sumatra
Island arc caused by subduction
Java
Volcanoes occur at the subduction zone
Eurasian Plate
A
A

Cross-section through Southeast Asia showing the subduction zone between the Indo-Australian and Eurasian plates and the island arc.

0 200 400 Km
0 200 400 Miles

The Arabian Shield and Iranian Plateau

Approximately five million years ago, rifting of the continental crust split the Arabian Plate from the African Plate and flooded the Red Sea. As this rift spread, the Arabian Plate collided with the Eurasian Plate, transforming part of the Tethys seabed into the Zagros Mountains which run northwest-southeast across western Iran.

The confluence of the Tigris and Euphrates on the Mesopotamian Depression
Folded sedimentary rock strata
Zagros Mountains
Iranian Plateau
B
B

Cross-section through southwestern Asia, showing the Mesopotamian Depression, the folded Zagros Mountains and the Iranian Plateau.

0 50 100 Km
0 50 100 Miles

East Asian Plains and Uplands

Several, small, isolated shield areas, such as the Shandong Peninsula, are found in east Asia. Between these stable shield areas, large river systems like the Yangtze and the Yellow River have deposited thick layers of sediment, forming extensive alluvial plains. The largest of these is the Great Plain of China, the relief of which does not rise above 300 ft (100 m).

Map Key

Elevation
6000m / 19,686ft
4000m / 13,124ft
3000m / 9843ft
2000m / 6562ft
1000m / 3281ft
500m / 1640ft
250m / 820ft
100m / 328ft
sea level

Plate margins
(for explanation see page xiv)
constructive
destructive
conservative
uncertain

physiographic regions
line of cross-section

Arctic Ocean · Chukchi Sea · Wrangel Island · Bering Sea · Gulf of Anadyr · East Siberian Sea · North American Plate · Eurasian Plate · Severnaya Zemlya · Laptev Sea · Kara Sea · Ozero Taymyr · Gulf of Ob · Yenisey · Central Siberian Plateau · Lena · East Siberian Mountains · Aldan · Sea of Okhotsk · Kamchatka · Kurile Islands · Pacific Ocean · Siberian Plateau & Plain · Siberia · Europe · Ural Mountains · Ob · West Siberian Plain · Sakhalin · Khrebet Sikhote-Alin · Amur · Lake Baikal · Hokkaido · Pacific Plate · Black Sea · Sea of Azov · Kirghiz Steppe · Irtysh · Ural · Caucasus · Caspian Sea · Aral Sea · Lake Balkhash · Altai Mountains · Plateau of Mongolia · Gobi · Liao He · Honshu · Sea of Japan · Turan Basin & Kazakh Uplands · Anatolia · Anatolian Plate · Arabian Plate · African Plate · Mediterranean Sea · Kara Kum · Amu Darya · Syr Darya · Tien Shan · Central Asian Plateaux & Basins · Shandong Peninsula · Korea Strait · Shikoku · Kyushu · Philippine Plate · Euphrates · Tigris · Syrian Desert · Africa · Takla Makan Desert · Qilian Shan · Yellow River · Great Plain of China · Yellow Sea · East China Sea · Arabian Shield · Iranian Plateau · Hindu Kush · Khyber Pass 1080m · K2 8611m · Kunlun Mountains · Plateau of Tibet · Sichuan Pendi · Yangtze · Poyang Hu · Ryukyu Islands · Red Sea · Zagros Mountains · The Gulf · Himalayas · Salween · Mekong · East Asian Plains & Uplands · Taiwan Strait · Taiwan · Arabian Peninsula · Gulf of Oman · Indus · Thar Desert · Mount Everest 8848m · Brahmaputra · Indian Shield & Himalayan System · Ganges · Red River · Xi Jiang · Luzon · Ar Rub' al Khali (Empty Quarter) · Indo-Australian Plate · Coastal Lowlands & Island Arcs · Hainan · Gulf of Aden · Socotra · Arabian Sea · Deccan · Western Ghats · Eastern Ghats · Bay of Bengal · Irrawaddy · South China Sea · Philippines · Philippine Sea · Caroline Plate · Andaman Islands · Andaman Sea · Gulf of Thailand · Palawan · Sulu Sea · Mindanao · Celebes Sea · Halmahera · New Guinea · Sri Lanka · Nicobar Islands · Indian Ocean · Malay Peninsula · Strait of Malacca · Natuna Islands · Moluccas · Borneo · Makassar Strait · Celebes · Seram · Banda Sea · Coral Sea · Arafura Sea · Sumatra · Greater Sunda Islands · Java Sea · Java · Flores Sea · Flores · Sumbawa · Lesser Sunda Islands · Timor · Timor Sea · Australia · A

The Indian Shield and Himalayan System

The large shield area beneath the Indian subcontinent is between 2.5 and 3.5 billion years old. As the floor of the southern Indian Ocean spread, it pushed the Indian Shield north. This was eventually driven beneath the Plateau of Tibet. This process closed up the ancient Tethys Sea and uplifted the world's highest mountain chain, the Himalayas. Much of the uplifted rock strata was from the seabed of the Tethys Sea, partly accounting for the weakness of the rocks and the high levels of erosion found in the Himalayas.

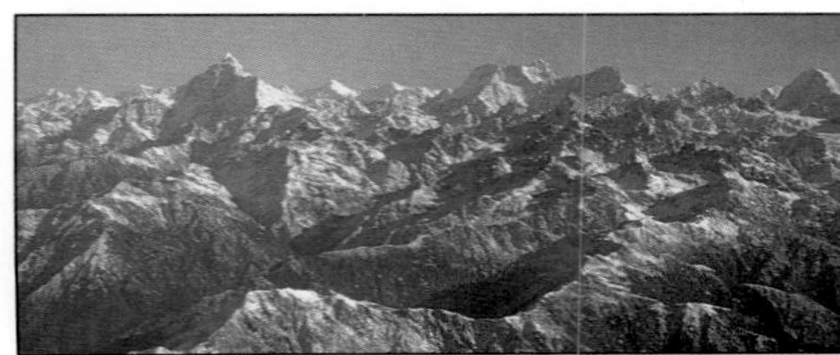

Indo-Gangetic Depression
Crushed sediment from seabed of the Tethys Sea
Himalayas
Thrust zone
Plateau of Tibet
C
C

Cross-section through the Himalayas showing thrust faulting of the rock strata.

0 50 100 Km
0 50 100 Miles

Scale 1:63,000,000
(projection: Lambert Azimuthal Equal Area)
Km 0 250 500 1000 1500
Miles 0 250 500 1000 1500

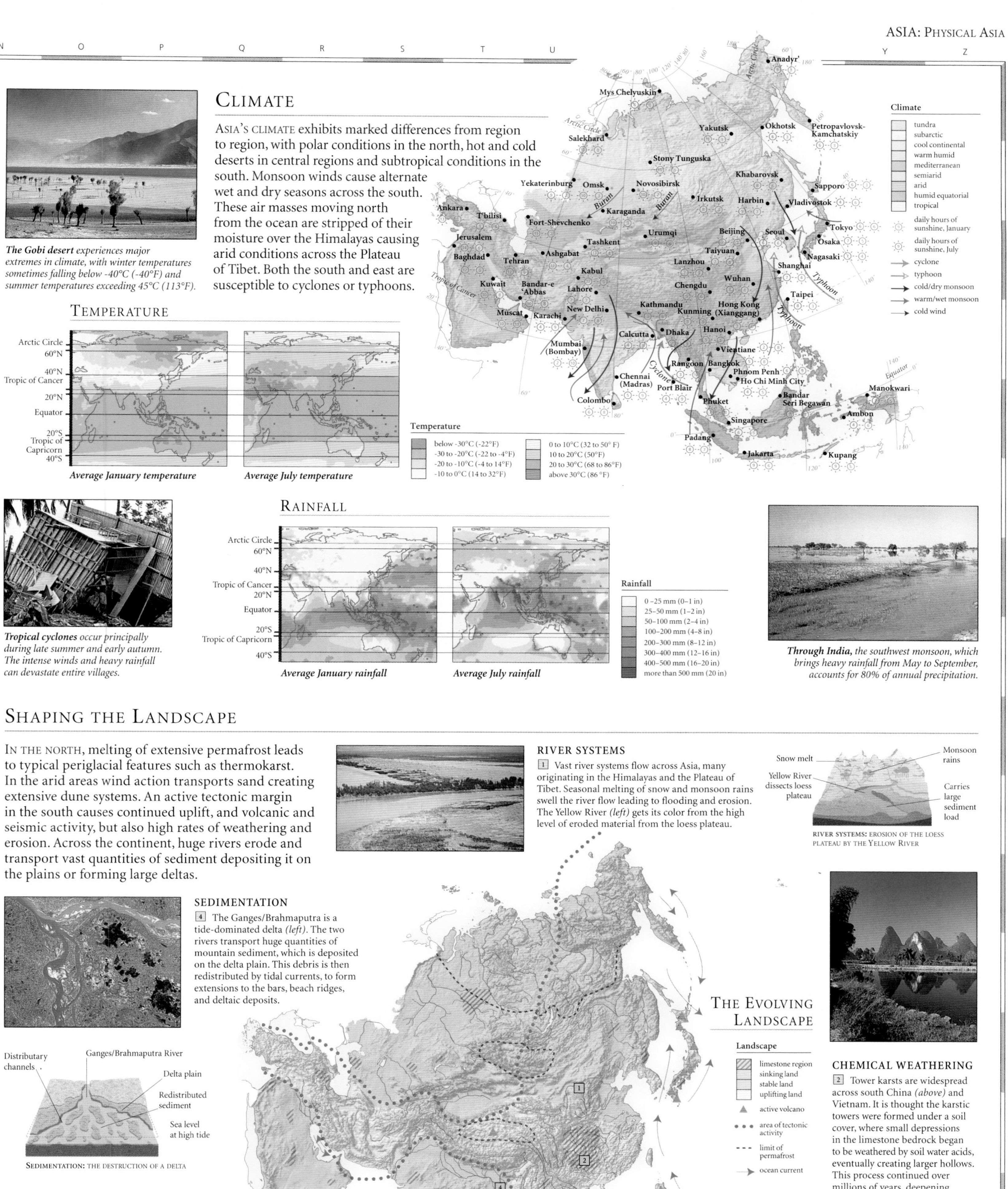

Climate
tundra
subarctic
cool continental
warm humid
mediterranean
semiarid
arid
humid equatorial
tropical
daily hours of sunshine, January
daily hours of sunshine, July
cyclone
typhoon
cold/dry monsoon
warm/wet monsoon
cold wind
Temperature
below -30°C (-22°F)
-30 to -20°C (-22 to -4°F)
-20 to -10°C (-4 to 14°F)
-10 to 0°C (14 to 32°F)
0 to 10°C (32 to 50° F)
10 to 20°C (50°F)
20 to 30°C (68 to 86°F)
above 30°C (86 °F)
Rainfall
0 -25 mm (0-1 in)
25-50 mm (1-2 in)
50-100 mm (2-4 in)
100-200 mm (4-8 in)
200-300 mm (8-12 in)
300-400 mm (12-16 in)
400-500 mm (16-20 in)
more than 500 mm (20 in)
Landscape
limestone region
sinking land
stable land
uplifting land
active volcano
area of tectonic activity
limit of permafrost
ocean current

Climate

The Gobi desert experiences major extremes in climate, with winter temperatures sometimes falling below -40°C (-40°F) and summer temperatures exceeding 45°C (113°F).

Asia's climate exhibits marked differences from region to region, with polar conditions in the north, hot and cold deserts in central regions and subtropical conditions in the south. Monsoon winds cause alternate wet and dry seasons across the south. These air masses moving north from the ocean are stripped of their moisture over the Himalayas causing arid conditions across the Plateau of Tibet. Both the south and east are susceptible to cyclones or typhoons.

Temperature

Average January temperature

Average July temperature

Rainfall

***Tropical cyclones** occur principally during late summer and early autumn. The intense winds and heavy rainfall can devastate entire villages.*

Average January rainfall

Average July rainfall

***Through India,** the southwest monsoon, which brings heavy rainfall from May to September, accounts for 80% of annual precipitation.*

Shaping the Landscape

In the north, melting of extensive permafrost leads to typical periglacial features such as thermokarst. In the arid areas wind action transports sand creating extensive dune systems. An active tectonic margin in the south causes continued uplift, and volcanic and seismic activity, but also high rates of weathering and erosion. Across the continent, huge rivers erode and transport vast quantities of sediment depositing it on the plains or forming large deltas.

River Systems

1 Vast river systems flow across Asia, many originating in the Himalayas and the Plateau of Tibet. Seasonal melting of snow and monsoon rains swell the river flow leading to flooding and erosion. The Yellow River *(left)* gets its color from the high level of eroded material from the loess plateau.

Snow melt
Monsoon rains
Yellow River dissects loess plateau
Carries large sediment load

River systems: erosion of the loess plateau by the Yellow River

Sedimentation

4 The Ganges/Brahmaputra is a tide-dominated delta *(left)*. The two rivers transport huge quantities of mountain sediment, which is deposited on the delta plain. This debris is then redistributed by tidal currents, to form extensions to the bars, beach ridges, and deltaic deposits.

Distributary channels
Ganges/Brahmaputra River
Delta plain
Redistributed sediment
Sea level at high tide

Sedimentation: the destruction of a delta

The Evolving Landscape

Chemical Weathering

2 Tower karsts are widespread across south China *(above)* and Vietnam. It is thought the karstic towers were formed under a soil cover, where small depressions in the limestone bedrock began to be weathered by soil water acids, eventually creating larger hollows. This process continued over millions of years, deepening the hollows and leaving steep-sided limestone hills.

Limestone hills
Old soil cover
Hollow being eroded by soil water acidity
Eroded hollow

Chemical weathering: formation of tower karst

Volcanic Activity

3 Volcanic eruptions occur frequently across Southeast Asia's island arcs *(below)*. Low-level eruptions occur when groundwater, superheated by underlying magma, becomes pressurized, forcing hot fluid and rocks up through cracks in the volcanic cone. This is known as a phreatic eruption.

Eruption within volcanic cone
Heat rising from the magma chamber
Fluid and rocks rising under pressure
Heated groundwater

Volcanic activity: a phreatic eruption

Political Asia

Asia is the world's largest continent, encompassing many different and discrete realms, from the desert Arab lands of the southwest to the subtropical archipelago of Indonesia; from the vast barren wastes of Siberia to the fertile river valleys of China and South Asia, seats of some of the world's most ancient civilizations. The collapse of the Soviet Union has fragmented the north of the continent into the Siberian portion of the Russian Federation, and the new republics of Central Asia. Strong religious traditions heavily influence the politics of South and Southwest Asia. Hindu and Muslim rivalries threaten to upset the political equilibrium in South Asia where India – in terms of population – remains the world's largest democracy. Communist China is the last great world empire; a population giant, but still relatively closed to the western world, while on its doorstep, the economically progressive and dynamic Pacific Rim countries, led by Japan, continue to assert their worldwide economic force.

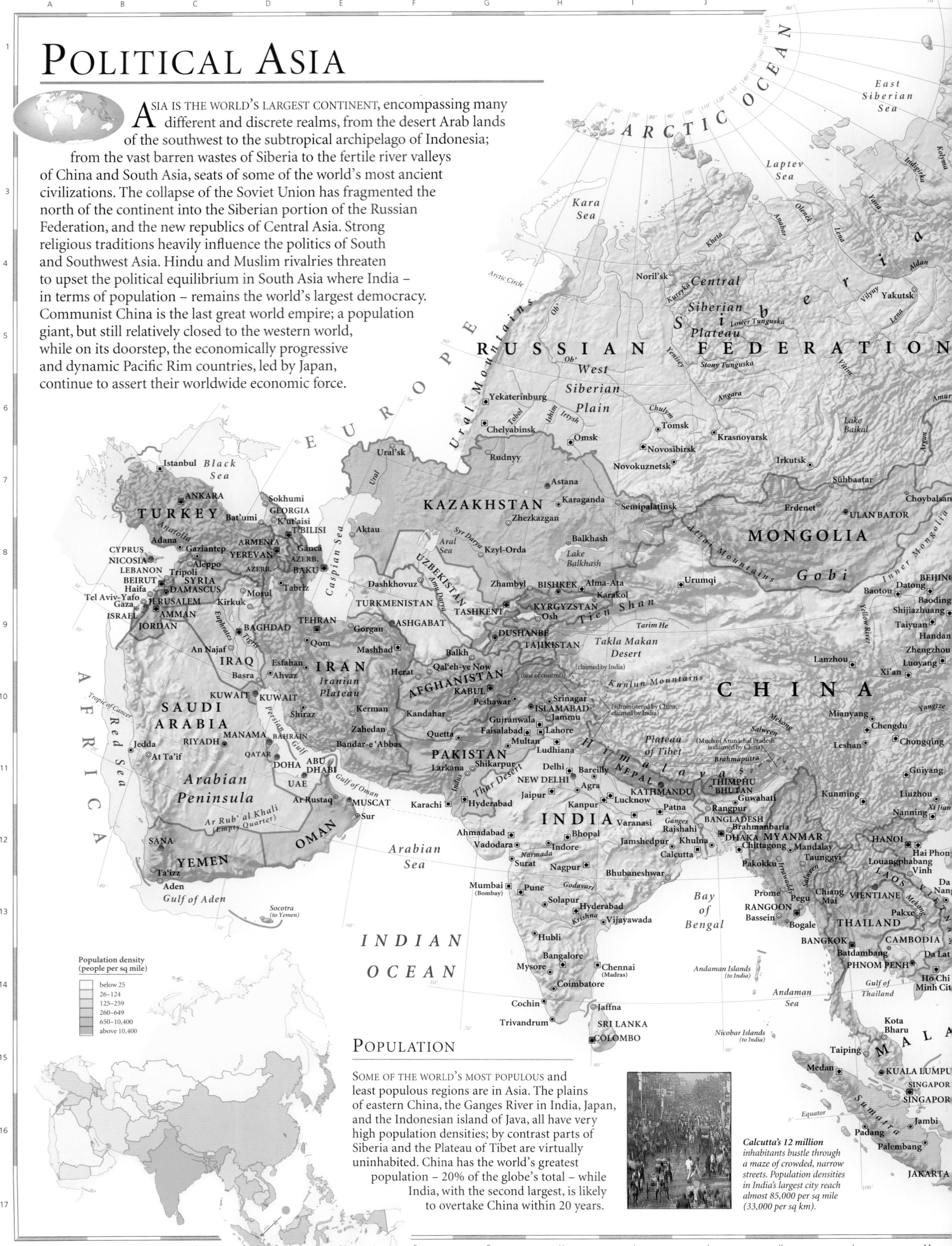

ARCTIC OCEAN
East Siberian Sea
Laptev Sea
Kara Sea
Arctic Circle
RUSSIAN FEDERATION
Siberia
Central Siberian Plateau
West Siberian Plain
EUROPE
Ural Mountains
Noril'sk
Yakutsk
Yekaterinburg
Chelyabinsk
Omsk
Tomsk
Novosibirsk
Krasnoyarsk
Novokuznetsk
Irkutsk
Lake Baikal
Ural'sk
Rudnyy
Astana
Karaganda
Semipalatinsk
KAZAKHSTAN
Zhezkazgan
Aral Sea
Kzyl-Orda
Balkhash
Lake Balkhash
MONGOLIA
ULAN BATOR
Erdenet
Sühbaatar
Choybalsan
Gobi
Altai Mountains
Urumqi
BISHKEK
Alma-Ata
Zhambyl
UZBEKISTAN
TASHKENT
KYRGYZSTAN
Osh
Tien Shan
TURKMENISTAN
ASHGABAT
Dashkhovuz
DUSHANBE
TAJIKISTAN
Takla Makan Desert
Kunlun Mountains
CHINA
Plateau of Tibet
Lanzhou
Xi'an
Luoyang
Zhengzhou
Taiyuan
Shijiazhuang
Baoding
BEIJING
Datong
Baotou
Mianyang
Chengdu
Chongqing
Leshan
Guiyang
Kunming
Liuzhou
Nanning
Istanbul
Black Sea
ANKARA
TURKEY
Anatolia
Adana
Gaziantep
Aleppo
CYPRUS
NICOSIA
LEBANON
BEIRUT
Tripoli
SYRIA
DAMASCUS
Haifa
Tel Aviv-Yafo
Gaza
JERUSALEM
ISRAEL
AMMAN
JORDAN
Sokhumi
GEORGIA
K'ut'aisi
T'BILISI
Bat'umi
ARMENIA
YEREVAN
Gäncä
AZERB.
BAKU
Aktau
Caspian Sea
Tabriz
Mosul
Kirkuk
BAGHDAD
IRAQ
An Najaf
Basra
TEHRAN
Qom
Gorgan
Mashhad
IRAN
Iranian Plateau
Esfahan
Ahvaz
Shiraz
Kerman
Zahedan
Bandar-e 'Abbas
KUWAIT
SAUDI ARABIA
RIYADH
Jedda
At Ta'if
MANAMA
BAHRAIN
QATAR
DOHA
ABU DHABI
UAE
Ar Rustaq
MUSCAT
Sur
OMAN
Gulf of Oman
Persian Gulf
Arabian Peninsula
Ar Rub' al Khali (Empty Quarter)
SANA
YEMEN
Ta'izz
Aden
Gulf of Aden
Socotra (to Yemen)
Red Sea
AFRICA
Tropic of Cancer
Herat
Qal'eh-ye Now
Balkh
AFGHANISTAN
KABUL
Kandahar
Quetta
Peshawar
ISLAMABAD
Srinagar
Jammu
Gujranwala
Faisalabad
Lahore
Multan
Ludhiana
PAKISTAN
Larkana
Shikarpur
Thar Desert
Karachi
Hyderabad
Himalaya
NEPAL
KATHMANDU
THIMPHU
BHUTAN
Delhi
NEW DELHI
Bareilly
Agra
Jaipur
Kanpur
Lucknow
Patna
Varanasi
INDIA
Ahmadabad
Vadodara
Bhopal
Indore
Surat
Nagpur
Jamshedpur
Rajshahi
Khulna
Calcutta
Guwahati
Rangpur
BANGLADESH
Brahmanbaria
DHAKA
Chittagong
Bhubaneshwar
Mumbai (Bombay)
Pune
Solapur
Hyderabad
Vijayawada
Hubli
Bangalore
Mysore
Chennai (Madras)
Coimbatore
Cochin
Trivandrum
Jaffna
SRI LANKA
COLOMBO
Arabian Sea
INDIAN OCEAN
Bay of Bengal
Andaman Islands (to India)
Andaman Sea
Nicobar Islands (to India)
MYANMAR
Mandalay
Taunggyi
Pakokku
Prome
Pegu
RANGOON
Bassein
Bogale
Chiang Mai
THAILAND
BANGKOK
VIENTIANE
LAOS
HANOI
Hai Phong
Louangphabang
Vinh
Pakxe
CAMBODIA
Batdambang
PHNOM PENH
Gulf of Thailand
Ho Chi Minh City
Kota Bharu
Taiping
Medan
KUALA LUMPUR
SINGAPORE
Sumatra
Equator
Padang
Jambi
Palembang
JAKARTA
Population density (people per sq mile)
below 25
26–124
125–259
260–649
650–10,400
above 10,400

Population

Some of the world's most populous and least populous regions are in Asia. The plains of eastern China, the Ganges River in India, Japan, and the Indonesian island of Java, all have very high population densities; by contrast parts of Siberia and the Plateau of Tibet are virtually uninhabited. China has the world's greatest population – 20% of the globe's total – while India, with the second largest, is likely to overtake China within 20 years.

Calcutta's 12 million *inhabitants bustle through a maze of crowded, narrow streets. Population densities in India's largest city reach almost 85,000 per sq mile (33,000 per sq km).*

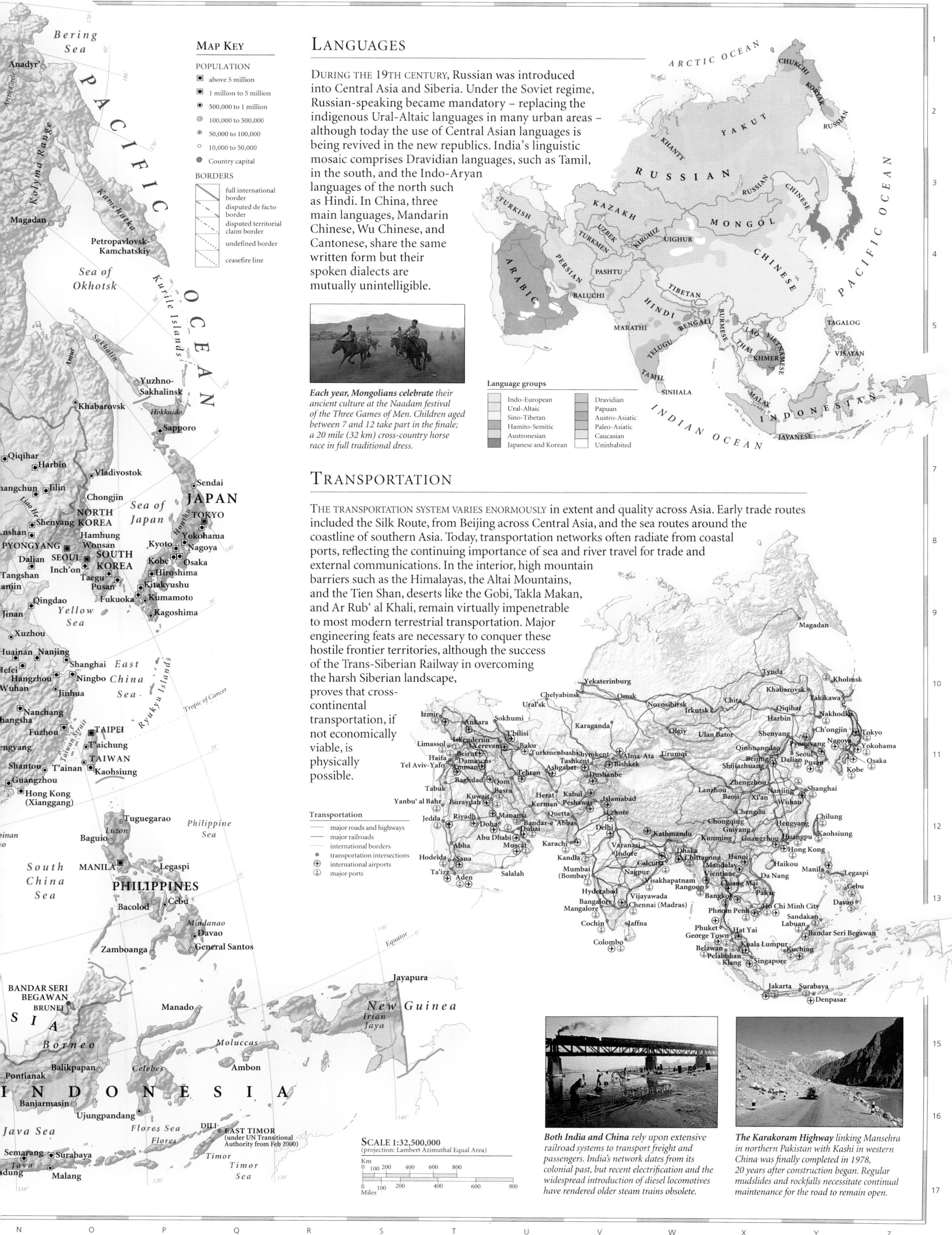
MAP KEY
POPULATION
above 5 million
1 million to 5 million
500,000 to 1 million
100,000 to 500,000
50,000 to 100,000
10,000 to 50,000
Country capital
BORDERS
full international border
disputed de facto border
disputed territorial claim border
undefined border
ceasefire line
Language groups
Indo-European
Ural-Altaic
Sino-Tibetan
Hamito-Semitic
Austronesian
Japanese and Korean
Dravidian
Papuan
Austro-Asiatic
Paleo-Asiatic
Caucasian
Uninhabited
Transportation
major roads and highways
major railroads
international borders
transportation intersections
international airports
major ports
SCALE 1:32,500,000
(projection: Lambert Azimuthal Equal Area)
Km 0 100 200 400 600 800
Miles 0 100 200 400 600 800

LANGUAGES

DURING THE 19TH CENTURY, Russian was introduced into Central Asia and Siberia. Under the Soviet regime, Russian-speaking became mandatory – replacing the indigenous Ural-Altaic languages in many urban areas – although today the use of Central Asian languages is being revived in the new republics. India's linguistic mosaic comprises Dravidian languages, such as Tamil, in the south, and the Indo-Aryan languages of the north such as Hindi. In China, three main languages, Mandarin Chinese, Wu Chinese, and Cantonese, share the same written form but their spoken dialects are mutually unintelligible.

***Each year, Mongolians celebrate** their ancient culture at the Naadam festival of the Three Games of Men. Children aged between 7 and 12 take part in the finale; a 20 mile (32 km) cross-country horse race in full traditional dress.*

TRANSPORTATION

THE TRANSPORTATION SYSTEM VARIES ENORMOUSLY in extent and quality across Asia. Early trade routes included the Silk Route, from Beijing across Central Asia, and the sea routes around the coastline of southern Asia. Today, transportation networks often radiate from coastal ports, reflecting the continuing importance of sea and river travel for trade and external communications. In the interior, high mountain barriers such as the Himalayas, the Altai Mountains, and the Tien Shan, deserts like the Gobi, Takla Makan, and Ar Rub' al Khali, remain virtually impenetrable to most modern terrestrial transportation. Major engineering feats are necessary to conquer these hostile frontier territories, although the success of the Trans-Siberian Railway in overcoming the harsh Siberian landscape, proves that cross-continental transportation, if not economically viable, is physically possible.

***Both India and China** rely upon extensive railroad systems to transport freight and passengers. India's network dates from its colonial past, but recent electrification and the widespread introduction of diesel locomotives have rendered older steam trains obsolete.*

***The Karakoram Highway** linking Mansehra in northern Pakistan with Kashi in western China was finally completed in 1978, 20 years after construction began. Regular mudslides and rockfalls necessitate continual maintenance for the road to remain open.*

A B C D E F G H I J K L M

Asian Resources

ALTHOUGH AGRICULTURE REMAINS THE ECONOMIC MAINSTAY of most Asian countries, the number of people employed in agriculture has steadily declined, as new industries have been developed during the past 30 years. China, Indonesia, Malaysia, Thailand, and Turkey have all experienced far-reaching structural change in their economies, while the breakup of the Soviet Union has created a new economic challenge in the Central Asian republics. The countries of the Persian Gulf illustrate the rapid transformation from rural nomadism to modern, urban society which oil wealth has brought to parts of the continent. Asia's most economically dynamic countries, Japan, Singapore, South Korea, and Taiwan, fringe the Pacific Ocean and are known as the Pacific Rim. In contrast, other Southeast Asian countries like Laos and Cambodia remain both economically and industrially underdeveloped.

Standard of Living

DESPITE JAPAN'S HIGH STANDARDS OF LIVING, and Southwest Asia's oil-derived wealth, immense disparities exist across the continent. Afghanistan remains one of the world's most underdeveloped nations, as do the mountain states of Nepal and Bhutan. Further rapid population growth is exacerbating poverty and overcrowding in many parts of India and Bangladesh.

Standard of Living
(UN Human Development Index)

- low
- high

Industry

JAPANESE INDUSTRY LEADS THE CONTINENT in both productivity and efficiency; electronics, hi-tech industries, car manufacture and shipbuilding are important. In recent years, the so-called economic "tigers" of the Pacific Rim such as Taiwan and South Korea are now challenging Japan's economic dominance. Heavy industries such as engineering, chemicals, and steel typify the industrial complexes along the corridor created by the Trans-Siberian Railway, the Fergana Valley in Central Asia, and also much of the huge industrial plain of east China. The discovery of oil in the Persian Gulf has brought immense wealth to countries that previously relied on subsistence agriculture on marginal desert land.

Industry

- aerospace
- brewing
- car/vehicle manufacture
- cement
- chemicals
- electronics
- engineering
- finance
- fish processing
- food processing
- hi-tech industry
- iron & steel
- pharmaceuticals
- printing & publishing
- shipbuilding
- sugar processing
- tea processing
- textiles
- timber processing
- tobacco processing
- coal
- oil
- gas
- industrial cities
- major industrial areas

ARCTIC OCEAN
PACIFIC OCEAN
RUSSIAN FEDERATION
Sea of Okhotsk
Yakutsk
Yekaterinburg
Chelyabinsk
Magnitogorsk
Omsk
Novosibirsk
Kemerovo
Krasnoyarsk
Novokuznetsk
Bratsk
Irkutsk
Khabarovsk
Vladivostok
Trans-Siberian Railway
Karaganda
KAZAKHSTAN
Aral Sea
UZBEKISTAN
Tashkent
KYRGYZSTAN
Farghona
Alma-Ata
Dushanbe
TAJIKISTAN
TURKMENISTAN
Ashgabat
AFGHANISTAN
Istanbul
Izmir
Ankara
TURKEY
GEORGIA
Tbilisi
ARMENIA
Yerevan
AZERB.
Baku
Caspian Sea
CYPRUS
LEBANON
Beirut
SYRIA
Damascus
Tel Aviv-Yafo
ISRAEL
Amman
JORDAN
Kirkuk
Baghdad
IRAQ
Tehran
Isfahan
IRAN
Basra
Kuwait
KUWAIT
SAUDI ARABIA
Red Sea
Jedda
Riyadh
Ad Damman
BAHRAIN
QATAR
Persian Gulf
Abu Dhabi
Dubai
UAE
Gulf of Oman
OMAN
YEMEN
Gulf of Aden
Arabian Sea
Rawalpindi
Lahore
PAKISTAN
Karachi
Delhi
NEPAL
Kanpur
INDIA
Ahmadabad
Indore
Jamshedpur
BANGLADESH
Dhaka
Calcutta
Chittagong
Mumbai (Bombay)
Nagpur
Bangalore
Chennai (Madras)
SRI LANKA
INDIAN OCEAN
BHUTAN
MYANMAR
Mandalay
Rangoon
Urumqi
MONGOLIA
Ulan Bator
CHINA
Harbin
Shenyang
Beijing
Tianjin
Taiyuan
Jinan
Lanzhou
Zhengzhou
Xi'an
Nanjing
Shanghai
Wuhan
Chengdu
Chongqing
Kunming
Guangzhou
Hong Kong
NORTH KOREA
Pyongyang
Dalian
Seoul
SOUTH KOREA
Pusan
Qingdao
JAPAN
Tokyo
Nagoya
Kobe
Taipei
TAIWAN
LAOS
Hanoi
VIETNAM
Da Nang
THAILAND
Bangkok
CAMBODIA
Ho Chi Minh City
South China Sea
Manila
PHILIPPINES
MALAYSIA
BRUNEI
Kuala Lumpur
Singapore
SINGAPORE
INDONESIA
Jakarta
Surabaya
EAST TIMOR (under UN Transitional Authority from Feb 2000)

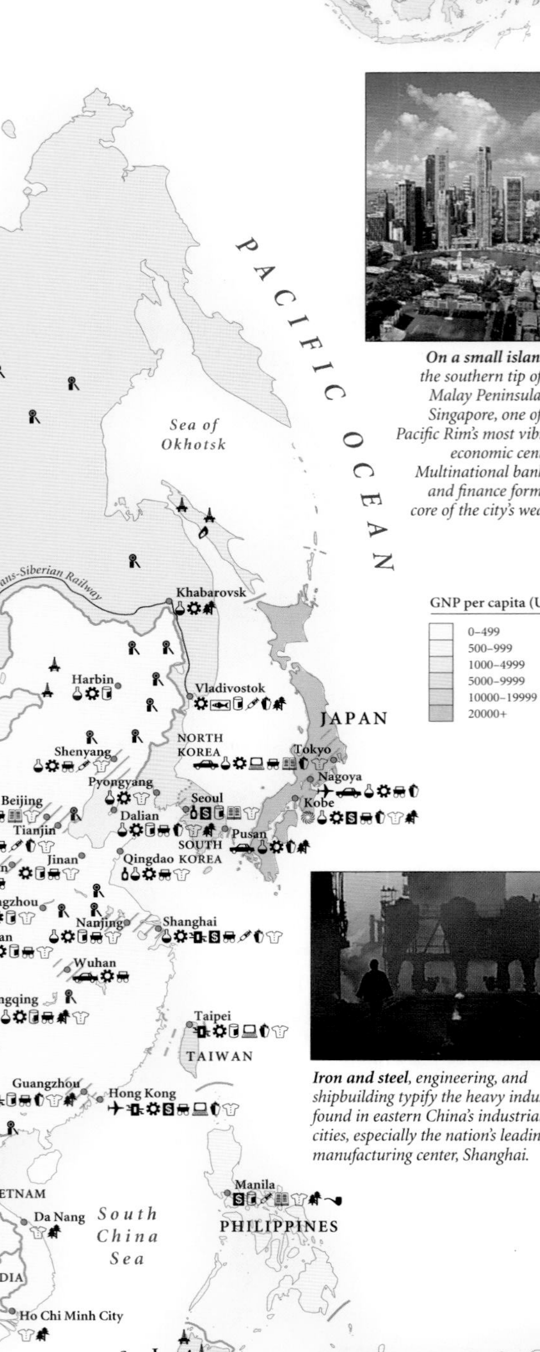

On a small island at the southern tip of the Malay Peninsula lies Singapore, one of the Pacific Rim's most vibrant economic centers. Multinational banking and finance form the core of the city's wealth.

GNP per capita (US$)

- 0–499
- 500–999
- 1000–4999
- 5000–9999
- 10000–19999
- 20000+

***Iron and steel**, engineering, and shipbuilding typify the heavy industry found in eastern China's industrial cities, especially the nation's leading manufacturing center, Shanghai.*

***Traditional industries** are still crucial to many rural economies across Asia. Here, on the Vietnamese coast, salt has been extracted from seawater by evaporation and is being loaded into a van to take to market.*

A B C D E F G M

ENVIRONMENTAL ISSUES

THE TRANSFORMATION OF UZBEKISTAN by the former Soviet Union into the world's second largest producer of cotton led to the diversion of several major rivers for irrigation. Starved of this water, the Aral Sea diminished in volume by over 50% in 30 years, irreversibly altering the ecology of the area. Heavy industries in eastern China have polluted coastal waters, rivers, and urban air, while in Myanmar, Malaysia, and Indonesia, ancient hardwood rain forests are felled faster than they can regenerate.

Environmental Issues

- tropical forest
- forest destroyed
- desert
- desertification
- acid rain
- polluted rivers
- marine pollution
- heavy marine pollution
- radioactive contamination
- poor urban air quality

***The long-term environmental** impact of the Gulf War (1991) is still uncertain. As Iraqi troops left Kuwait, equipment was abandoned to rust and thousands of oil wells were set alight, pouring crude oil into the Persian Gulf.*

***Although Siberia** remains a quintessentially frozen, inhospitable wasteland, vast untapped mineral reserves – especially the oil and gas of the West Siberian Plain – have lured industrial development to the area since the 1950s and 1960s.*

MINERAL RESOURCES

AT LEAST 60% OF THE WORLD'S known oil and gas deposits are found in Asia; notably the vast oil fields of the Persian Gulf, and the less-exploited oil and gas fields of the Ob' Basin in west Siberia. Immense coal reserves in Siberia and China have been utilized to support large steel industries. Southeast Asia has some of the world's largest deposits of tin, found in a belt running down the Malay Peninsula to Indonesia.

Mineral Resources

- oil field
- gas field
- coal field
- chromite
- copper
- gold
- iron
- lead
- nickel
- platinum
- tin
- wolfram

USING THE LAND AND SEA

VAST AREAS OF ASIA REMAIN UNCULTIVATED as a result of unsuitable climatic and soil conditions. In favorable areas such as river deltas, farming is intensive. Rice is the staple crop of most Asian countries, grown in paddy fields on waterlogged alluvial plains and terraced hillsides, and often irrigated for higher yields. Across the black earth region of the Eurasian steppe in southern Siberia and Kazakhstan, wheat farming is the dominant activity. Cash crops, like tea in Sri Lanka and dates in the Arabian Peninsula, are grown for export, and provide valuable income. The sovereignty of the rich fishing grounds in the South China Sea is disputed by China, Malaysia, Taiwan, the Philippines, and Vietnam, because of potential oil reserves.

Using the Land and Sea

- cropland
- desert
- forest
- mountain region
- pasture
- tundra
- wetland
- major conurbations
- cattle
- pigs
- goats
- sheep
- coconuts
- corn
- cotton
- dates
- fishing
- fruit
- jute
- peanuts
- rice
- rubber
- shellfish
- soybeans
- sugar beet
- sugar cane
- tea
- timber
- wheat

***Date palms** have been cultivated in oases throughout the Arabian Peninsula since antiquity. In addition to the fruit, palms are used for timber, fuel, rope, and for making vinegar, syrup, and a liquor known as arrack.*

***Rice terraces** blanket the landscape across the small Indonesian island of Bali. The large amounts of water needed to grow rice have resulted in Balinese farmers organizing water-control cooperatives.*

Turkey & the Caucasus

Armenia, Azerbaijan, Georgia, Turkey

This region occupies the fragmented junction between Europe, Asia, and the Russian Federation. Sunni Islam provides a common identity for the secular state of Turkey, which the revered leader Kemal Atatürk established from the remnants of the Ottoman Empire after the First World War. Turkey has a broad resource base and expanding trade links with Europe, but the east is relatively undeveloped and strife between the state and a large Kurdish minority has yet to be resolved. Georgia is similarly challenged by ethnic separatism, while the Christian state of Armenia and the mainly Muslim and oil-rich Azerbaijan are locked in conflict over the territory of Nagornyy Karabakh.

Transportation & Industry

Turkey leads the region's well-diversified economy. Petrochemicals, textiles, engineering, and food processing are the main industries. Azerbaijan is able to export oil, while the other states rely heavily on hydro-electric power and imported fuel. Georgia produces precision machinery. War and earthquake damage have devastated Armenia's infrastructure.

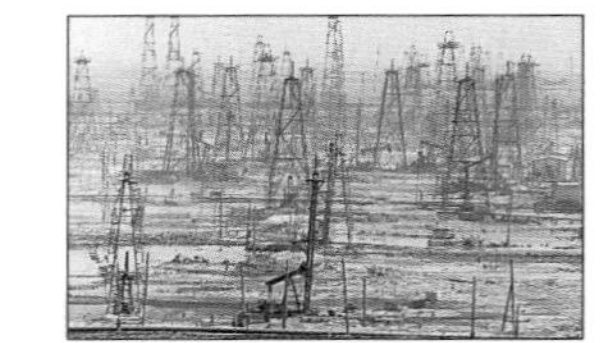

Azerbaijan has substantial oil reserves, located in and around the Caspian Sea. They were some of the earliest oilfields in the world to be exploited.

Major industry and infrastructure
- carpet weaving
- cement
- chemicals
- coal
- engineering
- food processing
- oil
- textiles
- tourism
- vehicle manufacture
- capital cities
- major towns
- international airports
- major roads
- major industrial areas

Transportation Network

- 76,289 miles (122,849 km)
- 7,74 miles (1,246 km)
- 9,047 miles (14,569 km)
- 745 miles (1,200 km)

Physical and political barriers have severely limited communications between Armenia, Georgia and Azerbaijan. Turkey has a relatively well-developed transportation network.

Using the Land and Sea

Turkey is largely self-sufficient in food. The irrigated Black Sea coastlands have the world's highest yields of hazelnuts. Tobacco, cotton, sultanas, tea, and figs are the region's main cash crops and a great range of fruit and vegetables are grown. Wine grapes are among the labor-intensive crops which allow full use of limited agricultural land in the Caucasus. Sturgeon fishing is particularly important in Azerbaijan.

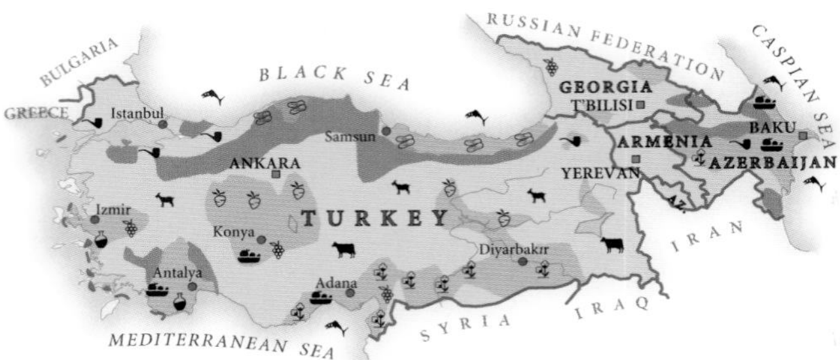

BULGARIA
GREECE
BLACK SEA
RUSSIAN FEDERATION
CASPIAN SEA
Istanbul
Samsun
GEORGIA
T'BILISI
ARMENIA
BAKU
AZERBAIJAN
YEREVAN
ANKARA
TURKEY
Izmir
Konya
Diyarbakır
Antalya
Adana
IRAN
IRAQ
SYRIA
MEDITERRANEAN SEA

Land use and agricultural distribution
- cattle
- goats
- cotton
- fishing
- fruit
- hazelnuts
- olives
- sugar beet
- tobacco
- vineyards
- capital cities
- major towns
- pasture
- cropland
- forest

The Urban/Rural Population Divide

urban 67% — rural 23%

0 10 20 30 40 50 60 70 80 90 100

Population Density	Total Land Area
218 people per sq mile (84 people per sq km)	368,912 sq miles (955,730 sq km)

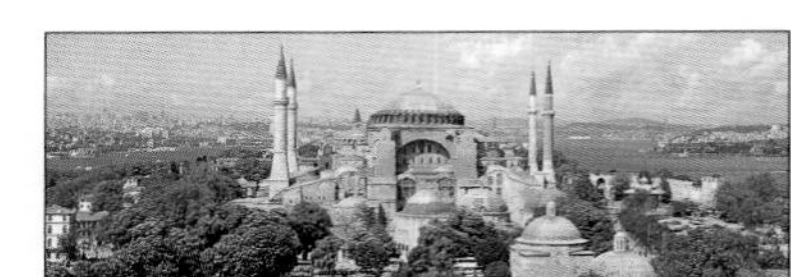

For many centuries, Istanbul has held tremendous strategic importance as a crucial gateway between Europe and Asia. Founded by the Greeks as Byzantium, the city became the center of the East Roman Empire and was known as Constantinople to the Romans. From the 15th century onward the city became the center of the great Ottoman Empire.

114

120

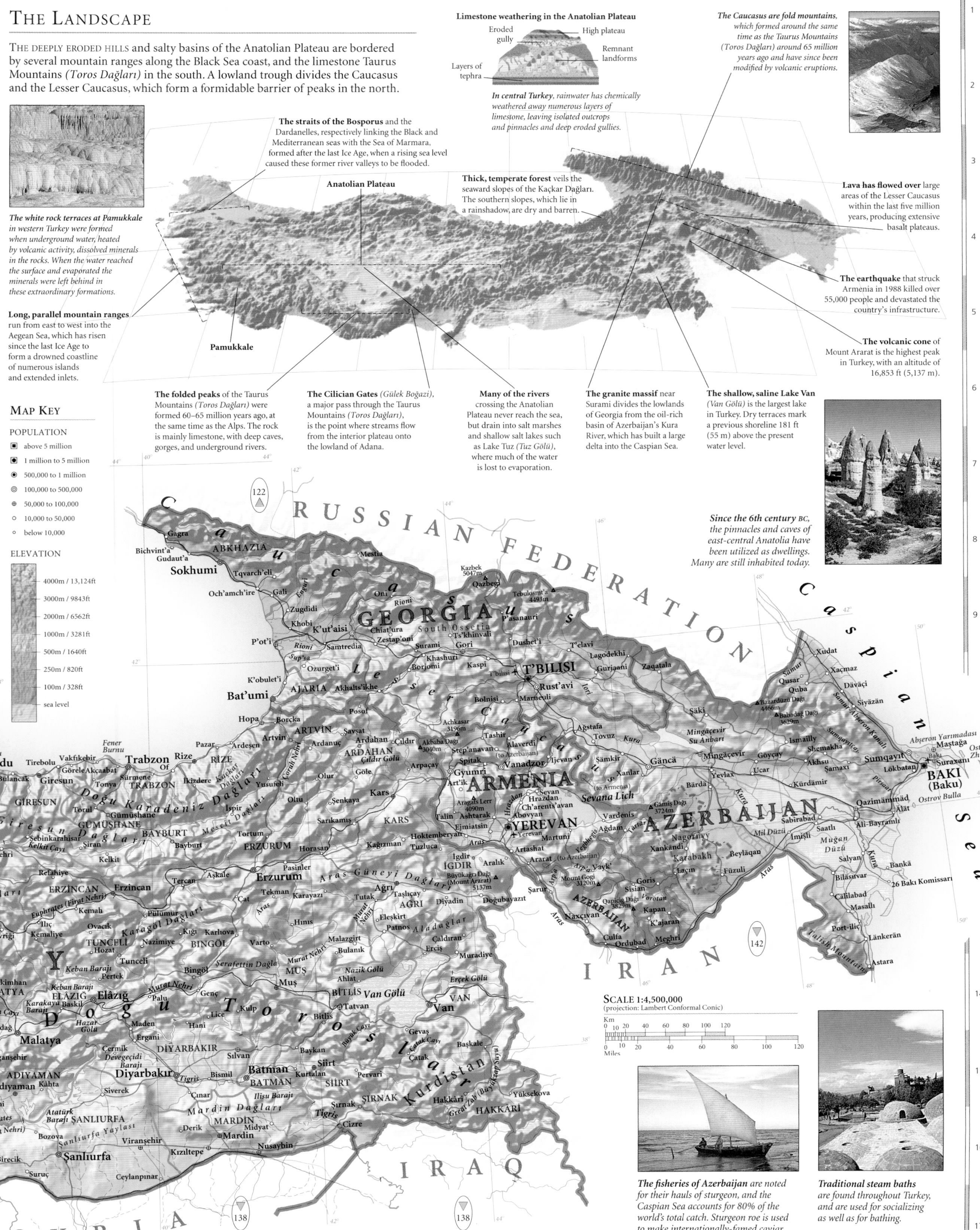

THE LANDSCAPE

THE DEEPLY ERODED HILLS and salty basins of the Anatolian Plateau are bordered by several mountain ranges along the Black Sea coast, and the limestone Taurus Mountains *(Toros Dağları)* in the south. A lowland trough divides the Caucasus and the Lesser Caucasus, which form a formidable barrier of peaks in the north.

Limestone weathering in the Anatolian Plateau

Eroded gully
High plateau
Remnant landforms
Layers of tephra

In central Turkey, rainwater has chemically weathered away numerous layers of limestone, leaving isolated outcrops and pinnacles and deep eroded gullies.

The Caucasus are fold mountains, which formed around the same time as the Taurus Mountains (Toros Dağları) around 65 million years ago and have since been modified by volcanic eruptions.

The white rock terraces at Pamukkale in western Turkey were formed when underground water, heated by volcanic activity, dissolved minerals in the rocks. When the water reached the surface and evaporated the minerals were left behind in these extraordinary formations.

The straits of the Bosporus and the Dardanelles, respectively linking the Black and Mediterranean seas with the Sea of Marmara, formed after the last Ice Age, when a rising sea level caused these former river valleys to be flooded.

Anatolian Plateau

Thick, temperate forest veils the seaward slopes of the Kaçkar Dağları. The southern slopes, which lie in a rainshadow, are dry and barren.

Lava has flowed over large areas of the Lesser Caucasus within the last five million years, producing extensive basalt plateaus.

The earthquake that struck Armenia in 1988 killed over 55,000 people and devastated the country's infrastructure.

Long, parallel mountain ranges run from east to west into the Aegean Sea, which has risen since the last Ice Age to form a drowned coastline of numerous islands and extended inlets.

Pamukkale

The volcanic cone of Mount Ararat is the highest peak in Turkey, with an altitude of 16,853 ft (5,137 m).

The folded peaks of the Taurus Mountains *(Toros Dağları)* were formed 60–65 million years ago, at the same time as the Alps. The rock is mainly limestone, with deep caves, gorges, and underground rivers.

The Cilician Gates *(Gülek Boğazi)*, a major pass through the Taurus Mountains *(Toros Dağları)*, is the point where streams flow from the interior plateau onto the lowland of Adana.

Many of the rivers crossing the Anatolian Plateau never reach the sea, but drain into salt marshes and shallow salt lakes such as Lake Tuz *(Tuz Gölü)*, where much of the water is lost to evaporation.

The granite massif near Surami divides the lowlands of Georgia from the oil-rich basin of Azerbaijan's Kura River, which has built a large delta into the Caspian Sea.

The shallow, saline Lake Van *(Van Gölü)* is the largest lake in Turkey. Dry terraces mark a previous shoreline 181 ft (55 m) above the present water level.

Since the 6th century BC, the pinnacles and caves of east-central Anatolia have been utilized as dwellings. Many are still inhabited today.

MAP KEY

POPULATION

- above 5 million
- 1 million to 5 million
- 500,000 to 1 million
- 100,000 to 500,000
- 50,000 to 100,000
- 10,000 to 50,000
- below 10,000

ELEVATION

- 4000m / 13,124ft
- 3000m / 9843ft
- 2000m / 6562ft
- 1000m / 3281ft
- 500m / 1640ft
- 250m / 820ft
- 100m / 328ft
- sea level

RUSSIAN FEDERATION
GEORGIA
ARMENIA
AZERBAIJAN
IRAN
IRAQ
SYRIA
Caspian Sea
T'BILISI
YEREVAN
BAKI (Baku)

122
142
138
138

SCALE 1:4,500,000
(projection: Lambert Conformal Conic)

The fisheries of Azerbaijan are noted for their hauls of sturgeon, and the Caspian Sea accounts for 80% of the world's total catch. Sturgeon roe is used to make internationally-famed caviar.

Traditional steam baths are found throughout Turkey, and are used for socializing as well as for bathing.

THE NEAR EAST

IRAQ, ISRAEL, JORDAN, LEBANON, SYRIA

SOME OF THE WORLD'S OLDEST CIVILIZATIONS developed in this region – the Fertile Crescent – which is venerated by Jews, Muslims, and Christians, but torn by competing religious, ethnic, and national claims to the land. Turkish Ottoman rule ended with World War I and the region was divided into areas administered by Britain and France. The UN endorsed calls for a Jewish homeland in what was then Palestine and in 1948 the state of Israel was declared. Hostility towards the Jewish state led to a series of wars but since 1977, and especially since 1993, a peace process between Israel and her neighbors has been evolving. Since independence, Syria has played a leading role in Middle Eastern politics. The once-prosperous state of Lebanon is emerging from a ruinous factional war, while Iraq's great oil wealth has funded military campaigns against Iran and Kuwait, and the stifling of internal dissent, leading to international ostracization.

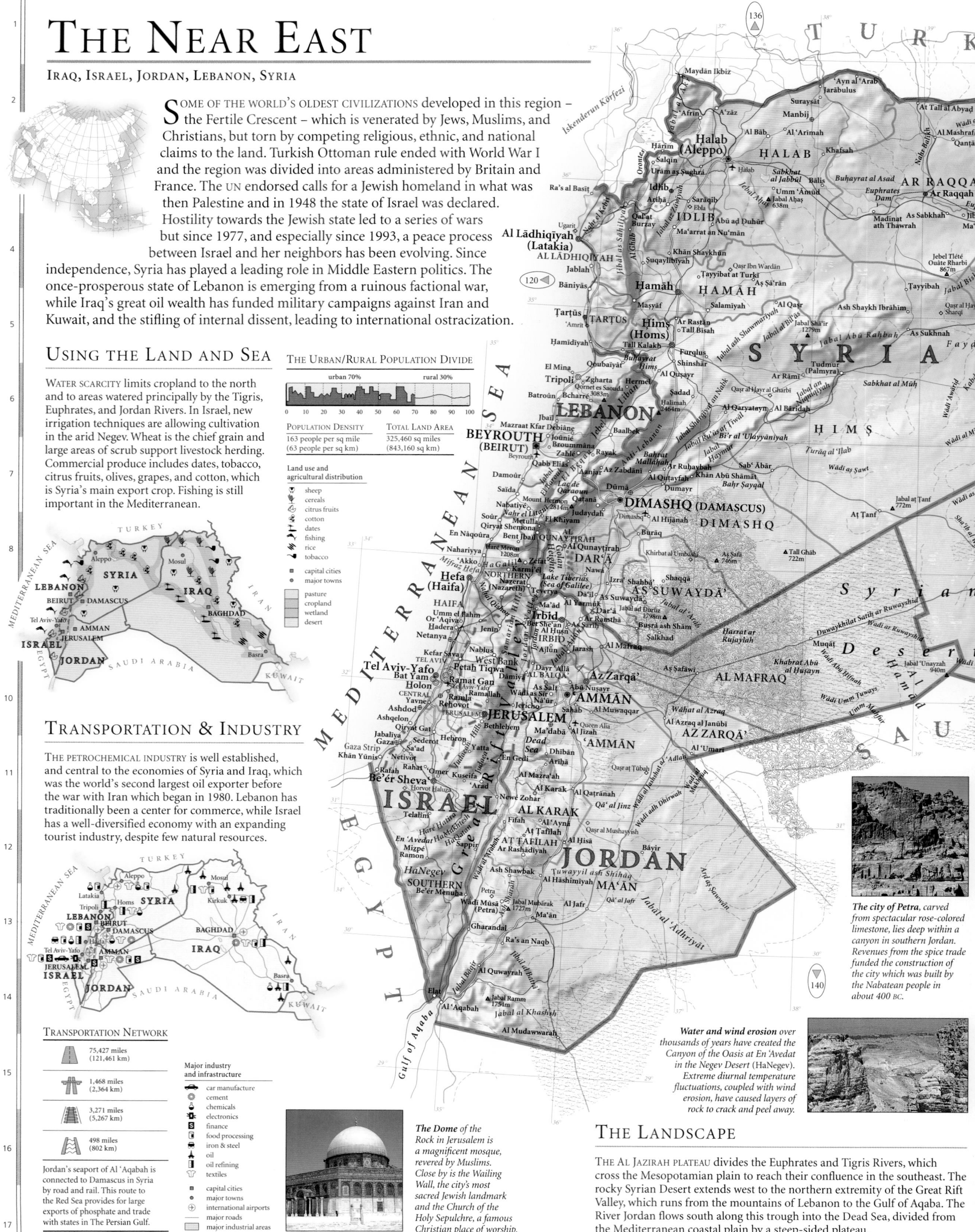

THE URBAN/RURAL POPULATION DIVIDE
urban 70%
rural 30%
0 10 20 30 40 50 60 70 80 90 100
POPULATION DENSITY
163 people per sq mile
(63 people per sq km)
TOTAL LAND AREA
325,460 sq miles
(843,160 sq km)
Land use and agricultural distribution
sheep
cereals
citrus fruits
cotton
dates
fishing
rice
tobacco
capital cities
major towns
pasture
cropland
wetland
desert
TRANSPORTATION NETWORK
75,427 miles
(121,461 km)
1,468 miles
(2,364 km)
3,271 miles
(5,267 km)
498 miles
(802 km)
Major industry and infrastructure
car manufacture
cement
chemicals
electronics
finance
food processing
iron & steel
oil
oil refining
textiles
capital cities
major towns
international airports
major roads
major industrial areas

USING THE LAND AND SEA

WATER SCARCITY limits cropland to the north and to areas watered principally by the Tigris, Euphrates, and Jordan Rivers. In Israel, new irrigation techniques are allowing cultivation in the arid Negev. Wheat is the chief grain and large areas of scrub support livestock herding. Commercial produce includes dates, tobacco, citrus fruits, olives, grapes, and cotton, which is Syria's main export crop. Fishing is still important in the Mediterranean.

TRANSPORTATION & INDUSTRY

THE PETROCHEMICAL INDUSTRY is well established, and central to the economies of Syria and Iraq, which was the world's second largest oil exporter before the war with Iran which began in 1980. Lebanon has traditionally been a center for commerce, while Israel has a well-diversified economy with an expanding tourist industry, despite few natural resources.

Jordan's seaport of Al 'Aqabah is connected to Damascus in Syria by road and rail. This route to the Red Sea provides for large exports of phosphate and trade with states in The Persian Gulf.

The Dome of the Rock in Jerusalem is a magnificent mosque, revered by Muslims. Close by is the Wailing Wall, the city's most sacred Jewish landmark and the Church of the Holy Sepulchre, a famous Christian place of worship.

The city of Petra, carved from spectacular rose-colored limestone, lies deep within a canyon in southern Jordan. Revenues from the spice trade funded the construction of the city which was built by the Nabatean people in about 400 BC.

Water and wind erosion over thousands of years have created the Canyon of the Oasis at En 'Avedat in the Negev Desert (HaNegev). Extreme diurnal temperature fluctuations, coupled with wind erosion, have caused layers of rock to crack and peel away.

THE LANDSCAPE

THE AL JAZIRAH PLATEAU divides the Euphrates and Tigris Rivers, which cross the Mesopotamian plain to reach their confluence in the southeast. The rocky Syrian Desert extends west to the northern extremity of the Great Rift Valley, which runs from the mountains of Lebanon to the Gulf of Aqaba. The River Jordan flows south along this trough into the Dead Sea, divided from the Mediterranean coastal plain by a steep-sided plateau.

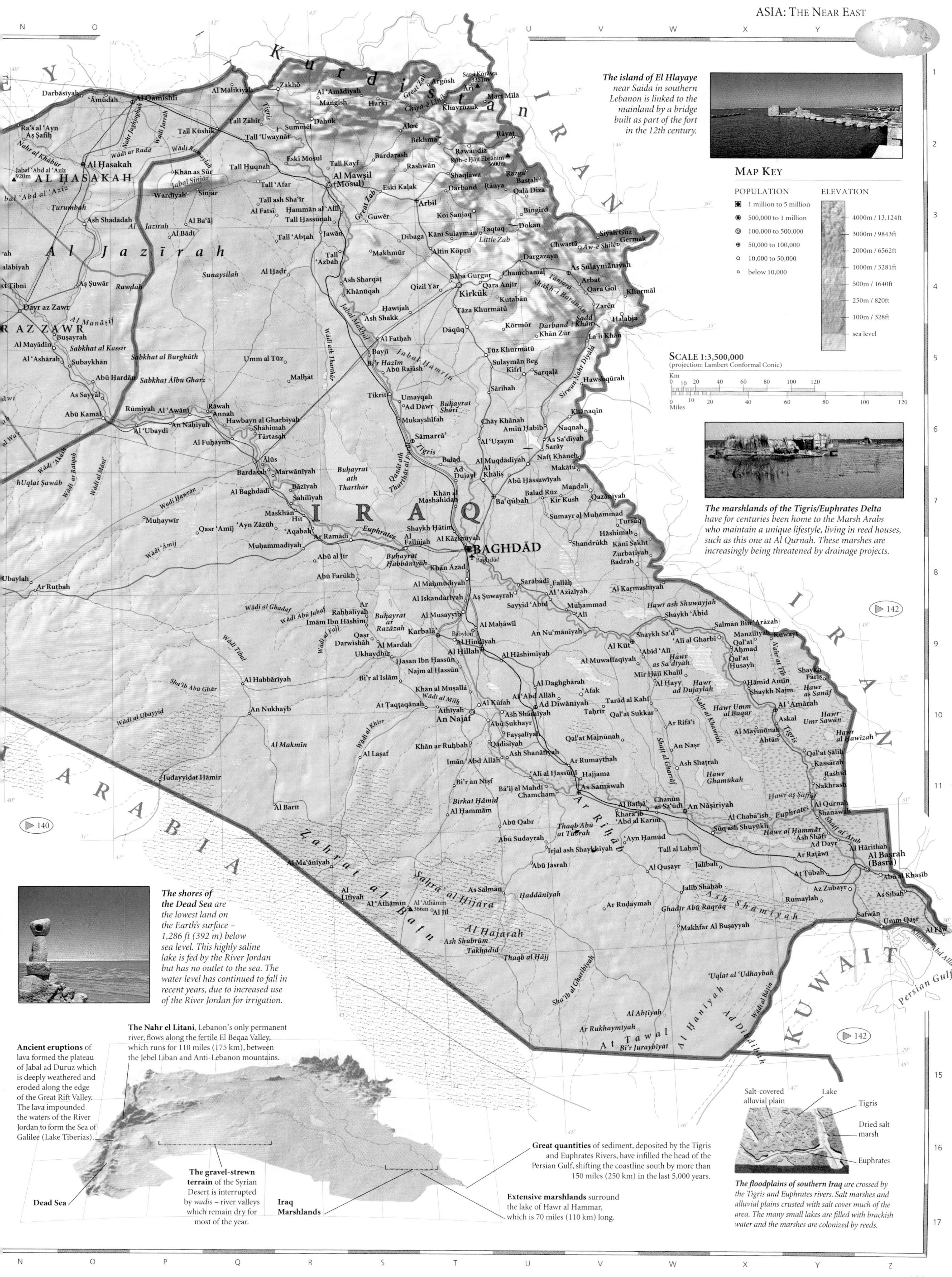

Map Key
POPULATION
1 million to 5 million
500,000 to 1 million
100,000 to 500,000
50,000 to 100,000
10,000 to 50,000
below 10,000
ELEVATION
4000m / 13,124ft
3000m / 9843ft
2000m / 6562ft
1000m / 3281ft
500m / 1640ft
250m / 820ft
100m / 328ft
sea level
SCALE 1:3,500,000
(projection: Lambert Conformal Conic)
Km
Miles
IRAQ
IRAN
KUWAIT
ARABIA
Kurdistan
Al Jazīrah
AL HASAKAH
BAGHDĀD
Al Mawşil (Mosul)
Kirkūk
Arbil
As Sulaymānīyah
Tikrīt
Sāmarrā'
Ar Ramādī
Al Fallūjah
Karbalā'
Al Ḩillah
An Najaf
Al Kūt
Al 'Amārah
An Nāşirīyah
Al Başrah (Başra)
Al Fāw
Umm Qaşr
Persian Gulf
Tigris
Euphrates
Great Zab
Little Zab
Shaţţ al 'Arab
Ar Ruţbah
Al Qāmishlī
Dayr az Zawr
Abū Kamāl
Zahrat al Baţn
Al Ḩajarah
Aş Şahrā' al Ḩijāra
Hawr al Hammār
Hawr al Ḩawīzah
Dead Sea
Iraq Marshlands
Salt-covered alluvial plain
Lake
Tigris
Dried salt marsh
Euphrates

The island of El Hlayaye *near Saida in southern Lebanon is linked to the mainland by a bridge built as part of the fort in the 12th century.*

The marshlands of the Tigris/Euphrates Delta *have for centuries been home to the Marsh Arabs who maintain a unique lifestyle, living in reed houses, such as this one at Al Qurnah. These marshes are increasingly being threatened by drainage projects.*

The shores of the Dead Sea *are the lowest land on the Earth's surface – 1,286 ft (392 m) below sea level. This highly saline lake is fed by the River Jordan but has no outlet to the sea. The water level has continued to fall in recent years, due to increased use of the River Jordan for irrigation.*

The Nahr el Litani, Lebanon's only permanent river, flows along the fertile El Beqaa Valley, which runs for 110 miles (175 km), between the Jebel Liban and Anti-Lebanon mountains.

Ancient eruptions of lava formed the plateau of Jabal ad Duruz which is deeply weathered and eroded along the edge of the Great Rift Valley. The lava impounded the waters of the River Jordan to form the Sea of Galilee (Lake Tiberias).

The gravel-strewn terrain of the Syrian Desert is interrupted by *wadis* – river valleys which remain dry for most of the year.

Great quantities of sediment, deposited by the Tigris and Euphrates Rivers, have infilled the head of the Persian Gulf, shifting the coastline south by more than 150 miles (250 km) in the last 5,000 years.

Extensive marshlands surround the lake of Hawr al Hammar, which is 70 miles (110 km) long.

***The floodplains of southern Iraq** are crossed by the Tigris and Euphrates rivers. Salt marshes and alluvial plains crusted with salt cover much of the area. The many small lakes are filled with brackish water and the marshes are colonized by reeds.*

140
142
142

The Arabian Peninsula

Bahrain, Kuwait, Oman, Qatar, Saudi Arabia, United Arab Emirates (UAE), Yemen

Huge expanses of desert cover much of the Arabian Peninsula, limiting settlement to oases, the mountains along the Red Sea and coastal belts. The most populous area is the fertile highlands of Yemen. The Islamic faith and Arabic language give the region a cultural and religious unity, and the Saudi city of Mecca *(Makkah)* is Islam's most holy place, visited by over two million pilgrims each year. More than half the world's oil reserves are contained in this region, and the exploitation of oil and gas has brought great wealth, particularly to Saudi Arabia. Yemen and Oman are the least developed of the Arabian states, with large rural populations. Within Saudi Arabia over two-thirds of the people live in urban areas.

Using the Land

Most of the Arabian Peninsula is unsuited to settled agriculture, making irrigation and land reclamation projects essential. The narrow coastal plain and isolated oases, commonly amounting to less than 1% of the land area, are used to cultivate grains, coffee, and exotic fruits. Goats, sheep, and camels are widespread throughout the region.

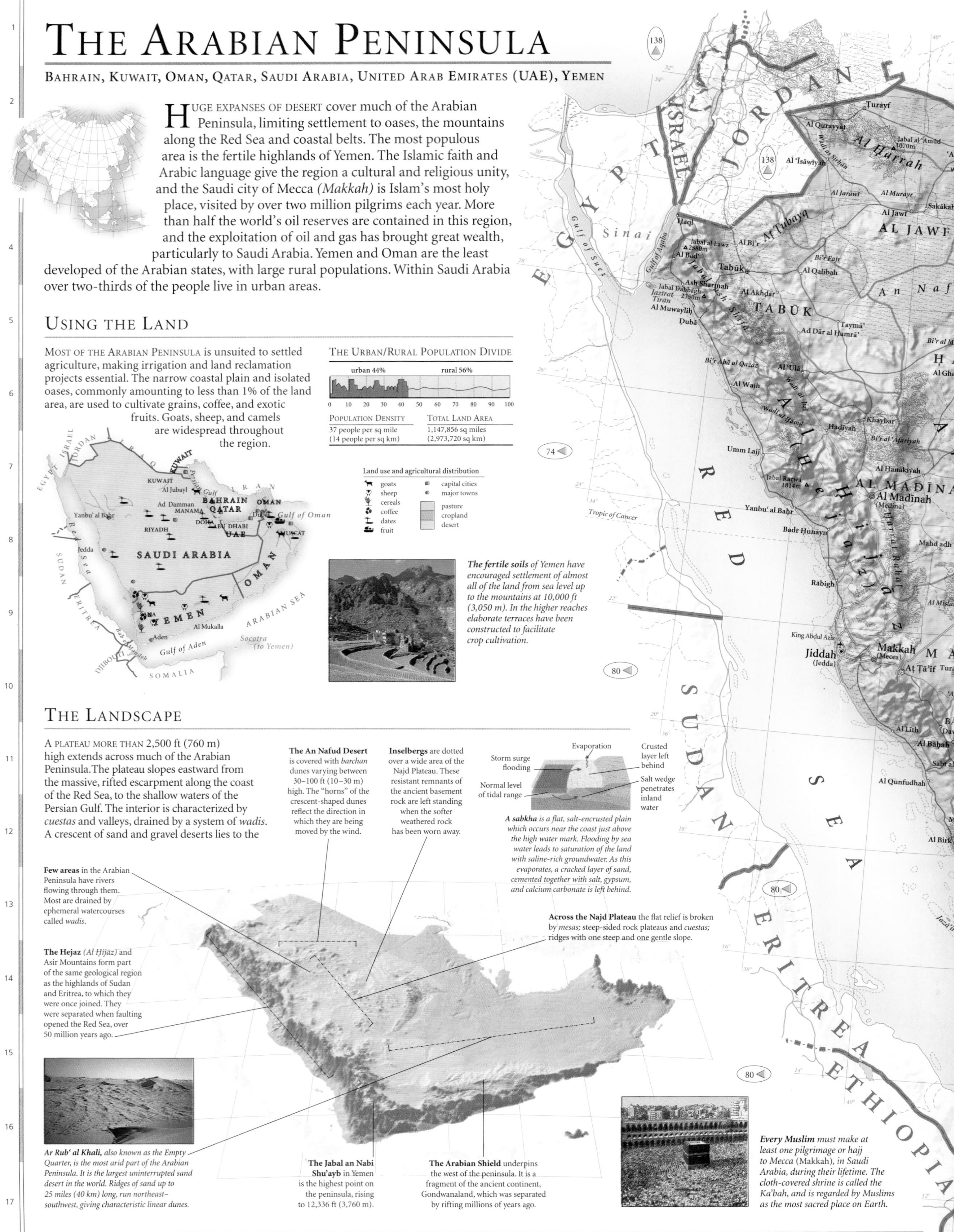

The Urban/Rural Population Divide
urban 44%
rural 56%
0 10 20 30 40 50 60 70 80 90 100
Population Density
37 people per sq mile
(14 people per sq km)
Total Land Area
1,147,856 sq miles
(2,973,720 sq km)
Land use and agricultural distribution
goats
sheep
cereals
coffee
dates
fruit
capital cities
major towns
pasture
cropland
desert
KUWAIT
Al Jubayl
Ad Damman
MANAMA
BAHRAIN
QATAR
DOHA
ABU DHABI
UAE
Dubai
MUSCAT
OMAN
Gulf of Oman
RIYADH
SAUDI ARABIA
Yanbu' al Bahr
Jedda
YEMEN
Al Mukalla
Aden
Gulf of Aden
Socotra (to Yemen)
ARABIAN SEA
SOMALIA
DJIBOUTI
ERITREA
SUDAN
EGYPT
ISRAEL
JORDAN
IRAQ
IRAN
Red Sea
Bab el Mandeb
Persian Gulf
Evaporation
Storm surge flooding
Normal level of tidal range
Crusted layer left behind
Salt wedge penetrates inland water
EGYPT
ISRAEL
JORDAN
Sinai
Gulf of Suez
Gulf of Aqaba
Turayf
Al Qurayyat
Wadi as Sirhan
Al Harrah
Jabal al 'Amud 1070m
Al 'Isawiyah
Al Jarawi
Al Murayr
Al Jawf
Sakakah
AL JAWF
At Tubayq
Haql
Jabal al Lawz 2580m
Al Bi'r
Al Bad'
Tabuk
Bi'r Fajr
Al Qalibah
An Nafud
Ash Sharmah
Jabal Dabbagh 2350m
Jazirat Tiran
Al Akhdar
TABUK
Al Muwaylih
Duba
Ad Dar al Hamra'
Tayma'
Bi'r Aba al Qazaz
Al 'Ula
Al Wajh
Wadi al Hamd
Hadiyah
Khaybar
Bi'r al 'Afariyah
Umm Lajj
Al Hanakiyah
Jabal Radwa 1814m
AL MADINAH
Al Madinah (Medina)
Yanbu' al Bahr
Badr Hunayn
Harrat Rahat
Mahd adh Dhahab
Rabigh
Al Mislah
King Abdul Aziz
Jiddah (Jedda)
Makkah (Mecca)
At Ta'if
Turabah
Al Lith
Al Bahah
Al Qunfudhah
Al Birk
Tropic of Cancer
RED SEA
SUDAN
ERITREA
ETHIOPIA
Jaza'ir Farasan
Al Hijaz

The fertile soils of Yemen have encouraged settlement of almost all of the land from sea level up to the mountains at 10,000 ft (3,050 m). In the higher reaches elaborate terraces have been constructed to facilitate crop cultivation.

138 74 80 80 80

The Landscape

A plateau more than 2,500 ft (760 m) high extends across much of the Arabian Peninsula. The plateau slopes eastward from the massive, rifted escarpment along the coast of the Red Sea, to the shallow waters of the Persian Gulf. The interior is characterized by *cuestas* and valleys, drained by a system of *wadis*. A crescent of sand and gravel deserts lies to the

The An Nafud Desert is covered with *barchan* dunes varying between 30–100 ft (10–30 m) high. The "horns" of the crescent-shaped dunes reflect the direction in which they are being moved by the wind.

Inselbergs are dotted over a wide area of the Najd Plateau. These resistant remnants of the ancient basement rock are left standing when the softer weathered rock has been worn away.

A sabkha is a flat, salt-encrusted plain which occurs near the coast just above the high water mark. Flooding by sea water leads to saturation of the land with saline-rich groundwater. As this evaporates, a cracked layer of sand, cemented together with salt, gypsum, and calcium carbonate is left behind.

Few areas in the Arabian Peninsula have rivers flowing through them. Most are drained by ephemeral watercourses called *wadis*.

Across the Najd Plateau the flat relief is broken by *mesas;* steep-sided rock plateaus and *cuestas;* ridges with one steep and one gentle slope.

The Hejaz *(Al Hijaz)* and Asir Mountains form part of the same geological region as the highlands of Sudan and Eritrea, to which they were once joined. They were separated when faulting opened the Red Sea, over 50 million years ago.

***Ar Rub' al Khali,** also known as the Empty Quarter, is the most arid part of the Arabian Peninsula. It is the largest uninterrupted sand desert in the world. Ridges of sand up to 25 miles (40 km) long, run northeast–southwest, giving characteristic linear dunes.*

The Jabal an Nabi Shu'ayb in Yemen is the highest point on the peninsula, rising to 12,336 ft (3,760 m).

The Arabian Shield underpins the west of the peninsula. It is a fragment of the ancient continent, Gondwanaland, which was separated by rifting millions of years ago.

***Every Muslim** must make at least one pilgrimage or hajj to Mecca (Makkah), in Saudi Arabia, during their lifetime. The cloth-covered shrine is called the Ka'bah, and is regarded by Muslims as the most sacred place on Earth.*

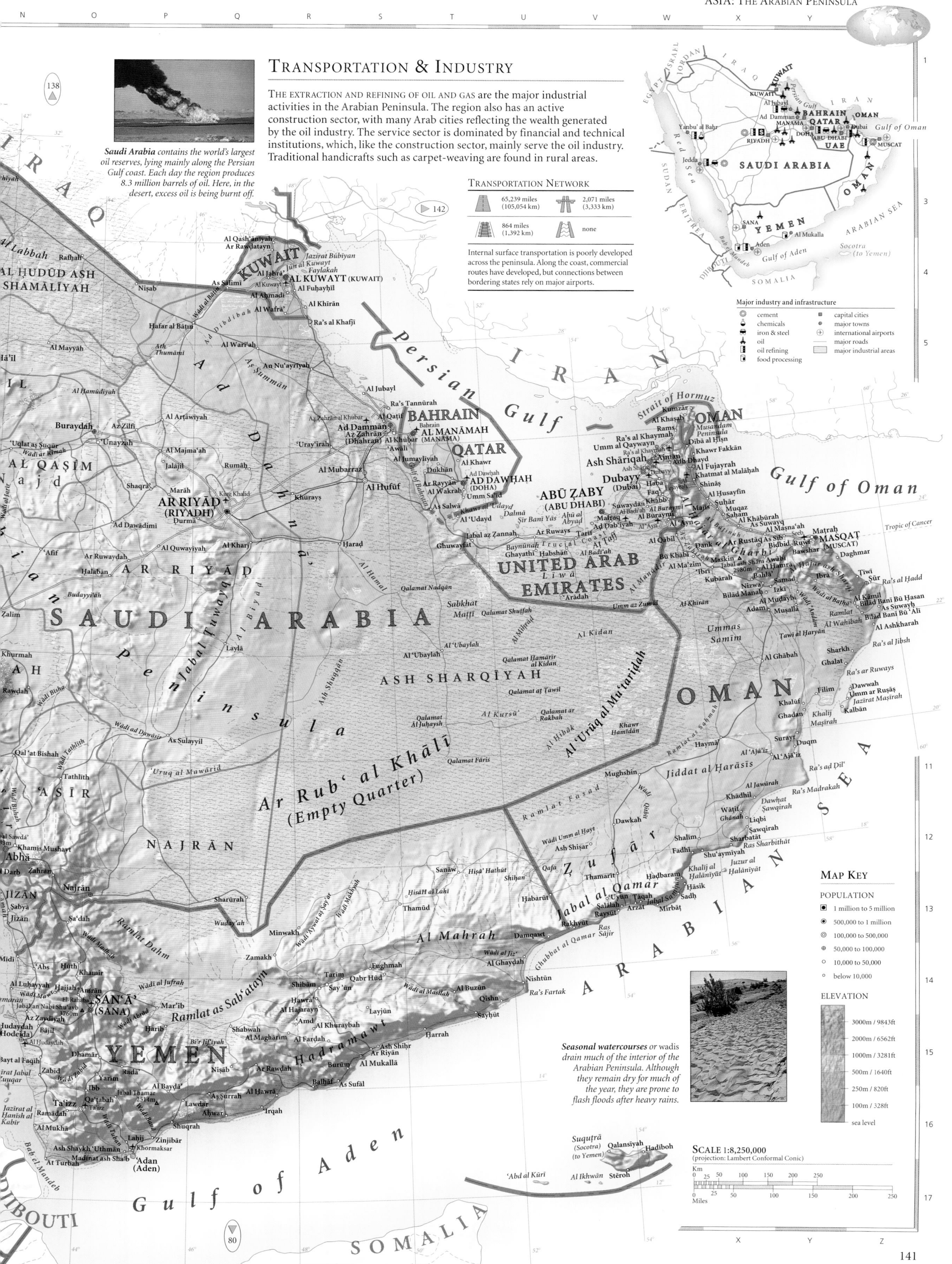

N O P Q R S T U V W X Y
138
142
80
IRAQ
KUWAIT
AL KUWAYT (KUWAIT)
BAHRAIN
AL MANĀMAH (MANAMA)
QATAR
AD DAWḤAH (DOHA)
AR RIYĀḌ (RIYADH)
SAUDI ARABIA
UNITED ARAB EMIRATES
ABŪ ẒABY (ABU DHABI)
Dubayy (Dubai)
OMAN
MASQAṬ (MUSCAT)
YEMEN
ṢAN'Ā' (SANA)
'Adan (Aden)
IRAN
Persian Gulf
Gulf of Oman
ARABIAN SEA
Gulf of Aden
SOMALIA
DJIBOUTI
Strait of Hormuz
Tropic of Cancer
Ar Rub' al Khālī (Empty Quarter)
Arabian Peninsula
ASH SHARQĪYAH
AR RIYĀḌ
NAJRĀN
'ASĪR
AL QAṢĪM
AL ḤUDŪD ASH SHAMĀLĪYAH
Ad Dahnā'
Jabal Ṭuwayq
Ramlat as Sab'atayn
Ḥaḍramawt
Al Mahrah
Ẓufār
Jiddat al Ḥarāsīs
Suquṭrā (Socotra) (to Yemen)
Transportation Network
65,239 miles (105,054 km)
2,071 miles (3,333 km)
864 miles (1,392 km)
none
Major industry and infrastructure
cement
chemicals
iron & steel
oil
oil refining
food processing
capital cities
major towns
international airports
major roads
major industrial areas
MAP KEY
POPULATION
1 million to 5 million
500,000 to 1 million
100,000 to 500,000
50,000 to 100,000
10,000 to 50,000
below 10,000
ELEVATION
3000m / 9843ft
2000m / 6562ft
1000m / 3281ft
500m / 1640ft
250m / 820ft
100m / 328ft
sea level
SCALE 1:8,250,000
(projection: Lambert Conformal Conic)

TRANSPORTATION & INDUSTRY

THE EXTRACTION AND REFINING OF OIL AND GAS are the major industrial activities in the Arabian Peninsula. The region also has an active construction sector, with many Arab cities reflecting the wealth generated by the oil industry. The service sector is dominated by financial and technical institutions, which, like the construction sector, mainly serve the oil industry. Traditional handicrafts such as carpet-weaving are found in rural areas.

***Saudi Arabia** contains the world's largest oil reserves, lying mainly along the Persian Gulf coast. Each day the region produces 8.3 million barrels of oil. Here, in the desert, excess oil is being burnt off.*

Internal surface transportation is poorly developed across the peninsula. Along the coast, commercial routes have developed, but connections between bordering states rely on major airports.

***Seasonal watercourses** or wadis drain much of the interior of the Arabian Peninsula. Although they remain dry for much of the year, they are prone to flash floods after heavy rains.*

IRAN & THE GULF STATES

BAHRAIN, IRAN, KUWAIT, QATAR, UNITED ARAB EMIRATES (UAE)

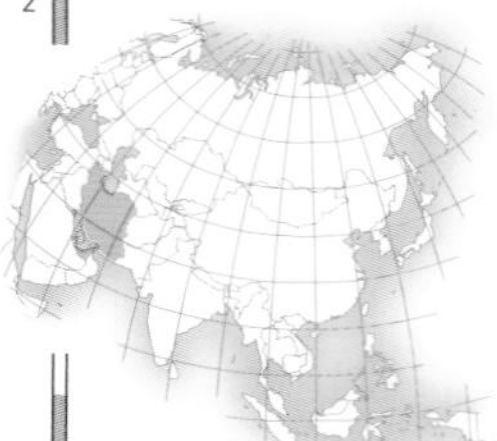

THE DISCOVERY OF OIL in the Persian Gulf in the 1930s brought great wealth to the surrounding states. The revenue was largely used to modernize industry and infrastructure, initiating great social change in these formerly agrarian countries. Today, over 80% of the people in the Gulf states live in urban areas, and foreign nationals make up a sizeable proportion of the population in Kuwait, Qatar ,and the United Arab Emirates. The importance of control of the oil reserves has led to a number of territorial disputes, including most recently the Iran–Iraq War and the Gulf War. Islam is practiced almost exclusively throughout the region and two distinct strands are found; Sunni Muslims in Qatar, Kuwait, and UAE, and Shi'a Muslims in Iran and Bahrain. In 1979 Iran became the world's largest theocracy.

THE LANDSCAPE

THE LAND RISES STEEPLY from the fragmented coastal lowlands bordering the Persian Gulf, to reach Iran's interior plateau, bounded by heavily-eroded mountain chains. An unstable plate boundary runs northwest to southeast across Iran causing frequent earthquakes. On the sandy west coast of the Persian Gulf, the relief is generally flat, with patches of salt marsh. Bahrain consists of two groups of islands, which are mostly small and rocky.

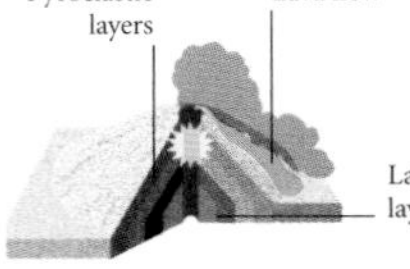

Pyroclastic layers

Lava flow

Lava flow layers

Qolleh-ye Damavand in the Elburz Mountains is a composite volcano. It comprises layers of lava and pyroclasts fragmentary rocks which accumulate on the slopes of the volcano after being ejected into the air.

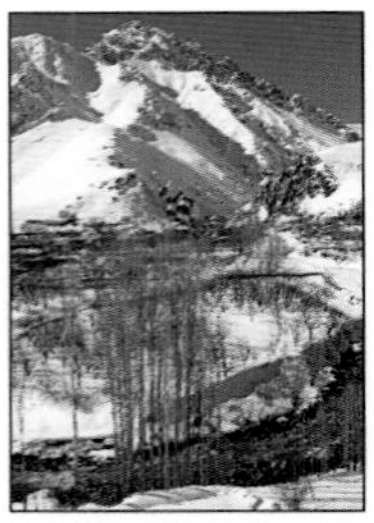

Marine sediments from deep beneath the ancient Tethys Sea have been uplifted to form the Elburz Mountains, which stretch along the shores of the Caspian Sea, northern Iran.

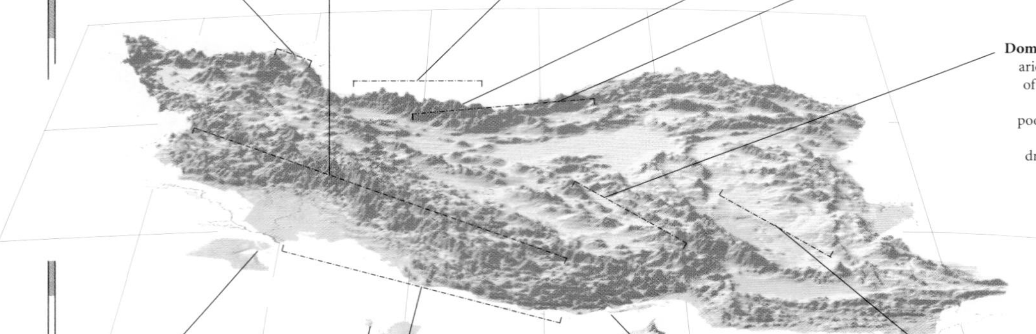

Lava and ash from previous volcanic activity covers a 200-mile (320-km) stretch from the border with Azerbaijan to the Caspian Sea.

Iran's two mountain chains, the Zagros and Elburz, were uplifted at the same time as the Alps in Europe, when the African Plate collided with the Eurasian Plate.

Caspian Sea

Qolleh-ye Damavand

Dominated by a vast, semi-arid interior plateau, most of Iran lies above 1,640 ft (500 m). The region is poorly drained with many of its basins remaining dry for months at a time.

The fierce Shamal wind affects much of this region. Every summer it blows dust south from the flood plains of the Tigris and Euphrates, reducing visibility to such an extent that Kuwait International Airport is frequently forced to close.

The oilfields of The Gulf are formed from marine shale deposits lying in sedimentary basins at the margins of the Zagros Mountains.

Autumn winds blowing across The Gulf can reach speeds of up to 95 mph (150 kmph) causing severe storms, squalls, and waterspouts.

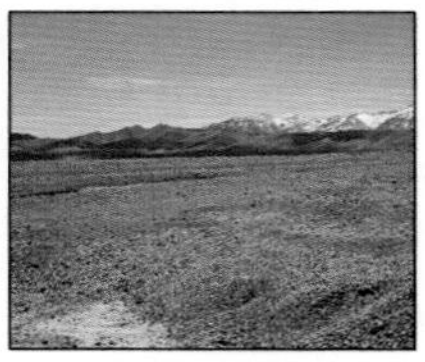

The Dasht-e Lut

Prolific springs tapping artesian water make cultivation possible across the north of Bahrain's main island. This provides a sharp contrast to the sandy plains in the south and west.

Numerous islands lie along the southern coast of the Persian Gulf. Some of these are salt domes, created when less dense salts were displaced and forced up to the surface by denser, overlying strata.

The Dasht-e Lut covers a large portion of eastern Iran with its dry, wind-eroded plain of scattered sandstone pillars and salty depressions. During the summer, temperatures soar, making it one of the world's hottest, driest places.

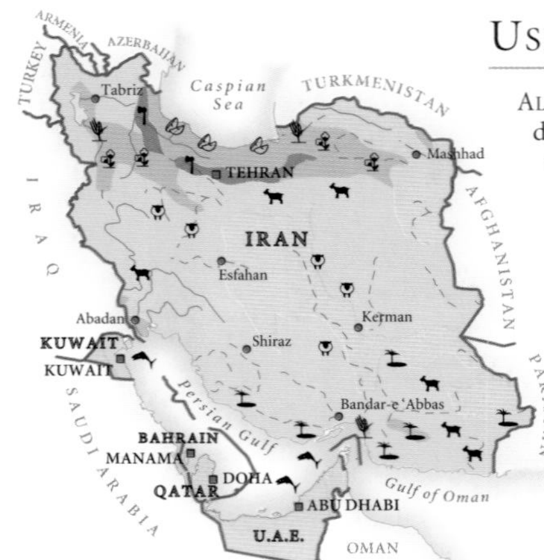

USING THE LAND AND SEA

ALONG THE COAST of the Caspian Sea, desalinated water allows fruits and vegetables to be produced, although water shortages and desert soils still limit farming. Sheep are the most important livestock raised in Iran and commercial forests cover the northwest of the country. Shrimp stocks were decimated by pollution during the Gulf War, but fishing remains important for domestic and export markets.

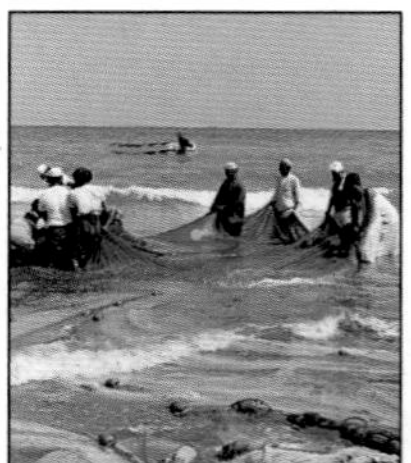

All of the Gulf states have commercial fishing fleets. Before the discovery of oil, fishing was the region's leading industry.

Land use and agricultural distribution

goats, sheep, cereals, citrus fruits, cotton, dates, fishing, timber

capital cities, major towns

pasture, cropland, forest, desert, wetland

THE URBAN/RURAL POPULATION DIVIDE

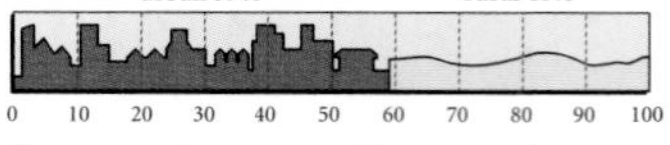

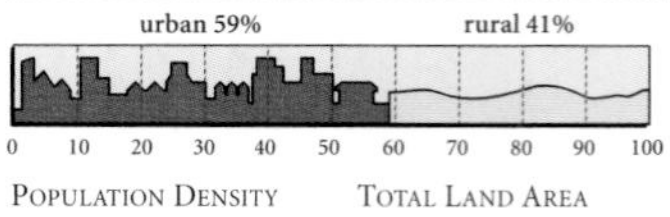

urban 59% — rural 41%

0 10 20 30 40 50 60 70 80 90 100

POPULATION DENSITY	TOTAL LAND AREA
118 people per sq mile (46 people per sq km)	642,883 sq miles (1,665,500 sq km)

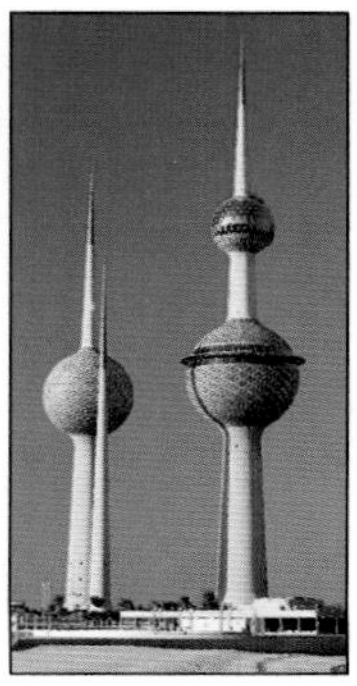

The Kuwait Towers in the centre of Kuwait are symbols of the vast wealth oil has brought to the country. Before 1960, the city had only one main street and was surrounded by a mud wall.

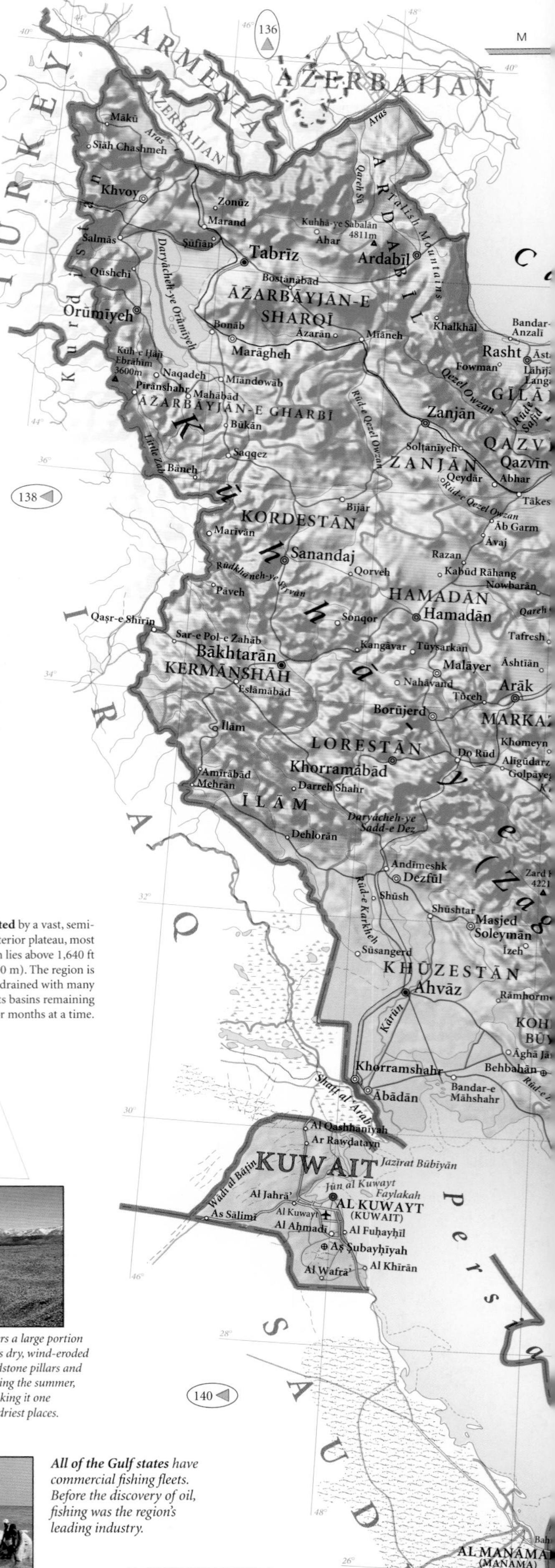

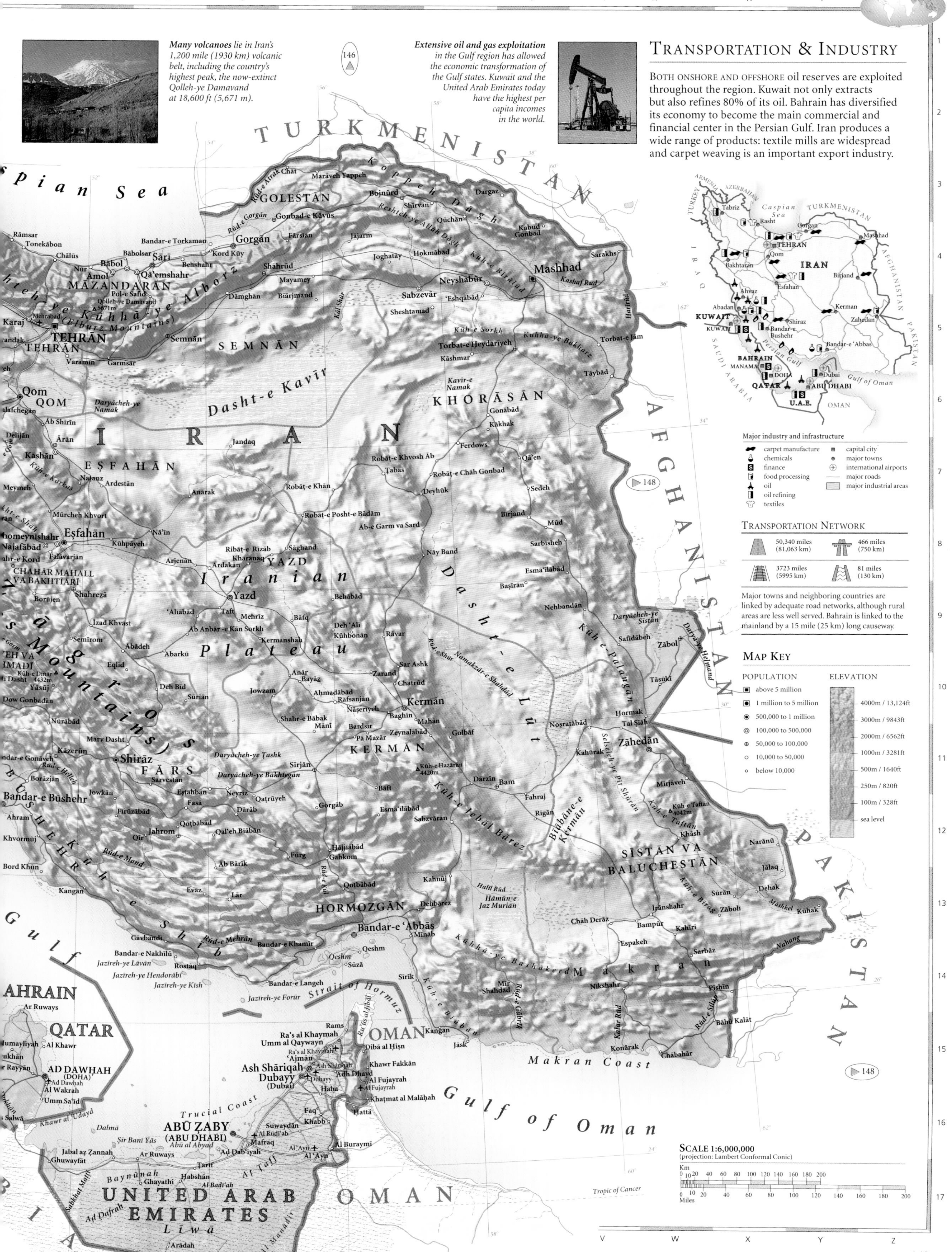
Many volcanoes lie in Iran's 1,200 mile (1930 km) volcanic belt, including the country's highest peak, the now-extinct Qolleh-ye Damavand at 18,600 ft (5,671 m).
Extensive oil and gas exploitation in the Gulf region has allowed the economic transformation of the Gulf states. Kuwait and the United Arab Emirates today have the highest per capita incomes in the world.
TRANSPORTATION & INDUSTRY
BOTH ONSHORE AND OFFSHORE oil reserves are exploited throughout the region. Kuwait not only extracts but also refines 80% of its oil. Bahrain has diversified its economy to become the main commercial and financial center in the Persian Gulf. Iran produces a wide range of products: textile mills are widespread and carpet weaving is an important export industry.
Major industry and infrastructure
carpet manufacture
chemicals
finance
food processing
oil
oil refining
textiles
capital city
major towns
international airports
major roads
major industrial areas
TRANSPORTATION NETWORK
50,340 miles (81,063 km)
466 miles (750 km)
3723 miles (5995 km)
81 miles (130 km)
Major towns and neighboring countries are linked by adequate road networks, although rural areas are less well served. Bahrain is linked to the mainland by a 15 mile (25 km) long causeway.
MAP KEY
POPULATION
above 5 million
1 million to 5 million
500,000 to 1 million
100,000 to 500,000
50,000 to 100,000
10,000 to 50,000
below 10,000
ELEVATION
4000m / 13,124ft
3000m / 9843ft
2000m / 6562ft
1000m / 3281ft
500m / 1640ft
250m / 820ft
100m / 328ft
sea level
SCALE 1:6,000,000
(projection: Lambert Conformal Conic)
TURKMENISTAN
Caspian Sea
IRAN
Iranian Plateau
Dasht-e Kavīr
Dasht-e Lūt
Zagros Mountains
Elburz Mountains
AFGHANISTAN
PAKISTAN
OMAN
QATAR
BAHRAIN
UNITED ARAB EMIRATES
Gulf of Oman
Strait of Hormuz
Makran Coast
Tehrān
Mashhad
Eşfahān
Shīrāz
Kermān
Zāhedān
Yazd
Bandar-e 'Abbās
Abū Zaby (Abu Dhabi)
Dubayy (Dubai)
Ad Dawhah (Doha)

A B C D E F G H I J K L M

KAZAKHSTAN

ABUNDANT NATURAL RESOURCES lie in the immense steppe grasslands, deserts, and central plateau of the former Soviet republic of Kazakhstan. An intensive program of industrial and agricultural development to exploit these resources during the Soviet era resulted in catastrophic industrial pollution, including fallout from nuclear testing and the shrinkage of the Aral Sea. Since independence, the government has encouraged foreign investment and liberalized the economy to promote growth. The adoption of Kazakh as the national language is intended to encourage a new sense of national identity in a state where living conditions for the majority remain harsh, both in cramped urban centers and impoverished rural areas.

USING THE LAND AND SEA

THE REARING OF LARGE HERDS of sheep and goats on the steppe grasslands forms the core of Kazakh agriculture. Arable cultivation and cotton-growing in pasture and desert areas was encouraged during the Soviet era, but relative yields are low. The heavy use of fertilizers and the diversion of natural water sources for irrigation has degraded much of the land.

THE URBAN/RURAL POPULATION DIVIDE

urban 60% | rural 40%

0 10 20 30 40 50 60 70 80 90 100

POPULATION DENSITY	TOTAL LAND AREA
16 people per sq mile (6 people per sq km)	1,048,878 sq miles (2,717,300 sq km)

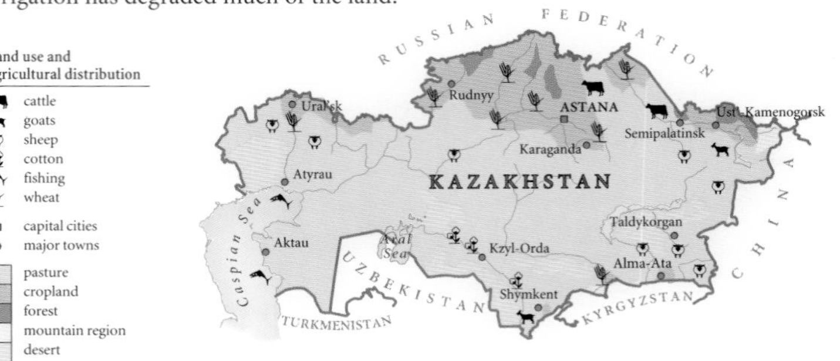

Land use and agricultural distribution
cattle
goats
sheep
cotton
fishing
wheat
capital cities
major towns
pasture
cropland
forest
mountain region
desert
RUSSIAN FEDERATION
KAZAKHSTAN
ASTANA
Rudnyy
Ural'sk
Ust'-Kamenogorsk
Semipalatinsk
Karaganda
Atyrau
Aktau
Aral Sea
Kzyl-Orda
Taldykorgan
Alma-Ata
Shymkent
Caspian Sea
UZBEKISTAN
TURKMENISTAN
KYRGYZSTAN
CHINA

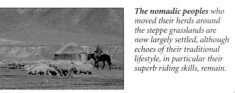

The nomadic peoples who moved their herds around the steppe grasslands are now largely settled, although echoes of their traditional lifestyle, in particular their superb riding skills, remain.

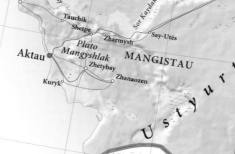

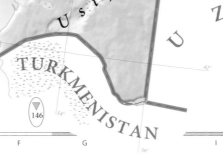

TRANSPORTATION & INDUSTRY

THE SINGLE MOST IMPORTANT INDUSTRY in Kazakhstan is mining, based around extensive oil deposits near the Caspian Sea, the world's largest chromium mine, and vast reserves of iron ore. Recent foreign investment has helped to develop industries including food processing and steel manufacture, and to expand the exploitation of mineral resources. The Russian space program is still based at Baykonur, near Zhezkazgan in central Kazakhstan.

Major industry and infrastructure

- chemicals
- engineering
- fish processing
- food processing
- iron & steel
- metallurgy
- mining
- oil
- capital cities
- major towns
- international airports
- major roads
- major industrial areas

TRANSPORTATION NETWORK

- 87,561 miles (141,000 km)
- none
- 8,483 miles (13,660 km)
- none

Industrial areas in the north and east are well-connected to Russia. Air and rail links with Germany and China have been established through foreign investment. Better access to Baltic ports is being sought.

An open-cast coal mine in Kazakhstan. Foreign investment is being actively sought by the Kazakh government in order to fully exploit the potential of the country's rich mineral reserves.

MAP KEY

POPULATION	ELEVATION
1 million to 5 million	4000m / 13,124ft
500,000 to 1 million	3000m / 9843ft
100,000 to 500,000	2000m / 6562ft
50,000 to 100,000	1000m / 3281ft
10,000 to 50,000	500m / 1640ft
below 10,000	250m / 820ft
	100m / 328ft
	sea level

SCALE 1:7,000,000 (projection: Lambert Conformal Conic)

Km 0 25 50 100 150 200 250

Miles 0 25 50 100 150 200 250

122 146

A B C D E F G H I J K L M

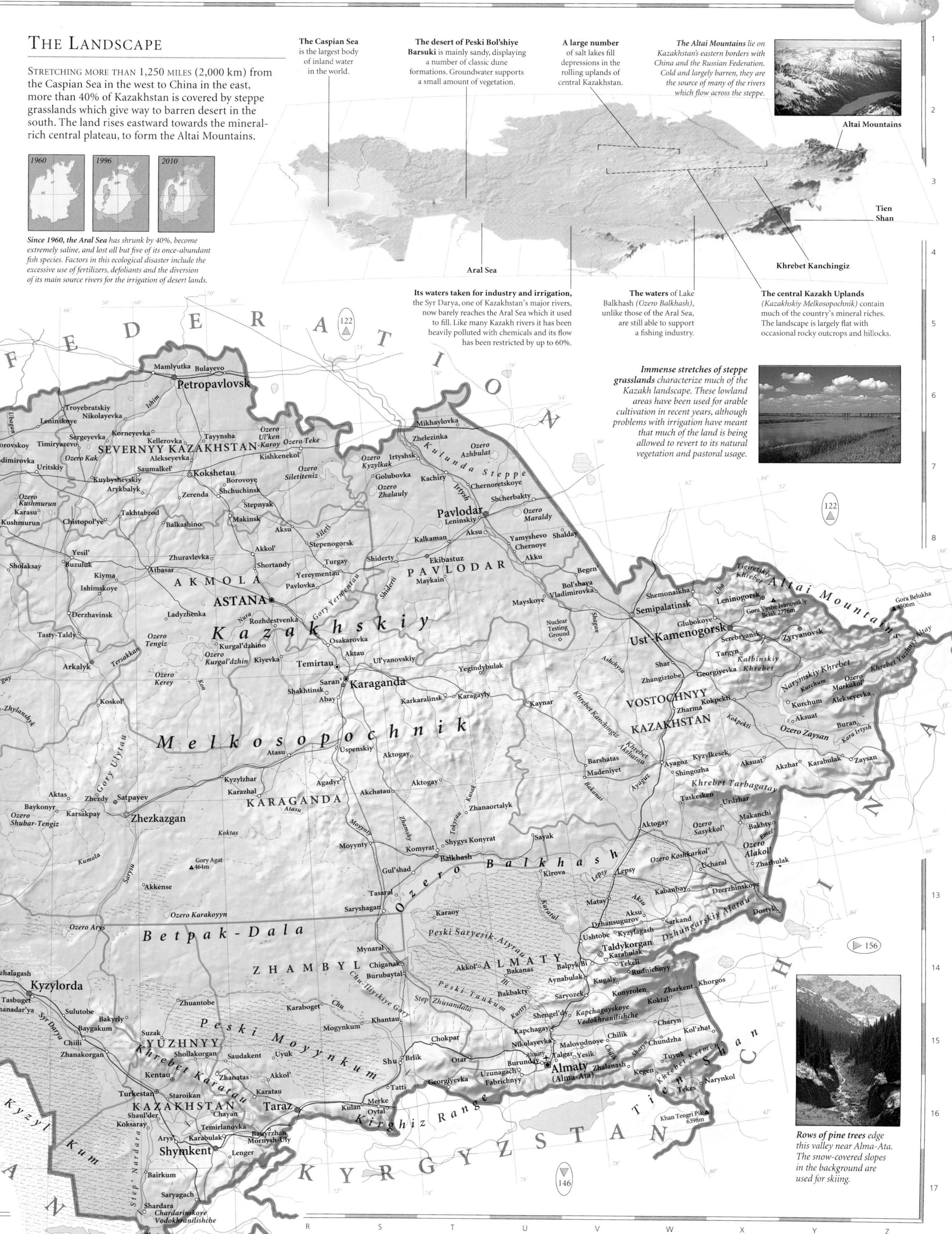
N O P Q R S T U V W X Y
1 2 3 4 5 6 7 8 13 14 15 16 17
1960
1996
2010
The Caspian Sea is the largest body of inland water in the world.
The desert of Peski Bol'shiye Barsuki is mainly sandy, displaying a number of classic dune formations. Groundwater supports a small amount of vegetation.
A large number of salt lakes fill depressions in the rolling uplands of central Kazakhstan.
The Altai Mountains lie on Kazakhstan's eastern borders with China and the Russian Federation. Cold and largely barren, they are the source of many of the rivers which flow across the steppe.
Altai Mountains
Tien Shan
Khrebet Kanchingiz
Aral Sea
Its waters taken for industry and irrigation, the Syr Darya, one of Kazakhstan's major rivers, now barely reaches the Aral Sea which it used to fill. Like many Kazakh rivers it has been heavily polluted with chemicals and its flow has been restricted by up to 60%.
The waters of Lake Balkhash (Ozero Balkhash), unlike those of the Aral Sea, are still able to support a fishing industry.
The central Kazakh Uplands (Kazakhskiy Melkosopochnik) contain much of the country's mineral riches. The landscape is largely flat with occasional rocky outcrops and hillocks.
Immense stretches of steppe grasslands characterize much of the Kazakh landscape. These lowland areas have been used for arable cultivation in recent years, although problems with irrigation have meant that much of the land is being allowed to revert to its natural vegetation and pastoral usage.
FEDERATION
122
Petropavlovsk
SEVERNYY KAZAKHSTAN
Kokshetau
Pavlodar
PAVLODAR
Kulunda Steppe
AKMOLA
ASTANA
Kazakhskiy
Melkosopochnik
Semipalatinsk
Ust'-Kamenogorsk
VOSTOCHNYY KAZAKHSTAN
Altai Mountains
Gora Belukha 4506m
Karaganda
Temirtau
KARAGANDA
Zhezkazgan
Ozero Balkhash
Balkhash
Betpak-Dala
ZHAMBYL
ALMATY
Taldykorgan
Kyzylorda
YUZHNYY KAZAKHSTAN
Peski Moyynkum
Taraz
Shymkent
Almaty (Alma-Ata)
Khan Tengri Pik 6398m
Tien Shan
Kirghiz Range
KYRGYZSTAN
CHINA
156
146
R S T U V W X Y Z

The Landscape

Stretching more than 1,250 miles (2,000 km) from the Caspian Sea in the west to China in the east, more than 40% of Kazakhstan is covered by steppe grasslands which give way to barren desert in the south. The land rises eastward towards the mineral-rich central plateau, to form the Altai Mountains.

Since 1960, the Aral Sea has shrunk by 40%, become extremely saline, and lost all but five of its once-abundant fish species. Factors in this ecological disaster include the excessive use of fertilizers, defoliants and the diversion of its main source rivers for the irrigation of desert lands.

Rows of pine trees edge this valley near Alma-Ata. The snow-covered slopes in the background are used for skiing.

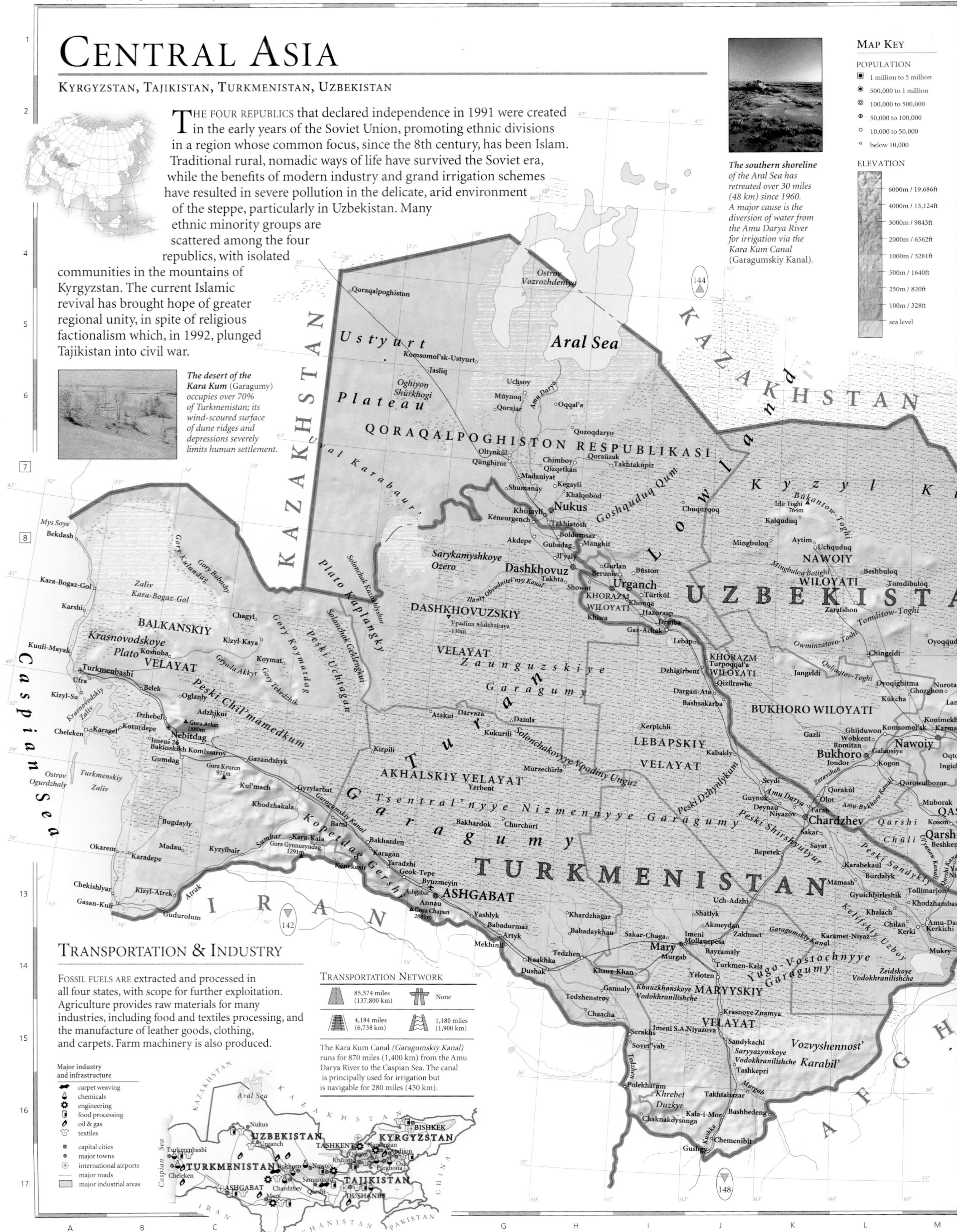

Map Key
Population
1 million to 5 million
500,000 to 1 million
100,000 to 500,000
50,000 to 100,000
10,000 to 50,000
below 10,000
Elevation
6000m / 19,686ft
4000m / 13,124ft
3000m / 9843ft
2000m / 6562ft
1000m / 3281ft
500m / 1640ft
250m / 820ft
100m / 328ft
sea level
KAZAKHSTAN
UZBEKISTAN
TURKMENISTAN
IRAN
AFGH.
Aral Sea
Caspian Sea
Ustyurt Plateau
QORAQALPOGHISTON RESPUBLIKASI
Turan Lowland
Garagumy
Kyzyl Kum
DASHKHOVUZSKIY VELAYAT
BALKANSKIY VELAYAT
AKHALSKIY VELAYAT
LEBAPSKIY VELAYAT
MARYYSKIY VELAYAT
KHORAZM WILOYATI
BUKHORO WILOYATI
NAWOIY WILOYATI
Nukus
Urganch
Dashkhovuz
Turkmenbashi
Nebitdag
ASHGABAT
Mary
Chardzhev
Bukhoro
Nawoiy
Qarshi
Transportation Network
85,574 miles (137,800 km)
None
4,184 miles (6,738 km)
1,180 miles (1,900 km)
Major industry and infrastructure
carpet weaving
chemicals
engineering
food processing
oil & gas
textiles
capital cities
major towns
international airports
major roads
major industrial areas
UZBEKISTAN
KYRGYZSTAN
TURKMENISTAN
TAJIKISTAN
BISHKEK
TASHKENT
DUSHANBE
ASHGABAT
CHINA
AFGHANISTAN
PAKISTAN

Central Asia

Kyrgyzstan, Tajikistan, Turkmenistan, Uzbekistan

The four republics that declared independence in 1991 were created in the early years of the Soviet Union, promoting ethnic divisions in a region whose common focus, since the 8th century, has been Islam. Traditional rural, nomadic ways of life have survived the Soviet era, while the benefits of modern industry and grand irrigation schemes have resulted in severe pollution in the delicate, arid environment of the steppe, particularly in Uzbekistan. Many ethnic minority groups are scattered among the four republics, with isolated communities in the mountains of Kyrgyzstan. The current Islamic revival has brought hope of greater regional unity, in spite of religious factionalism which, in 1992, plunged Tajikistan into civil war.

***The desert of the Kara Kum** (Garagumy) occupies over 70% of Turkmenistan; its wind-scoured surface of dune ridges and depressions severely limits human settlement.*

***The southern shoreline** of the Aral Sea has retreated over 30 miles (48 km) since 1960. A major cause is the diversion of water from the Amu Darya River for irrigation via the Kara Kum Canal* (Garagumskiy Kanal).

Transportation & Industry

Fossil fuels are extracted and processed in all four states, with scope for further exploitation. Agriculture provides raw materials for many industries, including food and textiles processing, and the manufacture of leather goods, clothing, and carpets. Farm machinery is also produced.

Transportation Network

The Kara Kum Canal *(Garagumskiy Kanal)* runs for 870 miles (1,400 km) from the Amu Darya River to the Caspian Sea. The canal is principally used for irrigation but is navigable for 280 miles (450 km).

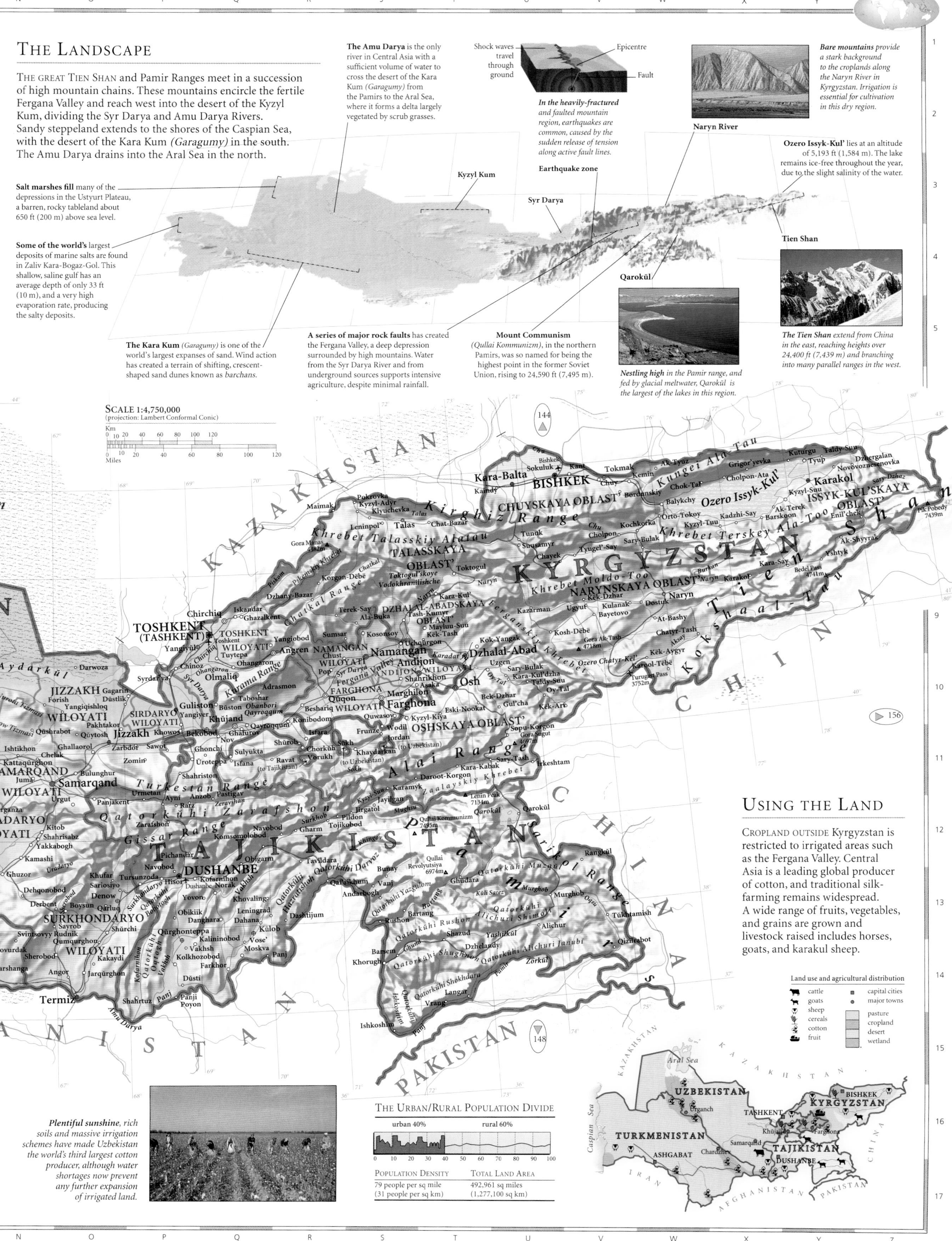
N O P Q R S T U V W X Y
THE LANDSCAPE
Shock waves travel through ground
Epicentre
Fault
Naryn River
Kyzyl Kum
Earthquake zone
Syr Darya
Tien Shan
Qarokŭl
SCALE 1:4,750,000
(projection: Lambert Conformal Conic)
KAZAKHSTAN
KYRGYZSTAN
TAJIKISTAN
CHINA
PAKISTAN
BISHKEK
TOSHKENT (TASHKENT)
DUSHANBE
Ozero Issyk-Kul'
Samarqand
Namangan
Andijon
Osh
Farghona
Khŭjand
Alai Range
Pamirs
Tien Shan
144
156
148
Land use and agricultural distribution
cattle
goats
sheep
cereals
cotton
fruit
capital cities
major towns
pasture
cropland
desert
wetland
UZBEKISTAN
TURKMENISTAN
ASHGABAT
IRAN
AFGHANISTAN
Aral Sea
Caspian Sea

THE LANDSCAPE

THE GREAT TIEN SHAN and Pamir Ranges meet in a succession of high mountain chains. These mountains encircle the fertile Fergana Valley and reach west into the desert of the Kyzyl Kum, dividing the Syr Darya and Amu Darya Rivers. Sandy steppeland extends to the shores of the Caspian Sea, with the desert of the Kara Kum *(Garagumy)* in the south. The Amu Darya drains into the Aral Sea in the north.

The Amu Darya is the only river in Central Asia with a sufficient volume of water to cross the desert of the Kara Kum *(Garagumy)* from the Pamirs to the Aral Sea, where it forms a delta largely vegetated by scrub grasses.

In the heavily-fractured *and faulted mountain region, earthquakes are common, caused by the sudden release of tension along active fault lines.*

Bare mountains *provide a stark background to the croplands along the Naryn River in Kyrgyzstan. Irrigation is essential for cultivation in this dry region.*

Ozero Issyk-Kul' lies at an altitude of 5,193 ft (1,584 m). The lake remains ice-free throughout the year, due to the slight salinity of the water.

Salt marshes fill many of the depressions in the Ustyurt Plateau, a barren, rocky tableland about 650 ft (200 m) above sea level.

Some of the world's largest deposits of marine salts are found in Zaliv Kara-Bogaz-Gol. This shallow, saline gulf has an average depth of only 33 ft (10 m), and a very high evaporation rate, producing the salty deposits.

The Kara Kum *(Garagumy)* is one of the world's largest expanses of sand. Wind action has created a terrain of shifting, crescent-shaped sand dunes known as *barchans*.

A series of major rock faults has created the Fergana Valley, a deep depression surrounded by high mountains. Water from the Syr Darya River and from underground sources supports intensive agriculture, despite minimal rainfall.

Mount Communism *(Qullai Kommunizm)*, in the northern Pamirs, was so named for being the highest point in the former Soviet Union, rising to 24,590 ft (7,495 m).

Nestling high *in the Pamir range, and fed by glacial meltwater, Qarokŭl is the largest of the lakes in this region.*

The Tien Shan *extend from China in the east, reaching heights over 24,400 ft (7,439 m) and branching into many parallel ranges in the west.*

USING THE LAND

CROPLAND OUTSIDE Kyrgyzstan is restricted to irrigated areas such as the Fergana Valley. Central Asia is a leading global producer of cotton, and traditional silk-farming remains widespread. A wide range of fruits, vegetables, and grains are grown and livestock raised includes horses, goats, and karakul sheep.

Plentiful sunshine, *rich soils and massive irrigation schemes have made Uzbekistan the world's third largest cotton producer, although water shortages now prevent any further expansion of irrigated land.*

THE URBAN/RURAL POPULATION DIVIDE

urban 40% — rural 60%

POPULATION DENSITY	TOTAL LAND AREA
79 people per sq mile (31 people per sq km)	492,961 sq miles (1,277,100 sq km)

AFGHANISTAN & PAKISTAN

PAKISTAN WAS CREATED by the partition of British India in 1947, becoming the western arm of a new Islamic state for Indian Muslims; the eastern sector, in Bengal, seceded to become the separate country of Bangladesh in 1971. Over half of Pakistan's 147 million people live in the Punjab, at the fertile head of the great Indus Basin. The river sustains a national economy based on irrigated agriculture, including cotton for the vital textiles industry. Afghanistan, a mountainous, landlocked country, with an ancient and independent culture, has been wracked by war since 1979, when calls for help from a beleaguered government led to a Soviet invasion. Despite the Soviet withdrawal, factional strife continues and five million Afghan refugees remain over the border in Pakistan.

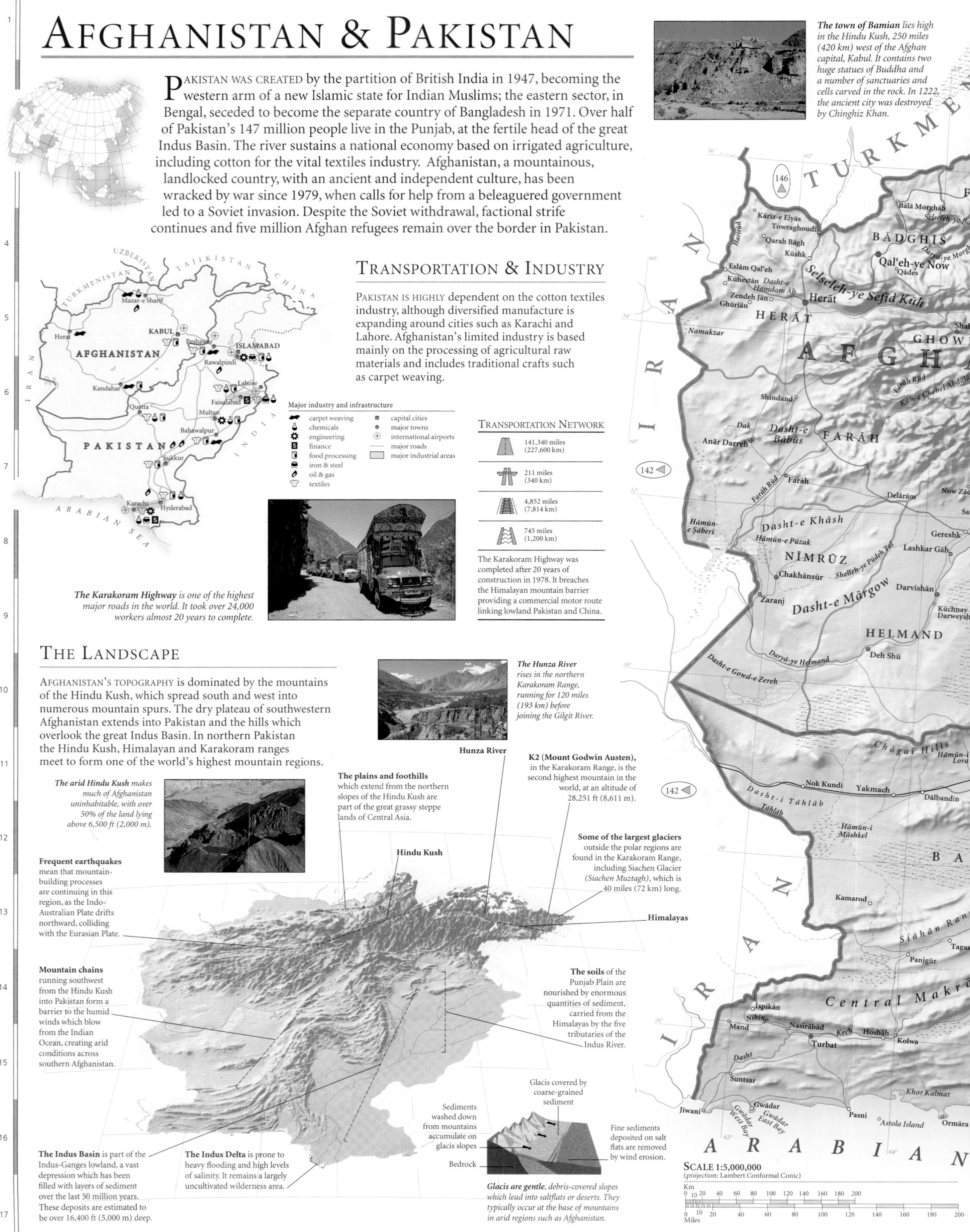

A B C D E F G H I J K L M
1 4 5 6 7 8 9 10 11 12 13 14 15 16 17
UZBEKISTAN
TAJIKISTAN
TURKMENISTAN
CHINA
IRAN
INDIA
ARABIAN SEA
AFGHANISTAN
PAKISTAN
Mazar-e Sharif
KABUL
Herat
Peshawar
ISLAMABAD
Rawalpindi
Kandahar
Lahore
Faisalabad
Quetta
Multan
Bahawalpur
Sukkur
Karachi
Hyderabad
Major industry and infrastructure
carpet weaving
chemicals
engineering
finance
food processing
iron & steel
oil & gas
textiles
capital cities
major towns
international airports
major roads
major industrial areas
Hunza River
Hindu Kush
Himalayas
Glacis covered by coarse-grained sediment
Sediments washed down from mountains accumulate on glacis slopes
Bedrock
Fine sediments deposited on salt flats are removed by wind erosion.
146
142
TURKMEN
Bālā Morghāb
Kārīz-e Elyās
Towraghoudī
Qarah Bāgh
Kūshk
BĀDGHĪS
Qal'eh-ye Now
Qādes
Eslām Qal'eh
Kūhestān
Dasht-e Hamdam Āb
Zendeh Jān
Ghūriān
Herāt
Selseleh-ye Sefīd Kūh
HERĀT
Namakzar
Shahrak
GHOWR
AFGHA
Farah Rūd
Kūh-e Chehel Abdālān
Shīndand
Dak
Anār Darreh
Dasht-e Bābūs
FARĀH
Farāh
Delārām
Now Zād
Sangin
Hāmūn-e Şāberī
Dasht-e Khāsh
Hāmūn-e Pūzak
NĪMRŪZ
Gereshk
Lashkar Gāh
Chakhānsūr
Shelleh-ye Pūdeh Tal
Zaranj
Dasht-e Mārgow
Darvīshān
Kūchnay Darweyshān
HELMAND
Daryā-ye Helmand
Deh Shū
Dasht-e Gowd-e Zereh
IRAN
Chāgai Hills
Hāmūn-i Lora
Nok Kundi
Yakmach
Dālbandin
Dasht-i Tāhlāb
Tāhlāb
Hāmūn-i Māshkel
BAL
Kamarod
Siāhān Range
Tagas
Panjgūr
Ispikān
Nihing
Central Makrān
Mand
Nasīrābād
Kech
Hoshāb
Turbat
Kolwa
Dasht
Suntsar
Khor Kalmat
Jiwani
Gwādar
Gwadar West Bay
Gwādar East Bay
Pasni
Astola Island
Ormāra
ARABIAN
SCALE 1:5,000,000
(projection: Lambert Conformal Conic)
Km
0 10 20 40 60 80 100 120 140 160 180 200
0 10 20 40 60 80 100 120 140 160 180 200
Miles

The town of Bamian lies high in the Hindu Kush, 250 miles (420 km) west of the Afghan capital, Kabul. It contains two huge statues of Buddha and a number of sanctuaries and cells carved in the rock. In 1222, the ancient city was destroyed by Chinghiz Khan.

TRANSPORTATION & INDUSTRY

PAKISTAN IS HIGHLY dependent on the cotton textiles industry, although diversified manufacture is expanding around cities such as Karachi and Lahore. Afghanistan's limited industry is based mainly on the processing of agricultural raw materials and includes traditional crafts such as carpet weaving.

TRANSPORTATION NETWORK

141,340 miles (227,600 km)

211 miles (340 km)

4,852 miles (7,814 km)

745 miles (1,200 km)

The Karakoram Highway was completed after 20 years of construction in 1978. It breaches the Himalayan mountain barrier providing a commercial motor route linking lowland Pakistan and China.

The Karakoram Highway is one of the highest major roads in the world. It took over 24,000 workers almost 20 years to complete.

THE LANDSCAPE

AFGHANISTAN'S TOPOGRAPHY is dominated by the mountains of the Hindu Kush, which spread south and west into numerous mountain spurs. The dry plateau of southwestern Afghanistan extends into Pakistan and the hills which overlook the great Indus Basin. In northern Pakistan the Hindu Kush, Himalayan and Karakoram ranges meet to form one of the world's highest mountain regions.

The Hunza River rises in the northern Karakoram Range, running for 120 miles (193 km) before joining the Gilgit River.

The arid Hindu Kush makes much of Afghanistan uninhabitable, with over 50% of the land lying above 6,500 ft (2,000 m).

The plains and foothills which extend from the northern slopes of the Hindu Kush are part of the great grassy steppe lands of Central Asia.

K2 (Mount Godwin Austen), in the Karakoram Range, is the second highest mountain in the world, at an altitude of 28,251 ft (8,611 m).

Some of the largest glaciers outside the polar regions are found in the Karakoram Range, including Siachen Glacier *(Siachen Muztagh)*, which is 40 miles (72 km) long.

Frequent earthquakes mean that mountain-building processes are continuing in this region, as the Indo-Australian Plate drifts northward, colliding with the Eurasian Plate.

Mountain chains running southwest from the Hindu Kush into Pakistan form a barrier to the humid winds which blow from the Indian Ocean, creating arid conditions across southern Afghanistan.

The soils of the Punjab Plain are nourished by enormous quantities of sediment, carried from the Himalayas by the five tributaries of the Indus River.

The Indus Basin is part of the Indus-Ganges lowland, a vast depression which has been filled with layers of sediment over the last 50 million years. These deposits are estimated to be over 16,400 ft (5,000 m) deep.

The Indus Delta is prone to heavy flooding and high levels of salinity. It remains a largely uncultivated wilderness area.

***Glacis are gentle,** debris-covered slopes which lead into saltflats or deserts. They typically occur at the base of mountains in arid regions such as Afghanistan.*

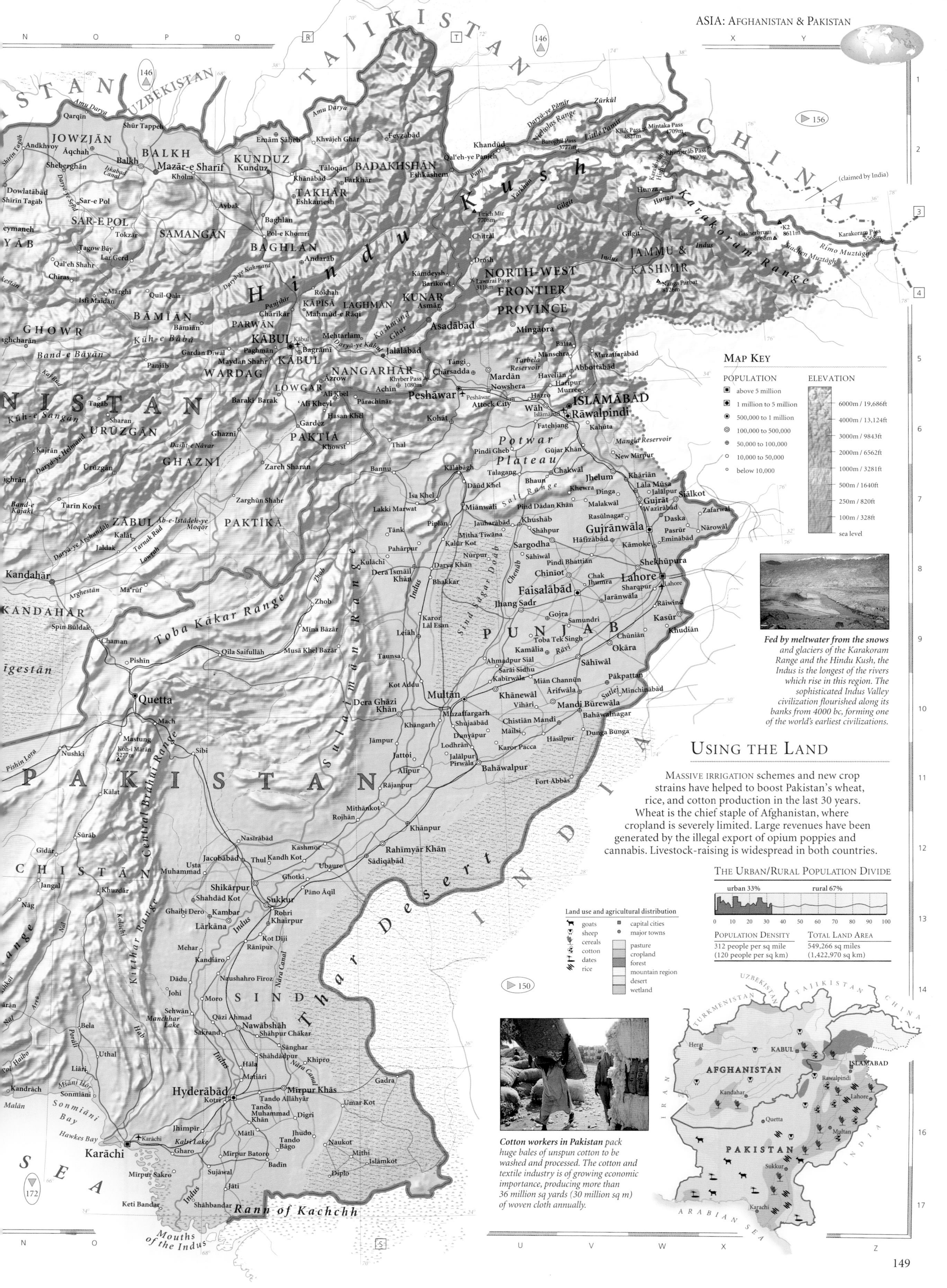

TAJIKISTAN
UZBEKISTAN
CHINA
INDIA
PAKISTAN
Hindu Kush
Karakoram Range
Thar Desert
ARABIAN SEA
NORTH-WEST FRONTIER PROVINCE
JAMMU & KASHMIR
PUNJAB
SIND
Kābul
Islāmābād
Rāwalpindi
Peshāwar
Lahore
Faisalābād
Multān
Quetta
Hyderābād
Karāchi
Kandahār
Mazār-e Sharīf
Indus
(claimed by India)
Map Key
POPULATION
above 5 million
1 million to 5 million
500,000 to 1 million
100,000 to 500,000
50,000 to 100,000
10,000 to 50,000
below 10,000
ELEVATION
6000m / 19,686ft
4000m / 13,124ft
3000m / 9843ft
2000m / 6562ft
1000m / 3281ft
500m / 1640ft
250m / 820ft
100m / 328ft
sea level
Land use and agricultural distribution
goats
sheep
cereals
cotton
dates
rice
capital cities
major towns
pasture
cropland
forest
mountain region
desert
wetland
AFGHANISTAN
KABUL
ISLAMABAD

Fed by meltwater from the snows and glaciers of the Karakoram Range and the Hindu Kush, the Indus is the longest of the rivers which rise in this region. The sophisticated Indus Valley civilization flourished along its banks from 4000 bc, forming one of the world's earliest civilizations.

Using the Land

Massive irrigation schemes and new crop strains have helped to boost Pakistan's wheat, rice, and cotton production in the last 30 years. Wheat is the chief staple of Afghanistan, where cropland is severely limited. Large revenues have been generated by the illegal export of opium poppies and cannabis. Livestock-raising is widespread in both countries.

The Urban/Rural Population Divide

urban 33% | rural 67%

0 10 20 30 40 50 60 70 80 90 100

Population Density	Total Land Area
312 people per sq mile (120 people per sq km)	549,266 sq miles (1,422,970 sq km)

Cotton workers in Pakistan pack huge bales of unspun cotton to be washed and processed. The cotton and textile industry is of growing economic importance, producing more than 36 million sq yards (30 million sq m) of woven cloth annually.

156 150 146 172

SOUTH ASIA

BANGLADESH, BHUTAN, INDIA, MALDIVES, NEPAL, PAKISTAN, SRI LANKA

MORE THAN ONE-FIFTH of the world's population lives in the south Asian subcontinent. Great cultural diversity has come from a long succession of foreign invaders, including Hindu Aryans, Islamic Moguls, and the British, whose empire incorporated the princely states of the Maharajas and extended to the borders of Nepal and Bhutan in the Himalayas. Half a century after independence, India is the world's largest democracy, and at the current rate of growth, may overtake China as the world's most populous country within the next century. There are points of tension in the region over claims for independence by the Sikhs in the Indian Punjab and the Tamil separatists in Sri Lanka, and the long-standing dispute with Pakistan over Jammu and Kashmir in the north.

THE LANDSCAPE

SOUTH ASIA is effectively isolated from the rest of Asia by desert along the western flank of Pakistan, and a continuous wall of mountains, dominated by the Himalayas, to the north and east. The great basins of the Indus and Ganges separate this mountain fringe from the rolling plateau of the Indian peninsula, which is bordered by a line of coastal hills, the Eastern and Western Ghats.

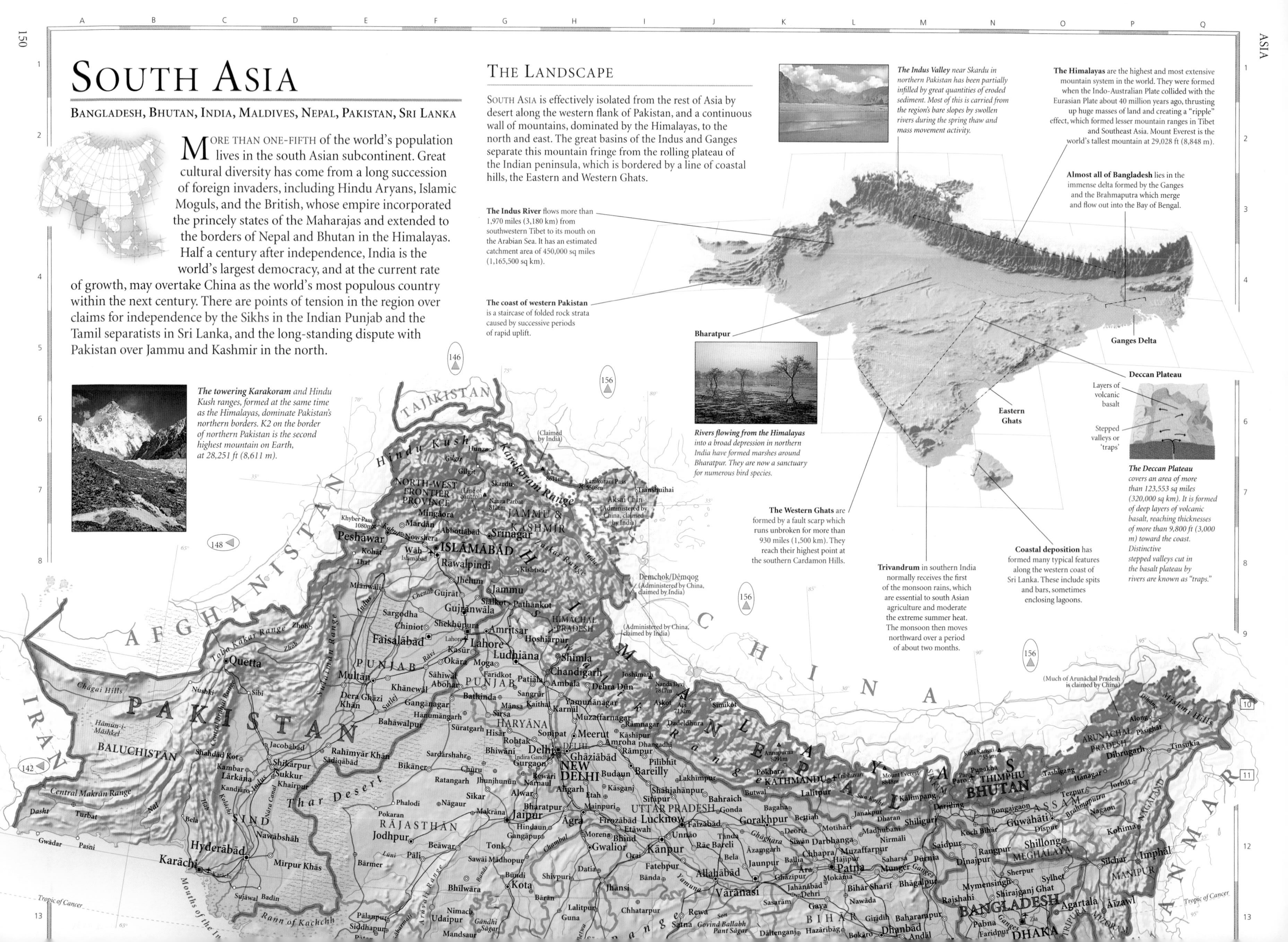
Bharatpur
Ganges Delta
Deccan Plateau
Layers of volcanic basalt
Stepped valleys or 'traps'
Eastern Ghats
AFGHANISTAN
PAKISTAN
IRAN
TAJIKISTAN
CHINA
NEPAL
BHUTAN
BANGLADESH
BALUCHISTAN
PUNJAB
SIND
RĀJASTHĀN
UTTAR PRADESH
HARYĀNA
HIMACHAL PRADESH
JAMMU & KASHMIR
NORTH-WEST FRONTIER PROVINCE
ASSAM
MEGHALAYA
MANIPUR
ARUNĀCHAL PRADESH
BIHĀR
NEW DELHI
ISLĀMĀBĀD
KATHMANDU
THIMPHU
DHAKA
Karāchi
Hyderābād
Quetta
Peshāwar
Lahore
Multān
Faisalābād
Rawalpindi
Srinagar
Ludhiāna
Amritsar
Jaipur
Agra
Lucknow
Kānpur
Allahābād
Vārānasi
Patna
Gwalior
Jodhpur
Karakoram Range
Hindu Kush
Thar Desert
Central Makrān Range
Rann of Kachchh
Mouths of the Indus
Tropic of Cancer
(Claimed by India)
(Administered by China, claimed by India)
Demchok/Dêmqog (Administered by China, claimed by India)
Aksai Chin (Administered by China, claimed by India)
(Much of Arunāchal Pradesh is claimed by China)

The towering Karakoram and Hindu Kush ranges, formed at the same time as the Himalayas, dominate Pakistan's northern borders. K2 on the border of northern Pakistan is the second highest mountain on Earth, at 28,251 ft (8,611 m).

The Indus River flows more than 1,970 miles (3,180 km) from southwestern Tibet to its mouth on the Arabian Sea. It has an estimated catchment area of 450,000 sq miles (1,165,500 sq km).

The coast of western Pakistan is a staircase of folded rock strata caused by successive periods of rapid uplift.

***The Indus Valley** near Skardu in northern Pakistan has been partially infilled by great quantities of eroded sediment. Most of this is carried from the region's bare slopes by swollen rivers during the spring thaw and mass movement activity.*

The Himalayas are the highest and most extensive mountain system in the world. They were formed when the Indo-Australian Plate collided with the Eurasian Plate about 40 million years ago, thrusting up huge masses of land and creating a "ripple" effect, which formed lesser mountain ranges in Tibet and Southeast Asia. Mount Everest is the world's tallest mountain at 29,028 ft (8,848 m).

Almost all of Bangladesh lies in the immense delta formed by the Ganges and the Brahmaputra which merge and flow out into the Bay of Bengal.

***Rivers flowing from the Himalayas** into a broad depression in northern India have formed marshes around Bharatpur. They are now a sanctuary for numerous bird species.*

The Western Ghats are formed by a fault scarp which runs unbroken for more than 930 miles (1,500 km). They reach their highest point at the southern Cardamon Hills.

Trivandrum in southern India normally receives the first of the monsoon rains, which are essential to south Asian agriculture and moderate the extreme summer heat. The monsoon then moves northward over a period of about two months.

Coastal deposition has formed many typical features along the western coast of Sri Lanka. These include spits and bars, sometimes enclosing lagoons.

***The Deccan Plateau** covers an area of more than 123,553 sq miles (320,000 sq km). It is formed of deep layers of volcanic basalt, reaching thicknesses of more than 9,800 ft (3,000 m) toward the coast. Distinctive stepped valleys cut in the basalt plateau by rivers are known as "traps."*

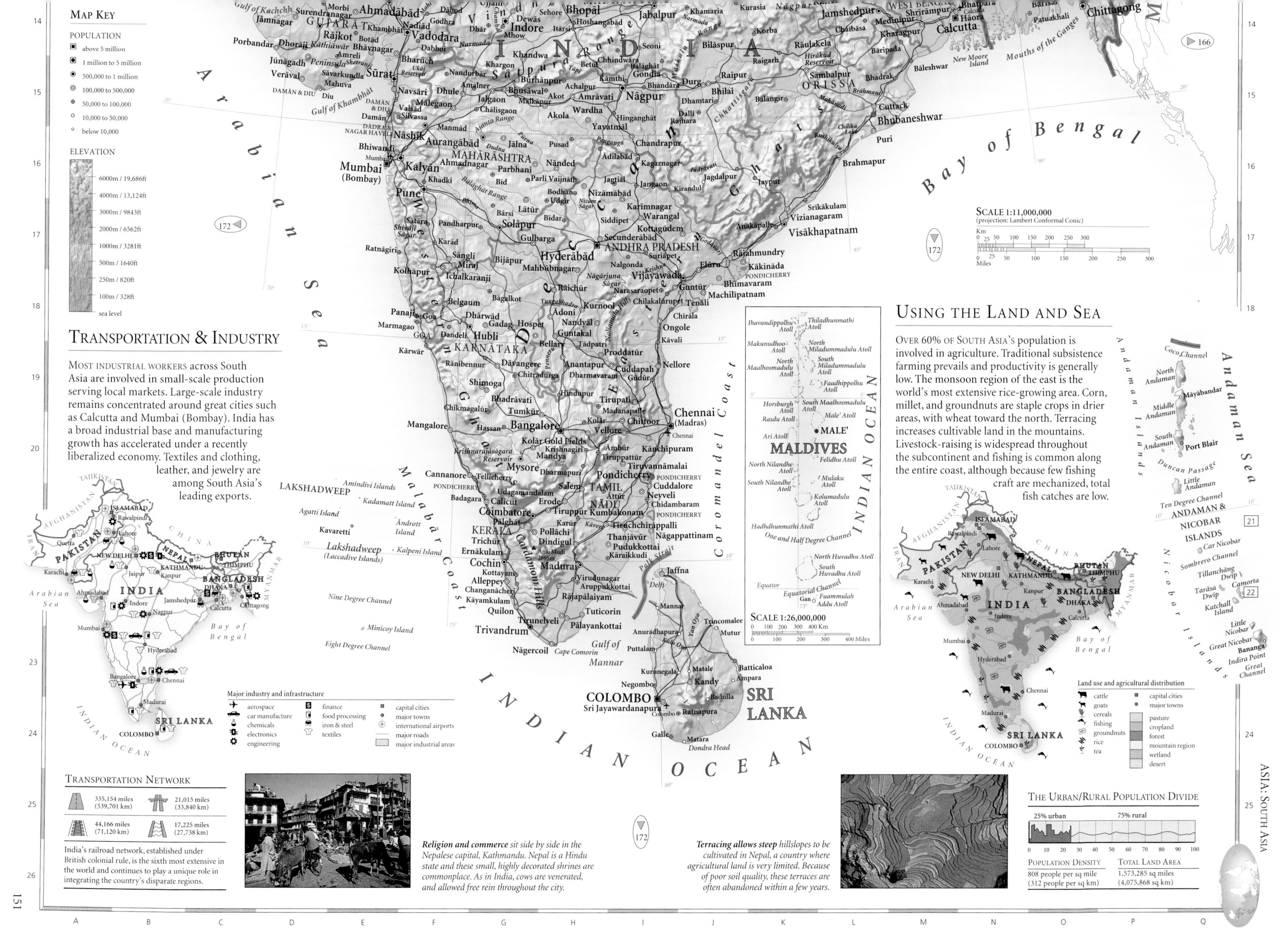
MAP KEY
POPULATION
above 5 million
1 million to 5 million
500,000 to 1 million
100,000 to 500,000
50,000 to 100,000
10,000 to 50,000
below 10,000
ELEVATION
6000m / 19,686ft
4000m / 13,124ft
3000m / 9843ft
2000m / 6562ft
1000m / 3281ft
500m / 1640ft
250m / 820ft
100m / 328ft
sea level
SCALE 1:11,000,000
(projection: Lambert Conformal Conic)
INDIA
Arabian Sea
Bay of Bengal
INDIAN OCEAN
SRI LANKA
MALDIVES
SCALE 1:26,000,000
LAKSHADWEEP
ANDAMAN & NICOBAR ISLANDS
Andaman Sea
Malabar Coast
Coromandel Coast
Mumbai (Bombay)
Chennai (Madras)
Calcutta
Hyderābād
Bangalore
COLOMBO
Sri Jayawardanapura
Major industry and infrastructure
aerospace
car manufacture
chemicals
electronics
engineering
finance
food processing
iron & steel
textiles
capital cities
major towns
international airports
major roads
major industrial areas
Land use and agricultural distribution
cattle
goats
cereals
fishing
groundnuts
rice
tea
capital cities
major towns
pasture
cropland
forest
mountain region
wetland
desert

Transportation & Industry

Most industrial workers across South Asia are involved in small-scale production serving local markets. Large-scale industry remains concentrated around great cities such as Calcutta and Mumbai (Bombay). India has a broad industrial base and manufacturing growth has accelerated under a recently liberalized economy. Textiles and clothing, leather, and jewelry are among South Asia's leading exports.

Using the Land and Sea

Over 60% of South Asia's population is involved in agriculture. Traditional subsistence farming prevails and productivity is generally low. The monsoon region of the east is the world's most extensive rice-growing area. Corn, millet, and groundnuts are staple crops in drier areas, with wheat toward the north. Terracing increases cultivable land in the mountains. Livestock-raising is widespread throughout the subcontinent and fishing is common along the entire coast, although because few fishing craft are mechanized, total fish catches are low.

Transportation Network

	335,154 miles (539,701 km)		21,015 miles (33,840 km)
	44,166 miles (71,120 km)		17,225 miles (27,738 km)

India's railroad network, established under British colonial rule, is the sixth most extensive in the world and continues to play a unique role in integrating the country's disparate regions.

Religion and commerce *sit side by side in the Nepalese capital, Kathmandu. Nepal is a Hindu state and these small, highly decorated shrines are commonplace. As in India, cows are venerated, and allowed free rein throughout the city.*

Terracing allows steep *hillslopes to be cultivated in Nepal, a country where agricultural land is very limited. Because of poor soil quality, these terraces are often abandoned within a few years.*

The Urban/Rural Population Divide

25% urban — 75% rural

Population Density	Total Land Area
808 people per sq mile (312 people per sq km)	1,573,285 sq miles (4,075,868 sq km)

Northern India & the Himalayan States

Bangladesh, Bhutan, Nepal, Arunachal Pradesh, Assam, Bihar, Chandigarh, Delhi, Haryana, Himachal Pradesh, Jammu & Kashmir, Manipur, Meghalaya, Mizoram, Nagaland, Punjab, Rajasthan, Sikkim, Tripura, Uttar Pradesh, West Bengal

The Ganges and Brahmaputra river basins and the massive mountain barrier of the Himalayas define this region's landscape and have served to reinforce potent cultural and religious differences among its people. Hinduism pervades most aspects of national life and is a growing political force within India, a secular country which also encompasses the center of Sikhism at Amritsar and the world's largest Muslim minority. Nepal is a crowded mountain state, which faces severe ecological problems from deforestation, while the tiny Himalayan Buddhist kingdom of Bhutan is emerging from long-term isolation, to welcome selected visitors. The Muslim state of Bangladesh, formerly East Pakistan, is one of the world's most densely populated countries and one of the poorest, with more than 120 million people living largely on the massive Ganges/Brahmaputra Delta. Many Bangladeshis live under threat of repeated, catastrophic floods.

***The Golden Temple** in Amritsar, the most sacred shrine of the Sikh religion, was the scene of violent clashes between Sikh separatists and government forces in 1984.*

Map Key

POPULATION

- 1 million to 5 million
- 500,000 to 1 million
- 100,000 to 500,000
- 50,000 to 100,000
- 10,000 to 50,000
- below 10,000

ELEVATION

- 6000m / 19,686ft
- 4000m / 13,124ft
- 3000m / 9843ft
- 2000m / 6562ft
- 1000m / 3281ft
- 500m / 1640ft
- 250m / 820ft
- 100m / 328ft
- sea level

SCALE 1:6,500,000 (projection: Lambert Conformal Conic)

Transportation & Industry

Textiles, engineering, chemicals, and electronics are leading industries in north India. The plateau of Chota Nagpur provides ore for iron and steel production in the major industrial region northeast of Calcutta. Bangladesh processes jute and Nepal has a small manufacturing sector based on agricultural produce, while Bhutan's limited industry is concentrated in the southern lowland area.

Major industry and infrastructure

- adventure tourism
- car manufacture
- chemicals
- coal
- electronics
- engineering
- finance
- food processing
- iron & steel
- jute processing
- oil
- tea processing
- textiles
- capital cities
- major towns
- international airports
- major roads
- major industrial areas

Transportation Network

Over 60% of Bangladesh's internal trade is carried by boat. The country has a very disjointed land transportation network, with no bridges over the Brahmaputra and few road crossings on the Ganges River.

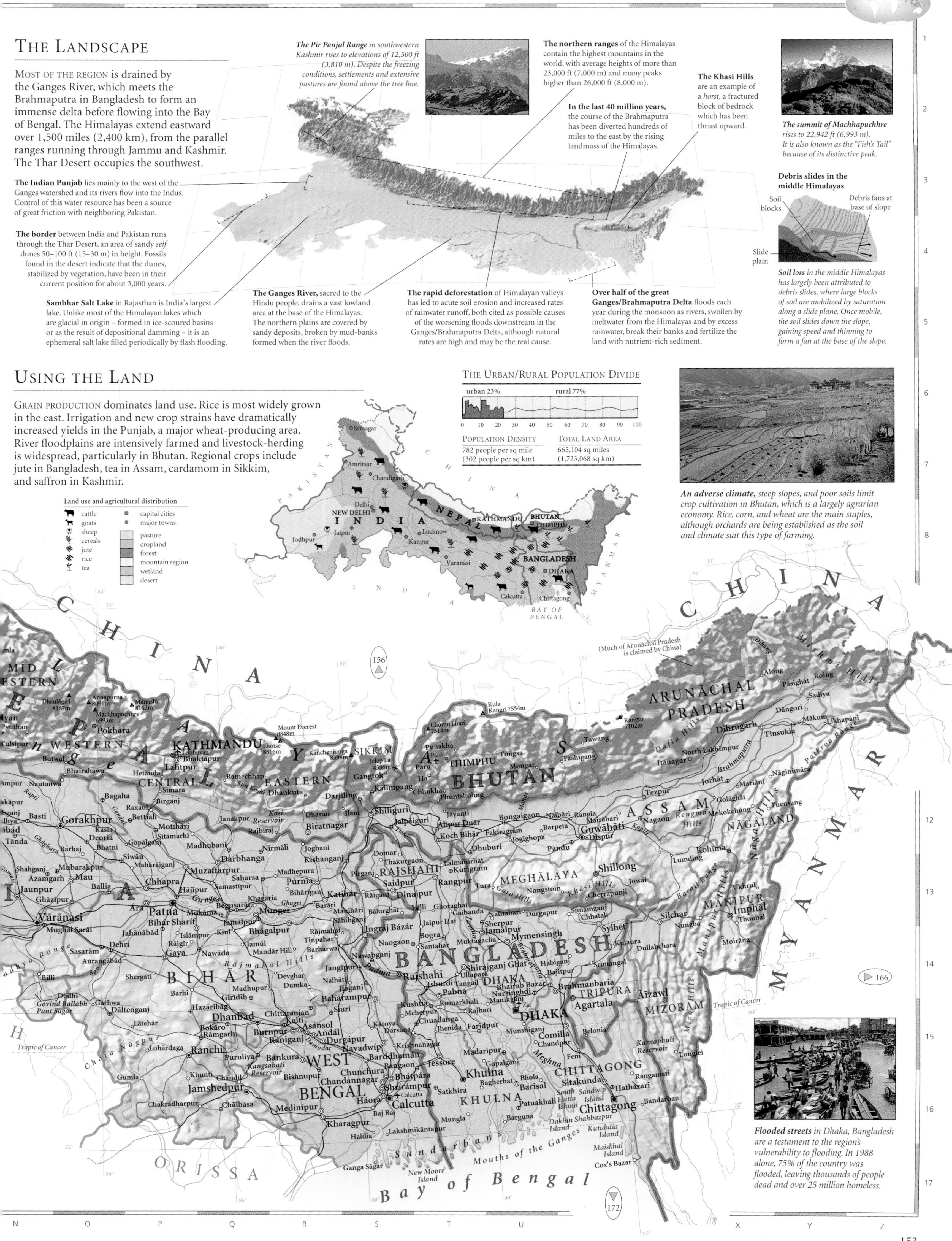

The Landscape

Most of the region is drained by the Ganges River, which meets the Brahmaputra in Bangladesh to form an immense delta before flowing into the Bay of Bengal. The Himalayas extend eastward over 1,500 miles (2,400 km), from the parallel ranges running through Jammu and Kashmir. The Thar Desert occupies the southwest.

The Pir Panjal Range in southwestern Kashmir rises to elevations of 12,500 ft (3,810 m). Despite the freezing conditions, settlements and extensive pastures are found above the tree line.

The northern ranges of the Himalayas contain the highest mountains in the world, with average heights of more than 23,000 ft (7,000 m) and many peaks higher than 26,000 ft (8,000 m).

In the last 40 million years, the course of the Brahmaputra has been diverted hundreds of miles to the east by the rising landmass of the Himalayas.

The Khasi Hills are an example of a *horst*, a fractured block of bedrock which has been thrust upward.

The summit of Machhapuchhre *rises to 22,942 ft (6,993 m). It is also known as the "Fish's Tail" because of its distinctive peak.*

Debris slides in the middle Himalayas

Soil blocks
Debris fans at base of slope
Slide plain

Soil loss *in the middle Himalayas has largely been attributed to debris slides, where large blocks of soil are mobilized by saturation along a slide plane. Once mobile, the soil slides down the slope, gaining speed and thinning to form a fan at the base of the slope.*

The Indian Punjab lies mainly to the west of the Ganges watershed and its rivers flow into the Indus. Control of this water resource has been a source of great friction with neighboring Pakistan.

The border between India and Pakistan runs through the Thar Desert, an area of sandy *seif* dunes 50–100 ft (15–30 m) in height. Fossils found in the desert indicate that the dunes, stabilized by vegetation, have been in their current position for about 3,000 years.

Sambhar Salt Lake in Rajasthan is India's largest lake. Unlike most of the Himalayan lakes which are glacial in origin – formed in ice-scoured basins or as the result of depositional damming – it is an ephemeral salt lake filled periodically by flash flooding.

The Ganges River, sacred to the Hindu people, drains a vast lowland area at the base of the Himalayas. The northern plains are covered by sandy deposits, broken by mud-banks formed when the river floods.

The rapid deforestation of Himalayan valleys has led to acute soil erosion and increased rates of rainwater runoff, both cited as possible causes of the worsening floods downstream in the Ganges/Brahmaputra Delta, although natural rates are high and may be the real cause.

Over half of the great Ganges/Brahmaputra Delta floods each year during the monsoon as rivers, swollen by meltwater from the Himalayas and by excess rainwater, break their banks and fertilize the land with nutrient-rich sediment.

Using the Land

Grain production dominates land use. Rice is most widely grown in the east. Irrigation and new crop strains have dramatically increased yields in the Punjab, a major wheat-producing area. River floodplains are intensively farmed and livestock-herding is widespread, particularly in Bhutan. Regional crops include jute in Bangladesh, tea in Assam, cardamom in Sikkim, and saffron in Kashmir.

Land use and agricultural distribution
cattle
goats
sheep
cereals
jute
rice
tea
capital cities
major towns
pasture
cropland
forest
mountain region
wetland
desert
Srinagar
Amritsar
Chandigarh
Delhi
NEW DELHI
INDIA
Jodhpur
Jaipur
Lucknow
Kanpur
Varanasi
Calcutta
Chittagong
NEPAL
KATHMANDU
BHUTAN
THIMPHU
BANGLADESH
DHAKA
PAKISTAN
CHINA
MYANMAR
BAY OF BENGAL

The Urban/Rural Population Divide

urban 23%
rural 77%
0 10 20 30 40 50 60 70 80 90 100

Population Density	Total Land Area
782 people per sq mile (302 people per sq km)	665,104 sq miles (1,723,068 sq km)

An adverse climate, *steep slopes, and poor soils limit crop cultivation in Bhutan, which is a largely agrarian economy. Rice, corn, and wheat are the main staples, although orchards are being established as the soil and climate suit this type of farming.*

CHINA
NEPAL
KATHMANDU
Mount Everest 8848m
Annapurna 8091m
Pokhara
SIKKIM
Gangtok
BHUTAN
THIMPHU
ARUNĀCHAL PRADESH
(Much of Arunāchal Pradesh is claimed by China)
ASSAM
NĀGĀLAND
MEGHĀLAYA
MANIPUR
MIZORAM
TRIPURA
BANGLADESH
DHAKA
Chittagong
Calcutta
WEST BENGAL
BIHĀR
ORISSA
MYANMAR
Bay of Bengal
Tropic of Cancer
Mouths of the Ganges
Sundarbans

156
166
172

Flooded streets *in Dhaka, Bangladesh are a testament to the region's vulnerability to flooding. In 1988 alone, 75% of the country was flooded, leaving thousands of people dead and over 25 million homeless.*

Southern India & Sri Lanka

Sri Lanka, Andhra Pradesh, Dadra & Nagar Haveli, Daman & Diu, Goa, Gujarat, Karnataka, Kerala, Lakshadweep, Madhya Pradesh, Maharashtra, Orissa, Pondicherry, Tamil Nadu

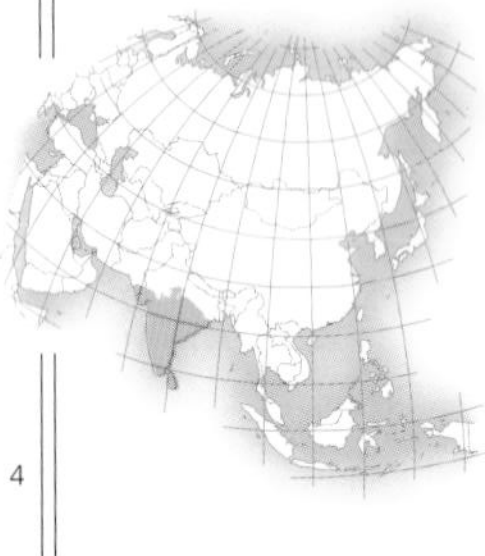

The unique and highly independent southern states reflect the diverse and decentralized nature of India, which has fourteen official languages. The southern half of the peninsula lay beyond the reach of early invaders from the north and retained the distinct and ancient culture of Dravidian peoples such as the Tamils, whose language is spoken in preference to Hindi throughout southern India. The interior plateau of southern India is less densely populated than the coastal lowlands, where the European colonial imprint is strongest. Urban and industrial growth is accelerating, but southern India's vast population remains predominantly rural. The island of Sri Lanka has two distinct cultural groups; the mainly Buddhist Sinhalese majority, and the Tamil minority whose struggle for a homeland in the northeast has led to prolonged civil war.

Using the Land and Sea

Rice is the main staple in the east, in Sri Lanka and along the humid Malabar Coast. Peanuts are grown on the Deccan Plateau, with wheat, corn, and chickpeas, toward the north. Sri Lanka is a leading exporter of tea, coconuts and rubber. Cotton plantations supply local mills around Nagpur and Mumbai (Bombay). Fishing supports many communities in Kerala and the Laccadive Islands.

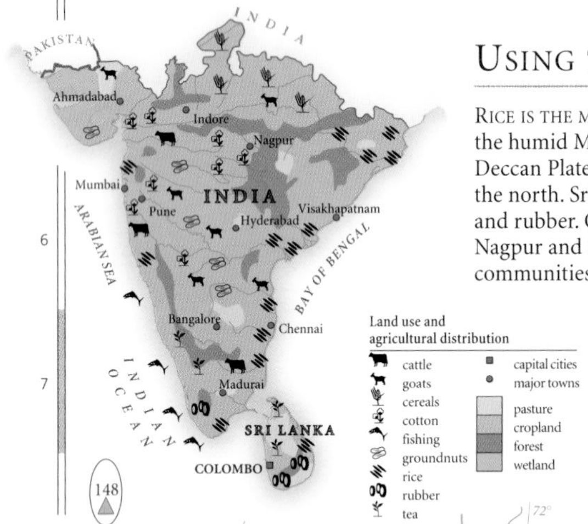

Land use and agricultural distribution: cattle, goats, cereals, cotton, fishing, groundnuts, rice, rubber, tea; capital cities, major towns; pasture, cropland, forest, wetland

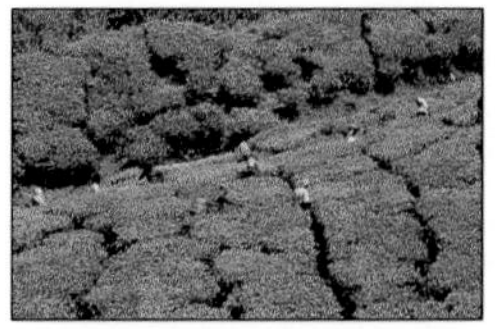

Commercial plantations, growing tea, (seen here), cardamom, coffee, coconuts, and rubber, occupy about half the agricultural land in Kerala, necessitating food imports for local consumption.

The Urban/Rural Population Divide

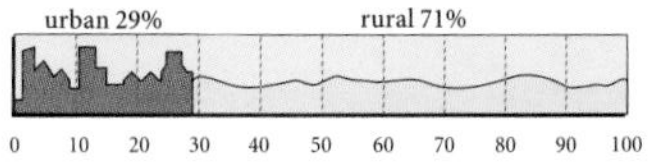

urban 29% — rural 71%

0 10 20 30 40 50 60 70 80 90 100

Population Density	Total Land Area
715 people per sq mile (276 people per sq km)	698,295 sq miles (1,809,054 sq km)

The Landscape

The undulating Deccan Plateau underlies most of southern India; it slopes gently down toward the east and is largely enclosed by the Ghats coastal hill ranges. The Western Ghats run continuously along the Arabian Sea coast, while the Eastern Ghats are interrupted by rivers which follow the slope of the plateau and flow across broad lowlands into the Bay of Bengal. The plateaus and basins of Sri Lanka's central highlands are surrounded by a broad plain.

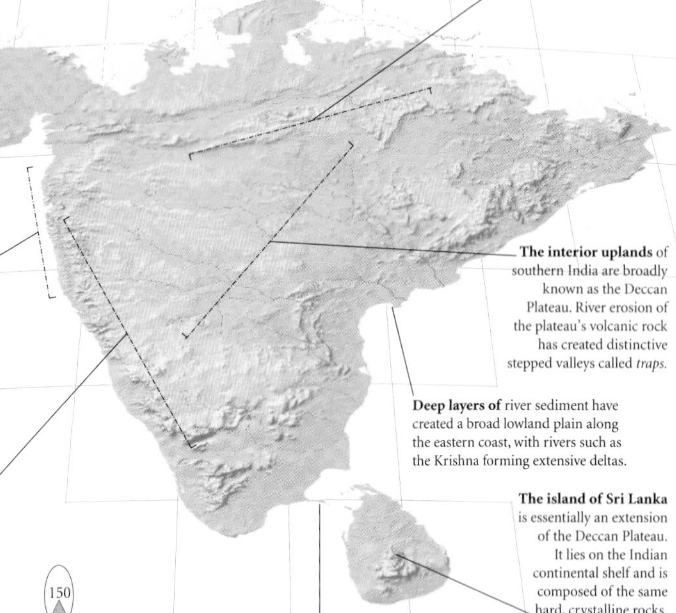

Along the northern boundary of the Deccan Plateau, old basement rocks are interspersed with younger sedimentary strata. This creates spectacular scarplands, cut by numerous waterfalls along the softer sedimentary strata.

The Rann of Kachchh tidal marshes encircle the low-lying Kachchh Peninsula. For several months during the rainy season the water level of the marshes rises and Kachchh becomes an island.

The Konkan coast, which runs between Daman and Goa, is characterized by rocky headlands, and bays with crescent-shaped beaches. Flooded river valleys known as *rias* extend inland.

The interior uplands of southern India are broadly known as the Deccan Plateau. River erosion of the plateau's volcanic rock has created distinctive stepped valleys called *traps.*

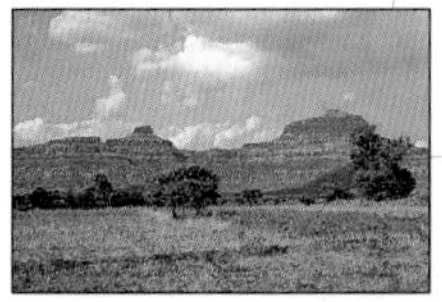

Deep layers of river sediment have created a broad lowland plain along the eastern coast, with rivers such as the Krishna forming extensive deltas.

***The Western Ghats** run north–south marking the western boundary of the Deccan Plateau. Their height rises to the south where their summits reach altitudes of 8,000 ft (2,500 m).*

The island of Sri Lanka is essentially an extension of the Deccan Plateau. It lies on the Indian continental shelf and is composed of the same hard, crystalline rocks.

Adam's Bridge

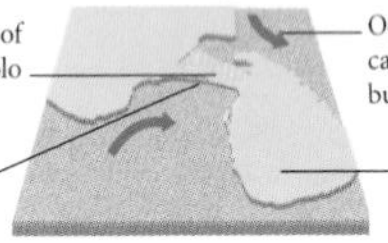

Relict of ancient tombolo; Adam's Bridge; Ocean currents cause sediment build up; Sri Lanka

***Adam's Bridge (Rama's Bridge)** is a chain of sandy shoals lying about 4 ft (1.2 m) under the sea between India and Sri Lanka. They once formed the world's longest tombolo, or land bridge, before the sea level began to rise several thousand years ago.*

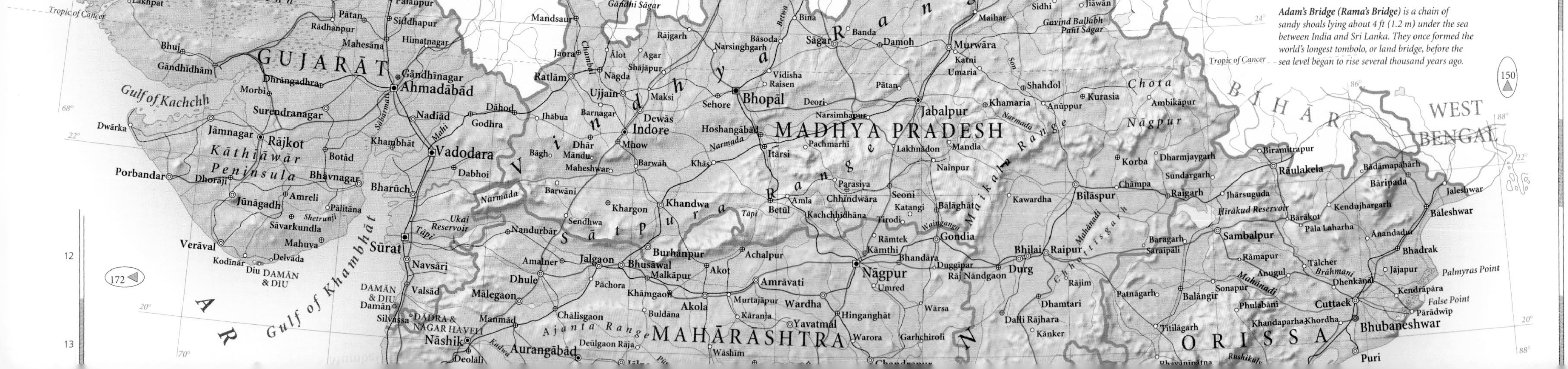

PAKISTAN · GUJARĀT · RĀJASTHĀN · UTTAR PRADESH · MADHYA PRADESH · MAHĀRĀSHTRA · ORISSA · BIHĀR · WEST BENGAL · Rann of Kachchh · Gulf of Kachchh · Gulf of Khambhāt · Kāthiāwār Peninsula · Vindhya Range · Sātpura Range · Ajanta Range · Maikala Range · Chota Nāgpur · Tropic of Cancer

148 150 150 150 172

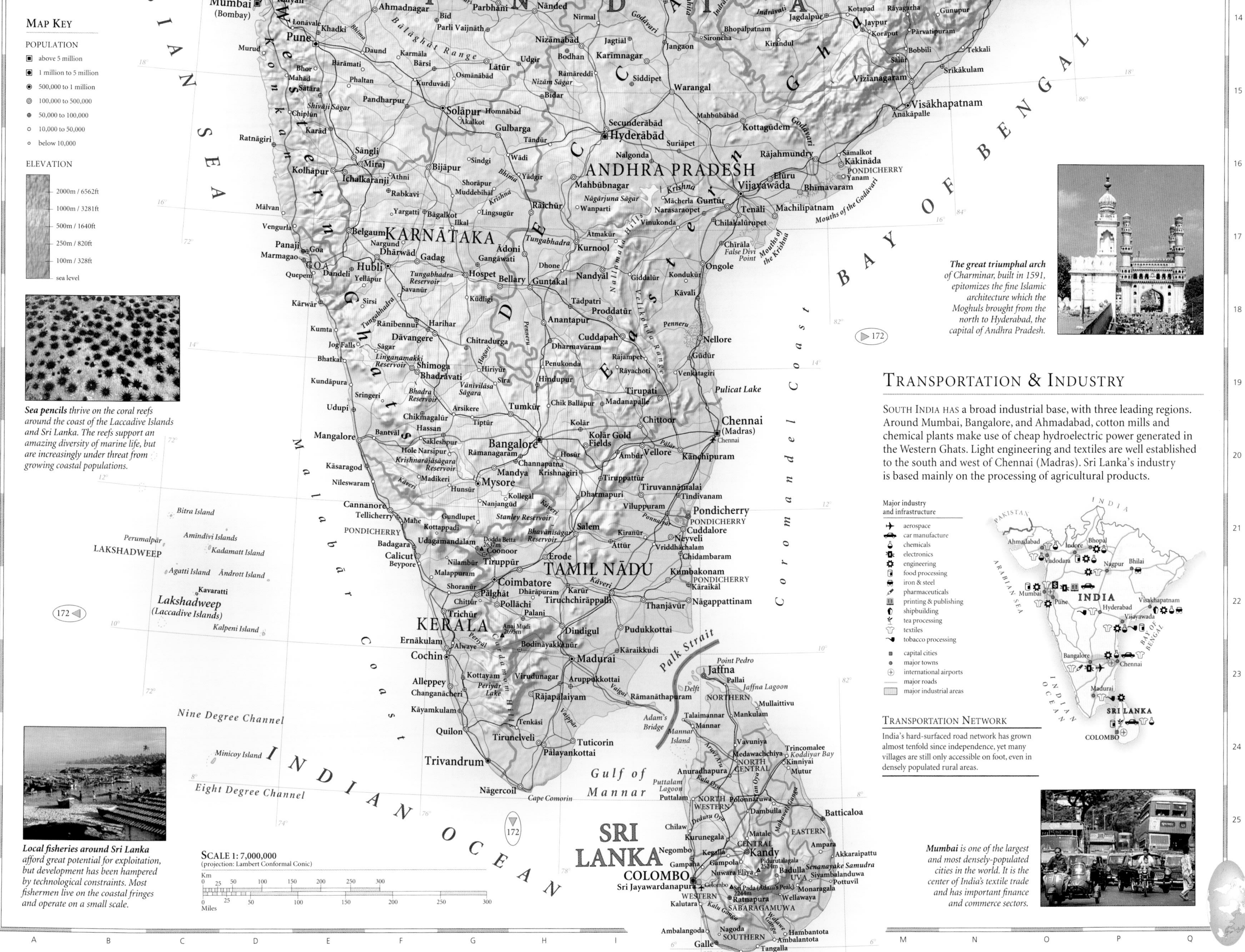
MAP KEY
POPULATION
above 5 million
1 million to 5 million
500,000 to 1 million
100,000 to 500,000
50,000 to 100,000
10,000 to 50,000
below 10,000
ELEVATION
2000m / 6562ft
1000m / 3281ft
500m / 1640ft
250m / 820ft
100m / 328ft
sea level
SCALE 1:7,000,000
(projection: Lambert Conformal Conic)
Major industry and infrastructure
aerospace
car manufacture
chemicals
electronics
engineering
food processing
iron & steel
pharmaceuticals
printing & publishing
shipbuilding
tea processing
textiles
tobacco processing
capital cities
major towns
international airports
major roads
major industrial areas

Sea pencils *thrive on the coral reefs around the coast of the Laccadive Islands and Sri Lanka. The reefs support an amazing diversity of marine life, but are increasingly under threat from growing coastal populations.*

Local fisheries around Sri Lanka *afford great potential for exploitation, but development has been hampered by technological constraints. Most fishermen live on the coastal fringes and operate on a small scale.*

The great triumphal arch *of Charminar, built in 1591, epitomizes the fine Islamic architecture which the Moghuls brought from the north to Hyderabad, the capital of Andhra Pradesh.*

TRANSPORTATION & INDUSTRY

SOUTH INDIA HAS a broad industrial base, with three leading regions. Around Mumbai, Bangalore, and Ahmadabad, cotton mills and chemical plants make use of cheap hydroelectric power generated in the Western Ghats. Light engineering and textiles are well established to the south and west of Chennai (Madras). Sri Lanka's industry is based mainly on the processing of agricultural products.

TRANSPORTATION NETWORK

India's hard-surfaced road network has grown almost tenfold since independence, yet many villages are still only accessible on foot, even in densely populated rural areas.

Mumbai *is one of the largest and most densely-populated cities in the world. It is the center of India's textile trade and has important finance and commerce sectors.*

MAINLAND EAST ASIA

CHINA, MONGOLIA, NORTH KOREA, SOUTH KOREA, TAIWAN

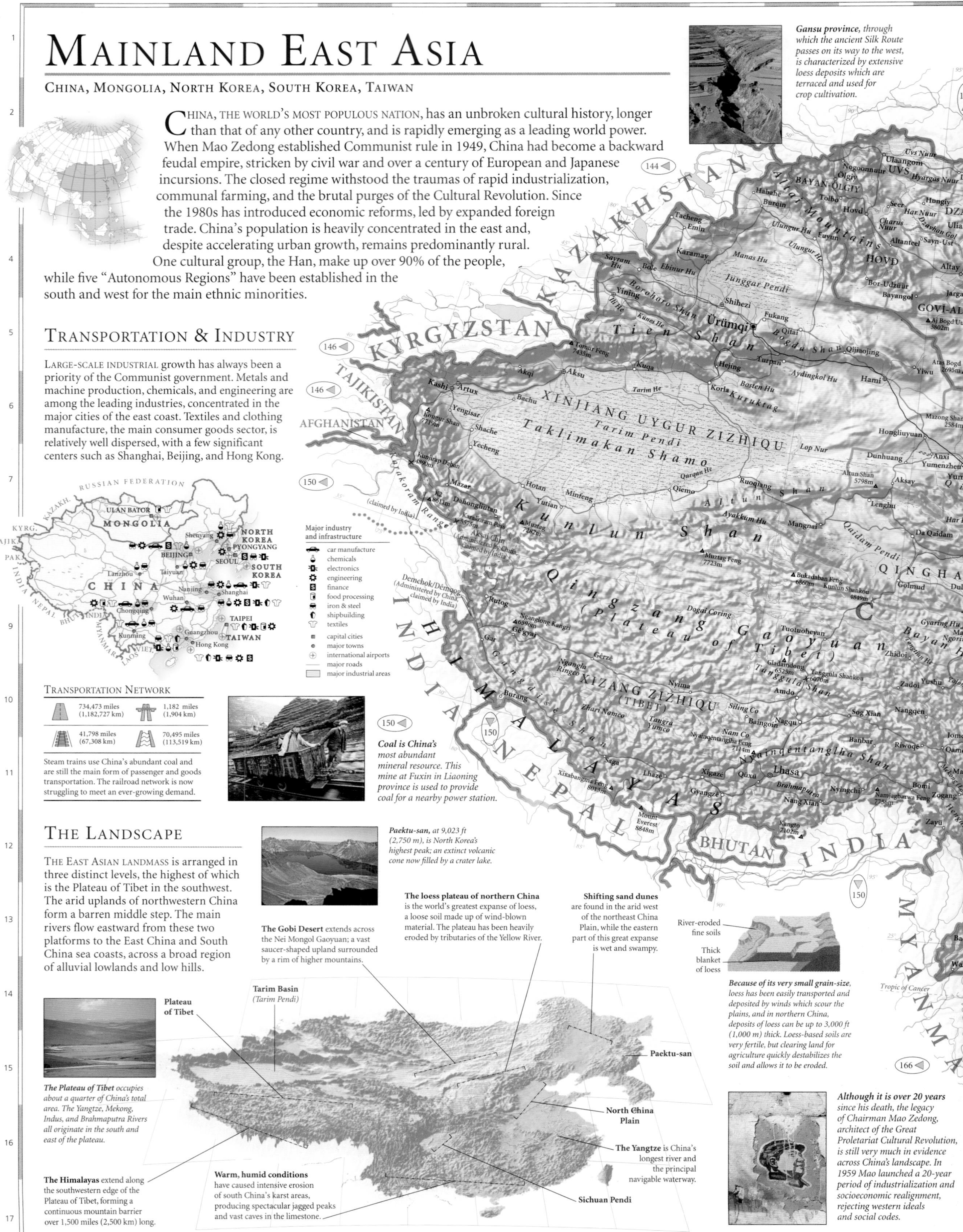

CHINA, THE WORLD'S MOST POPULOUS NATION, has an unbroken cultural history, longer than that of any other country, and is rapidly emerging as a leading world power. When Mao Zedong established Communist rule in 1949, China had become a backward feudal empire, stricken by civil war and over a century of European and Japanese incursions. The closed regime withstood the traumas of rapid industrialization, communal farming, and the brutal purges of the Cultural Revolution. Since the 1980s has introduced economic reforms, led by expanded foreign trade. China's population is heavily concentrated in the east and, despite accelerating urban growth, remains predominantly rural. One cultural group, the Han, make up over 90% of the people, while five "Autonomous Regions" have been established in the south and west for the main ethnic minorities.

Gansu province, through which the ancient Silk Route passes on its way to the west, is characterized by extensive loess deposits which are terraced and used for crop cultivation.

TRANSPORTATION & INDUSTRY

LARGE-SCALE INDUSTRIAL growth has always been a priority of the Communist government. Metals and machine production, chemicals, and engineering are among the leading industries, concentrated in the major cities of the east coast. Textiles and clothing manufacture, the main consumer goods sector, is relatively well dispersed, with a few significant centers such as Shanghai, Beijing, and Hong Kong.

Major industry and infrastructure
- car manufacture
- chemicals
- electronics
- engineering
- finance
- food processing
- iron & steel
- shipbuilding
- textiles
- capital cities
- major towns
- international airports
- major roads
- major industrial areas

TRANSPORTATION NETWORK

734,473 miles (1,182,727 km)	1,182 miles (1,904 km)
41,798 miles (67,308 km)	70,495 miles (113,519 km)

Steam trains use China's abundant coal and are still the main form of passenger and goods transportation. The railroad network is now struggling to meet an ever-growing demand.

***Coal is China's** most abundant mineral resource. This mine at Fuxin in Liaoning province is used to provide coal for a nearby power station.*

THE LANDSCAPE

THE EAST ASIAN LANDMASS is arranged in three distinct levels, the highest of which is the Plateau of Tibet in the southwest. The arid uplands of northwestern China form a barren middle step. The main rivers flow eastward from these two platforms to the East China and South China sea coasts, across a broad region of alluvial lowlands and low hills.

***Paektu-san,** at 9,023 ft (2,750 m), is North Korea's highest peak; an extinct volcanic cone now filled by a crater lake.*

The loess plateau of northern China is the world's greatest expanse of loess, a loose soil made up of wind-blown material. The plateau has been heavily eroded by tributaries of the Yellow River.

Shifting sand dunes are found in the arid west of the northeast China Plain, while the eastern part of this great expanse is wet and swampy.

River-eroded fine soils

Thick blanket of loess

***Because of its very small grain-size,** loess has been easily transported and deposited by winds which scour the plains, and in northern China, deposits of loess can be up to 3,000 ft (1,000 m) thick. Loess-based soils are very fertile, but clearing land for agriculture quickly destabilizes the soil and allows it to be eroded.*

The Gobi Desert extends across the Nei Mongol Gaoyuan; a vast saucer-shaped upland surrounded by a rim of higher mountains.

Tarim Basin *(Tarim Pendi)*

Plateau of Tibet

Paektu-san

North China Plain

The Yangtze is China's longest river and the principal navigable waterway.

Sichuan Pendi

***The Plateau of Tibet** occupies about a quarter of China's total area. The Yangtze, Mekong, Indus, and Brahmaputra Rivers all originate in the south and east of the plateau.*

The Himalayas extend along the southwestern edge of the Plateau of Tibet, forming a continuous mountain barrier over 1,500 miles (2,500 km) long.

Warm, humid conditions have caused intensive erosion of south China's karst areas, producing spectacular jagged peaks and vast caves in the limestone.

***Although it is over 20 years** since his death, the legacy of Chairman Mao Zedong, architect of the Great Proletariat Cultural Revolution, is still very much in evidence across China's landscape. In 1959 Mao launched a 20-year period of industrialization and socioeconomic realignment, rejecting western ideals and social codes.*

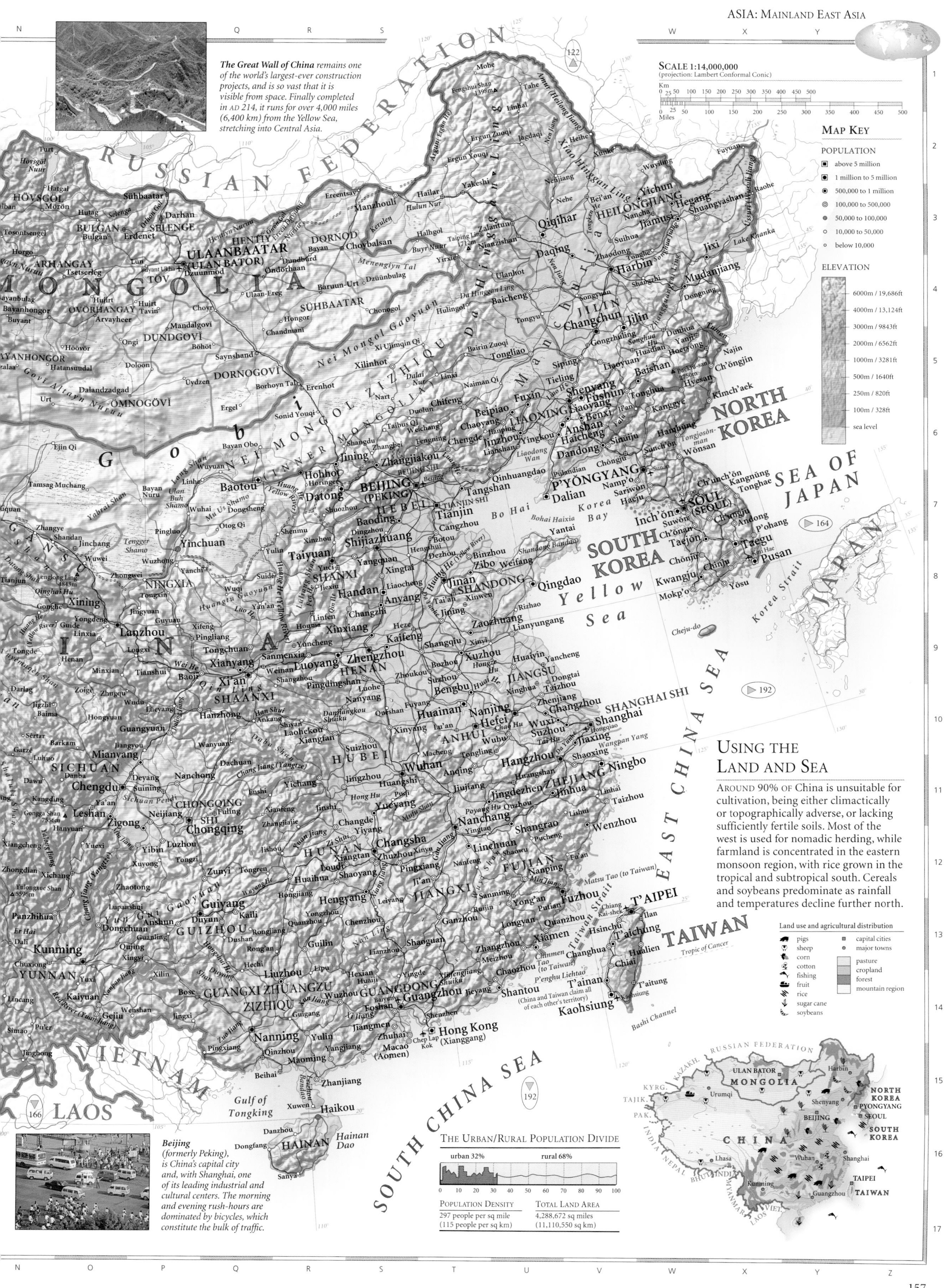
SCALE 1:14,000,000
(projection: Lambert Conformal Conic)
MAP KEY
POPULATION
above 5 million
1 million to 5 million
500,000 to 1 million
100,000 to 500,000
50,000 to 100,000
10,000 to 50,000
below 10,000
ELEVATION
6000m / 19,686ft
4000m / 13,124ft
3000m / 9843ft
2000m / 6562ft
1000m / 3281ft
500m / 1640ft
250m / 820ft
100m / 328ft
sea level
RUSSIAN FEDERATION
MONGOLIA
CHINA
NORTH KOREA
SOUTH KOREA
JAPAN
TAIWAN
VIETNAM
LAOS
SEA OF JAPAN
Yellow Sea
EAST CHINA SEA
SOUTH CHINA SEA
Gobi
ULAANBAATAR (ULAN BATOR)
BEIJING (PEKING)
P'YŎNGYANG
SOUL (SEOUL)
T'AIPEI
Shanghai
Hong Kong (Xianggang)
Macao (Aomen)
Tropic of Cancer
(China and Taiwan claim all of each other's territory)
Land use and agricultural distribution
pigs
sheep
corn
cotton
fishing
fruit
rice
sugar cane
soybeans
capital cities
major towns
pasture
cropland
forest
mountain region
THE URBAN/RURAL POPULATION DIVIDE
urban 32%
rural 68%
POPULATION DENSITY
297 people per sq mile
(115 people per sq km)
TOTAL LAND AREA
4,288,672 sq miles
(11,110,550 sq km)

The Great Wall of China remains one of the world's largest-ever construction projects, and is so vast that it is visible from space. Finally completed in AD 214, it runs for over 4,000 miles (6,400 km) from the Yellow Sea, stretching into Central Asia.

USING THE LAND AND SEA

AROUND 90% OF China is unsuitable for cultivation, being either climactically or topographically adverse, or lacking sufficiently fertile soils. Most of the west is used for nomadic herding, while farmland is concentrated in the eastern monsoon region, with rice grown in the tropical and subtropical south. Cereals and soybeans predominate as rainfall and temperatures decline further north.

Beijing (formerly Peking), is China's capital city and, with Shanghai, one of its leading industrial and cultural centers. The morning and evening rush-hours are dominated by bicycles, which constitute the bulk of traffic.

Western China

Gansu, Ningxia, Qinghai, Tibet, Xinjiang

The plateaus and basins of China's dry, desolate western domain are sparsely populated and largely undeveloped, although they have rich mineral reserves; they also form a critical buffer zone for China, in a geographically important and culturally sensitive part of the Asian continent. Across most of the west, the Han Chinese are outnumbered by a range of cultural groups, including the Uygur, the largest group of the various seminomadic Muslim peoples from Central Asia. The remote, inhospitable Plateau of Tibet is the world's coldest and highest plateau. It has been occupied by the Chinese since 1950. Tibet is one of western China's five "Autonomous Regions," but its reclusive Buddhist culture has been systematically undermined by the Chinese government.

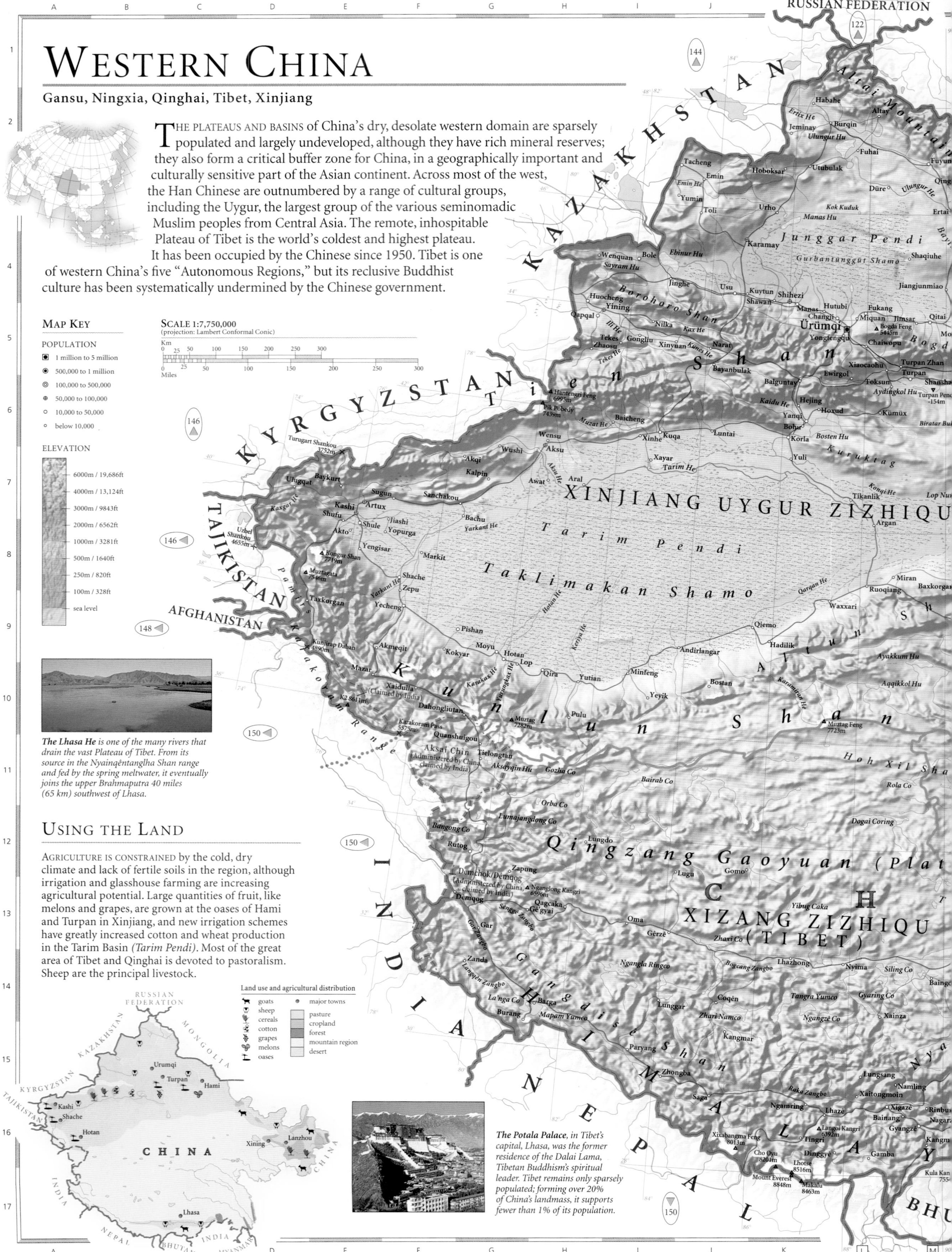

Map Key
POPULATION
1 million to 5 million
500,000 to 1 million
100,000 to 500,000
50,000 to 100,000
10,000 to 50,000
below 10,000
ELEVATION
6000m / 19,686ft
4000m / 13,124ft
3000m / 9843ft
2000m / 6562ft
1000m / 3281ft
500m / 1640ft
250m / 820ft
100m / 328ft
sea level
SCALE 1:7,750,000
(projection: Lambert Conformal Conic)
RUSSIAN FEDERATION
KAZAKHSTAN
KYRGYZSTAN
TAJIKISTAN
AFGHANISTAN
INDIA
NEPAL
XINJIANG UYGUR ZIZHIQU
XIZANG ZIZHIQU (TIBET)
Junggar Pendi
Tarim Pendi
Taklimakan Shamo
Tien Shan
Kunlun Shan
Altun Shan
Qingzang Gaoyuan (Plateau)
Gangdisê Shan
Himalaya
Karakoram Range
Pamirs
Aksai Chin (Administered by China, claimed by India)
Ürümqi
Turpan
Kashi
Hotan
Aksu
Karamay
Mount Everest 8848m
K2 8611m
Land use and agricultural distribution
goats
sheep
cereals
cotton
grapes
melons
oases
major towns
pasture
cropland
forest
mountain region
desert
CHINA

The Lhasa He is one of the many rivers that drain the vast Plateau of Tibet. From its source in the Nyainqêntanglha Shan range and fed by the spring meltwater, it eventually joins the upper Brahmaputra 40 miles (65 km) southwest of Lhasa.

Using the Land

Agriculture is constrained by the cold, dry climate and lack of fertile soils in the region, although irrigation and glasshouse farming are increasing agricultural potential. Large quantities of fruit, like melons and grapes, are grown at the oases of Hami and Turpan in Xinjiang, and new irrigation schemes have greatly increased cotton and wheat production in the Tarim Basin *(Tarim Pendi)*. Most of the great area of Tibet and Qinghai is devoted to pastoralism. Sheep are the principal livestock.

The Potala Palace, in Tibet's capital, Lhasa, was the former residence of the Dalai Lama, Tibetan Buddhism's spiritual leader. Tibet remains only sparsely populated; forming over 20% of China's landmass, it supports fewer than 1% of its population.

THE LANDSCAPE

THE HIMALAYAS MARK the southwestern edge of the Plateau of Tibet, an extreme mountain wilderness which occupies nearly a quarter of China's total area. A large structural depression, the Qaidam Pendi, lies at its northeastern edge. The Kunlun mountain chain isolates the plateau from the desert to the north, where the Tien Shan range forms a spur between the Tarim Basin *(Tarim Pendi)* and Dzungarian Basin *(Junggar Pendi)*.

The Tien Shan reach elevations of over 24,400 ft (7435 m) and have permanent ice fields, from which large glaciers extend.

Dzungarian Basin *(Junggar Pendi)*

The Bogda Shan*, an eastward arm of the Tien Shan range, rise high above the Turpan Depression* (Turpan Pendi).

The Turpan Depression *(Turpan Pendi)* is the lowest and hottest place in China. Temperatures can exceed 117°F (47°C) around the lake of Aydingkol Hu, which lies 505 ft (154 m) below sea level.

Northwestern China is largely a region of internal drainage. The Tarim He flows only as far as Lop Nur, where its water is lost by evapotranspiration from the lake and land surface.

A vast glacial lake filled much of the Tarim Basin *(Tarim Pendi)* during the last Ice Age. This area is now occupied by the Takla Makan Desert *(Taklimakan Shamo)*. A remnant of the lake, Lop Nur, forms the eastern margin, where it is fed by the Tarim He.

Sand dunes cover western parts of the the basin of Qaidam Pendi. Strong winds frequently carry the sands east, threatening the agricultural areas around the lake of Qinghai Hu.

The terrain of the Plateau of Tibet *consists of mountain peaks and open plateaus, dotted with brackish lakes. These are probably remnants of the Tethys Sea, which covered the area before it was uplifted following the collision of the Indo-Australian and Eurasian plates.*

Mount Everest is the world's highest peak, at 29,028 ft (8,848 m). The summit marks the border between China and Nepal.

Tarim Basin *(Tarim Pendi)*

Barchan sand dunes in Takla Makan Desert *(Taklimakan Shamo)*

Oases at edge of basin

Lop Nur

The Tarim Basin (Tarim Pendi) *has no permanent rivers. Rainfall from the surrounding Plateau of Tibet and Tien Shan ranges drains into the basin's sand and gravel floor.*

From its source*, high in eastern Qinghai, the Yellow River starts on a 3,395 mile (5,464 km) journey to the Yellow Sea.*

TRANSPORTATION & INDUSTRY

OIL EXTRACTION AT Yumen and in the Dzungarian and Qaidam basins has led to the growth of the petrochemical industry and a range of heavy manufacturing plants in the cities of Lanzhou and Urumqi. Tibet, and most of Xinjiang, have little industry beyond traditional handicrafts, especially textiles at Hotan and Kashi, located along the ancient Silk Route. Nuclear and space-research testing are carried out at Lop Nur in Xinjiang.

TRANSPORTATION NETWORK

The construction of roads connecting Lhasa in Tibet with Sichuan, Qinghai, and Xinjiang was achieved in the 1950s, in spite of the extreme physical conditions of the Plateau of Tibet.

Major industry and infrastructure

- agribusiness
- chemicals
- coal
- engineering
- food processing
- iron & steel
- nuclear testing
- oil
- textiles
- major towns
- major roads
- major industrial areas

EASTERN CHINA

TAIWAN, Anhui, Beijing, Fujian, Guangdong, Guangxi, Guizhou, Hainan, Hebei, Henan, Hubei, Hunan, Jiangsu, Jiangxi, Shaanxi, Shandong, Shanghai, Shanxi, Sichuan, Tianjin, Yunnan, Zhejiang

THE EAST IS CHINA'S HEARTLAND. Massive industrial development since 1949 has transformed much of the densely populated rural landscape, in a region still prone to flooding and drought. Over 20 cities have populations of over a million, including the giant metropolis of Shanghai and the capital Beijing, which has been China's cultural and political center since the 13th century. The ethnically diverse southwest and the oil-rich interior provinces of Sichuan and Shaanxi have largely missed out on the remarkable economic growth occurring in designated free-trade areas along the coasts of the South and East China seas. The republic of Taiwan was established in 1949 by Chinese nationalists ousted from the mainland by the victorious Communist forces. Taiwan now has one of the strongest economies in the world but its sovereignty is not recognized by China. Hong Kong provides a major international trade link for China; a 99-year "lease" period of British control was concluded in 1997.

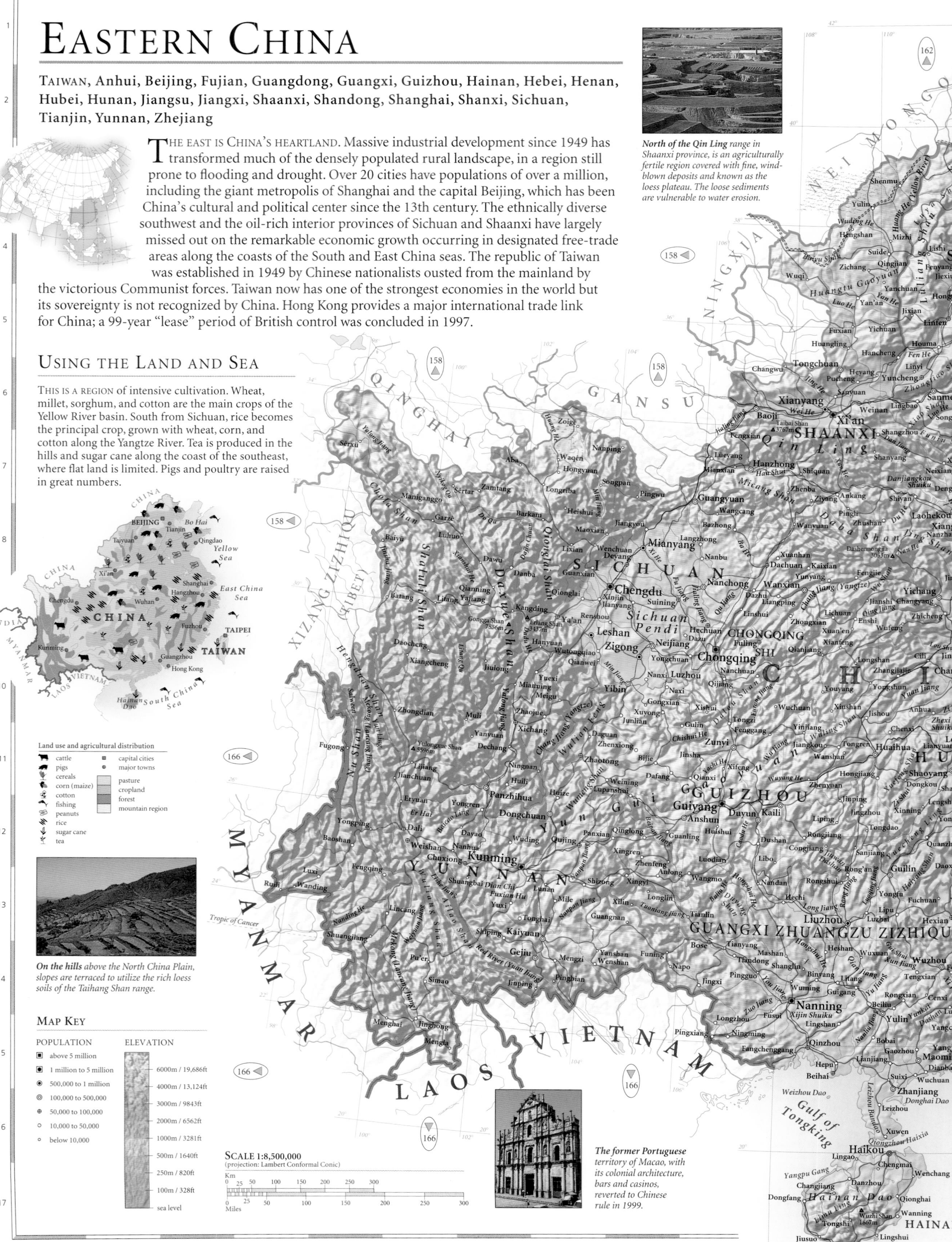

QINGHAI
GANSU
NINGXIA
NEI MONGOL
XIZANG ZIZHIQU (TIBET)
SICHUAN
SHAANXI
CHONGQING SHI
GUIZHOU
YUNNAN
GUANGXI ZHUANGZU ZIZHIQU
HAINAN
MYANMAR
LAOS
VIETNAM
Gulf of Tongking
Chengdu
Chongqing
Kunming
Guiyang
Nanning
Xi'an
Haikou
Hainan Dao
Qin Ling
Sichuan Pendi
Tropic of Cancer

North of the Qin Ling range in Shaanxi province, is an agriculturally fertile region covered with fine, wind-blown deposits and known as the loess plateau. The loose sediments are vulnerable to water erosion.

USING THE LAND AND SEA

THIS IS A REGION of intensive cultivation. Wheat, millet, sorghum, and cotton are the main crops of the Yellow River basin. South from Sichuan, rice becomes the principal crop, grown with wheat, corn, and cotton along the Yangtze River. Tea is produced in the hills and sugar cane along the coast of the southeast, where flat land is limited. Pigs and poultry are raised in great numbers.

Land use and agricultural distribution

- cattle
- pigs
- cereals
- corn (maize)
- cotton
- fishing
- peanuts
- rice
- sugar cane
- tea
- capital cities
- major towns
- pasture
- cropland
- forest
- mountain region

On the hills above the North China Plain, slopes are terraced to utilize the rich loess soils of the Taihang Shan range.

MAP KEY

POPULATION

- above 5 million
- 1 million to 5 million
- 500,000 to 1 million
- 100,000 to 500,000
- 50,000 to 100,000
- 10,000 to 50,000
- below 10,000

ELEVATION

- 6000m / 19,686ft
- 4000m / 13,124ft
- 3000m / 9843ft
- 2000m / 6562ft
- 1000m / 3281ft
- 500m / 1640ft
- 250m / 820ft
- 100m / 328ft
- sea level

SCALE 1:8,500,000
(projection: Lambert Conformal Conic)

The former Portuguese territory of Macao, with its colonial architecture, bars and casinos, reverted to Chinese rule in 1999.

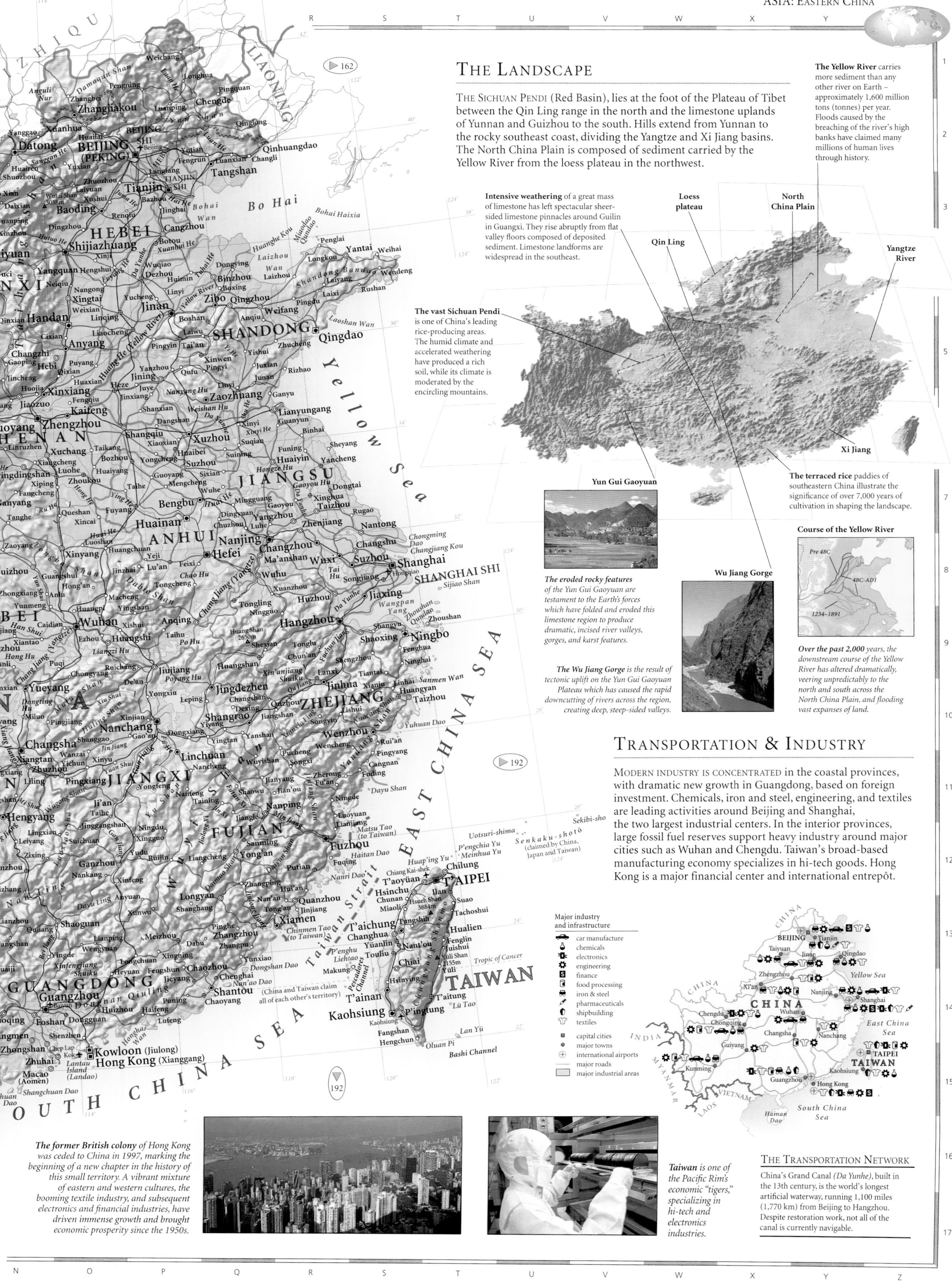
HEBEI
SHANDONG
JIANGSU
ANHUI
ZHEJIANG
JIANGXI
FUJIAN
GUANGDONG
TAIWAN
SHANGHAI SHI
Bo Hai
Yellow Sea
EAST CHINA SEA
SOUTH CHINA SEA
Taiwan Strait
Tropic of Cancer
Loess plateau
North China Plain
Qin Ling
Yangtze River
Xi Jiang
Yun Gui Gaoyuan
Wu Jiang Gorge
Course of the Yellow River
Pre 4BC
4BC-AD1
1234–1891
Major industry and infrastructure
car manufacture
chemicals
electronics
engineering
finance
food processing
iron & steel
pharmaceuticals
shipbuilding
textiles
capital cities
major towns
international airports
major roads
major industrial areas

The Landscape

The Sichuan Pendi (Red Basin), lies at the foot of the Plateau of Tibet between the Qin Ling range in the north and the limestone uplands of Yunnan and Guizhou to the south. Hills extend from Yunnan to the rocky southeast coast, dividing the Yangtze and Xi Jiang basins. The North China Plain is composed of sediment carried by the Yellow River from the loess plateau in the northwest.

The Yellow River carries more sediment than any other river on Earth – approximately 1,600 million tons (tonnes) per year. Floods caused by the breaching of the river's high banks have claimed many millions of human lives through history.

Intensive weathering of a great mass of limestone has left spectacular sheer-sided limestone pinnacles around Guilin in Guangxi. They rise abruptly from flat valley floors composed of deposited sediment. Limestone landforms are widespread in the southeast.

The vast Sichuan Pendi is one of China's leading rice-producing areas. The humid climate and accelerated weathering have produced a rich soil, while its climate is moderated by the encircling mountains.

The terraced rice paddies of southeastern China illustrate the significance of over 7,000 years of cultivation in shaping the landscape.

The eroded rocky features of the Yun Gui Gaoyuan are testament to the Earth's forces which have folded and eroded this limestone region to produce dramatic, incised river valleys, gorges, and karst features.

The Wu Jiang Gorge is the result of tectonic uplift on the Yun Gui Gaoyuan Plateau which has caused the rapid downcutting of rivers across the region, creating deep, steep-sided valleys.

Over the past 2,000 years, the downstream course of the Yellow River has altered dramatically, veering unpredictably to the north and south across the North China Plain, and flooding vast expanses of land.

Transportation & Industry

Modern industry is concentrated in the coastal provinces, with dramatic new growth in Guangdong, based on foreign investment. Chemicals, iron and steel, engineering, and textiles are leading activities around Beijing and Shanghai, the two largest industrial centers. In the interior provinces, large fossil fuel reserves support heavy industry around major cities such as Wuhan and Chengdu. Taiwan's broad-based manufacturing economy specializes in hi-tech goods. Hong Kong is a major financial center and international entrepôt.

The Transportation Network

China's Grand Canal (*Da Yunhe*), built in the 13th century, is the world's longest artificial waterway, running 1,100 miles (1,770 km) from Beijing to Hangzhou. Despite restoration work, not all of the canal is currently navigable.

The former British colony of Hong Kong was ceded to China in 1997, marking the beginning of a new chapter in the history of this small territory. A vibrant mixture of eastern and western cultures, the booming textile industry, and subsequent electronics and financial industries, have driven immense growth and brought economic prosperity since the 1950s.

Taiwan is one of the Pacific Rim's economic "tigers," specializing in hi-tech and electronics industries.

Northeastern China, Mongolia & Korea

Mongolia, North Korea, South Korea, Heilongjiang, Inner Mongolia, Jilin, Liaoning

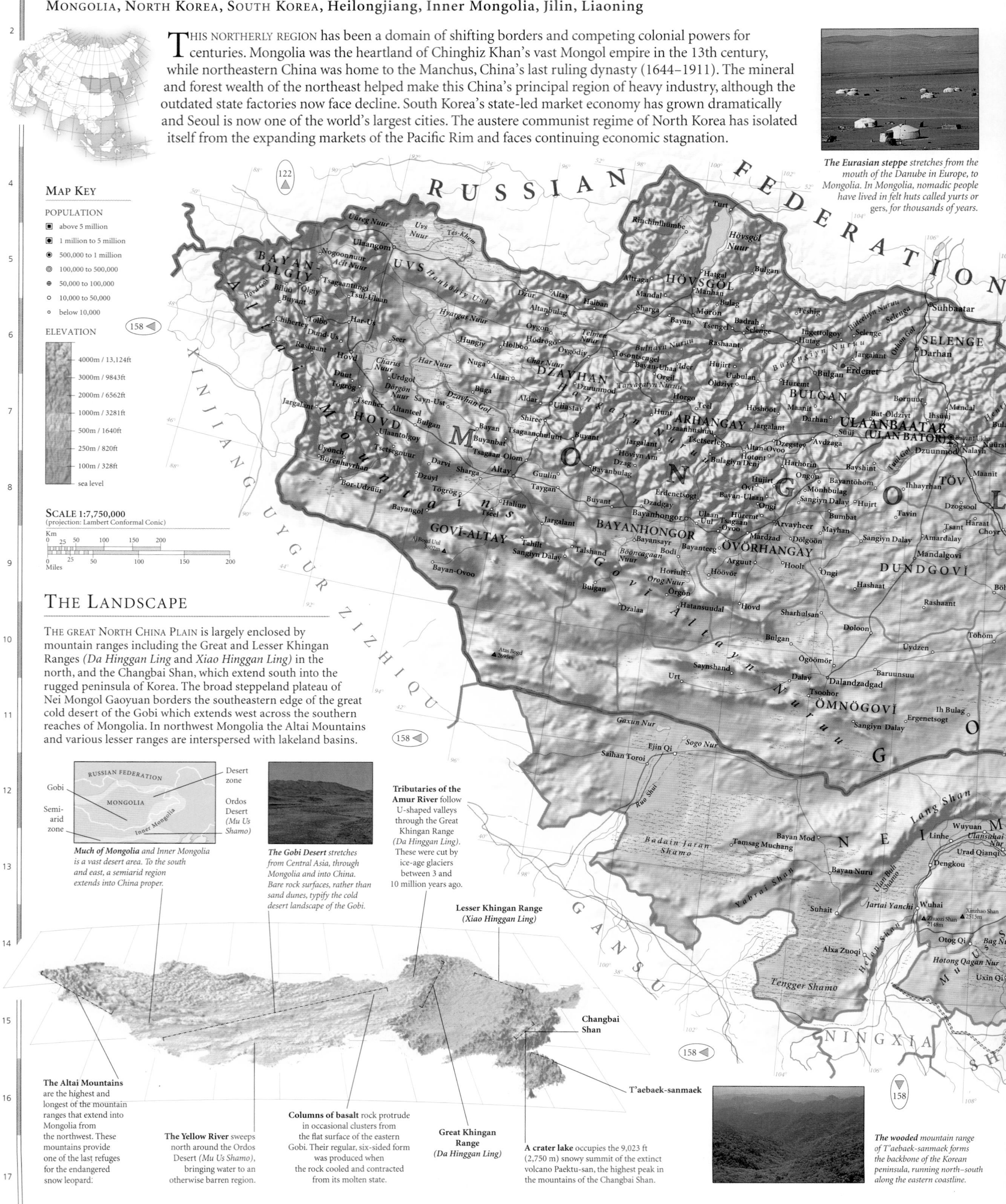
RUSSIAN FEDERATION
MONGOLIA
XINJIANG UYGUR ZIZHIQU
GANSU
NINGXIA
NEI
Altai Mountains
Govĭ Altayn Nuruu
Hangayn Nuruu
BAYAN-ÖLGIY
UVS
HÖVSGÖL
HOVD
DZAVHAN
ARHANGAY
BULGAN
SELENGE
GOVĬ-ALTAY
BAYANHONGOR
ÖVÖRHANGAY
TÖV
DUNDGOVĬ
ÖMNÖGOVĬ
ULAANBAATAR (ULAN BATOR)
Uvs Nuur
Hövsgöl Nuur
Har Nuur
Ulaangom
Hovd
Uliastay
Tsetserleg
Harhorin
Bayanhongor
Dalandzadgad
Sühbaatar
Darhan
Ejin Qi
Badain Jaran Shamo
Tengger Shamo
Yabrai Shan
Lang Shan
Wuhai
Alxa Zuoqi
Mu Us

Asia locator map.

THIS NORTHERLY REGION has been a domain of shifting borders and competing colonial powers for centuries. Mongolia was the heartland of Chinghiz Khan's vast Mongol empire in the 13th century, while northeastern China was home to the Manchus, China's last ruling dynasty (1644–1911). The mineral and forest wealth of the northeast helped make this China's principal region of heavy industry, although the outdated state factories now face decline. South Korea's state-led market economy has grown dramatically and Seoul is now one of the world's largest cities. The austere communist regime of North Korea has isolated itself from the expanding markets of the Pacific Rim and faces continuing economic stagnation.

The Eurasian steppe *stretches from the mouth of the Danube in Europe, to Mongolia. In Mongolia, nomadic people have lived in felt huts called yurts or gers, for thousands of years.*

Map Key

POPULATION
- above 5 million
- 1 million to 5 million
- 500,000 to 1 million
- 100,000 to 500,000
- 50,000 to 100,000
- 10,000 to 50,000
- below 10,000

ELEVATION
- 4000m / 13,124ft
- 3000m / 9843ft
- 2000m / 6562ft
- 1000m / 3281ft
- 500m / 1640ft
- 250m / 820ft
- 100m / 328ft
- sea level

SCALE 1:7,750,000
(projection: Lambert Conformal Conic)

Km 0 25 50 100 150 200
Miles 0 25 50 100 150 200

The Landscape

THE GREAT NORTH CHINA PLAIN is largely enclosed by mountain ranges including the Great and Lesser Khingan Ranges *(Da Hinggan Ling* and *Xiao Hinggan Ling)* in the north, and the Changbai Shan, which extend south into the rugged peninsula of Korea. The broad steppeland plateau of Nei Mongol Gaoyuan borders the southeastern edge of the great cold desert of the Gobi which extends west across the southern reaches of Mongolia. In northwest Mongolia the Altai Mountains and various lesser ranges are interspersed with lakeland basins.

RUSSIAN FEDERATION · MONGOLIA · Inner Mongolia · Gobi · Semi-arid zone · Desert zone · Ordos Desert (Mu Us Shamo)

Much of Mongolia and Inner Mongolia is a vast desert area. To the south and east, a semiarid region extends into China proper.

The Gobi Desert stretches from Central Asia, through Mongolia and into China. Bare rock surfaces, rather than sand dunes, typify the cold desert landscape of the Gobi.

Tributaries of the Amur River follow U-shaped valleys through the Great Khingan Range *(Da Hinggan Ling)*. These were cut by ice-age glaciers between 3 and 10 million years ago.

Lesser Khingan Range *(Xiao Hinggan Ling)*

Changbai Shan

T'aebaek-sanmaek

The Altai Mountains are the highest and longest of the mountain ranges that extend into Mongolia from the northwest. These mountains provide one of the last refuges for the endangered snow leopard.

The Yellow River sweeps north around the Ordos Desert *(Mu Us Shamo)*, bringing water to an otherwise barren region.

Columns of basalt rock protrude in occasional clusters from the flat surface of the eastern Gobi. Their regular, six-sided form was produced when the rock cooled and contracted from its molten state.

Great Khingan Range *(Da Hinggan Ling)*

A crater lake occupies the 9,023 ft (2,750 m) snowy summit of the extinct volcano Paektu-san, the highest peak in the mountains of the Changbai Shan.

***The wooded** mountain range of T'aebaek-sanmaek forms the backbone of the Korean peninsula, running north–south along the eastern coastline.*

TRANSPORTATION & INDUSTRY

NORTH KOREA'S CENTRALLY-PLANNED ECONOMY is strongly oriented toward heavy industry, while South Korea has a broad manufacturing base which includes textiles, steel, electronics, and one of the world's largest shipbuilding industries. Mongolia and Inner Mongolia's great mineral resource potential is largely undeveloped. The heavy industrial region around Shenyang produces iron, steel, chemicals, and cement on a massive scale.

Major industry and infrastructure

- car manufacture
- chemicals
- coal
- electronics
- engineering
- finance
- food processing
- iron & steel
- pharmaceuticals
- shipbuilding
- textiles
- capital cities
- major towns
- international airports
- major roads
- major industrial areas

TRANSPORTATION NETWORK

Liaoning has China's most comprehensive railroad network, the legacy of the Japanese occupation of Manchuria in the 20th century. The railroads are used primarily for freight transportation.

Ulan Bator, the Mongolian capital bears many of the hallmarks of Soviet-style central planning, the result of economic and industrial assistance from the Soviet Union following Mongolian independence in 1921.

While North Korea has remained politically and economically isolated from the rest of the world, South Korea has enjoyed immense economic growth. It has benefited considerably from US economic aid in the aftermath of the Korean war of 1950–1953.

USING THE LAND AND SEA

MONGOLIA AND INNER MONGOLIA rely heavily on livestock farming, with only about 1% of the land area cultivated. Northeastern China produces wheat, corn, soybeans, and sugar beet. The cool climate limits the range of crops and large upland areas of the northeast remain forested. Rice is the staple food of North and South Korea. The latter has become a leading ocean-fishing nation.

Land use and agricultural distribution

- goats
- pigs
- sheep
- corn
- fishing
- rice
- soybeans
- sugar beet
- wheat
- capital cities
- major towns
- pasture
- cropland
- forest
- mountain region
- desert

JAPAN

In the years since the end of the Second World War, Japan has become the world's most dynamic industrial nation. The country comprises a string of over 4,000 islands which lie in a great northeast to southwest arc in the northwest Pacific. Four major islands: Hokkaido, Honshu, Shikoku, and Kyushu are home to the great majority of Japan's population of 125.9 million people, although the mountainous terrain of the central region means that most cities are situated on the coast. A densely populated industrial belt stretches along much of Honshu's southern coast, including Japan's crowded capital, Tokyo. Alongside its spectacular economic growth and the increasing westernization of its cities, Japan still maintains a most singular culture, reflected in its traditional food, formal behavioural codes, unique Shinto religion, and the reverence for the emperor, who is officially regarded as a god.

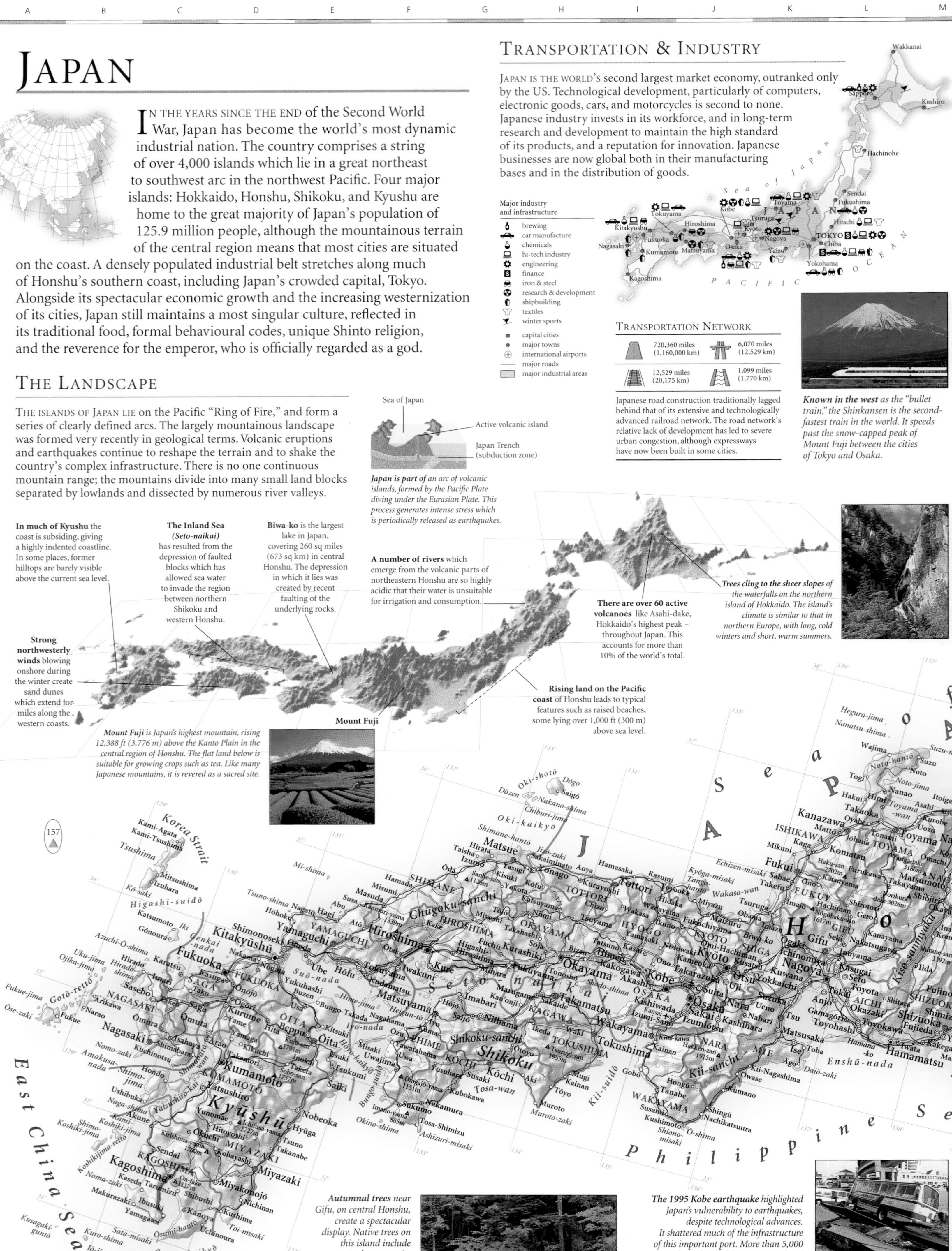

Sea of Japan
Active volcanic island
Japan Trench (subduction zone)
Mount Fuji
Major industry and infrastructure
brewing
car manufacture
chemicals
hi-tech industry
engineering
finance
iron & steel
research & development
shipbuilding
textiles
winter sports
capital cities
major towns
international airports
major roads
major industrial areas
Sea of Japan
Pacific Ocean
Philippine Sea
East China Sea
Korea Strait

The Landscape

The islands of Japan lie on the Pacific "Ring of Fire," and form a series of clearly defined arcs. The largely mountainous landscape was formed very recently in geological terms. Volcanic eruptions and earthquakes continue to reshape the terrain and to shake the country's complex infrastructure. There is no one continuous mountain range; the mountains divide into many small land blocks separated by lowlands and dissected by numerous river valleys.

***Japan is part of** an arc of volcanic islands, formed by the Pacific Plate diving under the Eurasian Plate. This process generates intense stress which is periodically released as earthquakes.*

In much of Kyushu the coast is subsiding, giving a highly indented coastline. In some places, former hilltops are barely visible above the current sea level.

The Inland Sea (*Seto-naikai*) has resulted from the depression of faulted blocks which has allowed sea water to invade the region between northern Shikoku and western Honshu.

Biwa-ko is the largest lake in Japan, covering 260 sq miles (673 sq km) in central Honshu. The depression in which it lies was created by recent faulting of the underlying rocks.

A number of rivers which emerge from the volcanic parts of northeastern Honshu are so highly acidic that their water is unsuitable for irrigation and consumption.

There are over 60 active volcanoes like Asahi-dake, Hokkaido's highest peak – throughout Japan. This accounts for more than 10% of the world's total.

***Trees cling to the sheer slopes** of the waterfalls on the northern island of Hokkaido. The island's climate is similar to that in northern Europe, with long, cold winters and short, warm summers.*

Strong northwesterly winds blowing onshore during the winter create sand dunes which extend for miles along the western coasts.

Rising land on the Pacific coast of Honshu leads to typical features such as raised beaches, some lying over 1,000 ft (300 m) above sea level.

***Mount Fuji** is Japan's highest mountain, rising 12,388 ft (3,776 m) above the Kanto Plain in the central region of Honshu. The flat land below is suitable for growing crops such as tea. Like many Japanese mountains, it is revered as a sacred site.*

Transportation & Industry

Japan is the world's second largest market economy, outranked only by the US. Technological development, particularly of computers, electronic goods, cars, and motorcycles is second to none. Japanese industry invests in its workforce, and in long-term research and development to maintain the high standard of its products, and a reputation for innovation. Japanese businesses are now global both in their manufacturing bases and in the distribution of goods.

Transportation Network

720,360 miles (1,160,000 km)	6,070 miles (12,529 km)
12,529 miles (20,175 km)	1,099 miles (1,770 km)

Japanese road construction traditionally lagged behind that of its extensive and technologically advanced railroad network. The road network's relative lack of development has led to severe urban congestion, although expressways have now been built in some cities.

***Known in the west** as the "bullet train," the Shinkansen is the second-fastest train in the world. It speeds past the snow-capped peak of Mount Fuji between the cities of Tokyo and Osaka.*

***Autumnal trees** near Gifu, on central Honshu, create a spectacular display. Native trees on this island include camphor, pasania, Japanese evergreen oak, camellia, and holly.*

***The 1995 Kobe earthquake** highlighted Japan's vulnerability to earthquakes, despite technological advances. It shattered much of the infrastructure of this important port. More than 5,000 people died as buildings and overhead highways collapsed and fires broke out.*

157

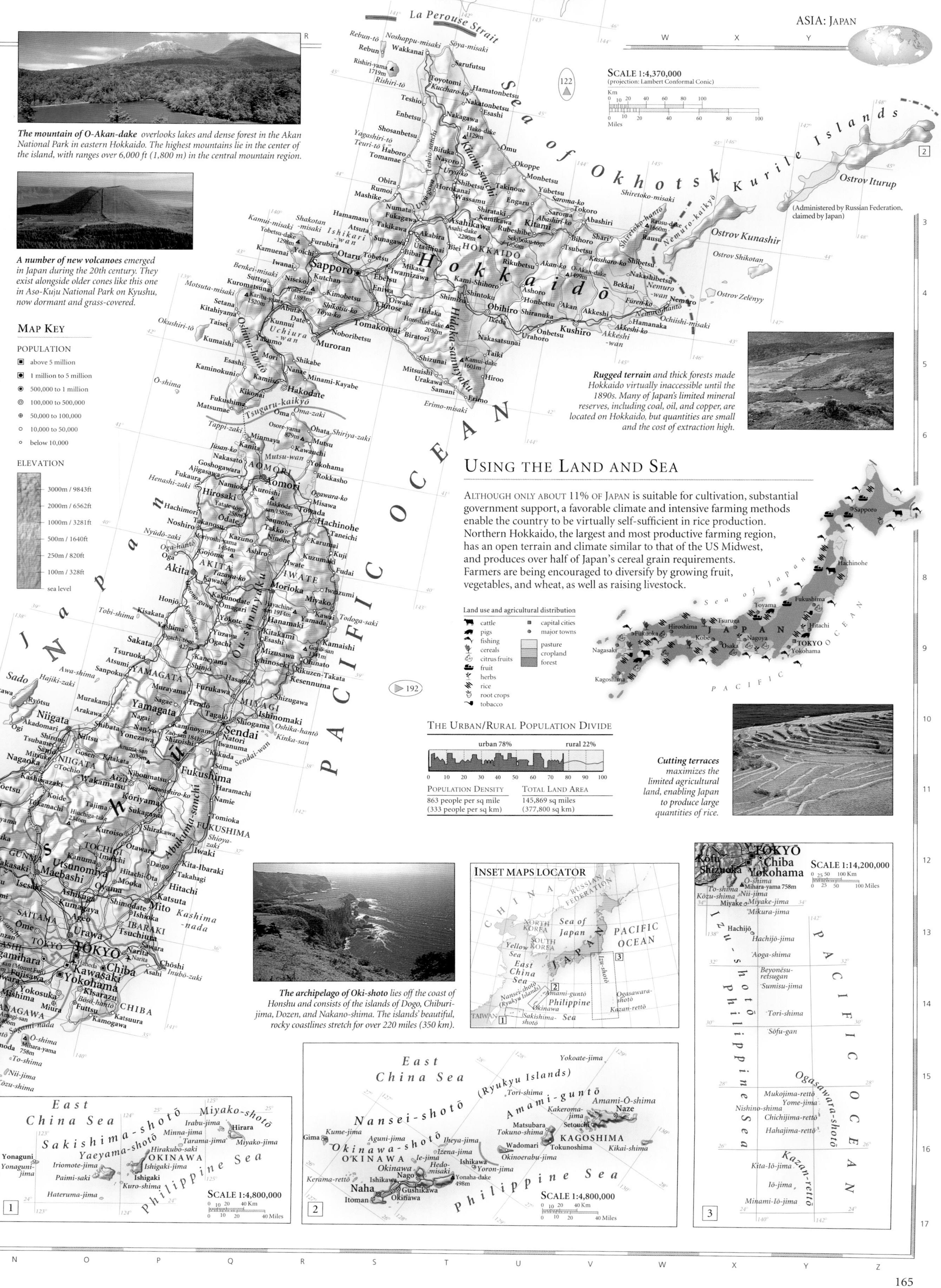
La Perouse Strait
Sea of Okhotsk
Kuril Islands
Ostrov Iturup
(Administered by Russian Federation, claimed by Japan)
Ostrov Kunashir
Ostrov Shikotan
Ostrov Zelënyy
Hokkaidō
HOKKAIDO
Sapporo
Asahikawa
Hakodate
Kushiro
Obihiro
Tomakomai
Muroran
Tsugaru-kaikyō
Sea of Japan
Honshū
Aomori
Hachinohe
Akita
Morioka
Sendai
Yamagata
Niigata
Fukushima
Kōriyama
Utsunomiya
Mito
Maebashi
TOKYO
Chiba
Kawasaki
Yokohama
PACIFIC OCEAN
Sado
SCALE 1:4,370,000
(projection: Lambert Conformal Conic)
Km
Miles
MAP KEY
POPULATION
above 5 million
1 million to 5 million
500,000 to 1 million
100,000 to 500,000
50,000 to 100,000
10,000 to 50,000
below 10,000
ELEVATION
3000m / 9843ft
2000m / 6562ft
1000m / 3281ft
500m / 1640ft
250m / 820ft
100m / 328ft
sea level
INSET MAPS LOCATOR
CHINA
RUSSIAN FEDERATION
NORTH KOREA
SOUTH KOREA
Sea of Japan
JAPAN
PACIFIC OCEAN
Yellow Sea
East China Sea
TAIWAN
Philippine Sea
1 East China Sea
Sakishima-shotō
Miyako-shotō
Yaeyama-shotō
OKINAWA
Philippine Sea
SCALE 1:4,800,000
2 East China Sea
(Ryukyu Islands)
Nansei-shotō
Amami-guntō
Okinawa-shotō
KAGOSHIMA
OKINAWA
Naha
Philippine Sea
SCALE 1:4,800,000
3 TOKYO
Chiba
Yokohama
SCALE 1:14,200,000
Izu-shotō
Philippine Sea
PACIFIC OCEAN
Ogasawara-shotō
Kazan-rettō

122

192

The mountain of O-Akan-dake *overlooks lakes and dense forest in the Akan National Park in eastern Hokkaido. The highest mountains lie in the center of the island, with ranges over 6,000 ft (1,800 m) in the central mountain region.*

A number of new volcanoes *emerged in Japan during the 20th century. They exist alongside older cones like this one in Aso-Kuju National Park on Kyushu, now dormant and grass-covered.*

Rugged terrain *and thick forests made Hokkaido virtually inaccessible until the 1890s. Many of Japan's limited mineral reserves, including coal, oil, and copper, are located on Hokkaido, but quantities are small and the cost of extraction high.*

Using the Land and Sea

ALTHOUGH ONLY ABOUT 11% OF JAPAN is suitable for cultivation, substantial government support, a favorable climate and intensive farming methods enable the country to be virtually self-sufficient in rice production. Northern Hokkaido, the largest and most productive farming region, has an open terrain and climate similar to that of the US Midwest, and produces over half of Japan's cereal grain requirements. Farmers are being encouraged to diversify by growing fruit, vegetables, and wheat, as well as raising livestock.

Land use and agricultural distribution
cattle
pigs
fishing
cereals
citrus fruits
fruit
herbs
rice
root crops
tobacco
capital cities
major towns
pasture
cropland
forest
Sapporo
Hachinohe
Sea of Japan
Toyama
Fukushima
Tsuruga
Hiroshima
Fukuoka
Kobe
JAPAN
Nagoya
Hitachi
TOKYO
Yokohama
Osaka
Nagasaki
Kagoshima
PACIFIC OCEAN

The Urban/Rural Population Divide

urban 78% | rural 22%

Population Density	Total Land Area
863 people per sq mile (333 people per sq km)	145,869 sq miles (377,800 sq km)

Cutting terraces *maximizes the limited agricultural land, enabling Japan to produce large quantities of rice.*

The archipelago of Oki-shoto *lies off the coast of Honshu and consists of the islands of Dogo, Chiburi-jima, Dozen, and Nakano-shima. The islands' beautiful, rocky coastlines stretch for over 220 miles (350 km).*

Mainland Southeast Asia

Cambodia, Laos, Myanmar, Thailand, Vietnam

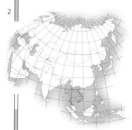

THICKLY FORESTED MOUNTAINS, intercut by the broad valleys of five great rivers characterize the landscape of Southeast Asia's mainland countries. Agriculture remains the main activity for much of the population, which is concentrated in the river flood plains and deltas. Linked ethnic and cultural roots give the region a distinct identity. Most people on the mainland are Theravada Buddhists. Foreign intervention began in the 16th century with the opening of the spice trade; Cambodia, Laos, and Vietnam were French colonies until the end of the Second World War, Myanmar was under British control. Only Thailand was never colonized. Today, Thailand is poised to play a leading role in the economic development of the Pacific Rim, and Laos and Vietnam have begun to mend the devastation of the Vietnam War, and to develop their economies. With continuing political instability and a shattered infrastructure, Cambodia faces an uncertain future, while Myanmar is seeking investment and the ending of its 38-year isolation from the world community.

The Irrawaddy River is Myanmar's vital central artery, watering the ricefields and providing a rich source of fish, as well as an important transportation link, particularly for local traffic.

The coastline of the Isthmus of Kra

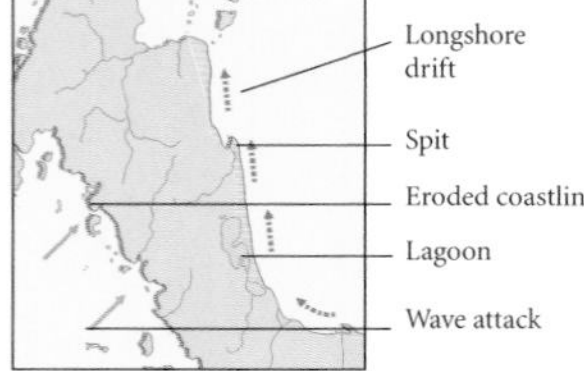

Longshore drift
Spit
Eroded coastline
Lagoon
Wave attack

The east and west coasts of the Isthmus of Kra differ greatly. The tectonically uplifted west coast is exposed to the harsh south-westerly monsoon and is heavily eroded. On the east coast, longshore currents produce depositional features such as spits and lagoons.

The Landscape

A SERIES OF MOUNTAIN RANGES runs north–south through the mainland, formed as the result of the collision between the Eurasian Plate and the Indian subcontinent, which created the Himalayas. They are interspersed by the valleys of a number of great rivers. On their passage to the sea these rivers have deposited sediment, forming huge, fertile floodplains and deltas.

Hkakabo Razi is the highest point in mainland Southeast Asia. It rises 19,300 ft (5,885 m) at the border between China and Myanmar.

Mountains dominate the Laotian landscape with more than 90% of the land lying more than 600 ft (180 m) above sea level. The mountains of the Chaine Annamitique form the country's eastern border.

The Irrawaddy River runs virtually north–south, draining Myanmar. The Irrawaddy Delta is the country's main rice-growing area.

The Red River Delta in northern Vietnam is fringed to the north by steep-sided, round-topped limestone hills, typical of karst scenery.

Salween River

Mekong River

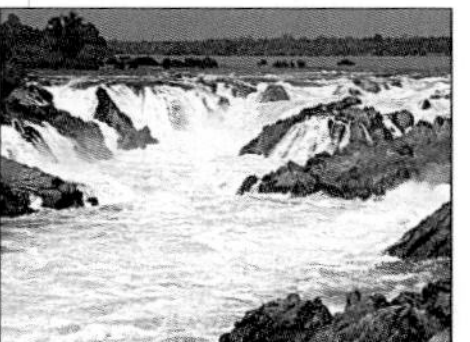

The fast-flowing waters of the Mekong River cascade over this waterfall in Champasak province in Laos. The force of the water erodes rocks at the base of the fall.

Isthmus of Kra

The coast of the Isthmus of Kra, in southeast Thailand has many small, precipitous islands like these, formed by chemical erosion on limestone, which is weathered along vertical cracks. The humidity of the climate in Southeast Asia increases the rate of weathering.

Malay Peninsula

Tonle Sap, a freshwater lake, drains into the Mekong Delta via the Mekong River. It is the largest lake in Southeast Asia.

The Mekong River flows through southern China and Myanmar, then for much of its length forms the border between Laos and Thailand, flowing through Cambodia before terminating in a vast delta on the southern Vietnamese coast.

Using the Land and Sea

THE FERTILE FLOODPLAINS of rivers such as the Mekong and Salween, and the humid climate, enable the production of rice throughout the region. Cambodia, Myanmar, and Laos still have substantial forests, producing hardwoods such as teak and rosewood. Cash crops include tropical fruits such as coconuts, bananas, and pineapples, rubber, oil palm, sugar cane and the jute substitute, kenaf. Pigs and cattle are the main livestock raised. Large quantities of marine and freshwater fish are caught throughout the region.

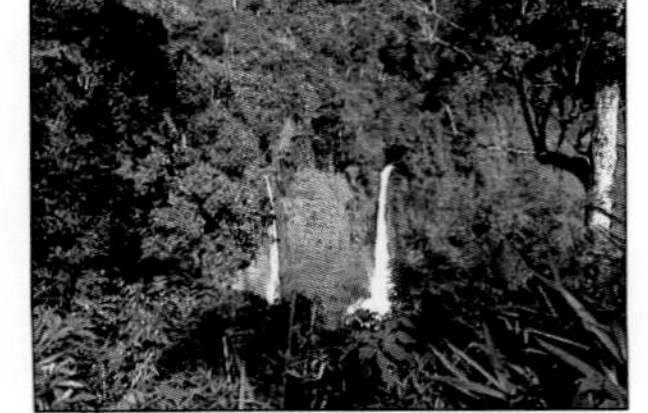

Commercial logging – still widespread in Myanmar – has now been stopped in Thailand because of overexploitation of the tropical rain forest.

The Urban/Rural Population Divide

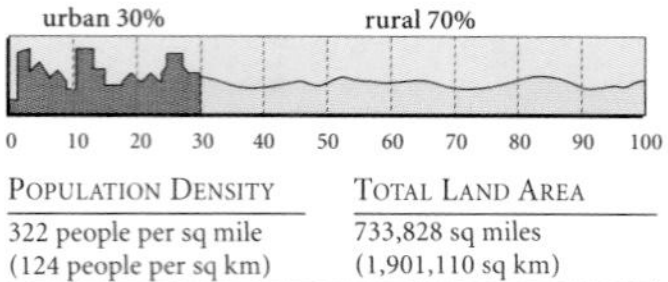

urban 30%
rural 70%
0 10 20 30 40 50 60 70 80 90 100

Population Density
322 people per sq mile (124 people per sq km)

Total Land Area
733,828 sq miles (1,901,110 sq km)

Land use and agricultural distribution: cattle, pigs, bananas, coconuts, fishing, oil palms, rice, rubber, sugar cane, timber; capital cities, major towns; pasture, cropland, forest, wetland

BURMA, THAILAND, LAOS, CAMBODIA, VIETNAM, HANOI, VIENTIANE, BANGKOK, PHNOM PENH, RANGOON, Mandalay, Hue, Ho Chi Minh City, Bay of Bengal, Andaman Sea, Gulf of Thailand, Gulf of Tongking, South China Sea, CHINA, INDIA, BANGLADESH, MALAYSIA

TRANSPORTATION & INDUSTRY

INDUSTRIAL MANUFACTURING has become increasingly important in Thailand and Vietnam in recent years. The assembling of component-based electrical and electronic goods is becoming more common throughout this region, with foreign companies benefiting from low labor costs and the upgrading of technology. The economies of Myanmar and Cambodia are still based on agricultural produce and the processing of raw materials. Tin is the region's most important metal, and nickel, copper, and chromite are also mined, although the quantities produced are not significant on a global scale. Thailand's successful tourist industry is the country's highest earner of foreign exchange.

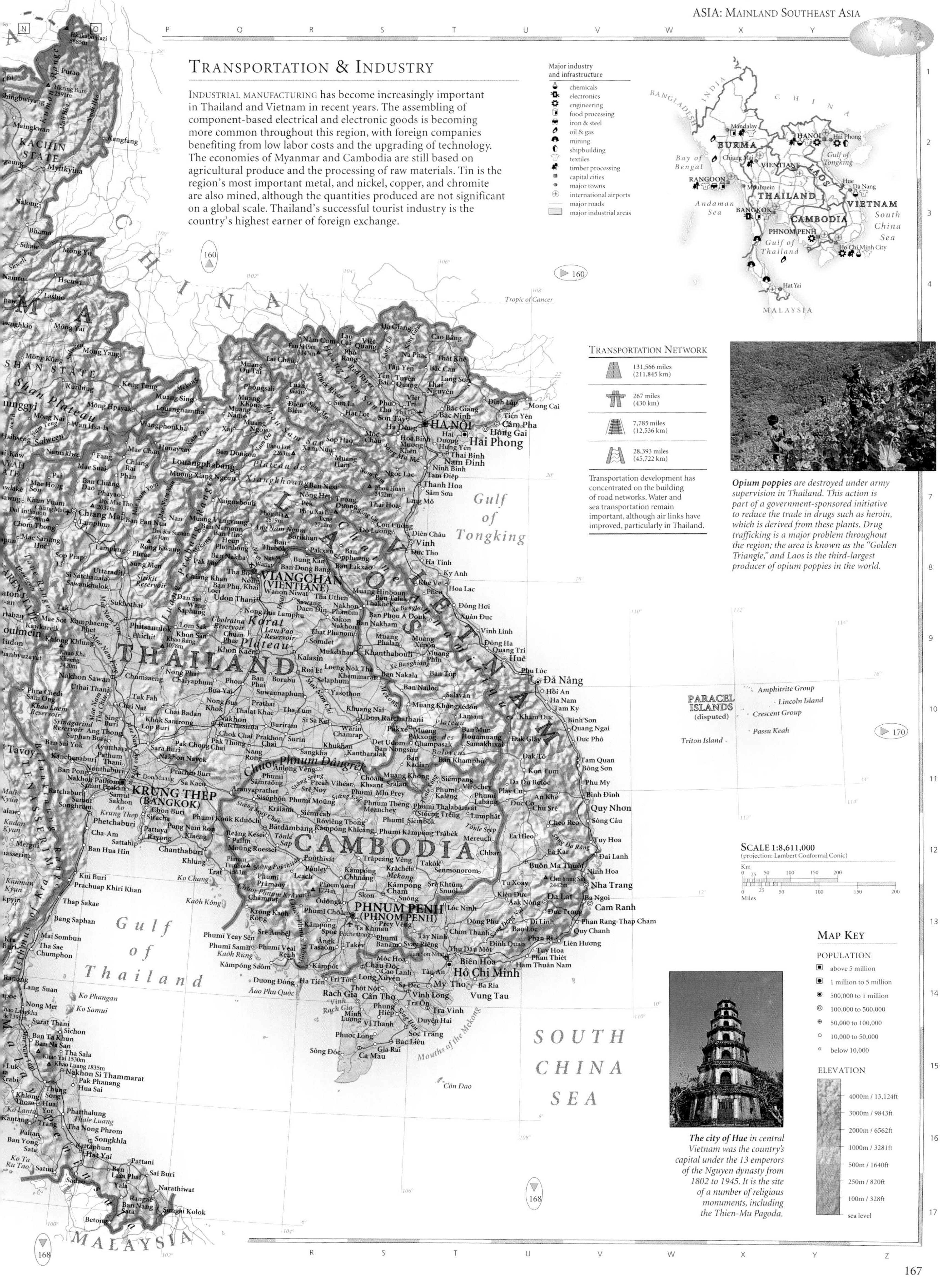

Major industry and infrastructure
chemicals
electronics
engineering
food processing
iron & steel
oil & gas
mining
shipbuilding
textiles
timber processing
capital cities
major towns
international airports
major roads
major industrial areas
BANGLADESH
INDIA
CHINA
BURMA
Mandalay
Bay of Bengal
Chiang Mai
VIENTIANE
HANOI
Hai Phong
Gulf of Tongking
LAOS
RANGOON
Moulmein
THAILAND
Hue
Da Nang
VIETNAM
Andaman Sea
BANGKOK
CAMBODIA
South China Sea
PHNOM PENH
Gulf of Thailand
Ho Chi Minh City
Hat Yai
MALAYSIA
TRANSPORTATION NETWORK
131,566 miles (211,845 km)
267 miles (430 km)
7,785 miles (12,536 km)
28,393 miles (45,722 km)
CHINA
THAILAND
LAOS
VIETNAM
CAMBODIA
MALAYSIA
Gulf of Tongking
Gulf of Thailand
SOUTH CHINA SEA
PARACEL ISLANDS (disputed)
Amphitrite Group
Lincoln Island
Crescent Group
Passu Keah
Triton Island
Tropic of Cancer
HANOI
Hai Phong
VIANGCHAN (VIENTIANE)
KRUNG THEP (BANGKOK)
PHNUM PENH (PHNOM PENH)
Hô Chi Minh
Đà Nâng
Huê
Chiang Mai
Korat Plateau
SCALE 1:8,611,000
(projection: Lambert Conformal Conic)
MAP KEY
POPULATION
above 5 million
1 million to 5 million
500,000 to 1 million
100,000 to 500,000
50,000 to 100,000
10,000 to 50,000
below 10,000
ELEVATION
4000m / 13,124ft
3000m / 9843ft
2000m / 6562ft
1000m / 3281ft
500m / 1640ft
250m / 820ft
100m / 328ft
sea level

Transportation development has concentrated on the building of road networks. Water and sea transportation remain important, although air links have improved, particularly in Thailand.

Opium poppies are destroyed under army supervision in Thailand. This action is part of a government-sponsored initiative to reduce the trade in drugs such as heroin, which is derived from these plants. Drug trafficking is a major problem throughout the region; the area is known as the "Golden Triangle," and Laos is the third-largest producer of opium poppies in the world.

The city of Hue in central Vietnam was the country's capital under the 13 emperors of the Nguyen dynasty from 1802 to 1945. It is the site of a number of religious monuments, including the Thien-Mu Pagoda.

Western Maritime Southeast Asia

Indonesia, Malaysia, Brunei, Singapore

The world's largest archipelago, Indonesia's myriad islands stretch 3,100 miles (5,000 km) eastwards across the Pacific, from the Malay Peninsula to western New Guinea. Only about 1,500 of the 13,677 islands are inhabited and the huge, predominently Muslim population is unevenly distributed, with some two-thirds crowded onto the western islands of Java, Madura, and Bali. The national government is trying to resettle large numbers of people from these islands to other parts of the country to reduce population pressure there. Malaysia, split between the mainland and the east Malaysian states of Sabah and Sarawak on Borneo, has a diverse population, as well as a fast-growing economy, although the pace of its development is still far outstripped by that of Singapore. This small island nation is the financial and commercial capital of Southeast Asia. The Sultanate of Brunei in northern Borneo, one of the world's last princely states, has an extremely high standard of living, based on its oil revenues.

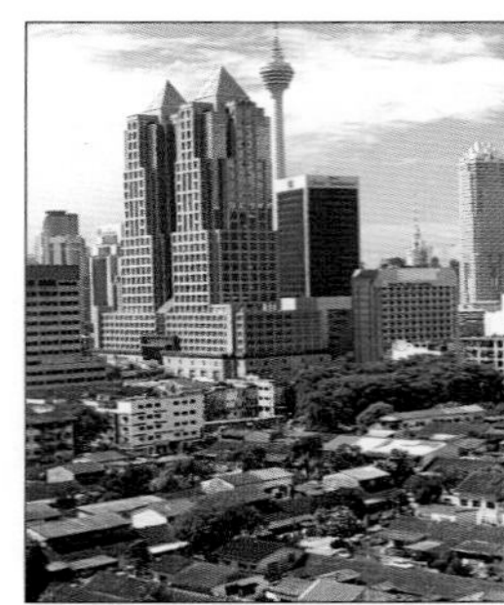

Ranks of gleaming skyscrapers, new highways, and infrastructure construction reflect the investment that is pouring into Southeast Asian cities like the Malaysian capital, Kuala Lumpur. Many of the city's inhabitants subsist at a level far removed from the prosperity implied by its outward modernity.

Transportation Network

160,350 miles (258,213 km)
188 miles (302 km)
5,482 miles (8,828 km)
8,827 miles (14,207,075 km)

Singapore's subway system is among the most efficient in the world. Malaysia has several fast, modern highways and most roads are paved. Java, Madura, and Sumatra have by far the most developed land transportation networks in Indonesia.

Major industry and infrastructure

aerospace
copra processing
chemicals
electronics
engineering
finance
food processing
iron & steel
oil
ship building
timber processing
textiles
capital cities
major towns
international airports
major roads
major industrial areas

Scale 1:8,750,000
(projection: Mercator)

The Landscape

Indonesia's western islands are characterized by rugged volcanic mountains cloaked with dense tropical forest, which slope down to coastal plains covered by thick alluvial swamps. The Sunda Shelf, an extension of the Eurasian Plate, lies between Java, Bali, Sumatra, and Borneo. These islands' mountains rise from a base below the sea, and they were once joined together by dry land, which has since been submerged by rising sea levels.

Danau (lake) Toba in Sumatra fills an enormous caldera 18 miles (30 km) wide and 62 miles (100 km) long – the largest in the world. It was formed through a combination of volcanic action and tectonic activity.

Borneo
Malay Peninsula
Sumatra
Drowned rivers
Broad, shallow valleys on sea floor
Present sea level
Quaternary sea level, 460 ft (140 m) below present sea level

***The Sunda Shelf underlies this whole region.** It is one of the largest submarine shelves in the world, covering an area of 714,285 sq miles (1,850,000 sq km). During the early Quaternary period, when sea levels were lower, the shelf was exposed.*

Malay Peninsula has a rugged east coast, but the west coast, fronting the Strait of Malacca, has many sheltered beaches and bays. The two coasts are divided by the Banjaran Titiwangsa, which run the length of the peninsula.

The third largest island in the world, Borneo has a total area of 292,222 sq miles (757,050 sq km). Although mountainous, it is one of the most stable of the Indonesian islands, with little volcanic activity.

Gunung Kinabalu is the highest peak in Malaysia, rising 13,455 ft (4,101 m)

Much of eastern Sumatra is a low-lying swampy forest that is difficult to penetrate, seriously impeding the development of the inland area.

The island of Krakatau (Palau Rakata), lying between Sumatra and Java, was all but destroyed in 1883, when the volcano erupted. The release of gas and dust into the atmosphere disrupted cloud cover and global weather patterns for several years.

Indonesia has around 220 active volcanoes and hundreds more that are considered extinct. They are strung out along the island arc from Sumatra and Java, then through the Lesser Sunda Islands and into the Moluccas and Sulawesi (see pages 170–171).

Sungai Mahakam River

A large part of Borneo is drained by navigable rivers, the main, and often the only, lifelines of trade and commerce. The river of Sungai Mahakam cuts through the island's central highlands.

166
172
172

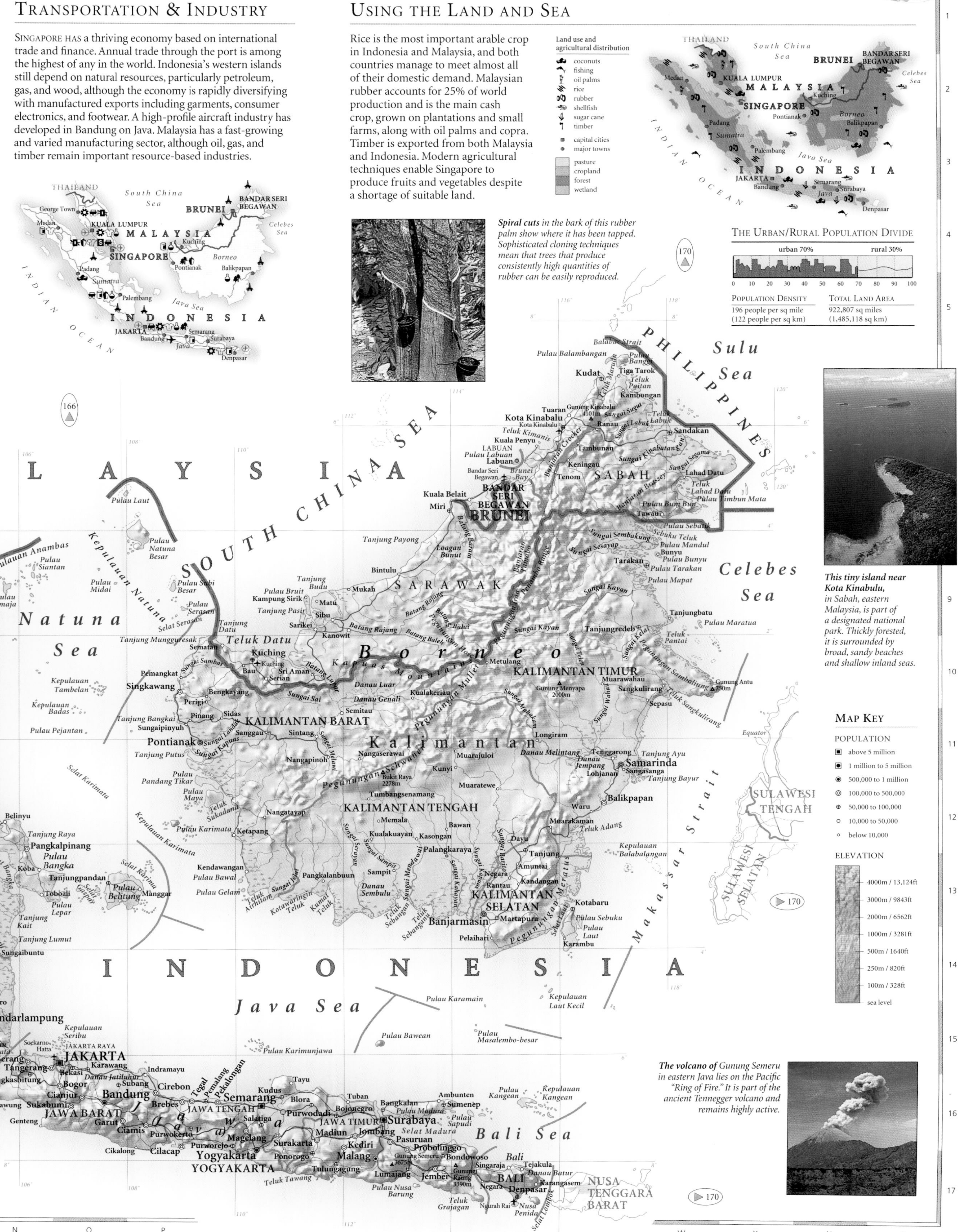

TRANSPORTATION & INDUSTRY

SINGAPORE HAS a thriving economy based on international trade and finance. Annual trade through the port is among the highest of any in the world. Indonesia's western islands still depend on natural resources, particularly petroleum, gas, and wood, although the economy is rapidly diversifying with manufactured exports including garments, consumer electronics, and footwear. A high-profile aircraft industry has developed in Bandung on Java. Malaysia has a fast-growing and varied manufacturing sector, although oil, gas, and timber remain important resource-based industries.

USING THE LAND AND SEA

Rice is the most important arable crop in Indonesia and Malaysia, and both countries manage to meet almost all of their domestic demand. Malaysian rubber accounts for 25% of world production and is the main cash crop, grown on plantations and small farms, along with oil palms and copra. Timber is exported from both Malaysia and Indonesia. Modern agricultural techniques enable Singapore to produce fruits and vegetables despite a shortage of suitable land.

Land use and agricultural distribution
coconuts
fishing
oil palms
rice
rubber
shellfish
sugar cane
timber
capital cities
major towns
pasture
cropland
forest
wetland

Spiral cuts in the bark of this rubber palm show where it has been tapped. Sophisticated cloning techniques mean that trees that produce consistently high quantities of rubber can be easily reproduced.

THE URBAN/RURAL POPULATION DIVIDE

urban 70%
rural 30%
0 10 20 30 40 50 60 70 80 90 100

POPULATION DENSITY	TOTAL LAND AREA
196 people per sq mile (122 people per sq km)	922,807 sq miles (1,485,118 sq km)

This tiny island near Kota Kinabulu, *in Sabah, eastern Malaysia, is part of a designated national park. Thickly forested, it is surrounded by broad, sandy beaches and shallow inland seas.*

MAP KEY

POPULATION
above 5 million
1 million to 5 million
500,000 to 1 million
100,000 to 500,000
50,000 to 100,000
10,000 to 50,000
below 10,000
ELEVATION
4000m / 13,124ft
3000m / 9843ft
2000m / 6562ft
1000m / 3281ft
500m / 1640ft
250m / 820ft
100m / 328ft
sea level
SOUTH CHINA SEA
Sulu Sea
Celebes Sea
Natuna Sea
Java Sea
Bali Sea
PHILIPPINES
MALAYSIA
INDONESIA
BRUNEI
SABAH
SARAWAK
Borneo
Kalimantan
KALIMANTAN BARAT
KALIMANTAN TENGAH
KALIMANTAN TIMUR
KALIMANTAN SELATAN
JAWA BARAT
JAWA TENGAH
JAWA TIMUR
YOGYAKARTA
BALI
NUSA TENGGARA BARAT
SULAWESI TENGAH
SULAWESI SELATAN
Makassar Strait
JAKARTA
BANDAR SERI BEGAWAN
Kota Kinabalu
Kuching
Pontianak
Samarinda
Balikpapan
Banjarmasin
Surabaya
Semarang
Bandung
Yogyakarta
Denpasar

The volcano of Gunung Semeru in eastern Java lies on the Pacific "Ring of Fire." It is part of the ancient Tennegger volcano and remains highly active.

166
170

Eastern Maritime Southeast Asia

Indonesia, East Timor, Philippines

The Philippines takes its name from Philip II of Spain who was king when the islands were colonized during the 16th century. Almost 400 years of Spanish, and later US, rule have left their mark on the country's culture; English is widely spoken and over 90% of the population is Christian. The Philippines' economy is agriculturally based – inadequate infrastructure and electrical power shortages have so far hampered faster industrial growth. Indonesia's eastern islands are less economically developed than the rest of the country. Irian Jaya, which constitutes the western portion of New Guinea, is one of the world's last great wildernesses. It accounts for more than 20% of Indonesia's total area but less than 1% of its population.

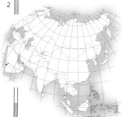

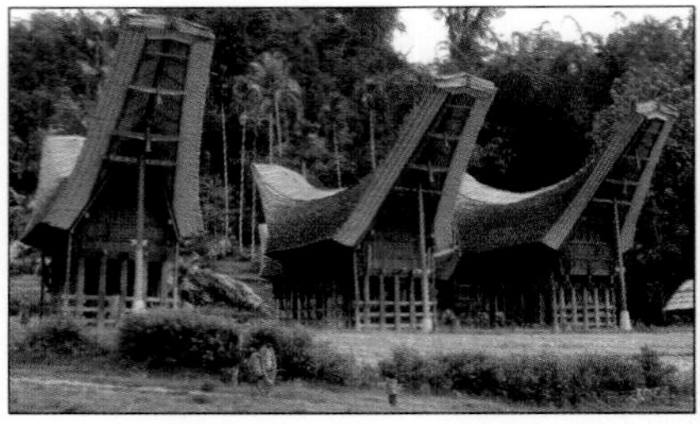

***The traditional** boat-shaped houses of the Toraja people in Sulawesi. Although now Christian, the Toraja still practice the animist traditions and rituals of their ancestors. They are famous for their elaborate funeral ceremonies and burial sites in cliffside caves.*

The Landscape

Located on the Pacific "Ring of Fire" the Philippines' 7,100 islands are subject to frequent earthquakes and volcanic activity. Their terrain is largely mountainous, with narrow coastal plains and interior valleys and plains. Luzon and Mindanao are by far the largest islands and comprise roughly 66% of the country's area. Indonesia's eastern islands are mountainous and dotted with volcanoes, both active and dormant.

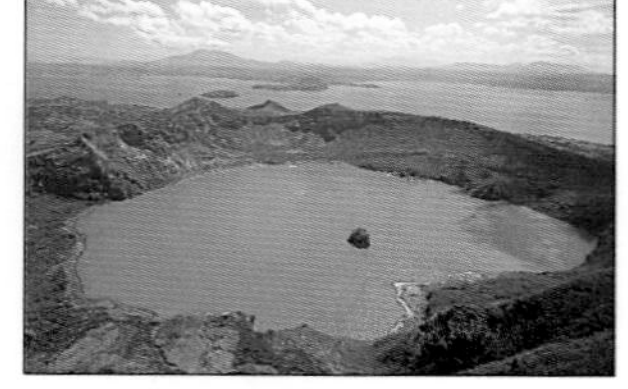

***Lake Taal** on the Philippines island of Luzon lies within the crater of an immense volcano that erupted twice in the 20th century, first in 1911 and again in 1965, causing the deaths of more than 3200 people.*

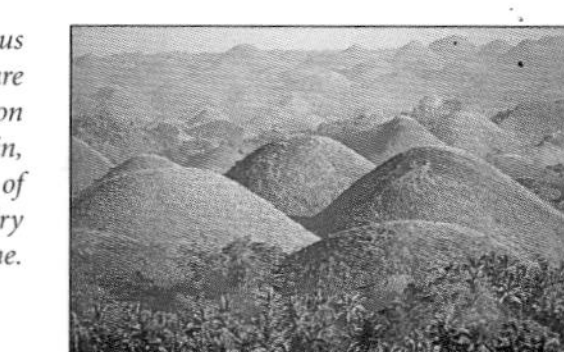

***Bohol in the southern Philippines** is famous for its so-called "chocolate hills." There are more than 1,000 of these regular mounds on the island. The hills are limestone in origin, the smoothed remains of an earlier cycle of erosion. Their brown appearance in the dry season gives them their name.*

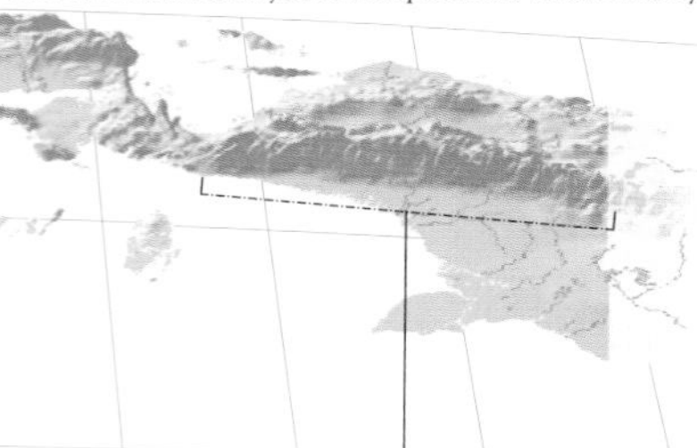

Mindanao has five mountain ranges many of which have large numbers of active volcanoes. Lying just west of the Philippines Trench, which forms the boundary between the colliding Philippine and Eurasian plates, the entire island chain is subject to earthquakes and volcanic activity.

The four-pronged island of Sulawesi is the product of complex tectonic activity that ruptured and then reattached small fragments of the Earth's crust to form the island's many peninsulas.

Coral islands such as Timor show evidence of very recent and dramatic movements of the Earth's plates. Reefs in Timor have risen by as much as 4,000 ft (1,300 m) in the last million years.

The 1,000 islands of the Moluccas are the fabled Spice Islands of history, whose produce attracted traders from around the globe. Most of the northern and central Moluccas have dense vegetation and rugged mountainous interiors where elevations often exceed 3,000 feet (9,144 m).

The Pegunungan Maoke range in central Irian Jaya contains the world's highest range of limestone mountains, some with peaks more than 16,400 ft (5,000 m) in height. Heavy rainfall and high temperatures, which promote rapid weathering, have led to the creation of large underground caves and river systems such as the river of Sungai Baliem.

Transportation & Industry

The Philippines' economy is primarily a mixture of agriculture and light industry. The manufacturing sector is still developing; many factories are licensees of foreign companies producing finished goods for export. Mining is also important – the country's chromite, nickel, and copper deposits are among the largest in the world. Agriculture is the main activity in eastern Indonesia. Most industry has a primary basis, including logging, food-processing, and mining. Nickel, the most important metal, is produced on Sulawesi, in Irian Jaya, and in the Moluccas.

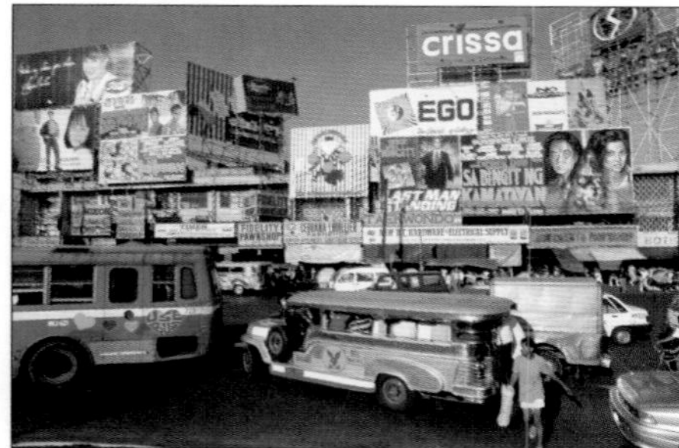
crissa
EGO

***Manila** is the Philippines' chief port and transportation center, and the focus of the country's commercial, industrial, and cultural activities. Much of the city lies below sea level, and it suffers from floods during the rainy summer season.*

Luzon Strait
Luzon
Philippine Sea
MANILA
South China Sea
PHILIPPINES
Cebu
Sulu Sea
Zamboanga
Mindanao
Davao
MALAYSIA
PACIFIC OCEAN
Celebes Sea
Manado
Halmahera
Maluku (Moluccas)
Celebes
Ceram
Jayapura
Ujungpandang
Banda Sea
New Guinea
PAPUA NEW GUINEA
INDONESIA
Arafura Sea
Lombok
Sumbawa
Flores
DILI
EAST TIMOR
Sumba
Timor
Kupang
Timor Sea
INDIAN OCEAN

Major industry and infrastructure
- copra processing
- chemicals
- finance
- food processing
- mining
- oil
- timber processing
- textiles
- capital cities
- major towns
- international airports
- major roads
- major industrial areas

Transportation Network

Roads	16,652 miles (26,800 km)
Motorways	None
Railways	500 miles (805 km)
Waterways	8704 miles (14,008 km)

Sulawesi has some good roads, but on Irian Jaya and the Moluccas there are few road interconnections between major settled areas. Water and sea transportation remain important although air links have improved in the Philippines.

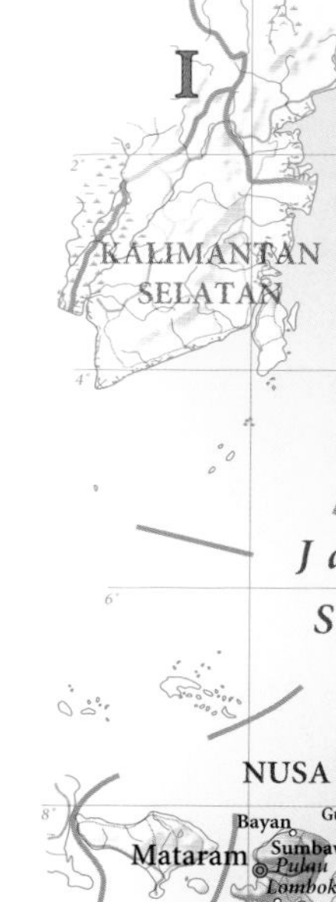
SOUTH CHINA SEA
SPRATLY ISLANDS
(disputed)
Palawan Passage
Quezon
Brooke's Point
Balabac Island
Balabac Strait
MALAYSIA
KALIMANTAN TIMUR
Equator
KALIMANTAN SELATAN
Makassar Strait
Java Sea
NUSA TENGGARA
Gunung Tambora 2821m
Bayan
Mataram
Sumbawabesar
Taliwang
Kuta
Gunung Takan 1400m

168
168
168

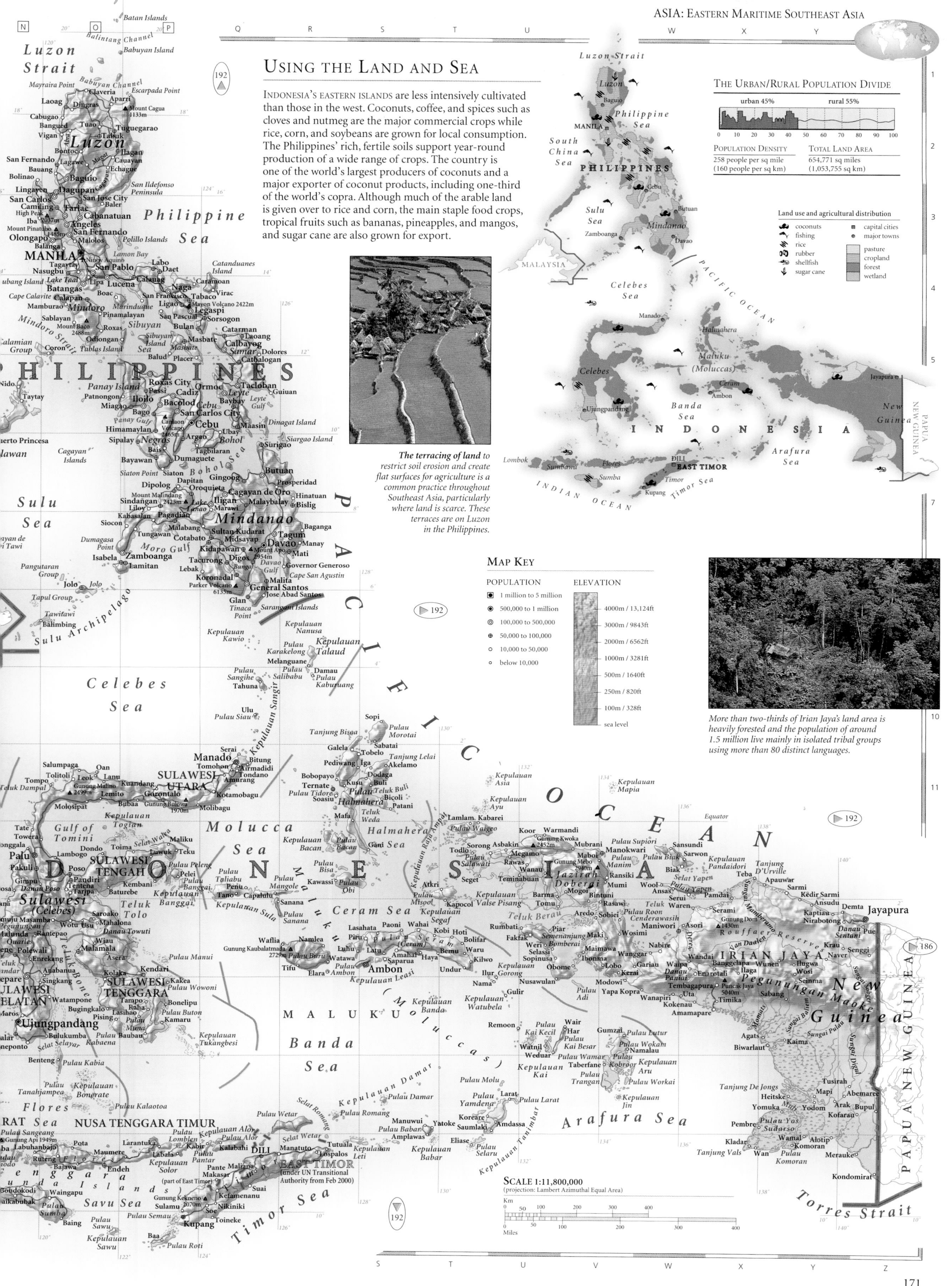

THE URBAN/RURAL POPULATION DIVIDE
urban 45%
rural 55%
POPULATION DENSITY
258 people per sq mile
(160 people per sq km)
TOTAL LAND AREA
654,771 sq miles
(1,053,755 sq km)
Land use and agricultural distribution
coconuts
fishing
rice
rubber
shellfish
sugar cane
capital cities
major towns
pasture
cropland
forest
wetland
MAP KEY
POPULATION
1 million to 5 million
500,000 to 1 million
100,000 to 500,000
50,000 to 100,000
10,000 to 50,000
below 10,000
ELEVATION
4000m / 13,124ft
3000m / 9843ft
2000m / 6562ft
1000m / 3281ft
500m / 1640ft
250m / 820ft
100m / 328ft
sea level
SCALE 1:11,800,000
(projection: Lambert Azimuthal Equal Area)

USING THE LAND AND SEA

INDONESIA'S EASTERN ISLANDS are less intensively cultivated than those in the west. Coconuts, coffee, and spices such as cloves and nutmeg are the major commercial crops while rice, corn, and soybeans are grown for local consumption. The Philippines' rich, fertile soils support year-round production of a wide range of crops. The country is one of the world's largest producers of coconuts and a major exporter of coconut products, including one-third of the world's copra. Although much of the arable land is given over to rice and corn, the main staple food crops, tropical fruits such as bananas, pineapples, and mangos, and sugar cane are also grown for export.

The terracing of land *to restrict soil erosion and create flat surfaces for agriculture is a common practice throughout Southeast Asia, particularly where land is scarce. These terraces are on Luzon in the Philippines.*

More than two-thirds of Irian Jaya's land area is heavily forested and the population of around 1.5 million live mainly in isolated tribal groups using more than 80 distinct languages.

THE INDIAN OCEAN

DESPITE BEING THE SMALLEST of the three major oceans, the evolution of the Indian Ocean was the most complex. The ocean basin was formed during the breakup of the supercontinent Gondwanaland, when the Indian subcontinent moved northeast, Africa moved west and Australia separated from Antarctica. Like the Pacific Ocean, the warm waters of the Indian Ocean are punctuated by coral atolls and islands. About one-fifth of the world's population – over a billion people – live on its shores. Those people living along the northern coasts are constantly threatened by flooding and typhoons caused by the monsoon winds.

THE LANDSCAPE

THE INDIAN OCEAN BEGAN FORMING about 150 million years ago, but in its present form it is relatively young, only about 36 million years old. Along the three subterranean mountain chains of its mid-ocean ridge the seafloor is still spreading. The Indian Ocean has fewer trenches than other oceans and only a narrow continental shelf around most of its surrounding land.

Sediments come from Ganges/Brahmaputra river system

Submarine canyons transport sediment to fan – some of these are more than 1,500 miles (2,500 km) long

Sri Lanka

The Ganges Fan is one of the world's largest submarine accumulations of sediment, extending far beyond Sri Lanka. It is fed by the Ganges/Brahmaputra River system, whose sediment is carried through a network of underwater canyons at the edge of the continental shelf.

The mid-oceanic ridge runs from the Arabian Sea. It diverges east of Madagascar. One arm runs southwest to join the Mid-Atlantic Ridge, the other branches southeast, joining the Pacific-Antarctic Ridge, southeast of Tasmania.

The Ninetyeast Ridge takes its name from the line of longitude it follows. It is the world's longest and straightest under-sea ridge.

Two of the world's largest rivers flow into the Indian Ocean; the Indus and the Ganges/Brahmaputra. Both have deposited enormous fans of sediment.

Indus River

***A large proportion** of the coast of Thailand, on the Isthmus of Kra, is stabilized by mangrove thickets. They act as an important breeding ground for wildlife.*

The Java Trench is the world's longest, it runs 1,600 miles (2,570 km) from the southwest of Java, but is only 50 miles (80 km) wide.

The relief of Madagascar rises from a low-lying coastal strip in the east, to the central plateau. The plateau is also a major watershed separating Madagascar's three main river basins.

***The central group** of the Seychelles are mountainous, granite islands. They have a narrow coastal belt and lush, tropical vegetation cloaks the highlands.*

The Kerguelen Islands in the Southern Ocean were created by a hot spot in the Earth's crust. The islands were formed in succession as the Antarctic Plate moved slowly over the hot spot.

The circulation in the northern Indian Ocean is controlled by the monsoon winds. Biannually these winds reverse their pattern, causing a reversal in the surface currents and alternative high and low pressure conditions over Asia and Australia.

MADAGASCAR

SCALE 1:12,250,000

RESOURCES

MANY OF THE SMALL ISLANDS in the Indian Ocean rely exclusively on tuna-fishing and tourism to maintain their economies. Most fisheries are artisanal, although large-scale tuna-fishing does take place in the Seychelles, Mauritius and the western Indian Ocean. Nonliving resources include oil in the Persian Gulf, pearls in the Red Sea, and tin from deposits off the shores of Myanmar, Thailand, and Indonesia.

Resources (including wildlife)

- fish
- penguins
- shellfish
- whales
- oil & gas
- tin deposits
- tourism
- major towns
- major ports

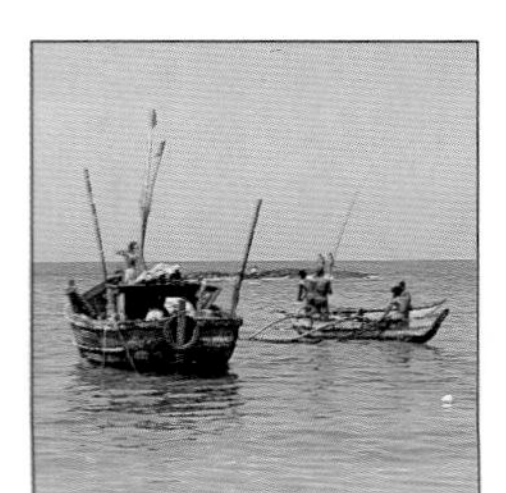

***The recent use** of large dragnets for tuna-fishing has not only threatened the livelihoods of many small-scale fisheries, but also caused widespread environmental concern about the potential impact on other marine species.*

COMOROS

SCALE 1:5,000,000

SEYCHELLES

SCALE 1:2,250,000

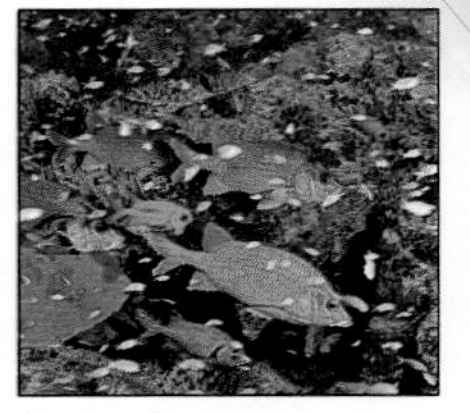

***Coral reefs** support an enormous diversity of animal and plant life. Many species of tiny tropical fish, like these squirrel fish, live and feed around the profusion of reefs and atolls in the Indian Ocean.*

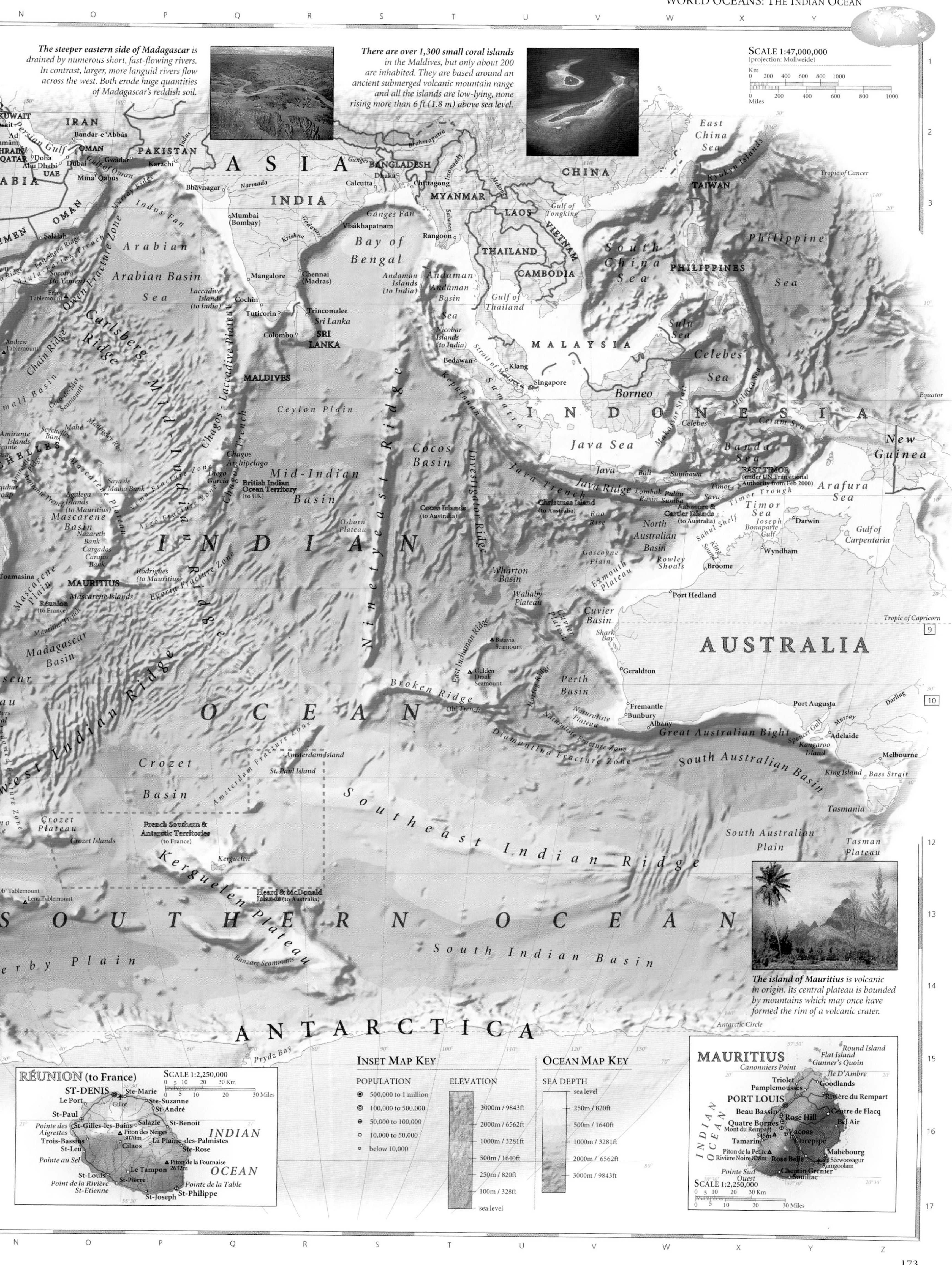

SCALE 1:47,000,000
(projection: Mollweide)
Km 0 200 400 600 800 1000
Miles 0 200 400 600 800 1000
N O P Q R S T U V W X Y Z
1 2 3 9 10 12 13 14 15 16 17
ASIA
IRAN
KUWAIT
QATAR
UAE
OMAN
PAKISTAN
INDIA
BANGLADESH
MYANMAR
CHINA
LAOS
VIETNAM
THAILAND
CAMBODIA
TAIWAN
PHILIPPINES
MALAYSIA
INDONESIA
SRI LANKA
MALDIVES
MAURITIUS
AUSTRALIA
New Guinea
Borneo
Sumatra
Java
Bali
Sumbawa
Lombok
Timor
Celebes
EAST TIMOR (under UN Transitional Authority from Feb 2000)
ANTARCTICA
INDIAN OCEAN
SOUTHERN OCEAN
Persian Gulf
Gulf of Oman
Arabian Sea
Bay of Bengal
Andaman Sea
Gulf of Thailand
Gulf of Tongking
South China Sea
Philippine Sea
East China Sea
Sulu Sea
Celebes Sea
Java Sea
Banda Sea
Ceram Sea
Timor Sea
Arafura Sea
Gulf of Carpentaria
Joseph Bonaparte Gulf
Great Australian Bight
Spencer Gulf
Bass Strait
Strait of Malacca
Makassar Strait
Molucca Sea
Tropic of Cancer
Equator
Tropic of Capricorn
Antarctic Circle
Bandar-e 'Abbās
Dubai
Doha
Abu Dhabi
Masqat
Gwādar
Karāchi
Bhāvnagar
Mumbai (Bombay)
Mangalore
Cochin
Tuticorin
Colombo
Trincomalee
Chennai (Madras)
Vishākhapatnam
Calcutta
Dhaka
Chittagong
Rangoon
Bedawan
Klang
Singapore
Salalah
Darwin
Wyndham
Broome
Port Hedland
Geraldton
Fremantle
Bunbury
Albany
Port Augusta
Adelaide
Melbourne
Tasmania
King Island
Kangaroo Island
Toamasina
Réunion (to France)
Mascarene Islands
Socotra (to Yemen)
Laccadive Islands (to India)
Andaman Islands (to India)
Nicobar Islands (to India)
Chagos Archipelago
Diego Garcia
British Indian Ocean Territory (to UK)
Cocos Islands (to Australia)
Christmas Island (to Australia)
Ashmore & Cartier Islands (to Australia)
Rodrigues (to Mauritius)
Agalega Islands (to Mauritius)
Amirante Islands
Seychelles Bank
Mahé
Cargados Carajos Bank
Nazareth Bank
Saya de Malha Bank
Amsterdam Island
St. Paul Island
French Southern & Antarctic Territories (to France)
Crozet Islands
Kerguelen
Heard & McDonald Islands (to Australia)
Indus
Narmada
Ganges
Brahmaputra
Irrawaddy
Salween
Mekong
Krishna
Godavari
Murray
Darling
Indus Fan
Ganges Fan
Murray Ridge
Carlsberg Ridge
Owen Fracture Zone
Chain Ridge
Somali Basin
Arabian Basin
Mid-Indian Ridge
Mid-Indian Basin
Chagos Trench
Chagos Laccadive Plateau
Ceylon Plain
Ninetyeast Ridge
Cocos Basin
Investigator Ridge
Java Trench
Java Ridge
Wharton Basin
Mascarene Basin
Mascarene Plateau
Mascarene Plain
Madagascar Basin
Madagascar Ridge
Mauritius Trench
Amirante Trench
Vema Fracture Zone
Argo Fracture Zone
Egeria Fracture Zone
Amsterdam Fracture Zone
Southwest Indian Ridge
Southeast Indian Ridge
Crozet Basin
Crozet Plateau
Kerguelen Plateau
Banzare Seamounts
South Indian Basin
Enderby Plain
Broken Ridge
Ob' Trench
Diamantina Fracture Zone
Naturaliste Plateau
Perth Basin
Cuvier Basin
Cuvier Plateau
Exmouth Plateau
Gascoyne Plain
Wallaby Plateau
North Australian Basin
Rowley Shoals
Roo Rise
Sahul Shelf
Timor Trough
East Indiaman Ridge
Batavia Seamount
Gulden Draak Seamount
Osborn Plateau
South Australian Basin
South Australian Plain
Tasman Plateau
Prydz Bay
Lena Tablemount
Ob' Tablemount
Andrew Tablemount
Error Tablemount
Coco-de-Mer Seamounts
Mauritius Trench
INSET MAP KEY
POPULATION
500,000 to 1 million
100,000 to 500,000
50,000 to 100,000
10,000 to 50,000
below 10,000
ELEVATION
3000m / 9843ft
2000m / 6562ft
1000m / 3281ft
500m / 1640ft
250m / 820ft
100m / 328ft
sea level
OCEAN MAP KEY
SEA DEPTH
sea level
250m / 820ft
500m / 1640ft
1000m / 3281ft
2000m / 6562ft
3000m / 9843ft
RÉUNION (to France)
SCALE 1:2,250,000
0 5 10 20 30 Km
0 5 10 20 30 Miles
ST-DENIS
Ste-Marie
Le Port
Gillot
Ste-Suzanne
St-André
St-Paul
St-Gilles-les-Bains
Salazie
St-Benoit
Pointe des Aigrettes
Piton des Neiges 3070m
Trois-Bassins
Cilaos
La Plaine-des-Palmistes
St-Leu
Ste-Rose
Pointe au Sel
Piton de la Fournaise 2632m
Le Tampon
St-Louis
St-Pierre
Point de la Rivière St-Etienne
Pointe de la Table
St-Joseph
St-Philippe
INDIAN OCEAN
MAURITIUS
Round Island
Flat Island
Gunner's Quoin
Canonniers Point
Île D'Ambre
Triolet
Pamplemousses
Goodlands
PORT LOUIS
Rivière du Rempart
Beau Bassin
Rose Hill
Centre de Flacq
Quatre Bornes
Bel Air
Mont du Rempart
Vacoas
Tamarin
Curepipe
Piton de la Petite Rivière Noire 828m
Mahebourg
Rose Belle
Seewoosagur Ramgoolam
Pointe Sud Ouest
Chemin Grenier
Souillac
SCALE 1:2,250,000
0 5 10 20 30 Km
0 5 10 20 30 Miles

The steeper eastern side of Madagascar is drained by numerous short, fast-flowing rivers. In contrast, larger, more languid rivers flow across the west. Both erode huge quantities of Madagascar's reddish soil.

There are over 1,300 small coral islands in the Maldives, but only about 200 are inhabited. They are based around an ancient submerged volcanic mountain range and all the islands are low-lying, none rising more than 6 ft (1.8 m) above sea level.

***The island of Mauritius** is volcanic in origin. Its central plateau is bounded by mountains which may once have formed the rim of a volcanic crater.*

AUSTRALASIA AND OCEANIA

AUSTRALASIA AND OCEANIA, COVERING A LAND AREA OF 3,285,048 SQ MILES (8,508,238 SQ KM), TAKES IN 14 COUNTRIES INCLUDING THE CONTINENT OF AUSTRALIA, NEW ZEALAND, PAPUA NEW GUINEA, AND MANY ISLAND GROUPS SCATTERED ACROSS THE PACIFIC OCEAN.

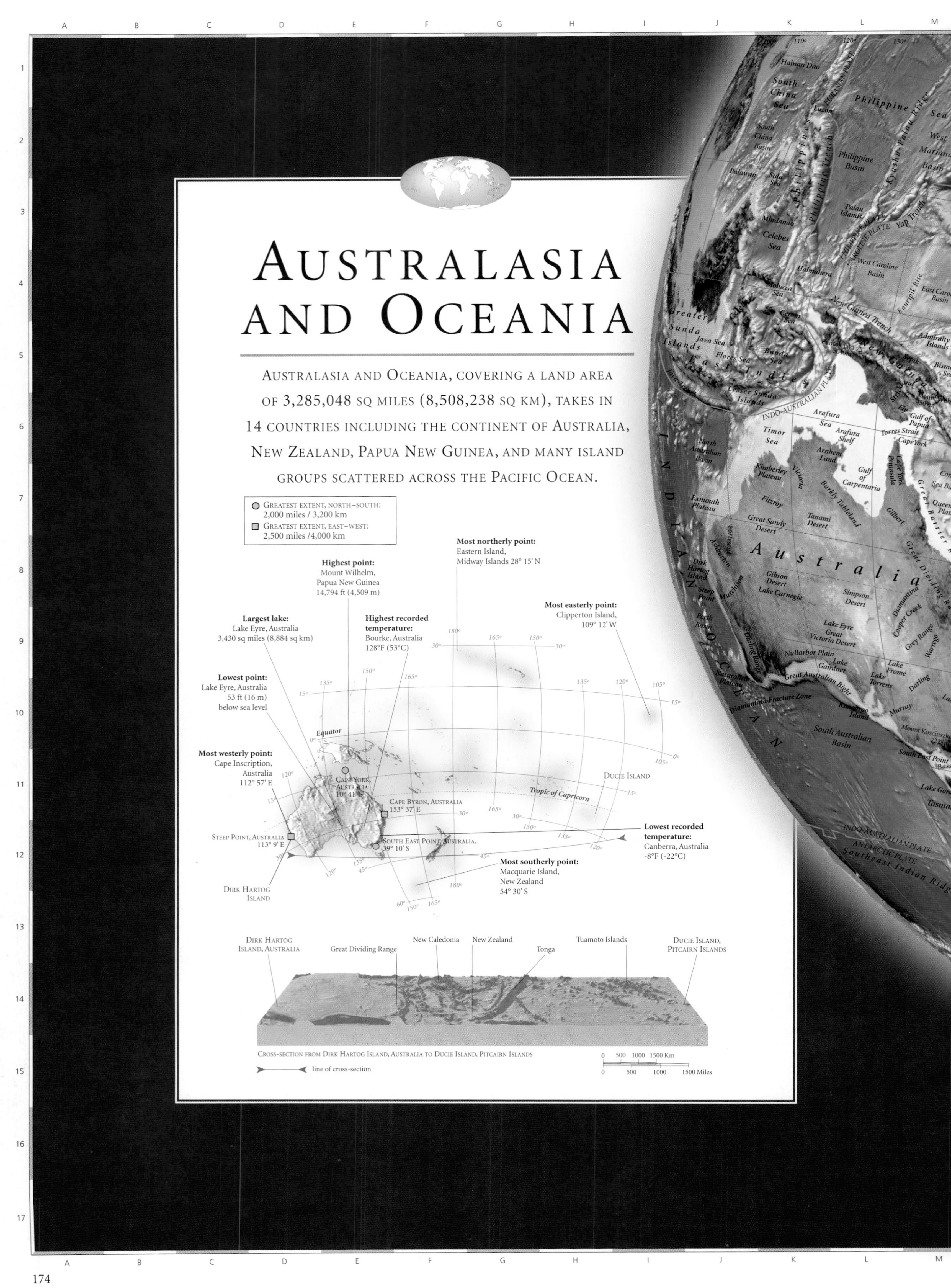

Greatest extent, north–south: 2,000 miles / 3,200 km
Greatest extent, east–west: 2,500 miles /4,000 km
Most northerly point: Eastern Island, Midway Islands 28° 15' N
Highest point: Mount Wilhelm, Papua New Guinea 14,794 ft (4,509 m)
Largest lake: Lake Eyre, Australia 3,430 sq miles (8,884 sq km)
Highest recorded temperature: Bourke, Australia 128°F (53°C)
Most easterly point: Clipperton Island, 109° 12' W
Lowest point: Lake Eyre, Australia 53 ft (16 m) below sea level
Equator
Most westerly point: Cape Inscription, Australia 112° 57' E
Cape York, Australia 10° 41' S
Cape Byron, Australia 153° 37' E
Ducie Island
Tropic of Capricorn
Steep Point, Australia 113° 9' E
South East Point, Australia, 39° 10' S
Lowest recorded temperature: Canberra, Australia -8°F (-22°C)
Most southerly point: Macquarie Island, New Zealand 54° 30' S
Dirk Hartog Island
Dirk Hartog Island, Australia
Great Dividing Range
New Caledonia
New Zealand
Tonga
Tuamoto Islands
Ducie Island, Pitcairn Islands
Cross-section from Dirk Hartog Island, Australia to Ducie Island, Pitcairn Islands
line of cross-section
0 500 1000 1500 Km
0 500 1000 1500 Miles
South China Sea
Philippine Sea
Philippine Basin
Celebes Sea
Java Sea
Banda Sea
Arafura Sea
Timor Sea
Gulf of Carpentaria
Arnhem Land
Kimberley Plateau
Great Sandy Desert
Tanami Desert
Gibson Desert
Simpson Desert
Australia
Great Victoria Desert
Nullarbor Plain
Great Australian Bight
Indian Ocean
South Australian Basin
Coral Sea
Tasmania

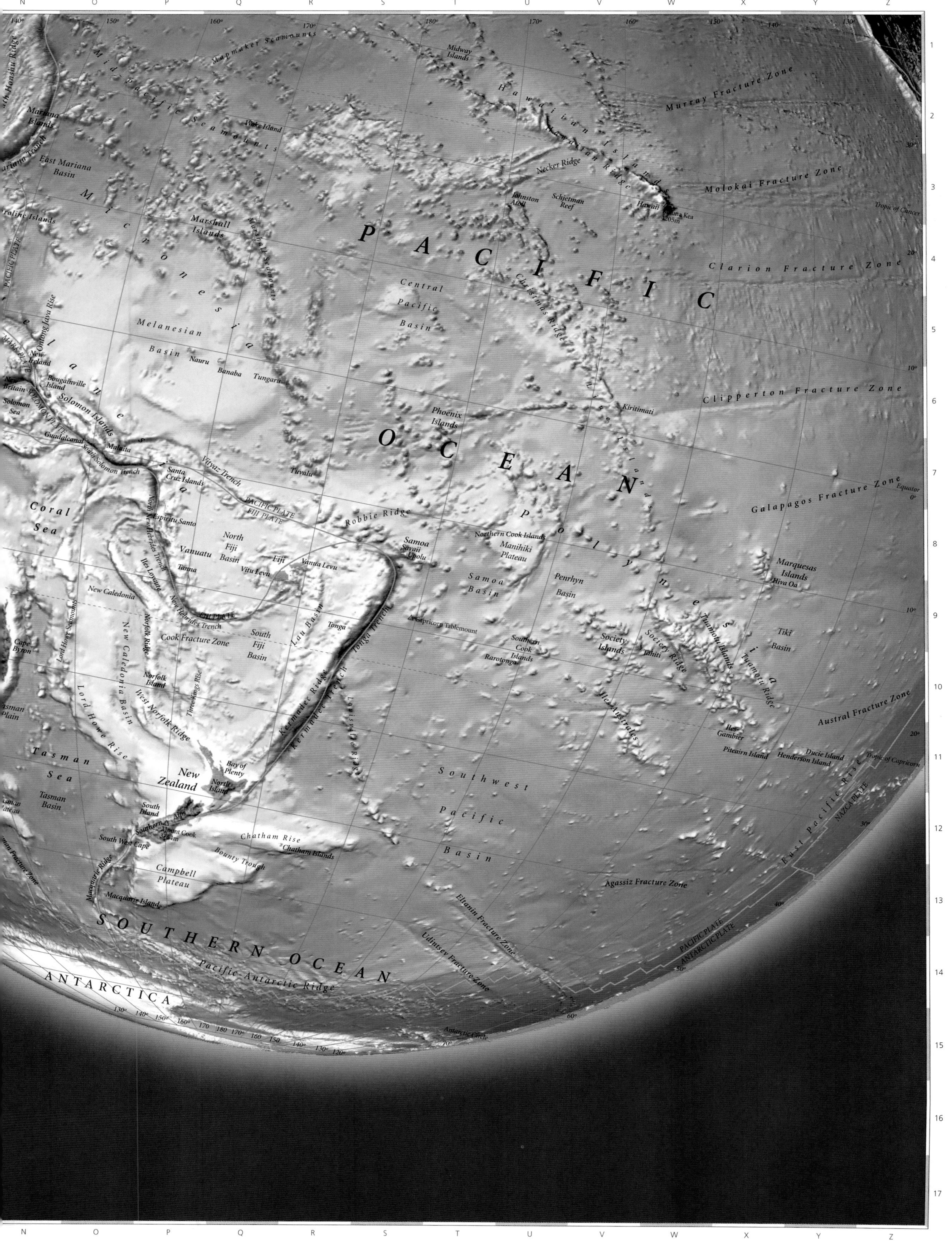

N O P Q R S T U V W X Y Z
1 2 3 4 5 6 7 8 9 10 11 12 13 14 15 16 17
PACIFIC OCEAN
SOUTHERN OCEAN
ANTARCTICA
Mapmaker Seamounts
Midpacific Seamounts
Midway Islands
Hawaiian Islands
Hawaiian Ridge
Murray Fracture Zone
Mariana Islands
Mariana Trench
Wake Island
East Mariana Basin
Necker Ridge
Molokai Fracture Zone
Micronesia
Johnston Atoll
Schjetman Reef
Hawaii
Tropic of Cancer
Caroline Islands
Marshall Islands
Marshall Seamounts
PACIFIC PLATE
Clarion Fracture Zone
Central Pacific Basin
Christmas Ridge
Ontong Java Rise
Melanesian Basin
Melanesia
New Ireland
Nauru
Banaba
Tungaru
Bougainville Island
New Britain
Solomon Sea
Solomon Islands
Clipperton Fracture Zone
Kiritimati
Line Islands
Phoenix Islands
Guadalcanal
Malaita
South Solomon Trench
Santa Cruz Islands
Vityaz Trench
Tuvalu
Coral Sea
PACIFIC PLATE
FIJI PLATE
Espiritu Santo
Robbie Ridge
Polynesia
Galapagos Fracture Zone
Equator
North Fiji Basin
Vanuatu
Fiji
Samoa
Savaii
Upolu
Northern Cook Islands
Manihiki Plateau
Marquesas Islands
Hiva Oa
Tanna
Viti Levu
Vanua Levu
Iles Loyauté
Samoa Basin
Penrhyn Basin
New Caledonia
New Hebrides Trench
Capricorn Tablemount
Norfolk Ridge
Cook Fracture Zone
South Fiji Basin
Lau Basin
Tonga
Tonga Trench
Southern Cook Islands
Rarotonga
Society Islands
Tahiti
Society Ridge
Tuamotu Islands
Tuamotu Ridge
Tiki Basin
Cape Byron
Lord Howe Seamounts
New Caledonia Basin
Norfolk Island
Three Kings Rise
West Norfolk Ridge
Lord Howe Rise
Kermadec Ridge
Kermadec Trench
Louisville Ridge
Iles Australes
Iles Gambier
Austral Fracture Zone
Pitcairn Island
Henderson Island
Ducie Island
Tropic of Capricorn
Tasman Plain
Tasman Sea
Tasman Basin
Bay of Plenty
New Zealand
North Island
South Island
Southern Alps
Mount Cook
Southwest Pacific Basin
East Pacific Rise
NAZCA PLATE
South West Cape
Chatham Rise
Chatham Islands
Bounty Trough
Campbell Plateau
Macquarie Ridge
Macquarie Island
Agassiz Fracture Zone
Eltanin Fracture Zone
Udintsev Fracture Zone
PACIFIC PLATE
ANTARCTIC PLATE
Pacific-Antarctic Ridge
Antarctic Circle

Political Australasia and Oceania

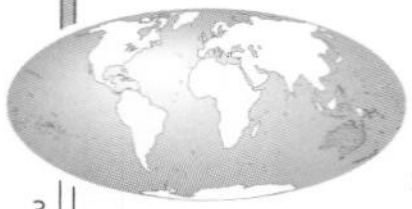

Vast expanses of ocean separate this geographically fragmented realm, characterized more by each country's isolation than by any political unity. Australia's and New Zealand's traditional ties with the United Kingdom, as members of the Commonwealth, are now being called into question as Australasian and Oceanian nations are increasingly looking to forge new relationships with neighboring Asian countries like Japan. External influences have featured strongly in the politics of the Pacific Islands; the various territories of Micronesia were largely under US control until the late 1980s, and France, New Zealand, the US, and the UK still have territories under colonial rule in Polynesia. Nuclear weapons-testing by Western superpowers was widespread during the Cold War period, but has now been discontinued.

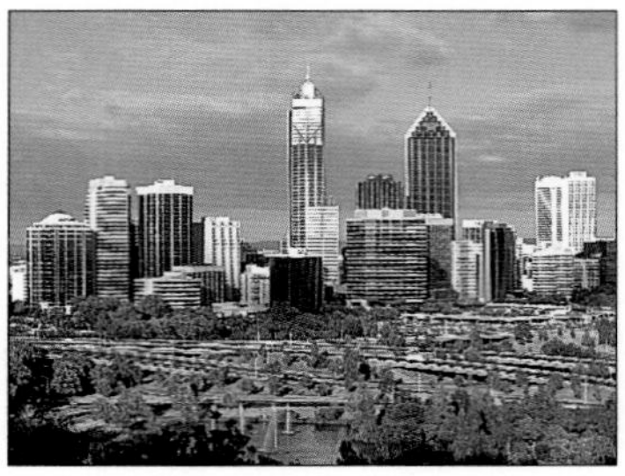

Western Australia's mineral wealth has transformed its state capital, Perth, into one of Australia's major cities. Perth is one of the world's most isolated cities – over 2,500 miles (4,000 km) from the population centers of the eastern seaboard.

Population

Density of settlement in the region is generally low. Australia is one of the least densely populated countries on Earth with over 80% of its population living within 25 miles (40 km) of the coast – mostly in the southeast of the country. New Zealand, and the island groups of Melanesia, Micronesia, and Polynesia, are much more densely populated, although many of the smaller islands remain uninhabited.

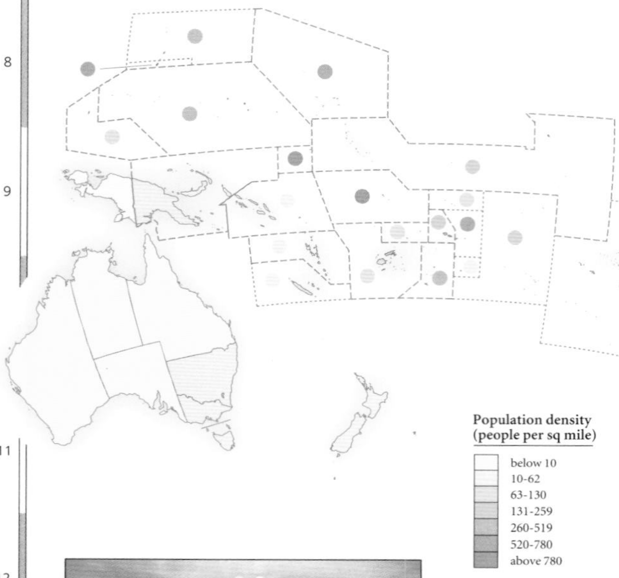

Population density (people per sq mile)
- below 10
- 10-62
- 63-130
- 131-259
- 260-519
- 520-780
- above 780

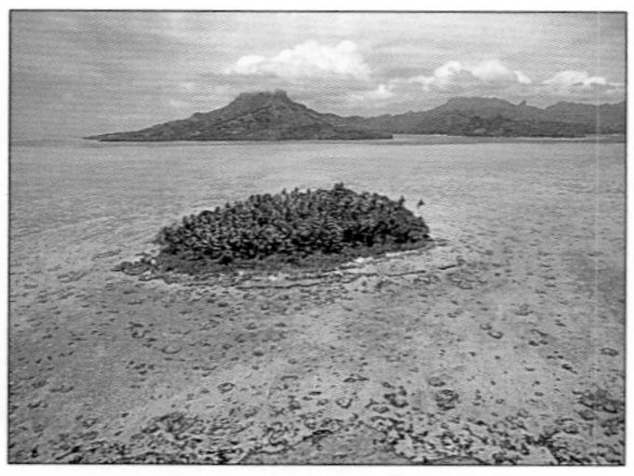

***The myriad of small coral islands** that are scattered across the Pacific Ocean are often uninhabited, as they offer little shelter from the weather, often no fresh water, and only limited food supplies.*

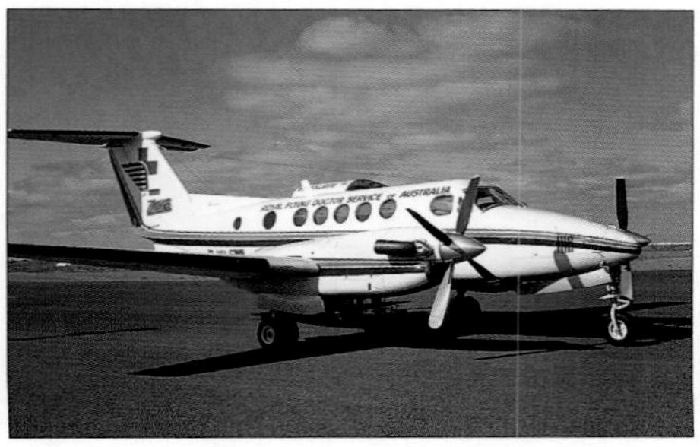

***The planes** of the Australian Royal Flying Doctor Service are able to cover large expanses of barren land quickly, bringing medical treatment to the most inaccessible and far-flung places.*

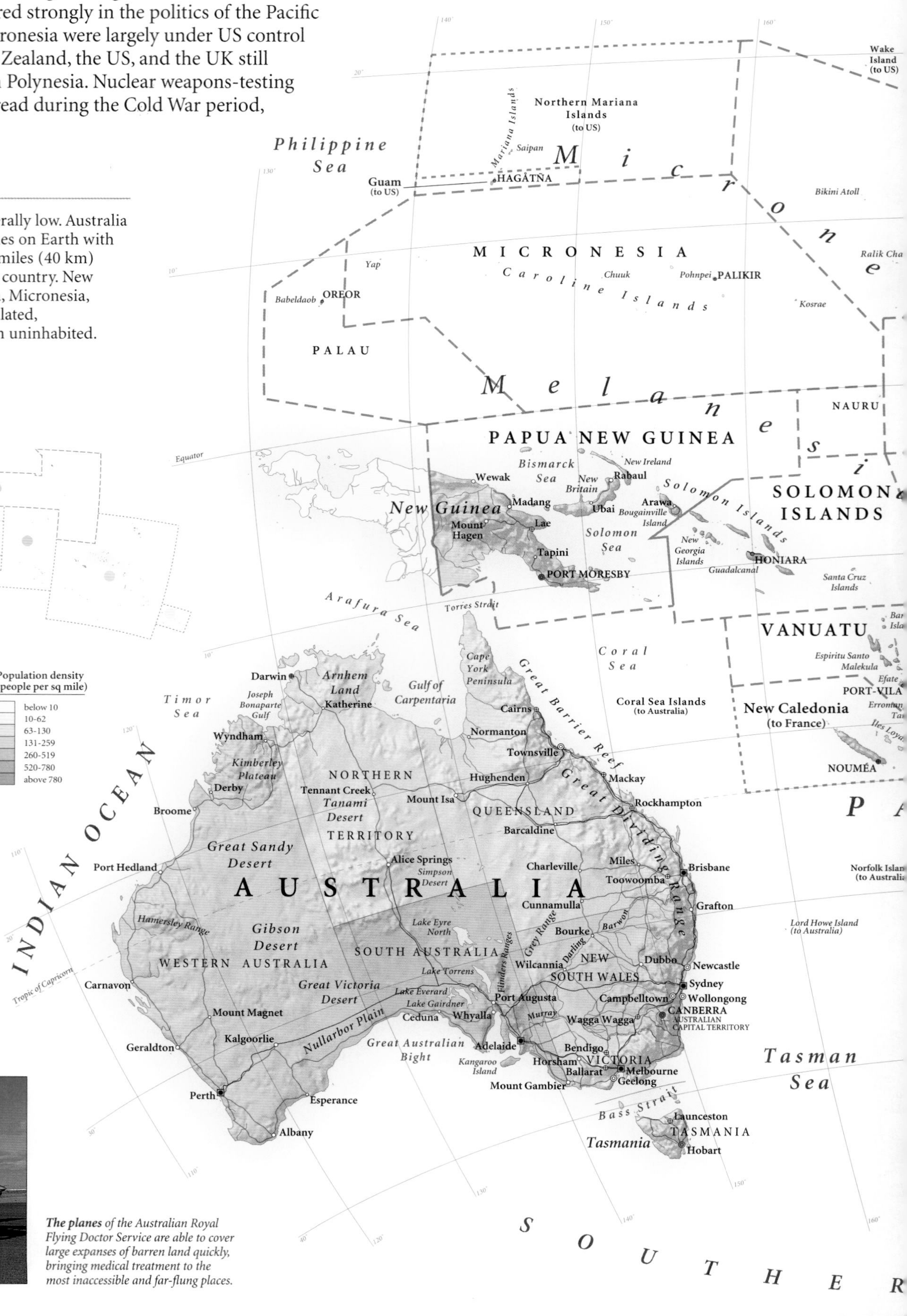

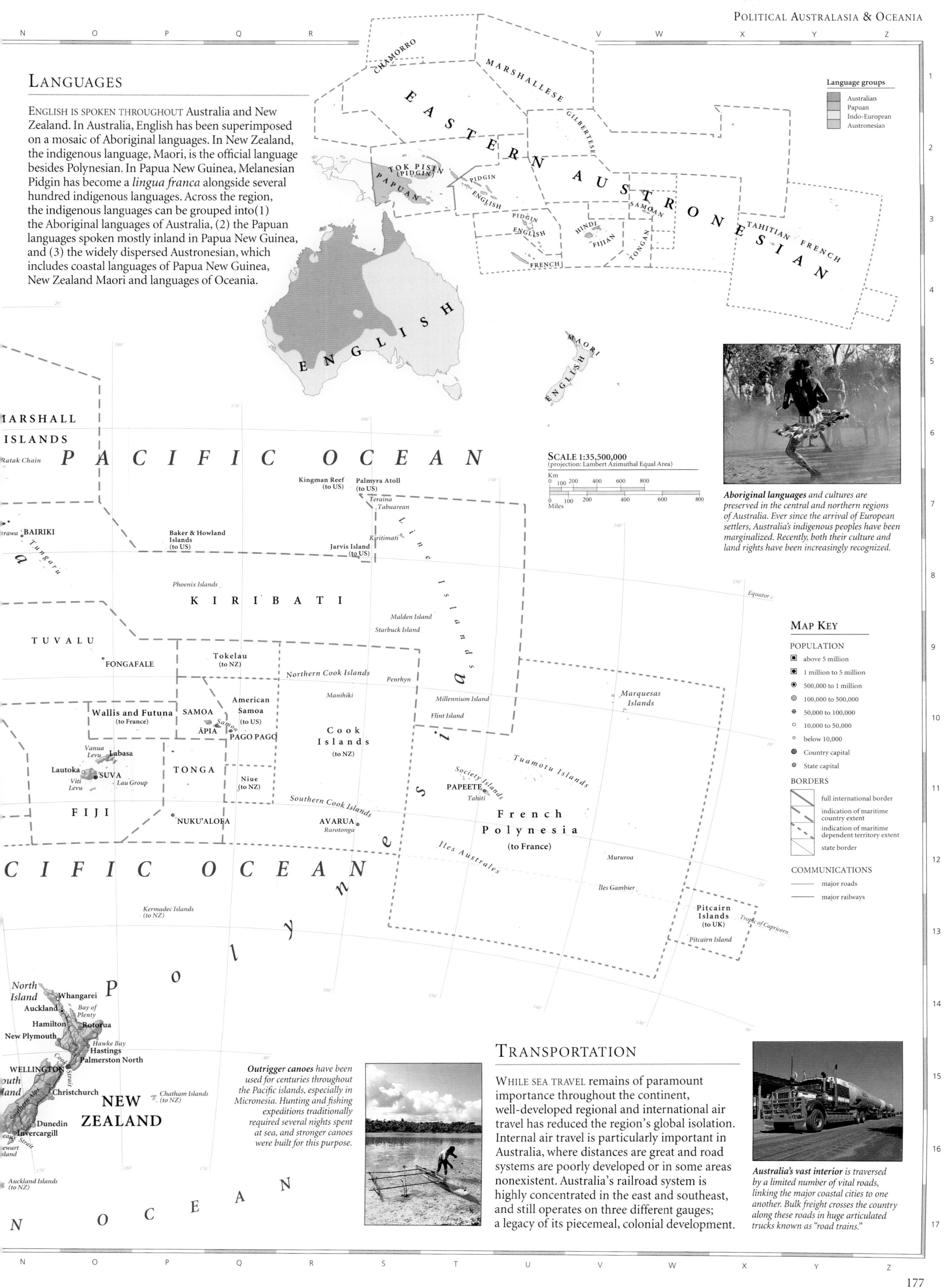
Language groups
Australian
Papuan
Indo-European
Austronesian
CHAMORRO
MARSHALLESE
GILBERTESE
EASTERN AUSTRONESIAN
TOK PISIN (PIDGIN)
PAPUAN
PIDGIN ENGLISH
SAMOAN
HINDI
FIJIAN
TONGAN
FRENCH
TAHITIAN FRENCH
ENGLISH
MAORI
ENGLISH
MARSHALL ISLANDS
Ratak Chain
PACIFIC OCEAN
Kingman Reef (to US)
Palmyra Atoll (to US)
Teraina
Tabuaerean
Kiritimati
Line Islands
BAIRIKI
Tungaru
Baker & Howland Islands (to US)
Jarvis Island (to US)
Phoenix Islands
KIRIBATI
Malden Island
Starbuck Island
TUVALU
FONGAFALE
Tokelau (to NZ)
Northern Cook Islands
Penrhyn
Manihiki
Millennium Island
Flint Island
Marquesas Islands
Wallis and Futuna (to France)
SAMOA
ĀPIA
Samoa
American Samoa (to US)
PAGO PAGO
Cook Islands (to NZ)
Vanua Levu
Labasa
Lautoka
SUVA
Viti Levu
Lau Group
TONGA
Niue (to NZ)
FIJI
NUKU'ALOFA
Southern Cook Islands
AVARUA
Rarotonga
Society Islands
PAPEETE
Tahiti
Tuamotu Islands
French Polynesia (to France)
Îles Australes
Mururoa
Îles Gambier
Pitcairn Islands (to UK)
Pitcairn Island
Tropic of Capricorn
Equator
PACIFIC OCEAN
Polynesia
Kermadec Islands (to NZ)
North Island
Whangarei
Auckland
Bay of Plenty
Hamilton
Rotorua
New Plymouth
Hawke Bay
Hastings
Palmerston North
WELLINGTON
Cook Strait
Christchurch
Southern Alps
Dunedin
Invercargill
Foveaux Strait
Stewart Island
Chatham Islands (to NZ)
NEW ZEALAND
Auckland Islands (to NZ)
OCEAN
SCALE 1:35,500,000
(projection: Lambert Azimuthal Equal Area)
Km 0 100 200 400 600 800
Miles 0 100 200 400 600 800
MAP KEY
POPULATION
above 5 million
1 million to 5 million
500,000 to 1 million
100,000 to 500,000
50,000 to 100,000
10,000 to 50,000
below 10,000
Country capital
State capital
BORDERS
full international border
indication of maritime country extent
indication of maritime dependent territory extent
state border
COMMUNICATIONS
major roads
major railways

LANGUAGES

ENGLISH IS SPOKEN THROUGHOUT Australia and New Zealand. In Australia, English has been superimposed on a mosaic of Aboriginal languages. In New Zealand, the indigenous language, Maori, is the official language besides Polynesian. In Papua New Guinea, Melanesian Pidgin has become a *lingua franca* alongside several hundred indigenous languages. Across the region, the indigenous languages can be grouped into(1) the Aboriginal languages of Australia, (2) the Papuan languages spoken mostly inland in Papua New Guinea, and (3) the widely dispersed Austronesian, which includes coastal languages of Papua New Guinea, New Zealand Maori and languages of Oceania.

***Aboriginal languages** and cultures are preserved in the central and northern regions of Australia. Ever since the arrival of European settlers, Australia's indigenous peoples have been marginalized. Recently, both their culture and land rights have been increasingly recognized.*

***Outrigger canoes** have been used for centuries throughout the Pacific islands, especially in Micronesia. Hunting and fishing expeditions traditionally required several nights spent at sea, and stronger canoes were built for this purpose.*

TRANSPORTATION

WHILE SEA TRAVEL remains of paramount importance throughout the continent, well-developed regional and international air travel has reduced the region's global isolation. Internal air travel is particularly important in Australia, where distances are great and road systems are poorly developed or in some areas nonexistent. Australia's railroad system is highly concentrated in the east and southeast, and still operates on three different gauges; a legacy of its piecemeal, colonial development.

***Australia's vast interior** is traversed by a limited number of vital roads, linking the major coastal cities to one another. Bulk freight crosses the country along these roads in huge articulated trucks known as "road trains."*

Australasian and Oceanian Resources

NATURAL RESOURCES ARE OF MAJOR ECONOMIC IMPORTANCE throughout Australasia and Oceania. Australia in particular is a major world exporter of raw materials such as coal, iron ore, and bauxite, while New Zealand's agricultural economy is dominated by sheep-raising. Trade with western Europe has declined significantly in the last 20 years, and the Pacific Rim countries of Southeast Asia are now the main trading partners, as well as a source of new settlers to the region. Australasia and Oceania's greatest resources are its climate and environment; tourism increasingly provides a vital source of income for the whole continent.

***The largely unpolluted** waters of the Pacific Ocean support rich and varied marine life, much of which is farmed commercially. Here, oysters are gathered for market off the coast of New Zealand's South Island.*

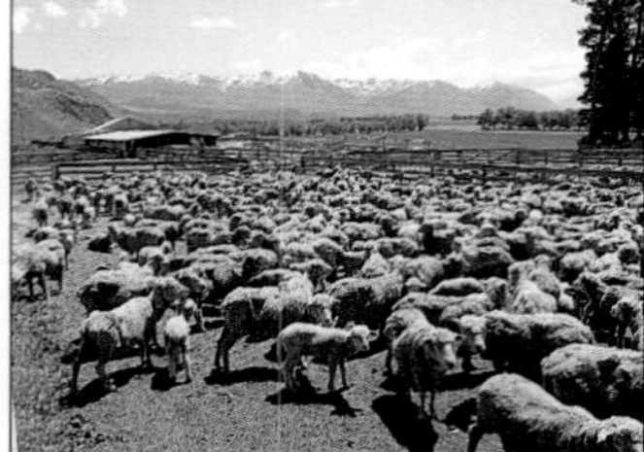

***Huge flocks of sheep** are a common sight in New Zealand, where they outnumber people by 20 to 1. New Zealand is one of the world's largest exporters of wool and frozen lamb.*

Standard of Living

IN MARKED CONTRAST TO ITS NEIGHBOR, Australia, with one of the world's highest life expectancies and standards of living, Papua New Guinea is one of the world's least developed countries. In addition, high population growth and urbanization rates throughout the Pacific islands contribute to overcrowding. In Australia and New Zealand, the Aboriginal and Maori people have been isolated, although recently their traditional land ownership rights have begun to be legally recognized in an effort to ease their social and economic isolation, and to improve living standards.

Standard of Living (UN Human Development Index)

- low
- high
- figures unavailable

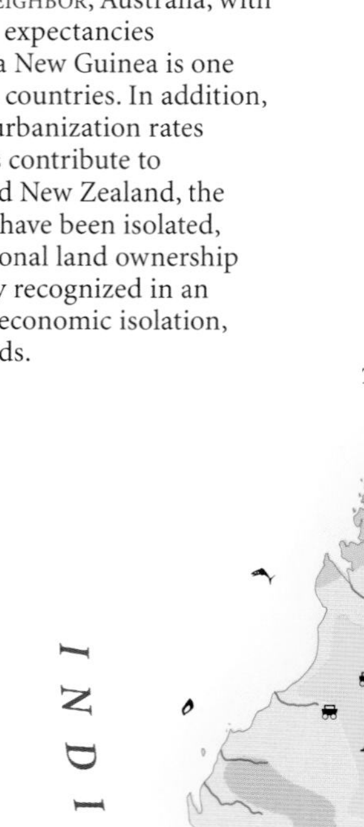

Environmental Issues

THE PROSPECT OF RISING SEA LEVELS poses a threat to many low-lying islands in the Pacific. The testing of nuclear weapons, once common throughout the region, was finally discontinued in 1996. Australia's ecological balance has been irreversibly altered by the introduction of alien species. Although it has the world's largest underground water reserve, the Great Artesian Basin, the availability of fresh water in Australia remains critical. Periodic droughts combined with overgrazing lead to desertification and increase the risk of devastating bush fires, and occasional flash floods.

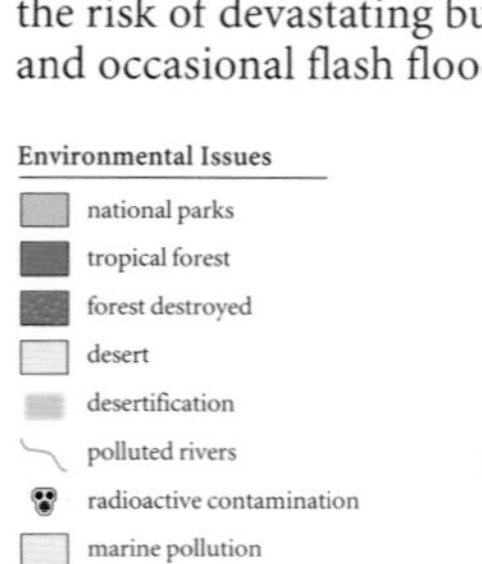

Environmental Issues

- national parks
- tropical forest
- forest destroyed
- desert
- desertification
- polluted rivers
- radioactive contamination
- marine pollution
- heavy marine pollution
- poor urban air quality

***In 1946 Bikini Atoll,** in the Marshall Islands, was chosen as the site for Operation Crossroads – investigating the effects of atomic bombs upon naval vessels. Further nuclear tests continued until the early 1990s. The long-term environmental effects are unknown.*

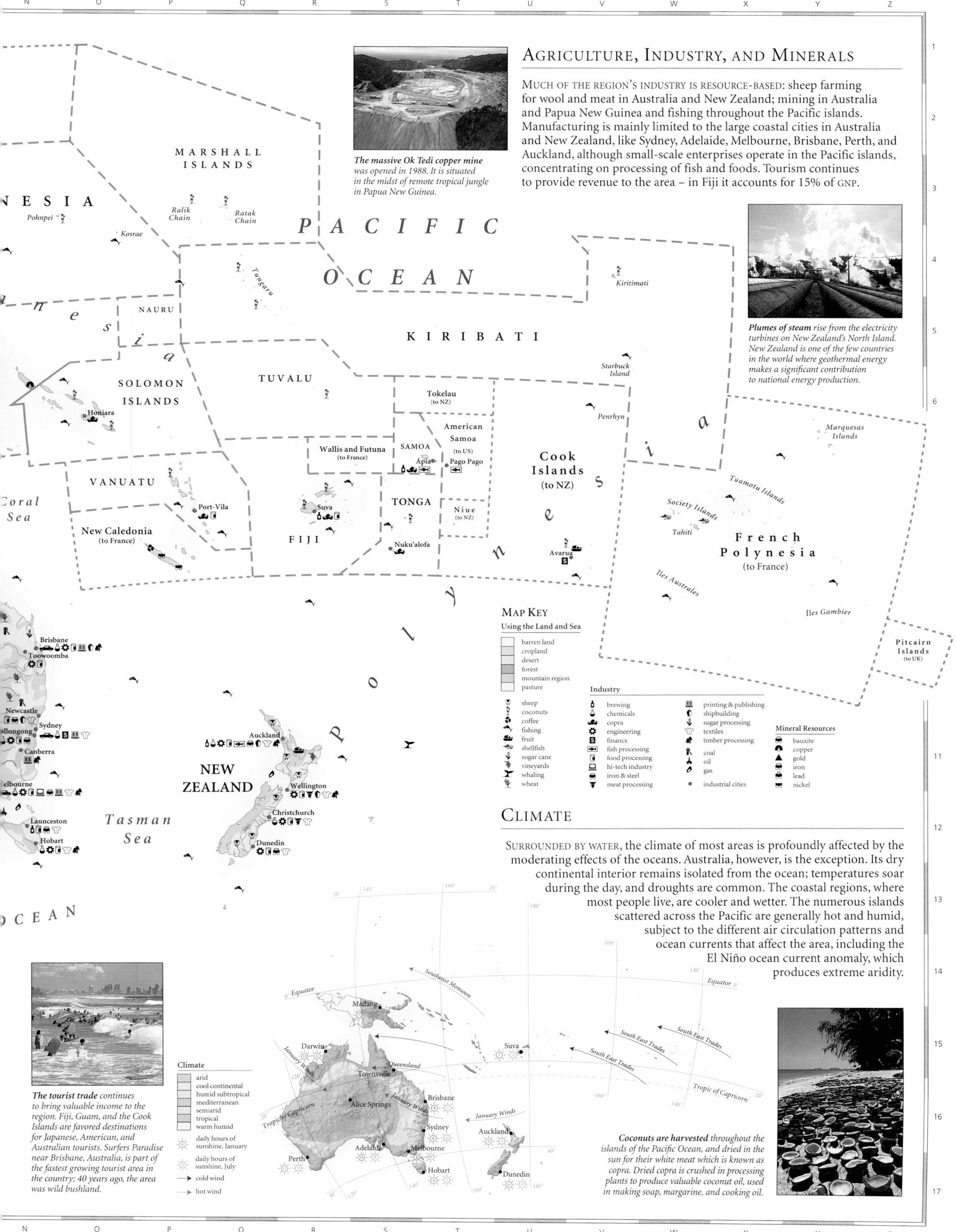
MARSHALL ISLANDS
Ralik Chain
Ratak Chain
Pohnpei
Kosrae
PACIFIC OCEAN
Tungaru
Kiritimati
NAURU
KIRIBATI
SOLOMON ISLANDS
Honiara
TUVALU
Tokelau (to NZ)
Starbuck Island
Penrhyn
Marquesas Islands
American Samoa (to US)
Pago Pago
SAMOA
Apia
Wallis and Futuna (to France)
Cook Islands (to NZ)
VANUATU
Port-Vila
Coral Sea
TONGA
Niue (to NZ)
Tuamotu Islands
Society Islands
Tahiti
French Polynesia (to France)
New Caledonia (to France)
FIJI
Suva
Nuku'alofa
Avarua
Îles Australes
Îles Gambier
Pitcairn Islands (to UK)
Brisbane
Toowoomba
Newcastle
Sydney
Wollongong
Canberra
Melbourne
Launceston
Hobart
Auckland
NEW ZEALAND
Wellington
Christchurch
Dunedin
Tasman Sea
OCEAN
MAP KEY
Using the Land and Sea
barren land
cropland
desert
forest
mountain region
pasture
sheep
coconuts
coffee
fishing
fruit
shellfish
sugar cane
vineyards
whaling
wheat
Industry
brewing
chemicals
copra
engineering
finance
fish processing
food processing
hi-tech industry
iron & steel
meat processing
printing & publishing
shipbuilding
sugar processing
textiles
timber processing
coal
oil
gas
industrial cities
Mineral Resources
bauxite
copper
gold
iron
lead
nickel
Climate
arid
cool continental
humid subtropical
mediterranean
semiarid
tropical
warm humid
daily hours of sunshine, January
daily hours of sunshine, July
cold wind
hot wind
Equator
Southeast Monsoon
Madang
Darwin
January Winds
Queensland
Townsville
Alice Springs
Tropic of Capricorn
Perth
Adelaide
Melbourne
Hobart
Brisbane
Sydney
Auckland
Dunedin
Suva
South East Trades

AGRICULTURE, INDUSTRY, AND MINERALS

MUCH OF THE REGION'S INDUSTRY IS RESOURCE-BASED: sheep farming for wool and meat in Australia and New Zealand; mining in Australia and Papua New Guinea and fishing throughout the Pacific islands. Manufacturing is mainly limited to the large coastal cities in Australia and New Zealand, like Sydney, Adelaide, Melbourne, Brisbane, Perth, and Auckland, although small-scale enterprises operate in the Pacific islands, concentrating on processing of fish and foods. Tourism continues to provide revenue to the area – in Fiji it accounts for 15% of GNP.

The massive Ok Tedi copper mine *was opened in 1988. It is situated in the midst of remote tropical jungle in Papua New Guinea.*

Plumes of steam *rise from the electricity turbines on New Zealand's North Island. New Zealand is one of the few countries in the world where geothermal energy makes a significant contribution to national energy production.*

CLIMATE

SURROUNDED BY WATER, the climate of most areas is profoundly affected by the moderating effects of the oceans. Australia, however, is the exception. Its dry continental interior remains isolated from the ocean; temperatures soar during the day, and droughts are common. The coastal regions, where most people live, are cooler and wetter. The numerous islands scattered across the Pacific are generally hot and humid, subject to the different air circulation patterns and ocean currents that affect the area, including the El Niño ocean current anomaly, which produces extreme aridity.

The tourist trade *continues to bring valuable income to the region. Fiji, Guam, and the Cook Islands are favored destinations for Japanese, American, and Australian tourists. Surfers Paradise near Brisbane, Australia, is part of the fastest growing tourist area in the country; 40 years ago, the area was wild bushland.*

Coconuts are harvested *throughout the islands of the Pacific Ocean, and dried in the sun for their white meat which is known as copra. Dried copra is crushed in processing plants to produce valuable coconut oil, used in making soap, margarine, and cooking oil.*

AUSTRALIA

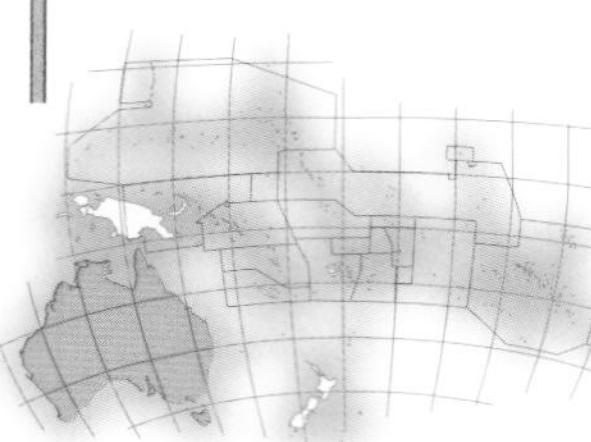

AUSTRALIA IS THE WORLD'S smallest continent, a stable landmass lying between the Indian and Pacific oceans. Previously home to its aboriginal peoples only, since the end of the 18th century immigration has transformed the face of the country. Initially settlers came mainly from western Europe, particularly the UK, and for years Australia remained wedded to its British colonial past. More recent immigrants have come from eastern Europe, and from Asian countries such as Japan, South Korea, and Indonesia. Australia is now forging strong trading links with these "Pacific Rim" countries and its economic future seems to lie with Asia and the Americas, rather than Europe, its traditional partner.

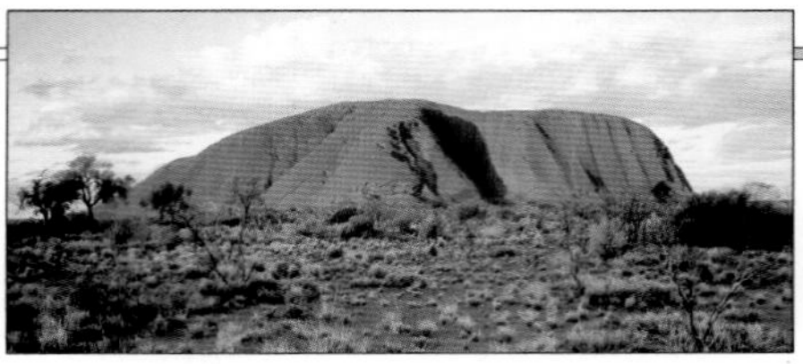

Uluru (Ayers Rock), the world's largest free-standing rock, is a massive outcrop of red sandstone in Australia's desert center. Wind and sandstorms have ground the rock into the smooth curves seen here. Uluru is revered as a sacred site by many aboriginal peoples.

SCALE 1:11,500,000
(projection: Lambert Conformal Conic)

MAP KEY

POPULATION	ELEVATION
1 million to 5 million	2000m / 6562ft
500,000 to 1 million	1000m / 3281ft
100,000 to 500,000	500m / 1640ft
50,000 to 100,000	250m / 820ft
10,000 to 50,000	100m / 328ft
below 10,000	sea level

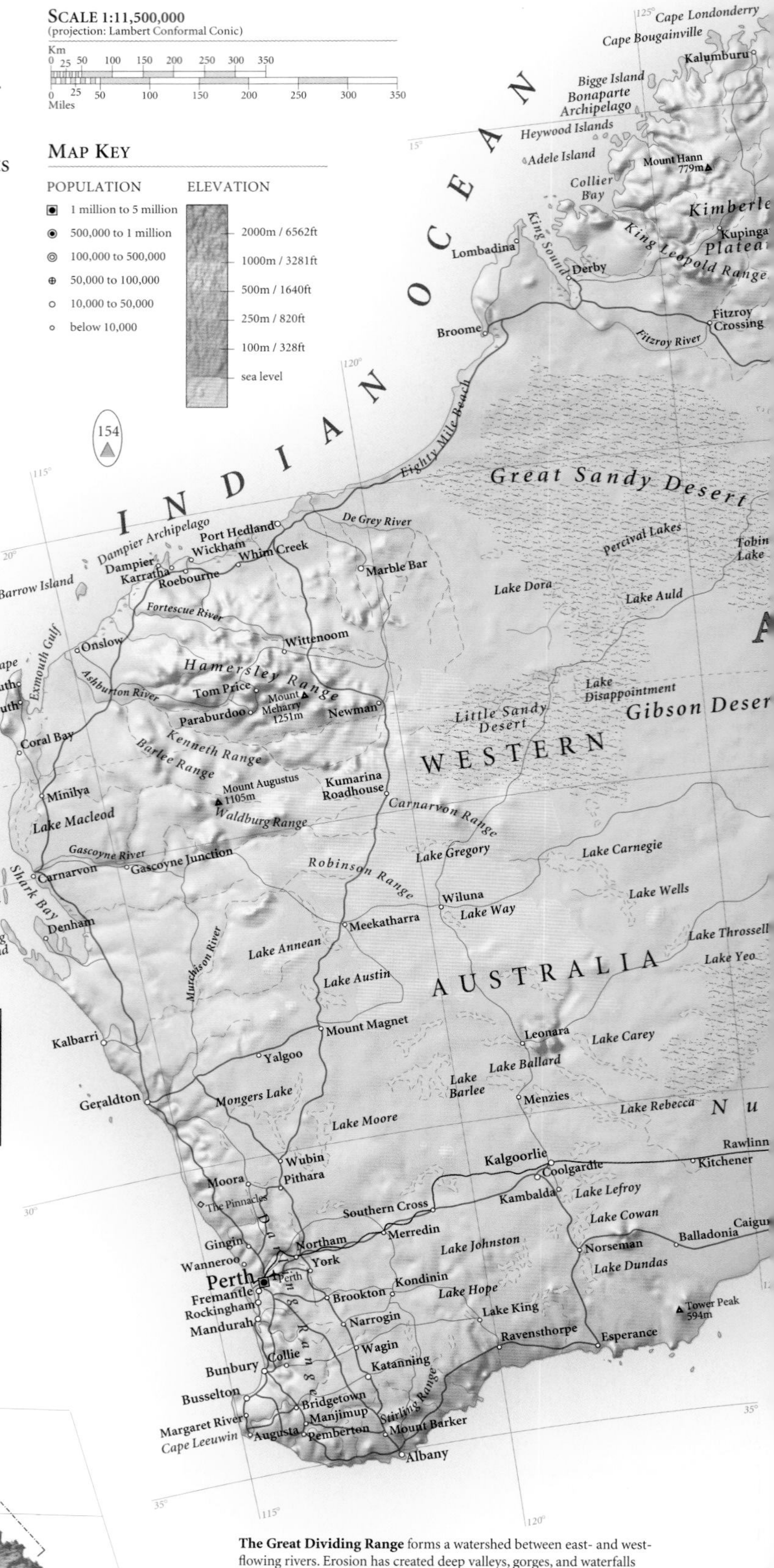

USING THE LAND

OVER 165 MILLION SHEEP are dispersed in vast herds around the country, contributing to a major export industry. Cattle-ranching is important, particularly in the west. Wheat, and grapes for Australia's wine industry, are grown mainly in the south. Much of the country is desert, unsuitable for agriculture unless irrigation is used.

THE URBAN/RURAL POPULATION DIVIDE

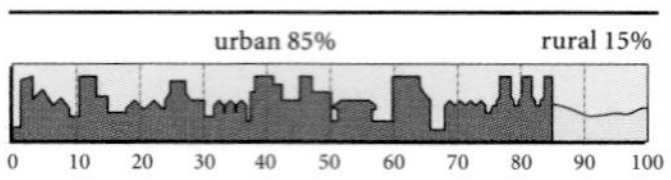

urban 85% | rural 15%

POPULATION DENSITY	TOTAL LAND AREA
6 people per sq mile (2 people per sq km)	2,967,893 sq miles (7,686,850 sq km)

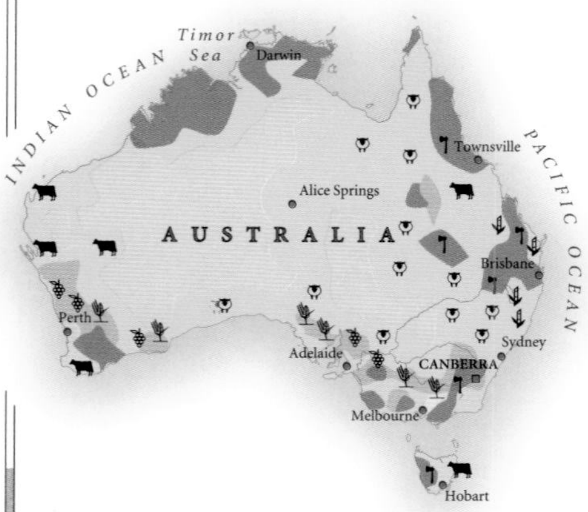

Land use and agricultural distribution

cattle, sheep, cereals, sugar cane, timber, vineyards; capital cities, major towns; pasture, cropland, forest, desert, mountain region

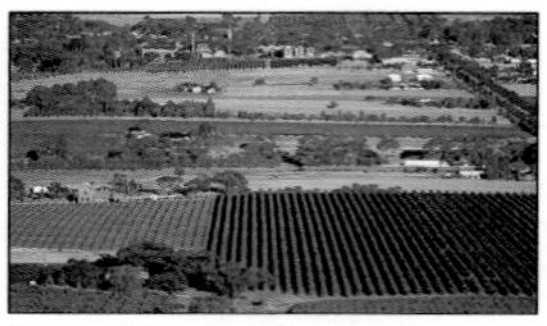

Lines of ripening vines stretch for miles in Barossa Valley, a major wine-growing region near Adelaide.

THE LANDSCAPE

AUSTRALIA CONSISTS OF MANY ERODED PLATEAUS, lying firmly in the middle of the Indo-Australian Plate. It is the world's flattest continent, and the driest, after Antarctica. The coasts tend to be more hilly and fertile, especially in the east. The mountains of the Great Dividing Range form a natural barrier between the eastern coastal areas and the flat, dry plains and desert regions of the Australian "outback."

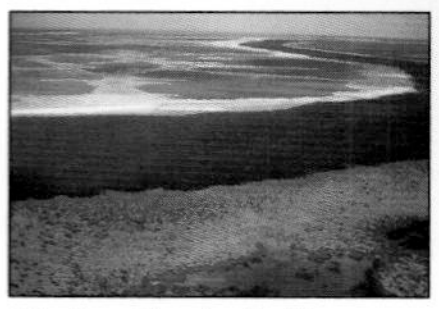

The Great Barrier Reef is the world's largest area of coral islands and reefs. It runs for about 1,240 miles (2,000 km) along the Queensland coast.

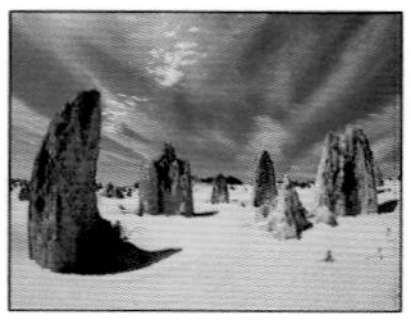

The Pinnacles are a series of rugged sandstone pillars. Their strange shapes have been formed by water and wind erosion.

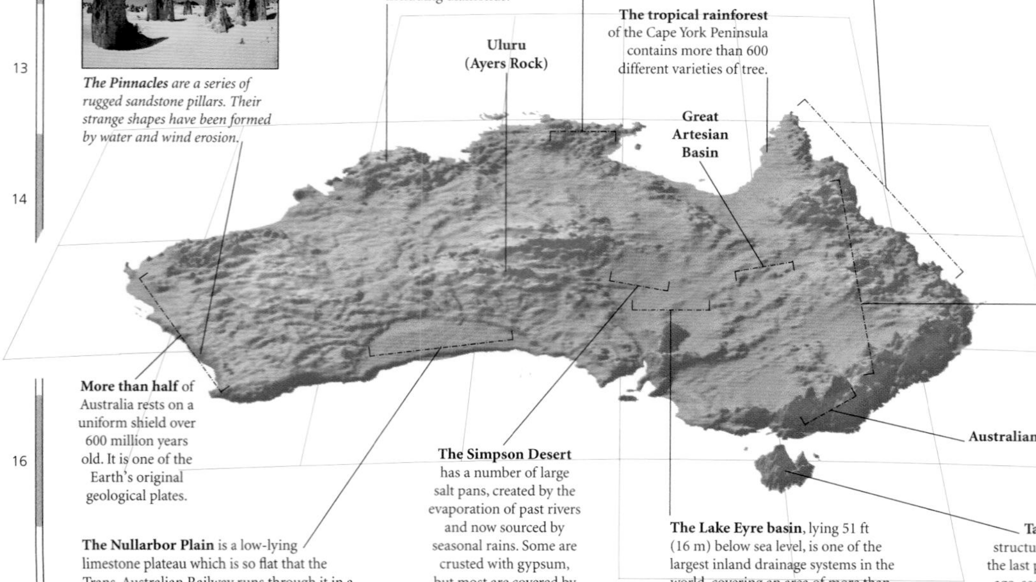

The ancient Kimberley Plateau is the source of some of Australia's richest mineral deposits, including diamonds.

Arnhem Land

Uluru (Ayers Rock)

The tropical rainforest of the Cape York Peninsula contains more than 600 different varieties of tree.

Great Artesian Basin

The Great Dividing Range forms a watershed between east- and west-flowing rivers. Erosion has created deep valleys, gorges, and waterfalls where rivers tumble over escarpments on their way to the sea.

More than half of Australia rests on a uniform shield over 600 million years old. It is one of the Earth's original geological plates.

The Nullarbor Plain is a low-lying limestone plateau which is so flat that the Trans-Australian Railway runs through it in a straight line for more than 300 miles (483 km).

The Simpson Desert has a number of large salt pans, created by the evaporation of past rivers and now sourced by seasonal rains. Some are crusted with gypsum, but most are covered by common salt crystals.

The Lake Eyre basin, lying 51 ft (16 m) below sea level, is one of the largest inland drainage systems in the world, covering an area of more than 500,000 sq miles (1,300,000 sq km).

Australian Alps

Tasmania has the same geological structure as the Australian Alps. During the last period of glaciation, 18,000 years ago, sea levels were some 300 ft (100 m) lower and it was joined to the mainland.

Great Artesian Basin

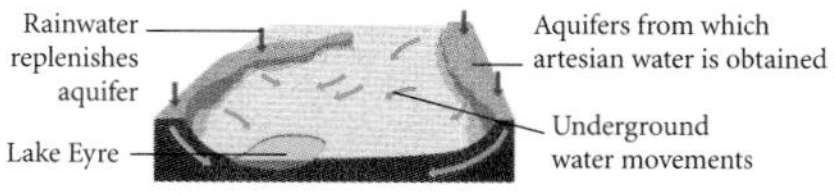

Rainwater replenishes aquifer; Lake Eyre; Aquifers from which artesian water is obtained; Underground water movements

The Great Artesian Basin underlies nearly 20% of the total area of Australia, providing a valuable store of underground water, essential to Australian agriculture. The ephemeral rivers which drain the northern part of the basin have highly braided courses and, in consequence, the area is known as "channel country."

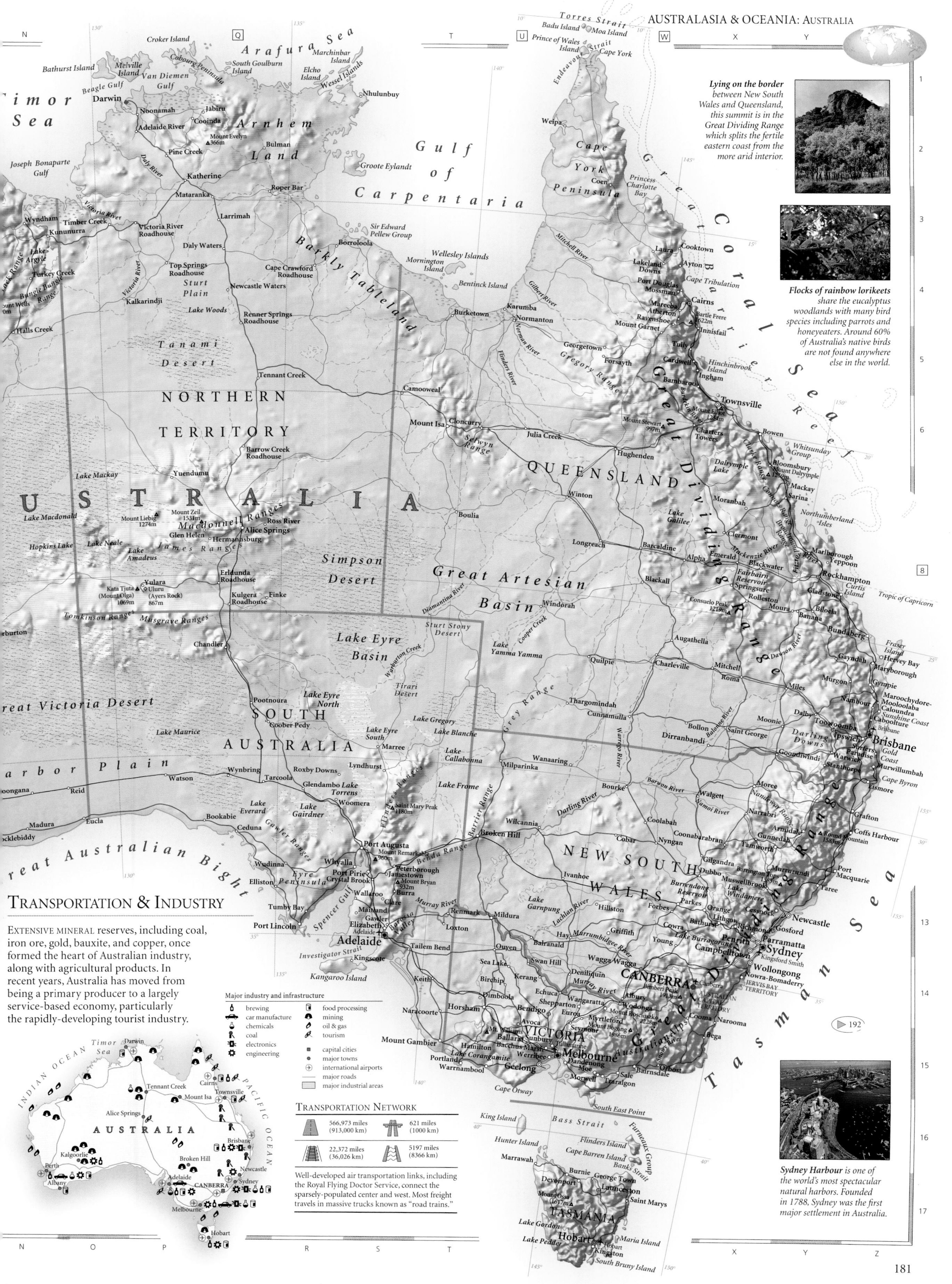

Timor Sea
Arafura Sea
Gulf of Carpentaria
Coral Sea
Great Barrier Reef
Tasman Sea
Great Australian Bight
Torres Strait
Bass Strait
Arnhem Land
Cape York Peninsula
Barkly Tableland
Tanami Desert
Simpson Desert
Great Artesian Basin
Lake Eyre Basin
Great Victoria Desert
Sturt Stony Desert
Great Dividing Range
Macdonnell Ranges
Musgrave Ranges
Flinders Ranges
NORTHERN TERRITORY
QUEENSLAND
SOUTH AUSTRALIA
NEW SOUTH WALES
VICTORIA
TASMANIA
AUSTRALIA
Darwin
Katherine
Tennant Creek
Alice Springs
Mount Isa
Cooktown
Cairns
Townsville
Mackay
Rockhampton
Brisbane
Gold Coast
Newcastle
Sydney
Wollongong
CANBERRA
Melbourne
Geelong
Adelaide
Port Augusta
Broken Hill
Hobart
Launceston
Tropic of Capricorn
Major industry and infrastructure
brewing
car manufacture
chemicals
coal
electronics
engineering
food processing
mining
oil & gas
tourism
capital cities
major towns
international airports
major roads
major industrial areas
INDIAN OCEAN
PACIFIC OCEAN
Timor Sea
Darwin
Tennant Creek
Mount Isa
Cairns
Townsville
Alice Springs
AUSTRALIA
Brisbane
Kalgoorlie
Broken Hill
Newcastle
Perth
Albany
Adelaide
CANBERRA
Sydney
Melbourne
Hobart

Lying on the border between New South Wales and Queensland, this summit is in the Great Dividing Range which splits the fertile eastern coast from the more arid interior.

Flocks of rainbow lorikeets share the eucalyptus woodlands with many bird species including parrots and honeyeaters. Around 60% of Australia's native birds are not found anywhere else in the world.

Transportation & Industry

EXTENSIVE MINERAL reserves, including coal, iron ore, gold, bauxite, and copper, once formed the heart of Australian industry, along with agricultural products. In recent years, Australia has moved from being a primary producer to a largely service-based economy, particularly the rapidly-developing tourist industry.

Transportation Network

566,973 miles (913,000 km)	621 miles (1000 km)
22,372 miles (36,026 km)	5197 miles (8366 km)

Well-developed air transportation links, including the Royal Flying Doctor Service, connect the sparsely-populated center and west. Most freight travels in massive trucks known as "road trains."

Sydney Harbour is one of the world's most spectacular natural harbors. Founded in 1788, Sydney was the first major settlement in Australia.

192

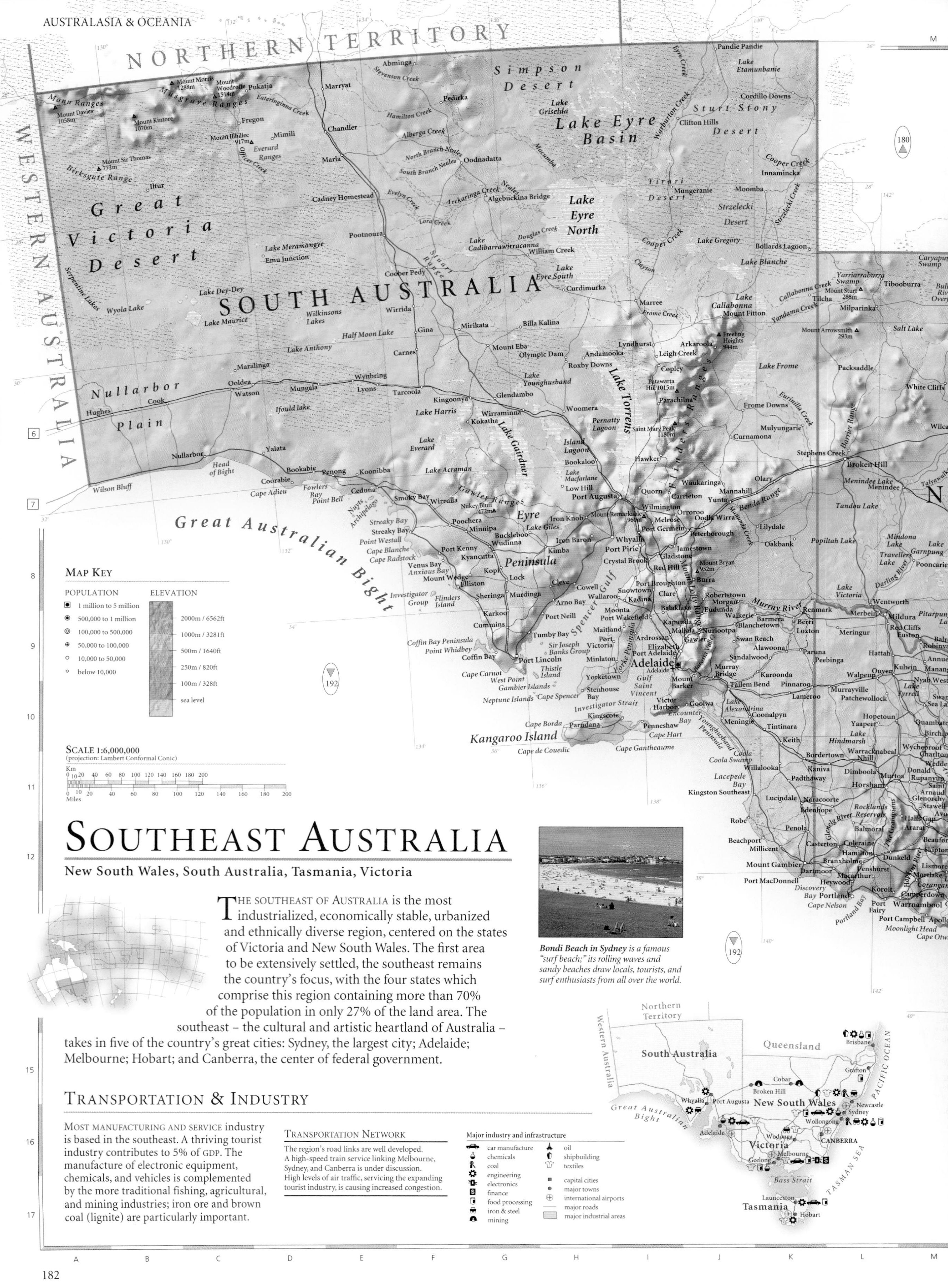
NORTHERN TERRITORY
WESTERN AUSTRALIA
SOUTH AUSTRALIA
Great Victoria Desert
Nullarbor Plain
Simpson Desert
Lake Eyre Basin
Sturt Stony Desert
Lake Eyre North
Lake Torrens
Flinders Ranges
Eyre Peninsula
Great Australian Bight
Kangaroo Island
Adelaide
Port Augusta
Whyalla
Port Lincoln
Broken Hill
Mount Gambier
Murray River
MAP KEY
POPULATION
1 million to 5 million
500,000 to 1 million
100,000 to 500,000
50,000 to 100,000
10,000 to 50,000
below 10,000
ELEVATION
2000m / 6562ft
1000m / 3281ft
500m / 1640ft
250m / 820ft
100m / 328ft
sea level
SCALE 1:6,000,000
(projection: Lambert Conformal Conic)
Km
Miles
Northern Territory
Western Australia
South Australia
Queensland
New South Wales
Victoria
Tasmania
CANBERRA
Brisbane
Sydney
Newcastle
Wollongong
Melbourne
Geelong
Hobart
Launceston
Bass Strait
TASMAN SEA
PACIFIC OCEAN
Major industry and infrastructure
car manufacture
chemicals
coal
engineering
electronics
finance
food processing
iron & steel
mining
oil
shipbuilding
textiles
capital cities
major towns
international airports
major roads
major industrial areas

SOUTHEAST AUSTRALIA

New South Wales, South Australia, Tasmania, Victoria

THE SOUTHEAST OF AUSTRALIA is the most industrialized, economically stable, urbanized and ethnically diverse region, centered on the states of Victoria and New South Wales. The first area to be extensively settled, the southeast remains the country's focus, with the four states which comprise this region containing more than 70% of the population in only 27% of the land area. The southeast – the cultural and artistic heartland of Australia – takes in five of the country's great cities: Sydney, the largest city; Adelaide; Melbourne; Hobart; and Canberra, the center of federal government.

Bondi Beach in Sydney *is a famous "surf beach;" its rolling waves and sandy beaches draw locals, tourists, and surf enthusiasts from all over the world.*

TRANSPORTATION & INDUSTRY

MOST MANUFACTURING AND SERVICE industry is based in the southeast. A thriving tourist industry contributes to 5% of GDP. The manufacture of electronic equipment, chemicals, and vehicles is complemented by the more traditional fishing, agricultural, and mining industries; iron ore and brown coal (lignite) are particularly important.

TRANSPORTATION NETWORK

The region's road links are well developed. A high-speed train service linking Melbourne, Sydney, and Canberra is under discussion. High levels of air traffic, servicing the expanding tourist industry, is causing increased congestion.

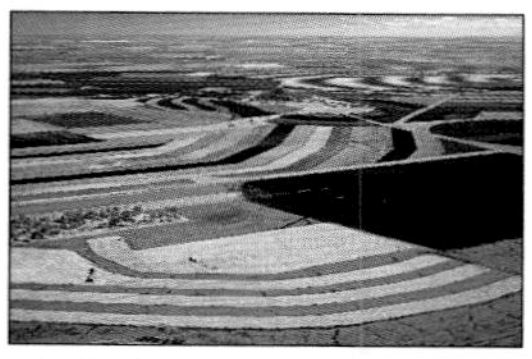

USING THE LAND AND SEA

THE WESTERN FLANKS of the Great Dividing Range and the northern deserts of South Australia support massive herds of sheep and cattle, while more intensive stockrearing occurs near the cities. Sugar cane is the most important industrial crop, and cereal grains including wheat, corn, barley, and sorghum are also grown. Grapes, citrus, and orchard fruits are among the wide range of fruit and vegetables cultivated in this region. Tasmania's forestry and fishing contributes to over one-third of the state's exports.

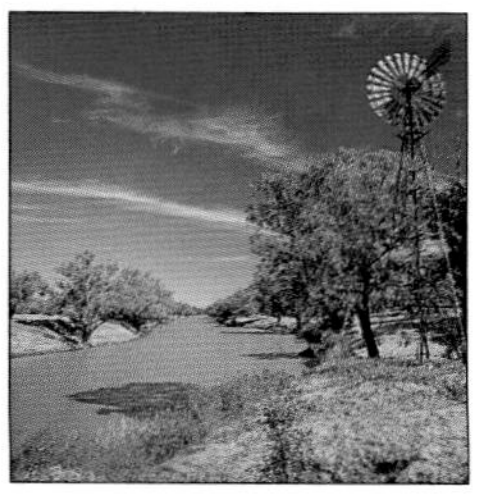

***The fertile Darling Downs**, known as the "breadbasket of Australia," support a wide range of crops including cereals, sugar cane, and fruit.*

***The Murray River** has its source in the eastern uplands of the Great Dividing Range. Fed by melting snow, it runs for 1,609 miles (2,589 km), and has sufficient volume to reach the ocean southeast of Adelaide despite a minimal gradient for most of its lower reaches.*

THE URBAN/RURAL POPULATION DIVIDE

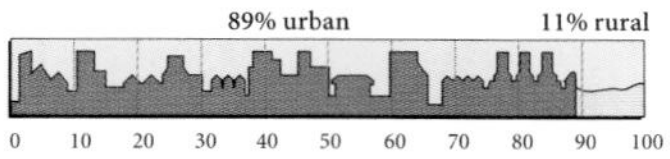

89% urban — 11% rural

0 10 20 30 40 50 60 70 80 90 100

POPULATION DENSITY	TOTAL LAND AREA
16 people per sq mile (6 people per sq km)	778,022 sq miles (2,015,600 sq km)

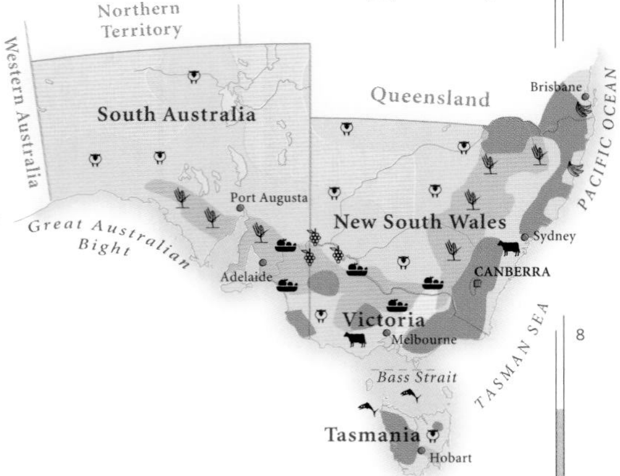

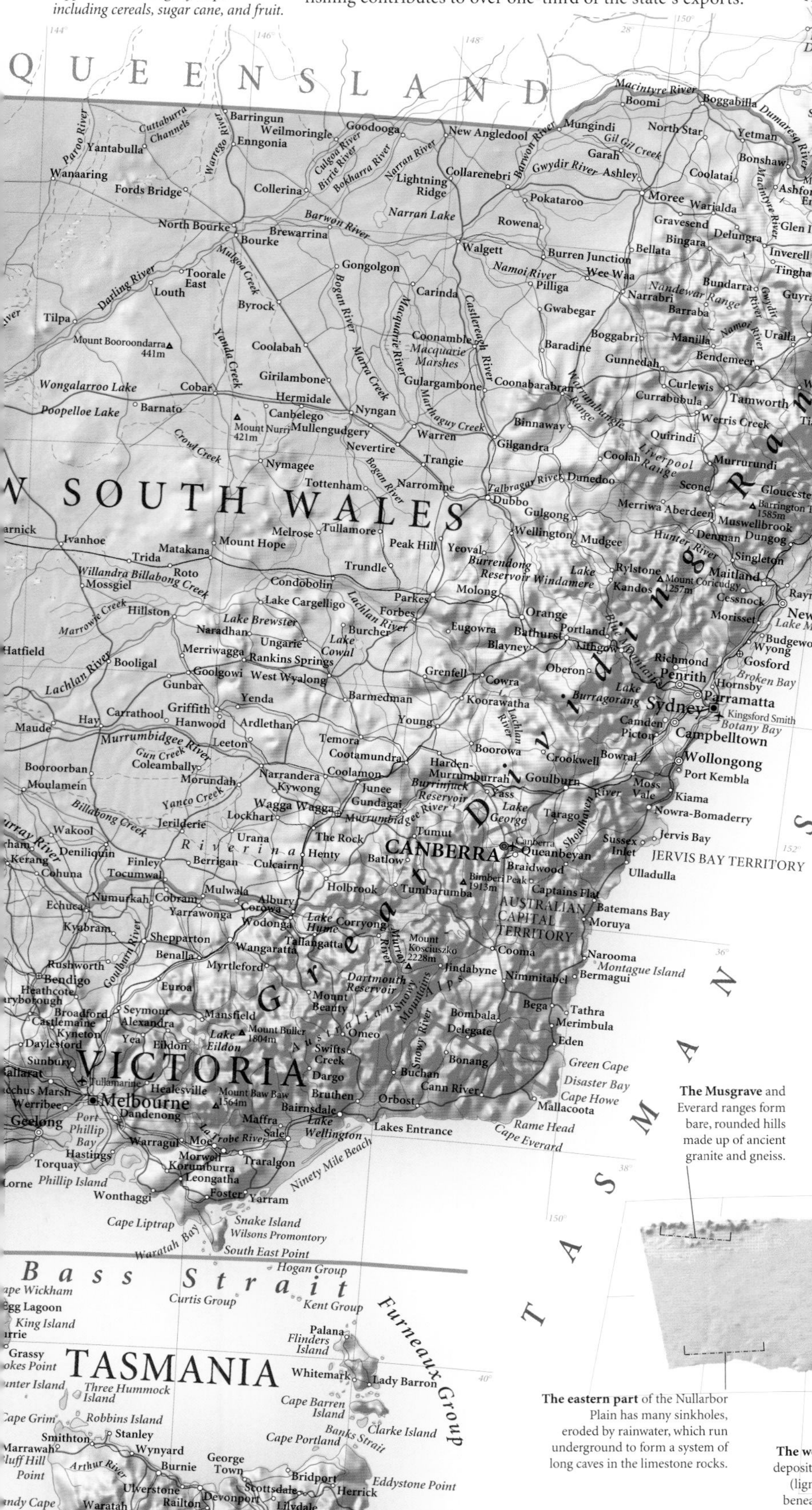

Land use and agricultural distribution

cattle, sheep, bananas, fishing, fruit, vineyards, wheat, capital cities, major towns, pasture, cropland, forest, desert, mountain region

Northern Territory, Western Australia, South Australia, Queensland, New South Wales, Victoria, Tasmania, Great Australian Bight, Port Augusta, Adelaide, Melbourne, CANBERRA, Sydney, Brisbane, Hobart, Bass Strait, PACIFIC OCEAN, TASMAN SEA

▶ 192

THE LANDSCAPE

THE SOUTHERN HALF of the Great Dividing Range runs parallel to the eastern coast of Victoria and New South Wales as far as Tasmania, which, though divided from the mainland is part of the same mountain chain. South Australia comprises the Australian Shield and half of the dry, flat Nullarbor Plain. The Murray/Darling River Basin is the only major river system.

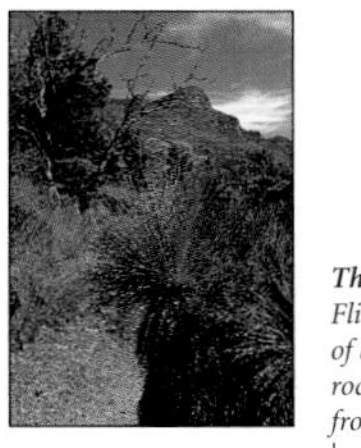

Shallow continental shelf — Past land link — Bass Strait — Tasmania

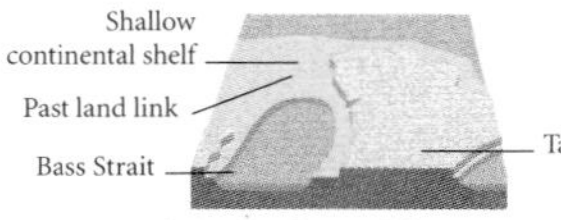

***Tasmania** is part of Australia's eastern highlands, separated from the mainland by 155 miles (250 km) of the Bass Strait. In the recent geological past, dry land links between Tasmania and Victoria would have been possible during periods of world-wide glaciation, when the sea level was more than 1,80 ft (55 m) below that of present sea levels.*

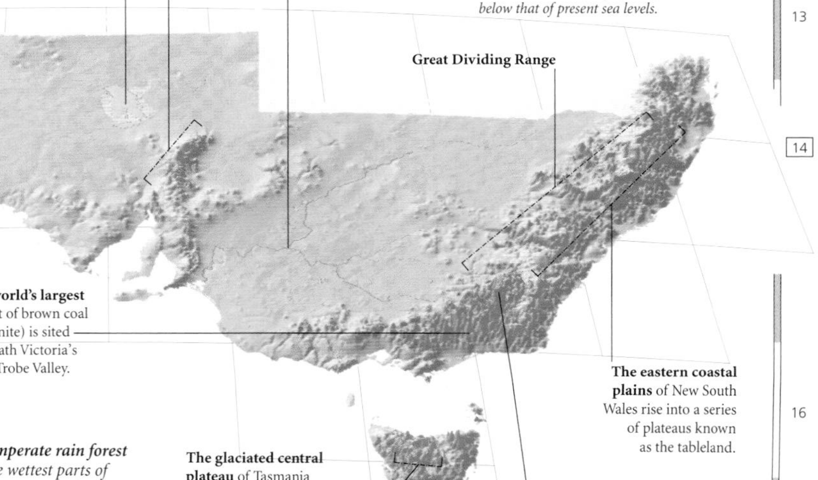

***The heavily folded** Flinders Range is part of an arc of sedimentary rocks reaching northward from Kangaroo Island.*

Lake Eyre is the largest of southern Australia's dry lakes. Lying -51 ft (-16 m) below sea level, it has flooded only three times in the last century.

The Musgrave and Everard ranges form bare, rounded hills made up of ancient granite and gneiss.

The Murray/Darling is Australia's longest river at 1,703 miles (2,739 km).

Great Dividing Range

The eastern part of the Nullarbor Plain has many sinkholes, eroded by rainwater, which run underground to form a system of long caves in the limestone rocks.

The world's largest deposit of brown coal (lignite) is sited beneath Victoria's La Trobe Valley.

The eastern coastal plains of New South Wales rise into a series of plateaus known as the tableland.

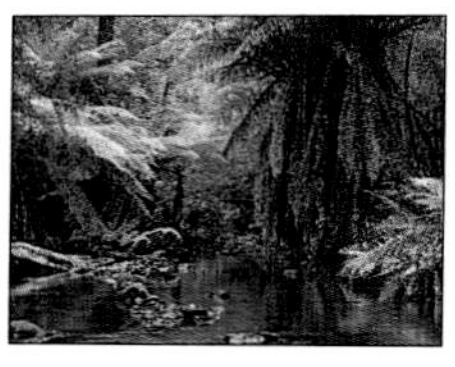

***Though temperate rain forest** grows in the wettest parts of Tasmania, extreme variations in the levels of rainfall over the island mean that some drier areas may experience forest fires.*

The glaciated central plateau of Tasmania has many lakes, including Lake St. Clair, a piedmont lake more than 700 ft (200 m) deep.

Mount Kosciuszko, the highest point in the Snowy Mountains, is the tallest mountain in Australia at 7,316 ft (2,228 m).

QUEENSLAND — NEW SOUTH WALES — VICTORIA — TASMANIA — Great Dividing Range — TASMAN SEA — Bass Strait — AUSTRALIAN CAPITAL TERRITORY — JERVIS BAY TERRITORY — CANBERRA — Sydney — Brisbane — Melbourne — Hobart — Newcastle — Wollongong

NEW ZEALAND

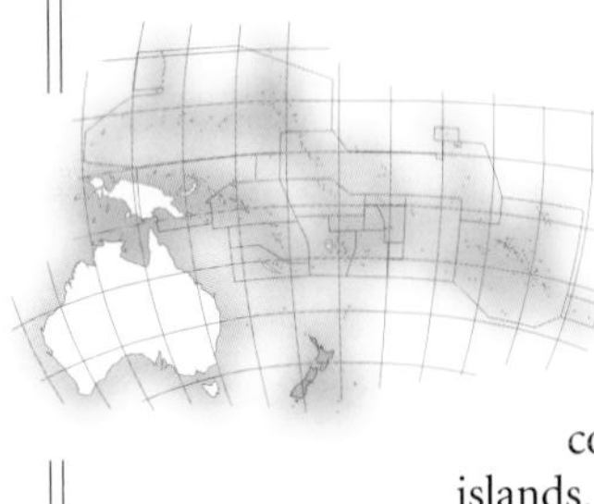

LYING 1,500 MILES EAST-SOUTHEAST OF AUSTRALIA, New Zealand was originally settled by the Maori people of Polynesia. It was visited by Europeans for the first time only as recently as the 1770s. The islands' rugged topography means that most settlement has concentrated in coastal areas. People of European origin make up more than 85% of the population of 3.7 million, following immigration which began in the 1920s. Many recent settlers have come from Asia, including India and China, and a number of the Pacific islands. The Maori now make up a minority of less than half a million. Their ancient claims to at least half of national territory, however, are gaining increasing legal credence.

THE LANDSCAPE

NEW ZEALAND comprises two large islands and many scattered smaller islands. On South Island the Alpine Fault marks the boundary between the Pacific and Indo-Australian plates. Tectonic activity has strongly influenced the formation of the Southern Alps, snowcapped mountains with several peaks over 9,800 ft (3,000 m). North Island has a lower and less extensive mountain region, containing forested hills, a central volcanic plateau, and downlands.

Mountain-building in the Southern Alps

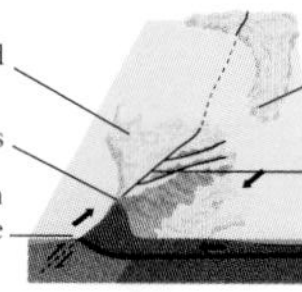

South Island
North Island
Southern Alps
Alpine Fault
Indo-Australian Plate
Pacific Plate

***The Southern Alps** have been formed by "slip" faulting. The Indo-Australian and Pacific plates run in opposite directions along the Alpine Fault. Although they slide past each other, they are also being thrust over one another, causing the continental crust of the Pacific Plate to be uplifted to form the Alps.*

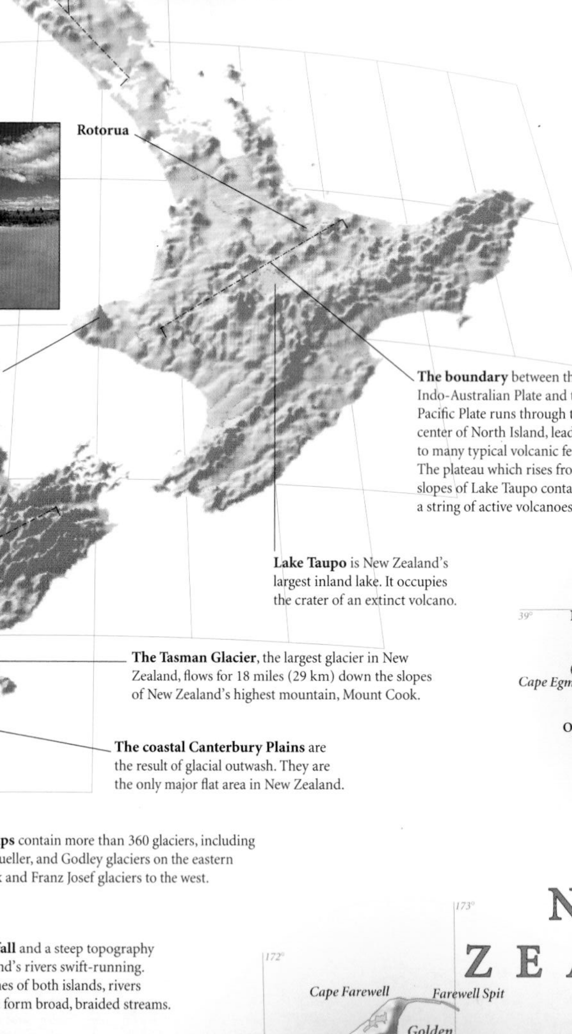

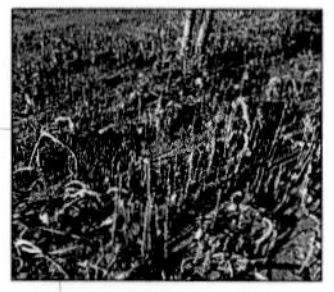

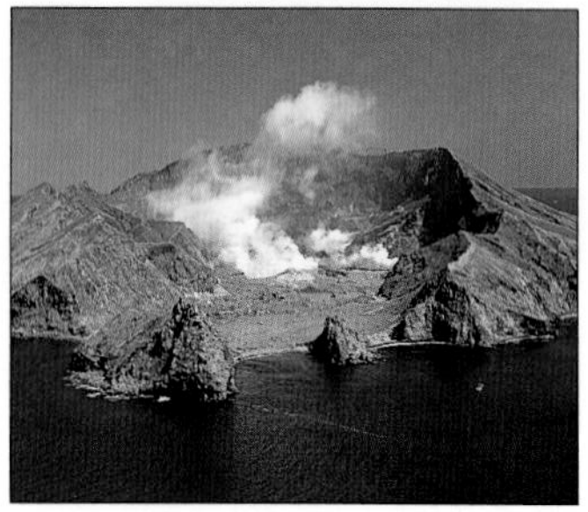

Clouds of steam rise from White Island, an active, offshore volcano lying in the Bay of Plenty, off the northern coast of North Island.

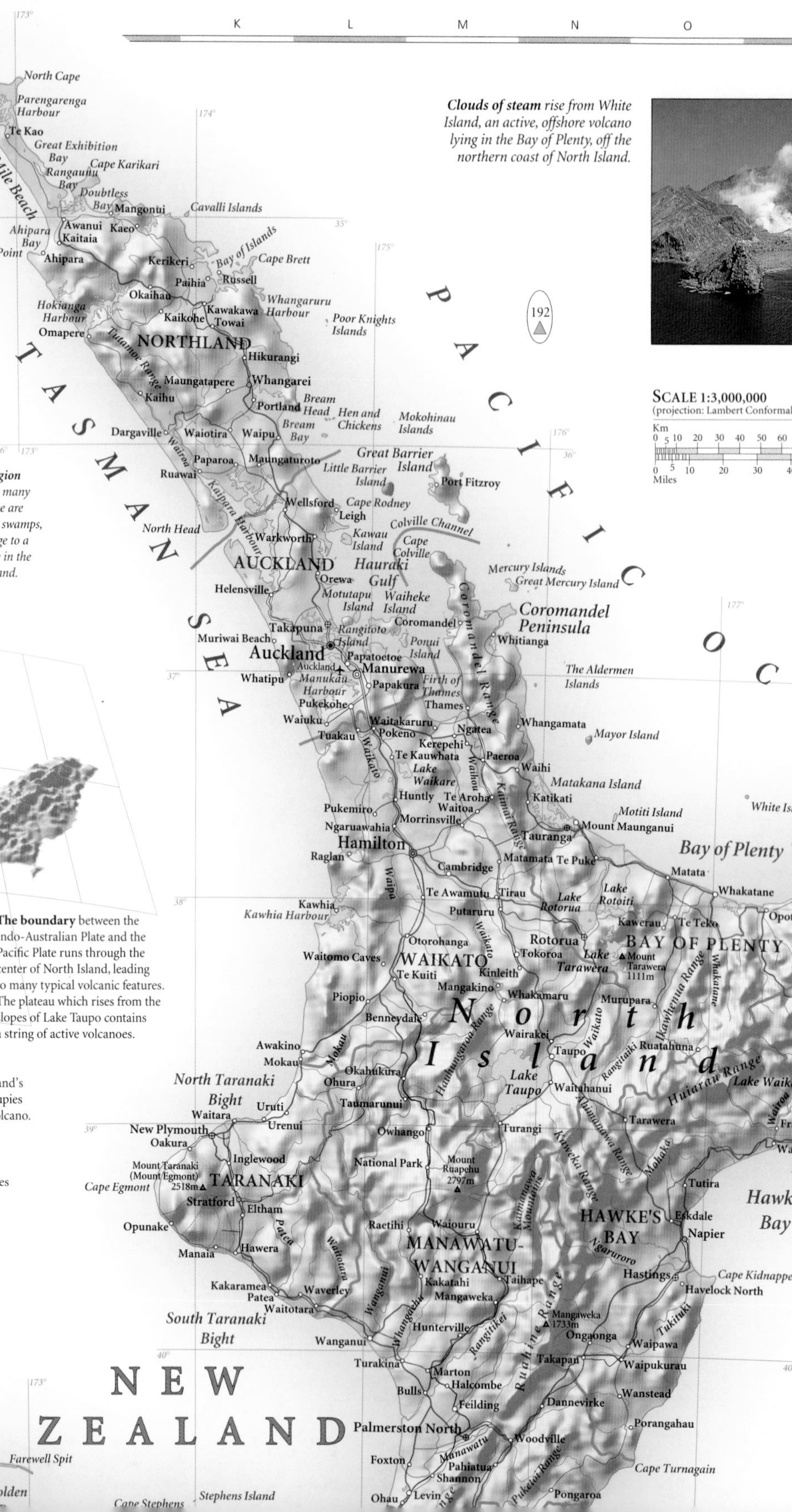

SCALE 1:3,000,000
(projection: Lambert Conformal Conic)

Northland

***The Northland region** is characterized by many coastal inlets. These are lined by mangrove swamps, signaling the change to a subtropical climate in the far north of the island.*

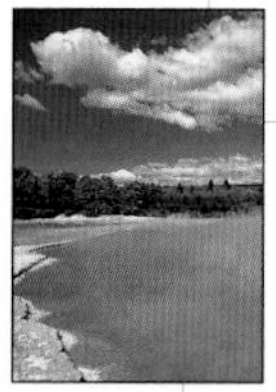

Rotorua

***The Rotorua and Taupo valleys** have some of the largest and most spectacular thermal springs in New Zealand. These occur when superheated groundwater rises to the surface through joints in the rocks.*

Mount Taranaki, rising 8,261 ft (2,518 m) is an isolated, dormant volcano.

The boundary between the Indo-Australian Plate and the Pacific Plate runs through the center of North Island, leading to many typical volcanic features. The plateau which rises from the slopes of Lake Taupo contains a string of active volcanoes.

Lake Taupo is New Zealand's largest inland lake. It occupies the crater of an extinct volcano.

The Southern Alps run for more than 300 miles, (483 km) forming the backbone of South Island. They were uplifted following the collision of the Pacific and Indo-Australian plates.

Probable location of Alpine Fault

Fiordland, in the far south west, contains a large number of flooded glacial valleys.

Sutherland Falls

The Tasman Glacier, the largest glacier in New Zealand, flows for 18 miles (29 km) down the slopes of New Zealand's highest mountain, Mount Cook.

The coastal Canterbury Plains are the result of glacial outwash. They are the only major flat area in New Zealand.

The Southern Alps contain more than 360 glaciers, including the Murchison, Mueller, and Godley glaciers on the eastern slopes and the Fox and Franz Josef glaciers to the west.

High levels of rainfall and a steep topography has made New Zealand's rivers swift-running. In the southern reaches of both islands, rivers such as the Mokoreta form broad, braided streams.

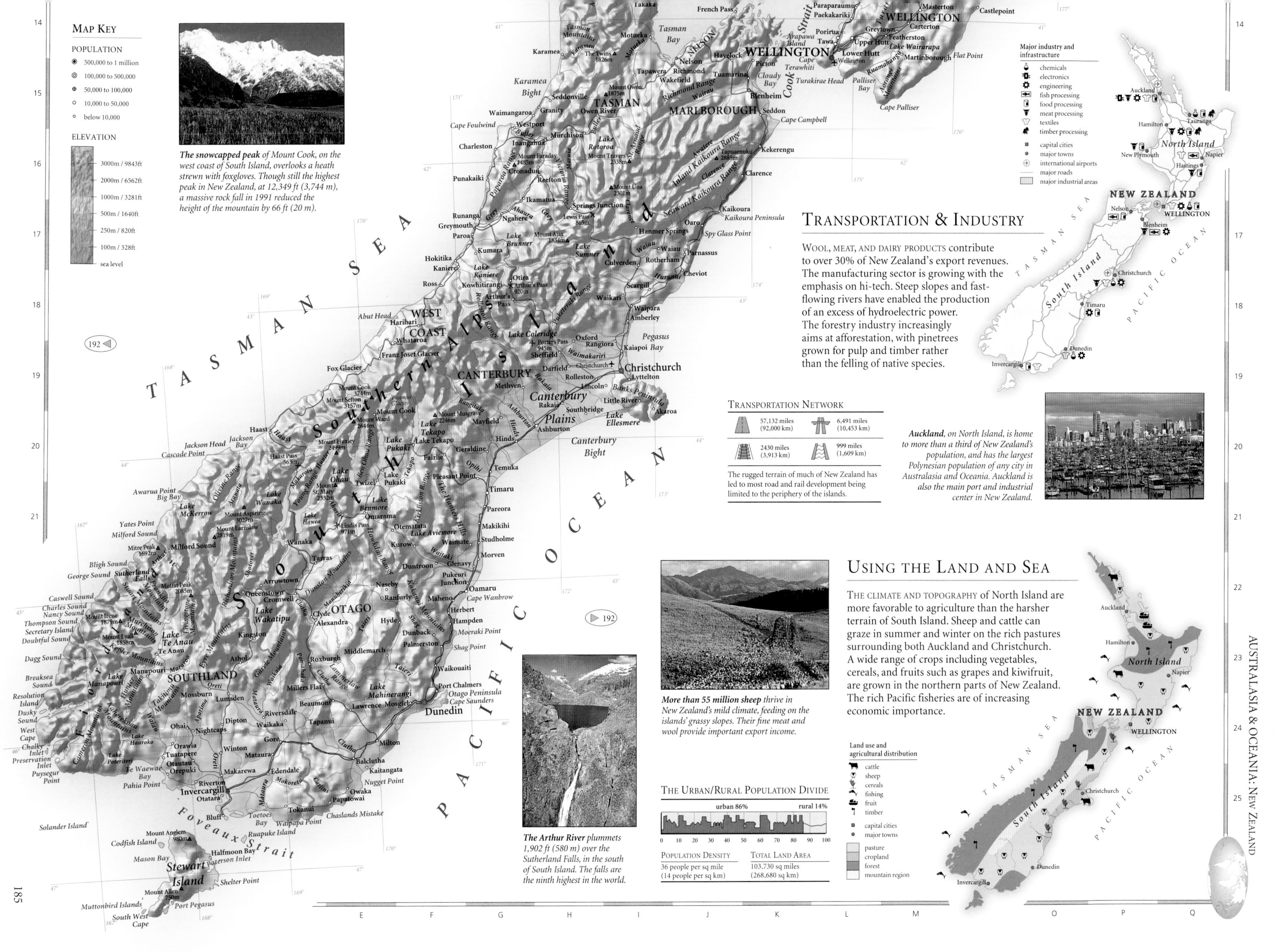
Map Key
Population
500,000 to 1 million
100,000 to 500,000
50,000 to 100,000
10,000 to 50,000
below 10,000
Elevation
3000m / 9843ft
2000m / 6562ft
1000m / 3281ft
500m / 1640ft
250m / 820ft
100m / 328ft
sea level
TASMAN SEA
PACIFIC OCEAN
South Island
Southern Alps
Fiordland
Foveaux Strait
Stewart Island
Christchurch
Dunedin
Invercargill
WELLINGTON
Cook Strait
CANTERBURY
OTAGO
SOUTHLAND
WEST COAST
TASMAN
MARLBOROUGH
NELSON
Canterbury Plains
Canterbury Bight
Major industry and infrastructure
chemicals
electronics
engineering
fish processing
food processing
meat processing
textiles
timber processing
capital cities
major towns
international airports
major roads
major industrial areas
NEW ZEALAND
North Island
Land use and agricultural distribution
cattle
sheep
cereals
fishing
fruit
timber
capital cities
major towns
pasture
cropland
forest
mountain region

The snowcapped peak *of Mount Cook, on the west coast of South Island, overlooks a heath strewn with foxgloves. Though still the highest peak in New Zealand, at 12,349 ft (3,744 m), a massive rock fall in 1991 reduced the height of the mountain by 66 ft (20 m).*

192 ◀

▶ 192

Transportation & Industry

Wool, meat, and dairy products contribute to over 30% of New Zealand's export revenues. The manufacturing sector is growing with the emphasis on hi-tech. Steep slopes and fast-flowing rivers have enabled the production of an excess of hydroelectric power. The forestry industry increasingly aims at afforestation, with pinetrees grown for pulp and timber rather than the felling of native species.

Transportation Network

57,132 miles (92,000 km)	6,491 miles (10,453 km)
2430 miles (3,913 km)	999 miles (1,609 km)

The rugged terrain of much of New Zealand has led to most road and rail development being limited to the periphery of the islands.

Auckland*, on North Island, is home to more than a third of New Zealand's population, and has the largest Polynesian population of any city in Australasia and Oceania. Auckland is also the main port and industrial center in New Zealand.*

The Arthur River *plummets 1,902 ft (580 m) over the Sutherland Falls, in the south of South Island. The falls are the ninth highest in the world.*

More than 55 million sheep *thrive in New Zealand's mild climate, feeding on the islands' grassy slopes. Their fine meat and wool provide important export income.*

Using the Land and Sea

The climate and topography of North Island are more favorable to agriculture than the harsher terrain of South Island. Sheep and cattle can graze in summer and winter on the rich pastures surrounding both Auckland and Christchurch. A wide range of crops including vegetables, cereals, and fruits such as grapes and kiwifruit, are grown in the northern parts of New Zealand. The rich Pacific fisheries are of increasing economic importance.

The Urban/Rural Population Divide

urban 86% — rural 14%

Population Density	Total Land Area
36 people per sq mile (14 people per sq km)	103,730 sq miles (268,680 sq km)

MELANESIA

PAPUA NEW GUINEA, FIJI, SOLOMON ISLANDS, VANUATU, *New Caledonia* (to France)

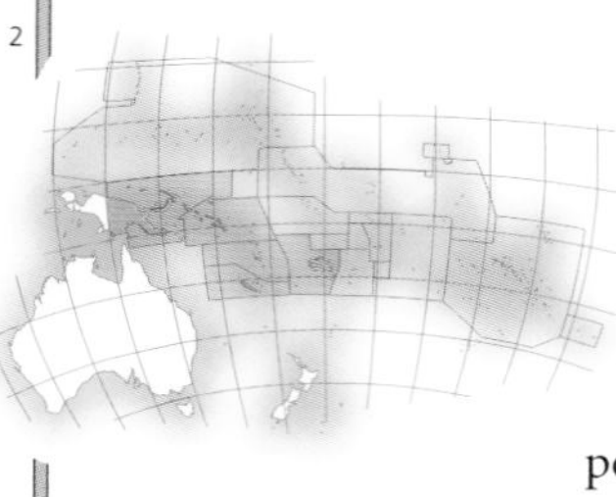

LYING IN THE SOUTHWEST PACIFIC OCEAN, northeast of Australia and south of the Equator, the islands of Melanesia form one of the three geographic divisions (along with Polynesia and Micronesia) of Oceania. Melanesia's name derives from the Greek *melas*, "black," and *nesoi*, "islands." Most of the larger islands are volcanic in origin. The smaller islands tend to be coral atolls and are mainly uninhabited. Rugged mountains, covered by dense rain forest, take up most of the land area. Melanesian's cultivate yams, taro, and sweet potatoes for local consumption and live in small, usually dispersed, homesteads.

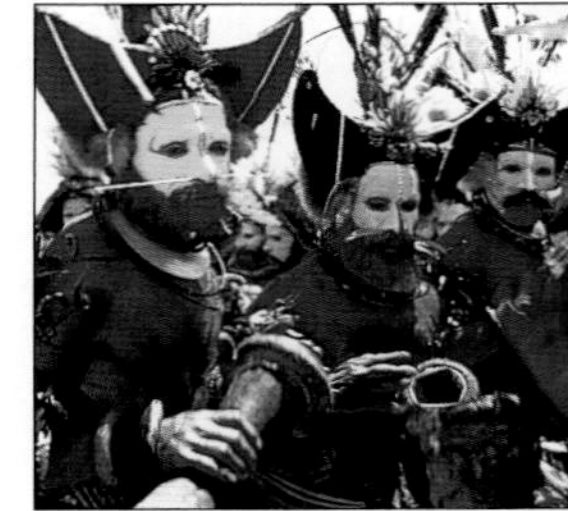

***Huli tribesmen** from Southern Highlands Province in Papua New Guinea parade in ceremonial dress, their powdered wigs decorated with exotic plumage and their faces and bodies painted with coloured pigments.*

MAP KEY

POPULATION

- 100,000 to 500,000
- 50,000 to 100,000
- 10,000 to 50,000
- below 10,000

ELEVATION

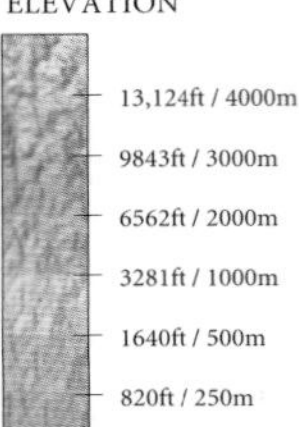

13,124ft / 4000m
9843ft / 3000m
6562ft / 2000m
3281ft / 1000m
1640ft / 500m
820ft / 250m
328ft / 100m
sea level

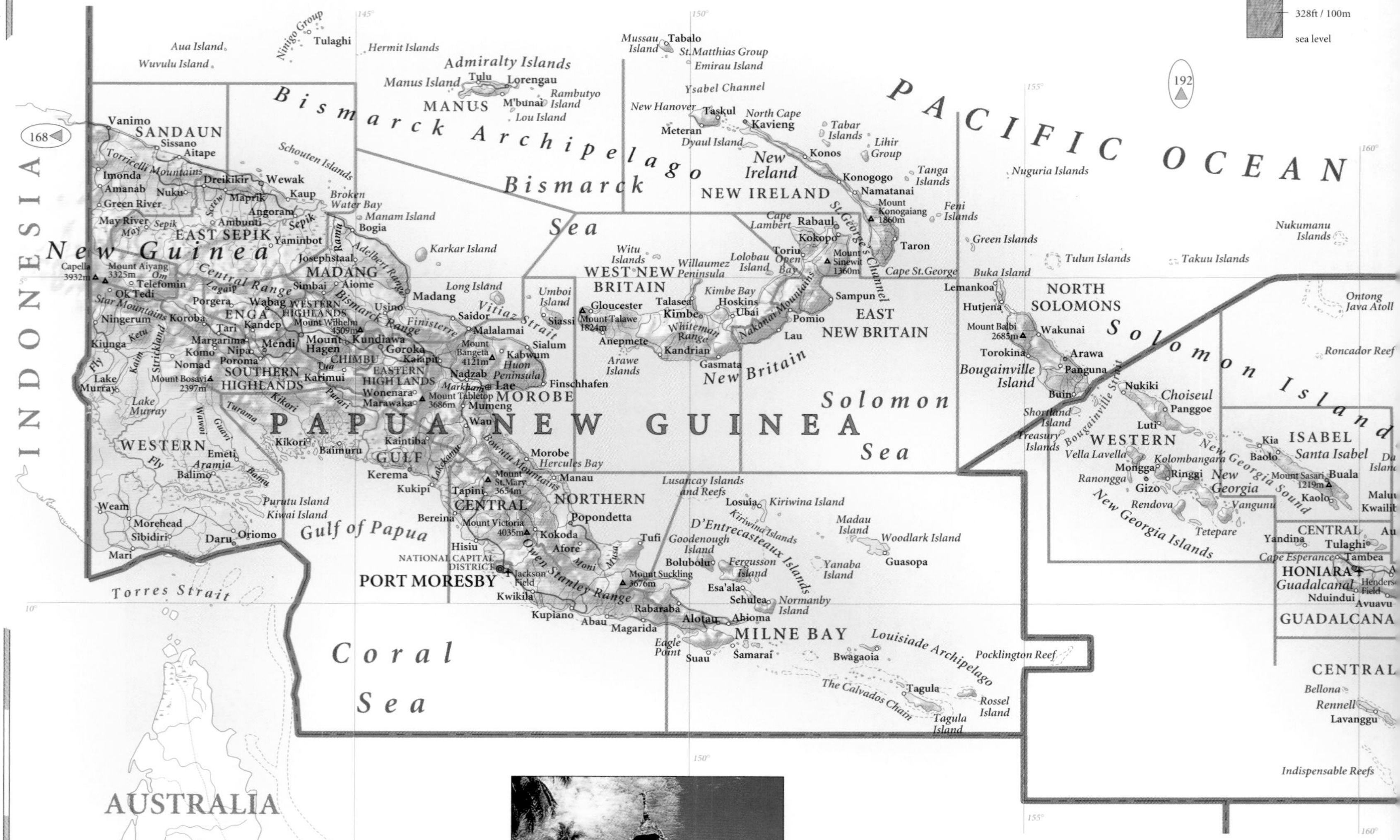

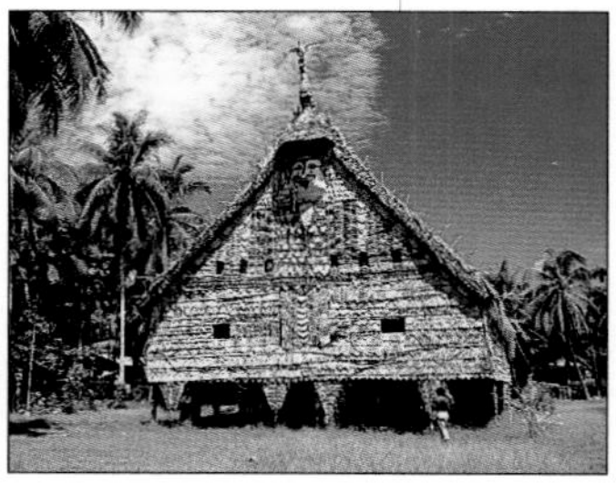

***Lying close to the banks** of the Sepik River in northern Papua New Guinea, this building is known as the Spirit House. It is constructed from leaves and twigs, ornately woven and trimmed into geometric patterns. The house is decorated with a mask and topped by a carved statue.*

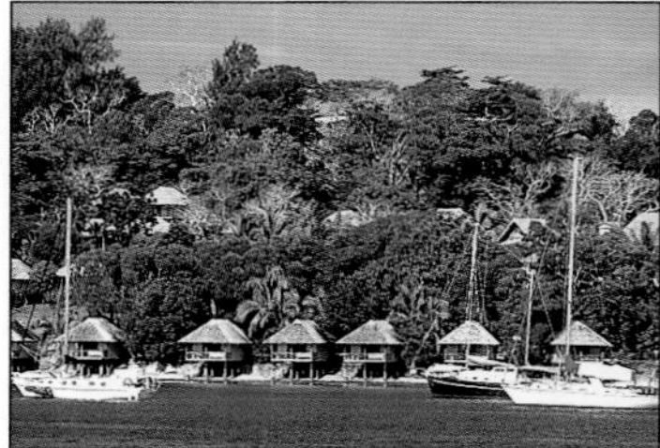

***On one of Vanuatu's many islands,** simple beach houses stand at the water's edge, surrounded by coconut palms and other tropical vegetation. The unspoilt beaches and tranquillity of its islands are drawing ever-larger numbers of tourists to Vanuatu.*

TRANSPORTATION & INDUSTRY

The processing of natural resources generates significant export revenue for the countries of Melanesia. The region relies mainly on copra, tuna, and timber exports, with some production of cocoa and palm oil. The islands have substantial mineral resources including the world's largest copper reserves on Bougainville Island; gold, and potential oil and natural gas. Tourism has become the fastest growing sector in most of the countries' economies.

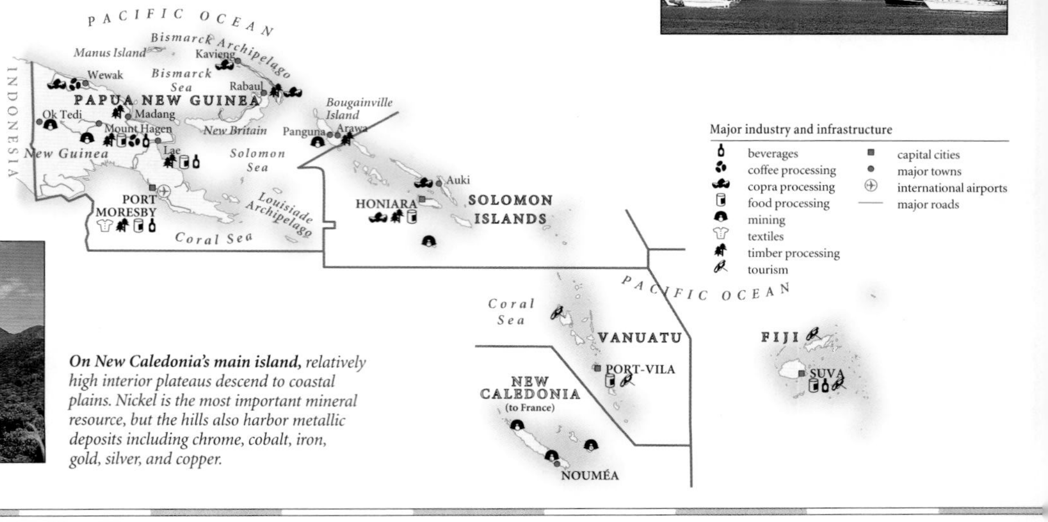

TRANSPORTATION NETWORK

1,236 miles (1,990 km)	None
370 miles (595 km)	6,924 miles (11,143 km)

As most of the islands of Melanesia lie off the major sea and air routes, services to and from the rest of the world are infrequent. Transportation by road on rugged terrain is difficult and expensive.

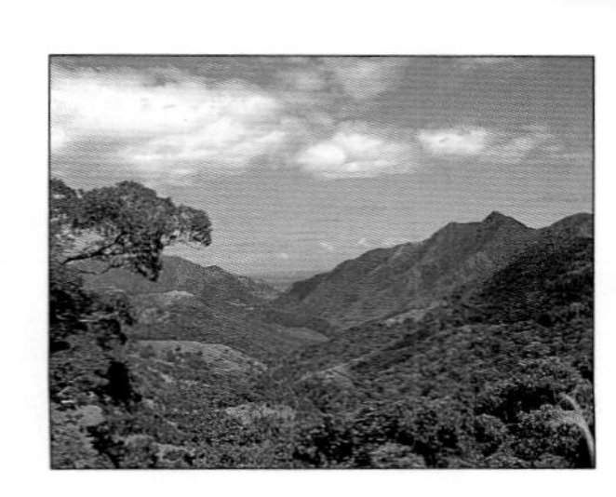

***On New Caledonia's main island,** relatively high interior plateaus descend to coastal plains. Nickel is the most important mineral resource, but the hills also harbor metallic deposits including chrome, cobalt, iron, gold, silver, and copper.*

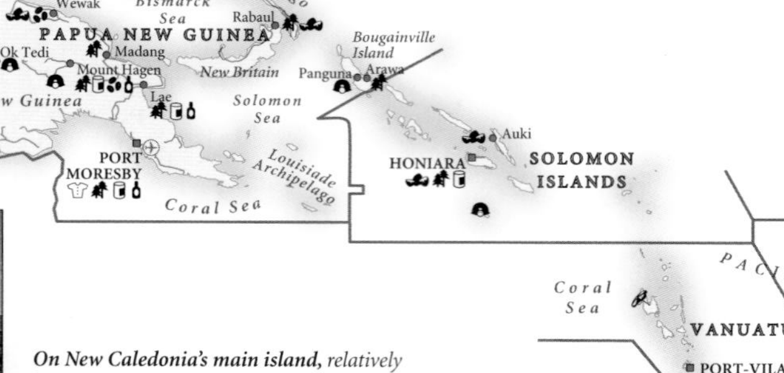

PACIFIC OCEAN
Bismarck Archipelago
Manus Island
Kavieng
Wewak
Bismarck Sea
Rabaul
INDONESIA
PAPUA NEW GUINEA
Bougainville Island
Ok Tedi
Madang
Mount Hagen
New Britain
Panguna
Arawa
New Guinea
Lae
Solomon Sea
PORT MORESBY
Louisiade Archipelago
Coral Sea
Auki
HONIARA
SOLOMON ISLANDS
PACIFIC OCEAN
Coral Sea
VANUATU
PORT-VILA
FIJI
SUVA
NEW CALEDONIA (to France)
NOUMÉA
Major industry and infrastructure
beverages
coffee processing
copra processing
food processing
mining
textiles
timber processing
tourism
capital cities
major towns
international airports
major roads

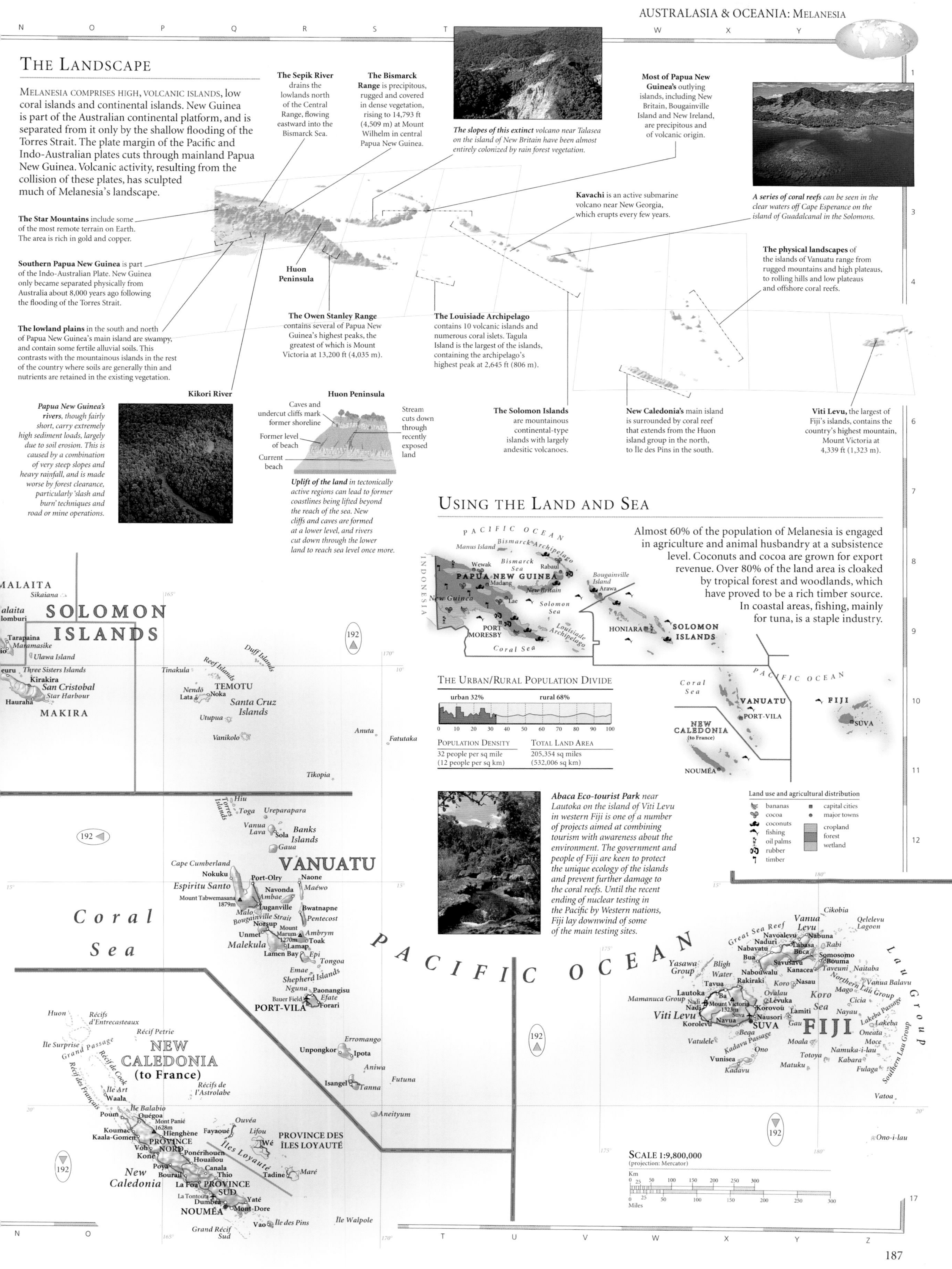

N O P Q R S T W X Y
Huon Peninsula
Caves and undercut cliffs mark former shoreline
Former level of beach
Current beach
Stream cuts down through recently exposed land
PACIFIC OCEAN
Manus Island
Bismarck Archipelago
Wewak
Bismarck Sea
Rabaul
PAPUA NEW GUINEA
Madang
New Britain
Bougainville Island
Arawa
INDONESIA
New Guinea
Lae
Solomon Sea
PORT MORESBY
Louisiade Archipelago
Coral Sea
HONIARA
SOLOMON ISLANDS
Coral Sea
VANUATU
PORT-VILA
FIJI
SUVA
NEW CALEDONIA (to France)
NOUMÉA
urban 32%
rural 68%
0 10 20 30 40 50 60 70 80 90 100
Land use and agricultural distribution
bananas
cocoa
coconuts
fishing
oil palms
rubber
timber
capital cities
major towns
cropland
forest
wetland
MALAITA
Sikaiana
SOLOMON ISLANDS
Tarapaina
Maramasike
Ulawa Island
Three Sisters Islands
Kirakira
San Cristobal
Star Harbour
Hauraha
MAKIRA
Tinakula
Reef Islands
Duff Islands
Nendö
Lata
Noka
TEMOTU
Santa Cruz Islands
Utupua
Vanikolo
Anuta
Fatutaka
Tikopia
192
Hiu
Torres Islands
Toga
Ureparapara
Vanua Lava
Sola
Banks Islands
Gaua
VANUATU
Cape Cumberland
Nokuku
Port-Olry
Naone
Espiritu Santo
Navonda
Maéwo
Mount Tabwemasana 1879m
Ambae
Luganville
Bwatnapne
Malo
Bougainville Strait
Pentecost
Norsup
Mount Marum 1270m
Ambrym
Unmet
Malekula
Toak
Lamap
Lamen Bay
Epi
Tongoa
Emae
Shepherd Islands
Nguna
Paonangisu
Bauer Field
Efate
PORT-VILA
Forari
Coral Sea
PACIFIC OCEAN
Erromango
Unpongkor
Ipota
Aniwa
Isangel
Tanna
Futuna
Aneityum
Huon
Récifs d'Entrecasteaux
Récif Petrie
Île Surprise
Grand Passage
Récif de Cook
Récifs des Français
NEW CALEDONIA (to France)
Récifs de l'Astrolabe
Île Art
Waala
Île Balabio
Poum
Ouégoa
Mont Panié 1628m
Hienghène
Koumac
Kaala-Gomen
PROVINCE NORD
Voh
Koné
Ponérihouen
Houaïlou
Poya
Bourail
Canala
Thio
New Caledonia
La Foa
PROVINCE SUD
La Tontouta
Dumbéa
Yaté
Mont-Dore
NOUMÉA
Grand Récif Sud
Vao
Île des Pins
Île Walpole
Ouvéa
Fayaoué
Lifou
Wé
PROVINCE DES ÎLES LOYAUTÉ
Îles Loyauté
Tadine
Maré
Yasawa Group
Bligh Water
Great Sea Reef
Vanua Levu
Cikobia
Qelelevu Lagoon
Navoalevu
Nabuna
Naduri
Nabavatu
Labasa
Rabi
Buca
Bua
Savusavu
Somosomo
Bouma
Taveuni
Naitaba
Nabouwalu
Kanacea
Lau Group
Tavua
Rakiraki
Koro
Nasau
Northern Lau Group
Vanua Balavu
Mago
Mamanuca Group
Lautoka
Ba
Ovalau
Levuka
Koro Sea
Cicia
Nadi
Mount Victoria 1323m
Korovou
Nayau
Viti Levu
Korolevu
Navua
Nausori
Lamiti
Lakeba Passage
Lakeba
SUVA
Gau
FIJI
Oneata
Vatulele
Beqa
Kadavu Passage
Moala
Moce
Ono
Namuka-i-lau
Vunisea
Kadavu
Totoya
Kabara
Matuku
Southern Lau Group
Fulaga
Vatoa
Ono-i-lau
SCALE 1:9,800,000
(projection: Mercator)
Km 0 25 50 100 150 200 250 300
Miles 0 25 50 100 150 200 250 300
T U V W X Y Z

The Landscape

Melanesia comprises high, volcanic islands, low coral islands and continental islands. New Guinea is part of the Australian continental platform, and is separated from it only by the shallow flooding of the Torres Strait. The plate margin of the Pacific and Indo-Australian plates cuts through mainland Papua New Guinea. Volcanic activity, resulting from the collision of these plates, has sculpted much of Melanesia's landscape.

The Sepik River drains the lowlands north of the Central Range, flowing eastward into the Bismarck Sea.

The Bismarck Range is precipitous, rugged and covered in dense vegetation, rising to 14,793 ft (4,509 m) at Mount Wilhelm in central Papua New Guinea.

The slopes of this extinct volcano near Talasea on the island of New Britain have been almost entirely colonized by rain forest vegetation.

Most of Papua New Guinea's outlying islands, including New Britain, Bougainville Island and New Ireland, are precipitous and of volcanic origin.

A series of coral reefs can be seen in the clear waters off Cape Esperance on the island of Guadalcanal in the Solomons.

The Star Mountains include some of the most remote terrain on Earth. The area is rich in gold and copper.

Kavachi is an active submarine volcano near New Georgia, which erupts every few years.

Southern Papua New Guinea is part of the Indo-Australian Plate. New Guinea only became separated physically from Australia about 8,000 years ago following the flooding of the Torres Strait.

Huon Peninsula

The physical landscapes of the islands of Vanuatu range from rugged mountains and high plateaus, to rolling hills and low plateaus and offshore coral reefs.

The lowland plains in the south and north of Papua New Guinea's main island are swampy, and contain some fertile alluvial soils. This contrasts with the mountainous islands in the rest of the country where soils are generally thin and nutrients are retained in the existing vegetation.

The Owen Stanley Range contains several of Papua New Guinea's highest peaks, the greatest of which is Mount Victoria at 13,200 ft (4,035 m).

The Louisiade Archipelago contains 10 volcanic islands and numerous coral islets. Tagula Island is the largest of the islands, containing the archipelago's highest peak at 2,645 ft (806 m).

Kikori River

*Papua New Guinea's **rivers**, though fairly short, carry extremely high sediment loads, largely due to soil erosion. This is caused by a combination of very steep slopes and heavy rainfall, and is made worse by forest clearance, particularly 'slash and burn' techniques and road or mine operations.*

Huon Peninsula

***Uplift of the land** in tectonically active regions can lead to former coastlines being lifted beyond the reach of the sea. New cliffs and caves are formed at a lower level, and rivers cut down through the lower land to reach sea level once more.*

The Solomon Islands are mountainous continental-type islands with largely andesitic volcanoes.

New Caledonia's main island is surrounded by coral reef that extends from the Huon island group in the north, to Île des Pins in the south.

Viti Levu, the largest of Fiji's islands, contains the country's highest mountain, Mount Victoria at 4,339 ft (1,323 m).

Using the Land and Sea

Almost 60% of the population of Melanesia is engaged in agriculture and animal husbandry at a subsistence level. Coconuts and cocoa are grown for export revenue. Over 80% of the land area is cloaked by tropical forest and woodlands, which have proved to be a rich timber source. In coastal areas, fishing, mainly for tuna, is a staple industry.

The Urban/Rural Population Divide

Population Density	Total Land Area
32 people per sq mile	205,354 sq miles
(12 people per sq km)	(532,006 sq km)

***Abaca Eco-tourist Park** near Lautoka on the island of Viti Levu in western Fiji is one of a number of projects aimed at combining tourism with awareness about the environment. The government and people of Fiji are keen to protect the unique ecology of the islands and prevent further damage to the coral reefs. Until the recent ending of nuclear testing in the Pacific by Western nations, Fiji lay downwind of some of the main testing sites.*

MICRONESIA

MARSHALL ISLANDS, MICRONESIA, NAURU, PALAU,
Guam, Northern Mariana Islands, Wake Island

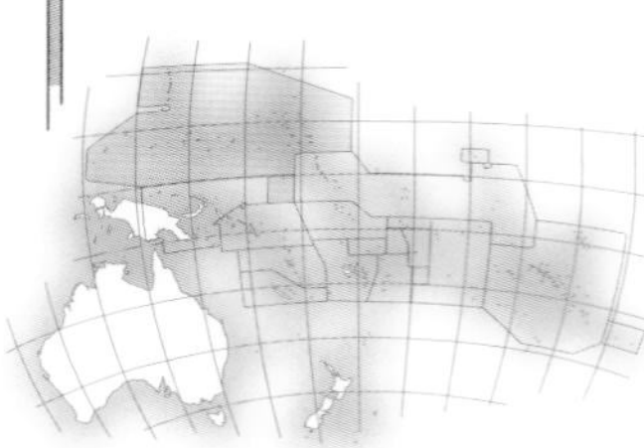

THE MICRONESIAN ISLANDS lie in the western reaches of the Pacific Ocean and are all part of the same volcanic zone. The Federated States of Micronesia is the largest group, with more than 600 atolls and forested volcanic islands in an area of more than 1,120 sq miles (2,900 sq km). Micronesia is a mixture of former colonies, overseas territories, and dependencies. Most of the region still relies on aid and subsidies to sustain economies limited by resources, isolation, and an emigrating population, drawn to New Zealand and Australia by the attractions of a western lifestyle.

PALAU

PALAU IS AN ARCHIPELAGO OF OVER 200 ISLANDS, only eight of which are inhabited. It was the last remaining UN trust territory in the Pacific, controlled by the US until 1994, when it became independent. The economy operates on a subsistence level, with coconuts and cassava the principal crops. Fishing licenses and tourism provide foreign currency.

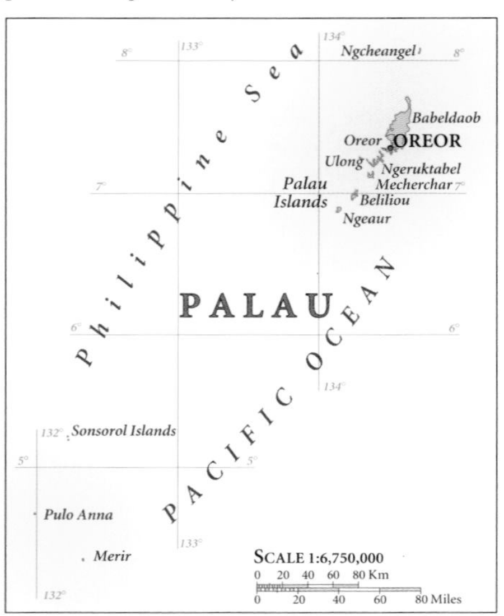
Philippine Sea
Ngcheangel
Babeldaob
Oreor
OREOR
Ulong
Ngeruktabel
Palau Islands
Mecherchar
Beliliou
Ngeaur
PALAU
PACIFIC OCEAN
Sonsorol Islands
Pulo Anna
Merir
SCALE 1:6,750,000
0 20 40 60 80 Km
0 20 40 60 80 Miles

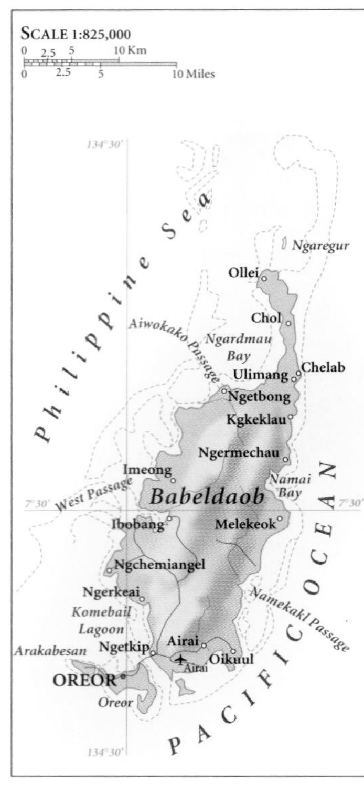
SCALE 1:825,000
0 2.5 5 10 Km
0 2.5 5 10 Miles
Philippine Sea
Ngaregur
Ollei
Aiwokako Passage
Ngardmau Bay
Chol
Ulimang
Chelab
Ngetbong
Kgkeklau
Ngermechau
Imeong
West Passage
Babeldaob
Namai Bay
Ibobang
Melekeok
Ngchemiangel
Ngerkeai
Komebail Lagoon
Namekakl Passage
Arakabesan
Ngetkip
Airai
Oikuul
OREOR
Oreor
PACIFIC OCEAN

NORTHERN MARIANA ISLANDS (to US)

A US COMMONWEALTH TERRITORY, the Northern Marianas comprise the whole of the Mariana archipelago except for Guam. The islands retain their close links with the US and continue to receive American aid. Tourism, though bringing in much-needed revenue, has speeded the decline of the traditional subsistence economy. Most of the population lives on Saipan.

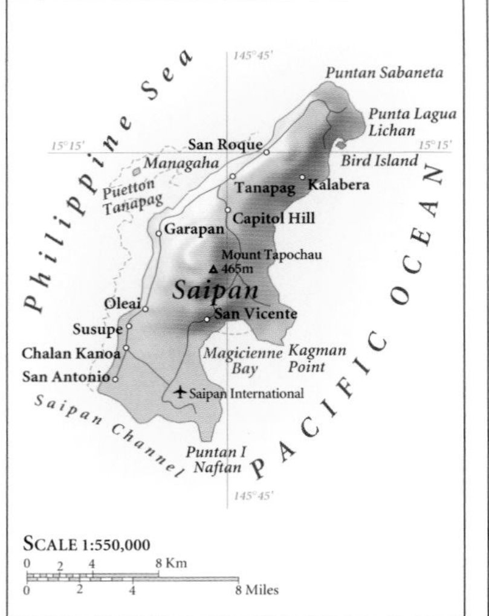
Philippine Sea
Puntan Sabaneta
Punta Lagua Lichan
San Roque
Managaha
Bird Island
Puetton Tanapag
Tanapag
Kalabera
Capitol Hill
Garapan
Mount Tapochau
465m
Saipan
Oleai
San Vicente
Susupe
Chalan Kanoa
San Antonio
Magicienne Bay
Kagman Point
Saipan International
Saipan Channel
Puntan I Naftan
PACIFIC OCEAN
SCALE 1:550,000
0 2 4 8 Km
0 2 4 8 Miles

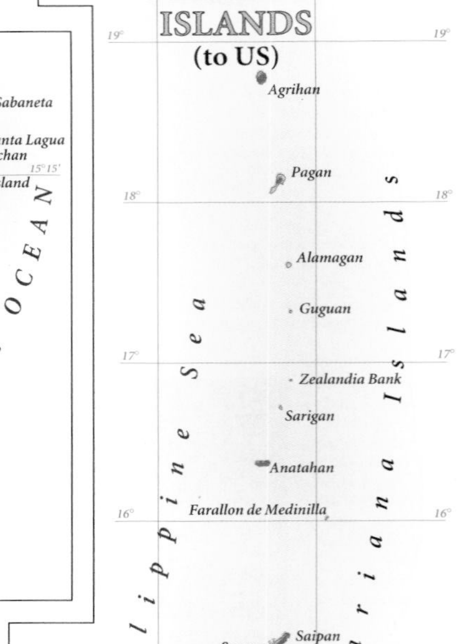
Farallon de Pajaros
Supply Reef
PACIFIC OCEAN
Maug Islands
Asuncion Island
NORTHERN MARIANA ISLANDS
(to US)
Agrihan
Pagan
Alamagan
Guguan
Zealandia Bank
Sarigan
Anatahan
Farallon de Medinilla
Philippine Sea
Mariana Islands

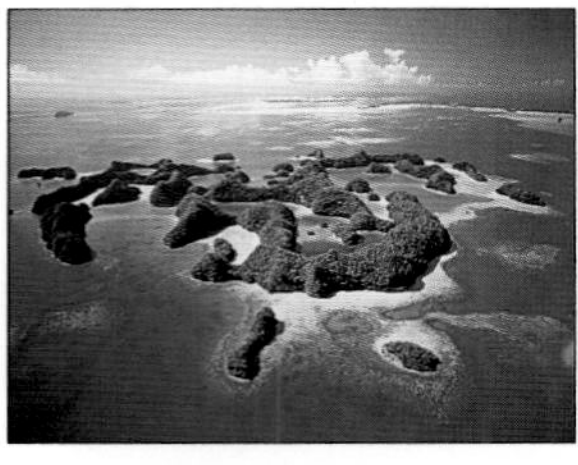

***The Palau Islands** have numerous hidden lakes and lagoons. These sustain their own ecosystems which have developed in isolation. This has produced adaptations in the animals and plants that are often unique to each lake.*

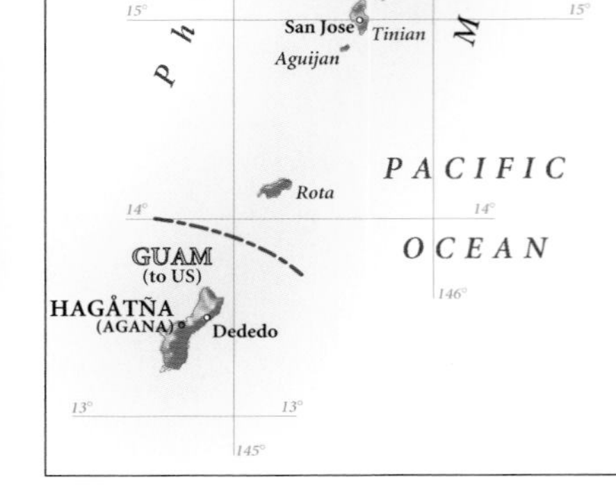
Saipan
Susupe
San Jose
Tinian
Aguijan
PACIFIC OCEAN
Rota
GUAM
(to US)
HAGÅTÑA
(AGANA)
Dededo

MICRONESIA

A MIXTURE OF HIGH VOLCANIC ISLANDS and low-lying coral atolls, the Federated States of Micronesia include all the Caroline Islands except Palau. Pohnpei, Kosrae, Chuuk, and Yap are the four main island cluster states, each of which has its own language, with English remaining the official language. Nearly half the population is concentrated on Pohnpei, the largest island. Independent since 1986, the islands continue to receive considerable aid from the US which supplements an economy based primarily on fishing and copra processing.

GUAM (to US)

LYING AT THE SOUTHERN END OF the Mariana Islands, Guam is an important US military base and tourist destination. Social and political life is dominated by the indigenous Chamorro, who make up just under half the population, although the increasing prevalence of western culture threatens Guam's traditional social stability.

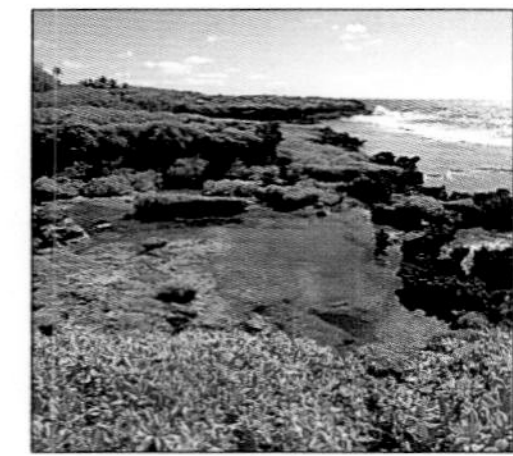

***The tranquillity** of these coastal lagoons, at Inarajan in southern Guam, belies the fact that the island lies in a region where typhoons are common.*

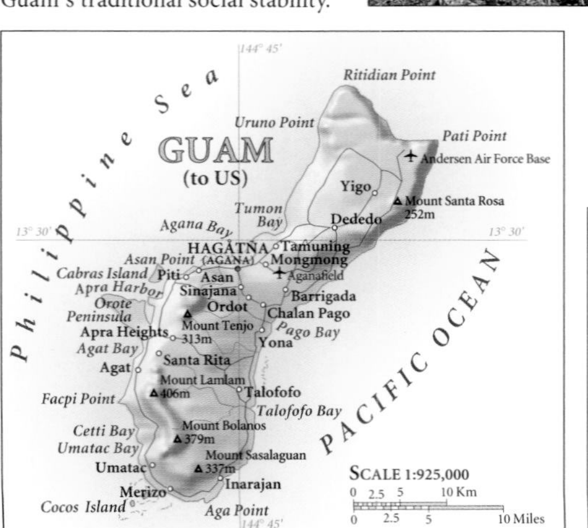
Philippine Sea
Ritidian Point
Uruno Point
GUAM
(to US)
Pati Point
Andersen Air Force Base
Yigo
Tumon Bay
Mount Santa Rosa
252m
Agana Bay
Dededo
HAGÅTÑA (AGANA)
Tamuning
Mongmong
Asan Point
Cabras Island
Piti
Asan
Apra Harbor
Sinajana
Orote Peninsula
Ordot
Barrigada
Apra Heights
Mount Tenjo
313m
Chalan Pago
Pago Bay
Agat Bay
Yona
Santa Rita
Agat
Mount Lamlam
406m
Facpi Point
Talofofo
Talofofo Bay
Cetti Bay
Mount Bolanos
379m
Umatac Bay
Umatac
Mount Sasalaguan
337m
Merizo
Inarajan
Cocos Island
Aga Point
PACIFIC OCEAN
SCALE 1:925,000
0 2.5 5 10 Km
0 2.5 5 10 Miles

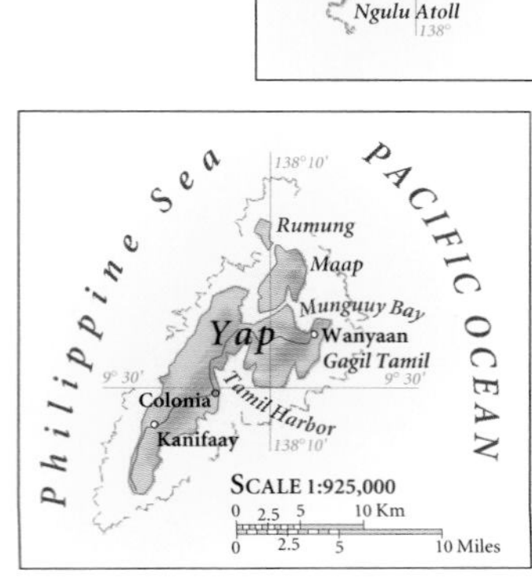
Philippine Sea
PACIFIC OCEAN
Rumung
Maap
Munguuy Bay
Yap
Wanyaan
Gagil Tamil
Colonia
Tamil Harbor
Kanifaay
SCALE 1:925,000
0 2.5 5 10 Km
0 2.5 5 10 Miles

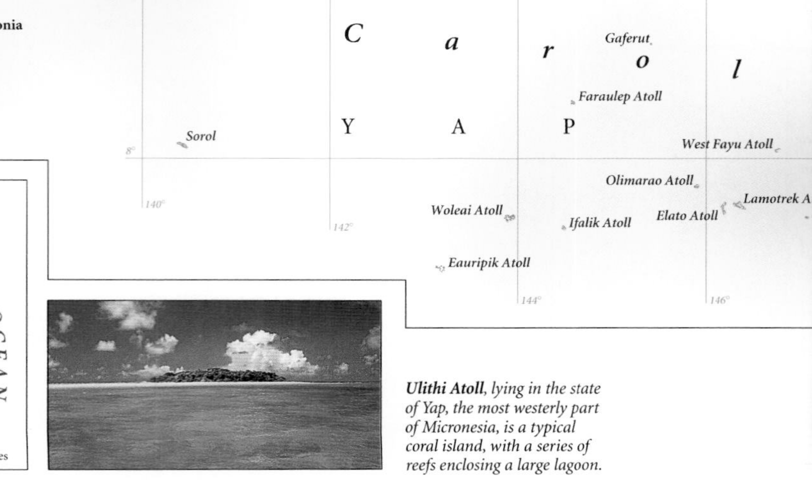
Philippine Sea
PACIFIC OCEAN
Ulithi Atoll
Fais
Yap
Colonia
CAROLINE
YAP
Gaferut
Faraulep Atoll
Ngulu Atoll
Sorol
West Fayu Atoll
Olimarao Atoll
Lamotrek Atoll
Woleai Atoll
Ifalik Atoll
Elato Atoll
Eauripik Atoll

***Ulithi Atoll**, lying in the state of Yap, the most westerly part of Micronesia, is a typical coral island, with a series of reefs enclosing a large lagoon.*

MARSHALL ISLANDS

A GROUP OF 34 WIDELY-SCATTERED ATOLLS in the central Pacific Ocean, the Marshall Islands include some of the largest atolls in the world, formed from low coral islands with sandy beaches and enclosing vast lagoons. Formerly under US protection as part of the UN Trust Territory of the Pacific Islands, and including the former US nuclear testing sites of Bikini Atoll and Enewetak Atoll, the Marshall Islands became self-governing in 1979. The economy is reliant on US aid and on the rent paid by the US for its missile base on Kwajalein Atoll.

NAURU

A FORMER BRITISH COLONY, the tiny island of Nauru, with an area of only 8.2 sq miles (21.2 sq km), has been exploited for its substantial phosphate deposits by the UK, Australia, and New Zealand. Since independence in 1968, the phosphate industry has made its citizens some of the wealthiest in the world, and scars from the vast mining operation pit the island's landscape. Phosphate reserves are now virtually exhausted and investment overseas will in future form the bulk of Nauru's income.

WAKE ISLAND (to US)

AN UNINCORPORATED TERRITORY of the US with a tiny population, Wake Island remains strategically important to US forces, and has been used as a base in several conflicts. Formed by the rim of an extinct underwater volcano, it is now used as an emergency airstrip for trans-Pacific flights, and as a stopover for cargo planes.

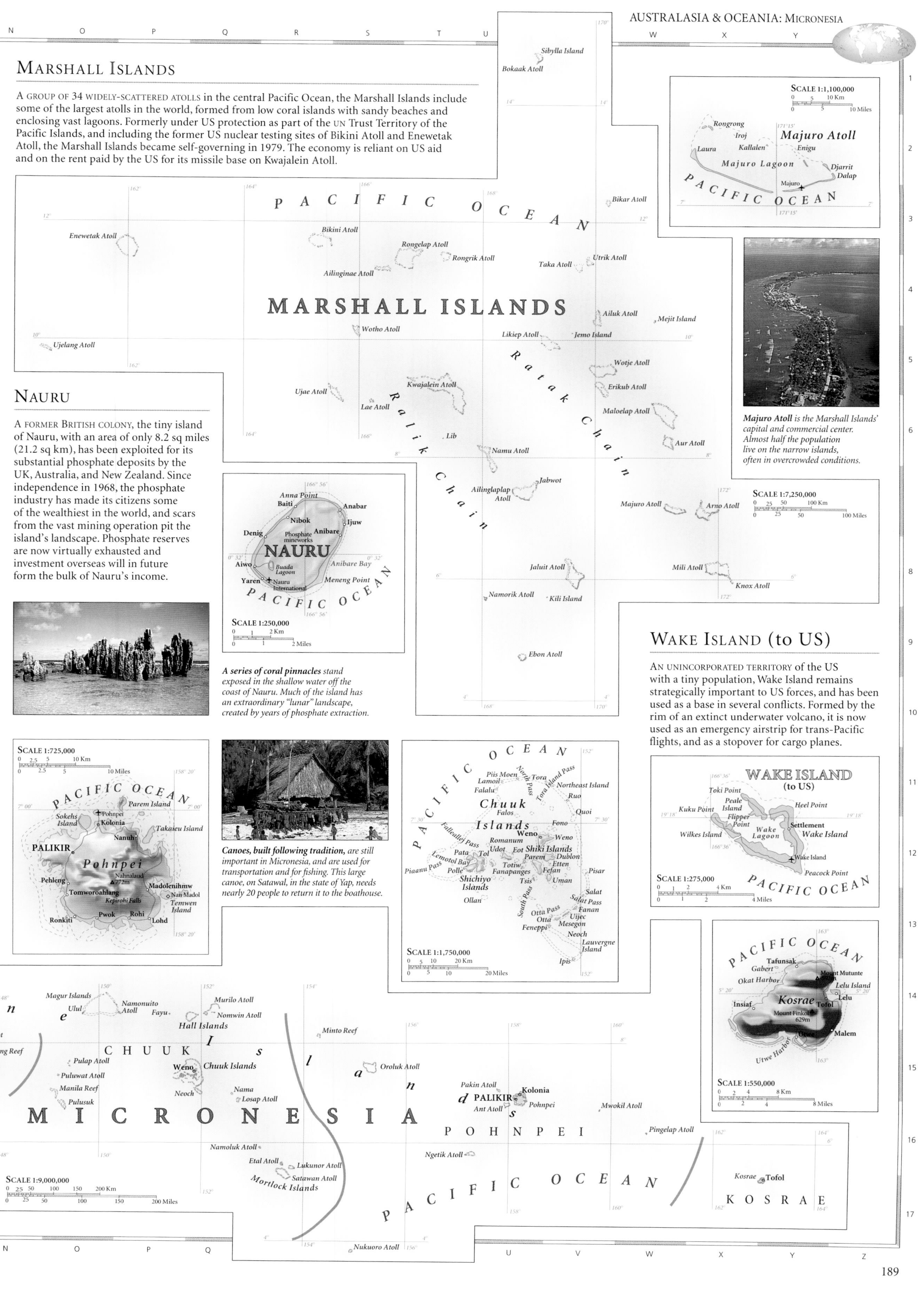

N O P Q R S T U W X Y
1 2 3 4 5 6 7 8 9 10 11 12 13 14 15 16 17
PACIFIC OCEAN
MARSHALL ISLANDS
Sibylla Island
Bokaak Atoll
Bikar Atoll
Enewetak Atoll
Bikini Atoll
Rongelap Atoll
Rongrik Atoll
Ailinginae Atoll
Taka Atoll
Utrik Atoll
Ailuk Atoll
Mejit Island
Wotho Atoll
Likiep Atoll
Jemo Island
Ujelang Atoll
Ratak Chain
Ralik Chain
Wotje Atoll
Erikub Atoll
Kwajalein Atoll
Ujae Atoll
Lae Atoll
Maloelap Atoll
Lib
Aur Atoll
Namu Atoll
Jabwot
Ailinglaplap Atoll
Majuro Atoll
Arno Atoll
Jaluit Atoll
Mili Atoll
Knox Atoll
Namorik Atoll
Kili Island
Ebon Atoll
SCALE 1:7,250,000
SCALE 1:1,100,000
Rongrong
Iroj
Majuro Atoll
Laura
Kallalen
Enigu
Majuro Lagoon
Djarrit
Dalap
Majuro
NAURU
Anna Point
Baiti
Anabar
Nibok
Ijuw
Denig
Phosphate mineworks
Anibare
Aiwo
Buada Lagoon
Anibare Bay
Yaren
Nauru International
Meneng Point
SCALE 1:250,000
SCALE 1:725,000
Parem Island
Sokehs Island
Pohnpei
Kolonia
Takaieu Island
Nanuh
PALIKIR
Pohnpei
Nahnalaud 772m
Pehleng
Madolenihmw
Nan Madol
Tomworoahlang
Kepirohi Falls
Temwen Island
Ronkiti
Pwok
Rohi
Lohd
Chuuk Islands
Piis Moen
Lamoil
Falalu
Tora
North Pass
Tora Island Pass
Northeast Island
Ruo
Falos
Quoi
Fono
Weno
Romanum
Udot
Eot
Shiki Islands
Dublon
Pata
Tol
Parem
Etten
Piaanu Pass
Polle
Totiw
Fanapanges
Fefan
Pisar
Shichiyo Islands
Tsis
Uman
Ollan
Salat
Salat Pass
Otta Pass
Otta
Fanan
Uijec
Feneppi
Mesegon
Neoch
Lauvergne Island
Ipis
SCALE 1:1,750,000
WAKE ISLAND (to US)
Toki Point
Peale Island
Kuku Point
Flipper Point
Heel Point
Wilkes Island
Wake Lagoon
Settlement
Wake Island
Peacock Point
SCALE 1:275,000
Tafunsak
Gabert
Okat Harbor
Mount Mutunte
Lelu Island
Lelu
Insiaf
Kosrae
Tofol
Mount Finkol 629m
Malem
Utwe Harbor
SCALE 1:550,000
Magur Islands
Ulul
Namonuito Atoll
Fayu
Murilo Atoll
Nomwin Atoll
Hall Islands
CHUUK
Pulap Atoll
Puluwat Atoll
Manila Reef
Pulusuk
Weno
Chuuk Islands
Neoch
Nama
Losap Atoll
Minto Reef
Oroluk Atoll
Pakin Atoll
PALIKIR
Kolonia
Pohnpei
Ant Atoll
Mwokil Atoll
MICRONESIA
Caroline Islands
POHNPEI
Pingelap Atoll
Namoluk Atoll
Etal Atoll
Lukunor Atoll
Satawan Atoll
Mortlock Islands
Ngetik Atoll
Kosrae
Tofol
KOSRAE
Nukuoro Atoll
SCALE 1:9,000,000

Majuro Atoll is the Marshall Islands' capital and commercial center. Almost half the population live on the narrow islands, often in overcrowded conditions.

A series of coral pinnacles *stand exposed in the shallow water off the coast of Nauru. Much of the island has an extraordinary "lunar" landscape, created by years of phosphate extraction.*

Canoes, built following tradition, *are still important in Micronesia, and are used for transportation and for fishing. This large canoe, on Satawal, in the state of Yap, needs nearly 20 people to return it to the boathouse.*

A B C D E F G H I J K L M

Polynesia

Kiribati, Tuvalu, ***Cook Islands, Easter Island, French Polynesia, Niue, Pitcairn Islands, Tokelau, Wallis & Futuna***

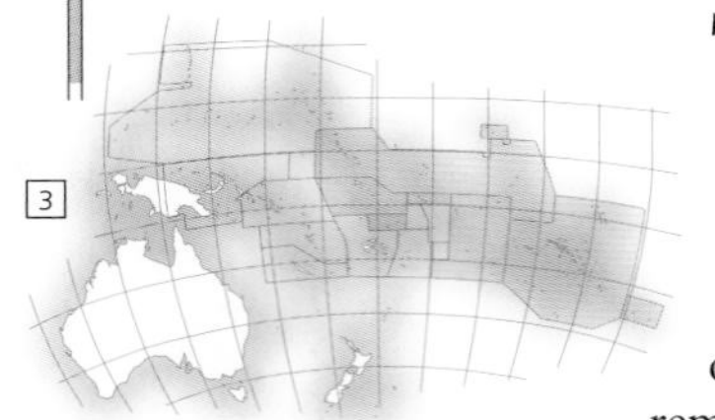

The numerous island groups of Polynesia lie to the east of Australia, scattered over a vast area in the south Pacific. The islands are a mixture of low-lying coral atolls, some of which enclose lagoons, and the tips of great underwater volcanoes. The populations on the islands are small, and most people are of Polynesian origin, as are the Maori of New Zealand. Local economies remain simple, relying mainly on subsistence crops, mineral deposits, many now exhausted, fishing, and tourism.

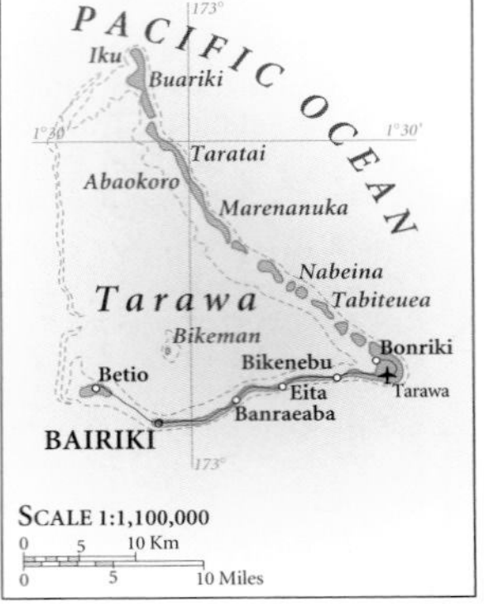

PACIFIC OCEAN
Iku
Buariki
Taratai
Abaokoro
Marenanuka
Nabeina
Tabiteuea
Tarawa
Bikeman
Bonriki
Betio
Bikenebu
Eita
Banraeaba
Tarawa
BAIRIKI
SCALE 1:1,100,000
0 5 10 Km
0 5 10 Miles

With the exception of Banaba all the islands in Kiribati's three groups are low-lying, coral atolls. This aerial view shows the sparsely vegetated islands, intercut by many small lagoons.

Kiribati

A former British colony, Kiribati became independent in 1979. Banaba's phosphate deposits ran out in 1980, following decades of exploitation by the British. Economic development remains slow and most agriculture is at a subsistence level, though coconuts provide export income, and underwater agriculture is being developed.

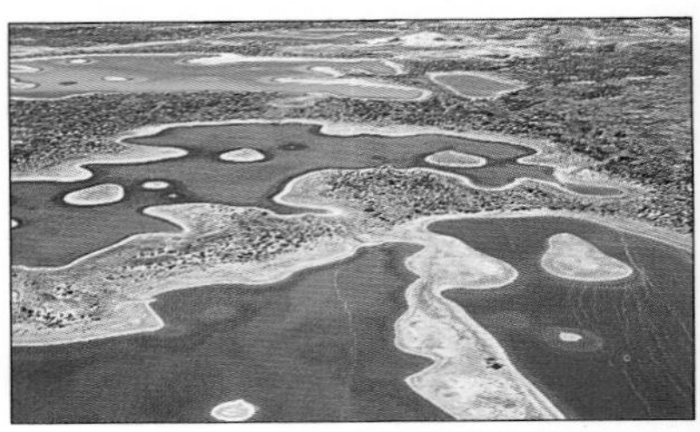

Tuvalu

A chain of nine coral atolls, 360 miles (579 km) long with a land area of just over 9 sq miles (23 sq km), Tuvalu is one of the world's smallest and most isolated states. As the Ellice Islands, Tuvalu was linked to the Gilbert Islands (now part of Kiribati) as a British colony until independence in 1978. Politically and socially conservative, Tuvaluans live by fishing and subsistence farming.

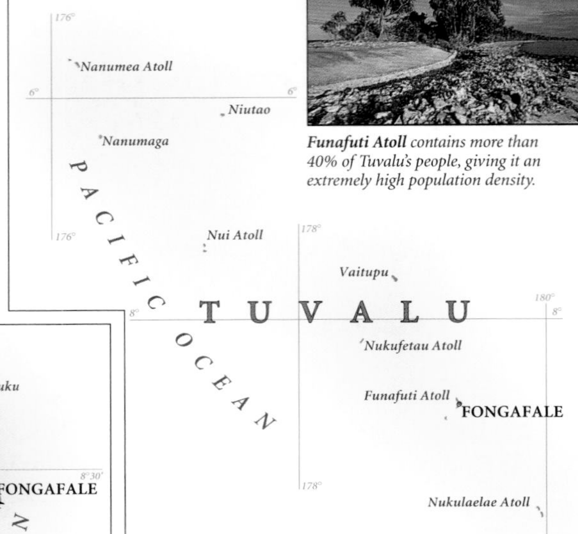

Nanumea Atoll
Niutao
Nanumaga
PACIFIC OCEAN
Nui Atoll
Vaitupu
TUVALU
Nukufetau Atoll
Funafuti Atoll
FONGAFALE
Nukulaelae Atoll
Niulakita
SCALE 1:6,750,000
0 10 20 40 60 80 Km
0 10 20 40 60 80 Miles

Funafuti Atoll contains more than 40% of Tuvalu's people, giving it an extremely high population density.

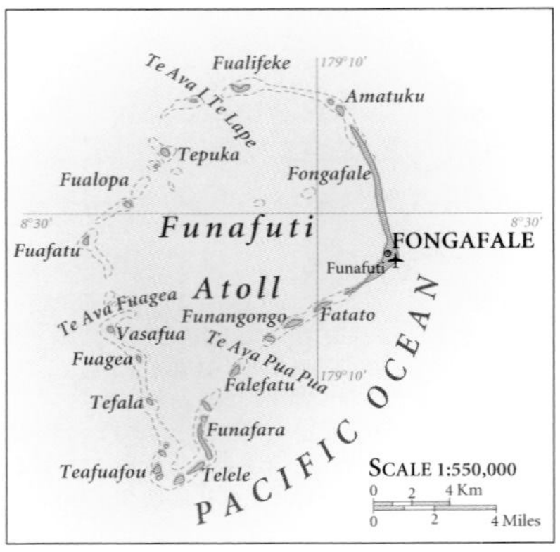

Te Ava I Te Lape
Fualifeke
Amatuku
Tepuka
Fualopa
Fongafale
Funafuti Atoll
Fuafatu
FONGAFALE
Funafuti
Te Ava Fuagea
Funangongo
Fatato
Vasafua
Te Ava Pua Pua
Fuagea
Falefatu
Tefala
Funafara
Teafuafou
Telele
PACIFIC OCEAN
SCALE 1:550,000
0 2 4 Km
0 2 4 Miles

Tokelau (to New Zealand)

A low-lying coral atoll, Tokelau is a dependent territory of New Zealand with few natural resources. Although a 1990 cyclone destroyed crops and infrastructure, a tuna cannery and the sale of fishing licenses have raised revenue and a catamaran link between the islands has increased their tourism potential. Tokelau's small size and economic weakness makes independence from New Zealand unlikely.

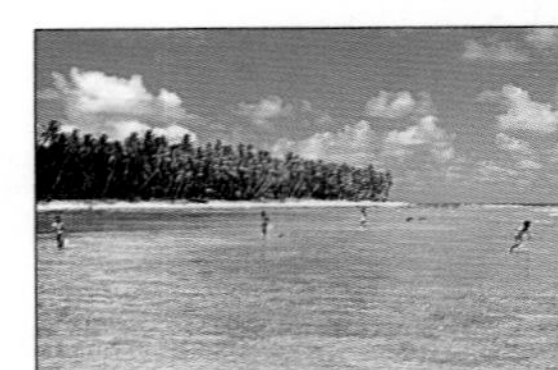

Fishermen cast their nets to catch small fish in the shallow waters off Atafu Atoll, the most westerly island in Tokelau.

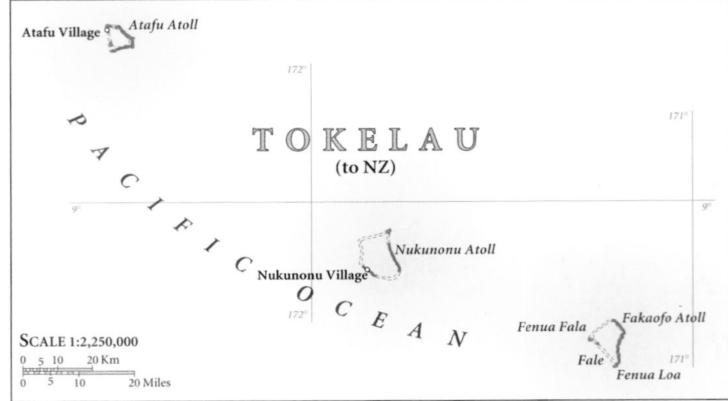

Atafu Village
Atafu Atoll
TOKELAU
(to NZ)
PACIFIC OCEAN
Nukunonu Atoll
Nukunonu Village
Fenua Fala
Fakaofo Atoll
Fale
Fenua Loa
SCALE 1:2,250,000
0 5 10 20 Km
0 5 10 20 Miles

Wallis & Futuna (to France)

In contrast to other French overseas territories in the south Pacific, the inhabitants of Wallis and Futuna have shown little desire for greater autonomy. A subsistence economy produces a variety of tropical crops, while foreign currency remittances come from expatriates and from the sale of licenses to Japanese and Korean fishing fleets.

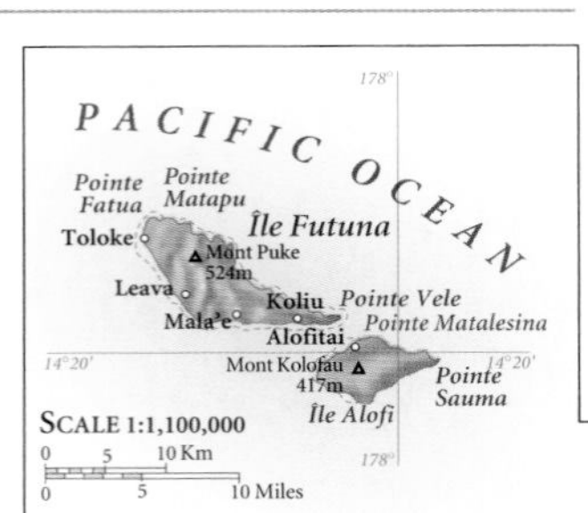

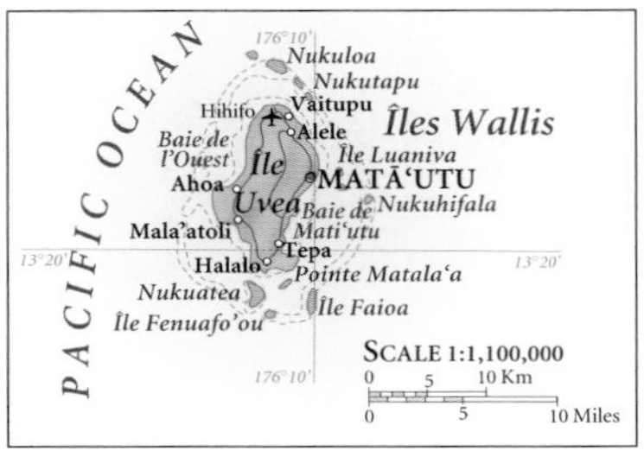

PACIFIC OCEAN
Pointe Fatua
Pointe Matapu
Île Futuna
Toloke
Mont Puke 524m
Leava
Mala'e
Koliu
Pointe Vele
Alofitai
Pointe Matalesina
Mont Kolofau 417m
Pointe Sauma
Île Alofi
SCALE 1:1,100,000
0 5 10 Km
0 5 10 Miles

PACIFIC OCEAN
Nukuloa
Nukutapu
Vaitupu
Hihifo
Alele
Îles Wallis
Baie de l'Ouest
Île Luaniva
Ahoa
Île Uvea
MATĀ'UTU
Baie de Mati'utu
Nukuhifala
Mala'atoli
Tepa
Halalo
Pointe Matala'a
Nukuatea
Île Faioa
Île Fenuafo'ou
SCALE 1:1,100,000
0 5 10 Km
0 5 10 Miles

Cook Islands (to New Zealand)

A mixture of coral atolls and volcanic peaks, the Cook Islands achieved self-government in 1965 but exist in free association with New Zealand. A diverse economy includes pearl and giant clam farming, and an ostrich farm, plus tourism and banking. A 1991 friendship treaty with France provides for French surveillance of territorial waters.

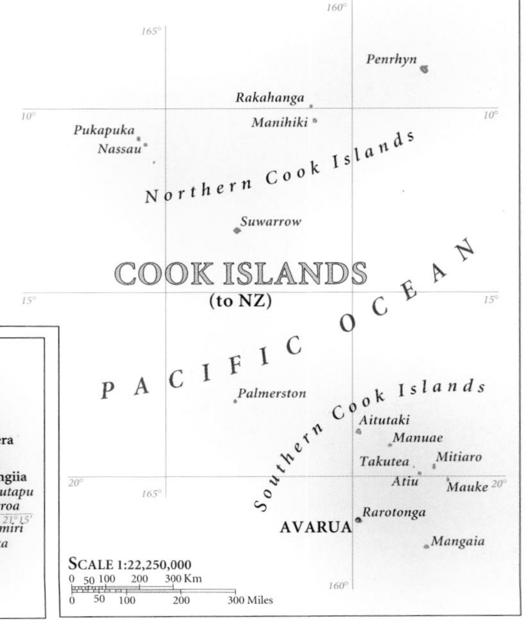

Penrhyn
Rakahanga
Manihiki
Pukapuka
Nassau
Northern Cook Islands
Suwarrow
COOK ISLANDS
(to NZ)
PACIFIC OCEAN
Palmerston
Southern Cook Islands
Aitutaki
Manuae
Takutea
Mitiaro
Atiu
Mauke
Rarotonga
AVARUA
Mangaia
SCALE 1:22,250,000
0 50 100 200 300 Km
0 50 100 200 300 Miles

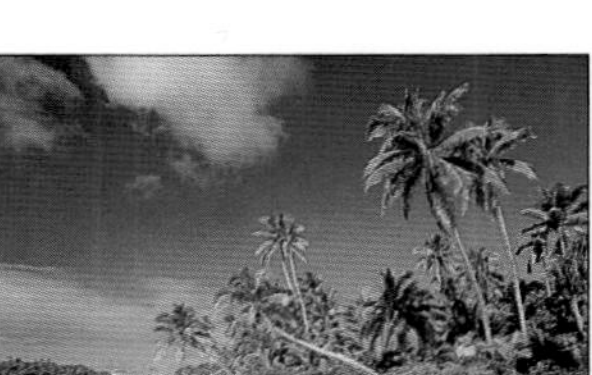

Palm trees fringe the white sands of a beach on Aitutaki in the Southern Cook Islands, where tourism is of increasing economic importance.

Niue (to New Zealand)

Niue, the world's largest coral island, is self-governing but exists in free association with New Zealand. Tropical fruits are grown for local consumption; tourism and the sale of postage stamps provide foreign currency. The lack of local job prospects has led more than 10,000 Niueans to emigrate to New Zealand, which has now invested heavily in Niue's economy in the hope of reversing this trend.

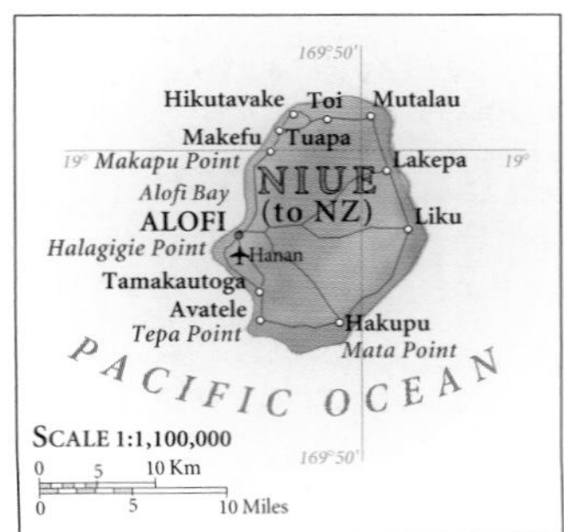

Hikutavake
Toi
Mutalau
Makefu
Tuapa
Makapu Point
Lakepa
Alofi Bay
NIUE
(to NZ)
ALOFI
Liku
Halagigie Point
Hanan
Tamakautoga
Avatele
Hakupu
Tepa Point
Mata Point
PACIFIC OCEAN
SCALE 1:1,100,000
0 5 10 Km
0 5 10 Miles

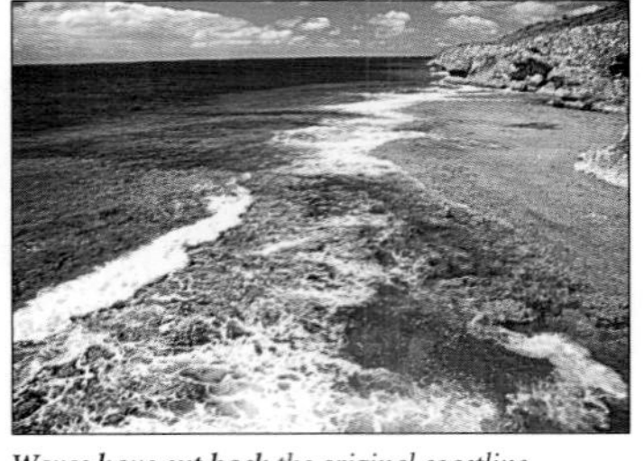

Waves have cut back the original coastline, exposing a sandy beach, near Mutalau in the northeast corner of Niue.

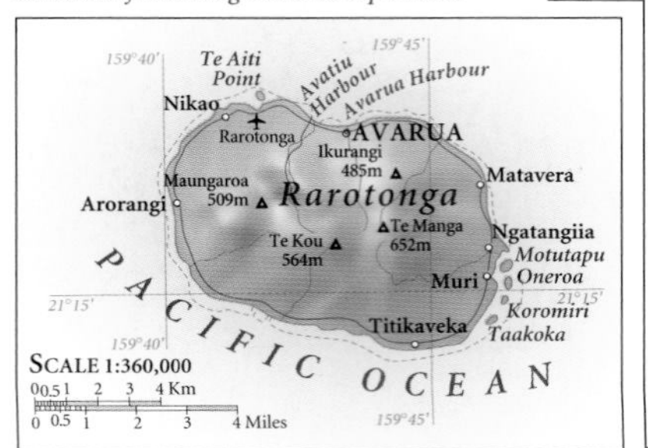

Te Aiti Point
Avatiu Harbour
Avarua Harbour
Nikao
Rarotonga
AVARUA
Ikurangi 485m
Maungaroa 509m
Rarotonga
Matavera
Arorangi
Te Kou 564m
Te Manga 652m
Ngatangiia
Motutapu
Oneroa
Muri
Koromiri
Titikaveka
Taakoka
PACIFIC OCEAN
SCALE 1:360,000
0 0.5 1 2 3 4 Km
0 0.5 1 2 3 4 Miles

A B C D E F G H I J K L M

N O P Q R S T U V W X Y

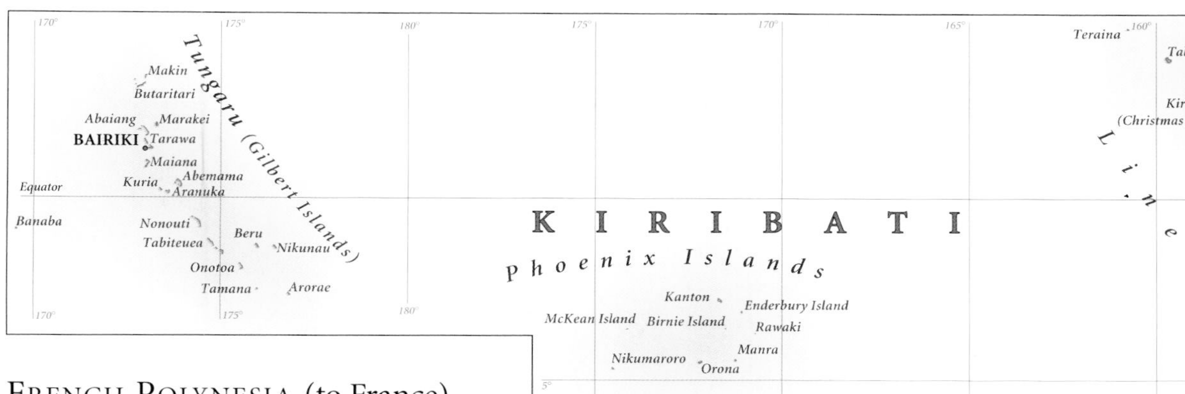
Tungaru (Gilbert Islands)
Makin
Butaritari
Abaiang
Marakei
BAIRIKI
Tarawa
Maiana
Abemama
Kuria
Aranuka
Equator
Banaba
Nonouti
Tabiteuea
Beru
Nikunau
Onotoa
Tamana
Arorae
KIRIBATI
Phoenix Islands
Kanton
Enderbury Island
McKean Island
Birnie Island
Rawaki
Manra
Nikumaroro
Orona
Teraina
Tabuaeran
Kiritimati (Christmas Island)
Line Islands
Equator
Malden Island
Starbuck Island

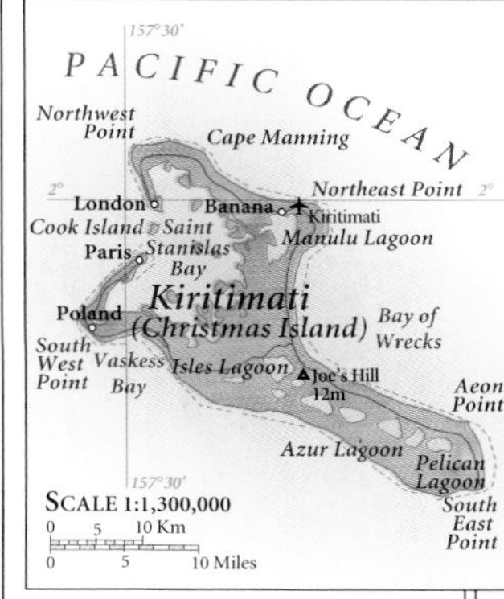
PACIFIC OCEAN
Northwest Point
Cape Manning
Northeast Point
London
Banana
Kiritimati
Cook Island
Saint Stanislas Bay
Manulu Lagoon
Paris
Poland
Kiritimati (Christmas Island)
Bay of Wrecks
South West Point
Vaskess Bay
Isles Lagoon
Joe's Hill 12m
Aeon Point
Azur Lagoon
Pelican Lagoon
South East Point
SCALE 1:1,300,000
0 5 10 Km
0 5 10 Miles

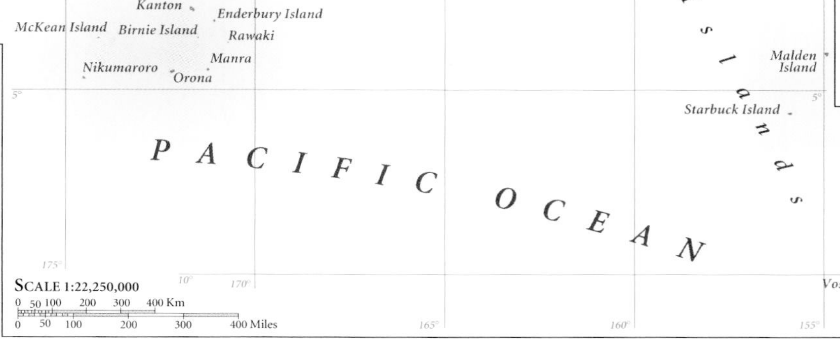
PACIFIC OCEAN
Millennium Island
Vostok Island
Flint Island
SCALE 1:22,250,000
0 50 100 200 300 400 Km
0 50 100 200 300 400 Miles

FRENCH POLYNESIA (to France)

THE 130 ISLANDS OF FRENCH POLYNESIA cover 4 million sq miles (10.5 million sq km). Nearly 75% of the people live on Tahiti. The use of Mururoa as a nuclear testing site by the French military transformed the economy, creating many jobs. The end of testing led to calls from the Polynesian majority for greater autonomy from France, the rebuilding of indigenous trade, and a reduction in tourism to stop the erosion of the islands' traditional culture.

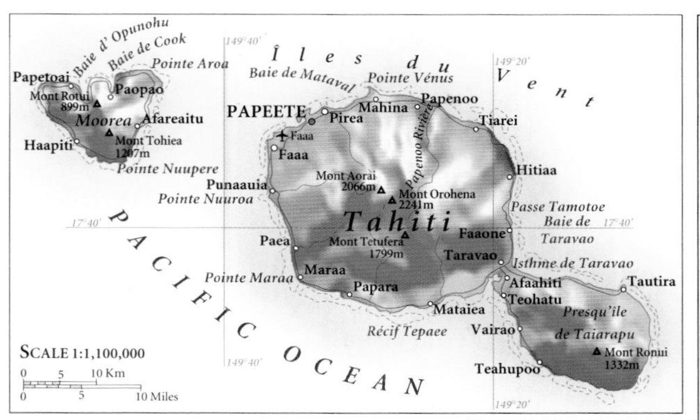
Îles du Vent
Baie d'Opunohu
Baie de Cook
Pointe Aroa
Baie de Matavai
Pointe Vénus
Papetoai
Paopao
Mont Rotui 899m
Moorea
Afareaitu
PAPEETE
Pirea
Mahina
Papenoo
Tiarei
Faaa
Haapiti
Mont Tohiea 1207m
Pointe Nuupere
Punaauia
Pointe Nuuroa
Mont Aorai 2066m
Mont Orohena 2241m
Hitiaa
Passe Tamotoe
Baie de Taravao
Tahiti
Paea
Mont Tetufera 1799m
Faaone
Taravao
Isthme de Taravao
Afaahiti
Tautira
Teohatu
Maraa
Papara
Pointe Maraa
Presqu'île de Taiarapu
Mataiea
Récif Tepaee
Vairao
Mont Ronui 1332m
Teahupoo
PACIFIC OCEAN
SCALE 1:1,100,000
0 5 10 Km
0 5 10 Miles

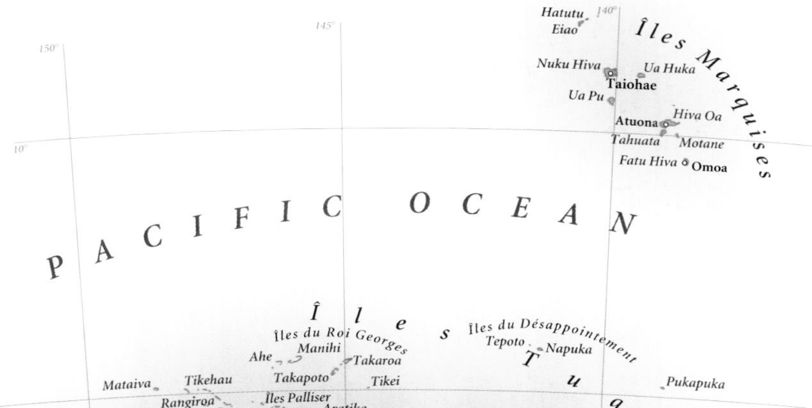
Hatutu
Eiao
Îles Marquises
Nuku Hiva
Ua Huka
Taiohae
Ua Pu
Atuona
Hiva Oa
Tahuata
Motane
Fatu Hiva
Omoa
PACIFIC OCEAN

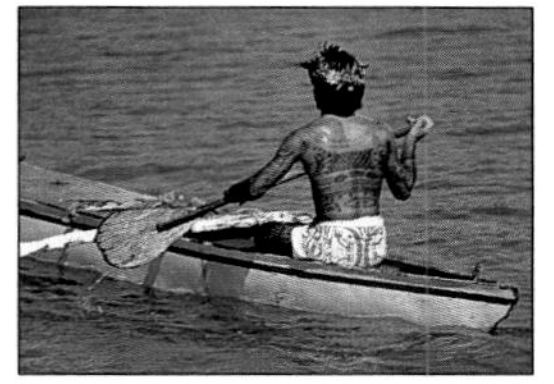
The traditional Tahitian welcome for visitors, who are greeted by parties of canoes, has become a major tourist attraction.

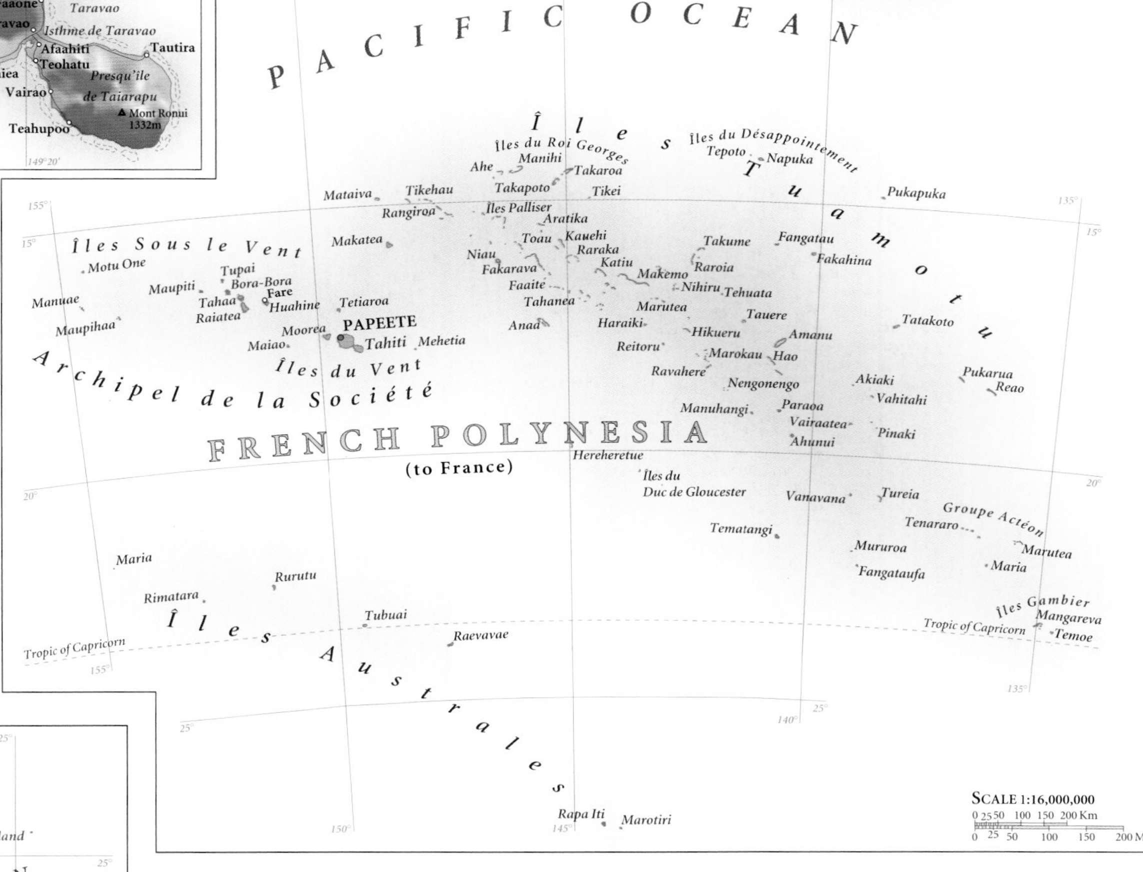
Îles Tuamotu
Îles du Roi Georges
Îles du Désappointement
Manihi
Ahe
Takaroa
Tepoto
Napuka
Mataiva
Tikehau
Takapoto
Tikei
Pukapuka
Rangiroa
Îles Palliser
Aratika
Îles Sous le Vent
Makatea
Toau
Kauehi
Raraka
Takume
Fangatau
Motu One
Niau
Fakarava
Katiu
Makemo
Raroia
Fakahina
Tupai
Bora-Bora
Maupiti
Fare
Faaite
Nihiru
Tehuata
Manuae
Tahaa
Huahine
Tetiaroa
Tahanea
Marutea
Tauere
Raiatea
PAPEETE
Anaa
Haraiki
Tatakoto
Maupihaa
Moorea
Tahiti
Mehetia
Hikueru
Amanu
Maiao
Reitoru
Marokau
Hao
Îles du Vent
Ravahere
Akiaki
Pukarua
Archipel de la Société
Nengonengo
Reao
Vahitahi
Manuhangi
Paraoa
Vairaatea
Ahunui
Pinaki
FRENCH POLYNESIA (to France)
Hereheretue
Îles du Duc de Gloucester
Vanavana
Tureia
Groupe Actéon
Tenararo
Tematangi
Marutea
Maria
Mururoa
Fangataufa
Maria
Rururu
Rimatara
Tubuai
Îles Gambier
Mangareva
Temoe
Tropic of Capricorn
Raevavae
Îles Australes
Rapa Iti
Marotiri
SCALE 1:16,000,000
0 25 50 100 150 200 Km
0 25 50 100 150 200 Miles

PITCAIRN ISLANDS (to UK)

BRITAIN'S MOST ISOLATED DEPENDENCY, Pitcairn Island was first populated by mutineers from the HMS *Bounty* in 1790. Emigration is further depleting the already limited gene pool of the island's inhabitants, with associated social and health problems. Barter, fishing, and subsistence farming form the basis of the economy although postage stamp sales provide foreign currency earnings, and offshore mineral exploitation may boost the economy in future.

PITCAIRN ISLANDS (to UK)
Oeno Island
Henderson Island
Ducie Island
Pitcairn Island
PACIFIC OCEAN
SCALE 1:11,000,000
0 25 50 100 Km
0 25 50 100 Miles

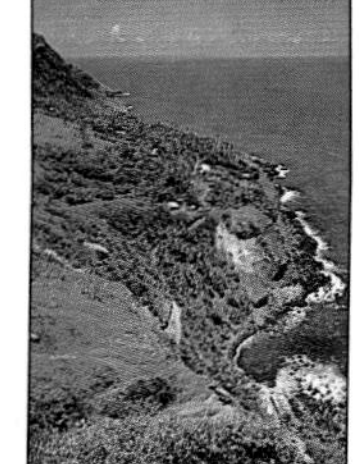
The Pitcairn Islanders rely on regular airdrops from New Zealand and periodic visits by supply vessels to provide them with basic commodities.

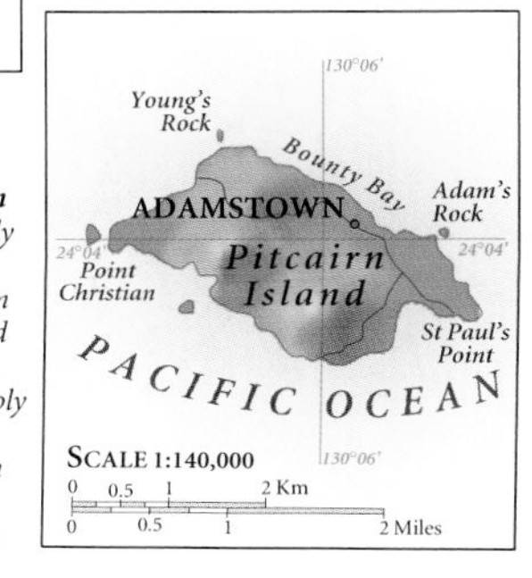
Young's Rock
Bounty Bay
Adam's Rock
ADAMSTOWN
Pitcairn Island
Point Christian
St Paul's Point
PACIFIC OCEAN
SCALE 1:140,000
0 0.5 1 2 Km
0 0.5 1 2 Miles

EASTER ISLAND (to Chile)

ONE OF THE MOST EASTERLY ISLANDS in Polynesia, Easter Island *(Isla de Pascua)* – also known as Rapa Nui, is part of Chile. The mainly Polynesian inhabitants support themselves by farming, which is mainly of a subsistence nature, and includes cattle rearing and crops such as sugar cane, bananas, corn, gourds, and potatoes. In recent years, tourism has become the most important source of income and the island sustains a small commercial airport.

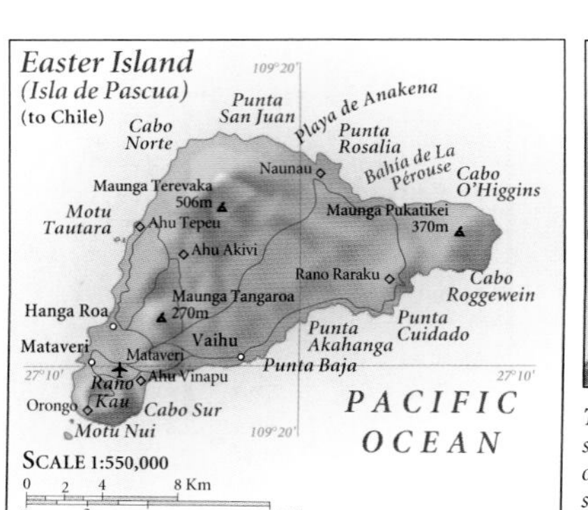
Easter Island (Isla de Pascua) (to Chile)
Punta San Juan
Playa de Anakena
Cabo Norte
Punta Rosalia
Bahía de La Pérouse
Naunau
Cabo O'Higgins
Maunga Terevaka 506m
Maunga Pukatikei 370m
Motu Tautara
Ahu Tepeu
Ahu Akivi
Rano Raraku
Cabo Roggewein
Maunga Tangaroa 270m
Hanga Roa
Punta Cuidado
Punta Akahanga
Mataveri
Vaihu
Ahu Vinapu
Punta Baja
Rano Kau
Orongo
Cabo Sur
Motu Nui
PACIFIC OCEAN
SCALE 1:550,000
0 2 4 8 Km
0 2 4 8 Miles

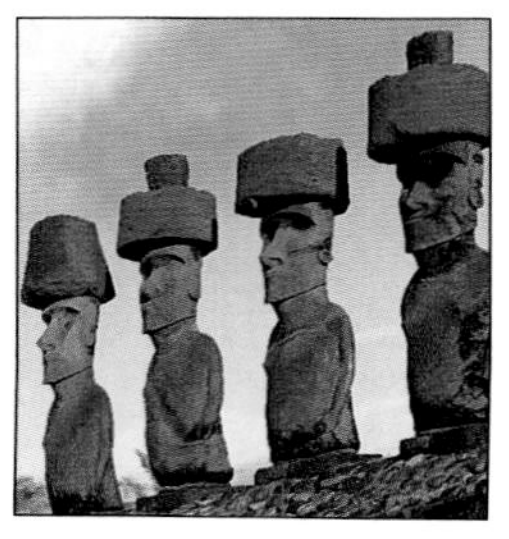
The Naunau, a series of huge stone statues overlook Playa de Anakena, on Easter Island. Carved from a soft volcanic rock, they were erected between 400 and 900 years ago.

N O P Q R S T U V W X Y Z

Pacific Ocean

The Pacific is the world's largest and deepest ocean. It is nearly twice the area of the Atlantic and contains almost three times as much water. The ocean is dotted with islands and surrounded by some of the world's most populous states; over half the world's population lives on its shores. The Pacific is bordered by active plate margins known as the "Ring of Fire," causing earthquakes and tsunamis, and creating volcanic islands and subterranean mountain chains. The largest underwater mountains break the surface as island arcs. The fisheries of the Pacific are some of the most productive in the world and provide a vital resource for many of the Pacific islands. Since the Second World War there has been a shift in trading patterns, with a considerable growth in trade between the United States and the countries of the Pacific Rim.

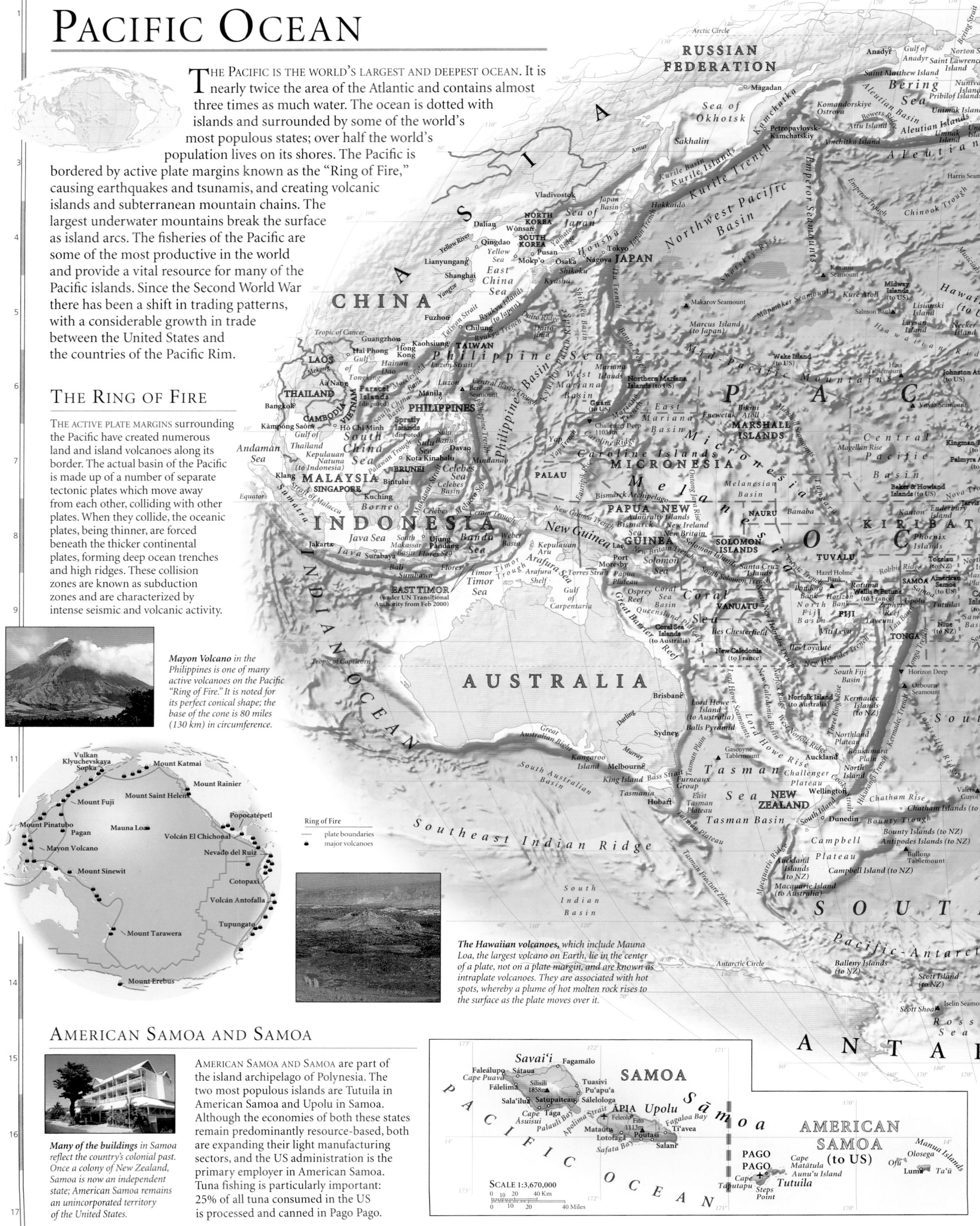

RUSSIAN FEDERATION
ASIA
CHINA
INDONESIA
MALAYSIA
PHILIPPINES
JAPAN
AUSTRALIA
NEW ZEALAND
PAPUA NEW GUINEA
SOLOMON ISLANDS
MICRONESIA
MARSHALL ISLANDS
KIRIBATI
TUVALU
VANUATU
FIJI
TONGA
PALAU
NAURU
EAST TIMOR
THAILAND
CAMBODIA
VIETNAM
LAOS
TAIWAN
NORTH KOREA
SOUTH KOREA
BRUNEI
SINGAPORE
Sea of Okhotsk
Bering Sea
Sea of Japan
East China Sea
South China Sea
Philippine Sea
Coral Sea
Tasman Sea
Java Sea
Banda Sea
Arafura Sea
Timor Sea
Andaman Sea
Solomon Sea
INDIAN OCEAN
Southeast Indian Ridge
Northwest Pacific Basin
Mid-Pacific Mountains
Emperor Seamounts
Kurile Trench
Aleutian Islands
Hawaiian Ridge
Tasman Basin
South Indian Basin
Tropic of Cancer
Tropic of Capricorn
Equator
Arctic Circle
Antarctic Circle
ANTARCTICA
Ring of Fire
plate boundaries
major volcanoes
Vulkan Klyuchevskaya Sopka
Mount Katmai
Mount Rainier
Mount Fuji
Mount Saint Helens
Mount Pinatubo
Pagan
Mauna Loa
Popocatépetl
Volcán El Chichonal
Mayon Volcano
Nevado del Ruiz
Mount Sinewit
Cotopaxi
Volcán Antofalla
Tupungato
Mount Tarawera
Mount Erebus
SAMOA
AMERICAN SAMOA (to US)
Savai'i
Upolu
Tutuila
Manua Islands
ĀPIA
PAGO PAGO
PACIFIC OCEAN
Sāmoa
SCALE 1:3,670,000

The Ring of Fire

The active plate margins surrounding the Pacific have created numerous land and island volcanoes along its border. The actual basin of the Pacific is made up of a number of separate tectonic plates which move away from each other, colliding with other plates. When they collide, the oceanic plates, being thinner, are forced beneath the thicker continental plates, forming deep ocean trenches and high ridges. These collision zones are known as subduction zones and are characterized by intense seismic and volcanic activity.

Mayon Volcano in the Philippines is one of many active volcanoes on the Pacific "Ring of Fire." It is noted for its perfect conical shape; the base of the cone is 80 miles (130 km) in circumference.

The Hawaiian volcanoes, which include Mauna Loa, the largest volcano on Earth, lie in the center of a plate, not on a plate margin, and are known as intraplate volcanoes. They are associated with hot spots, whereby a plume of hot molten rock rises to the surface as the plate moves over it.

American Samoa and Samoa

American Samoa and Samoa are part of the island archipelago of Polynesia. The two most populous islands are Tutuila in American Samoa and Upolu in Samoa. Although the economies of both these states remain predominantly resource-based, both are expanding their light manufacturing sectors, and the US administration is the primary employer in American Samoa. Tuna fishing is particularly important: 25% of all tuna consumed in the US is processed and canned in Pago Pago.

Many of the buildings in Samoa reflect the country's colonial past. Once a colony of New Zealand, Samoa is now an independent state; American Samoa remains an unincorporated territory of the United States.

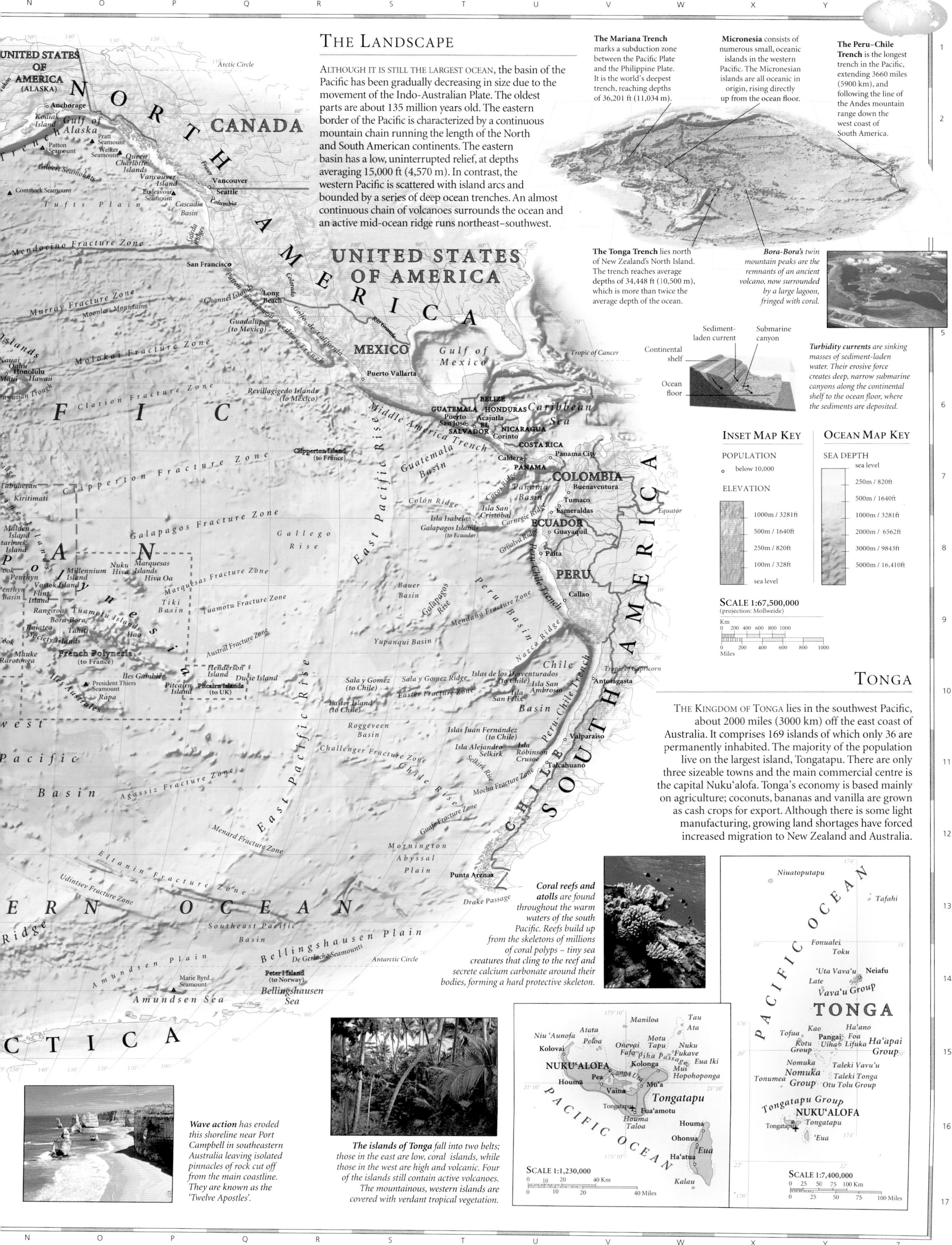
NORTH AMERICA
CANADA
UNITED STATES OF AMERICA
UNITED STATES OF AMERICA (ALASKA)
MEXICO
SOUTH AMERICA
COLOMBIA
ECUADOR
PERU
Gulf of Mexico
Caribbean Sea
East Pacific Rise
Peru-Chile Trench
Middle America Trench
Polynesia
French Polynesia (to France)
Southern Ocean
Antarctica
Amundsen Sea
Bellingshausen Sea
Drake Passage
Arctic Circle
Tropic of Cancer
Equator
Tropic of Capricorn
Antarctic Circle
Sediment-laden current
Submarine canyon
Continental shelf
Ocean floor
INSET MAP KEY
POPULATION
below 10,000
ELEVATION
1000m / 3281ft
500m / 1640ft
250m / 820ft
100m / 328ft
sea level
OCEAN MAP KEY
SEA DEPTH
sea level
250m / 820ft
500m / 1640ft
1000m / 3281ft
2000m / 6562ft
3000m / 9843ft
5000m / 16,410ft
SCALE 1:67,500,000
(projection: Mollweide)
NUKU'ALOFA
Tongatapu
PACIFIC OCEAN
SCALE 1:1,230,000
TONGA
Vava'u Group
Ha'apai Group
Nomuka Group
Tongatapu Group
SCALE 1:7,400,000

THE LANDSCAPE

ALTHOUGH IT IS STILL THE LARGEST OCEAN, the basin of the Pacific has been gradually decreasing in size due to the movement of the Indo-Australian Plate. The oldest parts are about 135 million years old. The eastern border of the Pacific is characterized by a continuous mountain chain running the length of the North and South American continents. The eastern basin has a low, uninterrupted relief, at depths averaging 15,000 ft (4,570 m). In contrast, the western Pacific is scattered with island arcs and bounded by a series of deep ocean trenches. An almost continuous chain of volcanoes surrounds the ocean and an active mid-ocean ridge runs northeast–southwest.

The Mariana Trench marks a subduction zone between the Pacific Plate and the Philippine Plate. It is the world's deepest trench, reaching depths of 36,201 ft (11,034 m).

Micronesia consists of numerous small, oceanic islands in the western Pacific. The Micronesian islands are all oceanic in origin, rising directly up from the ocean floor.

The Peru–Chile Trench is the longest trench in the Pacific, extending 3660 miles (5900 km), and following the line of the Andes mountain range down the west coast of South America.

The Tonga Trench lies north of New Zealand's North Island. The trench reaches average depths of 34,448 ft (10,500 m), which is more than twice the average depth of the ocean.

***Bora-Bora's** twin mountain peaks are the remnants of an ancient volcano, now surrounded by a large lagoon, fringed with coral.*

***Turbidity currents** are sinking masses of sediment-laden water. Their erosive force creates deep, narrow submarine canyons along the continental shelf to the ocean floor, where the sediments are deposited.*

TONGA

THE KINGDOM OF TONGA lies in the southwest Pacific, about 2000 miles (3000 km) off the east coast of Australia. It comprises 169 islands of which only 36 are permanently inhabited. The majority of the population live on the largest island, Tongatapu. There are only three sizeable towns and the main commercial centre is the capital Nuku'alofa. Tonga's economy is based mainly on agriculture; coconuts, bananas and vanilla are grown as cash crops for export. Although there is some light manufacturing, growing land shortages have forced increased migration to New Zealand and Australia.

***Coral reefs and atolls** are found throughout the warm waters of the south Pacific. Reefs build up from the skeletons of millions of coral polyps – tiny sea creatures that cling to the reef and secrete calcium carbonate around their bodies, forming a hard protective skeleton.*

***Wave action** has eroded this shoreline near Port Campbell in southeastern Australia leaving isolated pinnacles of rock cut off from the main coastline. They are known as the 'Twelve Apostles'.*

***The islands of Tonga** fall into two belts; those in the east are low, coral islands, while those in the west are high and volcanic. Four of the islands still contain active volcanoes. The mountainous, western islands are covered with verdant tropical vegetation.*

ANTARCTICA

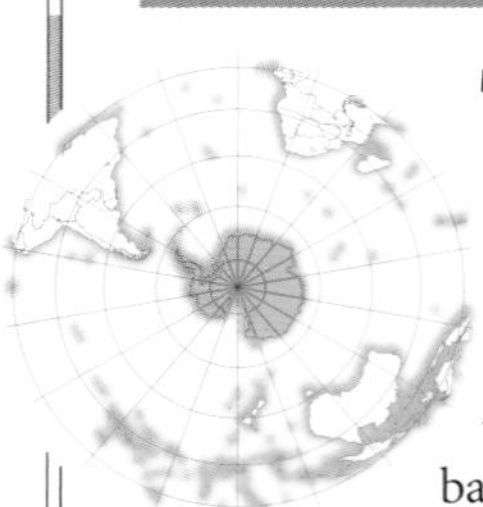

THE ICE-COVERED CONTINENT of Antarctica, which is the Earth's most southerly region, has drawn explorers and entrepreneurs seeking challenge and riches in its wintry lands for over 200 years. The extreme climate has deterred any large-scale settlement of the continent, and though commercial hunters built outposts in the past, habitation is now limited to scientific bases. The Antarctic Treaty, which came into force in 1961, provides for international governance and scientific cooperation in place of potential territorial conflict.

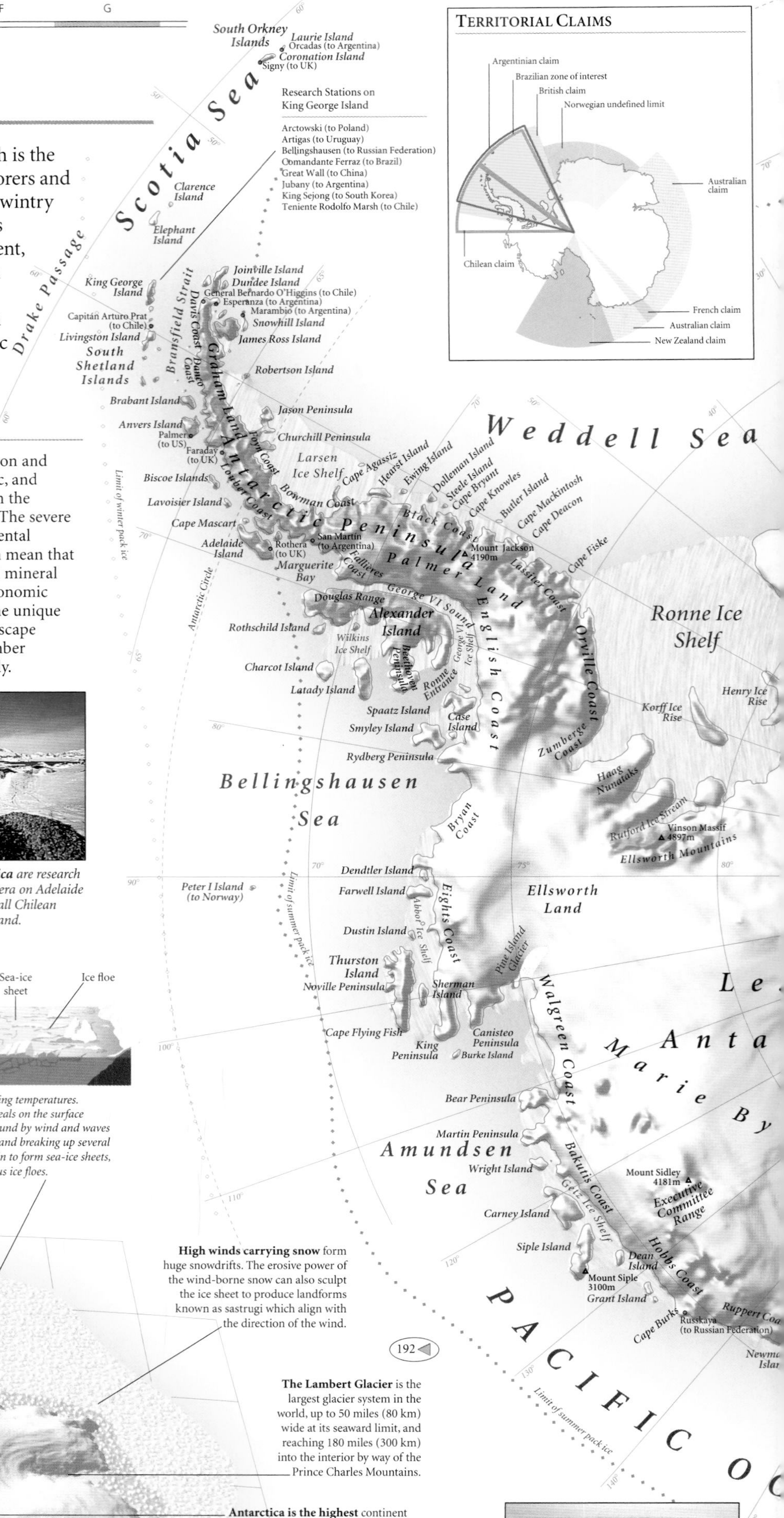

RESOURCES

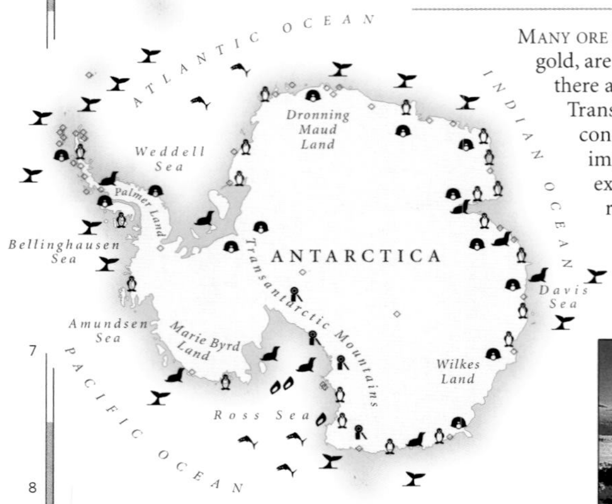

MANY ORE MINERALS, including iron and gold, are found in the Antarctic, and there are also coal reserves in the Transantarctic Mountains. The severe conditions and environmental importance of the region mean that exploitation of potential mineral resources is both uneconomic and undesirable. The unique wildlife and landscape draw a small number of tourists annually.

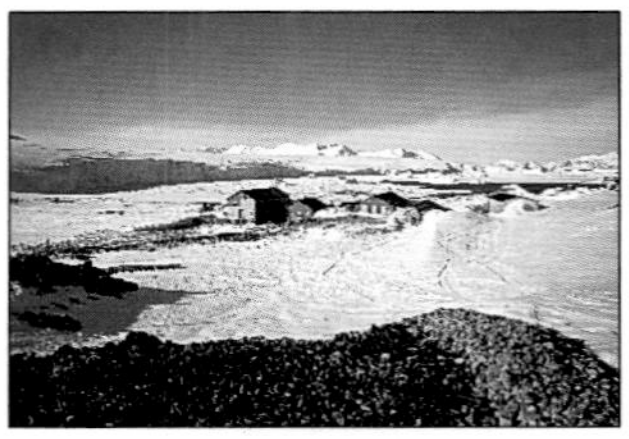

ATLANTIC OCEAN
INDIAN OCEAN
PACIFIC OCEAN
Dronning Maud Land
Weddell Sea
Palmer Land
Bellinghausen Sea
ANTARCTICA
Transantarctic Mountains
Davis Sea
Amundsen Sea
Marie Byrd Land
Wilkes Land
Ross Sea

Resources (including wildlife)
- coal
- fish
- minerals
- oil & gas
- penguins
- seals
- whales
- polar research base

Most settlements in Antarctica are research bases such as this one at Rothera on Adelaide Island, although there is a small Chilean settlement on King George Island.

THE LANDSCAPE

THERE ARE TWO DISTINCT PARTS to Antarctica: Lesser Antarctica, a series of ice-covered, mountainous islands, joined together by the ice; and the high plateau of Greater Antarctica. The Ross Sea and the Weddell Sea are outliers of the Atlantic and Pacific oceans – deep bays partially covered by thick ice shelves.

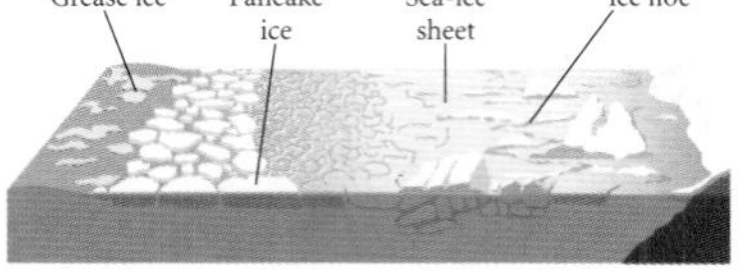

Grease ice
Pancake ice
Sea-ice sheet
Ice floe

***Pack ice forms out at sea** in freezing temperatures. At the outer limits, grease ice congeals on the surface of the ocean. This is then spun around by wind and waves into irregular "pancakes," freezing and breaking up several times before bonding together again to form sea-ice sheets, which finally cement into enormous ice floes.*

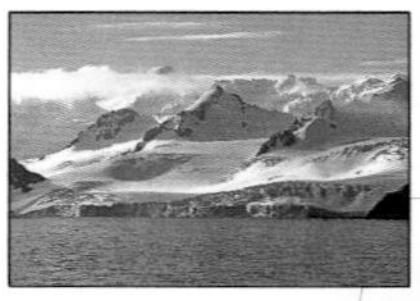

***On Elephant Island,** the coast is edged by glaciers, although the land is not permanently covered by ice.*

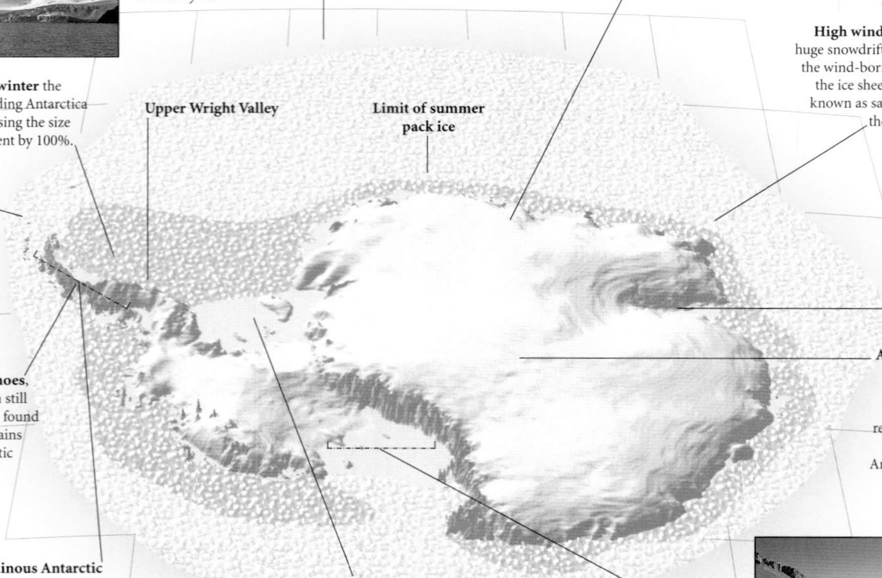

Limit of winter pack ice

Upper Wright Valley

Limit of summer pack ice

Elephant Island

During the winter the seas surrounding Antarctica freeze, increasing the size of the continent by 100%.

High winds carrying snow form huge snowdrifts. The erosive power of the wind-borne snow can also sculpt the ice sheet to produce landforms known as sastrugi which align with the direction of the wind.

The Lambert Glacier is the largest glacier system in the world, up to 50 miles (80 km) wide at its seaward limit, and reaching 180 miles (300 km) into the interior by way of the Prince Charles Mountains.

Many volcanoes, some of them still active, can be found in the mountains of the Antarctic Peninsula.

Antarctica is the highest continent on Earth, because of the great thickness of ice which overlays the land. In places the ice alone can reach up to 15,700 ft (4,800 m) thick. Much of the basement rock of west Antarctica lies below sea level, pushed down by the weight of the ice.

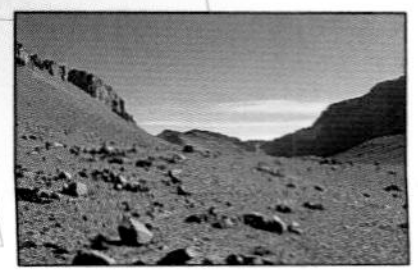

The mountainous Antarctic Peninsula is formed of rocks 65–225 million years old, overlain by more recent rocks and glacial deposits. It is connected to the Andes in South America by a submarine ridge.

Nearly half – 44% – of the Antarctic coastline is bounded by ice shelves, like the Ronne Ice Shelf, which float on the Ocean. These are joined to the inland ice sheet by dome-shaped ice "rises."

More than 30% of Antarctic ice is contained in the Ross Ice Shelf.

***The barren, flat-bottomed** Upper Wright Valley was once filled by a glacier, but is now dry, strewn with boulders and pebbles. In some dry valleys, there has been no rain for over 2 million years.*

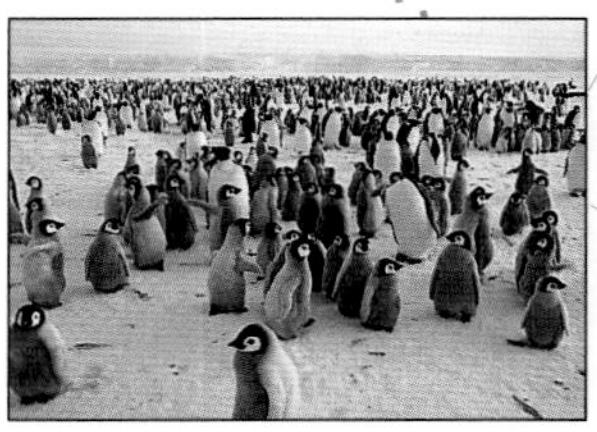

***Large colonies of seabirds** live in the extremely harsh Antarctic climate. The Emperor penguins seen here, the smaller Adélie penguin, the Antarctic petrel and the South Polar skua are the only birds that breed exclusively on the continent.*

TERRITORIAL CLAIMS

Argentinian claim
Brazilian zone of interest
British claim
Norwegian undefined limit
Australian claim
Chilean claim
French claim
Australian claim
New Zealand claim

South Orkney Islands
Laurie Island
Orcadas (to Argentina)
Coronation Island
Signy (to UK)

Research Stations on King George Island

Arctowski (to Poland)
Artigas (to Uruguay)
Bellingshausen (to Russian Federation)
Comandante Ferraz (to Brazil)
Great Wall (to China)
Jubany (to Argentina)
King Sejong (to South Korea)
Teniente Rodolfo Marsh (to Chile)

Scotia Sea
Drake Passage
Clarence Island
Elephant Island
King George Island
Capitán Arturo Prat (to Chile)
Livingston Island
South Shetland Islands
Joinville Island
Dundee Island
General Bernardo O'Higgins (to Chile)
Esperanza (to Argentina)
Marambio (to Argentina)
Snowhill Island
James Ross Island
Bransfield Strait
Davis Coast
Danco Coast
Graham Land
Robertson Island
Brabant Island
Anvers Island
Palmer (to US)
Faraday (to UK)
Jason Peninsula
Churchill Peninsula
Larsen Ice Shelf
Biscoe Islands
Lavoisier Island
Cape Mascart
Adelaide Island
Rothera (to UK)
San Martin (to Argentina)
Marguerite Bay
Foyn Coast
Oscar II Coast
Bowman Coast
Antarctic Peninsula
Cape Agassiz
Hearst Island
Ewing Island
Dolleman Island
Steele Island
Cape Bryant
Cape Knowles
Butler Island
Cape Mackintosh
Cape Deacon
Black Coast
Palmer Land
Mount Jackson 4190m
Lassiter Coast
Cape Fiske
Fallières Coast
Douglas Range
George VI Sound
Alexander Island
Rothschild Island
Wilkins Ice Shelf
Beethoven Peninsula
George VI Ice Shelf
English Coast
Charcot Island
Latady Island
Ronne Entrance
Spaatz Island
Smyley Island
Case Island
Rydberg Peninsula
Orville Coast
Weddell Sea
Ronne Ice Shelf
Henry Ice Rise
Korff Ice Rise
Zumberge Coast
Haag Nunataks
Rutford Ice Stream
Vinson Massif 4897m
Ellsworth Mountains
Bellingshausen Sea
Bryan Coast
Peter I Island (to Norway)
Dendtler Island
Farwell Island
Eights Coast
Abbot Ice Shelf
Ellsworth Land
Dustin Island
Thurston Island
Noville Peninsula
Sherman Island
Pine Island Glacier
Cape Flying Fish
King Peninsula
Canisteo Peninsula
Burke Island
Walgreen Coast
Lesser Antarctica
Marie Byrd Land
Bear Peninsula
Martin Peninsula
Amundsen Sea
Wright Island
Bakutis Coast
Getz Ice Shelf
Carney Island
Mount Sidley 4181m
Executive Committee Range
Siple Island
Dean Island
Hobbs Coast
Mount Siple 3100m
Grant Island
Cape Burks
Russkaya (to Russian Federation)
Ruppert Coast
PACIFIC OCEAN
Antarctic Circle
Limit of winter pack ice
Limit of summer pack ice

192

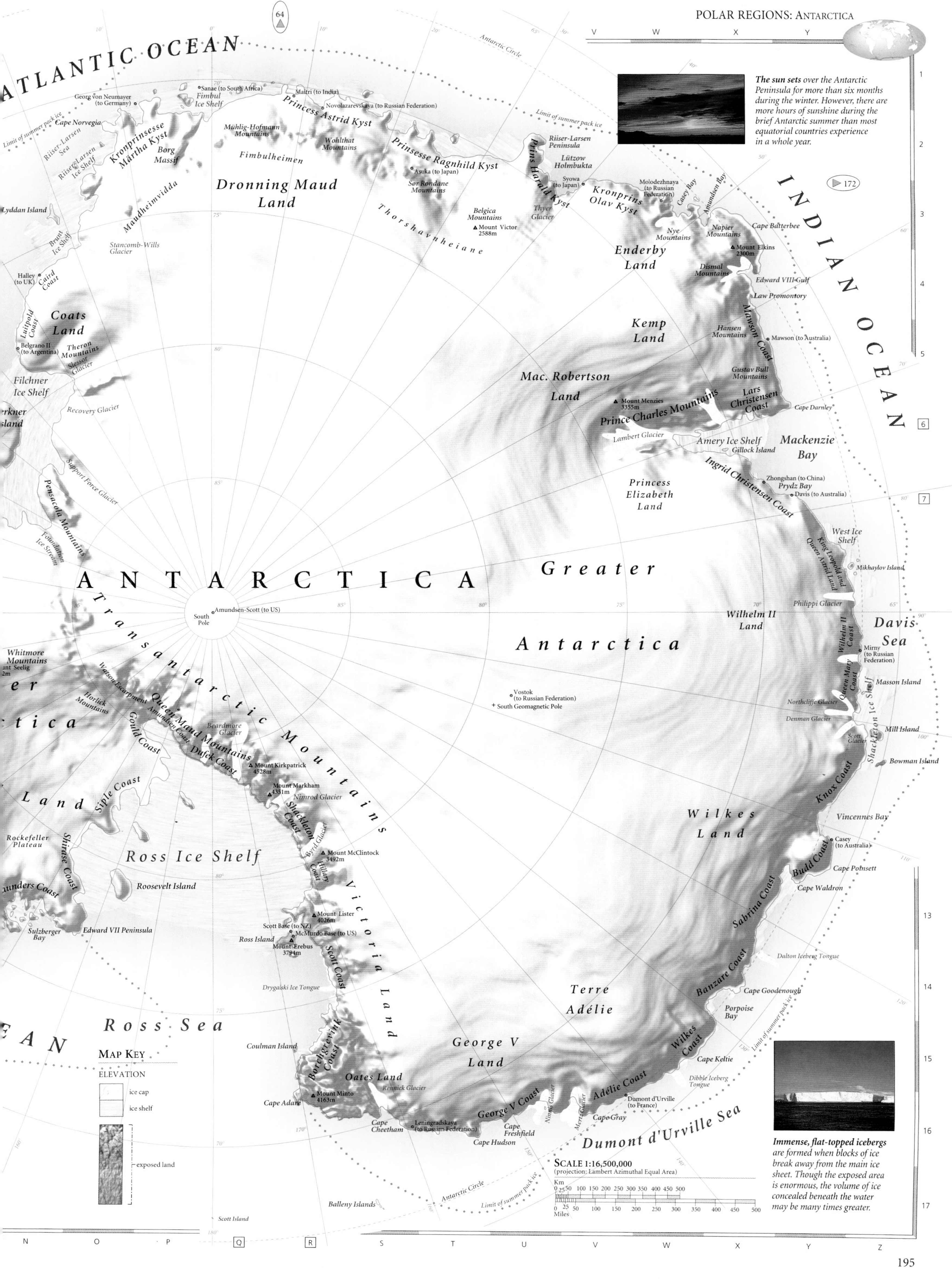
ATLANTIC OCEAN
INDIAN OCEAN
ANTARCTICA
Greater Antarctica
Dronning Maud Land
Enderby Land
Kemp Land
Mac. Robertson Land
Princess Elizabeth Land
Wilhelm II Land
Wilkes Land
Terre Adélie
George V Land
Oates Land
Victoria Land
Coats Land
Transantarctic Mountains
Ross Ice Shelf
Ross Sea
Davis Sea
Mackenzie Bay
Dumont d'Urville Sea
South Pole
Amundsen-Scott (to US)
Vostok (to Russian Federation)
South Geomagnetic Pole
Roosevelt Island
Ross Island
Amery Ice Shelf
Filchner Ice Shelf
Prince Charles Mountains
Queen Maud Mountains
Mount Kirkpatrick 4528m
Mount Markham 4351m
Mount McClintock 3492m
Mount Lister 4026m
Mount Erebus 3794m
Mount Minto 4163m
Mount Menzies 3355m
Mount Elkins 2300m
Mount Victor 2588m
Scott Base (to NZ)
McMurdo Base (to US)
Casey (to Australia)
Mawson (to Australia)
Davis (to Australia)
Mirny (to Russian Federation)
Dumont d'Urville (to France)
Leningradskaya (to Russian Federation)
Halley (to UK)
Belgrano II (to Argentina)
MAP KEY
ELEVATION
ice cap
ice shelf
exposed land
SCALE 1:16,500,000
(projection: Lambert Azimuthal Equal Area)

The sun sets over the Antarctic Peninsula for more than six months during the winter. However, there are more hours of sunshine during the brief Antarctic summer than most equatorial countries experience in a whole year.

Immense, flat-topped icebergs are formed when blocks of ice break away from the main ice sheet. Though the exposed area is enormous, the volume of ice concealed beneath the water may be many times greater.

The Arctic

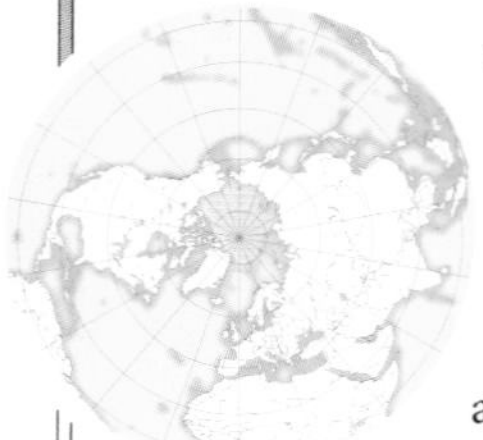

Three continents, Asia, North America, and Europe, reach into the Arctic Circle at their northernmost limits, almost entirely encircling the Arctic Ocean. Despite the region's extraordinarily harsh climate, it has been inhabited for thousands of years by peoples such as the European Lapps, the Russian Nenet, and the North American Inuit, who draw a living from fishing, herding, and hunting. More recently, particularly in the Russian Arctic, opportunities to exploit oil and other mineral reserves have encouraged immigration. Pollution of the Arctic's unique ecology and damage to the traditional lifestyles of many native peoples have been the unfortunate results of this activity, and international cooperation is needed to safeguard the future of the region.

Map Key

POPULATION
- above 5 million
- 1 million to 5 million
- 500,000 to 1 million
- 100,000 to 500,000
- 50,000 to 100,000
- 10,000 to 50,000
- below 10,000

SEA DEPTH
- sea level
- 250m / 820ft
- 500m / 1640ft
- 1000m / 3281ft
- 2000m / 6562ft
- 3000m / 9843ft

Scale 1:23,500,000
(projection: Lambert Azimuthal Equal Area)

Km 0 100 200 300 400 500 600
Miles 0 100 200 300 400 500 600

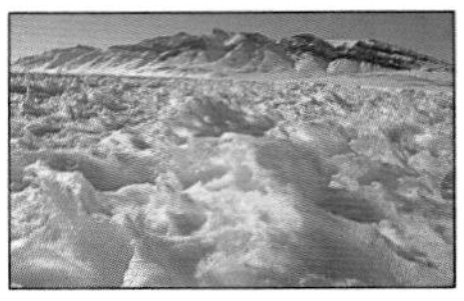

192

Windblown snow *etches deep patterns in the ice sheet known as sastrugi. They align with the direction of the wind*

8

Resources

Large quantities of coal, oil, and natural gas are to be found in the basins of the Arctic Ocean, and in northern Canada, Alaska and the Russian Federation. The cost and difficulty of extraction and, more recently, awareness of damage to the environment, have limited exploitation to coastal regions. The unfrozen waters have stocks of fish including cod, flounder, and haddock. Quotas have now been put in place to restrict the number of fish caught annually. Reindeer are herded in large numbers by many of the native Arctic peoples. Most grain and vegetables are imported from elsewhere.

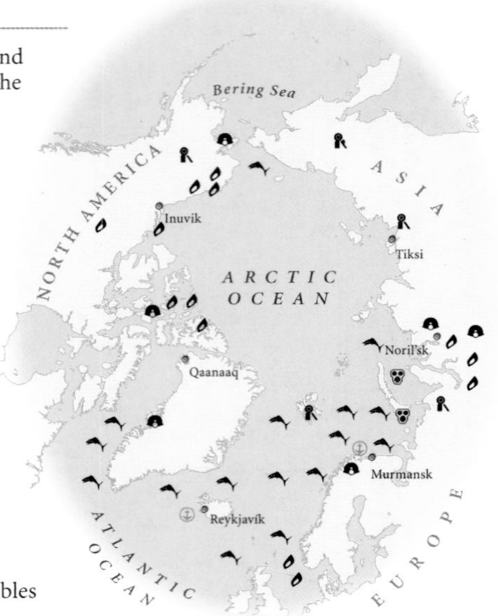

Resources
- coal
- fish
- mining
- oil & gas
- radioactive contamination
- major towns
- major ports

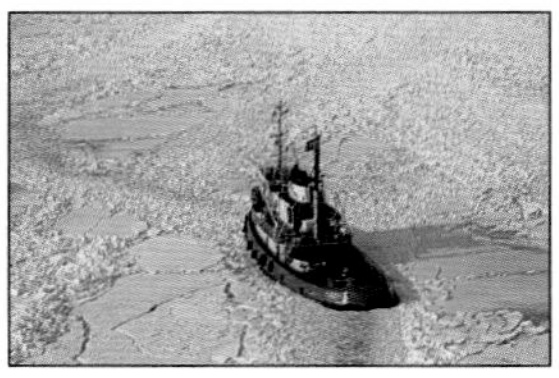

Icebreakers *are ships with specially strengthened hulls, designed to break a path through the ice. They are used to keep important routes open during the winter, when falling temperatures cause much of the Arctic Ocean to freeze over.*

8

The Landscape

The Arctic Ocean comprises two large ocean basins divided by three submarine ridges, the greatest of which, the Lomonosov Ridge, is a huge underwater mountain range which has an average height of more than 10,000 ft (3,000 m). The lands which encircle the Arctic Ocean are underlain by great shield areas of ancient rocks, which were heavily glaciated during the last Ice Age.

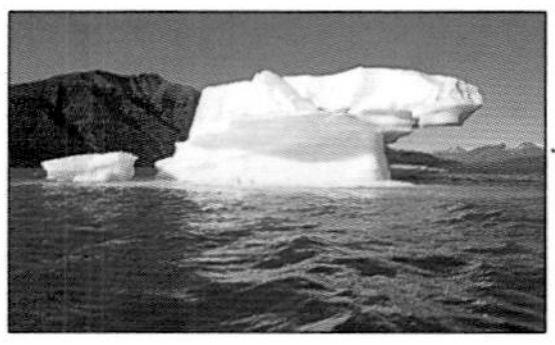

Icebergs *are constantly broken up and reshaped by wind and the oceans. This flat-topped iceberg has been undercut, leaving a craggy ice cliff.*

A complex and ancient mountain system, extending from the Queen Elizabeth Islands to eastern Greenland was formed more than 245 million years ago.

The Canadian Shield underlies almost all of the Canadian Arctic. It is a very stable plateau of ancient rock, now covered by glacial lakes and sediment, which supports tundra vegetation.

The Arctic Ocean is the world's smallest ocean with a total area of 5,440,000 sq miles (15,100,000 sq km).

At a latitude of more than 75° N, the Arctic Ocean is almost permanently covered by pack-ice, though high winds and the movement of the seas may cause the ice to crack and break up.

In the more southerly reaches of the Arctic, like Siberia, much of the land is covered by permafrost. In the summer, higher temperatures warm the frozen ground, causing a number of typical phenomena. These include solifluction, the fast downhill movement of top soil layers; freeze/thaw activity, which patterns the ground into regular polygonal shapes, and the formation of large domes with a frozen ice core, known as pingos.

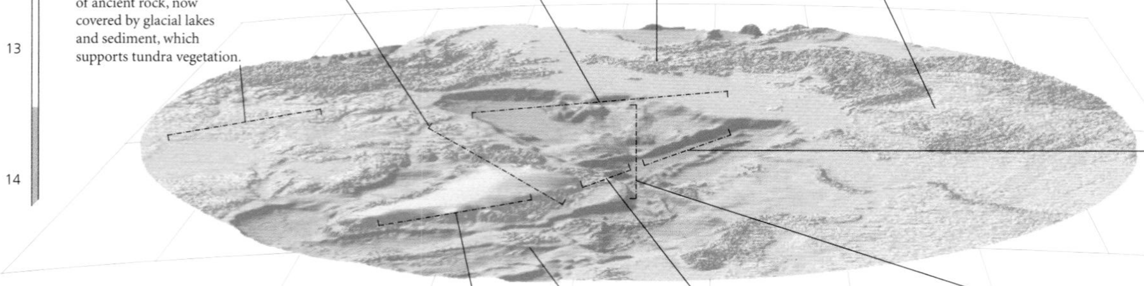

Lomonosov Ridge

Lomonosov Ridge

Arctic ice shelf

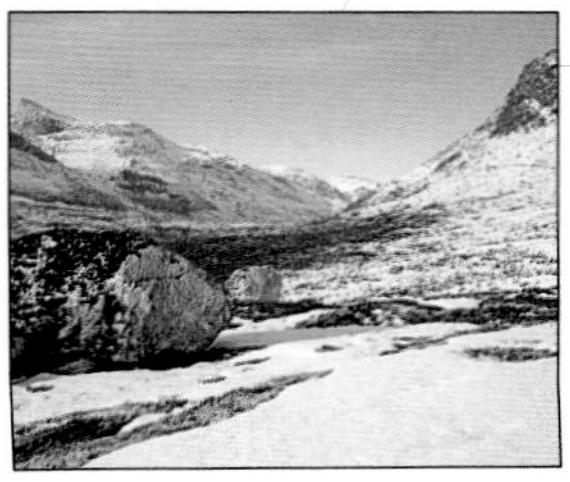

Much of Greenland *is covered by a massive ice sheet more than 650,000 sq miles (1,683,400 sq km) in extent. The weight of the ice has depressed the central land area to form a basin lying more than 1,000 ft (300 m) below sea level. Only at the edges of the island is bare rock visible.*

Iceland has five major glaciers, sustained by heavy snowfall. Parts of the ice cap cover active volcanoes, such as Bárdharbunga, which periodically erupt causing the melted ice to form a great lake at the glacier margins.

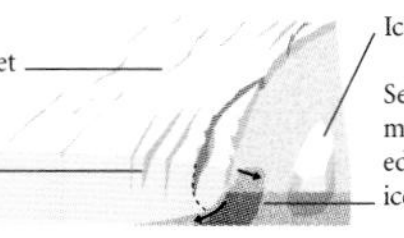

Ice sheet

Crevasses occur at the edge of the ice sheet

Iceberg

Sea water melts the edge of the ice sheet

At the boundary *of the Arctic ice shelves, sea water flows under the ice causing melting and forming crevasses on the surface. This eventually weakens blocks of ice which break away as icebergs. This process is known as calving.*

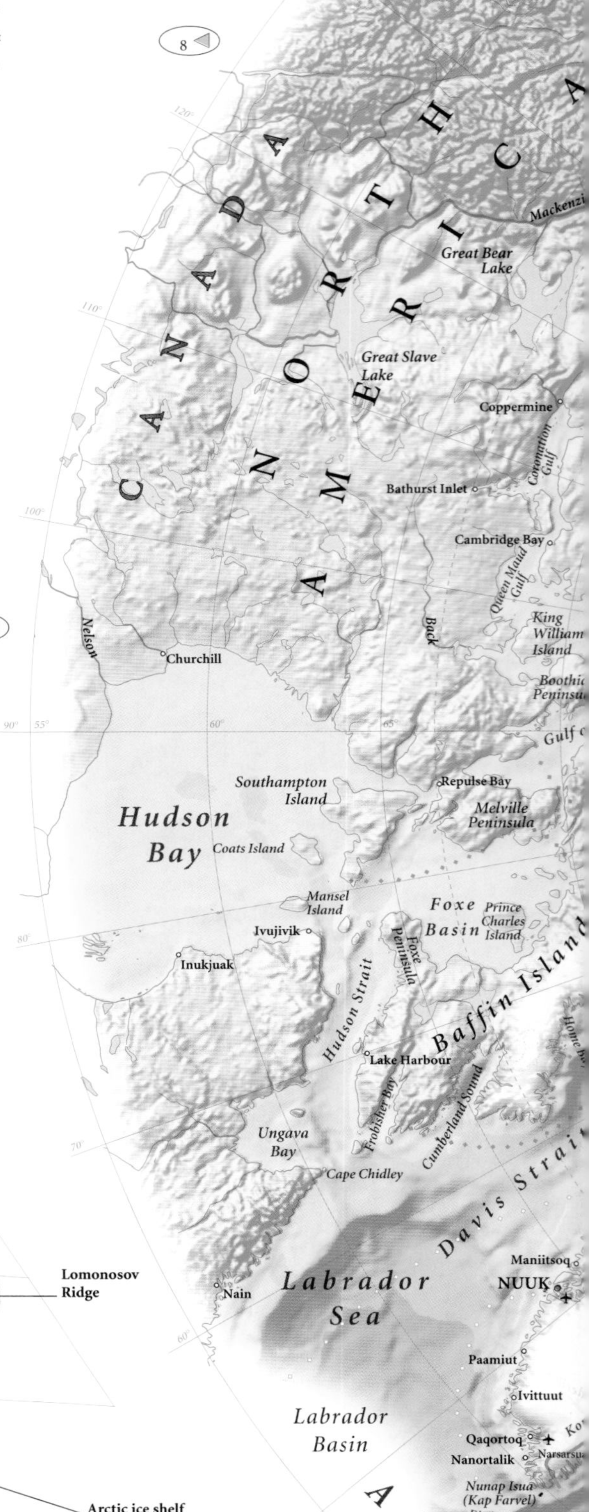

64

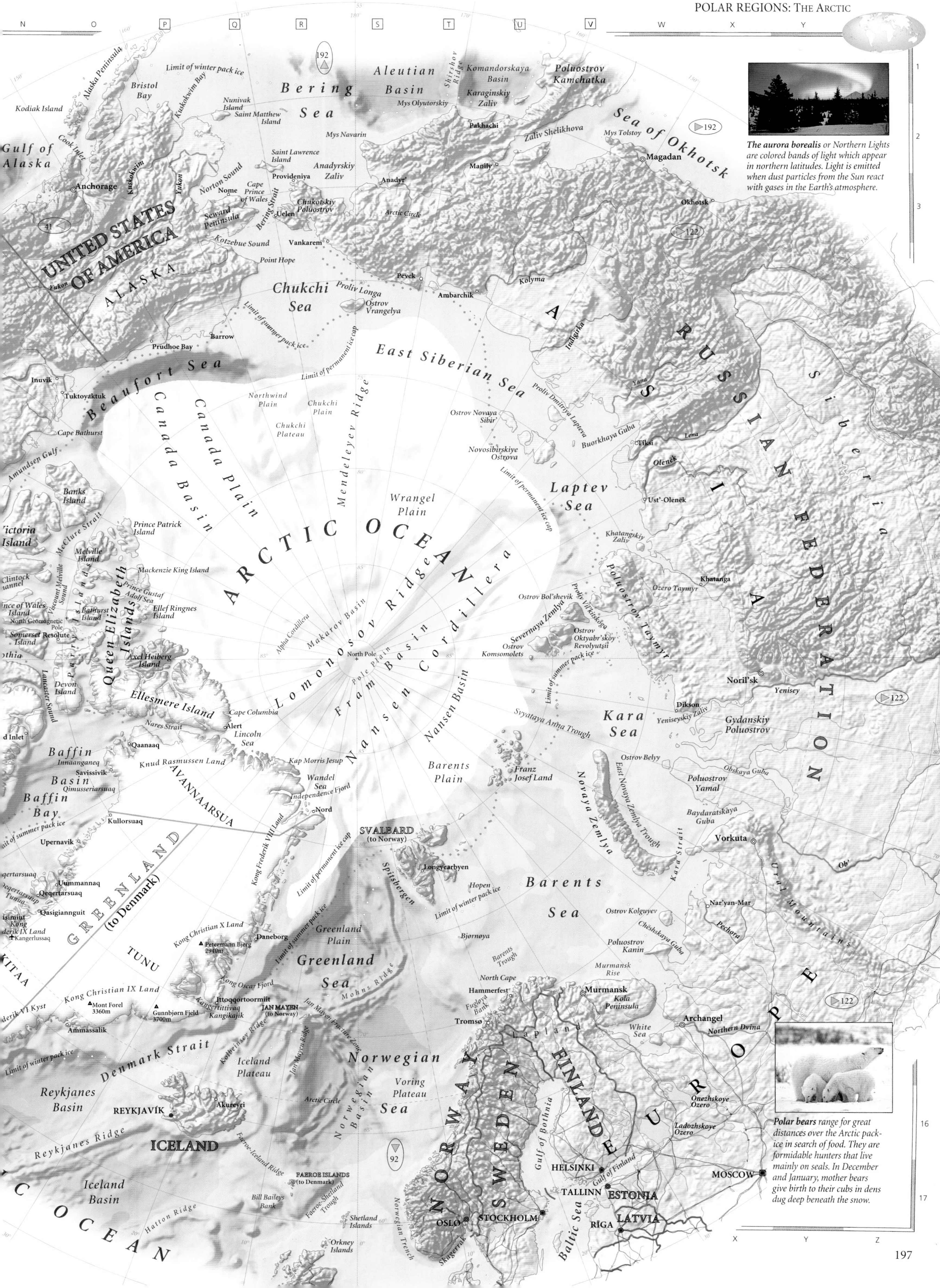

The aurora borealis *or Northern Lights are colored bands of light which appear in northern latitudes. Light is emitted when dust particles from the Sun react with gases in the Earth's atmosphere.*

Polar bears *range for great distances over the Arctic pack-ice in search of food. They are formidable hunters that live mainly on seals. In December and January, mother bears give birth to their cubs in dens dug deep beneath the snow.*

Geographical Comparisons

Largest Countries

Russian Federation	6,592,800 sq miles	(17,075,400 sq km)
Canada	3,851,788 sq miles	(9,976,140 sq km)
USA	3,681,760 sq miles	(9,372,610 sq km)
China	3,600,292 sq miles	(9,326,410 sq km)
Brazil	3,286,472 sq miles	(8,511,970 sq km)
Australia	2,967,893 sq miles	(7,686,850 sq km)
India	1,269,338 sq miles	(3,287,590 sq km)
Argentina	1,068,296 sq miles	(2,766,890 sq km)
Kazakhstan	1,049,150 sq miles	(2,717,300 sq km)
Sudan	967,493 sq miles	(2,505,815 sq km)

Smallest Countries

Vatican City	0.17 sq miles	(0.44 sq km)
Monaco	0.75 sq miles	(1.95 sq km)
Nauru	8.2 sq miles	(21.2 sq km)
Tuvalu	10 sq miles	(26 sq km)
San Marino	24 sq miles	(61 sq km)
Liechtenstein	62 sq miles	(160 sq km)
Marshall Islands	70 sq miles	(181 sq km)
Seychelles	108 sq miles	(280 sq km)
Maldives	116 sq miles	(300 sq km)
Malta	124 sq miles	(320 sq km)

Largest Islands

(TO THE NEAREST 1,000 - OR 100,000 FOR THE LARGEST)

Greenland	849,400 sq miles	(2,200,000 sq km)
New Guinea	312,000 sq miles	(808,000 sq km)
Borneo	292,222 sq miles	(757,050 sq km)
Madagascar	229,300 sq miles	(594,000 sq km)
Sumatra	202,300 sq miles	(524,000 sq km)
Baffin Island	183,800 sq miles	(476,000 sq km)
Honshu	88,800 sq miles	(230,000 sq km)
Britain	88,700 sq miles	(229,800 sq km)
Victoria Island	81,900 sq miles	(212,000 sq km)
Ellesmere Island	75,700 sq miles	(196,000 sq km)

Richest Countries

(GNP PER CAPITA, IN US$)

Luxembourg	45,360
Switzerland	44,350
Japan	40,940
Liechtenstein	40,000
Norway	34,510
Denmark	32,100
Singapore	30,550
Germany	28,870
Austria	28,110
USA	28,020

Poorest Countries

(GNP PER CAPITA, IN US$)

Mozambique	80
Somalia	100
Ethiopia	100
Eritrea	100
Congo (Zaire)	130
Chad	160
Tanzania	170
Burundi	170
Malawi	180
Rwanda	190
Sierra Leone	200
Niger	200

Most Populous Countries

China	1,255,100,000
India	935,700,000
USA	263,300,000
Indonesia	197,600,000
Brazil	165,800,000
Russian Federation	147,000,000
Pakistan	140,500,000
Japan	125,100,000
Bangladesh	120,400,000
Nigeria	111,700,000

Least Populous Countries

Vatican City	1,000
Tuvalu	9,000
Nauru	10,000
Palau	16,200
San Marino	24,000
Liechtenstein	30,630
Monaco	31,000
St Kitts & Nevis	44,000
Marshall Islands	52,000
Andorra	64,000
Dominica	71,000
Seychelles	73,000

Most Densely Populated Countries

Monaco	41,332 people per sq mile	(15,897 per sq km)
Singapore	11,894 people per sq mile	(4,590 per sq km)
Vatican City	5,890 people per sq mile	(2,273 per sq km)
Malta	3,239 people per sq mile	(1,250 per sq km)
Maldives	2,591 people per sq mile	(1,000 per sq km)
Bangladesh	2,330 people per sq mile	(899 per sq km)
Bahrain	2,286 people per sq mile	(882 per sq km)
Barbados	1,809 people per sq mile	(698 per sq km)
Taiwan	1,682 people per sq mile	(649 per sq km)
Mauritius	1,542 people per sq mile	(595 per sq km)

Most Sparsely Populated Countries

Australia	5 people per sq mile	(2 per sq km)
Mauritania	5 people per sq mile	(2 per sq km)
Mongolia	5 people per sq mile	(2 per sq km)
Namibia	5 people per sq mile	(2 per sq km)
Suriname	5 people per sq mile	(2 per sq km)
Botswana	8 people per sq mile	(3 per sq km)
Canada	8 people per sq mile	(3 per sq km)
Iceland	8 people per sq mile	(3 per sq km)
Libya	8 people per sq mile	(3 per sq km)
Guyana	10 people per sq mile	(4 per sq km)

Most Widely Spoken Languages

1. Chinese (Mandarin)	**6. Arabic**
2. English	**7. Bengali**
3. Hindi	**8. Portuguese**
4. Spanish	**9. Malay-Indonesian**
5. Russian	**10. French**

Countries With The Most Land Borders

14: China *(Afghanistan, Bhutan, Mynamar, India, Kazakhstan, Kyrgyzstan, Laos, Mongolia, Nepal, North Korea, Pakistan, Russian Federation, Tajikistan, Vietnam)*

14: Russian Federation *(Azerbaijan, Belarus, China, Estonia, Finland, Georgia, Kazakhstan, Latvia, Lithuania, Mongolia, North Korea, Norway, Poland, Ukraine)*

10: Brazil *(Argentina, Bolivia, Colombia, French Guiana, Guyana, Paraguay, Peru, Suriname, Uruguay, Venezuela)*

9: Congo (Zaire) *(Angola, Burundi, Central African Republic, Congo, Rwanda, Sudan, Tanzania, Uganda, Zambia)*

9: Germany *(Austria, Belgium, Czech Republic, Denmark, France, Luxembourg, Netherlands, Poland, Switzerland)*

9: Sudan *(Central African Republic, Chad, Congo (Zaire), Egypt, Eritrea, Ethiopia, Kenya, Libya, Uganda)*

8: Austria *(Czech Republic, Germany, Hungary, Italy, Liechtenstein, Slovakia, Slovenia, Switzerland)*
8: France *(Andorra, Belgium, Germany, Italy, Luxembourg, Monaco, Spain, Switzerland)*
8: Tanzania *(Burundi, Congo (Zaire), Kenya, Malawi, Mozambique, Rwanda, Uganda, Zambia)*
8: Turkey *(Armenia, Azerbaijan, Bulgaria, Georgia, Greece, Iran, Iraq, Syria)*
8: Zambia *(Angola, Botswana, Congo (Zaire), Malawi, Mozambique, Namibia, Tanzania, Zimbabwe)*

Longest Rivers

Nile (NE Africa) .... 4,160 miles ....(6,695 km)
Amazon (South America) .... 4,049 miles ....(6,516 km)
Yangtze (China).................... 3,915 miles ....(6,299 km)
Mississippi/Missouri (USA).......... 3,710 miles ....(5,969 km)
Ob'-Irtysh (Russian Federation) ...... 3,461 miles ....(5,570 km)
Yellow River (China)................ 3,395 miles ....(5,464 km)
Congo (Central Africa) .... 2,900 miles ....(4,667 km)
Mekong (Southeast Asia).............. 2,749 miles ....(4,425 km)
Lena (Russian Federation)............ 2,734 miles ....(4,400 km)
Mackenzie (Canada)................. 2,640 miles ....(4,250 km)
Yenisey (Russian Federation) .... 2,541 miles ....(4,090km)

Highest Mountains

(height above sea level)

Everest ....29,030 ft ....(8,848 m)
K2 ....28,253 ft ....(8,611 m)
Kanchenjunga I ....28,210 ft ....(8,598 m)
Makalu I ....27,767 ft ....(8,463 m)
Cho Oyu ....26,907 ft ....(8,201 m)
Dhaulagiri I ....26,796 ft ....(8,167 m)
Manaslu I ....26,783 ft ....(8,163 m)
Nanga Parbat I ....26,661 ft ....(8,126 m)
Annapurna I ....26,547 ft ....(8,091 m)
Gasherbrum I ....26,471 ft ....(8,068 m)

Largest Bodies of Inland Water

(with area and depth)

Caspian Sea .....143,243 sq miles (371,000 sq km) .....3,215 ft (980 m)
Lake Superior .....31,151 sq miles (83,270 sq km) .....1,289 ft (393 m)
Lake Victoria .....26,828 sq miles (69,484 sq km) ......328 ft (100 m)
Lake Huron ....23,436 sq miles (60,700 sq km) ......751 ft (229 m)
Lake Michigan ....22,402 sq miles (58,020 sq km) ......922 ft (281 m)
Lake Tanganyika ..12,703 sq miles (32,900 sq km) ....4,700 ft (1435 m)
Great Bear Lake ...12,274 sq miles (31,790 sq km) .....1,047 ft (319 m)
Lake Baikal ....11,776 sq miles (30,500 sq km) ....5,712 ft (1741 m)
Great Slave Lake ...10,981 sq miles (28,440 sq km) ......459 ft (140 m)
Lake Erie ....9,915 sq miles (25,680 sq km) ....197 ft (60 m)

Deepest Ocean Features

Challenger Deep, Marianas Trench (Pacific).......... 36,201 ft .....(11,034 m)
Vityaz III Depth, Tonga Trench (Pacific)............. 35,704 ft .....(10,882 m)
Vityaz Depth, Kurile-Kamchatka Trench (Pacific) .... 34,588 ft .....(10,542 m)
Cape Johnson Deep, Philippine Trench (Pacific)...... 34,441 ft .....(10,497 m)
Kermadec Trench (Pacific) .... 32,964 ft .....(10,047 m)
Ramapo Deep, Japan Trench (Pacific) .... 32,758 ft ......(9,984 m)
Milwaukee Deep, Puerto Rico Trench (Atlantic) ...... 30,185 ft ......(9,200 m)
Argo Deep, Torres Trench (Pacific).................. 30,070 ft ......(9,165 m)
Meteor Depth, South Sandwich Trench (Atlantic)..... 30,000 ft ......(9,144 m)
Planet Deep, New Britain Trench (Pacific) .... 29,988 ft ......(9,140 m)

Greatest Waterfalls

(Mean flow of water)

Boyoma (Congo (Zaire)) ....600,400 cu. ft/sec ..(17,000 cu.m/sec)
Khône (Laos/Cambodia) ....410,000 cu. ft/sec ..(11,600 cu.m/sec)
Niagara (USA/Canada) ....195,000 cu. ft/sec ...(5,500 cu.m/sec)
Grande (Uruguay) ....160,000 cu. ft/sec ...(4,500 cu.m/sec)
Paulo Afonso (Brazil) ....100,000 cu. ft/sec ...(2,800 cu.m/sec)
Urubupunga (Brazil) ....97,000 cu. ft/sec ...(2,750 cu.m/sec)
Iguaçu (Argentina/Brazil) ....62,000 cu. ft/sec ...(1,700 cu.m/sec)
Maribondo (Brazil) ....53,000 cu. ft/sec ...(1,500 cu.m/sec)
Victoria (Zimbabwe) ....39,000 cu. ft/sec ...(1,100 cu.m/sec)
Kabalega (Uganda) ....42,000 cu. ft/sec ...(1,200 cu.m/sec)
Churchill (Canada) ....35,000 cu. ft/sec ...(1,000 cu.m/sec)
Cauvery (India) ....33,000 cu. ft/sec .....(900 cu.m/sec)

Highest Waterfalls

Angel (Venezuela) ....3,212 ft ....(979 m)
Tugela (South Africa)...............3,110 ft ....(948 m)
Utigard (Norway) ....2,625 ft ....(800 m)
Mongefossen (Norway) ....2,539 ft ....(774 m)
Mtarazi (Zimbabwe) ....2,500 ft ....(762 m)
Yosemite (USA) ....2,425 ft ....(739 m)
Ostre Mardola Foss (Norway) ....2,156 ft ....(657 m)
Tyssestrengane (Norway)...........2,119 ft ....(646 m)
***Cuquenan** (Venezuela) ....2,001 ft ....(610 m)
Sutherland (New Zealand) ....1,903 ft ....(580 m)
***Kjellfossen** (Norway) ....1,841 ft ....(561 m)

** indicates that the total height is a single leap*

Largest Deserts

Sahara ....3,450,000 sq miles ......(9,065,000 sq km)
Gobi ....500,000 sq miles ......(1,295,000 sq km)
Ar Rub al Khali ....289,600 sq miles ....(750,000 sq km)
Great Victorian ....249,800 sq miles ....(647,000 sq km)
Sonoran ....120,000 sq miles ....(311,000 sq km)
Kalahari ....120,000 sq miles ....(310,800 sq km)
Kara Kum ....115,800 sq miles ....(300,000 sq km)
Takla Makan ....100,400 sq miles ....(260,000 sq km)
Namib ....52,100 sq miles ....(135,000 sq km)
Thar ....33,670 sq miles ....(130,000 sq km)

NB – Most of Antarctica is a polar desert, with only 50mm of precipitation annually

Hottest Inhabited Places

Djibouti (Djibouti)	86° F	(30 °C)
Timbouctou (Mali)	84.7° F	(29.3 °C)
Tirunelveli (India)		
Tuticorin (India)		
Nellore (India)	84.5° F	(29.2 °C)
Santa Marta (Colombia)		
Aden (Yemen)	84° F	(28.9 °C)
Madurai (India)		
Niamey (Niger)		
Hodeida (Yemen)	83.8° F	(28.8 °C)
Ouagadougou (Burkina)		
Thanjavur (India)		
Tiruchchirappalli (India)		

Driest Inhabited Places

Aswân (Egypt) ....0.02 in ....(0.5 mm)
Luxor (Egypt) ....0.03 in ....(0.7 mm)
Arica (Chile) ....0.04 in ....(1.1 mm)
Ica (Peru) ....0.1 in ....(2.3 mm)
Antofagasta (Chile) ....0.2 in ....(4.9 mm)
El Minya (Egypt) ....0.2 in ....(5.1 mm)
Asyût (Egypt) ....0.2 in ....(5.2 mm)
Callao (Peru) ....0.5 in ....(12.0 mm)
Trujillo (Peru) ....0.55 in ....(14.0 mm)
El Faiyûm (Egypt) ....0.8 in ....(19.0 mm)

Wettest Inhabited Places

Buenaventura (Colombia) ....265 in ....(6,743 mm)
Monrovia (Liberia) ....202 in ....(5,131 mm)
Pago Pago (American Samoa) ....196 in ....(4,990 mm)
Moulmein (Burma) ....191 in ....(4,852 mm)
Lae (Papua New Guinea) ....183 in ....(4,645 mm)
Baguio (Luzon Island, Philippines) ......180 in ....(4,573 mm)
Sylhet (Bangladesh) ....176 in ....(4,457 mm)
Padang (Sumatra, Indonesia) ....166 in ....(4,225 mm)
Bogor (Java, Indonesia) ....166 in ....(4,225 mm)
Conakry (Guinea) ....171 in ....(4,341 mm)

The Time Zones

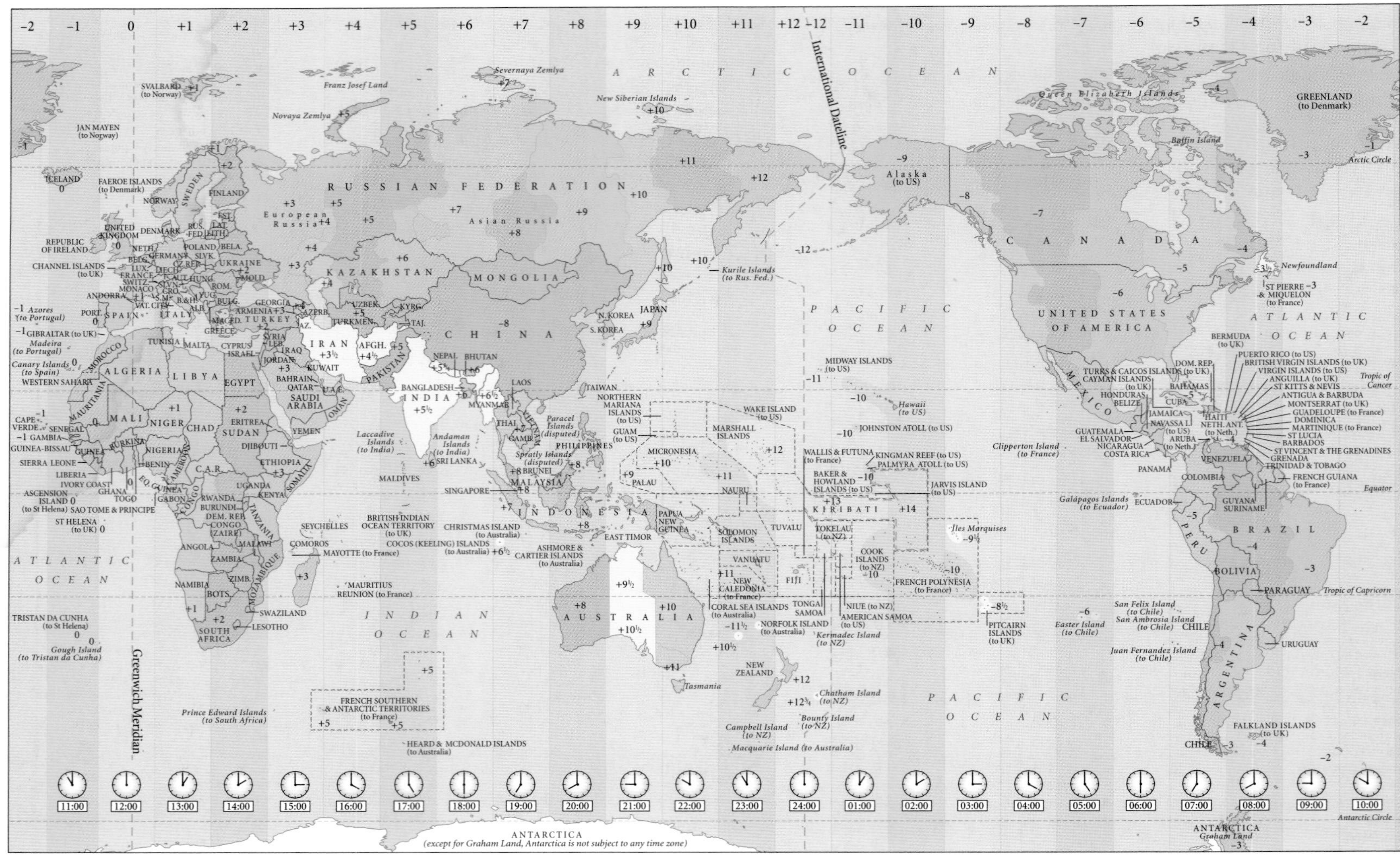
-2 -1 0 +1 +2 +3 +4 +5 +6 +7 +8 +9 +10 +11 +12 -12 -11 -10 -9 -8 -7 -6 -5 -4 -3 -2
International Dateline
Greenwich Meridian
ARCTIC OCEAN
RUSSIAN FEDERATION
CHINA
MONGOLIA
KAZAKHSTAN
CANADA
UNITED STATES OF AMERICA
GREENLAND (to Denmark)
PACIFIC OCEAN
ATLANTIC OCEAN
INDIAN OCEAN
AUSTRALIA
BRAZIL
ANTARCTICA
(except for Graham Land, Antarctica is not subject to any time zone)
11:00
12:00
13:00
14:00
15:00
16:00
17:00
18:00
19:00
20:00
21:00
22:00
23:00
24:00
01:00
02:00
03:00
04:00
05:00
06:00
07:00
08:00
09:00
10:00
Arctic Circle
Tropic of Cancer
Equator
Tropic of Capricorn
Antarctic Circle

The numbers at the top of the map indicate the number of hours each time zone is ahead or behind Greenwich Mean Time (GMT). The clocks and 24-hour times given at the bottom of the map show the time in each time zone when it is 12:00 hours noon GMT.

Time Zones

The present system of international timekeeping divides the world into 24 time zones by means of 24 standard meridians of longitude, each 15° apart. Time is measured in each zone as so many hours ahead or behind the time at the Greenwich Meridian (GMT). Countries, or parts of countries, falling in the vicinity of each zone, adopt its time as shown on the map above. Therefore, using the map, when it is 12:00 noon GMT, it will be 2:00 pm in Zambia; similarly, when it is 4:30 pm GMT, it will be 11:30 am in Peru.

Greenwich Mean Time (GMT)

Greenwich Mean Time (or Universal Time, as it is more correctly called) has been the internationally accepted basis for calculating solar time – measured in relation to the Earth's rotation around the Sun – since 1884. Greenwich Mean Time is specifically the solar time at the site of the former Royal Observatory in the London Borough of Greenwich, United Kingdom. The Greenwich Meridian is an imaginary line around the world that runs through the North and South poles. It corresponds to 0° of longitude, which lies on this site at Greenwich. Time is measured around the world in relation to the official time along the Meridian.

Standard Time

Standard time is the official time, designated by law, in any specific country or region. Standard time was initiated in 1884, after it became apparent that the practice of keeping various systems of local time was causing confusion – particularly in the US and Canada, where several railroad routes passed through scores of areas which calculated local time by different rules. The standard time of a particular region is calculated in reference to the longitudinal time zone in which it falls. In practice, these zones do not always match their longitudinal position; in some places the area of the zone has been altered in shape for the convenience of inhabitants, as can be seen in the map. For example, whilst Greenland occupies three time zones, the majority of the territory uses a standard time of -3 hours GMT. Similarly China, which spans five time zones, is standardized at -8 hours GMT.

The International Dateline

The International Dateline is an imaginary line that extends from pole to pole, and roughly corresponds to a line of 180° longitude for much of its length. This line is the arbitrary marker between calendar days. By moving from east to west across the line, a traveler will need to set their calendar back one day, whilst those traveling in the opposite direction will need to add a day. This is to compensate for the use of standard time around the world, which is based on the time at noon along the Greenwich Meridian, approximately halfway around the world. Wide deviations from 180° longitude occur through the Bering Strait – to avoid dividing Siberia into two separate calendar days – and in the Pacific Ocean – to allow certain Pacific islands the same calendar day as New Zealand. Changes were made to the International Dateline in 1995 that made Millennium Island (formerly Caroline Island) in Kiribati the first land area to witness the beginning of the year 2000.

Daylight Saving Time

Also known as summer time, daylight saving is a system of advancing clocks in order to extend the waking day during periods of later daylight hours. This normally means advancing clocks by one hour in early spring, and reverting back to standard time in early autumn. The system of daylight saving is used throughout much of Europe, the US, Australia, and many other countries worldwide, although there are no standardized dates for the changeover to summer time due to the differences in hours of daylight at different latitudes. Daylight saving was first introduced in certain countries during the First World War, to decrease the need for artificial light and heat – the system stayed in place after the war, as it proved practical. During the Second World War, some countries went so far as to keep their clocks an hour ahead of standard time continuously, and the UK temporarily introduced "double summer time," which advanced clocks two hours ahead of standard time during the summer months.

Countries of the World

There are currently 192 independent countries in the world – more than at any previous time – and 59 dependencies. Antarctica is the only land area on Earth that is not officially part of, and does not belong to, any single country.

In 1950, the world comprised 82 countries. In the decades following, many more states came into being as they achieved independence from their former colonial rulers. Most recently, the breakup of the former Soviet Union in 1991, and the former Yugoslavia in 1992, swelled the ranks of independent states.

Country Factfile Key

Formation Date of independence / date current borders were established
Population Total population / population density – based on total *land* area / percentage of urban-based population
Languages An asterisk (*) denotes the official language(s)
Calorie consumption Average number of calories consumed daily per person

Afghanistan
Central Asia

Official name Islamic State of Afghanistan
Formation 1919 / 1919
Capital Kabul
Population 23.4 million / 93 people per sq mile (36 people per sq km) / 20%
Total area 251,770 sq miles (652,090 sq km)
Languages Persian*, Pashtu*, Dari, Uzbek, Turkmen
Religions Sunni Muslim 84%, Shi'a Muslim 15%, other 1%
Ethnic mix Pashtun 38%, Tajik 25%, Hazara 19%, Uzbek 6%, other 12%
Government Mujahideen coalition
Currency Afghani = 100 puls
Literacy rate 31%
Calorie consumption 1,523 kilocalories

Albania
Southeastern Europe

Official name Republic of Albania
Formation 1912 / 1921
Capital Tiranë
Population 3.4 million / 321 people per sq mile (124 people per sq km) / 37%
Total area 11,100 sq miles (28,750 sq km)
Languages Albanian*, Greek, Macedonian
Religions Muslim 70%, Greek Orthodox 20%, Roman Catholic 10%
Ethnic mix Albanian 96%, Greek 2%, other (including Macedonian) 2%
Government Multiparty republic
Currency Lek = 100 qindars
Literacy rate 85%
Calorie consumption 2,605 kilocalories

Algeria
Northern Africa

Official name Democratic and Popular Republic of Algeria
Formation 1962 / 1962
Capital Algiers
Population 27.9 million / 33 people per sq mile (13 people per sq km) / 56%
Total area 919,590 sq miles (2,381,740 sq km)
Languages Arabic*, Berber, French
Religions Muslim 99%, Christian and Jewish 1%
Ethnic mix Arab and Berber 99%, European 1%
Government Multiparty republic
Currency Dinar = 100 centimes
Literacy rate 60%
Calorie consumption 2,897 kilocalories

Andorra
Southwestern Europe

Official name Principality of Andorra
Formation 1278 / 1278
Capital Andorra la Vella
Population 65,000 / 359 people per sq mile (139 people per sq km) / 63%
Total area 181 sq miles (468 sq km)
Languages Catalan*, Spanish, French, Portuguese
Religions Roman Catholic 94%, other 6%
Ethnic mix Catalan 61%, Spanish Castilian 30%, other 9%
Government Parliamentary democracy
Currency French franc, Spanish peseta
Literacy rate 100%
Calorie consumption 3,708 kilocalories

Angola
Southern Africa

Official name Republic of Angola
Formation 1975 / 1975
Capital Luanda
Population 12 million / 25 people per sq mile (10 people per sq km) / 32%
Total area 481,551 sq miles (1,246,700 sq km)
Languages Portuguese*, Umbundu, Kimbundu, Kongo
Religions Roman Catholic / Protestant 64%, traditional beliefs 34%, other 2%
Ethnic mix Ovimbundu 37%, Mbundu 25%, Bakongo 13%, other 25%
Government Multiparty republic
Currency Readjusted kwanza = 100 lwei
Literacy rate 45%
Calorie consumption 1,839 kilocalories

Antigua & Barbuda
West Indies

Official name Antigua and Barbuda
Formation 1981 / 1981
Capital St John's
Population 66,000 / 389 people per sq mile (150 people per sq km) / 36%
Total area 170 sq miles (440 sq km)
Languages English*, English patios
Religions Protestant 86%, Roman Catholic 10%, other 4%
Ethnic mix Black 98%, other 2%
Government Parliamentary democracy
Currency E. Caribbean dollar = 100 cents
Literacy rate 95%
Calorie consumption 2,458 kilocalories

Argentina
South America

Official name Republic of Argentina
Formation 1816 / 1816
Capital Buenos Aires
Population 36.1 million / 34 people per sq mile (13 people per sq km) / 87%
Total area 1,068,296 sq miles (2,766,890 sq km)
Languages Spanish*, Italian, English, German, French, Amerindian languages
Religions Roman Catholic 90%, Jewish 2%, other 8%
Ethnic mix European 85%, other (including *mestizo* and Indian) 15%
Government Multiparty republic
Currency Peso = 100 centavos
Literacy rate 96%
Calorie consumption 2,880 kilocalories

Armenia
Southwestern Asia

Official name Republic of Armenia
Formation 1991 / 1991
Capital Yerevan
Population 3.6 million / 313 people per sq mile (121 people per sq km) / 69%
Total area 11,505 sq miles (29,000 sq km)
Languages Armenian*, Azerbaijani, Russian, Kurdish
Religions Armenian Apostolic 90%, other Christian and Muslim 10%
Ethnic mix Armenian 93%, Azeri 3%, other 4%
Government Multiparty republic
Currency Dram = 100 louma
Literacy rate 99%
Calorie consumption Not available

Australia
Australasia & Oceania

Official name Commonwealth of Australia
Formation 1901 / 1901
Capital Canberra
Population 18.5 million / 6 people per sq mile (2 people per sq km) / 85%
Total area 2,967,893 sq miles (7,686,850 sq km)
Languages English*, Greek, Italian, Vietnamese, Aboriginal languages
Religions Protestant 38%, Roman Catholic 26%, other 36%
Ethnic mix European 95%, Asian 4%, Aboriginal and other 1%
Government Parliamentary democracy
Currency Australian dollar = 100 cents
Literacy rate 99%
Calorie consumption 3,179 kilocalories

Austria
Central Europe

Official name Republic of Austria
Formation 1918 / 1919
Capital Vienna
Population 8.2 million / 257 people per sq mile (99 people per sq km) / 56%
Total area 32,375 sq miles (83,850 sq km)
Languages German*, Croat, Slovene
Religions Roman Catholic 78%, Protestant 5%, other (including Jewish and Muslim) 17%
Ethnic mix German 93%, Croat, Slovene, Hungarian 6%, other 1%
Government Multiparty republic
Currency Austrian Schilling = 100 groschen
Literacy rate 99%
Calorie consumption 3,497 kilocalories

Azerbaijan
Southwestern Asia

Official name Azerbaijani Republic
Formation 1991 / 1991
Capital Baku
Population 7.7 million / 230 people per sq mile (89 people per sq km) / 56%
Total area 33,436 sq miles (86,600 sq km)
Languages Azerbaijani*, Russian, Armenian
Religions Muslim 83%, Armenian Apostolic and Russian Orthodox 17%
Ethnic mix Azeri 83%, Armenian 6%, Russian 5%, Daghestani 3%, other 3%
Government Multiparty republic
Currency Manat = 100 gopik
Literacy rate 96%
Calorie consumption Not available

Bahamas
West Indies

Official name Commonwealth of the Bahamas
Formation 1973 / 1973
Capital Nassau
Population 293,000 / 76 people per sq mile (29 people per sq km)/ 87%
Total area 5,359 sq miles (13,880 sq km)
Languages English*, English Creole,
Religions Protestant 64%, Roman Catholic 19%, other 17%
Ethnic mix Black 85%, White 15%
Government Parliamentary democracy
Currency Bahamian dollar = 100 cents
Literacy rate 96%
Calorie consumption 2,624 kilocalories

Bahrain
Southwestern Asia

Official name State of Bahrain
Formation 1971 / 1971
Capital Manama
Population 594,000 / 2,262 people per sq mile (874 people per sq km) / 90%
Total area 263 sq miles (680 sq km)
Languages Arabic*, English, Urdu
Religions Muslim (Shi'a majority) 85%, Christian 7%, other 8%
Ethnic mix Bahraini 70%, Iranian, Indian, Pakistani 24%, other Arab 4%, European 2%
Government Absolute monarchy (emirate)
Currency Bahrain dinar = 1,000 fils
Literacy rate 86%
Calorie consumption Not available

Bangladesh
Southern Asia

Official name People's Republic of Bangladesh
Formation 1971 / 1971
Capital Dhaka
Population 124 million / 2,400 people per sq mile (926 people per sq km) / 18%
Total area 55,598 sq miles (143,998 sq km)
Languages Bengali*, Urdu, Chakma, Marma, Garo, Khasi, Santhali, Tripuri, Mro
Religions Muslim 87%, Hindu 12%, other 1%
Ethnic mix Bengali 98%, other 2%
Government Multiparty republic
Currency Taka = 100 paisa
Literacy rate 40%
Calorie consumption 2,019 kilocalories

Barbados
West Indies

Official name Barbados
Formation 1966 / 1966
Capital Bridgetown
Population 263,000 / 1,584 people per sq mile (612 people per sq km) / 47%
Total area 166 sq miles (430 sq km)
Languages English*, English Creole
Religions Protestant 55%, Roman Catholic 4%, other 41%
Ethnic mix Black 80%, mixed 15%, White 4%, other 1%
Government Parliamentary democracy
Currency Barbados dollar = 100 cents
Literacy rate 97%
Calorie consumption 3,207 kilocalories

Belarus
Eastern Europe

Official name Republic of Belarus
Formation 1991 / 1991
Capital Minsk
Population 10.3 million / 129 people per sq mile (50 people per sq km) / 68%
Total area 80,154 sq miles (207,600 sq km)
Languages Belarusian*, Russian*
Religions Russian Orthodox 60%, Roman Catholic 8%, other 32%
Ethnic mix Belarusian 78%, Russian 13%, Polish 4%, other 5%
Government Multiparty republic
Currency Belarusian rouble = 100 kopeks
Literacy rate 99%
Calorie consumption Not available

Belgium
Northwestern Europe

Official name Kingdom of Belgium
Formation 1830 / 1919
Capital Brussels
Population 10.2 million / 805 people per sq mile (311 people per sq km) / 97%
Total area 12,780 sq miles (33,100 sq km)
Languages Flemish*, French*, German*
Religions Roman Catholic 88%, other 12%
Ethnic mix Fleming 58%, Walloon 33%, other 9%
Government Constitutional monarchy
Currency Belgian franc = 100 centimes
Literacy rate 99%
Calorie consumption: 3,681 kilocalories

Belize
Central America

Official name Belize
Formation 1981 / 1981
Capital Belmopan
Population 200,000 /23 people per sq mile (9 people per sq km) / 47%
Total area 8,865 sq miles (22,960 sq km)
Languages English*, English Creole, Spanish
Religions Christian 87%, other 13%
Ethnic mix *Mestizo* 44%, Creole 30%, Maya 11%, Asian Indian 4%, Garifuna 7%, other 4%
Government Parliamentary democracy
Currency Belizean dollar =100 cents
Literacy rate 75%
Calorie consumption 2,662 kilocalories

Benin
Western Africa

Official name Republic of Benin
Formation 1960 / 1960
Capital Porto-Novo
Population 5.9 million / 138 people per sq mile (53 people per sq km) / 31%
Total area 43,480 sq miles (112,620 sq km)
Languages French*, Fon, Bariba, Yoruba, Adja
Religions Traditional beliefs 70%, Muslim 15%, Christian 15%
Ethnic mix Fon 39%, Yoruba 12%, Adja 10%, other 39%
Government Multiparty republic
Currency CFA franc = 100 centimes
Literacy rate 34%
Calorie consumption 2,532 kilocalories

Bhutan
Southeastern Asia

Official name Kingdom of Bhutan
Formation 1656 / 1865
Capital Thimphu
Population 1.9 million / 105 people per sq mile (40 people per sq km) / 6%
Total area 18,147 sq miles (47,000 sq km)
Languages Dzongkha*, Nepali, Assamese
Religions Mahayana Buddhism 70%, Hindu 24%, Muslim 5%, other 1%
Ethnic mix Bhutia 61%, Gurung 15%, Assamese 13%, other 11%
Government Constitutional monarchy
Currency Ngultrum = 100 chetrum
Literacy rate 44%
Calorie consumption 2,553 kilocalories

Bolivia
South America

Official name Republic of Bolivia
Formation 1825 / 1938
Capitals Sucre (official)/La Paz (administrative)
Population 8 million / 19 people per sq mile (7 people per sq km) / 61%
Total area 424,162 sq miles (1,098,580 sq km)
Languages Spanish*, Quechua*, Aymará*
Religions Roman Catholic 93%, other 7%
Ethnic mix Quechua 37%, Aymará 32%, mixed 13%, European 10%, other 8%
Government Multiparty republic
Currency Boliviano = 100 centavos
Literacy rate 84%
Calorie consumption 2,094 kilocalories

Bosnia & Herzegovina
Southeastern Europe

Official name Republic of Bosnia and Herzegovina
Formation 1992 / 1992
Capital Sarajevo
Population 4 million / 203 people per sq mile (78 people per sq km) / 49%
Total area 19,741 sq miles (51,130 sq km)
Languages Serbian*, Croatian*
Religions Muslim 40%, Serbian Orthodox 31%, Roman Catholic 15%, other 14%
Ethnic mix Bosnian 44%, Serb 31%, Croat 17%, other 8%
Government Multiparty republic
Currency Maraka = 100 pfenniga
Literacy rate 93%
Calorie consumption Not available

Botswana
Southern Africa

Official name Republic of Botswana
Formation 1966 / 1966
Capital Gaborone
Population 1.6 million / 7 people per sq mile (3 people per sq km) / 28%
Total area 224,600 sq miles (581,730 sq km)
Languages English*, Tswana, Shona, San
Religions Traditional beliefs 50%, Christian 50%
Ethnic mix Tswana 98%, other 2%
Government Multiparty republic
Currency Pula = 100 thebe
Literacy rate 74%
Calorie consumption 2,266 kilocalories

Brazil
South America

Official name Federative Republic of Brazil
Formation 1822 / 1889
Capital Brasília
Population 165.2 million / 51 people per sq mile (20 people per sq km) / 78%
Total area 3,286,472 sq miles (8,511,970 sq km)
Languages Portuguese*, German, Italian
Religions Roman Catholic 89%, other 11%
Ethnic mix White (Portuguese, Italian, German, Japanese) 66%, mixed 22%, Black 12%
Government Multiparty republic
Currency Real = 100 centavos
Literacy rate 84%
Calorie consumption 2,824 kilocalories

Brunei
Southeastern Asia

Official name Sultanate of Brunei
Formation 1984 / 1984
Capital Bandar Seri Begawan
Population 313,000 / 154 people per sq mile (57 people per sq km) / 59%
Total area 2,228 sq miles (5,770 sq km)
Languages Malay*, English, Chinese
Religions Muslim 63%, Buddhist 14%, Christian 10%, other 13%
Ethnic mix Malay 67%, Chinese 16%, other 17%
Government Absolute monarchy
Currency Brunei dollar = 100 cents
Literacy rate 90%
Calorie consumption 2,745 kilocalories

Bulgaria
Southeastern Europe

Official name Republic of Bulgaria
Formation 1908 / 1947
Capital Sofia
Population 8.4 million / 197 people per sq mile (76 people per sq km) / 71%
Total area 42,822 sq miles (110,910 sq km)
Languages Bulgarian*, Turkish, Macedonian, Romany, Armenian, Russian
Religions Christian 85%, Muslim 13%, Jewish 1%, other 1%
Ethnic mix Bulgarian 85%, Turkish 9%, Macedonian 3%, Romany 3%
Government Multiparty republic
Currency Lev = 100 stoninki
Literacy rate 98%
Calorie consumption 2,831 kilocalories

Burkina
Western Africa

Official name Burkina Faso
Formation 1960 / 1960
Capital Ouagadougou
Population 11.4 million / 108 people per sq mile (42 people per sq km) / 27%
Total area 105,870 sq miles (274,200 sq km)
Languages French*, Mossi, Fulani
Religions Indigenous beliefs 55%, Muslim 35%, Christian 10%
Ethnic mix Mossi 45%, Mande 10%, Fulani 10%, other 35%
Government Multiparty republic
Currency CFA franc = 100 centimes
Literacy rate 21%
Calorie consumption 2,387 kilocalories

BURUNDI
Central Africa

Official name Republic of Burundi
Formation 1962 / 1962
Capital Bujumbura
Population 6.6 million / 666 people per sq mile (257 people per sq km) / 7%
Total area 10,750 sq miles (27,830 sq km)
Languages Kirundi*, French*, Swahili
Religions Christian 68%, Traditional beliefs 32%
Ethnic mix Hutu 85%, Tutsi 14%, Twa pygmy 1%
Government Multiparty republic
Currency Burundi franc = 100 centimes
Literacy rate 45%
Calorie consumption 1,941 kilocalories

CAMBODIA
Southeastern Asia

Official name Kingdom of Cambodia
Formation 1953 / 1953
Capital Phnom Penh
Population 10.8 million / 158 people per sq mile (61 people per sq km) /21%
Total area 69,000 sq miles (181,040 sq km)
Languages Khmer*, French, Chinese, Vietnamese
Religions Theravada Buddhist 88%, Muslim 2%, other 10%
Ethnic mix Khmer 94%, Chinese 4%, other 2%
Government Constitutional monarchy
Currency Riel = 100 sen
Literacy rate 66%
Calorie consumption 2,021 kilocalories

CAMEROON
Central Africa

Official name Republic of Cameroon
Formation 1960 / 1961
Capital Yaoundé
Population 14.3 million / 80 people per sq mile (31 people per sq km) / 45%
Total area 183,570 miles (475,440 sq km)
Languages English*, French*, Fang, Bulu, Yaundé, Duala
Religions Traditional beliefs 25%, Christian 53%, Muslim 22%
Ethnic mix Bamileke and Manum 20%, Fang 19%, other 61%
Government Multiparty republic
Currency CFA franc = 100 centimes
Literacy rate 72%
Calorie consumption 1,981 kilocalories

CANADA
North America

Official name Canada
Formation 1867 / 1949
Capital Ottawa
Population 30.2 million / 8 people per sq mile (3 people per sq km) / 77%
Total area 3,851,788 sq miles (9,976,140 sq km)
Languages English*, French*, Chinese, Italian, German, Portuguese, Inuit
Religions Roman Catholic 47%, Protestant 41%, other 12%
Ethnic mix British origin 44%, French origin 25%, other European 20%, other 11%
Government Parliamentary democracy
Currency Canadian dollar = 100 cents
Literacy rate 99%
Calorie consumption 3,094 kilocalories

CAPE VERDE
Atlantic Ocean

Official Name Republic of Cape Verde
Formation 1975 / 1975
Capital Praia
Population 417,000 / 268 people per sq mile (103 people per sq km) / 54%
Total area 1,556 sq miles (4,030 sq km)
Languages Portuguese*, Creole
Religions Roman Catholic 98%, Protestant 2%
Ethnic mix Mestico 60%, African 30%, other 10%
Government Multiparty republic
Currency Cape Verde escudo = 100 centavos
Literacy rate 71%
Calorie consumption 2,805 kilocalories

CENTRAL AFRICAN REPUBLIC
Central Africa

Official name Central African Republic
Formation 1960 / 1960
Capital Bangui
Population 3.5 million / 15 people per sq mile (6 people per sq km) / 39%
Total area 240,530 sq miles (622,980 sq km)
Languages French*, Sango, Banda, Gbaya
Religions Christian 50%, traditional beliefs 27%, Muslim 15%, other 8%
Ethnic mix Baya 34%, Banda 27%, Mandjia 21%, other 18%
Government Multiparty republic
Currency CFA franc = 100 centimes
Literacy rate 42%
Calorie consumption 1,690 kilocalories

CHAD
Central Africa

Official name Republic of Chad
Formation 1960 / 1960
Capital N'Djamena
Population 6.9 million / 14 people per sq mile (5 people per sq km) / 21%
Total area 495,752 sq miles (1,284,000 sq km)
Languages French*, Sara, Maba
Religions Muslim 50%, Traditional beliefs 43%, Christian 7%
Ethnic mix Bagirmi, Sara and Kreish 31%, Sudanic Arab 26%, Teda 7%, other 36%
Government Multiparty republic
Currency CFA franc = 100 centimes
Literacy rate 50%
Calorie consumption 1,989 kilocalories

CHILE
South America

Official name Republic of Chile
Formation 1818 / 1883
Capital Santiago
Population 14.8 million / 51 people per sq mile (20 people per sq km) / 84%
Total area 292,258 sq miles (756,950 sq km)
Languages Spanish*, Indian languages
Religions Roman Catholic 80%, Protestant and other 20%
Ethnic mix *Mestizo* and European 90%, Indian 10%
Government Multiparty republic
Currency Chilean peso = 100 centavos
Literacy rate 95%
Calorie consumption 2,582 kilocalories

CHINA
Eastern Asia

Official name People's Republic of China
Formation 1949 / 1999
Capital Beijing
Population 1.3 billion / 349 people per sq mile (135 people per sq km) / 30%
Total area 3,628,166 sq miles (9,396,960 sq km)
Languages Mandarin*, Wu, Cantonese, Hsiang, Min, Hakka, Kan
Religions Nonreligious 59%, Traditional beliefs 20%, Buddhist 6%, other 15%
Ethnic mix Han 93%, Zhaung 1%, other 6%
Government Single-party republic
Currency Yuan = 10 jiao = 100 fen
Literacy rate 84%
Calorie consumption 2,727 kilocalories

COLOMBIA
South America

Official name Republic of Colombia
Formation 1819 / 1922
Capital Bogotá
Population 37.7 million / 94 people per sq mile (36 people per sq km) / 73%
Total area 439,733 sq miles (1,138,910 sq km)
Languages Spanish*, Amerindian languages, English Creole
Religions Roman Catholic 95%, other 5%
Ethnic mix *Mestizo* 58%, White 20%, European-African 14%, other 8%
Government Multiparty republic
Currency Colombian peso = 100 centavos
Literacy rate 91%
Calorie consumption 2,677 kilocalories

COMOROS
Indian Ocean

Official name Federal Islamic Republic of the Comoros
Formation 1975 / 1975
Capital Moroni
Population 672,000 / 780 people per sq mile (301 people per sq km) / 29%
Total area 861 sq miles (2,230 sq km)
Languages Arabic*, French*, Comoran
Religions Muslim 98%, Roman Catholic 1%, other 1%
Ethnic mix Comorian 96%, other 4%
Government Islamic republic
Currency Comoros franc = 100 centimes
Literacy rate 55%
Calorie consumption 1,897 kilocalories

CONGO
Central Africa

Official name Republic of the Congo
Formation 1960 / 1960
Capital Brazzaville
Population 2.8 million / 21 people per sq km (8 people per sq km) / 59%
Total area 132,040 sq miles (342,000 sq km)
Languages French*, Kongo, Teke, Lingala
Religions Roman Catholic 50%, Traditional beliefs 48%, other 2%
Ethnic mix Bakongo 48%, Sangha 20%, Teke 17%, Mbochi 12%, other 3%
Government Multiparty republic
Currency CFA franc = 100 centimes
Literacy rate 77%
Calorie consumption 2,296 kilocalories

CONGO, DEM. REP. (ZAIRE)
Central Africa

Official name Democratic Republic of the Congo
Formation 1960 / 1960
Capital Kinshasa
Population 49.2 million / 56 people per sq mile (22 people per sq km) / 29%
Total area 905,563 sq miles (2,345,410 sq km)
Languages French*, Kiswahili, Tshiluba, Lingala
Religions Traditional beliefs 50%, Roman Catholic 37%, Protestant 13%
Ethnic mix Bantu 23%, Hamitic 23%, other 54%
Government Single-party republic
Currency Congolese franc = 100 centimes
Literacy rate 77%
Calorie consumption 2,060 kilocalories

COSTA RICA
Central America

Official name Republic of Costa Rica
Formation 1821 / 1838
Capital San José
Population 3.7 million / 188 people per sq mile (72 people per sq km) / 50%
Total area 19,730 miles (51,100 sq km)
Languages Spanish*, English Creole, Bribri, Cabecar
Religions Roman Catholic 76%, other 24%
Ethnic mix White and *mestizo* 96%, Black 2%, Indian 2%
Government Multiparty republic
Currency Costa Rica colón = 100 centimos
Literacy rate 95%
Calorie consumption 2,883 kilocalories

CROATIA
Southeastern Europe

Official name Republic of Croatia
Formation 1991 / 1991
Capital Zagreb
Population 4.5 million / 206 people per sq mile (80 people per sq km) / 64%
Total area 21,830 sq miles (56,540 sq km)
Languages Croatian*, Serbian, Hungarian (Magyar), Slovenian
Religions Roman Catholic 76%, Eastern Orthodox 11%, Protestant 1%, Muslim 1%, other 10%
Ethnic mix Croat 80%, Serb 12%, Hungarian, Slovenian, other 8%
Government Multiparty republic
Currency Kuna = 100 lipa
Literacy rate 98%
Calorie consumption NOT AVAILABLE

CUBA
West Indies

Official name Republic of Cuba
Formation 1902 / 1898
Capital Havana
Population 11.1 million / 259 people per sq mile (100 people per sq km) / 76%
Total area 42,803 sq miles (110,860 sq km)
Languages Spanish*, English, French
Religions Nonreligious 55%, Roman Catholic 40%, other 5%
Ethnic mix White 66%, European-African 22%, Black 12%
Government Socialist republic
Currency Cuban peso = 100 centavos
Literacy rate 96%
Calorie consumption 2,833 kilocalories

CYPRUS
Southeastern Europe

Official name Republic of Cyprus
Formation 1960 / 1983
Capital Nicosia
Population 766,000 / 218 people per sq mile (84 people per sq km) / 54%
Total area 3,572 sq miles (9,251 sq km)
Languages Greek*, Turkish, English
Religions Greek Orthodox 77%, Muslim 18%, other 5%
Ethnic mix Greek 77%, Turkish 18%, other (mainly British) 5%
Government Multiparty republic
Currency Cyprus pound / Turkish lira
Literacy rate 96%
Calorie consumption 3,779 kilocalories

CZECH REPUBLIC
Central Europe

Official name Czech Republic
Formation 1993 / 1993
Capital Prague
Population 10.2 million / 335 people per sq mile (129 people per sq km) / 65%
Total area 30,260 sq miles (78,370 sq km)
Languages Czech*, Slovak, Romany, Hungarian (Magyar)
Religions Roman Catholic 39%, nonreligious 40%, other 21%
Ethnic mix Czech 85%, Moravian 13%, other 2%
Government Multiparty republic
Currency Czech koruna = 100 halura
Literacy rate 99%
Calorie consumption 3,156 kilocalories

DENMARK
Northern Europe

Official name Kingdom of Denmark
Formation AD 960 / 1920
Capital Copenhagen
Population 5.3 million / 324 people per sq mile (125 people per sq km) / 85%
Total area 16,629 sq miles (43,069 sq km)
Languages Danish*, Faeroese, Inuit
Religions Evangelical Lutheran 89% other Christian 11%
Ethnic mix Danish 96%, Faeroese & Inuit 1%, other 3%
Government Constitutional monarchy
Currency Danish krone = 100 øre
Literacy rate 100%
Calorie consumption 3,664 kilocalories

DJIBOUTI
Eastern Africa

Official name Republic of Djibouti
Formation 1977 / 1977
Capital Djibouti
Population 652,000 / 73 people per sq mile (28 people per sq km) /83%
Total area 8,958 sq miles (23,200 sq km)
Languages Arabic*, French*, Somali, Afar
Religions Christian 87%, other 13%
Ethnic mix Issa 60%, Afar 35%, other 5%
Government Multiparty republic
Currency Djibouti franc = 100 centimes
Literacy rate 48%
Calorie consumption 2,338 kilocalories

DOMINICA
West Indies

Official name Commonwealth of Dominica
Formation 1978 / 1978
Capital Roseau
Population 74,000 / 256 people per sq mile (99 people per sq km)/ 69%
Total area 290 sq miles (750 sq km)
Languages English*, French Creole, Carib, Cocoy
Religions Roman Catholic 77%, Protestant 15%, other 8%
Ethnic mix Black 98%, Indian 2%
Government Multiparty republic
Currency East Caribbean dollar = 100 cents
Literacy rate 94%
Calorie consumption 2,778 kilocalories

DOMINICAN REPUBLIC
West Indies

Official name Dominican Republic
Formation 1865 / 1865
Capital Santo Domingo
Population 8.2 million / 439 people per sq mile (169 people per sq km) / 65%
Total area 18,815 sq miles (48,730 sq km)
Languages Spanish*, French Creole
Religions Roman Catholic 92%, other 8%
Ethnic mix European-African 73%, White 16%, Black 11%
Government Multiparty republic
Currency Dom. Republic peso = 100 centavos
Literacy rate 83%
Calorie consumption 2,286 kilocalories

ECUADOR
South America

Official name Republic of Ecuador
Formation 1830 / 1941
Capital Quito
Population 12.2 million / 114 people per sq mile (44 people per sq km) / 58%
Total area 109,483 sq miles (283,560 sq km)
Languages Spanish*, Quechua, other Amerindian languages
Religions Roman Catholic 95%, other 5%
Ethnic mix *Mestizo* 55%, Indian 25%, Black 10%, White 10%
Government Multiparty republic
Currency Sucre = 100 centavos
Literacy rate 91%
Calorie consumption 2,583 kilocalories

EGYPT
Northern Africa

Official name Arab Republic of Egypt
Formation 1936 / 1982
Capital Cairo
Population 65.7 million / 171 people per sq mile (66 people per sq km) / 45%
Total area 386,660 sq miles (1,001,450 sq km)
Languages Arabic*, French, English, Berber, Greek, Armenian
Religions Muslim 94%, other 6%
Ethnic mix Eastern Hamitic 90%, other (including Greek, Armenian) 10%
Government Multiparty republic
Currency Egyptian pound = 100 piastres
Literacy rate 53%
Calorie consumption 3,335 kilocalories

EL SALVADOR
Central America

Official name Republic of El Salvador
Formation 1856 / 1838
Capital San Salvador
Population 6.1 million / 763 people per sq mile (294 people per sq km) /45%
Total area 8,124 sq miles (21,040 sq km)
Languages Spanish*, Nahua
Religions Roman Catholic 80%, other 20%
Ethnic mix *Mestizo* 89%, Indian 10%, White 1%
Government Multiparty republic
Currency Salvadorean colón = 100 centavos
Literacy rate 73%
Calorie consumption 2,663 kilocalories

EQUATORIAL GUINEA
Central Africa

Official name Republic of Equatorial Guinea
Formation 1968 / 1968
Capital Malabo
Population 430,000 / 40 people per sq mile (15 people per sq km) / 42%
Total area 10,830 sq miles (28,050 sq km)
Languages Spanish*, Fang, Bubi
Religions Christian 90%, other 10%
Ethnic mix Fang 72%, Bubi 14%, Duala 3%, other 11%
Government Multiparty republic
Currency CFA franc = 100 centimes
Literacy rate 80%
Calorie consumption NOT AVAILABLE

ERITREA
Eastern Africa

Official name State of Eritrea
Formation 1993 / 1993
Capital Asmara
Population 3.5 million / 97 people per sq mile (37 people per sq km) / 17%
Total area 36,170 sq miles (93,680 sq km)
Languages Tigrinya*, Arabic*, Tigre
Religions Christian 45%, Muslim 45%, other 10%
Ethnic mix Nine main ethnic groups
Government Provisional military government
Currency Nakfa = 100 cents
Literacy rate 25%
Calorie consumption 1,610 kilocalories

ESTONIA
Northeastern Europe

Official name Republic of Estonia
Formation 1991 / 1991
Capital Tallinn
Population 1.4 million / 80 people per sq mile (31 people per sq km) / 73%
Total area 17,423 sq miles (45,125 sq km)
Languages Estonian*, Russian
Religions Evangelical Lutheran 98%, Eastern Orthodox, Baptist 2%
Ethnic mix Russian 62%, Estonian 30%, Ukrainian 3%, other 5%
Government Multiparty republic
Currency Kroon = 100 cents
Literacy rate 99%
Calorie consumption NOT AVAILABLE

ETHIOPIA
Eastern Africa

Official name Federal Democratic Republic of Ethiopia
Formation 1896 / 1993
Capital Addis Ababa
Population 62.1 million / 146 people per sq mile (56 people per sq km) / 13%
Total area 435,605 sq miles (1,128,221 sq km)
Languages Amharic*, English, Arabic
Religions Muslim 40%, Christian 40%, Traditional beliefs 15%, other 5%
Ethnic mix Oromo 40%, Amhara 25%, Sidamo 9%, Somali 6%, other 20%
Government Multiparty republic
Currency Ethiopian birr = 100 cents
Literacy rate 35%
Calorie consumption 1,610 kilocalories

FIJI
Australasia & Oceania

Official name Sovereign Democratic Republic of Fiji
Formation 1970 / 1970
Capital Suva
Population 822,000 / 117 people per sq mile (45 people per sq km) / 40%
Total area 7,054 sq miles (18,270 sq km)
Languages English*, Fijian, Hindu, Urdu
Religions Christian 46%, Hindu 38%, Muslim 8%, other 8%
Ethnic mix Native Fijian 49%, Indo-Fijian 46%, other 5%
Government Multiparty republic
Currency Fiji dollar = 100 cents
Literacy rate 92%
Calorie consumption 3,089 kilocalories

Finland
Northern Europe

Official name Republic of Finland
Formation 1917 / 1947
Capital Helsinki
Population 5.2 million / 44 people per sq mile (17 people per sq km) / 63%
Total area 130,552 sq miles (338,130 sq km)
Languages Finnish*, Swedish*, Lappish
Religions Evangelical Lutheran 89%, Finnish Orthodox 1%, other 10%
Ethnic mix Finnish 93%, Swedish 6%, other (including Sami) 1%
Government Multiparty republic
Currency Markka = 100 pennia
Literacy rate 99%
Calorie consumption 3,018 kilocalories

France
Western Europe

Official name French Republic
Formation 486 / 1919
Capital Paris
Population 58.7 million / 276 people per sq mile (107 people per sq km) / 73%
Total area 212,930 sq miles (551,500 sq km)
Languages French*, Provençal, Breton, Catalan, Basque
Religions Roman Catholic 88%, Muslim 8%, other 4%
Ethnic mix French 90%, North African 6%, German 2%, Breton 1%, other 1%
Government Multiparty republic
Currency Franc = 100 centimes
Literacy rate 99%
Calorie consumption 3,633 kilocalories

Gabon
Central Africa

Official name Gabonese Republic
Formation 1960 / 1960
Capital Libreville
Population 1.2 million / 12 people per sq mile (5 people per sq km) / 50%
Total area 103,347 sq miles (267,670 sq km)
Languages French*, Fang, Punu, Sira, Nzebi, Mpongwe
Religions Christian 96%, Muslim 2%, other 2%
Ethnic mix Fang 3%, Eshira 25%, other Bantu 25%, European and other African 9%
Government Multiparty republic
Currency CFA franc = 100 centimes
Literacy rate 66%
Calorie consumption 2,500 kilocalories

Gambia
Western Africa

Official name Republic of the Gambia
Formation 1965 / 1965
Capital Banjul
Population 1.9 million / 309 people per sq mile (119 people per sq km) / 26%
Total area 4,363 sq miles (11,300 sq km)
Languages English*, Mandinka, Fulani, Wolof, Diola, Soninke
Religions Muslim 85%, Christian 9%, Traditional beliefs 6%
Ethnic mix Mandingo 42%, Fulani 18% Wolof 16%, Jola 10%, Serahull 9%, other 5%
Government Multiparty republic
Currency Dalasi = 100 butut
Literacy rate 33%
Calorie consumption 2,360 kilocalories

Georgia
Southwestern Asia

Official name Republic of Georgia
Formation 1991 / 1991
Capital Tbilisi
Population 5.4 million / 201 people per sq mile (77 people per sq km) / 58%
Total area 26,911 sq miles (69,700 sq km)
Languages Georgian*, Russian
Religions Georgian Orthodox 70%, Russian Orthodox 10%, other 20%
Ethnic mix Georgian 70%, Armenian 8%, Russian 6%, Azeri 6%, other 10%
Government Multiparty republic
Currency Lari = 100 tetri
Literacy rate 99%
Calorie consumption NOT AVAILABLE

Germany
Northern Europe

Official name Federal Republic of Germany
Formation 1871 / 1990
Capital Berlin
Population 82.4 million / 611 people per sq mile (236 people per sq km) / 87%
Total area 137,800 sq miles (356,910 sq km)
Languages German*, Sorbian, Turkish
Religions Protestant 36%, Roman Catholic 35%, Muslim 2%, other 27%
Ethnic mix German 92%, other 8%
Government Multiparty republic
Currency Deutsche Mark = 100 pfennigs
Literacy rate 99%
Calorie consumption 3,344 kilocalories

Ghana
Western Africa

Official name Republic of Ghana
Formation 1957 / 1957
Capital Accra
Population 18.9 million / 213 people per sq mile (82 people per sq km) / 36%
Total area 92,100 sq miles (238,540 sq km)
Languages English*, Akan, Mossi, Ewe
Religions Traditional beliefs 38%, Christian 43%, Muslim 11%, other 8%
Ethnic mix Akan 52%, Mossi 15%, Ewe 12%, Ga 8%, other 13%
Government Multiparty republic
Currency Cedi = 100 pesewas
Literacy rate 66%
Calorie consumption 2,199 kilocalories

Greece
Southeastern Europe

Official name Hellenic Republic
Formation 1829 / 1947
Capital Athens
Population 10.6 million / 210 people per sq mile (81 people per sq km) / 65%
Total area 50,961 sq miles (131,990 sq km)
Languages Greek*, Turkish, Albanian, Macedonian
Religions Greek Orthodox 98%, Muslim 1%, other 1%
Ethnic mix Greek 98%, other 2%
Government Multiparty republic
Currency Drachma = 100 lepta
Literacy rate 96%
Calorie consumption 3,815 kilocalories

Grenada
West Indies

Official name Grenada
Formation 1974 / 1974
Capital St George's
Population 98,600 / 751 people per sq mile (290 people per sq km) / 37%
Total area 131 sq miles (340 sq km)
Languages English*, English Creole
Religions Roman Catholic 68%, Anglican 17%, other 15%
Ethnic mix Black 84%, European-African 13%, South Asian 3%
Government Parliamentary democracy
Currency East Caribbean dollar = 100 cents
Literacy rate 98%
Calorie consumption 2,402 kilocalories

Guatemala
Central America

Official name Republic of Guatemala
Formation 1838 / 1838
Capital Guatemala City
Population 11.6 million / 277 people per sq mile (107 people per sq km) / 41%
Total area 42,043 sq miles (108,890 sq km)
Languages Spanish*, Quiché, Mam, Kekchí
Religions Christian 99%, other 1%
Ethnic mix Indian 60%, *mestizo* 30%, other 10%
Government Multiparty republic
Currency Quetzal = 100 centavos
Literacy rate 66%
Calorie consumption 2,255 kilocalories

Guinea
Western Africa

Official name Republic of Guinea
Formation 1958 / 1958
Capital Conakry
Population 7.7 million / 81 people per sq mile (31 people per sq km) / 30%
Total area 94,926 sq miles (245,860 sq km)
Languages French*, Fulani, Malinke, Soussou, Kissi
Religions Muslim 85%, Christian 8%, Traditional beliefs 7%
Ethnic mix Fila (Fulani) 30%, Malinke 30%, Soussou 15%, Kissi 10% other 20%
Government Multiparty republic
Currency Franc = 100 centimes
Literacy rate 37%
Calorie consumption 2,389 kilocalories

Guinea-Bissau
Western Africa

Official name Republic of Guinea-Bissau
Formation 1974 / 1974
Capital Bissau
Population 1.1 million / 101 people per sq mile (39 people per sq km) / 22%
Total area 13,940 sq miles (36,120 sq km)
Languages Portuguese*, Balante, Fulani, Malinke
Religions Traditional beliefs 52%, Muslim 40%, Christian 8%
Ethnic mix Balante 30%, Fila (Fulani) 22%, Malinke 12%, other 36%
Government Multiparty republic
Currency Guinea peso = 100 centavos
Literacy rate 33%
Calorie consumption 2,556 kilocalories

Guyana
South America

Official name Cooperative Republic of Guyana
Formation 1966 / 1966
Capital Georgetown
Population 856,000 / 11 people per sq mile (4 people per sq km) / 36%
Total area 83,000 sq miles (214,970 sq km)
Languages English*, English Creole, Hindi, Tamil, English
Religions Christian 57%, Hindu 33%, Muslim 9%, other 1%
Ethnic mix East Indian 52%, Black African 38%, Indian 4%, other 6%
Government Multiparty republic
Currency Guyana dollar =100 cents
Literacy rate 98%
Calorie consumption 2,384 kilocalories

Haiti
West Indies

Official name Republic of Haiti
Formation 1804 / 1844
Capital Port-au-Prince
Population 7.5 million / 705 people per sq mile (272 people per sq km) / 32%
Total area 10,714 sq miles (27,750 sq km)
Languages French*, French Creole*,
Religions Roman Catholic 80%, Protestant 16%, other 4%
Ethnic mix Black 95%, European-African 5%
Government Multiparty republic
Currency Gourde = 100 centimes
Literacy rate 45%
Calorie consumption 1,706 kilocalories

Honduras
Central America

Official name Republic of Honduras
Formation 1838 / 1838
Capital Tegucigalpa
Population 6.1 million / 141 people per sq mile (55 people per sq km) / 44%
Total area 43,278 sq miles (112,090 sq km)
Languages Spanish*, English Creole, Garifuna, Indian languages
Religions Roman Catholic 97%, other 3%
Ethnic mix *Mestizo* 90%, Black African 5%, Indian 4%, White 1%
Government Multiparty republic
Currency Lempira = 100 centavos
Literacy rate 70%
Calorie consumption 2,305 kilocalories

Hungary
Central Europe

Official name Republic of Hungary
Formation 1918 / 1947
Capital Budapest
Population 9.9 million / 278 people per sq mile (107 people per sq km) / 65%
Total area 35,919 sq miles (93,030 sq km)
Languages Hungarian (Magyar)*, German, Slovak
Religions Roman Catholic 64%, Protestant 27%, other 7%
Ethnic mix Hungarian (Magyar) 90%, German 2%, other 8%
Government Multiparty republic
Currency Forint = 100 filler
Literacy rate 99%
Calorie consumption 3,503 kilocalories

Iceland
Northwestern Europe

Official name Republic of Iceland
Formation 1944 / 1944
Capital Reykjavík
Population 277,000 / 7 people per sq mile (3 people per sq km) / 92%
Total area 39,770 sq miles (103,000 sq km)
Languages Icelandic*, English
Religions Evangelical Lutheran 93%, nonreligious 6%, other Christian 1%
Ethnic mix Icelandic (Norwegian-Celtic descent) 98%, other 2%
Government Constitutional republic
Currency New Icelandic króna = 100 aurar
Literacy rate 99%
Calorie consumption 3,058 kilocalories

India
Southern Asia

Official name Republic of India
Formation 1947 / 1947
Capital New Delhi
Population 976 million / 850 people per sq mile (328 people per sq km) / 27%
Total area 1,269,338 sq miles (3,287,590 sq km)
Languages Hindi*, English*, Urdu, Bengali, Marathi, Telugu, Tamil, Bihari
Religions Hindu 83%, Muslim 11%, Christian 2%, Sikh 2%, other 2%
Ethnic mix Indo-Aryan 72%, Dravidian 25%, Mongoloid and other 3%
Government Multiparty republic
Currency Rupee = 100 paisa
Literacy rate 53%
Calorie consumption 2,395 kilocalories

Indonesia
Southeastern Asia

Official name Republic of Indonesia
Formation 1949 / 1963
Capital Jakarta
Population 206.5 million / 295 people per sq mile (114 people per sq km) / 35%
Total area 735,555 sq miles (1,904,570 sq km)
Languages Bahasa Indonesia*, 250 (est.) languages or dialects
Religions Muslim 87%, Christian 9%, Hindu 2%, Buddhist 1%, other 1%
Ethnic mix Javanese 45%, Sundanese 14%, Madurese 8%, Coastal Malays 8%, other 25%
Government Multiparty republic
Currency Rupiah = 100 sen
Literacy rate 82%
Calorie consumption 2,752 kilocalories

Iran
Southwestern Asia

Official name Islamic Republic of Iran
Formation 1906 / 1906
Capital Tehran
Population 73.1 million / 116 people per sq mile (45 people per sq km) / 59%
Total area 636,293 sq miles (1,648,000 sq km)
Languages Farsi (Persian)*, Azerbaijani, Gilaki, Mazanderani, Kurdish, Baluchi, Arabic
Religions Shi'a Muslim 95%, Sunni Muslim 4%, other 1%
Ethnic mix Persian 50%, Azeri 20%, Lur and Bakhtiari 10%, Kurd 8%, Arab 2%, other 10%
Government Islamic Republic
Currency Iranian rial = 100 dinars
Literacy rate 73%
Calorie consumption 2,860 kilocalories

Iraq
Southwestern Asia

Official name Republic of Iraq
Formation 1932 / 1991
Capital Baghdad
Population 21.8 million / 129 people per sq mile (50 people per sq km) / 73%
Total area 169,235 sq miles (438,320 sq km)
Languages Arabic*, Kurdish, Armenian, Assyrian
Religions Shi'a ithna Muslim 62%, Sunni Muslim 33%, other 5%
Ethnic mix Arab 79%, Kurdish 16%, Persian 3%, Turkoman 2%
Government Single-party republic
Currency Iraqi dinar = 1000 fils
Literacy rate 58%
Calorie consumption 2,121 kilocalories

Ireland
Northwestern Europe

Official name Republic of Ireland
Formation 1922 / 1922
Capital Dublin
Population 3.6 million / 135 people per sq mile (52 people per sq km) / 57%
Total area 27,155 sq miles (70,280 sq km)
Languages English*, Irish Gaelic*
Religions Roman Catholic 88%, Protestant 3%, other 9%
Ethnic mix Irish 95%, other 5%
Government Multiparty republic
Currency Punt = 100 pence
Literacy rate 99%
Calorie consumption 3,847 kilocalories

Israel
Southwestern Asia

Official name State of Israel
Formation 1948 / 1994
Capital Jerusalem
Population 5.9 million / 752 people per sq mile (290 people per sq km) / 91%
Total area 7,992 sq miles (20,700 sq km)
Languages Hebrew*, Arabic*, Yiddish
Religions Jewish 82%, Muslim 14%, Christian 2%, Druze and other 2%
Ethnic mix Jewish 82%, Arab 18%
Government Multiparty republic
Currency New Israeli shekel = 100 agorat
Literacy rate 95%
Calorie consumption 3,050 kilocalories

Italy
Southern Europe

Official name Italian Republic
Formation 1871 / 1954
Capital Rome
Population 57.2 million / 504 people per sq mile (195 people per sq km) / 67%
Total area 116,320 sq miles (301,270 sq km)
Languages Italian*, German, French, Rhaeto-Romanic, Sardinian
Religions Roman Catholic 83%, other 17%
Ethnic mix Italian 94%, other 6%
Government Multiparty republic
Currency Lira = 100 centesimi
Literacy rate 98%
Calorie consumption 3,561 kilocalories

Ivory Coast
Western Africa

Official name Republic of the Ivory Coast
Formation 1960 / 1960
Capital Yamoussoukro
Population 14.6 million / 119 people per sq mile (45 people per sq km) / 42%
Total area 124,503 sq miles (322,463 sq km)
Languages French*, Akran, Kru, Voltaic
Religions Traditional beliefs 63%, Muslim 25%, Christian 12%
Ethnic mix Baoulé 23%, Bété 18%, Kru 17%, Malinke 15%, other 27%
Government Multiparty republic
Currency CFA franc = 100 centimes
Literacy rate 54%
Calorie consumption 2,491 kilocalories

Jamaica
West Indies

Official name Jamaica
Formation 1962 / 1962
Capital Kingston
Population 2.5 million / 598 people per sq mile (231 people per sq km) / 54%
Total area 4,243 sq miles (10,990 sq km)
Languages English*, English Creole
Religions Christian 55%, other 45%
Ethnic mix Black 75%, mixed 15%, South Asian 5%, other 5%
Government Parliamentary democracy
Currency Jamaican dollar = 100 cents
Literacy rate 85%
Calorie consumption 2,607 kilocalories

Japan
Eastern Asia

Official name Japan
Formation 1600 / 1972
Capital Tokyo
Population 125.9 million / 866 people per sq mile (334 people per sq km) / 78%
Total area 145,869 sq miles (377,800 sq km)
Languages Japanese*, Korean, Chinese
Religions Shinto and Buddhist 76%, Buddhist 16%, other 8%
Ethnic mix Japanese 99%, other 1%
Government Constitutional monarchy
Currency Yen = 100 sen
Literacy rate 99%
Calorie consumption 2,903 kilocalories

Jordan
Southwestern Asia

Official name Hashemite Kingdom of Jordan
Formation 1946 / 1976
Capital Amman
Population 6 million / 175 people per sq mile (67 people per sq km) / 71%
Total area 34,440 sq miles (89,210 sq km)
Languages Arabic*
Religions Muslim 95%, Christian 5%
Ethnic mix Arab 98%, (40% Palestinian), Armenian 1%, Circassian 1%
Government Constitutional monarchy
Currency Jordanian dinar = 1,000 fils
Literacy rate 87%
Calorie consumption 3,022 kilocalories

Kazakhstan
Central Asia

Official Name Republic of Kazakhstan
Formation 1991 / 1991
Capital Astana
Population 16.9 million / 16 people per sq mile (6 people per sq km) / 60%
Total area 1,049,150 sq miles (2,717,300 sq km)
Languages Kazakh*, Russian, German
Religions Muslim 47%, other 53% (mostly Russian Orthodox and Lutheran)
Ethnic mix Kazakh 44%, Russian 38%, Ukrainian 6%, German 2%, other 14%
Government Multiparty republic
Currency Tenge = 100 tein
Literacy rate 99%
Calorie consumption NOT AVAILABLE

Kenya
East Africa

Official name Republic of Kenya
Formation 1963 / 1963
Capital Nairobi
Population 29 million / 132 people per sq mile (51 people per sq km) / 28%
Total area 224,081 sq miles (580,370 sq km)
Languages Swahili*, English, Kikuyu, Luo, Kamba
Religions Christian 60%, Traditional beliefs 25%, Muslim 6%, other 9%
Ethnic mix Kikuyu 21%, Luhya 14%, Luo 13%, Kalenjin 11% other 41%
Government Multiparty republic
Currency Kenya shilling = 100 cents
Literacy rate 79%
Calorie consumption 2,075 kilocalories

KIRIBATI
Australasia & Oceania

Official Name Republic of Kiribati
Formation 1979 / 1979
Capital Bairiki
Population 78,000 / 284 people per sq mile (110 people per sq km) / 36%
Total area 274 sq miles (710 sq km)
Languages English*, Kiribati
Religions Roman Catholic 53%, Protestant 39%, other 8%
Ethnic mix I-Kiribati 98%, other 2%
Government Multiparty republic
Currency Australian dollar = 100 cents
Literacy rate 98%
Calorie consumption 2,651 kilocalories

KUWAIT
Southwestern Asia

Official name State of Kuwait
Formation 1961 / 1961
Capital Kuwait
Population 1.8 million / 262 people per sq mile (101 people per sq km) / 97%
Total area 6,880 sq miles (17,820 sq km)
Languages Arabic*, English
Religions Muslim 92%, Christian 6%, other 2%
Ethnic mix Kuwaiti 45%, other Arab 35%, South Asian 9%, Iranian 4%, other 7%
Government Constitutional monarchy
Currency Dinar = 1,000 fils
Literacy rate 80%
Calorie consumption 2,523 kilocalories

KYRGYZSTAN
Central Asia

Official name Kyrgyz Republic
Formation 1991 / 1991
Capital Bishkek
Population 4.5 million / 59 people per sq mile (23 people per sq km) / 39%
Total area 76,640 sq miles (198,500 sq km)
Languages Kyrgyz*, Russian*, Uzbek
Religions Muslim 65%, other (mostly Russian Orthodox) 35%
Ethnic mix Kyrgyz 57%, Russian 19%, Uzbek 13%, Tatar, Ukrainian, other 11%
Government Multiparty republic
Currency Som =100 teen
Literacy rate 97%
Calorie consumption NOT AVAILABLE

LAOS
Southeastern Asia

Official name Lao People's Democratic Republic
Formation 1953 / 1953
Capital Vientiane
Population 5.4 million / 61 people per sq mile (23 people per sq km) / 22%
Total area 91,428 sq miles (236,800 sq km)
Languages Lao*, Miao, Yao
Religions Buddhist 85%, other (including Traditional beliefs) 15%
Ethnic mix Lao Loum 56%, Lao Theung 34%, Lao Soung 9%, other 1%
Government Single-party republic
Currency New kip = 100 cents
Literacy rate 58%
Calorie consumption 2,259 kilocalories

LATVIA
Northeastern Europe

Official name Republic of Latvia
Formation 1991 / 1991
Capital Riga
Population 2.4 million / 96 people per sq mile (37 people per sq km) / 73%
Total area 24,938 sq miles (64,589 sq km)
Languages Latvian*, Russian
Religions Evangelical Lutheran 85%, other Christian 15%
Ethnic mix Latvian 52%, Russian 34%, Belarusian 5%, Ukrainian 4%, other 5%
Government Multiparty republic
Currency Lats = 100 santimi
Literacy rate 99%
Calorie consumption NOT AVAILABLE

LEBANON
Southwestern Asia

Official name Republic of Lebanon
Formation 1944 / 1944
Capital Beirut
Population 3.2 million / 810 people per sq mile (313 people per sq km) / 87%
Total area 4015 sq miles (10,400 sq km)
Languages Arabic*, French, Armenian,
Religions Muslim (mainly Shi'a) 70%, Christian (mainly Maronite) 30%
Ethnic mix Arab 93% (Lebanese 83%, Palestinian 10%), other 7%
Government Multiparty republic
Currency Lebanese pound = 100 piastres
Literacy rate 84%
Calorie consumption 3,317 kilocalories

LESOTHO
Southern Africa

Official name Kingdom of Lesotho
Formation 1966 / 1966
Capital Maseru
Population 2.2 million / 188 people per sq mile (72 people per sq km) / 23%
Total area 11,718 sq miles (30,350 sq km)
Languages English*, Sesotho*, Zulu
Religions Christian 93%, other 7%
Ethnic mix Basotho 97%, European and Asian 3%
Government Constitutional monarchy
Currency Loti = 100 lisente
Literacy rate 82%
Calorie consumption 2,201 kilocalories

LIBERIA
Western Africa

Official name Republic of Liberia
Formation 1847 / 1947
Capital Monrovia
Population 2.7 million / 73 people per sq mile (28 people per sq km) / 45%
Total area 43,000 sq miles (111,370 sq km)
Languages English*, Kpelle, Bassa, Vai, Kru, Grebo, Kissi, Gola
Religions Traditional beliefs 70%, Muslim 20%, Christian 10%
Ethnic mix Indigenous tribes (16 main groups) 95%, Americo-Liberians 4%
Government Multiparty republic
Currency Liberian dollar = 100 cents
Literacy rate 38%
Calorie consumption 1,640 kilocalories

LIBYA
Northern Africa

Official name The Great Socialist People's Libyan Arab Jamahiriya
Formation 1951 / 1951
Capital Tripoli
Population 6 million / 9 people per sq mile (3 people per sq km) / 86%
Total area 679,358 sq miles (1,759,540 sq km)
Languages Arabic*, Tuareg
Religions Muslim (mainly Sunni) 97%, other 3%
Ethnic mix Arab and Berber 95%, other 5%
Government Single-party state
Currency Libyan dinar = 1,000 dirhams
Literacy rate 76%
Calorie consumption 3,308 kilocalories

LIECHTENSTEIN
Western Europe

Official name Principality of Liechtenstein
Formation 1719 / 1719
Capital Vaduz
Population 31,000 / 504 people per sq mile (195 people per sq km) / 87%
Total area 62 sq miles (160 sq km)
Languages German*, Alemannish, Italian
Religions Roman Catholic 81%, Protestant 7%, other 12%
Ethnic mix Liechtensteiner 63%, Swiss 15%, German 9%, other 13%
Government Constitutional monarchy
Currency Swiss franc = 100 centimes
Literacy rate 99%
Calorie consumption NOT AVAILABLE

LITHUANIA
Northeastern Europe

Official name Republic of Lithuania
Formation 1991 / 1991
Capital Vilnius
Population 3.7 million / 147 people per sq mile (57 people per sq km) / 72%
Total area 25,174 sq miles (65,200 sq km)
Languages Lithuanian*, Russian
Religions Roman Catholic 87%, Russian Orthodox 10%, other 3%
Ethnic mix Lithuanian 80%, Russian 9%, Polish 7%, Belarusian 2%, other 2%
Government Multiparty republic
Currency Litas = 100 centas
Literacy rate 98%
Calorie consumption NOT AVAILABLE

LUXEMBOURG
Northwest Europe

Official name Grand Duchy of Luxembourg
Formation 1867 / 1867
Capital Luxembourg
Population 422,000 / 423 people per sq mile (163 people per sq km) / 89%
Total area 998 sq miles (2,586 sq km)
Languages Letzeburgish*, French*, German*
Religions Roman Catholic 97%, other 3%
Ethnic mix Luxemburger 72%, Portuguese 9%, Italian 5%, other 14%
Government Constitutional monarchy
Currency Franc = 100 centimes
Literacy rate 99%
Calorie consumption 3,681 kilocalories

MACEDONIA
Southeastern Europe

Official name Former Yugoslav Republic of Macedonia
Formation 1991 / 1991
Capital Skopje
Population 2.2 million / 222 people per sq mile (86 people per sq km) / 60%
Total area 9,929 sq miles (25,715 sq km)
Languages Macedonian*, Serbo-Croatian
Religions Christian 80%, Muslim 20%
Ethnic mix Macedonian 67%, Albanian 23%, Turkish 4%, Serb 2%, Romany 2%, other 2%
Government Multiparty republic
Currency Macedonian denar = 100 deni
Literacy rate 89%
Calorie consumption NOT AVAILABLE

MADAGASCAR
Indian Ocean

Official name Democratic Republic of Madagascar
Formation 1960 / 1960
Capital Antananarivo
Population 16.3 million / 73 people per sq mile (28 people per sq km) / 27%
Total area 226,660 sq miles (587,040 sq km)
Languages Malagasy*, French*
Religions Traditional beliefs 52%, Christian 41%, Muslim 7%
Ethnic mix Merina 26%, Betsimisaraka 15%, Betsileo 12%, other 47%
Government Multiparty republic
Currency Franc = 100 centimes
Literacy rate 81%
Calorie consumption 2,135 kilocalories

MALAWI
Southern Africa

Official name Republic of Malawi
Formation 1964 / 1964
Capital Lilongwe
Population 10.4 million / 286 people per sq mile (111 people per sq km) / 14%
Total area 45,745 sq miles (118,480 sq km)
Languages English*, Chewa, Lomwe, Yao
Religions Christian 75%, Muslim 20% traditional beliefs 5%
Ethnic mix Maravi 55%, Lomwe 17%, Yao 13%, other 15%
Government Multiparty republic
Currency Malawi kwacha = 100 tambala
Literacy rate 57%
Calorie consumption 1,825 kilocalories

MALAYSIA
Southeastern Asia

Official name Malaysia
Formation 1963 / 1965
Capital Kuala Lumpur
Population 21.5 million / 169 people per sq mile (65 people per sq km) / 54%
Total area 127,317 sq miles (329,750 sq km)
Languages Malay*, English*, Chinese, Tamil
Religions Muslim 53%, Buddhist 19%, Chinese faiths 12%, Christian 7%, other 9%
Ethnic mix Malay 47%, Chinese 32%, Indigenous tribes 12%, Indian 8%, other 1%
Government Federal constitutional monarchy
Currency Ringgit = 100 cents
Literacy rate 85%
Calorie consumption 2,888 kilocalories

MALDIVES
Indian Ocean

Official name Republic of Maldives
Formation 1965 / 1965
Capital Male'
Population 282,000 / 2,435 people per sq mile (940 people per sq km) / 26%
Total area 116 sq miles (300 sq km)
Languages Dhivehi (Maldivian)*, Sinhala, Tamil
Religions Sunni Muslim 100%
Ethnic mix Maldivian 99%, other 1%
Government Republic
Currency Rufiyaa = 100 laari
Literacy rate 91%
Calorie consumption 2,580 kilocalories

MALI
Western Africa

Official name Republic of Mali
Formation 1960 / 1960
Capital Bamako
Population 11.8 million / 25 people per sq mile (10 people per sq km) / 27%
Total area 478,837 sq miles (1,240,190 sq km)
Languages French*, Bambara, Fulani, Senufo, Soninké
Religions Muslim 80%, Traditional beliefs 18%, Christian 2%
Ethnic mix Bambara 31%, Fulani 13%, Senufo 12%, other 44%
Government Multiparty republic
Currency CFA franc = 100 centimes
Literacy rate 35%
Calorie consumption 2,278 kilocalories

MALTA
Southern Europe

Official name Republic of Malta
Formation 1964 / 1964
Capital Valletta
Population 374,000 / 3,027 people per sq mile (1,169 people per sq km) / 89%
Total area 124 sq miles (320 sq km)
Languages Maltese*, English*
Religions Roman Catholic 98%, other (mostly Anglican) 2%
Ethnic mix Maltese (mixed Arab, Sicilian, Norman, Spanish, Italian, English) 98%, other 2%
Government Multiparty republic
Currency Maltese lira = 100 cents
Literacy rate 91%
Calorie consumption 3,486 kilocalories

MARSHALL ISLANDS
Australasia & Oceania

Official name Republic of the Marshall Islands
Formation 1986 / 1986
Capital Majuro
Population 59,000 / 848 people per sq mile (327 people per sq km) / 69%
Total area 70 sq miles (181 sq km)
Languages English*, Marshallese*
Religions Protestant 80%, Roman Catholic 15%, other 5%
Ethnic mix Micronesian 97%, other 3%
Government Multiparty republic
Currency US dollar = 100 cents
Literacy rate 91%
Calorie consumption NOT AVAILABLE

MAURITANIA
West Africa

Official name Islamic Republic of Mauritania
Formation 1960 / 1960
Capital Nouakchott
Population 2.5 million / 6 people per sq mile (2 people per sq km) / 54%
Total area 395,953 sq miles (1,025,520 sq km)
Languages French*, Arabic*, Wolof
Religions Muslim 100%
Ethnic mix Maure 80%, Wolof 7%, Tukulor 5%, other 8%
Government Multiparty republic
Currency Ouguiya = 5 khoums
Literacy rate 38%
Calorie consumption 2,685 kilocalories

MAURITIUS
Indian Ocean

Official name Republic of Mauritius
Formation 1968 / 1968
Capital Port Louis
Population 1.2 million / 1,680 people per sq mile (649 people per sq km) / 41%
Total area 718 sq miles (1,860 sq km)
Languages English*, French Creole, Hindi, Urdu, Tamil, Chinese
Religions Hindu 52%, Roman Catholic, 26%, Muslim 17%, other 5%
Ethnic mix Creole 55%, South Asian 40%, Chinese 3%, other 2%
Government Multiparty republic
Currency Mauritian rupee = 100 cents
Literacy rate 83%
Calorie consumption 2,690 kilocalories

MEXICO
North America

Official name United Mexican States
Formation 1836 / 1848
Capital Mexico City
Population 95.8 million / 130 people per sq mile (50 people per sq km) / 75%
Total area 756,061 sq miles (1,958,200 sq km)
Languages Spanish*, Mayan dialects
Religions Roman Catholic 95%, Protestant 1%, other 4%
Ethnic mix *Mestizo* 55%, Indigenous Indian 20%, European 16%, other 9%
Government Multiparty republic
Currency Mexican peso = 100 centavos
Literacy rate 90%
Calorie consumption 3,146 kilocalories

MICRONESIA
Australasia & Oceania

Official name Federated States of Micronesia
Formation 1986 / 1986
Capital Palikir
Population 109,000 / 403 people per sq mile (156 people per sq km) / 28%
Total area 1,120 sq miles (2,900 sq km)
Languages English*, Trukese, Pohnpeian, Mortlockese, Kosrean
Religions Roman Catholic 50%, Protestant 48%, other 2%
Ethnic mix Micronesian 99%, other 1%
Government Republic
Currency US dollar = 100 cents
Literacy rate 90%
Calorie consumption NOT AVAILABLE

MOLDOVA
Southeastern Europe

Official name Republic of Moldova
Formation 1991 / 1991
Capital Chişinău
Population 4.5 million / 346 people per sq mile (134 people per sq km) / 52%
Total area 13,000 sq miles (33,700 sq km)
Languages Romanian*, Moldovan, Russian
Religions Romanian Orthodox 98%, Jewish 1%, other 1%
Ethnic mix Moldovan 65%, Ukrainian 14%, Russian 13%, Gagauz 4%, other 4%
Government Multiparty republic
Currency Moldovan leu = 100 bani
Literacy rate 98%
Calorie consumption NOT AVAILABLE

MONACO
Southern Europe

Official name Principality of Monaco
Formation 1861 / 1861
Capital Monaco
Population 32,000 / 42,503 people per sq mile (16,410 people per sq km) / 100%
Total area 0.75 sq miles (1.95 sq km)
Languages French*, Italian, Monégasque, English
Religions Roman Catholic 89%, other 11%
Ethnic mix French 47%, Monégasque 17%, Italian 16%, other 20%
Government Constitutional monarchy
Currency French franc = 100 centimes
Literacy rate 99%
Calorie consumption NOT AVAILABLE

MONGOLIA
Eastern Asia

Official name Mongolia
Formation 1924 / 1924
Capital Ulan Bator
Population 2.6 million / 4 people per sq mile (2 people per sq km) / 61%
Total area 604,247 sq miles (1,565,000 sq km)
Languages Khalkha Mongol*, Turkic, Russian, Chinese
Religions Predominantly Tibetan Buddhist, with a Muslim minority
Ethnic mix Mongol 90%, Kazakh 4%, Chinese 2%, Russian 2%, other 2%
Government Multiparty republic
Currency Tughrik (togrog) = 100 möngös
Literacy rate 84%
Calorie consumption 1,899 kilocalories

MOROCCO
Northern Africa

Official name Kingdom of Morocco
Formation 1956 / 1956
Capital Rabat
Population 28 million / 162 people per sq mile (63 people per sq km) / 48%
Total area 269,757 sq miles (698,670 sq km)
Religions Muslim 98%, Jewish 1%, Christian 1%
Ethnic mix Arab and Berber 99%, European 1%
Government Constitutional monarchy
Currency Moroccan dirham = 100 centimes
Literacy rate 45%
Calorie consumption 2,984 kilocalories

MOZAMBIQUE
Southern Africa

Official name Republic of Mozambique
Formation 1975 / 1975
Capital Maputo
Population 18.7 million / 62 people per sq mile (24 people per sq km) / 34%
Total area 309,493 sq miles (801,590 sq km)
Languages Portuguese*, Makua, Tsonga, Sena
Religions Traditional beliefs 60%, Christian 30%, Muslim 10%
Ethnic mix Makua-Lomwe 47%, Thonga 23%, Malawi 12%, Shona 11%, Yao 4%, other 3%
Government Multiparty republic
Currency Metical = 100 centavos
Literacy rate 40%
Calorie consumption 1,680 kilocalories

MYANMAR
Southeastern Asia

Official name Union of Myanmar
Formation 1948 / 1948
Capital Rangoon
Population 47.6 million / 187 people per sq mile (72 people per sq km) / 26%
Total area 261,200 sq miles (676,550 sq km)
Languages Burmese*, Karen, Shan, Mon
Religions Buddhist 87%, Christian 6%, Muslim 4%, other 3%
Ethnic mix Burman 68%, Shan 9%, Karen 6%, Rakhine 4%, other 13%
Government Military regime
Currency Kyat = 100 pyas
Literacy rate 84%
Calorie consumption 2,598 kilocalories

NAMIBIA
Southern Africa

Official name Republic of Namibia
Formation 1990 / 1994
Capital Windhoek
Population 1.7 million / 5 people per sq mile (2 people per sq km) / 37%
Total area 318,260 sq miles (824,290 sq km)
Languages English*, Afrikaans, Ovambo, Kavango, Bergdama
Religions Christian 90%, other 10%
Ethnic mix Ovambo 50%, Kavango 9%, Herero 8%, Damara 8%, other 25%
Government Multiparty republic
Currency Namibian dollar = 100 cents
Literacy rate 79%
Calorie consumption 2,134 kilocalories

NAURU
Australasia & Oceania

Official name Republic of Nauru
Formation 1968 / 1968
Capital No official capital
Population 11,000 / 1332 people per sq mile (514 people per sq km) / 100%
Total area 8.2 sq miles (21.2 sq km)
Languages Nauruan*, English, Kiribati, Chinese, Tuvaluan
Religions Christian 95%, other 5%
Ethnic mix Nauruan 62%, other Pacific islanders 25%, Chinese 8%, European 5%
Government Parliamentary democracy
Currency Australian dollar = 100 cents
Literacy rate 99%
Calorie consumption NOT AVAILABLE

NEPAL
Southern Asia

Official name Kingdom of Nepal
Formation 1769 / 1769
Capital Kathmandu
Population 23.2 million / 439 people per sq mile (170 people per sq km) / 11%
Total area 54,363 sq miles (140,800 sq km)
Languages Nepali*, Maithilli, Bhojpuri
Religions Hindu 90%, Buddhist 4%, Muslim 3%, Christian 1%, other 2%
Ethnic mix Nepalese 58%, Bihari 19%, Tamang 6%, other 17%
Government Constitutional monarchy
Currency Nepalese rupee = 100 paisa
Literacy rate 38%
Calorie consumption 1,957 kilocalories

NETHERLANDS
Northwest Europe

Official name Kingdom of the Netherlands
Formation 1815 / 1839
Capitals Amsterdam, The Hague
Population 15.7 million / 1,199 people per sq mile (463 people per sq km) / 89%
Total area 14,410 sq miles (37,330 sq km)
Languages Dutch*, Frisian
Religions Roman Catholic 36%, Protestant 27%, Muslim 3%, other 34%
Ethnic mix Dutch 96%, other 4%
Government Constitutional monarchy
Currency Netherland guilder = 100 cents
Literacy rate 99%
Calorie consumption 3,222 kilocalories

NEW ZEALAND
Australasia & Oceania

Official name New Zealand
Formation 1947 / 1947
Capital Wellington
Population 3.7 million / 36 people per sq mile (14 people per sq km) / 86%
Total area 103,730 sq miles (268,680 sq km)
Languages English*, Maori
Religions Protestant 47%, Roman Catholic 15%, other 38%
Ethnic mix European 82%, Maori 9%, Pacific Islanders 3%, other 6%
Government Constitutional monarchy
Currency NZ dollar = 100 cents
Literacy rate 99%
Calorie consumption 3,669 kilocalories

NICARAGUA
Central America

Official name Republic of Nicaragua
Formation 1838 / 1838
Capital Managua
Population 4.5 million / 98 people per sq mile (38 people per sq km) / 63%
Total area 50,193 sq miles (130,000 sq km)
Languages Spanish*, English Creole, Miskito
Religions Roman Catholic 95%, other 5%
Ethnic mix *Mestizo* 69%, White 14%, Black 8%, Indigenous Indian 5%, Zambos 4%
Government Multiparty republic
Currency Córdoba ora = 100 pence
Literacy rate 63%
Calorie consumption 2,293 kilocalories

NIGER
Western Africa

Official name Republic of Niger
Formation 1960 / 1960
Capital Niamey
Population 10.1 million / 21 people per sq mile (8 people per sq km) / 17%
Total area 489,188 sq miles (1,267,000 sq km)
Languages French*, Hausa, Djerma, Fulani, Tuareg, Teda
Religions Muslim 85%, traditional beliefs 14%, Christian 1%
Ethnic mix Hausa 54%, Djerma and Songhal 21%, Fulani 10%, Tuareg 9%, other 6%
Government Multiparty republic
Currency CFA franc = 100 centimes
Literacy rate 14%
Calorie consumption 2,257 kilocalories

NIGERIA
Western Africa

Official name Federal Republic of Nigeria
Formation 1960 / 1961
Capital Abuja
Population 122 million / 346 people per sq mile (123 people per sq km) / 34%
Total area 356,668 sq miles (923,770 sq km)
Languages English*, Hausa, Yoruba, Ibo
Religions Muslim 50%, Christian 40%, Traditional beliefs 10%
Ethnic mix Hausa 21%, Yoruba 21%, Ibo 18%, Fulani 11%, other 29%
Government Multiparty republic
Currency Naira = 100 kobo
Literacy rate 59%
Calorie consumption 2,124 kilocalories

NORTH KOREA
Eastern Asia

Official name Democratic People's Republic of Korea
Formation 1948 / 1953
Capital Pyongyang
Population 23.2 million / 499 people per sq mile (193 people per sq km) / 61%
Total area 46,540 sq miles (120,540 sq km)
Languages Korean*, Chinese
Religions Traditional beliefs 16%, Ch'ondogyo 14%, Buddhist 2%, nonreligious 68%
Ethnic mix Korean 99%, other 1%
Government Single-party republic
Currency North Korean Won = 100 chon
Literacy rate 99%
Calorie consumption 2,833 kilocalories

NORWAY
Northern Europe

Official name Kingdom of Norway
Formation 1905 / 1905
Capital Oslo
Population 4.4 million / 37 people per sq mile (14 people per sq km) / 73%
Total area 125,060 sq miles (323,900 sq km)
Languages Norwegian* (Bokmal and *Nynorsk*), Lappish, Finnish
Religions Evangelical Lutheran 89%, Roman Catholic 1%, other and nonreligious 10%
Ethnic mix Norwegian 95%, Lapp 1%, other 4%
Government Constitutional monarchy
Currency Norwegian krone = 100 øre
Literacy rate 99%
Calorie consumption 3,244 kilocalories

OMAN
Southwestern Asia

Official name Sultanate of Oman
Formation 1951 / 1951
Capital Muscat
Population 2.5 million / 30 people per sq mile (12 people per sq km) / 13%
Total area 82,030 sq miles (212,460 sq km)
Languages Arab*, Baluchi
Religions Ibadi Muslim 75%, other Muslim 11%, Hindu 14%
Ethnic mix Arab 75%, Baluchi 15%, other 15%
Government Monarchy with Consultative Council
Currency Omani rial = 1,000 baizas
Literacy rate 67%
Calorie consumption 3,013 kilocalories

PAKISTAN
Southern Asia

Official name Islamic Republic of Pakistan
Formation 1947 / 1947
Capital Islamabad
Population 147.8 million / 497 people per sq mile (192 people per sq km) / 35%
Total area 307,374 sq miles (796,100 sq km)
Main languages Urdu*, Punjabi, Sindhi, Pashtu, Baluchi
Religions Sunni Muslim 77%, Shi'a Muslim 20%, Hindu 2%, Christian 1%
Ethnic mix Punjabi 50%, Sindhi 15%, Pashtu 15%, Mohajir 8%, Baluch 5%, other 7%
Government Multiparty republic
Currency Pakistani rupee = 100 paisa
Literacy rate 40%
Calorie consumption 2,315 kilocalories

PALAU
Australasia & Oceania

Official name Palau
Formation 1994 / 1994
Capital Oreor
Population 17,700 /90 people per sq mile (35 people per sq km) / 29%
Total area 192 sq miles (497 sq km)
Languages Palauan*, English*, Japanese
Religions Roman Catholic 66%, Modekngei 34%
Ethnic mix Palauan 99%, other 1%
Government Multiparty republic
Currency US dollar = 100 cents
Literacy rate 92%
Calorie consumption NOT AVAILABLE

PANAMA
Central America

Official name Republic of Panama
Formation 1903 / 1903
Capital Panama City
Population 2.8 million / 95 people per sq mile (37 people per sq km) / 53%
Total area 29,761 sq miles (77,080 sq km)
Languages Spanish*, English Creole, Indian languages
Religions Roman Catholic 93%, other 7%
Ethnic mix *Mestizo* 60%, White 14%, Black 12%, Indigenous Indian 8%, other 6%
Government Multiparty republic
Currency Balboa = 100 centesimos
Literacy rate 91%
Calorie consumption 2,242 kilocalories

PAPUA NEW GUINEA
Australasia & Oceania

Official name Independent State of Papua New Guinea
Formation 1975 / 1975
Capital Port Moresby
Population 4.6 million / 26 people per sq mile (10 people per sq km) / 16%
Total area 178,700 sq miles (462, 840 sq km)
Languages English*, Pidgin English, Papuan, Motu, 750 (estimated) native languages
Religions Christian 62%, Traditional beliefs 38%
Ethnic mix Papuan 85%, other 15%
Government Parliamentary democracy
Currency Kina = 100 toea
Literacy rate 73%
Calorie consumption 2,613 kilocalories

PARAGUAY
South America

Official name Paraguay
Formation 1811 / 1938
Capital Asunción
Population 5.2 million / 34 people per sq mile (13 people per sq km) / 53%
Total area 157,046 sq miles (406,750 sq km)
Languages Spanish*, Guaraní
Religions Roman Catholic 90%, other 10%
Ethnic mix *Mestizo* 90%, Indigenous Indian 2%, other 8%
Government Multiparty republic
Literacy rate 92%
Calorie consumption 2,670 kilocalories

PERU
South America

Official name Republic of Peru
Formation 1824 / 1941
Capital Lima
Population 24.8 million / 50 people per sq mile (19 people per sq km) / 72%
Total area 496,223 sq miles (1,285,220 sq km)
Languages Spanish*, Quechua*, Aymará
Religions Roman Catholic 95%, other 5%
Ethnic mix Indigenous Indian 54%, *mestizo* 32%, White 12%, other 2%
Government Multiparty republic
Currency New sol = 100 centimos
Literacy rate 88%
Calorie consumption 1,882 kilocalories

PHILIPPINES
Southwestern Asia

Official name Republic of the Philippines
Formation 1946 / 1946
Capital Manila
Population 72.2 million / 627 people per sq mile (242 people per sq km) / 54%
Total area 115,831 sq miles (300,000 sq km)
Languages Filipino*, English*, Cebuano, Hiligaynon, Samaran, Bikol, Ilocano
Religions Roman Catholic 83%, Protestant 9%, Muslim 5%, other 3%
Ethnic mix Malay 50%, Indonesian and Polynesian 30%, Chinese 10%, other 10%
Government Multiparty republic
Currency Philippine peso = 100 centavos
Literacy rate 94%
Calorie consumption 2,257 kilocalories

POLAND
Northern Europe

Official name Republic of Poland
Formation 1918 / 1945
Capital Warsaw
Population 38.7 million / 329 people per sq mile (127 people per sq km) / 65%
Total area 120,720 sq miles (312,680 sq km)
Languages Polish*, German
Religions Roman Catholic 93%, Eastern Orthodox 2%, other and nonreligious 5%
Ethnic mix Polish 98%, German 1%, other 1%
Government Multiparty republic
Currency Zloty = 100 groszy
Literacy rate 99%
Calorie consumption 3,301 kilocalories

PORTUGAL
Southwestern Europe

Official name Republic of Portugal
Formation 1140 / 1640
Capital Lisbon
Population 9.8 million / 276 people per sq mile (107 people per sq km) / 36%
Total area 35,670 sq miles (92,390 sq km)
Languages Portuguese*
Religions Roman Catholic 97%, Protestant 1%, other 2%
Ethnic mix Portuguese 99%, African 1%
Government Multiparty republic
Currency Escudo = 100 centavos
Literacy rate 90%
Calorie consumption 3,634 kilocalories

QATAR
Southwestern Asia

Official name State of Qatar
Formation 1971 / 1971
Capital Doha
Population 600,000 / 136 people per sq mile (53 people per sq km) / 91%
Total area 4,247 sq miles (11,000 sq km)
Languages Arabic*, Farsi (Persian), Urdu, Hindi, English
Religions Sunni Muslim 86%, Hindu 10%, Christian 4%
Ethnic mix Arab 40%, Pakistani 18%, Iranian 10% Indian 18%, other 14%
Government Absolute monarchy
Currency Qatar riyal = 100 dirhams
Literacy rate 80%
Calorie consumption NOT AVAILABLE

ROMANIA
Southeastern Europe

Official name Romania
Formation 1878 / 1947
Capital Bucharest
Population 22.6 million /254 people per sq mile (98 people per sq km) / 55%
Total area 91,700 sq miles (237,500 sq km)
Languages Romanian*, Hungarian, Romany
Religions Romanian Orthodox 70%, Roman Catholic 5%, Protestant 4%, other 21%
Ethnic mix Romanian 89%, Magyar 9%, Romany 1%, other 1%
Government Multiparty republic
Currency Leu = 100 bani
Literacy rate 97%
Calorie consumption 3,051 kilocalories

RUSSIAN FEDERATION
Europe / Asia

Official name Russian Federation
Formation 1991 / 1991
Capital Moscow
Population 147.2 million /22 people per sq mile (9 people per sq km) / 76%
Total area 6,592,800 sq miles (17,075,400 sq km)
Languages Russian*, Tatar, Ukrainian
Religions Russian Orthodox 75%, other (including Jewish, Muslim) 25%
Ethnic mix Russian 82%, Tatar 4%, Ukrainian 3%, Chuvash 1%, other 10%
Currency Rouble = 100 kopeks
Literacy rate 99%
Calorie consumption NOT AVAILABLE

RWANDA
Central Africa

Official name Rwandese Republic
Formation 1962 / 1962
Capital Kigali
Population 6.5 million / 675 people per sq mile (261 people per sq km) / 6%
Total area 10,170 sq miles (26,340 sq km)
Languages Kinyarwanda*, French*, Kiswahili, English
Religions Christian 74%, Traditional beliefs 25%, other 1%
Ethnic mix Hutu 90%, Tutsi 8%, Twa pygmy 2%
Government Multiparty republic
Currency Rwanda franc = 100 centimes
Literacy rate 63%
Calorie consumption 1,821 kilocalories

SAINT KITTS & NEVIS
West Indies

Official name Federation of Saint Christopher and Nevis
Formation 1983 / 1983
Capital Basseterre
Population 41,000 / 295 people per sq mile (114 people per sq km) / 42%
Total area 139 sq miles (360 sq km)
Languages English*, English Creole
Religions Protestant 71%, Roman Catholic 7%, other 22%
Ethnic mix Black 95%, mixed 5%
Government Parliamentary democracy
Currency E. Caribbean dollar = 100 cents
Literacy rate 90%
Calorie consumption 2,419 kilocalories

SAINT LUCIA
West Indies

Official name Saint Lucia
Formation 1979 / 1979
Capital Castries
Population 142,000 / 603 people per sq mile (233 people per sq km) / 48%
Total area 239 sq miles (620 sq km)
Languages English*, French Creole, Hindi, Urdu
Religions Roman Catholic 90%, other 10%
Ethnic mix Black 90%, African-European 6%, South Asian 4%
Government Parliamentary democracy
Currency E. Caribbean dollar = 100 cents
Literacy rate 93%
Calorie consumption 2,588 kilocalories

SAINT VINCENT & THE GRENADINES
West Indies

Official name Saint Vincent and the Grenadines
Formation 1979 / 1979
Capital Kingstown
Population 111,000 / 846 people per sq mile (327 people per sq km) / 46%
Total area 131 sq miles (340 sq km)
Languages English*, English Creole
Religions Protestant 62% Roman Catholic 19%, other 19%
Ethnic mix Black 82%, mixed 14%, White 3%, South Asian 1%
Government Parliamentary democracy
Currency E. Caribbean dollar = 100 cents
Literacy rate 82%
Calorie consumption 2,347 kilocalories

SAMOA
Australasia & Oceania

Official name Independent State of Samoa
Formation 1962 / 1962
Capital Apia
Population 170,000 / 156 people per sq mile (60 people per sq km) / 21%
Total area 1,027 sq miles (2,840 sq km)
Languages Samoan*, English*
Religions Protestant 74%, Roman Catholic 26%
Ethnic mix Samoan 90%, other 10%
Government Parliamentary state
Currency Tala = 100 sene
Literacy rate 98%
Calorie consumption 2,828 kilocalories

SAN MARINO
Southern Europe

Official name Republic of San Marino
Formation AD 301 / 301
Capital San Marino
Population 25,000 / 1,061 people per sq mile (410 people per sq km) / 94%
Total area 24 sq miles (61 sq km)
Languages *Italian
Religions Roman Catholic 93%, other and nonreligious 7%
Ethnic mix Sammarinese 95%, other 5%
Government Multiparty republic
Currency Lira = 100 centesimi
Literacy rate 96%
Calorie consumption 3,561 kilocalories

SAO TOME & PRINCIPE
Western Africa

Official name Democratic Republic of Sao Tome and Principe
Formation 1975 / 1975
Capital São Tomé
Population 131,000 / 354 people per sq mile (137 people per sq km) / 46%
Total area 372 sq miles (964 sq km)
Languages *Portuguese, Portuguese Creole
Religions Roman Catholic 90%, other Christian 10%
Ethnic mix Black 90%, Portuguese and Creole 10%
Government Multiparty republic
Currency Dobra = 100 centimos
Literacy rate 75%
Calorie consumption 2,129 kilocalories

SAUDI ARABIA
Southwestern Asia

Official name Kingdom of Saudi Arabia
Formation 1932 / 1935
Capital Riyadh
Population 20.2 million / 24 people per sq mile (8 people per sq km) / 80%
Total area 829,995 sq miles (2,149,690 sq km)
Languages Arabic*
Religions Sunni Muslim 85%, Shi'a Muslim 15%
Ethnic mix Arab 90%, Afroasian 10%
Government Absolute monarchy
Currency Saudi riyal = 100 malalah
Literacy rate 73%
Calorie consumption 2,735 kilocalories

SENEGAL
Western Africa

Official name Republic of Senegal
Formation 1960 / 1960
Capital Dakar
Population 9 million /121 people per sq mile (47 people per sq km) / 42%
Total area 75,950 sq miles (196,720 sq km)
Languages *French, Wolof, Fulani, Serer
Religions Muslim 90%, Traditional beliefs 5%, Christian 5%
Ethnic mix Wolof 46%, Fulani 25%, Serer 16%, other 13%
Government Multiparty republic
Currency CFA franc = 100 centimes
Literacy rate 35%
Calorie consumption 2,262 kilocalories

SEYCHELLES
Indian Ocean

Official name Republic of Seychelles
Formation 1976 / 1976
Capital Victoria
Population 75,000 / 722 people per sq mile (279 people per sq km) / 54%
Total area 108 sq miles (280 sq km)
Languages *French Creole, French, English
Religions Roman Catholic 90%, other 10%
Ethnic mix Seychellois (mixed African, South Asian and European) 95%, Chinese and South Asian 5%
Government Multiparty republic
Currency Seychelles rupee = 100 cents
Literacy rate 84%
Calorie consumption 2,287 kilocalories

SIERRA LEONE
Western Africa

Official name Republic of Sierra Leone
Formation 1961 / 1961
Capital Freetown
Population 4.6 million / 166 people per sq mile (64 people per sq km) / 36%
Total area 27,699 sq miles (71,740 sq km)
Languages English*, Krio (Creole), Mende, Temne
Religions Traditional beliefs 52%, Muslim 40%, Christian 8%
Ethnic mix Mende 35%, Temne 32%, Limba 8%, Kuranko 4%, other 21%
Government Multiparty republic
Currency Leone = 100 cents
Literacy rate 33%
Calorie consumption 1,694 kilocalories

SINGAPORE
Southeastern Asia

Official name Republic of Singapore
Formation 1965 / 1965
Capital Singapore
Population 3.5 million / 14,861 people per sq mile (5,738 people per sq km) / 100%
Total area 239 sq miles (620 sq km)
Languages Malay*, Chinese*, Tamil*, English*
Religions Buddhist 30%, Christian 20%, Muslim 17%, other 33%
Ethnic mix Chinese 78%, Malay 14%, Indian 6%, other 2%
Government Multiparty republic
Currency Singapore dollar = 100 cents
Literacy rate 91%
Calorie consumption 3,128 kilocalories

SLOVAKIA
Central Europe

Official name Slovak Republic
Formation 1993 / 1993
Capital Bratislava
Population 5.4 million / 285 people per sq mile (110 people per sq km) / 59%
Total area 19,100 sq miles (49,500 sq km)
Languages Slovak*, Hungarian (Magyar), Romany, Czech
Religions Roman Catholic 60%, Atheist 10%, Protestant 8%, Orthodox 4%, other 18%
Ethnic mix Slovak 85%, Hungarian 9%, Czech 1%, other 5%
Government Multiparty republic
Currency Koruna = 100 halierov
Literacy rate 99%
Calorie consumption 3,156 kilocalories

SLOVENIA
Central Europe

Official name Republic of Slovenia
Formation 1991 / 1991
Capital Ljubljana
Population 1.9 million / 243 people per sq mile (94 people per sq km) / 64%
Total area 7,820 sq miles (20,250 sq km)
Languages Slovene*, Serbian, Croatian
Religions Roman Catholic 96%, Muslim 1%, other 3%
Ethnic mix Slovene 88%, Croat 3%, Serb 2%, Bosniak 1%, other 4%
Government Multiparty republic
Currency Tolar = 100 stotins
Literacy rate 99%
Calorie consumption NOT AVAILABLE

SOLOMON ISLANDS
Australasia & Oceania

Official name Solomon Islands
Formation 1978 / 1978
Capital Honiara
Population 417,000 / 39 people per sq mile (15 people per sq km) / 17%
Total area 10,954 sq miles (28,370 sq km)
Languages English*, Pidgin English, Melanesian Pidgin
Religions Christian 91%, other 9%
Ethnic mix Melanesian 94%, other 6%
Government Parliamentary democracy
Currency Solomon Islands dollar = 100 cents
Literacy rate 62%
Calorie consumption 2,173 kilocalories

SOMALIA
Eastern Africa

Official name Somali Democratic Republic
Formation 1960 / 1960
Capital Mogadishu
Population 10.7 million / 39 people per sq mile (15 people per sq km) / 25%
Total area 246,200 sq miles (637,660 sq km)
Languages Somali*, Arabic*, English
Religions Sunni Muslim 98%, other (including Christian) 2%
Ethnic mix Somali 98%, Bantu, Arab and other 2%
Government Transitional
Currency Somaili shilling = 100 cents
Literacy rate 24%
Calorie consumption 1,499 kilocalories

SOUTH AFRICA
Southern Africa

Official name Republic of South Africa
Formation 1934 / 1994
Capitals Pretoria/Cape Town/Bloemfontein
Population 44.3 million / 94 people per sq mile (36 people per sq km) / 51%
Total area 471,443 sq miles (1,221,040 sq km)
Languages Afrikaans*, English*, 11 African languages
Religions Protestant 55%, Roman Catholic 9%, Hindu 1%, Muslim 1%, other 34%
Ethnic mix Other Black 38%, White 16%, Zulu 23%, mixed 10%, Xhosa 9%, other 4%
Government Multiparty republic
Currency Rand = 100 cents
Literacy rate 82%
Calorie consumption 2,695 kilocalories

SOUTH KOREA
Eastern Asia

Official name Republic of Korea
Formation 1948 / 1953
Capital Seoul
Population 46.1 million / 1209 people per sq mile (467 people per sq km) / 81%
Total area 38,232 sq miles (99,020 sq km)
Languages Korean*, Chinese
Religions Mahayana Buddhist 47%, Protestant 38%, Roman Catholic 11%, Confucianist 3%, other 1%
Ethnic mix Korean 100%
Government Multiparty republic
Currency Won = 100 chon
Literacy rate 97%
Calorie consumption 3,285 kilocalories

SPAIN
Southwestern Europe

Official name Kingdom of Spain
Formation 1492 / 1713
Capital Madrid
Population 39.8 million / 206 people per sq mile (80 people per sq km) / 76%
Total area 194,900 sq miles (504,780 sq km)
Languages Castilian Spanish*, Catalan*, Galician*, Basque*
Religions Roman Catholic 96%, other 4%
Ethnic mix Castilian Spanish 72%, Catalan 17%, Galician 6%, other 5%
Government Constitutional monarchy
Currency Spanish Peseta = 100 céntimos
Literacy rate 95%
Calorie consumption 3,708 kilocalories

SRI LANKA
Southern Asia

Official name Democratic Socialist Republic of Sri Lanka
Formation 1948 / 1948
Capital Colombo
Population 18.5 million / 740 people per sq mile (286 people per sq km) / 22%
Total area 25,332 sq miles (65,610 sq km)
Languages Sinhala*, Tamil, English
Religions Buddhist 70%, Hindu 15%, Christian 8%, Muslim 7%
Ethnic mix Sinhalese 74%, Tamil 18%, other 8%
Government Multiparty republic
Currency Sri Lanka rupee = 100 cents
Literacy rate 90%
Calorie consumption 2,273 kilocalories

SUDAN
Eastern Africa

Official name Republic of Sudan
Formation 1956 / 1956
Capital Khartoum
Population 28.5 million / 31 people per sq mile (12 people per sq km) / 25%
Total area 967,493 sq miles (2,505,815 sq km)
Languages Arabic*, Dinka, Nuer, Nubian, Beja, Zande, Bari, Fur
Religions Muslim 70%, Traditional beliefs 20%, Christian 9%, other 1%
Ethnic mix Arab 51%, Dinka 13%, Nuba 9%, Beja 7%, other 20%
Government Military regime
Currency Sudanese pound or dinar = 100 piastres
Literacy rate 53%
Calorie consumption 2,202 kilocalories

SURINAME
South America

Official name Republic of Suriname
Formation 1975 / 1975
Capital Paramaribo
Population 442,000 / 7 people per sq mile (3 people per sq km) / 50%
Total area 63,039 sq miles (163,270 sq km)
Languages Dutch*, Pidgin English (Taki-Taki), Hindi, Javanese, Carib
Religions Christian 48%, Hindu 27%, Muslim 20%, other 5%
Ethnic mix Hindustani 34%, Creole 34%, Javanese 18%, Black 9%, other 5%
Government Multiparty republic
Currency Suriname guilder = 100 cents
Literacy rate 93%
Calorie consumption 2547 kilocalories

SWAZILAND
Southern Africa

Official name Kingdom of Swaziland
Formation 1968 / 1968
Capital Mbabane
Population 900,000 / 140 people per sq mile (54 people per sq km) / 29%
Total area 6,703 sq miles (17,360 sq km)
Languages Siswati*, English*, Zulu
Religions Christian 60%, Traditional beliefs 40%
Ethnic mix Swazi 95%, other 5%
Government Executive monarchy
Currency Lilangeni = 100 cents
Literacy rate 77%
Calorie consumption 2,706 kilocalories

SWEDEN
Northern Europe

Official name Kingdom of Sweden
Formation 1809 / 1905
Capital Stockholm
Population 8.9 million / 56 people per sq mile (22 people per sq km) / 83%
Total area 173,730 sq miles (449,960 sq km)
Languages Swedish*, Finnish, Lappish
Religions Evangelical Lutheran 89%, Roman Catholic 2%, Muslim 1%, other 8%
Ethnic mix Swedish 91%, other European 6%, Finnish and Lapp 3%
Government Constitutional monarchy
Currency Swedish krona = 100 öre
Literacy rate 99%
Calorie consumption 2,972 kilocalories

SWITZERLAND
Central Europe

Official name Swiss Confederation
Formation 1291 / 1815
Capital Bern
Population 7.3 million / 475 people per sq mile (184 people per sq km) / 61%
Total area 15,940 sq miles (41,290 sq km)
Languages German*, French*, Italian*, Romansch
Religions Roman Catholic 48%, Protestant 44%, other 8%
Ethnic mix German 65%, French 18%, Italian 10%, other 7%
Government Federal republic
Currency Franc = 100 centimes
Literacy rate 99%
Calorie consumption 3,379 kilocalories

SYRIA
Southwest Asia

Official name Syrian Arab Republic
Formation 1946 / 1967
Capital Damascus
Population 15.3 million / 215 people per sq mile (83 people per sq km) / 52%
Total area 71,500 sq miles (185,180 sq km)
Languages Arabic*, French, Kurdish
Religions Sunni Muslim 74%, other Muslim 16%, Christian 10%
Ethnic mix Arab 89%, Kurdish 6%, Armenian, Turkmen, Circassian 2%, other 3%
Government Single-party republic
Currency Syrian pound = 100 piastres
Literacy rate 71%
Calorie consumption 3175 kilocalories

TAIWAN
East Asia

Official name Republic of China
Formation 1949 / 1949
Capital Taipei
Population 21.5 million / 1724 people per sq mile (666 people per sq km) / 69%
Total area 13,969 sq miles (36,179 sq km)
Languages Mandarin Chinese*, Amoy Chinese, Hakka Chinese
Religions Buddhist, Confucianist, Taoist 93%, Christian 5%, other 2%
Ethnic mix Indigenous Chinese, Mainland Chinese 14%, Aborigine 2%
Government Multiparty republic
Currency Taiwan dollar = 100 cents
Literacy rate 94%
Calorie consumption NOT AVAILABLE

TAJIKISTAN
Central Asia

Official name Republic of Tajikistan
Formation 1991 / 1991
Capital Dushanbe
Population 6.2 million / 112 people per sq mile (43 people per sq km) / 32%
Total area 55,251 sq miles (143,100 sq km)
Main languages Tajik*, Uzbek, Russian
Religions Sunni Muslim 80%, Shi'a Muslim 5%, other 15%
Ethnic mix Tajik 62%, Uzbek 24%, Russian 4%, Tatar 2%, other 8%
Government Multiparty republic
Currency Tajik rouble = 100 kopeks
Literacy rate 99%
Calorie consumption NOT AVAILABLE

TANZANIA
East Africa

Official name United Republic of Tanzania
Formation 1961 / 1964
Capital Dodoma
Population 32.2 million / 94 people per sq mile (36 people per sq km) / 24%
Total area 364,900 sq miles (945,090 sq km)
Languages English*, Swahili*, Sukuma, Chagga, Nyamwezi, Hehe, Makonde
Religions Muslim 33%, Christian 33%, Traditional beliefs 30%, other 4%
Ethnic mix 120 small ethnic Bantu groups 99%, other 1%
Government Multiparty republic
Currency Tanzanian shilling = 100 cents
Literacy rate 71%
Calorie consumption 2018 kilocalories

THAILAND
Southeastern Asia

Official name Kingdom of Thailand
Formation 1782 / 1907
Capital Bangkok
Population 59.6 million / 302 people per sq mile (117 people per sq km) / 20%
Total area 198,116 sq miles (513,120 sq km)
Languages Thai*, Chinese, Malay, Khmer, Mon, Karen
Religions Buddhist 95%, other 5%
Ethnic mix Thai 80%, Chinese 12%, Malay 4%, Khmer and other 4%
Government Constitutional monarchy
Currency Baht = 100 stangs
Literacy rate 94%
Calorie consumption 2432 kilocalories

TOGO
Western Africa

Official name Togolese Republic
Formation 1960 / 1960
Capital Lomé
Population 4.4 million /210 people per sq mile (81 people per sq km) / 31%
Total area 21,927 sq miles (56,790 sq km)
Languages French*, Ewe, Kabye, Gurma
Religions Traditional beliefs 50%, Christian 35%, Muslim 15%
Ethnic mix Ewe 43%, Kabye 26%, Gurma 16%, other 15%
Government Multiparty republic
Currency CFA franc = 100 centimes
Literacy rate 53%
Calorie consumption 2242 kilocalories

TONGA
Australasia & Oceania

Official name Kingdom of Tonga
Formation 1970 / 1970
Capital Nuku'alofa
Population 97,000 / 351 people per sq mile (135 people per sq km) / 21%
Total area 290 sq miles (750 sq km)
Languages Tongan*, English*
Religions Protestant 64%, Roman Catholic 15%, other 21%
Ethnic mix Tongan 98%, other 2%
Government Constitutional monarchy
Currency Pa'anga = 100 seniti
Literacy rate 99%
Calorie consumption 2,946 kilocalories

TRINIDAD & TOBAGO
West Indies

Official name Republic of Trinidad and Tobago
Formation 1962 / 1962
Capital Port-of-Spain
Population 1.3 million / 656 people per sq mile (253 people per sq km) / 72%
Total area 1,981 sq miles (5,130 sq km)
Languages English*, English Creole, Hindi, French, Spanish
Religions Christian 58%, Hindu 30%, Muslim 8%, other 4%
Ethnic mix Black 43%, Asian 40%, mixed 19%, White and Chinese 1%
Government Multiparty republic
Currency Trinidad & Tobago dollar = 100 cents
Literacy rate 98%
Calorie consumption 2,585 kilocalories

TUNISIA
Northern Africa

Official name Republic of Tunisia
Formation 1956 / 1956
Capital Tunis
Population 9.5 million / 158 people per sq mile (61 people per sq km) / 57%
Total area 63,170 sq miles (163,610 sq km)
Languages Arabic*, French
Religions Muslim 98%, Christian 1%, Jewish 1%
Ethnic mix Arab and Berber 98%, European 1%, other 1%
Government Multiparty republic
Currency Tunisian dinar = 1,000 millimes
Literacy rate 67%
Calorie consumption 3,330 kilocalories

TURKEY
Asia / Europe

Official name Republic of Turkey
Formation 1923 / 1939
Capital Ankara
Population 63.8 million / 215 people per sq mile (83 people per sq km) / 69%
Total area 300,950 sq miles (779,450 sq km)
Languages Turkish*, Kurdish, Arabic, Circassian, Armenian
Religions Muslim 99%, other 1%
Ethnic mix Turkish 70%, Kurdish 20%, other 8%, Arab 2%
Government Multiparty republic
Currency Turkish lira = 100 krural
Literacy rate 83%
Calorie consumption 3,429 kilocalories

TURKMENISTAN
Central Asia

Official name Turkmenistan
Formation 1991 / 1991
Capital Ashgabat
Population 4.3 million / 23 people per sq mile (9 people per sq km) / 45%
Total area 188,455 sq miles (488,100 sq km)
Languages Turkmen*, Uzbek, Russian
Religions Muslim 87%, Eastern Orthodox 11%, other 2%
Ethnic mix Turkmen 72%, Russian 9%, Uzbek 9%, other 10%
Government Multiparty republic
Currency Manat = 100 tenge
Literacy rate 98%
Calorie consumption NOT AVAILABLE

TUVALU
Australasia & Oceania

Official name Tuvalu
Formation 1978 / 1978
Capital Fongafale
Population 9000 / 976 people per sq mile (377 people per sq km) / 46%
Total area 10 sq miles (26 sq km)
Languages Tuvaluan*, Kiribati, English
Religions Protestant 97%, other 3%
Ethnic mix Polynesian 95% other 5%
Government Constitutional monarchy
Currency Australian dollar = 100 cents
Literacy rate 95%
Calorie consumption NOT AVAILABLE

Uganda
Eastern Africa

Official name Republic of Uganda
Formation 1962 / 1962
Capital Kampala
Population 21.3 million / 276 people per sq mile (107 people per sq km) / 13%
Total area 91,073 sq miles (235,880 sq km)
Languages English*, Luganda, Nkole, Chiga, Lango, Acholi, Teso
Religions Christian 71%, Traditional beliefs 13%, Muslim 5%, other (including Hindu) 11%
Ethnic mix Buganda 18%, Banyoro 14%, Teso 9%, other 59%
Government Multiparty republic
Currency New Uganda shilling = 100 cents
Literacy rate 64%
Calorie consumption 2,159 kilocalories

Ukraine
Eastern Europe

Official name Ukraine
Formation 1991 / 1991
Capital Kiev
Population 51.2 million / 220 people per sq mile (85 people per sq km) / 70%
Total area 223,090 sq miles (603,700 sq km)
Languages Ukrainian*, Russian, Tatar
Religions Mostly Ukrainian Orthodox, with Roman Catholic, Protestant and Jewish minorities
Ethnic mix Ukrainian 73%, Russian 22%, other (including Tatar) 5%
Government Multiparty republic
Currency Hryvna = 100 kopiykas
Literacy rate 98%
Calorie consumption NOT AVAILABLE

United Arab Emirates
Southwestern Asia

Official name United Arab Emirates
Formation 1971 / 1971
Capital Abu Dhabi
Population 2.4 million / 7 people per sq mile (29 people per sq km) / 84%
Total area 32,278 sq miles (83,600 sq km)
Languages Arabic*, Farsi (Persian), Urdu, Hindi, English
Religions Sunni Muslim 77%, Shi'a Muslim 19%, other 4%
Ethnic mix Asian 50%, Emirian 19%, other Arab 23%, other 8%
Government Federation of monarchs
Currency UAE dirham = 100 fils
Literacy rate 79%
Calorie consumption 3,384 kilocalories

United Kingdom
Northwestern Europe

Official name United Kingdom of Great Britain and Northern Ireland
Formation 1707 / 1922
Capital London
Population 58.2 million / 624 people per sq mile (241 people per sq km) / 89%
Total area 94,550 sq miles (244,880 sq km)
Languages English*, Welsh*, Scottish, Gaelic
Religions Protestant 52%, Roman Catholic 9%, Muslim 3%, other 36%
Ethnic mix English 80%, Scottish 10%, Northern Irish 4%, Welsh 2%, West Indian, Asian 4%
Government Constitutional monarchy
Currency Pound sterling = 100 pence
Literacy rate 99%
Calorie consumption 3,317 kilocalories

United States
North America

Official name United States of America
Formation 1787 / 1959
Capital Washington DC
Population 273.8 million / 77 people per sq mile (30 people per sq km) / 76%
Total area 3,681,760 sq miles (9,372,610 sq km)
Languages English*, Spanish, Italian, German, French, Polish, Chinese, Greek
Religions Protestant 61%, Roman Catholic 25%, Jewish 2%, other 12%
Ethnic mix White (including Hispanic) 84%, Black 12%, Chinese 1%, other 3%
Government Multiparty republic
Currency US dollar = 100 cents
Literacy rate 99%
Calorie consumption 3,732 kilocalories

Uruguay
South America

Official name Oriental Republic of Uruguay
Formation 1828 / 1828
Capital Montevideo
Population 3.2 million / 47 people per sq mile (18 people per sq km) / 90%
Total area 67,494 sq miles (174,810 sq km)
Languages Spanish*
Religions Roman Catholic 66%, Protestant 2%, Jewish 2%, other 30%
Ethnic mix White 90%, *mestizo* 6% Black 4%
Government Multiparty republic
Currency Uruguayan peso = 100 centimes
Literacy rate 97%
Calorie consumption 2,750 kilocalories

Uzbekistan
Central Asia

Official name Republic of Uzbekistan
Formation 1991 / 1991
Capital Tashkent
Population 24.1 million / 140 people per sq mile (54 people per sq km) / 41%
Total area 172,741 sq miles (447,400 sq km)
Languages Uzbek*, Russian
Religions Muslim 88%, other (mostly Eastern Orthodox) 9%, other 3%
Ethnic mix Uzbek 71%, Russian 8%, Tajik 5%, Kazakh 4%, other 12%
Government Multiparty republic
Currency Sum = 100 teen
Literacy rate 99%
Calorie consumption NOT AVAILABLE

Vanuatu
Australasia & Oceania

Official name Republic of Vanuatu
Formation 1980 / 1980
Capital Port-Vila
Population 200,000 / 42 people per sq mile (16 people per sq km) / 19%
Total area 4706 sq miles (12,190 sq km)
Languages Bislama*, English*, French*
Religions Protestant 77%, Roman Catholic 15%, Traditional beliefs 8%
Ethnic mix ni-Vanuatu 94%, other 6%
Government Multiparty republic
Currency Vatu = 100 centimes
Literacy rate 64%
Calorie consumption 2,739 kilocalories

Vatican City
Southern Europe

Official name Vatican City State
Formation 1929 / 1929
Capital Not applicable
Population 1,000 / 5,886 people per sq mile (2,273 people per sq km) /100%
Total area 0.17 sq miles (0.44 sq km)
Languages Italian*, Latin*
Religions Roman Catholic 100%
Ethnic mix Italian 90%, Swiss 10% (including the Swiss Guard, which is responsible for papal security)
Government Papal Commission
Currency Italian lira = 100 centesimi
Literacy rate 99%
Calorie consumption 3,561 kilocalories

Venezuela
South America

Official name Republic of Venezuela
Formation 1821 / 1930
Capital Caracas
Population 23.2 million / 68 people per sq mile (26 people per sq km) / 93%
Total area 352,143 sq miles (912,050 sq km)
Languages Spanish*, Indian languages *
Religions Roman Catholic 89%, Protestant and other 11%
Ethnic mix *Mestizo* 69%, White 20%, Black 9%, Indian 2%
Government Multiparty republic
Currency Bolívar = 100 centimos
Literacy rate 92%
Calorie consumption 2,618 kilocalories

Vietnam
Southeastern Asia

Official name Socialist Republic of Vietnam
Formation 1976 / 1976
Capital Hanoi
Population 77.9 million / 620 people per sq mile (239 people per sq km) / 21%
Total area 127,243 sq miles (329,560 sq km)
Languages Vietnamese*, Chinese, Thai, Khmer, Muong
Religions Buddhist 55%, Christian 7%, other and nonreligious 38%
Ethnic mix Vietnamese 88%, Chinese 4%, Thai 2%, other 6%
Government Single-party republic
Currency Dong = 10 hao = 100 xu
Literacy rate 91%
Calorie consumption 2,250 kilocalories

Yemen
Southwestern Asia

Official name Republic of Yemen
Formation 1990 / 1990
Capital Sana
Population 16.9 million / 82 people per sq mile (32 people per sq km) / 34%
Total area 203,849 sq miles (527,970 sq km)
Languages Arabic*, Hindi, Tamil, Urdu
Religions Shi'a Muslim 55%, Sunni Muslim 42%, Christian, Hindu, Jewish 3%
Ethnic mix Arab 95%, Afro-Arab 3%, Indian, Somali, European 2%
Government Multiparty republic
Currency Rial (North), Dinar (South) – both are legal currency
Literacy rate 42%
Calorie consumption 2,203 kilocalories

Yugoslavia (Serbia & Montenegro) *Europe*

Official name Federal Republic of Yugoslavia
Formation 1992 / 1992
Capital Belgrade
Population 10.4 million / 264 people per sq mile (102 people per sq km) / 57%
Total area 39,449 sq miles (102,173 sq km)
Languages Serbo-croat*, Albanian
Religions Roman Catholic, Eastern Orthodox 69%, Muslim 19%, Protestant 1%, other 11%
Ethnic mix Serb 62%, Albanian 17%, Montenegrin 5%, Magyar 3%, other 13%
Government Multiparty republic
Currency Dinar = 100 para
Literacy rate 93%
Calorie consumption NOT AVAILABLE

Zambia
Southern Africa

Official name Republic of Zambia
Formation 1964 / 1964
Capital Lusaka
Population 8.7 million / 30 people per sq mile (12 people per sq km) / 43%
Total area 285,992 sq miles (740,720 sq km)
Languages English*, Bemba, Nyanja, Tonga, Kaonde, Lunda
Religions Christian 63%, Traditional beliefs 36%, other 1%
Ethnic mix Bemba 36%, Maravi 18%, Tonga 15%, other 31%
Government Multiparty republic
Currency Kwacha = 100 ngwee
Literacy rate 75%
Calorie consumption 1,931 kilocalories

Zimbabwe
Southern Africa

Official name Republic of Zimbabwe
Formation 1980 / 1980
Capital Harare
Population 11.9 million / 80 people per sq mile (21 people per sq km) / 32%
Total area 150,800 sq miles (390,580 sq km)
Languages English*, Shona, Ndebele
Religions Syncretic (Christian and traditional beliefs) 50%, Christian 26%, Traditional beliefs 24%
Ethnic mix Shona 71%, Ndebele 16%, other African 11%, White, Asian 2%
Government Multiparty republic
Currency Zimbabwe dollar = 100 cents
Literacy rate 90%
Calorie consumption 1,985 kilocalories

GLOSSARY

THIS GLOSSARY lists all geographical, technical, and foreign language terms that appear in the text, followed by a brief definition of the term. Any acronyms used in the text are also listed in full. Terms in italics are for cross-reference and indicate that the word is separately defined in the glossary.

A

Aboriginal The original (*indigenous*) inhabitants of a country or continent. Especially used with reference to Australia.

Abyssal plain A broad *plain* found in the depths of the ocean, more than 10,000 ft (3,000 m) below sea level.

Acid rain Rain, sleet, snow, or mist which has absorbed waste gases from fossil-fueled power stations and vehicle exhausts, becoming more acid. It causes severe environmental damage.

Adaptation The gradual evolution of plants and animals so that they become better suited to survive and reproduce in their *environment*.

Afforestation The planting of new forest in areas that were once forested but have been cleared.

Agribusiness A term applied to activities such as the growing of crops, rearing of animals, or the manufacture of farm machinery, which eventually leads to the supply of agricultural produce at market.

Air mass A huge, homogeneous mass of air, within which horizontal patterns of temperature and *humidity* are consistent. Air masses are separated by *fronts*.

Alliance An agreement between two or more states, to work together to achieve common purposes.

Alluvial fan A large fan-shaped deposit of fine sediments deposited by a river as it emerges from a narrow, mountain valley onto a broad, open *plain*.

Alluvium Material deposited by rivers. Nowadays usually only applied to finer particles of silt and clay.

Alpine Mountain *environment*, between the *treeline* and the level of permanent snow cover.

Alpine mountains Ranges of mountains formed between 30 and 65 million years ago, by *folding*, in western and central Europe.

Amerindian A term applied to people *indigenous* to North, Central, and South America.

Animal husbandry The business of rearing animals.

Antarctic circle The parallel which lies at *latitude* of 66° 32′ S.

Anticline A geological *fold* that forms an arch shape, curving upward in the rock *strata*.

Anticyclone An area of relatively high atmospheric pressure.

Aquaculture Collective term for the farming of produce derived from the sea, including fish-farming, the cultivation of shellfish, and plants such as seaweed.

Aquifer A body of rock that can absorb water. Also applied to any rock strata that have sufficient porosity to yield *groundwater* through wells or springs.

Arable Land which has been plowed and is being used, or is suitable, for growing crops.

Archipelago A group or chain of islands.

Arctic Circle The parallel that lies at a *latitude* of 66° 32′ N.

Arête A thin, jagged mountain ridge that divides two adjacent *cirques*, found in regions where *glaciation* has occurred.

Arid Dry. An area of low rainfall, where the rate of *evaporation* may be greater than that of *precipitation*. Often defined as those areas that receive less than one inch (25 mm) of rain a year. In these areas only drought-resistant plants can survive.

Artesian well A naturally occurring source of underground water, stored in an *aquifer*.

Artisanal Small-scale, manual operation, such as fishing, using little or no machinery.

ASEAN Association of Southeast Asian Nations. Established in 1967 to promote economic, social, and cultural cooperation. Its members include Brunei, Indonesia, Malaysia, Philippines, Singapore, and Thailand.

Aseismic A region where *earthquake* activity has ceased.

Asteroid A minor planet circling the Sun, mainly between the orbits of Mars and Jupiter.

Asthenosphere A zone of hot, partially melted rock, which underlies the *lithosphere*, within the Earth's *crust*.

Atmosphere The envelope of odorless, colorless and tasteless gases surrounding the Earth, consisting of *oxygen* (23%), *nitrogen* (75%), argon (1%), *carbon dioxide* (0.03%), as well as tiny proportions of other gases.

Atmospheric pressure The pressure created by the action of gravity on the gases surrounding the Earth.

Atoll A ring-shaped island or *coral reef* often enclosing a *lagoon* of sea water.

Avalanche The rapid movement of a mass of snow and ice down a steep slope. Similar movements of other materials are described as *rock avalanches* or *landslides* and *sand avalanches*.

B

Badlands A landscape that has been heavily eroded and dissected by rainwater, and which has little or no vegetation.

Back slope The gentler windward slope of a sand *dune* or gentler slope of a *cuesta*.

Bajos An *alluvial fan* deposited by a river at the base of mountains and hills that encircle *desert* areas.

Bar, coastal An offshore strip of sand or shingle, either above or below the water. Usually parallel to the shore but sometimes crescent-shaped or at an oblique angle.

Barchan A crescent-shaped sand *dune*, formed where wind direction is very consistent. The horns of the crescent point downwind and where there is enough sand the barchan is mobile.

Barrio A Spanish term for the shantytowns – settlements of shacks – that are clustered around many South and Central American cities (*see also Favela*).

Basalt Dark, fine-grained *igneous rock* that is formed near the Earth's surface from fast-cooling *lava*.

Base level The level below which flowing water cannot erode the land.

Basement rock A mass of ancient rock often of *PreCambrian age*, covered by a layer of more recent *sedimentary rocks*. Commonly associated with *shield* areas.

Beach Lake or sea shore where waves break and there is an accumulation of loose sand, mud, gravel, or pebbles.

Bedrock Solid, consolidated and relatively unweathered rock, found on the surface of the land or just below a layer of soil or *weathered* rock.

Biodiversity The quantity of animal or plant species in a given area.

Biomass The total mass of organic matter – plants and animals – in a given area. It is usually measured in kilogrammes per square meter. Plant biomass is proportionally greater than that of animals, except in cities.

Biosphere The zone just above and below the Earth's surface, where all plants and animals live.

Blizzard A severe windstorm with snow and sleet. Visibility is often severely restricted.

Bluff The steep bank of a *meander*, formed by the erosive action of a river.

Boreal forest Tracts of mainly coniferous forest found in northern *latitudes*.

Breccia A type of rock composed of sharp fragments, cemented by a fine-grained material such as clay.

Butte An isolated, flat-topped hill with steep or vertical sides, buttes are the eroded remnants of a former land surface.

C

Caatinga Portuguese (Brazilian) term for thorny woodland growing in areas of pale granitic soils.

CACM Central American Common Market. Established in 1960 to further economic ties between its members, which are Costa Rica, El Salvador, Guatemala, Honduras, and Nicaragua.

Calcite Hexagonal crystals of calcium carbonate.

Caldera A huge volcanic vent, often containing a number of smaller vents, and sometimes a crater lake.

Carbon cycle The transfer of carbon to and from the *atmosphere*. This occurs on land through *photosynthesis*. In the sea, *carbon dioxide* is absorbed, some returning to the air and some taken up into the bodies of sea creatures.

Carbon dioxide A colorless, odorless gas (CO_2) that makes up 0.03% of the *atmosphere*.

Carbonation The process whereby rocks are broken down by carbonic acid. Carbon dioxide in the air dissolves in rainwater, forming carbonic acid. *Limestone* terrain can be rapidly eaten away.

Cash crop A single crop grown specifically for export sale, rather than for local use. Typical examples include coffee, tea, and citrus fruits.

Cassava A type of grain meal, used to produce tapioca. A staple crop in many parts of Africa.

Castle kopje Hill or rock outcrop, especially in southern Africa, where steep sides, and a summit composed of blocks, give a castle-like appearance.

Cataracts A series of stepped waterfalls created as a river flows over a band of hard, resistant rock.

Causeway A raised route through marshland or a body of water.

CEEAC Economic Community of Central African States. Established in 1983 to promote regional cooperation and if possible, establish a common market between 16 Central African nations.

Chemical weathering The chemical reactions leading to the decomposition of rocks. Types of chemical weathering include *carbonation*, *hydrolysis*, and *oxidation*.

Chernozem A fertile soil, also known as "black earth" consisting of a layer of dark topsoil, rich in decaying vegetation, overlying a lighter chalky layer.

Cirque Armchair-shaped basin, found in mountain regions, with a steep back, or rear, wall and a raised rock lip, often containing a lake (or *tarn*). The cirque floor has been eroded by a *glacier*, while the back wall is eroded both by the *glacier* and by *weathering*.

Climate The average weather conditions in a given area over a period of years, sometimes defined as 30 years or more.

Cold War A period of hostile relations between the US and the Soviet Union and their allies after the Second World War.

Composite volcano Also known as a strato-volcano, the volcanic cone is composed of alternating deposits of *lava* and *pyroclastic* material.

Compound A substance made up of *elements* chemically combined in a consistent way.

Condensation The process whereby a gas changes into a liquid. For example, water vapor in the *atmosphere* condenses around tiny airborne particles to form droplets of water.

Confluence The point at which two rivers meet.

Conglomerate Rock composed of large, water-worn or rounded pebbles, held together by a natural cement.

Coniferous forest A forest type containing trees which are generally, but not necessarily, *evergreen* and have slender, needlelike leaves. Coniferous trees reproduce by means of seeds contained in a cone.

Continental drift The theory that the continents of today are fragments of one or more prehistoric *supercontinents* which have moved across the Earth's surface, creating ocean basins. The theory has been superseded by a more sophisticated one – *plate tectonics*.

Continental shelf An area of the continental crust, below sea level, which slopes gently. It is separated from the deep ocean by a much more steeply inclined *continental slope*.

Continental slope A steep slope running from the edge of the *continental shelf* to the ocean floor.

Conurbation A vast metropolitan area created by the expansion of towns and cities into a virtually continuous urban area.

Cool continental A rainy *climate* with warm summers [warmest month below 76°F (22°C)] and often severe winters [coldest month below 32°F (0°C)].

Copra The dried, white kernel of a coconut, from which coconut oil is extracted.

Coral reef An underwater barrier created by colonies of the coral polyp. Polyps secrete a protective skeleton of calcium carbonate, and reefs develop as live polyps build on the skeletons of dead generations.

Core The center of the Earth, consisting of a dense mass of iron and nickel. It is thought that the outer core is molten or liquid, and that the inner core is solid due to extremely high pressures.

Coriolis effect A deflecting force caused by the rotation of the Earth. In the northern hemisphere a body, such as an *air mass* or ocean current, is deflected to the right, and in the southern hemisphere to the left. This prevents winds from blowing straight from areas of high to low pressure.

Coulées A US / Canadian term for a ravine formed by river *erosion*.

Craton A large block of the Earth's *crust* which has remained stable for a long period of *geological time*. It is made up of ancient *shield* rocks.

Cretaceous A period of *geological time* beginning about 145 million years ago and lasting until about 65 million years ago.

Crevasse A deep crack in a *glacier*.

Crust The hard, thin outer shell of the Earth. The crust floats on the *mantle*, which is softer and more dense. Under the oceans (oceanic crust) the crust is 3.7–6.8 miles (6–11 km) thick. Continental crust averages 18–24 miles (30–40 km).

Crystalline rock Rocks formed when molten *magma* crystallizes (*igneous rocks*) or when heat or pressure cause re-crystallization (*metamorphic rocks*). Crystalline rocks are distinct from *sedimentary rocks*.

Cuesta A hill which rises into a steep slope on one side but has a gentler gradient on its other slope.

Cyclone An area of low *atmospheric pressure*, occurring where the air is warm and relatively low in density, causing low level winds to spiral. *Hurricanes* and *typhoons* are tropical cyclones.

D

De facto
1 Government or other activity that takes place, or exists in actuality if not by right.
2 A border, which exists in practice, but which is not officially recognized by all the countries it adjoins.

Deciduous forest A forest of trees that shed their leaves annually at a particular time or season. In *temperate* climates the fall of leaves occurs in the autumn. Some *coniferous* trees, such as the larch, are deciduous. Deciduous vegetation contrasts with *evergreen*, which keeps its leaves for more than a year.

Defoliant Chemical spray used to remove foliage (leaves) from trees.

Deforestation The act of cutting down and clearing large areas of forest for human activities, such as agricultural land or urban development.

Delta Low-lying, fan-shaped area at a river mouth, formed by the *deposition* of successive layers of *sediment*. Slowing as it enters the sea, a river deposits sediment and may, as a result, split into numerous smaller channels, known as *distributaries*.

Denudation The combined effect of *weathering*, *erosion*, and *mass movement*, which, over long periods, exposes underlying rocks.

Deposition The laying down of material that has accumulated:
(*1*) after being *eroded* and then transported by physical forces such as wind, ice, or water;
(*2*) as organic remains, such as coal and coral;
(*3*) as the result of *evaporation* and chemical *precipitation*.

Depression
1 In climatic terms it is a large low pressure system.
2 A complex *fold*, producing a large valley, which incorporates both a *syncline* and an *anticline*.

Desert An *arid* region of low rainfall, with little vegetation or animal life, which is adapted to the dry conditions. The term is now applied not only to hot tropical and subtropical regions, but to arid areas of the continental interiors and to the ice deserts of the *Arctic* and *Antarctic*.

Desertification The gradual extension of *desert* conditions in *arid* or *semiarid* regions, as a result of climatic change or human activity, such as over-grazing and *deforestation*.

Despot A ruler with absolute power. Despots are often associated with oppressive regimes.

Detritus Piles of rock deposited by an erosive agent such as a river or *glacier*.

Distributary A minor branch of a river, which does not rejoin the main stream, common at *deltas*.

Diurnal Daily, something that occurs each day. Diurnal temperature refers to the variation in temperature over the course of a full day and night.

Divide A US term describing the area of high ground separating two *drainage basins*.

Donga A steep-sided *gully*, resulting from *erosion* by a river or by floods.

Dormant A term used to describe a *volcano* which is not currently erupting. They differ from extinct volcanoes as dormant volcanoes are still considered likely to erupt in the future.

Drainage basin The area drained by a single river system, its boundary is marked by a *watershed* or *divide*.

Drought A long period of continuously low rainfall.

Drumlin A long, streamlined hillock composed of material deposited by a *glacier*. They often occur in groups known as swarms.

Dune A mound or ridge of sand, shaped, and often moved, by the wind. They are found in hot *deserts* and on low-lying coasts where onshore winds blow across sandy beaches.

Dyke A wall constructed in low-lying areas to contain floodwaters or protect from high tides.

E

Earthflow The rapid movement of soil and other loose surface material down a slope, when saturated by water. Similar to a mudflow but not as fast-flowing, due to a lower percentage of water.

Earthquake Sudden movements of the Earth's *crust*, causing the ground to shake. Frequently occurring at *tectonic plate* margins. The shock, or series of shocks, spreads out from an *epicenter*.

EC The European Community (*see* EU).

Ecosystem A system of living organisms – plants and animals – interacting with their *environment*.

ECOWAS Economic Community of West African States. Established in 1975, it incorporates 16 West African states and aims to promote closer regional and economic cooperation.

Element
1 A constituent of the *climate* – *precipitation*, *humidity*, temperature, *atmospheric pressure*, or wind.
2 A substance that cannot be separated into simpler substances by chemical means.

El Niño A climatic phenomenon, the El Niño effect occurs about 14 times each century and leads to major shifts in global air circulation. It is associated with unusually warm currents off the coasts of Peru, Ecuador and Chile. The anomaly can last for up to two years.

Environment The conditions created by the surroundings (both natural and artificial) within which an organism lives. In human geography the word includes the surrounding economic, cultural, and social conditions.

Eon (aeon) Traditionally a long, but indefinite, period of *geological time*.

Ephemeral A nonpermanent feature, often used in connection with seasonal rivers or lakes in dry areas.

Epicenter The point on the Earth's surface directly above the underground origin – or focus – of an *earthquake*.

Equator The line of *latitude* which lies equidistant between the North and South Poles.

Erg An extensive area of sand *dunes*, particularly in the Sahara Desert.

Erosion The processes which wear away the surface of the land. *Glaciers*, wind, rivers, waves, and currents all carry debris which causes *erosion*. Some definitions also include *mass movement* due to gravity as an agent of erosion.

Escarpment A steep slope at the margin of a level, upland surface. In a landscape created by *folding*, escarpments (or scarps) frequently lie behind a more gentle backward slope.

Esker A narrow, winding ridge of sand and gravel deposited by streams of water flowing beneath or at the edge of a *glacier*.

Erratic A rock transported by a *glacier* and deposited some distance from its place of origin.

Eustacy A world-wide fall or rise in ocean levels.

EU The European Union. Established in 1965, it was formerly known as the EEC (European Economic Community) and then the EC (European Community). Its members are Austria, Belgium, Denmark, Finland, France, Germany, Greece, Ireland, Italy, Luxembourg, Netherlands, Portugal, Spain, Sweden, and UK. It seeks to establish an integrated European common market and eventual federation.

Evaporation The process whereby a liquid or solid is turned into a gas or vapor. Also refers to the diffusion of water vapor into the *atmosphere* from exposed water surfaces such as lakes and seas.

Evapotranspiration The loss of moisture from the Earth's surface through a combination of *evaporation*, and *transpiration* from the leaves of plants.

Evergreen Plants with long-lasting leaves, which are not shed annually or seasonally.

Exfoliation A kind of *weathering* whereby scalelike flakes of rock are peeled or broken off by the development of salt crystals in water within the rocks. *Groundwater*, which contains dissolved salts, seeps to the surface and evaporates, precipitating a film of salt crystals, which expands causing fine cracks. As these grow, flakes of rock break off.

Extrusive rock *Igneous* rock formed when molten material (*magma*) pours forth at the Earth's surface and cools rapidly. It usually has a glassy texture.

F

Factionalism The actions of one or more minority political group acting against the interests of the majority government.

Fault A fracture or crack in rock, where strains (*tectonic* movement) have caused blocks to move, vertically or laterally, relative to each other.

Fauna Collective name for the animals of a particular period of time, or region.

Favela Brazilian term for the shantytowns or temporary huts that have grown up around the edge of many South and Central American cities.

Ferrel cell A component in the global pattern of air circulation, which rises in the colder *latitudes* (60° N and S) and descends in warmer *latitudes* (30° N and S). The Ferrel cell forms part of the world's three-cell air circulation pattern, with the *Hadley* and Polar cells.

Fissure A deep crack in a rock or a *glacier*.

Fjord A deep, narrow inlet, created when the sea inundates the *U-shaped valley* created by a *glacier*.

Flash flood A sudden, short-lived rise in the water level of a river or stream, or surge of water down a dry river channel, or *wadi*, caused by heavy rainfall.

Flax A plant used to make linen.

Floodplain The broad, flat part of a river valley, adjacent to the river itself, formed by *sediment* deposited during flooding.

Flora The collective name for the plants of a particular period of time or region.

Flow The movement of a river within its banks, particularly in terms of the speed and volume of water.

Fold A bend in the rock *strata* of the Earth's *crust*, resulting from compression.

Fossil The remains, or traces, of a dead organism preserved in the Earth's *crust*.

Fossil dune A *dune* formed in a once-*arid* region which is now wetter. *Dunes* normally move with the wind, but in these cases vegetation makes them stable.

Fossil fuel Fuel – coal, natural gas or oil – composed of the fossilized remains of plants and animals.

Front The boundary between two *air masses*, which contrast sharply in temperature and *humidity*.

Frontal depression An area of low pressure caused by rising warm air. They are generally 600–1,200 miles (1,000–2,000 km) in diameter. Within *depressions* there are both warm and cold fronts.

Frost shattering A form of *weathering* where water freezes in cracks, causing expansion. As temperatures fluctuate and the ice melts and refreezes, it eventually causes the rocks to shatter and fragments of rock to break off.

G

Gaucho South American term for a stock herder or cowboy who works on the grassy *plains* of Paraguay, Uruguay, and Argentina.

Geological timescale The chronology of the Earth's history as revealed in its rocks. Geological time is divided into a number of periods: *eon*, era, period, epoch, age, and chron (the shortest). These units are not of uniform length.

Geosyncline A concave fold (*syncline*) or large depression in the Earth's *crust*, extending hundreds of miles. This basin contains a deep layer of sediment, especially at its center, from the land masses around it.

Geothermal energy Heat derived from hot rocks within the Earth's *crust* and resulting in hot springs, steam, or hot rocks at the surface. The energy is generated by rock movements, and from the breakdown of radioactive elements occurring under intense pressure.

GDP Gross Domestic Product. The total value of goods and services produced by a country excluding income from foreign countries.

Geyser A jet of steam and hot water that intermittently erupts from vents in the ground in areas that are, or were, *volcanic*. Some geysers occasionally reach heights of 196 ft (60 m).

Ghetto An area of a city or region occupied by an overwhelming majority of people from one racial or religious group, who may be subject to persecution or containment.

Glaciation The growth of *glaciers* and *ice sheets*, and their impact on the landscape.

Glacier A body of ice moving downslope under the influence of gravity and consisting of compacted and frozen snow. A glacier is distinct from an *ice sheet*, which is wider and less confined by features of the landscape.

Glacio-eustacy A world-wide change in the level of the oceans, caused when the formation of *ice sheets* takes up water or when their melting returns water to the ocean. The formation of ice sheets in the *Pleistocene* epoch, for example, caused sea level to drop by about 320 ft (100 m).

Glaciofluvial To do with glacial *meltwater*, the landforms it creates and its processes; *erosion*, transportation, and *deposition*. Glaciofluvial effects are more powerful and rapid where they occur within or beneath the *glacier*, rather than beyond its edge.

Glacis A gentle slope or *pediment*.

Global warming An increase in the average temperature of the Earth. At present the *greenhouse effect* is thought to contribute to this.

GNP Gross National Product. The total value of goods and services produced by a country.

Gondwanaland The *supercontinent* thought to have existed over 200 million years ago in the southern hemisphere. Gondwanaland is believed to have comprised today's Africa, Madagascar, Australia, parts of South America, *Antarctica*, and the Indian subcontinent.

Graben A block of rock let down between two parallel *faults*. Where the graben occurs within a valley, the structure is known as a *rift valley*.

Grease ice Slicks of ice which form in *Antarctic* seas, when ice crystals are bonded together by wind and wave action.

Greenhouse effect A change in the temperature of the *atmosphere*. Short-wave solar radiation travels through the *atmosphere* unimpeded to the Earth's surface, whereas outgoing, long-wave terrestrial radiation is absorbed by materials that reradiate it back to the Earth. Radiation trapped in this way, by water vapor, carbon dioxide, and other "greenhouse gases," keeps the Earth warm. As more *carbon dioxide* is released into the atmosphere by the burning of *fossil fuels*, the greenhouse effect may cause a global increase in temperature.

Groundwater Water that has seeped into the pores, cavities, and cracks of rocks or into soil and water held in an *aquifer*.

Gully A deep, narrow channel eroded in the landscape by *ephemeral* streams.

Guyot A small, flat-topped submarine mountain, formed as a result of subsidence which occurs during *sea-floor spreading*.

Gypsum A soft mineral *compound* (hydrated calcium sulphate), used as the basis of many forms of plaster, including plaster of Paris.

H

Hadley cell A large-scale component in the global pattern of air circulation. Warm air rises over the *Equator* and blows at high altitude toward the poles, sinking in subtropical regions (30° N and 30° S) and creating high pressure. The air then flows at the surface toward the *Equator* in the form of trade winds. There is one cell in each hemisphere. Named after G. Hadley, who published his theory in 1735.

Hamada An Arabic word for a plateau of bare rock in a *desert*.

Hanging valley A tributary valley that ends suddenly, high above the bed of the main valley. The effect is found where the main valley has been more deeply eroded by a *glacier*, than has the tributary valley. A stream in a hanging valley will descend to the floor of the main valley as a waterfall or *cataract*.

Headwards The action of a river eroding back upstream, as opposed to the normal process of downstream *erosion*. Headwards erosion is often associated with *gullying*.

Hoodos Pinnacles of rock that have been worn away by *weathering* in *semiarid* regions.

Horst A block of the Earth's *crust* which has been left upstanding by the sinking of adjoining blocks along fault lines.

Hot spot A region of the Earth's *crust* where high thermal activity occurs, often leading to volcanic eruptions. Hot spots often occur far from plate boundaries, but their movement is associated with *plate tectonics*.

Humid equatorial Rainy *climate* with no winter, where the coolest month is generally above 64°F (18°C).

Humidity The relative amount of moisture held in the Earth's *atmosphere*.

Hurricane
1 A tropical *cyclone* occurring in the Caribbean and western North Atlantic.
2 A wind of more than 65 knots (75 kmph).

Hydroelectric power Energy produced by harnessing the rapid movement of water down steep mountain slopes to drive turbines to generate electricity.

Hydrolysis The chemical breakdown of rocks in reaction with water, forming new compounds.

I

Ice Age A period in the Earth's history when surface temperatures in the temperate *latitudes* were much lower and *ice sheets* expanded considerably. There have been *ice ages* from *Pre-Cambrian* times onward. The most recent began two million years ago and ended 10,000 years ago.

Ice cap A permanent dome of ice in highland areas. The term ice cap is often seen as distinct from *ice sheet*, which denotes a much wider covering of ice; and is also used refer to the very extensive polar and Greenland ice caps.

Ice floe A large, flat mass of ice floating free on the ocean surface. It is usually formed after the break-up of winter ice by heavy storms.

Ice sheet A continuous, very thick layer of ice and snow. The term is usually used of ice masses which are continental in extent.

Ice shelf A floating mass of ice attached to the edge of a coast. The seaward edge is usually a sheer cliff up to 100 ft (30 m) high.

Ice wedge Massive blocks of ice up to 6.5 ft (2 m) wide at the top and extending 32 ft (10 m) deep. They are found in cracks in *polygonally-patterned* ground in *periglacial* regions.

Iceberg A large mass of ice in a lake or a sea, which has broken off from a floating *ice sheet* (an *ice shelf*) or from a *glacier*.

Igneous rock Rock formed when molten material, *magma*, from the hot, lower layers of the Earth's *crust*, cools, solidifies, and crystallizes, either within the Earth's *crust* (*intrusive*) or on the surface (*extrusive*).

IMF International Monetary Fund. Established in 1944 as a UN agency, it contains 182 members around the world and is concerned with world monetary stability and economic development.

Incised meander A *meander* where the river, following its original course, cuts deeply into *bedrock*. This may occur when a mature, meandering river begins to erode its bed much more vigorously after the surrounding land has been uplifted.

Indigenous People, plants, or animals native to a particular region.

Infrastructure The communications and services – roads, railroads, and telecommunications – necessary for the functioning of a country or region.

Inselberg An isolated, steep-sided hill, rising from a low *plain* in *semiarid* and *savannah* landscapes. Inselbergs are usually composed of a rock, such as granite, which resists *erosion*.

Interglacial A period of global *climate*, between two *ice ages*, when temperatures rise and *ice sheets* and *glaciers* retreat.

Intraplate volcano A *volcano* which lies in the centre of one of the Earth's *tectonic plates*, rather than, as is more common, at its edge. They are thought to have been formed by a *hot spot*.

Intrusion (intrusive igneous rock) Rock formed when molten material, *magma*, penetrates existing rocks below the Earth's surface before cooling and solidifying. These rocks cool more slowly than extrusive rock and therefore tend to have coarser grains.

Irrigation The artificial supply of agricultural water to dry areas, often involving the creation of canals and the diversion of natural watercourses.

Island arc A curved chain of islands. Typically, such an arc fringes an ocean trench, formed at the margin between two *tectonic plates*. As one plate overrides another, *earthquakes* and volcanic activity are common and the islands themselves are often volcanic cones.

Isostasy The state of equilibrium that the Earth's *crust* maintains as its lighter and heavier parts float on the denser underlying mantle.

Isthmus A narrow strip of land connecting two larger landmasses or islands.

J

Jet stream A narrow belt of westerly winds in the *troposphere*, at altitudes above 39,000 ft (12,000 m). Jet streams tend to blow more strongly in winter and include: the subtropical jet stream; the *polar* front jet stream in mid-*latitudes*; the *Arctic* jet stream; and the polar-night jet stream.

Joint A crack in a rock, formed where blocks of rock have not shifted relative to each other, as is the case with a *fault*. Joints are created by *folding*; by shrinkage in *igneous rock* as it cools or *sedimentary rock* as it dries out; and by the release of pressure in a rock mass when overlying materials are removed by *erosion*.

Jute A plant fiber used to make coarse ropes, sacks, and matting.

K

Kame A mound of stratified sand and gravel with steep sides, deposited in a *crevasse* by *meltwater* running over a *glacier*. When the ice retreats, this forms an undulating terrain of hummocks.

Karst A barren *limestone* landscape created by carbonic acid in streams and rainwater, in areas where *limestone* is close to the surface. Typical features include caverns, towerlike hills, *sinkholes*, and flat limestone pavements.

Kettle hole A round hollow formed in a glacial deposit by a detached block of glacial ice, which later melted. They can fill with water to form kettle-lakes.

L

Lagoon A shallow stretch of coastal salt-water behind a partial barrier such as a sandbank or *coral reef*. Lagoon is also used to describe the water encircled by an *atoll*.

LAIA Latin American Integration Association. Established in 1980, its members are Argentina, Bolivia, Brazil, Chile, Colombia, Ecuador, Mexico, Paraguay, Peru, Uruguay, and Venezuala. It aims to promote economic cooperation between member states.

Landslide The sudden downslope movement of a mass of rock or earth on a slope, caused either by heavy rain; the impact of waves; an *earthquake* or human activity.

Laterite A hard red deposit left by *chemical weathering* in tropical conditions, and consisting mainly of oxides of iron and aluminium.

Latitude The angular distance from the *Equator*, to a given point on the Earth's surface. Imaginary lines of *latitude* running parallel to the Equator encircle the Earth, and are measured in degrees north or south of the Equator. The Equator is 0°, the poles 90° South and North respectively. Also called parallels.

Laurasia In the theory of *continental drift*, the northern part of the great *supercontinent* of *Pangaea*. Laurasia is said to consist of N America, Greenland and all of Eurasia north of the Indian subcontinent.

Lava The molten rock, *magma*, which erupts onto the Earth's surface through a *volcano*, or through a *fault* or crack in the Earth's *crust*. Lava refers to the rock both in its molten and in its later, solidified form.

Leaching The process whereby water dissolves minerals and moves them down through layers of soil or rock.

Levée A raised bank alongside the channel of a river. Levées are either human-made or formed in times of flood when the river overflows its channel, slows and deposits much of its *sediment* load.

Lichen An organism which is the symbiotic product of an algae and a fungus. Lichens form in tight crusts on stones and trees, and are resistant to extreme cold. They are often found in tundra regions.

Lignite Low-grade coal, also known as brown coal. Found in large deposits in eastern Europe.

Limestone A porous *sedimentary* rock formed from carbonate materials.

Lingua franca The language adopted as the common language between speakers whose native languages are different. This is common in former colonial states.

Lithosphere The rigid upper layer of the Earth, comprising the *crust* and the upper part of the *mantle*.

Llanos Vast grassland *plains* of northern South America.

Loess Fine-grained, yellow deposits of unstratified silts and sands. Loess is believed to be wind-carried *sediment* created in the last *Ice Age*. Some deposits may later have been redistributed by rivers. Loess-derived soils are of high quality, fertile, and easy to work.

Longitude A division of the Earth which pinpoints how far east or west a given place is from the Prime Meridian (0°) which runs through the Royal Observatory at Greenwich, England (UK). Imaginary lines of longitude are drawn around the world from pole to pole. The world is divided into 360 degrees.

Longshore drift The movement of sand and silt along the coast, carried by waves hitting the beach at an angle.

M

Magma Underground, molten rock, which is very hot and highly charged with gas. It is generated at great pressure, at depths 10 miles (16 km) or more below the Earth's surface. It can issue as *lava* at the Earth's surface or, more often, solidify below the surface as *intrusive igneous rock*.

Mantle The layer of the Earth between the *crust* and the *core*. It is about 1,800 miles (2,900 km) thick. The uppermost layer of the mantle is the soft, 125-mile (200 km) thick *asthenosphere* on which the more rigid *lithosphere* floats.

Maquiladoras Factories on the Mexico side of the Mexico/US border, that are allowed to import raw materials and components duty-free and use low-cost labor to assemble the goods, finally exporting them for sale in the US.

Market gardening The intensive growing of fruit and vegetables close to large local markets.

Mass movement Downslope movement of weathered materials such as rock, often helped by rainfall or glacial *meltwater*. Mass movement may be a gradual process or rapid, as in a *landslide* or rockfall.

Massif A single very large mountain or an area of mountains with uniform characteristics and clearly-defined boundaries.

Meander A looplike bend in a river, which is found typically in the lower, mature reaches of a river but can form wherever the valley is wide and the slope gentle.

Mediterranean climate A temperate *climate* of hot, dry summers and warm, damp winters. This is typical of the western fringes of the world's continents in the warm temperate regions between *latitudes* of 30° and 40° (north and south).

Meltwater Water resulting from the melting of a *glacier* or *ice sheet*.

Mesa A broad, flat-topped hill, characteristic of *arid* regions.

Mesosphere A layer of the Earth's *atmosphere*, between the *stratosphere* and the *thermosphere*. Extending from about 25–50 miles (40–80 km) above the surface of the Earth.

Mestizo A person of mixed *Amerindian* and European origin.

Metallurgy The refining and working of metals.

Metamorphic rocks Rocks that have been altered from their original form, in terms of texture, composition, and structure by intense heat, pressure, or by the introduction of new chemical substances – or a combination of more than one of these.

Meteor A body of rock, metal or other material, that travels through space at great speeds. Meteors are visible as they enter the Earth's *atmosphere* as shooting stars and fireballs.

Meteorite The remains of a *meteor* that has fallen to Earth.

Meteoroid A *meteor* that is still traveling in space, outside the Earth's *atmosphere*.

Mezzogiorno A term applied to the southern portion of Italy.

Milankovitch hypothesis A theory suggesting that there are a series of cycles that slightly alter the Earth's position when rotating about the Sun. The cycles identified all affect the amount of *radiation* the Earth receives at different *latitudes*. The theory is seen as a key factor in the cause of *ice ages*.

Millet A grain-crop, forming part of the staple diet in much of Africa.

Mistral A strong, dry, cold northerly or north-westerly wind, which blows from the Massif Central of France to the Mediterranean Sea. It is common in winter and its cold blasts can cause crop damage in the Rhône Delta, in France.

Mohorovičić discontinuity (Moho) The structural divide at the margin between the Earth's *crust* and the *mantle*. On average it is 20 miles (35 km) below the continents and 6 miles (10 km) below the oceans. The different densities of the *crust* and the mantle cause *earthquake* waves to accelerate at this point.

Monarchy A form of government in which the head of state is a single hereditary monarch. The monarch may be a mere figurehead, or may retain significant authority.

Monsoon A wind that changes direction biannually. The change is caused by the reversal of pressure over landmasses and the adjacent oceans. Because the inflowing moist winds bring rain, the term monsoon is also used to refer to the rains themselves. The term is derived from and most commonly refers to the seasonal winds of south and east Asia.

Montaña Mountain areas along the west coast of South America.

Moraine Debris, transported and deposited by a *glacier* or *ice sheet* in unstratified, mixed, piles of rock, boulders, pebbles, and clay.

Mountain-building The formation of *fold* mountains by tectonic activity. Also known as orogeny, mountain-building often occurs on the margin where two *tectonic plates* collide. The periods when most mountain-building occurred are known as orogenic phases and lasted many millions of years.

Mudflow An *avalanche* of mud that occurs when a mass of soil is drenched by rain or melting snow. It is a type of *mass movement*, faster than an *earthflow* because it is lubricated by water.

N

Nappe A mass of rocks which has been overfolded by repeated thrust *faulting*.

NAFTA The North American Free Trade Association. Established in 1994 between Canada, Mexico, and the US to set up a free-trade zone.

NASA The North American Space Agency. It is a government body, established in 1958 to develop manned and unmanned space programs.

NATO The North Atlantic Treaty Organization. Established in 1949 to promote mutual defense and cooperation between its members, which are Belgium, Canada, Czech Republic, Denmark, France, Germany, Greece, Iceland, Italy, Luxembourg, the Netherlands, Norway, Portugal, Poland, Spain, Turkey, UK, and US.

Nitrogen The odorless, colorless gas that makes up 78% of the atmosphere. Within the soil, it is a vital nutrient for plants.

Nomads (nomadic) Wandering communities that move around in search of suitable pasture for their herds of animals.

Nuclear fusion A technique used to create a new nucleus by the merging of two lighter ones, resulting in the release of large quantities of energy.

O

Oasis A fertile area in the midst of a *desert*, usually watered by an underground *aquifer*.

Oceanic ridge A mid-ocean ridge formed, according to the theory of *plate tectonics*, when plates drift apart and hot *magma* pours through to form new oceanic *crust*.

Oligarchy The government of a state by a small, exclusive group of people – such as an elite class or a family group.

Onion-skin weathering The *weathering* away or *exfoliation* of a rock or outcrop by the peeling off of surface layers.

Oriente A flatter region lying to the east of the Andes in South America.

Outwash plain *Glaciofluvial* material (typically clay, sand, and gravel) carried beyond an ice sheet by *meltwater* streams, forming a broad, flat deposit.

Oxbow lake A crescent-shaped lake formed on a river *floodplain* when a river erodes the outside bend of a *meander*, making the neck of the *meander* narrower until the river cuts across the neck. The meander is cut off and is dammed off with sediment, creating an oxbow lake. Also known as a cut-off or mortlake.

Oxidation A form of *chemical weathering* where *oxygen* dissolved in water reacts with minerals in rocks – particularly iron – to form oxides. Oxidation causes brown or yellow staining on rocks, and eventually leads to the break down of the rock.

Oxygen A colorless, odorless gas which is one of the main constituents of the Earth's *atmosphere* and is essential to life on Earth.

Ozone layer A layer of enriched *oxygen* (0_3) within the stratosphere, mostly between 18–50 miles (30–80 km) above the Earth's surface. It is vital to the existence of life on Earth because it absorbs harmful shortwave ultraviolet radiation, while allowing beneficial longer wave ultraviolet radiation to penetrate to the Earth's surface.

P

Pacific Rim The name given to the economically-dynamic countries bordering the Pacific Ocean.

Pack ice Ice masses more than 10 ft (3 m) thick that form on the sea surface and are not attached to a landmass.

Pancake ice Thin discs of ice, up to 8 ft (2.4 m) wide which form when slicks of *grease ice* are tossed together by winds and stormy seas.

Pangaea In the theory of continental drift, Pangaea is the original great land mass which, about 190 million years ago, began to split into Gondwanaland in the south and Laurasia in the north, separated by the Tethys Sea.

Pastoralism Grazing of livestock– usually sheep, goats, or cattle. Pastoralists in many drier areas have traditionally been *nomadic*.

Parallel *see Latitude*.

Peat Ancient, partially-decomposed vegetation found in wet, boggy conditions where there is little *oxygen*. It is the first stage in the development of coal and is often dried for use as fuel. It is also used to improve soil quality.

Pediment A gently-sloping ramp of *bedrock* below a steeper slope, often found at mountain edges in *desert* areas, but also in other climatic zones. Pediments may include depositional elements such as *alluvial fans*.

Peninsula A thin strip of land surrounded on three of its sides by water. Large examples include Florida and Korea.

Per capita Latin term meaning "for each person."

Periglacial Regions on the edges of *ice sheets* or *glaciers* or, more commonly, cold regions experiencing intense frost action, *permafrost* or both. Periglacial climates bring long, freezing winters and short, mild summers.

Permafrost Permanently frozen ground, typical of *Arctic* regions. Although a layer of soil above the permafrost melts in summer, the melted water does not drain through the permafrost.

Permeable rocks Rocks through which water can seep, because they are either porous or cracked.

Pharmaceuticals The manufacture of medicinal drugs.

Phreatic eruption A volcanic eruption which occurs when *lava* combines with *groundwater*, superheating the water and causing a sudden emission of steam at the surface.

Physical weathering (mechanical weathering) The breakdown of rocks by physical, as opposed to chemical, processes. Examples include: changes in pressure or temperature; the effect of windblown sand; the pressure of growing salt crystals in cracks within rock; and the expansion and contraction of water within rock as it freezes and thaws.

Pingo A dome of earth with a core of ice, found in *tundra* regions. Pingos are formed either when *groundwater* freezes and expands, pushing up the land surface, or when trapped, freezing water in a lake expands and pushes up lake *sediments* to form the pingo dome.

Placer A belt of mineral-bearing rock *strata* lying at or close to the Earth's surface, from which minerals can be easily extracted.

Plain A flat, level region of land, often relatively low-lying.

Plateau A highland tract of flat land.

Plate *see Tectonic plates*.

Plate tectonics The study of *tectonic plates*, that helps to explain *continental drift*, mountain formation and volcanic activity. The movement of tectonic plates may be explained by the currents of rock rising and falling from within the Earth's *mantle*, as it heats up and then cools. The boundaries of the plates are known as plate margins and most mountains, *earthquakes*, and *volcanoes* occur at these margins. Constructive margins are moving apart; destructive margins are crunching together and conservative margins are sliding past one another.

Pleistocene A period of *geological time* spanning from about 5.2 million years ago to 1.6 million years ago.

Plutonic rock *Igneous* rocks found deep below the surface. They are coarse-grained because they cooled and solidified slowly.

Polar The zones within the *Arctic* and *Antarctic* circles.

Polje A long, broad *depression* found in *karst* (*limestone*) regions.

Polygonal patterning Typical ground patterning, found in areas where the soil is subject to severe frost action, often in *periglacial* regions.

Porosity A measure of how much water can be held within a rock or a soil. Porosity is measured as the percentage of holes or pores in a material, compared to its total volume. For example, the porosity of slate is less than 1%, whereas that of gravel is 25–35%.

Prairies Originally a French word for grassy *plains* with few or no trees.

Pre-Cambrian The earliest period of *geological time* dating from over 570 million years ago.

Precipitation The fall of moisture from the *atmosphere* onto the surface of the Earth, whether as dew, hail, rain, sleet, or snow.

Pyramidal peak A steep, isolated mountain summit, formed when the back walls of three or more *cirques* are cut back and move toward each other. The cliffs around such a horned peak, or horn, are divided by sharp *arêtes*. The Matterhorn in the Swiss Alps is an example.

Pyroclasts Fragments of rock ejected during volcanic eruptions.

Q

Quaternary The current period of *geological time*, which started about 1.6 million years ago.

R

Radiation The emission of energy in the form of particles or waves. Radiation from the sun includes heat, light, ultraviolet rays, gamma rays, and X-rays. Only some of the solar energy radiated into space reaches the Earth.

Rainforest Dense forests in tropical zones with high rainfall, temperature and *humidity*. Strictly, the term applies to the equatorial rain forest in tropical lowlands with constant rainfall and no seasonal change. The Congo and Amazon basins are examples. The term is applied more loosely to lush forest in other climates. Within rain forests organic life is dense and varied: at least 40% of all plant and animal species are found here and there may be as many as 100 tree species per hectare.

Rainshadow An area which experiences low rainfall, because of its position on the leeward side of a mountain range.

Reg A large area of stony *desert*, where tightly-packed gravel lies on top of clayey sand. A reg is formed where the wind blows away the finer sand.

Remote-sensing Method of obtaining information about the *environment* using unmanned equipment, such as a satellite, that relays the information to a point where it is collected and used.

Resistance The capacity of a rock to resist *denudation*, by processes such as *weathering* and *erosion*.

Ria A flooded *V-shaped river valley* or estuary, flooded by a rise in sea level (*eustacy*) or sinking land. It is shorter than a *fjord* and gets deeper as it meets the sea.

Rift valley A long, narrow depression in the Earth's *crust*, formed by the sinking of rocks between two *faults*.

River channel The trough which contains a river and is molded by the flow of water within it.

Roche moutonée A rock found in a glaciated valley. The side facing the flow of the *glacier* has been smoothed and rounded, while the other side has been left more rugged because the *glacier*, as it flows over it, has plucked out frozen fragments and carried them away.

Runoff Water draining from a land surface by flowing across it.

S

Sabkha The floor of an isolated *depression* that occurs in an *arid environment* – usually covered by salt deposits and devoid of vegetation.

SADC Southern African Development Community. Established in 1992 to promote economic integration between its member states, which are Angola, Botswana, Lesotho, Malawi, Mauritius, Mozambique, Namibia, South Africa, Swaziland, Tanzania, Zambia, and Zimbabwe.

Salt plug A rounded hill produced by the upward doming of rock *strata* caused by the movement of salt or other evaporite deposits under intense pressure.

Sastrugi Ice ridges formed by wind action. They lie parallel to the direction of the wind.

Savannah Open grassland found between the zone of *deserts*, and that of tropical *rain forests* in the tropics and subtropics. Scattered trees and shrubs are found in some kinds of savannah. A savannah *climate* usually has wet and dry seasons.

Scarp *see Escarpment*.

Scree Piles of rock fragments beneath a cliff or rock face, caused by mechanical *weathering*, especially *frost shattering*, where the expansion and contraction of freezing and thawing water within the rock, gradually breaks it up.

Sea-floor spreading The process whereby *tectonic plates* move apart, allowing hot *magma* to erupt and solidify. This forms a new sea floor and, ultimately, widens the ocean.

Seamount An isolated, submarine mountain or hill, probably of volcanic origin.

Season A period of time linked to regular changes in the weather, especially the intensity of solar *radiation*.

Sediment Grains of rock transported and deposited by rivers, sea, ice, or wind.

Sedimentary rocks Rocks formed from the debris of preexisting rocks or of organic material. They are found in many *environments* – on the ocean floor, on beaches, rivers, and *deserts*. Organically-formed sedimentary rocks include coal and chalk. Other sedimentary rocks, such as flint, are formed by chemical processes. Most of these rocks contain *fossils*, which can be used to date them.

Seif A sand *dune* which lies parallel to the direction of the prevailing wind. Seifs form steep-sided ridges, sometimes extending for miles.

Seismic activity Movement within the Earth, such as an *earthquake* or *tremor*.

Selva A region of wet forest found in the Amazon Basin.

Semiarid, semidesert The *climate* and landscape which lies between *savannah* and *desert* or between savannah and a *mediterranean* climate. In semiarid conditions there is a little more moisture than in a true *desert*; and more patches of drought-resistant vegetation can survive.

Shale (marine shale) A compacted *sedimentary rock*, with fine-grained particles. Marine shale is formed on the seabed. Fuel such as oil may be extracted from it.

Sheetwash Water that runs downhill in thin sheets without forming channels. It can cause *sheet erosion*.

Sheet erosion The washing away of soil by a thin film or sheet of water, known as *sheetwash*.

Shield A vast stable block of the Earth's *crust*, which has experienced little or no *mountain-building*.

Sierra The Spanish word for mountains.

Sinkhole A circular *depression* in a *limestone* region. They are formed by the collapse of an underground cave system or the *chemical weathering* of the *limestone*.

Sisal A plant-fiber used to make matting.

Slash and burn A farming technique involving the cutting down and burning of scrub forest, to create agricultural land. After a number of seasons this land is abandoned and the process is repeated. This practice is common in Africa and South America.

Slip face The steep leeward side of a sand *dune* or slope. Opposite side to a *back slope*.

Soil A thin layer of rock particles mixed with the remains of dead plants and animals. This occurs naturally on the surface of the Earth and provides a medium for plants to grow.

Soil creep The very gradual downslope movement of rock debris and soil, under the influence of gravity. This is a type of *mass movement*.

Soil erosion The wearing away of soil more quickly than it is replaced by natural processes. Soil can be carried away by wind as well as by water. Human activities, such as over-grazing and the clearing of land for farming, accelerate the process in many areas.

Solar energy Energy derived from the Sun. Solar energy is converted into other forms of energy. For example, the wind and waves, as well as the creation of plant material in photosynthesis, depend on solar energy.

Solifluction A kind of *soil creep*, where water in the surface layer has saturated the soil and rock debris which slips slowly downhill. It often happens where frozen top-layer deposits thaw, leaving frozen layers below them.

Sorghum A type of grass found in South America, similar to sugar cane. When refined it is used to make molasses.

Spit A thin linear deposit of sand or shingle extending from the sea shore. Spits are formed as angled waves shift sand along the beach, eventually extending a ridge of sand beyond a change in the angle of the coast. Spits are common where the coastline bends, especially at estuaries.

Squash A type of edible gourd.

Stack A tall, isolated pillar of rock near a coastline, created as wave action erodes away the adjacent rock.

Stalactite A tapering cylinder of mineral deposit, hanging from the roof of a cave in a *karst* area. It is formed by calcium carbonate, dissolved in water, which drips through the roof of a *limestone* cavern.

Stalagmite A cone of calcium carbonate, similar to a *stalactite*, rising from the floor of a *limestone* cavern and formed when drops of water fall from the roof of a *limestone* cave. If the water has dripped from a *stalactite* above the stalagmite, the two may join to form a continuous pillar.

Staple crop The main crop on which a country is economically and or physically reliant. For example, the major crop grown for large-scale local consumption in South Asia is rice.

Steppe Large areas of dry grassland in the northern hemisphere – particularly found in southeast Europe and central Asia.

Strata The plural of stratum, a distinct, virtually horizontal layer of deposited material, lying parallel to other layers.

Stratosphere A layer of the *atmosphere*, above the *troposphere*, extending from about 7–30 miles (11–50 km) above the Earth's surface. In the lower part of the stratosphere, the temperature is relatively stable and there is little moisture.

Strike-slip fault Occurs where plates move sideways past each other and blocks of rocks move horizontally in relation to each other, not up or down as in normal *faults*.

Subduction zone A region where two *tectonic plates* collide, forcing one beneath the other. Typically, a dense oceanic plate dips below a lighter continental plate, melting in the heat of the *asthenosphere*. This is why the zone is also called a destructive margins (*see Plate tectonics*). These zones are characterized by *earthquakes*, volcanoes, *mountain-building*, and the development of oceanic trenches and *island arcs*.

Submarine canyon A steep-sided valley, that extends along the *continental shelf* to the ocean floor. Often formed by *turbidity currents*.

Submarine fan Deposits of silt and *alluvium*, carried by large rivers forming great fan-shaped deposits on the ocean floor.

Subsistence agriculture An agricultural practice in which enough food is produced to support the farmer and his dependents, but not providing any surplus to generate an income.

Subtropical A term applied loosely to *climates* which are nearly tropical or tropical for a part of the year – areas north or south of the *tropics* but outside the *temperate zone*.

Supercontinent A large continent that breaks up to form smaller continents or that forms when smaller continents merge. In the theory of *continental drift*, the supercontinents are *Pangaea*, *Gondwanaland*, and *Laurasia*.

Sustainable development An approach to development, especially applied to economies across the world which exploit natural resources without destroying them or the *environment*.

Syncline A basin-shaped downfold in rock *strata*, created when the *strata* are compressed, for example where *tectonic plates* collide.

T

Tableland A highland area with a flat or gently undulating surface.

Taiga The belt of *coniferous* forest found in the north of Asia and North America. The conifers are adapted to survive low temperatures and long periods of snowfall.

Tarn A Scottish term for a small mountain lake, usually found at the head of a *glacier*.

Tectonic plates Plates, or tectonic plates, are the rigid slabs which form the Earth's outer shell, the *lithosphere*. Eight big plates and several smaller ones have been identified.

Temperate A moderate *climate* without extremes of temperature, typical of the mid-*latitudes* between the *tropics* and the *polar* circles.

Theocracy A state governed by religious laws – today Iran is the world's largest theocracy.

Thermokarst Subsidence created by the thawing of ground ice in *periglacial* areas, creating depressions.

Thermosphere A layer of the Earth's *atmosphere* which lies above the *mesosphere*, about 60–300 miles (100–500 km) above the Earth

Terraces Steps cut into steep slopes to create flat surfaces for cultivating crops. They also help reduce soil *erosion* on unconsolidated slopes. They are most common in heavily-populated parts of Southeast Asia.

Till Unstratified glacial deposits or drift left by a *glacier* or *ice sheet*. Till includes mixtures of clay, sand, gravel, and boulders.

Topography The typical shape and features of a given area such as land height and terrain.

Tombolo A large sand *spit* which attaches part of the mainland to an island.

Tornado A violent, spiraling windstorm, with a center of very low pressure. Wind speeds reach 200 mph (320 kmph) and there is often thunder and heavy rain.

Transform fault In *plate tectonics*, a *fault* of continental scale, occurring where two plates slide past each other, staying close together for example, the San Andreas Fault, USA. The jerky, uneven movement creates *earthquakes* but does not destroy or add to the Earth's *crust*

Transpiration The loss of water vapor through the pores (or stomata) of plants. The process helps to return moisture to the *atmosphere*.

Trap An area of fine-grained *igneous rock* that has been extruded and cooled on the Earth's surface in stages, forming a series of steps or terraces.

Treeline The line beyond which trees cannot grow, dependent on *latitude* and altitude, as well as local factors such as soil.

Tremor A slight *earthquake*.

Trench (oceanic trench) A long, deep trough in the ocean floor, formed, according to the theory of *plate tectonics*, when two plates collide and one dives under the other, creating a *subduction zone*.

Tropics The zone between the *Tropic of Cancer* and the *Tropic of Capricorn* where the *climate* is hot. Tropical climate is also applied to areas rather further north and south of the *Equator* where the climate is similar to that of the true tropics.

Tropic of Cancer A line of *latitude* or imaginary circle round the Earth, lying at 23° 28' N.

Tropic of Capricorn A line of *latitude* or imaginary circle round the Earth, lying at 23° 28' S.

Troposphere The lowest layer of the Earth's *atmosphere*. From the surface, it reaches a height of between 4–10 miles (7–16 km). It is the most turbulent zone of the atmosphere and accounts for the generation of most of the world's weather. The layer above it is called the *stratosphere*.

Tsunami A huge wave created by shock waves from an *earthquake* under the sea. Reaching speeds of up to 600 mph (960 kmph), the wave may increase to heights of 50 ft (15 m) on entering coastal waters; and it can cause great damage.

Tundra The treeless *plains* of the *Arctic Circle*, found south of the *polar* region of permanent ice and snow, and north of the belt of *coniferous* forests known as *taiga*. In this region of long, very cold winters, vegetation is usually limited to mosses, *lichens*, sedges, and rushes, although flowers and dwarf shrubs blossom in the brief summer.

Turbidity current An oceanic feature. A turbidity current is a mass of *sediment*-laden water that has substantial erosive power. Turbidity currents are thought to contribute to the formation of *submarine canyons*.

Typhoon A kind of *hurricane* (or tropical cyclone) bringing violent winds and heavy rain, a typhoon can do great damage. They occur in the South China Sea, especially around the Philippines.

U

U-shaped valley A river valley that has been deepened and widened by a *glacier*. They are characteristically flat-bottomed and steep-sided and generally much deeper than river valleys.

UN United Nations. Established in 1945, it contains 188 nations and aims to maintain international peace and security, and promote cooperation over economic, social, cultural, and humanitarian problems.

UNICEF United Nations Children's Fund. A UN organization set up to promote family and child related programs.

Urstromtäler A German word used to describe *meltwater* channels that flowed along the front edge of the advancing *ice sheet* during the last Ice Age, 18,000–20,000 years ago.

V

V-shaped valley A typical valley eroded by a river in its upper course.

Virgin rain forest Tropical *rain-forest* in its original state, untouched by human activity such as logging, clearance for agriculture, settlement, or roadbuilding.

Viticulture The cultivation of grapes for wine.

Volcano An opening or vent in the Earth's *crust* where molten rock, *magma*, erupts. Volcanoes tend to be conical but may also be a crack in the Earth's surface or a hole blasted through a mountain. The magma is accompanied by other materials such as gas, steam, and fragments of rock, or *pyroclasts*. They tend to occur on destructive or constructive tectonicplate margins.

W–Z

Wadi The dry bed left by a torrent of water. Also classified as a *ephemeral* stream, found in *arid* and *semiarid* regions, which are subject to sudden and often severe flash flooding.

Warm humid climate A rainy climate with warm summers and mild winters.

Water cycle The continuous circulation of water between the Earth's surface and the *atmosphere*. The processes include *evaporation* and *transpiration* of moisture into the atmosphere, and its return as *precipitation*, some of which flows into lakes and oceans.

Water table The upper level of *groundwater* saturation in permeable rock *strata*.

Watershed The dividing line between one *drainage basin* – an area where all streams flow into a single river system – and another. In the US, watershed also means the whole drainage basin of a single river system – its catchment area.

Waterspout A rotating column of water in the form of cloud, mist, and spray which form on open water. Often has the appearance of a small *tornado*.

Weathering The decay and breakup of rocks at or near the Earth's surface, caused by water, wind, heat or ice, organic material, or the *atmosphere*. *Physical weathering* includes the effects of frost and temperature changes. Biological weathering includes the effects of plant roots, burrowing animals and the acids produced by animals, especially as they decay after death. *Carbonation* and *hydrolysis* are among many kinds of *chemical weathering*.

GEOGRAPHICAL NAMES

THE FOLLOWING GLOSSARY lists all geographical terms occurring on the maps and in main-entry names in the Index-Gazetteer. These terms may precede, follow or be run together with the proper element of the name; where they precede it the term is reversed for indexing purposes – thus Poluostrov Yamal is indexed as Yamal, Poluostrov.

KEY
Geographical term *Language*, Term

A

Å *Danish, Norwegian*, River
Āb *Persian*, River
Adrar *Berber*, Mountains
Agía, Ágios *Greek*, Saint
Air *Indonesian*, River
Ákra *Greek*, Cape, point
Alpen *German*, Alps
Alt- *German*, Old
Altiplanicie *Spanish*, Plateau
Älve(en) *Swedish*, River
-ån *Swedish*, River
Anse *French*, Bay
'Aqabat *Arabic*, Pass
Archipiélago *Spanish*, Archipelago
Arcipelago *Italian*, Archipelago
Arquipélago *Portuguese*, Archipelago
Arrecife(s) *Spanish*, Reef(s)
Aru *Tamil*, River
Augstiene *Latvian*, Upland
Aukštuma *Lithuanian*, Upland
Aust- *Norwegian*, Eastern
Avtonomnyy Okrug *Russian*, Autonomous district
Āw *Kurdish*, River
'Ayn *Arabic*, Spring, well
'Ayoûn *Arabic*, Wells

B

Baelt *Danish*, Strait
Bahía *Spanish*, Bay
Baḥr *Arabic*, River
Baía *Portuguese*, Bay
Baie *French*, Bay
Bañado *Spanish*, Marshy land
Bandao *Chinese*, Peninsula
Banjaran *Malay*, Mountain range
Barajı *Turkish*, Dam
Barragem *Portuguese*, Reservoir
Bassin *French*, Basin
Batang *Malay*, Stream
Beinn, Ben *Gaelic*, Mountain
-berg *Afrikaans, Norwegian*, Mountain
Besar *Indonesian, Malay*, Big
Birkat, Birket *Arabic*, Lake, well, spring
Boğazi *Turkish*, Lake
Boka *Serbo-Croatian*, Bay
Bol'sh-aya, -iye, -oy, -oye *Russian*, Big
Botigh(i) *Uzbek*, Depression basin
-bre(en) *Norwegian*, Glacier
Bredning *Danish*, Bay
Bucht *German*, Bay
Bugt(en) *Danish*, Bay
Buḥayrat *Arabic*, Lake, reservoir
Buḥeiret *Arabic*, Lake
Bukit *Malay*, Mountain
-bukta *Norwegian*, Bay
bukten *Swedish*, Bay
Bulag *Mongolian*, Spring
Bulak *Uighur*, Spring
Burnu *Turkish*, Cape, point
Buuraha *Somali*, Mountains

C

Cabo *Portuguese*, Cape
Caka *Tibetan*, Salt lake
Canal *Spanish*, Channel
Cap *French*, Cape
Capo *Italian*, Cape, headland
Cascada *Portuguese*, Waterfall
Cayo(s) *Spanish*, Islet(s), rock(s)
Cerro *Spanish*, Mountain
Chaîne *French*, Mountain range
Chapada *Portuguese*, Hills, upland
Chau *Cantonese*, Island
Chāy *Turkish*, River
Chhâk *Cambodian*, Bay
Chhu *Tibetan*, River
-chŏsuji *Korean*, Reservoir
Chott *Arabic*, Depression, salt lake
Chūli *Uzbek*, Grassland, steppe
Ch'ün-tao *Chinese*, Island group
Chuŏr Phnum *Cambodian*, Mountains
Ciudad *Spanish*, City, town
Co *Tibetan*, Lake
Colline(s) *French*, Hill(s)
Cordillera *Spanish*, Mountain range
Costa *Spanish*, Coast
Côte *French*, Coast
Coxilha *Portuguese*, Mountains
Cuchilla *Spanish*, Mountains

D

Daban *Mongolian, Uighur*, Pass
Daği *Azerbaijani, Turkish*, Mountain
Dağlari *Azerbaijani, Turkish*, Mountains
-dake *Japanese*, Peak
-dal(en) *Norwegian*, Valley
Danau *Indonesian*, Lake
Dao *Chinese*, Island
Đao *Vietnamese*, Island
Daryā *Persian*, River
Daryācheh *Persian*, Lake
Dasht *Persian*, Desert, plain
Dawḥat *Arabic*, Bay
Denizi *Turkish*, Sea
Dere *Turkish*, Stream
Desierto *Spanish*, Desert
Dili *Azerbaijani*, Spit
-do *Korean*, Island
Dooxo *Somali*, Valley
Düzü *Azerbaijani*, Steppe
-dwīp *Bengali*, Island

E

-eilanden *Dutch*, Islands
Embalse *Spanish*, Reservoir
Ensenada *Spanish*, Bay
Erg *Arabic*, Dunes
Estany *Catalan*, Lake
Estero *Spanish*, Inlet
Estrecho *Spanish*, Strait
Étang *French*, Lagoon, lake
-ey *Icelandic*, Island
Ezero *Bulgarian, Macedonian*, Lake
Ezers *Latvian*, Lake

F

Feng *Chinese*, Peak
Fjord *Danish*, Fjord
-fjord(en) *Danish, Norwegian, Swedish*, fjord
-fjørdhur *Faeroese*, Fjord
Fleuve *French*, River
Fliegu *Maltese*, Channel
-fljór *Icelandic*, River
-flói *Icelandic*, Bay
Forêt *French*, Forest

G

-gan *Japanese*, Rock
-gang *Korean*, River
Ganga *Hindi, Nepali, Sinhala*, River
Gaoyuan *Chinese*, Plateau
Garagumy *Turkmen*, Sands
-gawa *Japanese*, River
Gebel *Arabic*, Mountain
-gebirge *German*, Mountain range
Ghadīr *Arabic*, Well
Ghubbat *Arabic*, Bay
Gjiri *Albanian*, Bay
Gol *Mongolian*, River
Golfe *French*, Gulf
Golfo *Italian, Spanish*, Gulf
Göl(ü) *Turkish*, Lake
Golyam, -a *Bulgarian*, Big
Gora *Russian, Serbo-Croatian*, Mountain
Góra *Polish*, Mountain
Gory *Russian*, Mountain
Gryada *Russian*, Ridge
Guba *Russian*, Bay
-gundo *Korean*, Island group
Gunung *Malay*, Mountain

H

Ḥadd *Arabic*, Spit
-haehyŏp *Korean*, Strait
Haff *German*, Lagoon
Hai *Chinese*, Bay, lake, sea
Haixia *Chinese*, Strait
Hamada *Arabic*, Plateau
Ḥammādat *Arabic*, Plateau
Hāmūn *Persian*, Lake
-hantō *Japanese*, Peninsula
Har, Haré *Hebrew*, Mountain
Ḥarrat *Arabic*, Lava-field
Hav(et) *Danish, Swedish*, Sea
Hawr *Arabic*, Lake
Hāyk' *Amharic*, Lake
He *Chinese*, River
-hegység *Hungarian*, Mountain range
Heide *German*, Heath, moorland
Helodrano *Malagasy*, Bay
Higashi- *Japanese*, East(ern)
Ḥiṣā' *Arabic*, Well
Hka *Burmese*, River
-ho *Korean*, Lake
Hô *Korean*, Reservoir
Ḥolot *Hebrew*, Dunes
Hora *Belorussian, Czech*, Mountain
Hrada *Belorussian*, Mountain, ridge
Hsi *Chinese*, River
Hu *Chinese*, Lake
Huk *Danish*, Point

I

Île(s) *French*, Island(s)
Ilha(s) *Portuguese*, Island(s)
Ilhéu(s) *Portuguese*, Islet(s)
Imeni *Russian*, In the name of
Inish- *Gaelic*, Island
Insel(n) *German*, Island(s)
Irmağı, Irmak *Turkish*, River
Isla(s) *Spanish*, Island(s)
Isola (Isole) *Italian*, Island(s)

J

Jabal *Arabic*, Mountain
Jāl *Arabic*, Ridge
-järv *Estonian*, Lake
-järvi *Finnish*, Lake
Jazā'ir *Arabic*, Islands
Jazīrat *Arabic*, Island
Jazīreh *Persian*, Island
Jebel *Arabic*, Mountain
Jezero *Serbo-Croatian*, Lake
Jezioro *Polish*, Lake
Jiang *Chinese*, River
-jima *Japanese*, Island
Jižní *Czech*, Southern
-jõgi *Estonian*, River
-joki *Finnish*, River
-jökull *Icelandic*, Glacier
Jūn *Arabic*, Bay
Juzur *Arabic*, Islands

K

Kaikyō *Japanese*, Strait
-kaise *Lappish*, Mountain
Kali *Nepali*, River
Kalnas *Lithuanian*, Mountain
Kalns *Latvian*, Mountain
Kang *Chinese*, Harbor
Kangri *Tibetan*, Mountain(s)
Kaôh *Cambodian*, Island
Kapp *Norwegian*, Cape
Káto *Greek*, Lower
Kavīr *Persian*, Desert
K'edi *Georgian*, Mountain range
Kediet *Arabic*, Mountain
Kepi *Albanian*, Cape, point
Kepulauan *Indonesian, Malay*, Island group
Khalig, Khalīj *Arabic*, Gulf
Khawr *Arabic*, Inlet
Khola *Nepali*, River
Khrebet *Russian*, Mountain range
Ko *Thai*, Island
-ko *Japanese*, Inlet, lake
Kólpos *Greek*, Bay
-kopf *German*, Peak
Körfäzi *Azerbaijani*, Bay
Körfezi *Turkish*, Bay
Kõrgustik *Estonian*, Upland
Kosa *Russian, Ukrainian*, Spit
Koshi *Nepali*, River
Kou *Chinese*, River-mouth
Kowtal *Persian*, Pass
Kray *Russian*, Region, territory
Kryazh *Russian*, Ridge
Kuduk *Uighur*, Well
Kūh(hā) *Persian*, Mountain(s)
-kul' *Russian*, Lake
Kŭl(i) *Tajik, Uzbek*, Lake
-kundo *Korean*, Island group
-kysten *Norwegian*, Coast
Kyun *Burmese*, Island

L

Laaq *Somali*, Watercourse
Lac *French*, Lake
Lacul *Romanian*, Lake
Lagh *Somali*, Stream
Lago *Italian, Portuguese, Spanish*, Lake
Lagoa *Portuguese*, Lagoon
Laguna *Italian, Spanish*, Lagoon, lake
Laht *Estonian*, Bay
Laut *Indonesian*, Bay
Lembalemba *Malagasy*, Plateau
Lerr *Armenian*, Mountain
Lerrnashght'a *Armenian*, Mountain range
Les *Czech*, Forest
Lich *Armenian*, Lake
Liehtao *Chinese*, Island group
Liqeni *Albanian*, Lake
Límni *Greek*, Lake
Ling *Chinese*, Mountain range
Llano *Spanish*, Plain, prairie
Lumi *Albanian*, River
Lyman *Ukrainian*, Estuary

M

Madīnat *Arabic*, City, town
Mae Nam *Thai*, River
-mägi *Estonian*, Hill
Maja *Albanian*, Mountain
Mal *Albanian*, Mountains
Mal-aya, -oye, -yy, *Russian*, Small
-man *Korean*, Bay
Mar *Spanish*, Lake
Marios *Lithuanian*, Lake
Massif *French*, Mountains
Meer *German*, Lake
-meer *Dutch*, Lake
Melkosopochnik *Russian*, Plain
-meri *Estonian*, Sea
Mifraz *Hebrew*, Bay
Minami- *Japanese*, South(ern)
-misaki *Japanese*, Cape, point
Monkhafad *Arabic*, Depression
Montagne(s) *French*, Mountain(s)
Montañas *Spanish*, Mountains
Mont(s) *French*, Mountain(s)
Monte *Italian, Portuguese*, Mountain
More *Russian*, Sea
Mörön *Mongolian*, River
Mys *Russian*, Cape, point

N

-nada *Japanese*, Open stretch of water
Nagor'ye *Russian*, Upland
Naḥal *Hebrew*, River
Nahr *Arabic*, River
Nam *Laotian*, River
Namakzār *Persian*, Salt desert
Né-a, -on, -os *Greek*, New
Nedre- *Norwegian*, Lower
-neem *Estonian*, Cape, point
Nehri *Turkish*, River
-nes *Norwegian*, Cape, point
Nevado *Spanish*, Mountain (snow-capped)
Nieder- *German*, Lower
Nishi- *Japanese*, West(ern)
-nísi *Greek*, Island
Nisoi *Greek*, Islands
Nizhn-eye, -iy, -iye, -yaya *Russian*, Lower
Nizmennost' *Russian*, Lowland, plain
Nord *Danish, French, German*, North
Norte *Portuguese, Spanish*, North
Nos *Bulgarian*, Point, spit
Nosy *Malagasy*, Island
Nov-a, -i, *Bulgarian, Serbo-Croatian*, New
Nov-aya, -o, -oye, -yy, -yye *Russian*, New
Now-a, -e, -y *Polish*, New
Nur *Mongolian*, Lake
Nuruu *Mongolian*, Mountains
Nuur *Mongolian*, Lake
Nyzovyna *Ukrainian*, Lowland, plain

O

-ø *Danish*, Island
Ober- *German*, Upper
Oblast' *Russian*, Province
Órmos *Greek*, Bay
Orol(i) *Uzbek*, Island
Øster- *Norwegian*, Eastern
Ostrov(a) *Russian*, Island(s)
Otok *Serbo-Croatian*, Island
Oued *Arabic*, Watercourse
-oy *Faeroese*, Island
-øy(a) *Norwegian*, Island
Oya *Sinhala*, River
Ozero *Russian, Ukrainian*, Lake

P

Passo *Italian*, Pass
Pegunungan *Indonesian, Malay*, Mountain range
Pélagos *Greek*, Sea
Pendi *Chinese*, Basin
Penisola *Italian*, Peninsula
Pertuis *French*, Strait
Peski *Russian*, Sands
Phanom *Thai*, Mountain
Phou *Laotian*, Mountain
Pi *Chinese*, Point
Pic *Catalan, French*, Peak
Pico *Portuguese, Spanish*, Peak
-piggen *Danish*, Peak
Pik *Russian*, Peak
Pivostriv *Ukrainian*, Peninsula
Planalto *Portuguese*, Plateau
Planina, Planini *Bulgarian, Macedonian, Serbo-Croatian*, Mountain range
Plato *Russian*, Plateau
Ploskogor'ye *Russian*, Upland
Poluostrov *Russian*, Peninsula
Ponta *Portuguese*, Point
Porthmós *Greek*, Strait
Pótamos *Greek*, River
Presa *Spanish*, Dam
Prokhod *Bulgarian*, Pass
Proliv *Russian*, Strait
Pulau *Indonesian, Malay*, Island
Pulu *Malay*, Island
Punta *Spanish*, Point
Pushcha *Belarussian*, Forest
Puszcza *Polish*, Forest

Q

Qā' *Arabic*, Depression
Qalamat *Arabic*, Well
Qatorkŭh(i) *Tajik*, Mountain
Qiuling *Chinese*, Hills
Qolleh *Persian*, Mountain
Qu *Tibetan*, Stream
Quan *Chinese*, Well
Qulla(i) *Tajik*, Peak
Qundao *Chinese*, Island group

R

Raas *Somali*, Cape
-rags *Latvian*, Cape
Ramlat *Arabic*, Sands
Ra's *Arabic*, Cape, headland, point
Ravnina *Bulgarian, Russian*, Plain
Récif *French*, Reef
Recife *Portuguese*, Reef
Reka *Bulgarian*, River
Represa (Rep.) *Portuguese, Spanish*, Reservoir
Reshteh *Persian*, Mountain range
Respublika *Russian*, Republic, first-order administrative division
Respublika(si) *Uzbek*, Republic, first-order administrative division
-retsugan *Japanese*, Chain of rocks
-rettō *Japanese*, Island chain
Riacho *Spanish*, Stream
Riban' *Malagasy*, Mountains
Rio *Portuguese*, River
Río *Spanish*, River
Riu *Catalan*, River
Rivier *Dutch*, River
Rivière *French*, River
Rowd *Pashtu*, River
Rt *Serbo-Croatian*, Point
Rūd *Persian*, River
Rūdkhāneh *Persian*, River
Rudohorie *Slovak*, Mountains
Ruisseau *French*, Stream

S

-saar *Estonian*, Island
-saari *Finnish*, Island
Sabkhat *Arabic*, Salt marsh
Sāgar(a) *Hindi*, Lake, reservoir
Ṣaḥrā' *Arabic*, Desert
Saint, Sainte *French*, Saint
Salar *Spanish*, Salt-pan
Salto *Portuguese, Spanish*, Waterfall
Samudra *Sinhala*, Reservoir
-san *Japanese, Korean*, Mountain
-sanchi *Japanese*, Mountains
-sandur *Icelandic*, Beach
Sankt *German, Swedish*, Saint
-sanmaek *Korean*, Mountain range
-sanmyaku *Japanese*, Mountain range
San, Santa, Santo *Italian, Portuguese, Spanish*, Saint
São *Portuguese*, Saint
Sarīr *Arabic*, Desert
Sebkha, Sebkhet *Arabic*, Depression, salt marsh
Sedlo *Czech*, Pass
See *German*, Lake
Selat *Indonesian*, Strait
Selatan *Indonesian*, Southern
-selkä *Finnish*, Lake, ridge
Selseleh *Persian*, Mountain range
Serra *Portuguese*, Mountain
Serranía *Spanish*, Mountain
-seto *Japanese*, Channel, strait
Sever-naya, -noye, -nyy, -o *Russian*, Northern
Sha'īb *Arabic*, Watercourse
Shākh *Kurdish*, Mountain
Shamo *Chinese*, Desert
Shan *Chinese*, Mountain(s)
Shankou *Chinese*, Pass
Shanmo *Chinese*, Mountain range
Shaṭṭ *Arabic*, Distributary
Shet' *Amharic*, River
Shi *Chinese*, Municipality
-shima *Japanese*, Island
Shiqqat *Arabic*, Depression
-shotō *Japanese*, Group of islands
Shuiku *Chinese*, Reservoir
Shūrkhog(i) *Uzbek*, Salt marsh
Sierra *Spanish*, Mountains
Sint *Dutch*, Saint
-sjø(en) *Norwegian*, Lake
-sjön *Swedish*, Lake
Solonchak *Russian*, Salt lake
Solonchakovyye Vpadiny *Russian*, Salt basin, wetlands
Son *Vietnamese*, Mountain
Sông *Vietnamese*, River
Sør- *Norwegian*, Southern
-spitze *German*, Peak
Star-á, -é *Czech*, Old
Star-aya, -oye, -yy, -yye *Russian*, Old
Stenó *Greek*, Strait
Step' *Russian*, Steppe
Štít *Slovak*, Peak
Stœng *Cambodian*, River
Stolovaya Strana *Russian*, Plateau
Stredné *Slovak*, Middle
Střední *Czech*, Middle
Stretto *Italian*, Strait
Su Anbari *Azerbaijani*, Reservoir
-suidō *Japanese*, Channel, strait
Sund *Swedish*, Sound, strait
Sungai *Indonesian, Malay*, River
Suu *Turkish*, River

T

Tal *Mongolian*, Plain
Tandavan' *Malagasy*, Mountain range
Tangorombohitr' *Malagasy*, Mountain massif
Tanjung *Indonesian, Malay*, Cape, point
Tao *Chinese*, Island
Ṭaraq *Arabic*, Hills
Tassili *Berber*, Mountain, plateau
Tau *Russian*, Mountain(s)
Taungdan *Burmese*, Mountain range
Techníti Límni *Greek*, Reservoir
Tekojärvi *Finnish*, Reservoir
Teluk *Indonesian, Malay*, Bay
Tengah *Indonesian*, Middle
Terara *Amharic*, Mountain
Timur *Indonesian*, Eastern
-tind(an) *Norwegian*, Peak
Tizma(si) *Uzbek*, Mountain range, ridge
-tō *Japanese*, Island
Tog *Somali*, Valley
-tōge *Japanese*, Pass
Togh(i) *Uzbek*, Mountain
Tônlé *Cambodian*, Lake
Top *Dutch*, Peak
-tunturi *Finnish*, Mountain
Ṭurāq *Arabic*, Hills
Tur'at *Arabic*, Channel

U

Udde(n) *Swedish*, Cape, point
'Uqlat *Arabic*, Well
Utara *Indonesian*, Northern
Uul *Mongolian*, Mountains

V

Väin *Estonian*, Strait
Vallée *French*, Valley
-vatn *Icelandic*, Lake
-vatnet *Norwegian*, Lake
Velayat *Turkmen*, Province
-vesi *Finnish*, Lake
Vestre- *Norwegian*, Western
-vidda *Norwegian*, Plateau
-vík *Icelandic*, Bay
-viken *Swedish*, Bay, inlet
Vinh *Vietnamese*, Bay
Víztárloló *Hungarian*, Reservoir
Vodaskhovishcha *Belarussian*, Reservoir
Vodokhranilishche (Vdkhr.) *Russian*, Reservoir
Vodoskhovyshche (Vdskh.) *Ukrainian*, Reservoir
Volcán *Spanish*, Volcano
Vostochn-o, yy *Russian*, Eastern
Vozvyshennost' *Russian*, Upland, plateau
Vozyera *Belarussian*, Lake
Vpadina *Russian*, Depression
Vrchovina *Czech*, Mountains
Vrha *Macedonian*, Peak
Vychodné *Slovak*, Eastern
Vysochyna *Ukrainian*, Upland
Vysočina *Czech*, Upland

W

Waadi *Somali*, Watercourse
Wādī *Arabic* Watercourse
Wāḥat, Wâhat *Arabic*, Oasis
Wald *German*, Forest
Wan *Chinese*, Bay
Way *Indonesian*, River
Webi *Somali*, River
Wenz *Amharic*, River
Wiloyat(i) *Uzbek*, Province
Wyżyna *Polish*, Upland
Wzgórza *Polish*, Upland
Wzvyshsha *Belarussian*, Upland

X

Xé *Laotian*, River
Xi *Chinese*, Stream

Y

-yama *Japanese*, Mountain
Yanchi *Chinese*, Salt lake
Yang *Chinese*, Bay
Yanhu *Chinese*, Salt lake
Yarımadası *Azerbaijani, Turkish*, Peninsula
Yaylası *Turkish*, Plateau
Yazovir *Bulgarian*, Reservoir
Yoma *Burmese*, Mountains
Ytre- *Norwegian*, Outer
Yü *Chinese*, Island
Yunhe *Chinese*, Canal
Yuzhn-o, -yy *Russian*, Southern

Z

-zaki *Japanese*, Cape, point
Zaliv *Bulgarian, Russian*, Bay
-zan *Japanese*, Mountain
Zangbo *Tibetan*, River
Zapadn-aya, -o, -yy *Russian*, Western
Západné *Slovak*, Western
Západní *Czech*, Western
Zatoka *Polish, Ukrainian*, Bay
-zee *Dutch*, Sea
Zemlya *Russian*, Earth, land
Zizhiqu *Chinese*, Autonomous region

Index

Glossary of Abbreviations

This glossary provides a comprehensive guide to the abbreviations used in this Atlas, and in the Index.

A
abbrev. abbreviated
AD Anno Domini
Afr. Afrikaans
Alb. Albanian
Amh. Amharic
anc. ancient
approx. approximately
Ar. Arabic
Arm. Armenian
ASEAN Association of South East Asian Nations
ASSR Autonomous Soviet Socialist Republic
Aust. Australian
Az. Azerbaijani
Azerb. Azerbaijan

B
Basq. Basque
BC before Christ
Bel. Belorussian
Ben. Bengali
Ber. Berber
B-H Bosnia-Herzegovina
bn billion (one thousand million)
BP British Petroleum
Bret. Breton
Brit. British
Bul. Bulgarian
Bur. Burmese

C
C central
C. Cape
°C degrees Centigrade
CACM Central America Common Market
Cam. Cambodian
Cant. Cantonese
CAR Central African Republic
Cast. Castilian
Cat. Catalan
CEEAC Central America Common Market
Chin. Chinese
CIS Commonwealth of Independent States
cm centimeter(s)
Cro. Croat
Cz. Czech
Czech Rep. Czech Republic

D
Dan. Danish
Div. Divehi
Dom. Rep. Dominican Republic
Dut. Dutch

E
E east
EC *see* EU
EEC *see* EU
ECOWAS Economic Community of West African States
ECU European Currency Unit
EMS European Monetary System
Eng. English
est estimated
Est. Estonian
EU European Union (previously European Community [EC], European Economic Community [EEC])

F
°F degrees Fahrenheit
Faer. Faeroese
Fij. Fijian
Fin. Finnish
Fr. French
Fris. Frisian
ft foot/feet
FYROM Former Yugoslav Republic of Macedonia

G
g gram(s)
Gael. Gaelic
Gal. Galician
GDP Gross Domestic Product (the total value of goods and services produced by a country excluding income from foreign countries)
Geor. Georgian
Ger. German
Gk Greek
GNP Gross National Product (the total value of goods and services produced by a country)

H
Heb. Hebrew
HEP hydroelectric power
Hind. Hindi
hist. historical
Hung. Hungarian

I
I. Island
Icel. Icelandic
in inch(es)
In. Inuit (Eskimo)
Ind. Indonesian
Intl International
Ir. Irish
Is Islands
It. Italian

J
Jap. Japanese

K
Kaz. Kazakh
kg kilogram(s)
Kir. Kirghiz
km kilometer(s)
km² square kilometer (singular)
Kor. Korean
Kurd. Kurdish

L
L. Lake
LAIA Latin American Integration Association
Lao. Laotian
Lapp. Lappish
Lat. Latin
Latv. Latvian
Liech. Liechtenstein
Lith. Lithuanian
Lux. Luxembourg

M
m million/meter(s)
Mac. Macedonian
Maced. Macedonia
Mal. Malay
Malg. Malagasy
Malt. Maltese
mi. mile(s)
Mong. Mongolian
Mt. Mountain
Mts Mountains

N
N north
NAFTA North American Free Trade Agreement
Nep. Nepali
Neth. Netherlands
Nic. Nicaraguan
Nor. Norwegian
NZ New Zealand

P
Pash. Pashtu
PNG Papua New Guinea
Pol. Polish
Poly. Polynesian
Port. Portuguese
prev. previously

R
Rep. Republic
Res. Reservoir
Rmsch Romansch
Rom. Romanian
Rus. Russian
Russ. Fed. Russian Federation

S
S south
SADC Southern Africa Development Community
SCr. Serbian/Croatian
Sinh. Sinhala
Slvk Slovak
Slvn. Slovene
Som. Somali
Sp. Spanish
St., St Saint
Strs Straits
Swa. Swahili
Swe. Swedish
Switz. Switzerland

T
Taj. Tajik
Th. Thai
Thai. Thailand
Tib. Tibetan
Turk. Turkish
Turkm. Turkmenistan

U
UAE United Arab Emirates
Uigh. Uighur
UK United Kingdom
Ukr. Ukrainian
UN United Nations
Urd. Urdu
US/USA United States of America
USSR Union of Soviet Socialist Republics
Uzb. Uzbek

V
var. variant
Vdkhr. Vodokhranilishche (Russian for reservoir)
Vdskh. Vodoskhovyshche (Ukrainian for reservoir)
Vtn. Vietnamese

W
W west
Wel. Welsh

Y
Yugo. Yugoslavia

This index lists all the placenames and features shown on the regional and continental maps in this Atlas. Placenames are referenced to the largest scale map on which they appear. The policy followed throughout the Atlas is to use the local spelling or local name at regional level; commonly-used English language names may occasionally be added (in parentheses) where this is an aid to identification e.g. Firenze (Florence). English names, where they exist, have been used for all international features e.g. oceans and country names; they are also used on the continental maps and in the introductory World Today section; these are then fully cross-referenced to the local names found on the regional maps. The index also contains commonly-found alternative names and variant spellings, which are also fully cross-referenced.

All main entry names are those of settlements unless otherwise indicated by the use of italicized definitions or representative symbols, which are keyed at the foot of each page.

1

25 de Mayo *see* Veinticinco de Mayo
137 *Y13* **26** *Bakı Komissarı* ***Rus.*** Imeni *26 Bakinskikh Komissarov. SE Azerbaijan*
26 *Baku Komissarlary Adyndaky* *see* Imeni 26 *Bakinskikh Komissarov*
10 *M16* **100** *Mile House* ***var.*** Hundred Mile House. British Columbia, SW Canada

A

Aa *see* Gauja
Aabenraa *see* Åbenrå
Aabybro *see* Åbybro
101 *C16* **Aachen** ***Dut.*** Aken, ***Fr.*** Aix-la-Chapelle; ***anc.*** Aquae Grani, Aquisgranum. Nordrhein-Westfalen, W Germany
Aaiún *see* Laâyoune
Aakirkeby *see* Åkirkeby
Aalborg *see* Ålborg
Aalborg Bugt *see* Ålborg Bugt
101 *J21* **Aalen** Baden-Württemberg, S Germany
Aalestrup *see* Ålestrup
98 *I11* **Aalsmeer** Noord-Holland, C Netherlands
99 *F18* **Aalst** ***Fr.*** Alost. Oost-Vlaanderen, C Belgium
99 *K18* **Aalst** Noord-Brabant, S Netherlands
98 *O12* **Aalten** Gelderland, E Netherlands
99 *D17* **Aalter** Oost-Vlaanderen, NW Belgium
Aanaar *see* Inari
Aanaarjävri *see* I narijärvi
93 *M17* **Äänekoski** Länsi-Suomi, W Finland
138 *H7* **Aanjar** ***var.*** 'Anjar. C Lebanon
83 *G21* **Aansluit** Northern Cape, N South Africa
Aar *see* Aare
108 *F7* **Aarau** Aargau, N Switzerland
108 *D8* **Aarberg** Bern, W Switzerland
99 *D16* **Aardenburg** Zeeland, SW Netherlands
108 *D8* **Aare** ***var.*** Aar. ~ W Switzerland
108 *F7* **Aargau** ***Fr.*** Argovie. ⬗ *canton* N Switzerland
Aarhus *see* Århus
Aarlen *see* Arlon
Aars *see* Års
99 *I17* **Aarschot** Vlaams Brabant, C Belgium
Aassi, Nahr el *see* Orontes
Aat *see* Ath
160 *G7* **Aba** ***prev.*** Ngawa. Sichuan, C China
77 *V17* **Aba** Abia, S Nigeria
79 *P16* **Aba** Orientale, NE Dem. Rep. Congo (Zaire)
140 *J6* **Abā al Qazāz, Bi'r** *well* NW Saudi Arabia
Abā as Su'ūd *see* Najrān
59 *G14* **Abacaxis, Rio** ~ NW Brazil
Abaco Island *see* Great Abaco/Little Abaco
Abaco Island *see* Great Abaco, N Bahamas
142 *K10* **Ābādān** Khūzestān, SW Iran
143 *O10* **Ābādeh** Fārs, C Iran
74 *H8* **Abadla** W Algeria
59 *M20* **Abaeté** Minas Gerais, SE Brazil
163 *Q10* **Abag Qi** ***var.*** Xin Hot. Nei Mongol Zizhiqu, N China
62 *P7* **Abaí** Caazapá, S Paraguay
191 *O2* **Abaiang** ***var.*** Apia; ***prev.*** Charlotte Island. *atoll* Tungaru, W Kiribati
Abaj *see* Abay
77 *U15* **Abaji** Federal Capital District, C Nigeria
37 *O7* **Abajo Peak** ▲ Utah, W USA
77 *V16* **Abakaliki** Ebonyi, SE Nigeria
122 *K13* **Abakan** Respublika Khakasiya, S Russian Federation
77 *S11* **Abala** Tillabéri, SW Niger
77 *U11* **Abalak** Tahoua, C Niger
119 *N14* **Abalyanka** ***Rus.*** Obolyanka. ~ N Belarus
122 *L12* **Aban** Krasnoyarskiy Kray, S Russian Federation
143 *P9* **Āb Anbār-e Kān Sorkh** Yazd, C Iran
57 *G16* **Abancay** Apurímac, SE Peru
190 *H2* **Abaokoro** *atoll* Tungaru, W Kiribati
Abariringa *see* Kanton
143 *P10* **Abarkū** Yazd, C Iran
165 *V3* **Abashiri** ***var.*** Abasiri. Hokkaidō, NE Japan
165 *U3* **Abashiri-ko** ◎ Hokkaidō, NE Japan
Abasiri *see* Abashiri
41 *P10* **Abasolo** Tamaulipas, C Mexico
186 *F9* **Abau** Central, S PNG
145 *R10* **Abay** ***var.*** Abaj. Karaganda, C Kazakhstan
81 *I15* **Ābaya Hāyk'** ***Eng.*** Lake Margherita, ***It.*** Abbaia. ◎ SW Ethiopia
Ābay Wenz *see* Blue Nile
122 *K13* **Abaza** Respublika Khakasiya, S Russian Federation
Abbaia *see* Ābaya Hāyk'
143 *Q13* **Āb Bārīk** Fārs, S Iran
107 *C18* **Abbasanta** Sardegna, Italy, C Mediterranean Sea
Abbatis Villa *see* Abbeville
30 *M3* **Abbaye, Point** *headland* Michigan, N USA
Abbazia *see* Opatija
Abbé, Lake *see* Abhe, Lake
103 *N2* **Abbeville** ***anc.*** Abbatis Villa. Somme, N France
23 *R7* **Abbeville** Alabama, S USA
23 *U6* **Abbeville** Georgia, SE USA
22 *I9* **Abbeville** Louisiana, S USA
21 *P12* **Abbeville** South Carolina, SE USA
97 *B20* **Abbeyfeale** ***Ir.*** Mainistir na Féile. SW Ireland
106 *D8* **Abbiategrasso** Lombardia, NW Italy
93 *I14* **Abborrträsk** Norrbotten, N Sweden
194 *J9* **Abbot Ice Shelf** *ice shelf* Antarctica
10 *M17* **Abbotsford** British Columbia, SW Canada
30 *K6* **Abbotsford** Wisconsin, N USA
149 *U5* **Abbottābād** North-West Frontier Province, NW Pakistan
119 *M14* **Abchuha** ***Rus.*** Obchuga. Minskaya Voblasts', NW Belarus
98 *I10* **Abcoude** Utrecht, C Netherlands
139 *N2* **'Abd al 'Azīz, Jabal** ▲ NE Syria
141 *U17* **'Abd al Kūrī** *island* SE Yemen
139 *Z13* **'Abd Allāh, Khawr** *bay* Iraq/Kuwait
129 *U6* **Abdulino** Orenburgskaya Oblast', W Russian Federation
78 *J10* **Abéché** ***var.*** Abécher, Abeshr. Ouaddaï, SE Chad
Abécher *see* Abéché
143 *S8* **Āb-e Garm va Sard** Khorāsān, E Iran
77 *R8* **Abeïbara** Kidal, NE Mali
105 *P5* **Abejar** Castilla-León, N Spain
54 *E9* **Abejorral** Antioquia, W Colombia
Abela *see* Ávila
Abellinum *see* Avellino
92 *Q2* **Abeløya** *island* Kong Karls Land, E Svalbard
80 *I13* **Ābeltī** Oromo, C Ethiopia
191 *O2* **Abemama** ***var.*** Apamama; ***prev.*** Roger Simpson Island. *atoll* Tungaru, W Kiribati
171 *Y15* **Abemaree** ***var.*** Abemarre. Irian Jaya, E Indonesia
77 *O16* **Abengourou** E Ivory Coast
95 *G24* **Åbenrå** ***var.*** Aabenraa, ***Ger.*** Apenrade. Sønderjylland, SW Denmark
101 *L22* **Abens** ~ SE Germany
77 *S16* **Abeokuta** Ogun, SW Nigeria
97 *I20* **Aberaeron** SW Wales, UK
Aberbrothock *see* Arbroath
Abercorn *see* Mbala
29 *R6* **Abercrombie** North Dakota, N USA
183 *T7* **Aberdeen** New South Wales, SE Australia
11 *T15* **Aberdeen** Saskatchewan, S Canada
83 *H25* **Aberdeen** Eastern Cape, S South Africa
96 *L9* **Aberdeen** ***anc.*** Devana. NE Scotland, UK
21 *X2* **Aberdeen** Maryland, NE USA
23 *N3* **Aberdeen** Mississippi, S USA
21 *T10* **Aberdeen** North Carolina, SE USA
29 *P8* **Aberdeen** South Dakota, N USA
32 *F8* **Aberdeen** Washington, NW USA
96 *K9* **Aberdeen** *cultural region* NE Scotland, UK
8 *L8* **Aberdeen Lake** ◎ Nunavut, NE Canada
96 *J10* **Aberfeldy** C Scotland, UK
97 *K21* **Abergavenny** ***anc.*** Gobannium. SE Wales, UK
Abergwaun *see* Fishguard
Abermarre *see* Abemaree
25 *N5* **Abernathy** Texas, SW USA
Abersee *see* Wolfgangsee
Abertawe *see* Swansea
Aberteifi *see* Cardigan
32 *I15* **Abert, Lake** ◎ Oregon, NW USA
97 *I20* **Aberystwyth** W Wales, UK
Abeshr *see* Abéché
106 *F10* **Abetone** Toscana, C Italy
127 *V5* **Abez'** Respublika Komi, NW Russian Federation
142 *M5* **Āb Garm** Qazvin, N Iran
141 *N12* **Abhā** 'Asīr, SW Saudi Arabia
142 *M5* **Abhar** Zanjān, NW Iran
Abhé Bad/Ābhē Bid Hāyk' *see* Abhe, Lake
80 *K12* **Abhe, Lake** ***var.*** Lake Abbé, ***Amh.*** Ābhē Bid Hāyk', ***Som.*** Abhé Bad. ◎ Djibouti/Ethiopia
77 *V17* **Abia** ⬗ *state* SE Nigeria
139 *V9* **'Abīd 'Alī** E Iraq
119 *O17* **Abidavichy** ***Rus.*** Obidovichi. Mahilyowskaya Voblasts', E Belarus
115 *L15* **Abide** Çanakkale, NW Turkey
77 *N17* **Abidjan** S Ivory Coast
Āb-i-Istāda *see* Īstādeh-ye Moqor, Āb-e-
27 *N4* **Abilene** Kansas, C USA
25 *Q7* **Abilene** Texas, SW USA
Abindonia *see* Abingdon
97 *M21* **Abingdon** ***anc.*** Abindonia. S England, UK
30 *K12* **Abingdon** Illinois, N USA
21 *P8* **Abingdon** Virginia, NE USA
Abingdon *see* Pinta, Isla
18 *J15* **Abington** Pennsylvania, NE USA
128 *K14* **Abinsk** Krasnodarskiy Kray, SW Russian Federation
37 *R9* **Abiquiu Reservoir** ▣ New Mexico, SW USA
92 *I10* **Abisko** Norrbotten, N Sweden
12 *G12* **Abitibi** ~ Ontario, S Canada
12 *H12* **Abitibi, Lac** ◎ Ontario/Quebec, S Canada
80 *J10* **Ābīy Ādī** Tigray, N Ethiopia
118 *H6* **Abja-Paluoja** Viljandimaa, S Estonia
137 *Q8* **Abkhazia** ⬗ *autonomous republic* NW Georgia
182 *F1* **Abminga** South Australia
75 *W9* **Abnûb** C Egypt
Åbo *see* Turku
152 *G9* **Abohar** Punjab, N India
77 *O17* **Aboisso** SE Ivory Coast
78 *H5* **Abo, Massif d'** ▲ NW Chad
77 *R16* **Abomey** S Benin
79 *F16* **Abong Mbang** Est, SE Cameroon
111 *L23* **Abony** Pest, C Hungary
78 *J11* **Abou-Déïa** Salamat, SE Chad
Aboudouhour *see* Abū aḍ Ḍuhūr
Abou Kémal *see* Abū Kamāl
Abou Simbel *see* Abu Simbel
137 *T12* **Abovyan** C Armenia
171 *O2* **Abra** ~ Luzon, N Philippines
141 *P15* **Abrād, Wādī** *seasonal river* W Yemen
Abraham Bay *see* The Carlton
104 *G10* **Abrantes** ***var.*** Abrántes. Santarém, C Portugal
62 *J4* **Abra Pampa** Jujuy, N Argentina
Abrashlare *see* Brezovo
54 *G7* **Abrego** Norte de Santander, N Colombia
Abrene *see* Pytalovo
40 *C7* **Abreojos, Punta** *headland* W Mexico
65 *J16* **Abrolhos Bank** *undersea feature* W Atlantic Ocean
119 *H19* **Abrova** ***Rus.*** Obrovo. Brestskaya Voblasts', SW Belarus
116 *G11* **Abrud** ***Ger.*** Gross-Schlatten, ***Hung.*** Abrudbánya. Alba, SW Romania
Abrudbánya *see* Abrud
118 *E6* **Abruka** *island* SW Estonia
107 *J15* **Abruzzese, Appennino** ▲ C Italy
107 *J14* **Abruzzo** ⬗ *region* C Italy
141 *N14* **'Abs** ***var.*** Sūq 'Abs. W Yemen
33 *T12* **Absaroka Range** ▲ Montana/Wyoming, NW USA
137 *Z11* **Abşeron Yarımadası** ***Rus.*** Apsheronskiy Poluostrov. *peninsula* E Azerbaijan
143 *N6* **Āb Shīrīn** Eşfahān, C Iran
139 *X10* **Abtān** SE Iraq
109 *R6* **Abtenau** Salzburg, NW Austria
164 *E12* **Abu** Yamaguchi, Honshū, SW Japan
152 *E14* **Ābu** Rājasthān, N India
138 *I4* **Abū aḍ Ḍuhūr** ***Fr.*** Aboudouhour. Idlib, NW Syria
143 *P17* **Abū al Abyaḍ** *island* C UAE
138 *K10* **Abū al Ḥuşayn, Khabrat** ◎ N Jordan
139 *R8* **Abū al Jīr** C Iraq
139 *Y12* **Abū al Khaşīb** ***var.*** Abul Khasib. SE Iraq
139 *U12* **Abū at Tubrah, Thaqb** *well* S Iraq
75 *V11* **Abu Balâs** ▲ SW Egypt
Abu Dhabi *see* Abū Ẓaby
139 *R8* **Abū Farūkh** C Iraq
80 *C12* **Abu Gabra** Southern Darfur, W Sudan
139 *P10* **Abū Ghār, Sha'īb** *dry watercourse* S Iraq
80 *G7* **Abu Hamed** River Nile, N Sudan
139 *O5* **Abū Ḥardān** ***var.*** Hajîne. Dayr az Zawr, E Syria
139 *T7* **Abū Ḥāssawīyah** E Iraq
138 *K10* **Abū Ḥifnah, Wādī** *dry watercourse* N Jordan
77 *V15* **Abuja** ● (Nigeria) Federal Capital District, C Nigeria
139 *R9* **Abū Jahaf, Wādī** *dry watercourse* C Iraq
56 *F12* **Abujao, Río** ~ E Peru
139 *U12* **Abū Jasrah** S Iraq
139 *O6* **Abū Kamāl** ***Fr.*** Abou Kémal. Dayr az Zawr, E Syria
165 *P12* **Abukuma-sanchi** ▲ Honshū, C Japan
Abula *see* Ávila
Abul Khasib *see* Abū al Khaşīb
79 *K16* **Abumombazi** ***var.*** Abumonbazi. Equateur, N Dem. Rep. Congo (Zaire)
Abumonbazi *see* Abumombazi
59 *D15* **Abunã** Rondônia, W Brazil
56 *K13* **Abunã, Rio** ***var.*** Río Abuná. ~ Bolivia/Brazil
138 *G10* **Abū Nuşayr** ***var.*** Abu Nuseir. 'Ammān, W Jordan
Abu Nuseir *see* Abū Nuşayr
139 *T12* **Abū Qabr** S Iraq
138 *K5* **Abū Raḩbah, Jabal** ▲ C Syria
139 *S5* **Abū Rajāsh** N Iraq

◆ Country ● Country Capital ◇ Dependent Territory ○ Dependent Territory Capital ⬗ Administrative Region ✈ International Airport ▲ Mountain ▲ Mountain Range ⛰ Volcano ~ River ◎ Lake ▣ Reservoir

139 W13 **Abū Raqrāq, Ghadīr** well S Iraq
152 E14 **Ābu Road** Rājasthān, N India
80 I6 **Abu Shagara, Ras** headland NE Sudan
75 W12 **Abu Simbel** var. Abou Simbel, Abū Sunbul. ancient monument S Egypt
139 U12 **Abū Sudayrah** S Iraq
139 T10 **Abū Şukhayr** S Iraq
Abū Sunbul see Abu Simbel
165 R4 **Abuta** Hokkaidō, NE Japan
185 E18 **Abut Head** headland South Island, NZ
80 E9 **Abu 'Urug** Northern Kordofan, C Sudan
80 K12 **Ābuyē Mēda** ▲ C Ethiopia
80 D11 **Abu Zabad** Western Kordofan, C Sudan
Abū Ẓabī see Abū Ẓaby
143 P16 **Abū Ẓaby** var. Abū Ẓabī, Eng. Abu Dhabi. ● (UAE) Abū Ẓaby, C UAE
75 X8 **Abu Zenima** E Egypt
95 N17 **Åby** Östergötland, S Sweden
Abyaḍ, Al Baḥr al see White Nile
95 G20 **Åbybro** var. Aabybro. Nordjylland, N Denmark
80 D13 **Abyei** Western Kordofan, S Sudan
Abyla see Ávila
Abymes see les Abymes
Abyssinia see Ethiopia
Acâba see Assaba
54 F11 **Acacias** Meta, C Colombia
58 L13 **Açailandia** Maranhão, E Brazil
Acaill see Achill Island
42 E8 **Acajutla** Sonsonate, W El Salvador
79 D17 **Acalayong** SW Equatorial Guinea
41 N13 **Acámbaro** Guanajuato, C Mexico
54 C6 **Acandí** Chocó, NW Colombia
104 H4 **A Cañiza** var. La Cañiza. Galicia, NW Spain
40 J11 **Acaponeta** Nayarit, C Mexico
40 J11 **Acaponeta, Río de** ≈ C Mexico
41 O16 **Acapulco** var. Acapulco de Juárez. Guerrero, S Mexico
Acapulco de Juárez see Acapulco
55 T13 **Acarai Mountains** Sp. Serra Acaraí. ⛰ Brazil/Guyana
Acaraí, Serra see Acarai Mountains
58 O13 **Acaraú** Ceará, NE Brazil
54 J6 **Acarigua** Portuguesa, N Venezuela
42 C6 **Acatenango, Volcán de** ☼ S Guatemala
41 Q15 **Acatlán** var. Acatlán de Osorio. Puebla, S Mexico
Acatlán de Osorio see Acatlán
41 S15 **Acayucan** var. Acayucán. Veracruz-Llave, E Mexico
Accho see 'Akko
21 Y5 **Accomac** Virginia, NE USA
77 Q17 **Accra** ● (Ghana) SE Ghana
97 L17 **Accrington** NW England, UK
61 B19 **Acebal** Santa Fe, C Argentina
101 H8 **Aceh** off. Daerah Istimewa Aceh, var. Acheen, Achin, Atchin, Atjeh. ◈ autonomous district NW Indonesia
107 M18 **Acerenza** Basilicata, S Italy
107 K17 **Acerra** anc. Acerrae. Campania, S Italy
Acerrae see Acerra
Ach'asar Lerr see Achkasar
57 J17 **Achacachi** La Paz, W Bolivia
54 K7 **Achaguas** Apure, C Venezuela
154 H12 **Achalpur** prev. Elichpur, Ellichpur. Mahārāshtra, C India
61 F18 **Achar** Tacuarembó, C Uruguay
115 H19 **Acharnés** var. Aharnes; prev. Akharnaí. Attikí, C Greece
Acheen see Aceh
99 K16 **Achel** Limburg, NE Belgium
115 D16 **Achelóos** var. Akhelóos, Aspropótamos; anc. Achelous. ≈ W Greece
Achelous see Achelóos
163 W8 **Acheng** Heilongjiang, NE China
109 N6 **Achenkirch** Tirol, W Austria
101 L24 **Achenpass** pass Austria/Germany
109 N7 **Achensee** ◎ W Austria
101 F22 **Achern** Baden-Württemberg, SW Germany
115 C16 **Acherón** ≈ W Greece
77 W11 **Achétinamou** ≈ S Niger
152 J12 **Achhnera** Uttar Pradesh, N India
42 C7 **Achiguate, Río** ≈ S Guatemala
97 A16 **Achill Head** Ir. Ceann Acla. headland W Ireland
97 A16 **Achill Island** Ir. Acaill. island W Ireland
100 H11 **Achim** Niedersachsen, NW Germany
149 S5 **Achin** Nangarhār, E Afghanistan
Achin see Aceh
122 K12 **Achinsk** Krasnoyarskiy Kray, S Russian Federation
162 E5 **Achit Nuur** ◎ NW Mongolia
137 T11 **Achkasar** Arm. Ach'asar Lerr. ▲ Armenia/Georgia
128 K13 **Achuyevo** Krasnodarskiy Kray, SW Russian Federation
81 F16 **Achwa** var. Aswa. ≈ N Uganda
136 E15 **Acıgöl** salt lake SW Turkey
107 L24 **Acireale** Sicilia, Italy, C Mediterranean Sea
Aciris see Agri
25 N7 **Ackerly** Texas, SW USA
22 M4 **Ackerman** Mississippi, S USA
29 W13 **Ackley** Iowa, C USA
44 J5 **Acklins Island** island SE Bahamas
Acla, Ceann see Achill Head
62 H11 **Aconcagua, Cerro** ▲ W Argentina
Açores/Açores, Arquipélago dos/Açores, Ilhas dos see Azores
104 G2 **A Coruña** Cast. La Coruña ◈ province Galicia, NW Spain
104 H2 **A Coruña** Cast. La Coruña, Eng. Corunna; anc. Caronium. Galicia, NW Spain
42 L10 **Acoyapa** Chontales, S Nicaragua
106 H13 **Acquapendente** Lazio, C Italy
106 J13 **Acquasanta Terme** Marche, C Italy
106 I13 **Acquasparta** Lazio, C Italy
106 C9 **Acqui Terme** Piemonte, NW Italy
Acrae see Palazzola Acreide
182 F7 **Acraman, Lake** salt lake South Australia
59 A15 **Acre** off. Estado do Acre. ◈ state W Brazil
Acre see 'Akko
59 C16 **Acre, Rio** ≈ W Brazil
107 N20 **Acri** Calabria, SW Italy
Acte see Ágion Óros
191 Y12 **Actéon, Groupe** island group Îles Tuamotu, SE French Polynesia
15 P12 **Acton-Vale** Quebec, SE Canada
41 P13 **Actopan** var. Actopán. Hidalgo, C Mexico
59 P14 **Açu** var. Assu. Rio Grande do Norte, E Brazil
Acunum Acusio see Montélimar
77 Q17 **Ada** SE Ghana
29 R5 **Ada** Minnesota, N USA
31 R12 **Ada** Ohio, N USA
27 O12 **Ada** Oklahoma, C USA
112 L8 **Ada** Serbia, N Yugoslavia
Ada Bazar see Adapazarı
40 D3 **Adair, Bahía de** bay NW Mexico
104 M7 **Adaja** ≈ N Spain
38 H17 **Adak Island** island Aleutian Islands, Alaska, USA
Adalia see Antalya
Adalia, Gulf of see Antalya Körfezi
141 X9 **Adam** N Oman
Adama see Nazrēt
60 I8 **Adamantina** São Paulo, S Brazil
79 E14 **Adamaoua** Eng. Adamawa. ◈ province N Cameroon
68 F11 **Adamaoua, Massif d'** Eng. Adamawa Highlands. plateau NW Cameroon
77 Y14 **Adamawa** ◈ state E Nigeria
Adamawa see Adamaoua
Adamawa Highlands see Adamaoua, Massif d'
106 F6 **Adamello** ▲ N Italy
81 J14 **Ādamī Tulu** Oromo, C Ethiopia
63 M23 **Adam, Mount** var. Monte Independencia. ▲ West Falkland, Falkland Islands
29 R16 **Adams** Nebraska, C USA
18 H8 **Adams** New York, NE USA
29 Q3 **Adams** North Dakota, N USA
155 I23 **Adam's Bridge** chain of shoals NW Sri Lanka
32 H10 **Adams, Mount** ▲ Washington, NW USA
Adam's Peak see Sri Pada
191 R16 **Adam's Rock** island Pitcairn Island, Pitcairn Islands
191 P16 **Adamstown** ○ (Pitcairn Islands) Pitcairn Island, Pitcairn Islands
20 G10 **Adamsville** Tennessee, S USA
25 S9 **Adamsville** Texas, SW USA
141 O17 **'Adan** Eng. Aden. SW Yemen
136 K16 **Adana** var. Seyhan. Adana, S Turkey
136 K16 **Adana** var. Seyhan. ◈ province S Turkey
Adâncata see Horlivka
169 V12 **Adang, Teluk** bay Borneo, C Indonesia
136 F11 **Adapazarı** prev. Ada Bazar. Sakarya, NW Turkey
80 H8 **Adarama** River Nile, NE Sudan
195 Q16 **Adare, Cape** headland Antarctica
106 E6 **Adda** anc. Addua. ≈ N Italy
80 A13 **Adda** ≈ W Sudan
143 Q17 **Aḍ Ḍab'īyah** Abū Ẓaby, C UAE
143 O18 **Aḍ Ḍafrah** desert S UAE
141 Q6 **Ad Dahnā'** desert E Saudi Arabia
74 A11 **Ad Dakhla** var. Dakhla. SW Western Sahara
Ad Dalanj see Dilling
Ad Damar see Ed Damer
Ad Damazīn see Ed Damazin
Ad Dāmir see Ed Damer
173 N2 **Ad Dammām** desert NE Saudi Arabia
141 R6 **Ad Dammān** var. Dammām. Ash Sharqīyah, NE Saudi Arabia
Ad Dāmūr see Damoûr
140 K5 **Ad Dār al Ḥamrā'** Tabūk, NW Saudi Arabia
140 M13 **Ad Darb** Jīzān, SW Saudi Arabia
141 O8 **Ad Dawādimī** Ar Riyāḍ, C Saudi Arabia
143 N16 **Ad Dawḥah** Eng. Doha. ● (Qatar) C Qatar
143 N16 **Ad Dawḥah** Eng. Doha. ✕ C Qatar
139 S6 **Ad Dawr** N Iraq
139 Y12 **Ad Dayr** var. Dayr, Shahbān. E Iraq
Addi Arkay see Ādī Ārk'ay
139 X15 **Ad Dibdibah** physical region Iraq/Kuwait
Aḍ Ḍiffah see Libyan Plateau
Addis Ababa see Ādīs Ābeba
Addison see Webster Springs
139 U10 **Ad Dīwānīyah** var. Diwaniyah. C Iraq
Addua see Adda
151 K22 **Addu Atoll** atoll S Maldives
Ad Dujail see Ad Dujayl
139 T7 **Ad Dujayl** var. Ad Dujail. N Iraq
Ad Duwaym/Ad Duwēm see Ed Dueim
99 D16 **Adegem** Oost-Vlaanderen, NW Belgium
23 U7 **Adel** Georgia, SE USA
29 U14 **Adel** Iowa, C USA
182 I9 **Adelaide** state capital South Australia
44 H2 **Adelaide** New Providence, N Bahamas
182 I9 **Adelaide** ✕ South Australia
194 H6 **Adelaide Island** island Antarctica
181 P2 **Adelaide River** Northern Territory, N Australia
76 M10 **'Adel Bagrou** Hodh ech Chargui, SE Mauritania
186 D6 **Adelbert Range** ⛰ N PNG
180 K3 **Adele Island** island Western Australia
107 O17 **Adelfia** Puglia, SE Italy
195 V16 **Adélie Coast** physical region Antarctica
195 V14 **Adélie, Terre** physical region Antarctica
Adelnau see Odolanów
Adelsberg see Postojna
Aden see 'Adan
141 Q17 **Aden, Gulf of** gulf SW Arabian Sea
77 V10 **Aderbissinat** Agadez, C Niger
Adhaim see Al 'Uẓaym
143 R16 **Adh Dhayd** var. Al Dhaid. Ash Shāriqah, NE UAE
140 M4 **'Adhfā'** spring/well NW Saudi Arabia
138 I13 **'Ādhriyāt, Jabāl al** ⛰ S Jordan
80 I10 **Ādī Ārk'ay** var. Addi Arkay. Amhara, N Ethiopia
182 C7 **Adieu, Cape** headland South Australia
106 H8 **Adige** Ger. Etsch. ≈ N Italy
80 J10 **Ādīgrat** Tigray, N Ethiopia
154 I13 **Ādilābād** var. Ādilābād. Andhra Pradesh, C India
35 P2 **Adin** California, W USA
171 V14 **Adi, Pulau** island E Indonesia
18 K8 **Adirondack Mountains** ⛰ New York, NE USA
80 J13 **Ādīs Ābeba** Eng. Addis Ababa. ● (Ethiopia) Ādīs Ābeba, C Ethiopia
80 J13 **Ādīs Ābeba** ✕ Ādīs Ābeba, C Ethiopia
80 I11 **Ādīs Zemen** Amhara, N Ethiopia
Adi Ugri see Mendefera
137 N15 **Adıyaman** Adıyaman, SE Turkey
137 N15 **Adıyaman** ◈ province S Turkey
116 L11 **Adjud** Vrancea, E Romania
45 T6 **Adjuntas** C Puerto Rico
Adjuntas, Presa de las see Vicente Guerrero, Presa
Ādkup see Erikub Atoll
128 L15 **Adler** Krasnodarskiy Kray, SW Russian Federation
Adler see Orlice
108 G7 **Adliswil** Zürich, NW Switzerland
32 G7 **Admiralty Inlet** inlet Washington, NW USA
39 X13 **Admiralty Island** island Alexander Archipelago, Alaska, USA
186 E5 **Admiralty Islands** island group N PNG
136 B14 **Adnan Menderes** ✕ (İzmir) İzmir, W Turkey
37 V6 **Adobe Creek Reservoir** ⊞ Colorado, C USA
77 T16 **Ado-Ekiti** Ekiti, SW Nigeria
Adola see Kibre Mengist
61 C23 **Adolfo González Chaues** Buenos Aires, E Argentina
155 H17 **Ādoni** Andhra Pradesh, C India
102 K15 **Adour** anc. Aturus. ≈ SW France
Adowa see Ādwa
105 O15 **Adra** Andalucía, S Spain
107 L24 **Adrano** Sicilia, Italy, C Mediterranean Sea
74 I9 **Adrar** C Algeria
76 K7 **Adrar** ◈ region C Mauritania
74 L11 **Adrar** ⛰ SE Algeria
74 A12 **Adrar Souttouf** ⛰ SW Western Sahara
Adrasman see Adrasmon
147 Q10 **Adrasmon** Rus. Adrasman. NW Tajikistan
78 K10 **Adré** Ouaddaï, E Chad
106 H9 **Adria** anc. Atria, Hadria, Hatria. Veneto, NE Italy
31 R10 **Adrian** Michigan, N USA
29 S11 **Adrian** Minnesota, N USA
27 R5 **Adrian** Missouri, C USA
24 M2 **Adrian** Texas, SW USA
21 S4 **Adrian** West Virginia, NE USA
Adrianople/Adrianopolis see Edirne
121 P7 **Adriatic Basin** undersea feature Adriatic Sea, N Mediterranean Sea
Adriatico, Mare see Adriatic Sea
106 L13 **Adriatic Sea** Alb. Deti Adriatik, It. Mare Adriatico, SCr. Jadransko More, Slvn. Jadransko Morje. sea N Mediterranean Sea
Adriatik, Deti see Adriatic Sea
Adua see Ādwa
Aduana del Sásabe see El Sásabe
79 O17 **Adusa** Orientale, NE Dem. Rep. Congo (Zaire)
118 J13 **Adutiškis** Švenčionys, E Lithuania
27 Y7 **Advance** Missouri, USA
65 D25 **Adventure Sound** bay East Falkland, Falkland Islands
80 J10 **Ādwa** var. Adowa, It. Adua. Tigray, N Ethiopia
123 Q8 **Adycha** ≈ NE Russian Federation
128 L14 **Adygeya, Respublika** ◈ autonomous republic SW Russian Federation
146 C11 **Adzhikui** Turkm. Ajyguyy. Balkanskiy Velayat, W Turkmenistan
77 N17 **Adzopé** SE Ivory Coast
127 U4 **Adz'va** ≈ NW Russian Federation
127 U5 **Adz'vavom** Respublika Komi, NW Russian Federation
Ædua see Autun
115 K19 **Aegean Islands** island group Greece/Turkey
Aegean North see Vóreion Aigaíon
115 I17 **Aegean Sea** Gk. Aigaíon Pélagos, Aigaío Pélagos, Turk. Ege Denizi. sea NE Mediterranean Sea
Aegean South see Nótion Aigaíon
118 H3 **Aegviidu** Ger. Charlottenhof. Harjumaa, NW Estonia
Aegyptus see Egypt
Aelana see Al 'Aqabah
Aelok see Ailuk Atoll
Aelōninae see Ailinginae Atoll
Aelōnļapļap see Ailinglaplap Atoll
Æmilia see Emilia-Romagna
Æmilianum see Millau
Aemona see Ljubljana
Aenaria see Ischia
Aeolian Islands see Eolie, Isole
191 Z3 **Aeon Point** headland Kiritimati, NE Kiribati
95 G24 **Ærø** Ger. Arrö. island C Denmark
95 H24 **Ærøskøbing** Fyn, C Denmark
Æsernia see Isernia
104 G3 **A Estrada** Galicia, NW Spain
115 C18 **Aetós** Itháki, Iónioi Nísoi, Greece, C Mediterranean Sea
191 Q8 **Afaahiti** Tahiti, W French Polynesia
139 U10 **'Afak** C Iraq
Afanasjevo see Afanas'yevo
127 T14 **Afanas'yevo** var. Afanasjevo. Kirovskaya Oblast', NW Russian Federation
Afándou see Afántou
115 O23 **Afántou** var. Afándou. Ródos, Dodekánisos, Greece, Aegean Sea
Afar Depression see Danakil Desert
80 K11 **Afar** ◈ region NE Ethiopia
191 O7 **Afareaitu** Moorea, W French Polynesia
140 L7 **'Afarīyah, Bi'r al** well NW Saudi Arabia
Afars et des Issas, Territoire Français des see Djibouti
83 D22 **Affenrücken** Karas, SW Namibia
Afghānestān, Dowlat-e Eslāmī-ye see Afghanistan
148 M6 **Afghanistan** off. Islamic State of Afghanistan, Per. Dowlat-e Eslāmī-ye Afghānestān; prev. Republic of Afghanistan. ◆ Islamic state C Asia
Afgoi see Afgooye
81 N17 **Afgooye** It. Afgoi. Shabeellaha Hoose, S Somalia
141 N8 **'Afīf** Ar Riyāḍ, C Saudi Arabia
77 V17 **Afikpo** Ebonyi, SE Nigeria
Afiun Karahissar see Afyon
94 H7 **Åfjord** Sør-Trøndelag, C Norway
109 V6 **Aflenz Kurort** Steiermark, E Austria
74 J6 **Aflou** N Algeria
81 L18 **Afmadow** Jubbada Hoose, S Somalia
39 Q14 **Afognak Island** island Alaska, USA
104 J2 **A Fonsagrada** Galicia, NW Spain
186 E9 **Afore** Northern, S PNG
59 O15 **Afrânio** Pernambuco, E Brazil
68-69 **Africa** continent
68 L11 **Africa, Horn of** physical region Ethiopia/Somalia
172 K11 **Africana Seamount** undersea feature SW Indian Ocean
86 A14 **African Plate** tectonic feature
138 I2 **'Afrīn** Ḥalab, N Syria
136 M15 **Afşin** Kahramanmaraş, C Turkey
98 J7 **Afsluitdijk** dam N Netherlands
29 U15 **Afton** Iowa, C USA
29 W9 **Afton** Minnesota, N USA
27 R8 **Afton** Oklahoma, C USA
136 F14 **Afyon** prev. Afyonkarahisar. Afyon, W Turkey
136 F14 **Afyon** var. Afiun Karahissar. ◈ province W Turkey
Afyonkarahisar see Afyon
Agadès see Agadez
77 V10 **Agadez** prev. Agadès. Agadez, C Niger
77 W8 **Agadez** ◈ department N Niger
74 E8 **Agadir** SW Morocco
64 M9 **Agadir Canyon** undersea feature SE Atlantic Ocean
145 R12 **Agadyr'** Zhezkazgan, C Kazakhstan
173 O7 **Agalega Islands** island group N Mauritius
42 K6 **Agalta, Sierra de** ⛰ E Honduras
122 I10 **Agan** ≈ C Russian Federation
Agana/Agaña see Hagåtña
188 B15 **Agana Bay** bay NW Guam
188 C16 **Agana Field** ✕ (Agana) C Guam
171 Kk13 **Agano-gawa** ≈ Honshū, C Japan
188 B17 **Aga Point** headland S Guam
154 G9 **Agar** Madhya Pradesh, C India
81 I14 **Āgaro** Oromo, C Ethiopia
153 V15 **Agartala** Tripura, NE India
194 I5 **Agassiz, Cape** headland Antarctica
9 N2 **Agassiz Ice Cap** ice feature Nunavut, N Canada
175 V13 **Agassiz Fracture Zone** tectonic feature S Pacific Ocean
188 B16 **Agat** W Guam
188 B16 **Agat Bay** bay W Guam
145 P13 **Agat, Gory** hill C Kazakhstan
Agatha see Agde
115 M20 **Agathónisi** island Dodekánisos, Greece, Aegean Sea
171 X14 **Agats** Irian Jaya, E Indonesia
155 C21 **Agatti Island** island Lakshadweep, India, N Indian Ocean
38 D16 **Agattu Island** island Aleutian Islands, Alaska, USA
38 D16 **Agattu Strait** strait Aleutian Islands, Alaska, USA
14 B8 **Agawa** ≈ Ontario, S Canada
14 B8 **Agawa Bay** lake bay Ontario, S Canada
77 N17 **Agboville** SE Ivory Coast
137 V12 **Ağdam** Rus. Agdam. SW Azerbaijan
103 P16 **Agde** anc. Agatha. Hérault, S France
103 P16 **Agde, Cap d'** headland S France
Agedabia see Ajdābiyā
102 L14 **Agen** anc. Aginnum. Lot-et-Garonne, SW France
Agendicum see Sens
165 O13 **Ageo** Saitama, Honshū, S Japan
109 R5 **Ager** ≈ N Austria
Agere Hiywet see Hāgere Hiywet
108 G8 **Ägerisee** ◎ W Switzerland
142 M10 **Āghā Jārī** Khūzestān, SW Iran
39 P15 **Aghiyuk Island** island Alaska, USA
74 B12 **Aghouinit** SE Western Sahara
Aghri Dagh see Büyükağrı Dağı
74 B10 **Aghzoumal, Sebkhet** var. Sebjet Agsumal. salt lake E Western Sahara
115 F15 **Agiá** var. Ayiá. Thessalía, C Greece
40 G7 **Agiabampo, Estero de** estuary NW Mexico
121 P3 **Agía Fýlaxis** var. Ayia Phyla. S Cyprus
Agialoúsa see Yenierenköy
115 M21 **Agía Marína** Léros, Dodekánisos, Greece, Aegean Sea
121 Q2 **Agía Nápa** var. Ayia Napa. E Cyprus
115 L16 **Agía Paraskeví** Lésvos, E Greece
115 J15 **Agías Eirínis, Akrotírio** headland Límnos, E Greece
115 L17 **Agiasós** var. Ayiásos, Ayiássos. Lésvos, E Greece
Aginnum see Agen
123 O14 **Aginskiy Buryatskiy Avtonomnyy Okrug** ◈ autonomous district S Russian Federation
123 O14 **Aginskoye** Aginskiy Buryatskiy Avtonomnyy Okrug, S Russian Federation
115 I14 **Ágion Óros** Eng. Mount Athos. ◈ monastic republic NE Greece
115 H14 **Ágion Óros** var. Akte, Aktí; anc. Acte. peninsula NE Greece
114 D13 **Ágios Achílleios** religious building Dytikí Makedonía, N Greece
115 J16 **Ágios Efstrátios** var. Áyios Evstrátios, Hagios Evstrátios. island E Greece
115 H20 **Ágios Geórgios** island Kykládes, Greece, Aegean Sea
115 Q23 **Ágios Geórgios** island SE Greece
115 E21 **Ágios Ilías** ▲ S Greece
115 K25 **Ágios Ioannis, Akrotírio** headland Kríti, Greece, E Mediterranean Sea
115 L20 **Ágios Kírykos** var. Áyios Kírikos. Ikaría, Dodekánisos, Greece, Aegean Sea
115 D16 **Ágios Nikolaos** Thessalía, C Greece
115 K25 **Ágios Nikólaos** var. Áyios Nikólaos. Kríti, Greece, E Mediterranean Sea
115 H14 **Agíou Órous, Kólpos** gulf N Greece
107 K24 **Agira** anc. Agyrium. Sicilia, Italy, C Mediterranean Sea
115 G20 **Agkístri** island S Greece
114 G12 **Agkístro** var. Angistro. ▲ NE Greece
103 O17 **Agly** ≈ S France
Agnetheln see Agnita
14 E10 **Agnew Lake** ◎ Ontario, S Canada
77 O16 **Agnibilékrou** E Ivory Coast
116 I11 **Agnita** Ger. Agnetheln, Hung. Szentágota. Sibiu, SW Romania
107 K15 **Agnone** Molise, C Italy
164 K14 **Ago** Mie, Honshū, SW Japan
106 C8 **Agogna** ≈ N Italy
Agoitz see Aoiz-Agoitz
77 P17 **Agona Swedru** var. Swedru. SE Ghana
Agordat see Akurdet
Agosta see Augusta
103 N15 **Agout** ≈ S France
152 J12 **Āgra** Uttar Pradesh, N India
Agra and Oudh, United Provinces of see Uttar Pradesh
Agram see Zagreb
105 U5 **Agramunt** Cataluña, NE Spain
105 Q5 **Agreda** Castilla-León, N Spain
137 S13 **Ağrı** var. Karaköse; prev. Karakılısse. Ağrı, NE Turkey
137 S13 **Ağrı** ◈ province NE Turkey
107 N19 **Agri** anc. Aciris. ≈ S Italy
Agri Dagi see Büyükağrı Dağı
107 J24 **Agrigento** Gk. Akragas; prev. Girgenti. Sicilia, Italy, C Mediterranean Sea
188 K4 **Agrihan** island N Northern Mariana Islands
115 D18 **Agrínio** prev. Agrinion. Dytikí Ellás, W Greece
Agrinion see Agrínio
115 G17 **Agriovótano** Évvoia, C Greece
107 L18 **Agropoli** Campania, S Italy
129 T3 **Agryz** Udmurtskaya Respublika, NW Russian Federation
137 U11 **Ağstafa** Rus. Akstafa. NW Azerbaijan
Agsumal, Sebjet see Aghzoumal, Sebkhet
40 J11 **Agua Brava, Laguna** lagoon W Mexico
54 F7 **Aguachica** Cesar, N Colombia
59 J20 **Água Clara** Mato Grosso do Sul, SW Brazil
44 D5 **Aguada de Pasajeros** Cienfuegos, C Cuba
54 J5 **Aguada Grande** Lara, N Venezuela
45 S5 **Aguadilla** W Puerto Rico
43 S16 **Aguadulce** Coclé, S Panama
104 L14 **Aguadulce** Andalucía, S Spain
41 O8 **Agualeguas** Nuevo León, NE Mexico
40 L9 **Aguanaval, Río** ≈ C Mexico
42 J5 **Aguán, Río** ≈ N Honduras
25 R16 **Agua Nueva** Texas, SW USA
60 J8 **Aguapeí, Rio** ≈ S Brazil
61 E14 **Aguapey, Río** ≈ NE Argentina
40 G3 **Agua Prieta** Sonora, NW Mexico
104 G5 **A Guardia** var. Laguardia, La Guardia. Galicia, NW Spain
56 E6 **Aguarico, Río** ≈ Ecuador/Peru
55 O6 **Aguasay** Monagas, NE Venezuela
40 M12 **Aguascalientes** Aguascalientes, C Mexico
40 L12 **Aguascalientes** ◈ state C Mexico
57 I18 **Aguas Calientes, Río** ≈ S Peru
105 R7 **Aguasvivas** ≈ NE Spain
60 J7 **Água Vermelha, Represa de** ⊞ S Brazil
56 E12 **Aguaytía** Ucayali, C Peru
104 I5 **A Gudiña** var. La Gudiña. Galicia, NW Spain
104 G7 **Águeda** Aveiro, N Portugal
104 J8 **Águeda** ≈ Portugal/Spain
77 Q8 **Aguelhok** Kidal, NE Mali
77 V12 **Aguié** Maradi, S Niger
188 K8 **Aguijan** island S Northern Mariana Islands
104 M14 **Aguilar** var. Aguilar de la Frontera. Andalucía, S Spain
104 M3 **Aguilar de Campóo** Castilla-León, N Spain
Aguilar de la Frontera see Aguilar
42 F7 **Aguilares** San Salvador, C El Salvador
105 Q14 **Aguilas** Murcia, SE Spain
40 L15 **Aguililla** Michoacán de Ocampo, SW Mexico
Agulhas see L'Agulhas
172 J11 **Agulhas Bank** undersea feature SW Indian Ocean
172 K11 **Agulhas Basin** undersea feature SW Indian Ocean
83 F26 **Agulhas, Cape** Afr. Kaap Agulhas. headland SW South Africa
Agulhas, Kaap see Agulhas, Cape
60 O9 **Agulhas Negras, Pico das** ▲ SE Brazil
172 K11 **Agulhas Plateau** undersea feature SW Indian Ocean
165 S16 **Aguni-jima** island Nansei-shotō, SW Japan
Agurain see Salvatierra
54 G5 **Agustín Codazzi** var. Codazzi. Cesar, N Colombia
Agyrium see Agira
74 L12 **Ahaggar** high plateau region SE Algeria
Ahal Welayaty see Akhalskiy Velayat
142 K2 **Ahar** Āzarbāyjān-e Khāvarī, NW Iran
Aharnes see Acharnés
138 J3 **Aḥaṣ, Jabal** ▲ NW Syria
138 J3 **Aḥaṣ, Jebal** ⛰ W Syria
185 G16 **Ahaura** ≈ South Island, NZ
100 E13 **Ahaus** Nordrhein-Westfalen, NW Germany
191 U9 **Ahe** atoll Îles Tuamotu, C French Polynesia
184 N10 **Ahimanawa Range** ⛰ North Island, NZ
119 I19 **Ahinski Kanal** Rus. Oginskiy Kanal. canal SW Belarus
186 G10 **Ahioma** SE PNG
184 I2 **Ahipara** Northland, North Island, NZ
184 I2 **Ahipara Bay** bay SE Tasman Sea
39 N13 **Ahklun Mountains** ⛰ Alaska, USA
137 R14 **Ahlat** Bitlis, E Turkey
101 F14 **Ahlen** Nordrhein-Westfalen, W Germany
154 D10 **Ahmadābād** var. Ahmedabad. Gujarāt, W India
143 R10 **Ahmadābād** Kermān, C Iran
Ahmadi see Al Aḥmadī
Ahmad Khel see Ḥasan Khēl
155 F14 **Ahmadnagar** var. Ahmednagar. Mahārāshtra, W India
149 T9 **Ahmadpur Siāl** Punjab, E Pakistan
77 N5 **Aḥmar, 'Erg el** desert N Mali
80 K13 **Ahmar Mountains** ⛰ C Ethiopia
Ahmedabad see Ahmadābād
Ahmednagar see Ahmadnagar
114 N12 **Ahmetbey** Kırklareli, NW Turkey
14 H12 **Ahmic Lake** ◎ Ontario, S Canada
190 G12 **Ahoa** Île Uvea, E Wallis and Futuna
40 G8 **Ahomé** Sinaloa, C Mexico
21 X8 **Ahoskie** North Carolina, SE USA
101 D17 **Ahr** ≈ W Germany
143 N12 **Ahram** var. Ahrom. Būshehr, S Iran
100 J9 **Ahrensburg** Schleswig-Holstein, N Germany
Ahrom see Ahram
93 L17 **Ähtäri** Länsi-Suomi, W Finland
40 K12 **Ahuacatlán** Nayarit, C Mexico
42 E7 **Ahuachapán** Ahuachapán, W El Salvador
42 A9 **Ahuachapán** ◈ department W El Salvador
191 V16 **Ahu Akivi** var. Siete Moai. ancient monument Easter Island, Chile, E Pacific Ocean

◆ Country ● Country Capital ◇ Dependent Territory ○ Dependent Territory Capital ◈ Administrative Region ✕ International Airport ▲ Mountain ⛰ Mountain Range ☼ Volcano ≈ River ◎ Lake ⊞ Reservoir

191 W11 Ahunui atoll Îles Tuamotu, C French Polynesia
185 E20 Ahuriri ≈ South Island, NZ
95 L22 Åhus Skåne, S Sweden
Ahu Tahira see Ahu Vinapu
191 V16 Ahu Tepeu ancient monument Easter Island, Chile, E Pacific Ocean
191 V17 Ahu Vinapu var. Ahu Tahira. ancient monument Easter Island, Chile, E Pacific Ocean
142 L9 Ahvāz var. Ahwāz; prev. Nāsiri. Khūzestān, SW Iran
Ahvenanmaa see Åland
141 Q16 Aḥwar SW Yemen
Ahwāz see Ahvāz
Aibak see Āybak
101 K22 Aichach Bayern, SE Germany
164 L14 Aichi off. Aichi-ken, var. Aiti. ❖ prefecture Honshū, SW Japan
Aïdin see Aydın
Aidussina see Ajdovščina
Aifir, Clochán an see Giant's Causeway
Aigaíon Pélagos/Aigaío Pélagos see Aegean Sea
109 S3 Aigen im Mühlkreis Oberösterreich, N Austria
115 G20 Aígina var. Aíyina, Egina. Aígina, C Greece
115 G20 Aígina island S Greece
115 E18 Aígio var. Egio; prev. Aíyion. Dytikí Ellás, S Greece
108 C10 Aigle Vaud, SW Switzerland
103 P14 Aigoual, Mont ▲ S France
173 O16 Aigrettes, Pointe des headland W Réunion
61 G19 Aiguá var. Aigua. Maldonado, S Uruguay
103 S13 Aigues ≈ SE France
103 N10 Aigurande Indre, C France
Ai-hun see Heihe
165 N10 Aikawa Niigata, Sado, C Japan
21 Q13 Aiken South Carolina, SE USA
25 N4 Aiken Texas, SW USA
160 F13 Ailao Shan ⛰ SW China
43 W14 Ailigandí San Blas, NE Panama
189 R4 Ailinginae Atoll var. Aelōninae. atoll Ralik Chain, SW Marshall Islands
189 T7 Ailinglaplap Atoll var. Aelōnlaplap. atoll Ralik Chain, S Marshall Islands
Aillionn, Loch see Allen, Lough
96 H13 Ailsa Craig island SW Scotland, UK
189 V5 Ailuk Atoll var. Aelok. atoll Ratak Chain, NE Marshall Islands
123 R11 Aim Khabarovskiy Kray, E Russian Federation
103 R11 Ain ❖ department E France
103 S10 Ain ≈ E France
118 G7 Ainaži Est. Heinaste, Ger. Hainasch. Limbaži, N Latvia
74 L6 Aïn Beida NE Algeria
76 K4 'Aïn Ben Tili Tiris Zemmour, N Mauritania
74 J5 Aïn Defla var. Aïn Eddefla. N Algeria
Aïn Eddefla see Aïn Defla
74 L5 Aïn El Bey × (Constantine) NE Algeria
115 C19 Aínos ▲ Kefallinía, Iónioi Nísoi, Greece, C Mediterranean Sea
105 T4 Ainsa Aragón, NE Spain
74 I7 Aïn Sefra NW Algeria
29 N13 Ainsworth Nebraska, C USA
Aintab see Gaziantep
74 H5 Aïn Témouchent N Algeria
186 C6 Aiome Madang, N PNG
Aïoun el Atrous/Aïoun el Atroûss see 'Ayoûn el 'Atroûs
54 E11 Aipe Huila, C Colombia
56 D9 Aipena, Río ≈ N Peru
57 L19 Aiquile Cochabamba, C Bolivia
Aïr see Aïr, Massif de l'
188 E10 Airai Babeldaob, C Palau
188 E10 Airai × (Oreor) Babeldaob, N Palau
168 I11 Airbangis Sumatera, NW Indonesia
11 Q16 Airdrie Alberta, SW Canada
96 I12 Airdrie S Scotland, UK
Air du Azbine see Aïr, Massif de l'
97 M17 Aire ≈ N England, UK
102 K15 Aire-sur-l'Adour Landes, SW France
103 O1 Aire-sur-la-Lys Pas-de-Calais, N France
9 Q6 Air Force Island island Baffin Island, Nunavut, NE Canada
169 Q13 Airhitam, Teluk bay Borneo, C Indonesia
171 Q11 Airmadidi Sulawesi, N Indonesia
77 V8 Aïr, Massif de l' var. Aïr, Air du Azbine, Asben. ⛰ NC Niger
108 G10 Airolo Ticino, S Switzerland
102 K9 Airvault Deux-Sèvres, W France
101 K19 Aisch ≈ S Germany
63 G20 Aisén off. Región Aisén del General Carlos Ibañez del Campo, var. Aysen. ❖ region S Chile
10 H7 Aishihik Lake ◎ Yukon Territory, W Canada
103 P3 Aisne ❖ department N France
103 R4 Aisne ≈ NE France
109 T4 Aist ≈ N Austria
114 K13 Aisými Anatolikí Makedonía kai Thráki, NE Greece
105 S11 Aitana ▲ E Spain
186 B5 Aitape var. Eitape. Sandaun, NW PNG
Aiti see Aichi
29 V6 Aitkin Minnesota, N USA
115 D18 Aitolikó var. Etoliko; prev. Aitolikón. Dytikí Ellás, C Greece
Aitolikón see Aitolikó
190 L15 Aitutaki island S Cook Islands
116 H11 Aiud Ger. Strassburg, Hung. Nagyenyed; prev. Engeten. Alba, SW Romania
118 I9 Aiviekste ≈ C Latvia
189 Q8 Aiwo SW Nauru
188 E8 Aiwokako Passage passage Babeldaob, N Palau
Aix see Aix-en-Provence
103 S15 Aix-en-Provence var. Aix; anc. Aquae Sextiae. Bouches-du-Rhône, SE France
Aix-la-Chapelle see Aachen
103 T11 Aix-les-Bains Savoie, E France
186 A6 Aiyang, Mount ▲ NW PNG
Aíyina see Aígina
Aíyion see Aígio
153 W15 Āizawl Mizoram, NE India
118 H9 Aizkraukle Aizkraukle, S Latvia
118 C9 Aizpute Liepāja, W Latvia
165 O11 Aizu-Wakamatsu var. Aizuwakamatu. Fukushima, Honshū, C Japan
Aizuwakamatu see Aizu-Wakamatsu
103 X15 Ajaccio Corse, France, C Mediterranean Sea
103 X15 Ajaccio, Golfe d' gulf Corse, France, C Mediterranean Sea
41 Q15 Ajalpán Puebla, S Mexico
154 F13 Ajanta Range ⛰ C India
137 R10 Ajaria ❖ autonomous republic SW Georgia
Ajastan see Armenia
93 G14 Ajaureforsen Västerbotten, N Sweden
185 H17 Ajax, Mount ▲ South Island, NZ
162 F9 Aj Bogd Uul ▲ SW Mongolia
75 R8 Ajdābiyā var. Agedabia, Ajdābiyah. NE Libya
Ajdābiyah see Ajdābiyā
109 S12 Ajdovščina Ger. Haidenschaft, It. Aidussina. W Slovenia
165 Q7 Ajigasawa Aomori, Honshū, C Japan
Ajjinena see El Geneina
111 H23 Ajka Veszprém, W Hungary
138 G9 'Ajlūn Irbid, N Jordan
138 H9 'Ajlūn, Jabal ⛰ W Jordan
143 R15 'Ajmān var. Ajman, 'Ujmān. 'Ajmān, NE UAE
152 G12 Ajmer var. Ajmere. Rājasthān, N India
36 J15 Ajo Arizona, SW USA
105 N2 Ajo, Cabo de headland N Spain
36 J16 Ajo Range ⛰ Arizona, SW USA
Ajyguyy see Adzhikui
Akaba see Al 'Aqabah
165 T3 Akabira Hokkaidō, NE Japan
165 N10 Akadomari Niigata, Sado, C Japan
81 E20 Akagera var. Kagera. ≈ Rwanda/Tanzania see also Kagera
191 W16 Akahanga, Punta headland Easter Island, Chile, E Pacific Ocean
80 J13 Āk'ak'i Oromo, C Ethiopia
155 G15 Akalkot Mahārāshtra, W India
Akamagaseki see Shimonoseki
165 U4 Akan Hokkaidō, NE Japan
165 U4 Akan-ko ◎ Hokkaidō, NE Japan
Akanthoú see Tatlısu
185 I19 Akaroa Canterbury, South Island, NZ
80 E6 Akasha Northern, N Sudan
164 I13 Akashi var. Akasi. Hyōgo, Honshū, SW Japan
139 N7 'Akāsh, Wādī var. Wādī 'Ukash. dry watercourse W Iraq
Akasi see Akashi
92 K11 Äkäsjokisuu Lappi, N Finland
137 S11 Akbaba Dağı ▲ Armenia/Turkey
136 B15 Akbük Limanı bay W Turkey
129 V8 Akbulak Orenburgskaya Oblast', W Russian Federation
137 O11 Akçaabat Trabzon, NE Turkey
137 N15 Akçadağ Malatya, C Turkey
136 G11 Akçakoca Bolu, NW Turkey
Akchakaya, Vpadina see Akdzhakaya, Vpadina
76 H7 Akchâr desert W Mauritania
145 S12 Akchatau Kaz. Aqshataū. Zhezkazgan, C Kazakhstan
136 L13 Akdağlar ⛰ C Turkey
136 E17 Ak Dağları ⛰ SW Turkey
136 K13 Akdağmadeni Yozgat, C Turkey
146 G8 Akdepe prev. Ak-Tepe, Leninsk, Turkm. Lenin. Dashkhovuzskiy Velayat, N Turkmenistan
Ak-Dere see Byala
121 P2 Akdoğan Gk. Lýsi. C Cyprus
122 D14 Ak-Dovurak Respublika Tyva, S Russian Federation
146 F9 Akdzhakaya, Vpadina var. Vpadina Akchakaya. depression N Turkmenistan
171 S11 Akelamo Pulau Halmahera, E Indonesia
Aken see Aachen
Akermanceaster see Bath
95 P15 Åkersberga Stockholm, C Sweden
95 H15 Akershus ❖ county S Norway
79 L16 Aketi Orientale, N Dem. Rep. Congo (Zaire)
Akgyr Erezi see Gryada Akkyr
146 E12 Akhalskiy Velayat Turkm. Ahal Welayaty. ❖ province C Turkmenistan
137 S10 Akhalts'ikhe SW Georgia
Akhangaran see Ohangaron
Akharnaí see Acharnés
75 R7 Akhḍar, Al Jabal al hill range NE Libya
Akhelóös see Achelóos
39 Q15 Akhiok Kodiak Island, Alaska, USA
136 C13 Akhisar Manisa, W Turkey
75 X10 Akhmīm anc. Panopolis. C Egypt
152 H6 Akhnūr Jammu and Kashmir, NW India
129 P11 Akhtuba ≈ SW Russian Federation
129 P11 Akhtubinsk Astrakhanskaya Oblast', SW Russian Federation
Akhtyrka see Okhtyrka
164 H14 Aki Kōchi, Shikoku, SW Japan
39 N12 Akiachak Alaska, USA
39 N12 Akiak Alaska, USA
191 X11 Akiaki atoll Îles Tuamotu, E French Polynesia
12 H9 Akimiski Island island Nunavut, C Canada
136 K17 Akıncı Burnu headland S Turkey
Akıncılar see Selçuk
117 U10 Akinovka Zaporiz'ka Oblast', S Ukraine
95 M24 Åkirkeby var. Aakirkeby. Bornholm, E Denmark
165 P8 Akita Akita, Honshū, C Japan
165 Q8 Akita off. Akita-ken. ❖ prefecture Honshū, C Japan
76 H8 Akjoujt prev. Fort-Repoux. Inchiri, W Mauritania
92 H11 Akkajaure ◎ N Sweden
Akkala see Oqqal'a
155 L25 Akkaraipattu Eastern Province, E Sri Lanka
92 H11 Akkavare ▲ N Sweden
145 P13 Akkense Zhezkazgan, C Kazakhstan
Akkerman see Bilhorod-Dnistrovs'kyy
129 W8 Akkermanovka Orenburgskaya Oblast', W Russian Federation
165 V4 Akkeshi Hokkaidō, NE Japan
165 V4 Akkeshi-ko ◎ Hokkaidō, NE Japan
165 V5 Akkeshi-wan bay NW Pacific Ocean
138 F8 'Akko Eng. Acre, Fr. Saint-Jean-d'Acre; Bibl. Accho, Ptolemaïs. Northern, N Israel
145 Q8 Akkol' Kaz. Aqköl; prev. Alekseyevka, Kaz. Alekseevka. Akmola, C Kazakhstan
145 T14 Akkol' Kaz. Aqköl. Almaty, SE Kazakhstan
145 Q16 Akkol' Kaz. Aqköl. Zhambyl, S Kazakhstan
144 M11 Akkol', Ozero prev. Ozero Zhaman-Akkol'. ◎ C Kazakhstan
98 L6 Akkrum Friesland, N Netherlands
145 U8 Akku prev. Lebyazh'ye. Pavlodar, NE Kazakhstan
144 F12 Akkystau Kaz. Aqqystaū. Atyrau, SW Kazakhstan
8 G6 Aklavik Northwest Territories, NW Canada
118 B9 Akmenrags headland W Latvia
158 E9 Akmeqit Xinjiang Uygur Zizhiqu, NW China
146 J14 Akmeydan Maryyskiy Velayat, C Turkmenistan
145 P9 Akmola off. Akmolinskaya Oblast', Kaz. Aqmola Oblysy; prev. Tselinogradskaya Oblast. ❖ province C Kazakhstan
Akmolinsk see Astana
Akmolinskaya Oblast' see Akmola
Aknavásár see Târgu Ocna
118 I11 Aknīste Jēkabpils, S Latvia
81 G14 Akobo Jonglei, SE Sudan
81 G14 Akobo var. Åkobowenz. ≈ Ethiopia/Sudan
Åkobowenz see Akobo
154 H12 Akola Mahārāshtra, C India
Akordat see Akurdet
77 Q16 Akosombo Dam dam SE Ghana
154 H12 Akot Mahārāshtra, C India
77 N16 Akoupé SE Ivory Coast
12 M3 Akpatok Island island Nunavut, E Canada
158 G7 Akqi Xinjiang Uygur Zizhiqu, NW China
138 I2 Akrād, Jabal al ⛰ N Syria
Akragas see Agrigento
92 H3 Akranes Vesturland, W Iceland
139 S2 Ākrē Ar. 'Aqrah. N Iraq
95 C16 Åkrehamn Rogaland, S Norway
77 V9 Akrérèb Agadez, C Niger
115 D22 Akrítas, Akrotírio headland S Greece
37 V3 Akron Colorado, C USA
29 R12 Akron Iowa, C USA
31 U12 Akron Ohio, N USA
Akrotiri see Akrotírion
Akrotiri Bay see Akrotírion, Kólpos
121 P3 Akrotírion var. Akrotiri. UK air base S Cyprus
121 P3 Akrotírion, Kólpos var. Akrotiri Bay. bay S Cyprus
121 O3 Akrotiri Sovereign Base Area UK military installation S Cyprus
158 F11 Aksai Chin Chin. Aksayqin. disputed region China/India
Aksaj see Aksay
136 I15 Aksaray Aksaray, C Turkey
136 I15 Aksaray ❖ province C Turkey
159 P8 Aksay var. Aksay Kazakzu Zizhixian. Gansu, N China
144 G8 Aksay var. Aksaj, Kaz. Aqsay. Zapadnyy Kazakhstan, NW Kazakhstan
129 O11 Aksay Volgogradskaya Oblast', SW Russian Federation
147 W10 Aksay var. Toxkan He. ≈ China/Kyrgyzstan
Aksay Kazakzu Zizhixian see Aksay
Aksayqin see Aksai Chin
158 G11 Aksayqin Hu ◎ NW China
136 G14 Akşehir Konya, W Turkey
136 G14 Akşehir Gölü ◎ C Turkey
136 G16 Akseki Antalya, SW Turkey
123 P13 Aksenovo-Zilovskoye Chitinskaya Oblast', S Russian Federation
145 V11 Akshatau, Khrebet ⛰ E Kazakhstan
147 Y8 Ak-Shyyrak Issyk-Kul'skaya Oblast', E Kyrgyzstan
Akstafa see Ağstafa
158 H7 Aksu Xinjiang Uygur Zizhiqu, NW China
145 R8 Aksu Kaz. Aqsū. Akmola, N Kazakhstan
145 T8 Aksu var. Jermak, Kaz. Ermak; prev. Yermak. Pavlodar, NE Kazakhstan
145 W13 Aksu Kaz. Aqsū. Almaty, SE Kazakhstan
145 V13 Aksu Kaz. Aqsū. ≈ SE Kazakhstan
145 X11 Aksuat Kaz. Aqsūat. Vostochnyy Kazakhstan, E Kazakhstan
145 Y11 Aksuat Kaz. Aqsūat. Vostochnyy Kazakhstan, SE Kazakhstan
129 S4 Aksubayevo Respublika Tatarstan, W Russian Federation
158 H7 Aksu He Rus. Sary-Dzhaz. ≈ China/Kyrgyzstan see also Sary-Dzhaz
80 J10 Āksum Tigray, N Ethiopia
145 O12 Aktas Kaz. Aqtas. Zhezkazgan, C Kazakhstan
Aktash see Oqtosh
147 V9 Ak-Tash, Gora ▲ C Kyrgyzstan
145 R10 Aktau Kaz. Aqtaū. Karaganda, C Kazakhstan
144 E11 Aktau Kaz. Aqtaū; prev. Shevchenko. Mangistau, W Kazakhstan
Aktau, Khrebet see Oqtogh, SW Tajikistan
Aktau, Khrebet see Oqtow Tizmasi, C Uzbekistan
Akte see Ágion Óros
Ak-Tepe see Akdepe
147 X7 Ak-Terek Issyk-Kul'skaya Oblast', E Kyrgyzstan
Aktí see Ágion Óros
158 E8 Akto Xinjiang Uygur Zizhiqu, NW China
145 V12 Aktogay Kaz. Aqtoghay. Vostochnyy Kazakhstan, E Kazakhstan
145 T12 Aktogay Kaz. Aqtoghay. Zhezkazgan, C Kazakhstan
119 M18 Aktsyabrski Rus. Oktyabr'skiy; prev. Karpilovka. Homyel'skaya Voblasts', SE Belarus
144 I10 Aktyubinsk Kaz. Aqtöbe. Aktyubinsk, NW Kazakhstan
144 H11 Aktyubinsk off. Aktyubinskaya Oblast', Kaz. Aqtöbe Oblysy. ❖ province W Kazakhstan
147 W7 Ak-Tyuz var. Aktyuz. Chuyskaya Oblast', N Kyrgyzstan
79 J17 Akula Equateur, NW Dem. Rep. Congo (Zaire)
164 C15 Akune Kagoshima, Kyūshū, SW Japan
38 L16 Akun Island island Aleutian Islands, Alaska, USA
80 J9 Akurdet var. Agordat, Akordat. C Eritrea
77 T16 Akure Ondo, SW Nigeria
92 J2 Akureyri Nordhurland Eystra, N Iceland
38 L17 Akutan Akutan Island, Alaska, USA
38 K17 Akutan Island island Aleutian Islands, Alaska, USA
77 V17 Akwa Ibom ❖ state SE Nigeria
Akyab see Sittwe
129 W7 Ak"yar Respublika Bashkortostan, W Russian Federation
145 Y11 Akzhar Kaz. Aqzhar. Vostochnyy Kazakhstan, E Kazakhstan
94 F13 Ål Buskerud, S Norway
119 N18 Ala Rus. Ola. ≈ SE Belarus
20 H11 Alabama off. State of Alabama; also known as Camellia State, Heart of Dixie, The Cotton State, Yellowhammer State. ❖ state S USA
23 P6 Alabama River ≈ Alabama, S USA
23 P4 Alabaster Alabama, S USA
139 U10 Al 'Abd Allāh var. Al Abdullah. S Iraq
Al Abdullah see Al 'Abd Allāh
139 W14 Al Abṭīyah well S Iraq
147 S9 Ala-Buka Dzhalal-Abadskaya Oblast', W Kyrgyzstan
136 J12 Alaca Çorum, N Turkey
136 K10 Alaçam Samsun, N Turkey
Alacant see Alicante
23 V9 Alachua Florida, SE USA
137 S13 Aladağlar ⛰ W Turkey
136 K15 Ala Dağları ⛰ C Turkey
129 O16 Alagir Respublika Severnaya Osetiya, SW Russian Federation
106 B6 Alagna Valsesia Valle d'Aosta, NW Italy
103 P12 Alagnon ≈ C France
59 P16 Alagoas off. Estado de Alagoas. ❖ state E Brazil
59 P17 Alagoinhas Bahia, E Brazil
105 R5 Alagón Aragón, NE Spain
104 J9 Alagón ≈ W Spain
93 K16 Alahärmä Länsi-Suomi, W Finland
al Ahdar see Al Akhḍar
142 K12 Al Aḥmadī var. Ahmadi. E Kuwait
Al Ain see Al 'Ayn
105 Z8 Alaior prev. Alayor. Menorca, Spain, W Mediterranean Sea
147 T11 Alai Range Rus. Alayskiy Khrebet. ⛰ Kyrgyzstan/Tajikistan
Alais see Alès
141 X11 Al 'Ajā'iz E Oman
141 X11 Al 'Ajā'iz oasis SE Oman
93 L16 Alajärvi Länsi-Suomi, W Finland
118 K4 Alajõe Ida-Virumaa, NE Estonia
42 M13 Alajuela Alajuela, C Costa Rica
42 L12 Alajuela off. Provincia de Alajuela. ❖ province N Costa Rica
43 T14 Alajuela, Lago ◎ C Panama
38 M11 Alakanuk Alaska, USA
140 K5 Al Akhḍar var. al Ahdar. Tabūk, NW Saudi Arabia
Alakol' see Alakol', Ozero
145 X13 Alakol', Ozero Kaz. Alaköl. ◎ SE Kazakhstan
126 I5 Alakurtti Murmanskaya Oblast', NW Russian Federation
38 F10 Alalakeiki Channel channel Hawaii, USA, C Pacific Ocean
Al 'Alamayn see El 'Alamein
139 R1 Al 'Amādīyah N Iraq
188 K5 Alamagan island C Northern Mariana Islands
139 X10 Al 'Amārah var. Amara. E Iraq
80 J11 Ālamat'ā Tigray, N Ethiopia
37 R11 Alameda New Mexico, SW USA
121 T13 'Alam el Rûm, Râs headland N Egypt
Alamícamba see Alamikamba
42 M8 Alamikamba var. Alamícamba. Región Autónoma Atlántico Norte, NE Nicaragua
24 K11 Alamito Creek ≈ Texas, SW USA
40 M8 Alamitos, Sierra de los ▲ NE Mexico
35 X9 Alamo Nevada, W USA
20 F9 Alamo Tennessee, S USA
41 Q12 Álamo Veracruz-Llave, C Mexico
37 S14 Alamogordo New Mexico, SW USA
36 J12 Alamo Lake ▣ Arizona, SW USA
40 H7 Alamos Sonora, NW Mexico
37 S7 Alamosa Colorado, C USA
93 J20 Åland var. Aland Islands, Fin. Ahvenanmaa. ❖ province SW Finland
93 J19 Åland Fin. Ahvenanmaa. island SW Finland
88 K9 Åland var. Aland Islands, Fin. Ahvenanmaa. island group SW Finland
Aland Islands see Åland
Aland Sea see Ålands Hav
95 Q14 Ålands Hav var. Aland Sea. strait Baltic Sea/Gulf of Bothnia
43 P16 Alanje Chiriquí, SW Panama
25 O2 Alanreed Texas, SW USA
136 G17 Alanya Antalya, S Turkey
23 U7 Alapaha River ≈ Florida/Georgia, SE USA
122 G10 Alapayevsk Sverdlovskaya Oblast', C Russian Federation
Alappuzha see Alleppey
138 F14 Al 'Aqabah var. Akaba, Aqaba, 'Aqaba; anc. Aelana, Elath. Ma'ān, SW Jordan
Al 'Arabīyah as Su'ūdīyah see Saudi Arabia
al Araïch see Larache
105 Q10 Alarcón Castilla-La Mancha, C Spain
105 Q9 Alarcón, Embalse de ▣ C Spain
138 J2 Al 'Arīmah Fr. Arime. Ḥalab, N Syria
Al 'Arīsh see El 'Arîsh
141 P6 Al Arṭāwīyah Ar Riyāḍ, N Saudi Arabia
Alasca, Golfo de see Alaska, Gulf of
136 D14 Alaşehir Manisa, W Turkey
139 N5 Al 'Ashārah var. Ashara. Dayr az Zawr, E Syria
Al Ashkhara see Al Ashkharah
141 Z9 Al Ashkharah var. Al Ashkhara. NE Oman
39 P8 Alaska off. State of Alaska; also known as Land of the Midnight Sun, The Last Frontier, Seward's Folly; prev. Russian America. ❖ state NW USA
39 T13 Alaska, Gulf of var. Golfo de Alasca. gulf Canada/USA
39 O15 Alaska Peninsula peninsula Alaska, USA
39 Q11 Alaska Range ⛰ Alaska, USA
Al-Asnam see Chlef
106 B10 Alassio Liguria, NW Italy
Alat see Olot
137 Y12 Älät Rus. Alyat; prev. Alyaty-Pristan'. SE Azerbaijan
139 S13 Al 'Athāmīn S Iraq
39 P7 Alatna River ≈ Alaska, USA
107 J15 Alatri Lazio, C Italy
Alattio see Alta
129 P5 Alatyr' Chuvashskaya Respublika, W Russian Federation
56 C7 Alausí Chimborazo, C Ecuador
105 O3 Álava Basq. Araba. ❖ province País Vasco, N Spain
137 T11 Alaverdi N Armenia
Alavo see Alavus
93 N14 Ala-Vuokki Oulu, E Finland
93 K17 Alavus Swe. Alavo. Länsi-Suomi, W Finland
Al 'Awābī see Awābī
139 P6 Al 'Awānī W Iraq
75 U12 Al Awaynāt SE Libya
Al Awaynāt see Al 'Uwaynāt
182 K9 Alawoona South Australia
Alaykel'/Alay-Kuu see Këk-Art
143 R17 Al 'Ayn var. Al Ain. Abū Ẓaby, E UAE
143 R17 Al 'Ayn var. Al Ain. × Abū Ẓaby, E UAE
138 G12 Al 'Aynā Al Karak, W Jordan
Alayor see Alaior
Alayskiy Khrebet see Alai Range
123 S6 Alazeya ≈ NE Russian Federation
139 U8 Al 'Azīzīyah var. Aziziya. E Iraq
120 M12 Al 'Azīzīyah NW Libya
138 I10 Al Azraq al Janūbī Az Zarqā', N Jordan
106 B9 Alba anc. Alba Pompeia. Piemonte, NW Italy
25 V6 Alba Texas, SW USA
116 G11 Alba ❖ county W Romania
139 P3 Al Ba'āj N Iraq
138 J2 Al Bāb Ḥalab, N Syria
116 G10 Albac Hung. Fehérvölgy; prev. Álbák. Alba, SW Romania
105 Q11 Albacete Castilla-La Mancha, C Spain
105 P11 Albacete ❖ province Castilla-La Mancha, C Spain
140 I4 Al Bad' Tabūk, NW Saudi Arabia
104 L7 Alba de Tormes Castilla-León, N Spain
139 P3 Al Bādī N Iraq
141 V8 Al Badī'ah × (Abū Ẓaby) Abū Ẓaby, C UAE
143 P17 Al Badī'ah var. Al Bedei'ah. spring/well C UAE
139 Q7 Al Baghdādī var. Khān al Baghdādī. SW Iraq
Al Bāha see Al Bāḥah
140 M11 Al Bāḥah var. Al Bāha. Al Bāḥah, SW Saudi Arabia
140 M11 Al Bāḥah off. Minṭaqat al Bāḥah. ❖ province W Saudi Arabia
Al Baḥrayn see Bahrain
105 S11 Albaida País Valenciano, E Spain
116 H11 Alba Iulia Ger. Weissenburg, Hung. Gyulafehérvár; prev. Bălgrad, Karlsburg, Károly-Fehérvár. Alba, W Romania
Álbák see Albac
138 G10 Al Balqā' off. Muḥāfaẓat al Balqā', var. Balqā'. ❖ governorate NW Jordan
14 F11 Alban Ontario, S Canada
103 O15 Alban Tarn, S France
12 K11 Albanel, Lac ◎ Quebec, SE Canada
113 L20 Albania off. Republic of Albania, Alb. Republika e Shqipërisë, Shqipëria; prev. People's Socialist Republic of Albania. ◆ republic SE Europe
Albania see Aubagne
107 H15 Albano Laziale Lazio, C Italy
180 J14 Albany Western Australia
23 S7 Albany Georgia, SE USA
31 P13 Albany Indiana, N USA
20 L8 Albany Kentucky, S USA
29 U7 Albany Minnesota, N USA
27 R2 Albany Missouri, C USA
18 L10 Albany state capital New York, NE USA
32 G12 Albany Oregon, NW USA
25 Q6 Albany Texas, SW USA
12 F10 Albany ≈ Ontario, S Canada
Alba Pompeia see Alba
Alba Regia see Székesfehérvár
138 J6 Al Bāridah var. Bāridah. Ḥimṣ, C Syria
139 Q11 Al Barīt S Iraq
105 R8 Albarracín Aragón, NE Spain
139 Y12 Al Baṣrah Eng. Basra; hist. Busra, Bussora. SE Iraq
139 V11 Al Baṭḥā' SE Iraq
141 X8 Al Bāṭinah var. Batinah. coastal region N Oman
(0) H16 Albatross Plateau undersea feature E Pacific Ocean
Al Batrūn see Batroûn
121 Q12 Al Bayḍā' var. Beida. NE Libya
141 P16 Al Bayḍā' var. Al Beida. SW Yemen
Al Bedei'ah see Al Badī'ah
Al Beida see Al Bayḍā'
21 S10 Albemarle var. Albermarle. North Carolina, SE USA
Albemarle Island see Isabela, Isla
21 N8 Albemarle Sound inlet W Atlantic Ocean
106 B10 Albenga Liguria, NW Italy
104 L8 Alberche ≈ C Spain
103 O17 Albères, Chaîne des var. les Albères, Montes Albères. ⛰ France/Spain
Albères, Montes see Albères, Chaîne des
182 F2 Alberga Creek seasonal river South Australia
104 G7 Albergaria-a-Velha Aveiro, N Portugal
105 S10 Alberic País Valenciano, E Spain
Albermarle see Albemarle
107 P18 Alberobello Puglia, SE Italy
108 J7 Alberschwende Vorarlberg, W Austria
103 O3 Albert Somme, N France
11 O12 Alberta ❖ province SW Canada
Albert Edward Nyanza see Edward, Lake
61 C20 Alberti Buenos Aires, E Argentina
111 K23 Albertirsa Pest, C Hungary
99 I16 Albertkanaal canal N Belgium
79 P17 Albert, Lake var. Albert Nyanza, Lac Mobutu Sese Seko. ◎ Uganda/Dem. Rep. Congo (Zaire)
29 V11 Albert Lea Minnesota, N USA
81 F16 Albert Nile ≈ NW Uganda
Albert Nyanza see Albert, Lake
103 T11 Albertville Savoie, E France
23 Q2 Albertville Alabama, S USA
Albertville see Kalemie
103 N15 Albi anc. Albiga. Tarn, S France
29 W15 Albia Iowa, C USA
Albiga see Albi
55 X9 Albina Marowijne, NE Suriname
83 A15 Albina, Ponta headland SW Angola
30 M16 Albion Illinois, N USA
31 P11 Albion Indiana, N USA
29 P14 Albion Nebraska, C USA
18 E9 Albion New York, NE USA
18 B12 Albion Pennsylvania, NE USA
Al Biqā' see El Beqaa
140 J4 Al Bi'r var. Bi'r Ibn Hirmās. Tabūk, NW Saudi Arabia
140 M12 Al Birk Makkah, SW Saudi Arabia
141 Q9 Al Biyāḍ desert C Saudi Arabia
98 H13 Alblasserdam Zuid-Holland, SW Netherlands

◆ Country ● Country Capital ◇ Dependent Territory ○ Dependent Territory Capital ❖ Administrative Region × International Airport ▲ Mountain ⛰ Mountain Range ⚠ Volcano ≈ River ◎ Lake ▣ Reservoir

105 T8 **Albocácer** *var.* Albocasser. País Valenciano, E Spain
Albocasser *see* Albocácer
95 H19 **Ålbæk** Nordjylland, N Denmark
Albona *see* Labin
105 O17 **Alborán, Isla de** *island* S Spain
Alborán, Mar de *see* Alboran Sea
105 N17 **Alboran Sea** *Sp.* Mar de Alborán. *sea* SW Mediterranean Sea
95 G20 **Ålborg** *var.* Aalborg, Ålborg-Nørresundby; *anc.* Alburgum. Nordjylland, N Denmark
95 H21 **Ålborg Bugt** *var.* Aalborg Bugt. *bay* N Denmark
Ålborg-Nørresundby *see* Ålborg
143 O5 **Alborz, Reshteh-ye Kūhhā-ye** *Eng.* Elburz Mountains. ▲ N Iran
105 Q14 **Albox** Andalucía, S Spain
101 H23 **Albstadt** Baden-Württemberg, SW Germany
104 G14 **Albufeira** Beja, S Portugal
139 P5 **Ālbū Gharz, Sabkhat** ◎ W Iraq
105 O15 **Albuñol** Andalucía, S Spain
37 Q11 **Albuquerque** New Mexico, SW USA
141 W8 **Al Buraymī** *var.* Buraimi. N Oman
143 R17 **Al Buraymī** *var.* Buraimi. *spring/well* Oman/UAE
Al Burayqah *see* Marsá al Burayqah
Alburgum *see* Ålborg
104 I10 **Alburquerque** Extremadura, W Spain
181 V14 **Albury** New South Wales, SE Australia
141 T14 **Al Buzūn** SE Yemen
93 G17 **Alby** Västernorrland, C Sweden
Albyn, Glen *see* Mor, Glen
104 G12 **Alcácer do Sal** Setúbal, W Portugal
Alcalá de Chisvert *see* Alcalà de Chivert
105 T8 **Alcalà de Chivert** *var.* Alcalá de Chisvert. País Valenciano, E Spain
104 K14 **Alcalá de Guadaira** Andalucía, S Spain
105 O8 **Alcalá de Henares** *Ar.* Alkal'a; *anc.* Complutum. Madrid, C Spain
104 K16 **Alcalá de los Gazules** Andalucía, S Spain
105 N14 **Alcalá La Real** Andalucía, S Spain
107 I23 **Alcamo** Sicilia, Italy, C Mediterranean Sea
105 T4 **Alcanadre** ≈ NE Spain
105 S12 **Alcanar** Cataluña, NE Spain
104 J5 **Alcañices** Castilla-León, N Spain
105 T7 **Alcañiz** Aragón, NE Spain
104 I9 **Alcántara** Extremadura, W Spain
104 J9 **Alcántara, Embalse de** ▣ W Spain
105 R13 **Alcantarilla** Murcia, SE Spain
105 P11 **Alcaraz** Castilla-La Mancha, C Spain
105 P12 **Alcaraz, Sierra de** ▲ C Spain
104 I12 **Alcarrache** ≈ SW Spain
105 T6 **Alcarràs** Cataluña, NE Spain
105 N14 **Alcaudete** Andalucía, S Spain
Alcázar *see* Ksar-el-Kebir
105 O10 **Alcázar de San Juan** *anc.* Alce. Castilla-La Mancha, C Spain
Alcazarquivir *see* Ksar-el-Kebir
Alce *see* Alcázar de San Juan
57 B17 **Alcebo, Volcán** ※ Galapagos Islands, Ecuador, E Pacific Ocean
139 X12 **Al Chabā'ish** *var.* Al Kaba'ish. SE Iraq
117 Y7 **Alchevs'k** *prev.* Kommunarsk, Voroshilovsk. Luhans'ka Oblast', E Ukraine
Alcira *see* Alzira
21 N9 **Alcoa** Tennessee, S USA
104 F9 **Alcobaça** Leiria, C Portugal
105 N8 **Alcobendas** Madrid, C Spain
Alcoi *see* Alcoy
105 P7 **Alcolea del Pinar** Castilla-La Mancha, C Spain
104 I11 **Alconchel** Extremadura, W Spain
105 S9 **Alcora** País Valenciano, E Spain
105 N8 **Alcorcón** Madrid, C Spain
105 S7 **Alcorisa** Aragón, NE Spain
61 B19 **Alcorta** Santa Fe, C Argentina
104 H14 **Alcoutim** Faro, S Portugal
33 W15 **Alcova** Wyoming, C USA
105 S11 **Alcoy** *var.* Alcoi. País Valenciano, E Spain
105 Y9 **Alcúdia, Badia d'** *bay* Mallorca, Spain, W Mediterranean Sea
172 M7 **Aldabra Group** *island group* SW Seychelles
139 U10 **Al Daghghārah** C Iraq
40 J5 **Aldama** Chihuahua, N Mexico
41 P11 **Aldama** Tamaulipas, C Mexico
123 Q11 **Aldan** Respublika Sakha (Yakutiya), NE Russian Federation
123 Q10 **Aldan** ≈ NE Russian Federation
162 G7 **Aldar** Dzavhan, W Mongolia
al Dar al Baida *see* Rabat
97 Q20 **Aldeburgh** E England, UK
105 P5 **Aldehuela de Calatañazor** Castilla-León, N Spain
Aldeia Nova *see* Aldeia Nova de São Bento
104 H13 **Aldeia Nova de São Bento** *var.* Aldeia Nova. Beja, S Portugal
29 V11 **Alden** Minnesota, N USA
184 N6 **Aldermen Islands, The** *island group* N NZ
97 L25 **Alderney** *island* Channel Islands
97 N22 **Aldershot** S England, UK
21 R6 **Alderson** West Virginia, NE USA
Al Dhaid *see* Adh Dhayd
30 J11 **Aledo** Illinois, N USA
76 H9 **Aleg** Brakna, SW Mauritania
64 Q10 **Alegranza** *island* Islas Canarias, Spain, NE Atlantic Ocean
37 P12 **Alegres Mountain** ▲ New Mexico, SW USA
61 F15 **Alegrete** Rio Grande do Sul, S Brazil
61 C16 **Alejandra** Santa Fe, C Argentina
193 T11 **Alejandro Selkirk, Isla** *island* Islas Juan Fernández, Chile, E Pacific Ocean
126 I12 **Alekhovshchina** Leningradskaya Oblast', NW Russian Federation
39 O13 **Aleknagik** Alaska, USA
Aleksandriya *see* Oleksandriya
Aleksandropol' *see* Gyumri
128 L3 **Aleksandrov** Vladimirskaya Oblast', W Russian Federation
113 N14 **Aleksandrovac** Serbia, C Yugoslavia
129 R9 **Aleksandrov Gay** Saratovskaya Oblast', W Russian Federation
129 U6 **Aleksandrovka** Orenburgskaya Oblast', W Russian Federation
Aleksandrovka *see* Oleksandrivka
114 J8 **Aleksandrovo** Lovech, N Bulgaria
127 V13 **Aleksandrovsk** Permskaya Oblast', NW Russian Federation
Aleksandrovsk *see* Zaporizhzhya
129 N14 **Aleksandrovskoye** Stavropol'skiy Kray, SW Russian Federation
123 T12 **Aleksandrovsk-Sakhalinskiy** Ostrov Sakhalin, Sakhalinskaya Oblast', SE Russian Federation
110 J10 **Aleksandrów Kujawski** Kujawsko-pomorskie, C Poland
110 K12 **Aleksandrów Łódzki** Łódzkie, C Poland
Alekseevka *see* Akkol'/Alekseyevka
126 L9 **Alekseyevka** Belgorodskaya Oblast', W Russian Federation
145 P7 **Alekseyevka** *Kaz.* Alekseevka. Severnyy Kazakhstan, N Kazakhstan
145 Z10 **Alekseyevka** *Kaz.* Alekseevka. Vostochnyy Kazakhstan, E Kazakhstan
129 S7 **Alekseyevka** Samarskaya Oblast', W Russian Federation
Alekseyevka *see* Akkol'
129 R4 **Alekseyevskoye** Respublika Tatarstan, W Russian Federation
128 K5 **Aleksin** Tul'skaya Oblast', W Russian Federation
113 O14 **Aleksinac** Serbia, SE Yugoslavia
190 G11 **Alele** Île Uvea, E Wallis and Futuna
95 N20 **Ålem** Kalmar, S Sweden
102 L6 **Alençon** Orne, N France
58 I12 **Alenquer** Pará, NE Brazil
38 G10 **Alenuihaha Channel** *channel* Hawaii, USA, C Pacific Ocean
Alep/Aleppo *see* Ḥalab
103 Y15 **Aléria** Corse, France, C Mediterranean Sea
197 Q11 **Alert** Ellesmere Island, Nunavut, N Canada
103 Q14 **Alès** *prev.* Alais. Gard, S France
116 G9 **Aleşd** *Hung.* Élesd. Bihor, SW Romania
106 C9 **Alessandria** *Fr.* Alexandrie. Piemonte, N Italy
95 G21 **Ålestrup** *var.* Aalestrup. Viborg, NW Denmark
94 D9 **Ålesund** Møre og Romsdal, S Norway
108 E10 **Aletschhorn** ▲ SW Switzerland
197 S1 **Aleutian Basin** *undersea feature* Bering Sea
38 H17 **Aleutian Islands** *island group* Alaska, USA
39 P14 **Aleutian Range** ▲ Alaska, USA
(0) B5 **Aleutian Trench** *undersea feature* S Bering Sea
123 T10 **Alevina, Mys** *headland* E Russian Federation
15 Q6 **Alex** ≈ Quebec, SE Canada
28 J3 **Alexander** North Dakota, N USA
39 W14 **Alexander Archipelago** *island group* Alaska, USA
Alexanderbaai *see* Alexander Bay
83 D23 **Alexander Bay** *Afr.* Alexanderbaai. Northern Cape, W South Africa
23 Q5 **Alexander City** Alabama, S USA
194 J6 **Alexander Island** *island* Antarctica
Alexander Range *see* Kirghiz Range
183 O12 **Alexandra** Victoria, SE Australia
185 D22 **Alexandra** Otago, South Island, NZ
115 F14 **Alexándreia** *var.* Alexándria. Kentrikí Makedonía, N Greece
Alexandretta *see* İskenderun
Alexandretta, Gulf of *see* İskenderun Körfezi
15 N13 **Alexandria** Ontario, SE Canada
121 U13 **Alexandria** *Ar.* Al Iskandarīyah. N Egypt
44 J12 **Alexandria** C Jamaica
116 J15 **Alexandria** Teleorman, S Romania
31 P13 **Alexandria** Indiana, N USA
20 M4 **Alexandria** Kentucky, S USA
22 H7 **Alexandria** Louisiana, S USA
29 T7 **Alexandria** Minnesota, N USA
29 Q11 **Alexandria** South Dakota, N USA
21 W4 **Alexandria** Virginia, NE USA
Alexándria *see* Alexándreia
18 I7 **Alexandria Bay** New York, NE USA
Alexandrie *see* Alessandria
182 J10 **Alexandrina, Lake** ◎ South Australia
114 K13 **Alexandroúpoli** *var.* Alexandroúpolis, *Turk.* Dedeagaç, Dedeagach. Anatolikí Makedonía kai Thráki, NE Greece
Alexandroúpolis *see* Alexandroúpoli
10 L15 **Alexis Creek** British Columbia, SW Canada
122 I13 **Aleysk** Altayskiy Kray, S Russian Federation
8 L15 **Alexis Creek** British Columbia, SW Canada
122 I13 **Aleysk** Altayskiy Kray, S Russian Federation
139 S8 **Al Fallūjah** *var.* Falluja. C Iraq
105 R8 **Alfambra** ≈ E Spain
Al Faqa *see* Faq'
141 R15 **Al Farḍah** C Yemen
105 Q4 **Alfaro** La Rioja, N Spain
105 U5 **Alfarràs** Cataluña, NE Spain
Al Fāshir *see* El Fasher
Al Fashn *see* El Fashn
114 M7 **Alfatar** Silistra, NE Bulgaria
139 S5 **Al Fatḥah** C Iraq
139 Q3 **Al Fatsī** N Iraq
139 Z13 **Al Fāw** *var.* Fao. SE Iraq
Al Fayyūm *see* El Faiyûm
115 D20 **Alfeiós** *prev.* Alfiós, *anc.* Alpheius, Alpheus. ≈ S Greece
100 I13 **Alfeld** Niedersachsen, C Germany
Alfiós *see* Alfeiós
Alföld *see* Great Hungarian Plain
94 C11 **Ålfotbreen** *glacier* S Norway
19 P9 **Alfred** Maine, NE USA
18 F11 **Alfred** New York, NE USA
61 K14 **Alfredo Vagner** Santa Catarina, S Brazil
94 M12 **Alfta** Gävleborg, C Sweden
140 K12 **Al Fuḥayḥīl** *var.* Fahaheel. SE Kuwait
139 Q6 **Al Fuḥaymī** C Iraq
143 S16 **Al Fujayrah** *Eng.* Fujairah. Al Fujayrah, NE UAE
143 S16 **Al Fujayrah** *Eng.* Fujairah. × Al Fujayrah, NE UAE
Al Furāt *see* Euphrates
144 J10 **Alga** *Kaz.* Algha. Aktyubinsk, NW Kazakhstan
144 G9 **Algabas** Zapadnyy Kazakhstan, NW Kazakhstan
95 C17 **Ålgård** Rogaland, S Norway
104 G14 **Algarve** *cultural region* S Portugal
182 G3 **Algebuckina Bridge** South Australia
104 K16 **Algeciras** Andalucía, SW Spain
105 S10 **Algemesí** País Valenciano, E Spain
Al-Genain *see* El Geneina
120 F9 **Alger** *var.* Algiers, El Djazaïr, Al Jazair. ● (Algeria) N Algeria
74 H9 **Algeria** *off.* Democratic and Popular Republic of Algeria. ◆ *republic* N Africa
120 J8 **Algerian Basin** *var.* Balearic Plain *undersea feature* W Mediterranean Sea
Algha *see* Alga
138 I4 **Al Ghāb** ◎ NW Syria
141 X10 **Al Ghābah** *var.* Ghaba. C Oman
141 U14 **Al Ghayḍah** E Yemen
140 M6 **Al Ghazālah** Ḥā'il, NW Saudi Arabia
107 B17 **Alghero** Sardegna, Italy, C Mediterranean Sea
95 M20 **Älghult** Kronoberg, S Sweden
Al Ghurdaqah *see* Hurghada
Algiers *see* Alger
105 S10 **Alginet** País Valenciano, E Spain
83 I26 **Algoa Bay** *bay* S South Africa
104 L15 **Algodonales** Andalucía, S Spain
105 N9 **Algodor** ≈ C Spain
Al Golea *see* El Goléa
31 N6 **Algoma** Wisconsin, N USA
29 U12 **Algona** Iowa, C USA
20 L8 **Algood** Tennessee, S USA
105 O2 **Algorta** País Vasco, N Spain
61 E18 **Algorta** Río Negro, W Uruguay
Al Haba *see* Haba
139 Q10 **Al Habbārīyah** S Iraq
Al Hadhar *see* Al Ḥaḍr
139 Q4 **Al Ḥaḍr** *var.* Al Hadhar; *anc.* Hatra. NW Iraq
139 T13 **Al Ḥajarah** *desert* S Iraq
141 W8 **Al Ḥajar al Gharbī** ▲ N Oman
141 Y8 **Al Ḥajar ash Sharqī** ▲ NE Oman
141 R15 **Al Hajarayn** C Yemen
138 L10 **Al Ḥamād** *desert* Jordan/Saudi Arabia
Al Hamad *see* Syrian Desert
75 N9 **Al Ḥamādah al Ḥamrā'** *var.* Al Ḥamrā'. *desert* NW Libya
105 N15 **Alhama de Granada** Andalucía, S Spain
105 R13 **Alhama de Murcia** Murcia, SE Spain
35 T15 **Alhambra** California, W USA
139 T12 **Al Ḥammām** S Iraq
141 X8 **Al Ḥamrā'** NE Oman
Al Ḥamrā' *see* Al Ḥamādah al Ḥamrā'
141 O6 **Al Ḥamūdīyah** *spring/well* N Saudi Arabia
140 M7 **Al Ḥanākīyah** Al Madīnah, W Saudi Arabia
139 W14 **Al Ḥanīyah** *escarpment* Iraq/Saudi Arabia
139 Y12 **Al Ḥārithah** SE Iraq
140 L3 **Al Ḥarrah** *desert* NW Saudi Arabia
75 Q10 **Al Harūj al Aswad** *desert* C Libya
Al Hasaifin *see* Al Ḥusayfin
139 N2 **Al Ḥasakah** *var.* Al Hasijah, El Haseke, *Fr.* Hassetché. Al Ḥasakah, NE Syria
139 O2 **Al Ḥasakah** *off.* Muḥāfaẓat al Ḥasakah, *var.* Al Hasakah, Āl Hasakah, Hasakah, Hassakeh. ◈ *governorate* NE Syria
139 T9 **Al Hāshimīyah** C Iraq
138 G13 **Al Hāshimīyah** Ma'ān, S Jordan
Al Hasijah *see* Al Ḥasakah
104 M15 **Alhaurín el Grande** Andalucía, S Spain
141 Q16 **Al Ḥawrā** S Yemen
139 V10 **Al Ḥayy** *var.* Kut al Hai, Kūt al Ḥayy. E Iraq
141 U11 **Al Ḥibāk** *desert* E Saudi Arabia
138 H8 **Al Hījānah** *var.* Hejanah, Hijanah. Dimashq, W Syria
140 K7 **Al Ḥijāz** *Eng.* Hejaz. *physical region* NW Saudi Arabia
Al Hilbeh *see* 'Ulayyānīyah, Bi'r al
139 T9 **Al Ḥillah** *var.* Hilla. C Iraq
139 T9 **Al Hindīyah** *var.* Hindiya. C Iraq
138 G12 **Al Ḥisā** Aṭ Ṭafīlah, W Jordan
74 G5 **Al-Hoceïma** *var.* al Hoceima, Al-Hoceima, Alhucemas; *prev.* Villa Sanjurjo. N Morocco
Alhucemas *see* Al-Hoceïma
105 N17 **Alhucemas, Peñon de** *island group* S Spain
141 N15 **Al Ḥudaydah** *Eng.* Hodeida. W Yemen
141 N15 **Al Ḥudaydah** *Eng.* Hodeida. × W Yemen
140 M4 **Al Ḥudūd ash Shamālīyah** *var.* Minṭaqat al Ḥudūd ash Shamālīyah, *Eng.* Northern Border Region. ◈ *province* N Saudi Arabia
141 S7 **Al Hufūf** *var.* Hofuf. Ash Sharqīyah, NE Saudi Arabia
al-Hurma *see* Al Khurmah
141 X7 **Al Ḥusayfin** *var.* Al Hasaifin. N Oman
138 G9 **Al Ḥuṣn** *var.* Husn. Irbid, N Jordan
139 U9 **'Alī** E Iraq
104 L10 **Alia** Extremadura, W Spain
143 P9 **'Alīābād** Yazd, C Iran
'Alīābad *see* Qā'emshahr
105 S7 **Aliaga** Aragón, NE Spain
136 B13 **Aliağa** İzmir, W Turkey
Aliákmon *see* Aliákmonas
115 F14 **Aliákmonas** *prev.* Aliákmon, *anc.* Haliacmon. ≈ N Greece
139 W9 **'Alī al Gharbī** E Iraq
139 U11 **'Alī al Ḥassūnī** S Iraq
115 G18 **Alíartos** Stereá Ellás, C Greece
137 Y12 **Äli-Bayramlı** *Rus.* Ali-Bayramly. SE Azerbaijan
Ali-Bayramly *see* Äli-Bayramlı
114 P12 **Alibey Barajı** ▣ NW Turkey
77 S13 **Alibori** ≈ N Benin
112 M10 **Alibunar** Serbia, NE Yugoslavia
105 S12 **Alicante** *Cat.* Alacant; *Lat.* Lucentum. País Valenciano, SE Spain
105 S12 **Alicante** ◈ *province* País Valenciano, SE Spain
105 S12 **Alicante** × Murcia, E Spain
83 I25 **Alice** Eastern Cape, S South Africa
25 S14 **Alice** Texas, SW USA
83 I25 **Alicedale** Eastern Cape, S South Africa
65 B25 **Alice, Mount** *hill* West Falkland, Falkland Islands
107 P20 **Alice, Punta** *headland* S Italy
181 Q7 **Alice Springs** Northern Territory, C Australia
23 N4 **Aliceville** Alabama, S USA
147 U13 **Alichur** SE Tajikistan
147 U14 **Alichuri Janubí, Qatorkŭhi** *Rus.* Yuzhno-Alichurskiy Khrebet. ▲ SE Tajikistan
147 U13 **Alichuri Shimolí, Qatorkŭhi** *Rus.* Severo-Alichurskiy Khrebet. ▲ SE Tajikistan
107 K22 **Alicudi, Isola** *island* Isole Eolie, S Italy
152 J11 **Alīgarh** Uttar Pradesh, N India
142 M7 **Alīgūdarz** Lorestān, W Iran
(0) F12 **Alijos, Islas** *island group* California, SW USA
149 R6 **'Alī Kbel** *Pash.* 'Alī Khēl. Paktīkā, E Afghanistan
Ali Khel *see* 'Alī Kheyl, Paktiā, Afghanistan
'Alī Khēl *see* 'Alī Kbel, Paktīkā, Afghanistan
149 R6 **'Alī Kheyl** *var.* Ali Khel, Jajı. Paktiā, SE Afghanistan
141 V17 **Al Ikhwān** *island group* SE Yemen
Aliki *see* Alykí
79 H19 **Alima** ≈ C Congo
Al Imārāt al 'Arabīyah al Muttaḥidah *see* United Arab Emirates
115 N23 **Alimia** *island* Dodekánisos, Greece, Aegean Sea
55 V12 **Alimimuni Piek** ▲ S Suriname
79 K15 **Alindao** Basse-Kotto, S Central African Republic
95 J18 **Alingsås** Västra Götaland, S Sweden
81 K18 **Alinjugul** *spring/well* E Kenya
149 S11 **Alīpur** Punjab, E Pakistan
153 T12 **Alīpur Duār** West Bengal, NE India
18 B14 **Aliquippa** Pennsylvania, NE USA
80 L12 **'Ali Sabieh** *var.* 'Alī Sabīḥ. S Djibouti
'Alī Sabīḥ *see* 'Ali Sabieh
140 K3 **Al 'Isāwīyah** Al Jawf, NW Saudi Arabia
104 J10 **Aliseda** Extremadura, W Spain
139 T8 **Al Iskandarīyah** C Iraq
Al Iskandarīyah *see* Alexandria
123 T6 **Aliskerovo** Chukotskiy Avtonomnyy Okrug, NE Russian Federation
114 H13 **Alistráti** Kentrikí Makedonía, NE Greece
39 P15 **Alitak Bay** *bay* Kodiak Island, Alaska, USA
Al Ittiḥād *see* Madīnat ash Sha'b
115 H18 **Alivéri** *var.* Alivérion. Évvoia, C Greece
Alivérion *see* Alivéri
Aliwal-Noord *see* Aliwal North
83 I24 **Aliwal North** *Afr.* Aliwal-Noord. Eastern Cape, SE South Africa
121 Q13 **Al Jabal al Akhḍar** ▲ NE Libya
138 H13 **Al Jafr** Ma'ān, S Jordan
75 T8 **Al Jaghbūb** NE Libya
142 K11 **Al Jahrā'** *var.* Al Jahrah, Jahra. C Kuwait
Al Jahrah *see* Al Jahrā'
Al Jamāhīrīyah al 'Arabīyah al Lībīyah ash Sha'bīyah al Ishtirāk *see* Libya
140 K3 **Al Jarāwī** *spring/well* NW Saudi Arabia
141 X11 **Al Jawārah** *oasis* SE Oman
140 L3 **Al Jawf** *var.* Jauf. Al Jawf, NW Saudi Arabia
140 L4 **Al Jawf** *off.* Minṭaqat al Jawf. ◈ *province* N Saudi Arabia
Al Jawlān *see* Golan Heights
Al Jazair *see* Alger
139 N4 **Al Jazīrah** *physical region* Iraq/Syria
104 F14 **Aljezur** Faro, S Portugal
139 S13 **Al Jil** S Iraq
138 G11 **Al Jīzah** *var.* Jiza. 'Ammān, N Jordan
Al Jīzah *see* El Gîza
Al Jubail *see* Al Jubayl
141 S6 **Al Jubayl** *var.* Al Jubail. Ash Sharqīyah, NE Saudi Arabia
141 T10 **Āl Juḥaysh, Qalamat** *well* SE Saudi Arabia
143 N15 **Al Jumaylīyah** N Qatar
Al Junaynah *see* El Geneina
104 G13 **Aljustrel** Beja, S Portugal
Al Kaba'ish *see* Al Chabā'ish
Al-Kadhimain *see* Al Kāẓimīyah
Al Kāf *see* El Kef
Alkal'a *see* Alcalá de Henares
35 W4 **Alkali Flat** *salt flat* Nevada, W USA
35 Q1 **Alkali Lake** ◎ Nevada, W USA
141 Z9 **Al Kāmil** NE Oman
138 G11 **Al Karak** *var.* El Kerak, Karak, Kerak; *anc.* Kir Moab, Kir of Moab. Al Karak, W Jordan
138 G12 **Al Karak** *off.* Muḥāfaẓat al Karak. ◈ *governorate* W Jordan
139 W8 **Al Karmashīyah** E Iraq
Al-Kashaniya *see* Al Qash'ānīyah
Al-Kasr al-Kebir *see* Ksar-el-Kebir
139 T8 **Al Kāẓimīyah** *var.* Al-Kadhimain, Kadhimain. C Iraq
99 J18 **Alken** Limburg, NE Belgium
141 X8 **Al Khābūrah** *var.* Khabura. N Oman
Al Khalīl *see* Hebron
139 T7 **Al Khāliṣ** C Iraq
Al Khaluf *see* Khalūf
Al Khārijah *see* El Khârga
141 Q8 **Al Kharj** Ar Riyāḍ, C Saudi Arabia
141 W6 **Al Khaṣab** *var.* Khasab. N Oman
Al Khaur *see* Al Khawr
143 N15 **Al Khawr** *var.* Al Khaur, Al Khor. N Qatar
142 K12 **Al Khīrān** *var.* Al Khiran. SE Kuwait
141 W9 **Al Khīrān** *spring/well* NW Oman
Al Khiyām *see* El Khiyam
Al-Khobar *see* Al Khubar
Al Khor *see* Al Khawr
141 S6 **Al Khubar** *var.* Al-Khobar. Ash Sharqīyah, NE Saudi Arabia
75 T11 **Al Khufrah** SE Libya
120 M12 **Al Khums** *var.* Homs, Khoms, Khums. NW Libya
141 R15 **Al Khuraybah** C Yemen
140 M9 **Al Khurmah** *var.* al-Hurma. Makkah, W Saudi Arabia
141 V9 **Al Kidan** *desert* NE Saudi Arabia
98 H9 **Alkmaar** Noord-Holland, NW Netherlands
139 T10 **Al Kūfah** *var.* Kufa. S Iraq
141 T10 **Al Kursū'** *desert* E Saudi Arabia
139 V9 **Al Kūt** *var.* Kūt al 'Amārah, Kut al Imara. E Iraq
Al-Kuwait *see* Al Kuwayt
Al Kuwayr *see* Guwēr
142 K11 **Al Kuwayt** *var.* Al-Kuwait, *Eng.* Kuwait, Kuwait City; *prev.* Qurein. ● (Kuwait) E Kuwait
142 K11 **Al Kuwayt** × C Kuwait
115 G19 **Alkyonidón, Kólpos** *gulf* C Greece
141 N4 **Al Labbah** *physical region* N Saudi Arabia
138 G4 **Al Lādhiqīyah** *Eng.* Latakia, *Fr.* Lattaquié; *anc.* Laodicea, Laodicea ad Mare. Al Lādhiqīyah, W Syria
138 H4 **Al Lādhiqīyah** *off.* Muḥāfaẓat al Lādhiqīyah, *var.* Al Lathqiyah, Latakia, Lattakia. ◈ *governorate* W Syria
19 R2 **Allagash River** ≈ Maine, NE USA
152 M13 **Allahābād** Uttar Pradesh, N India
143 S3 **Allāh Dāgh, Reshteh-ye** ▲ NE Iran
39 Q8 **Allakaket** Alaska, USA
11 T15 **Allan** Saskatchewan, S Canada
166 L6 **Allanmyo** Magwe, C Myanmar
83 I22 **Allanridge** Free State, C South Africa
104 H4 **Allariz** Galicia, NW Spain
139 R11 **Al Laṣaf** *var.* Al Lussuf. S Iraq
Al Lathqiyah *see* Al Lādhiqīyah
23 S2 **Allatoona Lake** ▣ Georgia, SE USA
83 J19 **Alldays** Northern, NE South Africa
Alle *see* Łyna
31 P10 **Allegan** Michigan, N USA
18 E14 **Allegheny Mountains** ▲ NE USA
18 E12 **Allegheny Plateau** ▲ New York/Pennsylvania, NE USA
18 D11 **Allegheny Reservoir** ▣ New York/Pennsylvania, NE USA
18 E12 **Allegheny River** ≈ New York/Pennsylvania, NE USA
22 K9 **Allemands, Lac des** ◎ Louisiana, S USA
25 U6 **Allen** Texas, SW USA
21 R14 **Allendale** South Carolina, SE USA
41 N6 **Allende** Coahuila de Zaragoza, NE Mexico
41 O9 **Allende** Nuevo León, NE Mexico
97 D16 **Allen, Lough** *Ir.* Loch Aillionn. ◎ NW Ireland
185 B26 **Allen, Mount** ▲ Stewart Island, Southland, SW NZ
109 V2 **Allensteig** Niederösterreich, N Austria
Allenstein *see* Olsztyn
18 I14 **Allentown** Pennsylvania, NE USA
155 G23 **Alleppey** *var.* Alappuzha; *prev.* Alleppi. Kerala, SW India
Alleppi *see* Alleppey
100 J12 **Aller** ≈ NW Germany
29 V16 **Allerton** Iowa, C USA
99 K19 **Alleur** Liège, E Belgium
101 J25 **Allgäuer Alpen** ▲ Austria/Germany
28 J13 **Alliance** Nebraska, C USA
31 U12 **Alliance** Ohio, N USA
103 O10 **Allier** ◈ *department* N France
139 R13 **Al Līfiyah** S Iraq
44 J13 **Alligator Pond** C Jamaica
21 Y9 **Alligator River** ≈ North Carolina, SE USA
29 W12 **Allison** Iowa, C USA
14 G14 **Alliston** Ontario, S Canada
140 L11 **Al Līth** Makkah, SW Saudi Arabia
Al Liwā' *see* Līwā
96 J12 **Alloa** C Scotland, UK
103 U14 **Allos** Alpes-de-Haute-Provence, SE France
108 D6 **Allschwil** Basel-Land, NW Switzerland
Al Lubnān *see* Lebanon
141 N14 **Al Luḥayyah** W Yemen
14 K12 **Allumettes, Île des** *island* Quebec, SE Canada
Al Lussuf *see* Al Laṣaf
109 S5 **Alm** ≈ N Austria
15 Q7 **Alma** Quebec, SE Canada
27 S10 **Alma** Arkansas, C USA
23 V7 **Alma** Georgia, SE USA
27 P4 **Alma** Kansas, C USA
31 Q8 **Alma** Michigan, N USA
29 O17 **Alma** Nebraska, C USA
30 I7 **Alma** Wisconsin, N USA
139 R12 **Al Ma'ānīyah** S Iraq
Alma-Ata *see* Almaty
Alma-Atinskaya Oblast' *see* Almaty
Almacellas *see* Almacelles
105 T5 **Almacelles** *var.* Almacellas. Cataluña, NE Spain
104 F11 **Almada** Setúbal, W Portugal
104 L11 **Almadén** Castilla-La Mancha, C Spain
66 L6 **Almadies, Pointe des** *headland* W Senegal
140 L7 **Al Madīnah** *Eng.* Medina. Al Madīnah, W Saudi Arabia
140 L7 **Al Madīnah** *off.* Minṭaqat al Madīnah. ◈ *province* W Saudi Arabia
138 H9 **Al Mafraq** *var.* Mafraq. Al Mafraq, N Jordan
138 J10 **Al Mafraq** *off.* Muḥāfaẓat al Mafraq. ◈ *governorate* NW Jordan
141 R15 **Al Maghārim** C Yemen
105 N11 **Almagro** Castilla-La Mancha, C Spain
Al Maḥallah al Kubrá *see* El Maḥalla el Kubra
139 T9 **Al Maḥāwīl** *var.* Khān al Maḥāwīl. C Iraq
Al Mahdīyah *see* Mahdia
139 T8 **Al Maḥmūdīyah** *var.* Mahmudiya. C Iraq
141 T14 **Al Mahrah** ▲ E Yemen
141 P7 **Al Majma'ah** Ar Riyāḍ, C Saudi Arabia
139 Q11 **Al Makmin** *well* S Iraq
139 Q1 **Al Mālikīyah** *var.* Malkiye. Al Ḥasakah, N Syria
Almalyk *see* Olmaliq
Al Mamlakah al Urdunīyah al Hāshimīyah *see* Jordan
Al Mamlakah *see* Morocco
143 Q18 **Al Manādir** *var.* Al Manadir. *desert* Oman/UAE
142 L15 **Al Manāmah** *Eng.* Manama. ● (Bahrain) N Bahrain
139 O5 **Al Manāṣif** ▲ E Syria
35 O4 **Almanor, Lake** ▣ California, W USA
105 R11 **Almansa** Castilla-La Mancha, C Spain
Al Manṣūrah *see* El Manṣûra
104 L3 **Almanza** Castilla-León, N Spain
104 L8 **Almanzor** ▲ W Spain
105 P14 **Almanzora** ≈ SE Spain
139 S9 **Al Mardah** C Iraq
Al-Mariyya *see* Almería
75 R7 **Al Marj** *var.* Barka, *It.* Barce. NE Libya
138 L2 **Al Mashrafah** Ar Raqqah, N Syria
141 X8 **Al Maṣna'ah** *var.* Al Muṣana'a. NE Oman
105 T9 **Almassora** País Valenciano, E Spain
Almatinskaya Oblast' *see* Almaty
145 U15 **Almaty** *var.* Alma-Ata. Almaty, SE Kazakhstan
145 S14 **Almaty** *off.* Almatinskaya Oblast', *Kaz.* Almaty Oblysy; *prev.* Alma-Atinskaya Oblast'. ◈ *province* SE Kazakhstan
145 U15 **Almaty** × Almaty, SE Kazakhstan
Almaty Oblysy *see* Almaty
al-Mawailih *see* Al Muwayliḥ
139 R3 **Al Mawṣil** *Eng.* Mosul. N Iraq

◆ Country ● Country Capital ◇ Dependent Territory ○ Dependent Territory Capital ◈ Administrative Region × International Airport ▲ Mountain ▲ Mountain Range ※ Volcano ≈ River ◎ Lake ▣ Reservoir

139 N5 **Al Mayādīn** var. Mayadin, Fr. Meyadine. Dayr az Zawr, E Syria
139 X10 **Al Maymūnah** var. Maimuna. SE Iraq
141 N5 **Al Mayyāh** Ḩā'il, N Saudi Arabia
Al Ma'zam see Al Ma'zim
105 P6 **Almazán** Castilla-León, N Spain
141 W8 **Al Ma'zim** var. Al Ma'zam. NW Oman
123 N11 **Almaznyy** Respublika Sakha (Yakutiya), NE Russian Federation
Al Mazra' see Al Mazra'ah
138 G11 **Al Mazra'ah** var. Al Mazra', Mazra'a. Al Karak, W Jordan
101 G15 **Alme** ≈ W Germany
104 I7 **Almeida** Guarda, N Portugal
104 G10 **Almeirim** Santarém, C Portugal
98 O10 **Almelo** Overijssel, E Netherlands
105 S9 **Almenara** País Valenciano, E Spain
105 P12 **Almenaras** ▲ S Spain
105 P5 **Almenar de Soria** Castilla-León, N Spain
104 J6 **Almendra, Embalse de** ⊡ Castilla-León, NW Spain
104 J11 **Almendralejo** Extremadura, W Spain
98 J10 **Almere** var. Almere-stad. Flevoland, C Netherlands
98 J10 **Almere-Buiten** Flevoland, C Netherlands
98 J10 **Almere-Haven** Flevoland, C Netherlands
Almere-stad see Almere
105 P15 **Almería** Ar. Al-Mariyya; anc. Unci, Lat. Portus Magnus. Andalucía, S Spain
105 P14 **Almería** ◆ province Andalucía, S Spain
105 P15 **Almería, Golfo de** gulf S Spain
129 S5 **Al'met'yevsk** Respublika Tatarstan, W Russian Federation
95 L21 **Älmhult** Kronoberg, S Sweden
141 U9 **Al Miḩrāḑ** desert NE Saudi Arabia
Al Mīnā' see El Mina
104 L17 **Almina, Punta** headland Ceuta, Spain, N Africa
Al Minyā see El Minya
Al Miqdādīyah see Al Muqdādīyah
43 P14 **Almirante** Bocas del Toro, NW Panama
Almirós see Almyrós
140 M9 **Al Mislaḩ** spring/well W Saudi Arabia
Almissa see Omiš
104 G13 **Almodôvar** var. Almodóvar. Beja, S Portugal
104 M11 **Almodóvar del Campo** Castilla-La Mancha, C Spain
105 Q9 **Almodóvar del Pinar** Castilla-La Mancha, C Spain
31 S9 **Almont** Michigan, N USA
14 L13 **Almonte** Ontario, SE Canada
104 J14 **Almonte** Andalucía, S Spain
104 K9 **Almonte** ≈ W Spain
152 K9 **Almora** Uttar Pradesh, N India
104 M8 **Almorox** Castilla-La Mancha, C Spain
141 S7 **Al Mubarraz** Ash Sharqīyah, E Saudi Arabia
Al Muḑaibī see Al Muḑaybī
138 G15 **Al Mudawwarah** Ma'ān, SW Jordan
141 Y9 **Al Muḑaybī** var. Al Muḑaibī. NE Oman
Almudébar see Almudévar
105 S5 **Almudévar** var. Almudébar. Aragón, NE Spain
141 S15 **Al Mukallā** var. Mukalla. SE Yemen
141 N16 **Al Mukhā** Eng. Mocha. SW Yemen
105 N15 **Almuñécar** Andalucía, S Spain
139 U7 **Al Muqdādīyah** var. Al Miqdādīyah. C Iraq
140 L3 **Al Murayr** spring/well NW Saudi Arabia
136 M12 **Almus** Tokat, N Turkey
Al Muşana'a see Al Maşna'ah
139 T9 **Al Musayyib** var. Musaiyib. C Iraq
139 V9 **Al Muwaffaqīyah** S Iraq
138 H10 **Al Muwaqqar** var. El Muwaqqar. 'Ammān, W Jordan
140 J5 **Al Muwayliḩ** var. al-Mawailih. Tabūk, NW Saudi Arabia
115 F17 **Almyrós** var. Almirós. Thessalía, C Greece
115 I24 **Almyroú, Órmos** bay Kriti, Greece, E Mediterranean Sea
Al Nūwfalīyah see An Nawfalīyah
96 L13 **Alnwick** N England, UK
Al Obayyid see El Obeid
Al Odaid see Al 'Udayd
190 B16 **Alofi** ○ (Niue) W Niue
190 A16 **Alofi Bay** bay W Niue, C Pacific Ocean
190 E13 **Alofi, Île** island S Wallis and Futuna
190 E13 **Alofitai** Île Alofi, W Wallis and Futuna
Aloha State see Hawaii
118 G7 **Aloja** Limbaži, N Latvia
153 X10 **Along** Arunāchal Pradesh, NE India
115 H16 **Alónnisos** island Vóreioi Sporádes, Greece, Aegean Sea
104 M15 **Álora** Andalucía, S Spain
171 Q16 **Alor, Kepulauan** island group E Indonesia
171 Q16 **Alor, Pulau** prev. Ombai. island Kepulauan Alor, E Indonesia
168 I7 **Alor Setar** var. Alor Star, Alur Setar. Kedah, Peninsular Malaysia
Alost see Aalst
154 F9 **Ālot** Madhya Pradesh, C India
186 G10 **Alotau** Milne Bay, SE PNG
171 Y16 **Alotip** Irian Jaya, E Indonesia
Al Oued see El Oued
35 R12 **Alpaugh** California, W USA
Alpen see Alps
31 R6 **Alpena** Michigan, N USA
Alpes see Alps
103 S14 **Alpes-de-Haute-Provence** ◆ department SE France
103 U14 **Alpes-Maritimes** ◆ department SE France
181 W8 **Alpha** Queensland, E Australia
197 R9 **Alpha Cordillera** var. Alpha Ridge. undersea feature Arctic Ocean
Alpha Ridge see Alpha Cordillera
Alpheius see Alfeiós
99 I15 **Alphen** Noord-Brabant, S Netherlands
98 H11 **Alphen aan den Rijn** var. Alphen. Zuid-Holland, C Netherlands
Alpheus see Alfeiós
Alpi see Alps
104 G10 **Alpiarça** Santarém, C Portugal
24 K10 **Alpine** Texas, SW USA
108 F8 **Alpnach** Unterwalden, W Switzerland
108 D11 **Alps** Fr. Alpes, Ger. Alpen, It. Alpi. ▲▲ C Europe
141 W8 **Al Qābil** var. Qabil. N Oman
Al Qaḑārif see Gedaref
75 P8 **Al Qaddāḩīyah** N Libya
Al Qāhirah see Cairo
140 K4 **Al Qalībah** Tabūk, NW Saudi Arabia
139 O1 **Al Qāmishlī** var. Kamishli, Qamishly. Al Ḩasakah, NE Syria
138 I6 **Al Qaryatayn** var. Qaryatayn, Fr. Qariateïne. Ḩimş, C Syria
142 K11 **Al Qash'ānīyah** var. Al-Kashaniya. NE Kuwait
141 N7 **Al Qaşīm** off. Minţaqat Qaşīm, Qassim. ◆ province C Saudi Arabia
138 J5 **Al Qaşr** Ḩimş, C Syria
Al Qaşr see El Qaşr
Al Qaşrayn see Kasserine
141 S6 **Al Qaţīf** Ash Sharqīyah, NE Saudi Arabia
138 G11 **Al Qaţrānah** var. El Qatrani, Qatrana. Al Karak, W Jordan
75 P11 **Al Qaţrūn** SW Libya
Al Qayrawān see Kairouan
Al-Qsar al-Kbir see Ksar-el-Kebir
Al Qubayyāt see Qoubaïyât
Al Quds/Al Quds ash Sharīf see Jerusalem
138 G8 **Al Qunayţirah** var. El Kuneitra, El Quneitra, Kuneitra, Qunaytra. Al Qunayţirah, SW Syria
138 G8 **Al Qunayţirah** off. Muḩāfaẓat al Qunayţirah, var. El Q'unayţirah, Qunaytirah, Fr. Kuneitra. ◆ governorate SW Syria
140 M11 **Al Qunfudhah** Makkah, SW Saudi Arabia
140 K2 **Al Qurayyāt** Al Jawf, NW Saudi Arabia
139 Y11 **Al Qurnah** var. Kurna. SE Iraq
139 V12 **Al Quşayr** S Iraq
138 I6 **Al Quşayr** var. El Quseir, Quşayr, Fr. Kousseir. Ḩimş, W Syria
Al Quşayr see Quseir
138 H7 **Al Quţayfah** var. Quţayfah, Qutayfe, Quteife, Fr. Kouteifé. Dimashq, W Syria
141 P8 **Al Quwayīyah** Ar Riyāḑ, C Saudi Arabia
Al Quwayr see Guwēr
138 F14 **Al Quwayrah** var. El Quweira. Ma'ān, SW Jordan
Al Rayyan see Ar Rayyān
Al Ruweis see Ar Ruways
95 G24 **Als** Ger. Alsen. island SW Denmark
103 U5 **Alsace** Ger. Elsass; anc. Alsatia. ◆ region NE France
11 R16 **Alsask** Saskatchewan, S Canada
Alsasua see Altsasu
Alsatia see Alsace
101 C16 **Alsdorf** Nordrhein-Westfalen, W Germany
10 G8 **Alsek** ≈ Canada/USA
Alsen see Als
101 F19 **Alsenz** ≈ W Germany
101 H17 **Alsfeld** Hessen, C Germany
119 K20 **Al'shany** Rus. Ol'shany. Brestskaya Voblasts', SW Belarus
Alsókubin see Dolný Kubín
118 C9 **Alsunga** Kuldīga, W Latvia
Alt see Olt
92 K9 **Alta** Fin. Alattio. Finnmark, N Norway
29 T12 **Alta** Iowa, C USA
108 I7 **Altach** Vorarlberg, W Austria
92 K9 **Altaelva** ≈ N Norway
92 J8 **Altafjorden** fjord NE Norwegian Sea
62 K10 **Alta Gracia** Córdoba, C Argentina
42 K11 **Alta Gracia** Rivas, SW Nicaragua
54 H4 **Altagracia** Zulia, NW Venezuela
54 M5 **Altagracia de Orituco** Guárico, N Venezuela
Altai see Altai Mountains
131 T7 **Altai Mountains** var. Altai, Chin. Altay Shan, Rus. Altay. ▲▲ Asia/Europe
23 V6 **Altamaha River** ≈ Georgia, SE USA
58 J13 **Altamira** Pará, NE Brazil
54 D12 **Altamira** Huila, S Colombia
42 M13 **Altamira** Alajuela, N Costa Rica
41 Q11 **Altamira** Tamaulipas, C Mexico
30 L15 **Altamont** Illinois, N USA
27 Q7 **Altamont** Kansas, C USA
32 H16 **Altamont** Oregon, NW USA
20 K10 **Altamont** Tennessee, S USA
23 X11 **Altamonte Springs** Florida, SE USA
107 O17 **Altamura** anc. Lupatia. Puglia, SE Italy
40 H9 **Altamura, Isla** island C Mexico
162 G7 **Altan** Dzavhan, W Mongolia
162 G6 **Altanbulag** Dzavhan, N Mongolia
Altan Emel see Xin Barag Youqi
162 J8 **Altan-Ovoo** Arhangay, C Mongolia
162 E7 **Altanteel** Hovd, W Mongolia
40 F3 **Altar** Sonora, NW Mexico
40 D2 **Altar, Desierto de** var. Sonoran Desert. desert Mexico/USA see also Sonoran Desert
105 Q8 **Alta, Sierra** ▲ N Spain
40 H9 **Altata** Sinaloa, C Mexico
42 D4 **Alta Verapaz** off. Departamento de Alta Verapaz. ◆ department C Guatemala
107 L18 **Altavilla Silentia** Campania, S Italy
21 T7 **Altavista** Virginia, NE USA
158 L2 **Altay** Xinjiang Uygur Zizhiqu, NW China
162 G5 **Altay** Dzavhan, N Mongolia
162 G8 **Altay** Govĭ-Altay, W Mongolia
Altay see Altai Mountains
122 J14 **Altay, Respublika** var. Gornyy Altay; prev. Gorno-Altayskaya Respublika. ◆ autonomous republic S Russian Federation
Altay Shan see Altai Mountains
123 I13 **Altayskiy Kray** ◆ territory S Russian Federation
Altbetsche see Bečej
101 L20 **Altdorf** Bayern, SE Germany
108 G8 **Altdorf** var. Altorf. Uri, C Switzerland
105 T11 **Altea** País Valenciano, E Spain
100 L10 **Alte Elde** ≈ N Germany
101 M16 **Altenburg** Thüringen, E Germany
Altenburg see București, Romania
Altenburg see Baia de Criş, Romania
100 P12 **Alte Oder** ≈ NE Germany
104 H10 **Alter do Chão** Portalegre, C Portugal
92 I10 **Altevatnet** ◎ N Norway
27 V12 **Altheimer** Arkansas, C USA
109 T9 **Althofen** Kärnten, S Austria
114 H7 **Altimir** Vratsa, NW Bulgaria
136 K11 **Altınkaya Barajı** ⊡ N Turkey
139 S3 **Altin Köprü** var. Altun Kupri. N Iraq
136 E13 **Altıntaş** Kütahya, W Turkey
57 K18 **Altiplano** physical region W South America
Altkanischa see Kanjiža
103 U7 **Altkirch** Haut-Rhin, NE France
Altlublau see Stará Ľubovňa
100 L12 **Altmark** cultural region N Germany
Altmoldowa see Moldova Veche
25 W8 **Alto** Texas, SW USA
104 H11 **Alto Alentejo** physical region S Portugal
59 I19 **Alto Araguaia** Mato Grosso, C Brazil
58 L12 **Alto Bonito** Pará, NE Brazil
83 O15 **Alto Molócuè** Zambézia, NE Mozambique
30 K15 **Alton** Illinois, N USA
27 W8 **Alton** Missouri, C USA
11 X17 **Altona** Manitoba, S Canada
18 E14 **Altoona** Pennsylvania, NE USA
30 J6 **Altoona** Wisconsin, N USA
62 N3 **Alto Paraguay** off. Departamento del Alto Paraguay. ◆ department N Paraguay
59 L17 **Alto Paraíso de Goiás** Goiás, S Brazil
62 P6 **Alto Paraná** off. Departamento del Alto Paraná. ◆ department E Paraguay
Alto Paraná see Paraná
59 L15 **Alto Parnaíba** Maranhão, E Brazil
56 H13 **Alto Purús, Río** ≈ E Peru
Altorf see Altdorf
63 H19 **Alto Río Senguer** var. Alto Río Senguerr. Chubut, S Argentina
41 Q13 **Altotonga** Veracruz-Llave, E Mexico
101 N23 **Altötting** Bayern, SE Germany
Altpasua see Stara Pazova
162 I5 **Altraga** Hövsgöl, N Mongolia
Alt-Schwanenburg see Gulbene
105 P3 **Altsasu** Cast. Alsasua. Navarra, N Spain
Altsohl see Zvolen
108 I7 **Altstätten** Sankt Gallen, NE Switzerland
42 G1 **Altun Ha** ruins Belize, N Belize
Altun Kupri see Altin Köprü
158 D8 **Altun Shan** ▲ C China
158 L9 **Altun Shan** var. Altyn Tagh. ▲▲ NW China
35 P2 **Alturas** California, W USA
26 K12 **Altus** Oklahoma, C USA
26 K11 **Altus Lake** ⊡ Oklahoma, C USA
Altvater see Praděd
Altyn Tagh see Altun Shan
Alu see Shortland Island
al-'Ubaila see Al 'Ubaylah
139 O6 **Al 'Ubaydī** W Iraq
141 T9 **Al 'Ubaylah** var. al-'Ubaila. Ash Sharqīyah, E Saudi Arabia
141 T9 **Al 'Ubaylah** spring/well E Saudi Arabia
Al Ubayyiḑ see El Obeid
141 T7 **Al 'Udayd** var. Al Odaid. Abū Ẓaby, W UAE
118 J8 **Alūksne** Ger. Marienburg. Alūksne, NE Latvia
140 K6 **Al 'Ulā** Al Madīnah, NW Saudi Arabia
173 N4 **Alula-Fartak Trench** var. Illaue Fartak Trench. undersea feature W Indian Ocean
138 I11 **Al 'Umarī** 'Ammān, E Jordan
31 S13 **Alum Creek Lake** ⊡ Ohio, N USA
63 H15 **Aluminé** Neuquén, C Argentina
95 O14 **Alunda** Uppsala, C Sweden
117 T14 **Alupka** Respublika Krym, S Ukraine
75 P8 **Al 'Uqaylah** N Libya
Al Uqşur see Luxor
Al Urdunn see Jordan
168 J9 **Alur Panal** bay Sumatera, W Indonesia
141 V10 **Al 'Urūq al Mu'tariḑah** salt lake SE Saudi Arabia
139 Q7 **Ālūs** C Iraq
117 T13 **Alushta** Respublika Krym, S Ukraine
75 N11 **Al 'Uwaynāt** var. Al Awaynāt. SW Libya
139 T6 **Al 'Uẓaym** var. Adhaim. E Iraq
26 L8 **Alva** Oklahoma, C USA
104 H8 **Alva** ≈ N Portugal
95 J18 **Älvängen** Västra Götaland, S Sweden
14 F14 **Alvanley** Ontario, S Canada
41 S14 **Alvarado** Veracruz-Llave, E Mexico
25 T7 **Alvarado** Texas, SW USA
58 D13 **Alvarães** Amazonas, NW Brazil
40 G6 **Alvaro Obregón, Presa** ⊡ W Mexico
94 H10 **Alvdal** Hedmark, S Norway
94 K12 **Älvdalen** Dalarna, C Sweden
61 E15 **Alvear** Corrientes, NE Argentina
104 F10 **Alverca do Ribatejo** Lisboa, C Portugal
95 L20 **Alvesta** Kronoberg, S Sweden
94 D13 **Ålvik** Hordaland, S Norway
25 W12 **Alvin** Texas, SW USA
94 O13 **Älvkarleby** Uppsala, C Sweden
25 S5 **Alvord** Texas, SW USA
93 G18 **Älvros** Jämtland, C Sweden
92 J13 **Älvsbyn** Norrbotten, N Sweden
142 K12 **Al Wafrā'** SE Kuwait
140 J6 **Al Wajh** Tabūk, NW Saudi Arabia
143 N16 **Al Wakrah** var. Wakra. C Qatar
138 M8 **al Walaj, Sha'īb** dry watercourse W Iraq
152 I11 **Alwar** Rājasthān, N India
141 Q5 **Al Wari'ah** Ash Sharqīyah, N Saudi Arabia
155 G22 **Alwaye** Kerala, SW India
162 K14 **Alxa Zuoqi** var. Ehen Hudag. Nei Mongol Zizhiqu, N China
Al Yaman see Yemen
138 G9 **Al Yarmūk** Irbid, N Jordan
Alyat/Alyaty-Pristan' see Älät
115 I14 **Alykí** var. Aliki. Thásos, N Greece
119 F14 **Alytus** Pol. Olita. Alytus, S Lithuania
101 N23 **Alz** ≈ SE Germany
33 Y11 **Alzada** Montana, NW USA
122 L12 **Alzamay** Irkutskaya Oblast', S Russian Federation
99 M25 **Alzette** ≈ S Luxembourg
105 S10 **Alzira** var. Alcira; anc. Saetabicula, Suero. País Valenciano, E Spain
Al Zubair see Az Zubayr
181 O8 **Amadeus, Lake** seasonal lake Northern Territory, C Australia
81 E15 **Amadi** Western Equatoria, SW Sudan
9 R7 **Amadjuak Lake** ◎ Baffin Island, Nunavut, N Canada
95 J23 **Amager** island E Denmark
165 N14 **Amagi-san** ▲ Honshū, S Japan
171 S13 **Amahai** var. Masohi. Pulau Seram, E Indonesia
38 M16 **Amak Island** island Alaska, USA
164 B14 **Amakusa-nada** gulf Kyūshū, SW Japan
95 J16 **Åmål** Västra Götaland, S Sweden
54 E8 **Amalfi** Antioquia, N Colombia
107 L18 **Amalfi** Campania, S Italy
115 D19 **Amaliáda** var. Amaliás. Dytikí Ellás, S Greece
Amaliás see Amaliáda
154 F12 **Amalner** Mahārāshtra, C India
171 W14 **Amamapare** Irian Jaya, E Indonesia
59 H21 **Amambaí, Serra de** var. Cordillera de Amambay, Serra de Amambay. ▲▲ Brazil/Paraguay see also Amambay, Cordillera de
62 P4 **Amambay** off. Departamento del Amambay. ◆ department E Paraguay
62 P5 **Amambay, Cordillera de** var. Serra de Amambaí, Serra de Amambay. ▲▲ Brazil/Paraguay see also Amambaí, Serra de
Amambay, Serra de see Amambaí, Serra de/Amambay, Cordillera de
165 U16 **Amami-guntō** island group SW Japan
165 V15 **Amami-Ō-shima** island S Japan
186 A5 **Amanab** Sandaun, NW PNG
106 J13 **Amandola** Marche, C Italy
107 N21 **Amantea** Calabria, SW Italy
191 W10 **Amanu** island Îles Tuamotu, C French Polynesia
58 J10 **Amapá** Amapá, NE Brazil
58 J11 **Amapá** off. Estado de Amapá; prev. Território de Amapá. ◆ state NE Brazil
42 H8 **Amapala** Valle, S Honduras
Amara see Al 'Amārah
104 H6 **Amarante** Porto, N Portugal
166 M5 **Amarapura** Mandalay, C Myanmar
162 L9 **Amardalay** Dundgovĭ, C Mongolia
104 I12 **Amareleja** Beja, S Portugal
35 V11 **Amargosa Range** ▲▲ California, W USA
25 N2 **Amarillo** Texas, SW USA
Amarinthos see Amárynthos
107 K15 **Amaro, Monte** ▲ C Italy
115 H18 **Amárynthos** var. Amarinthos. Évvoia, C Greece
Amasia see Amasya
136 K12 **Amasya** anc. Amasia. Amasya, N Turkey
136 K11 **Amasya** ◆ province N Turkey
42 F4 **Amatique, Bahía de** bay Gulf of Honduras, W Caribbean Sea
42 D6 **Amatitlán, Lago de** ◎ S Guatemala
107 J14 **Amatrice** Lazio, C Italy
190 C8 **Amatuku** atoll C Tuvalu
99 J20 **Amay** Liège, E Belgium
48 F7 **Amazon** Sp. Amazonas. ≈ Brazil/Peru
59 C14 **Amazonas** off. Estado do Amazonas. ◆ state N Brazil
54 G15 **Amazonas** off. Comisaria del Amazonas. ◆ province SE Colombia
56 C10 **Amazonas** off. Departamento de Amazonas. ◆ department N Peru
54 M12 **Amazonas** off. Territorio Amazonas. ◆ federal territory S Venezuela
Amazonas see Amazon
48 F7 **Amazon Basin** basin N South America
47 V5 **Amazon Fan** undersea feature W Atlantic Ocean
58 K11 **Amazon, Mouths of the** delta NE Brazil
187 R13 **Ambae** var. Aoba, Omba. island C Vanuatu
152 I9 **Ambāla** Haryāna, NW India
155 J26 **Ambalangoda** Southern Province, SW Sri Lanka
155 K26 **Ambalantota** Southern Province, S Sri Lanka
172 I6 **Ambalavao** Fianarantsoa, C Madagascar
54 E10 **Ambalema** Tolima, C Colombia
79 E17 **Ambam** Sud, S Cameroon
172 J2 **Ambanja** Antsirañana, N Madagascar
123 T6 **Ambarchik** Respublika Sakha (Yakutiya), NE Russian Federation
62 K9 **Ambargasta, Salinas de** salt lake C Argentina
126 J6 **Ambarnyy** Respublika Kareliya, NW Russian Federation
56 C7 **Ambato** Tungurahua, C Ecuador
172 I5 **Ambatolampy** Antananarivo, C Madagascar
172 H4 **Ambatomainty** Mahajanga, W Madagascar
172 J4 **Ambatondrazaka** Toamasina, C Madagascar
101 L20 **Amberg** var. Amberg in der Oberpfalz. Bayern, SE Germany
Amberg in der Oberpfalz see Amberg
42 H1 **Ambergris Cay** island NE Belize
103 S11 **Ambérieu-en-Bugey** Ain, E France
185 I18 **Amberley** Canterbury, South Island, NZ
103 P11 **Ambert** Puy-de-Dôme, C France
Ambianum see Amiens
76 J11 **Ambidédi** Kayes, SW Mali
154 M10 **Ambikāpur** Madhya Pradesh, C India
172 J2 **Ambilobe** Antsirañana, N Madagascar
39 O7 **Ambler** Alaska, USA
Amblève see Amel
Ambo see Hägere Hiywet
172 I8 **Amboasary** Toliara, S Madagascar
172 J4 **Ambodifotatra** var. Ambodifototra. Toamasina, E Madagascar
Amboenten see Ambunten
172 I5 **Ambohidratrimo** Antananarivo, C Madagascar
172 I6 **Ambohimahasoa** Fianarantsoa, SE Madagascar
172 K3 **Ambohitralanana** Antsirañana, NE Madagascar
Amboina see Ambon
102 M8 **Amboise** Indre-et-Loire, C France
171 S13 **Ambon** prev. Amboina, Amboyna. Pulau Ambon, E Indonesia
171 S13 **Ambon, Pulau** island E Indonesia
81 I20 **Amboseli, Lake** ◎ Kenya/Tanzania
172 I6 **Ambositra** Fianarantsoa, SE Madagascar
172 I8 **Ambovombe** Toliara, S Madagascar
35 W14 **Amboy** California, W USA
30 L11 **Amboy** Illinois, N USA
Amboyna see Ambon
Ambracia see Árta
18 B14 **Ambridge** Pennsylvania, NE USA
Ambrim see Ambrym
Ambrizete see N'Zeto
187 R13 **Ambrym** var. Ambrim. island C Vanuatu
8 K3 **Amund Ringnes Island** island Nunavut, N Canada
169 T16 **Ambunten** prev. Amboenten. Pulau Madura, E Indonesia
186 B6 **Ambunti** East Sepik, NW PNG
155 I20 **Āmbūr** Tamil Nādu, SE India
38 E17 **Amchitka Island** island Aleutian Islands, Alaska, USA
38 F17 **Amchitka Pass** strait Aleutian Islands, Alaska, USA
141 R15 **'Amd** C Yemen
78 J10 **Am Dam** Ouaddaï, E Chad
171 U16 **Amdassa** Pulau Yamdena, E Indonesia
127 U1 **Amderma** Nenetskiy Avtonomnyy Okrug, NW Russian Federation
159 N14 **Amdo** Xizang Zizhiqu, W China
40 K13 **Ameca** Jalisco, SW Mexico
41 P14 **Amecameca** var. Amecameca de Juárez. México, C Mexico
Amecameca de Juárez see Amecameca
61 A20 **Ameghino** Buenos Aires, E Argentina
99 M21 **Amel** Fr. Amblève. Liège, E Belgium
98 K4 **Ameland** Fris. It Amelân. island Waddeneilanden, N Netherlands
Amelân, It see Ameland
107 H14 **Amelia** Umbria, C Italy
21 V6 **Amelia Court House** Virginia, NE USA
23 W8 **Amelia Island** island Florida, SE USA
18 L12 **Amenia** New York, NE USA
America see United States of America
65 M21 **America-Antarctica Ridge** undersea feature S Atlantic Ocean
America in Miniature see Maryland
60 L9 **Americana** São Paulo, S Brazil
33 Q15 **American Falls** Idaho, NW USA
33 Q15 **American Falls Reservoir** ⊡ Idaho, NW USA
36 L3 **American Fork** Utah, W USA
192 K16 **American Samoa** ◇ US unincorporated territory W Polynesia
23 S6 **Americus** Georgia, SE USA
98 K12 **Amerongen** Utrecht, C Netherlands
98 K11 **Amersfoort** Utrecht, C Netherlands
97 N21 **Amersham** SE England, UK
30 I5 **Amery** Wisconsin, N USA
195 W6 **Amery Ice Shelf** ice shelf Antarctica
29 V13 **Ames** Iowa, C USA
19 P10 **Amesbury** Massachusetts, NE USA
Amestratus see Mistretta
115 F18 **Amfíkleia** var. Amfíklia. Stereá Ellás, C Greece
Amfíklia see Amfíkleia
115 D17 **Amfilochía** var. Amfilokhía. Dytikí Ellás, C Greece
Amfilokhía see Amfilochía
114 H13 **Amfípoli** anc. Amphipolis. site of ancient city Kentrikí Makedonía, NE Greece
115 F18 **Ámfissa** Stereá Ellás, C Greece
123 Q10 **Amga** Respublika Sakha (Yakutiya), NE Russian Federation
123 Q11 **Amga** ≈ NE Russian Federation
Amgalang see Xin Barag Zuoqi
123 V5 **Amguema** ≈ NE Russian Federation
123 S12 **Amgun'** ≈ SE Russian Federation
80 J12 **Amhara** ◆ region N Ethiopia
13 P15 **Amherst** Nova Scotia, SE Canada
18 M11 **Amherst** Massachusetts, NE USA
18 D10 **Amherst** New York, NE USA
24 M4 **Amherst** Texas, SW USA
21 U6 **Amherst** Virginia, NE USA
Amherst see Kyaikkami
14 C18 **Amherstburg** Ontario, S Canada
21 Q6 **Amherstdale** West Virginia, NE USA
14 K15 **Amherst Island** island Ontario, SE Canada
Amida see Diyarbakır
28 J6 **Amidon** North Dakota, N USA
103 O3 **Amiens** anc. Ambianum, Samarobriva. Somme, N France
139 P8 **'Āmij, Wādī** var. Wadi 'Amīq. dry watercourse W Iraq
136 L17 **Amik Ovası** ◎ S Turkey
76 E9 **Amilcar Cabral** ✕ Sal, NE Cape Verde
Amilḩayt, Wādī see Umm al Ḩayt, Wādī
Amíndaion/Amindeo see Amýntaio
155 C21 **Amīndīvi Islands** island group Lakshadweep, India, N Indian Ocean
139 U6 **Amīn Ḩabīb** E Iraq
83 E20 **Aminuis** Omaheke, E Namibia
'Amīq, Wadi see 'Āmij, Wādī
142 J7 **Amīrābād** Īlām, NW Iran
Amirante Bank see Amirante Ridge
173 N6 **Amirante Basin** undersea feature W Indian Ocean
173 N6 **Amirante Islands** var. Amirantes Group. island group C Seychelles
173 N7 **Amirante Ridge** var. Amirante Bank. undersea feature W Indian Ocean
Amirantes Group see Amirante Islands
173 N7 **Amirante Trench** undersea feature W Indian Ocean
11 U13 **Amisk Lake** ◎ Saskatchewan, C Canada
Amistad, Presa de la see Amistad Reservoir
25 O12 **Amistad Reservoir** var. Presa de la Amistad. ⊡ Mexico/USA
Amisus see Samsun
22 K8 **Amite** var. Amite City. Louisiana, S USA
Amite City see Amite
27 T12 **Amity** Arkansas, C USA
154 H11 **Amla** prev. Amulla. Madhya Pradesh, C India
38 I17 **Amlia Island** island Aleutian Islands, Alaska, USA
97 I18 **Amlwch** NW Wales, UK
Ammaia see Portalegre
138 H10 **'Ammān** var. Amman; anc. Philadelphia, Bibl. Rabbah Ammon, Rabbath Ammon. ● (Jordan) 'Ammān, NW Jordan

◆ Country ● Country Capital ◇ Dependent Territory ○ Dependent Territory Capital ◆ Administrative Region ✕ International Airport ▲ Mountain ▲▲ Mountain Range Volcano ≈ River ◎ Lake ⊡ Reservoir

138 H10 **'Ammān** *off.* Muḥāfaẓat 'Ammān. ◆ *governorate* NW Jordan
93 N14 **Ämmänsaari** Oulu, E Finland
92 H13 **Ammarnäs** Västerbotten, N Sweden
197 O15 **Ammassalik** *var.* Angmagssalik. Tunu, S Greenland
101 K24 **Ammer** ~ SE Germany
101 K24 **Ammersee** ◎ SE Germany
98 J13 **Ammerzoden** Gelderland, C Netherlands
Ammóchostos *see* Gazimağusa
Ammóchostos, Kólpos *see* Gazimağusa Körfezi
Amnok-kang *see* Yalu
Amoea *see* Portalegre
Amoentai *see* Amuntai
Amoerang *see* Amurang
143 O4 **Āmol** *var.* Amul. Māzandarān, N Iran
115 K21 **Amorgós** Amorgós, Kykládes, Greece, Aegean Sea
115 K22 **Amorgós** *island* Kykládes, Greece, Aegean Sea
23 N3 **Amory** Mississippi, S USA
12 I13 **Amos** Quebec, SE Canada
95 G15 **Åmot** Buskerud, S Norway
95 E15 **Åmot** Telemark, S Norway
95 J15 **Åmotfors** Värmland, C Sweden
76 L10 **Amourj** Hodh ech Chargui, SE Mauritania
Amoy *see* Xiamen
172 H7 **Ampanihy** Toliara, SW Madagascar
155 L25 **Ampara** *var.* Amparai. Eastern Province, E Sri Lanka
172 J4 **Amparafaravola** Toamasina, E Madagascar
Amparai *see* Ampara
60 M9 **Amparo** São Paulo, S Brazil
172 J5 **Ampasimanolotra** Toamasina, E Madagascar
57 H17 **Ampato, Nevado** ▲ S Peru
101 L23 **Amper** ~ SE Germany
64 M9 **Ampère Seamount** *undersea feature* E Atlantic Ocean
Amphipolis *see* Amfipoli
167 X10 **Amphitrite Group** *island group* N Paracel Islands
171 T16 **Amplawas** *var.* Emplawas. Pulau Babar, E Indonesia
105 U7 **Amposta** Cataluña, NE Spain
15 V7 **Amqui** Quebec, SE Canada
141 O14 **'Amrān** W Yemen
Amraoti *see* Amrāvati
154 H12 **Amrāvati** *prev.* Amraoti. Mahārāshtra, C India
154 C11 **Amreli** Gujarāt, W India
108 H6 **Amriswil** Thurgau, NE Switzerland
138 H5 **'Amrīt** *ruins* Ṭarṭūs, W Syria
152 H7 **Amritsar** Punjab, N India
152 J10 **Amroha** Uttar Pradesh, N India
100 G7 **Amrum** *island* NW Germany
93 I15 **Åmsele** Västerbotten, N Sweden
98 I10 **Amstelveen** Noord-Holland, C Netherlands
98 I10 **Amsterdam** ● (Netherlands) Noord-Holland, C Netherlands
18 K10 **Amsterdam** New York, NE USA
173 Q11 **Amsterdam Fracture Zone** *tectonic feature* S Indian Ocean
173 R11 **Amsterdam Island** *island* NE French Southern and Antarctic Territories
109 U4 **Amstetten** Niederösterreich, N Austria
78 J11 **Am Timan** Salamat, SE Chad
146 L12 **Amu-Bukhoro Kanali** *var.* Aral-Bukhorskiy Kanal. *canal* C Uzbekistan
139 O1 **'Āmūdah** *var.* Amude. Al Ḥasakah, N Syria
146 M14 **Amu-Dar'ya** Lebapskiy Velayat, NE Turkmenistan
147 O15 **Amu Darya** *Rus.* Amudar'ya, *Taj.* Dar"yoi Amu, *Turkm.* Amyderya, *Uzb.* Amudaryo; *anc.* Oxus. ~ C Asia
Amudar'ya/Amudaryo/Amu, Dar"yoi *see* Amu Darya
Amude *see* 'Āmūdah
140 L3 **'Amūd, Jabal al** ▲ NW Saudi Arabia
38 J17 **Amukta Island** *island* Aleutian Islands, Alaska, USA
38 I17 **Amukta Pass** *strait* Aleutian Islands, Alaska, USA
Amul *see* Āmol
Amulla *see* Amla
Amundsen Basin *see* Fram Basin
195 X3 **Amundsen Bay** *bay* Antarctica
195 P10 **Amundsen Coast** *physical region* Antarctica
8 I6 **Amundsen Gulf** *gulf* Northwest Territories, N Canada
193 O14 **Amundsen Plain** *undersea feature* S Pacific Ocean
195 Q9 **Amundsen-Scott** *US research station* Antarctica
194 J11 **Amundsen Sea** *sea* S Pacific Ocean
94 M12 **Amungen** ◎ C Sweden
169 U13 **Amuntai** *prev.* Amoentai. Borneo, C Indonesia
131 W6 **Amur** *Chin.* Heilong Jiang. ~ China/Russian Federation
171 Q11 **Amurang** *prev.* Amoerang. Sulawesi, C Indonesia
105 O3 **Amurrio** País Vasco, N Spain
123 S13 **Amursk** Khabarovskiy Kray, SE Russian Federation
123 Q12 **Amurskaya Oblast'** ◆ *province* SE Russian Federation
80 G7 **'Amur, Wadi** ~ NE Sudan
115 C17 **Amvrakikós Kólpos** *gulf* W Greece
Amvrosiyevka *see* Amvrosiyivka
117 X8 **Amvrosiyivka** *Rus.* Amvrosiyevka. Donets'ka Oblast', SE Ukraine
Amyderya *see* Amu Darya
114 E13 **Amýntaio** *var.* Amindeo; *prev.* Amíndaion. Dytikí Makedonía, N Greece
14 B6 **Amyot** Ontario, S Canada
191 U10 **Anaa** *atoll* Îles Tuamotu, C French Polynesia
Anabanoea *see* Anabanua
171 N14 **Anabanua** *prev.* Anabanoea. Sulawesi, C Indonesia
189 R8 **Anabar** NE Nauru
123 N8 **Anabar** ~ NE Russian Federation
An Abhainn Mhór *see* Blackwater
55 O6 **Anaco** Anzoátegui, NE Venezuela
33 Q10 **Anaconda** Montana, NW USA
32 H7 **Anacortes** Washington, NW USA
26 M11 **Anadarko** Oklahoma, C USA
114 N12 **Ana Dere** ~ NW Turkey
104 G8 **Anadia** Aveiro, N Portugal
Anadolu Dağları *see* Doğu Karadeniz Dağları
123 V6 **Anadyr'** Chukotskiy Avtonomnyy Okrug, NE Russian Federation
123 V6 **Anadyr'** ~ NE Russian Federation
Anadyr, Gulf of *see* Anadyrskiy Zaliv
131 X4 **Anadyrskiy Khrebet** *var.* Chukot Range. ▲ NE Russian Federation
123 W6 **Anadyrskiy Zaliv** *Eng.* Gulf of Anadyr. *gulf* NE Russian Federation
115 K22 **Anáfi** *anc.* Anaphe. *island* Kykládes, Greece, Aegean Sea
107 J15 **Anagni** Lazio, C Italy
'Ānah *see* 'Annah
35 T15 **Anaheim** California, W USA
10 L15 **Anahim Lake** British Columbia, SW Canada
38 B8 **Anahola** Kauai, Hawaii, USA, C Pacific Ocean
25 X11 **Anahuac** Texas, SW USA
41 O7 **Anáhuac** Nuevo León, NE Mexico
155 G22 **Anai Mudi** ▲ S India
Anaiza *see* 'Unayzah
155 M15 **Anakāpalle** Andhra Pradesh, E India
191 W15 **Anakena, Playa de** *beach* Easter Island, Chile, E Pacific Ocean
39 Q7 **Anaktuvuk Pass** Alaska, USA
39 Q6 **Anaktuvuk River** ~ Alaska, USA
172 J3 **Analalava** Mahajanga, NW Madagascar
44 F6 **Ana María, Golfo de** *gulf* C Cuba
Anambas Islands *see* Anambas, Kepulauan
169 N8 **Anambas, Kepulauan** *var.* Anambas Islands *island group* W Indonesia
77 U17 **Anambra** ◆ *state* SE Nigeria
29 N4 **Anamoose** North Dakota, N USA
29 Y13 **Anamosa** Iowa, C USA
136 H17 **Anamur** İçel, S Turkey
136 H17 **Anamur Burnu** *headland* S Turkey
154 O12 **Ānandadur** Orissa, E India
155 H18 **Anantapur** Andhra Pradesh, S India
152 H5 **Anantnāg** *var.* Islamabad. Jammu and Kashmir, NW India
Ananyev *see* Anan'yiv
117 O9 **Anan'yiv** *Rus.* Ananyev. Odes'ka Oblast', SW Ukraine
128 J14 **Anapa** Krasnodarskiy Kray, SW Russian Federation
Anaphe *see* Anáfi
59 K18 **Anápolis** Goiás, C Brazil
143 R10 **Anār** Kermān, C Iran
Anár *see* Inari
143 P7 **Anārak** Eşfahān, C Iran
Anar Dara *see* Anār Darreh
148 J7 **Anār Darreh** *var.* Anar Dara. Farāh, W Afghanistan
Anárjohka *see* Inarijoki
23 X9 **Anastasia Island** *island* Florida, SE USA
188 K7 **Anatahan** *island* C Northern Mariana Islands
130 M6 **Anatolia** *plateau* C Turkey
86 F14 **Anatolian Plate** *tectonic feature* Asia/Europe
114 H13 **Anatolikí Makedonía kai Thráki** *Eng.* Macedonia East and Thrace. ◆ *region* NE Greece
Anatom *see* Aneityum
62 L8 **Añatuya** Santiago del Estero, N Argentina
An Baile Meánach *see* Ballymena
An Bhearú *see* Barrow
An Bhóinn *see* Boyne
An Blascaod Mór *see* Great Blasket Island
An Cabhán *see* Cavan
An Caisleán Nua *see* Newcastle
An Caisleán Riabhach *see* Castlereagh, Northern Ireland, UK
An Caisleán Riabhach *see* Castlerea, Ireland
56 C13 **Ancash** *off.* Departamento de Ancash. ◆ *department* W Peru
An Cathair *see* Caher
102 J8 **Ancenis** Loire-Atlantique, NW France
An Chanáil Ríoga *see* Royal Canal
An Cheacha *see* Caha Mountains
39 R11 **Anchorage** Alaska, USA
39 R12 **Anchorage** ✕ Alaska, USA
39 Q13 **Anchor Point** Alaska, USA
An Chorr Chríochach *see* Cookstown
65 M24 **Anchorstack Point** *headland* W Tristan da Cunha
An Clár *see* Clare
An Clochán *see* Clifden
An Clochán Liath *see* Dunglow
23 U12 **Anclote Keys** *island group* Florida, SE USA
An Cóbh *see* Cobh
57 J17 **Ancohuma, Nevado de** ▲ W Bolivia
An Comar *see* Comber
57 D14 **Ancón** Lima, W Peru
106 J12 **Ancona** Marche, C Italy
Ancuabe *see* Ancuabi
82 Q13 **Ancuabi** *var.* Ancuabe. Cabo Delgado, NE Mozambique
63 F17 **Ancud** *prev.* San Carlos de Ancud. Los Lagos, S Chile
63 G17 **Ancud, Golfo de** *gulf* S Chile
Ancyra *see* Ankara
163 V8 **Anda** Heilongjiang, NE China
57 G16 **Andahuaylas** Apurímac, S Peru
An Daingean *see* Dingle
153 R15 **Andāl** West Bengal, NE India
94 E9 **Åndalsnes** Møre og Romsdal, S Norway
104 K13 **Andalucía** *Eng.* Andalusia. ◆ *autonomous community* S Spain
23 P7 **Andalusia** Alabama, S USA
Andalusia *see* Andalucía
151 Q21 **Andaman and Nicobar Islands** *var.* Andamans and Nicobars. ◆ *union territory* India, NE Indian Ocean
173 T4 **Andaman Basin** *undersea feature* NE Indian Ocean
151 P19 **Andaman Islands** *island group* India, NE Indian Ocean
173 T4 **Andaman Sea** *sea* NE Indian Ocean
57 K19 **Andamarca** Oruro, C Bolivia
182 H5 **Andamooka** South Australia
141 Y9 **'Andām, Wādī** *seasonal river* NE Oman
172 J3 **Andapa** Antsirañana, NE Madagascar
149 R4 **Andarāb** *var.* Banow. Baghlān, NE Afghanistan
Andarbag *see* Andarbogh
147 S13 **Andarbogh** *Rus.* Andarbag, Anderbak. S Tajikistan
109 Z5 **Andau** Burgenland, E Austria
108 I10 **Andeer** Graubünden, S Switzerland
92 H9 **Andenes** Nordland, C Norway
99 J20 **Andenne** Namur, SE Belgium
77 S11 **Andéramboukane** Gao, E Mali
Anderbak *see* Andarbogh
99 G18 **Anderlecht** Brussels, C Belgium
99 G21 **Anderlues** Hainaut, S Belgium
108 G9 **Andermatt** Uri, C Switzerland
101 E17 **Andernach** *anc.* Antunnacum. Rheinland-Pfalz, SW Germany
188 D15 **Andersen Air Force Base** *air base* NE Guam
39 R9 **Anderson** Alaska, USA
35 N4 **Anderson** California, W USA
31 P13 **Anderson** Indiana, N USA
27 R8 **Anderson** Missouri, C USA
21 P11 **Anderson** South Carolina, SE USA
25 V10 **Anderson** Texas, SW USA
95 K20 **Anderstorp** Jönköping, S Sweden
54 D9 **Andes** Antioquia, W Colombia
47 P7 **Andes** ▲ W South America
29 P12 **Andes, Lake** ◎ South Dakota, N USA
92 H9 **Andfjorden** *fjord* E Norwegian Sea
155 H16 **Andhra Pradesh** ◆ *state* E India
98 J8 **Andijk** Noord-Holland, NW Netherlands
147 S10 **Andijon** *Rus.* Andizhan. Andijon Wiloyati, E Uzbekistan
147 S10 **Andijon Wiloyati** *Rus.* Andizhanskaya Oblast'. ◆ *province* E Uzbekistan
Andikíthira *see* Antikýthira
172 J4 **Andilamena** Toamasina, C Madagascar
142 L8 **Andīmeshk** *var.* Andimishk; *prev.* Salehābād. Khūzestān, SW Iran
Andimishk *see* Andīmeshk
Andipáros *see* Antíparos
Andipaxi *see* Antípaxoi
Andípsara *see* Antípsara
136 L16 **Andırın** Kahramanmaraş, S Turkey
158 J8 **Andirlangar** Xinjiang Uygur Zizhiqu, NW China
Andírrion *see* Antírrio
Ándissa *see* Ántissa
Andizhan *see* Andijon
Andizhanskaya Oblast' *see* Andijon Wiloyati
149 N2 **Andkhvoy** Fāryāb, N Afghanistan
105 Q2 **Andoain** País Vasco, N Spain
163 Y15 **Andong** *Jap.* Antō. E South Korea
109 R4 **Andorf** Oberösterreich, N Austria
105 S7 **Andorra** Aragón, NE Spain
105 V4 **Andorra** *off.* Principality of Andorra, *Cat.* Valls d'Andorra, *Fr.* Vallée d'Andorre. ◆ *monarchy* SW Europe
Andorra *see* Andorra la Vella
105 V4 **Andorra la Vella** *var.* Andorra, *Fr.* Andorre la Vielle, *Sp.* Andorra la Vieja. ● (Andorra) C Andorra
Andorra la Vieja *see* Andorra la Vella
Andorra, Valls d'/Andorre, Vallée d' *see* Andorra
Andorre la Vielle *see* Andorra la Vella
97 M22 **Andover** S England, UK
27 N6 **Andover** Kansas, C USA
92 G10 **Andøya** *island* C Norway
60 I8 **Andradina** São Paulo, S Brazil
39 N10 **Andreafsky River** ~ Alaska, USA
38 H17 **Andreanof Islands** *island group* Aleutian Islands, Alaska, USA
126 H16 **Andreapol'** Tverskaya Oblast', W Russian Federation
Andreas, Cape *see* Zafer Burnu
Andreevka *see* Kabanbay
21 N10 **Andrews** North Carolina, SE USA
21 T13 **Andrews** South Carolina, SE USA
24 M7 **Andrews** Texas, SW USA
173 N5 **Andrew Tablemount** *var.* Gora Andryu. *undersea feature* W Indian Ocean
Andreyevka *see* Kabanbay
107 N17 **Andria** Puglia, SE Italy
113 K16 **Andrijevica** Montenegro, SW Yugoslavia
115 E20 **Andrítsaina** Pelopónnisos, S Greece
An Droichead Nua *see* Newbridge
Andropov *see* Rybinsk
115 J19 **Ándros** Ándros, Kykládes, Greece, Aegean Sea
115 J20 **Ándros** *island* Kykládes, Greece, Aegean Sea
19 O7 **Androscoggin River** ~ Maine/New Hampshire, NE USA
44 F3 **Andros Island** *island* NW Bahamas
129 R7 **Androsovka** Samarskaya Oblast', W Russian Federation
44 G3 **Andros Town** Andros Island, NW Bahamas
155 D21 **Āndrott Island** *island* Lakshadweep, India, N Indian Ocean
117 N5 **Andrushivka** Zhytomyrs'ka Oblast', N Ukraine
111 K17 **Andrychów** Małopolskie, S Poland
Andryu, Gora *see* Andrew Tablemount
92 I10 **Andselv** Troms, N Norway
79 O17 **Andudu** Orientale, NE Dem. Rep. Congo (Zaire)
105 N13 **Andújar** *anc.* Illiturgis. Andalucía, SW Spain
82 C12 **Andulo** Bié, W Angola
103 Q14 **Anduze** Gard, S France
An Earagail *see* Errigal Mountain
95 L19 **Aneby** Jönköping, S Sweden
Anécho *see* Aného
77 Q9 **Anéfis** Kidal, NE Mali
45 U8 **Anegada** *island* NE British Virgin Islands
61 B25 **Anegada, Bahía** *bay* E Argentina
45 U9 **Anegada Passage** *passage* Anguilla/British Virgin Islands
77 R17 **Aného** *var.* Anécho; *prev.* Petit-Popo. S Togo
197 D17 **Aneityum** *var.* Anatom; *prev.* Kéamu. *island* S Vanuatu
117 N10 **Anenii Noi** *Rus.* Novyye Aneny. C Moldova
186 F7 **Anepmete** New Britain, E PNG
105 U4 **Aneto** ▲ NE Spain
Änew *see* Annau
Änewetak *see* Enewetak Atoll
77 Y8 **Aney** Agadez, NE Niger
An Fheoir *see* Nore
122 L12 **Angara** ~ C Russian Federation
122 M13 **Angarsk** Irkutskaya Oblast', S Russian Federation
93 G17 **Ånge** Västernorrland, C Sweden
Angel *see* Úhlava
40 D4 **Ángel de la Guarda, Isla** *island* NW Mexico
171 O3 **Angeles** *off.* Angeles City. Luzon, N Philippines
Angeles City *see* Angeles
Angel Falls *see* Ángel, Salto
95 J22 **Ängelholm** Skåne, S Sweden
61 A17 **Angélica** Santa Fe, C Argentina
25 W8 **Angelina River** ~ Texas, SW USA
55 Q9 **Ángel, Salto** *Eng.* Angel Falls. *waterfall* E Venezuela
95 M15 **Ängelsberg** Västmanland, C Sweden
35 P8 **Angels Camp** California, W USA
109 W7 **Anger** Steiermark, SE Austria
Angerapp *see* Ozersk
Angerburg *see* Węgorzewo
93 H15 **Ångermanälven** ~ N Sweden
100 P11 **Angermünde** Brandenburg, NE Germany
102 K7 **Angers** *anc.* Juliomagus. Maine-et-Loire, NW France
15 W7 **Angers** ~ Quebec, SE Canada
93 J16 **Ängesön** *island* N Sweden
Angistro *see* Ágkistro
114 H13 **Angítis** ~ NE Greece
167 R13 **Ângk Tasaôm** *prev.* Angtassom. Takêv, S Cambodia
185 C25 **Anglem, Mount** ▲ Stewart Island, Southland, SW NZ
97 I18 **Anglesey** *cultural region* NW Wales, UK
97 I18 **Anglesey** *island* NW Wales, UK
102 I15 **Anglet** Pyrénées-Atlantiques, SW France
25 W12 **Angleton** Texas, SW USA
Anglia *see* England
14 H9 **Angliers** Quebec, SE Canada
Anglo-Egyptian Sudan *see* Sudan
Angmagssalik *see* Ammassalik
167 Q7 **Ang Nam Ngum** ◎ C Laos
79 N16 **Ango** Orientale, N Dem. Rep. Congo (Zaire)
83 Q15 **Angoche** Nampula, E Mozambique
63 G14 **Angol** Araucanía, C Chile
31 Q11 **Angola** Indiana, N USA
82 A9 **Angola** *off.* Republic of Angola; *prev.* People's Republic of Angola, Portuguese West Africa. ◆ *republic* SW Africa
65 P15 **Angola Basin** *undersea feature* E Atlantic Ocean
39 X13 **Angoon** Admiralty Island, Alaska, USA
147 O14 **Angor** Surkhondaryo Wiloyati, S Uzbekistan
Angora *see* Ankara
186 C6 **Angoram** East Sepik, NW PNG
40 H8 **Angostura** Sinaloa, C Mexico
Angostura *see* Ciudad Bolívar
41 U17 **Angostura, Presa de la** ⊠ SE Mexico
28 J11 **Angostura Reservoir** ⊠ South Dakota, N USA
102 L11 **Angoulême** *anc.* Iculisma. Charente, W France
102 K11 **Angoumois** *cultural region* W France
64 O2 **Angra do Heroísmo** Terceira, Azores, Portugal, NE Atlantic Ocean
60 O10 **Angra dos Reis** Rio de Janeiro, SE Brazil
Angra Pequena *see* Lüderitz
147 Q10 **Angren** Toshkent Wiloyati, E Uzbekistan
Angtassom *see* Ângk Tasaôm
167 O10 **Ang Thong** *var.* Angthong. Ang Thong, C Thailand
79 M16 **Angu** Orientale, N Dem. Rep. Congo (Zaire)
105 S5 **Angües** Aragón, NE Spain
45 U9 **Anguilla** ◇ *UK dependent territory* E West Indies
45 V9 **Anguilla** *island* E West Indies
44 F4 **Anguilla Cays** *islets* SW Bahamas
Angul *see* Anugul
161 N1 **Anguli Nur** ◎ E China
79 O18 **Angumu** Orientale, E Dem. Rep. Congo (Zaire)
14 G14 **Angus** Ontario, S Canada
96 J10 **Angus** *cultural region* E Scotland, UK
59 K19 **Anhangüera** Goiás, S Brazil
99 I21 **Anhée** Namur, S Belgium
95 I21 **Anholt** *island* C Denmark
160 M11 **Anhua** *prev.* Dongping. Hunan, S China
161 P8 **Anhui** *var.* Anhui Sheng, Anhwei, Wan. ◆ *province* E China
Anhui Sheng/Anhwei *see* Anhui
39 O11 **Aniak** Alaska, USA
39 O12 **Aniak River** ~ Alaska, USA
An Iarmhí *see* Westmeath
189 R8 **Anibare** E Nauru
189 R8 **Anibare Bay** *bay* E Nauru, W Pacific Ocean
Anicium *see* le Puy
115 K22 **Ánidro** *island* Kykládes, Greece, Aegean Sea
77 R15 **Anié** C Togo
77 Q15 **Anié** ~ C Togo
102 J16 **Anie, Pic d'** ▲ SW France
129 Y7 **Anikhovka** Orenburgskaya Oblast', W Russian Federation
14 G9 **Anima Nipissing Lake** ◎ Ontario, S Canada
37 O16 **Animas** New Mexico, SW USA
37 P16 **Animas Peak** ▲ New Mexico, SW USA
37 P16 **Animas Valley** *valley* New Mexico, SW USA
116 F13 **Anina** *Ger.* Steierdorf, *Hung.* Stájerlakanina; *prev.* Ştaierdorf-Anina, Steierdorf-Anina, Steyerlak-Anina. Caraş-Severin, SW Romania
29 U14 **Anita** Iowa, C USA
123 U14 **Aniva, Mys** *headland* Ostrov Sakhalin, SE Russian Federation
187 S15 **Aniwa** *island* S Vanuatu
93 M19 **Anjalankoski** Etelä-Suomi, S Finland
'Anjar *see* Aanjar
Anjiangying *see* Luanping
14 B8 **Anjigami Lake** ◎ Ontario, S Canada
164 K14 **Anjō** *var.* Anzyô. Aichi, Honshū, SW Japan
102 J8 **Anjou** *cultural region* NW France
172 I13 **Anjouan** *var.* Nzwani, Johanna Island. *island* SE Comoros
172 J4 **Anjozorobe** Antananarivo, C Madagascar
163 W13 **Anju** W North Korea
98 M5 **Anjum** *Fris.* Eanjum. Friesland, N Netherlands
172 G6 **Ankaboa, Tanjona** *headland* W Madagascar
160 L7 **Ankang** *prev.* Xing'an. Shaanxi, C China
136 I12 **Ankara** *prev.* Angora, *anc.* Ancyra. ● (Turkey) Ankara, C Turkey
136 H12 **Ankara** ◆ *province* C Turkey
95 N19 **Ankarsrum** Kalmar, S Sweden
172 H6 **Ankazoabo** Toliara, SW Madagascar
172 I4 **Ankazobe** Antananarivo, C Madagascar
29 V14 **Ankeny** Iowa, C USA
167 UU **An Khê** Gia Lai, C Vietnam
100 O9 **Anklam** Mecklenburg-Vorpommern, NE Germany
80 K13 **Änkober** Amhara, N Ethiopia
77 O17 **Ankobra** ~ S Ghana
79 N22 **Ankoro** Katanga, SE Dem. Rep. Congo (Zaire)
99 L24 **Anlier, Forêt d'** *forest* SE Belgium
160 I13 **Anlong** Guizhou, S China
An Longfort *see* Longford
167 R11 **Ânlong Vêng** Siĕmréab, NW Cambodia
An Lorgain *see* Lurgan
161 N8 **Anlu** Hubei, C China
An Mhí *see* Meath
An Mhuir Cheilteach *see* Celtic Sea
An Muileann gCearr *see* Mullingar
93 F16 **Ånn** Jämtland, C Sweden
128 M8 **Anna** Voronezhskaya Oblast', W Russian Federation
30 L17 **Anna** Illinois, N USA
25 U5 **Anna** Texas, SW USA
74 L5 **Annaba** *prev.* Bône. NE Algeria
An Nabatīyah at Taḥtā *see* Nabatîyé
101 N17 **Annaberg-Buchholz** Sachsen, E Germany
109 T9 **Annabichl** ✕ (Klagenfurt) Kärnten, S Austria
140 M5 **An Nafūd** *desert* NW Saudi Arabia
139 P6 **'Annah** *var.* 'Ānah. NW Iraq
139 P6 **An Nāḥiyah** W Iraq
139 T10 **An Najaf** *var.* Najaf. S Iraq
21 V5 **Anna, Lake** ◎ Virginia, NE USA
97 F16 **Annalee** ~ N Ireland
167 S9 **Annamitique, Chaîne** ▲ C Laos
97 J14 **Annan** S Scotland, UK
29 U8 **Annandale** Minnesota, N USA
21 W4 **Annandale** Virginia, NE USA
189 Q7 **Anna Point** *headland* N Nauru
21 X3 **Annapolis** *state capital* Maryland, NE USA
188 A10 **Anna, Pulo** *island* S Palau
153 O10 **Annapurna** ▲ C Nepal
An Nāqūrah *see* En Nâqoûra
31 R10 **Ann Arbor** Michigan, N USA
An Nás *see* Naas
139 W12 **An Nāşirīyah** *var.* Nasiriya. SE Iraq
139 W11 **An Naşr** E Iraq
146 F13 **Annau** *Turkm.* Änew. Akhalskiy Velayat, C Turkmenistan
121 O13 **An Nawfalīyah** *var.* Al Nūwfalīyah. N Libya
19 P10 **Ann, Cape** *headland* Massachusetts, NE USA
180 I10 **Annean, Lake** ◎ Western Australia
Anneciacum *see* Annecy
103 T11 **Annecy** *anc.* Anneciacum. Haute-Savoie, E France
103 T11 **Annecy, Lac d'** ◎ E France
103 T10 **Annemasse** Haute-Savoie, E France
39 Z14 **Annette Island** *island* Alexander Archipelago, Alaska, USA
An Nhon *see* Binh Đinh
An Nīl al Abyaḍ *see* White Nile
An Nīl al Azraq *see* Blue Nile
23 Q3 **Anniston** Alabama, S USA
79 A19 **Annobón** *island* W Equatorial Guinea
103 R12 **Annonay** Ardèche, E France
44 K12 **Annotto Bay** C Jamaica
141 R5 **An Nu'ayrīyah** *var.* Narıya. Ash Sharqīyah, NE Saudi Arabia
182 M9 **Annuello** Victoria, SE Australia
139 Q10 **An Nukhayb** S Iraq
139 U9 **An Nu'mānīyah** E Iraq
Áno Arkhánai *see* Epáno Archánes
115 J25 **Anógeia** *var.* Anogia, Anóyia. Kríti, Greece, E Mediterranean Sea
Anogia *see* Anógeia
29 V8 **Anoka** Minnesota, N USA
An Ómaigh *see* Omagh
172 I1 **Anorontany, Tanjona** *headland* N Madagascar
172 J5 **Anosibe An'Ala** Toamasina, E Madagascar
Anóyia *see* Anógeia
An Pointe *see* Warrenpoint
161 P9 **Anqing** Anhui, E China
161 Q5 **Anqiu** Shandong, E China
An Ráth *see* Ráth Luirc
An Ribhéar *see* Kenmare River
An Ros *see* Rush
99 K19 **Ans** Liège, E Belgium
Anşāb *see* Nişāb
171 W12 **Ansas** Irian Jaya, E Indonesia
101 J20 **Ansbach** Bayern, SE Germany
An Sciobairín *see* Skibbereen
An Scoil *see* Skull
An Seancheann *see* Old Head of Kinsale
45 Y5 **Anse-Bertrand** Grande Terre, N Guadeloupe
172 H17 **Anse Boileau** Mahé, NE Seychelles
45 S11 **Anse La Raye** NW Saint Lucia
54 D9 **Anserma** Caldas, W Colombia
109 T4 **Ansfelden** Oberösterreich, N Austria
163 U12 **Anshan** Liaoning, NE China
160 J12 **Anshun** Guizhou, S China
61 F17 **Ansina** Tacuarembó, C Uruguay
29 O15 **Ansley** Nebraska, C USA
25 P6 **Anson** Texas, SW USA
77 Q10 **Ansongo** Gao, E Mali
An Srath Bán *see* Strabane
21 R5 **Ansted** West Virginia, NE USA
171 Y13 **Ansudu** Irian Jaya, E Indonesia
57 G15 **Anta** Cusco, S Peru
57 G16 **Antabamba** Apurímac, C Peru
Antafalva *see* Kovačica
136 L17 **Antakya** *anc.* Antioch, Antiochia. Hatay, S Turkey
172 K3 **Antalaha** Antsirañana, NE Madagascar
136 F17 **Antalya** *prev.* Adalia, *anc.* Attaleia, *Bibl.* Attalia. Antalya, SW Turkey
136 F17 **Antalya** ◆ *province* SW Turkey
136 F16 **Antalya** ✕ Antalya, SW Turkey
121 U10 **Antalya Basin** *undersea feature* E Mediterranean Sea
Antalya, Gulf of *see* Antalya Körfezi
136 F16 **Antalya Körfezi** *var.* Gulf of Adalia, *Eng.* Gulf of Antalya. *gulf* SW Turkey
172 J5 **Antanambao Manampotsy** Toamasina, E Madagascar
172 I5 **Antananarivo** *prev.* Tananarive. ● (Madagascar) Antananarivo, C Madagascar

◆ Country ● Country Capital ◇ Dependent Territory ○ Dependent Territory Capital ◆ Administrative Region ✕ International Airport ▲ Mountain ▲ Mountain Range ⩘ Volcano ~ River ◎ Lake ⊠ Reservoir

172 I4 **Antananarivo** ◈ province C Madagascar
172 J5 **Antananarivo** ✕ Antananarivo, C Madagascar
An tAonach see Nenagh
204-205 **Antarctica** continent
194 I5 **Antarctic Peninsula** peninsula Antarctica
61 J15 **Antas, Rio das** ≈ S Brazil
189 U16 **Ant Atoll** atoll Caroline Islands, E Micronesia
An Teampall Mór see Templemore
Antep see Gaziantep
104 M15 **Antequera** anc. Anticaria, Antiquaria. Andalucía, S Spain
Antequera see Oaxaca
37 S5 **Antero Reservoir** ▣ Colorado, C USA
26 M7 **Anthony** Kansas, C USA
37 R16 **Anthony** New Mexico, SW USA
182 D5 **Anthony, Lake** salt lake South Australia
74 E8 **Anti-Atlas** ▲ SW Morocco
103 U15 **Antibes** anc. Antipolis. Alpes-Maritimes, SE France
103 U15 **Antibes, Cap d'** headland SE France
Anticaria see Antequera
13 Q11 **Anticosti, Île d'** Eng. Anticosti Island. island Quebec, E Canada
Anticosti Island see Anticosti, Île d'
102 K3 **Antifer, Cap d'** headland N France
30 L6 **Antigo** Wisconsin, N USA
13 Q15 **Antigonish** Nova Scotia, SE Canada
64 P11 **Antigua** Fuerteventura, Islas Canarias, NE Atlantic Ocean
45 X10 **Antigua** island S Antigua and Barbuda, Leeward Islands
Antigua see Antigua Guatemala
45 W9 **Antigua and Barbuda** ◆ commonwealth republic E West Indies
42 C6 **Antigua Guatemala** var. Antigua. Sacatepéquez, SW Guatemala
41 P11 **Antiguo Morelos** var. Antiguo-Morelos. Tamaulipas, C Mexico
115 F19 **Antíkyras, Kólpos** gulf C Greece
115 G24 **Antikýthira** var. Andikíthira. island S Greece
138 I7 **Anti-Lebanon** var. Jebel esh Sharqi, Ar. Al Jabal ash Sharqī, Fr. Anti-Liban. ▲ Lebanon/Syria
Anti-Liban see Anti-Lebanon
115 I22 **Antímilos** island Kykládes, Greece, Aegean Sea
36 L6 **Antimony** Utah, W USA
An tInbhear Mór see Arklow
30 M10 **Antioch** Illinois, N USA
Antioch see Antakya
102 I10 **Antioche, Pertuis d'** inlet W France
Antiochia see Antakya
54 D8 **Antioquia** Antioquia, C Colombia
54 E8 **Antioquia** off. Departamento de Antioquia. ◈ province C Colombia
115 J21 **Antíparos** var. Andipáros. island Kykládes, Greece, Aegean Sea
115 B17 **Antípaxoi** var. Andipaxi. island Iónioi Nísoi, Greece, C Mediterranean Sea
122 J8 **Antipayuta** Yamalo-Nenetskiy Avtonomnyy Okrug, N Russian Federation
192 L12 **Antipodes Islands** island group S NZ
Antipolis see Antibes
115 J18 **Antípsara** var. Andípsara. island E Greece
Antiquaria see Antequera
15 N10 **Antique, Lac** ◎ Quebec, SE Canada
115 E18 **Antírrio** var. Andírrion. Dytikí Ellás, C Greece
115 K16 **Ántissa** var. Ándissa. Lésvos, E Greece
An tIúr see Newry
Antivari see Bar
56 C6 **Antizana** ▲ N Ecuador
27 Q13 **Antlers** Oklahoma, C USA
93 J14 **Antnäs** Norrbotten, N Sweden
Antō see Andong
62 G5 **Antofagasta** Antofagasta, N Chile
62 G6 **Antofagasta** off. Región de Antofagasta. ◈ region N Chile
62 I7 **Antofalla, Salar de** salt lake NW Argentina
99 D20 **Antoing** Hainaut, SW Belgium
24 M5 **Anton** Texas, SW USA
43 S16 **Antón** Coclé, C Panama
37 T11 **Anton Chico** New Mexico, SW USA
60 K12 **Antonina** Paraná, S Brazil
103 O5 **Antony** Hauts-de-Seine, N France
Antratsit see Antratsyt
117 Y8 **Antratsyt** Rus. Antratsit. Luhans'ka Oblast', E Ukraine
97 G15 **Antrim** Ir. Aontroim. NE Northern Ireland, UK
97 G14 **Antrim** Ir. Aontroim. cultural region NE Northern Ireland, UK
97 G14 **Antrim Mountains** ▲ NE Northern Ireland, UK
172 H5 **Antsalova** Mahajanga, W Madagascar
Antserana see Antsirañana
An tSionainn see Shannon
172 J2 **Antsirañana** var. Antserana; prev. Antsirane, Diégo-Suarez. Antsirañana, N Madagascar
172 J2 **Antsirañana** ◈ province N Madagascar
Antsirane see Antsirañana
An tSiúir see Suir
118 I7 **Antsla** Ger. Anzen. Võrumaa, SE Estonia
An tSláine see Slaney
172 J3 **Antsohihy** Mahajanga, NW Madagascar
63 G14 **Antuco, Volcán** ▲ C Chile
169 W10 **Antu, Gunung** ▲ Borneo, N Indonesia
An Tullach see Tullow
An-tung see Dandong
Antunnacum see Andernach
Antwerp see Antwerpen
99 G16 **Antwerpen** Eng. Antwerp, Fr. Anvers. Antwerpen, N Belgium
99 H16 **Antwerpen** Eng. Antwerp. ◈ province N Belgium
An Uaimh see Navan
154 N12 **Anugul** var. Angul. Orissa, E India
152 F9 **Anūpgarh** Rājasthān, NW India
154 K10 **Anūppur** Madhya Pradesh, C India
155 K24 **Anuradhapura** North Central Province, C Sri Lanka
187 S11 **Anuta** island, E Soloman Islands
Anvers see Antwerpen
194 G4 **Anvers Island** island Antarctica
39 N11 **Anvik** Alaska, USA
39 N10 **Anvik River** ≈ Alaska, USA
38 F17 **Anvil Peak** ▲ Semisopochnoi Island, Alaska, USA
159 P7 **Anxi** Gansu, N China
182 F8 **Anxious Bay** bay South Australia
161 O5 **Anyang** Henan, C China
159 S11 **A'nyêmaqên Shan** ▲ C China
118 H12 **Anykščiai** Anykščiai, E Lithuania
161 P13 **Anyuan** Jiangxi, S China
123 T7 **Anyuysk** Chukotskiy Avtonomnyy Okrug, NE Russian Federation
123 T7 **Anyuyskiy Khrebet** ▲ NE Russian Federation
54 D8 **Anza** Antioquia, C Colombia
Anzen see Antsla
107 I16 **Anzio** Lazio, C Italy
55 O6 **Anzoátegui** off. Estado Anzoátegui. ◈ state NE Venezuela
147 P12 **Anzob** W Tajikistan
Anzyô see Anjō
165 X13 **Aoga-shima** island Izu-shotō, SE Japan
163 T12 **Aohan Qi** Nei Mongol Zizhiqu, N China
Aoiz see Aoiz-Agoitz
105 R3 **Aoiz-Agoitz** var. Agoitz, Aoiz. Navarra, N Spain
186 M9 **Aola** var. Tenaghau. Guadalcanal, C Solomon Islands
166 M15 **Ao Luk Nua** Krabi, SW Thailand
Aomen see Macao
172 N8 **Aomori** Aomori, Honshū, C Japan
165 Q6 **Aomori** off. Aomori-ken. ◈ prefecture Honshū, C Japan
Aontroim see Antrim
117 C15 **Aóos** var. Vijosa, Vijosë, Alb. Lumi i Vjosës,. ≈ Albania/Greece see also Vjosës, Lumi i
191 Q7 **Aorai, Mont** ✱ Tahiti, W French Polynesia
Aorangi see Cook, Mount
178 Ii13 **Aôral, Phnum** prev. Phnom Aural. ▲ W Cambodia
Aorangi see Cook, Mount
193 L15 **Aorangi Mountains** ▲ North Island, NZ
184 H13 **Aorere** ≈ South Island, NZ
106 A7 **Aosta** anc. Augusta Praetoria. Valle d'Aosta, NW Italy
77 O11 **Aougoundou, Lac** ◎ S Mali
76 K9 **Aoukâr** var. Aouker. plateau C Mauritania
78 J13 **Aouk, Bahr** ≈ Central African Republic/Chad
Aouker see Aoukâr
74 B11 **Aousard** SE Western Sahara
164 H12 **Aoya** Tottori, Honshū, SW Japan
78 H5 **Aozou** Borkou-Ennedi-Tibesti, N Chad
26 M11 **Apache** Oklahoma, C USA
36 L14 **Apache Junction** Arizona, SW USA
24 J9 **Apache Mountains** ▲ Texas, SW USA
36 M16 **Apache Peak** ▲ Arizona, SW USA
116 H10 **Apahida** Cluj, NW Romania
23 T9 **Apalachee Bay** bay Florida, SE USA
23 T3 **Apalachee River** ≈ Georgia, SE USA
23 S10 **Apalachicola** Florida, SE USA
23 S10 **Apalachicola Bay** bay Florida, SE USA
23 R9 **Apalachicola River** ≈ Florida, SE USA
Apam see Apan
Apamama see Abemama
41 P14 **Apan** var. Apam. Hidalgo, C Mexico
42 J8 **Apanás, Lago de** ◎ NW Nicaragua
54 H14 **Apaporis, Río** ≈ Brazil/Colombia
185 C23 **Aparima** ≈ South Island, NZ
171 O1 **Aparri** Luzon, N Philippines
112 J9 **Apatin** Serbia, NW Yugoslavia
126 J4 **Apatity** Murmanskaya Oblast', NW Russian Federation
55 X9 **Apatou** NW French Guiana
40 M14 **Apatzingán** var. Apatzingán de la Constitución. Michoacán de Ocampo, SW Mexico
171 X12 **Apauwar** Irian Jaya, E Indonesia
Apaxtla see Apaxtla de Castrejón
41 O15 **Apaxtla de Castrejón** var. Apaxtla. Guerrero, S Mexico
118 J7 **Ape** Alūksne, NE Latvia
98 L11 **Apeldoorn** Gelderland, E Netherlands
Apennines see Appennino
Apenrade see Åbenrå
57 L17 **Apere, Río** ≈ C Bolivia
55 W11 **Apetina** Sipaliwini, SE Suriname
21 U9 **Apex** North Carolina, SE USA
79 M16 **Api** Orientale, N Dem. Rep. Congo (Zaire)
152 M9 **Api** ▲ NW Nepal
Apia see Abaiang
192 H16 **Āpia** ● (Samoa) Upolu, SE Samoa
60 K11 **Apiaí** São Paulo, S Brazil
170 M16 **Api, Gunung** ▲ Pulau Sangeang, S Indonesia
187 N9 **Apio** Maramasike Island, N Solomon Islands
41 O15 **Apipilulco** Guerrero, S Mexico
41 P14 **Apizaco** Tlaxcala, S Mexico
104 I4 **A Pobla de Trives** Cast. Puebla de Trives. Galicia, NW Spain
55 U9 **Apoera** Sipaliwini, NW Suriname
115 O23 **Apolakkiá** Ródos, Dodekánisos, Greece, Aegean Sea
101 L16 **Apolda** Thüringen, C Germany
192 H16 **Apolima Strait** strait C Pacific Ocean
182 M13 **Apollo Bay** Victoria, SE Australia
Apollonia see Sozopol
57 J16 **Apolo** La Paz, W Bolivia
57 J16 **Apolobamba, Cordillera** ▲ Bolivia/Peru
171 Q8 **Apo, Mount** ✱ Mindanao, S Philippines
23 W11 **Apopka** Florida, SE USA
23 W11 **Apopka, Lake** ◎ Florida, SE USA
59 J19 **Aporé, Rio** ≈ SW Brazil
30 K2 **Apostle Islands** island group Wisconsin, N USA
Apostolas Andreas, Cape see Zafer Burnu
61 F14 **Apóstoles** Misiones, NE Argentina
Apostólou Andréa, Akrotíri see Zafer Burnu
117 S9 **Apostolove** Rus. Apostolovo. Dnipropetrovs'ka Oblast', E Ukraine
Apostolovo see Apostolove
17 S10 **Appalachian Mountains** ▲ E USA
95 K14 **Äppelbo** Dalarna, C Sweden
98 N7 **Appelscha** Fris. Appelskea. Friesland, N Netherlands
Appelskea see Appelscha
106 G11 **Appennino** Eng. Apennines. ▲ Italy/San Marino
107 L17 **Appennino Campano** ▲ C Italy
108 I7 **Appenzell** Appenzell, NW Switzerland
108 H7 **Appenzell** ◈ canton NE Switzerland
55 V12 **Appikalo** Sipaliwini, S Suriname
98 O5 **Appingedam** Groningen, NE Netherlands
25 X8 **Appleby** Texas, SW USA
97 L15 **Appleby-in-Westmorland** NW England, UK
30 K10 **Apple River** ≈ Illinois, N USA
30 I5 **Apple River** ≈ Wisconsin, N USA
25 W9 **Apple Springs** Texas, SW USA
29 S8 **Appleton** Minnesota, N USA
30 M7 **Appleton** Wisconsin, N USA
27 S5 **Appleton City** Missouri, C USA
35 U14 **Apple Valley** California, W USA
29 V9 **Apple Valley** Minnesota, N USA
21 U6 **Appomattox** Virginia, NE USA
188 B16 **Apra Harbour** harbour W Guam
188 B16 **Apra Heights** W Guam
106 F6 **Aprica, Passo dell'** pass N Italy
107 M15 **Apricena** anc. Hadria Picena. Puglia, SE Italy
128 L14 **Apsheronsk** Krasnodarskiy Kray, SW Russian Federation
Apsheronskiy Poluostrov see Abşeron Yarımadası
103 S15 **Apt** anc. Apta Julia. Vaucluse, SE France
Apta Julia see Apt
38 H12 **Apua Point** headland Hawaii, USA, C Pacific Ocean
60 I10 **Apucarana** Paraná, S Brazil
Apulia see Puglia
54 K8 **Apure** off. Estado Apure. ◈ state C Venezuela
54 J7 **Apure, Río** ≈ W Venezuela
57 F16 **Apurímac** off. Departamento de Apurímac. ◈ department C Peru
57 F15 **Apurímac, Río** ≈ S Peru
116 G10 **Apuseni, Munţii** ▲ W Romania
Aqaba/'Aqaba see Al 'Aqabah
138 F15 **Aqaba, Gulf of** var. Gulf of Elat, Ar. Khalīj al 'Aqabah; anc. Sinus Aelaniticus. gulf NE Red Sea
139 R7 **'Aqabah** C Iraq
'Aqabah, Khalīj al see Aqaba, Gulf of
149 O2 **Āqchah** var. Āqcheh. Jowzjān, N Afghanistan
Āqcheh see Āqchah
Aqköl see Akkol'
Aqmola see Astana
Aqmola Oblysy see Akmola
158 L10 **Aqqikkol Hu** ◎ NW China
Aqqystaū see Akkystau
'Aqrah see Ākrē
Aqsay see Aksay
Aqshataū see Akchatau
Aqsū see Aksu
Aqsūat see Aksuat
Aqtas see Aktas
Aqtaū see Aktau
Aqtöbe/Aqtöbe Oblysy see Aktyubinsk
Aqtoghay see Aktogay
Aquae Augustae see Dax
Aquae Calidae see Bath
Aquae Flaviae see Chaves
Aquae Grani see Aachen
Aquae Panoniae see Baden
Aquae Sextiae see Aix-en-Provence
Aquae Solis see Bath
Aquae Tarbelicae see Dax
36 J11 **Aquarius Mountains** ▲ Arizona, SW USA
62 O5 **Aquidabán, Río** ≈ E Paraguay
59 H20 **Aquidauana** Mato Grosso do Sul, S Brazil
40 L15 **Aquila** Michoacán de Ocampo, S Mexico
Aquila/Aquila degli Abruzzi see L'Aquila
25 T8 **Aquilla** Texas, SW USA
44 L9 **Aquin** S Haiti
Aquisgranum see Aachen
102 J13 **Aquitaine** ◈ region SW France
Aqzhar see Akzhar
153 P13 **Āra** prev. Arrah. Bihār, N India
105 S4 **Ara** ≈ NE Spain
23 P2 **Arab** Alabama, S USA
Araba see Álava
138 G12 **'Arabah, Wādī al** Heb. Ha'Arava. dry watercourse Israel/Jordan
117 U12 **Arabats'ka Strilka, Kosa** spit S Ukraine
117 U12 **Arabats'ka Zatoka** gulf S Ukraine
'Arab, Baḩr al see Arab, Bahr el
80 C12 **Arab, Bahr el** var. Baḩr al 'Arab. ≈ S Sudan
56 E7 **Arabela, Río** ≈ N Peru
173 O4 **Arabian Basin** undersea feature N Arabian Sea
Arabian Desert see Sahara el Sharqîya
141 N9 **Arabian Peninsula** peninsula SW Asia
85 P15 **Arabian Plate** tectonic feature Africa/Asia/Europe
141 W14 **Arabian Sea** sea NW Indian Ocean
Arabicus, Sinus see Red Sea
'Arabī, Khalīj al see Persian Gulf
Arabistan see Khūzestān
'Arabīyah as Su'ūdīyah, Al Mamlakah al see Saudi Arabia
'Arabīyah Jumhūrīyah, Mişr al see Egypt
138 I9 **'Arab, Jabal al** ▲ S Syria
Arab Republic of Egypt see Egypt
Arabs Gulf see 'Arab, Khalīg el
139 Y12 **'Arab, Shaţţ al** Eng. Shatt al Arab, Per. Arvand Rūd. ≈ Iran/Iraq
136 I11 **Araç** Kastamonu, N Turkey
59 P16 **Aracaju** state capital Sergipe, E Brazil
54 F5 **Aracataca** Magdalena, N Colombia
58 P13 **Aracati** Ceará, E Brazil
60 J8 **Araçatuba** São Paulo, S Brazil
104 J13 **Aracena** Andalucía, S Spain
115 F20 **Arachnaío** ▲ S Greece
115 D16 **Árachthos** var. Arta; prev. Árakhthos, anc. Arachthus. ≈ W Greece
Arachthus see Árachthos
59 N19 **Araçuaí** Minas Gerais, SE Brazil
136 I11 **Araç Çayı** ≈ N Turkey
138 F11 **'Arad** Southern, S Israel
116 F11 **Arad** Arad, W Romania
116 F11 **Arad** ◈ county W Romania
78 J9 **Arada** Biltine, NE Chad
143 P18 **'Arādah** Abū Z̧aby, S UAE
Aradhippou see Aradíppou
121 Q3 **Aradíppou** var. Aradhippou. SE Cyprus
174 K6 **Arafura Sea** Ind. Laut Arafuru. sea W Pacific Ocean
174 L6 **Arafura Shelf** undersea feature C Arafura Sea
Arafuru, Laut see Arafura Sea
59 J18 **Aragarças** Goiás, C Brazil
Aragats, Gora see Aragats Lerr
137 T12 **Aragats Lerr** Rus. Gora Aragats. ▲ W Armenia
32 E14 **Arago, Cape** headland Oregon, NW USA
105 R6 **Aragón** ◈ autonomous community E Spain
105 Q4 **Aragón** ≈ NE Spain
107 I24 **Aragona** Sicilia, Italy, C Mediterranean Sea
105 Q7 **Aragoncillo** ▲ C Spain
54 L5 **Aragua** off. Estado Aragua. ◈ state N Venezuela
55 N6 **Aragua de Barcelona** Anzoátegui, NE Venezuela
55 O5 **Aragua de Maturín** Monagas, NE Venezuela
59 K15 **Araguaia, Río** var. Araguaya. ≈ C Brazil
59 K19 **Araguari** Minas Gerais, SE Brazil
58 J11 **Araguari, Rio** ≈ SW Brazil
Araguaya see Araguaia, Río
104 K14 **Arahal** Andalucía, S Spain
165 N11 **Arai** Niigata, Honshū, C Japan
Árainn see Inishmore
Árainn Mhór see Aran Island
Ara Jovis see Aranjuez
74 J11 **Arak** C Algeria
171 Y15 **Arak** Irian Jaya, E Indonesia
142 M7 **Arāk** prev. Sultānābād. Markazī, W Iran
188 D10 **Arakabesan** island Palau Islands, N Palau
55 S7 **Arakaka** NW Guyana
166 K6 **Arakan State** var. Rakhine State. ◈ state W Myanmar
166 K5 **Arakan Yoma** ▲ W Myanmar
165 O10 **Arakawa** Niigata, Honshū, C Japan
Árakhthos see Árachthos
Araks/Arak's see Aras
158 H7 **Aral** Xinjiang Uygur Zizhiqu, NW China
Aral see Aral'sk, Kazakhstan
Aral see Vose', Tajikistan
Aral-Bukhorskiy Kanal see Amu-Bukhoro Kanali
137 T12 **Aralik** Iğdır, E Turkey
146 H5 **Aral Sea** Kaz. Aral Tengizi, Rus. Aral'skoye More, Uzb. Orol Dengizi. inland sea Kazakhstan/Uzbekistan
144 L13 **Aral'sk** Kaz. Aral. Kzylorda, SW Kazakhstan
Aral'skoye More/Aral Tengizi see Aral Sea
41 O10 **Aramberri** Nuevo León, NE Mexico
186 B8 **Aramia** ≈ SW PNG
143 N6 **Ārān** var. Golārā. Eşfahān, C Iran
105 N5 **Aranda de Duero** Castilla-León, N Spain
112 M12 **Aranđelovac** prev. Arandjelovac. Serbia, C Yugoslavia
Arandjelovac see Aranđelovac
97 J19 **Aran Fawddwy** ▲ NW Wales, UK
97 C14 **Aran Island** Ir. Árainn Mhór. island NW Ireland
97 A18 **Aran Islands** island group W Ireland
105 N9 **Aranjuez** anc. Ara Jovis. Madrid, C Spain
83 E20 **Aranos** Hardap, SE Namibia
25 U14 **Aransas Bay** inlet Texas, SW USA
25 T14 **Aransas Pass** Texas, SW USA
191 O3 **Aranuka** prev. Nanouki. atoll Tungaru, W Kiribati
167 Q11 **Aranyaprathet** Prachin Buri, S Thailand
Aranyosasztal see Zlatý Stôl
Aranyosgyéres see Câmpia Turzii
Aranyosmarót see Zlaté Moravce
164 C14 **Arao** Kumamoto, Kyūshū, SW Japan
77 O8 **Araouane** Tombouctou, N Mali
26 L10 **Arapaho** Oklahoma, C USA
29 N16 **Arapahoe** Nebraska, C USA
57 I16 **Arapa, Laguna** ◎ SE Peru
185 K14 **Arapawa Island** island C NZ
61 E17 **Arapey Grande, Río** ≈ N Uruguay
59 P16 **Arapiraca** Alagoas, E Brazil
140 M3 **'Ar'ar** Al Ḩudūd ash Shamālīyah, NW Saudi Arabia
54 G15 **Araracuara** Caquetá, S Colombia
61 K15 **Araranguá** Santa Catarina, S Brazil
60 L8 **Araraquara** São Paulo, S Brazil
59 O13 **Araras** Ceará, E Brazil
58 I14 **Araras** Pará, N Brazil
60 L9 **Araras** São Paulo, S Brazil
60 H11 **Araras, Serra das** ▲ S Brazil
137 U12 **Ararat** S Armenia
182 M12 **Ararat** Victoria, SE Australia
Ararat, Mount see Büyükağrı Dağı
140 M3 **'Ar'ar, Wādī** dry watercourse Iraq/Saudi Arabia
131 N7 **Aras** Arm. Arak's, Az. Araz Nehri, Per. Rūd-e Aras, Rus. Araks; prev. Araxes. ≈ SW Asia
105 R9 **Aras de Alpuente** País Valenciano, E Spain
137 S13 **Aras Güneyi Dağları** ▲ NE Turkey
Aras, Rūd-e see Aras
191 U9 **Aratika** atoll Îles Tuamotu, C French Polynesia
Aratürük see Yiwu
54 I8 **Arauca** Arauca, NE Colombia
54 I8 **Arauca** off. Intendencia de Arauca. ◈ province NE Colombia
63 G15 **Araucanía** off. Región de la Araucanía. ◈ region C Chile
54 L7 **Arauca, Río** ≈ Colombia/Venezuela
63 F14 **Arauco** Bío Bío, C Chile
63 F14 **Arauco, Golfo de** gulf S Chile
54 H8 **Arauquita** Arauca, C Colombia
Arausio see Orange
152 F13 **Arāvali Range** ▲ N India
186 J7 **Arawa** Bougainville Island, NE PNG
185 C20 **Arawata** ≈ South Island, NZ
186 F7 **Arawe Islands** island group E PNG
59 L20 **Araxá** Minas Gerais, SE Brazil
Araxes see Aras
55 O5 **Araya** Sucre, N Venezuela
105 R4 **Arba** ≈ N Spain
81 I15 **Ārba Minch'** Southern, S Ethiopia
139 U4 **Arbat** NE Iraq
107 D19 **Arbatax** Sardegna, Italy, C Mediterranean Sea
Arbe see Rab
Arbela see Arbīl
139 S3 **Arbīl** var. Erbil, Irbīl, Kurd. Hawlêr; anc. Arbela. N Iraq
95 M16 **Arboga** Västmanland, C Sweden
95 M16 **Arbogaån** ≈ C Sweden
103 S9 **Arbois** Jura, E France
54 D6 **Arboletes** Antioquia, NW Colombia
11 X15 **Arborg** Manitoba, S Canada
94 N12 **Arbrå** Gävleborg, C Sweden
96 K10 **Arbroath** anc. Aberbrothock. E Scotland, UK
35 N6 **Arbuckle** California, W USA
27 N12 **Arbuckle Mountains** ▲ Oklahoma, C USA
Arbuzinka see Arbyzynka
117 Q8 **Arbyzynka** Rus. Arbuzinka. Mykolayivs'ka Oblast', S Ukraine
103 U12 **Arc** ≈ E France
102 J13 **Arcachon** Gironde, SW France
102 J13 **Arcachon, Bassin d'** inlet SW France
18 E10 **Arcade** New York, NE USA
23 W14 **Arcadia** Florida, SE USA
22 H5 **Arcadia** Louisiana, S USA
30 J7 **Arcadia** Wisconsin, N USA
Arcae Remorum see Châlons-en-Champagne
44 L9 **Arcahaie** C Haiti
34 K3 **Arcata** California, W USA
35 U6 **Arc Dome** ▲ Nevada, W USA
107 J16 **Arce** Lazio, C Italy
41 O15 **Arcelia** Guerrero, S Mexico
99 M15 **Arcen** Limburg, SE Netherlands
Archangel see Arkhangel'sk
Archangel Bay see Chëshskaya Guba
115 O23 **Archángelos** var. Arhangelos, Arkhángelos. Ródos, Dodekánisos, Greece, Aegean Sea
114 F7 **Archar** ≈ NW Bulgaria
31 R11 **Archbold** Ohio, N USA
105 R12 **Archena** Murcia, SE Spain
25 R5 **Archer City** Texas, SW USA
104 M14 **Archidona** Andalucía, S Spain
65 B25 **Arch Islands** island group SW Falkland Islands
106 G13 **Arcidosso** Toscana, C Italy
103 Q5 **Arcis-sur-Aube** Aube, N France
182 F3 **Arckaringa Creek** seasonal river South Australia
106 G7 **Arco** Trentino-Alto Adige, N Italy
33 Q14 **Arco** Idaho, NW USA
30 M14 **Arcola** Illinois, N USA
105 P6 **Arcos de Jalón** Castilla-León, N Spain
104 K15 **Arcos de la Frontera** Andalucía, S Spain
104 G5 **Arcos de Valdevez** Viana do Castelo, N Portugal
59 P15 **Arcoverde** Pernambuco, E Brazil
102 H5 **Arcovest, Pointe de l'** headland NW France
Arctic-Mid Oceanic Ridge see Nansen Cordillera
197 R8 **Arctic Ocean** ocean
8 G7 **Arctic Red River** ≈ Northwest Territories/Yukon Territory, NW Canada
Arctic Red River see Tsiigehtchic
39 S6 **Arctic Village** Alaska, USA
194 H1 **Arctowski** Polish research station South Shetland Islands, Antarctica
114 I12 **Arda** var. Ardhas, Gk. Ardas. ≈ Bulgaria/Greece see also Ardas
142 L2 **Ardabīl** var. Ardebil. Ardabīl, NW Iran
142 L2 **Ardabīl** off. Ostān-e Ardabīl. ◈ province NW Iran
137 R11 **Ardahan** Ardahan, NE Turkey
137 S11 **Ardahan** ◈ province NE Turkey
143 P8 **Ardakān** Yazd, C Iran
94 E12 **Årdalstangen** Sogn og Fjordane, S Norway
137 R11 **Ardanuç** Artvin, NE Turkey
114 L12 **Ardas** var. Ardhas, Bul. Arda. ≈ Bulgaria/Greece see also Arda
138 I13 **Ard aş Şawwān** var. Ardh es Suwwān. plain S Jordan
129 P5 **Ardatov** Respublika Mordoviya, W Russian Federation
14 G12 **Ardbeg** Ontario, S Canada
Ardeal see Transylvania
Ardebil see Ardabīl
103 Q13 **Ardèche** ≈ C France
103 Q13 **Ardèche** ◈ department E France
97 F17 **Ardee** Ir. Baile Átha Fhirdhia. NE Ireland
103 Q3 **Ardennes** ◈ department NE France
99 J23 **Ardennes** physical region Belgium/France
137 Q11 **Ardeşen** Rize, NE Turkey
143 O7 **Ardestān** var. Ardistan. Eşfahān, C Iran
108 J9 **Ardez** Graubünden, SE Switzerland
Ardhas see Arda/Ardas
Ardh es Suwwān see Ard aş Şawwān
104 I12 **Ardila, Ribeira de** Sp. Ardilla. ≈ Portugal/Spain see also Ardilla
11 T17 **Ardill** Saskatchewan, S Canada
104 I12 **Ardilla** Port. Ribeira de Ardila. ≈ Portugal/Spain see also Ardila, Ribeira de
40 M11 **Ardilla, Cerro la** ▲ C Mexico
114 J12 **Ardino** Kŭrdzhali, S Bulgaria
Ardistan see Ardestān
183 P9 **Ardlethan** New South Wales, SE Australia
Ard Mhacha see Armagh
23 P1 **Ardmore** Alabama, S USA
27 N13 **Ardmore** Oklahoma, C USA
20 J10 **Ardmore** Tennessee, S USA
96 G10 **Ardnamurchan, Point of** headland N Scotland, UK
99 C17 **Ardooie** West-Vlaanderen, W Belgium
182 I9 **Ardrossan** South Australia
116 H9 **Ardusat** Hung. Erdőszáda. Maramureş, N Romania
93 F16 **Åre** Jämtland, C Sweden
79 P16 **Arebi** Orientale, NE Dem. Rep. Congo (Zaire)
45 T5 **Arecibo** C Puerto Rico
171 V13 **Aredo** Irian Jaya, E Indonesia
59 P14 **Areia Branca** Rio Grande do Norte, E Brazil
119 O14 **Arekhawsk** Rus. Orekhovsk. Vitsyebskaya Voblasts', N Belarus
Arel see Arlon
Arelas/Arelate see Arles
Arenal, Embalse de see Arenal Laguna
42 L12 **Arenal Laguna** var. Embalse de Arenal. ◎ NW Costa Rica
42 L13 **Arenal, Volcán** ✱ NW Costa Rica
34 K6 **Arena, Point** headland California, W USA
59 H17 **Arenápolis** Mato Grosso, W Brazil
40 G10 **Arena, Punta** headland W Mexico
104 L8 **Arenas de San Pedro** Castilla-León, N Spain

◆ Country ● Country Capital ◇ Dependent Territory ○ Dependent Territory Capital ◈ Administrative Region ✕ International Airport ▲ Mountain ▲ Mountain Range ✱ Volcano ≈ River ◎ Lake ▣ Reservoir

63 I24 **Arenas, Punta de** *headland* S Argentina
61 B20 **Arenaza** Buenos Aires, E Argentina
95 F17 **Arendal** Aust-Agder, S Norway
99 J16 **Arendonk** Antwerpen, N Belgium
43 T15 **Arenosa** Panamá, N Panama
Arensburg *see* Kuressaare
105 W5 **Arenys de Mar** Cataluña, NE Spain
106 C9 **Arenzano** Liguria, NW Italy
115 F22 **Areópoli** *prev.* Areópolis. Pelopónnisos, S Greece
Areópolis *see* Areópoli
57 H18 **Arequipa** Arequipa, SE Peru
57 G17 **Arequipa** *off.* Departamento de Arequipa. ◈ *department* SW Peru
61 B19 **Arequito** Santa Fe, C Argentina
104 M7 **Arévalo** Castilla-León, N Spain
106 H12 **Arezzo** *anc.* Arretium. Toscana, C Italy
105 Q4 **Arga** ≈ N Spain
Argaeus *see* Erciyes Dağı
115 G17 **Argalastí** Thessalía, C Greece
105 O10 **Argamasilla de Alba** Castilla-La Mancha, C Spain
158 L8 **Argan** Xinjiang Uygur Zizhiqu, NW China
105 O8 **Arganda** Madrid, C Spain
104 H8 **Arganil** Coimbra, N Portugal
171 P6 **Argao** Cebu, C Philippines
153 V15 **Argartala** Tripura, NE India
123 N9 **Arga-Sala** ≈ NE Russian Federation
103 P17 **Argelès-sur-Mer** Pyrénées-Orientales, S France
103 T15 **Argens** ≈ SE France
106 H9 **Argenta** Emilia-Romagna, N Italy
102 K5 **Argentan** Orne, N France
103 N12 **Argentat** Corrèze, C France
106 A9 **Argentera** Piemonte, NE Italy
103 N5 **Argenteuil** Val-d'Oise, N France
62 K13 **Argentina** *off.* Republic of Argentina. ◆ *republic* S South America
Argentina Basin *see* Argentine Basin
Argentine Abyssal Plain *see* Argentine Plain
65 I19 **Argentine Basin** *var.* Argentina Basin. *undersea feature* SW Atlantic Ocean
65 I20 **Argentine Plain** *var.* Argentine Abyssal Plain. *undersea feature* SW Atlantic Ocean
Argentine Rise *see* Falkland Plateau
63 H22 **Argentino, Lago** ◎ S Argentina
102 K8 **Argenton-Château** Deux-Sèvres, W France
102 M9 **Argenton-sur-Creuse** Indre, C France
Argentoratum *see* Strasbourg
116 I12 **Argeș** ◈ *county* S Romania
116 K14 **Argeș** ≈ S Romania
149 O8 **Arghandāb, Daryā-ye** ≈ SE Afghanistan
Arghastān *see* Arghestān
149 O8 **Arghestān** *Pash.* Arghastān. ≈ SE Afghanistan
Argirocastro *see* Gjirokastër
80 E7 **Argo** Northern, N Sudan
173 P7 **Argo Fracture Zone** *tectonic feature* C Indian Ocean
115 F20 **Argolikós Kólpos** *gulf* S Greece
103 R4 **Argonne** *physical region* NE France
115 F20 **Árgos** Pelopónnisos, S Greece
139 S1 **Argōsh** N Iraq
115 D14 **Árgos Orestikó** Dytikí Makedonía, N Greece
115 B19 **Argostóli** *var.* Argostólion. Kefallinía, Iónioi Nísoi, Greece, C Mediterranean Sea
Argostólion *see* Argostóli
Argovie *see* Aargau
35 O14 **Arguello, Point** *headland* California, W USA
129 P16 **Argun** Chechenskaya Respublika, SW Russian Federation
157 T2 **Argun** *Chin.* Ergun He, *Rus.* Argun'. ≈ China/Russian Federation
77 T12 **Argungu** Kebbi, NW Nigeria
162 J9 **Arguut** Övörhangay, C Mongolia
181 N3 **Argyle, Lake** *salt lake* Western Australia
96 G12 **Argyll** *cultural region* W Scotland, UK
Argyrokastron *see* Gjirokastër
162 I7 **Arhangay** ◈ *province* C Mongolia
Arhangelos *see* Archángelos
95 P14 **Arholma** Stockholm, C Sweden
95 G22 **Århus** *var.* Aarhus. Århus, C Denmark
95 G22 **Århus** ◈ *county* C Denmark
139 T1 **Ārī** E Iraq
Aria *see* Herāt
83 F22 **Ariamsvlei** Karas, SE Namibia
107 L17 **Ariano Irpino** Campania, S Italy
54 F11 **Ariari, Río** ≈ C Colombia
151 K19 **Ari Atoll** *atoll* C Maldives
77 P11 **Aribinda** N Burkina
62 G2 **Arica** *hist.* San Marcos de Arica. Tarapacá, N Chile
54 H16 **Arica** Amazonas, S Colombia
62 G2 **Arica** ✕ Tarapacá, N Chile
114 E13 **Aridaía** *var.* Aridea, Aridhaía. Dytikí Makedonía, N Greece
Aridea *see* Aridaía
172 I15 **Aride, Île** *island* Inner Islands, NE Seychelles
Aridhaía *see* Aridaía
103 N17 **Ariège** ◈ *department* S France
102 M16 **Ariège** *var.* la Riege. ≈ Andorra/France
116 H11 **Arieș** ≈ W Romania
149 U10 **Ārifwāla** Punjab, E Pakistan
Ariguaní *see* El Difícil
138 G11 **Arīḥā** Al Karak, W Jordan
138 I3 **Arīḥā** *var.* Arīhā. Idlib, W Syria
Arīḥā *see* Jericho
37 W4 **Arikaree River** ≈ Colorado/Nebraska, C USA
164 B14 **Arikawa** Nagasaki, Nakadōri-jima, SW Japan
112 L13 **Arilje** Serbia, W Yugoslavia
45 U14 **Arima** Trinidad, Trinidad and Tobago
Arime *see* Al 'Arīmah
Ariminum *see* Rimini
59 H16 **Arinos, Rio** ≈ W Brazil
40 M14 **Ario de Rosales** *var.* Ario de Rosáles. Michoacán de Ocampo, SW Mexico
118 F12 **Ariogala** Raseiniai, C Lithuania
47 T7 **Aripuanā** ≈ W Brazil
59 E15 **Ariquemes** Rondônia, W Brazil
121 W13 **'Arīsh, Wâdi el** ≈ NE Egypt
54 K6 **Arismendi** Barinas, C Venezuela
10 J14 **Aristazabal Island** *island* SW Canada
60 F13 **Aristóbulo del Valle** Misiones, NE Argentina
172 I5 **Arivonimamo** ✕ (Antananarivo) Antananarivo, C Madagascar
Arixang *see* Wenquan
105 Q6 **Ariza** Aragón, NE Spain
62 I6 **Arizaro, Salar de** *salt lake* NW Argentina
62 K13 **Arizona** San Luis, C Argentina
36 J12 **Arizona** *off.* State of Arizona; also known as Copper State, Grand Canyon State. ◈ *state* SW USA
40 G4 **Arizpe** Sonora, NW Mexico
95 J16 **Årjäng** Värmland, C Sweden
143 P8 **Arjenān** Yazd, C Iran
92 I13 **Arjeplog** Norrbotten, N Sweden
54 E5 **Arjona** Bolívar, N Colombia
105 N13 **Arjona** Andalucía, S Spain
123 S10 **Arka** Khabarovskiy Kray, E Russian Federation
22 L2 **Arkabutla Lake** ▣ Mississippi, S USA
129 O7 **Arkadak** Saratovskaya Oblast', W Russian Federation
27 T13 **Arkadelphia** Arkansas, C USA
115 J25 **Arkalochóri** *prev.* Arkalohori, Arkalokhórion. Kríti, Greece, E Mediterranean Sea
Arkalohori/ Arkalokhórion *see* Arkalochóri
145 O10 **Arkalyk** *Kaz.* Arqalyq. Kostanay, N Kazakhstan
27 U10 **Arkansas** *off.* State of Arkansas; also known as The Land of Opportunity. ◈ *state* S USA
27 W14 **Arkansas City** Arkansas, C USA
27 O7 **Arkansas City** Kansas, C USA
16 K11 **Arkansas River** ≈ C USA
182 J5 **Arkaroola** South Australia
Arkhángelos *see* Archángelos
126 L8 **Arkhangel'sk** *Eng.* Archangel. Arkhangel'skaya Oblast', NW Russian Federation
126 L9 **Arkhangel'skaya Oblast'** ◈ *province* NW Russian Federation
129 O14 **Arkhangel'skoye** Stavropol'skiy Kray, SW Russian Federation
123 R14 **Arkhara** Amurskaya Oblast', S Russian Federation
97 G19 **Arklow** *Ir.* An tInbhear Mór. SE Ireland
115 M20 **Arkoí** *island* Dodekánisos, Greece, Aegean Sea
27 R11 **Arkoma** Oklahoma, C USA
100 O7 **Arkona, Kap** *headland* NE Germany
95 N17 **Arkösund** Östergötland, S Sweden
122 J6 **Arkticheskogo Instituta, Ostrova** *island* N Russian Federation
95 O15 **Arlanda** ✕ (Stockholm) Stockholm, C Sweden
146 C11 **Arlan, Gora** ▲ W Turkmenistan
105 O5 **Arlanza** ≈ N Spain
105 N5 **Arlanzón** ≈ N Spain
103 R15 **Arles** *var.* Arles-sur-Rhône; *anc.* Arelas, Arelate. Bouches-du-Rhône, SE France
Arles-sur-Rhône *see* Arles
103 O17 **Arles-sur-Tech** Pyrénées-Orientales, S France
29 U9 **Arlington** Minnesota, N USA
29 R15 **Arlington** Nebraska, C USA
32 J11 **Arlington** Oregon, NW USA
29 R10 **Arlington** South Dakota, N USA
20 E10 **Arlington** Tennessee, S USA
25 T6 **Arlington** Texas, SW USA
21 W4 **Arlington** Virginia, NE USA
32 H7 **Arlington** Washington, NW USA
30 M10 **Arlington Heights** Illinois, N USA
77 U8 **Arlit** Agadez, C Niger
99 L24 **Arlon** *Dut.* Aarlen, *Ger.* Arel; *Lat.* Orolaunum. Luxembourg, SE Belgium
27 R7 **Arma** Kansas, C USA
97 F16 **Armagh** *Ir.* Ard Mhacha. S Northern Ireland, UK
97 F16 **Armagh** *cultural region* S Northern Ireland, UK
102 K15 **Armagnac** *cultural region* S France
103 Q7 **Armançon** ≈ C France
60 K10 **Armando Laydner, Represa** ▣ S Brazil
115 M24 **Armathía** *island* SE Greece
128 M14 **Armavir** Krasnodarskiy Kray, SW Russian Federation
54 E10 **Armenia** Quindío, W Colombia
137 T12 **Armenia** *off.* Republic of Armenia, *var.* Ajastan, *Arm.* Hayastani Hanrapetut'yun; *prev.* Armenian Soviet Socialist Republic. ◆ *republic* SW Asia
Armenierstadt *see* Gherla
103 O1 **Armentières** Nord, N France
40 K14 **Armería** Colima, SW Mexico
183 T5 **Armidale** New South Wales, SE Australia
29 P11 **Armour** South Dakota, N USA
61 B18 **Armstrong** Santa Fe, C Argentina
11 N16 **Armstrong** British Columbia, SW Canada
12 D11 **Armstrong** Ontario, S Canada
29 U11 **Armstrong** Iowa, C USA
25 S16 **Armstrong** Texas, SW USA
117 S11 **Armyans'k** *Rus.* Armyansk. Respublika Krym, S Ukraine
115 H14 **Arnaía** *var.* Arnea. Kentrikí Makedonía, N Greece
121 N2 **Arnaoúti, Akrotíri** *var.* Arnaoútis, Cape Arnaouti. *headland* W Cyprus
Arnaouti, Cape/Arnaoútis *see* Arnaoúti, Akrotíri
12 L4 **Arnaud** ≈ Quebec, E Canada
103 Q8 **Arnay-le-Duc** Côte d'Or, C France
Arnea *see* Arnaía
105 Q4 **Arnedo** La Rioja, N Spain
95 I14 **Årnes** Akershus, S Norway
95 E15 **Årnes** Sør-Trøndelag, S Norway
26 K9 **Arnett** Oklahoma, C USA
98 L12 **Arnhem** Gelderland, SE Netherlands
181 Q2 **Arnhem Land** *physical region* Northern Territory, N Australia
106 F11 **Arno** ≈ C Italy
Arno *see* Arno Atoll
189 W7 **Arno Atoll** *var.* Arno. *atoll* Ratak Chain, NE Marshall Islands
182 H8 **Arno Bay** South Australia
35 Q8 **Arnold** California, W USA
27 X5 **Arnold** Missouri, C USA
29 N15 **Arnold** Nebraska, C USA
109 R10 **Arnoldstein** *Slvn.* Pod Klošter. Kärnten, S Austria
103 N9 **Arnon** ≈ C France
45 P14 **Arnos Vale** ✕ (Kingstown) Saint Vincent, SE Saint Vincent and the Grenadines
92 I8 **Arnøy** *island* N Norway
14 L12 **Arnprior** Ontario, SE Canada
101 G15 **Arnsberg** Nordrhein-Westfalen, W Germany
101 K16 **Arnstadt** Thüringen, C Germany
Arnswalde *see* Choszczno
54 K5 **Aroa** Yaracuy, N Venezuela
83 E21 **Aroab** Karas, SE Namibia
115 E19 **Aroánia** ▲ S Greece
191 O6 **Aroa, Pointe** *headland* Moorea, W French Polynesia
Aroe Islands *see* Aru, Kepulauan
101 H15 **Arolsen** Niedersachsen, C Germany
106 C7 **Arona** Piemonte, NE Italy
19 R3 **Aroostook River** ≈ Canada/USA
Arop Island *see* Long Island
38 M12 **Aropuk Lake** ◎ Alaska, USA
191 P4 **Arorae** *atoll* Tungaru, W Kiribati
190 G16 **Arorangi** Rarotonga, S Cook Islands
108 I9 **Arosa** Graubünden, S Switzerland
104 F4 **Arousa, Ría de** *estuary* E Atlantic Ocean
184 P8 **Arowhana** ▲ North Island, NZ
137 V12 **Arp'a** *Az.* Arpaçay. ≈ Armenia/Azerbaijan
137 S11 **Arpaçay** Kars, NE Turkey
Arpaçay *see* Arp'a
Arqalyq *see* Arkalyk
149 N14 **Arra** ≈ SW Pakistan
Arrabona *see* Győr
Arrah *see* Āra
Ar Rahad *see* Er Rahad
139 R9 **Ar Raḥḥālīyah** C Iraq
60 Q10 **Arraial do Cabo** Rio de Janeiro, SE Brazil
104 H11 **Arraiolos** Évora, S Portugal
139 R8 **Ar Ramādī** *var.* Ramadi, Rumadiya. SW Iraq
138 J6 **Ar Rāmī** Ḥimṣ, C Syria
Ar Rams *see* Rams
138 H9 **Ar Ramthā** *var.* Ramtha. Irbid, N Jordan
96 H13 **Arran, Isle of** *island* SW Scotland, UK
138 L3 **Ar Raqqah** *var.* Rakka; *anc.* Nicephorium. Ar Raqqah, N Syria
138 L3 **Ar Raqqah** *off.* Muḥāfaẓat al Raqqah, *var.* Raqqah, *Fr.* Rakka. ◈ *governorate* N Syria
103 O2 **Arras** *anc.* Nemetocenna. Pas-de-Calais, N France
Arrasate *see* Mondragón
138 G12 **Ar Rashādīyah** Aṭ Ṭafīlah, W Jordan
138 I5 **Ar Rastān** *var.* Rastâne. Ḥimṣ, W Syria
139 X12 **Ar Raṭāwī** E Iraq
102 L15 **Arrats** ≈ S France
141 N10 **Ar Rawḍah** Makkah, S Saudi Arabia
141 Q15 **Ar Rawḍah** S Yemen
142 K11 **Ar Rawḍatayn** *var.* Raudhatain. N Kuwait
143 N16 **Ar Rayyān** *var.* Al Rayyan. C Qatar
102 L17 **Arreau** Hautes-Pyrénées, S France
64 Q11 **Arrecife** *var.* Arrecife de Lanzarote, Puerto Arrecife. Lanzarote, Islas Canarias, NE Atlantic Ocean
Arrecife de Lanzarote *see* Arrecife
43 P6 **Arrecife Edinburgh** *reef* NE Nicaragua
61 C19 **Arrecifes** Buenos Aires, E Argentina
102 F6 **Arrée, Monts d'** ▲ NW France
Ar Refā'ī *see* Ar Rifā'ī
Arretium *see* Arezzo
Arriaca *see* Guadalajara
109 S9 **Arriach** Kärnten, S Austria
41 T16 **Arriaga** Chiapas, SE Mexico
41 N12 **Arriaga** San Luis Potosí, C Mexico
139 W10 **Ar Rifā'ī** *var.* Ar Refā'ī. SE Iraq
139 V12 **Ar Riḥāb** *salt flat* S Iraq
104 L2 **Arriondas** Asturias, N Spain
141 Q7 **Ar Riyāḍ** *Eng.* Riyadh. ● (Saudi Arabia) Ar Riyāḍ, C Saudi Arabia
141 O8 **Ar Riyāḍ** *off.* Minṭaqat ar Riyāḍ. ◈ *province* C Saudi Arabia
141 S15 **Ar Riyān** S Yemen
Arrö *see* Ærø
61 H18 **Arroio Grande** Rio Grande do Sul, S Brazil
102 K15 **Arros** ≈ S France
103 Q9 **Arroux** ≈ C France
25 R5 **Arrowhead, Lake** ▣ Texas, SW USA
182 L5 **Arrowsmith, Mount** *hill* New South Wales, SE Australia
185 D21 **Arrowtown** Otago, South Island, NZ
61 D17 **Arroyo Barú** Entre Ríos, E Argentina
104 J10 **Arroyo de la Luz** Extremadura, W Spain
63 J16 **Arroyo de la Ventana** Río Negro, SE Argentina
35 P13 **Arroyo Grande** California, W USA
Ar Ru'ays *see* Ar Ruways
141 R11 **Ar Rub' al Khālī** *Eng.* Empty Quarter, Great Sandy Desert. *desert* SW Asia
139 V13 **Ar Rudaymah** S Iraq
61 A16 **Arrufó** Santa Fe, C Argentina
138 I7 **Ar Ruḥaybah** *var.* Ruhaybeh, *Fr.* Rouhaïbé. Dimashq, W Syria
139 V15 **Ar Rukhaymīyah** *well* S Iraq
139 U11 **Ar Rumaythah** *var.* Rumaitha. S Iraq
141 X8 **Ar Rustāq** *var.* Rostak, Rustaq. N Oman
139 N8 **Ar Ruṭbah** *var.* Rutba. SW Iraq
140 M3 **Ar Rūthīyah** *spring/well* NW Saudi Arabia
ar-Ruwaida *see* Ar Ruwayḍah
141 O8 **Ar Ruwayḍah** *var.* ar-Ruwaida. Jīzān, C Saudi Arabia
143 N15 **Ar Ruways** *var.* Al Ruweis, Ar Ru'ays, Ruwais. N Qatar
143 O17 **Ar Ruways** *var.* Ar Ru'ays, Ruwaisv. Abū Ẓaby, W UAE
95 G21 **Års** *var.* Aars. Nordjylland, N Denmark
Arsanias *see* Murat Nehri
123 S15 **Arsen'yev** Primorskiy Kray, SE Russian Federation
155 G19 **Arsikere** Karnātaka, W India
129 R3 **Arsk** Respublika Tatarstan, W Russian Federation
94 N10 **Årskogen** Gävleborg, C Sweden
121 O3 **Ársos** C Cyprus
94 N13 **Årsunda** Gävleborg, C Sweden
Arta *see* Árachthos
115 C17 **Árta** *anc.* Ambracia. Ípeiros, W Greece
137 T12 **Artashat** S Armenia
40 M15 **Arteaga** Michoacán de Ocampo, SW Mexico
123 S15 **Artem** Primorskiy Kray, SE Russian Federation
44 C4 **Artemisa** La Habana, W Cuba
117 W7 **Artemivs'k** Donets'ka Oblast', E Ukraine
122 K13 **Artemovsk** Krasnoyarskiy Kray, S Russian Federation
105 U5 **Artesa de Segre** Cataluña, NE Spain
37 U14 **Artesia** New Mexico, SW USA
25 Q14 **Artesia Wells** Texas, SW USA
108 G8 **Arth** Schwyz, C Switzerland
14 F15 **Arthur** Ontario, S Canada
30 M14 **Arthur** Illinois, N USA
28 L14 **Arthur** Nebraska, C USA
29 Q5 **Arthur** North Dakota, N USA
185 B21 **Arthur** ≈ South Island, NZ
18 B13 **Arthur, Lake** ▣ Pennsylvania, NE USA
183 N15 **Arthur River** ≈ Tasmania, SE Australia
185 G18 **Arthur's Pass** Canterbury, South Island, NZ
185 G17 **Arthur's Pass** *pass* South Island, NZ
44 I3 **Arthur's Town** Cat Island, C Bahamas
44 M9 **Artibonite, Rivière de l'** ≈ C Haiti
61 E16 **Artigas** *prev.* San Eugenio, San Eugenio del Cuareim. Artigas, N Uruguay
61 E16 **Artigas** ◈ *department* N Uruguay
194 H1 **Artigas** *Uruguayan research station* Antarctica
137 T11 **Art'ik** W Armenia
187 O16 **Art, Île** *island* Îles Belep, W New Caledonia
103 O2 **Artois** *cultural region* N France
136 L12 **Artova** Tokat, N Turkey
105 Y9 **Artrutx, Cap d'** *var.* Cabo Dartuch. *headland* Menorca, Spain, W Mediterranean Sea
Artsiz *see* Artsyz
117 N11 **Artsyz** *Rus.* Artsiz. Odes'ka Oblast', SW Ukraine
158 E7 **Artux** Xinjiang Uygur Zizhiqu, NW China
137 R11 **Artvin** Artvin, NE Turkey
137 R11 **Artvin** ◈ *province* NE Turkey
146 G14 **Artyk** Akhalskiy Velayat, C Turkmenistan
79 Q16 **Aru** Orientale, NE Dem. Rep. Congo (Zaire)
104 I4 **A Rúa** *var.* La Rúa. Galicia, NW Spain
81 E17 **Arua** NW Uganda
Aruângua *see* Luangwa
45 O15 **Aruba** *var.* Oruba. ◇ *Dutch autonomous region* S West Indies
47 Q4 **Aruba** *island* Aruba, Lesser Antilles
Aru Islands *see* Aru, Kepulauan
171 W15 **Aru, Kepulauan** *Eng.* Aru Islands; *prev.* Aroe Islands. *island group* E Indonesia
153 W10 **Arunāchal Pradesh** *prev.* North East Frontier Agency, North East Frontier Agency of Assam. ◈ *state* NE India
163 U7 **Arun Qi** Nei Mongol Zizhiqu, N China
155 H23 **Aruppukkottai** Tamil Nādu, SE India
81 I20 **Arusha** Arusha, N Tanzania
81 I21 **Arusha** ◈ *region* E Tanzania
81 I20 **Arusha** ✕ Arusha, N Tanzania
54 C9 **Arusí, Punta** *headland* NW Colombia
155 J23 **Aruvi Aru** ≈ NW Sri Lanka
79 M17 **Aruwimi** *var.* Ituri (upper course). ≈ NE Dem. Rep. Congo (Zaire)
Árva *see* Orava
37 T4 **Arvada** Colorado, C USA
Arvand Rūd *see* 'Arab, Shaṭṭ al
162 J8 **Arvayheer** Övörhangay, C Mongolia
9 O10 **Arviat** *prev.* Eskimo Point. Nunavut, C Canada
93 I14 **Arvidsjaur** Norrbotten, N Sweden
95 J15 **Arvika** Värmland, C Sweden
92 J8 **Årviksand** Troms, N Norway
35 S13 **Arvin** California, W USA
145 P7 **Arykbalyk** *Kaz.* Aryqbalyq. Severnyy Kazakhstan, N Kazakhstan
Aryqbalyq *see* Arykbalyk
145 P17 **Arys'** *Kaz.* Arys. Yuzhnyy Kazakhstan, S Kazakhstan
Arys *see* Orzysz
Arys Köli *see* Arys, Ozero
145 O14 **Arys, Ozero** *Kaz.* Arys Köli. ◎ C Kazakhstan
107 D16 **Arzachena** Sardegna, Italy, C Mediterranean Sea
129 O4 **Arzamas** Nizhegorodskaya Oblast', W Russian Federation
141 V13 **Arzāt** S Oman
104 H3 **Arzúa** Galicia, NW Spain
111 A16 **Aš** *Ger.* Asch. Karlovarský Kraj, W Czech Republic
95 H15 **Ås** Akershus, S Norway
95 H20 **Aså** Nordjylland, N Denmark
83 E21 **Asab** Karas, S Namibia
77 U16 **Asaba** Delta, S Nigeria
149 S4 **Asadābād** *var.* Asadābād; *prev.* Chaghasarāy. Kunar, E Afghanistan
138 K3 **Asad, Buḥayrat al** ◎ N Syria
63 H20 **Asador, Pampa del** *plain* S Argentina
165 P14 **Asahi** Chiba, Honshū, S Japan
164 M11 **Asahi** Toyama, Honshū, SW Japan
165 T3 **Asahi-dake** ▲ Hokkaidō, N Japan
165 T3 **Asahikawa** Hokkaidō, N Japan
147 S10 **Asaka** *Rus.* Assake; *prev.* Leninsk. Andijon Wiloyati, E Uzbekistan
77 P17 **Asamankese** SE Ghana
188 B15 **Asan** W Guam
188 B15 **Asan Point** *headland* W Guam
153 R15 **Āsānsol** West Bengal, NE India
80 K12 **Āsayita** Afar, NE Ethiopia
171 T12 **Asbakin** Irian Jaya, E Indonesia
Asben *see* Aïr, Massif de l'
15 Q12 **Asbestos** Quebec, SE Canada
29 Y13 **Asbury** Iowa, C USA
18 K15 **Asbury Park** New Jersey, NE USA
41 Z12 **Ascención, Bahiá de la** *bay* NW Caribbean Sea
40 I3 **Ascensión** Chihuahua, N Mexico
65 M14 **Ascension Fracture Zone** *tectonic feature* C Atlantic Ocean
65 G14 **Ascension Island** ◇ *dependency of St. Helena* C Atlantic Ocean
65 N16 **Ascension Island** *island* C Atlantic Ocean
Asch *see* Aš
109 S3 **Aschach an der Donau** Oberösterreich, N Austria
101 H18 **Aschaffenburg** Bayern, SW Germany
101 F14 **Ascheberg** Nordrhein-Westfalen, W Germany
101 L14 **Aschersleben** Sachsen-Anhalt, C Germany
106 G12 **Asciano** Toscana, C Italy
106 J13 **Ascoli Piceno** *anc.* Asculum Picenum. Marche, C Italy
107 M17 **Ascoli Satriano** *anc.* Asculub, Asculum Apulum. Puglia, SE Italy
108 G11 **Ascona** Ticino, S Switzerland
Asculub *see* Ascoli Satriano
Asculum Picenum *see* Ascoli Piceno
80 L11 **Aseb** *var.* Assab, *Amh.* Āseb. SE Eritrea
95 M20 **Åseda** Kronoberg, S Sweden
129 T6 **Asekeyevo** Orenburgskaya Oblast', W Russian Federation
81 J14 **Āsela** *var.* Asella, Aselle, Asselle. Oromo, C Ethiopia
93 H15 **Åsele** Västerbotten, N Sweden
Asella/Aselle *see* Āsela
94 K12 **Åsen** Dalarna, C Sweden
114 J11 **Asenovgrad** *prev.* Stanimaka. Plovdiv, C Bulgaria
171 O13 **Asera** Sulawesi, C Indonesia
95 E17 **Åseral** Vest-Agder, S Norway
118 J3 **Aseri** *var.* Asserien, *Ger.* Asserin. Ida-Virumaa, NE Estonia
40 J10 **Aserradero** Durango, NW Mexico
95 H16 **Åsgårdstrand** Vestfold, S Norway
Ashara *see* Al 'Ashārah
23 T6 **Ashburn** Georgia, SE USA
185 G19 **Ashburton** Canterbury, South Island, NZ
185 G19 **Ashburton** ≈ South Island, NZ
180 H8 **Ashburton River** ≈ Western Australia
145 V10 **Ashchysu** ≈ E Kazakhstan
10 M16 **Ashcroft** British Columbia, SW Canada
138 E10 **Ashdod** *anc.* Azotos, *Lat.* Azotus. Central, W Israel
27 S14 **Ashdown** Arkansas, C USA
21 T9 **Asheboro** North Carolina, SE USA
11 X15 **Ashern** Manitoba, S Canada
21 P10 **Asheville** North Carolina, SE USA
12 E8 **Asheweig** ≈ Ontario, C Canada
27 V9 **Ash Flat** Arkansas, C USA
183 T4 **Ashford** New South Wales, SE Australia
97 P22 **Ashford** SE England, UK
36 K11 **Ash Fork** Arizona, SW USA
146 F13 **Ashgabat** *prev.* Ashkhabad, Poltoratsk. ● (Turkmenistan) Akhalskiy Velayat, C Turkmenistan
146 F13 **Ashgabat** ✕ Akhalskiy Velayat, C Turkmenistan
27 T7 **Ash Grove** Missouri, C USA
165 O12 **Ashikaga** *var.* Asikaga. Tochigi, Honshū, S Japan
165 Q8 **Ashiro** Iwate, Honshū, C Japan
164 F15 **Ashizuri-misaki** *headland* Shikoku, SW Japan
Ashkelon *see* Ashqelon
Ashkhabad *see* Ashgabat
23 Q4 **Ashland** Alabama, S USA
26 K7 **Ashland** Kansas, C USA
21 P5 **Ashland** Kentucky, S USA
19 S2 **Ashland** Maine, NE USA
22 M1 **Ashland** Mississippi, S USA
27 U4 **Ashland** Missouri, C USA
29 S15 **Ashland** Nebraska, C USA
31 T12 **Ashland** Ohio, N USA
32 G15 **Ashland** Oregon, NW USA
21 W6 **Ashland** Virginia, NE USA
30 K3 **Ashland** Wisconsin, N USA
20 I8 **Ashland City** Tennessee, S USA
183 S4 **Ashley** New South Wales, SE Australia
29 O7 **Ashley** North Dakota, N USA
173 W7 **Ashmore and Cartier Islands** ◇ *Australian external territory* E Indian Ocean
119 I14 **Ashmyany** *Rus.* Oshmyany. Hrodzyenskaya Voblasts', W Belarus
18 K12 **Ashokan Reservoir** ▣ New York, NE USA
165 U4 **Ashoro** Hokkaidō, NE Japan
138 E10 **Ashqelon** *var.* Ashkelon. Southern, C Israel
Ashraf *see* Behshahr
139 O3 **Ash Shadādah** *var.* Ash Shaddādah, Jisr ash Shadadi, Shaddādī, Shedadi, Tell Shedadi. Al Ḥasakah, NE Syria
Ash Shaddādah *see* Ash Shadādah
139 Y12 **Ash Shāfī** E Iraq
139 R4 **Ash Shakk** *var.* Shaykh. C Iraq
Ash Sham/Ash Shām *see* Dimashq
139 T10 **Ash Shāmīyah** *var.* Shamiya. C Iraq
139 Y13 **Ash Shāmīyah** *var.* Al Bādiyah al Janūbīyah. *desert* S Iraq
139 T11 **Ash Shanāfīyah** *var.* Ash Shināfiyah. S Iraq
138 G13 **Ash Sharāh** *var.* Esh Sharā. ▲ W Jordan
143 R16 **Ash Shāriqah** *Eng.* Sharjah. Ash Shāriqah, NE UAE
143 R16 **Ash Shāriqah** *var.* Sharjah. ✕ Ash Shāriqah, NE UAE
140 I4 **Ash Sharmah** *var.* Šarma. Tabūk, NW Saudi Arabia
139 R4 **Ash Sharqāṭ** NW Iraq
141 S10 **Ash Sharqīyah** *off.* Al Minṭaqah ash Sharqīyah, *Eng.* Eastern Region. ◈ *province* E Saudi Arabia
139 W11 **Ash Shaṭrah** *var.* Shatra. SE Iraq
138 G13 **Ash Shawbak** Ma'ān, W Jordan
138 L5 **Ash Shaykh Ibrāhīm** Ḥimṣ, C Syria
141 O17 **Ash Shaykh 'Uthmān** SW Yemen
141 S15 **Ash Shiḥr** SE Yemen
Ash Shināfiyah *see* Ash Shanāfīyah
141 V12 **Ash Shiṣar** *var.* Shisur. SW Oman
139 S13 **Ash Shubrūm** *well* S Iraq
141 R10 **Ash Shuqqān** *desert* E Saudi Arabia
75 O9 **Ash Shuwayrif** *var.* Ash Shwayrif. N Libya
Ash Shwayrif *see* Ash Shuwayrif
31 U10 **Ashtabula** Ohio, N USA
29 Q5 **Ashtabula, Lake** ▣ North Dakota, N USA
137 T12 **Ashtarak** W Armenia
142 M6 **Āshtiān** *var.* Āshtiyān. Markazī, W Iran
Āshtiyān *see* Āshtiān
33 R13 **Ashton** Idaho, NW USA
13 O10 **Ashuanipi Lake** ◎ Newfoundland, E Canada
15 P6 **Ashuapmushuan** ≈ Quebec, SE Canada
23 Q3 **Ashville** Alabama, S USA
31 S14 **Ashville** Ohio, N USA
30 K3 **Ashwabay, Mount** *hill* Wisconsin, N USA
171 T11 **Asia, Kepulauan** *island group* E Indonesia
154 N13 **Āsika** Orissa, E India

◆ Country ● Country Capital ◇ Dependent Territory ○ Dependent Territory Capital ◈ Administrative Region ✕ International Airport ▲ Mountain ▲ Mountain Range Volcano ≈ River ◎ Lake ▣ Reservoir

Asikaga see Ashikaga
93 M18 **Asikkala** var. Vääksy. Etelä-Suomi, S Finland
74 G5 **Asilah** N Morocco
'Aṣī, Nahr al see Orontes
107 B16 **Asinara, Isola** island W Italy
122 J12 **Asino** Tomskaya Oblast', C Russian Federation
119 O14 **Asintorf** Rus. Osintorf. Vitsyebskaya Voblasts', N Belarus
119 L17 **Asipovichy** Rus. Osipovichi. Mahilyowskaya Voblasts', C Belarus
141 N12 **'Asīr** off. Minţaqat 'Asīr. ◆ province SW Saudi Arabia
140 M11 **'Asīr** Eng. Asir. ▲ SW Saudi Arabia
139 X10 **Askal** E Iraq
137 P13 **Aşkale** Erzurum, NE Turkey
117 T11 **Askaniya-Nova** Khersons'ka Oblast', S Ukraine
95 H15 **Asker** Akershus, S Norway
95 L17 **Askersund** Örebro, C Sweden
Askī Kalak see Eski Kaļak
95 I15 **Askim** Østfold, S Norway
129 V3 **Askino** Respublika Bashkortostan, W Russian Federation
115 D14 **Áskio** ▲ N Greece
152 L9 **Askot** Uttar Pradesh, N India
94 C12 **Askvoll** Sogn og Fjordane, S Norway
136 A13 **Aslan Burnu** headland W Turkey
136 L16 **Aslantaş Barajı** ⊠ S Turkey
149 S4 **Asmār** var. Bar Kunar. Kunar, E Afghanistan
80 I9 **Asmara** Amh. Āsmera. ● (Eritrea) C Eritrea
Āsmera see Asmara
95 L21 **Åsnen** ◎ S Sweden
115 F19 **Asopós** ⇝ S Greece
171 W13 **Asori** Irian Jaya, E Indonesia
80 G12 **Āsosa** Benishangul, W Ethiopia
32 M10 **Asotin** Washington, NW USA
Aspadana see Eşfahān
Aspang see Aspang Markt
109 X6 **Aspang Markt** var. Aspang. Niederösterreich, E Austria
105 S12 **Aspe** País Valenciano, E Spain
37 R5 **Aspen** Colorado, C USA
25 P6 **Aspermont** Texas, SW USA
Asphaltites, Lacus see Dead Sea
Aspinwall see Colón
185 C20 **Aspiring, Mount** ▲ South Island, NZ
115 B16 **Asprókavos, Akrotírio** headland Kérkyra, Iónioi Nísoi, Greece, C Mediterranean Sea
Aspropótamos see Achelóos
Assab see Aseb
76 J10 **Assaba** var. Açâba. ◆ region S Mauritania
138 L4 **As Sabkhah** var. Sabkha. Ar Raqqah, NE Syria
139 U6 **As Sa'dīyah** E Iraq
Assad, Lake see Asad, Buḩayrat al
138 I8 **Aş Şafā** ▲ S Syria
138 I10 **Aş Şafāwī** Al Mafraq, N Jordan
Aş Şaff see El Şaff
139 N2 **Aş Şafīḩ** Al Ḩasakah, N Syria
Aş Şaḩrā' al Gharbīyah see Sahara el Gharbîya
Aş Şaḩrā' ash Sharqīyah see Sahara el Sharqîya
Assake see Asaka
As Salamīyah see Salamīyah
141 Q4 **As Sālimī** var. Salemy. SW Kuwait
67 W7 **'Assal, Lac** ◎ C Djibouti
As Sallūm see Salûm
139 T13 **As Salmān** S Iraq
138 G10 **As Salţ** var. Salt. Al Balqā', NW Jordan
142 M16 **As Salwā** var. Salwa, Salwah. S Qatar
153 V12 **Assam** ◆ state NE India
Assamaka see Assamakka
77 T8 **Assamakka** var. Assamaka. Agadez, NW Niger
139 U11 **As Samāwah** var. Samawa. S Iraq
As Saqia al Hamra see Saguia al Hamra
138 J4 **Aş Şā'rān** Ḩamāh, C Syria
138 G9 **Aş Şarīḩ** Irbid, N Jordan
21 Z5 **Assateague Island** island Maryland, NE USA
139 O6 **As Sayyāl** var. Sayyāl. Dayr az Zawr, E Syria
99 G18 **Asse** Vlaams Brabant, C Belgium
99 D16 **Assebroek** West-Vlaanderen, NW Belgium
Asselle see Āsela
107 C20 **Assemini** Sardegna, Italy, C Mediterranean Sea
98 N7 **Assen** Drenthe, NE Netherlands
99 E16 **Assenede** Oost-Vlaanderen, NW Belgium
95 G24 **Assens** Fyn, C Denmark
Asserien/Asserin see Aseri
99 I21 **Assesse** Namur, SE Belgium
141 Y8 **As Sīb** var. Seeb. NE Oman
139 Z13 **As Sībah** var. Sibah. SE Iraq
11 T17 **Assiniboia** Saskatchewan, S Canada
11 V15 **Assiniboine** ⇝ Manitoba, S Canada
11 P16 **Assiniboine, Mount** ▲ Alberta/British Columbia, SW Canada
Assiout see Asyût
60 J9 **Assis** São Paulo, S Brazil
106 I13 **Assisi** Umbria, C Italy
Assiut see Asyût
Assling see Jesenice
Assouan see Aswân
Assu see Açu
Assuan see Aswân
142 K12 **Aş Şubayḩīyah** var. Subiyah. S Kuwait
141 R16 **As Sufāl** S Yemen
138 L5 **As Sukhnah** var. Sukhne, Fr. Soukhné. Ḩimş, C Syria
139 U4 **As Sulaymānīyah** var. Sulaimaniya, Kurd. Slēmānī. NE Iraq
141 P11 **As Sulayyil** Ar Riyāḑ, S Saudi Arabia
121 O13 **As Sulţān** N Libya
141 Q5 **Aş Şummān** desert N Saudi Arabia
141 Q16 **Aş Şurrah** SW Yemen
139 N4 **Aş Şuwār** var. Şuwār. Dayr az Zawr, E Syria
138 H9 **As Suwaydā'** var. El Suweida, Es Suweida, Suweida, Fr. Soueida. As Suwaydā', SW Syria
138 H9 **As Suwaydā'** off. Muḩāfaz̧at as Suwaydā', var. As Suwaydā, Suwaydá, Suweida, Fr. Soueida. ◆ governorate S Syria
141 Z9 **As Suwayḩ** NE Oman
141 X8 **As Suwayq** var. Suwaik. N Oman
139 T8 **Aş Şuwayrah** var. Suwaira. E Iraq
As Suways see Suez
Asta Colonia see Asti
Astacus see İzmit
115 M23 **Astakída** island SE Greece
145 Q9 **Astana** prev. Akmola, Akmolinsk, Tselinograd, Aqmola. ● (Kazakhstan) Akmola, N Kazakhstan
142 M3 **Āstāneh** Gīlān, NW Iran
Asta Pompeia see Asti
137 Y14 **Astara** S Azerbaijan
Astarabad see Gorgān
99 L15 **Asten** Noord-Brabant, SE Netherlands
Asterābād see Gorgān
106 C8 **Asti** anc. Asta Colonia, Asta Pompeia, Hasta Colonia, Hasta Pompeia. Piemonte, NW Italy
Astigi see Ecija
Astipálaia see Astypálaia
148 L16 **Astola Island** island SW Pakistan
152 H4 **Astor** Jammu and Kashmir, NW India
104 K4 **Astorga** anc. Asturica Augusta. Castilla-León, N Spain
32 F10 **Astoria** Oregon, NW USA
(0) F8 **Astoria Fan** undersea feature E Pacific Ocean
95 J22 **Åstorp** Skåne, S Sweden
Astrabad see Gorgān
129 Q13 **Astrakhan'** Astrakhanskaya Oblast', SW Russian Federation
Astrakhan-Bazar see Cälilabad
129 Q11 **Astrakhanskaya Oblast'** ◆ province SW Russian Federation
93 J15 **Åsträsk** Västerbotten, N Sweden
Astrida see Butare
65 O22 **Astrid Ridge** undersea feature S Atlantic Ocean
187 P15 **Astrolabe, Récifs de l'** reef C New Caledonia
121 P2 **Astromerítis** N Cyprus
115 F20 **Ástros** Pelopónnisos, S Greece
119 G16 **Astryna** Rus. Ostryna. Hrodzyenskaya Voblasts', W Belarus
104 J2 **Asturias** ◆ autonomous community NW Spain
Asturias see Oviedo
Asturica Augusta see Astorga
115 L22 **Astypálaia** var. Astipálaia, It. Stampalia. island Kykládes, Greece, Aegean Sea
192 G16 **Āsuisui, Cape** headland Savai'i, W Samoa
195 S2 **Asuka** Japanese research station Antarctica
62 O6 **Asunción** ● (Paraguay) Central, S Paraguay
62 O6 **Asunción** × Central, S Paraguay
188 K3 **Asuncion Island** island N Northern Mariana Islands
42 E6 **Asunción Mita** Jutiapa, SE Guatemala
Asunción Nochixtlán see Nochixtlán
40 E3 **Asunción, Río** ⇝ NW Mexico
95 M18 **Åsunden** ◎ S Sweden
118 K11 **Asvyeya** Rus. Osveya. Vitsyebskaya Voblasts', N Belarus
Aswa see Achwa
75 X11 **Aswân** var. Assouan, Assuan; anc. Syene. SE Egypt
75 X11 **Aswân High Dam** dam SE Egypt
75 W9 **Asyût** var. Assiout, Assiut, Siut; anc. Lycopolis. C Egypt
193 W15 **Ata** island Tongatapu Group, SW Tonga
62 G8 **Atacama** off. Región de Atacama. ◆ region C Chile
Atacama Desert see Atacama, Desierto de
62 H4 **Atacama, Desierto de** Eng. Atacama Desert. desert N Chile
62 I6 **Atacama, Puna de** ▲ NW Argentina
62 I5 **Atacama, Salar de** salt lake N Chile
54 E11 **Ataco** Tolima, C Colombia
190 H8 **Atafu Atoll** island NW Tokelau
190 H8 **Atafu Village** Atafu Atoll, NW Tokelau
74 K12 **Atakor** ▲ SE Algeria
77 R14 **Atakora, Chaîne de l'** var. Atakora Mountains. ▲ N Benin
Atakora Mountains see Atakora, Chaîne de l'
77 R16 **Atakpamé** C Togo
146 F11 **Atakui** Akhalskiy Velayat, C Turkmenistan
58 B13 **Atalaia do Norte** Amazonas, N Brazil
76 I7 **Atâr** Adrar, W Mauritania
162 G10 **Atas Bogd** ▲ SW Mongolia
35 P12 **Atascadero** California, W USA
25 S13 **Atascosa River** ⇝ Texas, SW USA
145 R11 **Atasu** Zhezkazgan, C Kazakhstan
145 R12 **Atasu** ⇝ C Kazakhstan
193 V15 **Atata** island Tongatapu Group, S Tonga
136 H10 **Atatürk** × (İstanbul) İstanbul, NW Turkey
137 N16 **Atatürk Barajı** ⊠ S Turkey
Atax see Aude
80 G8 **Atbara** var. 'Aţbārah. River Nile, NE Sudan
80 H8 **Atbara** var. Nahr 'Aţbarah. ⇝ Eritrea/Sudan
'Aţbārah/'Aţbarah, Nahr see Atbara
145 P9 **Atbasar** Akmola, N Kazakhstan
At-Bashi see At-Bashy
147 W9 **At-Bashy** var. At-Bashi. Narynskaya Oblast', C Kyrgyzstan
22 I10 **Atchafalaya Bay** bay Louisiana, S USA
22 I8 **Atchafalaya River** ⇝ Louisiana, S USA
Atchin see Aceh
27 Q3 **Atchison** Kansas, C USA
77 P16 **Atebubu** C Ghana
105 Q6 **Ateca** Aragón, NE Spain
40 K11 **Atengo, Río** ⇝ C Mexico
Aternum see Pescara
107 K15 **Atessa** Abruzzo, C Italy
Ateste see Este
99 E19 **Ath** var. Aat. Hainaut, SW Belgium
11 Q13 **Athabasca** Alberta, SW Canada
11 Q12 **Athabasca** var. Athabaska. ⇝ Alberta, SW Canada
11 R10 **Athabasca, Lake** ◎ Alberta/Saskatchewan, SW Canada
Athabaska see Athabasca
115 C16 **Athamánon** ▲ C Greece
97 F17 **Athboy** Ir. Baile Átha Buí. E Ireland
Athenae see Athína
97 C18 **Athenry** Ir. Baile Átha an Rí. W Ireland
23 P2 **Athens** Alabama, S USA
23 T3 **Athens** Georgia, SE USA
31 T14 **Athens** Ohio, N USA
20 M10 **Athens** Tennessee, S USA
25 V7 **Athens** Texas, SW USA
Athens see Athína
115 B18 **Athéras, Akrotírio** headland Kefallinía, Iónioi Nísoi, Greece, C Mediterranean Sea
181 W4 **Atherton** Queensland, NE Australia
81 I19 **Athi** ⇝ S Kenya
121 Q2 **Athíenou** SE Cyprus
115 H19 **Athína** Eng. Athens; prev. Athínai, anc. Athenae. ● (Greece) Attikí, C Greece
Athínai see Athína
139 S10 **Athīyah** C Iraq
97 D18 **Athlone** Ir. Baile Átha Luain. C Ireland
155 F16 **Athni** Karnātaka, W India
185 C23 **Athol** Southland, South Island, NZ
19 N11 **Athol** Massachusetts, NE USA
115 I15 **Áthos** ▲ NE Greece
Athos, Mount see Ágion Óros
Ath Thawrah see Madīnat ath Thawrah
141 P5 **Ath Thumāmī** spring/well N Saudi Arabia
99 L25 **Athus** Luxembourg, SE Belgium
97 E19 **Athy** Ir. Baile Átha Í. C Ireland
78 I10 **Ati** Batha, C Chad
81 F16 **Atiak** NW Uganda
57 G17 **Atico** Arequipa, SW Peru
105 O6 **Atienza** Castilla-La Mancha, C Spain
39 Q6 **Atigun Pass** pass Alaska, USA
12 B12 **Atikokan** Ontario, S Canada
13 O9 **Atikonak Lac** ◎ Newfoundland, E Canada
42 C6 **Atitlán, Lago de** ◎ W Guatemala
190 L16 **Atiu** island S Cook Islands
Atjeh see Aceh
123 T9 **Atka** Magadanskaya Oblast', E Russian Federation
38 H17 **Atka** Atka Island, Alaska, USA
38 H17 **Atka Island** island Aleutian Islands, Alaska, USA
129 O7 **Atkarsk** Saratovskaya Oblast', W Russian Federation
27 U11 **Atkins** Arkansas, C USA
29 O13 **Atkinson** Nebraska, C USA
171 T12 **Atkri** Irian Jaya, E Indonesia
41 O13 **Atlacomulco** var. Atlacomulco de Fabela. México, C Mexico
Atlacomulco de Fabela see Atlacomulco
23 S3 **Atlanta** state capital Georgia, SE USA
31 R6 **Atlanta** Michigan, N USA
25 X6 **Atlanta** Texas, SW USA
29 T15 **Atlantic** Iowa, C USA
21 Y10 **Atlantic** North Carolina, SE USA
23 W8 **Atlantic Beach** Florida, SE USA
18 J17 **Atlantic City** New Jersey, NE USA
172 L14 **Atlantic-Indian Basin** undersea feature SW Indian Ocean
172 K13 **Atlantic-Indian Ridge** undersea feature SW Indian Ocean
54 E4 **Atlántico** off. Departamento del Atlántico. ◆ province NW Colombia
66-67 **Atlantic Ocean** ocean
42 K7 **Atlántico Norte, Región Autónoma** prev. Zelaya Norte. ◆ autonomous region NE Nicaragua
42 L10 **Atlántico Sur, Región Autónoma** prev. Zelaya Sur. ◆ autonomous region SE Nicaragua
42 I5 **Atlántida** ◆ department N Honduras
77 Y15 **Atlantika Mountains** ▲ E Nigeria
64 J10 **Atlantis Fracture Zone** tectonic feature NW Atlantic Ocean
74 H7 **Atlas Mountains** ▲ NW Africa
123 V11 **Atlasova, Ostrov** island SE Russian Federation
123 V10 **Atlasovo** Kamchatskaya Oblast', E Russian Federation
120 G11 **Atlas Saharien** var. Saharan Atlas. ▲ Algeria/Morocco
Atlas, Tell see Atlas Tellien
120 H10 **Atlas Tellien** Eng. Tell Atlas. ▲ N Algeria
10 I9 **Atlin** British Columbia, W Canada
10 I9 **Atlin Lake** ◎ British Columbia, W Canada
41 P14 **Atlixco** Puebla, S Mexico
94 B11 **Atløyna** island S Norway
155 I17 **Ātmakūr** Andhra Pradesh, C India
23 O8 **Atmore** Alabama, S USA
101 J20 **Atmühl** ⇝ S Germany
94 H11 **Atna** ⇝ S Norway
164 E13 **Atō** Yamaguchi, Honshū, SW Japan
57 L21 **Atocha** Potosí, S Bolivia
27 P12 **Atoka** Oklahoma, C USA
27 O12 **Atoka Lake** var. Atoka Reservoir. ⊠ Oklahoma, C USA
Atoka Reservoir see Atoka Lake
33 Q14 **Atomic City** Idaho, NW USA
40 L10 **Atotonilco** Zacatecas, C Mexico
40 M13 **Atotonilco el Alto** var. Atotonilco. Jalisco, SW Mexico
77 N7 **Atouila, 'Erg** desert N Mali
41 N16 **Atoyac** var. Atoyac de Alvarez. Guerrero, S Mexico
Atoyac de Alvarez see Atoyac
41 P15 **Atoyac, Río** ⇝ S Mexico
39 O5 **Atqasuk** Alaska, USA
146 C13 **Atrak** Per. Rūd-e Atrak, Rus. Atrek, Turkm. Etrek. ⇝ Iran/Turkmenistan
Atrak, Rūd-e see Atrak
95 J20 **Ätran** ⇝ S Sweden
54 C7 **Atrato, Río** ⇝ NW Colombia
Atrek see Atrak
107 K14 **Atri** Abruzzo, C Italy
Atria see Adria
165 P9 **Atsumi** Yamagata, Honshū, C Japan
165 S3 **Atsuta** Hokkaidō, NE Japan
143 Q17 **Aţ Ţaff** desert C UAE
138 G12 **Aţ Ţafīlah** var. Et Tafila, Tafila. Aţ Ţafīlah, W Jordan
138 G12 **Aţ Ţafīlah** off. Muḩāfaz̧at aţ Ţafīlah. ◆ governorate W Jordan
140 L10 **Aţ Ţā'if** Makkah, W Saudi Arabia
Attaleia/Attalia see Antalya
23 Q3 **Attalla** Alabama, S USA
138 L2 **At Tall al Abyaḑ** var. Tall al Abyaḑ, Tell Abyad, Fr. Tell Abiad. Ar Raqqah, N Syria
138 L7 **Aţ Ţanf** Ḩimş, S Syria
Attapu see Samakhixai
139 S10 **At Taqtaqānah** C Iraq
115 O23 **Attávytos** ▲ Ródos, Dodekánisos, Greece, Aegean Sea
139 V15 **At Tawal** desert Iraq/Saudi Arabia
12 G9 **Attawapiskat** Ontario, C Canada
12 F9 **Attawapiskat** ⇝ Ontario, S Canada
12 D9 **Attawapiskat Lake** ◎ Ontario, C Canada
At Taybé see Ţayyibah
101 F16 **Attendorn** Nordrhein-Westfalen, W Germany
109 R5 **Attersee** Salzburg, NW Austria
109 R5 **Attersee** ◎ N Austria
99 L24 **Attert** Luxembourg, SE Belgium
138 M4 **At Tibnī** var. Tibnī. Dayr az Zawr, NE Syria
31 N13 **Attica** Indiana, N USA
18 E10 **Attica** New York, NE USA
Attica see Attikí
13 N7 **Attikamagen Lake** ◎ Newfoundland, E Canada
115 H20 **Attikí** Eng. Attica. ◆ region C Greece
19 O12 **Attleboro** Massachusetts, NE USA
109 R5 **Attnang** Oberösterreich, N Austria
149 U6 **Attock City** Punjab, E Pakistan
Attopeu see Samakhixai
25 X8 **Attoyac River** ⇝ Texas, SW USA
38 D16 **Attu** Attu Island, Alaska, USA
139 Y12 **Aţ Ţūbah** E Iraq
140 K4 **Aţ Ţubayq** plain Jordan/Saudi Arabia
38 C16 **Attu Island** island Aleutian Islands, Alaska, USA
Aţ Ţūr see El Ţûr
155 I21 **Āttūr** Tamil Nādu, SE India
141 N17 **At Turbah** SW Yemen
62 I12 **Atuel, Río** ⇝ C Argentina
Atugi see Atsugi
191 X7 **Atuona** Hiva Oa, NE French Polynesia
Aturus see Adour
95 M18 **Åtvidaberg** Östergötland, S Sweden
35 P9 **Atwater** California, W USA
29 T8 **Atwater** Minnesota, N USA
26 I2 **Atwood** Kansas, C USA
31 U12 **Atwood Lake** ⊠ Ohio, N USA
129 P5 **Atyashevo** Respublika Mordoviya, W Russian Federation
144 F12 **Atyrau** prev. Gur'yev. Atyrau, W Kazakhstan
144 E11 **Atyrau** off. Atyrauskaya Oblast', var. Kaz. Atyraū Oblysy; prev. Gur'yevskaya Oblast'. ◆ province W Kazakhstan
Atyraū Oblysy/Atyrauskaya Oblast' see Atyrau
108 J7 **Au** Vorarlberg, NW Austria
186 B4 **Aua Island** island NW PNG
103 S16 **Aubagne** anc. Albania. Bouches-du-Rhône, SE France
99 L25 **Aubange** Luxembourg, SE Belgium
103 Q6 **Aube** ◆ department N France
103 R6 **Aube** ⇝ N France
99 L19 **Aubel** Liège, E Belgium
103 Q13 **Aubenas** Ardèche, E France
103 O8 **Aubigny-sur-Nère** Cher, C France
103 O13 **Aubin** Aveyron, S France
103 O13 **Aubrac, Monts d'** ▲ S France
36 J10 **Aubrey Cliffs** cliff Arizona, SW USA
23 R5 **Auburn** Alabama, S USA
35 P6 **Auburn** California, W USA
30 K14 **Auburn** Illinois, N USA
31 Q11 **Auburn** Indiana, N USA
20 J7 **Auburn** Kentucky, S USA
19 P8 **Auburn** Maine, NE USA
19 N11 **Auburn** Massachusetts, NE USA
29 S16 **Auburn** Nebraska, C USA
18 H10 **Auburn** New York, NE USA
32 H8 **Auburn** Washington, NW USA
103 N11 **Aubusson** Creuse, C France
118 E10 **Auce** Ger. Autz. Dobele, SW Latvia
102 L15 **Auch** Lat. Augusta Auscorum, Elimberrum. Gers, S France
77 U16 **Auchi** Edo, S Nigeria
23 T9 **Aucilla River** ⇝ Florida/Georgia, SE USA
184 L6 **Auckland** Auckland, North Island, NZ
184 K5 **Auckland** off. Auckland Region. ◆ region North Island, NZ
184 L6 **Auckland** × Auckland, North Island, NZ
192 J12 **Auckland Islands** island group S NZ
103 O16 **Aude** ◆ department S France
103 N16 **Aude** anc. Atax. ⇝ S France
Audenarde see Oudenaarde
Audern see Audru
102 E6 **Audierne** Finistère, NW France
102 E6 **Audierne, Baie d'** bay NW France
103 U7 **Audincourt** Doubs, E France
118 G5 **Audru** Ger. Audern. Pärnumaa, SW Estonia
29 T14 **Audubon** Iowa, C USA
101 N17 **Aue** Sachsen, E Germany
100 H12 **Aue** ⇝ NW Germany
100 L9 **Auerbach** Bayern, SE Germany
101 M17 **Auerbach** Sachsen, E Germany
108 I10 **Auererrhein** ⇝ SW Switzerland
101 N17 **Auersberg** ▲ E Germany
181 W9 **Augathella** Queensland, E Australia
31 Q12 **Auglaize River** ⇝ Ohio, N USA
83 F22 **Augrabies Falls** waterfall W South Africa
31 R7 **Au Gres River** ⇝ Michigan, N USA
Augsbourg see Augsburg
101 K22 **Augsburg** Fr. Augsbourg; anc. Augusta Vindelicorum. Bayern, S Germany
180 I14 **Augusta** Western Australia
107 L25 **Augusta** It. Agosta. Sicilia, Italy, C Mediterranean Sea
27 W11 **Augusta** Arkansas, C USA
23 V3 **Augusta** Georgia, SE USA
27 O6 **Augusta** Kansas, C USA
19 Q7 **Augusta** state capital Maine, NE USA
33 Q8 **Augusta** Montana, NW USA
Augusta see London
Augusta Auscorum see Auch
Augusta Emerita see Mérida
Augusta Praetoria see Aosta
Augusta Suessionum see Soissons
Augusta Trajana see Stara Zagora
Augusta Treverorum see Trier
Augusta Vangionum see Worms
Augusta Vindelicorum see Augsburg
95 G24 **Augustenborg** Ger. Augustenburg. Sønderjylland, SW Denmark
Augustenburg see Augustenborg
39 Q13 **Augustine Island** island Alaska, USA
14 L9 **Augustines, Lac des** ◎ Quebec, SE Canada
Augustobona Tricassium see Troyes
Augustodunum see Autun
Augustodurum see Bayeux
Augustoritum Lemovicensium see Limoges
110 O8 **Augustów** Rus. Avgustov. Podlaskie, NE Poland
Augustow Canal see Augustowski, Kanał
110 O8 **Augustowski, Kanał** Eng. Augustow Canal, Rus. Avgustovskiy Kanal. canal NE Poland
180 I9 **Augustus, Mount** ▲ Western Australia
186 M9 **Auki** Malaita, N Solomon Islands
21 W8 **Aulander** North Carolina, SE USA
180 L7 **Auld, Lake** salt lake Western Australia
Aulie Ata/Auliye-Ata see Taraz
106 E10 **Aulla** Toscana, C Italy
102 F6 **Aulne** ⇝ NW France
Aulong see Ulong
37 T3 **Ault** Colorado, C USA
103 N3 **Aumale** Seine-Maritime, N France
Auminzatau, Gory see Owminzatovo-Toshi
77 T14 **Auna** Niger, W Nigeria
95 H21 **Auning** Århus, C Denmark
192 K17 **Aunu'u Island** island W American Samoa
83 E20 **Auob** var. Oup. ⇝ Namibia/South Africa
93 K19 **Aura** Länsi-Suomi, W Finland
109 R5 **Aurach** ⇝ N Austria
Aural, Phnom see Aôral, Phnum
153 O14 **Aurangābād** Bihār, N India
154 F13 **Aurangābād** Mahārāshtra, C India
189 V7 **Aur Atoll** atoll E Marshall Islands
102 G7 **Auray** Morbihan, NW France
94 G13 **Aurdal** Oppland, S Norway
94 F8 **Aure** Møre og Romsdal, S Norway
29 T12 **Aurelia** Iowa, C USA
Aurelia Aquensis see Baden-Baden
Aurelianum see Orléans
120 J10 **Aurès, Massif de l'** ▲ NE Algeria
100 F10 **Aurich** Niedersachsen, NW Germany
103 O13 **Aurillac** Cantal, C France
Aurine, Alpi see Zillertaler Alpen
Aurium see Ourense
14 H15 **Aurora** Ontario, S Canada
55 S8 **Aurora** NW Guyana
37 T4 **Aurora** Colorado, C USA
30 M11 **Aurora** Illinois, N USA
31 Q15 **Aurora** Indiana, N USA
29 W4 **Aurora** Minnesota, N USA
27 S8 **Aurora** Missouri, C USA
29 P16 **Aurora** Nebraska, C USA
36 J5 **Aurora** Utah, W USA
Aurora see Maéwo, Vanuatu
Aurora see San Francisco, Philippines
94 F10 **Aursjøen** ◎ S Norway
94 I9 **Aursunden** ◎ S Norway
83 D21 **Aus** Karas, SW Namibia
Ausa see Vic
14 E16 **Ausable** ⇝ Ontario, S Canada
31 O3 **Au Sable Point** headland Michigan, N USA
31 S7 **Au Sable Point** headland Michigan, N USA
31 R6 **Au Sable River** ⇝ Michigan, N USA
57 H16 **Ausangate, Nevado** ▲ C Peru
Auschwitz see Oświęcim
Ausculum Apulum see Ascoli Satriano
105 Q4 **Ausejo** La Rioja, N Spain
Aussig see Ústí nad Labem
95 F17 **Aust-Agder** ◆ county S Norway
92 P2 **Austfonna** glacier NE Svalbard
31 P15 **Austin** Indiana, N USA
29 W11 **Austin** Minnesota, N USA
35 U5 **Austin** Nevada, W USA
25 S10 **Austin** state capital Texas, S USA
180 J10 **Austin, Lake** salt lake Western Australia
31 V11 **Austintown** Ohio, N USA
25 V9 **Austonio** Texas, SW USA
Australes, Archipel des see Australes, Îles
Australes et Antarctiques Françaises, Terres see French Southern and Antarctic Territories
191 T14 **Australes, Îles** var. Archipel des Australes, Îles Tubuai, Tubuai Islands, Eng. Austral Islands. island group SW French Polynesia
175 Y11 **Austral Fracture Zone** tectonic feature S Pacific Ocean
181 O7 **Australia** off. Commonwealth of Australia. ◆ commonwealth republic
174 M8 **Australia** continent
183 Q12 **Australian Alps** ▲ SE Australia
183 R11 **Australian Capital Territory** prev. Federal Capital Territory. ◆ territory SE Australia
Australie, Bassin Nord de l' see North Australian Basin
Austral Islands see Australes, Îles
Austrava see Ostrov
109 T6 **Austria** off. Republic of Austria, Ger. Österreich. ◆ republic C Europe
92 K3 **Austurland** ◆ region SE Iceland
92 G10 **Austvågøya** island C Norway
Ausuituq see Grise Fiord
58 G13 **Autazes** Amazonas, N Brazil
102 M16 **Auterive** Haute-Garonne, S France
Autesiodorum see Auxerre
103 N2 **Authie** ⇝ N France
Autissiodorum see Auxerre
40 K14 **Autlán** var. Autlán de Navarro. Jalisco, SW Mexico
Autlán de Navarro see Autlán
Autricum see Chartres
103 Q9 **Autun** anc. Ædua, Augustodunum. Saône-et-Loire, C France
Autz see Auce
99 H20 **Auvelais** Namur, S Belgium
103 P11 **Auvergne** ◆ region C France
102 M12 **Auvézère** ⇝ W France
103 P7 **Auxerre** anc. Autesiodorum, Autissiodorum. Yonne, C France
103 N2 **Auxi-le-Château** Pas-de-Calais, N France
103 S8 **Auxonne** Côte d'Or, C France
55 P9 **Auyan Tebuy** ▲ SE Venezuela
103 O10 **Auzances** Creuse, C France
27 U8 **Ava** Missouri, C USA
142 M5 **Āvaj** Qazvīn, N Iran
95 C15 **Avaldsnes** Rogaland, S Norway
103 Q8 **Avallon** Yonne, C France
102 K6 **Avaloirs, Mont des** ▲ NW France
35 S16 **Avalon** Santa Catalina Island, California, W USA
18 J17 **Avalon** New Jersey, NE USA
13 V13 **Avalon Peninsula** peninsula Newfoundland, E Canada
197 Q11 **Avannaarsua** ◆ province N Greenland
60 K10 **Avaré** São Paulo, S Brazil
Avaricum see Bourges
190 H16 **Avarua** ○ (Cook Islands) Rarotonga, S Cook Islands
190 H16 **Avarua Harbour** harbour Rarotonga, S Cook Islands
Avasfelsőfalu see Negreşti-Oaş
38 L17 **Avatanak Island** island Aleutian Islands, Alaska, USA
190 B16 **Avatele** S Niue
190 H16 **Avatiu** Rarotonga, S Cook Islands

◆ Country ● Country Capital ◇ Dependent Territory ○ Dependent Territory Capital ◆ Administrative Region × International Airport ▲ Mountain ▲ Mountain Range ⚲ Volcano ⇝ River ◎ Lake ⊠ Reservoir

190 H15 Avatiu Harbour harbour Rarotonga, S Cook Islands
Avdeyevka see Avdiyivka
114 J13 Ávdira Anatolikí Makedonía kai Thráki, NE Greece
117 X8 Avdiyivka Rus. Avdeyevka. Donets'ka Oblast', SE Ukraine
162 K7 Avdzaga C Mongolia
104 G6 Ave ≈ N Portugal
104 G7 Aveiro anc. Talabriga. Aveiro, W Portugal
104 G7 Aveiro ◈ district N Portugal
Avela see Ávila
99 D18 Avelgem West-Vlaanderen, W Belgium
61 D20 Avellaneda Buenos Aires, E Argentina
107 L17 Avellino anc. Abellinum. Campania, S Italy
35 Q12 Avenal California, W USA
Avenio see Avignon
94 E8 Averoya island S Norway
107 K17 Aversa Campania, S Italy
33 N9 Avery Idaho, NW USA
25 W5 Avery Texas, SW USA
Aves, Islas de see Las Aves, Islas
Avesnes see Avesnes-sur-Helpe
103 Q2 Avesnes-sur-Helpe var. Avesnes. Nord, N France
64 G12 Aves Ridge undersea feature SE Caribbean Sea
95 M14 Avesta Dalarna, C Sweden
103 O14 Aveyron ◈ department S France
103 N14 Aveyron ≈ S France
107 J15 Avezzano Abruzzo, C Italy
115 D16 Avgó ▲ C Greece
Avgustov see Augustów
Avgustovskiy Kanal see Augustowski, Kanał
96 J9 Aviemore N Scotland, UK
185 F21 Aviemore, Lake ◎ South Island, NZ
103 R15 Avignon anc. Avenio. Vaucluse, SE France
104 M7 Ávila var. Avila; anc. Abela, Abula, Abyla, Avela. Castilla-León, C Spain
104 L8 Ávila ◈ province Castilla-León, C Spain
104 K2 Avilés Asturias, NW Spain
118 J4 Avinurme Ger. Awwinorm. Ida-Virumaa, NE Estonia
104 H10 Avis Portalegre, C Portugal
95 F22 Avlum Ringkøbing, C Denmark
182 M11 Avoca Victoria, SE Australia
29 T14 Avoca Iowa, C USA
182 M11 Avoca River ≈ Victoria, SE Australia
107 L25 Avola Sicilia, Italy, C Mediterranean Sea
18 F10 Avon New York, NE USA
29 P12 Avon South Dakota, N USA
97 M23 Avon ≈ S England, UK
97 L20 Avon ≈ C England, UK
66 K13 Avondale Arizona, SW USA
23 X13 Avon Park Florida, SE USA
102 J5 Avranches Manche, N France
103 O3 Avre ≈ N France
186 M6 Avuavu var. Kolotambu. Guadalcanal, C Solomon Islands
Avveel see Ivalo, Finland
Avveel see Ivalojoki, Finland
Avvil see Ivalo
77 O17 Awaaso var. Awaso. SW Ghana
141 X8 Awābī var. Al 'Awābī. NE Oman
184 L9 Awakino Waikato, North Island, NZ
142 M15 'Awālī C Bahrain
99 K19 Awans Liège, E Belgium
184 I2 Awanui Northland, North Island, NZ
148 M14 Awārān Baluchistān, SW Pakistan
81 K16 Awara Plain plain NE Kenya
80 M13 Āwarē Somali, E Ethiopia
138 M6 'Awāriḍ, Wādī dry watercourse E Syria
185 B20 Awarua Point headland South Island, NZ
81 J14 Āwasa Southern, S Ethiopia
80 K13 Āwash Afar, NE Ethiopia
80 K12 Āwash var. Hawash. ≈ C Ethiopia
Awaso see Awaaso
158 H7 Awat Xinjiang Uygur Zizhiqu, NW China
185 J15 Awatere ≈ South Island, NZ
75 O10 Awbārī SW Libya
75 N9 Awbāri, Idhān var. Edeyen d'Oubari. desert Algeria/Libya
80 C13 Aweil Northern Bahr el Ghazal, SW Sudan
96 H11 Awe, Loch ◎ W Scotland, UK
77 U16 Awka Anambra, SW Nigeria
39 O6 Awuna River ≈ Alaska, USA
Awwinorm see Avinurme
Ax see Dax
Axarfjördhur see Öxarfjördhur
103 N17 Axat Aude, S France
99 F16 Axel Zeeland, SW Netherlands
8 M2 Axel Heiberg Island var. Axel Heiburg. island Nunavut, N Canada
Axel Heiburg see Axel Heiberg Island
77 O17 Axim S Ghana
114 F13 Axiós var. Vardar. ≈ Greece/FYR Macedonia see also Vardar
103 N17 Ax-les-Thermes Ariège, S France
120 D11 Ayachi, Jbel ▲ C Morocco
61 D22 Ayacucho Buenos Aires, E Argentina
57 F15 Ayacucho Ayacucho, S Peru
57 E16 Ayacucho off. Departamento de Ayacucho. ◈ department SW Peru
145 W11 Ayagoz var. Ayaguz, Kaz. Ayaköz; prev. Sergiopol. Vostochnyy Kazakhstan, E Kazakhstan
145 V12 Ayagoz var. Ayaguz, Kaz. Ayaköz. ≈ E Kazakhstan
Ayaguz see Ayagoz
Ayakagytma see Oyoqighitma
Ayakkuduk see Oyoqquduq
158 L10 Ayakkum Hu ◎ NW China
Ayaköz see Ayagoz
104 H14 Ayamonte Andalucía, S Spain
123 S11 Ayan Khabarovskiy Kray, E Russian Federation
136 J10 Ayancık Sinop, N Turkey
55 S9 Ayanganna Mountain ▲ C Guyana
77 U16 Ayangba Kogi, C Nigeria
123 U7 Ayanka Koryakskiy Avtonomnyy Okrug, E Russian Federation
54 E7 Ayapel Córdoba, NW Colombia
136 H12 Ayaş Ankara, N Turkey
57 I16 Ayaviri Puno, S Peru
149 P3 Āybak var. Aibak, Haibak; prev. Samangān. Samangān, NE Afghanistan
147 N10 Aydarkŭl Rus. Ozero Aydarkul'. ◎ C Uzbekistan
Aydarkul', Ozero see Aydarkŭl
21 W10 Ayden North Carolina, SE USA
136 C15 Aydın var. Aïdin; anc. Tralles. Aydın, SW Turkey
136 C15 Aydın var. Aïdin. ◈ province SW Turkey
136 I17 Aydıncık İçel, S Turkey
136 C15 Aydın Dağları ▲ W Turkey
158 L6 Aydingkol Hu ◎ NW China
129 X7 Aydyrlinskiy Orenburgskaya Oblast', W Russian Federation
105 S4 Ayerbe Aragón, NE Spain
Ayers Rock see Uluru
Ayeyarwady see Irrawaddy
Ayiá see Agiá
Ayia Napa see Agía Nápa
Ayia Phyla see Agía Fýlaxis
Ayiásos/Ayiássos see Agiasós
Áyios Evstrátios see Ágios Efstrátios
Áyios Kírikos see Ágios Kírykos
Áyios Nikólaos see Ágios Nikólaos
Ayios Seryios see Yeniboğaziçi
80 I11 Āykel Amhara, N Ethiopia
123 N9 Aykhal Respublika Sakha (Yakutiya), NE Russian Federation
14 J12 Aylen Lake ◎ Ontario, SE Canada
97 N21 Aylesbury SE England, UK
105 O6 Ayllón Castilla-León, N Spain
14 F17 Aylmer Ontario, S Canada
14 L12 Aylmer Quebec, SE Canada
15 R12 Aylmer, Lac ◎ Quebec, SE Canada
8 L9 Aylmer Lake ◎ Northwest Territories, NW Canada
145 V14 Aynabulak Almaty, SE Kazakhstan
138 K2 'Ayn al 'Arab Ḥalab, N Syria
Aynayn see 'Aynīn
139 V12 'Ayn Ḥamūd S Iraq
147 P12 Ayni prev. Rus. Varzimanor Ayni. W Tajikistan
140 M10 'Aynīn var. Aynayn. spring/well SW Saudi Arabia
21 U12 Aynor South Carolina, SE USA
139 Q7 'Ayn Zāzūh C Iraq
153 N12 Ayodhya Uttar Pradesh, N India
123 S6 Ayon, Ostrov island NE Russian Federation
105 R11 Ayora País Valenciano, E Spain
77 Q11 Ayorou Tillabéri, W Niger
79 E16 Ayos Centre, S Cameroon
76 L5 'Ayoûn 'Abd el Mâlek well N Mauritania
76 K10 'Ayoûn el 'Atroûs var. Aïoun el Atrous, Aïoun el Atroûss. Hodh el Gharbi, SE Mauritania
96 I13 Ayr W Scotland, UK
96 I13 Ayr ≈ W Scotland, UK
96 I13 Ayrshire cultural region SW Scotland, UK
Aysen see Aisén
80 L12 Āysha Somali, E Ethiopia
144 L14 Ayteke Bi Kaz. Zhangaqazaly prev. Novokazalinsk. Kzylorda, SW Kazakhstan
146 K8 Aytim Nawoiy Wiloyati, N Uzbekistan
181 W4 Ayton Queensland, NE Australia
114 M9 Aytos Burgas, E Bulgaria
171 T11 Ayu, Kepulauan island group E Indonesia
A Yun Pa see Cheo Reo
169 V11 Ayu, Tanjung headland Borneo, N Indonesia
40 K13 Ayutla Jalisco, C Mexico
41 P16 Ayutlá var. Ayutla de los Libres. Guerrero, S Mexico
Ayutla de los Libres see Ayutlá
167 O11 Ayutthaya var. Phra Nakhon Si Ayutthaya. Phra Nakhon Si Ayutthaya, C Thailand
136 B13 Ayvalık Balıkesir, W Turkey
99 L20 Aywaille Liège, E Belgium
141 R13 'Aywat aş Şay'ar, Wādī seasonal river N Yemen
Azaffal see Azeffâl
105 T9 Azahar, Costa del coastal region E Spain
105 S6 Azaila Aragón, NE Spain
104 F10 Azambuja Lisboa, C Portugal
153 N13 Āzamgarh Uttar Pradesh, N India
77 O9 Azaouâd desert C Mali
77 S10 Azaouagh, Vallée de l' var. Azaouak. ≈ W Niger
Azaouak see Azaouagh, Vallée de l'
61 F14 Azara Misiones, NE Argentina
142 K3 Āzarān Āžarbāyjān-e Khāvarī, N Iran
Azärbaycan/Azärbaycan Respublikası see Azerbaijan
Āžarbāyjān-e Bākhtarī see Āžarbāyjān-e Gharbī
142 I4 Āžarbāyjān-e Gharbī off. Ostān-e Āžarbāyjān-e Gharbī Eng. West Azerbaijan prev. Āžarbāyjān-e Bākhtarī. ◈ province NW Iran
Āžarbāyjān-e Khāvarī see Āžarbāyjān-e Sharqī
142 J3 Āžarbāyjān-e Sharqī off. Ostān-e Āžarbāyjān-e Sharqī, Eng. East Azerbaijan; prev. Āžarbāyjān-e Sharqī. ◈ province NW Iran
77 W13 Azare Bauchi, N Nigeria
119 M19 Azarychy Rus. Ozarichi. Homyel'skaya Voblasts', SE Belarus
102 L8 Azay-le-Rideau Indre-et-Loire, C France
138 I2 A'zāz Ḥalab, NW Syria
76 H7 Azeffâl var. Azaffal. desert Mauritania/Western Sahara
137 V12 Azerbaijan off. Azerbaijani Republic, Az. Azärbaycan, Azärbaycan Respublikasi; prev. Azerbaijan SSR. ◆ republic SE Asia
145 T7 Azhbulat, Ozero ◎ NE Kazakhstan
74 F7 Azilal C Morocco
Azimabad see Patna
19 O6 Aziscohos Lake ⊟ Maine, NE USA
Azizbekov see Vayk'
Azizie see Telish
Aziziya see Al 'Azīzīyah
129 T4 Aznakayevo Respublika Tatarstan, W Russian Federation
56 C8 Azogues Cañar, S Ecuador
64 N2 Azores var. Açores, Ilhas dos Açores, Port. Arquipélago dos Açores. island group Portugal, NE Atlantic Ocean
64 L8 Azores-Biscay Rise undersea feature E Atlantic Ocean
Azotos/Azotus see Ashdod
78 K11 Azoum, Bahr seasonal river SE Chad
128 L12 Azov Rostovskaya Oblast', SW Russian Federation
128 J13 Azov, Sea of Rus. Azovskoye More, Ukr. Azovs'ke More. sea NE Black Sea
Azovs'ke More/Azovskoye More see Azov, Sea of
138 I10 Azraq, Wāḥat al oasis N Jordan
Āzro see Āzrow
74 G6 Azrou C Morocco
149 R5 Āzrow var. Āzro. Lowgar, E Afghanistan
37 P8 Aztec New Mexico, SW USA
36 M13 Aztec Peak ▲ Arizona, SW USA
45 N9 Azua var. Azua de Compostela. S Dominican Republic
Azua de Compostela see Azua
104 K12 Azuaga Extremadura, W Spain
56 B8 Azuay ◈ province W Ecuador
164 C13 Azuchi-Ō-shima island SW Japan
105 O11 Azuer ≈ C Spain
43 S17 Azuero, Península de peninsula S Panama
62 I6 Azufre, Volcán var. Volcán Lastarria. ▲ N Chile
116 J12 Azuga Prahova, SE Romania
61 C22 Azul Buenos Aires, E Argentina
62 I8 Azul, Cerro ▲ NW Argentina
56 E12 Azul, Cordillera ▲ C Peru
165 P11 Azuma-san ▲ Honshū, C Japan
103 V15 Azur, Côte d' coastal region SE France
191 Z3 Azur Lagoon ◎ Kiritimati, E Kiribati
'Azza see Gaza
Az Zāb al Kabīr see Great Zab
138 H7 Az Zabdānī var. Zabadani. Dimashq, W Syria
141 W8 Az Ẓāhirah desert NW Oman
141 S6 Aẓ Ẓahrān Eng. Dhahran. Ash Sharqīyah, NE Saudi Arabia
141 R6 Aẓ Ẓahrān al Khubar var. Dhahran Al Khobar. ✕ Ash Sharqīyah, NE Saudi Arabia
Az Zaqāzīq see Zagazig
138 H10 Az Zarqā' var. Zarqa. Az Zarqā', NW Jordan
138 I11 Az Zarqā' off. Muḥāfaẓat az Zarqā', var. Zarqa. ◈ governorate N Jordan
75 O7 Az Zāwiyah var. Zawia. NW Libya
141 N15 Az Zaydīyah W Yemen
74 I11 Azzel Matti, Sebkha var. Sebkra Azz el Matti. salt flat C Algeria
141 P6 Az Zilfī Ar Riyāḍ, N Saudi Arabia
139 Y13 Az Zubayr var. Al Zubair. SE Iraq
Az Zuqur see Jabal Zuuqar, Jazīrat

B

187 X15 Ba prev. Mba. Viti Levu, W Fiji
Ba see Đa Rằng
171 P17 Baa Pulau Rote, C Indonesia
138 H7 Baalbek var. Ba'labakk; anc. Heliopolis. E Lebanon
108 G8 Baar Zug, N Switzerland
81 L17 Baardheere var. Bardere, It. Bardera. Gedo, SW Somalia
80 Q12 Baargaal Bari, NE Somalia
99 I15 Baarle-Hertog Antwerpen, N Belgium
99 I15 Baarle-Nassau Noord-Brabant, S Netherlands
98 J11 Baarn Utrecht, C Netherlands
114 D13 Baba var. Buševa, Gk. Varnoús. ▲ FYR Macedonia/Greece
76 H10 Bababé Brakna, W Mauritania
136 G10 Baba Burnu headland NW Turkey
117 N13 Babadag Tulcea, SE Romania
137 X10 Babadağ Dağı ▲ NE Azerbaijan
Babadayhan see Babadaykhan
146 H14 Babadaykhan Turkm. Babadayhan; prev. Kirovsk. Akhalskiy Velayat, C Turkmenistan
146 G14 Babadurmaz Akhalskiy Velayat, C Turkmenistan
114 M12 Babaeski Kırklareli, NW Turkey
139 T4 Bāba Gurgur N Iraq
56 B7 Babahoyo prev. Bodegas. Los Ríos, C Ecuador
149 P5 Bābā, Kūh-e ▲ C Afghanistan
171 N12 Babana Sulawesi, C Indonesia
171 Q12 Babar, Kepulauan island group E Indonesia
171 T12 Babar, Pulau island Kepulauan Babar, E Indonesia
152 G4 Bābāsar Pass pass India/Pakistan
146 C9 Babashy ▲ W Turkmenistan
168 M13 Babat Sumatera, W Indonesia
Babatag, Khrebet see Bobotogh, Qatorkŭhi
81 H21 Babati Arusha, NE Tanzania
126 J13 Babayevo Vologodskaya Oblast', NW Russian Federation
129 Q15 Babayurt Respublika Dagestan, SW Russian Federation
33 P6 Babb Montana, NW USA
29 X4 Babbitt Minnesota, N USA
188 E9 Babeldaob var. Babeldaop, Babelthuap. island N Palau
Babeldaop see Babeldaob
141 N17 Bab el Mandeb strait Gulf of Aden/Red Sea
Babelthuap see Babeldaob
111 K17 Babia Góra var. Babia Hora. ▲ Slovakia/Poland
Babia Hora see Babia Góra
Babian Jiang see Black River
Babichi see Babichy
119 N19 Babichy Rus. Babichi. Homyel'skaya Voblasts', SE Belarus
112 I10 Babina Greda Vukovar-Srijem, E Croatia
10 K13 Babine Lake ◎ British Columbia, SW Canada
143 O4 Bābol var. Babul, Balfrush, Barfrush; prev. Barfurush. Māzandarān, N Iran
143 O4 Bābolsar var. Babulsar; prev. Meshed-i-Sar. Māzandarān, N Iran
36 L16 Baboquivari Peak ▲ Arizona, SW USA
79 G15 Baboua Nana-Mambéré, W Central African Republic
119 M17 Babruysk Rus. Bobruysk. Mahilyowskaya Voblasts', E Belarus
Babu see Hexian
Babul see Bābol
Babulsar see Bābolsar
113 O19 Babuna ≈ C FYR Macedonia
113 O19 Babuna ▲ C FYR Macedonia
148 K7 Bābūs, Dasht-e Pash. Bebas, Dasht-i. ▲ W Afghanistan
171 O1 Babuyan Channel channel N Philippines
171 O1 Babuyan Island island N Philippines
139 T9 Babylon site of ancient city C Iraq
112 J9 Bač Ger. Batsch. Serbia, NW Yugoslavia
58 M13 Bacabal Maranhão, E Brazil
41 Y14 Bacalar Quintana Roo, SE Mexico
41 Y14 Bacalar Chico, Boca strait SE Mexico
171 Q12 Bacan, Kepulauan island group E Indonesia
171 S12 Bacan, Pulau prev. Batjan. island Maluku, E Indonesia
116 L10 Bacău Hung. Bákó. Bacău, NE Romania
116 K11 Bacău ◈ county E Romania
Bắc Bộ, Vịnh see Tongking, Gulf of
167 T5 Bắc Can Bắc Thai, N Vietnam
103 T5 Baccarat Meurthe-et-Moselle, NE France
183 N12 Bacchus Marsh Victoria, SE Australia
40 H4 Bacerac Sonora, NW Mexico
116 L10 Băceşti Vaslui, E Romania
167 T6 Bắc Giang Ha Bắc, N Vietnam
54 I5 Bachaquero Zulia, NW Venezuela
Bacher see Pohorje
118 M13 Bacheykava Rus. Bocheykovo. Vitsyebskaya Voblasts', N Belarus
40 I5 Bachíniva Chihuahua, N Mexico
158 G8 Bachu Xinjiang Uygur Zizhiqu, NW China
9 N8 Back ≈ Nunavut, N Canada
112 K10 Bačka Palanka prev. Palanka. Serbia, NW Yugoslavia
112 K8 Bačka Topola Hung. Topolya; prev. Hung. Bácstopolya. Serbia, N Yugoslavia
95 J17 Bäckefors Västra Götaland, S Sweden
Bäckermühle Schulzenmühle see Żywiec
95 L16 Bäckhammar Värmland, C Sweden
112 K9 Bački Petrovac Hung. Petrőcz; prev. Petrovac, Petrovácz. Serbia, NW Yugoslavia
101 I21 Backnang Baden-Württemberg, SW Germany
167 S15 Bac Liêu var. Vinh Loi. Minh Hai, S Vietnam
167 T6 Bắc Ninh Ha Bắc, N Vietnam
40 G4 Bacoachi Sonora, NW Mexico
171 P6 Bacolod off. Bacolod City. Negros, C Philippines
171 O4 Baco, Mount ▲ Mindoro, N Philippines
111 K25 Bácsalmás Bács-Kiskun, S Hungary
Bácsjózseffalva see Žednik
111 J24 Bács-Kiskun off. Bács-Kiskun Megye. ◈ county S Hungary
Bácsszenttamás see Srbobran
Bácstopolya see Bačka Topola
Bactra see Balkh
155 F21 Badagara Kerala, SW India
101 M24 Bad Aibling Bayern, SE Germany
162 I13 Badain Jaran Shamo desert N China
104 I11 Badajoz anc. Pax Augusta. Extremadura, W Spain
104 J11 Badajoz ◈ province Extremadura, W Spain
149 S2 Badakhshān ◈ province NE Afghanistan
105 W6 Badalona anc. Baetulo. Cataluña, E Spain
154 O11 Bādāmapāhārh Orissa, E India
152 K8 Badarīnāth ▲ N India
169 O10 Badas, Kepulauan island group W Indonesia
109 S6 Bad Aussee Salzburg, E Austria
31 S8 Bad Axe Michigan, N USA
101 G16 Bad Berleburg Nordrhein-Westfalen, W Germany
101 L17 Bad Blankenburg Thüringen, C Germany
Bad Borseck see Borsec
101 G18 Bad Camberg Hessen, W Germany
100 L8 Bad Doberan Mecklenburg-Vorpommern, N Germany
101 N14 Bad Düben Sachsen, E Germany
109 X4 Baden var. Baden bei Wien; anc. Aquae Panoniae, Thermae Pannonicae. Niederösterreich, NE Austria
108 F9 Baden Aargau, N Switzerland
101 G21 Baden-Baden anc. Aurelia Aquensis. Baden-Württemberg, SW Germany
Baden bei Wien see Baden
101 G22 Baden-Württemberg Fr. Bade-Wurtemberg. ◈ state SW Germany
112 A10 Baderna Istra, NW Croatia
Bade-Wurtemberg see Baden-Württemberg
101 H20 Bad Fredrichshall Baden-Württemberg, S Germany
100 P11 Bad Freienwalde Brandenburg, NE Germany
109 Q8 Badgastein var. Gastein. Salzburg, NW Austria
Badger State see Wisconsin
148 L4 Bādghīs ◈ province NW Afghanistan
109 T5 Bad Hall Oberösterreich, N Austria
101 J14 Bad Harzburg Niedersachsen, C Germany
101 I16 Bad Hersfeld Hessen, C Germany
98 I10 Badhoevedorp Noord-Holland, C Netherlands
109 Q8 Bad Hofgastein Salzburg, NW Austria
Bad Homburg see Bad Homburg vor der Höhe
101 G18 Bad Homburg vor der Höhe var. Bad Homburg. Hessen, W Germany
101 E17 Bad Honnef Nordrhein-Westfalen, W Germany
149 Q17 Badīn Sind, SE Pakistan
21 S10 Badin Lake ◎ North Carolina, SE USA
40 I8 Badiraguato Sinaloa, C Mexico
109 R6 Bad Ischl Oberösterreich, N Austria
Badjawa see Bajawa
101 J18 Bad Kissingen Bayern, SE Germany
Bad Königswart see Lázně Kynžvart
101 F19 Bad Kreuznach Rheinland-Pfalz, SW Germany
101 F24 Bad Krozingen Baden-Württemberg, SW Germany
101 G16 Bad Laasphe Nordrhein-Westfalen, W Germany
28 J6 Badlands physical region North Dakota, N USA
101 K16 Bad Langensalza Thüringen, C Germany
109 T3 Bad Leonfelden Oberösterreich, N Austria
101 I20 Bad Mergentheim Baden-Württemberg, SW Germany
101 H17 Bad Nauheim Hessen, W Germany
101 E17 Bad Neuenahr-Arhweiler Rheinland-Pfalz, W Germany
Bad Neustadt see Bad Neustadt an der Saale
101 J18 Bad Neustadt an der Saale var. Bad Neustadt. Berlin, C Germany
Badnur see Betūl
100 H13 Bad Oeynhausen Nordrhein-Westfalen, NW Germany
100 J9 Bad Oldesloe Schleswig-Holstein, N Germany
77 Q16 Badou C Togo
Bad Polzin see Połczyn-Zdrój
100 H13 Bad Pyrmont Niedersachsen, C Germany
109 X9 Bad Radkersburg Steiermark, SE Austria
139 V8 Badrah E Iraq
162 J6 Badrah Hövsgöl, N Mongolia
101 N24 Bad Reichenhall Bayern, SE Germany
140 K8 Badr Ḥunayn Al Madīnah, W Saudi Arabia
28 M10 Bad River ≈ South Dakota, N USA
30 K4 Bad River ≈ Wisconsin, N USA
100 H13 Bad Salzuflen Nordrhein-Westfalen, NW Germany
101 J16 Bad Salzungen Thüringen, C Germany
109 V8 Bad Sankt Leonhard im Lavanttal Kärnten, S Austria
100 K9 Bad Schwartau Schleswig-Holstein, N Germany
101 L24 Bad Tölz Bayern, SE Germany
181 U1 Badu Island island Queensland, NE Australia
155 K25 Badulla Uva Province, C Sri Lanka
109 X5 Bad Vöslau Niederösterreich, NE Austria
101 I24 Bad Waldsee Baden-Württemberg, S Germany
35 U11 Badwater Basin depression California, W USA
101 J20 Bad Windsheim Bayern, C Germany
101 J23 Bad Wörishofen Bayern, S Germany
100 G10 Bad Zwischenahn Niedersachsen, NW Germany
104 M13 Baena Andalucía, S Spain
Baeterrae/Baeterrae Septimanorum see Béziers
Baetic Cordillera/Baetic Mountains see Béticos, Sistemas
Baetulo see Badalona
57 K18 Baeza Napo, NE Ecuador
105 N13 Baeza Andalucía, S Spain
79 D15 Bafang Ouest, W Cameroon
76 H12 Bafatá C Guinea-Bissau
149 U5 Baffa North-West Frontier Province, NW Pakistan
197 O11 Baffin Basin undersea feature N Labrador Sea
197 N12 Baffin Bay bay Canada/Greenland
25 T15 Baffin Bay inlet Texas, SW USA
196 M12 Baffin Island island Nunavut, NE Canada
79 E15 Bafia Centre, C Cameroon
77 R14 Bafilo NE Togo
76 J12 Bafing ≈ W Africa
76 J12 Bafoulabé Kayes, W Mali
79 D15 Bafoussam Ouest, W Cameroon
143 R9 Bāfq Yazd, C Iran
136 L10 Bafra Samsun, N Turkey
136 L10 Bafra Burnu headland N Turkey
143 S12 Bāft Kermān, S Iran
79 N18 Bafwabalinga Orientale, NE Dem. Rep. Congo (Zaire)
79 N18 Bafwaboli Orientale, NE Dem. Rep. Congo (Zaire)
79 N17 Bafwasende Orientale, NE Dem. Rep. Congo (Zaire)
42 K13 Bagaces Guanacaste, NW Costa Rica
153 O12 Bagaha Bihār, N India
155 F16 Bāgalkot Karnātaka, W India
81 J22 Bagamoyo Pwani, E Tanzania
168 J8 Bagan Datuk var. Bagan Datok. Perak, Peninsular Malaysia
171 R7 Baganga Mindanao, S Philippines
168 J9 Bagansiapiapi var. Pasirpangarayan. Sumatera, W Indonesia
Bagaria see Bagheria
77 T11 Bagaroua Tahoua, W Niger
79 I20 Bagata Bandundu, W Dem. Rep. Congo (Zaire)
Bagdad see Baghdād
123 O13 Bagdarin Respublika Buryatiya, S Russian Federation
61 G17 Bagé Rio Grande do Sul, S Brazil
Bagenalstown see Muine Bheag
Bagerhat see Bagherhat
103 P16 Bages et de Sigean, Étang de ◎ S France
33 W17 Baggs Wyoming, C USA
154 F11 Bāgh Madhya Pradesh, C India
139 T8 Baghdād var. Bagdad, Eng. Baghdad. ● (Iraq) C Iraq
139 T8 Baghdād ✕ C Iraq
153 T16 Bagherhat var. Bagerhat. Khulna, S Bangladesh
107 J23 Bagheria var. Bagaria. Sicilia, Italy, C Mediterranean Sea
143 S10 Bāghīn Kermān, C Iran
149 Q3 Baghlān Baghlān, NE Afghanistan
149 Q3 Baghlān var. Bāghlān. ◈ province NE Afghanistan
148 M7 Bāghrān Helmand, S Afghanistan
29 T4 Bagley Minnesota, N USA
106 H10 Bagnacavallo Emilia-Romagna, C Italy
102 K16 Bagnères-de-Bigorre Hautes-Pyrénées, S France
102 L17 Bagnères-de-Luchon Hautes-Pyrénées, S France
106 F11 Bagni di Lucca Toscana, C Italy
106 H11 Bagno di Romagna Emilia-Romagna, C Italy
103 R14 Bagnols-sur-Cèze Gard, S France
162 M14 Bag Nur ◎ N China
171 P6 Bago off. Bago City. Negros, C Philippines
Bago see Pegu
76 M13 Bagoé ≈ Ivory Coast/Mali
Bagrāmē see Bagrāmī
149 R5 Bagrāmī var. Bagrāmē. Kābul, E Afghanistan
119 B14 Bagrationovsk Ger. Preussisch Eylau. Kaliningradskaya Oblast', W Russian Federation
Bagrax see Bohu
Bagrax Hu see Bosten Hu
56 C10 Bagua Amazonas, NE Peru
171 O2 Baguio off. Baguio City. Luzon, N Philippines
77 V9 Bagzane, Monts ▲ N Niger
Bāḥah, Minṭaqat al see Al Bāḥah
Bahama Islands see Bahamas
44 H3 Bahamas off. Commonwealth of the Bahamas. ◆ commonwealth republic N West Indies
(0) L13 Bahamas var. Bahama Islands. island group N West Indies
153 S15 Baharampur prev. Berhampore. West Bengal, NE India
149 U10 Bahāwalnagar Punjab, E Pakistan
149 T11 Bahāwalpur Punjab, E Pakistan
136 L16 Bahçe Osmaniye, S Turkey

◆ Country ● Country Capital ◇ Dependent Territory ○ Dependent Territory Capital ◈ Administrative Region ✕ International Airport ▲ Mountain ▲ Mountain Range ✕ Volcano ≈ River ◎ Lake ⊟ Reservoir

160 J8 **Ba He** ≈ C China
Bäherden see Bakharden
59 N16 **Bahia** off. Estado da Bahia. ◈ state E Brazil
61 B24 **Bahía Blanca** Buenos Aires, E Argentina
40 L15 **Bahía Bufadero** Michoacán de Ocampo, SW Mexico
63 J19 **Bahía Bustamante** Chubut, SE Argentina
40 D5 **Bahía de los Ángeles** Baja California, NW Mexico
40 C6 **Bahía de Tortugas** Baja California Sur, W Mexico
42 J4 **Bahía, Islas de la** Eng. Bay Islands. island group N Honduras
40 E5 **Bahía Kino** Sonora, NW Mexico
40 E9 **Bahía Magdalena** var. Puerto Magdalena. Baja California Sur, W Mexico
54 C8 **Bahía Solano** var. Ciudad Mutis, Solano. Chocó, W Colombia
80 I11 **Bahir Dar** var. Bahr Dar, Bahrdar Giyorgis. Amhara, N Ethiopia
141 X8 **Bahlā'** var. Bahlah, Bahlat. NW Oman
Bāhla see Bālān
Bahlah/Bahlat see Bahlā'
152 M11 **Bahraich** Uttar Pradesh, N India
143 M14 **Bahrain** off. State of Bahrain, Dawlat al Bahrayn, Ar. Al Baḩrayn; prev. Bahrein, anc. Tylos or Tyros. ◆ monarchy SW Asia
142 M14 **Bahrain** ✕ C Bahrain
142 M15 **Bahrain, Gulf of** gulf Persian Gulf, NW Arabian Sea
138 I7 **Baḩrat Mallāḩah** ◎ W Syria
Bahrayn, Dawlat al see Bahrain
Bahr Dar/Bahrdar Giyorgis see Bahir Dar
Bahrein see Bahrain
81 E16 **Bahr el Gabel** ◈ state S Sudan
80 E13 **Bahr ez Zaref** ≈ C Sudan
67 R8 **Bahr Kameur** ≈ N Central African Republic
Bahr Tabariya, Sea of see Tiberias, Lake
143 W15 **Bāhū Kalāt** Sīstān va Balūchestān, SE Iran
118 N13 **Bahushewsk** Rus. Bogushëvsk. Vitsyebskaya Voblasts', NE Belarus
Bai see Tagow Bāy
116 G13 **Baia de Aramă** Mehedinți, SW Romania
116 G11 **Baia de Criş** Ger. Altenburg, Hung. Körösbánya. Hunedoara, SW Romania
83 A16 **Baia dos Tigres** Namibe, SW Angola
82 A13 **Baia Farta** Benguela, W Angola
116 H9 **Baia Mare** Ger. Frauenbach, Hung. Nagybánya; prev. Neustadt. Maramureş, NW Romania
116 H8 **Baia Sprie** Ger. Mittelstadt, Hung. Felsőbánya. Maramureş, NW Romania
78 G13 **Baïbokoum** Logone-Oriental, SW Chad
160 F12 **Baicao Ling** ▲▲ SW China
163 U9 **Baicheng** var. Pai-ch'eng; prev. T'aon-an. Jilin, NE China
158 I6 **Baicheng** var. Bay. Xinjiang Uygur Zizhiqu, NW China
116 J13 **Băicoi** Prahova, SE Romania
Baidoa see Baydhabo
15 U6 **Baie-Comeau** Quebec, SE Canada
15 T7 **Baie-des-Bacon** Quebec, SE Canada
15 S8 **Baie-des-Rochers** Quebec, SE Canada
15 U6 **Baie-des-Sables** Quebec, SE Canada
12 K11 **Baie-du-Poste** Quebec, SE Canada
172 H17 **Baie Lazare** Mahé, NE Seychelles
45 Y5 **Baie-Mahault** Basse Terre, C Guadeloupe
15 R9 **Baie-St-Paul** Quebec, SE Canada
15 V5 **Baie-Trinité** Quebec, SE Canada
13 T11 **Baie Verte** Newfoundland, SE Canada
163 X11 **Baihe** prev. Erdaobaihe. Jilin, NE China
Baiguan see Shangyu
139 U11 **Bā'ij al Mahdī** S Iraq
Baiji see Bayjī
Baikal, Lake see Baykal, Ozero
Bailādila see Kirandul
Baile an Chaistil see Ballycastle
Baile an Róba see Ballinrobe
Baile an tSratha see Ballintra
Baile Átha an Rí see Athenry
Baile Átha Buí see Athboy
Baile Átha Cliath see Dublin
Baile Átha Fhirdhia see Ardee
Baile Átha Í see Athy
Baile Átha Luain see Athlone
Baile Átha Troim see Trim
Baile Brigín see Balbriggan
Baile Easa Dara see Ballysadare
116 I13 **Băile Govora** Vâlcea, SW Romania
116 F13 **Băile Herculane** Ger. Herkulesbad, Hung. Herkulesfürdő. Caraş-Severin, SW Romania
Baile Locha Riach see Loughrea
Baile Mhistéala see Mitchelstown
Baile Monaidh see Ballymoney
105 N12 **Bailén** Andalucía, S Spain
Baile na hInse see Ballynahinch
Baile na Lorgan see Castleblayney
Baile na Mainistreach see Newtownabbey
Baile Nua na hArda see Newtownards
116 I12 **Băile Olăneşti** Vâlcea, SW Romania
116 H14 **Băileşti** Dolj, SW Romania
Bailingmiao see Darhan Muminggan Lianheqi
58 K11 **Bailique, Ilha** island NE Brazil
103 O1 **Bailleul** Nord, N France
78 H12 **Ba Illi** Chari-Baguirmi, SW Chad
159 V12 **Bailong Jiang** ≈ C China
82 C13 **Bailundo** Port. Vila Teixeira da Silva. Huambo, C Angola
159 T13 **Baima** var. Sêraitang. Qinghai, C China
186 C8 **Baimuru** Gulf, S PNG
158 M16 **Bainang** Xizang Zizhiqu, W China
23 S8 **Bainbridge** Georgia, SE USA
171 O17 **Baing** Pulau Sumba, SE Indonesia
158 M14 **Baingoin** Xizang Zizhiqu, W China
104 G2 **Baio Grande** Galicia, NW Spain
104 G4 **Baiona** Galicia, NW Spain
163 V7 **Baiquan** Heilongjiang, NE China
Bā'ir see Bāyir
158 I11 **Bairab Co** ◎ W China
25 Q7 **Baird** Texas, SW USA
39 N7 **Baird Mountains** ▲▲ Alaska, USA
Baireuth see Bayreuth
190 H3 **Bairiki** ● (Kiribati) Tarawa, NW Kiribati
163 S11 **Bairin Youqi** var. Daban. Nei Mongol Zizhiqu, N China
163 S10 **Bairin Zuoqi** var. Lindong. Nei Mongol Zizhiqu, N China
145 P17 **Bairkum** Kaz. Bayyrqum. Yuzhnyy Kazakhstan, S Kazakhstan
183 P12 **Bairnsdale** Victoria, SE Australia
171 P6 **Bais** Negros, S Philippines
102 L15 **Baïse** var. Baise. ≈ S France
163 W11 **Baishan** prev. Hunjiang. Jilin, NE China
118 F12 **Baisogala** Radviliškis, C Lithuania
189 Q7 **Baiti** N Nauru
104 G13 **Baixo Alentejo** physical region S Portugal
64 P5 **Baixo, Ilhéu de** island Madeira, Portugal, NE Atlantic Ocean
83 E15 **Baixo Longa** Cuando Cubango, SE Angola
159 V10 **Baiyin** Gansu, C China
160 E8 **Baiyü** Sichuan, C China
161 N14 **Baiyun** ✕ (Guangzhou) Guangdong, S China
160 K4 **Baiyu Shan** ▲▲ C China
111 J25 **Baja** Bács-Kiskun, S Hungary
40 C4 **Baja California** ◈ state NW Mexico
40 C4 **Baja California** Eng. Lower California. peninsula NW Mexico
40 E9 **Baja California Sur** ◈ state W Mexico
Bājah see Béja
Bajan see Bayan
191 V16 **Baja, Punta** headland Easter Island, Chile, E Pacific Ocean
40 B4 **Baja, Punta** headland NW Mexico
55 R5 **Baja, Punta** headland NE Venezuela
42 D5 **Baja Verapaz** off. Departamento de Baja Verapaz. ◈ department C Guatemala
171 N16 **Bajawa** prev. Badjawa. Flores, S Indonesia
153 S16 **Baj Baj** prev. Budge-Budge. West Bengal, E India
141 N15 **Bājil** W Yemen
183 U4 **Bajimba, Mount** ▲ New South Wales, SE Australia
112 K13 **Bajina Bašta** Serbia, W Yugoslavia
153 U14 **Bajitpur** Dhaka, E Bangladesh
112 K8 **Bajmok** Serbia, NW Yugoslavia
Bajo Boquete see Boquete
113 L17 **Bajram Curri** Kukës, N Albania
79 J14 **Bakala** Ouaka, C Central African Republic
129 T4 **Bakaly** Respublika Bashkortostan, W Russian Federation
Bakan see Shimonoseki
145 U14 **Bakanas** Kaz. Baqanas. Almaty, SE Kazakhstan
145 V12 **Bakanas** Kaz. Baqanas. ≈ E Kazakhstan
145 U14 **Bakbakty** Kaz. Baqbaqty. Almaty, SE Kazakhstan
122 J12 **Bakchar** Tomskaya Oblast', C Russian Federation
76 I11 **Bakel** E Senegal
35 W13 **Baker** California, W USA
22 J8 **Baker** Louisiana, S USA
33 Y9 **Baker** Montana, NW USA
32 L12 **Baker** Oregon, NW USA
192 L7 **Baker and Howland Islands** ◇ US unincorporated territory W Polynesia
36 L12 **Baker Butte** ▲ Arizona, SW USA
39 X15 **Baker Island** island Alexander Archipelago, Alaska, USA
9 N9 **Baker Lake** Nunavut, N Canada
9 N9 **Baker Lake** ◎ Nunavut, N Canada
32 H6 **Baker, Mount** ▲ Washington, NW USA
35 R13 **Bakersfield** California, W USA
24 M9 **Bakersfield** Texas, SW USA
21 P9 **Bakersville** North Carolina, SE USA
Bakhābī see Bū Khābī
146 E12 **Bakharden** Turkm. Bäherden; prev. Bakherden. Akhalskiy Velayat, C Turkmenistan
146 F12 **Bakhardok** Turkm. Bokurdak. Akhalskiy Velayat, C Turkmenistan
143 U5 **Bākharz, Kuhhā-ye** ▲▲ NE Iran
152 D13 **Bākhāsar** Rājasthān, NW India
Bakhchisaray see Bakhchysaray
117 T13 **Bakhchysaray** Rus. Bakhchisaray. Respublika Krym, S Ukraine
Bakherden see Bakharden
117 R3 **Bakhmach** Chernihivs'ka Oblast', N Ukraine
142 K6 **Bākhtarān** prev. Kermānshāh, Qahremānshahr. Kermānshāh, W Iran
Bākhtarān see Kermānshāh
143 Q11 **Bakhtegān, Daryācheh-ye** ◎ C Iran
145 X12 **Bakhty** Vostochnyy Kazakhstan, E Kazakhstan
137 Z11 **Bakı** Eng. Baku. ● (Azerbaijan) E Azerbaijan
137 Z11 **Bakı** ✕ E Azerbaijan
136 C13 **Bakır Çayı** ≈ W Turkey
92 L1 **Bakkafjördhur** Austurland, NE Iceland
92 L1 **Bakkaflói** sea area W Norwegian Sea
81 I15 **Bako** Southern, S Ethiopia
76 L15 **Bako** NW Ivory Coast
Bákó see Bacău
111 H23 **Bakony** Eng. Bakony Mountains, Ger. Bakonywald. ▲▲ W Hungary
Bakony Mountains/Bakonywald see Bakony
81 M16 **Bakool** off. Gobolka Bakool. ◈ region W Somalia
79 L15 **Bakouma** Mbomou, SE Central African Republic
129 N15 **Baksan** Kabardino-Balkarskaya Respublika, SW Russian Federation
119 I16 **Bakshty** Hrodzyenskaya Voblasts', W Belarus
Baku see Bakı
194 K12 **Bakutis Coast** physical region Antarctica
Bakwanga see Mbuji-Mayi
145 O15 **Bakyrly** Yuzhnyy Kazakhstan, S Kazakhstan
14 H13 **Bala** Ontario, S Canada
97 J19 **Bala** NW Wales, UK
136 I13 **Balā** Ankara, C Turkey
170 L7 **Balabac Island** island W Philippines
Balabac, Selat see Balabac Strait
169 V5 **Balabac Strait** var. Selat Balabac. strait Malaysia/Philippines
Ba'labakk see Baalbek
187 P16 **Balabio, Île** island Province Nord, W New Caledonia
116 I14 **Balaci** Teleorman, S Romania
139 S7 **Balad** N Iraq
139 U7 **Balad Rūz** E Iraq
154 J11 **Bālāghāt** Madhya Pradesh, C India
155 F14 **Bālāghāt Range** ▲▲ W India
103 X14 **Balagne** physical region Corse, France, C Mediterranean Sea
105 U5 **Balaguer** Cataluña, NE Spain
105 S3 **Balaïtous** var. Pic de Balaïtous, Pic de Balaïtous. ▲ France/Spain
Balaïtous, Pic de see Balaïtous
129 O3 **Balakhna** Nizhegorodskaya Oblast', W Russian Federation
122 L12 **Balakhta** Krasnoyarskiy Kray, S Russian Federation
182 I9 **Balaklava** South Australia
Balakleya see Balakliya
117 V6 **Balakliya** Rus. Balakleya. Kharkivs'ka Oblast', E Ukraine
129 Q7 **Balakovo** Saratovskaya Oblast', W Russian Federation
83 P14 **Balama** Cabo Delgado, N Mozambique
169 U6 **Balambangan, Pulau** island East Malaysia
148 L3 **Bālā Morghāb** Laghmān, NW Afghanistan
152 E11 **Bālān** prev. Bāhla. Rājasthān, NW India
116 J10 **Bălan** Hung. Balánbánya. Harghita, C Romania
Balánbánya see Bălan
171 O3 **Balanga** Luzon, N Philippines
154 M12 **Balāngīr** prev. Bolangir. Orissa, E India
129 N8 **Balashov** Saratovskaya Oblast', W Russian Federation
Balasore see Bāleshwar
111 K21 **Balassagyarmat** Nógrád, N Hungary
29 S10 **Balaton** Minnesota, N USA
111 H24 **Balaton** var. Lake Balaton, Ger. Plattensee. ◎ W Hungary
111 I23 **Balatonfüred** var. Füred. Veszprém, W Hungary
Balaton, Lake see Balaton
116 I11 **Bălăuşeri** Ger. Bladenmarkt, Hung. Balavásár. Mureş, C Romania
Balavásár see Bălăuşeri
105 Q11 **Balazote** Castilla-La Mancha, C Spain
Balázsfalva see Blaj
119 F14 **Balbieriškis** Prienai, S Lithuania
186 J7 **Balbi, Mount** ▲ Bougainville Island, NE PNG
58 F11 **Balbina, Represa** ⊞ NW Brazil
43 T15 **Balboa** Panamá, C Panama
97 G17 **Balbriggan** Ir. Baile Brigín. E Ireland
Balbunar see Kubrat
81 N17 **Balcad** Shabeellaha Dhexe, C Somalia
61 D23 **Balcarce** Buenos Aires, E Argentina
11 U16 **Balcarres** Saskatchewan, S Canada
114 O8 **Balchik** Dobrich, NE Bulgaria
185 E24 **Balclutha** Otago, South Island, NZ
25 Q12 **Balcones Escarpment** escarpment Texas, SW USA
18 F14 **Bald Eagle Creek** ≈ Pennsylvania, NE USA
Baldenburg see Biały Bór
21 V12 **Bald Head Island** island North Carolina, SE USA
27 W10 **Bald Knob** Arkansas, C USA
30 K17 **Bald Knob** hill Illinois, N USA
Baldohn see Baldone
118 G9 **Baldone** Ger. Baldohn. Rīga, W Latvia
22 I9 **Baldwin** Louisiana, S USA
31 P7 **Baldwin** Michigan, N USA
27 Q4 **Baldwin City** Kansas, C USA
39 N8 **Baldwin Peninsula** headland Alaska, USA
18 H9 **Baldwinsville** New York, NE USA
23 N2 **Baldwyn** Mississippi, S USA
11 W15 **Baldy Mountain** ▲ Manitoba, S Canada
33 T7 **Baldy Mountain** ▲ Montana, NW USA
37 O13 **Baldy Peak** ▲ Arizona, SW USA
Bâle see Basel
105 X9 **Baleares** ◈ autonomous community E Spain
105 X11 **Baleares, Islas** Eng. Balearic Islands. island group Spain, W Mediterranean Sea
Baleares Major see Mallorca
Balearic Islands see Baleares, Islas
Balearic Plain see Algerian Basin
Balearis Minor see Menorca
169 S9 **Baleh, Batang** ≈ East Malaysia
12 J8 **Baleine, Grande Rivière de la** ≈ Quebec, E Canada
12 K7 **Baleine, Petite Rivière de la** ≈ Quebec, SE Canada
13 N6 **Baleine, Rivière à la** ≈ Quebec, E Canada
99 J16 **Balen** Antwerpen, N Belgium
171 O3 **Baler** Luzon, N Philippines
154 P11 **Bāleshwar** prev. Balasore. Orissa, E India
77 S12 **Baléyara** Tillabéri, W Niger
129 T1 **Balezino** Udmurtskaya Respublika, NW Russian Federation
42 J4 **Balfate** Colón, N Honduras
11 O17 **Balfour** British Columbia, SW Canada
29 N3 **Balfour** North Dakota, N USA
Balfrush see Bābol
122 L14 **Balgazyn** Respublika Tyva, S Russian Federation
11 U16 **Balgonie** Saskatchewan, S Canada
Bălgrad see Alba Iulia
81 J19 **Balguda** spring/well S Kenya
158 K6 **Balguntay** Xinjiang Uygur Zizhiqu, NW China
141 R16 **Balḩāf** S Yemen
152 F13 **Bāli** Rājasthān, N India
169 U17 **Bali** ◈ province S Indonesia
169 T17 **Bali** island C Indonesia
111 K16 **Balice** ✕ (Kraków) Małopolskie, S Poland
171 Y14 **Baliem, Sungai** ≈ Irian Jaya, E Indonesia
136 C12 **Balıkesir** Balıkesir, W Turkey
136 C12 **Balıkesir** ◈ province NW Turkey
138 L3 **Balīkh, Nahr** ≈ N Syria
169 V12 **Balikpapan** Borneo, C Indonesia
Bali, Laut see Bali Sea
171 N9 **Balimbing** Tawitawi, SW Philippines
186 B8 **Balimo** Western, SW PNG
Bálinc see Balinţ
101 H23 **Balingen** Baden-Württemberg, SW Germany
116 F11 **Balinţ** Hung. Bálinc. Timiş, W Romania
171 O1 **Balintang Channel** channel N Philippines
138 K3 **Bālis** Ḩalab, N Syria
169 T16 **Bali Sea** Ind. Laut Bali. sea C Indonesia
98 K7 **Balk** Friesland, N Netherlands
121 R6 **Balkan Mountains** Bul./SCr. Stara Planina. ▲▲ Bulgaria/Yugoslavia
146 B9 **Balkanskiy Velayat** Turkm. Balkan Welaýaty. ◈ province W Turkmenistan
Balkan Welaýaty see Balkanskiy Velayat
145 P8 **Balkashino** Akmola, N Kazakhstan
149 O2 **Balkh** anc. Bactra. Balkh, N Afghanistan
149 P2 **Balkh** ◈ province N Afghanistan
145 T13 **Balkhash** Kaz. Balqash. Zhezkazgan, SE Kazakhstan
Balkhash, Lake see Balkhash, Ozero
145 T13 **Balkhash, Ozero** Eng. Lake Balkhash, Kaz. Balqash. ◎ SE Kazakhstan
Balla Balla see Mbalabala
96 H10 **Ballachulish** N Scotland, UK
180 M12 **Balladonia** Western Australia
97 C16 **Ballaghaderreen** Ir. Bealach an Doirín. C Ireland
92 H10 **Ballangen** Nordland, NW Norway
97 H14 **Ballantrae** W Scotland, UK
183 N12 **Ballarat** Victoria, SE Australia
180 K11 **Ballard, Lake** salt lake Western Australia
Ballari see Bellary
76 L11 **Ballé** Koulikoro, W Mali
40 D7 **Ballenas, Bahía de** bay W Mexico
40 D5 **Ballenas, Canal de** channel NW Mexico
195 R17 **Balleny Islands** island group Antarctica
40 J7 **Balleza** var. San Pablo Balleza. Chihuahua, N Mexico
114 M13 **Ballı** Tekirdağ, NW Turkey
153 O13 **Ballia** Uttar Pradesh, N India
183 V4 **Ballina** New South Wales, SE Australia
97 C16 **Ballina** Ir. Béal an Átha. W Ireland
97 D16 **Ballinamore** Ir. Béal an Átha Móir. NW Ireland
97 D18 **Ballinasloe** Ir. Béal Átha na Sluaighe. W Ireland
25 P8 **Ballinger** Texas, SW USA
97 C17 **Ballinrobe** Ir. Baile an Róba. W Ireland
97 A21 **Ballinskelligs Bay** Ir. Bá na Scealg. inlet SW Ireland
97 D15 **Ballintra** Ir. Baile an tSratha. NW Ireland
103 T7 **Ballon d'Alsace** ▲ NE France
Ballon de Guebwiller see Grand Ballon
113 K21 **Ballsh** var. Ballshi. Fier, SW Albania
Ballshi see Ballsh
98 K4 **Ballum** Friesland, N Netherlands
97 F16 **Ballybay** Ir. Béal Átha Beithe. N Ireland
97 E14 **Ballybofey** Ir. Bealach Féich. NW Ireland
97 G14 **Ballycastle** Ir. Baile an Chaistil. N Northern Ireland, UK
97 G15 **Ballyclare** Ir. Bealach Cláir. E Northern Ireland, UK
97 E16 **Ballyconnell** Ir. Béal Átha Conaill. N Ireland
97 C17 **Ballyhaunis** Ir. Béal Átha hAmhnais. W Ireland
97 G14 **Ballymena** Ir. An Baile Meánach. NE Northern Ireland, UK
97 F14 **Ballymoney** Ir. Baile Monaidh. NE Northern Ireland, UK
97 G15 **Ballynahinch** Ir. Baile na hInse. SE Northern Ireland, UK
97 D16 **Ballysadare** Ir. Baile Easa Dara. NW Ireland
97 D15 **Ballyshannon** Ir. Béal Átha Seanaidh. NW Ireland
63 H19 **Balmaceda** Aisén, S Chile
63 G23 **Balmaceda, Cerro** ▲ S Chile
111 N22 **Balmazújváros** Hajdú-Bihar, E Hungary
108 E10 **Balmhorn** ▲ SW Switzerland
182 L12 **Balmoral** Victoria, SE Australia
24 K9 **Balmorhea** Texas, SW USA
Balneario Claromecó see Claromecó
Balochistān see Baluchistān
82 B13 **Balombo** Port. Norton de Matos, Vila Norton de Matos. Benguela, W Angola
82 B13 **Balombo** ≈ W Angola
181 X10 **Balonne River** ≈ Queensland, E Australia
152 E13 **Bālotra** Rājasthān, N India
145 V14 **Balpyk Bi** prev. Kirovskiy Kaz. Kīrov. Almaty, SE Kazakhstan
Balqā'/Balqā', Muḩāfaẓat al see Al Balqā'
Balqash see Balkhash/Balkhash, Ozero
152 M12 **Balrāmpur** Uttar Pradesh, N India
182 M9 **Balranald** New South Wales, SE Australia
116 H14 **Balş** Olt, S Romania
14 H11 **Balsam Creek** Ontario, S Canada
30 I5 **Balsam Lake** Wisconsin, N USA
14 I14 **Balsam Lake** ◎ Ontario, SE Canada
59 M14 **Balsas** Maranhão, E Brazil
40 M15 **Balsas, Río** var. Río Mexcala. ≈ S Mexico
43 W16 **Balsas, Río** ≈ SE Panama
119 O18 **Bal'shavik** Rus. Bol'shevik. Homyel'skaya Voblasts', SE Belarus
95 O15 **Bålsta** Uppsala, C Sweden
108 E7 **Balsthal** Solothurn, NW Switzerland
117 O8 **Balta** Odes'ka Oblast', SW Ukraine
119 H14 **Baltaji Voke** Vilnius, SE Lithuania
105 N5 **Baltanás** Castilla-León, N Spain
61 E16 **Baltasar Brum** Artigas, N Uruguay
116 M9 **Bălţi** Rus. Bel'tsy. N Moldova
Baltic Port see Paldiski
118 B10 **Baltic Sea** Ger. Ostee, Rus. Baltiskoye More. sea N Europe
21 X3 **Baltimore** Maryland, NE USA
31 T13 **Baltimore** Ohio, N USA
21 X3 **Baltimore-Washington** ✕ Maryland, E USA
Baltischport/Baltiski see Paldiski
Baltiskoye More see Baltic Sea
119 A14 **Baltiysk** Ger. Pillau. Kaliningradskaya Oblast', W Russian Federation
Baltkrievija see Belarus
Balūchestān va Sīstān see Sīstān va Balūchestān
148 M12 **Baluchistān** var. Balochistān, Beluchistan. ◈ province SW Pakistan
171 P5 **Balud** Masbate, N Philippines
169 T9 **Balui, Batang** ≈ East Malaysia
153 S13 **Bālurghat** West Bengal, NE India
118 J8 **Balvi** Balvi, NE Latvia
147 W7 **Balykchy** Kir. Ysyk-Köl; prev. Issyk-Kul', Rybach'ye. Issyk-Kul'skaya Oblast', NE Kyrgyzstan
56 B7 **Balzar** Guayas, W Ecuador
108 I8 **Balzers** S Liechtenstein
143 T12 **Bam** Kermān, SE Iran
77 Y13 **Bama** Borno, NE Nigeria
76 L12 **Bamako** ● (Mali) Capital District, SW Mali
77 P10 **Bamba** Gao, C Mali
42 M8 **Bambana, Río** ≈ NE Nicaragua
79 J15 **Bambari** Ouaka, C Central African Republic
181 W5 **Bambaroo** Queensland, NE Australia
101 K19 **Bamberg** Bayern, SE Germany
21 R14 **Bamberg** South Carolina, SE USA
79 M16 **Bambesa** Orientale, N Dem. Rep. Congo (Zaire)
76 G11 **Bambey** W Senegal
79 H16 **Bambio** Sangha-Mbaéré, SW Central African Republic
83 I24 **Bamboesberge** ▲ South Africa
79 D14 **Bamenda** Nord-Ouest, W Cameroon
10 K17 **Bamfield** Vancouver Island, British Columbia, SW Canada
146 E12 **Bami** Turkm. Bamy. Akhalskiy Velayat, C Turkmenistan
149 P4 **Bāmīān** var. Bāmiān. Bāmīān, NE Afghanistan
149 O4 **Bāmīān** ◈ province C Afghanistan
79 J14 **Bamingui** Bamingui-Bangoran, C Central African Republic
78 J13 **Bamingui** ≈ N Central African Republic
78 J13 **Bamingui-Bangoran** ◈ prefecture N Central African Republic
143 V13 **Bampūr** Sīstān va Balūchestān, SE Iran
186 C8 **Bamu** ≈ SW PNG
Bamy see Bami
Bán see Bánovce nad Bebravou
81 N17 **Banaadir** off. Gobolka Banaadir. ◈ region S Somalia
191 N3 **Banaba** var. Ocean Island. island Tungaru, W Kiribati
59 O14 **Banabuiú, Açude** ⊞ NE Brazil
57 O19 **Bañados del Izozog** salt lake SE Bolivia
97 D18 **Banagher** Ir. Beannchar. C Ireland
79 M17 **Banalia** Orientale, N Dem. Rep. Congo (Zaire)
76 L12 **Banamba** Koulikoro, W Mali
40 G4 **Banámichi** Sonora, NW Mexico
181 Y9 **Banana** Queensland, E Australia
191 Z2 **Banana** prev. Main Camp. Kiritimati, E Kiribati
59 K16 **Bananal, Ilha do** island C Brazil
23 Y12 **Banana River** lagoon Florida, SE USA
151 Q22 **Bananga** Andaman and Nicobar Islands, India, NE Indian Ocean
Banaras see Vārānasi
114 N13 **Banarlı** Tekirdağ, NW Turkey
152 H12 **Banās** ≈ N India
75 Z11 **Banâs, Râs** headland E Egypt
112 N10 **Banatski Karlovac** Serbia, NE Yugoslavia
141 P16 **Banā, Wādī** dry watercourse SW Yemen
136 E14 **Banaz** Uşak, W Turkey
136 E14 **Banaz Çayı** ≈ W Turkey
159 P14 **Banbar** Xizang Zizhiqu, W China
97 G15 **Banbridge** Ir. Droichead na Banna. SE Northern Ireland, UK
Ban Bua Yai see Bua Yai
97 M21 **Banbury** S England, UK
167 O7 **Ban Chiang Dao** Chiang Mai, NW Thailand
96 K9 **Banchory** NE Scotland, UK
14 J13 **Bancroft** Ontario, SE Canada
33 R15 **Bancroft** Idaho, NW USA
29 U11 **Bancroft** Iowa, C USA
154 I9 **Banda** Madhya Pradesh, C India
152 L13 **Bānda** Uttar Pradesh, N India
168 F7 **Bandaaceh** var. Banda Atjeh; prev. Koetaradja, Kutaradja, Kutaraja. Sumatera, W Indonesia
Banda Atjeh see Bandaaceh
171 S14 **Banda, Kepulauan** island group E Indonesia
Banda, Laut see Banda Sea
77 N17 **Bandama** var. Bandama Fleuve. ≈ S Ivory Coast
77 N15 **Bandama Blanc** ≈ C Ivory Coast
Bandama Fleuve see Bandama
Bandar 'Abbās see Bandar-e 'Abbās
153 W16 **Bandarban** Chittagong, SE Bangladesh
80 Q13 **Bandarbeyla** var. Bender Beila, Bender Beyla. Bari, NE Somalia
143 R14 **Bandar-e 'Abbās** var. Bandar 'Abbās; prev. Gombroon. Hormozgān, S Iran
142 M3 **Bandar-e Anzalī** Gīlān, NW Iran
143 N12 **Bandar-e Būshehr** var. Būshehr, Eng. Bushire. Būshehr, S Iran
142 M11 **Bandar-e Gonāveh** var. Ganāveh; prev. Gonāveh. Būshehr, SW Iran
143 R14 **Bandar-e Khamīr** Hormozgān, S Iran
143 Q14 **Bandar-e Langeh** var. Bandar-e Lengeh, Lingeh. Hormozgān, S Iran
Bandar-e Lengeh see Bandar-e Langeh
142 L10 **Bandar-e Māhshahr** var. Māh-Shahr; prev. Bandar-e Ma'shūr. Khūzestān, SW Iran
Bandar-e Ma'shūr see Bandar-e Māhshahr
143 O14 **Bandar-e Nakhīlū** Hormozgān, S Iran
Bandar-e Shāh see Bandar-e Torkaman
143 P4 **Bandar-e Torkaman** var. Bandar-e Torkeman, Bandar-e Torkman; prev. Bandar-e Shāh. Golestān, N Iran
Bandar-e Torkeman/Bandar-e Torkman see Bandar-e Torkaman
Bandar Kassim see Boosaaso
168 M15 **Bandarlampung** prev. Tanjungkarang, Teloekbetoeng, Telukbetung. Sumatera, W Indonesia
Bandar Maharani see Muar
Bandar Masulipatnam see Machilipatnam
Bandar Penggaram see Batu Pahat
169 T7 **Bandar Seri Begawan** prev. Brunei Town. ● (Brunei) N Brunei

◆ Country ● Country Capital ◇ Dependent Territory ○ Dependent Territory Capital ◈ Administrative Region ✕ International Airport ▲ Mountain ▲▲ Mountain Range Volcano ≈ River ◎ Lake ⊞ Reservoir

169 T7 **Bandar Seri Begawan** ✈ N Brunei
171 R15 **Banda Sea** var. Laut Banda. sea E Indonesia
104 H5 **Bande** Galicia, NW Spain
59 G15 **Bandeirantes** Mato Grosso, W Brazil
59 N20 **Bandeira, Pico da** ▲ SE Brazil
83 K19 **Bandelierkop** Northern, NE South Africa
62 L8 **Bandera** Santiago del Estero, N Argentina
25 Q11 **Bandera** Texas, SW USA
40 J13 **Banderas, Bahía de** bay W Mexico
77 O11 **Bandiagara** Mopti, C Mali
152 I12 **Bāndīkūi** Rājasthān, N India
136 C11 **Bandırma** var. Penderma. Balıkesir, NW Turkey
Bandjarmasin see Banjarmasin
Bandoeng see Bandung
97 C21 **Bandon** Ir. Droicheadna Bandan. SW Ireland
32 E14 **Bandon** Oregon, NW USA
167 R8 **Ban Dong Bang** Nong Khai, E Thailand
167 Q6 **Ban Donkon** Oudômxai, N Laos
172 J14 **Bandrélé** SE Mayotte
79 H20 **Bandundu** prev. Banningville. Bandundu, W Dem. Rep. Congo (Zaire)
79 I21 **Bandundu** off. Région de Bandundu. ◆ region W Dem. Rep. Congo (Zaire)
169 O16 **Bandung** prev. Bandoeng. Jawa, C Indonesia
116 L15 **Băneasa** Constanța, SW Romania
142 J4 **Bāneh** Kordestān, N Iran
44 I7 **Banes** Holguín, E Cuba
11 P16 **Banff** Alberta, SW Canada
96 K8 **Banff** NE Scotland, UK
96 K8 **Banff** cultural region NE Scotland, UK
Bánffyhunyad see Huedin
77 N14 **Banfora** SW Burkina
155 H19 **Bangalore** Karnātaka, S India
153 S16 **Bangaon** West Bengal, NE India
79 L15 **Bangassou** Mbomou, SE Central African Republic
186 D7 **Bangeta, Mount** ▲ C PNG
171 P12 **Banggai, Kepulauan** island group C Indonesia
177 Q12 **Banggai, Pulau** island Kepulauan Banggai, N Indonesia
171 X13 **Banggelapa** Irian Jaya, E Indonesia
Banggi see Banggi, Pulau
169 V6 **Banggi, Pulau** var. Banggi. island East Malaysia
121 P13 **Banghāzī** Eng. Bengazi, Benghazi, It. Bengasi. NE Libya
Bang Hieng see Xé Banghiang
169 P11 **Bangkai, Tanjung** var. Bankai. headland Borneo, N Indonesia
169 S16 **Bangkalan** Pulau Madura, C Indonesia
169 N12 **Bangka, Pulau** island W Indonesia
169 N13 **Bangka, Selat** strait Sumatera, W Indonesia
168 J11 **Bangkinang** Sumatera, W Indonesia
168 K12 **Bangko** Sumatera, W Indonesia
Bangkok see Krung Thep
Bangkok, Bight of see Krung Thep, Ao
153 T14 **Bangladesh** off. People's Republic of Bangladesh; prev. East Pakistan. ◆ republic S Asia
167 V13 **Ba Ngoi** Khanh Hoa, S Vietnam
152 K5 **Bangong Co** var. Pangong Tso. ◎ China/India see also Pangong Tso
97 G15 **Bangor** Ir. Beannchar. E Northern Ireland, UK
97 I18 **Bangor** NW Wales, UK
19 R6 **Bangor** Maine, NE USA
18 I14 **Bangor** Pennsylvania, NE USA
67 R8 **Bangoran** ⤳ S Central African Republic
Bang Phra see Trat
Bang Pla Soi see Chon Buri
25 Q8 **Bangs** Texas, SW USA
167 N13 **Bang Saphan** var. Bang Saphan Yai. Prachuap Khiri Khan, SW Thailand
Bang Saphan Yai see Bang Saphan
36 I8 **Bangs, Mount** ▲ Arizona, SW USA
93 E15 **Bangsund** Nord-Trøndelag, C Norway
171 O2 **Bangued** Luzon, N Philippines
79 I15 **Bangui** ● (Central African Republic) Ombella-Mpoko, SW Central African Republic
79 I15 **Bangui** ✈ Ombella-Mpoko, SW Central African Republic
83 N16 **Bangula** Southern, S Malawi
Bangwaketse see Southern
82 K12 **Bangweulu, Lake** var. Lake Bengweulu. ◎ N Zambia
Banhā see Benha
Ban Hat Yai see Hat Yai
167 Q7 **Ban Hin Heup** Viangchan, C Laos
Ban Houayxay/Ban Houei Sai see Houayxay
167 O12 **Ban Hua Hin** var. Hua Hin. Prachuap Khiri Khan, SW Thailand
79 L14 **Bani** Haute-Kotto, E Central African Republic
77 N12 **Bani** ⤳ S Mali
45 O9 **Baní** S Dominican Republic
Banias see Bāniyās
77 S11 **Bani Bangou** Tillabéri, SW Niger
76 M12 **Banifing** var. Ngorolaka. ⤳ Burkina/Mali
77 R13 **Banikoara** N Benin
Banī Mazār see Beni Mazâr
114 K8 **Baniski Lom** ⤳ N Bulgaria
21 U7 **Banister River** ⤳ Virginia, NE USA
Banī Suwayf see Beni Suef
75 O8 **Banī Walīd** NW Libya
138 H5 **Bāniyās** var. Banias, Baniyas, Paneas. Tarṭūs, W Syria
113 K14 **Banja** Serbia, W Yugoslavia
Banjak, Kepulauan see Banyak, Kepulauan
112 J12 **Banja Koviljača** Serbia, W Yugoslavia
112 G11 **Banja Luka** Republika Srpska, NW Bosnia and Herzegovina
169 T13 **Banjarmasin** prev. Bandjarmasin. Borneo, C Indonesia
76 F11 **Banjul** prev. Bathurst. ● (Gambia) W Gambia
76 F11 **Banjul** ✈ W Gambia
Bank see Bankă
137 Y13 **Bankă** Rus. Bank. SE Azerbaijan
167 S11 **Ban Kadian** var. Ban Kadiene. Champasak, S Laos
Ban Kadiene see Ban Kadian
Bankai see Bangkai, Tanjung
166 M14 **Ban Kam Phuam** Phangnga, SW Thailand
Ban Kantang see Kantang
77 O11 **Bankass** Mopti, S Mali
95 L19 **Bankeryd** Jönköping, S Sweden
83 K16 **Banket** Mashonaland West, N Zimbabwe
167 T11 **Ban Khamphô** Attapu, S Laos
23 O4 **Bankhead Lake** ▣ Alabama, S USA
77 Q11 **Bankilaré** Tillabéri, SW Niger
Banks, Îles see Banks Islands
10 I14 **Banks Island** island British Columbia, SW Canada
187 R12 **Banks Islands** Fr. Îles Banks. island group N Vanuatu
23 U8 **Banks Lake** ◎ Georgia, SE USA
32 K8 **Banks Lake** ▣ Washington, NW USA
185 I19 **Banks Peninsula** peninsula South Island, NZ
183 Q15 **Banks Strait** strait SW Tasman Sea
Ban Kui Nua see Kui Buri
153 R16 **Bānkura** West Bengal, NE India
167 S8 **Ban Lakxao** var. Lak Sao. Bolikhamxai, C Laos
167 O16 **Ban Lam Phai** Songkhla, SW Thailand
Ban Mae Sot see Mae Sot
Ban Mae Suai see Mae Suai
Ban Mak Khaeng see Udon Thani
166 M3 **Banmauk** Sagaing, N Burma
Banmo see Bhamo
167 T10 **Ban Mun-Houamuang** S Laos
97 F14 **Bann** var. Lower Bann, Upper Bann. ⤳ N Northern Ireland, UK
167 S10 **Ban Nadou** Salavan, S Laos
167 S9 **Ban Nakala** Savannakhét, S Laos
167 Q8 **Ban Nakha** Viangchan, C Laos
167 S9 **Ban Nakham** Khammouan, S Laos
167 P7 **Ban Namoun** Xaignabouli, N Laos
167 O17 **Ban Nang Sata** Yala, SW Thailand
167 N15 **Ban Na San** Surat Thani, SW Thailand
167 R7 **Ban Nasi** Xiangkhoang, N Laos
44 I3 **Bannerman Town** Eleuthera Island, C Bahamas
35 V15 **Banning** California, W USA
Banningville see Bandundu
167 S11 **Ban Nongsim** Champasak, S Laos
149 S7 **Bannu** prev. Edwardesabad. North-West Frontier Province, NW Pakistan
Bañolas see Banyoles
56 C7 **Baños** Tungurahua, C Ecuador
Bánovce see Bánovce nad Bebravou
111 I19 **Bánovce nad Bebravou** var. Bánovce, Hung. Bán. Trenčiansky Kraj, W Slovakia
112 J12 **Banovići** Federacija Bosna I Hercegovina, E Bosnia and Herzegovina
Banow see Andarāb
Ban Pak Phanang see Pak Phanang
167 O7 **Ban Pan Nua** Lampang, NW Thailand
167 Q9 **Ban Phai** Khon Kaen, E Thailand
167 T9 **Ban Phou A Douk** Khammouan, C Laos
167 Q8 **Ban Phu** Uthai Thani, W Thailand
167 O11 **Ban Pong** Ratchaburi, W Thailand
190 I3 **Banraeaba** Tarawa, W Kiribati
167 N10 **Ban Sai Yok** Kanchanaburi, W Thailand
Ban Sattahip/Ban Sattahipp see Sattahip
Ban Sichon see Sichon
Ban Si Racha see Siracha
111 J19 **Banská Bystrica** Ger. Neusohl, Hung. Besztercebánya. Banskobystrický Kraj, C Slovakia
111 K20 **Banskobystrický Kraj** ◆ region C Slovakia
167 R8 **Ban Sôppheung** Bolikhamxai, C Laos
Ban Sop Prap see Sop Prap
152 G15 **Bānswāra** Rājasthān, N India
167 N15 **Ban Ta Khun** Surat Thani, SW Thailand
Ban Takua Pa see Takua Pa
167 S8 **Ban Talak** Khammouan, C Laos
77 R15 **Bantè** W Benin
167 Q8 **Ban Thabôk** Bolikhamxai, C Laos
167 T9 **Ban Tôp** Savannakhét, S Laos
97 B21 **Bantry** Ir. Beanntraí. SW Ireland
97 A21 **Bantry Bay** Ir. Bá Bheanntraí. bay SW Ireland
155 F19 **Bantvāl** var. Bantwāl. Karnātaka, E India
Bantwāl see Bantvāl
114 N9 **Banya** Burgas, E Bulgaria
168 G10 **Banyak, Kepulauan** prev. Kepulauan Banjak. island group NW Indonesia
105 U8 **Banya, La** headland E Spain
79 E14 **Banyo** Adamaoua, NW Cameroon
105 X4 **Banyoles** var. Bañolas. Cataluña, NE Spain
167 N16 **Ban Yong Sata** Trang, SW Thailand
195 X14 **Banzare Coast** physical region Antarctica
173 Q14 **Banzare Seamounts** undersea feature S Indian Ocean
Banzart see Bizerte
Baochang see Taibus Qi
161 O3 **Baoding** var. Pao-ting; prev. Tsingyuan. Hebei, E China
Baoebaoe see Baubau
Baoi, Oileán see Dursey Island
160 J6 **Baoji** var. Pao-chi, Paoki. Shaanxi, C China
186 L8 **Baolo** Santa Isabel, N Solomon Islands
167 U13 **Bao Lôc** Lâm Đông, S Vietnam
163 Z7 **Baoqing** Heilongjiang, NE China
Baoqing see Shaoyang
79 H15 **Baoro** Nana-Mambéré, W Central African Republic
160 E12 **Baoshan** var. Pao-shan. Yunnan, SW China
163 N13 **Baotou** var. Pao-t'ou, Paotow. Nei Mongol Zizhiqu, N China
76 L14 **Baoulé** ⤳ S Mali
76 K12 **Baoulé** ⤳ W Mali
103 O2 **Bapaume** Pas-de-Calais, N France
14 J13 **Baptiste Lake** ◎ Ontario, SE Canada
Baqanas see Bakanas
Baqbaqty see Bakbakty
159 P14 **Baqên** var. Dartang. Xizang Zizhiqu, W China
138 F14 **Bāqir, Jabal** ▲ S Jordan
139 T7 **Ba'qūbah** var. Qubba. C Iraq
62 H5 **Baquedano** Antofagasta, N Chile
116 M6 **Bar** Vinnyts'ka Oblast', C Ukraine
113 J18 **Bar** It. Antivari. Montenegro, SW Yugoslavia
80 E10 **Bara** Northern Kordofan, C Sudan
81 M18 **Baraawe** It. Brava. Shabeellaha Hoose, S Somalia
152 M12 **Bāra Banki** Uttar Pradesh, N India
30 L8 **Baraboo** Wisconsin, N USA
30 K8 **Baraboo Range** hill range Wisconsin, N USA
Baracaldo see San Vicente de Barakaldo
15 Y6 **Barachois** Quebec, SE Canada
44 J7 **Baracoa** Guantánamo, E Cuba
61 C19 **Baradero** Buenos Aires, E Argentina
183 R6 **Baradine** New South Wales, SE Australia
Baraf Daja Islands see Damar, Kepulauan
154 M12 **Baragarh** Orissa, E India
81 I17 **Baragoi** Rift Valley, W Kenya
45 N9 **Barahona** SW Dominican Republic
153 W13 **Barail Range** ▲▲ NE India
80 I9 **Baraka** var. Barka, Ar. Khawr Barakah. seasonal river Eritrea/Sudan
80 G10 **Barakat** Gezira, C Sudan
Barakī see Barakī Barak
149 Q6 **Barakī Barak** var. Barakī, Baraki Rajan. Lowgar, E Afghanistan
Baraki Rajan see Barakī Barak
154 N11 **Bārākot** Orissa, E India
55 S7 **Barama River** ⤳ N Guyana
155 E14 **Bārāmati** Mahārāshtra, W India
152 H5 **Bāramūla** Jammu and Kashmir, NW India
119 N14 **Baran'** Vitsyebskaya Voblasts', NE Belarus
152 I14 **Bārān** Rājasthān, N India
139 U4 **Bārānān, Shākh-i** ▲▲ E Iraq
119 I17 **Baranavichy** Pol. Baranowicze, Rus. Baranovichi. Brestskaya Voblasts', SW Belarus
123 T6 **Baranikha** Chukotskiy Avtonomnyy Okrug, NE Russian Federation
116 M4 **Baranivka** Zhytomyrs'ka Oblast', N Ukraine
39 W14 **Baranof Island** island Alexander Archipelago, Alaska, USA
Baranovichi/ Baranowicze see Baranavichy
111 N15 **Baranów Sandomierski** Podkarpackie, SE Poland
111 I26 **Baranya** off. Baranya Megye. ◆ county S Hungary
153 R13 **Barauni** Bihār, NE India
22 L10 **Barataria Bay** bay Louisiana, S USA
Barat Daya, Kepulauan see Damar, Kepulauan
118 L12 **Baravukha** Rus. Borovukha. Vitsyebskaya Voblasts', N Belarus
54 E11 **Baraya** Huila, C Colombia
59 M21 **Barbacena** Minas Gerais, SE Brazil
54 B13 **Barbacoas** Nariño, SW Colombia
54 L6 **Barbacoas** Aragua, N Venezuela
45 Z13 **Barbados** ◆ commonwealth republic SE West Indies
47 S3 **Barbados** island Barbados
105 U11 **Barbaria, Cap de** var. Cabo de Berberia. headland Formentera, E Spain
114 N13 **Barbaros** Tekirdağ, NW Turkey
74 A11 **Barbas, Cap** headland S Western Sahara
105 T5 **Barbastro** Aragón, NE Spain
104 K16 **Barbate** ⤳ SW Spain
104 K16 **Barbate de Franco** Andalucía, S Spain
9 N1 **Barbeau Peak** ▲ Nunavut, N Canada
83 K21 **Barberton** Mpumalanga, NE South Africa
31 U12 **Barberton** Ohio, N USA
102 K12 **Barbezieux-St-Hilaire** Charente, W France
54 G9 **Barbosa** Santander, C Colombia
21 N7 **Barbourville** Kentucky, S USA
45 W9 **Barbuda** island N Antigua and Barbuda
181 W8 **Barcaldine** Queensland, E Australia
Barcarozsnyó see Râşnov
104 I11 **Barcarrota** Extremadura, W Spain
Barcău see Berettyó
Barce see Al Marj
107 L23 **Barcellona** var. Barcellona Pozzo di Gotto. Sicilia, Italy, C Mediterranean Sea
Barcellona Pozzo di Gotto see Barcellona
105 W6 **Barcelona** anc. Barcino, Barcinona. Cataluña, E Spain
55 N5 **Barcelona** Anzoátegui, NE Venezuela
105 S5 **Barcelona** ◆ province Cataluña, NE Spain
105 W6 **Barcelona** ✈ Cataluña, E Spain
103 U14 **Barcelonnette** Alpes-de-Haute-Provence, SE France
58 E12 **Barcelos** Amazonas, N Brazil
104 G5 **Barcelos** Braga, N Portugal
110 I10 **Barcin** Ger. Bartschin. Kujawski-pomorskie, C Poland
Barcino/Barcinona see Barcelona
Barcoo see Cooper Creek
111 H26 **Barcs** Somogy, SW Hungary
137 W11 **Bärdä** Rus. Barda. C Azerbaijan
78 H5 **Bardaï** Borkou-Ennedi-Tibesti, N Chad
139 R2 **Bardaraṣh** N Iraq
139 Q7 **Bardasah** SW Iraq
153 S16 **Barddhamān** West Bengal, NE India
111 N18 **Bardejov** Ger. Bartfeld, Hung. Bártfa. Prešovský Kraj, E Slovakia
105 R4 **Bárdenas Reales** physical region N Spain
Bardera/Bardere see Baardheere
Bardesīr see Bardsīr
92 K3 **Bárðarbunga** ▲ C Iceland
Bardhë, Drini i see Beli Drim
106 E9 **Bardi** Emilia-Romagna, C Italy
106 A8 **Bardonecchia** Piemonte, W Italy
97 H19 **Bardsey Island** island NW Wales, UK
143 S11 **Bardsīr** var. Bardesīr, Mashīz. Kermān, C Iran
20 L6 **Bardstown** Kentucky, S USA
Barduli see Barletta
20 G7 **Bardwell** Kentucky, S USA
152 K11 **Bareilly** var. Bareli. Uttar Pradesh, N India
Bareli see Bareilly
98 H13 **Barendrecht** Zuid-Holland, SW Netherlands
102 M3 **Barentin** Seine-Maritime, N France
92 N3 **Barentsburg** Spitsbergen, W Svalbard
Barentsevo More/Barents Havet see Barents Sea
92 O3 **Barentsøya** island E Svalbard
197 T11 **Barents Plain** undersea feature N Barents Sea
127 P3 **Barents Sea** Nor. Barents Havet, Rus. Barentsevo More. sea Arctic Ocean
197 U14 **Barents Trough** undersea feature SW Barents Sea
80 I9 **Barentu** W Eritrea
102 J3 **Barfleur** Manche, N France
102 J3 **Barfleur, Pointe de** headland N France
Barfrush/Barfurush see Bābol
158 H14 **Barga** Xizang Zizhiqu, W China
105 N9 **Bargas** Castilla-La Mancha, C Spain
81 I15 **Bargē** Southern, S Ethiopia
106 A9 **Barge** Piemonte, NE Italy
153 U16 **Barguna** Khulna, S Bangladesh
Bärguşad see Vorotan
123 N13 **Barguzin** Respublika Buryatiya, S Russian Federation
153 O13 **Barhaj** Uttar Pradesh, N India
183 N10 **Barham** New South Wales, SE Australia
152 J12 **Barhan** Uttar Pradesh, N India
19 S7 **Bar Harbor** Mount Desert Island, Maine, NE USA
153 R14 **Barharwa** Bihār, NE India
153 P15 **Barhi** Bihār, N India
107 O17 **Bari** var. Bari delle Puglie; anc. Barium. Puglia, SE Italy
80 P12 **Bari** off. Gobolka Bari. ◆ region NE Somalia
167 T14 **Ba Ria** Ba Ria-Vung Tau, S Vietnam
Bāridah see Al Bāridah
Bari delle Puglie see Bari
Barikot see Barīkowṭ
149 T4 **Barīkowṭ** var. Barikot. Kunar, NE Afghanistan
42 C4 **Barillas** var. Santa Cruz Barillas. Huehuetenango, NW Guatemala
54 J6 **Barinas** Barinas, W Venezuela
54 I7 **Barinas** off. Estado Barinas; prev. Zamora. ◆ state C Venezuela
54 I6 **Barinitas** Barinas, NW Venezuela
154 P11 **Bāripada** Orissa, E India
60 K9 **Bariri** São Paulo, S Brazil
75 W11 **Bârîs** S Egypt
152 G14 **Bari Sādri** Rājasthān, N India
153 U16 **Barisal** Khulna, S Bangladesh
168 I10 **Barisan, Pegunungan** ▲▲ Sumatera, W Indonesia
169 T12 **Barito, Sungai** ⤳ Borneo, C Indonesia
Barium see Bari
Barka see Baraka
Barka see Al Marj
160 H8 **Barkam** Sichuan, C China
118 J9 **Barkava** Madona, C Latvia
10 M15 **Barkerville** British Columbia, SW Canada
14 J12 **Bark Lake** ◎ Ontario, SE Canada
20 H7 **Barkley, Lake** ▣ Kentucky/Tennessee, S USA
10 K17 **Barkley Sound** inlet British Columbia, W Canada
83 J24 **Barkly East** Afr. Barkly-Oos. Eastern Cape, SE South Africa
Barkly-Oos see Barkly East
181 S4 **Barkly Tableland** plateau Northern Territory/Queensland, N Australia
Barkly-Wes see Barkly West
83 H22 **Barkly West** Afr. Barkly-Wes. Northern Cape, N South Africa
159 O5 **Barkol** var. Barkol Kazak Zizhixian. Xinjiang Uygur Zizhiqu, NW China
159 O5 **Barkol Hu** ◎ NW China
Barkol Kazak Zizhixian see Barkol
30 J3 **Bark Point** headland Wisconsin, N USA
25 P11 **Barksdale** Texas, SW USA
Bar Kunar see Asmār
116 L11 **Bârlad** prev. Bîrlad. Vaslui, E Romania
116 M11 **Bârlad** prev. Bîrlad. ⤳ E Romania
76 D9 **Barlavento, Ilhas de** var. Windward Islands. island group N Cape Verde
103 R5 **Bar-le-Duc** var. Bar-sur-Ornain. Meuse, NE France
180 K11 **Barlee, Lake** ◎ Western Australia
180 H8 **Barlee Range** ▲▲ Western Australia
107 N16 **Barletta** anc. Barduli. Puglia, SE Italy
110 E10 **Barlinek** Ger. Berlinchen. Zachodniopomorskie, NW Poland
27 S11 **Barling** Arkansas, C USA
171 U12 **Barma** Irian Jaya, E Indonesia
183 Q9 **Barmedman** New South Wales, SE Australia
Barmen-Elberfeld see Wuppertal
152 D12 **Bārmer** Rājasthān, NW India
182 K9 **Barmera** South Australia
97 I19 **Barmouth** NW Wales, UK
154 F10 **Barnagar** Madhya Pradesh, C India
152 H9 **Barnāla** Punjab, NW India
97 L15 **Barnard Castle** N England, UK
183 O6 **Barnato** New South Wales, SE Australia
122 I13 **Barnaul** Altayskiy Kray, C Russian Federation
109 V8 **Bärnbach** Steiermark, SE Austria
18 K16 **Barnegat** New Jersey, NE USA
23 S4 **Barnesville** Georgia, SE USA
29 R6 **Barnesville** Minnesota, N USA
31 U13 **Barnesville** Ohio, N USA
98 K11 **Barneveld** var. Barnveld. Gelderland, C Netherlands
25 O9 **Barnhart** Texas, SW USA
27 P8 **Barnsdall** Oklahoma, C USA
97 M17 **Barnsley** N England, UK
19 Q12 **Barnstable** Massachusetts, NE USA
97 I23 **Barnstaple** SW England, UK
Barnveld see Barneveld
21 Q14 **Barnwell** South Carolina, SE USA
67 U8 **Baro** var. Baro Wenz. ⤳ Ethiopia/Sudan
77 U15 **Baro** Niger, C Nigeria
Baro see Baro Wenz
Baroda see Vadodara
149 U2 **Baroghil Pass** var. Kowtal-e Barowghīl. pass Afghanistan/Pakistan
119 Q17 **Baron'ki** Rus. Boron'ki. Mahilyowskaya Voblasts', E Belarus
182 J9 **Barossa Valley** valley South Australia
Baroui see Salisbury
81 H14 **Baro Wenz** var. Baro, Nahr Barū. ⤳ Ethiopia/Sudan
153 U12 **Barpeta** Assam, NE India
31 S7 **Barques, Pointe Aux** headland Michigan, N USA
54 I5 **Barquisimeto** Lara, NW Venezuela
59 N16 **Barra** Bahia, E Brazil
96 E9 **Barra** island NW Scotland, UK
183 T5 **Barraba** New South Wales, SE Australia
60 L9 **Barra Bonita** São Paulo, S Brazil
64 J12 **Barracuda Fracture Zone** var. Fifteen Twenty Fracture Zone. tectonic feature SW Atlantic Ocean
64 G11 **Barracuda Ridge** undersea feature N Atlantic Ocean
43 N12 **Barra del Colorado** Limón, NE Costa Rica
43 N9 **Barra de Río Grande** Región Autónoma Atlántico Sur, E Nicaragua
82 A11 **Barra do Cuanza** Luanda, NW Angola
60 O9 **Barra do Piraí** Rio de Janeiro, SE Brazil
61 D16 **Barra do Quaraí** Rio Grande do Sul, SE Brazil
59 G14 **Barra do São Manuel** Pará, N Brazil
83 N19 **Barra Falsa, Ponta da** headland S Mozambique
96 E10 **Barra Head** headland NW Scotland, UK
Barram see Baram, Batang
60 O9 **Barra Mansa** Rio de Janeiro, SE Brazil
57 D14 **Barranca** Lima, W Peru
54 F8 **Barrancabermeja** Santander, N Colombia
54 H4 **Barrancas** La Guajira, N Colombia
54 J6 **Barrancas** Barinas, NW Venezuela
55 Q6 **Barrancas** Monagas, NE Venezuela
54 F6 **Barranco de Loba** Bolívar, N Colombia
104 I12 **Barrancos** Beja, S Portugal
62 N7 **Barranqueras** Chaco, N Argentina
54 E4 **Barranquilla** Atlántico, N Colombia
83 N20 **Barra, Ponta da** headland S Mozambique
105 P11 **Barrax** Castilla-La Mancha, C Spain
19 N11 **Barre** Massachusetts, NE USA
18 M7 **Barre** Vermont, NE USA
59 M17 **Barreiras** Bahia, E Brazil
104 F11 **Barreiro** Setúbal, W Portugal
65 C26 **Barren Island** island S Falkland Islands
20 K7 **Barren River Lake** ▣ Kentucky, S USA
60 L7 **Barretos** São Paulo, S Brazil
11 P14 **Barrhead** Alberta, SW Canada
14 G14 **Barrie** Ontario, S Canada
11 N16 **Barrière** British Columbia, SW Canada
14 H8 **Barrière, Lac** ◎ Quebec, SE Canada
182 L6 **Barrier Range** hill range New South Wales, SE Australia
42 G3 **Barrier Reef** reef E Belize
188 C16 **Barrigada** C Guam
Barrington Island see Santa Fe, Isla
183 T7 **Barrington Tops** ▲ New South Wales, SE Australia
183 O4 **Barringun** New South Wales, SE Australia
59 K18 **Barro Alto** Goiás, S Brazil
59 N14 **Barro Duro** Piauí, NE Brazil
30 I5 **Barron** Wisconsin, N USA
14 J12 **Barron** ⤳ Ontario, SE Canada
61 H15 **Barros Cassal** Rio Grande do Sul, S Brazil
45 P14 **Barrouallie** Saint Vincent, W Saint Vincent and the Grenadines
39 O4 **Barrow** Alaska, USA
97 E20 **Barrow** Ir. An Bhearú. ⤳ SE Ireland
181 Q6 **Barrow Creek Roadhouse** Northern Territory, N Australia
97 J16 **Barrow-in-Furness** NW England, UK
180 G7 **Barrow Island** island Western Australia
39 O4 **Barrow, Point** headland Alaska, USA
11 V14 **Barrows** Manitoba, S Canada
97 J22 **Barry** S Wales, UK
14 J12 **Barry's Bay** Ontario, SE Canada
144 K14 **Barsakel'mes, Ostrov** island SW Kazakhstan
Baršć Łužyca see Forst
147 S14 **Barsem** S Tajikistan
145 V11 **Barshatas** Vostochnyy Kazakhstan, E Kazakhstan
155 F14 **Bārsi** Mahārāshtra, W India
100 I13 **Barsinghausen** Niedersachsen, C Germany
147 X8 **Barskoon** Issyk-Kul'skaya Oblast', E Kyrgyzstan
100 F10 **Barssel** Niedersachsen, NW Germany
35 U14 **Barstow** California, W USA
24 L8 **Barstow** Texas, SW USA
103 R6 **Bar-sur-Aube** Aube, NE France
Bar-sur-Ornain see Bar-le-Duc
103 Q6 **Bar-sur-Seine** Aube, N France
147 S13 **Bartang** S Tajikistan
147 T13 **Bartang** ⤳ SE Tajikistan
Bartenstein see Bartoszyce
Bártfa/Bartfeld see Bardejov
100 N7 **Barth** Mecklenburg-Vorpommern, NE Germany
27 W13 **Bartholomew, Bayou** ⤳ Arkansas/Louisiana, S USA
55 T8 **Bartica** N Guyana
136 H10 **Bartın** Bartin, NW Turkey
136 H10 **Bartın** ◆ province NW Turkey
181 W4 **Bartle Frere** ▲ Queensland, E Australia
27 P8 **Bartlesville** Oklahoma, C USA
29 P14 **Bartlett** Nebraska, C USA
20 E10 **Bartlett** Tennessee, S USA
25 T9 **Bartlett** Texas, SW USA
36 L13 **Bartlett Reservoir** ▣ Arizona, SW USA
19 N6 **Barton** Vermont, NE USA
110 L7 **Bartoszyce** Ger. Bartenstein. Warmińsko-Mazurskie, NE Poland,
23 W12 **Bartow** Florida, SE USA
Bartschin see Barcin
168 J10 **Barumun, Sungai** ⤳ Sumatera, W Indonesia
Barū, Nahr see Baro Wenz
169 S17 **Barung, Nusa** island S Indonesia
168 H9 **Barus** Sumatera, NW Indonesia
162 L10 **Baruunsuu** Ömnögovĭ, S Mongolia
163 P8 **Baruun-Urt** Sühbaatar, E Mongolia
43 P15 **Barú, Volcán** var. Volcán de Chiriquí. ⚠ W Panama
99 K21 **Barvaux** Luxembourg, SE Belgium
42 M13 **Barva, Volcán** ⚠ NW Costa Rica
117 W6 **Barvinkove** Kharkivs'ka Oblast', E Ukraine
154 G11 **Barwāh** Madhya Pradesh, C India
Bärwalde Neumark see Mieszkowice
154 F11 **Barwāni** Madhya Pradesh, C India
183 P5 **Barwon River** ⤳ New South Wales, SE Australia
119 L15 **Barysaw** Rus. Borisov. Minskaya Voblasts', NE Belarus
129 Q6 **Barysh** Ul'yanovskaya Oblast', W Russian Federation

117 Q4 **Baryshivka** Kyyivs'ka Oblast', N Ukraine
79 J17 **Basankusu** Equateur, NW Dem. Rep. Congo (Zaire)
117 N11 **Basarabeasca** *Rus.* Bessarabka. SE Moldova
116 M14 **Basarabi** Constanța, SW Romania
40 H6 **Basaseachic** Chihuahua, NW Mexico
105 O2 **Basauri** País Vasco, N Spain
61 D18 **Basavilbaso** Entre Ríos, E Argentina
79 F21 **Bas-Congo** *off.* Région du Bas-Congo; *prev.* Bas-Zaïre. ◆ *region* SW Dem. Rep. Congo (Zaire)
108 E6 **Basel** *Eng.* Basle, *Fr.* Bâle. Basel-Stadt, NW Switzerland
108 E7 **Basel** *Eng.* Basle, *Fr.* Bâle. ◆ *canton* NW Switzerland
143 T14 **Bashākerd, Kūhhā-ye** ⛰ SE Iran
11 Q15 **Bashaw** Alberta, SW Canada
146 K16 **Bashbedeng** Maryyskiy Velayat, S Turkmenistan
161 T15 **Bashi Channel** *Chin.* Pa-shih Hai-hsia. *channel* Philippines/Taiwan
Bashkiria *see* Bashkortostan, Respublika
122 F11 **Bashkortostan, Respublika** *prev.* Bashkiria. ◆ *autonomous republic* W Russian Federation
129 N6 **Bashmakovo** Penzenskaya Oblast', W Russian Federation
146 J10 **Bashsakarba** Lebapskiy Velayat, NE Turkmenistan
117 R9 **Bashtanka** Mykolayivs'ka Oblast', S Ukraine
22 H8 **Basile** Louisiana, S USA
107 M18 **Basilicata** ◆ *region* S Italy
33 V13 **Basin** Wyoming, C USA
97 N22 **Basingstoke** S England, UK
143 U8 **Başīrān** Khorāsān, E Iran
112 B10 **Baška** *It.* Bescanuova. Primorje-Gorski Kotar, NW Croatia
137 T15 **Başkale** Van, SE Turkey
14 L10 **Baskatong, Réservoir** ⊠ Quebec, SE Canada
137 O14 **Baskil** Elâzığ, E Turkey
Basle *see* Basel
154 H9 **Bāsoda** Madhya Pradesh, C India
79 L17 **Basoko** Orientale, N Dem. Rep. Congo (Zaire)
Basque Country, The *see* País Vasco
Basra *see* Al Başrah
103 U5 **Bas-Rhin** ◆ *department* NE France
Bassam *see* Grand-Bassam
9 Q16 **Bassano** Alberta, SW Canada
106 H7 **Bassano del Grappa** Veneto, NE Italy
77 Q15 **Bassar** *var.* Bassari. NW Togo
Bassari *see* Bassar
172 L9 **Bassas da India** *island group* W Madagascar
108 D7 **Bassecourt** Jura, W Switzerland
166 K8 **Bassein** *var.* Pathein. Irrawaddy, SW Myanmar
79 J15 **Basse-Kotto** ◆ *prefecture* S Central African Republic
105 V5 **Bassella** Cataluña, NE Spain
102 J5 **Basse-Normandie** *Eng.* Lower Normandy. ◆ *region* N France
45 Q11 **Basse-Pointe** N Martinique
76 H12 **Basse Santa Su** E Gambia
Basse-Saxe *see* Niedersachsen
45 X6 **Basse-Terre** ○ (Guadeloupe) Basse Terre, SW Guadeloupe
45 X6 **Basse Terre** *island* W Guadeloupe
45 V10 **Basseterre** ● (Saint Kitts and Nevis) Saint Kitts, Saint Kitts and Nevis
29 O13 **Bassett** Nebraska, C USA
21 S7 **Bassett** Virginia, NE USA
37 N15 **Bassett Peak** ▲ Arizona, SW USA
76 M10 **Bassikounou** Hodh ech Chargui, SE Mauritania
77 R15 **Bassila** W Benin
Bass, Îlots de *see* Marotiri
31 O11 **Bass Lake** Indiana, N USA
183 O14 **Bass Strait** *strait* SE Australia
100 H11 **Bassum** Niedersachsen, NW Germany
29 X3 **Basswood Lake** ◎ Canada/USA
95 J21 **Båstad** Skåne, S Sweden
139 U2 **Basṭah** E Iraq
153 N12 **Basti** Uttar Pradesh, N India
103 X14 **Bastia** Corse, France, C Mediterranean Sea
99 L23 **Bastogne** Luxembourg, SE Belgium
22 I5 **Bastrop** Louisiana, S USA
25 T11 **Bastrop** Texas, SW USA
93 J15 **Bastuträsk** Västerbotten, N Sweden
119 J19 **Bastyn'** *Rus.* Bostyn'. Brestskaya Voblasts', SW Belarus
Basuo *see* Dongfang
Basutoland *see* Lesotho
119 O15 **Basya** ≈ E Belarus
117 V8 **Basyl'kivka** Dnipropetrovs'ka Oblast', E Ukraine
79 D17 **Bata** NW Equatorial Guinea
79 D17 **Bata** ✕ S Equatorial Guinea
Batae Coritanorum *see* Leicester
123 Q8 **Batagay** Respublika Sakha (Yakutiya), NE Russian Federation
123 P8 **Batagay-Alyta** Respublika Sakha (Yakutiya), NE Russian Federation
112 L10 **Batajnica** Serbia, N Yugoslavia
136 H15 **Bataklık Gölü** ◎ S Turkey
114 H11 **Batak, Yazovir** ⊠ SW Bulgaria
152 H7 **Batāla** Punjab, N India
104 F9 **Batalha** Leiria, C Portugal
79 N17 **Batama** Orientale, NE Dem. Rep. Congo (Zaire)
123 Q10 **Batamay** Respublika Sakha (Yakutiya), NE Russian Federation
160 F9 **Batang** Sichuan, C China
79 I14 **Batangafo** Ouham, NW Central African Republic
171 P8 **Batangas** *off.* Batangas City. Luzon, N Philippines
Bătania *see* Battonya
171 Q10 **Batan Islands** *island group* N Philippines
60 L8 **Batatais** São Paulo, S Brazil
18 E10 **Batavia** New York, NE USA
Batavia *see* Jakarta
173 T9 **Batavia Seamount** *undersea feature* E Indian Ocean
128 L12 **Bataysk** Rostovskaya Oblast', SW Russian Federation
14 B9 **Batchawana** ≈ Ontario, S Canada
14 B9 **Batchawana Bay** Ontario, S Canada
167 Q12 **Bătdâmbâng** *prev.* Battambang. Bătdâmbâng, NW Cambodia
79 G20 **Batéké, Plateaux** *plateau* S Congo
183 S11 **Batemans Bay** New South Wales, SE Australia
21 Q13 **Batesburg** South Carolina, SE USA
28 K12 **Batesland** South Dakota, N USA
27 V10 **Batesville** Arkansas, C USA
31 Q14 **Batesville** Indiana, N USA
22 L2 **Batesville** Mississippi, S USA
25 Q13 **Batesville** Texas, SW USA
44 L13 **Bath** E Jamaica
97 L22 **Bath** *hist.* Akermanceaster, *anc.* Aquae Calidae, Aquae Solis. SW England, UK
19 Q8 **Bath** Maine, NE USA
18 F11 **Bath** New York, NE USA
Bath *see* Berkeley Springs
78 I10 **Batha** *off.* Préfecture du Batha. ◆ *prefecture* C Chad
78 I10 **Batha** *seasonal river* C Chad
141 Y8 **Baṭḥā', Wādī al** *dry watercourse* NE Oman
152 H9 **Bathinda** Punjab, NW India
98 M11 **Bathmen** Overijssel, E Netherlands
45 Z14 **Bathsheba** E Barbados
183 R8 **Bathurst** New South Wales, SE Australia
13 O13 **Bathurst** New Brunswick, SE Canada
Bathurst *see* Banjul
8 H6 **Bathurst, Cape** *headland* Northwest Territories, NW Canada
196 L8 **Bathurst Inlet** Nunavut, N Canada
8 L7 **Bathurst Inlet** *inlet* Nunavut, N Canada
8 k4 **Bathurst Island** *island* Northern Territory, N Australia
197 O9 **Bathurst Island** *island* Parry Islands, Nunavut, N Canada
77 O14 **Batié** SW Burkina
Batinah *see* Al Bāṭinah
141 Y9 **Bāṭin, Wādī al** *dry watercourse* SW Asia
15 P9 **Batiscan** ≈ Quebec, SE Canada
136 F16 **Batı Toroslar** ⛰ SW Turkey
Batjan *see* Bacan, Pulau
Batlle y Ordóñez *see* José Batlle y Ordóñez
183 Q10 **Batlow** New South Wales, SE Australia
137 Q15 **Batman** *var.* Iluh. Batman, SE Turkey
137 Q15 **Batman** ◆ *province* SE Turkey
74 L6 **Batna** NE Algeria
Batoe *see* Batu, Kepulauan
162 K7 **Bat-Öldziyt** Töv, C Mongolia
22 J8 **Baton Rouge** *state capital* Louisiana, S USA
79 G15 **Batouri** Est, E Cameroon
138 G14 **Baträ', Jibāl al** ⛰ S Jordan
138 G6 **Batroûn** *var.* Al Batrūn. N Lebanon
Batsch *see* Bač
Batsevichi *see* Batsevichy
119 M17 **Batsevichy** *Rus.* Batsevichi. Mahilyowskaya Voblasts', E Belarus
92 M7 **Båtsfjord** Finnmark, N Norway
Battambang *see* Bătdâmbâng
195 X3 **Batterbee, Cape** *headland* Antarctica
155 L24 **Batticaloa** Eastern Province, E Sri Lanka
99 L19 **Battice** Liège, E Belgium
107 L18 **Battipaglia** Campania, S Italy
11 R15 **Battle** ≈ Alberta/Saskatchewan, SW Canada
Battle Born State *see* Nevada
31 Q10 **Battle Creek** Michigan, N USA
27 T7 **Battlefield** Missouri, C USA
11 S15 **Battleford** Saskatchewan, S Canada
29 S6 **Battle Lake** Minnesota, N USA
35 U3 **Battle Mountain** Nevada, W USA
111 M25 **Battonya** *Rom.* Bătania. Békés, SE Hungary
168 D11 **Batu, Kepulauan** *prev.* Batoe. *island group* W Indonesia
137 Q10 **Bat'umi** W Georgia
168 K10 **Batu Pahat** *prev.* Bandar Penggaram. Johor, Peninsular Malaysia
171 O12 **Baturebe** Sulawesi, N Indonesia
122 J12 **Baturino** Tomskaya Oblast', C Russian Federation
117 R3 **Baturyn** Chernihivs'ka Oblast', N Ukraine
138 F10 **Bat Yam** Tel Aviv, C Israel
129 Q4 **Batyrevo** Chuvashskaya Respublika, W Russian Federation
Batys Qazaqstan Oblysy *see* Zapadnyy Kazakhstan
102 F5 **Batz, Île de** *island* NW France
169 Q10 **Bau** Sarawak, East Malaysia
171 N2 **Bauang** Luzon, N Philippines
171 P14 **Baubau** *var.* Baoebaoe. Pulau Buton, C Indonesia
77 W14 **Bauchi** Bauchi, NE Nigeria
77 W14 **Bauchi** ◆ *state* C Nigeria
102 H7 **Baud** Morbihan, NW France
29 T2 **Baudette** Minnesota, N USA
193 S9 **Bauer Basin** *undersea feature* E Pacific Ocean
187 R14 **Bauer Field** *var.* Port Vila. ✕ (Port-Vila) Éfaté, C Vanuatu
13 T9 **Bauld, Cape** *headland* Newfoundland, E Canada
103 T8 **Baume-les-Dames** Doubs, E France
101 I15 **Baunatal** Hessen, C Germany
107 D18 **Baunei** Sardegna, Italy, C Mediterranean Sea
57 M15 **Baures, Río** ≈ N Bolivia
60 K9 **Bauru** São Paulo, S Brazil
Baushar *see* Bawshar
118 G10 **Bauska** *Ger.* Bauske. Bauska, S Latvia
Bauske *see* Bauska
101 Q15 **Bautzen** *Lus.* Budyšin. Sachsen, E Germany
145 Q16 **Bauyrzhan Momysh-Uly** *Kaz.* Baūyrzhan Momyshuly; *prev.* Burnoye. Zhambyl, S Kazakhstan
Bauzanum *see* Bolzano
Bavaria *see* Bayern
109 N7 **Bavarian Alps** *Ger.* Bayrische Alpen. ⛰ Austria/Germany
Bavière *see* Bayern
40 H4 **Bavispe, Río** ≈ NW Mexico
129 T5 **Bavly** Respublika Tatarstan, W Russian Federation
169 P13 **Bawal, Pulau** *island* N Indonesia
169 T12 **Bawan** Borneo, C Indonesia
183 O12 **Baw Baw, Mount** ▲ Victoria, SE Australia
169 S15 **Bawean, Pulau** *island* S Indonesia
75 V9 **Bawīṭī** N Egypt
77 Q13 **Bawku** N Ghana
167 N7 **Bawlakè** Kayah State, C Myanmar
169 H11 **Bawo Ofuloa** Pulau Tanahmasa, W Indonesia
141 Y8 **Bawshar** *var.* Baushar. NE Oman
Ba Xian *see* Bazhou
158 M8 **Baxkorgan** Xinjiang Uygur Zizhiqu, W China
23 V6 **Baxley** Georgia, SE USA
159 R15 **Baxoi** Xizang Zizhiqu, W China
29 W14 **Baxter** Iowa, C USA
29 U6 **Baxter** Minnesota, N USA
27 R8 **Baxter Springs** Kansas, C USA
81 M17 **Bay** *off.* Gobolka Bay. ◆ *region* SW Somalia
Bay *see* Baicheng
44 H7 **Bayamo** Granma, E Cuba
45 U5 **Bayamón** E Puerto Rico
163 W8 **Bayan** Heilongjiang, NE China
170 L16 **Bayan** *prev.* Bajan. Pulau Lombok, C Indonesia
162 I6 **Bayan** Arhangay, C Mongolia
163 P7 **Bayan** Dornod, E Mongolia
163 N9 **Bayan** Dornogovĭ, SE Mongolia
162 F7 **Bayan** Govĭ-Altay, W Mongolia
163 O8 **Bayan** Hentiy, C Mongolia
152 I12 **Bayāna** Rājasthān, N India
149 N5 **Bāyān, Band-e** ⛰ C Afghanistan
162 H8 **Bayanbulag** Bayanhongor, C Mongolia
163 N7 **Bayanbulag** Hentiy, C Mongolia
158 J5 **Bayanbulak** Xinjiang Uygur Zizhiqu, W China
Bayan Gol *see* Dengkou
162 F8 **Bayangovĭ** Govĭ-Altay, SW Mongolia
159 R12 **Bayan Har Shan** *var.* Bayan Khar. ⛰ C China
162 I8 **Bayanhongor** Bayanhongor, C Mongolia
162 H9 **Bayanhongor** ◆ *province* C Mongolia
Bayan Khar *see* Bayan Har Shan
168 J7 **Bayan Lepas** ✕ (George Town) Pinang, Peninsular Malaysia
162 K13 **Bayan Mod** Nei Mongol Zizhiqu, N China
162 K13 **Bayan Nuru** Nei Mongol Zizhiqu, N China
163 N12 **Bayan Obo** Nei Mongol Zizhiqu, N China
43 V15 **Bayano, Lago** ◎ E Panama
162 C5 **Bayan-Ölgiy** ◆ *province* NW Mongolia
162 F9 **Bayan-Ovoo** Govĭ-Altay, SW Mongolia
162 H9 **Bayansayr** Bayanhongor, C Mongolia
159 Q9 **Bayan Shan** ▲ C China
162 J9 **Bayanteeg** Övörhangay, C Mongolia
162 L8 **Bayantöhöm** Töv, C Mongolia
162 H6 **Bayan-Uhaa** Dzavhan, C Mongolia
162 J8 **Bayan-Ulaan** Övörhangay, C Mongolia
Bayan Ul Hot *see* Xi Ujimqin Qi
28 J14 **Bayard** Nebraska, C USA
37 P15 **Bayard** New Mexico, SW USA
103 T13 **Bayard, Col** *pass* SE France
163 O8 **Bayasgalant** Sühbaatar, E Mongolia
136 J12 **Bayat** Çorum, N Turkey
171 P6 **Bayawan** Negros, C Philippines
143 R10 **Bayāz** Kermān, C Iran
171 Q6 **Baybay** Leyte, C Philippines
21 X10 **Bayboro** North Carolina, SE USA
137 P12 **Bayburt** Bayburt, NE Turkey
137 P12 **Bayburt** ◆ *province* NE Turkey
31 R8 **Bay City** Michigan, N USA
25 V12 **Bay City** Texas, SW USA
122 I7 **Baydaratskaya Guba** *var.* Baydarata Bay. *bay* N Russian Federation
81 M16 **Baydhabo** *var.* Baydhowa, Isha Baydhabo, *It.* Baidoa. Bay, SW Somalia
Baydhowa *see* Baydhabo
101 N21 **Bayerischer Wald** ⛰ SE Germany
101 K21 **Bayern** *Eng.* Bavaria, *Fr.* Bavière. ◆ *state* SE Germany
147 V9 **Bayetovo** Narynskaya Oblast', C Kyrgyzstan
102 K4 **Bayeux** *anc.* Augustodurum. Calvados, N France
14 E15 **Bayfield** ≈ Ontario, S Canada
145 O15 **Baygakum** *Kaz.* Bäygequm. Kzylorda, S Kazakhstan
Bäygequm *see* Baygakum
136 C14 **Bayındır** İzmir, SW Turkey
138 H12 **Bāyir** *var.* Bā'ir. Ma'ān, S Jordan
Bay Islands *see* Bahía, Islas de la
139 R5 **Bayjī** *var.* Baiji. N Iraq
Baykadam *see* Saudakent
123 N13 **Baykal, Ozero** *Eng.* Lake Baikal. ◎ S Russian Federation
123 M14 **Baykal'sk** Irkutskaya Oblast', S Russian Federation
137 R15 **Baykan** Siirt, SE Turkey
123 L11 **Baykit** Evenkiyskiy Avtonomnyy Okrug, C Russian Federation
Baykonur *see* Baykonyr
144 M14 **Baykonyr** *var.* Baykonur *Kaz.* Bayqongyr; *prev.* Leninsk. Kzylorda, S Kazakhstan
145 N12 **Baykonyr** *var.* Baykonur. Zhezkazgan, C Kazakhstan
158 E7 **Baykurt** Xinjiang Uygur Zizhiqu, W China
14 I9 **Bay, Lac** ◎ Quebec, SE Canada
129 W6 **Baymak** Respublika Bashkortostan, W Russian Federation
23 O8 **Bay Minette** Alabama, S USA
143 O17 **Baynūnah** *desert* W UAE
184 O8 **Bay of Plenty** *off.* Bay of Plenty Region. ◆ *region* North Island, NZ
191 Z3 **Bay of Wrecks** *bay* Kiritimati, E Kiribati
102 I15 **Bayonne** *anc.* Lapurdum. Pyrénées-Atlantiques, SW France
22 H4 **Bayou D'Arbonne Lake** ⊠ Louisiana, S USA
23 N9 **Bayou La Batre** Alabama, S USA
Bayou State *see* Mississippi
Bayqadam *see* Saudakent
Bayqongyr *see* Baykonyr
Bayram-Ali *see* Bayramaly
146 J14 **Bayramaly** *prev.* Bayram-Ali. Maryyskiy Velayat, S Turkmenistan
101 L19 **Bayreuth** *var.* Baireuth. Bayern, SE Germany
Bayrische Alpen *see* Bavarian Alps
Bayrūt *see* Beyrouth
22 L9 **Bay Saint Louis** Mississippi, S USA
Baysān *see* Bet She'an
162 L8 **Bayshint** Töv, C Mongolia
14 H13 **Bays, Lake of** ◎ Ontario, S Canada
22 M6 **Bay Springs** Mississippi, S USA
Bay State *see* Massachusetts
Baysun *see* Boysun
14 H13 **Baysville** Ontario, S Canada
141 N15 **Bayt al Faqīh** W Yemen
158 M4 **Baytik Shan** ⛰ China/Mongolia
Bayt Laḥm *see* Bethlehem
25 W11 **Baytown** Texas, SW USA
169 V11 **Bayur, Tanjung** *headland* Borneo, N Indonesia
121 N14 **Bayy al Kabīr, Wādī** *dry watercourse* NW Libya
Bayyrqum *see* Bairkum
105 P14 **Baza** Andalucía, S Spain
137 X10 **Bazardüzü Dağı** *Rus.* Gora Bazardyuzyu. ▲ N Azerbaijan
Bazardyuzyu, Gora *see* Bazardüzü Dağı
Bazargic *see* Dobrich
83 N18 **Bazaruto, Ilha do** *island* SE Mozambique
102 K14 **Bazas** Gironde, SW France
105 O14 **Baza, Sierra de** ⛰ S Spain
160 J8 **Bazhong** Sichuan, C China
161 P3 **Bazhou** *prev.* Baxian, Ba Xian. Hebei, E China
14 M9 **Bazin** ≈ Quebec, SE Canada
Bazin *see* Pezinok
139 Q7 **Bāziyah** C Iraq
138 H6 **Bcharré** *var.* Bcharreh, Bsharrī, Bsherri. NE Lebanon
Bcharreh *see* Bcharré
28 J5 **Beach** North Dakota, N USA
182 K12 **Beachport** South Australia
97 O23 **Beachy Head** *headland* SE England, UK
18 K13 **Beacon** New York, NE USA
63 J25 **Beagle Channel** *channel* Argentina/Chile
181 O1 **Beagle Gulf** *gulf* Northern Territory, N Australia
Bealach an Doirín *see* Ballaghaderreen
Bealach Cláir *see* Ballyclare
Bealach Féich *see* Ballybofey
172 J3 **Bealanana** Mahajanga, NE Madagascar
Béal an Átha *see* Ballina
Béal an Átha Móir *see* Ballinamore
Béal an Mhuirhead *see* Belmullet
Béal Átha Beithe *see* Ballybay
Béal Átha Conaill *see* Ballyconnell
Beál Átha hAmhnais *see* Ballyhaunis
Béal Átha na Sluaighe *see* Ballinasloe
Béal Átha Seanaidh *see* Ballyshannon
Bealdovuopmi *see* Peltovuoma
Béal Feirste *see* Belfast
Béal Tairbirt *see* Belturbet
Beanna Boirche *see* Mourne Mountains
Beannchar *see* Banagher, Ireland
Beannchar *see* Bangor, Northern Ireland, UK
Beanntraí *see* Bantry
23 N2 **Bear Creek** ≈ Alabama/Mississippi, S USA
30 J13 **Bear Creek** ≈ Illinois, N USA
27 U13 **Bearden** Arkansas, C USA
195 Q10 **Beardmore Glacier** *glacier* Antarctica
30 K13 **Beardstown** Illinois, N USA
28 L14 **Bear Hill** ▲ Nebraska, C USA
Bear Island *see* Bjørnøya
14 H12 **Bear Lake** Ontario, S Canada
36 M1 **Bear Lake** ◎ Idaho/Utah, NW USA
39 U11 **Bear, Mount** ▲ Alaska, USA
102 J16 **Béarn** *cultural region* SW France
194 J11 **Bear Peninsula** *peninsula* Antarctica
152 I7 **Beās** ≈ India/Pakistan
105 P3 **Beasain** País Vasco, N Spain
105 O12 **Beas de Segura** Andalucía, S Spain
45 N10 **Beata, Cabo** *headland* SW Dominican Republic
45 N10 **Beata, Isla** *island* SW Dominican Republic
64 F11 **Beata Ridge** *undersea feature* N Caribbean Sea
29 R17 **Beatrice** Nebraska, C USA
83 L16 **Beatrice** Mashonaland East, NE Zimbabwe
11 N11 **Beatton** ≈ British Columbia, W Canada
11 N11 **Beatton River** British Columbia, W Canada
35 V10 **Beatty** Nevada, W USA
21 N6 **Beattyville** Kentucky, S USA
173 X16 **Beau Bassin** W Mauritius
103 R15 **Beaucaire** Gard, S France
14 I8 **Beauchastel, Lac** ◎ Quebec, SE Canada
14 I10 **Beauchêne, Lac** ◎ Quebec, SE Canada
183 V3 **Beaudesert** Queensland, E Australia
182 M12 **Beaufort** Victoria, SE Australia
21 X11 **Beaufort** North Carolina, SE USA
21 R15 **Beaufort** South Carolina, SE USA
38 M11 **Beaufort Sea** *sea* Arctic Ocean
Beaufort-Wes *see* Beaufort West
83 G25 **Beaufort West** *Afr.* Beaufort-Wes. Western Cape, SW South Africa
103 N7 **Beaugency** Loiret, C France
19 R1 **Beau Lake** ⊠ Maine, NE USA
96 I8 **Beauly** N Scotland, UK
99 G21 **Beaumont** Hainaut, S Belgium
185 E23 **Beaumont** Otago, South Island, NZ
22 M7 **Beaumont** Mississippi, S USA
25 X10 **Beaumont** Texas, SW USA
102 M15 **Beaumont-de-Lomagne** Tarn-et-Garonne, S France
102 L6 **Beaumont-sur-Sarthe** Sarthe, NW France
103 R8 **Beaune** Côte d'Or, C France
15 R9 **Beaupré** Quebec, SE Canada
102 J8 **Beaupréau** Maine-et-Loire, NW France
99 I22 **Beauraing** Namur, SE Belgium
103 R12 **Beaurepaire** Isère, E France
11 Y16 **Beausejour** Manitoba, S Canada
103 N4 **Beauvais** *anc.* Bellovacum, Caesaromagus. Oise, N France
11 S13 **Beauval** Saskatchewan, C Canada
102 I9 **Beauvoir-sur-Mer** Vendée, NW France
39 R8 **Beaver** Alaska, USA
26 J8 **Beaver** Oklahoma, C USA
18 B14 **Beaver** Pennsylvania, NE USA
36 K6 **Beaver** Utah, W USA
10 L9 **Beaver** ≈ British Columbia/Yukon Territory, W Canada
11 S13 **Beaver** ≈ Saskatchewan, C Canada
29 N17 **Beaver City** Nebraska, C USA
10 G6 **Beaver Creek** Yukon Territory, W Canada
31 R14 **Beavercreek** Ohio, N USA
39 S8 **Beaver Creek** ≈ Alaska, USA
26 H3 **Beaver Creek** ≈ Kansas/Nebraska, C USA
28 J5 **Beaver Creek** ≈ Montana/North Dakota, N USA
29 Q14 **Beaver Creek** ≈ Nebraska, C USA
25 Q4 **Beaver Creek** ≈ Texas, SW USA
30 M8 **Beaver Dam** Wisconsin, N USA
30 M8 **Beaver Dam Lake** ◎ Wisconsin, N USA
18 B14 **Beaver Falls** Pennsylvania, NE USA
33 P12 **Beaverhead Mountains** ⛰ Idaho/Montana, NW USA
33 Q12 **Beaverhead River** ≈ Montana, NW USA
65 A25 **Beaver Island** *island* W Falkland Islands
31 P5 **Beaver Island** *island* Michigan, N USA
27 S9 **Beaver Lake** ⊠ Arkansas, C USA
11 N13 **Beaverlodge** Alberta, W Canada
18 I8 **Beaver River** ≈ New York, NE USA
26 J8 **Beaver River** ≈ Oklahoma, C USA
18 B13 **Beaver River** ≈ Pennsylvania, NE USA
65 A25 **Beaver Settlement** Beaver Island, W Falkland Islands
Beaver State *see* Oregon
14 H14 **Beaverton** Ontario, S Canada
32 G11 **Beaverton** Oregon, NW USA
152 G12 **Beāwar** Rājasthān, N India
Bebas, Dasht-i *see* Bābūs, Dasht-e
60 L8 **Bebedouro** São Paulo, S Brazil
101 I16 **Bebra** Hessen, C Germany
41 W12 **Becal** Campeche, SE Mexico
15 Q11 **Bécancour** ≈ Quebec, SE Canada
97 Q19 **Beccles** E England, UK
112 L9 **Bečej** *Ger.* Altbetsche, *Hung.* Óbecse, Rácz-Becse; *prev.* Magyar-Becse, Stari Bečej. Serbia, N Yugoslavia
104 I3 **Becerreá** Galicia, NW Spain
74 H7 **Béchar** *prev.* Colomb-Béchar. W Algeria
39 O14 **Becharof Lake** ◎ Alaska, USA
116 H15 **Bechet** *var.* Bechetu. Dolj, SW Romania
Bechetu *see* Bechet
21 R6 **Beckley** West Virginia, NE USA
101 G14 **Beckum** Nordrhein-Westfalen, W Germany
25 X7 **Beckville** Texas, SW USA
35 X4 **Becky Peak** ▲ Nevada, W USA
116 I9 **Beclean** *Hung.* Bethlen; *prev.* Betlen. Bistrița-Năsăud, N Romania
Bécs *see* Wien
111 H18 **Bečva** *Ger.* Betschau, *Pol.* Beczwa. ≈ E Czech Republic
Beczwa *see* Bečva
103 P15 **Bédarieux** Hérault, S France
120 B10 **Beddouza, Cap** *headland* W Morocco
80 I13 **Bedelē** Oromo, C Ethiopia
147 Y8 **Bedel Pass** *Rus.* Pereval Bedel. *pass* China/Kyrgyzstan
Bedel, Pereval *see* Bedel Pass
95 H22 **Beder** Århus, C Denmark
97 N20 **Bedford** E England, UK
31 O15 **Bedford** Indiana, N USA
29 U16 **Bedford** Iowa, C USA
20 L4 **Bedford** Kentucky, S USA
18 D15 **Bedford** Pennsylvania, NE USA
21 T6 **Bedford** Virginia, NE USA
97 N20 **Bedfordshire** *cultural region* E England, UK
129 N5 **Bednodem'yanovsk** Penzenskaya Oblast', W Russian Federation
98 N5 **Bedum** Groningen, NE Netherlands
27 V11 **Beebe** Arkansas, C USA
45 T9 **Beef Island** ✕ (Road Town) Tortola, E British Virgin Islands
Beehive State *see* Utah
99 L18 **Beek** Limburg, SE Netherlands
99 L18 **Beek** ✕ (Maastricht) Limburg, SE Netherlands
99 K14 **Beek-en-Donk** Noord-Brabant, S Netherlands
138 F13 **Be'er Menuḥa** *var.* Be'er Menukha. Southern, S Israel
Be'er Menukha *see* Be'ér Menuḥa
99 D16 **Beernem** West-Vlaanderen, NW Belgium
99 I16 **Beerse** Antwerpen, N Belgium
Beersheba *see* Be'er Sheva'
138 E11 **Be'er Sheva'** *var.* Beersheba, *Ar.* Bir es Saba. Southern, S Israel
98 J13 **Beesd** Gelderland, C Netherlands
99 M16 **Beesel** Limburg, SE Netherlands
83 J21 **Beestekraal** North-West, N South Africa
194 J7 **Beethoven Peninsula** *peninsula* Alexander Island, Antarctica
Beetstersweach *see* Beetsterzwaag
98 M6 **Beetsterzwaag** *Fris.* Beetstersweach. Friesland, N Netherlands
25 S13 **Beeville** Texas, SW USA
79 J18 **Befale** Equateur, NW Dem. Rep. Congo (Zaire)
Befandriana *see* Befandriana Avaratra
172 J3 **Befandriana Avaratra** *var.* Befandriana, Befandriana Nord. Mahajanga, NW Madagascar
Befandriana Nord *see* Befandriana Avaratra
79 K18 **Befori** Equateur, N Dem. Rep. Congo (Zaire)
172 I7 **Befotaka** Fianarantsoa, S Madagascar
183 R11 **Bega** New South Wales, SE Australia
102 G5 **Bégard** Côtes d'Armor, NW France
112 M9 **Begejski Kanal** *canal* NE Yugoslavia
145 V9 **Begen'** Vostochnyy Kazakhstan, E Kazakhstan
94 G13 **Begna** ≈ S Norway
Begoml' *see* Byahoml'
Begovat *see* Bekobod
153 Q13 **Begusarāi** Bihār, NE India
143 R9 **Behābād** Yazd, C Iran
Behagle *see* Laï
55 Z10 **Béhague, Pointe** *headland* E French Guiana
Behar *see* Bihār
142 M10 **Behbahān** *var.* Behbehān. Khūzestān, SW Iran
Behbehān *see* Behbahān
44 G3 **Behring Point** Andros Island, W Bahamas
143 P4 **Behshahr** *prev.* Ashraf. Māzandarān, N Iran
163 V6 **Bei'an** Heilongjiang, NE China
Beibunar *see* Sredishte
Beibu Wan *see* Tongking, Gulf of
Beida *see* Al Bayḍā'
80 H13 **Beigi** Oromo, C Ethiopia
160 L16 **Beihai** Guangxi Zhuangzu Zizhiqu, S China
159 Q10 **Bei Hulsan Hu** ◎ C China
161 N13 **Bei Jiang** ≈ S China
161 O2 **Beijing** *var.* Pei-ching, *Eng.* Peking; *prev.* Pei-p'ing. *country/municipality capital* (China) Beijing Shi, E China
161 P2 **Beijing** ✕ Beijing Shi, E China
Beijing *see* Beijing Shi
161 O2 **Beijing Shi** *var.* Beijing, Jing, Pei-ching, *Eng.* Peking; *prev.* Pei-p'ing. ◆ *municipality* E China

◆ Country ● Country Capital ◇ Dependent Territory ○ Dependent Territory Capital ◆ Administrative Region ✕ International Airport ▲ Mountain ⛰ Mountain Range ⚠ Volcano ≈ River ◎ Lake ⊠ Reservoir

76 G8 **Beïla** Trarza, W Mauritania
98 N7 **Beilen** Drenthe, NE Netherlands
160 L15 **Beiliu** Guangxi Zhuangzu Zizhiqu, S China
159 O12 **Beilu He** ≈ W China
Beilul see Beylul
96 H8 **Beinn Dearg** ▲ N Scotland, UK
Beinn MacDuibh see Ben Macdui
160 I12 **Beipan Jiang** ≈ S China
163 T12 **Beipiao** Liaoning, NE China
83 N17 **Beira** Sofala, C Mozambique
83 N17 **Beira** ✕ Sofala, C Mozambique
104 I7 **Beira Alta** former province N Portugal
104 H9 **Beira Baixa** former province C Portugal
104 G8 **Beira Litoral** former province N Portugal
Beirut see Beyrouth
Beisān see Bet She'an
9 Q16 **Beiseker** Alberta, SW Canada
83 K19 **Beitbridge** Matabeleland South, S Zimbabwe
116 G10 **Beiuş** Hung. Belényes. Bihor, NW Romania
163 U12 **Beizhen** Liaoning, NE China
104 H12 **Beja** anc. Pax Julia. Beja, SE Portugal
104 G13 **Beja** ◈ district S Portugal
74 M5 **Béja** var. Bājah. N Tunisia
120 I9 **Béjaïa** var. Bejaïa, Fr. Bougie; anc. Saldae. NE Algeria
104 K8 **Béjar** Castilla-León, N Spain
Bejraburi see Phetchaburi
Bekaa Valley see El Beqaa
Bekabad see Bekobod
Békás see Bicaz
169 O15 **Bekasi** Jawa, C Indonesia
Bek-Budi see Qarshi
146 A8 **Bekdash** Balkanskiy Velayat, NW Turkmenistan
147 T10 **Bek-Dzhar** Oshskaya Oblast', SW Kyrgyzstan
111 N24 **Békés** Rom. Bichiş. Békés, SE Hungary
111 M24 **Békés** off. Békés Megye. ◈ county SE Hungary
111 M24 **Békéscsaba** Rom. Bichiş-Ciaba. Békés, SE Hungary
139 S2 **Bēkhma** E Iraq
172 H7 **Bekily** Toliara, S Madagascar
165 W4 **Bekkai** Hokkaidō, NE Japan
147 Q11 **Bekobod** Rus. Bekabad; prev. Begovat. Toshkent Wiloyati, E Uzbekistan
129 O7 **Bekovo** Penzenskaya Oblast', W Russian Federation
Bél see Beliu
152 M13 **Bela** Uttar Pradesh, N India
149 N15 **Bela** Baluchistān, SW Pakistan
79 F15 **Bélabo** Est, C Cameroon
112 N10 **Bela Crkva** Ger. Weisskirchen, Hung. Fehértemplom. Serbia, W Yugoslavia
173 Y16 **Bel Air** var. Rivière Sèche. E Mauritius
104 L12 **Belalcázar** Andalucía, S Spain
113 P15 **Bela Palanka** Serbia, SE Yugoslavia
119 H16 **Belarus** off. Republic of Belarus, var. Belorussia, Latv. Baltkrievija; prev. Belorussian SSR, Rus. Belorusskaya SSR. ◆ republic E Europe
Belau see Palau
59 H21 **Bela Vista** Mato Grosso do Sul, SW Brazil
83 L21 **Bela Vista** Maputo, S Mozambique
168 I8 **Belawan** Sumatera, W Indonesia
Běla Woda see Weisswasser
129 U4 **Belaya** ≈ W Russian Federation
123 R7 **Belaya Gora** Respublika Sakha (Yakutiya), NE Russian Federation
128 M11 **Belaya Kalitiva** Rostovskaya Oblast', SW Russian Federation
127 R14 **Belaya Kholunitsa** Kirovskaya Oblast', NW Russian Federation
Belaya Tserkov' see Bila Tserkva
77 V11 **Belbédji** Zinder, S Niger
110 K13 **Bełchatów** var. Belchatow. Łodzkie, C Poland
Belcher, Îles see Belcher Islands
12 H7 **Belcher Islands** Fr. Îles Belcher. island group Nunavut, SE Canada
105 S6 **Belchite** Aragón, NE Spain
29 O2 **Belcourt** North Dakota, N USA
31 P9 **Belding** Michigan, N USA
129 U5 **Belebey** Respublika Bashkortostan, W Russian Federation
81 N16 **Beledweyne** var. Belet Huen, It. Belet Uen. Hiiraan, C Somalia
146 B10 **Belek** Balkanskiy Velayat, W Turkmenistan
58 L12 **Belém** var. Pará. state capital Pará, N Brazil
65 I14 **Belém Ridge** undersea feature C Atlantic Ocean
37 R12 **Belen** New Mexico, SW USA
62 I7 **Belén** Catamarca, NW Argentina
54 G9 **Belén** Boyacá, C Colombia
42 J11 **Belén** Rivas, SW Nicaragua
62 O5 **Belén** Concepción, C Paraguay
61 D16 **Belén** Salto, N Uruguay
61 D20 **Belén de Escobar** Buenos Aires, E Argentina
114 J7 **Belene** Pleven, N Bulgaria
114 J7 **Belene, Ostrov** island N Bulgaria
43 R15 **Belén, Río** ≈ C Panama
Belényes see Beiuş
104 H3 **Belesar, Embalse de** ▣ NW Spain
Belet Huen/Belet Uen see Beledweyne
128 J5 **Belëv** Tul'skaya Oblast', W Russian Federation
97 G15 **Belfast** Ir. Béal Feirste. ◐ E Northern Ireland, UK
19 R7 **Belfast** Maine, NE USA
97 G15 **Belfast** ✕ E Northern Ireland, UK
97 G15 **Belfast Lough** Ir. Loch Lao inlet E Northern Ireland, UK
28 K5 **Belfield** North Dakota, N USA
103 U7 **Belfort** Territoire-de-Belfort, E France
Belgard see Białogard
155 E17 **Belgaum** Karnātaka, W India
Belgian Congo see Congo (Democratic Republic of)
195 T3 **Belgica Mountains** ▲▲ Antarctica
België/Belgique see Belgium
99 F20 **Belgium** off. Kingdom of Belgium, Dut. België, Fr. Belgique. ◆ monarchy NW Europe
128 J8 **Belgorod** Belgorodskaya Oblast', W Russian Federation
Belgorod-Dnestrovskiy see Bilhorod-Dnistrovs'kyy
128 J8 **Belgorodskaya Oblast'** ◈ province W Russian Federation
Belgrad see Beograd
29 T8 **Belgrade** Minnesota, N USA
33 S11 **Belgrade** Montana, NW USA
Belgrade see Beograd
195 N5 **Belgrano II** Argentinian research station Antarctica
Belgrano, Cabo see Meredith, Cape
21 X9 **Belhaven** North Carolina, SE USA
107 I23 **Belice** anc. Hypsas. ≈ Sicilia, Italy, C Mediterranean Sea
Belice see Belize/Belize City
113 M16 **Beli Drim** Alb. Drini i Bardhë. ≈ Albania/Yugoslavia
Beligrad see Berat
188 C8 **Beliliou** prev. Peleliu. island S Palau
114 L8 **Beli Lom, Yazovir** ▣ NE Bulgaria
112 I8 **Beli Manastir** Hung. Pélmonostor; prev. Monostor. Osijek-Baranja, NE Croatia
102 J13 **Belin-Béliet** Gironde, SW France
79 F17 **Bélinga** Ogooué-Ivindo, NE Gabon
21 S4 **Belington** West Virginia, NE USA
129 O6 **Belinskiy** Penzenskaya Oblast', W Russian Federation
169 N12 **Belinyu** Pulau Bangka, W Indonesia
169 O13 **Belitung, Pulau** island W Indonesia
116 F10 **Beliu** Hung. Bel. Arad, W Romania
114 I9 **Beli Vit** ≈ NW Bulgaria
42 G2 **Belize** Sp. Belice; prev. British Honduras, Colony of Belize. ◆ commonwealth republic Central America
42 F2 **Belize** Sp. Belice. ◈ district NE Belize
42 G2 **Belize** ≈ Belize/Guatemala
Belize see Belize City
42 G2 **Belize City** var. Belize, Sp. Belice. Belize, NE Belize
42 G2 **Belize City** ✕ Belize, NE Belize
Beljak see Villach
39 N16 **Belkofski** Alaska, USA
123 O6 **Bel'kovskiy, Ostrov** island Novosibirskiye Ostrova, NE Russian Federation
14 J8 **Bell** ≈ Quebec, SE Canada
10 J15 **Bella Bella** British Columbia, SW Canada
102 M10 **Bellac** Haute-Vienne, C France
10 K15 **Bella Coola** British Columbia, SW Canada
106 D6 **Bellagio** Lombardia, N Italy
31 P6 **Bellaire** Michigan, N USA
106 D6 **Bellano** Lombardia, N Italy
155 G17 **Bellary** var. Ballari. Karnātaka, S India
183 S5 **Bellata** New South Wales, SE Australia
61 D16 **Bella Unión** Artigas, N Uruguay
61 C14 **Bella Vista** Corrientes, NE Argentina
62 J7 **Bella Vista** Tucumán, N Argentina
62 P4 **Bella Vista** Amambay, C Paraguay
56 B10 **Bellavista** Cajamarca, N Peru
56 D11 **Bellavista** San Martín, N Peru
183 U6 **Bellbrook** New South Wales, SE Australia
27 V5 **Belle** Missouri, C USA
21 Q5 **Belle** West Virginia, NE USA
31 R13 **Bellefontaine** Ohio, N USA
18 F14 **Bellefonte** Pennsylvania, NE USA
28 J9 **Belle Fourche** South Dakota, N USA
28 J9 **Belle Fourche Reservoir** ▣ South Dakota, N USA
28 K9 **Belle Fourche River** ≈ South Dakota/Wyoming, N USA
103 S10 **Bellegarde-sur-Valserine** Ain, E France
23 Y14 **Belle Glade** Florida, SE USA
102 G8 **Belle Île** island NW France
13 T9 **Belle Isle** island Belle Isle, Newfoundland, E Canada
13 S10 **Belle Isle, Strait of** strait Newfoundland, E Canada
Bellenz see Bellinzona
29 W14 **Belle Plaine** Iowa, C USA
29 V9 **Belle Plaine** Minnesota, N USA
14 I9 **Belleterre** Quebec, SE Canada
14 J15 **Belleville** Ontario, SE Canada
103 R10 **Belleville** Rhône, E France
30 K15 **Belleville** Illinois, N USA
27 N3 **Belleville** Kansas, C USA
29 Z13 **Bellevue** Iowa, C USA
29 S15 **Bellevue** Nebraska, C USA
31 S11 **Bellevue** Ohio, N USA
25 S5 **Bellevue** Texas, SW USA
32 H8 **Bellevue** Washington, NW USA
55 Y11 **Bellevue de l'Inini, Montagnes** ▲▲ S French Guiana
103 S11 **Belley** Ain, E France
Bellin see Kangirsuk
183 V6 **Bellingen** New South Wales, SE Australia
97 L14 **Bellingham** N England, UK
32 H6 **Bellingham** Washington, NW USA
Belling Hausen Mulde see Southeast Pacific Basin
194 H2 **Bellingshausen** Russian research station South Shetland Islands, Antarctica
Bellingshausen see Motu One
Bellingshausen Abyssal Plain see Bellingshausen Plain
196 R14 **Bellingshausen Plain** var. Bellingshausen Abyssal Plain. undersea feature SE Pacific Ocean
194 I8 **Bellingshausen Sea** sea Antarctica
98 P6 **Bellingwolde** Groningen, NE Netherlands
108 H11 **Bellinzona** Ger. Bellenz. Ticino, S Switzerland
25 T8 **Bellmead** Texas, SW USA
54 E8 **Bello** Antioquia, W Colombia
61 B21 **Bellocq** Buenos Aires, E Argentina
Bello Horizonte see Belo Horizonte
186 L10 **Bellona** var. Mungiki. island S Solomon Islands
Bellovacum see Beauvais
182 D7 **Bell, Point** headland South Australia
20 F9 **Bells** Tennessee, S USA
25 U5 **Bells** Texas, SW USA
92 N3 **Bellsund** inlet SW Svalbard
106 H6 **Belluno** Veneto, NE Italy
62 L11 **Bell Ville** Córdoba, C Argentina
83 E26 **Bellville** Western Cape, SW South Africa
25 U11 **Bellville** Texas, SW USA
104 L12 **Belmez** Andalucía, S Spain
29 V12 **Belmond** Iowa, C USA
18 E11 **Belmont** New York, NE USA
21 R10 **Belmont** North Carolina, SE USA
59 O18 **Belmonte** Bahia, E Brazil
104 I8 **Belmonte** Castelo Branco, C Portugal
105 P10 **Belmonte** Castilla-La Mancha, C Spain
42 G2 **Belmopan** ● (Belize) Cayo, C Belize
97 B16 **Belmullet** Ir. Béal an Mhuirhead. W Ireland
123 R13 **Belogorsk** Amurskaya Oblast', SE Russian Federation
Belogorsk see Bilohirs'k
114 F7 **Belogradchik** Vidin, NW Bulgaria
172 H8 **Beloha** Toliara, S Madagascar
59 M20 **Belo Horizonte** prev. Bello Horizonte. state capital Minas Gerais, SE Brazil
26 M3 **Beloit** Kansas, C USA
30 L9 **Beloit** Wisconsin, N USA
Belokorovichi see Bilokorovychi
126 J8 **Belomorsk** Respublika Kareliya, NW Russian Federation
126 J8 **Belomorsko-Baltiyskiy Kanal** Eng. White Sea-Baltic Canal, White Sea Canal. canal NW Russian Federation
153 V15 **Belonia** Tripura, NE India
Belopol'ye see Bilopillya
105 O4 **Belorado** Castilla-León, N Spain
128 L14 **Belorechensk** Krasnodarskiy Kray, SW Russian Federation
129 W5 **Beloretsk** Respublika Bashkortostan, W Russian Federation
Belorussia/Belorussian SSR see Belarus
Belorusskaya Gryada see Byelaruskaya Hrada
Belorusskaya SSR see Belarus
Beloshchel'ye see Nar'yan-Mar
114 N8 **Beloslav** Varna, E Bulgaria
Belostok see Białystok
172 H5 **Belo Tsiribihina** var. Belo-sur-Tsiribihina. Toliara, W Madagascar
Belovár see Bjelovar
Belovezhskaya Pushcha see Białowieska, Puszcza/Byelavyezhskaya Pushcha
114 H10 **Belovo** Pazardzhik, C Bulgaria
Belovodsk see Bilovods'k
122 H9 **Beloyarskiy** Khanty-Mansiyskiy Avtonomnyy Okrug, N Russian Federation
126 K7 **Beloye More** Eng. White Sea. sea NW Russian Federation
126 K13 **Beloye, Ozero** ◎ NW Russian Federation
114 J10 **Belozem** Plovdiv, C Bulgaria
126 K13 **Belozërsk** Vologodskaya Oblast', NW Russian Federation
99 E20 **Belœil** Hainaut, SW Belgium
108 D8 **Belp** Bern, W Switzerland
108 D8 **Belp** ✕ (Bern) Bern, C Switzerland
107 L24 **Belpasso** Sicilia, Italy, C Mediterranean Sea
31 U14 **Belpre** Ohio, N USA
98 M8 **Belterwijde** ◎ N Netherlands
27 R4 **Belton** Missouri, C USA
21 P11 **Belton** South Carolina, SE USA
25 T9 **Belton** Texas, SW USA
25 S9 **Belton Lake** ▣ Texas, SW USA
Bel'tsy see Bălţi
97 E16 **Belturbet** Ir. Béal Tairbirt. N Ireland
Beluchistan see Baluchistān
145 Z9 **Belukha, Gora** ▲ Kazakhstan/Russian Federation
107 M20 **Belvedere Marittimo** Calabria, SW Italy
30 L10 **Belvidere** Illinois, N USA
18 J14 **Belvidere** New Jersey, NE USA
Bely see Belyy
129 V8 **Belyayevka** Orenburgskaya Oblast', W Russian Federation
Belynichi see Byalynichy
126 H17 **Belyy** var. Bely, Beyj. Tverskaya Oblast', W Russian Federation
128 I6 **Belyye Berega** Bryanskaya Oblast', W Russian Federation
122 J6 **Belyy, Ostrov** island N Russian Federation
122 J11 **Belyy Yar** Tomskaya Oblast', C Russian Federation
100 N13 **Belzig** Brandenburg, NE Germany
22 K4 **Belzoni** Mississippi, S USA
172 H4 **Bemaraha** var. Plateau du Bemaraha. ▲▲ W Madagascar
82 B10 **Bembe** Uíge, NW Angola
77 S14 **Bembèrèkè** var. Bimbéréké. N Benin
104 K12 **Bembézar** ≈ SW Spain
104 J3 **Bembibre** Castilla-León, N Spain
29 T4 **Bemidji** Minnesota, N USA
98 L12 **Bemmel** Gelderland, SE Netherlands
171 T13 **Bemu** Pulau Seram, E Indonesia
Benāb see Bonāb
105 T5 **Benabarre** var. Benavarn. Aragón, NE Spain
Benaco see Garda, Lago di
79 L20 **Bena-Dibele** Kasai Oriental, C Dem. Rep. Congo (Zaire)
105 R9 **Benageber, Embalse de** ▣ E Spain
183 O11 **Benalla** Victoria, SE Australia
104 M14 **Benamejí** Andalucía, S Spain
Benares see Vārānasi
Benavarn see Benabarre
104 F10 **Benavente** Santarém, C Portugal
104 K5 **Benavente** Castilla-León, N Spain
25 S15 **Benavides** Texas, SW USA
96 F8 **Benbecula** island NW Scotland, UK
Bencovazzo see Benkovac
32 H13 **Bend** Oregon, NW USA
182 K7 **Benda Range** ▲▲ South Australia
183 T6 **Bendemeer** New South Wales, SE Australia
Bender see Tighina
Bender Beila/Bender Beyla see Bandarbeyla
Bender Cassim/Bender Qaasim see Boosaaso
Bendery see Tighina
183 N11 **Bendigo** Victoria, SE Australia
118 E10 **Bēne** Dobele, SW Latvia
98 K13 **Beneden-Leeuwen** Gelderland, C Netherlands
101 L24 **Benediktenwand** ▲ S Germany
Benemérita de San Cristóbal see San Cristóbal
77 N12 **Bénéna** Ségou, S Mali
172 I7 **Benenitra** Toliara, S Madagascar
Beneschau see Benešov
Beneški Zaliv see Venice, Gulf of
111 D17 **Benešov** Ger. Beneschau. Středočeský Kraj, W Czech Republic
123 Q5 **Benetta, Ostrov** island Novosibirskiye Ostrova, NE Russian Federation
107 L17 **Benevento** anc. Beneventum, Malventum. Campania, S Italy
Beneventum see Benevento
173 S3 **Bengal, Bay of** bay N Indian Ocean
79 M17 **Bengamisa** Orientale, N Dem. Rep. Congo (Zaire)
Bengasi see Banghāzī
Bengazi see Banghāzī
161 P7 **Bengbu** var. Peng-pu. Anhui, E China
32 L9 **Benge** Washington, NW USA
Benghazi see Banghāzī
168 K10 **Bengkalis** Pulau Bengkalis, W Indonesia
168 K10 **Bengkalis, Pulau** island W Indonesia
169 Q10 **Bengkayang** Borneo, C Indonesia
Bengkoelen/Bengkoeloe see Bengkulu
168 K14 **Bengkulu** prev. Bengkoeloe, Benkoelen, Benkulen. Sumatera, W Indonesia
168 J13 **Bengkulu** off. Propinsi Bengkulu; prev. Bengkoelen, Benkoelen, Benkulen. ◈ province W Indonesia
82 A11 **Bengo** ◈ province W Angola
95 J16 **Bengtsfors** Västra Götaland, S Sweden
82 B13 **Benguela** var. Benguella. Benguela, W Angola
83 A14 **Benguela** ◈ province W Angola
Benguella see Benguela
Bengweulu, Lake see Bangweulu, Lake
121 V13 **Benha** var. Banhā. N Egypt
192 F6 **Benham Seamount** undersea feature W Philippine Sea
96 H6 **Ben Hope** ▲ N Scotland, UK
79 P18 **Beni** Nord Kivu, NE Dem. Rep. Congo (Zaire)
57 L15 **Beni** var. El Beni. ◈ department N Bolivia
74 H8 **Beni Abbès** W Algeria
105 T8 **Benicarló** País Valenciano, E Spain
105 T9 **Benicasim** País Valenciano, E Spain
105 T12 **Benidorm** País Valenciano, SE Spain
75 W9 **Beni Mazâr** var. Banī Mazār. C Egypt
120 C11 **Beni-Mellal** C Morocco
77 R14 **Benin** off. Republic of Benin; prev. Dahomey. ◆ republic W Africa
77 S17 **Benin, Bight of** gulf W Africa
77 U16 **Benin City** Edo, SW Nigeria
57 K16 **Beni, Río** ≈ N Bolivia
120 F10 **Beni Saf** var. Beni-Saf. NW Algeria
80 H12 **Benishangul** ◈ region W Ethiopia
105 T11 **Benissa** País Valenciano, E Spain
121 V14 **Beni Suef** var. Banī Suwayf. N Egypt
11 V15 **Benito** Manitoba, S Canada
Benito see Uolo, Río
61 C23 **Benito Juárez** Buenos Aires, E Argentina
41 P14 **Benito Juaréz Internacional** ✕ (México) México, S Mexico
25 P5 **Benjamin** Texas, SW USA
58 B13 **Benjamin Constant** Amazonas, N Brazil
40 F4 **Benjamín Hill** Sonora, NW Mexico
63 F19 **Benjamín, Isla** island Archipiélago de los Chonos, S Chile
165 Q4 **Benkei-misaki** headland Hokkaidō, NE Japan
28 L17 **Benkelman** Nebraska, C USA
96 I7 **Ben Klibreck** ▲ N Scotland, UK
Benkoelen see Bengkulu
112 D13 **Benkovac** It. Bencovazzo. Zadar, SW Croatia
Benkulen see Bengkulu
96 I11 **Ben Lawers** ▲ C Scotland, UK
96 J9 **Ben Macdui** var. Beinn MacDuibh. ▲ C Scotland, UK
96 G11 **Ben More** ▲ W Scotland, UK
96 I11 **Ben More** ▲ C Scotland, UK
96 H7 **Ben More Assynt** ▲ N Scotland, UK
185 E20 **Benmore, Lake** ◎ South Island, NZ
98 L12 **Bennekom** Gelderland, SE Netherlands
21 T11 **Bennettsville** South Carolina, SE USA
96 H10 **Ben Nevis** ▲ N Scotland, UK
184 M9 **Benneydale** Waikato, North Island, NZ
Bennichab see Bennichchâb
76 H8 **Bennichchâb** var. Bennichab. Inchiri, W Mauritania
18 L10 **Bennington** Vermont, NE USA
185 E20 **Ben Ohau Range** ▲▲ South Island, NZ
83 J21 **Benoni** Gauteng, NE South Africa
172 J2 **Be, Nosy** var. Nossi-Bé. island NW Madagascar
Bénoué see Benue
42 F2 **Benque Viejo del Carmen** Cayo, W Belize
101 G19 **Bensheim** Hessen, W Germany
37 N16 **Benson** Arizona, SW USA
29 S8 **Benson** Minnesota, N USA
21 U10 **Benson** North Carolina, SE USA
171 N15 **Benteng** Pulau Selayar, C Indonesia
83 A14 **Bentiaba** Namibe, SW Angola
181 T4 **Bentinck Island** island Wellesley Islands, Queensland, N Australia
80 E13 **Bentiu** Wahda, S Sudan
138 G8 **Bent Jbaïl** var. Bint Jubayl. S Lebanon
11 Q15 **Bentley** Alberta, SW Canada
61 I15 **Bento Gonçalves** Rio Grande do Sul, S Brazil
27 U12 **Benton** Arkansas, C USA
30 L16 **Benton** Illinois, N USA
20 H7 **Benton** Kentucky, S USA
22 G5 **Benton** Louisiana, S USA
27 Y7 **Benton** Missouri, C USA
20 M10 **Benton** Tennessee, S USA
31 O10 **Benton Harbor** Michigan, N USA
27 S9 **Bentonville** Arkansas, C USA
77 V16 **Benue** ◈ state SE Nigeria
78 F13 **Benue** Fr. Bénoué. ≈ Cameroon/Nigeria
163 V12 **Benxi** prev. Pen-ch'i, Penhsihu, Penki. Liaoning, NE China
Benyakoni see Byenyakoni
112 K10 **Beočin** Serbia, N Yugoslavia
Beodericsworth see Bury St Edmunds
112 M11 **Beograd** Eng. Belgrade, Ger. Belgrad; anc. Singidunum. ● (Yugoslavia) Serbia, N Yugoslavia
112 L11 **Beograd** Eng. Belgrade. ✕ Serbia, N Yugoslavia
76 M16 **Béoumi** C Ivory Coast
35 V3 **Beowawe** Nevada, W USA
164 E14 **Beppu** Ōita, Kyūshū, SW Japan
187 X15 **Beqa** prev. Mbengga. island W Fiji
Beqa Barrier Reef see Kavukavu Reef
45 Y14 **Bequia** island C Saint Vincent and the Grenadines
113 L16 **Berane** prev. Ivangrad. Montenegro, SW Yugoslavia
113 L21 **Berat** var. Berati, SCr. Beligrad. Berat, C Albania
113 L21 **Berat** ◈ district C Albania
Berătău see Berettyó
Berati see Berat
Beraun see Berounka, Czech Republic
Beraun see Beroun, Czech Republic
171 U13 **Berau, Teluk** var. MacCluer Gulf. bay Irian Jaya, E Indonesia
80 G8 **Berber** River Nile, NE Sudan
80 N12 **Berbera** Woqooyi Galbeed, NW Somalia
79 H16 **Berbérati** Mambéré-Kadéï, SW Central African Republic
Berberia, Cabo de see Barbaria, Cap de
55 T9 **Berbice River** ≈ NE Guyana
Berchid see Berrechid
103 N2 **Berck-Plage** Pas-de-Calais, N France
25 T13 **Berclair** Texas, SW USA
117 W10 **Berda** ≈ SE Ukraine
Berdichev see Berdychiv
123 P10 **Berdigestyakh** Respublika Sakha (Yakutiya), NE Russian Federation
122 J12 **Berdsk** Novosibirskaya Oblast', C Russian Federation
117 W10 **Berdyans'k** Rus. Berdyansk; prev. Osipenko. Zaporiz'ka Oblast', SE Ukraine
117 W10 **Berdyans'ka Kosa** spit SE Ukraine
117 V10 **Berdyans'ka Zatoka** gulf S Ukraine
117 N5 **Berdychiv** Rus. Berdichev. Zhytomyrs'ka Oblast', N Ukraine
20 M6 **Berea** Kentucky, S USA
Beregovo/Beregszász see Berehove
116 G8 **Berehove** Cz. Berehovo, Hung. Beregszász, Rus. Beregovo. Zakarpats'ka Oblast', W Ukraine
Berehovo see Berehove
186 D8 **Bereina** Central, S PNG
45 O12 **Berekua** S Dominica
77 O16 **Berekum** W Ghana
75 Y11 **Berenice** var. Mînâ Baranîs. SE Egypt
9 O14 **Berens** ≈ Manitoba/Ontario, C Canada
11 X14 **Berens River** Manitoba, C Canada
29 R12 **Beresford** South Dakota, N USA
116 J4 **Berestechko** Volyns'ka Oblast', NW Ukraine
116 M11 **Bereşti** Galaţi, E Romania
117 U6 **Berestova** ≈ E Ukraine
Beretău see Berettyó
111 N23 **Berettyó** Rom. Barcău; prev. Berătău, Beretău. ≈ Hungary/Romania
111 N23 **Berettyóújfalu** Hajdú-Bihar, E Hungary
Berëza/Bereza Kartuska see Byaroza
117 Q4 **Berezan'** Kyyivs'ka Oblast', N Ukraine
117 Q10 **Berezanka** Mykolayivs'ka Oblast', S Ukraine
116 J6 **Berezhany** Pol. Brzeżany. Ternopil's'ka Oblast', W Ukraine
Berezina see Byerezino
Berezino see Byarezina
117 P10 **Berezivka** Rus. Berezovka. Odes'ka Oblast', SW Ukraine
117 Q2 **Berezna** Chernihivs'ka Oblast', NE Ukraine
116 L3 **Berezne** Rivnens'ka Oblast', NW Ukraine
117 R9 **Bereznehuvate** Mykolayivs'ka Oblast', S Ukraine
127 N10 **Bereznik** Arkhangel'skaya Oblast', NW Russian Federation
127 U13 **Berezniki** Permskaya Oblast', NW Russian Federation
Berezovka see Berezivka
122 H9 **Berezovo** Khanty-Mansiyskiy Avtonomnyy Okrug, N Russian Federation
129 O9 **Berezovskaya** Volgogradskaya Oblast', SW Russian Federation
123 S13 **Berezovyy** Khabarovskiy Kray, E Russian Federation
83 E25 **Berg** ≈ W South Africa
Berg see Berg bei Rohrbach
105 V4 **Berga** Cataluña, NE Spain
95 N20 **Berga** Kalmar, S Sweden
136 B13 **Bergama** İzmir, W Turkey
106 E7 **Bergamo** anc. Bergomum. Lombardia, N Italy
105 P3 **Bergara** País Vasco, N Spain
109 S3 **Berg bei Rohrbach** var. Berg. Oberösterreich, N Austria
100 O6 **Bergen** Mecklenburg-Vorpommern, NE Germany
101 I11 **Bergen** Niedersachsen, NW Germany
98 H8 **Bergen** Noord-Holland, NW Netherlands
94 C13 **Bergen** Hordaland, S Norway
Bergen see Mons
55 W9 **Berg en Dal** Brokopondo, C Suriname
99 G15 **Bergen op Zoom** Noord-Brabant, S Netherlands
102 L13 **Bergerac** Dordogne, SW France
99 J16 **Bergeyk** Noord-Brabant, S Netherlands
101 D16 **Bergheim** Nordrhein-Westfalen, W Germany
55 X10 **Bergi** Sipaliwini, E Suriname
101 E16 **Bergisch Gladbach** Nordrhein-Westfalen, W Germany
101 F14 **Bergkamen** Nordrhein-Westfalen, W Germany
95 N21 **Bergkvara** Kalmar, S Sweden
Bergomum see Bergamo
98 K13 **Bergse Maas** ≈ S Netherlands
95 P15 **Bergshamra** Stockholm, C Sweden
94 N10 **Bergsjö** Gävleborg, C Sweden
93 J14 **Bergsviken** Norrbotten, N Sweden
98 L6 **Bergum** Fris. Burgum. Friesland, N Netherlands
98 M6 **Bergumer Meer** ◎ N Netherlands
94 N12 **Bergviken** ◎ C Sweden
168 M11 **Berhala, Selat** strait Sumatera, W Indonesia
Berhampore see Baharampur
123 W9 **Beringa, Ostrov** island E Russian Federation
99 J17 **Beringen** Limburg, NE Belgium
39 T12 **Bering Glacier** glacier Alaska, USA
Beringov Proliv see Bering Strait
123 W6 **Beringovskiy** Chukotskiy Avtonomnyy Okrug, NE Russian Federation

◆ Country ● Country Capital ◇ Dependent Territory ○ Dependent Territory Capital ◈ Administrative Region ✕ International Airport ▲ Mountain ▲▲ Mountain Range ⩙ Volcano ≈ River ◎ Lake ▣ Reservoir

192 L2 **Bering Sea** *sea* N Pacific Ocean
38 L9 **Bering Strait** *Rus.* Beringov Proliv. *strait* Bering Sea/Chukchi Sea
Berislav *see* Beryslav
105 O15 **Berja** Andalucía, S Spain
94 H9 **Berkåk** Sør-Trøndelag, S Norway
98 N11 **Berkel** ≈ Germany/Netherlands
35 N8 **Berkeley** California, W USA
65 E24 **Berkeley Sound** *sound* NE Falkland Islands
21 V2 **Berkeley Springs** *var.* Bath. West Virginia, NE USA
195 N6 **Berkner Island** *island* Antarctica
114 G8 **Berkovitsa** Montana, NW Bulgaria
97 M22 **Berkshire** *cultural region* S England, UK
99 H17 **Berlaar** Antwerpen, N Belgium
Berlanga *see* Berlanga de Duero
105 P6 **Berlanga de Duero** *var.* Berlanga. Castilla-León, N Spain
(0) I16 **Berlanga Rise** *undersea feature* E Pacific Ocean
99 F17 **Berlare** Oost-Vlaanderen, NW Belgium
104 E9 **Berlenga, Ilha da** *island* C Portugal
92 M7 **Berlevåg** Finnmark, N Norway
100 O12 **Berlin** ● (Germany) Berlin, NE Germany
21 Z4 **Berlin** Maryland, NE USA
19 O7 **Berlin** New Hampshire, NE USA
18 D16 **Berlin** Pennsylvania, NE USA
30 L7 **Berlin** Wisconsin, N USA
100 O12 **Berlin** ◈ *state* NE Germany
Berlinchen *see* Barlinek
31 U12 **Berlin Lake** ▣ Ohio, N USA
183 R11 **Bermagui** New South Wales, SE Australia
40 L8 **Bermejillo** Durango, C Mexico
62 M6 **Bermejo (viejo), Río** ≈ N Argentina
62 L5 **Bermejo, Río** ≈ N Argentina
62 I10 **Bermejo, Río** ≈ W Argentina
105 P2 **Bermeo** País Vasco, N Spain
104 K6 **Bermillo de Sayago** Castilla-León, N Spain
106 E6 **Bermina, Pizzo** *Rmsch.* Piz Bernina. ▲ Italy/Switzerland *see also* Bernina, Piz
64 A12 **Bermuda** *var.* Bermuda Islands, Bermudas; *prev.* Somers Islands. ◇ *UK crown colony* NW Atlantic Ocean
1 N11 **Bermuda** *var.* Great Bermuda, Long Island, Main Island. *island* Bermuda
Bermuda Islands *see* Bermuda
Bermuda-New England Seamount Arc *see* New England Seamounts
1 N11 **Bermuda Rise** *undersea feature* C Sargasso Sea
Bermudas *see* Bermuda
108 D8 **Bern** *Fr.* Berne. ● (Switzerland) Bern, W Switzerland
108 D9 **Bern** *Fr.* Berne. ◈ *canton* W Switzerland
37 R11 **Bernalillo** New Mexico, SW USA
14 H12 **Bernard Lake** ◎ Ontario, S Canada
61 B18 **Bernardo de Irigoyen** Santa Fe, NE Argentina
18 J14 **Bernardsville** New Jersey, NE USA
63 K14 **Bernasconi** La Pampa, C Argentina
100 O12 **Bernau** Brandenburg, NE Germany
102 L4 **Bernay** Eure, N France
101 L14 **Bernburg** Sachsen-Anhalt, C Germany
109 X5 **Berndorf** Niederösterreich, NE Austria
31 Q12 **Berne** Indiana, N USA
Berne *see* Bern
108 D10 **Berner Alpen** *var.* Berner Oberland, *Eng.* Bernese Oberland. ▲ SW Switzerland
Berner Oberland/Bernese Oberland *see* Berner Alpen
109 Y2 **Bernhardsthal** Niederösterreich, N Austria
22 H4 **Bernice** Louisiana, S USA
27 Y8 **Bernie** Missouri, C USA
180 G9 **Bernier Island** *island* Western Australia
Bernina Pass *see* Bernina, Passo del
108 J10 **Bernina, Passo del** *Eng.* Bernina Pass. *pass* SE Switzerland
108 J10 **Bernina, Piz** *It.* Pizzo Bernina. ▲ Italy/Switzerland *see also* Bermina, Pizzo
99 E20 **Bernissart** Hainaut, SW Belgium
101 E18 **Bernkastel-Kues** Rheinland-Pfalz, W Germany
Beroea *see* Ḥalab
172 H6 **Beroroha** Toliara, SW Madagascar
Béroubouay *see* Gbéroubouè
111 C17 **Beroun** *Ger.* Beraun. Středočeský Kraj, W Czech Republic
111 C16 **Berounka** *Ger.* Beraun. ≈ W Czech Republic
113 Q18 **Berovo** E FYR Macedonia
74 F6 **Berrechid** *var.* Berchid. W Morocco
103 R15 **Berre, Étang de** ◎ SE France
103 S15 **Berre-l'Étang** Bouches-du-Rhône, SE France
182 K9 **Berri** South Australia
31 O10 **Berrien Springs** Michigan, N USA
183 O10 **Berrigan** New South Wales, SE Australia
103 N9 **Berry** *cultural region* C France
35 N7 **Berryessa, Lake** ◎ California, W USA
44 G2 **Berry Islands** *island group* N Bahamas
27 T9 **Berryville** Arkansas, C USA
21 V3 **Berryville** Virginia, NE USA
83 D21 **Berseba** Karas, S Namibia
117 O8 **Bershad'** Vinnyts'ka Oblast', C Ukraine
28 L3 **Berthold** North Dakota, N USA
37 T3 **Berthoud** Colorado, C USA
37 S4 **Berthoud Pass** *pass* Colorado, C USA
79 F15 **Bertoua** Est, E Cameroon
25 S10 **Bertram** Texas, SW USA
63 G22 **Bertrand, Cerro** ▲ S Argentina
99 J23 **Bertrix** Luxembourg, SE Belgium
191 P3 **Beru** *var.* Peru. *atoll* Tungaru, W Kiribati
Beruni *see* Beruniy
146 I9 **Beruniy** *var.* Biruni, *Rus.* Beruni. Qoraqalpoghiston Respublikasi, W Uzbekistan
58 F13 **Beruri** Amazonas, NW Brazil
18 H14 **Berwick** Pennsylvania, NE USA
96 K12 **Berwick** *cultural region* SE Scotland, UK
96 L12 **Berwick-upon-Tweed** N England, UK
117 S10 **Beryslav** *Rus.* Berislav. Khersons'ka Oblast', S Ukraine
Berytus *see* Beyrouth
172 H4 **Besalampy** Mahajanga, W Madagascar
103 T8 **Besançon** *anc.* Besontium, Vesontio. Doubs, E France
103 P10 **Besbre** ≈ C France
Bescanuova *see* Baška
Besdan *see* Bezdan
Besed' *see* Byesyedz'
147 R10 **Beshariq** *Rus.* Besharyk; *prev.* Kirovo. Farghona Wiloyati, E Uzbekistan
Besharyk *see* Beshariq
146 L9 **Beshbuloq** *Rus.* Beshulak. Nawoiy Wiloyati, N Uzbekistan
Beshenkovichi *see* Byeshankovichy
146 M13 **Beshkent** Qashqadaryo Wiloyati, S Uzbekistan
Beshulak *see* Beshbuloq
112 L10 **Beška** Serbia, N Yugoslavia
Beskra *see* Biskra
129 O16 **Beslan** Respublika Severnaya Osetiya, SW Russian Federation
113 P16 **Besna Kobila** ▲ SE Yugoslavia
137 N16 **Besni** Adıyaman, S Turkey
Besontium *see* Besançon
121 Q2 **Beşparmak Dağları** *Eng.* Kyrenia Mountains. ▲ N Cyprus
Bessarabka *see* Basarabeasca
92 O2 **Bessels, Kapp** *headland* C Svalbard
23 P4 **Bessemer** Alabama, S USA
30 K3 **Bessemer** Michigan, N USA
21 Q10 **Bessemer City** North Carolina, SE USA
102 M10 **Bessines-sur-Gartempe** Haute-Vienne, C France
99 K15 **Best** Noord-Brabant, S Netherlands
25 N9 **Best** Texas, SW USA
127 O11 **Bestuzhevo** Arkhangel'skaya Oblast', NW Russian Federation
123 M11 **Bestyakh** Respublika Sakha (Yakutiya), NE Russian Federation
Beszterce *see* Bistrița
Besztercebánya *see* Banská Bystrica
172 I5 **Betafo** Antananarivo, C Madagascar
104 H2 **Betanzos** Galicia, NW Spain
104 G2 **Betanzos, Ría de** *estuary* NW Spain
79 G15 **Bétaré Oya** Est, E Cameroon
105 S9 **Bétera** País Valenciano, E Spain
77 R15 **Bétérou** C Benin
83 K21 **Bethal** Mpumalanga, NE South Africa
30 K15 **Bethalto** Illinois, N USA
83 D21 **Bethanie** *var.* Bethanien, Bethany. Karas, S Namibia
Bethanien *see* Bethanie
27 S2 **Bethany** Missouri, C USA
27 N10 **Bethany** Oklahoma, C USA
Bethany *see* Bethanie
39 N12 **Bethel** Alaska, USA
19 P7 **Bethel** Maine, NE USA
21 W9 **Bethel** North Carolina, SE USA
18 B15 **Bethel Park** Pennsylvania, NE USA
21 W3 **Bethesda** Maryland, NE USA
83 J22 **Bethlehem** Free State, C South Africa
18 I14 **Bethlehem** Pennsylvania, NE USA
138 F10 **Bethlehem** *Ar.* Bayt Laḥm, *Heb.* Bet Leḥem. C West Bank
Bethlen *see* Beclean
83 I24 **Bethulie** Free State, C South Africa
103 O1 **Béthune** Pas-de-Calais, N France
102 M3 **Béthune** ≈ N France
104 M14 **Béticos, Sistemas** *var.* Sistema Penibético, *Eng.* Baetic Cordillera, Baetic Mountains. ▲ S Spain
54 I6 **Betijoque** Trujillo, NW Venezuela
59 M20 **Betim** Minas Gerais, SE Brazil
190 H3 **Betio** Tarawa, W Kiribati
172 H7 **Betioky** Toliara, S Madagascar
Bet Leḥem *see* Bethlehem
Betlen *see* Beclean
167 O17 **Betong** Yala, SW Thailand
79 I16 **Bétou** La Likouala, N Congo
145 P14 **Betpak-Dala** *Kaz.* Betpaqdala. *plateau* S Kazakhstan
Betpaqdala *see* Betpak-Dala
172 H7 **Betroka** Toliara, S Madagascar
Betschau *see* Bečva
138 G9 **Bet She'an** *Ar.* Baysān, Beisān; *anc.* Scythopolis. Northern, N Israel
15 T6 **Betsiamites** Quebec, SE Canada
15 T6 **Betsiamites** ≈ Quebec, SE Canada
172 I4 **Betsiboka** ≈ N Madagascar
99 M25 **Bettembourg** Luxembourg, S Luxembourg
99 M23 **Bettendorf** Diekirch, NE Luxembourg
29 Z14 **Bettendorf** Iowa, C USA
75 R13 **Bette, Pic** *var.* Bikkū Bīttī, *It.* Picco Bette. ▲ S Libya
Bette, Picco *see* Bette, Pic
153 P12 **Bettiah** Bihār, N India
39 Q7 **Bettles** Alaska, USA
95 N17 **Bettna** Södermanland, C Sweden
154 H11 **Betūl** *prev.* Badnur. Madhya Pradesh, C India
154 H9 **Betwa** ≈ C India
101 F16 **Betzdorf** Rheinland-Pfalz, W Germany
82 C9 **Béu** Uíge, NW Angola
31 P6 **Beulah** Michigan, N USA
28 L5 **Beulah** North Dakota, N USA
98 M8 **Beulakerwijde** ◎ N Netherlands
98 L13 **Beuningen** Gelderland, SE Netherlands
Beuthen *see* Bytom
103 N7 **Beuvron** ≈ C France
99 F16 **Beveren** Oost-Vlaanderen, N Belgium
21 T9 **B.Everett Jordan Reservoir** *var.* Jordan Lake. ▣ North Carolina, SE USA
97 N17 **Beverley** E England, UK
Beverley *see* Beverly
99 J17 **Beverlo** Limburg, NE Belgium
19 P11 **Beverly** Massachusetts, NE USA
32 J9 **Beverly** *var.* Beverley. Washington, NW USA
35 S15 **Beverly Hills** California, W USA
101 I14 **Beverungen** Nordrhein-Westfalen, C Germany
98 H9 **Beverwijk** Noord-Holland, W Netherlands
108 C10 **Bex** Vaud, W Switzerland
97 P23 **Bexhill** *var.* Bexhill-on-Sea. SE England, UK
Bexhill-on-Sea *see* Bexhill
136 E17 **Bey Dağları** ▲ SW Turkey
Beyj *see* Belyy
136 E10 **Beykoz** İstanbul, NW Turkey
76 K15 **Beyla** Guinée-Forestière, SE Guinea
137 X12 **Beyläqan** *prev.* Zhdanov. SW Azerbaijan
80 L10 **Beylul** *var.* Beilul. SE Eritrea
144 H14 **Beyneu** *Kaz.* Beyneū. Mangistau, SW Kazakhstan
Beyneū *see* Beyneu
165 X14 **Beyonēsu-retsugan** *Eng.* Bayonnaise Rocks. *island group* SE Japan
136 G12 **Beypazarı** Ankara, NW Turkey
155 F21 **Beypore** Kerala, SW India
138 G7 **Beyrouth** *var.* Bayrūt, *Eng.* Beirut; *anc.* Berytus. ● (Lebanon) W Lebanon
138 G7 **Beyrouth** ✕ W Lebanon
136 G15 **Beyşehir** Konya, SW Turkey
136 G15 **Beyşehir Gölü** ◎ C Turkey
108 J7 **Bezau** Vorarlberg, NW Austria
112 J8 **Bezdan** *Ger.* Besdan, *Hung.* Bezdán. Serbia, NW Yugoslavia
Bezdezh *see* Byezdzyezh
126 G15 **Bezhanitsy** Pskovskaya Oblast', W Russian Federation
126 K15 **Bezhetsk** Tverskaya Oblast', W Russian Federation
103 P16 **Béziers** *anc.* Baeterrae, Baeterrae Septimanorum, Julia Beterrae. Hérault, S France
Bezmein *see* Byuzmeyin
Bezwada *see* Vijayawāda
154 P12 **Bhadrak** *var.* Bhadrakh. Orissa, E India
Bhadrakh *see* Bhadrak
155 F19 **Bhadra Reservoir** ▣ SW India
155 F18 **Bhadrāvati** Karnātaka, SW India
153 R14 **Bhāgalpur** Bihār, NE India
Bhairab *see* Bhairab Bazar
153 U14 **Bhairab Bazar** *var.* Bhairab. Dhaka, C Bangladesh
153 O11 **Bhairahawa** Western, S Nepal
149 S8 **Bhakkar** Punjab, E Pakistan
153 P11 **Bhaktapur** Central, C Nepal
167 N3 **Bhamo** *var.* Banmo. Kachin State, N Myanmar
Bhāmragad *see* Bhāmragarh
154 K13 **Bhāmragarh** *var.* Bhāmragad. Mahārāshtra, C India
154 J12 **Bhandāra** Mahārāshtra, C India
Bhārat *see* India
152 J12 **Bharatpur** *prev.* Bhurtpore. Rājasthān, N India
154 D11 **Bharūch** Gujarāt, W India
155 E18 **Bhatkal** Karnātaka, W India
153 O13 **Bhatni** *var.* Bhatni Junction. Uttar Pradesh, N India
Bhatni Junction *see* Bhatni
153 S16 **Bhātpāra** West Bengal, NE India
149 U7 **Bhaun** Punjab, E Pakistan
Bhaunagar *see* Bhāvnagar
154 M13 **Bhavānīpātna** Orissa, E India
155 H21 **Bhavānīsāgar Reservoir** ▣ S India
154 D11 **Bhāvnagar** *prev.* Bhaunagar. Gujarāt, W India
Bheanntraí, Bá *see* Bantry Bay
Bheara, Béal an *see* Gweebarra Bay
154 K12 **Bhilai** Madhya Pradesh, C India
152 G13 **Bhīlwāra** Rājasthān, N India
155 E14 **Bhīma** ≈ S India
155 K16 **Bhīmavaram** Andhra Pradesh, E India
154 I7 **Bhind** Madhya Pradesh, C India
152 E13 **Bhīnmāl** Rājasthān, N India
Bhir *see* Bīd
154 D13 **Bhiwandi** Mahārāshtra, W India
152 H10 **Bhiwāni** Haryāna, N India
152 L13 **Bhognīpur** Uttar Pradesh, N India
153 U16 **Bhola** Khulna, S Bangladesh
154 H10 **Bhopāl** Madhya Pradesh, C India
155 J14 **Bhopālpatnam** Madhya Pradesh, C India
155 E14 **Bhor** Mahārāshtra, W India
154 O12 **Bhubaneshwar** *prev.* Bhubaneswar, Bhuvaneshwar. Orissa, E India
Bhubaneswar *see* Bhubaneshwar
154 B9 **Bhuj** Gujarāt, W India
Bhuket *see* Phuket
Bhurtpore *see* Bharatpur
Bhusawal *see* Bhusāwal
154 G12 **Bhusāwal** *prev.* Bhusaval. Mahārāshtra, C India
153 T12 **Bhutan** *off.* Kingdom of Bhutan, *var.* Druk-yul. ◆ *monarchy* S Asia
Bhuvaneshwar *see* Bhubaneshwar
143 T15 **Bīābān, Kūh-e** ▲ S Iran
77 V18 **Biafra, Bight of** *var.* Bight of Bonny. *bay* W Africa
171 W12 **Biak** Irian Jaya, E Indonesia
171 W12 **Biak, Pulau** *island* E Indonesia
110 P12 **Biała Podlaska** Lubelskie, E Poland
110 F7 **Białogard** *Ger.* Belgard. Zachodniopomorskie, NW Poland
110 P10 **Białowieska, Puszcza** *Bel.* Byelavyezhskaya Pushcha, *Rus.* Belovezhskaya Pushcha. *physical region* Belarus/Poland *see also* Byelavyezhskaya Pushcha
110 G8 **Biały Bór** *Ger.* Baldenburg. Zachodniopomorskie, NW Poland
110 P9 **Białystok** *Rus.* Belostok, Bielostok. Podlaskie, NE Poland
107 L24 **Biancavilla** *prev.* Inessa. Sicilia, Italy, C Mediterranean Sea
Bianco, Monte *see* Blanc, Mont
76 L15 **Biankouma** W Ivory Coast
167 R7 **Bia, Phou** *var.* Pou Bia. ▲ C Laos
Bia, Pou *see* Bia, Phou
143 R5 **Biārjmand** Semnān, N Iran
105 P4 **Biarra** ≈ NE Spain
102 I15 **Biarritz** Pyrénées-Atlantiques, SW France
108 H10 **Biasca** Ticino, S Switzerland
61 E17 **Biassini** Salto, N Uruguay
165 S3 **Bibai** Hokkaidō, NE Japan
83 B15 **Bibala** *Port.* Vila Arriaga. Namibe, SW Angola
104 I4 **Bibéi** ≈ NW Spain
Biberach *see* Biberach an der Riss
101 I23 **Biberach an der Riss** *var.* Biberach, *Ger.* Biberach an der Riß. Baden-Württemberg, S Germany
108 E7 **Biberist** Solothurn, NW Switzerland
77 O16 **Bibiani** SW Ghana
112 C13 **Bibinje** Zadar, SW Croatia
Biblical Gebal *see* Jbaïl
116 I5 **Bibrka** *Pol.* Bóbrka, *Rus.* Bobrka. L'vivs'ka Oblast', NW Ukraine
117 N10 **Bîc** ≈ S Moldova
113 M18 **Bicaj** Kukës, NE Albania
116 K10 **Bicaz** *Hung.* Békás. Neamț, NE Romania
183 Q16 **Bicheno** Tasmania, SE Australia
Bichiş *see* Békés
Bichiş-Ciaba *see* Békéscsaba
Bichitra *see* Phichit
137 P8 **Bichvint'a** *Rus.* Pitsunda. NW Georgia
15 T7 **Bic, Île du** *island* Quebec, SE Canada
32 J10 **Bickleton** Washington, NW USA
36 L6 **Bicknell** Utah, W USA
171 S11 **Bicoli** Pulau Halmahera, E Indonesia
111 J22 **Bicske** Fejér, C Hungary
155 F14 **Bīd** *prev.* Bhir. Mahārāshtra, W India
77 U15 **Bida** Niger, C Nigeria
155 H15 **Bīdar** Karnātaka, C India
141 Y8 **Bidbid** NE Oman
19 P9 **Biddeford** Maine, NE USA
98 L9 **Biddinghuizen** Flevoland, C Netherlands
33 X11 **Biddle** Montana, NW USA
97 J23 **Bideford** SW England, UK
82 D13 **Bié** ◈ *province* C Angola
35 O2 **Bieber** California, W USA
110 O9 **Biebrza** ≈ NE Poland
165 T3 **Biei** Hokkaidō, NE Japan
108 D8 **Biel** *Fr.* Bienne. Bern, W Switzerland
100 G13 **Bielefeld** Nordrhein-Westfalen, NW Germany
108 D8 **Bieler See** *Fr.* Lac de Bienne. ◎ W Switzerland
Bielitz/Bielitz-Biala *see* Bielsko-Biała
106 C7 **Biella** Piemonte, N Italy
Bielostok *see* Białystok
111 J17 **Bielsko-Biała** *Ger.* Bielitz, Bielitz-Biala. Śląskie, S Poland
110 P10 **Bielsk Podlaski** Białystok, E Poland
Bien Bien *see* Điên Biên
Biên Đông *see* South China Sea
9 V17 **Bienfait** Saskatchewan, S Canada
167 T14 **Biên Hoa** Đông Nai, S Vietnam
Bienne *see* Biel
Bienne, Lac de *see* Bieler See
12 K8 **Bienville, Lac** ◎ Quebec, C Canada
82 D13 **Bié, Planalto do** *var.* Bié Plateau. *plateau* C Angola
Bié Plateau *see* Bié, Planalto do
108 B9 **Bière** Vaud, W Switzerland
98 O4 **Bierum** Groningen, NE Netherlands
98 I13 **Biesbos** *var.* Biesbosch. *wetland* S Netherlands
Biesbosch *see* Biesbos
99 H21 **Biesme** Namur, S Belgium
101 H21 **Bietigheim-Bissingen** Baden-Württemberg, SW Germany
99 I23 **Bièvre** Namur, SE Belgium
79 D18 **Bifoun** Moyen-Ogooué, NW Gabon
165 T2 **Bifuka** Hokkaidō, NE Japan
136 C11 **Biga** Çanakkale, NW Turkey
136 C13 **Bigadiç** Balıkesir, W Turkey
26 J7 **Big Basin** *basin* Kansas, C USA
185 B20 **Big Bay** *bay* South Island, NZ
31 O5 **Big Bay de Noc** ◎ Michigan, N USA
31 N3 **Big Bay Point** *headland* Michigan, N USA
33 R10 **Big Belt Mountains** ▲ Montana, NW USA
29 N10 **Big Bend Dam** *dam* South Dakota, N USA
24 K12 **Big Bend National Park** *national park* Texas, S USA
22 K5 **Big Black River** ≈ Mississippi, S USA
27 O3 **Big Blue River** ≈ Kansas/Nebraska, C USA
24 M10 **Big Canyon** ≈ Texas, SW USA
33 N12 **Big Creek** Idaho, NW USA
23 N8 **Big Creek Lake** ▣ Alabama, S USA
23 X15 **Big Cypress Swamp** *wetland* Florida, SE USA
39 S9 **Big Delta** Alaska, USA
30 K6 **Big Eau Pleine Reservoir** ▣ Wisconsin, N USA
19 P5 **Bigelow Mountain** ▲ Maine, NE USA
29 U3 **Big Falls** Minnesota, N USA
33 P8 **Bigfork** Montana, NW USA
29 U3 **Big Fork River** ≈ Minnesota, N USA
11 S15 **Biggar** Saskatchewan, S Canada
180 L3 **Bigge Island** *island* Western Australia
35 O5 **Biggs** California, W USA
32 I11 **Biggs** Oregon, NW USA
14 K13 **Big Gull Lake** ◎ Ontario, SE Canada
37 P16 **Big Hachet Peak** ▲ New Mexico, SW USA
33 P11 **Big Hole River** ≈ Montana, NW USA
33 V13 **Bighorn Basin** *basin* Wyoming, C USA
33 U11 **Bighorn Lake** ◎ Montana/Wyoming, N USA
33 W13 **Bighorn Mountains** ▲ Wyoming, C USA
36 J13 **Big Horn Peak** ▲ Arizona, SW USA
33 V11 **Bighorn River** ≈ Montana/Wyoming, NW USA
9 S7 **Big Island** *island* Nunavut, NE Canada
39 O16 **Big Koniuji Island** *island* Shumagin Islands, Alaska, USA
25 N9 **Big Lake** Texas, SW USA
19 T5 **Big Lake** ◎ Maine, NE USA
30 I3 **Big Manitou Falls** *waterfall* Wisconsin, N USA
35 R2 **Big Mountain** ▲ Nevada, W USA
108 G10 **Bignasco** Ticino, S Switzerland
29 R16 **Big Nemaha River** ≈ Nebraska, C USA
76 G12 **Bignona** SW Senegal
Bigorra *see* Tarbes
Bigosovo *see* Bihosava
35 S10 **Big Pine** California, W USA
35 Q14 **Big Pine Mountain** ▲ California, W USA
27 V6 **Big Piney Creek** ≈ Missouri, C USA
65 M24 **Big Point** *headland* N Tristan da Cunha
31 P8 **Big Rapids** Michigan, N USA
30 K6 **Big Rib River** ≈ Wisconsin, N USA
14 L14 **Big Rideau Lake** ◎ Ontario, SE Canada
11 T14 **Big River** Saskatchewan, C Canada
27 X5 **Big River** ≈ Missouri, C USA
31 N7 **Big Sable Point** *headland* Michigan, N USA
33 S7 **Big Sandy** Montana, NW USA
25 W6 **Big Sandy** Texas, SW USA
37 V5 **Big Sandy Creek** ≈ Colorado, C USA
29 Q16 **Big Sandy Creek** ≈ Nebraska, C USA
29 V5 **Big Sandy Lake** ◎ Minnesota, N USA
36 J11 **Big Sandy River** ≈ Arizona, SW USA
21 P5 **Big Sandy River** ≈ S USA
23 V6 **Big Satilla Creek** ≈ Georgia, SE USA
29 R12 **Big Sioux River** ≈ Iowa/South Dakota, N USA
35 U7 **Big Smoky Valley** *valley* Nevada, W USA
25 N7 **Big Spring** Texas, SW USA
19 Q5 **Big Squaw Mountain** ▲ Maine, NE USA
21 O7 **Big Stone Gap** Virginia, NE USA
29 Q8 **Big Stone Lake** ◎ Minnesota/South Dakota, N USA
22 K4 **Big Sunflower River** ≈ Mississippi, S USA
33 T11 **Big Timber** Montana, NW USA
12 D8 **Big Trout Lake** Ontario, C Canada
14 I12 **Big Trout Lake** ◎ Ontario, SE Canada
35 O2 **Big Valley Mountains** ▲ California, W USA
25 Q13 **Big Wells** Texas, SW USA
14 F11 **Bigwood** Ontario, S Canada
112 D11 **Bihać** Federacija Bosna I Hercegovina, NW Bosnia and Herzegovina
153 P14 **Bihār** *prev.* Behar. ◈ *state* N India
Bihār *see* Bihār Sharīf
81 F20 **Biharamulo** Kagera, NW Tanzania
153 R13 **Bihārīganj** Bihār, NE India
153 P14 **Bihār Sharīf** *var.* Bihār. Bihār, N India
116 F10 **Bihor** ◈ *county* NW Romania
165 V3 **Bihoro** Hokkaidō, NE Japan
118 K11 **Bihosava** *Rus.* Bigosovo. Vitsyebskaya Voblasts', NW Belarus
Bijagos Archipelago *see* Bijagós, Arquipélago dos
76 G13 **Bijagós, Arquipélago dos** *var.* Bijagos Archipelago. *island group* W Guinea-Bissau
155 F16 **Bijāpur** Karnātaka, C India
142 K5 **Bījār** Kordestān, W Iran
112 J11 **Bijeljina** Republika Srpska, NE Bosnia and Herzegovina
113 K15 **Bijelo Polje** Montenegro, SW Yugoslavia
160 I11 **Bijie** Guizhou, S China
152 J10 **Bijnor** Uttar Pradesh, N India
152 F11 **Bikāner** Rājasthān, NW India
189 V3 **Bikar Atoll** *var.* Pikaar. *atoll* Ratak Chain, N Marshall Islands
190 H3 **Bikeman** *atoll* Tungaru, W Kiribati
190 I3 **Bikenebu** Tarawa, W Kiribati
123 S14 **Bikin** Khabarovskiy Kray, SE Russian Federation
123 S14 **Bikin** ≈ SE Russian Federation
189 R3 **Bikini Atoll** *var.* Pikinni. *atoll* Ralik Chain, NW Marshall Islands
83 L17 **Bikita** Masvingo, E Zimbabwe
Bikkū Bīttī *see* Bette, Pic
79 I19 **Bikoro** Equateur, W Dem. Rep. Congo (Zaire)
141 Z9 **Bilād Banī Bū 'Alī** NE Oman
141 Z9 **Bilād Banī Bū Ḥasan** NE Oman
141 X9 **Bilād Manaḥ** *var.* Manaḥ. NE Oman
77 Q12 **Bilanga** C Burkina
152 F12 **Bilāra** Rājasthān, N India
152 K10 **Bilāri** Uttar Pradesh, N India
138 J5 **Bil'ās, Jabal al** ▲ C Syria
152 I8 **Bilāspur** Himāchal Pradesh, N India
154 L11 **Bilāspur** Madhya Pradesh, C India
168 J9 **Bila, Sungai** ≈ Sumatera, W Indonesia
137 Y13 **Biläsuvar** *Rus.* Bilyasuvar; *prev.* Pushkino. SE Azerbaijan
117 O5 **Bila Tserkva** *Rus.* Belaya Tserkov'. Kyyivs'ka Oblast', N Ukraine
167 N11 **Bilauktaung Range** *var.* Thanintari Taungdan. ▲ Myanmar/Thailand
105 O2 **Bilbao** *Basq.* Bilbo. País Vasco, N Spain
Bilbo *see* Bilbao
92 H2 **Bíldudalur** Vestfirdhir, NW Iceland
113 I16 **Bileća** Republika Srpska, S Bosnia and Herzegovina
136 E12 **Bilecik** Bilecik, NW Turkey
136 F12 **Bilecik** ◈ *province* NW Turkey
116 E11 **Biled** *Ger.* Billed, *Hung.* Billéd. Timiș, W Romania
111 O15 **Biłgoraj** Lubelskie, E Poland
117 P11 **Bilhorod-Dnistrovs'kyy** *Rus.* Belgorod-Dnestrovskiy, *Rom.* Cetatea Albă; *prev.* Akkerman, *anc.* Tyras. Odes'ka Oblast', SW Ukraine
79 M16 **Bili** Orientale, N Dem. Rep. Congo (Zaire)
123 T6 **Bilibino** Chukotskiy Avtonomnyy Okrug, NE Russian Federation
166 M8 **Bilin** Mon State, S Myanmar
113 N21 **Bilisht** *var.* Bilishti. Korçë, SE Albania
Bilishti *see* Bilisht
183 N10 **Billabong Creek** *var.* Moulamein Creek. *seasonal river* New South Wales, SE Australia
182 G4 **Billa Kalina** South Australia
197 Q17 **Bill Baileys Bank** *undersea feature* N Atlantic Ocean
Billed/Billéd *see* Biled
153 N14 **Billi** Uttar Pradesh, N India
97 M15 **Billingham** N England, UK
33 U11 **Billings** Montana, NW USA
95 J16 **Billingsfors** Västra Götaland, S Sweden
Bill of Cape Clear, The *see* Clear, Cape
28 L9 **Billsburg** South Dakota, N USA
95 F23 **Billund** Ribe, W Denmark
36 L11 **Bill Williams Mountain** ▲ Arizona, SW USA
36 I12 **Bill Williams River** ≈ Arizona, SW USA
77 Y8 **Bilma** Agadez, NE Niger
77 Y8 **Bilma, Grand Erg de** *desert* NE Niger
181 Y9 **Biloela** Queensland, E Australia
112 G8 **Bilo Gora** ▲ N Croatia
117 U13 **Bilohirs'k** *Rus.* Belogorsk; *prev.* Karasubazar. Respublika Krym, S Ukraine
116 M3 **Bilokorovychi** *Rus.* Belokorovichi. Zhytomyrs'ka Oblast', N Ukraine
117 X5 **Bilokurakine** Luhans'ka Oblast', E Ukraine
117 T3 **Bilopillya** *Rus.* Belopol'ye. Sums'ka Oblast', NE Ukraine
117 Y6 **Bilovods'k** *Rus.* Belovodsk. Luhans'ka Oblast', E Ukraine
22 M9 **Biloxi** Mississippi, S USA
117 R10 **Bilozerka** Khersons'ka Oblast', S Ukraine
117 W7 **Bilozers'ke** Donets'ka Oblast', E Ukraine
98 J11 **Bilthoven** Utrecht, C Netherlands
78 K9 **Biltine** Biltine, E Chad
78 J9 **Biltine** *off.* Préfecture de Biltine. ◈ *prefecture* E Chad
162 D5 **Bilüü** Bayan-Ölgiy, W Mongolia
Bilwi *see* Puerto Cabezas
Bilyasuvar *see* Biläsuvar
117 O11 **Bilyayivka** Odes'ka Oblast', SW Ukraine

99 K18 **Bilzen** Limburg, NE Belgium
Bimbéréké see Bembèrèkè
183 R10 **Bimberi Peak** ▲ New South Wales, SE Australia
77 Q15 **Bimbila** E Ghana
79 I15 **Bimbo** Ombella-Mpoko, SW Central African Republic
44 F2 **Bimini Islands** island group W Bahamas
154 I9 **Bīna** Madhya Pradesh, C India
143 T4 **Bīnālūd, Kūh-e** ▲ NE Iran
99 F20 **Binche** Hainaut, S Belgium
Bindloe Island see Marchena, Isla
83 L16 **Bindura** Mashonaland Central, NE Zimbabwe
105 T5 **Binefar** Aragón, NE Spain
83 J16 **Binga** Matabeleland North, W Zimbabwe
183 T5 **Bingara** New South Wales, SE Australia
101 F18 **Bingen am Rhein** Rheinland-Pfalz, SW Germany
26 M11 **Binger** Oklahoma, C USA
Bingerau see Węgrów
Bin Ghalfān, Jazā'ir see Ḥalāniyāt, Juzur al
19 Q6 **Bingham** Maine, NE USA
18 H11 **Binghamton** New York, NE USA
Bin Ghanīmah, Jabal see Bin Ghunaymah, Jabal
75 P11 **Bin Ghunaymah, Jabal** var. Jabal Bin Ghanīmah. ▲ C Libya
139 U3 **Bingird** NE Iraq
137 P14 **Bingöl** Bingöl, E Turkey
137 P14 **Bingöl** ◆ province E Turkey
161 R6 **Binhai** var. Binhai Xian, Dongkan. Jiangsu, E China
Binhai Xian see Binhai
167 V11 **Binh Đinh** var. An Nhon. Binh Đinh, C Vietnam
167 U10 **Binh Sơn** var. Châu Ô. Quang Ngai, C Vietnam
Binimani see Bintimani
168 I8 **Binjai** Sumatera, W Indonesia
183 R6 **Binnaway** New South Wales, SE Australia
108 E6 **Binningen** Basel-Land, NW Switzerland
168 J8 **Bintang, Banjaran** ▲ Peninsular Malaysia
168 M10 **Bintan, Pulau** island Kepulauan Riau, W Indonesia
76 J14 **Bintimani** var. Binimani. ▲ NE Sierra Leone
Bint Jubayl see Bent Jbaïl
169 S9 **Bintulu** Sarawak, East Malaysia
171 V12 **Bintuni** prev. Steenkool. Irian Jaya, E Indonesia
163 W8 **Bin Xian** Heilongjiang, NE China
160 K14 **Binyang** Guangxi Zhuangzu Zizhiqu, S China
161 Q4 **Binzhou** Shandong, E China
63 G14 **Bío Bío** off. Región del Bío Bío. ◆ region C Chile
63 G14 **Bío Bío, Río** ≈ C Chile
79 C16 **Bioco, Isla de** var. Bioko, Eng. Fernando Po, Sp. Fernando Póo; prev. Macías Nguema Biyogo. island NW Equatorial Guinea
112 D13 **Biograd na Moru** It. Zaravecchia. Zadar, SW Croatia
Bioko see Bioco, Isla de
113 F14 **Biokovo** ▲ S Croatia
Biorra see Birr
Bipontium see Zweibrücken
143 W13 **Bīrag, Kūh-e** ▲ SE Iran
75 O10 **Birāk** var. Brak. C Libya
139 S10 **Bi'r al Islām** C Iraq
154 N11 **Biramitrapur** Orissa, E India
139 T11 **Bi'r an Nişf** S Iraq
78 L12 **Birao** Vakaga, NE Central African Republic
158 M6 **Biratar Bulak** well NW China
153 R12 **Biratnagar** Eastern, SE Nepal
165 R5 **Biratori** Hokkaidō, NE Japan
39 S8 **Birch Creek** Alaska, USA
38 M11 **Birch Creek** ≈ Alaska, USA
11 T14 **Birch Hills** Saskatchewan, S Canada
182 M10 **Birchip** Victoria, SE Australia
29 X4 **Birch Lake** ◎ Minnesota, N USA
11 Q11 **Birch Mountains** ▲ Alberta, W Canada
11 V15 **Birch River** Manitoba, S Canada
44 H12 **Birchs Hill** hill W Jamaica
39 R11 **Birchwood** Alaska, USA
188 I5 **Bird Island** island S Northern Mariana Islands
137 N16 **Birecik** Şanlıurfa, S Turkey
152 M10 **Birendranagar** var. Surkhet. Mid Western, W Nepal
Bir es Saba see Be'ér Sheva'
74 A12 **Bir-Gandouz** SW Western Sahara
153 P12 **Birganj** Central, C Nepal
81 B14 **Biri** ≈ W Sudan
Bi'r Ibn Hirmās see Al Bi'r
143 U8 **Bīrjand** Khorāsān, E Iran
139 T11 **Birkat Ḥāmid** well S Iraq
95 F18 **Birkeland** Aust-Agder, S Norway
101 E19 **Birkenfeld** Rheinland-Pfalz, SW Germany
97 K18 **Birkenhead** NW England, UK
109 W7 **Birkfeld** Steiermark, SE Austria
182 A2 **Birksgate Range** ▲ South Australia
Birlad see Bârlad
97 K20 **Birmingham** C England, UK
23 P4 **Birmingham** Alabama, S USA
97 M20 **Birmingham** × C England, UK
Bir Moghreïn see Bîr Mogreïn
76 J4 **Bîr Mogreïn** var. Bir Moghreïn; prev. Fort-Trinquet. Tiris Zemmour, N Mauritania
191 S4 **Birnie Island** atoll Phoenix Islands, C Kiribati
Birni-Ngaouré see Birnin Gaouré
77 S12 **Birnin Gaouré** var. Birni-Ngaouré. Dosso, SW Niger
77 S12 **Birnin Kebbi** Kebbi, NW Nigeria
Birni-Nkonni see Birnin Konni
77 T12 **Birnin Konni** var. Birni-Nkonni. Tahoua, SW Niger
77 W13 **Birnin Kudu** Jigawa, N Nigeria
123 S16 **Birobidzhan** Yevreyskaya Avtonomnaya Oblast', SE Russian Federation
97 D18 **Birr** var. Parsonstown, Ir. Biorra. C Ireland
183 P4 **Birrie River** ≈ New South Wales/Queensland, SE Australia
108 D7 **Birse** ≈ NW Switzerland
Birsen see Biržai
108 E6 **Birsfelden** Basel-Land, NW Switzerland
129 U4 **Birsk** Respublika Bashkortostan, W Russian Federation
119 F14 **Birštonas** Prienai, C Lithuania
159 P14 **Biru** Xinjiang Uygur Zizhiqu, W China
Biruni see Beruniy
122 L12 **Biryusa** ≈ C Russian Federation
122 L12 **Biryusinsk** Irkutskaya Oblast', C Russian Federation
118 G10 **Biržai** Ger. Birsen. Biržai, NE Lithuania
121 P16 **Birżebbuġa** SE Malta
Bisanthe see Tekirdağ
171 R12 **Bisa, Pulau** island Maluku, E Indonesia
37 N17 **Bisbee** Arizona, SW USA
29 O2 **Bisbee** North Dakota, N USA
Biscaia, Baía de see Biscay, Bay of
102 I13 **Biscarrosse et de Parentis, Étang de** ◎ SW France
104 M1 **Biscay, Bay of** Sp. Golfo de Vizcaya, Port. Baía de Biscaia. bay France/Spain
23 Z16 **Biscayne Bay** bay Florida, SE USA
64 M7 **Biscay Plain** undersea feature SE Bay of Biscay
107 N17 **Bisceglie** Puglia, SE Italy
Bischoflack see Škofja Loka
Bischofsburg see Biskupiec
109 Q7 **Bischofshofen** Salzburg, NW Austria
101 P15 **Bischofswerda** Sachsen, E Germany
103 V5 **Bischwiller** Bas-Rhin, NE France
21 T10 **Biscoe** North Carolina, SE USA
194 G5 **Biscoe Islands** island group Antarctica
14 E9 **Biscotasi Lake** ◎ Ontario, S Canada
14 E9 **Biscotasing** Ontario, S Canada
54 J6 **Biscucuy** Portuguesa, NW Venezuela
114 K11 **Biser** Khaskovo, S Bulgaria
113 D15 **Biševo** It. Busi. island SW Croatia
141 N12 **Bishah, Wādī** dry watercourse C Saudi Arabia
147 U7 **Bishkek** var. Pishpek; prev. Frunze. ● (Kyrgyzstan) Chuyskaya Oblast', N Kyrgyzstan
147 U7 **Bishkek** × Chuyskaya Oblast', N Kyrgyzstan
153 R16 **Bishnupur** West Bengal, NE India
83 J25 **Bisho** Eastern Cape, S South Africa
35 S9 **Bishop** California, W USA
25 S15 **Bishop** Texas, SW USA
97 L15 **Bishop Auckland** N England, UK
Bishop's Lynn see King's Lynn
97 O21 **Bishop's Stortford** E England, UK
21 S12 **Bishopville** South Carolina, SE USA
138 M5 **Bishrī, Jabal** ▲ E Syria
163 U4 **Bishui** Heilongjiang, NE China
81 G17 **Bisina, Lake** prev. Lake Salisbury. ◎ E Uganda
Biskara see Biskra
74 L6 **Biskra** var. Beskra, Biskara. NE Algeria
110 M8 **Biskupiec** Ger. Bischofsburg. Warmińsko-Mazurskie, NE Poland
171 R7 **Bislig** Mindanao, S Philippines
27 X6 **Bismarck** Missouri, C USA
28 M5 **Bismarck** state capital North Dakota, N USA
186 D5 **Bismarck Archipelago** island group NE PNG
131 Z16 **Bismarck Plate** tectonic feature W Pacific Ocean
186 D7 **Bismarck Range** ▲ N PNG
186 E6 **Bismarck Sea** sea W Pacific Ocean
137 P15 **Bismil** Diyarbakır, SE Turkey
43 N6 **Bismuna, Laguna** lagoon NE Nicaragua
Bisnulok see Phitsanulok
171 R10 **Bisoa, Tanjung** headland Pulau Halmahera, N Indonesia
28 K7 **Bison** South Dakota, N USA
93 H17 **Bispfors** Jämtland, C Sweden
76 G13 **Bissau** ● (Guinea-Bissau) W Guinea-Bissau
76 G13 **Bissau** × W Guinea-Bissau
99 M24 **Bissen** Luxembourg, C Luxembourg
76 G12 **Bissorã** W Guinea-Bissau
11 O10 **Bistcho Lake** ◎ Alberta, W Canada
22 G5 **Bistineau, Lake** ⊠ Louisiana, S USA
Bistrica see Ilirska Bistrica
116 I9 **Bistrița** Ger. Bistritz, Hung. Beszterce; prev. Nösen. Bistrița-Năsăud, N Romania
116 K10 **Bistrița** Ger. Bistritz. ≈ NE Romania
116 I9 **Bistrița-Năsăud** ◆ county N Romania
Bistritz see Bistrița
Bistritz ober Pernstein see Bystřice nad Pernštejnem
152 L11 **Biswān** Uttar Pradesh, N India
110 M7 **Bisztynek** Warmińsko-Mazurskie, NE Poland
79 E17 **Bitam** Woleu-Ntem, N Gabon
101 D18 **Bitburg** Rheinland-Pfalz, SW Germany
103 U4 **Bitche** Moselle, NE France
78 I11 **Bitkine** Guéra, C Chad
137 R15 **Bitlis** Bitlis, SE Turkey
137 R14 **Bitlis** ◆ province E Turkey
Bitoeng see Bitung
113 N20 **Bitola** Turk. Monastir; prev. Bitolj. S FYR Macedonia
Bitolj see Bitola
107 O17 **Bitonto** anc. Butuntum. Puglia, SE Italy
77 Q13 **Bitou** var. Bittou. SE Burkina
155 C20 **Bitra Island** island Lakshadweep, India, N Indian Ocean
101 M14 **Bitterfeld** Sachsen-Anhalt, E Germany
32 O9 **Bitterroot Range** ▲ Idaho/Montana, NW USA
33 P10 **Bitterroot River** ≈ Montana, NW USA
107 D18 **Bitti** Sardegna, Italy, C Mediterranean Sea
Bittou see Bitou
171 Q11 **Bitung** prev. Bitoeng. Sulawesi, C Indonesia
60 I12 **Bituruna** Paraná, S Brazil
77 Y13 **Biu** Borno, E Nigeria
Biumba see Byumba
164 J13 **Biwa-ko** ◎ Honshū, SW Japan
171 X14 **Biwarlaut** Irian Jaya, E Indonesia
27 P10 **Bixby** Oklahoma, C USA
122 J13 **Biya** ≈ S Russian Federation
Biy-Khem see Bol'shoy Yenisey
122 J13 **Biysk** Altayskiy Kray, S Russian Federation
164 H13 **Bizen** Okayama, Honshū, SW Japan
Bizerta see Bizerte
120 K10 **Bizerte** Ar. Banzart, Eng. Bizerta. N Tunisia
Bizkaia see Vizcaya
92 G2 **Bjargtangar** headland W Iceland
Bjärnå see Perniö
95 K22 **Bjärnum** Skåne, S Sweden
93 I16 **Bjästa** Västernorrland, C Sweden
113 I14 **Bjelašnica** ▲ SE Bosnia and Herzegovina
112 C10 **Bjelolasica** ▲ NW Croatia
112 F8 **Bjelovar** Hung. Belovár. Bjelovar-Bilogora, N Croatia
112 F8 **Bjelovar-Bilogora** off. Bjelovarsko-Bilogorska Županija. ◆ province NE Croatia
Bjelovarsko-Bilogorska Županija see Bjelovar-Bilogora
92 H10 **Bjerkvik** Nordland, C Norway
95 G21 **Bjerringbro** Viborg, NW Denmark
Bjeshkët e Namuna see North Albanian Alps
95 L14 **Björbo** Dalarna, C Sweden
95 I15 **Bjørkelangen** Akershus, S Norway
95 O14 **Björklinge** Uppsala, C Sweden
93 I14 **Björksele** Västerbotten, N Sweden
93 I16 **Björna** Västernorrland, C Sweden
95 C14 **Bjørnafjorden** fjord S Norway
95 L16 **Björneborg** Värmland, C Sweden
Björneborg see Pori
95 E14 **Bjornesfjorden** ◎ S Norway
92 M9 **Bjørnevatn** Finnmark, N Norway
197 T13 **Bjørnøya** Eng. Bear Island. island N Norway
93 I15 **Bjurholm** Västerbotten, N Sweden
95 J22 **Bjuv** Skåne, S Sweden
76 M12 **Bla** Ségou, W Mali
181 W8 **Blackall** Queensland, E Australia
29 V2 **Black Bay** lake bay Minnesota, N USA
27 N9 **Black Bear Creek** ≈ Oklahoma, C USA
97 K17 **Blackburn** NW England, UK
45 W10 **Blackburne** × (Plymouth) E Montserrat
39 T11 **Blackburn, Mount** ▲ Alaska, USA
35 N5 **Black Butte Lake** ⊠ California, W USA
194 J5 **Black Coast** physical region Antarctica
11 Q16 **Black Diamond** Alberta, SW Canada
18 K11 **Black Dome** ▲ New York, NE USA
113 L18 **Black Drin** Alb. Lumi i Drinit të Zi, SCr. Crni Drim. ≈ Albania/FYR Macedonia
12 D6 **Black Duck** ≈ Ontario, C Canada
29 U4 **Blackduck** Minnesota, N USA
33 R14 **Blackfoot** Idaho, NW USA
33 P9 **Blackfoot River** ≈ Montana, NW USA
Black Forest see Schwarzwald
28 J10 **Blackhawk** South Dakota, N USA
28 I10 **Black Hills** ▲ South Dakota/Wyoming, N USA
11 T10 **Black Lake** ◎ Saskatchewan, C Canada
31 Q5 **Black Lake** ◎ Michigan, N USA
18 I7 **Black Lake** ◎ New York, NE USA
22 G6 **Black Lake** ⊠ Louisiana, S USA
26 F7 **Black Mesa** ▲ Oklahoma, C USA
21 P10 **Black Mountain** North Carolina, SE USA
35 P13 **Black Mountain** ▲ California, W USA
37 Q2 **Black Mountain** ▲ Colorado, C USA
21 O7 **Black Mountain** ▲ Kentucky, E USA
96 K1 **Black Mountains** ▲ SE Wales, UK
36 H10 **Black Mountains** ▲ Arizona, SW USA
33 Q16 **Black Pine Peak** ▲ Idaho, NW USA
97 K17 **Blackpool** NW England, UK
37 Q14 **Black Range** ▲ New Mexico, SW USA
44 I12 **Black River** W Jamaica
14 J14 **Black River** ≈ Ontario, SE Canada
131 U12 **Black River** Chin. Babian Jiang, Lixian Jiang, Fr. Rivière Noire, Vtn. Sông Đa. ≈ China/Vietnam
44 I12 **Black River** ≈ W Jamaica
39 T7 **Black River** ≈ Alaska, USA
37 N13 **Black River** ≈ Arizona, SW USA
27 X7 **Black River** ≈ Arkansas/Missouri, C USA
22 I7 **Black River** ≈ Louisiana, S USA
31 S8 **Black River** ≈ Michigan, N USA
31 Q5 **Black River** ≈ Michigan, N USA
18 I8 **Black River** ≈ New York, NE USA
21 T13 **Black River** ≈ South Carolina, SE USA
30 J7 **Black River** ≈ Wisconsin, N USA
30 J7 **Black River Falls** Wisconsin, N USA
35 R3 **Black Rock Desert** desert Nevada, W USA
Black Sand Desert see Garagumy
21 S7 **Blacksburg** Virginia, NE USA
136 H10 **Black Sea** var. Euxine Sea, Bul. Cherno More, Rom. Marea Neagră, Rus. Chernoye More, Turk. Karadeniz, Ukr. Chorne More. sea Asia/Europe
117 Q10 **Black Sea Lowland** Ukr. Prychornomors'ka Nyzovyna. depression SE Europe
33 S17 **Blacks Fork** ≈ Wyoming, C USA
23 V7 **Blackshear** Georgia, SE USA
23 S6 **Blackshear, Lake** ⊠ Georgia, SE USA
97 A16 **Blacksod Bay** Ir. Cuan an Fhóid Duibh. inlet W Ireland
21 V7 **Blackstone** Virginia, NE USA
77 O14 **Black Volta** var. Borongo, Mouhoun, Moun Hou, Fr. Volta Noire. ≈ W Africa
23 O5 **Black Warrior River** ≈ Alabama, S USA
181 X8 **Blackwater** Queensland, E Australia
97 D20 **Blackwater** Ir. An Abhainn Mhór. ≈ S Ireland
27 T4 **Blackwater River** ≈ Missouri, C USA
21 W7 **Blackwater River** ≈ Virginia, NE USA
Blackwater State see Nebraska
27 N8 **Blackwell** Oklahoma, C USA
25 P7 **Blackwell** Texas, SW USA
99 J15 **Bladel** Noord-Brabant, S Netherlands
Bladenmarkt see Bălăuşeri
114 G11 **Blagoevgrad** prev. Gorna Dzhumaya. Blagoevgrad, SW Bulgaria
114 G11 **Blagoevgrad** ◆ province SW Bulgaria
123 Q14 **Blagoveshchensk** Amurskaya Oblast', SE Russian Federation
129 V4 **Blagoveshchensk** Respublika Bashkortostan, W Russian Federation
102 I7 **Blain** Loire-Atlantique, NW France
29 V8 **Blaine** Minnesota, N USA
32 H6 **Blaine** Washington, NW USA
11 T15 **Blaine Lake** Saskatchewan, S Canada
29 S14 **Blair** Nebraska, C USA
96 J10 **Blairgowrie** C Scotland, UK
18 C15 **Blairsville** Pennsylvania, NE USA
116 H11 **Blaj** Ger. Blasendorf, Hung. Balázsfalva. Alba, SW Romania
64 F9 **Blake-Bahama Ridge** undersea feature W Atlantic Ocean
23 S7 **Blakely** Georgia, SE USA
64 E10 **Blake Plateau** var. Blake Terrace. undersea feature W Atlantic Ocean
30 M1 **Blake Point** headland Michigan, N USA
Blake Terrace see Blake Plateau
61 B24 **Blanca, Bahía** bay E Argentina
56 C12 **Blanca, Cordillera** ▲ W Peru
105 T12 **Blanca, Costa** physical region SE Spain
37 S7 **Blanca Peak** ▲ Colorado, C USA
24 I9 **Blanca, Sierra** ▲ Texas, SW USA
120 K9 **Blanc, Cap** headland N Tunisia
Blanc, Cap see Nouâdhibou, Râs
31 R12 **Blanchard River** ≈ Ohio, N USA
182 E8 **Blanche, Cape** headland South Australia
182 J4 **Blanche, Lake** ◎ South Australia
31 R14 **Blanchester** Ohio, N USA
182 J9 **Blanchetown** South Australia
45 U13 **Blanchisseuse** Trinidad, Trinidad and Tobago
103 T11 **Blanc, Mont** It. Monte Bianco. ▲ France/Italy
25 R11 **Blanco** Texas, SW USA
42 K14 **Blanco, Cabo** headland NW Costa Rica
32 D14 **Blanco, Cape** headland Oregon, NW USA
62 H10 **Blanco, Río** ≈ W Argentina
56 F10 **Blanco, Río** ≈ NE Peru
15 O9 **Blanc, Réservoir** ⊠ Quebec, SE Canada
21 R7 **Bland** Virginia, NE USA
92 I2 **Blanda** ≈ N Iceland
37 O7 **Blanding** Utah, W USA
105 X5 **Blanes** Cataluña, NE Spain
103 N3 **Blangy-sur-Bresle** Seine-Maritime, N France
111 C18 **Blanice** Ger. Blanitz. ≈ SE Czech Republic
Blanitz see Blanice
99 C16 **Blankenberge** West-Vlaanderen, NW Belgium
101 D17 **Blankenheim** Nordrhein-Westfalen, W Germany
25 R8 **Blanket** Texas, SW USA
55 O3 **Blanquilla, Isla** var. La Blanquilla. island N Venezuela
Blanquilla, La see Blanquilla, Isla
61 F18 **Blanquillo** Durazno, C Uruguay
111 G18 **Blansko** Ger. Blanz. Brněnský Kraj, SE Czech Republic
83 N15 **Blantyre** var. Blantyre-Limbe. Southern, S Malawi
83 N15 **Blantyre** × Southern, S Malawi
Blantyre-Limbe see Blantyre
Blanz see Blansko
98 J10 **Blaricum** Noord-Holland, C Netherlands
Blasendorf see Blaj
Blatnitsa see Durankulak
113 F15 **Blato** It. Blatta. Dubrovnik-Neretva, S Croatia
Blatta see Blato
108 E10 **Blatten** Valais, SW Switzerland
101 J20 **Blaufelden** Baden-Württemberg, SW Germany
95 E23 **Blåvands Huk** headland W Denmark
102 G6 **Blavet** ≈ NW France
102 J12 **Blaye** Gironde, SW France
183 R8 **Blayney** New South Wales, SE Australia
65 D25 **Bleaker Island** island SE Falkland Islands
109 T10 **Bled** Ger. Veldes. NW Slovenia
99 D20 **Bléharies** Hainaut, SW Belgium
109 U9 **Bleiburg** Slvn. Pliberk. Kärnten, S Austria
101 L17 **Bleiloch-Stausee** ⊠ C Germany
98 H12 **Bleiswijk** Zuid-Holland, W Netherlands
95 L22 **Blekinge** ◆ county S Sweden
14 D17 **Blenheim** Ontario, S Canada
185 K15 **Blenheim** Marlborough, South Island, NZ
99 M15 **Blerick** Limburg, SE Netherlands
Blesae see Blois
25 V13 **Blessing** Texas, SW USA
14 I10 **Bleu, Lac** ◎ Quebec, SE Canada
Blibba see Blitta
120 H10 **Blida** var. El Boulaida, El Boulaïda. N Algeria
95 P15 **Blidö** Stockholm, C Sweden
95 K18 **Blidsberg** Västra Götaland, S Sweden
185 A21 **Bligh Sound** sound South Island, NZ
187 X14 **Bligh Water** strait NW Fiji
14 D11 **Blind River** Ontario, S Canada
31 R11 **Blissfield** Michigan, N USA
77 R15 **Blitta** prev. Blibba. C Togo
19 O13 **Block Island** island Rhode Island, NE USA
19 O13 **Block Island Sound** sound Rhode Island, NE USA
98 H10 **Bloemendaal** Noord-Holland, W Netherlands
83 H23 **Bloemfontein** var. Mangaung. ● (South Africa-judicial capital) Free State, C South Africa
83 I22 **Bloemhof** North-West, NW South Africa
102 M7 **Blois** anc. Blesae. Loir-et-Cher, C France
98 L8 **Blokzijl** Overijssel, N Netherlands
95 N20 **Blomstermåla** Kalmar, S Sweden
92 I2 **Blönduós** Nordhurland Vestra, N Iceland
110 L11 **Błonie** Mazowieckie, C Poland
97 C14 **Bloody Foreland** Ir. Cnoc Fola. headland NW Ireland
31 N15 **Bloomfield** Indiana, N USA
29 X16 **Bloomfield** Iowa, C USA
27 Y8 **Bloomfield** Missouri, C USA
37 P9 **Bloomfield** New Mexico, SW USA
25 U7 **Blooming Grove** Texas, SW USA
29 W10 **Blooming Prairie** Minnesota, N USA
30 L13 **Bloomington** Illinois, N USA
31 O15 **Bloomington** Indiana, N USA
29 V9 **Bloomington** Minnesota, N USA
25 U13 **Bloomington** Texas, SW USA
18 H14 **Bloomsburg** Pennsylvania, NE USA
181 X7 **Bloomsbury** Queensland, NE Australia
169 R16 **Blora** Jawa, C Indonesia
18 G12 **Blossburg** Pennsylvania, NE USA
25 V5 **Blossom** Texas, SW USA
123 T5 **Blossom, Mys** headland Ostrov Vrangelya, NE Russian Federation
23 R8 **Blountstown** Florida, SE USA
21 P8 **Blountville** Tennessee, S USA
21 Q9 **Blowing Rock** North Carolina, SE USA
108 J8 **Bludenz** Vorarlberg, W Austria
36 L6 **Blue Bell Knoll** ▲ Utah, W USA
23 Y12 **Blue Cypress Lake** ◎ Florida, SE USA
29 U11 **Blue Earth** Minnesota, N USA
21 Q7 **Bluefield** Virginia, NE USA
21 R7 **Bluefield** West Virginia, NE USA
43 N10 **Bluefields** Región Autónoma Atlántico Sur, SE Nicaragua
43 N10 **Bluefields, Bahía de** bay W Caribbean Sea
29 Z14 **Blue Grass** Iowa, C USA
Bluegrass State see Kentucky
Blue Hen State see Delaware
19 S7 **Blue Hill** Maine, NE USA
29 P16 **Blue Hill** Nebraska, C USA
30 J5 **Blue Hills** hill range Wisconsin, N USA
34 L3 **Blue Lake** California, W USA
Blue Law State see Connecticut
37 Q6 **Blue Mesa Reservoir** ⊠ Colorado, C USA
27 S12 **Blue Mountain** ▲ Arkansas, C USA
19 O6 **Blue Mountain** ▲ New Hampshire, NE USA
18 K8 **Blue Mountain** ▲ New York, NE USA
18 H15 **Blue Mountain** ridge Pennsylvania, NE USA
44 H10 **Blue Mountain Peak** ▲ E Jamaica
183 S8 **Blue Mountains** ▲ New South Wales, SE Australia
32 L11 **Blue Mountains** ▲ Oregon/Washington, NW USA
80 G12 **Blue Nile** ◆ state E Sudan
80 H12 **Blue Nile** var. Abai, Bahr el Azraq, Amh. Åbay Wenz, Ar. An Nīl al Azraq. ≈ Ethiopia/Sudan
8 J7 **Bluenose Lake** ◎ Nunavut, NW Canada
27 O3 **Blue Rapids** Kansas, C USA
23 S1 **Blue Ridge** Georgia, SE USA
17 S11 **Blue Ridge** var. Blue Ridge Mountains. ▲ North Carolina/Virginia, E USA
23 S1 **Blue Ridge Lake** ⊠ Georgia, SE USA
Blue Ridge Mountains see Blue Ridge
9 N15 **Blue River** British Columbia, SW Canada
27 O12 **Blue River** ≈ Oklahoma, C USA
27 R4 **Blue Springs** Missouri, C USA
21 R6 **Bluestone Lake** ⊠ West Virginia, NE USA
185 C25 **Bluff** Southland, South Island, NZ
37 O8 **Bluff** Utah, W USA
21 P8 **Bluff City** Tennessee, S USA
65 E24 **Bluff Cove** East Falkland, Falkland Islands
25 S7 **Bluff Dale** Texas, SW USA
183 N15 **Bluff Hill Point** headland Tasmania, SE Australia
31 Q12 **Bluffton** Indiana, N USA
31 R12 **Bluffton** Ohio, N USA
25 T7 **Blum** Texas, SW USA
101 G24 **Blumberg** Baden-Württemberg, SW Germany
60 K13 **Blumenau** Santa Catarina, S Brazil
29 N9 **Blunt** South Dakota, N USA
32 H15 **Bly** Oregon, NW USA
39 R13 **Blying Sound** sound Alaska, USA
97 M14 **Blyth** N England, UK
35 Y16 **Blythe** California, W USA
27 Y9 **Blytheville** Arkansas, C USA
117 V7 **Blyznyuky** Kharkivs'ka Oblast', E Ukraine
76 I15 **Bo** S Sierra Leone
95 G16 **Bø** Telemark, S Norway
171 O4 **Boac** Marinduque, N Philippines
42 K10 **Boaco** Boaco, S Nicaragua
42 J10 **Boaco** ◆ department C Nicaragua
79 I15 **Boali** Ombella-Mpoko, SW Central African Republic
Boalsert see Bolsward
31 V12 **Boardman** Ohio, N USA
32 J11 **Boardman** Oregon, NW USA
14 F13 **Boat Lake** ◎ Ontario, S Canada
58 F10 **Boa Vista** state capital Roraima, NW Brazil
76 D9 **Boa Vista** island Ilhas de Barlavento, E Cape Verde
23 Q2 **Boaz** Alabama, S USA
160 L15 **Bobai** Guangxi Zhuangzu Zizhiqu, S China
172 J1 **Bobaomby, Tanjona** Fr. Cap d'Ambre. headland N Madagascar
155 M14 **Bobbili** Andhra Pradesh, E India
106 D9 **Bobbio** Emilia-Romagna, C Italy
14 I14 **Bobcaygeon** Ontario, SE Canada
Bober see Bóbr
103 O5 **Bobigny** Seine-St-Denis, N France
77 N13 **Bobo-Dioulasso** SW Burkina
110 G8 **Bobolice** Ger. Bublitz. Zachodniopomorskie, NW Poland
171 R11 **Bobopayo** Pulau Halmahera, E Indonesia
147 P13 **Bobotogh, Qatorkŭhi** Rus. Khrebet Babatag. ▲ Tajikistan/Uzbekistan
114 G10 **Bobovdol** Kyustendil, W Bulgaria
119 M15 **Bobr** Minskaya Voblasts', NW Belarus
119 M15 **Bobr** ≈ C Belarus
111 E14 **Bóbr** Eng. Bobrawa, Ger. Bober. ≈ SW Poland
Bobrawa see Bóbr
Bobrik see Bobryk
Bobrinets see Bobrynets'
Bobrka/Bóbrka see Bibrka
128 L8 **Bobrov** Voronezhskaya Oblast', W Russian Federation
117 Q4 **Bobrovytsya** Chernihivs'ka Oblast', N Ukraine
Bobruysk see Babruysk
119 J19 **Bobryk** Rus. Bobrik. ≈ SW Belarus
117 Q8 **Bobrynets'** Rus. Bobrinets. Kirovohrads'ka Oblast', C Ukraine

14 K14 **Bobs Lake** ◎ Ontario, SE Canada
54 I6 **Bobures** Zulia, NW Venezuela
42 H1 **Boca Bacalar Chico** *headland* N Belize
112 G11 **Bočac** Republika Srpska, NW Bosnia and Herzegovina
41 R14 **Boca del Río** Veracruz-Llave, S Mexico
55 O4 **Boca de Pozo** Nueva Esparta, NE Venezuela
59 C15 **Boca do Acre** Amazonas, N Brazil
55 N12 **Boca Mavaca** Amazonas, S Venezuela
79 G14 **Bocaranga** Ouham-Pendé, W Central African Republic
23 Z15 **Boca Raton** Florida, SE USA
43 P14 **Bocas del Toro** Bocas del Toro, NW Panama
43 P15 **Bocas del Toro** *off.* Provincia de Bocas del Toro. ◆ *province* NW Panama
43 P15 **Bocas del Toro, Archipiélago de** *island group* NW Panama
42 L7 **Bocay** Jinotega, N Nicaragua
105 N6 **Boceguillas** Castilla-León, N Spain
Bocheykovo *see* Bacheykava
111 L17 **Bochnia** Małopolskie, SE Poland
99 K16 **Bocholt** Limburg, NE Belgium
101 D14 **Bocholt** Nordrhein-Westfalen, W Germany
101 E15 **Bochum** Nordrhein-Westfalen, W Germany
103 Y15 **Bocognano** Corse, France, C Mediterranean Sea
54 I6 **Boconó** Trujillo, NW Venezuela
116 F12 **Bocşa** *Ger.* Bokschen, *Hung.* Boksánbánya. Caraş-Severin, SW Romania
79 H15 **Boda** Lobaye, SW Central African Republic
94 L12 **Böda** Dalarna, C Sweden
95 O20 **Böda** Kalmar, S Sweden
95 L19 **Bodafors** Jönköping, S Sweden
123 O12 **Bodaybo** Irkutskaya Oblast', E Russian Federation
22 G5 **Bodcau, Bayou** *var.* Bodcau Creek. ≈ Louisiana, S USA
Bodcau Creek *see* Bodcau, Bayou
44 D8 **Bodden Town** *var.* Boddentown. Grand Cayman, SW Cayman Islands
101 K14 **Bode** ≈ C Germany
34 L7 **Bodega Head** *headland* California, W USA
Bodegas *see* Babahoyo
98 H11 **Bodegraven** Zuid-Holland, C Netherlands
78 H8 **Bodélé** *depression* W Chad
92 J13 **Boden** Norrbotten, N Sweden
Bodensee *see* Constance, Lake, C Europe
65 M15 **Bode Verde Fracture Zone** *tectonic feature* E Atlantic Ocean
155 H14 **Bodhan** Andhra Pradesh, C India
162 I9 **Bodĭ** Bayanhongor, C Mongolia
155 H22 **Bodināyakkanūr** Tamil Nādu, SE India
108 H10 **Bodio** Ticino, S Switzerland
97 I24 **Bodmin** SW England, UK
97 I24 **Bodmin Moor** *moorland* SW England, UK
92 G12 **Bodø** Nordland, C Norway
59 H20 **Bodoquena, Serra da** ▲ SW Brazil
136 B16 **Bodrum** Muğla, SW Turkey
Bodzafordulő *see* Întorsura Buzăului
99 L14 **Boekel** Noord-Brabant, SE Netherlands
Boeloekoemba *see* Bulukumba
103 Q11 **Boën** Loire, E France
79 K18 **Boende** Equateur, C Dem. Rep. Congo (Zaire)
25 R11 **Boerne** Texas, SW USA
Boeroe *see* Buru, Pulau
Boetoeng *see* Buton, Pulau
22 I5 **Boeuf River** ≈ Arkansas/Louisiana, S USA
76 H14 **Boffa** Guinée-Maritime, W Guinea
Bó Finne, Inis *see* Inishbofin
Boga *see* Bogë
166 L9 **Bogale** Irrawaddy, SW Myanmar
22 L8 **Bogalusa** Louisiana, S USA
77 Q12 **Bogandé** C Burkina
79 I15 **Bogangolo** Ombella-Mpoko, C Central African Republic
183 Q7 **Bogan River** ≈ New South Wales, SE Australia
25 W5 **Bogata** Texas, SW USA
111 D14 **Bogatynia** *Ger.* Reichenau. Dolnośląskie, SW Poland
136 K13 **Boğazlıyan** Yozgat, C Turkey
79 J17 **Bogbonga** Equateur, NW Dem. Rep. Congo (Zaire)
158 J14 **Bogcang Zangbo** ≈ W China
158 L5 **Bogda Feng** ▲ NW China
114 I9 **Bogdan** ▲ C Bulgaria
113 Q20 **Bogdanci** SE FYR Macedonia
158 M5 **Bogda Shan** *var.* Po-ko-to Shan. ▲ NW China
113 K17 **Bogë** *var.* Boga. Shkodër, N Albania
Bogendorf *see* Łuków
95 G23 **Bogense** Fyn, C Denmark
183 T3 **Boggabilla** New South Wales, SE Australia
183 S6 **Boggabri** New South Wales, SE Australia
186 D6 **Bogia** Madang, N PNG
97 N23 **Bognor Regis** SE England, UK
Bogodukhov *see* Bohodukhiv
181 V15 **Bogong, Mount** ▲ Victoria, SE Australia
169 O16 **Bogor** *Dut.* Buitenzorg. Jawa, C Indonesia
128 L5 **Bogoroditsk** Tul'skaya Oblast', W Russian Federation
129 O3 **Bogorodsk** Nizhegorodskaya Oblast', W Russian Federation
Bogorodskoje *see* Bogorodskoye
123 S12 **Bogorodskoye** Khabarovskiy Kray, SE Russian Federation
127 R15 **Bogorodskoye** *var.* Bogorodskoje. Kirovskaya Oblast', NW Russian Federation
54 F10 **Bogotá** *prev.* Santa Fe, Santa Fe de Bogotá. ● (Colombia) Cundinamarca, C Colombia
153 T14 **Bogra** Rajshahi, N Bangladesh
Bogschan *see* Boldu
122 L12 **Boguchany** Krasnoyarskiy Kray, C Russian Federation
128 M9 **Boguchar** Voronezhskaya Oblast', W Russian Federation
76 H10 **Bogué** Brakna, SW Mauritania
22 K8 **Bogue Chitto** ≈ Louisiana/Mississippi, S USA
Bogushëvsk *see* Bahushewsk
Boguslav *see* Bohuslav
44 K12 **Bog Walk** C Jamaica
161 Q3 **Bo Hai** *var.* Gulf of Chihli. *gulf* NE China
161 R3 **Bohai Haixia** *strait* NE China
161 Q3 **Bohai Wan** *bay* NE China
111 C17 **Bohemia** *Cz.* Čechy, *Ger.* Böhmen. *cultural and historical region* W Czech Republic
111 B18 **Bohemian Forest** *Cz.* Ceský Les, Šumava, *Ger.* Böhmerwald. ▲ C Europe
Bohemian-Moravian Highlands *see* Českomoravská Vrchovina
77 R16 **Bohicon** S Benin
109 S11 **Bohinjska Bistrica** *Ger.* Wocheiner Feistritz. NW Slovenia
Bohkká *see* Pokka
Böhmen *see* Bohemia
Böhmerwald *see* Bohemian Forest
Böhmisch-Krumau *see* Český Krumlov
Böhmisch-Leipa *see* Česká Lípa
Böhmisch-Mährische Höhe *see* Českomoravská Vrchovina
Böhmisch-Trübau *see* Česká Třebová
117 U5 **Bohodukhiv** *Rus.* Bogodukhov. Kharkivs'ka Oblast', E Ukraine
171 Q6 **Bohol** *island* C Philippines
171 Q7 **Bohol Sea** *var.* Mindanao Sea. *sea* S Philippines
116 I7 **Bohorodchany** Ivano-Frankivs'ka Oblast', W Ukraine
162 M9 **Böhöt** Dundgovĭ, C Mongolia
158 K6 **Bohu** *var.* Bagrax. Xinjiang Uygur Zizhiqu, NW China
111 I17 **Bohumín** *Ger.* Oderberg; *prev.* Neuoderberg, Nový Bohumín. Ostravský Kray, E Czech Republic
117 P6 **Bohuslav** *Rus.* Boguslav. Kyyivs'ka Oblast', N Ukraine
58 F11 **Boiaçu** Roraima, N Brazil
107 K16 **Boiano** Molise, C Italy
15 R8 **Boilleau** Quebec, SE Canada
59 O17 **Boipeba, Ilha de** *island* SE Brazil
104 G3 **Boiro** Galicia, NW Spain
31 Q5 **Bois Blanc Island** *island* Michigan, N USA
29 R7 **Bois de Sioux River** ≈ Minnesota, N USA
33 N14 **Boise** *var.* Boise City. *state capital* Idaho, NW USA
26 G8 **Boise City** Oklahoma, C USA
33 N14 **Boise River, Middle Fork** ≈ Idaho, NW USA
Bois, Lac des *see* Woods, Lake of the
Bois-le-Duc *see* 's-Hertogenbosch
9 W17 **Boissevain** Manitoba, S Canada
15 T7 **Boisvert, Pointe au** *headland* Quebec, SE Canada
100 K10 **Boizenburg** Mecklenburg-Vorpommern, N Germany
Bojador *see* Boujdour
113 K18 **Bojana** *Alb.* Bunë. ≈ Albania/Yugoslavia *see also* Bunë
143 S3 **Bojnūrd** *var.* Bujnurd. Khorāsān, N Iran
169 R16 **Bojonegoro** *prev.* Bodjonegoro. Jawa, C Indonesia
189 T1 **Bokaak Atoll** *var.* Bokak, Taongi. *atoll* Ratak Chain, NE Marshall Islands
Bokak *see* Bokaak Atoll
153 Q15 **Bokāro** Bihār, N India
79 I18 **Bokatola** Equateur, NW Dem. Rep. Congo (Zaire)
76 H13 **Boké** Guinée-Maritime, W Guinea
Bokhara *see* Bukhoro
183 Q4 **Bokharra River** ≈ New South Wales/Queensland, SE Australia
95 C16 **Boknafjorden** *fjord* S Norway
78 H11 **Bokoro** Chari-Baguirmi, W Chad
79 K19 **Bokota** Equateur, NW Dem. Rep. Congo (Zaire)
167 N13 **Bokpyin** Tenasserim, S Myanmar
Boksánbánya/Bokschen *see* Bocşa
83 F21 **Bokspits** Kgalagadi, SW Botswana
79 K18 **Bokungu** Equateur, C Dem. Rep. Congo (Zaire)
Bokurdak *see* Bakhardok
78 G10 **Bol** Lac, W Chad
76 G13 **Bolama** SW Guinea-Bissau
Bolangir *see* Balāngīr
Bolanos *see* Bolanos, Mount, Guam
Bolaños *see* Bolaños de Calatrava, Spain
105 N11 **Bolaños de Calatrava** *var.* Bolaños. Castilla-La Mancha, C Spain
188 B17 **Bolanos, Mount** *var.* Bolanos. ▲ S Guam
40 L12 **Bolaños, Río** ≈ C Mexico
115 M14 **Bolayır** Çanakkale, NW Turkey
102 L3 **Bolbec** Seine-Maritime, N France
116 L13 **Boldu** *var.* Bogschan. Buzău, SE Romania
146 H8 **Boldumsaz** *prev.* Kalinin, Kalininsk, Porsy. Dashkhovuzskiy Velayat, N Turkmenistan
158 I4 **Bole** *var.* Bortala. Xinjiang Uygur Zizhiqu, NW China
77 O15 **Bole** NW Ghana
79 J19 **Boleko** Equateur, W Dem. Rep. Congo (Zaire)
111 E14 **Bolesławiec** *Ger.* Bunzlau. Dolnośląskie, SW Poland
129 R4 **Bolgar** *prev.* Kuybyshev. Respublika Tatarstan, W Russian Federation
77 P14 **Bolgatanga** N Ghana
Bolgrad *see* Bolhrad
117 N12 **Bolhrad** *Rus.* Bolgrad. Odes'ka Oblast', SW Ukraine
163 Y8 **Boli** Heilongjiang, NE China
79 I19 **Bolia** Bandundu, W Dem. Rep. Congo (Zaire)
93 J14 **Boliden** Västerbotten, N Sweden
171 T13 **Bolifar** Pulau Seram, E Indonesia
171 N2 **Bolinao** Luzon, N Philippines
27 T6 **Bolivar** Missouri, C USA
20 F10 **Bolivar** Tennessee, S USA
54 C12 **Bolívar** Cauca, SW Colombia
54 F7 **Bolívar** *off.* Departmento de Bolívar. ◆ *province* N Colombia
56 A13 **Bolívar** ◆ *province* C Ecuador
55 N9 **Bolívar** *off.* Estado Bolívar. ◆ *state* SE Venezuela
25 X12 **Bolivar Peninsula** *headland* Texas, SW USA
54 I6 **Bolívar, Pico** ▲ W Venezuela
57 K17 **Bolivia** *off.* Republic of Bolivia. ◆ *republic* W South America
112 O13 **Boljevac** Serbia, E Yugoslavia
Bolkenhain *see* Bolków
128 J5 **Bolkhov** Orlovskaya Oblast', W Russian Federation
111 F14 **Bolków** *Ger.* Bolkenhain. Dolnośląskie, SW Poland
182 K3 **Bollards Lagoon** South Australia
103 R14 **Bollène** Vaucluse, SE France
94 N12 **Bollnäs** Gävleborg, C Sweden
181 W10 **Bollon** Queensland, C Australia
192 L12 **Bollons Tablemount** *undersea feature* S Pacific Ocean
93 H17 **Bollstabruk** Västernorrland, C Sweden
Bolluilos de Par del Condado *see* Bolluilos Par del Condado
104 J14 **Bollulos Par del Condado** *var.* Bolluilos de Par del Condado. Andalucía, S Spain
95 K21 **Bolmen** ◎ S Sweden
137 T10 **Bolnisi** S Georgia
79 H19 **Bolobo** Bandundu, W Dem. Rep. Congo (Zaire)
123 R12 **Bolodek** Khabarovskiy Kray, SE Russian Federation
106 G10 **Bologna** Emilia-Romagna, N Italy
126 I15 **Bologoye** Tverskaya Oblast', W Russian Federation
79 J18 **Bolomba** Equateur, NW Dem. Rep. Congo (Zaire)
41 X13 **Bolónchén de Rejón** *var.* Bolonchén de Rejón. Campeche, SE Mexico
114 J13 **Boloústra, Akrotírio** *headland* NE Greece
167 L8 **Bolovens, Plateau des** *plateau* S Laos
106 H13 **Bolsena** Lazio, C Italy
107 G14 **Bolsena, Lago di** ◎ C Italy
128 B3 **Bol'shakovo** *Ger.* Kreuzingen; *prev.* Gross-Skaisgirren. Kaliningradskaya Oblast', W Russian Federation
Bol'shaya Berëstovitsa *see* Vyalikaya Byerastavitsa
129 S7 **Bol'shaya Chernigovka** Samarskaya Oblast', W Russian Federation
129 S7 **Bol'shaya Glushitsa** Samarskaya Oblast', W Russian Federation
144 H9 **Bol'shaya Khobda** *Kaz.* Ülkenqobda. ≈ Kazakhstan/Russian Federation
128 M12 **Bol'shaya Martynovka** Rostovskaya Oblast', SW Russian Federation
122 K12 **Bol'shaya Murta** Krasnoyarskiy Kray, C Russian Federation
127 V4 **Bol'shaya Rogovaya** ≈ NW Russian Federation
127 U7 **Bol'shaya Synya** ≈ NW Russian Federation
145 V9 **Bol'shaya Vladimirovka** Vostochnyy Kazakhstan, E Kazakhstan
123 V11 **Bol'sheretsk** Kamchatskaya Oblast', E Russian Federation
129 W3 **Bol'sheust'ikinskoye** Respublika Bashkortostan, W Russian Federation
Bol'shevik *see* Bal'shavik
122 L5 **Bol'shevik, Ostrov** *island* Severnaya Zemlya, N Russian Federation
127 U4 **Bol'shezemel'skaya Tundra** *physical region* NW Russian Federation
144 J13 **Bol'shiye Barsuki, Peski** *desert* SW Kazakhstan
123 T7 **Bol'shoy Anyuy** ≈ NE Russian Federation
123 N7 **Bol'shoy Begichev, Ostrov** *island* NE Russian Federation
129 O4 **Bol'shoye Murashkino** Nizhegorodskaya Oblast', W Russian Federation
129 W4 **Bol'shoy Iremel'** ▲ W Russian Federation
129 R7 **Bol'shoy Irgiz** ≈ W Russian Federation
123 Q6 **Bol'shoy Lyakhovskiy, Ostrov** *island* NE Russian Federation
123 Q11 **Bol'shoy Nimnyr** Respublika Sakha (Yakutiya), NE Russian Federation
Bol'shoy Rozhan *see* Vyaliki Rozhan
144 E10 **Bol'shoy Uzen'** *Kaz.* Ülkenözen. ≈ Kazakhstan/Russian Federation
40 K6 **Bolson de Mapimi** ▲ NW Mexico
98 K6 **Bolsward** *Fris.* Boalsert. Friesland, N Netherlands
105 T4 **Boltaña** Aragón, NE Spain
14 G15 **Bolton** Ontario, S Canada
97 K17 **Bolton** *prev.* Bolton-le-Moors. NW England, UK
21 V12 **Bolton** North Carolina, SE USA
Bolton-le-Moors *see* Bolton
136 G11 **Bolu** Bolu, NW Turkey
136 G11 **Bolu** ◆ *province* NW Turkey
186 G9 **Bolubolu** Goodenough Island, S PNG
92 H1 **Bolungarvík** Vestfirdhir, NW Iceland
159 O10 **Boluntay** Qinghai, W China
136 F14 **Bolvadin** Afyon, W Turkey
114 M10 **Bolyarovo** *prev.* Pashkeni. Yambol, E Bulgaria
106 G6 **Bolzano** *Ger.* Bozen; *anc.* Bauzanum. Trentino-Alto Adige, N Italy
79 F22 **Boma** Bas-Congo, W Dem. Rep. Congo (Zaire)
183 R12 **Bombala** New South Wales, SE Australia
104 F10 **Bombarral** Leiria, C Portugal
Bombay *see* Mumbai
171 U13 **Bomberai, Semenanjung** *headland* Irian Jaya, E Indonesia
81 F18 **Bombo** S Uganda
79 I17 **Bomboma** Equateur, NW Dem. Rep. Congo (Zaire)
59 I14 **Bom Futuro** Pará, N Brazil
159 Q15 **Bomi** *var.* Bowo, Zhamo. Xizang Zizhiqu, W China
79 N17 **Bomili** Orientale, NE Dem. Rep. Congo (Zaire)
59 N17 **Bom Jesus da Lapa** Bahia, E Brazil
60 Q8 **Bom Jesus do Itabapoana** Rio de Janeiro, SE Brazil
95 C15 **Bømlafjorden** *fjord* S Norway
95 B15 **Bømlo** *island* S Norway
123 Q12 **Bomnak** Amurskaya Oblast', SE Russian Federation
79 I17 **Bomongo** Equateur, NW Dem. Rep. Congo (Zaire)
61 K14 **Bom Retiro** Santa Catarina, S Brazil
79 L15 **Bomu** *var.* Mbomou, Mbomu, M'Bomu. ≈ Central African Republic/Dem. Rep. Congo (Zaire)
142 J3 **Bonāb** *var.* Benāb, Bunab. Āžarbāyjān-e Khāvarī, N Iran
45 Q16 **Bonaire** *island* E Netherlands Antilles
39 U11 **Bona, Mount** ▲ Alaska, USA
183 Q12 **Bonang** Victoria, SE Australia
42 L7 **Bonanza** Región Autónoma Atlántico Norte, NE Nicaragua
37 O4 **Bonanza** Utah, W USA
45 O9 **Bonao** C Dominican Republic
180 L3 **Bonaparte Archipelago** *island group* Western Australia
32 K6 **Bonaparte, Mount** ▲ Washington, NW USA
39 N11 **Bonasila Dome** ▲ Alaska, USA
92 H11 **Bonåsjøen** Nordland, C Norway
45 T15 **Bonasse** Trinidad, Trinidad and Tobago
15 X7 **Bonaventure** Quebec, SE Canada
15 X7 **Bonaventure** ≈ Quebec, SE Canada
13 V11 **Bonavista** Newfoundland, SE Canada
13 U11 **Bonavista Bay** *inlet* NW Atlantic Ocean
79 E19 **Bonda** Ogooué-Lolo, C Gabon
129 N6 **Bondari** Tambovskaya Oblast', W Russian Federation
106 G9 **Bondeno** Emilia-Romagna, C Italy
30 L4 **Bond Falls Flowage** ◎ Michigan, N USA
79 L16 **Bondo** Orientale, N Dem. Rep. Congo (Zaire)
171 N17 **Bondokodi** Pulau Sumba, S Indonesia
77 O15 **Bondoukou** E Ivory Coast
Bondoukui/Bondoukuy *see* Boundoukui
169 T17 **Bondowoso** Jawa, C Indonesia
33 S14 **Bondurant** Wyoming, C USA
Bone *see* Watampone, Indonesia
Bône *see* Annaba, Algeria
30 I5 **Bone Lake** ◎ Wisconsin, N USA
171 P14 **Bonelipu** Pulau Buton, C Indonesia
171 O15 **Bonerate, Kepulauan** *var.* Macan. *island group* C Indonesia
29 O12 **Bonesteel** South Dakota, N USA
62 I8 **Bonete, Cerro** ▲ N Argentina
171 O14 **Bone, Teluk** *bay* Sulawesi, C Indonesia
108 D6 **Bonfol** Jura, NW Switzerland
153 U12 **Bongaigaon** Assam, NE India
79 K17 **Bongandanga** Equateur, NW Dem. Rep. Congo (Zaire)
78 L13 **Bongo, Massif des** *var.* Chaîne des Mongos. ▲ NE Central African Republic
78 G12 **Bongor** Mayo-Kébbi, SW Chad
77 N16 **Bongouanou** E Ivory Coast
167 V11 **Bông Sơn** *var.* Hoai Nhơn. Binh Đinh, C Vietnam
25 U5 **Bonham** Texas, SW USA
Bonhard *see* Bonyhád
103 U6 **Bonhomme, Col du** *pass* NE France
103 Y16 **Bonifacio** Corse, France, C Mediterranean Sea
Bonifacio, Bocche de/Bonifacio, Bouches de *see* Bonifacio, Strait of
103 Y16 **Bonifacio, Strait of** *Fr.* Bouches de Bonifacio, *It.* Bocche de Bonifacio. *strait* C Mediterranean Sea
23 Q8 **Bonifay** Florida, SE USA
Bonin Islands *see* Ogasawara-shotō
192 H5 **Bonin Trench** *undersea feature* NW Pacific Ocean
23 W15 **Bonita Springs** Florida, SE USA
42 I5 **Bonito, Pico** ▲ N Honduras
101 E17 **Bonn** Nordrhein-Westfalen, W Germany
14 J12 **Bonnechere** Ontario, SE Canada
14 J12 **Bonnechere** ≈ Ontario, SE Canada
33 N7 **Bonners Ferry** Idaho, NW USA
27 R4 **Bonner Springs** Kansas, C USA
102 L6 **Bonnétable** Sarthe, NW France
27 X6 **Bonne Terre** Missouri, C USA
10 J5 **Bonnet Plume** ≈ Yukon Territory, NW Canada
102 M6 **Bonneval** Eure-et-Loir, C France
103 T10 **Bonneville** Haute-Savoie, E France
36 J3 **Bonneville Salt Flats** *salt flat* Utah, W USA
77 U18 **Bonny** Rivers, S Nigeria
Bonny, Bight of *see* Biafra, Bight of
37 W4 **Bonny Reservoir** ▣ Colorado, C USA
11 R14 **Bonnyville** Alberta, SW Canada
107 C18 **Bono** Sardegna, Italy, C Mediterranean Sea
Bononia *see* Vidin, Bulgaria
Bononia *see* Boulogne-sur-Mer, France
107 B18 **Bonorva** Sardegna, Italy, C Mediterranean Sea
30 M15 **Bonpas Creek** ≈ Illinois, N USA
190 I3 **Bonriki** Tarawa, W Kiribati
183 T4 **Bonshaw** New South Wales, SE Australia
76 I16 **Bonthe** SW Sierra Leone
171 N2 **Bontoc** Luzon, N Philippines
25 Y9 **Bon Wier** Texas, SW USA
111 J25 **Bonyhád** *Ger.* Bonhard. Tolna, S Hungary
Bonzabaai *see* Bonza Bay
83 J25 **Bonza Bay** *Afr.* Bonzabaai. Eastern Cape, S South Africa
182 D7 **Bookabie** South Australia
182 H6 **Bookaloo** South Australia
37 P5 **Book Cliffs** *cliff* Colorado/Utah, W USA
25 P1 **Booker** Texas, SW USA
76 K15 **Boola** Guinée-Forestière, SE Guinea
183 O8 **Booligal** New South Wales, SE Australia
99 G17 **Boom** Antwerpen, N Belgium
43 N6 **Boom** *var.* Boon. Región Autónoma Atlántico Norte, NE Nicaragua
183 S3 **Boomi** New South Wales, SE Australia
Boon *see* Boom
29 V13 **Boone** Iowa, C USA
21 Q8 **Boone** North Carolina, SE USA
27 S11 **Booneville** Arkansas, C USA
21 N6 **Booneville** Kentucky, S USA
23 N2 **Booneville** Mississippi, S USA
21 V3 **Boonsboro** Maryland, NE USA
162 H9 **Böön Tsagaan Nuur** ◎ S Mongolia
34 L6 **Boonville** California, W USA
31 N16 **Boonville** Indiana, N USA
27 U4 **Boonville** Missouri, C USA
18 I9 **Boonville** New York, NE USA
80 M12 **Booraama** Woqooyi Galbeed, NW Somalia
183 O6 **Booroondarra, Mount** *hill* New South Wales, SE Australia
183 N9 **Booroorban** New South Wales, SE Australia
183 R9 **Boorowa** New South Wales, SE Australia
99 H17 **Boortmeerbeek** Vlaams Brabant, C Belgium
80 P11 **Boosaaso** *var.* Bandar Kassim, Bender Qaasim, Bosaso, *It.* Bender Cassim. Bari, N Somalia
19 Q8 **Boothbay Harbor** Maine, NE USA
Boothia Felix *see* Boothia Peninsula
9 N6 **Boothia, Gulf of** *gulf* Nunavut, NE Canada
8 M6 **Boothia Peninsula** *prev.* Boothia Felix. *peninsula* Nunavut, NE Canada
79 E18 **Booué** Ogooué-Ivindo, NE Gabon
101 J21 **Bopfingen** Baden-Württemberg, S Germany
101 F18 **Boppard** Rheinland-Pfalz, W Germany
62 M4 **Boquerón** *off.* Departamento de Boquerón. ◆ *department* W Paraguay
43 P15 **Boquete** *var.* Bajo Boquete. Chiriquí, W Panama
40 J6 **Boquilla, Presa de la** ▣ N Mexico
40 L5 **Boquillas** *var.* Boquillas del Carmen. Coahuila de Zaragoza, NE Mexico
Boquillas del Carmen *see* Boquillas
81 F15 **Bor** Jonglei, S Sudan
95 L20 **Bor** Jönköping, S Sweden
136 J15 **Bor** Niğde, S Turkey
112 P12 **Bor** Serbia, E Yugoslavia
191 S10 **Bora-Bora** *island* Îles Sous le Vent, W French Polynesia
167 Q9 **Borabu** Maha Sarakham, E Thailand
33 P13 **Borah Peak** ▲ Idaho, NW USA
Boralday *see* Burunday
95 J19 **Borås** Västra Götaland, S Sweden
143 N11 **Borāzjān** *var.* Borazjān. Būshehr, S Iran
Borazjan *see* Borāzjān
58 G13 **Borba** Amazonas, N Brazil
104 H11 **Borba** Évora, S Portugal
Borbetomagus *see* Worms
55 O7 **Borbón** Bolívar, E Venezuela
59 Q15 **Borborema, Planalto da** *plateau* NE Brazil
116 M14 **Borcea, Braţul** ≈ S Romania
Borchalo *see* Marneuli
195 R15 **Borchgrevink Coast** *physical region* Antarctica
137 Q11 **Borçka** Artvin, NE Turkey
98 N11 **Borculo** Gelderland, E Netherlands
182 G10 **Borda, Cape** *headland* South Australia
102 K13 **Bordeaux** *anc.* Burdigala. Gironde, SW France
11 T15 **Borden** Saskatchewan, S Canada
14 D8 **Borden Lake** ◎ Ontario, S Canada
9 N4 **Borden Peninsula** *peninsula* Baffin Island, Nunavut, NE Canada
182 K11 **Bordertown** South Australia
92 H2 **Bordheyri** Vestfirdhir, NW Iceland
95 B18 **Bordhoy** *Dan.* Bordø *Island* Faeroe Islands
106 B11 **Bordighera** Liguria, NW Italy
74 K5 **Bordj-Bou-Arreridj** *var.* Bordj Bou Arreridj, Bordj Bou Arréridj. N Algeria
74 L10 **Bordj Omar Driss** E Algeria
143 N13 **Bord Khūn** Hormozgān, S Iran
147 V7 **Bordunskiy** Chuyskaya Oblast', N Kyrgyzstan
95 M17 **Borensberg** Östergötland, S Sweden
Borgå *see* Porvoo
92 L2 **Borgarfjördhur** Austurland, NE Iceland
92 H3 **Borgarnes** Vesturland, W Iceland
93 G14 **Børgefjellet** ▲ C Norway
98 O7 **Borger** Drenthe, NE Netherlands
25 N2 **Borger** Texas, SW USA
95 N20 **Borgholm** Kalmar, S Sweden
107 N22 **Borgia** Calabria, SW Italy
99 J18 **Borgloon** Limburg, NE Belgium
195 P2 **Borg Massif** ▲ Antarctica
22 L9 **Borgne, Lake** ◎ Louisiana, S USA
106 C7 **Borgomanero** Piemonte, NE Italy
106 G10 **Borgo Panigale** ✕ (Bologna) Emilia-Romagna, N Italy
107 J15 **Borgorose** Lazio, C Italy
106 A9 **Borgo San Dalmazzo** Piemonte, N Italy
106 G11 **Borgo San Lorenzo** Toscana, C Italy
106 C7 **Borgosesia** Piemonte, NE Italy
106 E9 **Borgo Val di Taro** Emilia-Romagna, C Italy
106 G6 **Borgo Valsugana** Trentino-Alto Adige, N Italy
163 O11 **Borhoyn Tal** Dornogovĭ, SE Mongolia
167 R8 **Borikhan** *var.* Borikhane. Bolikhamxai, C Laos
Borikhane *see* Borikhan
Borislav *see* Boryslav
129 N8 **Borisoglebsk** Voronezhskaya Oblast', W Russian Federation
Borisov *see* Barysaw
Borisovgrad *see* Pŭrvomay
Borispol' *see* Boryspil'
172 I3 **Boriziny** Mahajanga, NW Madagascar
105 Q5 **Borja** Aragón, NE Spain
Borjas Blancas *see* Les Borges Blanques
137 S10 **Borjomi** *Rus.* Borzhomi. C Georgia
118 L12 **Borkavichy** *Rus.* Borkovichi. Vitsyebskaya Voblasts', N Belarus
101 H16 **Borken** Hessen, C Germany
101 E14 **Borken** Nordrhein-Westfalen, W Germany
92 H10 **Borkenes** Troms, N Norway
78 H7 **Borkou-Ennedi-Tibesti** *off.* Préfecture du Borkou-Ennedi-Tibesti. ◆ *prefecture* N Chad
Borkovichi *see* Borkavichy
100 E9 **Borkum** *island* NW Germany
81 K17 **Bor, Lagh** *var.* Lak Bor. *dry watercourse* NE Kenya
Bor, Lak *see* Bor, Lagh
95 M14 **Borlänge** Dalarna, C Sweden
106 C9 **Bormida** ≈ NW Italy
106 F6 **Bormio** Lombardia, N Italy
101 M16 **Borna** Sachsen, E Germany
98 O10 **Borne** Overijssel, E Netherlands
99 F17 **Bornem** Antwerpen, N Belgium
169 S10 **Borneo** *island* Brunei/Indonesia/Malaysia
101 E16 **Bornheim** Nordrhein-Westfalen, W Germany
95 L24 **Bornholm** ◆ *county* E Denmark
95 L24 **Bornholm** *island* E Denmark
77 Y13 **Borno** ◆ *state* NE Nigeria
104 K15 **Bornos** Andalucía, S Spain

◆ Country ● Country Capital ◇ Dependent Territory ○ Dependent Territory Capital ◆ Administrative Region ✕ International Airport ▲ Mountain ▲ Mountain Range Volcano ≈ River ◎ Lake ▣ Reservoir

162 L7 **Bornuur** Töv, C Mongolia
117 O4 **Borodyanka** Kyyivs'ka Oblast', N Ukraine
158 I5 **Borohoro Shan** ▲▲ NW China
77 O13 **Boromo** SW Burkina
35 T13 **Boron** California, W USA
Borongo see Black Volta
Boron'ki see Baron'ki
Borosjenő see Ineu
Borossebes see Sebiş
76 L15 **Borotou** NW Ivory Coast
117 W6 **Borova** Kharkivs'ka Oblast', E Ukraine
114 H8 **Borovan** Vratsa, NW Bulgaria
126 I14 **Borovichi** Novgorodskaya Oblast', W Russian Federation
Borovlje see Ferlach
112 J9 **Borovo** Vukovar-Srijem, NE Croatia
145 Q7 **Borovoye** Kaz. Būrabay. Severnyy Kazakhstan, N Kazakhstan
128 K4 **Borovsk** Kaluzhskaya Oblast', W Russian Federation
145 N7 **Borovskoy** Kostanay, N Kazakhstan
Borovukha see Baravukha
95 L23 **Borrby** Skåne, S Sweden
181 R3 **Borroloola** Northern Territory, N Australia
116 F9 **Bors** Bihor, NW Romania
116 I9 **Borşa** Hung. Borsa. Maramureş, N Romania
116 J10 **Borsec** Ger. Bad Borseck, Hung. Borszék. Harghita, C Romania
92 K8 **Børselv** Finnmark, N Norway
113 L23 **Borsh** var. Borshi. Vlorë, S Albania
Borshchev see Borshchiv
116 K7 **Borshchiv** Pol. Borszczów, Rus. Borshchev. Ternopil's'ka Oblast', W Ukraine
Borshi see Borsh
111 L20 **Borsod-Abaúj-Zemplén** off. Borsod-Abaúj-Zemplén Megye. ◆ county NE Hungary
99 E15 **Borssele** Zeeland, SW Netherlands
Borszczów see Borshchiv
Borszék see Borsec
Bortala see Bole
103 O12 **Bort-les-Orgues** Corrèze, C France
Bor u České Lípy see Nový Bor
162 E8 **Bor-Udzüür** Hovd, W Mongolia
143 N9 **Borūjen** Chahār Maḩall va Bakhtīārī, C Iran
142 L7 **Borūjerd** var. Burujird. Lorestān, W Iran
116 H6 **Boryslav** Pol. Borysław, Rus. Borislav. L'vivs'ka Oblast', NW Ukraine
Borysław see Boryslav
117 P4 **Boryspil'** Rus. Borispol'. Kyyivs'ka Oblast', N Ukraine
117 P4 **Boryspil'** Rus. Borispol'. × (Kyyiv) Kyyivs'ka Oblast', N Ukraine
Borzhomi see Borjomi
117 R3 **Borzna** Chernihivs'ka Oblast', NE Ukraine
123 O14 **Borzya** Chitinskaya Oblast', S Russian Federation
107 B18 **Bosa** Sardegna, Italy, C Mediterranean Sea
112 F10 **Bosanska Dubica** var. Kozarska Dubica. Republika Srpska, NW Bosnia and Herzegovina
112 G10 **Bosanska Gradiška** var. Gradiška. Republika Srpska, N Bosnia and Herzegovina
112 F10 **Bosanska Kostajnica** var. Srpska Kostajnica. Republika Srpska, NW Bosnia and Herzegovina
112 E11 **Bosanska Krupa** var. Krupa, Krupa na Uni. Federacija Bosna I Hercegovina, NW Bosnia and Herzegovina
112 H10 **Bosanski Brod** var. Srpski Brod. Republika Srpska, N Bosnia and Herzegovina
112 E10 **Bosanski Novi** var. Novi Grad. Republika Srpska, NW Bosnia and Herzegovina
112 E11 **Bosanski Petrovac** var. Petrovac. Federacija Bosna I Hercegovina, NW Bosnia and Herzegovina
112 N12 **Bosanski Petrovac** Serbia, E Yugoslavia
112 I10 **Bosanski Šamac** var. Šamac. Republika Srpska, N Bosnia and Herzegovina
112 E12 **Bosansko Grahovo** var. Grahovo, Hrvatsko Grahovo. Federacija Bosna I Hercegovina, W Bosnia and Herzegovina
Bosaso see Boosaaso
186 B7 **Bosavi, Mount** ※ W PNG
160 J14 **Bose** Guangxi Zhuangzu Zizhiqu, S China
161 Q5 **Boshan** Shandong, E China
113 P16 **Bosilegrad** prev. Bosiljgrad. Serbia, SE Yugoslavia
Bosiljgrad see Bosilegrad
Bösing see Pezinok
98 H12 **Boskoop** Zuid-Holland, C Netherlands
111 G18 **Boskovice** Ger. Boskowitz. Brněnský Kraj, SE Czech Republic
Boskowitz see Boskovice
112 I10 **Bosna** ≈ N Bosnia and Herzegovina
113 G14 **Bosna I Hercegovina, Federacija** ◆ republic Bosnia and Herzegovina
112 H12 **Bosnia and Herzegovina** off. Republic of Bosnia and Herzegovina. ◆ republic SE Europe
79 J16 **Bosobolo** Equateur, NW Dem. Rep. Congo (Zaire)
165 O14 **Bōsō-hantō** peninsula Honshū, S Japan
Bosora see Buşrá ash Shām
Bosphorus/Bosporus see İstanbul Boğazı
Bosporus Cimmerius see Kerch Strait
Bosporus Thracius see İstanbul Boğazı
Bosra see Buşrá ash Shām
79 H14 **Bossangoa** Ouham, C Central African Republic
Bossé Bangou see Bossey Bangou
79 I15 **Bossembélé** Ombella-Mpoko, C Central African Republic
79 H15 **Bossentélé** Ouham-Pendé, W Central African Republic
77 R12 **Bossey Bangou** var. Bossé Bangou. Tillabéri, SW Niger
22 G5 **Bossier City** Louisiana, S USA
83 D20 **Bossiesvlei** Hardap, S Namibia
77 Y11 **Bosso** Diffa, SE Niger
61 F15 **Bossoroca** Rio Grande do Sul, S Brazil
158 J10 **Bostan** Xinjiang Uygur Zizhiqu, W China
142 K3 **Bostānābād** Āzarbāyjān-e Khāvarī, N Iran
158 K6 **Bosten Hu** var. Bagrax Hu. ◎ NW China
97 O18 **Boston** prev. St.Botolph's Town. E England, UK
19 O11 **Boston** state capital Massachusetts, NE USA
10 M17 **Boston Bar** British Columbia, SW Canada
27 T10 **Boston Mountains** ▲▲ Arkansas, C USA
15 P8 **Bostonnais** ≈ Quebec, SE Canada
Bostyn' see Bastyn'
112 J10 **Bosut** ≈ E Croatia
154 C11 **Botād** Gujarāt, W India
183 T9 **Botany Bay** inlet New South Wales, SE Australia
83 G18 **Boteti** var. Botletle. ≈ N Botswana
114 J9 **Botev** ▲ C Bulgaria
114 H9 **Botevgrad** prev. Orkhaniye. Sofiya, W Bulgaria
93 J16 **Bothnia, Gulf of** Fin. Pohjanlahti, Swe. Bottniska Viken. gulf N Baltic Sea
183 P17 **Bothwell** Tasmania, SE Australia
104 H5 **Boticas** Vila Real, N Portugal
55 W10 **Boti-Pasi** Sipaliwini, C Suriname
Botletle see Boteti
129 P16 **Botlikh** Chechenskaya Respublika, SW Russian Federation
117 N10 **Botna** ≈ E Moldova
116 J9 **Botoşani** Hung. Botosány. Botoşani, NE Romania
116 K8 **Botoşani** ◆ county NE Romania
Botosány see Botoşani
161 P4 **Botou** prev. Bozhen. Hebei, E China
99 M20 **Botrange** ▲ E Belgium
107 O21 **Botricello** Calabria, SW Italy
83 I23 **Botshabelo** Free State, C South Africa
93 J15 **Botsmark** Västerbotten, N Sweden
83 G19 **Botswana** off. Republic of Botswana. ◆ republic S Africa
29 N2 **Bottineau** North Dakota, N USA
Bottniska Viken see Bothnia, Gulf of
60 L9 **Botucatu** São Paulo, S Brazil
76 M16 **Bouaflé** C Ivory Coast
77 N16 **Bouaké** var. Bwake. C Ivory Coast
79 G14 **Bouar** Nana-Mambéré, W Central African Republic
74 H7 **Bouarfa** NE Morocco
111 B19 **Boubín** ▲ SW Czech Republic
79 I14 **Bouca** Ouham, W Central African Republic
15 T5 **Boucher** ≈ Quebec, SE Canada
103 R15 **Bouches-du-Rhône** ◆ department SE France
74 C9 **Bou Craa** var. Bu Craa. NW Western Sahara
77 O9 **Boû Djébéha** oasis C Mali
108 C8 **Boudry** Neuchâtel, W Switzerland
180 L2 **Bougainville, Cape** headland Western Australia
65 E24 **Bougainville, Cape** headland East Falkland, Falkland Islands
Bougainville, Détroit de see Bougainville Strait, Vanuatu
186 J7 **Bougainville Island** island NE PNG
186 Q13 **Bougainville Strait** strait N Solomon Islands
197 B12 **Bougainville Strait** Fr. Détroit de Bougainville. strait C Vanuatu
120 I9 **Bougaroun, Cap** headland NE Algeria
77 R8 **Boughessa** Kidal, NE Mali
Bougie see Béjaïa
76 L13 **Bougouni** Sikasso, SW Mali
99 J24 **Bouillon** Luxembourg, SE Belgium
74 K5 **Bouira** var. Bouïra. N Algeria
74 D8 **Bou-Izakarn** SW Morocco
74 B9 **Boujdour** var. Bojador. W Western Sahara
74 G5 **Boukhalef** × (Tanger) N Morocco
Boukombé see Boukoumbé
77 R14 **Boukoumbé** var. Boukombé. C Benin
76 G6 **Boû Lanouâr** Dakhlet Nouâdhibou, W Mauritania
37 T4 **Boulder** Colorado, C USA
33 R10 **Boulder** Montana, NW USA
35 X12 **Boulder City** Nevada, W USA
181 T7 **Boulia** Queensland, C Australia
15 N10 **Boullé** ≈ Quebec, SE Canada
102 J9 **Boulogne** ≈ NW France
Boulogne see Boulogne-sur-Mer
102 L16 **Boulogne-sur-Gesse** Haute-Garonne, S France
103 N1 **Boulogne-sur-Mer** var. Boulogne; anc. Bononia, Gesoriacum, Gessoriacum. Pas-de-Calais, N France
77 Q12 **Boulsa** C Burkina
77 W11 **Boultoum** Zinder, C Niger
187 Y14 **Bouma** Taveuni, N Fiji
79 G16 **Boumba** ≈ SE Cameroon
76 J9 **Boûmdeïd** var. Boumdeït. Assaba, S Mauritania
Boumdeït see Boûmdeïd
115 C17 **Boumistós** ▲ W Greece
77 O15 **Bouna** NE Ivory Coast
19 P4 **Boundary Bald Mountain** ▲ Maine, NE USA
35 S8 **Boundary Peak** ▲ Nevada, W USA
76 M14 **Boundiali** N Ivory Coast
79 G19 **Boundji** Cuvette, C Congo
77 O13 **Boundoukui** var. Bondoukui, Bondoukuy. W Burkina
36 L2 **Bountiful** Utah, W USA
Bounty Basin see Bounty Trough
191 Q16 **Bounty Bay** bay Pitcairn Island, C Pacific Ocean
192 L12 **Bounty Islands** island group S NZ
175 Q13 **Bounty Trough** var. Bounty Basin. undersea feature S Pacific Ocean
187 P17 **Bourail** Province Sud, C New Caledonia
27 V5 **Bourbeuse River** ≈ Missouri, C USA
103 Q9 **Bourbon-Lancy** Saône-et-Loire, C France
31 N11 **Bourbonnais** Illinois, N USA
103 O10 **Bourbonnais** cultural region C France
103 S7 **Bourbonne-les-Bains** Haute-Marne, N France
Bourbon Vendée see la Roche-sur-Yon
74 M8 **Bourdj Messaouda** E Algeria
77 Q10 **Bourem** Gao, C Mali
Bourg see Bourg-en-Bresse
103 N11 **Bourganeuf** Creuse, C France
Bourgas see Burgas
Bourge-en-Bresse see Bourg-en-Bresse
103 S10 **Bourg-en-Bresse** var. Bourg, Bourge-en-Bresse. Ain, E France
103 O8 **Bourges** anc. Avaricum. Cher, C France
103 T11 **Bourget, Lac du** ◎ E France
103 P8 **Bourgogne** Eng. Burgundy. ◆ region E France
103 S11 **Bourgoin-Jallieu** Isère, E France
103 R14 **Bourg-St-Andéol** Ardèche, E France
103 U11 **Bourg-St-Maurice** Savoie, E France
108 C11 **Bourg St.Pierre** Valais, SW Switzerland
76 H8 **Boû Rjeïmât** well W Mauritania
183 P5 **Bourke** New South Wales, SE Australia
97 M24 **Bournemouth** S England, UK
99 M23 **Bourscheid** Diekirch, NE Luxembourg
74 K6 **Bou Saâda** var. Bou Saada. N Algeria
36 I13 **Bouse Wash** ≈ Arizona, SW USA
103 N10 **Boussac** Creuse, C France
102 M16 **Boussens** Haute-Garonne, S France
78 H12 **Bousso** prev. Fort-Bretonnet. Chari-Baguirmi, S Chad
76 H9 **Boutilimit** Trarza, SW Mauritania
65 D21 **Bouvet Island** ◇ Norwegian dependency S Atlantic Ocean
77 U11 **Bouza** Tahoua, SW Niger
109 R10 **Bovec** Ger. Flitsch, It. Plezzo. NW Slovenia
98 J8 **Bovenkarspel** Noord-Holland, NW Netherlands
29 V5 **Bovey** Minnesota, N USA
32 M9 **Bovill** Idaho, NW USA
24 L4 **Bovina** Texas, SW USA
107 M17 **Bovino** Puglia, SE Italy
61 C17 **Bovril** Entre Ríos, E Argentina
28 L2 **Bowbells** North Dakota, N USA
11 Q16 **Bow City** Alberta, SW Canada
29 O8 **Bowdle** South Dakota, N USA
181 X6 **Bowen** Queensland, NE Australia
192 L2 **Bowers Ridge** undersea feature S Bering Sea
25 S5 **Bowie** Texas, SW USA
11 R17 **Bow Island** Alberta, SW Canada
Bowkān see Būkān
20 J7 **Bowling Green** Kentucky, S USA
27 V3 **Bowling Green** Missouri, C USA
31 R11 **Bowling Green** Ohio, N USA
21 W5 **Bowling Green** Virginia, NE USA
28 J6 **Bowman** North Dakota, N USA
9 Q7 **Bowman Bay** bay NW Atlantic Ocean
194 I5 **Bowman Coast** physical region Antarctica
28 J7 **Bowman-Haley Lake** ⊡ North Dakota, N USA
195 Z11 **Bowman Island** island Antarctica
Bowo see Bomi
183 S9 **Bowral** New South Wales, SE Australia
186 E8 **Bowutu Mountains** ▲▲ C PNG
83 I16 **Bowwood** Southern, S Zambia
28 I12 **Box Butte Reservoir** ⊡ Nebraska, C USA
28 J10 **Box Elder** South Dakota, N USA
95 M18 **Boxholm** Östergötland, S Sweden
Bo Xian/Boxian see Bozhou
161 Q4 **Boxing** Shandong, E China
99 L14 **Boxmeer** Noord-Brabant, SE Netherlands
99 J14 **Boxtel** Noord-Brabant, S Netherlands
136 J10 **Boyabat** Sinop, N Turkey
54 F9 **Boyacá** off. Departamento de Boyacá. ◆ province C Colombia
117 O4 **Boyarka** Kyyivs'ka Oblast', N Ukraine
22 H7 **Boyce** Louisiana, S USA
33 U11 **Boyd** Montana, NW USA
25 S6 **Boyd** Texas, SW USA
21 V8 **Boydton** Virginia, NE USA
Boyer Ahmadī va Kohkīlūyeh see Kohkīlūyeh va Būyer Aḩmadī
29 T13 **Boyer River** ≈ Iowa, C USA
21 W8 **Boykins** Virginia, NE USA
11 Q13 **Boyle** Alberta, SW Canada
97 D16 **Boyle** Ir. Mainistirna Búille. C Ireland
97 F17 **Boyne** Ir. An Bhóinn. ≈ E Ireland
31 Q5 **Boyne City** Michigan, N USA
23 Z14 **Boynton Beach** Florida, SE USA
147 O13 **Boysun** Rus. Baysun. Surkhondaryo Wiloyati, S Uzbekistan
Bozau see Întorsura Buzăului
136 B12 **Bozcaada** island Çanakkale, NW Turkey
136 C14 **Boz Dağları** ▲▲ W Turkey
33 S11 **Bozeman** Montana, NW USA
Bozen see Bolzano
79 J16 **Bozene** Equateur, NW Dem. Rep. Congo (Zaire)
161 P7 **Bozhou** var. Boxian, Bo Xian. Anhui, E China
136 H16 **Bozkır** Konya, S Turkey
136 K13 **Bozok Yaylası** plateau C Turkey
79 H14 **Bozoum** Ouham-Pendé, W Central African Republic
137 N16 **Bozova** Sanlıurfa, S Turkey
Bozrah see Buşrá ash Shām
136 E12 **Bozüyük** Bilecik, NW Turkey
106 B9 **Bra** Piemonte, NW Italy
194 G4 **Brabant Island** island Antarctica
99 I20 **Brabant Wallon** ◆ province C Belgium
113 F15 **Brač** var. Brach, It. Brazza; anc. Brattia. island S Croatia
Bracara Augusta see Braga
107 H15 **Bracciano** Lazio, C Italy
107 H14 **Bracciano, Lago di** ◎ C Italy
14 H13 **Bracebridge** Ontario, S Canada
Brach see Brač
93 G17 **Bräcke** Jämtland, C Sweden
25 P12 **Brackettville** Texas, SW USA
97 N22 **Bracknell** S England, UK
61 K14 **Braço do Norte** Santa Catarina, S Brazil
116 G11 **Brad** Hung. Brád. Hunedoara, SW Romania
107 N18 **Bradano** ≈ S Italy
23 V13 **Bradenton** Florida, SE USA
14 H14 **Bradford** Ontario, S Canada
97 L17 **Bradford** N England, UK
27 W10 **Bradford** Arkansas, C USA
18 D12 **Bradford** Pennsylvania, NE USA
27 T15 **Bradley** Arkansas, C USA
25 P7 **Bradshaw** Texas, SW USA
25 Q9 **Brady** Texas, SW USA
25 Q9 **Brady Creek** ≈ Texas, SW USA
96 J10 **Braemar** NE Scotland, UK
116 K8 **Brăeşti** Botoşani, NW Romania
104 G5 **Braga** anc. Bracara Augusta. Braga, NW Portugal
104 G5 **Braga** ◆ district N Portugal
116 J15 **Bragadiru** Teleorman, S Romania
61 C20 **Bragado** Buenos Aires, E Argentina
104 J5 **Bragança** Eng. Braganza; anc. Julio Briga. Bragança, NE Portugal
104 I5 **Bragança** ◆ district N Portugal
60 N9 **Bragança Paulista** São Paulo, S Brazil
Braganza see Bragança
Bragin see Brahin
29 V7 **Braham** Minnesota, N USA
Brahe see Brda
Brahestad see Raahe
119 O20 **Brahin** Rus. Bragin. Homyel'skaya Voblasts', SE Belarus
153 U15 **Brahmanbaria** Chittagong, E Bangladesh
154 O12 **Brāhmani** ≈ E India
154 N13 **Brahmapur** Orissa, E India
131 S10 **Brahmaputra** var. Padma, Tsangpo, Ben. Jamuna, Chin. Yarlung Zangbo Jiang, Ind. Bramaputra, Dihang, Siang. ≈ S Asia
97 H19 **Braich y Pwll** headland NW Wales, UK
183 R10 **Braidwood** New South Wales, SE Australia
30 M11 **Braidwood** Illinois, N USA
116 M13 **Brăila** Brăila, E Romania
116 L13 **Brăila** ◆ county SE Romania
99 G19 **Braine-l'Alleud** Brabant Wallon, C Belgium
99 F19 **Braine-le-Comte** Hainaut, SW Belgium
29 U6 **Brainerd** Minnesota, N USA
99 J19 **Braives** Liège, E Belgium
83 H23 **Brak** ≈ C South Africa
Brak see Birāk
99 E18 **Brakel** Oost-Vlaanderen, SW Belgium
98 J13 **Brakel** Gelderland, C Netherlands
76 H9 **Brakna** ◆ region S Mauritania
95 J17 **Brålanda** Västra Götaland, S Sweden
Bramaputra see Brahmaputra
95 F23 **Bramming** Ribe, W Denmark
14 G15 **Brampton** Ontario, S Canada
100 F12 **Bramsche** Niedersachsen, NW Germany
116 J12 **Bran** Ger. Törzburg, Hung. Törcsvár. Braşov, S Romania
29 W8 **Branch** Minnesota, N USA
21 R14 **Branchville** South Carolina, SE USA
47 Y6 **Branco, Cabo** headland E Brazil
58 F11 **Branco, Rio** ≈ N Brazil
108 J8 **Brand** Vorarlberg, W Austria
83 B18 **Brandberg** ▲ NW Namibia
95 H14 **Brandbu** Oppland, S Norway
95 F22 **Brande** Ringkøbing, W Denmark
Brandebourg see Brandenburg
100 M12 **Brandenburg** var. Brandenburg an der Havel. Brandenburg, NE Germany
20 K5 **Brandenburg** Kentucky, S USA
100 N12 **Brandenburg** off. Freie und Hansestadt Hamburg, Fr. Brandebourg. ◆ state NE Germany
Brandenburg an der Havel see Brandenburg
83 I23 **Brandfort** Free State, C South Africa
11 W16 **Brandon** Manitoba, S Canada
23 V12 **Brandon** Florida, SE USA
22 L6 **Brandon** Mississippi, S USA
97 A20 **Brandon Mountain** Ir. Cnoc Bréanainn. ▲ SW Ireland
Brandsen see Coronel Brandsen
95 I14 **Brandval** Hedmark, S Norway
83 F24 **Brandvlei** Northern Cape, W South Africa
23 U9 **Branford** Florida, SE USA
110 K7 **Braniewo** Ger. Braunsberg. Warmińsko-Mazurskie, NE Poland
194 H3 **Bransfield Strait** strait Antarctica
37 U8 **Branson** Colorado, C USA
27 T8 **Branson** Missouri, C USA
14 G16 **Brantford** Ontario, S Canada
102 L12 **Brantôme** Dordogne, SW France
182 L12 **Branxholme** Victoria, SE Australia
Brasil see Brazil
59 C16 **Brasiléia** Acre, W Brazil
59 K18 **Brasília** ● (Brazil) Distrito Federal, C Brazil
Braslav see Braslaw
118 J12 **Braslaw** Pol. Brasław, Rus. Braslav. Vitsyebskaya Voblasts', N Belarus
116 J12 **Braşov** Ger. Kronstadt, Hung. Brassó; prev. Oraşul Stalin. Braşov, C Romania
116 I12 **Braşov** ◆ county C Romania
77 U18 **Brass** Bayelsa, S Nigeria
99 H16 **Brasschaat** var. Brasschaet. Antwerpen, N Belgium
Brasschaet see Brasschaat
169 V8 **Brassey, Banjaran** var. Brassey Range. ▲▲ East Malaysia
Brassey Range see Brassey, Banjaran
Brassó see Braşov
23 T1 **Brasstown Bald** ▲ Georgia, SE USA
113 K22 **Brataj** Vlorë, SW Albania
114 J10 **Bratan** var. Morozov. ▲ C Bulgaria
111 F21 **Bratislava** Ger. Pressburg, Hung. Pozsony. ● (Slovakia) Bratislavský Kraj, W Slovakia
111 H21 **Bratislavský Kraj** ◆ region W Slovakia
114 H10 **Bratiya** ▲ C Bulgaria
122 M12 **Bratsk** Irkutskaya Oblast', C Russian Federation
117 Q8 **Brats'ke** Mykolayivs'ka Oblast', S Ukraine
122 M13 **Bratskoye Vodokhranilishche** Eng. Bratsk Reservoir. ⊡ S Russian Federation
Bratsk Reservoir see Bratskoye Vodokhranilishche
Brattia see Brač
94 D9 **Brattvåg** Møre og Romsdal, S Norway
112 K12 **Bratunac** Republika Srpska, E Bosnia and Herzegovina
114 J10 **Bratya Daskalovi** prev. Grozdovo. Stara Zagora, C Bulgaria
109 U2 **Braunau** ≈ N Austria
Braunau see Braunau am Inn
109 Q4 **Braunau am Inn** var. Braunau. Oberösterreich, N Austria
Braunsberg see Braniewo
100 J13 **Braunschweig** Eng./Fr. Brunswick. Niedersachsen, N Germany
Brava see Baraawe
105 Y6 **Brava, Costa** coastal region NE Spain
43 V16 **Brava, Punta** headland E Panama
95 N17 **Bråviken** inlet S Sweden
56 B10 **Bravo, Cerro** ▲ N Peru
Bravo del Norte, Río/Bravo, Río see Grande, Rio
35 X17 **Brawley** California, W USA
97 G18 **Bray** Ir. Bré. E Ireland
59 G16 **Brazil** off. Federative Republic of Brazil, Port. República Federativa do Brasil, Sp. Brasil; prev. United States of Brazil. ◆ federal republic South America
65 K15 **Brazil Basin** var. Brazilian Basin, Brazil'skaya Kotlovina. undersea feature W Atlantic Ocean
Brazilian Basin see Brazil Basin
Brazilian Highlands see Central, Planalto
Brazil'skaya Kotlovina see Brazil Basin
25 U10 **Brazos River** ≈ Texas, SW USA
Brazza see Brač
79 G21 **Brazzaville** ● (Congo) Capital District, S Congo
79 G21 **Brazzaville** × Le Pool, S Congo
112 J11 **Brčko** Republika Srpska, NE Bosnia and Herzegovina
110 H8 **Brda** Ger. Brahe. ≈ N Poland
Bré see Bray
185 A23 **Breaksea Sound** sound South Island, NZ
184 L4 **Bream Bay** bay North Island, NZ
184 L4 **Bream Head** headland North Island, NZ
Bréanainn, Cnoc see Brandon Mountain
45 S6 **Brea, Punta** headland W Puerto Rico
22 I9 **Breaux Bridge** Louisiana, S USA
116 J13 **Breaza** Prahova, SE Romania
169 P16 **Brebes** Jawa, C Indonesia
96 K10 **Brechin** E Scotland, UK
99 H15 **Brecht** Antwerpen, N Belgium
37 S4 **Breckenridge** Colorado, C USA
29 R6 **Breckenridge** Minnesota, N USA
25 R6 **Breckenridge** Texas, SW USA
97 J21 **Brecknock** cultural region SE Wales, UK
63 G25 **Brecknock, Península** headland S Chile
111 G19 **Břeclav** Ger. Lundenburg. Brněnský Kraj, SE Czech Republic
97 J21 **Brecon** E Wales, UK
97 J21 **Brecon Beacons** ▲▲ S Wales, UK
99 I14 **Breda** Noord-Brabant, S Netherlands
95 K20 **Bredaryd** Jönköping, S Sweden
83 F26 **Bredasdorp** Western Cape, SW South Africa
93 H16 **Bredbyn** Västernorrland, N Sweden
122 F11 **Bredy** Chelyabinskaya Oblast', C Russian Federation
99 K17 **Bree** Limburg, NE Belgium
67 T15 **Breede** ≈ S South Africa
98 I7 **Breezand** Noord-Holland, NW Netherlands
113 P18 **Bregalnica** ≈ E FYR Macedonia
108 I6 **Bregenz** anc. Brigantium. Vorarlberg, W Austria
108 J7 **Bregenzer Wald** ▲▲ W Austria
114 F6 **Bregovo** Vidin, NW Bulgaria
102 H5 **Bréhat, Île de** island NW France
92 H2 **Breidhafjördhur** bay W Iceland
92 L3 **Breidhdalsvík** Austurland, E Iceland
108 H9 **Breil** Ger. Brigels. Graubünden, S Switzerland
92 J8 **Breivikbotn** Finnmark, N Norway
94 I9 **Brekken** Sør-Trøndelag, S Norway
94 G7 **Brekstad** Sør-Trøndelag, S Norway
94 B10 **Bremangerlandet** island S Norway
Brême see Bremen
100 H11 **Bremen** Fr. Brême. Bremen, NW Germany
23 R3 **Bremen** Georgia, SE USA
31 O11 **Bremen** Indiana, N USA
100 H10 **Bremen** off. Freie Hansestadt Bremen, Fr. Brême. ◆ state N Germany
100 G9 **Bremerhaven** Bremen, NW Germany
Bremersdorp see Manzini
32 G8 **Bremerton** Washington, NW USA
100 H10 **Bremervörde** Niedersachsen, NW Germany
25 U9 **Bremond** Texas, SW USA
25 U10 **Brenham** Texas, SW USA
108 M8 **Brenner** Tirol, W Austria
Brenner, Col du/Brennero, Passo del see Brenner Pass
108 M8 **Brenner Pass** var. Brenner Sattel, Fr. Col du Brenner, Ger. Brennerpass, It. Passo del Brennero. pass Austria/Italy
Brenner Sattel see Brenner Pass
108 G10 **Brenno** ≈ SW Switzerland
106 F7 **Breno** Lombardia, N Italy
23 O5 **Brent** Alabama, S USA
106 H7 **Brenta** ≈ NE Italy
97 P21 **Brentwood** E England, UK
18 L14 **Brentwood** Long Island, New York, NE USA
106 F7 **Brescia** anc. Brixia. Lombardia, N Italy
99 D15 **Breskens** Zeeland, SW Netherlands
Breslau see Dolnośląskie
106 H5 **Bressanone** Ger. Brixen. Trentino-Alto Adige, N Italy
96 M2 **Bressay** island NE Scotland, UK
102 K9 **Bressuire** Deux-Sèvres, W France
119 F20 **Brest** Pol. Brześć nad Bugiem, Rus. Brest-Litovsk; prev. Brześć Litewski. Brestskaya Voblasts', SW Belarus
102 F5 **Brest** Finistère, NW France
Brest-Litovsk see Brest
112 A10 **Brestova** Istra, NW Croatia
Brestskaya Oblast' see Brestskaya Voblasts'
119 G19 **Brestskaya Voblasts'** prev. Rus. Brestskaya Oblast'. ◆ province SW Belarus
102 G6 **Bretagne** Eng. Brittany; Lat. Britannia Minor. ◆ region NW France
116 G12 **Bretea-Română** Hung. Oláhbrettye; prev. Bretea-Romînă. Hunedoara, W Romania
Bretea-Romînă see Bretea-Română
103 O3 **Breteuil** Oise, N France
102 I10 **Breton, Pertuis** inlet W France
22 L10 **Breton Sound** sound Louisiana, S USA
184 K2 **Brett, Cape** headland North Island, NZ
101 G21 **Bretten** Baden-Württemberg, SW Germany
99 K15 **Breugel** Noord-Brabant, S Netherlands
106 B6 **Breuil-Cervinia** It. Cervinia. Valle d'Aosta, NW Italy
98 I11 **Breukelen** Utrecht, C Netherlands
21 P10 **Brevard** North Carolina, SE USA
38 L9 **Brevig Mission** Alaska, USA

95 G16 Brevik Telemark, S Norway
183 P5 Brewarrina New South Wales, SE Australia
19 R6 Brewer Maine, NE USA
29 T11 Brewster Minnesota, N USA
29 N14 Brewster Nebraska, C USA
31 U12 Brewster Ohio, N USA
183 O8 Brewster, Lake ◎ New South Wales, SE Australia
23 P7 Brewton Alabama, S USA
Brezhnev see Naberezhnyye Chelny
109 W12 Brežice Ger. Rann. E Slovenia
114 G9 Breznik Pernik, W Bulgaria
111 K19 Brezno Ger. Bries, Briesen, Hung. Breznóbánya; prev. Brezno nad Hronom. Banskobystrický Kraj, C Slovakia
Breznóbánya/Brezno nad Hronom see Brezno
116 I12 Brezoi Vâlcea, SW Romania
114 J10 Brezovo prev. Abrashlare. Plovdiv, C Bulgaria
79 K14 Bria Haute-Kotto, C Central African Republic
103 U13 Briançon anc. Brigantio. Hautes-Alpes, SE France
36 K7 Brian Head ▲ Utah, W USA
103 O7 Briare Loiret, C France
183 V2 Bribie Island island Queensland, E Australia
43 O14 Bribrí Limón, E Costa Rica
116 L8 Briceni var. Brinceni, Rus. Brichany. N Moldova
Bricgstow see Bristol
Brichany see Briceni
99 M24 Bridel Luxembourg, C Luxembourg
97 J22 Bridgend S Wales, UK
14 I14 Bridgenorth Ontario, SE Canada
23 Q1 Bridgeport Alabama, S USA
35 R8 Bridgeport California, W USA
18 L13 Bridgeport Connecticut, NE USA
31 N15 Bridgeport Illinois, N USA
28 J14 Bridgeport Nebraska, C USA
25 S6 Bridgeport Texas, SW USA
21 S3 Bridgeport West Virginia, NE USA
25 S5 Bridgeport, Lake ⊡ Texas, SW USA
33 U11 Bridger Montana, NW USA
18 I17 Bridgeton New Jersey, NE USA
180 J14 Bridgetown Western Australia
45 Y14 Bridgetown ● (Barbados) SW Barbados
183 P17 Bridgewater Tasmania, SE Australia
13 P16 Bridgewater Nova Scotia, SE Canada
19 P12 Bridgewater Massachusetts, NE USA
29 Q11 Bridgewater South Dakota, N USA
21 U5 Bridgewater Virginia, NE USA
19 P8 Bridgton Maine, NE USA
97 K23 Bridgwater SW England, UK
97 K22 Bridgwater Bay bay SW England, UK
97 O16 Bridlington E England, UK
97 O16 Bridlington Bay bay E England, UK
183 P15 Bridport Tasmania, SE Australia
97 K24 Bridport S England, UK
103 O5 Brie cultural region N France
Brieg see Brzeg
Briel see Brielle
98 G12 Brielle var. Briel, Bril, Eng. The Brill. Zuid-Holland, SW Netherlands
108 E9 Brienz Bern, C Switzerland
108 E9 Brienzer See ◎ SW Switzerland
Bries/Briesen see Brezno
Brietzig see Brzesko
103 S4 Briey Meurthe-et-Moselle, NE France
108 E10 Brig Fr. Brigue, It. Briga. Valais, SW Switzerland
Briga see Brig
101 G24 Brigach ⁓ S Germany
18 K17 Brigantine New Jersey, NE USA
Brigantio see Briançon
Brigantium see Bregenz
Brigels see Breil
25 S9 Briggs Texas, SW USA
36 L1 Brigham City Utah, W USA
14 J15 Brighton Ontario, SE Canada
97 O23 Brighton SE England, UK
37 T4 Brighton Colorado, C USA
30 K15 Brighton Illinois, N USA
103 T16 Brignoles Var, W France
Brigue see Brig
105 O7 Brihuega Castilla-La Mancha, C Spain
112 A10 Brijuni It. Brioni. island group NW Croatia
76 G12 Brikama W Gambia
Bril see Brielle
Brill, The see Brielle
101 G15 Brilon Nordrhein-Westfalen, W Germany
Brinceni see Briceni
107 Q18 Brindisi anc. Brundisium, Brundusium. Puglia, SE Italy
27 W11 Brinkley Arkansas, C USA
Brioni see Brijuni
103 P12 Brioude anc. Brivas. Haute-Loire, C France
Briovera see St-Lô
183 U2 Brisbane state capital Queensland, E Australia
183 V2 Brisbane ✕ Queensland, E Australia
25 P2 Briscoe Texas, SW USA
106 H10 Brisighella Emilia-Romagna, C Italy
108 G11 Brissago Ticino, S Switzerland
97 K22 Bristol anc. Bricgstow. SW England, UK
18 M12 Bristol Connecticut, NE USA
23 R9 Bristol Florida, SE USA
19 N9 Bristol New Hampshire, NE USA
29 Q8 Bristol South Dakota, N USA
21 P8 Bristol Tennessee, S USA
18 M8 Bristol Vermont, NE USA
39 N14 Bristol Bay bay Alaska, USA
97 I22 Bristol Channel inlet England/Wales, UK
35 W14 Bristol Lake ◎ California, W USA
27 P10 Bristow Oklahoma, C USA
86 C10 Britain var. Great Britain. island UK
Britannia Minor see Bretagne
10 L12 British Columbia Fr. Colombie-Britannique. ◆ province SW Canada
British Guiana see Guyana
British Honduras see Belize
173 Q7 British Indian Ocean Territory ◇ UK dependent territory C Indian Ocean
86 B9 British Isles island group NW Europe
10 I1 British Mountains ▲ Yukon Territory, NW Canada
British North Borneo see Sabah
British Solomon Islands Protectorate see Solomon Islands
45 S8 British Virgin Islands var. Virgin Islands. ◇ UK dependent territory E West Indies
83 J21 Brits North-West, N South Africa
83 H24 Britstown Northern Cape, W South Africa
14 F12 Britt Ontario, S Canada
29 V12 Britt Iowa, C USA
Brittany see Bretagne
29 Q7 Britton South Dakota, N USA
Briva Curretia see Brive-la-Gaillarde
Briva Isarae see Pontoise
Brivas see Brioude
Brive see Brive-la-Gaillarde
102 M12 Brive-la-Gaillarde prev. Brive, anc. Briva Curretia. Corrèze, C France
105 O4 Briviesca Castilla-León, N Spain
Brixen see Bressanone
Brixia see Brescia
145 S15 Brlik prev. Novotroickoje, Novotroitskoye. Zhambyl, SE Kazakhstan
111 G19 Brněnský Kraj ◆ region SE Czech republic
111 G18 Brno Ger. Brünn. Brněnský Kraj, SE Czech Republic
96 G7 Broad Bay bay NW Scotland, UK
25 X8 Broaddus Texas, SW USA
183 O12 Broadford Victoria, SE Australia
96 G9 Broadford N Scotland, UK
96 J13 Broad Law ▲ S Scotland, UK
23 U3 Broad River ⁓ Georgia, SE USA
21 N8 Broad River ⁓ North Carolina/South Carolina, SE USA
181 Y8 Broadsound Range ▲ Queensland, E Australia
33 X11 Broadus Montana, NW USA
21 U4 Broadway Virginia, NE USA
118 E9 Brocēni Saldus, SW Latvia
11 U11 Brochet Manitoba, C Canada
11 U10 Brochet, Lac ◎ Manitoba, C Canada
15 S5 Brochet, Lac au ◎ Quebec, SE Canada
101 K14 Brocken ▲ C Germany
19 O12 Brockton Massachusetts, NE USA
14 L14 Brockville Ontario, SE Canada
18 D13 Brockway Pennsylvania, NE USA
Brod/Bród see Slavonski Brod
9 N5 Brodeur Peninsula peninsula Baffin Island, Nunavut, NE Canada
96 H13 Brodick W Scotland, UK
Brod na Savi see Slavonski Brod
110 K9 Brodnica Ger. Buddenbrock. Kujawski-pomorskie, C Poland
112 G10 Brod-Posavina off. Brodsko-Posavska Županija. ◆ province NE Croatia
116 J5 Brody L'vivs'ka Oblast', NW Ukraine
95 G22 Brædstrup Vejle, C Denmark
98 I10 Broek-in-Waterland Noord-Holland, C Netherlands
32 L13 Brogan Oregon, NW USA
110 N10 Brok Mazowieckie, C Poland
27 P9 Broken Arrow Oklahoma, C USA
183 T9 Broken Bay bay New South Wales, SE Australia
29 N15 Broken Bow Nebraska, C USA
27 R13 Broken Bow Oklahoma, C USA
27 R12 Broken Bow Lake ⊡ Oklahoma, C USA
182 L6 Broken Hill New South Wales, SE Australia
173 S10 Broken Ridge undersea feature S Indian Ocean
186 C6 Broken Water Bay bay W Bismarck Sea
55 W10 Brokopondo Brokopondo, NE Suriname
55 W10 Brokopondo ◆ district C Suriname
Bromberg see Bydgoszcz
95 L22 Bromölla Skåne, S Sweden
97 L20 Bromsgrove W England, UK
95 G20 Brønderslev Nordjylland, N Denmark
106 D8 Broni Lombardia, N Italy
10 K11 Bronlund Peak ▲ British Columbia, W Canada
93 F14 Brønnøysund Nordland, C Norway
23 V10 Bronson Florida, SE USA
31 Q11 Bronson Michigan, N USA
25 X8 Bronson Texas, SW USA
107 L24 Bronte Sicilia, Italy, C Mediterranean Sea
25 P8 Bronte Texas, SW USA
25 Y9 Brookeland Texas, SW USA
170 M7 Brooke's Point Palawan, W Philippines
27 T3 Brookfield Missouri, C USA
22 K7 Brookhaven Mississippi, S USA
32 E16 Brookings Oregon, NW USA
29 R10 Brookings South Dakota, N USA
29 W14 Brooklyn Iowa, C USA
29 U8 Brooklyn Park Minnesota, N USA
21 U7 Brookneal Virginia, NE USA
11 R16 Brooks Alberta, SW Canada
25 V11 Brookshire Texas, SW USA
38 L8 Brooks Mountain ▲ Alaska, USA
38 M11 Brooks Range ▲ Alaska, USA
31 O12 Brookston Indiana, N USA
23 V11 Brooksville Florida, SE USA
23 N4 Brooksville Mississippi, S USA
180 J13 Brookton Western Australia
31 Q14 Brookville Indiana, N USA
18 D13 Brookville Pennsylvania, NE USA
31 Q14 Brookville Lake ⊡ Indiana, N USA
180 K5 Broome Western Australia
37 S4 Broomfield Colorado, C USA
Broos see Orăştie
96 J7 Brora N Scotland, UK
96 I7 Brora ⁓ N Scotland, UK
95 F23 Brørup Ribe, W Denmark
95 L23 Brösarp Skåne, S Sweden
116 J9 Broşteni Suceava, NE Romania
102 M6 Brou Eure-et-Loir, C France
Broucsella see Brussel/Bruxelles
Broughton Bay see Tongjosŏn-man
9 R5 Broughton Island Nunavut, NE Canada
138 G7 Broummâna C Lebanon
22 I9 Broussard Louisiana, S USA
98 E13 Brouwersdam dam SW Netherlands
98 E13 Brouwershaven Zeeland, SW Netherlands
117 P4 Brovary Kyyivs'ka Oblast', N Ukraine
95 G20 Brovst Nordjylland, N Denmark
31 S8 Brown City Michigan, N USA
24 M6 Brownfield Texas, SW USA
33 Q7 Browning Montana, NW USA
33 R6 Brown, Mount ▲ Montana, NW USA
(0) M9 Browns Bank undersea feature NW Atlantic Ocean
31 O14 Brownsburg Indiana, N USA
18 J16 Browns Mills New Jersey, NE USA
44 J12 Browns Town C Jamaica
31 P15 Brownstown Indiana, N USA
29 R8 Browns Valley Minnesota, N USA
20 K7 Brownsville Kentucky, S USA
20 F9 Brownsville Tennessee, S USA
25 T17 Brownsville Texas, SW USA
55 W10 Brownsweg Brokopondo, C Suriname
29 U9 Brownton Minnesota, N USA
19 R5 Brownville Junction Maine, NE USA
25 R8 Brownwood Texas, SW USA
25 R8 Brownwood Lake ⊡ Texas, SW USA
104 I9 Brozas Extremadura, W Spain
119 M18 Brozha Mahilyowskaya Voblasts', E Belarus
103 O2 Bruay-en-Artois Pas-de-Calais, N France
103 P2 Bruay-sur-l'Escaut Nord, N France
14 F13 Bruce Peninsula peninsula Ontario, S Canada
20 H9 Bruceton Tennessee, S USA
25 T9 Bruceville Texas, SW USA
101 G21 Bruchsal Baden-Württemberg, SW Germany
109 Q7 Bruck Salzburg, NW Austria
Bruck see Bruck an der Mur
109 Y4 Bruck an der Leitha Niederösterreich, NE Austria
109 V7 Bruck an der Mur var. Bruck. Steiermark, C Austria
101 M24 Bruckmühl Bayern, SE Germany
168 E7 Brueuh, Pulau island NW Indonesia
Bruges see Brugge
108 F6 Brugg Aargau, NW Switzerland
99 C16 Brugge Fr. Bruges. West-Vlaanderen, NW Belgium
109 R9 Bruggen Kärnten, S Austria
101 E16 Brühl Nordrhein-Westfalen, W Germany
99 F14 Bruinisse Zeeland, SW Netherlands
169 R9 Bruit, Pulau island East Malaysia
14 K10 Brûlé, Lac ◎ Quebec, SE Canada
30 M4 Brule River ⁓ Michigan/Wisconsin, N USA
99 H23 Brûly Namur, S Belgium
59 N17 Brumado Bahia, E Brazil
98 M11 Brummen Gelderland, E Netherlands
94 H13 Brumunddal Hedmark, S Norway
23 Q6 Brundidge Alabama, S USA
Brundisium/Brundusium see Brindisi
33 N15 Bruneau River ⁓ Idaho, NW USA
Bruneck see Brunico
169 T8 Brunei off. Sultanate of Brunei, Mal. Negara Brunei Darussalam. ● monarchy SE Asia
169 T7 Brunei Bay var. Teluk Brunei. bay N Brunei
Brunei, Teluk see Brunei Bay
Brunei Town see Bandar Seri Begawan
106 H5 Brunico Ger. Bruneck. Trentino-Alto Adige, N Italy
Brünn see Brno
185 G17 Brunner, Lake ◎ South Island, NZ
99 M18 Brunssum Limburg, SE Netherlands
23 W7 Brunswick Georgia, SE USA
19 Q8 Brunswick Maine, NE USA
21 V3 Brunswick Maryland, NE USA
27 T3 Brunswick Missouri, C USA
31 T11 Brunswick Ohio, N USA
Brunswick see Braunschweig
63 H24 Brunswick, Peninsula headland S Chile
111 H17 Bruntál Ger. Freudenthal. Ostravský Kraj, E Czech Republic
195 N3 Brunt Ice Shelf ice shelf Antarctica
Brusa see Bursa
37 U3 Brush Colorado, C USA
42 M5 Brus Laguna Gracias a Dios, E Honduras
60 K13 Brusque Santa Catarina, S Brazil
Brussa see Bursa
99 E18 Brussel var. Brussels, Fr. Bruxelles, Ger. Brüssel; anc. Broucsella. ● (Belgium) Brussels, C Belgium see also Bruxelles
Brüssel/Brussels see Brussel/Bruxelles
117 O5 Brusyliv Zhytomyrs'ka Oblast', N Ukraine
183 Q12 Bruthen Victoria, SE Australia
Bruttium see Calabria
Brüx see Most
99 E18 Bruxelles var. Brussels, Dut. Brussel, Ger. Brüssel; anc. Broucsella. ● (Belgium) Brussels, C Belgium see also Brussel
54 J7 Bruzual Apure, W Venezuela
31 Q11 Bryan Ohio, N USA
25 U10 Bryan Texas, SW USA
194 J4 Bryan Coast physical region Antarctica
122 L11 Bryanka Krasnoyarskiy Kray, C Russian Federation
117 Y7 Bryanka Luhans'ka Oblast', E Ukraine
182 J8 Bryan, Mount ▲ South Australia
128 I6 Bryansk Bryanskaya Oblast', W Russian Federation
128 H6 Bryanskaya Oblast' ◆ province W Russian Federation
194 J5 Bryant, Cape headland Antarctica
27 U8 Bryant Creek ⁓ Missouri, C USA
36 K8 Bryce Canyon canyon Utah, W USA
119 O15 Bryli Rus. Bryli. Mahilyowskaya Voblasts', E Belarus
95 C17 Bryne Rogaland, S Norway
25 R6 Bryson Texas, SW USA
21 N10 Bryson City North Carolina, SE USA
14 K11 Bryson, Lac ◎ Quebec, SE Canada
128 K13 Bryukhovetskaya Krasnodarskiy Kray, SW Russian Federation
111 H15 Brzeg Ger. Brieg; anc. Civitas Altae Ripae. Opolskie, S Poland
111 G14 Brzeg Dolny Ger. Dyhernfurth. Dolnośląskie, SW Poland
Brześć Litewski/Brześć nad Bugiem see Brest
111 L17 Brzesko Ger. Brietzig. Małopolskie, S Poland
Brzeżany see Berezhany
110 K12 Brzeziny Łódzkie, C Poland
Brzostowica Wielka see Vyalikaya Byerastavitsa
111 O17 Brzozów Podkarpackie, SE Poland
Bsharrī/Bsherri see Bcharré
187 X14 Bua Vanua Levu, N Fiji
95 J20 Bua Halland, S Sweden
82 M13 Bua ⁓ C Malawi
Bua see Čiovo
81 L18 Bu'aale It. Buale. Jubbada Dhexe, SW Somalia
189 Q8 Buada Lagoon lagoon Nauru, C Pacific Ocean
186 M8 Buala Santa Isabel, E Solomon Islands
Buale see Bu'aale
190 H1 Buariki atoll Tungaru, W Kiribati
167 Q10 Bua Yai var. Ban Bua Yai. Nakhon Ratchasima, E Thailand
75 P8 Bu'ayrāt al Ḩasūn var. Buwayrāt al Hasūn. C Libya
76 H13 Buba S Guinea-Bissau
171 P11 Bubaa Sulawesi, N Indonesia
81 D20 Bubanza NW Burundi
83 K18 Bubi prev. Bubye. ⁓ S Zimbabwe
142 L11 Būbīyan, Jazīrat island E Kuwait
Bublitz see Bobolice
Bubye see Bubi
187 Y13 Buca prev. Mbutha. Vanua Levu, N Fiji
136 F16 Bucak Burdur, SW Turkey
54 G8 Bucaramanga Santander, N Colombia
107 M18 Buccino Campania, S Italy
116 K9 Bucecea Botoşani, NE Romania
116 J6 Buchach Pol. Buczacz. Ternopil's'ka Oblast', W Ukraine
183 Q12 Buchan Victoria, SE Australia
76 J17 Buchanan prev. Grand Bassa. SW Liberia
23 R3 Buchanan Georgia, SE USA
31 O11 Buchanan Michigan, N USA
21 T6 Buchanan Virginia, NE USA
25 R10 Buchanan Dam Texas, SW USA
25 R10 Buchanan, Lake ⊡ Texas, SW USA
96 L8 Buchan Ness headland NE Scotland, UK
13 T12 Buchans Newfoundland, SE Canada
Bucharest see Bucureşti
101 H20 Buchen Baden-Württemberg, SW Germany
100 I10 Buchholz in der Nordheide Niedersachsen, NW Germany
108 F7 Buchs Aargau, N Switzerland
108 I8 Buchs Sankt Gallen, NE Switzerland
100 H13 Bückeburg Niedersachsen, NW Germany
36 K14 Buckeye Arizona, SW USA
Buckeye State see Ohio
21 S4 Buckhannon West Virginia, NE USA
25 T9 Buckholts Texas, SW USA
96 K8 Buckie NE Scotland, UK
14 M12 Buckingham Quebec, SE Canada
21 U6 Buckingham Virginia, NE USA
97 N21 Buckinghamshire cultural region SE England, UK
39 N8 Buckland Alaska, USA
182 G7 Buckleboo South Australia
26 K7 Bucklin Kansas, C USA
27 T3 Bucklin Missouri, C USA
36 I12 Buckskin Mountains ▲ Arizona, SW USA
19 R7 Bucksport Maine, NE USA
82 A9 Buco Zau Cabinda, NW Angola
Bu Craa see Bou Craa
116 K14 Bucureşti Eng. Bucharest, Ger. Bukarest; prev. Altenburg, anc. Cetatea Damboviţei. ● (Romania) Bucureşti, S Romania
31 S12 Bucyrus Ohio, N USA
Buczacz see Buchach
94 E9 Bud Møre og Romsdal, S Norway
25 S11 Buda Texas, SW USA
119 O18 Buda-Kashalyova Rus. Buda-Koshelëvo. Homyel'skaya Voblasts', SE Belarus
Buda-Koshelëvo see Buda-Kashalyova
166 L4 Budalin Sagaing, C Myanmar
111 J22 Budapest off. Budapest Főváros, SCr. Budimpešta. ● (Hungary) Pest, N Hungary
152 K11 Budaun Uttar Pradesh, N India
141 O9 Budayyi'ah oasis C Saudi Arabia
195 Y12 Budd Coast physical region Antarctica
Buddenbrock see Brodnica
107 C17 Budduso Sardegna, Italy, C Mediterranean Sea
97 I23 Bude SW England, UK
22 J7 Bude Mississippi, S USA
111 C18 Budějovický Kraj ◆ region S Czech Republic
99 K16 Budel Noord-Brabant, SE Netherlands
100 I8 Büdelsdorf Schleswig-Holstein, N Germany
129 O14 Budënnovsk Stavropol'skiy Kray, SW Russian Federation
116 K14 Budeşti Călăraşi, SE Romania
Budgewoi see Budgewoi Lake
183 T8 Budgewoi Lake var. Budgewoi. New South Wales, SE Australia
92 I2 Búdhardalur Vesturland, W Iceland
Budimpešta see Budapest
79 J16 Budjala Equateur, NW Dem. Rep. Congo (Zaire)
106 G10 Budrio Emilia-Romagna, C Italy
Budslav see Budslaw
119 K14 Budslaw Rus. Budslav. Minskaya Voblasts', N Belarus
Budua see Budva
169 R9 Budu, Tanjung headland East Malaysia
113 J17 Budva It. Budua. Montenegro, SW Yugoslavia
Budweis see České Budějovice
Budyšin see Bautzen
79 D16 Buea Sud-Ouest, SW Cameroon
103 S13 Buëch ⁓ SE France
18 J17 Buena New Jersey, NE USA
62 K12 Buena Esperanza San Luis, C Argentina
54 C11 Buenaventura Valle del Cauca, W Colombia
40 I4 Buenaventura Chihuahua, N Mexico
57 M18 Buena Vista Santa Cruz, C Bolivia
40 G10 Buenavista Baja California Sur, W Mexico
37 S5 Buena Vista Colorado, C USA
23 S5 Buena Vista Georgia, SE USA
21 T6 Buena Vista Virginia, NE USA
44 F5 Buena Vista, Bahia de bay N Cuba
35 R13 Buena Vista Lake Bed ◎ California, W USA
105 P8 Buendía, Embalse de ⊡ C Spain
63 F16 Bueno, Río ⁓ S Chile
62 N12 Buenos Aires hist. Santa Maria del Buen Aire. ● (Argentina) Buenos Aires, E Argentina
43 O15 Buenos Aires Puntarenas, SE Costa Rica
61 C20 Buenos Aires off. Provincia de Buenos Aires. ◆ province E Argentina
63 H19 Buenos Aires, Lago var. Lago General Carrera. ◎ Argentina/Chile
54 C13 Buesaco Nariño, SW Colombia
29 U8 Buffalo Minnesota, N USA
26 T6 Buffalo Missouri, C USA
18 D10 Buffalo New York, NE USA
27 K8 Buffalo Oklahoma, C USA
28 J7 Buffalo South Dakota, N USA
25 V8 Buffalo Texas, SW USA
33 W12 Buffalo Wyoming, C USA
29 U11 Buffalo Center Iowa, C USA
24 M3 Buffalo Lake ⊡ Texas, SW USA
30 K7 Buffalo Lake ⊡ Wisconsin, N USA
11 S12 Buffalo Narrows Saskatchewan, C Canada
27 U9 Buffalo River ⁓ Arkansas, C USA
29 R5 Buffalo River ⁓ Minnesota, N USA
20 I10 Buffalo River ⁓ Tennessee, S USA
30 J6 Buffalo River ⁓ Wisconsin, N USA
44 L12 Buff Bay E Jamaica
23 T3 Buford Georgia, SE USA
28 J3 Buford North Dakota, N USA
33 Y17 Buford Wyoming, C USA
116 J14 Buftea Bucureşti, S Romania
84 I9 Bug Bel. Zakhodni Buh, Eng. Western Bug, Rus. Zapadnyy Bug, Ukr. Zakhidnyy Buh. ⁓ E Europe
54 D11 Buga Valle del Cauca, W Colombia
162 F7 Buga Dzavhan, W Mongolia
103 O17 Bugarach, Pic du ▲ S France
146 B12 Bugdayly Balkanskiy Velayat, W Turkmenistan
Buggs Island Lake see John H.Kerr Reservoir
Bughotu see Santa Isabel
171 O14 Bugingkalo Sulawesi, C Indonesia
64 P6 Bugio island Madeira, Portugal, NE Atlantic Ocean
92 M8 Bugøynes Finnmark, N Norway
127 Q3 Bugrino Nenetskiy Avtonomnyy Okrug, NW Russian Federation
129 T5 Bugul'ma Respublika Tatarstan, W Russian Federation
Bügür see Luntai
129 T6 Buguruslan Orenburgskaya Oblast', W Russian Federation
159 R9 Buh He ⁓ C China
33 O15 Buhl Idaho, NW USA
101 F22 Bühl Baden-Württemberg, SW Germany
116 K10 Buhuşi Bacău, E Romania
Buie d'Istria see Buje
97 J20 Builth Wells E Wales, UK
186 J8 Buin Bougainville Island, NE PNG
108 I9 Buin, Piz ▲ Austria/Switzerland
129 Q4 Buinsk Chuvashskaya Respublika, W Russian Federation
129 Q4 Buinsk Respublika Tatarstan, W Russian Federation
163 R8 Buir Nur Mong. Buyr Nuur. ◎ China/Mongolia see also Buyr Nuur
98 M5 Buitenpost Fris. Bûtenpost. Friesland, N Netherlands
Buitenzorg see Bogor
83 F19 Buitepos Omaheke, E Namibia
105 N7 Buitrago del Lozoya Madrid, C Spain
Buj see Buy
104 M13 Bujalance Andalucía, S Spain
113 O17 Bujanovac Serbia, SE Yugoslavia
105 S6 Bujaraloz Aragón, NE Spain
112 A9 Buje It. Buie d'Istria. Istra, NW Croatia
Bujnurd see Bojnūrd
81 D21 Bujumbura prev. Usumbura. ● (Burundi) W Burundi
81 D20 Bujumbura ✕ W Burundi
159 N11 Bukadaban Feng ▲ C China
186 J6 Buka Island island NE PNG
81 F18 Bukakata S Uganda
79 N24 Bukama Katanga, SE Dem. Rep. Congo (Zaire)
142 J4 Būkān var. Bowkān. Āzarbāyjān-e Bākhtarī, NW Iran
Bukantau, Gory see Bŭkantov-Toghi
146 K8 Bŭkantow-Toghi Rus. Gory Bukantau. ▲ N Uzbekistan
Bukarest see Bucureşti
79 O19 Bukavu prev. Costermansville. Sud Kivu, E Dem. Rep. Congo (Zaire)
81 F21 Bukene Tabora, NW Tanzania
141 W8 Bū Khābī var. Bakhābī. NW Oman
Bukhara see Bukhoro
Bukharskaya Oblast' see Bukhoro Wiloyati
146 L11 Bukhoro var. Bokhara, Rus. Bukhara. Bukhoro Wiloyati, C Uzbekistan
146 J11 Bukhoro Wiloyati Rus. Bukharskaya Oblast'. ◆ province C Uzbekistan
168 M14 Bukitkemuning Sumatera, W Indonesia
168 I11 Bukittinggi prev. Fort de Kock. Sumatera, W Indonesia
111 L21 Bükk ▲ NE Hungary
81 F19 Bukoba Kagera, NW Tanzania
113 N20 Bukovo S FYR Macedonia
108 G6 Bülach Zürich, NW Switzerland
Bülaevo see Bulayevo
162 I6 Bulag Hövsgöl, N Mongolia
162 M7 Bulag Töv, C Mongolia
162 I8 Bulagiyn Denj Arhangay, C Mongolia
183 U7 Bulahdelah New South Wales, SE Australia
171 P4 Bulan Luzon, N Philippines

● Country
● Country Capital
◇ Dependent Territory
○ Dependent Territory Capital
◆ Administrative Region
✕ International Airport
▲ Mountain
▲ Mountain Range
Volcano
⁓ River
◎ Lake
⊡ Reservoir

137 N11 **Bulancak** Giresun, N Turkey
152 J10 **Bulandshahr** Uttar Pradesh, N India
137 R14 **Bulanık** Muş, E Turkey
129 V7 **Bulanovo** Orenburgskaya Oblast', W Russian Federation
83 J17 **Bulawayo** var. Buluwayo. Matabeleland North, SW Zimbabwe
83 J17 **Bulawayo** ✕ Matabeleland North, SW Zimbabwe
145 Q6 **Bulayevo** Kaz. Būlaevo. Severnyy Kazakhstan, N Kazakhstan
136 D15 **Buldan** Denizli, SW Turkey
154 G12 **Buldāna** Mahārāshtra, C India
38 E16 **Buldir Island** island Aleutian Islands, Alaska, USA
Buldur see Burdur
162 H9 **Bulgan** Bayanhongor, C Mongolia
162 K6 **Bulgan** Bulgan, N Mongolia
162 F7 **Bulgan** Hovd, W Mongolia
162 J5 **Bulgan** Hövsgöl, N Mongolia
162 J10 **Bulgan** Ömnögovĭ, S Mongolia
162 J7 **Bulgan** ◈ province N Mongolia
114 H10 **Bulgaria** off. Republic of Bulgaria, Bul. Bŭlgariya; prev. People's Republic of Bulgaria. ◆ republic SE Europe
Bŭlgariya see Bulgaria
114 L9 **Bŭlgarka** ▲ E Bulgaria
171 S11 **Buli** Pulau Halmahera, E Indonesia
171 S11 **Buli, Teluk** bay Pulau Halmahera, E Indonesia
160 J13 **Buliu He** ↝ S China
Bullange see Büllingen
104 M11 **Bullaque** ↝ C Spain
105 Q13 **Bullas** Murcia, SE Spain
80 M12 **Bullaxaar** Woqooyi Galbeed, NW Somalia
108 C9 **Bulle** Fribourg, SW Switzerland
185 G15 **Buller** ↝ South Island, NZ
183 P12 **Buller, Mount** ▲ Victoria, SE Australia
36 H11 **Bullhead City** Arizona, SW USA
99 N21 **Büllingen** Fr. Bullange. Liège, E Belgium
Bullion State see Missouri
21 T14 **Bull Island** island South Carolina, SE USA
182 M4 **Bulloo River Overflow** wetland New South Wales, SE Australia
184 M12 **Bulls** Manawatu-Wanganui, North Island, NZ
21 T14 **Bulls Bay** bay South Carolina, SE USA
27 U9 **Bull Shoals Lake** ⊠ Arkansas/Missouri, C USA
181 Q2 **Bulman** Northern Territory, N Australia
162 I6 **Bulnayn Nuruu** ▲ N Mongolia
171 O11 **Bulowa, Gunung** ▲ Sulawesi, N Indonesia
Bulqiza see Bulqizë
113 L19 **Bulqizë** var. Bulqiza. Dibër, C Albania
Bulsar see Valsād
171 N14 **Bulukumba** prev. Boeloekoemba. Sulawesi, C Indonesia
147 O11 **Bulunghur** Rus. Bulungur; prev. Krasnogvardeysk. Samarqand Wiloyati, C Uzbekistan
79 I21 **Bulungu** Bandundu, SW Dem. Rep. Congo (Zaire)
Bulungur see Bulunghur
Buluwayo see Bulawayo
79 K17 **Bumba** Equateur, N Dem. Rep. Congo (Zaire)
121 R12 **Bumbah, Khalīj al** gulf N Libya
162 K8 **Bumbat** Övörhangay, C Mongolia
81 F19 **Bumbire Island** island N Tanzania
169 V8 **Bum Bun, Pulau** island East Malaysia
81 J17 **Buna** North Eastern, NE Kenya
25 Y10 **Buna** Texas, SW USA
Bunab see Bonāb
Bunai see M'bunai
147 S13 **Bunay** S Tajikistan
180 I13 **Bunbury** Western Australia
97 E14 **Buncrana** Ir. Bun Cranncha. NW Ireland
Bun Cranncha see Buncrana
181 Z9 **Bundaberg** Queensland, E Australia
183 T5 **Bundarra** New South Wales, SE Australia
100 G13 **Bünde** Nordrhein-Westfalen, NW Germany
152 H13 **Būndi** Rājasthān, N India
Bun Dobhráin see Bundoran
97 D15 **Bundoran** Ir. Bun Dobhráin. NW Ireland
113 K18 **Bunë** SCr. Bojana. ↝ Albania/Yugoslavia see also Bojana
171 Q8 **Bunga** ↝ Mindanao, S Philippines
168 I12 **Bungalaut, Selat** strait W Indonesia
167 R8 **Bung Kan** Nong Khai, E Thailand
181 N4 **Bungle Bungle Range** ▲ Western Australia
82 C10 **Bungo** Uíge, NW Angola
81 G18 **Bungoma** Western, W Kenya
164 F15 **Bungo-suidō** strait SW Japan
164 E14 **Bungo-Takada** Ōita, Kyūshū, SW Japan
100 K8 **Bungsberg** hill N Germany
Bungur see Bunyu
79 P17 **Bunia** Orientale, NE Dem. Rep. Congo (Zaire)
35 U6 **Bunker Hill** ▲ Nevada, W USA
22 I7 **Bunkie** Louisiana, S USA
23 X10 **Bunnell** Florida, SE USA
105 S10 **Buñol** País Valenciano, E Spain
98 K11 **Bunschoten** Utrecht, C Netherlands
136 K14 **Bünyan** Kayseri, C Turkey
169 W8 **Bunyu** var. Bungur. Borneo, N Indonesia
169 W8 **Bunyu, Pulau** island N Indonesia
Bunzlau see Bolesławiec
Buoddobohki see Patoniva
123 P7 **Buorkhaya Guba** bay N Russian Federation
171 Z15 **Bupul** Irian Jaya, E Indonesia
81 K19 **Bura** Coast, SE Kenya
80 P12 **Buraan** Sanaag, N Somalia
Būrabay see Borovoye
Buraida see Buraydah
Buraimi see Al Buraymī
145 Y11 **Buran** Vostochnyy Kazakhstan, E Kazakhstan
158 G15 **Burang** Xizang Zizhiqu, W China
Burao see Burco
138 H8 **Burāq** Dar'ā, S Syria
141 O6 **Buraydah** var. Buraida. Al Qaşīm, N Saudi Arabia
35 S15 **Burbank** California, W USA
31 N11 **Burbank** Illinois, N USA
183 Q8 **Burcher** New South Wales, SE Australia
80 N13 **Burco** var. Burao, Bur'o. Togdheer, NW Somalia
146 L13 **Burdalyk** Lebapskiy Velayat, E Turkmenistan
181 W6 **Burdekin River** ↝ Queensland, NE Australia
27 O7 **Burden** Kansas, C USA
Burdigala see Bordeaux
136 E15 **Burdur** var. Buldur. Burdur, SW Turkey
136 E15 **Burdur** var. Buldur. ◈ province SW Turkey
136 E15 **Burdur Gölü** salt lake SW Turkey
65 H21 **Burdwood Bank** undersea feature SW Atlantic Ocean
80 I12 **Burē** Amhara, N Ethiopia
80 H13 **Burē** Oromo, C Ethiopia
93 J15 **Bureå** Västerbotten, N Sweden
101 G14 **Büren** Nordrhein-Westfalen, W Germany
162 K6 **Bürengiyn Nuruu** ▲ N Mongolia
162 E8 **Bürenhayrhan** Hovd, W Mongolia
Būrewāla see Mandi Būrewāla
92 J9 **Burfjord** Troms, N Norway
100 L13 **Burg** var. Burg an der Ihle, Burg bei Magdeburg. Sachsen-Anhalt, C Germany
Burg an der Ihle see Burg
114 N10 **Burgas** var. Bourgas. Burgas, E Bulgaria
114 N9 **Burgas** ✕ Burgas, E Bulgaria
114 M10 **Burgas** ◈ province E Bulgaria
114 N10 **Burgaski Zaliv** gulf E Bulgaria
114 M10 **Burgasko Ezero** lagoon E Bulgaria
21 V11 **Burgaw** North Carolina, SE USA
Burg bei Magdeburg see Burg
108 E8 **Burgdorf** Bern, NW Switzerland
109 Y7 **Burgenland** off. Land Burgenland. ◈ state SE Austria
13 S13 **Burgeo** Newfoundland, SE Canada
83 I24 **Burgersdorp** Eastern Cape, SE South Africa
83 K20 **Burgersfort** Mpumalanga, NE South Africa
101 N23 **Burghausen** Bayern, SE Germany
139 O5 **Burghūth, Sabkhat al** ◎ E Syria
101 M20 **Burglengenfeld** Bayern, SE Germany
41 P9 **Burgos** Tamaulipas, C Mexico
105 N4 **Burgos** Castilla-León, N Spain
105 N4 **Burgos** ◈ province Castilla-León, N Spain
Burgstadlberg see Hradiště
95 P20 **Burgsvik** Gotland, SE Sweden
Burgum see Bergum
Burgundy see Bourgogne
159 Q11 **Burhan Budai Shan** ▲ C China
136 B12 **Burhaniye** Balıkesir, W Turkey
154 G12 **Burhānpur** Madhya Pradesh, C India
129 W7 **Buribay** Respublika Bashkortostan, W Russian Federation
43 O17 **Burica, Punta** headland Costa Rica/Panama
167 Q10 **Buriram** var. Buri Ram, Puriramya. Buri Ram, E Thailand
105 S10 **Burjassot** País Valenciano, E Spain
81 N16 **Burka Giibi** Hiiraan, C Somalia
147 X8 **Burkan** ↝ E Kyrgyzstan
25 R4 **Burkburnett** Texas, SW USA
29 O12 **Burke** South Dakota, N USA
10 K15 **Burke Channel** channel British Columbia, W Canada
194 J10 **Burke Island** island Antarctica
20 L7 **Burkesville** Kentucky, S USA
181 T4 **Burketown** Queensland, NE Australia
25 Q8 **Burkett** Texas, SW USA
25 Y9 **Burkeville** Texas, SW USA
21 V7 **Burkeville** Virginia, NE USA
77 O12 **Burkina** off. Burkina Faso; prev. Upper Volta. ◆ republic W Africa
Burkina Faso see Burkina
194 L13 **Burks, Cape** headland Antarctica
14 H12 **Burk's Falls** Ontario, S Canada
101 H23 **Burladingen** Baden-Württemberg, S Germany
25 T7 **Burleson** Texas, SW USA
33 P15 **Burley** Idaho, NW USA
144 G8 **Burlin** Zapadnyy Kazakhstan, NW Kazakhstan
14 G16 **Burlington** Ontario, S Canada
37 W4 **Burlington** Colorado, C USA
29 Y15 **Burlington** Iowa, C USA
27 P5 **Burlington** Kansas, C USA
21 T9 **Burlington** North Carolina, SE USA
28 M3 **Burlington** North Dakota, N USA
18 L7 **Burlington** Vermont, NE USA
30 M9 **Burlington** Wisconsin, N USA
27 Q1 **Burlington Junction** Missouri, C USA
Burma see Myanmar
10 L17 **Burnaby** British Columbia, SW Canada
117 O12 **Burnas, Ozero** ◎ SW Ukraine
25 S10 **Burnet** Texas, SW USA
35 O3 **Burney** California, W USA
183 O16 **Burnie** Tasmania, SE Australia
97 L17 **Burnley** NW England, UK
Burnoye see Bauyrzhan Momysh-Uly
153 R15 **Burnpur** West Bengal, NE India
32 K14 **Burns** Oregon, NW USA
26 K11 **Burns Flat** Oklahoma, C USA
20 M7 **Burnside** Kentucky, S USA
8 K8 **Burnside** ↝ Nunavut, NW Canada
32 L15 **Burns Junction** Oregon, NW USA
10 L13 **Burns Lake** British Columbia, SW Canada
29 V9 **Burnsville** Minnesota, N USA
21 P9 **Burnsville** North Carolina, SE USA
21 R4 **Burnsville** West Virginia, NE USA
14 I13 **Burnt River** ↝ Ontario, SE Canada
14 I11 **Burntroot Lake** ◎ Ontario, SE Canada
11 W12 **Burntwood** ↝ Manitoba, C Canada
Bur'o see Burco
158 L2 **Burqin** Xinjiang Uygur Zizhiqu, NW China
182 J8 **Burra** South Australia
183 S9 **Burragorang, Lake** ⊠ New South Wales, SE Australia
96 K5 **Burray** island NE Scotland, UK
113 L19 **Burrel** var. Burreli. Dibër, C Albania
Burreli see Burrel
183 R8 **Burrendong Reservoir** ⊠ New South Wales, SE Australia
183 R5 **Burren Junction** New South Wales, SE Australia
105 T9 **Burriana** País Valenciano, E Spain
183 R10 **Burrinjuck Reservoir** ⊠ New South Wales, SE Australia
36 J12 **Burro Creek** ↝ Arizona, SW USA
40 M5 **Burro, Serranías del** ▲ NW Mexico
62 K7 **Burruyacú** Tucumán, N Argentina
136 E12 **Bursa** var. Brussa; prev. Brusa, anc. Prusa. Bursa, NW Turkey
136 D12 **Bursa** var. Brusa, Brussa. ◈ province NW Turkey
75 Y9 **Būr Safāga** var. Būr Safājah. E Egypt
Būr Safājah see Būr Safāga
Būr Sa'īd see Port Said
81 O14 **Bur Tinle** Mudug, C Somalia
31 Q5 **Burt Lake** ◎ Michigan, N USA
Burtnieks see Burtnieku Ezers
118 H7 **Burtnieku Ezers** var. Burtnieks. ◎ N Latvia
31 Q9 **Burton** Michigan, N USA
Burton on Trent see Burton upon Trent
97 M19 **Burton upon Trent** var. Burton on Trent, Burton-upon-Trent. C England, UK
93 J15 **Burträsk** Västerbotten, N Sweden
145 S14 **Burubaytal** prev. Burylbaytal. Zhambyl, SE Kazakhstan
Burujird see Borūjerd
Burultokay see Fuhai
141 R15 **Burūm** SE Yemen
145 U16 **Burunday** Kaz. Boralday. Almaty, SE Kazakhstan
81 D21 **Burundi** off. Republic of Burundi; prev. Kingdom of Burundi, Urundi. ◆ republic C Africa
171 R13 **Buru, Pulau** prev. Boeroe. island E Indonesia
77 T17 **Burutu** Delta, S Nigeria
10 G7 **Burwash Landing** Yukon Territory, W Canada
29 O14 **Burwell** Nebraska, C USA
97 L17 **Bury** NW England, UK
123 N13 **Buryatiya, Respublika** prev. Buryatskaya ASSR. ◈ autonomous republic S Russian Federation
Buryatskaya ASSR see Buryatiya, Respublika
Burylbaytal see Burubaytal
117 S3 **Buryn'** Sums'ka Oblast', NE Ukraine
97 P20 **Bury St Edmunds** hist. Beodericsworth. E England, UK
114 G8 **Bŭrziya** ↝ NW Bulgaria
106 D9 **Busalla** Liguria, NW Italy
Busan see Pusan
139 N5 **Buşayrah** Dayr az Zawr, E Syria
Buševa see Baba
143 N12 **Būshehr** off. Ostān-e Būshehr. ◈ province SW Iran
Būshehr/Bushire see Bandar-e Būshehr
25 N2 **Bushland** Texas, SW USA
30 J12 **Bushnell** Illinois, N USA
Busi see Biševo
81 G18 **Busia** SE Uganda
Busiasch see Buziaş
79 K16 **Businga** Equateur, NW Dem. Rep. Congo (Zaire)
79 J18 **Busira** ↝ NW Dem. Rep. Congo (Zaire)
116 I5 **Bus'k** Rus. Busk. L'vivs'ka Oblast', W Ukraine
95 E14 **Buskerud** ◈ county S Norway
113 F14 **Buško Jezero** ⊠ SW Bosnia and Herzegovina
111 M15 **Busko-Zdrój** Świętokrzyskie, C Poland
Busra see Al Başrah, Iraq
Buşrá see Buşrá ash Shām, Syria
138 H9 **Buşrá ash Shām** var. Bosora, Bosra, Bozrah, Buşrá. Dar'ā, S Syria
180 I13 **Busselton** Western Australia
81 C14 **Busseri** ↝ W Sudan
106 E9 **Busseto** Emilia-Romagna, C Italy
106 A8 **Bussoleno** Piemonte, NE Italy
Bussora see Al Başrah
98 J10 **Bussum** Noord-Holland, C Netherlands
41 N7 **Bustamante** Nuevo León, NE Mexico
63 I23 **Bustamante, Punta** headland S Argentina
Bustan see Bŭston
116 J12 **Buşteni** Prahova, SE Romania
106 D7 **Busto Arsizio** Lombardia, N Italy
147 Q10 **Bŭston** Rus. Buston. NW Tajikistan
146 I9 **Bŭston** Rus. Bustan. Qoraqalpoghiston Respublikasi, W Uzbekistan
100 H8 **Büsum** Schleswig-Holstein, N Germany
79 M16 **Buta** Orientale, N Dem. Rep. Congo (Zaire)
81 E20 **Butare** prev. Astrida. S Rwanda
191 O2 **Butaritari** atoll Tungaru, W Kiribati
Butawal see Butwal
96 H13 **Bute** cultural region SW Scotland, UK
162 K6 **Büteeliyn Nuruu** ▲ N Mongolia
10 L16 **Bute Inlet** fjord British Columbia, W Canada
96 H12 **Bute, Island of** island SW Scotland, UK
79 P18 **Butembo** Nord Kivu, NE Dem. Rep. Congo (Zaire)
Bûtenpost see Buitenpost
107 K25 **Butera** Sicilia, Italy, C Mediterranean Sea
99 M20 **Bütgenbach** Liège, E Belgium
Butha Qi see Zalantun
166 J5 **Buthidaung** Arakan State, W Myanmar
61 I16 **Butiá** Rio Grande do Sul, S Brazil
81 F17 **Butiaba** NW Uganda
23 N6 **Butler** Alabama, S USA
23 S5 **Butler** Georgia, SE USA
31 Q11 **Butler** Indiana, N USA
27 R5 **Butler** Missouri, C USA
18 B14 **Butler** Pennsylvania, NE USA
194 K5 **Butler Island** island Antarctica
21 U8 **Butner** North Carolina, SE USA
171 P14 **Buton, Pulau** var. Pulau Butung; prev. Boetoeng. island C Indonesia
Bütow see Bytów
113 L23 **Butrintit, Liqeni i** ◎ S Albania
23 N3 **Buttahatchee River** ↝ Alabama/Mississippi, S USA
33 Q10 **Butte** Montana, NW USA
29 O12 **Butte** Nebraska, C USA
168 J7 **Butterworth** Pinang, Peninsular Malaysia
83 J25 **Butterworth** var. Gcuwa. Eastern Cape, SE South Africa
13 O3 **Button Islands** island group Nunavut, NE Canada
35 R13 **Buttonwillow** California, W USA
171 Q7 **Butuan** off. Butuan City. Mindanao, S Philippines
Butung, Pulau see Buton, Pulau
Butuntum see Bitonto
128 M8 **Buturlinovka** Voronezhskaya Oblast', W Russian Federation
153 O11 **Butwal** var. Butawal. Western, C Nepal
101 G17 **Butzbach** Hessen, W Germany
100 L9 **Bützow** Mecklenburg-Vorpommern, N Germany
80 N13 **Buuhoodle** Togdheer, N Somalia
81 N16 **Buulobarde** var. Buulo Berde. Hiiraan, C Somalia Africa
Buulo Berde see Buulobarde
80 P12 **Buuraha Cal Miskaat** ▲ NE Somalia
81 L19 **Buur Gaabo** Jubbada Hoose, S Somalia
99 M22 **Buurgplaatz** ▲ N Luxembourg
Buwayrāt al Hasūn see Bu'ayrāt al Ḩasūn
100 I10 **Buxtehude** Niedersachsen, NW Germany
97 L18 **Buxton** C England, UK
126 M14 **Buy** var. Buj. Kostromskaya Oblast', NW Russian Federation
162 G7 **Buyanbat** Govĭ-Altay, W Mongolia
162 H8 **Buyant** Bayanhongor, C Mongolia
162 D6 **Buyant** Bayan-Ölgiy, W Mongolia
162 H7 **Buyant** Dzavhan, C Mongolia
163 N9 **Buyant** Hentiy, C Mongolia
163 N10 **Buyant-Uhaa** Dornogovĭ, SE Mongolia
162 M7 **Buyant Ukha** ✕ (Ulaanbaatar) Töv, N Mongolia
129 Q16 **Buynaksk** Respublika Dagestan, SW Russian Federation
119 L20 **Buynavichy** Rus. Buynovichi. Homyel'skaya Voblasts', SE Belarus
Buynovichi see Buynavichy
76 L16 **Buyo** SW Ivory Coast
76 L16 **Buyo, Lac de** ⊠ W Ivory Coast
163 R7 **Buyr Nuur** var. Buir Nur. ◎ China/Mongolia see also Buir Nur
137 T13 **Büyükağrı Dağı** var. Aghri Dagh, Agri Dagi, Koh I Noh, Masis, Eng. Great Ararat, Mount Ararat. ▲ E Turkey
137 R15 **Büyük Çayı** ↝ NE Turkey
114 O13 **Büyük Çekmece** İstanbul, NW Turkey
114 N12 **Büyükkarıştıran** Kırklareli, NW Turkey
115 L14 **Büyükkemikli Burnu** headland NW Turkey
136 E15 **Büyükmenderes Nehri** ↝ SW Turkey
Büyükzap Suyu see Great Zab
102 M9 **Buzançais** Indre, C France
116 K13 **Buzău** Buzău, SE Romania
116 K13 **Buzău** ◈ county SE Romania
116 L12 **Buzău** ↝ E Romania
75 S11 **Buzaymah** var. Bzīmah. SE Libya
164 E13 **Buzen** Fukuoka, Kyūshū, SW Japan
116 F12 **Buziaş** Ger. Busiasch, Hung. Buziásfürdő; prev. Buziás. Timiş, W Romania
Buziásfürdő see Buziaş
83 M18 **Búzi, Rio** ↝ C Mozambique
117 Q10 **Buz'kyy Lyman** bay S Ukraine
Büzmeyin see Byuzmeyin
145 O8 **Buzuluk** Akmola, C Kazakhstan
129 T6 **Buzuluk** Orenburgskaya Oblast', W Russian Federation
129 N8 **Buzuluk** ↝ SW Russian Federation
19 P12 **Buzzards Bay** Massachusetts, NE USA
19 P13 **Buzzards Bay** bay Massachusetts, NE USA
83 G16 **Bwabata** Caprivi, NE Namibia
186 H10 **Bwagaoia** Misima Island, SE PNG
Bwake see Bouaké
187 R13 **Bwatnapne** Pentecost, C Vanuatu
119 K14 **Byahoml'** Rus. Begoml'. Vitsyebskaya Voblasts', N Belarus
114 J8 **Byala** Ruse, N Bulgaria
114 N9 **Byala** prev. Ak-Dere. Varna, E Bulgaria
Byala Reka see Erydropótamos
114 H8 **Byala Slatina** Vratsa, NW Bulgaria
119 N15 **Byalynichy** Rus. Belynichi. Mahilyowskaya Voblasts', E Belarus
119 G19 **Byaroza** Pol. Bereza Kartuska, Rus. Berëza. Brestskaya Voblasts', SW Belarus
Bybles see Jbaïl
111 O14 **Bychawa** Lubelskie, SE Poland
Bychikha see Bychykha
118 N11 **Bychykha** Rus. Bychikha. Vitsyebskaya Voblasts', NE Belarus
111 I14 **Byczyna** Ger. Pitschen. Opolskie, S Poland
110 I10 **Bydgoszcz** Ger. Bromberg. Kujawski-pomorskie, C Poland
119 I17 **Byelaruskaya Hrada** Rus. Belorusskaya Gryada. ridge N Belarus
119 G18 **Byelavyezhskaya Pushcha** Pol. Puszcza Białowieska, Rus. Belovezhskaya Pushcha. forest Belarus/Poland see also Białowieska, Puszcza
119 H15 **Byenyakoni** Rus. Benyakoni. Hrodzyenskaya Voblasts', W Belarus
119 M16 **Byerazino** Rus. Berezino. Minskaya Voblasts', C Belarus
118 L13 **Byerazino** Rus. Berezino. Vitsyebskaya Voblasts', N Belarus
119 L14 **Byerezino** Rus. Berezina. ↝ C Belarus
118 M13 **Byeshankovichy** Rus. Beshenkovichi. Vitsyebskaya Voblasts', N Belarus
31 U13 **Byesville** Ohio, N USA
119 P18 **Byesyedz'** Rus. Besed'. ↝ SE Belarus
119 H19 **Byezdzyezh** Rus. Bezdezh. Brestskaya Voblasts', SW Belarus
93 J15 **Bygdeå** Västerbotten, N Sweden
94 F12 **Bygdin** ◎ S Norway
93 J15 **Bygdsiljum** Västerbotten, N Sweden
95 E17 **Bygland** Aust-Agder, S Norway
95 E17 **Byglandsfjord** Aust-Agder, S Norway
119 N16 **Bykhaw** Rus. Bykhov. Mahilyowskaya Voblasts', E Belarus
Bykhov see Bykhaw
129 P9 **Bykovo** Volgogradskaya Oblast', SW Russian Federation
123 P7 **Bykovskiy** Respublika Sakha (Yakutiya), NE Russian Federation
195 R12 **Byrd Glacier** glacier Antarctica
14 K10 **Byrd, Lac** ◎ Quebec, SE Canada
183 P5 **Byrock** New South Wales, SE Australia
30 L10 **Byron** Illinois, N USA
183 V4 **Byron Bay** New South Wales, SE Australia
183 V4 **Byron, Cape** headland New South Wales, E Australia
63 F21 **Byron, Isla** island S Chile
Byron Island see Nikunau
65 B24 **Byron Sound** sound NW Falkland Islands
122 M6 **Byrranga, Gora** ▲ N Russian Federation
93 J14 **Byske** Västerbotten, N Sweden
111 K18 **Bystrá** ▲ N Slovakia
111 F18 **Bystřice nad Pernštejnem** Ger. Bistritz ober Pernstein. Jihlavský Kraj, C Czech Republic
Bystrovka see Kemin
111 G16 **Bystrzyca Kłodzka** Ger. Habelschwerdt. Wałbrzych, SW Poland
111 I18 **Bytča** Žilinský Kraj, N Slovakia
119 L15 **Bytcha** Rus. Bytcha. Minskaya Voblasts', NE Belarus
Byteń/Byten' see Bytsyen'
111 J16 **Bytom** Ger. Beuthen. Śląskie, S Poland
110 H7 **Bytów** Ger. Bütow. Pomorskie, N Poland
119 H18 **Bytsyen'** Pol. Byteń, Rus. Byten'. Brestskaya Voblasts', SW Belarus
81 E19 **Byumba** var. Biumba. N Rwanda
146 F13 **Byuzmeyin** Turkm. Büzmeyin; prev. Bezmein. Akhalskiy Velayat, C Turkmenistan
119 O20 **Byval'ki** Homyel'skaya Voblasts', SE Belarus
95 O20 **Byxelkrok** Kalmar, S Sweden
Byzantium see İstanbul
Bzīmah see Buzaymah

C

62 O6 **Caacupé** Cordillera, S Paraguay
62 P6 **Caaguazú** off. Departamento de Caaguazú. ◈ department C Paraguay
82 C13 **Caála** var. Kaala, Port. Vila Robert Williams. Huambo, C Angola
62 P7 **Caazapá** Caazapá, S Paraguay
62 P7 **Caazapá** off. Departamento de Caazapá. ◈ department SE Paraguay
81 P15 **Cabaad, Raas** headland C Somalia
55 N10 **Cabadisocaña** Amazonas, S Venezuela
44 F5 **Cabaiguán** Sancti Spíritus, C Cuba
Caballeria, Cabo see Cavalleria, Cap de
37 Q14 **Caballo Reservoir** ⊠ New Mexico, SW USA
40 L6 **Caballos Mesteños, Llano de los** plain N Mexico
104 L2 **Cabañaquinta** Asturias, N Spain
42 B9 **Cabañas** ◈ department E El Salvador
171 O3 **Cabanatuan** off. Cabanatuan City. Luzon, N Philippines
15 T8 **Cabano** Quebec, SE Canada
104 L11 **Cabeza del Buey** Extremadura, W Spain
45 V5 **Cabezas de San Juan** headland E Puerto Rico
105 N2 **Cabezón de la Sal** Cantabria, N Spain
Cabhán see Cavan
61 B23 **Cabildo** Buenos Aires, E Argentina
Cabillonum see Chalon-sur-Saône
54 H5 **Cabimas** Zulia, NW Venezuela
82 A9 **Cabinda** var. Kabinda. Cabinda, NW Angola
82 A9 **Cabinda** var. Kabinda. ◈ province NW Angola
33 N7 **Cabinet Mountains** ▲ Idaho/Montana, NW USA
82 B11 **Cabiri** Bengo, NW Angola
63 J20 **Cabo Blanco** Santa Cruz, SE Argentina
82 P13 **Cabo Delgado** off. Província de Capo Delgado. ◈ province NE Mozambique
14 L9 **Cabonga, Réservoir** ⊠ Quebec, SE Canada
27 V7 **Cabool** Missouri, C USA
183 V2 **Caboolture** Queensland, E Australia
Cabora Bassa, Lake see Cahora Bassa, Albufeira de
40 F3 **Caborca** Sonora, NW Mexico
Cabo San Lucas see San Lucas
27 V11 **Cabot** Arkansas, C USA
14 F12 **Cabot Head** headland Ontario, S Canada
9 Y11 **Cabot Strait** strait E Canada
Cabo Verde, Ilhas do see Cape Verde
104 M14 **Cabra** Andalucía, S Spain
107 B19 **Cabras** Sardegna, Italy, C Mediterranean Sea
188 A15 **Cabras Island** island W Guam
45 O8 **Cabrera** N Dominican Republic
105 X10 **Cabrera** anc. Capraria. island Islas Baleares, Spain, W Mediterranean Sea
104 J4 **Cabrera** ↝ NW Spain
105 Q15 **Cabrera, Sierra** ▲ S Spain
11 S16 **Cabri** Saskatchewan, S Canada
105 R10 **Cabriel** ↝ E Spain
54 M7 **Cabruta** Guárico, C Venezuela
171 N2 **Cabugao** Luzon, N Philippines
54 G10 **Cabuyaro** Meta, C Colombia
60 I13 **Caçador** Santa Catarina, S Brazil
42 G8 **Cacaguatique, Cordillera** var. Cordillera. ▲ NE El Salvador
112 L13 **Čačak** Serbia, C Yugoslavia
55 Y10 **Cacao** NE French Guiana
61 H16 **Caçapava do Sul** Rio Grande do Sul, S Brazil
21 U3 **Cacapon River** ↝ West Virginia, NE USA
107 J23 **Caccamo** Sicilia, Italy, C Mediterranean Sea
107 A17 **Caccia, Capo** headland Sardegna, Italy, C Mediterranean Sea
59 G18 **Cáceres** Mato Grosso, W Brazil
104 J10 **Cáceres** Ar. Qazris. Extremadura, W Spain
104 J9 **Cáceres** ◈ province Extremadura, W Spain
Cachacrou see Scotts Head Village
61 C21 **Cacharí** Buenos Aires, E Argentina

◆ Country ● Country Capital ◇ Dependent Territory ○ Dependent Territory Capital ◈ Administrative Region ✕ International Airport ▲ Mountain ▲ Mountain Range ▲ Volcano ↝ River ◎ Lake ⊠ Reservoir

26 L12 **Cache** Oklahoma, C USA
10 M16 **Cache Creek** British Columbia, SW Canada
35 N6 **Cache Creek** ≈ California, W USA
37 S3 **Cache La Poudre River** ≈ Colorado, C USA
Cacheo *see* Cacheu
27 W11 **Cache River** ≈ Arkansas, C USA
30 L17 **Cache River** ≈ Illinois, N USA
76 G12 **Cacheu** *var.* Cacheo. W Guinea-Bissau
59 I15 **Cachimbo** Pará, NE Brazil
59 H15 **Cachimbo, Serra do** ⛰ C Brazil
82 D13 **Cachingues** Bié, C Angola
54 G7 **Cáchira** Norte de Santander, N Colombia
61 H16 **Cachoeira do Sul** Rio Grande do Sul, S Brazil
59 O20 **Cachoeiro de Itapemirim** Espírito Santo, SE Brazil
82 E12 **Cacolo** Lunda Sul, NE Angola
83 C14 **Caconda** Huíla, C Angola
82 A9 **Cacongo** Cabinda, NW Angola
35 U9 **Cactus Peak** ▲ Nevada, W USA
82 A11 **Cacuaco** Luanda, NW Angola
83 B14 **Cacula** Huíla, SW Angola
67 R12 **Caculuvar** ≈ SW Angola
59 O19 **Caçumba, Ilha** *island* SE Brazil
55 N10 **Cacuri** Amazonas, S Venezuela
81 N17 **Cadale** Shabeellaha Dhexe, E Somalia
105 X4 **Cadaqués** Cataluña, NE Spain
111 J18 **Čadca** *Hung.* Csaca. Žilinský Kraj, N Slovakia
27 P13 **Caddo** Oklahoma, C USA
25 R6 **Caddo** Texas, SW USA
25 X6 **Caddo Lake** ▣ Louisiana/Texas, SW USA
27 S12 **Caddo Mountains** ⛰ Arkansas, C USA
41 O8 **Cadereyta** Nuevo León, NE Mexico
97 J19 **Cader Idris** ▲ NW Wales, United Kingodm
182 F3 **Cadibarrawirracanna, Lake** *salt lake* South Australia
14 I7 **Cadillac** Quebec, SE Canada
11 T17 **Cadillac** Saskatchewan, S Canada
102 K13 **Cadillac** Gironde, SW France
31 P7 **Cadillac** Michigan, N USA
105 V4 **Cadí, Torre de** ▲ NE Spain
171 P5 **Cadiz** *off.* Cadiz City. Negros, C Philippines
20 H7 **Cadiz** Kentucky, S USA
31 U13 **Cadiz** Ohio, N USA
104 J15 **Cádiz** *anc.* Gades, Gadier, Gadir, Gadire. Andalucía, SW Spain
104 K15 **Cádiz** ◈ *province* Andalucía, SW Spain
104 I15 **Cadiz, Bahía de** *bay* SW Spain
Cadiz City *see* Cadiz
104 H15 **Cádiz, Golfo de** *Eng.* Gulf of Cadiz. *gulf* Portugal/Spain
Cadiz, Gulf of *see* Cádiz, Golfo de
35 X14 **Cadiz Lake** ◎ California, W USA
182 E2 **Cadney Homestead** South Australia
Cadurcum *see* Cahors
83 F17 **Caecae** Ngamiland, NW Botswana
102 K4 **Caen** Calvados, N France
Caene/Caenepolis *see* Qena
Caerdydd *see* Cardiff
Caer Glou *see* Gloucester
Caer Gybi *see* Holyhead
Caerleon *see* Chester
Caer Luel *see* Carlisle
97 I18 **Caernarfon** *var.* Caernarvon, Carnarvon. NW Wales, UK
97 H18 **Caernarfon Bay** *bay* NW Wales, UK
97 I19 **Caernarvon** *cultural region* NW Wales, UK
Caernarvon *see* Caernarfon
Caesaraugusta *see* Zaragoza
Caesarea Mazaca *see* Kayseri
Caesarobriga *see* Talavera de la Reina
Caesarodunum *see* Tours
Caesaromagus *see* Beauvais
Caesena *see* Cesena
59 N17 **Caetité** Bahia, E Brazil
62 J6 **Cafayate** Salta, N Argentina
171 O2 **Cagayan** ≈ Luzon, N Philippines
171 Q7 **Cagayan de Oro** *off.* Cagayan de Oro City. Mindanao, S Philippines
170 M8 **Cagayan de Tawi Tawi** *island* S Philippines
171 N6 **Cagayan Islands** *island group* C Philippines
31 O14 **Cagles Mill Lake** ▣ Indiana, N USA
106 I12 **Cagli** Marche, C Italy
107 C20 **Cagliari** *anc.* Caralis. Sardegna, Italy, C Mediterranean Sea
107 C20 **Cagliari, Golfo di** *gulf* Sardegna, Italy, C Mediterranean Sea
103 U15 **Cagnes-sur-Mer** Alpes-Maritimes, SE France
54 L5 **Cagua** Aragua, N Venezuela
171 O1 **Cagua, Mount** ▲ Luzon, N Philippines
54 F13 **Caguán, Río** ≈ SW Colombia
45 U6 **Caguas** E Puerto Rico
23 P5 **Cahaba River** ≈ Alabama, S USA
42 E5 **Cahabón, Río** ≈ C Guatemala
83 B15 **Cahama** Cunene, SW Angola
97 B21 **Caha Mountains** *Ir.* An Cheacha. ⛰ SW Ireland
97 D20 **Caher** *Ir.* An Cathair. S Ireland
97 A21 **Cahersiveen** *Ir.* Cathair Saidhbhín. SW Ireland
30 K15 **Cahokia** Illinois, N USA
83 L15 **Cahora Bassa, Albufeira de** *var.* Lake Cabora Bassa. ▣ NW Mozambique
97 G20 **Cahore Point** *Ir.* Rinn Chathóir. *headland* SE Ireland
102 M14 **Cahors** *anc.* Cadurcum. Lot, S France
56 D9 **Cahuapanas, Río** ≈ N Peru
116 M12 **Cahul** *Rus.* Kagul. S Moldova
Cahul, Lacul *see* Kahul, Ozero
83 N16 **Caia** Sofala, C Mozambique
59 J19 **Caiapó, Serra do** ⛰ C Brazil
44 F5 **Caibarién** Villa Clara, C Cuba
55 O5 **Caicara** Monagas, NE Venezuela
54 L5 **Caicara del Orinoco** Bolívar, C Venezuela
59 P14 **Caicó** Rio Grande do Norte, E Brazil
44 M6 **Caicos Islands** *island group* W Turks and Caicos Islands
44 L5 **Caicos Passage** *strait* Bahamas/Turks and Caicos Islands
161 O9 **Caidian** *prev.* Hanyang. Hubei, C China
Caiffa *see* Hefa
180 M12 **Caiguna** Western Australia
Caillí, Ceann *see* Hag's Head
40 J11 **Caimanero, Laguna del** *var.* Laguna del Camaronero. *lagoon* E Pacific Ocean
117 N10 **Căinari** *Rus.* Kaynary. C Moldova
57 L19 **Caine, Río** ≈ C Bolivia
Caiphas *see* Hefa
195 N4 **Caird Coast** *physical region* Antarctica
96 J9 **Cairn Gorm** ▲ C Scotland, UK
96 J9 **Cairngorm Mountains** ⛰ C Scotland, UK
39 P12 **Cairn Mountain** ▲ Alaska, USA
181 W4 **Cairns** Queensland, NE Australia
121 V13 **Cairo** *Ar.* Al Qāhirah, *var.* El Qâhira. ● (Egypt) N Egypt
23 T8 **Cairo** Georgia, SE USA
30 L17 **Cairo** Illinois, N USA
75 V8 **Cairo** ✕ C Egypt
Caiseal *see* Cashel
Caisleán an Bharraigh *see* Castlebar
Caisleán na Finne *see* Castlefinn
96 J6 **Caithness** *cultural region* N Scotland, UK
83 D15 **Caiundo** Cuando Cubango, S Angola
56 C11 **Cajamarca** *prev.* Caxamarca. Cajamarca, NW Peru
56 B11 **Cajamarca** *off.* Departamento de Cajamarca. ◈ *department* N Peru
103 N14 **Cajarc** Lot, S France
42 G6 **Cajón, Represa El** ▣ NW Honduras
58 N12 **Caju, Ilha do** *island* NE Brazil
Cakaubalavu Reef *see* Kavukavu Reef
159 R10 **Caka Yanhu** ◎ C China
112 E7 **Čakovec** *Ger.* Csakathurn, *Hung.* Csáktornya; *prev. Ger.* Tschakathurn. Međimurje, N Croatia
77 V17 **Calabar** Cross River, S Nigeria
14 K13 **Calabogie** Ontario, SE Canada
54 L6 **Calabozo** Guárico, C Venezuela
107 N20 **Calabria** *anc.* Bruttium. ◈ *region* SW Italy
104 M16 **Calaburra, Punta de** *headland* S Spain
116 G14 **Calafat** Dolj, SW Romania
Calafate *see* El Calafate
105 Q4 **Calahorra** La Rioja, N Spain
103 N1 **Calais** Pas-de-Calais, N France
19 T5 **Calais** Maine, NE USA
Calais, Pas de *see* Dover, Strait of
Calalen *see* Kallalen
62 H4 **Calama** Antofagasta, N Chile
Calamianes *see* Calamian Group
170 M5 **Calamian Group** *var.* Calamianes. *island group* W Philippines
105 R7 **Calamocha** Aragón, NE Spain
29 N14 **Calamus River** ≈ Nebraska, C USA
116 G12 **Călan** *Ger.* Kalan, *Hung.* Pusztakalán. Hunedoara, SW Romania
105 S7 **Calanda** Aragón, NE Spain
168 F9 **Calang** Sumatera, W Indonesia
171 N4 **Calapan** Mindoro, N Philippines
Călăras *see* Călărași
116 M9 **Călărași** *var.* Călăras, *Rus.* Kalarash. C Moldova
116 L14 **Călărași** Călărași, SE Romania
116 K14 **Călărași** ◈ *county* SE Romania
54 E10 **Calarca** Quindío, W Colombia
105 Q12 **Calasparra** Murcia, SE Spain
107 I23 **Calatafimi** Sicilia, Italy, C Mediterranean Sea
105 Q6 **Calatayud** Aragón, NE Spain
171 O4 **Calauag** Luzon, N Philippines
35 P8 **Calaveras River** ≈ California, W USA
171 N4 **Calavite, Cape** *headland* Mindoro, N Philippines
171 Q8 **Calbayog** *off.* Calbayog City. Samar, C Philippines
22 G9 **Calcasieu Lake** ◎ Louisiana, S USA
22 H8 **Calcasieu River** ≈ Louisiana, S USA
56 B6 **Calceta** Manabí, W Ecuador
61 B16 **Calchaquí** Santa Fe, C Argentina
62 J6 **Calchaquí, Río** ≈ NW Argentina
58 J10 **Calçoene** Amapá, NE Brazil
153 S16 **Calcutta** West Bengal, NE India
153 S16 **Calcutta** ✕ West Bengal, N India
54 E9 **Caldas** *off.* Departamento de Caldas. ◈ *province* W Colombia
104 F10 **Caldas da Rainha** Leiria, W Portugal
104 G3 **Caldas de Reis** *var.* Caldas de Reyes. Galicia, NW Spain
Caldas de Reyes *see* Caldas de Reis
58 F13 **Caldeirão** Amazonas, NW Brazil
62 G7 **Caldera** Atacama, N Chile
42 L14 **Caldera** Puntarenas, W Costa Rica
105 N10 **Calderina** ▲ C Spain
137 T13 **Çaldıran** Van, E Turkey
32 M14 **Caldwell** Idaho, NW USA
27 N8 **Caldwell** Kansas, C USA
14 G15 **Caledon** Ontario, S Canada
83 I23 **Caledon** *var.* Mohokare. ≈ Lesotho/South Africa
42 G1 **Caledonia** Corozal, N Belize
14 G16 **Caledonia** Ontario, S Canada
29 X11 **Caledonia** Minnesota, N USA
105 X5 **Calella** *var.* Calella de la Costa. Cataluña, NE Spain
Calella de la Costa *see* Calella
23 P4 **Calera** Alabama, S USA
63 I19 **Caleta Olivia** Santa Cruz, SE Argentina
35 X17 **Calexico** California, W USA
97 H16 **Calf of Man** *island* SW Isle of Man
11 Q16 **Calgary** Alberta, SW Canada
11 Q16 **Calgary** ✕ Alberta, SW Canada
37 U5 **Calhan** Colorado, C USA
64 O5 **Calheta** Madeira, Portugal, NE Atlantic Ocean
23 R2 **Calhoun** Georgia, SE USA
20 I6 **Calhoun** Kentucky, S USA
22 M3 **Calhoun City** Mississippi, S USA
21 P12 **Calhoun Falls** South Carolina, SE USA
54 D11 **Cali** Valle del Cauca, W Colombia
27 V9 **Calico Rock** Arkansas, C USA
155 F21 **Calicut** *var.* Kozhikode. Kerala, SW India
35 Y9 **Caliente** Nevada, W USA
27 U5 **California** Missouri, C USA
18 B15 **California** Pennsylvania, NE USA
35 Q12 **California** *off.* State of California; also known as El Dorado, The Golden State. ◈ *state* W USA
35 P11 **California Aqueduct** *aqueduct* California, W USA
35 T13 **California City** California, W USA
40 F6 **California, Golfo de** *Eng.* Gulf of California; *prev.* Sea of Cortez. *gulf* W Mexico
California, Gulf of *see* California, Golfo de
137 Y13 **Cälilabad** *Rus.* Dzhalilabad; *prev.* Astrakhan-Bazar. S Azerbaijan
116 I12 **Călimănești** Vâlcea, SW Romania
116 J9 **Călimani, Munții** ⛰ N Romania
Calinisc *see* Cupcina
35 X17 **Calipatria** California, W USA
Calisia *see* Kalisz
34 M7 **Calistoga** California, W USA
83 G25 **Calitzdorp** Western Cape, SW South Africa
41 W12 **Calkiní** Campeche, E Mexico
182 K4 **Callabonna Creek** *var.* Tilcha Creek. *seasonal river* New South Wales/South Australia
182 J4 **Callabonna, Lake** ◎ South Australia
102 G5 **Callac** Côtes d'Armor, NW France
35 U5 **Callaghan, Mount** ▲ Nevada, W USA
Callain *see* Callan
97 E19 **Callan** *Ir.* Callain. S Ireland
14 H11 **Callander** Ontario, S Canada
96 I11 **Callander** C Scotland, UK
98 H7 **Callantsoog** Noord-Holland, NW Netherlands
57 D14 **Callao** Callao, W Peru
57 D15 **Callao** *off.* Departamento del Callao. ◈ *constitutional province* W Peru
56 F11 **Callaria, Río** ≈ E Peru
Callatis *see* Mangalia
9 Q13 **Calling Lake** Alberta, W Canada
Callosa de Ensarriá *see* Callosa d'En Sarrià
105 T11 **Callosa d'En Sarrià** *var.* Callosa de Ensarriá. País Valenciano, E Spain
105 S12 **Callosa de Segura** País Valenciano, E Spain
29 X11 **Calmar** Iowa, C USA
Calmar *see* Kalmar
43 R16 **Calobre** Veraguas, C Panama
23 X14 **Caloosahatchee River** ≈ Florida, SE USA
183 V2 **Caloundra** Queensland, E Australia
105 T11 **Calpe** País Valenciano, E Spain
41 P14 **Calpulalpan** Tlaxcala, S Mexico
107 K25 **Caltagirone** Sicilia, Italy, C Mediterranean Sea
107 J24 **Caltanissetta** Sicilia, Italy, C Mediterranean Sea
82 E11 **Caluango** Lunda Norte, NE Angola
82 C12 **Calucinga** Bié, W Angola
82 B12 **Calulo** Cuanza Sul, NW Angola
83 B14 **Caluquembe** Huíla, W Angola
80 Q11 **Caluula** Bari, NE Somalia
102 K4 **Calvados** ◈ *department* N France
186 I10 **Calvados Chain, The** *island group* SE PNG
25 U9 **Calvert** Texas, SW USA
20 H7 **Calvert City** Kentucky, S USA
103 X14 **Calvi** Corse, France, C Mediterranean Sea
40 L12 **Calvillo** Aguascalientes, C Mexico
83 F24 **Calvinia** Northern Cape, W South Africa
104 K8 **Calvitero** ▲ W Spain
101 G22 **Calw** Baden-Württemberg, SW Germany
Calydon *see* Kalydón
105 N11 **Calzada de Calatrava** Castilla-La Mancha, C Spain
Cama *see* Kama
82 C11 **Camabatela** Cuanza Norte, NW Angola
64 Q5 **Camacha** Porto Santo, Madeira, Portugal, NE Atlantic Ocean
14 L8 **Camachigama, Lac** ◎ Quebec, SE Canada
40 M9 **Camacho** Zacatecas, C Mexico
82 D13 **Camacupa** *var.* General Machado, *Port.* Vila General Machado. Bié, C Angola
54 L7 **Camaguán** Guárico, C Venezuela
44 G6 **Camagüey** *prev.* Puerto Príncipe. Camagüey, C Cuba
44 G5 **Camagüey, Archipiélago de** *island group* C Cuba
40 D5 **Camalli, Sierra de** ▲ NW Mexico
57 G18 **Camana** *var.* Camaná. Arequipa, SW Peru
29 Z14 **Camanche** Iowa, C USA
35 P8 **Camanche Reservoir** ▣ California, W USA
61 I16 **Camaquã** Rio Grande do Sul, S Brazil
61 H16 **Camaquã, Rio** ≈ S Brazil
64 P6 **Câmara de Lobos** Madeira, Portugal, NE Atlantic Ocean
103 U16 **Camarat, Cap** *headland* SE France
41 O8 **Camargo** Tamaulipas, C Mexico
103 R15 **Camargue** *physical region* SE France
104 F2 **Camariñas** Galicia, NW Spain
Camaronero, Laguna del *see* Caimanero, Laguna del
63 J18 **Camarones** Chaco, S Argentina
63 J18 **Camarones, Bahía** *bay* S Argentina
104 J14 **Camas** Andalucía, S Spain
167 S15 **Ca Mau** *prev.* Quan Long. Minh Hai, S Vietnam
82 E11 **Camaxilo** Lunda Norte, NE Angola
104 G3 **Cambados** Galicia, NW Spain
Cambay, Gulf of *see* Khambhāt, Gulf of
Camberia *see* Chambéry
97 N22 **Camberley** SE England, UK
167 R12 **Cambodia** *off.* Kingdom of Cambodia, *var.* Democratic Kampuchea, Roat Kampuchea, *Cam.* Kampuchea; *prev.* People's Democratic Republic of Kampuchea. ◆ *republic* SE Asia
102 I16 **Cambo-les-Bains** Pyrénées-Atlantiques, SW France
103 P2 **Cambrai** *Flem.* Kambryk; *prev.* Cambray, *anc.* Cameracum. Nord, N France
Cambray *see* Cambrai
104 H2 **Cambre** Galicia, NW Spain
35 O12 **Cambria** California, W USA
97 J20 **Cambrian Mountains** ⛰ C Wales, UK
14 G16 **Cambridge** Ontario, S Canada
44 I12 **Cambridge** W Jamaica
184 M8 **Cambridge** Waikato, North Island, NZ
97 O20 **Cambridge** *Lat.* Cantabrigia. E England, UK
32 M12 **Cambridge** Idaho, NW USA
30 K11 **Cambridge** Illinois, N USA
21 Y4 **Cambridge** Maryland, NE USA
19 O11 **Cambridge** Massachusetts, NE USA
29 V7 **Cambridge** Minnesota, N USA
29 N16 **Cambridge** Nebraska, C USA
31 U13 **Cambridge** Ohio, NE USA
8 L7 **Cambridge Bay** Victoria Island, Nunavut, NW Canada
97 O20 **Cambridgeshire** *cultural region* E England, UK
105 U6 **Cambrils de Mar** Cataluña, NE Spain
Cambundi-Catembo *see* Nova Gaia
137 N11 **Çam Burnu** *headland* N Turkey
183 S9 **Camden** New South Wales, SE Australia
23 O6 **Camden** Alabama, S USA
27 U14 **Camden** Arkansas, C USA
21 Y3 **Camden** Delaware, NE USA
19 R7 **Camden** Maine, NE USA
18 I16 **Camden** New Jersey, NE USA
18 I9 **Camden** New York, NE USA
21 R12 **Camden** South Carolina, SE USA
20 H8 **Camden** Tennessee, S USA
25 X9 **Camden** Texas, SW USA
39 S5 **Camden Bay** *bay* S Beaufort Sea
27 U6 **Camdenton** Missouri, C USA
Camellia State *see* Alabama
18 M7 **Camels Hump** ▲ Vermont, NE USA
117 N8 **Camenca** *Rus.* Kamenka. N Moldova
Cameracum *see* Cambrai
22 G9 **Cameron** Louisiana, S USA
25 T9 **Cameron** Texas, SW USA
30 J5 **Cameron** Wisconsin, N USA
10 M12 **Cameron** ≈ British Columbia, W Canada
185 A24 **Cameron Mountains** ⛰ South Island, NZ
79 D15 **Cameroon** *off.* Republic of Cameroon, *Fr.* Cameroun. ◆ *republic* W Africa
79 D15 **Cameroon Mountain** ▲ SW Cameroon
Cameroon Ridge *see* Camerounaise, Dorsale
Cameroun *see* Cameroon
79 E14 **Camerounaise, Dorsale** *Eng.* Cameroon Ridge. *ridge* NW Cameroon
171 N3 **Camiling** Luzon, N Philippines
23 T7 **Camilla** Georgia, SE USA
104 G5 **Caminha** Viana do Castelo, N Portugal
35 P7 **Camino** California, W USA
136 B15 **Çamiçi Gölü** ◎ SW Turkey
107 J24 **Cammarata** Sicilia, Italy, C Mediterranean Sea
42 K10 **Camoapa** Boaco, S Nicaragua
58 O13 **Camocim** Ceará, E Brazil
106 D10 **Camogli** Liguria, NW Italy
181 S5 **Camooweal** Queensland, C Australia
55 Y11 **Camopi** E French Guiana
151 Q22 **Camorta** *island* Nicobar Islands, India, NE Indian Ocean
42 I6 **Campamento** Olancho, C Honduras
61 D19 **Campana** Buenos Aires, E Argentina
63 F21 **Campana, Isla** *island* S Chile
104 K11 **Campanario** Extremadura, W Spain
107 L17 **Campania** *Eng.* Champagne. ◈ *region* S Italy
27 Y8 **Campbell** Missouri, C USA
185 K15 **Campbell, Cape** *headland* South Island, NZ
14 J14 **Campbellford** Ontario, SE Canada
31 R13 **Campbell Hill** *hill* Ohio, N USA
192 K13 **Campbell Island** *island* S NZ
175 P13 **Campbell Plateau** *undersea feature* SW Pacific Ocean
10 K17 **Campbell River** Vancouver Island, British Columbia, SW Canada
20 L6 **Campbellsville** Kentucky, S USA
13 O13 **Campbellton** New Brunswick, SE Canada
183 P16 **Campbell Town** Tasmania, SE Australia
183 S9 **Campbelltown** New South Wales, SE Australia
96 G13 **Campbeltown** W Scotland, UK
41 W13 **Campeche** Campeche, SE Mexico
41 W14 **Campeche** ◈ *state* SE Mexico
41 T14 **Campeche, Bahía de** *Eng.* Bay of Campeche. *bay* E Mexico
Campeche, Banco de *see* Campeche Bank
64 C11 **Campeche Bank** *Sp.* Banco de Campeche, Sonda de Campeche. *undersea feature* S Gulf of Mexico
Campeche, Bay of *see* Campeche, Bahía de
Campeche, Sonda de *see* Campeche Bank
44 H7 **Campechuela** Granma, E Cuba
182 M13 **Camperdown** Victoria, SE Australia
167 U6 **Câm Pha** Quang Ninh, N Vietnam
116 H10 **Câmpia Turzii** *Ger.* Jerischmarkt, *Hung.* Aranyosgyéres; *prev.* Cîmpia Turzii, Ghiriș, Gyéres. Cluj, NW Romania
104 K12 **Campillo de Llerena** Extremadura, W Spain
104 L15 **Campillos** Andalucía, S Spain
116 J13 **Câmpina** *prev.* Cîmpina. Prahova, SE Romania
59 Q15 **Campina Grande** Paraíba, E Brazil
60 L9 **Campinas** São Paulo, S Brazil
38 L10 **Camp Kulowiye** Saint Lawrence Island, Alaska, USA
79 D17 **Campo** *var.* Kampo. Sud, SW Cameroon
Campo *see* Ntem
59 N15 **Campo Alegre de Lourdes** Bahia, E Brazil
107 L16 **Campobasso** Molise, C Italy
107 H24 **Campobello di Mazara** Sicilia, Italy, C Mediterranean Sea
Campo Criptana *see* Campo de Criptana
105 O10 **Campo de Criptana** *var.* Campo Criptana. Castilla-La Mancha, C Spain
59 I16 **Campo de Diauarum** *var.* Pôsto Diuarum. Mato Grosso, W Brazil
54 E5 **Campo de la Cruz** Atlántico, N Colombia
105 P11 **Campo de Montiel** *physical region* C Spain
Campo dos Goitacazes *see* Campos
60 H12 **Campo Erê** Santa Catarina, S Brazil
62 L7 **Campo Gallo** Santiago del Estero, N Argentina
59 I20 **Campo Grande** *state capital* Mato Grosso do Sul, SW Brazil
60 K12 **Campo Largo** Paraná, S Brazil
58 N13 **Campo Maior** Piauí, E Brazil
104 I10 **Campo Maior** Portalegre, C Portugal
60 H10 **Campo Mourão** Paraná, S Brazil
60 Q9 **Campos** *var.* Campo dos Goitacazes. Rio de Janeiro, SE Brazil
59 L17 **Campos Belos** Goiás, S Brazil
60 N9 **Campos do Jordão** São Paulo, S Brazil
60 I13 **Campos Novos** Santa Catarina, S Brazil
59 O14 **Campos Sales** Ceará, E Brazil
25 Q9 **Camp San Saba** Texas, SW USA
21 N6 **Campton** Kentucky, S USA
116 I13 **Câmpulung** *prev.* Câmpulung-Mușcel, Cîmpulung. Argeș, S Romania
116 J9 **Câmpulung Moldovenesc** *var.* Cîmpulung Moldovenesc, *Ger.* Kimpolung, *Hung.* Hosszúmezjő. Suceava, NE Romania
Câmpulung-Mușcel *see* Câmpulung
Campus Stellae *see* Santiago
36 L12 **Camp Verde** Arizona, SW USA
25 P11 **Camp Wood** Texas, SW USA
167 V13 **Cam Ranh** Khanh Hoa, S Vietnam
11 Q15 **Camrose** Alberta, SW Canada
Camulodunum *see* Colchester
136 B12 **Çan** Çanakkale, NW Turkey
18 L12 **Canaan** Connecticut, NE USA
9 O13 **Canada** ◆ *commonwealth republic* N North America
197 P6 **Canada Basin** *undersea feature* Arctic Ocean
61 B18 **Cañada de Gómez** Santa Fe, C Argentina
197 P6 **Canada Plain** *undersea feature* Arctic Ocean
61 A18 **Cañada Rosquín** Santa Fe, C Argentina
25 P1 **Canadian** Texas, SW USA
16 K12 **Canadian River** ≈ SW USA
8 L12 **Canadian Shield** *physical region* Canada
63 I18 **Cañadón Grande, Sierra** ⛰ S Argentina
55 P9 **Canaima** Bolívar, SE Venezuela
136 B11 **Çanakkale** *var.* Dardanelli; *prev.* Chanak, Kale Sultanie. Çanakkale, W Turkey
136 B12 **Çanakkale** ◈ *province* NW Turkey
136 B11 **Çanakkale Boğazı** *Eng.* Dardanelles. *strait* NW Turkey
187 Q17 **Canala** Province Nord, C New Caledonia
59 A15 **Canamari** Amazonas, W Brazil
18 G10 **Canandaigua** New York, NE USA
18 F10 **Canandaigua Lake** ◎ New York, NE USA
40 G3 **Cananea** Sonora, NW Mexico
56 B8 **Cañar** ◈ *province* C Ecuador
64 N10 **Canarias, Islas** *Eng.* Canary Islands. ◈ *autonomous community* Spain, NE Atlantic Ocean
Canaries Basin *see* Canary Basin
44 C6 **Canarreos, Archipiélago de los** *island group* W Cuba
66 K3 **Canary Basin** *var.* Canaries Basin, Monaco Basin. *undersea feature* E Atlantic Ocean
Canary Islands *see* Canarias, Islas
42 L13 **Cañas** Guanacaste, NW Costa Rica
18 I10 **Canastota** New York, NE USA
40 K9 **Canatlán** Durango, C Mexico
104 J9 **Cañaveral** Extremadura, W Spain
23 Y11 **Canaveral, Cape** *headland* Florida, SE USA
59 O18 **Canavieiras** Bahia, E Brazil
43 R16 **Cañazas** Veraguas, W Panama
106 H6 **Canazei** Trentino-Alto Adige, N Italy
183 P6 **Canbelego** New South Wales, SE Australia
183 R10 **Canberra** ● (Australia) Australian Capital Territory, SE Australia
183 R10 **Canberra** ✕ Australian Capital Territory, SE Australia
35 P2 **Canby** California, W USA
29 S9 **Canby** Minnesota, N USA
103 N2 **Canche** ≈ N France
102 L13 **Cancon** Lot-et-Garonne, SW France
41 Z11 **Cancún** Quintana Roo, SE Mexico
104 K2 **Candás** Asturias, N Spain
102 J7 **Cande** Maine-et-Loire, NW France
41 W14 **Candelaria** Campeche, SE Mexico
24 J11 **Candelaria** Texas, SW USA
41 W15 **Candelaria, Río** ≈ Guatemala/Mexico
104 L8 **Candeleda** Castilla-León, N Spain
Candia *see* Irákleio
41 P8 **Cándido Aguilar** Tamaulipas, C Mexico
39 N8 **Candle** Alaska, USA
11 T14 **Candle Lake** Saskatchewan, C Canada
18 L13 **Candlewood, Lake** ▣ Connecticut, NE USA
29 O3 **Cando** North Dakota, N USA
Canea *see* Chaniá
45 O12 **Canefield** ✕ (Roseau) SW Dominica
61 F20 **Canelones** *prev.* Guadalupe. Canelones, S Uruguay
61 E20 **Canelones** ◈ *department* S Uruguay
Canendiyú *see* Canindeyú
63 F14 **Cañete** Bío Bío, C Chile
105 Q9 **Cañete** Castilla-La Mancha, C Spain
Cañete *see* San Vicente de Cañete
27 P8 **Caney** Kansas, C USA
27 P8 **Caney River** ≈ Kansas/Oklahoma, C USA

◆ Country
● Country Capital
◇ Dependent Territory
○ Dependent Territory Capital
◈ Administrative Region
✕ International Airport
▲ Mountain
⛰ Mountain Range
Volcano
≈ River
◎ Lake
▣ Reservoir

105 S3 **Canfranc-Estación** Aragón, NE Spain
83 E14 **Cangamba** Port. Vila de Aljustrel. Moxico, E Angola
82 C12 **Cangandala** Malanje, NW Angola
104 G4 **Cangas** Galicia, NW Spain
104 J2 **Cangas del Narcea** Asturias, N Spain
104 L2 **Cangas de Onís** Asturias, N Spain
161 S11 **Cangnan** prev. Lingxi. Zhejiang, SE China
82 C10 **Cangola** Uíge, NW Angola
83 E14 **Cangombe** Moxico, E Angola
63 H21 **Cangrejo, Cerro** ▲ S Argentina
61 H17 **Canguçu** Rio Grande do Sul, S Brazil
161 P3 **Cangzhou** Hebei, E China
12 M7 **Caniapiscau** ≈ Quebec, E Canada
12 M8 **Caniapiscau, Réservoir de** ⊟ Quebec, C Canada
107 J24 **Canicattì** Sicilia, Italy, C Mediterranean Sea
136 L11 **Canik Dağları** ▲ N Turkey
105 P14 **Caniles** Andalucía, S Spain
59 B16 **Canindé** Acre, W Brazil
62 P6 **Canindeyú** var. Canendiyú, Canindiyú. ◐ department E Paraguay
Canindiyú see Canindeyú
194 J10 **Canisteo Peninsula** peninsula Antarctica
18 F11 **Canisteo River** ≈ New York, NE USA
40 M10 **Cañitas** var. Cañitas de Felipe Pescador. Zacatecas, C Mexico
Cañitas de Felipe Pescador see Cañitas
105 P15 **Canjáyar** Andalucía, S Spain
136 I12 **Çankırı** var. Chankiri; anc. Gangra, Germanicopolis. Çankın, N Turkey
136 I11 **Çankırı** var. Chankiri. ◐ province N Turkey
171 P6 **Canlaon Volcano** ▲ Negros, C Philippines
11 P16 **Canmore** Alberta, SW Canada
96 F9 **Canna** island NW Scotland, UK
155 F20 **Cannanore** var. Kananur, Kannur. Kerala, SW India
31 O17 **Cannelton** Indiana, N USA
103 U15 **Cannes** Alpes-Maritimes, SE France
39 R5 **Canning River** ≈ Alaska, USA
106 C6 **Cannobio** Piemonte, NE Italy
97 L19 **Cannock** C England, UK
28 M6 **Cannonball River** ≈ North Dakota, N USA
29 W9 **Cannon Falls** Minnesota, N USA
18 I11 **Cannonsville Reservoir** ⊟ New York, NE USA
183 R12 **Cann River** Victoria, SE Australia
61 I16 **Canoas** Rio Grande do Sul, S Brazil
61 I14 **Canoas, Rio** ≈ S Brazil
14 I12 **Canoe Lake** ◎ Ontario, SE Canada
60 J12 **Canoinhas** Santa Catarina, S Brazil
37 T6 **Canon City** Colorado, C USA
55 P8 **Caño Negro** Bolívar, SE Venezuela
173 X15 **Canonniers Point** headland N Mauritius
23 W6 **Canoochee River** ≈ Georgia, SE USA
11 V15 **Canora** Saskatchewan, S Canada
45 Y14 **Canouan** island S Saint Vincent and the Grenadines
13 R15 **Canso** Nova Scotia, SE Canada
104 M3 **Cantabria** ◐ autonomous community N Spain
104 K3 **Cantábrica, Cordillera** ▲ N Spain
Cantabrigia see Cambridge
103 O12 **Cantal** ◐ department C France
105 N6 **Cantalejo** Castilla-León, N Spain
103 O12 **Cantal, Monts du** ▲ C France
104 G8 **Cantanhede** Coimbra, C Portugal
Cantaño see Cataño
55 O6 **Cantaura** Anzoátegui, NE Venezuela
116 M11 **Cantemir** Rus. Kantemir. S Moldova
97 Q22 **Canterbury** hist. Cantwaraburh, anc. Durovernum, Lat. Cantuaria. SE England, UK
185 F19 **Canterbury** off. Canterbury Region. ◐ region South Island, NZ
185 H20 **Canterbury Bight** bight South Island, NZ
185 H19 **Canterbury Plains** plain South Island, NZ
167 S14 **Cần Thơ** Cần Thơ, S Vietnam
104 K13 **Cantillana** Andalucía, S Spain
59 N15 **Canto do Buriti** Piauí, NE Brazil
23 S2 **Canton** Georgia, SE USA
30 K12 **Canton** Illinois, N USA
22 L5 **Canton** Mississippi, S USA
27 V2 **Canton** Missouri, C USA
18 J7 **Canton** New York, NE USA
21 O10 **Canton** North Carolina, SE USA
31 U12 **Canton** Ohio, N USA
26 L9 **Canton** Oklahoma, C USA
18 G12 **Canton** Pennsylvania, NE USA
29 R11 **Canton** South Dakota, N USA
25 V7 **Canton** Texas, SW USA
Canton see Guangzhou
Canton Island see Kanton
26 L9 **Canton Lake** ⊟ Oklahoma, C USA
106 D7 **Cantù** Lombardia, N Italy
Cantuaria/Cantwaraburh see Canterbury
39 R10 **Cantwell** Alaska, USA
59 O16 **Canudos** Bahia, E Brazil
47 T7 **Canumã, Rio** ≈ N Brazil
Canusium see Puglia, Canosa di
24 G7 **Canutillo** Texas, SW USA
25 N3 **Canyon** Texas, SW USA
33 Y12 **Canyon** Wyoming, C USA
32 K13 **Canyon City** Oregon, NW USA
33 R10 **Canyon Ferry Lake** ◎ Montana, NW USA
25 S11 **Canyon Lake** ⊟ Texas, SW USA
167 T5 **Cao Băng** var. Caobang. Cao Băng, N Vietnam
160 J12 **Caodu He** ≈ S China
167 S14 **Cao Lanh** Đông Thap, S Vietnam
82 C11 **Caombo** Malanje, NW Angola
Caorach, Cuan na g see Sheep Haven
Caozhou see Heze
171 Q12 **Capalulu** Pulau Mangole, E Indonesia
54 K8 **Capanaparo, Río** ≈ Colombia/Venezuela
58 L12 **Capanema** Pará, NE Brazil
60 L10 **Capão Bonito** São Paulo, S Brazil
60 I13 **Capão Doce, Morro do** ▲ S Brazil
54 I4 **Capatárida** Falcón, N Venezuela
102 I15 **Capbreton** Landes, SW France
Cap-Breton, Île du see Cape Breton Island
15 W6 **Cap-Chat** Quebec, SE Canada
15 P11 **Cap-de-la-Madeleine** Quebec, SE Canada
103 N13 **Capdenac** Aveyron, S France
183 Q15 **Cape Barren Island** island Furneaux Group, Tasmania, SE Australia
65 O18 **Cape Basin** undersea feature S Atlantic Ocean
13 R14 **Cape Breton Island** Fr. Île du Cap-Breton. island Nova Scotia, SE Canada
23 Y11 **Cape Canaveral** Florida, SE USA
21 Y6 **Cape Charles** Virginia, NE USA
77 P17 **Cape Coast** prev. Cape Coast Castle. S Ghana
Cape Coast Castle see Cape Coast
19 Q12 **Cape Cod Bay** bay Massachusetts, NE USA
23 W15 **Cape Coral** Florida, SE USA
181 R4 **Cape Crawford Roadhouse** Northern Territory, N Australia
9 Q7 **Cape Dorset** Baffin Island, Nunavut, NE Canada
21 N8 **Cape Fear River** ≈ North Carolina, SE USA
27 Y7 **Cape Girardeau** Missouri, C USA
21 T14 **Cape Island** island South Carolina, SE USA
186 A6 **Capella** ▲ NW PNG
98 H12 **Capelle aan den IJssel** Zuid-Holland, SW Netherlands
83 C15 **Capelongo** Huíla, C Angola
18 J17 **Cape May** New Jersey, NE USA
18 J17 **Cape May Court House** New Jersey, NE USA
Cape Palmas see Harper
8 I6 **Cape Parry** Northwest Territories, N Canada
65 P19 **Cape Rise** undersea feature SW Indian Ocean
Cape Saint Jacques see Vung Tau
Capesterre see Capesterre-Belle-Eau
45 Y6 **Capesterre-Belle-Eau** var. Capesterre. Basse Terre, S Guadeloupe
83 D26 **Cape Town** var. Ekapa, Afr. Kaapstad, Kapstad. ● (South Africa-legislative capital) Western Cape, SW South Africa
83 E26 **Cape Town** ✕ Western Cape, SW South Africa
76 D9 **Cape Verde** off. Republic of Cape Verde, Port. Cabo Verde, Ilhas do Cabo Verde. ◆ republic E Atlantic Ocean
64 L11 **Cape Verde Basin** undersea feature E Atlantic Ocean
66 K5 **Cape Verde Islands** island group E Atlantic Ocean
64 L10 **Cape Verde Plain** undersea feature E Atlantic Ocean
Cape Verde Plateau/Cape Verde Rise see Cape Verde Terrace
64 L11 **Cape Verde Terrace** var. Cape Verde Plateau, Cape Verde Rise. undersea feature E Atlantic Ocean
181 V2 **Cape York Peninsula** peninsula Queensland, N Australia
44 M8 **Cap-Haïtien** var. Le Cap. N Haiti
43 T15 **Capira** Panamá, C Panama
14 K8 **Capitachouane** ≈ Quebec, SE Canada
14 L8 **Capitachouane, Lac** ◎ Quebec, SE Canada
37 T13 **Capitan** New Mexico, SW USA
194 G3 **Capitán Arturo Prat** Chilean research station South Shetland Islands, Antarctica
37 S13 **Capitan Mountains** ▲ New Mexico, SW USA
62 M3 **Capitán Pablo Lagerenza** var. Mayor Pablo Lagerenza. Chaco, N Paraguay
37 T13 **Capitan Peak** ▲ New Mexico, SW USA
188 H5 **Capitol Hill** Saipan, S Northern Mariana Islands
60 I9 **Capivara, Represa** ⊟ S Brazil
61 J16 **Capivari** Rio Grande do Sul, S Brazil
113 H15 **Čapljina** Federacija Bosna I Hercegovina, S Bosnia and Herzegovina
83 M15 **Capoche** var. Kapoche. ≈ Mozambique/Zambia
Capo Delgado, Província de see Cabo Delgado
107 K17 **Capodichino** ✕ (Napoli) Campania, S Italy
Capodistria see Koper
106 E12 **Capraia, Isola** island Archipelago Toscano, C Italy
107 B16 **Caprara, Punta** var. Punta dello Scorno. headland Isola Asinara, W Italy
Capraria, Isola di to Capraia, Isola see Cabrera
14 F10 **Capreol** Ontario, S Canada
107 K18 **Capri** Campania, S Italy
175 S9 **Capricorn Tablemount** undersea feature W Pacific Ocean
107 J18 **Capri, Isola di** island S Italy
83 G16 **Caprivi** ◐ district NE Namibia
Caprivi Concession see Caprivi Strip
83 F16 **Caprivi Strip** Ger. Caprivizipfel; prev. Caprivi Concession. cultural region NE Namibia
Caprivizipfel see Caprivi Strip
25 O5 **Cap Rock Escarpment** cliffs Texas, SW USA
15 R10 **Cap-Rouge** Quebec, SE Canada
Cap Saint-Jacques see Vung Tau
38 F12 **Captain Cook** Hawaii, USA, C Pacific Ocean
183 R10 **Captains Flat** New South Wales, SE Australia
102 K14 **Captieux** Gironde, SW France
107 K17 **Capua** Campania, S Italy
54 F14 **Caquetá** off. Departamento del Caquetá. ◐ province S Colombia
54 E13 **Caquetá, Río** var. Rio Japurá, Yapurá. ≈ Brazil/Colombia see also Japurá, Rio
CAR see Central African Republic
Cara see Kara
57 I16 **Carabaya, Cordillera** ▲ E Peru
54 K5 **Carabobo** off. Estado Carabobo. ◐ state N Venezuela
116 I14 **Caracal** Olt, S Romania
58 F10 **Caracaraí** Rondônia, W Brazil
54 L5 **Caracas** ● (Venezuela) Distrito Federal, N Venezuela
54 I5 **Carache** Trujillo, N Venezuela
60 N10 **Caraguatatuba** São Paulo, S Brazil
48 I7 **Carajás, Serra dos** ▲ N Brazil
Caralis see Cagliari
54 E9 **Caramanta** Antioquia, W Colombia
171 P4 **Caramoan** Catanduanes Island, N Philippines
Caramurat see Mihail Kogălniceanu
116 F12 **Caransebeş** Ger. Karansebesch, Hung. Karánsebes. Caraş-Severin, SW Romania
Carapella see Carapelle
107 M16 **Carapelle** var. Carapella. ≈ SE Italy
55 O9 **Carapo** Bolívar, SE Venezuela
13 P13 **Caraquet** New Brunswick, SE Canada
Caras see Caraz
116 F12 **Caraşova** Hung. Krassóvár. Caraş-Severin, SW Romania
116 F12 **Caraş-Severin** ◐ county SW Romania
42 M5 **Caratasca, Laguna de** lagoon NE Honduras
58 C13 **Carauari** Amazonas, NW Brazil
Caravaca see Caravaca de la Cruz
105 Q12 **Caravaca de la Cruz** var. Caravaca. Murcia, SE Spain
106 E7 **Caravaggio** Lombardia, N Italy
107 C18 **Caravai, Passo di** pass Sardegna, Italy, C Mediterranean Sea
59 O19 **Caravelas** Bahia, E Brazil
56 C12 **Caraz** var. Caras. Ancash, W Peru
61 H14 **Carazinho** Rio Grande do Sul, S Brazil
42 J11 **Carazo** ◐ department SW Nicaragua
Carballiño see O Carballiño
104 G2 **Carballo** Galicia, NW Spain
11 W16 **Carberry** Manitoba, S Canada
40 F4 **Carbó** Sonora, NW Mexico
107 C20 **Carbonara, Capo** headland Sardegna, Italy, C Mediterranean Sea
37 Q5 **Carbondale** Colorado, C USA
30 L17 **Carbondale** Illinois, N USA
27 Q4 **Carbondale** Kansas, C USA
18 I13 **Carbondale** Pennsylvania, NE USA
13 V12 **Carbonear** Newfoundland, SE Canada
105 Q9 **Carboneras de Guadazaón** var. Carboneras de Guadazón. Castilla-La Mancha, C Spain
Carboneras de Guadazón see Carboneras de Guadazaón
23 O3 **Carbon Hill** Alabama, S USA
107 B20 **Carbonia** var. Carbonia Centro. Sardegna, Italy, C Mediterranean Sea
Carbonia Centro see Carbonia
105 S10 **Carcaixent** País Valenciano, E Spain
Carcaso see Carcassonne
65 B24 **Carcass Island** island NW Falkland Islands
103 O16 **Carcassonne** anc. Carcaso. Aude, S France
105 R12 **Carche** ▲ S Spain
56 A13 **Carchi** ◐ province N Ecuador
10 I8 **Carcross** Yukon Territory, W Canada
Cardamomes, Chaîne des see Krâvanh, Chuŏr Phnum
155 G22 **Cardamom Hills** ▲ SW India
Cardamom Mountains see Krâvanh, Chuŏr Phnum
104 M12 **Cardeña** Andalucía, S Spain
44 D4 **Cárdenas** Matanzas, W Cuba
41 O11 **Cárdenas** San Luis Potosí, C Mexico
41 U15 **Cárdenas** Tabasco, SE Mexico
63 H21 **Cardiel, Lago** ◎ S Argentina
97 K22 **Cardiff** Wel. Caerdydd. ◉ S Wales, UK
97 J22 **Cardiff-Wales** ✕ S Wales, UK
97 I21 **Cardigan** Wel. Aberteifi. SW Wales, UK
97 I20 **Cardigan** cultural region W Wales, UK
97 I20 **Cardigan Bay** bay W Wales, UK
19 N8 **Cardigan, Mount** ▲ New Hampshire, NE USA
14 M13 **Cardinal** Ontario, SE Canada
105 V5 **Cardona** Cataluña, NE Spain
61 E19 **Cardona** Soriano, SW Uruguay
105 V4 **Cardoner** ≈ NE Spain
11 Q17 **Cardston** Alberta, SW Canada
181 W5 **Cardwell** Queensland, NE Australia
116 G8 **Carei** Ger. Gross-Karol, Karol, Hung. Nagykároly; prev. Careii-Mari. Satu Mare, NW Romania
Careii-Mari see Carei
58 F13 **Careiro** Amazonas, NW Brazil
102 J4 **Carentan** Manche, N France
42 M2 **Cares** ≈ N Spain
33 P14 **Carey** Idaho, NW USA
31 S12 **Carey** Ohio, N USA
25 P4 **Carey** Texas, SW USA
180 L11 **Carey, Lake** ◎ Western Australia
173 O8 **Cargados Carajos Bank** undersea feature C Indian Ocean
102 G6 **Carhaix-Plouguer** Finistère, NW France
61 A22 **Carhué** Buenos Aires, E Argentina
55 O5 **Cariaco** Sucre, NE Venezuela
107 O20 **Cariati** Calabria, SW Italy
2 H17 **Caribbean Plate** tectonic feature
44 I11 **Caribbean Sea** sea W Atlantic Ocean
11 N15 **Cariboo Mountains** ▲ British Columbia, SW Canada
11 W9 **Caribou** Manitoba, C Canada
19 S2 **Caribou** Maine, NE USA
11 P10 **Caribou Mountains** ▲ Alberta, SW Canada
Caribrod see Dimitrovgrad
40 I6 **Carichic** Chihuahua, N Mexico
103 R3 **Carignan** Ardennes, N France
183 Q5 **Carinda** New South Wales, SE Australia
105 R6 **Cariñena** Aragón, NE Spain
107 I23 **Carini** Sicilia, Italy, C Mediterranean Sea
107 K17 **Carinola** Campania, S Italy
Carinthi see Kärnten
55 O5 **Caripe** Monagas, NE Venezuela
55 P5 **Caripito** Monagas, NE Venezuela
15 W7 **Carleton** Quebec, SE Canada
31 S10 **Carleton** Michigan, N USA
13 O14 **Carleton, Mount** ▲ New Brunswick, SE Canada
14 L13 **Carleton Place** Ontario, SE Canada
35 V3 **Carlin** Nevada, W USA
30 K14 **Carlinville** Illinois, N USA
97 K14 **Carlisle** anc. Caer Luel, Luguvallium, Luguvallum. NW England, UK
27 V11 **Carlisle** Arkansas, C USA
31 N15 **Carlisle** Indiana, N USA
29 V14 **Carlisle** Iowa, C USA
21 N5 **Carlisle** Kentucky, S USA
18 F15 **Carlisle** Pennsylvania, NE USA
21 Q11 **Carlisle** South Carolina, SE USA
38 J17 **Carlisle Island** island Aleutian Islands, Alaska, USA
27 R7 **Carl Junction** Missouri, C USA
107 A20 **Carloforte** Sardegna, Italy, C Mediterranean Sea
Carlopago see Karlobag
61 B21 **Carlos Casares** Buenos Aires, E Argentina
61 E18 **Carlos Reyles** Durazno, C Uruguay
61 A21 **Carlos Tejedor** Buenos Aires, E Argentina
97 F19 **Carlow** Ir. Ceatharlach. SE Ireland
97 F19 **Carlow** Ir. Cheatharlach. cultural region SE Ireland
96 F7 **Carloway** NW Scotland, UK
Carlsbad see Karlovy Vary
35 U17 **Carlsbad** California, W USA
37 U15 **Carlsbad** New Mexico, SW USA
131 N13 **Carlsberg Ridge** undersea feature S Arabian Sea
Carlsruhe see Karlsruhe
29 W6 **Carlton** Minnesota, N USA
11 V17 **Carlyle** Saskatchewan, S Canada
30 L15 **Carlyle** Illinois, N USA
30 L15 **Carlyle Lake** ⊟ Illinois, N USA
10 H7 **Carmacks** Yukon Territory, W Canada
106 B9 **Carmagnola** Piemonte, NW Italy
11 X16 **Carman** Manitoba, S Canada
Carmana/Carmania see Kermān
97 I21 **Carmarthen** SW Wales, UK
97 I21 **Carmarthen** cultural region SW Wales, UK
97 I22 **Carmarthen Bay** inlet SW Wales, UK
103 N14 **Carmaux** Tarn, S France
35 N11 **Carmel** California, W USA
31 O13 **Carmel** Indiana, N USA
18 L13 **Carmel** New York, NE USA
97 H18 **Carmel Head** headland NW Wales, UK
42 E2 **Carmelita** Petén, N Guatemala
61 D19 **Carmelo** Colonia, SW Uruguay
41 V14 **Carmen** var. Ciudad del Carmen. Campeche, SE Mexico
61 A25 **Carmen de Patagones** Buenos Aires, E Argentina
40 F8 **Carmen, Isla** island W Mexico
40 M5 **Carmen, Sierra del** ▲ NW Mexico
30 M16 **Carmi** Illinois, N USA
35 O7 **Carmichael** California, W USA
Carmiel see Karmi'él
25 U11 **Carmine** Texas, SW USA
104 K14 **Carmona** Andalucía, S Spain
Carmona see Uíge
Carnaro see Kvarner
14 I13 **Carnarvon** Ontario, SE Canada
83 G24 **Carnarvon** Northern Cape, W South Africa
Carnarvon see Caernarfon
180 K9 **Carnarvon Range** ▲ Western Australia
180 G9 **Carnarvon** Western Australia
Carn Domhnach see Carndonagh
96 E13 **Carndonagh** Ir. Carn Domhnach. NW Ireland
11 V17 **Carnduff** Saskatchewan, S Canada
26 L11 **Carnegie** Oklahoma, C USA
180 L9 **Carnegie, Lake** salt lake Western Australia
193 U8 **Carnegie Ridge** undersea feature E Pacific Ocean
96 H9 **Carn Eige** ▲ N Scotland, UK
182 F5 **Carnes** South Australia
194 J12 **Carney Island** island Antarctica
18 H16 **Carneys Point** New Jersey, NE USA
Carniche, Alpi see Karnische Alpen
151 Q21 **Car Nicobar** island Nicobar Islands, India, NE Indian Ocean
79 H15 **Carnot** Mambéré-Kadéï, W Central African Republic
182 F10 **Carnot, Cape** headland South Australia
96 K11 **Carnoustie** E Scotland, UK
97 F20 **Carnsore Point** Ir. Ceann an Chairn. headland SE Ireland
8 H7 **Carnwath** ≈ Northwest Territories, NW Canada
31 R8 **Caro** Michigan, N USA
23 Z15 **Carol City** Florida, SE USA
59 L14 **Carolina** Maranhão, E Brazil
45 U5 **Carolina** E Puerto Rico
21 V12 **Carolina Beach** North Carolina, SE USA
Caroline Island see Millennium Island
189 N15 **Caroline Islands** island group C Micronesia
131 Z14 **Caroline Plate** tectonic feature
192 H7 **Caroline Ridge** undersea feature E Philippine Sea
Carolopois see Châlons-en-Champagne
45 V14 **Caroni Arena Dam** ⊟ Trinidad, Trinidad and Tobago
Caronie, Monti see Nebrodi, Monti
55 P7 **Caroní, Río** ≈ E Venezuela
45 U14 **Caroni River** ≈ Trinidad, Trinidad and Tobago
Caronium see A Coruña
54 J5 **Carora** Lara, N Venezuela
86 F12 **Carpathian Mountains** var. Carpathians, Cz./Pol. Karpaty, Ger. Karpaten. ▲ E Europe
Carpathians see Carpathian Mountains
Carpathos/Carpathus see Kárpathos
116 H12 **Carpaţii Meridionali** var. Alpi Transilvaniei, Carpaţii Sudici, Eng. South Carpathians, Transylvanian Alps, Ger. Südkarpaten, Transsylvanische Alpen, Hung. Déli-Kárpátok, Erdélyi-Havasok. ▲ C Romania
Carpaţii Sudici see Carpaţii Meridionali
174 L7 **Carpentaria, Gulf of** gulf N Australia
Carpentoracte see Carpentras
103 R14 **Carpentras** anc. Carpentoracte. Vaucluse, SE France
106 F9 **Carpi** Emilia-Romagna, N Italy
116 E11 **Cărpiniş** Hung. Gyertyámos. Timiş, W Romania
35 R14 **Carpinteria** California, W USA
23 S9 **Carrabelle** Florida, SE USA
Carraig Aonair see Fastnet Rock
Carraig Fhearghais see Carrickfergus
Carraig Mhachaire Rois see Carrickmacross
Carraig na Siúire see Carrick-on-Suir
Carrantual see Carrauntoohil
106 E10 **Carrara** Toscana, C Italy
61 F20 **Carrasco** ✕ (Montevideo) Canelones, S Uruguay
105 P9 **Carrascosa del Campo** Castilla-La Mancha, C Spain
54 H4 **Carrasquero** Zulia, NW Venezuela
183 O9 **Carrathool** New South Wales, SE Australia
Carrauntohil see Carrauntoohil
97 B21 **Carrauntoohil** Ir. Carrantual, Carrauntohil, Corrán Tuathail. ▲ SW Ireland
45 Y15 **Carriacou** island N Grenada
97 G15 **Carrickfergus** Ir. Carraig Fhearghais. NE Northern Ireland, UK
97 F16 **Carrickmacross** Ir. Carraig Mhachaire Rois. N Ireland
97 D16 **Carrick-on-Shannon** Ir. Cora Droma Rúisc. NW Ireland
97 E20 **Carrick-on-Suir** Ir. Carraig na Siúire. S Ireland
182 I7 **Carrieton** South Australia
40 L7 **Carrillo** Chihuahua, N Mexico
29 O4 **Carrington** North Dakota, N USA
104 M4 **Carrión** ≈ N Spain
104 M4 **Carrión de los Condes** Castilla-León, N Spain
25 P13 **Carrizo Springs** Texas, SW USA
37 S13 **Carrizozo** New Mexico, SW USA
29 T13 **Carroll** Iowa, C USA
23 N4 **Carrollton** Alabama, S USA
23 R3 **Carrollton** Georgia, SE USA
30 K14 **Carrollton** Illinois, N USA
20 L4 **Carrollton** Kentucky, S USA
31 R8 **Carrollton** Michigan, N USA
27 T3 **Carrollton** Missouri, C USA
31 U12 **Carrollton** Ohio, N USA
25 T6 **Carrollton** Texas, SW USA
11 U14 **Carrot** ≈ Saskatchewan, S Canada
11 U14 **Carrot River** Saskatchewan, C Canada
18 J7 **Carry Falls Reservoir** ⊟ New York, NE USA
136 L11 **Çarşamba** Samsun, N Turkey
28 L6 **Carson** North Dakota, N USA
35 Q6 **Carson City** state capital Nevada, W USA
35 R6 **Carson River** ≈ Nevada, W USA
35 S5 **Carson Sink** salt flat Nevada, W USA
11 Q16 **Carstairs** Alberta, SW Canada
Carstensz, Puntjak see Jaya, Puncak
54 E5 **Cartagena** var. Cartagena de los Indes. Bolívar, NW Colombia
105 R13 **Cartagena** anc. Carthago Nova. Murcia, SE Spain
Cartagena de los Indes see Cartagena
54 D10 **Cartago** Valle del Cauca, W Colombia
43 N14 **Cartago** Cartago, C Costa Rica
42 M14 **Cartago** off. Provincia de Cartago. ◐ province C Costa Rica
25 O11 **Carta Valley** Texas, SW USA
104 F10 **Cartaxo** Santarém, C Portugal
104 I14 **Cartaya** Andalucía, S Spain
Carteret Islands see Tulun Islands
29 S15 **Carter Lake** Iowa, C USA
23 S3 **Cartersville** Georgia, SE USA
185 M14 **Carterton** Wellington, North Island, NZ
30 J13 **Carthage** Illinois, N USA
22 L5 **Carthage** Mississippi, S USA
27 R7 **Carthage** Missouri, C USA
18 I8 **Carthage** New York, NE USA
21 T10 **Carthage** North Carolina, SE USA
20 K8 **Carthage** Tennessee, S USA
25 X7 **Carthage** Texas, SW USA
74 M5 **Carthage** ✕ (Tunis) N Tunisia
Carthago Nova see Cartagena
14 E10 **Cartier** Ontario, S Canada
54 E13 **Cartogena de Chaira** Caquetá, S Colombia
13 S8 **Cartwright** Newfoundland, E Canada
55 P9 **Caruana de Montaña** Bolívar, SE Venezuela
59 Q15 **Caruaru** Pernambuco, E Brazil
55 P5 **Carúpano** Sucre, NE Venezuela
Carusbur see Cherbourg
58 M12 **Carutapera** Maranhão, E Brazil
27 Y9 **Caruthersville** Missouri, C USA
103 O1 **Carvin** Pas-de-Calais, N France
58 E12 **Carvoeiro** Amazonas, NW Brazil
104 E10 **Carvoeiro, Cabo** headland C Portugal
21 U9 **Cary** North Carolina, SE USA
182 M3 **Caryapundy Swamp** wetland New South Wales/Queensland, SE Australia
65 E24 **Carysfort, Cape** headland East Falkland, Falkland Islands
74 F6 **Casablanca** Ar. Dar-el-Beida. NW Morocco
60 M8 **Casa Branca** São Paulo, S Brazil
36 L14 **Casa Grande** Arizona, SW USA
106 C8 **Casale Monferrato** Piemonte, NW Italy
106 E8 **Casalpusterlengo** Lombardia, N Italy
54 H10 **Casanare** off. Intendencia de Casanare. ◐ province C Colombia
55 P5 **Casanay** Sucre, NE Venezuela
24 K11 **Casa Piedra** Texas, SW USA
107 Q19 **Casarano** Puglia, SE Italy
42 J11 **Casares** Carazo, W Nicaragua
105 R10 **Casas Ibáñez** Castilla-La Mancha, C Spain
61 I14 **Casca** Rio Grande do Sul, S Brazil
172 I17 **Cascade** Mahé, NE Seychelles
33 N13 **Cascade** Idaho, NW USA
29 Y13 **Cascade** Iowa, C USA

◆ Country ● Country Capital ◇ Dependent Territory ○ Dependent Territory Capital ◐ Administrative Region ✕ International Airport ▲ Mountain ▲ Mountain Range ▲ Volcano ≈ River ◎ Lake ⊟ Reservoir

33 R9 **Cascade** Montana, NW USA
185 B20 **Cascade Point** headland South Island, NZ
32 G13 **Cascade Range** ▲ Oregon/Washington, NW USA
33 N12 **Cascade Reservoir** ▣ Idaho, NW USA
0 E8 **Cascadia Basin** undersea feature NE Pacific Ocean
104 E11 **Cascais** Lisboa, C Portugal
15 W7 **Cascapédia** ≈ Quebec, SE Canada
59 I22 **Cascavel** Ceará, E Brazil
60 G11 **Cascavel** Paraná, S Brazil
106 I13 **Cascia** Umbria, C Italy
106 F11 **Cascina** Toscana, C Italy
19 Q8 **Casco Bay** bay Maine, NE USA
194 J7 **Case Island** island Antarctica
106 B8 **Caselle** × (Torino) Piemonte, NW Italy
107 K17 **Caserta** Campania, S Italy
15 N8 **Casey** Quebec, SE Canada
30 M14 **Casey** Illinois, N USA
195 Y12 **Casey** Australian research station Antarctica
195 W3 **Casey Bay** bay Antarctica
80 Q11 **Caseyr, Raas** headland NE Somalia
97 D20 **Cashel** Ir. Caiseal. S Ireland
54 G6 **Casigua** Zulia, W Venezuela
61 B19 **Casilda** Santa Fe, C Argentina
Casim see General Toshevo
183 V4 **Casino** New South Wales, SE Australia
Casinum see Cassino
111 E17 **Čáslav** Ger. Tschaslau. Střední Čechy, C Czech Republic
56 C13 **Casma** Ancash, C Peru
167 S7 **Ca, Sông** ≈ N Vietnam
107 K17 **Casoria** Campania, S Italy
105 T6 **Caspe** Aragón, NE Spain
33 X15 **Casper** Wyoming, C USA
84 M10 **Caspian Depression** Kaz. Kaspīy Mangy Oypaty, Rus. Prikaspiyskaya Nizmennost'. depression Kazakhstan/Russian Federation
138 Kk9 **Caspian Sea** Az. Xäzär Dänizi, Kaz. Kaspiy Tengizi, Per. Baḩr-e Khazar, Daryā-ye Khazar, Rus. Kaspiyskoye More. inland sea Asia/Europe
83 L14 **Cassacatiza** Tete, NW Mozambique
Cassai see Kasai
82 F13 **Cassamba** Moxico, E Angola
107 N20 **Cassano allo Ionio** Calabria, SE Italy
31 S8 **Cass City** Michigan, N USA
Cassel see Kassel
14 M13 **Casselman** Ontario, SE Canada
29 R5 **Casselton** North Dakota, N USA
59 M16 **Cássia** var. Santa Rita de Cassia. Bahia, E Brazil
10 J9 **Cassiar** British Columbia, W Canada
10 K10 **Cassiar Mountains** ▲ British Columbia, W Canada
83 C15 **Cassinga** Huíla, SW Angola
107 J16 **Cassino** prev. San Germano; anc. Casinum. Lazio, C Italy
29 T4 **Cass Lake** Minnesota, N USA
29 T4 **Cass Lake** ◎ Minnesota, N USA
31 P10 **Cassopolis** Michigan, N USA
31 S8 **Cass River** ≈ Michigan, N USA
27 S8 **Cassville** Missouri, C USA
Castamoni see Kastamonu
58 L12 **Castanhal** Pará, NE Brazil
104 G8 **Castanheira de Pêra** Leiria, C Portugal
41 N7 **Castaños** Coahuila de Zaragoza, NE Mexico
108 I10 **Castasegna** Graubünden, SE Switzerland
106 D8 **Casteggio** Lombardia, N Italy
107 K23 **Castelbuono** Sicilia, Italy, C Mediterranean Sea
107 K15 **Castel di Sangro** Abruzzo, C Italy
106 H7 **Castelfranco Veneto** Veneto, NE Italy
102 K14 **Casteljaloux** Lot-et-Garonne, SW France
107 L18 **Castellabate** var. Santa Maria di Castellabate. Campania, S Italy
107 I23 **Castellammare del Golfo** Sicilia, Italy, C Mediterranean Sea
107 H22 **Castellammare, Golfo di** gulf Sicilia, Italy, C Mediterranean Sea
103 U15 **Castellane** Alpes-de-Haute-Provence, SE France
107 O18 **Castellaneta** Puglia, SE Italy
106 E9 **Castell'Arquato** Emilia-Romagna, C Italy
61 E21 **Castelli** Buenos Aires, E Argentina
105 T9 **Castelló de la Plana** var. Castellón. País Valenciano, E Spain
105 S8 **Castellón** ◆ province País Valenciano, E Spain
Castellón see Castelló de la Plana
105 S7 **Castellote** Aragón, NE Spain
103 N16 **Castelnaudary** Aude, S France
102 L16 **Castelnau-Magnoac** Hautes-Pyrénées, S France
106 F10 **Castelnovo ne' Monti** Emilia-Romagna, C Italy
Castelnuovo see Herceg-Novi
104 H9 **Castelo Branco** Castelo Branco, C Portugal
104 H8 **Castelo Branco** ◆ district C Portugal
104 I10 **Castelo de Vide** Portalegre, C Portugal
104 G9 **Castelo do Bode, Barragem do** ▣ C Portugal
106 G10 **Castel San Pietro Terme** Emilia-Romagna, C Italy
107 B17 **Castelsardo** Sardegna, Italy, C Mediterranean Sea
102 M14 **Castelsarrasin** Tarn-et-Garonne, S France
107 I24 **Casteltermini** Sicilia, Italy, C Mediterranean Sea
107 H24 **Castelvetrano** Sicilia, Italy, C Mediterranean Sea
182 L12 **Casterton** Victoria, SE Australia
102 J15 **Castets** Landes, SW France
106 H12 **Castiglione del Lago** Umbria, C Italy
106 F13 **Castiglione della Pescaia** Toscana, C Italy
106 F8 **Castiglione delle Stiviere** Lombardia, N Italy
104 M9 **Castilla-La Mancha** ◆ autonomous community NE Spain
104 L5 **Castilla-León** var. Castillia y Leon. ◆ autonomous community NW Spain
105 N10 **Castilla Nueva** cultural region C Spain
105 N6 **Castilla Vieja** cultural region N Spain
Castillia y Leon see Castilla-León
Castillo de Locubim see Castillo de Locubín
105 N14 **Castillo de Locubín** var. Castillo de Locubim. Andalucía, S Spain
102 K13 **Castillon-la-Bataille** Gironde, SW France
63 I19 **Castillo, Pampa del** plain S Argentina
61 G19 **Castillos** Rocha, SE Uruguay
97 B16 **Castlebar** Ir. Caisleán an Bharraigh. W Ireland
97 F16 **Castleblayney** Ir. Baile na Lorgan. N Ireland
45 O11 **Castle Bruce** E Dominica
36 M5 **Castle Dale** Utah, W USA
36 I14 **Castle Dome Peak** ▲ Arizona, SW USA
97 J14 **Castle Douglas** S Scotland, UK
97 E14 **Castlefinn** Ir. Caisleán na Finne. NW Ireland
97 M17 **Castleford** N England, UK
11 O17 **Castlegar** British Columbia, SW Canada
64 B12 **Castle Harbour** inlet Bermuda, NW Atlantic Ocean
21 V12 **Castle Hayne** North Carolina, SE USA
97 B20 **Castleisland** Ir. Oileán Ciarraí. SW Ireland
183 N12 **Castlemaine** Victoria, SE Australia
37 R5 **Castle Peak** ▲ Colorado, C USA
33 O13 **Castle Peak** ▲ Idaho, NW USA
184 N13 **Castlepoint** Wellington, North Island, NZ
97 D17 **Castlerea** Ir. An Caisleán Riabhach. W Ireland
97 G15 **Castlereagh** Ir. An Caisleán Riabhach. N Northern Ireland, UK
183 R6 **Castlereagh River** ≈ New South Wales, SE Australia
37 T5 **Castle Rock** Colorado, C USA
30 K7 **Castle Rock Lake** ▣ Wisconsin, N USA
65 G25 **Castle Rock Point** headland S Saint Helena
97 I16 **Castletown** SE Isle of Man
29 R9 **Castlewood** South Dakota, N USA
11 R15 **Castor** Alberta, SW Canada
14 M13 **Castor** ≈ Ontario, SE Canada
27 X7 **Castor River** ≈ Missouri, C USA
Castra Albiensium see Castres
Castra Regina see Regensburg
103 N15 **Castres** anc. Castra Albiensium. Tarn, S France
98 H9 **Castricum** Noord-Holland, W Netherlands
45 S11 **Castries** ● (Saint Lucia) N Saint Lucia
60 J11 **Castro** Paraná, S Brazil
63 F17 **Castro** Los Lagos, W Chile
104 H7 **Castro Daire** Viseu, N Portugal
104 M13 **Castro del Río** Andalucía, S Spain
Castrogiovanni see Enna
104 H14 **Castro Marim** Faro, S Portugal
104 J2 **Castropol** Asturias, N Spain
105 O2 **Castro-Urdiales** var. Castro Urdiales. Cantabria, N Spain
104 G13 **Castro Verde** Beja, S Portugal
107 N19 **Castrovillari** Calabria, SW Italy
35 N10 **Castroville** California, W USA
25 R12 **Castroville** Texas, SW USA
104 K11 **Castuera** Extremadura, W Spain
61 F19 **Casupá** Florida, S Uruguay
185 A22 **Caswell Sound** sound South Island, NZ
137 Q13 **Çat** Erzurum, NE Turkey
42 K6 **Catacamas** Olancho, C Honduras
56 A10 **Catacaos** Piura, NW Peru
22 I7 **Catahoula Lake** ◎ Louisiana, S USA
137 S15 **Çatak** Van, SE Turkey
137 S15 **Çatak Çayi** ≈ SE Turkey
114 O12 **Çatalca** İstanbul, NW Turkey
114 O12 **Çatalca Yarımadası** physical region NW Turkey
62 H6 **Catalina** Antofagasta, N Chile
Catalonia see Cataluña
105 U5 **Cataluña** Cat. Catalunya; Eng. Catalonia. ◆ autonomous community N Spain
Catalunya see Cataluña
62 I7 **Catamarca** off. Provincia de Catamarca. ◆ province NW Argentina
Catamarca see San Fernando del Valle de Catamarca
83 M16 **Catandica** Manica, C Mozambique
171 P4 **Catanduanes Island** island N Philippines
60 K8 **Catanduva** São Paulo, S Brazil
107 L24 **Catania** Sicilia, Italy, C Mediterranean Sea
107 M24 **Catania, Golfo di** gulf Sicilia, Italy, C Mediterranean Sea
45 U5 **Cataño** var. Cantaño. E Puerto Rico
107 O21 **Catanzaro** Calabria, SW Italy
107 O22 **Catanzaro Marina** var. Marina di Catanzaro. Calabria, S Italy
25 Q14 **Catarina** Texas, SW USA
171 Q5 **Catarman** Samar, C Philippines
105 S10 **Catarroja** País Valenciano, E Spain
21 R11 **Catawba River** ≈ North Carolina/South Carolina, SE USA
171 Q5 **Catbalogan** Samar, C Philippines
14 I14 **Catchacoma** Ontario, SE Canada
41 S15 **Catemaco** Veracruz-Llave, SE Mexico
Cathair na Mart see Westport
Cathair Saidhbhín see Cahersiveen
31 P5 **Cat Head Point** headland Michigan, N USA
23 Q2 **Cathedral Caverns** cave Alabama, S USA
35 V16 **Cathedral City** California, W USA
24 K10 **Cathedral Mountain** ▲ Texas, SW USA
32 G10 **Cathlamet** Washington, NW USA
76 G13 **Catió** S Guinea-Bissau
55 O10 **Catisimiña** Bolívar, SE Venezuela
44 J3 **Cat Island** island C Bahamas
12 B9 **Cat Lake** Ontario, S Canada
21 P5 **Catlettsburg** Kentucky, S USA
185 D24 **Catlins** ≈ South Island, NZ
35 R1 **Catnip Mountain** ▲ Nevada, W USA
41 Z11 **Catoche, Cabo** headland SE Mexico
27 P9 **Catoosa** Oklahoma, C USA
41 N10 **Catorce** San Luis Potosí, C Mexico
63 I14 **Catriel** Río Negro, C Argentina
62 K13 **Catriló** La Pampa, C Argentina
58 F11 **Catrimani** Roraima, N Brazil
58 E10 **Catrimani, Rio** ≈ N Brazil
18 K11 **Catskill** New York, NE USA
18 K11 **Catskill Creek** ≈ New York, NE USA
18 J11 **Catskill Mountains** ▲ New York, NE USA
18 D11 **Cattaraugus Creek** ≈ New York, NE USA
Cattaro see Kotor
Cattaro, Bocche di see Kotorska, Boka
107 I24 **Cattolica Eraclea** Sicilia, Italy, C Mediterranean Sea
83 B14 **Catumbela** ≈ W Angola
83 N14 **Catur** Niassa, N Mozambique
82 C10 **Cauale** ≈ NE Angola
171 O2 **Cauayan** Luzon, N Philippines
54 C12 **Cauca** off. Departamento del Cauca. ◆ province SW Colombia
47 P5 **Cauca** ≈ SE Venezuela
58 P13 **Caucaia** Ceará, E Brazil
54 E7 **Cauca, Río** ≈ N Colombia
54 E7 **Caucasia** Antioquia, NW Colombia
137 Q8 **Caucasus** Rus. Kavkaz. ▲ Georgia/Russian Federation
62 I10 **Caucete** San Juan, W Argentina
105 R11 **Caudete** Castilla-La Mancha, C Spain
103 P2 **Caudry** Nord, N France
82 D11 **Caungula** Lunda Norte, NE Angola
62 G13 **Cauquenes** Maule, C Chile
55 N8 **Caura, Río** ≈ C Venezuela
15 V7 **Causapscal** Quebec, SE Canada
117 N10 **Căuşeni** Rus. Kaushany. E Moldova
102 M14 **Caussade** Tarn-et-Garonne, S France
102 K17 **Cauterets** Hautes-Pyrénées, S France
8 J15 **Caution, Cape** headland British Columbia, SW Canada
44 H7 **Cauto** ≈ E Cuba
Cauvery see Kāveri
102 L3 **Caux, Pays de** physical region N France
107 L18 **Cava dei Tirreni** Campania, S Italy
104 G6 **Cávado** ≈ N Portugal
Cavaia see Kavajë
103 R15 **Cavaillon** Vaucluse, SE France
103 U16 **Cavalaire-sur-Mer** Var, SE France
106 G6 **Cavalese** Ger. Gablös. Trentino-Alto Adige, N Italy
29 Q2 **Cavalier** North Dakota, N USA
76 L17 **Cavalla** var. Cavally, Cavally Fleuve. ≈ Ivory Coast/Liberia
105 Y8 **Cavalleria, Cap de** var. Cabo Caballeria. headland Menorca, Spain, W Mediterranean Sea
184 K2 **Cavalli Islands** island group N NZ
Cavally/Cavally Fleuve see Cavalla
97 E16 **Cavan** Ir. Cabhán. N Ireland
97 E16 **Cavan** Ir. An Cabhán. cultural region N Ireland
106 H8 **Cavarzere** Veneto, NE Italy
27 W9 **Cave City** Arkansas, C USA
20 K7 **Cave City** Kentucky, S USA
65 M25 **Cave Point** headland S Tristan da Cunha
21 N5 **Cave Run Lake** ▣ Kentucky, S USA
58 K11 **Caviana de Fora, Ilha** var. Ilha Caviana. island N Brazil
Caviana, Ilha see Caviana de Fora, Ilha
113 I16 **Cavtat** It. Ragusavecchia. Dubrovnik-Neretva, SE Croatia
Cawnpore see Kānpur
Caxamarca see Cajamarca
58 A13 **Caxias** Amazonas, W Brazil
58 N13 **Caxias** Maranhão, E Brazil
61 I15 **Caxias do Sul** Rio Grande do Sul, S Brazil
42 J4 **Caxinas, Punta** headland N Honduras
82 B11 **Caxito** Bengo, NW Angola
136 F14 **Çay** Afyon, W Turkey
40 L15 **Cayacal, Punta** var. Punta Mongrove. headland S Mexico
56 C6 **Cayambe** Pichincha, N Ecuador
56 C6 **Cayambe** ▲ N Ecuador
21 R12 **Cayce** South Carolina, SE USA
55 Y10 **Cayenne** ○ (French Guiana) NE French Guiana
55 Y10 **Cayenne** × NE French Guiana
44 K10 **Cayes** var. Les Cayes. SW Haiti
45 U6 **Cayey** C Puerto Rico
45 U6 **Cayey, Sierra de** ▲ E Puerto Rico
103 N14 **Caylus** Tarn-et-Garonne, S France
44 E8 **Cayman Brac** island E Cayman Islands
44 D8 **Cayman Islands** ◇ UK dependent territory W West Indies
64 D11 **Cayman Trench** undersea feature NW Caribbean Sea
47 O3 **Cayman Trough** undersea feature NW Caribbean Sea
80 O13 **Caynabo** Togdheer, N Somalia
42 F3 **Cayo** ◆ district SW Belize
Cayo see San Ignacio
43 N9 **Cayos Guerrero** reef E Nicaragua
43 O9 **Cayos King** reef E Nicaragua
44 E4 **Cay Sal** islet SW Bahamas
14 G16 **Cayuga** Ontario, S Canada
25 V8 **Cayuga** Texas, SW USA
18 G10 **Cayuga Lake** ◎ New York, NE USA
104 K13 **Cazalla de la Sierra** Andalucía, S Spain
116 L14 **Căzănești** Ialomița, SE Romania
102 M16 **Cazères** Haute-Garonne, S France
112 E10 **Cazin** Federacija Bosna I Hercegovina, NW Bosnia and Herzegovina
82 G13 **Cazombo** Moxico, E Angola
105 O13 **Cazorla** Andalucía, S Spain
Cazza see Sušac
104 L4 **Cea** ≈ NW Spain
Ceadâr-Lunga see Ciadîr-Lunga
Ceanannas see Kells
Ceann Toirc see Kanturk
58 O13 **Ceará** off. Estado do Ceará. ◆ state C Brazil
Ceará see Fortaleza
Ceara Abyssal Plain see Ceará Plain
59 Q14 **Ceará Mirim** Rio Grande do Norte, E Brazil
64 J13 **Ceará Plain** var. Ceara Abyssal Plain. undersea feature W Atlantic Ocean
64 I13 **Ceará Ridge** undersea feature C Atlantic Ocean
Ceatharlach see Carlow
43 Q17 **Cébaco, Isla** island SW Panama
40 K7 **Ceballos** Durango, C Mexico
61 G19 **Cebollatí** Rocha, E Uruguay
61 G19 **Cebollatí, Río** ≈ E Uruguay
105 P5 **Cebollera** ▲ N Spain
104 M8 **Cebreros** Castilla-León, N Spain
171 P6 **Cebu** off. Cebu City. Cebu, C Philippines
171 P6 **Cebu** island C Philippines
107 J16 **Ceccano** Lazio, C Italy
Čechy see Bohemia
106 F12 **Cecina** Toscana, C Italy
26 K4 **Cedar Bluff Reservoir** ▣ Kansas, C USA
30 M8 **Cedarburg** Wisconsin, N USA
36 J7 **Cedar City** Utah, W USA
25 T11 **Cedar Creek** Texas, SW USA
28 L7 **Cedar Creek** ≈ North Dakota, N USA
25 U7 **Cedar Creek Reservoir** ▣ Texas, SW USA
29 W13 **Cedar Falls** Iowa, C USA
31 N8 **Cedar Grove** Wisconsin, N USA
21 Y6 **Cedar Island** island Virginia, NE USA
23 U11 **Cedar Key** Cedar Keys, Florida, SE USA
23 U11 **Cedar Keys** island group Florida, SE USA
11 V14 **Cedar Lake** ◎ Manitoba, C Canada
14 I11 **Cedar Lake** ◎ Ontario, SE Canada
24 M6 **Cedar Lake** ◎ Texas, SW USA
29 X13 **Cedar Rapids** Iowa, C USA
29 X14 **Cedar River** ≈ Iowa/Minnesota, C USA
29 O14 **Cedar River** ≈ Nebraska, C USA
31 P8 **Cedar Springs** Michigan, N USA
23 R3 **Cedartown** Georgia, SE USA
27 O7 **Cedar Vale** Kansas, C USA
35 Q2 **Cedarville** California, W USA
104 H1 **Cedeira** Galicia, NW Spain
42 H8 **Cedeño** Choluteca, S Honduras
41 N10 **Cedral** San Luis Potosí, C Mexico
42 I6 **Cedros** Francisco Morazán, C Honduras
40 M9 **Cedros** Zacatecas, C Mexico
40 B5 **Cedros, Isla** island W Mexico
193 R5 **Cedros Trench** undersea feature E Pacific Ocean
182 E7 **Ceduna** South Australia
110 D10 **Cedynia** Ger. Zehden. Zachodniopomorskie, W Poland
80 P12 **Ceelaayo** Sanaag, N Somalia
81 O16 **Ceel Buur** It. El Bur; Galguduud, C Somalia
81 N15 **Ceel Dheere** var. Ceel Dher, It. El Dere. Galguduud, C Somalia
Ceel Dher see Ceel Dheere
81 P14 **Ceel Xamure** Mudug, E Somalia
80 O12 **Ceerigaabo** var. Erigabo, Erigavo. Sanaag, N Somalia
107 J23 **Cefalu** anc. Cephaloedium. Sicilia, Italy, C Mediterranean Sea
105 N6 **Cega** ≈ N Spain
111 K23 **Cegléd** prev. Czegléd. Pest, C Hungary
113 N18 **Čegrane** W FYR Macedonia
105 Q13 **Cehegín** Murcia, SE Spain
136 K12 **Çekerek** Yozgat, N Turkey
107 J15 **Celano** Abruzzo, C Italy
104 H4 **Celanova** Galicia, NW Spain
42 F6 **Celaque, Cordillera de** ▲ W Honduras
41 N13 **Celaya** Guanajuato, C Mexico
Celebes see Sulawesi
192 F7 **Celebes Basin** undersea feature SE South China Sea
192 F7 **Celebes Sea** Ind. Laut Sulawesi. sea Indonesia/Philippines
41 W12 **Celestún** Yucatán, E Mexico
31 Q12 **Celina** Ohio, N USA
20 L8 **Celina** Tennessee, S USA
25 U5 **Celina** Texas, SW USA
112 G11 **Čelinac Donji** Republika Srpska, N Bosnia and Herzegovina
109 V10 **Celje** Ger. Cilli. C Slovenia
111 G23 **Celldömölk** Vas, W Hungary
100 J12 **Celle** var. Zelle. Niedersachsen, N Germany
99 D19 **Celles** Hainaut, SW Belgium
104 I7 **Celorico da Beira** Guarda, N Portugal
Celovec see Klagenfurt
64 M7 **Celtic Sea** Ir. An Mhuir Cheilteach. sea SW British Isles
64 N7 **Celtic Shelf** undersea feature E Atlantic Ocean
114 L13 **Çeltik Gölu** ◎ NW Turkey
113 M14 **Čemerno** ▲ C Yugoslavia
105 Q12 **Cenajo, Embalse del** ▣ S Spain
171 V13 **Cenderawasih, Teluk** var. Teluk Irian, Teluk Sarera. bay W Pacific Ocean
105 P4 **Cenicero** La Rioja, N Spain
106 E9 **Ceno** ≈ NW Italy
102 K13 **Cenon** Gironde, SW France
14 K13 **Centennial Lake** ◎ Ontario, SE Canada
Centennial State see Colorado
37 S7 **Center** Colorado, C USA
29 Q13 **Center** Nebraska, C USA
28 M5 **Center** North Dakota, N USA
25 X8 **Center** Texas, SW USA
29 W8 **Center City** Minnesota, N USA
36 L5 **Centerfield** Utah, W USA
20 K9 **Center Hill Lake** ▣ Tennessee, S USA
29 X13 **Center Point** Iowa, C USA
25 R11 **Center Point** Texas, SW USA
29 W16 **Centerville** Iowa, C USA
27 W7 **Centerville** Missouri, C USA
29 R12 **Centerville** South Dakota, N USA
20 I9 **Centerville** Tennessee, S USA
25 V9 **Centerville** Texas, SW USA
40 M5 **Centinela, Picacho del** ▲ NE Mexico
106 G9 **Cento** Emilia-Romagna, N Italy
Centrafricaine, République see Central African Republic
39 S8 **Central** Alaska, USA
37 P15 **Central** New Mexico, SW USA
83 H18 **Central** ◆ district E Botswana
138 E10 **Central** ◆ district C Israel
81 I19 **Central** ◆ province C Kenya
82 M13 **Central** ◆ region C Malawi
153 P12 **Central** ◆ zone C Nepal
186 E9 **Central** ◆ province S PNG
63 I21 **Central** ◆ department C Paraguay
186 M9 **Central** off. Central Province. ◆ province S Solomon Islands
83 J14 **Central** ◆ province C Zambia
117 P11 **Central** × (Odesa) Odes'ka Oblast', SW Ukraine
Central see Centre
79 H14 **Central African Republic** var. République Centrafricaine, abbrev. CAR; prev. Ubangi-Shari, Oubangui-Chari, Territoire de l'Oubangui-Chari. ◆ republic C Africa
192 G6 **Central Basin Trough** undersea feature W Pacific Ocean
Central Borneo see Kalimantan Tengah
149 P12 **Central Brāhui Range** ▲ W Pakistan
Central Celebes see Sulawesi Tengah
29 Y13 **Central City** Iowa, C USA
20 I6 **Central City** Kentucky, S USA
29 P15 **Central City** Nebraska, C USA
48 D6 **Central, Cordillera** ▲ W Bolivia
54 D11 **Central, Cordillera** ▲ W Colombia
42 M13 **Central, Cordillera** ▲ C Costa Rica
45 N9 **Central, Cordillera** ▲ C Dominican Republic
43 R16 **Central, Cordillera** ▲ C Panama
45 S6 **Central, Cordillera** ▲ Puerto Rico
42 H7 **Central District** var. Tegucigalpa. ◆ district C Honduras
30 L15 **Centralia** Illinois, N USA
27 U4 **Centralia** Missouri, C USA
32 G9 **Centralia** Washington, NW USA
Central Indian Ridge see Mid-Indian Ridge
Central Java see Jawa Tengah
Central Kalimantan see Kalimantan Tengah
148 L14 **Central Makrān Range** ▲ W Pakistan
192 K7 **Central Pacific Basin** undersea feature C Pacific Ocean
59 M19 **Central, Planalto** var. Brazilian Highlands. ▲ E Brazil
32 F15 **Central Point** Oregon, NW USA
155 K25 **Central Province** ◆ province C Sri Lanka
Central Provinces and Berar see Madhya Pradesh
186 B6 **Central Range** ▲ NW PNG
Central Russian Upland see Srednerusskaya Vozvyshennost'
Central Siberian Plateau/Central Siberian Uplands see Srednesibirskoye Ploskogor'ye
104 K8 **Central, Sistema** ▲ C Spain
Central Sulawesi see Sulawesi Tengah
35 N3 **Central Valley** California, W USA
35 P8 **Central Valley** valley California, W USA
23 Q3 **Centre** Alabama, S USA
79 E15 **Centre** Eng. Central. ◆ province C Cameroon
102 M8 **Centre** ◆ region N France
173 Y16 **Centre de Flacq** E Mauritius
55 Y9 **Centre Spatial Guyanais** space station N French Guiana
23 O5 **Centreville** Alabama, S USA
21 X3 **Centreville** Maryland, NE USA
22 J7 **Centreville** Mississippi, S USA
Centum Cellae see Civitavecchia
160 M14 **Cenxi** Guangxi Zhuangzu Zizhiqu, S China
Ceos see Kéa
Cephaloedium see Cefalu
112 I9 **Čepin** Hung. Csepén. Osijek-Baranja, E Croatia
Ceram see Seram, Pulau
171 R13 **Ceram Sea** Ind. Laut Seram. sea E Indonesia
192 G8 **Ceram Trough** undersea feature W Pacific Ocean
Cerasus see Giresun
36 I10 **Cerbat Mountains** ▲ Arizona, SW USA
103 P17 **Cerbère, Cap** headland S France
104 F13 **Cercal do Alentejo** Setúbal, S Portugal
111 A18 **Čerchov** Ger. Czerkow. ▲ W Czech Republic
103 O13 **Cère** ≈ C France
61 A16 **Ceres** Santa Fe, C Argentina
59 K18 **Ceres** Goiás, C Brazil
Ceresio see Lugano, Lago di
103 O17 **Céret** Pyrénées-Orientales, S France
54 E6 **Cereté** Córdoba, NW Colombia
172 I17 **Cerf, Île au** island Inner Islands, NE Seychelles
99 G22 **Cerfontaine** Namur, S Belgium
Cergy-Pontoise see Pontoise
107 N16 **Cerignola** Puglia, SE Italy
Cerigo see Kýthira
103 O9 **Cérilly** Allier, C France
136 I11 **Çerkeş** Çankırı, N Turkey
136 D10 **Çerkezköy** Tekirdağ, NW Turkey
109 T12 **Cerknica** Ger. Zirknitz. SW Slovenia
109 S11 **Cerkno** W Slovenia
116 F10 **Cermei** Hung. Csermő. Arad, W Romania
137 O15 **Çermik** Dıyarbakır, SE Turkey
112 I10 **Cerna** Vukovar-Srijem, E Croatia
Cernăuți see Chernivtsi
116 M14 **Cernavodă** Constanța, SW Romania
103 U7 **Cernay** Haut-Rhin, NE France
Černice see Schwarzach
41 O8 **Cerralvo** Nuevo León, NE Mexico
40 G9 **Cerralvo, Isla** island W Mexico
107 L16 **Cerreto Sannita** Campania, S Italy
113 L20 **Cërrik** var. Cerriku. Elbasan, C Albania
Cerriku see Cërrik
41 O11 **Cerritos** San Luis Potosí, C Mexico
60 K11 **Cerro Azul** Paraná, S Brazil
61 F18 **Cerro Chato** Treinta y Tres, E Uruguay
61 F19 **Cerro Colorado** Florida, S Uruguay
56 E13 **Cerro de Pasco** Pasco, C Peru
61 G18 **Cerro Largo** ◆ department NE Uruguay
61 G14 **Cêrro Largo** Rio Grande do Sul, S Brazil
42 E7 **Cerrón Grande, Embalse** ▣ N El Salvador
63 I14 **Cerros Colorados, Embalse** ◎ W Argentina
105 V5 **Cervera** Cataluña, NE Spain
104 M3 **Cervera del Pisuerga** Castilla-León, N Spain
105 Q5 **Cervera del Río Alhama** La Rioja, N Spain
107 H15 **Cerveteri** Lazio, C Italy
106 H10 **Cervia** Emilia-Romagna, N Italy
106 J7 **Cervignano del Friuli** Friuli-Venezia Giulia, NE Italy
107 L17 **Cervinara** Campania, S Italy
Cervinia see Breuil-Cervinia
106 B6 **Cervino, Monte** var. Matterhorn. ▲ Italy/Switzerland see also Matterhorn

◆ Country ● Country Capital ◇ Dependent Territory ○ Dependent Territory Capital ◆ Administrative Region × International Airport ▲ Mountain ▲ Mountain Range Volcano ≈ River ◎ Lake ▣ Reservoir

103 Y14 **Cervione** Corse, France, C Mediterranean Sea
104 I1 **Cervo** Galicia, NW Spain
54 F5 **Cesar** *off.* Departamento del Cesar. ◆ *province* N Colombia
106 H10 **Cesena** *anc.* Caesena. Emilia-Romagna, N Italy
106 I10 **Cesenatico** Emilia-Romagna, N Italy
118 H8 **Cēsis** *Ger.* Wenden. Cēsis, C Latvia
111 D15 **Česká Lípa** *Ger.* Böhmisch-Leipa. Liberecký Kraj, N Czech Republic
Česká Republika *see* Czech Republic
111 F17 **Česká Třebová** *Ger.* Böhmisch-Trübau. Pardubický Kraj, C Czech Republic
111 D19 **České Budějovice** *Ger.* Budweis. Budějovický Kraj, S Czech Republic
111 D19 **České Velenice** Budějovický Kraj, S Czech Republic
111 E18 **Českomoravská Vrchovina** *var.* Českomoravská Vysočina, *Eng.* Bohemian-Moravian Highlands, *Ger.* Böhmisch-Mährische Höhe. ▲ S Czech Republic
Českomoravská Vysočina *see* Českomoravská Vrchovina
111 C19 **Český Krumlov** *var.* Böhmisch-Krumau, *Ger.* Krummau. Budějovický Kraj, S Czech Republic
Ceský Les *see* Bohemian Forest
112 F8 **Česma** ≈ N Croatia
136 A14 **Çeşme** İzmir, W Turkey
Cess *see* Cestos
183 T8 **Cessnock** New South Wales, SE Australia
76 K17 **Cestos** *var.* Cess. ≈ S Liberia
118 I9 **Cesvaine** Madona, E Latvia
116 G14 **Cetate** Dolj, SW Romania
Cetatea Albă *see* Bilhorod-Dnistrovs'kyy
113 J17 **Cetinje** *It.* Cettigne. Montenegro, SW Yugoslavia
107 N20 **Cetraro** Calabria, S Italy
Cette *see* Sète
188 A17 **Cetti Bay** *bay* SW Guam
Cettigne *see* Cetinje
104 L17 **Ceuta** *var.* Sebta. Ceuta, Spain, N Africa
88 C15 **Ceuta** *enclave* Spain, N Africa
106 B9 **Ceva** Piemonte, NE Italy
103 P14 **Cévennes** ▲ S France
108 G10 **Cevio** Ticino, S Switzerland
136 K16 **Ceyhan** Adana, S Turkey
136 K17 **Ceyhan Nehri** ≈ S Turkey
137 P17 **Ceylanpınar** Şanlıurfa, SE Turkey
Ceylon *see* Sri Lanka
173 R6 **Ceylon Plain** *undersea feature* N Indian Ocean
Ceyre to the Caribs *see* Marie-Galante
103 Q14 **Cèze** ≈ S France
146 H15 **Chaacha** *Turkm.* Chäche. Akhalskiy Velayat, S Turkmenistan
129 P6 **Chaadayevka** Penzenskaya Oblast', W Russian Federation
167 O12 **Cha-Am** Phetchaburi, SW Thailand
143 W15 **Chābahār** *var.* Chāh Bahār, Chahbar. Sīstān va Balūchestān, SE Iran
61 B19 **Chabas** Santa Fe, C Argentina
103 T10 **Chablais** *physical region* E France
61 B20 **Chacabuco** Buenos Aires, E Argentina
42 K8 **Chachagón, Cerro** ▲ N Nicaragua
56 C10 **Chachapoyas** Amazonas, NW Peru
Chäche *see* Chaacha
119 O18 **Chachersk** *Rus.* Chechersk. Homyel'skaya Voblasts', SE Belarus
119 N16 **Chachevichy** *Rus.* Chechevichi. Mahilyowskaya Voblasts', E Belarus
61 B14 **Chaco** *off.* Provincia de Chaco. ◆ *province* NE Argentina
Chaco *see* Gran Chaco
62 M6 **Chaco Austral** *physical region* N Argentina
62 M3 **Chaco Boreal** *physical region* N Paraguay
62 M6 **Chaco Central** *physical region* N Argentina
39 Y15 **Chacon, Cape** *headland* Prince of Wales Island, Alaska, USA
78 H9 **Chad** *off.* Republic of Chad, *Fr.* Tchad. ◆ *republic* C Africa
122 K14 **Chadan** Respublika Tyva, S Russian Federation
21 U12 **Chadbourn** North Carolina, SE USA
83 L14 **Chadiza** Eastern, E Zambia
67 Q7 **Chad, Lake** *Fr.* Lac Tchad. ◎ C Africa
28 J12 **Chadron** Nebraska, C USA
Chadyr-Lunga *see* Ciadîr-Lunga
163 W14 **Chaeryŏng** SW North Korea
105 P17 **Chafarinas, Islas** *island group* S Spain
27 Y7 **Chaffee** Missouri, C USA
148 L12 **Chāgai Hills** *var.* Chāh Gay. ▲ Afghanistan/Pakistan
123 Q11 **Chagda** Respublika Sakha (Yakutiya), NE Russian Federation
Chaghasarāy *see* Asadābād
149 N5 **Chaghcharān** *var.* Chakhcharan, Cheghcheran, Qala Āhangarān. Ghowr, C Afghanistan
103 R9 **Chagny** Saône-et-Loire, C France
173 Q7 **Chagos Archipelago** *var.* Oil Islands. *island group* British Indian Ocean Territory
131 O15 **Chagos Bank** *undersea feature* C Indian Ocean
131 O14 **Chagos-Laccadive Plateau** *undersea feature* N Indian Ocean
173 Q7 **Chagos Trench** *undersea feature* N Indian Ocean
43 T14 **Chagres, Río** ≈ C Panama
45 U14 **Chaguanas** Trinidad, Trinidad and Tobago
54 M6 **Chaguaramas** Guárico, N Venezuela
146 C9 **Chagyl** Balkanskiy Velayat, NW Turkmenistan
Chahārmahāl and Bakhtiyāri *see* Chahār Maḩall va Bakhtiārī
142 M9 **Chahār Maḩall va Bakhtiārī** *off.* Ostān-e Chahār Maḩall va Bakhtiārī, *var.* Chahārmahāl and Bakhtiyāri. ◆ *province* SW Iran
Chāh Bahār/Chahbar *see* Chābahār
143 V13 **Chāh Derāz** Sīstān va Balūchestān, SE Iran
Chāh Gay *see* Chāgai Hills
167 P10 **Chai Badan** Lop Buri, C Thailand
153 Q16 **Chāībāsa** Bihār, N India
79 E19 **Chaillu, Massif du** ▲ C Gabon
167 O10 **Chai Nat** *var.* Chainat, Jainat, Jayanath. Chai Nat, C Thailand
65 M14 **Chain Fracture Zone** *tectonic feature* E Atlantic Ocean
173 N5 **Chain Ridge** *undersea feature* W Indian Ocean
Chairn, Ceann an *see* Carnsore Point
158 L5 **Chaiwopu** Xinjiang Uygur Zizhiqu, W China
167 Q10 **Chaiyaphum** *var.* Jayabum. Chaiyaphum, C Thailand
62 N10 **Chajarí** Entre Ríos, E Argentina
42 C5 **Chajul** Quiché, W Guatemala
83 K16 **Chakari** Mashonaland West, N Zimbabwe
148 J9 **Chakhānsūr** Nīmrūz, SW Afghanistan
Chakhānsūr *see* Nīmrūz
Chakhcharan *see* Chaghcharān
149 V8 **Chak Jhumra** *var.* Jhumra. Punjab, E Pakistan
146 I16 **Chaknakdysonga** Akhalskiy Velayat, S Turkmenistan
153 P16 **Chakradharpur** Bihār, N India
152 J8 **Chakrāta** Uttar Pradesh, N India
149 U7 **Chakwāl** Punjab, NE Pakistan
57 F17 **Chala** Arequipa, SW Peru
102 K12 **Chalais** Charente, W France
108 D10 **Chalais** Valais, SW Switzerland
115 J20 **Chalándri** *var.* Halandri; *prev.* Khalándrion. *prehistoric site* Sýros, Kykládes, Greece, Aegean Sea
188 H6 **Chalan Kanoa** Saipan, S Northern Mariana Islands
188 C16 **Chalan Pago** C Guam
Chalap Dalam/Chalap Dalan *see* Chehel Abdālān, Kūh-e
42 F7 **Chalatenango** Chalatenango, N El Salvador
42 A9 **Chalatenango** ◆ *department* NW El Salvador
83 P15 **Chalaua** Nampula, NE Mozambique
81 I16 **Chalbi Desert** *desert* N Kenya
42 D7 **Chalchuapa** Santa Ana, W El Salvador
Chalcidice *see* Chalkidikí
Chalcis *see* Chalkída
103 N6 **Châlette-sur-Loing** Loiret, C France
15 X8 **Chaleur Bay** *Fr.* Baie des Chaleurs. *bay* New Brunswick/Quebec, E Canada
Chaleurs, Baie des *see* Chaleur Bay
57 G16 **Chalhuanca** Apurímac, S Peru
154 F12 **Chālisgaon** Mahārāshtra, C India
115 N23 **Chálki** *island* Dodekánisos, Greece, Aegean Sea
115 F16 **Chalkiádes** Thessalía, C Greece
115 H18 **Chalkída** *var.* Halkida; *prev.* Khalkís, *anc.* Chalcis. Evvoia, E Greece
115 G14 **Chalkidikí** *var.* Khalkidhikí; *anc.* Chalcidice. *peninsula* NE Greece
185 A24 **Chalky Inlet** *inlet* South Island, NZ
39 S7 **Chalkyitsik** Alaska, USA
102 I9 **Challans** Vendée, NW France
57 K19 **Challapata** Oruro, SW Bolivia
192 H6 **Challenger Deep** *undersea feature* W Pacific Ocean
193 S11 **Challenger Fracture Zone** *tectonic feature* SE Pacific Ocean
192 K11 **Challenger Plateau** *undersea feature* E Tasman Sea
33 P13 **Challis** Idaho, NW USA
22 L9 **Chalmette** Louisiana, S USA
126 J11 **Chalna** Respublika Kareliya, NW Russian Federation
103 Q5 **Châlons-en-Champagne** *prev.* Châlons-sur-Marne, *hist.* Arcae Remorum, *anc.* Carolopois. Marne, NE France
Châlons-sur-Marne *see* Châlons-en-Champagne
103 R9 **Chalon-sur-Saône** *anc.* Cabillonum. Saône-et-Loire, C France
Chaltel, Cerro *see* Fitzroy, Monte
143 N4 **Chālūs** Māzandarān, N Iran
102 M11 **Châlus** Haute-Vienne, C France
101 N20 **Cham** Bayern, SE Germany
108 F7 **Cham** Zug, N Switzerland
37 R8 **Chama** New Mexico, SW USA
Cha Mai *see* Thung Song
83 E22 **Chamaites** Karas, S Namibia
149 O9 **Chaman** Baluchistān, SW Pakistan
37 R9 **Chama, Rio** ≈ New Mexico, SW USA
152 I6 **Chamba** Himāchal Pradesh, N India
81 I25 **Chamba** Ruvuma, S Tanzania
150 H12 **Chambal** ≈ C India
11 U16 **Chamberlain** Saskatchewan, S Canada
29 O11 **Chamberlain** South Dakota, N USA
19 R3 **Chamberlain Lake** ◎ Maine, NE USA
39 S5 **Chamberlin, Mount** ▲ Alaska, USA
37 O11 **Chambers** Arizona, SW USA
18 F16 **Chambersburg** Pennsylvania, NE USA
31 N5 **Chambers Island** *island* Wisconsin, N USA
103 T11 **Chambéry** *anc.* Camberia. Savoie, E France
82 L12 **Chambeshi** Northern, NE Zambia
82 L12 **Chambeshi** ≈ NE Zambia
74 M6 **Chambi, Jebel** *var.* Jabal ash Sha'nabī. ▲ W Tunisia
15 Q7 **Chambord** Quebec, SE Canada
139 U11 **Chamcham** S Iraq
139 T4 **Chamchamāl** N Iraq
40 J14 **Chamela** Jalisco, SW Mexico
42 G5 **Chamelecón, Río** ≈ NW Honduras
62 J9 **Chamical** La Rioja, C Argentina
115 L23 **Chamilí** *island* Kykládes, Greece, Aegean Sea
167 Q13 **Châmnar** Kaôh Kông, SW Cambodia
152 K9 **Chamoli** Uttar Pradesh, N India
103 U11 **Chamonix-Mont-Blanc** Haute-Savoie, E France
154 L11 **Chāmpa** Madhya Pradesh, C India
8 H8 **Champagne** Yukon Territory, W Canada
103 Q5 **Champagne** *cultural region* N France
Champagne *see* Campania
103 Q5 **Champagne-Ardenne** ◆ *region* N France
103 S9 **Champagnole** Jura, E France
30 M13 **Champaign** Illinois, N USA
167 S10 **Champasak** Champasak, S Laos
103 U6 **Champ de Feu** ▲ NE France
13 O7 **Champdoré, Lac** ◎ Quebec, NE Canada
42 B6 **Champerico** Retalhuleu, SW Guatemala
108 C11 **Champéry** Valais, SW Switzerland
18 L6 **Champlain** New York, NE USA
18 L9 **Champlain Canal** *canal* New York, NE USA
15 P13 **Champlain, Lac** ◎ Quebec, SE Canada
18 L7 **Champlain, Lake** ◎ Canada/USA
103 S7 **Champlitte** Haute-Saône, E France
41 W13 **Champotón** Campeche, SE Mexico
104 G10 **Chamusca** Santarém, C Portugal
119 O20 **Chamyarysy** *Rus.* Chemerisy. Homyel'skaya Voblasts', SE Belarus
129 P5 **Chamzinka** Respublika Mordoviya, W Russian Federation
Chanáil Mhór, An *see* Grand Canal
Chanak *see* Çanakkale
64 G7 **Chañaral** Atacama, N Chile
104 H13 **Chança, Rio** *var.* Chanza. ≈ Portugal/Spain
57 D14 **Chancay** Lima, W Peru
Chan-chiang/Chanchiang *see* Zhanjiang
64 G13 **Chanco** Maule, Chile
39 R7 **Chandalar** Alaska, USA
39 R6 **Chandalar River** ≈ Alaska, USA
152 L10 **Chandan Chauki** Uttar Pradesh, N India
153 S16 **Chandannagar** *prev.* Chandernagore. West Bengal, E India
152 K10 **Chandausi** Uttar Pradesh, N India
22 M10 **Chandeleur Islands** *island group* Louisiana, S USA
22 M9 **Chandeleur Sound** *sound* N Gulf of Mexico
152 I8 **Chandīgarh** Punjab, N India
153 Q16 **Chāndil** Bihār, NE India
182 D2 **Chandler** South Australia
15 Y7 **Chandler** Quebec, SE Canada
36 L14 **Chandler** Arizona, SW USA
27 O10 **Chandler** Oklahoma, C USA
25 V7 **Chandler** Texas, SW USA
39 Q6 **Chandler River** ≈ Alaska, USA
56 H13 **Chandles, Río** ≈ E Peru
163 N9 **Chandmanī** Dornogovĭ, SE Mongolia
14 J13 **Chandos Lake** ◎ Ontario, SE Canada
153 U15 **Chandpur** Chittagong, C Bangladesh
154 I13 **Chandrapur** Mahārāshtra, C India
83 J15 **Changa** Southern, S Zambia
Changan *see* Xi'an, Shaanxi, China
Chang'an *see* Rong'an, Guangxi Zhuangzu Zizhiqu, China
155 G23 **Changanācheri** Kerala, SW India
83 M19 **Changane** ≈ S Mozambique
83 M16 **Changara** Tete, NW Mozambique
163 X11 **Changbai** *var.* Changbai Chaoxianzu Zizhixian. Jilin, NE China
Changbai Chaoxianzu Zizhixian *see* Changbai
163 X11 **Changbai Shan** ▲ NE China
163 V10 **Changchun** *var.* Ch'angch'un, Ch'ang-ch'un; *prev.* Hsinking. Jilin, NE China
160 M10 **Changde** Hunan, S China
161 S13 **Changhua** *Jap.* Shōka. C Taiwan
168 L10 **Changi** × (Singapore) E Singapore
158 L5 **Changji** Xinjiang Uygur Zizhiqu, NW China
157 O13 **Chang Jiang** *var.* Yangtze Kiang, *Eng.* Yangtze. ≈ C China
160 L17 **Changjiang** *prev.* Shiliu. Hainan, S China
161 S8 **Changjiang Kou** *delta* E China
167 P12 **Chang, Ko** *island* S Thailand
161 Q2 **Changli** Hebei, E China
163 V10 **Changling** Jilin, NE China
161 N11 **Changsha** *var.* Ch'angsha, Ch'ang-sha. Hunan, S China
161 Q10 **Changshan** Zhejiang, SE China
163 V14 **Changshan Qundao** *island group* NE China
161 S8 **Changshu** *var.* Ch'ang-shu. Jiangsu, E China
163 V11 **Changtu** Liaoning, NE China
43 P14 **Changuinola** Bocas del Toro, NW Panama
159 N9 **Changweiliang** Qinghai, W China
160 K6 **Changwu** Shaanxi, C China
163 U13 **Changxing Dao** *island* N China
160 M9 **Changyang** Hubei, C China
163 W14 **Changyŏn** SW North Korea
161 N5 **Changzhi** Shanxi, C China
161 R8 **Changzhou** Jiangsu, E China
115 H24 **Chaniá** *var.* Hania, Khaniá, *Eng.* Canea; *anc.* Cydonia. Kríti, Greece, E Mediterranean Sea
62 J5 **Chañi, Nevado de** ▲ NW Argentina
115 H24 **Chanión, Kólpos** *gulf* Kríti, Greece, E Mediterranean Sea
Chankiri *see* Çankırı
30 M11 **Channahon** Illinois, N USA
155 H20 **Channapatna** Karnātaka, E India
97 K26 **Channel Islands** *Fr.* Îles Normandes. *island group* S English Channel
35 R16 **Channel Islands** *island group* California, W USA
13 S13 **Channel-Port aux Basques** Newfoundland, SE Canada
Channel, The *see* English Channel
97 Q23 **Channel Tunnel** *tunnel* France/UK
24 M2 **Channing** Texas, SW USA
Chantabun/Chantaburi *see* Chanthaburi
104 H3 **Chantada** Galicia, NW Spain
167 P12 **Chanthaburi** *var.* Chantabun, Chantaburi. Chantaburi, S Thailand
103 O4 **Chantilly** Oise, N France
139 V12 **Chanūn as Sa'ūdī** S Iraq
27 Q6 **Chanute** Kansas, C USA
Chanza *see* Chança, Rio
Ch'ao-an/Chaochow *see* Chaozhou
161 P8 **Chao Hu** ◎ E China
167 P11 **Chao Phraya, Mae Nam** ≈ C Thailand
163 T8 **Chaor He** ≈ NE China
Chaouèn *see* Chefchaouen
161 P14 **Chaoyang** Guangdong, S China
163 T12 **Chaoyang** Liaoning, NE China
Chaoyang *see* Huinan, Jilin, China
Chaoyang *see* Jiayin, Heilongjiang, China
161 Q14 **Chaozhou** *var.* Chaoan, Chao'an, Ch'ao-an; *prev.* Chaochow. Guangdong, SE China
58 N13 **Chapadinha** Maranhão, E Brazil
12 K12 **Chapais** Quebec, SE Canada
40 L13 **Chapala** Jalisco, SW Mexico
40 L13 **Chapala, Lago de** ◎ C Mexico
146 F13 **Chapan, Gora** ▲ C Turkmenistan
57 M18 **Chapare, Río** ≈ C Bolivia
54 E11 **Chaparral** Tolima, C Colombia
144 F9 **Chapayevo** Zapadnyy Kazakhstan, NW Kazakhstan
123 O11 **Chapayevo** Respublika Sakha (Yakutiya), NE Russian Federation
129 R6 **Chapayevsk** Samarskaya Oblast', W Russian Federation
60 H13 **Chapecó** Santa Catarina, S Brazil
60 I13 **Chapecó, Rio** ≈ S Brazil
20 J9 **Chapel Hill** Tennessee, S USA
44 J12 **Chapelton** C Jamaica
14 C8 **Chapleau** Ontario, SE Canada
14 D7 **Chapleau** ≈ Ontario, S Canada
11 T16 **Chaplin** Saskatchewan, S Canada
128 M6 **Chaplygin** Lipetskaya Oblast', W Russian Federation
117 S11 **Chaplynka** Khersons'ka Oblast', S Ukraine
9 O6 **Chapman, Cape** *headland* Nunavut, NE Canada
25 T15 **Chapman Ranch** Texas, SW USA
Chapman's *see* Okwa
21 P5 **Chapmanville** West Virginia, NE USA
28 K15 **Chappell** Nebraska, C USA
Chapra *see* Chhapra
56 D9 **Chapuli, Río** ≈ N Peru
76 I6 **Châr** *well* N Mauritania
123 P12 **Chara** Chitinskaya Oblast', S Russian Federation
123 O11 **Chara** ≈ C Russian Federation
54 G8 **Charala** Santander, C Colombia
41 N10 **Charcas** San Luis Potosí, C Mexico
25 T13 **Charco** Texas, SW USA
194 H7 **Charcot Island** *island* Antarctica
64 M8 **Charcot Seamounts** *undersea feature* E Atlantic Ocean
Chardara *see* Shardara
145 P17 **Chardarinskoye Vodokhranilishche** ▣ S Kazakhstan
31 U11 **Chardon** Ohio, N USA
44 K9 **Chardonnières** SW Haiti
146 K12 **Chardzhev** *prev.* Chardzhou, Chardzhui, Leninsk-Turkmenski, *Turkm.* Chärjew. Lebapskiy Velayat, E Turkmenistan
Chardzhevskaya Oblast' *see* Lebapskiy Velayat
Chardzhou/Chardzhui *see* Chardzhev
102 L11 **Charente** ◆ *department* W France
102 J11 **Charente** ≈ W France
102 J10 **Charente-Maritime** ◆ *department* W France
137 U12 **Ch'arents'avan** C Armenia
78 I12 **Chari** *var.* Shari. ≈ Central African Republic/Chad
78 G11 **Chari-Baguirmi** *off.* Préfecture du Chari-Baguirmi. ◆ *prefecture* SW Chad
149 Q4 **Chārīkār** Parwān, NE Afghanistan
29 V15 **Chariton** Iowa, C USA
27 U3 **Chariton River** ≈ Missouri, C USA
55 T7 **Charity** NW Guyana
31 R7 **Charity Island** *island* Michigan, N USA
Chärjew *see* Chardzhev
Chärjew Oblasty *see* Lebapskiy Velayat
Charkhlik/Charkhliq *see* Ruoqiang
99 G20 **Charleroi** Hainaut, S Belgium
11 V12 **Charles** Manitoba, C Canada
15 R10 **Charlesbourg** Quebec, SE Canada
21 Y7 **Charles, Cape** *headland* Virginia, NE USA
29 W12 **Charles City** Iowa, C USA
21 W6 **Charles City** Virginia, NE USA
103 O5 **Charles de Gaulle** × (Paris) Seine-et-Marne, N France
12 K1 **Charles Island** *island* Nunavut, NE Canada
Charles Island *see* Santa María, Isla
30 K9 **Charles Mound** *hill* Illinois, N USA
185 A22 **Charles Sound** *sound* South Island, NZ
185 G15 **Charleston** West Coast, South Island, NZ
27 S11 **Charleston** Arkansas, C USA
30 M14 **Charleston** Illinois, N USA
22 L3 **Charleston** Mississippi, S USA
27 Z7 **Charleston** Missouri, C USA
21 T15 **Charleston** South Carolina, SE USA
21 Q5 **Charleston** *state capital* West Virginia, NE USA
14 L14 **Charleston Lake** ◎ Ontario, SE Canada
35 W11 **Charleston Peak** ▲ Nevada, W USA
45 W10 **Charlestown** Nevis, Saint Kitts and Nevis
31 P16 **Charlestown** Indiana, N USA
18 M9 **Charlestown** New Hampshire, NE USA
21 V3 **Charles Town** West Virginia, NE USA
181 W9 **Charleville** Queensland, E Australia
103 R3 **Charleville-Mézières** Ardennes, N France
31 P5 **Charlevoix** Michigan, N USA
31 Q6 **Charlevoix, Lake** ◎ Michigan, N USA
39 T9 **Charley River** ≈ Alaska, USA
64 J6 **Charlie-Gibbs Fracture Zone** *tectonic feature* N Atlantic Ocean
103 Q10 **Charlieu** Loire, E France
31 Q9 **Charlotte** Michigan, N USA
21 R10 **Charlotte** North Carolina, SE USA
20 I8 **Charlotte** Tennessee, S USA
25 R13 **Charlotte** Texas, SW USA
21 R10 **Charlotte** × North Carolina, SE USA
45 T9 **Charlotte Amalie** *prev.* Saint Thomas. ○ (Virgin Islands (US)) Saint Thomas, N Virgin Islands (US)
21 U7 **Charlotte Court House** Virginia, NE USA
23 W14 **Charlotte Harbor** *inlet* Florida, SE USA
Charlotte Island *see* Abaiang
95 J15 **Charlottenberg** Värmland, C Sweden
Charlottenhof *see* Aegviidu
21 U5 **Charlottesville** Virginia, NE USA
Charlotte Town *see* Roseau, Dominica
Charlotte Town *see* Gouyave, Grenada
13 Q14 **Charlottetown** Prince Edward Island, Prince Edward Island, SE Canada
45 Z16 **Charlotteville** Tobago, Trinidad and Tobago
182 M11 **Charlton** Victoria, SE Australia
12 H10 **Charlton Island** *island* Nunavut, C Canada
103 T6 **Charmes** Vosges, NE France
119 F19 **Charnawchytsy** *Rus.* Chernavchitsy. Brestskaya Voblasts', SW Belarus
15 R10 **Charny** Quebec, SE Canada
149 T5 **Chārsadda** North-West Frontier Province, NW Pakistan
146 M14 **Charshanga** *prev.* Charshangy, *Turkm.* Charshangngy. Lebapskiy Velayat, E Turkmenistan
Charshangngy/Charshangy *see* Charshanga
Charsk *see* Shar
181 W6 **Charters Towers** Queensland, NE Australia
15 R12 **Chartierville** Quebec, SE Canada
102 M6 **Chartres** *anc.* Autricum, Civitas Carnutum. Eure-et-Loir, C France
145 W15 **Charyn** *Kaz.* Sharyn. Almaty, SE Kazakhstan
61 D21 **Chascomús** Buenos Aires, E Argentina
11 N16 **Chase** British Columbia, SW Canada
21 U7 **Chase City** Virginia, NE USA
19 S4 **Chase, Mount** ▲ Maine, NE USA
118 M13 **Chashniki** *Rus.* Chashniki. Vitsyebskaya Voblasts', N Belarus
115 D15 **Chásia** ▲ C Greece
29 V9 **Chaska** Minnesota, N USA
185 D25 **Chaslands Mistake** *headland* South Island, NZ
127 R11 **Chasovo** Respublika Komi, NW Russian Federation
Chasovo *see* Vazhgort
126 H14 **Chastova** Novgorodskaya Oblast', NW Russian Federation
143 R3 **Chāt** Golestān, N Iran
Chatak *see* Chhatak
39 R9 **Chatanika** Alaska, USA
39 R9 **Chatanika River** ≈ Alaska, USA
147 T8 **Chat-Bazar** Talasskaya Oblast', NW Kyrgyzstan
45 Y14 **Chateaubelair** Saint Vincent, W Saint Vincent and the Grenadines
102 J7 **Châteaubriant** Loire-Atlantique, NW France
103 Q8 **Château-Chinon** Nièvre, C France
108 C10 **Château d'Oex** Vaud, W Switzerland
102 L7 **Château-du-Loir** Sarthe, NW France
102 M6 **Châteaudun** Eure-et-Loir, C France
102 K7 **Château-Gontier** Mayenne, NW France
15 O13 **Châteauguay** Quebec, SE Canada
102 F6 **Châteaulin** Finistère, NW France
103 N9 **Châteaumeillant** Cher, C France
102 K11 **Châteauneuf-sur-Charente** Charente, W France
102 M7 **Château-Renault** Indre-et-Loire, C France
103 N9 **Châteauroux** *prev.* Indreville. Indre, C France
103 T5 **Château-Salins** Moselle, NE France
103 P4 **Château-Thierry** Aisne, N France
99 H21 **Châtelet** Hainaut, S Belgium
Châtelherault *see* Châtellerault
102 L9 **Châtellerault** *var.* Châtelherault. Vienne, W France
29 X10 **Chatfield** Minnesota, N USA
13 O14 **Chatham** New Brunswick, SE Canada
14 D17 **Chatham** Ontario, S Canada
97 P22 **Chatham** SE England, UK
30 K14 **Chatham** Illinois, N USA
21 T7 **Chatham** Virginia, NE USA
63 F22 **Chatham, Isla** *island* S Chile
175 R12 **Chatham Island** *island* Chatham Islands, NZ
Chatham Island *see* San Cristóbal, Isla
Chatham Island Rise *see* Chatham Rise
192 L12 **Chatham Islands** *island group* NZ, SW Pacific Ocean
175 Q12 **Chatham Rise** *var.* Chatham Island Rise. *undersea feature* S Pacific Ocean
39 X13 **Chatham Strait** *strait* Alaska, USA
Chathóir, Rinn *see* Cahore Point
102 M9 **Châtillon-sur-Indre** Indre, C France
103 Q7 **Châtillon-sur-Seine** Côte d'Or, C France
147 S8 **Chatkal** *Uzb.* Chotqol. ≈ Kyrgyzstan/Uzbekistan
147 R9 **Chatkal Range** *Rus.* Chatkal'skiy Khrebet. ▲ Kyrgyzstan/Uzbekistan
Chatkal'skiy Khrebet *see* Chatkal Range
23 N7 **Chatom** Alabama, S USA
Chatrapur *see* Chhatrapur
143 S10 **Chatrūd** Kermān, C Iran
23 S2 **Chatsworth** Georgia, SE USA
Chāttagām *see* Chittagong
23 S8 **Chattahoochee** Florida, SE USA
23 R8 **Chattahoochee River** ≈ SE USA
20 L10 **Chattanooga** Tennessee, S USA
147 V10 **Chatyr-Kël', Ozero** ◎ C Kyrgyzstan
147 W9 **Chatyr-Tash** Narynskaya Oblast', C Kyrgyzstan
15 R12 **Chaudière** ≈ Quebec, SE Canada
167 S14 **Châu Đốc** *var.* Chauphu, Chau Phu. An Giang, S Vietnam
152 D13 **Chauhtan** *prev.* Chohtan. Rājasthān, NW India
115 Ff5 **Chauk** Magwe, W Burma
103 R6 **Chaumont** *prev.* Chaumont-en-Bassigny. Haute-Marne, N France
Chaumont-en-Bassigny *see* Chaumont
123 T5 **Chaunskaya Guba** *bay* NE Russian Federation
103 P3 **Chauny** Aisne, N France
Châu Ô *see* Binh Sơn
Chau Phu *see* Châu Đôc
102 I5 **Chausey, Îles** *island group* N France
Chausy *see* Chavusy
18 C11 **Chautauqua Lake** ◎ New York, NE USA
102 L9 **Chauvigny** Vienne, W France
126 L6 **Chavan'ga** Murmanskaya Oblast', NW Russian Federation
14 K10 **Chavannes, Lac** ◎ Quebec, SE Canada

◆ Country
● Country Capital
◇ Dependent Territory
○ Dependent Territory Capital
◆ Administrative Region
× International Airport
▲ Mountain
▲ Mountain Range
Volcano
≈ River
◎ Lake
▣ Reservoir

Chavantes, Represa de see Xavantes, Represa de
61 D15 **Chavarría** Corrientes, NE Argentina
Chavash Respubliki see Chuvashskaya Respublika
104 I5 **Chaves** anc. Aquae Flaviae. Vila Real, N Portugal
Chávez, Isla see Santa Cruz, Isla
82 G13 **Chavuma** North Western, NW Zambia
119 O16 **Chavusy** Rus. Chausy. Mahilyowskaya Voblasts', E Belarus
145 Q16 **Chayan** Yuzhnyy Kazakhstan, S Kazakhstan
147 U8 **Chayek** Narynskaya Oblast', C Kyrgyzstan
139 T6 **Chāy Khānah** E Iraq
127 T16 **Chaykovskiy** Permskaya Oblast', NW Russian Federation
167 T12 **Chbar** Môndól Kiri, E Cambodia
23 Q4 **Cheaha Mountain** ▲ Alabama, S USA
Cheatharlach see Carlow
21 S2 **Cheat River** ≈ NE USA
111 A16 **Cheb** Ger. Eger. Karlovarský Kraj, W Czech Republic
129 Q3 **Cheboksary** Chuvashskaya Respublika, W Russian Federation
31 Q5 **Cheboygan** Michigan, N USA
Chechaouèn see Chefchaouen
Chechenia see Chechenskaya Respublika
129 O15 **Chechenskaya Respublika** Eng. Chechenia, Chechnia, Rus. Chechnya. ⬖ autonomous republic SW Russian Federation
67 N4 **Chech, Erg** desert Algeria/Mali
Chechersk see Chachersk
Chechevichi see Chachevichy
Che-chiang see Zhejiang
Chechnia/Chechnya see Chechenskaya Respublika
163 Y15 **Chech'ŏn** Jap. Teisen. N South Korea
111 L15 **Chęciny** Świętokrzyskie, S Poland
27 Q10 **Checotah** Oklahoma, C USA
13 R15 **Chedabucto Bay** inlet Nova Scotia, E Canada
166 J7 **Cheduba Island** island W Burma
37 T5 **Cheesman Lake** ⊞ Colorado, C USA
195 S16 **Cheetham, Cape** headland Antarctica
74 G5 **Chefchaouen** var. Chaouèn, Chechaouèn, Sp. Xauen. N Morocco
Chefoo see Yantai
38 M12 **Chefornak** Alaska, USA
123 R13 **Chegdomyn** Khabarovskiy Kray, SE Russian Federation
76 M4 **Chegga** Tiris Zemmour, NE Mauritania
Cheghcheran see Chaghcharān
32 G9 **Chehalis** Washington, NW USA
32 G9 **Chehalis River** ≈ Washington, NW USA
148 M6 **Chehel Abdālān, Kūh-e** var. Chalap Dalam, Pash. Chalap Dalan. ▲ C Afghanistan
115 D14 **Cheimadítis, Límni** ◎ N Greece
103 U15 **Cheiron, Mont** ▲ SE France
163 X17 **Cheju** Jap. Saishū. S South Korea
163 Y17 **Cheju** × S South Korea
163 Y17 **Cheju-do** Jap. Saishū; prev. Quelpart. island S South Korea
163 X17 **Cheju-haehyŏp** strait S South Korea
Chekiang see Zhejiang
Chekichler see Chekishlyar
146 B13 **Chekishlyar** Turkm. Chekichler. Balkanskiy Velayat, W Turkmenistan
188 F8 **Chelab** Babeldaob, N Palau
147 N11 **Chelak** Rus. Chelek. Samarqand Wiloyati, C Uzbekistan
32 J7 **Chelan, Lake** ⊞ Washington, NW USA
Chelek see Chelak
146 A11 **Cheleken** Balkanskiy Velayat, W Turkmenistan
Chélif/Chéliff see Chelif, Oued
74 J5 **Chelif, Oued** var. Chélif, Chéliff, Chellif, Shellif. ≈ N Algeria
144 K12 **Chelkar** Aktyubinsk, W Kazakhstan
Chelkar, Ozero see Shalkar, Ozero
Chellif see Chelif, Oued
111 P14 **Chełm** Rus. Kholm. Lubelskie, SE Poland
110 I9 **Chełmno** Ger. Culm, Kulm. Kujawski-pomorskie, C Poland
14 F10 **Chelmsford** Ontario, S Canada
97 P21 **Chelmsford** E England, UK
110 J9 **Chełmża** Ger. Culmsee, Kulmsee. Kujawski-pomorskie, C Poland
27 Q8 **Chelsea** Oklahoma, C USA
18 M8 **Chelsea** Vermont, NE USA
97 L21 **Cheltenham** C England, UK
105 R9 **Chelva** País Valenciano, E Spain
122 G11 **Chelyabinsk** Chelyabinskaya Oblast', C Russian Federation
122 F11 **Chelyabinskaya Oblast'** ⬖ province C Russian Federation
123 N5 **Chelyuskin, Mys** headland N Russian Federation
41 Y12 **Chemax** Yucatán, SE Mexico
83 N16 **Chemba** Sofala, C Mozambique
82 J13 **Chembe** Luapula, NE Zambia
146 J17 **Chemenibit** Maryyskiy Velayat, S Turkmenistan
Chemerisy see Chamyarysy
116 K7 **Chemerivtsi** Khmel'nyts'ka Oblast', W Ukraine
102 J8 **Chemillé** Maine-et-Loire, NW France
173 X17 **Chemin Grenier** S Mauritius
101 N16 **Chemnitz** prev. Karl-Marx-Stadt. Sachsen, E Germany
Chemulpo see Inch'ŏn
32 H14 **Chemult** Oregon, NW USA
18 G12 **Chemung River** ≈ New York/Pennsylvania, NE USA
149 U8 **Chenāb** ≈ India/Pakistan
39 S9 **Chena Hot Springs** Alaska, USA
18 I11 **Chenango River** ≈ New York, NE USA
168 J7 **Chenderoh, Tasik** ◎ Peninsular Malaysia
15 Q11 **Chêne, Rivière du** ≈ Quebec, SE Canada
32 L8 **Cheney** Washington, NW USA
26 M6 **Cheney Reservoir** ⊞ Kansas, C USA
Chengchiatun see Liaoyuan
Ch'eng-chou/Chengchow see Zhengzhou
161 P1 **Chengde** var. Jehol. Hebei, E China
160 I9 **Chengdu** var. Chengtu, Ch'eng-tu. Sichuan, C China
161 Q14 **Chenghai** Guangdong, S China
Chenghsien see Zhengzhou
160 L17 **Chengmai** Hainan, S China
Chengtu/Ch'eng-tu see Chengdu
159 W12 **Chengxian** var. Cheng Xian. Gansu, C China
Chenkiang see Zhenjiang
155 J19 **Chennai** prev. Madras. Tamil Nādu, S India
155 J19 **Chennai** × Tamil Nādu, S India
103 R8 **Chenôve** Côte d'Or, C France
Chenstokhov see Częstochowa
160 L11 **Chenxi** Hunan, S China
Chen Xian/Chenxian/Chen Xiang see Chenzhou
161 N12 **Chenzhou** var. Chenxian, Chen Xian, Chen Xiang. Hunan, S China
167 U12 **Cheo Reo** var. A Yun Pa. Gia Lai, S Vietnam
114 I11 **Chepelare** Smolyan, S Bulgaria
114 I11 **Chepelarska Reka** ≈ S Bulgaria
56 B11 **Chepén** La Libertad, C Peru
62 J10 **Chepes** La Rioja, C Argentina
161 O15 **Chep Lap Kok** × (Hong Kong) S China
43 U14 **Chepo** Panamá, C Panama
Chepping Wycombe see High Wycombe
127 R14 **Cheptsa** ≈ NW Russian Federation
30 K3 **Chequamegon Point** headland Wisconsin, N USA
103 O8 **Cher** ⬖ department C France
102 M8 **Cher** ≈ C France
Cherangani Hills see Cherangany Hills
81 H17 **Cherangany Hills** var. Cherangani Hills. ▲ W Kenya
21 S11 **Cheraw** South Carolina, SE USA
102 I3 **Cherbourg** anc. Carusbur. Manche, N France
129 R5 **Cherdakly** Ul'yanovskaya Oblast', W Russian Federation
127 U12 **Cherdyn'** Permskaya Oblast', NW Russian Federation
126 J14 **Cherekha** ≈ W Russian Federation
122 M13 **Cheremkhovo** Irkutskaya Oblast', S Russian Federation
Cheren see Keren
126 K14 **Cherepovets** Vologodskaya Oblast', NW Russian Federation
127 O11 **Cherevkovo** Arkhangel'skaya Oblast', NW Russian Federation
74 I6 **Chergui, Chott ech** salt lake NW Algeria
Cherikov see Cherykaw
117 P6 **Cherkas'ka Oblast'** var. Cherkasy, Rus. Cherkasskaya Oblast'. ⬖ province C Ukraine
Cherkasskaya Oblast' see Cherkas'ka Oblast'
Cherkassy see Cherkasy
117 Q6 **Cherkasy** Rus. Cherkassy. Cherkas'ka Oblast', C Ukraine
Cherkasy see Cherkas'ka Oblast'
128 M15 **Cherkessk** Karachayevo-Cherkesskaya Respublika, SW Russian Federation
122 H12 **Cherlak** Omskaya Oblast', C Russian Federation
122 H12 **Cherlakskiy** Omskaya Oblast', C Russian Federation
127 U13 **Chermoz** Permskaya Oblast', NW Russian Federation
Chernavchitsy see Charnawchytsy
127 T3 **Chernaya** Nenetskiy Avtonomnyy Okrug, NW Russian Federation
127 T4 **Chernaya** ≈ NW Russian Federation
Chernigov see Chernihiv
Chernigovskaya Oblast' see Chernihivs'ka Oblast'
117 Q2 **Chernihiv** Rus. Chernigov. Chernihivs'ka Oblast', NE Ukraine
Chernihiv see Chernihivs'ka Oblast'
117 V9 **Chernihivka** Zaporiz'ka Oblast', SE Ukraine
117 P2 **Chernihivs'ka Oblast'** var. Chernihiv, Rus. Chernigovskaya Oblast'. ⬖ province NE Ukraine
114 I9 **Cherni Osŭm** ≈ N Bulgaria
116 J8 **Chernivets'ka Oblast'** var. Chernivtsi, Rus. Chernovitskaya Oblast'. ⬖ province W Ukraine
114 I9 **Cherni Vit** ≈ NW Bulgaria
114 G10 **Cherni Vrŭkh** ▲ W Bulgaria
116 K8 **Chernivtsi** Ger. Czernowitz, Rom. Cernăuţi, Rus. Chernovtsy. Chernivets'ka Oblast', W Ukraine
116 M7 **Chernivtsi** Vinnyts'ka Oblast', C Ukraine
Chernivtsi see Chernivets'ka Oblast'
Chernobyl' see Chornobyl'
Cherno More see Black Sea
Chernomorskoye see Chornomors'ke
145 T7 **Chernoretskoye** Pavlodar, NE Kazakhstan
Chernovitskaya Oblast' see Chernivets'ka Oblast'
Chernovtsy see Chernivtsi
145 U8 **Chernoye** Pavlodar, NE Kazakhstan
Chernoye More see Black Sea
127 U16 **Chernushka** Permskaya Oblast', NW Russian Federation
117 N4 **Chernyakhiv** Rus. Chernyakhov. Zhytomyrs'ka Oblast', N Ukraine
Chernyakhov see Chernyakhiv
119 C14 **Chernyakhovsk** Ger. Insterburg. Kaliningradskaya Oblast', W Russian Federation
128 K8 **Chernyanka** Belgorodskaya Oblast', W Russian Federation
127 V5 **Chernyshëva, Gryada** ▲ NW Russian Federation
144 J14 **Chernyshëva, Zaliv** gulf SW Kazakhstan
123 O10 **Chernyshevskiy** Respublika Sakha (Yakutiya), NE Russian Federation
129 P13 **Chërnyye Zemli** plain SW Russian Federation
Chërnyy Irtysh see Ertix He
129 V7 **Chernyy Otrog** Orenburgskaya Oblast', W Russian Federation
29 T12 **Cherokee** Iowa, C USA
26 M8 **Cherokee** Oklahoma, C USA
25 R9 **Cherokee** Texas, SW USA
21 O8 **Cherokee Lake** ⊞ Tennessee, S USA
Cherokees, Lake O' The see Grand Lake O' The Cherokees
44 H1 **Cherokee Sound** Great Abaco, N Bahamas
153 V13 **Cherrapunji** Meghālaya, NE India
28 L9 **Cherry Creek** ≈ South Dakota, N USA
18 J16 **Cherry Hill** New Jersey, NE USA
27 Q7 **Cherryvale** Kansas, C USA
21 Q10 **Cherryville** North Carolina, SE USA
Cherski Range see Cherskogo, Khrebet
123 T6 **Cherskiy** Respublika Sakha (Yakutiya), NE Russian Federation
123 R8 **Cherskogo, Khrebet** var. Cherski Range. ▲ NE Russian Federation
Cherso see Cres
128 L10 **Chertkovo** Rostovskaya Oblast', SW Russian Federation
Cherven' see Chervyen'
114 H8 **Cherven Bryag** Pleven, N Bulgaria
116 M4 **Chervonoarmiys'k** Zhytomyrs'ka Oblast', N Ukraine
Chervonograd see Chervonohrad
116 I4 **Chervonohrad** Rus. Chervonograd. L'vivs'ka Oblast', NW Ukraine
117 W6 **Chervonooskil's'ke Vodoskhovyshche** Rus. Krasnooskol'skoye Vodokhranilishche. ⊞ NE Ukraine
Chervonoye, Ozero see Chyrvonaye, Vozyera
117 S4 **Chervonozavods'ke** Poltavs'ka Oblast', C Ukraine
119 L16 **Chervyen'** Rus. Cherven'. Minskaya Voblasts', C Belarus
119 P16 **Cherykaw** Rus. Cherikov. Mahilyowskaya Voblasts', E Belarus
31 R9 **Chesaning** Michigan, N USA
21 X5 **Chesapeake Bay** inlet NE USA
Cheshevlya see Tsyeshawlya
97 K18 **Cheshire** cultural region C England, UK
127 P5 **Chëshskaya Guba** var. Archangel Bay, Chesha Bay, Dvina Bay. bay NW Russian Federation
14 F14 **Chesley** Ontario, S Canada
21 Q10 **Chesnee** South Carolina, SE USA
97 K18 **Chester** Wel. Caerleon; hist. Legaceaster, Lat. Deva, Devana Castra. C England, UK
35 O4 **Chester** California, W USA
30 K16 **Chester** Illinois, N USA
33 S7 **Chester** Montana, NW USA
18 I16 **Chester** Pennsylvania, NE USA
21 R1 **Chester** South Carolina, SE USA
25 X9 **Chester** Texas, SW USA
21 W6 **Chester** Virginia, NE USA
21 R11 **Chester** West Virginia, NE USA
97 M18 **Chesterfield** C England, UK
21 S11 **Chesterfield** South Carolina, SE USA
21 W6 **Chesterfield** Virginia, NE USA
192 J9 **Chesterfield, Îles** island group NW New Caledonia
9 O9 **Chesterfield Inlet** Nunavut, NW Canada
9 O9 **Chesterfield Inlet** inlet Nunavut, N Canada
21 Y3 **Chester River** ≈ Delaware/Maryland, NE USA
21 X3 **Chestertown** Maryland, NE USA
19 R4 **Chesuncook Lake** ◎ Maine, NE USA
30 J5 **Chetek** Wisconsin, N USA
13 R14 **Chéticamp** Nova Scotia, SE Canada
27 Q8 **Chetopa** Kansas, C USA
41 Y14 **Chetumal** var. Payo Obispo. Quintana Roo, SE Mexico
Chetumal, Bahia/Chetumal, Bahía de see Chetumal Bay
42 G1 **Chetumal Bay** var. Bahia Chetumal, Bahía de Chetumal. bay Belize/Mexico
8 M13 **Chetwynd** British Columbia, W Canada
38 M11 **Chevak** Alaska, USA
36 M12 **Chevelon Creek** ≈ Arizona, SW USA
185 J17 **Cheviot** Canterbury, South Island, NZ
96 L13 **Cheviot Hills** hill range England/Scotland, UK
96 L13 **Cheviot, The** ▲ NE England, UK
14 M11 **Chevreuil, Lac du** ◎ Quebec, SE Canada
81 I16 **Ch'ew Bahir** var. Lake Stefanie. ◎ Ethiopia/Kenya
32 L7 **Chewelah** Washington, NW USA
26 K10 **Cheyenne** Oklahoma, C USA
33 Z17 **Cheyenne** state capital Wyoming, C USA
26 L5 **Cheyenne Bottoms** ◎ Kansas, C USA
16 J8 **Cheyenne River** ≈ South Dakota/Wyoming, N USA
37 W5 **Cheyenne Wells** Colorado, C USA
108 C9 **Cheyres** Vaud, W Switzerland
Chezdi-Oşorheiu see Târgu Secuiesc
153 P13 **Chhapra** prev. Chapra. Bihār, N India
153 V13 **Chhatak** var. Chatak. Chittagong, NE Bangladesh
154 J9 **Chhatarpur** Madhya Pradesh, C India
154 N13 **Chhatrapur** prev. Chatrapur; Orissa, E India
154 L12 **Chhattisgarh** plain C India
154 I11 **Chhindwāra** Madhya Pradesh, C India
153 T12 **Chhukha** SW Bhutan
161 S14 **Chiai** var. Chia-i, Chiayi, Kiayi, Jiayi, Jap. Kagi. C Taiwan
Chia-mu-ssu see Jiamusi
83 B15 **Chiange** Port. Vila de Almoster. Huíla, SW Angola
Chiang-hsi see Jiangxi
161 S12 **Chiang Kai-shek** × (T'aipei) N Taiwan
167 P8 **Chiang Khan** Loei, E Thailand
167 O7 **Chiang Mai** var. Chiangmai, Chiengmai, Kiangmai. Chiang Mai, NW Thailand
167 O7 **Chiang Mai** × Chiang Mai, NW Thailand
167 O6 **Chiang Rai** var. Chianpai, Chienrai, Muang Chiang Rai. Chiang Rai, NW Thailand
Chiang-su see Jiangsu
Chianning/Chian-ning see Nanjing
Chianpai see Chiang Rai
106 G12 **Chianti** cultural region C Italy
Chiapa see Chiapa de Corzo
41 U16 **Chiapa de Corzo** var. Chiapa. Chiapas, SE Mexico
41 V16 **Chiapas** ⬖ state SE Mexico
106 J12 **Chiaravalle** Marche, C Italy
107 N22 **Chiaravalle Centrale** Calabria, SW Italy
106 E7 **Chiari** Lombardia, N Italy
108 H12 **Chiasso** Ticino, S Switzerland
137 S9 **Chiat'ura** C Georgia
41 P15 **Chiautla** var. Chiautla de Tapia. Puebla, S Mexico
Chiautla de Tapia see Chiautla
106 D10 **Chiavari** Liguria, NW Italy
106 E6 **Chiavenna** Lombardia, N Italy
Chiayi see Chiai
Chiazza see Piazza Armerina
165 O13 **Chiba** var. Tiba. Chiba, Honshū, S Japan
165 O14 **Chiba** off. Chiba-ken, var. Tiba. ⬖ prefecture Honshū, S Japan
83 M18 **Chibabava** Sofala, C Mozambique
83 B15 **Chibia** Port. João de Almeida, Vila João de Almeida. Huíla, SW Angola
83 M18 **Chiboma** Sofala, C Mozambique
82 J12 **Chibondo** Luapula, N Zambia
82 K11 **Chibote** Luapula, NE Zambia
12 K12 **Chibougamau** Quebec, SE Canada
164 H11 **Chiburi-jima** island Oki-shotō, SW Japan
83 M20 **Chibuto** Gaza, S Mozambique
31 N11 **Chicago** Illinois, N USA
31 N11 **Chicago Heights** Illinois, N USA
15 W6 **Chic-Chocs, Monts** Eng. Shickshock Mountains. ▲ Quebec, SE Canada
39 W13 **Chichagof Island** island Alexander Archipelago, Alaska, USA
57 K20 **Chichas, Cordillera de** ▲ SW Bolivia
41 X12 **Chichén-Itzá, Ruinas** ruins Yucatán, SE Mexico
97 N23 **Chichester** SE England, UK
42 C5 **Chichicastenango** Quiché, W Guatemala
42 I9 **Chichigalpa** Chinandega, NW Nicaragua
Ch'i-ch'i-ha-erh see Qiqihar
165 X16 **Chichijima-rettō** Eng. Beechy Group. island group SE Japan
54 K4 **Chichiriviche** Falcón, N Venezuela
39 R11 **Chickaloon** Alaska, USA
20 L10 **Chickamauga Lake** ⊞ Tennessee, S USA
23 N7 **Chickasawhay River** ≈ Mississippi, S USA
26 M11 **Chickasha** Oklahoma, C USA
39 T9 **Chicken** Alaska, USA
104 J16 **Chiclana de la Frontera** Andalucía, S Spain
56 B11 **Chiclayo** Lambayeque, NW Peru
35 N5 **Chico** California, W USA
83 L15 **Chicoa** Tete, NW Mozambique
83 M20 **Chicomo** Gaza, S Mozambique
18 M11 **Chicopee** Massachusetts, NE USA
63 I19 **Chico, Río** ≈ SE Argentina
63 I21 **Chico, Río** ≈ S Argentina
27 W14 **Chicot, Lake** ◎ Arkansas, C USA
15 R7 **Chicoutimi** Quebec, SE Canada
15 Q8 **Chicoutimi** ≈ Quebec, SE Canada
83 L19 **Chicualacuala** Gaza, SW Mozambique
83 B14 **Chicuma** Benguela, C Angola
155 J21 **Chidambaram** Tamil Nādu, SE India
196 K13 **Chidley, Cape** headland Newfoundland, E Canada
101 N24 **Chiemsee** ◎ SE Germany
Chiengmai see Chiang Mai
Chienrai see Chiang Rai
106 B8 **Chieri** Piemonte, NW Italy
106 F8 **Chiese** ≈ N Italy
107 K14 **Chieti** var. Teate. Abruzzo, C Italy
99 E19 **Chièvres** Hainaut, SW Belgium
163 S12 **Chifeng** var. Ulanhad. Nei Mongol Zizhiqu, N China
82 F13 **Chifumage** ≈ E Angola
82 M13 **Chifunda** Eastern, NE Zambia
145 S14 **Chiganak** var. Čiganak. Zhambyl, SE Kazakhstan
39 P15 **Chiginagak, Mount** ▲ Alaska, USA
Chigirin see Chyhyryn
41 P13 **Chignahuapan** Puebla, S Mexico
39 O15 **Chignik** Alaska, USA
83 M19 **Chigombe** ≈ S Mozambique
54 D7 **Chigorodó** Antioquia, NW Colombia
83 M19 **Chigubo** Gaza, S Mozambique
162 D6 **Chihertey** Bayan-Ölgiy, W Mongolia
Chih-fu see Yantai
Chihli see Hebei
Chihli, Gulf of see Bo Hai
40 J6 **Chihuahua** Chihuahua, NW Mexico
40 I6 **Chihuahua** ⬖ state N Mexico
145 O15 **Chiili** Kzylorda, S Kazakhstan
26 M7 **Chikaskia River** ≈ Kansas/Oklahoma, C USA
155 H19 **Chik Ballāpur** Karnātaka, W India
126 G15 **Chikhachevo** Pskovskaya Oblast', W Russian Federation
155 F19 **Chikmagalūr** Karnātaka, W India
131 V7 **Chikoy** ≈ C Russian Federation
83 J15 **Chikumbi** Lusaka, C Zambia
82 M13 **Chikwa** Eastern, NE Zambia
Chikwana see Chikwawa
83 N15 **Chikwawa** var. Chikwana. Southern, S Malawi
155 J16 **Chilakalūrupet** Andhra Pradesh, E India
146 L14 **Chilan** Lebapskiy Velayat, E Turkmenistan
Chilapa see Chilapa de Alvarez
41 P16 **Chilapa de Alvarez** var. Chilapa. Guerrero, S Mexico
155 J25 **Chilaw** North Western Province, W Sri Lanka
57 D15 **Chilca** Lima, W Peru
23 Q4 **Childersburg** Alabama, S USA
25 P4 **Childress** Texas, SW USA
63 G14 **Chile** off. Republic of Chile. ◆ republic SW South America
47 R10 **Chile Basin** undersea feature E Pacific Ocean
63 H20 **Chile Chico** Aisén, W Chile
62 I9 **Chilecito** La Rioja, NW Argentina
62 H12 **Chilecito** Mendoza, W Argentina
83 L14 **Chilembwe** Eastern, E Zambia
193 S11 **Chile Rise** undersea feature SE Pacific Ocean
117 N13 **Chilia Braţul** ≈ SE Romania
Chilia-Nouă see Kiliya
145 V15 **Chilik** Almaty, SE Kazakhstan
145 V15 **Chilik** ≈ SE Kazakhstan
154 O13 **Chilika Lake** var. Chilka Lake. ◎ E India
82 J13 **Chililabombwe** Copperbelt, C Zambia
Chi-lin see Jilin
Chilka Lake see Chilika Lake
8 H9 **Chilkoot Pass** pass British Columbia, W Canada
Chill Ala, Cuan see Killala Bay
62 G13 **Chillán** Bío Bío, C Chile
61 C22 **Chillar** Buenos Aires, E Argentina
Chill Chiaráin, Cuan see Kilkieran Bay
30 K12 **Chillicothe** Illinois, N USA
27 S3 **Chillicothe** Missouri, C USA
31 S14 **Chillicothe** Ohio, N USA
25 Q4 **Chillicothe** Texas, SW USA
10 M17 **Chilliwack** British Columbia, SW Canada
Chill Mhantáin, Ceann see Wicklow Head
Chill Mhantáin, Sléibhte see Wicklow Mountains
108 C10 **Chillon** Vaud, W Switzerland
146 C11 **Chil'mamedkum, Peski** Turkm. Chilmämetgum. desert W Turkmenistan
Chilmämetgum see Chil'mamedkum, Peski
63 F17 **Chiloé, Isla de** var. Isla Grande de Chiloé. island W Chile
32 H15 **Chiloquin** Oregon, NW USA
41 O16 **Chilpancingo** var. Chilpancingo de los Bravos. Guerrero, S Mexico
Chilpancingo de los Bravos see Chilpancingo
97 N21 **Chiltern Hills** hill range S England, UK
30 M7 **Chilton** Wisconsin, N USA
82 F11 **Chiluage** Lunda Sul, NE Angola
82 N12 **Chilumba** prev. Deep Bay. Northern, N Malawi
161 T12 **Chilung** var. Keelung, Jap. Kirun, Kirun'; prev. Sp. Santissima Trinidad. N Taiwan
83 N15 **Chilwa, Lake** var. Lago Chirua, Lake Shirwa. ◎ SE Malawi
167 R10 **Chi, Mae Nam** ≈ E Thailand
42 C6 **Chimaltenango** Chimaltenango, C Guatemala
42 A2 **Chimaltenango** off. Departamento de Chimaltenango. ⬖ department S Guatemala
43 V15 **Chimán** Panamá, E Panama
83 M17 **Chimanimani** prev. Mandidzudzure, Melsetter. Manicaland, E Zimbabwe
99 G22 **Chimay** Hainaut, S Belgium
37 S10 **Chimayo** New Mexico, SW USA
Chimbay see Chimboy
56 A13 **Chimborazo** ⬖ province C Ecuador
56 C7 **Chimborazo** ⚶ C Ecuador
56 C12 **Chimbote** Ancash, W Peru
146 H7 **Chimboy** Rus. Chimbay. Qoraqalpoghiston Respublikasi, NW Uzbekistan
186 D7 **Chimbu** ⬖ province C PNG
54 F6 **Chimichagua** Cesar, N Colombia
Chimishliya see Cimişlia
Chimkent see Shymkent
Chimkentskaya Oblast' see Yuzhnyy Kazakhstan
28 I14 **Chimney Rock** rock Nebraska, C USA
83 M17 **Chimoio** Manica, C Mozambique
82 K11 **Chimpembe** Northern, NE Zambia
41 O8 **China** Nuevo León, NE Mexico
156 M9 **China** off. People's Republic of China, Chin. Chung-hua Jen-min Kung-ho-kuo, Zhonghua Renmin Gongheguo; prev. Chinese Empire. ◆ republic E Asia
19 Q7 **China Lake** ◎ Maine, NE USA
42 F8 **Chinameca** San Miguel, E El Salvador
Chi-nan/Chinan see Jinan
42 H9 **Chinandega** Chinandega, NW Nicaragua
42 H9 **Chinandega** ⬖ department NW Nicaragua
China, People's Republic of see China
China, Republic of see Taiwan
24 J11 **Chinati Mountains** ▲ Texas, SW USA
Chinaz see Chinoz
57 E15 **Chincha Alta** Ica, SW Peru
11 N11 **Chinchaga** ≈ Alberta, SW Canada
Chin-chiang see Quanzhou
Chinchilla see Chinchilla de Monte Aragón
105 Q11 **Chinchilla de Monte Aragón** var. Chinchilla. Castilla-La Mancha, C Spain
54 D10 **Chinchiná** Caldas, W Colombia
105 O8 **Chinchón** Madrid, C Spain
41 Z14 **Chinchorro, Banco** island SE Mexico
Chin-chou/Chinchow see Jinzhou
21 Z5 **Chincoteague** Assateague Island, Virginia, NE USA
83 O17 **Chinde** Zambézia, NE Mozambique
163 X17 **Chin-do** Jap. Chin-tō. island SW South Korea
159 R13 **Chindu** Qinghai, C China
166 M2 **Chindwin** ≈ N Burma
Chinese Empire see China
146 L10 **Chingeldi** Rus. Chingildi. Nawoiy Wiloyati, N Uzbekistan
Ch'ing Hai see Qinghai Hu
Chinghai see Qinghai
Chingildi see Chingeldi
144 H9 **Chingirlau** Kaz. Shyngghyrlaū. Zapadnyy Kazakhstan, W Kazakhstan
82 J13 **Chingola** Copperbelt, C Zambia
Ching-Tao/Ch'ing-tao see Qingdao
82 C13 **Chinguar** Huambo, C Angola
76 I7 **Chinguețți** var. Chinguetti. Adrar, C Mauritania
163 Z16 **Chinhae** Jap. Chinkai. S South Korea
166 K4 **Chin Hills** ▲ W Burma
83 K16 **Chinhoyi** prev. Sinoia. Mashonaland West, N Zimbabwe
Chinhsien see Jinzhou
39 Q14 **Chiniak, Cape** headland Kodiak Island, Alaska, USA
14 G10 **Chiniguchi Lake** ◎ Ontario, S Canada
149 U8 **Chiniot** Punjab, NE Pakistan
163 Y16 **Chinju** Jap. Shinshū. S South Korea
Chinkai see Chinhae
78 M13 **Chinko** ≈ E Central African Republic
37 O9 **Chinle** Arizona, SW USA
161 R13 **Chinmen Tao** var. Jinmen Dao, Quemoy. island W Taiwan
Chinnchâr see Shinshār
Chinnereth see Tiberias, Lake
164 C12 **Chino** var. Tino. Nagano, Honshū, S Japan

◆ Country ● Country Capital ◇ Dependent Territory ○ Dependent Territory Capital ⬖ Administrative Region × International Airport ▲ Mountain ▲ Mountain Range ⚶ Volcano ≈ River ◎ Lake ⊞ Reservoir

102 L8 **Chinon** Indre-et-Loire, C France
33 T7 **Chinook** Montana, NW USA
Chinook State see Washington
192 L4 **Chinook Trough** undersea feature N Pacific Ocean
36 K11 **Chino Valley** Arizona, SW USA
147 P10 **Chinoz** Rus. Chinaz. Toshkent Wiloyati, E Uzbekistan
82 L12 **Chinsali** Northern, NE Zambia
166 K5 **Chin State** ◈ state W Burma
Chinsura see Chunchura
Chin-tō see Chin-do
54 E6 **Chinú** Córdoba, NW Colombia
99 K24 **Chiny, Forêt de** forest SE Belgium
83 M15 **Chioco** Tete, NW Mozambique
106 H8 **Chioggia** anc. Fossa Claudia. Veneto, NE Italy
114 H12 **Chionótrypa** ▲ NE Greece
115 L18 **Chíos** var. Hios, Khíos, It. Scio, Turk. Sakiz-Adasi. Chíos, E Greece
115 K18 **Chíos** var. Khíos. island E Greece
83 M14 **Chipata** prev. Fort Jameson. Eastern, E Zambia
83 C14 **Chipindo** Huíla, C Angola
23 R8 **Chipley** Florida, SE USA
155 D15 **Chiplūn** Mahārāshtra, W India
81 H22 **Chipogolo** Dodoma, C Tanzania
23 R8 **Chipola River** ≈ Florida, SE USA
97 L22 **Chippenham** S England, UK
30 J6 **Chippewa Falls** Wisconsin, N USA
30 J4 **Chippewa, Lake** ◎ Wisconsin, N USA
31 Q8 **Chippewa River** ≈ Michigan, N USA
30 I6 **Chippewa River** ≈ Wisconsin, N USA
Chipping Wycombe see High Wycombe
114 G8 **Chiprovtsi** Montana, NW Bulgaria
19 T4 **Chiputneticook Lakes** lakes Canada/USA
56 D13 **Chiquián** Ancash, W Peru
41 Y11 **Chiquilá** Quintana Roo, SE Mexico
42 E6 **Chiquimula** Chiquimula, SE Guatemala
42 A3 **Chiquimula** off. Departamento de Chiquimula. ◈ department SE Guatemala
42 D7 **Chiquimulilla** Santa Rosa, S Guatemala
54 F9 **Chiquinquirá** Boyacá, C Colombia
155 J17 **Chīrāla** Andhra Pradesh, E India
149 N4 **Chīras** Ghowr, N Afghanistan
152 H11 **Chirāwa** Rājasthān, N India
Chirchik see Chirchiq
147 Q9 **Chirchiq** Rus. Chirchik. Toshkent Wiloyati, E Uzbekistan
147 P10 **Chirchiq** ≈ E Uzbekistan
Chire see Shire
83 L18 **Chiredzi** Masvingo, SE Zimbabwe
25 X8 **Chireno** Texas, SW USA
77 X7 **Chirfa** Agadez, NE Niger
37 O16 **Chiricahua Mountains** ⛰ Arizona, SW USA
37 O16 **Chiricahua Peak** ▲ Arizona, SW USA
54 F6 **Chiriguaná** Cesar, N Colombia
39 P15 **Chirikof Island** island Alaska, USA
43 P16 **Chiriquí** off. Provincia de Chiriquí. ◈ province SW Panama
43 P17 **Chiriquí, Golfo de** Eng. Chiriqui Gulf. gulf SW Panama
43 P15 **Chiriquí Grande** Bocas del Toro, W Panama
Chiriqui Gulf see Chiriquí, Golfo de
43 P15 **Chiriquí, Laguna de** lagoon NW Panama
43 O16 **Chiriquí Viejo, Río** ≈ W Panama
Chiriquí, Volcán de see Barú, Volcán
83 N15 **Chiromo** Southern, S Malawi
114 J10 **Chirpan** Stara Zagora, C Bulgaria
43 N14 **Chirripó Atlántico, Río** ≈ E Costa Rica
Chirripó, Cerro see Chirripó Grande, Cerro
43 N14 **Chirripó Grande, Cerro** var. Cerro Chirripó. ▲ SE Costa Rica
43 N13 **Chirripó, Río** var. Río Chirripó del Pacífico. ≈ NE Costa Rica
Chirua, Lago see Chilwa, Lake
83 J15 **Chirundu** Southern, S Zambia
29 W8 **Chisago City** Minnesota, N USA
83 J14 **Chisamba** Central, C Zambia
39 T10 **Chisana** Alaska, USA
82 I13 **Chisasa** North Western, NW Zambia
12 I9 **Chisasibi** Quebec, C Canada
42 D4 **Chisec** Alta Verapaz, C Guatemala
129 U5 **Chishmy** Respublika Bashkortostan, W Russian Federation
29 V4 **Chisholm** Minnesota, N USA
160 I11 **Chishui He** ≈ C China
Chisimaio/Chisimayu see Kismaayo
117 N10 **Chişinău** Rus. Kishinev. ● (Moldova) C Moldova
117 N10 **Chişinău** × S Moldova
Chişinău-Criş see Chişineu-Criş
116 F10 **Chişineu-Criş** Hung. Kisjenő; prev. Chişinău-Criş. Arad, W Romania
83 K14 **Chisomo** Central, C Zambia
106 A8 **Chisone** ≈ NW Italy
24 K12 **Chisos Mountains** ⛰ Texas, SW USA
149 U10 **Chistiān Mandi** Punjab, E Pakistan
39 T10 **Chistochina** Alaska, USA
129 R4 **Chistopol'** Respublika Tatarstan, W Russian Federation
145 O8 **Chistopol'ye** Severnyy Kazakhstan, N Kazakhstan
123 O13 **Chita** Chitinskaya Oblast', S Russian Federation
83 B16 **Chitado** Cunene, SW Angola
Chitaldroog/Chitaldrug see Chitradurga
83 C15 **Chitanda** ≈ S Angola
Chitangwiza see Chitungwiza
82 F10 **Chitato** Lunda Norte, NE Angola
83 C14 **Chitembo** Bié, C Angola
39 T11 **Chitina** Alaska, USA
39 T11 **Chitina River** ≈ Alaska, USA
123 O12 **Chitinskaya Oblast'** ◈ province S Russian Federation
82 M11 **Chitipa** Northern, NW Malawi
165 S4 **Chitose** var. Titose. Hokkaidō, NE Japan
155 G18 **Chitradurga** prev. Chitaldroog, Chitaldrug. Karnātaka, W India
149 T3 **Chitrāl** North-West Frontier Province, NW Pakistan
43 S16 **Chitré** Herrera, S Panama
153 V16 **Chittagong** Ben. Chāttagām. Chittagong, SE Bangladesh
153 U16 **Chittagong** ◈ division E Bangladesh
153 Q15 **Chittaranjan** West Bengal, NE India
152 G14 **Chittaurgarh** Rājasthān, N India
155 I19 **Chittoor** Andhra Pradesh, E India
155 G21 **Chittūr** Kerala, SW India
83 K16 **Chitungwiza** prev. Chitangwiza. Mashonaland East, NE Zimbabwe
62 H4 **Chiuchiu** Antofagasta, N Chile
82 F12 **Chiumbe** var. Tshiumbe. ≈ Angola/Dem. Rep. Congo (Zaire)
83 F15 **Chiume** Moxico, E Angola
82 K13 **Chiundaponde** Northern, NE Zambia
106 H13 **Chiusi** Toscana, C Italy
54 J5 **Chivacoa** Yaracuy, N Venezuela
106 B8 **Chivasso** Piemonte, NW Italy
83 L17 **Chivhu** prev. Enkeldoorn. Midlands, C Zimbabwe
61 C20 **Chivilcoy** Buenos Aires, E Argentina
82 N12 **Chiweta** Northern, N Malawi
42 D4 **Chixoy, Río** var. Río Negro, Río Salinas. ≈ Guatemala/Mexico
82 H13 **Chizela** North Western, NW Zambia
127 O5 **Chizha** Nenetskiy Avtonomnyy Okrug, NW Russian Federation
164 I12 **Chizu** Tottori, Honshū, SW Japan
Chkalov see Orenburg
74 J5 **Chlef** var. Ech Cheliff, Ech Chleff; prev. Al-Asnam, El Asnam, Orléansville. NW Algeria
115 G18 **Chlómo** ▲ C Greece
111 M15 **Chmielnik** Świętokrzyskie, C Poland
167 S11 **Chŏâm Khsant** Preăh Vihéar, N Cambodia
62 G10 **Choapa, Río** var. Choapo. ≈ C Chile
Choapas see Las Choapas
Choarta see Chwārtā
83 H17 **Chobe** ◈ district NE Botswana
67 T13 **Chobe** ≈ N Botswana
14 K8 **Chochocouane** ≈ Quebec, SE Canada
110 E13 **Chocianów** Ger. Kotzenan. Dolnośląskie, SW Poland
54 C9 **Chocó** off. Departamento del Chocó. ◈ province W Colombia
35 X16 **Chocolate Mountains** ⛰ California, W USA
21 W9 **Chocowinity** North Carolina, SE USA
27 N10 **Choctaw** Oklahoma, C USA
23 Q8 **Choctawhatchee Bay** bay Florida, SE USA
23 Q8 **Choctawhatchee River** ≈ Florida, SE USA
Chodau see Chodov
163 V14 **Chŏ-do** island SW North Korea
Chodorów see Khodoriv
111 A16 **Chodov** Ger. Chodau. Karlovarský Kraj, W Czech Republic
110 G10 **Chodzież** Wielkopolskie, C Poland
63 J15 **Choele Choel** Río Negro, C Argentina
83 L14 **Chofombo** Tete, NW Mozambique
Chohtan see Chauhtan
11 U14 **Choiceland** Saskatchewan, C Canada
186 K8 **Choiseul** var. Lauru. island NW Solomon Islands
63 M23 **Choiseul Sound** sound East Falkland, Falkland Islands
40 H7 **Choix** Sinaloa, C Mexico
110 D10 **Chojna** Zachodniopomorskie, W Poland
110 H8 **Chojnice** Ger. Konitz. Pomorskie, N Poland
111 F14 **Chojnów** Ger. Hainau, Haynau. Dolnośląskie, SW Poland
167 Q10 **Chok Chai** Nakhon Ratchasima, C Thailand
80 I12 **Ch'ok'ē** var. Choke Mountains. ⛰ NW Ethiopia
25 R13 **Choke Canyon Lake** ⊡ Texas, SW USA
Choke Mountains see Ch'ok'ē
145 T15 **Chokpar** Kaz. Shoqpar. Zhambyl, S Kazakhstan
147 W7 **Chok-Tal** var. Choktal. Issyk-Kul'skaya Oblast', E Kyrgyzstan
Chókué see Chokwé
123 R7 **Chokurdakh** Respublika Sakha (Yakutiya), NE Russian Federation
83 L20 **Chokwé** var. Chókué. Gaza, S Mozambique
188 F8 **Chol** Babeldaob, N Palau
160 E8 **Chola Shan** ⛰ C China
102 J8 **Cholet** Maine-et-Loire, NW France
63 H17 **Cholila** Chubut, W Argentina
Cholo see Thyolo
147 V8 **Cholpon** Narynskaya Oblast', C Kyrgyzstan
147 X7 **Cholpon-Ata** Issyk-Kul'skaya Oblast', E Kyrgyzstan
41 P14 **Cholula** Puebla, S Mexico
42 I8 **Choluteca** Choluteca, S Honduras
42 H8 **Choluteca** ◈ department S Honduras
42 G6 **Choluteca, Río** ≈ SW Honduras
83 I15 **Choma** Southern, S Zambia
153 T11 **Chomo Lhari** ▲ NW Bhutan
167 N7 **Chom Thong** Chiang Mai, NW Thailand
111 B15 **Chomutov** Ger. Komotau. Ústecký Kraj, NW Czech Republic
123 N11 **Chona** ≈ C Russian Federation
163 X15 **Ch'ŏnan** Jap. Tenan. W South Korea
167 P11 **Chon Buri** prev. Bang Pla Soi. Chon Buri, S Thailand
56 B6 **Chone** Manabí, W Ecuador
163 W13 **Ch'ŏngch'ŏn-gang** ≈ W North Korea
163 Y11 **Ch'ŏngjin** NE North Korea
163 W13 **Chŏngju** W North Korea
161 S8 **Chongming Dao** island E China
160 J10 **Chongqing** var. Ch'ung-ching, Ch'ung-ch'ing, Chungking, Pahsien, Tchongking, Yuzhou. Chongqing Shi, C China
Chŏngup see Chŏnju
161 O10 **Chongyang** Hubei, C China
163 Y16 **Chŏnju** prev. Chŏngup, Jap. Seiyu. SW South Korea
163 Y15 **Chŏnju** Jap. Zenshū. SW South Korea
Chonnacht see Connaught
163 Q9 **Chonogol** Sühbaatar, E Mongolia
63 F19 **Chonos, Archipiélago de los** island group S Chile
42 K10 **Chontales** ◈ department S Nicaragua
167 T13 **Chơn Thanh** Sông Be, S Vietnam
158 K17 **Cho Oyu** var. Qowowuyag. ▲ China/Nepal
116 G7 **Chop** Cz. Čop, Hung. Csap. Zakarpats'ka Oblast', W Ukraine
21 Y3 **Choptank River** ≈ Maryland, NE USA
Chorcaí, Cuan see Cork Harbour
43 P15 **Chorcha, Cerro** ▲ W Panama
Chorku see Chorkŭh
147 R11 **Chorkŭh** Rus. Chorku. N Tajikistan
97 K17 **Chorley** NW England, UK
Chorne More see Black Sea
117 R5 **Chornobay** Cherkas'ka Oblast', C Ukraine
117 O3 **Chornobyl'** Rus. Chernobyl'. Kyyivs'ka Oblast', N Ukraine
117 R12 **Chornomors'ke** Rus. Chernomorskoye. Respublika Krym, S Ukraine
117 R4 **Chornukhy** Poltavs'ka Oblast', C Ukraine
Chorokh/Chorokhi see Çoruh Nehri
110 O9 **Choroszcz** Podlaskie, NE Poland
116 K6 **Chortkiv** Rus. Chortkov. Ternopil's'ka Oblast', W Ukraine
Chortkov see Chortkiv
Chorum see Çorum
110 M9 **Chorzele** Mazowieckie, C Poland
111 J16 **Chorzów** Ger. Königshütte; prev. Królewska Huta. Śląskie, S Poland
163 W12 **Ch'osan** N North Korea
Chōsen-kaikyō see Korea Strait
164 P14 **Chōshi** var. Tyôsi. Chiba, Honshū, S Japan
63 H14 **Chos Malal** Neuquén, W Argentina
Chosŏn-minjujuŭi-inmin-kanghwaguk see North Korea
110 E9 **Choszczno** Ger. Arnswalde. Zachodniopomorskie, NW Poland
153 O15 **Chota Nāgpur** plateau N India
33 R8 **Choteau** Montana, NW USA
Chotqol see Chatkal
14 M8 **Chouart** ≈ Quebec, SE Canada
76 I7 **Choûm** Adrar, C Mauritania
27 Q9 **Chouteau** Oklahoma, C USA
21 X8 **Chowan River** ≈ North Carolina, SE USA
35 Q10 **Chowchilla** California, W USA
163 P7 **Choybalsan** Dornod, E Mongolia
162 M9 **Choyr** Dornogovĭ, C Mongolia
185 I19 **Christchurch** Canterbury, South Island, NZ
97 M24 **Christchurch** S England, UK
185 I18 **Christchurch** × Canterbury, South Island, NZ
44 J12 **Christiana** C Jamaica
83 H22 **Christiana** Free State, C South Africa
115 J23 **Christiáni** island Kykládes, Greece, Aegean Sea
Christiania see Oslo
14 G13 **Christian Island** island Ontario, S Canada
191 P16 **Christian, Point** headland Pitcairn Island, Pitcairn Islands
38 M11 **Christian River** ≈ Alaska, USA
Christiansand see Kristiansand
21 S7 **Christiansburg** Virginia, NE USA
95 G23 **Christiansfeld** Sønderjylland, SW Denmark
Christianshåb see Qasigiannguit
39 X14 **Christian Sound** inlet Alaska, USA
45 T9 **Christiansted** Saint Croix, S Virgin Islands (US)
Christiansund see Kristiansund
25 R13 **Christine** Texas, SW USA
173 U7 **Christmas Island** ◇ Australian external territory E Indian Ocean
131 T17 **Christmas Island** island E Indian Ocean
Christmas Island see Kiritimati
192 M7 **Christmas Ridge** undersea feature C Pacific Ocean
30 L16 **Christopher** Illinois, N USA
25 P9 **Christoval** Texas, SW USA
111 E17 **Chrudim** Pardubický Kraj, C Czech Republic
115 K25 **Chrýsi** island SE Greece
121 N2 **Chrysochoú, Kólpos** var. Khrysokhou Bay. bay E Mediterranean Sea
114 I13 **Chrysoúpoli** var. Hrisoupoli; prev. Khrisoúpolis. Anatolikí Makedonía kai Thráki, NE Greece
111 K16 **Chrzanów** var. Chrzanow, Ger. Zaumgarten. Śląskie, S Poland
131 Q7 **Chu** Kaz. Shū. ≈ Kazakhstan/Kyrgyzstan
42 C5 **Chuacús, Sierra de** ⛰ W Guatemala
153 S15 **Chuadanga** Khulna, W Bangladesh
Chuan see Sichuan
Ch'uan-chou see Quanzhou
39 O11 **Chuathbaluk** Alaska, USA
Chubek see Moskva
63 I17 **Chubut** off. Provincia de Chubut. ◈ province S Argentina
63 I17 **Chubut, Río** ≈ SE Argentina
43 V15 **Chucanti, Cerro** ▲ E Panama
Ch'u-chiang see Shaoguan
43 W15 **Chucunaque, Río** ≈ E Panama
Chudin see Chudzin
116 M5 **Chudniv** Zhytomyrs'ka Oblast', N Ukraine
126 H13 **Chudovo** Novgorodskaya Oblast', W Russian Federation
Chudskoye Ozero see Peipus, Lake
119 J18 **Chudzin** Rus. Chudin. Brestskaya Voblasts', SW Belarus
39 Q13 **Chugach Islands** island group Alaska, USA
39 S11 **Chugach Mountains** ⛰ Alaska, USA
164 G12 **Chūgoku-sanchi** ⛰ Honshū, SW Japan
Chuguyev see Chuhuyiv
117 V5 **Chuhuyiv** var. Chuguyev. Kharkivs'ka Oblast', E Ukraine
61 H19 **Chuí** Rio Grande do Sul, S Brazil
Chuí see Chuy
145 S15 **Chu-Iliyskiye Gory** Kaz. Shū-Ile Taūlary. ⛰ S Kazakhstan
Chukai see Cukai
Chukchi Avtonomnyy Okrug see Chukotskiy Avtonomnyy Okrug
Chukchi Peninsula see Chukotskiy Poluostrov
197 R6 **Chukchi Plain** undersea feature Arctic Ocean
197 R6 **Chukchi Plateau** undersea feature Arctic Ocean
197 R4 **Chukchi Sea** Rus. Chukotskoye More. sea Arctic Ocean
127 N14 **Chukhloma** Kostromskaya Oblast', NW Russian Federation
Chukotka see Chukotskiy Avtonomnyy Okrug
Chukot Range see Anadyrskiy Khrebet
123 V6 **Chukotskiy Avtonomnyy Okrug** var. Chukchi Avtonomnyy Okrug, Chukotka. ◈ autonomous district NE Russian Federation
123 W5 **Chukotskiy, Mys** headland NE Russian Federation
123 V5 **Chukotskiy Poluostrov** Eng. Chukchi Peninsula. peninsula NE Russian Federation
Chukotskoye More see Chukchi Sea
Chukurkak see Chuqurqoq
Chulakkurgan see Shollakorgan
35 U17 **Chula Vista** California, W USA
123 Q12 **Chul'man** Respublika Sakha (Yakutiya), NE Russian Federation
56 B9 **Chulucanas** Piura, NW Peru
122 J12 **Chulym** ≈ C Russian Federation
152 K6 **Chumar** Jammu and Kashmir, N India
114 K9 **Chumerna** ▲ C Bulgaria
123 R12 **Chumikan** Khabarovskiy Kray, E Russian Federation
167 Q9 **Chum Phae** Khon Kaen, C Thailand
167 N13 **Chumphon** var. Jumporn. Chumphon, SW Thailand
167 O9 **Chumsaeng** var. Chum Saeng. Nakhon Sawan, C Thailand
122 L12 **Chuna** ≈ C Russian Federation
161 R9 **Chun'an** var. Pailing. Zhejiang, SE China
161 S13 **Chunan** N Taiwan
163 Y14 **Ch'unch'ŏn** Jap. Shunsen. N South Korea
153 S16 **Chunchura** prev. Chinsura. West Bengal, NE India
145 W15 **Chundzha** Almaty, SE Kazakhstan
Ch'ung-ch'ing/Ch'ung-ching see Chongqing
Chung-hua Jen-min Kung-ho-kuo see China
163 Y15 **Ch'ungju** Jap. Chūshū. C South Korea
Chungking see Chongqing
161 T14 **Chungyang Shanmo** Chin. Taiwan Shan. ⛰ C Taiwan
149 V9 **Chūniān** Punjab, E Pakistan
122 L12 **Chunskiy** Irkutskaya Oblast', S Russian Federation
122 M11 **Chunya** ≈ C Russian Federation
126 J6 **Chupa** Respublika Kareliya, NW Russian Federation
127 P8 **Chuprovo** Respublika Komi, NW Russian Federation
57 G17 **Chuquibamba** Arequipa, SW Peru
62 H4 **Chuquicamata** Antofagasta, N Chile
57 L21 **Chuquisaca** ◈ department S Bolivia
Chuquisaca see Sucre
146 I8 **Chuqurqoq** Rus. Chukurkak. Qoraqalpoghiston Respublikasi, NW Uzbekistan
129 T2 **Chur** Udmurtskaya Respublika, NW Russian Federation
108 I9 **Chur** Fr. Coire, It. Coira, Rmsch. Cuera, Quera; anc. Curia Rhaetorum. Graubünden, E Switzerland
123 Q10 **Churapcha** Respublika Sakha (Yakutiya), NE Russian Federation
11 V16 **Churchbridge** Saskatchewan, S Canada
21 O8 **Church Hill** Tennessee, S USA
11 X9 **Churchill** Manitoba, C Canada
11 X10 **Churchill** ≈ Manitoba/Saskatchewan, C Canada
13 P9 **Churchill** ≈ Newfoundland, E Canada
11 Y9 **Churchill, Cape** headland Manitoba, C Canada
13 P9 **Churchill Falls** Newfoundland, E Canada
11 S12 **Churchill Lake** ◎ Saskatchewan, C Canada
19 Q3 **Churchill Lake** ⊡ Maine, NE USA
194 I5 **Churchill Peninsula** peninsula Antarctica
22 H8 **Church Point** Louisiana, S USA
29 O3 **Churchs Ferry** North Dakota, N USA
146 G12 **Churchuri** Akhalskiy Velayat, C Turkmenistan
21 T5 **Churchville** Virginia, NE USA
152 G10 **Chūru** Rājasthān, NW India
54 J4 **Churuguara** Falcón, N Venezuela
144 J12 **Chushkakul, Gory** ⛰ SW Kazakhstan
Chūshū see Ch'ungju
37 O9 **Chuska Mountains** ⛰ Arizona/New Mexico, SW USA
Chu, Sông see Sam, Nam
127 V14 **Chusovoy** Permskaya Oblast', NW Russian Federation
167 U11 **Chư Srê** Gia Lai, C Vietnam
147 R10 **Chust** Namangan Wiloyati, E Uzbekistan
Chust see Khust
15 U6 **Chute-aux-Outardes** Quebec, SE Canada
117 U5 **Chutove** Poltavs'ka Oblast', C Ukraine
189 O15 **Chuuk** var. Truk. ◈ state C Micronesia
189 P15 **Chuuk Islands** var. Hogoley Islands; prev. Truk Islands. island group Caroline Islands, C Micronesia
Chuvashia see Chuvashskaya Respublika
129 P4 **Chuvashskaya Respublika** var. Chavash Respubliki, Eng. Chuvashia. ◈ autonomous republic W Russian Federation
Chuwārtah see Chwārtā
Chu Xian/Chuxian see Chuzhou
160 G13 **Chuxiong** Yunnan, SW China
147 V7 **Chuy** Chuyskaya Oblast', N Kyrgyzstan
61 H19 **Chuy** var. Chuí. Rocha, E Uruguay
123 O11 **Chuya** Respublika Sakha (Yakutiya), NE Russian Federation
Chüy Oblasty see Chuyskaya Oblast'
147 U8 **Chuyskaya Oblast'** Kir. Chüy Oblasty. ◈ province N Kyrgyzstan
161 Q7 **Chuzhou** var. Chuxian, Chu Xian. Anhui, E China
139 U3 **Chwārtā** var. Choarta, Chuwārtah. NE Iraq
119 N16 **Chyhirynskaye Vodaskhovishcha** ⊡ E Belarus
117 R6 **Chyhyryn** Rus. Chigirin. Cherkas'ka Oblast', N Ukraine
Chyrvonaya Slabada see Krasnaya Slabada
119 L19 **Chyrvonaye, Vozyera** Rus. Ozero Chervonoye. ◎ SE Belarus
117 N11 **Ciadîr-Lunga** var. Ceadâr-Lunga, Rus. Chadyr-Lunga. S Moldova
169 P16 **Ciamis** prev. Tjiamis. Jawa, C Indonesia
107 I16 **Ciampino** × Lazio, C Italy
169 N16 **Cianjur** prev. Tjiandjoer. Jawa, C Indonesia
60 H10 **Cianorte** Paraná, S Brazil
Ciarraí see Kerry
112 N13 **Ćićevac** Serbia, E Yugoslavia
187 Z14 **Cicia** prev. Thithia. island Lau Group, E Fiji
105 P4 **Cidacos** ≈ N Spain
136 I10 **Cide** Kastamonu, N Turkey
110 L10 **Ciechanów** prev. Zichenau. Mazowieckie, C Poland
110 O10 **Ciechanowiec** Ger. Rudelstadt. Podlaskie, E Poland
110 J10 **Ciechocinek** Kujawsko-pomorskie, C Poland
44 F6 **Ciego de Ávila** Ciego de Ávila, C Cuba
54 F4 **Ciénaga** Magdalena, N Colombia
54 E6 **Ciénaga de Oro** Córdoba, NW Colombia
44 E5 **Cienfuegos** Cienfuegos, C Cuba
104 F4 **Cíes, Illas** island group NW Spain
111 P16 **Cieszanów** Podkarpackie, SE Poland
111 J17 **Cieszyn** Cz. Těšín, Ger. Teschen. Śląskie, S Poland
105 R12 **Cieza** Murcia, SE Spain
136 F13 **Çifteler** Eskişehir, W Turkey
105 P7 **Cifuentes** Castilla-La Mancha, C Spain
Čiganak see Chiganak
105 P9 **Cigüela** ≈ C Spain
136 H14 **Cihanbeyli** Konya, C Turkey
136 H14 **Cihanbeyli Yaylası** plateau C Turkey
104 L10 **Cíjara, Embalse de** ⊡ C Spain
169 P16 **Cikalong** Jawa, S Indonesia
169 N16 **Cikawung** Jawa, S Indonesia
187 Y13 **Cikobia** prev. Thikombia. island N Fiji
169 P17 **Cilacap** prev. Tjilatjap. Jawa, C Indonesia
173 O16 **Cilaos** C Réunion
137 S11 **Çıldır** Ardahan, NE Turkey
137 S11 **Çıldır Gölü** ◎ NE Turkey
160 M10 **Cili** Hunan, S China
121 V10 **Cilicia Trough** undersea feature E Mediterranean Sea
Cill Airne see Killarney
Cill Chainnigh see Kilkenny
Cill Chaoi see Kilkee
Cill Choca see Kilcock
Cill Dara see Kildare
105 N3 **Cilleruelo de Bezana** Castilla-León, N Spain
Cilli see Celje
Cill Mhantáin see Wicklow
Cill Rois see Kilrush
26 J6 **Cimarron** Kansas, C USA
37 T9 **Cimarron** New Mexico, SW USA
26 M9 **Cimarron River** ≈ Kansas/Oklahoma, C USA
117 N11 **Cimişlia** Rus. Chimishliya. S Moldova
Cîmpia Turzii see Câmpia Turzii
Cîmpina see Câmpina
Cîmpulung see Câmpulung
Cîmpulung Moldovenesc see Câmpulung Moldovenesc
137 P15 **Çınar** Diyarbakır, SE Turkey
54 J8 **Cinaruco, Río** ≈ Colombia/Venezuela
Cina Selatan, Laut see South China Sea
105 T5 **Cinca** ≈ NE Spain
112 G13 **Cincar** ▲ SW Bosnia and Herzegovina
31 Q15 **Cincinnati** Ohio, N USA
21 M4 **Cincinnati** × Kentucky, S USA
Cinco de Outubro see Xá-Muteba
136 C15 **Çine** Aydın, SW Turkey
99 J21 **Ciney** Namur, SE Belgium
104 H6 **Cinfães** Viseu, N Portugal
106 J12 **Cingoli** Marche, C Italy
41 U16 **Cintalapa** var. Cintalapa de Figueroa. Chiapas, SE Mexico
Cintalapa de Figueroa see Cintalapa
103 X14 **Cinto, Monte** ▲ Corse, France, C Mediterranean Sea
Cintra see Sintra
105 Q5 **Cintruénigo** Navarra, N Spain
Cionn tSáile see Kinsale
116 K13 **Ciorani** Prahova, SE Romania
113 E14 **Čiovo** It. Bua. island S Croatia
Cipiúr see Kippure
63 I15 **Cipolletti** Río Negro, C Argentina
120 L7 **Circeo, Capo** headland C Italy
39 S8 **Circle** var. Circle City. Alaska, USA
33 X8 **Circle** Montana, NW USA
Circle City see Circle
31 S14 **Circleville** Ohio, N USA
36 K6 **Circleville** Utah, W USA
169 P16 **Cirebon** prev. Tjirebon. Jawa, S Indonesia
97 L21 **Cirencester** anc. Corinium, Corinium Dobunorum. C England, UK
Cirkvenica see Crikvenica
107 O20 **Ciro** Calabria, SW Italy
107 O20 **Ciro Marina** Calabria, S Italy
102 K14 **Ciron** ≈ SW France
Cirquenizza see Crikvenica
25 R7 **Cisco** Texas, SW USA
116 I12 **Cisnădie** Ger. Heltau, Hung. Nagydisznód. Sibiu, SW Romania
63 G18 **Cisnes, Río** ≈ S Chile
25 T11 **Cistern** Texas, SW USA
104 L3 **Cistierna** Castilla-León, N Spain
Citharista see la Ciotat
Citlaltépetl see Orizaba, Volcán Pico de
55 X10 **Citron** NW French Guiana
23 N7 **Citronelle** Alabama, S USA
35 O7 **Citrus Heights** California, W USA
106 H7 **Cittadella** Veneto, NE Italy
106 H13 **Città della Pieve** Umbria, C Italy
106 H12 **Città di Castello** Umbria, C Italy
107 I14 **Cittaducale** Lazio, C Italy
107 N22 **Cittanova** Calabria, SW Italy

◆ Country
● Country Capital
◇ Dependent Territory
○ Dependent Territory Capital
◈ Administrative Region
× International Airport
▲ Mountain
⛰ Mountain Range
Ѫ Volcano
≈ River
◎ Lake
⊡ Reservoir

Cittavecchia see Starigrad
116 G10 **Ciucea** *Hung.* Csucsa. Cluj, NW Romania
116 M13 **Ciucurova** Tulcea, SE Romania
Ciudad Acuña see Villa Acuña
41 N15 **Ciudad Altamirano** Guerrero, S Mexico
42 G7 **Ciudad Barrios** San Miguel, NE El Salvador
54 I7 **Ciudad Bolívar** Barinas, NW Venezuela
55 N7 **Ciudad Bolívar** *prev.* Angostura. Bolívar, E Venezuela
40 K6 **Ciudad Camargo** Chihuahua, N Mexico
40 E8 **Ciudad Constitución** Baja California Sur, W Mexico
Ciudad Cortés see Cortés
41 V17 **Ciudad Cuauhtémoc** Chiapas, SE Mexico
42 J9 **Ciudad Darío** *var.* Dario. Matagalpa, W Nicaragua
Ciudad de Dolores Hidalgo see Dolores Hidalgo
42 C6 **Ciudad de Guatemala** *Eng.* Guatemala City; *prev.* Santiago de los Caballeros. ● (Guatemala) Guatemala, C Guatemala
Ciudad del Carmen see Carmen
62 Q6 **Ciudad del Este** *prev.* Cuidad Presidente Stroessner, Presidente Stroessner, Puerto Presidente Stroessner. Alto Paraná, SE Paraguay
62 K5 **Ciudad de Libertador General San Martín** *var.* Libertador General San Martín. Jujuy, C Argentina
Ciudad Delicias see Delicias
41 O11 **Ciudad del Maíz** San Luis Potosí, C Mexico
Ciudad de México see México
54 J7 **Ciudad de Nutrias** Barinas, NW Venezuela
Ciudad de Panamá see Panamá
55 P7 **Ciudad Guayana** *prev.* San Tomé de Guayana, Santo Tomé de Guayana. Bolívar, NE Venezuela
40 K14 **Ciudad Guzmán** Jalisco, SW Mexico
41 V17 **Ciudad Hidalgo** Chiapas, SE Mexico
41 N14 **Ciudad Hidalgo** Michoacán de Ocampo, SW Mexico
40 J3 **Ciudad Juárez** Chihuahua, N Mexico
40 L8 **Ciudad Lerdo** Durango, C Mexico
41 Q11 **Ciudad Madero** *var.* Villa Cecilia. Tamaulipas, C Mexico
41 P11 **Ciudad Mante** Tamaulipas, C Mexico
42 F2 **Ciudad Melchor de Mencos** *var.* Melchor de Mencos. Petén, NE Guatemala
41 P8 **Ciudad Miguel Alemán** Tamaulipas, C Mexico
Ciudad Mutis see Bahía Solano
40 G6 **Ciudad Obregón** Sonora, NW Mexico
54 I5 **Ciudad Ojeda** Zulia, NW Venezuela
55 P7 **Ciudad Piar** Bolívar, E Venezuela
Ciudad Porfirio Díaz see Piedras Negras
Ciudad Quesada see Quesada
105 N11 **Ciudad Real** Castilla-La Mancha, C Spain
105 N11 **Ciudad Real** ◆ *province* Castilla-La Mancha, C Spain
104 J7 **Ciudad-Rodrigo** Castilla-León, N Spain
42 A6 **Ciudad Tecún Umán** San Marcos, SW Guatemala
Ciudad Trujillo see Santo Domingo
41 P12 **Ciudad Valles** San Luis Potosí, C Mexico
41 O10 **Ciudad Victoria** Tamaulipas, C Mexico
42 C6 **Ciudad Vieja** Suchitepéquez, S Guatemala
116 L8 **Ciuhuru** *var.* Reuţel. ≈ N Moldova
Ciutadella see Ciutadella de Menorca
105 Z8 **Ciutadella de Menorca** *var.* Ciutadella. Menorca, Spain, W Mediterranean Sea
136 L11 **Civa Burnu** *headland* N Turkey
106 J7 **Cividale del Friuli** Friuli-Venezia Giulia, NE Italy
107 H14 **Civita Castellana** Lazio, C Italy
106 J12 **Civitanova Marche** Marche, C Italy
Civitas Altae Ripae see Brzeg
Civitas Carnutum see Chartres
Civitas Eburovicum see Évreux
Civitas Nemetum see Speyer
107 G15 **Civitavecchia** *anc.* Centum Cellae, Trajani Portus. Lazio, C Italy
102 L10 **Civray** Vienne, W France
136 E14 **Çivril** Denizli, W Turkey
161 O5 **Cixian** Hebei, E China
137 R16 **Cizre** Şırnak, SE Turkey
Clacton see Clacton-on-Sea
97 Q21 **Clacton-on-Sea** *var.* Clacton. E England, UK
22 H5 **Claiborne, Lake** ⊟ Louisiana, S USA
102 L10 **Clain** ≈ W France
11 Q11 **Claire, Lake** ◎ Alberta, C Canada
25 O6 **Clairemont** Texas, SW USA
34 M3 **Clair Engle Lake** ⊟ California, W USA
18 B15 **Clairton** Pennsylvania, NE USA
32 F7 **Clallam Bay** Washington, NW USA
103 P8 **Clamecy** Nièvre, C France
25 P5 **Clanton** Alabama, S USA
61 D17 **Clara** Entre Ríos, E Argentina
97 E18 **Clara** *Ir.* Clóirtheach. C Ireland
29 T9 **Clara City** Minnesota, N USA
61 D23 **Claraz** Buenos Aires, E Argentina
Clár Chlainne Mhuiris see Claremorris
182 I8 **Clare** South Australia
97 C19 **Clare** *Ir.* An Clár. *cultural region* W Ireland
97 C18 **Clare** ≈ W Ireland
97 A16 **Clare Island** *Ir.* Cliara. *island* W Ireland
44 J12 **Claremont** C Jamaica
29 W10 **Claremont** Minnesota, N USA
19 N9 **Claremont** New Hampshire, NE USA
27 Q9 **Claremore** Oklahoma, C USA
97 C17 **Claremorris** *Ir.* Clár Chlainne Mhuiris. W Ireland
185 J16 **Clarence** Canterbury, South Island, NZ
185 J16 **Clarence** ≈ South Island, NZ
65 F15 **Clarence Bay** *bay* Ascension Island, C Atlantic Ocean
63 H25 **Clarence, Isla** *island* S Chile
194 H2 **Clarence Island** *island* South Shetland Islands, Antarctica
183 V5 **Clarence River** ≈ New South Wales, SE Australia
44 J5 **Clarence Town** Long Island, C Bahamas
27 W12 **Clarendon** Arkansas, C USA
25 O3 **Clarendon** Texas, SW USA
13 U12 **Clarenville** Newfoundland, SE Canada
11 Q17 **Claresholm** Alberta, SW Canada
29 T16 **Clarinda** Iowa, C USA
55 N5 **Clarines** Anzoátegui, NE Venezuela
29 V12 **Clarion** Iowa, C USA
18 C13 **Clarion** Pennsylvania, NE USA
193 O6 **Clarion Fracture Zone** *tectonic feature* NE Pacific Ocean
18 D13 **Clarion River** ≈ Pennsylvania, NE USA
29 Q9 **Clark** South Dakota, N USA
36 K11 **Clarkdale** Arizona, SW USA
15 W4 **Clarke City** Quebec, SE Canada
183 Q15 **Clarke Island** *island* Furneaux Group, Tasmania, SE Australia
181 X6 **Clarke Range** ▲▲ Queensland, E Australia
23 T2 **Clarkesville** Georgia, SE USA
29 S9 **Clarkfield** Minnesota, N USA
33 N7 **Clark Fork** Idaho, NW USA
33 N8 **Clark Fork** ≈ Idaho/Montana, NW USA
39 Q12 **Clark, Lake** ◎ Alaska, USA
35 W12 **Clark Mountain** ▲ California, W USA
37 S3 **Clark Peak** ▲ Colorado, C USA
14 D14 **Clark, Point** *headland* Ontario, S Canada
21 S3 **Clarksburg** West Virginia, NE USA
22 K2 **Clarksdale** Mississippi, S USA
33 U12 **Clarks Fork Yellowstone River** ≈ Montana/Wyoming, NW USA
21 P13 **Clark Hill Lake** *var.* J.Storm Thurmond Reservoir. ⊟ Georgia/South Carolina, SE USA
29 R14 **Clarkson** Nebraska, C USA
39 O13 **Clarks Point** Alaska, USA
18 I13 **Clarks Summit** Pennsylvania, NE USA
32 M10 **Clarkston** Washington, NW USA
44 J12 **Clark's Town** C Jamaica
27 T10 **Clarksville** Arkansas, C USA
31 P13 **Clarksville** Indiana, N USA
20 I8 **Clarksville** Tennessee, S USA
25 W5 **Clarksville** Texas, SW USA
21 U8 **Clarksville** Virginia, NE USA
21 U11 **Clarkton** North Carolina, SE USA
61 C24 **Claromecó** *var.* Balneario Claromecó. Buenos Aires, E Argentina
25 N3 **Claude** Texas, SW USA
Clausentum see Southampton
171 O1 **Claveria** Luzon, N Philippines
99 J20 **Clavier** Liège, E Belgium
23 W6 **Claxton** Georgia, SE USA
21 R4 **Clay** West Virginia, NE USA
27 N3 **Clay Center** Kansas, C USA
29 P16 **Clay Center** Nebraska, C USA
21 Y2 **Claymont** Delaware, NE USA
36 M14 **Claypool** Arizona, SW USA
23 R6 **Clayton** Alabama, S USA
23 T1 **Clayton** Georgia, SE USA
22 J5 **Clayton** Louisiana, S USA
27 X5 **Clayton** Missouri, C USA
37 V9 **Clayton** New Mexico, SW USA
21 V9 **Clayton** North Carolina, SE USA
27 Q12 **Clayton** Oklahoma, C USA
182 I4 **Clayton River** *seasonal river* South Australia
21 R7 **Claytor Lake** ⊟ Virginia, NE USA
27 P13 **Clear Boggy Creek** ≈ Oklahoma, C USA
97 B22 **Clear, Cape** *var.* The Bill of Cape Clear, *Ir.* Ceann Cléire. *headland* SW Ireland
36 M12 **Clear Creek** ≈ Arizona, SW USA
39 S12 **Cleare, Cape** *headland* Montague Island, Alaska, USA
18 E13 **Clearfield** Pennsylvania, NE USA
36 L2 **Clearfield** Utah, W USA
25 Q6 **Clear Fork Brazos River** ≈ Texas, SW USA
31 T12 **Clear Fork Reservoir** ⊟ Ohio, N USA
11 N12 **Clear Hills** ▲▲ Alberta, SW Canada
29 V12 **Clear Lake** Iowa, C USA
29 R9 **Clear Lake** South Dakota, N USA
34 M6 **Clear Lake** ◎ California, W USA
22 G6 **Clear Lake** ⊟ Louisiana, S USA
34 M6 **Clearlake** California, W USA
35 P1 **Clear Lake Reservoir** ⊟ California, W USA
11 N16 **Clearwater** British Columbia, SW Canada
23 U12 **Clearwater** Florida, SE USA
11 R12 **Clearwater** ≈ Alberta/Saskatchewan, C Canada
27 W7 **Clearwater Lake** ⊟ Missouri, C USA
33 N10 **Clearwater Mountains** ▲▲ Idaho, NW USA
33 N10 **Clearwater River** ≈ Idaho, NW USA
29 S4 **Clearwater River** ≈ Minnesota, N USA
25 T7 **Cleburne** Texas, SW USA
32 I9 **Cle Elum** Washington, NW USA
97 O17 **Cleethorpes** E England, UK
Cléire, Ceann see Clear, Cape
21 O11 **Clemson** South Carolina, SE USA
21 Q4 **Clendenin** West Virginia, NE USA
26 M9 **Cleo Springs** Oklahoma, C USA
Clerk Island see Onotoa
181 X8 **Clermont** Queensland, E Australia
15 S8 **Clermont** Quebec, SE Canada
103 O4 **Clermont** Oise, N France
29 X12 **Clermont** Iowa, C USA
103 P11 **Clermont-Ferrand** Puy-de-Dôme, C France
103 Q15 **Clermont-l'Hérault** Hérault, S France
99 M22 **Clervaux** Diekirch, N Luxembourg
106 G6 **Cles** Trentino-Alto Adige, N Italy
182 H8 **Cleve** South Australia
Cleve see Kleve
23 T2 **Cleveland** Georgia, SE USA
22 K3 **Cleveland** Mississippi, S USA
31 T11 **Cleveland** Ohio, N USA
27 O9 **Cleveland** Oklahoma, C USA
20 L10 **Cleveland** Tennessee, S USA
25 W10 **Cleveland** Texas, SW USA
31 N7 **Cleveland** Wisconsin, N USA
31 O4 **Cleveland Cliffs Basin** ◎ Michigan, N USA
31 U11 **Cleveland Heights** Ohio, N USA
33 P6 **Cleveland, Mount** ▲ Montana, NW USA
Cleves see Kleve
97 B16 **Clew Bay** *Ir.* Cuan Mó. *inlet* W Ireland
23 Y14 **Clewiston** Florida, SE USA
Cliara see Clare Island
97 A17 **Clifden** *Ir.* An Clochán. W Ireland
37 O14 **Clifton** Arizona, SW USA
18 K14 **Clifton** New Jersey, NE USA
25 S8 **Clifton** Texas, SW USA
21 S6 **Clifton Forge** Virginia, NE USA
182 I1 **Clifton Hills** South Australia
11 S17 **Climax** Saskatchewan, S Canada
21 O8 **Clinch River** ≈ Tennessee/Virginia, S USA
25 P12 **Cline** Texas, SW USA
21 N10 **Clingmans Dome** ▲ North Carolina/Tennessee, SE USA
24 H8 **Clint** Texas, SW USA
10 M16 **Clinton** British Columbia, SW Canada
14 E15 **Clinton** Ontario, S Canada
27 U10 **Clinton** Arkansas, C USA
30 L10 **Clinton** Illinois, N USA
29 Z14 **Clinton** Iowa, C USA
20 G7 **Clinton** Kentucky, S USA
22 J8 **Clinton** Louisiana, S USA
19 N11 **Clinton** Massachusetts, NE USA
31 R10 **Clinton** Michigan, N USA
22 K5 **Clinton** Mississippi, S USA
27 S5 **Clinton** Missouri, C USA
21 V10 **Clinton** North Carolina, SE USA
26 L10 **Clinton** Oklahoma, C USA
21 Q12 **Clinton** South Carolina, SE USA
21 M9 **Clinton** Tennessee, S USA
8 L9 **Clinton-Colden Lake** ◎ Northwest Territories, NW Canada
10 H5 **Clinton Creek** Yukon Territory, NW Canada
30 L13 **Clinton Lake** ⊟ Illinois, N USA
27 Q4 **Clinton Lake** ⊟ Kansas, N USA
21 T11 **Clio** South Carolina, SE USA
193 O7 **Clipperton Fracture Zone** *tectonic feature* E Pacific Ocean
193 Q7 **Clipperton Island** ◇ *French dependency of French Polynesia* E Pacific Ocean
46 K6 **Clipperton Island** *island* E Pacific Ocean
(0) F16 **Clipperton Seamounts** *undersea feature* E Pacific Ocean
102 J8 **Clisson** Loire-Atlantique, NW France
62 K7 **Clodomira** Santiago del Estero, N Argentina
Cloich na Coillte see Clonakilty
Clóirtheach see Clara
97 C21 **Clonakilty** *Ir.* Cloich na Coillte. SW Ireland
181 T6 **Cloncurry** Queensland, C Australia
97 F18 **Clondalkin** *Ir.* Cluain Dolcáin. E Ireland
97 E16 **Clones** *Ir.* Cluain Eois. N Ireland
97 D20 **Clonmel** *Ir.* Cluain Meala. S Ireland
100 G11 **Cloppenburg** Niedersachsen, NW Germany
29 W6 **Cloquet** Minnesota, N USA
37 S14 **Cloudcroft** New Mexico, SW USA
33 W12 **Cloud Peak** ▲ Wyoming, C USA
185 K14 **Cloudy Bay** *inlet* South Island, NZ
21 R10 **Clover** South Carolina, SE USA
34 M6 **Cloverdale** California, W USA
20 J5 **Cloverport** Kentucky, S USA
35 Q10 **Clovis** California, W USA
37 W12 **Clovis** New Mexico, SW USA
14 K13 **Cloyne** Ontario, SE Canada
Cluain Dolcáin see Clondalkin
Cluain Eois see Clones
Cluainín see Manorhamilton
Cluain Meala see Clonmel
116 H10 **Cluj** ◆ *county* NW Romania
Cluj see Cluj-Napoca
116 H10 **Cluj-Napoca** *Ger.* Klausenburg, *Hung.* Kolozsvár; *prev.* Cluj. Cluj, NW Romania
Clunia see Feldkirch
103 R10 **Cluny** Saône-et-Loire, C France
103 T10 **Cluses** Haute-Savoie, E France
106 E7 **Clusone** Lombardia, N Italy
25 W12 **Clute** Texas, SW USA
185 D23 **Clutha** ≈ South Island, NZ
97 J18 **Clwyd** *cultural region* NE Wales, UK
185 D22 **Clyde** Otago, South Island, NZ
27 N3 **Clyde** Kansas, C USA
29 P2 **Clyde** North Dakota, N USA
31 S11 **Clyde** Ohio, N USA
25 Q7 **Clyde** Texas, SW USA
14 K13 **Clyde** ≈ Ontario, SE Canada
96 J13 **Clyde** ≈ W Scotland, UK
96 H12 **Clydebank** S Scotland, UK
96 H13 **Clyde, Firth of** *inlet* S Scotland, UK
33 S11 **Clyde Park** Montana, NW USA
104 I7 **Côa, Rio** ≈ N Portugal
35 W16 **Coachella** California, W USA
35 W16 **Coachella Canal** *canal* California, W USA
40 I9 **Coacoyole** Durango, C Mexico
25 N7 **Coahoma** Texas, SW USA
10 K8 **Coal** ≈ Yukon Territory, NW Canada
40 L14 **Coalcomán** *var.* Coalcomán de Matamoros. Michoacán de Ocampo, S Mexico
Coalcomán de Matamoros see Coalcomán
39 T8 **Coal Creek** Alaska, USA
11 Q17 **Coaldale** Alberta, SW Canada
27 P12 **Coalgate** Oklahoma, C USA
35 P11 **Coalinga** California, W USA
10 L9 **Coal River** British Columbia, W Canada
21 Q6 **Coal River** ≈ West Virginia, NE USA
36 M2 **Coalville** Utah, W USA
58 E13 **Coari** Amazonas, N Brazil
59 D14 **Coari, Rio** ≈ NW Brazil
81 J20 **Coast** ◆ *province* SE Kenya
Coast see Pwani
8 G12 **Coast Mountains** *Fr.* Chaîne Côtière. ▲▲ Canada/USA
16 C7 **Coast Ranges** ▲▲ W USA
96 I12 **Coatbridge** S Scotland, UK
42 B6 **Coatepeque** Quezaltenango, SW Guatemala
18 H16 **Coatesville** Pennsylvania, NE USA
15 Q13 **Coaticook** Quebec, SE Canada
9 P9 **Coats Island** *island* Nunavut, NE Canada
195 O4 **Coats Land** *physical region* Antarctica
41 T14 **Coatzacoalcos** *var.* Quetzalcoalco; *prev.* Puerto México. Veracruz-Llave, E Mexico
41 S14 **Coatzacoalcos, Río** ≈ SE Mexico
116 M15 **Cobadin** Constanţa, SW Romania
14 H9 **Cobalt** Ontario, S Canada
42 D5 **Cobán** Alta Verapaz, C Guatemala
183 O6 **Cobar** New South Wales, SE Australia
18 F12 **Cobb Hill** ▲ Pennsylvania, NE USA
(0) D8 **Cobb Seamount** *undersea feature* E Pacific Ocean
14 K12 **Cobden** Ontario, SE Canada
97 D21 **Cobh** *Ir.* An Cóbh; *prev.* Cove of Cork, Queenstown. SW Ireland
57 J14 **Cobija** Pando, NW Bolivia
Coblence/Coblenz see Koblenz
18 J10 **Cobleskill** New York, NE USA
14 I15 **Cobourg** Ontario, SE Canada
181 P1 **Cobourg Peninsula** *headland* Northern Territory, N Australia
183 O10 **Cobram** Victoria, SE Australia
82 N13 **Cóbuè** Niassa, N Mozambique
101 K18 **Coburg** Bayern, SE Germany
19 Q5 **Coburn Mountain** ▲ Maine, NE USA
Coca see Puerto Francisco de Orellana
57 H18 **Cocachacra** Arequipa, SW Peru
59 J17 **Cocalinho** Mato Grosso, W Brazil
Cocanada see Kākināda
105 S11 **Cocentaina** País Valenciano, E Spain
57 L18 **Cochabamba** *hist.* Oropeza. Cochabamba, C Bolivia
57 K18 **Cochabamba** ◆ *department* C Bolivia
57 L18 **Cochabamba, Cordillera de** ▲▲ C Bolivia
101 E18 **Cochem** Rheinland-Pfalz, W Germany
37 R6 **Cochetopa Hills** ▲▲ Colorado, C USA
155 G22 **Cochin** *var.* Kochi. Kerala, SW India
44 D5 **Cochinos, Bahía de** *Eng.* Bay of Pigs. *bay* SE Cuba
37 O16 **Cochise Head** ▲ Arizona, SW USA
23 U5 **Cochran** Georgia, SE USA
11 P16 **Cochrane** Alberta, SW Canada
12 G12 **Cochrane** Ontario, S Canada
63 G20 **Cochrane** Aisén, S Chile
11 U10 **Cochrane** ≈ Manitoba/Saskatchewan, C Canada
Cochrane, Lago see Pueyrredón, Lago
Cocibolca see Nicaragua, Lago de
Cockade State see Maryland
44 M6 **Cockburn Harbour** South Caicos, S Turks and Caicos Islands
14 C11 **Cockburn Island** *island* Ontario, S Canada
44 J3 **Cockburn Town** San Salvador, E Bahamas
21 X2 **Cockeysville** Maryland, NE USA
181 N12 **Cocklebiddy** Western Australia
44 I12 **Cockpit Country, The** *physical region* W Jamaica
43 S16 **Coclé** *off.* Provincia de Coclé. ◆ *province* C Panama
43 S15 **Coclé del Norte** Colón, C Panama
23 Y12 **Cocoa** Florida, SE USA
23 Y12 **Cocoa Beach** Florida, SE USA
79 D17 **Cocobeach** Estuaire, NW Gabon
44 G5 **Coco, Cayo** *island* C Cuba
151 Q19 **Coco Channel** *strait* Andaman Sea/Bay of Bengal
173 N6 **Coco-de-Mer Seamounts** *undersea feature* W Indian Ocean
36 K10 **Coconino Plateau** *plain* Arizona, SW USA
43 N6 **Coco, Río** *var.* Río Wanki, Segoviao Wangkí. ≈ Honduras/Nicaragua
173 T8 **Cocos (Keeling) Islands** ◇ *Australian external territory* E Indian Ocean
173 T7 **Cocos Basin** *undersea feature* E Indian Ocean
188 B17 **Cocos Island** *island* S Guam
Cocos Island Ridge see Cocos Ridge
131 S17 **Cocos Islands** *island group* E Indian Ocean
(0) G15 **Cocos Plate** *tectonic feature*
193 T7 **Cocos Ridge** *var.* Cocos Island Ridge. *undersea feature* E Pacific Ocean
40 K13 **Cocula** Jalisco, SW Mexico
107 D17 **Coda Cavallo, Capo** *headland* Sardegna, Italy, C Mediterranean Sea
58 E13 **Codajás** Amazonas, N Brazil
Codazzi see Agustín Codazzi
19 Q12 **Cod, Cape** *headland* Massachusetts, NE USA
185 B25 **Codfish Island** *island* SW NZ
106 H9 **Codigoro** Emilia-Romagna, N Italy
13 P5 **Cod Island** *island* Newfoundland, E Canada
116 J12 **Codlea** *Ger.* Zeiden, *Hung.* Feketehalom. Braşov, C Romania
58 M13 **Codó** Maranhão, E Brazil
106 E8 **Codogno** Lombardia, N Italy
116 M10 **Codrii** *hill range* C Moldova
45 W9 **Codrington** Barbuda, Antigua and Barbuda
106 J7 **Codroipo** Friuli-Venezia Giulia, NE Italy
28 M12 **Cody** Nebraska, C USA
33 U12 **Cody** Wyoming, C USA
21 P7 **Coeburn** Virginia, NE USA
54 E10 **Coello** Tolima, W Colombia
Coemba see Cuemba
181 V2 **Coen** Queensland, NE Australia
101 E14 **Coesfeld** Nordrhein-Westfalen, W Germany
32 M8 **Coeur d'Alene** Idaho, NW USA
32 M8 **Coeur d'Alene Lake** ⊟ Idaho, NW USA
98 O8 **Coevorden** Drenthe, NE Netherlands
10 H6 **Coffee Creek** Yukon Territory, W Canada
30 L15 **Coffeen Lake** ⊟ Illinois, N USA
22 L3 **Coffeeville** Mississippi, S USA
27 Q8 **Coffeyville** Kansas, C USA
182 G9 **Coffin Bay** South Australia
182 F9 **Coffin Bay Peninsula** *peninsula* South Australia
183 V5 **Coffs Harbour** New South Wales, SE Australia
105 R10 **Cofrentes** País Valenciano, E Spain
Cogîlnic see Kohyl'nyk
102 K11 **Cognac** *anc.* Compniacum. Charente, W France
106 B7 **Cogne** Valle d'Aosta, NW Italy
103 U16 **Cogolin** Var, SE France
105 O7 **Cogolludo** Castilla-La Mancha, C Spain
Cohalm see Rupea
92 L8 **Čohkará##a** *var.* Cuokkarašša. ▲ N Norway
F11 **Cohocton River** ≈ New York, NE USA
18 L10 **Cohoes** New York, NE USA
183 N10 **Cohuna** Victoria, SE Australia
43 P17 **Coiba, Isla de** *island* SW Panama
63 H23 **Coig, Río** ≈ S Argentina
63 G19 **Coihaique** *var.* Coyhaique. Aisén, S Chile
155 G21 **Coimbatore** Tamil Nādu, S India
104 G8 **Coimbra** *anc.* Conimbria, Conimbriga. Coimbra, W Portugal
104 G8 **Coimbra** ◆ *district* N Portugal
104 L15 **Coín** Andalucía, S Spain
57 J20 **Coipasa, Laguna** ◎ W Bolivia
57 J20 **Coipasa, Salar de** *salt lake* W Bolivia
Coira/Coire see Chur
Coirib, Loch see Corrib, Lough
54 K6 **Cojedes** *off.* Estado Cojedes. ◆ *state* N Venezuela
42 F7 **Cojutepeque** Cuscatlán, C El Salvador
33 S16 **Cokeville** Wyoming, C USA
182 M13 **Colac** Victoria, SE Australia
59 O20 **Colatina** Espírito Santo, SE Brazil
27 O13 **Colbert** Oklahoma, C USA
100 L12 **Colbitz-Letzinger Heide** *heathland* N Germany
26 I3 **Colby** Kansas, C USA
57 H17 **Colca, Río** ≈ SW Peru
97 P21 **Colchester** *hist.* Colneceaste, *anc.* Camulodunum. E England, UK
19 N13 **Colchester** Connecticut, NE USA
38 M16 **Cold Bay** Alaska, USA
11 R14 **Cold Lake** Alberta, SW Canada
11 R13 **Cold Lake** ◎ Alberta/Saskatchewan, S Canada
29 U8 **Cold Spring** Minnesota, N USA
25 W10 **Coldspring** Texas, SW USA
11 N17 **Coldstream** British Columbia, SW Canada
96 L13 **Coldstream** SE Scotland, UK
14 H13 **Coldwater** Ontario, S Canada
26 K7 **Coldwater** Kansas, C USA
31 Q10 **Coldwater** Michigan, N USA
25 N1 **Coldwater Creek** ≈ Oklahoma/Texas, SW USA
22 K2 **Coldwater River** ≈ Mississippi, S USA
183 O9 **Coleambally** New South Wales, SE Australia
19 O6 **Colebrook** New Hampshire, NE USA
27 T5 **Cole Camp** Missouri, C USA
39 T6 **Coleen River** ≈ Alaska, USA
11 P17 **Coleman** Alberta, SW Canada
25 Q8 **Coleman** Texas, SW USA
Çölemerik see Hakkâri
83 K22 **Colenso** KwaZulu/Natal, E South Africa
182 L12 **Coleraine** Victoria, SE Australia
97 F14 **Coleraine** *Ir.* Cúil Raithin. N Northern Ireland, UK
185 G18 **Coleridge, Lake** ◎ South Island, NZ
83 H24 **Colesberg** Northern Cape, C South Africa
22 H7 **Colfax** Louisiana, S USA
32 L9 **Colfax** Washington, NW USA
30 J6 **Colfax** Wisconsin, N USA
63 I19 **Colhué Huapí, Lago** ◎ S Argentina
45 Z6 **Colibris, Pointe des** *headland* Grande Terre, E Guadeloupe
106 D6 **Colico** Lombardia, N Italy
99 E14 **Colijnsplaat** Zeeland, SW Netherlands
40 L14 **Colima** Colima, S Mexico
40 K14 **Colima** ◆ *state* SW Mexico
40 L14 **Colima, Nevado de** ⛰ C Mexico
59 M14 **Colinas** Maranhão, E Brazil
96 F10 **Coll** *island* W Scotland, UK
105 N7 **Collado Villalba** *var.* Villalba. Madrid, C Spain
183 R4 **Collarenebri** New South Wales, SE Australia
37 P5 **Collbran** Colorado, C USA
106 G12 **Colle di Val d'Elsa** Toscana, C Italy
39 R9 **College** Alaska, USA
32 K10 **College Place** Washington, NW USA
25 U10 **College Station** Texas, SW USA
183 P4 **Collerina** New South Wales, SE Australia
180 I13 **Collie** Western Australia
180 L4 **Collier Bay** *bay* Western Australia
21 F10 **Collierville** Tennessee, S USA
106 F11 **Collina, Passo della** *pass* C Italy
14 G14 **Collingwood** Ontario, S Canada
184 I13 **Collingwood** Tasman, South Island, NZ
22 L7 **Collins** Mississippi, S USA
30 K15 **Collinsville** Illinois, N USA
27 P9 **Collinsville** Oklahoma, C USA
20 H10 **Collinwood** Tennessee, S USA
Collipo see Leiria
63 G14 **Collipulli** Araucanía, C Chile
97 D16 **Collooney** *Ir.* Cúil Mhuine. NW Ireland
29 R10 **Colman** South Dakota, N USA
103 U6 **Colmar** *Ger.* Kolmar. Haut-Rhin, NE France
104 M15 **Colmenar** Andalucía, S Spain
Colmenar see Colmenar de Oreja
105 O9 **Colmenar de Oreja** *var.* Colmenar. Madrid, C Spain
105 N7 **Colmenar Viejo** Madrid, C Spain
25 X9 **Colmesneil** Texas, SW USA
Cöln see Köln
Colneceaste see Colchester

◆ COUNTRY ● COUNTRY CAPITAL ◇ DEPENDENT TERRITORY ○ DEPENDENT TERRITORY CAPITAL ◆ ADMINISTRATIVE REGION ✕ INTERNATIONAL AIRPORT ▲ MOUNTAIN ▲▲ MOUNTAIN RANGE ⛰ VOLCANO ≈ RIVER ◎ LAKE ⊟ RESERVOIR

40 C3 Colnet Baja California, NW Mexico
59 G15 Colniza Mato Grosso, W Brazil
Cologne see Köln
42 B6 Colomba Quezaltenango, SW Guatemala
Colomb-Béchar see Béchar
54 E11 Colombia Huila, C Colombia
54 G10 Colombia off. Republic of Colombia. ◆ republic N South America
64 E12 Colombian Basin undersea feature SW Caribbean Sea
Colombie-Britannique see British Columbia
15 T6 Colombier Quebec, SE Canada
155 J25 Colombo ● (Sri Lanka) Western Province, W Sri Lanka
155 J25 Colombo × Western Province, SW Sri Lanka
29 N11 Colome South Dakota, N USA
61 D18 Colon Entre Ríos, E Argentina
61 B19 Colón Buenos Aires, E Argentina
44 D5 Colón Matanzas, C Cuba
43 T14 Colón prev. Aspinwall. Colón, C Panama
42 K5 Colón ◐ department NE Honduras
43 S15 Colón off. Provincia de Colón. ◐ province N Panama
57 A16 Colón, Archipiélago de var. Islas de los Galápagos, Eng. Galapagos Islands, Tortoise Islands. island group Ecuador, E Pacific Ocean
44 K5 Colonel Hill Crooked Island, SE Bahamas
40 B3 Colonet, Cabo headland NW Mexico
188 G14 Colonia Yap, W Micronesia
61 D19 Colonia ◐ department SW Uruguay
Colonia see Kolonia, Micronesia
Colonia see Colonia del Sacramento, Uruguay
Colonia Agrippina see Köln
61 D20 Colonia del Sacramento var. Colonia. Colonia, SW Uruguay
62 L8 Colonia Dora Santiago del Estero, N Argentina
Colonia Julia Fanestris see Fano
21 W5 Colonial Beach Virginia, NE USA
21 V6 Colonial Heights Virginia, NE USA
193 S7 Colón Ridge undersea feature E Pacific Ocean
96 F12 Colonsay island W Scotland, UK
57 K22 Colorada, Laguna ⊚ SW Bolivia
37 R6 Colorado off. State of Colorado; also known as Centennial State, Silver State. ◐ state C USA
63 H22 Colorado, Cerro ▲ S Argentina
25 O7 Colorado City Texas, SW USA
36 M7 Colorado Plateau plateau W USA
61 A24 Colorado, Río ~ E Argentina
43 N12 Colorado, Río ~ NE Costa Rica
Colorado, Río see Colorado River
16 F12 Colorado River var. Río Colorado. ~ Mexico/USA
16 K14 Colorado River ~ Texas, SW USA
35 W15 Colorado River Aqueduct aqueduct California, W USA
44 A4 Colorados, Archipiélago de los island group NW Cuba
62 J9 Colorados, Desagües de los ⊚ W Argentina
37 T5 Colorado Springs Colorado, C USA
40 L11 Colotlán Jalisco, SW Mexico
57 L19 Colquechaca Potosí, C Bolivia
23 S7 Colquitt Georgia, SE USA
29 R11 Colton South Dakota, N USA
32 M10 Colton Washington, NW USA
35 P8 Columbia California, W USA
30 K16 Columbia Illinois, N USA
20 L7 Columbia Kentucky, S USA
22 I6 Columbia Louisiana, S USA
21 W3 Columbia Maryland, NE USA
22 L7 Columbia Mississippi, S USA
27 U4 Columbia Missouri, C USA
21 Y9 Columbia North Carolina, SE USA
18 G16 Columbia Pennsylvania, NE USA
21 Q12 Columbia state capital South Carolina, SE USA
20 I9 Columbia Tennessee, S USA
(0) F9 Columbia ~ Canada/USA
32 K9 Columbia Basin basin Washington, NW USA
197 Q10 Columbia, Cape headland Ellesmere Island, Nunavut, NE Canada
31 Q12 Columbia City Indiana, N USA
21 W3 Columbia, District of ◐ federal district NE USA
33 P7 Columbia Falls Montana, NW USA
11 O15 Columbia Icefield icefield Alberta/British Columbia, S Canada
11 O15 Columbia, Mount ▲ Alberta/British Columbia, SW Canada
11 N15 Columbia Mountains ▲ British Columbia, SW Canada
23 P4 Columbiana Alabama, S USA
31 V12 Columbiana Ohio, N USA
32 M14 Columbia Plateau plateau Idaho/Oregon, NW USA
29 P7 Columbia Road Reservoir ⊠ South Dakota, N USA
65 K16 Columbia Seamount undersea feature C Atlantic Ocean
83 D25 Columbine, Cape headland SW South Africa
105 U9 Columbretes, Islas island group E Spain
23 R5 Columbus Georgia, SE USA
31 P14 Columbus Indiana, N USA
27 R7 Columbus Kansas, C USA
23 N4 Columbus Mississippi, S USA
33 U11 Columbus Montana, NW USA
29 Q15 Columbus Nebraska, C USA
37 Q16 Columbus New Mexico, SW USA
21 P10 Columbus North Carolina, SE USA
28 K2 Columbus North Dakota, N USA
31 S13 Columbus state capital Ohio, N USA
25 U11 Columbus Texas, SW USA
30 L8 Columbus Wisconsin, N USA
31 R12 Columbus Grove Ohio, N USA
29 Y15 Columbus Junction Iowa, C USA
44 J3 Columbus Point headland Cat Island, C Bahamas
35 T8 Columbus Salt Marsh salt marsh Nevada, W USA
35 N6 Colusa California, W USA
32 L7 Colville Washington, NW USA
184 M5 Colville, Cape headland North Island, NZ
184 M5 Colville Channel channel North Island, NZ
39 P6 Colville River ~ Alaska, USA
97 J18 Colwyn Bay N Wales, UK
106 H9 Comacchio var. Commachio; anc. Comactium. Emilia-Romagna, N Italy
106 H9 Comacchio, Valli di lagoon Adriatic Sea, N Mediterranean Sea
Comactium see Comacchio
41 V17 Comalapa Chiapas, SE Mexico
41 U15 Comalcalco Tabasco, SE Mexico
63 H16 Comallo Río Negro, SW Argentina
26 M12 Comanche Oklahoma, C USA
25 R8 Comanche Texas, SW USA
194 H2 Comandante Ferraz Brazilian research station Antarctica
62 N6 Comandante Fontana Formosa, N Argentina
63 I22 Comandante Luis Peidra Buena Santa Cruz, S Argentina
59 O18 Comandatuba Bahia, SE Brazil
116 K11 Comănești Hung. Kománfalva. Bacău, SW Romania
57 M19 Comarapa Santa Cruz, C Bolivia
116 J13 Comarnic Prahova, SE Romania
42 H6 Comayagua Comayagua, W Honduras
42 H6 Comayagua ◐ department W Honduras
42 I6 Comayagua, Montañas de ▲ C Honduras
21 R15 Combahee River ~ South Carolina, SE USA
62 G10 Combarbalá Coquimbo, C Chile
103 S7 Combeaufontaine Haute-Saône, E France
97 G15 Comber Ir. An Comar. E Northern Ireland, UK
99 K20 Comblain-au-Pont Liège, E Belgium
102 I6 Combourg Ille-et-Vilaine, NW France
44 M9 Comendador prev. Elías Piña. W Dominican Republic
Comer See see Como, Lago di
25 R11 Comfort Texas, SW USA
153 V15 Comilla Ben. Kumillā. Chittagong, E Bangladesh
99 B18 Comines Hainaut, W Belgium
121 O15 Comino Malt. Kemmuna. island C Malta
107 D18 Comino, Capo headland Sardegna, Italy, C Mediterranean Sea
107 K25 Comiso Sicilia, Italy, C Mediterranean Sea
41 V16 Comitán var. Comitán de Domínguez. Chiapas, SE Mexico
Comitán de Domínguez see Comitán
Commachio see Comacchio
Commander Islands see Komandorskiye Ostrova
103 O10 Commentry Allier, C France
23 T2 Commerce Georgia, SE USA
27 R8 Commerce Oklahoma, C USA
25 V5 Commerce Texas, SW USA
37 T4 Commerce City Colorado, C USA
103 S5 Commercy Meuse, NE France
55 W9 Commewijne var. Commewyne. ◐ district NE Suriname
Commewyne see Commewijne
15 P8 Commissaires, Lac des ⊚ Quebec, SE Canada
64 A12 Commissioner's Point headland W Bermuda
9 O7 Committee Bay bay Nunavut, N Canada
106 D7 Como anc. Comum. Lombardia, N Italy
63 J19 Comodoro Rivadavia Chubut, SE Argentina
106 D6 Como, Lago di var. Lario, Eng. Lake Como, Ger. Comer See. ⊚ N Italy
Como, Lake see Como, Lago di
40 E7 Comondú Baja California Sur, W Mexico
116 F12 Comorâște Hung. Komornok. Caraș-Severin, SW Romania
Comores, République Fédérale Islamique des see Comoros
155 G24 Comorin, Cape headland SE India
172 M8 Comoro Basin undersea feature SW Indian Ocean
172 I14 Comoro Islands island group W Indian Ocean
172 H13 Comoros off. Federal Islamic Republic of the Comoros, Fr. République Fédérale Islamique des Comores. ◆ republic W Indian Ocean
10 L17 Comox Vancouver Island, British Columbia, SW Canada
103 O4 Compiègne Oise, N France
Complutum see Alcalá de Henares
Compniacum see Cognac
40 K12 Compostela Nayarit, C Mexico
Compostella see Santiago
60 L11 Comprida, Ilha island S Brazil
117 N11 Comrat Rus. Komrat. S Moldova
25 O11 Comstock Texas, SW USA
31 P9 Comstock Park Michigan, N USA
193 N3 Comstock Seamount undersea feature N Pacific Ocean
Comum see Como
159 N17 Cona Xizang Zizhiqu, W China
76 H14 Conakry ● (Guinea) Conakry, SW Guinea
76 H14 Conakry × Conakry, SW Guinea
Conamara see Connemara
Conca see Cuenca
25 Q12 Concan Texas, SW USA
102 F6 Concarneau Finistère, NW France
83 O17 Conceição Sofala, C Mozambique
59 K15 Conceição do Araguaia Pará, NE Brazil
58 F10 Conceição do Maú Roraima, W Brazil
61 D14 Concepción var. Concepcion. Corrientes, NE Argentina
62 J8 Concepción Tucumán, N Argentina
57 O17 Concepción Santa Cruz, E Bolivia
62 G13 Concepción Bío Bío, C Chile
54 E14 Concepción Putumayo, S Colombia
62 O5 Concepción var. Villa Concepción. Concepción, C Paraguay
62 O5 Concepción off. Departamento de Concepción. ◐ department E Paraguay
Concepción see La Concepción
Concepción de la Vega see La Vega
41 N9 Concepción del Oro Zacatecas, C Mexico
61 D18 Concepción del Uruguay Entre Ríos, E Argentina
42 K11 Concepción, Volcán ⛰ SW Nicaragua
44 J4 Conception Island island C Bahamas
35 P14 Conception, Point headland California, W USA
54 H6 Concha Zulia, W Venezuela
60 L9 Conchas São Paulo, S Brazil
37 U11 Conchas Dam New Mexico, SW USA
37 U10 Conchas Lake ⊠ New Mexico, SW USA
102 M5 Conches-en-Ouche Eure, N France
37 N12 Concho Arizona, SW USA
40 J5 Conchos, Río ~ NW Mexico
41 O8 Conchos, Río ~ C Mexico
108 C8 Concise Vaud, W Switzerland
35 N8 Concord California, W USA
19 O9 Concord state capital New Hampshire, NE USA
21 R10 Concord North Carolina, SE USA
61 D17 Concordia Entre Ríos, E Argentina
54 D9 Concordia Antioquia, W Colombia
40 J10 Concordia Sinaloa, C Mexico
57 I19 Concordia Tacna, SW Peru
27 N3 Concordia Kansas, C USA
27 S4 Concordia Missouri, C USA
60 I13 Concórdia Santa Catarina, S Brazil
167 S7 Con Cuông Nghê An, N Vietnam
167 T15 Côn Đao var. Con Son. island S Vietnam
Condate see St-Claude, Jura, France
Condate see Rennes, Ille-et-Vilaine, France
Condate see Montereau-Faut-Yonne, Seine-St-Denis, France
29 P8 Conde South Dakota, N USA
42 J8 Condega Estelí, NW Nicaragua
103 P2 Condé-sur-l'Escaut Nord, N France
102 K5 Condé-sur-Noireau Calvados, N France
Condivincum see Nantes
183 P8 Condobolin New South Wales, SE Australia
102 L15 Condom Gers, S France
32 J11 Condon Oregon, NW USA
54 D9 Condoto Chocó, W Colombia
23 P7 Conecuh River ~ Alabama/Florida, SE USA
106 H7 Conegliano Veneto, NE Italy
61 C19 Conesa Buenos Aires, E Argentina
14 F15 Conestogo ~ Ontario, S Canada
Confluentes see Koblenz
102 L10 Confolens Charente, W France
36 J4 Confusion Range ▲ Utah, W USA
62 N6 Confuso, Río ~ C Paraguay
21 R12 Congaree River ~ South Carolina, SE USA
Công Hoa Xa Hôi Chu Nghia Viêt Nam see Vietnam
160 K12 Congjiang prev. Bingmei. Guizhou, S China
79 K19 Congo off. Democratic Republic of Congo; prev. Zaire, Belgian Congo, Congo (Kinshasa). ◆ republic C Africa
79 G18 Congo off. Republic of the Congo, Fr. Moyen-Congo; prev. Middle Congo. ◆ republic C Africa
67 T11 Congo var. Kongo, Fr. Zaire. ~ C Africa
Congo see Zaire (province, Angola)
Congo/Congo (Kinshasa) see Congo (Democratic Republic of)
79 K18 Congo Basin drainage basin W Dem. Rep. Congo (Zaire)
67 Q11 Congo Canyon var. Congo Seavalley, Congo Submarine Canyon. undersea feature E Atlantic Ocean
Congo Cone see Congo Fan
65 P15 Congo Fan var. Congo Cone. undersea feature E Atlantic Ocean
Coni see Cuneo
63 H18 Cónico, Cerro ▲ SW Argentina
Conimbria/Conimbriga see Coimbra
Conjeeveram see Kānchīpuram
11 R13 Conklin Alberta, C Canada
24 M1 Conlen Texas, SW USA
Con, Loch see Conn, Lough
Connacht see Connaught
97 B17 Connaught var. Connacht, Ir. Chonnacht, Cúige. cultural region W Ireland
31 V10 Conneaut Ohio, N USA
18 L13 Connecticut off. State of Connecticut; also known as Blue Law State, Constitution State, Land of Steady Habits, Nutmeg State. ◐ state NE USA
19 N8 Connecticut ~ Canada/USA
19 O6 Connecticut Lakes lakes New Hampshire, NE USA
32 K9 Connell Washington, NW USA
97 B17 Connemara Ir. Conamara. region W Ireland
31 Q14 Connersville Indiana, N USA
97 B16 Conn, Lough Ir. Loch Con. ⊚ W Ireland
35 X6 Connors Pass pass Nevada, W USA
181 X7 Connors Range ▲ Queensland, E Australia
56 E7 Cononaco, Río ~ E Ecuador
29 W13 Conrad Iowa, C USA
33 R7 Conrad Montana, NW USA
25 W10 Conroe Texas, SW USA
25 V10 Conroe, Lake ⊠ Texas, SW USA
61 C17 Conscripto Bernardi Entre Ríos, E Argentina
59 M20 Conselheiro Lafaiete Minas Gerais, SE Brazil
Consentia see Cosenza
97 L14 Consett N England, UK
44 B5 Consolación del Sur Pinar del Río, W Cuba
Con Son see Côn Đao
11 R15 Consort Alberta, SW Canada
Constance see Konstanz
108 I6 Constance, Lake Ger. Bodensee. ⊚ C Europe
104 G9 Constância Santarém, C Portugal
117 N14 Constanța var. Küstendje, Eng. Constanza, Ger. Konstanza, Turk. Küstence. Constanța, SE Romania
116 L14 Constanța ◐ county SE Romania
Constantia see Coutances, France
Constantia see Konstanz, Germany
104 K13 Constantina Andalucía, S Spain
74 L5 Constantine var. Qacentina, Ar. Qoussantîna. NE Algeria
39 O14 Constantine, Cape headland Alaska, USA
Constantinople see İstanbul
Constantiola see Oltenișa
Constanz see Konstanz
Constanza see Constanța
62 G13 Constitución Maule, C Chile
61 D17 Constitución Salto, N Uruguay
Constitution State see Connecticut
105 N10 Consuegra Castilla-La Mancha, C Spain
181 X9 Consuelo Peak ▲ Queensland, E Australia
56 E11 Contamana Loreto, N Peru
Contrasto, Colle del see Contrasto, Portella del
107 K23 Contrasto, Portella del var. Colle del Contrasto. pass Sicilia, Italy, C Mediterranean Sea
54 G8 Contratación Santander, C Colombia
102 M8 Contres Loir-et-Cher, C France
107 O17 Conversano Puglia, SE Italy
27 U11 Conway Arkansas, C USA
19 O8 Conway New Hampshire, NE USA
21 U13 Conway South Carolina, SE USA
25 N2 Conway Texas, SW USA
27 U11 Conway, Lake ⊠ Arkansas, C USA
27 N7 Conway Springs Kansas, C USA
97 J18 Conwy N Wales, UK
23 T3 Conyers Georgia, SE USA
Coo see Kos
182 F4 Coober Pedy South Australia
181 P2 Cooinda Northern Territory, N Australia
182 B6 Cook South Australia
29 W4 Cook Minnesota, N USA
191 N6 Cook, Baie de bay Moorea, W French Polynesia
10 J16 Cook, Cape headland Vancouver Island, British Columbia, SW Canada
37 Q15 Cookes Peak ▲ New Mexico, SW USA
20 L8 Cookeville Tennessee, S USA
175 P9 Cook Fracture Zone tectonic feature S Pacific Ocean
Cook, Grand Récif de see Cook, Récif de
39 Q12 Cook Inlet inlet Alaska, USA
191 X2 Cook Island island Line Islands, E Kiribati
190 J14 Cook Islands ◇ territory in free association with NZ S Pacific Ocean
185 E19 Cook, Mount prev. Aoraki, Aorangi. ▲ South Island, NZ
187 O15 Cook, Récif de var. Grand Récif de Cook. reef S New Caledonia
14 G14 Cookstown Ontario, S Canada
97 F15 Cookstown Ir. An Chorr Chríochach. C Northern Ireland, UK
185 K14 Cook Strait var. Raukawa. strait NZ
181 W3 Cooktown Queensland, NE Australia
183 P6 Coolabah New South Wales, SE Australia
182 J11 Coola Coola Swamp wetland South Australia
183 S7 Coolah New South Wales, SE Australia
183 P9 Coolamon New South Wales, SE Australia
183 T4 Coolatai New South Wales, SE Australia
180 K12 Coolgardie Western Australia
36 L14 Coolidge Arizona, SW USA
25 U8 Coolidge Texas, SW USA
183 Q11 Cooma New South Wales, SE Australia
Coomassie see Kumasi
183 R6 Coonabarabran New South Wales, SE Australia
182 J10 Coonalpyn South Australia
183 R6 Coonamble New South Wales, SE Australia
Coondapoor see Kundāpura
155 G21 Coonoor Tamil Nādu, SE India
29 U14 Coon Rapids Iowa, C USA
29 V8 Coon Rapids Minnesota, N USA
25 V5 Cooper Texas, SW USA
181 U9 Cooper Creek var. Barcoo, Cooper's Creek. seasonal river Queensland/South Australia
39 R12 Cooper Landing Alaska, USA
21 T14 Cooper River ~ South Carolina, SE USA
Cooper's Creek see Cooper Creek
44 H1 Coopers Town Great Abaco, N Bahamas
18 J10 Cooperstown New York, NE USA
29 P4 Cooperstown North Dakota, N USA
31 P9 Coopersville Michigan, N USA
182 D7 Coorabie South Australia
23 Q3 Coosa River ~ Alabama/Georgia, S USA
32 E14 Coos Bay Oregon, NW USA
183 Q9 Cootamundra New South Wales, SE Australia
97 E16 Cootehill Ir. Muinchille. N Ireland
Čop see Chop
57 J17 Copacabana La Paz, W Bolivia
63 H14 Copahué, Volcán ▲ C Chile
41 U16 Copainalá Chiapas, SE Mexico
32 F8 Copalis Beach Washington, NW USA
42 F6 Copán ◐ department W Honduras
Copán see Copán Ruinas
25 T14 Copano Bay bay NW Gulf of Mexico
42 F6 Copán Ruinas var. Copán. Copán, W Honduras
Copenhagen see København
107 Q19 Copertino Puglia, SE Italy
62 H7 Copiapó Atacama, N Chile
62 G8 Copiapó, Bahía bay N Chile
62 G7 Copiapó, Río ~ N Chile
114 M12 Çöpköy Edirne, NW Turkey
182 I5 Copley South Australia
106 H9 Copparo Emilia-Romagna, C Italy
55 V10 Coppename Rivier var. Koppename. ~ C Suriname
25 S9 Copperas Cove Texas, SW USA
82 J13 Copperbelt ◐ province C Zambia
39 S11 Copper Center Alaska, USA
Coppermine see Kugluktuk
8 K8 Coppermine ~ Northwest Territories/Nunavut, N Canada
39 T11 Copper River ~ Alaska, USA
Copper State see Arizona
116 I11 Copșa Mică Ger. Kleinkopisch, Hung. Kiskapus. Sibiu, C Romania
158 J14 Coqên Xizang Zizhiqu, W China
Coquilhatville see Mbandaka
32 E14 Coquille Oregon, NW USA
62 G9 Coquimbo Coquimbo, N Chile
62 G9 Coquimbo off. Región de Coquimbo. ◐ region C Chile
116 I15 Corabia Olt, S Romania
57 F17 Coracora Ayacucho, SW Peru
Cora Droma Rúisc see Carrick-on-Shannon
44 K9 Corail SW Haiti
183 V4 Coraki New South Wales, SE Australia
180 G8 Coral Bay Western Australia
23 Y16 Coral Gables Florida, SE USA
9 P8 Coral Harbour Southampton Island, Northwest Territories, NE Canada
192 I9 Coral Sea sea SW Pacific Ocean
174 M7 Coral Sea Basin undersea feature N Coral Sea
192 H9 Coral Sea Islands ◇ Australian external territory SW Pacific Ocean
182 M12 Corangamite, Lake ⊚ Victoria, SE Australia
Corantijn Rivier see Courantyne River
18 B14 Coraopolis Pennsylvania, NE USA
107 N17 Corato Puglia, SE Italy
103 O17 Corbières ▲ S France
103 P8 Corbigny Nièvre, C France
21 N7 Corbin Kentucky, S USA
104 L14 Corbones ~ SW Spain
Corcaigh see Cork
35 R11 Corcoran California, W USA
47 T14 Corcovado, Golfo gulf S Chile
63 G18 Corcovado, Volcán ▲ S Chile
104 F3 Corcubión Galicia, NW Spain
Corcyra Nigra see Korčula
60 Q9 Cordeiro Rio de Janeiro, SE Brazil
23 T6 Cordele Georgia, SE USA
26 L11 Cordell Oklahoma, C USA
103 N14 Cordes Tarn, S France
62 O6 Cordillera off. Departamento de la Cordillera. ◐ department C Paraguay
182 K1 Cordillo Downs South Australia
62 K10 Córdoba Córdoba, C Argentina
41 R14 Córdoba Veracruz-Llave, E Mexico
104 M13 Córdoba var. Cordoba, Eng. Cordova; anc. Corduba. Andalucía, SW Spain
62 K11 Córdoba off. Provincia de Córdoba. ◐ province C Argentina
54 D7 Córdoba off. Departamento de Córdoba. ◐ province NW Colombia
104 L13 Córdoba ◐ province Andalucía, S Spain
62 K10 Córdoba, Sierras de ▲ C Argentina
23 O3 Cordova Alabama, S USA
39 S12 Cordova Alaska, USA
Cordova/Corduba see Córdoba
Corentyne River see Courantyne River
Corfu see Kérkyra
104 J9 Coria Extremadura, W Spain
104 J14 Coria del Río Andalucía, S Spain
183 S8 Coricudgy, Mount ▲ New South Wales, SE Australia
107 N20 Corigliano Calabro Calabria, SW Italy
Corinium/Corinium Dobunorum see Cirencester
23 N1 Corinth Mississippi, S USA
Corinth see Kórinthos
Corinth Canal see Dióryga Korinthou
Corinth, Gulf of/Corinthiacus Sinus see Korinthiakós Kólpos
Corinthus see Kórinthos
42 I9 Corinto Chinandega, NW Nicaragua
97 C21 Cork Ir. Corcaigh. S Ireland
97 C21 Cork Ir. Corcaigh. cultural region SW Ireland
97 C21 Cork × SW Ireland
97 D21 Cork Harbour Ir. Cuan Chorcaí. inlet SW Ireland
107 I23 Corleone Sicilia, Italy, C Mediterranean Sea
114 N13 Çorlu Tekirdağ, NW Turkey
114 N12 Çorlu Çayı ~ NW Turkey
Cormaiore see Courmayeur
11 V13 Cormorant Manitoba, C Canada
23 T2 Cornelia Georgia, SE USA
60 J10 Cornélio Procópio Paraná, S Brazil
55 V9 Corneliskondre Sipaliwini, N Suriname
30 J5 Cornell Wisconsin, N USA
13 S12 Corner Brook Newfoundland, E Canada
Corner Rise Seamounts see Corner Seamounts
64 I9 Corner Seamounts var. Corner Rise Seamounts. undersea feature NW Atlantic Ocean
116 M9 Cornești Rus. Korneshty. C Moldova
Corneto see Tarquinia
Cornhusker State see Nebraska
27 X8 Corning Arkansas, C USA
35 N5 Corning California, W USA
29 U15 Corning Iowa, C USA
18 G11 Corning New York, NE USA
Corn Islands see Maíz, Islas del
107 J14 Corno Grande ▲ C Italy
15 N13 Cornwall Ontario, SE Canada
97 H25 Cornwall cultural region SW England, UK
97 G25 Cornwall, Cape headland SW England, UK
54 J4 Coro prev. Santa Ana de Coro. Falcón, NW Venezuela
57 J18 Corocoro La Paz, W Bolivia
57 K17 Coroico La Paz, W Bolivia
184 M5 Coromandel Waikato, North Island, NZ
155 K20 Coromandel Coast coast E India
184 M5 Coromandel Peninsula peninsula North Island, NZ

184 M6 **Coromandel Range** ▲ North Island, NZ
171 N5 **Coron** Busuanga Island, W Philippines
35 T15 **Corona** California, W USA
37 T12 **Corona** New Mexico, SW USA
11 U17 **Coronach** Saskatchewan, S Canada
35 U17 **Coronado** California, W USA
43 N15 **Coronado, Bahía de** *bay* S Costa Rica
11 R15 **Coronation** Alberta, SW Canada
8 K7 **Coronation Gulf** *gulf* Nunavut, N Canada
194 I1 **Coronation Island** *island* Antarctica
39 X14 **Coronation Island** *island* Alexander Archipelago, Alaska, USA
61 B18 **Coronda** Santa Fe, C Argentina
63 F14 **Coronel** Bío Bío, C Chile
61 D20 **Coronel Brandsen** *var.* Brandsen. Buenos Aires, E Argentina
62 K4 **Coronel Cornejo** Salta, N Argentina
61 B24 **Coronel Dorrego** Buenos Aires, E Argentina
62 P6 **Coronel Oviedo** Caaguazú, SE Paraguay
61 B23 **Coronel Pringles** Buenos Aires, E Argentina
61 B23 **Coronel Suárez** Buenos Aires, E Argentina
61 E22 **Coronel Vidal** Buenos Aires, E Argentina
55 V9 **Coronie** ◈ *district* NW Suriname
57 G17 **Coropuna, Nevado** ▲ S Peru
Çorovoda *see* Çorovodë
113 L22 **Çorovodë** *var.* Çorovoda. Berat, S Albania
183 P11 **Corowa** New South Wales, SE Australia
42 G1 **Corozal** Corozal, N Belize
54 E6 **Corozal** Sucre, NW Colombia
42 G1 **Corozal** ◈ *district* N Belize
25 T14 **Corpus Christi** Texas, SW USA
25 T14 **Corpus Christi Bay** *inlet* Texas, SW USA
25 R14 **Corpus Christi, Lake** ▣ Texas, SW USA
63 F16 **Corral** Los Lagos, C Chile
105 O9 **Corral de Almaguer** Castilla-La Mancha, C Spain
104 K6 **Corrales** Castilla-León, N Spain
37 R11 **Corrales** New Mexico, SW USA
Corrán Tuathail *see* Carrauntoohil
106 F9 **Correggio** Emilia-Romagna, C Italy
59 M16 **Corrente** Piauí, E Brazil
59 I19 **Correntes, Rio** ≈ SW Brazil
103 N12 **Corrèze** ◈ *department* C France
97 C17 **Corrib, Lough** *Ir.* Loch Coirib. ◎ W Ireland
61 C14 **Corrientes** Corrientes, NE Argentina
61 D15 **Corrientes** *off.* Provincia de Corrientes. ◈ *province* NE Argentina
44 A5 **Corrientes, Cabo** *headland* W Cuba
40 I13 **Corrientes, Cabo** *headland* SW Mexico
Corrientes, Provincia de *see* Corrientes
61 C16 **Corrientes, Río** ≈ NE Argentina
56 E8 **Corrientes, Río** ≈ Ecuador/Peru
25 W9 **Corrigan** Texas, SW USA
55 U9 **Corriverton** E Guyana
Corriza *see* Korçë
183 Q11 **Corryong** Victoria, SE Australia
103 Y12 **Corse** *Eng.* Corsica. ◈ *region* France, C Mediterranean Sea
103 X13 **Corse** *Eng.* Corsica. *island* France, C Mediterranean Sea
105 Y13 **Corse, Cap** *headland* Corse, France, C Mediterranean Sea
105 X15 **Corse-du-Sud** ◈ *department* Corse, France, C Mediterranean Sea
29 P11 **Corsica** South Dakota, N USA
Corsica *see* Corse
25 U7 **Corsicana** Texas, SW USA
103 Y15 **Corte** Corse, France, C Mediterranean Sea
63 G16 **Corte Alto** Los Lagos, S Chile
104 I13 **Cortegana** Andalucía, S Spain
43 N15 **Cortés** *var.* Ciudad Cortés. Puntarenas, SE Costa Rica
42 G5 **Cortés** ◈ *department* NW Honduras
37 P8 **Cortez** Colorado, C USA
Cortez, Sea of *see* California, Golfo de
106 H6 **Cortina d'Ampezzo** Veneto, NE Italy
18 H11 **Cortland** New York, NE USA
31 V11 **Cortland** Ohio, N USA
106 H12 **Cortona** Toscana, C Italy
76 H13 **Corubal, Rio** ≈ E Guinea-Bissau
104 G10 **Coruche** Santarém, C Portugal
Çoruh *see* Rize
137 R11 **Çoruh Nehri** *Geor.* Chorokhi, *Rus.* Chorokh. ≈ Georgia/Turkey
136 K12 **Çorum** *var.* Chorum. Çorum, N Turkey
136 J12 **Çorum** *var.* Chorum. ◈ *province* N Turkey
59 H19 **Corumbá** Mato Grosso do Sul, S Brazil
14 D16 **Corunna** Ontario, S Canada
Corunna *see* A Coruña
32 F12 **Corvallis** Oregon, NW USA
64 M1 **Corvo** *var.* Ilha do Corvo. *island* Azores, Portugal, NE Atlantic Ocean
Corvo, Ilha do *see* Corvo
31 O16 **Corydon** Indiana, N USA
29 V16 **Corydon** Iowa, C USA
Cos *see* Kos
40 I9 **Cosalá** Sinaloa, C Mexico
41 R15 **Cosamaloapan** *var.* Cosamaloapan de Carpio. Veracruz-Llave, E Mexico
Cosamaloapan de Carpio *see* Cosamaloapan
107 N21 **Cosenza** *anc.* Consentia. Calabria, SW Italy
31 T13 **Coshocton** Ohio, N USA
42 H9 **Cosigüina, Punta** *headland* NW Nicaragua
29 T9 **Cosmos** Minnesota, N USA
103 O8 **Cosne-sur-Loire** Nièvre, C France
108 B9 **Cossonay** Vaud, W Switzerland
Cossyra *see* Pantelleria
47 R4 **Costa, Cordillera de la** *var.* Cordillera de Venezuela. ▲ N Venezuela
42 K13 **Costa Rica** *off.* Republic of Costa Rica. ◆ *republic* Central America
43 N15 **Costeña, Fila** ▲ S Costa Rica
Costermansville *see* Bukavu
116 I14 **Costeşti** Argeş, SW Romania
37 S8 **Costilla** New Mexico, SW USA
35 O7 **Cosumnes River** ≈ California, W USA
101 O16 **Coswig** Sachsen, E Germany
101 M14 **Coswig** Sachsen-Anhalt, E Germany
Cosyra *see* Pantelleria
171 Q7 **Cotabato** Mindanao, S Philippines
56 C5 **Cotacachi** ▲ N Ecuador
57 L21 **Cotagaita** Potosí, S Bolivia
103 V15 **Côte d'Azur** *prev.* Nice. ✕ (Nice) Alpes-Maritimes, SE France
Côte d'Ivoire *see* Ivory Coast
103 R8 **Côte d'Or** *cultural region* C France
103 R7 **Côte d'Or** ◈ *department* E France
Côte Française des Somalis *see* Djibouti
102 J4 **Cotentin** *peninsula* N France
102 G6 **Côtes d'Armor** *prev.* Côtes-du-Nord. ◈ *department* NW France
Côtes-du-Nord *see* Côtes d'Armor
Cöthen *see* Köthen
Côtière, Chaîne *see* Coast Mountains
40 M13 **Cotija** *var.* Cotija de la Paz. Michoacán de Ocampo, SW Mexico
Cotija de la Paz *see* Cotija
77 R16 **Cotonou** *var.* Kotonu. S Benin
77 R16 **Cotonou** ✕ S Benin
56 B6 **Cotopaxi** *prev.* León. ◈ *province* C Ecuador
56 C6 **Cotopaxi** ⛰ N Ecuador
Cotrone *see* Crotone
97 L21 **Cotswold Hills** *var.* Cotswolds. *hill range* S England, UK
Cotswolds *see* Cotswold Hills
32 F13 **Cottage Grove** Oregon, NW USA
21 S14 **Cottageville** South Carolina, SE USA
101 P14 **Cottbus** *prev.* Kottbus. Brandenburg, E Germany
27 U9 **Cotter** Arkansas, C USA
106 A9 **Cottian Alps** *Fr.* Alpes Cottiennes, *It.* Alpi Cozie. ▲ France/Italy
Cottiennes, Alpes *see* Cottian Alps
Cotton State, The *see* Alabama
22 G4 **Cotton Valley** Louisiana, S USA
36 L12 **Cottonwood** Arizona, SW USA
32 M10 **Cottonwood** Idaho, NW USA
29 S9 **Cottonwood** Minnesota, N USA
25 Q7 **Cottonwood** Texas, SW USA
27 O5 **Cottonwood Falls** Kansas, C USA
36 L3 **Cottonwood Heights** Utah, W USA
29 S10 **Cottonwood River** ≈ Minnesota, N USA
45 O9 **Cotuí** C Dominican Republic
25 Q13 **Cotulla** Texas, SW USA
Cotyora *see* Ordu
102 I11 **Coubre, Pointe de la** *headland* W France
18 E12 **Coudersport** Pennsylvania, NE USA
15 S9 **Coudres, Île aux** *island* Quebec, SE Canada
182 G11 **Couedic, Cape de** *headland* South Australia
Couentrey *see* Coventry
102 I6 **Couesnon** ≈ NW France
32 H10 **Cougar** Washington, NW USA
102 L10 **Couhé** Vienne, W France
32 K8 **Coulee City** Washington, NW USA
195 Q15 **Coulman Island** *island* Antarctica
103 P5 **Coulommiers** Seine-et-Marne, N France
14 K11 **Coulonge** ≈ Quebec, SE Canada
14 K11 **Coulonge Est** ≈ Quebec, SE Canada
35 Q9 **Coulterville** California, W USA
38 M9 **Council** Alaska, USA
32 M12 **Council** Idaho, NW USA
29 S15 **Council Bluffs** Iowa, C USA
27 O5 **Council Grove** Kansas, C USA
27 O5 **Council Grove Lake** ▣ Kansas, C USA
32 G7 **Coupeville** Washington, NW USA
55 U12 **Courantyne River** *var.* Corantijn Rivier, Corentyne River. ≈ Guyana/Suriname
99 G21 **Courcelles** Hainaut, S Belgium
108 C7 **Courgenay** Jura, NW Switzerland
128 B2 **Courland Lagoon** *Ger.* Kurisches Haff, *Rus.* Kurskiy Zaliv. *lagoon* Lithuania/Russian Federation
118 B12 **Courland Spit** *Lith.* Kuršių Nerija, *Rus.* Kurshskaya Kosa. *spit* Lithuania/Russian Federation
106 A6 **Courmayeur** *prev.* Cormaiore. Valle d'Aosta, NW Italy
108 D7 **Courroux** Jura, NW Switzerland
10 K17 **Courtenay** Vancouver Island, British Columbia, SW Canada
21 W7 **Courtland** Virginia, NE USA
25 V10 **Courtney** Texas, SW USA
30 J4 **Court Oreilles, Lac** ◎ Wisconsin, N USA
Courtrai *see* Kortrijk
99 H19 **Court-Saint-Étienne** Wallon Brabant, C Belgium
22 G6 **Coushatta** Louisiana, S USA
172 I16 **Cousin** *island* Inner Islands, NE Seychelles
172 I16 **Cousine** *island* Inner Islands, NE Seychelles
102 J4 **Coutances** *anc.* Constantia. Manche, N France
102 K12 **Coutras** Gironde, SW France
45 U14 **Couva** Trinidad, Trinidad and Tobago
108 B8 **Couvet** Neuchâtel, W Switzerland
99 H22 **Couvin** Namur, S Belgium
116 K12 **Covasna** *Ger.* Kowasna, *Hung.* Kovászna. Covasna, E Romania
116 J11 **Covasna** ◈ *county* E Romania
14 E12 **Cove Island** *island* Ontario, S Canada
34 M5 **Covelo** California, W USA
97 M20 **Coventry** *anc.* Couentrey. C England, UK
Cove of Cork *see* Cobh
21 U5 **Covesville** Virginia, NE USA
104 I8 **Covilhã** Castelo Branco, E Portugal
23 T3 **Covington** Georgia, SE USA
31 N13 **Covington** Indiana, N USA
20 M3 **Covington** Kentucky, S USA
22 K8 **Covington** Louisiana, S USA
31 Q13 **Covington** Ohio, N USA
20 F9 **Covington** Tennessee, S USA
21 S6 **Covington** Virginia, NE USA
183 Q8 **Cowal, Lake** *seasonal lake* New South Wales, SE Australia
11 W15 **Cowan** Manitoba, S Canada
18 F12 **Cowanesque River** ≈ New York/Pennsylvania, NE USA
180 L12 **Cowan, Lake** ◎ Western Australia
15 P13 **Cowansville** Quebec, SE Canada
182 H8 **Cowell** South Australia
97 M23 **Cowes** S England, UK
27 Q10 **Coweta** Oklahoma, C USA
(0) D6 **Cowie Seamount** *undersea feature* NE Pacific Ocean
32 G10 **Cowlitz River** ≈ Washington, NW USA
21 Q11 **Cowpens** South Carolina, SE USA
183 R8 **Cowra** New South Wales, SE Australia
Coxen Hole *see* Roatán
59 I19 **Coxim** Mato Grosso do Sul, S Brazil
59 I19 **Coxim, Rio** ≈ SW Brazil
Coxin Hole *see* Roatán
153 V17 **Cox's Bazar** Chittagong, S Bangladesh
76 H14 **Coyah** Conakry, W Guinea
40 K5 **Coyame** Chihuahua, N Mexico
24 L9 **Coyanosa Draw** ≈ Texas, SW USA
Coyhaique *see* Coihaique
42 C7 **Coyolate, Río** ≈ S Guatemala
Coyote State *see* South Dakota
40 I10 **Coyotitán** Sinaloa, C Mexico
41 N15 **Coyuca** *var.* Coyuca de Catalán. Guerrero, S Mexico
41 O16 **Coyuca** *var.* Coyuca de Benítez. Guerrero, S Mexico
Coyuca de Benítez/Coyuca de Catalán *see* Coyuca
29 N15 **Cozad** Nebraska, C USA
Cozie, Alpi *see* Cottian Alps
Cozmeni *see* Kitsman'
40 E3 **Cozón, Cerro** ▲ NW Mexico
41 Z12 **Cozumel** Quintana Roo, E Mexico
41 Z12 **Cozumel, Isla** *island* SE Mexico
32 K8 **Crab Creek** ≈ Washington, NW USA
44 H12 **Crab Pond Point** *headland* W Jamaica
Cracovia/Cracow *see* Małopolskie
83 I25 **Cradock** Eastern Cape, S South Africa
39 Y14 **Craig** Prince of Wales Island, Alaska, USA
37 Q3 **Craig** Colorado, C USA
97 F15 **Craigavon** C Northern Ireland, UK
21 T5 **Craigsville** Virginia, NE USA
101 J21 **Crailsheim** Baden-Württemberg, S Germany
116 H14 **Craiova** Dolj, SW Romania
10 K12 **Cranberry Junction** British Columbia, SW Canada
18 J8 **Cranberry Lake** ◎ New York, NE USA
11 V13 **Cranberry Portage** Manitoba, C Canada
11 P17 **Cranbrook** British Columbia, SW Canada
30 M5 **Crandon** Wisconsin, N USA
32 K14 **Crane** Oregon, NW USA
24 M9 **Crane** Texas, SW USA
Crane *see* The Crane
25 S8 **Cranfills Gap** Texas, SW USA
19 O12 **Cranston** Rhode Island, NE USA
Cranz *see* Zelenogradsk
59 L15 **Craolândia** Tocantins, E Brazil
102 J7 **Craon** Mayenne, NW France
195 V16 **Crary, Cape** *headland* Antarctica
Crasna *see* Kraszna
32 G14 **Crater Lake** ◎ Oregon, NW USA
33 P14 **Craters of the Moon National Monument** *national park* Idaho, NW USA
59 O14 **Crateús** Ceará, E Brazil
Crathis *see* Crati
107 N20 **Crati** *anc.* Crathis. ≈ S Italy
11 U16 **Craven** Saskatchewan, S Canada
54 I8 **Cravo Norte** Arauca, E Colombia
28 J12 **Crawford** Nebraska, C USA
25 T8 **Crawford** Texas, SW USA
11 O17 **Crawford Bay** British Columbia, SW Canada
65 M19 **Crawford Seamount** *undersea feature* S Atlantic Ocean
31 O13 **Crawfordsville** Indiana, N USA
23 S9 **Crawfordville** Florida, SE USA
97 O23 **Crawley** SE England, UK
33 S10 **Crazy Mountains** ▲ Montana, NW USA
11 T11 **Cree** ≈ Saskatchewan, C Canada
37 R7 **Creede** Colorado, C USA
40 I6 **Creel** Chihuahua, N Mexico
11 S11 **Cree Lake** ◎ Saskatchewan, C Canada
11 V13 **Creighton** Saskatchewan, C Canada
29 Q13 **Creighton** Nebraska, C USA
103 O4 **Creil** Oise, N France
106 E8 **Crema** Lombardia, N Italy
106 E8 **Cremona** Lombardia, N Italy
Creole State *see* Louisiana
112 M10 **Crepaja** *Hung.* Cserépalja. Serbia, N Yugoslavia
103 O4 **Crépy-en-Valois** Oise, N France
112 B10 **Cres** *It.* Cherso. Primorje-Gorski Kotar, NW Croatia
112 A11 **Cres** *It.* Cherso; *anc.* Crexa. *island* W Croatia
32 H14 **Crescent** Oregon, NW USA
34 K1 **Crescent City** California, W USA
23 W10 **Crescent City** Florida, SE USA
167 X10 **Crescent Group** *island group* C Paracel Islands
23 W10 **Crescent Lake** ◎ Florida, SE USA
29 X11 **Cresco** Iowa, C USA
61 B18 **Crespo** Entre Ríos, E Argentina
54 E5 **Crespo** ✕ (Cartagena) Bolívar, NW Colombia
103 R13 **Crest** Drôme, E France
37 R5 **Crested Butte** Colorado, C USA
31 S12 **Crestline** Ohio, N USA
11 O17 **Creston** British Columbia, SW Canada
29 U15 **Creston** Iowa, C USA
33 V16 **Creston** Wyoming, C USA
37 S7 **Crestone Peak** ▲ Colorado, C USA
23 P8 **Crestview** Florida, SE USA
121 R10 **Cretan Trough** *undersea feature* Aegean Sea, C Mediterranean Sea
29 R16 **Crete** Nebraska, C USA
Crete *see* Kríti
103 O5 **Créteil** Val-de-Marne, N France
Crete, Sea of/Creticum, Mare *see* Kritikó Pélagos
105 X4 **Creus, Cap de** *headland* NE Spain
103 N10 **Creuse** ◈ *department* C France
102 L9 **Creuse** ≈ C France
103 T4 **Creutzwald** Moselle, NE France
105 S12 **Crevillente** País Valenciano, E Spain
97 L18 **Crewe** C England, UK
21 V7 **Crewe** Virginia, NE USA
Crexa *see* Cres
43 Q15 **Cricamola, Río** ≈ NW Panama
61 K14 **Criciúma** Santa Catarina, S Brazil
96 J11 **Crieff** C Scotland, UK
112 B10 **Crikvenica** *It.* Cirquenizza; *prev.* Cirkvenica, Crjkvenica. Primorje-Gorski Kotar, NW Croatia
Crimea/Crimean Oblast *see* Krym, Respublika
101 M16 **Crimmitschau** *var.* Krimmitschau. Sachsen, E Germany
116 G11 **Crişcior** *Hung.* Kristyor. Hunedoara, W Romania
21 Y5 **Crisfield** Maryland, NE USA
31 P3 **Crisp Point** *headland* Michigan, N USA
59 L19 **Cristalina** Goiás, C Brazil
44 J7 **Cristal, Sierra del** ▲ E Cuba
43 T14 **Cristóbal** Colón, C Panama
54 F4 **Cristóbal Colón, Pico** ▲ N Colombia
Cristur/Cristuru Săcuiesc *see* Cristuru Secuiesc
116 I11 **Cristuru Secuiesc** *prev.* Cristur, Cristuru Săcuiesc, Sitaş Cristuru, *Ger.* Kreutz, *Hung.* Székelykeresztúr, Szitás-Keresztúr. Harghita, C Romania
116 F10 **Crişul Alb** *var.* Weisse Kreisch, *Ger.* Weisse Körös, *Hung.* Fehér-Körös. ≈ Hungary/Romania
116 F10 **Crişul Negru** *Ger.* Schwarze Körös, *Hung.* Fekete-Körös. ≈ Hungary/Romania
116 G10 **Crişul Repede** *var.* Schnelle Kreisch, *Ger.* Schnelle Körös, *Hung.* Sebes-Körös. ≈ Hungary/Romania
117 N10 **Criuleni** *Rus.* Kriulyany. C Moldova
Crivadia Vulcanului *see* Vulcan
Crjkvenica *see* Crikvenica
113 O17 **Crna Gora** ▲ FYR Macedonia/Yugoslavia
Crna Gora *see* Montenegro
113 O20 **Crna Reka** ≈ S FYR Macedonia
Crni Drim *see* Black Drin
109 V10 **Črni Vrh** ▲ NE Slovenia
109 V13 **Črnomelj** *Ger.* Tschernembl. SE Slovenia
97 A17 **Croagh Patrick** *Ir.* Cruach Phádraig. ▲ W Ireland
112 D9 **Croatia** *off.* Republic of Croatia, *Ger.* Kroatien, *SCr.* Hrvatska. ◆ *republic* SE Europe
Croce, Picco di *see* Wilde Kreuzspitze
15 P8 **Croche** ≈ Quebec, SE Canada
169 V7 **Crocker, Banjaran** *var.* Crocker Range. ▲ East Malaysia
Crocker Range *see* Crocker, Banjaran
25 V9 **Crockett** Texas, SW USA
67 V14 **Crocodile** *var.* Krokodil. ≈ N South Africa
Crocodile *see* Limpopo
20 I7 **Crofton** Kentucky, S USA
29 Q12 **Crofton** Nebraska, C USA
Croia *see* Krujë
103 R16 **Croisette, Cap** *headland* SE France
102 G8 **Croisic, Pointe du** *headland* NW France
103 S13 **Croix Haute, Col de la** *pass* E France
15 U5 **Croix, Pointe à la** *headland* Quebec, SE Canada
14 F13 **Croker, Cape** *headland* Ontario, S Canada
181 P1 **Croker Island** *island* Northern Territory, N Australia
96 I8 **Cromarty** N Scotland, UK
99 M21 **Crombach** Liège, E Belgium
97 Q18 **Cromer** E England, UK
185 D22 **Cromwell** Otago, South Island, NZ
185 H16 **Cronadun** West Coast, South Island, NZ
39 O11 **Crooked Creek** Alaska, USA
44 K5 **Crooked Island** *island* SE Bahamas
44 J5 **Crooked Island Passage** *channel* SE Bahamas
32 I13 **Crooked River** ≈ Oregon, NW USA
29 R4 **Crookston** Minnesota, N USA
28 I10 **Crooks Tower** ▲ South Dakota, N USA
31 T14 **Crooksville** Ohio, N USA
183 R9 **Crookwell** New South Wales, SE Australia
14 L14 **Crosby** Ontario, SE Canada
97 K17 **Crosby** *var.* Great Crosby. NW England, UK
29 U6 **Crosby** Minnesota, N USA
28 K2 **Crosby** North Dakota, N USA
25 O5 **Crosbyton** Texas, SW USA
77 V16 **Cross** ≈ Cameroon/Nigeria
23 U10 **Cross City** Florida, SE USA
Crossen *see* Krosno Odrzańskie
27 V14 **Crossett** Arkansas, C USA
97 K15 **Cross Fell** ▲ N England, UK
11 P16 **Crossfield** Alberta, SW Canada
21 Q12 **Cross Hill** South Carolina, SE USA
19 U6 **Cross Island** *island* Maine, NE USA
11 X13 **Cross Lake** Manitoba, C Canada
22 F5 **Cross Lake** ▣ Louisiana, S USA
36 I12 **Crossman Peak** ▲ Arizona, SW USA
25 Q7 **Cross Plains** Texas, SW USA
77 V17 **Cross River** ◈ *state* SE Nigeria
20 L9 **Crossville** Tennessee, S USA
31 S8 **Croswell** Michigan, N USA
14 K13 **Crotch Lake** ◎ Ontario, SE Canada
Croton/Crotona *see* Crotone
107 O21 **Crotone** *var.* Cotrone; *anc.* Croton, Crotona. Calabria, SW Italy
33 V11 **Crow Agency** Montana, NW USA
183 U7 **Crowdy Head** *headland* New South Wales, SE Australia
25 Q4 **Crowell** Texas, SW USA
183 O6 **Crowl Creek** *seasonal river* New South Wales, SE Australia
22 H9 **Crowley** Louisiana, S USA
35 S9 **Crowley, Lake** ▣ California, W USA
27 X10 **Crowleys Ridge** *hill range* Arkansas, C USA
31 N11 **Crown Point** Indiana, N USA
37 P10 **Crownpoint** New Mexico, SW USA
33 R10 **Crow Peak** ▲ Montana, NW USA
11 P17 **Crowsnest Pass** *pass* Alberta/British Columbia, SW Canada
29 T6 **Crow Wing River** ≈ Minnesota, N USA
97 O22 **Croydon** SE England, UK
173 P11 **Crozet Basin** *undersea feature* S Indian Ocean
173 O12 **Crozet Islands** *island group* French Southern and Antarctic Territories
173 N12 **Crozet Plateau** *var.* Crozet Plateaus. *undersea feature* SW Indian Ocean
Crozet Plateaus *see* Crozet Plateau
102 E6 **Crozon** Finistère, NW France
Cruacha Dubha, Na *see* Macgillycuddy's Reeks
Cruach Phádraig *see* Croagh Patrick
116 M14 **Crucea** Constanţa, SE Romania
44 E5 **Cruces** Cienfuegos, C Cuba
107 O20 **Crucoli Torretta** Calabria, SW Italy
41 P9 **Cruillas** Tamaulipas, C Mexico
64 K9 **Cruiser Tablemount** *undersea feature* E Atlantic Ocean
61 G14 **Cruz Alta** Rio Grande do Sul, S Brazil
44 G8 **Cruz, Cabo** *headland* S Cuba
60 N9 **Cruzeiro** São Paulo, S Brazil
60 H10 **Cruzeiro do Oeste** Paraná, S Brazil
59 A15 **Cruzeiro do Sul** Acre, W Brazil
23 U11 **Crystal Bay** *bay* Florida, SE USA
182 I8 **Crystal Brook** South Australia
11 X17 **Crystal City** Manitoba, S Canada
27 X5 **Crystal City** Missouri, C USA
25 P13 **Crystal City** Texas, SW USA
30 M4 **Crystal Falls** Michigan, N USA
23 Q8 **Crystal Lake** Florida, SE USA
31 O6 **Crystal Lake** ◎ Michigan, N USA
23 V11 **Crystal River** Florida, SE USA
37 Q5 **Crystal River** ≈ Colorado, C USA
22 K6 **Crystal Springs** Mississippi, S USA
Csaca *see* Čadca
Csakathurn/Csáktornya *see* Čakovec
Csap *see* Chop
Csepén *see* Čepin
Cserépalja *see* Crepaja
Csermő *see* Cermei
Csíkszereda *see* Miercurea-Ciuc
111 L24 **Csongrád** Csongrád, SE Hungary
111 L24 **Csongrád** *off.* Csongrád Megye. ◈ *county* SE Hungary
111 H22 **Csorna** Győr-Moson-Sopron, NW Hungary
Csucsa *see* Ciucea
111 G25 **Csurgó** Somogy, SW Hungary
Csurog *see* Čurug
54 L5 **Cúa** Miranda, N Venezuela
82 C11 **Cuale** Malanje, NW Angola
67 T12 **Cuando** *var.* Kwando. ≈ S Africa
83 E15 **Cuando Cubango** *var.* Kuando-Kubango. ◈ *province* SE Angola
83 E16 **Cuangar** Cuando Cubango, S Angola
82 D11 **Cuango** Lunda Norte, NE Angola
82 C10 **Cuango** Uíge, NW Angola
82 C10 **Cuango** *var.* Kwango. ≈ Angola/Dem. Rep. Congo (Zaire) **see also** Kwango
Cuan, Loch *see* Strangford Lough
82 C12 **Cuanza** *var.* Kwanza. ≈ C Angola
82 B11 **Cuanza Norte** *var.* Kuanza Norte. ◈ *province* NE Angola
82 B12 **Cuanza Sul** *var.* Kuanza Sul. ◈ *province* NE Angola
61 E16 **Cuareim, Río** *var.* Rio Quaraí. ≈ Brazil/Uruguay **see also** Quaraí, Rio
83 D15 **Cuatir** ≈ S Angola
40 M7 **Cuatro Ciénegas** *var.* Cuatro Ciénegas de Carranza. Coahuila de Zaragoza, NE Mexico
Cuatro Ciénegas de Carranza *see* Cuatro Ciénegas
40 I6 **Cuauhtémoc** Chihuahua, N Mexico
41 P14 **Cuautla** Morelos, S Mexico
104 H12 **Cuba** Beja, S Portugal
27 W6 **Cuba** Missouri, C USA
37 R10 **Cuba** New Mexico, SW USA
44 E6 **Cuba** *off.* Republic of Cuba. ◆ *republic* W West Indies
47 O2 **Cuba** *island* W West Indies
82 B13 **Cubal** Benguela, W Angola
83 C15 **Cubango** *var.* Kuvango, *Port.* Vila Artur de Paiva, Vila da Ponte. Huíla, SW Angola
83 D16 **Cubango** *var.* Kavango, Kavengo, Kubango, Okavango, Okavanggo. ≈ S Africa **see also** Okavango
54 H8 **Cubará** Boyacá, N Colombia
136 I12 **Çubuk** Ankara, N Turkey
83 D14 **Cuchi** Cuando Cubango, C Angola
42 C5 **Cuchumatanes, Sierra de los** ▲ W Guatemala
Cuculaya, Rio *see* Kukalaya, Rio
82 E12 **Cucumbi** *prev.* Trás-os-Montes. Lunda Sul, NE Angola
54 G7 **Cúcuta** *var.* San José de Cúcuta. Norte de Santander, N Colombia
31 N9 **Cudahy** Wisconsin, N USA
155 J21 **Cuddalore** Tamil Nādu, SE India
155 I18 **Cuddapah** Andhra Pradesh, S India
104 M6 **Cuéllar** Castilla-León, N Spain
82 D13 **Cuemba** *var.* Coemba. Bié, C Angola
56 B8 **Cuenca** Azuay, S Ecuador
105 Q9 **Cuenca** *anc.* Conca. Castilla-La Mancha, C Spain
105 P9 **Cuenca** ◈ *province* Castilla-La Mancha, C Spain
40 L9 **Cuencamé** *var.* Cuencamé de Ceniceros. Durango, C Mexico
Cuencamé de Ceniceros *see* Cuencamé
105 Q8 **Cuenca, Serranía de** ▲ C Spain
Cuera *see* Chur
105 P5 **Cuerda del Pozo, Embalse de la** ▣ N Spain
41 O14 **Cuernavaca** Morelos, S Mexico
25 T12 **Cuero** Texas, SW USA
44 I7 **Cueto** Holguín, E Cuba
41 Q13 **Cuetzalán** *var.* Cuetzalán del Progreso. Puebla, S Mexico
Cuetzalán del Progreso *see* Cuetzalán

◆ Country ● Country Capital ◇ Dependent Territory ○ Dependent Territory Capital ◈ Administrative Region ✕ International Airport ▲ Mountain ▲ Mountain Range ⛰ Volcano ≈ River ◎ Lake ▣ Reservoir

105 Q14 **Cuevas de Almanzora** Andalucía, S Spain
105 T8 **Cuevas de Vinromá** País Valenciano, E Spain
116 H12 **Cugir** *Hung.* Kudzsir. Alba, SW Romania
59 H18 **Cuiabá** *prev.* Cuyabá. *state capital* Mato Grosso, SW Brazil
59 H19 **Cuiabá, Rio** ≈ SW Brazil
41 R15 **Cuicatlán** *var.* San Juan Bautista Cuicatlán. Oaxaca, SE Mexico
191 W16 **Cuidado, Punta** *headland* Easter Island, Chile, E Pacific Ocean
Cuidad Presidente Stroessner *see* Ciudad del Este
Cúige *see* Connaught
Cúige Laighean *see* Leinster
Cúige Mumhan *see* Munster
98 L13 **Cuijck** Noord-Brabant, SE Netherlands
Cúil an tSúdaire *see* Portarlington
42 D7 **Cuilapa** Santa Rosa, S Guatemala
42 B5 **Cuilco, Río** ≈ W Guatemala
Cúil Mhuine *see* Collooney
Cúil Raithin *see* Coleraine
83 C14 **Cuima** Huambo, C Angola
83 E16 **Cuito** *var.* Kwito. ≈ SE Angola
83 E15 **Cuíto Cuanavale** Cuando Cubango, E Angola
41 N14 **Cuitzeo, Lago de** ◎ C Mexico
27 W4 **Cuivre River** ≈ Missouri, C USA
Çuka *see* Çukë
168 L8 **Cukai** *var.* Chukai, Kemaman. Terengganu, Peninsular Malaysia
113 L23 **Çukë** *var.* Çuka. Vlorë, S Albania
Cularo *see* Grenoble
33 Y7 **Culbertson** Montana, NW USA
28 M16 **Culbertson** Nebraska, C USA
183 P10 **Culcairn** New South Wales, SE Australia
45 W5 **Culebra** *var.* Dewey. E Puerto Rico
45 W6 **Culebra, Isla de** *island* E Puerto Rico
37 T8 **Culebra Peak** ▲ Colorado, C USA
104 J5 **Culebra, Sierra de la** ▲▲ NW Spain
98 J12 **Culemborg** Gelderland, C Netherlands
137 V14 **Culfa** *Rus.* Dzhul'fa. SW Azerbaijan
183 P4 **Culgoa River** ≈ New South Wales/Queensland, SE Australia
40 I9 **Culiacán** *var.* Culiacán Rosales, Culiacán-Rosales. Sinaloa, C Mexico
Culiacán-Rosales/Culiacán Rosales *see* Culiacán
105 P14 **Cúllar-Baza** Andalucía, S Spain
105 S10 **Cullera** País Valenciano, E Spain
23 P3 **Cullman** Alabama, S USA
108 B10 **Cully** Vaud, W Switzerland
Culm *see* Chełmno
Culmsee *see* Chełmża
21 V4 **Culpeper** Virginia, NE USA
185 I17 **Culverden** Canterbury, South Island, NZ
55 N5 **Cumaná** Sucre, NE Venezuela
55 O5 **Cumanacoa** Sucre, NE Venezuela
54 C13 **Cumbal, Nevado de** *elevation* S Colombia
21 O7 **Cumberland** Kentucky, S USA
21 U2 **Cumberland** Maryland, NE USA
21 V6 **Cumberland** Virginia, NE USA
187 P12 **Cumberland, Cape** *var.* Cape Nahoi. *headland* Espiritu Santo, N Vanuatu
11 V14 **Cumberland House** Saskatchewan, C Canada
23 W8 **Cumberland Island** *island* Georgia, SE USA
20 L7 **Cumberland, Lake** ⊞ Kentucky, S USA
9 R5 **Cumberland Peninsula** *peninsula* Baffin Island, Nunavut, NE Canada
2 N9 **Cumberland Plateau** *plateau* E USA
30 L1 **Cumberland Point** *headland* Michigan, N USA
21 O7 **Cumberland River** ≈ Kentucky/Tennessee, S USA
9 S6 **Cumberland Sound** *inlet* Baffin Island, Nunavut, NE Canada
96 I12 **Cumbernauld** S Scotland, UK
97 K15 **Cumbria** *cultural region* NW England, UK
97 K15 **Cumbrian Mountains** ▲▲ NW England, UK
23 S2 **Cumming** Georgia, SE USA
Cummin in Pommern *see* Kamień Pomorski
182 G9 **Cummins** South Australia
96 I13 **Cumnock** W Scotland, UK
40 G4 **Cumpas** Sonora, NW Mexico
136 H16 **Çumra** Konya, C Turkey
63 G15 **Cunco** Araucanía, C Chile
54 E9 **Cundinamarca** *off.* Departamento de Cundinamarca. ◈ *province* C Colombia
41 U15 **Cunduacán** Tabasco, SE Mexico
83 C16 **Cunene** ◈ *province* S Angola
83 A16 **Cunene** *var.* Kunene. ≈ Angola/Namibia *see also* Kunene
106 A9 **Cuneo** *Fr.* Coni. Piemonte, NW Italy
83 E15 **Cunjamba** Cuando Cubango, E Angola
181 V10 **Cunnamulla** Queensland, E Australia
Cuokkarašša *see* Čohkarášša
106 B7 **Cuorgne** Piemonte, NE Italy
96 K11 **Cupar** E Scotland, UK
116 L8 **Cupcina** *Rus.* Kupchino; *prev.* Calinisc, Kalinisk. N Moldova
54 C8 **Cupica** Chocó, W Colombia
54 C8 **Cupica, Golfo de** *gulf* W Colombia
112 N13 **Ćuprija** Serbia, E Yugoslavia
Cura *see* Villa de Cura
45 P16 **Curaçao** *island* Netherlands Antilles
56 H13 **Curanja, Río** ≈ E Peru
56 F7 **Curaray, Rio** ≈ Ecuador/Peru
116 K14 **Curcani** Călăraşi, SE Romania
182 H4 **Curdimurka** South Australia
103 P7 **Cure** ≈ C France
173 Y16 **Curepipe** C Mauritius
55 R6 **Curiapo** Delta Amacuro, NE Venezuela
Curia Rhaetorum *see* Chur
62 G12 **Curicó** Maule, C Chile
Curieta *see* Krk
172 I15 **Curieuse** *island* Inner Islands, NE Seychelles
59 C16 **Curitiba** Acre, W Brazil
60 K12 **Curitiba** *prev.* Curytiba. *state capital* Paraná, S Brazil
60 J13 **Curitibanos** Santa Catarina, S Brazil
183 S6 **Curlewis** New South Wales, SE Australia
182 J6 **Curnamona** South Australia
83 A15 **Curoca** ≈ SW Angola
183 T6 **Currabubula** New South Wales, SE Australia
59 Q14 **Currais Novos** Rio Grande do Norte, E Brazil
35 W7 **Currant** Nevada, W USA
35 W6 **Currant Mountain** ▲ Nevada, W USA
44 H2 **Current** Eleuthera Island, C Bahamas
27 W8 **Current River** ≈ Arkansas/Missouri, C USA
182 M14 **Currie** Tasmania, SE Australia
21 Y8 **Currituck** North Carolina, SE USA
21 Y8 **Currituck Sound** *sound* North Carolina, SE USA
39 R11 **Curry** Alaska, USA
Curtbunar *see* Tervel
116 I13 **Curtea de Argeş** *var.* Curtea-de-Arges. Argeş, S Romania
116 E10 **Curtici** *Ger.* Kurtitsch, *Hung.* Kürtös. Arad, W Romania
28 M16 **Curtis** Nebraska, C USA
104 H2 **Curtis-Estación** Galicia, NW Spain
183 O14 **Curtis Group** *island group* Tasmania, SE Australia
181 Y8 **Curtis Island** *island* Queensland, SE Australia
58 K11 **Curuá, Ilha do** *island* NE Brazil
47 U7 **Curuá, Rio** ≈ N Brazil
59 A14 **Curuçá, Rio** ≈ NW Brazil
112 L9 **Čurug** *Hung.* Csurog. Serbia, N Yugoslavia
61 D16 **Curuzú Cuatiá** Corrientes, NE Argentina
59 M19 **Curvelo** Minas Gerais, SE Brazil
18 E14 **Curwensville** Pennsylvania, NE USA
30 M3 **Curwood, Mount** ▲ Michigan, N USA
Curytiba *see* Curitiba
Curzola *see* Korčula
42 A10 **Cuscatlán** ◈ *department* C El Salvador
57 H15 **Cusco** *var.* Cuzco. Cusco, C Peru
57 H15 **Cusco** *off.* Departamento de Cusco; *var.* Cuzco. ◈ *department* C Peru
27 O9 **Cushing** Oklahoma, C USA
25 W8 **Cushing** Texas, SW USA
40 I6 **Cusihuiriachic** Chihuahua, N Mexico
103 P10 **Cusset** Allier, C France
23 S6 **Cusseta** Georgia, SE USA
28 J10 **Custer** South Dakota, N USA
Cüstrin *see* Kostrzyn
33 Q7 **Cut Bank** Montana, NW USA
Cutch, Gulf of *see* Kachchh, Gulf of
23 S6 **Cuthbert** Georgia, SE USA
11 S15 **Cut Knife** Saskatchewan, S Canada
23 Y16 **Cutler Ridge** Florida, SE USA
22 K10 **Cut Off** Louisiana, S USA
63 I15 **Cutral-Có** Neuquén, C Argentina
107 O21 **Cutro** Calabria, SW Italy
183 O4 **Cuttaburra Channels** *seasonal river* New South Wales, SE Australia
154 O12 **Cuttack** Orissa, E India
83 C15 **Cuvelai** Cunene, SW Angola
79 G18 **Cuvette** *var.* Région de la Cuvette. ◈ *province* C Congo
173 V9 **Cuvier Basin** *undersea feature* E Indian Ocean
173 U9 **Cuvier Plateau** *undersea feature* E Indian Ocean
82 B12 **Cuvo** ≈ W Angola
100 H9 **Cuxhaven** Niedersachsen, NW Germany
Cuyabá *see* Cuiabá
Cuyuni, Río *see* Cuyuni River
55 S8 **Cuyuni River** *var.* Río Cuyuni. ≈ Guyana/Venezuela
Cuzco *see* Cusco
97 K22 **Cwmbran** *Wel.* Cwmbrân. SW Wales, UK
28 K15 **C.W.McConaughy, Lake** ⊞ Nebraska, C USA
81 D20 **Cyangugu** SW Rwanda
110 D11 **Cybinka** *Ger.* Ziebingen. Lubuskie, W Poland
Cyclades *see* Kykládes
Cydonia *see* Chaniá
Cymru *see* Wales
20 M5 **Cynthiana** Kentucky, S USA
11 S17 **Cypress Hills** ▲▲ Alberta/Saskatchewan, SW Canada
Cypro-Syrian Basin *see* Cyprus Basin
121 U11 **Cyprus** *off.* Republic of Cyprus, *Gk.* Kypros, *Turk.* Kıbrıs, Kıbrıs Cumhuriyeti. ◆ *republic* E Mediterranean Sea
84 L14 **Cyprus** *Gk.* Kypros, *Turk.* Kıbrıs. *island* E Mediterranean Sea
121 W11 **Cyprus Basin** *var.* Cypro-Syrian Basin. *undersea feature* E Mediterranean Sea
Cythera *see* Kýthira
Cythnos *see* Kýthnos
110 F9 **Czaplinek** *Ger.* Tempelburg. Zachodniopomorskie, NW Poland
Czarna Woda *see* Wda
110 G8 **Czarne** Pomorskie, N Poland
110 G10 **Czarnków** Wielkopolskie, C Poland
111 E17 **Czech Republic** *Cz.* Česká Republika. ◆ *republic* C Europe
Czegléd *see* Cegléd
110 G12 **Czempiń** Wielkolpolskie, C Poland
Czenstochau *see* Częstochowa
Czerkow *see* Čerchov
Czernowitz *see* Chernivtsi
110 I8 **Czersk** Pomorskie, N Poland
111 J15 **Częstochowa** *Ger.* Czenstochau, Tschenstochau, *Rus.* Chenstokhov. Śląskie, S Poland
110 F10 **Człopa** *Ger.* Schloppe. Zachodniopomorskie, NW Poland
110 H8 **Człuchów** *Ger.* Schlochau. Pomorskie, NW Poland

D

163 V9 **Da'an** *var.* Dalai. Jilin, NE China
15 S10 **Daaquam** Quebec, SE Canada
Daawo, Webi *see* Dawa Wenz
54 I4 **Dabajuro** Falcón, NW Venezuela
77 N15 **Dabakala** NE Ivory Coast
Daban *see* Bairin Youqi
111 K23 **Dabas** Pest, C Hungary
160 L8 **Daba Shan** ▲▲ C China
140 J5 **Dabbāgh, Jabal** ▲ NW Saudi Arabia
54 D8 **Dabeiba** Antioquia, NW Colombia
154 E11 **Dabhoi** Gujarāt, W India
161 P8 **Dabie Shan** ▲▲ C China
76 J13 **Dabola** Haute-Guinée, C Guinea
77 N17 **Dabou** S Ivory Coast
110 P8 **Dąbrowa Białostocka** Podlaskie, NE Poland
111 M16 **Dąbrowa Tarnowska** Małopolskie, S Poland
119 M20 **Dabryn'** *Rus.* Dobryn'. Homyel'skaya Voblasts', SE Belarus
159 P10 **Dabsan Hu** ◎ C China
161 Q13 **Dabu** *prev.* Huliao. Guangdong, S China
116 H15 **Dăbuleni** Dolj, SW Romania
Dacca *see* Dhaka
101 L23 **Dachau** Bayern, SE Germany
160 K8 **Dachuan** *prev.* Daxian, Da Xian. Sichuan, C China
Dacia Bank *see* Dacia Seamount
64 M10 **Dacia Seamount** *var.* Dacia Bank. *undersea feature* E Atlantic Ocean
37 T3 **Dacono** Colorado, C USA
Đắc Tô *see* Đak Tô
Dacura *see* Dákura
23 W12 **Dade City** Florida, SE USA
152 L10 **Dadeldhura** *var.* Dandeldhura. Far Western, W Nepal
23 Q5 **Dadeville** Alabama, S USA
103 N15 **Dadou** ≈ S France
154 D12 **Dādra and Nagar Haveli** ◈ *union territory* W India
149 P14 **Dādu** Sind, SE Pakistan
167 U11 **Da Du Boloc** Kon Tum, C Vietnam
160 G9 **Dadu He** ≈ C China
Daegu *see* Taegu
Daerah Istimewa Aceh *see* Aceh
171 P4 **Daet** Luzon, N Philippines
160 I11 **Dafang** Guizhou, S China
153 W11 **Dafla Hills** ▲▲ NE India
11 U15 **Dafoe** Saskatchewan, S Canada
76 G10 **Dagana** N Senegal
Dagana *see* Dahana, Tajikistan
Dagana *see* Massakory, Chad
118 K11 **Dagda** Krāslava, SE Latvia
Dagden *see* Hiiumaa
Dagden-Sund *see* Soela Väin
129 P16 **Dagestan, Respublika** *prev.* Dagestanskaya ASSR, *Eng.* Daghestan. ◈ *autonomous republic* SW Russian Federation
Dagestanskaya ASSR *see* Dagestan, Respublika
129 R17 **Dagestanskiye Ogni** Respublika Dagestan, SW Russian Federation
185 A23 **Dagg Sound** *sound* South Island, NZ
Daghestan *see* Dagestan, Respublika
141 Y8 **Daghmar** NE Oman
Dağliq Quarabağ *see* Nagornyy Karabakh
Dagö *see* Hiiumaa
54 D11 **Dagua** Valle del Cauca, W Colombia
160 H11 **Daguan** Yunnan, SW China
171 N3 **Dagupan** *off.* Dagupan City. Luzon, N Philippines
159 N16 **Dagzê** Xizang Zizhiqu, W China
147 Q13 **Dahana** *Rus.* Dagana, Dakhana. SW Tajikistan
163 V10 **Dahei Shan** ▲ N China
163 T7 **Da Hinggan Ling** *Eng.* Great Khingan Range. ▲▲ NE China
Dahlac Archipelago *see* Dahlak Archipelago
80 K9 **Dahlak Archipelago** *var.* Dahlac Archipelago. *island group* E Eritrea
23 T2 **Dahlonega** Georgia, SE USA
101 O14 **Dahme** Brandenburg, E Germany
100 O13 **Dahme** ≈ E Germany
141 O14 **Dahm, Ramlat** *desert* NW Yemen
154 E10 **Dāhod** *prev.* Dohad. Gujarāt, W India
Dahomey *see* Benin
158 G10 **Dahongliutan** Xinjiang Uygur Zizhiqu, NW China
Dahra *see* Dara
139 R2 **Dahūk** *var.* Dohuk, *Kurd.* Dihōk. N Iraq
116 J15 **Daia** Giurgiu, S Romania
165 P12 **Daigo** Ibaraki, Honshū, S Japan
163 O13 **Dai Hai** ◎ N China
Daihoku *see* T'aipei
186 M8 **Dai Island** *island* N Solomon Islands
166 M8 **Daik-u** Pegu, SW Burma
138 H9 **Dā'il** Dar'ā, S Syria
167 U12 **Đại Lanh** Khanh Hoa, S Vietnam
161 Q13 **Daimao Shan** ▲▲ SE China
105 N11 **Daimiel** Castilla-La Mancha, C Spain
115 F22 **Daimoniá** Pelopónnisos, S Greece
Dainan *see* T'ainan
25 W6 **Daingerfield** Texas, SW USA
Daingin, Bá an *see* Dingle Bay
159 R13 **Dainkognubma** Xizang Zizhiqu, W China
164 K14 **Daiō-zaki** *headland* Honshū, SW Japan
Dairbhre *see* Valencia Island
61 B22 **Daireaux** Buenos Aires, E Argentina
Dairen *see* Dalian
75 W9 **Dairûṭ** *var.* Dayrūṭ. C Egypt
25 X10 **Daisetta** Texas, SW USA
192 G5 **Daitō-jima** *island group* SW Japan
192 G5 **Daitō Ridge** *undersea feature* N Philippine Sea
161 N3 **Daixian** *var.* Dai Xian. Shanxi, C China
161 Q12 **Daiyun Shan** ▲▲ SE China
44 M8 **Dajabón** NW Dominican Republic
160 G8 **Dajin Chuan** ≈ C China
148 J6 **Dak** ◎ W Afghanistan
76 F11 **Dakar** ● (Senegal) W Senegal
76 F11 **Dakar** × W Senegal
167 U10 **Đak Glây** Kon Tum, C Vietnam
Dakhana *see* Dahana
153 U16 **Dakhin Shahbazpur Island** *island* S Bangladesh
Dakhla *see* Ad Dakhla
76 F7 **Dakhlet Nouâdhibou** ◈ *region* NW Mauritania
Đak Lap *see* Kiên Đưc
167 U13 **Đak Nông** Đắc Lắc, S Vietnam
77 U11 **Dakoro** Maradi, S Niger
29 U12 **Dakota City** Iowa, C USA
29 R13 **Dakota City** Nebraska, C USA
113 M17 **Đakovica** *var.* Djakovica, *Alb.* Gjakovë. Serbia, S Yugoslavia
112 I10 **Đakovo** *var.* Djakovo, *Hung.* Diakovár. Osijek-Baranja, E Croatia
Dakshin *see* Deccan
167 U11 **Đak Tô** *var.* Đắc Tô. Kon Tum, C Vietnam
43 N7 **Dákura** *var.* Dacura. Región Autónoma Atlántico Norte, NE Nicaragua
95 I14 **Dal** Akershus, S Norway
82 E12 **Dala** Lunda Sul, E Angola
108 J8 **Dalaas** Vorarlberg, W Austria
76 I13 **Dalaba** Moyenne-Guinée, W Guinea
Dalai *see* Da'an
Dalain Hob *see* Ejin Qi
Dalai Nor *see* Hulun Nur
163 Q11 **Dalai Nur** *salt lake* N China
Dala-Jarna *see* Järna
95 M14 **Dalälven** ≈ C Sweden
136 C16 **Dalaman** Muğla, SW Turkey
136 C16 **Dalaman** × Muğla, SW Turkey
136 D16 **Dalaman Çayı** ≈ SW Turkey
162 K11 **Dalandzadgad** Ömnögovĭ, S Mongolia
95 D17 **Dalane** *physical region* S Norway
189 Z2 **Dalap-Uliga-Djarrit** *var.* Delap-Uliga-Darrit, D-U-D. *island group* Ratak Chain, SE Marshall Islands
94 J12 **Dalarna** *prev.* Kopparberg ◈ *county* C Sweden
94 L13 **Dalarna** *prev. Eng.* Dalecarlia. *cultural region* C Sweden
95 P16 **Dalarö** Stockholm, C Sweden
167 U13 **Đa Lat** Lâm Đông, S Vietnam
162 J11 **Dalay** Ömnögovĭ, S Mongolia
148 L12 **Dālbandīn** *var.* Dāl Bandin. Baluchistān, SW Pakistan
95 J17 **Dalbosjön** *lake bay* S Sweden
181 Y10 **Dalby** Queensland, E Australia
94 D13 **Dale** Hordaland, S Norway
94 C12 **Dale** Sogn og Fjordane, S Norway
32 K12 **Dale** Oregon, NW USA
25 T11 **Dale** Texas, SW USA
Dalecarlia *see* Dalarna
21 W4 **Dale City** Virginia, NE USA
20 L8 **Dale Hollow Lake** ⊞ Kentucky/Tennessee, S USA
98 O8 **Dalen** Drenthe, NE Netherlands
95 E15 **Dalen** Telemark, S Norway
166 K14 **Daletme** Chin State, W Burma
23 Q7 **Daleville** Alabama, S USA
98 M9 **Dalfsen** Overijssel, E Netherlands
24 M1 **Dalhart** Texas, SW USA
13 O13 **Dalhousie** New Brunswick, SE Canada
152 I6 **Dalhousie** Himāchal Pradesh, N India
160 F12 **Dali** *var.* Xiaguan. Yunnan, SW China
Dali *see* Idálion
163 U14 **Dalian** *var.* Dairen, Dalien, Lüda, Ta-lien, *Rus.* Dalny. Liaoning, NE China
105 O15 **Dalías** Andalucía, S Spain
Dalien *see* Dalian
Dalijan *see* Delījān
112 J9 **Dalj** *Hung.* Dalja. Osijek-Baranja, E Croatia
Dalja *see* Dalj
32 F12 **Dallas** Oregon, NW USA
25 U6 **Dallas** Texas, SW USA
25 T7 **Dallas-Fort Worth** × Texas, SW USA
154 K12 **Dalli Rājhara** Madhya Pradesh, C India
39 X15 **Dall Island** *island* Alexander Archipelago, Alaska, USA
38 M12 **Dall Lake** ◎ Alaska, USA
77 S12 **Dallol Bosso** *seasonal river* W Niger
141 U7 **Dalmā** *island* W UAE
113 E14 **Dalmacija** *Eng.* Dalmatia, *Ger.* Dalmatien, *It.* Dalmazia. *cultural region* S Croatia
Dalmatia/Dalmatien/Dalmazia *see* Dalmacija
123 S15 **Dal'negorsk** Primorskiy Kray, SE Russian Federation
Dalny *see* Dalian
76 M16 **Daloa** C Ivory Coast
160 J11 **Dalou Shan** ▲▲ S China
181 X7 **Dalrymple Lake** ◎ Queensland, E Australia
14 H14 **Dalrymple Lake** ◎ Ontario, S Canada
181 X7 **Dalrymple, Mount** ▲ Queensland, E Australia
93 K20 **Dalsbruk** *Fin.* Taalintehdas. Länsi-Suomi, W Finland
95 K19 **Dalsjöfors** Västra Götaland, S Sweden
95 J17 **Dals Långed** *var.* Långed. Västra Götaland, S Sweden
153 O15 **Dāltenganj** *prev.* Daltonganj. Bihār, N India
23 R2 **Dalton** Georgia, SE USA
Daltonganj *see* Dāltenganj
195 X14 **Dalton Iceberg Tongue** *ice feature* Antarctica
92 J1 **Dalvík** Nordhurland Eystra, N Iceland
35 N8 **Daly City** California, W USA
181 P2 **Daly River** ≈ Northern Territory, N Australia
181 Q3 **Daly Waters** Northern Territory, N Australia
119 F20 **Damachava** *var.* Damachova, *Pol.* Domaczewo, *Rus.* Domachëvo. Brestskaya Voblasts', SW Belarus
Damachova *see* Damachava
77 W11 **Damagaram Takaya** Zinder, S Niger
154 D12 **Damān** Damān and Diu, W India
154 B12 **Damān and Diu** ◈ *union territory* W India
75 V7 **Damanhûr** *anc.* Hermopolis Parva. N Egypt
Damão *see* Damān
161 O1 **Damaqun Shan** ▲▲ E China
79 I15 **Damara** Ombella-Mpoko, S Central African Republic
83 D18 **Damaraland** *physical region* C Namibia
171 S15 **Damar, Kepulauan** *var.* Baraf Daja Islands, Kepulauan Barat Daya. *island group* C Indonesia
168 J8 **Damar Laut** Perak, Peninsular Malaysia
171 S15 **Damar, Pulau** *island* Maluku, E Indonesia
Damas *see* Dimashq
77 Y12 **Damasak** Borno, NE Nigeria
Damasco *see* Dimashq
21 Q8 **Damascus** Virginia, NE USA
Damascus *see* Dimashq
77 X13 **Damaturu** Yobe, NE Nigeria
171 R9 **Damau** Pulau Kaburuang, N Indonesia
143 O5 **Damāvand, Qolleh-ye** ▲ N Iran
82 B10 **Damba** Uíge, NW Angola
114 M12 **Dambaslar** Tekirdağ, NW Turkey
116 J13 **Dâmboviţa** *prev.* Dîmboviţa. ◈ *county* SE Romania
116 J13 **Dâmboviţa** *prev.* Dîmboviţa. ≈ S Romania
173 Y15 **D'Ambre, Île** *island* NE Mauritius
155 K24 **Dambulla** Central Province, C Sri Lanka
44 K9 **Dame-Marie** SW Haiti
44 J9 **Dame Marie, Cap** *headland* SW Haiti
143 Q4 **Dāmghān** Semnān, N Iran
Damietta *see* Dumyāt
138 G10 **Dāmiyā** Al Balqā', NW Jordan
146 G11 **Damla** Dashkhovuzskiy Velayat, N Turkmenistan
Dammām *see* Ad Dammān
100 G12 **Damme** Niedersachsen, NW Germany
153 R15 **Dāmodar** ≈ NE India
154 J9 **Damoh** Madhya Pradesh, C India
77 P15 **Damongo** NW Ghana
138 G7 **Damour** *var.* Ad Dāmūr. W Lebanon
171 N11 **Dampal, Teluk** *bay* Sulawesi, C Indonesia
180 H7 **Dampier** Western Australia
180 H6 **Dampier Archipelago** *island group* Western Australia
141 U14 **Damqawt** *var.* Damqut. E Yemen
159 O13 **Dam Qu** ≈ C China
Damqut *see* Damqawt
167 R13 **Dâmrei, Chuŏr Phmun** *Fr.* Chaîne de l'Éléphant. ▲▲ SW Cambodia
108 C7 **Damvant** Jura, NW Switzerland
Damwâld *see* Damwoude
98 L5 **Damwoude** *Fris.* Damwâld. Friesland, N Netherlands
159 N15 **Damxung** Xizang Zizhiqu, W China
80 K11 **Danakil Desert** *var.* Afar Depression, Danakil Plain. *desert* E Africa
Danakil Plain *see* Danakil Desert
35 R8 **Dana, Mount** ▲ California, W USA
76 L16 **Danané** W Ivory Coast
167 U10 **Đà Nẵng** *prev.* Tourane. Quang Nam-Đa Nẵng, C Vietnam
160 G9 **Danba** Sichuan, C China
Danborg *see* Daneborg
18 L13 **Danbury** Connecticut, NE USA
25 W12 **Danbury** Texas, SW USA
35 X15 **Danby Lake** ◎ California, W USA
194 H4 **Danco Coast** *physical region* Antarctica
82 B11 **Dande** ≈ NW Angola
Dandeldhura *see* Dadeldhura
155 E17 **Dandeli** Karnātaka, W India
183 O12 **Dandenong** Victoria, SE Australia
163 V13 **Dandong** *var.* Tan-tung; *prev.* An-tung. Liaoning, NE China
197 Q14 **Daneborg** *var.* Danborg. Tunu, N Greenland
25 V12 **Danevang** Texas, SW USA
Dänew *see* Deynau
14 L12 **Danford Lake** Quebec, SE Canada
19 T4 **Danforth** Maine, NE USA
37 P3 **Danforth Hills** ▲ Colorado, C USA
Dangara *see* Danghara
159 V12 **Dangchang** Gansu, C China
Dangchengwan *see* Subei
82 B10 **Dange** Uíge, NW Angola
Dangerous Archipelago *see* Tuamotu, Îles
83 E26 **Danger Point** *headland* SW South Africa
147 Q13 **Danghara** *Rus.* Dangara. SW Tajikistan
159 P8 **Danghe Nanshan** ▲▲ W China
80 I12 **Dangila** *var.* Dānglā. Amhara, NW Ethiopia
159 P8 **Dangjin Shankou** *pass* N China
Dangla *see* Tanggula Shan
Dānglā *see* Dangila, NW Ethiopia
Dangme Chu *see* Manās
153 Y11 **Dāngori** Assam, NE India
Dang Raek, Phanom/Dangrek, Chaîne des *see* Dângrêk, Chuŏr Phnum
167 S11 **Dângrêk, Chuŏr Phnum** *var.* Phanom Dang Raek, Phanom Dong Rak, *Fr.* Chaîne des Dangrek. ▲▲ Cambodia/Thailand
42 G3 **Dangriga** *prev.* Stann Creek. Stann Creek, E Belize
161 P6 **Dangshan** Anhui, E China
33 T15 **Daniel** Wyoming, C USA
83 H22 **Daniëlskuil** Northern Cape, N South Africa
19 N12 **Danielson** Connecticut, NE USA
126 M15 **Danilov** Yaroslavskaya Oblast', W Russian Federation
129 O9 **Danilovka** Volgogradskaya Oblast', SW Russian Federation
Danish West Indies *see* Virgin Islands (US)
160 L7 **Dan Jiang** ≈ C China
160 M7 **Danjiangkou Shuiku** ⊞ C China
141 W8 **Ḑank** *var.* Dhank. NW Oman
152 J7 **Dankhar** Himāchal Pradesh, N India
128 L6 **Dankov** Lipetskaya Oblast', W Russian Federation
42 J7 **Danlí** El Paraíso, S Honduras
Danmark *see* Denmark
Danmarksstraedet *see* Denmark Strait
95 O14 **Dannemora** Uppsala, C Sweden
18 L6 **Dannemora** New York, NE USA
100 K11 **Dannenberg** Niedersachsen, N Germany
184 N12 **Dannevirke** Manawatu-Wanganui, North Island, NZ
21 U8 **Dan River** ≈ Virginia, NE USA
167 P8 **Dan Sai** Loei, C Thailand
18 F10 **Dansville** New York, NE USA
Dantzig *see* Gdańsk
86 E12 **Danube** *Bul.* Dunav, *Cz.* Dunaj, *Ger.* Donau, *Hung.* Duna, *Rom.* Dunărea. ≈ C Europe
Danubian Plain *see* Dunavska Ravnina
166 L8 **Danubyu** Irrawaddy, SW Burma
Danum *see* Doncaster
19 P11 **Danvers** Massachusetts, NE USA
27 T11 **Danville** Arkansas, C USA
31 N13 **Danville** Illinois, N USA
31 O14 **Danville** Indiana, N USA
29 Y15 **Danville** Iowa, C USA
20 M6 **Danville** Kentucky, S USA
18 G14 **Danville** Pennsylvania, NE USA
21 T6 **Danville** Virginia, NE USA
Danxian/Dan Xian *see* Danzhou
160 L17 **Danzhou** *prev.* Danxian, Dan Xian, Nada. Hainan, S China
Danzig *see* Gdańsk
Danziger Bucht *see* Danzig, Gulf of
110 J6 **Danzig, Gulf of** *var.* Gulf of Gdańsk, *Ger.* Danziger Bucht, *Pol.* Zakota Gdańska, *Rus.* Gdan'skaya Bukhta. *gulf* N Poland
160 F10 **Daocheng** Sichuan, C China
Daokou *see* Huaxian
104 H7 **Dão, Rio** ≈ N Portugal
Daosa *see* Dausa
77 Y7 **Dao Timmi** Agadez, NE Niger
160 M13 **Daoxian** *var.* Dao Xian. Hunan, S China
77 Q14 **Dapaong** N Togo
23 N8 **Daphne** Alabama, S USA
171 P7 **Dapitan** Mindanao, S Philippines

◆ Country ● Country Capital ◇ Dependent Territory ○ Dependent Territory Capital ◈ Administrative Region × International Airport ▲ Mountain ▲▲ Mountain Range Volcano ≈ River ◎ Lake ⊞ Reservoir

159 P9 **Da Qaidam** Qinghai, C China
163 V8 **Daqing** Heilongjiang, NE China
163 O13 **Daqing Shan** ▲ N China
Daqm *see* Duqm
139 T5 **Dāqūq** *var.* Tāwūq. N Iraq
76 G10 **Dara** *var.* Dahra. NW Senegal
138 H9 **Dar'ā** *var.* Der'a, *Fr.* Déraa. Dar'ā, SW Syria
138 H8 **Dar'ā** *off.* Muḥāfaẓat Dar'ā, *var.* Darā, Derá, Derrá. ◆ *governorate* S Syria
143 Q12 **Dārāb** Fārs, S Iran
116 K8 **Darabani** Botoşani, NW Romania
Daraj *see* Dirj
142 M8 **Dārān** Eşfahān, W Iran
167 U12 **Đa Răng, Sông** *var.* Ba. ~ S Vietnam
Daraut-Kurgan *see* Daroot-Korgon
77 W13 **Darazo** Bauchi, E Nigeria
139 S3 **Darband** N Iraq
139 V4 **Darband-i Khān, Sadd** *dam* NE Iraq
139 N1 **Darbāsīyah** *var.* Derbisīye. Al Ḥasakah, N Syria
118 C11 **Darbėnai** Kretinga, NW Lithuania
153 Q13 **Darbhanga** Bihār, N India
38 M9 **Darby, Cape** *headland* Alaska, USA
112 I9 **Darda** *Hung.* Dárda. Osijek-Baranja, E Croatia
27 T11 **Dardanelle** Arkansas, C USA
27 S11 **Dardanelle, Lake** ▣ Arkansas, C USA
Dardanelles *see* Çanakkale Boğazı
Dardanelli *see* Çanakkale
Dar-el-Beida *see* Casablanca
136 M14 **Darende** Malatya, C Turkey
81 J22 **Dar es Salaam** Dar es Salaam, E Tanzania
81 J22 **Dar es Salaam** ✕ Pwani, E Tanzania
185 H18 **Darfield** Canterbury, South Island, NZ
106 F7 **Darfo** Lombardia, N Italy
80 B10 **Darfur** *var.* Darfur Massif. *cultural region* W Sudan
Darfur Massif *see* Darfur
146 J10 **Dargan-Ata** *var.* Darganata. Lebapskiy Velayat, NE Turkmenistan
Darganata *see* Dargan-Ata
143 T3 **Dargaz** *var.* Darreh Gaz; *prev.* Moḥammadābād. Khorāsān, NE Iran
139 U4 **Dargazayn** NE Iraq
183 P12 **Dargo** Victoria, SE Australia
162 K7 **Darhan** Bulgan, C Mongolia
163 N8 **Darhan** Hentiy, C Mongolia
162 L6 **Darhan** Selenge, N Mongolia
163 N12 **Darhan Muminggan Lianheqi** *var.* Bailingmiao. Nei Mongol Zizhiqu, N China
23 W7 **Darien** Georgia, SE USA
43 W16 **Darién** *off.* Provincia del Darién. ◆ *province* SE Panama
Darién, Golfo del *see* Darien, Gulf of
43 X14 **Darien, Gulf of** *Sp.* Golfo del Darién. *gulf* S Caribbean Sea
Darien, Isthmus of *see* Panamá, Istmo de
42 K9 **Dariense, Cordillera** ▲ C Nicaragua
43 W15 **Darién, Serranía del** ▲ Colombia/Panama
Dario *see* Ciudad Darío
Dariorigum *see* Vannes
Dariv *see* Darvi
Darj *see* Dirj
Darjeeling *see* Darjiling
153 S12 **Darjiling** *prev.* Darjeeling. West Bengal, NE India
Darkehnen *see* Ozersk
159 S12 **Darlag** Qinghai, C China
183 T3 **Darling Downs** *hill range* Queensland, E Australia
28 M2 **Darling, Lake** ▣ North Dakota, N USA
180 I12 **Darling Range** ▲ Western Australia
182 L8 **Darling River** ~ New South Wales, SE Australia
97 M15 **Darlington** N England, UK
21 T12 **Darlington** South Carolina, SE USA
30 K9 **Darlington** Wisconsin, N USA
110 G7 **Darłowo** Zachodniopomorskie, NW Poland
101 G19 **Darmstadt** Hessen, SW Germany
75 S7 **Darnah** *var.* Dérna. NE Libya
103 S6 **Darney** Vosges, NE France
182 M7 **Darnick** New South Wales, SE Australia
195 Y6 **Darnley, Cape** *headland* Antarctica
105 R7 **Daroca** Aragón, NE Spain
147 S11 **Daroot-Korgon** *var.* Daraut-Kurgan. Oshskaya Oblast', SW Kyrgyzstan
61 A23 **Darragueira** *var.* Darregueira. Buenos Aires, E Argentina
Darregueira *see* Darragueira
Darreh Gaz *see* Dargaz
142 K7 **Darreh Shahr** *var.* Darreh-ye Shahr. Īlām, W Iran
Darreh-ye Shahr *see* Darreh Shahr
32 I7 **Darrington** Washington, NW USA
25 P1 **Darrouzett** Texas, SW USA
153 S15 **Darsana** *var.* Darshana. Khulna, N Bangladesh
Darshana *see* Darsana
100 M7 **Darss** *peninsula* NE Germany
100 M7 **Darsser Ort** *headland* NE Germany
97 J24 **Dart** ~ SW England, UK
Dartang *see* Baqên
97 P22 **Dartford** SE England, UK
182 L12 **Dartmoor** Victoria, SE Australia
97 I24 **Dartmoor** *moorland* SW England, UK
13 Q15 **Dartmouth** Nova Scotia, SE Canada
97 J24 **Dartmouth** SW England, UK
15 Y6 **Dartmouth** ~ Quebec, SE Canada
183 Q11 **Dartmouth Reservoir** ◎ Victoria, SE Australia
Dartuch, Cabo *see* Artrutx, Cap d'
186 C9 **Daru** Western, SW PNG
112 G9 **Daruvar** *Hung.* Daruvár. Bjelovar-Bilogora, NE Croatia
146 F10 **Darvaza** *Turkm.* Derweze. Akhalskiy Velayat, C Turkmenistan
Darvaza *see* Darwoza
Darvazskiy Khrebet *see* Darvoz, Qatorkŭhi
162 F8 **Darvi** *var.* Dariv. Govĭ-Altay, W Mongolia
148 L9 **Darvīshān** *var.* Darweshan, Garmser. Helmand, S Afghanistan
147 R13 **Darvoz, Qatorkŭhi** *Rus.* Darvazskiy Khrebet. ▲ C Tajikistan
Darweshan *see* Darvīshān
63 J15 **Darwin** Río Negro, S Argentina
181 O1 **Darwin** *prev.* Palmerston, Port Darwin. *territory capital* Northern Territory, N Australia
65 D24 **Darwin** *var.* Darwin Settlement. East Falkland, Falkland Islands
62 H8 **Darwin, Cordillera** ▲ N Chile
57 B17 **Darwin, Volcán** ✱ Galapagos Islands, Ecuador, E Pacific Ocean
147 O10 **Darwoza** *Rus.* Darvaza. Jizzakh Wiloyati, C Uzbekistan
149 S8 **Darya Khān** Punjab, E Pakistan
145 O15 **Dar'yalyktakyr, Ravnina** *plain* S Kazakhstan
143 T11 **Dārzīn** Kermān, S Iran
160 L8 **Dashennongjia** ▲ C China
Dashhowuz *see* Dashkhovuz
Dashhowuz Welayaty *see* Dashkhovuzskiy Velayat
119 O16 **Dashkawka** *Rus.* Dashkovka. Mahilyowskaya Voblasts', E Belarus
146 H8 **Dashkhovuz** *Turkm.* Dashhowuz; *prev.* Tashauz. Dashkhovuzskiy Velayat, N Turkmenistan
Dashkhovuz *see* Dashkhovuzskiy Velayat
146 E9 **Dashkhovuzskiy Velayat** *var.* Dashkhovuz, *Turkm.* Dashhowuz Welayaty. ◆ *province* N Turkmenistan
Dashköpri *see* Tashkepri
Dashkovka *see* Dashkawka
148 J15 **Dasht** ~ SW Pakistan
Dashtidzhum *see* Dashtijum
147 R13 **Dashtijum** *Rus.* Dashtidzhum. SW Tajikistan
149 W7 **Daska** Punjab, NE Pakistan
Đa, Sông *see* Black River
77 R15 **Dassa** *var.* Dassa-Zoumé. S Benin
Dassa-Zoumé *see* Dassa
29 U8 **Dassel** Minnesota, N USA
152 H3 **Dastegil Sar** *var.* Disteghil Sār. ▲ N India
136 C16 **Datça** Muğla, SW Turkey
165 R4 **Date** Hokkaidō, NE Japan
154 I8 **Datia** *prev.* Duttia. Madhya Pradesh, C India
159 T10 **Datong** Qinghai, C China
161 N2 **Datong** *var.* Tatung, Ta-t'ung. Shanxi, C China
159 S9 **Datong He** ~ C China
159 S9 **Datong Shan** ▲ C China
169 O10 **Datu, Tanjung** *headland* Indonesia/Malaysia
Daua *see* Dawa Wenz
172 H16 **Dauban, Mount** ▲ Silhouette, NE Seychelles
149 T7 **Dāūd Khel** Punjab, E Pakistan
119 G15 **Daugai** Alytus, S Lithuania
Daugava *see* Western Dvina
118 J11 **Daugavpils** *Ger.* Dünaburg; *prev. Rus.* Dvinsk. *municipality* Daugvapils, SE Latvia
Dauka *see* Dawkah
Daulatabad *see* Malāyer
101 D18 **Daun** Rheinland-Pfalz, W Germany
155 E14 **Daund** *prev.* Dhond. Mahārāshtra, W India
166 M12 **Daung Kyun** *island* S Burma
11 W15 **Dauphin** Manitoba, S Canada
103 S13 **Dauphiné** *cultural region* E France
23 N9 **Dauphin Island** *island* Alabama, S USA
11 X15 **Dauphin River** Manitoba, S Canada
77 V12 **Daura** Katsina, N Nigeria
152 H12 **Dausa** *prev.* Daosa. Rājasthān, N India
Dauwa *see* Dawwah
137 Y10 **Däväçi** *Rus.* Divichi. NE Azerbaijan
155 F18 **Dāvangere** Karnātaka, W India
171 Q8 **Davao** *off.* Davao City. Mindanao, S Philippines
171 Q8 **Davao Gulf** *gulf* Mindanao, S Philippines
15 Q11 **Daveluyville** Quebec, SE Canada
29 Z14 **Davenport** Iowa, C USA
32 L8 **Davenport** Washington, NW USA
43 P16 **David** Chiriquí, W Panama
15 O11 **David** ~ Quebec, SE Canada
29 R15 **David City** Nebraska, C USA
David-Gorodok *see* Davyd-Haradok
11 T16 **Davidson** Saskatchewan, S Canada
21 R10 **Davidson** North Carolina, SE USA
26 K12 **Davidson** Oklahoma, C USA
39 S6 **Davidson Mountains** ▲ Alaska, USA
172 M8 **Davie Ridge** *undersea feature* W Indian Ocean
182 A1 **Davies, Mount** ▲ South Australia
35 O7 **Davis** California, W USA
27 N12 **Davis** Oklahoma, C USA
195 Y7 **Davis** *Australian research station* Antarctica
194 H3 **Davis Coast** *physical region* Antarctica
18 C16 **Davis, Mount** ▲ Pennsylvania, NE USA
24 K9 **Davis Mountains** ▲ Texas, SW USA
195 Z9 **Davis Sea** *sea* Antarctica
65 O20 **Davis Seamounts** *undersea feature* S Atlantic Ocean
196 M13 **Davis Strait** *strait* Baffin Bay/Labrador Sea
129 U5 **Davlekanovo** Respublika Bashkortostan, W Russian Federation
108 J9 **Davos** *Rmsch.* Tavau. Graubünden, E Switzerland
119 J20 **Davyd-Haradok** *Pol.* Dawidgródek, *Rus.* David-Gorodok. Brestskaya Voblasts', SW Belarus
163 U12 **Dawa** Liaoning, NE China
141 O11 **Dawāsir, Wādī ad** *dry watercourse* S Saudi Arabia
81 K15 **Dawa Wenz** *var.* Daua, Webi Daawo. ~ E Africa
Dawaymah, Birkat ad *see* Umm al Baqar, Hawr
Dawei *see* Tavoy
119 K14 **Dawhinava** *Rus.* Dolginovo. Minskaya Voblasts', N Belarus
Dawidgródek *see* Davyd-Haradok
141 V12 **Dawkah** *var.* Dauka. SW Oman
Dawlat Qaṭar *see* Qatar
24 M3 **Dawn** Texas, SW USA
140 M11 **Daws** Al Bāḥah, SW Saudi Arabia
10 H5 **Dawson** *var.* Dawson City. Yukon Territory, NW Canada
23 S6 **Dawson** Georgia, SE USA
29 S9 **Dawson** Minnesota, N USA
Dawson City *see* Dawson
11 N13 **Dawson Creek** British Columbia, W Canada
8 H7 **Dawson Range** ▲ Yukon Territory, W Canada
181 Y9 **Dawson River** ~ Queensland, E Australia
10 J15 **Dawsons Landing** British Columbia, SW Canada
20 I7 **Dawson Springs** Kentucky, S USA
23 S2 **Dawsonville** Georgia, SE USA
160 G8 **Dawu** Sichuan, C China
Dawu *see* Maqên
Dawukou *see* Shizuishan
141 Y10 **Dawwah** *var.* Dauwa. W Oman
102 J15 **Dax** *var.* Ax; *anc.* Aquae Augustae, Aquae Tarbelicae. Landes, SW France
Da Xian/Daxian *see* Dachuan
160 G9 **Daxue Shan** ▲ C China
160 G12 **Dayao** Yunnan, SW China
Dayishan *see* Gaoyou
183 N12 **Daylesford** Victoria, SE Australia
35 U10 **Daylight Pass** *pass* California, W USA
61 D17 **Daymán, Río** ~ N Uruguay
Dayr *see* Ad Dayr
138 G10 **Dayr 'Allā** *var.* Deir 'Alla. Al Balqā', N Jordan
139 N4 **Dayr az Zawr** *var.* Deir ez Zor. Dayr az Zawr, E Syria
138 M5 **Dayr az Zawr** *off.* Muḥāfaẓat Dayr az Zawr, *var.* Dayr Az-Zor. ◆ *governorate* E Syria
Dayr Az-Zor *see* Dayr az Zawr
Dayrūṭ *see* Dairûṭ
11 Q15 **Daysland** Alberta, SW Canada
31 R14 **Dayton** Ohio, N USA
20 L10 **Dayton** Tennessee, S USA
25 W11 **Dayton** Texas, SW USA
32 L10 **Dayton** Washington, NW USA
23 X10 **Daytona Beach** Florida, SE USA
169 U12 **Dayu** Borneo, C Indonesia
161 O13 **Dayu Ling** ▲ S China
161 R7 **Da Yunhe** *Eng.* Grand Canal. *canal* E China
161 S11 **Dayu Shan** *island* SE China
160 J9 **Dazhu** Sichuan, C China
160 J9 **Dazu** Chongqing Shi, C China
83 H24 **De Aar** Northern Cape, C South Africa
194 K5 **Deacon, Cape** *headland* Antarctica
39 R5 **Deadhorse** Alaska, USA
33 T12 **Dead Indian Peak** ▲ Wyoming, C USA
23 R9 **Dead Lake** ◎ Florida, SE USA
44 J4 **Deadman's Cay** Long Island, C Bahamas
138 G11 **Dead Sea** *var.* Bahret Lut, Lacus Asphaltites, *Ar.* Al Baḥr al Mayyit, Baḥrat Lūt, *Heb.* Yam HaMelaḥ. *salt lake* Israel/Jordan
28 J9 **Deadwood** South Dakota, N USA
97 Q22 **Deal** SE England, UK
83 I22 **Dealesville** Free State, C South Africa
Dealnu *see* Tana/Teno
161 P10 **De'an** Jiangxi, S China
62 K9 **Deán Funes** Córdoba, C Argentina
194 L12 **Dean Island** *island* Antarctica
31 S10 **Dearborn** Michigan, N USA
27 R3 **Dearborn** Missouri, C USA
32 K9 **Deary** Idaho, NW USA
32 M9 **Deary** Washington, NW USA
10 J10 **Dease** ~ British Columbia, W Canada
10 J10 **Dease Lake** British Columbia, W Canada
35 U11 **Death Valley** California, W USA
35 U11 **Death Valley** *valley* California, W USA
102 L4 **Deauville** Calvados, N France
117 X7 **Debal'tseve** *Rus.* Debal'tsevo. Donets'ka Oblast', SE Ukraine
Debal'tsevo *see* Debal'tseve
113 M19 **Debar** *Ger.* Dibra, *Turk.* Debre. W FYR Macedonia
39 O9 **Debauch Mountain** ▲ Alaska, USA
De Behagle *see* Laï
25 X7 **De Berry** Texas, SW USA
129 T2 **Debesy** Udmurtskaya Respublika, NW Russian Federation
111 N16 **Dębica** Podkarpackie, SE Poland
De Bildt *see* De Bilt
98 J11 **De Bilt** *var.* De Bildt. Utrecht, C Netherlands
123 T9 **Debin** Magadanskaya Oblast', E Russian Federation
110 N13 **Dęblin** *Rus.* Ivangorod. Lubelskie, E Poland
110 D10 **Dębno** Zachodniopomorskie, NW Poland
39 S10 **Deborah, Mount** ▲ Alaska, USA
33 N8 **De Borgia** Montana, NW USA
Debra Birhan *see* Debre Birhan
Debra Marcos *see* Debre Mark'os
Debra Tabor *see* Debre Tabor
Debre *see* Debar
80 J13 **Debre Birhan** *var.* Debra Birhan. Amhara, N Ethiopia
111 N22 **Debrecen** *Ger.* Debreczin, *Rom.* Debreţin; *prev.* Debreczen. Hajdú-Bihar, E Hungary
Debreczen/Debreczin *see* Debrecen
80 I12 **Debre Mark'os** *var.* Debra Marcos. Amhara, N Ethiopia
113 N19 **Debrešte** SW FYR Macedonia
80 J11 **Debre Tabor** *var.* Debra Tabor. Amhara, N Ethiopia
Debreţin *see* Debrecen
80 J13 **Debre Zeyt** Oromo, C Ethiopia
113 L16 **Dečani** Serbia, S Yugoslavia
23 P2 **Decatur** Alabama, S USA
23 S3 **Decatur** Georgia, SE USA
30 L13 **Decatur** Illinois, N USA
31 Q12 **Decatur** Indiana, N USA
22 M5 **Decatur** Mississippi, S USA
29 S14 **Decatur** Nebraska, C USA
25 S6 **Decatur** Texas, SW USA
20 H9 **Decaturville** Tennessee, S USA
103 O13 **Decazeville** Aveyron, S France
155 H17 **Deccan** *Hind.* Dakshin. *plateau* C India
14 J8 **Decelles, Réservoir** ▣ Quebec, SE Canada
12 K2 **Déception** Quebec, NE Canada
160 G11 **Dechang** Sichuan, C China
111 C15 **Děčín** *Ger.* Tetschen. Ústecký Kraj, NW Czech Republic
103 P9 **Decize** Nièvre, C France
98 I6 **De Cocksdorp** Noord-Holland, NW Netherlands
29 X11 **Decorah** Iowa, C USA
Dedeagaç/Dedeagach *see* Alexandroúpoli
188 C15 **Dededo** N Guam
98 N9 **Dedemsvaart** Overijssel, E Netherlands
19 O11 **Dedham** Massachusetts, NE USA
63 H19 **Dedo, Cerro** ▲ SW Argentina
77 O13 **Dédougou** W Burkina
126 G15 **Dedovichi** Pskovskaya Oblast', W Russian Federation
163 V6 **Dedu** *var.* Qingshan. Heilongjiang, NE China
155 J24 **Deduru Oya** ~ W Sri Lanka
83 N14 **Dedza** Central, S Malawi
83 N14 **Dedza Mountain** ▲ C Malawi
97 J19 **Dee** *Wel.* Afon Dyfrdwy. ~ England/Wales, UK
96 K9 **Dee** ~ NE Scotland, UK
Deep Bay *see* Chilumba
21 T3 **Deep Creek Lake** ▣ Maryland, NE USA
36 J4 **Deep Creek Range** ▲ Utah, W USA
27 P10 **Deep Fork** ~ Oklahoma, C USA
14 J11 **Deep River** Ontario, SE Canada
21 T10 **Deep River** ~ North Carolina, SE USA
183 U4 **Deepwater** New South Wales, SE Australia
31 S14 **Deer Creek Lake** ◎ Ohio, N USA
23 Z15 **Deerfield Beach** Florida, SE USA
39 N8 **Deering** Alaska, USA
38 M16 **Deer Island** *island* Alaska, USA
19 S7 **Deer Isle** *island* Maine, NE USA
13 S11 **Deer Lake** Newfoundland, SE Canada
99 D18 **Deerlijk** West-Vlaanderen, W Belgium
33 Q10 **Deer Lodge** Montana, NW USA
32 L8 **Deer Park** Washington, NW USA
29 U5 **Deer River** Minnesota, N USA
Deés *see* Dej
31 R11 **Defiance** Ohio, N USA
23 Q8 **De Funiak Springs** Florida, SE USA
95 L23 **Degeberga** Skåne, S Sweden
104 H12 **Degebe, Ribeira** ~ S Portugal
80 M13 **Degeh Bur** Somali, E Ethiopia
15 U9 **Dégelis** Quebec, SE Canada
77 U17 **Degema** Rivers, S Nigeria
95 L16 **Degerfors** Örebro, C Sweden
193 R14 **De Gerlache Seamounts** *undersea feature* SE Pacific Ocean
101 N21 **Deggendorf** Bayern, SE Germany
80 I11 **Degoma** Amhara, N Ethiopia
De Gordyk *see* Gorredijk
27 T12 **De Gray Lake** ▣ Arkansas, C USA
180 J6 **De Grey River** ~ Western Australia
128 M10 **Degtevo** Rostovskaya Oblast', SW Russian Federation
143 X13 **Dehak** Sīstān va Balūchestān, SE Iran
143 R9 **Deh 'Alī** Kermān, C Iran
143 S13 **Dehbārez** *var.* Rūdān. Hormozgān, S Iran
143 P10 **Deh Bīd** Fārs, C Iran
142 M10 **Deh Dasht** Kohkīlūyeh va Būyer Aḥmadī, SW Iran
75 N8 **Dehibat** SE Tunisia
Dehli *see* Delhi
142 K8 **Dehlorān** Īlām, W Iran
147 N13 **Dehqonobod** *Rus.* Dekhkanabad. Qashqadaryo Wiloyati, S Uzbekistan
152 J9 **Dehra Dūn** Uttar Pradesh, N India
153 O14 **Dehri** Bihār, N India
148 K10 **Deh Shū** *var.* Deshu. Helmand, S Afghanistan
99 D17 **Deinze** Oost-Vlaanderen, NW Belgium
Deir 'Alla *see* Dayr 'Allā
Deir ez Zor *see* Dayr az Zawr
Deirgeirt, Loch *see* Derg, Lough
116 H9 **Dej** *Hung.* Dés; *prev.* Deés. Cluj, NW Romania
95 K15 **Deje** Värmland, C Sweden
171 Y15 **De Jongs, Tanjung** *headland* Irian Jaya, SE Indonesia
De Jouwer *see* Joure
30 M10 **De Kalb** Illinois, N USA
22 M5 **De Kalb** Mississippi, S USA
25 W5 **De Kalb** Texas, SW USA
Dekéleia *see* Dhekélia
79 K20 **Dekese** Kasai Occidental, C Dem. Rep. Congo (Zaire)
Dekhkanabad *see* Dehqonobod
79 I14 **Dékoa** Kémo, 243C Central African Republic
98 H6 **De Koog** Noord-Holland, NW Netherlands
30 M9 **Delafield** Wisconsin, N USA
61 C23 **De La Garma** Buenos Aires, E Argentina
14 K10 **Delahey, Lac** ◎ Quebec, SE Canada
80 E11 **Delami** Southern Kordofan, C Sudan
23 X11 **De Land** Florida, SE USA
35 R12 **Delano** California, W USA
29 V8 **Delano** Minnesota, N USA
36 K6 **Delano Peak** ▲ Utah, W USA
Delap-Uliga-Darrit *see* Dalap-Uliga-Djarrit
148 L7 **Delārām** Farāh, SW Afghanistan
38 F17 **Delarof Islands** *island group* Aleutian Islands, Alaska, USA
30 M9 **Delavan** Wisconsin, N USA
31 S13 **Delaware** Ohio, N USA
18 I17 **Delaware** *off.* State of Delaware; also known as Blue Hen State, Diamond State, First State. ◆ *state* NE USA
18 I17 **Delaware Bay** *bay* NE USA
24 J8 **Delaware Mountains** ▲ Texas, SW USA
18 I12 **Delaware River** ~ NE USA
27 Q3 **Delaware River** ~ Kansas, C USA
18 J14 **Delaware Water Gap** *valley* New Jersey/Pennsylvania, NE USA
101 G14 **Delbrück** Nordrhein-Westfalen, W Germany
11 Q15 **Delburne** Alberta, SW Canada
172 M12 **Del Cano Rise** *undersea feature* SW Indian Ocean
113 Q18 **Delčevo** NE FYR Macedonia
Delcommune, Lac *see* Nzilo, Lac
98 O10 **Delden** Overijssel, E Netherlands
183 R12 **Delegate** New South Wales, SE Australia
De Lemmer *see* Lemmer
108 D7 **Delémont** *Ger.* Delsberg. Jura, NW Switzerland
25 R7 **De Leon** Texas, SW USA
115 F18 **Delfoí** Stereá Ellás, C Greece
98 G12 **Delft** Zuid-Holland, W Netherlands
155 J23 **Delft** *island* NW Sri Lanka
98 O5 **Delfzijl** Groningen, NE Netherlands
(0) E9 **Delgada Fan** *undersea feature* NE Pacific Ocean
42 F7 **Delgado** San Salvador, SW El Salvador
82 Q12 **Delgado, Cabo** *headland* N Mozambique
80 E6 **Delgo** Northern, N Sudan
159 R10 **Delhi** *var.* Delingha. Qinghai, C China
152 I10 **Delhi** *var.* Dehli, *Hind.* Dilli; *hist.* Shahjahanabad. Delhi, N India
22 J5 **Delhi** Louisiana, S USA
18 J11 **Delhi** New York, NE USA
152 I10 **Delhi** ◆ *union territory* NW India
136 J17 **Deli Burnu** *headland* S Turkey
55 X10 **Délices** C French Guiana
136 J12 **Delice Çayı** ~ C Turkey
40 J6 **Delicias** *var.* Ciudad Delicias. Chihuahua, N Mexico
143 N7 **Delījān** *var.* Dalijan, Dilijan. Markazī, W Iran
112 P12 **Deli Jovan** ▲ E Yugoslavia
Déli-Kárpátok *see* Carpaţii Meridionali
8 I8 **Déline** *prev.* Fort Franklin. Northwest Territories, NW Canada
Delingha *see* Delhi
15 Q7 **Delisle** Quebec, SE Canada
11 T15 **Delisle** Saskatchewan, S Canada
101 M15 **Delitzsch** Sachsen, E Germany
33 Q12 **Dell** Montana, NW USA
24 I7 **Dell City** Texas, SW USA
103 U7 **Delle** Territoire-de-Belfort, E France
36 J9 **Dellenbaugh, Mount** ▲ Arizona, SW USA
29 R11 **Dell Rapids** South Dakota, N USA
21 Y4 **Delmar** Maryland, NE USA
18 K11 **Delmar** New York, NE USA
100 G11 **Delmenhorst** Niedersachsen, NW Germany
112 C9 **Delnice** Primorje-Gorski Kotar, NW Croatia
37 R7 **Del Norte** Colorado, C USA
39 N6 **De Long Mountains** ▲ Alaska, USA
183 P16 **Deloraine** Tasmania, SE Australia
11 W17 **Deloraine** Manitoba, S Canada
31 O12 **Delphi** Indiana, N USA
31 Q12 **Delphos** Ohio, N USA
23 Z15 **Delray Beach** Florida, SE USA
25 O12 **Del Rio** Texas, SW USA
Delsberg *see* Delémont
94 N11 **Delsbo** Gävleborg, C Sweden
37 P6 **Delta** Colorado, C USA
36 K5 **Delta** Utah, W USA
77 T17 **Delta** ◆ *state* S Nigeria
55 Q6 **Delta Amacuro** *off.* Territorio Delta Amacuro. ◆ *federal district* NE Venezuela
39 S9 **Delta Junction** Alaska, USA
23 X11 **Deltona** Florida, SE USA
183 T5 **Delungra** New South Wales, SE Australia
154 C12 **Delvāda** Gujarāt, W India
61 B21 **Del Valle** Buenos Aires, E Argentina
Delvina *see* Delvinë
115 C15 **Delvináki** *var.* Dhelvinákion; *prev.* Pogónion. Ípeiros, W Greece
113 L23 **Delvinë** *var.* Delvina, *It.* Delvino. Vlorë, S Albania
Delvino *see* Delvinë
116 I7 **Delyatyn** Ivano-Frankivs'ka Oblast', W Ukraine
129 U5 **Dëma** ~ W Russian Federation
105 O5 **Demanda, Sierra de la** ▲ W Spain
39 T5 **Demarcation Point** *headland* Alaska, USA
79 K21 **Demba** Kasai Occidental, C Dem. Rep. Congo (Zaire)
172 H13 **Dembéni** Grande Comore, NW Comoros
79 M15 **Dembia** Mbomou, SE Central African Republic
Dembidollo *see* Dembī Dolo
80 H13 **Dembī Dolo** *var.* Dembidollo. Oromo, C Ethiopia
152 K6 **Demchok** *var.* Dêmqog. China/India **see also** Dêmqog
152 L6 **Demchok** *var.* Dêmqog. *disputed region* China/India **see also** Dêmqog
98 I12 **De Meern** Utrecht, C Netherlands
99 I17 **Demer** ~ C Belgium
64 H12 **Demerara Plain** *undersea feature* W Atlantic Ocean
64 H12 **Demerara Plateau** *undersea feature* W Atlantic Ocean
55 T9 **Demerara River** ~ NE Guyana
128 H3 **Demidov** Smolenskaya Oblast', W Russian Federation
37 Q15 **Deming** New Mexico, SW USA
32 H6 **Deming** Washington, NW USA
58 E10 **Demini, Rio** ~ NW Brazil
136 D13 **Demirci** Manisa, W Turkey
113 P19 **Demir Kapija** *prev.* Železna Vrata. SE FYR Macedonia
114 N11 **Demirköy** Kırklareli, NW Turkey
100 N9 **Demmin** Mecklenburg-Vorpommern, NE Germany
23 O5 **Demopolis** Alabama, S USA
31 N11 **Demotte** Indiana, N USA
158 F13 **Dêmqog** *var.* Demchok. China/India **see also** Demchok
152 L6 **Dêmqog** *var.* Demchok. *disputed region* China/India **see also** Demchok
171 Y13 **Demta** Irian Jaya, E Indonesia
122 H11 **Dem'yanka** ~ C Russian Federation
126 H15 **Demyansk** Novgorodskaya Oblast', W Russian Federation
122 H10 **Dem'yanskoye** Tyumenskaya Oblast', C Russian Federation
103 P2 **Denain** Nord, N France
39 S10 **Denali** Alaska, USA
Denali *see* McKinley, Mount
81 M14 **Denan** Somali, E Ethiopia
Denau *see* Denow
97 J18 **Denbigh** *Wel.* Dinbych. NE Wales, UK
97 J18 **Denbigh** *cultural region* N Wales, UK
98 I6 **Den Burg** Noord-Holland, NW Netherlands
99 F18 **Dender** *Fr.* Dendre. ~ W Belgium
99 F18 **Denderleeuw** Oost-Vlaanderen, NW Belgium
99 F17 **Dendermonde** *Fr.* Termonde. Oost-Vlaanderen, NW Belgium
Dendre *see* Dender
194 I9 **Dendtler Island** *island* Antarctica
98 P10 **Denekamp** Overijssel, E Netherlands
77 W12 **Dengas** Zinder, S Niger
Dêngkagoin *see* Têwo
162 L13 **Dengkou** *var.* Bayan Gol. Nei Mongol Zizhiqu, N China
159 Q14 **Dêngqên** Xizang Zizhiqu, W China
Deng Xian *see* Dengzhou
160 M7 **Dengzhou** *prev.* Deng Xian. Henan, C China
Dengzhou *see* Penglai
Den Haag *see* 's-Gravenhage
98 N9 **Den Ham** Overijssel, E Netherlands
180 H10 **Denham** Western Australia
44 J12 **Denham, Mount** ▲ C Jamaica
22 J8 **Denham Springs** Louisiana, S USA

◆ Country ◇ Dependent Territory ◆ Administrative Region ▲ Mountain ✱ Volcano ◎ Lake
● Country Capital ○ Dependent Territory Capital ✕ International Airport ▲ Mountain Range ~ River ▣ Reservoir

98 I7 **Den Helder** Noord-Holland, NW Netherlands
105 T11 **Denia** País Valenciano, E Spain
189 Q8 **Denig** W Nauru
183 N10 **Deniliquin** New South Wales, SE Australia
29 T14 **Denison** Iowa, C USA
25 U5 **Denison** Texas, SW USA
136 D15 **Denizli** Denizli, SW Turkey
136 D15 **Denizli** ◈ *province* SW Turkey
Denjong *see* Sikkim
183 S7 **Denman** New South Wales, SE Australia
195 Y10 **Denman Glacier** *glacier* Antarctica
21 R14 **Denmark** South Carolina, SE USA
95 G23 **Denmark** *off.* Kingdom of Denmark, *Dan.* Danmark; *anc.* Hafnia. ◆ *monarchy* N Europe
92 H1 **Denmark Strait** *var.* Danmarksstraedet. *strait* Greenland/Iceland
45 T11 **Dennery** E Saint Lucia
98 I7 **Den Oever** Noord-Holland, NW Netherlands
147 O13 **Denow** *Rus.* Denau. Surkhondaryo Wiloyati, S Uzbekistan
169 U17 **Denpasar** *prev.* Paloe. Bali, C Indonesia
116 E12 **Denta** Timiş, W Romania
21 Y3 **Denton** Maryland, NE USA
25 T6 **Denton** Texas, SW USA
186 G9 **D'Entrecasteaux Islands** *island group* SE PNG
37 T4 **Denver** *state capital* Colorado, C USA
16 I10 **Denver** × Colorado, C USA
24 L6 **Denver City** Texas, SW USA
152 J9 **Deoband** Uttar Pradesh, N India
Deoghar *see* Devghar
154 E13 **Deolāli** Mahārāshtra, W India
154 I10 **Deori** Madhya Pradesh, C India
153 O12 **Deoria** Uttar Pradesh, N India
99 A17 **De Panne** West-Vlaanderen, W Belgium
54 M5 **Dependencia Federal** *off.* Territorio Dependencia Federal. ◈ *federal dependency* N Venezuela
Dependencia Federal, Territorio *see* Dependencia Federal
30 M7 **De Pere** Wisconsin, N USA
18 D10 **Depew** New York, NE USA
99 E17 **De Pinte** Oost-Vlaanderen, NW Belgium
25 V5 **Deport** Texas, SW USA
123 Q8 **Deputatskiy** Respublika Sakha (Yakutiya), NE Russian Federation
27 S13 **De Queen** Arkansas, C USA
22 G8 **De Quincy** Louisiana, S USA
81 J20 **Dera** *spring/well* S Kenya
Der'a/Derá/Déraa *see* Dar'ā
149 S10 **Dera Ghāzi Khān** *var.* Dera Ghāzikhān. Punjab, C Pakistan
149 S8 **Dera Ismāīl Khān** North-West Frontier Province, C Pakistan
113 L16 **Deravica** ▲ S Yugoslavia
116 L6 **Derazhnya** Khmel'nyts'ka Oblast', W Ukraine
129 R17 **Derbent** Respublika Dagestan, SW Russian Federation
147 N13 **Derbent** Surkhondaryo Wiloyati, S Uzbekistan
Derbisīye *see* Darbāsīyah
79 M15 **Derbissaka** Mbomou, SE Central African Republic
180 L4 **Derby** Western Australia
97 M19 **Derby** C England, UK
27 N7 **Derby** Kansas, C USA
97 L18 **Derbyshire** *cultural region* C England, UK
112 O11 **Đerdap** *physical region* E Yugoslavia
Derelí *see* Gónnoi
171 W13 **Derew** ≈ Irian Jaya, E Indonesia
129 R8 **Dergachi** Saratovskaya Oblast', W Russian Federation
Dergachi *see* Derhachi
97 C19 **Derg, Lough** *Ir.* Loch Deirgeirt. ◎ W Ireland
117 V5 **Derhachi** *Rus.* Dergachi. Kharkivs'ka Oblast', E Ukraine
22 G8 **De Ridder** Louisiana, S USA
137 P16 **Derik** Mardin, SE Turkey
83 E20 **Derm** Hardap, C Namibia
144 M14 **Dermentobe** *prev.* Dyurmen'tyube. Kzylorda, S Kazakhstan
27 W14 **Dermott** Arkansas, C USA
Dérna *see* Darnah
Dernberg, Cape *see* Dolphin Head
22 J11 **Dernieres, Isles** *island group* Louisiana, S USA
Dernis *see* Drniš
102 I4 **Déroute, Passage de la** *strait* Channel Islands/France
Derrá *see* Dar'ā
Derry *see* Londonderry
Dertona *see* Tortona
Dertosa *see* Tortosa
80 H8 **Derudeb** Red Sea, NE Sudan
112 H10 **Derventa** Republika Srpska, N Bosnia and Herzegovina
183 O16 **Derwent Bridge** Tasmania, SE Australia
183 O17 **Derwent, River** ≈ Tasmania, SE Australia
Derweze *see* Darvaza
Deržavinsk *see* Derzhavinsk
145 O9 **Derzhavinsk** *var.* Deržavinsk. Akmola, C Kazakhstan
Dés *see* Dej
57 J18 **Desaguadero** Puno, S Peru
57 J18 **Desaguadero, Río** ≈ Bolivia/Peru
191 W9 **Désappointement, Îles du** *island group* Îles Tuamotu, C French Polynesia
27 W11 **Des Arc** Arkansas, C USA
14 C10 **Desbarats** Ontario, S Canada
62 H13 **Descabezado Grande, Volcán** ⩙ C Chile
40 B2 **Descanso** Baja California, NW Mexico
102 L9 **Descartes** Indre-et-Loire, C France
11 T13 **Deschambault Lake** ◎ Saskatchewan, C Canada
Deschnaer Koppe *see* Velká Deštná
32 I11 **Deschutes River** ≈ Oregon, NW USA
80 J12 **Desē** *var.* Desse, *It.* Dessie. Amhara, N Ethiopia
63 I20 **Deseado, Río** ≈ S Argentina
106 F8 **Desenzano del Garda** Lombardia, N Italy
36 K3 **Deseret Peak** ▲ Utah, W USA
64 P6 **Deserta Grande** *island* Madeira, Portugal, NE Atlantic Ocean
64 P6 **Desertas, Ilhas** *island group* Madeira, Portugal, NE Atlantic Ocean
35 X16 **Desert Center** California, W USA
35 V15 **Desert Hot Springs** California, W USA
14 K10 **Désert, Lac** ◎ Quebec, SE Canada
36 J2 **Desert Peak** ▲ Utah, W USA
31 R11 **Deshler** Ohio, N USA
Deshu *see* Deh Shū
Desiderii Fanum *see* St-Dizier
106 D7 **Desio** Lombardia, N Italy
115 E15 **Deskáti** *var.* Dheskáti. Dytikí Makedonía, N Greece
28 L2 **Des Lacs River** ≈ North Dakota, N USA
27 X6 **Desloge** Missouri, C USA
11 Q12 **Desmarais** Alberta, W Canada
29 Q10 **De Smet** South Dakota, N USA
29 V14 **Des Moines** *state capital* Iowa, C USA
17 N9 **Des Moines River** ≈ C USA
117 P4 **Desna** ≈ Russian Federation/Ukraine
116 G14 **Desnățui** ≈ S Romania
63 F24 **Desolación, Isla** *island* S Chile
29 V14 **De Soto** Iowa, C USA
23 Q4 **De Soto Falls** *waterfall* Alabama, S USA
83 I25 **Despatch** Eastern Cape, S South Africa
105 N12 **Despeñaperros, Desfiladero de** *pass* S Spain
31 N10 **Des Plaines** Illinois, N USA
115 J21 **Despotikó** *island* Kykládes, Greece, Aegean Sea
112 N12 **Despotovac** Serbia, E Yugoslavia
101 M14 **Dessau** Sachsen-Anhalt, E Germany
Desse *see* Desē
99 J16 **Dessel** Antwerpen, N Belgium
Dessie *see* Desē
Destêrro *see* Florianópolis
23 P9 **Destin** Florida, SE USA
Deštná *see* Velká Deštná
193 T10 **Desventurados, Islas de los** *island group* W Chile
103 N1 **Desvres** Pas-de-Calais, N France
116 E12 **Deta** *Ger.* Detta. Timiş, W Romania
101 H14 **Detmold** Nordrhein-Westfalen, W Germany
31 S10 **Detroit** Michigan, N USA
25 W5 **Detroit** Texas, SW USA
31 S10 **Detroit** ≈ Canada/USA
29 S6 **Detroit Lakes** Minnesota, N USA
31 S10 **Detroit Metropolitan** × Michigan, N USA
Detta *see* Deta
167 S10 **Det Udom** Ubon Ratchathani, E Thailand
111 K20 **Detva** *Hung.* Gyeva. Banskobystrický Kraj, C Slovakia
154 G13 **Deūlgaon Rāja** Mahārāshtra, C India
99 L15 **Deurne** Noord-Brabant, SE Netherlands
99 H16 **Deurne** × (Antwerpen) Antwerpen, N Belgium
Deutsch-Brod *see* Havlíčkův Brod
Deutschendorf *see* Poprad
Deutsch-Eylau *see* Iława
109 Y6 **Deutschkreutz** Burgenland, E Austria
Deutsch Krone *see* Wałcz
Deutschland/Deutschland, Bundesrepublik *see* Germany
109 V9 **Deutschlandsberg** Steiermark, SE Austria
Deutsch-Südwestafrika *see* Namibia
109 Y3 **Deutsch-Wagram** Niederösterreich, E Austria
Deux-Ponts *see* Zweibrücken
14 I11 **Deux Rivieres** Ontario, SE Canada
102 K9 **Deux-Sèvres** ◈ *department* W France
116 G11 **Deva** *Ger.* Diemrich, *Hung.* Déva. Hunedoara, W Romania
Deva *see* Chester
Devana *see* Aberdeen
Devana Castra *see* Chester
Đevđelija *see* Gevgelija
136 L12 **Deveci Dağları** ▲ N Turkey
137 P15 **Devegeçidi Barajı** ▣ SE Turkey
136 K15 **Develi** Kayseri, C Turkey
98 M11 **Deventer** Overijssel, E Netherlands
15 O10 **Devenyns, Lac** ◎ Quebec, SE Canada
96 K8 **Deveron** ≈ NE Scotland, UK
153 R14 **Devghar** *prev.* Deoghar. Bihār, NE India
27 R10 **Devil's Den** *plateau* Arkansas, C USA
35 R7 **Devils Gate** *pass* California, W USA
30 J2 **Devils Island** *island* Apostle Islands, Wisconsin, N USA
Devil's Island *see* Diable, Île du
29 P3 **Devils Lake** North Dakota, N USA
31 R10 **Devils Lake** ◎ Michigan, N USA
29 O3 **Devils Lake** ◎ North Dakota, N USA
35 W13 **Devils Playground** *desert* California, W USA
25 O11 **Devils River** ≈ Texas, SW USA
33 Y12 **Devils Tower** ▲ Wyoming, C USA
114 I11 **Devin** *prev.* Dovlen. Smolyan, SW Bulgaria
25 R12 **Devine** Texas, SW USA
152 H13 **Devli** Rājasthān, N India
Devne *see* Devnya
114 N8 **Devnya** *prev.* Devne. Varna, E Bulgaria
31 U14 **Devola** Ohio, N USA
Devoll *see* Devollit, Lumi i
113 M21 **Devollit, Lumi i** *var.* Devoll. ≈ SE Albania
11 Q14 **Devon** Alberta, SW Canada
97 I23 **Devon** *cultural region* SW England, UK
9 O4 **Devon Ice Cap** *ice feature* Nunavut, N Canada
8 N4 **Devon Island** *prev.* North Devon Island. *island* Parry Islands, Nunavut, NE Canada
183 O16 **Devonport** Tasmania, SE Australia
136 H11 **Devrek** Zonguldak, N Turkey
154 G10 **Dewās** Madhya Pradesh, C India
De Westerein *see* Zwaagwesteinde
27 P8 **Dewey** Oklahoma, C USA
Dewey *see* Culebra
98 M8 **De Wijk** Drenthe, NE Netherlands
27 W12 **De Witt** Arkansas, C USA
29 Z14 **De Witt** Iowa, C USA
29 R16 **De Witt** Nebraska, C USA
97 M17 **Dewsbury** N England, UK
161 Q10 **Dexing** Jiangxi, S China
27 Y8 **Dexter** Missouri, C USA
37 U14 **Dexter** New Mexico, SW USA
160 I8 **Deyang** Sichuan, C China
182 C4 **Dey-Dey, Lake** *salt lake* South Australia
143 S7 **Deyhūk** Khorāsān, E Iran
146 K12 **Deynau** *var.* Dyanev, *Turkm.* Dänew. Lebapskiy Velayat, NE Turkmenistan
142 L8 **Dezfūl** *var.* Dizful. Khūzestān, SW Iran
131 X4 **Dezhneva, Mys** *headland* NE Russian Federation
161 P4 **Dezhou** Shandong, E China
Dezh Shāhpūr *see* Marīvān
Dhahran *see* Aẓ Ẓahrān
Dhahran Al Khobar *see* Aẓ Ẓahrān al Khubar
153 U14 **Dhaka** *prev.* Dacca. ● (Bangladesh) Dhaka, C Bangladesh
153 T15 **Dhaka** ◈ *division* C Bangladesh
Dhali *see* Idálion
141 O15 **Dhamār** W Yemen
Dhambul *see* Taraz
154 K12 **Dhamtari** Madhya Pradesh, C India
153 Q15 **Dhanbād** Bihār, NE India
152 L10 **Dhangadhi** *var.* Dhangarhi. Far Western, W Nepal
Dhangarhi *see* Dhangadhi
Dhank *see* Ḍank
153 R12 **Dhankuta** Eastern, E Nepal
152 I6 **Dhaola Dhār** ▲ NE India
154 F10 **Dhār** Madhya Pradesh, C India
153 R12 **Dharan** *var.* Dharan Bazar. Eastern, E Nepal
155 H21 **Dhārāpuram** Tamil Nādu, SE India
155 H20 **Dharmapuri** Tamil Nādu, SE India
155 H18 **Dharmavaram** Andhra Pradesh, E India
154 M11 **Dharmjaygarh** Madhya Pradesh, C India
Dharmsāla *see* Dharmshāla
152 I7 **Dharmshāla** *prev.* Dharmsāla. Himāchal Pradesh, N India
155 F17 **Dhārwād** *prev.* Dharwar. Karnātaka, SW India
Dharwar *see* Dhārwād
153 O10 **Dhaulāgiri** ▲ C Nepal
81 L18 **Dheere Laaq** *var.* Lak Dera, *It.* Lach Dera. *seasonal river* Kenya/Somalia
121 Q3 **Dhekéleia Sovereign Base Area** *UK military installation* E Cyprus
121 Q3 **Dhekélia** *Eng.* Dhekelia. *Gk.* Dekéleia. *UK air base* SE Cyprus
Dhelvinákion *see* Delvináki
113 M22 **Dhëmbelit, Majae** ▲ S Albania
154 O12 **Dhenkānāl** Orissa, E India
Dheskáti *see* Deskáti
138 G11 **Dhībān** 'Ammān, NW Jordan
Dhidhimótikhon *see* Didymóteicho
Dhíkti Ori *see* Díkti
138 I12 **Dhirwah, Wādī adh** *dry watercourse* C Jordan
Dhístomon *see* Dístomo
Dhodhekánisos *see* Dodekánisos
Dhodhóni *see* Dodóni
Dhofar *see* Ẓufār
Dhomokós *see* Domokós
Dhond *see* Daund
155 H17 **Dhone** Andhra Pradesh, C India
154 B11 **Dhorāji** Gujarāt, W India
Dhráma *see* Dráma
154 C10 **Dhrāngadhra** Gujarāt, W India
Dhrepanon, Akrotírio *see* Drépano, Akrotírio
153 T13 **Dhuburi** Assam, NE India
154 F12 **Dhule** *prev.* Dhulia. Mahārāshtra, C India
Dhulia *see* Dhule
Dhún Dealgan, Cuan *see* Dundalk Bay
Dhún Droma, Cuan *see* Dundrum Bay
Dhún na nGall, Bá *see* Donegal Bay
Dhū Shaykh *see* Qazānīyah
80 Q13 **Dhuudo** Bari, NE Somalia
81 N15 **Dhuusa Marreeb** *var.* Dusa Marreb, *It.* Dusa Mareb. Galguduud, C Somalia
115 J24 **Día** *island* SE Greece
55 Y9 **Diable, Île du** *var.* Devil's Island. *island* N French Guiana
15 N12 **Diable, Rivière du** ≈ Quebec, SE Canada
35 N8 **Diablo, Mount** ▲ California, W USA
35 O9 **Diablo Range** ▲ California, W USA
24 I8 **Diablo, Sierra** ▲ Texas, SW USA
45 O11 **Diablotins, Morne** ▲ N Dominica
77 N11 **Diafarabé** Mopti, C Mali
77 N11 **Diaka** ≈ SW Mali
Diakovár *see* Đakovo
76 I12 **Dialakoto** S Senegal
61 B18 **Diamante** Entre Ríos, E Argentina
62 I12 **Diamante, Río** ≈ C Argentina
59 M19 **Diamantina** Minas Gerais, SE Brazil
59 N17 **Diamantina, Chapada** ▲ E Brazil
173 U11 **Diamantina Fracture Zone** *tectonic feature* E Indian Ocean
181 T8 **Diamantina River** ≈ Queensland/South Australia
38 D9 **Diamond Head** *headland* Oahu, Hawaii, USA, C Pacific Ocean
37 P2 **Diamond Peak** ▲ Colorado, C USA
35 W5 **Diamond Peak** ▲ Nevada, W USA
Diamond State *see* Delaware
76 J11 **Diamou** Kayes, SW Mali
95 I23 **Dianalund** Vestsjælland, C Denmark
65 G25 **Diana's Peak** ▲ C Saint Helena
160 M16 **Dianbai** Guangdong, S China
160 G13 **Dian Chi** ▣ SW China
106 B10 **Diano Marina** Liguria, NW Italy
77 R13 **Diapaga** E Burkina
Diarbekr *see* Diyarbakır
107 J15 **Diavolo, Passo del** *pass* C Italy
61 B18 **Díaz** Santa Fe, C Argentina
141 W6 **Dibā al Ḥiṣn** *var.* Dibāh, Dibba. Ash Shāriqah, NE UAE
139 S3 **Dībaga** N Iraq
Dibāh *see* Dibā al Ḥiṣn
79 L22 **Dibaya** Kasai Occidental, S Dem. Rep. Congo (Zaire)
Dibba *see* Dibā al Ḥiṣn
195 W15 **Dibble Iceberg Tongue** *ice feature* Antarctica
113 L19 **Dibër** ◈ *district* E Albania
83 I20 **Dibete** Central, SE Botswana
25 W9 **Diboll** Texas, SW USA
Dibra *see* Debar
153 X11 **Dibrugarh** Assam, NE India
54 G4 **Dibulla** La Guajira, N Colombia
25 O5 **Dickens** Texas, SW USA
19 R2 **Dickey** Maine, NE USA
30 K9 **Dickeyville** Wisconsin, N USA
28 K5 **Dickinson** North Dakota, N USA
(0) E6 **Dickins Seamount** *undersea feature* NE Pacific Ocean
27 O13 **Dickson** Oklahoma, C USA
20 I9 **Dickson** Tennessee, S USA
Dicle *see* Tigris
Dicsőszentmárton *see* Târnăveni
98 M12 **Didam** Gelderland, E Netherlands
163 Y8 **Didao** Heilongjiang, NE China
76 L12 **Didiéni** Koulikoro, W Mali
Didimo *see* Dídymo
Didimotiho *see* Didymóteicho
81 K17 **Didimtu** *spring/well* NE Kenya
67 U9 **Didinga Hills** ▲ S Sudan
11 Q16 **Didsbury** Alberta, SW Canada
152 G11 **Dīdwāna** Rājasthān, N India
115 G20 **Dídymo** *var.* Didimo. ▲ S Greece
114 L12 **Didymóteicho** *var.* Dhidhimótikhon, Didimotiho. Anatolikí Makedonía kai Thráki, NE Greece
103 S13 **Die** Drôme, E France
77 O13 **Diébougou** SW Burkina
Diedenhofen *see* Thionville
11 S16 **Diefenbaker, Lake** ▣ Saskatchewan, S Canada
Diemrich *see* Deva
62 H7 **Diego de Almagro** Atacama, N Chile
63 F23 **Diego de Almagro, Isla** *island* S Chile
61 A20 **Diego de Alvear** Santa Fe, C Argentina
173 Q7 **Diego Garcia** *island* S British Indian Ocean Territory
Diégo-Suarez *see* Antsirañana
99 M23 **Diekirch** Diekirch, C Luxembourg
99 L23 **Diekirch** ◈ *district* N Luxembourg
76 K11 **Diéma** Kayes, W Mali
101 H15 **Diemel** ≈ W Germany
98 I10 **Diemen** Noord-Holland, C Netherlands
Diemrich *see* Deva
167 R6 **Điện Biên** *var.* Bien Bien, Dien Bien Phu. Lai Châu, N Vietnam
Dien Bien Phu *see* Điện Biên
167 S7 **Diên Châu** Nghê An, N Vietnam
99 K18 **Diepenbeek** Limburg, NE Belgium
98 N11 **Diepenheim** Overijssel, E Netherlands
98 M10 **Diepenveen** Overijssel, E Netherlands
100 G12 **Diepholz** Niedersachsen, NW Germany
102 M3 **Dieppe** Seine-Maritime, N France
98 M12 **Dieren** Gelderland, E Netherlands
27 S13 **Dierks** Arkansas, C USA
99 J17 **Diest** Vlaams Brabant, C Belgium
108 F7 **Dietikon** Zürich, NW Switzerland
103 R13 **Dieulefit** Drôme, E France
103 T5 **Dieuze** Moselle, NE France
119 H15 **Dieveniškės** Šalčininkai, SE Lithuania
98 N7 **Diever** Drenthe, NE Netherlands
101 F17 **Diez** Rheinland-Pfalz, W Germany
77 Y12 **Diffa** Diffa, SE Niger
77 Y10 **Diffa** ◈ *department* SE Niger
99 L25 **Differdange** Luxembourg, SW Luxembourg
13 O16 **Digby** Nova Scotia, SE Canada
26 J5 **Dighton** Kansas, C USA
Dignano d'Istria *see* Vodnjan
103 T14 **Digne** *var.* Digne-les-Bains. Alpes-de-Haute-Provence, SE France
Digne-les-Bains *see* Digne
Digoel *see* Digul, Sungai
103 Q10 **Digoin** Saône-et-Loire, C France
171 Q8 **Digos** Mindanao, S Philippines
149 Q16 **Digri** Sind, SE Pakistan
171 Y14 **Digul Barat, Sungai** ≈ Irian Jaya, E Indonesia
171 Y15 **Digul, Sungai** *prev.* Digoel. ≈ Irian Jaya, E Indonesia
171 Z14 **Digul Timur, Sungai** ≈ Irian Jaya, E Indonesia
Dihang *see* Brahmaputra
153 X10 **Dihāng** ≈ NE India
Dihōk *see* Dahūk
81 L17 **Diinsoor** Bay, S Somalia
Dijlah *see* Tigris
99 H17 **Dijle** ≈ C Belgium
103 R8 **Dijon** *anc.* Dibio. Côte d'Or, C France
93 H14 **Dikanäs** Västerbotten, N Sweden
80 L12 **Dikhil** SW Djibouti
136 B13 **Dikili** İzmir, W Turkey
99 B17 **Diksmuide** *var.* Dixmuide, *Fr.* Dixmude. West-Vlaanderen, W Belgium
122 K7 **Dikson** Taymyrskiy (Dolgano-Nenetskiy) Avtonomnyy Okrug, N Russian Federation
115 K25 **Díkti** *var.* Dhíkti Ori. ▲ Kríti, Greece, E Mediterranean Sea
77 Z13 **Dikwa** Borno, NE Nigeria
81 J15 **Dīla** Southern, S Ethiopia
99 G18 **Dilbeek** Vlaams Brabant, C Belgium
171 Q16 **Dili** *var.* Dilli, Dilly. ○ (East Timor) N East Timor
77 Y11 **Dilia** *var.* Dillia. ≈ SE Niger
Dilijan *see* Delijan
167 U13 **Di Linh** Lâm Đông, S Vietnam
101 G16 **Dillenburg** Hessen, W Germany
25 Q13 **Dilley** Texas, SW USA
Dilli *see* Delhi, India
Dilli *see* Dili, East Timor
Dillia *see* Dilia
80 E11 **Dilling** *var.* Ad Dalanj. Southern Kordofan, C Sudan
101 D20 **Dillingen** Saarland, SW Germany
Dillingen *see* Dillingen an der Donau
101 J22 **Dillingen an der Donau** *var.* Dillingen. Bayern, S Germany
39 O13 **Dillingham** Alaska, USA
33 Q12 **Dillon** Montana, NW USA
21 T12 **Dillon** South Carolina, SE USA
31 T13 **Dillon Lake** ▣ Ohio, N USA
Dilly *see* Dili
Dilman *see* Salmās
79 K24 **Dilolo** Katanga, S Dem. Rep. Congo (Zaire)
115 J20 **Dílos** *island* Kykládes, Greece, Aegean Sea
141 Y11 **Ḍil', Ra's aḍ** *headland* E Oman
29 R5 **Dilworth** Minnesota, N USA
138 H7 **Dimashq** *var.* Ash Shām, Esh Sham, *Eng.* Damascus, *Fr.* Damas, *It.* Damasco. ● (Syria) Dimashq, SW Syria
138 I8 **Dimashq** *off.* Muḥāfaẓat Dimashq, *var.* Damascus, *Ar.* Ash Sham, Ash Shām, Damasco, Esh Sham, *Fr.* Damas. ◈ *governorate* S Syria
138 I7 **Dimashq** × Dimashq, S Syria
79 L21 **Dimbelenge** Kasai Occidental, C Dem. Rep. Congo (Zaire)
77 N16 **Dimbokro** E Ivory Coast
182 L11 **Dimboola** Victoria, SE Australia
Dîmbovița *see* Dâmbovița
Dimitrov *see* Dymytrov
114 K11 **Dimitrovgrad** Khaskovo, S Bulgaria
129 R5 **Dimitrovgrad** Ul'yanovskaya Oblast', W Russian Federation
113 Q15 **Dimitrovgrad** *prev.* Caribrod. Serbia, SE Yugoslavia
Dimitrovo *see* Pernik
Dimlang *see* Vogel Peak
24 M3 **Dimmitt** Texas, SW USA
114 F7 **Dimovo** Vidin, NW Bulgaria
59 A16 **Dimpolis** Acre, W Brazil
115 O23 **Dimyliá** Ródos, Dodekánisos, Greece, Aegean Sea
171 Q6 **Dinagat Island** *island* S Philippines
153 S13 **Dinajpur** Rajshahi, NW Bangladesh
102 I6 **Dinan** Côtes d'Armor, NW France
99 I21 **Dinant** Namur, S Belgium
136 E15 **Dinar** Afyon, SW Turkey
112 F13 **Dinara** ▲ W Croatia
Dinara *see* Dinaric Alps
102 I5 **Dinard** Ille-et-Vilaine, NW France
112 F13 **Dinaric Alps** *var.* Dinara. ▲ Bosnia and Herzegovina/Croatia
143 N10 **Dīnār, Kūh-e** ▲ C Iran
Dinbych *see* Denbigh
155 H22 **Dindigul** Tamil Nādu, SE India
83 M19 **Dindiza** Gaza, S Mozambique
149 V7 **Dinga** Punjab, E Pakistan
79 H21 **Dinga** Bandundu, SW Dem. Rep. Congo (Zaire)
158 L16 **Dinggyê** Xizang Zizhiqu, W China
97 A20 **Dingle** *Ir.* An Daingean. SW Ireland
97 A20 **Dingle Bay** *Ir.* Bá an Daingin. *bay* SW Ireland
18 I13 **Dingmans Ferry** Pennsylvania, NE USA
101 N22 **Dingolfing** Bayern, SE Germany
171 O1 **Dingras** Luzon, N Philippines
76 J13 **Dinguiraye** Haute-Guinée, N Guinea
96 I8 **Dingwall** N Scotland, UK
159 V10 **Dingxi** Gansu, C China
161 Q7 **Dingyuan** Anhui, E China
161 O3 **Dingzhou** *prev.* Ding Xian. Hebei, E China
167 U6 **Đinh Lâp** Lang Sơn, N Vietnam
167 T13 **Đinh Quan** Đông Nai, S Vietnam
100 E13 **Dinkel** ≈ Germany/Netherlands
101 J21 **Dinkelsbühl** Bayern, S Germany
101 D14 **Dinslaken** Nordrhein-Westfalen, W Germany
35 R11 **Dinuba** California, W USA
21 W7 **Dinwiddie** Virginia, NE USA
98 N13 **Dinxperlo** Gelderland, E Netherlands
115 F14 **Dió** *anc.* Dium. *site of ancient city* Kentrikí Makedonía, N Greece
Diófás *see* Nucet
76 M12 **Dioïla** Koulikoro, W Mali
115 G19 **Dióryga Korinthou** *Eng.* Corinth Canal. *canal* S Greece
76 G12 **Diouloulou** SW Senegal
77 N11 **Dioura** Mopti, W Mali
76 G11 **Diourbel** W Senegal
152 L10 **Dipayal** Far Western, W Nepal
121 R1 **Dipkarpaz** *Gk.* Rizokarpaso, Rizokárpason. NE Cyprus
149 R17 **Diplo** Sind, SE Pakistan
171 P7 **Dipolog** *var.* Dipolog City. Mindanao, S Philippines
185 C23 **Dipton** Southland, South Island, NZ
77 O10 **Diré** Tombouctou, C Mali
80 L13 **Dirē Dawa** Dirē Dawa, E Ethiopia
Dirfis *see* Dírfys
115 H18 **Dírfys** *var.* Dirfis. ▲ Évvioa, C Greece
75 N9 **Dirj** *var.* Daraj, Darj. W Libya
180 G10 **Dirk Hartog Island** *island* Western Australia
77 Y8 **Dirkou** Agadez, NE Niger
181 X11 **Dirranbandi** Queensland, E Australia
81 O16 **Dirri** Galguduud, C Somalia
Dirschau *see* Tczew
37 N6 **Dirty Devil River** ≈ Utah, W USA
32 E10 **Disappointment, Cape** *headland* Washington, NW USA
180 L8 **Disappointment, Lake** *salt lake* Western Australia
183 R12 **Disaster Bay** *bay* New South Wales, SE Australia
44 J11 **Discovery Bay** C Jamaica
182 K13 **Discovery Bay** *inlet* SE Australia
67 Y15 **Discovery II Fracture Zone** *tectonic feature* SW Indian Ocean
Discovery Seamount/Discovery Seamounts *see* Discovery Tablemount
65 O19 **Discovery Tablemount** *var.* Discovery Seamount, Discovery Seamounts. *undersea feature* SW Indian Ocean
108 G9 **Disentis** *Rmsch.* Mustér. Graubünden, S Switzerland
39 O10 **Dishna River** ≈ Alaska, USA
195 X4 **Dismal Mountains** ▲ Antarctica
28 M14 **Dismal River** ≈ Nebraska, C USA
Disna *see* Dzisna
99 L19 **Dison** Liège, E Belgium
153 V12 **Dispur** Assam, NE India
15 R11 **Disraeli** Quebec, SE Canada
115 F18 **Dístomo** *prev.* Dhístomon. Stereá Ellás, C Greece
115 H18 **Dístos, Límni** ◎ Évvoia, C Greece
59 L18 **Distrito Federal** *Eng.* Federal District. ◈ *federal district* C Brazil
41 P14 **Distrito Federal** ◈ *federal district* S Mexico
54 L4 **Distrito Federal** *off.* Territorio Distrito Federal. ◈ *federal district* N Venezuela
Distrito Federal, Territorio *see* Distrito Federal
116 J10 **Ditrău** *Hung.* Ditró. Harghita, C Romania
Ditró *see* Ditrău
154 B12 **Diu** Damān and Diu, W India
Dium *see* Dió
109 S13 **Divača** SW Slovenia
102 K5 **Dives** ≈ N France
Divichi *see* Däväçi
33 Q11 **Divide** Montana, NW USA
Divin *see* Dzivin
83 N18 **Divinhe** Sofala, E Mozambique
59 L20 **Divinópolis** Minas Gerais, SE Brazil
129 N13 **Divnoye** Stavropol'skiy Kray, SW Russian Federation
76 M17 **Divo** S Ivory Coast
Divodurum Mediomatricum *see* Metz
137 N13 **Divriği** Sivas, C Turkey
Diwaniyah *see* Ad Dīwānīyah
14 J10 **Dix Milles, Lac** ◎ Quebec, SE Canada
14 M8 **Dix Milles, Lac des** ◎ Quebec, SE Canada
Dixmude/Dixmuide *see* Diksmuide

35 N7 **Dixon** California, W USA
30 L10 **Dixon** Illinois, N USA
20 I6 **Dixon** Kentucky, S USA
27 V6 **Dixon** Missouri, C USA
37 S9 **Dixon** New Mexico, SW USA
39 Y15 **Dixon Entrance** *strait* Canada/USA
18 D14 **Dixonville** Pennsylvania, NE USA
137 T13 **Diyadin** Ağrı, E Turkey
139 V5 **Diyālá, Nahr** *var.* Rudkhaneh-ye Sīrvān, Sirwan. ≈ Iran/Iraq *see also* Sīrvān, Rudkhaneh-ye
137 P15 **Diyarbakır** *var.* Diarbekr; *anc.* Amida. Diyarbakır, SE Turkey
137 P15 **Diyarbakır** *var.* Diarbekr. ◆ *province* SE Turkey
Dizful *see* Dezfūl
79 F16 **Dja** ≈ SE Cameroon
Djadié *see* Zadié
77 X7 **Djado** Agadez, NE Niger
77 X6 **Djado, Plateau du** ▲ NE Niger
Djailolo *see* Halmahera, Pulau
Djajapura *see* Jayapura
Djakarta *see* Jakarta
Djakovica *see* Đakovica
Djakovo *see* Đakovo
79 G20 **Djambala** Plateaux, C Congo
Djambi *see* Jambi
Djambi *see* Hari, Batang, Sumatera, W Indonesia
74 M9 **Djanet** E Algeria
74 M11 **Djanet** *prev.* Fort Charlet. SE Algeria
Djatiwangi *see* Jatiwangi
Djaul *see* Dyaul Island
Djawa *see* Jawa
Djéblé *see* Jablah
78 I10 **Djédaa** Batha, C Chad
74 J6 **Djelfa** *var.* El Djelfa. N Algeria
79 M14 **Djéma** Haut-Mbomou, E Central African Republic
Djeneponto *see* Jeneponto
77 N12 **Djenné** *var.* Jenné. Mopti, C Mali
Djérablous *see* Jarābulus
Djerba *see* Jerba, Île de
79 F15 **Djérem** ≈ C Cameroon
Djevdjelija *see* Gevgelija
77 P11 **Djibo** N Burkina
80 L12 **Djibouti** *var.* Jibuti. ● (Djibouti) E Djibouti
80 L12 **Djibouti** *off.* Republic of Djibouti, *var.* Jibuti; *prev.* French Somaliland, French Territory of the Afars and Issas, *Fr.* Côte Française des Somalis, Territoire Français des Afars et des Issas. ◆ *republic* E Africa
80 L12 **Djibouti** × C Djibouti
Djidjel/Djidjelli *see* Jijel
55 W10 **Djoemoe** Sipaliwini, C Suriname
Djokjakarta *see* Yogyakarta
79 K21 **Djoku-Punda** Kasai Occidental, S Dem. Rep. Congo (Zaire)
79 K18 **Djolu** Equateur, N Dem. Rep. Congo (Zaire)
Djorče Petrov *see* Đorče Petrov
79 F17 **Djoua** ≈ Congo/Gabon
77 R14 **Djougou** W Benin
79 F16 **Djoum** Sud, S Cameroon
78 I8 **Djourab, Erg du** *dunes* N Chad
79 P17 **Djugu** Orientale, NE Dem. Rep. Congo (Zaire)
Djumbir *see* Ďumbier
92 L3 **Djúpivogur** Austurland, SE Iceland
94 L13 **Djura** Dalarna, C Sweden
Djurdjevac *see* Đurđevac
83 G18 **D'Kar** Ghanzi, NW Botswana
197 U6 **Dmitriya Lapteva, Proliv** *strait* N Russian Federation
128 J7 **Dmitriyev-L'govskiy** Kurskaya Oblast', W Russian Federation
Dmitriyevsk *see* Makiyivka
128 K3 **Dmitrov** Moskovskaya Oblast', W Russian Federation
Dmitrovichi *see* Dzmitravichy
128 J6 **Dmitrovsk-Orlovskiy** Orlovskaya Oblast', W Russian Federation
117 R3 **Dmytrivka** Chernihivs'ka Oblast', N Ukraine
Dnepr *see* Dnieper
Dneprodzerzhinsk *see* Dniprodzerzhyns'k
Dneprodzerzhinskoye Vodokhranilishche *see* Dniprodzerzhyns'ke Vodoskhovyshche
Dnepropetrovsk *see* Dnipropetrovs'k
Dnepropetrovskaya Oblast' *see* Dnipropetrovs'ka Oblast'
Dneprorudnoye *see* Dniprorudne
Dneprovskiy Liman *see* Dniprovs'kyy Lyman
Dneprovsko-Bugskiy Kanal *see* Dnyaprowska-Buhski, Kanal
Dnestr *see* Dniester
Dnestrovskiy Liman *see* Dnistrovs'kyy Lyman
86 H11 **Dnieper** *Bel.* Dnyapro, *Rus.* Dnepr, *Ukr.* Dnipro. ≈ E Europe
117 P3 **Dnieper Lowland** *Bel.* Prydnyaprowskaya Nizina, *Ukr.* Prydniprovs'ka Nyzovyna. *lowlands* Belarus/Ukraine
116 M8 **Dniester** *Rom.* Nistru, *Rus.* Dnestr, *Ukr.* Dnister; *anc.* Tyras. ≈ Moldova/Ukraine
Dnipro *see* Dnieper
117 T7 **Dniprodzerzhyns'k** *Rus.* Dneprodzerzhinsk; *prev.* Kamenskoye. Dnipropetrovs'ka Oblast', E Ukraine
117 T7 **Dniprodzerzhyns'ke Vodoskhovyshche** *Rus.* Dneprodzerzhinskoye Vodokhranilishche. ▣ C Ukraine
117 U7 **Dnipropetrovs'k** *Rus.* Dnepropetrovsk; *prev.* Yekaterinoslav. Dnipropetrovs'ka Oblast', E Ukraine
117 U8 **Dnipropetrovs'k** × Dnipropetrovs'ka Oblast', S Ukraine
Dnipropetrovs'k *see* Dnipropetrovs'ka Oblast'
117 T7 **Dnipropetrovs'ka Oblast'** *var.* Dnipropetrovs'k, *Rus.* Dnepropetrovskaya Oblast'. ◆ *province* E Ukraine
117 U9 **Dniprorudne** *Rus.* Dneprorudnoye. Zaporiz'ka Oblast', SE Ukraine
117 Q11 **Dniprovs'kyy Lyman** *Rus.* Dneprovskiy Liman. *bay* S Ukraine
Dnister *see* Dniester
117 O11 **Dnistrovs'kyy Lyman** *Rus.* Dnestrovskiy Liman. *inlet* S Ukraine
126 G14 **Dno** Pskovskaya Oblast', W Russian Federation
Dnyapro *see* Dnieper
119 H20 **Dnyaprowska-Buhski, Kanal** *Rus.* Dneprovsko-Bugskiy Kanal. *canal* SW Belarus
13 O14 **Doaktown** New Brunswick, SE Canada
78 H13 **Doba** Logone-Oriental, S Chad
118 E9 **Dobele** *Ger.* Doblen. Dobele, W Latvia
101 N16 **Döbeln** Sachsen, E Germany
171 U12 **Doberai, Jazirah** *Dut.* Vogelkop. *peninsula* Irian Jaya, E Indonesia
110 F10 **Dobiegniew** *Ger.* Lubuskie, W Poland
Doblen *see* Dobele
81 K18 **Dobli** *spring/well* SW Somalia
112 H11 **Doboj** Republika Srpska, N Bosnia and Herzegovina
110 L8 **Dobre Miasto** *Ger.* Guttstadt. Warmińsko-Mazurskie, NE Poland
114 N7 **Dobrich** *Rom.* Bazargic; *prev.* Tolbukhin. Dobrich, NE Bulgaria
114 N7 **Dobrich** ◆ *province* NE Bulgaria
128 M8 **Dobrinka** Lipetskaya Oblast', W Russian Federation
128 M7 **Dobrinka** Volgogradskaya Oblast', SW Russian Federation
Dobrla Vas *see* Eberndorf
111 I15 **Dobrodzień** *Ger.* Guttentag. Opolskie, S Poland
Dobrogea *see* Dobruja
117 W7 **Dobropillya** *Rus.* Dobropol'ye. Donets'ka Oblast', SE Ukraine
Dobropol'ye *see* Dobropillya
117 P8 **Dobrovelychkivka** Kirovohrads'ka Oblast', C Ukraine
Dobrudja/Dobrudzha *see* Dobruja
114 O7 **Dobruja** *var.* Dobrudja, *Bul.* Dobrudzha, *Rom.* Dobrogea. *physical region* Bulgaria/Romania
119 P19 **Dobrush** Homyel'skaya Voblasts', SE Belarus
127 U14 **Dobryanka** Permskaya Oblast', NW Russian Federation
117 P2 **Dobryanka** Chernihivs'ka Oblast', N Ukraine
Dobryn' *see* Dabryn'
21 R8 **Dobson** North Carolina, SE USA
59 N20 **Doce, Rio** ≈ SE Brazil
93 I16 **Docksta** Västernorrland, C Sweden
41 N10 **Doctor Arroyo** Nuevo León, NE Mexico
62 L4 **Doctor Pedro P. Peña** Boquerón, W Paraguay
171 S11 **Dodaga** Pulau Halmahera, E Indonesia
155 G21 **Dodda Betta** ▲ S India
Dodecanese *see* Dodekánisos
115 M22 **Dodekánisos** *var.* Nóties Sporádes, *Eng.* Dodecanese; *prev.* Dhodhekánisos. *island group* SE Greece
26 J6 **Dodge City** Kansas, C USA
30 K9 **Dodgeville** Wisconsin, N USA
97 H25 **Dodman Point** *headland* SW England, UK
81 J14 **Dodola** Oromo, C Ethiopia
81 H22 **Dodoma** ● (Tanzania) Dodoma, C Tanzania
81 H22 **Dodoma** ◆ *region* C Tanzania
115 C16 **Dodóni** *var.* Dhodhóni. *site of ancient city* Ípeiros, W Greece
33 U7 **Dodson** Montana, NW USA
25 P3 **Dodson** Texas, SW USA
98 M12 **Doesburg** Gelderland, E Netherlands
98 N12 **Doetinchem** Gelderland, E Netherlands
158 L12 **Dogai Coring** *var.* Lake Montcalm. ◎ W China
137 N15 **Doğanşehir** Malatya, C Turkey
84 E9 **Dogger Bank** *undersea feature* C North Sea
23 S10 **Dog Island** *island* Florida, SE USA
14 C7 **Dog Lake** ◎ Ontario, S Canada
106 B9 **Dogliani** Piemonte, NE Italy
164 H11 **Dōgo** *island* Oki-shotō, SW Japan
Do Gonbadān *see* Dow Gonbadān
77 S12 **Dogondoutchi** Dosso, SW Niger
Dogrular *see* Pravda
137 T13 **Doğubayazıt** Ağrı, E Turkey
137 P12 **Doğu Karadeniz Dağları** *var.* Anadolu Dağları. ▲ NE Turkey
Doha *see* Ad Dawḩah
Dohad *see* Dāhod
Dohuk *see* Dahūk
159 N16 **Doilungdêqên** Xizang Zizhiqu, W China
114 F12 **Doïranis, Límnis** *Bul.* Ezero Doyransko. ◎ N Greece
Doire *see* Londonderry
99 H22 **Doische** Namur, S Belgium
59 P17 **Dois de Julho** × (Salvador) Bahia, NE Brazil
60 H12 **Dois Vizinhos** Paraná, S Brazil
80 H10 **Doka** Gedaref, E Sudan
Doka *see* Kéita, Bahr
139 T3 **Dokan** *var.* Dūkān. E Iraq
94 H13 **Dokka** Oppland, S Norway
98 L5 **Dokkum** Friesland, N Netherlands
98 L5 **Dokkumer Ee** ≈ N Netherlands
76 K13 **Doko** Haute-Guinée, NE Guinea
Dokshitsy *see* Dokshytsy
118 K13 **Dokshytsy** *Rus.* Dokshitsy. Vitsyebskaya Voblasts', N Belarus
117 X8 **Dokuchayevs'k** *var.* Dokuchayevsk. Donets'ka Oblast', SE Ukraine
Dolak, Pulau *see* Yos Sudarso, Pulau
29 P9 **Doland** South Dakota, N USA
63 J18 **Dolavón** Chaco, S Argentina
15 P6 **Dolbeau** Quebec, SE Canada
102 I5 **Dol-de-Bretagne** Ille-et-Vilaine, NW France
64 J13 **Doldrums Fracture Zone** *tectonic feature* W Atlantic Ocean
103 S8 **Dôle** Jura, E France
97 J19 **Dolgellau** NW Wales, UK
Dolginovo *see* Dawhinava
Dolgi, Ostrov *see* Dolgiy, Ostrov
127 U2 **Dolgiy, Ostrov** *var.* Ostrov Dolgi. *island* NW Russian Federation
162 J9 **Dölgöön** Övörhangay, C Mongolia
107 C20 **Dolianova** Sardegna, Italy, C Mediterranean Sea
Dolina *see* Dolyna
123 T13 **Dolinsk** Ostrov Sakhalin, Sakhalinskaya Oblast', SE Russian Federation
Dolinskaya *see* Dolyns'ka
79 F21 **Dolisie** *prev.* Loubomo. Le Niari, S Congo
116 G14 **Dolj** ◆ *county* SW Romania
98 P5 **Dollard** *bay* NW Germany
194 J5 **Dolleman Island** *island* Antarctica
114 I8 **Dolni Dŭbnik** Pleven, N Bulgaria
114 F8 **Dolni Lom** Vidin, NW Bulgaria
Dolnja Lendava *see* Lendava
114 K9 **Dolno Panicherevo** *var.* Panicherevo. Sliven, C Bulgaria
111 F14 **Dolnośląskie** ◆ *province* SW Poland
111 K18 **Dolný Kubín** *Hung.* Alsókubin. Žilinský Kraj, N Slovakia
106 H8 **Dolo** Veneto, NE Italy
Dolomites/Dolomiti *see* Dolomitiche, Alpi
106 H6 **Dolomitiche, Alpi** *var.* Dolomiti, *Eng.* Dolomites. ▲ NE Italy
Dolonnur *see* Duolun
162 K10 **Doloon** Ömnögovĭ, S Mongolia
61 E21 **Dolores** Buenos Aires, E Argentina
42 E3 **Dolores** Petén, N Guatemala
171 Q5 **Dolores** Samar, C Philippines
105 S12 **Dolores** País Valenciano, E Spain
61 D19 **Dolores** Soriano, SW Uruguay
41 N12 **Dolores Hidalgo** *var.* Ciudad de Dolores Hidalgo. Guanajuato, C Mexico
8 J7 **Dolphin and Union Strait** *strait* Northwest Territories / Nunavut, N Canada
65 D23 **Dolphin, Cape** *headland* East Falkland, Falkland Islands
44 H12 **Dolphin Head** *hill* W Jamaica
83 B21 **Dolphin Head** *var.* Cape Dernberg. *headland* SW Namibia
110 G12 **Dolsk** *Ger.* Dolzig. Wielkolpolskie, C Poland
167 S8 **Đô Lương** Nghê An, N Vietnam
116 I6 **Dolyna** *Rus.* Dolina. Ivano-Frankivs'ka Oblast', W Ukraine
117 R8 **Dolyns'ka** *Rus.* Dolinskaya. Kirovohrads'ka Oblast', S Ukraine
Dolzig *see* Dolsk
Domachëvo/Domaczewo *see* Damachava
117 P9 **Domanivka** Mykolayivs'ka Oblast', S Ukraine
153 S13 **Domar** Rajshahi, N Bangladesh
108 I9 **Domat/Ems** Graubünden, SE Switzerland
111 A18 **Domažlice** *Ger.* Taus. Plzeňský Kraj, W Czech Republic
129 X8 **Dombarovskiy** Orenburgskaya Oblast', W Russian Federation
94 G10 **Dombås** Oppland, S Norway
83 M17 **Dombe** Manica, C Mozambique
82 A13 **Dombe Grande** Benguela, C Angola
103 R10 **Dombes** *physical region* E France
111 I25 **Dombóvár** Tolna, S Hungary
99 D14 **Domburg** Zeeland, SW Netherlands
58 L13 **Dom Eliseu** Pará, NE Brazil
Domel Island *see* Letsôk-aw Kyun
103 O11 **Dôme, Puy de** ▲ C France
36 H13 **Dome Rock Mountains** ▲ Arizona, SW USA
Domesnes, Cape *see* Kolkasrags
62 G8 **Domeyko** Atacama, N Chile
62 H5 **Domeyko, Cordillera** ▲ N Chile
102 K5 **Domfront** Orne, N France
171 X13 **Dom, Gunung** ▲ Irian Jaya, E Indonesia
45 X11 **Dominica** *off.* Commonwealth of Dominica. ◆ *republic* E West Indies
47 S3 **Dominica** *island* Dominica
Dominica Channel *see* Martinique Passage
43 N15 **Dominical** Puntarenas, SE Costa Rica
45 Q8 **Dominican Republic** ◆ *republic* C West Indies
45 X11 **Dominica Passage** *passage* E Caribbean Sea
99 K14 **Dommel** ≈ S Netherlands
81 O14 **Domo** Somali, E Ethiopia
128 L4 **Domodedovo** × (Moskva) Moskovskaya Oblast', W Russian Federation
106 C6 **Domodossola** Piemonte, NE Italy
115 F17 **Domokós** *var.* Dhomokós. Stereá Ellás, C Greece
172 I14 **Domoni** Anjouan, SE Comoros
61 G16 **Dom Pedrito** Rio Grande do Sul, S Brazil
Dompoe *see* Dompu
170 M16 **Dompu** *prev.* Dompoe. Sumbawa, C Indonesia
Domschale *see* Domžale
62 H13 **Domuyo, Volcán** ▲ W Argentina
109 U11 **Domžale** *Ger.* Domschale. C Slovenia
129 O10 **Don** *var.* Duna, Tanais. ≈ SW Russian Federation
96 K9 **Don** ≈ NE Scotland, UK
182 M11 **Donald** Victoria, SE Australia
22 J9 **Donaldsonville** Louisiana, S USA
23 S8 **Donalsonville** Georgia, SE USA
Donau *see* Danube
101 G23 **Donaueschingen** Baden-Württemberg, SW Germany
101 K22 **Donaumoos** *wetland* S Germany
101 K22 **Donauwörth** Bayern, S Germany
109 U7 **Donawitz** Steiermark, SE Austria
117 X7 **Donbass** *industrial region* Russian Federation/Ukraine
104 K11 **Don Benito** Extremadura, W Spain
97 M17 **Doncaster** *anc.* Danum. N England, UK
44 K12 **Don Christophers Point** *headland* C Jamaica
55 V9 **Donderkamp** Sipaliwini, NW Suriname
82 B12 **Dondo** Cuanza Norte, NW Angola
171 O12 **Dondo** Sulawesi, N Indonesia
83 N17 **Dondo** Sofala, C Mozambique
155 K26 **Dondra Head** *headland* S Sri Lanka
Donduşani *see* Donduşeni
116 M8 **Donduşeni** *var.* Donduşani, *Rus.* Dondyushany. N Moldova
Dondyushany *see* Donduşeni
97 D15 **Donegal** *Ir.* Dún na nGall. NW Ireland
97 D14 **Donegal** *Ir.* Dún na nGall. *cultural region* NW Ireland
97 C15 **Donegal Bay** *Ir.* Bá Dhún na nGall. *bay* NW Ireland
84 K10 **Donets** ≈ Russian Federation/Ukraine
117 X8 **Donets'k** *Rus.* Donetsk; *prev.* Stalino. Donets'ka Oblast', E Ukraine
117 W8 **Donets'k** × Donets'ka Oblast', E Ukraine
Donets'k *see* Donets'ka Oblast'
117 W8 **Donets'ka Oblast'** *var.* Donets'k, *Rus.* Donetskaya Oblast'; *prev. Rus.* Stalinskaya Oblast'. ◆ *province* SE Ukraine
Donetskaya Oblast' *see* Donets'ka Oblast'
67 P8 **Donga** ≈ Cameroon/Nigeria
157 O13 **Dongchuan** Yunnan, SW China
99 I14 **Dongen** Noord-Brabant, S Netherlands
160 K17 **Dongfang** *var.* Basuo. Hainan, S China
163 Z7 **Dongfanghong** Heilongjiang, NE China
163 W11 **Dongfeng** Jilin, NE China
171 N12 **Donggala** Sulawesi, C Indonesia
163 V13 **Donggou** Liaoning, NE China
161 O14 **Dongguan** Guangdong, S China
167 T9 **Đông Ha** Quang Tri, C Vietnam
Dong Hai *see* East China Sea
160 M16 **Donghai Dao** *island* S China
167 T9 **Đông Hơi** Quang Binh, C Vietnam
108 H10 **Dongio** Ticino, S Switzerland
Dongkan *see* Binhai
160 L11 **Dongkou** Hunan, S China
Dongliao *see* Liaoyuan
Dong-nai *see* Đông Nai, Sông
167 U13 **Đông Nai, Sông** *var.* Dong-nai, Dong Noi, Donnai. ≈ S Vietnam
161 O14 **Dongnan Qiuling** *plateau* SE China
163 Y9 **Dongning** Heilongjiang, NE China
Dong Noi *see* Đông Nai, Sông
83 C14 **Dongo** Huíla, C Angola
80 E7 **Dongola** *var.* Donqola, Dunqulah. Northern, N Sudan
79 I17 **Dongou** La Likouala, NE Congo
167 T13 **Đông Phu** Sông Be, S Vietnam
Dong Rak, Phanom *see* Dângrêk, Chuŏr Phnum
161 Q14 **Dongshan Dao** *island* SE China
163 N14 **Dongsheng** Nei Mongol Zizhiqu, N China
161 R7 **Dongtai** Jiangsu, E China
161 N10 **Dongting Hu** *var.* Tung-t'ing Hu. ◎ S China
161 P10 **Dongxiang** Jiangxi, S China
161 Q4 **Dongying** Shandong, E China
27 X8 **Doniphan** Missouri, C USA
10 G7 **Donjek** ≈ Yukon Territory, W Canada
112 E11 **Donji Lapac** Lika-Senj, W Croatia
112 H8 **Donji Miholjac** Osijek-Baranja, NE Croatia
112 P12 **Donji Milanovac** Serbia, E Yugoslavia
112 G12 **Donji Vakuf** *var.* Srbobran, Federacija Bosna I Hercegovina, C Bosnia & Herzegovina
98 M6 **Donkerbroek** Friesland, N Netherlands
167 P11 **Don Muang** × (Krung Thep) Nonthaburi, C Thailand
25 S17 **Donna** Texas, SW USA
15 Q10 **Donnacona** Quebec, SE Canada
Donnai *see* Đông Nai, Sông
29 Y16 **Donnellson** Iowa, C USA
11 O13 **Donnelly** Alberta, W Canada
35 H6 **Donner Pass** *pass* California, W USA
101 F19 **Donnersberg** ▲ W Germany
Donoso *see* Miguel de la Borda
105 P2 **Donostia-San Sebastián** País Vasco, N Spain
115 K21 **Donoússa** *island* Kykládes, Greece, Aegean Sea
35 P8 **Don Pedro Reservoir** ▣ California, W USA
Donqola *see* Dongola
128 L5 **Donskoy** Tul'skaya Oblast', W Russian Federation
81 L16 **Doolow** Somali, E Ethiopia
39 Q7 **Doonerak, Mount** ▲ Alaska, USA
98 J12 **Doorn** Utrecht, C Netherlands
Doornik *see* Tournai
31 N6 **Door Peninsula** *peninsula* Wisconsin, N USA
80 P13 **Dooxo Nugaaleed** *var.* Nogal Valley. *valley* E Somalia
160 G8 **Do Qu** ≈ C China
106 B7 **Dora Baltea** *anc.* Duria Major. ≈ NW Italy
180 K7 **Dora, Lake** *salt lake* Western Australia
106 A8 **Dora Riparia** *anc.* Duria Minor. ≈ NW Italy
Dorbiljin *see* Emin
163 V8 **Dorbod** *var.* Dorbod Mongolzu Zizhixian, Talkang. Heilongjiang, NE China
Dorbod Mongolzu Zizhixian *see* Dorbod
113 N18 **Đorče Petrov** *var.* Djorče Petrov, Gorče Petrov. N FYR Macedonia
14 F16 **Dorchester** Ontario, S Canada
97 L24 **Dorchester** *anc.* Durnovaria. S England, UK
9 P7 **Dorchester, Cape** *headland* Baffin Island, Nunavut, NE Canada
83 D19 **Dordabis** Khomas, C Namibia
102 L12 **Dordogne** ◆ *department* SW France
103 N12 **Dordogne** ≈ W France
98 H13 **Dordrecht** *var.* Dordt, Dort. Zuid-Holland, SW Netherlands
Dordt *see* Dordrecht
103 P11 **Dore** ≈ C France
11 S13 **Doré Lake** Saskatchewan, C Canada
103 O12 **Dore, Monts** ▲ C France
101 M23 **Dorfen** Bayern, SE Germany
107 D18 **Dorgali** Sardegna, Italy, C Mediterranean Sea
162 F7 **Dörgön Nuur** ◎ NW Mongolia
77 Q12 **Dori** N Burkina
83 E24 **Doring** ≈ S South Africa
101 E16 **Dormagen** Nordrhein-Westfalen, W Germany
103 P4 **Dormans** Marne, N France
108 E6 **Dornach** Solothurn, NW Switzerland
Dorna Watra *see* Vatra Dornei
108 J7 **Dornbirn** Vorarlberg, W Austria
96 I7 **Dornoch** N Scotland, UK
96 J7 **Dornoch Firth** *inlet* N Scotland, UK
163 P7 **Dornod** ◆ *province* E Mongolia
163 N10 **Dornogovĭ** ◆ *province* SE Mongolia
77 P10 **Doro** Tombouctou, S Mali
116 L14 **Dorobanţu** Călăraşi, S Romania
111 J22 **Dorog** Komárom-Esztergom, N Hungary
128 I4 **Dorogobuzh** Smolenskaya Oblast', W Russian Federation
116 K8 **Dorohoi** Botoşani, NE Romania
93 H15 **Dorotea** Västerbotten, N Sweden
Dorpat *see* Tartu
180 G10 **Dorre Island** *island* Western Australia
183 U5 **Dorrigo** New South Wales, SE Australia
35 N1 **Dorris** California, W USA
14 H13 **Dorset** Ontario, SE Canada
97 K23 **Dorset** *cultural region* S England, UK
101 E14 **Dorsten** Nordrhein-Westfalen, W Germany
Dort *see* Dordrecht
101 F15 **Dortmund** Nordrhein-Westfalen, W Germany
100 F12 **Dortmund-Ems-Kanal** *canal* W Germany
136 L17 **Dörtyol** Hatay, S Turkey
142 L7 **Do Rūd** *var.* Dow Rūd, Durud. Lorestān, W Iran
79 O15 **Doruma** Orientale, N Dem. Rep. Congo (Zaire)
15 O12 **Dorval** × (Montréal) Quebec, SE Canada
45 T5 **Dos Bocas, Lago** ◎ C Puerto Rico
104 K14 **Dos Hermanas** Andalucía, S Spain
Dospad Dagh *see* Rhodope Mountains
35 P10 **Dos Palos** California, W USA
114 I11 **Dospat** Smolyan, S Bulgaria
114 H11 **Dospat, Yazovir** ▣ SW Bulgaria
100 M11 **Dosse** ≈ NE Germany
77 S12 **Dosso** Dosso, SW Niger
77 S12 **Dosso** ◆ *department* SW Niger
144 G12 **Dossor** Atyrau, SW Kazakhstan
147 V9 **Dostuk** Narynskaya Oblast', C Kyrgyzstan
145 X13 **Dostyk** *prev.* Druzhba. Almaty, SE Kazakhstan
23 R7 **Dothan** Alabama, S USA
39 T9 **Dot Lake** Alaska, USA
118 F12 **Dotnuva** Kėdainiai, C Lithuania
99 D19 **Dottignies** Hainaut, W Belgium
103 P2 **Douai** *prev.* Douay, *anc.* Duacum. Nord, N France
14 L9 **Douaire, Lac** ◎ Quebec, SE Canada
79 D16 **Douala** *var.* Duala. Littoral, W Cameroon
79 D16 **Douala** × Littoral, W Cameroon
102 F6 **Douarnenez** Finistère, NW France
102 E6 **Douarnenez, Baie de** *bay* NW France
Douay *see* Douai
25 O6 **Double Mountain Fork Brazos River** ≈ Texas, SW USA
23 O3 **Double Springs** Alabama, S USA
103 T8 **Doubs** ◆ *department* E France
108 C8 **Doubs** ≈ France/Switzerland
185 A22 **Doubtful Sound** *sound* South Island, NZ
184 J2 **Doubtless Bay** *bay* North Island, NZ
25 X9 **Doucette** Texas, SW USA
102 K8 **Doué-la-Fontaine** Maine-et-Loire, NW France
77 O11 **Douentza** Mopti, S Mali
65 D24 **Douglas** East Falkland, Falkland Islands
97 I16 **Douglas** ○ (Isle of Man) E Isle of Man
83 H23 **Douglas** Northern Cape, C South Africa
39 X13 **Douglas** Alexander Archipelago, Alaska, USA
37 O17 **Douglas** Arizona, SW USA
23 U7 **Douglas** Georgia, SE USA
33 Y15 **Douglas** Wyoming, C USA
38 L9 **Douglas, Cape** *headland* Alaska USA
10 J14 **Douglas Channel** *channel* British Columbia, W Canada
182 G3 **Douglas Creek** *seasonal river* South Australia
31 P5 **Douglas Lake** ◎ Michigan, N USA
21 O9 **Douglas Lake** ▣ Tennessee, S USA
39 Q13 **Douglas, Mount** ▲ Alaska, USA
194 I6 **Douglas Range** ▲ Alexander Island, Antarctica
121 P9 **Doukáto, Akrotírio** *headland* Lefkáda, W Greece
103 O2 **Doullens** Somme, N France
Douma *see* Dūmā
79 F15 **Doumé** Est, E Cameroon
99 E21 **Dour** Hainaut, S Belgium
59 K18 **Dourada, Serra** ▲ S Brazil
59 I21 **Dourados** Mato Grosso do Sul, S Brazil
103 N5 **Dourdan** Essonne, N France
104 I6 **Douro** *Sp.* Duero. ≈ Portugal/Spain *see also* Duero
104 G6 **Douro Litoral** *former province* N Portugal
Douvres *see* Dover
102 K15 **Douze** ≈ SW France
183 P17 **Dover** Tasmania, SE Australia
97 Q22 **Dover** *Fr.* Douvres; *Lat.* Dubris Portus. SE England, UK
17 U9 **Dover** *state capital* Delaware, NE USA
19 P9 **Dover** New Hampshire, NE USA
18 J14 **Dover** New Jersey, NE USA
31 U12 **Dover** Ohio, N USA
20 H8 **Dover** Tennessee, S USA
97 Q23 **Dover, Strait of** *var.* Straits of Dover, *Fr.* Pas de Calais. *strait* England, UK/France
Dover, Straits of *see* Dover, Strait of
Dovlen *see* Devin
94 G11 **Dovre** Oppland, S Norway
94 G10 **Dovrefjell** *plateau* S Norway
Dovsk *see* Dowsk
83 M14 **Dowa** Central, C Malawi
31 O10 **Dowagiac** Michigan, N USA
143 N10 **Dow Gonbadān** *var.* Do Gonbadān, Gonbadān. Kohkīlūyeh va Būyer Aḩmadī, SW Iran
148 M2 **Dowlatābād** Fāryāb, N Afghanistan
97 G16 **Down** *cultural region* SE Northern Ireland, UK
33 R16 **Downey** Idaho, NW USA
35 P5 **Downieville** California, W USA
97 G16 **Downpatrick** *Ir.* Dún Pádraig. SE Northern Ireland, UK
26 M3 **Downs** Kansas, C USA
18 J12 **Downsville** New York, NE USA
Dow Rūd *see* Do Rūd
29 V12 **Dows** Iowa, C USA
119 O17 **Dowsk** *Rus.* Dovsk. Homyel'skaya Voblasts', SE Belarus
35 Q4 **Doyle** California, W USA
18 I15 **Doylestown** Pennsylvania, NE USA
Doyransko, Ezero *see* Doïranis, Límnis
114 I8 **Doyrentsi** Lovech, N Bulgaria
164 G11 **Dōzen** *island* Oki-shotō, SW Japan

◆ Country ● Country Capital ◇ Dependent Territory ○ Dependent Territory Capital ◆ Administrative Region × International Airport ▲ Mountain ▲ Mountain Range ▲ Volcano ≈ River ◎ Lake ▣ Reservoir

14 K9 **Dozois, Réservoir** ⊞ Quebec, SE Canada
74 D9 **Drâa** *seasonal river* S Morocco
Drâa, Hammada du *see* Dra, Hamada du
Drabble *see* José Enrique Rodó
117 Q5 **Drabiv** Cherkas'ka Oblast', C Ukraine
Drable *see* José Enrique Rodó
103 S13 **Drac** ≈ E France
Drač/Draç *see* Durrës
60 I8 **Dracena** São Paulo, S Brazil
98 M6 **Drachten** Friesland, N Netherlands
92 H11 **Drag** Nordland, C Norway
116 L14 **Dragalina** Călărași, SE Romania
116 J14 **Drăgănești-Vlașca** Teleorman, S Romania
116 I13 **Drăgășani** Vâlcea, SW Romania
114 G9 **Dragoman** Sofiya, W Bulgaria
115 L25 **Dragonáda** *island* SE Greece
Dragonera, Isla *see* Sa Dragonera
45 T14 **Dragon's Mouths, The** *strait* Trinidad and Tobago/Venezuela
95 J23 **Dragør** København, E Denmark
114 F10 **Dragovishitsa** Kyustendil, W Bulgaria
103 U15 **Draguignan** Var, SE France
74 E9 **Dra, Hamada du** *var.* Hammada du Drâa, Haut Plateau du Dra. *plateau* W Algeria
Dra, Haut Plateau du *see* Dra, Hamada du
119 H19 **Drahichyn** *Pol.* Drohiczyn Poleski, *Rus.* Drogichin. Brestskaya Voblasts', SW Belarus
29 N4 **Drake** North Dakota, N USA
83 K23 **Drakensberg** ▲ Lesotho/South Africa
194 F3 **Drake Passage** *passage* Atlantic Ocean/Pacific Ocean
114 L8 **Dralfa** Tŭrgovishte, N Bulgaria
114 I12 **Dráma** *var.* Dhráma. Anatolikí Makedonía kai Thráki, NE Greece
Dramburg *see* Drawsko Pomorskie
95 H15 **Drammen** Buskerud, S Norway
95 H15 **Drammensfjorden** *fjord* S Norway
92 H1 **Drangajökull** ▲ NW Iceland
95 F16 **Drangedal** Telemark, S Norway
92 I2 **Drangsnes** Vestfirdhir, NW Iceland
Drann *see* Dravinja
109 T10 **Drau** *var.* Drava, *Eng.* Drave, *Hung.* Dráva. ≈ C Europe *see also* Drava
84 I11 **Drava** *var.* Drau, *Eng.* Drave, *Hung.* Dráva. ≈ C Europe *see also* Drau
Dráva *see* Drau/Drava
Drave *see* Drau/Drava
109 W10 **Dravinja** *Ger.* Drann. ≈ NE Slovenia
109 V9 **Dravograd** *Ger.* Unterdrauburg; *prev.* Spodnji Dravograd. N Slovenia
110 F10 **Drawa** ≈ NW Poland
110 F9 **Drawno** Zachodniopomorskie, NW Poland
110 F9 **Drawsko Pomorskie** *Ger.* Dramburg. Zachodniopomorskie, NW Poland
29 R3 **Drayton** North Dakota, N USA
11 P14 **Drayton Valley** Alberta, SW Canada
186 B6 **Dreikikir** East Sepik, NW PNG
Dreikirchen *see* Teiuș
98 N7 **Drenthe** ◆ *province* NE Netherlands
115 H15 **Drépano, Akrotírio** *var.* Akra Dhrepanon. *headland* N Greece
Drepanum *see* Trapani
14 D17 **Dresden** Ontario, S Canada
101 O16 **Dresden** Sachsen, E Germany
20 G8 **Dresden** Tennessee, S USA
118 M11 **Dretun'** *Rus.* Dretun'. Vitsyebskaya Voblasts', N Belarus
102 M5 **Dreux** *anc.* Drocae, Durocasses. Eure-et-Loir, C France
94 I11 **Drevsjø** Hedmark, S Norway
22 K3 **Drew** Mississippi, S USA
110 F10 **Drezdenko** *Ger.* Driesen. Lubuskie, W Poland
98 J12 **Driebergen** *var.* Driebergen-Rijsenburg. Utrecht, C Netherlands
Driebergen-Rijsenburg *see* Driebergen
Driesen *see* Drezdenko
97 N16 **Driffield** E England, UK
65 D25 **Driftwood Point** *headland* East Falkland, Falkland Islands
33 S14 **Driggs** Idaho, NW USA
Drin *see* Drinit, Lumi i
112 K12 **Drina** ≈ Bosnia and Herzegovina/Yugoslavia
Drin, Gulf of *see* Drinit, Gjiri i
113 K18 **Drinit, Gjiri i** *var.* Pellg i Drinit, *Eng.* Gulf of Drin. *gulf* NW Albania
113 L17 **Drinit, Lumi i** *var.* Drin. ≈ NW Albania
Drinit, Pellg i *see* Drinit, Gjiri i
Drinit të Zi, Lumi i *see* Black Drin
113 L22 **Dríno** *var.* Drino, Drínos Pótamos, *Alb.* Lumi i Drinos. ≈ Albania/Greece
Drinos, Lumi i/Drínos Pótamos *see* Dríno
25 S11 **Dripping Springs** Texas, SW USA
25 S15 **Driscoll** Texas, SW USA
22 H5 **Driskill Mountain** ▲ Louisiana, S USA
Drissa *see* Drysa
94 G10 **Driva** ≈ S Norway
112 E13 **Drniš** *It.* Šibenik-Knin, S Croatia
95 H15 **Drøbak** Akershus, S Norway
116 G13 **Drobeta-Turnu Severin** *prev.* Turnu Severin. Mehedinți, SW Romania
Drocae *see* Dreux
116 M8 **Drochia** *Rus.* Drokiya. N Moldova
97 F17 **Drogheda** *Ir.* Droichead Átha. NE Ireland
Drogichin *see* Drahichyn
Drogobych *see* Drohobych
Drohiczyn Poleski *see* Drahichyn
116 H6 **Drohobych** *Pol.* Drohobycz, *Rus.* Drogobych. L'vivs'ka Oblast', NW Ukraine
Drohobycz *see* Drohobych
Droichead Átha *see* Drogheda
Droicheadna Bandan *see* Bandon
Droichead na Banna *see* Banbridge
Droim Mór *see* Dromore
Drokiya *see* Drochia
103 R13 **Drôme** ◆ *department* E France
103 S13 **Drôme** ≈ E France
97 G15 **Dromore** *Ir.* Droim Mór. SE Northern Ireland, UK
106 A9 **Dronero** Piemonte, NE Italy
102 L12 **Dronne** ≈ SW France
195 Q3 **Dronning Maud Land** *physical region* Antarctica
98 K6 **Dronrijp** *Fris.* Dronryp. Friesland, N Netherlands
Dronryp *see* Dronrijp
98 L9 **Dronten** Flevoland, C Netherlands
Drontheim *see* Trondheim
102 L13 **Dropt** ≈ SW France
149 T4 **Drosh** North-West Frontier Province, NW Pakistan
Drossen *see* Ośno Lubuskie
Drug *see* Durg
146 I9 **Drujba** *Rus.* Druzhba. Khorazm Wiloyati, W Uzbekistan
118 I12 **Drūkšiai** ◎ NE Lithuania
Druk-yul *see* Bhutan
11 Q16 **Drumheller** Alberta, SW Canada
33 Q10 **Drummond** Montana, NW USA
31 R4 **Drummond Island** *island* Michigan, N USA
Drummond Island *see* Tabiteuea
21 X7 **Drummond, Lake** ◎ Virginia, NE USA
15 P12 **Drummondville** Quebec, SE Canada
39 T11 **Drum, Mount** ▲ Alaska, USA
27 O9 **Drumright** Oklahoma, C USA
99 J14 **Drunen** Noord-Brabant, S Netherlands
Druskienniki *see* Druskininkai
119 F15 **Druskininkai** *Pol.* Druskienniki. Druskininkai, S Lithuania
98 K13 **Druten** Gelderland, SE Netherlands
118 K11 **Druya** Vitsyebskaya Voblasts', NW Belarus
117 S2 **Druzhba** Sums'ka Oblast', NE Ukraine
Druzhba *see* Dostyk, Kazakhstan
Druzhba *see* Drujba, Uzbekistan
123 R7 **Druzhina** Respublika Sakha (Yakutiya), NE Russian Federation
117 X7 **Druzhkivka** Donets'ka Oblast', E Ukraine
112 E12 **Drvar** Federacija Bosna I Hercegovina, Bosnia and Herzegovina
113 G15 **Drvenik** Split-Dalmacija, SE Croatia
114 K9 **Dryanovo** Gabrovo, N Bulgaria
26 G7 **Dry Cimarron River** ≈ Kansas/Oklahoma, C USA
12 B11 **Dryden** Ontario, C Canada
24 M11 **Dryden** Texas, SW USA
195 Q14 **Drygalski Ice Tongue** *ice feature* Antarctica
118 L11 **Drysa** *Rus.* Drissa. ≈ N Belarus
23 V17 **Dry Tortugas** *island* Florida, SE USA
79 D15 **Dschang** Ouest, W Cameroon
54 J5 **Duaca** Lara, N Venezuela
Duacum *see* Douai
Duala *see* Douala
45 N9 **Duarte, Pico** ▲ C Dominican Republic
140 J5 **Ḍubā** Tabūk, NW Saudi Arabia
Dubai *see* Dubayy
117 N9 **Dubăsari** *Rus.* Dubossary. NE Moldova
117 N9 **Dubăsari Reservoir** ⊞ NE Moldova
8 M10 **Dubawnt** ≈ Nunavut, NW Canada
8 L9 **Dubawnt Lake** ◎ Northwest Territories/Nunavut, N Canada
30 L6 **Du Bay, Lake** ⊞ Wisconsin, N USA
141 U7 **Dubayy** *Eng.* Dubai. Dubayy, NE UAE
141 W7 **Dubayy** *Eng.* Dubai. ✕ Dubayy, NE UAE
183 R7 **Dubbo** New South Wales, SE Australia
108 G7 **Dübendorf** Zürich, NW Switzerland
97 F18 **Dublin** *Ir.* Baile Átha Cliath; *anc.* Eblana. ● (Ireland), E Ireland
23 U5 **Dublin** Georgia, SE USA
25 R7 **Dublin** Texas, SW USA
97 G18 **Dublin** *Ir.* Baile Átha Cliath; *anc.* Eblana. *cultural region* E Ireland
97 G18 **Dublin Airport** ✕ E Ireland
189 V12 **Dublon** *var.* Tonoas. *island* Chuuk Islands, C Micronesia
128 K2 **Dubna** Moskovskaya Oblast', W Russian Federation
111 G19 **Dubňany** *Ger.* Dubnian. Brněnský Kraj, SE Czech Republic
Dubnian *see* Dubňany
111 I19 **Dubnica nad Váhom** *Hung.* Máriatölgyes; *prev.* Dubnicz. Trenčiansky Kraj, W Slovakia
Dubnicz *see* Dubnica nad Váhom
116 K4 **Dubno** Rivnens'ka Oblast', NW Ukraine
18 D13 **Du Bois** Pennsylvania, NE USA
33 R13 **Dubois** Idaho, NW USA
33 T14 **Dubois** Wyoming, C USA
Dubossary *see* Dubăsari
129 O10 **Dubovka** Volgogradskaya Oblast', SW Russian Federation
76 H14 **Dubréka** Guinée-Maritime, SW Guinea
14 B7 **Dubreuilville** Ontario, S Canada
Dubris Portus *see* Dover
119 L20 **Dubrova** *Rus.* Dubrova. Homyel'skaya Voblasts', SE Belarus
128 I5 **Dubrovka** Bryanskaya Oblast', W Russian Federation
113 H16 **Dubrovnik** *It.* Ragusa. Dubrovnik-Neretva, SE Croatia
113 I16 **Dubrovnik** ✕ Dubrovnik-Neretva, SE Croatia
113 F16 **Dubrovnik-Neretva** *off.* Dubrovačko-Neretvanska Županija. ◆ *province* SE Croatia
Dubrovno *see* Dubrowna
116 L2 **Dubrovytsya** Rivnens'ka Oblast', NW Ukraine
119 O14 **Dubrowna** *Rus.* Dubrovno. Vitsyebskaya Voblasts', N Belarus
29 Z13 **Dubuque** Iowa, C USA
118 E12 **Dubysa** ≈ C Lithuania
167 U11 **Đức Cơ** Gia Lai, C Vietnam
191 V12 **Duc de Gloucester, Îles du** *Eng.* Duke of Gloucester Islands. *island group* C French Polynesia
111 C15 **Duchcov** *Ger.* Dux. Ústecký Kraj, NW Czech Republic
37 N3 **Duchesne** Utah, W USA
191 P17 **Ducie Island** *atoll* E Pitcairn Islands
11 W15 **Duck Bay** Manitoba, S Canada
23 X17 **Duck Key** *island* Florida Keys, Florida, SE USA
11 T14 **Duck Lake** Saskatchewan, S Canada
11 V15 **Duck Mountain** ▲ Manitoba, S Canada
20 I9 **Duck River** ≈ Tennessee, S USA
20 M10 **Ducktown** Tennessee, S USA
167 U10 **Đức Phổ** Quang Ngai, C Vietnam
167 T8 **Đức Thọ** Ha Tinh, N Vietnam
167 U13 **Đức Trọng** *var.* Liên Nghia. Lâm Đồng, S Vietnam
D-U-D *see* Dalap-Uliga-Djarrit
99 M25 **Dudelange** *var.* Forge du Sud, *Ger.* Dudelingen. Luxembourg, S Luxembourg
Dudelingen *see* Dudelange
101 J15 **Duderstadt** Niedersachsen, C Germany
153 N15 **Dūdhi** Uttar Pradesh, N India
122 K8 **Dudinka** Taymyrskiy (Dolgano-Nenetskiy) Avtonomnyy Okrug, N Russian Federation
97 L20 **Dudley** C England, UK
154 G13 **Dudna** ≈ C India
76 L16 **Duékoué** W Ivory Coast
104 M5 **Dueñas** Castilla-León, N Spain
104 K4 **Duerna** ≈ NW Spain
105 O6 **Duero** *Port.* Douro. ≈ Portugal/Spain *see also* Douro
Duesseldorf *see* Düsseldorf
21 P12 **Due West** South Carolina, SE USA
195 P11 **Dufek Coast** *physical region* Antarctica
99 H17 **Duffel** Antwerpen, C Belgium
35 S2 **Duffer Peak** ▲ Nevada, W USA
187 Q9 **Duff Islands** *island group* E Solomon Islands
Dufour, Pizzo/Dufour, Punta *see* Dufour Spitze
108 E12 **Dufour Spitze** *It.* Pizzo Dufour, Punta Dufour. ▲ Italy/Switzerland
112 D9 **Duga Resa** Karlovac, C Croatia
22 H5 **Dugdemona River** ≈ Louisiana, S USA
154 J12 **Duggipar** Mahārāshtra, C India
112 B13 **Dugi Otok** *var.* Isola Grossa, *It.* Isola Lunga. *island* W Croatia
113 F14 **Dugopolje** Split-Dalmacija, S Croatia
160 L8 **Du He** ≈ C China
54 M11 **Duida, Cerro** ▲ S Venezuela
Duinekerke *see* Dunkerque
101 E15 **Duisburg** *prev.* Duisburg-Hamborn. Nordrhein-Westfalen, W Germany
Duisburg-Hamborn *see* Duisburg
99 F14 **Duiveland** *island* SW Netherlands
98 M12 **Duiven** Gelderland, E Netherlands
139 W10 **Dujaylah, Hawr ad** ◎ S Iraq
81 L18 **Dujuuma** Shabeellaha Hoose, S Somalia
Dūkān *see* Dokan
39 Z14 **Duke Island** *island* Alexander Archipelago, Alaska, USA
Dukelský Priesmy/Dukelský Průsmyk *see* Dukla Pass
Duke of Gloucester Islands *see* Duc de Gloucester, Îles du
81 F14 **Duk Faiwil** Jonglei, SE Sudan
141 T7 **Dukhān** C Qatar
Dukhan Heights *see* Dukhān, Jabal
143 N16 **Dukhān, Jabal** *var.* Dukhan Heights. *hill range* S Qatar
129 Q7 **Dukhovnitskoye** Saratovskaya Oblast', W Russian Federation
128 H4 **Dukhovshchina** Smolenskaya Oblast', W Russian Federation
Dukielska, Przełęcz *see* Dukla Pass
111 N17 **Dukla** Podkarpackie, SE Poland
Duklai Hág *see* Dukla Pass
111 N18 **Dukla Pass** *Cz.* Dukelský Průsmyk, *Ger.* Dukla-Pass, *Hung.* Duklai Hág, *Pol.* Przełęcz Dukielska, *Slvk.* Dukelský Priesmy. *pass* Poland/Slovakia
Dukou *see* Panzhihua
118 I12 **Dūkštas** Ignalina, E Lithuania
162 M8 **Dulaan** Hentiy, C Mongolia
159 R10 **Dulan** *var.* Qagan Us. Qinghai, C China
37 R8 **Dulce** New Mexico, SW USA
43 N16 **Dulce, Golfo** *gulf* S Costa Rica
Dulce, Golfo *see* Izabal, Lago de
42 K6 **Dulce Nombre de Culmí** Olancho, C Honduras
62 L9 **Dulce, Río** ≈ C Argentina
123 Q9 **Dulgalakh** ≈ NE Russian Federation
114 M8 **Dŭlgopol** Varna, E Bulgaria
153 V14 **Dullabchara** Assam, NE India
20 D3 **Dulles** ✕ (Washington DC) Virginia, NE USA
101 E14 **Dülmen** Nordrhein-Westfalen, W Germany
114 M7 **Dulovo** Silistra, NE Bulgaria
29 W5 **Duluth** Minnesota, N USA
138 H7 **Dūmā** *Fr.* Douma. Dimashq, SW Syria
171 O8 **Dumagasa Point** *headland* Mindanao, S Philippines
171 P6 **Dumaguete** *var.* Dumaguete City. Negros, C Philippines
168 J10 **Dumai** Sumatera, W Indonesia
183 T4 **Dumaresq River** ≈ New South Wales/Queensland, SE Australia
27 W13 **Dumas** Arkansas, C USA
25 N1 **Dumas** Texas, SW USA
138 I7 **Ḍumayr** Dimashq, W Syria
96 I12 **Dumbarton** W Scotland, UK
96 I12 **Dumbarton** *cultural region* C Scotland, UK
187 Q17 **Dumbéa** Province Sud, S New Caledonia
111 K19 **Ďumbier** *Ger.* Djumbir, *Hung.* Gyömbér. ▲ C Slovakia
116 I11 **Dumbrăveni** *Ger.* Elisabethstedt, *Hung.* Erzsébetváros; *prev.* Ebesfalva, Eppeschdorf, Ibașfalău. Sibiu, C Romania
116 L12 **Dumbrăveni** Vrancea, E Romania
97 J14 **Dumfries** S Scotland, UK
97 J14 **Dumfries** *cultural region* SW Scotland, UK
153 R15 **Dumka** Bihār, NE India
Dümmer *see* Dümmersee
100 G12 **Dümmersee** *var.* Dümmer. ◎ NW Germany
14 J11 **Dumoine** ≈ Quebec, SE Canada
14 J10 **Dumoine, Lac** ◎ Quebec, SE Canada
195 V16 **Dumont d'Urville** *French research station* Antarctica
195 W15 **Dumont d'Urville Sea** S Pacific Ocean
14 K11 **Dumont, Lac** ◎ Quebec, SE Canada
75 W7 **Dumyāṭ** *Eng.* Damietta. N Egypt
Duna *see* Don, Russian Federation
Duna *see* Danube, C Europe
Düna *see* Western Dvina
Dünaburg *see* Daugavpils
111 J24 **Dunaföldvár** Tolna, C Hungary
Dunaj *see* Wien, Austria
Dunaj *see* Danube, C Europe
111 L18 **Dunajec** ≈ S Poland
111 H21 **Dunajská Streda** *Hung.* Dunaszerdahely. Trnavský Kraj, W Slovakia
Dunapentele *see* Dunaújváros
Dunărea *see* Danube
116 M13 **Dunărea Veche, Brațul** ≈ SE Romania
117 N13 **Dunării, Delta** *delta* SE Romania
Dunaszerdahely *see* Dunajská Streda
111 J23 **Dunaújváros** *prev.* Dunapentele, Sztálinváros. Fejér, C Hungary
Dunav *see* Danube
114 J8 **Dunavska Ravnina** *Eng.* Danubian Plain. *plain* N Bulgaria
114 G7 **Dunavtsi** Vidin, NW Bulgaria
Dunayevtsy *see* Dunayivtsi
116 L7 **Dunayivtsi** *Rus.* Dunayevtsy. Khmel'nyts'ka Oblast', NW Ukraine
185 F22 **Dunback** Otago, South Island, NZ
10 L17 **Duncan** Vancouver Island, British Columbia, SW Canada
37 O15 **Duncan** Arizona, SW USA
26 M12 **Duncan** Oklahoma, C USA
Duncan Island *see* Pinzón, Isla
151 Q20 **Duncan Passage** *strait* Andaman Sea/Bay of Bengal
96 K6 **Duncansby Head** *headland* N Scotland, UK
14 G12 **Dunchurch** Ontario, S Canada
118 D7 **Dundaga** Talsi, NW Latvia
14 G14 **Dundalk** Ontario, S Canada
97 F16 **Dundalk** *Ir.* Dún Dealgan. NE Ireland
21 X3 **Dundalk** Maryland, NE USA
97 F16 **Dundalk Bay** *Ir.* Cuan Dhún Dealgan. *bay* NE Ireland
14 G16 **Dundas** Ontario, S Canada
180 L12 **Dundas, Lake** *salt lake* Western Australia
163 O7 **Dundbürd** Hentiy, E Mongolia
Dún Dealgan *see* Dundalk
15 N13 **Dundee** Quebec, SE Canada
83 K22 **Dundee** KwaZulu/Natal, E South Africa
96 K11 **Dundee** E Scotland, UK
31 R10 **Dundee** Michigan, N USA
25 R5 **Dundee** Texas, SW USA
194 H3 **Dundee Island** *island* Antarctica
162 L9 **Dundgovĭ** ◆ *province* C Mongolia
97 G16 **Dundrum Bay** *Ir.* Cuan Dhún Droma. *inlet* NW Irish Sea
11 T15 **Dundurn** Saskatchewan, S Canada
162 E6 **Dund-Us** Hovd, W Mongolia
185 F23 **Dunedin** Otago, South Island, NZ
183 R7 **Dunedoo** New South Wales, SE Australia
97 D14 **Dunfanaghy** *Ir.* Dún Fionnachaidh. NW Ireland
96 J12 **Dunfermline** C Scotland, UK
Dún Fionnachaidh *see* Dunfanaghy
149 V10 **Dunga Bunga** Punjab, E Pakistan
97 F15 **Dungannon** *Ir.* Dún Geanainn. C Northern Ireland, UK
Dun Garbháin *see* Dungarvan
152 F15 **Dūngarpur** Rājasthān, N India
97 E21 **Dungarvan** *Ir.* Dun Garbháin. S Ireland
101 N21 **Dungau** *cultural region* SE Germany
Dún Geanainn *see* Dungannon
97 P23 **Dungeness** *headland* SE England, UK
63 I23 **Dungeness, Punta** *headland* S Argentina
Dungloe *see* Dunglow
97 D14 **Dunglow** *var.* Dungloe, *Ir.* An Clochán Liath. NW Ireland
183 T7 **Dungog** New South Wales, SE Australia
79 O16 **Dungu** Orientale, NE Dem. Rep. Congo (Zaire)
168 L8 **Dungun** *var.* Kuala Dungun. Terengganu, Peninsular Malaysia
80 I6 **Dungûnab** Red Sea, NE Sudan
15 P13 **Dunham** Quebec, SE Canada
Dunheved *see* Launceston
Dunholme *see* Durham
163 X10 **Dunhua** Jilin, NE China
159 P8 **Dunhuang** Gansu, N China
182 L12 **Dunkeld** Victoria, SE Australia
103 O1 **Dunkerque** *Eng.* Dunkirk, *Flem.* Duinekerke; *prev.* Dunquerque. Nord, N France
97 K23 **Dunkery Beacon** ▲ SW England, UK
18 C11 **Dunkirk** New York, NE USA
Dunkirk *see* Dunkerque
77 P17 **Dunkwa** SW Ghana
97 G18 **Dún Laoghaire** *Eng.* Dunleary; *prev.* Kingstown. E Ireland
29 S14 **Dunlap** Iowa, C USA
20 L10 **Dunlap** Tennessee, S USA
Dunleary *see* Dún Laoghaire
Dún Mánmhaí *see* Dunmanway
97 B21 **Dunmanway** *Ir.* Dún Mánmhaí. SW Ireland
18 I13 **Dunmore** Pennsylvania, NE USA
21 U10 **Dunn** North Carolina, SE USA
Dún na nGall *see* Donegal
23 V11 **Dunnellon** Florida, SE USA
96 J6 **Dunnet Head** *headland* N Scotland, UK
29 N14 **Dunning** Nebraska, C USA
65 B24 **Dunnose Head Settlement** West Falkland, Falkland Islands
14 G17 **Dunnville** Ontario, S Canada
Dún Pádraig *see* Downpatrick
Dunquerque *see* Dunkerque
Dunqulah *see* Dongola
96 L12 **Duns** SE Scotland, UK
29 N2 **Dunseith** North Dakota, N USA
35 N2 **Dunsmuir** California, W USA
97 N21 **Dunstable** *Lat.* Durocobrivae. E England, UK
185 D21 **Dunstan Mountains** ▲ South Island, NZ
103 O9 **Dun-sur-Auron** Cher, C France
185 F21 **Duntroon** Canterbury, South Island, NZ
149 T10 **Dunyāpur** Punjab, E Pakistan
163 U5 **Duobukur He** ≈ NE China
163 R12 **Duolun** *var.* Dolonnur. Nei Mongol Zizhiqu, N China
167 Q14 **Dương Đông** Kiên Giang, S Vietnam
114 G10 **Dupnitsa** *prev.* Marek, Stanke Dimitrov. Kyustendil, W Bulgaria
28 L8 **Dupree** South Dakota, N USA
33 Q7 **Dupuyer** Montana, NW USA
141 Y11 **Duqm** *var.* Daqm. E Oman
63 F23 **Duque de York, Isla** *island* S Chile
181 N4 **Durack Range** ▲ Western Australia
136 K10 **Durağan** Sinop, N Turkey
103 S15 **Durance** ≈ SE France
31 R9 **Durand** Michigan, N USA
30 I6 **Durand** Wisconsin, N USA
40 K10 **Durango** *var.* Victoria de Durango. Durango, W Mexico
105 P3 **Durango** País Vasco, N Spain
37 Q8 **Durango** Colorado, C USA
40 J9 **Durango** ◆ *state* C Mexico
114 O7 **Durankulak** *Rom.* Răcari; *prev.* Blatnitsa, Duranulac. Dobrich, NE Bulgaria
22 L4 **Durant** Mississippi, S USA
27 P13 **Durant** Oklahoma, C USA
Duranulac *see* Durankulak
105 N6 **Duratón** ≈ N Spain
61 E19 **Durazno** *var.* San Pedro de Durazno. Durazno, C Uruguay
61 E19 **Durazno** ◆ *department* C Uruguay
Durazzo *see* Durrës
83 K23 **Durban** *var.* Port Natal. KwaZulu/Natal, E South Africa
83 K23 **Durban** ✕ KwaZulu/Natal, E South Africa
118 C9 **Durbe** *Ger.* Durben. Liepāja, W Latvia
Durben *see* Durbe
99 K21 **Durbuy** Luxembourg, SE Belgium
105 N15 **Dúrcal** Andalucía, S Spain
112 F8 **Đurđevac** *Ger.* Sankt Georgen, *Hung.* Szentgyörgy; *prev.* Djurdjevac, Gjurgjevac. Koprivnica-Križevci, N Croatia
113 K15 **Đurđevica Tara** ▲ Montenegro, SW Yugoslavia
97 L24 **Durdle Door** *natural arch* S England, UK
158 L3 **Düre** Xinjiang Uygur Zizhiqu, W China
101 D16 **Düren** *anc.* Marcodurum. Nordrhein-Westfalen, W Germany
154 K12 **Durg** *prev.* Drug. Madhya Pradesh, C India
153 U13 **Durgapur** Dhaka, N Bangladesh
153 R15 **Durgāpur** West Bengal, NE India
14 F14 **Durham** Ontario, S Canada
97 M14 **Durham** *hist.* Dunholme. N England, UK
21 U9 **Durham** North Carolina, SE USA
97 L15 **Durham** *cultural region* N England, UK
168 J10 **Duri** Sumatera, W Indonesia
Duria Major *see* Dora Baltea
Duria Minor *see* Dora Riparia
Durlas *see* Thurles
141 P8 **Ḍurmā** Ar Riyāḍ, C Saudi Arabia
113 J15 **Durmitor** ▲ N Yugoslavia
96 H6 **Durness** N Scotland, UK
109 Y3 **Dürnkrut** Niederösterreich, E Austria
Durnovaria *see* Dorchester
Durobrivae *see* Rochester
Durocasses *see* Dreux
Durocobrivae *see* Dunstable
Durocortorum *see* Reims
Durostorum *see* Silistra
Durovernum *see* Canterbury
113 K20 **Durrës** *var.* Durrësi, Dursi, *It.* Durazzo, *SCr.* Drač, *Turk.* Draç. Durrës, W Albania
113 K19 **Durrës** ◆ *district* W Albania
Durrësi *see* Durrës
97 A21 **Dursey Island** *Ir.* Oileán Baoi. *island* SW Ireland
Dursi *see* Durrës
Durud *see* Do Rūd
114 P12 **Durusu** İstanbul, NW Turkey
114 O12 **Durusu Gölü** ◎ NW Turkey
138 I9 **Durūz, Jabal ad** ▲ SW Syria
184 K13 **D'Urville Island** *island* C NZ
171 X12 **D'Urville, Tanjung** *headland* Irian Jaya, E Indonesia
Dusa Mareb/Dusa Marreb *see* Dhuusa Marreeb
118 I11 **Dusetos** Zarasai, NE Lithuania
146 H14 **Dushak** Akhalskiy Velayat, S Turkmenistan
160 K12 **Dushan** Guizhou, S China
147 P13 **Dushanbe** *var.* Dyushambe; *prev.* Stalinabad, *Taj.* Stalinobod. ● (Tajikistan) W Tajikistan
147 P13 **Dushanbe** ✕ W Tajikistan
137 T9 **Dushet'i** E Georgia
18 H13 **Dushore** Pennsylvania, NE USA
185 A23 **Dusky Sound** *sound* South Island, NZ
101 E15 **Düsseldorf** *var.* Duesseldorf. Nordrhein-Westfalen, W Germany
147 P14 **Dŭstí** *Rus.* Dusti. SW Tajikistan
194 I9 **Dustin Island** *island* Antarctica
147 O10 **Dŭstlik** Jizzakh Wiloyati, C Uzbekistan
Dutch East Indies *see* Indonesia
Dutch Guiana *see* Suriname
38 L17 **Dutch Harbor** Unalaska Island, Alaska, USA
36 J3 **Dutch Mount** ▲ Utah, W USA
Dutch New Guinea *see* Irian Jaya
Dutch West Indies *see* Netherlands Antilles
83 H20 **Dutlwe** Kweneng, S Botswana
67 V16 **Du Toit Fracture Zone** *tectonic feature* SW Indian Ocean
127 U8 **Dutovo** Respublika Komi, NW Russian Federation
77 V13 **Dutsan Wai** *var.* Dutsen Wai. Kaduna, C Nigeria
77 W13 **Dutse** Jigawa, N Nigeria
Dutsen Wai *see* Dutsan Wai
Duttia *see* Datia
14 E17 **Dutton** Ontario, S Canada
36 L7 **Dutton, Mount** ▲ Utah, W USA

◆ Country
● Country Capital
◇ Dependent Territory
○ Dependent Territory Capital
◆ Administrative Region
✕ International Airport
▲ Mountain
▲ Mountain Range
▲ Volcano
≈ River
◎ Lake
⊞ Reservoir

162 E7 Duut Hovd, W Mongolia
14 K11 Duval, Lac ◎ Quebec, SE Canada
129 W3 Duvan Respublika Bashkortostan, W Russian Federation
138 L9 Duwaykhilat Satih ar Ruwayshid seasonal river SE Jordan
Dux see Duchcov
160 J13 Duyang Shan ▲ S China
167 T14 Duyên Hai Tra Vinh, S Vietnam
160 K12 Duyun Guizhou, S China
136 G11 Düzce Bolu, NW Turkey
Duzdab see Zāhedān
Duzenkyr, Khrebet see Duzkyr, Khrebet
146 I16 Duzkyr, Khrebet prev. Khrebet Duzenkyr. ▲ S Turkmenistan
Dvina Bay see Chëshskaya Guba
Dvinsk see Daugavpils
126 L7 Dvinskaya Guba bay NW Russian Federation
112 E10 Dvor Sisak-Moslavina, C Croatia
117 W5 Dvorichna Kharkivs'ka Oblast', E Ukraine
111 F16 Dvůr Králové nad Labem Ger. Königinhof an der Elbe. Hradecký Kraj, NE Czech Republic
154 A10 Dwārka Gujarāt, W India
30 M12 Dwight Illinois, N USA
98 N8 Dwingeloo Drenthe, NE Netherlands
33 N10 Dworshak Reservoir ▣ Idaho, NW USA
Dyal see Dyaul Island
Dyanev see Deynau
Dyatlovo see Dzyatlava
186 G5 Dyaul Island var. Djaul, Dyal. island NE PNG
20 G8 Dyer Tennessee, S USA
9 S5 Dyer, Cape headland Baffin Island, Nunavut, NE Canada
20 F8 Dyersburg Tennessee, S USA
29 Y13 Dyersville Iowa, C USA
97 I21 Dyfed cultural region SW Wales, UK
Dyfrdwy, Afon see Dee
Dyhernfurth see Brzeg Dolny
111 E19 Dyje var. Thaya. ≈ Austria/Czech Republic see also Thaya
117 T5 Dykanska Poltavs'ka Oblast', C Ukraine
129 N16 Dykhtau ▲ SW Russian Federation
111 A16 Dyleń Ger. Tillenberg. ▲ NW Czech Republic
110 K9 Dylewska Góra ▲ N Poland
117 O4 Dymer Kyyivs'ka Oblast', N Ukraine
117 W7 Dymytrov Rus. Dimitrov. Donets'ka Oblast', SE Ukraine
111 O17 Dynów Podkarpackie, SE Poland
29 X13 Dysart Iowa, C USA
Dysna see Dzisna
115 D18 Dytikí Ellás Eng. Greece West. ◆ region C Greece
115 C14 Dytikí Makedonía Eng. Macedonia West. ◆ region N Greece
Dyurmen'tyube see Dermentobe
129 U4 Dyurtyuli Respublika Bashkortostan, W Russian Federation
Dyushambe see Dushanbe
162 I7 Dzaanhushuu Arhangay, C Mongolia
Dza Chu see Mekong
162 I8 Dzadgay Bayanhongor, C Mongolia
162 H8 Dzag Bayanhongor, C Mongolia
162 H10 Dzalaa Bayanhongor, C Mongolia
172 J14 Dzaoudzi E Mayotte
Dzaudzhikau see Vladikavkaz
162 G7 Dzavhan ◆ province NW Mongolia
162 G7 Dzavhan Gol ≈ NW Mongolia
162 J7 Dzegstey Arhangay, C Mongolia
129 O3 Dzerzhinsk Nizhegorodskaya Oblast', W Russian Federation
Dzerzhinsk see Dzyarzhynsk, Belarus
Dzerzhinsk see Dzerzhyns'k, Ukraine
Dzerzhinskiy see Nar'yan-Mar
145 W13 Dzerzhinskoye Almaty, SE Kazakhstan
117 X7 Dzerzhyns'k Rus. Dzerzhinsk. Donets'ka Oblast', SE Ukraine
116 M5 Dzerzhyns'k Zhytomyrs'ka Oblast', N Ukraine
Dzhailgan see Jayilgan
145 N14 Dzhalagash Kaz. Zhalashash. Kzylorda, S Kazakhstan
147 T10 Dzhalal-Abad Kir. Jalal-Abad. Dzhalal-Abadskaya Oblast', W Kyrgyzstan
147 S9 Dzhalal-Abadskaya Oblast' Kir. Jalal-Abad Oblasty. ◆ province W Kyrgyzstan
Dzhalilabad see Cälilabad
144 G9 Dzhambeyty Kaz. Zhympity. Zapadnyy Kazakhstan, W Kazakhstan
Dzhambulskaya Oblast' see Zhambyl
Dzhankel'dy see Jangeldi
117 T12 Dzhankoy Respublika Krym, S Ukraine
145 V14 Dzhansugurov Kaz. Zhansügirov. Almaty, SE Kazakhstan
147 R9 Dzhany-Bazar var. Yangibazar. Dzhalal-Abadskaya Oblast', W Kyrgyzstan
144 D9 Dzhanybek Kaz. Zhänibek. Zapadnyy Kazakhstan, W Kazakhstan
123 P8 Dzhardzhan Respublika Sakha (Yakutiya), NE Russian Federation
Dzharkurgan see Jarqŭrghon
117 S11 Dzharylhats'ka Zatoka gulf S Ukraine
Dzhayilgan see Jayilgan
146 B11 Dzhebel Turkm. Jebel. Balkanskiy Velayat, W Turkmenistan
147 T14 Dzhelandy SE Tajikistan
147 Y7 Dzhergalan Kir. Jyrgalan. Issyk-Kul'skaya Oblast', NE Kyrgyzstan
144 L8 Dzhetygara Kaz. Zhetiqara. Kostanay, NW Kazakhstan
Dzhetysay see Zhetysay.
Dzhezkazgan see Zhezqazghan
146 J10 Dzhigirbent Turkm. Jigerbent. Lebapskiy Velayat, NE Turkmenistan
Dzhirgatal' see Jirgatol
Dzhizak see Jizzakh
Dzhizakskaya Oblast' see Jizzakh Wiloyati
123 P8 Dzhugdzhur, Khrebet ▲ E Russian Federation
Dzhul'fa see Culfa
Dzhuma see Juma
145 W14 Dzhungarskiy Alatau ▲ China/Kazakhstan
144 M14 Dzhusaly Kaz. Zholsaly. Kzylorda, SW Kazakhstan
146 J12 Dzhynlykum, Peski desert E Turkmenistan
110 L9 Działdowo Warmińsko-Mazurskie, C Poland
111 L16 Działoszyce Świętokrzyskie, C Poland
41 X11 Dzidzantún Yucatán, E Mexico
111 G15 Dzierżoniów Ger. Reichenbach. Dolnośląskie, SW Poland
41 X11 Dzilam de Bravo Yucatán, E Mexico
118 L12 Dzisna Rus. Disna. Vitsyebskaya Voblasts', N Belarus
118 K12 Dzisna Lith. Dysna, Rus. Disna. ≈ Belarus/Lithuania
119 G20 Dzivin Rus. Divin. Brestskaya Voblasts', SW Belarus
119 M15 Dzmitravichy Rus. Dmitrovichi. Minskaya Voblasts', C Belarus
162 M8 Dzogsool Töv, C Mongolia
131 S8 Dzungaria var. Sungaria, Zungaria. physical region W China
Dzungarian Basin see Junggar Pendi
162 G5 Dzür Dzavhan, W Mongolia
163 Q8 Dzüünbulag Dornod, E Mongolia
163 O8 Dzüünbulag Sühbaatar, E Mongolia
162 H7 Dzuunmod Dzavhan, C Mongolia
162 L8 Dzuunmod Töv, C Mongolia
Dzüün Soyonĭ Nuruu see Eastern Sayans
162 F8 Dzüyl Govĭ-Altay, SW Mongolia
Dzvina see Western Dvina
119 J16 Dzyarzhynsk Rus. Dzerzhinsk; prev. Kaydanovo. Minskaya Voblasts', C Belarus
119 H17 Dzyatlava Pol. Zdzięcioł, Rus. Dyatlovo. Hrodzyenskaya Voblasts', W Belarus

E

E see Hubei
Éadan Doire see Edenderry
37 W6 Eads Colorado, C USA
37 O13 Eagar Arizona, SW USA
39 T8 Eagle Alaska, USA
13 S8 Eagle ≈ Newfoundland, E Canada
10 I3 Eagle ≈ Yukon Territory, NW Canada
29 T7 Eagle Bend Minnesota, N USA
28 M8 Eagle Butte South Dakota, N USA
29 V12 Eagle Grove Iowa, C USA
19 R2 Eagle Lake Maine, NE USA
25 U11 Eagle Lake Texas, SW USA
12 A11 Eagle Lake ◎ Ontario, S Canada
35 P3 Eagle Lake ◎ California, W USA
19 R3 Eagle Lake ◎ Maine, NE USA
29 Y3 Eagle Mountain ▲ Minnesota, N USA
25 T6 Eagle Mountain Lake ▣ Texas, SW USA
37 S9 Eagle Nest Lake ▣ New Mexico, SW USA
25 P13 Eagle Pass Texas, SW USA
65 C25 Eagle Passage passage SW Atlantic Ocean
35 R8 Eagle Peak ▲ California, W USA
35 Q2 Eagle Peak ▲ California, W USA
37 P13 Eagle Peak ▲ New Mexico, SW USA
10 I4 Eagle Plain Yukon Territory, NW Canada
32 G15 Eagle Point Oregon, NW USA
186 F10 Eagle Point headland SE PNG
39 R11 Eagle River Alaska, USA
30 M2 Eagle River Michigan, N USA
30 L4 Eagle River Wisconsin, N USA
21 S6 Eagle Rock Virginia, NE USA
36 J13 Eagletail Mountains ▲ Arizona, SW USA
167 U12 Ea Hleo Đăc Lăc, S Vietnam
167 U12 Ea Kar Đăc Lăc, S Vietnam
Eanjum see Anjum
Eanodat see Enontekiö
12 B10 Ear Falls Ontario, C Canada
27 X10 Earle Arkansas, C USA
35 R12 Earlimart California, W USA
20 I6 Earlington Kentucky, S USA
14 H8 Earlton Ontario, S Canada
29 T13 Early Iowa, C USA
96 J11 Earn ≈ N Scotland, UK
185 C21 Earnslaw, Mount ▲ South Island, NZ
24 M4 Earth Texas, SW USA
21 P11 Easley South Carolina, SE USA
East see Est
East Açores Fracture Zone see East Azores Fracture Zone
97 P19 East Anglia physical region E England, UK
15 Q12 East Angus Quebec, SE Canada
East Antarctica see Greater Antarctica
18 E10 East Aurora New York, NE USA
East Australian Basin see Tasman Basin
East Azerbaijan see Āzarbāyjān-e Sharqī
64 L9 East Azores Fracture Zone var. East Açores Fracture Zone. tectonic feature E Atlantic Ocean
22 M11 East Bay bay Louisiana, S USA
25 V11 East Bernard Texas, SW USA
29 V8 East Bethel Minnesota, N USA
East Borneo see Kalimantan Timur
97 P23 Eastbourne SE England, UK
15 R11 East-Broughton Quebec, SE Canada
44 M6 East Caicos island E Turks and Caicos Islands
184 R7 East Cape headland North Island, NZ
174 M4 East Caroline Basin undersea feature SW Pacific Ocean
192 F4 East China Sea Chin. Dong Hai. sea W Pacific Ocean
97 P19 East Dereham E England, UK
30 J9 East Dubuque Illinois, N USA
11 S17 Eastend Saskatchewan, S Canada
193 S10 Easter Fracture Zone tectonic feature E Pacific Ocean
Easter Island see Pascua, Isla de
81 J18 Eastern ◆ province Kenya
153 Q12 Eastern ◆ zone E Nepal
82 L13 Eastern ◆ province E Zambia
83 H24 Eastern Cape off. Eastern Cape Province, Afr. Oos-Kaap. ◆ province SE South Africa
Eastern Desert see Sahara el Sharqîya
81 F15 Eastern Equatoria ◆ state SE Sudan
Eastern Euphrates see Murat Nehri
155 J17 Eastern Ghats ▲ SE India
186 E7 Eastern Highlands ◆ province C PNG
155 K25 Eastern Province ◆ province E Sri Lanka
Eastern Region see Ash Sharqīyah
122 L13 Eastern Sayans Mong. Dzüün Soyonĭ Nuruu, Rus. Vostochnyy Sayan. ▲ Mongolia/Russian Federation
Eastern Scheldt see Oosterschelde
Eastern Sierra Madre see Madre Oriental, Sierra
Eastern Transvaal see Mpumalanga
11 W14 Easterville Manitoba, C Canada
Easterwâlde see Oosterwolde
63 M23 East Falkland var. Isla Soledad. island E Falkland Islands
19 P12 East Falmouth Massachusetts, NE USA
East Fayu see Fayu
East Flanders see Oost-Vlaanderen
39 S6 East Fork Chandalar River ≈ Alaska, USA
29 U12 East Fork Des Moines River ≈ Iowa/Minnesota, C USA
East Frisian Islands see Ostfriesische Inseln
18 K10 East Glenville New York, NE USA
29 R4 East Grand Forks Minnesota, N USA
97 O23 East Grinstead SE England, UK
18 M12 East Hartford Connecticut, NE USA
18 M13 East Haven Connecticut, NE USA
173 T9 East Indiaman Ridge undersea feature E Indian Ocean
131 V16 East Indies island group SE Asia
East Java see Jawa Timur
31 Q6 East Jordan Michigan, N USA
East Kalimantan see Kalimantan Timur
East Kazakhstan see Vostochnyy Kazakhstan
96 I12 East Kilbride S Scotland, UK
25 R7 Eastland Texas, SW USA
31 Q9 East Lansing Michigan, N USA
35 X11 East Las Vegas Nevada, W USA
97 M23 Eastleigh S England, UK
31 V12 East Liverpool Ohio, N USA
83 J25 East London Afr. Oos-Londen; prev. Emonti, Port Rex. Eastern Cape, S South Africa
96 K12 East Lothian cultural region SE Scotland, UK
12 I10 Eastmain Quebec, E Canada
12 J10 Eastmain ≈ Quebec, C Canada
15 P13 Eastman Quebec, SE Canada
23 U6 Eastman Georgia, SE USA
175 O3 East Mariana Basin undersea feature W Pacific Ocean
30 K11 East Moline Illinois, N USA
186 H7 East New Britain ◆ province E PNG
29 T15 East Nishnabotna River ≈ Iowa, C USA
197 V12 East Novaya Zemlya Trough var. Novaya Zemlya Trough. undersea feature W Kara Sea
East Nusa Tenggara see Nusa Tenggara Timur
21 X4 Easton Maryland, NE USA
18 I14 Easton Pennsylvania, NE USA
193 R16 East Pacific Rise undersea feature E Pacific Ocean
East Pakistan see Bangladesh
31 V12 East Palestine Ohio, N USA
30 L12 East Peoria Illinois, N USA
23 S3 East Point Georgia, SE USA
19 U6 Eastport Maine, NE USA
27 Z8 East Prairie Missouri, C USA
19 O12 East Providence Rhode Island, NE USA
20 L11 East Ridge Tennessee, S USA
97 N16 East Riding cultural region N England, UK
18 F9 East Rochester New York, NE USA
30 K15 East Saint Louis Illinois, N USA
65 K21 East Scotia Basin undersea feature SE Scotia Sea
East Sea see Japan, Sea of
186 B6 East Sepik ◆ province NW PNG
173 N4 East Sheba Ridge undersea feature W Arabian Sea
East Siberian Sea see Vostochno-Sibirskoye More
18 I14 East Stroudsburg Pennsylvania, NE USA
East Tasmanian Rise/East Tasmania Plateau/East Tasmania Rise see East Tasman Plateau
192 I12 East Tasman Plateau var. East Tasmanian Rise, East Tasmania Plateau, East Tasmania Rise. undersea feature SW Tasman Sea
64 L7 East Thulean Rise undersea feature N Atlantic Ocean
171 R16 East Timor var Loro Sae prev. Portuguese Timor, Timor Timur ◇ disputed territory SE Asia
21 Y6 Eastville Virginia, NE USA
35 R7 East Walker River ≈ California/Nevada, W USA
182 D1 Eateringinna Creek ≈ South Australia
37 T3 Eaton Colorado, C USA
15 Q12 Eaton ≈ Quebec, SE Canada
11 S16 Eatonia Saskatchewan, S Canada
31 Q10 Eaton Rapids Michigan, N USA
23 U4 Eatonton Georgia, SE USA
32 H9 Eatonville Washington, NW USA
30 J6 Eau Claire Wisconsin, N USA
Eau Claire, Lac à L' see St.Clair, Lake
12 J7 Eau Claire, Lac à l' ◎ Quebec, SE Canada
30 L6 Eau Claire River ≈ Wisconsin, N USA
188 J16 Eauripik Atoll atoll Caroline Islands, C Micronesia
192 H7 Eauripik Rise undersea feature W Pacific Ocean
102 K15 Eauze Gers, S France
41 P11 Ébano San Luis Potosí, C Mexico
97 K21 Ebbw Vale SE Wales, UK
79 E17 Ebebiyin NE Equatorial Guinea
95 H22 Ebeltoft Århus, C Denmark
109 X5 Ebenfurth Niederösterreich, E Austria
18 D14 Ebensburg Pennsylvania, NE USA
109 S5 Ebensee Oberösterreich, N Austria
101 H20 Eberbach Baden-Württemberg, SW Germany
121 U8 Eber Gölü salt lake C Turkey
109 U9 Eberndorf Slvn. Dobrla Vas. Kärnten, S Austria
109 R4 Eberschwang Oberösterreich, N Austria
100 O11 Eberswalde-Finow Brandenburg, E Germany
Ebesfalva see Dumbrăveni
165 T4 Ebetsu var. Ebetu. Hokkaidō, NE Japan
Ebetu see Ebetsu
Ebinayon see Evinayong
158 I4 Ebinur Hu ◎ NW China
138 I3 Ebla Ar. Tell Mardīkh. site of ancient city Idlib, NW Syria
Eblana see Dublin
108 H7 Ebnat Sankt Gallen, NE Switzerland
107 L18 Eboli Campania, S Italy
79 E16 Ebolowa Sud, S Cameroon
79 N21 Ebombo Kasai Oriental, C Dem. Rep. Congo (Zaire)
189 T9 Ebon Atoll var. Epoon. atoll Ralik Chain, S Marshall Islands
Ebora see Évora
Eboracum see York
Eborodunum see Yverdon
101 J19 Ebrach Bayern, C Germany
109 X5 Ebreichsdorf Niederösterreich, E Austria
105 S6 Ebro ≈ NE Spain
105 N3 Ebro, Embalse del ▣ N Spain
120 G7 Ebro Fan undersea feature W Mediterranean Sea
Eburacum see York
Ebusus see Eivissa
99 F20 Écaussinnes-d'Enghien Hainaut, SW Belgium
Ecbatana see Hamadān
21 Q6 Eccles West Virginia, NE USA
115 L14 Eceabat Çanakkale, NW Turkey
171 O2 Echague Luzon, N Philippines
Ech Cheliff/Ech Chleff see Chlef
Echeng see Ezhou
115 C18 Echinádes island group W Greece
114 J12 Echínos var. Ehinos, Ekhínos. Anatolikí Makedonía kai Thráki, NE Greece
164 J12 Echizen-misaki headland Honshū, SW Japan
Echmiadzin see Ejmiatsin
8 J8 Echo Bay Northwest Territories, NW Canada
35 Y11 Echo Bay Nevada, W USA
36 L9 Echo Cliffs cliff Arizona, SW USA
14 C10 Echo Lake ◎ Ontario, S Canada
35 Q7 Echo Summit ▲ California, W USA
14 L8 Échouani, Lac ◎ Quebec, SE Canada
99 L17 Echt Limburg, SE Netherlands
101 H22 Echterdingen ✕ (Stuttgart) Baden-Württemberg, SW Germany
99 N24 Echternach Grevenmacher, E Luxembourg
183 N11 Echuca Victoria, SE Australia
104 L14 Écija anc. Astigi. Andalucía, SW Spain
Eckengraf see Viesīte
100 I7 Eckernförde Schleswig-Holstein, N Germany
100 J7 Eckernförder Bucht inlet N Germany
102 L7 Écommoy Sarthe, NW France
14 L10 Écorce, Lac de l' ◎ Quebec, SE Canada
15 Q8 Écorces, Rivière aux ≈ Quebec, SE Canada
56 C7 Ecuador off. Republic of Ecuador. ◆ republic NW South America
80 L10 Ed var. Edd. SE Eritrea
95 I17 Ed Västra Götaland, S Sweden
98 I9 Edam Noord-Holland, C Netherlands
96 K4 Eday island NE Scotland, UK
25 S17 Edcouch Texas, SW USA
Edd see Ed
80 C11 Ed Da'ein Southern Darfur, W Sudan
80 G11 Ed Damazin var. Ad Damazīn. Blue Nile, E Sudan
80 G8 Ed Damer var. Ad Damar, Ad Dāmir. River Nile, NE Sudan
80 E8 Ed Debba Northern, N Sudan
80 F10 Ed Dueim var. Ad Duwaym, Ad Duwēm. White Nile, C Sudan
183 Q16 Eddystone Point headland Tasmania, SE Australia
97 I25 Eddystone Rocks rocks SW England, UK
29 W15 Eddyville Iowa, C USA
20 H7 Eddyville Kentucky, S USA
98 L12 Ede Gelderland, C Netherlands
77 T16 Ede Osun, SW Nigeria
79 D16 Edéa Littoral, SW Cameroon
111 M20 Edelény Borsod-Abaúj-Zemplén, NE Hungary
183 R12 Eden New South Wales, SE Australia
21 T8 Eden North Carolina, SE USA
25 P9 Eden Texas, SW USA
97 K14 Eden ≈ NW England, UK
83 I23 Edenburg Free State, C South Africa
185 D24 Edendale Southland, South Island, NZ
97 E18 Edenderry Ir. Éadan Doire. C Ireland
182 L11 Edenhope Victoria, SE Australia
21 X8 Edenton North Carolina, SE USA
101 G16 Eder ≈ NW Germany
101 H15 Edersee ◎ W Germany
Edessa see Şanlıurfa
114 E13 Édessa var. Édhessa. Kentrikí Makedonía, N Greece
Edfu see Idfu
29 P16 Edgar Nebraska, C USA
19 P13 Edgartown Martha's Vineyard, Massachusetts, NE USA
39 X13 Edgecumbe, Mount ▲ Baranof Island, Alaska, USA
21 Q13 Edgefield South Carolina, SE USA
29 P6 Edgeley North Dakota, N USA
28 J11 Edgemont South Dakota, N USA
92 O3 Edgeøya island S Svalbard
27 Q4 Edgerton Kansas, C USA
29 S10 Edgerton Minnesota, N USA
21 X3 Edgewood Maryland, NE USA
25 V6 Edgewood Texas, SW USA
Édhessa see Édessa
29 V9 Edina Minnesota, N USA
27 U2 Edina Missouri, C USA
25 S17 Edinburg Texas, SW USA
65 M24 Edinburgh var. Settlement of Edinburgh. ○ (Tristan da Cunha) NW Tristan da Cunha
96 J12 Edinburgh ● S Scotland, UK
31 P14 Edinburgh Indiana, N USA
96 J12 Edinburgh ✕ S Scotland, UK
116 L8 Edineţ var. Edineţi, Rus. Yedintsy. NW Moldova
Edineţi see Edineţ
Edingen see Enghien
136 B9 Edirne Eng. Adrianople; anc. Adrianopolis, Hadrianopolis. Edirne, NW Turkey
136 B11 Edirne ◆ province NW Turkey
18 K15 Edison New Jersey, NE USA
21 S15 Edisto Island South Carolina, SE USA
21 R14 Edisto River ≈ South Carolina, SE USA
33 S10 Edith, Mount ▲ Montana, NW USA
27 N10 Edmond Oklahoma, C USA
32 H8 Edmonds Washington, NW USA
11 Q14 Edmonton Alberta, SW Canada
20 K7 Edmonton Kentucky, S USA
11 Q14 Edmonton ✕ Alberta, SW Canada
29 P3 Edmore North Dakota, N USA
13 N13 Edmundston New Brunswick, SE Canada
25 U12 Edna Texas, SW USA
39 X14 Edna Bay Kosciusko Island, Alaska, USA
77 U16 Edo ◆ state S Nigeria
106 F6 Edolo Lombardia, N Italy
64 L6 Edoras Bank undersea feature C Atlantic Ocean
96 G7 Edrachillis Bay bay NW Scotland, UK
136 B12 Edremit Balıkesir, NW Turkey
136 B12 Edremit Körfezi gulf NW Turkey
95 P14 Edsbro Stockholm, C Sweden
95 N18 Edsbruk Kalmar, S Sweden
94 M12 Edsbyn Gävleborg, C Sweden
11 O14 Edson Alberta, SW Canada
62 K13 Eduardo Castex La Pampa, C Argentina
58 F12 Eduardo Gomes ✕ (Manaus) Amazonas, NW Brazil
Edwardesabad see Bannu
67 U9 Edward, Lake var. Albert Edward Nyanza, Edward Nyanza, Lac Idi Amin, Lake Rutanzige. ◎ Uganda/Dem. Rep. Congo (Zaire)
Edward Nyanza see Edward, Lake
22 K5 Edwards Mississippi, S USA
25 O10 Edwards Plateau plain Texas, SW USA
30 J11 Edwards River ≈ Illinois, N USA
30 K15 Edwardsville Illinois, N USA
195 O13 Edward VII Peninsula peninsula Antarctica
195 X4 Edward VIII Gulf bay Antarctica
10 J11 Edziza, Mount ▲ British Columbia, W Canada
8 K10 Edzo prev. Rae-Edzo. Northwest Territories, NW Canada
39 N12 Eek Alaska, USA
99 D16 Eeklo var. Eekloo. Oost-Vlaanderen, NW Belgium
Eekloo see Eeklo
39 N12 Eek River ≈ Alaska, USA
98 N6 Eelde Drenthe, NE Netherlands
34 L5 Eel River ≈ California, W USA
31 P12 Eel River ≈ Indiana, N USA
Eems see Ems
98 O4 Eemshaven Groningen, NE Netherlands
98 O5 Eems Kanaal canal NE Netherlands
98 M11 Eerbeek Gelderland, E Netherlands
99 C17 Eernegem West-Vlaanderen, W Belgium
99 J15 Eersel Noord-Brabant, S Netherlands
Eesti Vabariik see Estonia
187 R14 Efate var. Éfaté, Fr. Vaté prev. Sandwich Island. island C Vanuatu
109 S4 Eferding Oberösterreich, N Austria
30 M15 Effingham Illinois, N USA
117 N15 Eforie-Nord Constanţa, SE Romania
117 N15 Eforie Sud Constanţa, E Romania
Efyrnwy, Afon see Vyrnwy
163 N7 Eg Hentiy, N Mongolia
107 G23 Egadi, Isole island group S Italy
35 X6 Egan Range ▲ Nevada, W USA
14 K12 Eganville Ontario, SE Canada
Ege Denizi see Aegean Sea
39 O14 Egegik Alaska, USA
111 L21 Eger Ger. Erlau. Heves, NE Hungary
Eger see Cheb, Czech Republic
Eger see Ohre, Czech Republic/Germany
173 P8 Egeria Fracture Zone tectonic feature W Indian Ocean
95 C17 Egersund Rogaland, S Norway
108 J7 Egg Vorarlberg, NW Austria
101 H14 Egge-gebirge ▲ C Germany
109 Q4 Eggelsberg Oberösterreich, N Austria
109 W2 Eggenburg Niederösterreich, NE Austria
101 N22 Eggenfelden Bayern, SE Germany
18 J17 Egg Harbor City New Jersey, NE USA
65 G25 Egg Island island W Saint Helena
183 N14 Egg Lagoon Tasmania, SE Australia
99 I20 Éghezée Namur, C Belgium
92 L2 Egilsstadhir Austurland, E Iceland
Egina see Aígina
Egindibulaq see Yegindybulak
Egio see Aígio
103 N12 Égletons Corrèze, C France
98 H9 Egmond aan Zee Noord-Holland, NW Netherlands
Egmont see Taranaki, Mount
184 J10 Egmont, Cape headland North Island, NZ
Egoli see Johannesburg
Eğri Palanka see Kriva Palanka
95 G23 Egtved Vejle, C Denmark
123 U5 Egvekinot Chukotskiy Avtonomnyy Okrug, NE Russian Federation

◆ Country ● Country Capital ◇ Dependent Territory ○ Dependent Territory Capital ◆ Administrative Region ✕ International Airport ▲ Mountain ▲ Mountain Range ⛰ Volcano ≈ River ◎ Lake ▣ Reservoir

75 V9 **Egypt** off. Arab Republic of Egypt, Ar. Jumhūrīyah Miṣr al 'Arabīyah; prev. United Arab Republic, anc. Aegyptus. ◆ republic NE Africa
30 L17 **Egypt, Lake Of** ⊟ Illinois, N USA
Ehen Hudag see Alxa Zuoqi
164 F14 **Ehime** off. Ehime-ken. ◆ prefecture Shikoku, SW Japan
101 I23 **Ehingen** Baden-Württemberg, S Germany
Ehinos see Echínos
21 R14 **Ehrhardt** South Carolina, SE USA
108 L7 **Ehrwald** Tirol, W Austria
191 W6 **Eiao** island Îles Marquises, NE French Polynesia
105 P2 **Eibar** País Vasco, N Spain
98 O11 **Eibergen** Gelderland, E Netherlands
109 V9 **Eibiswald** Steiermark, SE Austria
109 P8 **Eichham** ▲ SW Austria
101 J15 **Eichsfeld** hill range C Germany
101 K21 **Eichstätt** Bayern, SE Germany
100 H8 **Eider** ≈ N Germany
94 E13 **Eidfjord** Hordaland, S Norway
94 D13 **Eidfjorden** fjord S Norway
94 F9 **Eidsvåg** Møre og Romsdal, S Norway
95 I14 **Eidsvoll** Akershus, S Norway
92 N2 **Eidsvollfjellet** ▲ NW Svalbard
Eier-Berg see Suur Munamägi
101 D18 **Eifel** plateau W Germany
108 E9 **Eiger** ▲ C Switzerland
96 G10 **Eigg** island W Scotland, UK
155 D24 **Eight Degree Channel** channel India/Maldives
44 G1 **Eight Mile Rock** Grand Bahama Island, N Bahamas
194 J9 **Eights Coast** physical region Antarctica
180 K6 **Eighty Mile Beach** beach Western Australia
99 L18 **Eijsden** Limburg, SE Netherlands
95 G15 **Eikeren** ◎ S Norway
Eil see Eyl
Eilat see Elat
183 O12 **Eildon** Victoria, SE Australia
183 O12 **Eildon, Lake** ◎ Victoria, SE Australia
80 E8 **Eilei** Northern Kordofan, C Sudan
101 N15 **Eilenburg** Sachsen, E Germany
94 H13 **Eina** Oppland, S Norway
Ein 'Avedat see En 'Avedat
101 I14 **Einbeck** Niedersachsen, C Germany
99 K15 **Eindhoven** Noord-Brabant, S Netherlands
108 G8 **Einsiedeln** Schwyz, NE Switzerland
Eipel see Ipeľ
Éire see Ireland, Republic of
Éireann, Muir see Irish Sea
Eirik Outer Ridge see Eirik Ridge
64 I6 **Eirik Ridge** var. Eirik Outer Ridge. undersea feature E Labrador Sea
92 I3 **Eiríksjökull** ▲ C Iceland
59 B14 **Eirunepé** Amazonas, N Brazil
99 L17 **Eisden** Limburg, NE Belgium
83 F18 **Eiseb** ≈ Botswana/Namibia
Eisen see Yŏngch'ŏn
101 J16 **Eisenach** Thüringen, C Germany
Eisenburg see Vasvár
109 U6 **Eisenerz** Steiermark, SE Austria
100 Q13 **Eisenhüttenstadt** Brandenburg, E Germany
109 U10 **Eisenkappel** Slvn. Železna Kapela. Kärnten, S Austria
Eisenmarkt see Hunedoara
109 Y5 **Eisenstadt** Burgenland, E Austria
Eishū see Yŏngju
119 H15 **Eišiškės** Šalčininkai, SE Lithuania
101 L15 **Eisleben** Sachsen-Anhalt, C Germany
190 I3 **Eita** Tarawa, W Kiribati
Eitape see Aitape
105 V11 **Eivissa** var. Iviza, Cast. Ibiza; anc. Ebusus. Eivissa, Spain, W Mediterranean Sea
105 V10 **Eivissa** var. Iviza, Cast. Ibiza; anc. Ebusus. island Islas Baleares, Spain, W Mediterranean Sea
105 R4 **Ejea de los Caballeros** Aragón, NE Spain
40 E8 **Ejido Insurgentes** Baja California Sur, W Mexico
162 I12 **Ejin Qi** var. Dalain Hob. Nei Mongol Zizhiqu, N China
Ejmiadzin see Ejmiatsin
137 T12 **Ejmiatsin** var. Ejmiadzin, Etchmiadzin, Rus. Echmiadzin. W Armenia
77 P16 **Ejura** C Ghana
41 R16 **Ejutla** var. Ejutla de Crespo. Oaxaca, SE Mexico
Ejutla de Crespo see Ejutla
33 Y10 **Ekalaka** Montana, NW USA
Ekapa see Cape Town
128 **Ekaterinodar** see Krasnodar
93 L20 **Ekenäs** Fin. Tammisaari. Etelä-Suomi, SW Finland
Ekerem see Okarem
184 M13 **Eketahuna** Manawatu-Wanganui, North Island, NZ
Ekhínos see Echínos
123 U5 **Ekiatapskiy Khrebet** ▲ NE Russian Federation
145 T8 **Ekibastuz** Pavlodar, NE Kazakhstan
123 R13 **Ekimchan** Amurskaya Oblast', SE Russian Federation
95 O15 **Ekoln** ◎ C Sweden
80 I7 **Ekowit** Red Sea, NE Sudan
95 L19 **Eksjö** Jönköping, S Sweden
93 I15 **Ekträsk** Västerbotten, N Sweden
39 O13 **Ekuk** Alaska, USA
12 F9 **Ekwan** ≈ Ontario, C Canada
39 O13 **Ekwok** Alaska, USA
166 M6 **Ela** Mandalay, C Burma
El Aaiun see El Ayoun
81 N15 **Ēl Ābrēd** Somali, E Ethiopia
115 F22 **Elafónisos** island S Greece
115 F22 **Elafonísou, Porthmós** strait S Greece
El-Aïoun see El Ayoun
75 U8 **El 'Alamein** var. Al 'Alamayn. N Egypt
41 Q12 **El Alazán** Veracruz-Llave, C Mexico
57 J18 **El Alto** var. La Paz. ✕ (La Paz) La Paz, W Bolivia
Elam see Īlām
El Amparo see El Amparo de Apure
54 I8 **El Amparo de Apure** var. El Amparo. Apure, C Venezuela
171 R13 **Elara** Pulau Ambelau, E Indonesia
El Araïch/El Araïche see Larache
40 D6 **El Arco** Baja California, NW Mexico
75 X7 **El 'Arîsh** var. Al 'Arīsh. NE Egypt
115 L25 **Elása** island SE Greece
El Asnam see Chlef
Elassón see Elassóna
115 E15 **Elassóna** prev. Elassón. Thessalía, C Greece
105 N2 **El Astillero** Cantabria, N Spain
138 F14 **Elat** var. Eilat, Elath. Southern, S Israel
Elat, Gulf of see Aqaba, Gulf of
Elath see Elat, Israel
Elath see Al 'Aqabah, Jordan
115 C17 **Eláti** ▲ Lefkáda, Iónioi Nísoi, Greece, C Mediterranean Sea
188 L16 **Elato Atoll** atoll Caroline Islands, C Micronesia
80 C7 **El'Atrun** Northern Darfur, NW Sudan
74 H6 **El Ayoun** var. El Aaiun, El-Aïoun, La Youne. NE Morocco
137 N14 **Elâzığ** var. Elâziz. Elâzığ, E Turkey
137 O14 **Elâzığ** var. Elâziz. ◆ province C Turkey
Elâziz see Elâzığ
Azraq, Bahr el see Blue Nile
23 Q7 **Elba** Alabama, S USA
106 E13 **Elba, Isola d'** island Archipelago Toscano, C Italy
54 F6 **El Banco** Magdalena, N Colombia
El Barco see O Barco
104 L8 **El Barco de Ávila** Castilla-León, N Spain
El Barco de Valdeorras see O Barco
138 H7 **El Barouk, Jabal** ▲ C Lebanon
113 L20 **Elbasan** var. Elbasani. Elbasan, C Albania
113 L20 **Elbasan** ◆ district C Albania
Elbasani see Elbasan
54 K6 **El Baúl** Cojedes, C Venezuela
86 D11 **Elbe** Cz. Labe. ≈ Czech Republic/Germany
100 L13 **Elbe-Havel-Kanal** canal E Germany
100 K9 **Elbe-Lübeck-Kanal** canal N Germany
El Beni see Beni
138 H7 **El Beqaa** var. Al Biqā', Bekaa Valley. valley E Lebanon
25 R6 **Elbert** Texas, SW USA
37 R5 **Elbert, Mount** ▲ Colorado, C USA
23 U3 **Elberton** Georgia, SE USA
100 K11 **Elbe-Seiten-Kanal** canal N Germany
102 M4 **Elbeuf** Seine-Maritime, N France
Elbing see Elbląg
136 M15 **Elbistan** Kahramanmaraş, S Turkey
110 K7 **Elbląg** var. Elblag, Ger. Elbing. Warmińsko-Mazurskie, NE Poland
43 N10 **El Bluff** Región Autónoma Atlántico Sur, SE Nicaragua
63 H17 **El Bolsón** Río Negro, W Argentina
105 P11 **El Bonillo** Castilla-La Mancha, C Spain
El Bordo see Patía
El Boulaida/El Boulaïda see Blida
11 T16 **Elbow** Saskatchewan, S Canada
29 S7 **Elbow Lake** Minnesota, N USA
129 N16 **El'brus** var. Gora El'brus. ▲ SW Russian Federation
El'brus, Gora see El'brus
128 M15 **El'brusskiy** Karachayevo-Cherkesskaya Respublika, SW Russian Federation
81 D14 **El Buhayrat** var. Lakes State. ◆ state S Sudan
El Bur see Ceel Buur
98 L10 **Elburg** Gelderland, E Netherlands
105 O6 **El Burgo de Osma** Castilla-León, C Spain
Elburz Mountains see Alborz, Reshteh-ye Kūhhā-ye
35 V17 **El Cajon** California, W USA
63 H22 **El Calafate** var. Calafate. Santa Cruz, S Argentina
55 Q8 **El Callao** Bolívar, E Venezuela
25 U12 **El Campo** Texas, SW USA
54 I7 **El Cantón** Barinas, W Venezuela
35 Q8 **El Capitan** ▲ California, W USA
54 H5 **El Carmelo** Zulia, NW Venezuela
62 J5 **El Carmen** Jujuy, NW Argentina
54 E5 **El Carmen de Bolívar** Bolívar, NW Colombia
55 O8 **El Casabe** Bolívar, SE Venezuela
42 M12 **El Castillo de La Concepción** Río San Juan, SE Nicaragua
El Cayo see San Ignacio
35 X17 **El Centro** California, W USA
55 N6 **El Chaparro** Anzoátegui, NE Venezuela
105 S12 **Elche** var. Elx-Elche; anc. Ilici, Lat. Illicis. País Valenciano, E Spain
105 Q12 **Elche de la Sierra** Castilla-La Mancha, C Spain
41 U15 **El Chichonal, Volcán** ▲ SE Mexico
40 C2 **El Chinero** Baja California, NW Mexico
181 R1 **Elcho Island** island Wessel Islands, Northern Territory, N Australia
63 H18 **El Corcovado** Chubut, SW Argentina
105 R12 **Elda** País Valenciano, E Spain
100 M10 **Elde** ≈ NE Germany
98 L12 **Elden** Gelderland, E Netherlands
81 J16 **El Der** spring/well S Ethiopia
El Dere see Ceel Dheere
40 E3 **El Desemboque** Sonora, NW Mexico
54 F5 **El Difícil** var. Ariguaní. Magdalena, N Colombia
123 R10 **El'dikan** Respublika Sakha (Yakutiya), NE Russian Federation
El Djazaïr see Alger
El Djelfa see Djelfa
29 X15 **Eldon** Iowa, C USA
27 U5 **Eldon** Missouri, C USA
54 E13 **El Doncello** Caquetá, S Colombia
29 W13 **Eldora** Iowa, C USA
60 G12 **Eldorado** Misiones, NE Argentina
40 I9 **El Dorado** Sinaloa, C Mexico
27 U14 **El Dorado** Arkansas, C USA
30 M17 **Eldorado** Illinois, N USA
27 O6 **El Dorado** Kansas, C USA
26 K12 **Eldorado** Oklahoma, C USA
25 O9 **Eldorado** Texas, SW USA
55 Q8 **El Dorado** Bolívar, E Venezuela
54 F10 **El Dorado** ✕ (Bogotá) Cundinamarca, C Colombia
El Dorado see California
27 O6 **El Dorado Lake** ⊟ Kansas, C USA
27 S6 **El Dorado Springs** Missouri, C USA
81 H18 **Eldoret** Rift Valley, W Kenya
29 Z14 **Eldridge** Iowa, C USA
95 J21 **Eldsberga** Halland, S Sweden
25 R4 **Electra** Texas, SW USA
37 Q7 **Electra Lake** ⊟ Colorado, C USA
38 B8 **Eleele** Haw. 'Ele'ele. Kauai, Hawaii, USA, C Pacific Ocean
Elefantes see Olifants
115 H19 **Elefsína** prev. Elevsís. Attikí, C Greece
115 G19 **Eléftheres** anc. Eleutherae. site of ancient city Attikí/Stereá Ellás, C Greece
114 I13 **Eleftheroúpoli** prev. Elevtheroúpolis. Anatolikí Makedonía kai Thráki, NE Greece
74 F10 **El Eglab** ▲ SW Algeria
118 F10 **Eleja** Jelgava, C Latvia
Elek see Ilek
119 G14 **Elektrėnai** Kaišiadorys, SE Lithuania
128 L3 **Elektrostal'** Moskovskaya Oblast', W Russian Federation
81 H15 **Elemi Triangle** disputed region Kenya/Sudan
54 G16 **El Encanto** Amazonas, S Colombia
37 R14 **Elephant Butte Reservoir** ⊟ New Mexico, SW USA
Éléphant, Chaîne de l' see Dâmrei, Chuŏr Phnum
194 G2 **Elephant Island** island South Shetland Islands, Antarctica
Elephant River see Olifants
El Escorial see San Lorenzo de El Escorial
Élesd see Aleşd
114 F11 **Eleshnitsa** ≈ W Bulgaria
137 S13 **Eleşkirt** Ağrı, E Turkey
42 F5 **El Estor** Izabal, E Guatemala
Eleutherae see Eléftheres
44 I2 **Eleuthera Island** island N Bahamas
37 S5 **Elevenmile Canyon Reservoir** ⊟ Colorado, C USA
27 W8 **Eleven Point River** ≈ Arkansas/Missouri, C USA
Elevsís see Elefsína
Elevtheroúpolis see Eleftheroúpoli
75 W8 **El Faiyûm** var. Al Fayyūm. N Egypt
80 B10 **El Fasher** var. Al Fāshir. Northern Darfur, W Sudan
75 W8 **El Fashn** var. Al Fashn. C Egypt
El Ferrol/El Ferrol del Caudillo see Ferrol
39 W13 **Elfin Cove** Chichagof Island, Alaska, USA
105 W4 **El Fluvià** ≈ NE Spain
40 H7 **El Fuerte** Sinaloa, W Mexico
80 D11 **El Fula** Western Kordofan, C Sudan
El Gedaref see Gedaref
80 A10 **El Geneina** var. Ajjinena, Al-Genain, Al Junaynah. Western Darfur, W Sudan
96 J8 **Elgin** NE Scotland, UK
30 M10 **Elgin** Illinois, N USA
29 P14 **Elgin** Nebraska, C USA
35 Y9 **Elgin** Nevada, W USA
28 L6 **Elgin** North Dakota, N USA
26 M12 **Elgin** Oklahoma, C USA
25 T10 **Elgin** Texas, SW USA
123 R9 **El'ginskiy** Respublika Sakha (Yakutiya), NE Russian Federation
75 W8 **El Gîza** var. Al Jīzah, Gîza, Gizeh. N Egypt
74 J8 **El Goléa** var. Al Golea. C Algeria
40 D2 **El Golfo de Santa Clara** Sonora, NW Mexico
81 G18 **Elgon, Mount** ▲ E Uganda
94 I10 **Elgpiggen** ▲ S Norway
105 T4 **El Grado** Aragón, NE Spain
40 L6 **El Guaje, Laguna** ⊟ NE Mexico
54 H6 **El Guayabo** Zulia, W Venezuela
77 O6 **El Guettâra** oasis N Mali
76 J6 **El Hammâmi** desert N Mauritania
76 M5 **El Hank** cliff N Mauritania
El Haseke see Al Ḩasakah
80 H10 **El Hawata** Gedaref, E Sudan
El Higo see Higos
171 T16 **Eliase** Pulau Selaru, E Indonesia
Elías Piña see Comendador
25 R6 **Eliasville** Texas, SW USA
Elichpur see Achalpur
37 V13 **Elida** New Mexico, SW USA
115 F18 **Elikónas** ▲ C Greece
67 T10 **Elila** ≈ W Dem. Rep. Congo (Zaire)
39 N9 **Elim** Alaska, USA
Elimberrum see Auch
Eliocroca see Lorca
61 B16 **Elisa** Santa Fe, C Argentina
Elisabethstedt see Dumbrăveni
Élisabethville see Lubumbashi
129 O13 **Elista** Respublika Kalmykiya, SW Russian Federation
182 I9 **Elizabeth** South Australia
21 Q3 **Elizabeth** West Virginia, NE USA
19 Q9 **Elizabeth, Cape** headland Maine, NE USA
21 Y8 **Elizabeth City** North Carolina, SE USA
21 P8 **Elizabethton** Tennessee, S USA
30 M17 **Elizabethtown** Illinois, N USA
20 K6 **Elizabethtown** Kentucky, S USA
18 L7 **Elizabethtown** New York, NE USA
21 U11 **Elizabethtown** North Carolina, SE USA
18 G15 **Elizabethtown** Pennsylvania, NE USA
74 E6 **El-Jadida** prev. Mazagan. W Morocco
El Jafr see Jafr, Qā' al
80 F11 **El Jebelein** White Nile, E Sudan
110 N8 **Ełk** Ger. Lyck. Warmińsko-Mazurskie, NE Poland
110 O8 **Ełk** ≈ NE Poland
29 Y12 **Elkader** Iowa, C USA
80 G9 **El Kamlin** Gezira, C Sudan
33 N11 **Elk City** Idaho, NW USA
26 K10 **Elk City** Oklahoma, C USA
27 P7 **Elk City Lake** ⊟ Kansas, C USA
34 M5 **Elk Creek** California, W USA
28 J10 **Elk Creek** ≈ South Dakota, N USA
74 M5 **El Kef** var. Al Kāf, Le Kef. NW Tunisia
74 F7 **El Kelâa Srarhna** var. Kal al Sraghna. C Morocco
El Kerak see Al Karak
11 P17 **Elkford** British Columbia, SW Canada
El Khalil see Hebron
80 E7 **El Khandaq** Northern, N Sudan
75 W10 **El Khârga** var. Al Khārijah. C Egypt
31 P11 **Elkhart** Indiana, N USA
26 H7 **Elkhart** Kansas, C USA
25 V8 **Elkhart** Texas, SW USA
30 M7 **Elkhart Lake** ◎ Wisconsin, N USA
El Khartûm see Khartoum
37 Q3 **Elkhead Mountains** ▲ Colorado, C USA
18 I12 **Elk Hill** ▲ Pennsylvania, NE USA
138 G8 **El Khiyam** var. Al Khiyām, Khiam. S Lebanon
29 S15 **Elkhorn** Nebraska, C USA
30 M9 **Elkhorn** Wisconsin, N USA
29 R14 **Elkhorn River** ≈ Nebraska, C USA
129 O16 **El'khotovo** Respublika Severnaya Osetiya, SW Russian Federation
114 L10 **Elkhovo** prev. Kizilagach. Yambol, E Bulgaria
21 R8 **Elkin** North Carolina, SE USA
21 S4 **Elkins** West Virginia, NE USA
195 X3 **Elkins, Mount** ▲ Antarctica
14 G8 **Elk Lake** Ontario, S Canada
31 P6 **Elk Lake** ◎ Michigan, N USA
18 F12 **Elkland** Pennsylvania, NE USA
35 W3 **Elko** Nevada, W USA
11 R14 **Elk Point** Alberta, SW Canada
29 R12 **Elk Point** South Dakota, N USA
29 V8 **Elk River** Minnesota, N USA
20 J10 **Elk River** ≈ Alabama/Tennessee, S USA
21 R4 **Elk River** ≈ West Virginia, NE USA
20 I7 **Elkton** Kentucky, S USA
21 Y2 **Elkton** Maryland, NE USA
29 R10 **Elkton** South Dakota, N USA
20 I10 **Elkton** Tennessee, S USA
21 U5 **Elkton** Virginia, NE USA
El Kuneitra see Al Qunayṭirah
81 L15 **El Kure** Somali, E Ethiopia
80 D12 **El Lagowa** Western Kordofan, C Sudan
39 S12 **Ellamar** Alaska, USA
Ellás see Greece
23 S6 **Ellaville** Georgia, SE USA
8 I3 **Ellef Ringnes Island** island Nunavut, N Canada
29 V10 **Ellendale** Minnesota, N USA
29 P7 **Ellendale** North Dakota, N USA
36 M6 **Ellen, Mount** ▲ Utah, W USA
32 I9 **Ellensburg** Washington, NW USA
18 K12 **Ellenville** New York, NE USA
Ellep see Lib
21 T10 **Ellerbe** North Carolina, SE USA
9 N2 **Ellesmere Island** island Queen Elizabeth Islands, Nunavut, N Canada
185 H19 **Ellesmere, Lake** ◎ South Island, NZ
97 K18 **Ellesmere Port** C England, UK
31 O14 **Ellettsville** Indiana, N USA
99 E19 **Ellezelles** Hainaut, SW Belgium
8 L7 **Ellice** ≈ Nunavut, NE Canada
Ellice Islands see Tuvalu
Ellichpur see Achalpur
21 W3 **Ellicott City** Maryland, NE USA
23 S2 **Ellijay** Georgia, SE USA
27 W7 **Ellington** Missouri, C USA
26 L5 **Ellinwood** Kansas, C USA
83 J24 **Elliot** Eastern Cape, SE South Africa
14 D10 **Elliot Lake** Ontario, S Canada
181 X6 **Elliot, Mount** ▲ Queensland, E Australia
21 T5 **Elliott Knob** ▲ Virginia, NE USA
26 K4 **Ellis** Kansas, C USA
182 F8 **Elliston** South Australia
22 M7 **Ellisville** Mississippi, S USA
105 V5 **El Llobregat** ≈ NE Spain
96 L9 **Ellon** NE Scotland, UK
Ellore see Elūru
21 S13 **Elloree** South Carolina, SE USA
26 M4 **Ellsworth** Kansas, C USA
19 S7 **Ellsworth** Maine, NE USA
30 I6 **Ellsworth** Wisconsin, N USA
26 M11 **Ellsworth, Lake** ⊟ Oklahoma, C USA
194 K9 **Ellsworth Land** physical region Antarctica
194 L9 **Ellsworth Mountains** ▲ Antarctica
101 J21 **Ellwangen** Baden-Württemberg, S Germany
18 B14 **Ellwood City** Pennsylvania, NE USA
108 H8 **Elm** Glarus, NE Switzerland
32 G9 **Elma** Washington, NW USA
121 V13 **El Maḥalla el Kubra** var. Al Maḥallah al Kubrá, Mahalla el Kubra. N Egypt
74 E9 **El Mahbas** var. Mahbés. SW Western Sahara
63 H17 **El Maitén** Chubut, W Argentina
136 E16 **Elmalı** Antalya, SW Turkey
80 G10 **El Manaqil** Gezira, C Sudan
54 M12 **El Mango** Amazonas, S Venezuela
75 W7 **El Manṣûra** var. Al Manṣūrah, Manṣūra. N Egypt
55 P8 **El Manteco** Bolívar, E Venezuela
29 O16 **Elm Creek** Nebraska, C USA
El Mediyya see Médéa
77 V9 **Elméki** Agadez, C Niger
108 K7 **Elmen** Tirol, W Austria
18 J16 **Elmer** New Jersey, NE USA
138 G6 **El Mina** var. Al Mīnā'. N Lebanon
75 W9 **El Minya** var. Al Minyā, Minya. C Egypt
14 F15 **Elmira** Ontario, S Canada
18 G11 **Elmira** New York, NE USA
36 K13 **El Mirage** Arizona, SW USA
29 O7 **Elm Lake** ⊟ South Dakota, N USA
El Mojón see San Rafael
105 N7 **El Molar** Madrid, C Spain
76 L7 **El Mrâyer** well C Mauritania
76 L5 **El Mreiti** well N Mauritania
76 L8 **El Mreyyé** desert E Mauritania
29 P8 **Elm River** ≈ North Dakota/South Dakota, N USA
100 I9 **Elmshorn** Schleswig-Holstein, N Germany
80 D12 **El Muglad** Western Kordofan, C Sudan
El Muwaqqar see Al Muwaqqar
14 G14 **Elmvale** Ontario, S Canada
30 K12 **Elmwood** Illinois, N USA
26 J8 **Elmwood** Oklahoma, C USA
103 P17 **Elne** anc. Illiberis. Pyrénées-Orientales, S France
54 F11 **El Nevado, Cerro** elevation C Colombia
171 N5 **El Nido** Palawan, W Philippines
62 I12 **El Nihuil** Mendoza, W Argentina
75 W7 **El Nouzha** ✕ (Alexandria) N Egypt
80 E10 **El Obeid** var. Al Obayyid, Al Ubayyiḍ. Northern Kordofan, C Sudan
41 O13 **El Oro** México, S Mexico
56 B8 **El Oro** ◆ province SW Ecuador
61 B19 **Elortondo** Santa Fe, C Argentina
54 J8 **Elorza** Apure, C Venezuela
El Ouâdi see El Oued
74 L7 **El Oued** var. Al Oued, El Ouâdi, El Wad. NE Algeria
36 L15 **Eloy** Arizona, SW USA
55 Q7 **El Palmar** Bolívar, E Venezuela
40 K8 **El Palmito** Durango, W Mexico
55 P7 **El Pao** Bolívar, E Venezuela
54 K5 **El Pao** Cojedes, N Venezuela
42 J7 **El Paraíso** El Paraíso, S Honduras
42 I7 **El Paraíso** ◆ department SE Honduras
30 L12 **El Paso** Illinois, N USA
24 G8 **El Paso** Texas, SW USA
24 G8 **El Paso** ✕ Texas, SW USA
105 U7 **El Perello** Cataluña, NE Spain
55 P5 **El Pilar** Sucre, NE Venezuela
42 F7 **El Pital, Cerro** ▲ El Salvador/Honduras
35 Q9 **El Portal** California, W USA
40 J3 **El Porvenir** Chihuahua, N Mexico
43 U14 **El Porvenir** San Blas, N Panama
105 W6 **El Prat de Llobregat** Cataluña, NE Spain
42 H5 **El Progreso** Yoro, NW Honduras
42 A2 **El Progreso** off. Departamento de El Progreso. ◆ department C Guatemala
El Progreso see Guastatoya
104 L9 **El Puente del Arzobispo** Castilla-La Mancha, C Spain
104 J15 **El Puerto de Santa María** Andalucía, S Spain
62 I8 **El Puesto** Catamarca, NW Argentina
El Qâhira see Cairo
75 V10 **El Qaṣr** var. Al Qaṣr. C Egypt
El Qatrani see Al Qaṭrānah
40 I10 **El Quelite** Sinaloa, C Mexico
62 G9 **Elqui, Río** ≈ N Chile
El Quneitra see Al Qunayṭirah
El Quseir see Al Quṣayr
El Quweira see Al Quwayrah
141 O15 **El-Rahaba** ✕ (Ṣan'ā') W Yemen
42 M10 **El Rama** Región Autónoma Atlántico Sur, SE Nicaragua
43 W16 **El Real** var. El Real de Santa María. Darién, SE Panama
El Real de Santa María see El Real
26 M10 **El Reno** Oklahoma, C USA
40 K9 **El Rodeo** Durango, C Mexico
104 J13 **El Ronquillo** Andalucía, S Spain
11 S16 **Elrose** Saskatchewan, S Canada
30 K8 **Elroy** Wisconsin, N USA
25 S17 **Elsa** Texas, SW USA
75 W8 **El Ṣaff** var. Aṣ Ṣaff. N Egypt
40 J10 **El Salto** Durango, C Mexico
42 D8 **El Salvador** off. Republica de El Salvador. ◆ republic Central America
54 K7 **El Samán de Apure** Apure, C Venezuela
14 D7 **Elsas** Ontario, S Canada
40 F3 **El Sásabe** var. Aduana del Sásabe. Sonora, NW Mexico
Elsass see Alsace
40 J5 **El Sáuz** Chihuahua, N Mexico
27 W4 **Elsberry** Missouri, C USA
45 P9 **El Seibo** var. Santa Cruz de El Seibo, Santa Cruz del Seibo. E Dominican Republic
42 B7 **El Semillero Barra Nahualate** Escuintla, SW Guatemala
Elsene see Ixelles
159 N11 **Elsen Nur** ◎ C China
36 L6 **Elsinore** Utah, W USA
Elsinore see Helsingør
99 L18 **Elsloo** Limburg, SE Netherlands
60 G13 **El Soberbio** Misiones, NE Argentina
55 N6 **El Socorro** Guárico, C Venezuela
54 L6 **El Sombrero** Guárico, N Venezuela
98 L10 **Elspeet** Gelderland, E Netherlands
98 L12 **Elst** Gelderland, E Netherlands
101 O15 **Elsterwerda** Brandenburg, E Germany
40 J4 **El Sueco** Chihuahua, N Mexico
El Suweida see As Suwaydā'
El Suweis see Suez
54 D12 **El Tambo** Cauca, SW Colombia
175 T13 **Eltanin Fracture Zone** tectonic feature SE Pacific Ocean
105 X5 **El Ter** ≈ NE Spain
184 K11 **Eltham** Taranaki, North Island, NZ
55 O6 **El Tigre** Anzoátegui, NE Venezuela
El Tigrito see San José de Guanipa
54 J5 **El Tocuyo** Lara, N Venezuela
129 Q10 **El'ton** Volgogradskaya Oblast', SW Russian Federation
32 K10 **Eltopia** Washington, NW USA
61 A18 **El Trébol** Santa Fe, C Argentina
40 J13 **El Tuito** Jalisco, SW Mexico
75 X8 **El Ṭûr** var. Aṭ Ṭūr. NE Egypt
155 K16 **Elūru** prev. Ellore. Andhra Pradesh, E India
118 H13 **Elva** Ger. Elwa. Tartumaa, SE Estonia
37 R9 **El Vado Reservoir** ⊟ New Mexico, SW USA
43 S15 **El Valle** Coclé, C Panama
104 I11 **Elvas** Portalegre, C Portugal
54 K7 **El Venado** Apure, C Venezuela
105 V6 **El Vendrell** Cataluña, NE Spain
94 I13 **Elverum** Hedmark, S Norway
42 I9 **El Viejo** Chinandega, NW Nicaragua
54 G7 **El Viejo, Cerro** ▲ C Colombia
54 H6 **El Vigía** Mérida, NW Venezuela
105 Q4 **El Villar de Arnedo** La Rioja, N Spain
59 A14 **Elvira** Amazonas, W Brazil
Elwa see Elva
El Wad see El Oued
81 K17 **El Wak** North Eastern, NE Kenya
33 R7 **Elwell, Lake** ⊟ Montana, NW USA
31 P13 **Elwood** Indiana, N USA
27 R3 **Elwood** Kansas, C USA
29 N16 **Elwood** Nebraska, C USA
Elx-Elche see Elche
97 O20 **Ely** E England, UK
29 X4 **Ely** Minnesota, N USA
35 X6 **Ely** Nevada, W USA
El Yopal see Yopal
31 T11 **Elyria** Ohio, N USA
45 S9 **El Yunque** ▲ E Puerto Rico
101 F23 **Elz** ≈ SW Germany
187 R14 **Emae** island Shepherd Islands, C Vanuatu
118 I5 **Emajõgi** Ger. Embach. ≈ SE Estonia
Emāmrūd see Shāhrūd
149 Q2 **Emām Ṣāḥeb** var. Emam Saheb, Hazarat Imam. Kunduz, NE Afghanistan
Emāmshahr see Shāhrūd
95 M20 **Emån** ≈ S Sweden

◆ Country ● Country Capital ◇ Dependent Territory ○ Dependent Territory Capital ◆ Administrative Region ✕ International Airport ▲ Mountain ▲ Mountain Range ▲ Volcano ≈ River ◎ Lake ⊟ Reservoir

144 J11 **Emba** Kaz. Embi. Aktyubinsk, W Kazakhstan
144 H12 **Emba** Kaz. Zhem. ≈ W Kazakhstan
Embach see Emajõgi
62 K5 **Embarcación** Salta, N Argentina
30 M15 **Embarras River** ≈ Illinois, N USA
Embi see Emba
81 I19 **Embu** Eastern, C Kenya
100 E10 **Emden** Niedersachsen, NW Germany
29 Q4 **Emerado** North Dakota, N USA
181 X8 **Emerald** Queensland, E Australia
Emerald Isle see Montserrat
57 J15 **Emero, Río** ≈ W Bolivia
11 Y17 **Emerson** Manitoba, S Canada
29 T15 **Emerson** Iowa, C USA
29 R13 **Emerson** Nebraska, C USA
36 M5 **Emery** Utah, W USA
Emesa see Ḥimṣ
136 E13 **Emet** Kütahya, W Turkey
186 B8 **Emeti** Western, SW PNG
35 V3 **Emigrant Pass** pass Nevada, W USA
78 I6 **Emi Koussi** ▲ N Chad
Emilia see Emilia-Romagna
41 V15 **Emiliano Zapata** Chiapas, SE Mexico
106 E9 **Emilia-Romagna** prev. Emilia, anc. Æmilia. ◈ region N Italy
158 J3 **Emin** var. Dorbiljin. Xinjiang Uygur Zizhiqu, NW China
149 W8 **Eminābād** Punjab, E Pakistan
21 L5 **Eminence** Kentucky, S USA
27 W7 **Eminence** Missouri, C USA
114 N9 **Emine, Nos** headland E Bulgaria
158 I3 **Emin He** ≈ NW China
186 G4 **Emirau Island** island N PNG
136 F13 **Emirdağ** Afyon, W Turkey
95 M21 **Emmaboda** Kalmar, S Sweden
118 E5 **Emmaste** Hiiumaa, W Estonia
18 I15 **Emmaus** Pennsylvania, NE USA
183 U4 **Emmaville** New South Wales, SE Australia
108 E9 **Emme** ≈ W Switzerland
98 L8 **Emmeloord** Flevoland, N Netherlands
98 O8 **Emmen** Drenthe, NE Netherlands
108 F8 **Emmen** Luzern, C Switzerland
101 F23 **Emmendingen** Baden-Württemberg, SW Germany
98 P8 **Emmer-Compascuum** Drenthe, NE Netherlands
101 D14 **Emmerich** Nordrhein-Westfalen, W Germany
29 U12 **Emmetsburg** Iowa, C USA
32 M14 **Emmett** Idaho, NW USA
38 M10 **Emmonak** Alaska, USA
Emona see Ljubljana
Emonti see East London
24 L12 **Emory Peak** ▲ Texas, SW USA
40 F6 **Empalme** Sonora, NW Mexico
83 L23 **Empangeni** KwaZulu/Natal, E South Africa
61 C14 **Empedrado** Corrientes, NE Argentina
192 K3 **Emperor Seamounts** undersea feature NW Pacific Ocean
192 L3 **Emperor Trough** undersea feature N Pacific Ocean
35 R4 **Empire** Nevada, W USA
Empire State of the South see Georgia
Emplawas see Amplawas
106 F11 **Empoli** Toscana, C Italy
27 P5 **Emporia** Kansas, C USA
21 W7 **Emporia** Virginia, NE USA
18 E13 **Emporium** Pennsylvania, NE USA
Empty Quarter see Ar Rub' al Khālī
100 E10 **Ems** Dut. Eems. ≈ NW Germany
100 F13 **Emsdetten** Nordrhein-Westfalen, NW Germany
Ems-Hunte Canal see Küstenkanal
100 F10 **Ems-Jade-Kanal** canal NW Germany
100 F11 **Emsland** cultural region NW Germany
182 D3 **Emu Junction** South Australia
163 T3 **Emur He** ≈ NE China
55 R8 **Enachu Landing** NW Guyana
93 F16 **Enafors** Jämtland, C Sweden
94 N11 **Enånger** Gävleborg, C Sweden
96 G7 **Enard Bay** bay NW Scotland, UK
Enareträsk see Inarijärvi
171 X14 **Enarotali** Irian Jaya, E Indonesia
138 E12 **En 'Avedat** var. Ein 'Avedat, well S Israel
165 T2 **Enbetsu** Hokkaidō, NE Japan
61 H16 **Encantadas, Serra das** ▲ S Brazil
40 E7 **Encantado, Cerro** ▲ NW Mexico
62 P7 **Encarnación** Itapúa, S Paraguay
40 M12 **Encarnación de Díaz** Jalisco, SW Mexico
77 O17 **Enchi** SW Ghana
25 Q14 **Encinal** Texas, SW USA
35 U17 **Encinitas** California, W USA
25 S16 **Encino** Texas, SW USA
54 H6 **Encontrados** Zulia, NW Venezuela
182 I10 **Encounter Bay** inlet South Australia
61 F15 **Encruzilhada** Rio Grande do Sul, S Brazil
61 H16 **Encruzilhada do Sul** Rio Grande do Sul, S Brazil
111 M20 **Encs** Borsod-Abaúj-Zemplén, NE Hungary
193 P3 **Endeavour Seamount** undersea feature N Pacific Ocean
181 V1 **Endeavour Strait** strait Queensland, NE Australia
171 O16 **Endeh** Flores, S Indonesia
95 G23 **Endelave** island C Denmark
191 T4 **Enderbury Island** atoll Phoenix Islands, C Kiribati
11 N16 **Enderby** British Columbia, SW Canada
195 W4 **Enderby Land** physical region Antarctica
173 N14 **Enderby Plain** undersea feature S Indian Ocean
29 Q6 **Enderlin** North Dakota, N USA
Endersdorf see Jędrzejów
28 K16 **Enders Reservoir** ▣ Nebraska, C USA
18 H11 **Endicott** New York, NE USA
39 P7 **Endicott Mountains** ▲ Alaska, USA
118 I5 **Endla Raba** wetland C Estonia
117 T9 **Enerhodar** Zaporiz'ka Oblast', SE Ukraine
57 F14 **Ene, Río** ≈ C Peru
189 N4 **Enewetak Atoll** var. Ānewetak, Eniwetok. atoll Ralik Chain, W Marshall Islands
114 L13 **Enez** Edirne, NW Turkey
21 W8 **Enfield** North Carolina, SE USA
186 B7 **Enga** ◈ province W PNG
45 Q9 **Engaño, Cabo** headland E Dominican Republic
164 U3 **Engaru** Hokkaidō, NE Japan
138 F11 **'En Gedi** Southern, E Israel
108 F9 **Engelberg** Unterwalden, C Switzerland
21 Y9 **Engelhard** North Carolina, SE USA
129 P8 **Engel's** Saratovskaya Oblast', W Russian Federation
101 G24 **Engen** Baden-Württemberg, SW Germany
Engeten see Aiud
168 K15 **Enggano, Pulau** island W Indonesia
80 I8 **Enghershatu** ▲ N Eritrea
99 F19 **Enghien** Dut. Edingen. Hainaut, SW Belgium
27 V12 **England** Arkansas, C USA
97 M20 **England** Lat. Anglia. national region UK
14 H8 **Englehart** Ontario, S Canada
37 T4 **Englewood** Colorado, C USA
31 O16 **English** Indiana, N USA
39 Q13 **English Bay** Alaska, USA
English Bazar see Ingrāj Bāzār
97 N25 **English Channel** var. The Channel, Fr. la Manche. channel NW Europe
194 J7 **English Coast** physical region Antarctica
105 S11 **Enguera** País Valenciano, E Spain
118 E8 **Engure** Tukums, W Latvia
118 E8 **Engures Ezers** ◎ NW Latvia
137 R9 **Enguri** Rus. Inguri. ≈ NW Georgia
Engyum see Gangi
26 M9 **Enid** Oklahoma, C USA
22 L3 **Enid Lake** ▣ Mississippi, S USA
189 Y2 **Enigu** island Ratak Chain, SE Marshall Islands
Enikale Strait see Kerch Strait
147 Z8 **Enil'chek** Issyk-Kul'skaya Oblast', E Kyrgyzstan
115 F17 **Enipéfs** ≈ C Greece
165 S4 **Eniwa** Hokkaidō, NE Japan
Eniwetok see Enewetak Atoll
Enkeldoorn see Chivhu
123 S11 **Enken, Mys** headland NE Russian Federation
98 J8 **Enkhuizen** Noord-Holland, NW Netherlands
109 Q4 **Enknach** ≈ N Austria
95 N15 **Enköping** Uppsala, C Sweden
107 K24 **Enna** var. Castrogiovanni, Henna. Sicilia, Italy, C Mediterranean Sea
80 D11 **En Nahud** Western Kordofan, C Sudan
138 F8 **En Nâqoûra** var. An Nāqūrah. SW Lebanon
En Nazira see Nazerat
78 K8 **Ennedi** plateau E Chad
101 E15 **Ennepetal** Nordrhein-Westfalen, W Germany
183 P4 **Enngonia** New South Wales, SE Australia
97 C19 **Ennis** Ir. Inis. W Ireland
33 R11 **Ennis** Montana, NW USA
25 U7 **Ennis** Texas, SW USA
97 F20 **Enniscorthy** Ir. Inis Córthaidh. SE Ireland
97 E15 **Enniskillen** var. Inniskilling, Ir. Inis Ceithleann. SW Northern Ireland, UK
97 B19 **Ennistimon** Ir. Inis Díomáin. W Ireland
109 T4 **Enns** Oberösterreich, N Austria
109 T4 **Enns** ≈ C Austria
93 O16 **Eno** Itä-Suomi, E Finland
24 M5 **Enochs** Texas, SW USA
93 N17 **Enonkoski** Isä-Suomi, E Finland
92 K10 **Enontekiö** Lapp. Eanodat. Lappi, N Finland
21 Q11 **Enoree** South Carolina, SE USA
21 P11 **Enoree River** ≈ South Carolina, SE USA
18 M6 **Enosburg Falls** Vermont, NE USA
171 N13 **Enrekang** Sulawesi, C Indonesia
45 N10 **Enriquillo** SW Dominican Republic
45 N9 **Enriquillo, Lago** ◎ SW Dominican Republic
98 L9 **Ens** Flevoland, N Netherlands
98 P11 **Enschede** Overijssel, E Netherlands
40 B2 **Ensenada** Baja California, NW Mexico
101 E20 **Ensheim** × (Saarbrücken) Saarland, W Germany
160 L9 **Enshi** Hubei, C China
164 L14 **Enshū-nada** gulf SW Japan
23 O8 **Ensley** Florida, SE USA
Enso see Svetogorsk
81 F18 **Entebbe** S Uganda
81 F18 **Entebbe** × C Uganda
101 M18 **Entenbühl** ▲ Czech Republic/Germany
98 N10 **Enter** Overijssel, E Netherlands
23 Q7 **Enterprise** Alabama, S USA
32 L11 **Enterprise** Oregon, NW USA
36 J7 **Enterprise** Utah, W USA
32 J8 **Entiat** Washington, NW USA
105 P15 **Entinas, Punta de las** headland S Spain
108 F8 **Entlebuch** Luzern, W Switzerland
108 F8 **Entlebuch** valley C Switzerland
63 I22 **Entrada, Punta** headland S Argentina
103 O13 **Entraygues-sur-Truyère** Aveyron, S France
187 O14 **Entrecasteaux, Récifs d'** reef N New Caledonia
61 C17 **Entre Ríos** off. Provincia de Entre Ríos. ◈ province NE Argentina
42 K7 **Entre Ríos, Cordillera** ▲ Honduras/Nicaragua
104 G9 **Entroncamento** Santarém, C Portugal
77 V16 **Enugu** Enugu, S Nigeria
77 U16 **Enugu** ◈ state SE Nigeria
123 V5 **Enurmino** Chukotskiy Avtonomnyy Okrug, NE Russian Federation
54 E9 **Envigado** Antioquia, W Colombia
59 B15 **Envira** Amazonas, W Brazil
Enyélé see Enyellé
79 I16 **Enyellé** var. Enyélé. La Likouala, NE Congo
101 H21 **Enz** ≈ SW Germany
165 N13 **Enzan** Yamanashi, Honshū, S Japan
104 I2 **Eo** ≈ NW Spain
Eochaill see Youghal
Eochaille, Cuan see Youghal Bay
107 K22 **Eolie, Isole** var. Isole Eolie, Eng. Aeolian Islands, Lipari Islands. island group S Italy
189 U12 **Eot** island Chuuk, C Micronesia
115 J25 **Epáno Archánes** var. Áno Arkhánai; prev. Epáno Arkhánai. Kríti, Greece, E Mediterranean Sea
Epáno Arkhánai see Epáno Archánes
115 G14 **Epanomí** Kentrikí Makedonía, N Greece
98 M10 **Epe** Gelderland, E Netherlands
77 S16 **Epe** Lagos, S Nigeria
79 I17 **Epéna** La Likouala, NE Congo
Eperies/Eperjes see Prešov
103 Q4 **Épernay** anc. Sparnacum. Marne, N France
36 L5 **Ephraim** Utah, W USA
18 H15 **Ephrata** Pennsylvania, NE USA
32 J8 **Ephrata** Washington, NW USA
187 R14 **Epi** var. Épi. island C Vanuatu
105 R6 **Épila** Aragón, NE Spain
103 T6 **Épinal** Vosges, NE France
Epiphania see Ḥamāh
Epirus see Ípeiros
121 P3 **Episkopí** SW Cyprus
Episkopi Bay see Episkopí, Kólpos
121 P3 **Episkopí, Kólpos** var. Episkopi Bay. bay SE Cyprus
Epitoli see Pretoria
Epoon see Ebon Atoll
Eporedia see Ivrea
Eppeschdorf see Dumbrăveni
101 H21 **Eppingen** Baden-Württemberg, SW Germany
83 E18 **Epukiro** Omaheke, E Namibia
29 Y13 **Epworth** Iowa, C USA
143 O10 **Eqlīd** var. Iqlid. Fārs, C Iran
Equality State see Wyoming
79 J18 **Equateur** off. Région de l' Equateur. ◈ region N Dem. Rep. Congo (Zaire)
151 K22 **Equatorial Channel** channel S Maldives
79 B17 **Equatorial Guinea** off. Republic of Equatorial Guinea. ◆ republic C Africa
121 V11 **Eratosthenes Tablemount** undersea feature E Mediterranean Sea
Erautini see Johannesburg
136 L12 **Erbaa** Tokat, N Turkey
101 E19 **Erbeskopf** ▲ W Germany
Erbil see Arbīl
121 P2 **Ercan** × (Nicosia) N Cyprus
Ercegnovi see Herceg-Novi
137 T14 **Erçek Gölü** ◎ E Turkey
137 S14 **Erciş** Van, E Turkey
136 K14 **Erciyes Dağı** anc. Argaeus. ▲ C Turkey
111 J22 **Érd** Ger. Hanselbeck. Pest, C Hungary
Erdaobaihe see Baihe
159 O12 **Erdaogou** Qinghai, W China
163 X11 **Erdao Jiang** ≈ NE China
Erdăt-Sângeorz see Sângeorgiu de Pădure
136 C11 **Erdek** Balıkesir, NW Turkey
Erdély see Transylvania
Erdélyi-Havasok see Carpații Meridionali
136 J17 **Erdemli** İçel, S Turkey
162 K6 **Erdenet** Bulgan, N Mongolia
162 I8 **Erdenetsogt** Bayanhongor, C Mongolia
78 K7 **Erdi** plateau NE Chad
78 L7 **Erdi Ma** desert NE Chad
101 M23 **Erding** Bayern, SE Germany
Erdőszáda see Ardusat
Erdőszentgyörgy see Sângeorgiu de Pădure
102 I7 **Erdre** ≈ NW France
195 R13 **Erebus, Mount** ▲ Ross Island, Antarctica
61 H14 **Erechim** Rio Grande do Sul, S Brazil
163 O7 **Ereen Davaanī Nuruu** ▲ NE Mongolia
163 Q6 **Ereentsav** Dornod, NE Mongolia
136 I16 **Ereğli** Konya, S Turkey
136 I15 **Ereğli Gölü** ◎ W Turkey
115 A15 **Ereíkoussa** island Iónioi Nísoi, Greece, C Mediterranean Sea
163 O11 **Erenhot** var. Erlian. Nei Mongol Zizhiqu, NE China
104 M6 **Eresma** ≈ N Spain
115 K17 **Eresós** var. Eressós. Lésvos, E Greece
Eressós see Eresós
Erevan see Yerevan
Ereymentau see Yereymentau
99 K21 **Érezée** Luxembourg, SE Belgium
74 G7 **Erfoud** SE Morocco
101 D16 **Erft** ≈ W Germany
101 K16 **Erfurt** Thüringen, C Germany
137 P15 **Ergani** Dıyarbakır, SE Turkey
163 N11 **Ergel** Dornogovĭ, SE Mongolia
Ergene Irmağı see Ergene Çayı
162 L11 **Ergenetsogt** Ömnögovĭ, S Mongolia
136 C10 **Ergene Çayı** var. Ergene Irmağı. ≈ NW Turkey
118 I9 **Ērgli** Madona, C Latvia
78 H11 **Erguig, Bahr** ≈ SW Chad
Ergun He see Argun
163 S5 **Ergun Youqi** Nei Mongol Zizhiqu, N China
163 T5 **Ergun Zuoqi** Nei Mongol Zizhiqu, N China
160 F12 **Er Hai** ◎ SW China
102 G4 **Er, Îles d'** island group NW France
106 K4 **Ería** ≈ NW Spain
80 H8 **Eriba** Kassala, NE Sudan
96 I6 **Eriboll, Loch** inlet NW Scotland, UK
65 Q18 **Erica Seamount** undersea feature SW Indian Ocean
107 H23 **Erice** Sicilia, Italy, C Mediterranean Sea
104 E10 **Ericeira** Lisboa, C Portugal
96 H10 **Ericht, Loch** ◎ C Scotland, UK
26 J11 **Erick** Oklahoma, C USA
18 B11 **Erie** Pennsylvania, NE USA
18 E9 **Erie Canal** canal New York, NE USA
Érié, Lac see Erie, Lake
31 T10 **Erie, Lake** Fr. Lac Érié. ◎ Canada/USA
77 N8 **'Erigât** desert N Mali
Erigavo see Ceerigaabo
92 P2 **Erik Eriksenstretet** strait E Svalbard
11 X15 **Eriksdale** Manitoba, S Canada
189 V6 **Erikub Atoll** var. Ādkup. atoll Ratak Chain, C Marshall Islands
Erimanthos see Erýmanthos
165 T6 **Erimo** Hokkaidō, NE Japan
165 T6 **Erimo-misaki** headland Hokkaidō, NE Japan
20 H8 **Erin** Tennessee, S USA
96 E9 **Eriskay** island NW Scotland, UK
Erithraí see Erythrés
80 I9 **Eritrea** off. State of Eritrea, Tig. Ērtra. ◆ transitional government E Africa
Erivan see Yerevan
101 D16 **Erkelenz** Nordrhein-Westfalen, W Germany
95 P15 **Erken** ◎ C Sweden
101 K19 **Erlangen** Bayern, S Germany
160 G9 **Erlang Shan** ▲ C China
Erlau see Eger
109 V5 **Erlauf** ≈ NE Austria
181 Q8 **Erldunda Roadhouse** Northern Territory, N Australia
Erlian see Erenhot
27 T15 **Erling, Lake** ▣ Arkansas, USA
109 O8 **Erlsbach** Tirol, W Austria
Ermak see Aksu
98 K10 **Ermelo** Gelderland, C Netherlands
83 K21 **Ermelo** Mpumalanga, NE South Africa
136 H17 **Ermenek** Karaman, S Turkey
Érmihályfalva see Valea lui Mihai
115 G20 **Ermióni** Pelopónnisos, S Greece
115 J20 **Ermoúpoli** var. Hermoupolis; prev. Ermoúpolis. Sýros, Kykládes, Greece, Aegean Sea
Ermoúpolis see Ermoúpoli
Ernabella see Pukatja
155 G22 **Ernākulam** Kerala, SW India
102 J6 **Ernée** Mayenne, NW France
61 H14 **Ernestina, Barragem** ▣ S Brazil
54 E4 **Ernesto Cortissoz** × (Barranquilla) Atlántico, N Colombia
155 H21 **Erode** Tamil Nādu, SE India
Eroj see Iroj
83 C19 **Erongo** ◈ district W Namibia
99 F21 **Erquelinnes** Hainaut, S Belgium
74 G7 **Er-Rachidia** var. Ksar al Soule. E Morocco
80 E11 **Er Rahad** var. Ar Rahad. Northern Kordofan, C Sudan
Er Ramle see Ramla
83 O15 **Errego** Zambézia, NE Mozambique
Errenteria see Rentería
Er Rif/Er Riff see Rif
97 D14 **Errigal Mountain** Ir. An Earagail. ▲ N Ireland
97 A15 **Erris Head** Ir. Ceann Iorrais. headland W Ireland
187 S15 **Erromango** island S Vanuatu
Error Guyot see Error Tablemount
173 O4 **Error Tablemount** var. Error Guyot. undersea feature W Indian Ocean
80 G11 **Er Roseires** Blue Nile, E Sudan
Erseka see Ersekë
113 M22 **Ersekë** var. Erseka, Kolonjë. Korçë, SE Albania
Érsekújvár see Nové Zámky
29 S4 **Erskine** Minnesota, N USA
103 V6 **Erstein** Bas-Rhin, NE France
108 G9 **Erstfeld** Uri, C Switzerland
158 M3 **Ertai** Xinjiang Uygur Zizhiqu, NW China
128 M7 **Ertil'** Voronezhskaya Oblast', W Russian Federation
Ertis see Irtysh, C Asia
Ertis see Irtyshsk, Kazakhstan
158 K2 **Ertix He** Rus. Chërnyy Irtysh. ≈ China/Kazakhstan
Ērtra see Eritrea
21 P9 **Erwin** North Carolina, SE USA
114 L12 **Erydropótamos** Bul. Byala Reka. ≈ Bulgaria/Greece
115 E19 **Erýmanthos** var. Erimanthos. ▲ S Greece
115 G19 **Erythrés** prev. Erithraí. Stereá Ellás, C Greece
160 F12 **Eryuan** Yunnan, SW China
109 U6 **Erzbach** ≈ W Austria
Erzerum see Erzurum
101 N17 **Erzgebirge** Cz. Krušné Hory, Eng. Ore Mountains. ▲ Czech Republic/Germany see also Krušné Hory
122 L14 **Erzin** Respublika Tyva, S Russian Federation
137 O13 **Erzincan** var. Erzinjan. Erzincan, E Turkey
137 N13 **Erzincan** var. Erzinjan. ◈ province NE Turkey
Erzinjan see Erzincan
Erzsébetváros see Dumbrăveni
137 Q13 **Erzurum** prev. Erzerum. Erzurum, NE Turkey
137 Q12 **Erzurum** prev. Erzerum. ◈ province NE Turkey
186 G9 **Esa'ala** Normanby Island, SE PNG
165 T2 **Esashi** Hokkaidō, NE Japan
165 Q9 **Esashi** var. Esasi. Iwate, Honshū, C Japan
165 Q5 **Esashi** Hokkaidō, N Japan
Esasi see Esashi
95 F23 **Esbjerg** Ribe, W Denmark
Esbo see Espoo
36 L7 **Escalante** Utah, W USA
36 M7 **Escalante River** ≈ Utah, W USA
14 L12 **Escalier, Réservoir l'** ▣ Quebec, SE Canada
40 K7 **Escalón** Chihuahua, N Mexico
104 M8 **Escalona** Castilla-La Mancha, C Spain
23 O8 **Escambia River** ≈ Florida, SE USA
31 N5 **Escanaba** Michigan, N USA
31 N4 **Escanaba River** ≈ Michigan, N USA
105 R8 **Escandón, Puerto de** pass E Spain
41 W14 **Escárcega** Campeche, SE Mexico
171 O1 **Escarpada Point** headland Luzon, N Philippines
23 N8 **Escatawpa River** ≈ Alabama/Mississippi, S USA
103 P2 **Escaut** ≈ N France
Escaut see Scheldt
99 M25 **Esch-sur-Alzette** Luxembourg, S Luxembourg
101 J15 **Eschwege** Hessen, C Germany
101 D16 **Eschweiler** Nordrhein-Westfalen, W Germany
Esclaves, Grand Lac des see Great Slave Lake
45 O8 **Escocesa, Bahía** bay N Dominican Republic
43 W15 **Escocés, Punta** headland NE Panama
35 U17 **Escondido** California, W USA
42 M10 **Escondido, Río** ≈ SE Nicaragua
15 S7 **Escoumins, Rivière des** ≈ Quebec, SE Canada
37 O13 **Escudilla Mountain** ▲ Arizona, SW USA
40 J11 **Escuinapa** var. Escuinapa de Hidalgo. Sinaloa, C Mexico
Escuinapa de Hidalgo see Escuinapa
42 C6 **Escuintla** Escuintla, S Guatemala
41 V17 **Escuintla** Chiapas, SE Mexico
42 A2 **Escuintla** off. Departamento de Escuintla. ◈ department S Guatemala
15 W7 **Escuminac** ≈ Quebec, SE Canada
79 D16 **Eséka** Centre, SW Cameroon
136 I12 **Esenboğa** × (Ankara) Ankara, C Turkey
Esenguly see Gasan-Kuli
136 D17 **Eşen Çayı** ≈ SW Turkey
105 T4 **Ésera** ≈ NE Spain
143 N8 **Eşfahān** Eng. Isfahan; anc. Aspadana. Eşfahān, C Iran
143 O7 **Eşfahān** off. Ostān-e Eşfahān. ◈ province C Iran
105 N5 **Esgueva** ≈ N Spain
149 Q3 **Eshkamesh** Takhār, NE Afghanistan
149 T2 **Eshkāshem** Badakhshān, NE Afghanistan
83 L23 **Eshowe** KwaZulu/Natal, E South Africa
143 T5 **'Eshqābād** Khorāsān, NE Iran
Esh Sham see Dimashq
Esh Sharā see Ash Sharāh
Esik see Yesik
Esil see Ishim, Kazakhstan/Russian Federation
Esil see Yesil', Kazakhstan
183 V2 **Esk** Queensland, E Australia
184 O11 **Eskdale** Hawke's Bay, North Island, NZ
Eski Dzhumaya see Türgovishte
92 L2 **Eskifjördhur** Austurland, E Iceland
139 S3 **Eski Kaļak** var. Askī Kalak, Kalak. N Iraq
95 N16 **Eskilstuna** Södermanland, C Sweden
8 H6 **Eskimo Lakes** lakes Northwest Territories, NW Canada
0 O10 **Eskimo Point** headland Nunavut, E Canada
Eskimo Point see Arviat
139 Q2 **Eski Mosul** N Iraq
147 T10 **Eski-Nookat** var. Iski-Nauket. Oshskaya Oblast', SW Kyrgyzstan
136 F12 **Eskişehir** var. Eskishehr. Eskişehir, W Turkey
136 F13 **Eskişehir** var. Eski shehr. ◈ province NW Turkey
Eskishehr see Eskişehir
104 K5 **Esla** ≈ NW Spain
142 J6 **Eslāmābād** var. Eslāmābād-e Gharb; prev. Harunabad, Shāhābād. Kermānshāhān, W Iran
Eslāmābād-e Gharb see Eslāmābād
148 J4 **Eslām Qal'eh** Pash. Islam Qala. Herāt, W Afghanistan
95 K23 **Eslöv** Skåne, S Sweden
143 S12 **Esmā'īlābād** Kermān, S Iran
143 U8 **Esmā'īlābād** Khorāsān, E Iran
136 D14 **Eşme** Uşak, W Turkey
44 G6 **Esmeralda** Camagüey, E Cuba
63 F21 **Esmeralda, Isla** island S Chile
56 B5 **Esmeraldas** Esmeraldas, N Ecuador
56 B5 **Esmeraldas** ◈ province NW Ecuador
Esna see Isna
14 B6 **Esnagi Lake** ◎ Ontario, S Canada
143 V14 **Espakeh** Sīstān va Balūchestān, SE Iran
103 O13 **Espalion** Aveyron, S France
España see Spain
14 E11 **Espanola** Ontario, S Canada
37 S10 **Espanola** New Mexico, SW USA
57 C18 **Española, Isla** var. Hood Island. island Galapagos Islands, Ecuador, E Pacific Ocean
104 M13 **Espejo** Andalucía, S Spain
94 C13 **Espeland** Hordaland, S Norway
100 G12 **Espelkamp** Nordrhein-Westfalen, NW Germany
38 M8 **Espenberg, Cape** headland Alaska, USA
180 L13 **Esperance** Western Australia
186 L9 **Esperance, Cape** headland Guadacanal, C Solomon Islands
57 P18 **Esperancita** Santa Cruz, E Bolivia
61 B17 **Esperanza** Santa Fe, C Argentina
40 G6 **Esperanza** Sonora, NW Mexico
24 H9 **Esperanza** Texas, SW USA
194 H3 **Esperanza** Argentinian research station Antarctica
104 E12 **Espichel, Cabo** headland S Portugal
54 E10 **Espinal** Tolima, C Colombia
48 K10 **Espinhaço, Serra do** ▲ SE Brazil
104 G6 **Espinho** Aveiro, N Portugal
59 N18 **Espinosa** Minas Gerais, SE Brazil
103 O15 **Espinouse** ▲ S France
60 Q8 **Espírito Santo** off. Estado do Espírito Santo. ◈ state E Brazil
187 P13 **Espiritu Santo** var. Santo. island W Vanuatu
41 Z13 **Espíritu Santo, Bahía del** bay SE Mexico
40 F9 **Espíritu Santo, Isla del** island W Mexico
41 Y12 **Espita** Yucatán, SE Mexico
15 Y7 **Espoir, Cap d'** headland Quebec, SE Canada
Esponsede/Esponsende see Esposende
93 L20 **Espoo** Swe. Esbo. Etelä-Suomi, S Finland
104 G5 **Esposende** var. Esponsede, Esponsende. Braga, N Portugal
83 M18 **Espungabera** Manica, SW Mozambique
63 H17 **Esquel** Chubut, SW Argentina
10 L17 **Esquimalt** Vancouver Island, British Columbia, SW Canada
61 C16 **Esquina** Corrientes, NE Argentina
42 E6 **Esquipulas** Chiquimula, SE Guatemala
42 K9 **Esquipulas** Matagalpa, C Nicaragua
94 I8 **Essandjøen** ◎ S Norway
74 E7 **Essaouira** prev. Mogador. W Morocco
Esseg see Osijek
Es Semara see Smara
99 G15 **Essen** Antwerpen, N Belgium
101 E15 **Essen** var. Essen an der Ruhr. Nordrhein-Westfalen, W Germany
Essen an der Ruhr see Essen
74 I5 **Es Senia** × (Oran) NW Algeria
55 T8 **Essequibo Islands** island group N Guyana
55 T11 **Essequibo River** ≈ C Guyana
14 C18 **Essex** Ontario, S Canada
29 T16 **Essex** Iowa, C USA
97 P21 **Essex** cultural region E England, UK
31 R8 **Essexville** Michigan, N USA
101 H22 **Esslingen** var. Esslingen am Neckar. Baden-Württemberg, SW Germany
Esslingen am Neckar see Esslingen
103 N6 **Essonne** ◈ department N France
Es Suweida see As Suwaydā'
79 F16 **Est** Eng. East. ◈ province SE Cameroon
104 I1 **Estaca de Bares, Punta da** point NW Spain
24 M5 **Estacado, Llano** plain New Mexico/Texas, SW USA
63 K25 **Estados, Isla de los** prev. Eng. Staten Island. island S Argentina
143 P12 **Eşţahbān** Fārs, S Iran
14 F11 **Estaire** Ontario, S Canada
37 S12 **Estancia** New Mexico, SW USA
59 P16 **Estância** Sergipe, E Brazil
104 G7 **Estarreja** Aveiro, N Portugal
102 M17 **Estats, Pic d'** Sp. Pico d'Estats. ▲ France/Spain

◆ Country ● Country Capital ◇ Dependent Territory ○ Dependent Territory Capital ◈ Administrative Region × International Airport ▲ Mountain ▲ Mountain Range ⌅ Volcano ≈ River ◎ Lake ▣ Reservoir

Estats, Pico d' see Estats, Pic d'
83 K23 **Estcourt** KwaZulu/Natal, E South Africa
106 H8 **Este** anc. Ateste. Veneto, NE Italy
42 J9 **Estelí** Estelí, NW Nicaragua
42 J9 **Estelí** ◐ department NW Nicaragua
Estella see Estella-Lizarra
105 Q4 **Estella-Lizarra** Bas. Lizarra var Estella Navarra, N Spain
29 R9 **Estelline** South Dakota, N USA
25 P4 **Estelline** Texas, SW USA
104 L14 **Estepa** Andalucía, S Spain
104 L16 **Estepona** Andalucía, S Spain
39 R9 **Ester** Alaska, USA
11 V16 **Esterhazy** Saskatchewan, S Canada
37 S3 **Estes Park** Colorado, C USA
11 V17 **Estevan** Saskatchewan, S Canada
29 T11 **Estherville** Iowa, C USA
21 R15 **Estill** South Carolina, SE USA
103 Q6 **Estissac** Aube, N France
15 T9 **Est, Lac de l'** ◎ Quebec, SE Canada
Estland see Estonia
11 S16 **Eston** Saskatchewan, S Canada
118 G5 **Estonia** off. Republic of Estonia, Est. Eesti Vabariik, Ger. Estland, Latv. Igaunija; prev. Estonian SSR, Rus. Estonskaya SSR. ◆ republic NE Europe
Estonskaya SSR see Estonia
104 E11 **Estoril** Lisboa, W Portugal
59 L14 **Estreito** Maranhão, E Brazil
104 I8 **Estrela, Serra da** ▲▲ C Portugal
40 D3 **Estrella, Punta** headland NW Mexico
Estremadura see Extremadura
104 F10 **Estremadura** cultural and historical region W Portugal
104 H11 **Estremoz** Évora, S Portugal
79 D18 **Estuaire** off. Province de l'Estuaire, var. L'Estuaire. ◐ province NW Gabon
Eszék see Osijek
111 I22 **Esztergom** Ger. Gran; anc. Strigonium. Komárom-Esztergom, N Hungary
152 K11 **Etah** Uttar Pradesh, N India
189 R17 **Etal Atoll** atoll Mortlock Islands, C Micronesia
99 K24 **Étalle** Luxembourg, SE Belgium
103 N6 **Étampes** Essonne, N France
182 J1 **Etamunbanie, Lake** salt lake South Australia
103 N1 **Étaples** Pas-de-Calais, N France
152 K12 **Etāwah** Uttar Pradesh, N India
15 R10 **Etchemin** ≈ Quebec, SE Canada
Etchmiadzin see Ejmiatsin
40 G7 **Etchojoa** Sonora, NW Mexico
93 L19 **Etelä-Suomi** ◐ province S Finland
83 B16 **Etengua** Kunene, NW Namibia
99 K25 **Éthe** Luxembourg, SE Belgium
11 W15 **Ethelbert** Manitoba, S Canada
80 H12 **Ethiopia** off. Federal Democratic Republic of Ethiopia; prev. Abyssinia, People's Democratic Republic of Ethiopia. ◆ republic E Africa
80 I13 **Ethiopian Highlands** var. Ethiopian Plateau. plateau N Ethiopia
Ethiopian Plateau see Ethiopian Highlands
34 M2 **Etna** California, W USA
18 B14 **Etna** Pennsylvania, NE USA
94 G12 **Etna** ≈ S Norway
107 L24 **Etna, Monte** Eng. Mount Etna. ✕ Sicilia, Italy, C Mediterranean Sea
Etna, Mount see Etna, Monte
95 C15 **Etne** Hordaland, S Norway
Etoliko see Aitolikó
39 Y14 **Etolin Island** island Alexander Archipelago, Alaska, USA
38 L12 **Etolin Strait** strait Alaska, USA
83 C17 **Etosha Pan** salt lake N Namibia
79 G18 **Etoumbi** Cuvette, NW Congo
20 M10 **Etowah** Tennessee, S USA
23 S2 **Etowah River** ≈ Georgia, SE USA
Etrek see Atrak
102 L3 **Étretat** Seine-Maritime, N France
114 H9 **Etropole** Sofiya, W Bulgaria
Etsch see Adige
Et Tafila see Aṭ Ṭafīlah
99 M23 **Ettelbrück** Diekirch, C Luxembourg
189 V12 **Etten** atoll Chuuk Islands, C Micronesia
99 H14 **Etten-Leur** Noord-Brabant, S Netherlands
76 G7 **Et Tîdra** var. Ile Tîdra. island Dakhlet Nouâdhibou, NW Mauritania
101 G21 **Ettlingen** Baden-Württemberg, SW Germany
102 M2 **Eu** Seine-Maritime, N France
193 W16 **'Eua** prev. Middleburg Island. island Tongatapu Group, SE Tonga
193 W15 **Eua Iki** island Tongatapu Group, S Tonga
Euboea see Évvoia
181 O12 **Eucla** Western Australia
31 U11 **Euclid** Ohio, N USA
27 W14 **Eudora** Arkansas, C USA
27 Q4 **Eudora** Kansas, C USA
182 J9 **Eudunda** South Australia
23 R6 **Eufaula** Alabama, S USA
27 Q11 **Eufaula** Oklahoma, C USA
27 Q11 **Eufaula Lake** var. Eufaula Reservoir. ▣ Oklahoma, C USA
Eufaula Reservoir see Eufaula Lake
32 F13 **Eugene** Oregon, NW USA
40 B6 **Eugenia, Punta** headland W Mexico
183 Q8 **Eugowra** New South Wales, SE Australia
104 I2 **Eume** ≈ NW Spain
104 H2 **Eume, Embalse do** ▣ NW Spain
Eumolpias see Plovdiv
59 O18 **Eunápolis** Bahia, SE Brazil
22 H8 **Eunice** Louisiana, S USA
37 W15 **Eunice** New Mexico, SW USA
99 M19 **Eupen** Liège, E Belgium
138 J9 **Euphrates** Ar. Al Furāt, Turk. Firat Nehri. ≈ SW Asia
138 L3 **Euphrates Dam** dam N Syria
22 M4 **Eupora** Mississippi, S USA
93 K19 **Eura** Länsi-Suomi, W Finland
93 K19 **Eurajoki** Länsi-Suomi, W Finland
84 **Eurasian Plate** tectonic feature
102 L4 **Eure** ◐ department N France
102 M4 **Eure** ≈ N France
102 M6 **Eure-et-Loir** ◐ department C France
34 K3 **Eureka** California, W USA
27 P6 **Eureka** Kansas, C USA
33 O6 **Eureka** Montana, NW USA
35 V5 **Eureka** Nevada, W USA
29 O7 **Eureka** South Dakota, N USA
36 L4 **Eureka** Utah, W USA
32 K10 **Eureka** Washington, NW USA
27 S9 **Eureka Springs** Arkansas, C USA
182 K6 **Eurinilla Creek** seasonal river South Australia
183 O11 **Euroa** Victoria, SE Australia
172 M9 **Europa** island W Madagascar
104 L3 **Europa, Picos de** ▲▲ N Spain
104 L16 **Europa Point** headland S Gibraltar
86-87 **Europe** continent
98 F12 **Europoort** Zuid-Holland, W Netherlands
Euskadi see País Vasco
101 D17 **Euskirchen** Nordrhein-Westfalen, W Germany
23 W11 **Eustis** Florida, SE USA
182 M9 **Euston** New South Wales, SE Australia
23 N5 **Eutaw** Alabama, S USA
100 K8 **Eutin** Schleswig-Holstein, N Germany
10 K14 **Eutsuk Lake** ▣ British Columbia, SW Canada
Euxine Sea see Black Sea
83 C16 **Evale** Cunene, SW Angola
37 T3 **Evans** Colorado, C USA
11 P14 **Evansburg** Alberta, SW Canada
29 X13 **Evansdale** Iowa, C USA
183 V4 **Evans Head** New South Wales, SE Australia
12 J11 **Evans, Lac** ◎ Quebec, SE Canada
37 S5 **Evans, Mount** ▲ Colorado, C USA
9 Q8 Nunavut, N Canada
31 N10 **Evanston** Illinois, N USA
33 S17 **Evanston** Wyoming, C USA
14 D11 **Evansville** Manitoulin Island, Ontario, S Canada
31 N16 **Evansville** Indiana, N USA
30 L9 **Evansville** Wisconsin, N USA
25 S8 **Evant** Texas, SW USA
143 P13 **Evaz** Fārs, S Iran
29 W4 **Eveleth** Minnesota, N USA
182 E3 **Evelyn Creek** seasonal river South Australia
181 Q2 **Evelyn, Mount** ▲ Northern Territory, N Australia
122 K10 **Evenkiyskiy Avtonomnyy Okrug** ◐ autonomous district N Russian Federation
183 R13 **Everard, Cape** headland Victoria, SE Australia
182 F6 **Everard, Lake** salt lake South Australia
182 C2 **Everard Ranges** ▲▲ South Australia
153 R11 **Everest, Mount** Chin. Qomolangma Feng, Nep. Sagarmatha. ▲ China/Nepal
18 E15 **Everett** Pennsylvania, NE USA
32 H7 **Everett** Washington, NW USA
99 E17 **Evergem** Oost-Vlaanderen, NW Belgium
23 X16 **Everglades City** Florida, SE USA
23 Y16 **Everglades, The** wetland Florida, SE USA
23 P7 **Evergreen** Alabama, S USA
37 T4 **Evergreen** Colorado, C USA
Evergreen State see Washington
97 L21 **Evesham** C England, UK
103 T10 **Évian-les-Bains** Haute-Savoie, E France
93 K16 **Evijärvi** Länsi-Suomi, W Finland
79 D17 **Evinayong** var. Ebinayon, Evinayoung. C Equatorial Guinea
Evinayoung see Evinayong
115 E18 **Évinos** ≈ C Greece
95 E17 **Evje** Aust-Agder, S Norway
Evmolpia see Plovdiv
104 H11 **Évora** anc. Ebora, Lat. Liberalitas Julia. Évora, C Portugal
104 G11 **Évora** ◐ district S Portugal
102 M4 **Évreux** anc. Civitas Eburovicum. Eure, N France
102 K6 **Évron** Mayenne, NW France
114 L13 **Évros** Bul. Maritsa, Turk. Meriç; anc. Hebrus. ≈ SE Europe see also Maritsa/Meriç
115 F21 **Evrótas** ≈ S Greece
103 O5 **Évry** Essonne, N France
25 O8 **E.V.Spence Reservoir** ▣ Texas, SW USA
115 I18 **Évvoia** Lat. Euboea. island C Greece
38 D9 **Ewa Beach** Oahu, Hawaii, USA, C Pacific Ocean
32 L9 **Ewan** Washington, NW USA
44 K12 **Ewarton** C Jamaica
81 J18 **Ewaso Ng'iro** var. Nyiro. ≈ C Kenya
29 P13 **Ewing** Nebraska, C USA
194 J5 **Ewing Island** island Antarctica
65 P17 **Ewing Seamount** undersea feature E Atlantic Ocean
158 L6 **Ewirgol** Xinjiang Uygur Zizhiqu, W China
79 G19 **Ewo** Cuvette, W Congo
27 S3 **Excelsior Springs** Missouri, C USA
97 J23 **Exe** ≈ SW England, UK
194 L12 **Executive Committee Range** ▲▲ Antarctica
14 E16 **Exeter** Ontario, S Canada
97 J24 **Exeter** anc. Isca Damnoniorum. SW England, UK
35 R11 **Exeter** California, W USA
19 P10 **Exeter** New Hampshire, NE USA
Exin see Kcynia
29 T14 **Exira** Iowa, C USA
97 J23 **Exmoor** moorland SW England, UK
21 Y6 **Exmore** Virginia, NE USA
180 G8 **Exmouth** Western Australia
97 J24 **Exmouth** SW England, UK
180 G8 **Exmouth Gulf** gulf Western Australia
173 V8 **Exmouth Plateau** undersea feature E Indian Ocean
115 J20 **Exompourgo** ancient monument Tínos, Kykládes, Greece, Aegean Sea
104 I10 **Extremadura** var. Estremadura. ◐ autonomous community W Spain
78 F12 **Extrême-Nord** Eng. Extreme North. ◐ province N Cameroon
Extreme North see Extrême-Nord
44 I3 **Exuma Cays** islets C Bahamas
44 I3 **Exuma Sound** sound C Bahamas
81 H20 **Eyasi, Lake** ◎ N Tanzania
95 F17 **Eydehavn** Aust-Agder, S Norway
96 L12 **Eyemouth** SE Scotland, UK
96 G7 **Eye Peninsula** peninsula NW Scotland, UK
80 Q13 **Eyl** It. Eil. Nugaal, E Somalia
103 N11 **Eymoutiers** Haute-Vienne, C France
Eyo (lower course) see Uolo, Río
29 X10 **Eyota** Minnesota, N USA
182 H2 **Eyre Basin, Lake** salt lake South Australia
182 I1 **Eyre Creek** seasonal river Northern Territory/South Australia
174 L9 **Eyre, Lake** salt lake South Australia
185 C22 **Eyre Mountains** ▲▲ South Island, NZ
182 H3 **Eyre North, Lake** salt lake South Australia
182 G7 **Eyre Peninsula** peninsula South Australia
182 H4 **Eyre South, Lake** salt lake South Australia
95 B18 **Eysturoy** Dan. Østerø Island Faeroe Islands
61 D20 **Ezeiza** × (Buenos Aires) Buenos Aires, E Argentina
Ezeres see Ezeriş
116 F12 **Ezeriş** Hung. Ezeres. Caraş-Severin, W Romania
161 O9 **Ezhou** prev. Echeng. Hubei, C China
127 R11 **Ezhva** Respublika Komi, NW Russian Federation
136 B12 **Ezine** Çanakkale, NW Turkey
Ezo see Hokkaidō
Ezra/Ezraa see Izra'

F

191 P7 **Faaa** Tahiti, W French Polynesia
191 P7 **Faaa** × (Papeete) Tahiti, W French Polynesia
Faaborg see Fåborg
151 K19 **Faadhippolhu Atoll** var. Fadiffolu, Lhaviyani Atoll. atoll N Maldives
191 U10 **Faaite** atoll Îles Tuamotu, C French Polynesia
191 Q8 **Faaone** Tahiti, W French Polynesia
24 H8 **Fabens** Texas, SW USA
94 H12 **Fåberg** Oppland, S Norway
95 H24 **Fåborg** var. Faaborg. Fyn, C Denmark
106 I12 **Fabriano** Marche, C Italy
145 U16 **Fabrichnyy** Almaty, SE Kazakhstan
54 F10 **Facatativá** Cundinamarca, C Colombia
77 X9 **Fachi** Agadez, C Niger
188 B16 **Facpi Point** headland W Guam
18 I13 **Factoryville** Pennsylvania, NE USA
78 K8 **Fada** Borkou-Ennedi-Tibesti, E Chad
77 Q13 **Fada-Ngourma** E Burkina
123 N6 **Faddeya, Zaliv** bay N Russian Federation
123 Q5 **Faddeyevskiy, Ostrov** island Novosibirskiye Ostrova, NE Russian Federation
141 W12 **Fadhī** S Oman
106 H10 **Faenza** anc. Faventia. Emilia-Romagna, N Italy
64 M5 **Faeroe-Iceland Ridge** undersea feature NW Norwegian Sea
64 M5 **Faeroe Islands** Dan. Færøerne, Faer. Føroyar. ◇ Danish external territory N Atlantic Ocean
86 C8 **Faeroe Islands** island group N Atlantic Ocean
Færøerne see Faeroe Islands
64 N6 **Faeroe-Shetland Trough** undersea feature NE Atlantic Ocean
104 H6 **Fafe** Braga, N Portugal
80 K13 **Fafen Shet'** ≈ E Ethiopia
193 V15 **Fafo** island Tongatapu Group, S Tonga
192 I16 **Fagaloa Bay** bay Upolu, E Samoa
192 H15 **Fagamālo** Savai'i, N Samoa
116 I12 **Făgăraş** Ger. Fogarasch, Hung. Fogaras. Braşov, C Romania
95 M20 **Fagerhult** Kalmar, S Sweden
94 G13 **Fagernes** Oppland, S Norway
92 I9 **Fagernes** Troms, N Norway
95 M14 **Fagersta** Västmanland, C Sweden
77 W13 **Faggo** var. Foggo. Bauchi, N Nigeria
Faghman see Fughmah
Fagibina, Lake see Faguibine, Lac
63 J25 **Fagnano, Lago** ◎ S Argentina
99 G22 **Fagne** hill range S Belgium
77 N10 **Faguibine, Lac** var. Lake Fagibina. ◎ NW Mali
Fahaheel see Al Fuḥayḥīl
Fahlun see Falun
143 U12 **Fahraj** Kermān, SE Iran
64 P5 **Faial** Madeira, Portugal, NE Atlantic Ocean
64 N2 **Faial** var. Ilha do Faial. island Azores, Portugal, NE Atlantic Ocean
Faial, Ilha do see Faial
108 G10 **Faido** Ticino, S Switzerland
Faifo see Hôi An
Failaka Island see Faylakah
190 G12 **Faioa, Île** island N Wallis and Futuna
181 W8 **Fairbairn Reservoir** ▣ Queensland, E Australia
39 R9 **Fairbanks** Alaska, USA
21 U12 **Fair Bluff** North Carolina, SE USA
31 R14 **Fairborn** Ohio, N USA
23 S3 **Fairburn** Georgia, SE USA
30 M12 **Fairbury** Illinois, N USA
29 Q17 **Fairbury** Nebraska, C USA
29 T9 **Fairfax** Minnesota, N USA
27 O8 **Fairfax** Oklahoma, C USA
21 R14 **Fairfax** South Carolina, SE USA
35 N8 **Fairfield** California, W USA
33 O14 **Fairfield** Idaho, NW USA
30 M16 **Fairfield** Illinois, N USA
29 X15 **Fairfield** Iowa, C USA
33 R8 **Fairfield** Montana, NW USA
31 Q14 **Fairfield** Ohio, N USA
25 U8 **Fairfield** Texas, SW USA
27 T7 **Fair Grove** Missouri, C USA
19 P12 **Fairhaven** Massachusetts, NE USA
23 N8 **Fairhope** Alabama, S USA
96 L4 **Fair Isle** island NE Scotland, UK
185 F20 **Fairlie** Canterbury, South Island, NZ
29 U11 **Fairmont** Minnesota, N USA
29 Q16 **Fairmont** Nebraska, C USA
21 S3 **Fairmont** West Virginia, NE USA
31 P13 **Fairmount** Indiana, N USA
18 H10 **Fairmount** New York, NE USA
29 R7 **Fairmount** North Dakota, N USA
37 S5 **Fairplay** Colorado, C USA
18 F9 **Fairport** New York, NE USA
11 O12 **Fairview** Alberta, W Canada
26 L9 **Fairview** Oklahoma, C USA
36 L4 **Fairview** Utah, W USA
35 T6 **Fairview Peak** ▲ Nevada, W USA
188 H14 **Fais** atoll Caroline Islands, W Micronesia
149 U8 **Faisalābād** prev. Lyallpur. Punjab, NE Pakistan
Faisaliya see Fayṣalīyah
28 L8 **Faith** South Dakota, N USA
153 N12 **Faizābād** Uttar Pradesh, N India
Faizabad/Faizābād see Feyzābād
45 S9 **Fajardo** E Puerto Rico
139 R9 **Fajj, Wādī al** dry watercourse S Iraq
140 K4 **Fajr, Bi'r** well NW Saudi Arabia
191 W10 **Fakahina** atoll Îles Tuamotu, C French Polynesia
190 L10 **Fakaofo Atoll** island SE Tokelau
191 U10 **Fakarava** atoll Îles Tuamotu, C French Polynesia
129 T2 **Fakel** Udmurtskaya Respublika, NW Russian Federation
97 P19 **Fakenham** E England, UK
171 U13 **Fakfak** Irian Jaya, E Indonesia
153 T12 **Fakīragrām** Assam, NE India
114 M10 **Fakiyska Reka** ≈ SE Bulgaria
95 J24 **Fakse** Storstrøm, SE Denmark
95 J24 **Fakse Bugt** bay SE Denmark
95 J24 **Fakse Ladeplads** Storstrøm, SE Denmark
163 V11 **Faku** Liaoning, NE China
76 J14 **Falaba** N Sierra Leone
102 K5 **Falaise** Calvados, N France
114 H12 **Falakró** ▲▲ NE Greece
189 T12 **Falalu** island Chuuk, C Micronesia
166 L4 **Falam** Chin State, W Burma
143 N8 **Falāvarjān** Eşfahān, C Iran
116 M11 **Fălciu** Vaslui, E Romania
54 I4 **Falcón** off. Estado Falcón. ◐ state NW Venezuela
106 J12 **Falconara Marittima** Marche, C Italy
Falcone, Capo del see Falcone, Punta del
107 A16 **Falcone, Punta del** var. Capo del Falcone. headland Sardegna, Italy, C Mediterranean Sea
11 Y16 **Falcon Lake** Manitoba, S Canada
Falcon Lake see Falcón, Presa/Falcon Reservoir
41 O7 **Falcón, Presa** var. Falcon Lake, Falcon Reservoir. ▣ Mexico/USA see also Falcon Reservoir
25 Q16 **Falcon Reservoir** var. Falcon Lake, Presa Falcón. ▣ Mexico/USA see also Falcón, Presa
190 L10 **Fale** island Fakaofo Atoll, SE Tokelau
192 F15 **Faleālupo** Savai'i, NW Samoa
190 B10 **Falefatu** island Funafuti Atoll, C Tuvalu
192 G15 **Fālelima** Savai'i, NW Samoa
95 N18 **Falerum** Östergötland, S Sweden
Faleshty see Făleşti
116 M9 **Făleşti** Rus. Faleshty. NW Moldova
25 S15 **Falfurrias** Texas, SW USA
11 O13 **Falher** Alberta, W Canada
Falkenau an der Eger see Sokolov
95 J21 **Falkenberg** Halland, S Sweden
Falkenberg see Niemodlin
Falkenburg in Pommern see Złocieniec
100 N12 **Falkensee** Brandenburg, NE Germany
96 J12 **Falkirk** C Scotland, UK
65 I20 **Falkland Escarpment** undersea feature SW Atlantic Ocean
63 K24 **Falkland Islands** var. Falklands, Islas Malvinas. ◇ UK dependent territory SW Atlantic Ocean
47 W14 **Falkland Islands** island group SW Atlantic Ocean
65 I20 **Falkland Plateau** var. Argentine Rise. undersea feature SW Atlantic Ocean
Falklands see Falkland Islands
63 M23 **Falkland Sound** var. Estrecho de San Carlos. strait C Falkland Islands
Falknov nad Ohří see Sokolov
115 H21 **Falkonéra** island S Greece
95 K18 **Falköping** Västra Götaland, S Sweden
139 U8 **Fallāḥ** E Iraq
35 U16 **Fallbrook** California, W USA
189 U12 **Falleallej Pass** passage Chuuk Islands, C Micronesia
93 J14 **Fällfors** Västerbotten, N Sweden
194 I6 **Fallières Coast** physical region Antarctica
100 I11 **Fallingbostel** Niedersachsen, NW Germany
33 X9 **Fallon** Montana, NW USA
35 S5 **Fallon** Nevada, W USA
19 O12 **Fall River** Massachusetts, NE USA
27 P6 **Fall River Lake** ▣ Kansas, C USA
35 O3 **Fall River Mills** California, W USA
21 W4 **Falls Church** Virginia, NE USA
29 S17 **Falls City** Nebraska, C USA
25 S12 **Falls City** Texas, SW USA
Falluja see Al Fallūjah
77 S12 **Falmey** Dosso, SW Niger
45 W10 **Falmouth** Antigua, Antigua and Barbuda
44 J11 **Falmouth** W Jamaica
97 H25 **Falmouth** SW England, UK
20 M4 **Falmouth** Kentucky, S USA
19 P13 **Falmouth** Massachusetts, NE USA
21 W5 **Falmouth** Virginia, NE USA
189 U12 **Falos** island Chuuk, C Micronesia
83 E26 **False Bay** Afr. Valsbaai. bay SW South Africa
155 K17 **False Divi Point** headland E India
38 M16 **False Pass** Unimak Island, Alaska, USA
154 P12 **False Point** headland E India
105 U6 **Falset** Cataluña, NE Spain
95 I25 **Falster** island SE Denmark
95 J23 **Falsterbo** Skåne, S Sweden
116 K9 **Fălticeni** Hung. Falticsén. Suceava, NE Romania
Falticsén see Fălticeni
94 M13 **Falun** var. Fahlun. Dalarna, C Sweden
Famagusta see Gazimağusa
Famagusta Bay see Gazimağusa Körfezi
62 I8 **Famatina** La Rioja, NW Argentina
99 J21 **Famenne** physical region SE Belgium
113 D22 **Fan** var. Fani. ≈ N Albania
77 X15 **Fan** ≈ E Nigeria
76 M12 **Fana** Koulikoro, SW Mali
115 K19 **Fána** ancient harbor Chíos, SE Greece
189 V13 **Fanan** island Chuuk, C Micronesia
189 U12 **Fanapanges** island Chuuk, C Micronesia
115 L20 **Fanári, Akrotírio** headland Ikaría, Dodekánisos, Greece, Aegean Sea
45 Q13 **Fancy** Saint Vincent, Saint Vincent and the Grenadines
172 I5 **Fandriana** Fianarantsoa, SE Madagascar
167 O6 **Fang** Chiang Mai, NW Thailand
80 E13 **Fangak** Jonglei, SE Sudan
191 W10 **Fangatau** atoll Îles Tuamotu, C French Polynesia
191 X12 **Fangataufa** island Îles Tuamotu, SE French Polynesia
193 V15 **Fanga Uta** bay S Tonga
161 N7 **Fangcheng** Henan, C China
160 K15 **Fangchenggang** var. Fangcheng Gezu Zizhixian; prev. Fangcheng. Guangxi Zhuangzu Zizhiqu, S China
161 S15 **Fangshan** S Taiwan
163 X8 **Fangzheng** Heilongjiang, NE China
Fani see Fan
119 K16 **Fanipal'** Rus. Fanipol'. Minskaya Voblasts', C Belarus
Fanipol' see Fanipal'
25 T13 **Fannin** Texas, SW USA
Fanning Island see Tabuaeran
94 G8 **Fannrem** Sør-Trøndelag, S Norway
106 I11 **Fano** anc. Colonia Julia Fanestris, Fanum Fortunae. Marche, C Italy
95 E23 **Fanø** island W Denmark
167 R5 **Fan Si Pan** ▲ N Vietnam
Fanum Fortunae see Fano
Fao see Al Fāw
141 W7 **Faq'** var. Al Faqa. Dubayy, E UAE
146 K12 **Farab** Turkm. Farap. Lebapskiy Velayat, NE Turkmenistan
194 H5 **Faraday** UK research station Antarctica
185 G16 **Faraday, Mount** ▲ South Island, NZ
79 P16 **Faradje** Orientale, NE Dem. Rep. Congo (Zaire)
Faradofay see Tôlañaro
172 I7 **Farafangana** Fianarantsoa, SE Madagascar
148 J7 **Farāh** var. Farah, Fararud. Farāh, W Afghanistan
148 K7 **Farāh** ◐ province W Afghanistan
148 J7 **Farāh Rūd** ≈ W Afghanistan
188 K7 **Farallon de Medinilla** island C Northern Mariana Islands
188 J2 **Farallon de Pajaros** var. Uracas. island N Northern Mariana Islands
76 J14 **Faranah** Haute-Guinée, S Guinea
Farap see Farab
Fararud see Farāh
140 M13 **Farasān, Jazā'ir** island group SW Saudi Arabia
172 I5 **Faratsiho** Antananarivo, C Madagascar
188 K15 **Faraulep Atoll** atoll Caroline Islands, C Micronesia
99 H20 **Farciennes** Hainaut, S Belgium
105 O14 **Fardes** ≈ S Spain
191 S10 **Fare** Huahine, W French Polynesia
97 M23 **Fareham** S England, UK
39 P11 **Farewell** Alaska, USA
184 H13 **Farewell, Cape** headland South Island, NZ
Farewell, Cape see Nunap Isua
184 I13 **Farewell Spit** spit South Island, NZ
95 I17 **Färgelanda** Västra Götaland, S Sweden
147 S10 **Farghona** Rus. Fergana; prev. Novyy Margilan. Farghona Wiloyati, E Uzbekistan
Farghona Valley see Fergana Valley
147 R10 **Farghona Wiloyati** Rus. Ferganskaya Oblast'. ◐ province E Uzbekistan
Farghona, Wodii/Farghona Wodiysi see Fergana Valley
23 V8 **Fargo** Georgia, SE USA
29 R5 **Fargo** North Dakota, N USA
29 V10 **Faribault** Minnesota, N USA
152 J11 **Farīdābād** Haryāna, N India
152 H8 **Farīdkot** Punjab, NW India
153 T15 **Faridpur** Dhaka, C Bangladesh
121 P14 **Fārigh, Wādī al** ≈ N Libya
172 I4 **Farihy Alaotra** ◎ C Madagascar
94 M11 **Färila** Gävleborg, C Sweden
104 E9 **Farilhões** island C Portugal
76 G12 **Farim** NW Guinea-Bissau
Farish see Forish
141 T11 **Fāris, Qalamat** well SE Saudi Arabia
95 N21 **Färjestaden** Kalmar, S Sweden
149 R2 **Farkhār** Takhār, NE Afghanistan
147 Q14 **Farkhor** Rus. Parkhar. SW Tajikistan
116 F12 **Fârliug** prev. Fîrliug, Hung. Furluk. Caraş-Severin, SW Romania
115 M21 **Farmakonísi** island Dodekánisos, Greece, Aegean Sea
30 M13 **Farmer City** Illinois, N USA
31 N14 **Farmersburg** Indiana, N USA
25 U6 **Farmersville** Texas, SW USA
22 H5 **Farmerville** Louisiana, S USA
29 X16 **Farmington** Iowa, C USA
19 Q6 **Farmington** Maine, NE USA
29 V9 **Farmington** Minnesota, N USA
27 X6 **Farmington** Missouri, C USA
19 O9 **Farmington** New Hampshire, NE USA
37 P9 **Farmington** New Mexico, SW USA
36 L2 **Farmington** Utah, W USA
21 W9 **Farmville** North Carolina, SE USA
21 U6 **Farmville** Virginia, NE USA
97 N22 **Farnborough** S England, UK
97 N22 **Farnham** S England, UK
10 J7 **Faro** Yukon Territory, W Canada
104 G14 **Faro** Faro, S Portugal
104 G14 **Faro** ◐ district S Portugal
104 G14 **Faro** × Faro, S Portugal
78 F13 **Faro** ≈ Cameroon/Nigeria
95 Q18 **Fårö** Gotland, SE Sweden
Faro, Punta del see Peloro, Capo
95 Q18 **Fårösund** Gotland, SE Sweden
173 N7 **Farquhar Group** island group S Seychelles
18 B13 **Farrell** Pennsylvania, NE USA
152 K11 **Farrukhābād** Uttar Pradesh, N India
143 P11 **Fārs** off. Ostān-e Fārs; anc. Persis. ◐ province S Iran
115 F16 **Fársala** Thessalía, C Greece
143 R4 **Fārsīān** Golestān, N Iran
Fars, Khalīj-e see The Gulf
95 G21 **Farsø** Nordjylland, N Denmark
95 D18 **Farsund** Vest-Agder, S Norway
141 U14 **Fartak, Ra's** headland E Yemen
60 H13 **Fartura, Serra da** ▲▲ S Brazil
Farvel, Kap see Nunap Isua
24 L4 **Farwell** Texas, SW USA
194 I9 **Farwell Island** island Antarctica

◆ Country
● Country Capital
◇ Dependent Territory
○ Dependent Territory Capital
◐ Administrative Region
× International Airport
▲ Mountain
▲▲ Mountain Range
✕ Volcano
≈ River
◎ Lake
▣ Reservoir

152 L9 **Far Western** ◆ zone W Nepal
148 M3 **Fāryāb** ◆ province N Afghanistan
143 P12 **Fasā** Fārs, S Iran
141 U12 **Fasad, Ramlat** desert SW Oman
107 P17 **Fasano** Puglia, SE Italy
92 L3 **Fáskrúdhsfjördhur** Austurland, E Iceland
117 O5 **Fastiv** Rus. Fastov. Kyyivs'ka Oblast', NW Ukraine
97 B22 **Fastnet Rock** Ir. Carraig Aonair. island SW Ireland
Fastov see Fastiv
190 C9 **Fatato** island Funafuti Atoll, C Tuvalu
152 K12 **Fatehgarh** Uttar Pradesh, N India
149 U6 **Fatehjang** Punjab, E Pakistan
152 G11 **Fatehpur** Rājasthān, N India
152 L13 **Fatehpur** Uttar Pradesh, N India
128 J7 **Fatezh** Kurskaya Oblast', W Russian Federation
76 G11 **Fatick** W Senegal
104 G9 **Fátima** Santarém, W Portugal
136 M11 **Fatsa** Ordu, N Turkey
Fatshan see Foshan
190 D12 **Fatua, Pointe** var. Pointe Nord. headland Île Futuna, S Wallis and Futuna
191 X7 **Fatu Hiva** island Îles Marquises, NE French Polynesia
Fatunda see Fatundu
79 H21 **Fatundu** var. Fatunda. Bandundu, W Dem. Rep. Congo (Zaire)
187 S11 **Fatutaka** island, E Soloman Islands
29 O8 **Faulkton** South Dakota, N USA
116 L13 **Făurei** prev. Filimon Sîrbu. Brăila, SE Romania
92 G12 **Fauske** Nordland, C Norway
11 P13 **Faust** Alberta, W Canada
99 L23 **Fauvillers** Luxembourg, SE Belgium
107 J24 **Favara** Sicilia, Italy, C Mediterranean Sea
Faventia see Faenza
107 G23 **Favignana, Isola** island Isole Egadi, S Italy
12 D8 **Fawn** ≈ Ontario, SE Canada
Faxa Bay see Faxaflói
92 H3 **Faxaflói** Eng. Faxa Bay. bay W Iceland
78 I7 **Faya** prev. Faya-Largeau, Largeau. Borkou-Ennedi-Tibesti, N Chad
Faya-Largeau see Faya
187 Q16 **Fayaoué** Province des Îles Loyauté, C New Caledonia
138 M5 **Fayḍāt** hill range E Syria
23 O3 **Fayette** Alabama, S USA
29 X12 **Fayette** Iowa, C USA
22 J6 **Fayette** Mississippi, S USA
27 U4 **Fayette** Missouri, C USA
27 S9 **Fayetteville** Arkansas, C USA
21 U10 **Fayetteville** North Carolina, SE USA
20 J10 **Fayetteville** Tennessee, S USA
25 U11 **Fayetteville** Texas, SW USA
21 R5 **Fayetteville** West Virginia, NE USA
141 R4 **Faylakah** var. Failaka Island. island E Kuwait
139 T10 **Fayṣalīyah** var. Faisaliya. S Iraq
189 P15 **Fayu** var. East Fayu. island Hall Islands, C Micronesia
152 G8 **Fāzilka** Punjab, NW India
Fdérick see Fdérik
76 I6 **Fdérik** var. Fdérick, Fr. Fort Gouraud. Tiris Zemmour, NW Mauritania
Feabhail, Loch see Foyle, Lough
97 B20 **Feale** ≈ SW Ireland
21 V12 **Fear, Cape** headland Bald Head Island, North Carolina, SE USA
35 O6 **Feather River** ≈ California, W USA
185 M14 **Featherston** Wellington, North Island, NZ
102 L3 **Fécamp** Seine-Maritime, N France
Fédala see Mohammedia
61 D17 **Federación** Entre Ríos, E Argentina
61 D17 **Federal** Entre Ríos, E Argentina
77 T15 **Federal Capital District** ◆ capital territory C Nigeria
Federal Capital Territory see Australian Capital Territory
Federal District see Distrito Federal
21 Y4 **Federalsburg** Maryland, NE USA
74 M6 **Fedjaj, Chott el** var. Chott el Fejaj, Shaṭṭ al Fijāj. salt lake C Tunisia
94 B13 **Fedje** island S Norway
144 M7 **Fedorovka** Kostanay, N Kazakhstan
129 U6 **Fedorovka** Respublika Bashkortostan, W Russian Federation
Fëdory see Fyadory
117 U11 **Fedotova Kosa** spit SE Ukraine
189 V13 **Fefan** atoll Chuuk Islands, C Micronesia
111 O21 **Fehérgyarmat** Szabolcs-Szatmár-Bereg, E Hungary
Fehér-Körös see Crişul Alb
Fehértemplom see Bela Crkva
Fehérvölgy see Albac
100 L7 **Fehmarn** island N Germany
Fehmarnbelt see Femerbælt
109 X8 **Fehring** Steiermark, SE Austria
59 B15 **Feijó** Acre, W Brazil
184 M12 **Feilding** Manawatu-Wanganui, North Island, NZ
Feira see Feira de Santana
59 O17 **Feira de Santana** var. Feira. Bahia, E Brazil
109 X7 **Feistritz** ≈ SE Austria
Feistritz see Ilirska Bistrica
161 P8 **Feixi** prev. Shangpaihe. Anhui, E China
Fejaj, Chott el see Fedjaj, Chott el
111 I23 **Fejér** off. Fejér Megye. ◆ county W Hungary
95 I24 **Fejø** island SE Denmark
136 K15 **Feke** Adana, S Turkey
Feketehalom see Codlea
Fekete-Körös see Crişul Negru
109 T3 **Feldaist** ≈ N Austria
109 W8 **Feldbach** Steiermark, SE Austria
101 F24 **Feldberg** ▲ SW Germany
116 J12 **Feldioara** Ger. Marienburg, Hung. Földvár. Braşov, C Romania
108 I7 **Feldkirch** anc. Clunia. Vorarlberg, W Austria
109 S9 **Feldkirchen in Kärnten** Slvn. Trg. Kärnten, S Austria
Félegyháza see Kiskunfélegyháza
192 H16 **Feleolo** ✖ (Āpia) Upolu, C Samoa
104 H6 **Felgueiras** Porto, N Portugal
Felicitas Julia see Lisboa
172 J16 **Félicité** island Inner Islands, NE Seychelles
151 K20 **Felidhu Atoll** atoll C Maldives
41 Y13 **Felipe Carrillo Puerto** Quintana Roo, SE Mexico
97 Q21 **Felixstowe** E England, UK
103 N11 **Felletin** Creuse, C France
Fellin see Viljandi
Felsőbánya see Baia Sprie
Felsőmuzslya see Mužlja
Felsővisó see Vişeu de Sus
35 N10 **Felton** California, W USA
106 H7 **Feltre** Veneto, NE Italy
95 H25 **Femerbælt** Ger. Fehmarnbelt. strait Denmark/Germany
95 I24 **Femø** island SE Denmark
94 I10 **Femunden** ◎ S Norway
104 H2 **Fene** Galicia, NW Spain
14 I14 **Fenelon Falls** Ontario, SE Canada
189 U13 **Feneppi** atoll Chuuk Islands, C Micronesia
137 O11 **Fener Burnu** headland N Turkey
115 J14 **Fengári** ▲ Samothráki, E Greece
163 V13 **Fengcheng** var. Feng-cheng, Fenghwangcheng. Liaoning, NE China
160 K11 **Fenggang** prev. Longquan. Guizhou, S China
161 S9 **Fenghua** Zhejiang, SE China
Fenghwangcheng see Fengcheng
160 L9 **Fengjie** Sichuan, C China
160 M14 **Fengkai** prev. Jiankou. Guangdong, S China
161 T13 **Fenglin** Jap. Hōrin. C Taiwan
161 P1 **Fengning** prev. Dagezhen. Hebei, E China
160 E13 **Fengqing** Yunnan, SW China
161 O6 **Fengqiu** Henan, C China
161 Q2 **Fengrun** Hebei, E China
163 T4 **Fengshui Shan** ▲ NE China
161 P14 **Fengshun** Guangdong, S China
Fengtien see Liaoning, China
Fengtien see Shenyang, China
160 J7 **Fengxian** var. Feng Xian; prev. Shuangshipu. Shaanxi, C China
Fengxiang see Luobei
163 P13 **Fengzhen** Nei Mongol Zizhiqu, N China
160 M6 **Fen He** ≈ C China
153 V15 **Feni** Chittagong, E Bangladesh
186 I6 **Feni Islands** island group NE PNG
38 H17 **Fenimore Pass** strait Aleutian Islands, Alaska, USA
84 B9 **Feni Ridge** undersea feature N Atlantic Ocean
Fennern see Vändra
30 J9 **Fennimore** Wisconsin, N USA
172 J4 **Fenoarivo** Toamasina, E Madagascar
95 I24 **Fensmark** Storstrøm, SE Denmark
97 O19 **Fens, The** wetland E England, UK
31 R9 **Fenton** Michigan, N USA
190 K10 **Fenua Fala** island SE Tokelau
190 F12 **Fenuafo'ou, Île** island E Wallis and Futuna
190 L10 **Fenua Loa** island Fakaofo Atoll, E Tokelau
160 M4 **Fenyang** Shanxi, C China
117 U13 **Feodosiya** var. Kefe, It. Kaffa; anc. Theodosia. Respublika Krym, S Ukraine
94 I10 **Feragen** ◎ S Norway
74 L5 **Fer, Cap de** headland NE Algeria
31 O16 **Ferdinand** Indiana, N USA
Ferdinand see Montana, Bulgaria
Ferdinand see Mihail Kogălniceanu, Romania
Ferdinandsberg see Oţelu Roşu
143 T7 **Ferdows** var. Firdaus; prev. Tūn. Khorāsān, E Iran
103 Q5 **Fère-Champenoise** Marne, N France
Ferencz-Jósef Csúcs see Gerlachovský štít
107 J16 **Ferentino** Lazio, C Italy
114 L13 **Féres** Anatolikí Makedonía kai Thráki, NE Greece
Fergana see Farghona
147 S10 **Fergana Valley** var. Farghona Valley, Rus. Ferganskaya Dolina, Taj. Wodii Farghona, Uzb. Farghona Wodiysi. basin Tajikistan/Uzbekistan
Ferganskaya Dolina see Fergana Valley
Ferganskaya Oblast' see Farghona Wiloyati
147 U9 **Ferganskiy Khrebet** ▲ C Kyrgyzstan
14 F15 **Fergus** Ontario, S Canada
29 S6 **Fergus Falls** Minnesota, N USA
186 G9 **Fergusson Island** var. Kaluwawa. island SE PNG
111 K22 **Ferihegy** ✖ (Budapest) Budapest, C Hungary
Ferizaj see Uroševac
77 N14 **Ferkessédougou** N Ivory Coast
109 T10 **Ferlach** Slvn. Borovlje. Kärnten, S Austria
97 E16 **Fermanagh** cultural region SW Northern Ireland, UK
106 J13 **Fermo** anc. Firmum Picenum. Marche, C Italy
104 J6 **Fermoselle** Castilla-León, N Spain
97 D20 **Fermoy** Ir. Mainistir Fhear Maí. SW Ireland
23 W8 **Fernandina Beach** Amelia Island, Florida, SE USA
57 A17 **Fernandina, Isla** var. Narborough Island. island Galapagos Islands, Ecuador, E Pacific Ocean
47 Y5 **Fernando de Noronha** island E Brazil
Fernando Po/Fernando Póo see Bioco, Isla de
60 J7 **Fernandópolis** São Paulo, S Brazil
104 M13 **Fernán Núñez** Andalucía, S Spain
83 Q14 **Fernão Veloso, Baia de** bay NE Mozambique
34 K3 **Ferndale** California, W USA
32 H6 **Ferndale** Washington, NW USA
11 P17 **Fernie** British Columbia, SW Canada
35 R5 **Fernley** Nevada, W USA
Ferozepore see Firozpur
107 N18 **Ferrandina** Basilicata, S Italy
106 G9 **Ferrara** anc. Forum Alieni. Emilia-Romagna, N Italy
120 F9 **Ferrat, Cap** headland NW Algeria
107 D20 **Ferrato, Capo** headland Sardegna, Italy, C Mediterranean Sea
104 G12 **Ferreira do Alentejo** Beja, S Portugal
56 B11 **Ferreñafe** Lambayeque, W Peru
108 C12 **Ferret** Valais, SW Switzerland
102 I13 **Ferret, Cap** headland W France
22 I6 **Ferriday** Louisiana, S USA
Ferro see Hierro
107 D16 **Ferro, Capo** headland Sardegna, Italy, C Mediterranean Sea
104 H2 **Ferrol** var. El Ferrol; prev. El Ferrol del Caudillo. Galicia, NW Spain
56 B12 **Ferrol, Península de** peninsula W Peru
36 M5 **Ferron** Utah, W USA
21 S7 **Ferrum** Virginia, NE USA
23 O8 **Ferry Pass** Florida, SE USA
Ferryville see Menzel Bourguiba
29 S4 **Fertile** Minnesota, N USA
Fertő see Neusiedler See
98 L5 **Ferwerd** Fris. Ferwert. Friesland, N Netherlands
Ferwert see Ferwerd
74 G6 **Fès** Eng. Fez. N Morocco
79 I22 **Feshi** Bandundu, SW Dem. Rep. Congo (Zaire)
29 O4 **Fessenden** North Dakota, N USA
Festenberg see Twardogóra
27 X5 **Festus** Missouri, C USA
116 M14 **Feteşti** Ialomiţa, SE Romania
136 D17 **Fethiye** Muğla, SW Turkey
96 M1 **Fetlar** island NE Scotland, UK
95 I15 **Fetsund** Akershus, S Norway
12 L5 **Feuilles, Lac aux** ◎ Quebec, E Canada
12 L5 **Feuilles, Rivière aux** ≈ Quebec, E Canada
99 M23 **Feulen** Diekirch, C Luxembourg
103 Q11 **Feurs** Loire, E France
95 F18 **Fevik** Aust-Agder, S Norway
123 R13 **Fevral'sk** Amurskaya Oblast', SE Russian Federation
149 S2 **Feyẓābād** var. Faizabad, Faizābād, Feyzābād, Fyzabad. Badakhshān, NE Afghanistan
Fez see Fès
97 J19 **Ffestiniog** NW Wales, UK
Fhóid Duibh, Cuan an see Blacksod Bay
62 I8 **Fiambalá** Catamarca, NW Argentina
172 I6 **Fianarantsoa** Fianarantsoa, C Madagascar
172 H6 **Fianarantsoa** ◆ province SE Madagascar
78 G12 **Fianga** Mayo-Kébbi, SW Chad
Ficce see Fichē
80 J12 **Fichē** It. Ficce. Oromo, C Ethiopia
101 N17 **Fichtelberg** ▲ Czech Republic/Germany
101 M18 **Fichtelgebirge** ▲ SE Germany
101 M19 **Fichtelnaab** ≈ SE Germany
106 E9 **Fidenza** Emilia-Romagna, N Italy
113 K21 **Fier** var. Fieri. Fier, SW Albania
113 K21 **Fier** ◆ district W Albania
Fieri see Fier
Fierza see Fierzë
113 L17 **Fierzë** var. Fierza. Shkodër, N Albania
113 L17 **Fierzës, Liqeni i** ◎ N Albania
108 F10 **Fiesch** Valais, SW Switzerland
106 G11 **Fiesole** Toscana, C Italy
138 G12 **Fifah** Aṭ Ṭafīlah, W Jordan
96 K11 **Fife** var. Kingdom of Fife. cultural region E Scotland, UK
96 K11 **Fife Ness** headland E Scotland, UK
Fifteen Twenty Fracture Zone see Barracuda Fracture Zone
103 N13 **Figeac** Lot, S France
95 N19 **Figeholm** Kalmar, SE Sweden
Figig see Figuig
83 J18 **Figtree** Matabeleland South, SW Zimbabwe
104 F8 **Figueira da Foz** Coimbra, W Portugal
105 X4 **Figueres** Cataluña, E Spain
74 H7 **Figuig** var. Figig. E Morocco
Fijāj, Shaṭṭ al see Fedjaj, Chott el
187 Y15 **Fiji** off. Sovereign Democratic Republic of Fiji, Fij. Viti. ◆ republic SW Pacific Ocean
192 K9 **Fiji** island group SW Pacific Ocean
175 Q8 **Fiji Plate** tectonic feature
105 P14 **Filabres, Sierra de los** ▲ SE Spain
83 K18 **Filabusi** Matabeleland South, S Zimbabwe
42 K13 **Filadelfia** Guanacaste, W Costa Rica
111 K20 **Fil'akovo** Hung. Fülek. Banskobystrický Kraj, C Slovakia
195 N5 **Filchner Ice Shelf** ice shelf Antarctica
14 J11 **Fildegrand** ≈ Quebec, SE Canada
33 O15 **Filer** Idaho, NW USA
Filevo see Vŭrbitsa
116 H14 **Filiaşi** Dolj, SW Romania
115 B16 **Filiátes** Ípeiros, W Greece
115 D21 **Filiatrá** Pelopónnisos, S Greece
107 K22 **Filicudi, Isola** island Isole Eolie, S Italy
141 Y10 **Filim** E Oman
Filimon Sîrbu see Făurei
77 S11 **Filingué** Tillabéri, W Niger
114 K13 **Filiourí** ≈ NE Greece
114 I13 **Fílippoi** anc. Philippi. site of ancient city Anatolikí Makedonía kai Thráki, NE Greece
95 L15 **Filipstad** Värmland, C Sweden
108 I9 **Filisur** Graubünden, S Switzerland
94 E12 **Fillefjell** ▲ S Norway
35 R14 **Fillmore** California, W USA
36 K5 **Fillmore** Utah, W USA
14 J10 **Fils, Lac du** ◎ Quebec, SE Canada
136 H11 **Filyos Çayı** ≈ N Turkey
195 Q2 **Fimbulheimen** physical region Antarctica
195 Q1 **Fimbul Ice Shelf** ice shelf Antarctica
106 G9 **Finale Emilia** Emilia-Romagna, C Italy
106 C10 **Finale Ligure** Liguria, NW Italy
105 P14 **Fiñana** Andalucía, S Spain
172 I6 **Finandrahana** Fianarantsoa, SE Madagascar
21 S6 **Fincastle** Virginia, NE USA
99 M25 **Findel** ✖ (Luxembourg) Luxembourg, C Luxembourg
96 J9 **Findhorn** ≈ N Scotland, UK
31 R12 **Findlay** Ohio, N USA
83 G11 **Finger Lakes** lakes New York, NE USA
83 L14 **Fingoè** Tete, NW Mozambique
136 E17 **Finike** Antalya, SW Turkey
102 F6 **Finistère** ◆ department NW France
186 D7 **Finisterre Range** ▲ N PNG
181 Q8 **Finke** Northern Territory, N Australia
109 S10 **Finkenstein** Kärnten, S Austria
189 Y15 **Finkol, Mount** var. Mount Crozer. ▲ Kosrae, E Micronesia
93 L17 **Finland** off. Republic of Finland, Fin. Suomen Tasavalta, Suomi. ◆ republic N Europe
126 F12 **Finland, Gulf of** Est. Soome Laht, Fin. Suomenlahti, Ger. Finnischer Meerbusen, Rus. Finskiy Zaliv, Swe. Finska Viken. gulf E Baltic Sea
10 L11 **Finlay** ≈ British Columbia, W Canada
183 O10 **Finley** New South Wales, SE Australia
29 Q4 **Finley** North Dakota, N USA
Finnischer Meerbusen see Finland, Gulf of
92 K9 **Finnmark** ◆ county N Norway
92 K9 **Finnmarksvidda** physical region N Norway
92 I9 **Finnsnes** Troms, N Norway
186 E7 **Finschhafen** Morobe, C PNG
94 E13 **Finse** Hordaland, S Norway
Finska Viken/Finskiy Zaliv see Finland, Gulf of
95 M17 **Finspång** Östergötland, S Sweden
108 F10 **Finsteraarhorn** ▲ Switzerland
101 O14 **Finsterwalde** Brandenburg, E Germany
185 A23 **Fiordland** physical region South Island, NZ
106 E9 **Fiorenzuola d'Arda** Emilia-Romagna, C Italy
Firat Nehri see Euphrates
Firdaus see Ferdows
18 M14 **Fire Island** island New York, NE USA
106 G11 **Firenze** Eng. Florence; anc. Florentia. Toscana, C Italy
106 G10 **Firenzuola** Toscana, C Italy
14 C6 **Fire River** Ontario, S Canada
Firliug see Fârliug
61 B19 **Firmat** Santa Fe, C Argentina
103 Q12 **Firminy** Loire, E France
Firmum Picenum see Fermo
152 J12 **Fīrozābād** Uttar Pradesh, N India
152 G8 **Fīrozpur** var. Ferozepore. Punjab, NW India
First State see Delaware
143 O12 **Fīrūzābād** Fārs, S Iran
Fischamend see Fischamend Markt
109 Y4 **Fischamend Markt** var. Fischamend. Niederösterreich, NE Austria
109 W6 **Fischbacher Alpen** ▲ E Austria
Fischhausen see Primorsk
83 D21 **Fish** var. Vis. ≈ S Namibia
83 F24 **Fish** Afr. Vis. ≈ SW South Africa
11 X15 **Fisher Branch** Manitoba, S Canada
11 X15 **Fisher River** Manitoba, S Canada
19 N13 **Fishers Island** island New York, NE USA
37 U8 **Fishers Peak** ▲ Colorado, C USA
9 P9 **Fisher Strait** strait Nunavut, N Canada
97 H21 **Fishguard** Wel. Abergwaun. SW Wales, UK
19 R2 **Fish River Lake** ◎ Maine, NE USA
194 K6 **Fiske, Cape** headland Antarctica
103 P4 **Fismes** Marne, N France
104 F3 **Fisterra, Cabo** headland NW Spain
19 N11 **Fitchburg** Massachusetts, NE USA
96 L3 **Fitful Head** headland NE Scotland, UK
95 C14 **Fitjar** Hordaland, S Norway
192 H16 **Fito** ▲ Upolu, C Samoa
23 U6 **Fitzgerald** Georgia, SE USA
180 M5 **Fitzroy Crossing** Western Australia
63 G21 **Fitzroy, Monte** var. Cerro Chaltel. ▲ S Argentina
181 Y8 **Fitzroy River** ≈ Queensland, E Australia
180 L5 **Fitzroy River** ≈ Western Australia
14 E12 **Fitzwilliam Island** island Ontario, S Canada
107 J15 **Fiuggi** Lazio, C Italy
Fiume see Rijeka
107 H15 **Fiumicino** Lazio, C Italy
Fiumicino see Leonardo da Vinci
106 E10 **Fivizzano** Toscana, C Italy
79 O21 **Fizi** Sud Kivu, E Dem. Rep. Congo (Zaire)
Fizuli see Füzuli
92 I11 **Fjällåsen** Norrbotten, N Sweden
95 G20 **Fjerritslev** Nordjylland, N Denmark
F.J.S. see Franz Josef Strauss
95 L16 **Fjugesta** Örebro, C Sweden
Fladstrand see Frederikshavn
37 V5 **Flagler** Colorado, C USA
23 X10 **Flagler Beach** Florida, SE USA
36 L11 **Flagstaff** Arizona, SW USA
65 H24 **Flagstaff Bay** bay Saint Helena, C Atlantic Ocean
19 P5 **Flagstaff Lake** ◎ Maine, NE USA
94 E13 **Flåm** Sogn og Fjordane, S Norway
15 O8 **Flamand** ≈ Quebec, SE Canada
30 J5 **Flambeau River** ≈ Wisconsin, N USA
97 O16 **Flamborough Head** headland E England, UK
100 N13 **Fläming** hill range NE Germany
16 H8 **Flaming Gorge Reservoir** ▣ Utah/Wyoming, NW USA
99 B18 **Flanders** Dut. Vlaanderen, Fr. Flandre. cultural region Belgium/France
Flandre see Flanders
29 R10 **Flandreau** South Dakota, N USA
96 D6 **Flannan Isles** island group NW Scotland, UK
28 M6 **Flasher** North Dakota, N USA
93 G15 **Flåsjön** ◎ N Sweden
39 O11 **Flat** Alaska, USA
92 H1 **Flateyri** Vestfirdhir, Nw Iceland
33 P8 **Flathead Lake** ◎ Montana, NW USA
173 Y15 **Flat Island** Fr. Île Plate. island N Mauritius
25 T11 **Flatonia** Texas, SW USA
185 M14 **Flat Point** headland North Island, NZ
27 X6 **Flat River** Missouri, C USA
31 P8 **Flat River** ≈ Michigan, N USA
31 P14 **Flatrock River** ≈ Indiana, N USA
32 E6 **Flattery, Cape** headland Washington, NW USA
64 B12 **Flatts Village** var. The Flatts Village. C Bermuda
108 H7 **Flawil** Sankt Gallen, NE Switzerland
97 N22 **Fleet** S England, UK
97 K16 **Fleetwood** NW England, UK
18 H15 **Fleetwood** Pennsylvania, NE USA
95 D18 **Flekkefjord** Vest-Agder, S Norway
21 N5 **Flemingsburg** Kentucky, S USA
18 J15 **Flemington** New Jersey, NE USA
64 J7 **Flemish Cap** undersea feature NW Atlantic Ocean
95 N16 **Flen** Södermanland, C Sweden
100 I6 **Flensburg** Schleswig-Holstein, N Germany
100 J6 **Flensburger Förde** inlet Denmark/Germany
102 K5 **Flers** Orne, N France
95 C14 **Flesland** ✖ (Bergen) Hordaland, S Norway
Flessingue see Vlissingen
21 P10 **Fletcher** North Carolina, SE USA
31 R6 **Fletcher Pond** ◎ Michigan, N USA
102 L15 **Fleurance** Gers, S France
108 B8 **Fleurier** Neuchâtel, W Switzerland
99 H20 **Fleurus** Hainaut, S Belgium
103 N7 **Fleury-les-Aubrais** Loiret, C France
98 K10 **Flevoland** ◆ province C Netherlands
Flickertail State see North Dakota
108 H9 **Flims** Glarus, NE Switzerland
182 F8 **Flinders Island** island Investigator Group, South Australia
183 P14 **Flinders Island** island Furneaux Group, Tasmania, SE Australia
182 I6 **Flinders Ranges** ▲ South Australia
181 U5 **Flinders River** ≈ Queensland, NE Australia
11 V13 **Flin Flon** Manitoba, C Canada
97 K18 **Flint** NE Wales, UK
31 R9 **Flint** Michigan, N USA
97 J18 **Flint** cultural region NE Wales, UK
27 O7 **Flint Hills** hill range Kansas, C USA
191 Y6 **Flint Island** island Line Islands, E Kiribati
23 S4 **Flint River** ≈ Georgia, SE USA
31 R9 **Flint River** ≈ Michigan, N USA
189 X12 **Flipper Point** headland C Wake Island
94 I13 **Flisa** Hedmark, S Norway
94 J13 **Flisa** ≈ S Norway
122 J5 **Flissingskiy, Mys** headland Novaya Zemlya, NW Russian Federation
Flitsch see Bovec
105 U6 **Flix** Cataluña, NE Spain
95 J19 **Floda** Västra Götaland, S Sweden
101 O16 **Flöha** ≈ E Germany
25 O4 **Flomot** Texas, SW USA
29 V5 **Floodwood** Minnesota, N USA
30 M15 **Flora** Illinois, N USA
103 P14 **Florac** Lozère, S France
23 Q8 **Florala** Alabama, S USA
103 S4 **Florange** Moselle, NE France
Floreana, Isla see Santa María, Isla
23 O2 **Florence** Alabama, S USA
36 L14 **Florence** Arizona, SW USA
37 T6 **Florence** Colorado, C USA
27 O5 **Florence** Kansas, C USA
20 M4 **Florence** Kentucky, S USA
32 E13 **Florence** Oregon, NW USA
21 T12 **Florence** South Carolina, SE USA
25 S9 **Florence** Texas, SW USA
Florence see Firenze
54 E13 **Florencia** Caquetá, S Colombia
99 H21 **Florennes** Namur, S Belgium
Florentia see Firenze
63 J18 **Florentino Ameghino, Embalse** ◎ S Argentina
99 J24 **Florenville** Luxembourg, SE Belgium
42 E3 **Flores** Petén, N Guatemala
61 E19 **Flores** ◆ department S Uruguay
171 O16 **Flores** island Nusa Tenggara, C Indonesia
64 M1 **Flores** island Azores, Portugal, NE Atlantic Ocean
Floreshty see Floreşti
Flores, Lago de see Petén Itzá, Lago
Flores, Laut see Flores Sea
171 N15 **Flores Sea** Ind. Laut Flores. sea C Indonesia
116 M8 **Floreşti** Rus. Floreshty. N Moldova
25 S12 **Floresville** Texas, SW USA
59 N14 **Floriano** Piauí, E Brazil
61 K14 **Florianópolis** prev. Destêrro. state capital Santa Catarina, S Brazil
44 G6 **Florida** Camagüey, C Cuba
61 F19 **Florida** Florida, S Uruguay
61 F19 **Florida** ◆ department S Uruguay
23 U9 **Florida** off. State of Florida; also known as Peninsular State, Sunshine State. ◆ state SE USA
23 Y17 **Florida Bay** bay Florida, SE USA
54 G8 **Floridablanca** Santander, N Colombia
23 Y17 **Florida Keys** island group Florida, SE USA
37 Q16 **Florida Mountains** ▲ New Mexico, SW USA
64 D10 **Florida, Straits of** strait Atlantic Ocean/Gulf of Mexico
114 D13 **Flórina** var. Phlórina. Dytikí Makedonía, N Greece
27 X4 **Florissant** Missouri, C USA
94 C11 **Florø** Sogn og Fjordane, S Norway
115 L22 **Floúda, Akrotírio** headland Astypálaia, Kykládes, Greece, Aegean Sea
21 S7 **Floyd** Virginia, NE USA
25 N4 **Floydada** Texas, SW USA
Flüela Wisshorn see Weisshorn
98 K7 **Fluessen** ◎ N Netherlands
105 S5 **Flúmen** ≈ NE Spain
107 C20 **Flumendosa** ≈ Sardegna, Italy, C Mediterranean Sea
31 R9 **Flushing** Michigan, N USA
Flushing see Vlissingen
25 O6 **Fluvanna** Texas, SW USA
186 B8 **Fly** ≈ Indonesia/PNG
194 I10 **Flying Fish, Cape** headland Thurston Island, Antarctica
Flylân see Vlieland
193 Y15 **Foa** island Ha'apai Group, C Tonga
11 U15 **Foam Lake** Saskatchewan, S Canada
113 J14 **Foča** var Srbinje, Republika Srpska, Bosnia and Herzegovina
116 L12 **Focşani** Vrancea, E Romania
Fogaras/Fogarasch see Făgăraş
107 M16 **Foggia** Puglia, SE Italy
Foggo see Faggo
76 D10 **Fogo** island Ilhas de Sotavento, SW Cape Verde
13 U11 **Fogo Island** island Newfoundland, E Canada
109 U7 **Fohnsdorf** Steiermark, SE Austria
100 G7 **Föhr** island NW Germany
104 F14 **Fóia** ▲ S Portugal
14 I10 **Foins, Lac aux** ◎ Quebec, SE Canada
103 N17 **Foix** Ariège, S France
128 I5 **Fokino** Bryanskaya Oblast', W Russian Federation
Fola, Cnoc see Bloody Foreland
94 E13 **Folarskardnuten** ▲ S Norway
92 G11 **Folda** fjord C Norway
93 E14 **Foldafjorden** fjord C Norway
Földvár see Feldioara
93 F14 **Foldereid** Nord-Trøndelag, C Norway
115 J22 **Folégandros** island Kykládes, Greece, Aegean Sea
23 O9 **Foley** Alabama, S USA
29 U7 **Foley** Minnesota, N USA
14 E7 **Foleyet** Ontario, S Canada
95 D14 **Folgefonni** glacier S Norway

◆ Country ● Country Capital ◇ Dependent Territory ○ Dependent Territory Capital ◆ Administrative Region ✖ International Airport ▲ Mountain ▲ Mountain Range Volcano ≈ River ◎ Lake ▣ Reservoir

106 I13 **Foligno** Umbria, C Italy
97 Q23 **Folkestone** SE England, UK
23 W8 **Folkston** Georgia, SE USA
94 H10 **Folldal** Hedmark, S Norway
25 P1 **Follett** Texas, SW USA
106 F13 **Follonica** Toscana, C Italy
21 T15 **Folly Beach** South Carolina, SE USA
35 O7 **Folsom** California, W USA
116 M12 **Folteşti** Galaţi, E Romania
172 H14 **Fomboni** Mohéli, S Comoros
18 K10 **Fonda** New York, NE USA
11 S10 **Fond-du-Lac** Saskatchewan, C Canada
30 M8 **Fond du Lac** Wisconsin, N USA
11 T10 **Fond-du-Lac** ~ Saskatchewan, C Canada
190 C9 **Fongafale** *var.* Funafuti. • (Tuvalu) Funafuti Atoll, SE Tuvalu
190 G8 **Fongafale** *atoll* C Tuvalu
107 C18 **Fonni** Sardegna, Italy, C Mediterranean Sea
189 V12 **Fono** *island* Chuuk, C Micronesia
54 G4 **Fonseca** La Guajira, N Colombia
Fonseca, Golfo de *see* Fonseca, Gulf of
42 H8 **Fonseca, Gulf of** *Sp.* Golfo de Fonseca. *gulf* Central America
103 O6 **Fontainebleau** Seine-et-Marne, N France
63 G19 **Fontana, Lago** ⊚ W Argentina
21 N10 **Fontana Lake** ⊠ North Carolina, SE USA
107 L24 **Fontanarossa** ✕ (Catania) Sicilia, Italy, C Mediterranean Sea
11 N11 **Fontas** ~ British Columbia, W Canada
58 D12 **Fonte Boa** Amazonas, N Brazil
102 J10 **Fontenay-le-Comte** Vendée, NW France
33 T16 **Fontenelle Reservoir** ⊠ Wyoming, C USA
193 Y14 **Fonualei** *island* Vava'u Group, N Tonga
111 H24 **Fonyód** Somogy, W Hungary
Foochow *see* Fuzhou
39 Q10 **Foraker, Mount** ▲ Alaska, USA
187 R14 **Forari** Éfaté, C Vanuatu
103 U4 **Forbach** Moselle, NE France
183 Q8 **Forbes** New South Wales, SE Australia
77 T17 **Forcados** Delta, S Nigeria
103 S14 **Forcalquier** Alpes-de-Haute-Provence, SE France
101 K19 **Forchheim** Bayern, SE Germany
35 R13 **Ford City** California, W USA
94 D11 **Førde** Sogn og Fjordane, S Norway
31 N4 **Ford River** ~ Michigan, N USA
183 O4 **Fords Bridge** New South Wales, SE Australia
20 J6 **Fordsville** Kentucky, S USA
27 U13 **Fordyce** Arkansas, C USA
76 I14 **Forécariah** Guinée-Maritime, SW Guinea
197 O14 **Forel, Mont** ▲ SE Greenland
11 R17 **Foremost** Alberta, SW Canada
14 D16 **Forest** Ontario, S Canada
22 L5 **Forest** Mississippi, S USA
31 S12 **Forest** Ohio, N USA
29 V11 **Forest City** Iowa, C USA
21 Q10 **Forest City** North Carolina, SE USA
32 G11 **Forest Grove** Oregon, NW USA
183 P17 **Forestier Peninsula** *peninsula* Tasmania, SE Australia
29 V8 **Forest Lake** Minnesota, N USA
23 S3 **Forest Park** Georgia, SE USA
29 Q3 **Forest River** ~ North Dakota, N USA
15 T6 **Forestville** Quebec, SE Canada
103 Q11 **Forez, Monts du** ▲ C France
96 K10 **Forfar** E Scotland, UK
26 J8 **Forgan** Oklahoma, C USA
Forge du Sud *see* Dudelange
101 J24 **Forggensee** ⊚ S Germany
147 N10 **Forish** *Rus.* Farish. Jizzakh Wiloyati, C Uzbekistan
20 F9 **Forked Deer River** ~ Tennessee, S USA
32 F7 **Forks** Washington, NW USA
92 N2 **Forlandsundet** *sound* W Svalbard
106 H10 **Forlì** *anc.* Forum Livii. Emilia-Romagna, N Italy
29 Q7 **Forman** North Dakota, N USA
97 K17 **Formby** NW England, UK
105 V11 **Formentera** *anc.* Ophiusa, *Lat.* Frumentum. *island* Islas Baleares, Spain, W Mediterranean Sea
Formentor, Cabo de *see* Formentor, Cap de
105 Y9 **Formentor, Cap de** *var.* Cabo de Formentor, Cape Formentor. *headland* Mallorca, Spain, W Mediterranean Sea
Formentor, Cape *see* Formentor, Cap de
107 J16 **Formia** Lazio, C Italy
62 O7 **Formosa** Formosa, NE Argentina
62 M6 **Formosa** *off.* Provincia de Formosa. ◈ *province* NE Argentina
Formosa/Formo'sa *see* Taiwan
59 I17 **Formosa, Serra** ▲ C Brazil
Formosa Strait *see* Taiwan Strait
95 H15 **Fornebu** ✕ (Oslo) Akershus, S Norway
25 U6 **Forney** Texas, SW USA
95 H21 **Fornæs** *headland* C Denmark
106 E9 **Fornovo di Taro** Emilia-Romagna, C Italy
117 T14 **Foros** Respublika Krym, S Ukraine
Føroyar *see* Faeroe Islands
96 J8 **Forres** NE Scotland, UK
27 X11 **Forrest City** Arkansas, C USA
39 Y15 **Forrester Island** *island* Alexander Archipelago, Alaska, USA
25 N7 **Forsan** Texas, SW USA
181 V5 **Forsayth** Queensland, NE Australia
95 L19 **Forserum** Jönköping, S Sweden
95 K15 **Forshaga** Värmland, C Sweden
93 L19 **Forssa** Etelä-Suomi, S Finland
101 Q14 **Forst** *Lus.* Baršć Łužyca. Brandenburg, E Germany
183 U7 **Forster-Tuncurry** New South Wales, SE Australia
23 T4 **Forsyth** Georgia, SE USA
27 T8 **Forsyth** Missouri, C USA
33 W10 **Forsyth** Montana, NW USA
149 U11 **Fort Abbās** Punjab, E Pakistan
12 G10 **Fort Albany** Ontario, C Canada
56 L13 **Fortaleza** Pando, N Bolivia
58 P13 **Fortaleza** *prev.* Ceará. *state capital* Ceará, NE Brazil
59 D16 **Fortaleza** Rondônia, W Brazil
56 C13 **Fortaleza, Río** ~ W Peru
Fort-Archambault *see* Sarh
21 U3 **Fort Ashby** West Virginia, NE USA
96 I9 **Fort Augustus** N Scotland, UK
Fort-Bayard *see* Zhanjiang
33 S8 **Fort Benton** Montana, NW USA
35 Q1 **Fort Bidwell** California, W USA
34 L5 **Fort Bragg** California, W USA
31 N16 **Fort Branch** Indiana, N USA
Fort-Bretonnet *see* Bousso
33 T17 **Fort Bridger** Wyoming, C USA
Fort-Cappolani *see* Tidjikja
Fort Charlet *see* Djanet
Fort-Chimo *see* Kuujjuaq
11 R10 **Fort Chipewyan** Alberta, C Canada
Fort Cobb Lake *see* Fort Cobb Reservoir
26 L11 **Fort Cobb Reservoir** *var.* Fort Cobb Lake. ⊠ Oklahoma, C USA
37 T3 **Fort Collins** Colorado, C USA
14 K12 **Fort-Coulonge** Quebec, SE Canada
Fort-Crampel *see* Kaga Bandoro
Fort-Dauphin *see* Tôlanaro
24 K10 **Fort Davis** Texas, SW USA
37 O10 **Fort Defiance** Arizona, SW USA
45 Q12 **Fort-de-France** *prev.* Fort-Royal. ○ (Martinique) W Martinique
45 P12 **Fort-de-France, Baie de** *bay* W Martinique
Fort de Kock *see* Bukittinggi
23 P6 **Fort Deposit** Alabama, S USA
29 U13 **Fort Dodge** Iowa, C USA
13 S10 **Forteau** Quebec, E Canada
106 E11 **Forte dei Marmi** Toscana, C Italy
14 H17 **Fort Erie** Ontario, S Canada
180 H7 **Fortescue River** ~ Western Australia
19 S2 **Fort Fairfield** Maine, NE USA
Fort-Foureau *see* Kousséri
12 A11 **Fort Frances** Ontario, S Canada
Fort Franklin *see* Déljne
23 R7 **Fort Gaines** Georgia, SE USA
37 T8 **Fort Garland** Colorado, C USA
21 P5 **Fort Gay** West Virginia, NE USA
Fort George *see* La Grande Rivière
27 Q10 **Fort Gibson** Oklahoma, C USA
27 Q9 **Fort Gibson Lake** ⊠ Oklahoma, C USA
8 H7 **Fort Good Hope** *var.* Good Hope. Northwest Territories, NW Canada
23 V4 **Fort Gordon** Georgia, SE USA
Fort Gouraud *see* Fdérik
96 I11 **Forth** ~ C Scotland, UK
Fort Hall *see* Murang'a
24 H8 **Fort Hancock** Texas, SW USA
Fort Hertz *see* Putao
96 K12 **Forth, Firth of** *estuary* E Scotland, UK
14 L14 **Forthton** Ontario, SE Canada
14 M8 **Fortier** ~ Quebec, SE Canada
Fortín General Eugenio Garay *see* General Eugenio A. Garay
Fort Jameson *see* Chipata
Fort Johnston *see* Mangochi
19 R1 **Fort Kent** Maine, NE USA
Fort-Lamy *see* Ndjamena
23 Z15 **Fort Lauderdale** Florida, SE USA
21 R11 **Fort Lawn** South Carolina, SE USA
8 H10 **Fort Liard** *var.* Liard. Northwest Territories, W Canada
44 M8 **Fort-Liberté** NE Haiti
21 N9 **Fort Loudoun Lake** ⊠ Tennessee, S USA
37 T3 **Fort Lupton** Colorado, C USA
11 R12 **Fort MacKay** Alberta, C Canada
11 Q17 **Fort Macleod** *var.* MacLeod. Alberta, SW Canada
29 Y16 **Fort Madison** Iowa, C USA
Fort Manning *see* Mchinji
25 P9 **Fort McKavett** Texas, SW USA
11 R12 **Fort McMurray** Alberta, C Canada
8 G7 **Fort McPherson** *var.* McPherson. Northwest Territories, NW Canada
21 R11 **Fort Mill** South Carolina, SE USA
Fort-Millot *see* Ngouri
37 U3 **Fort Morgan** Colorado, C USA
23 W14 **Fort Myers** Florida, SE USA
23 W15 **Fort Myers Beach** Florida, SE USA
10 M10 **Fort Nelson** British Columbia, W Canada
10 M10 **Fort Nelson** ~ British Columbia, W Canada
Fort Norman *see* Tulita.
23 Q2 **Fort Payne** Alabama, S USA
33 W7 **Fort Peck** Montana, NW USA
33 V8 **Fort Peck Lake** ⊠ Montana, NW USA
23 Y13 **Fort Pierce** Florida, SE USA
29 N10 **Fort Pierre** South Dakota, N USA
81 E18 **Fort Portal** SW Uganda
8 J10 **Fort Providence** *var.* Providence. Northwest Territories, W Canada
11 U16 **Fort Qu'Appelle** Saskatchewan, S Canada
Fort-Repoux *see* Akjoujt
8 K10 **Fort Resolution** *var.* Resolution. Northwest Territories, W Canada
33 T13 **Fortress Mountain** ▲ Wyoming, C USA
Fort Rosebery *see* Mansa
Fort-Rousset *see* Owando
Fort-Royal *see* Fort-de-France
12 I10 **Fort Rupert** *prev.* Rupert House. Quebec, SE Canada
8 H13 **Fort St.James** British Columbia, SW Canada
11 N12 **Fort St.John** British Columbia, W Canada
Fort Sandeman *see* Zhob
11 Q14 **Fort Saskatchewan** Alberta, SW Canada
27 R6 **Fort Scott** Kansas, C USA
12 E6 **Fort Severn** Ontario, C Canada
31 R12 **Fort Shawnee** Ohio, N USA
144 E14 **Fort-Shevchenko** Mangistau, W Kazakhstan
Fort-Sibut *see* Sibut
8 I10 **Fort Simpson** *var.* Simpson. Northwest Territories, W Canada
8 K11 **Fort Smith** *district capital* Northwest Territories, W Canada
27 R10 **Fort Smith** Arkansas, C USA
37 T13 **Fort Stanton** New Mexico, SW USA
24 L9 **Fort Stockton** Texas, SW USA
37 U12 **Fort Sumner** New Mexico, SW USA
26 K8 **Fort Supply** Oklahoma, C USA
26 K8 **Fort Supply Lake** ⊠ Oklahoma, C USA
29 O10 **Fort Thompson** South Dakota, N USA
Fort-Trinquet *see* Bîr Mogreïn
105 R12 **Fortuna** Murcia, SE Spain
34 K3 **Fortuna** California, W USA
28 J2 **Fortuna** North Dakota, N USA
23 T5 **Fort Valley** Georgia, SE USA
11 P11 **Fort Vermilion** Alberta, W Canada
Fort Victoria *see* Masvingo
31 P13 **Fortville** Indiana, N USA
23 P9 **Fort Walton Beach** Florida, SE USA
31 P12 **Fort Wayne** Indiana, N USA
96 H10 **Fort William** N Scotland, UK
25 T6 **Fort Worth** Texas, SW USA
28 M7 **Fort Yates** North Dakota, N USA
39 S7 **Fort Yukon** Alaska, USA
Forum Alieni *see* Ferrara
Forum Julii *see* Fréjus
Forum Livii *see* Forlì
143 Q15 **Forūr, Jazīreh-ye** *island* S Iran
94 H7 **Fosen** *physical region* S Norway
161 N14 **Foshan** *var.* Fatshan, Foshan, Namhoi. Guangdong, S China
Fossa Claudia *see* Chioggia
106 B9 **Fossano** Piemonte, NW Italy
99 H21 **Fosses-la-Ville** Namur, S Belgium
32 J12 **Fossil** Oregon, NW USA
Foss Lake *see* Foss Reservoir
106 I11 **Fossombrone** Marche, C Italy
26 K10 **Foss Reservoir** *var.* Foss Lake. ⊠ Oklahoma, C USA
29 S4 **Fosston** Minnesota, N USA
183 O13 **Foster** Victoria, SE Australia
11 T12 **Foster Lakes** ⊚ Saskatchewan, C Canada
31 S12 **Fostoria** Ohio, N USA
79 D19 **Fougamou** Ngounié, C Gabon
102 J6 **Fougères** Ille-et-Vilaine, NW France
Fou-hsin *see* Fuxin
27 S14 **Fouke** Arkansas, C USA
96 K2 **Foula** *island* NE Scotland, UK
65 D24 **Foul Bay** *bay* East Falkland, Falkland Islands
97 P21 **Foulness Island** *island* SE England, UK
185 F15 **Foulwind, Cape** *headland* South Island, NZ
79 E15 **Foumban** Ouest, NW Cameroon
172 H13 **Foumbouni** Grande Comore, NW Comoros
195 N8 **Foundation Ice Stream** *glacier* Antarctica
37 T6 **Fountain** Colorado, C USA
36 L4 **Fountain Green** Utah, W USA
21 P11 **Fountain Inn** South Carolina, SE USA
27 S11 **Fourche LaFave River** ~ Arkansas, C USA
33 Z13 **Four Corners** Wyoming, C USA
103 Q2 **Fourmies** Nord, N France
38 J17 **Four Mountains, Islands of** *island group* Aleutian Islands, Alaska, USA
173 P17 **Fournaise, Piton de la** ▲ SE Réunion
14 J8 **Fournière, Lac** ⊚ Quebec, SE Canada
115 L20 **Foúrnoi** *island* Dodekánisos, Greece, Aegean Sea
64 K13 **Four North Fracture Zone** *tectonic feature* W Atlantic Ocean
Fouron-Saint-Martin *see* Sint-Martens-Voeren
30 L3 **Fourteen Mile Point** *headland* Michigan, N USA
76 I13 **Fouta Djallon** *var.* Futa Jallon. ▲ W Guinea
185 C25 **Foveaux Strait** *strait* S NZ
35 Q11 **Fowler** California, W USA
37 U6 **Fowler** Colorado, C USA
31 N12 **Fowler** Indiana, N USA
182 D7 **Fowlers Bay** *bay* South Australia
25 R13 **Fowlerton** Texas, SW USA
142 M3 **Fowman** *var.* Fuman, Fumen. Gīlān, NW Iran
65 C25 **Fox Bay East** West Falkland, Falkland Islands
65 C25 **Fox Bay West** West Falkland, Falkland Islands
14 J14 **Foxboro** Ontario, SE Canada
11 O14 **Fox Creek** Alberta, W Canada
64 G5 **Foxe Basin** *sea* Nunavut, N Canada
64 G5 **Foxe Channel** *channel* Nunavut, N Canada
95 I16 **Foxen** ⊚ C Sweden
9 Q7 **Foxe Peninsula** *peninsula* Baffin Island, Nunavut, NE Canada
185 E19 **Fox Glacier** West Coast, South Island, NZ
38 L17 **Fox Islands** *island* Aleutian Islands, Alaska, USA
30 M10 **Fox Lake** Illinois, N USA
11 V12 **Fox Mine** Manitoba, C Canada
35 R3 **Fox Mountain** ▲ Nevada, W USA
65 E25 **Fox Point** *headland* East Falkland, Falkland Islands
30 M11 **Fox River** ~ Illinois/Wisconsin, N USA
30 L7 **Fox River** ~ Wisconsin, N USA
184 L13 **Foxton** Manawatu-Wanganui, North Island, NZ
11 S16 **Fox Valley** Saskatchewan, S Canada
11 W16 **Foxwarren** Manitoba, S Canada
97 E14 **Foyle, Lough** *Ir.* Loch Feabhail. *inlet* N Ireland
194 H5 **Foyn Coast** *physical region* Antarctica
104 I2 **Foz** Galicia, NW Spain
60 I12 **Foz do Areia, Represa de** ⊠ S Brazil
59 A16 **Foz do Breu** Acre, W Brazil
83 A16 **Foz do Cunene** Namibe, SW Angola
60 G12 **Foz do Iguaçu** Paraná, S Brazil
58 C12 **Foz do Mamoriá** Amazonas, NW Brazil
105 T6 **Fraga** Aragón, NE Spain
44 F5 **Fragoso, Cayo** *island* C Cuba
61 G18 **Fraile Muerto** Cerro Largo, NE Uruguay
99 H21 **Fraire** Namur, S Belgium
99 L21 **Fraiture, Baraque de** *hill* SE Belgium
Frakštát *see* Hlohovec
197 S10 **Fram Basin** *var.* Amundsen Basin. *undersea feature* Arctic Ocean
99 F20 **Frameries** Hainaut, S Belgium
19 O11 **Framingham** Massachusetts, NE USA
60 L7 **Franca** São Paulo, S Brazil
187 O15 **Français, Récif des** *reef* W New Caledonia
107 K14 **Francavilla al Mare** Abruzzo, C Italy
107 P18 **Francavilla Fontana** Puglia, SE Italy
102 M8 **France** *off.* French Republic, *It./Sp.* Francia; *prev.* Gaul, Gaule, *Lat.* Gallia. ◆ *republic* W Europe
45 O8 **Francés Viejo, Cabo** *headland* NE Dominican Republic
79 F19 **Franceville** *var.* Massoukou, Masuku. Haut-Ogooué, E Gabon
79 F19 **Franceville** ✕ Haut-Ogooué, E Gabon
Francfort *see* Frankfurt am Main
103 T8 **Franche-Comté** ◈ *region* E France
Francia *see* France
29 O11 **Francis Case, Lake** ⊠ South Dakota, N USA
60 H12 **Francisco Beltrão** Paraná, S Brazil
Francisco l. Madero *see* Villa Madero
61 A21 **Francisco Madero** Buenos Aires, E Argentina
42 H6 **Francisco Morazán** *prev.* Tegucigalpa. ◈ *department* C Honduras
83 J18 **Francistown** North East, NE Botswana
Franconian Forest *see* Frankenwald
Franconian Jura *see* Fränkische Alb
98 K6 **Franeker** *Fris.* Frjentsjer. Friesland, N Netherlands
Frankenalb *see* Fränkische Alb
101 H16 **Frankenberg** Hessen, C Germany
101 J20 **Frankenhöhe** *hill range* C Germany
31 R8 **Frankenmuth** Michigan, N USA
101 F20 **Frankenstein** *hill* W Germany
Frankenstein/Frankenstein in Schlesien *see* Ząbkowice Śląskie
101 G20 **Frankenthal** Rheinland-Pfalz, W Germany
101 L18 **Frankenwald** *Eng.* Franconian Forest. ▲ C Germany
44 J12 **Frankfield** C Jamaica
14 J14 **Frankford** Ontario, SE Canada
31 O13 **Frankfort** Indiana, N USA
27 O3 **Frankfort** Kansas, C USA
20 L5 **Frankfort** *state capital* Kentucky, S USA
Frankfort on the Main *see* Frankfurt am Main
Frankfurt *see* Słubice, Poland
Frankfurt *see* Frankfurt am Main, Germany
101 G18 **Frankfurt am Main** *var.* Frankfurt, *Fr.* Francfort; *prev. Eng.* Frankfort on the Main. Hessen, SW Germany
100 Q12 **Frankfurt an der Oder** Brandenburg, E Germany
101 L21 **Fränkische Alb** *var.* Frankenalb, *Eng.* Franconian Jura. ▲ S Germany
101 I18 **Fränkische Saale** ~ C Germany
101 L19 **Fränkische Schweiz** *hill range* C Germany
23 R4 **Franklin** Georgia, SE USA
31 P14 **Franklin** Indiana, N USA
20 J7 **Franklin** Kentucky, S USA
22 I9 **Franklin** Louisiana, S USA
29 O17 **Franklin** Nebraska, C USA
21 N10 **Franklin** North Carolina, SE USA
18 C13 **Franklin** Pennsylvania, NE USA
20 J9 **Franklin** Tennessee, S USA
25 U9 **Franklin** Texas, SW USA
21 X7 **Franklin** Virginia, NE USA
21 T4 **Franklin** West Virginia, NE USA
30 M9 **Franklin** Wisconsin, N USA
8 I6 **Franklin Bay** *inlet* Northwest Territories, N Canada
32 K7 **Franklin D.Roosevelt Lake** ⊠ Washington, NW USA
35 W4 **Franklin Lake** ⊚ Nevada, W USA
185 B22 **Franklin Mountains** ▲ South Island, NZ
39 R5 **Franklin Mountains** ▲ Alaska, USA
39 N4 **Franklin, Point** *headland* Alaska, USA
183 O17 **Franklin River** ~ Tasmania, SE Australia
22 K8 **Franklinton** Louisiana, S USA
21 U9 **Franklinton** North Carolina, SE USA
Frankstadt *see* Frenštát pod Radhoštěm
25 V7 **Frankston** Texas, SW USA
33 U12 **Frannie** Wyoming, C USA
15 U5 **Franquelin** Quebec, SE Canada
15 U5 **Franquelin** ~ Quebec, SE Canada
83 C18 **Fransfontein** Kunene, NW Namibia
93 H17 **Fränsta** Västernorrland, C Sweden
122 J3 **Frantsa-Iosifa, Zemlya** *Eng.* Franz Josef Land. *island group* N Russian Federation
185 E18 **Franz Josef Glacier** West Coast, South Island, NZ
Franz Josef Land *see* Frantsa-Iosifa, Zemlya
Franz-Josef Spitze *see* Gerlachovský štít
101 L23 **Franz Josef Strauss** *abbrev.* F.J.S. ✕ (München) Bayern, SE Germany
107 A19 **Frasca, Capo della** *headland* Sardegna, Italy, C Mediterranean Sea
107 I15 **Frascati** Lazio, C Italy
11 N14 **Fraser** ~ British Columbia, SW Canada
83 G24 **Fraserburg** Western Cape, SW South Africa
96 L8 **Fraserburgh** NE Scotland, UK
181 Z9 **Fraser Island** *var.* Great Sandy Island. *island* Queensland, E Australia
10 L14 **Fraser Lake** British Columbia, SW Canada
10 L15 **Fraser Plateau** *plateau* British Columbia, SW Canada
184 P10 **Frasertown** Hawke's Bay, North Island, NZ
99 E19 **Frasnes-lez-Buissenal** Hainaut, SW Belgium
108 I7 **Frastanz** Vorarlberg, NW Austria
14 B8 **Frater** Ontario, S Canada
Frauenbach *see* Baia Mare
Frauenburg *see* Saldus, Latvia
Frauenburg *see* Frombork, Poland
108 H6 **Frauenfeld** Thurgau, NE Switzerland
109 Z5 **Frauenkirchen** Burgenland, E Austria
61 D19 **Fray Bentos** Río Negro, W Uruguay
61 F19 **Fray Marcos** Florida, S Uruguay
29 S6 **Frazee** Minnesota, N USA
104 M5 **Frechilla** Castilla-León, N Spain
30 I4 **Frederic** Wisconsin, N USA
95 G23 **Fredericia** Vejle, C Denmark
21 W3 **Frederick** Maryland, NE USA
26 L12 **Frederick** Oklahoma, C USA
29 P7 **Frederick** South Dakota, N USA
29 X12 **Fredericksburg** Iowa, C USA
25 R10 **Fredericksburg** Texas, SW USA
21 W5 **Fredericksburg** Virginia, NE USA
39 X13 **Frederick Sound** *sound* Alaska, USA
27 X6 **Fredericktown** Missouri, C USA
60 H13 **Frederico Westphalen** Rio Grande do Sul, S Brazil
13 O15 **Fredericton** New Brunswick, SE Canada
95 I22 **Frederiksborg** *off.* Frederiksborgs Amt. ◈ *county* E Denmark
Frederikshåb *see* Paamiut
95 H19 **Frederikshavn** *prev.* Fladstrand. Nordjylland, N Denmark
95 J22 **Frederikssund** Frederiksborg, E Denmark
45 T9 **Frederiksted** Saint Croix, S Virgin Islands (US)
95 I22 **Frederiksværk** *var.* Frederiksværk og Hanehoved. Frederiksborg, E Denmark
Frederiksværk og Hanehoved *see* Frederiksværk
54 E9 **Fredonia** Antioquia, W Colombia
36 K8 **Fredonia** Arizona, SW USA
27 P7 **Fredonia** Kansas, C USA
18 C11 **Fredonia** New York, NE USA
35 P4 **Fredonyer Pass** *pass* California, W USA
93 I15 **Fredrika** Västerbotten, N Sweden
95 L14 **Fredriksberg** Dalarna, C Sweden
Fredrikshald *see* Halden
Fredrikshamn *see* Hamina
95 H16 **Fredrikstad** Østfold, S Norway
30 K16 **Freeburg** Illinois, N USA
18 K15 **Freehold** New Jersey, NE USA
18 H14 **Freeland** Pennsylvania, NE USA
182 J5 **Freeling Heights** ▲ South Australia
35 Q7 **Freel Peak** ▲ California, W USA
9 Z9 **Freels, Cape** *headland* Newfoundland, E Canada
29 Q11 **Freeman** South Dakota, N USA
44 G1 **Freeport** Grand Bahama Island, N Bahamas
30 L10 **Freeport** Illinois, N USA
25 W12 **Freeport** Texas, SW USA
44 G1 **Freeport** ✕ Grand Bahama Island, N Bahamas
25 R14 **Freer** Texas, SW USA
83 I22 **Free State** *off.* Free State Province; *prev.* Orange Free State, *Afr.* Oranje Vrystaat. ◈ *province* C South Africa
Free State *see* Maryland
76 G15 **Freetown** • (Sierra Leone) W Sierra Leone
172 J16 **Frégate** *island* Inner Islands, NE Seychelles
104 J12 **Fregenal de la Sierra** Extremadura, W Spain
182 C2 **Fregon** South Australia
102 H5 **Fréhel, Cap** *headland* NW France
94 F8 **Frei** Møre og Romsdal, S Norway
101 O16 **Freiberg** Sachsen, E Germany
101 O16 **Freiberger Mulde** ~ E Germany
Freiburg *see* Fribourg, Switzerland
Freiburg *see* Freiburg im Breisgau, Germany
101 F23 **Freiburg im Breisgau** *var.* Freiburg, *Fr.* Fribourg-en-Brisgau. Baden-Württemberg, SW Germany
Freiburg in Schlesien *see* Świebodzice
Freie Hansestadt Bremen *see* Bremen
Freie und Hansestadt Hamburg *see* Brandenburg
101 L22 **Freising** Bayern, SE Germany
109 T3 **Freistadt** Oberösterreich, N Austria
Freistadtl *see* Hlohovec
101 O16 **Freital** Sachsen, E Germany
Freiwaldau *see* Jeseník
104 J6 **Freixo de Espada à Cinta** Bragança, N Portugal
103 U15 **Fréjus** *anc.* Forum Julii. Var, SE France
180 I13 **Fremantle** Western Australia
35 N9 **Fremont** California, W USA
31 Q11 **Fremont** Indiana, N USA
29 W15 **Fremont** Iowa, C USA
31 P8 **Fremont** Michigan, N USA
29 R15 **Fremont** Nebraska, C USA
31 S11 **Fremont** Ohio, N USA
33 T14 **Fremont Peak** ▲ Wyoming, C USA
36 M6 **Fremont River** ~ Utah, W USA
21 O9 **French Broad River** ~ Tennessee, S USA
21 N5 **Frenchburg** Kentucky, S USA
18 C12 **French Creek** ~ Pennsylvania, NE USA
32 K15 **Frenchglen** Oregon, NW USA
55 Y10 **French Guiana** *var.* Guiana, Guyane. ◇ *French overseas department* N South America
French Guinea *see* Guinea
31 O15 **French Lick** Indiana, N USA
185 J14 **French Pass** Marlborough, South Island, NZ
191 T11 **French Polynesia** ◇ *French overseas territory* C Polynesia
French Republic *see* France
14 F11 **French River** ~ Ontario, S Canada
French Somaliland *see* Djibouti
173 P12 **French Southern and Antarctic Territories** *Fr.* Terres Australes et Antarctiques Françaises. ◇ *French overseas territory* S Indian Ocean
French Sudan *see* Mali
French Territory of the Afars and Issas *see* Djibouti
French Togoland *see* Togo
74 J6 **Frenda** NW Algeria
111 I18 **Frenštát pod Radhoštěm** *Ger.* Frankstadt. Ostravský Kraj E Czech Republic
76 M17 **Fresco** S Ivory Coast
195 U16 **Freshfield, Cape** *headland* Antarctica
40 L10 **Fresnillo** *var.* Fresnillo de González Echeverría. Zacatecas, C Mexico
Fresnillo de González Echeverría *see* Fresnillo

◆ Country • Country Capital ◇ Dependent Territory ○ Dependent Territory Capital ◈ Administrative Region ✕ International Airport ▲ Mountain ▲ Mountain Range ⋀ Volcano ~ River ⊚ Lake ⊠ Reservoir

35 Q10 **Fresno** California, W USA
Freu, Cabo del see Freu, Cap des
105 Y9 **Freu, Cap des** var. Cabo del Freu. headland Mallorca, Spain, W Mediterranean Sea
101 G22 **Freudenstadt** Baden-Württemberg, SW Germany
Freudenthal see Bruntál
183 Q17 **Freycinet Peninsula** peninsula Tasmania, SE Australia
76 H14 **Fria** Guinée-Maritime, W Guinea
83 A17 **Fria, Cape** headland NW Namibia
35 Q10 **Friant** California, W USA
62 K8 **Frías** Catamarca, N Argentina
108 D9 **Fribourg** Ger. Freiburg. Fribourg, W Switzerland
108 C9 **Fribourg** Ger. Freiburg. ◈ canton W Switzerland
Fribourg-en-Brisgau see Freiburg im Breisgau
32 G7 **Friday Harbor** San Juan Islands, Washington, NW USA
Friedau see Ormož
101 K23 **Friedberg** Bayern, S Germany
101 H18 **Friedberg** Hessen, W Germany
Friedeberg Neumark see Strzelce Krajeńskie
Friedek-Mistek see Frýdek-Místek
Friedland see Pravdinsk
101 I24 **Friedrichshafen** Baden-Württemberg, S Germany
Friedrichstadt see Jaunjelgava
29 Q16 **Friend** Nebraska, C USA
Friendly Islands see Tonga
55 V9 **Friendship** Coronie, N Suriname
30 L7 **Friendship** Wisconsin, N USA
109 T8 **Friesach** Kärnten, S Austria
Friesche Eilanden see Frisian Islands
101 F22 **Friesenheim** Baden-Württemberg, SW Germany
Friesische Inseln see Frisian Islands
98 K6 **Friesland** ◈ province N Netherlands
60 Q10 **Frio, Cabo** headland SE Brazil
24 M3 **Friona** Texas, SW USA
42 L12 **Frío, Río** ≈ N Costa Rica
25 R13 **Frio River** ≈ Texas, SW USA
99 M25 **Frisange** Luxembourg, S Luxembourg
Frisches Haff see Vistula Lagoon
36 J6 **Frisco Peak** ▲ Utah, W USA
84 F9 **Frisian Islands** Dut. Friesche Eilanden, Ger. Friesische Inseln. island group N Europe
18 L12 **Frissell, Mount** ▲ Connecticut, NE USA
95 J19 **Fristad** Västra Götaland, S Sweden
25 N2 **Fritch** Texas, SW USA
95 J19 **Fritsla** Västra Götaland, S Sweden
101 H16 **Fritzlar** Hessen, C Germany
106 H6 **Friuli-Venezia Giulia** ◈ region NE Italy
Frjentsjer see Franeker
196 L13 **Frobisher Bay** inlet Baffin Island, Nunavut, NE Canada
Frobisher Bay see Iqaluit
11 S12 **Frobisher Lake** ◎ Saskatchewan, C Canada
94 G7 **Frohavet** sound C Norway
Frohenbruck see Veselí nad Lužnicí
109 V7 **Frohnleiten** Steiermark, SE Austria
99 G22 **Froidchapelle** Hainaut, S Belgium
129 O9 **Frolovo** Volgogradskaya Oblast', SW Russian Federation
110 K7 **Frombork** Ger. Frauenburg. Warmińsko-Mazurskie, NE Poland
97 L22 **Frome** SW England, UK
182 I4 **Frome Creek** seasonal river South Australia
182 J6 **Frome Downs** South Australia
182 J5 **Frome, Lake** salt lake South Australia
Fronicken see Wronki
104 H10 **Fronteira** Portalegre, C Portugal
40 M7 **Frontera** Coahuila de Zaragoza, NE Mexico
41 U14 **Frontera** Tabasco, SE Mexico
40 G3 **Fronteras** Sonora, NW Mexico
103 Q16 **Frontignan** Hérault, S France
54 D8 **Frontino** Antioquia, NW Colombia
21 V4 **Front Royal** Virginia, NE USA
107 J16 **Frosinone** anc. Frusino. Lazio, C Italy
107 K16 **Frosolone** Molise, C Italy
25 U7 **Frost** Texas, SW USA
21 U2 **Frostburg** Maryland, NE USA
23 X13 **Frostproof** Florida, SE USA
Frostviken see Kvarnbergsvattnet
95 M15 **Frövi** Örebro, C Sweden
94 F7 **Frøya** island W Norway
37 P5 **Fruita** Colorado, C USA
28 J9 **Fruitdale** South Dakota, N USA
23 W11 **Fruitland Park** Florida, SE USA
Frumentum see Formentera
147 S11 **Frunze** Oshskaya Oblast', SW Kyrgyzstan
Frunze see Bishkek
117 O9 **Frunzivka** Odes'ka Oblast', SW Ukraine
Frusino see Frosinone
108 E9 **Frutigen** Bern, W Switzerland
111 I17 **Frýdek-Místek** Ger. Friedek-Mistek. Ostravský Kraj, E Czech Republic
193 V16 **Fua'amotu** Tongatapu, S Tonga
190 A9 **Fuafatu** island Funafuti Atoll, C Tuvalu
190 A9 **Fuagea** island Funafuti Atoll, C Tuvalu
190 B8 **Fualifeke** atoll C Tuvalu
190 A8 **Fualopa** island Funafuti Atoll, C Tuvalu
151 K22 **Fuammulah** var. Gnaviyani Atoll. atoll S Maldives
161 R11 **Fu'an** Fujian, SE China
Fu-chien see Fujian
Fu-chou see Fuzhou
164 G13 **Fuchū** var. Hutyû. Hiroshima, Honshū, SW Japan
160 M13 **Fuchuan** Guangxi Zhuangzu Zizhiqu, S China
165 R8 **Fudai** Iwate, Honshū, C Japan
161 S11 **Fuding** Fujian, SE China
81 J20 **Fudua** spring/well S Kenya
104 M16 **Fuengirola** Andalucía, S Spain
104 J12 **Fuente de Cantos** Extremadura, W Spain
104 J11 **Fuente del Maestre** Extremadura, W Spain
104 L12 **Fuente Obejuna** Andalucía, S Spain
104 L6 **Fuentesaúco** Castilla-León, N Spain
62 O3 **Fuerte Olimpo** var. Olimpo. Alto Paraguay, NE Paraguay
40 H8 **Fuerte, Río** ≈ C Mexico
64 Q11 **Fuerteventura** island Islas Canarias, Spain, NE Atlantic Ocean
141 S14 **Fughmah** var. Faghman, Fugma. C Yemen
92 M2 **Fuglehuken** headland W Svalbard
95 B18 **Fugloy** Dan. Fuglø Island Faeroe Islands
197 T15 **Fugløya Bank** undersea feature E Norwegian Sea
166 E11 **Fugong** Yunnang, SW China
Fugma see Fughmah
81 K16 **Fugugo** spring/well N Kenya
158 L2 **Fuhai** var. Burultokay. Xinjiang Uygur Zizhiqu, NW China
161 P10 **Fu He** ≈ S China
Fuhkien see Fujian
100 J9 **Fuhlsbüttel** ✈ (Hamburg) Hamburg, N Germany
101 L14 **Fuhne** ≈ C Germany
Fu-hsin see Fuxin
Fujairah see Al Fujayrah
164 M14 **Fuji** var. Huzi. Shizuoka, Honshū, S Japan
161 Q12 **Fujian** var. Fu-chien, Fuhkien, Fujian Sheng, Fukien, Min. ◈ province SE China
160 I9 **Fu Jiang** ≈ C China
Fujian Sheng see Fujian
164 M14 **Fujieda** var. Huzieda. Shizuoka, Honshū, S Japan
Fuji, Mount/Fujiyama see Fuji-san
163 Y7 **Fujin** Heilongjiang, NE China
164 M13 **Fujinomiya** var. Huzinomiya. Shizuoka, Honshū, S Japan
164 N13 **Fuji-san** var. Fujiyama, Eng. Mount Fuji. ▲ Honshū, SE Japan
165 N14 **Fujisawa** var. Huzisawa. Kanagawa, Honshū, S Japan
165 T3 **Fukagawa** var. Hukagawa. Hokkaidō, NE Japan
158 L5 **Fukang** Xinjiang Uygur Zizhiqu, W China
165 P7 **Fukaura** Aomori, Honshū, C Japan
193 W15 **Fukave** island Tongatapu Group, S Tonga
Fukien see Fujian
164 J13 **Fukuchiyama** var. Hukutiyama. Kyōto, Honshū, SW Japan
164 A14 **Fukue** var. Hukue. Nagasaki, Fukue-jima, SW Japan
164 A13 **Fukue-jima** island Gotō-rettō, SW Japan
164 K12 **Fukui** var. Hukui. Fukui, Honshū, SW Japan
164 K12 **Fukui** off. Fukui-ken, var. Hukui. ◈ prefecture Honshū, SW Japan
164 D13 **Fukuoka** var. Hukuoka; hist. Najima. Fukuoka, Kyūshū, SW Japan
164 D13 **Fukuoka** off. Fukuoka-ken, var. Hukuoka. ◈ prefecture Kyūshū, SW Japan
165 P11 **Fukushima** var. Hukusima. Fukushima, Honshū, C Japan
165 Q6 **Fukushima** Hokkaidō, NE Japan
165 Q12 **Fukushima** off. Fukushima-ken, var. Hukusima. ◈ prefecture Honshū, C Japan
164 G13 **Fukuyama** var. Hukuyama. Hiroshima, Honshū, SW Japan
76 G13 **Fulacunda** C Guinea-Bissau
131 P8 **Fūlādī, Kūh-e** ▲ E Afghanistan
187 Z15 **Fulaga** island Lau Group, E Fiji
101 I17 **Fulda** Hessen, C Germany
29 S10 **Fulda** Minnesota, N USA
101 I16 **Fulda** ≈ C Germany
Fülek see Fil'akovo
Fulin see Hanyuan
160 K10 **Fuling** Chongqing Shi, C China
35 T15 **Fullerton** California, SE USA
29 P15 **Fullerton** Nebraska, C USA
108 M8 **Fulpmes** Tirol, W Austria
20 G8 **Fulton** Kentucky, S USA
23 N2 **Fulton** Mississippi, S USA
27 V4 **Fulton** Missouri, C USA
18 H9 **Fulton** New York, NE USA
Fuman/Fumen see Fowman
103 R3 **Fumay** Ardennes, N France
102 M13 **Fumel** Lot-et-Garonne, SW France
190 B10 **Funafara** atoll C Tuvalu
190 C9 **Funafuti** ✈ Funafuti Atoll, C Tuvalu
Funafuti see Fongafale
190 F8 **Funafuti Atoll** atoll C Tuvalu
190 B9 **Funangongo** atoll C Tuvalu
93 F17 **Funäsdalen** Jämtland, C Sweden
64 O6 **Funchal** Madeira, Portugal, NE Atlantic Ocean
64 P5 **Funchal** ✈ Madeira, Portugal, NE Atlantic Ocean
54 F5 **Fundación** Magdalena, N Colombia
104 I8 **Fundão** var. Fundáo. Castelo Branco, C Portugal
13 O16 **Fundy, Bay of** bay Canada/USA
Fünen see Fyn
54 C13 **Fúnes** Nariño, SW Colombia
Fünfkirchen see Pécs
83 M19 **Funhalouro** Inhambane, S Mozambique
161 R6 **Funing** Jiangsu, E China
160 I14 **Funing** Yunnan, SW China
160 M7 **Funiu Shan** ⛰ C China
77 U13 **Funtua** Katsina, N Nigeria
161 R12 **Fuqing** Fujian, SE China
83 M14 **Furancungo** Tete, NW Mozambique
116 I15 **Furculeşti** Teleorman, S Romania
Füred see Balatonfüred
165 W4 **Füren-ko** ◎ Hokkaidō, NE Japan
143 R12 **Fūrg** Fārs, S Iran
Furluk see Fârliug
Fürmanov/Furmanovka see Moyynkum
Furmanovo see Zhalpaktal
59 L20 **Furnas, Represa de** ⊞ SE Brazil
183 Q14 **Furneaux Group** island group Tasmania, SE Australia
Furnes see Veurne
160 I10 **Furong Jiang** ≈ S China
138 I5 **Furqlus** Ḩimş, W Syria
100 F12 **Fürstenau** Niedersachsen, NW Germany
109 X8 **Fürstenfeld** Steiermark, SE Austria
101 L23 **Fürstenfeldbruck** Bayern, S Germany
100 P12 **Fürstenwalde** Brandenburg, NE Germany
101 K20 **Fürth** Bayern, S Germany
109 W3 **Furth bei Göttweig** Niederösterreich, NW Austria
165 R3 **Furubira** Hokkaidō, NE Japan
94 L12 **Furudal** Dalarna, C Sweden
164 L12 **Furukawa** Gifu, Honshū, SW Japan
165 Q10 **Furukawa** var. Hurukawa. Miyagi, Honshū, C Japan
54 F10 **Fusagasugá** Cundinamarca, C Colombia
Fusan see Pusan
Fushë-Arëzi/Fushë-Arrësi see Fushë-Arrëz
113 L18 **Fushë-Arrëz** var. Fushë-Arëzi, Fushë-Arrësi. Shkodër, N Albania
Fushë-Kruja see Fushë-Krujë
113 K19 **Fushë-Krujë** var. Fushë-Kruja. Durrës, C Albania
163 V12 **Fushun** var. Fou-shan, Fu-shun. Liaoning, NE China
Fusin see Fuxin
108 G10 **Fusio** Ticino, S Switzerland
163 X11 **Fusong** Jilin, NE China
101 K24 **Füssen** Bayern, S Germany
160 K15 **Fusui** prev. Funan. Guangxi Zhuangzu Zizhiqu, S China
Futa Jallon see Fouta Djallon
63 G18 **Futaleufú** Los Lagos, S Chile
112 K10 **Futog** Serbia, NW Yugoslavia
165 O14 **Futtsu** var. Huttu. Chiba, Honshū, S Japan
187 S15 **Futuna** island S Vanuatu
190 D12 **Futuna, Île** island S Wallis and Futuna
161 Q11 **Futun Xi** ≈ SE China
160 L5 **Fuxian** var. Fu Xian. Shaanxi, C China
Fuxian see Wafangdian
160 G13 **Fuxian Hu** ◎ SW China
163 U12 **Fuxin** var. Fou-hsin, Fu-hsin, Fusin. Liaoning, NE China
Fuxing see Wangmo
161 P7 **Fuyang** Anhui, E China
161 O4 **Fuyang He** ≈ E China
163 U7 **Fuyu** Heilongjiang, NE China
Fuyu/Fu-yü see Songyuan
163 Z6 **Fuyuan** Heilongjiang, NE China
158 M3 **Fuyun** var. Koktokay. Xinjiang Uygur Zizhiqu, NW China
111 L22 **Füzesabony** Heves, E Hungary
161 R12 **Fuzhou** var. Foochow, Fu-chou. Fujian, SE China
Fuzhou see Linchuan
137 W13 **Füzuli** Rus. Fizuli. SW Azerbaijan
119 I20 **Fyadory** Rus. Fëdory. Brestskaya Voblasts', SW Belarus
95 G24 **Fyn** off. Fyns Amt, var. Fünen. ◈ county C Denmark
95 G23 **Fyn** Ger. Fünen. island C Denmark
96 H12 **Fyne, Loch** inlet W Scotland, UK
95 E16 **Fyresvatnet** ◎ S Norway
FYR Macedonia/FYROM see Macedonia, FYR
Fyzabad see Feyzābād

G

81 O14 **Gaalkacyo** var. Galka'yo, It. Galcaio. Mudug, C Somalia
Gabakly see Kabakly
114 H8 **Gabare** Vratsa, NW Bulgaria
102 K15 **Gabas** ≈ SW France
35 T7 **Gabbs** Nevada, W USA
82 B12 **Gabela** Cuanza Sul, W Angola
Gaberones see Gaborone
189 X14 **Gabert** island Caroline Islands, E Micronesia
74 M7 **Gabès** var. Qābis. E Tunisia
74 M6 **Gabès, Golfe de** Ar. Khalīj Qābis. gulf E Tunisia
Gablonz an der Neisse see Jablonec nad Nisou
Gablös see Cavalese
79 E18 **Gabon** off. Gabonese Republic. ◆ republic C Africa
83 I20 **Gaborone** prev. Gaberones. ● (Botswana) South East, SE Botswana
83 I20 **Gaborone** ✈ South East, SE Botswana
104 K8 **Gabriel y Galán, Embalse de** ⊞ W Spain
143 U15 **Gābrīk, Rūd-e** ≈ SE Iran
114 J9 **Gabrovo** Gabrovo, N Bulgaria
114 J9 **Gabrovo** ◈ province N Bulgaria
76 H12 **Gabú** prev. Nova Lamego. E Guinea-Bissau
29 O6 **Gackle** North Dakota, N USA
113 I15 **Gacko** Republika Srpska, Bosnia and Herzegovina
155 F17 **Gadag** Karnātaka, W India
93 G15 **Gäddede** Jämtland, C Sweden
159 S12 **Gadê** Qinghai, C China
Gades/Gadier/Gadir/Gadire see Cádiz
105 P15 **Gádor, Sierra de** ⛰ S Spain
149 S15 **Gadra** Sind, SE Pakistan
23 Q3 **Gadsden** Alabama, S USA
36 H15 **Gadsden** Arizona, SW USA
Gadyach see Hadyach
79 H15 **Gadzi** Mambéré-Kadéï, SW Central African Republic
116 J13 **Găeşti** Dâmboviţa, S Romania
107 J17 **Gaeta** Lazio, C Italy
107 J17 **Gaeta, Golfo di** var. Gulf of Gaeta. gulf C Italy
188 L14 **Gaferut** atoll Caroline Islands, W Micronesia
21 Q10 **Gaffney** South Carolina, SE USA
Gäfle see Gävle
Gäfleborg see Gävleborg
74 M6 **Gafsa** var. Qafşah. W Tunisia
Gafurov see Ghafurov
128 J3 **Gagarin** Smolenskaya Oblast', W Russian Federation
147 O10 **Gagarin** Jizzakh Wiloyati, C Uzbekistan
101 G21 **Gaggenau** Baden-Württemberg, SW Germany
188 F16 **Gagil Tamil** var. Gagil-Tomil. island Caroline Islands, W Micronesia
Gagil-Tomil see Gagil Tamil
129 O4 **Gagino** Nizhegorodskaya Oblast', W Russian Federation
107 Q19 **Gagliano del Capo** Puglia, SE Italy
94 L13 **Gagnef** Dalarna, C Sweden
76 M17 **Gagnoa** C Ivory Coast
13 N10 **Gagnon** Quebec, E Canada
Gago Coutinho see Lumbala N'Guimbo
137 P8 **Gagra** NW Georgia
31 S13 **Gahanna** Ohio, N USA
143 R13 **Gahkom** Hormozgān, S Iran
Gahnpa see Ganta
57 Q19 **Gaíba, Laguna** ◎ E Bolivia
153 T13 **Gaibanda** var. Gaibandah. Rajshahi, NW Bangladesh
Gaibandah see Gaibanda
Gaibhlte, Cnoc Mór na n see Galtymore Mountain
109 R9 **Gail** ≈ S Austria
101 I21 **Gaildorf** Baden-Württemberg, S Germany
103 N15 **Gaillac** var. Gaillac-sur-Tarn. Tarn, S France
Gaillac-sur-Tarn see Gaillac
Gaillimh see Galway
Gaillimhe, Cuan na see Galway Bay
109 Q9 **Gailtaler Alpen** ⛰ S Austria
63 J17 **Gaimán** Chaco, S Argentina
20 K8 **Gainesboro** Tennessee, S USA
23 V10 **Gainesville** Florida, SE USA
23 T2 **Gainesville** Georgia, SE USA
27 U8 **Gainesville** Missouri, C USA
25 T5 **Gainesville** Texas, SW USA
109 X5 **Gainfarn** Niederösterreich, NE Austria
97 N18 **Gainsborough** E England, UK
182 G6 **Gairdner, Lake** salt lake South Australia
Gaissane see Gáissát
92 L8 **Gáissát** var. Gaissane ⛰ N Norway
43 T15 **Gaital, Cerro** ▲ C Panama
21 W3 **Gaithersburg** Maryland, NE USA
163 U13 **Gaizhou** Liaoning, NE China
Gaiziņ see Gaiziņa Kalns
118 I9 **Gaiziņa Kalns** var. Gaiziņ. ▲ E Latvia
Gajac see Villeneuve-sur-Lot
39 S10 **Gakona** Alaska, USA
Galaassiya see Galaosiye
Galāğil see Jalājil
Galam, Pulau see Gelam, Pulau
62 J6 **Galán, Cerro** ▲ NW Argentina
111 H21 **Galanta** Hung. Galánta. Trnavský Kraj, W Slovakia
146 L11 **Galaosiye** Rus. Galaassiya. Bukhoro Wiloyati, C Uzbekistan
57 B17 **Galápagos** off. Provincia de Galápagos. ◈ province Ecuador, E Pacific Ocean
193 P8 **Galapagos Fracture Zone** tectonic feature E Pacific Ocean
193 S9 **Galapagos Rise** undersea feature E Pacific Ocean
96 K13 **Galashiels** SE Scotland, UK
116 M12 **Galaţi** Ger. Galatz. Galaţi, E Romania
116 L12 **Galaţi** ◈ county E Romania
107 Q19 **Galatina** Puglia, SE Italy
107 Q19 **Galatone** Puglia, SE Italy
Galatz see Galaţi
21 R8 **Galax** Virginia, NE USA
Galaymor see Kala-i-Mor
Galcaio see Gaalkacyo
64 P11 **Gáldar** Gran Canaria, Islas Canarias, NE Atlantic Ocean
94 F11 **Galdhøpiggen** ▲ S Norway
40 I4 **Galeana** Chihuahua, N Mexico
41 O9 **Galeana** Nuevo León, NE Mexico
60 P9 **Galeão** ✈ (Rio de Janeiro) Rio de Janeiro, SE Brazil
171 R10 **Galela** Pulau Halmahera, E Indonesia
39 O9 **Galena** Alaska, USA
30 K10 **Galena** Illinois, N USA
27 R7 **Galena** Kansas, C USA
27 T8 **Galena** Missouri, C USA
45 V15 **Galeota Point** headland Trinidad, Trinidad and Tobago
105 P13 **Galera** Andalucía, S Spain
45 Y16 **Galera Point** headland Trinidad, Trinidad and Tobago
56 A5 **Galera, Punta** headland NW Ecuador
30 K12 **Galesburg** Illinois, N USA
30 J7 **Galesville** Wisconsin, N USA
18 F12 **Galeton** Pennsylvania, NE USA
116 H9 **Gâlgău** Hung. Galgó; prev. Gilgău. Sălaj, NW Romania
Galgó see Gâlgău
Galgóc see Hlohovec
81 N15 **Galguduud** off. Gobolka Galguduud. ◈ region E Somalia
137 Q9 **Gali** W Georgia
127 N14 **Galich** Kostromskaya Oblast', NW Russian Federation
114 H7 **Galiche** Vratsa, NW Bulgaria
104 H3 **Galicia** anc. Gallaecia. ◈ autonomous community NW Spain
64 M8 **Galicia Bank** undersea feature E Atlantic Ocean
Galilee see HaGalil
181 W7 **Galilee, Lake** ◎ Queensland, NE Australia
Galilee, Sea of see Tiberias, Lake
106 E11 **Galileo Galilei** ✈ (Pisa) Toscana, C Italy
31 S12 **Galion** Ohio, N USA
Galka'yo see Gaalkacyo
80 H11 **Gallabat** Gedaref, E Sudan
Gallaecia see Galicia
106 C7 **Gallarate** Lombardia, NW Italy
27 S2 **Gallatin** Missouri, C USA
20 J8 **Gallatin** Tennessee, S USA
33 R11 **Gallatin Peak** ▲ Montana, NW USA
33 R12 **Gallatin River** ≈ Montana/Wyoming, NW USA
155 J26 **Galle** prev. Point de Galle. Southern Province, SW Sri Lanka
105 S5 **Gállego** ≈ NE Spain
193 Q8 **Gallego Rise** undersea feature E Pacific Ocean
Gallegos see Río Gallegos
63 H23 **Gallegos, Río** ≈ Argentina/Chile
Gallia see France
22 K10 **Galliano** Louisiana, S USA
114 G13 **Gallikós** ≈ N Greece
37 S12 **Gallinas Peak** ▲ New Mexico, SW USA
54 H3 **Gallinas, Punta** headland NE Colombia
37 T11 **Gallinas River** ≈ New Mexico, SW USA
107 Q19 **Gallipoli** Puglia, SE Italy
Gallipoli see Gelibolu
Gallipoli Peninsula see Gelibolu Yarımadası
31 T15 **Gallipolis** Ohio, N USA
92 J12 **Gällivare** Norrbotten, N Sweden
109 T4 **Gallneukirchen** Oberösterreich, N Austria
105 Q7 **Gallo** ≈ C Spain
93 G17 **Gällö** Jämtland, C Sweden
107 I23 **Gallo, Capo** headland Sicilia, Italy, C Mediterranean Sea
37 P13 **Gallo Mountains** ⛰ New Mexico, SW USA
18 G8 **Galloo Island** island New York, NE USA
97 H15 **Galloway, Mull of** headland S Scotland, UK
37 P10 **Gallup** New Mexico, SW USA
105 R5 **Gallur** Aragón, NE Spain
Gâlma see Guelma
35 O8 **Galt** California, W USA
74 C10 **Galtat-Zemmour** C Western Sahara
95 G22 **Galten** Århus, C Denmark
97 D20 **Galtymore Mountain** Ir. Cnoc Mór na nGaibhlte. ▲ S Ireland
97 D20 **Galty Mountains** Ir. Na Gaibhlte. ⛰ S Ireland
30 K11 **Galva** Illinois, N USA
25 X12 **Galveston** Texas, SW USA
25 W11 **Galveston Bay** inlet Texas, SW USA
25 W12 **Galveston Island** island Texas, SW USA
61 B18 **Gálvez** Santa Fe, C Argentina
97 C18 **Galway** Ir. Gaillimh. W Ireland
97 B18 **Galway** Ir. Gaillimh. cultural region W Ireland
97 B18 **Galway Bay** Ir. Cuan na Gaillimhe. bay W Ireland
83 F18 **Gam** Otjozondjupa, NE Namibia
164 L14 **Gamagōri** Aichi, Honshū, SW Japan
54 F7 **Gamarra** Cesar, N Colombia
Gámas see Kaamanen
158 L17 **Gamba** Xizang Zizhiqu, W China
77 P14 **Gambaga** NE Ghana
80 G13 **Gambēla** Gambēla, W Ethiopia
83 H14 **Gambēla** ◈ region, W Ethiopia
38 K10 **Gambell** Saint Lawrence Island, Alaska, USA
76 E12 **Gambia** off. Republic of The Gambia, The Gambia. ◆ republic W Africa
76 I12 **Gambia** Fr. Gambie. ≈ W Africa
64 K12 **Gambia Plain** undersea feature E Atlantic Ocean
Gambie see Gambia
31 T13 **Gambier** Ohio, N USA
191 Y13 **Gambier, Îles** island group E French Polynesia
182 G10 **Gambier Islands** island group South Australia
79 H19 **Gamboma** Plateaux, E Congo
79 G16 **Gamboula** Mambéré-Kadéï, SW Central African Republic
37 P10 **Gamerco** New Mexico, SW USA
137 V12 **Gamiş Dağı** ▲ W Azerbaijan
Gamlakarleby see Kokkola
95 N18 **Gamleby** Kalmar, S Sweden
Gammelstad see Gammelstaden
93 J14 **Gammelstaden** var. Gammelstad. Norrbotten, N Sweden
Gammouda see Sidi Bouzid
155 J25 **Gampaha** Western Province, W Sri Lanka
155 K25 **Gampola** Central Province, C Sri Lanka
167 S5 **Gâm, Sông** ≈ N Vietnam
92 L7 **Gamvik** Finnmark, N Norway
150 H13 **Gan** Addu Atoll, C Maldives
Gan see Gansu, China
Gan see Jiangxi, China
Ganaane see Juba
37 O10 **Ganado** Arizona, SW USA
25 U12 **Ganado** Texas, SW USA
14 L14 **Gananoque** Ontario, SE Canada
Ganāveh see Bandar-e Gonāveh
137 V11 **Gäncä** Rus. Gyandzha; prev. Kirovabad, Yelisavetpol. W Azerbaijan
Ganchi see Ghonchí
Gand see Gent
82 B13 **Ganda** var. Mariano Machado, Port. Vila Mariano Machado. Benguela, W Angola
79 L22 **Gandajika** Kasai Oriental, S Dem. Rep. Congo (Zaire)
153 O12 **Gandak** Nep. Nārāyāni. ≈ India/Nepal
13 U11 **Gander** Newfoundland, SE Canada
13 U11 **Gander** ✈ Newfoundland, E Canada
100 G11 **Ganderkesee** Niedersachsen, NW Germany
105 T7 **Gandesa** Cataluña, NE Spain
154 B10 **Gāndhīdhām** Gujarāt, W India
154 D10 **Gāndhīnagar** Gujarāt, W India
154 F9 **Gāndhi Sāgar** ◎ C India
105 T11 **Gandía** País Valenciano, E Spain
159 O10 **Gang** Qinghai, W China
152 G9 **Gangānagar** Rājasthān, NW India
152 I12 **Gangāpur** Rājasthān, N India
153 S17 **Ganga Sāgar** West Bengal, NE India
Gangavathi see Gangāwati
155 G17 **Gangāwati** var. Gangavathi. Karnātaka, C India
159 S9 **Gangca** var. Shaliuhe. Qinghai, C China
158 H14 **Gangdisê Shan** Eng. Kailas Range. ⛰ W China
103 Q15 **Ganges** Hérault, S France
153 P13 **Ganges** Ben. Padma. ≈ Bangladesh/India see also Padma
Ganges Cone see Ganges Fan
173 S3 **Ganges Fan** var. Ganges Cone. undersea feature N Bay of Bengal
153 U17 **Ganges, Mouths of the** delta Bangladesh/India
107 K23 **Gangi** anc. Engyum. Sicilia, Italy, C Mediterranean Sea
152 K8 **Gangotri** Uttar Pradesh, N India
Gangra see Çankırı
153 S11 **Gangtok** Sikkim, N India
159 W11 **Gangu** Gansu, C China
163 U5 **Gan He** ≈ NE China
171 S12 **Gani** Pulau Halmahera, E Indonesia
161 O12 **Gan Jiang** ≈ S China
146 H15 **Gannaly** Akhalskiy Velayat, S Turkmenistan
163 U7 **Gannan** Heilongjiang, NE China
103 P10 **Gannat** Allier, C France
33 T14 **Gannett Peak** ▲ Wyoming, C USA
29 O10 **Gannvalley** South Dakota, N USA
109 Y3 **Gänserndorf** Niederösterreich, NE Austria
Gansos, Lago dos see Goose Lake
159 T9 **Gansu** var. Gan, Gansu Sheng, Kansu. ◈ province N China
Gansu Sheng see Gansu
76 K16 **Ganta** var. Gahnpa. NE Liberia
182 H11 **Gantheaume, Cape** headland South Australia
Gantsevichi see Hantsavichy
161 Q6 **Ganyu** var. Qingkou. Jiangsu, E China
144 D12 **Ganyushkino** Atyrau, SW Kazakhstan
161 O12 **Ganzhou** Jiangxi, S China
77 Q10 **Gao** Gao, E Mali
77 R10 **Gao** ◈ region SE Mali
161 O10 **Gao'an** Jiangxi, S China
161 N5 **Gaoping** Shanxi, C China
159 S8 **Gaotai** Gansu, N China
Gaoth Dobhair see Gweedore
77 O14 **Gaoua** SW Burkina
76 I13 **Gaoual** Moyenne-Guinée, N Guinea
Gaoxiong see Kaohsiung
161 R7 **Gaoyou** var. Dayishan. Jiangsu, E China
161 R7 **Gaoyou Hu** ◎ E China
160 M15 **Gaozhou** Guangdong, S China
103 T13 **Gap** anc. Vapincum. Hautes-Alpes, SE France
158 G13 **Gar** var. Gar Xincun. Xizang Zizhiqu, W China
Garabekevyul/Garabekewül see Karabekaul
Garabogazköl see Kara-Bogaz-Gol

◆ Country ● Country Capital ◇ Dependent Territory ○ Dependent Territory Capital ◈ Administrative Region ✈ International Airport ▲ Mountain ⛰ Mountain Range ⁂ Volcano ≈ River ◎ Lake ⊞ Reservoir

43 V16 **Garachiné** Darién, SE Panama
43 V16 **Garachiné, Punta** *headland* SE Panama
Garagan *see* Karagan
54 G10 **Garagoa** Boyacá, C Colombia
Garagöl *see* Karagel'
Garagum *see* Garagumy
Garagum Kanaly *see* Garagumskiy Kanal
146 E12 **Garagumskiy Kanal** *var.* Kara Kum Canal, Karakumskiy Kanal, *Turkm.* Garagum Kanaly. *canal* C Turkmenistan
146 F12 **Garagumy** *var.* Qara Qum, *Eng.* Black Sand Desert, Kara Kum, *Turkm.* Garagum; *prev.* Peski Karakumy. *desert* C Turkmenistan
183 S4 **Garah** New South Wales, SE Australia
64 O11 **Garajonay** ▲ Gomera, Islas Canarias, NE Atlantic Ocean
114 M8 **Gara Khitrino** Shumen, NE Bulgaria
76 L13 **Garalo** Sikasso, SW Mali
Garam *see* Hron
Garamäbnyyaz *see* Karamet-Niyaz
Garamszentkereszt *see* Žiar nad Hronom
77 Q13 **Garango** S Burkina
59 Q15 **Garanhuns** Pernambuco, E Brazil
188 H5 **Garapan** Saipan, S Northern Mariana Islands
Gárassavon *see* Kaaresuvanto
78 J13 **Garba** Bamingui-Bangoran, N Central African Republic
81 L16 **Garbahaarrey** *It.* Garba Harre. Gedo, SW Somalia
Garba Harre *see* Garbahaarrey
81 J18 **Garba Tula** Eastern, C Kenya
27 N9 **Garber** Oklahoma, C USA
34 L4 **Garberville** California, W USA
100 I12 **Garbsen** Niedersachsen, N Germany
60 K9 **Garça** São Paulo, S Brazil
104 L10 **García de Solá, Embalse de** ⊠ C Spain
103 Q14 **Gard** ❖ *department* S France
103 Q14 **Gard** ≈ S France
106 F7 **Garda, Lago di** *var.* Benaco, *Eng.* Lake Garda, *Ger.* Gardasee. ◎ NE Italy
Garda, Lake *see* Garda, Lago di
Gardan Divāl *see* Gardan Dīwāl
149 Q5 **Gardan Dīwāl** *var.* Gardan Divāl. Wardag, C Afghanistan
103 S15 **Gardanne** Bouches-du-Rhône, SE France
Gardasee *see* Garda, Lago di
100 L12 **Gardelegen** Sachsen-Anhalt, C Germany
14 B10 **Garden** ≈ Ontario, S Canada
23 X6 **Garden City** Georgia, SE USA
26 I6 **Garden City** Kansas, C USA
27 S5 **Garden City** Missouri, C USA
25 N8 **Garden City** Texas, SW USA
23 P3 **Gardendale** Alabama, S USA
31 P5 **Garden Island** *island* Michigan, N USA
22 M11 **Garden Island Bay** *bay* Louisiana, S USA
31 O5 **Garden Peninsula** *peninsula* Michigan, N USA
Garden State *see* New Jersey
95 I14 **Gardermoen** Akershus, S Norway
Gardeyz *see* Gardēz
149 Q6 **Gardēz** *var.* Gardeyz, Gordiaz. Paktīā, E Afghanistan
93 G14 **Gardiken** ◎ N Sweden
19 Q7 **Gardiner** Maine, NE USA
33 S12 **Gardiner** Montana, NW USA
19 N13 **Gardiners Island** *island* New York, NE USA
Gardner Island *see* Nikumaroro
19 T6 **Gardner Lake** ◎ Maine, NE USA
35 Q6 **Gardnerville** Nevada, W USA
Gardo *see* Qardho
106 F7 **Gardone Val Trompia** Lombardia, N Italy
Garegegasnjárga *see* Karigasniemi
38 F17 **Gareloi Island** *island* Aleutian Islands, Alaska, USA
106 B10 **Garessio** Piemonte, NE Italy
32 M9 **Garfield** Washington, NW USA
31 U11 **Garfield Heights** Ohio, N USA
Gargaliani *see* Gargaliánoi
115 D21 **Gargaliánoi** *var.* Gargaliani. Pelopónnisos, S Greece
107 N15 **Gargano, Promontorio del** *headland* SE Italy
108 J8 **Gargellen** Graubünden, W Switzerland
93 I14 **Gargnäs** Västerbotten, N Sweden
118 C11 **Gargždai** Gargždai, W Lithuania
154 J13 **Garhchiroli** Mahārāshtra, C India
153 O15 **Garhwa** Bihār, N India
171 V13 **Gariau** Irian Jaya, E Indonesia
83 E24 **Garies** Northern Cape, W South Africa
109 K17 **Garigliano** ≈ C Italy
81 K19 **Garissa** Coast, E Kenya
21 V11 **Garland** North Carolina, SE USA
25 T6 **Garland** Texas, SW USA
36 L1 **Garland** Utah, W USA
106 D8 **Garlasco** Lombardia, N Italy
119 F14 **Garliava** Kaunas, S Lithuania
Garm *see* Gharm
142 M9 **Garm, Āb-e** *var.* Rūd-e Khersān. ≈ SW Iran
101 K25 **Garmisch-Partenkirchen** Bayern, S Germany
143 O5 **Garmsār** *prev.* Qishlaq. Semnān, N Iran
Garmser *see* Darvīshān
29 V12 **Garner** Iowa, C USA
21 U9 **Garner** North Carolina, SE USA
27 Q5 **Garnett** Kansas, C USA
99 M25 **Garnich** Luxembourg, SW Luxembourg
182 M8 **Garnpung, Lake** *salt lake* New South Wales, SE Australia
Garoe *see* Garoowe
Garoet *see* Garut
153 U13 **Gāro Hills** *hill range* NE India
102 K13 **Garonne** *anc.* Garumna. ≈ S France
80 P13 **Garoowe** *var.* Garoe. Nugaal, N Somalia
78 F12 **Garoua** *var.* Garua. Nord, N Cameroon
79 G14 **Garoua Boulaï** Est, E Cameroon
77 O10 **Garou, Lac** ◎ C Mali
95 L16 **Garphyttan** Örebro, C Sweden
29 R11 **Garretson** South Dakota, N USA
31 Q11 **Garrett** Indiana, N USA
33 Q10 **Garrison** Montana, NW USA
28 M4 **Garrison** North Dakota, N USA
25 X8 **Garrison** Texas, SW USA
28 L4 **Garrison Dam** *dam* North Dakota, N USA
104 J9 **Garrovillas** Extremadura, W Spain
Garrygala *see* Kara-Kala
8 L8 **Garry Lake** ◎ Nunavut, N Canada
Gars *see* Gars am Kamp
109 W3 **Gars am Kamp** *var.* Gars. Niederösterreich, NE Austria
81 K20 **Garsen** Coast, S Kenya
Garshy *see* Karshi
14 F10 **Garson** Ontario, S Canada
109 T5 **Garsten** Oberösterreich, N Austria
Gartar *see* Qianning
102 M10 **Gartempe** ≈ C France
Gartog *see* Markam
Garua *see* Garoua
83 D21 **Garub** Karas, SW Namibia
Garumna *see* Garonne
169 P16 **Garut** *prev.* Garoet. Jawa, C Indonesia
185 C20 **Garvie Mountains** ▲ South Island, NZ
110 N12 **Garwolin** Mazowieckie, E Poland
25 U12 **Garwood** Texas, SW USA
Gar Xincun *see* Gar
31 N11 **Gary** Indiana, N USA
25 X7 **Gary** Texas, SW USA
158 G13 **Gar Zangbo** ≈ W China
160 F8 **Garzê** Sichuan, C China
54 E12 **Garzón** Huila, S Colombia
146 B13 **Gasan-Kuli** *var.* Esenguly. Balkanskiy Velayat, W Turkmenistan
31 P13 **Gas City** Indiana, N USA
102 K15 **Gascogne** *Eng.* Gascony. *cultural region* S France
Gascogne, Golfe de *see* Gascony, Gulf of
26 V5 **Gasconade River** ≈ Missouri, C USA
Gascony *see* Gascogne
180 H9 **Gascoyne Junction** Western Australia
173 V8 **Gascoyne Plain** *undersea feature* E Indian Ocean
180 H9 **Gascoyne River** ≈ Western Australia
192 J11 **Gascoyne Tablemount** *undersea feature* N Tasman Sea
67 U6 **Gash** *var.* Nahr al Qāsh. ≈ W Sudan
149 X3 **Gasherbrum** ▲ NE Pakistan
159 N9 **Gas Hu** ◎ C China
77 X12 **Gashua** Yobe, NE Nigeria
186 G7 **Gasmata** New Britain, E PNG
23 V14 **Gasparilla Island** *island* Florida, SE USA
169 O13 **Gaspar, Selat** *strait* W Indonesia
15 Y6 **Gaspé** Quebec, SE Canada
15 Z6 **Gaspé, Cap de** *headland* Quebec, SE Canada
15 X6 **Gaspé, Péninsule de** *var.* Péninsule de la Gaspésie. *peninsula* Quebec, SE Canada
Gaspésie, Péninsule de la *see* Gaspé, Péninsule de
77 W15 **Gassol** Taraba, E Nigeria
Gastein *see* Badgastein
21 R10 **Gastonia** North Carolina, SE USA
21 V8 **Gaston, Lake** ⊠ North Carolina/Virginia, SE USA
115 D19 **Gastoúni** Dytikí Ellás, S Greece
63 I17 **Gastre** Chubut, S Argentina
Gat *see* Ghāt
105 P15 **Gata, Cabo de** *headland* S Spain
Gata, Cape *see* Gátas, Akrotíri
105 T11 **Gata de Gorgos** País Valenciano, E Spain
116 E12 **Gătaia** *Ger.* Gataja, *Hung.* Gátalja; *prev.* Gáttája. Timiş, W Romania
Gataja/Gátalja *see* Gătaia
121 P3 **Gátas, Akrotíri** *var.* Cape Gata. *headland* S Cyprus
104 J8 **Gata, Sierra de** ▲ W Spain
126 G13 **Gatchina** Leningradskaya Oblast', NW Russian Federation
21 P8 **Gate City** Virginia, NE USA
97 M14 **Gateshead** NE England, UK
21 X8 **Gatesville** North Carolina, SE USA
25 S8 **Gatesville** Texas, SW USA
14 L12 **Gatineau** Quebec, SE Canada
14 L11 **Gatineau** ≈ Ontario/Quebec, SE Canada
21 N9 **Gatlinburg** Tennessee, S USA
Gatooma *see* Kadoma
Gáttája *see* Gătaia
43 T14 **Gatún, Lago** ⊠ C Panama
59 N14 **Gaturiano** Piauí, NE Brazil
97 O22 **Gatwick** ✕ (London) SE England, UK
187 Y14 **Gau** *prev.* Ngau. *island* C Fiji
187 R12 **Gaua** *var* Santa Maria, *island* Banks Islands, N Vanuatu
104 L16 **Gaucín** Andalucía, S Spain
Gauhāti *see* Guwāhāti
118 I8 **Gauja** *Ger.* Aa. ≈ Estonia/Latvia
118 I7 **Gaujiena** Alūksne, NE Latvia
Gaul/Gaule *see* France
94 H9 **Gauldalen** *valley* S Norway
21 R5 **Gauley River** ≈ West Virginia, NE USA
99 D19 **Gaurain-Ramecroix** Hainaut, SW Belgium
95 F15 **Gausta** ▲ S Norway
83 J21 **Gauteng** *off.* Gauteng Province; *prev.* Pretoria-Witwatersrand-Vereeniging. ❖ *province* NE South Africa
Gauteng *see* Germiston, South Africa
Gauteng *see* Johannesburg, South Africa
143 P14 **Gāvbandī** Hormozgān, S Iran
115 H25 **Gavdopoúla** *island* SE Greece
115 H26 **Gávdos** *island* SE Greece
102 K16 **Gave de Pau** *var.* Gave-de-Pay. ≈ SW France
Gave-de-Pay *see* Gave de Pau
102 J16 **Gave d'Oloron** ≈ SW France
99 E18 **Gavere** Oost-Vlaanderen, NW Belgium
94 N13 **Gävle** *var.* Gäfle; *prev.* Gefle. Gävleborg, C Sweden
94 M11 **Gävleborg** *var.* Gäfleborg, Gefleborg. ❖ *county* C Sweden
94 O13 **Gävlebukten** *bay* C Sweden
126 L16 **Gavrilov-Yam** Yaroslavskaya Oblast', W Russian Federation
182 I9 **Gawler** South Australia
182 G7 **Gawler Ranges** *hill range* South Australia
Gawso *see* Goaso
162 H11 **Gaxun Nur** ◎ N China
153 P14 **Gaya** Bihār, N India
77 S13 **Gaya** Dosso, SW Niger
Gaya *see* Kyjov
31 Q6 **Gaylord** Michigan, N USA
29 U9 **Gaylord** Minnesota, N USA
181 Y9 **Gayndah** Queensland, E Australia
127 T12 **Gayny** Komi-Permyatskiy Avtonomnyy Okrug, NW Russian Federation
Gaysin *see* Haysyn
Gayvorno *see* Hayvoron
138 E11 **Gaza** *Ar.* Ghazzah, *Heb.* 'Azza. NE Gaza Strip
83 L20 **Gaza** *off.* Província de Gaza. ❖ *province* SW Mozambique
146 I9 **Gaz-Achak** *Turkm.* Gazojak. Lebapskiy Velayat, NE Turkmenistan
Gazalkent *see* Ghazalkent
146 C11 **Gazandzhyk** *Turkm.* Gazanjyk; *prev.* Kazandzhik. Balkanskiy Velayat, W Turkmenistan
Gazanjyk *see* Gazandzhyk
77 V12 **Gazaoua** Maradi, S Niger
138 E11 **Gaza Strip** *Ar.* Qiṭā' Ghazzah. *disputed region* SW Asia
Gazgan *see* Ghozghon
Gazi Antep *see* Gaziantep
136 M16 **Gaziantep** *var.* Gazi Antep; *prev.* Aintab, Antep. Gaziantep, S Turkey
136 M17 **Gaziantep** *var.* Gazi Antep. ❖ *province* S Turkey
114 M13 **Gaziköy** Tekirdağ, NW Turkey
121 Q2 **Gazimağusa** *var.* Famagusta, *Gk.* Ammóchostos. E Cyprus
121 Q2 **Gazimağusa Körfezi** *var.* Famagusta Bay, *Gk.* Kólpos Ammóchostos. *bay* E Cyprus
146 K11 **Gazli** Bukhoro Wiloyati, C Uzbekistan
Gazojak *see* Gaz-Achak
79 K15 **Gbadolite** Equateur, NW Dem. Rep. Congo (Zaire)
76 K16 **Gbanga** *var.* Gbarnga. N Liberia
Gbarnga *see* Gbanga
77 S14 **Gbéroubouè** *var.* Béroubouay. N Benin
77 W16 **Gboko** Benue, S Nigeria
Gcuwa *see* Butterworth
110 J7 **Gdańsk** *Fr.* Dantzig, *Ger.* Danzig. Pomorskie, N Poland
Gdan'skaya Bukhta/Gdańsk, Gulf of *see* Danzig, Gulf of
Gdańska, Zakota *see* Danzig, Gulf of
Gdingen *see* Gdynia
126 F13 **Gdov** Pskovskaya Oblast', W Russian Federation
110 I6 **Gdynia** *Ger.* Gdingen. Pomorskie, N Poland
26 M10 **Geary** Oklahoma, C USA
Geavvú *see* Kevo
76 H12 **Gêba, Rio** ≈ C Guinea-Bissau
136 E11 **Gebze** Kocaeli, NW Turkey
80 H10 **Gedaref** *var.* Al Qaḍārif, El Gedaref. Gedaref, E Sudan
80 H10 **Gedaref** ❖ *state* E Sudan
80 B11 **Gedid Ras el Fil** Southern Darfur, W Sudan
101 I23 **Gedinne** Namur, SE Belgium
136 E13 **Gediz** Kütahya, W Turkey
136 C14 **Gediz Nehri** ≈ W Turkey
81 N14 **Gedlegubē** Somali, E Ethiopia
81 L17 **Gedo** *off.* Gobolka Gedo. ❖ *region* SW Somalia
95 I25 **Gedser** Storstrøm, SE Denmark
99 I16 **Geel** *var.* Gheel. Antwerpen, N Belgium
183 N13 **Geelong** Victoria, SE Australia
Ge'e'mu *see* Golmud
99 I14 **Geertruidenberg** Noord-Brabant, S Netherlands
100 H10 **Geeste** ≈ NW Germany
100 J10 **Geesthacht** Schleswig-Holstein, N Germany
183 P17 **Geeveston** Tasmania, SE Australia
Gefle *see* Gävle
Gefleborg *see* Gävleborg
158 G13 **Gê'gyai** Xizang Zizhiqu, W China
77 X12 **Geidam** Yobe, NE Nigeria
11 T11 **Geikie** ≈ Saskatchewan, C Canada
94 F13 **Geilo** Buskerud, S Norway
94 E10 **Geiranger** Møre og Romsdal, S Norway
101 I22 **Geislingen** *var.* Geislingen an der Steige. Baden-Württemberg, SW Germany
Geislingen an der Steige *see* Geislingen
81 F20 **Geita** Mwanza, NW Tanzania
95 G15 **Geithus** Buskerud, S Norway
160 H14 **Gejiu** *var.* Kochiu. Yunnan, S China
Gëkdepe *see* Geok-Tepe
146 E9 **Geklengkui, Solonchak** *var.* Solonchak Goklenkuy. *salt marsh* NW Turkmenistan
81 D14 **Gel** ≈ W Sudan
107 K25 **Gela** *prev.* Terranova di Sicilia. Sicilia, Italy, C Mediterranean Sea
Gëladaindong *see* Geladandong
81 N14 **Geladī** Somali, E Ethiopia
169 P13 **Gelam, Pulau** *var.* Pulau Galam. *island* N Indonesia
98 L11 **Gelderland** *prev. Eng.* Guelders. ❖ *province* E Netherlands
98 J13 **Geldermalsen** Gelderland, C Netherlands
101 D14 **Geldern** Nordrhein-Westfalen, W Germany
99 K15 **Geldrop** Noord-Brabant, SE Netherlands
99 L17 **Geleen** Limburg, SE Netherlands
128 K14 **Gelendzhik** Krasnodarskiy Kray, SW Russian Federation
Gelib *see* Jilib
136 B11 **Gelibolu** *Eng.* Gallipoli. Çanakkale, NW Turkey
115 L14 **Gelibolu Yarımadası** *Eng.* Gallipoli Peninsula. *peninsula* NW Turkey
81 O14 **Gellinsor** Mudug, C Somalia
101 H18 **Gelnhausen** Hessen, C Germany
101 E14 **Gelsenkirchen** Nordrhein-Westfalen, W Germany
83 C20 **Geluk** Hardap, SW Namibia
99 H20 **Gembloux** Namur, Belgium
79 J16 **Gemena** Equateur, NW Dem. Rep. Congo (Zaire)
99 L14 **Gemert** Noord-Brabant, SE Netherlands
136 E11 **Gemlik** Bursa, NW Turkey
Gem of the Mountains *see* Idaho
106 J6 **Gemona del Friuli** Friuli-Venezia Giulia, NE Italy
Gem State *see* Idaho
Genalē Wenz *see* Juba
169 R10 **Genali, Danau** ◎ Borneo, N Indonesia
99 G19 **Genappe** Wallon Brabant, C Belgium
137 P14 **Genç** Bingöl, E Turkey
Genck *see* Genk
98 M9 **Genemuiden** Overijssel, E Netherlands
63 K14 **General Acha** La Pampa, C Argentina
61 C21 **General Alvear** Buenos Aires, E Argentina
62 I12 **General Alvear** Mendoza, W Argentina
61 B20 **General Arenales** Buenos Aires, E Argentina
61 D21 **General Belgrano** Buenos Aires, E Argentina
194 H3 **General Bernardo O'Higgins** *Chilean research station* Antarctica
41 O8 **General Bravo** Nuevo León, NE Mexico
62 M7 **General Capdevila** Chaco, N Argentina
General Carrera, Lago *see* Buenos Aires, Lago
41 N9 **General Cepeda** Coahuila de Zaragoza, NE Mexico
63 K15 **General Conesa** Río Negro, E Argentina
61 G18 **General Enrique Martínez** Treinta y Tres, E Uruguay
62 L3 **General Eugenio A. Garay** *var.* Fortín General Eugenio Garay; *prev.* Yrendagüé. Nueva Asunción, NW Paraguay
61 C18 **General Galarza** Entre Ríos, E Argentina
61 E22 **General Guido** Buenos Aires, E Argentina
General José F.Uriburu *see* Zárate
61 E22 **General Juan Madariaga** Buenos Aires, E Argentina
41 O16 **General Juan N Alvarez** ✕ (Acapulco) Guerrero, S Mexico
61 B22 **General La Madrid** Buenos Aires, E Argentina
61 E21 **General Lavalle** Buenos Aires, E Argentina
General Machado *see* Camacupa
62 I8 **General Manuel Belgrano, Cerro** ▲ W Argentina
41 O8 **General Mariano Escobero** ✕ (Monterrey) Nuevo León, NE Mexico
61 B20 **General O'Brien** Buenos Aires, E Argentina
62 K13 **General Pico** La Pampa, C Argentina
62 M7 **General Pinedo** Chaco, N Argentina
61 B20 **General Pinto** Buenos Aires, E Argentina
61 E22 **General Pirán** Buenos Aires, E Argentina
43 N15 **General, Río** ≈ S Costa Rica
63 I15 **General Roca** Río Negro, C Argentina
171 Q8 **General Santos** *off.* General Santos City. Mindanao, S Philippines
41 O9 **General Terán** Nuevo León, NE Mexico
114 N7 **General Toshevo** *Rom.* I.G.Duca, *prev.* Casim, Kasimköj. Dobrich, NE Bulgaria
61 B20 **General Viamonte** Buenos Aires, E Argentina
61 A20 **General Villegas** Buenos Aires, E Argentina
Gênes *see* Genova
18 E11 **Genesee River** ≈ New York/Pennsylvania, NE USA
30 K11 **Geneseo** Illinois, N USA
18 F10 **Geneseo** New York, NE USA
57 L14 **Geneshuaya, Río** ≈ N Bolivia
23 Q8 **Geneva** Alabama, S USA
30 M10 **Geneva** Illinois, N USA
29 Q16 **Geneva** Nebraska, C USA
18 G10 **Geneva** New York, NE USA
31 U10 **Geneva** Ohio, NE USA
Geneva *see* Genève
108 B10 **Geneva, Lake** *Fr.* Lac de Genève, Lac Léman, le Léman, *Ger.* Genfer See. ◎ France/Switzerland
108 A10 **Genève** *Eng.* Geneva, *Ger.* Genf, *It.* Ginevra. Genève, SW Switzerland
108 A11 **Genève** *Eng.* Geneva, *Ger.* Genf, *It.* Ginevra. ❖ *canton* SW Switzerland
108 A10 **Genève** *var.* Geneva. ✕ Vaud, SW Switzerland
Genève, Lac de *see* Geneva, Lake
Genf *see* Genève
Genfer See *see* Geneva, Lake
163 S5 **Gen He** ≈ NE China
Genichesk *see* Heniches'k
104 L14 **Genil** ≈ S Spain
99 K18 **Genk** *var.* Genck. Limburg, NE Belgium
164 C13 **Genkai-nada** *gulf* Kyūshū, SW Japan
107 C19 **Gennargentu, Monti del** ▲ Sardegna, Italy, C Mediterranean Sea
99 M14 **Gennep** Limburg, SE Netherlands
30 M10 **Genoa** Illinois, N USA
29 Q15 **Genoa** Nebraska, C USA
Genoa *see* Genova
Genoa, Gulf of *see* Genova, Golfo di
106 D10 **Genova** *Eng.* Genoa, *Fr.* Gênes; *anc.* Genua. Liguria, NW Italy
106 D10 **Genova, Golfo di** *Eng.* Gulf of Genoa. *gulf* NW Italy
57 C17 **Genovesa, Isla** *var.* Tower Island. *island* Galapagos Islands, Ecuador, E Pacific Ocean
Genshū *see* Wŏnju
99 E17 **Gent** *Eng.* Ghent, *Fr.* Gand. Oost-Vlaanderen, NW Belgium
169 N16 **Genteng** Jawa, C Indonesia
100 M12 **Genthin** Sachsen-Anhalt, E Germany
27 R9 **Gentry** Arkansas, C USA
Genua *see* Genova
107 I15 **Genzano di Roma** Lazio, C Italy
Geokchay *see* Göyçay
146 F13 **Geok-Tepe** *var.* Gëkdepe, *Turkm.* Gökdepe. Akhalskiy Velayat, C Turkmenistan
122 I3 **Georga, Zemlya** *Eng.* George Land. *island* Zemlya Frantsa-Iosifa, N Russian Federation
83 G26 **George** Western Cape, S South Africa
29 S11 **George** Iowa, C USA
AA O5 **George** ≈ Newfoundland/Quebec, E Canada
65 C25 **George Island** *island* S Falkland Islands
183 R10 **George, Lake** ◎ New South Wales, SE Australia
81 E18 **George, Lake** ◎ SW Uganda
23 W10 **George, Lake** ◎ Florida, SE USA
18 L8 **George, Lake** ⊠ New York, NE USA
George Land *see* Georga, Zemlya
Georgenburg *see* Jurbarkas
George River *see* Kangiqsualujjuaq
64 G8 **Georges Bank** *undersea feature* W Atlantic Ocean
185 A21 **George Sound** *sound* South Island, NZ
65 F15 **Georgetown** ○ (Ascension Island) NW Ascension Island
181 V5 **Georgetown** Queensland, NE Australia
183 P15 **George Town** Tasmania, SE Australia
44 I4 **George Town** Great Exuma Island, C Bahamas
44 D8 **George Town** *var.* Georgetown. ○ (Cayman Islands) Grand Cayman, SW Cayman Islands
76 H12 **Georgetown** E Gambia
55 T8 **Georgetown** ● (Guyana) N Guyana
168 I7 **George Town** *var.* Penang, Pinang. Pinang, Peninsular Malaysia
45 Y14 **Georgetown** Saint Vincent, Saint Vincent and the Grenadines
21 Y4 **Georgetown** Delaware, NE USA
23 R6 **Georgetown** Georgia, SE USA
20 M5 **Georgetown** Kentucky, S USA
21 T13 **Georgetown** South Carolina, SE USA
25 S10 **Georgetown** Texas, SW USA
55 T8 **Georgetown** ✕ N Guyana
195 U16 **George V Coast** *physical region* Antarctica
195 T15 **George V Land** *physical region* Antarctica
194 J7 **George VI Ice Shelf** *ice shelf* Antarctica
194 J6 **George VI Sound** *sound* Antarctica
25 S14 **George West** Texas, SW USA
137 R9 **Georgia** *off.* Republic of Georgia, *Geor.* Sak'art'velo, *Rus.* Gruzinskaya SSR, Gruziya; *prev.* Georgian SSR. ◆ *republic* SW Asia
23 S5 **Georgia** *off.* State of Georgia; also known as Empire State of the South, Peach State. ❖ *state* SE USA
14 F12 **Georgian Bay** *lake bay* Ontario, S Canada
10 L17 **Georgia, Strait of** *strait* British Columbia, W Canada
Georgi Dimitrov *see* Kostenets
Georgi Dimitrov, Yazovir *see* Koprinka, Yazovir
114 M9 **Georgi Traykov, Yazovir** ⊠ NE Bulgaria
Georgiu-Dezh *see* Liski
145 W10 **Georgiyevka** Vostochnyy Kazakhstan, E Kazakhstan
Georgiyevka *see* Korday
129 N15 **Georgiyevsk** Stavropol'skiy Kray, SW Russian Federation
100 G13 **Georgsmarienhütte** Niedersachsen, NW Germany
195 O1 **Georg von Neumayer** *German research station* Antarctica
101 M16 **Gera** Thüringen, E Germany
101 K16 **Gera** ≈ C Germany
99 E19 **Geraardsbergen** Oost-Vlaanderen, SW Belgium
115 F21 **Geráki** Pelopónnisos, S Greece
27 W5 **Gerald** Missouri, C USA
47 V8 **Geral de Goiás, Serra** ▲ E Brazil
185 G20 **Geraldine** Canterbury, South Island, NZ
180 H11 **Geraldton** Western Australia
12 E11 **Geraldton** Ontario, S Canada
60 J12 **Geral, Serra** ▲ S Brazil
103 U6 **Gérardmer** Vosges, NE France
Gerasa *see* Jarash
Gerdauen *see* Zheleznodorozhnyy
39 Q11 **Gerdine, Mount** ▲ Alaska, USA
136 H11 **Gerede** Bolu, N Turkey
136 H11 **Gerede Çayı** ≈ N Turkey
148 M8 **Gereshk** Helmand, SW Afghanistan
101 L24 **Geretsried** Bayern, S Germany
105 P14 **Gérgal** Andalucía, S Spain
28 I14 **Gering** Nebraska, C USA
35 R3 **Gerlach** Nevada, W USA
Gerlachfalvi Csúcs/Gerlachovka *see* Gerlachovský štít
111 L18 **Gerlachovský štít** *var.* Gerlachovka, *Ger.* Gerlsdorfer Spitze, *Hung.* Gerlachfalvi Csúcs; *prev.* Stalinov Štít, *Ger.* Franz-Josef Spitze, *Hung.* Ferencz-Jósef Csúcs. ▲ N Slovakia
108 E8 **Gerlafingen** Solothurn, NW Switzerland
Gerlsdorfer Spitze *see* Gerlachovský štít
139 V3 **Germak** E Iraq
German East Africa *see* Tanzania
Germanicopolis *see* Çankırı
Germanicum, Mare/German Ocean *see* North Sea
Germanovichi *see* Hyermanavichy
German Southwest Africa *see* Namibia
20 E10 **Germantown** Tennessee, S USA
101 I15 **Germany** *off.* Federal Republic of Germany, *Ger.* Bundesrepublik Deutschland, Deutschland. ◆ *federal republic* N Europe
101 L23 **Germering** Bayern, S Germany
83 J21 **Germiston** *var.* Gauteng. Gauteng, NE South Africa
Gernika *see* Gernika-Lumo
105 P2 **Gernika-Lumo** *var.* Gernika, Guernica, Guernica y Lumo. País Vasco, N Spain
164 L12 **Gero** Gifu, Honshū, SW Japan
115 F22 **Geroliménas** Pelopónnisos, S Greece
Gerona *see* Girona
99 H21 **Gerpinnes** Hainaut, S Belgium
102 L15 **Gers** ❖ *department* S France
102 L14 **Gers** ≈ S France
Gerunda *see* Girona
136 K10 **Gerze** Sinop, N Turkey
158 I13 **Gêrzê** Xizang Zizhiqu, W China
Gesoriacum/Gessoriacum *see* Boulogne-sur-Mer
99 J21 **Gesves** Namur, SE Belgium
93 J20 **Geta** Åland, SW Finland
105 N8 **Getafe** Madrid, C Spain
95 J21 **Getinge** Halland, S Sweden
18 F16 **Gettysburg** Pennsylvania, NE USA
29 N8 **Gettysburg** South Dakota, N USA
194 K12 **Getz Ice Shelf** *ice shelf* Antarctica
137 S15 **Gevaş** Van, SE Turkey
Gevgeli *see* Gevgelija
113 Q20 **Gevgelija** *var.* Đevđelija, Djevdjelija, *Turk.* Gevgeli. SE FYR Macedonia
103 T10 **Gex** Ain, E France
92 I3 **Geysir** *physical region* SW Iceland
136 F11 **Geyve** Sakarya, NW Turkey
80 G10 **Gezira** ❖ *state* E Sudan
109 V3 **Gföhl** Niederösterreich, N Austria
83 H22 **Ghaap Plateau** *Afr.* Ghaapplato. *plateau* C South Africa
Ghaapplato *see* Ghaap Plateau
Ghaba *see* Al Ghābah
138 J8 **Ghāb, Tall** ▲ SE Syria
139 Q9 **Ghadaf, Wādī al** *dry watercourse* C Iraq
Ghadamès *see* Ghadāmis
74 M9 **Ghadāmis** *var.* Ghadamès, Rhadames. W Libya
141 Y10 **Ghadan** E Oman
75 O10 **Ghaddūwah** C Libya
147 Q11 **Ghafurov** *Rus.* Gafurov; *prev.* Sovetabad. NW Tajikistan
153 N12 **Ghāghara** ≈ S Asia
149 P13 **Ghaibi Dero** Sind, SE Pakistan

◆ Country ● Country Capital ◇ Dependent Territory ○ Dependent Territory Capital ❖ Administrative Region ✕ International Airport ▲ Mountain ▲ Mountain Range ▲ Volcano ≈ River ◎ Lake ⊠ Reservoir

141 Y10 **Ghalat** E Oman
147 O11 **Ghallaorol** Jizzakh Wiloyati, C Uzbekistan
139 W11 **Ghamūkah, Hawr** ◎ S Iraq
77 P15 **Ghana** *off.* Republic of Ghana. ◆ *republic* W Africa
141 X12 **Ghānah** *spring/well* S Oman
Ghanongga *see* Ranongga
Ghansi/Ghansiland *see* Ghanzi
83 F18 **Ghanzi** *var.* Khanzi. Ghanzi, W Botswana
83 G19 **Ghanzi** *var.* Ghansi, Ghansiland, Khanzi. ◆ *district* C Botswana
67 T14 **Ghanzi** *var.* Knanzi. ≈ Botswana/South Africa
Ghap'an *see* Kapan
138 F13 **Gharandal** Ma'ān, SW Jordan
Gharbt, Jabal al *see* Liban, Jebel
74 K7 **Ghardaïa** N Algeria
139 U14 **Gharibīyah, Sha'īb al** ≈ S Iraq
147 R12 **Gharm** *Rus.* Garm. C Tajikistan
149 P17 **Gharo** Sind, SE Pakistan
139 W10 **Gharrāf, Shaṭṭ al** ≈ S Iraq
Gharvān *see* Gharyān
75 O7 **Gharyān** *var.* Gharvān. NW Libya
74 M11 **Ghāt** *var.* Gat. SW Libya
Ghawdex *see* Gozo
141 U8 **Ghayathi** Abū Ẓaby, W UAE
Ghazāl, Baḥr al *see* Ghazal, Bahr el
78 H9 **Ghazal, Bahr el** *var.* Soro. *seasonal river* C Chad
80 E13 **Ghazal, Bahr el** *var.* Baḥr al Ghazāl. ≈ S Sudan
147 Q9 **Ghazalkent** *Rus.* Gazalkent. Toshkent Wiloyati, E Uzbekistan
74 H6 **Ghazaouet** NW Algeria
152 J10 **Ghāziābād** Uttar Pradesh, N India
153 O13 **Ghāzīpur** Uttar Pradesh, N India
149 Q6 **Ghaznī** *var.* Ghazni. Ghaznī, E Afghanistan
149 P7 **Ghaznī** ◆ *province* SE Afghanistan
Ghazzah *see* Gaza
Gheel *see* Geel
Ghelîzâne *see* Relizane
Ghent *see* Gent
Gheorghe Braţul *see* Sfântu Gheorghe, Braţul
Gheorghe Gheorghiu-Dej *see* Oneşti
116 J10 **Gheorgheni** *prev.* Gheorghieni, Sînt-Miclăuş, *Ger.* Niklasmarkt, *Hung.* Gyergyószentmiklós. Harghita, C Romania
Gheorghieni *see* Gheorgheni
116 H10 **Gherla** *Ger.* Neuschliss, *Hung.* Szamosújvár; *prev.* Armenierstadt. Cluj, NW Romania
Gheweifat *see* Ghuwayfāt
146 L11 **Ghijduwon** *Rus.* Gizhduvan. Bukhoro Wiloyati, C Uzbekistan
Ghilan *see* Gīlān
107 C18 **Ghilarza** Sardegna, Italy, C Mediterranean Sea
Ghilizane *see* Relizane
Ghimbi *see* Gīmbī
Ghiriş *see* Câmpia Turzii
103 Y15 **Ghisonaccia** Corse, France, C Mediterranean Sea
147 Q11 **Ghonchí** *Rus.* Ganchi. NW Tajikistan
Ghor *see* Ghowr
153 T13 **Ghoraghat** Rajshahi, NW Bangladesh
149 R13 **Ghotki** Sind, SE Pakistan
148 M5 **Ghowr** *var.* Ghor. ◆ *province* C Afghanistan
146 M10 **Ghozghon** *Rus.* Gazgan. Nawoiy Wiloyati, C Uzbekistan
147 T13 **Ghŭdara** *var.* Gudara, *Rus.* Kudara. SE Tajikistan
153 R13 **Ghugri** ≈ N India
147 S14 **Ghund** *Rus.* Gunt. ≈ SE Tajikistan
Ghurdaqah *see* Hurghada
148 J5 **Ghūriān** Herāt, W Afghanistan
141 T8 **Ghuwayfāt** *var.* Gheweifat. Abū Ẓaby, W UAE
121 O14 **Ghuzayyil, Sabkhat** *salt lake* N Libya
147 N13 **Ghuzor** *Rus.* Guzar. Qashqadaryo Wiloyati, S Uzbekistan
115 G17 **Giáltra** Évvoia, C Greece
Giamame *see* Jamaame
114 F13 **Giannitsá** *var.* Yiannitsá. Kentrikí Makedonía, N Greece
107 F14 **Giannutri, Isola di** *island* Archipelago Toscano, C Italy
96 F13 **Giant's Causeway** *Ir.* Clochán an Aifir. *lava flow* N Northern Ireland, UK
167 S15 **Gia Rai** Minh Hai, S Vietnam
107 L24 **Giarre** Sicilia, Italy, C Mediterranean Sea
44 I7 **Gibara** Holguín, E Cuba
29 O16 **Gibbon** Nebraska, C USA
32 K11 **Gibbon** Oregon, NW USA
33 P11 **Gibbonsville** Idaho, NW USA
64 A13 **Gibb's Hill** *hill* S Bermuda
92 I9 **Gibostad** Troms, N Norway
104 I14 **Gibraleón** Andalucía, S Spain
104 L16 **Gibraltar** ○ (Gibraltar) S Gibraltar
104 L16 **Gibraltar** ◇ *UK dependent territory* SW Europe
Gibraltar, Détroit de/Gibraltar, Estrecho de *see* Gibraltar, Strait of
104 J17 **Gibraltar, Strait of** *Fr.* Détroit de Gibraltar, *Sp.* Estrecho de Gibraltar. *strait* Atlantic Ocean/ Mediterranean Sea
31 S11 **Gibsonburg** Ohio, N USA
30 M13 **Gibson City** Illinois, N USA
180 L8 **Gibson Desert** *desert* Western Australia
10 L17 **Gibsons** British Columbia, SW Canada
149 N12 **Gīdār** Baluchistān, SW Pakistan
155 I17 **Giddalūr** Andhra Pradesh, E India
24 U10 **Giddings** Texas, SW USA
27 Y8 **Gideon** Missouri, C USA
81 I15 **Gīdolē** Southern, S Ethiopia
118 H13 **Giedraičiai** Molėtai, E Lithuania
103 O7 **Gien** Loiret, C France
101 G17 **Giessen** Hessen, W Germany
98 O6 **Gieten** Drenthe, NE Netherlands
23 Y13 **Gifford** Florida, SE USA
9 O5 **Gifford** ≈ Baffin Island, Nunavut, NE Canada
100 J12 **Gifhorn** Niedersachsen, N Germany
11 P13 **Gift Lake** Alberta, W Canada
164 K13 **Gifu** *var.* Gihu. Gifu, Honshū, SW Japan
164 L13 **Gifu** *off.* Gifu-ken, *var.* Gihu. ◆ *prefecture* Honshū, SW Japan
128 M13 **Gigant** Rostovskaya Oblast', SW Russian Federation
40 E8 **Giganta, Sierra de la** ▲ W Mexico
54 E12 **Gigante** Huila, S Colombia
114 I7 **Gigen** Pleven, N Bulgaria
Giggiga *see* Jijiga
96 G12 **Gigha Island** *island* SW Scotland, UK
107 E14 **Giglio, Isola del** *island* Archipelago Toscano, C Italy
Gihu *see* Gifu
104 L2 **Gijón** *var.* Xixón. Asturias, NW Spain
81 D20 **Gikongoro** SW Rwanda
36 K14 **Gila Bend** Arizona, SW USA
36 J14 **Gila Bend Mountains** ▲ Arizona, SW USA
37 N14 **Gila Mountains** ▲ Arizona, SW USA
36 I15 **Gila Mountains** ▲ Arizona, SW USA
142 M4 **Gīlān** *off.* Ostān-e Gīlān; *var.* Ghilan, Guilan. ◆ *province* NW Iran
Gilani *see* Gnjilane
36 L14 **Gila River** ≈ Arizona, SW USA
29 W4 **Gilbert** Minnesota, N USA
Gilbert Islands *see* Tungaru
10 L16 **Gilbert, Mount** ▲ British Columbia, SW Canada
181 U4 **Gilbert River** ≈ Queensland, NE Australia
(0) C6 **Gilbert Seamounts** *undersea feature* NE Pacific Ocean
33 S7 **Gildford** Montana, NW USA
83 P15 **Gilé** Zambézia, NE Mozambique
30 K4 **Gile Flowage** ◎ Wisconsin, N USA
182 G7 **Giles, Lake** *salt lake* South Australia
75 U12 **Gilf Kebir Plateau** *Ar.* Haḍabat al Jilf al Kabīr. *plateau* SW Egypt
183 R6 **Gilgandra** New South Wales, SE Australia
Gilgāu *see* Gâlgău
81 I19 **Gilgil** Rift Valley, SW Kenya
183 S4 **Gil Gil Creek** ≈ New South Wales, SE Australia
149 V3 **Gilgit** Jammu and Kashmir, NE Pakistan
149 V3 **Gilgit** ≈ N Pakistan
11 X11 **Gillam** Manitoba, C Canada
95 J22 **Gilleleje** Frederiksborg, E Denmark
30 K14 **Gillespie** Illinois, N USA
27 W13 **Gillett** Arkansas, C USA
33 X12 **Gillette** Wyoming, C USA
97 P22 **Gillingham** SE England, UK
195 X6 **Gillock Island** *island* Antarctica
173 O16 **Gillot** ✕ (St-Denis) N Réunion
65 H25 **Gill Point** *headland* E Saint Helena
30 M12 **Gilman** Illinois, N USA
25 W6 **Gilmer** Texas, SW USA
Gilolo *see* Halmahera, Pulau
81 G14 **Gilo Wenz** ≈ SW Ethiopia
35 O10 **Gilroy** California, W USA
123 Q12 **Gilyuy** ≈ SE Russian Federation
99 I14 **Gilze** Noord-Brabant, S Netherlands
165 R16 **Gima** Okinawa, Kume-jima, SW Japan
80 H13 **Gimbi** *It.* Ghimbi. Oromo, C Ethiopia
45 T12 **Gimie, Mount** ▲ C Saint Lucia
11 X16 **Gimli** Manitoba, S Canada
Gimma *see* Jīma
95 O14 **Gimo** Uppsala, C Sweden
102 L15 **Gimone** ≈ S France
Gimpoe *see* Gimpu
171 N12 **Gimpu** *prev.* Gimpoe. Sulawesi, C Indonesia
182 F5 **Gina** South Australia
Ginevra *see* Genève
99 J19 **Gingelom** Limburg, NE Belgium
180 I12 **Gingin** Western Australia
171 Q7 **Gingoog** Mindanao, S Philippines
81 K14 **Gīnīr** Oromo, C Ethiopia
Giohar *see* Jawhar
107 O17 **Gioia del Colle** Puglia, SE Italy
107 M22 **Gioia, Golfo di** *gulf* S Italy
Giona *see* Gkióna
115 I16 **Gioúra** *island* Vóreioi Sporádes, Greece, Aegean Sea
107 O17 **Giovinazzo** Puglia, SE Italy
Gipeswic *see* Ipswich
Gipuzkoa *see* Guipúzcoa
Giran *see* Ilan
30 K14 **Girard** Illinois, N USA
27 R7 **Girard** Kansas, C USA
25 O6 **Girard** Texas, SW USA
54 E10 **Girardot** Cundinamarca, C Colombia
172 M7 **Giraud Seamount** *undersea feature* SW Indian Ocean
83 A15 **Giraul** ≈ SW Angola
96 L9 **Girdle Ness** *headland* NE Scotland, UK
137 N11 **Giresun** *var.* Kerasunt; *anc.* Cerasus, Pharnacia. Giresun, NE Turkey
137 N12 **Giresun** *var.* Kerasunt. ◆ *province* NE Turkey
137 N12 **Giresun Dağları** ▲ N Turkey
75 X10 **Girga** *var.* Girgeh, Jirjā. C Egypt
Girgeh *see* Girga
Girgenti *see* Agrigento
153 Q15 **Girīdīh** Bihār, NE India
183 P6 **Girilambone** New South Wales, SE Australia
Girin *see* Jilin
121 W10 **Girne** *Gk.* Kerýneia, Kyrenia. N Cyprus
105 X5 **Girona** *var.* Gerona; *anc.* Gerunda. Cataluña, NE Spain
105 W5 **Girona** *var.* Gerona ◆ *province* Cataluña, NE Spain
102 J12 **Gironde** ◆ *department* SW France
102 J11 **Gironde** *estuary* SW France
105 V5 **Gironella** Cataluña, NE Spain
103 N15 **Girou** ≈ S France
97 H14 **Girvan** W Scotland, UK
24 M9 **Girvin** Texas, SW USA
184 Q9 **Gisborne** Gisborne, North Island, NZ
184 P9 **Gisborne** *off.* Gisborne District. ◆ *unitary authority* North Island, NZ
Giseifu *see* Ŭijŏngbu
Gisenye *see* Gisenyi
81 D19 **Gisenyi** *var.* Gisenye. NW Rwanda
95 K20 **Gislaved** Jönköping, S Sweden
103 N4 **Gisors** Eure, N France
Gissar *see* Hisor
147 P12 **Gissar Range** *Rus.* Gissarskiy Khrebet. ▲ Tajikistan/Uzbekistan
Gissarskiy Khrebet *see* Gissar Range
99 B16 **Gistel** West-Vlaanderen, W Belgium
108 F9 **Giswil** Unterwalden, C Switzerland
115 B16 **Gitánes** *ancient monument* Ípeiros, W Greece
81 E20 **Gitarama** C Rwanda
81 E20 **Gitega** C Burundi
Githio *see* Gýtheio
108 H11 **Giubiasco** Ticino, S Switzerland
106 K13 **Giulianova** Abruzzo, C Italy
Giulie, Alpi *see* Julian Alps
Giumri *see* Gyumri
116 M13 **Giurgeni** Ialomiţa, SE Romania
116 J15 **Giurgiu** Giurgiu, S Romania
116 J14 **Giurgiu** ◆ *county* SE Romania
95 F22 **Give** Vejle, C Denmark
103 R2 **Givet** Ardennes, N France
103 R11 **Givors** Rhône, E France
83 K19 **Giyani** Northern, NE South Africa
80 I13 **Giyon** Oromo, C Ethiopia
Giza/Gizeh *see* El Gîza
75 V8 **Giza, Pyramids of** *ancient monument* N Egypt
Gizhduvan *see* Ghijduwon
123 U8 **Gizhiga** Magadanskaya Oblast', E Russian Federation
123 T9 **Gizhiginskaya Guba** *bay* E Russian Federation
186 K8 **Gizo** Gizo, NW Solomon Islands
110 N7 **Giżycko** *Ger.* Lötzen. Warmińsko-Mazurskie, NE Poland
Gizymałów *see* Hrymayliv
Gjakovë *see* Đakovica
94 F12 **Gjende** ◎ S Norway
95 F17 **Gjerstad** Aust-Agder, S Norway
Gjilan *see* Gnjilane
Gjinokastër *see* Gjirokastër
113 L23 **Gjirokastër** *var.* Gjirokastra; *prev.* Gjinokastër, *Gk.* Argyrokastron, *It.* Argirocastro. Gjirokastër, S Albania
113 L22 **Gjirokastër** ◆ *district* S Albania
8 M7 **Gjoa Haven** King William Island, Nunavut, NW Canada
94 H13 **Gjøvik** Oppland, S Norway
113 J22 **Gjuhëzës, Kepi i** *headland* SW Albania
Gjurgjevac *see* Đurđevac
115 E18 **Gkióna** *var.* Giona. ▲ C Greece
121 R3 **Gkréko, Akrotíri** *var.* Cape Greco, Pidálion. *headland* E Cyprus
99 I18 **Glabbeek-Zuurbemde** Vlaams Brabant, C Belgium
13 R14 **Glace Bay** Cape Breton Island, Nova Scotia, SE Canada
11 O16 **Glacier** British Columbia, SW Canada
39 W12 **Glacier Bay** *inlet* Alaska, USA
32 I7 **Glacier Peak** ▲ Washington, NW USA
159 N13 **Gladaindong** *var.* Gèladaindong. ▲ C China
21 Q7 **Glade Spring** Virginia, NE USA
25 W7 **Gladewater** Texas, SW USA
181 Y8 **Gladstone** Queensland, E Australia
182 I8 **Gladstone** South Australia
11 X16 **Gladstone** Manitoba, S Canada
31 O5 **Gladstone** Michigan, N USA
27 R4 **Gladstone** Missouri, C USA
31 Q7 **Gladwin** Michigan, N USA
95 J15 **Glafsfjorden** ◎ C Sweden
92 H2 **Gláma** *physical region* NW Iceland
94 I12 **Gláma** *var.* Glommen, Glomma. ≈ S Norway
112 F13 **Glamoč** Federacija Bosna I Hercegovina, NE Bosnia and Herzegovina
97 J22 **Glamorgan** *cultural region* S Wales, UK
95 G24 **Glamsbjerg** Fyn, C Denmark
171 Q8 **Glan** Mindanao, S Philippines
95 M17 **Glan** ◎ S Sweden
109 T9 **Glan** ≈ SE Austria
101 F19 **Glan** ≈ W Germany
Glaris *see* Glarus
108 H9 **Glarner Alpen** *Eng.* Glarus Alps. ▲ E Switzerland
108 H8 **Glarus** Glarus, E Switzerland
108 H9 **Glarus** *Fr.* Glaris. ◆ *canton* C Switzerland
Glarus Alps *see* Glarner Alpen
27 N3 **Glasco** Kansas, C USA
96 I12 **Glasgow** S Scotland, UK
20 K7 **Glasgow** Kentucky, S USA
27 T4 **Glasgow** Missouri, C USA
33 W7 **Glasgow** Montana, NW USA
21 T6 **Glasgow** Virginia, NE USA
96 I12 **Glasgow** ✕ W Scotland, UK
11 S14 **Glaslyn** Saskatchewan, S Canada
18 I16 **Glassboro** New Jersey, NE USA
24 L10 **Glass Mountains** ▲ Texas, SW USA
97 K23 **Glastonbury** SW England, UK
Glatz *see* Kłodzko
101 N16 **Glauchau** Sachsen, E Germany
Glavn'a Morava *see* Velika Morava
113 N16 **Glavnik** Serbia, S Yugoslavia
129 T1 **Glazov** Udmurtskaya Respublika, NW Russian Federation
Głda *see* Gwda
109 U8 **Gleinalpe** ▲ SE Austria
109 W8 **Gleisdorf** Steiermark, SE Austria
Gleiwitz *see* Gliwice
39 S11 **Glenallen** Alaska, USA
102 F7 **Glénan, Îles** *island group* NW France
185 G21 **Glenavy** Canterbury, South Island, NZ
10 H5 **Glenboyle** Yukon Territory, NW Canada
21 X3 **Glen Burnie** Maryland, NE USA
36 L8 **Glen Canyon** *canyon* Utah, W USA
36 L8 **Glen Canyon Dam** *dam* Arizona, SW USA
30 K15 **Glen Carbon** Illinois, N USA
14 E17 **Glencoe** Ontario, S Canada
83 K22 **Glencoe** KwaZulu/Natal, E South Africa
29 U9 **Glencoe** Minnesota, N USA
96 H10 **Glen Coe** *valley* N Scotland, UK
36 K13 **Glendale** Arizona, SW USA
35 S15 **Glendale** California, W USA
182 G5 **Glendambo** South Australia
33 Y8 **Glendive** Montana, NW USA
33 Y15 **Glendo** Wyoming, C USA
55 S10 **Glendor Mountians** ▲ C Guyana
182 K12 **Glenelg River** ≈ South Australia/Victoria, SE Australia
29 P4 **Glenfield** North Dakota, N USA
25 V12 **Glen Flora** Texas, SW USA
181 P7 **Glen Helen** Northern Territory, N Australia
183 U5 **Glen Innes** New South Wales, SE Australia
31 P6 **Glen Lake** ◎ Michigan, N USA
10 I7 **Glenlyon Peak** ▲ Yukon Territory, W Canada
37 N16 **Glenn, Mount** ▲ Arizona, SW USA
33 N15 **Glenns Ferry** Idaho, NW USA
23 W6 **Glennville** Georgia, SE USA
10 J10 **Glenora** British Columbia, W Canada
182 M11 **Glenorchy** Victoria, SE Australia
183 V5 **Glenreagh** New South Wales, SE Australia
33 X15 **Glenrock** Wyoming, C USA
96 K11 **Glenrothes** E Scotland, UK
18 L9 **Glens Falls** New York, NE USA
97 D14 **Glenties** *Ir.* Na Gleannta. NW Ireland
28 L5 **Glen Ullin** North Dakota, N USA
21 R4 **Glenville** West Virginia, NE USA
27 T12 **Glenwood** Arkansas, C USA
29 S15 **Glenwood** Iowa, C USA
29 T7 **Glenwood** Minnesota, N USA
36 L5 **Glenwood** Utah, W USA
30 I5 **Glenwood City** Wisconsin, N USA
37 Q4 **Glenwood Springs** Colorado, C USA
108 F10 **Gletsch** Valais, S Switzerland
Glevum *see* Gloucester
29 U14 **Glidden** Iowa, C USA
112 E9 **Glina** Sisak-Moslavina, NE Croatia
94 F11 **Glittertind** ▲ S Norway
111 J16 **Gliwice** *Ger.* Gleiwitz. Śląskie, S Poland
36 M14 **Globe** Arizona, SW USA
Globino *see* Hlobyne
108 L9 **Glockturm** ▲ SW Austria
116 L9 **Glodeni** *Rus.* Glodyany. N Moldova
109 S9 **Glödnitz** Kärnten, S Austria
Glodyany *see* Glodeni
Glogau *see* Głogów
109 W6 **Gloggnitz** Niederösterreich, E Austria
110 F13 **Głogów** *Ger.* Glogau, Glogow. Dolnośląskie, SW Poland
111 I16 **Głogówek** *Ger.* Oberglogau. Opolskie, S Poland
92 G12 **Glomfjord** Nordland, C Norway
Glommen *see* Gláma
93 I14 **Glommersträsk** Norrbotten, N Sweden
172 I1 **Glorieuses, Nosy** *island group* N Madagascar
65 C25 **Glorious Hill** *hill* East Falkland, Falkland Islands
38 J12 **Glory of Russia Cape** *headland* Saint Matthew Island, Alaska, USA
22 J7 **Gloster** Mississippi, S USA
183 U7 **Gloucester** New South Wales, SE Australia
186 F7 **Gloucester** New Britain, E PNG
97 L21 **Gloucester** *hist.* Caer Glou, *Lat.* Glevum. C England, UK
19 P10 **Gloucester** Massachusetts, NE USA
21 X6 **Gloucester** Virginia, NE USA
97 K21 **Gloucestershire** *cultural region* C England, UK
31 T14 **Glouster** Ohio, N USA
42 H3 **Glovers Reef** *reef* E Belize
18 K10 **Gloversville** New York, NE USA
110 K12 **Głowno** Łódź, C Poland
111 H16 **Głubczyce** *Ger.* Leobschütz. Opolskie, S Poland
128 L11 **Glubokiy** Rostovskaya Oblast', SW Russian Federation
145 W9 **Glubokoye** Vostochnyy Kazakhstan, E Kazakhstan
Glubokoye *see* Hlybokaye
111 H16 **Głuchołazy** *Ger.* Ziegenhais. Opolskie, S Poland
100 I9 **Glückstadt** Schleswig-Holstein, N Germany
Glukhov *see* Hlukhiv
Glushkevichi *see* Hlushkavichy
Glusk/Glussk *see* Hlusk
Glybokaya *see* Hlyboka
95 F21 **Glyngøre** Viborg, NW Denmark
129 Q9 **Gmelinka** Volgogradskaya Oblast', SW Russian Federation
109 R8 **Gmünd** Kärnten, S Austria
109 U2 **Gmünd** Niederösterreich, N Austria
Gmünd *see* Schwäbisch Gmünd
109 S5 **Gmunden** Oberösterreich, N Austria
Gmundner See *see* Traunsee
94 N10 **Gnarp** Gävleborg, C Sweden
109 W8 **Gnas** Steiermark, SE Austria
Gnesen *see* Gniezno
95 O16 **Gnesta** Södermanland, C Sweden
110 H11 **Gniezno** *Ger.* Gnesen. Wielkolpolskie, C Poland
113 O17 **Gnjilane** *var.* Gilani, *Alb.* Gjilan. Serbia, S Yugoslavia
95 K20 **Gnosjö** Jönköping, S Sweden
155 E17 **Goa** *prev.* Old Goa, Vela Goa, Velha Goa. Goa, W India
155 E17 **Goa** *var.* Old Goa. ◆ *state* W India
42 H7 **Goascorán, Río** ≈ El Salvador/Honduras
77 O16 **Goaso** *var.* Gawso. W Ghana
81 K14 **Goba** *It.* Oromo, S Ethiopia
83 C20 **Gobabed** Erongo, W Namibia
83 E19 **Gobabis** Omaheke, E Namibia
Gobannium *see* Abergavenny
64 M7 **Goban Spur** *undersea feature* NW Atlantic Ocean
Gobbà *see* Goba
63 H21 **Gobernador Gregores** Santa Cruz, S Argentina
61 F14 **Gobernador Ingeniero Virasoro** Corrientes, NE Argentina
162 L12 **Gobi** *desert* China/Mongolia
164 I14 **Gobō** Wakayama, Honshū, SW Japan
101 D14 **Goch** Nordrhein-Westfalen, W Germany
83 E20 **Gochas** Hardap, S Namibia
155 I14 **Godāvari** *var.* Godavari. ≈ C India
155 L16 **Godāvari, Mouths of the** *delta* E India
15 V5 **Godbout** Quebec, SE Canada
15 U5 **Godbout** ≈ Quebec, SE Canada
15 U5 **Godbout Est** ≈ Quebec, SE Canada
27 N6 **Goddard** Kansas, C USA
14 E15 **Goderich** Ontario, S Canada
Godhavn *see* Qeqertarsuaq
154 E10 **Godhra** Gujarāt, W India
Göding *see* Hodonín
111 K22 **Gödöllő** Pest, N Hungary
62 H11 **Godoy Cruz** Mendoza, W Argentina
11 Y11 **Gods** ≈ Manitoba, C Canada
11 Y13 **Gods Lake** Manitoba, C Canada
11 X13 **Gods Lake** ◎ Manitoba, C Canada
Godthaab/Godthåb *see* Nuuk
Godwin Austen, Mount *see* K2
Goede Hoop, Kaap de *see* Good Hope, Cape of
Goedgegun *see* Nhlangano
Goeie Hoop, Kaap die *see* Good Hope, Cape of
13 O7 **Goélands, Lac aux** ◎ Quebec, SE Canada
98 E13 **Goeree** *island* SW Netherlands
99 F15 **Goes** Zeeland, SW Netherlands
Goettingen *see* Göttingen
19 O10 **Goffstown** New Hampshire, NE USA
14 E8 **Gogama** Ontario, S Canada
30 L3 **Gogebic, Lake** ◎ Michigan, N USA
30 K3 **Gogebic Range** *hill range* Michigan/Wisconsin, N USA
137 V13 **Gogi, Mount** *Arm.* Gogi Lerr, *Az.* Küküdağ. ▲ Armenia/Azerbaijan
126 F12 **Gogland, Ostrov** *island* NW Russian Federation
111 I15 **Gogolin** Opolskie, S Poland
Gogonou *see* Gogounou
77 S14 **Gogounou** *var.* Gogonou. N Benin
152 I10 **Gohāna** Haryāna, N India
59 K18 **Goianésia** Goiás, C Brazil
59 K18 **Goiânia** *prev.* Goyania. *state capital* Goiás, C Brazil
59 K18 **Goiás** Goiás, C Brazil
59 J18 **Goiás** *off.* Estado de Goiás; *prev.* Goiaz, Goyaz. ◆ *state* C Brazil
Goiaz *see* Goiás
159 R14 **Goinsargoin** Xizang Zizhiqu, W China
60 H10 **Goio-Erê** Paraná, SW Brazil
99 I15 **Goirle** Noord-Brabant, S Netherlands
104 H8 **Góis** Coimbra, N Portugal
165 Q8 **Gojōme** Akita, Honshū, NW Japan
149 U9 **Gojra** Punjab, E Pakistan
136 A11 **Gökçeada** *var.* Imroz Adası, *Gk.* Imbros. *island* NW Turkey
Gökçeada *see* İmroz
Gökdepe *see* Geok-Tepe
136 I10 **Gökırmak** ≈ N Turkey
Goklenkuy, Solonchak *see* Geklengkui, Solonchak
136 C16 **Gökova Körfezi** *gulf* SW Turkey
136 K15 **Göksu** ≈ S Turkey
136 L15 **Göksun** Kahramanmaraş, C Turkey
136 I17 **Göksu Nehri** ≈ S Turkey
83 J16 **Gokwe** Midlands, NW Zimbabwe
94 F13 **Gol** Buskerud, S Norway
153 X12 **Golāghāt** Assam, NE India
110 H10 **Gołańcz** Wielkopolskie, C Poland
138 G8 **Golan Heights** *Ar.* Al Jawlān, *Heb.* HaGolan. ▲ SW Syria
Golārā *see* Ārān
Golaya Pristan *see* Hola Prystan'
143 T11 **Golbāf** Kermān, C Iran
136 M15 **Gölbaşı** Adıyaman, S Turkey
109 P9 **Gölbner** ▲ SW Austria
30 M17 **Golconda** Illinois, N USA
35 T3 **Golconda** Nevada, W USA
136 E11 **Gölcük** Kocaeli, NW Turkey
108 I7 **Goldach** Sankt Gallen, NE Switzerland
110 N7 **Gołdap** *Ger.* Goldap. Warmińsko-Mazurskie, NE Poland
32 E15 **Gold Beach** Oregon, NW USA
Goldberg *see* Złotoryja
68 D11 **Gold Coast** *coastal region* S Ghana
183 V3 **Gold Coast** *cultural region* Queensland, E Australia
39 R10 **Gold Creek** Alaska, USA
11 O16 **Golden** British Columbia, SW Canada
37 T4 **Golden** Colorado, C USA
184 I13 **Golden Bay** *bay* South Island, NZ
27 R7 **Golden City** Missouri, C USA
32 I11 **Goldendale** Washington, NW USA
Goldener Tisch *see* Zlatý Stôl
44 L13 **Golden Grove** E Jamaica
14 J12 **Golden Lake** ◎ Ontario, SE Canada
22 K10 **Golden Meadow** Louisiana, S USA
45 V10 **Golden Rock** ✕ (Basseterre) Saint Kitts, Saint Kitts and Nevis
Golden State, The *see* California
83 K16 **Golden Valley** Mashonaland West, N Zimbabwe
35 U9 **Goldfield** Nevada, W USA
Goldingen *see* Kuldīga
Goldmarkt *see* Zlatna
10 K17 **Gold River** Vancouver Island, British Columbia, SW Canada
21 V10 **Goldsboro** North Carolina, SE USA
24 M8 **Goldsmith** Texas, SW USA
25 R8 **Goldthwaite** Texas, SW USA
137 R11 **Göle** Ardahan, NE Turkey
Golema Ada *see* Ostrovo
114 H9 **Golema Planina** ▲ W Bulgaria
114 F9 **Golemi Vrŭkh** ▲ W Bulgaria
110 D8 **Goleniów** *Ger.* Gollnow. Zachodniopomorskie, NW Poland
149 R3 **Golestān** ◆ *province* N Iran
35 Q14 **Goleta** California, W USA
43 O16 **Golfito** Puntarenas, SE Costa Rica
25 T13 **Goliad** Texas, SW USA
113 L14 **Golija** ▲ SW Yugoslavia
113 O16 **Goljak** ▲ SE Yugoslavia
136 M12 **Gölköy** Ordu, N Turkey
Gollel *see* Lavumisa
109 X3 **Göllersbach** ≈ NE Austria
Gollnow *see* Goleniów
Golmo *see* Golmud
159 P10 **Golmud** *var.* Ge'e'mu, Golmo, *Chin.* Ko-erh-mu. Qinghai, C China
103 Y14 **Golo** ≈ Corse, France, C Mediterranean Sea
Golovanevsk *see* Holovanivs'k
Golovchin *see* Halowchyn
39 N9 **Golovin** Alaska, USA
142 M7 **Golpāyegān** *var.* Gulpaigan. Eşfahān, W Iran
Golshan *see* Ṭabas
Gol'shany *see* Hal'shany
96 J7 **Golspie** N Scotland, UK
112 O11 **Golubac** Serbia, NE Yugoslavia
110 J9 **Golub-Dobrzyń** Kujawski-pomorskie, C Poland
145 S7 **Golubovka** Pavlodar, N Kazakhstan
82 B11 **Golungo Alto** Cuanza Norte, NW Angola
114 M8 **Golyama Kamchiya** ≈ E Bulgaria
114 L8 **Golyama Reka** ≈ N Bulgaria
114 H11 **Golyama Syutkya** ▲ SW Bulgaria
114 I12 **Golyam Perelik** ▲ S Bulgaria
114 I11 **Golyam Persenk** ▲ S Bulgaria
79 P19 **Goma** Nord Kivu, NE Dem. Rep. Congo (Zaire)
Gomati *see* Gumti
77 X14 **Gombe** Gombe, E Nigeria
67 U10 **Gombe** *var.* Igombe. ≈ E Tanzania
77 Y14 **Gombi** Adamawa, E Nigeria
Gombroon *see* Bandar-e 'Abbās
Gomel' *see* Homyel'
Gomel'skaya Oblast' *see* Homyel'skaya Voblasts'

◆ Country ● Country Capital ◇ Dependent Territory ○ Dependent Territory Capital ◆ Administrative Region ✕ International Airport ▲ Mountain ▲ Mountain Range Volcano ≈ River ◎ Lake Reservoir

64 N11 **Gomera** *island* Islas Canarias, Spain, NE Atlantic Ocean
40 I5 **Gómez Farias** Chihuahua, N Mexico
40 L8 **Gómez Palacio** Durango, C Mexico
158 J13 **Gomo** Xizang Zizhiqu, W China
143 T6 **Gonābād** *var.* Gunabad. Khorāsān, NE Iran
44 L8 **Gonaïves** *var.* Les Gonaïves. N Haiti
123 Q12 **Gonam** ≈ NE Russian Federation
44 L9 **Gonâve, Canal de la** *var.* Canal de Sud. *channel* N Caribbean Sea
44 K9 **Gonâve, Golfe de la** *gulf* N Caribbean Sea
Gonāveh *see* Bandar-e Gonāveh
44 K9 **Gonâve, Île de la** *island* C Haiti
Gonbadān *see* Dow Gonbadān
143 Q3 **Gonbad-e Kāvūs** *var.* Gunbad-i-Qawus. Golestān, N Iran
152 M12 **Gonda** Uttar Pradesh, N India
Gondar *see* Gonder
80 I11 **Gonder** *var.* Gondar. Amhara, N Ethiopia
78 J13 **Gondey** Moyen-Chari, S Chad
154 J12 **Gondia** Mahārāshtra, C India
104 G6 **Gondomar** Porto, NW Portugal
136 C12 **Gönen** Balıkesir, W Turkey
136 C12 **Gönen Çayı** ≈ NW Turkey
159 O15 **Gongbo'gyamda** Xizang Zizhiqu, W China
159 N16 **Gonggar** Xizang Zizhiqu, W China
160 G9 **Gongga Shan** ▲ C China
159 T10 **Gonghe** Qinghai, C China
158 I5 **Gongliu** *var.* Tokkuztara. Xinjiang Uygur Zizhiqu, NW China
77 W14 **Gongola** ≈ E Nigeria
Gongoleh State *see* Jonglei
183 P5 **Gongolgon** New South Wales, SE Australia
159 Q6 **Gongpoquan** Gansu, N China
160 I10 **Gongxian** *var.* Gong Xian. Sichuan, C China
157 V10 **Gongzhuling** *prev.* Huaide. Jilin, NE China
159 S14 **Gonjo** Xizang Zizhiqu, W China
107 B20 **Gonnesa** Sardegna, Italy, C Mediterranean Sea
Gonni/Gónnos *see* Gónnoi
115 F15 **Gónnoi** *var.* Gonni, Gónnos; *prev.* Derelí. Thessalía, C Greece
164 C13 **Gōnoura** Nagasaki, Iki, SW Japan
35 O11 **Gonzales** California, W USA
22 J9 **Gonzales** Louisiana, S USA
25 T12 **Gonzales** Texas, SW USA
41 P11 **González** Tamaulipas, C Mexico
21 V6 **Goochland** Virginia, NE USA
195 X14 **Goodenough, Cape** *headland* Antarctica
186 F9 **Goodenough Island** *var.* Morata. *island* SE PNG
Good Hope *see* Fort Good Hope
39 N8 **Goodhope Bay** *bay* Alaska, USA
83 D26 **Good Hope, Cape of** *Afr.* Kaap de Goede Hoop, Kaap die Goeie Hoop. *headland* SW South Africa
10 K10 **Good Hope Lake** British Columbia, W Canada
83 E23 **Goodhouse** Northern Cape, W South Africa
33 O15 **Gooding** Idaho, NW USA
26 H3 **Goodland** Kansas, C USA
173 Y15 **Goodlands** NW Mauritius
20 J8 **Goodlettsville** Tennessee, S USA
39 N13 **Goodnews** Alaska, USA
25 O3 **Goodnight** Texas, SW USA
183 Q4 **Goodooga** New South Wales, SE Australia
29 N4 **Goodrich** North Dakota, N USA
25 W10 **Goodrich** Texas, SW USA
29 X10 **Goodview** Minnesota, N USA
26 H8 **Goodwell** Oklahoma, C USA
97 N17 **Goole** E England, UK
183 O8 **Goolgowi** New South Wales, SE Australia
182 I10 **Goolwa** South Australia
181 Y11 **Goondiwindi** Queensland, E Australia
98 O11 **Goor** Overijssel, E Netherlands
Goose Bay *see* Happy Valley-Goose Bay
33 V13 **Gooseberry Creek** ≈ Wyoming, C USA
21 S14 **Goose Creek** South Carolina, SE USA
63 M23 **Goose Green** *var.* Prado del Ganso. East Falkland, Falkland Islands
16 D8 **Goose Lake** *var.* Lago dos Gansos. ◎ California/Oregon, W USA
29 Q4 **Goose River** ≈ North Dakota, N USA
153 T16 **Gopalganj** Dhaka, S Bangladesh
153 O12 **Gopālganj** Bihār, N India
Gopher State *see* Minnesota
101 I22 **Göppingen** Baden-Württemberg, SW Germany
110 G13 **Góra** *Ger.* Guhrau. Dolnośląskie, SW Poland
110 M12 **Góra Kalwaria** Mazowieckie, C Poland
153 O12 **Gorakhpur** Uttar Pradesh, N India
Gorany *see* Harany
113 J14 **Goražde** Federacija Bosna I Hercegovina, Bosnia and Herzegovina
Gorbovichi *see* Harbavichy
Gorče Petrov *see* Đorče Petrov
(0) E9 **Gorda Ridges** *undersea feature* NE Pacific Ocean
Gordiaz *see* Gardēz
78 K12 **Gordil** Vakaga, N Central African Republic
23 U5 **Gordon** Georgia, SE USA
28 K12 **Gordon** Nebraska, C USA
25 R7 **Gordon** Texas, SW USA
28 L13 **Gordon Creek** ≈ Nebraska, C USA
63 I25 **Gordon, Isla** *island* S Chile
183 O17 **Gordon, Lake** ◎ Tasmania, SE Australia
183 O17 **Gordon River** ≈ Tasmania, SE Australia
21 V5 **Gordonsville** Virginia, NE USA
80 H13 **Gorē** Oromo, C Ethiopia
185 D24 **Gore** Southland, South Island, NZ
78 H13 **Goré** Logone-Oriental, S Chad
14 D11 **Gore Bay** Manitoulin Island, Ontario, S Canada
25 Q5 **Goree** Texas, SW USA
137 O11 **Görele** Giresun, NE Turkey
19 N6 **Gore Mountain** ▲ Vermont, NE USA
39 R13 **Gore Point** *headland* Alaska, USA
37 R4 **Gore Range** ▲▲ Colorado, C USA
97 F19 **Gorey** *Ir.* Guaire. SE Ireland
143 R12 **Gorgāb** Kermān, S Iran
143 Q4 **Gorgān** *var.* Astarabad, Astrabad, Gurgan; *prev.* Asterābād, *anc.* Hyrcania. Golestān, N Iran
143 Q4 **Gorgān, Rūd-e** ≈ N Iran
76 I10 **Gorgol** ◈ *region* S Mauritania
106 D12 **Gorgona, Isola di** *island* Archipelago Toscano, C Italy
19 P8 **Gorham** Maine, NE USA
137 T10 **Gori** C Georgia
98 I13 **Gorinchem** *var.* Gorkum. Zuid-Holland, C Netherlands
137 V13 **Goris** SE Armenia
126 K16 **Goritsy** Tverskaya Oblast', W Russian Federation
106 J7 **Gorizia** *Ger.* Görz. Friuli-Venezia Giulia, NE Italy
116 G13 **Gorj** ◈ *county* SW Romania
109 W12 **Gorjanci** *var.* Uskočke Planine, Žumberak, Žumberačko Gorje, *Ger.* Uskokengebirge; *prev.* Sichelburger Gerbirge. ▲▲ Croatia/Slovenia *see also* Žumberačko Gorje
Görkau *see* Jirkov
Gorki *see* Horki
Gor'kiy *see* Nizhniy Novgorod
Gor'kiy Reservoir *see* Gor'kovskoye Vodokhranilishche
Gorkum *see* Gorinchem
95 I23 **Gørlev** Vestsjælland, E Denmark
111 M17 **Gorlice** Małopolskie, S Poland
101 Q15 **Görlitz** Sachsen, E Germany
Görlitz *see* Zgorzelec
Gorlovka *see* Horlivka
25 R7 **Gorman** Texas, SW USA
21 T3 **Gormania** West Virginia, NE USA
Gorna Dzhumaya *see* Blagoevgrad
114 K8 **Gorna Oryakhovitsa** Veliko Tŭrnovo, N Bulgaria
114 J8 **Gorna Studena** Veliko Tŭrnovo, N Bulgaria
Gornja Mužlja *see* Mužlja
109 X9 **Gornja Radgona** *Ger.* Oberradkersburg. NE Slovenia
112 M13 **Gornji Milanovac** Serbia, C Yugoslavia
112 G13 **Gornji Vakuf** *var.* Uskoplje. Federacija Bosna I Hercegovina, W Bosnia and Herzegovina
122 J13 **Gorno-Altaysk** Respublika Altay, S Russian Federation
Gorno-Altayskaya Respublika *see* Altay, Respublika
123 N12 **Gorno-Chuyskiy** Irkutskaya Oblast', C Russian Federation
127 V14 **Gornozavodsk** Permskaya Oblast', NW Russian Federation
122 I13 **Gornyak** Altayskiy Kray, S Russian Federation
129 R8 **Gornyy** Saratovskaya Oblast', W Russian Federation
Gornyy Altay *see* Altay, Respublika
129 O10 **Gornyy Balykley** Volgogradskaya Oblast', SW Russian Federation
80 I13 **Goroch'an** ▲ W Ethiopia
Gorodenka *see* Horodenka
129 O3 **Gorodets** Nizhegorodskaya Oblast', W Russian Federation
Gorodets *see* Haradzyets
Gorodeya *see* Haradzyeya
129 P6 **Gorodishche** Penzenskaya Oblast', W Russian Federation
Gorodishche *see* Horodyshche
Gorodnya *see* Horodnya
Gorodok *see* Haradok
Gorodok/Gorodok Yagellonski *see* Horodok
128 M13 **Gorodovikovsk** Respublika Kalmykiya, SW Russian Federation
186 D7 **Goroka** Eastern Highlands, C PNG
Gorokhov *see* Horokhiv
129 N3 **Gorokhovets** Vladimirskaya Oblast', W Russian Federation
77 Q11 **Gorom-Gorom** NE Burkina
171 U13 **Gorong, Kepulauan** *island group* E Indonesia
83 M17 **Gorongosa** Sofala, C Mozambique
171 P11 **Gorontalo** Sulawesi, C Indonesia
Gorontalo, Teluk *see* Tomini, Gulf of
110 L7 **Górowo Iławeckie** *Ger.* Landsberg. Warmińsko-Mazurskie, NE Poland,
98 M7 **Gorredijk** *Fris.* De Gordyk. Friesland, N Netherlands
84 C14 **Gorringe Ridge** *undersea feature* E Atlantic Ocean
98 M11 **Gorssel** Gelderland, E Netherlands
109 T8 **Görtschitz** ≈ S Austria
Goryn *see* Horyn'
Görz *see* Gorizia
110 E10 **Gorzów Wielkopolski** *Ger.* Landsberg, Landsberg an der Warthe. Lubuskie, W Poland
108 G9 **Göschenen** Uri, C Switzerland
165 O11 **Gosen** Niigata, Honshū, C Japan
183 T8 **Gosford** New South Wales, SE Australia
31 P11 **Goshen** Indiana, N USA
18 K13 **Goshen** New York, NE USA
Goshoba *see* Koshoba
165 Q7 **Goshogawara** *var.* Gosyogawara. Aomori, Honshū, C Japan
146 I8 **Goshquduq Qum** *var.* Tosquduq Qumlari, *Rus.* Peski Taskuduk. *desert* W Uzbekistan
101 J14 **Goslar** Niedersachsen, C Germany
27 Y9 **Gosnell** Arkansas, C USA
112 C11 **Gospić** Lika-Senj, C Croatia
97 N23 **Gosport** S England, UK
94 D9 **Gossa** *island* S Norway
108 H7 **Gossau** Sankt Gallen, NE Switzerland
99 G20 **Gosselies** *var.* Goss'lies. Hainaut, S Belgium
77 P10 **Gossi** Tombouctou, C Mali
Goss'lies *see* Gosselies
113 N18 **Gostivar** W FYR Macedonia
Gostomel' *see* Hostomel'
110 G12 **Gostyń** *var.* Gostyn. Wielkopolskie, C Poland
110 K11 **Gostynin** Mazowieckie, C Poland
Gosyogawara *see* Goshogawara
95 J18 **Göta Älv** ≈ S Sweden
95 N17 **Göta kanal** *canal* S Sweden
95 K18 **Götaland** *cultural region* S Sweden
95 H17 **Göteborg** *Eng.* Gothenburg. Västra Götaland, S Sweden
77 X16 **Gotel Mountains** ▲▲ E Nigeria
95 K17 **Götene** Västra Götaland, S Sweden
Gotera *see* San Francisco
101 K16 **Gotha** Thüringen, C Germany
29 N15 **Gothenburg** Nebraska, C USA
Gothenburg *see* Göteborg
77 R12 **Gothèye** Tillabéri, SW Niger
Gothland *see* Gotland
95 P19 **Gotland** *var.* Gothland, Gottland. ◈ *county* SE Sweden
95 O18 **Gotland** *island* SE Sweden
164 B13 **Gotō-rettō** *island group* SW Japan
114 H12 **Gotse Delchev** *prev.* Nevrokop. Blagoevgrad, SW Bulgaria
95 P17 **Gotska Sandön** *island* SE Sweden
101 I15 **Göttingen** *var.* Goettingen. Niedersachsen, C Germany
Gottland *see* Gotland
93 I16 **Gottne** Västernorrland, C Sweden
Gottschee *see* Kočevje
Gottwaldov *see* Zlín
Gôtu *see* Gōtsu
Goturdepe *see* Koturdepe
108 I7 **Götzis** Vorarlberg, NW Austria
98 H12 **Gouda** Zuid-Holland, C Netherlands
76 I11 **Goudiri** *var.* Goudiry. E Senegal
Goudiry *see* Goudiri
77 X12 **Goudoumaria** Diffa, S Niger
15 R9 **Gouffre, Rivière du** ≈ Quebec, SE Canada
65 M19 **Gough Fracture Zone** *tectonic feature* S Atlantic Ocean
65 M19 **Gough Island** *island* Tristan da Cunha, S Atlantic Ocean
15 N8 **Gouin, Réservoir** ⊞ Quebec, SE Canada
14 B10 **Goulais River** Ontario, S Canada
183 R9 **Goulburn** New South Wales, SE Australia
183 O11 **Goulburn River** ≈ Victoria, SE Australia
195 O10 **Gould Coast** *physical region* Antarctica
Goulimime *see* Guelmime
114 F13 **Gouménissa** Kentrikí Makedonía, N Greece
77 O10 **Goundam** Tombouctou, NW Mali
78 H12 **Goundi** Moyen-Chari, S Chad
78 G12 **Gounou-Gaya** Mayo-Kébbi, SW Chad
77 O12 **Gourci** *var.* Gourcy. NW Burkina
Gourcy *see* Gourci
102 M13 **Gourdon** Lot, S France
77 W11 **Gouré** Zinder, SE Niger
102 G6 **Gourin** Morbihan, NW France
77 P10 **Gourma-Rharous** Tombouctou, C Mali
103 N4 **Gournay-en-Bray** Seine-Maritime, N France
78 J6 **Gouro** Borkou-Ennedi-Tibesti, N Chad
104 H8 **Gouveia** Guarda, N Portugal
18 I7 **Gouverneur** New York, NE USA
99 L21 **Gouvy** Luxembourg, E Belgium
45 R14 **Gouyave** *var.* Charlotte Town. NW Grenada
Goverla, Gora *see* Hoverla, Hora
59 N20 **Governador Valadares** Minas Gerais, SE Brazil
171 R8 **Governor Generoso** Mindanao, S Philippines
44 I2 **Governor's Harbour** Eleuthera Island, C Bahamas
162 F9 **Govĭ-Altay** ◈ *province* SW Mongolia
162 I10 **Govĭ Altayn Nuruu** ▲▲ S Mongolia
154 L9 **Govind Ballabh Pant Sāgar** ⊞ C India
152 J7 **Govind Sāgar** ⊞ NE India
147 N14 **Govurdak** *Turkm.* Gowurdak; *prev.* Guardak. Lebapskiy Velayat, E Turkmenistan
18 D11 **Gowanda** New York, NE USA
148 J10 **Gowd-e Zereh, Dasht-e** *var.* Guad-i-Zirreh. *marsh* SW Afghanistan
14 F8 **Gowganda** Ontario, S Canada
14 G8 **Gowganda Lake** ◎ Ontario, S Canada
29 U13 **Gowrie** Iowa, C USA
Gowurdak *see* Govurdak
61 C15 **Goya** Corrientes, NE Argentina
Goyania *see* Goiânia
137 X11 **Göyçay** *Rus.* Geokchay. C Azerbaijan
Goymat *see* Koymat
Goymatdag *see* Koymatdag, Gory
136 F12 **Göynük** Bolu, NW Turkey
165 R9 **Goyō-san** ▲ Honshū, C Japan
78 K11 **Goz Beïda** Ouaddaï, SE Chad
158 H11 **Gozha Co** ◎ W China
121 O15 **Gozo** *Malt.* Ghawdex. *island* N Malta
80 H9 **Gōz Regeb** Kassala, NE Sudan
Gozyô *see* Gojō
83 H25 **Graaff-Reinet** Eastern Cape, S South Africa
Graasten *see* Gråsten
76 L17 **Grabo** SW Ivory Coast
112 P11 **Grabovica** Serbia, E Yugoslavia
110 I13 **Grabów nad Prosną** Wielkopolskie, C Poland
108 I8 **Grabs** Sankt Gallen, NE Switzerland
112 D12 **Gračac** Zadar, C Croatia
112 I11 **Gračanica** Federacija Bosna I Hercegovina, NE Bosnia and Herzegovina
14 L11 **Gracefield** Quebec, SE Canada
99 K19 **Grâce-Hollogne** Liège, E Belgium
23 R8 **Graceville** Florida, SE USA
29 R8 **Graceville** Minnesota, N USA
42 G6 **Gracias** Lempira, W Honduras
Gracias *see* Lempira
42 L5 **Gracias a Dios** ◈ *department* E Honduras
43 O6 **Gracias a Dios, Cabo de** *headland* Honduras/Nicaragua
64 O2 **Graciosa** *var.* Ilha Graciosa. *island* Azores, Portugal, NE Atlantic Ocean
64 Q11 **Graciosa** *island* Islas Canarias, Spain, NE Atlantic Ocean
Graciosa, Ilha *see* Graciosa
112 I11 **Gradačac** Federacija Bosna I Hercegovina, N Bosnia and Herzegovina
59 J15 **Gradaús, Serra dos** ▲▲ C Brazil
104 L3 **Gradefes** Castilla-León, N Spain
Gradiška *see* Bosanska Gradiška
Gradizhsk *see* Hradyz'k
106 J7 **Grado** Friuli-Venezia Giulia, NE Italy
104 K2 **Grado** Asturias, N Spain
113 P19 **Gradsko** C FYR Macedonia
37 V11 **Grady** New Mexico, SW USA
29 T12 **Graettinger** Iowa, C USA
101 M23 **Grafing** Bayern, SE Germany
25 S6 **Graford** Texas, SW USA
183 V5 **Grafton** New South Wales, SE Australia
29 Q3 **Grafton** North Dakota, N USA
21 S3 **Grafton** West Virginia, NE USA
21 T9 **Graham** North Carolina, SE USA
25 R6 **Graham** Texas, SW USA
Graham Bell Island *see* Greem-Bell, Ostrov
10 I13 **Graham Island** *island* Queen Charlotte Islands, British Columbia, SW Canada
19 S6 **Graham Lake** ◎ Maine, NE USA
194 H4 **Graham Land** *physical region* Antarctica
37 N15 **Graham, Mount** ▲ Arizona, SW USA
Grahamstad *see* Grahamstown
83 I25 **Grahamstown** *Afr.* Grahamstad. Eastern Cape, S South Africa
Grahovo *see* Bosansko Grahovo
68 C11 **Grain Coast** *coastal region* S Liberia
169 S17 **Grajagan, Teluk** *bay* Jawa, S Indonesia
59 L14 **Grajaú** Maranhão, E Brazil
58 M13 **Grajaú, Rio** ≈ NE Brazil
110 O8 **Grajewo** Podlaskie, NE Poland
95 F24 **Gram** Sønderjylland, SW Denmark
103 N13 **Gramat** Lot, S France
22 H5 **Grambling** Louisiana, S USA
115 C14 **Grámmos** ▲ Albania/Greece
96 I9 **Grampian Mountains** ▲▲ C Scotland, UK
182 L12 **Grampians, The** ▲▲ Victoria, SE Australia
98 O9 **Gramsbergen** Overijssel, E Netherlands
113 L21 **Gramsh** *var.* Gramshi. Elbasan, C Albania
Gramshi *see* Gramsh
Gran *see* Hron, Slovakia
Gran *see* Esztergom, N Hungary
54 F11 **Granada** Meta, C Colombia
42 J10 **Granada** Granada, SW Nicaragua
105 N14 **Granada** Andalucía, S Spain
37 W6 **Granada** Colorado, C USA
42 J11 **Granada** ◈ *department* SW Nicaragua
105 N14 **Granada** ◈ *province* Andalucía, S Spain
63 I21 **Gran Altiplanicie Central** *plain* S Argentina
97 E17 **Granard** *Ir.* Gránárd. C Ireland
63 J20 **Gran Bajo** *basin* S Argentina
63 J15 **Gran Bajo del Gualicho** *basin* E Argentina
63 I21 **Gran Bajo de San Julián** *basin* SE Argentina
25 S7 **Granbury** Texas, SW USA
15 P12 **Granby** Quebec, SE Canada
27 S8 **Granby** Missouri, C USA
37 S3 **Granby, Lake** ⊞ Colorado, C USA
64 O12 **Gran Canaria** *var.* Grand Canary. *island* Islas Canarias, Spain, NE Atlantic Ocean
47 T11 **Gran Chaco** *var.* Chaco. *lowland plain* South America
45 R14 **Grand Anse** SW Grenada
Grand-Anse *see* Portsmouth
44 G1 **Grand Bahama Island** *island* N Bahamas
Grand Balé *see* Tui
103 U7 **Grand Ballon** *Ger.* Ballon de Guebwiller. ▲ NE France
13 T13 **Grand Bank** Newfoundland, SE Canada
64 I7 **Grand Banks of Newfoundland** *undersea feature* NW Atlantic Ocean
Grand Bassa *see* Buchanan
77 N17 **Grand-Bassam** *var.* Bassam. SE Ivory Coast
14 E16 **Grand Bend** Ontario, S Canada
76 L17 **Grand-Bérébi** *var.* Grand-Béréby. SW Ivory Coast
Grand-Béréby *see* Grand-Bérébi
45 X11 **Grand-Bourg** Marie-Galante, SE Guadeloupe
44 M6 **Grand Caicos** *var.* Middle Caicos. *island* C Turks and Caicos Islands
14 K12 **Grand Calumet, Île du** *island* Quebec, SE Canada
97 E18 **Grand Canal** *Ir.* An Chanáil Mhór. *canal* C Ireland
Grand Canary *see* Gran Canaria
36 K10 **Grand Canyon** Arizona, SW USA
36 J9 **Grand Canyon** *canyon* Arizona, SW USA
Grand Canyon State *see* Arizona
44 D8 **Grand Cayman** *island* SW Cayman Islands
11 R14 **Grand Centre** Alberta, SW Canada
76 L17 **Grand Cess** SE Liberia
108 D12 **Grand Combin** ▲ S Switzerland
32 K8 **Grand Coulee** Washington, NW USA
32 J8 **Grand Coulee** *valley* Washington, NW USA
45 X5 **Grand Cul-de-Sac Marin** *bay* N Guadeloupe
Grand Duchy of Luxembourg *see* Luxembourg
63 I22 **Grande, Bahía** *bay* S Argentina
11 N14 **Grande Cache** Alberta, W Canada
103 U12 **Grande Casse** ▲ E France
172 G12 **Grande Comore** *var.* Njazidja, Great Comoro. *island* NW Comoros
61 G18 **Grande, Cuchilla** *hill range* E Uruguay
45 S5 **Grande de Añasco, Río** ≈ W Puerto Rico
Grande de Chiloé, Isla *see* Chiloé, Isla de
58 J12 **Grande de Gurupá, Ilha** *river island* NE Brazil
57 K21 **Grande de Lipez, Río** ≈ SW Bolivia
45 U6 **Grande de Loíza, Río** ≈ E Puerto Rico
45 T5 **Grande de Manatí, Río** ≈ C Puerto Rico
42 L9 **Grande de Matagalpa, Río** ≈ C Nicaragua
40 K12 **Grande de Santiago, Río** *var.* Santiago. ≈ C Mexico
43 O15 **Grande de Térraba, Río** *var.* Río Térraba. ≈ SE Costa Rica
12 J9 **Grande Deux, Réservoir la** ⊞ Quebec, E Canada
60 O10 **Grande, Ilha** *island* SE Brazil
11 O13 **Grande Prairie** Alberta, W Canada
74 I8 **Grand Erg Occidental** *desert* W Algeria
74 L9 **Grand Erg Oriental** *desert* Algeria/Tunisia
59 J20 **Grande, Rio** ≈ S Brazil
2 F15 **Grande, Rio** *var.* Río Bravo, *Sp.* Río Bravo del Norte, Bravo del Norte. ≈ Mexico/USA
57 M18 **Grande, Río** ≈ C Bolivia
15 Y7 **Grande-Rivière** Quebec, SE Canada
15 Y6 **Grande Rivière** ≈ Quebec, SE Canada
44 M8 **Grande-Rivière-du-Nord** N Haiti
62 K9 **Grande, Salina** *var.* Gran Salitral. *salt lake* C Argentina
15 S7 **Grandes-Bergeronnes** Quebec, SE Canada
47 W6 **Grande, Serra** ▲▲ W Brazil
40 K4 **Grande, Sierra** ▲▲ N Mexico
103 S12 **Grandes Rousses** ▲▲ E France
63 K17 **Grandes, Salinas** *salt lake* E Argentina
45 Y5 **Grande Terre** *island* E West Indies
15 X5 **Grande-Vallée** Quebec, SE Canada
45 Y5 **Grande Vigie, Pointe de la** *headland* Grande Terre, N Guadeloupe
13 N14 **Grand Falls** New Brunswick, SE Canada
13 T11 **Grand Falls** Newfoundland, SE Canada
24 L9 **Grandfalls** Texas, SW USA
21 P9 **Grandfather Mountain** ▲ North Carolina, SE USA
26 L13 **Grandfield** Oklahoma, C USA
11 N17 **Grand Forks** British Columbia, SW Canada
29 R4 **Grand Forks** North Dakota, N USA
31 O9 **Grand Haven** Michigan, N USA
Grandichi *see* Hrandzichy
29 P15 **Grand Island** Nebraska, C USA
31 O3 **Grand Island** *island* Michigan, N USA
22 K10 **Grand Isle** Louisiana, S USA
65 A23 **Grand Jason** *island* Jason Islands, NW Falkland Islands
37 P5 **Grand Junction** Colorado, C USA
20 F10 **Grand Junction** Tennessee, S USA
14 J9 **Grand-Lac-Victoria** Quebec, SE Canada
14 J9 **Grand lac Victoria** ◎ Quebec, SE Canada
77 N17 **Grand-Lahou** *var.* Grand Lahu. S Ivory Coast
Grand Lahu *see* Grand-Lahou
37 S3 **Grand Lake** Colorado, C USA
13 S11 **Grand Lake** ◎ Newfoundland, E Canada
22 G9 **Grand Lake** ◎ Louisiana, S USA
31 R5 **Grand Lake** ◎ Michigan, N USA
31 Q13 **Grand Lake** ⊞ Ohio, N USA
27 R9 **Grand Lake O' The Cherokees** *var.* Lake O' The Cherokees. ⊞ Oklahoma, C USA
31 Q9 **Grand Ledge** Michigan, N USA
102 I8 **Grand-Lieu, Lac de** ◎ NW France
19 U6 **Grand Manan Channel** *channel* Canada/USA
13 O15 **Grand Manan Island** *island* New Brunswick, SE Canada
29 Y4 **Grand Marais** Minnesota, N USA
15 P10 **Grand-Mère** Quebec, SE Canada
37 P5 **Grand Mesa** ▲ Colorado, C USA
108 C10 **Grand Muveran** ▲ W Switzerland
104 G12 **Grândola** Setúbal, S Portugal
Grand Paradis *see* Gran Paradiso
187 O15 **Grand Passage** *passage* N New Caledonia
77 R16 **Grand-Popo** S Benin
29 Z3 **Grand Portage** Minnesota, N USA
25 T6 **Grand Prairie** Texas, SW USA
11 W14 **Grand Rapids** Manitoba, C Canada
31 P9 **Grand Rapids** Michigan, N USA
29 V5 **Grand Rapids** Minnesota, N USA
14 L10 **Grand-Remous** Quebec, SE Canada
14 F15 **Grand River** ≈ Ontario, S Canada
31 P9 **Grand River** ≈ Michigan, N USA
27 T3 **Grand River** ≈ Missouri, C USA
28 M7 **Grand River** ≈ South Dakota, N USA
45 Q11 **Grand' Rivière** N Martinique
32 F11 **Grand Ronde** Oregon, NW USA
32 L11 **Grand Ronde River** ≈ Oregon/Washington, NW USA
Grand-Saint-Bernard, Col du *see* Great Saint Bernard Pass
25 V6 **Grand Saline** Texas, SW USA
55 X10 **Grand-Santi** W French Guiana
Grandsee *see* Grandson
108 B9 **Grandson** *prev.* Grandsee. Vaud, W Switzerland
172 J16 **Grand Sœur** *island* Les Sœurs, NE Seychelles
33 S14 **Grand Teton** ▲ Wyoming, C USA
31 P5 **Grand Traverse Bay** *lake bay* Michigan, N USA
45 N6 **Grand Turk** ○ (Turks and Caicos Islands) Grand Turk Island, S Turks and Caicos Islands
45 N6 **Grand Turk Island** *island* SE Turks and Caicos Islands
103 S13 **Grand Veymont** ▲ E France
11 W15 **Grandview** Manitoba, S Canada
27 R4 **Grandview** Missouri, C USA
36 I10 **Grand Wash Cliffs** *cliff* Arizona, SW USA
14 J8 **Granet, Lac** ◎ Quebec, SE Canada
95 L14 **Grangärde** Dalarna, C Sweden
44 H12 **Grange Hill** W Jamaica
96 J12 **Grangemouth** C Scotland, UK
25 T10 **Granger** Texas, SW USA
32 J10 **Granger** Washington, NW USA
33 T17 **Granger** Wyoming, C USA
Granges *see* Grenchen
95 L14 **Grängesberg** Dalarna, C Sweden
33 N11 **Grangeville** Idaho, NW USA
10 K13 **Granisle** British Columbia, SW Canada
30 K15 **Granite City** Illinois, N USA
29 S9 **Granite Falls** Minnesota, N USA
21 Q9 **Granite Falls** North Carolina, SE USA
36 K12 **Granite Mountain** ▲ Arizona, SW USA
33 T12 **Granite Peak** ▲ Montana, NW USA
35 T2 **Granite Peak** ▲ Nevada, W USA
36 J3 **Granite Peak** ▲ Utah, W USA

Granite State see New Hampshire
107 H24 **Granitola, Capo** *headland* Sicilia, Italy, C Mediterranean Sea
185 H15 **Granity** West Coast, South Island, NZ
Gran Lago see Nicaragua, Lago de
63 J18 **Gran Laguna Salada** ⊚ S Argentina
Gran Malvina, Isla see West Falkland
95 L18 **Gränna** Jönköping, S Sweden
105 W5 **Granollers** *var.* Granollérs. Cataluña, NE Spain
106 A7 **Gran Paradiso** *Fr.* Grand Paradis. ▲ NW Italy
Gran Pilastro see Hochfeiler
Gran Salitral see Grande, Salina
Gran San Bernardo, Passo di see Great Saint Bernard Pass
Gran Santiago see Santiago
107 J14 **Gran Sasso d'Italia** ▲ C Italy
100 N11 **Gransee** Brandenburg, NE Germany
28 L15 **Grant** Nebraska, C USA
27 R1 **Grant City** Missouri, C USA
97 N19 **Grantham** E England, UK
65 D24 **Grantham Sound** *sound* East Falkland, Falkland Islands
194 K13 **Grant Island** *island* Antarctica
45 Z14 **Grantley Adams** ✕ (Bridgetown) SE Barbados
35 S7 **Grant, Mount** ▲ Nevada, W USA
96 J9 **Grantown-on-Spey** N Scotland, UK
35 W8 **Grant Range** ▲ Nevada, W USA
37 Q11 **Grants** New Mexico, SW USA
30 I4 **Grantsburg** Wisconsin, N USA
32 F15 **Grants Pass** Oregon, NW USA
36 K3 **Grantsville** Utah, W USA
21 R4 **Grantsville** West Virginia, NE USA
102 I5 **Granville** Manche, N France
11 V12 **Granville Lake** ⊚ Manitoba, C Canada
25 V8 **Grapeland** Texas, SW USA
25 T6 **Grapevine** Texas, SW USA
83 K20 **Graskop** Mpumalanga, NE South Africa
95 P14 **Gräsö** Uppsala, C Sweden
93 I19 **Gräsö** *island* C Sweden
103 U15 **Grasse** Alpes-Maritimes, SE France
18 E14 **Grassflat** Pennsylvania, NE USA
33 U9 **Grassrange** Montana, NW USA
18 J6 **Grass River** ⁓ New York, NE USA
35 P6 **Grass Valley** California, W USA
183 N14 **Grassy** Tasmania, SE Australia
28 K4 **Grassy Butte** North Dakota, N USA
21 R5 **Grassy Knob** ▲ West Virginia, NE USA
95 G24 **Gråsten** *var.* Graasten. Sønderjylland, SW Denmark
95 J18 **Grästorp** Västra Götaland, S Sweden
Gratianopolis see Grenoble
109 V8 **Gratwein** Steiermark, SE Austria
Gratz see Graz
108 I9 **Graubünden** *Fr.* Grisons, *It.* Grigioni. ◆ *canton* SE Switzerland
Graudenz see Grudziądz
103 N15 **Graulhet** Tarn, S France
105 T4 **Graus** Aragón, NE Spain
61 I16 **Gravataí** Rio Grande do Sul, S Brazil
98 L13 **Grave** Noord-Brabant, SE Netherlands
11 T17 **Gravelbourg** Saskatchewan, S Canada
103 N1 **Gravelines** Nord, N France
Graven see Grez-Doiceau
14 H13 **Gravenhurst** Ontario, S Canada
33 O10 **Grave Peak** ▲ Idaho, NW USA
102 I11 **Grave, Pointe de** *headland* W France
183 S4 **Gravesend** New South Wales, SE Australia
97 P22 **Gravesend** SE England, UK
107 N17 **Gravina di Puglia** *Eng.* Gravina in Puglia. Puglia, SE Italy
Gravina in Puglia see Gravina di Puglia
103 S8 **Gray** Haute-Saône, E France
23 T4 **Gray** Georgia, SE USA
195 V16 **Gray, Cape** *headland* Antarctica,
32 F9 **Grayland** Washington, NW USA
39 N10 **Grayling** Alaska, USA
31 Q6 **Grayling** Michigan, N USA
32 F9 **Grays Harbor** *inlet* Washington, NW USA
21 O5 **Grayson** Kentucky, S USA
37 S4 **Grays Peak** ▲ Colorado, C USA
30 M16 **Grayville** Illinois, N USA
109 V8 **Graz** *prev.* Gratz. Steiermark, SE Austria
104 L15 **Grazalema** Andalucía, S Spain
113 P15 **Grdelica** Serbia, SE Yugoslavia
44 H1 **Great Abaco** *var.* Abaco Island. *island* N Bahamas
Great Admiralty Island see Manus Island
Great Alfold see Great Hungarian Plain
Great Ararat see Büyükağrı Dağı
181 U8 **Great Artesian Basin** *lowlands* Queensland, C Australia
181 O12 **Great Australian Bight** *bight* S Australia
64 E11 **Great Bahama Bank** *undersea feature* E Gulf of Mexico
184 M4 **Great Barrier Island** *island* N NZ
181 X4 **Great Barrier Reef** *reef* Queensland, NE Australia
18 L11 **Great Barrington** Massachusetts, NE USA
(0) F10 **Great Basin** *basin* W USA
8 I8 **Great Bear Lake** *Fr.* Grand Lac de l'Ours. ⊚ Northwest Territories, NW Canada
Great Belt see Storebælt
26 L5 **Great Bend** Kansas, C USA
Great Bermuda see Bermuda
97 A20 **Great Blasket Island** *Ir.* An Blascaod Mór. *island* SW Ireland
Great Britain see Britain
151 Q23 **Great Channel** *channel* Andaman Sea/Indian Ocean
166 J10 **Great Coco Island** *island* SW Burma
Great Crosby see Crosby
21 X7 **Great Dismal Swamp** *wetland* North Carolina/Virginia, SE USA
33 V16 **Great Divide Basin** *basin* Wyoming, C USA
181 W7 **Great Dividing Range** ▲ NE Australia
14 D12 **Great Duck Island** *island* Ontario, S Canada
Great Elder Reservoir see Waconda Lake
195 V8 **Greater Antarctica** *var.* East Antarctica. *physical region* Antarctica
44 G8 **Greater Antilles** *island group* West Indies
131 V16 **Greater Sunda Islands** *var.* Sunda Islands. *island group* Indonesia
184 I1 **Great Exhibition Bay** *inlet* North Island, NZ
44 H4 **Great Exuma Island** *island* C Bahamas
33 R8 **Great Falls** Montana, NW USA
21 R11 **Great Falls** South Carolina, SE USA
84 F9 **Great Fisher Bank** *undersea feature* C North Sea
Great Glen see Mor, Glen
Great Grimsby see Grimsby
44 I4 **Great Guana Cay** *island* C Bahamas
64 I5 **Great Hellefiske Bank** *undersea feature* N Atlantic Ocean
111 L24 **Great Hungarian Plain** *var.* Great Alfold, Plain of Hungary, *Hung.* Alföld. *plain* SE Europe
44 L7 **Great Inagua** *var.* Inagua Islands. *island* S Bahamas
Great Indian Desert see Thar Desert
83 G25 **Great Karoo** *var.* Great Karroo, High Veld, *Afr.* Groot Karoo, Hoë Karoo. *plateau region* S South Africa
Great Karroo see Great Karoo
Great Kei see Groot-Kei
Great Khingan Range see Da Hinggan Ling
14 E11 **Great La Cloche Island** *island* Ontario, S Canada
183 P16 **Great Lake** ⊚ Tasmania, SE Australia
Great Lake see Tônlé Sap
9 R15 **Great Lakes** *lakes* Ontario, Canada/USA
Great Lakes State see Michigan
97 L20 **Great Malvern** W England, UK
184 M5 **Great Mercury Island** *island* N NZ
Great Meteor Seamount see Great Meteor Tablemount
64 K10 **Great Meteor Tablemount** *var.* Great Meteor Seamount. *undersea feature* E Atlantic Ocean
31 Q14 **Great Miami River** ⁓ Ohio, N USA
151 Q24 **Great Nicobar** *island* Nicobar Islands, India, NE Indian Ocean
97 O19 **Great Ouse** *var.* Ouse. ⁓ E England, UK
183 Q17 **Great Oyster Bay** *bay* Tasmania, SE Australia
44 I13 **Great Pedro Bluff** *headland* W Jamaica
21 T12 **Great Pee Dee River** ⁓ North Carolina/South Carolina, SE USA
131 W9 **Great Plain of China** *plain* E China
(0) F12 **Great Plains** *var.* High Plains. *plains* Canada/USA
37 W6 **Great Plains Reservoirs** ⊠ Colorado, C USA
19 Q13 **Great Point** *headland* Nantucket Island, Massachusetts, NE USA
68 I13 **Great Rift Valley** *var.* Rift Valley. *depression* Asia/Africa
81 I23 **Great Ruaha** ⁓ S Tanzania
18 K10 **Great Sacandaga Lake** ⊠ New York, NE USA
108 C12 **Great Saint Bernard Pass** *Fr.* Col du Grand-Saint-Bernard, *It.* Passo di Gran San Bernardo. *pass* Italy/Switzerland
44 F1 **Great Sale Cay** *island* N Bahamas
Great Salt Desert see Kavīr, Dasht-e
36 K1 **Great Salt Lake** *salt lake* Utah, W USA
36 J3 **Great Salt Lake Desert** *plain* Utah, W USA
26 M8 **Great Salt Plains Lake** ⊠ Oklahoma, C USA
75 T9 **Great Sand Sea** *desert* Egypt/Libya
180 L6 **Great Sandy Desert** *desert* Western Australia
Great Sandy Desert see Ar Rub' al Khālī
Great Sandy Island see Fraser Island
187 Y13 **Great Sea Reef** *reef* Vanua Levu, N Fiji
38 H17 **Great Sitkin Island** *island* Aleutian Islands, Alaska, USA
8 J10 **Great Slave Lake** *Fr.* Grand Lac des Esclaves. ⊚ Northwest Territories, NW Canada
21 O10 **Great Smoky Mountains** ▲ North Carolina/Tennessee, SE USA
10 L11 **Great Snow Mountain** ▲ British Columbia, W Canada
64 A12 **Great Sound** *bay* Bermuda, NW Atlantic Ocean
180 M10 **Great Victoria Desert** *desert* South Australia/Western Australia
194 H2 **Great Wall** *Chinese research station* South Shetland Islands, Antarctica
19 T7 **Great Wass Island** *island* Maine, NE USA
97 Q19 **Great Yarmouth** *var.* Yarmouth. E England, UK
139 S1 **Great Zab** *Ar.* Az Zāb al Kabīr, *Kurd.* Zē-i Bādinān, *Turk.* Büyükzap Suyu. ⁓ Iraq/Turkey
95 I17 **Grebbestad** Västra Götaland, S Sweden
Grebenka see Hrebinka
42 M13 **Grecia** Alajuela, C Costa Rica
61 E18 **Greco** Río Negro, W Uruguay
Greco, Cape see Gkréko, Akrotíri
104 L8 **Gredos, Sierra de** ▲ W Spain
18 F9 **Greece** New York, NE USA
115 E17 **Greece** *off.* Hellenic Republic, *Gk.* Ellás; *anc.* Hellas. ◆ *republic* SE Europe
Greece Central see Stereá Ellás
Greece West see Dytikí Ellás
37 T3 **Greeley** Colorado, C USA
29 P14 **Greeley** Nebraska, C USA
122 K3 **Greem-Bell, Ostrov** *Eng.* Graham Bell Island. *island* Zemlya Frantsa-Iosifa, N Russian Federation
30 M6 **Green Bay** Wisconsin, N USA
31 N6 **Green Bay** *lake bay* Michigan/Wisconsin, N USA
21 S5 **Greenbrier River** ⁓ West Virginia, NE USA
29 S2 **Greenbush** Minnesota, N USA
183 R12 **Green Cape** *headland* New South Wales, SE Australia
31 O14 **Greencastle** Indiana, N USA
18 F16 **Greencastle** Pennsylvania, NE USA
27 T2 **Green City** Missouri, C USA
21 O9 **Greeneville** Tennessee, S USA
35 O11 **Greenfield** California, W USA
31 P14 **Greenfield** Indiana, N USA
29 U15 **Greenfield** Iowa, C USA
18 M11 **Greenfield** Massachusetts, NE USA
27 S7 **Greenfield** Missouri, C USA
31 S14 **Greenfield** Ohio, N USA
20 G8 **Greenfield** Tennessee, S USA
30 M9 **Greenfield** Wisconsin, N USA
27 T9 **Green Forest** Arkansas, C USA
37 T7 **Greenhorn Mountain** ▲ Colorado, C USA
Green Island see Lü Tao
186 I6 **Green Islands** *var.* Nissan Islands. *island group* NE PNG
11 S14 **Green Lake** Saskatchewan, C Canada
30 L8 **Green Lake** ⊚ Wisconsin, N USA
197 O14 **Greenland** *Dan.* Grønland, *Inuit* Kalaallit Nunaat. ◇ *Danish external territory* NE North America
84 D4 **Greenland** *island* NE North America
197 R13 **Greenland Plain** *undersea feature* N Greenland Sea
197 R14 **Greenland Sea** *sea* Arctic Ocean
37 R4 **Green Mountain Reservoir** ⊠ Colorado, C USA
18 M8 **Green Mountains** ▲ Vermont, NE USA
Green Mountain State see Vermont
96 H12 **Greenock** W Scotland, UK
39 T5 **Greenough, Mount** ▲ Alaska, USA
16 G10 **Green River** Sandaun, NW PNG
37 N5 **Green River** Utah, W USA
33 U17 **Green River** Wyoming, C USA
16 H9 **Green River** ⁓ W USA
30 K11 **Green River** ⁓ Illinois, N USA
20 J7 **Green River** ⁓ Kentucky, S USA
28 K5 **Green River** ⁓ North Dakota, N USA
37 N6 **Green River** ⁓ Utah, W USA
33 T16 **Green River** ⁓ Wyoming, C USA
20 L7 **Green River Lake** ⊠ Kentucky, S USA
23 O5 **Greensboro** Alabama, S USA
23 U3 **Greensboro** Georgia, SE USA
21 T9 **Greensboro** North Carolina, SE USA
31 P14 **Greensburg** Indiana, N USA
26 K6 **Greensburg** Kansas, C USA
20 L7 **Greensburg** Kentucky, S USA
18 C15 **Greensburg** Pennsylvania, NE USA
37 O13 **Greens Peak** ▲ Arizona, SW USA
21 V12 **Green Swamp** *wetland* North Carolina, SE USA
21 O4 **Greenup** Kentucky, S USA
36 M16 **Green Valley** Arizona, SW USA
76 K17 **Greenville** *var.* Sino, Sinoe. SE Liberia
23 P6 **Greenville** Alabama, S USA
23 T8 **Greenville** Florida, SE USA
23 S4 **Greenville** Georgia, SE USA
30 L15 **Greenville** Illinois, N USA
20 I7 **Greenville** Kentucky, S USA
19 Q5 **Greenville** Maine, NE USA
31 P9 **Greenville** Michigan, N USA
22 J4 **Greenville** Mississippi, S USA
21 W9 **Greenville** North Carolina, SE USA
31 Q13 **Greenville** Ohio, N USA
19 O12 **Greenville** Rhode Island, NE USA
21 P11 **Greenville** South Carolina, SE USA
25 U6 **Greenville** Texas, SW USA
31 T12 **Greenwich** Ohio, N USA
27 S11 **Greenwood** Arkansas, C USA
31 O14 **Greenwood** Indiana, N USA
22 K4 **Greenwood** Mississippi, S USA
21 P12 **Greenwood** South Carolina, SE USA
21 Q12 **Greenwood, Lake** ⊠ South Carolina, SE USA
21 P11 **Greer** South Carolina, SE USA
27 V10 **Greers Ferry Lake** ⊠ Arkansas, C USA
27 S13 **Greeson, Lake** ⊠ Arkansas, C USA
29 O12 **Gregory** South Dakota, N USA
182 J3 **Gregory, Lake** *salt lake* South Australia
180 J9 **Gregory Lake** ⊚ Western Australia
181 V5 **Gregory Range** ▲ Queensland, E Australia
Greifenberg/Greifenberg in Pommern see Gryfice
Greifenhagen see Gryfino
100 O8 **Greifswald** Mecklenburg-Vorpommern, NE Germany
100 O8 **Greifswalder Bodden** *bay* NE Germany
109 U4 **Grein** Oberösterreich, N Austria
101 M17 **Greiz** Thüringen, C Germany
Gremicha/Gremiha see Gremikha
126 M4 **Gremikha** *var.* Gremicha, Gremiha. Murmanskaya Oblast', NW Russian Federation
127 V14 **Gremyachinsk** Permskaya Oblast', NW Russian Federation
95 H21 **Grenå** *var.* Grenaa. Århus, C Denmark
Grenaa see Grenå
22 L3 **Grenada** Mississippi, S USA
45 W15 **Grenada** ◆ *commonwealth republic* SE West Indies
47 S4 **Grenada** *island* Grenada
47 R4 **Grenada Basin** *undersea feature* W Atlantic Ocean
22 L3 **Grenada Lake** ⊠ Mississippi, S USA
45 Y14 **Grenadines, The** *island group* Grenada/St Vincent and the Grenadines
108 D7 **Grenchen** *Fr.* Granges. Solothurn, NW Switzerland
183 Q9 **Grenfell** New South Wales, SE Australia
11 V16 **Grenfell** Saskatchewan, S Canada
92 J1 **Grenivík** Nordhurland Eystra, N Iceland
103 S12 **Grenoble** *anc.* Cularo, Gratianopolis. Isère, E France
28 J2 **Grenora** North Dakota, N USA
92 N8 **Grense-Jakobselv** Finnmark, N Norway
45 S14 **Grenville** E Grenada
32 G11 **Gresham** Oregon, NW USA
Gresk see Hresk
106 B7 **Gressoney-St-Jean** Valle d'Aosta, NW Italy
22 K9 **Gretna** Louisiana, S USA
21 T7 **Gretna** Virginia, NE USA
98 F13 **Grevelingen** *inlet* S North Sea
100 F13 **Greven** Nordrhein-Westfalen, NW Germany
115 D15 **Grevená** Dytikí Makedonía, N Greece
101 D16 **Grevenbroich** Nordrhein-Westfalen, W Germany
99 N24 **Grevenmacher** Grevenmacher, E Luxembourg
99 M24 **Grevenmacher** ◆ *district* E Luxembourg
100 K9 **Grevesmühlen** Mecklenburg-Vorpommern, N Germany
185 H16 **Grey** ⁓ South Island, NZ
33 V12 **Greybull** Wyoming, C USA
33 U13 **Greybull River** ⁓ Wyoming, C USA
65 A24 **Grey Channel** *sound* Falkland Islands
Greyerzer See see Gruyère, Lac de la
13 T10 **Grey Islands** *island group* Newfoundland, E Canada
18 L10 **Greylock, Mount** ▲ Massachusetts, NE USA
185 G17 **Greymouth** West Coast, South Island, NZ
181 U10 **Grey Range** ▲ New South Wales/Queensland, E Australia
97 G18 **Greystones** *Ir.* Na Clocha Liatha. E Ireland
185 M14 **Greytown** Wellington, North Island, NZ
83 K23 **Greytown** KwaZulu/Natal, E South Africa
Greytown see San Juan del Norte
99 H19 **Grez-Doiceau** *Dut.* Graven. Wallon Brabant, C Belgium
115 J19 **Griá, Akrotírio** *headland* Ándros, Kykládes, Greece, Aegean Sea
129 N8 **Gribanovskiy** Voronezhskaya Oblast', W Russian Federation
78 I13 **Gribingui** ⁓ N Central African Republic
35 O6 **Gridley** California, W USA
83 G23 **Griekwastad** Northern Cape, C South Africa
23 S4 **Griffin** Georgia, SE USA
183 O9 **Griffith** New South Wales, SE Australia
14 F13 **Griffith Island** *island* Ontario, S Canada
21 W10 **Grifton** North Carolina, SE USA
Grigioni see Graubünden
119 H14 **Grigiškes** Trakai, SE Lithuania
117 N10 **Grigoriopol** C Moldova
147 X7 **Grigor'yevka** Issyk-Kul'skaya Oblast', E Kyrgyzstan
193 U8 **Grijalva Ridge** *undersea feature* E Pacific Ocean
41 U15 **Grijalva, Río** *var.* Tabasco. ⁓ Guatemala/Mexico
98 N5 **Grijpskerk** Groningen, NE Netherlands
83 C22 **Grillenthal** Karas, SW Namibia
79 J15 **Grimari** Ouaka, C Central African Republic
Grimaylov see Hrymayliv
99 G18 **Grimbergen** Vlaams Brabant, C Belgium
183 N15 **Grim, Cape** *headland* Tasmania, SE Australia
100 N8 **Grimmen** Mecklenburg-Vorpommern, NE Germany
14 G16 **Grimsby** Ontario, S Canada
97 O17 **Grimsby** *prev.* Great Grimsby. E England, UK
92 J1 **Grímsey** *var.* Grimsey. *island* N Iceland
11 O12 **Grimshaw** Alberta, W Canada
95 F18 **Grimstad** Aust-Agder, S Norway
92 H4 **Grindavík** Reykjanes, W Iceland
108 F9 **Grindelwald** Bern, S Switzerland
95 F23 **Grindsted** Ribe, W Denmark
29 W14 **Grinnell** Iowa, C USA
8 K4 **Grinnell Peninsula** *peninsula* Nunavut, N Canada
109 U10 **Grintovec** ▲ N Slovenia
9 N3 **Grise Fiord** *var.* Ausuittuq. Nunavut, N Canada
182 H1 **Griselda, Lake** *salt lake* South Australia
Grisons see Graubünden
95 P14 **Grisslehamn** Stockholm, C Sweden
29 T15 **Griswold** Iowa, C USA
102 M1 **Griz Nez, Cap** *headland* N France
112 P13 **Grljan** Serbia, E Yugoslavia
112 E11 **Grmeč** ▲ NW Bosnia and Herzegovina
99 H16 **Grobbendonk** Antwerpen, N Belgium
Grobin see Grobiņa
118 C10 **Grobiņa** *Ger.* Grobin. Liepāja, W Latvia
83 K20 **Groblersdal** Mpumalanga, NE South Africa
83 G23 **Groblershoop** Northern Cape, W South Africa
Gródek Jagielloński see Horodok
109 Q6 **Grödig** Salzburg, W Austria
111 H15 **Grodków** Opolskie, S Poland
Grodnenskaya Oblast' see Hrodzyenskaya Voblasts'
Grodno see Hrodna
110 L12 **Grodzisk Mazowiecki** Mazowieckie, C Poland
110 F12 **Grodzisk Wielkopolski** Wielkolpolskie, C Poland
Grodzyanka see Hradzyanka
98 O12 **Groenlo** Gelderland, E Netherlands
83 E22 **Groenrivier** Karas, SE Namibia
25 U8 **Groesbeck** Texas, SW USA
98 L13 **Groesbeek** Gelderland, SE Netherlands
102 G7 **Groix, Îles de** *island group* NW France
110 M12 **Grójec** Mazowieckie, C Poland
65 K15 **Gröll Seamount** *undersea feature* C Atlantic Ocean
100 E13 **Gronau** *var.* Gronau in Westfalen. Nordrhein-Westfalen, NW Germany
Gronau in Westfalen see Gronau
93 F15 **Grong** Nord-Trøndelag, C Norway
95 N22 **Grönhögen** Kalmar, S Sweden
98 N5 **Groningen** Groningen, NE Netherlands
55 W9 **Groningen** Saramacca, N Suriname
98 N5 **Groningen** ◆ *province* NE Netherlands
Grønland see Greenland
108 H11 **Grono** Graubünden, S Switzerland
95 M20 **Grönskåra** Kalmar, S Sweden
25 O2 **Groom** Texas, SW USA
35 W9 **Groom Lake** ⊚ Nevada, W USA
83 H25 **Groot** ⁓ S South Africa
181 S2 **Groote Eylandt** *island* Northern Territory, N Australia
98 M6 **Grootegast** Groningen, NE Netherlands
83 D17 **Grootfontein** Otjozondjupa, N Namibia
83 E22 **Groot Karasberge** ▲ S Namibia
Groot Karoo see Great Karoo
83 J25 **Groot-Kei** *Eng.* Great Kei. ⁓ S South Africa
45 T10 **Gros Islet** N Saint Lucia
44 L8 **Gros-Morne** NW Haiti
13 S11 **Gros Morne** ▲ Newfoundland, E Canada
103 R9 **Grosne** ⁓ C France
45 S12 **Gros Piton** ▲ SW Saint Lucia
Grossa, Isola see Dugi Otok
Grossbetschkerek see Zrenjanin
Grosse Isper see Grosse Ysper
Grosse Kokel see Târnava Mare
101 M21 **Grosse Laaber** *var.* Grosse Laber. ⁓ SE Germany
Grosse Laber see Grosse Laaber
Grosse Morava see Velika Morava
101 O15 **Grossenhain** Sachsen, E Germany
109 Y4 **Grossenzersdorf** Niederösterreich, NE Austria
101 O21 **Grosser Arber** ▲ SE Germany
101 K17 **Grosser Beerberg** ▲ C Germany
101 G18 **Grosser Feldberg** ▲ W Germany
109 O8 **Grosser Löffler** *It.* Monte Lovello. ▲ Austria/Italy
109 N8 **Grosser Möseler** *var.* Mesule. ▲ Austria/Italy
100 J8 **Grosser Plöner See** ⊚ N Germany
101 O21 **Grosser Rachel** ▲ SE Germany
Grosser Sund see Suur Väin
15 V6 **Grosses-Roches** Quebec, SE Canada
109 P8 **Grosses Weiesbachhorn** *var.* Wiesbachhorn. ▲ W Austria
106 F13 **Grosseto** Toscana, C Italy
101 M22 **Grosse Vils** ⁓ SE Germany
109 U4 **Grosse Ysper** *var.* Grosse Isper. ⁓ N Austria
101 G19 **Gross-Gerau** Hessen, W Germany
109 U3 **Gross Gerungs** Niederösterreich, N Austria
109 P8 **Grossglockner** ▲ W Austria
Grosskanizsa see Nagykanizsa
Gross-Karol see Carei
Grosskikinda see Kikinda
109 W9 **Grossklein** Steiermark, SE Austria
Grosskoppe see Velká Deštná
Grossmeseritsch see Velké Meziříčí
Grossmichel see Michalovce
101 H19 **Grossostheim** Bayern, C Germany
109 X7 **Grosspetersdorf** Burgenland, SE Austria
109 T5 **Grossraming** Oberösterreich, C Austria
101 P14 **Grossräschen** Brandenburg, E Germany
Grossrauschenbach see Revúca
Gross-Sankt-Johannis see Suure-Jaani
Gross-Schlatten see Abrud
109 V2 **Gross-Siegharts** Niederösterreich, N Austria
Gross-Skaisgirren see Bol'shakovo
Gross-Steffelsdorf see Rimavská Sobota
Gross Strehlitz see Strzelce Opolskie
109 O8 **Grossvenediger** ▲ W Austria
Grosswardein see Oradea
Gross Wartenberg see Syców
109 U11 **Grosuplje** C Slovenia
99 H17 **Grote Nete** ⁓ N Belgium
94 E10 **Grotli** Oppland, S Norway
19 N13 **Groton** Connecticut, NE USA
29 P8 **Groton** South Dakota, N USA
107 P18 **Grottaglie** Puglia, SE Italy
107 L17 **Grottaminarda** Campania, S Italy
106 K13 **Grottammare** Marche, C Italy
21 U5 **Grottoes** Virginia, NE USA
Grou see Grouw
13 N10 **Groulx, Monts** ▲ Quebec, E Canada
14 E7 **Groundhog** ⁓ Ontario, S Canada
36 J1 **Grouse Creek** Utah, W USA
36 J1 **Grouse Creek Mountains** ▲ Utah, W USA
98 L6 **Grouw** *Fris.* Grou. Friesland, N Netherlands
27 R8 **Grove** Oklahoma, C USA
31 S13 **Grove City** Ohio, N USA
18 B13 **Grove City** Pennsylvania, NE USA
23 O6 **Grove Hill** Alabama, S USA
33 S15 **Grover** Wyoming, C USA
35 P13 **Grover City** California, W USA
25 Y11 **Groves** Texas, SW USA
19 O7 **Groveton** New Hampshire, NE USA
25 W9 **Groveton** Texas, SW USA
36 J15 **Growler Mountains** ▲ Arizona, SW USA
Grozdovo see Bratya Daskalovi
129 P16 **Groznyy** Chechenskaya Respublika, SW Russian Federation
Grubeshov see Hrubieszów
112 G9 **Grubišno Polje** Bjelovar-Bilogora, NE Croatia
Grudovo see Sredets
110 J9 **Grudziądz** *Ger.* Graudenz. Kujawsko-pomorskie, C Poland
25 R17 **Grulla** *var.* La Grulla. Texas, SW USA
40 K14 **Grullo** Jalisco, SW Mexico
67 V10 **Grumeti** ⁓ N Tanzania
95 K16 **Grums** Värmland, C Sweden
109 S5 **Grünau im Almtal** Oberösterreich, N Austria
101 H17 **Grünberg** Hessen, W Germany
Grünberg/Grünberg in Schlesien see Zielona Góra
Grünberg in Schlesien see Zielona Góra
92 H3 **Grundarfjördhur** Vestfirdhir, W Iceland
21 P7 **Grundy** Virginia, NE USA
29 W13 **Grundy Center** Iowa, C USA
Grüneberg see Zielona Góra
25 N1 **Gruver** Texas, SW USA
108 C9 **Gruyère, Lac de la** *Ger.* Greyerzer See. ⊚ SW Switzerland
108 C9 **Gruyères** Fribourg, W Switzerland
118 E11 **Gruzdžiai** Šiauliai, N Lithuania
Gruzinskaya SSR/Gruziya see Georgia
146 C10 **Gryada Akkyr** *Turkm.* Akgyr Erezi. *hill range* NW Turkmenistan
128 L7 **Gryazi** Lipetskaya Oblast', W Russian Federation
126 M14 **Gryazovets** Vologodskaya Oblast', NW Russian Federation
111 M17 **Grybów** Małopolskie, SE Poland
94 M13 **Grycksbo** Dalarna, C Sweden

◆ Country ● Country Capital ◇ Dependent Territory ○ Dependent Territory Capital ◆ Administrative Region ✕ International Airport ▲ Mountain ▲ Mountain Range ⚠ Volcano ⁓ River ⊚ Lake ⊠ Reservoir

110 E8 **Gryfice** *Ger.* Greifenberg, Greifenberg in Pommern. Zachodniopomorskie, NW Poland
110 D9 **Gryfino** *Ger.* Greifenhagen. Zachodniopomorskie, NW Poland
92 H9 **Gryllefjord** Troms, N Norway
95 L15 **Grythyttan** Örebro, C Sweden
108 D10 **Gstaad** Bern, W Switzerland
43 P14 **Guabito** Bocas del Toro, NW Panama
44 G7 **Guacanayabo, Golfo de** *gulf* S Cuba
40 I7 **Guachochi** Chihuahua, N Mexico
104 J11 **Guadajira** ⩫ SW Spain
104 M13 **Guadajoz** ⩫ S Spain
40 L13 **Guadalajara** Jalisco, C Mexico
105 O8 **Guadalajara** *Ar.* Wad Al-Hajarah; *anc.* Arriaca. Castilla-La Mancha, C Spain
105 O7 **Guadalajara** ◆ *province* Castilla-La Mancha, C Spain
104 K12 **Guadalcanal** Andalucía, S Spain
186 L10 **Guadalcanal** *off.* Guadalcanal Province. ◆ *province* C Solomon Islands
186 M9 **Guadalcanal** *island* C Solomon Islands
105 O12 **Guadalén** ⩫ S Spain
105 R13 **Guadalentín** ⩫ SE Spain
104 K15 **Guadalete** ⩫ SW Spain
105 O13 **Guadalimar** ⩫ S Spain
105 P12 **Guadalmena** ⩫ S Spain
104 L11 **Guadalmez** ⩫ W Spain
105 S7 **Guadalope** ⩫ E Spain
104 K13 **Guadalquivir** ⩫ W Spain
104 J14 **Guadalquivir, Marismas del** *var.* Las Marismas. *wetland* SW Spain
40 M11 **Guadalupe** Zacatecas, C Mexico
57 E16 **Guadalupe** Ica, W Peru
104 L10 **Guadalupe** Extremadura, W Spain
36 L14 **Guadalupe** Arizona, SW USA
35 P13 **Guadalupe** California, W USA
193 P5 **Guadalupe** *island* NW Mexico
Guadalupe *see* Canelones
40 J3 **Guadalupe Bravos** Chihuahua, N Mexico
40 A4 **Guadalupe, Isla** *island* NW Mexico
37 U15 **Guadalupe Mountains** ▲ New Mexico/Texas, SW USA
24 J8 **Guadalupe Peak** ▲ Texas, SW USA
25 R11 **Guadalupe River** ⩫ SW USA
104 K10 **Guadalupe, Sierra de** ▲ W Spain
40 K9 **Guadalupe Victoria** Durango, C Mexico
40 I8 **Guadalupe y Calvo** Chihuahua, N Mexico
105 N7 **Guadarrama** Madrid, C Spain
105 N7 **Guadarrama** ⩫ C Spain
104 M7 **Guadarrama, Puerto de** *pass* C Spain
105 N9 **Guadarrama, Sierra de** ▲ C Spain
105 Q9 **Guadazaón** ⩫ C Spain
45 X10 **Guadeloupe** ◇ *French overseas department* E West Indies
47 S3 **Guadeloupe** *island group* E West Indies
45 W10 **Guadeloupe Passage** *passage* E Caribbean Sea
104 H13 **Guadiana** ⩫ Portugal/Spain
105 O13 **Guadiana Menor** ⩫ S Spain
105 Q8 **Guadiela** ⩫ C Spain
105 O14 **Guadix** Andalucía, S Spain
Guad-i-Zirreh *see* Gowd-e Zereh, Dasht-e
193 T12 **Guafo Fracture Zone** *tectonic feature* SE Pacific Ocean
63 F18 **Guafo, Isla** *island* S Chile
42 I6 **Guaimaca** Francisco Morazán, C Honduras
54 J12 **Guainía** *off.* Comisaría del Guainía. ◆ *province* E Colombia
54 K12 **Guainía, Río** ⩫ Colombia/Venezuela
55 O9 **Guaiquinima, Cerro** *elevation* SE Venezuela
62 O7 **Guairá** *off.* Departamento del Guairá. ◆ *department* S Paraguay
60 G10 **Guaíra** Paraná, S Brazil
60 L7 **Guaíra** São Paulo, S Brazil
Guaire *see* Gorey
63 F18 **Guaiteca, Isla** *island* S Chile
44 G6 **Guajaba, Cayo** *headland* C Cuba
59 D16 **Guajará-Mirim** Rondônia, W Brazil
Guajira *see* La Guajira
54 H3 **Guajira, Península de la** *peninsula* N Colombia
42 J6 **Gualaco** Olancho, C Honduras
34 L7 **Gualala** California, W USA
42 E5 **Gualán** Zacapa, C Guatemala
61 C19 **Gualeguay** Entre Ríos, E Argentina
61 D18 **Gualeguaychú** Entre Ríos, E Argentina
61 C18 **Gualeguay, Río** ⩫ E Argentina
63 K16 **Gualicho, Salina del** *salt lake* E Argentina
188 B15 **Guam** ◇ *US unincorporated territory* W Pacific Ocean
63 F19 **Guamblin, Isla** *island* Archipiélago de los Chonos, S Chile
61 A22 **Guaminí** Buenos Aires, E Argentina
40 H8 **Guamúchil** Sinaloa, C Mexico
54 H4 **Guana** *var.* Misión de Guana. Zulia, NW Venezuela
44 C4 **Guanabacoa** La Habana, W Cuba
42 K13 **Guanacaste** *off.* Provincia de Guanacaste. ◆ *province* NW Costa Rica
42 K12 **Guanacaste, Cordillera de** ▲ NW Costa Rica
40 J8 **Guanaceví** Durango, C Mexico
44 A5 **Guanahacabibes, Golfo de** *gulf* W Cuba
42 K4 **Guanaja, Isla de** *island* Islas de la Bahía, N Honduras
44 C4 **Guanajay** La Habana, W Cuba
41 N12 **Guanajuato** Guanajuato, C Mexico
40 M12 **Guanajuato** ◆ *state* C Mexico
54 J6 **Guanare** Portuguesa, N Venezuela
54 K7 **Guanare, Río** ⩫ W Venezuela
54 J6 **Guanarito** Portuguesa, NW Venezuela
160 M3 **Guancen Shan** ▲ C China
62 I9 **Guandacol** La Rioja, W Argentina
44 A5 **Guane** Pinar del Río, W Cuba
161 N14 **Guangdong** *var.* Guangdong Sheng, Kuang-tung, Kwangtung, Yue. ◆ *province* S China
Guangdong Sheng *see* Guangdong
Guanghua *see* Laohekou
Guangju *see* Kwangju
160 I13 **Guangnan** Yunnan, SW China
161 N8 **Guangshui** *prev.* Yingshan. Hubei, C China
Guangxi *see* Guangxi Zhuangzu Zizhiqu
160 K14 **Guangxi Zhuangzu Zizhiqu** *var.* Guangxi, Gui, Kuang-hsi, Kwangsi, *Eng.* Kwangsi Chuang Autonomous Region. ◆ *autonomous region* S China
160 J8 **Guangyuan** *var.* Kuang-yuan, Kwangyuan. Sichuan, C China
161 N14 **Guangzhou** *var.* Kuang-chou, Kwangchow, *Eng.* Canton. Guangdong, S China
59 N19 **Guanhães** Minas Gerais, SE Brazil
160 I12 **Guanling** *var.* Guanling Bouyeizu Miaozu Zizhixian. Guizhou, S China
Guanling Bouyeizu Miaozu Zizhixian *see* Guanling
55 N5 **Guanta** Anzoátegui, NE Venezuela
44 J8 **Guantánamo** Guantánamo, SE Cuba
160 H9 **Guanxian** *var.* Guan Xian. Sichuan, C China
161 Q6 **Guanyun** Jiangsu, E China
54 C12 **Guapí** Cauca, SW Colombia
43 N13 **Guápiles** Limón, NE Costa Rica
61 I15 **Guaporé** Rio Grande do Sul, S Brazil
47 S8 **Guaporé, Rio** *var.* Río Iténez. ⩫ Bolivia/Brazil *see also* Iténez, Río
56 B7 **Guaranda** Bolívar, C Ecuador
60 H11 **Guaraniaçu** Paraná, S Brazil
59 O20 **Guarapari** Espírito Santo, SE Brazil
60 I12 **Guarapuava** Paraná, S Brazil
60 J8 **Guararapes** São Paulo, S Brazil
105 S4 **Guara, Sierra de** ▲ NE Spain
60 N10 **Guaratinguetá** São Paulo, S Brazil
104 I7 **Guarda** Guarda, N Portugal
104 I7 **Guarda** ◆ *district* N Portugal
Guardak *see* Govurdak
104 M3 **Guardo** Castilla-León, N Spain
104 K11 **Guareña** Extremadura, W Spain
60 J11 **Guaricana, Pico** ▲ S Brazil
54 L6 **Guárico** *off.* Estado Guárico. ◆ *state* N Venezuela
44 J7 **Guarico, Punta** *headland* E Cuba
54 L7 **Guárico, Río** ⩫ C Venezuela
60 M10 **Guarujá** São Paulo, SE Brazil
61 L22 **Guarulhos** ✕ (São Paulo) São Paulo, S Brazil
43 R17 **Guarumal** Veraguas, S Panama
Guasapa *see* Guasopa
40 H8 **Guasave** Sinaloa, C Mexico
54 I8 **Guasdualito** Apure, C Venezuela
55 Q7 **Guasipati** Bolívar, E Venezuela
186 I9 **Guasopa** *var.* Guasapa. Woodlark Island, SE PNG
106 F9 **Guastalla** Emilia-Romagna, C Italy
42 D6 **Guastatoya** *var.* El Progreso. El Progreso, C Guatemala
42 D5 **Guatemala** *off.* Republic of Guatemala. ◆ *republic* Central America
42 A2 **Guatemala** *off.* Departamento de Guatemala. ◆ *department* S Guatemala
193 S7 **Guatemala Basin** *undersea feature* E Pacific Ocean
Guatemala City *see* Ciudad de Guatemala
45 V14 **Guatuaro Point** *headland* Trinidad, Trinidad and Tobago
186 B8 **Guavi** ⩫ SW PNG
54 G13 **Guaviare** *off.* Comisaría Guaviare. ◆ *province* S Colombia
54 J11 **Guaviare, Río** ⩫ E Colombia
61 E15 **Guaviravi** Corrientes, NE Argentina
54 G12 **Guayabero, Río** ⩫ SW Colombia
45 U6 **Guayama** E Puerto Rico
42 J7 **Guayambre, Río** ⩫ S Honduras
Guayanas, Macizo de las *see* Guiana Highlands
45 V6 **Guayanés, Punta** *headland* E Puerto Rico
42 J6 **Guayape, Río** ⩫ C Honduras
56 B7 **Guayaquil** *var.* Santiago de Guayaquil. Guayas, SW Ecuador
Guayaquil *see* Simon Bolivar
56 A8 **Guayaquil, Golfo de** *var.* Gulf of Guayaquil. *gulf* SW Ecuador
Guayaquil, Gulf of *see* Guayaquil, Golfo de
56 A7 **Guayas** ◆ *province* W Ecuador
62 N7 **Guaycurú, Río** ⩫ NE Argentina
40 F6 **Guaymas** Sonora, NW Mexico
45 U5 **Guaynabo** E Puerto Rico
80 H12 **Guba** Benishangul, W Ethiopia
146 H8 **Gubadag** *Turkm.* Tel'man; *prev.* Tel'mansk. Dashkhovuzskiy Velayat, N Turkmenistan
127 T1 **Guba Dolgaya** Nenetskiy Avtonomnyy Okrug, NW Russian Federation
127 V13 **Gubakha** Permskaya Oblast', NW Russian Federation
106 I12 **Gubbio** Umbria, C Italy
100 Q13 **Guben** *var.* Wilhelm-Pieck-Stadt. Brandenburg, E Germany
Guben *see* Gubin
110 D12 **Gubin** *Ger.* Guben. Lubuskie, W Poland
128 K8 **Gubkin** Belgorodskaya Oblast', W Russian Federation
Gudara *see* Ghŭdara
105 S8 **Gúdar, Sierra de** ▲ Spain
137 P8 **Gudaut'a** NW Georgia
94 G12 **Gudbrandsdalen** *valley* S Norway
95 G21 **Gudenå** *var.* Gudenaa. ⩫ C Denmark
Gudenaa *see* Gudenå
129 P16 **Gudermes** Chechenskaya Respublika, SW Russian Federation
155 J18 **Gūdūr** Andhra Pradesh, E India
146 B13 **Gudurolum** Balkanskiy Velayat, W Turkmenistan
94 D13 **Gudvangen** Sogn og Fjordane, S Norway
103 U7 **Guebwiller** Haut-Rhin, NE France
Guéckédou *see* Guékédou
14 K8 **Guéguen, Lac** ◎ Quebec, SE Canada
76 J15 **Guékédou** *var.* Guéckédou. Guinée-Forestière, S Guinea
41 R16 **Guelatao** Oaxaca, SE Mexico
Guelders *see* Gelderland
78 G11 **Guélengdeng** Mayo-Kébbi, W Chad
74 L5 **Guelma** *var.* Gâlma. NE Algeria
74 D8 **Guelmime** *var.* Goulimime. SW Morocco
14 G15 **Guelph** Ontario, S Canada
102 I7 **Guémené-Penfao** Loire-Atlantique, NW France
102 H6 **Guer** Morbihan, NW France
78 I11 **Guéra** *off.* Préfecture du Guéra. ◆ *prefecture* S Chad
102 H8 **Guérande** Loire-Atlantique, NW France
78 K9 **Guéréda** Biltine, E Chad
103 N10 **Guéret** Creuse, C France
Guernica/Guernica y Lumo *see* Gernika-Lumo
33 Z15 **Guernsey** Wyoming, C USA
97 K25 **Guernsey** *island* Channel Islands, NW Europe
76 J10 **Guérou** Assaba, S Mauritania
25 R16 **Guerra** Texas, SW USA
41 O15 **Guerrero** ◆ *state* S Mexico
40 D6 **Guerrero Negro** Baja California Sur, NW Mexico
103 P9 **Gueugnon** Saône-et-Loire, C France
76 M17 **Guéyo** S Ivory Coast
107 L15 **Guglionesi** Molise, C Italy
188 K5 **Guguan** *island* C Northern Mariana Islands
Guhrau *see* Góra
Gui *see* Guangxi Zhuangzu Zizhiqu
Guiana *see* French Guiana
47 V4 **Guiana Basin** *undersea feature* W Atlantic Ocean
48 G6 **Guiana Highlands** *var.* Macizo de las Guayanas. ▲ N South America
Guiba *see* Juba
102 I7 **Guichen** Ille-et-Vilaine, NW France
61 E18 **Guichón** Paysandú, W Uruguay
77 U12 **Guidan-Roumji** Maradi, S Niger
Guidder *see* Guider
159 T10 **Guide** Qinghai, C China
78 F12 **Guider** *var.* Guidder. Nord, N Cameroon
76 I11 **Guidimaka** ◆ *region* S Mauritania
77 W12 **Guidimouni** Zinder, S Niger
76 G10 **Guier, Lac de** *var.* Lac de Guiers. ◎ N Senegal
160 L14 **Guigang** *prev.* Guixian, Gui Xian. Guangxi Zhuangzu Zizhiqu, S China
76 L16 **Guiglo** W Ivory Coast
54 L5 **Güigüe** Carabobo, N Venezuela
83 M20 **Guijá** Gaza, S Mozambique
42 E7 **Güija, Lago de** ◎ El Salvador/Guatemala
104 K8 **Guijuelo** Castilla-León, N Spain
Guilan *see* Gīlān
97 N22 **Guildford** SE England, UK
19 R5 **Guildford** Maine, NE USA
19 O7 **Guildhall** Vermont, NE USA
103 R13 **Guilherand** Ardèche, E France
160 L13 **Guilin** *var.* Kuei-lin, Kweilin. Guangxi Zhuangzu Zizhiqu, S China
12 J6 **Guillaume-Delisle, Lac** ◎ Quebec, NE Canada
103 U13 **Guillestre** Hautes-Alpes, SE France
104 H6 **Guimarães** *var.* Guimaráes. Braga, N Portugal
58 D11 **Guimarães Rosas, Pico** ▲ NW Brazil
23 N3 **Guin** Alabama, S USA
Güina *see* Wina
76 I14 **Guinea** *off.* Republic of Guinea, *var.* Guinée; *prev.* French Guinea, People's Revolutionary Republic of Guinea. ◆ *republic* W Africa
64 N13 **Guinea Basin** *undersea feature* E Atlantic Ocean
76 E12 **Guinea-Bissau** *off.* Republic of Guinea-Bissau, *Fr.* Guinée-Bissau, *Port.* Guiné-Bissau; *prev.* Portuguese Guinea. ◆ *republic* W Africa
66 K7 **Guinea Fracture Zone** *tectonic feature* E Atlantic Ocean
64 O13 **Guinea, Gulf of** *Fr.* Golfe de Guinée. *gulf* E Atlantic Ocean
Guiné-Bissau *see* Guinea-Bissau
Guinée *see* Guinea
Guinée-Bissau *see* Guinea-Bissau
76 K15 **Guinée-Forestière** ◆ *state* SE Guinea
Guinée, Golfe de *see* Guinea, Gulf of
76 H13 **Guinée-Maritime** ◆ *state* W Guinea
44 C4 **Güines** La Habana, W Cuba
102 G5 **Guingamp** Côtes d'Armor, NW France
105 P3 **Guipúzcoa** *Basq.* Gipuzkoa. ◆ *province* País Vasco, N Spain
44 C5 **Güira de Melena** La Habana, W Cuba
74 G8 **Guir, Hamada du** *desert* Algeria/Morocco
55 P5 **Güiria** Sucre, NE Venezuela
160 L14 **Gui Shui** ⩫ S China
104 H2 **Guitiriz** Galicia, NW Spain
77 N17 **Guitri** S Ivory Coast
171 Q5 **Guiuan** Samar, C Philippines
Gui Xian/Guixian *see* Guigang
160 J12 **Guiyang** *var.* Kuei-Yang, Kuei-yang, Kueyang, Kweiyang; *prev.* Kweichu. Guizhou, S China
160 J12 **Guizhou** *var.* Guizhou Sheng, Kuei-chou, Kweichow, Qian. ◆ *province* S China
Guizhou Sheng *see* Guizhou
102 J13 **Gujan-Mestras** Gironde, SW France
154 B10 **Gujarāt** *var.* Gujerat. ◆ *state* W India
149 V6 **Gujar Khān** Punjab, E Pakistan
Gujerat *see* Gujarāt
149 V7 **Gujrānwāla** Punjab, NE Pakistan
149 V7 **Gujrāt** Punjab, E Pakistan
159 U9 **Gulang** Gansu, C China
183 R6 **Gulargambone** New South Wales, SE Australia
155 G15 **Gulbarga** Karnātaka, C India
118 J8 **Gulbene** *Ger.* Alt-Schwanenburg. Gulbene, NE Latvia
147 U10 **Gul'cha** *Kir.* Gülchö. Oshskaya Oblast', SW Kyrgyzstan
Gülchö *see* Gul'cha
173 T10 **Gulden Draak Seamount** *undersea feature* E Indian Ocean
136 J16 **Gülek Boğazı** *var.* Cilician Gates. *pass* S Turkey
186 D8 **Gulf** ◆ *province* S PNG
23 O9 **Gulf Breeze** Florida, SE USA
23 V13 **Gulfport** Florida, SE USA
22 M9 **Gulfport** Mississippi, S USA
23 O9 **Gulf Shores** Alabama, S USA
141 T5 **The Gulf** *var.* Persian Gulf *Ar.* Khalīj al 'Arabī, *Per.* Khalīj-e Fars. *gulf* SW Asia
183 R7 **Gulgong** New South Wales, SE Australia
160 I11 **Gulin** Sichuan, C China
171 U14 **Gulir** Pulau Kasiui, E Indonesia
Gulistan *see* Guliston
147 P10 **Guliston** *Rus.* Gulistan. Sirdaryo Wiloyati, E Uzbekistan
163 T6 **Guliya Shan** ▲ NE China
Gulja *see* Yining
39 S11 **Gulkana** Alaska, USA
11 S17 **Gull Lake** Saskatchewan, S Canada
31 P10 **Gull Lake** ◎ Michigan, N USA
29 T6 **Gull Lake** ◎ Minnesota, N USA
95 L16 **Gullspång** Västra Götaland, S Sweden
152 H5 **Gulmarg** Jammu and Kashmir, NW India
Gulpaigan *see* Golpāyegān
99 L18 **Gulpen** Limburg, SE Netherlands
145 S13 **Gul'shad** *Kaz.* Gulshat. Zhezkazgan, E Kazakhstan
Gulshat *see* Gul'shad
81 F17 **Gulu** N Uganda
114 K10 **Gŭlŭbovo** Stara Zagora, C Bulgaria
114 I7 **Gulyantsi** Pleven, N Bulgaria
Gulyaypole *see* Hulyaypole
Guma *see* Pishan
79 K16 **Gumba** Equateur, NW Dem. Rep. Congo (Zaire)
Gumbinnen *see* Gusev
81 H24 **Gumbiro** Ruvuma, S Tanzania
146 B11 **Gumdag** *prev.* Kum-Dag. Balkanskiy Velayat, W Turkmenistan
77 W12 **Gumel** Jigawa, N Nigeria
105 N5 **Gumiel de Hizán** Castilla-León, N Spain
Gumire *see* Gumine
153 P16 **Gumla** Bihār, N India
Gumma *see* Gunma
101 F16 **Gummersbach** Nordrhein-Westfalen, W Germany
77 T13 **Gummi** Zamfara, NW Nigeria
Gumpolds *see* Humpolec
153 N13 **Gumti** *var.* Gomati. ⩫ N India
Gümülcine/Gümüljina *see* Komotiní
Gümüşane *see* Gümüşhane
137 O12 **Gümüşhane** *var.* Gümüşane, Gumushkhane. Gümüşhane, NE Turkey
137 O12 **Gümüşhane** *var.* Gümüşane, Gumushkhane. ◆ *province* NE Turkey
Gumushkhane *see* Gümüşhane
171 V14 **Gumzai** Pulau Kola, E Indonesia
154 H9 **Guna** Madhya Pradesh, C India
Gunabad *see* Gonābād
Gunbad-i-Qawus *see* Gonbad-e Kāvūs
183 O9 **Gunbar** New South Wales, SE Australia
183 O9 **Gun Creek** *seasonal river* New South Wales, SE Australia
183 Q10 **Gundagai** New South Wales, SE Australia
79 K17 **Gundji** Equateur, N Dem. Rep. Congo (Zaire)
155 G20 **Gundlupet** Karnātaka, W India
136 G16 **Gündoğmuş** Antalya, S Turkey
137 O14 **Güney Doğu Toroslar** ▲ SE Turkey
79 J21 **Gungu** Bandundu, SW Dem. Rep. Congo (Zaire)
129 P17 **Gunib** Respublika Dagestan, SW Russian Federation
112 J11 **Gunja** Vukovar-Srijem, E Croatia
31 P9 **Gun Lake** ◎ Michigan, N USA
165 N12 **Gunma** *off.* Gunma-ken, *var.* Gumma. ◆ *prefecture* Honshū, S Japan
197 P15 **Gunnbjørn Fjeld** *var.* Gunnbjörns Bjerge. ▲ C Greenland
183 S6 **Gunnedah** New South Wales, SE Australia
173 Y15 **Gunner's Quoin** *var.* Coin de Mire. *island* N Mauritius
37 R6 **Gunnison** Colorado, C USA
36 L5 **Gunnison** Utah, W USA
37 P5 **Gunnison River** ⩫ Colorado, C USA
21 X2 **Gunpowder River** ⩫ Maryland, NE USA
Güns *see* Kőszeg
Gunsan *see* Kunsan
109 S4 **Gunskirchen** Oberösterreich, N Austria
Gunt *see* Ghund
155 H17 **Guntakal** Andhra Pradesh, C India
23 Q2 **Guntersville** Alabama, S USA
23 Q2 **Guntersville Lake** ⊠ Alabama, S USA
109 X4 **Guntramsdorf** Niederösterreich, E Austria
155 J16 **Guntūr** *var.* Guntur. Andhra Pradesh, SE India
168 H10 **Gunungsitoli** Pulau Nias, W Indonesia
155 M14 **Gunupur** Orissa, E India
101 J23 **Günz** ⩫ S Germany
Gunzan *see* Kunsan
101 J22 **Günzburg** Bayern, S Germany
101 K21 **Gunzenhausen** Bayern, S Germany
161 P7 **Guoyang** Anhui, E China
116 G11 **Gurahonţ** *Hung.* Honctő. Arad, W Romania
Gurahumora *see* Gura Humorului
116 K9 **Gura Humorului** *Ger.* Gurahumora. Suceava, NE Romania
158 K4 **Gurbantünggüt Shamo** *desert* W China
152 H7 **Gurdāspur** Punjab, N India
27 T13 **Gurdon** Arkansas, C USA
Gurdzhaani *see* Gurjaani
Gurgan *see* Gorgān
152 I10 **Gurgaon** Haryāna, N India
59 M15 **Gurguéia, Rio** ⩫ NE Brazil
55 Q7 **Guri, Embalse de** ⊠ E Venezuela
137 V10 **Gurjaani** *Rus.* Gurdzhaani. E Georgia
109 T8 **Gurk** Kärnten, S Austria
109 T9 **Gurk** *Slvn.* Krka. ⩫ S Austria
Gurkfeld *see* Krško
114 K9 **Gurkovo** *prev.* Kolupchii. Stara Zagora, C Bulgaria
109 S9 **Gurktaler Alpen** ▲ S Austria
146 H8 **Gurlan** *Rus.* Gurlen. Khorazm Wiloyati, W Uzbekistan
Gurlen *see* Gurlan
83 M16 **Guro** Manica, C Mozambique
136 M13 **Gürün** Sivas, C Turkey
59 K16 **Gurupi** Tocantins, C Brazil
58 L12 **Gurupi, Rio** ⩫ NE Brazil
152 E14 **Guru Sikhar** ▲ NW India
Gur'yev/Gur'yevskaya Oblast' *see* Atyrau
77 U13 **Gusau** Zamfara, NW Nigeria
128 C3 **Gusev** *Ger.* Gumbinnen. Kaliningradskaya Oblast', W Russian Federation
146 J17 **Gushgy** *prev.* Kushka. Maryyskiy Velayat, S Turkmenistan
Gushiago *see* Gushiegu
77 Q14 **Gushiegu** *var.* Gushiago. NE Ghana
165 S17 **Gushikawa** Okinawa, Okinawa, SW Japan
113 L16 **Gusinje** Montenegro, SW Yugoslavia
128 M4 **Gus'-Khrustal'nyy** Vladimirskaya Oblast', W Russian Federation
107 B19 **Guspini** Sardegna, Italy, C Mediterranean Sea
109 X8 **Güssing** Burgenland, SE Austria
109 V6 **Gusswerk** Steiermark, E Austria
92 O2 **Gustav Adolf Land** *physical region* NE Svalbard
195 X5 **Gustav Bull Mountains** ▲ Antarctica
39 W13 **Gustavus** Alaska, USA
92 O1 **Gustav V Land** *physical region* NE Svalbard
35 P9 **Gustine** California, W USA
25 R8 **Gustine** Texas, SW USA
100 M9 **Güstrow** Mecklenburg-Vorpommern, NE Germany
95 N18 **Gusum** Östergötland, S Sweden
Guta/Gúta *see* Kolárovo
Gutenstein *see* Ravne na Koroškem
101 G14 **Gütersloh** Nordrhein-Westfalen, W Germany
27 N10 **Guthrie** Oklahoma, C USA
25 P5 **Guthrie** Texas, SW USA
29 U14 **Guthrie Center** Iowa, C USA
41 Q13 **Gutiérrez Zamora** Veracruz-Llave, E Mexico
Gutta *see* Kolárovo
29 Y12 **Guttenberg** Iowa, C USA
Guttentag *see* Dobrodzień
Guttstadt *see* Dobre Miasto
162 G8 **Guulin** Govĭ-Altay, C Mongolia
153 V12 **Guwāhāti** *prev.* Gauhāti. Assam, NE India
139 R3 **Guwēr** *var.* Al Kuwayr, Al Quwayr, Quwair. N Iraq
Guwlumayak *see* Kuuli-Mayak
55 R9 **Guyana** *off.* Cooperative Republic of Guyana; *prev.* British Guiana. ◆ *republic* N South America
21 P5 **Guyandotte River** ⩫ West Virginia, NE USA
Guyane *see* French Guiana
Guyi *see* Sanjiang
26 H8 **Guymon** Oklahoma, C USA
146 K12 **Guynuk** Lebapskiy Velayat, NE Turkmenistan
21 O9 **Guyot, Mount** ▲ North Carolina/Tennessee, SE USA
183 U5 **Guyra** New South Wales, SE Australia
159 W10 **Guyuan** Ningxia, N China
Guzar *see* Ghuzor
121 P2 **Güzelyurt** *Gk.* Mórfou, Morphou. W Cyprus
121 N2 **Güzelyurt Körfezi** *var.* Morfou Bay, Morphou Bay, *Gk.* Kólpos Mórfou. *bay* W Cyprus
40 I3 **Guzmán** Chihuahua, N Mexico
119 B14 **Gvardeysk** *Ger.* Tapaiu. Kaliningradskaya Oblast', W Russian Federation
Gvardeyskoye *see* Hvardiys'ke
183 R5 **Gwabegar** New South Wales, SE Australia
148 J16 **Gwādar** *var.* Gwadur. Baluchistān, SW Pakistan
148 J16 **Gwādar East Bay** *bay* SW Pakistan
148 J16 **Gwādar West Bay** *bay* SW Pakistan
Gwadur *see* Gwādar
83 J17 **Gwai** Matabeleland North, W Zimbabwe
154 I7 **Gwalior** Madhya Pradesh, C India
83 J18 **Gwanda** Matabeleland South, SW Zimbabwe
79 N15 **Gwane** Orientale, N Dem. Rep. Congo (Zaire)
83 I17 **Gwayi** ⩫ W Zimbabwe
110 G8 **Gwda** *var.* Głda, *Ger.* Küddow. ⩫ NW Poland
97 C14 **Gweebarra Bay** *Ir.* Béal an Bheara. *inlet* W Ireland
97 D14 **Gweedore** *Ir.* Gaoth Dobhair. NW Ireland
Gwelo *see* Gweru
97 K21 **Gwent** *cultural region* S Wales, UK
83 K17 **Gweru** *prev.* Gwelo. Midlands, C Zimbabwe
29 Q7 **Gwinner** North Dakota, N USA
77 Y13 **Gwoza** Borno, NE Nigeria
Gwy *see* Wye
183 R4 **Gwydir River** ⩫ New South Wales, SE Australia
97 I19 **Gwynedd** *var.* Gwyneth. *cultural region* NW Wales, UK
Gwyneth *see* Gwynedd
159 O16 **Gyaca** Xizang Zizhiqu, W China
Gya'gya *see* Saga
115 M22 **Gyalí** *var.* Yialí. *island* Dodekánisos, Greece, Aegean Sea
Gyandzha *see* Gäncä
158 M16 **Gyangzê** Xizang Zizhiqu, W China
158 L14 **Gyaring Co** ◎ W China
159 Q12 **Gyaring Hu** ◎ C China
115 I20 **Gyáros** *var.* Yioúra. *island* Kykládes, Greece, Aegean Sea
122 J7 **Gyda** Yamalo-Nenetskiy Avtonomnyy Okrug, N Russian Federation
122 J7 **Gydanskiy Poluostrov** *Eng.* Gyda Peninsula. *peninsula* N Russian Federation
Gyda Peninsula *see* Gydanskiy Poluostrov
Gyéres *see* Câmpia Turzii
Gyergyószentmiklós *see* Gheorgheni
Gyergyótölgyes *see* Tulgheş
Gyertyámos *see* Cărpiniş
Gyeva *see* Detva
Gyigang *see* Zayü
95 I23 **Gyldenløves Høy** *hill range* C Denmark
181 Z10 **Gympie** Queensland, E Australia
166 L7 **Gyobingauk** Pegu, SW Myanmar
111 M23 **Gyomaendrőd** Békés, SE Hungary
Gyömbér *see* Ďumbier
111 L22 **Gyöngyös** Heves, NE Hungary
111 H22 **Győr** *Ger.* Raab; *Lat.* Arrabona. Győr-Moson-Sopron, NW Hungary
111 G22 **Győr-Moson-Sopron** *off.* Győr-Moson-Sopron Megye. ◆ *county* NW Hungary
11 X15 **Gypsumville** Manitoba, S Canada
12 M4 **Gyrfalcon Islands** *island group* Nunavut, NE Canada
95 N14 **Gysinge** Gävleborg, C Sweden
115 F22 **Gýtheio** *var.* Githio; *prev.* Yíthion. Pelopónnisos, S Greece
146 L13 **Gyuichbirleshik** Lebapskiy Velayat, E Turkmenistan
111 N24 **Gyula** *Rom.* Jula. Békés, SE Hungary
Gyulafehérvár *see* Alba Iulia
Gyulovo *see* Roza

◆ Country ◇ Dependent Territory ◆ Administrative Region ▲ Mountain ▲ Volcano ◎ Lake
● Country Capital ○ Dependent Territory Capital ✕ International Airport ▲ Mountain Range ⩫ River ⊠ Reservoir

137 T11 Gyumri var. Giumri, Rus. Kumayri; prev. Aleksandropol', Leninakan. W Armenia
146 D13 Gyunuzyndag, Gora ▲ W Turkmenistan
146 D12 Gyzylarbat prev. Kizyl-Arvat. Balkanskiy Velayat, W Turkmenistan
Gyzylbaydak see Krasnoye Znamya
Gyzyletrek see Kizyl-Atrek
Gyzylgaya see Kizyl-Kaya
Gyzylsu see Kizyl-Su

H

159 T12 Ha W Bhutan
Haabai see Ha'apai Group
99 H17 Haacht Vlaams Brabant, C Belgium
109 T4 Haag Niederösterreich, NE Austria
194 L8 Haag Nunataks ▲ Antarctica
92 N2 Haakon VII Land physical region NW Svalbard
98 O11 Haaksbergen Overijssel, E Netherlands
99 E14 Haamstede Zeeland, SW Netherlands
193 Y15 Ha'ano island Ha'apai Group, C Tonga
193 Y15 Ha'apai Group var. Haabai. island group C Tonga
93 L15 Haapajärvi Oulu, C Finland
93 L17 Haapamäki Länsi-Suomi, W Finland
93 L15 Haapavesi Oulu, C Finland
191 N7 Haapiti Moorea, W French Polynesia
118 F4 Haapsalu Ger. Hapsal. Läänemaa, W Estonia
Ha'Arava see 'Arabah, Wādī al
Haarby see Hårby
98 H10 Haarlem prev. Harlem. Noord-Holland, W Netherlands
185 D19 Haast West Coast, South Island, NZ
185 C20 Haast ∽ South Island, NZ
185 D20 Haast Pass pass South Island, NZ
193 W16 Ha'atua 'Eau, E Tonga
149 P15 Hab ∽ SW Pakistan
141 W7 Haba var. Al Haba. Dubayy, NE UAE
158 K2 Habahe var. Kaba. Xinjiang Uygur Zizhiqu, NW China
141 U13 Ḩabarūt var. Habrut. SW Oman
81 J18 Habaswein North Eastern, NE Kenya
99 L24 Habay-la-Neuve Luxembourg, SE Belgium
139 S8 Ḩabbānīyah, Buḩayrat ◎ C Iraq
Habelschwerdt see Bystrzyca Kłodzka
153 V14 Habiganj Chittagong, NE Bangladesh
163 Q12 Habirag Nei Mongol Zizhiqu, N China
95 L19 Habo Västra Götaland, S Sweden
123 V14 Habomai Islands island group Kuril'skiye Ostrova, SE Russian Federation
165 S2 Haboro Hokkaidō, NE Japan
153 S16 Habra West Bengal, NE India
Habrut see Ḩabarūt
143 P17 Ḩabshān Abū Ẓaby, C UAE
54 E14 Hacha Putumayo, S Colombia
165 X13 Hachijō Tōkyō, Hachijō-jima, SE Japan
165 X13 Hachijō-jima var. Hatizyô Zima. island Izu-shotō, SE Japan
164 L12 Hachiman Gifu, Honshū, SW Japan
165 P7 Hachimori Akita, Honshū, C Japan
165 R7 Hachinohe Aomori, Honshū, C Japan
93 G17 Hackås Jämtland, C Sweden
18 K14 Hackensack New Jersey, NE USA
Hadama see Nazrēt
141 W13 Ḩadbaram S Oman
139 U13 Ḩaddānīyah well S Iraq
96 K12 Haddington SE Scotland, UK
141 Z8 Ḩadd, Ra's al headland NE Oman
Haded see Xadeed
77 W12 Hadejia Jigawa, N Nigeria
77 W12 Hadejia ∽ N Nigeria
138 F9 Hadera var. Khadera. Haifa, C Israel
Hadersleben see Haderslev
95 G24 Haderslev Ger. Hadersleben. Sønderjylland, SW Denmark
151 J21 Hadhdhunmathi Atoll var. Haddummati Atoll, Laamu Atoll. atoll S Maldives
Hadhramaut see Ḩaḑramawt
141 W17 Hadīboh Suquṭrā, SE Yemen
158 K9 Hadilik Xinjiang Uygur Zizhiqu, W China
136 H16 Hadım Konya, S Turkey
140 K7 Hadīyah Al Madīnah, W Saudi Arabia
8 L5 Hadley Bay bay Victoria Island, Nunavut, N Canada
167 S6 Ha Đông var. Hadong. Ha Tây, N Vietnam
141 R15 Ḩaḑramawt Eng. Hadhramaut. ▲▲ S Yemen
Hadria see Adria
Hadrianopolis see Edirne
Hadria Picena see Apricena
95 G22 Hadsten Århus, C Denmark
95 G21 Hadsund Nordjylland, N Denmark
117 S4 Hadyach Rus. Gadyach. Poltavs'ka Oblast', NE Ukraine
112 I13 Hadžići Federacija Bosna I Hercegovina, SE Bosnia and Herzegovina
163 W14 Haeju S North Korea
Haerbin/Haerhpin/Ha-erh-pin see Harbin
141 P5 Ḩafar al Bāṭin Ash Sharqīyah, N Saudi Arabia
11 T15 Hafford Saskatchewan, S Canada
136 M13 Hafik Sivas, N Turkey
149 V8 Hāfizābād Punjab, E Pakistan
92 H4 Hafnarfjördhur Reykjanes, W Iceland
Hafnia see København, Denmark
Hafnia see Denmark
Hafren see Severn
Hafun see Xaafuun
Hafun, Ras see Xaafuun, Raas
80 G10 Hag 'Abdullah Sinnar, E Sudan
81 K18 Hagadera North Eastern, E Kenya
138 G8 HaGalil Eng. Galilee. ▲▲ N Israel
14 G10 Hagar Ontario, S Canada
155 G18 Hagari var. Vedāvati. ∽ W India
188 B16 Hagåtña var. Agana, Agaña. ○ (Guam) NW Guam
100 M13 Hagelberg hill NE Germany
39 N14 Hagemeister Island island Alaska, USA
101 F15 Hagen Nordrhein-Westfalen, W Germany
100 K10 Hagenow Mecklenburg-Vorpommern, N Germany
10 K15 Hagensborg British Columbia, SW Canada
80 I13 Hägere Hiywet var. Agere Hiywet, Ambo. Oromo, C Ethiopia
33 O15 Hagerman Idaho, NW USA
37 U14 Hagerman New Mexico, SW USA
21 V2 Hagerstown Maryland, NE USA
14 G16 Hagersville Ontario, S Canada
102 J15 Hagetmau Landes, SW France
95 K14 Hagfors Värmland, C Sweden
93 G16 Häggenås Jämtland, C Sweden
164 E12 Hagi Yamaguchi, Honshū, SW Japan
167 S5 Ha Giang Ha Giang, N Vietnam
Hagios Evstrátios see Ágios Efstrátios
HaGolan see Golan Heights
103 T4 Hagondange Moselle, NE France
97 B18 Hag's Head Ir. Ceann Caillí. headland W Ireland
102 I3 Hague, Cap de la headland N France
103 V5 Haguenau Bas-Rhin, NE France
165 X16 Hahajima-rettō island group SE Japan
15 R8 Há Há, Lac ◎ Quebec, SE Canada
172 H13 Hahaya ✕ (Moroni) Grande Comore, NW Comoros
22 K9 Hahnville Louisiana, S USA
83 E22 Haib Karas, S Namibia
Haibak see Āybak
149 N15 Haibo ∽ SW Pakistan
163 U12 Haicheng Liaoning, NE China
Haida see Nový Bor
Haidarabad see Hyderābād
Haidenschaft see Ajdovščina
167 T6 Hai Dương Hai Hưng, N Vietnam
138 F9 Haifa ◈ district NW Israel
Haifa see Hefa
Haifa, Bay of see Hefa, Mifraz
161 P14 Haifeng Guangdong, S China
Haifong see Hai Phong
161 P3 Hai He ∽ E China
Haikang see Leizhou
160 L17 Haikou var. Hai-k'ou, Hoihow, Fr. Hoï-Hao. Hainan, S China
140 M6 Ḩā'il Ḩā'il, NW Saudi Arabia
141 N5 Ḩā'il off. Minṭaqah Ḩā'il. ◈ province N Saudi Arabia
Hai-la-erh see Hailar
163 S6 Hailar var. Hai-la-erh; prev. Hulun. Nei Mongol Zizhiqu, N China
163 S6 Hailar He ∽ NE China
33 P14 Hailey Idaho, NW USA
14 H9 Haileybury Ontario, S Canada
163 X9 Hailin Heilongjiang, NE China
Ḩā'il, Minṭaqah see Ḩā'il
Hailong see Meihekou
93 K14 Hailuoto Swe. Karlö. island W Finland
Haima see Haymā'
Haimen see Taizhou
160 M17 Hainan var. Hainan Sheng, Qiong. ◈ province S China
160 K17 Hainan Dao island S China
Hainan Sheng see Hainan
Hainan Strait see Qiongzhou Haixia
Hainasch see Ainaži
Hainau see Chojnów
99 E20 Hainaut ◈ province SW Belgium
Hainburg see Hainburg an der Donau
109 Z4 Hainburg an der Donau var. Hainburg. Niederösterreich, NE Austria
39 W12 Haines Alaska, USA
32 L12 Haines Oregon, NW USA
23 W12 Haines City Florida, SE USA
10 H8 Haines Junction Yukon Territory, W Canada
109 W4 Hainfeld Niederösterreich, NE Austria
101 N16 Hainichen Sachsen, E Germany
167 T6 Hai Phong var. Haifong, Haiphong. N Vietnam
161 S12 Haitan Dao island SE China
44 K8 Haiti off. Republic of Haiti. ◆ republic C West Indies
35 T11 Haiwee Reservoir ⊡ California, W USA
80 I7 Haiya Red Sea, NE Sudan
159 T10 Haiyan Qinghai, W China
160 M13 Haiyang Shan ▲▲ S China
159 V10 Haiyuan Ningxia, N China
Hajda see Nový Bor
111 M22 Hajdú-Bihar off. Hajdú-Bihar Megye. ◈ county E Hungary
111 N22 Hajdúböszörmény Hajdú-Bihar, E Hungary
111 N22 Hajdúhadház Hajdú-Bihar, E Hungary
111 N21 Hajdúnánás Hajdú-Bihar, E Hungary
111 N22 Hajdúszoboszló Hajdú-Bihar, E Hungary
142 I3 Ḩājī Ebrāhīm, Kūh-e ▲ Iran/Iraq
165 O9 Hajiki-zaki headland Sado, C Japan
Hajîne see Abû Ḩardân
153 P13 Hājīpur Bihār, N India
141 N14 Ḩajjah W Yemen
139 U11 Ḩajjama S Iraq
143 R12 Ḩājjīābād Hormozgān, C Iran
139 U14 Ḩājj, Thaqb al well S Iraq
113 L16 Hajla ▲▲ SW Yugoslavia
110 P10 Hajnówka Ger. Hermhausen. Podlaskie, NE Poland
166 K4 Haka Chin State, W Myanmar
Hakapehi see Punaauia
Hakâri see Hakkâri
137 T16 Hakkâri var. Çölemerik, Hakâri. Hakkâri, SE Turkey
137 T16 Hakkâri var. Hakkari. ◈ province SE Turkey
92 J12 Hakkas Norrbotten, N Sweden
164 J14 Hakken-zan ▲ Honshū, SW Japan
165 R7 Hakkōda-san ▲ Honshū, C Japan
165 T2 Hako-dake ▲ Hokkaidō, NE Japan
165 R5 Hakodate Hokkaidō, NE Japan
164 L11 Hakui Ishikawa, Honshū, SW Japan
190 B16 Hakupu SE Niue
164 L12 Haku-san ▲ Honshū, SW Japan
Hal see Halle
149 Q15 Hāla Sind, SE Pakistan
138 J3 Ḩalab Eng. Aleppo, Fr. Alep; anc. Beroea. Ḩalab, NW Syria
138 J3 Ḩalab off. Muḩāfaẓat Ḩalab, var. Aleppo, Halab. ◈ governorate NW Syria
138 J3 Ḩalab ✕ Ḩalab, NW Syria
141 O8 Ḩalabān var. Halibān. Ar Riyāḑ, C Saudi Arabia
139 V4 Ḩalabja NE Iraq
190 A16 Halagigie Point headland W Niue
75 Z11 Halaib SE Egypt
190 G12 Halalo Île Uvea, N Wallis and Futuna
Halandri see Chalándri
141 X13 Ḩalāniyāt, Juzur al var. Jazā'ir Bin Ghalfān, Eng. Kuria Muria Islands. island group S Oman
141 W13 Ḩalānīyāt, Khalīj al Eng. Kuria Muria Bay. bay S Oman
Halas see Kiskunhalas
38 G11 Halawa Haw. Hālawa. Hawaii, USA, C Pacific Ocean
38 F9 Halawa, Cape headland Molokai, Hawaii, USA, C Pacific Ocean
162 H6 Halban Hövsgöl, N Mongolia
101 K14 Halberstadt Sachsen-Anhalt, C Germany
184 M12 Halcombe Manawatu-Wanganui, North Island, NZ
95 I16 Halden prev. Fredrikshald. Østfold, S Norway
100 L13 Haldensleben Sachsen-Anhalt, C Germany
Håldi see Halti
153 S17 Haldia West Bengal, NE India
152 K10 Haldwāni Uttar Pradesh, N India
38 F10 Haleakala crater Maui, Hawaii, USA, C Pacific Ocean
25 N4 Hale Center Texas, SW USA
99 J18 Halen Limburg, NE Belgium
23 O2 Haleyville Alabama, S USA
77 O17 Half Assini SW Ghana
35 R8 Half Dome ▲ California, W USA
185 C25 Halfmoon Bay var. Oban. Stewart Island, Southland, NZ
182 E5 Half Moon Lake salt lake South Australia
163 R7 Halhgol Dornod, E Mongolia
Haliacmon see Aliákmonas
Halibān see Ḩalabān
14 I13 Haliburton Ontario, SE Canada
14 I12 Haliburton Highlands var. Madawaska Highlands. hill range Ontario, SE Canada
13 Q15 Halifax Nova Scotia, SE Canada
97 L17 Halifax N England, UK
21 W8 Halifax North Carolina, SE USA
21 U7 Halifax Virginia, NE USA
13 Q15 Halifax ✕ Nova Scotia, SE Canada
143 T13 Halīl Rūd seasonal river SE Iran
138 I6 Ḩalīmah ▲ Lebanon/Syria
162 G8 Haliun Govĭ-Altay, W Mongolia
118 I3 Haljala Ger. Halljal. Lääne-Virumaa, N Estonia
39 Q4 Halkett, Cape headland Alaska, USA
Halkida see Chalkída
96 J6 Halkirk N Scotland, UK
15 X7 Hall ∽ Quebec, SE Canada
Hall see Schwäbisch Hall
93 H15 Hälla Västerbotten, N Sweden
96 J6 Halladale ∽ N Scotland, UK
95 J21 Halland ◈ county S Sweden
23 Z15 Hallandale Florida, SE USA
95 K22 Hallandsås physical region S Sweden
9 P6 Hall Beach Nunavut, N Canada
99 G19 Halle Fr. Hal. Vlaams Brabant, C Belgium
101 M15 Halle var. Halle an der Saale. Sachsen-Anhalt, C Germany
Halle an der Saale see Halle
35 W3 Halleck Nevada, W USA
95 L15 Hällefors Örebro, C Sweden
95 N16 Hälleforsnäs Södermanland, C Sweden
109 Q6 Hallein Salzburg, N Austria
101 L15 Halle-Neustadt Sachsen-Anhalt, C Germany
25 U12 Hallettsville Texas, SW USA
195 N4 Halley UK research station Antarctica
28 L4 Halliday North Dakota, N USA
37 S2 Halligan Reservoir ⊡ Colorado, C USA
100 G7 Halligen island group N Germany
94 G13 Hallingdal valley S Norway
38 J12 Hall Island island Alaska, USA
Hall Island see Maiana
189 P15 Hall Islands island group C Micronesia
118 H6 Halliste ∽ S Estonia
Halljal see Haljala
93 I15 Hällnäs Västerbotten, N Sweden
29 R2 Hallock Minnesota, N USA
9 S6 Hall Peninsula peninsula Baffin Island, Nunavut, NE Canada
20 F9 Halls Tennessee, S USA
95 M16 Hallsberg Örebro, C Sweden
181 N5 Halls Creek Western Australia
182 L12 Halls Gap Victoria, SE Australia
95 N15 Hallstahammar Västmanland, C Sweden
109 R6 Hallstatt Salzburg, W Austria
109 R6 Hallstatter See ◎ C Austria
95 P14 Hallstavik Stockholm, C Sweden
24 X7 Hallsville Texas, SW USA
103 P1 Halluin Nord, N France
Halmahera, Laut see Halmahera Sea
171 R11 Halmahera, Pulau prev. Djailolo, Gilolo, Jailolo. island E Indonesia
171 S12 Halmahera Sea Ind. Laut Halmahera. sea E Indonesia
95 J21 Halmstad Halland, S Sweden
119 N15 Halowchyn Rus. Golovchin. Mahilyowskaya Voblasts', E Belarus
95 H20 Hals Nordjylland, N Denmark
94 F8 Halsa Møre og Romsdal, S Norway
119 I15 Hal'shany Rus. Gol'shany. Hrodzyenskaya Voblasts', W Belarus
Hälsingborg see Helsingborg
29 R5 Halstad Minnesota, N USA
27 N6 Halstead Kansas, C USA
99 G15 Halsteren Noord-Brabant, S Netherlands
93 L16 Halsua Länsi-Suomi, W Finland
101 E14 Haltern Nordrhein-Westfalen, W Germany
92 J9 Halti var. Haltiatunturi, Lapp. Háldi. ▲ Finland/Norway
Haltiatunturi see Halti
116 J6 Halych Ivano-Frankivs'ka Oblast', W Ukraine
Halycus see Platani
103 P3 Ham Somme, N France
Hama see Ḩamāh
164 F12 Hamada Shimane, Honshū, SW Japan
142 L6 Hamadān anc. Ecbatana. Hamadān, W Iran
142 L6 Hamadān off. Ostān-e Hamadān. ◈ province W Iran
138 I5 Ḩamāh var. Hama; anc. Epiphania, Bibl. Hamath. Ḩamāh, W Syria
138 I5 Ḩamāh off. Muḩāfaẓat Ḩamāh, var. Hama. ◈ governorate C Syria
165 S3 Hamamasu Hokkaidō, NE Japan
164 L14 Hamamatsu var. Hamamatu. Shizuoka, Honshū, S Japan
Hamamatu see Hamamatsu
165 W14 Hamanaka Hokkaidō, NE Japan
164 L14 Hamana-ko ◎ Honshū, S Japan
94 I13 Hamar prev. Storhammer. Hedmark, S Norway
141 U10 Ḩamārīr al Kidan, Qalamat well E Saudi Arabia
164 I12 Hamasaka Hyōgo, Honshū, SW Japan
Hamath see Ḩamāh
165 T1 Hamatonbetsu Hokkaidō, NE Japan
155 K26 Hambantota Southern Province, SE Sri Lanka
Hambourg see Hamburg
100 J9 Hamburg Hamburg, N Germany
27 V14 Hamburg Arkansas, C USA
29 S16 Hamburg Iowa, C USA
18 D10 Hamburg New York, NE USA
100 I10 Hamburg Fr. Hambourg. ◈ state N Germany
148 K5 Hamdam Āb, Dasht-e Pash. Dasht-i Hamdamab. ▲▲ W Afghanistan
Hamdamab, Dasht-i see Hamdam Āb, Dasht-e
18 M13 Hamden Connecticut, NE USA
140 K6 Ḩamḑ, Wādī al dry watercourse W Saudi Arabia
93 K18 Hämeenkyrö Länsi-Suomi, W Finland
93 L19 Hämeenlinna Swe. Tavastehus. Etelä-Suomi, S Finland
HaMelah, Yam see Dead Sea
Hamelin see Hameln
100 I13 Hameln Eng. Hamelin. Niedersachsen, N Germany
180 I8 Hamersley Range ▲▲ Western Australia
163 Y12 Hamgyŏng-sanmaek ▲▲ N North Korea
163 X13 Hamhŭng C North Korea
159 O6 Hami var. Ha-mi, Uigh. Kumul, Qomul. Xinjiang Uygur Zizhiqu, NW China
139 X10 Ḩamīd Amīn E Iraq
141 W11 Hamīdān, Khawr oasis SE Saudi Arabia
138 H5 Ḩamīdīyah var. Hamīdīyé. Ṭarṭūs, W Syria
114 L12 Hamidiye Edirne, NW Turkey
Hamīdīyé see Ḩamīdīyah
182 L12 Hamilton Victoria, SE Australia
64 B12 Hamilton ○ (Bermuda) C Bermuda
14 G16 Hamilton Ontario, S Canada
184 M7 Hamilton Waikato, North Island, NZ
96 I12 Hamilton S Scotland, UK
23 N3 Hamilton Alabama, S USA
38 M10 Hamilton Alaska, USA
30 J13 Hamilton Illinois, N USA
27 S3 Hamilton Missouri, C USA
33 P10 Hamilton Montana, NW USA
25 S8 Hamilton Texas, SW USA
14 G16 Hamilton ✕ Ontario, SE Canada
64 I6 Hamilton Bank undersea feature SE Labrador Sea
182 E1 Hamilton Creek seasonal river South Australia
13 R8 Hamilton Inlet inlet Newfoundland, E Canada
27 T12 Hamilton, Lake ⊡ Arkansas, C USA
35 W6 Hamilton, Mount ▲ Nevada, W USA
75 S8 Ḩamīm, Wādī al ∽ NE Libya
93 N19 Hamina Swe. Fredrikshamn. Etelä-Suomi, S Finland
11 W16 Hamiota Manitoba, S Canada
152 L13 Hamīrpur Uttar Pradesh, N India
Hamīs Musait see Khamīs Mushayt
21 T11 Hamlet North Carolina, SE USA
25 P6 Hamlin Texas, SW USA
21 P5 Hamlin West Virginia, NE USA
31 O7 Hamlin Lake ◎ Michigan, N USA
101 F14 Hamm var. Hamm in Westfalen. Nordrhein-Westfalen, W Germany
Ḩammāmāt, Khalīj al see Hammamet, Golfe de
75 N5 Hammamet, Golfe de Ar. Khalīj al Ḩammāmāt. gulf NE Tunisia
139 R3 Ḩammān al 'Alīl N Iraq
139 X12 Ḩammār, Hawr al ◎ SE Iraq
93 J20 Hammarland Åland, SW Finland
93 H16 Hammarstrand Jämtland, C Sweden
93 O17 Hammaslahti Itä-Suomi, E Finland
99 F17 Hamme Oost-Vlaanderen, NW Belgium
100 H10 Hamme ∽ NW Germany
95 G22 Hammel Århus, C Denmark
101 I18 Hammelburg Bayern, C Germany
99 H18 Hamme-Mille Wallon Brabant, C Belgium
100 H10 Hamme-Oste-Kanal canal NW Germany
93 G16 Hammerdal Jämtland, C Sweden
92 K8 Hammerfest Finnmark, N Norway
101 D14 Hamminkeln Nordrhein-Westfalen, W Germany
Hamm in Westfalen see Hamm
26 K10 Hammon Oklahoma, C USA
31 N11 Hammond Indiana, N USA
22 K8 Hammond Louisiana, S USA
99 K20 Hamoir Liège, E Belgium
99 J21 Hamois Namur, SE Belgium
99 K16 Hamont Limburg, NE Belgium
185 F22 Hampden Otago, South Island, NZ
19 R6 Hampden Maine, NE USA
97 M23 Hampshire cultural region S England, UK
13 O15 Hampton New Brunswick, SE Canada
27 U14 Hampton Arkansas, C USA
29 V12 Hampton Iowa, C USA
19 P10 Hampton New Hampshire, NE USA
21 R14 Hampton South Carolina, SE USA
21 P8 Hampton Tennessee, S USA
21 X7 Hampton Virginia, NE USA
94 L11 Hamra Gävleborg, C Sweden
80 D10 Hamrat esh Sheikh Northern Kordofan, C Sudan
139 S5 Ḩamrīn, Jabal ▲ N Iraq
121 P16 Hamrun C Malta
167 U14 Ham Thuân Nam Bình Thuân, S Vietnam
Hāmūn, Daryācheh-ye see Şāberī, Hāmūn-e/Sīstān, Daryācheh-ye
Hamwih see Southampton
38 G10 Hana Haw. Hāna. Maui, Hawaii, USA, C Pacific Ocean
21 S14 Hanahan South Carolina, SE USA
38 B8 Hanalei Kauai, Hawaii, USA, C Pacific Ocean
167 U10 Ha Nam Quang Nam-Đa Nâng, C Vietnam
165 Q9 Hanamaki Iwate, Honshū, C Japan
38 F10 Hanamanioa, Cape headland Maui, Hawaii, USA, C Pacific Ocean
190 B16 Hanan ✕ (Alofi) SW Niue
101 H18 Hanau Hessen, W Germany
8 L9 Hanbury ∽ Northwest Territories, NW Canada
Hâncești see Hîncești
10 M15 Hanceville British Columbia, SW Canada
23 P3 Hanceville Alabama, S USA
Hancewicze see Hantsavichy
160 L6 Hancheng Shaanxi, C China
21 V2 Hancock Maryland, NE USA
30 M3 Hancock Michigan, N USA
29 S8 Hancock Minnesota, N USA
18 I12 Hancock New York, NE USA
80 Q12 Handa Bari, NE Somalia
161 O5 Handan var. Han-tan. Hebei, E China
95 P16 Handen Stockholm, C Sweden
81 J22 Handeni Tanga, E Tanzania
37 Q7 Handies Peak ▲ Colorado, C USA
111 J19 Handlová Ger. Krickerhäu, Hung. Nyitrabánya; prev. Ger. Kriegerhaj. Trenčiansky Kraj, W Slovakia
165 O13 Haneda ✕ (Tōkyō) Tōkyō, Honshū, S Japan
138 F13 HaNegev Eng. Negev. desert S Israel
35 Q11 Hanford California, W USA
191 V16 Hanga Roa Easter Island, Chile, E Pacific Ocean
162 H7 Hangayn Nuruu ▲▲ C Mongolia
Hang-chou/Hangchow see Hangzhou
95 K20 Hånger Jönköping, S Sweden
Hangö see Hanko
161 R9 Hangzhou var. Hang-chou, Hangchow. Zhejiang, SE China
162 F5 Hanhöhiy Uul ▲▲ NW Mongolia
Hanhowuz see Khauz-Khan
137 P15 Hani Dıyarbakır, SE Turkey
Hania see Chaniá
141 R11 Ḩanīsh al Kabīr, Jazīrat al island SW Yemen
Hanka, Lake see Khanka, Lake
93 M17 Hankasalmi Länsi-Suomi, W Finland
29 R7 Hankinson North Dakota, N USA
93 K20 Hanko Swe. Hangö. Etelä-Suomi, SW Finland
Han-kou/Han-k'ou/Hankow see Wuhan
36 M6 Hanksville Utah, W USA
152 K6 Hanle Jammu and Kashmir, NW India
185 I17 Hanmer Springs Canterbury, South Island, NZ
11 R16 Hanna Alberta, SW Canada
27 V3 Hannibal Missouri, C USA
180 M3 Hann, Mount ▲ Western Australia
100 I12 Hannover Eng. Hanover. Niedersachsen, NW Germany
99 J19 Hannut Liège, C Belgium
95 L22 Hanöbukten bay S Sweden
167 T6 Ha Nôi Eng. Hanoi, Fr. Ha noï. ● (Vietnam) N Vietnam
14 F14 Hanover Ontario, S Canada
31 P15 Hanover Indiana, N USA
18 G16 Hanover Pennsylvania, NE USA
21 W6 Hanover Virginia, NE USA
Hanover see Hannover
63 G23 Hanover, Isla island S Chile
Hanselbeck see Érd
195 X5 Hansen Mountains ▲▲ Antarctica
160 M8 Han Shui ∽ C China
152 H10 Hānsi Haryāna, NW India
95 F20 Hanstholm Viborg, NW Denmark
Han-tan see Handan
158 H6 Hantengri Feng var. Pik Khan-Tengri. ▲ China/Kazakhstan see also Khan-Tengri, Pik
119 I18 Hantsavichy Pol. Hancewicze, Rus. Gantsevichi. Brestskaya Voblasts', SW Belarus
9 Q6 Hantzsch ∽ Baffin Island, Nunavut, NE Canada
152 G9 Hanumāngarh Rājasthān, NW India
183 O9 Hanwood New South Wales, SE Australia
Hanyang see Caidian
Hanyang see Wuhan
160 H10 Hanyuan var. Fulin. Sichuan, C China
160 J7 Hanzhong Shaanxi, C China
191 W11 Hao atoll Îles Tuamotu, C French Polynesia
153 S16 Hāora prev. Howrah. West Bengal, NE India
78 K8 Haouach, Ouadi dry watercourse E Chad
92 K13 Haparanda Norrbotten, N Sweden
25 N3 Happy Texas, SW USA
34 M1 Happy Camp California, W USA
13 Q9 Happy Valley-Goose Bay prev. Goose Bay. Newfoundland, E Canada
Hapsal see Haapsalu
152 J10 Hāpur Uttar Pradesh, N India
138 F12 HaQatan, HaMakhtesh ▲▲ S Israel
140 I4 Ḩaql Tabūk, NW Saudi Arabia
171 U14 Har Pulau Kai Besar, E Indonesia
162 M8 Haraat Dundgovĭ, C Mongolia
141 R8 Ḩaraḑ var. Haradh. Ash Sharqīyah, E Saudi Arabia
Haradh see Ḩaraḑ
118 N12 Haradok Rus. Gorodok. Vitsyebskaya Voblasts', N Belarus
92 J13 Harads Norrbotten, N Sweden
119 G19 Haradzyets Rus. Gorodets. Brestskaya Voblasts', SW Belarus
119 J17 Haradzyeya Rus. Gorodeya. Minskaya Voblasts', C Belarus
191 V10 Haraiki atoll Îles Tuamotu, C French Polynesia
165 Q11 Haramachi Fukushima, Honshū, E Japan
118 M12 Harany Rus. Gorany. Vitsyebskaya Voblasts', N Belarus
83 L16 Harare prev. Salisbury. ● (Zimbabwe) Mashonaland East, NE Zimbabwe
83 L16 Harare ✕ Mashonaland East, NE Zimbabwe
78 J10 Haraz-Djombo Batha, C Chad
119 O16 Harbavichy Rus. Gorbovichi. Mahilyowskaya Voblasts', E Belarus

◆ Country
● Country Capital
◇ Dependent Territory
○ Dependent Territory Capital
◈ Administrative Region
✕ International Airport
▲ Mountain
▲▲ Mountain Range
Volcano
∽ River
◎ Lake
⊡ Reservoir

76 J16 **Harbel** W Liberia
163 W8 **Harbin** *var.* Haerbin, Ha-erh-pin, Kharbin; *prev.* Haerhpin, Pingkiang, Pinkiang. Heilongjiang, NE China
31 S7 **Harbor Beach** Michigan, N USA
13 T13 **Harbour Breton** Newfoundland, E Canada
65 D25 **Harbours, Bay of** *bay* East Falkland, Falkland Islands
95 G24 **Hårby** *var.* Haarby. Fyn, C Denmark
36 I13 **Harcuvar Mountains** ▲ Arizona, SW USA
108 I7 **Hard** Vorarlberg, NW Austria
154 H11 **Harda Khās** Madhya Pradesh, C India
95 D14 **Hardanger** *physical region* S Norway
95 D14 **Hardangerfjorden** *fjord* S Norway
94 E13 **Hardangerjøkulen** *glacier* S Norway
95 E14 **Hardangervidda** *plateau* S Norway
83 D20 **Hardap** ◈ *district* S Namibia
21 R15 **Hardeeville** South Carolina, SE USA
98 L5 **Hardegarijp** *Fris.* Hurdegaryp. Friesland, N Netherlands
98 O9 **Hardenberg** Overijssel, E Netherlands
183 Q9 **Harden-Murrumburrah** New South Wales, SE Australia
98 K10 **Harderwijk** Gelderland, C Netherlands
30 J14 **Hardin** Illinois, N USA
33 V11 **Hardin** Montana, NW USA
23 R5 **Harding, Lake** ▣ Alabama/Georgia, SE USA
20 J6 **Hardinsburg** Kentucky, S USA
98 I13 **Hardinxveld-Giessendam** Zuid-Holland, C Netherlands
11 R15 **Hardisty** Alberta, SW Canada
152 L12 **Hardoi** Uttar Pradesh, N India
23 U4 **Hardwick** Georgia, SE USA
27 W9 **Hardy** Arkansas, C USA
94 D10 **Hareid** Møre og Romsdal, S Norway
8 H7 **Hare Indian** ∿ Northwest Territories, NW Canada
99 D18 **Harelbeke** *var.* Harlebeke. West-Vlaanderen, W Belgium
Harem *see* Ḩārim
100 E11 **Haren** Niedersachsen, NW Germany
98 N6 **Haren** Groningen, NE Netherlands
80 L13 **Hārer** Hārer, E Ethiopia
95 P14 **Harg** Uppsala, C Sweden
Hargeisa *see* Hargeysa
80 M13 **Hargeysa** *var.* Hargeisa. Woqooyi Galbeed, NW Somalia
116 J10 **Harghita** ◈ *county* NE Romania
25 S17 **Hargill** Texas, SW USA
162 J8 **Harhorin** Övörhangay, C Mongolia
159 Q9 **Har Hu** ◎ C China
Hariana *see* Haryāna
141 P15 **Ḩarīb** W Yemen
168 M12 **Hari, Batang** *prev.* Djambi. ∿ Sumatera, W Indonesia
152 J9 **Haridwār** *prev.* Hardwar. Uttar Pradesh, N India
155 F18 **Harihar** Karnātaka, W India
185 F18 **Harihari** West Coast, South Island, NZ
138 I3 **Ḩārim** *var.* Harem. Idlib, W Syria
98 F13 **Haringvliet** *channel* SW Netherlands
98 F13 **Haringvlietdam** *dam* SW Netherlands
149 U5 **Harīpur** North-West Frontier Province, NW Pakistan
148 J4 **Harīrūd** *var.* Tedzhen, *Turkm.* Tejen. ∿ Afghanistan/Iran *see also* Tedzhen
94 J11 **Härjåhågnen** *Swe.* Härjahågen, Härjehågna. ▲ Norway/Sweden
93 K18 **Harjavalta** Länsi-Suomi, W Finland
Härjehågna *see* Härjåhågnen
118 G4 **Harjumaa** *off.* Harju Maakond. ◈ *province* NW Estonia
21 X11 **Harkers Island** North Carolina, SE USA
139 S1 **Harki** N Iraq
29 T14 **Harlan** Iowa, C USA
21 O7 **Harlan** Kentucky, S USA
29 N17 **Harlan County Lake** ▣ Nebraska, C USA
116 L9 **Hârlău** *var.* Hîrlău. Iaşi, NE Romania
Harlebeke *see* Harelbeke
33 U7 **Harlem** Montana, NW USA
Harlem *see* Haarlem
95 G22 **Harlev** Århus, C Denmark
98 K6 **Harlingen** *Fris.* Harns. Friesland, N Netherlands
25 T17 **Harlingen** Texas, SW USA
97 O21 **Harlow** E England, UK
33 T10 **Harlowton** Montana, NW USA
94 N11 **Harmånger** Gävleborg, C Sweden
98 I11 **Harmelen** Utrecht, C Netherlands
29 X11 **Harmony** Minnesota, N USA
32 J14 **Harney Basin** *basin* Oregon, NW USA
(0) F9 **Harney Basin** ▲ Oregon, NW USA
32 J14 **Harney Lake** ◎ Oregon, NW USA
28 J10 **Harney Peak** ▲ South Dakota, N USA
93 H17 **Härnösand** *var.* Hernösand. Västernorrland, C Sweden
Harns *see* Harlingen
162 F6 **Har Nuur** ◎ NW Mongolia
105 P4 **Haro** La Rioja, N Spain
40 F6 **Haro, Cabo** *headland* NW Mexico
94 D9 **Harøy** *island* S Norway
97 N21 **Harpenden** E England, UK
76 L18 **Harper** *var.* Cape Palmas. NE Liberia
26 M7 **Harper** Kansas, C USA
32 L13 **Harper** Oregon, NW USA
25 Q10 **Harper** Texas, SW USA
35 U13 **Harper Lake** *salt flat* California, W USA
39 T9 **Harper, Mount** ▲ Alaska, USA
95 J21 **Harplinge** Halland, S Sweden
36 J13 **Harquahala Mountains** ▲ Arizona, SW USA
141 T15 **Ḩarrah** SE Yemen
12 H11 **Harricana** ∿ Quebec, SE Canada
20 M9 **Harriman** Tennessee, S USA
13 R11 **Harrington Harbour** Quebec, E Canada
64 B12 **Harrington Sound** *bay* Bermuda, NW Atlantic Ocean
96 F8 **Harris** *physical region* NW Scotland, UK
27 X10 **Harrisburg** Arkansas, C USA
30 M17 **Harrisburg** Illinois, N USA
28 I14 **Harrisburg** Nebraska, C USA
32 F12 **Harrisburg** Oregon, NW USA
18 G15 **Harrisburg** *state capital* Pennsylvania, NE USA
182 F6 **Harris, Lake** ◎ South Australia
23 W11 **Harris, Lake** ◎ Florida, SE USA
83 J22 **Harrismith** Free State, E South Africa
27 T9 **Harrison** Arkansas, C USA
31 Q7 **Harrison** Michigan, N USA
28 I12 **Harrison** Nebraska, C USA
39 Q5 **Harrison Bay** *inlet* Alaska, USA
22 I6 **Harrisonburg** Louisiana, S USA
21 U4 **Harrisonburg** Virginia, NE USA
13 R7 **Harrison, Cape** *headland* Newfoundland, E Canada
27 R5 **Harrisonville** Missouri, C USA
Harris Ridge *see* Lomonosov Ridge
192 M3 **Harris Seamount** *undersea feature* N Pacific Ocean
96 F8 **Harris, Sound of** *strait* NW Scotland, UK
31 R6 **Harrisville** Michigan, N USA
21 R3 **Harrisville** West Virginia, NE USA
20 M6 **Harrodsburg** Kentucky, S USA
97 M16 **Harrogate** N England, UK
25 Q4 **Harrold** Texas, SW USA
27 S5 **Harry S.Truman Reservoir** ▣ Missouri, C USA
100 G13 **Harsewinkel** Nordrhein-Westfalen, W Germany
116 M14 **Hârşova** *prev.* Hîrşova. Constanţa, SE Romania
92 H10 **Harstad** Troms, N Norway
31 O8 **Hart** Michigan, N USA
24 M4 **Hart** Texas, SW USA
10 I5 **Hart** ∿ Yukon Territory, NW Canada
83 F23 **Hartbees** ∿ C South Africa
109 X7 **Hartberg** Steiermark, SE Austria
182 I10 **Hart, Cape** *headland* South Australia
95 E14 **Hårteigen** ▲ S Norway
23 Q7 **Hartford** Alabama, S USA
27 R11 **Hartford** Arkansas, C USA
18 M12 **Hartford** *state capital* Connecticut, NE USA
20 J6 **Hartford** Kentucky, S USA
31 P10 **Hartford** Michigan, N USA
29 R11 **Hartford** South Dakota, N USA
30 M8 **Hartford** Wisconsin, N USA
31 P13 **Hartford City** Indiana, N USA
29 Q13 **Hartington** Nebraska, C USA
13 N14 **Hartland** New Brunswick, SE Canada
97 H23 **Hartland Point** *headland* SW England, UK
97 M15 **Hartlepool** N England, UK
29 T12 **Hartley** Iowa, C USA
24 M1 **Hartley** Texas, SW USA
32 J15 **Hart Mountain** ▲ Oregon, NW USA
173 U10 **Hartog Ridge** *undersea feature* W Indian Ocean
93 M18 **Hartola** Etelä-Suomi, S Finland
67 U14 **Harts** *var.* Hartz. ∿ N South Africa
23 P2 **Hartselle** Alabama, S USA
23 S3 **Hartsfield Atlanta** ✕ Georgia, SE USA
27 Q11 **Hartshorne** Oklahoma, C USA
21 S12 **Hartsville** South Carolina, SE USA
20 K8 **Hartsville** Tennessee, S USA
27 U7 **Hartville** Missouri, C USA
23 U2 **Hartwell** Georgia, SE USA
21 O11 **Hartwell Lake** ▣ Georgia/South Carolina, SE USA
Hartz *see* Harts
Harunabad *see* Eslāmābād
162 E6 **Har-Us** Hovd, W Mongolia
162 E6 **Har Us Nuur** ◎ NW Mongolia
30 M10 **Harvard** Illinois, N USA
29 P16 **Harvard** Nebraska, C USA
37 R5 **Harvard, Mount** ▲ Colorado, C USA
31 N11 **Harvey** Illinois, N USA
29 N4 **Harvey** North Dakota, N USA
97 Q21 **Harwich** E England, UK
152 H10 **Haryāna** *var.* Hariana. ◈ *state* N India
141 Y9 **Ḩaryān, Ţawī al** *spring/well* NE Oman
101 J14 **Harz** ▲ C Germany
Hasakah *see* Al Ḩasakah
165 Q9 **Hasama** Miyagi, Honshū, C Japan
136 J15 **Hasan Dağı** ▲ C Turkey
139 T9 **Ḩasan Ibn Ḩassūn** C Iraq
149 R6 **Ḩasan Khēl** *var.* Ahmad Khel. Paktīā, SE Afghanistan
100 F12 **Hase** ∿ NW Germany
Haselberg *see* Krasnoznamensk
100 F12 **Haselünne** Niedersachsen, NW Germany
162 K9 **Hashaat** Dundgovĭ, C Mongolia
Hashemite Kingdom of Jordan *see* Jordan
139 V8 **Hāshimah** E Iraq
141 W13 **Ḩāsik** S Oman
149 U10 **Hāsilpur** Punjab, E Pakistan
Hasimoto *see* Hashimoto
27 Q10 **Haskell** Oklahoma, C USA
25 Q6 **Haskell** Texas, SW USA
114 M11 **Hasköy** Edirne, NW Turkey
95 L24 **Hasle** Bornholm, E Denmark
97 N23 **Haslemere** SE England, UK
102 I16 **Hasparren** Pyrénées-Atlantiques, SW France
Hassakeh *see* Al Ḩasakah
155 G19 **Hassan** Karnātaka, W India
36 J13 **Hassayampa River** ∿ Arizona, SW USA
101 J18 **Hassberge** *hill range* C Germany
94 N10 **Hassela** Gävleborg, C Sweden
99 J18 **Hasselt** Limburg, NE Belgium
98 M9 **Hasselt** Overijssel, E Netherlands
Hassetché *see* Al Ḩasakah
101 J18 **Hassfurt** Bayern, C Germany
74 L9 **Hassi Bel Guebbour** E Algeria
74 L8 **Hassi Messaoud** E Algeria
95 K22 **Hässleholm** Skåne, S Sweden
Hasta Colonia/Hasta Pompeia *see* Asti
183 O13 **Hastings** Victoria, SE Australia
184 O11 **Hastings** Hawke's Bay, North Island, NZ
97 P23 **Hastings** SE England, UK
31 P9 **Hastings** Michigan, N USA
29 W9 **Hastings** Minnesota, N USA
29 P16 **Hastings** Nebraska, C USA
95 K22 **Hästveda** Skåne, S Sweden
92 J8 **Hasvik** Finnmark, N Norway
37 V6 **Haswell** Colorado, C USA
162 I10 **Hatansuudal** Bayanhongor, C Mongolia
163 P9 **Hatavch** Sühbaatar, E Mongolia
136 K17 **Hatay** ◈ *province* S Turkey
37 R15 **Hatch** New Mexico, SW USA
36 K7 **Hatch** Utah, W USA
20 F9 **Hatchie River** ∿ Tennessee, S USA
116 G12 **Haţeg** *Ger.* Wallenthal, *Hung.* Hátszeg; *prev.* Hatzeg, Hötzing. Hunedoara, SW Romania
165 O17 **Hateruma-jima** *island* Yaeyama-shotō, SW Japan
183 N8 **Hatfield** New South Wales, SE Australia
162 I5 **Hatgal** Hövsgöl, N Mongolia
153 V16 **Hathazari** Chittagong, SE Bangladesh
141 T13 **Hathūt, Hişā'** *oasis* NE Yemen
167 R14 **Ha Tiên** Kiên Giang, S Vietnam
167 T8 **Ha Tinh** Ha Tinh, N Vietnam
Hatiôzi *see* Hachiōji
138 F12 **Ḥatira, Haré** *hill range* S Israel
167 R6 **Hat Lot** Sơn La, N Vietnam
45 P16 **Hato Airport** ✕ (Willemstad) Curaçao, SW Netherlands Antilles
54 H9 **Hato Corozal** Casanare, C Colombia
Hato del Volcán *see* Volcán
45 P9 **Hato Mayor** E Dominican Republic
Hatra *see* Al Ḩaḑr
Hatria *see* Adria
Hátszeg *see* Haţeg
143 R16 **Ḩattā** Dubayy, NE UAE
182 L9 **Hattah** Victoria, SE Australia
98 M9 **Hattem** Gelderland, E Netherlands
21 Z10 **Hatteras** Hatteras Island, North Carolina, SE USA
21 Rr10 **Hatteras, Cape** *headland* North Carolina, SE USA
21 Z9 **Hatteras Island** *island* North Carolina, SE USA
64 F10 **Hatteras Plain** *undersea feature* W Atlantic Ocean
93 G14 **Hattfjelldal** Troms, N Norway
22 M7 **Hattiesburg** Mississippi, S USA
29 Q4 **Hatton** North Dakota, N USA
Hatton Bank *see* Hatton Ridge
64 L6 **Hatton Ridge** *var.* Hatton Bank. *undersea feature* N Atlantic Ocean
191 W6 **Hatutu** *island* Îles Marquises, NE French Polynesia
111 K22 **Hatvan** Heves, NE Hungary
167 O16 **Hat Yai** *var.* Ban Hat Yai. Songkhla, SW Thailand
Hatzeg *see* Haţeg
Hatzfeld *see* Jimbolia
80 N13 **Haud** *plateau* Ethiopia/Somalia
95 D18 **Hauge** Rogaland, S Norway
95 C15 **Haugesund** Rogaland, S Norway
109 X2 **Haugsdorf** Niederösterreich, NE Austria
184 M9 **Hauhungaroa Range** ▲ North Island, NZ
95 E15 **Haukeligrend** Telemark, S Norway
93 L14 **Haukipudas** Oulu, C Finland
93 M17 **Haukivesi** ◎ SE Finland
93 M17 **Haukivuori** Isä-Suomi, E Finland
Hauptkanal *see* Havelländ Grosse
187 N10 **Hauraha** San Cristobal, SE Solomon Islands
184 L5 **Hauraki Gulf** *gulf* North Island, NZ
185 B24 **Hauroko, Lake** ◎ South Island, NZ
167 S14 **Hâu, Sông** ∿ S Vietnam
92 N12 **Hautajärvi** Lappi, NE Finland
74 F7 **Haut Atlas** *Eng.* High Atlas. ▲ C Morocco
79 M17 **Haut-Congo** *off.* Région du Haut-Congo; *prev.* Haut-Zaïre. ◈ *region* NE Dem. Rep. Congo (Zaire)
103 Y14 **Haute-Corse** ◈ *department* Corse, France, C Mediterranean Sea
102 L16 **Haute-Garonne** ◈ *department* S France
76 J13 **Haute-Guinée** ◈ *state* NE Guinea
79 K14 **Haute-Kotto** ◈ *prefecture* E Central African Republic
103 P12 **Haute-Loire** ◈ *department* C France
103 R6 **Haute-Marne** ◈ *department* N France
102 M3 **Haute-Normandie** ◈ *region* N France
15 U6 **Hauterive** Quebec, SE Canada
103 T13 **Hautes-Alpes** ◈ *department* SE France
103 S7 **Haute-Saône** ◈ *department* E France
103 T10 **Haute-Savoie** ◈ *department* E France
99 M20 **Hautes Fagnes** *Ger.* Hohes Venn. ▲ E Belgium
102 K16 **Hautes-Pyrénées** ◈ *department* S France
99 L23 **Haute Sûre, Lac de la** ▣ NW Luxembourg
102 M11 **Haute-Vienne** ◈ *department* C France
19 S8 **Haut, Isle au** *island* Maine, NE USA
79 M14 **Haut-Mbomou** ◈ *préfecture* SE Central African Republic
103 Q2 **Hautmont** Nord, N France
79 F19 **Haut-Ogooué** *off.* Province du Haut-Ogooué, *var.* Le Haut-Ogooué. ◈ *province* SE Gabon
Haut-Ogooué, Le *see* Haut-Ogooué
103 U7 **Haut-Rhin** ◈ *department* NE France
74 I6 **Hauts Plateaux** *plateau* Algeria/Morocco
38 D9 **Hauula** *Haw.* Hau'ula. Oahu, Hawaii, USA, C Pacific Ocean
101 O22 **Hauzenberg** Bayern, SE Germany
30 K13 **Havana** Illinois, N USA
Havana *see* La Habana
97 N23 **Havant** S England, UK
35 Y14 **Havasu, Lake** ▣ Arizona/California, W USA
95 J23 **Havdrup** Roskilde, E Denmark
100 N10 **Havel** ∿ NE Germany
99 J21 **Havelange** Namur, SE Belgium
100 M11 **Havelberg** Sachsen-Anhalt, NE Germany
149 U5 **Haveliān** North-West Frontier Province, NW Pakistan
100 N12 **Havelländ Grosse** *var.* Hauptkanal. *canal* NE Germany
14 J14 **Havelock** Ontario, SE Canada
185 J14 **Havelock** Marlborough, South Island, NZ
21 X11 **Havelock** North Carolina, SE USA
184 O11 **Havelock North** Hawke's Bay, North Island, NZ
98 M8 **Havelte** Drenthe, NE Netherlands
27 N6 **Haven** Kansas, C USA
97 H21 **Haverfordwest** SW Wales, UK
97 P20 **Haverhill** E England, UK
19 O10 **Haverhill** Massachusetts, NE USA
93 G17 **Haverö** Västernorrland, C Sweden
111 I17 **Havířov** Ostravský Kraj, E Czech Republic
111 E17 **Havlíčkův Brod** *Ger.* Deutsch-Brod; *prev.* Německý Brod. Jihlavský Kraj, C Czech Republic
92 K7 **Havøysund** Finnmark, N Norway
33 T7 **Havre** Montana, NW USA
Havre *see* le Havre
99 F20 **Havré** Hainaut, S Belgium
13 P11 **Havre-St-Pierre** Quebec, E Canada
136 B10 **Havsa** Edirne, NW Turkey
38 D8 **Hawaii** *off.* State of Hawaii; also known as Aloha State, Paradise of the Pacific. ◈ *state* USA, C Pacific Ocean
38 G12 **Hawaii** *Haw.* Hawai'i. *island* Hawaiian Islands, USA, C Pacific Ocean
192 M5 **Hawaiian Islands** *prev.* Sandwich Islands. *island group* Hawaii, USA, C Pacific Ocean
192 L5 **Hawaiian Ridge** *undersea feature* N Pacific Ocean
193 N6 **Hawaiian Trough** *undersea feature* N Pacific Ocean
29 R12 **Hawarden** Iowa, C USA
Hawash *see* Āwash
139 P6 **Hawbayn al Gharbīyah** C Iraq
185 D21 **Hawea, Lake** ◎ South Island, NZ
184 K11 **Hawera** Taranaki, North Island, NZ
20 J5 **Hawesville** Kentucky, S USA
38 G11 **Hawi** *Haw.* Hāwī. Hawaii, USA, C Pacific Ocean
96 K13 **Hawick** SE Scotland, UK
139 S4 **Ḩawījah** C Iraq
139 Y10 **Ḩawīzah, Hawr al** ◎ S Iraq
185 E21 **Hawkdun Range** ▲ South Island, NZ
184 P10 **Hawke Bay** *bay* North Island, NZ
182 I6 **Hawker** South Australia
184 N11 **Hawke's Bay** *off.* Hawkes Bay Region. ◈ *region* North Island, NZ
149 O16 **Hawkes Bay** *bay* SE Pakistan
15 N12 **Hawkesbury** Ontario, SE Canada
Hawkeye State *see* Iowa
23 T5 **Hawkinsville** Georgia, SE USA
14 B7 **Hawk Junction** Ontario, S Canada
21 N10 **Haw Knob** ▲ North Carolina/Tennessee, SE USA
21 Q9 **Hawksbill Mountain** ▲ North Carolina, SE USA
33 Z16 **Hawk Springs** Wyoming, C USA
Hawlēr *see* Arbīl
29 S5 **Hawley** Minnesota, N USA
25 P7 **Hawley** Texas, SW USA
141 R14 **Ḩawrā'** C Yemen
139 P7 **Ḩawrān, Wadi** *dry watercourse* W Iraq
21 T9 **Haw River** ∿ North Carolina, SE USA
139 U5 **Hawshqūrah** E Iraq
35 S7 **Hawthorne** Nevada, W USA
37 W3 **Haxtun** Colorado, C USA
183 N9 **Hay** New South Wales, SE Australia
11 O10 **Hay** ∿ W Canada
171 S13 **Haya** Pulau Seram, E Indonesia
165 R9 **Hayachine-san** ▲ Honshū, C Japan
103 S4 **Hayange** Moselle, NE France
HaYarden *see* Jordan
Hayastani Hanrapetut'yun *see* Armenia
Hayasui-seto *see* Hōyo-kaikyō
39 N9 **Haycock** Alaska, USA
36 M14 **Hayden** Arizona, SW USA
37 Q3 **Hayden** Colorado, C USA
28 M10 **Hayes** South Dakota, N USA
11 X13 **Hayes** ∿ Manitoba, C Canada
9 P12 **Hayes** ∿ Nunavut, NE Canada
28 M16 **Hayes Center** Nebraska, C USA
39 S10 **Hayes, Mount** ▲ Alaska, USA
21 N11 **Hayesville** North Carolina, SE USA
35 X10 **Hayford Peak** ▲ Nevada, W USA
34 M3 **Hayfork** California, W USA
Hayir, Qasr al *see* Ḩayr al Gharbī, Qaşr al
163 P8 **Haylaastay** Sühbaatar, E Mongolia
14 I12 **Hay Lake** ◎ Ontario, SE Canada
141 X11 **Haymā'** *var.* Haima. C Oman
136 H13 **Haymana** Ankara, C Turkey
138 J7 **Ḩaymūr, Jabal** ▲ W Syria
Haynau *see* Chojnów
22 G4 **Haynesville** Louisiana, S USA
23 P6 **Hayneville** Alabama, S USA
114 M12 **Hayrabolu** Tekirdağ, NW Turkey
136 C10 **Hayrabolu Deresi** ∿ NW Turkey
138 J6 **Ḩayr al Gharbī, Qaşr al** *var.* Qasr al Hayir, Qasr al Hir al Gharbi. *ruins* Ḩimş, C Syria
138 L5 **Ḩayr ash Sharqī, Qaşr al** *var.* Qasr al Hir Ash Sharqī. *ruins* Ḩimş, C Syria
8 J10 **Hay River** Northwest Territories, W Canada
26 K4 **Hays** Kansas, C USA
28 K12 **Hay Springs** Nebraska, C USA
65 H25 **Haystack, The** ▲ NE Saint Helena
27 N7 **Haysville** Kansas, C USA
117 O7 **Haysyn** *Rus.* Gaysin. Vinnyts'ka Oblast', C Ukraine
27 Y9 **Hayti** Missouri, C USA
29 Q9 **Hayti** South Dakota, N USA
117 O8 **Hayvoron** *Rus.* Gayvorno. Kirovohrads'ka Oblast', C Ukraine
35 N9 **Hayward** California, W USA
30 J4 **Hayward** Wisconsin, N USA
97 O23 **Haywards Heath** SE England, UK
143 S11 **Hazārān, Kūh-e** *var.* Kūh-e ā Hazr. ▲ SE Iran
Hazarat Imam *see* Emām Şāḩeb
21 O7 **Hazard** Kentucky, S USA
137 O15 **Hazar Gölü** ◎ C Turkey
153 P15 **Hazārībāg** *var.* Hazārībāgh. Bihār, N India
Hazārībāgh *see* Hazārībāg
103 O1 **Hazebrouck** Nord, N France
30 K9 **Hazel Green** Wisconsin, N USA
192 K9 **Hazel Holme Bank** *undersea feature* S Pacific Ocean
10 K13 **Hazelton** British Columbia, SW Canada
29 N6 **Hazelton** North Dakota, N USA
35 R5 **Hazen** Nevada, W USA
28 L5 **Hazen** North Dakota, N USA
38 L12 **Hazen Bay** *bay* E Bering Sea
9 N1 **Hazen, Lake** ◎ Nunavut, N Canada
139 S5 **Hazīm, Bi'r** *well* C Iraq
23 V6 **Hazlehurst** Georgia, SE USA
22 K6 **Hazlehurst** Mississippi, S USA
18 K15 **Hazlet** New Jersey, NE USA
146 I9 **Hazorasp** *Rus.* Khazarosp. Khorazm Wiloyati, W Uzbekistan
147 R13 **Hazratishoh, Qatorkŭhi** *var.* Khrebet Khazretishi, *Rus.* Khrebet Khozretishi. ▲ S Tajikistan
Hazr, Kūh-e ā *see* Hazārān, Kūh-e
149 U6 **Hazro** Punjab, E Pakistan
23 R7 **Headland** Alabama, S USA
182 C6 **Head of Bight** *headland* South Australia
33 N10 **Headquarters** Idaho, NW USA
34 M7 **Healdsburg** California, W USA
27 N13 **Healdton** Oklahoma, C USA
183 O12 **Healesville** Victoria, SE Australia
39 R10 **Healy** Alaska, USA
173 R13 **Heard and McDonald Islands** ◇ *Australian external territory* S Indian Ocean
173 R13 **Heard Island** *island* Heard and McDonald Islands, S Indian Ocean
25 U9 **Hearne** Texas, SW USA
12 F12 **Hearst** Ontario, S Canada
194 J5 **Hearst Island** *island* Antarctica
Heart of Dixie *see* Alabama
28 L5 **Heart River** ∿ North Dakota, N USA
31 T13 **Heath** Ohio, N USA
183 N11 **Heathcote** Victoria, SE Australia
97 N22 **Heathrow** ✕ (London)SE England, UK
21 X5 **Heathsville** Virginia, NE USA
27 R11 **Heavener** Oklahoma, C USA
25 R15 **Hebbronville** Texas, SW USA
163 Q13 **Hebei** *var.* Hebei Sheng, Hopeh, Hopei, Ji; *prev.* Chihli. ◈ *province* E China
Hebei Sheng *see* Hebei
36 M3 **Heber City** Utah, W USA
27 V10 **Heber Springs** Arkansas, C USA
161 N5 **Hebi** Henan, C China
32 F11 **Hebo** Oregon, NW USA
96 F9 **Hebrides, Sea of the** *sea* NW Scotland, UK
13 P5 **Hebron** Newfoundland, E Canada
31 N11 **Hebron** Indiana, N USA
29 Q17 **Hebron** Nebraska, C USA
28 L5 **Hebron** North Dakota, N USA
138 F11 **Hebron** *var.* Al Khalīl, El Khalil, *Heb.* Hevron; *anc.* Kiriath-Arba. S West Bank
Hebrus *see* Évros/Maritsa/Meriç
95 N14 **Heby** Västmanland, C Sweden
10 I14 **Hecate Strait** *strait* British Columbia, W Canada
41 W12 **Hecelchakán** Campeche, SE Mexico
160 K13 **Hechi** *var.* Jinchengjiang. Guangxi Zhuangzu Zizhiqu, S China
101 H23 **Hechingen** Baden-Württemberg, S Germany
99 K17 **Hechtel** Limburg, NE Belgium
160 J9 **Hechuan** Chongqing Shi, C China
29 P7 **Hecla** South Dakota, N USA
9 N1 **Hecla, Cape** *headland* Nunavut, N Canada
29 T9 **Hector** Minnesota, N USA
93 F17 **Hede** Jämtland, C Sweden
95 M14 **Hedemora** Dalarna, C Sweden
92 K13 **Hedenäset** Norrbotten, N Sweden
95 G23 **Hedensted** Vejle, C Denmark
95 N14 **Hedesunda** Gävleborg, C Sweden
95 N14 **Hedesundafjord** ◎ C Sweden
25 O3 **Hedley** Texas, SW USA
94 I12 **Hedmark** ◈ *county* S Norway
165 T16 **Hedo-misaki** *headland* Okinawa, SW Japan
29 X15 **Hedrick** Iowa, C USA
99 L16 **Heel** Limburg, SE Netherlands
189 Y12 **Heel Point** *point* Wake Island
98 H9 **Heemskerk** Noord-Holland, W Netherlands
98 M10 **Heerde** Gelderland, E Netherlands
98 L7 **Heerenveen** *Fris.* It Hearrenfean. Friesland, N Netherlands
98 I8 **Heerhugowaard** Noord-Holland, NW Netherlands
92 O3 **Heer Land** *physical region* C Svalbard
99 M18 **Heerlen** Limburg, SE Netherlands
99 J19 **Heers** Limburg, NE Belgium
Heerwegen *see* Polkowice
98 K13 **Heesch** Noord-Brabant, S Netherlands
99 K15 **Heeze** Noord-Brabant, SE Netherlands
138 F8 **Ḥefa** *var.* Haifa; *hist.* Caiffa, Caiphas, *anc.* Sycaminum. Haifa, N Israel
138 F8 **Ḥefa, Mifraz** *Eng.* Bay of Haifa. *bay* N Israel
161 Q8 **Hefei** *var.* Hofei; *hist.* Luchow. Anhui, E China
23 R3 **Heflin** Alabama, S USA
163 X7 **Hegang** Heilongjiang, NE China
164 L10 **Hegura-jima** *island* SW Japan
Heguri-jima *see* Heigun-tō
Hei *see* Heilongjiang
100 H8 **Heide** Schleswig-Holstein, N Germany
101 G20 **Heidelberg** Baden-Württemberg, SW Germany
83 J21 **Heidelberg** Gauteng, NE South Africa
22 M6 **Heidelberg** Mississippi, S USA
Heidenheim *see* Heidenheim an der Brenz
101 J22 **Heidenheim an der Brenz** *var.* Heidenheim. Baden-Württemberg, S Germany
109 U2 **Heidenreichstein** Niederösterreich, N Austria
164 F14 **Heigun-tō** *var.* Heguri-jima. *island* SW Japan
163 W5 **Heihe** *prev.* Ai-hun. Heilongjiang, NE China
Hei-ho *see* Nagqu
83 J22 **Heilbron** Free State, N South Africa
101 H21 **Heilbronn** Baden-Württemberg, SW Germany
Heiligenbeil *see* Mamonovo
109 Q8 **Heiligenblut** Tirol, W Austria
100 K7 **Heiligenhafen** Schleswig-Holstein, N Germany
Heiligenkreuz *see* Žiar nad Hronom
101 J15 **Heiligenstadt** Thüringen, C Germany
Heilong Jiang *see* Amur

◆ Country
● Country Capital
◇ Dependent Territory
○ Dependent Territory Capital
◈ Administrative Region
✕ International Airport
▲ Mountain
▲ Mountain Range
▲ Volcano
∿ River
◎ Lake
▣ Reservoir

163 W8 **Heilongjiang** var. Hei, Heilongjiang Sheng, Hei-lung-chiang, Heilungkiang. ◐ province NE China
Heilongjiang Sheng see Heilongjiang
98 H9 **Heiloo** Noord-Holland, NW Netherlands
Heilsberg see Lidzbark Warmiński
Hei-lung-chiang/Heilungkiang see Heilongjiang
92 I4 **Heimaey** var. Heimaæy. island S Iceland
94 H8 **Heimdal** Sør-Trøndelag, S Norway
Heinaste see Ainaži
93 N17 **Heinävesi** Itä-Suomi, E Finland
99 M22 **Heinerscheid** Diekirch, N Luxembourg
98 M10 **Heino** Overijssel, E Netherlands
93 M18 **Heinola** Etelä-Suomi, S Finland
101 C16 **Heinsberg** Nordrhein-Westfalen, W Germany
163 U12 **Heishan** Liaoning, NE China
160 H8 **Heishui** Sichuan, C China
99 H17 **Heist-op-den-Berg** Antwerpen, C Belgium
Heitō see P'ingtung
171 X15 **Heitske** Irian Jaya, E Indonesia
Hejanah see Al Hījānah
Hejaz see Al Ḥijāz
160 M14 **He Jiang** ≈ S China
158 K6 **Hejing** Xinjiang Uygur Zizhiqu, NW China
Héjjasfalva see Vânători
159 S11 **Heka** Qinghai, W China
137 N14 **Hekimhan** Malatya, C Turkey
92 J4 **Hekla** ▲ S Iceland
110 J6 **Hel** Ger. Hela. Pomorskie, N Poland
Hela see Hel
93 F17 **Helagsfjället** ▲ C Sweden
159 W8 **Helan** var. Xigang. Ningxia, N China
162 K14 **Helan Shan** ▲ N China
99 M16 **Helden** Limburg, SE Netherlands
27 X12 **Helena** Arkansas, C USA
33 R10 **Helena** state capital Montana, NW USA
96 H12 **Helensburgh** W Scotland, UK
184 K5 **Helensville** Auckland, North Island, NZ
95 L20 **Helgasjön** ◎ S Sweden
100 G8 **Helgoland** Eng. Heligoland. island NW Germany
Helgoland Bay see Helgoländer Bucht
100 G8 **Helgoländer Bucht** var. Helgoland Bay, Heligoland Bight. bay NW Germany
Heligoland see Helgoland
Heligoland Bight see Helgoländer Bucht
Heliopolis see Baalbek
92 I4 **Hella** Sudhurland, SW Iceland
Hellas see Greece
143 N11 **Ḥelleh, Rūd-e** ≈ S Iran
98 N10 **Hellendoorn** Overijssel, E Netherlands
Hellenic Republic see Greece
121 Q10 **Hellenic Trough** undersea feature Aegean Sea, C Mediterranean Sea
94 E10 **Hellesylt** Møre og Romsdal, S Norway
98 F13 **Hellevoetsluis** Zuid-Holland, SW Netherlands
105 Q12 **Hellín** Castilla-La Mancha, C Spain
115 H19 **Hellinikon** ✕ (Athína) Attikí, C Greece
32 M12 **Hells Canyon** valley Idaho/Oregon, NW USA
148 L9 **Helmand** ◐ province S Afghanistan
148 K10 **Helmand, Daryā-ye** var. Rūd-e Hīrmand. ≈ Afghanistan/Iran see also Hīrmand, Rūd-e
Helmantica see Salamanca
101 K15 **Helme** ≈ C Germany
99 L15 **Helmond** Noord-Brabant, S Netherlands
96 J7 **Helmsdale** N Scotland, UK
101 K13 **Helmstedt** Niedersachsen, N Germany
163 Y10 **Helong** Jilin, NE China
36 M4 **Helper** Utah, W USA
100 O10 **Helpter Berge** hill NE Germany
95 J22 **Helsingborg** prev. Hälsingborg. Skåne, S Sweden
Helsingfors see Helsinki
95 J22 **Helsingør** Eng. Elsinore. Frederiksborg, E Denmark
93 M20 **Helsinki** Swe. Helsingfors. ● (Finland) Etelä-Suomi, S Finland
97 H25 **Helston** SW England, UK
Heltau see Cisnădie
61 C17 **Helvecia** Santa Fe, C Argentina
97 K15 **Helvellyn** ▲ NW England, UK
Helvetia see Switzerland
75 W8 **Helwân** var. Hilwân, Hulwan, Hulwân. N Egypt
97 N21 **Hemel Hempstead** E England, UK
35 U16 **Hemet** California, W USA
28 J13 **Hemingford** Nebraska, C USA
21 T13 **Hemingway** South Carolina, SE USA
92 G13 **Hemnesberget** Nordland, C Norway
25 Y8 **Hemphill** Texas, SW USA
25 V11 **Hempstead** Texas, SW USA
95 P20 **Hemse** Gotland, SE Sweden
94 F13 **Hemsedal** valley S Norway
159 T11 **Henan** var. Henan Mongolzu Zizhixian, Yêgainnyin. Qinghai, C China
161 N6 **Henan** var. Henan Sheng, Honan, Yu. ◐ province C China
184 L4 **Hen and Chickens** island group N NZ
Henan Mongolzu Zizhixian/Henan Sheng see Henan
105 O7 **Henares** ≈ C Spain
165 P7 **Henashi-zaki** headland Honshū, C Japan
102 I16 **Hendaye** Pyrénées-Atlantiques, SW France
136 F11 **Hendek** Sakarya, NW Turkey
61 B21 **Henderson** Buenos Aires, E Argentina
20 I5 **Henderson** Kentucky, S USA
35 X11 **Henderson** Nevada, W USA
21 V8 **Henderson** North Carolina, SE USA
20 G10 **Henderson** Tennessee, S USA
25 W7 **Henderson** Texas, SW USA
30 J12 **Henderson Creek** ≈ Illinois, N USA
186 M9 **Henderson Field** ✕ (Honiara) Guadalcanal, C Solomon Islands
191 O17 **Henderson Island** atoll N Pitcairn Islands
21 O10 **Hendersonville** North Carolina, SE USA
20 J8 **Hendersonville** Tennessee, S USA
143 O14 **Hendorābī, Jazīreh-ye** island S Iran
55 V10 **Hendrik Top** var. Hendriktop. elevation C Surinam
Hendū Kosh see Hindu Kush
14 L12 **Heney, Lac** ◎ Quebec, SE Canada
Hengchow see Hengyang
161 S15 **Hengchun** S Taiwan
159 R16 **Hengduan Shan** ▲ SW China
98 N12 **Hengelo** Gelderland, E Netherlands
98 O10 **Hengelo** Overijssel, E Netherlands
Hengnan see Hengyang
161 N11 **Hengshan** Hunan, S China
160 L4 **Hengshan** Shaanxi, C China
161 O4 **Hengshui** Hebei, E China
161 N12 **Hengyang** var. Hengnan, Heng-yang; prev. Hengchow. Hunan, S China
117 U11 **Heniches'k** Rus. Genichesk. Khersons'ka Oblast', S Ukraine
21 Z4 **Henlopen, Cape** headland Delaware, NE USA
Henna see Enna
94 M10 **Hennan** Gävleborg, C Sweden
102 G7 **Hennebont** Morbihan, NW France
30 L11 **Hennepin** Illinois, N USA
26 M9 **Hennessey** Oklahoma, C USA
100 N12 **Hennigsdorf** var. Hennigsdorf bei Berlin. Brandenburg, NE Germany
Hennigsdorf bei Berlin see Hennigsdorf
19 N9 **Henniker** New Hampshire, NE USA
25 S5 **Henrietta** Texas, SW USA
Henrique de Carvalho see Saurimo
30 L12 **Henry** Illinois, N USA
21 Y7 **Henry, Cape** headland Virginia, NE USA
27 P10 **Henryetta** Oklahoma, C USA
194 M7 **Henry Ice Rise** ice cap Antarctica
9 Q5 **Henry Kater, Cape** headland Baffin Island, Nunavut, NE Canada
33 R13 **Henrys Fork** ≈ Idaho, NW USA
14 E15 **Hensall** Ontario, S Canada
100 J9 **Henstedt-Ulzburg** Schleswig-Holstein, N Germany
163 N7 **Hentiy** ◐ province N Mongolia
162 M7 **Hentiyn Nuruu** ▲ N Mongolia
183 P10 **Henty** New South Wales, SE Australia
166 L8 **Henzada** Irrawaddy, SW Myanmar
101 G19 **Heppenheim** Hessen, W Germany
32 J11 **Heppner** Oregon, NW USA
160 L15 **Hepu** prev. Lianzhou. Guangxi Zhuangzu Zizhiqu, S China
92 J2 **Heradhsvötn** ≈ C Iceland
Herakleion see Irákleio
148 K5 **Herāt** var. Herat; anc. Aria. Herāt, W Afghanistan
148 J5 **Herāt** ◐ province W Afghanistan
103 P14 **Hérault** ◐ department S France
103 P15 **Hérault** ≈ S France
11 T16 **Herbert** Saskatchewan, S Canada
185 F22 **Herbert** Otago, South Island, NZ
38 J17 **Herbert Island** island Aleutian Islands, Alaska, USA
Herbertshöhe see Kokopo
15 Q7 **Hérbertville** Quebec, SE Canada
101 G17 **Herborn** Hessen, W Germany
113 I17 **Herceg-Novi** It. Castelnuovo; prev. Ercegnovi. Montenegro, SW Yugoslavia
11 X10 **Herchmer** Manitoba, C Canada
186 E8 **Hercules Bay** bay E PNG
92 K2 **Herdhubreidh** ▲ C Iceland
42 M13 **Heredia** Heredia, C Costa Rica
42 M12 **Heredia** off. Provincia de Heredia. ◐ province N Costa Rica
97 K21 **Hereford** W England, UK
24 M3 **Hereford** Texas, SW USA
15 Q13 **Hereford, Mont** ▲ Quebec, SE Canada
97 K21 **Herefordshire** cultural region W England, UK
191 U11 **Hereheretue** atoll Îles Tuamotu, C French Polynesia
105 N10 **Herencia** Castilla-La Mancha, C Spain
99 H18 **Herent** Vlaams Brabant, C Belgium
99 I16 **Herentals** var. Herenthals. Antwerpen, N Belgium
Herenthals see Herentals
99 H17 **Herenthout** Antwerpen, N Belgium
95 J23 **Herfølge** Roskilde, E Denmark
100 G13 **Herford** Nordrhein-Westfalen, NW Germany
27 O5 **Herington** Kansas, C USA
108 H7 **Herisau** Fr. Hérisau. Appenzell Ausser Rhoden, NE Switzerland
Héristal see Herstal
99 J18 **Herk-de-Stad** Limburg, NE Belgium
Herkulesbad/Herkulesfürdő see Băile Herculane
Herlen Gol/Herlen He see Kerulen
35 Q4 **Herlong** California, W USA
97 L26 **Herm** island Channel Islands
109 R9 **Hermagor** Slvn. Šmohor. Kärnten, S Austria
29 S7 **Herman** Minnesota, N USA
96 L1 **Herma Ness** headland NE Scotland, UK
27 V4 **Hermann** Missouri, C USA
181 Q8 **Hermannsburg** Northern Territory, N Australia
Hermannstadt see Sibiu
94 E12 **Hermansverk** Sogn og Fjordane, S Norway
138 H6 **Hermel** var. Hirmil. NE Lebanon
Hermhausen see Hajnówka
183 P6 **Hermidale** New South Wales, SE Australia
55 X9 **Herminadorp** Sipaliwini, NE Surinam
32 K11 **Hermiston** Oregon, NW USA
27 T6 **Hermitage** Missouri, C USA
186 D4 **Hermit Islands** island group N PNG
25 O7 **Hermleigh** Texas, SW USA
138 G7 **Hermon, Mount** Ar. Jabal ash Shaykh. ▲ S Syria
Hermopolis Parva see Damanhûr
28 J10 **Hermosa** South Dakota, N USA
40 F5 **Hermosillo** Sonora, NW Mexico
Hermoupolis see Ermoúpoli
111 N20 **Hernád** var. Hornád, Ger. Kundert. ≈ Hungary/Slovakia
61 C18 **Hernández** Entre Ríos, E Argentina
23 V11 **Hernando** Florida, SE USA
22 L1 **Hernando** Mississippi, S USA
105 Q2 **Hernani** País Vasco, N Spain
99 F19 **Herne** Vlaams Brabant, C Belgium
101 E14 **Herne** Nordrhein-Westfalen, W Germany
95 F22 **Herning** Ringkøbing, W Denmark
Hernösand see Härnösand
121 U11 **Herodotus Basin** undersea feature E Mediterranean Sea
121 Q12 **Herodotus Trough** undersea feature C Mediterranean Sea
29 T11 **Heron Lake** Minnesota, N USA
Herowābād see Khalkhāl
95 G16 **Herre** Telemark, S Norway
29 N7 **Herreid** South Dakota, N USA
101 H22 **Herrenberg** Baden-Württemberg, S Germany
104 L14 **Herrera** Andalucía, S Spain
43 R17 **Herrera** off. Provincia de Herrera. ◐ province S Panama
104 L10 **Herrera del Duque** Extremadura, W Spain
104 M4 **Herrera de Pisuerga** Castilla-León, N Spain
41 Z13 **Herrero, Punta** headland SE Mexico
183 P16 **Herrick** Tasmania, SE Australia
30 L17 **Herrin** Illinois, N USA
20 M6 **Herrington Lake** ▣ Kentucky, S USA
95 K18 **Herrljunga** Västra Götaland, S Sweden
103 N16 **Hers** ≈ S France
10 I1 **Herschel Island** island Yukon Territory, NW Canada
99 I17 **Herselt** Antwerpen, C Belgium
18 G15 **Hershey** Pennsylvania, NE USA
99 K19 **Herstal** Fr. Héristal. Liège, E Belgium
97 O21 **Hertford** E England, UK
21 X8 **Hertford** North Carolina, SE USA
97 O21 **Hertfordshire** cultural region E England, UK
181 Z9 **Hervey Bay** Queensland, E Australia
101 O14 **Herzberg** Brandenburg, E Germany
99 E18 **Herzele** Oost-Vlaanderen, NW Belgium
101 K20 **Herzogenaurach** Bayern, SE Germany
109 W4 **Herzogenburg** Niederösterreich, NE Austria
Herzogenbusch see 's-Hertogenbosch
103 N2 **Hesdin** Pas-de-Calais, N France
160 K14 **Heshan** Guangxi Zhuangzu Zizhiqu, S China
159 X10 **Heshui** var. Xihuachi. Gansu, C China
99 M25 **Hespérange** Luxembourg, SE Luxembourg
35 U14 **Hesperia** California, W USA
37 P7 **Hesperus Mountain** ▲ Colorado, C USA
10 J6 **Hess** ≈ Yukon Territory, NW Canada
Hesse see Hessen
101 J21 **Hesselberg** ▲ S Germany
95 I22 **Hesselo** island E Denmark
101 H17 **Hessen** Eng./Fr. Hesse. ◐ state C Germany
192 L6 **Hess Tablemount** undersea feature C Pacific Ocean
27 N6 **Hesston** Kansas, C USA
93 G15 **Hestskjølen** ▲ C Norway
97 K18 **Heswall** NW England, UK
153 P12 **Hetauda** Central, C Nepal
Hétfalu see Săcele
28 K7 **Hettinger** North Dakota, N USA
101 L14 **Hettstedt** Sachsen-Anhalt, C Germany
92 P3 **Heuglin, Kapp** headland SE Svalbard
187 N10 **Heuru** San Cristobal, SE Solomon Islands
99 J17 **Heusden** Limburg, NE Belgium
98 J13 **Heusden** Noord-Brabant, S Netherlands
102 K3 **Hève, Cap de la** headland N France
99 H18 **Heverlee** Vlaams Brabant, C Belgium
111 L22 **Heves** Heves, NE Hungary
111 L22 **Heves** off. Heves Megye. ◐ county NE Hungary
Hevron see Hebron
45 Y13 **Hewanorra** ✕ (Saint Lucia) S Saint Lucia
160 M13 **Hexian** var. Babu, He Xian. Guangxi Zhuangzu Zizhiqu, S China
160 L6 **Heyang** Shaanxi, C China
Heydebrech see Kędzierzyn-Kozle
Heydekrug see Šilutė
97 K16 **Heysham** NW England, UK
161 O14 **Heyuan** Guangdong, S China
182 L12 **Heywood** Victoria, SE Australia
180 K3 **Heywood Islands** island group Western Australia
161 O6 **Heze** var. Caozhou. Shandong, E China
159 U11 **Hezheng** Gansu, C China
159 U11 **Hezuozhen** Gansu, C China
23 Z16 **Hialeah** Florida, SE USA
27 Q3 **Hiawatha** Kansas, C USA
36 M4 **Hiawatha** Utah, W USA
29 V4 **Hibbing** Minnesota, N USA
183 N17 **Hibbs, Point** headland Tasmania, SE Australia
Hibernia see Ireland
20 F8 **Hickman** Kentucky, S USA
21 Q9 **Hickory** North Carolina, SE USA
21 Q9 **Hickory, Lake** ◎ North Carolina, SE USA
184 Q7 **Hicks Bay** Gisborne, North Island, NZ
25 S8 **Hico** Texas, SW USA
165 T4 **Hidaka** Hokkaidō, NE Japan
164 I12 **Hidaka** Hyōgo, Honshū, SW Japan
165 T5 **Hidaka-sanmyaku** ▲ Hokkaidō, NE Japan
41 O6 **Hidalgo** var. Villa Hidalgo. Coahuila de Zaragoza, NE Mexico
41 N8 **Hidalgo** Nuevo León, NE Mexico
41 O10 **Hidalgo** Tamaulipas, C Mexico
41 O13 **Hidalgo** ◐ state C Mexico
40 J7 **Hidalgo del Parral** var. Parral. Chihuahua, N Mexico
100 N7 **Hiddensee** island NE Germany
80 G6 **Hidiglib, Wadi** ≈ NE Sudan
109 U6 **Hieflau** Salzburg, E Austria
187 P16 **Hienghène** Province Nord, C New Caledonia
Hierosolyma see Jerusalem
64 N12 **Hierro** var. Ferro. island Islas Canarias, Spain, NE Atlantic Ocean
164 G13 **Higashi-Hiroshima** var. Higasihirosima. Hiroshima, Honshū, SW Japan
164 C12 **Higashi-suidō** strait SW Japan
Higasihirosima see Higashi-Hiroshima
Higasine see Higashine
25 P1 **Higgins** Texas, SW USA
31 P7 **Higgins Lake** ◎ Michigan, N USA
27 S4 **Higginsville** Missouri, C USA
High Atlas see Haut Atlas
30 M5 **High Falls Reservoir** ▣ Wisconsin, N USA
44 K12 **Highgate** C Jamaica
25 X11 **High Island** Texas, SW USA
31 O5 **High Island** island Michigan, N USA
30 K15 **Highland** Illinois, N USA
31 N10 **Highland Park** Illinois, N USA
21 O10 **Highlands** North Carolina, SE USA
11 O11 **High Level** Alberta, W Canada
29 O9 **Highmore** South Dakota, N USA
171 N3 **High Peak** ▲ Luzon, N Philippines
High Plains see Great Plains
21 S9 **High Point** North Carolina, SE USA
18 J13 **High Point** hill New Jersey, NE USA
11 P13 **High Prairie** Alberta, W Canada
11 Q16 **High River** Alberta, SW Canada
21 S9 **High Rock Lake** ▣ North Carolina, SE USA
23 V9 **High Springs** Florida, SE USA
High Veld see Great Karoo
97 J24 **High Willhays** ▲ SW England, UK
97 N22 **High Wycombe** prev. Chepping Wycombe, Chipping Wycombe. SE England, UK
41 P12 **Higos** var. El Higo. Veracruz-Llave, E Mexico
102 I16 **Higuer, Cap** headland NE Spain
45 R5 **Higüero, Punta** headland W Puerto Rico
45 P9 **Higüey** var. Salvaleón de Higüey. E Dominican Republic
190 G11 **Hihifo** ✕ (Matā'utu) Île Uvea, N Wallis and Futuna
81 N16 **Hiiraan** off. Gobolka Hiiraan. ◐ region C Somalia
118 E4 **Hiiumaa** off. Hiiumaa Maakond. ◐ province W Estonia
118 D4 **Hiiumaa** Ger. Dagden, Swe. Dagö. island W Estonia
Hijanah see Al Hījānah
105 S6 **Híjar** Aragón, NE Spain
191 V10 **Hikueru** atoll Îles Tuamotu, C French Polynesia
184 K3 **Hikurangi** Northland, North Island, NZ
184 Q8 **Hikurangi** ▲ North Island, NZ
192 L11 **Hikurangi Trench** var. Hikurangi Trough. undersea feature SW Pacific Ocean
Hikurangi Trough see Hikurangi Trench
190 B15 **Hikutavake** NW Niue
121 Q12 **Hilāl, Ra's al** headland N Libya
61 A24 **Hilario Ascasubi** Buenos Aires, E Argentina
101 K17 **Hildburghausen** Thüringen, C Germany
101 E15 **Hilden** Nordrhein-Westfalen, W Germany
100 I13 **Hildesheim** Niedersachsen, N Germany
33 T9 **Hilger** Montana, NW USA
Hili see Hilli
Hilla see Al Ḥillah
45 O14 **Hillaby, Mount** ▲ N Barbados
95 K19 **Hillared** Västra Götaland, S Sweden
195 R12 **Hillary Coast** physical region Antarctica
42 G2 **Hill Bank** Orange Walk, N Belize
33 O14 **Hill City** Idaho, NW USA
26 K3 **Hill City** Kansas, C USA
29 V5 **Hill City** Minnesota, N USA
28 J10 **Hill City** South Dakota, N USA
65 C24 **Hill Cove Settlement** West Falkland, Falkland Islands
98 H10 **Hillegom** Zuid-Holland, W Netherlands
95 J22 **Hillerød** Frederiksborg, E Denmark
36 M7 **Hillers, Mount** ▲ Utah, W USA
153 S13 **Hilli** var. Hili. Rajshahi, NW Bangladesh
29 R11 **Hills** Minnesota, N USA
30 L14 **Hillsboro** Illinois, N USA
27 N5 **Hillsboro** Kansas, C USA
27 X5 **Hillsboro** Missouri, C USA
19 N10 **Hillsboro** New Hampshire, NE USA
37 Q14 **Hillsboro** New Mexico, SW USA
29 R4 **Hillsboro** North Dakota, N USA
31 R14 **Hillsboro** Ohio, N USA
32 G11 **Hillsboro** Oregon, NW USA
25 T8 **Hillsboro** Texas, SW USA
30 K8 **Hillsboro** Wisconsin, N USA
23 Y14 **Hillsboro Canal** canal Florida, SE USA
45 Y15 **Hillsborough** Carriacou, N Grenada
97 G15 **Hillsborough** E Northern Ireland, UK
21 U9 **Hillsborough** North Carolina, SE USA
31 Q10 **Hillsdale** Michigan, N USA
183 O8 **Hillston** New South Wales, SE Australia
21 R7 **Hillsville** Virginia, NE USA
96 L2 **Hillswick** NE Scotland, UK
Hill Tippera see Tripura
38 H11 **Hilo** Hawaii, USA, C Pacific Ocean
18 F9 **Hilton** New York, NE USA
14 C10 **Hilton Beach** Ontario, S Canada
21 R16 **Hilton Head Island** South Carolina, SE USA
21 R16 **Hilton Head Island** island South Carolina, SE USA
99 J15 **Hilvarenbeek** Noord-Brabant, S Netherlands
98 J11 **Hilversum** Noord-Holland, C Netherlands
Hilwân see Helwân
152 J7 **Himāchal Pradesh** ◐ state NW India
Himalaya/Himalaya Shan see Himalayas
152 M9 **Himalayas** var. Himalaya, Chin. Himalaya Shan. ▲ S Asia
171 P6 **Himamaylan** Negros, C Philippines
93 K15 **Himanka** Länsi-Suomi, W Finland
Himara see Himarë
113 L23 **Himarë** var. Himara. Vlorë, S Albania
138 M2 **Ḥimār, Wādī al** dry watercourse N Syria
154 D9 **Himatnagar** Gujarāt, W India
109 Y4 **Himberg** Niederösterreich, E Austria
164 I13 **Himeji** var. Himezi. Hyōgo, Honshū, SW Japan
164 E14 **Hime-jima** island SW Japan
Himezi see Himeji
164 L13 **Himi** Toyama, Honshū, SW Japan
109 S9 **Himmelberg** Kärnten, S Austria
138 I5 **Ḥimṣ** var. Homs; anc. Emesa. Ḥimṣ, C Syria
138 K6 **Ḥimṣ** off. Muḥāfaẓat Ḥimṣ, var. Homs. ◐ governorate C Syria
138 I5 **Ḥimṣ, Buḥayrat** var. Buḥayrat Qaṭṭīnah. ◎ W Syria
171 R7 **Hinatuan** Mindanao, S Philippines
117 N10 **Hinceşti** var. Hânceşti; prev. Kotovsk. C Moldova
44 M9 **Hinche** C Haiti
181 X5 **Hinchinbrook Island** island Queensland, NE Australia
39 S12 **Hinchinbrook Island** island Alaska, USA
97 M19 **Hinckley** C England, UK
29 V7 **Hinckley** Minnesota, N USA
36 K5 **Hinckley** Utah, W USA
18 J9 **Hinckley Reservoir** ▣ New York, NE USA
152 I12 **Hindaun** Rājasthān, N India
Hindenburg/Hindenburg in Oberschlesien see Zabrze
Hindiya see Al Hindīyah
21 O6 **Hindman** Kentucky, S USA
182 L10 **Hindmarsh, Lake** ◎ Victoria, SE Australia
185 G19 **Hinds** Canterbury, South Island, NZ
185 G19 **Hinds** ≈ South Island, NZ
95 H23 **Hindsholm** island C Denmark
149 S4 **Hindu Kush** Per. Hendū Kosh. ▲ Afghanistan/Pakistan
155 H19 **Hindupur** Andhra Pradesh, E India
11 O12 **Hines Creek** Alberta, W Canada
23 W6 **Hinesville** Georgia, SE USA
154 I12 **Hinganghāt** Mahārāshtra, C India
149 N15 **Hingol** ≈ SW Pakistan
154 H13 **Hingoli** Mahārāshtra, C India
137 R13 **Hınıs** Erzurum, E Turkey
92 O2 **Hinlopenstretet** strait N Svalbard
92 G10 **Hinnøya** island C Norway
108 H10 **Hinterrhein** ≈ SW Switzerland
11 O14 **Hinton** Alberta, SW Canada
26 M10 **Hinton** Oklahoma, C USA
21 R6 **Hinton** West Virginia, NE USA
Hios see Chíos
41 N8 **Hipolito** Coahuila de Zaragoza, NE Mexico
Hipponium see Vibo Valentia
164 B13 **Hirado** Nagasaki, Hirado-shima, SW Japan
164 B13 **Hirado-shima** island SW Japan
165 P16 **Hirakubo-saki** headland Ishigaki-jima, SW Japan
154 M11 **Hirākud Reservoir** ▣ E India
Hir al Gharbi, Qasr al see Ḥayr al Gharbī, Qaṣr al
165 Q16 **Hirara** Okinawa, Miyako-jima, SW Japan
Qasr al Hir Ash Sharqī see Ḥayr ash Sharqī, Qaṣr al
164 G12 **Hirata** Shimane, Honshū, SW Japan
Hiratuka see Hiratsuka
136 I13 **Hirfanlı Barajı** ▣ C Turkey
155 G18 **Hiriyūr** Karnātaka, W India
Hîrlău see Hârlău
148 K10 **Hirmand, Rūd-e** var. Daryā-ye Helmand. ≈ Afghanistan/Iran see also Helmand, Daryā-ye
Hirmil see Hermel
165 T5 **Hiroo** Hokkaidō, NE Japan
165 Q7 **Hirosaki** Aomori, Honshū, C Japan
164 F13 **Hiroshima** var. Hirosima. Hiroshima, Honshū, SW Japan
164 G13 **Hiroshima** off. Hiroshima-ken, var. Hirosima. ◐ prefecture Honshū, SW Japan
Hirosima see Hiroshima
Hirschberg/Hirschberg im Riesengebirge/Hirschberg in Schlesien see Jelenia Góra
103 Q3 **Hirson** Aisne, N France
Hirşova see Hârşova
95 G19 **Hirtshals** Nordjylland, N Denmark
152 H10 **Hisār** Haryāna, NW India
186 E9 **Hisiu** Central, SW PNG
147 P13 **Hisor** Rus. Gissar. W Tajikistan
Hispalis see Sevilla
Hispana/Hispania see Spain
44 M7 **Hispaniola** island Dominion Republic/Haiti
64 F11 **Hispaniola Basin** var. Hispaniola Trough. undersea feature SW Atlantic Ocean
Hispaniola Trough see Hispaniola Basin
Histonium see Vasto
139 R7 **Hīt** SW Iraq
165 P14 **Hita** Ōita, Kyūshū, SW Japan
165 P12 **Hitachi** var. Hitati. Ibaraki, Honshū, S Japan
165 P12 **Hitachi-Ōta** var. Hitatiôta. Ibaraki, Honshū, S Japan
Hitati see Hitachi
Hitatiôta see Hitachi-Ōta
97 O21 **Hitchin** E England, UK
191 Q7 **Hitiaa** Tahiti, W French Polynesia
164 D15 **Hitoyoshi** var. Hitoyosi. Kumamoto, Kyūshū, SW Japan
Hitoyosi see Hitoyoshi
94 F7 **Hitra** prev. Hitteren. island S Norway
Hitteren see Hitra
187 Q11 **Hiu** island Torres Islands, N Vanuatu
165 O11 **Hiuchiga-take** ▲ Honshū, C Japan
191 X7 **Hiva Oa** island Îles Marquises, N French Polynesia
20 M10 **Hiwassee Lake** ▣ North Carolina, SE USA
20 M10 **Hiwassee River** ≈ SE USA
95 H20 **Hjallerup** Nordjylland, N Denmark
95 M16 **Hjälmaren** Eng. Lake Hjalmar. ◎ C Sweden
Hjalmar, Lake see Hjälmaren
95 C14 **Hjellestad** Hordaland, S Norway
95 D16 **Hjelmeland** Rogaland, S Norway
94 G10 **Hjerkinn** Oppland, S Norway
95 L18 **Hjo** Västra Götaland, S Sweden
95 G19 **Hjørring** Nordjylland, N Denmark
167 O1 **Hkakabo Razi** ▲ Myanmar/China
167 N1 **Hkring Bum** ▲ N Myanmar
83 L21 **Hlathikulu** var. Hlatikulu. S Swaziland
Hlatikulu see Hlathikulu
Hliboka see Hlyboka
111 F17 **Hlinsko** var. Hlinsko v Čechách. Pardubický Kraj, C Czech Republic
Hlinsko v Čechách see Hlinsko
117 S6 **Hlobyne** Rus. Globino. Poltavs'ka Oblast', NE Ukraine
111 H20 **Hlohovec** Ger. Freistadt, Hung. Galgóc; prev. Frakštát. Trnavský Kraj, W Slovakia
83 J23 **Hlotse** var. Leribe. NW Lesotho

◆ Country ● Country Capital ◇ Dependent Territory ○ Dependent Territory Capital ◐ Administrative Region ✕ International Airport ▲ Mountain ▲ Mountain Range ⩋ Volcano ≈ River ◎ Lake ▣ Reservoir

111 I17 **Hlučín** Ger. Hultschin, Pol. Hulczyn. Ostravský Kraj, E Czech Republic
117 S2 **Hlukhiv** Rus. Glukhov. Sums'ka Oblast', NE Ukraine
119 K21 **Hlushkavichy** Rus. Glushkevichi. Homyel'skaya Voblasts', SE Belarus
119 L18 **Hlusk** Rus. Glusk, Glussk. Mahilyowskaya Voblasts', E Belarus
116 K8 **Hlyboka** Ger. Hliboka, Rus. Glybokaya. Chernivets'ka Oblast', W Ukraine
118 K13 **Hlybokaye** Rus. Glubokoye. Vitsyebskaya Voblasts', N Belarus
77 Q16 **Ho** SE Ghana
167 S6 **Hoa Binh** Hoa Binh, N Vietnam
83 E20 **Hoachanas** Hardap, C Namibia
Hoai Nhơn see Bồng Sơn
167 T8 **Hoa Lac** Quang Binh, C Vietnam
167 S5 **Hoang Liên Sơn** ▲▲ N Vietnam
83 B17 **Hoanib** ≈ NW Namibia
33 S15 **Hoback Peak** ▲ Wyoming, C USA
183 P17 **Hobart** prev. Hobarton, Hobart Town. state capital Tasmania, SE Australia
26 L11 **Hobart** Oklahoma, C USA
183 P17 **Hobart** ✈ Tasmania, SE Australia
Hobarton/Hobart Town see Hobart
37 W14 **Hobbs** New Mexico, SW USA
194 L12 **Hobbs Coast** physical region Antarctica
23 Z14 **Hobe Sound** Florida, SE USA
Hobicaurikány see Uricani
54 E12 **Hobo** Huila, S Colombia
99 G16 **Hoboken** Antwerpen, N Belgium
158 K3 **Hoboksar** var. Hoboksar Mongol Zizhixian. Xinjiang Uygur Zizhiqu, NW China
Hoboksar Mongol Zizhixian see Hoboksar
95 G21 **Hobro** Nordjylland, N Denmark
21 X10 **Hobucken** North Carolina, SE USA
95 O20 **Hoburgen** headland SE Sweden
81 P15 **Hobyo** It. Obbia. Mudug, E Somalia
109 R8 **Hochalmspitze** ▲ SW Austria
109 Q4 **Hochburg** Oberösterreich, N Austria
108 F8 **Hochdorf** Luzern, N Switzerland
109 N8 **Hochfeiler** It. Gran Pilastro. ▲ Austria/Italy
167 T14 **Hô Chi Minh** var. Ho Chi Minh City; prev. Saigon. S Vietnam
Ho Chi Minh City see Hô Chi Minh
108 I7 **Höchst** Vorarlberg, NW Austria
Höchstadt see Höchstadt an der Aisch
101 K19 **Höchstadt an der Aisch** var. Höchstadt. Bayern, C Germany
108 L9 **Hochwilde** It. L'Altissima. ▲ Austria/Italy
109 S7 **Hochwildstelle** ▲ C Austria
31 T14 **Hocking River** ≈ Ohio, N USA
Hoctúm see Hoctún
41 X12 **Hoctún** var. Hoctúm. Yucatán, E Mexico
Hodeida see Al Ḥudaydah
20 K6 **Hodgenville** Kentucky, S USA
11 T17 **Hodgeville** Saskatchewan, S Canada
76 L9 **Hodh ech Chargui** ◈ region E Mauritania
Hodh el Garbi see Hodh el Gharbi
76 J10 **Hodh el Gharbi** var. Hodh el Garbi. ◈ region S Mauritania
111 L25 **Hódmezővásárhely** Csongrád, SE Hungary
74 J6 **Hodna, Chott El** var. Chott el-Hodna, Ar. Shatt al-Hodna. salt lake N Algeria
Hodna, Shatt al- see Hodna, Chott El
111 G19 **Hodonín** Ger. Göding. Brněnský Kraj, SE Czech Republic
162 G6 **Hödrögö** Dzavhan, N Mongolia
Hodság/Hodschag see Odžaci
39 R7 **Hodzana River** ≈ Alaska, USA
Hoei see Huy
99 H19 **Hoeilaart** Vlaams Brabant, C Belgium
Hoë Karoo see Great Karoo
98 F12 **Hoek van Holland** Eng. Hook of Holland. Zuid-Holland, W Netherlands
98 L11 **Hoenderloo** Gelderland, E Netherlands
99 L18 **Hoensbroek** Limburg, SE Netherlands
163 Y11 **Hoeryŏng** NE North Korea
99 K18 **Hoeselt** Limburg, NE Belgium
98 K11 **Hoevelaken** Gelderland, C Netherlands
Hoey see Huy
101 M18 **Hof** Bayern, SE Germany
Höfðakaupstadhur see Skagaströnd
Hofei see Hefei
101 G18 **Hofheim am Taunus** Hessen, W Germany
Hofmarkt see Odorheiu Secuiesc
92 L3 **Höfn** Austurland, SE Iceland
94 N13 **Hofors** Gävleborg, C Sweden
92 J6 **Hofsjökull** glacier C Iceland
92 J1 **Hofsós** Nordhurland Vestra, N Iceland
164 E13 **Hōfu** Yamaguchi, Honshū, SW Japan
Hofuf see Al Hufūf
95 J22 **Höganäs** Skåne, S Sweden
183 P14 **Hogan Group** island group Tasmania, SE Australia
23 R4 **Hogansville** Georgia, SE USA
39 P8 **Hogatza River** ≈ Alaska, USA
28 I14 **Hogback Mountain** ▲ Nebraska, C USA
95 G14 **Høgevarde** ▲ S Norway
Högfors see Karkkila
31 P5 **Hog Island** island Michigan, N USA
21 Y6 **Hog Island** island Virginia, NE USA
Hogoley Islands see Chuuk Islands
95 N20 **Högsby** Kalmar, S Sweden
36 K1 **Hogup Mountains** ▲▲ Utah, W USA
101 E17 **Hohe Acht** ▲ W Germany
Hohenelbe see Vrchlabí
108 I7 **Hohenems** Vorarlberg, W Austria
Hohenmauth see Vysoké Mýto
Hohensalza see Inowrocław
Hohenstadt see Zábřeh
Hohenstein in Ostpreussen see Olsztynek
20 I9 **Hohenwald** Tennessee, S USA
101 L17 **Hohenwarte-Stausee** ▣ C Germany
Hohes Venn see Hautes Fagnes
109 Q8 **Hohe Tauern** ▲▲ W Austria
163 O13 **Hohhot** var. Huhehot, Huhuohaote, Mong. Kukukhoto; prev. Kweisui, Kwesui. Nei Mongol Zizhiqu, N China
103 U6 **Hohneck** ▲ NE France
77 Q16 **Hohoe** E Ghana
164 E12 **Hōhoku** Yamaguchi, Honshū, SW Japan
159 O11 **Hoh Sai Hu** ◎ C China
159 N11 **Hoh Xil Hu** ◎ C China
158 L11 **Hoh Xil Shan** ▲▲ W China
167 U10 **Hôi An** prev. Faifo. Quang Nam-Đa Nẵng, C Vietnam
Hoï-Hao/Hoihow see Haikou
81 F17 **Hoima** W Uganda
26 L5 **Hoisington** Kansas, C USA
Hojagala see Khodzhakala
Hojambaz see Khodzhambas
95 H23 **Højby** Fyn, C Denmark
95 F24 **Højer** Sønderjylland, SW Denmark
164 E14 **Hōjō** var. Hôzyô. Ehime, Shikoku, SW Japan
184 J3 **Hokianga Harbour** inlet SE Tasman Sea
185 F17 **Hokitika** West Coast, South Island, NZ
165 U4 **Hokkai-dō** ◈ territory Hokkaidō, NE Japan
165 T3 **Hokkaidō** prev. Ezo, Yeso, Yezo. island NE Japan
95 G15 **Hokksund** Buskerud, S Norway
143 S4 **Hokmābād** Khorāsān, N Iran
Hokō see P'ohang
Hoko-guntō/Hoko-shotō see P'enghu Liehtao
137 T12 **Hoktemberyan** Rus. Oktemberyan. SW Armenia
94 F13 **Hol** Buskerud, S Norway
117 R11 **Hola Prystan'** Rus. Golaya Pristan. Khersons'ka Oblast', S Ukraine
95 I23 **Holbæk** Vestsjælland, E Denmark
162 G6 **Holboo** Dzavhan, W Mongolia
183 P10 **Holbrook** New South Wales, SE Australia
37 N11 **Holbrook** Arizona, SW USA
27 S5 **Holden** Missouri, C USA
36 K5 **Holden** Utah, W USA
27 O11 **Holdenville** Oklahoma, C USA
29 O16 **Holdrege** Nebraska, C USA
35 X3 **Hole in the Mountain Peak** ▲ Nevada, W USA
155 G20 **Hole Narsipur** Karnātaka, W India
111 H18 **Holešov** Ger. Holleschau. Zlínský Kraj, E Czech Republic
45 N14 **Holetown** prev. Jamestown. W Barbados
31 Q12 **Holgate** Ohio, N USA
44 I7 **Holguín** Holguín, SE Cuba
23 V12 **Holiday** Florida, SE USA
39 O12 **Holitna River** ≈ Alaska, USA
94 I13 **Höljes** Värmland, C Sweden
109 X3 **Hollabrunn** Niederösterreich, NE Austria
36 L3 **Holladay** Utah, W USA
11 X16 **Holland** Manitoba, S Canada
31 O9 **Holland** Michigan, N USA
25 T9 **Holland** Texas, SW USA
Holland see Netherlands
22 K4 **Hollandale** Mississippi, S USA
Hollandia see Jayapura
Hollandsch Diep see Hollands Diep
99 H14 **Hollands Diep** var. Hollandsch Diep. channel SW Netherlands
Holleschau see Holešov
25 R5 **Holliday** Texas, SW USA
18 E15 **Hollidaysburg** Pennsylvania, NE USA
21 S6 **Hollins** Virginia, NE USA
26 J12 **Hollis** Oklahoma, C USA
35 O10 **Hollister** California, W USA
27 T8 **Hollister** Missouri, C USA
93 M19 **Hollola** Etelä-Suomi, S Finland
98 K4 **Hollum** Friesland, N Netherlands
95 J23 **Höllviksnäs** Skåne, S Sweden
37 W6 **Holly** Colorado, C USA
31 R9 **Holly** Michigan, N USA
21 S14 **Holly Hill** South Carolina, SE USA
21 W11 **Holly Ridge** North Carolina, SE USA
22 L1 **Holly Springs** Mississippi, S USA
23 Z15 **Hollywood** Florida, SE USA
8 J6 **Holman** Victoria Island, Northwest Territories, N Canada
92 I2 **Hólmavík** Vestfirdhir, NW Iceland
30 J7 **Holmen** Wisconsin, N USA
23 R8 **Holmes Creek** ≈ Alabama/Florida, SE USA
95 H16 **Holmestrand** Vestfold, S Norway
93 J16 **Holmön** island N Sweden
95 E22 **Holmsland Klit** beach W Denmark
93 J16 **Holmsund** Västerbotten, N Sweden
95 Q18 **Holmudden** headland SE Sweden
138 F10 **Holon** var. Kholon. Tel Aviv, C Israel
117 P8 **Holovanivs'k** Rus. Golovanevsk. Kirovohrads'ka Oblast', C Ukraine
95 F21 **Holstebro** Ringkøbing, W Denmark
95 F23 **Holsted** Ribe, W Denmark
29 T13 **Holstein** Iowa, C USA
Holsteinborg/Holsteinsborg/Holstenborg/Holstensborg see Sisimiut
21 O8 **Holston River** ≈ Tennessee, S USA
31 Q9 **Holt** Michigan, N USA
98 N10 **Holten** Overijssel, E Netherlands
27 P3 **Holton** Kansas, C USA
27 U5 **Holts Summit** Missouri, C USA
35 X17 **Holtville** California, W USA
98 L5 **Holwerd** Fris. Holwert. Friesland, N Netherlands
Holwert see Holwerd
39 O11 **Holy Cross** Alaska, USA
37 R4 **Holy Cross, Mount Of The** ▲ Colorado, C USA
97 I18 **Holyhead** Wel. Caer Gybi. NW Wales, UK
97 H18 **Holy Island** island NW Wales, UK
96 L12 **Holy Island** island NE England, UK
37 W3 **Holyoke** Colorado, C USA
18 M11 **Holyoke** Massachusetts, NE USA
101 I14 **Holzminden** Niedersachsen, C Germany
81 G19 **Homa Bay** Nyanza, W Kenya
Homāyūnshahr see Khomeynīshahr
77 P11 **Hombori** Mopti, S Mali
101 E20 **Homburg** Saarland, SW Germany
9 Q5 **Home Bay** bay Baffin Bay, Nunavut, NE Canada
Homenau see Humenné
39 Q13 **Homer** Alaska, USA
22 H4 **Homer** Louisiana, S USA
18 H10 **Homer** New York, NE USA
23 V7 **Homerville** Georgia, SE USA
23 Y16 **Homestead** Florida, SE USA
27 O9 **Hominy** Oklahoma, C USA
94 H8 **Hommelvik** Sør-Trøndelag, S Norway
95 C16 **Hommersåk** Rogaland, S Norway
155 H15 **Homnābād** Karnātaka, C India
22 J7 **Homochitto River** ≈ Mississippi, S USA
83 N20 **Homoine** Inhambane, SE Mozambique
112 O12 **Homoljske Planine** ▲ E Yugoslavia
Homonna see Humenné
Homs see Al Khums, Libya
Homs see Ḥimṣ, Syria
119 P19 **Homyel'** Rus. Gomel'. Homyel'skaya Voblasts', SE Belarus
118 L12 **Homyel'** Vitsyebskaya Voblasts', N Belarus
119 L19 **Homyel'skaya Voblasts'** prev. Rus. Gomel'skaya Oblast'. ◈ province SE Belarus
Honan see Henan, China
Honan see Luoyang, China
165 U4 **Honbetsu** Hokkaidō, NE Japan
Honctö see Gurahonț
54 E9 **Honda** Tolima, C Colombia
83 D24 **Hondeklip** Afr. Hondeklipbaai. Northern Cape, W South Africa
Hondeklipbaai see Hondeklip
11 Q13 **Hondo** Alberta, W Canada
164 C15 **Hondo** Kumamoto, Shimo-jima, SW Japan
25 Q12 **Hondo** Texas, SW USA
42 G1 **Hondo** ≈ Central America
Hondo see Honshū
42 G6 **Honduras** off. Republic of Honduras. ◆ republic Central America
Honduras, Golfo de see Honduras, Gulf of
42 H4 **Honduras, Gulf of** Sp. Golfo de Honduras. gulf W Caribbean Sea
11 V12 **Hone** Manitoba, C Canada
21 P12 **Honea Path** South Carolina, SE USA
95 H14 **Hønefoss** Buskerud, S Norway
31 S12 **Honey Creek** ≈ Ohio, N USA
25 V5 **Honey Grove** Texas, SW USA
35 Q4 **Honey Lake** ◎ California, W USA
102 L4 **Honfleur** Calvados, N France
Hon Gai see Hông Gai
161 O8 **Hong'an** prev. Huang'an. Hubei, C China
Hongay see Hông Gai
167 T6 **Hông Gai** var. Hon Gai, Hongay. Quang Ninh, N Vietnam
161 O15 **Honghai Wan** bay N South China Sea
Hông Hà, Sông see Red River
161 O7 **Hong He** ≈ C China
161 N9 **Hong Hu** ◎ C China
160 L11 **Hongjiang** Hunan, S China
161 O15 **Hong Kong** Chin. Xianggang. S China
159 P7 **Hongliuyuan** Gansu, N China
163 O9 **Hongor** Dornogovĭ, SE Mongolia
161 S8 **Hongqiao** ✈ (Shanghai) Shanghai Shi, E China
160 K14 **Hongshui He** ≈ S China
160 M5 **Hongtong** Shanxi, C China
164 J15 **Hongū** Wakayama, Honshū, SW Japan
Honguedo, Détroit d' see Honguedo Passage
15 Y5 **Honguedo Passage** var. Honguedo Strait, Fr. Détroit d'Honguedo. strait Quebec, E Canada
Honguedo Strait see Honguedo Passage
Hongwan see Sunan
163 X13 **Hongwŏn** E North Korea
160 H7 **Hongyuan** prev. Hurama. Sichuan, C China
161 Q7 **Hongze Hu** var. Hung-tse Hu. ◎ E China
186 L9 **Honiara** ● (Solomon Islands) Guadalcanal, C Solomon Islands
165 P8 **Honjō** var. Honzyô. Akita, Honshū, C Japan
93 K18 **Honkajoki** Länsi-Suomi, W Finland
92 K7 **Honningsvåg** Finnmark, N Norway
95 I19 **Hönö** Västra Götaland, S Sweden
38 G11 **Honokaa** Haw. Honoka'a. Hawaii, USA, C Pacific Ocean
38 G11 **Honokohau** Haw. Honokōhau. Hawaii, USA, C Pacific Ocean
38 D9 **Honolulu** ● Oahu, Hawaii, USA, C Pacific Ocean
38 H11 **Honomu** Haw. Honomū. Hawaii, USA, C Pacific Ocean
105 P10 **Honrubia** Castilla-La Mancha, C Spain
164 M12 **Honshū** var. Hondo, Honsyû. island SW Japan
Honsyû see Honshū
Honte see Westerschelde
Honzyô see Honjō
8 K8 **Hood** ≈ Nunavut, NW Canada
Hood Island see Española, Isla
32 H11 **Hood, Mount** ▲ Oregon, NW USA
32 H11 **Hood River** Oregon, NW USA
98 H10 **Hoofddorp** Noord-Holland, W Netherlands
99 G15 **Hoogerheide** Noord-Brabant, S Netherlands
98 N8 **Hoogeveen** Drenthe, NE Netherlands
98 O6 **Hoogezand-Sappemeer** Groningen, NE Netherlands
98 J8 **Hoogkarspel** Noord-Holland, NW Netherlands
98 N5 **Hoogkerk** Groningen, NE Netherlands
98 G13 **Hoogvliet** Zuid-Holland, SW Netherlands
26 I8 **Hooker** Oklahoma, C USA
97 E21 **Hook Head** Ir. Rinn Duáin. headland SE Ireland
Hook of Holland see Hoek van Holland
162 J9 **Hoolt** Övörhangay, C Mongolia
39 W13 **Hoonah** Chichagof Island, Alaska, USA
38 L11 **Hooper Bay** Alaska, USA
31 N13 **Hoopeston** Illinois, N USA
95 K22 **Höör** Skåne, S Sweden
98 I9 **Hoorn** Noord-Holland, NW Netherlands
18 L10 **Hoosic River** ≈ New York, NE USA
Hoosier State see Indiana
35 Y11 **Hoover Dam** dam Arizona/Nevada, W USA
162 I9 **Höövör** Övörhangay, C Mongolia
137 Q11 **Hopa** Artvin, NE Turkey
18 J14 **Hopatcong** New Jersey, NE USA
10 M17 **Hope** British Columbia, SW Canada
39 R12 **Hope** Alaska, USA
27 T14 **Hope** Arkansas, C USA
31 P14 **Hope** Indiana, N USA
29 Q5 **Hope** North Dakota, N USA
13 Q7 **Hopedale** Newfoundland, NE Canada
Hopeh/Hopei see Hebei
180 K13 **Hope, Lake** salt lake Western Australia
41 X13 **Hopelchén** Campeche, SE Mexico
21 U11 **Hope Mills** North Carolina, SE USA
183 O7 **Hope, Mount** New South Wales, SE Australia
92 P4 **Hopen** island SE Svalbard
197 Q4 **Hope, Point** headland Alaska, USA
12 M3 **Hopes Advance, Cap** headland Quebec, NE Canada
182 L10 **Hopetoun** Victoria, SE Australia
83 H23 **Hopetown** Northern Cape, W South Africa
21 W6 **Hopewell** Virginia, NE USA
109 O7 **Hopfgarten-im-Brixental** Tirol, W Austria
181 N8 **Hopkins Lake** salt lake Western Australia
182 M12 **Hopkins River** ≈ Victoria, SE Australia
20 I7 **Hopkinsville** Kentucky, S USA
34 M6 **Hopland** California, W USA
95 G24 **Hoptrup** Sønderjylland, SW Denmark
32 F9 **Hoquiam** Washington, NW USA
29 R6 **Horace** North Dakota, N USA
137 R12 **Horasan** Erzurum, NE Turkey
101 G22 **Horb am Neckar** Baden-Württemberg, S Germany
95 K23 **Hörby** Skåne, S Sweden
43 P16 **Horconcitos** Chiriquí, W Panama
95 C14 **Hordaland** ◈ county S Norway
116 H13 **Horezu** Vâlcea, SW Romania
108 G7 **Horgen** Zürich, N Switzerland
162 I7 **Horgo** Arhangay, C Mongolia
Hörin see Fenglin
163 O13 **Horinger** Nei Mongol Zizhiqu, N China
162 I9 **Horiult** Bayanhongor, C Mongolia
11 U17 **Horizon** Saskatchewan, S Canada
192 K9 **Horizon Bank** undersea feature S Pacific Ocean
192 L10 **Horizon Deep** undersea feature W Pacific Ocean
95 L14 **Hörken** Örebro, S Sweden
119 O15 **Horki** Rus. Gorki. Mahilyowskaya Voblasts', E Belarus
195 O10 **Horlick Mountains** ▲▲ Antarctica
117 X7 **Horlivka** Rom. Adâncata, Rus. Gorlovka. Donets'ka Oblast', E Ukraine
143 V11 **Ḩormak** Sīstān va Balūchestān, SE Iran
143 R13 **Hormozgān** off. Ostān-e Hormozgān. ◈ province S Iran
Hormoz, Tangeh-ye see Hormuz, Strait of
141 W6 **Hormuz, Strait of** var. Strait of Ormuz, Per. Tangeh-ye Hormoz. strait Iran/Oman
109 W2 **Horn** Niederösterreich, NE Austria
95 M18 **Horn** Östergötland, S Sweden
8 J9 **Horn** ≈ Northwest Territories, NW Canada
Hornád see Hernád
8 I6 **Hornaday** ≈ Northwest Territories, NW Canada
92 H13 **Hornavan** ◎ N Sweden
65 C24 **Hornby Mountains** hill range West Falkland, Falkland Islands
Horn, Cape see Hornos, Cabo de
97 O18 **Horncastle** E England, UK
95 N14 **Horndal** Dalarna, C Sweden
93 I16 **Hörnefors** Västerbotten, N Sweden
18 F11 **Hornell** New York, NE USA
Horné Nové Mesto see Kysucké Nové Mesto
12 F12 **Hornepayne** Ontario, S Canada
94 D10 **Hornindalsvatnet** ◎ S Norway
101 G22 **Hornisgrinde** ▲ SW Germany
22 M9 **Horn Island** island Mississippi, S USA
63 J26 **Hornos, Cabo de** Eng. Cape Horn. headland S Chile
117 S10 **Hornostayivka** Khersons'ka Oblast', S Ukraine
183 T9 **Hornsby** New South Wales, SE Australia
97 O16 **Hornsea** E England, UK
94 O11 **Hornslandet** peninsula C Sweden
95 H22 **Hornslet** Århus, C Denmark
92 O4 **Hornsundtind** ▲ S Svalbard
Horochów see Horokhiv
116 J7 **Horodenka** Rus. Gorodenka. Ivano-Frankivs'ka Oblast', W Ukraine
117 Q2 **Horodnya** Rus. Gorodnya. Chernihivs'ka Oblast', NE Ukraine
116 K6 **Horodok** Khmel'nyts'ka Oblast', W Ukraine
116 H5 **Horodok** Pol. Gródek Jagielloński, Rus. Gorodok, Gorodok Yagellonski. L'vivs'ka Oblast', NW Ukraine
117 Q6 **Horodyshche** Rus. Gorodishche. Cherkas'ka Oblast', C Ukraine
165 T3 **Horokanai** Hokkaidō, NE Japan
116 J4 **Horokhiv** Pol. Horochów, Rus. Gorokhov. Volyns'ka Oblast', NW Ukraine
165 T4 **Horoshiri-dake** var. Horosiri Dake. ▲ Hokkaidō, N Japan
Horosiri Dake see Horoshiri-dake
111 C17 **Hořovice** Ger. Horowitz. Středočeský Kraj, W Czech Republic
Horowitz see Hořovice
163 T9 **Horqin Youyi Zhongqi** Nei Mongol Zizhiqu, NE China
163 U11 **Horqin Zuoyi Houqi** Nei Mongol Zizhiqu, N China
163 T9 **Horqin Zuoyi Zhongqi** Nei Mongol Zizhiqu, N China
62 O5 **Horqueta** Concepción, C Paraguay
55 O12 **Horqueta Minas** Amazonas, S Venezuela
95 J20 **Horred** Västra Götaland, S Sweden
151 J19 **Horsburgh Atoll** atoll N Maldives
20 K7 **Horse Cave** Kentucky, S USA
37 V6 **Horse Creek** ≈ Colorado, C USA
27 S6 **Horse Creek** ≈ Missouri, C USA
18 G11 **Horseheads** New York, NE USA
37 P13 **Horse Mount** ▲ New Mexico, SW USA
95 G22 **Horsens** Vejle, C Denmark
65 F25 **Horse Pasture Point** headland W Saint Helena
33 N13 **Horseshoe Bend** Idaho, NW USA
36 L13 **Horseshoe Reservoir** ▣ Arizona, SW USA
64 M9 **Horseshoe Seamounts** undersea feature E Atlantic Ocean
182 L11 **Horsham** Victoria, SE Australia
97 O23 **Horsham** SE England, UK
99 M15 **Horst** Limburg, SE Netherlands
64 N2 **Horta** Faial, Azores, Portugal, NE Atlantic Ocean
95 H16 **Horten** Vestfold, S Norway
111 M23 **Hortobágy-Berettyó** ≈ E Hungary
27 Q3 **Horton** Kansas, C USA
8 I7 **Horton** ≈ Northwest Territories, NW Canada
95 I23 **Hørve** Vestsjælland, E Denmark
95 L22 **Hörvik** Blekinge, S Sweden
138 E11 **Horvot Haluza** var. Khorvot Khalutsa. ruins Southern, S Israel
14 E7 **Horwood Lake** ◎ Ontario, S Canada
116 K4 **Horyn'** Rus. Goryn. ≈ NW Ukraine
81 I14 **Hosa'ina** var. Hosseina, It. Hosanna. Southern, S Ethiopia
Hosanna see Hosa'ina
101 H18 **Hösbach** Bayern, C Germany
Hose Mountains see Hose, Pegunungan
169 T9 **Hose, Pegunungan** var. Hose Mountains. ▲▲ East Malaysia
148 L15 **Hoshāb** Baluchistān, SW Pakistan
154 H10 **Hoshangābād** Madhya Pradesh, C India
116 L4 **Hoshcha** Rivnens'ka Oblast', NW Ukraine
152 I7 **Hoshiārpur** Punjab, NW India
162 J7 **Höshööt** Arhangay, C Mongolia
99 M23 **Hosingen** Diekirch, NE Luxembourg
186 G7 **Hoskins** New Britain, E PNG
155 G17 **Hospet** Karnātaka, C India
104 K4 **Hospital de Orbigo** Castilla-León, N Spain
Hospitalet see L'Hospitalet de Llobregat
92 N13 **Hossa** Oulu, E Finland
Hosseina see Hosa'ina
Hosszúmezjő see Câmpulung Moldovenesc
63 I25 **Hoste, Isla** island S Chile
117 O4 **Hostomel'** Rus. Gostomel'. Kyyivs'ka Oblast', N Ukraine
155 H20 **Hosūr** Tamil Nādu, SE India
167 N8 **Hot** Chiang Mai, NW Thailand
158 G10 **Hotan** var. Khotan, Chin. Ho-t'ien. Xinjiang Uygur Zizhiqu, NW China
158 H9 **Hotan He** ≈ NW China
83 G22 **Hotazel** Northern Cape, N South Africa
37 Q5 **Hotchkiss** Colorado, C USA
35 V7 **Hot Creek Range** ▲▲ Nevada, W USA
Hote see Hoti
171 T13 **Hoti** var. Hote. Pulau Seram, E Indonesia
Ho-t'ien see Hotan
Hotin see Khotyn
93 H15 **Hoting** Jämtland, C Sweden
162 L14 **Hotong Qagan Nur** ◎ N China
162 J8 **Hotont** Arhangay, C Mongolia
27 T12 **Hot Springs** Arkansas, C USA
28 J11 **Hot Springs** South Dakota, N USA
21 S5 **Hot Springs** Virginia, NE USA
35 Q4 **Hot Springs Peak** ▲ California, W USA
27 T12 **Hot Springs Village** Arkansas, C USA
Hotspur Bank see Hotspur Seamount
65 J16 **Hotspur Seamount** var. Hotspur Bank. undersea feature C Atlantic Ocean
8 J8 **Hottah Lake** ◎ Northwest Territories, NW Canada
44 K9 **Hotte, Massif de la** ▲▲ SW Haiti
99 K21 **Hotton** Luxembourg, SE Belgium
Hötzing see Hațeg
187 P17 **Houaïlou** Province Nord, C New Caledonia
74 K5 **Houari Boumediène** ✈ (Alger) N Algeria
167 P6 **Houayxay** var. Ban Houayxay, Ban Houei Sai. Bokèo, N Laos
103 N5 **Houdan** Yvelines, N France
99 F20 **Houdeng-Goegnies** var. Houdeng-Gœgnies. Hainaut, S Belgium
102 K14 **Houeillès** Lot-et-Garonne, SW France
99 L22 **Houffalize** Luxembourg, SE Belgium
30 M3 **Houghton** Michigan, N USA
31 Q7 **Houghton Lake** Michigan, N USA
31 Q7 **Houghton Lake** ◎ Michigan, N USA
19 T3 **Houlton** Maine, NE USA
160 M5 **Houma** Shanxi, C China
193 U15 **Houma** 'Eua, C Tonga
193 U16 **Houma** Tongatapu, S Tonga
22 J10 **Houma** Louisiana, S USA
196 V16 **Houma Taloa** headland Tongatapu, S Tonga
77 O13 **Houndé** SW Burkina
102 J12 **Hourtin-Carcans, Lac d'** ◎ SW France
36 J5 **House Range** ▲▲ Utah, W USA
10 K13 **Houston** British Columbia, SW Canada
39 R11 **Houston** Alaska, USA
29 X10 **Houston** Minnesota, N USA
22 M3 **Houston** Mississippi, S USA
27 V7 **Houston** Missouri, C USA
25 W11 **Houston** Texas, SW USA
25 W11 **Houston** ✈ Texas, SW USA
98 J12 **Houten** Utrecht, C Netherlands
99 K17 **Houthalen** Limburg, NE Belgium
99 I22 **Houyet** Namur, SE Belgium
95 H22 **Hov** Århus, C Denmark
95 L17 **Hova** Västra Götaland, S Sweden
162 E6 **Hovd** var. Khovd. Hovd, W Mongolia
162 J10 **Hovd** Övörhangay, C Mongolia
162 E7 **Hovd** ◈ province W Mongolia
162 C5 **Hovd Gol** ≈ NW Mongolia
97 O23 **Hove** SE England, UK
29 N8 **Hoven** South Dakota, N USA
116 I8 **Hoverla, Hora** Rus. Gora Goverla. ▲ W Ukraine
162 H8 **Höviyn Am** Bayanhongor, C Mongolia
95 M21 **Hovmantorp** Kronoberg, S Sweden
163 N11 **Hövsgöl** Dornogovĭ, SE Mongolia
162 I5 **Hövsgöl** ◈ province N Mongolia
Hovsgol, Lake see Hövsgöl Nuur

◆ Country ● Country Capital ◇ Dependent Territory ○ Dependent Territory Capital ◈ Administrative Region ✈ International Airport ▲ Mountain ▲▲ Mountain Range Volcano ≈ River ◎ Lake ▣ Reservoir

162 J5 **Hövsgöl Nuur** *var.* Lake Hovsgöl. ◎ N Mongolia
78 L9 **Howa, Ouadi** *var.* Wādi Howar. ∽ Chad/Sudan *see also* Howar, Wādi
27 P7 **Howard** Kansas, C USA
29 Q10 **Howard** South Dakota, N USA
25 N10 **Howard Draw** *valley* Texas, SW USA
29 U8 **Howard Lake** Minnesota, N USA
80 B8 **Howar, Wādi** *var.* Ouadi Howa. ∽ Chad/Sudan *see also* Howa, Ouadi
25 U5 **Howe** Texas, SW USA
183 R12 **Howe, Cape** *headland* New South Wales/Victoria, SE Australia
31 R9 **Howell** Michigan, N USA
28 L9 **Howes** South Dakota, N USA
83 K23 **Howick** KwaZulu/Natal, E South Africa
Howrah *see* Hāora
27 W9 **Hoxie** Arkansas, C USA
26 J3 **Hoxie** Kansas, C USA
101 I14 **Höxter** Nordrhein-Westfalen, W Germany
158 K6 **Hoxud** Xinjiang Uygur Zizhiqu, NW China
96 J5 **Hoy** *island* N Scotland, UK
43 S17 **Hoya, Cerro** ▲ S Panama
94 D12 **Høyanger** Sogn og Fjordane, S Norway
101 P15 **Hoyerswerda** Sachsen, E Germany
164 E14 **Hōyo-kaikyō** *var.* Hayasui-seto. *strait* SW Japan
104 J8 **Hoyos** Extremadura, W Spain
29 W4 **Hoyt Lakes** Minnesota, N USA
87 V2 **Hoyvík** Streymoy, N Faeroe Islands
137 O14 **Hozat** Tunceli, E Turkey
Hôzyô *see* Hōjō
111 F16 **Hradec Králové** *Ger.* Königgrätz. Hradecký Kraj, N Czech Republic
111 E16 **Hradecký Kraj** ◈ *region* N Czech Republic
111 B16 **Hradiště** *Ger.* Burgstadlberg. ▲ NW Czech Republic
117 R6 **Hradyz'k** *Rus.* Gradizhsk. Poltavs'ka Oblast', NE Ukraine
119 M16 **Hradzyanka** *Rus.* Grodzyanka. Mahilyowskaya Voblasts', E Belarus
119 F16 **Hrandzichy** *Rus.* Grandichi. Hrodzyenskaya Voblasts', W Belarus
111 H18 **Hranice** *Ger.* Mährisch-Weisskirchen. Olomoucký Kraj, E Czech Republic
112 I13 **Hrasnica** Federacija Bosna I Hercegovina, SE Bosnia and Herzegovina
109 V11 **Hrastnik** C Slovenia
137 U12 **Hrazdan** *Rus.* Razdan. C Armenia
137 T12 **Hrazdan** *var.* Zanga, *Rus.* Razdan. ∽ C Armenia
117 R5 **Hrebinka** *Rus.* Grebenka. Poltavs'ka Oblast', NE Ukraine
119 K17 **Hresk** *Rus.* Gresk. Minskaya Voblasts', C Belarus
Hrisoupoli *see* Chrysoúpoli
119 F16 **Hrodna** *Pol.* Grodno. Hrodzyenskaya Voblasts', W Belarus
119 F16 **Hrodzyenskaya Voblasts'** *prev. Rus.* Grodnenskaya Oblast'. ◈ *province* W Belarus
111 J21 **Hron** *Ger.* Gran, *Hung.* Garam. ∽ C Slovakia
111 Q14 **Hrubieszów** *Rus.* Grubeshov. Lubelskie, E Poland
112 F13 **Hrvace** Split-Dalmacija, SE Croatia
Hrvatska *see* Croatia
112 F10 **Hrvatska Kostajnica** *var.* Kostajnica. Sisak-Moslavina, C Croatia
Hrvatsko Grahovo *see* Bosansko Grahovo
116 K6 **Hrymayliv** *Pol.* Gizymałów, *Rus.* Grimaylov. Ternopil's'ka Oblast', W Ukraine
167 N4 **Hsenwi** Shan State, E Myanmar
Hsia-men *see* Xiamen
Hsiang-t'an *see* Xiangtan
Hsi Chiang *see* Xi Jiang
167 N6 **Hsihseng** Shan State, C Myanmar
161 S13 **Hsinchu** *municipality* N Taiwan
Hsing-k'ai Hu *see* Khanka, Lake
Hsi-ning/Hsining *see* Xining
Hsinking *see* Changchun
Hsin-yang *see* Xinyang
161 S14 **Hsinying** *var.* Sinying, *Jap.* Shinei. C Taiwan
167 N4 **Hsipaw** Shan State, C Myanmar
Hsu-chou *see* Xuzhou
161 S13 **Hsüeh Shan** ▲ N Taiwan
Hu *see* Shanghai Shi
83 B18 **Huab** ∽ W Namibia
57 M21 **Huacaya** Chuquisaca, S Bolivia
57 J19 **Huachacalla** Oruro, SW Bolivia
159 X9 **Huachi** *var.* Rouyuanchengzi. Gansu, C China
57 N16 **Huachi, Laguna** ◎ N Bolivia
57 D14 **Huacho** Lima, W Peru
163 Y8 **Huachuan** Heilongjiang, NE China
163 P12 **Huade** Nei Mongol Zizhiqu, N China
163 W10 **Huadian** Jilin, NE China
56 E13 **Huagaruncho, Cordillera** ▲ C Peru
Hua Hin *see* Ban Hua Hin
191 S10 **Huahine** *island* Îles Sous le Vent, W French Polynesia
Huahua, Rio *see* Wawa, Río
167 R8 **Huai** ∽ E Thailand
161 P6 **Huaibei** Anhui, E China
Huaide *see* Gongzhuling
157 T10 **Huai He** ∽ C China
160 L11 **Huaihua** Hunan, S China
161 N14 **Huaiji** Guangdong, S China
161 O2 **Huailai** *prev.* Shacheng. Hebei, E China
161 P7 **Huainan** *var.* Huai-nan, Hwainan. Anhui, E China
161 N2 **Huairen** Shanxi, C China
161 O7 **Huaiyang** Henan, C China
161 Q7 **Huaiyin** *var.* Qingjiang. Jiangsu, E China
167 N16 **Huai Yot** Trang, SW Thailand
41 Q15 **Huajuapan** *var.* Huajuapan de León. Oaxaca, SE Mexico
Huajuapan de León *see* Huajuapan
41 O9 **Hualahuises** Nuevo León, NE Mexico
36 I11 **Hualapai Mountains** ▲ Arizona, SW USA
36 I11 **Hualapai Peak** ▲ Arizona, SW USA
62 J7 **Hualfín** Catamarca, N Argentina
161 T13 **Hualien** *var.* Hwalien, *Jap.* Karen. C Taiwan
56 E10 **Huallaga, Río** ∽ N Peru
56 C11 **Huamachuco** La Libertad, C Peru
41 Q14 **Huamantla** Tlaxcala, S Mexico
82 C13 **Huambo** *Port.* Nova Lisboa. Huambo, C Angola
82 B13 **Huambo** ◈ *province* C Angola
41 P15 **Huamuxtitlán** Guerrero, S Mexico
63 H17 **Huancache, Sierra** ▲ SW Argentina
57 I17 **Huancané** Puno, SE Peru
57 F16 **Huancapi** Ayacucho, C Peru
57 E15 **Huancavelica** Huancavelica, SW Peru
57 E15 **Huancavelica** *off.* Departamento de Huancavelica. ◈ *department* W Peru
57 E14 **Huancayo** Junín, C Peru
57 K20 **Huanchaca, Cerro** ▲ S Bolivia
56 C12 **Huandoy, Nevado** ▲ W Peru
161 O8 **Huangchuan** Henan, C China
Huang Hai *see* Yellow Sea
157 Q8 **Huang He** *var.* Yellow River. ∽ C China
161 Q4 **Huanghe Kou** *delta* E China
160 L5 **Huangling** Shaanxi, C China
161 O9 **Huangpi** Hubei, C China
161 P13 **Huangqi Hai** ◎ N China
161 Q9 **Huang Shan** ▲ Anhui, E China
161 Q9 **Huangshan** *var.* Tunxi. Anhui, E China
161 O9 **Huangshi** *var.* Huang-shih, Hwangshih. Hubei, C China
Huang-shih *see* Huangshi
160 L5 **Huangtu Gaoyuan** *plateau* C China
61 B22 **Huanguelén** Buenos Aires, E Argentina
161 S10 **Huangyan** Zhejiang, SE China
159 T10 **Huangyuan** Qinghai, C China
159 T10 **Huangzhong** Qinghai, C China
163 W12 **Huanren** Liaoning, NE China
57 F15 **Huanta** Ayacucho, C Peru
56 E13 **Huánuco** Huánuco, C Peru
56 D13 **Huánuco** *off.* Departamento de Huánuco. ◈ *department* C Peru
57 K19 **Huanuni** Oruro, W Bolivia
159 X10 **Huan Xian** Gansu, C China
161 S12 **Huap'ing Yu** *island* N Taiwan
62 H3 **Huara** Tarapacá, N Chile
57 D14 **Huaral** Lima, W Peru
Huarás *see* Huaraz
56 D13 **Huaraz** *var.* Huarás. Ancash, W Peru
57 I16 **Huari Huari, Río** ∽ S Peru
56 C13 **Huarmey** Ancash, W Peru
40 H4 **Huásabas** Sonora, NW Mexico
56 D8 **Huasaga, Río** ∽ Ecuador/Peru
167 O15 **Hua Sai** Nakhon Si Thammarat, SW Thailand
56 D12 **Huascarán, Nevado** ▲ W Peru
62 G8 **Huasco** Atacama, N Chile
62 G8 **Huasco, Río** ∽ C Chile
159 S11 **Huashixia** Qinghai, W China
40 G7 **Huatabampo** Sonora, NW Mexico
159 W10 **Huating** Gansu, C China
167 S7 **Huatt, Phou** ▲ N Vietnam
41 Q14 **Huatusco** *var.* Huatusco de Chicuellar. Veracruz-Llave, C Mexico
Huatusco de Chicuellar *see* Huatusco
41 P13 **Huauchinango** Puebla, S Mexico
Huaunta *see* Wounta
41 R15 **Huautla** *var.* Huautla de Jiménez. Oaxaca, SE Mexico
Huautla de Jiménez *see* Huautla
161 O5 **Huaxian** *var.* Daokou, Hua Xian. Henan, C China
29 V13 **Hubbard** Iowa, C USA
25 U8 **Hubbard** Texas, SW USA
25 Q6 **Hubbard Creek Lake** ⊡ Texas, SW USA
31 R6 **Hubbard Lake** ◎ Michigan, N USA
160 M9 **Hubei** *var.* E, Hubei Sheng, Hupeh, Hupei. ◈ *province* C China
Hubei Sheng *see* Hubei
109 P8 **Huben** Tirol, W Austria
31 R13 **Huber Heights** Ohio, N USA
155 F17 **Hubli** Karnātaka, SW India
163 X12 **Huch'ang** N North Korea
97 M18 **Hucknall** C England, UK
97 L17 **Huddersfield** N England, UK
95 O16 **Huddinge** Stockholm, C Sweden
94 N11 **Hudiksvall** Gävleborg, C Sweden
29 W13 **Hudson** Iowa, C USA
19 O11 **Hudson** Massachusetts, NE USA
31 Q11 **Hudson** Michigan, N USA
30 H6 **Hudson** Wisconsin, N USA
11 V14 **Hudson Bay** Saskatchewan, S Canada
12 G6 **Hudson Bay** *bay* NE Canada
195 T16 **Hudson, Cape** *headland* Antarctica
Hudson, Détroit d' *see* Hudson Strait
27 Q9 **Hudson, Lake** ⊡ Oklahoma, C USA
18 K9 **Hudson River** ∽ New Jersey/New York, NE USA
10 M12 **Hudson's Hope** British Columbia, W Canada
12 L2 **Hudson Strait** *Fr.* Détroit d'Hudson. *strait* Nunavut/Quebec, NE Canada
Hudūd ash Shamālīyah, Minṭaqat al *see* Al Ḥudūd ash Shamālīyah
Hudur *see* Xuddur
167 U9 **Huê** Thưa Thiên-Huê, C Vietnam
104 J7 **Huebra** ∽ W Spain
24 H8 **Hueco Mountains** ▲ Texas, SW USA
116 G10 **Huedin** *Hung.* Bánffyhunyad. Cluj, NW Romania
40 J10 **Huehuento, Cerro** ▲ C Mexico
42 B5 **Huehuetenango** Huehuetenango, W Guatemala
42 B4 **Huehuetenango** *off.* Departamento de Huehuetenango. ◈ *department* W Guatemala
40 L11 **Huejuquilla** Jalisco, SW Mexico
41 P12 **Huejutla** *var.* Huejutla de Reyes. Hidalgo, C Mexico
Huejutla de Reyes *see* Huejutla
102 G6 **Huelgoat** Finistère, NW France
105 O13 **Huelma** Andalucía, S Spain
104 I14 **Huelva** *anc.* Onuba. Andalucía, SW Spain
104 I13 **Huelva** ◈ *province* Andalucía, S Spain
104 J13 **Huelva** ∽ SW Spain
105 Q14 **Huercal-Overa** Andalucía, S Spain
37 Q9 **Huerfano Mountain** ▲ New Mexico, SW USA
37 T7 **Huerfano River** ∽ Colorado, C USA
105 S12 **Huertas, Cabo** *headland* SE Spain
105 R6 **Huerva** ∽ N Spain
105 S4 **Huesca** *anc.* Osca. Aragón, NE Spain
105 T4 **Huesca** ◈ *province* Aragón, NE Spain
105 P13 **Huéscar** Andalucía, S Spain
41 N15 **Huetamo** *var.* Huetamo de Núñez. Michoacán de Ocampo, SW Mexico
Huetamo de Núñez *see* Huetamo
105 P8 **Huete** Castilla-La Mancha, C Spain
23 P4 **Hueytown** Alabama, S USA
28 L16 **Hugh Butler Lake** ⊡ Nebraska, C USA
181 V6 **Hughenden** Queensland, NE Australia
182 A6 **Hughes** South Australia
39 P8 **Hughes** Alaska, USA
27 X11 **Hughes** Arkansas, C USA
25 W6 **Hughes Springs** Texas, SW USA
37 V5 **Hugo** Colorado, C USA
27 Q13 **Hugo** Oklahoma, C USA
27 Q13 **Hugo Lake** ⊡ Oklahoma, C USA
26 H7 **Hugoton** Kansas, C USA
Huhehot/Huhuohaote *see* Hohhot
161 R13 **Hui'an** Fujian, SE China
184 O9 **Huiarau Range** ▲ North Island, NZ
83 D22 **Huib-Hoch Plateau** *plateau* S Namibia
41 O13 **Huichapán** Hidalgo, C Mexico
Huicheng *see* Shexian
163 W13 **Hŭich'ŏn** C North Korea
54 E12 **Huila** *off.* Departamento del Huila. ◈ *province* S Colombia
83 B15 **Huíla** ◈ *province* SW Angola
54 D11 **Huila, Nevado del** *elevation* C Colombia
83 B15 **Huíla Plateau** *plateau* S Angola
160 G12 **Huili** Sichuan, C China
161 P4 **Huimin** Shandong, E China
163 W11 **Huinan** *var.* Chaoyang. Jilin, NE China
62 K12 **Huinca Renancó** Córdoba, C Argentina
159 V10 **Huining** Gansu, C China
160 J12 **Huishui** Guizhou, S China
102 L6 **Huisne** ∽ NW France
98 L12 **Huissen** Gelderland, SE Netherlands
159 N11 **Huiten Nur** ◎ C China
93 K19 **Huittinen** Länsi-Suomi, W Finland
41 O15 **Huitzuco** *var.* Huitzuco de los Figueroa. Guerrero, S Mexico
Huitzuco de los Figueroa *see* Huitzuco
159 W11 **Huixian** *var.* Hui Xian. Gansu, C China
41 V17 **Huixtla** Chiapas, SE Mexico
160 H12 **Huize** Yunnan, SW China
98 J10 **Huizen** Noord-Holland, C Netherlands
161 O14 **Huizhou** Guangdong, S China
162 J6 **Hujirt** Arhangay, C Mongolia
162 J8 **Hujirt** Övörhangay, C Mongolia
162 K8 **Hujrt** Töv, C Mongolia
Hukagawa *see* Fukagawa
Hŭksan-chedo *see* Hŭksan-gundo
163 W17 **Hŭksan-gundo** *var.* Hŭksan-chedo. *island group* SW South Korea
Hukue *see* Fukue
Hukui *see* Fukui
83 G20 **Hukuntsi** Kgalagadi, SW Botswana
Hukuoka *see* Fukuoka
Hukusima *see* Fukushima
Hukutiyama *see* Fukuchiyama
Hukuyama *see* Fukuyama
163 W8 **Hulan** Heilongjiang, NE China
163 W8 **Hulan He** ∽ NE China
31 Q4 **Hulbert Lake** ◎ Michigan, N USA
Hulczyn *see* Hlučín
163 Z8 **Hulin** Heilongjiang, NE China
163 S9 **Hulingol** *prev.* Huolin Gol. Nei Mongol Zizhiqu, N China
14 L12 **Hull** Quebec, SE Canada
29 S12 **Hull** Iowa, C USA
Hull *see* Kingston upon Hull
Hull Island *see* Orona
99 F16 **Hulst** Zeeland, SW Netherlands
163 Q7 **Hulstay** Dornod, NE Mongolia
Hultschin *see* Hlučín
95 M19 **Hultsfred** Kalmar, S Sweden
Hulun *see* Hailar
Hu-lun Ch'ih *see* Hulun Nur
163 Q6 **Hulun Nur** *var.* Hu-lun Ch'ih; *prev.* Dalai Nor. ◎ NE China
Hulwan/Hulwân *see* Helwân
117 V8 **Hulyaypole** *Rus.* Gulyaypole. Zaporiz'ka Oblast', SE Ukraine
163 V4 **Huma** Heilongjiang, NE China
45 V6 **Humacao** E Puerto Rico
163 U4 **Huma He** ∽ NE China
62 J5 **Humahuaca** Jujuy, N Argentina
59 E14 **Humaitá** Amazonas, N Brazil
62 N7 **Humaitá** Ñeembucú, S Paraguay
83 H26 **Humansdorp** Eastern Cape, S South Africa
27 S6 **Humansville** Missouri, C USA
40 I8 **Humaya, Río** ∽ C Mexico
83 C16 **Humbe** Cunene, SW Angola
97 N17 **Humber** *estuary* E England, UK
97 N17 **Humberside** *cultural region* E England, UK
Humberto *see* Umberto
25 W11 **Humble** Texas, SW USA
11 U15 **Humboldt** Saskatchewan, S Canada
29 U12 **Humboldt** Iowa, C USA
27 Q6 **Humboldt** Kansas, C USA
29 S17 **Humboldt** Nebraska, C USA
35 S3 **Humboldt** Nevada, W USA
20 G9 **Humboldt** Tennessee, S USA
34 K3 **Humboldt Bay** *bay* California, W USA
35 S4 **Humboldt Lake** ◎ Nevada, W USA
35 S4 **Humboldt River** ∽ Nevada, W USA
35 T5 **Humboldt Salt Marsh** *wetland* Nevada, W USA
183 P11 **Hume, Lake** ◎ New South Wales/Victoria, SE Australia
111 N19 **Humenné** *Ger.* Homenau, *Hung.* Homonna. Prešovský Kraj, E Slovakia
29 V15 **Humeston** Iowa, C USA
54 J5 **Humocaro Bajo** Lara, N Venezuela
29 Q14 **Humphrey** Nebraska, C USA
35 S9 **Humphreys, Mount** ▲ California, W USA
36 L11 **Humphreys Peak** ▲ Arizona, SW USA
111 E17 **Humpolec** *Ger.* Gumpolds, Humpoletz. Jihlavský Kraj, C Czech Republic
Humpoletz *see* Humpolec
93 K19 **Humppila** Etelä-Suomi, S Finland
32 F8 **Humptulips** Washington, NW USA
42 H7 **Humuya, Río** ∽ W Honduras
75 P9 **Hūn** N Libya
Hunabasi *see* Funabashi
92 I1 **Húnaflói** *bay* NW Iceland
160 M11 **Hunan** *var.* Hunan Sheng, Xiang. ◈ *province* S China
Hunan Sheng *see* Hunan
163 Y10 **Hunchun** Jilin, NE China
95 I22 **Hundested** Frederiksborg, E Denmark
Hundred Mile House *see* 100 Mile House
116 G12 **Hunedoara** *Ger.* Eisenmarkt, *Hung.* Vajdahunyad. Hunedoara, SW Romania
116 G12 **Hunedoara** ◈ *county* W Romania
101 I17 **Hünfeld** Hessen, C Germany
111 H23 **Hungary** *off.* Republic of Hungary, *Ger.* Ungarn, *Hung.* Magyarország, *Rom.* Ungaria, *SCr.* Mađarska, *Ukr.* Uhorshchyna; *prev.* Hungarian People's Republic. ◆ *republic* C Europe
Hungary, Plain of *see* Great Hungarian Plain
162 F6 **Hungiy** Dzavhan, W Mongolia
163 X13 **Hŭngnam** E North Korea
33 P8 **Hungry Horse Reservoir** ⊡ Montana, NW USA
Hungt'ou *see* Lan Yü
Hung-tse Hu *see* Hongze Hu
167 T6 **Hưng Yên** Hai Hưng, N Vietnam
Hunjiang *see* Baishan
95 I18 **Hunnebostrand** Västra Götaland, S Sweden
101 E19 **Hunsrück** ▲ W Germany
97 P18 **Hunstanton** E England, UK
155 G20 **Hunsūr** Karnātaka, E India
162 I7 **Hunt** Arhangay, C Mongolia
100 G12 **Hunte** ∽ NW Germany
29 Q5 **Hunter** North Dakota, N USA
25 S11 **Hunter** Texas, SW USA
185 D20 **Hunter** ∽ South Island, NZ
183 N15 **Hunter Island** *island* Tasmania, SE Australia
18 K11 **Hunter Mountain** ▲ New York, NE USA
185 B23 **Hunter Mountains** ▲ South Island, NZ
183 S7 **Hunter River** ∽ New South Wales, SE Australia
32 L7 **Hunters** Washington, NW USA
185 F20 **Hunters Hills, The** *hill range* South Island, NZ
184 M12 **Hunterville** Manawatu-Wanganui, North Island, NZ
31 N16 **Huntingburg** Indiana, N USA
97 O20 **Huntingdon** E England, UK
18 E15 **Huntingdon** Pennsylvania, NE USA
20 G9 **Huntingdon** Tennessee, S USA
97 O20 **Huntingdonshire** *cultural region* C England, UK
31 P12 **Huntington** Indiana, N USA
32 L13 **Huntington** Oregon, NW USA
25 X9 **Huntington** Texas, SW USA
36 M5 **Huntington** Utah, W USA
21 P5 **Huntington** West Virginia, NE USA
35 T16 **Huntington Beach** California, W USA
35 W4 **Huntington Creek** ∽ Nevada, W USA
184 L7 **Huntly** Waikato, North Island, NZ
96 K8 **Huntly** NE Scotland, UK
10 K8 **Hunt, Mount** ▲ Yukon Territory, NW Canada
14 H12 **Huntsville** Ontario, S Canada
23 P2 **Huntsville** Alabama, S USA
27 S9 **Huntsville** Arkansas, C USA
27 U3 **Huntsville** Missouri, C USA
20 M8 **Huntsville** Tennessee, S USA
25 V10 **Huntsville** Texas, SW USA
36 L2 **Huntsville** Utah, W USA
41 W12 **Hunucmá** Yucatán, SE Mexico
149 W3 **Hunza** *var.* Karīmābād. Jammu and Kashmir, NE Pakistan
149 W3 **Hunza** ∽ NE Pakistan
Hunze *see* Oostermoers Vaart
158 H4 **Huocheng** *var.* Shuiding. Xinjiang Uygur Zizhiqu, NW China
161 N6 **Huojia** Henan, C China
Huolin Gol *see* Hulingol
186 N14 **Huon** *reef* N New Caledonia
186 E7 **Huon Peninsula** *headland* C PNG
Huoshao Dao *see* Lü Tao
Huoshao Tao *see* Lan Yü
Hupeh/Hupei *see* Hubei
Hurano *see* Furano
95 H14 **Hurdalssjøen** ◎ S Norway
14 E13 **Hurd, Cape** *headland* Ontario, S Canada
Hurdegaryp *see* Hardegarijp
29 N4 **Hurdsfield** North Dakota, N USA
162 J7 **Hüremt** Bulgan, C Mongolia
162 J8 **Hüremt** Övörhangay, C Mongolia
75 X9 **Hurghada** *var.* Al Ghurdaqah, Ghurdaqah. E Egypt
67 V9 **Huri Hills** ▲ NW Kenya
37 P15 **Hurley** New Mexico, SW USA
30 K4 **Hurley** Wisconsin, N USA
21 Y4 **Hurlock** Maryland, NE USA
29 P10 **Huron** South Dakota, N USA
31 S6 **Huron, Lake** ◎ Canada/USA
31 N3 **Huron Mountains** *hill range* Michigan, N USA
36 J8 **Hurricane** Utah, W USA
21 P5 **Hurricane** West Virginia, NE USA
36 J8 **Hurricane Cliffs** *cliff* Arizona, SW USA
23 V6 **Hurricane Creek** ∽ Georgia, SE USA
94 E12 **Hurrungane** ▲ S Norway
101 E16 **Hürth** Nordrhein-Westfalen, W Germany
Hurukawa *see* Furukawa
185 I17 **Hurunui** ∽ South Island, NZ
95 F21 **Hurup** Viborg, NW Denmark
117 T14 **Hurzuf** Respublika Krym, S Ukraine
Huş *see* Huşi
95 B19 **Húsavík** *Dan.* Husevig Faeroe Islands
92 K1 **Húsavík** Nordhurland Eystra, NE Iceland
116 M10 **Huşi** *var.* Huş. Vaslui, E Romania
95 L19 **Huskvarna** Jönköping, S Sweden
39 P8 **Huslia** Alaska, USA
Husn *see* Al Ḥuṣn
95 C15 **Husnes** Hordaland, S Norway
94 D8 **Hustadvika** *sea area* S Norway
Husté *see* Khust
100 H7 **Husum** Schleswig-Holstein, N Germany
93 I16 **Husum** Västernorrland, C Sweden
116 K6 **Husyatyn** Ternopil's'ka Oblast', W Ukraine
Huszt *see* Khust
162 K6 **Hutag** Bulgan, N Mongolia
26 M6 **Hutchinson** Kansas, C USA
29 U9 **Hutchinson** Minnesota, N USA
23 Y13 **Hutchinson Island** *island* Florida, SE USA
36 L11 **Hutch Mountain** ▲ Arizona, SW USA
141 O14 **Ḩūth** NW Yemen
186 I7 **Hutjena** Buka Island, NE PNG
109 T8 **Hüttenberg** Kärnten, S Austria
25 T10 **Hutto** Texas, SW USA
Huttu *see* Futtsu
108 E8 **Huttwil** Bern, W Switzerland
158 K5 **Hutubi** Xinjiang Uygur Zizhiqu, NW China
161 N4 **Hutuo He** ∽ C China
Hutyû *see* Fuchū
185 E20 **Huxley, Mount** ▲ South Island, NZ
99 J20 **Huy** *Dut.* Hoei, Hoey. Liège, E Belgium
161 R8 **Huzhou** *var.* Wuxing. Zhejiang, SE China
Huzi *see* Fuji
Huzieda *see* Fujieda
Huzinomiya *see* Fujinomiya
Huzisawa *see* Fujisawa
Huziyosida *see* Fuji-Yoshida
92 I2 **Hvammstangi** Nordhurland Vestra, N Iceland
92 K4 **Hvannadalshnúkur** ▲ S Iceland
113 E15 **Hvar** *It.* Lesina. Split-Dalmacija, S Croatia
113 F15 **Hvar** *It.* Lesina; *anc.* Pharus. *island* S Croatia
117 T13 **Hvardiys'ke** *Rus.* Gvardeyskoye. Respublika Krym, S Ukraine
92 I4 **Hveragerdhi** Sudhurland, SW Iceland
95 E22 **Hvide Sande** Ringkøbing, W Denmark
92 I3 **Hvítá** ∽ C Iceland
95 G15 **Hvittingfoss** Buskerud, S Norway
92 I4 **Hvolsvöllur** Sudhurland, SW Iceland
Hwach'ŏn-chŏsuji *see* P'aro-ho
Hwainan *see* Huainan
Hwalien *see* Hualien
83 I16 **Hwange** *prev.* Wankie. Matabeleland North, W Zimbabwe
Hwang-Hae *see* Yellow Sea
Hwangshih *see* Huangshi
83 L17 **Hwedza** Mashonaland East, E Zimbabwe
63 G20 **Hyades, Cerro** ▲ S Chile
19 Q12 **Hyannis** Massachusetts, NE USA
28 L13 **Hyannis** Nebraska, C USA
162 F6 **Hyargas Nuur** ◎ NW Mongolia
Hybla/Hybla Major *see* Paternò
39 Y14 **Hydaburg** Prince of Wales Island, Alaska, USA
185 F22 **Hyde** Otago, South Island, NZ
21 O7 **Hyden** Kentucky, S USA
18 K12 **Hyde Park** New York, NE USA
39 Z14 **Hyder** Alaska, USA
155 I15 **Hyderābād** *var.* Haidarabad. Andhra Pradesh, C India
149 Q16 **Hyderābād** *var.* Haidarabad. Sind, SE Pakistan
103 T16 **Hyères** Var, SE France
103 T16 **Hyères, Îles d'** *island group* S France
118 K12 **Hyermanavichy** *Rus.* Germanovichi. Vitsyebskaya Voblasts', N Belarus
163 X12 **Hyesan** NE North Korea
10 K8 **Hyland** ∽ Yukon Territory, NW Canada
95 K20 **Hyltebruk** Halland, S Sweden
18 D16 **Hyndman** Pennsylvania, NE USA
33 P14 **Hyndman Peak** ▲ Idaho, NW USA
164 I13 **Hyōgo** *off.* Hyōgo-ken. ◈ *prefecture* Honshū, SW Japan
Hypanis *see* Kuban'
Hypsas *see* Belice
Hyrcania *see* Gorgān
36 L1 **Hyrum** Utah, W USA
93 N14 **Hyrynsalmi** Oulu, C Finland
33 V10 **Hysham** Montana, NW USA
11 N13 **Hythe** Alberta, W Canada
97 Q23 **Hythe** SE England, UK
164 D15 **Hyūga** Miyazaki, Kyūshū, SW Japan
Hyvinge *see* Hyvinkää
93 L19 **Hyvinkää** *Swe.* Hyvinge. Etelä-Suomi, S Finland

I

118 J9 **Iacobeni** *Ger.* Jakobeny. Suceava, NE Romania
Iader *see* Zadar
172 I7 **Iakora** Fianarantsoa, SE Madagascar
116 K14 **Ialomița** *var.* Jalomitsa. ◈ *county* SE Romania
116 K14 **Ialomița** ∽ SE Romania
117 N10 **Ialoveni** *Rus.* Yaloveny. C Moldova
117 N11 **Ialpug** *var.* Ialpugul Mare, *Rus.* Yalpug. ∽ Moldova/Ukraine
Ialpugul Mare *see* Ialpug
23 T8 **Iamonia, Lake** ◎ Florida, SE USA
116 L13 **Ianca** Brăila, SE Romania
116 M10 **Iaşi** *Ger.* Jassy. Iaşi, NE Romania
116 L9 **Iaşi** *Ger.* Jassy, Yassy. ◈ *county* NE Romania
114 J13 **Íasmos** Anatolikí Makedonía kai Thráki, NE Greece
22 H6 **Iatt, Lake** ⊡ Louisiana, S USA
58 B11 **Iauaretê** Amazonas, NW Brazil
171 N3 **Iba** Luzon, N Philippines
77 S16 **Ibadan** Oyo, SW Nigeria
54 E10 **Ibagué** Tolima, C Colombia
60 J10 **Ibaiti** Paraná, S Brazil
36 J4 **Ibapah Peak** ▲ Utah, W USA
113 M15 **Ibar** *Alb.* Ibër. ∽ C Yugoslavia
165 P13 **Ibaraki** *off.* Ibaraki-ken. ◈ *prefecture* Honshū, S Japan
56 C5 **Ibarra** *var.* San Miguel de Ibarra. Imbabura, N Ecuador
Ibaşfalău *see* Dumbrăveni
141 O16 **Ibb** W Yemen
100 F13 **Ibbenbüren** Nordrhein-Westfalen, NW Germany
79 H16 **Ibenga** ∽ N Congo
Ibër *see* Ibar
57 I14 **Iberia** Madre de Dios, E Peru
Iberia *see* Spain
66 M1 **Iberian Basin** *undersea feature* E Atlantic Ocean
Iberian Mountains *see* Ibérico, Sistema
84 D12 **Iberian Peninsula** *physical region* Portugal/Spain

◆ Country ◇ Dependent Territory ◈ Administrative Region ▲ Mountain ☒ Volcano ◎ Lake
● Country Capital ○ Dependent Territory Capital ✕ International Airport ▲ Mountain Range ∽ River ⊡ Reservoir

64 M8 **Iberian Plain** undersea feature E Atlantic Ocean
Ibérica, Cordillera see Ibérico, Sistema
105 P6 **Ibérico, Sistema** var. Cordillera Ibérica, Eng. Iberian Mountains. ▲ NE Spain
12 K7 **Iberville Lac d'** ◎ Quebec, NE Canada
77 T14 **Ibeto** Niger, W Nigeria
77 W15 **Ibi** Taraba, C Nigeria
105 S11 **Ibi** País Valenciano, E Spain
59 L20 **Ibiá** Minas Gerais, SE Brazil
61 F15 **Ibicuí, Rio** ≈ S Brazil
61 C19 **Ibicuy** Entre Ríos, E Argentina
61 F16 **Ibirapuitã** ≈ S Brazil
Ibiza see Eivissa
138 J4 **Ibn Wardān, Qaṣr** ruins Ḥamāh, C Syria
Ibo see Sassandra
188 E9 **Ibobang** Babeldaob, N Palau
171 V13 **Ibonma** Irian Jaya, E Indonesia
59 N17 **Ibotirama** Bahia, E Brazil
141 Y8 **Ibrā** NE Oman
129 Q4 **Ibresi** Chuvashskaya Respublika, W Russian Federation
141 X8 **'Ibrī** NW Oman
164 C16 **Ibusuki** Kagoshima, Kyūshū, SW Japan
57 E16 **Ica** Ica, SW Peru
57 E16 **Ica** off. Departamento de Ica. ◈ department SW Peru
58 C11 **Içana** Amazonas, NW Brazil
Icaria see Ikaría
58 B13 **Içá, Rio** var. Río Putumayo. ≈ NW South America see also Putumayo, Río
136 I17 **İçel** var. Ichili. ◈ province S Turkey
92 I3 **Iceland** off. Republic of Iceland, Dan. Island, Icel. Ísland. ◆ republic N Atlantic Ocean
86 B7 **Iceland** island N Atlantic Ocean
64 L5 **Iceland Basin** undersea feature N Atlantic Ocean
Icelandic Plateau see Iceland Plateau
197 Q15 **Iceland Plateau** var. Icelandic Plateau. undersea feature S Greenland Sea
155 E16 **Ichalkaranji** Mahārāshtra, W India
164 D15 **Ichifusa-yama** ▲ Kyūshū, SW Japan
Ichili see İçel
164 K13 **Ichinomiya** var. Itinomiya. Aichi, Honshū, SW Japan
165 Q9 **Ichinoseki** var. Itinoseki. Iwate, Honshū, C Japan
117 R3 **Ichnya** Chernihivs'ka Oblast', NE Ukraine
57 L17 **Ichoa, Río** ≈ C Bolivia
I-ch'un see Yichun
Iconium see Konya
Iculisma see Angoulême
39 U12 **Icy Bay** inlet Alaska, USA
39 N5 **Icy Cape** headland Alaska, USA
39 W13 **Icy Strait** strait Alaska, USA
27 R13 **Idabel** Oklahoma, C USA
29 T13 **Ida Grove** Iowa, C USA
77 U16 **Idah** Kogi, S Nigeria
33 N13 **Idaho** off. State of Idaho; also known as Gem of the Mountains, Gem State. ◈ state NW USA
33 N14 **Idaho City** Idaho, NW USA
33 R14 **Idaho Falls** Idaho, NW USA
121 P2 **Idálion** var. Dali, Dhali. C Cyprus
25 N5 **Idalou** Texas, SW USA
104 I9 **Idanha-a-Nova** Castelo Branco, C Portugal
101 E19 **Idar-Oberstein** Rheinland-Pfalz, SW Germany
118 J3 **Ida-Virumaa** off. Ida-Viru Maakond. ◈ province NE Estonia
126 J8 **Idel'** Respublika Kareliya, NW Russian Federation
79 C15 **Idenao** Sud-Ouest, SW Cameroon
Idenburg-rivier see Taritatu, Sungai
Idensalmi see Iisalmi
162 I6 **Ider** Hövsgöl, C Mongolia
75 X10 **Idfu** var. Edfu. SE Egypt
Ídhi Óros see Ídi
Ídhra see Ýdra
168 H7 **Idi** Sumatera, W Indonesia
115 I25 **Ídi** var. Ídhi Óros. ▲ Kríti, Greece, E Mediterranean Sea
Idi Amin, Lac see Edward, Lake
106 G10 **Idice** ≈ N Italy
76 G9 **Idini** Trarza, W Mauritania
79 J21 **Idiofa** Bandundu, SW Dem. Rep. Congo (Zaire)
39 O10 **Iditarod River** ≈ Alaska, USA
95 M14 **Idkerberget** Dalarna, C Sweden
138 I3 **Idlib** Idlib, NW Syria
138 I4 **Idlib** off. Muḥāfaẓat Idlib. ◈ governorate NW Syria
Idra see Ýdra
94 J11 **Idre** Dalarna, C Sweden
Idria see Idrija
109 S11 **Idrija** It. Idria. W Slovenia
101 G18 **Idstein** Hessen, W Germany
83 J25 **Idutywa** Eastern Cape, SE South Africa
Idzhevan see Ijevan
118 G9 **Iecava** Bauska, S Latvia
165 T16 **Ie-jima** var. Ii-shima. island Nansei-shotō, SW Japan
99 B18 **Ieper** Fr. Ypres. West-Vlaanderen, W Belgium
115 K25 **Ierápetra** Kríti, Greece, E Mediterranean Sea
115 G22 **Iérax, Akrotírio** headland S Greece
Ierisós see Ierissós
115 H14 **Ierissós** var. Ierisós. Kentrikí Makedonía, N Greece
116 I11 **Iernut** Hung. Radnót. Mureş, C Romania
106 J12 **Iesi** var. Jesi. Marche, C Italy
92 K9 **Iešjávri** var. Jiesjavrre. ◎ N Norway
Iesolo see Jesolo
188 K16 **Ifalik Atoll** atoll Caroline Islands, C Micronesia
172 I6 **Ifanadiana** Fianarantsoa, SE Madagascar
77 T16 **Ife** Osun, SW Nigeria
77 V8 **Iferouâne** Agadez, N Niger
Iferten see Yverdon
92 L8 **Ifjord** Finnmark, N Norway
77 R8 **Ifôghas, Adrar des** var. Adrar des Iforas. ▲ NE Mali
Iforas, Adrar des see Ifôghas, Adrar des
182 D6 **Ifould lake** salt lake South Australia
74 G6 **Ifrane** C Morocco
171 S11 **Iga** Pulau Halmahera, E Indonesia
81 G18 **Iganga** SE Uganda
60 L7 **Igarapava** São Paulo, S Brazil
122 K9 **Igarka** Krasnoyarskiy Kray, N Russian Federation
Igaunija see Estonia
I.G.Duca see General Toshevo
Igel see Jihlava
137 T12 **Iğdır** ◈ province E Turkey
94 N11 **Iggesund** Gävleborg, C Sweden
39 P7 **Igikpak, Mount** ▲ Alaska, USA
39 P13 **Igiugig** Alaska, USA
Iglau/Iglawa/Igława see Jihlava
107 B20 **Iglesias** Sardegna, Italy, C Mediterranean Sea
129 V4 **Iglino** Respublika Bashkortostan, W Russian Federation
Igló see Spišská Nová Ves
9 O6 **Igloolik** Nunavut, N Canada
12 B11 **Ignace** Ontario, S Canada
118 I12 **Ignalina** Ignalina, E Lithuania
129 Q5 **Ignatovka** Ul'yanovskaya Oblast', W Russian Federation
126 K12 **Ignatovo** Vologodskaya Oblast', NW Russian Federation
114 N11 **İğneada** Kırklareli, NW Turkey
121 S7 **İğneada Burnu** headland NW Turkey
Igombe see Gombe
115 B16 **Igoumenítsa** Ípeiros, W Greece
129 T2 **Igra** Udmurtskaya Respublika, NW Russian Federation
122 H9 **Igrim** Khanty-Mansiyskiy Avtonomnyy Okrug, N Russian Federation
60 G12 **Iguaçu, Rio** Sp. Río Iguazú. ≈ Argentina/Brazil see also Iguazú, Río
59 I22 **Iguaçu, Salto do** Sp. Cataratas del Iguazú; prev. Victoria Falls. waterfall Argentina/Brazil see also Iguazú, Cataratas del
41 O15 **Iguala** var. Iguala de la Independencia. Guerrero, S Mexico
105 V5 **Igualada** Cataluña, NE Spain
Iguala de la Independencia see Iguala
60 G12 **Iguazú, Cataratas del** Port. Salto do Iguaçu, prev. Victoria Falls. waterfall Argentina/Brazil see also Iguaçu, Salto do
62 Q6 **Iguazú, Río** Port. Rio Iguaçu. ≈ Argentina/Brazil see also Iguaçu, Rio
79 D19 **Iguéla** Ogooué-Maritime, SW Gabon
Iguid, Erg see Iguîdi, 'Erg
67 M5 **Iguîdi, 'Erg** var. Erg Iguid. desert Algeria/Mauritania
172 K2 **Iharaña** prev. Vohémar. Antsiranana, NE Madagascar
151 K18 **Ihavandippolhu Atoll** var. Ihavandiffulu Atoll. atoll N Maldives
162 M11 **Ih Bulag** Ömnögovĭ, S Mongolia
165 T16 **Iheya-jima** island Nansei-shotō, SW Japan
162 L8 **Ihhayrhan** Töv, C Mongolia
172 I6 **Ihosy** Fianarantsoa, S Madagascar
162 L7 **Ihsüüj** Töv, C Mongolia
93 L14 **Ii** Oulu, C Finland
164 M13 **Iida** Nagano, Honshū, S Japan
93 M14 **Iijoki** ≈ C Finland
118 J4 **Iisaku** Ger. Isaak. Ida-Virumaa, NE Estonia
93 M16 **Iisalmi** var. Idensalmi. Itä-Suomi, C Finland
165 N11 **Iiyama** Nagano, Honshū, S Japan
77 S16 **Ijebu-Ode** Ogun, SW Nigeria
137 U11 **Ijevan** Rus. Idzhevan. N Armenia
98 H9 **IJmuiden** Noord-Holland, W Netherlands
98 M12 **IJssel** var. Yssel. ≈ Netherlands/Germany
98 J8 **IJsselmeer** prev. Zuider Zee. ◎ N Netherlands
98 L9 **IJsselmuiden** Overijssel, E Netherlands
98 I12 **IJsselstein** Utrecht, C Netherlands
61 G14 **Ijuí** Rio Grande do Sul, S Brazil
61 G14 **Ijuí, Rio** ≈ S Brazil
189 R8 **Ijuw** NE Nauru
99 E16 **IJzendijke** Zeeland, SW Netherlands
99 A18 **Ijzer** ≈ W Belgium
93 K18 **Ikaalinen** Länsi-Suomi, W Finland
172 I6 **Ikalamavony** Fianarantsoa, SE Madagascar
185 G16 **Ikamatua** West Coast, South Island, NZ
77 U16 **Ikare** Ondo, SW Nigeria
115 L20 **Ikaría** var. Kariot, Nicaria, Nikaria; anc. Icaria. island Dodekánisos, Greece, Aegean Sea
95 F22 **Ikast** Ringkøbing, W Denmark
184 O9 **Ikawhenua Range** ▲ North Island, NZ
165 U4 **Ikeda** Hokkaidō, NE Japan
164 H14 **Ikeda** Tokushima, Shikoku, SW Japan
77 S16 **Ikeja** Lagos, SW Nigeria
79 L19 **Ikela** Equateur, C Dem. Rep. Congo (Zaire)
114 H10 **Ikhtiman** Sofiya, W Bulgaria
164 C13 **Iki** island SW Japan
129 O13 **Iki Burul** Respublika Kalmykiya, SW Russian Federation
137 P11 **İkizdere** Rize, NE Turkey
39 P14 **Ikolik, Cape** headland Kodiak Island, Alaska, USA
77 V17 **Ikom** Cross River, SE Nigeria
172 I6 **Ikongo** prev. Fort-Carnot. Fianarantsoa, SE Madagascar
39 P5 **Ikpikpuk River** ≈ Alaska, USA
190 H1 **Iku** prev. Lone Tree Islet. atoll Tungaru, W Kiribati
164 I12 **Ikuno** Hyōgo, Honshū, SW Japan
190 H16 **Ikurangi** ▲ Rarotonga, S Cook Islands
171 X14 **Ilaga** Irian Jaya, E Indonesia
171 O2 **Ilagan** Luzon, N Philippines
153 R12 **Ilam** Eastern, E Nepal
142 J7 **Īlām** var. Elam. Īlām, W Iran
142 J8 **Īlām** off. Ostān-e Īlām. ◈ province W Iran
161 T13 **Ilan** Jap. Giran. N Taiwan
146 G11 **Ilanly Obvodnitel'nyy Kanal** canal N Turkmenistan
122 L12 **Ilanskiy** Krasnoyarskiy Kray, S Russian Federation
108 H9 **Ilanz** Graubünden, S Switzerland
77 S16 **Ilaro** Ogun, SW Nigeria
57 I17 **Ilave** Puno, S Peru
110 K8 **Iława** Ger. Deutsch-Eylau. Warmińsko-Mazurskie, NE Poland
123 P10 **Il'benge** Respublika Sakha (Yakutiya), NE Russian Federation
Ile see Ili
11 S13 **Île-à-la-Crosse** Saskatchewan, C Canada
79 J21 **Ilebo** prev. Port-Francqui. Kasai Occidental, W Dem. Rep. Congo (Zaire)
103 N5 **Île-de-France** ◈ region N France
144 I9 **Ilek** Kaz. Elek. ≈ Kazakhstan/Russian Federation
Ilerda see Lleida
77 T16 **Ilesha** Osun, SW Nigeria
187 Q16 **Îles Loyauté, Province des** ◈ province E New Caledonia
11 X12 **Ilford** Manitoba, C Canada
97 I23 **Ilfracombe** SW England, UK
136 I11 **Ilgaz Dağları** ▲ N Turkey
136 G15 **Ilgın** Konya, W Turkey
60 I7 **Ilha Solteira** São Paulo, S Brazil
104 G7 **Ílhavo** Aveiro, N Portugal
59 O18 **Ilhéus** Bahia, E Brazil
131 R7 **Ili** Kaz. Ile, Rus. Reka Ili. ≈ China/Kazakhstan
Ili see Ili He
116 G11 **Ilia** Hung. Marosillye. Hunedoara, SW Romania
39 P13 **Iliamna** Alaska, USA
39 P13 **Iliamna Lake** ◎ Alaska, USA
137 N13 **İliç** Erzincan, C Turkey
Il'ichevsk see Şărur, Azerbaijan
Il'ichevsk see Illichivs'k, Ukraine
Ilici see Elche
37 V2 **Iliff** Colorado, C USA
171 Q7 **Iligan** off. Iligan City. Mindanao, S Philippines
171 Q7 **Iligan Bay** bay S Philippines
158 I5 **Ili He** Rus. Ili. ≈ China/Kazakhstan
56 C6 **Iliniza** ▲ N Ecuador
Ilinski see Il'inskiy
127 U14 **Il'inskiy** Permskaya Oblast', NW Russian Federation
123 T13 **Il'inskiy** Ostrov Sakhalin, Sakhalinskaya Oblast', SE Russian Federation
18 I10 **Ilion** New York, NE USA
38 E9 **Ilio Point** headland Molokai, Hawaii, USA, C Pacific Ocean
109 T13 **Ilirska Bistrica** prev. Bistrica, Ger. Feistritz, Illyrisch-Feistritz, It. Villa del Nevoso. SW Slovenia
137 Q16 **Ilısu Barajı** ▣ SE Turkey
155 G17 **Ilkal** Karnātaka, C India
97 M19 **Ilkeston** C England, UK
121 O16 **Il-Kullana** headland SW Malta
108 J8 **Ill** ≈ W Austria
103 U6 **Ill** ≈ NE France
62 G10 **Illapel** Coquimbo, C Chile
Illaue Fartak Trench see Alula-Fartak Trench
182 C2 **Illbillee, Mount** ▲ South Australia
102 I6 **Ille-et-Vilaine** ◈ department NW France
77 T11 **Illéla** Tahoua, SW Niger
101 J24 **Iller** ≈ S Germany
101 J23 **Illertissen** Bayern, S Germany
105 N8 **Illescas** Castilla-La Mancha, C Spain
Ille-sur-la-Têt see Ille-sur-Têt
103 O17 **Ille-sur-Têt** var. Ille-sur-la-Têt. Pyrénées-Orientales, S France
Illiberis see Elne
117 P11 **Illichivs'k** Rus. Il'ichevsk. Odes'ka Oblast', SW Ukraine
Illicis see Elche
102 M6 **Illiers-Combray** Eure-et-Loir, C France
30 K12 **Illinois** off. State of Illinois; also known as Prairie State, Sucker State. ◈ state C USA
30 J13 **Illinois River** ≈ Illinois, N USA
117 N6 **Illintsi** Vinnyts'ka Oblast', C Ukraine
Illiturgis see Andújar
74 M10 **Illizi** SE Algeria
27 Y7 **Illmo** Missouri, C USA
Illur co see Lorca
Illuro see Mataró
Illyrisch-Feistritz see Ilirska Bistrica
101 K16 **Ilm** ≈ C Germany
101 K17 **Ilmenau** Thüringen, C Germany
126 H14 **Il'men', Ozero** ◎ NW Russian Federation
57 H18 **Ilo** Moquegua, SW Peru
171 O6 **Iloilo** off. Iloilo City. Panay Island, C Philippines
112 K10 **Ilok** Hung. Újlak. Serbia, NW Yugoslavia
93 O16 **Ilomantsi** Itä-Suomi, E Finland
42 F8 **Ilopango, Lago de** volcanic lake C El Salvador
77 T15 **Ilorin** Kwara, W Nigeria
117 X8 **Ilovays'k** Rus. Ilovaysk. Donets'ka Oblast', SE Ukraine
129 O10 **Ilovlya** Volgogradskaya Oblast', SW Russian Federation
129 O10 **Ilovlya** ≈ SW Russian Federation
123 V8 **Il'pyrskiy** Koryakskiy Avtonomnyy Okrug, E Russian Federation
128 K14 **Il'skiy** Krasnodarskiy Kray, SW Russian Federation
182 B2 **Iltur** South Australia
171 Y13 **Ilugwa** Irian Jaya, E Indonesia
Iluh see Batman
118 I11 **Ilūkste** Daugavpils, SE Latvia
171 U14 **Ilur** Pulau Gorong, E Indonesia
32 F10 **Ilwaco** Washington, NW USA
146 H8 **Il'yaly** var. Yylanly. Dashkhovuzskiy Velayat, N Turkmenistan
Ilyasbaba Burnu see Tekke Burnu
127 U9 **Ilych** ≈ NW Russian Federation
101 O21 **Ilz** ≈ SE Germany
111 M14 **Iłża** Radom, SE Poland
164 G13 **Imabari** var. Imaharu. Ehime, Shikoku, SW Japan
Imaharu see Imabari
165 O12 **Imaichi** var. Imaiti. Tochigi, Honshū, S Japan
Imaiti see Imaichi
164 K12 **Imajō** Fukui, Honshū, SW Japan
139 R9 **Imām Ibn Hāshim** C Iraq
139 T11 **Imān 'Abd Allāh** S Iraq
126 J4 **Imandra, Ozero** ◎ NW Russian Federation
164 F15 **Imano-yama** ▲ Shikoku, SW Japan
164 C13 **Imari** Saga, Kyūshū, SW Japan
Imarssuak Mid-Ocean Seachannel see Imarssuak Seachannel
64 J6 **Imarssuak Seachannel** var. Imarssuak Mid-Ocean Seachannel. channel N Atlantic Ocean
93 N18 **Imatra** Etelä-Suomi, S Finland
164 K13 **Imazu** Shiga, Honshū, SW Japan
56 C6 **Imbabura** ◈ province N Ecuador
55 R9 **Imbaimadai** W Guyana
61 K14 **Imbituba** Santa Catarina, S Brazil
27 W9 **Imboden** Arkansas, C USA
Imbros see Gökçeada
146 B11 **Imeni 26 Bakinskikh Komissarov** Turkm. 26 Baku Komissarlary Adyndaky. Balkanskiy Velayat, W Turkmenistan
Imeni 26 Bakinskikh Komissarov see 26 Bakı Komissarı
127 N13 **Imeni Babushkina** Vologodskaya Oblast', NW Russian Federation
128 J7 **Imeni Karla Libknekhta** Kurskaya Oblast', W Russian Federation
146 I14 **Imeni Mollanepesa** Maryyskiy Velayat, S Turkmenistan
146 J15 **Imeni S.A.Niyazova** Maryyskiy Velayat, S Turkmenistan
Imeni Sverdlova Rudnik see Sverdlovs'k
188 E9 **Imeong** Babeldaob, N Palau
81 L14 **Īmī** Somali, E Ethiopia
115 M21 **Imia** Turk. Kardak. island Dodekánisos, Greece, Aegean Sea
Imishli see İmişli
137 X12 **İmişli** Rus. Imishli. C Azerbaijan
163 X14 **Imjin-gang** ≈ North Korea/South Korea
35 S3 **Imlay** Nevada, W USA
31 S9 **Imlay City** Michigan, N USA
23 X15 **Immokalee** Florida, SE USA
77 U17 **Imo** ◈ state SE Nigeria
106 G10 **Imola** Emilia-Romagna, N Italy
186 A5 **Imonda** Sandaun, NW PNG
Imoschi see Imotski
113 G14 **Imotski** It. Imoschi. Split-Dalmacija, SE Croatia
59 L14 **Imperatriz** Maranhão, NE Brazil
106 B10 **Imperia** Liguria, NW Italy
57 E15 **Imperial** Lima, W Peru
35 X17 **Imperial** California, W USA
28 L16 **Imperial** Nebraska, C USA
24 M9 **Imperial** Texas, SW USA
35 Y17 **Imperial Dam** dam California, W USA
79 I17 **Impfondo** La Likouala, NE Congo
153 X14 **Imphāl** Manipur, NE India
103 P9 **Imphy** Nièvre, C France
106 G11 **Impruneta** Toscana, C Italy
115 K15 **İmroz** var. Gökçeada. Çanakkale, NW Turkey
Imroz Adası see Gökçeada
108 L7 **Imst** Tirol, W Austria
40 F3 **Imuris** Sonora, NW Mexico
164 M13 **Ina** Nagano, Honshū, S Japan
65 M18 **Inaccessible Island** island W Tristan da Cunha
115 F20 **Ínachos** ≈ S Greece
188 H6 **I Naftan, Puntan** headland Saipan, S Northern Mariana Islands
Inagua Islands see Great Inagua/Little Inagua
185 H15 **Inangahua** West Coast, South Island, NZ
57 I14 **Iñapari** Madre de Dios, E Peru
188 B17 **Inarajan** SE Guam
92 L10 **Inari** Lapp. Anár, Aanaar. Lappi, N Finland
92 L10 **Inarijärvi** Lapp. Aanaarjävri, Swe. Enareträsk. ◎ N Finland
92 L9 **Inarijoki** Lapp. Anárjohka. ≈ Finland/Norway
Inău see Ineu
165 P11 **Inawashiro-ko** var. Inawasiro Ko. ◎ Honshū, C Japan
Inawasiro Ko see Inawashiro-ko
62 H7 **Inca de Oro** Atacama, N Chile
115 J15 **İnce Burnu** headland NW Turkey
136 K9 **İnce Burnu** headland N Turkey
136 I17 **İncekum Burnu** headland S Turkey
76 G7 **Inchiri** ◈ region NW Mauritania
163 X15 **Inch'ŏn** off. Inch'ŏn-gwangyŏksi, Jap. Jinsen; prev. Chemulpo. NW South Korea
83 M17 **Inchope** Manica, C Mozambique
Incoronata see Kornat
103 Y15 **Incudine, Monte** ▲ Corse, France, C Mediterranean Sea
60 M10 **Indaiatuba** São Paulo, S Brazil
93 H17 **Indal** Västernorrland, C Sweden
93 H17 **Indalsälven** ≈ C Sweden
40 K8 **Inde** Durango, C Mexico
Indefatigable Island see Santa Cruz, Isla
35 S10 **Independence** California, W USA
29 X13 **Independence** Iowa, C USA
27 P7 **Independence** Kansas, C USA
20 M4 **Independence** Kentucky, S USA
27 R4 **Independence** Missouri, C USA
21 R8 **Independence** Virginia, NE USA
30 J7 **Independence** Wisconsin, N USA
197 R12 **Independence Fjord** fjord N Greenland
Independence Island see Malden Island
35 W2 **Independence Mountains** ▲ Nevada, W USA
57 K18 **Independencia** Cochabamba, C Bolivia
57 E16 **Independencia, Bahía de la** bay W Peru
Independencia, Monte see Adam, Mount
116 M12 **Independenţa** Galaţi, SE Romania
Inderagiri see Indragiri, Sungai
Inderbor see Inderborskiy
144 F11 **Inderborskiy** Kaz. Inderbor. Atyrau, W Kazakhstan
151 I14 **India** off. Republic of India, var. Indian Union, Union of India, Hind. Bhārat. ◆ republic S Asia
India see Inđija
18 D14 **Indiana** Pennsylvania, NE USA
31 N13 **Indiana** off. State of Indiana; also known as The Hoosier State. ◈ state N USA
31 O14 **Indianapolis** state capital Indiana, N USA
11 O10 **Indian Cabins** Alberta, W Canada
42 G1 **Indian Church** Orange Walk, N Belize
Indian Desert see Thar Desert
11 U16 **Indian Head** Saskatchewan, S Canada
31 O4 **Indian Lake** ◎ Michigan, N USA
18 K9 **Indian Lake** ◎ New York, NE USA
31 R13 **Indian Lake** ▣ Ohio, N USA
180-181 **Indian Ocean** ocean
29 V15 **Indianola** Iowa, C USA
22 K4 **Indianola** Mississippi, S USA
36 J6 **Indian Peak** ▲ Utah, W USA
23 Y13 **Indian River** lagoon Florida, SE USA
35 W10 **Indian Springs** Nevada, W USA
23 Y14 **Indiantown** Florida, SE USA
59 K19 **Indiara** Goiás, S Brazil
127 Q4 **Indiga** Nenetskiy Avtonomnyy Okrug, NW Russian Federation
123 R9 **Indigirka** ≈ NE Russian Federation
112 L10 **Inđija** Hung. India; prev. Indjija. Serbia, N Yugoslavia
35 V16 **Indio** California, W USA
42 M12 **Indio, Río** ≈ SE Nicaragua
152 I10 **Indira Gandhi International** ✕ (Delhi) Delhi, N India
151 Q23 **Indira Point** headland Andaman and Nicobar Islands, India, NE Indian Ocean
Indjija see Inđija
131 Q13 **Indo-Australian Plate** tectonic feature
173 N11 **Indomed Fracture Zone** tectonic feature SW Indian Ocean
170 L12 **Indonesia** off. Republic of Indonesia, Ind. Republik Indonesia; prev. Dutch East Indies, Netherlands East Indies, United States of Indonesia. ◆ republic SE Asia
Indonesian Borneo see Kalimantan
154 G10 **Indore** Madhya Pradesh, C India
168 L11 **Indragiri, Sungai** var. Batang Kuantan, Inderagiri. ≈ Sumatera, W Indonesia
Indramajoe/Indramaju see Indramayu
169 P15 **Indramayu** prev. Indramajoe, Indramaju. Jawa, C Indonesia
155 K14 **Indrāvati** ≈ S India
103 N9 **Indre** ◈ department C France
102 M8 **Indre** ≈ C France
102 L8 **Indre-et-Loire** ◈ department C France
Indreville see Châteauroux
152 G3 **Indus** Chin. Yindu He; prev. Yin-tu Ho. ≈ S Asia
Indus Cone see Indus Fan
173 P3 **Indus Fan** var. Indus Cone. undersea feature N Arabian Sea
149 P17 **Indus, Mouths of the** delta S Pakistan
83 I24 **Indwe** Eastern Cape, SE South Africa
136 I10 **İnebolu** Kastamonu, N Turkey
77 P8 **I-n-Échaï** oasis C Mali
114 M13 **İnecik** Tekirdağ, NW Turkey
136 E12 **İnegöl** Bursa, NW Turkey
Inessa see Biancavilla
116 F10 **Ineu** Hung. Borosjenő; prev. Inău. Arad, W Romania
Ineul/Ineu, Vârful see Ineu, Vârful
116 J9 **Ineu, Vârful** var. Ineul; prev. Vîrful Ineu. ▲ N Romania
21 P6 **Inez** Kentucky, S USA
74 E8 **Inezgane** ✕ (Agadir) W Morocco
41 T17 **Inferior, Laguna** lagoon S Mexico
40 M15 **Infiernillo, Presa del** ▣ S Mexico
104 L2 **Infiesto** Asturias, N Spain
93 L20 **Ingå** Fin. Inkoo. Etelä-Suomi, S Finland
77 U10 **Ingal** var. I-n-Gall. Agadez, C Niger
I-n-Gall see Ingal
99 C18 **Ingelmunster** West-Vlaanderen, W Belgium
79 I18 **Ingende** Equateur, W Dem. Rep. Congo (Zaire)
62 L5 **Ingeniero Guillermo Nueva Juárez** Formosa, N Argentina
63 H16 **Ingeniero Jacobacci** Río Negro, C Argentina
14 F16 **Ingersoll** Ontario, S Canada
162 K6 **Ingettolgoy** Bulgan, N Mongolia
181 W5 **Ingham** Queensland, NE Australia
146 M11 **Ingichka** Samarqand Wiloyati, C Uzbekistan
97 L16 **Ingleborough** ▲ N England, UK
25 T14 **Ingleside** Texas, SW USA
184 K10 **Inglewood** Taranaki, North Island, NZ
35 S15 **Inglewood** California, W USA
101 L21 **Ingolstadt** Bayern, S Germany
33 V9 **Ingomar** Montana, NW USA
13 R14 **Ingonish Beach** Cape Breton Island, Nova Scotia, SE Canada
153 S14 **Ingrāj Bāzār** prev. English Bazar. West Bengal, NE India
25 Q11 **Ingram** Texas, SW USA
195 X7 **Ingrid Christensen Coast** physical region Antarctica
74 K14 **I-n-Guezzam** S Algeria
Ingulets see Inhulets'
Inguri see Enguri
Ingushetia/Ingushetiya, Respublika see Ingushskaya Respublika
129 O15 **Ingushskaya Respublika** var. Respublika Ingushetiya, Eng. Ingushetia. ◈ autonomous republic SW Russian Federation
83 N20 **Inhambane** Inhambane, SE Mozambique
83 M20 **Inhambane** off. Província de Inhambane. ◈ province S Mozambique
83 N17 **Inhaminga** Sofala, C Mozambique
83 N20 **Inharrime** Inhambane, SE Mozambique
83 M18 **Inhassoro** Inhambane, E Mozambique
117 S9 **Inhulets'** Rus. Ingulets. Dnipropetrovs'ka Oblast', E Ukraine
117 R10 **Inhulets'** Rus. Ingulets. ≈ S Ukraine
105 Q10 **Iniesta** Castilla-La Mancha, C Spain
I-ning see Yining
54 K11 **Inírida, Río** ≈ E Colombia
Inis see Ennis
Inis Ceithleann see Enniskillen
Inis Córthaidh see Enniscorthy
Inis Díomáin see Ennistimon
97 A17 **Inishbofin** Ir. Inis Bó Finne. island W Ireland
97 B18 **Inisheer** var. Inishere, Ir. Inis Oírr. island W Ireland
Inishere see Inisheer
97 B18 **Inishmaan** Ir. Inis Meáin. island W Ireland
97 A18 **Inishmore** Ir. Árainn. island W Ireland
96 E13 **Inishtrahull** Ir. Inis Trá Tholl. island NW Ireland
97 A17 **Inishturk** Ir. Inis Toirc. island W Ireland
Inkoo see Ingå
185 J16 **Inland Kaikoura Range** ▲ South Island, NZ
Inland Sea see Seto-naikai
21 P11 **Inman** South Carolina, SE USA
108 L7 **Inn** ≈ C Europe
197 O11 **Innaanganeq** var. Kap York. headland NW Greenland
182 K2 **Innamincka** South Australia
94 I12 **Innbygda** ≈ Hedmark, S Norway
92 G12 **Inndyr** Nordland, C Norway
42 G3 **Inner Channel** inlet SE Belize
96 F11 **Inner Hebrides** island group W Scotland, UK
172 H15 **Inner Islands** var. Central Group. island group NE Seychelles
Inner Mongolia/Inner Mongolian Autonomous Region see Nei Mongol Zizhiqu
96 G8 **Inner Sound** strait NW Scotland, UK
100 J13 **Innerste** ≈ C Germany
181 W5 **Innisfail** Queensland, NE Australia
11 Q15 **Innisfail** Alberta, SW Canada
Inniskilling see Enniskillen

39 O11 **Innoko River** ≈ Alaska, USA
Innosima see Innoshima
Innsbruch see Innsbruck
108 M7 **Innsbruck** var. Innsbruch. Tirol, W Austria
79 I19 **Inongo** Bandundu, W Dem. Rep. Congo (Zaire)
Inoucdjouac see Inukjuak
Inowrazlaw see Inowrocław
110 I10 **Inowrocław** Ger. Hohensalza; prev. Inowrazlaw. Kujawski-pomorskie, C Poland
57 K18 **Inquisivi** La Paz, W Bolivia
Inrin see Yüanlin
77 O8 **I-n-Sâkâne, 'Erg** desert N Mali
74 J10 **I-n-Salah** var. In Salah. C Algeria
129 O5 **Insar** Respublika Mordoviya, W Russian Federation
189 X15 **Insiaf** Kosrae, E Micronesia
94 L13 **Insjön** Dalarna, C Sweden
Insterburg see Chernyakhovsk
Insula see Lille
116 L13 **Însurăţei** Brăila, SE Romania
127 V6 **Inta** Respublika Komi, NW Russian Federation
77 R9 **I-n-Tebezas** Kidal, E Mali
Interamna see Teramo
Interamna Nahars see Terni
28 L11 **Interior** South Dakota, N USA
108 E9 **Interlaken** Bern, SW Switzerland
29 V2 **International Falls** Minnesota, N USA
167 O7 **Inthanon, Doi** ▲ NW Thailand
42 G7 **Intibucá** ◈ department SW Honduras
42 G8 **Intipucá** La Unión, SE El Salvador
61 B15 **Intiyaco** Santa Fe, C Argentina
116 K12 **Întorsura Buzăului** Ger. Bozau, Hung. Bodzafordulő. Covasna, E Romania
22 H9 **Intracoastal Waterway** inland waterway system Louisiana, S USA
25 V13 **Intracoastal Waterway** inland waterway system Texas, SW USA
108 G11 **Intragna** Ticino, S Switzerland
165 P14 **Inubō-zaki** headland Honshū, S Japan
164 E14 **Inukai** Ōita, Kyūshū, SW Japan
12 I5 **Inukjuak** var. Inoucdjouac; prev. Port Harrison. Quebec, NE Canada
63 I24 **Inútil, Bahía** bay S Chile
Inuuvik see Inuvik
9 R8 **Inuvik** var. Inuuvik. Northwest Territories, NW Canada
164 L13 **Inuyama** Aichi, Honshū, SW Japan
56 G13 **Inuya, Río** ≈ E Peru
127 U13 **In'va** ≈ NW Russian Federation
96 H11 **Inveraray** W Scotland, UK
185 C24 **Invercargill** Southland, South Island, NZ
183 T5 **Inverell** New South Wales, SE Australia
96 I8 **Invergordon** N Scotland, UK
11 P16 **Invermere** British Columbia, SW Canada
13 R14 **Inverness** Cape Breton Island, Nova Scotia, SE Canada
96 I8 **Inverness** N Scotland, UK
23 V11 **Inverness** Florida, SE USA
96 I9 **Inverness** cultural region NW Scotland, UK
96 K9 **Inverurie** NE Scotland, UK
182 F8 **Investigator Group** island group South Australia
173 T7 **Investigator Ridge** undersea feature E Indian Ocean
182 H10 **Investigator Strait** strait South Australia
29 R11 **Inwood** Iowa, C USA
123 S10 **Inya** ≈ E Russian Federation
Inyanga see Nyanga
83 M16 **Inyangani** ▲ NE Zimbabwe
83 J17 **Inyathi** Matabeleland North, SW Zimbabwe
35 T12 **Inyokern** California, W USA
35 T10 **Inyo Mountains** ▲ California, W USA
129 P6 **Inza** Ul'yanovskaya Oblast', W Russian Federation
129 W5 **Inzer** Respublika Bashkortostan, W Russian Federation
129 N7 **Inzhavino** Tambovskaya Oblast', W Russian Federation
115 C16 **Ioánnina** var. Janina, Yannina. Ípeiros, W Greece
164 B17 **Iō-jima** var. Iwojima. island Nansei-shotō, SW Japan
126 L4 **Iokan'ga** ≈ NW Russian Federation
27 Q6 **Iola** Kansas, C USA
Iolcus see Iolkós
115 G16 **Iolkós** anc. Iolcus. site of ancient city Thessalía, C Greece
Iolotan' see Yëloten
83 A16 **Iona** Namibe, SW Angola
96 F11 **Iona** island W Scotland, UK
116 M15 **Ion Corvin** Constanţa, SE Romania
35 P7 **Ione** California, W USA
116 I13 **Ioneşti** Vâlcea, SW Romania
31 Q9 **Ionia** Michigan, N USA
Ionia Basin see Ionian Basin
121 O10 **Ionian Basin** var. Ionia Basin. undersea feature Ionian Sea, C Mediterranean Sea
Ionian Islands see Iónioi Nísoi
121 O10 **Ionian Sea** Gk. Iónio Pélagos, It. Mar Ionio. sea C Mediterranean Sea
115 B17 **Iónioi Nísoi** Eng. Ionian Islands. ◈ region W Greece
115 B17 **Iónioi Nísoi** Eng. Ionian Islands. island group W Greece
Ionio, Mar/Iónio Pélagos see Ionian Sea
Iordan see Jordan
137 U10 **Iori** var. Qabırrı. ≈ Azerbaijan/Georgia
Iorrais, Ceann see Erris Head
115 J22 **Íos** Íos, Kykládes, Greece, Aegean Sea
115 J22 **Íos** var. Nio. island Kykládes, Greece, Aegean Sea
22 G9 **Iowa** Louisiana, S USA
29 V13 **Iowa** off. State of Iowa; also known as The Hawkeye State. ◈ state C USA
29 Y14 **Iowa City** Iowa, C USA
29 V13 **Iowa Falls** Iowa, C USA
25 R4 **Iowa Park** Texas, SW USA
29 Y14 **Iowa River** ≈ Iowa, C USA
119 M19 **Ipa** Rus. Ipa. ≈ SE Belarus
59 N20 **Ipatinga** Minas Gerais, SE Brazil
129 N13 **Ipatovo** Stavropol'skiy Kray, SW Russian Federation
115 C16 **Ípeiros** Eng. Epirus. ◈ region W Greece
Ipek see Peć
111 J21 **Ipel'** var. Ipoly, Ger. Eipel. ≈ Hungary/Slovakia
54 C13 **Ipiales** Nariño, SW Colombia
189 V14 **Ipis** atoll Chuuk Islands, C Micronesia
59 A14 **Ipixuna** Amazonas, W Brazil
168 J8 **Ipoh** Perak, Peninsular Malaysia
Ipoly see Ipel'
187 S15 **Ipota** Erromango, S Vanuatu
79 K14 **Ippy** Ouaka, C Central African Republic
114 L13 **İpsala** Edirne, NW Turkey
Ipsario see Ypsário
183 V3 **Ipswich** Queensland, E Australia
97 Q20 **Ipswich** hist. Gipeswic. E England, UK
29 O8 **Ipswich** South Dakota, N USA
Iput' see Iputs'
119 P18 **Iputs'** Rus. Iput'. ≈ Belarus/Russian Federation
9 R7 **Iqaluit** prev. Frobisher Bay. Baffin Island, Nunavut, NE Canada
159 P9 **Iqe** Qinghai, W China
159 P9 **Iqe He** ≈ C China
Iqlid see Eqlīd
62 G3 **Iquique** Tarapacá, N Chile
56 G8 **Iquitos** Loreto, N Peru
25 N9 **Iraan** Texas, SW USA
79 K14 **Ira Banda** Haute-Kotto, E Central African Republic
165 P16 **Irabu-jima** island Miyako-shotō, SW Japan
55 Y9 **Iracoubo** N French Guiana
60 H13 **Iraí** Rio Grande do Sul, S Brazil
114 G12 **Irákleia** Kentrikí Makedonía, N Greece
115 J21 **Irákleia** island Kykládes, Greece, Aegean Sea
115 J25 **Irákleio** var. Herakleion, Eng. Candia; prev. Iráklion. Kríti, Greece, E Mediterranean Sea
115 J25 **Irákleio** ✕ Kríti, Greece, E Mediterranean Sea
115 F15 **Irákleio** anc. Heracleum. castle Kentrikí Makedonía, N Greece
Iráklion see Irákleio
143 O7 **Iran** off. Islamic Republic of Iran; prev. Persia. ◆ republic SW Asia
58 F13 **Iranduba** Amazonas, NW Brazil
85 P13 **Iranian Plate** tectonic feature
143 Q9 **Iranian Plateau** var. Plateau of Iran. plateau N Iran
169 U9 **Iran, Pegunungan** var. Iran Mountains. ▲ Indonesia/Malaysia
Iran, Plateau of see Iranian Plateau
143 W13 **Īrānshahr** Sīstān va Balūchestān, SE Iran
55 P5 **Irapa** Sucre, NE Venezuela
41 N13 **Irapuato** Guanajuato, C Mexico
139 R7 **Iraq** off. Republic of Iraq, Ar. 'Irāq. ◆ republic SW Asia
60 J12 **Irati** Paraná, S Brazil
105 R3 **Irati** ≈ N Spain
127 T8 **Irayël'** Respublika Komi, NW Russian Federation
43 N13 **Irazú, Volcán** ▲ C Costa Rica
Irbenskiy Zaliv/Irbes Šaurums see Irbe Strait
118 D7 **Irbe Strait** Est. Kura Kurk, Latv. Irbes Šaurums, Rus. Irbenskiy Zaliv; prev. Est. Irbe Väin. strait Estonia/Latvia
Irbe Väin see Irbe Strait
138 G9 **Irbid** Irbid, N Jordan
138 G9 **Irbid** off. Muḥāfaẓat Irbid. ◈ governorate N Jordan
Irbīl see Arbīl
109 S6 **Irdning** Steiermark, SE Austria
79 I18 **Irebu** Equateur, W Dem. Rep. Congo (Zaire)
84 C9 **Ireland** Lat. Hibernia. island Ireland/UK
Ireland see Ireland, Republic of
64 A12 **Ireland Island North** island W Bermuda
64 A12 **Ireland Island South** island W Bermuda
97 D17 **Ireland, Republic of** off. Republic of Ireland, var. Ireland, Ir. Éire. ◆ republic NW Europe
127 V15 **Iren'** ≈ NW Russian Federation
185 A22 **Irene, Mount** ▲ South Island, NZ
Irgalem see Yirga 'Alem
144 L11 **Irgiz** Aktyubinsk, C Kazakhstan
Irian see New Guinea
Irian Barat see Irian Jaya
171 X13 **Irian Jaya** var. Irian Barat, West Irian, West New Guinea, West Papua ; prev. Dutch New Guinea, Netherlands New Guinea. ◈ province E Indonesia
Irian, Teluk see Cenderawasih, Teluk
78 K9 **Iriba** Biltine, NE Chad
129 X7 **Iriklinskoye Vodokhranilishche** ⊠ W Russian Federation
81 H23 **Iringa** Iringa, C Tanzania
81 H23 **Iringa** ◈ region S Tanzania
165 O16 **Iriomote-jima** island Sakishima-shotō, SW Japan
42 L4 **Iriona** Colón, NE Honduras
47 U7 **Iriri** ≈ N Brazil
58 I13 **Iriri, Rio** ≈ C Brazil
Iris see Yeşilırmak
35 W9 **Irish, Mount** ▲ Nevada, W USA
97 H17 **Irish Sea** Ir. Muir Éireann. sea C British Isles
139 U12 **Irjal ash Shaykhīyah** S Iraq
147 U11 **Irkeshtam** Oshskaya Oblast', SW Kyrgyzstan
122 M13 **Irkutsk** Irkutskaya Oblast', S Russian Federation
122 M12 **Irkutskaya Oblast'** ◈ province S Russian Federation
Irlir, Gora see Irlir Toghi
146 K8 **Irlir Toghi** var. Gora Irlir. ▲ N Uzbekistan
Irminger Basin see Reykjanes Basin
21 R12 **Irmo** South Carolina, SE USA
102 E6 **Iroise** sea NW France
189 X2 **Iroj** var. Eroj. island Ratak Chain, SE Marshall Islands
182 H7 **Iron Baron** South Australia
14 C10 **Iron Bridge** Ontario, S Canada
20 H10 **Iron City** Tennessee, S USA
14 I13 **Irondale** ≈ Ontario, SE Canada
182 H7 **Iron Knob** South Australia
30 M5 **Iron Mountain** Michigan, N USA
30 M4 **Iron River** Michigan, N USA
30 J3 **Iron River** Wisconsin, N USA
27 X6 **Ironton** Missouri, C USA
31 S15 **Ironton** Ohio, N USA
30 K4 **Ironwood** Michigan, N USA
12 H12 **Iroquois Falls** Ontario, S Canada
31 N12 **Iroquois River** ≈ Illinois/Indiana, N USA
164 M15 **Irō-zaki** headland Honshū, S Japan
Irpen' see Irpin'
117 O4 **Irpin'** Rus. Irpen'. Kyyivs'ka Oblast', N Ukraine
117 O4 **Irpin'** Rus. Irpen'. ≈ N Ukraine
141 Q16 **'Irqah** SW Yemen
166 K8 **Irrawaddy** var. Ayeyarwady. ◈ division SW Myanmar
166 L6 **Irrawaddy** var. Ayeyarwady. ≈ W Myanmar
166 K8 **Irrawaddy, Mouths of the** delta SW Myanmar
117 N4 **Irsha** ≈ N Ukraine
116 H7 **Irshava** Zakarpats'ka Oblast', W Ukraine
107 N18 **Irsina** Basilicata, S Italy
Irtish see Irtysh
131 R5 **Irtysh** var. Irtish, Kaz. Ertis. ≈ C Asia
145 S7 **Irtyshsk** Kaz. Ertis. Pavlodar, NE Kazakhstan
79 P17 **Irumu** Orientale, E Dem. Rep. Congo (Zaire)
105 Q2 **Irún** País Vasco, N Spain
Iruña see Pamplona
105 Q3 **Irurtzun** Navarra, N Spain
96 I13 **Irvine** W Scotland, UK
21 N6 **Irvine** Kentucky, S USA
25 T6 **Irving** Texas, SW USA
20 K5 **Irvington** Kentucky, S USA
Isaak see Iisaku
28 L8 **Isabel** South Dakota, N USA
186 L8 **Isabel** off. Isabel Province. ◈ province N Solomon Islands
171 O8 **Isabela** Basilan Island, SW Philippines
45 S5 **Isabela** W Puerto Rico
45 N8 **Isabela, Cabo** headland NW Dominican Republic
57 A18 **Isabela, Isla** var. Albemarle Island. island Galapagos Islands, Ecuador, E Pacific Ocean
40 I12 **Isabela, Isla** island C Mexico
42 K9 **Isabella, Cordillera** ▲ NW Nicaragua
35 S12 **Isabella Lake** ⊠ California, W USA
31 N2 **Isabelle, Point** headland Michigan, N USA
Isabel Segunda see Vieques
116 M13 **Isaccea** Tulcea, E Romania
92 H1 **Ísafjarðardjúp** inlet NW Iceland
92 H1 **Ísafjördhur** Vestfirdhir, NW Iceland
164 C14 **Isahaya** Nagasaki, Kyūshū, SW Japan
149 S7 **Isa Khel** Punjab, E Pakistan
172 H7 **Isalo** var. Massif de L'Isalo. ▲ SW Madagascar
Isalo, Massif de L' see Isalo
79 K20 **Isandja** Kasai Occidental, C Dem. Rep. Congo (Zaire)
187 R15 **Isangel** Tanna, S Vanuatu
79 M18 **Isangi** Orientale, C Dem. Rep. Congo (Zaire)
101 L24 **Isar** ≈ Austria/Germany
101 M23 **Isar-Kanal** canal SE Germany
Isbarta see Isparta
Isca Damnoniorum see Exeter
107 K18 **Ischia** var. Isola d'Ischia; anc. Aenaria. Campania, S Italy
107 J18 **Ischia, Isola d'** island S Italy
54 B12 **Iscuandé** var. Santa Bárbara. Nariño, SW Colombia
164 K14 **Ise** Mie, Honshū, SW Japan
100 J12 **Ise** ≈ N Germany
95 I23 **Isefjord** fjord E Denmark
Iseghem see Izegem
192 M14 **Iselin Seamount** undersea feature S Pacific Ocean
Isenhof see Püssi
106 E7 **Iseo** Lombardia, N Italy
103 U12 **Iseran, Col de l'** pass E France
103 S11 **Isère** ◈ department E France
103 S12 **Isère** ≈ E France
101 F15 **Iserlohn** Nordrhein-Westfalen, W Germany
107 K16 **Isernia** var. Æsernia. Molise, C Italy
165 N12 **Isesaki** Gunma, Honshū, S Japan
131 Q5 **Iset'** ≈ C Russian Federation
77 S15 **Iseyin** Oyo, W Nigeria
Isfahan see Eşfahān
147 Q11 **Isfana** Oshskaya Oblast', SW Kyrgyzstan
147 R11 **Isfara** N Tajikistan
149 O4 **Isfi Maidān** Ghowr, N Afghanistan
92 O3 **Isfjorden** fjord W Svalbard
Isha Baydhabo see Baydhabo
127 V11 **Isherim, Gora** ▲ NW Russian Federation
129 Q5 **Isheyevka** Ul'yanovskaya Oblast', W Russian Federation
165 P16 **Ishigaki** Okinawa, Ishigaki-jima, SW Japan
165 P16 **Ishigaki-jima** var. Isigaki Zima. island Sakishima-shotō, SW Japan
165 R3 **Ishikari-wan** bay Hokkaidō, NE Japan
165 S16 **Ishikawa** var. Isikawa. Okinawa, Okinawa, SW Japan
164 K11 **Ishikawa** off. Ishikawa-ken, var. Isikawa. ◈ prefecture Honshū, SW Japan
122 H11 **Ishim** Tyumenskaya Oblast', C Russian Federation
131 R6 **Ishim** Kaz. Esil. ≈ Kazakhstan/Russian Federation
129 V6 **Ishimbay** Respublika Bashkortostan, W Russian Federation
145 O9 **Ishimskoye** Akmola, C Kazakhstan
165 Q10 **Ishinomaki** var. Isinomaki. Miyagi, Honshū, C Japan
165 P13 **Ishioka** var. Isioka. Ibaraki, Honshū, S Japan
Ishkashim see Ishkoshim
Ishkashimskiy Khrebet see Ishkoshim, Qatorkŭhi
147 S15 **Ishkoshim** Rus. Ishkashim. S Tajikistan
147 S15 **Ishkoshim, Qatorkŭhi** Rus. Ishkashimskiy Khrebet. ▲ SE Tajikistan
31 N4 **Ishpeming** Michigan, N USA
147 N11 **Ishtikhon** Rus. Ishtykhan. Samarqand Wiloyati, C Uzbekistan
Ishtykhan see Ishtikhon
153 T15 **Ishurdi** var. Iswardi. Rajshahi, W Bangladesh
61 G17 **Isidoro Noblia** Cerro Largo, NE Uruguay
102 J4 **Isigny-sur-Mer** Calvados, N France
Isikari Gawa see Ishikari-gawa
Isikawa see Ishikawa
136 C11 **Işıklar Dağı** ▲ NW Turkey
107 C19 **Isili** Sardegna, Italy, C Mediterranean Sea
122 H12 **Isil'kul'** Omskaya Oblast', C Russian Federation
Isinomaki see Ishinomaki
Isioka see Ishioka
81 I18 **Isiolo** Eastern, C Kenya
79 O16 **Isiro** Orientale, NE Dem. Rep. Congo (Zaire)
92 P2 **Isispynten** headland NE Svalbard
123 P11 **Isit** Respublika Sakha (Yakutiya), NE Russian Federation
149 O2 **Iskabad Canal** canal N Afghanistan
147 Q9 **Iskandar** Rus. Iskander. Toshkent Wiloyati, E Uzbekistan
Iskander see Iskandar
Iskär see Iskŭr
121 Q2 **Iskele** var. Trikomo, Gk. Tríkomon. E Cyprus
136 K17 **İskenderun** Eng. Alexandretta. Hatay, S Turkey
138 H2 **İskenderun Körfezi** Eng. Gulf of Alexandretta. gulf S Turkey
136 J11 **İskilip** Çorum, N Turkey
Iski-Nauket see Eski-Nookat
114 J11 **Iskra** prev. Popovo. Kŭrdzhali, S Bulgaria
114 G10 **Iskŭr** var. Iskär. ≈ NW Bulgaria
114 H10 **Iskŭr, Yazovir** prev. Yazovir Stalin. ⊠ W Bulgaria
41 S15 **Isla** Veracruz-Llave, SE Mexico
119 J15 **Islach** Rus. Isloch'. ≈ C Belarus
104 H14 **Isla Cristina** Andalucía, S Spain
Isla de León see San Fernando
149 U6 **Islāmābād** ● (Pakistan) Federal Capital Territory Islāmābād, NE Pakistan
149 V6 **Islāmābād** ✕ Federal Capital Territory Islāmābād, NE Pakistan
Islamabad see Anantnāg
149 R17 **Islāmkot** Sind, SE Pakistan
23 Y17 **Islamorada** Florida Keys, Florida, SE USA
153 P14 **Islāmpur** Bihār, N India
Islam Qala see Eslām Qal'eh
Island/Ísland see Iceland
18 K16 **Island Beach** spit New Jersey, NE USA
19 S4 **Island Falls** Maine, NE USA
182 H6 **Island Lagoon** ⊚ South Australia
11 Y13 **Island Lake** ⊚ Manitoba, C Canada
29 W5 **Island Lake Reservoir** ⊠ Minnesota, N USA
33 R13 **Island Park** Idaho, NW USA
19 N6 **Island Pond** Vermont, NE USA
184 K2 **Islands, Bay of** inlet North Island, NZ
103 R7 **Is-sur-Tille** Côte d'Or, C France
42 J3 **Islas de la Bahía** ◈ department N Honduras
65 L20 **Islas Orcadas Rise** undersea feature S Atlantic Ocean
96 F12 **Islay** island SW Scotland, UK
116 I15 **Islaz** Teleorman, S Romania
29 V7 **Isle** Minnesota, N USA
102 M12 **Isle** ≈ W France
97 I16 **Isle of Man** ◇ UK crown dependency NW Europe
21 X7 **Isle of Wight** Virginia, NE USA
97 M24 **Isle of Wight** cultural region S England, UK
191 Y3 **Isles Lagoon** ⊚ Kiritimati, E Kiribati
37 R11 **Isleta Pueblo** New Mexico, SW USA
Isloch' see Islach
61 E19 **Ismael Cortinas** Flores, S Uruguay
Ismailia see Ismâ'ilîya
75 W7 **Ismâ'ilîya** var. Ismailia. N Egypt
Ismid see İzmit
75 X10 **Isna** var. Esna. SE Egypt
93 K18 **Isojoki** Länsi-Suomi, W Finland
82 M12 **Isoka** Northern, NE Zambia
Isola d'Ischia see Ischia
Isola d'Istria see Izola
Isonzo see Soča
15 U4 **Isoukustouc** ≈ Quebec, SE Canada
136 F15 **Isparta** var. Isbarta. Isparta, SW Turkey
136 F15 **Isparta** var. Isbarta. ◈ province SW Turkey
114 M7 **Isperikh** prev. Kemanlar. Razgrad, N Bulgaria
107 L26 **Ispica** Sicilia, Italy, C Mediterranean Sea
148 J14 **Ispikān** Baluchistān, SW Pakistan
137 Q12 **İspir** Erzurum, NE Turkey
138 E12 **Israel** off. State of Israel, var. Medinat Israel, Heb. Yisrael, Yisra'el. ◆ republic SW Asia
Issa see Vis
55 S9 **Issano** C Guyana
76 M16 **Issia** SW Ivory Coast
Issiq Köl see Issyk-Kul', Ozero
103 P11 **Issoire** Puy-de-Dôme, C France
103 N9 **Issoudun** anc. Uxellodunum. Indre, C France
81 H22 **Issuna** Singida, C Tanzania
Issyk see Yesik
Issyk-Kul' see Balykchy
147 X7 **Issyk-Kul', Ozero** var. Issiq Köl, Kir. Ysyk-Köl. ⊚ E Kyrgyzstan
147 X7 **Issyk-Kul'skaya Oblast'** Kir. Ysyk-Köl Oblasty. ◈ province E Kyrgyzstan
149 Q7 **Īstādeh-ye Moqor, Āb-e-** var. Āb-i-Istāda. ⊚ SE Afghanistan
136 D11 **İstanbul** Bul. Tsarigrad, Eng. Istanbul; prev. Constantinople, anc. Byzantium. İstanbul, NW Turkey
114 P12 **İstanbul** ◈ province NW Turkey
114 P12 **İstanbul Boğazı** var. Bosporus Thracius, Eng. Bosphorus, Bosporus, Turk. Karadeniz Boğazı. strait NW Turkey
Istarska Županija see Istra
115 G19 **Isthmía** Pelopónnisos, S Greece
115 G17 **Istiaía** Évvoia, C Greece
54 D9 **Istmina** Chocó, W Colombia
23 W13 **Istokpoga, Lake** ⊚ Florida, SE USA
112 A9 **Istra** off. Istarska županija. ◈ province NW Croatia
112 I10 **Istra** Eng. Istria, Ger. Istrien. cultural region NW Croatia
103 R15 **Istres** Bouches-du-Rhône, SE France
Istria/Istrien see Istra
Iswardi see Ishurdi
129 V7 **Isyangulovo** Respublika Bashkortostan, W Russian Federation
62 O6 **Itá** Central, S Paraguay
59 O17 **Itaberaba** Bahia, E Brazil
59 M20 **Itabira** prev. Presidente Vargas. Minas Gerais, SE Brazil
59 O18 **Itabuna** Bahia, E Brazil
59 J18 **Itacaiu** Mato Grosso, S Brazil
58 G12 **Itacoatiara** Amazonas, N Brazil
54 D9 **Itagüí** Antioquia, W Colombia
60 D13 **Itá Ibaté** Corrientes, NE Argentina
60 G11 **Itaipú, Represa de** ⊠ Brazil/Paraguay
58 H13 **Itaituba** Pará, NE Brazil
60 K13 **Itajaí** Santa Catarina, S Brazil
Italia/Italiana, Republica/Italian Republic, The see Italy
Italian Somaliland see Somalia
25 T7 **Italy** Texas, SW USA
106 G12 **Italy** off. The Italian Republic, It. Italia, Republica Italiana. ◆ republic S Europe
59 O19 **Itamaraju** Bahia, E Brazil
59 C14 **Itamarati** Amazonas, W Brazil
59 M19 **Itambé, Pico de** ▲ SE Brazil
164 J13 **Itami** ✕ (Ōsaka) Ōsaka, Honshū, SW Japan
115 H15 **Ítamos** ▲ N Greece
153 W11 **Itānagar** Arunāchal Pradesh, NE India
Itany see Litani
59 N19 **Itaobim** Minas Gerais, SE Brazil
59 P15 **Itaparica, Represa de** ⊠ E Brazil
58 M13 **Itapecuru-Mirim** Maranhão, E Brazil
60 Q8 **Itaperuna** Rio de Janeiro, SE Brazil
59 O18 **Itapetinga** Bahia, E Brazil
60 L10 **Itapetininga** São Paulo, S Brazil
60 K10 **Itapeva** São Paulo, S Brazil
47 W6 **Itapicuru, Rio** ≈ NE Brazil
58 O13 **Itapipoca** Ceará, E Brazil
60 M9 **Itapira** São Paulo, S Brazil
60 K8 **Itápolis** São Paulo, S Brazil
60 K10 **Itaporanga** São Paulo, S Brazil
62 P7 **Itapúa** off. Departamento de Itapúa. ◈ department SE Paraguay
59 E15 **Itapuã do Oeste** Rondônia, W Brazil
61 E15 **Itaqui** Rio Grande do Sul, S Brazil
60 K10 **Itararé** São Paulo, S Brazil
60 K10 **Itararé, Rio** ≈ S Brazil
154 H11 **Itārsi** Madhya Pradesh, C India
25 T7 **Itasca** Texas, SW USA
Itassi see Vieille Case
93 N17 **Itä-Suomi** ◈ province E Finland
60 D13 **Itatí** Corrientes, NE Argentina
60 K10 **Itatinga** São Paulo, S Brazil
115 F18 **Itéas, Kólpos** gulf C Greece
57 N15 **Iténez, Río** var. Rio Guaporé. ≈ Bolivia/Brazil **see also** Guaporé, Rio
54 H11 **Iteviate, Río** ≈ C Colombia
100 I13 **Ith** hill range C Germany
31 Q8 **Ithaca** Michigan, N USA
18 H11 **Ithaca** New York, NE USA
115 C18 **Itháki** Itháki, Iónioi Nísoi, Greece, C Mediterranean Sea
115 C18 **Itháki** island Iónioi Nísoi, Greece, C Mediterranean Sea
It Hearrenfean see Heerenveen
79 L17 **Itimbiri** ≈ N Dem. Rep. Congo (Zaire)
Itinomiya see Ichinomiya
Itinoseki see Ichinoseki
39 Q5 **Itkilik River** ≈ Alaska, USA
164 M11 **Itoigawa** Niigata, Honshū, C Japan
15 R6 **Itomamo, Lac** ⊚ Quebec, SE Canada
165 S17 **Itoman** Okinawa, SW Japan
102 M5 **Iton** ≈ N France
57 M16 **Itonamas Río** ≈ NE Bolivia
Itoupé, Mont see Sommet Tabulaire
Itseqqortoormiit see Ittoqqortoormiit
22 K4 **Itta Bena** Mississippi, S USA
107 B17 **Ittiri** Sardegna, Italy, C Mediterranean Sea
197 Q14 **Ittoqqortoormiit** var. Itseqqortoormiit, Dan. Scoresbysund, Eng. Scoresby Sound. Tunu, C Greenland
60 M10 **Itu** São Paulo, S Brazil
54 D8 **Ituango** Antioquia, NW Colombia
59 A14 **Ituí, Rio** ≈ NW Brazil
79 O20 **Itula** Sud Kivu, E Dem. Rep. Congo (Zaire)
59 K19 **Itumbiara** Goiás, C Brazil
55 T9 **Ituni** E Guyana
41 X13 **Iturbide** Campeche, SE Mexico
Ituri see Aruwimi
123 V13 **Iturup, Ostrov** island Kuril'skiye Ostrova, SE Russian Federation
60 L7 **Ituverava** São Paulo, S Brazil
59 C15 **Ituxi, Rio** ≈ W Brazil
61 E14 **Ituzaingó** Corrientes, NE Argentina
101 K18 **Itz** ≈ C Germany
100 I9 **Itzehoe** Schleswig-Holstein, N Germany
23 N2 **Iuka** Mississippi, S USA
60 I11 **Ivaiporã** Paraná, S Brazil
60 I11 **Ivaí, Rio** ≈ S Brazil
92 L10 **Ivalo** Lapp. Avveel, Avvil. Lappi, N Finland
92 L10 **Ivalojoki** Lapp. Avreel. ≈ N Finland
119 H20 **Ivanava** Pol. Janów, Janów Poleski, Rus. Ivanovo. Brestskaya Voblasts', SW Belarus
Ivangorod see Dęblin
Ivangrad see Berane
183 N7 **Ivanhoe** New South Wales, SE Australia
29 S9 **Ivanhoe** Minnesota, N USA
14 D8 **Ivanhoe** ≈ Ontario, S Canada
112 E8 **Ivanić-Grad** Sisak-Moslavina, N Croatia
117 T10 **Ivanivka** Khersons'ka Oblast', S Ukraine
117 P10 **Ivanivka** Odes'ka Oblast', SW Ukraine
113 L14 **Ivanjica** Serbia, C Yugoslavia
112 G11 **Ivanjska** var. Potkozarje. Republika Srpska, NW Bosnia & Herzegovina
111 H21 **Ivanka** ✕ (Bratislava) Bratislavský Kraj, W Slovakia
117 O3 **Ivankiv** Rus. Ivankov. Kyyivs'ka Oblast', N Ukraine
Ivankov see Ivankiv
39 O15 **Ivanof Bay** Alaska, USA
116 J7 **Ivano-Frankivs'k** Ger. Stanislau, Pol. Stanisławów, Rus. Ivano-Frankovsk; prev. Stanislav. Ivano-Frankivs'ka Oblast', W Ukraine
Ivano-Frankivs'k see Ivano-Frankivs'ka Oblast'
116 I7 **Ivano-Frankivs'ka Oblast'** var. Ivano-Frankivs'k, Rus. Ivano-Frankovskaya Oblast'; prev. Stanislavskaya Oblast'. ◈ province W Ukraine
Ivano-Frankovsk see Ivano-Frankivs'k
Ivano-Frankovskaya Oblast' see Ivano-Frankivs'ka Oblast'
126 M16 **Ivanovo** Ivanovskaya Oblast', W Russian Federation
Ivanovo see Ivanava
126 M16 **Ivanovskaya Oblast'** ◈ province W Russian Federation
35 X12 **Ivanpah Lake** ⊚ California, W USA
112 E7 **Ivanščica** ▲ NE Croatia
114 M8 **Ivanski** Shumen, NE Bulgaria
129 R7 **Ivanteyevka** Saratovskaya Oblast', W Russian Federation
Ivantsevichi/Ivatsevichi see Ivatsevichy
116 I4 **Ivanychi** Volyns'ka Oblast', NW Ukraine
119 H18 **Ivatsevichy** Pol. Iwacewicze, Rus. Ivantsevichi, Ivatsevichi. Brestskaya Voblasts', SW Belarus
114 L12 **Ivaylovgrad** Khaskovo, S Bulgaria

◆ Country ● Country Capital ◇ Dependent Territory ○ Dependent Territory Capital ◈ Administrative Region ✕ International Airport ▲ Mountain ▲ Mountain Range ▲ Volcano ≈ River ⊚ Lake ⊠ Reservoir

114 K11 **Ivaylovgrad, Yazovir** ⊞ S Bulgaria
122 G9 **Ivdel'** Sverdlovskaya Oblast', C Russian Federation
Ivenets see Ivyanyets
116 L12 **Iveşti** Galaţi, E Romania
Ivigtut see Ivittuut
79 F18 **Ivindo** ≈ Congo/Gabon
59 I21 **Ivinheima** Mato Grosso do Sul, SW Brazil
196 M15 **Ivittuut** var. Ivigtut. Kitaa, S Greenland
Iviza see Eivissa
172 I6 **Ivohibe** Fianarantsoa, SE Madagascar
Ivoire, Côte d' see Ivory Coast
76 L15 **Ivory Coast** off. Republic of the Ivory Coast, Fr. Côte d'Ivoire, République de la Côte d'Ivoire. ◆ republic W Africa
68 C11 **Ivory Coast** Fr. Côte d'Ivoire. coastal region S Ivory Coast
95 L22 **Ivösjön** ◎ S Sweden
106 B7 **Ivrea** anc. Eporedia. Piemonte, NW Italy
12 J2 **Ivujivik** Quebec, NE Canada
119 J16 **Ivyanyets** Rus. Ivenets. Minskaya Voblasts', C Belarus
Iv'ye see Iwye
Iwacewicze see Ivatsevichy
165 R8 **Iwaizumi** Iwate, Honshū, NE Japan
165 P12 **Iwaki** Fukushima, Honshū, N Japan
164 F13 **Iwakuni** Yamaguchi, Honshū, SW Japan
165 S4 **Iwamizawa** Hokkaidō, NE Japan
165 R4 **Iwanai** Hokkaidō, NE Japan
165 Q10 **Iwanuma** Miyagi, Honshū, C Japan
164 L14 **Iwata** Shizuoka, Honshū, S Japan
165 R8 **Iwate** Iwate, Honshū, N Japan
165 R8 **Iwate** off. Iwate-ken. ◆ prefecture Honshū, C Japan
Iwje see Iwye
77 S16 **Iwo** Oyo, SW Nigeria
Iwojima see Iō-jima
119 I16 **Iwye** Pol. Iwje, Rus. Iv'ye. Hrodzyenskaya Voblasts', W Belarus
42 C4 **Ixcán, Río** ≈ Guatemala/Mexico
99 G18 **Ixelles** Dut. Elsene. Brussels, C Belgium
57 J16 **Ixiamas** La Paz, NW Bolivia
41 O13 **Ixmiquilpan** var. Ixmiquilpán. Hidalgo, C Mexico
83 K23 **Ixopo** KwaZulu/Natal, E South Africa
Ixtaccíhuatal, Volcán see Iztaccíhuatl, Volcán
40 M16 **Ixtapa** Guerrero, S Mexico
41 S16 **Ixtepec** Oaxaca, SE Mexico
40 K12 **Ixtlán** var. Ixtlán del Río. Nayarit, C Mexico
Ixtlán del Río see Ixtlán
122 H11 **Iyevlevo** Tyumenskaya Oblast', C Russian Federation
164 F14 **Iyo** Ehime, Shikoku, SW Japan
Iyomishima see Iyomishima
164 E14 **Iyo-nada** sea S Japan
42 E4 **Izabal** off. Departamento de Izabal. ◆ department E Guatemala
42 F5 **Izabal, Lago de** prev. Golfo Dulce. ◎ E Guatemala
143 O9 **Izad Khvāst** Fārs, C Iran
41 X12 **Izamal** Yucatán, SE Mexico
129 Q16 **Izberbash** Respublika Dagestan, SW Russian Federation
99 C18 **Izegem** prev. Iseghem. West-Vlaanderen, W Belgium
142 M9 **Īzeh** Khūzestān, SW Iran
165 T16 **Izena-jima** island Nansei-shotō, SW Japan
114 N10 **Izgrev** Burgas, E Bulgaria
129 T2 **Izhevsk** prev. Ustinov. Udmurtskaya Respublika, NW Russian Federation
127 S7 **Izhma** Respublika Komi, NW Russian Federation
127 S7 **Izhma** ≈ NW Russian Federation
141 X8 **Izkī** NE Oman
Izmail see Izmayil
117 N13 **Izmayil** Rus. Izmail. Odes'ka Oblast', SW Ukraine
136 B14 **İzmir** prev. Smyrna. İzmir, W Turkey
136 C14 **İzmir** prev. Smyrna. ◆ province W Turkey
136 E11 **İzmit** var. Ismid; anc. Astacus. Kocaeli, NW Turkey
104 M14 **Iznájar** Andalucía, S Spain
104 M14 **Iznajar, Embalse de** ⊞ S Spain
105 N14 **Iznalloz** Andalucía, S Spain
136 E11 **İznik** Bursa, NW Turkey
136 E12 **İznik Gölü** ◎ NW Turkey
128 M14 **Izobil'nyy** Stavropol'skiy Kray, SW Russian Federation
109 S13 **Izola** It. Isola d'Istria. SW Slovenia
138 H9 **Izra'** var. Ezra, Ezraa. Dar'ā, S Syria
41 P14 **Iztaccíhuatl, Volcán** var. Volcán Ixtaccíhuatal. ⛰ S Mexico
42 C7 **Iztapa** Escuintla, SE Guatemala
Izúcar de Matamoros see Matamoros
165 N14 **Izu-hantō** peninsula Honshū, S Japan
164 C12 **Izuhara** Nagasaki, Tsushima, SW Japan
164 J14 **Izumiōtsu** Ōsaka, Honshū, SW Japan
164 I14 **Izumi-Sano** Ōsaka, Honshū, SW Japan
164 G12 **Izumo** Shimane, Honshū, SW Japan
Izu Shichito see Izu-shotō
192 H5 **Izu Trench** undersea feature NW Pacific Ocean
122 K6 **Izvestiy TsIK, Ostrova** island N Russian Federation
114 G10 **Izvor** Pernik, W Bulgaria
116 L5 **Izyaslav** Khmel'nyts'ka Oblast', W Ukraine
117 W6 **Izyum** Kharkivs'ka Oblast', E Ukraine

J

95 M18 **Jaala** Etelä-Suomi, S Finland
140 J5 **Jabal ash Shifā** desert NW Saudi Arabia
141 U8 **Jabal az Zannah** var. Jebel Dhanna. Abū Ẓaby, W UAE
138 E11 **Jabalīya** var. Jabāliyah. NE Gaza Strip
Jabāliyah see Jabalīya
105 N11 **Jabalón** ≈ C Spain
154 J10 **Jabalpur** prev. Jubbulpore. Madhya Pradesh, C India
141 N15 **Jabal Zuuqar, Jazīrat** var. Az Zuqur. island SW Yemen
Jabat see Jabwot
138 J3 **Jabbūl, Sabkhat al** salt flat NW Syria
181 P1 **Jabiru** Northern Territory, N Australia
138 H4 **Jablah** var. Jeble, Fr. Djéblé. Al Lādhiqīyah, W Syria
112 C11 **Jablanac** Lika-Senj, W Croatia
113 H14 **Jablanica** Federacija Bosna I Hercegovina, SW Bosnia and Herzegovina
113 M20 **Jablanica** Alb. Mali i Jabllanicës, var. Malet e Jabllanicës. ▲ Albania/FYR Macedonia see also Jabllanicës, Mali i
Jabllanicës, Malet e see Jablanica/Jabllanicës, Mali i
113 M20 **Jabllanicës, Mali i** var. Malet e Jabllanicës, Mac. Jablanica. ▲ Albania/FYR Macedonia see also Jablanica
111 E15 **Jablonec nad Nisou** Ger. Gablonz an der Neisse. Liberecký Kraj, N Czech Republic
Jabłonków/Jablunkau see Jablunkov
110 J9 **Jabłonowo Pomorskie** Kujawski-pomorskie, C Poland
111 J17 **Jablunkov** Ger. Jablunkau, Pol. Jabłonków. Ostravský Kraj, E Czech Republic
59 Q15 **Jaboatão** Pernambuco, E Brazil
60 L8 **Jaboticabal** São Paulo, S Brazil
189 U7 **Jabwot** var. Jabat, Jebat, Jōwat. island Ralik Chain, S Marshall Islands
105 S4 **Jaca** Aragón, NE Spain
42 B4 **Jacaltenango** Huehuetenango, W Guatemala
59 G14 **Jacaré-a-Canga** Pará, NE Brazil
60 N10 **Jacareí** São Paulo, S Brazil
59 I18 **Jaciara** Mato Grosso, W Brazil
59 E15 **Jaciparaná** Rondônia, W Brazil
19 P5 **Jackman** Maine, NE USA
35 X1 **Jackpot** Nevada, W USA
20 M8 **Jacksboro** Tennessee, S USA
25 S6 **Jacksboro** Texas, SW USA
23 N7 **Jackson** Alabama, S USA
35 P7 **Jackson** California, W USA
23 T4 **Jackson** Georgia, SE USA
21 O6 **Jackson** Kentucky, S USA
22 J8 **Jackson** Louisiana, S USA
31 Q10 **Jackson** Michigan, N USA
29 T11 **Jackson** Minnesota, N USA
22 K5 **Jackson** state capital Mississippi, S USA
27 Y7 **Jackson** Missouri, C USA
21 W8 **Jackson** North Carolina, SE USA
31 T15 **Jackson** Ohio, NE USA
20 G9 **Jackson** Tennessee, S USA
33 S14 **Jackson** Wyoming, C USA
185 C19 **Jackson Bay** bay South Island, NZ
186 E9 **Jackson Field** ✈ (Port Moresby) Central/National Capital District, S PNG
185 C20 **Jackson Head** headland South Island, NZ
23 S8 **Jackson, Lake** ◎ Florida, SE USA
33 S13 **Jackson Lake** ◎ Wyoming, C USA
194 J6 **Jackson, Mount** ▲ Antarctica
37 U3 **Jackson Reservoir** ◎ Colorado, C USA
23 Q3 **Jacksonville** Alabama, S USA
27 V11 **Jacksonville** Arkansas, C USA
23 W8 **Jacksonville** Florida, SE USA
30 K14 **Jacksonville** Illinois, N USA
21 W11 **Jacksonville** North Carolina, SE USA
25 W7 **Jacksonville** Texas, SW USA
23 X9 **Jacksonville Beach** Florida, SE USA
44 L9 **Jacmel** var. Jaquemel. S Haiti
Jacob see Nkayi
149 Q12 **Jacobābād** Sind, SE Pakistan
55 T11 **Jacobs Ladder Falls** waterfall S Guyana
45 O11 **Jaco, Pointe** headland N Dominica
15 Q9 **Jacques-Cartier** ≈ Quebec, SE Canada
13 P11 **Jacques-Cartier, Détroit de** var. Jacques-Cartier Passage. strait Gulf of St. Lawrence/St. Lawrence River
15 W6 **Jacques-Cartier, Mont** ▲ Quebec, SE Canada
Jacques-Cartier Passage see Jacques-Cartier, Détroit de
61 H16 **Jacuí, Rio** ≈ S Brazil
60 L11 **Jacupiranga** São Paulo, S Brazil
100 G10 **Jade** ≈ NW Germany
100 G10 **Jadebusen** bay NW Germany
Jadotville see Likasi
Jadransko More/Jadransko Morje see Adriatic Sea
105 O7 **Jadraque** Castilla-La Mancha, C Spain
56 C10 **Jaén** Cajamarca, N Peru
105 N13 **Jaén** Andalucía, SW Spain
105 N13 **Jaén** ◆ province Andalucía, S Spain
155 J23 **Jaffna** Northern Province, N Sri Lanka
155 K23 **Jaffna Lagoon** lagoon N Sri Lanka
19 N10 **Jaffrey** New Hampshire, NE USA
138 H13 **Jafr, Qā' al** var. El Jafr. salt pan S Jordan
152 J9 **Jagādhri** Haryāna, N India
118 H4 **Jägala** var. Jägala Jõgi, Ger. Jaggowal. ≈ NW Estonia
Jägala Jõgi see Jägala
Jagannath see Puri
155 L14 **Jagdalpur** Madhya Pradesh, C India
163 U5 **Jagdaqi** Nei Mongol Zizhiqu, N China
Jägerndorf see Krnov
Jaggowal see Jägala
139 O2 **Jaghjaghah, Nahr** ≈ N Syria
112 N13 **Jagodina** prev. Svetozarevo. Serbia, C Yugoslavia
112 K12 **Jagodnja** ▲ W Yugoslavia
101 I20 **Jagst** ≈ SW Germany
155 I14 **Jagtiāl** Andhra Pradesh, C India
61 H18 **Jaguarão** Rio Grande do Sul, S Brazil
61 H18 **Jaguarão, Rio** var. Río Yaguarón. ≈ Brazil/Uruguay
60 K11 **Jaguariaíva** Paraná, S Brazil
44 D5 **Jagüey Grande** Matanzas, W Cuba
153 P14 **Jahānābād** Bihār, N India
Jahra see Al Jahrā'
143 P12 **Jahrom** var. Jahrum. Fārs, S Iran
Jahrum see Jahrom
Jailolo see Halmahera, Pulau
Jainat see Chai Nat
Jainti see Jayanti
152 H12 **Jaipur** prev. Jeypore. Rājasthān, N India
153 T14 **Jaipur Hat** Rajshahi, NW Bangladesh
152 D11 **Jaisalmer** Rājasthān, NW India
154 O12 **Jājapur** Orissa, E India
143 R4 **Jājarm** Khorāsān, NE Iran
112 G12 **Jajce** Federacija Bosna I Hercegovina, W Bosnia and Herzegovina
Jajı see 'Alī Kheyl
83 D17 **Jakalsberg** Otjozondjupa, N Namibia
169 O15 **Jakarta** prev. Djakarta, Dut. Batavia. ● (Indonesia) Jawa, C Indonesia
10 I8 **Jakes Corner** Yukon Territory, W Canada
152 H9 **Jākhal** Haryāna, NW India
Jakobeny see Iacobeni
93 K16 **Jakobstad** Fin. Pietarsaari. Länsi-Suomi, W Finland
Jakobstadt see Jēkabpils
113 O18 **Jakupica** ▲ C FYR Macedonia
37 W15 **Jal** New Mexico, SW USA
141 P7 **Jalājil** var. Ğalāğıl. Ar Riyāḍ, C Saudi Arabia
Jalal-Abad see Dzhalal-Abad, Dzhalal-Abadskaya Oblast', W Kyrgyzstan
149 S5 **Jalālābād** var. Jalalabad, Jelalabad. Nangarhār, E Afghanistan
Jalal-Abad Oblasty see Dzhalal-Abadskaya Oblast'
149 V7 **Jalālpur** Punjab, E Pakistan
149 T11 **Jalālpur Pīrwāla** Punjab, E Pakistan
152 H8 **Jalandhar** prev. Jullundur. Punjab, N India
42 J7 **Jalán, Río** ≈ S Honduras
42 E6 **Jalapa** Jalapa, C Guatemala
42 J7 **Jalapa** Nueva Segovia, NW Nicaragua
42 A3 **Jalapa** off. Departamento de Jalapa. ◆ department SE Guatemala
42 E6 **Jalapa, Río** ≈ SE Guatemala
143 X13 **Jālaq** Sīstān va Balūchestān, SE Iran
93 K17 **Jalasjärvi** Länsi-Suomi, W Finland
149 O8 **Jaldak** Zābul, SE Afghanistan
60 J7 **Jales** São Paulo, S Brazil
154 P11 **Jaleshwar** var. Jaleswar. Orissa, NE India
Jaleswar see Jaleshwar
154 F12 **Jalgaon** Mahārāshtra, C India
139 W12 **Jalībah** S Iraq
139 W13 **Jalīb Shahāb** S Iraq
77 X15 **Jalingo** Taraba, E Nigeria
40 K13 **Jalisco** ◆ state SW Mexico
154 G13 **Jālna** Mahārāshtra, W India
Jalomitsa see Ialomiţa
105 R5 **Jalón** ≈ N Spain
152 E13 **Jālor** Rājasthān, N India
112 K11 **Jalovik** Serbia, W Yugoslavia
40 L12 **Jalpa** Zacatecas, C Mexico
153 S12 **Jalpāiguri** West Bengal, NE India
41 O12 **Jalpán** var. Jalpan. Querétaro de Arteaga, C Mexico
67 P2 **Jalta** island N Tunisia
75 S9 **Jālū** var. Jūlā. NE Libya
189 U8 **Jaluit Atoll** var. Jālwōj. atoll Ralik Chain, S Marshall Islands
Jālwōj see Jaluit Atoll
81 L18 **Jamaame** It. Giamame; prev. Margherita. Jubbada Hoose, S Somalia
77 W13 **Jamaare** ≈ NE Nigeria
44 G9 **Jamaica** ◆ commonwealth republic W West Indies
47 P3 **Jamaica** island W West Indies
44 I9 **Jamaica Channel** channel Haiti/Jamaica
153 T14 **Jamalpur** Dhaka, N Bangladesh
153 Q14 **Jamālpur** Bihār, NE India
168 L9 **Jamaluang** var. Jemaluang. Johor, Peninsular Malaysia
59 I14 **Jamanxim, Rio** ≈ C Brazil
56 B8 **Jambeli, Canal de** channel S Ecuador
99 I20 **Jambes** Namur, SE Belgium
168 Hh9 **Jambi** var. Telanaipura; prev. Djambi. Sumatera, W Indonesia
GG H9 **Jambi** off. Propinsi Jambi, var. Djambi. ◆ province W Indonesia
Jamdena see Yamdena, Pulau
12 H8 **James Bay** bay Ontario/Quebec, E Canada
63 F19 **James, Isla** island Archipiélago de los Chonos, S Chile
181 Q8 **James Ranges** ▲ Northern Territory, C Australia
29 P8 **James River** ≈ North Dakota/South Dakota, N USA
21 X7 **James River** ≈ Virginia, NE USA
194 H4 **James Ross Island** island Antarctica
182 I8 **Jamestown** South Australia
65 G25 **Jamestown** ○ (Saint Helena) NW Saint Helena
35 P8 **Jamestown** California, W USA
20 L7 **Jamestown** Kentucky, S USA
18 D11 **Jamestown** New York, NE USA
29 P5 **Jamestown** North Dakota, N USA
20 L8 **Jamestown** Tennessee, S USA
Jamestown see Holetown
15 N10 **Jamet** ≈ Quebec, SE Canada
41 Q17 **Jamiltepec** var. Santiago Jamiltepec. Oaxaca, SE Mexico
95 F20 **Jammerbugten** bay Skagerrak, E North Sea
152 H6 **Jammu** prev. Jummoo. Jammu and Kashmir, NW India
152 I5 **Jammu and Kashmir** var. Jammu-Kashmir, Kashmir. ◆ state NW India
149 V4 **Jammu and Kashmir** disputed region India/Pakistan
154 B10 **Jāmnagar** prev. Navanagar. Gujarāt, W India
149 S11 **Jāmpur** Punjab, E Pakistan
93 L18 **Jämsä** Länsi-Suomi, W Finland
93 L18 **Jämsänkoski** Länsi-Suomi, W Finland
153 Q16 **Jamshedpur** Bihār, NE India
94 K9 **Jämtland** ◆ county C Sweden
153 Q14 **Jamūi** Bihār, NE India
153 T14 **Jamuna** ≈ N Bangladesh
Jamuna see Brahmaputra
Jamundá see Nhamundá, Rio
54 D11 **Jamundí** Valle del Cauca, SW Colombia
153 Q12 **Janakpur** Central, C Nepal
59 N18 **Janaúba** Minas Gerais, SE Brazil
58 K11 **Janaucu, Ilha** island NE Brazil
143 Q7 **Jandaq** Eşfahān, C Iran
64 Q11 **Jandia, Punta de** headland Fuerteventura, Islas Canarias, Spain, NE Atlantic Ocean
59 B14 **Jandiatuba, Rio** ≈ NW Brazil
105 N12 **Jándula** ≈ S Spain
29 V10 **Janesville** Minnesota, N USA
30 L9 **Janesville** Wisconsin, N USA
149 N13 **Jangal** Baluchistān, SW Pakistan
83 N20 **Jangamo** Inhambane, SE Mozambique
155 J14 **Jangaon** Andhra Pradesh, C India
146 K10 **Jangeldi** Rus. Dzhankel'dy. Bukhoro Wiloyati, C Uzbekistan
153 S14 **Jangīpur** West Bengal, NE India
Janina see Ioánnina
Janischken see Joniškis
112 J11 **Janja** Republika Srpska, NE Bosnia and Herzegovina
Jankovac see Jánoshalma
197 Q15 **Jan Mayen** ◇ Norwegian dependency N Atlantic Ocean
84 D5 **Jan Mayen** island N Atlantic Ocean
197 R15 **Jan Mayen Fracture Zone** tectonic feature Greenland Sea/Norwegian Sea
197 R15 **Jan Mayen Ridge** undersea feature Greenland Sea/Norwegian Sea
40 H3 **Janos** Chihuahua, N Mexico
111 K25 **Jánoshalma** SCr. Jankovac. Bács-Kiskun, S Hungary
Janow/Janów see Jonava, Lithuania
Janów see Ivanava, Belarus
110 H10 **Janowiec Wielkopolski** Ger. Janowitz. Kujawski-pomorskie, C Poland
Janowitz see Janowiec Wielkopolski
111 O15 **Janów Lubelski** Lubelskie, E Poland
Janów Poleski see Ivanava
83 H25 **Jansenville** Eastern Cape, S South Africa
59 M18 **Januária** Minas Gerais, SE Brazil
Janūbīyah, Al Bādiyah al see Ash Shāmīyah
102 I7 **Janzé** Ille-et-Vilaine, NW France
154 F10 **Jaora** Madhya Pradesh, C India
164 K11 **Japan** var. Nippon, Jap. Nihon. ◆ monarchy E Asia
131 Y9 **Japan** island group E Asia
192 H4 **Japan Basin** undersea feature N Sea of Japan
131 Y8 **Japan, Sea of** var. East Sea, Rus. Yapanskoye More. sea NW Pacific Ocean
192 H4 **Japan Trench** undersea feature NW Pacific Ocean
Japen see Yapen, Pulau
59 A15 **Japiim** var. Máncio Lima. Acre, W Brazil
58 D12 **Japurá** Amazonas, N Brazil
58 C12 **Japurá, Rio** var. Río Caquetá, Yapurá. ≈ Brazil/Colombia see also Caquetá, Río
43 W17 **Jaqué** Darién, SE Panama
Jaquemel see Jacmel
Jarablos see Jarābulus
138 K2 **Jarābulus** var. Jarablos, Jerablus, Fr. Djérablous. Ḥalab, N Syria
60 K13 **Jaraguá do Sul** Santa Catarina, S Brazil
104 K9 **Jaraicejo** Extremadura, W Spain
104 K9 **Jaráiz de la Vera** Extremadura, W Spain
105 O7 **Jarama** ≈ C Spain
63 J20 **Jaramillo** Santa Cruz, SE Argentina
Jarandilla de la Vega see Jarandilla de la Vera
104 K8 **Jarandilla de la Vera** var. Jarandilla de la Vega. Extremadura, W Spain
149 V9 **Jarānwāla** Punjab, E Pakistan
138 G9 **Jarash** var. Jerash; anc. Gerasa. Irbid, NW Jordan
Jarbah, Jazīrat see Jerba, Île de
94 N13 **Järbo** Gävleborg, C Sweden
44 F7 **Jardines de la Reina, Archipiélago de los** island group C Cuba
162 J7 **Jargalant** Arhangay, C Mongolia
162 I8 **Jargalant** Bayanhongor, C Mongolia
162 D7 **Jargalant** Bayan-Ölgiy, W Mongolia
162 K6 **Jargalant** Bulgan, N Mongolia
162 G9 **Jargalant** Govĭ-Altay, W Mongolia
Jarīd, Shaṭṭ al see Jerid, Chott el
58 I11 **Jari, Rio** var. Jary. ≈ N Brazil
141 N7 **Jarīr, Wādī al** dry watercourse C Saudi Arabia
Jarja see Yur'ya
94 L13 **Järna** var. Dala-Jarna. Dalarna, C Sweden
95 O16 **Järna** Stockholm, C Sweden
102 K11 **Jarnac** Charente, W France
110 H12 **Jarocin** Wielkopolskie, C Poland
111 F16 **Jaroměř** Ger. Jermer. Hradecký Kraj, N Czech Republic
Jaroslau see Jarosław
111 O16 **Jarosław** Ger. Jaroslau, Rus. Yaroslav. Podkarpackie, SE Poland
93 F16 **Järpen** Jämtland, C Sweden
147 O14 **Jarqŭrghon** Rus. Dzharkurgan. Surkhondaryo Wiloyati, S Uzbekistan
139 P2 **Jarrāh, Wadi** dry watercourse NE Syria
Jars, Plain of see Xiangkhoang, Plateau de
162 K14 **Jartai Yanchi** ◎ N China
59 E16 **Jaru** Rondônia, W Brazil
163 T10 **Jarud Qi** Nei Mongol Zizhiqu, N China
118 I4 **Järva-Jaani** Ger. Sankt-Johannis. Järvamaa, N Estonia
118 G5 **Järvakandi** Ger. Jerwakant. Raplamaa, NW Estonia
118 H4 **Järvamaa** off. Järva Maakond. ◆ province N Estonia
93 L19 **Järvenpää** Etelä-Suomi, S Finland
14 G17 **Jarvis** Ontario, S Canada
177 R8 **Jarvis Island** ◇ US unincorporated territory C Pacific Ocean
94 M11 **Järvsö** Gävleborg, C Sweden
Jary see Jari, Rio
112 M9 **Jaša Tomić** Serbia, NE Yugoslavia
112 D12 **Jasenice** Zadar, SW Croatia
138 I11 **Jashshat al 'Adlah, Wādī al** dry watercourse C Jordan
77 Q16 **Jasikan** E Ghana
143 T15 **Jāsk** Hormozgān, SE Iran
146 F6 **Jasliq** Rus. Zhaslyk. Qoraqalpoghiston Respublikasi, NW Uzbekistan
111 N17 **Jasło** Podkarpackie, SE Poland
11 U16 **Jasmin** Saskatchewan, S Canada
65 A23 **Jason Islands** island group NW Falkland Islands
194 I4 **Jason Peninsula** peninsula Antarctica
31 N15 **Jasonville** Indiana, N USA
11 O15 **Jasper** Alberta, SW Canada
14 L13 **Jasper** Ontario, SE Canada
23 O3 **Jasper** Alabama, S USA
27 T9 **Jasper** Arkansas, C USA
23 U8 **Jasper** Florida, SE USA
31 N16 **Jasper** Indiana, N USA
29 R11 **Jasper** Minnesota, N USA
27 S7 **Jasper** Missouri, C USA
20 K10 **Jasper** Tennessee, S USA
25 Y9 **Jasper** Texas, SW USA
11 O15 **Jasper National Park** national park Alberta/British Columbia, SW Canada
Jassy see Iaşi
113 N14 **Jastrebac** ▲ SE Yugoslavia
112 D9 **Jastrebarsko** Zagreb, N Croatia
Jastrow see Jastrowie
110 G9 **Jastrowie** Ger. Jastrow. Wielkopolskie, C Poland
111 J17 **Jastrzębie-Zdrój** Śląskie, S Poland
111 L22 **Jászapáti** Jász-Nagykun-Szolnok, E Hungary
111 L22 **Jászberény** Jász-Nagykun-Szolnok, E Hungary
111 L23 **Jász-Nagykun-Szolnok** off. Jász-Nagykun-Szolnok Megye. ◆ county E Hungary
59 J19 **Jataí** Goiás, C Brazil
58 G12 **Jatapu, Serra do** ▲ N Brazil
41 W16 **Jatate, Río** ≈ SE Mexico
149 P17 **Jāti** Sind, SE Pakistan
44 F6 **Jatibonico** Sancti Spíritus, C Cuba
169 O16 **Jatiluhur, Danau** ◎ Jawa, S Indonesia
Jativa see Xátiva
149 S11 **Jattoi** Punjab, E Pakistan
60 L9 **Jaú** São Paulo, S Brazil
58 F11 **Jauaperi, Rio** ≈ N Brazil
99 I19 **Jauche** Wallon Brabant, C Belgium
Jauer see Jawor
Jauf see Al Jawf
149 U7 **Jauharābād** Punjab, E Pakistan
57 E14 **Jauja** Junín, C Peru
41 O10 **Jaumave** Tamaulipas, C Mexico
118 H10 **Jaunjelgava** Ger. Friedrichstadt. Aizkraukle, S Latvia
Jaunlatgale see Pytalovo
118 I8 **Jaunpiebalga** Gulbene, NE Latvia
118 E9 **Jaunpils** Tukums, C Latvia
153 N13 **Jaunpur** Uttar Pradesh, N India
29 N8 **Java** South Dakota, N USA
Java see Jawa
105 R9 **Javalambre** ▲ E Spain
173 V7 **Java Ridge** undersea feature E Indian Ocean
59 A14 **Javari, Rio** var. Yavarí. ≈ Brazil/Peru
163 O7 **Javarthushuu** Dornod, NE Mongolia
169 Q15 **Java Sea** Ind. Laut Jawa. sea W Indonesia
173 U7 **Java Trench** var. Sunda Trench. undersea feature E Indian Ocean
105 T11 **Jávea** var. Xàbia. País Valenciano, E Spain
163 O7 **Javhlant** Hentiy, E Mongolia
63 G20 **Javier, Isla** island S Chile
113 L14 **Javor** ▲ Bosnia and Herzegovina/Yugoslavia
111 K20 **Javorie** Hung. Jávoros. ▲ S Slovakia
Jávoros see Javorie
93 J14 **Jävre** Norrbotten, N Sweden
192 E8 **Jawa** Eng. Java; prev. Djawa. island C Indonesia
169 O16 **Jawa Barat** off. Propinsi Jawa Barat, Eng. West Java. ◆ province S Indonesia
Jawa, Laut see Java Sea
139 R3 **Jawān** NW Iraq
169 P16 **Jawa Tengah** off. Propinsi Jawa Tengah, Eng. Central Java. ◆ province S Indonesia
169 R16 **Jawa Timur** off. Propinsi Jawa Timur, Eng. East Java. ◆ province S Indonesia
81 N17 **Jawhar** var. Jowhar, It. Giohar. Shabeellaha Dhexe, S Somalia
111 F14 **Jawor** Ger. Jauer. Dolnośląskie, SW Poland
Jaworów see Yavoriv
111 J16 **Jaworzno** Śląskie, S Poland
Jaxartes see Syr Darya
27 R9 **Jay** Oklahoma, C USA
Jayabum see Chaiyaphum
Jayanath see Chai Nat
153 T12 **Jayanti** prev. Jainti. West Bengal, NE India
171 X14 **Jaya, Puncak** prev. Puntjak Carstensz, Puntjak Sukarno. ▲ Irian Jaya, E Indonesia
171 Z13 **Jayapura** var. Djajapura, Dut. Hollandia; prev. Kotabaru, Sukarnapura. Irian Jaya, E Indonesia
Jay Dairen see Dalian
Jayhawker State see Kansas
147 S12 **Jayilgan** Rus. Dzhailgan, Dzhayilgan. C Tajikistan
155 L14 **Jaypur** var. Jeypore, Jeypur. Orissa, E India
25 O6 **Jayton** Texas, SW USA
143 U13 **Jaz Murian, Hāmūn-e** ◎ SE Iran
138 M4 **Jazrah** Ar Raqqah, C Syria
138 G6 **Jbaïl** var. Jebeil, Jubayl, Jubeil; anc. Biblical Gebal, Bybles. W Lebanon
25 O7 **J.B.Thomas, Lake** ⊞ Texas, SW USA
Jdaïdé see Judaydah
35 X12 **Jean** Nevada, W USA
22 I9 **Jeanerette** Louisiana, S USA
44 L8 **Jean-Rabel** NW Haiti
143 T12 **Jebāl Bārez, Kūh-e** ▲ SE Iran
Jebat see Jabwot
77 T15 **Jebba** Kwara, W Nigeria
Jebeil see Jbaïl
116 E12 **Jebel** Hung. Széphely; prev. Hung. Zsebely. Timiş, W Romania
Jebel see Dzhebel
Jebel, Bahr el see White Nile
Jebel Dhanna see Jabal az Zannah
Jeble see Jablah
96 K13 **Jedburgh** SE Scotland, UK
Jedda see Jiddah
111 L15 **Jędrzejów** Ger. Endersdorf. Świętokrzyskie, C Poland
100 K12 **Jeetze** var. Jeetzel. ≈ C Germany
Jeetzel see Jeetze
29 U14 **Jefferson** Iowa, C USA
21 Q8 **Jefferson** North Carolina, SE USA
25 X6 **Jefferson** Texas, SW USA
30 M9 **Jefferson** Wisconsin, N USA
27 U5 **Jefferson City** state capital Missouri, C USA
33 R10 **Jefferson City** Montana, NW USA
21 N9 **Jefferson City** Tennessee, S USA
35 U7 **Jefferson, Mount** ▲ Nevada, W USA
32 H12 **Jefferson, Mount** ▲ Oregon, NW USA
20 L5 **Jeffersontown** Kentucky, S USA
31 P16 **Jeffersonville** Indiana, N USA
33 V15 **Jeffrey City** Wyoming, C USA
77 T13 **Jega** Kebbi, NW Nigeria
Jehol see Chengde
62 P5 **Jejui-Guazú, Río** ≈ E Paraguay
118 I10 **Jēkabpils** Ger. Jakobstadt. Jēkabpils, S Latvia
23 W7 **Jekyll Island** island Georgia, SE USA
169 R13 **Jelai, Sungai** ≈ Borneo, N Indonesia
Jelalabad see Jalālābād
111 H14 **Jelcz-Laskowice** Dolnośląskie, SW Poland
111 E14 **Jelenia Góra** Ger. Hirschberg, Hirschberg im Riesengebirge, Hirschberg in Riesengebirge, Hirschberg in Schlesien. Dolnośląskie, SW Poland
153 S11 **Jelep La** pass N India
118 F9 **Jelgava** Ger. Mitau. Jelgava, C Latvia
112 L13 **Jelica** ▲ C Yugoslavia
20 M8 **Jellico** Tennessee, S USA
95 G23 **Jelling** Vejle, C Denmark
169 N9 **Jemaja, Pulau** island W Indonesia
Jemaluang see Jamaluang
99 E20 **Jemappes** Hainaut, S Belgium
169 S17 **Jember** prev. Djember. Jawa, C Indonesia

◆ Country ● Country Capital ◇ Dependent Territory ○ Dependent Territory Capital ◆ Administrative Region ✈ International Airport ▲ Mountain ▲ Mountain Range ⛰ Volcano ≈ River ◎ Lake ⊞ Reservoir

99 I20 **Jemeppe-sur-Sambre** Namur, S Belgium
37 R10 **Jemez Pueblo** New Mexico, SW USA
158 K2 **Jeminay** Xinjiang Uygur Zizhiqu, NW China
189 U5 **Jemo Island** *atoll* Ratak Chain, C Marshall Islands
169 U11 **Jempang, Danau** ◎ Borneo, N Indonesia
101 L16 **Jena** Thüringen, C Germany
22 I6 **Jena** Louisiana, S USA
108 I8 **Jenaz** Graubünden, SE Switzerland
109 N7 **Jenbach** Tirol, W Austria
171 N15 **Jeneponto** *prev.* Djeneponto. Sulawesi, C Indonesia
138 F9 **Jenīn** N West Bank
21 P7 **Jenkins** Kentucky, S USA
27 P9 **Jenks** Oklahoma, C USA
Jenné *see* Djenné
109 X8 **Jennersdorf** Burgenland, SE Austria
22 H9 **Jennings** Louisiana, S USA
9 N7 **Jenny Lind Island** *island* Nunavut, N Canada
23 Y13 **Jensen Beach** Florida, SE USA
9 P6 **Jens Munk Island** *island* Nunavut, NE Canada
59 O17 **Jequié** Bahia, E Brazil
59 O18 **Jequitinhonha, Rio** ≈ E Brazil
Jerablus *see* Jarābulus
74 H6 **Jerada** NE Morocco
Jerash *see* Jarash
75 N7 **Jerba, Île de** *var.* Djerba, Jazīrat Jarbah. *island* E Tunisia
44 K9 **Jérémie** SW Haiti
Jerez *see* Jeréz de la Frontera, Spain
Jeréz *see* Jerez de García Salinas, Mexico
40 L11 **Jerez de García Salinas** *var.* Jeréz. Zacatecas, C Mexico
104 J15 **Jeréz de la Frontera** *var.* Jerez; *prev.* Xeres. Andalucía, SW Spain
104 I12 **Jeréz de los Caballeros** Extremadura, W Spain
Jergucati *see* Jorgucat
138 G10 **Jericho** *Ar.* Arīḩā, *Heb.* Yeriḩo. E West Bank
74 M7 **Jerid, Chott el** *var.* Shaţţ al Jarīd. *salt lake* SW Tunisia
183 O10 **Jerilderie** New South Wales, SE Australia
Jerischmarkt *see* Câmpia Turzii
92 K11 **Jerisjärvi** ◎ NW Finland
Jermentau *see* Yereymentau
Jermer *see* Jaroměř
36 K11 **Jerome** Arizona, SW USA
33 O15 **Jerome** Idaho, NW USA
97 L26 **Jersey** *island* Channel Islands, NW Europe
18 K14 **Jersey City** New Jersey, NE USA
18 F13 **Jersey Shore** Pennsylvania, NE USA
30 K14 **Jerseyville** Illinois, N USA
104 K8 **Jerte** ≈ W Spain
138 F10 **Jerusalem** *Ar.* Al Quds, Al Quds ash Sharīf, *Heb.* Yerushalayim; *anc.* Hierosolyma. ● (Israel) Jerusalem, NE Israel
138 G10 **Jerusalem** ◈ *district* E Israel
183 S10 **Jervis Bay** New South Wales, SE Australia
183 S10 **Jervis Bay Territory** ◈ *territory* SE Australia
Jerwakant *see* Järvakandi
109 S10 **Jesenice** *Ger.* Assling. NW Slovenia
111 H16 **Jeseník** *Ger.* Freiwaldau. Olomoucký Kraj, E Czech Republic
Jesi *see* Iesi
106 I8 **Jesolo** *var.* Iesolo. Veneto, NE Italy
Jesselton *see* Kota Kinabalu
95 I14 **Jessheim** Akershus, S Norway
153 T15 **Jessore** Khulna, W Bangladesh
23 W6 **Jesup** Georgia, SE USA
41 S15 **Jesús Carranza** Veracruz-Llave, SE Mexico
62 K10 **Jesús María** Córdoba, C Argentina
26 K6 **Jetmore** Kansas, C USA
103 Q2 **Jeumont** Nord, N France
95 H14 **Jevnaker** Oppland, S Norway
Jewe *see* Jõhvi
25 V9 **Jewett** Texas, SW USA
19 N12 **Jewett City** Connecticut, NE USA
Jewish Autonomous Oblast *see* Yevreyskaya Avtonomnaya Oblast'
Jeypore/Jeypur *see* Jaypur, Orissa, India
Jeypore *see* Jaipur, Rājasthān, India
113 L17 **Jezercës, Maja e** ▲ N Albania
111 B18 **Jezerní Hora** ▲ SW Czech Republic
154 F10 **Jhābua** Madhya Pradesh, C India
152 H14 **Jhālāwār** Rājasthān, N India
Jhang/Jhang Sadar *see* Jhang Sadr
149 U9 **Jhang Sadr** *var.* Jhang, Jhang Sadar. Punjab, NE Pakistan
152 J13 **Jhānsi** Uttar Pradesh, N India
154 M11 **Jhārsuguda** Orissa, E India
149 V7 **Jhelum** Punjab, NE Pakistan
131 P9 **Jhelum** ≈ E Pakistan
Jhenaidaha *see* Jhenida
153 T15 **Jhenida** *var.* Jhenaidaha. Dhaka, W Bangladesh
149 P16 **Jhimpīr** Sind, SE Pakistan
Jhind *see* Jīnd
149 R16 **Jhudo** Sind, SE Pakistan
Jhumra *see* Chak Jhumra
152 H11 **Jhunjhunūn** Rājasthān, N India
Ji *see* Hebei, China
Ji *see* Jilin, China
153 S14 **Jiāganj** West Bengal, NE India
160 J7 **Jialing Jiang** ≈ C China
163 Y7 **Jiamusi** *var.* Chia-mu-ssu, Kiamusze. Heilongjiang, NE China
161 O11 **Ji'an** Jiangxi, S China
163 W12 **Ji'an** Jilin, NE China
163 T13 **Jianchang** Liaoning, NE China
160 F11 **Jianchuan** Yunnan, SW China
158 M4 **Jiangjunmiao** Xinjiang Uygur Zizhiqu, W China
160 K11 **Jiangkou** Guizhou, S China
161 Q12 **Jiangle** Fujian, SE China
161 N15 **Jiangmen** Guangdong, S China
161 Q10 **Jiangshan** Zhejiang, SE China
161 Q7 **Jiangsu** *var.* Chiang-su, Jiangsu Sheng, Kiangsu, Su. ◈ *province* E China
Jiangsu Sheng *see* Jiangsu
161 O11 **Jiangxi** *var.* Chiang-hsi, Gan, Jiangxi Sheng, Kiangsi. ◈ *province* S China
Jiangxi Sheng *see* Jiangxi
160 I8 **Jiangyou** *prev.* Zhongba. Sichuan, C China
161 N9 **Jianli** Hubei, C China
161 Q11 **Jian'ou** Fujian, SE China
163 S12 **Jianping** Liaoning, NE China
160 L9 **Jianshi** Hubei, C China
131 V11 **Jian Xi** ≈ SE China
161 Q11 **Jianyang** Fujian, SE China
160 I9 **Jianyang** Sichuan, C China
163 X10 **Jiaohe** Jilin, NE China
Jiaojiang *see* Taizhou
161 N6 **Jiaozuo** Henan, C China
Jiashan *see* Mingguang
158 F8 **Jiashi** *var.* Payzawat. Xinjiang Uygur Zizhiqu, NW China
154 L9 **Jiāwān** Madhya Pradesh, C India
161 S9 **Jiaxing** Zhejiang, SE China
Jiayi *see* Chiai
163 X6 **Jiayin** *var.* Chaoyang. Heilongjiang, NE China
159 R8 **Jiayuguan** Gansu, N China
138 M4 **Jibli** Ar Raqqah, C Syria
116 H9 **Jibou** *Hung.* Zsibó. Sălaj, NW Romania
141 Z9 **Jibsh, Ra's al** *headland* E Oman
Jibuti *see* Djibouti
111 E15 **Jičín** *Ger.* Jitschin. Hradecký Kraj, N Czech Republic
140 K10 **Jiddah** *Eng.* Jedda. Makkah, W Saudi Arabia
141 W11 **Jiddat al Ḩarāsīs** *desert* C Oman
Jiesjavrre *see* Iešjávri
160 M4 **Jiexiu** Shanxi, C China
161 P14 **Jieyang** Guangdong, S China
119 F14 **Jieznas** Prienai, S Lithuania
Jifa', Bi'r *see* Jif'iyah, Bi'r
141 P15 **Jif'iyah, Bi'r** *var.* Bi'r Jifa'. *well* C Yemen
77 W13 **Jigawa** ◈ *state* N Nigeria
Jigerbent *see* Dzhigirbent
44 I7 **Jiguaní** Granma, E Cuba
159 T12 **Jigzhi** Qinghai, C China
Jih-k'a-tse *see* Xigazê
111 E18 **Jihlava** *Ger.* Iglau, *Pol.* Igława. Jihlavský Kraj, C Czech Republic
111 E18 **Jihlava** *var.* Igel, *Ger.* Iglawa. ≈ S Czech Republic
111 E18 **Jihlavský kraj** ◈ *region* C Czech Republic
74 L5 **Jijel** *var.* Djidjel; *prev.* Djidjelli. NE Algeria
116 L9 **Jijia** ≈ N Romania
80 L13 **Jijiga** *It.* Giggiga. Somali, E Ethiopia
105 S12 **Jijona** *var.* Xixona. País Valenciano, E Spain
Jilf al Kabīr, Haḑabat al *see* Gilf Kebir Plateau
81 L18 **Jilib** *It.* Gelib. Jubbada Dhexe, S Somalia
163 W10 **Jilin** *var.* Chi-lin, Girin, Kirin; *prev.* Yungki, Yunki. Jilin, NE China
163 W10 **Jilin** *var.* Chi-lin, Girin, Ji, Jilin Sheng, Kirin. ◈ *province* NE China
163 W11 **Jilin Hada Ling** ▲ NE China
Jilin Sheng *see* Jilin
163 W8 **Jiliu He** ≈ NE China
105 Q6 **Jiloca** ≈ N Spain
81 I14 **Jīma** *var.* Jimma, *It.* Gimma. Oromo, C Ethiopia
44 M9 **Jimaní** W Dominican Republic
116 E11 **Jimbolia** *Ger.* Hatzfeld, *Hung.* Zsombolya. Timiş, W Romania
104 K16 **Jimena de la Frontera** Andalucía, S Spain
40 K7 **Jiménez** Chihuahua, N Mexico
41 N5 **Jiménez** Coahuila de Zaragoza, NE Mexico
41 P9 **Jiménez** *var.* Santander Jiménez. Tamaulipas, C Mexico
40 L10 **Jiménez del Teul** Zacatecas, C Mexico
77 Y14 **Jimeta** Adamawa, E Nigeria
Jimma *see* Jīma
158 M5 **Jimsar** Xinjiang Uygur Zizhiqu, NW China
18 I14 **Jim Thorpe** Pennsylvania, NE USA
Jin *see* Shanxi, China
Jin *see* Tianjin Shi, China
161 P5 **Jinan** *var.* Chinan, Chi-nan, Tsinan. Shandong, E China
159 T8 **Jinchang** Gansu, N China
161 N5 **Jincheng** Shanxi, C China
Jinchengjiang *see* Hechi
152 I9 **Jīnd** *prev.* Jhind. Haryāna, NW India
183 Q11 **Jindabyne** New South Wales, SE Australia
111 O18 **Jindřichův Hradec** *Ger.* Neuhaus. Budějovický Kraj, S Czech Republic
Jing *see* Beijing Shi, China
Jing *see* Jinghe, China
159 X10 **Jingchuan** Gansu, C China
161 Q10 **Jingdezhen** Jiangxi, S China
161 O12 **Jinggangshan** Jiangxi, S China
161 P3 **Jinghai** Tianjin Shi, E China
160 K6 **Jing He** ≈ C China
158 I4 **Jinghe** *var.* Jing. Xinjiang Uygur Zizhiqu, NW China
160 F15 **Jinghong** *var.* Yunjinghong. Yunnan, SW China
160 M9 **Jingmen** Hubei, C China
163 X10 **Jingpo Hu** ◎ NE China
160 M8 **Jing Shan** ▲ C China
159 V9 **Jingtai** *var.* Yitiaoshan. Gansu, C China
160 J14 **Jingxi** Guangxi Zhuangzu Zizhiqu, S China
Jing Xian *see* Jingzhou
163 W11 **Jingyu** Jilin, NE China
159 V10 **Jingyuan** Gansu, C China
160 L12 **Jingzhou** *var.* Jing Xian. Hunan, S China
160 M9 **Jingzhou** *prev.* Shahi, Shashih, Shasi. Hubei, C China
161 R10 **Jinhua** Zhejiang, SE China
163 P13 **Jining** Nei Mongol Zizhiqu, N China
161 P5 **Jining** Shandong, E China
81 G18 **Jinja** S Uganda
161 O11 **Jin Jiang** ≈ S China
161 R13 **Jinjiang** *var.* Qingyang. Fujian, SE China
171 V15 **Jin, Kepulauan** *island group* E Indonesia
Jinmen Dao *see* Chinmen Tao
42 J9 **Jinotega** Jinotega, NW Nicaragua
42 K7 **Jinotega** ◈ *department* N Nicaragua
42 J11 **Jinotepe** Carazo, SW Nicaragua
160 L13 **Jinping** *prev.* Sanjiang. Guizhou, S China
160 H14 **Jinping** Yunnan, SW China
Jinsen *see* Inch'ŏn
160 J11 **Jinsha** Guizhou, S China
157 N12 **Jinsha Jiang** ≈ SW China
160 M10 **Jinshi** Hunan, S China
159 R7 **Jinta** Gansu, N China
161 Q12 **Jin Xi** ≈ SE China
Jinxi *see* Lianshan
Jinxian *see* Jinzhou
161 P6 **Jinxiang** Shandong, E China
161 P8 **Jinzhai** *prev.* Meishan. Anhui, E China
163 U14 **Jinzhou** *prev.* Jinxian. Liaoning, NE China
163 T12 **Jinzhou** *var.* Chin-chou, Chinchow; *prev.* Chinhsien. Liaoning, NE China
138 H12 **Jinz, Qā' al** ◎ C Jordan
47 S8 **Jiparaná, Rio** ≈ W Brazil
56 A7 **Jipijapa** Manabí, W Ecuador
42 F8 **Jiquilisco** Usulután, S El Salvador
147 S12 **Jirgatol** *Rus.* Dzhirgatal'. C Tajikistan
Jirjā *see* Girga
111 B15 **Jirkov** *Ger.* Görkau. Ústecký Kraj, NW Czech Republic
Jiroft *see* Sabzvārān
160 L11 **Jishou** Hunan, S China
Jisr ash Shadadi *see* Ash Shadādah
116 I14 **Jitaru** Olt, S Romania
Jitschin *see* Jičín
116 H14 **Jiu** *Ger.* Schil, Schyl, *Hung.* Zsil, Zsily. ≈ S Romania
161 R11 **Jiufeng Shan** ▲ SE China
161 P9 **Jiujiang** Jiangxi, S China
161 O10 **Jiuling Shan** ▲ S China
160 G10 **Jiulong** Sichuan, C China
161 Q13 **Jiulong Jiang** ≈ SE China
161 Q12 **Jiulong Xi** ≈ SE China
159 R8 **Jiuquan** Gansu, N China
160 K17 **Jiusuo** Hainan, S China
163 W10 **Jiutai** Jilin, NE China
160 K13 **Jiuwan Dashan** ▲ S China
148 I16 **Jiwani** Baluchistān, SW Pakistan
163 Y8 **Jixi** Heilongjiang, NE China
163 Y7 **Jixian** Heilongjiang, NE China
160 M5 **Jixian** *var.* Ji Xian. Shanxi, C China
Jiza *see* Al Jīzah
141 N13 **Jīzān** *var.* Qīzān. Jīzān, SW Saudi Arabia
141 N13 **Jīzān** *var.* Minţaqat Jīzān. ◈ *province* SW Saudi Arabia
140 K6 **Jizl, Wādī al** *dry watercourse* W Saudi Arabia
164 H12 **Jizō-zaki** *headland* Honshū, SW Japan
141 U14 **Jiz', Wādī al** *dry watercourse* E Yemen
147 O11 **Jizzakh** *Rus.* Dzhizak. Jizzakh Wiloyati, C Uzbekistan
147 N10 **Jizzakh Wiloyati** *Rus.* Dzhizakskaya Oblast'. ◈ *province* C Uzbekistan
60 I13 **Joaçaba** Santa Catarina, S Brazil
Joal *see* Joal-Fadiout
76 F11 **Joal-Fadiout** *prev.* Joal. W Senegal
76 E10 **João Barrosa** Boa Vista, E Cape Verde
João Belo *see* Xai-Xai
João de Almeida *see* Chibia
59 Q15 **João Pessoa** *prev.* Paraíba. *state capital* Paraíba, E Brazil
25 X7 **Joaquin** Texas, SW USA
62 K6 **Joaquín V.González** Salta, N Argentina
Joazeiro *see* Juazeiro
Jo'burg *see* Johannesburg
109 O7 **Jochberger Ache** ≈ W Austria
Jo-ch'iang *see* Ruoqiang
92 K12 **Jock** Norrbotten, N Sweden
42 I5 **Jocón** Yoro, N Honduras
105 O13 **Jódar** Andalucía, S Spain
152 F12 **Jodhpur** Rājasthān, NW India
99 I19 **Jodoigne** Wallon Brabant, C Belgium
95 I22 **Jægerspris** Frederiksborg, E Denmark
93 O16 **Joensuu** Itä-Suomi, E Finland
95 C17 **Jæren** *physical region* S Norway
37 W4 **Joes** Colorado, C USA
191 Z3 **Joe's Hill** *hill* Kiritimati, NE Kiribati
165 N11 **Jōetsu** *var.* Zyôetu. Niigata, Honshū, C Japan
83 M18 **Jofane** Inhambane, S Mozambique
153 R12 **Jogbani** Bihār, NE India
118 I5 **Jõgeva** *Ger.* Laisholm. Jõgevamaa, E Estonia
118 I4 **Jõgevamaa** *off.* Jõgeva Maakond. ◈ *province* E Estonia
155 E18 **Jog Falls** *waterfall* Karnātaka, W India
143 S4 **Joghatāy** Khorāsān, NE Iran
153 U12 **Jogīghopa** Assam, NE India
152 I7 **Jogindarnagar** Himāchal Pradesh, N India
Jogjakarta *see* Yogyakarta
164 L11 **Jōhana** Toyama, Honshū, SW Japan
83 J21 **Johannesburg** *var.* Egoli, Erautini, Gauteng, *abbrev.* Jo'burg. Gauteng, NE South Africa
35 T13 **Johannesburg** California, W USA
83 I21 **Johannesburg** × Gauteng, NE South Africa
Johannisburg *see* Pisz
149 P14 **Johi** Sind, SE Pakistan
55 T13 **Johi Village** S Guyana
32 K13 **John Day** Oregon, NW USA
32 I11 **John Day River** ≈ Oregon, NW USA
18 L14 **John F Kennedy** × (New York) Long Island, New York, NE USA
21 V8 **John H.Kerr Reservoir** *var.* Buggs Island Lake, Kerr Lake. ⊡ North Carolina/Virginia, SE USA
37 V6 **John Martin Reservoir** ⊡ Colorado, C USA
96 K6 **John o'Groats** N Scotland, UK
27 P5 **John Redmond Reservoir** ⊡ Kansas, C USA
39 Q7 **John River** ≈ Alaska, USA
26 H6 **Johnson** Kansas, C USA
18 M7 **Johnson** Vermont, NE USA
18 D13 **Johnsonburg** Pennsylvania, NE USA
18 H11 **Johnson City** New York, NE USA
21 P8 **Johnson City** Tennessee, S USA
25 R10 **Johnson City** Texas, SW USA
35 S12 **Johnsondale** California, W USA
10 I8 **Johnsons Crossing** Yukon Territory, W Canada
21 T13 **Johnsonville** South Carolina, SE USA
21 Q13 **Johnston** South Carolina, SE USA
192 M6 **Johnston Atoll** ◇ *US unincorporated territory* C Pacific Ocean
175 Q3 **Johnston Atoll** *atoll* C Pacific Ocean
30 L17 **Johnston City** Illinois, N USA
180 K12 **Johnston, Lake** *salt lake* Western Australia
31 S13 **Johnstown** Ohio, N USA
18 D15 **Johnstown** Pennsylvania, NE USA
168 L10 **Johor** *var.* Johore. ◈ *state* Peninsular Malaysia
Johor Baharu *see* Johor Bahru
168 K10 **Johor Bahru** *var.* Johor Baharu, Johore Bahru. Johor, Peninsular Malaysia
Johore *see* Johor
Johore Bahru *see* Johor Bahru
118 K3 **Jõhvi** *Ger.* Jewe. Ida-Virumaa, NE Estonia
103 P7 **Joigny** Yonne, C France
Joinvile *see* Joinville
60 K12 **Joinville** *var.* Joinvile. Santa Catarina, S Brazil
103 R6 **Joinville** Haute-Marne, N France
194 H3 **Joinville Island** *island* Antarctica
41 O15 **Jojutla** *var.* Jojutla de Juárez. Morelos, S Mexico
Jojutla de Juárez *see* Jojutla
92 I12 **Jokkmokk** Norrbotten, N Sweden
92 L2 **Jökulsá á Dal** ≈ E Iceland
92 K2 **Jökulsá á Fjöllum** ≈ NE Iceland
Jokyakarta *see* Yogyakarta
30 M11 **Joliet** Illinois, N USA
15 O11 **Joliette** Quebec, SE Canada
171 O8 **Jolo** Jolo Island, SW Philippines
94 D11 **Jølstervatnet** ◎ S Norway
169 S16 **Jombang** *prev.* Djombang. Jawa, S Indonesia
159 R14 **Jomda** Xizang Zizhiqu, W China
56 A6 **Jome, Punta de** *headland* W Ecuador
118 G13 **Jonava** *Ger.* Janow, *Pol.* Janów. Jonava, C Lithuania
146 L11 **Jondor** *Rus.* Zhondor. Bukhoro Wiloyati, C Uzbekistan
159 V11 **Jonê** Gansu, C China
27 X9 **Jonesboro** Arkansas, C USA
23 S4 **Jonesboro** Georgia, SE USA
30 L17 **Jonesboro** Illinois, N USA
22 H5 **Jonesboro** Louisiana, S USA
21 P8 **Jonesboro** Tennessee, S USA
19 T6 **Jonesport** Maine, NE USA
9 N4 **Jones Sound** *channel* Nunavut, N Canada
22 I6 **Jonesville** Louisiana, S USA
31 Q10 **Jonesville** Michigan, N USA
21 Q11 **Jonesville** South Carolina, SE USA
81 F14 **Jonglei** Jonglei, SE Sudan
81 F14 **Jonglei** *var.* Gongoleh State. ◈ *state* SE Sudan
81 F14 **Jonglei Canal** *canal* S Sudan
118 F11 **Joniškėlis** Pasvalys, N Lithuania
118 F10 **Joniškis** *Ger.* Janischken. Joniškis, N Lithuania
95 L19 **Jönköping** Jönköping, S Sweden
95 K20 **Jönköping** ◈ *county* S Sweden
15 Q7 **Jonquière** Quebec, SE Canada
41 V15 **Jonuta** Tabasco, SE Mexico
102 K12 **Jonzac** Charente-Maritime, W France
27 R7 **Joplin** Missouri, C USA
33 W8 **Jordan** Montana, NW USA
147 S11 **Jordan** *var.* Iordan, *Rus.* Jardan. Farghona Wiloyati, E Uzbekistan
138 H12 **Jordan** *off.* Hashemite Kingdom of Jordan, *Ar.* Al Mamlakah al Urdunīyah al Hāshimīyah, Al Urdunn; *prev.* Transjordan. ◆ *monarchy* SW Asia
138 G9 **Jordan** *Ar.* Urdunn, *Heb.* HaYarden. ≈ SW Asia
Jordan Lake *see* B.Everett Jordan Reservoir
111 K17 **Jordanów** Małopolskie, S Poland
32 M15 **Jordan Valley** Oregon, NW USA
138 G9 **Jordan Valley** *valley* N Israel
57 D15 **Jorge Chávez International** *var.* Lima. × (Lima) Lima, W Peru
113 L23 **Jorgucat** *var.* Jergucati, Jorgucati. Gjirokastër, S Albania
Jorgucati *see* Jorgucat
153 X12 **Jorhāt** Assam, NE India
93 J14 **Jörn** Västerbotten, N Sweden
37 R14 **Jornada Del Muerto** *valley* New Mexico, SW USA
93 N17 **Joroinen** Isä-Suomi, E Finland
95 C16 **Jørpeland** Rogaland, S Norway
77 W14 **Jos** Plateau, C Nigeria
171 Q8 **Jose Abad Santos** *var.* Trinidad. Mindanao, S Philippines
61 F19 **José Batlle y Ordóñez** *var.* Batlle y Ordóñez. Florida, C Uruguay
63 H18 **José de San Martín** Chubut, S Argentina
61 E19 **José Enrique Rodó** *var.* Rodó, José E.Rodo; *prev.* Drabble, Drable. Soriano, SW Uruguay
José E.Rodo *see* José Enrique Rodó
Josefsdorf *see* Žabalj
44 C4 **José Martí** × (La Habana) Cuidad de La Habana, N Cuba
61 F19 **José Pedro Varela** *var.* José P.Varela. Lavalleja, S Uruguay
181 N2 **Joseph Bonaparte Gulf** *gulf* N Australia
37 N11 **Joseph City** Arizona, SW USA
13 O9 **Joseph, Lake** ◎ Newfoundland, E Canada
14 G13 **Joseph, Lake** ◎ Ontario, S Canada
186 C6 **Josephstaal** Madang, N PNG
José P.Varela *see* José Pedro Varela
59 J14 **José Rodrigues** Pará, N Brazil
152 K9 **Joshīmath** Uttar Pradesh, N India
25 T7 **Joshua** Texas, SW USA
35 V15 **Joshua Tree** California, W USA
77 V14 **Jos Plateau** *plateau* C Nigeria
102 H6 **Josselin** Morbihan, NW France
Jos Sudarso *see* Yos Sudarso, Pulau
94 E11 **Jostedalsbreen** *glacier* S Norway
94 F12 **Jotunheimen** ▲ S Norway
138 G7 **Joûnié** *var.* Juniyah. W Lebanon
25 R13 **Jourdanton** Texas, SW USA
98 L7 **Joure** *Fris.* De Jouwer. Friesland, N Netherlands
93 M18 **Joutsa** Länsi-Suomi, W Finland
93 N18 **Joutseno** Etelä-Suomi, S Finland
92 M12 **Joutsijärvi** Lappi, NE Finland
108 A9 **Joux, Lac de** ◎ W Switzerland
44 D5 **Jovellanos** Matanzas, W Cuba
153 V13 **Jowai** Meghālaya, NE India
Jowat *see* Jabwot
Jowhar *see* Jawhar
143 O12 **Jowkān** Fārs, S Iran
143 Q10 **Jowzam** Kermān, C Iran
149 N2 **Jowzjān** ◈ *province* N Afghanistan
Józseffalva *see* Žabalj
J.Storm Thurmond Reservoir *see* Clark Hill Lake
45 T6 **Juana Díaz** C Puerto Rico
40 L9 **Juan Aldama** Zacatecas, C Mexico
(0) E9 **Juan de Fuca Plate** *tectonic feature*
32 F7 **Juan de Fuca, Strait of** *strait* Canada/USA
Juan Fernandez Islands *see* Juan Fernández, Islas
193 S11 **Juan Fernández, Islas** *Eng.* Juan Fernandez Islands. *island group* W Chile
55 O4 **Juangriego** Nueva Esparta, NE Venezuela
56 D11 **Juanjuí** *var.* Juanjuy. San Martín, N Peru
Juanjuy *see* Juanjuí
93 N16 **Juankoski** Itä-Suomi, C Finland
Juan Lacaze *see* Juan L.Lacaze
61 E20 **Juan L.Lacaze** *var.* Juan Lacaze, Puerto Sauce; *prev.* Sauce. Colonia, SW Uruguay
62 L5 **Juan Solá** Salta, N Argentina
63 F21 **Juan Stuven, Isla** *island* S Chile
59 H16 **Juará** Mato Grosso, W Brazil
41 N7 **Juárez** *var.* Villa Juárez. Coahuila de Zaragoza, NE Mexico
40 C2 **Juárez, Sierra de** ▲ NW Mexico
59 O15 **Juazeiro** *prev.* Joazeiro. Bahia, E Brazil
59 P14 **Juazeiro do Norte** Ceará, E Brazil
81 F15 **Juba** *var.* Jūbā. Bahr el Gabel, S Sudan
81 L17 **Juba** *Amh.* Genalē Wenz, *It.* Guiba, *Som.* Ganaane, Webi Jubba. ≈ Ethiopia/Somalia
194 H2 **Jubany** *Argentinian research station* Antarctica
Jubayl *see* Jbail
81 L18 **Jubbada Dhexe** *off.* Gobolka Jubbada Dhexe. ◈ *region* SW Somalia
81 K18 **Jubbada Hoose** ◈ *region* SW Somalia
Jubba, Webi *see* Juba
Jubbulpore *see* Jabalpur
Jubeil *see* Jbail
74 B9 **Juby, Cap** *headland* SW Morocco
105 R10 **Júcar** *var.* Jucar. ≈ C Spain
40 L12 **Juchipila** Zacatecas, C Mexico
41 S16 **Juchitán** *var.* Juchitán de Zaragosa. Oaxaca, SE Mexico
Juchitán de Zaragosa *see* Juchitán
138 G11 **Judaea** *cultural region* Israel/West Bank
138 F11 **Judaean Hills** *Heb.* Haré Yehuda. *hill range* E Israel
138 H8 **Judaydah** *Fr.* Jdaïdé. Dimashq, W Syria
139 P11 **Judayyidat Hāmir** S Iraq
109 U8 **Judenburg** Steiermark, C Austria
27 V11 **Judith River** ≈ Montana, NW USA
27 V11 **Judsonia** Arkansas, C USA
141 P14 **Jufrah, Wādī al** *dry watercourse* NW Yemen
Jugoslavija/Jugoslavija, Savezna Republika *see* Serbia and Montenegro
42 K10 **Juigalpa** Chontales, S Nicaragua
161 T13 **Juishui** C Taiwan
100 E9 **Juist** *island* NW Germany
59 M21 **Juiz de Fora** Minas Gerais, SE Brazil
62 J5 **Jujuy** *off.* Provincia de Jujuy. ◈ *province* N Argentina
Jujuy *see* San Salvador de Jujuy
92 J11 **Jukkasjärvi** Norrbotten, N Sweden
Jula *see* Gyula, Hungary
Jūlā *see* Jālū, Libya
37 W2 **Julesburg** Colorado, C USA
Julia Beterrae *see* Béziers
57 I17 **Juliaca** Puno, SE Peru
181 U6 **Julia Creek** Queensland, C Australia
35 V17 **Julian** California, W USA
98 H7 **Julianadorp** Noord-Holland, NW Netherlands
109 S11 **Julian Alps** *Ger.* Julische Alpen, *It.* Alpi Giulie, *Slvn.* Julijske Alpe. ▲ Italy/Slovenia
55 V11 **Juliana Top** ▲ C Surinam
Julianehåb *see* Qaqortoq
Julijske Alpe *see* Julian Alps
40 J6 **Julimes** Chihuahua, N Mexico
Julio Briga *see* Bragança, Portugal
Juliobriga *see* Logroño, Spain
61 G15 **Júlio de Castilhos** Rio Grande do Sul, S Brazil
Juliomagus *see* Angers
Julische Alpen *see* Julian Alps
Jullundur *see* Jalandhar
147 N11 **Juma** *Rus.* Dzhuma. Samarqand Wiloyati, C Uzbekistan
161 O3 **Juma He** ≈ E China
81 L18 **Jumboo** Jubbada Hoose, S Somalia
35 Y11 **Jumbo Peak** ▲ Nevada, W USA
105 R12 **Jumilla** Murcia, SE Spain
153 N10 **Jumla** Mid Western, NW Nepal
Jummoo *see* Jammu
Jumna *see* Yamuna
Jumporn *see* Chumphon
30 K5 **Jump River** ≈ Wisconsin, N USA
154 B11 **Jūnāgadh** *var.* Junagarh. Gujarāt, W India
Junagarh *see* Jūnāgadh
161 Q6 **Junan** *prev.* Shizilu. Shandong, E China
62 G11 **Juncal, Cerro** ▲ C Chile
25 Q10 **Junction** Texas, SW USA
36 K6 **Junction** Utah, W USA
27 O4 **Junction City** Kansas, C USA
32 F13 **Junction City** Oregon, NW USA
60 M10 **Jundiaí** São Paulo, S Brazil
39 X12 **Juneau** *state capital* Alaska, USA
30 M8 **Juneau** Wisconsin, N USA
105 U6 **Juneda** Cataluña, NE Spain
183 Q9 **Junee** New South Wales, SE Australia
35 R8 **June Lake** California, W USA
Jungbunzlau *see* Mladá Boleslav
158 L4 **Junggar Pendi** *Eng.* Dzungarian Basin. *basin* NW China
99 N24 **Junglinster** Grevenmacher, C Luxembourg
18 F14 **Juniata River** ≈ Pennsylvania, NE USA
61 B20 **Junín** Buenos Aires, E Argentina
57 E14 **Junín** Junín, C Peru
57 F14 **Junín** *off.* Departamento de Junín. ◈ *department* C Peru
63 H15 **Junín de los Andes** Neuquén, W Argentina
57 D14 **Junín, Lago de** ◎ C Peru
Juniyah *see* Joûnié
Junkseylon *see* Phuket
160 I11 **Junlian** Sichuan, C China
25 O11 **Juno** Texas, SW USA
92 J11 **Junosuando** Norrbotten, N Sweden
93 H16 **Junsele** Västernorrland, C Sweden
Junten *see* Sunch'ŏn
32 L14 **Juntura** Oregon, NW USA
93 N14 **Juntusranta** Oulu, E Finland
118 H11 **Juodupė** Rokiškis, NE Lithuania
119 H14 **Juozapinės Kalnas** ▲ SE Lithuania
99 K19 **Juprelle** Liège, E Belgium
80 D13 **Jur** ≈ C Sudan
103 S9 **Jura** ◈ *department* E France
108 C7 **Jura** ◈ *canton* NW Switzerland
108 B8 **Jura** *var.* Jura Mountains. ▲ France/Switzerland
96 G12 **Jura** *island* SW Scotland, UK
Juraciszki *see* Yuratsishki
54 C8 **Juradó** Chocó, NW Colombia
Jura Mountains *see* Jura
96 G12 **Jura, Sound of** *strait* W Scotland, UK
139 V15 **Jurayblyāt, Bi'r** *well* S Iraq
118 E13 **Jurbarkas** *Ger.* Georgenburg, Jurburg. Jurbarkas, W Lithuania
99 F20 **Jurbise** Hainaut, SW Belgium
Jurburg *see* Jurbarkas
118 F9 **Jūrmala** Riga, C Latvia
58 D13 **Juruá** Amazonas, NW Brazil

◆ Country ● Country Capital ◇ Dependent Territory ○ Dependent Territory Capital ◈ Administrative Region × International Airport ▲ Mountain ▲ Mountain Range ⛰ Volcano ≈ River ◎ Lake ⊡ Reservoir

48 F7 **Juruá, Rio** *var.* Río Yuruá. ≈ Brazil/Peru
59 G16 **Juruena** Mato Grosso, W Brazil
59 G16 **Juruena** ≈ W Brazil
165 Q6 **Jūsan-ko** ◎ Honshū, C Japan
25 O6 **Justiceburg** Texas, SW USA
Justinianopolis *see* Kirşehir
62 K11 **Justo Daract** San Luis, C Argentina
59 C14 **Jutaí** Amazonas, W Brazil
58 C13 **Jutaí, Rio** ≈ NW Brazil
100 N13 **Jüterbog** Brandenburg, E Germany
42 E6 **Jutiapa** Jutiapa, S Guatemala
42 A3 **Jutiapa** *off.* Departamento de Jutiapa. ◈ *department* SE Guatemala
42 J6 **Juticalpa** Olancho, C Honduras
82 I13 **Jutila** North Western, NW Zambia
Jutland *see* Jylland
84 F8 **Jutland Bank** *undersea feature* SE North Sea
93 N16 **Juuka** Itä-Suomi, E Finland
93 N17 **Juva** Isä-Suomi, SE Finland
Juvavum *see* Salzburg
44 A6 **Juventud, Isla de la** *var.* Isla de Pinos, *Eng.* Isle of Youth; *prev.* The Isle of the Pines. *island* W Cuba
Ju Xian *see* Juxian
161 Q5 **Juxian** *var.* Ju Xian. Shandong, E China
161 P6 **Juye** Shandong, E China
113 O15 **Južna Morava** *Ger.* Südliche Morava. ≈ SE Yugoslavia
95 I23 **Jyderup** Vestsjælland, E Denmark
95 F22 **Jylland** *Eng.* Jutland. *peninsula* W Denmark
Jyrgalan *see* Dzhergalan
93 M17 **Jyväskylä** Länsi-Suomi, W Finland

K

155 X3 **K2** *Chin.* Qogir Feng, *Eng.* Mount Godwin Austen. ▲ China/Pakistan
38 D9 **Kaaawa** *Haw.* Ka'a'wa. Oahu, Hawaii, USA, C Pacific Ocean
81 G16 **Kaabong** NE Uganda
Kaaden *see* Kadaň
55 V9 **Kaaimanston** Sipaliwini, N Surinam
146 G14 **Kaakhka** *var.* Kaka. Akhalskiy Velayat, S Turkmenistan
Kaala *see* Caála
187 O16 **Kaala-Gomen** Province Nord, W New Caledonia
92 L9 **Kaamanen** *Lapp.* Gámas. Lappi, N Finland
Kaapstad *see* Cape Town
Kaarasjoki *see* Karasjok
Kaaresuanto *see* Karesuando
92 J10 **Kaaresuvanto** *Lapp.* Gárassavon. Lappi, N Finland
93 K19 **Kaarina** Länsi-Suomi, W Finland
99 I14 **Kaatsheuvel** Noord-Brabant, S Netherlands
93 N16 **Kaavi** Itä-Suomi, C Finland
Ka'a'wa *see* Kaaawa
Kaba *see* Habahe
171 O14 **Kabaena, Pulau** *island* C Indonesia
146 J11 **Kabakly** *Turkm.* Gabakly. Lebapskiy Velayat, NE Turkmenistan
76 J14 **Kabala** N Sierra Leone
81 E19 **Kabale** SW Uganda
55 U10 **Kabalebo Rivier** ≈ W Surinam
79 N22 **Kabalo** Katanga, SE Dem. Rep. Congo (Zaire)
145 W13 **Kabanbay** *Kaz.* Qabanbay *prev.* Andreyevka, *Kaz.* Andreevka. Almaty, SE Kazakhstan
79 O21 **Kabambare** Maniema, E Dem. Rep. Congo (Zaire)
187 Y15 **Kabara** *prev.* Kambara. *island* Lau Group, E Fiji
Kabardino-Balkaria *see* Kabardino-Balkarskaya Respublika
128 M15 **Kabardino-Balkarskaya Respublika** *Eng.* Kabardino-Balkaria. ◈ *autonomous republic* SW Russian Federation
79 O19 **Kabare** Sud Kivu, E Dem. Rep. Congo (Zaire)
171 T11 **Kabarei** Irian Jaya, E Indonesia
171 P7 **Kabasalan** Mindanao, S Philippines
77 U15 **Kabba** Kogi, S Nigeria
92 I13 **Kåbdalis** Norrbotten, N Sweden
138 M6 **Kabd aş Şārim** *hill range* E Syria
14 B7 **Kabenung Lake** ◎ Ontario, S Canada
29 W3 **Kabetogama Lake** ◎ Minnesota, N USA
Kabia, Pulau *see* Kabin, Pulau
79 M22 **Kabinda** Kasai Oriental, SE Dem. Rep. Congo (Zaire)
Kabinda *see* Cabinda
171 O15 **Kabin, Pulau** *var.* Pulau Kabia. *island* W Indonesia
171 P16 **Kabir** Pulau Pantar, S Indonesia
149 T10 **Kabīrwāla** Punjab, E Pakistan
78 I13 **Kabo** Ouham, NW Central African Republic
Kābol *see* Kābul
83 H14 **Kabompo** North Western, W Zambia
83 H14 **Kabompo** ≈ W Zambia
79 M22 **Kabongo** Katanga, SE Dem. Rep. Congo (Zaire)
120 K11 **Kaboudia, Rass** *headland* E Tunisia
126 J14 **Kabozha** Novgorodskaya Oblast', W Russian Federation
143 U4 **Kabūd Gonbad** Khorāsān, NE Iran
142 L5 **Kabūd Rāhang** Hamadān, W Iran
82 L12 **Kabuko** Northern, NE Zambia
149 Q5 **Kābul** *var.* Kabul, *Per.* Kābol. ● (Afghanistan) Kābul, E Afghanistan
149 Q5 **Kābul** *Eng.* Kabul, *Per.* Kābol. ◈ *province* E Afghanistan
149 Q5 **Kābul** × Kābul, E Afghanistan
149 R5 **Kabul** *var.* Daryā-ye Kābul. ≈ Afghanistan/Pakistan *see also* Kābul, Daryā-ye
149 S5 **Kābul, Daryā-ye** *var.* Kabul. ≈ Afghanistan/Pakistan *see also* Kabul
79 O25 **Kabunda** Katanga, SE Dem. Rep. Congo (Zaire)
171 R9 **Kaburuang, Pulau** *island* Kepulauan Talaud, N Indonesia
80 G8 **Kabushiya** River Nile, NE Sudan
83 J14 **Kabwe** Central, C Zambia
186 E7 **Kabwum** Morobe, C PNG
113 N17 **Kačanik** Serbia, S Yugoslavia
118 F13 **Kačerginė** Kaunas, C Lithuania
117 S13 **Kacha** Respublika Krym, S Ukraine
154 A10 **Kachchh, Gulf of** *var.* Gulf of Cutch, Gulf of Kutch. *gulf* W India
154 I11 **Kachchhīdhāna** Madhya Pradesh, C India
149 Q11 **Kachchh, Rann of** *var.* Rann of Kachh, Rann of Kutch. *salt marsh* India/Pakistan
39 Q13 **Kachemak Bay** *bay* Alaska, USA
Kachh, Rann of *see* Kachchh, Rann of
77 V14 **Kachia** Kaduna, C Nigeria
167 N2 **Kachin State** ◈ *state* N Myanmar
145 T7 **Kachiry** Pavlodar, NE Kazakhstan
137 Q11 **Kaçkar Dağları** ⛰ NE Turkey
155 C21 **Kadamatt Island** *island* Lakshadweep, India, N Indian Ocean
111 B15 **Kadaň** *Ger.* Kaaden.Ústecký Kraj, NW Czech Republic
167 N11 **Kadan Kyun** *prev.* King Island. *island* Mergui Archipelago, S Myanmar
187 X15 **Kadavu** *prev.* Kandavu. *island* S Fiji
187 X15 **Kadavu Passage** *channel* S Fiji
79 G16 **Kadéï** ≈ Cameroon/Central African Republic
Kadhimain *see* Al Kāẓimīyah
Kadijica *see* Kadiytsa
114 M13 **Kadıköy Barajı** ▣ NW Turkey
182 I8 **Kadina** South Australia
136 H15 **Kadınhanı** Konya, C Turkey
76 M14 **Kadiolo** Sikasso, S Mali
136 L16 **Kadirli** Osmaniye, S Turkey
114 G11 **Kadiytsa** *Mac.* Kadijica. ▲ Bulgaria/FYR Macedonia
28 L10 **Kadoka** South Dakota, N USA
129 N5 **Kadom** Ryazanskaya Oblast', W Russian Federation
83 K16 **Kadoma** *prev.* Gatooma. Mashonaland West, C Zimbabwe
80 E12 **Kadugli** Southern Kordofan, S Sudan
77 V14 **Kaduna** Kaduna, C Nigeria
77 V14 **Kaduna** ◈ *state* C Nigeria
77 V15 **Kaduna** ≈ N Nigeria
126 K14 **Kaduy** Vologodskaya Oblast', NW Russian Federation
154 E13 **Kadwa** ≈ W India
123 S9 **Kadykchan** Magadanskaya Oblast', E Russian Federation
Kadzharan *see* K'ajaran
127 T7 **Kadzherom** Respublika Komi, NW Russian Federation
147 X8 **Kadzhi-Say** *Kir.* Kajisay. Issyk-Kul'skaya Oblast', NE Kyrgyzstan
76 I10 **Kaédi** Gorgol, S Mauritania
78 G12 **Kaélé** Extrême-Nord, N Cameroon
38 C9 **Kaena Point** *headland* Oahu, Hawaii, USA, C Pacific Ocean
184 J2 **Kaeo** Northland, North Island, NZ
163 X14 **Kaesŏng** *var.* Kaesŏng-si. S North Korea
Kaesŏng-si *see* Kaesŏng
Kaewieng *see* Kavieng
79 L24 **Kafakumba** Katanga, S Dem. Rep. Congo (Zaire)
Kafan *see* Kapan
77 V14 **Kafanchan** Kaduna, C Nigeria
Kaffa *see* Feodosiya
76 G11 **Kaffrine** C Senegal
Kafiau *see* Kofiau, Pulau
115 I19 **Kafiréas, Akrotírio** *headland* Évvoia, C Greece
115 I19 **Kafiréos, Stenó** *strait* Évvoia/Kykládes, Greece, Aegean Sea
Kafirnigan *see* Kofarnihon
Kafo *see* Kafu
Kafr ash Shaykh/Kafrel Sheik *see* Kafr el Sheikh
75 W7 **Kafr el Sheikh** *var.* Kafr ash Shaykh, Kafrel Sheik. N Egypt
81 F17 **Kafu** *var.* Kafo. ≈ W Uganda
83 J15 **Kafue** Lusaka, SE Zambia
83 I14 **Kafue** ≈ C Zambia
67 T13 **Kafue Flats** *plain* C Zambia
164 K12 **Kaga** Ishikawa, Honshū, SW Japan
79 J14 **Kaga Bandoro** *prev.* Fort-Crampel. Nana-Grébizi, C Central African Republic
81 E18 **Kagadi** W Uganda
38 H17 **Kagalaska Island** *island* Aleutian Islands, Alaska, USA
Kagan *see* Kogon
Kaganovichabad *see* Kolkhozobod
Kagarlyk *see* Kaharlyk
164 H14 **Kagawa** *off.* Kagawa-ken. ◈ *prefecture* Shikoku, SW Japan
154 J13 **Kagaznagar** Andhra Pradesh, C India
93 J14 **Kåge** Västerbotten, N Sweden
81 E19 **Kagera** *var.* Ziwa Magharibi, *Eng.* West Lake. ◈ *region* NW Tanzania
81 E19 **Kagera** *var.* Akagera. ≈ Rwanda/Tanzania *see also* Akagera
76 L5 **Kâgheṭ** *var.* Karet. *physical region* N Mauritania
Kagi *see* Chiai
137 S12 **Kağızman** Kars, NE Turkey
188 I6 **Kagman Point** *headland* Saipan, S Northern Mariana Islands
164 C16 **Kagoshima** *var.* Kagosima. Kagoshima, Kyūshū, SW Japan
164 C16 **Kagoshima** *off.* Kagoshima-ken, *var.* Kagosima. ◈ *prefecture* Kyūshū, SW Japan
Kagosima *see* Kagoshima
Kagul *see* Cahul
Kagul, Ozero *see* Kahul, Ozero
38 B8 **Kahala Point** *headland* Kauai, Hawaii, USA, C Pacific Ocean
38 G12 **Kahaluu** *Haw.* Kahalu'u. Hawaii, USA, C Pacific Ocean
81 F21 **Kahama** Shinyanga, NW Tanzania
117 P5 **Kaharlyk** *Rus.* Kagarlyk. Kyyivs'ka Oblast', N Ukraine
169 T13 **Kahayan, Sungai** ≈ Borneo, C Indonesia
79 I22 **Kahemba** Bandundu, SW Dem. Rep. Congo (Zaire)
185 A23 **Kaherekoau Mountains** ⛰ South Island, NZ
143 W14 **Kahīrī** *var.* Kūhīrī. Sīstān va Balūchestān, SE Iran
101 L16 **Kahla** Thüringen, C Germany
101 G15 **Kahler Asten** ▲ W Germany
149 Q4 **Kahmard, Daryā-ye** *prev.* Darya-i-Surkhab. ≈ NE Afghanistan
143 T13 **Kahnūj** Kermān, SE Iran
27 V1 **Kahoka** Missouri, C USA
38 E10 **Kahoolawe** *island* Hawaii, USA, C Pacific Ocean
136 M16 **Kahramanmaraş** *var.* Kahraman Maraş, Maraş, Marash. Kahramanmaraş, S Turkey
136 L15 **Kahramanmaraş** *var.* Kahraman Maraş, Maraş, Marash. ◈ *province* C Turkey
Kahror/Kahror Pakka *see* Karor Pacca
137 N15 **Kâhta** Adıyaman, S Turkey
38 D8 **Kahuku** Oahu, Hawaii, USA, C Pacific Ocean
38 D8 **Kahuku Point** *headland* Oahu, Hawaii, USA, C Pacific Ocean
116 M12 **Kahul, Ozero** *var.* Lacul Cahul, *Rus.* Ozero Kagul. ◎ Moldova/Ukraine
143 V11 **Kahūrak** Sīstān va Balūchestān, SE Iran
184 G13 **Kahurangi Point** *headland* South Island, NZ
149 V6 **Kahūta** Punjab, E Pakistan
77 S14 **Kaiama** Kwara, W Nigeria
186 D7 **Kaiapit** Morobe, C PNG
185 I18 **Kaiapoi** Canterbury, South Island, NZ
36 K9 **Kaibab Plateau** *plain* Arizona, SW USA
171 U14 **Kai Besar, Pulau** *island* Kepulauan Kai, E Indonesia
36 L9 **Kaibito Plateau** *plain* Arizona, SW USA
158 K6 **Kaidu He** *var.* Karaxahar. ≈ NW China
55 S10 **Kaieteur Falls** *waterfall* C Guyana
161 O6 **Kaifeng** Henan, C China
184 J3 **Kaihu** Northland, North Island, NZ
171 U14 **Kai Kecil, Pulau** *island* Kepulauan Kai, E Indonesia
169 U16 **Kai, Kepulauan** *prev.* Kei Islands. *island group* Maluku, SE Indonesia
184 J3 **Kaikohe** Northland, North Island, NZ
185 J16 **Kaikoura** Canterbury, South Island, NZ
185 J16 **Kaikoura Peninsula** *peninsula* South Island, NZ
Kailas Range *see* Gangdisê Shan
160 K12 **Kaili** Guizhou, S China
38 F10 **Kailua** Maui, Hawaii, USA, C Pacific Ocean
38 G11 **Kailua** *var.* Kailua-Kona, Kona. Hawaii, USA, C Pacific Ocean
Kailua-Kona *see* Kailua
186 B7 **Kaim** ≈ W PNG
171 X14 **Kaima** Irian Jaya, E Indonesia
184 M7 **Kaimai Range** ⛰ North Island, NZ
114 E13 **Kaïmaktsalán** ▲ Greece/FYR Macedonia
185 C20 **Kaimanawa Mountains** ⛰ North Island, NZ
118 E4 **Käina** *Ger.* Keinis; *prev.* Keina. Hiiumaa, W Estonia
109 V7 **Kainach** ≈ SE Austria
164 I14 **Kainan** Tokushima, Shikoku, SW Japan
164 H15 **Kainan** Wakayama, Honshū, SW Japan
147 U7 **Kaindy** *Kir.* Kayyngdy. Chuyskaya Oblast', N Kyrgyzstan
77 T14 **Kainji Dam** *dam* W Nigeria
Kainji Lake *see* Kainji Reservoir
77 T14 **Kainji Reservoir** *var.* Kainji Lake. ▣ W Nigeria
186 D8 **Kaintiba** *var.* Kamina. Gulf, S PNG
92 K12 **Kainulaisjärvi** Norrbotten, N Sweden
184 K5 **Kaipara Harbour** *harbour* North Island, NZ
152 I10 **Kairāna** Uttar Pradesh, N India
74 M6 **Kairouan** *var.* Al Qayrawān. E Tunisia
Kaisaria *see* Kayseri
101 F20 **Kaiserslautern** Rheinland-Pfalz, SW Germany
118 G13 **Kaišiadorys** Kaišiadorys, S Lithuania
184 I2 **Kaitaia** Northland, North Island, NZ
185 E24 **Kaitangata** Otago, South Island, NZ
152 I9 **Kaithal** Haryāna, NW India
169 N13 **Kait, Tanjung** *headland* Sumatera, W Indonesia
38 E9 **Kaiwi Channel** *channel* Hawaii, USA, C Pacific Ocean
160 K9 **Kaixian** *var.* Kai Xian. Sichuan, C China
163 V11 **Kaiyuan** *var.* K'ai-yüan. Liaoning, NE China
160 H14 **Kaiyuan** Yunnan, SW China
39 O9 **Kaiyuh Mountains** ⛰ Alaska, USA
93 M15 **Kajaani** *Swe.* Kajana. Oulu, C Finland
149 N7 **Kajakī, Band-e** ◎ C Afghanistan
Kajan *see* Kayan, Sungai
Kajana *see* Kajaani
137 V13 **K'ajaran** *Rus.* Kadzharan. SE Armenia
Kajisay *see* Kadzhi-Say
113 O20 **Kajmakčalan** ▲ S FYR Macedonia
Kajnar *see* Kaynar
149 N6 **Kajrān** Urūzgān, C Afghanistan
149 N5 **Kaj Rūd** ≈ C Afghanistan
Kaka *see* Kaakhka
12 C12 **Kakabeka Falls** Ontario, S Canada
83 F23 **Kakamas** Northern Cape, W South Africa
81 H18 **Kakamega** Western, W Kenya
112 H13 **Kakanj** Federacija Bosna I Hercegovina, Bosnia and Herzegovina
185 F22 **Kakanui Mountains** ⛰ South Island, NZ
184 K11 **Kakaramea** Taranaki, North Island, NZ
76 J16 **Kakata** C Liberia
184 M11 **Kakatahi** Manawatu-Wanganui, North Island, NZ
113 M23 **Kakavi** Gjirokastër, S Albania
147 O14 **Kakaydi** Surkhondaryo Wiloyati, S Uzbekistan
164 F13 **Kake** Hiroshima, Honshū, SW Japan
39 X13 **Kake** Kupreanof Island, Alaska, USA
171 P14 **Kakea** Pulau Wowoni, C Indonesia
164 M14 **Kakegawa** Shizuoka, Honshū, S Japan
165 V16 **Kakeromajima** Kagoshima, SW Japan
143 T6 **Kākhak** *var.* Kākhk. Khorāsān, E Iran
118 L11 **Kakhanavichy** *Rus.* Kokhanovichi. Vitsyebskaya Voblasts', N Belarus
39 P13 **Kakhonak** Alaska, USA
117 S10 **Kakhovka** Khersons'ka Oblast', S Ukraine
117 U9 **Kakhovs'ka Vodoskhovyshche** *Rus.* Kakhovskoye Vodokhranilishche. ▣ SE Ukraine
Kakhovskoye Vodokhranilishche *see* Kakhovs'ka Vodoskhovyshche
117 T11 **Kakhovs'kyy Kanal** *canal* S Ukraine
Kakia *see* Khakhea
155 L16 **Kākināda** *prev.* Cocanada. Andhra Pradesh, E India
Käkisalmi *see* Priozersk
164 I13 **Kakogawa** Hyōgo, Honshū, SW Japan
81 F18 **Kakoge** C Uganda
145 O7 **Kak, Ozero** ◎ N Kazakhstan
Ka-Krem *see* Malyy Yenisey
Kakshaal-Too, Khrebet *see* Kokshaal-Tau
39 S5 **Kaktovik** Alaska, USA
165 Q11 **Kakuda** Miyagi, Honshū, C Japan
165 Q8 **Kakunodate** Akita, Honshū, C Japan
Kalaallit Nunaat *see* Greenland
149 T7 **Kālābāgh** Punjab, E Pakistan
171 Q16 **Kalabahi** Pulau Alor, S Indonesia
188 I5 **Kalabera** Saipan, S Northern Mariana Islands
83 G14 **Kalabo** Western, W Zambia
128 M9 **Kalach** Voronezhskaya Oblast', W Russian Federation
129 N10 **Kalach-na-Donu** Volgogradskaya Oblast', SW Russian Federation
166 K5 **Kaladan** ≈ W Myanmar
14 K14 **Kaladar** Ontario, SE Canada
38 G13 **Ka Lae** *var.* South Cape, South Point. *headland* Hawaii, USA, C Pacific Ocean
83 G19 **Kalahari Desert** *desert* Southern Africa
38 B8 **Kalaheo** *Haw.* Kalāheo. Kauai, Hawaii, USA, C Pacific Ocean
Kalaikhum *see* Qal'aikhum
146 J16 **Kala-i-Mor** *Turkm.* Galaymor. Maryyskiy Velayat, S Turkmenistan
93 K15 **Kalajoki** Oulu, W Finland
Kalak *see* Eski Kalak
Kal al Sraghna *see* El Kelâa Srarhna
32 G10 **Kalama** Washington, NW USA
Kalámai *see* Kalámata
115 G14 **Kalamariá** Kentrikí Makedonía, N Greece
115 E21 **Kalámata** *prev.* Kalámai. Pelopónnisos, S Greece
31 P10 **Kalamazoo** Michigan, N USA
31 P9 **Kalamazoo River** ≈ Michigan, N USA
Kalambaka *see* Kalampáka
117 S13 **Kalamits'ka Zatoka** *Rus.* Kalamitskiy Zaliv. *gulf* S Ukraine
Kalamitskiy Zaliv *see* Kalamits'ka Zatoka
115 H18 **Kálamos** Attikí, C Greece
115 C18 **Kálamos** *island* Iónioi Nísoi, Greece, C Mediterranean Sea
115 D15 **Kalampáka** *var.* Kalambaka. Thessalía, C Greece
Kalan *see* Călan, Romania
Kalan *see* Tunceli, Turkey
117 S11 **Kalanchak** Khersons'ka Oblast', S Ukraine
171 O15 **Kalaotoa, Pulau** *island* W Indonesia
155 J24 **Kala Oya** ≈ NW Sri Lanka
Kalarash *see* Călăraşi
93 H17 **Kälarne** Jämtland, C Sweden
143 V15 **Kalar Rūd** ≈ SE Iran
167 R9 **Kalasin** *var.* Muang Kalasin. Kalasin, E Thailand
149 O8 **Kalāt** *Per.* Qalāt. Zābul, S Afghanistan
149 O11 **Kālat** *var.* Kelat, Khelat. Baluchistān, SW Pakistan
115 J14 **Kalathriá, Akrotírio** *headland* Samothráki, NE Greece
193 W17 **Kalau** *island* Tongatapu Group, SE Tonga
38 E9 **Kalaupapa** Molokai, Hawaii, USA, C Pacific Ocean
129 N13 **Kalaus** ≈ SW Russian Federation
Kalávrita *see* Kalávryta
115 E19 **Kalávryta** *var.* Kalávrita. Dytikí Ellás, S Greece
141 Y10 **Kalbān** W Oman
180 H11 **Kalbarri** Western Australia
145 X10 **Kalbinskiy Khrebet** *Kaz.* Qalba Zhotasy. ⛰ E Kazakhstan
144 G10 **Kaldygayty** ≈ W Kazakhstan
136 I12 **Kalecik** Ankara, N Turkey
79 O19 **Kalehe** Sud Kivu, E Dem. Rep. Congo (Zaire)
79 P22 **Kalemie** *prev.* Albertville. Katanga, SE Dem. Rep. Congo (Zaire)
166 L4 **Kalemyo** Sagaing, W Myanmar
82 H12 **Kalene Hill** North Western, NW Zambia
Kale Sultanie *see* Çanakkale
126 I7 **Kalevala** Respublika Kareliya, NW Russian Federation
166 L4 **Kalewa** Sagaing, C Myanmar
Kalgan *see* Zhangjiakou
39 Q12 **Kalgin Island** *island* Alaska, USA
180 L12 **Kalgoorlie** Western Australia
Kali *see* Sārda
115 E17 **Kaliakoúda** ▲ C Greece
114 O8 **Kaliakra, Nos** *headland* NE Bulgaria
115 F19 **Kaliánoi** Pelopónnisos, S Greece
115 N24 **Kalí Límni** ▲ Kárpathos, SE Greece
79 N20 **Kalima** Maniema, E Dem. Rep. Congo (Zaire)
169 S11 **Kalimantan** *Eng.* Indonesian Borneo. *geopolitical region* Borneo, C Indonesia
169 Q11 **Kalimantan Barat** *off.* Propinsi Kalimantan Barat, *Eng.* West Borneo, West Kalimantan. ◈ *province* N Indonesia
169 T13 **Kalimantan Selatan** *off.* Propinsi Kalimantan Selatan, *Eng.* South Borneo, South Kalimantan. ◈ *province* N Indonesia
169 R12 **Kalimantan Tengah** *off.* Propinsi Kalimantan Tengah, *Eng.* Central Borneo, Central Kalimantan. ◈ *province* N Indonesia
169 U10 **Kalimantan Timur** *off.* Propinsi Kalimantan Timur, *Eng.* East Borneo, East Kalimantan. ◈ *province* N Indonesia
Kálimnos *see* Kálymnos
153 S12 **Kālimpang** West Bengal, NE India
Kalinin *see* Tver', Russian Federation
Kalinin *see* Boldumsaz, Turkmenistan
Kalininabad *see* Kalininobod
128 B3 **Kaliningrad** Kaliningradskaya Oblast', W Russian Federation
Kaliningrad *see* Kaliningradskaya Oblast'
128 A3 **Kaliningradskaya Oblast'** *var.* Kaliningrad. ◈ *province and enclave* W Russian Federation
Kalinino *see* Tashir
147 P14 **Kalininobod** *Rus.* Kalininabad. SW Tajikistan
129 O8 **Kalininsk** Saratovskaya Oblast', W Russian Federation
Kalininsk *see* Boldumsaz
Kalinisk *see* Cupcina
119 M19 **Kalinkavichy** *Rus.* Kalinkovichi. Homyel'skaya Voblasts', SE Belarus
Kalinkovichi *see* Kalinkavichy
81 G18 **Kaliro** SE Uganda
Kalisch/Kalish *see* Kalisz
33 O7 **Kalispell** Montana, NW USA
110 I13 **Kalisz** *Ger.* Kalisch, *Rus.* Kalish; *anc.* Calisia. Wielkopolskie, C Poland
110 F9 **Kalisz Pomorski** *Ger.* Kallies. Zachodniopomorskie, NW Poland
128 M10 **Kalitva** ≈ SW Russian Federation
81 F21 **Kaliua** Tabora, C Tanzania
92 K13 **Kalix** Norrbotten, N Sweden
92 K12 **Kalixälven** ≈ N Sweden
92 J11 **Kalixfors** Norrbotten, N Sweden
145 T8 **Kalkaman** Pavlodar, NE Kazakhstan
Kalkandelen *see* Tetovo
181 O4 **Kalkarindji** Northern Territory, N Australia
31 P6 **Kalkaska** Michigan, N USA
93 F16 **Kall** Jämtland, C Sweden
189 X2 **Kallalen** *var.* Calalen. *island* Ratak Chain, SE Marshall Islands
118 J5 **Kallaste** *Ger.* Krasnogor. Tartumaa, SE Estonia
93 N16 **Kallavesi** ◎ SE Finland
115 F17 **Kallídromo** ⛰ C Greece
Kallies *see* Kalisz Pomorski
95 M22 **Kallinge** Blekinge, S Sweden
115 L16 **Kalloní** Lésvos, E Greece
93 F16 **Kallsjön** ◎ C Sweden
95 N21 **Kalmar** *var.* Calmar. Kalmar, S Sweden
95 M19 **Kalmar** *var.* Calmar. ◈ *county* S Sweden
95 N20 **Kalmarsund** *strait* S Sweden
148 L16 **Kalmat, Khor** *Eng.* Kalmat Lagoon. *lagoon* SW Pakistan
Kalmat Lagoon *see* Kalmat, Khor
117 X9 **Kal'mius** ≈ E Ukraine
99 H15 **Kalmthout** Antwerpen, N Belgium
Kalmykia/Kalmykiya-Khal'mg Tangch, Respublika *see* Kalmykiya, Respublika
129 O12 **Kalmykiya, Respublika** *var.* Respublika Kalmykiya-Khal'mg Tangch, *Eng.* Kalmykia; *prev.* Kalmytskaya ASSR. ◈ *autonomous republic* SW Russian Federation
Kalmytskaya ASSR *see* Kalmykiya, Respublika
118 F9 **Kalnciems** Jelgava, C Latvia
114 L10 **Kalnitsa** ≈ SE Bulgaria
111 J24 **Kalocsa** Bács-Kiskun, S Hungary
114 J9 **Kalofer** Plovdiv, C Bulgaria
38 E10 **Kalohi Channel** *channel* C Pacific Ocean
83 I16 **Kalomo** Southern, S Zambia
29 X14 **Kalona** Iowa, C USA
115 K22 **Kalotási, Akrotírio** *headland* Amorgós, Kykládes, Greece, Aegean Sea
152 J8 **Kalpa** Himāchal Pradesh, N India
115 C15 **Kalpáki** Ípeiros, W Greece
155 C22 **Kalpeni Island** *island* Lakshadweep, India, N Indian Ocean
152 K13 **Kālpi** Uttar Pradesh, N India
158 G7 **Kalpin** Xinjiang Uygur Zizhiqu, NW China
146 K8 **Kalquduq** *Rus.* Kulkuduk. Nawoiy Wiloyati, N Uzbekistan
149 P16 **Kalri Lake** ◎ SE Pakistan
143 R5 **Kāl Shūr** N Iran
39 N11 **Kalskag** Alaska, USA
95 B18 **Kalsoy** *Dan.* Kalsø *Island* Faeroe Islands
39 O9 **Kaltag** Alaska, USA
108 H7 **Kaltbrunn** Sankt Gallen, NE Switzerland
Kaltdorf *see* Pruszków
77 X14 **Kaltungo** Gombe, E Nigeria
128 K4 **Kaluga** Kaluzhskaya Oblast', W Russian Federation
155 J26 **Kalu Ganga** ≈ S Sri Lanka
82 J13 **Kalulushi** Copperbelt, C Zambia
180 M2 **Kalumburu** Western Australia
95 H23 **Kalundborg** Vestsjælland, E Denmark
82 K11 **Kalungwishi** ≈ N Zambia
149 T8 **Kalūr Kot** Punjab, E Pakistan
116 I6 **Kalush** *Pol.* Kałusz. Ivano-Frankivs'ka Oblast', W Ukraine
Kałusz *see* Kalush
110 N11 **Kałuszyn** Mazowieckie, C Poland
155 J26 **Kalutara** Western Province, SW Sri Lanka
Kaluwawa *see* Fergusson Island
128 I5 **Kaluzhskaya Oblast'** ◈ *province* W Russian Federation
119 E14 **Kalvarija** *Pol.* Kalwaria. Marijampolė, S Lithuania
93 K15 **Kälviä** Länsi-Suomi, W Finland
109 U6 **Kalwang** Steiermark, E Austria
Kalwaria *see* Kalvarija
154 D13 **Kalyān** Mahārāshtra, W India
126 K16 **Kalyazin** Tverskaya Oblast', W Russian Federation
115 D18 **Kalydón** *anc.* Calydon. *site of ancient city* Dytikí Ellás, C Greece
115 M21 **Kálymnos** *var.* Kálimnos. Kálymnos, Dodekánisos, Greece, Aegean Sea
115 M21 **Kálymnos** *var.* Kálimnos. *island* Dodekánisos, Greece, Aegean Sea
117 O5 **Kalynivka** Kyyivs'ka Oblast', N Ukraine
117 N6 **Kalynivka** Vinnyts'ka Oblast', C Ukraine
42 M10 **Kama** *var.* Cama. Región Autónoma Atlántico Sur, SE Nicaragua
165 R9 **Kamaishi** *var.* Kamaisi. Iwate, Honshū, C Japan
Kamaisi *see* Kamaishi
118 H13 **Kamajai** Molėtai, E Lithuania
118 H11 **Kamajai** Rokiškis, NE Lithuania
149 U9 **Kamālia** Punjab, NE Pakistan
83 I14 **Kamalondo** North Western, NW Zambia
136 I13 **Kaman** Kirşehir, C Turkey
79 O20 **Kamanyola** Sud Kivu, E Dem. Rep. Congo (Zaire)
141 N14 **Kamarān** *island* W Yemen
55 R9 **Kamarang** W Guyana
Kāmāreddi/Kamareddy *see* Rāmāreddi
Kama Reservoir *see* Kamskoye Vodokhranilishche
148 K13 **Kamarod** Baluchistān, SW Pakistan
171 P14 **Kamaru** Pulau Buton, C Indonesia
147 N12 **Kamashi** Qashqadaryo Wiloyati, S Uzbekistan
77 S13 **Kamba** Kebbi, NW Nigeria
Kambaeng Petch *see* Kamphaeng Phet
180 L12 **Kambalda** Western Australia

◆ Country ● Country Capital ◇ Dependent Territory ○ Dependent Territory Capital ◈ Administrative Region × International Airport ▲ Mountain ⛰ Mountain Range Volcano ≈ River ◎ Lake ▣ Reservoir

149 P13 **Kambar** *var.* Qambar. Sind, SE Pakistan
Kambara *see* Kabara
76 I14 **Kambia** W Sierra Leone
Kambos *see* Kámpos
79 N25 **Kambove** Katanga, SE Dem. Rep. Congo (Zaire)
Kambryk *see* Cambrai
123 V10 **Kamchatka** ≈ E Russian Federation
Kamchatka *see* Kamchatka, Poluostrov
Kamchatka Basin *see* Komandorskaya Basin
123 U10 **Kamchatka, Poluostrov** *Eng.* Kamchatka. *peninsula* E Russian Federation
123 V10 **Kamchatskaya Oblast'** ◈ *province* E Russian Federation
123 V10 **Kamchatskiy Zaliv** *gulf* E Russian Federation
114 N9 **Kamchiya** ≈ E Bulgaria
114 L9 **Kamchiya, Yazovir** ▣ E Bulgaria
Kamdesh *see* Kāmdeysh
149 T4 **Kāmdeysh** *var.* Kamdesh. Kunar, E Afghanistan
118 M13 **Kamen'** *Rus.* Kamen'. Vitsyebskaya Voblasts', N Belarus
Kamenets *see* Kam"yanyets
Kamenets-Podol'skaya Oblast' *see* Khmel'nyts'ka Oblast'
Kamenets-Podol'skiy *see* Kam"yanets'-Podil's'kyy
113 Q18 **Kamenica** NE FYR Macedonia
112 A11 **Kamenjak, Rt** *headland* NW Croatia
144 F8 **Kamenka** Zapadnyy Kazakhstan, NW Kazakhstan
127 O6 **Kamenka** Arkhangel'skaya Oblast', NW Russian Federation
128 O6 **Kamenka** Penzenskaya Oblast', W Russian Federation
129 L8 **Kamenka** Voronezhskaya Oblast', W Russian Federation
Kamenka *see* Camenca, Moldova
Kamenka *see* Kam"yanka, Ukraine
Kamenka-Bugskaya *see* Kam"yanka-Buz'ka
Kamenka Dneprovskaya *see* Kam"yanka-Dniprovs'ka
Kamen Kashirskiy *see* Kamin'-Kashyrs'kyy
1028L15 **Kamennomostskiy** Respublika Adygeya, SW Russian Federation
128 L11 **Kamenolomni** Rostovskaya Oblast', SW Russian Federation
129 P8 **Kamenskiy** Saratovskaya Oblast', W Russian Federation
Kamenskoye *see* Dniprodzerzhyns'k
128 L11 **Kamensk-Shakhtinskiy** Rostovskaya Oblast', SW Russian Federation
101 P15 **Kamenz** Sachsen, E Germany
164 J13 **Kameoka** Kyōto, Honshū, SW Japan
128 M3 **Kameshkovo** Vladimirskaya Oblast', W Russian Federation
164 C11 **Kami-Agata** Nagasaki, Tsushima, SW Japan
33 N10 **Kamiah** Idaho, NW USA
Kamień Koszyrski *see* Kamin'-Kashyrs'kyy
110 H9 **Kamień Krajeński** *Ger.* Kamin in Westpreussen. Kujawsko-pomorskie, C Poland
111 F15 **Kamienna Góra** *Ger.* Landeshut, Landeshut in Schlesien. Dolnośląskie, SW Poland
110 D8 **Kamień Pomorski** *Ger.* Cummin in Pommern. Zachodniopomorskie, NW Poland
165 R5 **Kamiiso** Hokkaidō, NE Japan
79 L22 **Kamiji** Kasai Oriental, S Dem. Rep. Congo (Zaire)
165 T3 **Kamikawa** Hokkaidō, NE Japan
164 B15 **Kami-Koshiki-jima** *island* SW Japan
79 M23 **Kamina** Katanga, S Dem. Rep. Congo (Zaire)
Kamina *see* Kaintiba
42 C6 **Kaminaljuyú** *ruins* Guatemala, C Guatemala
Kamin in Westpreussen *see* Kamień Krajeński
116 J2 **Kamin'-Kashyrs'kyy** *Pol.* Kamień Koszyrski, *Rus.* Kamen Kashirskiy. Volyns'ka Oblast', NW Ukraine
165 Q5 **Kaminokuni** Hokkaidō, NE Japan
165 P10 **Kaminoyama** Yamagata, Honshū, C Japan
39 Q13 **Kamishak Bay** *bay* Alaska, USA
165 U4 **Kami-Shihoro** Hokkaidō, NE Japan
Kamishli *see* Al Qāmishlī
Kamissar *see* Kamsar
164 C11 **Kami-Tsushima** Nagasaki, Tsushima, SW Japan
79 O20 **Kamituga** Sud Kivu, E Dem. Rep. Congo (Zaire)
164 B17 **Kamiyaku** Kagoshima, Yaku-shima, SW Japan
11 N16 **Kamloops** British Columbia, SW Canada
107 G25 **Kamma** Sicilia, Italy, C Mediterranean Sea
192 K4 **Kammu Seamount** *undersea feature* N Pacific Ocean
109 U11 **Kamnik** *Ger.* Stein. C Slovenia
Kamniške Alpe *see* Kamniško-Savinjske Alpe
109 T10 **Kamniško-Savinjske Alpe** *var.* Kamniške Alpe, Sanntaler Alpen, *Ger.* Steiner Alpen. ▲ N Slovenia
165 O14 **Kamogawa** Chiba, Honshū, S Japan
149 W8 **Kāmoke** Punjab, E Pakistan
82 L13 **Kamoto** Eastern, E Zambia
109 V3 **Kamp** ≈ N Austria
81 F18 **Kampala** ● (Uganda) S Uganda
168 K11 **Kampar, Sungai** ≈ Sumatera, W Indonesia
98 L9 **Kampen** Overijssel, E Netherlands
79 N20 **Kampene** Maniema, E Dem. Rep. Congo (Zaire)
29 Q9 **Kampeska, Lake** ◎ South Dakota, N USA
167 O9 **Kamphaeng Phet** *var.* Kambaeng Petch. Kamphaeng Phet, W Thailand
Kampo *see* Campo, Cameroon
Kampo *see* Ntem, Cameroon/Equatorial Guinea
167 S12 **Kâmpóng Cham** *prev.* Kompong Cham. Kâmpóng Cham, C Cambodia
167 R12 **Kâmpóng Chhnăng** *prev.* Kompong. Kâmpóng Chhnăng, C Cambodia
167 R12 **Kâmpóng Khleăng** *prev.* Kompong Kleang. Siĕmréab, NW Cambodia
167 Q14 **Kâmpóng Saôm** *prev.* Kompong Som, Sihanoukville. Kâmpóng Saôm, SW Cambodia
167 R13 **Kâmpóng Spoe** *prev.* Kompong Speu. Kâmpóng Spœ, S Cambodia
121 O2 **Kámpos** *var.* Kambos. NW Cyprus
167 R14 **Kâmpôt** Kâmpôt, SW Cambodia
Kamptee *see* Kāmthi
77 O14 **Kampti** SW Burkina
Kampuchea *see* Cambodia
169 Q9 **Kampung Sirik** Sarawak, East Malaysia
11 V15 **Kamsack** Saskatchewan, S Canada
76 H13 **Kamsar** *var.* Kamissar. Guinée-Maritime, W Guinea
129 R4 **Kamskoye Ust'ye** Respublika Tatarstan, W Russian Federation
127 U14 **Kamskoye Vodokhranilishche** *var.* Kama Reservoir. ▣ NW Russian Federation
154 I12 **Kāmthi** *prev.* Kamptee. Mahārāshtra, C India
Kamuela *see* Waimea
165 R3 **Kamuenai** Hokkaidō, NE Japan
165 T5 **Kamui-dake** ※ Hokkaidō, NE Japan
165 R3 **Kamui-misaki** *headland* Hokkaidō, NE Japan
43 O15 **Kámuk, Cerro** ▲ SE Costa Rica
116 K7 **Kam"yanets'-Podil's'kyy** *Rus.* Kamenets-Podol'skiy. Khmel'nyts'ka Oblast', W Ukraine
117 Q6 **Kam"yanka** *Rus.* Kamenka. Cherkas'ka Oblast', C Ukraine
116 I5 **Kam"yanka-Buz'ka** *Rus.* Kamenka-Bugskaya. L'vivs'ka Oblast', NW Ukraine
117 T9 **Kam"yanka-Dniprovs'ka** *Rus.* Kamenka Dneprovskaya. Zaporiz'ka Oblast', SE Ukraine
119 F19 **Kamyanyets** *Rus.* Kamenets. Brestskaya Voblasts', SW Belarus
129 P9 **Kamyshin** Volgogradskaya Oblast', SW Russian Federation
129 Q13 **Kamyzyak** Astrakhanskaya Oblast', SW Russian Federation
12 K8 **Kanaaupscow** ≈ Quebec, C Canada
36 K8 **Kanab** Utah, W USA
36 K9 **Kanab Creek** ≈ Arizona/Utah, SW USA
187 Y14 **Kanacea** *prev.* Kanathea. Taveuni, N Fiji
38 G17 **Kanaga Island** *island* Aleutian Islands, Alaska, USA
38 G17 **Kanaga Volcano** ▲ Kanaga Island, Alaska, USA
165 N14 **Kanagawa** *off.* Kanagawa-ken. ◈ *prefecture* Honshū, S Japan
13 Q8 **Kanairiktok** ≈ Newfoundland, E Canada
Kanaky *see* New Caledonia
79 K22 **Kananga** *prev.* Luluabourg. Kasai Occidental, S Dem. Rep. Congo (Zaire)
Kananur *see* Cannanore
Kanara *see* Karnātaka
36 J7 **Kanarraville** Utah, W USA
129 Q4 **Kanash** Chuvashskaya Respublika, W Russian Federation
Kanathea *see* Kanacea
21 Q4 **Kanawha River** ≈ West Virginia, NE USA
164 L13 **Kanayama** Gifu, Honshū, SW Japan
164 L11 **Kanazawa** Ishikawa, Honshū, SW Japan
166 M4 **Kanbalu** Sagaing, C Myanmar
166 L8 **Kanbe** Yangon, SW Myanmar
167 O11 **Kanchanaburi** Kanchanaburi, W Thailand
Kānchenjunga *see* Kangchenjunga
145 V11 **Kanchingiz, Khrebet** ▲ E Kazakhstan
155 J19 **Kānchīpuram** *prev.* Conjeeveram. Tamil Nādu, SE India
149 N8 **Kandahār** *Per.* Qandahār. Kandahār, S Afghanistan
149 N9 **Kandahār** *Per.* Qandahār. ◈ *province* SE Afghanistan
Kandalakša *see* Kandalaksha
126 I5 **Kandalaksha** *var.* Kandalakša, *Fin.* Kantalahti. Murmanskaya Oblast', NW Russian Federation
Kandalaksha Gulf/Kandalakshskaya Guba *see* Kandalakshskiy Zaliv
126 K6 **Kandalakshskiy Zaliv** *var.* Kandalakshskaya Guba, *Eng.* Kandalaksha Gulf. *bay* NW Russian Federation
Kandalangodi *see* Kandalengoti
83 G17 **Kandalengoti** *var.* Kandalangodi. Ngamiland, NW Botswana
169 U13 **Kandangan** Borneo, C Indonesia
Kandau *see* Kandava
118 E8 **Kandava** *Ger.* Kandau. Tukums, W Latvia
Kandavu *see* Kadavu
77 R14 **Kandé** *var.* Kanté. NE Togo
101 F23 **Kandel** ▲ SW Germany
186 C7 **Kandep** Enga, W PNG
149 R12 **Kandh Kot** Sind, SE Pakistan
77 S13 **Kandi** N Benin
149 P14 **Kandiāro** Sind, SE Pakistan
136 F11 **Kandıra** Kocaeli, NW Turkey
183 S8 **Kandos** New South Wales, SE Australia
148 M16 **Kandrāch** *var.* Kanrach. Baluchistān, SW Pakistan
172 I4 **Kandreho** Mahajanga, C Madagascar
186 F7 **Kandrian** New Britain, E PNG
Kandukur *see* Kondukūr
155 K25 **Kandy** Central Province, C Sri Lanka
144 I10 **Kandyagash** *Kaz.* Qandyaghash; *prev.* Oktyabr'sk. Aktyubinsk, W Kazakhstan
18 D12 **Kane** Pennsylvania, NE USA
64 I11 **Kane Fracture Zone** *tectonic feature* NW Atlantic Ocean
Kanëka *see* Kanëvka
78 G9 **Kanem** *off.* Préfecture du Kanem. ◈ *prefecture* W Chad
38 D9 **Kaneohe** *Haw.* Kāne'ohe. Oahu, Hawaii, USA, C Pacific Ocean
Kanestron, Akrotírio *see* Palioúri, Akrotírio
Kanëv *see* Kaniv
126 M5 **Kanëvka** *var.* Kanëka. Murmanskaya Oblast', NW Russian Federation
128 K13 **Kanevskaya** Krasnodarskiy Kray, SW Russian Federation
Kanevskoye Vodokhranilishche *see* Kanivs'ke Vodoskhovyshche
165 P9 **Kaneyama** Yamagata, Honshū, C Japan
83 G20 **Kang** Kgalagadi, C Botswana
76 L13 **Kangaba** Koulikoro, SW Mali
136 M13 **Kangal** Sivas, C Turkey
143 O13 **Kangān** Būshehr, S Iran
143 S15 **Kangān** Hormozgān, SE Iran
168 J6 **Kangar** Perlis, Peninsular Malaysia
76 L13 **Kangaré** Sikasso, S Mali
182 F10 **Kangaroo Island** *island* South Australia
93 M17 **Kangasniemi** Itä-Suomi, E Finland
142 K6 **Kangāvar** *var.* Kangāwar. Kermānshāh, W Iran
Kangāwar *see* Kangāvar
153 S11 **Kangchenjunga** *var.* Kānchenjunga. ▲ NE India
160 G9 **Kangding** Sichuan, C China
169 U16 **Kangean, Kepulauan** *island group* S Indonesia
169 T16 **Kangean, Pulau** *island* Kepulauan Kangean, S Indonesia
67 U8 **Kangen** *var.* Kengen. ≈ SE Sudan
197 N14 **Kangerlussuaq** *Dan.* Sondre Strømfjord ✕ Kitaa, W Greenland
197 Q15 **Kangertittivaq** *Dan.* Scoresby Sund. *fjord* E Greenland
167 O2 **Kangfang** Kachin State, N Myanmar
163 X12 **Kanggye** N North Korea
197 P15 **Kangikajik** *var.* Kap Brewster. *headland* E Greenland
13 N5 **Kangiqsualujjuaq** *prev.* George River, Port-Nouveau-Québec. Quebec, E Canada
12 L2 **Kangiqsujuaq** *prev.* Maricourt, Wakeham Bay. Quebec, NE Canada
12 M4 **Kangirsuk** *prev.* Bellin, Payne. Quebec, E Canada
158 J15 **Kangmar** Xizang Zizhiqu, W China
158 M16 **Kangmar** Xizang Zizhiqu, W China
163 Y14 **Kangnŭng** *Jap.* Kōryō. NE South Korea
79 D18 **Kango** Estuaire, NW Gabon
152 I7 **Kāngra** Himāchal Pradesh, NW India
153 Q16 **Kangsabati Reservoir** ▣ N India
159 O17 **Kangto** ▲ China/India
159 W12 **Kangxian** *var.* Kang Xian, Zuitaizi. Gansu, C China
166 L4 **Kani** Sagaing, C Myanmar
76 M15 **Kani** NW Ivory Coast
79 M23 **Kaniama** Katanga, S Dem. Rep. Congo (Zaire)
Kanibadam *see* Konibodom
169 V6 **Kanibongan** Sabah, East Malaysia
185 F17 **Kaniere** West Coast, South Island, NZ
185 G17 **Kaniere, Lake** ◎ South Island, NZ
188 E17 **Kanifaay** Yap, W Micronesia
127 O4 **Kanin Kamen'** ▲ NW Russian Federation
127 N3 **Kanin Nos** Nenetskiy Avtonomnyy Okrug, NW Russian Federation
127 N3 **Kanin Nos, Mys** *headland* NW Russian Federation
127 O5 **Kanin, Poluostrov** *peninsula* NW Russian Federation
139 V8 **Kānī Sakht** E Iraq
139 T3 **Kānī Sulaymān** N Iraq
165 Q6 **Kanita** Aomori, Honshū, C Japan
117 Q5 **Kaniv** *Rus.* Kanëv. Cherkas'ka Oblast', C Ukraine
182 K11 **Kaniva** Victoria, SE Australia
117 Q5 **Kanivs'ke Vodoskhovyshche** *Rus.* Kanevskoye Vodokhranilishche. ▣ C Ukraine
112 L8 **Kanjiža** *Ger.* Altkanischa, *Hung.* Magyarkanizsa, Ókanizsa; *prev.* Stara Kanjiža. Serbia, N Yugoslavia
93 K18 **Kankaanpää** Länsi-Suomi, W Finland
30 M12 **Kankakee** Illinois, N USA
31 O11 **Kankakee River** ≈ Illinois/Indiana, N USA
76 K14 **Kankan** Haute-Guinée, E Guinea
154 K13 **Kānker** Madhya Pradesh, C India
76 J10 **Kankossa** Assaba, S Mauritania
167 N12 **Kanmaw Kyun** *var.* Kisseraing, Kithareng. *island* Mergui Archipelago, S Myanmar
164 F12 **Kanmuri-yama** ▲ Kyūshū, SW Japan
21 R10 **Kannapolis** North Carolina, SE USA
93 L16 **Kannonkoski** Länsi-Suomi, W Finland
Kannur *see* Cannanore
93 K15 **Kannus** Länsi-Suomi, W Finland
77 V13 **Kano** Kano, N Nigeria
77 V13 **Kano** ◈ *state* N Nigeria
77 V13 **Kano** ✕ Kano, N Nigeria
164 G14 **Kan'onji** *var.* Kanonzi. Kagawa, Shikoku, SW Japan
Kanonzi *see* Kan'onji
26 M5 **Kanopolis Lake** ▣ Kansas, C USA
36 K5 **Kanosh** Utah, W USA
169 R9 **Kanowit** Sarawak, East Malaysia
164 C16 **Kanoya** Kagoshima, Kyūshū, SW Japan
152 L13 **Kānpur** *Eng.* Cawnpore. Uttar Pradesh, N India
Kanrach *see* Kandrāch
164 I14 **Kansai** ✕ (Ōsaka) Ōsaka, Honshū, SW Japan
27 R9 **Kansas** Oklahoma, C USA
26 L5 **Kansas** *off.* State of Kansas; also known as Jayhawker State, Sunflower State. ◈ *state* C USA
27 R4 **Kansas City** Kansas, C USA
27 R4 **Kansas City** Missouri, C USA
27 R3 **Kansas City** ✕ Missouri, C USA
27 P4 **Kansas River** ≈ Kansas, C USA
122 L14 **Kansk** Krasnoyarskiy Kray, S Russian Federation
Kansu *see* Gansu
147 V7 **Kant** Chuyskaya Oblast', N Kyrgyzstan
Kantalahti *see* Kandalaksha
167 N16 **Kantang** *var.* Ban Kantang. Trang, SW Thailand
115 H25 **Kántanos** Kríti, Greece, E Mediterranean Sea
77 R12 **Kantchari** E Burkina
Kanté *see* Kandé
Kantemir *see* Cantemir
128 L9 **Kantemirovka** Voronezhskaya Oblast', W Russian Federation
167 R11 **Kantharalak** Si Sa Ket, E Thailand
Kantipur *see* Kathmandu
39 Q9 **Kantishna River** ≈ Alaska, USA
191 S3 **Kanton** *var.* Abariringa, Canton Island; *prev.* Mary Island. *atoll* Phoenix Islands, C Kiribati
97 C20 **Kanturk** *Ir.* Ceann Toirc. SW Ireland
55 T11 **Kanuku Mountains** ▲ S Guyana
165 O12 **Kanuma** Tochigi, Honshū, S Japan
83 H20 **Kanye** Southern, SE Botswana
83 H17 **Kanyu** Ngamiland, C Botswana
166 M7 **Kanyutkwin** Pegu, C Myanmar
79 M24 **Kanzenze** Katanga, SE Dem. Rep. Congo (Zaire)
193 Y15 **Kao** *island* Kotu Group, W Tonga
161 S14 **Kaohsiung** *var.* Gaoxiong, *Jap.* Takao, Takow. S Taiwan
161 S14 **Kaohsiung** ✕ S Taiwan
Kaokaona *see* Kirakira
83 B17 **Kaoko Veld** ▲ N Namibia
76 G11 **Kaolack** *var.* Kaolak. W Senegal
Kaolak *see* Kaolack
Kaolan *see* Lanzhou
186 M8 **Kaolo** San Jorge, N Solomon Islands
83 H14 **Kaoma** Western, W Zambia
38 B8 **Kapaa** *Haw.* Kapa'a. Kauai, Hawaii, USA, C Pacific Ocean
113 J16 **Kapa Moračka** ▲ SW Yugoslavia
137 V13 **Kapan** *Rus.* Kafan; *prev.* Ghap'an. SE Armenia
82 L13 **Kapandashila** Northern, NE Zambia
79 L23 **Kapanga** Katanga, S Dem. Rep. Congo (Zaire)
145 U15 **Kapchagay** *Kaz.* Kapshagay. Almaty, SE Kazakhstan
145 V15 **Kapchagayskoye Vodokhranilishche** *Kaz.* Qapshagay Böyeni. ▣ SE Kazakhstan
99 F15 **Kapelle** Zeeland, SW Netherlands
99 G16 **Kapellen** Antwerpen, N Belgium
95 P15 **Kapellskär** Stockholm, C Sweden
81 H18 **Kapenguria** Rift Valley, W Kenya
109 V6 **Kapfenberg** Steiermark, C Austria
83 J14 **Kapiri Mposhi** Central, C Zambia
149 R4 **Kāpīsā** ◈ *province* E Afghanistan
12 G10 **Kapiskau** ≈ Ontario, C Canada
184 K13 **Kapiti Island** *island* C NZ
78 K9 **Kapka, Massif du** ▲ E Chad
Kaplamada *see* Kaubalatmada, Gunung
22 H9 **Kaplan** Louisiana, S USA
146 E9 **Kaplangky, Plato** *ridge* Turkmenistan/Uzbekistan
111 D19 **Kaplice** *Ger.* Kaplitz. Budějovický Kraj , S Czech Republic
Kaplitz *see* Kaplice
Kapoche *see* Capoche
171 T12 **Kapocol** Irian Jaya, E Indonesia
167 N14 **Kapoe** Ranong, SW Thailand
Kapoeas *see* Kapuas, Sungai
81 G15 **Kapoeta** Eastern Equatoria, SE Sudan
111 I25 **Kapos** ≈ S Hungary
111 H25 **Kaposvár** Somogy, SW Hungary
94 H13 **Kapp** Oppland, S Norway
100 I7 **Kappeln** Schleswig-Holstein, N Germany
Kaproncza *see* Koprivnica
109 P7 **Kaprun** Salzburg, C Austria
Kapshaghay *see* Kapchagay
Kapstad *see* Cape Town
Kapsukas *see* Marijampolė
171 Y13 **Kaptiau** Irian Jaya, E Indonesia
119 L19 **Kaptsevichy** *Rus.* Koptsevichi. Homyel'skaya Voblasts', SE Belarus
Kapuas Hulu, Banjaran/Kapuas Hulu, Pegunungan *see* Kapuas Mountains
169 S10 **Kapuas Mountains** *Ind.* Banjaran Kapuas Hulu, Pegunungan Kapuas Hulu. ▲ Indonesia/Malaysia
169 P11 **Kapuas, Sungai** ≈ Borneo, N Indonesia
169 T13 **Kapuas, Sungai** *prev.* Kapoeas. ≈ Borneo, C Indonesia
182 J9 **Kapunda** South Australia
152 H8 **Kapūrthala** Punjab, N India
12 G12 **Kapuskasing** Ontario, S Canada
14 D6 **Kapuskasing** ≈ Ontario, S Canada
129 P11 **Kapustin Yar** Astrakhanskaya Oblast', SW Russian Federation
82 K11 **Kaputa** Northern, NE Zambia
111 G22 **Kapuvár** Győr-Moson-Sopron, NW Hungary
Kapydzhik, Gora *see* Qapiciğ Dağı
119 J17 **Kapyl'** *Rus.* Kopyl'. Minskaya Voblasts', C Belarus
43 N9 **Kara** *var.* Cara. Región Autónoma Atlántico Sur, E Nicaragua
77 R14 **Kara** *var.* Lama-Kara. NE Togo
77 Q14 **Kara** ≈ N Togo
147 U7 **Kara-Balta** Chuyskaya Oblast', N Kyrgyzstan
144 G11 **Karabau** Atyrau, W Kazakhstan
146 E7 **Karabaur', Uval** *Kaz.* Korabavur Pastligi, *Uzb.* Qorabowur Kirlari. *physical region* Kazakhstan/Uzbekistan
146 L13 **Karabekaul** *var.* Garabekevyul, *Turkm.* Garabekewül. Lebapskiy Velayat, E Turkmenistan
146 K15 **Karabil', Vozvyshennost'** ▲ S Turkmenistan
146 A9 **Kara-Bogaz-Gol** *Turkm.* Garabogazköl. Balkanskiy Velayat, NW Turkmenistan
146 B9 **Kara-Bogaz-Gol, Zaliv** *bay* NW Turkmenistan
145 R15 **Karaboget** *Kaz.* Qaraböget. Zhambyl, S Kazakhstan
136 H11 **Karabük** Karabük, NW Turkey
136 H11 **Karabük** ◈ *province* NW Turkey
122 L12 **Karabula** Krasnoyarskiy Kray, C Russian Federation
145 V14 **Karabulak** *Kaz.* Qarabulaq. Almaty, SE Kazakhstan
145 Y11 **Karabulak** *Kaz.* Qarabulaq. Vostochnyy Kazakhstan, E Kazakhstan
145 Q17 **Karabulak** *Kaz.* Qarabulaq. Yuzhnyy Kazakhstan, S Kazakhstan
136 C17 **Kara Burnu** *headland* SW Turkey
144 K10 **Karabutak** *Kaz.* Qarabutaq. Aktyubinsk, W Kazakhstan
136 D12 **Karacabey** Bursa, NW Turkey
114 O12 **Karacaköy** İstanbul, NW Turkey
114 M12 **Karacaoğlan** Kırklareli, NW Turkey
Karachay-Cherkessia *see* Karachayevo-Cherkesskaya Respublika
128 L15 **Karachayevo-Cherkesskaya Respublika** *Eng.* Karachay-Cherkessia. ◈ *autonomous republic* SW Russian Federation
128 M15 **Karachayevsk** Karachayevo-Cherkesskaya Respublika, SW Russian Federation
128 J6 **Karachev** Bryanskaya Oblast', W Russian Federation
149 O16 **Karāchi** Sind, SE Pakistan
149 O16 **Karāchi** ✕ Sind, S Pakistan
Karácsonkő *see* Piatra-Neamț
155 E15 **Karād** Mahārāshtra, W India
136 H16 **Karadağ** ▲ S Turkey
147 T10 **Karadar'ya** *Uzb.* Qoradaryo. ≈ Kyrgyzstan/Uzbekistan
Karadeniz *see* Black Sea
Karadeniz Boğazı *see* İstanbul Boğazı
146 B13 **Karadepe** Balkanskiy Velayat, W Turkmenistan
Karadzhar *see* Qorajar
Karaferiye *see* Véroia
146 E13 **Karagan** *Turkm.* Garagan. Akhalskiy Velayat, C Turkmenistan
145 R10 **Karaganda** *Kaz.* Qaraghandy. Karaganda, C Kazakhstan
145 R10 **Karaganda** *off.* Karagandinskaya Oblast', *Kaz.* Qaraghandy Oblysy. ◈ *province* C Kazakhstan
Karagandinskaya Oblast' *see* Karaganda
145 T10 **Karagayly** *Kaz.* Qaraghayly. Karaganda, C Kazakhstan
146 A11 **Karagel'** *Turkm.* Garagöl. Balkanskiy Velayat, W Turkmenistan
123 U9 **Karaginskiy, Ostrov** *island* E Russian Federation
197 T1 **Karaginskiy Zaliv** *bay* E Russian Federation
137 P13 **Karagöl Dağları** ▲ NE Turkey
114 L13 **Karahisar** Edirne, NW Turkey
129 V3 **Karaidel'** Respublika Bashkortostan, W Russian Federation
129 V3 **Karaidel'skiy** Respublika Bashkortostan, W Russian Federation
114 L13 **Karaidemir Barajı** ▣ NW Turkey
155 J21 **Kāraikāl** Pondicherry, SE India
155 I22 **Kāraikkudi** Tamil Nādu, SE India
145 Y11 **Kara Irtysh** *Rus.* Chërnyy Irtysh. ≈ NE Kazakhstan
143 N5 **Karaj** Tehrān, N Iran
168 K8 **Karak** Pahang, Peninsular Malaysia
Karak *see* Al Karak
147 T11 **Kara-Kabak** Oshskaya Oblast', SW Kyrgyzstan
146 D12 **Kara-Kala** *var.* Garrygala. Balkanskiy Velayat, W Turkmenistan
Karakala *see* Oqqal'a
Karakalpakstan, Respublika *see* Qoraqalpoghiston Respublikasi
Karakalpakya *see* Qoraqalpoghiston
Karakax *see* Moyu
158 G10 **Karakax He** ≈ NW China
121 X8 **Karakaya Barajı** ▣ C Turkey
171 Q9 **Karakelang, Pulau** *island* N Indonesia
Karakılısse *see* Ağrı
Karak, Muḩāfaẓat al *see* Al Karak
Kara-Köl *see* Kara-Kul'
147 Y7 **Karakol** *prev.* Przheval'sk. Issyk-Kul'skaya Oblast', NE Kyrgyzstan
147 X8 **Karakol** *var.* Karakolka. Issyk-Kul'skaya Oblast', NE Kyrgyzstan
Karakolka *see* Karakol
149 W2 **Karakoram Highway** *road* China/Pakistan
149 Z3 **Karakoram Pass** *Chin.* Karakoram Shankou. *pass* C Asia
152 I3 **Karakoram Range** ▲ C Asia
Karakoram Shankou *see* Karakoram Pass
Karaköse *see* Ağrı
145 P14 **Karakoyyn, Ozero** *Kaz.* Qaraqoyyn. ◎ C Kazakhstan
83 F19 **Karakubis** Ghanzi, W Botswana
147 T9 **Kara-Kul'** *Kir.* Kara-Köl. Dzhalal-Abadskaya Oblast', W Kyrgyzstan
Karakul' *see* Qarokŭl, Tajikistan
Karakul' *see* Qorakŭl, Uzbekistan
147 U10 **Kara-Kul'dzha** Oshskaya Oblast', SW Kyrgyzstan
129 T3 **Karakulino** Udmurtskaya Respublika, NW Russian Federation
Karakul', Ozero *see* Qarokŭl
Kara Kum *see* Garagumy
Kara Kum Canal/Karakumskiy Kanal *see* Garagumskiy Kanal
Karakumy, Peski *see* Garagumy
83 E17 **Karakuwisa** Okavango, NE Namibia
122 M13 **Karam** Irkutskaya Oblast', S Russian Federation
Karamai *see* Karamay
169 T14 **Karamain, Pulau** *island* N Indonesia
136 I16 **Karaman** Karaman, S Turkey
136 H16 **Karaman** ◈ *province* S Turkey
114 M8 **Karamandere** ≈ NE Bulgaria
158 J4 **Karamay** *var.* Karamai, Kelamayi, *prev. Chin.* K'o-la-ma-i. Xinjiang Uygur Zizhiqu, NW China
169 U14 **Karambu** Borneo, N Indonesia
185 H14 **Karamea** West Coast, South Island, NZ
185 H14 **Karamea** ≈ South Island, NZ
185 G15 **Karamea Bight** *gulf* South Island, NZ
146 L14 **Karamet-Niyaz** *Turkm.* Garamäbnyyaz. Lebapskiy Velayat, E Turkmenistan
158 K10 **Karamiran He** ≈ NW China
147 S11 **Karamyk** Oshskaya Oblast', SW Kyrgyzstan
169 U17 **Karangasem** Bali, S Indonesia
154 H12 **Kāranja** Mahārāshtra, C India
Karanpur *see* Karanpura
152 F9 **Karanpura** *var.* Karanpur. Rājasthān, NW India
Karánsebes/Karansebesch *see* Caransebeș
145 T14 **Karaoy** *Kaz.* Qaraoy. Almaty, SE Kazakhstan
114 N7 **Karapelit** *Rom.* Stejarul. Dobrich, NE Bulgaria
136 I15 **Karapınar** Konya, C Turkey
83 D22 **Karas** ◈ *district* S Namibia
147 Y8 **Kara-Say** Issyk-Kul'skaya Oblast', NE Kyrgyzstan
83 E22 **Karasburg** Karas, S Namibia
Kara Sea *see* Karskoye More
92 K9 **Kárášjohka** *var.* Karašjokka. ≈ N Norway
92 L9 **Karasjok** *Fin.* Kaarasjoki. Finnmark, N Norway
Karašjokka *see* Kárášjohka
Kara Strait *see* Karskiye Vorota, Proliv
Kara Su *see* Mesta/Néstos
145 N8 **Karasu** *Kaz.* Qarasū. Kostanay, N Kazakhstan

◆ Country ● Country Capital ◇ Dependent Territory ○ Dependent Territory Capital ◈ Administrative Region ✕ International Airport ▲ Mountain ▲ Mountain Range ※ Volcano ≈ River ◎ Lake ▣ Reservoir

136 F11 **Karasu** Sakarya, NW Turkey
Karasubazar see Bilohirs'k
122 I12 **Karasuk** Novosibirskaya Oblast', C Russian Federation
145 U13 **Karatal** Kaz. Qaratal. ≈ SE Kazakhstan
136 K17 **Karataş** Adana, S Turkey
145 Q16 **Karatau** Kaz. Qaratau. Zhambyl, S Kazakhstan
Karatau see Karatau, Khrebet
145 P16 **Karatau, Khrebet** var. Karatau, Kaz. Qaratau. ▲▲ S Kazakhstan
144 G13 **Karaton** Kaz. Qaraton. Atyrau, W Kazakhstan
164 C13 **Karatsu** var. Karatu. Saga, Kyūshū, SW Japan
Karatu see Karatsu
122 K8 **Karaul** Taymyrskiy (Dolgano-Nenetskiy) Avtonomnyy Okrug, N Russian Federation
Karaulbazar see Qorowulbozor
Karauzyak see Qoraŭzak
115 D16 **Karáva** ▲ C Greece
Karavanke see Karawanken
115 F22 **Karavás** Kýthira, S Greece
113 J20 **Karavastasë, Laguna e** var. Kënet' e Karavastas, Kravasta Lagoon. lagoon W Albania
Karavastas, Kënet' e see Karavastasë, Laguna e
118 I5 **Karavere** Tartumaa, E Estonia
115 L23 **Karavonísia** island Kykládes, Greece, Aegean Sea
169 O15 **Karawang** prev. Krawang. Jawa, C Indonesia
109 T10 **Karawanken** Slvn. Karavanke. ▲▲ Austria/Yugoslavia
Karaxahar see Kaidu He
137 R13 **Karayazı** Erzurum, NE Turkey
145 Q12 **Karazhal** Zhezkazgan, C Kazakhstan
139 S9 **Karbalā'** var. Kerbala, Kerbela. S Iraq
94 L11 **Kårböle** Gävleborg, C Sweden
111 M23 **Karcag** Jász-Nagykun-Szolnok, E Hungary
Kardak see Imia
114 N7 **Kardam** Dobrich, NE Bulgaria
115 M22 **Kardámaina** Kos, Dodekánisos, Greece, Aegean Sea
Kardamila see Kardámyla
115 L18 **Kardámyla** var. Kardamila, Kardhámila. Chíos, E Greece
Kardeljevo see Ploče
Kardh see Qardho
Kardhámila see Kardámyla
Kardhítsa see Kardítsa
115 E16 **Kardítsa** var. Kardhítsa. Thessalía, C Greece
118 E4 **Kärdla** Ger. Kertel. Hiiumaa, W Estonia
Karelia see Kareliya, Respublika
119 I16 **Karelichy** Pol. Korelicze, Rus. Korelichi. Hrodzyenskaya Voblasts', W Belarus
126 I10 **Kareliya, Respublika** prev. Karel'skaya ASSR, Eng. Karelia. ◈ autonomous republic NW Russian Federation
Karel'skaya ASSR see Kareliya, Respublika
81 E22 **Karema** Rukwa, W Tanzania
Karen see Hualien
83 I14 **Karenda** Central, C Zambia
167 N8 **Karen State** var. Kawthule State, Kayin State. ◈ state S Myanmar
92 J10 **Karesuando** Lapp. Kaaresuanto. Norrbotten, N Sweden
Karet see Kâgheț
Kareyz-e-Elyās/Kārez Iliās see Kārīz-e Elyās
122 J11 **Kargasok** Tomskaya Oblast', C Russian Federation
122 I12 **Kargat** Novosibirskaya Oblast', C Russian Federation
136 J11 **Kargı** Çorum, N Turkey
152 I5 **Kargil** Jammu and Kashmir, NW India
Kargilik see Yecheng
126 L11 **Kargopol'** Arkhangel'skaya Oblast', NW Russian Federation
110 F12 **Kargowa** Ger. Unruhstadt. Lubuskie, W Poland
77 X13 **Kari** Bauchi, E Nigeria
83 J15 **Kariba** Mashonaland West, N Zimbabwe
83 J16 **Kariba, Lake** ▣ Zambia/Zimbabwe
165 Q4 **Kariba-yama** ▲ Hokkaidō, NE Japan
83 C19 **Karibib** Erongo, C Namibia
Karies see Karyés
92 L9 **Karigasniemi** Lapp. Garegegasnjárga. Lappi, N Finland
184 J2 **Karikari, Cape** headland North Island, NZ
Karīmābād see Hunza
169 P12 **Karimata, Kepulauan** island group N Indonesia
169 P12 **Karimata, Pulau** island Kepulauan Karimata, N Indonesia
169 O11 **Karimata, Selat** strait W Indonesia
155 I14 **Karīmnagar** Andhra Pradesh, C India
186 C7 **Karimui** Chimbu, C PNG
169 Q15 **Karimunjawa, Pulau** island S Indonesia
80 N12 **Karin** Woqooyi Galbeed, N Somalia
Kariot see Ikaría
93 L20 **Karis** Fin. Karjaa. Etelä-Suomi, SW Finland
Káristos see Kárystos
148 J4 **Kārīz-e Elyās** var. Kareyz-e-Elyās, Kārez Iliās. Herāt, NW Afghanistan
Karjaa see Karis
145 T10 **Karkaralinsk** Kaz. Qarqaraly. Karaganda, E Kazakhstan
186 D6 **Karkar Island** island N PNG
143 N7 **Karkas, Kūh-e** ▲▲ C Iran
142 K8 **Karkheh, Rūd-e** ≈ SW Iran
115 L20 **Karkinágrio** Ikaría, Dodekánisos, Greece, Aegean Sea
117 R12 **Karkinits'ka Zatoka** Rus. Karkinitskiy Zaliv. gulf S Ukraine
Karkinitskiy Zaliv see Karkinits'ka Zatoka
93 L19 **Karkkila** Swe. Högfors. Etelä-Suomi, S Finland
93 M19 **Kärkölä** Etelä-Suomi, S Finland
182 G9 **Karkoo** South Australia
Karkūk see Kirkūk
118 D5 **Kärla** Ger. Kergel. Saaremaa, W Estonia
Karleby see Kokkola
110 F7 **Karlino** Ger. Körlin an der Persante. Zachodniopomorskie, NW Poland
137 Q13 **Karlıova** Bingöl, E Turkey
117 U6 **Karlivka** Poltavs'ka Oblast', C Ukraine
Karl-Marx-Stadt see Chemnitz
Karlö see Hailuoto
112 C11 **Karlobag** It. Carlopago. Lika-Senj, W Croatia
112 D9 **Karlovac** Ger. Karlstadt, Hung. Károlyváros. Karlovac, C Croatia
112 C10 **Karlovac** off. Karlovačka Županija. ◈ province C Croatia
Karlovačka Županija see Karlovac
111 A16 **Karlovarský Kraj** ◈ W Czech Republic
114 J9 **Karlovo** prev. Levskigrad. Plovdiv, C Bulgaria
111 A16 **Karlovy Vary** Ger. Karlsbad; prev. Eng. Carlsbad. Karlovarský Kraj, W Czech Republic
Karlsbad see Karlovy Vary
95 L17 **Karlsborg** Västra Götaland, S Sweden
Karlsburg see Alba Iulia
95 L22 **Karlshamn** Blekinge, S Sweden
95 L16 **Karlskoga** Örebro, C Sweden
95 M22 **Karlskrona** Blekinge, S Sweden
101 G21 **Karlsruhe** var. Carlsruhe. Baden-Württemberg, SW Germany
95 K16 **Karlstad** Värmland, C Sweden
29 R3 **Karlstad** Minnesota, N USA
101 I18 **Karlstadt** Bayern, C Germany
Karlstadt see Karlovac
39 Q14 **Karluk** Kodiak Island, Alaska, USA
Karluk see Qarluq
119 O17 **Karma** Rus. Korma. Homyel'skaya Voblasts', SE Belarus
155 F14 **Karmāla** Mahārāshtra, W India
146 M11 **Karmana** Nawoiy Wiloyati, C Uzbekistan
138 G8 **Karmi'él** var. Carmiel. Northern, N Israel
95 B16 **Karmøy** island S Norway
152 I9 **Karnāl** Haryāna, N India
153 W15 **Karnaphuli Reservoir** ▣ NE India
155 F17 **Karnātaka** var. Kanara; prev. Maisur, Mysore. ◈ state W India
25 S13 **Karnes City** Texas, SW USA
109 P9 **Karnische Alpen** It. Alpi Carniche. ▲▲ Austria/Italy
114 M9 **Karnobat** Burgas, E Bulgaria
109 Q9 **Kärnten** off. Land Kärnten, Eng. Carinthia, Slvn. Koroška. ◈ state S Austria
Karnul see Kurnool
83 K16 **Karoi** Mashonaland West, N Zimbabwe
Karol see Carei
Károly-Fehérvár see Alba Iulia
Károlyváros see Karlovac
82 M12 **Karonga** Northern, N Malawi
147 W10 **Karool-Tëbë** Narynskaya Oblast', C Kyrgyzstan
182 J9 **Karoonda** South Australia
149 S9 **Karor Lāl Esan** Punjab, E Pakistan
149 T11 **Karor Pacca** var. Kahror, Kahror Pakka. Punjab, E Pakistan
171 N12 **Karosa** Sulawesi, C Indonesia
Karpaten see Carpathian Mountains
115 L22 **Karpáthio Pélagos** sea Dodekánisos, Greece, Aegean Sea
115 N24 **Kárpathos** Kárpathos, SE Greece
115 N24 **Kárpathos** It. Scarpanto; anc. Carpathos, Carpathus. island SE Greece
Karpathos Strait see Karpathou, Stenó
115 N24 **Karpathou, Stenó** var. Karpathos Strait, Scarpanto Strait. strait Dodekánisos, Greece, Aegean Sea
Karpaty see Carpathian Mountains
115 E17 **Karpenísi** prev. Karpenísion. Stereá Ellás, C Greece
Karpenísion see Karpenísi
Karpilovka see Aktsyabrski
127 O8 **Karpogory** Arkhangel'skaya Oblast', NW Russian Federation
180 I7 **Karratha** Western Australia
137 S12 **Kars** var. Qars. Kars, NE Turkey
137 S12 **Kars** var. Qars. ◈ province NE Turkey
145 O12 **Karsakpay** Kaz. Qarsaqbay. Zhezkazgan, C Kazakhstan
93 L15 **Kärsämäki** Oulu, C Finland
Karsau see Kārsava
118 K9 **Kārsava** Ger. Karsau; prev. Rus. Korsovka. Ludza, E Latvia
146 A9 **Karshi** Turkm. Garshy. Balkanskiy Velayat, NW Turkmenistan
Karshi see Qarshi
Karshinskaya Step see Qarshi Chŭli
Karshinskiy Kanal see Qarshi Kanali
84 I5 **Karskiye Vorota, Proliv** Eng. Kara Strait. strait N Russian Federation
122 J6 **Karskoye More** Eng. Kara Sea. sea Arctic Ocean
93 L17 **Karstula** Länsi-Suomi, W Finland
129 Q5 **Karsun** Ul'yanovskaya Oblast', W Russian Federation
122 F11 **Kartaly** Chelyabinskaya Oblast', C Russian Federation
18 E13 **Karthaus** Pennsylvania, NE USA
110 I7 **Kartuzy** Pomorskie, NW Poland
165 R8 **Karumai** Iwate, Honshū, C Japan
181 U4 **Karumba** Queensland, NE Australia
142 L10 **Kārūn** var. Rūd-e Kārūn. ≈ SW Iran
92 K13 **Karungi** Norrbotten, N Sweden
92 K13 **Karunki** Lappi, N Finland
Kārūn, Rūd-e see Kārūn
155 H21 **Karūr** Tamil Nādu, SE India
93 K17 **Karvia** Länsi-Suomi, W Finland
111 J17 **Karviná** Ger. Karwin, Pol. Karwina; prev. Nová Karvinná. Ostravský Kraj, E Czech Republic
155 E17 **Kārwār** Karnātaka, W India
108 M7 **Karwendelgebirge** ▲▲ Austria/Germany
Karwin/Karwina see Karviná
115 I14 **Karyés** var. Karies. Ágion Óros, N Greece
115 I19 **Kárystos** var. Káristos. Évvoia, C Greece
136 E17 **Kaş** Antalya, SW Turkey
39 Y14 **Kasaan** Prince of Wales Island, Alaska, USA
164 I13 **Kasai** Hyōgo, Honshū, SW Japan
79 K21 **Kasai** var. Cassai, Kassai. ≈ Angola/Dem. Rep. Congo (Zaire)
79 K22 **Kasai Occidental** off. Région Kasai Occidental. ◈ region S Dem. Rep. Congo (Zaire)
79 L21 **Kasai Oriental** off. Région Kasai Oriental. ◈ region C Dem. Rep. Congo (Zaire)
79 L24 **Kasaji** Katanga, S Dem. Rep. Congo (Zaire)
82 L12 **Kasama** Northern, N Zambia
Kasan see Koson
83 H16 **Kasane** Chobe, NE Botswana
81 E23 **Kasanga** Rukwa, W Tanzania
79 G21 **Kasangulu** Bas-Congo, W Dem. Rep. Congo (Zaire)
Kasansay see Kosonsoy
Kasargen see Kasari
155 E20 **Kāsargod** Kerala, SW India
118 P13 **Kasari** var. Kasari Jõgi, Ger. Kasargen. ≈ W Estonia
Kasari Jõgi see Kasari
8 L11 **Kasba Lake** ◎ Northwest Territories/Nunavut, N Canada
Kaschau see Košice
164 B16 **Kaseda** Kagoshima, Kyūshū, SW Japan
83 I14 **Kasempa** North Western, NW Zambia
79 O24 **Kasenga** Katanga, SE Dem. Rep. Congo (Zaire)
79 P17 **Kasenye** var. Kasenyi. Orientale, NE Dem. Rep. Congo (Zaire)
Kasenyi see Kasenye
81 E18 **Kasese** SW Uganda
79 O19 **Kasese** Maniema, E Dem. Rep. Congo (Zaire)
152 J11 **Kāsganj** Uttar Pradesh, N India
143 U4 **Kashaf Rūd** ≈ NE Iran
143 N7 **Kāshān** Eşfahān, C Iran
128 M10 **Kashary** Rostovskaya Oblast', SW Russian Federation
39 O12 **Kashegelok** Alaska, USA
Kashgar see Kashi
158 E7 **Kashi** Chin. Kaxgar, K'o-shih, Uigh. Kashgar. Xinjiang Uygur Zizhiqu, NW China
164 J14 **Kashihara** var. Kasihara. Nara, Honshū, SW Japan
165 P13 **Kashima-nada** gulf S Japan
126 K15 **Kashin** Tverskaya Oblast', W Russian Federation
152 K10 **Kāshīpur** Uttar Pradesh, N India
128 L4 **Kashira** Moskovskaya Oblast', W Russian Federation
165 N11 **Kashiwazaki** var. Kasiwazaki. Niigata, Honshū, C Japan
Kashkadar'inskaya Oblast' see Qashqadaryo Wiloyati
143 T5 **Kāshmar** var. Turshiz; prev. Solṭānābād, Torshiz. Khorāsān, NE Iran
Kashmir see Jammu and Kashmir
149 R12 **Kashmor** Sind, SE Pakistan
149 S5 **Kashmūnd Ghar** Eng. Kashmund Range. ▲▲ E Afghanistan
Kashmund Range see Kashmūnd Ghar
Kasi see Vārānasi
153 O12 **Kasia** Uttar Pradesh, N India
39 N12 **Kasigluk** Alaska, USA
Kasihara see Kashihara
39 R12 **Kasilof** Alaska, USA
Kasima see Kashima
Kasimköj see General Toshevo
128 M4 **Kasimov** Ryazanskaya Oblast', W Russian Federation
79 P18 **Kasindi** Nord Kivu, E Dem. Rep. Congo (Zaire)
82 M12 **Kasitu** ≈ N Malawi
Kasiwa see Kashiwa
Kasiwazaki see Kashiwazaki
30 L14 **Kaskaskia River** ≈ Illinois, N USA
93 J17 **Kaskinen** Swe. Kaskö. Länsi-Suomi, W Finland
Kaskö see Kaskinen
Kas Kong see Kŏng, Kaôh
11 O17 **Kaslo** British Columbia, SW Canada
Käsmark see Kežmarok
169 T12 **Kasongan** Borneo, C Indonesia
79 N21 **Kasongo** Maniema, E Dem. Rep. Congo (Zaire)
79 H22 **Kasongo-Lunda** Bandundu, SW Dem. Rep. Congo (Zaire)
115 M24 **Kásos** island S Greece
Kasos Strait see Kasou, Stenó
115 M25 **Kasou, Stenó** var. Kasos Strait. strait Dodekánisos/Kríti, Greece, Aegean Sea
137 T10 **Kaspi** C Georgia
114 M8 **Kaspichan** Shumen, NE Bulgaria
Kaspīy Mangy Oypaty see Caspian Depression
129 Q16 **Kaspiysk** Respublika Dagestan, SW Russian Federation
Kaspiyskiy see Lagan'
Kaspiyskoye More/Kaspiy Tengizi see Caspian Sea
Kassa see Košice
Kassai see Kasai
80 I9 **Kassala** Kassala, E Sudan
80 H9 **Kassala** ◈ state NE Sudan
115 G15 **Kassándra** prev. Pallíni; anc. Pallene. peninsula NE Greece
115 G15 **Kassándras, Akrotírio** headland N Greece
115 H15 **Kassándras, Kólpos** var. Kólpos Toronaíos. gulf N Greece
139 Y11 **Kassārah** E Iraq
101 I15 **Kassel** prev. Cassel. Hessen, C Germany
74 M6 **Kasserine** var. Al Qaşrayn. W Tunisia
14 J14 **Kasshabog Lake** ◎ Ontario, SE Canada
139 O5 **Kassīr, Sabkhat al** ◎ E Syria
29 W10 **Kasson** Minnesota, N USA
115 C17 **Kassópi** site of ancient city Ípeiros, W Greece
115 N24 **Kastállou, Akrotírio** headland Kárpathos, SE Greece
136 I11 **Kastamonu** var. Castamoni, Kastamuni. Kastamonu, N Turkey
136 I10 **Kastamonu** var. Kastamuni. ◈ province N Turkey
Kastamuni see Kastamonu
115 E14 **Kastaneá** Kentrikí Makedonía, N Greece
115 H24 **Kastélli** Kríti, Greece, E Mediterranean Sea
Kastellórizon see Megísti
95 N21 **Kastlösa** Kalmar, S Sweden
115 D14 **Kastoría** Dytikí Makedonía, N Greece
128 K7 **Kastornoye** Kurskaya Oblast', W Russian Federation
115 I21 **Kástro** Sífnos, Kykládes, Greece, Aegean Sea
95 J23 **Kastrup** ✈ (København) København, E Denmark
119 Q17 **Kastsyukovichy** Rus. Kostyukovichi. Mahilyowskaya Voblasts', E Belarus
119 O18 **Kastsyukowka** Rus. Kostyukovka. Homyel'skaya Voblasts', SE Belarus
164 D13 **Kasuga** Fukuoka, Kyūshū, SW Japan
164 L13 **Kasugai** Aichi, Honshū, SW Japan
81 E21 **Kasulu** Kigoma, W Tanzania
164 I12 **Kasumi** Hyōgo, Honshū, SW Japan
129 R17 **Kasumkent** Respublika Dagestan, SW Russian Federation
82 M13 **Kasungu** Central, C Malawi
149 W9 **Kasūr** Punjab, E Pakistan
83 G15 **Kataba** Western, W Zambia
19 R4 **Katahdin, Mount** ▲ Maine, NE USA
79 M20 **Katako-Kombe** Kasai Oriental, C Dem. Rep. Congo (Zaire)
39 T12 **Katalla** Alaska, USA
Katana see Qaṭanā
79 L24 **Katanga** off. Région du Katanga; prev. Shaba. ◈ region SE Dem. Rep. Congo (Zaire)
122 M11 **Katanga** ≈ C Russian Federation
154 J11 **Katangi** Madhya Pradesh, C India
180 J13 **Katanning** Western Australia
189 P8 **Kata Tjuta** var. Mount Olga ▲ Northern Territory, C Australia
Katawaz see Zarghūn Shahr
151 Q22 **Katchall Island** island Nicobar Islands, India, NE Indian Ocean
115 F14 **Kateríni** Kentrikí Makedonía, N Greece
117 P7 **Katerynopil'** Cherkas'ka Oblast', C Ukraine
166 M3 **Katha** Sagaing, N Myanmar
181 P2 **Katherine** Northern Territory, N Australia
154 B11 **Kāthiāwār Peninsula** peninsula W India
153 P11 **Kathmandu** prev. Kantipur. ● (Nepal) Central, C Nepal
152 H7 **Kathua** Jammu and Kashmir, NW India
76 L12 **Kati** Koulikoro, SW Mali
153 R13 **Katihār** Bihār, NE India
184 N7 **Katikati** Bay of Plenty, North Island, NZ
83 H16 **Katima Mulilo** Caprivi, NE Namibia
77 N15 **Katiola** C Ivory Coast
191 V10 **Katiu** atoll Îles Tuamotu, C French Polynesia
117 N12 **Katlabukh, Ozero** ◎ SW Ukraine
39 P14 **Katmai, Mount** ▲ Alaska, USA
154 J9 **Katni** Madhya Pradesh, C India
115 D19 **Káto Achaïa** var. Kato Ahaia, Káto Akhaía. Dytikí Ellás, S Greece
Kato Ahaia/Káto Akhaía see Káto Achaïa
121 P2 **Kato Lakatámeia** var. Kato Lakatamia. C Cyprus
Kato Lakatamia see Kato Lakatámeia
79 N22 **Katompi** Katanga, SE Dem. Rep. Congo (Zaire)
83 K14 **Katondwe** Lusaka, C Zambia
114 H12 **Káto Nevrokópi** prev. Káto Nevrokópion. Anatolikí Makedonía kai Thráki, NE Greece
Káto Nevrokópion see Káto Nevrokópi
81 E18 **Katonga** ≈ S Uganda
115 F15 **Káto Ólympos** ▲▲ C Greece
115 D17 **Katoúna** Dytikí Ellás, C Greece
115 E19 **Káto Vlasiá** Dytikí Makedonía, S Greece
111 J16 **Katowice** Ger. Kattowitz. Śląskie, S Poland
153 S15 **Kātoya** West Bengal, NE India
136 E16 **Katrançik Dağı** ▲▲ SW Turkey
95 N16 **Katrineholm** Södermanland, C Sweden
96 I11 **Katrine, Loch** ◎ C Scotland, UK
77 V12 **Katsina** Katsina, N Nigeria
77 U12 **Katsina** ◈ state N Nigeria
67 P8 **Katsina Ala** ≈ S Nigeria
164 C13 **Katsumoto** Nagasaki, Iki, SW Japan
165 P13 **Katsuta** var. Katuta. Ibaraki, Honshū, S Japan
165 O14 **Katsuura** var. Katuura. Chiba, Honshū, S Japan
164 K12 **Katsuyama** var. Katuyama. Fukui, Honshū, SW Japan
164 H12 **Katsuyama** Okayama, Honshū, SW Japan
Kattakurgan see Kattaqŭrghon
147 N11 **Kattaqŭrghon** Rus. Kattakurgan. Samarqand Wiloyati, C Uzbekistan
115 O23 **Kattavía** Ródos, Dodekánisos, Greece, Aegean Sea
95 I21 **Kattegat** Dan. Kattegatt. strait N Europe
Kattegatt see Kattegat
95 P19 **Katthammarsvik** Gotland, SE Sweden
Kattowitz see Katowice
122 J13 **Katun'** ≈ S Russian Federation
Katuta see Katsuta
Katuura see Katsuura
Katuyama see Katsuyama
Katwijk see Katwijk aan Zee
98 G11 **Katwijk aan Zee** var. Katwijk. Zuid-Holland, W Netherlands
38 B8 **Kauai** Haw. Kaua'i. island Hawaiian Islands, Hawaii, USA, C Pacific Ocean
38 C8 **Kauai Channel** channel Hawaii, USA, C Pacific Ocean
171 R13 **Kaubalatmada, Gunung** var. Kaplamada. ▲ Pulau Buru, E Indonesia
191 U10 **Kauehi** atoll Îles Tuamotu, C French Polynesia
Kauen see Kaunas
101 K24 **Kaufbeuren** Bayern, S Germany
25 U7 **Kaufman** Texas, SW USA
101 I15 **Kaufungen** Hessen, C Germany
93 K17 **Kauhajoki** Länsi-Suomi, W Finland
93 K16 **Kauhava** Länsi-Suomi, W Finland
30 M7 **Kaukauna** Wisconsin, N USA
92 L11 **Kaukonen** Lappi, N Finland
38 A8 **Kaulakahi Channel** channel Hawaii, USA, C Pacific Ocean
38 E9 **Kaunakakai** Molokai, Hawaii, USA, C Pacific Ocean
38 F12 **Kauna Point** headland Hawaii, USA, C Pacific Ocean
118 F13 **Kaunas** Ger. Kauen, Pol. Kowno; prev. Rus. Kovno. Kaunas, C Lithuania
186 C6 **Kaup** East Sepik, NW PNG
77 U12 **Kaura Namoda** Zamfara, NW Nigeria
Kaushany see Căuşeni
93 K16 **Kaustinen** Länsi-Suomi, W Finland
99 M23 **Kautenbach** Diekirch, NE Luxembourg
92 K10 **Kautokeino** Finnmark, N Norway
Kavadar see Kavadarci
113 P19 **Kavadarci** Turk. Kavadar. C FYR Macedonia
Kavaja see Kavajë
113 K20 **Kavajë** It. Cavaia, Kavaja. Tiranë, W Albania
114 M13 **Kavak Çayı** ≈ NW Turkey
Kavakli see Topolovgrad
114 I13 **Kavála** prev. Kaválla. Anatolikí Makedonía kai Thráki, NE Greece
114 I13 **Kaválas, Kólpos** gulf Aegean Sea, NE Mediterranean Sea
155 J17 **Kāvali** Andhra Pradesh, E India
Kaválla see Kavála
Kavango see Cubango/Okavango
155 C21 **Kavaratti** Lakshadweep, SW India
114 O8 **Kavarna** Dobrich, NE Bulgaria
118 G12 **Kavarskas** Anykščiai, E Lithuania
76 I13 **Kavendou** ▲ C Guinea
Kavengo see Cubango/Okavango
155 F20 **Kāveri** var. Cauvery. ≈ S India
186 G5 **Kavieng** var. Kaewieng. NE PNG
83 H16 **Kavimba** Chobe, NE Botswana
83 I15 **Kavingu** Southern, S Zambia
143 Q6 **Kavīr, Dasht-e** var. Great Salt Desert. salt pan N Iran
Kavirondo Gulf see Winam Gulf
Kavkaz see Caucasus
95 K23 **Kävlinge** Skåne, S Sweden
82 G12 **Kavungo** Moxico, E Angola
165 Q8 **Kawabe** Akita, Honshū, C Japan
165 R9 **Kawai** Iwate, Honshū, C Japan
38 A8 **Kawaihoa Point** headland Niihau, Hawaii, USA, C Pacific Ocean
184 K3 **Kawakawa** Northland, North Island, NZ
82 I13 **Kawama** North Western, NW Zambia
82 K11 **Kawambwa** Luapula, N Zambia
154 K11 **Kawardha** Madhya Pradesh, C India
14 I14 **Kawartha Lakes** ◎ Ontario, SE Canada
165 O13 **Kawasaki** Kanagawa, Honshū, S Japan
171 R12 **Kawassi** Pulau Obi, E Indonesia
165 R6 **Kawauchi** Aomori, Honshū, C Japan
184 L5 **Kawau Island** island N NZ
184 N10 **Kaweka Range** ▲▲ North Island, NZ
Kawelecht see Puhja
184 O8 **Kawerau** Bay of Plenty, North Island, NZ
184 L8 **Kawhia** Waikato, North Island, NZ
184 K8 **Kawhia Harbour** inlet North Island, NZ
35 V8 **Kawich Peak** ▲ Nevada, W USA
35 V9 **Kawich Range** ▲▲ Nevada, W USA
14 G12 **Kawigamog Lake** ◎ Ontario, S Canada
171 P9 **Kawio, Kepulauan** island group N Indonesia
167 N9 **Kawkareik** Karen State, S Myanmar
27 O8 **Kaw Lake** ▣ Oklahoma, C USA
166 M3 **Kawlin** Sagaing, N Myanmar
Kawm Umbū see Kôm Ombo
Kawthule State see Karen State
Kaxgar see Kashi
158 D7 **Kaxgar He** ≈ NW China
158 J5 **Kax He** ≈ NW China
77 P12 **Kaya** C Burkina
167 N6 **Kayah State** ◈ state C Myanmar
39 T12 **Kayak Island** island Alaska, USA
114 M11 **Kayalıköy Barajı** ▣ NW Turkey
155 G23 **Kāyamkulam** Kerala, SW India
166 M8 **Kayan** Yangon, SW Myanmar
169 V9 **Kayan, Sungai** prev. Kajan. ≈ Borneo, C Indonesia
144 F14 **Kaydak, Sor** salt flat SW Kazakhstan
Kaydanovo see Dzyarzhynsk
37 N9 **Kayenta** Arizona, SW USA
76 J11 **Kayes** Kayes, W Mali
76 J11 **Kayes** ◈ region SW Mali
Kayin State see Karen State
145 U10 **Kaynar** var. Kajnar. Vostochnyy Kazakhstan, E Kazakhstan
Kaynary see Căinari
83 H15 **Kayoya** Western, W Zambia
Kayrakkum see Qayroqqum
Kayrakkumskoye Vodokhranilishche see Qayroqqum, Obanbori
136 K14 **Kayseri** var. Kaisaria; anc. Caesarea Mazaca, Mazaca. Kayseri, C Turkey
136 K14 **Kayseri** var. Kaisaria. ◈ province C Turkey
36 L2 **Kaysville** Utah, W USA
Kayyngdy see Kaindy
14 L11 **Kazabazua** Quebec, SE Canada
14 L12 **Kazabazua** ≈ Quebec, SE Canada
123 Q7 **Kazach'ye** Respublika Sakha (Yakutiya), NE Russian Federation
Kazakdar'ya see Qozoqdaryo
146 E9 **Kazakhlyshor, Solonchak** var. Solonchak Shorkazakhly. salt marsh NW Turkmenistan
Kazakhskaya SSR/Kazakh Soviet Socialist Republic see Kazakhstan
145 R9 **Kazakhskiy Melkosopochnik** Eng. Kazakh Uplands, Kirghiz Steppe, Kaz. Saryarqa. uplands C Kazakhstan
144 L12 **Kazakhstan** off. Republic of Kazakhstan, var. Kazakstan, Kaz. Qazaqstan, Qazaqstan Respublikasy; prev. Kazakh Soviet Socialist Republic, Rus. Kazakhskaya SSR. ◆ republic C Asia
Kazakh Uplands see Kazakhskiy Melkosopochnik
Kazakstan see Kazakhstan
144 L14 **Kazalinsk** Kzylorda, S Kazakhstan
129 R4 **Kazan'** Respublika Tatarstan, W Russian Federation
129 R4 **Kazan'** ✈ Respublika Tatarstan, W Russian Federation
8 M10 **Kazan** ≈ Nunavut, NW Canada
Kazandzhik see Gazandzhyk
117 R8 **Kazanka** Mykolayivs'ka Oblast', S Ukraine
Kazanketken see Qizqetkan
Kazanlik see Kazanlŭk
114 J9 **Kazanlŭk** prev. Kazanlik. Stara Zagora, C Bulgaria
165 Y16 **Kazan-rettō** Eng. Volcano Islands. island group SE Japan
117 V12 **Kazantip, Mys** headland S Ukraine
147 U9 **Kazarman** Narynskaya Oblast', C Kyrgyzstan
Kazatin see Kozyatyn
Kazbegi see Kazbek
Kazbegi see Qazbegi

◆ Country ● Country Capital ◇ Dependent Territory ○ Dependent Territory Capital ◈ Administrative Region ✈ International Airport ▲ Mountain ▲▲ Mountain Range Volcano ≈ River ◎ Lake ▣ Reservoir

137 T9 **Kazbek** *var.* Kazbegi, *Geor.* Mqinvartsveri. ▲ N Georgia
82 M13 **Kazembe** Eastern, NE Zambia
143 N11 **Kāzerūn** Fārs, S Iran
127 R12 **Kazhym** Respublika Komi, NW Russian Federation
Kazi Ahmad *see* Qāzi Ahmad
Kazi Magomed *see* Qazimämmäd
136 H16 **Kazımkarabekir** Karaman, S Turkey
111 M20 **Kazincbarcika** Borsod-Abaúj-Zemplén, NE Hungary
119 H17 **Kazlowshchyna** *Pol.* Kozlowszczyzna, *Rus.* Kozlovshchina. Hrodzyenskaya Voblasts', W Belarus
119 E14 **Kazlų Rūda** Marijampolė, S Lithuania
144 E9 **Kaztalovka** Zapadnyy Kazakhstan, W Kazakhstan
79 K22 **Kazumba** Kasai Occidental, S Dem. Rep. Congo (Zaire)
165 Q8 **Kazuno** Akita, Honshū, C Japan
Kazvin *see* Qazvīn
118 J12 **Kaz'yany** *Rus.* Koz'yany. Vitsyebskaya Voblasts', NW Belarus
122 H9 **Kazym** ≈ N Russian Federation
110 H10 **Kcynia** *Ger.* Exin. Kujawsko-pomorskie, C Poland
115 I20 **Kéa** Kéa, Kykládes, Greece, Aegean Sea
115 I20 **Kéa** *prev.* Kéos, *anc.* Ceos. *island* Kykládes, Greece, Aegean Sea
38 H11 **Keaau** *Haw.* Kea'au. Hawaii, USA, C Pacific Ocean
38 F11 **Keahole Point** *headland* Hawaii, USA, C Pacific Ocean
38 G12 **Kealakekua** Hawaii, USA, C Pacific Ocean
38 H11 **Kea, Mauna** ▲ Hawaii, USA, C Pacific Ocean
37 N10 **Keams** Arizona, SW USA
Kéamu *see* Aneityum
29 O16 **Kearney** Nebraska, C USA
36 L3 **Kearns** Utah, W USA
115 H20 **Kéas, Stenó** *strait* SE Greece
137 O14 **Keban Barajı** *dam* C Turkey
137 O14 **Keban Barajı** ⊠ C Turkey
77 S13 **Kebbi** ◈ *state* NW Nigeria
76 G10 **Kébémèr** NW Senegal
74 M7 **Kebili** *var.* Qibilī. C Tunisia
138 H4 **Kebir, Nahr el** ≈ NW Syria
80 A10 **Kebkabiya** Northern Darfur, W Sudan
92 I11 **Kebnekaise** ▲ N Sweden
81 M14 **K'ebrī Dehar** Somali, E Ethiopia
148 K15 **Kech** ≈ SW Pakistan
10 K10 **Kechika** ≈ British Columbia, W Canada
111 K23 **Kecskemét** Bács-Kiskun, C Hungary
168 J6 **Kedah** ◈ *state* Peninsular Malaysia
118 F12 **Kėdainiai** Kėdainiai, C Lithuania
Kedder *see* Kehra
13 N13 **Kedgwick** New Brunswick, SE Canada
169 R16 **Kediri** Jawa, C Indonesia
171 Y13 **Kedir Sarmi** Irian Jaya, E Indonesia
163 V7 **Kedong** Heilongjiang, NE China
76 I12 **Kédougou** SE Senegal
122 I11 **Kedrovyy** Tomskaya Oblast', C Russian Federation
111 H16 **Kędzierzyn-Kozle** *Ger.* Heydebrech. Opolskie, S Poland
8 H8 **Keele** ≈ Northwest Territories, NW Canada
10 K6 **Keele Peak** ▲ Yukon Territory, NW Canada
Keelung *see* Chilung
19 N10 **Keene** New Hampshire, NE USA
99 H17 **Keerbergen** Vlaams Brabant, C Belgium
83 E21 **Keetmanshoop** Karas, S Namibia
12 A11 **Keewatin** Ontario, S Canada
29 V4 **Keewatin** Minnesota, N USA
115 B18 **Kefallinía** *var.* Kefallonía. *island* Iónioi Nísoi, Greece, C Mediterranean Sea
Kefallonía *see* Kefallinía
115 M22 **Kéfalos** Kos, Dodekánisos, Greece, Aegean Sea
171 Q17 **Kefamenanu** Timor, C Indonesia
138 F10 **Kefar Sava** *var.* Kfar Saba. Central, C Israel
Kefe *see* Feodosiya
77 V15 **Keffi** Nassarawa, C Nigeria
92 H4 **Keflavík** ✕ (Reykjavík) Reykjanes, W Iceland
92 H4 **Keflavík** Reykjanes, W Iceland
Kegalee *see* Kegalla
155 J25 **Kegalla** *var.* Kegalee, Kegalle. Sabaragamuwa Province, C Sri Lanka
Kegalle *see* Kegalla
146 H7 **Kegayli** *Rus.* Kegeyli. Qoraqalpoghiston Respublikasi, W Uzbekistan
Kegel *see* Keila
145 W16 **Kegen** Almaty, SE Kazakhstan
Kegeyli *see* Kegayli
101 F22 **Kehl** Baden-Württemberg, SW Germany
118 H3 **Kehra** *Ger.* Kedder. Harjumaa, NW Estonia
117 U6 **Kehychivka** Kharkivs'ka Oblast', E Ukraine
97 L17 **Keighley** N England, UK
Kei Islands *see* Kai, Kepulauan
Keijō *see* Sŏul
118 G3 **Keila** *Ger.* Kegel. Harjumaa, NW Estonia
Keilberg *see* Klínovec
83 F23 **Keimoes** Northern Cape, W South Africa
Keina/Keinis *see* Käina
Keishū *see* Kyŏngju
77 T11 **Keïta** Tahoua, C Niger
78 J12 **Kéita, Bahr** *var.* Doka. ≈ S Chad
93 M16 **Keitele** ◎ C Finland
182 K10 **Keith** South Australia
96 K8 **Keith** NE Scotland, UK
26 K3 **Keith Sebelius Lake** ⊠ Kansas, C USA
32 G11 **Keizer** Oregon, NW USA
38 A8 **Kekaha** Kauai, Hawaii, USA, C Pacific Ocean
147 U10 **Këk-Art** *prev.* Alaykel', Alay-Kuu. Oshskaya Oblast', SW Kyrgyzstan
147 W10 **Këk-Aygyr** *var.* Keyaygyr. Narynskaya Oblast', C Kyrgyzstan
147 V9 **Këk-Dzhar** Narynskaya Oblast', C Kyrgyzstan
14 L8 **Kekek** ≈ Quebec, SE Canada
185 K15 **Kekerengu** Canterbury, South Island, NZ
111 L21 **Kékes** ▲ N Hungary
171 P17 **Kekneno, Gunung** ▲ Timor, S Indonesia
147 S9 **Këk-Tash** *Kir.* Kök-Tash. Dzhalal-Abadskaya Oblast', W Kyrgyzstan
81 M15 **K'elafo** Somali, E Ethiopia
169 U10 **Kelai, Sungai** ≈ Borneo, N Indonesia
Kelamayi *see* Karamay
Kelang *see* Klang
168 K7 **Kelantan** ◈ *state* Peninsular Malaysia
Kelantan *see* Kelantan, Sungai
168 K7 **Kelantan, Sungai** *var.* Kelantan. ≈ Peninsular Malaysia
Kelat *see* Kālat
Këlcyra *see* Këlcyrë
113 L22 **Këlcyrë** *var.* Këlcyra. Gjirokastër, S Albania
146 L14 **Kelifskiy Uzboy** *salt marsh* E Turkmenistan
137 O12 **Kelkit** Gümüşhane, NE Turkey
136 M12 **Kelkit Çayı** ≈ N Turkey
77 W11 **Kellé** Zinder, S Niger
79 G18 **Kéllé** Cuvette, W Congo
145 P7 **Kellerovka** Severnyy Kazakhstan, N Kazakhstan
8 I5 **Kellett, Cape** *headland* Banks Island, Northwest Territories, NW Canada
31 S11 **Kelleys Island** *island* Ohio, N USA
33 N8 **Kellogg** Idaho, NW USA
92 M12 **Kelloselkä** Lappi, N Finland
97 F17 **Kells** *Ir.* Ceanannas. E Ireland
118 E12 **Kelmė** Kelmė, C Lithuania
99 M19 **Kelmis** *var.* La Calamine. Liège, E Belgium
78 H12 **Kélo** Tandjilé, SW Chad
83 I14 **Kelongwa** North Western, NW Zambia
11 N17 **Kelowna** British Columbia, SW Canada
11 X12 **Kelsey** Manitoba, C Canada
34 M6 **Kelseyville** California, W USA
96 K13 **Kelso** SE Scotland, UK
32 G10 **Kelso** Washington, NW USA
195 W15 **Keltie, Cape** *headland* Antarctica
Keltsy *see* Kielce
168 L9 **Keluang** *var.* Kluang. Johor, Peninsular Malaysia
168 M11 **Kelume** Pulau Lingga, W Indonesia
11 U15 **Kelvington** Saskatchewan, S Canada
126 J7 **Kem'** Respublika Kareliya, NW Russian Federation
126 I7 **Kem'** ≈ NW Russian Federation
137 O13 **Kemah** Erzincan, E Turkey
137 N13 **Kemaliye** Erzincan, C Turkey
Kemaman *see* Cukai
Kemanlar *see* Isperikh
10 K14 **Kemano** British Columbia, SW Canada
Kemarat *see* Khemmarat
171 P12 **Kembani** Pulau Peleng, N Indonesia
136 F17 **Kemer** Antalya, SW Turkey
122 J12 **Kemerovo** *prev.* Shcheglovsk. Kemerovskaya Oblast', C Russian Federation
122 K12 **Kemerovskaya Oblast'** ◈ *province* S Russian Federation
92 L13 **Kemi** Lappi, NW Finland
92 M12 **Kemijärvi** *Swe.* Kemiträsk. Lappi, N Finland
92 M12 **Kemijärvi** ◎ N Finland
92 L13 **Kemijoki** ≈ NW Finland
147 V7 **Kemin** *prev.* Bystrovka. Chuyskaya Oblast', N Kyrgyzstan
92 L13 **Keminmaa** Lappi, NW Finland
Kemins Island *see* Nikumaroro
Kemiö *see* Kimito
Kemiträsk *see* Kemijärvi
129 P5 **Kemlya** Respublika Mordoviya, W Russian Federation
99 B18 **Kemmel** West-Vlaanderen, W Belgium
33 S16 **Kemmerer** Wyoming, C USA
Kemmuna *see* Comino
79 I14 **Kémo** ◈ *prefecture* S Central African Republic
25 U7 **Kemp** Texas, SW USA
93 L14 **Kempele** Oulu, C Finland
101 D15 **Kempen** Nordrhein-Westfalen, W Germany
25 Q5 **Kemp, Lake** ◎ Texas, SW USA
195 W5 **Kemp Land** *physical region* Antarctica
25 S9 **Kempner** Texas, SW USA
44 H3 **Kemp's Bay** Andros Island, W Bahamas
183 U6 **Kempsey** New South Wales, SE Australia
101 J24 **Kempten** Bayern, S Germany
15 N9 **Kempt, Lac** ◎ Quebec, SE Canada
183 P17 **Kempton** Tasmania, SE Australia
154 J9 **Ken** ≈ C India
39 R12 **Kenai** Alaska, USA
(0) D5 **Kenai Mountains** ⛰ Alaska, USA
39 R12 **Kenai Peninsula** *peninsula* Alaska, USA
21 V11 **Kenansville** North Carolina, SE USA
121 U13 **Kenâyis, Râs el-** *headland* N Egypt
97 K16 **Kendal** NW England, UK
23 Y16 **Kendall** Florida, SE USA
9 O8 **Kendall, Cape** *headland* Nunavut, E Canada
18 J15 **Kendall Park** New Jersey, NE USA
31 Q11 **Kendallville** Indiana, N USA
171 P14 **Kendari** Sulawesi, C Indonesia
169 Q13 **Kendawangan** Borneo, C Indonesia
154 O12 **Kendrāpāra** *var.* Kendrāparha. Orissa, E India
Kendrāparha *see* Kendrāpāra
154 O11 **Kendujhargarh** *prev.* Keonjihargarh. Orissa, E India
25 S13 **Kenedy** Texas, SW USA
146 E13 **Kënekesir** *Turkm.* Könekesir. Balkanskiy Velayat, W Turkmenistan
76 J15 **Kenema** SE Sierra Leone
29 P16 **Kenesaw** Nebraska, C USA
146 G8 **Këneurgench** *Turkm.* Köneürgench; *prev.* Kunya-Urgench. Dashkhovuzskiy Velayat, N Turkmenistan
79 H21 **Kenge** Bandundu, SW Dem. Rep. Congo (Zaire)
Kengen *see* Kangen
167 O5 **Keng Tung** *var.* Kentung. Shan State, E Myanmar
83 F23 **Kenhardt** Northern Cape, W South Africa
76 J12 **Kéniéba** Kayes, W Mali
Kenimekh *see* Konimekh
169 U7 **Keningau** Sabah, East Malaysia
74 F6 **Kénitra** *prev.* Port-Lyautey. NW Morocco
21 V9 **Kenly** North Carolina, SE USA
97 B21 **Kenmare** *Ir.* Neidín. S Ireland
28 L2 **Kenmare** North Dakota, N USA
97 A21 **Kenmare River** *Ir.* An Ribhéar. *inlet* NE Atlantic Ocean
18 D10 **Kenmore** New York, NE USA
25 W8 **Kennard** Texas, SW USA
29 N10 **Kennebec** South Dakota, N USA
19 Q7 **Kennebec River** ≈ Maine, NE USA
19 P9 **Kennebunk** Maine, NE USA
39 R13 **Kennedy Entrance** *strait* Alaska, USA
166 L3 **Kennedy Peak** ▲ W Myanmar
22 K9 **Kenner** Louisiana, S USA
180 I8 **Kenneth Range** ⛰ Western Australia
27 Y9 **Kennett** Missouri, C USA
18 I16 **Kennett Square** Pennsylvania, NE USA
32 K10 **Kennewick** Washington, NW USA
12 E11 **Kenogami** ≈ Ontario, S Canada
15 Q7 **Kénogami, Lac** ◎ Quebec, SE Canada
14 G8 **Kenogami Lake** Ontario, S Canada
14 F7 **Kenogamissi Lake** ◎ Ontario, S Canada
10 I6 **Keno Hill** Yukon Territory, NW Canada
12 A11 **Kenora** Ontario, S Canada
31 N9 **Kenosha** Wisconsin, N USA
13 P14 **Kensington** Prince Edward Island, SE Canada
26 L3 **Kensington** Kansas, C USA
32 I11 **Kent** Oregon, NW USA
24 J9 **Kent** Texas, SW USA
32 H8 **Kent** Washington, NW USA
97 P22 **Kent** *cultural region* SE England, UK
145 P16 **Kentau** Yuzhnyy Kazakhstan, S Kazakhstan
183 P14 **Kent Group** *island group* Tasmania, SE Australia
31 N12 **Kentland** Indiana, N USA
31 R12 **Kenton** Ohio, N USA
8 K7 **Kent Peninsula** *peninsula* Nunavut, N Canada
115 F14 **Kentrikí Makedonía** *Eng.* Macedonia Central. ◈ *region* N Greece
20 J6 **Kentucky** *off.* Commonwealth of Kentucky; also known as The Bluegrass State. ◈ *state* C USA
20 H8 **Kentucky Lake** ⊠ Kentucky/Tennessee, S USA
Kentung *see* Keng Tung
13 P15 **Kentville** Nova Scotia, SE Canada
22 K8 **Kentwood** Louisiana, S USA
31 P9 **Kentwood** Michigan, N USA
81 H17 **Kenya** *off.* Republic of Kenya. ◆ *republic* E Africa
Kenya, Mount *see* Kirinyaga
168 L7 **Kenyir, Tasik** *var.* Tasek Kenyir. ◎ Peninsular Malaysia
29 W10 **Kenyon** Minnesota, N USA
29 Y16 **Keokuk** Iowa, C USA
Keonjihargarh *see* Kendujhargarh
Kéos *see* Kéa
29 X16 **Keosauqua** Iowa, C USA
29 X15 **Keota** Iowa, C USA
21 O11 **Keowee, Lake** ⊠ South Carolina, SE USA
126 I7 **Kepa** *var.* Kepe. Respublika Kareliya, NW Russian Federation
Kepe *see* Kepa
189 O13 **Kepirohi Falls** *waterfall* Pohnpei, E Micronesia
185 B22 **Kepler Mountains** ⛰ South Island, NZ
111 I14 **Kępno** Wielkopolskie, C Poland
65 C24 **Keppel Island** *island* N Falkland Islands
Keppel Island *see* Niuatoputapu
65 C23 **Keppel Sound** *sound* N Falkland Islands
136 D12 **Kepsut** Balıkesir, NW Turkey
171 V13 **Kerai** Irian Jaya, E Indonesia
Kerak *see* Al Karak
155 F22 **Kerala** ◈ *state* S India
165 R16 **Kerama-rettō** *island group* SW Japan
183 N10 **Kerang** Victoria, SE Australia
Kerasunt *see* Giresun
115 H19 **Keratéa** *var.* Keratea. Attikí, C Greece
93 M19 **Kerava** *Swe.* Kervo. Etelä-Suomi, S Finland
Kerbala/Kerbela *see* Karbalā'
32 F15 **Kerby** Oregon, NW USA
117 W12 **Kerch** *Rus.* Kerch'. Respublika Krym, SE Ukraine
Kerchens'ka Protoka/Kerchenskiy Proliv *see* Kerch Strait
117 V13 **Kerchens'kyy Pivostriv** *peninsula* S Ukraine
121 V4 **Kerch Strait** *var.* Bosporus Cimmerius, Enikale Strait, *Rus.* Kerchenskiy Proliv, *Ukr.* Kerchens'ka Protska. *strait* Black Sea/Sea of Azov
152 K8 **Kerdārnāth** Uttar Pradesh, N India
Kerdilio *see* Kerdýlio
114 H13 **Kerdýlio** *var.* Kerdilio. ▲ N Greece
186 D8 **Kerema** Gulf, S PNG
Keremitlik *see* Lyulyakovo
136 I9 **Kerempe Burnu** *headland* N Turkey
80 J9 **Keren** *var.* Cheren. C Eritrea
25 U7 **Kerens** Texas, SW USA
184 M6 **Kerepehi** Waikato, North Island, NZ
145 P10 **Kerey, Ozero** ◎ C Kazakhstan
Kergel *see* Kärla
173 Q12 **Kerguelen** *island* C French Southern and Antarctic Territories
173 Q13 **Kerguelen Plateau** *undersea feature* S Indian Ocean
115 C20 **Kerí** Zákynthos, Iónioi Nísoi, Greece, C Mediterranean Sea
81 H19 **Kericho** Rift Valley, W Kenya
184 K2 **Kerikeri** Northland, North Island, NZ
93 O17 **Kerimäki** Isä-Suomi, E Finland
168 K12 **Kerinci, Gunung** ▲ Sumatera, W Indonesia
Keriya *see* Yutian
158 H9 **Keriya He** ≈ NW China
98 J9 **Kerkbuurt** Noord-Holland, C Netherlands
98 J13 **Kerkdriel** Gelderland, C Netherlands
75 N6 **Kerkenah, Îles de** *var.* Kerkenna Islands, *Ar.* Juzur Qarqannah. *island group* E Tunisia
Kerkenna Islands *see* Kerkenah, Îles de
115 M20 **Kerketévs** ▲ Sámos, Dodekánisos, Greece, Aegean Sea
29 T8 **Kerkhoven** Minnesota, N USA
146 M14 **Kerki** Lebapskiy Velayat, E Turkmenistan
146 M14 **Kerkichi** Lebapskiy Velayat, E Turkmenistan
115 F16 **Kerkíneo** *prehistoric site* Thessalía, C Greece
114 G12 **Kerkinitis, Límni** ◎ N Greece
Kérkira *see* Kérkyra
99 M18 **Kerkrade** Limburg, SE Netherlands
Kerkuk *see* Kirkūk
115 B16 **Kérkyra** ✕ Kérkyra, Iónioi Nísoi, Greece, C Mediterranean Sea
115 B16 **Kérkyra** *var.* Kérkira, *Eng.* Corfu. Kérkyra, Iónioi Nísoi, Greece, C Mediterranean Sea
115 A16 **Kérkyra** *var.* Kérkira, *Eng.* Corfu. *island* Iónioi Nísoi, Greece, C Mediterranean Sea
192 K10 **Kermadec Islands** *island group* NZ, SW Pacific Ocean
175 R10 **Kermadec Ridge** *undersea feature* SW Pacific Ocean
175 R11 **Kermadec Trench** *undersea feature* SW Pacific Ocean
143 S10 **Kermān** *var.* Kirman; *anc.* Carmana. Kermān, C Iran
143 R11 **Kermān** *off.* Ostān-e Kermān, *var.* Kirman; *anc.* Carmania. ◈ *province* SE Iran
143 U12 **Kermān, Bīābān-e** *var.* Kerman Desert. *desert* SE Iran
Kerman Desert *see* Kermān, Bīābān-e
143 Q9 **Kermānshāh** Yazd, C Iran
142 J6 **Kermānshāh** *off.* Ostān-e Kermānshāh; *prev.* Bākhtarān, Kermānshāhān. ◈ *province* W Iran
Kermānshāhān *see* Kermānshāh
114 L10 **Kermen** Sliven, C Bulgaria
24 L8 **Kermit** Texas, SW USA
21 P6 **Kermit** West Virginia, NE USA
21 S9 **Kernersville** North Carolina, SE USA
35 S12 **Kern River** ≈ California, W USA
35 S12 **Kernville** California, W USA
115 K21 **Kéros** *island* Kykládes, Greece, Aegean Sea
76 K14 **Kérouané** Haute-Guinée, SE Guinea
101 D16 **Kerpen** Nordrhein-Westfalen, W Germany
146 I11 **Kerpichli** Lebapskiy Velayat, NE Turkmenistan
24 M1 **Kerrick** Texas, SW USA
Kerr Lake *see* John H.Kerr Reservoir
11 S15 **Kerrobert** Saskatchewan, S Canada
25 Q11 **Kerrville** Texas, SW USA
97 B20 **Kerry** *Ir.* Ciarraí. *cultural region* SW Ireland
21 S11 **Kershaw** South Carolina, SE USA
Kertel *see* Kärdla
95 H23 **Kerteminde** Fyn, C Denmark
163 Q7 **Kerulen** *Chin.* Herlen He, *Mong.* Herlen Gol. ≈ China/Mongolia
Kervo *see* Kerava
Kerýneia *see* Girne
12 H11 **Kesagami Lake** ◎ Ontario, SE Canada
93 O17 **Kesälahti** Itä-Suomi, E Finland
136 B11 **Keşan** Edirne, NW Turkey
165 R9 **Kesennuma** Miyagi, Honshū, C Japan
163 V7 **Keshan** Heilongjiang, NE China
30 M6 **Keshena** Wisconsin, N USA
136 I13 **Keskin** Kırıkkale, C Turkey
Késmárk *see* Kežmarok
126 I6 **Kesten'ga** *var.* Kest Enga. Respublika Kareliya, NW Russian Federation
98 K12 **Kesteren** Gelderland, C Netherlands
14 H14 **Keswick** Ontario, S Canada
97 K15 **Keswick** NW England, UK
111 H24 **Keszthely** Zala, SW Hungary
122 K11 **Ket'** ≈ C Russian Federation
77 R17 **Keta** SE Ghana
169 Q12 **Ketapang** Borneo, C Indonesia
129 O12 **Ketchenery** *prev.* Sovetskoye. Respublika Kalmykiya, SW Russian Federation
39 Y14 **Ketchikan** Revillagigedo Island, Alaska, USA
33 O14 **Ketchum** Idaho, NW USA
Kete/Kete Krakye *see* Kete-Krachi
77 Q15 **Kete-Krachi** *var.* Kete, Kete Krakye. E Ghana
98 L9 **Ketelmeer** *channel* E Netherlands
149 P17 **Keti Bandar** Sind, SE Pakistan
145 W16 **Ketmen', Khrebet** ⛰ SE Kazakhstan
77 S16 **Kétou** SE Benin
110 M7 **Kętrzyn** *Ger.* Rastenburg. Warmińsko-Mazurskie, NE Poland,
97 N20 **Kettering** C England, UK
31 R14 **Kettering** Ohio, N USA
18 F13 **Kettle Creek** ≈ Pennsylvania, NE USA
32 L7 **Kettle Falls** Washington, NW USA
14 D16 **Kettle Point** *headland* Ontario, S Canada
29 V6 **Kettle River** ≈ Minnesota, N USA
186 B7 **Ketu** ≈ W PNG
18 G10 **Keuka Lake** ◎ New York, NE USA
Keupriya *see* Primorsko
93 L17 **Keuruu** Länsi-Suomi, W Finland
Kevevára *see* Kovin
92 L9 **Kevo** *Lapp.* Geavvú. Lappi, N Finland
44 M6 **Kew** North Caicos, N Turks and Caicos Islands
30 K11 **Kewanee** Illinois, N USA
31 N7 **Kewaunee** Wisconsin, N USA
30 M3 **Keweenaw Bay** ◎ Michigan, N USA
31 N2 **Keweenaw Peninsula** *peninsula* Michigan, N USA
31 N2 **Keweenaw Point** *headland* Michigan, N USA
29 N12 **Keya Paha River** ≈ Nebraska/South Dakota, N USA
Keyaygyr *see* Këk-Aygyr
23 Z16 **Key Biscayne** Florida, SE USA
26 G8 **Keyes** Oklahoma, C USA
23 Y17 **Key Largo** Key Largo, Florida, SE USA
21 U3 **Keyser** West Virginia, NE USA
27 O9 **Keystone Lake** ⊠ Oklahoma, C USA
36 L16 **Keystone Peak** ▲ Arizona, SW USA
Keystone State *see* Pennsylvania
21 U7 **Keysville** Virginia, NE USA
27 T3 **Keytesville** Missouri, C USA
23 W17 **Key West** Florida Keys, Florida, SE USA
129 T1 **Kez** Udmurtskaya Respublika, NW Russian Federation
Kezdivásárhely *see* Târgu Secuiesc
122 M12 **Kezhma** Krasnoyarskiy Kray, C Russian Federation
111 L18 **Kežmarok** *Ger.* Käsmark, *Hung.* Késmárk. Prešovský Kraj, E Slovakia
Kfar Saba *see* Kefar Sava
83 F20 **Kgalagadi** ◈ *district* SW Botswana
83 I20 **Kgatleng** ◈ *district* SE Botswana
188 F8 **Kgkeklau** Babeldaob, N Palau
127 R6 **Khabarikha** *var.* Chabaricha. Respublika Komi, NW Russian Federation
123 S14 **Khabarovsk** Khabarovskiy Kray, SE Russian Federation
123 R11 **Khabarovskiy Kray** ◈ *territory* E Russian Federation
141 W7 **Khabb** Abū Ẓaby, E UAE
Khabour, Nahr al *see* Khābūr, Nahr al
Khabura *see* Al Khābūrah
139 N2 **Khābūr, Nahr al** *var.* Nahr al Khabour. ≈ Syria/Turkey
Khachmas *see* Xaçmaz
80 B12 **Khadari** ≈ W Sudan
Khadera *see* Ḥadera
141 X12 **Khādhil** *var.* Khudal. SE Oman
155 E14 **Khadki** *prev.* Kirkee. Mahārāshtra, W India
128 L14 **Khadyzhensk** Krasnodarskiy Kray, SW Russian Federation
114 N9 **Khadzhiyska Reka** ≈ E Bulgaria
117 P10 **Khadzhybeys'kyy Lyman** ◎ SW Ukraine
138 K3 **Khafsah** Ḥalab, N Syria
152 M13 **Khāga** Uttar Pradesh, N India
153 Q13 **Khagaria** Bihār, NE India
149 Q13 **Khairpur** Sind, SE Pakistan
122 K13 **Khakasiya, Respublika** *prev.* Khakasskaya Avtonomnaya Oblast', *Eng.* Khakassia. ◈ *autonomous republic* C Russian Federation
Khakassia/Khakasskaya Avtonomnaya Oblast' *see* Khakasiya, Respublika
167 N9 **Kha Khaeng, Khao** ▲ W Thailand
83 G20 **Khakhea** *var.* Kakia. Southern, S Botswana
146 L13 **Khalach** Lebapskiy Velayat, E Turkmenistan
Khalándrion *see* Chalándri
129 W7 **Khalilovo** Orenburgskaya Oblast', W Russian Federation
Khalkabad *see* Khalqobod
142 L3 **Khalkhāl** *prev.* Herowābād. Ardabīl, NW Iran
Khalkidhikí *see* Chalkidikí
Khalkís *see* Chalkída
127 W3 **Khal'mer-Yu** Respublika Komi, NW Russian Federation
119 M14 **Khalopyenichy** *Rus.* Kholopenichi. Minskaya Voblasts', NE Belarus
146 H7 **Khalqobod** *Rus.* Khalkabad. Qoraqalpoghiston Respublikasi, W Uzbekistan
Khalturin *see* Orlov
141 Y10 **Khalūf** *var.* Al Khaluf. E Oman
154 K10 **Khamaria** Madhya Pradesh, C India
154 D11 **Khambhāt** Gujarāt, W India
154 C12 **Khambhāt, Gulf of** *Eng.* Gulf of Cambay. *gulf* W India
167 U10 **Khâm Đuc** Quang Nam-Đa Nẵng, C Vietnam
154 G12 **Khāmgaon** Mahārāshtra, C India
141 O14 **Khamir** *var.* Khamr. W Yemen
141 N12 **Khamīs Mushayt** *var.* Hamīs Musait. 'Asīr, SW Saudi Arabia
123 P10 **Khampa** Respublika Sakha (Yakutiya), NE Russian Federation
Khamr *see* Khamir
83 C19 **Khan** ≈ W Namibia
149 Q2 **Khānābād** Kunduz, NE Afghanistan
Khân Abou Châmâte/Khan Abou Ech Cham *see* Khān Abū Shāmāt
138 I7 **Khān Abū Shāmāt** *var.* Khân Abou Châmâte, Khan Abou Ech Cham. Dimashq, W Syria
Khān al Baghdādī *see* Al Baghdādī
Khān al Maḥāwīl *see* Al Maḥāwīl
139 T7 **Khān al Mashāhidah** C Iraq
139 T10 **Khān al Muṣallá** S Iraq
139 U6 **Khānaqīn** E Iraq
139 T11 **Khān ar Ruḥbah** S Iraq
139 P2 **Khān as Sūr** N Iraq
139 T8 **Khān Āzād** C Iraq
154 N13 **Khandaparha** *prev.* Khandpara. Orissa, E India
Khandpara *see* Khandaparha
149 T2 **Khandūd** *var.* Khandud, Wakhan. Badakhshān, NE Afghanistan
154 G11 **Khandwa** Madhya Pradesh, C India
123 R10 **Khandyga** Respublika Sakha (Yakutiya), NE Russian Federation
149 T10 **Khānewāl** Punjab, NE Pakistan
149 S10 **Khāngarh** Punjab, E Pakistan
Khanh Hung *see* Soc Trăng
Khaniá *see* Chaniá
Khanka *see* Khonqa
163 Z8 **Khanka, Lake** *var.* Hsing-k'ai Hu, Lake Hanka, *Chin.* Xingkai Hu, *Rus.* Ozero Khanka. ◎ China/Russian Federation
Khanka, Ozero *see* Khanka, Lake
Khankendi *see* Xankändi
Khanlar *see* Xanlar
123 O9 **Khannya** ≈ NE Russian Federation
149 S12 **Khānpur** Punjab, SE Pakistan
149 S12 **Khānpur** Punjab, E Pakistan
138 I4 **Khān Shaykhūn** *var.* Khan Sheikhun. Idlib, NW Syria
Khan Sheikhun *see* Khān Shaykhūn
145 S15 **Khantau** Zhambyl, S Kazakhstan
145 W16 **Khan Tengri, Pik** ▲ SE Kazakhstan
167 S9 **Khanthabouli** *prev.* Savannakhét. Savannakhét, S Laos
127 V8 **Khanty-Mansiyskiy Avtonomnyy Okrug** ◈ *autonomous district* C Russian Federation
139 R4 **Khānūqah** C Iraq
138 E11 **Khān Yūnis** *var.* Khān Yūnus. S Gaza Strip
Khān Yūnus *see* Khān Yūnis
Khanzi *see* Ghanzi
139 U5 **Khān Zūr** E Iraq
167 N10 **Khao Laem Reservoir** ⊠ W Thailand
123 O14 **Khapcheranga** Chitinskaya Oblast', S Russian Federation
129 Q12 **Kharabali** Astrakhanskaya Oblast', SW Russian Federation
153 R16 **Kharagpur** West Bengal, NE India
139 V11 **Kharā'ib 'Abd al Karīm** S Iraq
143 Q8 **Kharānaq** Yazd, C Iran
Kharbin *see* Harbin
146 H13 **Khardzhagaz** Akhalskiy Velayat, C Turkmenistan
Khārga Oasis *see* Great Oasis, The
154 F11 **Khargon** Madhya Pradesh, C India
149 V7 **Khāriān** Punjab, NE Pakistan
117 X8 **Kharisyz'k** Donets'ka Oblast', E Ukraine
117 V5 **Kharkiv** *Rus.* Khar'kov. Kharkivs'ka Oblast', NE Ukraine
117 V5 **Kharkiv** ✕ Kharkivs'ka Oblast', E Ukraine
Kharkiv *see* Kharkivs'ka Oblast'

◆ Country ● Country Capital ◇ Dependent Territory ○ Dependent Territory Capital ◈ Administrative Region ✕ International Airport ▲ Mountain ⛰ Mountain Range Volcano ≈ River ◎ Lake ⊠ Reservoir

117 U5 **Kharkivs'ka Oblast'** var. Kharkiv, Rus. Khar'kovskaya Oblast'. ◈ province E Ukraine
Khar'kov see Kharkiv
Khar'kovskaya Oblast' see Kharkivs'ka Oblast'
126 L3 **Kharlovka** Murmanskaya Oblast', NW Russian Federation
114 K11 **Kharmanli** Khaskovo, S Bulgaria
114 K11 **Kharmanliyska Reka** ≈ S Bulgaria
126 M13 **Kharovsk** Vologodskaya Oblast', NW Russian Federation
80 F9 **Khartoum** var. El Khartûm, Khartum. ● (Sudan) Khartoum, C Sudan
80 F9 **Khartoum** ◈ state NE Sudan
80 F9 **Khartoum** ✈ Khartoum, C Sudan
80 F9 **Khartoum North** Khartoum, C Sudan
117 X8 **Khartsyz'k** Rus. Khartsyzsk. Donets'ka Oblast', SE Ukraine
Khartsyzsk see Khartsyz'k
Khartum see Khartoum
Khasab see Al Khaşab
123 S15 **Khasan** Primorskiy Kray, SE Russian Federation
129 P16 **Khasavyurt** Respublika Dagestan, SW Russian Federation
143 W12 **Khāsh** prev. Vāsht. Sīstān va Balūchestān, SE Iran
148 K8 **Khāsh, Dasht-e** Eng. Khash Desert. desert SW Afghanistan
Khash Desert see Khāsh, Dasht-e
Khashim Al Qirba/Khashm al Qirbah see Khashm el Girba
80 H9 **Khashm el Girba** var. Khashim Al Qirba, Khashm al Qirbah. Kassala, E Sudan
138 G14 **Khashsh, Jabal al** ▲ S Jordan
137 S10 **Khashuri** C Georgia
153 V13 **Khāsi Hills** hill range NE India
114 K11 **Khaskovo** Khaskovo, S Bulgaria
114 K11 **Khaskovo** ◈ province S Bulgaria
122 M7 **Khatanga** ≈ N Russian Federation
Khatanga, Gulf of see Khatangskiy Zaliv
123 N7 **Khatangskiy Zaliv** var. Gulf of Khatanga. bay N Russian Federation
141 W7 **Khatmat al Malāḥah** N Oman
143 S16 **Khaṭmat al Malāḥah** Ash Shāriqah, E UAE
123 V7 **Khatyrka** Chukotskiy Avtonomnyy Okrug, NE Russian Federation
146 I14 **Khauz-Khan** Turkm. Hanhowuz. Akhalskiy Velayat, S Turkmenistan
146 I14 **Khauzkhanskoye Vodokhranilishche** ⊞ S Turkmenistan
Khavaling see Khovaling
Khavast see Khowos
139 W10 **Khawrah, Nahr al** ≈ S Iraq
Khawr Barakah see Baraka
141 W7 **Khawr Fakkān** var. Khor Fakkan. Ash Shāriqah, NE UAE
140 L6 **Khaybar** Al Madīnah, NW Saudi Arabia
Khaybar, Kowtal-e see Khyber Pass
147 S11 **Khaydarkan** var. Khaydarken. Oshskaya Oblast', SW Kyrgyzstan
Khaydarken see Khaydarkan
127 U2 **Khaypudyrskaya Guba** bay NW Russian Federation
139 S1 **Khayrūzuk** E Iraq
Khazar, Baḥr-e/Khazar, Daryā-ye see Caspian Sea
Khazarosp see Hazorasp
Khazretishi, Khrebet see Hazratishoh, Qatorkŭhi
Khelat see Kālat
74 F6 **Khemisset** NW Morocco
167 R10 **Khemmarat** var. Kemarat. Ubon Ratchathani, E Thailand
74 L6 **Khenchela** var. Khenchla. NE Algeria
Khenchla see Khenchela
74 G7 **Khénifra** C Morocco
Khersān, Rūd-e see Garm, Āb-e
117 R10 **Kherson** Khersons'ka Oblast', S Ukraine
Kherson see Khersons'ka Oblast'
117 S14 **Khersones, Mys** Rus. Mys Khersonesskiy. headland S Ukraine
Khersonesskiy, Mys see Khersones, Mys
117 R10 **Khersons'ka Oblast'** var. Kherson, Rus. Khersonskaya Oblast'. ◈ province S Ukraine
Khersonskaya Oblast' see Khersons'ka Oblast'
122 L8 **Kheta** ≈ N Russian Federation
167 S8 **Khe Ve** Quang Binh, C Vietnam
149 U7 **Khewra** Punjab, E Pakistan
Khiam see El Khiyam
126 J4 **Khibiny** ▲ NW Russian Federation
128 K3 **Khimki** Moskovskaya Oblast', W Russian Federation
147 S12 **Khingov** Rus. Obi-Khingou. ≈ C Tajikistan
Khíos see Chíos
149 R15 **Khipro** Sind, SE Pakistan
139 S10 **Khirr, Wādī al** dry watercourse S Iraq
114 I10 **Khisarya** Plovdiv, C Bulgaria
Khiva see Khiwa
146 H9 **Khiwa** Rus. Khiva. Khorazm Wiloyati, W Uzbekistan
167 N9 **Khlong Khlung** Kamphaeng Phet, W Thailand
167 N15 **Khlong Thom** Krabi, SW Thailand
167 P12 **Khlung** Chantaburi, S Thailand
Khmel'nik see Khmil'nyk
Khmel'nitskaya Oblast' see Khmel'nyts'ka Oblast'
Khmel'nitskiy see Khmel 'nyts'kyy
116 K5 **Khmel'nyts'ka Oblast'** var. Khmel'nyts'kyy, Rus. Khmel'nitskaya Oblast'; prev. Kamenets-Podol'skaya Oblast'. ◈ province NW Ukraine
116 L6 **Khmel 'nyts'kyy** Rus. Khmel'nitskiy; prev. Proskurov. Khmel'nyts'ka Oblast', W Ukraine
Khmel'nyts'kyy see Khmel'nyts'ka Oblast'
116 M6 **Khmil'nyk** Rus. Khmel'nik. Vinnyts'ka Oblast', C Ukraine
137 R9 **Khobi** W Georgia
119 P15 **Khodasy** Rus. Khodosy. Mahilyowskaya Voblasts', E Belarus
116 I6 **Khodoriv** Pol. Chodorów, Rus. Khodorov. L'vivs'ka Oblast', NW Ukraine
Khodorov see Khodoriv
Khodosy see Khodasy
146 D12 **Khodzhakala** Turkm. Hojagala. Balkanskiy Velayat, W Turkmenistan
146 M13 **Khodzhambas** Turkm. Hojambaz. Lebapskiy Velayat, E Turkmenistan
Khodzhent see Khŭjand
Khodzheyli see Khŭjayli
Khoi see Khvoy
Khojend see Khŭjand
Khokand see Qŭqon
128 L8 **Khokhol'skiy** Voronezhskaya Oblast', W Russian Federation
167 P10 **Khok Samrong** Lop Buri, C Thailand
149 P2 **Kholm** var. Tashqurghan, Pash. Khulm. Balkh, N Afghanistan
126 H15 **Kholm** Novgorodskaya Oblast', W Russian Federation
Kholm see Chełm
Kholmech' see Kholmyech
123 T13 **Kholmsk** Ostrov Sakhalin, Sakhalinskaya Oblast', SE Russian Federation
119 O19 **Kholmyech** Rus. Kholmech'. Homyel'skaya Voblasts', SE Belarus
Kholon see Holon
Kholopenichi see Khalopyenichy
83 D19 **Khomas** ◈ district C Namibia
83 D19 **Khomas Hochland** var. Khomasplato. plateau C Namibia
Khomasplato see Khomas Hochland
Khomein see Khomeyn
142 M7 **Khomeyn** var. Khomein, Khumain. Markazī, W Iran
143 N8 **Khomeynīshahr** prev. Homāyūnshahr. Eşfahān, C Iran
Khoms see Al Khums
Khong Sedone see Muang Khôngxédôn
167 Q9 **Khon Kaen** var. Muang Khon Kaen. Khon Kaen, E Thailand
146 I9 **Khonqa** Rus. Khanka. Khorazm Wiloyati, W Uzbekistan
167 Q9 **Khon San** Khon Kaen, E Thailand
123 R8 **Khonuu** Respublika Sakha (Yakutiya), NE Russian Federation
129 N8 **Khopër** var. Khoper. ≈ SW Russian Federation
123 S14 **Khor** Khabarovskiy Kray, SE Russian Federation
143 S6 **Khorāsān** off. Ostān-e Khorāsān, var. Khorassan, Khurasan. ◈ province NE Iran
Khorassan see Khorāsān
Khorat see Nakhon Ratchasima
146 H9 **Khorazm Wiloyati** Rus. Khorezmskaya Oblast'. ◈ province W Uzbekistan
154 O13 **Khordha** prev. Khurda. Orissa, E India
127 U4 **Khorey-Ver** Nenetskiy Avtonomnyy Okrug, NW Russian Federation
Khorezmskaya Oblast' see Khorazm Wiloyati
Khor Fakkan see Khawr Fakkān
145 W15 **Khorgos** Almaty, SE Kazakhstan
123 N13 **Khorinsk** Respublika Buryatiya, S Russian Federation
83 C18 **Khorixas** Kunene, NW Namibia
141 O17 **Khormaksar** var. Aden. ✈ ('Adan) SW Yemen
Khormal see Khurmāl
Khormuj see Khvormūj
Khorog see Khorugh
117 S5 **Khorol** Poltavs'ka Oblast', NE Ukraine
142 L7 **Khorramābād** var. Khurramabad. Lorestān, W Iran
142 K10 **Khorramshahr** var. Khurramshahr, Muhammerah; prev. Mohammerah. Khūzestān, SW Iran
147 S14 **Khorugh** Rus. Khorog. S Tajikistan
129 Q12 **Khosheutovo** Astrakhanskaya Oblast', SW Russian Federation
Khotan see Hotan
Khorvot Khalutsa see Horvot Haluza
Khotimsk see Khotsimsk
Khotin see Khotyn
119 R16 **Khotsimsk** Rus. Khotimsk. Mahilyowskaya Voblasts', E Belarus
116 K7 **Khotyn** Rom. Hotin, Rus. Khotin. Chernivets'ka Oblast', W Ukraine
74 F7 **Khouribga** C Morocco
147 Q13 **Khovaling** Rus. Khavaling. SW Tajikistan
Khovd see Hovd
147 P11 **Khowos** var. Ursat'yevskaya, Rus. Khavast. Sirdaryo Wiloyati, E Uzbekistan
149 R6 **Khowst** Paktīā, E Afghanistan
Khoy see Khvoy
119 N20 **Khoyniki** Rus. Khoyniki. Homyel'skaya Voblasts', SE Belarus
Khozretishi, Khrebet see Hazratishoh, Qatorkŭhi
Khrisoúpolis see Chrysoúpoli
144 J10 **Khromtau** Kaz. Khromtaū. Aktyubinsk, W Kazakhstan
Khrysokhou Bay see Chrysochoú, Kólpos
117 O7 **Khrystynivka** Cherkas'ka Oblast', C Ukraine
167 R10 **Khuang Nai** Ubon Ratchathani, E Thailand
Khudal see Khādhil
Khudat see Xudat
149 W9 **Khudiān** Punjab, E Pakistan
Khudzhand see Khŭjand
147 O13 **Khufar** Surkhondaryo Wiloyati, S Uzbekistan
83 G21 **Khuis** Kgalagadi, SW Botswana
147 Q11 **Khŭjand** var. Khodzhent, Khojend, Rus. Khudzhand; prev. Leninabad, Taj. Leninobod. N Tajikistan
146 H8 **Khŭjayli** Rus. Khodzheyli. Qoraqalpoghiston Respublikasi, W Uzbekistan
167 R11 **Khukhan** Si Sa Ket, E Thailand
Khulm see Kholm
153 T16 **Khulna** Khulna, SW Bangladesh
153 T16 **Khulna** ◈ division SW Bangladesh
Khumain see Khomeyn
Khums see Al Khums
149 W2 **Khunjerāb Pass** Chin. Kunjirap Daban. pass China/Pakistan **see also** Kunjirap Daban
153 P16 **Khunti** Bihār, N India
167 N7 **Khun Yuam** Mae Hong Son, NW Thailand
Khurais see Khurays
Khurasan see Khorāsān
141 R7 **Khurays** var. Khurais. Ash Sharqīyah, C Saudi Arabia
Khurda see Khordha
152 J11 **Khurja** Uttar Pradesh, N India
139 V4 **Khurmāl** var. Khormal. NE Iraq
Khurramabad see Khorramābād
Khurramshahr see Khorramshahr
149 U7 **Khushāb** Punjab, NE Pakistan
116 H8 **Khust** Cz. Chust, Husté, Hung. Huszt. Zakarpats'ka Oblast', W Ukraine
80 D11 **Khuwei** Western Kordofan, C Sudan
149 O13 **Khuzdār** Baluchistān, SW Pakistan
142 L9 **Khūzestān** off. Ostān-e Khūzestān, var. Khuzistan; prev. Arabistan, anc. Susiana. ◈ province SW Iran
Khuzistan see Khūzestān
149 R2 **Khvājeh Ghār** var. Khwajaghar, Khwaja-i-Ghar. Takhār, NE Afghanistan
129 Q7 **Khvalynsk** Saratovskaya Oblast', W Russian Federation
143 N12 **Khvormūj** var. Khormuj. Būshehr, S Iran
142 I2 **Khvoy** var. Khoi, Khoy. Āzarbāyjān-e Bākhtarī, NW Iran
Khwajaghar/Khwaja-i-Ghar see Khvājeh Ghār
149 S5 **Khyber Pass** var. Kowtal-e Khaybar. pass Afghanistan/Pakistan
186 L8 **Kia** Santa Isabel, N Solomon Islands
183 S10 **Kiama** New South Wales, SE Australia
79 O22 **Kiambi** Katanga, SE Dem. Rep. Congo (Zaire)
27 Q12 **Kiamichi Mountains** ▲ Oklahoma, C USA
27 Q12 **Kiamichi River** ≈ Oklahoma, C USA
14 M10 **Kiamika, Réservoir** ⊞ Quebec, SE Canada
Kiamusze see Jiamusi
39 N7 **Kiana** Alaska, USA
Kiangmai see Chiang Mai
Kiang-ning see Nanjing
Kiangsi see Jiangxi
Kiangsu see Jiangsu
93 M14 **Kiantajärvi** ⊚ E Finland
115 F19 **Kiáto** prev. Kiáton. Pelopónnisos, S Greece
Kiáton see Kiáto
Kiayi see Chiai
67 T9 **Kibali** var. Uele (upper course). ≈ NE Dem. Rep. Congo (Zaire)
79 E20 **Kibangou** Le Niari, SW Congo
Kibarty see Kybartai
92 M8 **Kiberg** Finnmark, N Norway
95 F22 **Kibæk** Ringkøbing, W Denmark
79 N20 **Kibombo** Maniema, E Dem. Rep. Congo (Zaire)
81 E20 **Kibondo** Kigoma, NW Tanzania
81 J15 **Kibre Mengist** var. Adola. Oromo, C Ethiopia
Kıbrıs/Kıbrıs Cumhuriyeti see Cyprus
81 E20 **Kibungo** var. Kibungu. SE Rwanda
Kibungu see Kibungo
113 N19 **Kičevo** SW FYR Macedonia
127 P13 **Kichmengskiy Gorodok** Vologodskaya Oblast', NW Russian Federation
30 J8 **Kickapoo River** ≈ Wisconsin, N USA
11 P16 **Kicking Horse Pass** pass Alberta/British Columbia, SW Canada
77 R9 **Kidal** Kidal, C Mali
77 Q8 **Kidal** ◈ region NE Mali
171 Q7 **Kidapawan** Mindanao, S Philippines
97 L20 **Kidderminster** C England, UK
76 I11 **Kidira** E Senegal
184 O11 **Kidnappers, Cape** headland North Island, NZ
100 J8 **Kiel** Schleswig-Holstein, N Germany
111 L15 **Kielce** Rus. Keltsy. Świętokrzyskie, C Poland
100 K7 **Kieler Bucht** bay N Germany
100 J7 **Kieler Förde** inlet N Germany
167 U13 **Kiên Đưc** var. Đak Lap. Đăc Lăc, S Vietnam
79 N24 **Kienge** Katanga, SE Dem. Rep. Congo (Zaire)
100 Q12 **Kietz** Brandenburg, NE Germany
Kiev see Kyyiv
Kiev Reservoir see Kyyivs'ke Vodoskhovyshche
76 J10 **Kiffa** Assaba, S Mauritania
115 H19 **Kifisiá** Attikí, C Greece
115 F18 **Kifisós** ≈ C Greece
139 U5 **Kifrī** N Iraq
81 D20 **Kigali** ● (Rwanda) C Rwanda
81 E20 **Kigali** ✈ C Rwanda
137 P13 **Kiğı** Bingöl, E Turkey
81 E21 **Kigoma** Kigoma, W Tanzania
81 E21 **Kigoma** ◈ region W Tanzania
38 F10 **Kihei** Haw. Kihei. Maui, Hawaii, USA, C Pacific Ocean
93 K17 **Kihniö** Länsi-Suomi, W Finland
118 F6 **Kihnu** var. Kihnu Saar, Ger. Kühnö. island SW Estonia
Kihnu Saar see Kihnu
38 A8 **Kii Landing** Niihau, Hawaii, USA, C Pacific Ocean
93 L14 **Kiiminki** Oulu, C Finland
164 J14 **Kii-Nagashima** var. Nagashima. Mie, Honshū, SW Japan
164 J14 **Kii-sanchi** ▲ Honshū, SW Japan
92 L11 **Kiistala** Lappi, N Finland
164 I15 **Kii-suidō** strait S Japan
165 V16 **Kikai-shima** var. Kikaiga-shima. island Nansei-shotō, SW Japan
112 M8 **Kikinda** Ger. Grosskikinda, Hung. Nagykikinda; prev. Velika Kikinda. Serbia, N Yugoslavia
Kikládhes see Kykládes
165 Q5 **Kikonai** Hokkaidō, NE Japan
186 C8 **Kikori** Gulf, S PNG
186 C8 **Kikori** ≈ W PNG
165 O14 **Kikuchi** var. Kikuti. Kumamoto, Kyūshū, SW Japan
Kikuti see Kikuchi
129 N8 **Kikvidze** Volgogradskaya Oblast', SW Russian Federation
14 I10 **Kikwissi, Lac** ⊚ Quebec, SE Canada
79 I21 **Kikwit** Bandundu, W Dem. Rep. Congo (Zaire)
95 K15 **Kil** Värmland, C Sweden
94 N12 **Kilafors** Gävleborg, C Sweden
38 B8 **Kilauea** Haw. Kilauea. Kauai, Hawaii, USA, C Pacific Ocean
38 H12 **Kilauea Caldera** crater Hawaii, USA, C Pacific Ocean
109 V4 **Kilb** Niederösterreich, C Austria
39 O12 **Kilbuck Mountains** ▲ Alaska, USA
163 Y12 **Kilchu** NE North Korea
97 F18 **Kilcock** Ir. Cill Choca. E Ireland
183 V2 **Kilcoy** Queensland, E Australia
97 F18 **Kildare** Ir. Cill Dara. E Ireland
97 F18 **Kildare** Ir. Cill Dara. cultural region E Ireland
126 K2 **Kil'din, Ostrov** island NW Russian Federation
25 W7 **Kilgore** Texas, SW USA
Kilien Mountains see Qilian Shan
114 K9 **Kilifarevo** Veliko Tŭrnovo, N Bulgaria
81 K20 **Kilifi** Coast, SE Kenya
189 U9 **Kili Island** var. Kōle. island Ralik Chain, S Marshall Islands
149 V2 **Kilik Pass** pass Afghanistan/China
Kilimane see Quelimane
81 I21 **Kilimanjaro** ◈ region E Tanzania
81 I20 **Kilimanjaro** var. Uhuru Peak. ▲ NE Tanzania
Kilimbangara see Kolombangara
Kilinailau Islands see Tulun Islands
81 K23 **Kilindoni** Pwani, E Tanzania
118 H6 **Kilingi-Nõmme** Ger. Kurkund. Pärnumaa, SW Estonia
136 M17 **Kilis** Kilis, S Turkey
136 M16 **Kilis** ◈ province S Turkey
117 N12 **Kiliya** Rom. Chilia-Nouă. Odes'ka Oblast', SW Ukraine
97 B19 **Kilkee** Ir. Cill Chaoi. W Ireland
97 E19 **Kilkenny** Ir. Cill Chainnigh. S Ireland
97 E19 **Kilkenny** Ir. Cill Chainnigh. cultural region S Ireland
97 B18 **Kilkieran Bay** Ir. Cuan Chill Chiaráin. bay W Ireland
114 G13 **Kilkís** Kentrikí Makedonía, N Greece
97 C15 **Killala Bay** Ir. Cuan Chill Ala. inlet NW Ireland
11 R15 **Killam** Alberta, SW Canada
183 U3 **Killarney** Queensland, E Australia
11 W17 **Killarney** Manitoba, S Canada
14 E11 **Killarney** Ontario, S Canada
97 B20 **Killarney** Ir. Cill Airne. SW Ireland
28 K4 **Killdeer** North Dakota, N USA
28 J4 **Killdeer Mountains** ▲ North Dakota, N USA
45 V15 **Killdeer River** ≈ Trinidad, Trinidad and Tobago
25 S9 **Killeen** Texas, SW USA
39 P6 **Killik River** ≈ Alaska, USA
9 T7 **Killinek Island** island Nunavut, NE Canada
Killini see Kyllíni
115 C19 **Killínis, Akrotírio** headland S Greece
97 D15 **Killybegs** Ir. Na Cealla Beaga. NW Ireland
Kilmain see Quelimane
96 I13 **Kilmarnock** W Scotland, UK
21 X6 **Kilmarnock** Virginia, NE USA
127 S16 **Kil'mez'** Kirovskaya Oblast', NW Russian Federation
129 S2 **Kil'mez'** Udmurtskaya Respublika, NW Russian Federation
127 R16 **Kil'mez'** ≈ NW Russian Federation
67 V11 **Kilombero** ≈ S Tanzania
92 J10 **Kilpisjarvi** Lappi, N Finland
97 B19 **Kilrush** Ir. Cill Rois. W Ireland
79 O24 **Kilwa** Katanga, SE Dem. Rep. Congo (Zaire)
Kilwa see Kilwa Kivinje
81 J24 **Kilwa Kivinje** var. Kilwa. Lindi, SE Tanzania
81 J24 **Kilwa Masoko** Lindi, SE Tanzania
171 T13 **Kilwo** Pulau Seram, E Indonesia
114 P12 **Kilyos** Istanbul, NW Turkey
37 V8 **Kim** Colorado, C USA
169 U7 **Kimanis, Teluk** bay Sabah, East Malaysia
182 H8 **Kimba** South Australia
28 I15 **Kimball** Nebraska, C USA
29 O11 **Kimball** South Dakota, N USA
79 I21 **Kimbao** Bandundu, SW Dem. Rep. Congo (Zaire)
186 F7 **Kimbe** New Britain, E PNG
186 G7 **Kimbe Bay** inlet New Britain, E PNG
11 P17 **Kimberley** British Columbia, SW Canada
83 H23 **Kimberley** Northern Cape, C South Africa
180 M4 **Kimberley Plateau** plateau Western Australia
33 P15 **Kimberly** Idaho, NW USA
163 Y12 **Kimch'aek** prev. Sŏngjin. E North Korea
163 Y15 **Kimch'ŏn** C South Korea
163 Z16 **Kim Hae** var. Pusan. ✈ (Pusan) SE South Korea
Kími see Kými
93 K20 **Kimito** Swe. Kemiö. Länsi-Suomi, W Finland
165 R4 **Kimobetsu** Hokkaidō, NE Japan
115 I21 **Kímolos** island Kykládes, Greece, Aegean Sea
115 I21 **Kímolou Sífnou, Stenó** strait Kykládes, Greece, Aegean Sea
128 L5 **Kimovsk** Tul'skaya Oblast', W Russian Federation
163 X15 **Kimpo** ✈ (Sŏul) NW South Korea
Kimpolung see Câmpulung Moldovenesc
126 K16 **Kimry** Tverskaya Oblast', W Russian Federation
79 H21 **Kimvula** Bas-Congo, SW Dem. Rep. Congo (Zaire)
169 U6 **Kinabalu, Gunung** ▲ East Malaysia
Kinabatangan see Kinabatangan, Sungai
169 V7 **Kinabatangan, Sungai** var. Kinabatangan. ≈ East Malaysia
115 L21 **Kínaros** island Kykládes, Greece, Aegean Sea
11 O15 **Kinbasket Lake** ⊞ British Columbia, SW Canada
96 I7 **Kinbrace** N Scotland, UK
14 E14 **Kincardine** Ontario, S Canada
96 K10 **Kincardine** cultural region E Scotland, UK
79 K21 **Kinda** Kasai Occidental, SE Dem. Rep. Congo (Zaire)
79 M24 **Kinda** Katanga, SE Dem. Rep. Congo (Zaire)
166 L3 **Kindat** Sagaing, N Myanmar
109 V6 **Kindberg** Steiermark, C Austria
22 H8 **Kinder** Louisiana, S USA
98 H13 **Kinderdijk** Zuid-Holland, SW Netherlands
97 M17 **Kinder Scout** ▲ C England, UK
11 S16 **Kindersley** Saskatchewan, S Canada
76 I14 **Kindia** Guinée-Maritime, SW Guinea
64 B11 **Kindley Field** air base E Bermuda
29 R6 **Kindred** North Dakota, N USA
79 N20 **Kindu** prev. Kindu-Port-Empain. Maniema, C Dem. Rep. Congo (Zaire)
Kindu-Port-Empain see Kindu
129 S6 **Kinel'** Samarskaya Oblast', W Russian Federation
127 N15 **Kineshma** Ivanovskaya Oblast', W Russian Federation
King see King William's Town
140 K10 **King Abdul Aziz** ✈ (Makkah) Makkah, W Saudi Arabia
21 X6 **King and Queen Court House** Virginia, NE USA
King Charles Islands see Kong Karls Land
King Christian IX Land see Kong Christian IX Land
King Christian X Land see Kong Christian X Land
35 O11 **King City** California, W USA
27 R2 **King City** Missouri, C USA
38 M16 **King Cove** Alaska, USA
26 M10 **Kingfisher** Oklahoma, C USA
King Frederik VI Coast see Kong Frederik VI Kyst
King Frederik VIII Land see Kong Frederik VIII Land
65 B24 **King George Bay** bay West Falkland, Falkland Islands
194 G3 **King George Island** var. King George Land. island South Shetland Islands, Antarctica
12 I6 **King George Islands** island group Nunavut, C Canada
King George Land see King George Island
126 G13 **Kingisepp** Leningradskaya Oblast', NW Russian Federation
183 N14 **King Island** island Tasmania, SE Australia
10 J15 **King Island** island British Columbia, SW Canada
King Island see Kadan Kyun
Kingissepp see Kuressaare
141 Q7 **King Khalid** ✈ (Ar Riyāḍ) Ar Riyāḍ, C Saudi Arabia
35 S2 **King Lear Peak** ▲ Nevada, W USA
195 Y8 **King Leopold and Queen Astrid Land** physical region Antarctica
180 M4 **King Leopold Ranges** ▲ Western Australia
36 I11 **Kingman** Arizona, SW USA
26 M6 **Kingman** Kansas, C USA
192 L7 **Kingman Reef** ◇ US territory C Pacific Ocean
79 N20 **Kingombe** Maniema, E Dem. Rep. Congo (Zaire)
182 F5 **Kingoonya** South Australia
194 J10 **King Peninsula** peninsula Antarctica
39 P13 **King Salmon** Alaska, USA
35 Q6 **Kings Beach** California, W USA
35 R11 **Kingsburg** California, W USA
182 I10 **Kingscote** South Australia
King's County see Offaly
194 H2 **King Sejong** South Korean research station Antarctica
183 T9 **Kingsford Smith** ✈ (Sydney) New South Wales, SE Australia
11 P17 **Kingsgate** British Columbia, SW Canada
23 W8 **Kingsland** Georgia, SE USA
29 S13 **Kingsley** Iowa, C USA
97 O19 **King's Lynn** var. Bishop's Lynn, Kings Lynn, Lynn, Lynn Regis. E England, UK
21 Q10 **Kings Mountain** North Carolina, SE USA
180 K4 **King Sound** sound Western Australia
37 N2 **Kings Peak** ▲ Utah, W USA
21 O8 **Kingsport** Tennessee, S USA
35 R11 **Kings River** ≈ California, W USA
183 P17 **Kingston** Tasmania, SE Australia
14 K14 **Kingston** Ontario, SE Canada
44 K13 **Kingston** ● (Jamaica) E Jamaica
185 C22 **Kingston** Otago, South Island, NZ
19 P12 **Kingston** Massachusetts, NE USA
27 S3 **Kingston** Missouri, C USA
18 K12 **Kingston** New York, NE USA
31 S14 **Kingston** Ohio, N USA
19 O13 **Kingston** Rhode Island, NE USA
20 M9 **Kingston** Tennessee, S USA
35 W12 **Kingston Peak** ▲ California, W USA
182 J11 **Kingston Southeast** South Australia
97 N17 **Kingston upon Hull** var. Hull. E England, UK
97 N22 **Kingston upon Thames** SE England, UK
45 P14 **Kingstown** ● (Saint Vincent and the Grenadines) Saint Vincent, Saint Vincent and the Grenadines
Kingstown see Dún Laoghaire
21 T13 **Kingstree** South Carolina, SE USA
64 L8 **Kings Trough** undersea feature E Atlantic Ocean
14 C18 **Kingsville** Ontario, S Canada
25 S15 **Kingsville** Texas, SW USA
21 W6 **King William** Virginia, NE USA
8 M7 **King William Island** island Nunavut, N Canada Arctic Ocean
83 I25 **King William's Town** var. King, Kingwilliamstown. Eastern Cape, S South Africa
21 T3 **Kingwood** West Virginia, NE USA
136 C13 **Kınık** İzmir, W Turkey
79 G21 **Kinkala** Le Pool, S Congo
165 R10 **Kinka-san** headland Honshū, C Japan
184 M8 **Kinleith** Waikato, North Island, NZ
95 J19 **Kinna** Västra Götaland, S Sweden
96 L8 **Kinnaird Head** var. Kinnairds Head. headland NE Scotland, UK
95 K20 **Kinnared** Halland, S Sweden
Kinneret, Yam see Tiberias, Lake
155 K24 **Kinniyai** Eastern Province, NE Sri Lanka
93 L16 **Kinnula** Länsi-Suomi, W Finland
14 I8 **Kinojévis** ≈ Quebec, SE Canada
164 I14 **Kino-kawa** ≈ Honshū, SW Japan
11 U11 **Kinoosao** Saskatchewan, C Canada
99 L17 **Kinrooi** Limburg, NE Belgium
96 J11 **Kinross** C Scotland, UK
96 J11 **Kinross** cultural region C Scotland, UK
97 C21 **Kinsale** Ir. Cionn tSáile. SW Ireland
95 D14 **Kinsarvik** Hordaland, S Norway
79 G21 **Kinshasa** prev. Léopoldville. ● (Zaire) Kinshasa, W Dem. Rep. Congo (Zaire)
79 G21 **Kinshasa** off. Ville de Kinshasa, var. Kinshasa City. ◈ region SW Dem. Rep. Congo (Zaire)

◆ Country ● Country Capital ◇ Dependent Territory ○ Dependent Territory Capital ◈ Administrative Region ✈ International Airport ▲ Mountain ▲ Mountain Range Volcano ≈ River ⊚ Lake ⊞ Reservoir

79 G21 **Kinshasa** ✈ Kinshasa, SW Dem. Rep. Congo (Zaire)
Kinshasa City *see* Kinshasa
117 U9 **Kins'ka** ≈ SE Ukraine
26 K6 **Kinsley** Kansas, C USA
21 W10 **Kinston** North Carolina, SE USA
77 P15 **Kintampo** W Ghana
182 B1 **Kintore, Mount** ▲ South Australia
96 G13 **Kintyre** *peninsula* W Scotland, UK
96 G13 **Kintyre, Mull of** *headland* W Scotland, UK
166 M4 **Kin-u** Sagaing, C Myanmar
12 G8 **Kinushseo** ≈ Ontario, C Canada
11 P13 **Kinuso** Alberta, W Canada
154 I13 **Kinwat** Mahārāshtra, C India
81 F16 **Kinyeti** ▲ S Sudan
101 I17 **Kinzig** ≈ SW Germany
Kioga, Lake *see* Kyoga, Lake
26 M8 **Kiowa** Kansas, C USA
27 P12 **Kiowa** Oklahoma, C USA
Kiparissía *see* Kyparissía
14 H10 **Kipawa, Lac** ◎ Quebec, SE Canada
81 G24 **Kipengere Range** ⛰ SW Tanzania
81 E23 **Kipili** Rukwa, W Tanzania
81 K20 **Kipini** Coast, SE Kenya
11 V16 **Kipling** Saskatchewan, S Canada
38 M13 **Kipnuk** Alaska, USA
97 F18 **Kippure** *Ir.* Cipiúr. ▲ E Ireland
79 N25 **Kipushi** Katanga, SE Dem. Rep. Congo (Zaire)
187 N10 **Kirakira** *var.* Kaokaona. San Cristobal, SE Solomon Islands
155 K14 **Kirandul** *var.* Bailādila. Madhya Pradesh, C India
155 I21 **Kiranūr** Tamil Nādu, SE India
119 N21 **Kiraw** *Rus.* Kirovo. Homyel'skaya Voblasts', SE Belarus
119 M17 **Kirawsk** *Rus.* Kirovsk; *prev.* Startsy. Mahilyowskaya Voblasts', E Belarus
118 F5 **Kirbla** Läänemaa, W Estonia
25 Y9 **Kirbyville** Texas, SW USA
114 M12 **Kırcasalih** Edirne, NW Turkey
109 W8 **Kirchbach** *var.* Kirchbach in Steiermark. Steiermark, SE Austria
Kirchbach in Steiermark *see* Kirchbach
108 H7 **Kirchberg** Sankt Gallen, NE Switzerland
109 S5 **Kirchdorf an der Krems** Oberösterreich, N Austria
Kirchheim *see* Kirchheim unter Teck
101 I22 **Kirchheim unter Teck** *var.* Kirchheim. Baden-Württemberg, SW Germany
Kirdzhali *see* Kŭrdzhali
123 N13 **Kirenga** ≈ S Russian Federation
123 N12 **Kirensk** Irkutskaya Oblast', C Russian Federation
Kirghizia *see* Kyrgyzstan
145 S16 **Kirghiz Range** *Rus.* Kirgizskiy Khrebet; *prev.* Alexander Range. ⛰ Kazakhstan/Kyrgyzstan
Kirghiz SSR *see* Kyrgyzstan
Kirghiz Steppe *see* Kazakhskiy Melkosopochnik
Kirgizskaya SSR *see* Kyrgyzstan
Kirgizskiy Khrebet *see* Kirghiz Range
79 I19 **Kiri** Bandundu, W Dem. Rep. Congo (Zaire)
Kiriath-Arba *see* Hebron
191 R3 **Kiribati** *off.* Republic of Kiribati. ◆ *republic* C Pacific Ocean
136 L17 **Kırıkhan** Hatay, S Turkey
136 I13 **Kırıkkale** Kırıkkale, C Turkey
136 C10 **Kırıkkale** ◈ *province* C Turkey
126 L13 **Kirillov** Vologodskaya Oblast', NW Russian Federation
Kirin *see* Jilin
81 I18 **Kirinyaga** *prev.* Mount Kenya. ✱ C Kenya
126 H13 **Kirishi** *var.* Kirisi. Leningradskaya Oblast', NW Russian Federation
164 C16 **Kirishima-yama** ▲ Kyūshū, SW Japan
Kirisi *see* Kirishi
191 Y2 **Kiritimati** ✈ Kiritimati, E Kiribati
191 Y2 **Kiritimati** *prev.* Christmas Island. *atoll* Line Islands, E Kiribati
186 G9 **Kiriwina Island** *Eng.* Trobriand Island. *island* SE PNG
186 G9 **Kiriwina Islands** *var.* Trobriand Islands. *island group* S PNG
96 K12 **Kirkcaldy** E Scotland, UK
97 I14 **Kirkcudbright** S Scotland, UK
97 I14 **Kirkcudbright** *cultural region* S Scotland, UK
Kirkee *see* Khadki
92 M8 **Kirkenes** *var.* Kirkkoniemi. Finnmark, N Norway
95 I14 **Kirkenær** Hedmark, S Norway
92 J4 **Kirkjubæjarklaustur** Sudhurland, S Iceland
Kirk-Kilissa *see* Kırklareli
Kirkkoniemi *see* Kirkenes
93 L20 **Kirkkonummi** *Swe.* Kyrkslätt. Etelä-Suomi, S Finland
14 G7 **Kirkland Lake** Ontario, S Canada
136 C9 **Kırklareli** *prev.* Kirk-Kilissa. Kırklareli, NW Turkey
136 I13 **Kırklareli** ◈ *province* NW Turkey
185 F20 **Kirkliston Range** ⛰ South Island, NZ
14 D10 **Kirkpatrick Lake** ◎ Ontario, S Canada
195 Q11 **Kirkpatrick, Mount** ▲ Antarctica
27 U2 **Kirksville** Missouri, C USA
139 T4 **Kirkūk** *var.* Karkūk, Kerkuk. N Iraq
139 U7 **Kir Kush** E Iraq
96 K5 **Kirkwall** NE Scotland, UK
83 H25 **Kirkwood** Eastern Cape, S South Africa
27 X5 **Kirkwood** Missouri, C USA
Kirman *see* Kermān
Kir Moab/Kir of Moab *see* Al Karak
128 I5 **Kirov** Kaluzhskaya Oblast', W Russian Federation
127 R14 **Kirov** *prev.* Vyatka. Kirovskaya Oblast', NW Russian Federation
Kīrov *see* Balpyk Bi, Kazakhstan
Kīrov *see* Kirova, Almaty, Kazakhstan
145 U13 **Kirova** *Kaz.* Kīrov. Almaty, SE Kazakhstan
Kirovabad *see* Gäncä, Azerbaijan
Kirovabad *see* Panj, Tajikistan
Kirovakan *see* Vanadzor
Kirovo *see* Kiraw, Belarus
Kirovo/Kirovograd *see* Kirovohrad, Ukraine
Kirovo *see* Beshariq, Uzbekistan
127 R14 **Kirovo-Chepetsk** Kirovskaya Oblast', NW Russian Federation
Kirovogradskaya Oblast'/Kirovohrad *see* Kirovohrads'ka Oblast'
117 R7 **Kirovohrad** *Rus.* Kirovograd; *prev.* Kirovo, Yelizavetgrad, Zinov'yevsk. Kirovohrads'ka Oblast', C Ukraine
117 P7 **Kirovohrads'ka Oblast'** *var.* Kirovohrad, *Rus.* Kirovogradskaya Oblast'. ◈ *province* C Ukraine
126 J4 **Kirovsk** Murmanskaya Oblast', NW Russian Federation
Kirovsk *see* Babadaykhan, Turkmenistan
Kirovsk *see* Kirawsk, Belarus
117 X7 **Kirovs'k** Luhans'ka Oblast', E Ukraine
122 E9 **Kirovskaya Oblast'** ◈ *province* NW Russian Federation
117 X8 **Kirov'ske** Donets'ka Oblast', E Ukraine
117 U13 **Kirovs'ke** *Rus.* Kirovskoye. Respublika Krym, S Ukraine
123 V10 **Kirovskiy** Kamchatskaya Oblast', E Russian Federation
Kirovskiy *see* Balpyk Bi
Kirovskoye *see* Kyzyl-Adyr
Kirovskoye *see* Kirovs'ke
146 E11 **Kirpili** Akhalskiy Velayat, C Turkmenistan
96 K10 **Kirriemuir** E Scotland, UK
127 S13 **Kirs** Kirovskaya Oblast', NW Russian Federation
129 N7 **Kirsanov** Tambovskaya Oblast', W Russian Federation
136 J14 **Kırşehir** *anc.* Justinianopolis. Kirşehir, C Turkey
136 I13 **Kırşehir** ◈ *province* C Turkey
149 P4 **Kīrthar Range** ⛰ S Pakistan
37 P9 **Kirtland** New Mexico, SW USA
Kirun/Kirun' *see* Chilung
92 J11 **Kiruna** Norrbotten, N Sweden
79 M18 **Kirundu** Orientale, NE Dem. Rep. Congo (Zaire)
26 L3 **Kirwin Reservoir** ⊞ Kansas, C USA
129 Q4 **Kirya** Chuvashskaya Respublika, W Russian Federation
Kiryat Gat *see* Qiryat Gat
95 M18 **Kisa** Östergötland, S Sweden
165 P9 **Kisakata** Akita, Honshū, C Japan
Kisalföld *see* Little Alföld
79 L18 **Kisangani** *prev.* Stanleyville. Orientale, NE Dem. Rep. Congo (Zaire)
39 N12 **Kisaralik River** ≈ Alaska, USA
165 O14 **Kisarazu** Chiba, Honshū, S Japan
111 I22 **Kisbér** Komárom-Esztergom, NW Hungary
11 V17 **Kisbey** Saskatchewan, S Canada
122 J13 **Kiselevsk** Kemerovskaya Oblast', S Russian Federation
153 R13 **Kishanganj** Bihār, NE India
152 G12 **Kishangarh** Rājasthān, N India
Kishegyes *see* Mali Idoš
77 S15 **Kishi** Oyo, W Nigeria
Kishinev *see* Chişinău
Kishiözen *see* Malyy Uzen'
164 I14 **Kishiwada** *var.* Kisiwada. Ōsaka, Honshū, SW Japan
143 P14 **Kīsh, Jazīreh-ye** *var.* Qeys. *island* S Iran
145 R7 **Kishkenekol'** *prev.* Kzyltu. *Kaz.* Qyzyltu; Severnyy Kazakhstan, N Kazakhstan
152 I6 **Kishtwār** Jammu and Kashmir, NW India
81 H19 **Kisii** Nyanza, SW Kenya
81 J23 **Kisiju** Pwani, E Tanzania
Kisiwada *see* Kishiwada
Kisjenő *see* Chişineu-Criş
38 E17 **Kiska Island** *island* Aleutian Islands, Alaska, USA
Kiskapus *see* Copşa Mică
111 M22 **Kiskörei-víztároló** ⊞ E Hungary
Kis-Küküllo *see* Târnava Mică
111 L24 **Kiskunfélegyháza** *var.* Félegyháza. Bács-Kiskun, C Hungary
111 K25 **Kiskunhalas** *var.* Halas. Bács-Kiskun, S Hungary
111 K24 **Kiskunmajsa** Bács-Kiskun, S Hungary
129 N15 **Kislovodsk** Stavropol'skiy Kray, SW Russian Federation
81 L18 **Kismaayo** *var.* Chisimayu, Kismayu, *It.* Chisimaio. Jubbada Hoose, S Somalia
Kismayu *see* Kismaayo
164 M13 **Kiso-sanmyaku** ⛰ Honshū, S Japan
Kisseraing *see* Kanmaw Kyun
76 K14 **Kissidougou** Guinée-Forestière, S Guinea
23 X12 **Kissimmee** Florida, SE USA
23 X12 **Kissimmee, Lake** ◎ Florida, SE USA
23 X13 **Kissimmee River** ≈ Florida, SE USA
11 V13 **Kississing Lake** ◎ Manitoba, C Canada
111 L24 **Kistelek** Csongrád, SE Hungary
Kistna *see* Krishna
111 M23 **Kisújszállás** Jász-Nagykun-Szolnok, E Hungary
164 G12 **Kisuki** Shimane, Honshū, SW Japan
81 H18 **Kisumu** *prev.* Port Florence. Nyanza, W Kenya
Kisutzaneustadtl *see* Kysucké Nové Mesto
111 O20 **Kisvárda** *Ger.* Kleinwardein. Szabolcs-Szatmár-Bereg, E Hungary
81 J24 **Kiswere** Lindi, SE Tanzania
Kiszucaújhely *see* Kysucké Nové Mesto
76 K12 **Kita** Kayes, W Mali
207 N14 **Kitaa** ◈ *province* W Greenland
Kitab *see* Kitob
165 Q4 **Kitahiyama** Hokkaidō, NE Japan
165 P12 **Kita-Ibaraki** Ibaraki, Honshū, S Japan
165 X16 **Kita-Iō-jima** *Eng.* San Alessandro. *island* SE Japan
165 Q9 **Kitakami** Iwate, Honshū, C Japan
165 P11 **Kitakata** Fukushima, Honshū, C Japan
164 D13 **Kitakyūshū** *var.* Kitakyûsyû. Fukuoka, Kyūshū, SW Japan
Kitakyûsyû *see* Kitakyūshū
81 H18 **Kitale** Rift Valley, W Kenya
165 U3 **Kitami** Hokkaidō, NE Japan
165 T2 **Kitami-sanchi** ⛰ Hokkaidō, NE Japan
37 W5 **Kit Carson** Colorado, C USA
180 M12 **Kitchener** Western Australia
14 F16 **Kitchener** Ontario, S Canada
93 O17 **Kitee** Itä-Suomi, E Finland
81 G16 **Kitgum** N Uganda
Kithareng *see* Kanmaw Kyun
Kíthira *see* Kýthira
Kíthnos *see* Kýthnos
10 J13 **Kitimat** British Columbia, SW Canada
92 L11 **Kitinen** ≈ N Finland
147 N12 **Kitob** *Rus.* Kitab. Qashqadaryo Wiloyati, S Uzbekistan
116 K7 **Kitsman'** *Ger.* Kotzman, *Rom.* Cozmeni, *Rus.* Kitsman. Chernivets'ka Oblast', W Ukraine
164 E14 **Kitsuki** *var.* Kituki. Ōita, Kyūshū, SW Japan
18 C14 **Kittanning** Pennsylvania, NE USA
19 P10 **Kittery** Maine, NE USA
92 L11 **Kittilä** Lappi, N Finland
109 Z4 **Kittsee** Burgenland, E Austria
81 J19 **Kitui** Eastern, S Kenya
Kituki *see* Kitsuki
81 G22 **Kitunda** Tabora, C Tanzania
10 K13 **Kitwanga** British Columbia, SW Canada
82 J13 **Kitwe** *var.* Kitwe-Nkana. Copperbelt, C Zambia
Kitwe-Nkana *see* Kitwe
109 O7 **Kitzbühel** Tirol, W Austria
109 O7 **Kitzbüheler Alpen** ⛰ W Austria
101 J19 **Kitzingen** Bayern, SE Germany
153 Q14 **Kiul** Bihār, NE India
186 A7 **Kiunga** Western, SW PNG
93 M16 **Kiuruvesi** Itä-Suomi, C Finland
38 M7 **Kivalina** Alaska, USA
92 L13 **Kivalo** *ridge* C Finland
116 J3 **Kivertsi** *Pol.* Kiwerce, *Rus.* Kivertsy. Volyns'ka Oblast', NW Ukraine
Kivertsy *see* Kivertsi
93 L16 **Kivijärvi** Länsi-Suomi, W Finland
95 L23 **Kivik** Skåne, S Sweden
118 J3 **Kiviõli** Ida-Virumaa, NE Estonia
Kivu, Lac *see* Kivu, Lake
67 U10 **Kivu, Lake** *Fr.* Lac Kivu. ◎ Rwanda/Dem. Rep. Congo (Zaire)
186 C9 **Kiwai Island** *island* SW PNG
39 N8 **Kiwalik** Alaska, USA
Kiwerce *see* Kivertsi
Kiyev *see* Kyyiv
145 R10 **Kiyevka** Karaganda, C Kazakhstan
Kiyevskaya Oblast' *see* Kyyivs'ka Oblast'
Kiyevskoye Vodokhranilishche *see* Kyyivs'ke Vodoskhovyshche
136 D10 **Kıyıköy** Kırklareli, NW Turkey
145 O9 **Kiyma** Akmola, C Kazakhstan
127 V13 **Kizel** Permskaya Oblast', NW Russian Federation
127 O12 **Kizema** *var.* Kizëma. Arkhangel'skaya Oblast', NW Russian Federation
Kizilagach *see* Elkhovo
136 H12 **Kızılcahamam** Ankara, N Turkey
136 J10 **Kızıl Irmak** ≈ C Turkey
Kızılkoca *see* Şefaatli
Kizil Kum *see* Kyzyl Kum
137 P16 **Kızıltepe** Mardin, SE Turkey
Ki Zil Uzen *see* Qezel Owzan
129 Q16 **Kizilyurt** Respublika Dagestan, SW Russian Federation
129 Q15 **Kizlyar** Respublika Dagestan, SW Russian Federation
129 S3 **Kizner** Udmurtskaya Respublika, NW Russian Federation
Kizyl-Arvat *see* Gyzylarbat
146 B13 **Kizyl-Atrek** *Turkm.* Gyzyletrek. Balkanskiy Velayat, W Turkmenistan
146 D10 **Kizyl-Kaya** *Turkm.* Gyzylgaya. Balkanskiy Velayat, NW Turkmenistan
146 A10 **Kizyl-Su** *Turkm.* Gyzylsu. Balkanskiy Velayat, W Turkmenistan
95 H16 **Kjerkøy** *island* S Norway
Kjølen *see* Kölen
92 L7 **Kjøllefjord** Finnmark, N Norway
92 H11 **Kjøpsvik** Nordland, C Norway
169 N12 **Klabat, Teluk** *bay* Pulau Bangka, W Indonesia
112 I12 **Kladanj** Federacija Bosan I Hercegovina, C Bosnia and Herzegovina
171 X16 **Kladar** Irian Jaya, E Indonesia
111 C16 **Kladno** Středočeský Kraj, NW Czech Republic
112 P11 **Kladovo** Serbia, E Yugoslavia
167 P12 **Klaeng** Rayong, S Thailand
109 T9 **Klagenfurt** *Slvn.* Celovec. Kärnten, S Austria
118 B11 **Klaipėda** *Ger.* Memel. Klaipėda, NW Lithuania
95 B18 **Klaksvík** *Dan.* Klaksvig Faeroe Islands
34 L2 **Klamath** California, W USA
32 H16 **Klamath Falls** Oregon, NW USA
34 M1 **Klamath Mountains** ⛰ California/Oregon, W USA
34 L2 **Klamath River** ≈ California/Oregon, W USA
168 K9 **Klang** *var.* Kelang; *prev.* Port Swettenham. Selangor, Peninsular Malaysia
94 J13 **Klarälven** ≈ Norway/Sweden
111 B15 **Klášterec nad Ohří** *Ger.* Klösterle an der Eger. Ústecký Kraj, NW Czech Republic
111 B18 **Klatovy** *Ger.* Klattau. Plzeňský Kraj, W Czech Republic
Klattau *see* Klatovy
Klausenburg *see* Cluj-Napoca
39 Y14 **Klawock** Prince of Wales Island, Alaska, USA
98 P8 **Klazienaveen** Drenthe, NE Netherlands
Kleck *see* Klyetsk
110 H11 **Klecko** Wielkolpolskie, C Poland
110 I11 **Kleczew** Wielkopolskie, C Poland
10 L15 **Kleena Kleene** British Columbia, SW Canada
83 D20 **Klein Aub** Hardap, C Namibia
Kleine Donau *see* Mosoni-Duna
101 O14 **Kleine Elster** ≈ E Germany
Kleine Kokel *see* Târnava Mică
99 I16 **Kleine Nete** ≈ N Belgium
Kleines Ungarisches Tiefland *see* Little Alföld
83 E22 **Klein Karas** Karas, S Namibia
Kleinkopisch *see* Copşa Mică
Klein-Marien *see* Väike-Maarja
Kleinschlatten *see* Zlatna
83 D23 **Kleinsee** Northern Cape, W South Africa
Kleinwardein *see* Kisvárda
115 C16 **Kleisoúra** Ípeiros, W Greece
95 C17 **Klepp** Rogaland, S Norway
83 I22 **Klerksdorp** North-West, N South Africa
128 I5 **Kletnya** Bryanskaya Oblast', W Russian Federation
Kletsk *see* Klyetsk
101 D14 **Kleve** *Eng.* Cleves, *Fr.* Clèves; *prev.* Cleve. Nordrhein-Westfalen, W Germany
113 J16 **Kličevo** Montenegro, SW Yugoslavia
119 M16 **Klichaw** *Rus.* Klichev. Mahilyowskaya Voblasts', E Belarus
Klichev *see* Klichaw
119 Q16 **Klimavichy** *Rus.* Klimovichi. Mahilyowskaya Voblasts', E Belarus
114 M7 **Kliment** Shumen, NE Bulgaria
Klimovichi *see* Klimavichy
93 G14 **Klimpfjäll** Västerbotten, N Sweden
128 K3 **Klin** Moskovskaya Oblast', W Russian Federation
113 M16 **Klina** Serbia, S Yugoslavia
111 B15 **Klínovec** *Ger.* Keilberg. ▲ NW Czech Republic
95 P19 **Klintehamn** Gotland, SE Sweden
129 R8 **Klintsovka** Saratovskaya Oblast', W Russian Federation
128 H6 **Klintsy** Bryanskaya Oblast', W Russian Federation
95 K22 **Klippan** Skåne, S Sweden
92 G13 **Klippen** Västerbotten, N Sweden
121 P2 **Klírou** W Cyprus
114 I9 **Klisura** Plovdiv, C Bulgaria
95 F20 **Klitmøller** Viborg, NW Denmark
112 F11 **Ključ** Federacija Bosna I Hercegovina, NW Bosnia and Herzegovina
111 J14 **Kłobuck** Śląskie, S Poland
110 J11 **Kłodawa** Wielkopolskie, C Poland
111 G16 **Kłodzko** *Ger.* Glatz. Dolnośląskie, SW Poland
95 I14 **Kløfta** Akershus, S Norway
112 P12 **Klokočevac** Serbia, E Yugoslavia
118 G3 **Klooga** *Ger.* Lodensee. Harjumaa, NW Estonia
99 F15 **Kloosterzande** Zeeland, SW Netherlands
113 L19 **Klos** *var.* Klosi. Dibër, C Albania
Klosi *see* Klos
Klösterle an der Eger *see* Klášterec nad Ohří
109 X3 **Klosterneuburg** Niederösterreich, NE Austria
108 J9 **Klosters** Graubünden, SE Switzerland
108 G7 **Kloten** Zürich, N Switzerland
108 G7 **Kloten** ✈ (Zürich) Zürich, N Switzerland
100 K12 **Klötze** Sachsen-Anhalt, C Germany
12 K3 **Klotz, Lac** ◎ Quebec, NE Canada
101 O15 **Klotzsche** ✈ (Dresden) Sachsen, E Germany
10 H7 **Kluane Lake** ◎ Yukon Territory, W Canada
Kluang *see* Keluang
111 I14 **Kluczbork** *Ger.* Kreuzburg, Kreuzburg in Oberschlesien. Opolskie, S Poland
39 W12 **Klukwan** Alaska, USA
Klyastitsy *see* Klyastsitsy
118 L11 **Klyastsitsy** *Rus.* Klyastitsy. Vitsyebskaya Voblasts', N Belarus
129 T5 **Klyavlino** Samarskaya Oblast', W Russian Federation
84 K9 **Klyaz'in** ≈ W Russian Federation
129 N3 **Klyaz'ma** ≈ W Russian Federation
119 J17 **Klyetsk** *Pol.* Kleck, *Rus.* Kletsk. Minskaya Voblasts', SW Belarus
147 S8 **Klyuchevka** Talasskaya Oblast', NW Kyrgyzstan
123 V10 **Klyuchevskaya Sopka, Vulkan** ✱ E Russian Federation
95 D17 **Knaben** Vest-Agder, S Norway
Knanzi *see* Ghanzi
95 K21 **Knäred** Halland, S Sweden
97 M16 **Knaresborough** N England, UK
114 H8 **Knezha** Vratsa, NW Bulgaria
25 O9 **Knickerbocker** Texas, SW USA
28 K5 **Knife River** ≈ North Dakota, N USA
10 K16 **Knight Inlet** *inlet* British Columbia, W Canada
39 S12 **Knight Island** *island* Alaska, USA
97 K20 **Knighton** E Wales, UK
35 O7 **Knights Landing** California, W USA
112 E13 **Knin** Šibenik-Knin, S Croatia
25 Q12 **Knippal** Texas, SW USA
109 U7 **Knittelfeld** Steiermark, C Austria
95 O15 **Knivsta** Uppsala, C Sweden
113 P14 **Knjaževac** Serbia, E Yugoslavia
27 S4 **Knob Noster** Missouri, C USA
99 D15 **Knokke-Heist** West-Vlaanderen, NW Belgium
95 H20 **Knøsen** *hill* N Denmark
Knosós *see* Knossos
115 J25 **Knossos** *Gk.* Knosós. *prehistoric site* Kríti, Greece, E Mediterranean Sea
25 N7 **Knott** Texas, SW USA
194 K5 **Knowles, Cape** *headland* Antarctica
31 O11 **Knox** Indiana, N USA
29 O3 **Knox** North Dakota, N USA
18 C13 **Knox** Pennsylvania, NE USA
189 X8 **Knox Atoll** *var.* Ņadikdik, Narikrik. *atoll* Ratak Chain, SE Marshall Islands
10 H13 **Knox, Cape** *headland* Graham Island, British Columbia, SW Canada
25 P5 **Knox City** Texas, SW USA
195 Y11 **Knox Coast** *physical region* Antarctica
31 T12 **Knox Lake** ⊞ Ohio, N USA
23 T5 **Knoxville** Georgia, SE USA
30 K12 **Knoxville** Illinois, N USA
29 W15 **Knoxville** Iowa, C USA
21 N9 **Knoxville** Tennessee, S USA
197 P11 **Knud Rasmussen Land** *physical region* N Greenland
Knüll *see* Knüllgebirge
101 I16 **Knüllgebirge** *var.* Knüll. ⛰ C Germany
Knyazhevo *see* Sredishte
Knyazhitsy *see* Knyazhytsy
119 O15 **Knyazhytsy** *Rus.* Knyazhitsy. Mahilyowskaya Voblasts', E Belarus
83 G26 **Knysna** Western Cape, SW South Africa
Koartac *see* Quaqtaq
169 N13 **Koba** Pulau Bangka, W Indonesia
164 D16 **Kobayashi** *var.* Kobayasi. Miyazaki, Kyūshū, SW Japan
Kobayasi *see* Kobayashi
164 I13 **Kōbe** Hyōgo, Honshū, SW Japan
Kobelyaki *see* Kobelyaky
117 T6 **Kobelyaky** *Rus.* Kobelyaki. Poltavs'ka Oblast', NE Ukraine
95 J22 **København** *Eng.* Copenhagen; *anc.* Hafnia. ● (Denmark) Sjælland, København, E Denmark
95 J23 **København** *off.* Københavns Amt. ◈ *county* E Denmark
76 K10 **Kobenni** Hodh el Gharbi, S Mauritania
171 T13 **Kobi** Pulau Seram, E Indonesia
101 F17 **Koblenz** *prev.* Coblenz, *Fr.* Coblence, *anc.* Confluentes. Rheinland-Pfalz, W Germany
108 F6 **Koblenz** Aargau, N Switzerland
Kobrin *see* Kobryn
171 V15 **Kobroor, Pulau** *island* Kepulauan Aru, E Indonesia
119 G19 **Kobryn** *Pol.* Kobryn, *Rus.* Kobrin. Brestskaya Voblasts', SW Belarus
39 O7 **Kobuk** Alaska, USA
39 O7 **Kobuk River** ≈ Alaska, USA
137 Q10 **K'obulet'i** W Georgia
123 P10 **Kobyay** Respublika Sakha (Yakutiya), NE Russian Federation
136 E11 **Kocaeli** ◈ *province* NW Turkey
113 P18 **Kočani** NE FYR Macedonia
112 K12 **Koceljevo** Serbia, W Yugoslavia
109 U12 **Kočevje** *Ger.* Gottschee. S Slovenia
153 T12 **Koch Bihār** West Bengal, NE India
122 M9 **Kochechum** ≈ N Russian Federation
101 I20 **Kocher** ≈ SW Germany
127 T13 **Kochevo** Komi-Permyatskiy Avtonomnyy Okrug, NW Russian Federation
164 G14 **Kōchi** *var.* Kôti. Kōchi, Shikoku, SW Japan
164 G14 **Kōchi** *off.* Kōchi-ken, *var.* Kôti. ◈ *prefecture* Shikoku, SW Japan
Kochi *see* Cochin
Kochiu *see* Gejiu
Kochkor *see* Kochkorka
147 V8 **Kochkorka** *Kir.* Kochkor. Narynskaya Oblast', C Kyrgyzstan
127 V5 **Kochmes** Respublika Komi, NW Russian Federation
129 P15 **Kochubey** Respublika Dagestan, SW Russian Federation
115 I17 **Kochýlas** ▲ Skýros, Vóreioi Sporádes, Greece, Aegean Sea
110 O13 **Kock** Lubelskie, E Poland
81 J19 **Kodacho** *spring/well* S Kenya
155 K24 **Koddiyar Bay** *bay* NE Sri Lanka
39 Q14 **Kodiak** Kodiak Island, Alaska, USA
39 Q14 **Kodiak Island** *island* Alaska, USA
154 B12 **Kodīnār** Gujarāt, W India
126 M9 **Kodino** Arkhangel'skaya Oblast', NW Russian Federation
122 M12 **Kodinsk** Krasnoyarskiy Kray, C Russian Federation
80 F12 **Kodok** Upper Nile, SE Sudan
117 N8 **Kodyma** Odes'ka Oblast', SW Ukraine
99 B17 **Koekelare** West-Vlaanderen, W Belgium
Koeln *see* Köln
Koepang *see* Kupang
Ko-erh-mu *see* Golmud
99 J17 **Koersel** Limburg, NE Belgium
83 E21 **Koës** Karas, SE Namibia
Koetai *see* Mahakam, Sungai
Koetaradja *see* Bandaaceh
36 I14 **Kofa Mountains** ⛰ Arizona, SW USA
171 Y15 **Kofarau** Irian Jaya, E Indonesia
147 P13 **Kofarnihon** *Rus.* Kofarnikhon; *prev.* Ordzhonikidzeabad, *Taj.* Orjonikidzeobod, Yangi-Bazar. W Tajikistan
147 P14 **Kofarnihon** *Rus.* Kafirnigan. ≈ SW Tajikistan
Kofarnikhon *see* Kofarnihon
114 M11 **Kofçaz** Kırklareli, NW Turkey
115 J25 **Kófinas** ▲ Kríti, Greece, E Mediterranean Sea
121 P3 **Kofínou** *var.* Kophinou. S Cyprus
109 V8 **Köflach** Steiermark, SE Austria
77 Q17 **Koforidua** SE Ghana
164 H12 **Kōfu** Tottori, Honshū, SW Japan
164 M13 **Kōfu** *var.* Kôhu. Yamanashi, Honshū, S Japan
81 F22 **Koga** Tabora, C Tanzania
Kogălniceanu *see* Mihail Kogălniceanu
13 P6 **Kogaluk** ≈ Newfoundland, E Canada
12 J4 **Kogaluk** ≈ Quebec, NE Canada
122 I10 **Kogalym** Khanty-Mansiyskiy Avtonomnyy Okrug, C Russian Federation
95 J23 **Køge** Roskilde, E Denmark
95 J23 **Køge Bugt** *bay* E Denmark
77 U16 **Kogi** ◈ *state* C Nigeria
146 L11 **Kogon** *Rus.* Kagan. Bukhoro Wiloyati, C Uzbekistan
163 Y17 **Kōgŭm-do** *island* S South Korea
Kōhalom *see* Rupea
149 T6 **Kohāt** North-West Frontier Province, NW Pakistan
118 G4 **Kohila** *Ger.* Koil. Raplamaa, NW Estonia
153 X13 **Kohīma** Nāgāland, E India
Koh I Noh *see* Büyükağrı Dağı
142 L10 **Kohkīlūyeh va Būyer Aḥmadī** *off.* Ostān-e Kohkīlūyeh va Būyer Aḥmadī, *var.* Boyer Ahmadī va Kohkīlūyeh. ◈ *province* SW Iran
Kohsān *see* Kūhestān
118 J3 **Kohtla-Järve** Ida-Virumaa, NE Estonia
Kôhu *see* Kōfu
117 N10 **Kohyl'nyk** *Rom.* Cogîlnic. ≈ Moldova/Ukraine
165 N11 **Koide** Niigata, Honshū, C Japan
10 G7 **Koidern** Yukon Territory, W Canada
76 J15 **Koidu** E Sierra Leone
118 I4 **Koigi** Järvamaa, C Estonia
Koil *see* Kohila
172 H13 **Koimbani** Grande Comore, NW Comoros
139 T3 **Koi Sanjaq** *var.* Koysanjaq, Küysanjaq. N Iraq
93 O16 **Koitere** ◎ E Finland
Koivisto *see* Primorsk
163 Z16 **Kōje-do** *Jap.* Kyōsai-tō. *island* S South Korea
80 J13 **K'ok'a Hāyk'** ◎ C Ethiopia
Kokand *see* Qŭqon
182 F6 **Kokatha** South Australia
Kokcha *see* Kŭkcha
Kokchetav *see* Kokshetau
93 K18 **Kokemäenjoki** ≈ SW Finland
171 W14 **Kokenau** *var.* Kokonau. Irian Jaya, E Indonesia
83 E22 **Kokerboom** Karas, SE Namibia
119 N14 **Kokhanava** *Rus.* Kokhanovo. Vitsyebskaya Voblasts', NE Belarus
Kokhanovichi *see* Kakhanavichy
Kokhanovo *see* Kokhanava

◆ Country ● Country Capital ◇ Dependent Territory ○ Dependent Territory Capital ◈ Administrative Region ✈ International Airport ▲ Mountain ⛰ Mountain Range ✱ Volcano ≈ River ◎ Lake ⊞ Reservoir

Kök-Janggak see Kok-Yangak
93 K16 **Kokkola** Swe. Karleby; prev. Swe. Gamlakarleby. Länsi-Suomi, W Finland
158 L3 **Kok Kuduk** well N China
118 H9 **Koknese** Aizkraukle, C Latvia
77 T13 **Koko** Kebbi, W Nigeria
186 E9 **Kokoda** Northern, S PNG
76 K12 **Kokofata** Kayes, W Mali
39 N6 **Kokolik River** ≈ Alaska, USA
31 O13 **Kokomo** Indiana, N USA
Kokonau see Kokenau
Koko Nor see Qinghai Hu, China
Koko Nor see Qinghai, China
186 H6 **Kokopo** var. Kopopo; prev. Herbertshöhe. New Britain, E PNG
145 X10 **Kokpekti** Kaz. Kökpekti. Vostochnyy Kazakhstan, E Kazakhstan
145 X11 **Kokpekti** ≈ E Kazakhstan
39 P9 **Kokrines** Alaska, USA
39 P9 **Kokrines Hills** ▲ Alaska, USA
145 P17 **Koksaray** Yuzhnyy Kazakhstan, S Kazakhstan
147 X9 **Kokshaal-Tau** Rus. Khrebet Kakshaal-Too. ▲ China/Kyrgyzstan
145 P7 **Kokshetau** Kaz. Kökshetaū; prev. Kokchetav. Severnyy Kazakhstan, N Kazakhstan
99 A17 **Koksijde** West-Vlaanderen, W Belgium
12 M5 **Koksoak** ≈ Quebec, E Canada
83 K24 **Kokstad** KwaZulu/Natal, E South Africa
145 W15 **Koktal** Kaz. Köktal. Almaty, SE Kazakhstan
145 Q12 **Koktas** ≈ C Kazakhstan
Kök-Tash see Kĕk-Tash
Koktokay see Fuyun
147 T9 **Kok-Yangak** Kir. Kök-Janggak. Dzhalal-Abadskaya Oblast', W Kyrgyzstan
158 F9 **Kokyar** Xinjiang Uygur Zizhiqu, W China
149 O13 **Kolāchi** var. Kulachi. ≈ SW Pakistan
76 J15 **Kolahun** N Liberia
171 O14 **Kolaka** Sulawesi, C Indonesia
Kolam see Quilon
K'o-la-ma-i see Karamay
Kola Peninsula see Kol'skiy Poluostrov
155 H19 **Kolār** Karnātaka, E India
155 H19 **Kolār Gold Fields** Karnātaka, E India
92 K11 **Kolari** Lappi, NW Finland
111 I21 **Kolárovo** Ger. Gutta; prev. Guta, Hung. Gúta. Nitriansky Kraj, SW Slovakia
113 K16 **Kolašin** Montenegro, SW Yugoslavia
152 F11 **Kolāyat** Rājasthān, NW India
95 N15 **Kolbäck** Västmanland, C Sweden
Kolbcha see Kowbcha
197 Q15 **Kolbeinsey Ridge** undersea feature Denmark Strait/Norwegian Sea
Kolberg see Kołobrzeg
95 H15 **Kolbotn** Akershus, S Norway
111 N16 **Kolbuszowa** Podkarpackie, SE Poland
128 L3 **Kol'chugino** Vladimirskaya Oblast', W Russian Federation
76 H12 **Kolda** S Senegal
95 G23 **Kolding** Vejle, C Denmark
79 M17 **Kole** Orientale, N Dem. Rep. Congo (Zaire)
79 K20 **Kole** Kasai Oriental, SW Dem. Rep. Congo (Zaire)
Kōle see Kili Island
84 F6 **Kölen** Nor. Kjølen. ▲ Norway/Sweden
Kolepom, Pulau see Yos Sudarso, Pulau
118 H3 **Kolga Laht** Ger. Kolko-Wiek. bay N Estonia
127 Q3 **Kolguyev, Ostrov** island NW Russian Federation
155 E16 **Kolhāpur** Mahārāshtra, SW India
151 K21 **Kolhumadulu Atoll** var. Kolumadulu Atoll, Thaa Atoll. atoll S Maldives
93 O16 **Koli** var. Kolinkylä. Itä-Suomi, E Finland
39 O13 **Koliganek** Alaska, USA
111 E16 **Kolín** Ger. Kolin. Středočeský Kraj, C Czech Republic
Kolinkylä see Koli
190 E12 **Koliu** Île Futuna, W Wallis and Futuna
118 E7 **Kolka** Talsi, NW Latvia
118 E7 **Kolkasrags** prev. Eng. Cape Domesnes. headland NW Latvia
Kolkhozabad see Kolkhozobod
147 P14 **Kolkhozobod** Rus. Kolkhozabad; prev. Kaganovichabad, Tugalan. SW Tajikistan
Kolki/Kołki see Kolky
Kolko-Wiek see Kolga Laht
116 K3 **Kolky** Pol. Kołki, Rus. Kolki. Volyns'ka Oblast', NW Ukraine
Kollam see Quilon
155 G20 **Kollegāl** Karnātaka, W India
98 M5 **Kollum** Friesland, N Netherlands
Kolmar see Colmar
101 E16 **Köln** var. Koeln, Eng./Fr. Cologne; prev. Cöln, anc. Colonia Agrippina, Oppidum Ubiorum. Nordrhein-Westfalen, W Germany
110 N9 **Kolno** Podlaskie, NE Poland
110 J12 **Koło** Wielkopolskie, C Poland
38 B8 **Koloa** Haw. Kōloa. Kauai, Hawaii, USA, C Pacific Ocean
110 E7 **Kołobrzeg** Ger. Kolberg. Zachodniopomorskie, NW Poland
128 H4 **Kolodnya** Smolenskaya Oblast', W Russian Federation
190 E13 **Kolofau, Mont** ▲ Île Alofi, S Wallis and Futuna
127 O14 **Kologriv** Kostromskaya Oblast', NW Russian Federation
76 L12 **Kolokani** Koulikoro, W Mali
77 N13 **Koloko** W Burkina
186 K8 **Kolombangara** var. Kilimbangara, Nduke. island New Georgia Islands, NW Solomon Islands
Kolomea see Kolomyya
128 L4 **Kolomna** Moskovskaya Oblast', W Russian Federation
116 J7 **Kolomyya** Ger. Kolomea. Ivano-Frankivs'ka Oblast', W Ukraine
76 M13 **Kolondiéba** Sikasso, SW Mali
193 V15 **Kolonga** Tongatapu, S Tonga
189 U16 **Kolonia** var. Colonia. Pohnpei, E Micronesia
Kolonja see Kolonjë
113 K21 **Kolonjë** var. Kolonja. Fier, C Albania
Kolonjë see Ersekë
Kolotambu see Avuavu
193 U15 **Kolovai** Tongatapu, S Tonga
Kolozsvár see Cluj-Napoca
112 C9 **Kolpa** Ger. Kulpa, SCr. Kupa. ≈ Croatia/Slovenia
122 J11 **Kolpashevo** Tomskaya Oblast', C Russian Federation
126 H13 **Kolpino** Leningradskaya Oblast', NW Russian Federation
100 M10 **Kölpinsee** ◎ NE Germany
126 K5 **Kol'skiy Poluostrov** Eng. Kola Peninsula. peninsula NW Russian Federation
129 T6 **Koltubanovskiy** Orenburgskaya Oblast', W Russian Federation
112 L11 **Kolubara** ≈ C Yugoslavia
Kolupchii see Gurkovo
110 K13 **Koluszki** Łodzkie, C Poland
127 T6 **Kolva** ≈ NW Russian Federation
93 E14 **Kolvereid** Nord-Trøndelag, W Norway
148 L15 **Kolwa** Baluchistān, SW Pakistan
79 M24 **Kolwezi** Katanga, S Dem. Rep. Congo (Zaire)
123 S7 **Kolyma** ≈ NE Russian Federation
Kolyma Lowland see Kolymskaya Nizmennost'
Kolyma Range/Kolymskiy, Khrebet see Kolymskoye Nagor'ye
123 S7 **Kolymskaya Nizmennost'** Eng. Kolyma Lowland. lowlands NE Russian Federation
123 S7 **Kolymskoye** Respublika Sakha (Yakutiya), NE Russian Federation
123 U8 **Kolymskoye Nagor'ye** var. Khrebet Kolymskiy, Eng. Kolyma Range. ▲ E Russian Federation
123 V5 **Kolyuchinskaya Guba** bay NE Russian Federation
145 W15 **Kol'zhat** Almaty, SE Kazakhstan
114 G8 **Kom** ▲ NW Bulgaria
80 I13 **Koma** Oromo, C Ethiopia
77 X12 **Komadugu Gana** ≈ NE Nigeria
164 M13 **Komagane** Nagano, Honshū, S Japan
79 P17 **Komanda** Orientale, NE Dem. Rep. Congo (Zaire)
197 U1 **Komandorskaya Basin** var. Kamchatka Basin. undersea feature SW Bering Sea
127 Pp9 **Komandorskiye Ostrova** Eng. Commander Islands. island group E Russian Federation
Kománfalva see Comănești
111 I22 **Komárno** Ger. Komorn, Hung. Komárom. Nitriansky Kraj, SW Slovakia
111 I22 **Komárom** Komárom-Esztergom, NW Hungary
Komárom see Komárno
111 I22 **Komárom-Esztergom** off. Komárom-Esztergom Megye. ◈ county N Hungary
164 K11 **Komatsu** var. Komatu. Ishikawa, Honshū, SW Japan
Komatu see Komatsu
83 D17 **Kombat** Otjozondjupa, N Namibia
Kombissiguiri see Kombissiri
77 P13 **Kombissiri** var. Kombissiguiri. C Burkina
188 E10 **Komebail Lagoon** lagoon N Palau
81 F20 **Kome Island** island N Tanzania
Komeyo see Wandai
117 P10 **Kominternivs'ke** Odes'ka Oblast', SW Ukraine
127 R12 **Komi-Permyatskiy Avtonomnyy Okrug** ◈ autonomous district W Russian Federation
127 R8 **Komi, Respublika** ◈ autonomous republic NW Russian Federation
111 I25 **Komló** Baranya, SW Hungary
Kommunarsk see Alchevs'k
147 S12 **Kommunizm, Qullai** ▲ E Tajikistan
186 B7 **Komo** Southern Highlands, W PNG
170 M16 **Komodo, Pulau** island Nusa Tenggara, S Indonesia
77 N15 **Komoé** var. Komoé Fleuve. ≈ E Ivory Coast
Komoé Fleuve see Komoé
75 X11 **Kôm Ombo** var. Kawm Umbū. SE Egypt
79 F20 **Komono** La Lékoumou, SW Congo
171 Y16 **Komoran** Irian Jaya, E Indonesia
171 Y16 **Komoran, Pulau** island E Indonesia
Komorn see Komárno
Komornok see Comorâște
Komosolabad see Komsomolobod
Komotau see Chomutov
114 K13 **Komotiní** var. Gümüljina, Turk. Gümülcine. Anatolikí Makedonía kai Thráki, NE Greece
113 K16 **Komovi** ▲ SW Yugoslavia
117 R8 **Kompaniyivka** Kirovohrads'ka Oblast', C Ukraine
Kompong see Kâmpóng Chhnăng
Kompong Cham see Kâmpóng Cham
Kompong Kleang see Kâmpóng Khleăng
Kompong Som see Kâmpóng Saôm
Kompong Speu see Kâmpóng Spoe
Komrat see Comrat
Komsomol see Komsomol'skiy, Atyrau, Kazakhstan
Komsomol see Komsomolets, Kostanay, Kazakhstan
144 L7 **Komsomolets** Kaz. Komsomol. Kostanay, N Kazakhstan
122 K14 **Komsomolets, Ostrov** island Severnaya Zemlya, N Russian Federation
144 F13 **Komsomolets, Zaliv** lake gulf SW Kazakhstan
147 Q12 **Komsomolobod** Rus. Komosolabad. C Tajikistan
126 M16 **Komsomol'sk** Ivanovskaya Oblast', W Russian Federation
117 S6 **Komsomol's'k** Poltavs'ka Oblast', C Ukraine
146 M11 **Komsomol'sk** Nawoiy Wiloyati, N Uzbekistan
144 G12 **Komsomol'skiy** Kaz. Komsomol. Atyrau, W Kazakhstan
127 W4 **Komsomol'skiy** Respublika Komi, NW Russian Federation
123 S13 **Komsomol'sk-na-Amure** Khabarovskiy Kray, SE Russian Federation
Komsomol'sk-na-Ustyurte see Komsomol'sk-Ustyurt
144 K10 **Komsomol'skoye** Aktyubinsk, NW Kazakhstan
129 Q8 **Komsomol'skoye** Saratovskaya Oblast', W Russian Federation
146 G6 **Komsomol'sk-Ustyurt** Rus. Komsomol'sk-na-Ustyurte. Qoraqalpoghiston Respublikasi, NW Uzbekistan
145 P10 **Kon** ≈ C Kazakhstan
Kona see Kailua
126 K16 **Konakovo** Tverskaya Oblast', W Russian Federation
143 V15 **Konārak** Sīstān va Balūchestān, SE Iran
Konarhā see Kunar
27 O11 **Konawa** Oklahoma, C USA
122 H10 **Konda** ≈ C Russian Federation
154 L13 **Kondagaon** Madhya Pradesh, C India
14 K10 **Kondiaronk, Lac** ◎ Quebec, SE Canada
180 J13 **Kondinin** Western Australia
81 H21 **Kondoa** Dodoma, C Tanzania
129 P6 **Kondol'** Penzenskaya Oblast', W Russian Federation
114 N10 **Kondolovo** Burgas, E Bulgaria
171 Z16 **Kondomirat** Irian Jaya, E Indonesia
126 J10 **Kondopoga** Respublika Kareliya, NW Russian Federation
Kondoz see Kunduz
155 J17 **Kondukūr** var. Kandukur. Andhra Pradesh, E India
Kondūz see Kunduz
187 P16 **Koné** Province Nord, W New Caledonia
Könekesir see Kënekesir
Köneürgench see Këneurgench
77 N15 **Kong** N Ivory Coast
39 S5 **Kongakut River** ≈ Alaska, USA
197 O14 **Kong Christian IX Land** Eng. King Christian IX Land. physical region SE Greenland
197 P13 **Kong Christian X Land** Eng. King Christian X Land. physical region E Greenland
197 N13 **Kong Frederik IX Land** Eng. King Frederik IX Land. physical region SW Greenland
197 Q12 **Kong Frederik VIII Land** Eng. King Frederik VIII Land. physical region NE Greenland
197 N15 **Kong Frederik VI Kyst** Eng. King Frederik VI Coast. physical region SE Greenland
167 P13 **Kông, Kaôh** prev. Kas Kong. island SW Cambodia
92 P2 **Kong Karls Land** Eng. King Charles Islands. island group SE Svalbard
81 G14 **Kong Kong** ≈ SE Sudan
Kongo see Congo (river)
83 G16 **Kongola** Caprivi, NE Namibia
79 N21 **Kongolo** Katanga, E Dem. Rep. Congo (Zaire)
81 F14 **Kongor** Jonglei, SE Sudan
197 Q14 **Kong Oscar Fjord** fjord E Greenland
77 P12 **Kongoussi** N Burkina
95 G15 **Kongsberg** Buskerud, S Norway
92 Q2 **Kongsøya** island Kong Karls Land, E Svalbard
95 I14 **Kongsvinger** Hedmark, S Norway
167 T11 **Kông, Tônle** Lao. Xê Kong. ≈ Cambodia/Laos
158 E8 **Kongur Shan** ▲ NW China
81 I22 **Kongwa** Dodoma, C Tanzania
Kong, Xê see Kông, Tônle
Konia see Konya
147 R11 **Konibodom** Rus. Kanibadam. N Tajikistan
111 K15 **Koniecpol** Śląskie, S Poland
Konieh see Konya
Königgrätz see Hradec Králové
Königinhof an der Elbe see Dvůr Králové nad Labem
101 K23 **Königsbrunn** Bayern, S Germany
Königshütte see Chorzów
101 O24 **Königssee** ◎ SE Germany
109 S8 **Königstuhl** ▲ S Austria
109 U3 **Königswiesen** Oberösterreich, N Austria
101 E17 **Königswinter** Nordrhein-Westfalen, W Germany
146 M11 **Konimekh** Rus. Kenimekh. Nawoiy Wiloyati, N Uzbekistan
110 I12 **Konin** Ger. Kuhnau. Wielkopolskie, C Poland
Koninkrijk der Nederlanden see Netherlands
113 L24 **Konispol** var. Konispoli. Vlorë, S Albania
Konispoli see Konispol
115 C15 **Kónitsa** Ípeiros, W Greece
Konitz see Chojnice
108 D8 **Köniz** Bern, W Switzerland
113 H14 **Konjic** Federacija Bosna I Hercegovina, C Bosnia and Herzegovina
92 J10 **Könkämäälven** ≈ Finland/Sweden
155 D14 **Konkan** W India
83 D22 **Konkiep** ≈ S Namibia
76 I14 **Konkouré** ≈ W Guinea
77 O11 **Konna** Mopti, S Mali
186 H6 **Konogaiang, Mount** ▲ New Ireland, NE PNG
186 H5 **Konogogo** New Ireland, NE PNG
108 E9 **Konolfingen** Bern, W Switzerland
77 P16 **Konongo** C Ghana
186 H5 **Konos** New Ireland, NE PNG
126 M12 **Konosha** Arkhangel'skaya Oblast', NW Russian Federation
117 R3 **Konotop** Sums'ka Oblast', NE Ukraine
158 L7 **Konqi He** ≈ NW China
111 L14 **Końskie** Świętokrzyskie, C Poland
Konstantinovka see Kostyantynivka
128 M11 **Konstantinovsk** Rostovskaya Oblast', SW Russian Federation
101 H24 **Konstanz** var. Constanz, Eng. Constance; hist. Kostnitz, anc. Constantia. Baden-Württemberg, S Germany
Konstanza see Constanța
77 T14 **Kontagora** Niger, W Nigeria
78 E13 **Kontcha** Nord, N Cameroon
99 G17 **Kontich** Antwerpen, N Belgium
93 O16 **Kontiolahti** Itä-Suomi, E Finland
93 M15 **Kontiomäki** Oulu, C Finland
167 U11 **Kon Tum** var. Kontum. Kon Tum, C Vietnam
Konur see Sulakyurt
136 H15 **Konya** var. Konieh; prev. Konia, anc. Iconium. Konya, C Turkey
136 H15 **Konya** var. Konia, Konieh. ◈ province C Turkey
145 T13 **Konyrat** var. Kounradskiy, Kaz. Qongyrat. Karaganda, C Kazakhstan
145 W15 **Konyrolen** Almaty, SE Kazakhstan
81 I19 **Konza** Eastern, S Kenya
98 I9 **Koog aan den Zaan** Noord-Holland, C Netherlands
182 E7 **Koonibba** South Australia
31 O11 **Koontz Lake** Indiana, N USA
171 U12 **Koor** Irian Jaya, E Indonesia
183 R9 **Koorawatha** New South Wales, SE Australia
118 J5 **Koosa** Tartumaa, E Estonia
33 N7 **Kootenai** var. Kootenay. ≈ Canada/USA see also Kootenay
11 P17 **Kootenay** var. Kootenai. ≈ Canada/USA see also Kootenai
83 F24 **Kootjieskolk** Northern Cape, W South Africa
113 M15 **Kopaonik** ▲ S Yugoslavia
Kopar see Koper
92 K1 **Kópasker** Nordhurland Eystra, N Iceland
92 H4 **Kópavogur** Reykjanes, W Iceland
109 S13 **Koper** It. Capodistria; prev. Kopar. SW Slovenia
95 C16 **Kopervik** Rogaland, S Norway
Kopetdag, Khrebet see Koppeh Dāgh
Kophinou see Kofínou
182 G8 **Kopi** South Australia
Kopiago see Lake Copiago
153 W12 **Kopili** ≈ NE India
95 M15 **Köping** Västmanland, C Sweden
113 K17 **Koplik** var. Kopliku. Shkodër, NW Albania
Kopliku see Koplik
Kopopo see Kokopo
94 I11 **Koppang** Hedmark, S Norway
Kopparberg see Dalarna
143 S3 **Koppeh Dāgh** var. Khrebet Kopetdag. ▲ Iran/Turkmenistan
Koppename see Coppename Rivier
95 J15 **Koppom** Värmland, C Sweden
Kopreinitz see Koprivnica
114 K9 **Koprinka, Yazovir** prev. Yazovir Georgi Dimitrov. ⊡ C Bulgaria
112 F7 **Koprivnica** Ger. Kopreinitz, Hung. Kaproncza. Koprivnica-Križevci, N Croatia
112 F8 **Koprivnica-Križevci** off. Koprivničko-Križevačka Županija. ◈ province N Croatia
111 I17 **Kopřivnice** Ger. Nesselsdorf. Ostravský Kraj, E Czech Republic
Köprülü see Veles
Koptsevichi see Kaptsevichy
Kopyl' see Kapyl'
119 O14 **Kopys'** Rus. Kopys'. Vitsyebskaya Voblasts', NE Belarus
113 M18 **Korab** ▲ Albania/FYR Macedonia
Korabavur Pastligi see Karabaur', Uval
81 M14 **K'orahē** Somali, E Ethiopia
115 L16 **Kórakas, Akrotírio** headland Lésvos, E Greece
112 D9 **Korana** ≈ C Croatia
155 L14 **Korāput** Orissa, E India
Korat see Nakhon Ratchasima
167 Q9 **Korat Plateau** plateau E Thailand
139 T1 **Korāwa, Sar-i** ▲ NE Iraq
154 L11 **Korba** Madhya Pradesh, C India
101 H15 **Korbach** Hessen, C Germany
Korça see Korçë
113 M21 **Korçë** var. Korça, Gk. Korytsa, It. Coritza; prev. Koritsa. Korçë, SE Albania
113 M21 **Korçë** ◈ district SE Albania
113 G15 **Korčula** It. Curzola. Dubrovnik-Neretva, S Croatia
113 F15 **Korčula** It. Curzola; anc. Corcyra Nigra. island S Croatia
113 F15 **Korčulanski Kanal** channel S Croatia
145 T6 **Korday** prev. Georgiyevka. Zhambyl, SE Kazakhstan
142 J5 **Kordestān** off. Ostān-e Kordestān, var. Kurdestan. ◈ province W Iran
143 P4 **Kord Kūy** var. Kurd Kui. Golestān, N Iran
163 V13 **Korea Bay** bay China/North Korea
Korea, Democratic People's Republic of see North Korea
171 T15 **Koreare** Pulau Yamdena, E Indonesia
Korea, Republic of see South Korea
163 Z17 **Korea Strait** Jap. Chōsen-kaikyō, Kor. Taehan-haehyŏp. channel Japan/South Korea
Korelichi/Korelicze see Karelichy
80 J11 **Korem** Tigray, N Ethiopia
77 U11 **Korén Adoua** ≈ C Niger
128 I7 **Korenevo** Kurskaya Oblast', W Russian Federation
128 L13 **Korenovsk** Krasnodarskiy Kray, SW Russian Federation
116 L4 **Korets'** Pol. Korzec, Rus. Korets. Rivnens'ka Oblast', NW Ukraine
194 L7 **Korff Ice Rise** ice cap Antarctica
92 G13 **Korgen** Troms, N Norway
147 R9 **Korgon-Dĕbĕ** Dzhalal-Abadskaya Oblast', W Kyrgyzstan
76 M14 **Korhogo** N Ivory Coast
115 F19 **Korinthiakós Kólpos** Eng. Gulf of Corinth; anc. Corinthiacus Sinus. gulf C Greece
115 F19 **Kórinthos** Eng. Corinth; anc. Corinthus. Pelopónnisos, S Greece
113 M18 **Koritnik** ▲ S Yugoslavia
Koritsa see Korçë
165 P11 **Kōriyama** Fukushima, Honshū, C Japan
136 E16 **Korkuteli** Antalya, SW Turkey
158 K6 **Korla** Chin. K'u-erh-lo. Xinjiang Uygur Zizhiqu, NW China
122 J10 **Korliki** Khanty-Mansiyskiy Avtonomnyy Okrug, C Russian Federation
Körlin an der Persante see Karlino
Korma see Karma
14 D8 **Kormak** Ontario, S Canada
Kormakíti, Akrotíri/Kormakiti, Cape/Kormakítis see Koruçam Burnu
111 G23 **Körmend** Vas, W Hungary
139 T5 **Kōrmōr** E Iraq
112 C13 **Kornat** It. Incoronata. island W Croatia
Korneshty see Cornești
109 X3 **Korneuburg** Niederösterreich, NE Austria
145 P7 **Korneyevka** Severnyy Kazakhstan, N Kazakhstan
95 I17 **Kornsjø** Østfold, S Norway
77 O11 **Koro** Mopti, S Mali
187 Y14 **Koro** island C Fiji
186 B7 **Koroba** Southern Highlands, W PNG
128 K8 **Korocha** Belgorodskaya Oblast', W Russian Federation
136 H12 **Köroğlu Dağları** ▲ C Turkey
183 V6 **Korogoro Point** headland New South Wales, SE Australia
81 J21 **Korogwe** Tanga, E Tanzania
182 L13 **Koroit** Victoria, SE Australia
187 X15 **Korolevu** Viti Levu, W Fiji
190 I17 **Koromiri** island S Cook Islands
171 Q8 **Koronadal** Mindanao, S Philippines
115 E22 **Koróni** Pelopónnisos, S Greece
114 G13 **Korónia, Límni** ◎ N Greece
110 I9 **Koronowo** Ger. Krone an der Brahe. Kujawski-pomorskie, C Poland
117 R2 **Korop** Chernihivs'ka Oblast', N Ukraine
115 H19 **Koropí** Attikí, C Greece
Koror see Oreor
Kőrös see Križevci
111 L23 **Körös** ≈ E Hungary
Kőrösbánya see Baia de Criș
187 Y14 **Koro Sea** sea C Fiji
Koroška see Kärnten
117 N3 **Korosten'** Zhytomyrs'ka Oblast', NW Ukraine
Korostyshev see Korostyshiv
117 N4 **Korostyshiv** Rus. Korostyshev. Zhytomyrs'ka Oblast', N Ukraine
127 V3 **Korotaikha** ≈ NW Russian Federation
122 J9 **Korotchayevo** Yamalo-Nenetskiy Avtonomnyy Okrug, N Russian Federation
78 I8 **Koro Toro** Borkou-Ennedi-Tibesti, N Chad
39 N16 **Korovin Island** island Shumagin Islands, Alaska, USA
187 X14 **Korovou** Viti Levu, W Fiji
93 M17 **Korpilahti** Länsi-Suomi, W Finland
92 K12 **Korpilombolo** Norrbotten, N Sweden
123 T13 **Korsakov** Ostrov Sakhalin, Sakhalinskaya Oblast', SE Russian Federation
93 J16 **Korsholm** Fin. Mustasaari. Länsi-Suomi, W Finland
95 I23 **Korsør** Vestsjælland, E Denmark
Korsovka see Kārsava
117 P6 **Korsun'-Shevchenkivs'kyy** Rus. Korsun'-Shevchenkovskiy. Cherkas'ka Oblast', C Ukraine
Korsun'-Shevchenkovskiy see Korsun'-Shevchenkivs'kyy
99 C17 **Kortemark** West-Vlaanderen, W Belgium
99 H18 **Kortenberg** Vlaams Brabant, C Belgium
99 K18 **Kortessem** Limburg, NE Belgium
99 E14 **Kortgene** Zeeland, SW Netherlands
80 F8 **Korti** Northern, N Sudan
99 C18 **Kortrijk** Fr. Courtrai. West-Vlaanderen, W Belgium
121 O2 **Koruçam Burnu** var. Cape Kormakiti, Kormakítis, Gk. Akrotíri Kormakíti. headland N Cyprus
183 O13 **Korumburra** Victoria, SE Australia
Koryak Range see Koryakskoye Nagor'ye
123 V8 **Koryakskiy Avtonomnyy Okrug** ◈ autonomous district E Russian Federation
Koryakskiy Khrebet see Koryakskoye Nagor'ye
123 V7 **Koryakskoye Nagor'ye** var. Koryakskiy Khrebet, Eng. Koryak Range. ▲ NE Russian Federation
127 P11 **Koryazhma** Arkhangel'skaya Oblast', NW Russian Federation
Kōryō see Kangnŭng
Korytsa see Korçë
117 Q2 **Koryukivka** Chernihivs'ka Oblast', N Ukraine
Korzec see Korets'
115 N21 **Kos** Kos, Dodekánisos, Greece, Aegean Sea
115 M21 **Kos** It. Coo; anc. Cos. island Dodekánisos, Greece, Aegean Sea
127 T12 **Kosa** Komi-Permyatskiy Avtonomnyy Okrug, NW Russian Federation
127 T13 **Kosa** ≈ NW Russian Federation
164 B12 **Kō-saki** headland Nagasaki, Tsushima, SW Japan
163 X13 **Kosan** SE North Korea
119 H18 **Kosava** Rus. Kosovo. Brestskaya Voblasts', SW Belarus
Kosch see Kose
144 G12 **Koschagyl** Kaz. Qosshaghyl. Atyrau, W Kazakhstan
110 G12 **Kościan** Ger. Kosten. Wielkopolskie, C Poland
110 I7 **Kościerzyna** Pomorskie, NW Poland
22 L4 **Kosciusko** Mississippi, S USA
Kosciusko, Mount see Kosciuszko, Mount
183 R11 **Kosciuszko, Mount** prev. Mount Kosciusko ▲ New South Wales, SE Australia
118 H4 **Kose** Ger. Kosch. Harjumaa, NW Estonia
114 G6 **Koshava** Vidin, NW Bulgaria
147 U9 **Kosh-Dĕbĕ** var. Koshtebĕ. Narynskaya Oblast', C Kyrgyzstan
K'o-shih see Kashi
164 B16 **Koshikijima-rettō** var. Kosikizima Rettô. island group SW Japan
145 W13 **Koshkarkol', Ozero** ◎ SE Kazakhstan
30 L9 **Koshkonong, Lake** ◎ Wisconsin, N USA
146 B10 **Koshoba** Turkm. Goshoba. Balkanskiy Velayat, NW Turkmenistan
164 M12 **Kōshoku** var. Kôsyoku. Nagano, Honshū, S Japan
Koshtebĕ see Kosh-Dĕbĕ
Kōshū see Kwangju
111 N19 **Košice** Ger. Kaschau, Hung. Kassa. Košický Kraj, E Slovakia
111 M20 **Košický Kraj** ◈ region E Slovakia
Kosigaya see Koshigaya
Kosikizima Rettô see Koshikijima-rettō
153 R12 **Kosi Reservoir** ⊡ E Nepal
116 J8 **Kosiv** Ivano-Frankivs'ka Oblast', W Ukraine
145 O11 **Koskol'** Zhezkazgan, C Kazakhstan
127 Q9 **Koslan** Respublika Komi, NW Russian Federation
Köslin see Koszalin
146 M12 **Koson** Rus. Kasan. Qashqadaryo Wiloyati, S Uzbekistan
163 Y13 **Kosŏng** SE North Korea
147 S9 **Kosonsoy** Rus. Kasansay. Namangan Wiloyati, E Uzbekistan
113 M16 **Kosovo** prev. Autonomous Province of Kosovo and Metohija. region S Yugoslavia
Kosovo see Kosava
Kosovo and Metohija, Autonomous Province of see Kosovo
113 N16 **Kosovo Polje** Serbia, S Yugoslavia
113 O16 **Kosovska Kamenica** Serbia, SE Yugoslavia
113 M16 **Kosovska Mitrovica** Alb. Mitrovicë; prev. Mitrovica, Titova Mitrovica. Serbia, S Yugoslavia

◆ Country ● Country Capital ◇ Dependent Territory ○ Dependent Territory Capital ◈ Administrative Region ✕ International Airport ▲ Mountain ▲ Mountain Range ▲ Volcano ≈ River ◎ Lake ⊡ Reservoir

189 X17 **Kosrae** ◈ state E Micronesia
189 Y14 **Kosrae** prev. Kusaie. island Caroline Islands, E Micronesia
25 U9 **Kosse** Texas, SW USA
109 P6 **Kössen** Tirol, W Austria
76 M16 **Kossou, Lac de** ◎ C Ivory Coast
Kossukavak see Krumovgrad
Kostajnica see Hrvatska Kostajnica
150 M7 **Kostanay** var. Kustanay, Kaz. Qostanay. N Kazakhstan
150 L8 **Kostanay** var. Kostanayskaya Oblast, Kaz. Qostanay Oblysy. ◈ province N Kazakhstan
Kostanayskaya Oblast see Kostanay
Kostamus see Kostomuksha
Kosten see Kościan
114 H10 **Kostenets** prev. Georgi Dimitrov. Sofiya, W Bulgaria
80 F10 **Kosti** White Nile, C Sudan
Kostnitz see Konstanz
126 H7 **Kostomuksha** Fin. Kostamus. Respublika Kareliya, NW Russian Federation
116 K3 **Kostopil'** Rus. Kostopol'. Rivnens'ka Oblast', NW Ukraine
Kostopol' see Kostopil'
126 M15 **Kostroma** Kostromskaya Oblast', NW Russian Federation
127 N14 **Kostroma** ≈ NW Russian Federation
127 N14 **Kostromskaya Oblast'** ◈ province NW Russian Federation
110 D11 **Kostrzyn** Ger. Cüstrin, Küstrin. Lubuskie, W Poland
110 H11 **Kostrzyn** Wielkolpolskie, C Poland
117 X7 **Kostyantynivka** Rus. Konstantinovka. Donets'ka Oblast', SE Ukraine
Kostyukovichi see Kastsyukovichy
Kostyukovka see Kastsyukowka
Kôsyoku see Kōshoku
127 U6 **Kos'yu** Respublika Komi, NW Russian Federation
127 U6 **Kos'yu** ≈ NW Russian Federation
110 F7 **Koszalin** Ger. Köslin. Koszalin, NW Poland
111 F22 **Kőszeg** Ger. Güns. Vas, W Hungary
152 H13 **Kota** prev. Kotah. Rājasthān, N India
168 K12 **Kota Baru** Sumatera, W Indonesia
169 U13 **Kotabaru** Pulau Laut, C Indonesia
Kotabaru see Jayapura
168 K6 **Kota Bharu** var. Kota Baharu, Kota Bahru. Kelantan, Peninsular Malaysia
Kotaboemi see Kotabumi
168 M14 **Kotabumi** prev. Kotaboemi. Sumatera, W Indonesia
149 S10 **Kot Addu** Punjab, E Pakistan
Kotah see Kota
169 U7 **Kota Kinabalu** prev. Jesselton. Sabah, East Malaysia
169 U7 **Kota Kinabalu** × Sabah, East Malaysia
92 M12 **Kotala** Lappi, N Finland
Kotamobagoe see Kotamobagu
171 Q11 **Kotamobagu** prev. Kotamobagoe. Sulawesi, C Indonesia
155 L14 **Kotapad** var. Kotapārh. Orissa, E India
Kotapārh see Kotapad
166 N17 **Ko Ta Ru Tao** island SW Thailand
169 R13 **Kotawaringin, Teluk** bay Borneo, C Indonesia
149 Q13 **Kot Diji** Sind, SE Pakistan
152 K9 **Kotdwāra** Uttar Pradesh, N India
127 Q14 **Kotel'nich** Kirovskaya Oblast', NW Russian Federation
129 N12 **Kotel'nikovo** Volgogradskaya Oblast', SW Russian Federation
123 Q6 **Kotel'nyy, Ostrov** island Novosibirskiye Ostrova, N Russian Federation
117 T5 **Kotel'va** Poltavs'ka Oblast', C Ukraine
101 M14 **Köthen** var. Cöthen. Sachsen-Anhalt, C Germany
Kôti see Kōchi
81 G17 **Kotido** NE Uganda
93 N19 **Kotka** Etelä-Suomi, S Finland
127 P11 **Kotlas** Arkhangel'skaya Oblast', NW Russian Federation
38 M10 **Kotlik** Alaska, USA
77 Q17 **Kotoka** × (Accra) S Ghana
Kotonu see Cotonou
113 J17 **Kotor** It. Cattaro. Montenegro, SW Yugoslavia
Kotor see Kotoriba
112 F7 **Kotoriba** Hung. Kotor. Medimurje, N Croatia
113 I17 **Kotorska, Boka** It. Bocche di Cattaro. bay Montenegro, SW Yugoslavia
112 H11 **Kotorsko** Republika Srpska, N Bosnia and Herzegovina
112 G11 **Kotor Varoš** Republika Srpska, N Bosnia and Herzegovina
Koto Sho/Kotosho see Lan Yü
128 M7 **Kotovsk** Tambovskaya Oblast', W Russian Federation
117 O9 **Kotovs'k** Rus. Kotovsk. Odes'ka Oblast', SW Ukraine
Kotovsk see Hînceşti
119 G16 **Kotra** Rus. Kotra. ≈ W Belarus
149 P16 **Kotri** Sind, SE Pakistan
109 Q9 **Kötschach** Kärnten, S Austria
155 K15 **Kottagūdem** Andhra Pradesh, E India
155 F21 **Kottappadi** Kerala, SW India
155 G23 **Kottayam** Kerala, SW India
Kottbus see Cottbus
Kotte see Sri Jayawardanapura
79 K15 **Kotto** ≈ Central African Republic/Dem. Rep. Congo (Zaire)
193 X15 **Kotu Group** island group W Tonga
146 B11 **Koturdepe** Turkm. Goturdepe. Balkanskiy Velayat, W Turkmenistan
122 M9 **Kotuy** ≈ N Russian Federation
83 M16 **Kotwa** Mashonaland East, NE Zimbabwe
39 N7 **Kotzebue** Alaska, USA
38 M7 **Kotzebue Sound** inlet Alaska, USA
Kotzenan see Chocianów
Kotzman see Kitsman'
77 R14 **Kouandé** NW Benin
79 J15 **Kouango** Ouaka, S Central African Republic
77 O13 **Koudougou** C Burkina
98 K7 **Koudum** Friesland, N Netherlands
115 L25 **Koufonísi** island SE Greece
115 K21 **Koufonísi** island Kykládes, Greece, Aegean Sea
38 M8 **Kougarok Mountain** ▲ Alaska, USA
79 E20 **Kouilou** ≈ S Congo
121 O3 **Koúklia** SW Cyprus
79 E19 **Koulamoutou** Ogooué-Lolo, C Gabon
76 L12 **Koulikoro** Koulikoro, SW Mali
76 L11 **Koulikoro** ◈ region SW Mali
187 P16 **Koumac** Province Nord, W New Caledonia
165 N12 **Koumi** Nagano, Honshū, S Japan
78 I13 **Koumra** Moyen-Chari, S Chad
Kounadougou see Koundougou
76 M15 **Kounahiri** C Ivory Coast
76 I12 **Koundâra** Moyenne-Guinée, NW Guinea
77 N13 **Koundougou** var. Kounadougou. C Burkina
76 H11 **Koungheul** C Senegal
Kounradskiy see Konyrat
25 X10 **Kountze** Texas, SW USA
77 Q13 **Koupéla** C Burkina
77 N13 **Kouri** Sikasso, SW Mali
55 Y9 **Kourou** N French Guiana
114 J12 **Kouroú** ≈ NE Greece
76 K14 **Kouroussa** Haute-Guinée, C Guinea
Kousseir see Al Quşayr
78 G11 **Kousséri** prev. Fort-Foureau. Extrême-Nord, NE Cameroon
Kouteifé see Al Quţayfah
76 M13 **Koutiala** Sikasso, S Mali
76 M14 **Kouto** NW Ivory Coast
93 M19 **Kouvola** Etelä-Suomi, S Finland
79 G18 **Kouyou** ≈ C Congo
112 M10 **Kovačica** Hung. Antafalva; prev. Kovacsicza. Serbia, N Yugoslavia
Kovacsicza see Kovačica
Kővárhosszúfalu see Satulung
Kovászna see Covasna
126 I4 **Kovdor** Murmanskaya Oblast', NW Russian Federation
126 I5 **Kovdozero, Ozero** ◎ NW Russian Federation
116 J3 **Kovel'** Pol. Kowel. Volyns'ka Oblast', NW Ukraine
112 M11 **Kovin** Hung. Kevevára; prev. Temes-Kubin. Serbia, NE Yugoslavia
Kovno see Kaunas
129 N3 **Kovrov** Vladimirskaya Oblast', W Russian Federation
129 O5 **Kovylkino** Respublika Mordoviya, W Russian Federation
110 J11 **Kowal** Kujawsko-pomorskie, C Poland
110 J9 **Kowalewo Pomorskie** Ger. Schönsee. Kujawsko-pomorskie, C Poland
Kowasna see Covasna
119 M16 **Kowbcha** Rus. Kolbcha. Mahilyowskaya Voblasts', E Belarus
Koweit see Kuwait
Kowel see Kovel'
185 F17 **Kowhitirangi** West Coast, South Island, NZ
161 O15 **Kowloon** Chin. Jiulong. Hong Kong, S China
Kowno see Kaunas
159 N7 **Kox Kuduk** well NW China
136 D16 **Köyceğiz** Muğla, SW Turkey
127 N6 **Koyda** Arkhangel'skaya Oblast', NW Russian Federation
146 D10 **Koymat** Turkm. Goymat. Balkanskiy Velayat, NW Turkmenistan
146 D10 **Koymatdag, Gory** Turkm. Goymatdag. hill range NW Turkmenistan
Koyna Reservoir see Shivāji Sāgar
165 P9 **Koyoshi-gawa** ≈ Honshū, C Japan
Koysanjaq see Koi Sanjaq
Koytash see Qŭytosh
39 N9 **Koyuk** Alaska, USA
39 N9 **Koyuk River** ≈ Alaska, USA
39 O9 **Koyukuk** Alaska, USA
39 O9 **Koyukuk River** ≈ Alaska, USA
136 J13 **Kozaklı** Nevşehir, C Turkey
136 K16 **Kozan** Adana, S Turkey
115 E14 **Kozáni** Dytikí Makedonía, N Greece
112 F10 **Kozara** ▲ NW Bosnia and Herzegovina
Kozarska Dubica see Bosanska Dubica
117 P3 **Kozelets'** Rus. Kozelets. Chernihivs'ka Oblast', NE Ukraine
117 S6 **Kozel'shchyna** Poltavs'ka Oblast', C Ukraine
128 J5 **Kozel'sk** Kaluzhskaya Oblast', W Russian Federation
Kozhikode see Calicut
127 V9 **Kozhimiz, Gora** ▲ NW Russian Federation
126 L9 **Kozhozero, Ozero** ◎ NW Russian Federation
127 T7 **Kozhva** var. Kozya. Respublika Komi, NW Russian Federation
127 T7 **Kozhva** ≈ NW Russian Federation
127 U6 **Kozhym** Respublika Komi, NW Russian Federation
110 N13 **Kozienice** Mazowieckie, C Poland
109 S13 **Kozina** SW Slovenia
114 H7 **Kozloduy** Vratsa, NW Bulgaria
129 Q3 **Kozlovka** Chuvashskaya Respublika, W Russian Federation
Kozlovshchina/Kozlowszczyzna see Kazlowshchyna
129 P3 **Koz'modem'yansk** Respublika Mariy El, W Russian Federation
116 J6 **Kozova** Ternopil's'ka Oblast', W Ukraine
113 P20 **Kožuf** ▲ S FYR Macedonia
165 N15 **Kōzu-shima** island E Japan
Kozya see Kozhva
117 N5 **Kozyatyn** Rus. Kazatin. Vinnyts'ka Oblast', C Ukraine
77 Q16 **Kpalimé** var. Palimé. SW Togo
77 Q16 **Kpandu** E Ghana
99 F15 **Krabbendijke** Zeeland, SW Netherlands
167 N15 **Krabi** var. Muang Krabi. Krabi, SW Thailand
167 N13 **Kra Buri** Ranong, SW Thailand
167 S12 **Krâchéh** prev. Kratie. Krâchéh, E Cambodia
95 G17 **Kragerø** Telemark, S Norway
112 M13 **Kragujevac** Serbia, C Yugoslavia
Krainburg see Kranj
166 N13 **Kra, Isthmus of** isthmus Malaysia/Thailand
112 D12 **Krajina** cultural region SW Croatia
Krakatau, Pulau see Rakata, Pulau
Krakau see Małopolskie
111 L16 **Kraków** Eng. Cracow, Ger. Krakau; anc. Cracovia. Małopolskie, S Poland
100 L9 **Krakower See** ◎ NE Germany
167 Q11 **Krâlănh** Siĕmréab, NW Cambodia
45 Q16 **Kralendijk** Bonaire, E Netherlands Antilles
112 B10 **Kraljevica** It. Porto Re. Primorje-Gorski Kotar, NW Croatia
112 M13 **Kraljevo** prev. Rankovićevo. Serbia, C Yugoslavia
Kralup an der Moldau see Kralupy nad Vltavou
111 C16 **Kralupy nad Vltavou** Ger. Kralup an der Moldau. Středočeský Kraj, NW Czech Republic
117 W7 **Kramators'k** Rus. Kramatorsk. Donets'ka Oblast', SE Ukraine
93 H17 **Kramfors** Västernorrland, C Sweden
115 D15 **Kranéa** Dytikí Makedonía, N Greece
108 M7 **Kranebitten** × (Innsbruck) Tirol, W Austria
115 G20 **Kranídi** Pelopónnisos, S Greece
109 T11 **Kranj** Ger. Krainburg. NW Slovenia
115 F16 **Krannón** battleground Thessalía, C Greece
Kranz see Zelenogradsk
112 D7 **Krapina** Krapina-Zagorje, N Croatia
112 E8 **Krapina** ≈ N Croatia
112 D8 **Krapina-Zagorje** off. Krapinsko-Zagorska Županija. ◈ province N Croatia
114 L7 **Krapinets** ≈ NE Bulgaria
111 I15 **Krapkowice** Ger. Krappitz. Opolskie, S Poland
Krappitz see Krapkowice
127 O12 **Krasavino** Vologodskaya Oblast', NW Russian Federation
122 H6 **Krasino** Novaya Zemlya, Arkhangel'skaya Oblast', N Russian Federation
123 S15 **Kraskino** Primorskiy Kray, SE Russian Federation
118 J11 **Krāslava** Krāslava, SE Latvia
119 M14 **Krasnaluki** Rus. Krasnoluki. Vitsyebskaya Voblasts', N Belarus
119 P17 **Krasnapollye** Rus. Krasnopol'ye. Mahilyowskaya Voblasts', E Belarus
128 L15 **Krasnaya Polyana** Krasnodarskiy Kray, SW Russian Federation
119 J18 **Krasnaya Slabada** var. Chyrvonaya Slabada, Rus. Krasnaya Sloboda. Minskaya Voblasts', S Belarus
Krasnaya Sloboda see Krasnaya Slabada
119 J15 **Krasnaye** Rus. Krasnoye. Minskaya Voblasts', C Belarus
111 O14 **Kraśnik** Ger. Kratznick. Lubelskie, E Poland
111 O14 **Kraśnik Fabryczny** Lubelskie, SE Poland
117 O9 **Krasni Okny** Odes'ka Oblast', SW Ukraine
145 P7 **Krasnoarmeysk** Severnyy Kazakhstan, N Kazakhstan
129 P8 **Krasnoarmeysk** Saratovskaya Oblast', W Russian Federation
Krasnoarmeysk see Krasnoarmiys'k/Tayynsha
123 T6 **Krasnoarmeyskiy** Chukotskiy Avtonomnyy Okrug, NE Russian Federation
117 W7 **Krasnoarmiys'k** Rus. Krasnoarmeysk. Donets'ka Oblast', SE Ukraine
127 P11 **Krasnoborsk** Arkhangel'skaya Oblast', NW Russian Federation
128 K14 **Krasnodar** prev. Ekaterinodar, Yekaterinodar. Krasnodarskiy Kray, SW Russian Federation
128 K13 **Krasnodarskiy Kray** ◈ territory SW Russian Federation
117 Z7 **Krasnodon** Luhans'ka Oblast', E Ukraine
Krasnogor see Kallaste
129 T2 **Krasnogorskoye** Latv. Sarkaņi. Udmurtskaya Respublika, NW Russian Federation
Krasnograd see Krasnohrad
Krasnogvardeysk see Bulunghur
128 M13 **Krasnogvardeyskoye** Stavropol'skiy Kray, SW Russian Federation
Krasnogvardeyskoye see Krasnohvardiys'ke
117 U6 **Krasnohrad** Rus. Krasnograd. Kharkivs'ka Oblast', E Ukraine
117 S12 **Krasnohvardiys'ke** Rus. Krasnogvardeyskoye. Respublika Krym, S Ukraine
123 P14 **Krasnokamensk** Chitinskaya Oblast', S Russian Federation
127 U14 **Krasnokamsk** Permskaya Oblast', W Russian Federation
129 U8 **Krasnokholm** Orenburgskaya Oblast', W Russian Federation
117 U5 **Krasnokuts'k** Rus. Krasnokutsk. Kharkivs'ka Oblast', E Ukraine
128 L7 **Krasnolesnyy** Voronezhskaya Oblast', W Russian Federation
Krasnoluki see Krasnaluki
Krasnoosol'skoye Vodokhranilishche see Chervonooskil's'ke Vodoskhovyshche
117 S11 **Krasnoperekops'k** Rus. Krasnoperekopsk. Respublika Krym, S Ukraine
117 U4 **Krasnopillya** Sums'ka Oblast', NE Ukraine
Krasnopol'ye see Krasnapollye
126 L5 **Krasnoshchel'ye** Murmanskaya Oblast', NW Russian Federation
129 O5 **Krasnoslobodsk** Respublika Mordoviya, W Russian Federation
129 O12 **Krasnoslobodsk** Volgogradskaya Oblast', SW Russian Federation
Krasnostav see Krasnystaw
129 V5 **Krasnousol'skiy** Respublika Bashkortostan, W Russian Federation
127 U12 **Krasnovishersk** Permskaya Oblast', NW Russian Federation
Krasnovodsk see Turkmenbashi
146 A10 **Krasnovodskiy Zaliv** Turkm. Krasnowodsk Aylagy. lake gulf W Turkmenistan
146 B10 **Krasnovodskoye Plato** Turkm. Krasnowodsk Platosy. plateau NW Turkmenistan
Krasnowodsk Aylagy see Krasnovodskiy Zaliv
Krasnowodsk Platosy see Krasnovodskoye Plato
122 K12 **Krasnoyarsk** Krasnoyarskiy Kray, S Russian Federation
129 X7 **Krasnoyarskiy** Orenburgskaya Oblast', W Russian Federation
122 K11 **Krasnoyarskiy Kray** ◈ territory C Russian Federation
Krasnoye see Krasnaye
146 J15 **Krasnoye Znamya** Turkm. Gyzylbaydak. Maryyskiy Velayat, S Turkmenistan
127 R11 **Krasnozatonskiy** Respublika Komi, NW Russian Federation
118 D13 **Krasnoznamensk** prev. Lasdehnen, Ger. Haselberg. Kaliningradskaya Oblast', W Russian Federation
117 R11 **Krasnoznam"yans'kyy Kanal** canal S Ukraine
111 P14 **Krasnystaw** Rus. Krasnostav. Lubelskie, SE Poland
128 H4 **Krasnyy** Smolenskaya Oblast', W Russian Federation
129 P2 **Krasnyye Baki** Nizhegorodskaya Oblast', W Russian Federation
129 Q13 **Krasnyye Barrikady** Astrakhanskaya Oblast', SW Russian Federation
126 K15 **Krasnyy Kholm** Tverskaya Oblast', W Russian Federation
129 Q8 **Krasnyy Kut** Saratovskaya Oblast', W Russian Federation
Krasnyy Liman see Krasnyy Lyman
117 Y7 **Krasnyy Luch** prev. Krindachevka. Luhans'ka Oblast', E Ukraine
117 X6 **Krasnyy Lyman** Rus. Krasnyy Liman. Donets'ka Oblast', SE Ukraine
129 R3 **Krasnyy Steklovar** Respublika Mariy El, W Russian Federation
129 P8 **Krasnyy Tekstil'shchik** Saratovskaya Oblast', W Russian Federation
129 R13 **Krasnyy Yar** Astrakhanskaya Oblast', SW Russian Federation
Krassóvár see Caraşova
116 L5 **Krasyliv** Khmel'nyts'ka Oblast', W Ukraine
111 O21 **Kraszna** Rom. Crasna. ≈ Hungary/Romania
Kratie see Krâchéh
113 P17 **Kratovo** NE FYR Macedonia
Kratznick see Kraśnik
171 Y13 **Krau** Irian Jaya, E Indonesia
167 Q13 **Krâvanh, Chuŏr Phnum** Eng. Cardamom Mountains, Fr. Chaîne des Cardamomes. ▲ W Cambodia
Kravasta Lagoon see Karavastasë, Laguna e
Krawang see Karawang
Kraxatau see Rakata, Pulau
129 Q15 **Kraynovka** Respublika Dagestan, SW Russian Federation
118 D12 **Kražiai** Kelmė, C Lithuania
27 P11 **Krebs** Oklahoma, C USA
101 D15 **Krefeld** Nordrhein-Westfalen, W Germany
Kreisstadt see Krosno Odrzańskie
115 D17 **Kremastón, Technití Límni** ▣ C Greece
Kremenchug see Kremenchuk
Kremenchugskoye Vodokhranilishche/Kremenchuk Reservoir see Kremenchuts'ke Vodoskhovyshche
117 S6 **Kremenchuk** Rus. Kremenchug. Poltavs'ka Oblast', NE Ukraine
117 R6 **Kremenchuts'ke Vodoskhovyshche** Eng. Kremenchuk Reservoir, Rus. Kremenchugskoye Vodokhranilishche. ▣ C Ukraine
116 K5 **Kremenets'** Pol. Krzemieniec, Rus. Kremenets. Ternopil's'ka Oblast', W Ukraine
Kremennaya see Kreminna
117 X6 **Kreminna** Rus. Kremennaya. Luhans'ka Oblast', E Ukraine
37 R4 **Kremmling** Colorado, C USA
109 V3 **Krems** ≈ NE Austria
Krems see Krems an der Donau
109 W3 **Krems an der Donau** var. Krems. Niederösterreich, N Austria
Kremsier see Kroměříž
109 S4 **Kremsmünster** Oberösterreich, N Austria
38 M17 **Krenitzin Islands** island Aleutian Islands, Alaska, USA
Kresena see Kresna
114 G11 **Kresna** var. Kresena. Blagoevgrad, SW Bulgaria
112 O12 **Krespoljin** Serbia, E Yugoslavia
25 N4 **Kress** Texas, SW USA
123 V6 **Kresta, Zaliv** bay E Russian Federation
115 D20 **Kréstena** prev. Selinoús. Dytikí Ellás, S Greece
126 H14 **Kresttsy** Novgorodskaya Oblast', W Russian Federation
Kretikon Delagos see Kritikó Pélagos
118 C11 **Kretinga** Ger. Krottingen. Kretinga, NW Lithuania
Kreutz see Cristuru Secuiesc
Kreuz see Križevci, Croatia
Kreuz see Risti, Estonia
Kreuzburg/Kreuzburg in Oberschlesien see Kluczbork
Kreuzingen see Bol'shakovo
108 H6 **Kreuzlingen** Thurgau, NE Switzerland
101 K25 **Kreuzspitze** ▲ S Germany
101 F16 **Kreuztal** Nordrhein-Westfalen, W Germany
119 I15 **Kreva** Rus. Krevo. Hrodzyenskaya Voblasts', W Belarus
Krevo see Kreva
Kría Vrísi see Krýa Vrýsi
79 D16 **Kribi** Sud, SW Cameroon
Krichëv see Krychaw
Krickerhäu/Kriegerhaj see Handlová
109 W6 **Krieglach** Steiermark, E Austria
108 F8 **Kriens** Luzern, W Switzerland
Krimmitschau see Crimmitschau
98 H12 **Krimpen aan den IJssel** Zuid-Holland, SW Netherlands
Krindachevka see Krasnyy Luch
115 G25 **Kríos, Akrotírio** headland Kríti, Greece, E Mediterranean Sea
155 J16 **Krishna** prev. Kistna. ≈ C India
155 H20 **Krishnagiri** Tamil Nādu, SE India
155 K17 **Krishna, Mouths of the** delta SE India
153 S15 **Krishnanagar** West Bengal, N India
155 G20 **Krishnarājāsāgara Reservoir** ▣ W India
95 N19 **Kristdala** Kalmar, S Sweden
Kristiania see Oslo
95 E18 **Kristiansand** var. Christiansand. Vest-Agder, S Norway
95 L22 **Kristianstad** Skåne, S Sweden
94 F8 **Kristiansund** var. Christiansund. Møre og Romsdal, S Norway
Kristiinankaupunki see Kristinestad
93 I14 **Kristineberg** Västerbotten, N Sweden
95 L16 **Kristinehamn** Värmland, C Sweden
93 J17 **Kristinestad** Fin. Kristiinankaupunki. Länsi-Suomi, W Finland
Kristyor see Crişcior
115 J25 **Kríti** Eng. Crete. ◈ region Greece, Aegean Sea
115 J24 **Kríti** Eng. Crete. island Greece, Aegean Sea
115 J23 **Kritikó Pélagos** var. Kretikon Delagos, Eng. Sea of Crete; anc. Mare Creticum. sea Greece, Aegean Sea
Kriulyany see Criuleni
112 I12 **Krivaja** ≈ NE Bosnia and Herzegovina
Krivaja see Mali Iđoš
113 P17 **Kriva Palanka** Turk. Eğri Palanka. NE FYR Macedonia
Krivichi see Kryvychy
114 H8 **Krivodol** Vratsa, NW Bulgaria
128 M10 **Krivorozh'ye** Rostovskaya Oblast', SW Russian Federation
Krivoshin see Kryvoshyn
Krivoy Rog see Kryvyy Rih
112 F7 **Križevci** Ger. Kreuz, Hung. Kőrös. Varaždin, NE Croatia
112 B10 **Krk** It. Veglia. Primorje-Gorski Kotar, NW Croatia
112 B10 **Krk** It. Veglia; anc. Curieta. island NW Croatia
109 V12 **Krka** ≈ SE Slovenia
Krka see Gurk
109 R11 **Krn** ▲ NW Slovenia
111 H16 **Krnov** Ger. Jägerndorf. Ostravský Kraj, E Czech Republic
Kroatien see Croatia
95 G14 **Krøderen** Buskerud, S Norway
95 G14 **Krøderen** ◎ S Norway
Kroi see Krui
95 N17 **Krokek** Östergötland, S Sweden
Krokodil see Crocodile
93 G16 **Krokom** Jämtland, C Sweden
117 S2 **Krolevets'** Rus. Krolevets. Sums'ka Oblast', NE Ukraine
Królewska Huta see Chorzów
111 H18 **Kroměříž** Ger. Kremsier. Zlínský Kraj, E Czech Republic
98 I9 **Krommenie** Noord-Holland, C Netherlands
128 J6 **Kromy** Orlovskaya Oblast', W Russian Federation
101 L18 **Kronach** Bayern, E Germany
Krone an der Brahe see Koronowo
167 Q13 **Krŏng Kaôh Kŏng** Kaôh Kŏng, SW Cambodia
95 K21 **Kronoberg** ◈ county S Sweden
123 V10 **Kronotskiy Zaliv** bay E Russian Federation
195 O2 **Kronprinsesse Märtha Kyst** physical region Antarctica
195 V3 **Kronprins Olav Kyst** physical region Antarctica
126 G12 **Kronshtadt** Leningradskaya Oblast', NW Russian Federation
Kronstadt see Braşov
83 I22 **Kroonstad** Free State, C South Africa
123 O12 **Kropotkin** Irkutskaya Oblast', C Russian Federation
128 L14 **Kropotkin** Krasnodarskiy Kray, SW Russian Federation
110 J11 **Krośniewice** Łódzkie, C Poland
111 N17 **Krosno** Ger. Krossen. Podkarpackie, SE Poland
110 E12 **Krosno Odrzańskie** Ger. Crossen, Kreisstadt. Lubuskie, W Poland
Krossen see Krosno
Krotoschin see Krotoszyn
110 H13 **Krotoszyn** Ger. Krotoschin. Wielkopolskie, C Poland
Krottingen see Kretinga
Krousón see Krousónas
115 J25 **Krousónas** prev. Krousón, Kroussón. Kríti, Greece, E Mediterranean Sea
Kroussón see Krousónas
Krraba see Krrabë
113 L20 **Krrabë** var. Krraba. Tiranë, C Albania
113 L17 **Krrabit, Mali i** ▲ N Albania
109 W12 **Krško** Ger. Gurkfeld; prev. Videm-Krško. E Slovenia
83 K19 **Kruger National Park** national park Northern, N South Africa
83 J21 **Krugersdorp** Gauteng, NE South Africa
38 D16 **Krugloi Point** headland Agattu Island, Alaska, USA
Krugloye see Kruhlaye
119 N15 **Kruhlaye** Rus. Krugloye. Mahilyowskaya Voblasts', E Belarus
168 L15 **Krui** var. Kroi. Sumatera, SW Indonesia
99 G16 **Kruibeke** Oost-Vlaanderen, N Belgium
83 G25 **Kruidfontein** Western Cape, SW South Africa
99 F15 **Kruiningen** Zeeland, SW Netherlands
Kruja see Krujë
113 L19 **Krujë** var. Kruja, It. Croia. Durrës, C Albania
Krulevshchina see Krulewshchyna
118 K13 **Krulewshchyna** Rus. Krulevshchina. Vitsyebskaya Voblasts', N Belarus
25 T6 **Krum** Texas, SW USA
101 J23 **Krumbach** Bayern, S Germany
113 M17 **Krumë** Kukës, NE Albania
Krummau see Český Krumlov
114 K12 **Krumovgrad** prev. Kossukavak. Kŭrdzhali, S Bulgaria
114 K12 **Krumovitsa** ≈ S Bulgaria
114 L10 **Krumovo** Yambol, E Bulgaria
167 O11 **Krung Thep** var. Krung Thep Mahanakhon, Eng. Bangkok. ● (Thailand) Bangkok, C Thailand
167 O11 **Krung Thep, Ao** var. Bight of Bangkok. bay S Thailand
Krung Thep Mahanakhon see Krung Thep
Krupa/Krupa na Uni see Bosanska Krupa
119 M15 **Krupki** Rus. Krupki. Minskaya Voblasts', C Belarus
95 G24 **Kruså** var. Krusaa. Sønderjylland, SW Denmark
Krusaa see Kruså
113 N14 **Kruševac** Serbia, C Yugoslavia
113 N19 **Kruševo** SW FYR Macedonia
111 A15 **Krušné Hory** Eng. Ore Mountains, Ger. Erzgebirge. ▲ Czech Republic/Germany see also Erzgebirge
39 W13 **Kruzof Island** island Alexander Archipelago, Alaska, USA
114 F13 **Krýa Vrýsi** var. Kría Vrísi. Kentrikí Makedonía, N Greece
119 P16 **Krychaw** Rus. Krichëv. Mahilyowskaya Voblasts', E Belarus
64 K11 **Krylov Seamount** undersea feature E Atlantic Ocean
Krym see Krym, Respublika
117 S13 **Krym, Respublika** var. Krym, Eng. Crimea, Crimean Oblast; prev. Rus. Krymskaya ASSR, Krymskaya Oblast'. ◈ province SE Ukraine
128 K14 **Krymsk** Krasnodarskiy Kray, SW Russian Federation

◆ Country ● Country Capital ◇ Dependent Territory ○ Dependent Territory Capital ◈ Administrative Region × International Airport ▲ Mountain ▲ Mountain Range Volcano ≈ River ◎ Lake ▣ Reservoir

Krymskaya ASSR/Krymskaya Oblast' see Krym, Respublika
117 T13 **Kryms'ki Hory** ▲ S Ukraine
117 T13 **Kryms'kyy Pivostriv** peninsula S Ukraine
111 M18 **Krynica** Ger. Tannenhof. Małopolskie, S Poland
117 P8 **Kryve Ozero** Odes'ka Oblast', SW Ukraine
119 I18 **Kryvoshyn** Rus. Krivoshin. Brestskaya Voblasts', SW Belarus
119 K14 **Kryvychy** Rus. Krivichi. Minskaya Voblasts', C Belarus
117 S8 **Kryvyy Rih** Rus. Krivoy Rog. Dnipropetrovs'ka Oblast', SE Ukraine
117 N8 **Kryzhopil'** Vinnyts'ka Oblast', C Ukraine
Krzemieniec see Kremenets'
111 J14 **Krzepice** Śląskie, S Poland
110 F10 **Krzyż Wielkopolski** Wielkopolskie, C Poland
Ksar al Kabir see Ksar-el-Kebir
Ksar al Soule see Er-Rachidia
74 J5 **Ksar El Boukhari** N Algeria
74 G5 **Ksar-el-Kebir** var. Alcázar, Ksar al Kabir, Ksar-al-Kébir, Ar. Al-Kasr al-Kebir, Al-Qsar al-Kbir, Sp. Alcazarquivir. NW Morocco
110 H12 **Książ Wielkopolski** Ger. Xions. Wielkolpolskie, C Poland
129 O3 **Kstovo** Nizhegorodskaya Oblast', W Russian Federation
169 T8 **Kuala Belait** W Brunei
Kuala Dungun see Dungun
169 S10 **Kualakerian** Borneo, C Indonesia
169 S12 **Kualakuayan** Borneo, C Indonesia
168 K8 **Kuala Lipis** Pahang, Peninsular Malaysia
168 K9 **Kuala Lumpur** ● (Malaysia) Kuala Lumpur, Peninsular Malaysia
Kuala Pelabohan Kelang see Pelabuhan Klang
169 U7 **Kuala Penyu** Sabah, East Malaysia
38 E9 **Kualapuu** Haw. Kualapu'u. Molokai, Hawaii, USA, C Pacific Ocean
168 L7 **Kuala Terengganu** var. Kuala Trengganu. Terengganu, Peninsular Malaysia
168 L11 **Kualatungkal** Sumatera, W Indonesia
171 P11 **Kuandang** Sulawesi, N Indonesia
163 V12 **Kuandian** Liaoning, NE China
Kuando-Kubango see Cuando Cubango
Kuang-chou see Guangzhou
Kuang-hsi see Guangxi Zhuangzu Zizhiqu
Kuang-tung see Guangdong
Kuang-yuan see Guangyuan
Kuantan, Batang see Indragiri, Sungai
Kuanza Norte see Cuanza Norte
Kuanza Sul see Cuanza Sul
Kuba see Quba
Kubango see Cubango/Okavango
141 X8 **Kubārah** NW Oman
93 H16 **Kubbe** Västernorrland, C Sweden
80 A11 **Kubbum** Southern Darfur, W Sudan
126 L13 **Kubenskoye, Ozero** ◎ NW Russian Federation
164 G15 **Kubokawa** Kōchi, Shikoku, SW Japan
114 L7 **Kubrat** prev. Balbunar. Razgrad, N Bulgaria
112 O13 **Kučajske Planine** ▲ E Yugoslavia
165 T1 **Kuccharo-ko** ◎ Hokkaidō, N Japan
112 O11 **Kučevo** Serbia, NE Yugoslavia
Kuchan see Qūchān
169 Q10 **Kuching** prev. Sarawak. Sarawak, East Malaysia
169 Q10 **Kuching** ✕ Sarawak, East Malaysia
164 B17 **Kuchinoerabu-jima** island Nansei-shotō, SW Japan
164 C14 **Kuchinotsu** Nagasaki, Kyūshū, SW Japan
109 Q6 **Kuchl** Salzburg, NW Austria
148 L9 **Küchnay Darweyshān** Helmand, S Afghanistan
Kuchurgan see Kuchurhan
117 O9 **Kuchurhan** Rus. Kuchurgan. ≈ NE Ukraine
Kuçova see Kuçovë
113 L21 **Kuçovë** var. Kuçova; prev. Qyteti Stalin. Berat, C Albania
136 D11 **Küçük Çekmece** İstanbul, NW Turkey
164 F14 **Kudamatsu** var. Kudamatu. Yamaguchi, Honshū, SW Japan
Kudamatu see Kudamatsu
Kudara see Ghŭdara
169 V6 **Kudat** Sabah, East Malaysia
Küddow see Gwda
155 G17 **Kūdligi** Karnātaka, W India
Kudowa see Kudowa-Zdrój
111 F16 **Kudowa-Zdrój** Ger. Kudowa. Wałbrzych, SW Poland
117 P9 **Kudryavtsivka** Mykolayivs'ka Oblast', S Ukraine
169 R16 **Kudus** prev. Koedoes. Jawa, C Indonesia
127 T13 **Kudymkar** Komi-Permyatskiy Avtonomnyy Okrug, NW Russian Federation
Kudzsir see Cugir
Kuei-chou see Guizhou
Kuei-lin see Guilin
Kuei-yang see Guiyang
K'u-erh-lo see Korla
Kueyang see Guiyang
Kufa see Al Kūfah
136 E14 **Küfiçayı** ≈ C Turkey
109 O6 **Kufstein** Tirol, W Austria
145 V14 **Kugaly** Kaz. Qoghaly. Almaty, SE Kazakhstan
8 K8 **Kugluktuk** var. Qurlurtuuq prev. Coppermine. Nunavut, NW Canada
143 Y13 **Kūhak** Sīstān va Balūchestān, SE Iran
143 R9 **Kūhbonān** Kermān, C Iran
148 J5 **Kūhestān** var. Kohsān. Herāt, W Afghanistan
93 N15 **Kuhmo** Oulu, E Finland
93 L18 **Kuhmoinen** Länsi-Suomi, W Finland
Kuhnau see Konin
Kühnö see Kihnu
143 O8 **Kūhpāyeh** Eşfahān, C Iran
167 O12 **Kui Buri** var. Ban Kui Nua. Prachuap Khiri Khan, SW Thailand
Kuibyshev see Kuybyshevskoye Vodokhranilishche
82 D13 **Kuito** Port. Silva Porto. Bié, C Angola
39 X14 **Kuiu Island** island Alexander Archipelago, Alaska, USA
92 L13 **Kuivaniemi** Oulu, C Finland
77 V14 **Kujama** Kaduna, C Nigeria
110 I10 **Kujawsko-pomorskie** ◈ province, C Poland
165 R8 **Kuji** var. Kuzi. Iwate, Honshū, C Japan
Kujto, Ozero see Kuyto, Ozero
Kujū-renzan see Kujū-san
164 D14 **Kujū-san** var. Kujū-renzan. ▲ Kyūshū, SW Japan
43 N7 **Kukalaya, Rio** var. Rio Cuculaya, Rio Kukulaya. ≈ NE Nicaragua
113 O16 **Kukavica** var. Vlajna. ▲ SE Yugoslavia
146 M10 **Kükcha** Rus. Kokcha. Bukhoro Wiloyati, C Uzbekistan
113 M18 **Kukës** var. Kukësi. Kukës, NE Albania
113 L18 **Kukës** ◈ district NE Albania
Kukësi see Kukës
186 D8 **Kukipi** Gulf, S PNG
129 S3 **Kukmor** Respublika Tatarstan, W Russian Federation
Kukong see Shaoguan
39 N6 **Kukpowruk River** ≈ Alaska, USA
38 M6 **Kukpuk River** ≈ Alaska, USA
Kukukhoto see Hohhot
Kukulaya, Rio see Kukalaya, Rio
189 W12 **Kuku Point** headland NW Wake Island
146 G11 **Kukurtli** Akhalskiy Velayat, C Turkmenistan
Kül see Kül, Rūd-e
114 F7 **Kula** Vidin, NW Bulgaria
136 D14 **Kula** Manisa, W Turkey
112 K9 **Kula** Serbia, NW Yugoslavia
149 S8 **Kulāchi** North-West Frontier Province, NW Pakistan
Kulachi see Kolāchi
144 F11 **Kulagino** Kaz. Kūlagino. Atyrau, W Kazakhstan
168 L10 **Kulai** Johor, Peninsular Malaysia
114 M7 **Kulak** ≈ NE Bulgaria
153 T11 **Kula Kangri** var. Kulhakangri. ▲ Bhutan/China
144 E13 **Kulaly, Ostrov** island SW Kazakhstan
147 V9 **Kulanak** Narynskaya Oblast', C Kyrgyzstan
146 B8 **Kulandag** ▲ W Turkmenistan
145 S16 **Kulan** Kaz. Qulan; prev. Lugovoy, Lugovoye. Zhambyl, S Kazakhstan
153 V14 **Kulaura** Chittagong, NE Bangladesh
118 D9 **Kuldīga** Ger. Goldingen. Kuldīga, W Latvia
Kuldja see Yining
Kul'dzhuktau, Gory see Quljuqtov-Toghi
129 N4 **Kulebaki** Nizhegorodskaya Oblast', W Russian Federation
112 E11 **Kulen Vakuf** var. Spasovo. Federacija Bosna I Hercegovina, NW Bosnia and Herzegovina
181 Q9 **Kulgera Roadhouse** Northern Territory, N Australia
Kulhakangri see Kula Kangri
129 T1 **Kuliga** Udmurtskaya Respublika, NW Russian Federation
Kulkuduk see Kalquduq
118 G4 **Kullamaa** Läänemaa, W Estonia
197 O12 **Kullorsuaq** var. Kuvdlorssuak. Kitaa, C Greenland
29 O6 **Kulm** North Dakota, N USA
Kulm see Chełmno
146 D12 **Kul'mach** Balkanskiy Velayat, W Turkmenistan
101 L18 **Kulmbach** Bayern, SE Germany
Kulmsee see Chełmża
147 Q14 **Kŭlob** Rus. Kulyab. SW Tajikistan
92 M13 **Kuloharju** Lappi, N Finland
127 N7 **Kuloy** Arkhangel'skaya Oblast', NW Russian Federation
127 N7 **Kuloy** ≈ NW Russian Federation
137 Q14 **Kulp** Dıyarbakır, SE Turkey
Kulpa see Kolpa
77 P14 **Kulpawn** ≈ N Ghana
143 R13 **Kül, Rūd-e** var. Kül. ≈ S Iran
144 G12 **Kul'sary** Kaz. Qulsary. Atyrau, W Kazakhstan
153 R15 **Kulti** West Bengal, NE India
93 G16 **Kultsjön** ◎ N Sweden
136 I14 **Kulu** Konya, W Turkey
123 S9 **Kulu** ≈ E Russian Federation
122 I13 **Kulunda** Altayskiy Kray, S Russian Federation
145 T7 **Kulunda Steppe** Kaz. Qulyndy Zhazyghy, Rus. Kulundinskaya Ravnina. grassland Kazakhstan/Russian Federation
Kulundinskaya Ravnina see Kulunda Steppe
182 M9 **Kulwin** Victoria, SE Australia
Kulyab see Kŭlob
117 Q3 **Kulykivka** Chernihivs'ka Oblast', N Ukraine
Kum see Qom
164 F14 **Kuma** Ehime, Shikoku, SW Japan
129 P14 **Kuma** ≈ SW Russian Federation
165 O12 **Kumagaya** Saitama, Honshū, S Japan
165 Q5 **Kumaishi** Hokkaidō, NE Japan
169 R13 **Kumai, Teluk** bay Borneo, C Indonesia
129 Y7 **Kumak** Orenburgskaya Oblast', W Russian Federation
164 C14 **Kumamoto** Kumamoto, Kyūshū, SW Japan
164 D15 **Kumamoto** off. Kumamoto-ken. ◈ prefecture Kyūshū, SW Japan
164 J15 **Kumano** Mie, Honshū, SW Japan
Kumanova see Kumanovo
113 O17 **Kumanovo** Turk. Kumanova. N FYR Macedonia
185 G17 **Kumara** West Coast, South Island, NZ
180 J8 **Kumarina Roadhouse** Western Australia
153 T15 **Kumarkhali** Khulna, W Bangladesh
77 P16 **Kumasi** prev. Coomassie. C Ghana
Kumayri see Gyumri
79 D15 **Kumba** Sud-Ouest, W Cameroon
114 N13 **Kumbağ** Tekirdağ, NW Turkey
155 J21 **Kumbakonam** Tamil Nādu, SE India
Kum-Dag see Gumdag
165 R16 **Kume-jima** island Nansei-shotō, SW Japan
129 V6 **Kumertau** Respublika Bashkortostan, W Russian Federation
35 R4 **Kumiva Peak** ▲ Nevada, W USA
159 N8 **Kum Kuduk** well NW China
159 N7 **Kumkuduk** Xinjiang Uygur Zizhiqu, W China
Kumkurgan see Qumqurghon
95 M16 **Kumla** Örebro, C Sweden
136 E17 **Kumluca** Antalya, SW Turkey
100 N9 **Kummerower See** ◎ NE Germany
77 X14 **Kumo** Gombe, E Nigeria
145 O13 **Kumola** ≈ C Kazakhstan
167 N1 **Kumon Range** ▲ N Myanmar
83 F22 **Kums** Karas, SE Namibia
155 E18 **Kumta** Karnātaka, W India
158 L6 **Kümük** Xinjiang Uygur Zizhiqu, W China
38 H12 **Kumukahi, Cape** headland Hawaii, USA, C Pacific Ocean
129 Q17 **Kumukh** Respublika Dagestan, SW Russian Federation
Kumul see Hami
129 N9 **Kumylzhenskaya** Volgogradskaya Oblast', SW Russian Federation
141 W6 **Kumzār** N Oman
149 S4 **Kunar** Per. Konarhā. ◈ province E Afghanistan
Kunashiri see Kunashir, Ostrov
123 U14 **Kunashir, Ostrov** var. Kunashiri. island Kuril'skiye Ostrova, SE Russian Federation
118 I3 **Kunda** Lääne-Virumaa, NE Estonia
152 M13 **Kunda** Uttar Pradesh, N India
155 E19 **Kundāpura** var. Coondapoor. Karnātaka, W India
79 O24 **Kundelungu, Monts** ▲ S Dem. Rep. Congo (Zaire)
Kundert see Hernád
186 D7 **Kundiawa** Chimbu, W PNG
Kundla see Sāvarkundla
168 L10 **Kundur, Pulau** island W Indonesia
149 Q2 **Kunduz** var. Kondoz, Kundūz, Qondūz, Per. Kondūz. Kunduz, NE Afghanistan
149 Q2 **Kunduz** Per. Kondūz. ◈ province NE Afghanistan
Kuneitra see Al Qunayţirah
83 B18 **Kunene** ◈ district NE Namibia
83 A16 **Kunene** var. Cunene. ≈ Angola/Namibia see also Cunene
Künes see Xinyuan
158 J5 **Künes He** ≈ NW China
95 I19 **Kungälv** Västra Götaland, S Sweden
147 W7 **Kungei Ala-Tau** Rus. Khrebet Kyungëy Ala-Too, Kir. Küngöy Ala-Too. ▲ Kazakhstan/Kyrgyzstan
Küngöy Ala-Too see Kungei Ala-Tau
Kungrad see Qŭnghirot
95 J19 **Kungsbacka** Halland, S Sweden
95 I18 **Kungshamn** Västra Götaland, S Sweden
95 M16 **Kungsör** Västmanland, C Sweden
79 J16 **Kungu** Equateur, NW Dem. Rep. Congo (Zaire)
127 V15 **Kungur** Permskaya Oblast', NW Russian Federation
166 L9 **Kungyangon** Yangon, SW Myanmar
111 M22 **Kunhegyes** Jász-Nagykun-Szolnok, E Hungary
167 O5 **Kunhing** Shan State, E Myanmar
158 D9 **Kunjirap Daban** var. Khūnjerāb Pass. pass China/Pakistan see also Khūnjerāb Pass
Kunlun Mountains see Kunlun Shan
158 H10 **Kunlun Shan** Eng. Kunlun Mountains. ▲ NW China
159 P11 **Kunlun Shankou** pass C China
160 G13 **Kunming** var. K'un-ming; prev. Yunnan. Yunnan, SW China
165 R4 **Kunnui** Hokkaidō, NE Japan
95 B18 **Kunoy** Dan. Kunø Island Faeroe Islands
163 X16 **Kunsan** var. Gunsan, Jap. Gunzan. W South Korea
111 L24 **Kunszentmárton** Jász-Nagykun-Szolnok, E Hungary
111 J23 **Kunszentmiklós** Bács-Kiskun, C Hungary
181 N3 **Kununurra** Western Australia
Kunya-Urgench see Këneurgench
Kunyé see Pins, Île des
169 T11 **Kunyi** Borneo, C Indonesia
101 I20 **Künzelsau** Baden-Württemberg, S Germany
161 S10 **Kuocang Shan** ▲ SE China
126 H5 **Kuoloyarvi** var. Luolajarvi. Murmanskaya Oblast', NW Russian Federation
93 N16 **Kuopio** Itä-Suomi, C Finland
93 K17 **Kuortane** Länsi-Suomi, W Finland
93 M18 **Kuortti** Itä-Suomi, E Finland
Kupa see Kolpa
171 P17 **Kupang** prev. Koepang. Timor, C Indonesia
39 Q5 **Kuparuk River** ≈ Alaska, USA
Kupchino see Cupcina
186 E9 **Kupiano** Central, S PNG
180 M4 **Kupingarri** Western Australia
122 I12 **Kupino** Novosibirskaya Oblast', C Russian Federation
118 H11 **Kupiškis** Kupiškis, NE Lithuania
114 L13 **Küplü** Edirne, NW Turkey
39 X13 **Kupreanof Island** island Alexander Archipelago, Alaska, USA
39 O16 **Kupreanof Point** headland Alaska, USA
112 G13 **Kupres** Federacija Bosna I Hercegovina, SW Bosnia and Herzegovina
117 W5 **Kup"yans'k** Rus. Kupyansk. Kharkivs'ka Oblast', E Ukraine
117 W5 **Kup"yans'k-Vuzlovyy** Kharkivs'ka Oblast', E Ukraine
158 I6 **Kuqa** Xinjiang Uygur Zizhiqu, NW China
Kür see Kura
137 W11 **Kura** Az. Kür, Geor. Mtkvari, Turk. Kura Nehri. ≈ SW Asia
55 R8 **Kuracki** NW Guyana
Kura Kurk see Irbe Strait
147 Q10 **Kurama Range** Rus. Kuraminskiy Khrebet. ▲ Tajikistan/Uzbekistan
Kuraminskiy Khrebet see Kurama Range
Kura Nehri see Kura
119 J14 **Kuranyets** Rus. Kurenets. Minskaya Voblasts', C Belarus
164 H13 **Kurashiki** var. Kurasiki. Okayama, Honshū, SW Japan
154 L10 **Kurasia** Madhya Pradesh, C India
Kurasiki see Kurashiki
164 H12 **Kurayoshi** var. Kurayosi. Tottori, Honshū, SW Japan
Kurayosi see Kurayoshi
163 X6 **Kurbin He** ≈ NE China
145 X10 **Kurchum** Kaz. Kürshim. Vostochnyy Kazakhstan, E Kazakhstan
145 Y10 **Kurchum** ≈ E Kazakhstan
137 X11 **Kürdämir** Rus. Kyurdamir. C Azerbaijan
Kurdestan see Kordestān
139 S1 **Kurdistan** cultural region SW Asia
Kurd Kui see Kord Küy
155 F15 **Kurduvādi** Mahārāshtra, W India
114 J11 **Kŭrdzhali** var. Kirdzhali. Kŭrdzhali, S Bulgaria
114 K11 **Kŭrdzhali** ◈ province S Bulgaria
114 J11 **Kŭrdzhali, Yazovir** ⊡ S Bulgaria
164 F13 **Kure** Hiroshima, Honshū, SW Japan
192 K5 **Kure Atoll** var. Ocean Island. atoll Hawaiian Islands, Hawaii, USA, C Pacific Ocean
136 J10 **Küre Dağları** ▲ N Turkey
Kurenets see Kuranyets
118 E6 **Kuressaare** Ger. Arensburg; prev. Kingissepp. Saaremaa, W Estonia
122 K9 **Kureyka** Krasnoyarskiy Kray, N Russian Federation
122 K9 **Kureyka** ≈ N Russian Federation
145 P10 **Kurgal'dzhin, Ozero** ◎ C Kazakhstan
145 Q10 **Kurgal'dzhinskiy** see Kurgal'dzhino
145 Q10 **Kurgal'dzhino** var. Kurgal'dzhinskiy, Kaz. Qorgazhyn. Akmola, C Kazakhstan
122 G11 **Kurgan** Kurganskaya Oblast', C Russian Federation
128 L14 **Kurganinsk** Krasnodarskiy Kray, SW Russian Federation
122 G11 **Kurganskaya Oblast'** ◈ province C Russian Federation
Kurgan-Tyube see Qŭrghonteppa
191 O2 **Kuria** prev. Woodle Island. island Tungaru, W Kiribati
Kuria Muria Bay see Ḩalāniyāt, Khalīj al
Kuria Muria Islands see Ḩalāniyāt, Juzur al
153 T13 **Kurigram** Rajshahi, N Bangladesh
93 K17 **Kurikka** Länsi-Suomi, W Finland
192 I3 **Kurile Basin** undersea feature NW Pacific Ocean
Kurile Islands see Kuril'skiye Ostrova
Kurile-Kamchatka Depression see Kurile Trench
192 J3 **Kurile Trench** var. Kurile-Kamchatka Depression. undersea feature NW Pacific Ocean
129 Q9 **Kurilovka** Saratovskaya Oblast', W Russian Federation
123 U13 **Kuril'sk** Kuril'skiye Ostrova, Sakhalinskaya Oblats', SE Russian Federation
122 G11 **Kuril'skiye Ostrova** Eng. Kurile Islands. island group SE Russian Federation
42 M9 **Kurinwas, Río** ≈ E Nicaragua
Kurisches Haff see Courland Lagoon
Kurkund see Kilingi-Nõmme
128 M4 **Kurlovskiy** Vladimirskaya Oblast', W Russian Federation
80 G12 **Kurmuk** Blue Nile, SE Sudan
Kurna see Al Qurnah
155 H17 **Kurnool** var. Karnul. Andhra Pradesh, S India
164 M11 **Kurobe** Toyama, Honshū, SW Japan
165 Q7 **Kuroishi** var. Kuroisi. Aomori, Honshū, C Japan
Kuroisi see Kuroishi
165 O12 **Kuroiso** Tochigi, Honshū, S Japan
165 Q4 **Kuromatsunai** Hokkaidō, NE Japan
164 B17 **Kuro-shima** island SW Japan
185 F21 **Kurow** Canterbury, South Island, NZ
129 N15 **Kursavka** Stavropol'skiy Kray, SW Russian Federation
118 E11 **Kuršėnai** Šiauliai, N Lithuania
Kürshim see Kurchum
Kurshskaya Kosa/Kuršių Nerija see Courland Spit
128 J7 **Kursk** Kurskaya Oblast', W Russian Federation
128 I7 **Kurskaya Oblast'** ◈ province W Russian Federation
Kurskiy Zaliv see Courland Lagoon
113 N15 **Kuršumlija** Serbia, S Yugoslavia
137 R15 **Kurtalan** Siirt, SE Turkey
Kurtbunar see Tervel
Kurt-Dere see Vŭlchidol
Kurtitsch/Kürtös see Curtici
145 U15 **Kurtty** ≈ SE Kazakhstan
93 L18 **Kuru** Länsi-Suomi, W Finland
80 C13 **Kuru** ≈ W Sudan
114 M13 **Kuru Dağı** ▲ NW Turkey
158 L7 **Kuruktag** ▲ NW China
83 G22 **Kuruman** Northern Cape, N South Africa
67 T14 **Kuruman** ≈ W South Africa
164 D14 **Kurume** Fukuoka, Kyūshū, SW Japan
123 N13 **Kurumkan** Respublika Buryatiya, S Russian Federation
155 J25 **Kurunegala** North Western Province, C Sri Lanka
55 T10 **Kurupukari** C Guyana
127 U10 **Kur"ya** Respublika Komi, NW Russian Federation
144 E15 **Kuryk** prev. Yeraliyev. Mangistau, SW Kazakhstan
136 B15 **Kuşadası** Aydın, SW Turkey
115 M19 **Kuşadası Körfezi** gulf SW Turkey
164 A17 **Kusagaki-guntō** island SW Japan
Kusaie see Kosrae
145 T12 **Kusak** ≈ C Kazakhstan
Kusary see Qusar
167 P7 **Ku Sathan, Doi** ▲ NW Thailand
164 J13 **Kusatsu** var. Kusatu. Shiga, Honshū, SW Japan
Kusatu see Kusatsu
138 F11 **Kuseifa** Southern, C Israel
136 C12 **Kuş Gölü** ◎ NW Turkey
128 L12 **Kushchevskaya** Krasnodarskiy Kray, SW Russian Federation
164 D16 **Kushima** var. Kusima. Miyazaki, Kyūshū, SW Japan
164 I15 **Kushimoto** Wakayama, Honshū, SW Japan
165 V4 **Kushiro** var. Kusiro. Hokkaidō, NE Japan
148 K4 **Kūshk** Herāt, W Afghanistan
146 J17 **Kushka** ≈ S Turkmenistan
Kushka see Gushgy
145 N8 **Kushmurun** Kaz. Qusmuryn. Kostanay, N Kazakhstan
145 N8 **Kushmurun, Ozero** Kaz. Qusmuryn. ◎ N Kazakhstan
129 U4 **Kushnarenkovo** Respublika Bashkortostan, W Russian Federation
Kushrabat see Qŭshrabot
153 T15 **Kushtia** var. Kustia. Khulna, W Bangladesh
Kusikino see Kushikino
Kusima see Kushima
Kusiro see Kushiro
38 M13 **Kuskokwim Bay** bay Alaska, USA
39 P11 **Kuskokwim Mountains** ▲ Alaska, USA
39 N12 **Kuskokwim River** ≈ Alaska, USA
108 G7 **Küsnacht** Zürich, N Switzerland
165 V4 **Kussharo-ko** var. Kussyaro. ◎ Hokkaidō, NE Japan
Küssnacht see Küssnacht am Rigi
108 F8 **Küssnacht am Rigi** var. Küssnacht. Schwyz, C Switzerland
Kussyaro see Kussharo-ko
Kustanay see Kostanay
Küstence/Küstendje see Constanţa
100 F11 **Küstenkanal** var. Ems-Hunte Canal. canal NW Germany
Küstrin see Kostrzyn
Kustia see Kushtia
171 R11 **Kusu** Pulau Halmahera, E Indonesia
170 L16 **Kuta** Pulau Lombok, S Indonesia
139 T4 **Kutabān** N Iraq
136 E13 **Kütahya** prev. Kutaia. Kütahya, W Turkey
136 E13 **Kütahya** var. Kutaia. ◈ province W Turkey
Kutai see Mahakam, Sungai
Kutaia see Kütahya
137 R9 **K'ut'aisi** W Georgia
Kūt al 'Amārah see Al Kūt
Kut al Hai/Kūt al Ḩayy see Al Ḩayy
Kut al Imara see Al Kūt
123 Q11 **Kutana** Respublika Sakha (Yakutiya), NE Russian Federation
Kutaradja/Kutaraja see Bandaaceh
165 R4 **Kutchan** Hokkaidō, NE Japan
Kutch, Gulf of see Kachchh, Gulf of
Kutch, Rann of see Kachchh, Rann of
112 F9 **Kutina** Sisak-Moslavina, NE Croatia
112 H9 **Kutjevo** Požega-Slavonija, NE Croatia
111 E17 **Kutná Hora** Ger. Kuttenberg. Středočeský Kraj, C Czech Republic
110 K12 **Kutno** Łódzkie, C Poland
Kuttenberg see Kutná Hora
79 I20 **Kutu** Bandundu, W Dem. Rep. Congo (Zaire)
153 V17 **Kutubdia Island** island SE Bangladesh
80 B10 **Kutum** Northern Darfur, W Sudan
147 Y7 **Kuturgu** Issyk-Kul'skaya Oblast', E Kyrgyzstan
12 M5 **Kuujjuaq** prev. Fort-Chimo. Quebec, E Canada
12 I7 **Kuujjuarapik** Quebec, C Canada
146 A10 **Kuuli-Mayak** Turkm. Guwlumayak. Balkanskiy Velayat, NW Turkmenistan
118 I6 **Kuulse magi** ▲ S Estonia
92 N13 **Kuusamo** Oulu, E Finland
93 M19 **Kuusankoski** Etelä-Suomi, S Finland
129 W7 **Kuvandyk** Orenburgskaya Oblast', W Russian Federation
Kuvango see Cubango
Kuvasay see Quwasoy
Kuvdlorssuak see Kullorsuaq
126 I16 **Kuvshinovo** Tverskaya Oblast', W Russian Federation
141 Q4 **Kuwait** off. State of Kuwait, var. Dawlat al Kuwait, Koweit, Kuweit. ◆ monarchy SW Asia
Kuwait see Al Kuwayt
Kuwait Bay see Kuwayt, Jūn al
Kuwait City see Al Kuwayt
Kuwait, Dawlat al see Kuwait
Kuwajleen see Kwajalein Atoll
164 K13 **Kuwana** Mie, Honshū, SW Japan
139 X9 **Kuwayt** E Iraq
142 K11 **Kuwayt, Jūn al** var. Kuwait Bay. bay E Kuwait
Kuweit see Kuwait
117 P10 **Kuyal'nyts'kyy Lyman** ◎ SW Ukraine
122 I12 **Kuybyshev** Novosibirskaya Oblast', C Russian Federation
Kuybyshev see Bolgar, Respublika Tatarstan, Russian Federation
Kuybyshev see Samara
117 W9 **Kuybysheve** Rus. Kuybyshevo. Zaporiz'ka Oblast', SE Ukraine
Kuybyshevo see Kuybysheve
Kuybyshev Reservoir see Kuybyshevskoye Vodokhranilishche
Kuybyshevskaya Oblast' see Samarskaya Oblast'
145 O7 **Kuybyshevskiy** Severnyy Kazakhstan, N Kazakhstan
129 R4 **Kuybyshevskoye Vodokhranilishche** var. Kuibyshev, Eng. Kuybyshev Reservoir. ⊡ W Russian Federation
123 S9 **Kuydusun** Respublika Sakha (Yakutiya), NE Russian Federation
127 U16 **Kuyeda** Permskaya Oblast', NW Russian Federation
Küysanjaq see Koi Sanjaq
126 I7 **Kuyto, Ozero** var. Ozero Kujto. ◎ NW Russian Federation
158 J4 **Kuytun** Xinjiang Uygur Zizhiqu, NW China
122 M13 **Kuytun** Irkutskaya Oblast', S Russian Federation
55 S12 **Kuyuwini Landing** S Guyana
Kuzi see Kuji
38 M9 **Kuzitrin River** ≈ Alaska, USA
129 P6 **Kuznetsk** Penzenskaya Oblast', W Russian Federation
116 K3 **Kuznetsovs'k** Rivnens'ka Oblast', NW Ukraine
126 K6 **Kuzomen'** Murmanskaya Oblast', NW Russian Federation
165 R8 **Kuzumaki** Iwate, Honshū, C Japan
92 H9 **Kvaløya** island N Norway
92 K8 **Kvalsund** Finnmark, N Norway
94 G11 **Kvam** Oppland, S Norway
129 X7 **Kvarkeno** Orenburgskaya Oblast', W Russian Federation
93 G15 **Kvarnbergsvattnet** var. Frostviken. ◎ N Sweden
112 A11 **Kvarner** var. Carnaro, It. Quarnero. gulf W Croatia
112 B11 **Kvarnerić** channel W Croatia
39 O14 **Kvichak Bay** bay Alaska, USA
92 H12 **Kvikkjokk** Norrbotten, N Sweden
95 D17 **Kvina** ≈ S Norway
92 Q1 **Kvitøya** island NE Svalbard
95 F16 **Kvitseid** Telemark, S Norway
95 H24 **Kværndrup** Fyn, C Denmark
79 H20 **Kwa** ≈ W Dem. Rep. Congo (Zaire)
77 Q15 **Kwadwokurom** C Ghana

◆ Country ● Country Capital ◇ Dependent Territory ○ Dependent Territory Capital ◈ Administrative Region ✕ International Airport ▲ Mountain ▲ Mountain Range Volcano ≈ River ◎ Lake ⊡ Reservoir

186 M8 **Kwailibesi** Malaita, N Solomon Islands
189 S6 **Kwajalein Atoll** *var.* Kuwajleen. *atoll* Ralik Chain, C Marshall Islands
55 W9 **Kwakoegron** Brokopondo, N Surinam
81 J21 **Kwale** Coast, S Kenya
77 U17 **Kwale** Delta, S Nigeria
79 H20 **Kwamouth** Bandundu, W Dem. Rep. Congo (Zaire)
Kwando *see* Cuando
Kwangchow *see* Guangzhou
Kwangchu *see* Kwangju
163 X16 **Kwangju** *off.* Kwangju-gwangyŏksi, *var.* Guangju, Kwangchu, *Jap.* Kōshū. SW South Korea
79 H20 **Kwango** *Port.* Cuango. ⤳ Angola/Dem. Rep. Congo (Zaire) *see also* Cuango
Kwangsi/Kwangsi Chuang Autonomous Region *see* Guangxi Zhuangzu Zizhiqu
Kwangtung *see* Guangdong
Kwangyuan *see* Guangyuan
81 F17 **Kwania, Lake** ◎ C Uganda
Kwanza *see* Cuanza
77 S15 **Kwara** ◆ *state* SW Nigeria
83 K22 **KwaZulu/Natal** *off.* KwaZulu/Natal Province; *prev.* Natal. ◆ *province* E South Africa
Kweichow *see* Guizhou
Kweichu *see* Guiyang
Kweilin *see* Guilin
Kweisui *see* Hohhot
Kweiyang *see* Guiyang
83 K17 **Kwekwe** *prev.* Que Que. Midlands, C Zimbabwe
83 G20 **Kweneng** ◆ *district* S Botswana
Kwesui *see* Hohhot
39 N12 **Kwethluk** Alaska, USA
39 N12 **Kwethluk River** ⤳ Alaska, USA
110 J8 **Kwidzyń** *Ger.* Marienwerder. Pomorskie, N Poland
38 M13 **Kwigillingok** Alaska, USA
186 E9 **Kwikila** Central, S PNG
79 I20 **Kwilu** ⤳ W Dem. Rep. Congo (Zaire)
Kwito *see* Cuito
171 U12 **Kwoka, Gunung** ▲ Irian Jaya, E Indonesia
78 I12 **Kyabé** Moyen-Chari, S Chad
183 O11 **Kyabram** Victoria, SE Australia
166 M9 **Kyaikkami** *prev.* Amherst. Mon State, S Myanmar
166 L9 **Kyaiklat** Irrawaddy, SW Myanmar
166 M8 **Kyaikto** Mon State, S Myanmar
123 N14 **Kyakhta** Respublika Buryatiya, S Russian Federation
182 G8 **Kyancutta** South Australia
167 T8 **Ky Anh** Ha Tinh, N Vietnam
166 L5 **Kyaukpadaung** Mandalay, C Myanmar
166 J6 **Kyaukpyu** Arakan State, W Myanmar
166 M5 **Kyaukse** Mandalay, C Myanmar
166 L8 **Kyaunggon** Irrawaddy, SW Myanmar
119 E14 **Kybartai** *Pol.* Kibarty. Vilkaviškis, S Lithuania
152 I7 **Kyelang** Himāchal Pradesh, NW India
111 G19 **Kyjov** *Ger.* Gaya. Brněnský Kraj, SE Czech Republic
115 J21 **Kykládes** *var.* Kikládhes, *Eng.* Cyclades. *island group* SE Greece
25 S11 **Kyle** Texas, SW USA
96 G9 **Kyle of Lochalsh** N Scotland, UK
101 D18 **Kyll** ⤳ W Germany
115 F19 **Kyllíni** *var.* Killini. ▲ S Greece
93 M19 **Kymijoki** ⤳ S Finland
115 H18 **Kýmis, Akrotírio** *headland* Évvoia, C Greece
127 W14 **Kyn** Permskaya Oblast', NW Russian Federation
183 N12 **Kyneton** Victoria, SE Australia
81 G17 **Kyoga, Lake** *var.* Lake Kioga. ◎ C Uganda
164 J12 **Kyōga-misaki** *headland* Honshū, SW Japan
183 V4 **Kyogle** New South Wales, SE Australia
163 W15 **Kyŏnggi-man** *bay* NW South Korea
163 Z16 **Kyŏngju** *Jap.* Keishū. SE South Korea
Kyŏngsŏng *see* Sŏul
Kyōsai-tō *see* Kŏje-do
81 F19 **Kyotera** S Uganda
164 J13 **Kyōto** Kyōto, Honshū, SW Japan
164 J13 **Kyōto** *off.* Kyōto-fu, *var.* Kyōto Hu. ◆ *urban prefecture* Honshū, SW Japan
Kyōto-fu/Kyōto Hu *see* Kyōto
115 D21 **Kyparissía** *var.* Kiparissía. Pelopónnisos, S Greece
115 D20 **Kyparissiakós Kólpos** *gulf* S Greece
Kyperounda *see* Kyperoúnta
121 P3 **Kyperoúnta** *var.* Kyperounda. C Cyprus
Kypros *see* Cyprus
115 H16 **Kyrá Panagía** *island* Vóreioi Sporádes, Greece, Aegean Sea
Kyrenia *see* Girne
Kyrenia Mountains *see* Beşparmak Dağları
Kyrgyz Republic *see* Kyrgyzstan
147 U9 **Kyrgyzstan** *off.* Kyrgyz Republic, *var.* Kirghizia; *prev.* Kirgizskaya SSR, Kirghiz SSR, Republic of Kyrgyzstan. ◆ *republic* C Asia
100 M11 **Kyritz** Brandenburg, NE Germany
Kyrkslätt *see* Kirkkonummi
94 G8 **Kyrksæterøra** Sør-Trøndelag, S Norway
127 U8 **Kyrta** Respublika Komi, NW Russian Federation
111 J18 **Kysucké Nové Mesto** *prev.* Horné Nové Mesto, *Ger.* Kisutzaneustadtl, Oberneustadtl, *Hung.* Kiszucaújhely. Žilinský Kraj, N Slovakia
117 N12 **Kytay, Ozero** ◎ SW Ukraine
115 F23 **Kýthira** *var.* Kíthira, *It.* Cerigo; *Lat.* Cythera. Kýthira, S Greece
115 F23 **Kýthira** *var.* Kíthira, *It.* Cerigo; *Lat.* Cythera. *island* S Greece
115 I20 **Kýthnos** Kýthnos, Kykládes, Greece, Aegean Sea
115 I20 **Kýthnos** *var.* Kíthnos, Thermiá, *It.* Termia; *anc.* Cythnos. *island* Kykládes, Greece, Aegean Sea
115 I20 **Kýthnou, Stenó** *strait* Kykládes, Greece, Aegean Sea
Kyungëy Ala-Too, Khrebet *see* Kungei Ala-Tau
Kyurdamir *see* Kürdämir
146 C11 **Kyuren, Gora** ▲ W Turkmenistan
164 D15 **Kyūshū** *var.* Kyûsyû. *island* SW Japan
192 H6 **Kyushu-Palau Ridge** *var.* Kyusyu-Palau Ridge. *undersea feature* W Pacific Ocean
114 F10 **Kyustendil** *anc.* Pautalia. Kyustendil, W Bulgaria
114 G11 **Kyustendil** ◆ *province* W Bulgaria
Kyûsyû *see* Kyūshū
Kyusyu-Palau Ridge *see* Kyushu-Palau Ridge
123 P8 **Kyusyur** Respublika Sakha (Yakutiya), NE Russian Federation
183 P10 **Kywong** New South Wales, SE Australia
117 P4 **Kyyiv** *Eng.* Kiev, *Rus.* Kiyev. ● (Ukraine) Kyyivs'ka Oblast', N Ukraine
Kyyiv *see* Kyyivs'ka Oblast'
117 O4 **Kyyivs'ka Oblast'** *var.* Kyyiv, *Rus.* Kiyevskaya Oblast'. ◆ *province* N Ukraine
117 P3 **Kyyivs'ke Vodoskhovyshche** *Eng.* Kiev Reservoir, *Rus.* Kiyevskoye Vodokhranilishche. ⊠ N Ukraine
93 L16 **Kyyjärvi** Länsi-Suomi, W Finland
122 K14 **Kyzyl** Respublika Tyva, C Russian Federation
147 S8 **Kyzyl-Adyr** *prev.* Kirovskoye. Talasskaya Oblast', NW Kyrgyzstan
145 V14 **Kyzylagash** Almaty, SE Kazakhstan
146 C13 **Kyzylbair** Balkanskiy Velayat, W Turkmenistan
Kyzyl-Dzhiik, Pereval *see* Uzbel Shankou
145 S7 **Kyzylkak, Ozero** ◎ NE Kazakhstan
145 X11 **Kyzylkesek** Vostochnyy Kazakhstan, E Kazakhstan
147 S10 **Kyzyl-Kiya** *Kir.* Kyzyl-Kyya. Oshskaya Oblast', SW Kyrgyzstan
144 L11 **Kyzylkol', Ozero** ◎ C Kazakhstan
151 N15 **Kyzylorda** *var.* Kzyl-Orda, Qizil Orda *Kaz.* Qyzylorda; *prev.* Perovsk. Kyzylorda, S Kazakhstan
150 L14 **Kyzylorda** *off.* Kyzylordinskaya Oblast' *Kaz.* Qyzylorda Oblysy. ◆ *province* S Kazakhstan
122 K14 **Kyzyl Kum** *var.* Kizil Kum, Qizil Qum, *Uzb.* Qizilqum. *desert* Kazakhstan/ Uzbekistan
Kyzyl-Kyya *see* Kyzyl-Kiya
Kyzylrabat *see* Qizilrawbe
Kyzylrabot *see* Qizilrabot
Kyzylsu *see* Kyzyl-Suu
147 X7 **Kyzyl-Suu** *prev.* Pokrovka. Issyk-Kul'skaya Oblast', NE Kyrgyzstan
147 S12 **Kyzyl-Suu** *var.* Kyzylsu. ⤳ Kyrgyzstan/Tajikistan
147 X8 **Kyzyl-Tuu** Issyk-Kul'skaya Oblast', E Kyrgyzstan
145 Q12 **Kyzylzhar** *Kaz.* Qyzylzhar. Zhezkazgan, C Kazakhstan
Kzyl-Orda *see* Kyzylorda
Kzylordinskaya Oblast' *see* Kyzylorda
Kzyltu *see* Kishkenekol'

L

109 X2 **Laa an der Thaya** Niederösterreich, NE Austria
63 K15 **La Adela** La Pampa, SE Argentina
Laagen *see* Numedalslågen
109 S5 **Laakirchen** Oberösterreich, N Austria
Laaland *see* Lolland
104 I11 **La Albuera** Extremadura, W Spain
105 O7 **La Alcarria** *physical region* C Spain
104 K14 **La Algaba** Andalucía, S Spain
105 P9 **La Almarcha** Castilla-La Mancha, C Spain
105 R6 **La Almunia de Doña Godina** Aragón, NE Spain
41 N5 **La Amistad, Presa** ⊠ NW Mexico
118 F4 **Läänemaa** *off.* Lääne Maakond. ◆ *province* NW Estonia
118 I3 **Lääne-Virumaa** *off.* Lääne-Viru Maakond. ◆ *province* NE Estonia
62 J9 **La Antigua, Salina** *salt lake* W Argentina
99 E17 **Laarne** Oost-Vlaanderen, NW Belgium
80 O13 **Laas Caanood** Nugaal, N Somalia
41 O9 **La Ascensión** Nuevo León, NE Mexico
80 N12 **Laas Dhaareed** Woqooyi Galbeed, N Somalia
55 O4 **La Asunción** Nueva Esparta, NE Venezuela
Laatokka *see* Ladozhskoye Ozero
100 I13 **Laatzen** Niedersachsen, NW Germany
38 E9 **Laau Point** *headland* Molokai, Hawaii, USA, C Pacific Ocean
42 D6 **La Aurora** ✕ (Ciudad de Guatemala) Guatemala, C Guatemala
74 C9 **Laâyoune** *var.* Aaiún. ○ (Western Sahara) NW Western Sahara
128 L14 **Laba** ⤳ SW Russian Federation
40 M6 **La Babia** Coahuila de Zaragoza, NE Mexico
15 R7 **La Baie** Quebec, SE Canada
171 P16 **Labala** Pulau Lomblen, S Indonesia
62 K8 **La Banda** Santiago del Estero, N Argentina
La Banda Oriental *see* Uruguay
104 K4 **La Bañeza** Castilla-León, N Spain
40 M13 **La Barca** Jalisco, SW Mexico
40 K14 **La Barra de Navidad** Jalisco, C Mexico
171 P16 **Labasa** *prev.* Lambasa. Vanua Levu, N Fiji
102 H8 **la Baule-Escoublac** Loire-Atlantique, NW France
Labe *see* Elbe
76 I13 **Labé** Moyenne-Guinée, NW Guinea
23 X14 **La Belle** Florida, SE USA
15 N11 **Labelle** Quebec, SE Canada
10 H7 **Laberge, Lake** ◎ Yukon Territory, W Canada
Labes *see* Łobez
Labiau *see* Polessk
112 A10 **Labin** *It.* Albona. Istra, NW Croatia
128 L14 **Labinsk** Krasnodarskiy Kray, SW Russian Federation
105 X5 **La Bisbal d'Empordà** Cataluña, NE Spain
119 P16 **Labkovichy** *Rus.* Lobkovichi. Mahilyowskaya Voblasts', E Belarus
15 S4 **La Blache, Lac de** ◎ Quebec, SE Canada
171 P4 **Labo** Luzon, N Philippines
Laboehanbadjo *see* Labuhanbajo
Laborca *see* Laborec
111 N18 **Laborec** *Hung.* Laborca. ⤳ E Slovakia
108 D11 **La Borgne** ⤳ S Switzerland
45 T12 **Laborie** SW Saint Lucia
79 F21 **La Bouenza** ◆ *province* S Congo
102 J14 **Labouheyre** Landes, SW France
62 L12 **Laboulaye** Córdoba, C Argentina
13 Q7 **Labrador** *cultural region* Newfoundland, SW Canada
64 I6 **Labrador Basin** *var.* Labrador Sea Basin. *undersea feature* Labrador Sea
13 N9 **Labrador City** Newfoundland, E Canada
13 Q5 **Labrador Sea** *sea* NW Atlantic Ocean
Labrador Sea Basin *see* Labrador Basin
Labrang *see* Xiahe
54 G9 **Labranzagrande** Boyacá, C Colombia
45 U15 **La Brea** Trinidad, Trinidad and Tobago
59 D14 **Lábrea** Amazonas, N Brazil
15 S6 **Labrieville** Quebec, SE Canada
102 K14 **Labrit** Landes, SW France
108 C9 **La Broye** ⤳ SW Switzerland
103 N15 **Labruguière** Tarn, S France
168 M11 **Labu** Pulau Singkep, W Indonesia
169 T7 **Labuan** *var.* Victoria. Labuan, East Malaysia
169 T7 **Labuan** ◆ *federal territory* East Malaysia
Labuan *see* Labuan, Pulau
169 T7 **Labuan, Pulau** *var.* Labuan. *island* East Malaysia
171 N16 **Labuhanbajo** *prev.* Laboehanbadjo. Flores, S Indonesia
168 J9 **Labuhanbilik** Sumatera, N Indonesia
168 G8 **Labuhanhaji** Sumatera, W Indonesia
Labuk *see* Labuk, Sungai
Labuk Bay *see* Labuk, Teluk
169 V7 **Labuk, Sungai** *var.* Labuk. ⤳ East Malaysia
169 W6 **Labuk, Teluk** *var.* Labuk Bay, Telukan Labuk. *bay* S Sulu Sea
Labuk, Telukan *see* Labuk, Teluk
166 K9 **Labutta** Irrawaddy, SW Myanmar
122 I8 **Labytnangi** Yamalo-Nenetskiy Avtonomnyy Okrug, N Russian Federation
78 F10 **Lac** *off.* Préfecture du Lac. ◆ *prefecture* W Chad
113 K19 **Laç** *var.* Laci. Lezhë, C Albania
57 K19 **Lacajahuira, Rio** ⤳ W Bolivia
La Calamine *see* Kelmis
62 G11 **La Calera** Valparaíso, C Chile
13 P11 **Lac-Allard** Quebec, E Canada
104 L13 **La Campana** Andalucía, S Spain
102 J12 **Lacanau** Gironde, SW France
42 C2 **Lacandón, Sierra del** ▲ Guatemala/Mexico
La Cañiza *see* A Cañiza
41 W16 **Lacantún, Río** ⤳ SE Mexico
103 Q3 **la Capelle** Aisne, N France
112 K10 **Laćarak** Serbia, NW Yugoslavia
62 L11 **La Carlota** Córdoba, C Argentina
104 L13 **La Carlota** Andalucía, S Spain
105 N12 **La Carolina** Andalucía, S Spain
103 O15 **Lacaune** Tarn, S France
15 P7 **Lac-Bouchette** Quebec, SE Canada
Laccadive Islands/Laccadive Minicoy and Amindivi Islands, the *see* Lakshadweep
11 Y16 **Lac du Bonnet** Manitoba, S Canada
30 L4 **Lac du Flambeau** Wisconsin, N USA
15 P8 **Lac-Édouard** Quebec, SE Canada
42 I4 **La Ceiba** Atlántida, N Honduras
54 E9 **La Ceja** Antioquia, W Colombia
182 J11 **Lacepede Bay** *bay* South Australia
32 G9 **Lacey** Washington, NW USA
103 P12 **la Chaise-Dieu** Haute-Loire, C France
114 G13 **Lachanás** Kentrikí Makedonía, N Greece
126 L11 **Lacha, Ozero** ◎ NW Russian Federation
103 O8 **la Charité-sur-Loire** Nièvre, C France
103 N9 **la Châtre** Indre, C France
108 C8 **La Chaux-de-Fonds** Neuchâtel, W Switzerland
Lach Dera *see* Dheere Laaq
108 G8 **Lachen** Schwyz, C Switzerland
183 Q8 **Lachlan River** ⤳ New South Wales, SE Australia
43 T15 **La Chorrera** Panamá, C Panama
15 V7 **Lac-Humqui** Quebec, SE Canada
15 N12 **Lachute** Quebec, SE Canada
Lachyn *see* Laçın
Laci *see* Laç
137 W13 **Laçın** *Rus.* Lachyn. SW Azerbaijan
103 S16 **la Ciotat** *anc.* Citharista. Bouches-du-Rhône, SE France
18 D10 **Lackawanna** New York, NE USA
11 Q13 **Lac La Biche** Alberta, SW Canada
Lac La Martre *see* Wha Ti
15 R12 **Lac-Mégantic** *var.* Mégantic. Quebec, SE Canada
Lacobriga *see* Lagos
40 G5 **La Colorada** Sonora, NW Mexico
11 Q15 **Lacombe** Alberta, SW Canada
30 L12 **Lacon** Illinois, N USA
43 P16 **La Concepción** *var.* Concepción. Chiriquí, W Panama
54 H5 **La Concepción** Zulia, NW Venezuela
54 H5 **La Concepción** Zulia, NW Venezuela
107 C19 **Laconi** Sardegna, Italy, C Mediterranean Sea
19 O9 **Laconia** New Hampshire, NE USA
61 H19 **La Coronilla** Rocha, E Uruguay
La Coruña *see* A Coruña
103 O11 **la Courtine** Creuse, C France
102 J16 **Lacq** Pyrénées-Atlantiques, SW France
15 P9 **La Croche** Quebec, SE Canada
29 X3 **la Croix, Lac** ◎ Canada/USA
26 K5 **La Crosse** Kansas, C USA
21 V7 **La Crosse** Virginia, NE USA
32 L9 **La Crosse** Washington, NW USA
30 J7 **La Crosse** Wisconsin, N USA
54 C13 **La Cruz** Nariño, SW Colombia
42 K12 **La Cruz** Guanacaste, NW Costa Rica
40 I10 **La Cruz** Sinaloa, W Mexico
61 F19 **La Cruz** Florida, S Uruguay
42 M9 **La Cruz de Río Grande** Región Autónoma Atlántico Sur, E Nicaragua
54 J4 **La Cruz de Taratara** Falcón, N Venezuela
15 Q10 **Lac-St-Charles** Quebec, SE Canada
40 M6 **La Cuesta** Coahuila de Zaragoza, NE Mexico
57 A17 **La Cumbra, Volcán** ⚶ Galapagos Islands, Ecuador, E Pacific Ocean
152 J5 **Ladākh Range** ▲ NE India
26 I5 **Ladder Creek** ⤳ Kansas, C USA
45 X10 **la Désirade** *atoll* E Guadeloupe
Lādhiqīyah, Muḩāfaẓat al *see* Al Lādhiqīyah
83 F25 **Ladismith** Western Cape, SW South Africa
152 G11 **Lādnūn** Rājasthān, NW India
Ladoga, Lake *see* Ladozhskoye Ozero
115 E19 **Ládon** ⤳ S Greece
54 E9 **La Dorada** Caldas, C Colombia
126 H11 **Ladozhskoye Ozero** *Eng.* Lake Ladoga, *Fin.* Laatokka. ◎ NW Russian Federation
37 R12 **Ladron Peak** ▲ New Mexico, SW USA
126 J11 **Ladva-Vetka** Respublika Kareliya, NW Russian Federation
183 Q15 **Lady Barron** Tasmania, SE Australia
14 G9 **Lady Evelyn Lake** ◎ Ontario, S Canada
23 W11 **Lady Lake** Florida, SE USA
10 L17 **Ladysmith** Vancouver Island, British Columbia, SW Canada
83 J22 **Ladysmith** KwaZulu/Natal, E South Africa
30 J5 **Ladysmith** Wisconsin, N USA
145 P9 **Ladyzhenka** Akmola, C Kazakhstan
186 E7 **Lae** Morobe, W PNG
189 R6 **Lae Atoll** *atoll* Ralik Chain, W Marshall Islands
40 C3 **La Encantada, Cerro de** ▲ NW Mexico
94 E12 **Lærdalsøyri** Sogn og Fjordane, S Norway
55 N11 **La Esmeralda** Amazonas, S Venezuela
42 G7 **La Esperanza** Intibucá, SW Honduras
30 K8 **La Farge** Wisconsin, N USA
23 R5 **Lafayette** Alabama, S USA
37 T4 **Lafayette** Colorado, C USA
23 R2 **La Fayette** Georgia, SE USA
31 O13 **Lafayette** Indiana, N USA
22 I9 **Lafayette** Louisiana, S USA
20 K8 **Lafayette** Tennessee, S USA
19 N7 **Lafayette, Mount** ▲ New Hampshire, NE USA
La Fe *see* Santa Fé
103 P3 **la Fère** Aisne, N France
102 L6 **la Ferté-Bernard** Sarthe, NW France
102 K5 **la Ferté-Macé** Orne, N France
103 N7 **la Ferté-St-Aubin** Loiret, C France
103 P5 **la Ferté-sous-Jouarre** Seine-et-Marne, N France
77 V15 **Lafia** Nassarawa, C Nigeria
77 T15 **Lafiagi** Kwara, W Nigeria
11 T17 **Lafleche** Saskatchewan, S Canada
102 K7 **la Flèche** Sarthe, NW France
109 X7 **Lafnitz** *Hung.* Lapines. ⤳ Austria/Hungary
187 P17 **La Foa** Province Sud, S New Caledonia
20 M8 **La Follette** Tennessee, S USA
15 N12 **Lafontaine** Quebec, SE Canada
22 K10 **Lafourche, Bayou** ⤳ Louisiana, S USA
62 K6 **La Fragua** Santiago del Estero, N Argentina
54 H7 **La Fría** Táchira, NW Venezuela
104 J7 **La Fuente de San Esteban** Castilla-León, N Spain
186 C7 **Lagaip** ⤳ W PNG
61 B15 **La Gallareta** Santa Fe, C Argentina
129 Q14 **Lagan'** *prev.* Kaspiyskiy. Respublika Kalmykiya, SW Russian Federation
95 L20 **Lagan** Kronoberg, S Sweden
95 K21 **Lågan** ⤳ S Sweden
92 L2 **Lagarfljót** *var.* Lögurinn. ◎ E Iceland
37 R7 **La Garita Mountains** ▲ Colorado, C USA
171 O2 **Lagawe** Luzon, N Philippines
78 F13 **Lagdo** Nord, N Cameroon
78 F13 **Lagdo, Lac de** ◎ N Cameroon
100 H13 **Lage** Nordrhein-Westfalen, W Germany
94 H12 **Lågen** ⤳ S Norway
61 J14 **Lages** Santa Catarina, S Brazil
149 R4 **Laghmān** ◆ *province* E Afghanistan
74 J6 **Laghouat** N Algeria
105 Q10 **La Gineta** Castilla-La Mancha, C Spain
115 E21 **Lagkáda** *var.* Langada. Pelopónnisos, S Greece
114 G13 **Lagkadás** *var.* Langades, Langadhás. Kentrikí Makedonía, N Greece
115 E20 **Lagkádia** *var.* Langádhia, Langadia. Pelopónnisos, S Greece
54 F6 **La Gloria** Cesar, N Colombia
41 O7 **La Gloria** Nuevo León, NE Mexico
92 N3 **Lågneset** *headland* W Svalbard
104 G14 **Lagoa** Faro, S Portugal
La Goagira *see* La Guajira
61 I14 **Lagoa Vermelha** Rio Grande do Sul, S Brazil
137 V10 **Lagodekhi** SE Georgia
42 C7 **La Gomera** Escuintla, S Guatemala
Lagone *see* Logone
107 M19 **Lagonegro** Basilicata, S Italy
63 G16 **Lago Ranco** Los Lagos, S Chile
77 S16 **Lagos** Lagos, SW Nigeria
104 F14 **Lagos** *anc.* Lacobriga. Faro, S Portugal
77 S16 **Lagos** ◆ *state* SW Nigeria
40 M12 **Lagos de Moreno** Jalisco, SW Mexico
Lagosta *see* Lastovo
74 A12 **Lagouira** SW Western Sahara
92 O1 **Lågøya** *island* N Svalbard
32 L11 **La Grande** Oregon, NW USA
103 Q14 **la Grande-Combe** Gard, S France
12 K9 **La Grande Rivière** *var.* Fort George. ⤳ Quebec, SE Canada
23 R4 **La Grange** Georgia, SE USA
31 P11 **Lagrange** Indiana, N USA
20 L5 **La Grange** Kentucky, S USA
27 V2 **La Grange** Missouri, C USA
21 V10 **La Grange** North Carolina, SE USA
25 U11 **La Grange** Texas, SW USA
105 N7 **La Granja** Castilla-León, N Spain
55 Q9 **La Gran Sabana** *grassland* E Venezuela
54 H7 **La Grita** Táchira, NW Venezuela
La Grulla *see* Grulla
15 R11 **La Guadeloupe** Quebec, SE Canada
64 F12 **La Guaira** Distrito Federal, N Venezuela
54 G4 **La Guajira** *off.* Departamento de La Guajira, *var.* Guajira, La Goagira. ◆ *province* NE Colombia
188 I4 **Lagua Lichan, Punta** *headland* Saipan, S Northern Mariana Islands
18 K14 **La Guardia** ✕ (New York) Long Island, New York, NE USA
La Guardia/Laguardia *see* A Guardia
105 P4 **Laguardia** País Vasco, N Spain
La Gudiña *see* A Gudiña
103 O9 **la Guerche-sur-l'Aubois** Cher, C France
103 O13 **Laguiole** Aveyron, S France
83 F26 **L'Agulhas** *var.* Agulhas. W Cape, SW South Africa
61 K14 **Laguna** Santa Catarina, S Brazil
37 Q11 **Laguna** New Mexico, SW USA
35 T16 **Laguna Beach** California, W USA
35 Y17 **Laguna Dam** *dam* Arizona/California, W USA
40 L7 **Laguna El Rey** Coahuila de Zaragoza, N Mexico
35 V17 **Laguna Mountains** ▲ California, W USA
61 B17 **Laguna Paiva** Santa Fe, C Argentina
62 H3 **Lagunas** Tarapacá, N Chile
56 E9 **Lagunas** Loreto, N Peru
57 M20 **Lagunillas** Santa Cruz, SE Bolivia
54 H6 **Lagunillas** Mérida, NW Venezuela
44 C4 **La Habana** *var.* Havana. ● (Cuba) Ciudad de La Habana, W Cuba
169 W7 **Lahad Datu** Sabah, East Malaysia
169 W7 **Lahad Datu, Teluk** *var.* Telukan Lahad Datu, Teluk Darvel, Teluk Datu; *prev.* Darvel Bay. *bay* Sabah, East Malaysia
38 F10 **Lahaina** Maui, Hawaii, USA, C Pacific Ocean
168 L14 **Lahat** Sumatera, W Indonesia
La Haye *see* 's-Gravenhage
Lahej *see* Laḩij
62 G9 **La Higuera** Coquimbo, N Chile
141 S13 **Laḩī, Ḩisā' al** *spring/well* NE Yemen
141 O16 **Laḩij** *var.* Laḩj, *Eng.* Lahej. SW Yemen
142 M3 **Lāhījān** Gīlān, NW Iran
119 I19 **Lahishyn** *Pol.* Lohiszyn, *Rus.* Logishin. Brestskaya Voblasts', SW Belarus
Laḩj *see* Laḩij
101 F18 **Lahn** ⤳ W Germany
Lähn *see* Wleń
95 J21 **Laholm** Halland, S Sweden
95 J21 **Laholmsbukten** *bay* S Sweden
35 R6 **Lahontan Reservoir** ⊠ Nevada, W USA
149 W8 **Lahore** Punjab, NE Pakistan
149 W8 **Lahore** ✕ Punjab, E Pakistan
55 Q6 **La Horqueta** Delta Amacuro, NE Venezuela
119 K15 **Lahoysk** *Rus.* Logoysk. Minskaya Voblasts', C Belarus
101 F22 **Lahr** Baden-Württemberg, S Germany
93 M19 **Lahti** *Swe.* Lahtis. Etelä-Suomi, S Finland
Lahtis *see* Lahti
40 M14 **La Huacana** Michoacán de Ocampo, SW Mexico
40 K14 **La Huerta** Jalisco, SW Mexico
78 H12 **Laï** *prev.* Behagle, De Behagle. Tandjilé, S Chad
Laibach *see* Ljubljana
167 Q5 **Lai Châu** Lai Châu, N Vietnam
38 D9 **Laie** *Haw.* Lā'ie. Oahu, Hawaii, USA, C Pacific Ocean
102 L5 **l'Aigle** Orne, N France
103 Q7 **Laignes** Côte d'Or, C France
93 K17 **Laihia** Länsi-Suomi, W Finland
Laila *see* Laylā
83 F25 **Laingsburg** Western Cape, SW South Africa
109 U2 **Lainsitz** *Cz.* Lužnice. ⤳ Austria/Czech Republic
96 I7 **Lairg** N Scotland, UK
81 I17 **Laisamis** Eastern, N Kenya
Laisberg *see* Leisi
129 R4 **Laishevo** Respublika Tatarstan, W Russian Federation
Laisholm *see* Jõgeva
92 H13 **Laisvall** Norrbotten, N Sweden
93 K19 **Laitila** Länsi-Suomi, W Finland
161 P5 **Laiwu** Shandong, E China
161 R4 **Laixi** *var.* Shuiji. Shandong, E China
161 R4 **Laiyang** Shandong, E China
161 O3 **Laiyuan** Hebei, E China
161 R4 **Laizhou** *var.* Ye Xian. Shandong, E China
161 Q4 **Laizhou Wan** *var.* Laichow Bay. *bay* E China
37 S8 **La Jara** Colorado, C USA
61 I15 **Lajeado** Rio Grande do Sul, S Brazil
112 L12 **Lajkovac** Serbia, C Yugoslavia
111 K23 **Lajosmizse** Bács-Kiskun, C Hungary
Lajta *see* Leitha
40 I6 **La Junta** Chihuahua, N Mexico
37 V7 **La Junta** Colorado, C USA
92 J13 **Lakaträsk** Norrbotten, N Sweden
Lak Dera *see* Dheere Laaq
Lakeamu *see* Lakekamu
29 P12 **Lake Andes** South Dakota, N USA
22 H9 **Lake Arthur** Louisiana, S USA
187 Z15 **Lakeba** *prev.* Lakemba. *island* Lau Group, E Fiji
187 Z14 **Lakeba Passage** *channel* E Fiji
29 S10 **Lake Benton** Minnesota, N USA
23 V9 **Lake Butler** Florida, SE USA
183 P8 **Lake Cargelligo** New South Wales, SE Australia
22 G9 **Lake Charles** Louisiana, S USA
27 X9 **Lake City** Arkansas, C USA
37 Q7 **Lake City** Colorado, C USA
23 V9 **Lake City** Florida, SE USA
29 U13 **Lake City** Iowa, C USA
31 P7 **Lake City** Michigan, N USA
29 W9 **Lake City** Minnesota, N USA
21 T13 **Lake City** South Carolina, SE USA
29 Q7 **Lake City** South Dakota, N USA
20 M8 **Lake City** Tennessee, S USA
10 L17 **Lake Cowichan** Vancouver Island, British Columbia, SW Canada
29 U10 **Lake Crystal** Minnesota, N USA
25 T6 **Lake Dallas** Texas, SW USA
97 K15 **Lake District** *physical region* NW England, UK
18 D10 **Lake Erie Beach** New York, NE USA
29 T11 **Lakefield** Minnesota, N USA
25 V6 **Lake Fork Reservoir** ◎ Texas, SW USA
30 M9 **Lake Geneva** Wisconsin, N USA
18 L9 **Lake George** New York, NE USA

◆ Country ● Country Capital ◇ Dependent Territory ○ Dependent Territory Capital ◆ Administrative Region ✕ International Airport ▲ Mountain ▲ Mountain Range ⚶ Volcano ⤳ River ◎ Lake ⊠ Reservoir

9 R7 **Lake Harbour** Baffin Island, Nunavut, NE Canada
36 I12 **Lake Havasu City** Arizona, SW USA
25 W12 **Lake Jackson** Texas, SW USA
186 D8 **Lakekamu** var. Lakeamu. ≈ S PNG
180 K13 **Lake King** Western Australia
23 V12 **Lakeland** Florida, SE USA
23 U7 **Lakeland** Georgia, SE USA
181 W4 **Lakeland Downs** Queensland, NE Australia
11 P16 **Lake Louise** Alberta, SW Canada
Lakemba see Lakeba
29 V11 **Lake Mills** Iowa, C USA
39 Q10 **Lake Minchumina** Alaska, USA
Lakemti see Nek'emtē
186 A7 **Lake Murray** Western, SW PNG
80 F5 **Lake Nasser** var. Buhayrat Nasir, Buḩayrat Nāşir, Buḩeiret Nâşir. ◎ Egypt/Sudan
31 R9 **Lake Orion** Michigan, N USA
190 B16 **Lakepa** NE Niue
29 T11 **Lake Park** Iowa, C USA
18 K7 **Lake Placid** New York, NE USA
18 K9 **Lake Pleasant** New York, NE USA
34 M6 **Lakeport** California, W USA
29 Q10 **Lake Preston** South Dakota, N USA
22 J5 **Lake Providence** Louisiana, S USA
185 E20 **Lake Pukaki** Canterbury, South Island, NZ
183 Q12 **Lakes Entrance** Victoria, SE Australia
37 N12 **Lakeside** Arizona, SW USA
35 V17 **Lakeside** California, W USA
23 S9 **Lakeside** Florida, SE USA
28 K13 **Lakeside** Nebraska, C USA
32 E13 **Lakeside** Oregon, NW USA
21 W6 **Lakeside** Virginia, NE USA
Lakes State see El Buhayrat
Lake State see Michigan
185 F20 **Lake Tekapo** Canterbury, South Island, NZ
21 O10 **Lake Toxaway** North Carolina, SE USA
29 T13 **Lake View** Iowa, C USA
32 I16 **Lakeview** Oregon, NW USA
25 O3 **Lakeview** Texas, SW USA
27 W14 **Lake Village** Arkansas, C USA
23 W12 **Lake Wales** Florida, SE USA
37 T4 **Lakewood** Colorado, C USA
18 K15 **Lakewood** New Jersey, NE USA
18 C11 **Lakewood** New York, NE USA
31 T11 **Lakewood** Ohio, N USA
23 Y13 **Lakewood Park** Florida, SE USA
23 Z14 **Lake Worth** Florida, SE USA
152 H4 **Lake Wular** ◎ NE India
126 H11 **Lakhdenpokh'ya** Respublika Kareliya, NW Russian Federation
152 L11 **Lakhīmpur** Uttar Pradesh, N India
154 J11 **Lakhnādon** Madhya Pradesh, C India
Lakhnau see Lucknow
154 A9 **Lakhpat** Gujarāt, W India
119 K19 **Lakhva** Rus. Lakhva. Brestskaya Voblasts', SW Belarus
26 I6 **Lakin** Kansas, C USA
149 S7 **Lakki Marwat** North-West Frontier Province, NW Pakistan
115 F21 **Lakonía** historical region S Greece
115 F22 **Lakonikós Kólpos** gulf S Greece
76 M17 **Lakota** S Ivory Coast
29 U11 **Lakota** Iowa, C USA
29 P3 **Lakota** North Dakota, N USA
Lak Sao see Ban Lakxao
92 L8 **Laksefjorden** fjord N Norway
92 K8 **Lakselv** Finnmark, N Norway
155 B21 **Lakshadweep** prev. the Laccadive, Minicoy and Amindivi Islands. ⬖ union territory India, N Indian Ocean
155 C22 **Lakshadweep** Eng. Laccadive Islands. island group India, N Indian Ocean
153 S17 **Lakshmikāntapur** West Bengal, NE India
112 G11 **Laktaši** Republika Srpska, N Bosnia and Herzegovina
149 V7 **Lāla Mūsa** Punjab, NE Pakistan
la Laon see Laon
114 M11 **Lalapaşa** Edirne, NW Turkey
83 P14 **Lalaua** Nampula, N Mozambique
105 S10 **L'Alcúdia** var. L'Alcudia. País Valenciano, E Spain
80 J11 **Lalibela** Amhara, N Ethiopia,
153 T12 **Lalmanirhat** Rajshahi, N Bangladesh
79 F20 **La Lékoumou** ⬖ province SW Congo
42 E8 **La Libertad** La Libertad, SW El Salvador
42 E3 **La Libertad** Petén, N Guatemala
42 H6 **La Libertad** Comayagua, SW Honduras
40 E4 **La Libertad** var. Puerto Libertad. Sonora, NW Mexico
42 K10 **La Libertad** Chontales, S Nicaragua
42 A9 **La Libertad** ⬖ department SW El Salvador
56 B11 **La Libertad** off. Departamento de La Libertad. ⬖ department W Peru
62 G11 **La Ligua** Valparaíso, C Chile
139 U5 **La'li Khān** E Iraq
79 H16 **La Likouala** ⬖ province NE Congo
104 H3 **Lalín** Galicia, NW Spain
102 L13 **Lalinde** Dordogne, SW France
104 K16 **La Línea** var. La Línea de la Concepción. Andalucía, S Spain
La Línea de la Concepción see La Línea
152 J14 **Lalitpur** Uttar Pradesh, N India
153 P11 **Lalitpur** Central, C Nepal
152 K10 **Lālkua** Uttar Pradesh, N India
11 R12 **La Loche** Saskatchewan, C Canada
102 M6 **la Loupe** Eure-et-Loir, C France
99 G20 **La Louvière** Hainaut, S Belgium
L'Altissima see Hochwilde
104 L14 **La Luisiana** Andalucía, S Spain
37 S14 **La Luz** New Mexico, SW USA
107 D16 **la Maddalena** Sardegna, Italy, C Mediterranean Sea
62 J7 **La Madrid** Tucumán, N Argentina
Lama-Kara see Kara
15 S8 **La Malbaie** Quebec, SE Canada
167 T10 **Lamam** Xékong, S Laos
105 P10 **La Mancha** physical region C Spain
la Manche see English Channel
187 R13 **Lamap** Malekula, C Vanuatu
37 W6 **Lamar** Colorado, C USA
27 S7 **Lamar** Missouri, C USA
21 S12 **Lamar** South Carolina, SE USA
107 C19 **La Marmora, Punta** ▲ Sardegna, Italy, C Mediterranean Sea
8 I9 **La Martre, Lac** ◎ Northwest Territories, NW Canada
56 D10 **Lamas** San Martín, N Peru
42 J5 **La Masica** Atlántida, NW Honduras
103 R12 **Lamastre** Ardèche, E France
La Matepec see Santa Ana, Volcán de
44 I7 **La Maya** Santiago de Cuba, E Cuba
109 S5 **Lambach** Oberösterreich, N Austria
168 I11 **Lambak** Pulau Pini, W Indonesia
102 H5 **Lamballe** Côtes d'Armor, NW France
79 D18 **Lambaréné** Moyen-Ogooué, W Gabon
Lambasa see Labasa
56 B11 **Lambayeque** Lambayeque, W Peru
56 A10 **Lambayeque** off. Departamento de Lambayeque. ⬖ department NW Peru
97 G17 **Lambay Island** Ir. Reachrainn. island E Ireland
186 G6 **Lambert, Cape** headland New Britain, E PNG
195 W6 **Lambert Glacier** glacier Antarctica
29 T10 **Lamberton** Minnesota, N USA
27 X4 **Lambert-Saint Louis** × Missouri, C USA
31 R11 **Lambertville** Michigan, N USA
18 J15 **Lambertville** New Jersey, NE USA
171 N12 **Lambogo** Sulawesi, N Indonesia
106 D8 **Lambro** ≈ N Italy
33 W11 **Lame Deer** Montana, NW USA
104 H6 **Lamego** Viseu, N Portugal
187 Q14 **Lamen Bay** Épi, C Vanuatu
45 X6 **Lamentin** Basse Terre, N Guadeloupe
Lamentin see le Lamentin
182 K10 **Lameroo** South Australia
54 F10 **La Mesa** Cundinamarca, C Colombia
35 U17 **La Mesa** California, W USA
37 R16 **La Mesa** New Mexico, SW USA
25 N6 **Lamesa** Texas, SW USA
115 F17 **Lamía** Stereá Ellás, C Greece
171 O8 **Lamitan** Basilan Island, SW Philippines
187 Y14 **Lamiti** Gau, C Fiji
171 T11 **Lamlam** Irian Jaya, E Indonesia
188 B16 **Lamlam, Mount** ▲ SW Guam
109 Q6 **Lammer** ≈ E Austria
185 E23 **Lammerlaw Range** ▲ South Island, NZ
95 L20 **Lammhult** Kronoberg, S Sweden
93 L18 **Lammi** Etelä-Suomi, S Finland
189 U11 **Lamoil** island Chuuk, C Micronesia
35 W3 **Lamoille** Nevada, W USA
18 M7 **Lamoille River** ≈ Vermont, NE USA
30 J13 **La Moine River** ≈ Illinois, N USA
171 P4 **Lamon Bay** bay Luzon, N Philippines
29 V16 **Lamoni** Iowa, C USA
35 R13 **Lamont** California, W USA
27 N8 **Lamont** Oklahoma, C USA
54 E13 **La Montañita** var. Montañita. Caquetá, S Colombia
43 N8 **La Mosquitia** var. Miskito Coast, Eng. Mosquito Coast. coastal region E Nicaragua
102 I9 **la Mothe-Achard** Vendée, NW France
188 L15 **Lamotrek Atoll** atoll Caroline Islands, C Micronesia
29 P6 **La Moure** North Dakota, N USA
167 O8 **Lampang** var. Muang Lampang. Lampang, NW Thailand
167 R9 **Lam Pao Reservoir** ⊞ E Thailand
25 S9 **Lampasas** Texas, SW USA
25 S9 **Lampasas River** ≈ Texas, SW USA
41 N7 **Lampazos** var. Lampazos de Naranjo. Nuevo León, NE Mexico
Lampazos de Naranjo see Lampazos
115 E19 **Lámpeia** Dytikí Ellás, S Greece
101 G19 **Lampertheim** Hessen, W Germany
97 I20 **Lampeter** SW Wales, UK
167 O7 **Lamphun** var. Lampun, Muang Lamphun. Lamphun, NW Thailand
11 X10 **Lamprey** Manitoba, C Canada
Lampun see Lamphun
168 M15 **Lampung** off. Propinsi Lampung. ⬖ province SW Indonesia
128 K6 **Lamskoye** Lipetskaya Oblast', W Russian Federation
81 K20 **Lamu** Coast, SE Kenya
43 N14 **La Muerte, Cerro** ▲ C Costa Rica
103 S13 **la Mure** Isère, E France
37 S10 **Lamy** New Mexico, SW USA
119 J18 **Lan'** Rus. Lan'. ≈ C Belarus
38 E10 **Lanai** Haw. Lāna'i. island Hawaii, USA, C Pacific Ocean
38 E10 **Lanai City** Lanai, Hawaii, USA, C Pacific Ocean
99 L18 **Lanaken** Limburg, NE Belgium
171 Q7 **Lanao, Lake** var. Lake Sultan Alonto. ◎ Mindanao, S Philippines
96 J12 **Lanark** S Scotland, UK
96 I13 **Lanark** cultural region C Scotland, UK
104 L9 **La Nava de Ricomalillo** Castilla-La Mancha, C Spain
166 M13 **Lanbi Kyun** prev. Sullivan Island. island Mergui Archipelago, S Myanmar
Lancang Jiang see Mekong
97 K17 **Lancashire** cultural region NW England, UK
15 N13 **Lancaster** Ontario, SE Canada
97 K16 **Lancaster** NW England, UK
35 T14 **Lancaster** California, W USA
20 M6 **Lancaster** Kentucky, S USA
27 U1 **Lancaster** Missouri, C USA
19 O7 **Lancaster** New Hampshire, NE USA
18 D10 **Lancaster** New York, NE USA
31 T14 **Lancaster** Ohio, N USA
18 H16 **Lancaster** Pennsylvania, NE USA
21 R11 **Lancaster** South Carolina, SE USA
25 U7 **Lancaster** Texas, SW USA
21 X5 **Lancaster** Virginia, NE USA
30 J9 **Lancaster** Wisconsin, N USA
9 O4 **Lancaster Sound** sound Nunavut, N Canada
Lan-chou/Lan-chow/Lanchow see Lanzhou
107 K14 **Lanciano** Abruzzo, C Italy
111 O16 **Łańcut** Podkarpackie, SE Poland
169 Q11 **Landak, Sungai** ≈ Borneo, N Indonesia
Landao see Lantau Island
Landau see Landau an der Isar, Bayern, Germany
Landau see Landau in der Pfalz, Rheinland-Pfalz, Germany
101 N22 **Landau an der Isar** var. Landau. Bayern, SE Germany
101 F20 **Landau in der Pfalz** var. Landau. Rheinland-Pfalz, SW Germany
Land Burgenland see Burgenland
108 K8 **Landeck** Tirol, W Austria
99 J19 **Landen** Vlaams Brabant, C Belgium
33 U15 **Lander** Wyoming, C USA
102 F5 **Landerneau** Finistère, NW France
95 K20 **Landeryd** Halland, S Sweden
102 J15 **Landes** ⬖ department SW France
Landeshut/Landeshut in Schlesien see Kamienna Góra
105 R9 **Landete** Castilla-La Mancha, C Spain
99 M18 **Landgraaf** Limburg, SE Netherlands
102 F5 **Landivisiau** Finistère, NW France
Land of Enchantment see New Mexico
Land of Opportunity see Arkansas
Land of Steady Habits see Connecticut
Land of the Midnight Sun see Alaska
108 I8 **Landquart** Graubünden, SE Switzerland
108 J9 **Landquart** ≈ Austria/Switzerland
21 P10 **Landrum** South Carolina, SE USA
Landsberg see Górowo Iławeckie, Warmińsko-Mazurskie, NE Poland
Landsberg see Gorzów Wielkopolski, Gorzów, Poland
101 K23 **Landsberg am Lech** Bayern, S Germany
Landsberg an der Warthe see Gorzów Wielkopolski
8 J4 **Lands End** headland Northwest Territories, NW Canada
97 G25 **Land's End** headland SW England, UK
101 M22 **Landshut** Bayern, SE Germany
Landskron see Lanškroun
95 J22 **Landskrona** Skåne, S Sweden
98 I10 **Landsmeer** Noord-Holland, C Netherlands
95 J19 **Landvetter** × (Göteborg) Västra Götaland, S Sweden
Landwarów see Lentvaris
23 R5 **Lanett** Alabama, S USA
108 C8 **La Neuveville** var. Neuveville, Ger. Neuenstadt. Neuchâtel, W Switzerland
95 G21 **Langå** var. Langaa. Århus, C Denmark
Langaa see Langå
158 G14 **La'nga Co** ◎ W China
Langada see Lagkáda
Langades/Langadhás see Lagkadás
Langádhia/Langadia see Lagkádia
147 T14 **Langar** Rus. Lyangar. SE Tajikistan
146 M10 **Langar** Rus. Lyangar. Nawoiy Wiloyati, C Uzbekistan
142 M3 **Langarūd** Gīlān, NW Iran
11 V16 **Langbank** Saskatchewan, S Canada
29 P2 **Langdon** North Dakota, N USA
103 P12 **Langeac** Haute-Loire, C France
102 L8 **Langeais** Indre-et-Loire, C France
80 I8 **Langeb, Wadi** ≈ NE Sudan
Långed see Dals Långed
95 G25 **Langeland** island S Denmark
99 B18 **Langemark** West-Vlaanderen, W Belgium
101 G18 **Langen** Hessen, W Germany
101 J22 **Langenau** Baden-Württemberg, S Germany
11 V16 **Langenburg** Saskatchewan, S Canada
101 E16 **Langenfeld** Nordrhein-Westfalen, W Germany
108 L8 **Längenfeld** Tirol, W Austria
100 I12 **Langenhagen** Niedersachsen, N Germany
100 I12 **Langenhagen** × (Hannover) Niedersachsen, NW Germany
109 W3 **Langenlois** Niederösterreich, NE Austria
108 E7 **Langenthal** Bern, NW Switzerland
109 W6 **Langenwang** Steiermark, E Austria
109 X3 **Langenzersdorf** Niederösterreich, E Austria
100 F9 **Langeoog** island NW Germany
95 H23 **Langeskov** Fyn, C Denmark
95 G16 **Langesund** Telemark, S Norway
95 G17 **Langesundsfjorden** fjord S Norway
94 D10 **Langevågen** Møre og Romsdal, S Norway
161 P3 **Langfang** Hebei, E China
94 E9 **Langfjorden** fjord S Norway
29 Q8 **Langford** South Dakota, N USA
168 I10 **Langgapayung** Sumatera, W Indonesia
106 E9 **Langhirano** Emilia-Romagna, C Italy
97 K14 **Langholm** S Scotland, UK
92 I3 **Langjökull** glacier C Iceland
168 I6 **Langkawi, Pulau** island Peninsular Malaysia
166 M14 **Langkha Tuk, Khao** ▲ SW Thailand
14 L8 **Langlade** Quebec, SE Canada
10 M17 **Langley** British Columbia, SW Canada
167 S7 **Lang Mô** Thanh Hoa, N Vietnam
Langnau see Langnau im Emmental
108 E8 **Langnau im Emmental** var. Langnau. Bern, W Switzerland
103 Q13 **Langogne** Lozère, S France
158 K16 **Langoi Kangri** ▲ W China
102 K13 **Langon** Gironde, SW France
La Ngounié see Ngounié
92 G10 **Langøya** island C Norway
158 G14 **Langqên Zangbo** ≈ China/India
104 K2 **Langreo** var. Sama de Langreo. Asturias, N Spain
103 S7 **Langres** Haute-Marne, N France
103 R8 **Langres, Plateau de** plateau C France
168 H8 **Langsa** Sumatera, W Indonesia
93 H16 **Långsele** Västernorrland, C Sweden
162 L12 **Lang Shan** ▲ N China
95 M14 **Långshyttan** Dalarna, C Sweden
167 T5 **Lang Sơn** var. Langson. Lang Sơn, N Vietnam
167 N14 **Lang Suan** Chumphon, SW Thailand
93 J14 **Långträsk** Norrbotten, N Sweden
25 N11 **Langtry** Texas, SW USA
103 P16 **Languedoc** cultural region S France
103 P15 **Languedoc-Roussillon** ⬖ region S France
27 X10 **L'Anguille River** ≈ Arkansas, C USA
93 I16 **Långviksmon** Västernorrland, N Sweden
101 K22 **Langweid** Bayern, S Germany
160 J8 **Langzhong** Sichuan, C China
Lan Hsü see Lan Yü
11 U15 **Lanigan** Saskatchewan, S Canada
116 K5 **Lanivtsi** Ternopil's'ka Oblast', W Ukraine
137 Y13 **Länkäran** Rus. Lenkoran'. S Azerbaijan
102 L16 **Lannemezan** Hautes-Pyrénées, S France
102 G5 **Lannion** Côtes d'Armor, NW France
14 M11 **L'Annonciation** Quebec, SE Canada
105 V5 **L'Anoia** ≈ NE Spain
18 I15 **Lansdale** Pennsylvania, NE USA
14 L14 **Lansdowne** Ontario, SE Canada
152 K9 **Lansdowne** Uttar Pradesh, N India
30 M3 **L'Anse** Michigan, N USA
15 S7 **L'Anse-St-Jean** Quebec, SE Canada
93 K18 **Länsi-Suomi** ⬖ province W Finland
29 Y11 **Lansing** Iowa, C USA
27 R4 **Lansing** Kansas, C USA
31 Q9 **Lansing** state capital Michigan, N USA
92 J12 **Lansjärv** Norrbotten, N Sweden
111 G17 **Lanškroun** Ger. Landskron. Pardubický Kraj, C Czech Republic
167 N16 **Lanta, Ko** island S Thailand
161 O15 **Lantau Island** Cant. Tai Yue Shan, Chin. Landao. island Hong Kong, S China
Lan-ts'ang Chiang see Mekong
171 O11 **Lanu** Sulawesi, N Indonesia
107 D19 **Lanusei** Sardegna, Italy, C Mediterranean Sea
102 H7 **Lanvaux, Landes de** physical region NW France
163 W8 **Lanxi** Heilongjiang, NE China
161 R10 **Lanxi** Zhejiang, SE China
La Nyanga see Nyanga
161 T15 **Lan Yü** var. Huoshao Tao, var. Hungt'ou, Lan Hsü, Lanyü, Eng. Orchid Island; prev. Kotosho, Koto Sho. island SE Taiwan
64 P11 **Lanzarote** island Islas Canarias, Spain, NE Atlantic Ocean
159 V10 **Lanzhou** var. Lan-chou, Lanchow, Lan-chow; prev. Kaolan. Gansu, C China
106 B8 **Lanzo Torinese** Piemonte, NE Italy
171 O1 **Laoag** Luzon, N Philippines
171 Q5 **Laoang** Samar, C Philippines
167 R5 **Lao Cai** Lao Cai, N Vietnam
Laodicea/Laodicea ad Mare see Al Lādhiqīyah
Laoet see Laut, Pulau
163 T11 **Laoha He** ≈ NE China
160 M8 **Laohekou** prev. Guanghua. Hubei, C China
Laoi, An see Lee
97 E19 **Laois** prev. Leix, Queen's County. cultural region C Ireland
Laojunmiao see Yumen
163 W12 **Lao Ling** ▲ N China
64 Q11 **La Oliva** var. Oliva. Fuerteventura, Islas Canarias, Spain, NE Atlantic Ocean
Lao, Loch see Belfast Lough
Lao Mangnai see Mangnai
103 P3 **Laon** var. la Laon; anc. Laudunum. Aisne, N France
Lao People's Democratic Republic see Laos
54 M3 **La Orchila, Isla** island N Venezuela
64 O11 **La Orotava** Tenerife, Islas Canarias, Spain, NE Atlantic Ocean
57 E14 **La Oroya** Junín, C Peru
167 Q7 **Laos** off. Lao People's Democratic Republic. ◆ republic SE Asia
161 R5 **Laoshan Wan** bay E China
163 Y10 **Laoye Ling** ▲ NE China
60 J12 **Lapa** Paraná, S Brazil
103 P10 **Lapalisse** Allier, C France
54 F9 **La Palma** Cundinamarca, C Colombia
42 F7 **La Palma** Chalatenango, N El Salvador
43 W16 **La Palma** Darién, SE Panama
64 N11 **La Palma** island Islas Canarias, Spain, NE Atlantic Ocean
104 J14 **La Palma del Condado** Andalucía, S Spain
61 F18 **La Paloma** Durazno, C Uruguay
61 G20 **La Paloma** Rocha, E Uruguay
61 A21 **La Pampa** off. Provincia de La Pampa. ⬖ province C Argentina
55 P8 **La Paragua** Bolívar, E Venezuela
119 O16 **Lapatsichy** Rus. Lopatichi. Mahilyowskaya Voblasts', E Belarus
61 C16 **La Paz** Entre Ríos, E Argentina
62 I11 **La Paz** Mendoza, C Argentina
57 J18 **La Paz** var. La Paz de Ayacucho. ● (Bolivia-legislative and administrative capital) La Paz, W Bolivia
42 H6 **La Paz** La Paz, SW Honduras
40 F9 **La Paz** Baja California Sur, NW Mexico
61 F20 **La Paz** Canelones, S Uruguay
57 J16 **La Paz** ⬖ department W Bolivia
42 B9 **La Paz** ⬖ department S El Salvador
42 G7 **La Paz** ⬖ department SW Honduras
La Paz see El Alto, Bolivia
La Paz see Robles, Colombia
La Paz see La Paz Centro, Nicaragua
40 F9 **La Paz, Bahía de** bay W Mexico
42 I10 **La Paz Centro** var. La Paz. León, W Nicaragua
La Paz de Ayacucho see La Paz
54 J15 **La Pedrera** Amazonas, SE Colombia
31 S9 **Lapeer** Michigan, N USA
40 K6 **La Perla** Chihuahua, N Mexico
165 T1 **La Perouse Strait** Jap. Sōya-kaikyō, Rus. Proliv Laperuza. strait Japan/Russian Federation
63 I14 **La Perra, Salitral de** salt lake C Argentina
Laperuza, Proliv see La Perouse Strait
41 Q10 **La Pesca** Tamaulipas, C Mexico
40 M13 **La Piedad Cavadas** Michoacán de Ocampo, C Mexico
Lapines see Lafnitz
93 M16 **Lapinlahti** Itä-Suomi, C Finland
Lápithos see Lapta
22 K9 **Laplace** Louisiana, S USA
45 X12 **La Plaine** SE Dominica
173 P16 **la Plaine-des-Palmistes** C Réunion
92 K11 **Lapland** Fin. Lappi, Swe. Lappland. cultural region N Europe
28 M8 **La Plant** South Dakota, N USA
61 D20 **La Plata** Buenos Aires, E Argentina
54 D12 **La Plata** Huila, SW Colombia
21 W4 **La Plata** Maryland, NE USA
La Plata see Sucre
45 U6 **la Plata, Río de** ≈ C Puerto Rico
105 W4 **La Pobla de Lillet** Cataluña, NE Spain
105 U4 **La Pobla de Segur** Cataluña, NE Spain
15 S9 **La Pocatière** Quebec, SE Canada
104 L3 **La Pola de Gordón** Castilla-León, N Spain
31 O11 **La Porte** Indiana, N USA
18 H13 **Laporte** Pennsylvania, NE USA
29 X13 **La Porte City** Iowa, C USA
62 J8 **La Posta** Catamarca, C Argentina
40 E8 **La Poza Grande** Baja California Sur, W Mexico
93 K16 **Lappajärvi** Länsi-Suomi, W Finland
93 L16 **Lappajärvi** ◎ W Finland
93 N18 **Lappeenranta** Swe. Villmanstrand. Etelä-Suomi, S Finland
93 J17 **Lappfjärd** Fin. Lapväärtti. Länsi-Suomi, W Finland
92 L12 **Lappi** Swe. Lappland. ⬖ province N Finland
Lappi see Lapland
Lappland see Lappi
Lappland see Lapland, N Europe
Lappo see Lapua
61 C23 **Laprida** Buenos Aires, E Argentina
25 P13 **La Pryor** Texas, SW USA
136 B11 **Lâpseki** Çanakkale, NW Turkey
121 P2 **Lapta** Gk. Lápithos. NW Cyprus
Laptev Sea see Laptevykh, More
122 N6 **Laptevykh, More** Eng. Laptev Sea. sea Arctic Ocean
93 K16 **Lapua** Swe. Lappo. Länsi-Suomi, W Finland
105 P3 **La Puebla de Arganzón** País Vasco, N Spain
104 L14 **La Puebla de Cazalla** Andalucía, S Spain
104 M9 **La Puebla de Montalbán** Castilla-La Mancha, C Spain
54 I6 **La Puerta** Trujillo, NW Venezuela
Lapurdum see Bayonne
40 E7 **La Purísima** Baja California Sur, W Mexico
Lapväärtti see Lappfjärd
110 O10 **Łapy** Podlaskie, NE Poland
80 D6 **Laqiya Arba'in** Northern, NW Sudan
62 J4 **La Quiaca** Jujuy, N Argentina
107 J14 **L'Aquila** var. Aquila, Aquila degli Abruzzo. Abruzzo, C Italy
143 Q13 **Lār** Fārs, S Iran
54 J5 **Lara** off. Estado Lara. ⬖ state NW Venezuela
104 G2 **Laracha** Galicia, NW Spain
74 G5 **Larache** var. al Araïch, El Araïch, El Araïche, anc. Lixus. NW Morocco
103 T14 **Laragne-Montéglin** Hautes-Alpes, SE France
104 M13 **La Rambla** Andalucía, S Spain
33 Y17 **Laramie** Wyoming, C USA
33 X15 **Laramie Mountains** ▲ Wyoming, C USA
33 Y16 **Laramie River** ≈ Wyoming, C USA
60 H12 **Laranjeiras do Sul** Paraná, S Brazil
Larantoeka see Larantuka
171 P16 **Larantuka** prev. Larantoeka. Flores, C Indonesia
171 U15 **Larat** Pulau Larat, E Indonesia
171 U15 **Larat, Pulau** island Kepulauan Tanimbar, E Indonesia
95 P19 **Lärbro** Gotland, SE Sweden
106 A9 **Larche, Col de** pass France/Italy
14 H8 **Larder Lake** Ontario, S Canada
105 O2 **Laredo** Cantabria, N Spain
25 Q15 **Laredo** Texas, SW USA
40 H9 **La Reforma** Sinaloa, W Mexico
98 N11 **Laren** Gelderland, E Netherlands
98 J11 **Laren** Noord-Holland, C Netherlands
102 K13 **la Réole** Gironde, SW France
La Réunion see Réunion
Largeau see Faya
103 U13 **l'Argentière-la-Bessée** Hautes-Alpes, SE France
149 O4 **Lar Gerd** var. Largird. Balkh, N Afghanistan
Largird see Lar Gerd
23 V12 **Largo** Florida, SE USA
37 Q9 **Largo, Canon** valley New Mexico, SW USA
44 D6 **Largo, Cayo** island W Cuba
23 Z17 **Largo, Key** island Florida Keys, Florida, SE USA
96 H12 **Largs** W Scotland, UK
102 I16 **la Rhune** var. Larrún. ▲ France/Spain see also Larrún
la Riege see Ariège
29 Q4 **Larimore** North Dakota, N USA
107 L15 **Larino** Molise, C Italy
Lario see Como, Lago di
62 J9 **La Rioja** La Rioja, NW Argentina
62 I9 **La Rioja** off. Provincia de La Rioja. ⬖ province NW Argentina
105 O4 **La Rioja** ⬖ autonomous community N Spain
115 F16 **Lárisa** var. Larissa. Thessalía, C Greece
Larissa see Lárisa
149 Q13 **Lārkāna** var. Larkhana. Sind, SE Pakistan
Larkhana see Lārkāna
Larnaca see Lárnaka
121 Q3 **Lárnaka** var. Larnaca, Larnax. SE Cyprus
121 Q3 **Lárnaka** × SE Cyprus
Larnax see Lárnaka
97 G14 **Larne** Ir. Latharna. E Northern Ireland, UK
26 L5 **Larned** Kansas, C USA
104 L3 **La Robla** Castilla-León, N Spain

◆ Country ● Country Capital ◇ Dependent Territory ○ Dependent Territory Capital ⬖ Administrative Region × International Airport ▲ Mountain ▲ Mountain Range Volcano ≈ River ◎ Lake ⊞ Reservoir

104 J10 La Roca de la Sierra Extremadura, W Spain
99 K22 La Roche-en-Ardenne Luxembourg, SE Belgium
102 L11 la Rochefoucauld Charente, W France
102 J10 la Rochelle anc. Rupella. Charente-Maritime, W France
102 I9 la Roche-sur-Yon prev. Bourbon Vendée, Napoléon-Vendée. Vendée, NW France
105 Q10 La Roda Castilla-La Mancha, C Spain
104 L14 La Roda de Andalucía Andalucía, S Spain
45 P9 La Romana E Dominican Republic
11 T13 La Ronge Saskatchewan, C Canada
11 U13 La Ronge, Lac ◎ Saskatchewan, C Canada
22 K10 Larose Louisiana, S USA
42 M7 La Rosita Región Autónoma Atlántico Norte, NE Nicaragua
181 Q3 Larrimah Northern Territory, N Australia
62 N11 Larroque Entre Ríos, E Argentina
105 Q2 Larrún Fr. la Rhune. ▲ France/Spain see also la Rhune
195 X6 Lars Christensen Coast physical region Antarctica
39 Q14 Larsen Bay Kodiak Island, Alaska, USA
194 I5 Larsen Ice Shelf ice shelf Antarctica
8 M6 Larsen Sound sound Nunavut, N Canada
La Rúa see A Rúa
102 K16 Laruns Pyrénées-Atlantiques, SW France
95 G16 Larvik Vestfold, S Norway
La-sa see Lhasa
171 S13 Lasahata Pulau Seram, E Indonesia
Lasahau see Lasihao
37 O6 La Sal Utah, W USA
14 C17 La Salle Ontario, S Canada
30 L11 La Salle Illinois, N USA
45 O9 Las Americas ✕ (Santo Domingo) S Dominican Republic
79 G17 La Sangha ◆ province N Congo
37 V6 Las Animas Colorado, C USA
108 D10 La Sarine var. Sarine. ∿ SW Switzerland
108 B9 La Sarraz Vaud, W Switzerland
12 H12 La Sarre Quebec, SE Canada
54 L3 Las Aves, Islas var. Islas de Aves. island group N Venezuela
55 N7 Las Bonitas Bolívar, C Venezuela
104 K15 Las Cabezas de San Juan Andalucía, S Spain
61 G19 Lascano Rocha, E Uruguay
62 I5 Lascar, Volcán ▲ N Chile
41 T15 Las Choapas var. Choapas. Veracruz-Llave, SE Mexico
37 R15 Las Cruces New Mexico, SW USA
Lasdehnen see Krasnoznamensk
105 V4 La See d'Urgel var. La Seu d'Urgell, Seo de Urgel. Cataluña, NE Spain
La Selle see Selle, Pic de la
62 G9 La Serena Coquimbo, C Chile
104 K11 La Serena physical region W Spain
La Seu d'Urgell see La See d'Urgel
103 T16 la Seyne-sur-Mer Var, SE France
61 D21 Las Flores Buenos Aires, E Argentina
62 H9 Las Flores San Juan, W Argentina
11 S14 Lashburn Saskatchewan, S Canada
62 I11 Las Heras Mendoza, W Argentina
167 N4 Lashio Shan State, E Myanmar
148 M8 Lashkar Gāh var. Lash-Kar-Gar'. Helmand, S Afghanistan
Lash-Kar-Gar' see Lashkar Gāh
171 P14 Lasihao var. Lasahau. Pulau Muna, C Indonesia
107 N21 La Sila ▲ SW Italy
63 H23 La Silueta, Cerro ▲ S Chile
42 L9 La Sirena Región Autónoma Atlántico Sur, E Nicaragua
110 J13 Łask Łódzkie, C Poland
109 V11 Laško Ger. Tüffer. C Slovenia
63 H14 Las Lajas Neuquén, W Argentina
63 H15 Las Lajas, Cerro ▲ W Argentina
62 M6 Las Lomitas Formosa, N Argentina
41 V16 Las Margaritas Chiapas, SE Mexico
Las Marismas see Guadalquivir, Marismas del
54 M6 Las Mercedes Guárico, N Venezuela
42 F6 Las Minas, Cerro ▲ W Honduras
105 O11 La Solana Castilla-La Mancha, C Spain
45 Q14 La Soufrière ✱ Saint Vincent, Saint Vincent and the Grenadines
102 M10 la Souterraine Creuse, C France
62 N7 Las Palmas Chaco, N Argentina
43 Q16 Las Palmas Veraguas, W Panama
64 P12 Las Palmas var. Las Palmas de Gran Canaria. Gran Canaria, Islas Canarias, Spain, NE Atlantic Ocean
64 P12 Las Palmas ◆ province Islas Canarias, Spain, NE Atlantic Ocean
64 Q12 Las Palmas ✕ Gran Canaria, Islas Canarias, Spain, NE Atlantic Ocean
Las Palmas de Gran Canaria see Las Palmas
40 D6 Las Palomas Baja California Sur, W Mexico
105 P10 Las Pedroñeras Castilla-La Mancha, C Spain
106 E10 La Spezia Liguria, NW Italy
61 F20 Las Piedras Canelones, S Uruguay
63 J18 Las Plumas Chubut, S Argentina
61 B18 Las Rosas Santa Fe, C Argentina
Lassa see Lhasa
35 O4 Lassen Peak ▲ California, W USA
194 K6 Lassiter Coast physical region Antarctica
109 V9 Lassnitz ∿ SE Austria
15 O12 L'Assomption Quebec, SE Canada
15 N11 L'Assomption ∿ Quebec, SE Canada
43 S17 Las Tablas Los Santos, S Panama
Lastarria, Volcán see Azufre, Volcán
37 V4 Last Chance Colorado, C USA
Last Frontier, The see Alaska
11 U16 Last Mountain Lake ◎ Saskatchewan, S Canada
62 H9 Las Tórtolas, Cerro ▲ W Argentina
61 C14 Las Toscas Santa Fe, C Argentina
79 F19 Lastoursville Ogooué-Lolo, E Gabon
113 F16 Lastovo It. Lagosta. island SW Croatia
113 F16 Lastovski Kanal channel SW Croatia
40 E6 Las Tres Vírgenes, Volcán ✱ W Mexico
40 F4 Las Trincheras Sonora, NW Mexico
55 N8 Las Trincheras Bolívar, E Venezuela
44 H7 Las Tunas var. Victoria de las Tunas. Las Tunas, E Cuba
La Suisse see Switzerland
40 I5 Las Varas Chihuahua, N Mexico
40 J12 Las Varas Nayarit, C Mexico
62 L10 Las Varillas Córdoba, E Argentina
35 X11 Las Vegas Nevada, W USA
37 T10 Las Vegas New Mexico, SW USA
187 P10 Lata Nendö, Solomon Islands
13 R10 La Tabatière Quebec, E Canada
56 C6 Latacunga Cotopaxi, C Ecuador
194 I7 Latady Island island Antarctica
54 E14 La Tagua Putumayo, S Colombia
Latakia see Al Lādhiqīyah
92 J10 Lätäseno ∿ NW Finland
14 H9 Latchford Ontario, S Canada
14 J13 Latchford Bridge Ontario, SE Canada
193 Y14 Late island Vava'u Group, N Tonga
153 P15 Lātehār Bihār, N India
15 R7 Laterrière Quebec, SE Canada
102 J13 la Teste Gironde, SW France
25 V8 Latexo Texas, SW USA
18 L10 Latham New York, NE USA
Latharna see Larne
108 B9 La Thielle var. Thièle. ∿ W Switzerland
27 R3 Lathrop Missouri, C USA
107 I16 Latina prev. Littoria. Lazio, C Italy
41 R14 La Tinaja Veracruz-Llave, S Mexico
106 J7 Latisana Friuli-Venezia Giulia, NE Italy
Latium see Lazio
115 K25 Lató site of ancient city Kríti, Greece, E Mediterranean Sea
187 Q17 La Tontouta ✕ (Noumea) Province Sud, S New Caledonia
55 N4 La Tortuga, Isla var. Isla Tortuga. island N Venezuela
108 C10 La Tour-de-Peilz var. La Tour de Peilz. Vaud, SW Switzerland
103 S11 la Tour-du-Pin Isère, E France
102 J11 la Tremblade Charente-Maritime, W France
102 L10 la Trimouille Vienne, W France
42 J9 La Trinidad Estelí, NW Nicaragua
41 V16 La Trinitaria Chiapas, SE Mexico
45 Q11 la Trinité E Martinique
15 U7 La Trinité-des-Monts Quebec, SE Canada
18 C15 Latrobe Pennsylvania, NE USA
183 P13 La Trobe River ∿ Victoria, SE Australia
Lattakia/Lattaquié see Al Lādhiqīyah
171 S13 Latu Pulau Seram, E Indonesia
15 P9 La Tuque Quebec, SE Canada
155 G14 Lātūr Mahārāshtra, C India
118 G8 Latvia off. Republic of Latvia, Ger. Lettland, Latv. Latvija, Latvijas Republika; prev. Latvian SSR, Rus. Latviyskaya SSR. ◆ republic NE Europe
Latvian SSR/Latvija/Latvijas Republika/Latviyskaya SSR see Latvia
186 H7 Lau New Britain, E PNG
175 R9 Lau Basin undersea feature S Pacific Ocean
101 O15 Lauchhammer Brandenburg, E Germany
Laudunum see Laon
Laudus see St-Lô
Lauenburg/Lauenburg in Pommern see Lębork
101 L20 Lauf an der Pegnitz Bayern, SE Germany
108 D7 Laufen Basel, NW Switzerland
109 P5 Lauffen Salzburg, NW Austria
92 I2 Laugarbakki Nordhurland Vestra, N Iceland
92 I4 Laugarvatn Sudhurland, SW Iceland
31 O3 Laughing Fish Point headland Michigan, N USA
187 Z14 Lau Group island group E Fiji
Lauis see Lugano
93 M17 Laukaa Länsi-Suomi, W Finland
118 D12 Laukuva Šilalė, W Lithuania
Laun see Louny
183 P16 Launceston Tasmania, SE Australia
97 I24 Launceston anc. Dunheved. SW England, UK
54 C13 La Unión Nariño, SW Colombia
42 H8 La Unión La Unión, SE El Salvador
42 I6 La Unión Olancho, C Honduras
40 M15 La Unión Guerrero, S Mexico
41 Y14 La Unión Quintana Roo, E Mexico
105 S13 La Unión Murcia, SE Spain
54 L7 La Unión Barinas, C Venezuela
42 B10 La Unión ◆ department E El Salvador
38 H11 Laupahoehoe Haw. Laupāhoehoe. Hawaii, USA, C Pacific Ocean
101 I23 Laupheim Baden-Württemberg, S Germany
181 W3 Laura Queensland, NE Australia
189 X2 Laura atoll Majuro Atoll, SE Marshall Islands
Laurana see Lovran
54 L8 La Urbana Bolívar, C Venezuela
21 Y4 Laurel Delaware, NE USA
23 V14 Laurel Florida, SE USA
21 W3 Laurel Maryland, NE USA
22 M6 Laurel Mississippi, S USA
33 U11 Laurel Montana, NW USA
29 R13 Laurel Nebraska, C USA
18 H15 Laureldale Pennsylvania, NE USA
18 C16 Laurel Hill ridge Pennsylvania, NE USA
29 T12 Laurens Iowa, C USA
21 P11 Laurens South Carolina, SE USA
Laurentian Highlands see Laurentian Mountains
15 P10 Laurentian Mountains var. Laurentian Highlands, Fr. Les Laurentides. plateau Newfoundland/Quebec, Canada
15 O12 Laurentides Quebec, SE Canada
Laurentides, Les see Laurentian Mountains
107 M19 Lauria Basilicata, S Italy
194 I1 Laurie Island island Antarctica
21 T11 Laurinburg North Carolina, SE USA
30 M2 Laurium Michigan, N USA
Lauru see Choiseul
108 B9 Lausanne It. Losanna. Vaud, SW Switzerland
101 Q16 Lausche Cz. Luže. ▲ Czech Republic/Germany see also Luže
101 Q16 Lausitzer Bergland var. Lausitzer Gebirge, Cz. Gory Lužycke, Lužické Hory, Eng. Lusatian Mountains. ▲ E Germany
Lausitzer Gebirge see Lausitzer Bergland
Lausitzer Neisse see Neisse
103 T12 Lautaret, Col du pass SE France
63 G15 Lautaro Araucanía, C Chile
101 F21 Lauter ∿ W Germany
108 I7 Lauterach Vorarlberg, NW Austria
101 I17 Lauterbach Hessen, C Germany
108 E9 Lauterbrunnen Bern, C Switzerland
169 U14 Laut Kecil, Kepulauan island group N Indonesia
187 X14 Lautoka Viti Levu, W Fiji
169 O8 Laut, Pulau prev. Laoet. island Borneo, C Indonesia
169 V14 Laut, Pulau island Kepulauan Natuna, W Indonesia
169 U13 Laut, Selat strait Borneo, C Indonesia
168 H8 Laut Tawar, Danau ◎ Sumatera, NW Indonesia
189 V14 Lauvergne Island island Chuuk, C Micronesia
98 M5 Lauwers Meer ◎ N Netherlands
98 M4 Lauwersoog Groningen, NE Netherlands
102 M14 Lauzerte Tarn-et-Garonne, S France
25 U13 Lavaca Bay bay Texas, SW USA
25 U12 Lavaca River ∿ Texas, SW USA
15 O12 Laval Quebec, SE Canada
102 J6 Laval Mayenne, NW France
15 T6 Laval ∿ Quebec, SE Canada
61 F19 Lavalleja ◆ department S Uruguay
15 O12 Lavaltrie Quebec, SE Canada
186 M10 Lavanggu Rennell, S Solomon Islands
143 O14 Lāvān, Jazīreh-ye island S Iran
109 U8 Lavant ∿ S Austria
118 G5 Lavassaare Ger. Lawassaar. Pärnumaa, SW Estonia
104 L3 La Vecilla de Curueño Castilla-León, N Spain
45 N8 La Vega var. Concepción de la Vega. C Dominican Republic
La Vela see La Vela de Coro
54 J4 La Vela de Coro var. La Vela. Falcón, N Venezuela
103 N17 Lavelanet Ariège, S France
107 M17 Lavello Basilicata, S Italy
36 J8 La Verkin Utah, W USA
26 J8 Laverne Oklahoma, C USA
25 S12 La Vernia Texas, SW USA
93 K18 Lavia Länsi-Suomi, W Finland
14 I12 Lavieille, Lake ◎ Ontario, SE Canada
94 C12 Lavik Sogn og Fjordane, S Norway
La Vila Jojosa see Villajoyosa
33 U10 Lavina Montana, NW USA
194 H5 Lavoisier Island island Antarctica
23 U2 Lavonia Georgia, SE USA
103 R13 la Voulte-sur-Rhône Ardèche, E France
123 W5 Lavrentiya Chukotskiy Avtonomnyy Okrug, NE Russian Federation
115 H20 Lávrio prev. Lávrion. Attikí, C Greece
Lávrion see Lávrio
83 L22 Lavumisa prev. Gollel. SE Swaziland
149 T4 Lawarai Pass pass N Pakistan
Lawassaar see Lavassaare
141 P16 Lawdar SW Yemen
25 Q7 Lawn Texas, SW USA
195 Y4 Law Promontory headland Antarctica
77 O14 Lawra NW Ghana
185 E23 Lawrence Otago, South Island, NZ
31 P14 Lawrence Indiana, N USA
27 Q4 Lawrence Kansas, C USA
19 O10 Lawrence Massachusetts, NE USA
20 L5 Lawrenceburg Kentucky, S USA
20 I10 Lawrenceburg Tennessee, S USA
23 T3 Lawrenceville Georgia, SE USA
31 N15 Lawrenceville Illinois, N USA
21 V7 Lawrenceville Virginia, NE USA
27 S3 Lawson Missouri, C USA
26 L12 Lawton Oklahoma, C USA
140 I4 Lawz, Jabal al ▲ NW Saudi Arabia
95 L16 Laxå Örebro, C Sweden
127 T5 Laya ∿ NW Russian Federation
57 I19 La Yarada Tacna, SW Peru
141 S15 Layjūn C Yemen
141 Q9 Laylā var. Laila. Ar Riyāḍ, C Saudi Arabia
23 P4 Lay Lake ⊞ Alabama, S USA
45 P14 Layou Saint Vincent, Saint Vincent and the Grenadines
La Youne see El Ayoun
192 L5 Laysan Island island Hawaiian Islands, Hawaii, USA, C Pacific Ocean
36 L2 Layton Utah, W USA
34 L5 Laytonville California, W USA
172 H17 Lazare, Pointe headland Mahé, NE Seychelles
123 T12 Lazarev Khabarovskiy Kray, SE Russian Federation
112 L12 Lazarevac Serbia, C Yugoslavia
65 N22 Lazarev Sea sea Antarctica
40 M15 Lázaro Cárdenas Michoacán de Ocampo, SW Mexico
119 F15 Lazdijai Lazdijai, S Lithuania
107 H15 Lazio anc. Latium. ◆ region C Italy
111 A16 Lázně Kynžvart Ger. Bad Königswart. Karlovarský Kraj, W Czech Republic
Lazovsk see Sîngerei
167 R12 Leach Poŭthĭsăt, W Cambodia
27 X9 Leachville Arkansas, C USA
28 I9 Lead South Dakota, N USA
11 S16 Leader Saskatchewan, S Canada
19 S6 Lead Mountain ▲ Maine, NE USA
37 R5 Leadville Colorado, C USA
11 V12 Leaf Rapids Manitoba, C Canada
22 M7 Leaf River ∿ Mississippi, S USA
25 W11 League City Texas, SW USA
23 N7 Leakesville Mississippi, S USA
25 Q11 Leakey Texas, SW USA
Leal see Lihula
83 G15 Lealui Western, W Zambia
Leamhcán see Lucan
14 C18 Leamington Ontario, S Canada
Leamington/Leamington Spa see Royal Leamington Spa
Leammi see Lemmenjoki
25 S10 Leander Texas, SW USA
60 F13 Leandro N.Alem Misiones, NE Argentina
97 A20 Leane, Lough Ir. Loch Léin. ◎ SW Ireland
180 G8 Learmouth Western Australia
Leau see Zoutleeuw
L'Eau d'Heure see Plate Taille, Lac de la
190 D12 Leava Île Futuna, S Wallis and Futuna
27 R3 Leavenworth Kansas, C USA
32 I8 Leavenworth Washington, NW USA
92 L8 Leavvajohka var. Levajok, Lævvajok. Finnmark, N Norway
27 R4 Leawood Kansas, C USA
110 H6 Łeba Ger. Leba. Pomorskie, N Poland
110 I6 Łeba Ger. Leba. ∿ N Poland
101 D20 Lebach Saarland, SW Germany
Łeba, Jezioro see Łebsko, Jezioro
171 P8 Lebak Mindanao, S Philippines
31 O13 Lebanon Indiana, N USA
20 L6 Lebanon Kentucky, S USA
27 U6 Lebanon Missouri, C USA
19 N9 Lebanon New Hampshire, NE USA
32 G12 Lebanon Oregon, NW USA
18 H15 Lebanon Pennsylvania, NE USA
20 J8 Lebanon Tennessee, S USA
21 P7 Lebanon Virginia, NE USA
138 G6 Lebanon off. Republic of Lebanon, Ar. Al Lubnān, Fr. Liban. ◆ republic SW Asia
20 K6 Lebanon Junction Kentucky, S USA
Lebanon, Mount see Liban, Jebel
146 J10 Lebap Lebapskiy Velayat, NE Turkmenistan
146 H11 Lebapskiy Velayat Turkm. Lebap Welayaty; prev. Rus. Chardzhevskaya Oblast', Turkm. Chärjew Oblasty. ◆ province E Turkmenistan
Lebap Welayaty see Lebapskiy Velayat
Lebasee see Łebsko, Jezioro
99 F17 Lebbeke Oost-Vlaanderen, NW Belgium
35 S14 Lebec California, W USA
Lebedin see Lebedyn
123 Q11 Lebedinyy Respublika Sakha (Yakutiya), NE Russian Federation
128 L6 Lebedyan' Lipetskaya Oblast', W Russian Federation
117 T4 Lebedyn Rus. Lebedin. Sums'ka Oblast', NE Ukraine
12 I12 Lebel-sur-Quévillon Quebec, SE Canada
92 L8 Lebesby Finnmark, N Norway
102 M9 le Blanc Indre, C France
27 P5 Lebo Kansas, C USA
79 L15 Lebo Orientale, N Dem. Rep. Congo (Zaire)
110 H6 Lębork var. Lęborg, Ger. Lauenburg, Lauenburg in Pommern. Pomorskie, N Poland
103 O17 le Boulou Pyrénées-Orientales, S France
108 A9 Le Brassus Vaud, W Switzerland
104 J15 Lebrija Andalucía, S Spain
110 G6 Łebsko, Jezioro Ger. Lebasee; prev. Jezioro Łeba. ◎ N Poland
63 F14 Lebu Bío Bío, C Chile
Lebyazh'ye see Akku
104 F6 Leça da Palmeira Porto, N Portugal
103 U15 le Cannet Alpes-Maritimes, SE France
Le Cap see Cap-Haïtien
103 P2 le Cateau-Cambrésis Nord, N France
107 Q18 Lecce Puglia, SE Italy
106 D7 Lecco Lombardia, N Italy
29 V10 Le Center Minnesota, N USA
108 J7 Lech Vorarlberg, W Austria
101 K22 Lech ∿ Austria/Germany
115 D19 Lechainá var. Lehena, Lekhainá. Dytikí Ellás, S Greece
102 J11 le Château d'Oléron Charente-Maritime, W France
103 R3 le Chesne Ardennes, N France
103 R13 le Cheylard Ardèche, E France
108 K7 Lechtaler Alpen ▲ W Austria
100 H6 Leck Schleswig-Holstein, N Germany
14 L9 Lecointre, Lac ◎ Quebec, SE Canada
22 H7 Lecompte Louisiana, S USA
103 Q9 le Creusot Saône-et-Loire, C France
Lecumberri see Lekunberri
110 P13 Łęczna Lubelskie, E Poland
110 J12 Łęczyca Ger. Lentschiza, Rus. Lenchitsa. Łódzkie, C Poland
100 F10 Leda ∿ NW Germany
99 F17 Lede Oost-Vlaanderen, NW Belgium
104 K6 Ledesma Castilla-León, N Spain
45 Q12 le Diamant SW Martinique
172 J16 Le Digue island Inner Islands, NE Seychelles
103 Q10 le Donjon Allier, C France
102 M10 le Dorat Haute-Vienne, C France
Ledo Salinarius see Lons-le-Saunier
11 Q14 Leduc Alberta, SW Canada
123 V7 Ledyanaya, Gora ▲ E Russian Federation
97 C21 Lee Ir. An Laoi. ∿ SW Ireland
29 U5 Leech Lake ◎ Minnesota, N USA
26 K10 Leedey Oklahoma, C USA
97 M17 Leeds N England, UK
23 P4 Leeds Alabama, S USA
29 O3 Leeds North Dakota, N USA
98 N6 Leek Groningen, NE Netherlands
99 K15 Leende Noord-Brabant, SE Netherlands
100 F10 Leer Niedersachsen, NW Germany
98 J13 Leerdam Zuid-Holland, C Netherlands
98 K12 Leersum Utrecht, C Netherlands
23 W11 Leesburg Florida, SE USA
21 V3 Leesburg Virginia, NE USA
27 R4 Lees Summit Missouri, C USA
22 G7 Leesville Louisiana, S USA
25 S12 Leesville Texas, SW USA
31 U13 Leesville Lake ⊞ Ohio, N USA
Leesville Lake see Smith Mountain Lake
183 P9 Leeton New South Wales, SE Australia
98 L6 Leeuwarden Fris. Ljouwert. Friesland, N Netherlands
180 I14 Leeuwin, Cape headland Western Australia
35 R8 Lee Vining California, W USA
45 V8 Leeward Islands island group E West Indies
Leeward Islands see Vent, Îles Sous le, W French Polynesia
Leeward Islands see Sotavento, Ilhas de, Cape Verde
79 G20 Léfini ∿ SE Congo
Léfka see Lefke
115 C17 Lefkáda prev. Levkás. Lefkáda, Iónioi Nísoi, Greece, C Mediterranean Sea
115 B17 Lefkáda It. Santa Maura; prev. Levkás, anc. Leucas. island Iónioi Nísoi, Greece, C Mediterranean Sea
115 H25 Lefká Óri ▲ Kríti, Greece, E Mediterranean Sea
115 B16 Lefkímmi var. Levkímmi. Kérkyra, Iónioi Nísoi, Greece, C Mediterranean Sea
Lefkoşa/Lefkosía see Nicosia
25 O2 Lefors Texas, SW USA
45 R12 le François E Martinique
180 L12 Lefroy, Lake salt lake Western Australia
Legaceaster see Chester
105 N8 Leganés Madrid, C Spain
171 P4 Legaspi off. Legaspi City. Luzon, N Philippines
Leghorn see Livorno
110 M11 Legionowo Mazowieckie, C Poland
99 K24 Léglise Luxembourg, SE Belgium
106 G8 Legnago Lombardia, NE Italy
106 D7 Legnano Veneto, NE Italy
111 F14 Legnica Ger. Liegnitz. Dolnośląskie, SW Poland
35 Q9 Le Grand California, W USA
103 Q15 le Grau-du-Roi Gard, S France
183 U3 Legume New South Wales, SE Australia
102 L4 le Havre Eng. Havre; prev. le Havre-de-Grâce. Seine-Maritime, N France
le Havre-de-Grâce see le Havre
Lehena see Lechainá
36 L3 Lehi Utah, W USA
18 I14 Lehighton Pennsylvania, NE USA
29 O6 Lehr North Dakota, N USA
38 A8 Lehua Island island Hawaiian Islands, Hawaii, USA, C Pacific Ocean
149 S9 Leiāh Punjab, NE Pakistan
109 W9 Leibnitz Steiermark, SE Austria
97 M19 Leicester Lat. Batae Coritanorum. C England, UK
97 M19 Leicestershire cultural region C England, UK
98 H11 Leiden prev. Leyden, anc. Lugdunum Batavorum. Zuid-Holland, W Netherlands
98 H11 Leiderdorp Zuid-Holland, W Netherlands
98 G11 Leidschendam Zuid-Holland, W Netherlands
99 D18 Leie Fr. Lys. ∿ Belgium/France
Leifear see Lifford
184 L4 Leigh Auckland, North Island, NZ
97 K17 Leigh NW England, UK
182 I5 Leigh Creek South Australia
23 O2 Leighton Alabama, S USA
97 M21 Leighton Buzzard E England, UK
Léim an Bhradáin see Leixlip
Léim an Mhadaidh see Limavady
Léime, Ceann see Loop Head, Ireland
Léime, Ceann see Slyne Head, Ireland
101 G20 Leimen Baden-Württemberg, SW Germany
100 I13 Leine ∿ NW Germany
101 J15 Leinefelde Thüringen, C Germany
Léin, Loch see Leane, Lough
97 D19 Leinster Ir. Cúige Laighean. cultural region E Ireland
97 F19 Leinster, Mount Ir. Stua Laighean. ▲ SE Ireland
119 F15 Leipalingis Lazdijai, S Lithuania
92 J12 Leipojärvi Norrbotten, N Sweden
31 R12 Leipsic Ohio, N USA
Leipsic see Leipzig
115 M20 Leipsoí island Dodekánisos, Greece, Aegean Sea
101 M15 Leipzig Pol. Lipsk; hist. Leipsic, anc. Lipsia. Sachsen, E Germany
101 M15 Leipzig Halle ✕ Sachsen, E Germany
104 G9 Leiria anc. Collipo. Leiria, C Portugal
104 F9 Leiria ◆ district C Portugal
95 C15 Leirvik Hordaland, S Norway
118 E5 Leisi Ger. Laisberg. Saaremaa, W Estonia
104 J3 Leitariegos, Puerto de pass NW Spain
20 J6 Leitchfield Kentucky, S USA
109 Y5 Leitha Hung. Lajta. ∿ Austria/Hungary
Leitir Ceanainn see Letterkenny
Leitmeritz see Litoměřice
Leitomischl see Litomyšl
97 D16 Leitrim Ir. Liatroim. cultural region NW Ireland
115 F18 Leivádia prev. Levádhia. Stereá Ellás, C Greece
Leix see Laois
97 F18 Leixlip Eng. Salmon Leap, Ir. Léim an Bhradáin. E Ireland
64 N8 Leixões Porto, N Portugal
161 N12 Leiyang Hunan, S China
160 L16 Leizhou var. Haikang. Guangdong, S China
160 L16 Leizhou Bandao var. Luichow Peninsula. peninsula S China
98 H13 Lek ∿ SW Netherlands
114 I13 Lekánis ▲ NE Greece
172 H13 Le Kartala ▲ Grande Comore, NW Comoros
Le Kef see El Kef
79 G20 Lékéti, Monts de la ▲ S Congo
Lekhainá see Lechainá
114 H8 Lekhchevo Montana, NW Bulgaria
92 G11 Leknes Nordland, C Norway
79 E21 Le Kouilou ◆ province SW Congo
94 L13 Leksand Dalarna, C Sweden
126 H8 Leksozero, Ozero ◎ NW Russian Federation
105 Q3 Lekunberri var. Lecumberri. Navarra, N Spain
171 S11 Lelai, Tanjung headland Pulau Halmahera, N Indonesia
45 Q12 le Lamentin var. Lamentin. C Martinique
45 Q12 le Lamentin ✕ (Fort-de-France) C Martinique
31 P6 Leland Michigan, N USA
22 J4 Leland Mississippi, S USA
95 J16 Lelång var. Lelången. ◎ S Sweden

◆ Country ● Country Capital ◇ Dependent Territory ○ Dependent Territory Capital ◆ Administrative Region ✕ International Airport ▲ Mountain ▲ Mountain Range ✱ Volcano ∿ River ◎ Lake ⊞ Reservoir

Lelången see Lelång
Lel'chitsy see Lyel'chytsy
le Léman see Geneva, Lake
25 O3 **Lelia Lake** Texas, SW USA
113 I14 **Lelija** ▲ SE Bosnia and Herzegovina
108 C8 **Le Locle** Neuchâtel, W Switzerland
189 Y14 **Lelu** Kosrae, E Micronesia
Lelu see Lelu Island
189 Y14 **Lelu Island** *var.* Lelu. *island* Kosrae, E Micronesia
55 W9 **Lelydorp** Wanica, N Surinam
98 K9 **Lelystad** Flevoland, C Netherlands
63 K25 **Le Maire, Estrecho de** *strait* S Argentina
168 L10 **Lemang** Pulau Rangsang, W Indonesia
186 I7 **Lemankoa** Buka Island, NE PNG
Léman, Lac see Geneva, Lake
102 L6 **le Mans** Sarthe, NW France
29 S12 **Le Mars** Iowa, C USA
109 S3 **Lembach im Mühlkreis** Oberösterreich, N Austria
101 G23 **Lemberg** ▲ SW Germany
Lemberg see L'viv
Lemdiyya see Médéa
121 P3 **Lemesós** *var.* Limassol. SW Cyprus
100 H13 **Lemgo** Nordrhein-Westfalen, W Germany
33 P13 **Lemhi Range** ▲ Idaho, NW USA
9 S6 **Lemieux Islands** *island group* Nunavut, NE Canada
171 O11 **Lemito** Sulawesi, N Indonesia
92 L10 **Lemmenjoki** *Lapp.* Leammi. ≈ NE Finland
98 L7 **Lemmer** *Fris.* De Lemmer. Friesland, N Netherlands
28 L7 **Lemmon** South Dakota, N USA
36 M15 **Lemmon, Mount** ▲ Arizona, SW USA
Lemnos see Límnos
31 O14 **Lemon, Lake** ◎ Indiana, N USA
102 J5 **le Mont St-Michel** *castle* Manche, N France
35 Q11 **Lemoore** California, W USA
189 T13 **Lemotol Bay** *bay* Chuuk Islands, C Micronesia
45 Y5 **le Moule** *var.* Moule. Grande Terre, NE Guadeloupe
Lemovices see Limoges
Le Moyen-Ogooué see Moyen-Ogooué
12 M6 **le Moyne, Lac** ◎ Quebec, E Canada
93 L18 **Lempäälä** Länsi-Suomi, W Finland
42 E7 **Lempa, Río** ≈ Central America
42 F7 **Lempira** *prev.* Gracias. ◆ *department* SW Honduras
Lemsalu see Limbaži
107 N17 **Le Murge** ▲ SE Italy
127 V6 **Lemva** ≈ NW Russian Federation
95 F21 **Lemvig** Ringkøbing, W Denmark
166 K8 **Lemyethna** Irrawaddy, SW Myanmar
30 K10 **Lena** Illinois, N USA
131 V4 **Lena** ≈ NE Russian Federation
173 N13 **Lena Tablemount** *undersea feature* S Indian Ocean
Lenchitsa see Łęczyca
59 N17 **Lençóis** Bahia, E Brazil
60 K9 **Lençóis Paulista** São Paulo, S Brazil
109 Y9 **Lendava** *Hung.* Lendva, *Ger.* Unterlimbach; *prev.* Dolnja Lendava. NE Slovenia
83 F20 **Lendepas** Hardap, SE Namibia
126 H9 **Lendery** Respublika Kareliya, NW Russian Federation
Lendum see Lens
Lendva see Lendava
27 R4 **Lenexa** Kansas, C USA
109 Q5 **Lengau** Oberösterreich, N Austria
145 Q17 **Lenger** Yuzhnyy Kazakhstan, S Kazakhstan
159 O9 **Lenghu** Qinghai, C China
159 T9 **Lenglong Ling** ▲ N China
108 D7 **Lengnau** Bern, W Switzerland
160 M12 **Lengshuitan** Hunan, S China
95 M20 **Lenhovda** Kronoberg, S Sweden
79 E20 **Le Niari** ◆ *province* SW Congo
Lenīn see Leninskoye, Kazakhstan
Lenin see Akdepe, Turkmenistan
Leninabad see Khŭjand
Leninakan see Gyumri
Lenina, Pik see Lenin Peak
117 V12 **Lenine** *Rus.* Lenino. Respublika Krym, S Ukraine
Lenīngor see Leninogorsk
147 Q13 **Leningrad** *Rus.* Leningradskiy; *prev.* Mŭ'minobod, *Rus.* Muminabad. SW Tajikistan
Leningrad see Sankt-Peterburg
128 L13 **Leningradskaya** Krasnodarskiy Kray, SW Russian Federation
195 S16 **Leningradskaya** *Russian research station* Antarctica
126 H12 **Leningradskaya Oblast'** ◆ *province* NW Russian Federation
Leningradskiy see Leningrad
Lenino see Lenine, Ukraine
Lenino see Lyenina, Belarus
Leninobod see Khŭjand
145 X9 **Leninogorsk** *Kaz.* Lenīngor. Vostochnyy Kazakhstan, E Kazakhstan
129 T5 **Leninogorsk** Respublika Tatarstan, W Russian Federation
147 T12 **Lenin Peak** *Rus.* Pik Lenina, *Taj.* Qullai Lenin. ▲ Kyrgyzstan/Tajikistan
147 S8 **Leninpol'** Talasskaya Oblast', NW Kyrgyzstan
Lenin, Qullai see Lenin Peak
129 P11 **Leninsk** Volgogradskaya Oblast', SW Russian Federation
Leninsk see Akdepe, Turkmenistan
Leninsk see Asaka, Uzbekistan
Leninsk see Baykonyr, Kazakhstan
145 T8 **Leninskiy** Pavlodar, E Kazakhstan
122 I13 **Leninsk-Kuznetskiy** Kemerovskaya Oblast', S Russian Federation
145 N7 **Leninskoye** *Kaz.* Lenin. Kostanay, N Kazakhstan
127 P15 **Leninskoye** Kirovskaya Oblast', NW Russian Federation
Leninsk-Turkmenski see Chardzhev
Leninváros see Tiszaújváros
Lenkoran' see Länkäran
101 F15 **Lenne** ≈ W Germany
101 G16 **Lennestadt** Nordrhein-Westfalen, W Germany
29 R11 **Lennox** South Dakota, N USA
63 J25 **Lennox, Isla** *Eng.* Lennox Island. *island* S Chile
Lennox Island see Lennox, Isla
21 Q9 **Lenoir** North Carolina, SE USA
20 M9 **Lenoir City** Tennessee, S USA
108 C7 **Le Noirmont** Jura, NW Switzerland
14 L9 **Lenôtre, Lac** ◎ Quebec, SE Canada
29 U15 **Lenox** Iowa, C USA
103 O2 **Lens** *anc.* Lendum, Lentium. Pas-de-Calais, N France
123 O11 **Lensk** Respublika Sakha (Yakutiya), NE Russian Federation
111 F24 **Lenti** Zala, SW Hungary
Lentia see Linz
93 N14 **Lentiira** Oulu, E Finland
107 L25 **Lentini** *anc.* Leontini. Sicilia, Italy, C Mediterranean Sea
Lentium see Lens
Lentschiza see Łęczyca
93 N15 **Lentua** ◎ E Finland
119 H14 **Lentvaris** *Pol.* Landwarów. Trakai, SE Lithuania
108 F7 **Lenzburg** Aargau, N Switzerland
109 R5 **Lenzing** Oberösterreich, N Austria
77 P13 **Léo** SW Burkina
109 V7 **Leoben** Steiermark, C Austria
Leobschütz see Głubczyce
44 L9 **Léogâne** S Haiti
171 O11 **Leok** Sulawesi, N Indonesia
29 O7 **Leola** South Dakota, N USA
97 K20 **Leominster** W England, UK
19 N11 **Leominster** Massachusetts, NE USA
29 V16 **Leon** Iowa, C USA
40 M12 **León** *var.* León de los Aldamas. Guanajuato, C Mexico
42 I10 **León** León, NW Nicaragua
104 L4 **León** Castilla-León, NW Spain
42 I9 **León** ◆ *department* W Nicaragua
104 K4 **León** ◆ *province* Castilla-León, NW Spain
León see Cotopaxi
102 I15 **Léon** Landes, SW France
25 V9 **Leona** Texas, SW USA
180 K11 **Leonara** Western Australia
25 U5 **Leonard** Texas, SW USA
107 H15 **Leonardo da Vinci** *prev.* Fiumicino. × (Roma) Lazio, C Italy
21 X5 **Leonardtown** Maryland, NE USA
25 Q13 **Leona River** ≈ Texas, SW USA
41 Z11 **Leona Vicario** Quintana Roo, SE Mexico
101 H21 **Leonberg** Baden-Württemberg, SW Germany
62 M3 **León, Cerro** ▲ NW Paraguay
León de los Aldamas see León
109 T4 **Leonding** Oberösterreich, N Austria
107 I14 **Leonessa** Lazio, C Italy
107 K24 **Leonforte** Sicilia, Italy, C Mediterranean Sea
183 O13 **Leongatha** Victoria, SE Australia
115 F21 **Leonídi** Pelopónnisos, S Greece
104 J4 **León, Montes de** ▲ NW Spain
25 S8 **Leon River** ≈ Texas, SW USA
Leontini see Lentini
Léopold II, Lac see Mai-Ndombe, Lac
99 J17 **Leopoldsburg** Limburg, NE Belgium
Léopoldville see Kinshasa
26 I5 **Leoti** Kansas, C USA
116 M11 **Leova** *Rus.* Leovo. SW Moldova
Leovo see Leova
102 G8 **le Palais** Morbihan, NW France
27 X10 **Lepanto** Arkansas, C USA
169 N13 **Lepar, Pulau** *island* W Indonesia
104 I14 **Lepe** Andalucía, S Spain
Lepel' see Lyepyel'
83 I19 **Lephepe** Kweneng, SE Botswana
161 Q10 **Leping** Jiangxi, S China
Lépontiennes, Alpes/Lepontine, Alpi see Lepontine Alps
108 G10 **Lepontine Alps** *Fr.* Alpes Lépontiennes, *It.* Alpi Lepontine. ▲ Italy/Switzerland
79 G20 **Le Pool** ◆ *province* S Congo
173 O16 **le Port** NW Réunion
103 N1 **le Portel** Pas-de-Calais, N France
93 N17 **Leppävirta** Itä-Suomi, C Finland
45 Q11 **le Prêcheur** NW Martinique
Lepsi see Lepsy
145 V13 **Lepsy** *Kaz.* Lepsi. Almaty, SE Kazakhstan
145 V13 **Lepsy** *Kaz.* Lepsi. ≈ SE Kazakhstan
Le Puglie see Puglia
103 Q12 **le Puy** *prev.* le Puy-en-Velay, *hist.* Anicium, Podium Anicensis. Haute-Loire, C France
le Puy-en-Velay see le Puy
Le Raizet see le Raizet
45 X11 **le Raizet** *var.* Le Raizet. × (Pointe-à-Pitre) Grande Terre, C Guadeloupe
107 J24 **Lercara Friddi** Sicilia, Italy, C Mediterranean Sea
78 G12 **Léré** Mayo-Kébbi, SW Chad
Leribe see Hlotse
106 E10 **Lerici** Liguria, NW Italy
54 I14 **Lérida** Vaupés, SE Colombia
Lérida see Lleida
105 N5 **Lerma** Castilla-León, N Spain
40 M13 **Lerma, Río** ≈ C Mexico
115 F20 **Lérna** *prehistoric site* Pelopónnisos, S Greece
45 R11 **le Robert** E Martinique
115 M21 **Léros** *island* Dodekánisos, Greece, Aegean Sea
30 L13 **Le Roy** Illinois, N USA
27 Q6 **Le Roy** Kansas, C USA
29 W11 **Le Roy** Minnesota, N USA
18 E10 **Le Roy** New York, NE USA
Lerrnayin Gharabakh see Nagornyy Karabakh
95 J19 **Lerum** Västra Götaland, S Sweden
96 M2 **Lerwick** NE Scotland, UK
45 Y6 **les Abymes** *var.* Abymes. Grande Terre, C Guadeloupe
les Albères see Albères, Chaîne des
102 M4 **les Andelys** Eure, N France
45 Q12 **les Anses-d'Arlets** SW Martinique
105 U6 **Les Borges Blanques** *var.* Borjas Blancas. Cataluña, NE Spain
Lesbos see Lésvos
Les Cayes see Cayes
31 Q4 **Les Cheneaux Islands** *island* Michigan, N USA
103 T12 **les Écrins** ▲ E France
108 C10 **Le Sépey** Vaud, W Switzerland
15 T7 **Les Escoumins** Quebec, SE Canada
Les Gonaïves see Gonaïves
Lesh/Leshi see Lezhë
160 H9 **Leshan** Sichuan, C China
108 D11 **Les Haudères** Valais, SW Switzerland
102 J9 **les Herbiers** Vendée, NW France
127 O8 **Leshukonskoye** Arkhangel'skaya Oblast', NW Russian Federation
Lesina see Hvar
107 M15 **Lesina, Lago di** ◎ SE Italy
114 K13 **Lesítse** ▲ NE Greece
94 G10 **Lesja** Oppland, S Norway
95 L15 **Lesjöfors** Värmland, C Sweden
111 O18 **Lesko** Podkarpackie, SE Poland
113 O15 **Leskovac** Serbia, SE Yugoslavia
113 M22 **Leskovik** *var.* Leskoviku. Korçë, S Albania
Leskoviku see Leskovik
33 P14 **Leslie** Idaho, NW USA
31 Q10 **Leslie** Michigan, N USA
Leśna/Lesnaya see Lyasnaya
102 F5 **Lesneven** Finistère, NW France
112 J11 **Lešnica** Serbia, W Yugoslavia
127 S13 **Lesnoy** Kirovskaya Oblast', NW Russian Federation
122 K12 **Lesosibirsk** Krasnoyarskiy Kray, C Russian Federation
83 J23 **Lesotho** *off.* Kingdom of Lesotho; *prev.* Basutoland. ◆ *monarchy* S Africa
102 J12 **Lesparre-Médoc** Gironde, SW France
108 C8 **Les Ponts-de-Martel** Neuchâtel, W Switzerland
102 I9 **les Sables-d'Olonne** Vendée, NW France
103 P1 **Lesquin** × Nord, N France
109 S7 **Lessach** *var.* Lessachbach. ≈ E Austria
Lessachbach see Lessach
45 W11 **les Saintes** *var.* Îles des Saintes. *island group* S Guadeloupe
74 L5 **Les Salines** × (Annaba) NE Algeria
99 J22 **Lesse** ≈ SE Belgium
95 M21 **Lessebo** Kronoberg, S Sweden
194 M10 **Lesser Antarctica** *var.* West Antarctica. *physical region* Antarctica
45 P15 **Lesser Antilles** *island group* E West Indies
137 T10 **Lesser Caucasus** *Rus.* Malyy Kavkaz. ▲ SW Asia
Lesser Khingan Range see Xiao Hinggan Ling
11 P13 **Lesser Slave Lake** ◎ Alberta, W Canada
Lesser Sunda Islands see Nusa Tenggara
99 E19 **Lessines** Hainaut, SW Belgium
103 R16 **les Stes-Maries-de-la-Mer** Bouches-du-Rhône, SE France
14 G15 **Lester B.Pearson** *var.* Toronto. × (Toronto) Ontario, S Canada
29 U9 **Lester Prairie** Minnesota, N USA
93 L16 **Lestijärvi** Länsi-Suomi, W Finland
L'Estuaire see Estuaire
29 U9 **Le Sueur** Minnesota, N USA
108 B8 **Les Verrières** Neuchâtel, W Switzerland
115 L17 **Lésvos** *anc.* Lesbos. *island* E Greece
110 G12 **Leszno** *Ger.* Lissa. Wielkopolskie, C Poland
83 L20 **Letaba** Northern, NE South Africa
173 P17 **le Tampon** SW Réunion
97 O21 **Letchworth** E England, UK
111 G25 **Letenye** Zala, SW Hungary
11 Q17 **Lethbridge** Alberta, SW Canada
55 S11 **Lethem** S Guyana
83 H18 **Letiahau** ≈ W Botswana
54 J18 **Leticia** Amazonas, S Colombia
171 S16 **Leti, Kepulauan** *island group* E Indonesia
83 I18 **Letlhakane** Central, C Botswana
83 H20 **Letlhakeng** Kweneng, SE Botswana
114 J8 **Letnitsa** Lovech, N Bulgaria
103 N1 **le Touquet-Paris-Plage** Pas-de-Calais, N France
166 L8 **Letpadan** Pegu, SW Myanmar
166 K6 **Letpan** Arakan State, W Myanmar
102 M2 **le Tréport** Seine-Maritime, N France
166 M12 **Letsôk-aw Kyun** *var.* Letsutan Island; *prev.* Domel Island. *island* Mergui Archipelago, S Myanmar
Letsutan Island see Letsôk-aw Kyun
97 E14 **Letterkenny** *Ir.* Leitir Ceanainn. NW Ireland
Lettland see Latvia
116 M6 **Letychiv** Khmel'nyts'ka Oblast', W Ukraine
Lëtzebuerg see Luxembourg
116 H14 **Leu** Dolj, SW Romania
Leucas see Lefkáda
103 P17 **Leucate** Aude, S France
103 P17 **Leucate, Étang de** ◎ S France
108 E10 **Leuk** Valais, SW Switzerland
108 E10 **Leukerbad** Valais, SW Switzerland
Leusden see Leusden-Centrum
98 K11 **Leusden-Centrum** *var.* Leusden. Utrecht, C Netherlands
Leutensdorf see Litvínov
Leutschau see Levoča
99 H18 **Leuven** *Fr.* Louvain, *Ger.* Löwen. Vlaams Brabant, C Belgium
99 I20 **Leuze** Namur, C Belgium
Leuze see Leuze-en-Hainaut
99 E19 **Leuze-en-Hainaut** *var.* Leuze. Hainaut, SW Belgium
Léva see Levice
Levádhia see Leivádia
Levajok see Leavvajohka
36 L4 **Levan** Utah, W USA
93 E16 **Levanger** Nord-Trøndelag, C Norway
121 S12 **Levantine Basin** *undersea feature* E Mediterranean Sea
106 D10 **Levanto** Liguria, W Italy
107 H23 **Levanzo, Isola di** *island* Isole Egadi, S Italy
129 Q17 **Levashi** Respublika Dagestan, SW Russian Federation
24 M5 **Levelland** Texas, SW USA
39 P13 **Levelock** Alaska, USA
101 E16 **Leverkusen** Nordrhein-Westfalen, W Germany
111 J21 **Levice** *Ger.* Lewentz, Lewenz, *Hung.* Léva. Nitriansky Kraj, SW Slovakia
106 G6 **Levico Terme** Trentino-Alto Adige, N Italy
115 E20 **Levídi** Pelopónnisos, S Greece
103 P14 **le Vigan** Gard, S France
184 L13 **Levin** Manawatu-Wanganui, North Island, NZ
15 R10 **Lévis** *var.* Levis. Quebec, SE Canada
21 P6 **Levisa Fork** ≈ Kentucky/Virginia, S USA
115 L21 **Levítha** *island* Kykládes, Greece, Aegean Sea
18 L14 **Levittown** Long Island, New York, NE USA
18 J15 **Levittown** Pennsylvania, NE USA
Levkás see Lefkáda
Levkímmi see Lefkímmi
111 L19 **Levoča** *Ger.* Leutschau, *Hung.* Lőcse. Prešovský Kraj, E Slovakia
Lévrier, Baie du see Nouâdhibou, Dakhlet
103 N9 **Levroux** Indre, C France
114 J8 **Levski** Pleven, N Bulgaria
Levskigrad see Karlovo
128 L6 **Lev Tolstoy** Lipetskaya Oblast', W Russian Federation
187 X14 **Levuka** Ovalau, C Fiji
166 L6 **Lewe** Mandalay, C Myanmar
Lewentz/Lewenz see Levice
97 O23 **Lewes** SE England, UK
21 Z4 **Lewes** Delaware, NE USA
29 Q12 **Lewis and Clark Lake** ⊠ Nebraska/South Dakota, N USA
18 G14 **Lewisburg** Pennsylvania, NE USA
20 J10 **Lewisburg** Tennessee, S USA
21 S6 **Lewisburg** West Virginia, NE USA
96 F6 **Lewis, Butt of** *headland* NW Scotland, UK
96 F7 **Lewis, Isle of** *island* NW Scotland, UK
35 U4 **Lewis, Mount** ▲ Nevada, W USA
185 H16 **Lewis Pass** *pass* South Island, NZ
33 P7 **Lewis Range** ▲ Montana, NW USA
23 O3 **Lewis Smith Lake** ⊠ Alabama, S USA
32 M10 **Lewiston** Idaho, NW USA
19 P7 **Lewiston** Maine, NE USA
29 X10 **Lewiston** Minnesota, N USA
18 D9 **Lewiston** New York, NE USA
36 L1 **Lewiston** Utah, W USA
30 K13 **Lewistown** Illinois, N USA
33 T9 **Lewistown** Montana, NW USA
27 T14 **Lewisville** Arkansas, C USA
25 T6 **Lewisville** Texas, SW USA
25 T6 **Lewisville, Lake** ⊠ Texas, SW USA
Le Woleu-Ntem see Woleu-Ntem
23 U3 **Lexington** Georgia, SE USA
20 M5 **Lexington** Kentucky, S USA
22 L4 **Lexington** Mississippi, S USA
27 S4 **Lexington** Missouri, C USA
29 N16 **Lexington** Nebraska, C USA
20 S9 **Lexington** North Carolina, SE USA
27 N11 **Lexington** Oklahoma, C USA
21 R12 **Lexington** South Carolina, SE USA
20 G9 **Lexington** Tennessee, S USA
25 T10 **Lexington** Texas, SW USA
21 T6 **Lexington** Virginia, NE USA
21 X5 **Lexington Park** Maryland, NE USA
Leyden see Leiden
102 J14 **Leyre** ≈ SW France
171 Q5 **Leyte** *island* C Philippines
171 Q6 **Leyte Gulf** *gulf* E Philippines
111 O16 **Leżajsk** Podkarpackie, SE Poland
Lezha see Lezhë
113 K18 **Lezhë** *var.* Lezha; *prev.* Lesh, Leshi. Lezhë, NW Albania
113 K18 **Lezhë** ◆ *district* NW Albania
103 O16 **Lézignan-Corbières** Aude, S France
128 J7 **L'gov** Kurskaya Oblast', W Russian Federation
159 P15 **Lhari** Xizang Zizhiqu, W China
159 N16 **Lhasa** *var.* La-sa, Lassa. Xizang Zizhiqu, W China
159 O15 **Lhasa He** ≈ W China
158 K16 **Lhazê** Xizang Zizhiqu, W China
158 K14 **Lhazhong** Xizang Zizhiqu, W China
168 H7 **Lhoksukon** Sumatera, W Indonesia
159 Q15 **Lhorong** Xizang Zizhiqu, W China
105 W6 **L'Hospitalet de Llobregat** *var.* Hospitalet. Cataluña, NE Spain
153 R11 **Lhotse** ▲ China/Nepal
159 N17 **Lhozhag** Xizang Zizhiqu, W China
159 O16 **Lhünzê** Xizang Zizhiqu, W China
159 N15 **Lhünzhub** *var.* Poindo. Xizang Zizhiqu, W China
167 N8 **Li** Lamphun, NW Thailand
Liancheng see Qinglong
161 P12 **Liancheng** Fujian, SE China
160 K9 **Liangping** Chongqing Shi, C China
Liangzhou see Wuwei
161 O9 **Liangzi Hu** ◎ C China
161 R12 **Lianjiang** Fujian, SE China
160 L15 **Lianjiang** Guangdong, S China
161 O13 **Lianping** Guangdong, S China
163 T13 **Lianshan** *prev.* Jinxi. Liaoning, NE China
Lian Xian see Lianzhou
160 M11 **Lianyuan** *prev.* Lantian. Hunan, S China
161 Q6 **Lianyungang** *var.* Xinpu. Jiangsu, E China
161 N13 **Lianzhou** *var.* Linxian; *prev.* Lian Xian. Guangdong, S China
Liao see Liaoning
161 P5 **Liaocheng** Shandong, E China
163 U13 **Liaodong Bandao** *var.* Liaotung Peninsula. *peninsula* NE China
163 T13 **Liaodong Wan** *Eng.* Gulf of Lantung, Gulf of Liaotung. *gulf* NE China
163 U11 **Liao He** ≈ NE China
163 W12 **Liao Ling** ▲ NE China
163 U12 **Liaoning** *var.* Liao, Liaoning Sheng, Shengking; *hist.* Fengtien, Shenking. ◆ *province* NE China
Liaoning Sheng see Liaoning
Liaotung, Gulf of see Liaodong Wan
Liaotung Peninsula see Liaodong Bandao
163 V12 **Liaoyang** *var.* Liao-yang. Liaoning, NE China
163 V11 **Liaoyuan** *var.* Dongliao, Shuang-liao, *Jap.* Chengchiatun. Jilin, NE China
163 U12 **Liaozhong** Liaoning, NE China
Liaqatabad see Piplān
10 M10 **Liard** ≈ W Canada
Liard see Fort Liard
10 L10 **Liard River** British Columbia, W Canada
149 O15 **Liāri** Baluchistān, SW Pakistan
Liatroim see Leitrim
189 S6 **Lib** *var.* Ellep. *island* Ralik Chain, C Marshall Islands
Liban see Lebanon
138 H6 **Liban, Jebel** *Ar.* Jabal al Gharbt, Jabal Lubnān, *Eng.* Mount Lebanon. ▲ C Lebanon
Libau see Liepāja
33 N7 **Libby** Montana, NW USA
79 I16 **Libenge** Equateur, NW Dem. Rep. Congo (Zaire)
26 I7 **Liberal** Kansas, C USA
27 R7 **Liberal** Missouri, C USA
Liberalitas Julia see Évora
111 D15 **Liberec** *Ger.* Reichenberg. Liberecký Kraj, N Czech Republic
111 D15 **Liberecký Kraj** ◆ *region* N Czech Republic
42 K12 **Liberia** Guanacaste, NW Costa Rica
76 K17 **Liberia** *off.* Republic of Liberia. ◆ *republic* W Africa
61 D16 **Libertad** Corrientes, NE Argentina
61 E20 **Libertad** San José, S Uruguay
54 I7 **Libertad** Barinas, NW Venezuela
54 K6 **Libertad** Cojedes, N Venezuela
62 G12 **Libertador** *off.* Región del Libertador General Bernardo O'Higgins. ◆ *region* C Chile
Libertador General San Martín see Ciudad de Libertador General San Martín
20 L6 **Liberty** Kentucky, S USA
22 J7 **Liberty** Mississippi, S USA
27 R4 **Liberty** Missouri, C USA
18 J12 **Liberty** New York, NE USA
21 T9 **Liberty** North Carolina, SE USA
Libian Desert see Libyan Desert
99 J23 **Libin** Luxembourg, SE Belgium
160 K13 **Libo** Guizhou, S China
Libohova see Libohovë
113 L23 **Libohovë** *var.* Libohova. Gjirokastër, S Albania
81 K18 **Liboi** North Eastern, E Kenya
102 K13 **Libourne** Gironde, SW France
99 K23 **Libramont** Luxembourg, SE Belgium
113 M20 **Librazhd** *var.* Librazhdi. Elbasan, E Albania
Librazhdi see Librazhd
79 C18 **Libreville** ● (Gabon) Estuaire, NW Gabon
75 P10 **Libya** *off.* Socialist People's Libyan Arab Jamahiriya, *Ar.* Al Jamāhīrīyah al 'Arabīyah al Lībīyah ash Sha'bīyah al Ishtirākīyah; *prev.* Libyan Arab Republic. ◆ *Islamic state* N Africa
75 T11 **Libyan Desert** *var.* Libian Desert, *Ar.* Aş Şahrā' al Lībīyah. *desert* N Africa
75 T8 **Libyan Plateau** *var.* Aḍ Diffah. *plateau* Egypt/Libya
Lībīyah, Aş Şahrā' al see Libyan Desert
62 G12 **Licantén** Maule, C Chile
107 J25 **Licata** *anc.* Phintias. Sicilia, Italy, C Mediterranean Sea
137 P14 **Lice** Diyarbakır, SE Turkey
97 L19 **Lichfield** C England, UK
83 N14 **Lichinga** Niassa, N Mozambique
109 V3 **Lichtenau** Niederösterreich, N Austria
83 I21 **Lichtenburg** North-West, N South Africa
101 K18 **Lichtenfels** Bayern, SE Germany
98 O12 **Lichtenvoorde** Gelderland, E Netherlands
Lichtenwald see Sevnica
99 C17 **Lichtervelde** West-Vlaanderen, W Belgium
160 L9 **Lichuan** Hubei, C China
27 V7 **Licking** Missouri, C USA
20 M4 **Licking River** ≈ Kentucky, S USA
112 C11 **Lički Osik** Lika-Senj, C Croatia
Ličko-Senjska Županija see Lika-Senj
107 K19 **Licosa, Punta** *headland* S Italy
119 H16 **Lida** *Rus.* Lida. Hrodzyenskaya Voblasts', W Belarus
93 H17 **Liden** Västernorrland, C Sweden
29 R7 **Lidgerwood** North Dakota, N USA
Lidhorikíon see Lidoríki
95 K21 **Lidhult** Kronoberg, S Sweden
95 P16 **Lidingö** Stockholm, C Sweden
95 K17 **Lidköping** Västra Götaland, S Sweden
Lido di Iesolo see Lido di Jesolo
106 I8 **Lido di Jesolo** *var.* Lido di Iesolo. Veneto, NE Italy
107 H15 **Lido di Ostia** Lazio, C Italy
Lidokhorikion see Lidoríki
115 E18 **Lidoríki** *prev.* Lidhorikíon, Lidokhorikion. Stereá Ellás, C Greece
110 K9 **Lidzbark** Warmińsko-Mazurskie, NE Poland
110 L7 **Lidzbark Warmiński** *Ger.* Heilsberg. Warmińsko-Mazurskie, NE Poland
109 U3 **Liebenau** Oberösterreich, N Austria
181 P7 **Liebig, Mount** ▲ Northern Territory, C Australia
109 V8 **Lieboch** Steiermark, SE Austria
108 I8 **Liechtenstein** *off.* Principality of Liechtenstein. ◆ *principality* C Europe
99 F18 **Liedekerke** Vlaams Brabant, C Belgium
99 K19 **Liège** *Dut.* Luik, *Ger.* Lüttich. Liège, E Belgium
99 K20 **Liège** *Dut.* Luik. ◆ *province* E Belgium
Liegnitz see Legnica
93 O16 **Lieksa** Itä-Suomi, E Finland
118 F10 **Lielupe** ≈ Latvia/Lithuania
118 G9 **Lielvārde** Ogre, C Latvia
167 U13 **Liên Hương** *var.* Tuy Phong. Binh Thuân, S Vietnam
Liên Nghia see Đuc Trong
109 P9 **Lienz** Tirol, W Austria
118 B10 **Liepāja** *Ger.* Libau. Liepāja, W Latvia
99 H17 **Lier** *Fr.* Lierre. Antwerpen, N Belgium
95 H15 **Lierbyen** Buskerud, S Norway
99 L21 **Lierneux** Liège, E Belgium
Lierre see Lier
101 D18 **Lieser** ≈ W Germany
109 U7 **Liesing** ≈ E Austria
108 E6 **Liestal** Basel-Land, N Switzerland
Lietuva see Lithuania
Lievenhof see Līvāni
103 O2 **Liévin** Pas-de-Calais, N France
14 M9 **Lièvre, Rivière du** ≈ Quebec, SE Canada
109 T6 **Liezen** Steiermark, C Austria
97 E14 **Lifford** *Ir.* Leifear. NW Ireland
187 Q16 **Lifou** *island* Îles Loyauté, E New Caledonia
193 Y15 **Lifuka** *island* Ha'apai Group, C Tonga
171 P4 **Ligao** Luzon, N Philippines
Liger see Loire
42 H2 **Lighthouse Reef** *reef* E Belize
183 Q4 **Lightning Ridge** New South Wales, SE Australia
103 N9 **Lignières** Cher, C France
103 S5 **Ligny-en-Barrois** Meuse, NE France
83 P15 **Ligonha** ≈ NE Mozambique
31 P11 **Ligonier** Indiana, N USA
81 I25 **Ligunga** Ruvuma, S Tanzania
106 D9 **Ligure, Appennino** *Eng.* Ligurian Mountains. ▲ NW Italy
Ligure, Mar see Ligurian Sea
106 C9 **Liguria** ◆ *region* NW Italy
Ligurian Mountains see Ligure, Appennino
120 K6 **Ligurian Sea** *Fr.* Mer Ligurienne, *It.* Mar Ligure. *sea* N Mediterranean Sea

◆ Country ● Country Capital ◇ Dependent Territory ○ Dependent Territory Capital ◆ Administrative Region × International Airport ▲ Mountain ▲ Mountain Range ⚠ Volcano ≈ River ◎ Lake ⊠ Reservoir

Ligurienne, Mer see Ligurian Sea
186 H5 **Lihir Group** island group NE PNG
38 B8 **Līhue** Haw. Lihu'e. Kauai, Hawaii, USA, C Pacific Ocean
118 F5 **Lihula** Ger. Leal. Läänemaa, W Estonia
126 I2 **Liinakhamari** var. Linacmamari. Murmanskaya Oblast', NW Russian Federation
Liivi Laht see Riga, Gulf of
160 F11 **Lijiang** var. Dayan, Lijiang Naxizu Zizhixian. Yunnan, SW China
112 C11 **Lika-Senj** off. Ličko-Senjska Županija. ◆ province W Croatia
79 N25 **Likasi** prev. Jadotville. Katanga, SE Dem. Rep. Congo (Zaire)
79 L16 **Likati** Orientale, N Dem. Rep. Congo (Zaire)
10 M15 **Likely** British Columbia, SW Canada
153 Y11 **Likhapāni** Assam, NE India
126 J16 **Likhoslavl'** Tverskaya Oblast', W Russian Federation
189 U5 **Likiep Atoll** atoll Ratak Chain, C Marshall Islands
95 D18 **Liknes** Vest-Agder, S Norway
79 H18 **Likouala** ~ N Congo
79 H18 **Likouala aux Herbes** ~ E Congo
190 B16 **Liku** E Niue
Likupang, Selat see Bangka, Selat
27 Y8 **Lilbourn** Missouri, C USA
103 X14 **l'Île-Rousse** Corse, France, C Mediterranean Sea
109 W5 **Lilienfeld** Niederösterreich, NE Austria
161 N11 **Liling** Hunan, S China
95 J18 **Lilla Edet** Västra Götaland, S Sweden
103 P1 **Lille** var. l'Isle, Dut. Rijssel, Flem. Ryssel; prev. Lisle, anc. Insula. Nord, N France
95 G24 **Lillebælt** var. Lille Bælt, Eng. Little Belt. strait S Denmark
102 L3 **Lillebonne** Seine-Maritime, N France
94 H12 **Lillehammer** Oppland, S Norway
103 O1 **Lillers** Pas-de-Calais, N France
95 F18 **Lillesand** Aust-Agder, S Norway
95 I15 **Lillestrøm** Akershus, S Norway
93 F18 **Lillhärdal** Jämtland, C Sweden
21 U10 **Lillington** North Carolina, SE USA
105 O9 **Lillo** Castilla-La Mancha, C Spain
10 M16 **Lillooet** British Columbia, SW Canada
83 M14 **Lilongwe** ● (Malawi) Central, W Malawi
83 M14 **Lilongwe** ✕ Central, W Malawi
83 M14 **Lilongwe** ~ W Malawi
171 P7 **Liloy** Mindanao, S Philippines
Lilybaeum see Marsala
182 J7 **Lilydale** South Australia
183 P16 **Lilydale** Tasmania, SE Australia
113 J14 **Lim** ~ Bosnia and Herzegovina/Yugoslavia
57 D15 **Lima** ● (Peru) Lima, W Peru
94 K13 **Lima** Dalarna, C Sweden
31 R12 **Lima** Ohio, NE USA
57 D14 **Lima** ◆ department W Peru
Lima see Jorge Chávez International
104 G5 **Lima, Rio** Sp. Limia ~ Portugal/Spain see also Limia
111 L17 **Limanowa** Małopolskie, S Poland
168 M11 **Limas** Pulau Sebangka, W Indonesia
Limassol see Lemesós
97 F14 **Limavady** Ir. Léim an Mhadaidh. NW Northern Ireland, UK
63 J14 **Limay Mahuida** La Pampa, C Argentina
63 H15 **Limay, Río** ~ W Argentina
101 N16 **Limbach-Oberfrohna** Sachsen, E Germany
81 F22 **Limba Limba** ~ C Tanzania
107 C17 **Limbara, Monte** ▲ Sardegna, Italy, C Mediterranean Sea
118 G7 **Limbaži** Est. Lemsalu. Limbaži, N Latvia
44 M8 **Limbé** N Haiti
99 L19 **Limbourg** Liège, E Belgium
99 K17 **Limburg** ◆ province NE Belgium
99 L16 **Limburg** ◆ province SE Netherlands
101 F17 **Limburg an der Lahn** Hessen, W Germany
94 K13 **Limedsforsen** Dalarna, C Sweden
60 L9 **Limeira** São Paulo, S Brazil
97 C19 **Limerick** Ir. Luimneach. SW Ireland
97 C20 **Limerick** Ir. Luimneach. cultural region SW Ireland
19 S2 **Limestone** Maine, NE USA
25 U9 **Limestone, Lake** ⊚ Texas, SW USA
39 P12 **Lime Village** Alaska, USA
95 F20 **Limfjorden** fjord N Denmark
95 J23 **Limhamn** Skåne, S Sweden
104 H5 **Limia** Port. Rio Lima ~ Portugal/ Spain see also Lima, Rio
93 L14 **Liminka** Oulu, C Finland
Limín Vathéos see Sámos
115 G17 **Límni** Évvoia, C Greece
115 J15 **Límnos** anc. Lemnos. island E Greece
102 M11 **Limoges** anc. Augustoritum Lemovicensium, Lemovices. Haute-Vienne, C France
37 U5 **Limon** Colorado, C USA
43 O13 **Limón** var. Puerto Limón. Limón, E Costa Rica
42 K4 **Limón** Colón, NE Honduras
43 N13 **Limón** off. Provincia de Limón. ◆ province E Costa Rica
106 A10 **Limone Piemonte** Piemonte, NE Italy
Limones see Valdéz
Limonum see Poitiers
103 N11 **Limousin** ◆ region C France
103 N16 **Limoux** Aude, S France
83 L19 **Limpopo** var. Crocodile. ~ S Africa
160 K17 **Limu Ling** ▲ S China
113 M20 **Lin** var. Lini. Elbasan, E Albania
Linacmamari see Liinakhamari
62 G13 **Linares** Maule, C Chile
54 C13 **Linares** Nariño, SW Colombia
41 O9 **Linares** Nuevo León, NE Mexico
105 N12 **Linares** Andalucía, S Spain
107 G15 **Linaro, Capo** headland C Italy
106 D8 **Linate** ✕ (Milano) Lombardia, N Italy
160 F13 **Lincang** Yunnan, SW China
161 P11 **Linchuan** var. Fuzhou. Jiangxi, S China
61 B20 **Lincoln** Buenos Aires, E Argentina
185 H19 **Lincoln** Canterbury, South Island, NZ
97 N18 **Lincoln** anc. Lindum, Lindum Colonia. E England, UK
35 O6 **Lincoln** California, W USA
30 L13 **Lincoln** Illinois, N USA
26 M4 **Lincoln** Kansas, C USA
19 S5 **Lincoln** Maine, NE USA
27 T5 **Lincoln** Missouri, C USA
29 R16 **Lincoln** state capital Nebraska, C USA
32 F11 **Lincoln City** Oregon, NW USA
167 X10 **Lincoln Island** island E Paracel Islands
197 Q11 **Lincoln Sea** sea Arctic Ocean
97 N18 **Lincolnshire** cultural region E England, UK
21 R10 **Lincolnton** North Carolina, SE USA
25 V7 **Lindale** Texas, SW USA
101 I25 **Lindau** var. Lindau am Bodensee. Bayern, S Germany
Lindau am Bodensee see Lindau
123 P9 **Linde** ~ NE Russian Federation
55 T9 **Linden** E Guyana
23 O6 **Linden** Alabama, S USA
20 H9 **Linden** Tennessee, S USA
25 X6 **Linden** Texas, SW USA
18 J16 **Lindenwold** New Jersey, NE USA
95 M15 **Lindesberg** Örebro, C Sweden
95 D18 **Lindesnes** headland S Norway
Líndhos see Líndos
81 K24 **Lindi** Lindi, SE Tanzania
81 J24 **Lindi** ◆ region SE Tanzania
79 N17 **Lindi** ~ NE Dem. Rep. Congo (Zaire)
163 V7 **Lindian** Heilongjiang, NE China
185 E21 **Lindis Pass** pass South Island, NZ
83 J22 **Lindley** Free State, C South Africa
95 J19 **Lindome** Västra Götaland, S Sweden
Lindong see Bairin Zuoqi
115 O23 **Líndos** var. Líndhos. Ródos, Dodekánisos, Greece, Aegean Sea
14 I14 **Lindsay** Ontario, SE Canada
35 R11 **Lindsay** California, W USA
33 X8 **Lindsay** Montana, NW USA
27 N11 **Lindsay** Oklahoma, C USA
27 N5 **Lindsborg** Kansas, C USA
95 N21 **Lindsdal** Kalmar, S Sweden
Lindum/Lindum Colonia see Lincoln
191 W3 **Line Islands** island group E Kiribati
Linëvo see Linova
160 M5 **Linfen** var. Lin-fen. Shanxi, C China
155 F18 **Linganamakki Reservoir** ⊡ SW India
160 L17 **Lingao** Hainan, S China
171 N3 **Lingayen** Luzon, N Philippines
160 M6 **Lingbao** var. Guolüezhen. Henan, C China
94 N12 **Lingbo** Gävleborg, C Sweden
Lingeh see Bandar-e Langeh
100 E12 **Lingen** var. Lingen an der Ems. Niedersachsen, NW Germany
Lingen an der Ems see Lingen
168 M11 **Lingga, Kepulauan** island group W Indonesia
168 L11 **Lingga, Pulau** island Kepulauan Lingga, W Indonesia
14 J14 **Lingham Lake** ⊚ Ontario, SE Canada
94 M13 **Linghed** Dalarna, C Sweden
33 Z15 **Lingle** Wyoming, C USA
18 G15 **Linglestown** Pennsylvania, NE USA
79 K18 **Lingomo II** Equateur, NW Dem. Rep. Congo (Zaire)
160 L15 **Lingshan** Guangxi Zhuangzu Zizhiqu, S China
160 L17 **Lingshui** Hainan, S China
155 G16 **Lingsugūr** Karnātaka, C India
107 L23 **Linguaglossa** Sicilia, Italy, C Mediterranean Sea
76 H10 **Linguère** N Senegal
159 W8 **Lingwu** Ningxia, N China
Lingxi see Yongshun
161 O12 **Lingxian** var. Ling Xian. Hunan, S China
163 S12 **Lingyuan** Liaoning, NE China
163 U4 **Linhai** Heilongjiang, NE China
161 S10 **Linhai** var. Taizhou. Zhejiang, SE China
59 O20 **Linhares** Espírito Santo, SE Brazil
162 M13 **Linhe** Nei Mongol Zizhiqu, N China
Lini see Lin
139 S1 **Līnik, Chiyā-ē** ▲ N Iraq
95 M18 **Linköping** Östergötland, S Sweden
163 Y8 **Linkou** Heilongjiang, NE China
118 F11 **Linkuva** Pakruojis, N Lithuania
27 V5 **Linn** Missouri, C USA
25 S16 **Linn** Texas, SW USA
27 T2 **Linneus** Missouri, C USA
96 H10 **Linnhe, Loch** inlet W Scotland, UK
119 G19 **Linova** Rus. Linëvo. Brestskaya Voblasts', SW Belarus
161 O5 **Linqing** Shandong, E China
161 N6 **Linruzhen** Henan, C China
60 K8 **Lins** São Paulo, S Brazil
93 F17 **Linsell** Jämtland, C Sweden
160 J9 **Linshui** Sichuan, C China
44 K12 **Linstead** C Jamaica
159 U11 **Lintan** Gansu, N China
159 V11 **Lintao** Gansu, C China
15 S12 **Lintère** ~ Quebec, SE Canada
108 H8 **Linth** ~ NW Switzerland
108 H8 **Linthal** Glarus, NE Switzerland
31 N15 **Linton** Indiana, N USA
29 N6 **Linton** North Dakota, N USA
163 R11 **Linxi** Nei Mongol Zizhiqu, N China
159 U11 **Linxia** var. Linxia Huizu Zizhizhou. Gansu, C China
Linxia Huizu Zizhizhou see Linxia
Linxian see Lianzhou
161 Q6 **Linyi** Shandong, S China
161 P4 **Linyi** Shandong, E China
160 M6 **Linyi** Shanxi, C China
109 T4 **Linz** anc. Lentia. Oberösterreich, N Austria
159 S8 **Linze** var. Shahepu. Gansu, N China
44 J13 **Lionel Town** C Jamaica
103 Q16 **Lion, Golfe du** Eng. Gulf of Lion, Gulf of Lions; anc. Sinus Gallicus. gulf S France
Lion, Gulf of/Lions, Gulf of see Lion, Golfe du
83 K16 **Lions Den** Mashonaland West, N Zimbabwe
14 F13 **Lion's Head** Ontario, S Canada
Lios Ceannúir, Bá see Liscannor Bay
Lios Mór see Lismore
Lios na gCearrbhach see Lisburn
Lios Tuathail see Listowel
79 G17 **Liouesso** La Sangha, N Congo
Liozno see Lyozna
171 O4 **Lipa** off. Lipa City. Luzon, N Philippines
25 S7 **Lipan** Texas, SW USA
Lipari Islands/Lipari, Isole see Eolie, Isole
107 L22 **Lipari, Isola** island Isole Eolie, S Italy
116 L8 **Lipcani** Rus. Lipkany. N Moldova
93 N17 **Liperi** Itä-Suomi, E Finland
128 L7 **Lipetsk** Lipetskaya Oblast', W Russian Federation
128 K6 **Lipetskaya Oblast'** ◆ province W Russian Federation
57 K22 **Lipez, Cordillera de** ▲ SW Bolivia
110 E10 **Lipiany** Ger. Lippehne. Zachodniopomorskie, W Poland
112 G9 **Lipik** Požega-Slavonija, NE Croatia
126 L12 **Lipin Bor** Vologodskaya Oblast', NW Russian Federation
160 L12 **Liping** Guizhou, S China
Lipkany see Lipcani
119 H15 **Lipnishki** Rus. Lipnishki. Hrodzyenskaya Voblasts', W Belarus
110 J10 **Lipno** Kujawsko-pomorskie, C Poland
116 F11 **Lipova** Hung. Lippa. Arad, W Romania
Lipovets see Lypovets'
Lippa see Lipova
101 E14 **Lippe** ~ W Germany
Lippehne see Lipiany
101 G14 **Lippstadt** Nordrhein-Westfalen, W Germany
25 P1 **Lipscomb** Texas, SW USA
Lipsia/Lipsk see Leipzig
Liptau-Sankt-Nikolaus/Liptószentmiklós see Liptovský Mikuláš
111 K19 **Liptovský Mikuláš** Ger. Liptau-Sankt-Nikolaus, Hung. Liptószentmiklós. Žilinský Kraj, N Slovakia
183 O13 **Liptrap, Cape** headland Victoria, SE Australia
160 L13 **Lipu** Guangxi Zhuangzu Zizhiqu, S China
141 X12 **Liqbi** S Oman
81 G17 **Lira** N Uganda
57 F15 **Lircay** Huancavelica, C Peru
107 J15 **Liri** ~ C Italy
144 M8 **Lisakovsk** Kostanay, NW Kazakhstan
79 K17 **Lisala** Equateur, N Dem. Rep. Congo (Zaire)
104 F11 **Lisboa** Eng. Lisbon; anc. Felicitas Julia, Olisipo. ● (Portugal) Lisboa, W Portugal
104 F10 **Lisboa** ◆ Eng. Lisbon. district C Portugal
19 N7 **Lisbon** New Hampshire, NE USA
29 Q6 **Lisbon** North Dakota, N USA
Lisbon see Lisboa
19 Q8 **Lisbon Falls** Maine, NE USA
97 G15 **Lisburn** Ir. Lios na gCearrbhach. E Northern Ireland, UK
38 L6 **Lisburne, Cape** headland Alaska, USA
97 B19 **Liscannor Bay** Ir. Bá Lios Ceannúir. inlet W Ireland
113 Q18 **Lisec** ▲ E FYR Macedonia
160 F13 **Lishe Jiang** ~ SW China
160 M4 **Lishi** Shanxi, C China
163 V10 **Lishu** Jilin, NE China
161 R10 **Lishui** Zhejiang, SE China
192 L5 **Lisianski Island** island Hawaiian Islands, Hawaii, USA, C Pacific Ocean
Lisichansk see Lysychans'k
102 L4 **Lisieux** anc. Noviomagus. Calvados, N France
128 L8 **Liski** prev. Georgiu-Dezh. Voronezhskaya Oblast', W Russian Federation
Lisle/l'Isle see Lille
103 N4 **l'Isle-Adam** Val-d'Oise, N France
103 R15 **l'Isle-sur-la-Sorgue** Vaucluse, SE France
15 S9 **L'Islet** Quebec, SE Canada
182 M12 **Lismore** Victoria, SE Australia
97 D20 **Lismore** Ir. Lios Mór. S Ireland
Lissa see Vis, Croatia
Lissa see Leszno, Poland
98 H11 **Lisse** Zuid-Holland, W Netherlands
95 D18 **Lista** peninsula S Norway
95 D18 **Listafjorden** fjord S Norway
195 R13 **Lister, Mount** ▲ Antarctica
128 M8 **Listopadovka** Voronezhskaya Oblast', W Russian Federation
14 F15 **Listowel** Ontario, S Canada
97 B20 **Listowel** Ir. Lios Tuathail. SW Ireland
160 L14 **Litang** Guangxi Zhuangzu Zizhiqu, S China
160 F9 **Litang** Sichuan, C China
160 F10 **Litang Qu** ~ C China
55 X12 **Litani** var. Itany. ~ French Guiana/Surinam
138 G8 **Lītani, Nahr el** var. Nahr al Litant. ~ C Lebanon
Litant, Nahr al see Lītani, Nahr el
Litauen see Lithuania
30 K14 **Litchfield** Illinois, N USA
29 U8 **Litchfield** Minnesota, N USA
36 K13 **Litchfield Park** Arizona, SW USA
183 S8 **Lithgow** New South Wales, SE Australia
115 I26 **Líthino, Akrotírio** headland Kríti, Greece, E Mediterranean Sea
118 D12 **Lithuania** off. Republic of Lithuania, Ger. Litauen, Lith. Lietuva, Pol. Litwa, Rus. Litva; prev. Lithuanian SSR, Rus. Litovskaya SSR. ◆ republic NE Europe
Lithuanian SSR see Lithuania
109 U11 **Litija** Ger. Littai. C Slovenia
18 H15 **Lititz** Pennsylvania, NE USA
115 F15 **Litóchoro** var. Litohoro, Litókhoron. Kentrikí Makedonía, N Greece
Litohoro/Litókhoron see Litóchoro
111 C15 **Litoměřice** Ger. Ústecký Kraj, NW Czech Republic
111 F17 **Litomyšl** Ger. Pardubický Kraj, C Czech Republic
111 G17 **Litovel** Ger. Littau. Olomoucký Kraj, E Czech Republic
123 S13 **Litovko** Khabarovskiy Kray, SE Russian Federation
Litovskaya SSR see Lithuania
Littai see Litija
Littau see Litovel
44 G1 **Little Abaco** var. Abaco Island. island N Bahamas
111 I21 **Little Alföld** Ger. Kleines Ungarisches Tiefland, Hung. Kisalföld, Slvk. Podunajská Rovina. plain Hungary/Slovakia
151 Q20 **Little Andaman** island Andaman Islands, India, NE Indian Ocean
26 M5 **Little Arkansas River** ~ Kansas, C USA
184 L4 **Little Barrier Island** island N NZ
Little Belt see Lillebælt
38 M11 **Little Black River** ~ Alaska, USA
27 O2 **Little Blue River** ~ Kansas/Nebraska, C USA
44 D8 **Little Cayman** island E Cayman Islands
11 X11 **Little Churchill** ~ Manitoba, C Canada
166 J10 **Little Coco Island** island SW Myanmar
36 L10 **Little Colorado River** ~ Arizona, SW USA
14 E11 **Little Current** Manitoulin Island, Ontario, S Canada
12 E11 **Little Current** ~ Ontario, S Canada
38 L8 **Little Diomede Island** island Alaska, USA
44 I4 **Little Exuma** island C Bahamas
29 U7 **Little Falls** Minnesota, N USA
18 J10 **Little Falls** New York, NE USA
24 M5 **Littlefield** Texas, SW USA
29 V3 **Littlefork** Minnesota, N USA
29 V3 **Little Fork River** ~ Minnesota, N USA
11 N16 **Little Fort** British Columbia, SW Canada
11 Y14 **Little Grand Rapids** Manitoba, C Canada
97 N23 **Littlehampton** SE England, UK
35 T2 **Little Humboldt River** ~ Nevada, W USA
44 K6 **Little Inagua** var. Inagua Islands. island S Bahamas
21 Q4 **Little Kanawha River** ~ West Virginia, NE USA
83 F25 **Little Karoo** plateau S South Africa
39 O16 **Little Koniuji Island** island Shumagin Islands, Alaska, USA
44 H12 **Little London** W Jamaica
13 R10 **Little Mecatina** Fr. Rivière du Petit Mécatina. ~ Newfoundland/Quebec, E Canada
96 F8 **Little Minch, The** strait NW Scotland, UK
27 T13 **Little Missouri River** ~ Arkansas, USA
28 J7 **Little Missouri River** ~ NW USA
28 J3 **Little Muddy River** ~ North Dakota, N USA
151 Q22 **Little Nicobar** island Nicobar Islands, India, NE Indian Ocean
27 R6 **Little Osage River** ~ Missouri, C USA
97 P20 **Little Ouse** ~ E England, UK
149 V2 **Little Pamir** Pash. Pāmīr-e Khord, Rus. Malyy Pamir. ▲ Afghanistan/Tajikistan
21 U12 **Little Pee Dee River** ~ North Carolina/South Carolina, SE USA
27 V10 **Little Red River** ~ Arkansas, C USA
Little Rhody see Rhode Island
185 I19 **Little River** Canterbury, South Island, NZ
21 U12 **Little River** South Carolina, SE USA
27 Y9 **Little River** ~ Arkansas/Missouri, C USA
27 R13 **Little River** ~ Arkansas/Oklahoma, USA
23 T7 **Little River** ~ Georgia, SE USA
22 H6 **Little River** ~ Louisiana, S USA
25 T10 **Little River** ~ Texas, SW USA
27 V12 **Little Rock** state capital Arkansas, C USA
31 N8 **Little Sable Point** headland Michigan, N USA
103 U11 **Little Saint Bernard Pass** Fr. Col du Petit St-Bernard, It. Colle di Piccolo San Bernardo. pass France/Italy
36 K7 **Little Salt Lake** ⊚ Utah, W USA
180 K8 **Little Sandy Desert** desert Western Australia
29 S13 **Little Sioux River** ~ Iowa, C USA
38 E17 **Little Sitkin Island** island Aleutian Islands, Alaska, USA
11 O13 **Little Smoky** Alberta, W Canada
11 O14 **Little Smoky** ~ Alberta, W Canada
37 P3 **Little Snake River** ~ Colorado, C USA
64 A12 **Little Sound** bay Bermuda, NW Atlantic Ocean
37 T4 **Littleton** Colorado, C USA
19 N7 **Littleton** New Hampshire, NE USA
18 D11 **Little Valley** New York, NE USA
30 M15 **Little Wabash River** ~ Illinois, N USA
14 D10 **Little White River** ~ Ontario, S Canada
28 M12 **Little White River** ~ South Dakota, N USA
25 R5 **Little Wichita River** ~ Texas, SW USA
142 I4 **Little Zab** Ar. Nahraz Zāb aş Şaghīr, Kurd. Zē-i Kōya, Per. Rūdkhāneh-ye Zāb-e Kūchek. ~ Iran/Iraq
79 D15 **Littoral** ◆ province W Cameroon
Littoria see Latina
Litva/Litwa see Lithuania
111 B15 **Litvínov** Ger. Ústecký Kraj, NW Czech Republic
116 M6 **Lityn** Vinnyts'ka Oblast', C Ukraine
Liu-chou/Liuchow see Liuzhou
163 W11 **Liuhe** Jilin, NE China
83 Q15 **Liúpo** Nampula, NE Mozambique
83 G14 **Liuwa Plain** plain W Zambia
160 L13 **Liuzhou** var. Liu-chou, Liuchow. Guangxi Zhuangzu Zizhiqu, S China
116 H8 **Livada** Hung. Sárköz. Satu Mare, NW Romania
115 J20 **Liváda, Akrotírio** headland Tínos, Kykládes, Greece, Aegean Sea
115 L21 **Livádi** island Kykládes, Greece, Aegean Sea
Livanátai see Livanátes
115 G18 **Livanátes** prev. Livanátai. Stereá Ellás, C Greece
118 I10 **Līvāni** Ger. Lievenhof. Preiļi, SE Latvia
65 E25 **Lively Island** island SE Falkland Islands
65 D25 **Lively Sound** sound SE Falkland Islands
39 R8 **Livengood** Alaska, USA
106 I7 **Livenza** ~ NE Italy
35 O6 **Live Oak** California, W USA
23 U9 **Live Oak** Florida, SE USA
35 O9 **Livermore** California, W USA
20 I6 **Livermore** Kentucky, S USA
19 Q7 **Livermore Falls** Maine, NE USA
24 J10 **Livermore, Mount** ▲ Texas, SW USA
97 K17 **Liverpool** NW England, UK
183 S7 **Liverpool Range** ▲ New South Wales, SE Australia
96 J12 **Livingston** C Scotland, UK
23 N5 **Livingston** Alabama, S USA
35 P9 **Livingston** California, W USA
22 J8 **Livingston** Louisiana, S USA
33 S11 **Livingston** Montana, NW USA
20 L8 **Livingston** Tennessee, S USA
25 W9 **Livingston** Texas, SW USA
42 F4 **Livingston** Izabal, E Guatemala
83 I16 **Livingstone** var. Maramba. Southern, S Zambia
185 B22 **Livingstone Mountains** ▲ South Island, NZ
80 K13 **Livingstone Mountains** ▲ S Tanzania
82 N12 **Livingstonia** Northern, N Malawi
194 G4 **Livingston Island** island Antarctica
25 W9 **Livingston, Lake** ⊡ Texas, SW USA
112 F13 **Livno** Federacija Bosna I Hercegovina, SW Bosnia and Herzegovina
128 K7 **Livny** Orlovskaya Oblast', W Russian Federation
93 M14 **Livojoki** ~ C Finland
31 R10 **Livonia** Michigan, N USA
106 E11 **Livorno** Eng. Leghorn. Toscana, C Italy
Livramento see Santana do Livramento
141 U8 **Liwā** var. Al Liwā'. oasis region S UAE
81 I24 **Liwale** Lindi, SE Tanzania
159 W9 **Liwangbu** Ningxia, N China
83 N15 **Liwonde** Southern, S Malawi
159 V11 **Lixian** var. Li Xian. Gansu, C China
160 H8 **Lixian** var. Li Xian; prev. Zagunao. Sichuan, C China
Lixian Jiang see Black River
115 B18 **Lixoúri** prev. Lixoúrion. Kefallinía, Iónioi Nísoi, Greece, C Mediterranean Sea
Lixoúrion see Lixoúri
Lixus see Larache
Lizarra see Estella-Lizarra
33 U15 **Lizard Head Peak** ▲ Wyoming, C USA
97 H25 **Lizard Point** headland SW England, UK
112 L12 **Ljig** Serbia, C Yugoslavia
Ljouwert see Leeuwarden
Ljubelj see Loibl Pass
109 U11 **Ljubljana** Ger. Laibach, It. Lubiana; anc. Aemona, Emona. ● (Slovenia) C Slovenia
109 T11 **Ljubljana** ✕ C Slovenia
113 N17 **Ljuboten** ▲ S Yugoslavia
95 P19 **Ljugarn** Gotland, SE Sweden
84 G7 **Ljungan** ~ N Sweden
93 F17 **Ljungan** ~ C Sweden
95 K21 **Ljungby** Kronoberg, S Sweden
95 M17 **Ljungsbro** Östergötland, S Sweden
95 I18 **Ljungskile** Västra Götaland, S Sweden
94 M11 **Ljusdal** Gävleborg, C Sweden
94 M11 **Ljusnan** ~ C Sweden
94 N12 **Ljusne** Gävleborg, C Sweden
95 P15 **Ljusterö** Stockholm, C Sweden
109 X9 **Ljutomer** Ger. Luttenberg. NE Slovenia
63 G15 **Llaima, Volcán** ▲ S Chile
105 X4 **Llançà** var. Llansá. Cataluña, NE Spain
97 J21 **Llandovery** C Wales, UK
97 J20 **Llandrindod Wells** E Wales, UK
97 J18 **Llandudno** N Wales, UK
97 I21 **Llanelli** prev. Llanelly. SW Wales, UK
Llanelly see Llanelli
104 M2 **Llanes** Asturias, N Spain
97 K19 **Llangollen** NE Wales, UK
25 R10 **Llano** Texas, SW USA
25 Q10 **Llano River** ~ Texas, SW USA
54 I9 **Llanos** physical region Colombia/Venezuela
63 G16 **Llanquihue, Lago** ⊚ S Chile
Llansá see Llançà
105 U5 **Lleida** Cast. Lérida; anc. Ilerda. Cataluña, NE Spain
105 U5 **Lleida** Cast. Lérida ◆ province Cataluña, NE Spain
104 K12 **Llerena** Extremadura, W Spain
105 S9 **Llíria** País Valenciano, E Spain
105 W4 **Llivia** Cataluña, NE Spain
105 O3 **Llodio** País Vasco, N Spain
105 X5 **Lloret de Mar** Cataluña, NE Spain
Llorri see Tossal de l'Orri
10 L11 **Lloyd George, Mount** ▲ British Columbia, W Canada
11 R14 **Lloydminster** Alberta/Saskatchewan, SW Canada
36 L6 **Loa** Utah, W USA
169 S8 **Loagan Bunut** ⊚ East Malaysia
38 G12 **Loa, Mauna** ▲ Hawaii, USA, C Pacific Ocean
Loanda see Luanda
79 J22 **Loange** ~ S Dem. Rep. Congo (Zaire)
79 E21 **Loango** Le Kouilou, S Congo
106 B10 **Loano** Liguria, NW Italy
62 H4 **Loa, Río** ~ N Chile
83 I20 **Lobatse** var. Lobatsi. Kgatleng, SE Botswana
Lobatsi see Lobatse
101 Q15 **Löbau** Sachsen, E Germany
79 H16 **Lobaye** ◆ prefecture SW Central African Republic
79 I16 **Lobaye** ~ SW Central African Republic
99 G21 **Lobbes** Hainaut, S Belgium
61 D23 **Lobería** Buenos Aires, E Argentina
110 F8 **Łobez** Ger. Labes. Zachodniopomorskie, NW Poland
82 A13 **Lobito** Benguela, W Angola
Lobkovichi see Labkovichy
Lob Nor see Lop Nur
171 V13 **Lobo** Irian Jaya, E Indonesia
104 J11 **Lobón** Extremadura, W Spain
61 D20 **Lobos** Buenos Aires, E Argentina
40 E4 **Lobos, Cabo** headland NW Mexico
40 F6 **Lobos, Isla** island NW Mexico
Lobositz see Lovosice
Lobsens see Łobżenica
Loburi see Lop Buri
110 H9 **Łobżenica** Ger. Lobsens. Wielkopolskie, C Poland
108 G11 **Locarno** Ger. Luggarus. Ticino, S Switzerland
96 E9 **Lochboisdale** NW Scotland, UK
98 N11 **Lochem** Gelderland, E Netherlands
102 M8 **Loches** Indre-et-Loire, C France
Loch Garman see Wexford
96 H12 **Lochgilphead** W Scotland, UK
96 H7 **Lochinver** N Scotland, UK
96 F8 **Lochmaddy** NW Scotland, UK
96 J10 **Lochnagar** ▲ C Scotland, UK
99 E17 **Lochristi** Oost-Vlaanderen, NW Belgium
96 H9 **Lochy, Loch** ⊚ N Scotland, UK
182 G8 **Lock** South Australia
97 J14 **Lockerbie** S Scotland, UK
27 S13 **Lockesburg** Arkansas, C USA
183 P10 **Lockhart** New South Wales, SE Australia
25 S11 **Lockhart** Texas, SW USA

◆ Country ● Country Capital ◇ Dependent Territory ○ Dependent Territory Capital ◆ Administrative Region ✕ International Airport ▲ Mountain ▲ Mountain Range Volcano ~ River ⊚ Lake ⊡ Reservoir

18 F13 **Lock Haven** Pennsylvania, NE USA
25 N4 **Lockney** Texas, SW USA
100 O12 **Löcknitz** ∽ NE Germany
18 E9 **Lockport** New York, NE USA
167 T13 **Lôc Ninh** Sông Be, S Vietnam
107 N23 **Locri** Calabria, SW Italy
Locse see Levoča
27 T2 **Locust Creek** ∽ Missouri, C USA
23 P3 **Locust Fork** ∽ Alabama, S USA
27 Q9 **Locust Grove** Oklahoma, C USA
94 E11 **Lodalskåpa** ▲ S Norway
183 N10 **Loddon River** ∽ Victoria, SE Australia
Lodensee see Klooga
103 P15 **Lodève** anc. Luteva. Hérault, S France
126 I12 **Lodeynoye Pole** Leningradskaya Oblast', NW Russian Federation
33 V11 **Lodge Grass** Montana, NW USA
28 J15 **Lodgepole Creek** ∽ Nebraska/Wyoming, C USA
149 T11 **Lodhrān** Punjab, E Pakistan
106 D8 **Lodi** Lombardia, NW Italy
35 O8 **Lodi** California, W USA
31 T12 **Lodi** Ohio, N USA
92 H10 **Lødingen** Nordland, C Norway
79 L20 **Lodja** Kasai Oriental, C Dem. Rep. Congo (Zaire)
37 O3 **Lodore, Canyon of** canyon Colorado, C USA
105 Q4 **Lodosa** Navarra, N Spain
81 H16 **Lodwar** Rift Valley, NW Kenya
110 K13 **Łódź** Rus. Lodz. Łódź, C Poland
110 J13 **Łódzkie** ◈ province C Poland
167 P8 **Loei** var. Loey, Muang Loei. Loei, C Thailand
98 I11 **Loenen** Utrecht, C Netherlands
167 R9 **Loeng Nok Tha** Yasothon, E Thailand
83 F24 **Loeriesfontein** Northern Cape, W South Africa
95 H20 **Læsø** island N Denmark
Loewoek see Luwuk
Loey see Loei
76 J16 **Lofa** ∽ N Liberia
109 P6 **Lofer** Salzburg, C Austria
92 F11 **Lofoten** var. Lofoten Islands. island group C Norway
Lofoten Islands see Lofoten
95 N18 **Loftahammar** Kalmar, S Sweden
129 O10 **Log** Volgogradskaya Oblast', SW Russian Federation
77 S12 **Loga** Dosso, SW Niger
29 S14 **Logan** Iowa, C USA
26 K3 **Logan** Kansas, C USA
31 T14 **Logan** Ohio, N USA
36 L1 **Logan** Utah, W USA
21 P6 **Logan** West Virginia, NE USA
35 Y10 **Logandale** Nevada, W USA
19 O11 **Logan International** ✕ (Boston) Massachusetts, NE USA
11 N16 **Logan Lake** British Columbia, SW Canada
23 Q4 **Logan Martin Lake** ⊡ Alabama, S USA
10 G8 **Logan, Mount** ▲ Yukon Territory, W Canada
32 I7 **Logan, Mount** ▲ Washington, NW USA
33 P7 **Logan Pass** pass Montana, NW USA
31 O12 **Logansport** Indiana, N USA
22 F6 **Logansport** Louisiana, S USA
Logar see Lowgar
67 R11 **Loge** ∽ NW Angola
Logishin see Lahishyn
Log na Coille see Lugnaquillia Mountain
78 G11 **Logone** var. Lagone. ∽ Cameroon/Chad
78 G13 **Logone-Occidental** off. Préfecture du Logone-Occidental. ◈ prefecture SW Chad
78 H13 **Logone Occidental** ∽ SW Chad
78 G13 **Logone-Oriental** off. Préfecture du Logone-Oriental. ◈ prefecture SW Chad
78 H13 **Logone Oriental** ∽ SW Chad
Logone Oriental see Pendé
L'Ogooué-Ivindo see Ogooué-Ivindo
L'Ogooué-Lolo see Ogooué-Lolo
L'Ogooué-Maritime see Ogooué-Maritime
Logoysk see Lahoysk
105 P4 **Logroño** anc. Vareia, Lat. Juliobriga. La Rioja, N Spain
104 L10 **Logrosán** Extremadura, W Spain
95 G20 **Løgstør** Nordjylland, N Denmark
95 H22 **Løgten** Århus, C Denmark
95 F24 **Løgumkloster** Sønderjylland, SW Denmark
Lögurinn see Lagarfljót
153 P15 **Lohārdaga** Bihār, N India
152 H10 **Lohāru** Haryāna, N India
101 D15 **Lohausen** ✕ (Düsseldorf) Nordrhein-Westfalen, W Germany
189 O14 **Lohd** Pohnpei, E Micronesia
92 L12 **Lohiniva** Lappi, N Finland
Lohiszyn see Lahishyn
93 L20 **Lohja** var. Lojo. Etelä-Suomi, S Finland
169 V11 **Lohjanan** Borneo, C Indonesia
25 Q9 **Lohn** Texas, SW USA
100 G12 **Lohne** Niedersachsen, NW Germany
Lohr see Lohr am Main
101 I18 **Lohr am Main** var. Lohr. Bayern, C Germany
109 T10 **Loibl Pass** Ger. Loiblpass, Slvn. Ljubelj. pass Austria/Slovenia
167 N6 **Loi-Kaw** Kayah State, C Myanmar
93 K19 **Loimaa** Länsi-Suomi, W Finland
103 O6 **Loing** ∽ C France
167 R6 **Loi, Phou** ▲ N Laos
102 L7 **Loir** ∽ C France
103 Q11 **Loire** ◈ department E France
102 M7 **Loire** var. Liger. ∽ C France
102 I7 **Loire-Atlantique** ◈ department NW France
103 O7 **Loiret** ◈ department C France
102 M8 **Loir-et-Cher** ◈ department C France
101 L24 **Loisach** ∽ SE Germany
56 B9 **Loja** Loja, S Ecuador
104 M14 **Loja** Andalucía, S Spain
56 B9 **Loja** ◈ province S Ecuador
Lojo see Lohja
116 J4 **Lokachi** Volyns'ka Oblast', NW Ukraine
79 M20 **Lokandu** Maniema, C Dem. Rep. Congo (Zaire)
92 M11 **Lokan Tekojärvi** ◎ NE Finland
137 Z11 **Lökbatan** Rus. Lokbatan. E Azerbaijan
99 F17 **Lokeren** Oost-Vlaanderen, NW Belgium
Lokhvitsa see Lokhvytsya
117 S4 **Lokhvytsya** Rus. Lokhvitsa. Poltavs'ka Oblast', NE Ukraine
81 H17 **Lokichar** Rift Valley, NW Kenya
81 G16 **Lokichokio** Rift Valley, NW Kenya
81 H16 **Lokitaung** Rift Valley, NW Kenya
92 M11 **Lokka** Lappi, N Finland
94 G8 **Løkken Verk** Sør-Trøndelag, S Norway
126 G16 **Loknya** Pskovskaya Oblast', W Russian Federation
77 V15 **Loko** Nassarawa, C Nigeria
77 U15 **Lokoja** Kogi, C Nigeria
81 H17 **Lokori** Rift Valley, W Kenya
77 R16 **Lokossa** S Benin
118 I3 **Loksa** Ger. Loxa. Harjumaa, NW Estonia
9 T7 **Loks Land** island Nunavut, NE Canada
80 C13 **Lol** ∽ S Sudan
76 K15 **Lola** Guinée-Forestière, SE Guinea
35 Q5 **Lola, Mount** ▲ California, W USA
81 H20 **Loliondo** Arusha, NE Tanzania
95 H25 **Lolland** prev. Laaland. island S Denmark
186 G6 **Lolobau Island** island E PNG
79 E16 **Lolodorf** Sud, SW Cameroon
114 G7 **Lom** prev. Lom-Palanka. Oblast Montana, NW Bulgaria
114 G7 **Lom** ∽ Montana, NW Bulgaria
79 M19 **Lomami** ∽ C Dem. Rep. Congo (Zaire)
57 F17 **Lomas** Arequipa, SW Peru
63 I23 **Lomas, Bahía** bay S Chile
61 D20 **Lomas de Zamora** Buenos Aires, E Argentina
61 D20 **Loma Verde** Buenos Aires, E Argentina
180 K4 **Lombadina** Western Australia
106 E6 **Lombardia** Eng. Lombardy. ◈ region N Italy
Lombardy see Lombardia
102 M15 **Lombez** Gers, S France
171 Q16 **Lomblen, Pulau** island Nusa Tenggara, S Indonesia
173 W7 **Lombok Basin** undersea feature E Indian Ocean
170 L16 **Lombok, Pulau** island Nusa Tenggara, C Indonesia
77 Q16 **Lomé** ● (Togo) S Togo
77 Q16 **Lomé** ✕ S Togo
79 L19 **Lomela** Kasai Oriental, C Dem. Rep. Congo (Zaire)
25 R9 **Lometa** Texas, SW USA
79 F16 **Lomié** Est, SE Cameroon
30 M8 **Lomira** Wisconsin, N USA
95 K23 **Lomma** Skåne, S Sweden
99 J16 **Lommel** Limburg, N Belgium
96 I11 **Lomond, Loch** ◎ C Scotland, UK
197 R9 **Lomonosov Ridge** var. Harris Ridge, Rus. Khrebet Lomonsova. undersea feature Arctic Ocean
Lomonsova, Khrebet see Lomonosov Ridge
Lom-Palanka see Lom
Lomphat see Lumphăt
35 P14 **Lompoc** California, W USA
167 P9 **Lom Sak** var. Muang Lom Sak. Phetchabun, C Thailand
110 N9 **Łomża** Rus. Lomzha. Podlaskie, NE Poland
Lomzha see Łomża
155 D14 **Lonāvale** prev. Lonauli. Mahārāshtra, W India
63 G15 **Loncoche** Araucanía, C Chile
63 H14 **Loncopue** Neuquén, W Argentina
99 G17 **Londerzeel** Vlaams Brabant, C Belgium
Londinium see London
14 E16 **London** Ontario, S Canada
191 Y2 **London** Kiritimati, E Kiribati
97 O22 **London** anc. Augusta, Lat. Londinium. ● (UK) SE England, UK
21 N7 **London** Kentucky, S USA
31 S13 **London** Ohio, NE USA
25 Q10 **London** Texas, SW USA
97 O22 **London City** ✕ SE England, UK
97 E14 **Londonderry** var. Derry, Ir. Doire. NW Northern Ireland, UK
97 F14 **Londonderry** cultural region NW Northern Ireland, UK
180 M2 **Londonderry, Cape** headland Western Australia
63 H25 **Londonderry, Isla** island S Chile
43 O7 **Londres, Cayos** reef NE Nicaragua
60 I10 **Londrina** Paraná, S Brazil
27 N13 **Lone Grove** Oklahoma, C USA
14 E12 **Lonely Island** island Ontario, S Canada
35 T8 **Lone Mountain** ▲ Nevada, W USA
25 V6 **Lone Oak** Texas, SW USA
35 T11 **Lone Pine** California, W USA
Lone Star State see Texas
83 D14 **Longa** Cuando Cubango, C Angola
82 B12 **Longa** ∽ W Angola
83 E15 **Longa** ∽ SE Angola
163 W11 **Longang Shan** ▲▲ NE China
197 S4 **Longa, Proliv** Eng. Long Strait. strait NE Russian Federation
44 J13 **Long Bay** bay W Jamaica
21 V13 **Long Bay** bay North Carolina/South Carolina, E USA
35 T16 **Long Beach** California, W USA
22 M9 **Long Beach** Mississippi, S USA
18 L14 **Long Beach** Long Island, New York, NE USA
32 F9 **Long Beach** Washington, NW USA
18 K16 **Long Beach Island** island New Jersey, NE USA
65 M25 **Longbluff** headland SW Tristan da Cunha
23 U13 **Longboat Key** island Florida, SE USA
18 K15 **Long Branch** New Jersey, NE USA
44 J5 **Long Cay** island SE Bahamas
161 P14 **Longchuan** prev. Laolong. Guangdong, S China
Longchuan Jiang see Shweli
32 K12 **Long Creek** Oregon, NW USA
159 W10 **Longde** Ningxia, N China
183 P16 **Longford** Tasmania, SE Australia
97 D17 **Longford** Ir. An Longfort. C Ireland
97 E17 **Longford** Ir. An Longfort. cultural region C Ireland
161 P1 **Longhua** Hebei, E China
169 U11 **Longiram** Borneo, C Indonesia
44 J4 **Long Island** island C Bahamas
12 H8 **Long Island** island Nunavut, C Canada
186 D7 **Long Island** var. Arop Island. island N PNG
18 L14 **Long Island** island New York, NE USA
Long Island see Bermuda
18 M14 **Long Island Sound** sound NE USA
160 K13 **Long Jiang** ∽ S China
163 U7 **Longjiang** Heilongjiang, NE China
163 Y10 **Longjing** var. Yanji. Jilin, NE China
161 R4 **Longkou** Shandong, E China
12 E11 **Longlac** Ontario, S Canada
19 S1 **Long Lake** ◎ Maine, NE USA
31 O6 **Long Lake** ◎ Michigan, N USA
31 R5 **Long Lake** ◎ Michigan, N USA
29 N6 **Long Lake** ◎ North Dakota, N USA
30 J4 **Long Lake** ⊡ Wisconsin, N USA
99 K23 **Longlier** Luxembourg, SE Belgium
160 I13 **Longlin** var. Longlin Gezu Zizhixian. Guangxi Zhuangzu Zizhiqu, S China
37 T3 **Longmont** Colorado, C USA
29 N13 **Long Pine** Nebraska, C USA
Longping see Luodian
14 F17 **Long Point** headland Ontario, S Canada
14 K15 **Long Point** headland Ontario, SE Canada
184 P10 **Long Point** headland North Island, NZ
30 L2 **Long Point** headland Michigan, N USA
14 G17 **Long Point Bay** lake bay Ontario, S Canada
29 T7 **Long Prairie** Minnesota, N USA
13 S11 **Long Range Mountains** hill range Newfoundland, E Canada
65 H25 **Long Range Point** headland SE Saint Helena
181 V8 **Longreach** Queensland, E Australia
160 H7 **Longriba** Sichuan, C China
160 L10 **Longshan** Hunan, S China
37 S3 **Longs Peak** ▲ Colorado, C USA
Long Strait see Longa, Proliv
102 K8 **Longué** Maine-et-Loire, NW France
13 P11 **Longue-Pointe** Quebec, E Canada
103 S4 **Longuyon** Meurthe-et-Moselle, NE France
25 W7 **Longview** Texas, SW USA
32 G10 **Longview** Washington, NW USA
65 H25 **Longwood** C Saint Helena
25 P7 **Longworth** Texas, SW USA
103 S3 **Longwy** Meurthe-et-Moselle, NE France
159 V11 **Longxi** Gansu, C China
167 S14 **Long Xuyên** var. Longxuyen. An Giang, S Vietnam
161 Q13 **Longyan** Fujian, SE China
92 O3 **Longyearbyen** ○ (Svalbard) Spitsbergen, W Svalbard
160 J15 **Longzhou** Guangxi Zhuangzu Zizhiqu, S China
100 F12 **Löningen** Niedersachsen, NW Germany
27 V11 **Lonoke** Arkansas, C USA
95 L21 **Lönsboda** Skåne, S Sweden
103 S9 **Lons-le-Saunier** anc. Ledo Salinarius. Jura, E France
31 O15 **Loogootee** Indiana, N USA
31 Q9 **Looking Glass River** ∽ Michigan, N USA
21 X11 **Lookout, Cape** headland North Carolina, SE USA
39 O6 **Lookout Ridge** ridge Alaska, USA
181 N11 **Loongana** Western Australia
99 I14 **Loon op Zand** Noord-Brabant, S Netherlands
97 A19 **Loop Head** Ir. Ceann Léime. headland W Ireland
109 V4 **Loosdorf** Niederösterreich, NE Austria
158 G10 **Lop** Xinjiang Uygur Zizhiqu, NW China
112 J11 **Lopare** Republika Srpska, NE Bosnia and Herzegovina
Lopatichi see Lapatsichy
129 Q15 **Lopatin** Respublika Dagestan, SW Russian Federation
129 P7 **Lopatino** Penzenskaya Oblast', W Russian Federation
167 P10 **Lop Buri** var. Loburi. Lop Buri, C Thailand
25 R16 **Lopeno** Texas, SW USA
79 C18 **Lopez, Cap** headland W Gabon
98 I12 **Lopik** Utrecht, C Netherlands
Lop Nor see Lop Nur
158 M7 **Lop Nur** var. Lob Nor, Lop Nor, Lo-pu Po. seasonal lake NW China
Lopnur see Yuli
79 K17 **Lopori** ∽ NW Dem. Rep. Congo (Zaire)
98 O5 **Loppersum** Groningen, NE Netherlands
92 I8 **Lopphavet** sound N Norway
Lo-pu Po see Lop Nur
Lora see Lowrah
182 F3 **Lora Creek** seasonal river South Australia
104 K13 **Lora del Río** Andalucía, S Spain
148 M11 **Lora, Hāmūn-i** wetland SW Pakistan
31 T11 **Lorain** Ohio, N USA
25 O7 **Loraine** Texas, SW USA
31 R13 **Loramie, Lake** ⊡ Ohio, N USA
105 Q13 **Lorca** Ar. Lurka; anc. Eliocroca, Lat. Illur co. Murcia, S Spain
192 I10 **Lord Howe Island** island E Australia
Lord Howe Island see Ontong Java Atoll
175 O10 **Lord Howe Rise** undersea feature SW Pacific Ocean
192 J10 **Lord Howe Seamounts** undersea feature W Pacific Ocean
37 P15 **Lordsburg** New Mexico, SW USA
186 E5 **Lorengau** var. Lorungau. Manus Island, N PNG
25 N5 **Lorenzo** Texas, SW USA
142 K7 **Lorestān** off. Ostān-e Lorestān, var. Luristan. ◈ province W Iran
57 M17 **Loreto** Beni, N Bolivia
106 J12 **Loreto** Marche, C Italy
40 F8 **Loreto** Baja California Sur, W Mexico
40 M11 **Loreto** Zacatecas, C Mexico
56 E9 **Loreto** off. Departamento de Loreto. ◈ department NE Peru
81 K18 **Lorian Swamp** swamp E Kenya
54 E6 **Lorica** Córdoba, NW Colombia
102 G7 **Lorient** prev. l'Orient. Morbihan, NW France
111 K22 **Lőrinci** Heves, NE Hungary
14 G11 **Loring** Ontario, S Canada
33 V6 **Loring** Montana, NW USA
103 R13 **Loriol-sur-Drôme** Drôme, E France
21 U12 **Loris** South Carolina, SE USA
57 I18 **Loriscota, Laguna** ◎ S Peru
183 N13 **Lorne** Victoria, SE Australia
96 G11 **Lorn, Firth of** inlet W Scotland, UK
Loro Sae see East Timor
101 F24 **Lörrach** Baden-Württemberg, S Germany
103 T5 **Lorraine** ◈ region NE France
Lorungau see Lorengau
94 L11 **Los** Gävleborg, C Sweden
35 P14 **Los Alamos** California, W USA
37 S10 **Los Alamos** New Mexico, SW USA
42 F5 **Los Amates** Izabal, E Guatemala
35 S15 **Los Angeles** California, W USA
35 S15 **Los Angeles** ✕ California, W USA
63 G14 **Los Ángeles** Bío Bío, C Chile
35 T13 **Los Angeles Aqueduct** aqueduct California, W USA
Losanna see Lausanne
63 H20 **Los Antiguos** Santa Cruz, SW Argentina
189 Q16 **Losap Atoll** atoll C Micronesia
35 P10 **Los Banos** California, W USA
104 K16 **Los Barrios** Andalucía, S Spain
62 L5 **Los Blancos** Salta, N Argentina
42 L12 **Los Chiles** Alajuela, NW Costa Rica
105 O2 **Los Corrales de Buelna** Cantabria, N Spain
25 T17 **Los Fresnos** Texas, SW USA
35 N9 **Los Gatos** California, W USA
110 O11 **Łosice** Mazowieckie, E Poland
112 B11 **Lošinj** Ger. Lussin, It. Lussino. island W Croatia
Los Jardines see Ngetik Atoll
63 G15 **Los Lagos** Los Lagos, C Chile
63 F17 **Los Lagos** off. Región de los Lagos. ◈ region C Chile
Loslau see Wodzisław Śląski
64 N11 **Los Llanos** var. Los Llanos de Aridane. La Palma, Islas Canarias, Spain, NE Atlantic Ocean
Los Llanos de Aridane see Los Llanos
37 R11 **Los Lunas** New Mexico, SW USA
63 I16 **Los Menucos** Río Negro, C Argentina
40 H8 **Los Mochis** Sinaloa, C Mexico
35 N4 **Los Molinos** California, W USA
104 M9 **Los Navalmorales** Castilla-La Mancha, C Spain
25 S15 **Los Olmos Creek** ∽ Texas, SW USA
Losonc/Losontz see Lučenec
167 S5 **Lô, Sông** Chin. Panlong Jiang. ∽ China/Vietnam
44 B5 **Los Palacios** Pinar del Río, W Cuba
104 K14 **Los Palacios y Villafranca** Andalucía, S Spain
171 R16 **Lospalos** E East Timor
37 R12 **Los Pinos Mountains** ▲▲ New Mexico, SW USA
37 R11 **Los Ranchos De Albuquerque** New Mexico, SW USA
40 M14 **Los Reyes** Michoacán de Ocampo, SW Mexico
56 B7 **Los Ríos** ◈ province C Ecuador
64 O11 **Los Rodeos** ✕ (Santa Cruz de Tenerife) Tenerife, Islas Canarias, Spain, NE Atlantic Ocean
54 L4 **Los Roques, Islas** island group N Venezuela
43 S17 **Los Santos** Los Santos, S Panama
43 S17 **Los Santos** off. Provincia de Los Santos. ◈ province S Panama
Los Santos see Los Santos de Maimona
104 J12 **Los Santos de Maimona** var. Los Santos. Extremadura, W Spain
98 P10 **Losser** Overijssel, E Netherlands
96 J8 **Lossiemouth** NE Scotland, UK
61 B14 **Los Tábanos** Santa Fe, C Argentina
54 J4 **Los Taques** Falcón, N Venezuela
14 G11 **Lost Channel** Ontario, S Canada
54 L5 **Los Teques** Miranda, N Venezuela
35 Q12 **Lost Hills** California, W USA
36 I7 **Lost Peak** ▲ Utah, W USA
33 P11 **Lost Trail Pass** pass Montana, NW USA
186 G9 **Losuia** Kiriwina Island, SE PNG
62 G10 **Los Vilos** Coquimbo, C Chile
105 N10 **Los Yébenes** Castilla-La Mancha, C Spain
103 N13 **Lot** ◈ department S France
103 N13 **Lot** ∽ S France
63 F14 **Lota** Bío Bío, C Chile
81 G15 **Lotagipi Swamp** wetland Kenya/Sudan
102 K14 **Lot-et-Garonne** ◈ department SW France
83 K21 **Lothair** Mpumalanga, NE South Africa
33 R7 **Lothair** Montana, NW USA
79 L20 **Loto** Kasai Oriental, C Dem. Rep. Congo (Zaire)
192 H16 **Lotofagā** Upolu, SE Samoa
108 E10 **Lötschbergtunnel** tunnel Valais, SW Switzerland
25 T9 **Lott** Texas, SW USA
126 H3 **Lotta** var. Lutto. ∽ Finland/Russian Federation
184 Q7 **Lottin Point** headland North Island, NZ
Lötzen see Giżycko
Loualaba see Lualaba
167 P6 **Louangnamtha** var. Luong Nam Tha. Louang Namtha, N Laos
167 Q7 **Louangphabang** var. Louangphrabang, Luang Prabang. Louangphabang, N Laos
Louangphrabang see Louangphabang
194 H5 **Loubet Coast** physical region Antarctica
Loubomo see Dolisie
Louch see Loukhi
102 H6 **Loudéac** Côtes d'Armor, NW France
160 M11 **Loudi** Hunan, S China
79 F21 **Loudima** La Bouenza, S Congo
20 M9 **Loudon** Tennessee, S USA
31 T12 **Loudonville** Ohio, N USA
102 L8 **Loudun** Vienne, W France
102 K7 **Loué** Sarthe, NW France
76 G10 **Louga** NW Senegal
97 M19 **Loughborough** C England, UK
8 L4 **Lougheed Island** island Nunavut, N Canada
97 C18 **Loughrea** Ir. Baile Locha Riach. W Ireland
103 S9 **Louhans** Saône-et-Loire, C France
21 P5 **Louisa** Kentucky, S USA
21 V5 **Louisa** Virginia, NE USA
21 V9 **Louisburg** North Carolina, SE USA
25 U12 **Louise** Texas, SW USA
15 P11 **Louiseville** Quebec, SE Canada
27 W3 **Louisiana** Missouri, C USA
22 G8 **Louisiana** off. State of Louisiana; also known as Creole State, Pelican State. ◈ state S USA
186 E5 **Lou Island** island N PNG
83 K19 **Louis Trichardt** Northern, NE South Africa
23 V4 **Louisville** Georgia, SE USA
30 M15 **Louisville** Illinois, N USA
20 K5 **Louisville** Kentucky, S USA
22 M4 **Louisville** Mississippi, S USA
29 S15 **Louisville** Nebraska, C USA
192 L11 **Louisville Ridge** undersea feature S Pacific Ocean
126 J6 **Loukhi** var. Louch. Respublika Kareliya, NW Russian Federation
79 H19 **Loukoléla** Cuvette, E Congo
104 G14 **Loulé** Faro, S Portugal
111 C16 **Louny** Ger. Laun. Ústecký kraj NW Czech Republic
29 O15 **Loup City** Nebraska, C USA
29 P15 **Loup River** ∽ Nebraska, C USA
15 S9 **Loup, Rivière du** ∽ Quebec, SE Canada
12 K7 **Loups Marins, Lacs des** lakes Quebec, NE Canada
102 K16 **Lourdes** Hautes-Pyrénées, S France
Lourenço Marques see Maputo
104 F11 **Loures** Lisboa, C Portugal
104 F10 **Lourinhã** Lisboa, C Portugal
115 C16 **Loúros** ∽ W Greece
104 G8 **Lousã** Coimbra, N Portugal
160 M10 **Lou Shui** ∽ C China
183 O5 **Louth** New South Wales, SE Australia
97 O18 **Louth** E England, UK
97 F17 **Louth** Ir. Lú. cultural region NE Ireland
115 H15 **Loutrá** Kentrikí Makedonía, N Greece
115 G19 **Loutráki** Pelopónnisos, S Greece
Louvain see Leuven
99 H19 **Louvain-la Neuve** Wallon Brabant, C Belgium
14 J8 **Louvicourt** Quebec, SE Canada
102 M4 **Louviers** Eure, N France
30 K14 **Lou Yaeger, Lake** ⊡ Illinois, N USA
93 J15 **Lövånger** Västerbotten, N Sweden
126 J14 **Lovat'** ∽ NW Russian Federation
113 J17 **Lovćen** ▲ S Yugoslavia
114 I8 **Lovech** Lovech, N Bulgaria
114 I9 **Lovech** ◈ province N Bulgaria
25 V9 **Lovelady** Texas, SW USA
37 T3 **Loveland** Colorado, C USA
33 U12 **Lovell** Wyoming, C USA
Lovello, Monte see Grosser Löffler
35 S4 **Lovelock** Nevada, W USA
106 E7 **Lovere** Lombardia, N Italy
30 L10 **Loves Park** Illinois, N USA
26 M2 **Lovewell Reservoir** ⊡ Kansas, C USA
93 M19 **Loviisa** Swe. Lovisa. Etelä-Suomi, S Finland
37 V15 **Loving** New Mexico, SW USA
21 U6 **Lovingston** Virginia, NE USA
37 V14 **Lovington** New Mexico, SW USA
Lovisa see Loviisa
111 C15 **Lovosice** Ger. Lobositz. Ústecký Kraj, NW Czech Republic
126 K4 **Lovozero** Murmanskaya Oblast', NW Russian Federation
126 K4 **Lovozero, Ozero** ◎ NW Russian Federation
112 B9 **Lovran** It. Laurana. Primorje-Gorski Kotar, NW Croatia
116 E11 **Lovrin** Ger. Lowrin. Timiș, W Romania
82 E10 **Lóvua** Lunda Norte, NE Angola
82 G12 **Lóvua** Moxico, E Angola
65 D25 **Low Bay** bay East Falkland, Falkland Islands
9 P9 **Low, Cape** headland Nunavut, E Canada
33 N10 **Lowell** Idaho, NW USA
19 O10 **Lowell** Massachusetts, NE USA
Löwen see Leuven
Löwenberg in Schlesien see Lwówek Śląski
Lower Austria see Niederösterreich
Lower Bann see Bann
Lower California see Baja California
Lower Danube see Niederösterreich
185 L14 **Lower Hutt** Wellington, North Island, NZ
39 N11 **Lower Kalskag** Alaska, USA
35 O1 **Lower Klamath Lake** ◎ California, W USA
35 Q2 **Lower Lake** ◎ California/Nevada, W USA
97 E15 **Lower Lough Erne** ◎ SW Northern Ireland, UK
Lower Lusatia see Niederlausitz
Lower Normandy see Basse-Normandie, France
10 K9 **Lower Post** British Columbia, W Canada
29 T4 **Lower Red Lake** ◎ Minnesota, N USA
Lower Rhine see Neder Rijn
Lower Saxony see Niedersachsen
Lower Tunguska see Nizhnyaya Tunguska
97 Q19 **Lowestoft** E England, UK
149 Q5 **Lowgar** var. Logar. ◈ province E Afghanistan
182 H7 **Low Hill** South Australia
110 K12 **Łowicz** Łódzkie, C Poland
33 N13 **Lowman** Idaho, NW USA
149 P8 **Lowrah** var. Lora. ∽ SE Afghanistan
Lowrin see Lovrin
183 N17 **Low Rocky Point** headland Tasmania, SE Australia
18 I8 **Lowville** New York, NE USA
Loxa see Loksa
182 K9 **Loxton** South Australia
81 G21 **Loya** Tabora, C Tanzania
30 K6 **Loyal** Wisconsin, N USA
18 G13 **Loyalsock Creek** ∽ Pennsylvania, NE USA
35 Q5 **Loyalton** California, W USA
Lo-yang see Luoyang
187 Q16 **Loyauté, Îles** island group S New Caledonia
Loyev see Loyew
119 O20 **Loyew** Rus. Loyev. Homyel'skaya Voblasts', SE Belarus
127 S13 **Loyno** Kirovskaya Oblast', NW Russian Federation
103 P13 **Lozère** ◈ department S France
103 Q14 **Lozère, Mont** ▲ S France
112 J11 **Loznica** Serbia, W Yugoslavia
117 V7 **Lozova** Rus. Lozovaya. Kharkivs'ka Oblast', E Ukraine
Lozovaya see Lozova
105 N7 **Lozoyuela** Madrid, C Spain
Lœvvajok see Leavvajohka
Lu see Shandong, China
Lú see Louth, Ireland
82 F12 **Luacano** Moxico, E Angola
79 N21 **Lualaba** Fr. Loualaba. ∽ SE Dem. Rep. Congo (Zaire)
83 H14 **Luampa** Western, NW Zambia
83 H15 **Luampa Kuta** Western, W Zambia
161 P8 **Lu'an** Anhui, E China
104 K2 **Luanco** Asturias, N Spain
82 A11 **Luanda** var. Loanda, Port. São Paulo de Loanda. ● (Angola) Luanda, NW Angola
82 A11 **Luanda** ◈ province NW Angola

◆ Country ● Country Capital ◇ Dependent Territory ○ Dependent Territory Capital ◈ Administrative Region ✕ International Airport ▲ Mountain ▲▲ Mountain Range ☒ Volcano ∽ River ◎ Lake ⊡ Reservoir

82 A11 **Luanda** × Luanda, NW Angola
82 D12 **Luando** ≈ C Angola
Luang see Tapi, Mae Nam
83 G14 **Luanginga** var. Luanguinga. ≈ Angola/Zambia
167 N15 **Luang, Khao** ▲ SW Thailand
Luang Prabang see Louangphabang
167 P8 **Luang Prabang Range** Th. Thiukhaoluang Phrahang. ⛰ Laos/Thailand
167 N16 **Luang, Thale** lagoon S Thailand
Luangua, Rio see Luangwa
82 E11 **Luangue** ≈ NE Angola
Luanguinga see Luanginga
83 K15 **Luangwa** var. Aruângua. Lusaka, C Zambia
83 K14 **Luangwa** var. Aruângua, Rio Luangua. ≈ Mozambique/Zambia
161 Q2 **Luan He** ≈ E China
190 G11 **Luaniva, Île** island E Wallis and Futuna
161 P2 **Luanping** var. Anjiangying. Hebei, E China
82 J13 **Luanshya** Copperbelt, C Zambia
62 K13 **Luan Toro** La Pampa, C Argentina
161 Q2 **Luanxian** var. Luan Xian. Hebei, E China
82 J12 **Luapula** ◈ province N Zambia
79 O25 **Luapula** ≈ Dem. Rep. Congo (Zaire)/Zambia
104 J2 **Luarca** Asturias, N Spain
169 R10 **Luar, Danau** ◎ Borneo, N Indonesia
79 L25 **Luashi** Katanga, S Dem. Rep. Congo (Zaire)
82 G12 **Luau** Port. Vila Teixeira de Sousa. Moxico, NE Angola
79 C16 **Luba** prev. San Carlos. Isla de Bioco, NW Equatorial Guinea
42 F4 **Lubaantun** ruins Toledo, S Belize
111 P16 **Lubaczów** var. Lúbaczów. Podkarpackie, SE Poland
Lubale see Lubalo
82 E11 **Lubalo** Lunda Norte, NE Angola
82 E11 **Lubalo** var. Lubale. ≈ Angola/Zaire
118 J9 **Lubāna** Madona, E Latvia
Lubānas Ezers see Lubāns
171 N4 **Lubang Island** island N Philippines
83 B15 **Lubango** Port. Sá da Bandeira. Huíla, SW Angola
118 J9 **Lubāns** var. Lubānas Ezers. ◎ E Latvia
79 M21 **Lubao** Kasai Oriental, C Dem. Rep. Congo (Zaire)
110 O13 **Lubartów** Ger. Qumälisch. Lubelskie, E Poland
100 G13 **Lübbecke** Nordrhein-Westfalen, NW Germany
100 O13 **Lübben** Brandenburg, E Germany
101 P14 **Lübbenau** Brandenburg, E Germany
25 N5 **Lubbock** Texas, SW USA
Lubcz see Lyubcha
19 U6 **Lubec** Maine, NE USA
100 K9 **Lübeck** Schleswig-Holstein, N Germany
100 K8 **Lübecker Bucht** bay N Germany
79 M21 **Lubefu** Kasai Oriental, C Dem. Rep. Congo (Zaire)
111 O14 **Lubelska, Wyżyna** plateau SE Poland
111 O14 **Lubelskie** ◈ province E Poland
Lubembe see Luembe
Lüben see Lubin
144 H9 **Lubenka** Zapadnyy Kazakhstan, W Kazakhstan
79 P18 **Lubero** Nord Kivu, E Dem. Rep. Congo (Zaire)
79 L22 **Lubi** ≈ S Dem. Rep. Congo (Zaire)
Lubiana see Ljubljana
110 J11 **Lubień Kujawski** Kujawsko-pomorskie, C Poland
67 T11 **Lubilandji** ≈ S Dem. Rep. Congo (Zaire)
110 F13 **Lubin** Ger. Lüben. Dolnośląskie, SW Poland
111 O14 **Lublin** Rus. Lyublin. Lubelskie, E Poland
111 J15 **Lubliniec** Śląskie, S Poland
Lubnān, Jabal see Liban, Jebel
117 R5 **Lubny** Poltavs'ka Oblast', NE Ukraine
Luboml see Lyuboml'
110 G11 **Luboń** Ger. Peterhof. Wielkolpolskie, C Poland
110 D12 **Lubsko** Ger. Sommerfeld. Lubuskie, W Poland
79 N24 **Lubudi** Katanga, SE Dem. Rep. Congo (Zaire)
168 L13 **Lubuklinggau** Sumatera, W Indonesia
79 N25 **Lubumbashi** prev. Élisabethville. Katanga, SE Dem. Rep. Congo (Zaire)
83 I14 **Lubungu** Central, C Zambia
110 E12 **Lubuskie** ◈ province W Poland
79 N18 **Lubutu** Maniema, E Dem. Rep. Congo (Zaire)
Luca see Lucca
82 C11 **Lucala** ≈ W Angola
14 E16 **Lucan** Ontario, S Canada
97 F18 **Lucan** Ir. Leamhcán. E Ireland
Lucanian Mountains see Lucano, Appennino
107 M18 **Lucano, Appennino** Eng. Lucanian Mountains. ⛰ S Italy
82 F11 **Lucapa** var. Lukapa. Lunda Norte, NE Angola
29 V15 **Lucas** Iowa, C USA
61 C18 **Lucas González** Entre Ríos, E Argentina
65 C25 **Lucas Point** headland West Falkland, Falkland Islands
31 S15 **Lucasville** Ohio, N USA
106 F11 **Lucca** anc. Luca. Toscana, C Italy
44 H12 **Lucea** W Jamaica
97 H15 **Luce Bay** inlet SW Scotland, UK
22 M8 **Lucedale** Mississippi, S USA
171 O4 **Lucena** off. Lucena City. Luzon, N Philippines
104 M14 **Lucena** Andalucía, S Spain
105 S8 **Lucena del Cid** País Valenciano, E Spain
111 D15 **Lučenec** Ger. Losontz, Hung. Losonc. Banskobystrický Kraj, C Slovakia
Lucentum see Alicante
107 M16 **Lucera** Puglia, SE Italy
Lucerna/Lucerne see Luzern
Lucerne, Lake of see Vierwaldstätter See
40 J4 **Lucero** Chihuahua, N Mexico
123 S14 **Luchegorsk** Primorskiy Kray, SE Russian Federation
105 Q13 **Luchena** ≈ SE Spain
82 N13 **Lucheringo** var. Luchulingo. ≈ N Mozambique
Luchesa see Luchosa
Luchin see Luchyn
118 N13 **Luchosa** Rus. Luchesa. ≈ N Belarus
Luchow see Hefei
100 K11 **Lüchow** Mecklenburg-Vorpommern, N Germany
Luchulingo see Lucheringo
119 N17 **Luchyn** Rus. Luchin. Homyel'skaya Voblasts', SE Belarus
55 U11 **Lucie Rivier** ≈ W Surinam
182 K11 **Lucindale** South Australia
83 A14 **Lucira** Namibe, SW Angola
Łuck see Luts'k
101 O14 **Luckau** Brandenburg, E Germany
100 N13 **Luckenwalde** Brandenburg, E Germany
14 E15 **Lucknow** Ontario, S Canada
152 L12 **Lucknow** var. Lakhnau. Uttar Pradesh, N India
102 J10 **Luçon** Vendée, NW France
44 I7 **Lucrecia, Cabo** headland E Cuba
82 F13 **Lucusse** Moxico, E Angola
Lüda see Dalian
114 M9 **Luda Kamchiya** ≈ E Bulgaria
Ludasch see Luduş
114 I10 **Luda Yana** ≈ C Bulgaria
112 F7 **Ludbreg** Varaždin, N Croatia
29 P7 **Ludden** North Dakota, N USA
101 F15 **Lüdenscheid** Nordrhein-Westfalen, W Germany
83 C21 **Lüderitz** prev. Angra Pequena. Karas, SW Namibia
152 H8 **Ludhiāna** Punjab, N India
31 O7 **Ludington** Michigan, N USA
97 K20 **Ludlow** W England, UK
35 W14 **Ludlow** California, W USA
28 J7 **Ludlow** South Dakota, N USA
18 M9 **Ludlow** Vermont, NE USA
114 L7 **Ludogorie** physical region NE Bulgaria
23 W6 **Ludowici** Georgia, SE USA
Ludsan see Ludza
116 I10 **Luduş** Ger. Ludasch, Hung. Marosludas. Mureş, C Romania
95 M14 **Ludvika** Dalarna, C Sweden
101 H21 **Ludwigsburg** Baden-Württemberg, SW Germany
100 O13 **Ludwigsfelde** Brandenburg, NE Germany
101 G20 **Ludwigshafen** var. Ludwigshafen am Rhein. Rheinland-Pfalz, W Germany
Ludwigshafen am Rhein see Ludwigshafen
101 L20 **Ludwigskanal** canal SE Germany
100 L10 **Ludwigslust** Mecklenburg-Vorpommern, N Germany
118 K10 **Ludza** Ger. Ludsan. Ludza, E Latvia
79 K21 **Luebo** Kasai Occidental, SW Dem. Rep. Congo (Zaire)
25 Q6 **Lueders** Texas, SW USA
79 N20 **Lueki** Maniema, C Dem. Rep. Congo (Zaire)
82 F10 **Luembe** var. Lubembe. ≈ Angola/Dem. Rep. Congo (Zaire)
82 E13 **Luena** var. Lwena, Port. Luso. Moxico, E Angola
79 M24 **Luena** Katanga, SE Dem. Rep. Congo (Zaire)
82 K12 **Luena** Northern, NE Zambia
82 F13 **Luena** ≈ E Angola
83 F16 **Luengue** ≈ SE Angola
67 V13 **Luenha** ≈ W Mozambique
83 G15 **Lueti** ≈ Angola/Zambia
160 J7 **Lüeyang** Shaanxi, C China
161 P14 **Lufeng** Guangdong, S China
79 N24 **Lufira** ≈ SE Dem. Rep. Congo (Zaire)
79 N25 **Lufira, Lac de Retenue de la** var. Lac Tshangalele. ◎ SE Dem. Rep. Congo (Zaire)
25 W8 **Lufkin** Texas, SW USA
82 L11 **Lufubu** ≈ N Zambia
126 G14 **Luga** Leningradskaya Oblast', NW Russian Federation
126 G13 **Luga** ≈ NW Russian Federation
Luganer See see Lugano, Lago di
108 H11 **Lugano** Ger. Lauis. Ticino, S Switzerland
108 H12 **Lugano, Lago di** var. Ceresio, Ger. Luganer See. ◎ S Switzerland
Lugansk see Luhans'k
187 Q13 **Luganville** Espiritu Santo, C Vanuatu
Lugdunum see Lyon
Lugdunum Batavorum see Leiden
83 O15 **Lugela** Zambézia, NE Mozambique
83 O16 **Lugela** ≈ C Mozambique
82 P13 **Lugenda, Rio** ≈ N Mozambique
Luggarus see Locarno
Lugh Ganana see Luuq
97 G19 **Lugnaquillia Mountain** Ir. Log na Coille. ▲ E Ireland
106 H10 **Lugo** Emilia-Romagna, N Italy
104 I3 **Lugo** anc. Lugus Augusti. Galicia, NW Spain
104 I3 **Lugo** ◈ province Galicia, NW Spain
21 R12 **Lugoff** South Carolina, SE USA
116 F12 **Lugoj** Ger. Lugosch, Hung. Lugos. Timiş, W Romania
Lugos/Lugosch see Lugoj
Lugovoy/Lugovoye see Kulan
158 I13 **Lugu** Xizang Zizhiqu, W China
Lugus Augusti see Lugo
Luguvallium/Luguvallum see Carlisle
117 Y7 **Luhans'k** Rus. Lugansk; prev. Voroshilovgrad. Luhans'ka Oblast', E Ukraine
117 Y7 **Luhans'k** × Luhans'ka Oblast', E Ukraine
117 X6 **Luhans'ka Oblast'** var. Luhans'k; prev. Voroshilovgrad, Rus. Voroshilovgradskaya Oblast'. ◈ province E Ukraine
161 Q7 **Luhe** Jiangsu, E China
171 S13 **Luhu** Pulau Seram, E Indonesia
160 G8 **Luhuo** var. Zhaggo. Sichuan, C China
116 M3 **Luhyny** Zhytomyrs'ka Oblast', N Ukraine
83 G15 **Lui** ≈ W Zambia
83 G16 **Luiana** ≈ SE Angola
83 L15 **Luia, Rio** var. Ruya. ≈ Mozambique/Zimbabwe
Luichow Peninsula see Leizhou Bandao
Luik see Liège
82 C13 **Luimbale** Huambo, C Angola
Luimneach see Limerick
106 D6 **Luino** Lombardia, N Italy
82 E13 **Luio** ≈ E Angola
92 L11 **Luiro** ≈ NE Finland
79 N25 **Luishia** Katanga, SE Dem. Rep. Congo (Zaire)
59 M19 **Luislândia do Oeste** Minas Gerais, SE Brazil
40 K5 **Luis L.León, Presa** ▣ N Mexico
Luis Muñoz Marin see San Juan
195 N5 **Luitpold Coast** physical region Antarctica
79 K22 **Luiza** Kasai Occidental, S Dem. Rep. Congo (Zaire)
61 D20 **Luján** Buenos Aires, E Argentina
79 N24 **Lukafu** Katanga, SE Dem. Rep. Congo (Zaire)
Lukapa see Lucapa
112 I11 **Lukavac** Federacija Bosna I Hercegovina, NE Bosnia and Herzegovina
79 I20 **Lukenie** ≈ C Dem. Rep. Congo (Zaire)
79 H19 **Lukolela** Equateur, W Dem. Rep. Congo (Zaire)
119 M14 **Lukoml'skaye, Vozyera** Rus. Ozero Lukoml'skoye. ◎ N Belarus
Lukoml'skoye, Ozero see Lukoml'skaye, Vozyera
114 I8 **Lukovit** Lovech, N Bulgaria
110 O12 **Łuków** Ger. Bogendorf. Lubelskie, E Poland
129 O4 **Lukoyanov** Nizhegorodskaya Oblast', W Russian Federation
79 N22 **Lukuga** ≈ SE Dem. Rep. Congo (Zaire)
79 F21 **Lukula** Bas-Congo, SW Dem. Rep. Congo (Zaire)
83 G14 **Lukulu** Western, NW Zambia
189 R17 **Lukunor Atoll** atoll Mortlock Islands, C Micronesia
82 J12 **Lukwesa** Luapula, NE Zambia
93 K14 **Luleå** Norrbotten, N Sweden
92 J13 **Luleälven** ≈ N Sweden
136 C10 **Lüleburgaz** Kırklareli, NW Turkey
160 M4 **Lüliang Shan** ⛰ C China
79 O21 **Lulimba** Maniema, E Dem. Rep. Congo (Zaire)
22 K9 **Luling** Louisiana, S USA
25 T11 **Luling** Texas, SW USA
79 I18 **Lulonga** ≈ NW Dem. Rep. Congo (Zaire)
79 K22 **Lulua** ≈ S Dem. Rep. Congo (Zaire)
Luluabourg see Kananga
192 L17 **Luma** Ta'ū, E American Samoa
169 S17 **Lumajang** Jawa, C Indonesia
158 G12 **Lumajangdong Co** ◎ W China
82 G13 **Lumbala Kaquengue** Moxico, E Angola
83 F14 **Lumbala N'Guimbo** var. Nguimbo, Port. Gago Coutinho, Vila Gago Coutinho. Moxico, E Angola
21 T11 **Lumber River** ≈ North Carolina/South Carolina, SE USA
Lumber State see Maine
22 L8 **Lumberton** Mississippi, S USA
21 U11 **Lumberton** North Carolina, SE USA
105 R4 **Lumbier** Navarra, N Spain
83 Q15 **Lumbo** Nampula, NE Mozambique
126 M4 **Lumbovka** Murmanskaya Oblast', NW Russian Federation
104 J7 **Lumbrales** Castilla-León, N Spain
153 W13 **Lumding** Assam, NE India
82 F12 **Lumege** var. Lumeje. Moxico, E Angola
Lumeje see Lumege
99 J17 **Lummen** Limburg, NE Belgium
93 J20 **Lumparland** Åland, SW Finland
167 T11 **Lumphăt** prev. Lomphat. Rôtânôkiri, NE Cambodia
11 U16 **Lumsden** Saskatchewan, S Canada
185 C23 **Lumsden** Southland, South Island, NZ
169 N14 **Lumut, Tanjung** headland Sumatera, W Indonesia
157 P4 **Lün** Töv, C Mongolia
160 H13 **Lunan** var. Lunan Yizu Zizhixian. Yunnan, SW China
Lunan Yizu Zizhixian see Lunan
116 I13 **Lunca Corbului** Argeş, S Romania
95 K23 **Lund** Skåne, S Sweden
35 X6 **Lund** Nevada, W USA
82 D11 **Lunda Norte** ◈ province NE Angola
82 E12 **Lunda Sul** ◈ province NE Angola
82 M13 **Lundazi** Eastern, NE Zambia
95 G16 **Lunde** Telemark, S Norway
Lundenburg see Břeclav
95 C17 **Lundevatnet** ◎ S Norway
Lundi see Runde
97 I23 **Lundy** island SW England, UK
100 J10 **Lüneburg** Niedersachsen, N Germany
100 J11 **Lüneburger Heide** heathland NW Germany
103 Q15 **Lunel** Hérault, S France
101 F14 **Lünen** Nordrhein-Westfalen, W Germany
13 P16 **Lunenburg** Nova Scotia, SE Canada
21 V7 **Lunenburg** Virginia, NE USA
103 T5 **Lunéville** Meurthe-et-Moselle, NE France
83 I14 **Lunga** ≈ C Zambia
Lunga, Isola see Dugi Otok
158 H12 **Lungdo** Xizang Zizhiqu, W China
158 I14 **Lunggar** Xizang Zizhiqu, W China
76 I15 **Lungi** × (Freetown) W Sierra Leone
Lungkiang see Qiqihar
Lungleh see Lunglei
153 W15 **Lunglei** prev. Lungleh. Mizoram, NE India
158 L15 **Lungsang** Xizang Zizhiqu, W China
82 E13 **Lungué-Bungo** var. Lungwebungu. ≈ Angola/Zambia see also Lungwebungu
83 G14 **Lungwebungu** var. Lungué-Bungo. ≈ Angola/Zambia see also Lungué-Bungo
152 F12 **Lūni** Rājasthān, N India
152 F12 **Lūni** ≈ N India
Luninets see Luninyets
35 S7 **Luning** Nevada, W USA
Łuniniec see Luninyets
129 P6 **Lunino** Penzenskaya Oblast', W Russian Federation
119 J19 **Luninyets** Pol. Łuniniec, Rus. Luninets. Brestskaya Voblasts', SW Belarus
152 F10 **Lūnkaransar** Rājasthān, NW India
119 G17 **Lunna** Pol. Łunna, Rus. Lunna. Hrodzyenskaya Voblasts', W Belarus
76 I15 **Lunsar** W Sierra Leone
83 K14 **Lunsemfwa** ≈ C Zambia
158 J6 **Luntai** var. Bügür. Xinjiang Uygur Zizhiqu, NW China
98 K11 **Lunteren** Gelderland, C Netherlands
109 U5 **Lunz am See** Niederösterreich, C Austria
163 Y7 **Luobei** var. Fengxiang. Heilongjiang, NE China
160 J13 **Luodian** var. Longping. Guizhou, S China
160 M15 **Luoding** Guangdong, S China
160 M6 **Luo He** ≈ C China
160 L5 **Luo He** ≈ C China
161 N7 **Luohe** Henan, C China
Luolajarvi see Kuoloyarvi
Luong Nam Tha see Louangnamtha
160 L13 **Luoqing Jiang** ≈ S China
161 O8 **Luoshan** Henan, C China
161 O12 **Luoxiao Shan** ⛰ S China
161 N6 **Luoyang** var. Honan, Lo-yang. Henan, C China
161 R12 **Luoyuan** Fujian, SE China
79 F21 **Luozi** Bas-Congo, W Dem. Rep. Congo (Zaire)
83 J17 **Lupane** Matabeleland North, W Zimbabwe
160 I12 **Lupanshui** prev. Shuicheng. Guizhou, S China
169 R10 **Lupar, Batang** ≈ East Malaysia
Lupatia see Altamura
116 G12 **Lupeni** Hung. Lupény. Hunedoara, SW Romania
Lupény see Lupeni
82 N13 **Lupiliche** Niassa, N Mozambique
83 E14 **Lupire** Cuando Cubango, E Angola
79 L22 **Luputa** Kasai Oriental, S Dem. Rep. Congo (Zaire)
121 P16 **Luqa** × (Valletta) S Malta
159 U11 **Luqu** Gansu, C China
45 U5 **Luquillo, Sierra de** ⛰ E Puerto Rico
26 L4 **Luray** Kansas, C USA
21 U4 **Luray** Virginia, NE USA
103 T7 **Lure** Haute-Saône, E France
82 D11 **Luremo** Lunda Norte, NE Angola
97 F15 **Lurgan** Ir. An Lorgain. S Northern Ireland, UK
57 K18 **Luribay** La Paz, W Bolivia
83 Q14 **Lúrio** Nampula, NE Mozambique
83 P14 **Lúrio, Rio** ≈ NE Mozambique
Luristan see Lorestān
Lurka see Lorca
83 J15 **Lusaka** ● (Zambia) Lusaka, SE Zambia
83 J15 **Lusaka** ◈ province C Zambia
83 J15 **Lusaka** × Lusaka, C Zambia
79 L21 **Lusambo** Kasai Oriental, C Dem. Rep. Congo (Zaire)
186 F8 **Lusancay Islands and Reefs** island group SE PNG
79 I21 **Lusanga** Bandundu, SW Dem. Rep. Congo (Zaire)
79 N21 **Lusangi** Maniema, E Dem. Rep. Congo (Zaire)
Lusatian Mountains see Lausitzer Bergland
Lushnja see Lushnjë
113 K21 **Lushnjë** var. Lushnja. Fier, C Albania
81 J21 **Lushoto** Tanga, E Tanzania
102 L10 **Lusignan** Vienne, W France
33 Z15 **Lusk** Wyoming, C USA
Luso see Luena
102 L10 **Lussac-les-Châteaux** Vienne, W France
Lussin/Lussino see Lošinj
Lussinpiccolo see Mali Lošinj
108 I7 **Lustenau** Vorarlberg, W Austria
161 T14 **Lü Tao** var. Huoshao Dao, Lütao, Eng. Green Island. island SE Taiwan
Lūt, Baḩrat/Lut, Bahret see Dead Sea
22 K9 **Lutcher** Louisiana, S USA
143 T9 **Lūt, Dasht-e** var. Kavīr-e Lūt. desert E Iran
83 F14 **Lutembo** Moxico, E Angola
Lutetia/Lutetia Parisiorum see Paris
Luteva see Lodève
14 G15 **Luther Lake** ◎ Ontario, S Canada
186 K8 **Luti** Choiseul Island, NW Solomon Islands
Lūt, Kavīr-e see Lūt, Dasht-e
97 N21 **Luton** SE England, UK
97 N21 **Luton** × (London) SE England, UK
108 B10 **Lutry** Vaud, SW Switzerland
8 K10 **Lutselk'e** prev. Snowdrift. Northwest Territories, W Canada
29 Y4 **Lutsen** Minnesota, N USA
116 J4 **Luts'k** Pol. Łuck, Rus. Lutsk. Volyns'ka Oblast', NW Ukraine
Luttenberg see Ljutomer
Lüttich see Liège
83 G25 **Luttig** Western Cape, SW South Africa
Lutto see Lotta
82 E13 **Lutuai** Moxico, E Angola
117 Y7 **Lutuhyne** Luhans'ka Oblast', E Ukraine
171 V14 **Lutur, Pulau** island Kepulauan Aru, E Indonesia
23 V12 **Lutz** Florida, SE USA
Lützow-Holm Bay see Lützow-Holmbukta
195 V2 **Lützow Holmbukta** var. Lutzow-Holm Bay. bay Antarctica
81 L16 **Luuq** It. Lugh Ganana. Gedo, SW Somalia
92 M12 **Luusua** Lappi, NE Finland
23 Q6 **Luverne** Alabama, S USA
29 S11 **Luverne** Minnesota, N USA
79 O22 **Luvua** ≈ SE Dem. Rep. Congo (Zaire)
82 F13 **Luvuei** Moxico, E Angola
81 H24 **Luwego** ≈ S Tanzania
82 K12 **Luwingu** Northern, NE Zambia
171 P12 **Luwuk** prev. Loewoek. Sulawesi, C Indonesia
23 N3 **Luxapallila Creek** ≈ Alabama/Mississippi, S USA
99 M25 **Luxembourg** ● (Luxembourg) Luxembourg, S Luxembourg
99 M25 **Luxembourg** off. Grand Duchy of Luxembourg, var. Lëtzebeurg, Luxemburg. ◆ monarchy NW Europe
99 J23 **Luxembourg** ◈ province SE Belgium
99 L24 **Luxembourg** ◈ district S Luxembourg
31 N6 **Luxemburg** Wisconsin, N USA
Luxemburg see Luxembourg
103 U7 **Luxeuil-les-Bains** Haute-Saône, E France
160 E13 **Luxi** prev. Mangshi. Yunnan, SW China
82 E10 **Luxico** ≈ Angola/Dem. Rep. Congo (Zaire)
75 X10 **Luxor** Ar. Al Uqşur. E Egypt
75 X10 **Luxor** × C Egypt
160 M4 **Luya Shan** ⛰ C China
102 J15 **Luy de Béarn** ≈ SW France
102 J15 **Luy de France** ≈ SW France
127 P12 **Luza** Kirovskaya Oblast', NW Russian Federation
127 Q12 **Luza** ≈ NW Russian Federation
104 I16 **Luz, Costa de la** coastal region SW Spain
111 K20 **Luže** var. Lausche. ▲ Czech Republic/Germany see also Lausche
108 F8 **Luzern** Fr. Lucerne, It. Lucerna. Luzern, C Switzerland
108 E8 **Luzern** Fr. Lucerne. ◈ canton C Switzerland
160 L13 **Luzhai** Guangxi Zhuangzu Zizhiqu, S China
118 K12 **Luzhki** Rus. Luzhki. Vitsyebskaya Voblasts', N Belarus
160 I10 **Luzhou** Sichuan, C China
Lužická Nisa see Neisse
Lužické Hory see Lausitzer Bergland
Lužnice see Lainsitz
171 O2 **Luzon** island N Philippines
171 N1 **Luzon Strait** strait Philippines/Taiwan
116 I5 **L'viv** Ger. Lemberg, Pol. Lwów, Rus. L'vov. L'vivs'ka Oblast', W Ukraine
L'viv see L'vivs'ka Oblast'
116 I4 **L'vivs'ka Oblast'** var. L'viv, Rus. L'vovskaya Oblast'. ◈ province NW Ukraine
L'vov see L'viv
L'vovskaya Oblast' see L'vivs'ka Oblast'
Lwena see Luena
Lwów see L'viv
110 F11 **Lwówek** Ger. Neustadt bei Pinne. Wielkolpolskie, C Poland
111 E14 **Lwówek Śląski** Ger. Löwenberg in Schlesien. Dolnośląskie, SW Poland
119 I18 **Lyakhavichy** Rus. Lyakhovichi. Brestskaya Voblasts', SW Belarus
Lyakhovichi see Lyakhavichy
185 B22 **Lyall, Mount** ▲ South Island, NZ
Lyallpur see Faisalābād
Lyangar see Langar
126 H11 **Lyaskelya** Respublika Kareliya, NW Russian Federation
119 I18 **Lyasnaya** Rus. Lesnaya. Brestskaya Voblasts', SW Belarus
119 F19 **Lyasnaya** Pol. Leśna, Rus. Lesnaya. ≈ SW Belarus
126 H15 **Lychkovo** Novgorodskaya Oblast', W Russian Federation
Lyck see Ełk
93 I15 **Lycksele** Västerbotten, N Sweden
18 G13 **Lycoming Creek** ≈ Pennsylvania, NE USA
Lycopolis see Asyūt
195 N3 **Lyddan Island** island Antarctica
83 K20 **Lydenburg** Mpumalanga, NE South Africa
119 L20 **Lyel'chytsy** Rus. Lel'chitsy. Homyel'skaya Voblasts', SE Belarus
119 P14 **Lyenina** Rus. Lenino. Mahilyowskaya Voblasts', E Belarus
118 L13 **Lyepyel'** Rus. Lepel'. Vitsyebskaya Voblasts', N Belarus
25 S17 **Lyford** Texas, SW USA
95 E17 **Lygna** ≈ S Norway
18 G14 **Lykens** Pennsylvania, NE USA
115 E21 **Lykódimo** ▲ S Greece
97 K24 **Lyme Bay** bay S England, UK
97 K24 **Lyme Regis** S England, UK
110 L7 **Łyna** Ger. Alle. ≈ N Poland
29 P12 **Lynch** Nebraska, C USA
20 J10 **Lynchburg** Tennessee, S USA
21 T6 **Lynchburg** Virginia, NE USA
21 T12 **Lynches River** ≈ South Carolina, SE USA
32 H6 **Lynden** Washington, NW USA
182 I5 **Lyndhurst** South Australia
27 Q5 **Lyndon** Kansas, C USA
19 N7 **Lyndonville** Vermont, NE USA
95 D18 **Lyngdal** Vest-Agder, S Norway
92 I9 **Lyngen** inlet Arctic Ocean
95 G17 **Lyngør** Aust-Agder, S Norway
92 I9 **Lyngseidet** Troms, N Norway
19 P11 **Lynn** Massachusetts, NE USA
Lynn see King's Lynn
23 R9 **Lynn Haven** Florida, SE USA
11 V11 **Lynn Lake** Manitoba, C Canada
Lynn Regis see King's Lynn
118 I13 **Lyntupy** Rus. Lyntupy. Vitsyebskaya Voblasts', NW Belarus
103 R11 **Lyon** Eng. Lyons; anc. Lugdunum. Rhône, E France
8 I6 **Lyon, Cape** headland Northwest Territories, NW Canada
18 K6 **Lyon Mountain** ▲ New York, NE USA
103 Q11 **Lyonnais, Monts du** ⛰ C France
65 N25 **Lyon Point** headland SE Tristan da Cunha
182 E5 **Lyons** South Australia
37 T3 **Lyons** Colorado, C USA
23 V6 **Lyons** Georgia, SE USA
26 M5 **Lyons** Kansas, C USA
29 R14 **Lyons** Nebraska, C USA
18 G10 **Lyons** New York, NE USA
Lyons see Lyon
118 O13 **Lyozna** Rus. Liozno. Vitsyebskaya Voblasts', NE Belarus
117 S4 **Lypova Dolyna** Sums'ka Oblast', NE Ukraine
117 N6 **Lypovets'** Rus. Lipovets. Vinnyts'ka Oblast', C Ukraine
Lys see Leie
111 I18 **Lysá Hora** ▲ E Czech Republic
95 D16 **Lysefjorden** fjord S Norway
95 I18 **Lysekil** Västra Götaland, S Sweden
Lýsi see Akdoğan
33 V14 **Lysite** Wyoming, C USA
129 P3 **Lyskovo** Nizhegorodskaya Oblast', W Russian Federation
108 D8 **Lyss** Bern, W Switzerland
95 H22 **Lystrup** Århus, C Denmark
127 V14 **Lys'va** Permskaya Oblast', NW Russian Federation
117 P6 **Lysyanka** Cherkas'ka Oblast', C Ukraine
117 X6 **Lysychans'k** Rus. Lisichansk. Luhans'ka Oblast', E Ukraine
97 K17 **Lytham St Anne's** NW England, UK
185 I19 **Lyttelton** Canterbury, South Island, NZ
10 M17 **Lytton** British Columbia, SW Canada
119 L18 **Lyuban'** Rus. Lyuban'. Minskaya Voblasts', S Belarus
119 L18 **Lyubanskaye Vodaskhovishcha** ▣ C Belarus
116 M5 **Lyubar** Zhytomyrs'ka Oblast', N Ukraine
Lyubashëvka see Lyubashivka
117 O8 **Lyubashivka** Rus. Lyubashëvka. Odes'ka Oblast', SW Ukraine
119 I16 **Lyubcha** Pol. Lubcz, Rus. Lyubcha. Hrodzyenskaya Voblasts', W Belarus
128 L4 **Lyubertsy** Moskovskaya Oblast', W Russian Federation
116 K2 **Lyubeshiv** Volyns'ka Oblast', NW Ukraine
126 M14 **Lyubim** Yaroslavskaya Oblast', NW Russian Federation
114 K11 **Lyubimets** Khaskovo, S Bulgaria
Lyublin see Lublin
116 I3 **Lyuboml'** Pol. Luboml. Volyns'ka Oblast', NW Ukraine
Lyubotin see Lyubotyn
117 U5 **Lyubotyn** Rus. Lyubotin. Kharkivs'ka Oblast', E Ukraine
128 I5 **Lyudinovo** Kaluzhskaya Oblast', W Russian Federation
129 T2 **Lyuk** Udmurtskaya Respublika, NW Russian Federation
114 M9 **Lyulyakovo** prev. Keremitlik. Burgas, E Bulgaria
119 I18 **Lyusina** Rus. Lyusino. Brestskaya Voblasts', SW Belarus
Lyusino see Lyusina

M

138 G9 **Ma'ād** Irbid, N Jordan
Maalahti see Malax
Maale see Male'

◆ Country ● Country Capital ◇ Dependent Territory ○ Dependent Territory Capital ◈ Administrative Region × International Airport ▲ Mountain ⛰ Mountain Range ✻ Volcano ≈ River ◎ Lake ▣ Reservoir

138 G13 **Ma'ān** Ma'ān, SW Jordan
138 H13 **Ma'ān** *off.* Muḥāfaẓat Ma'ān, *var.* Ma'an, Ma'ān. ◈ *governorate* S Jordan
93 M16 **Maaninka** Itä-Suomi, C Finland
162 K7 **Maanĭt** Bulgan, C Mongolia
162 M8 **Maanĭt** Töv, C Mongolia
93 N15 **Maanselkä** Oulu, C Finland
161 Q8 **Ma'anshan** Anhui, E China
188 F16 **Maap** *island* Caroline Islands, W Micronesia
118 H3 **Maardu** *Ger.* Maart. Harjumaa, NW Estonia
Ma'aret-en-Nu'man *see* Ma'arrat an Nu'mān
99 K16 **Maarheeze** Noord-Brabant, SE Netherlands
Maarianhamina *see* Mariehamn
138 I4 **Ma'arrat an Nu'mān** *var.* Ma'aret-en-Nu'man, *Fr.* Maarret enn Naamâne. Idlib, NW Syria
Maarret enn Naamâne *see* Ma'arrat an Nu'mān
98 I11 **Maarssen** Utrecht, C Netherlands
Maart *see* Maardu
99 L17 **Maas** *Fr.* Meuse. ≈ W Europe *see also* Meuse
99 M15 **Maasbree** Limburg, SE Netherlands
99 L17 **Maaseik** *prev.* Maeseyck. Limburg, NE Belgium
171 Q6 **Maasin** Leyte, C Philippines
99 L17 **Maasmechelen** Limburg, NE Belgium
98 G12 **Maassluis** Zuid-Holland, SW Netherlands
99 L18 **Maastricht** *var.* Maestricht; *anc.* Traiectum ad Mosam, Traiectum Tungorum. Limburg, SE Netherlands
183 N18 **Maatsuyker Group** *island group* Tasmania, SE Australia
Maba *see* Qujiang
83 L20 **Mabalane** Gaza, S Mozambique
25 V7 **Mabank** Texas, SW USA
97 O18 **Mablethorpe** E England, UK
171 V12 **Maboi** Irian Jaya, E Indonesia
83 M19 **Mabote** Inhambane, S Mozambique
32 J10 **Mabton** Washington, NW USA
Mabuchi-gawa *see* Mabechi-gawa
83 H20 **Mabutsane** Southern, S Botswana
63 G19 **Macá, Cerro** ▲ S Chile
60 Q9 **Macaé** Rio de Janeiro, SE Brazil
82 N13 **Macaloge** Niassa, N Mozambique
Macan *see* Bonerate, Kepulauan
161 N15 **Macao** *Chin.* Aomen, *Port.* Macau. S China
104 H9 **Mação** Santarém, C Portugal
58 J11 **Macapá** *state capital* Amapá, N Brazil
43 S17 **Macaracas** Los Santos, S Panama
55 P6 **Macare, Caño** ≈ NE Venezuela
55 Q6 **Macareo, Caño** ≈ NE Venezuela
Macarsca *see* Makarska
MacArthur *see* Ormoc
182 L12 **Macarthur** Victoria, SE Australia
56 C7 **Macas** Morona Santiago, SE Ecuador
Macassar *see* Ujungpandang
59 Q14 **Macau** Rio Grande do Norte, E Brazil
Macau *see* Macao
Macău *see* Makó, Hungary
65 E24 **Macbride Head** *headland* East Falkland, Falkland Islands
23 V9 **Macclenny** Florida, SE USA
97 L18 **Macclesfield** C England, UK
192 F6 **Macclesfield Bank** *undersea feature* N South China Sea
MacCluer Gulf *see* Berau, Teluk
181 N7 **Macdonald, Lake** *salt lake* Western Australia
181 Q7 **Macdonnell Ranges** ▲▲ Northern Territory, C Australia
96 K8 **Macduff** NE Scotland, UK
104 I6 **Macedo de Cavaleiros** Bragança, N Portugal
Macedonia Central *see* Kentrikí Makedonía
Macedonia East and Thrace *see* Anatolikí Makedonía kai Thráki
113 O19 **Macedonia, FYR** *off.* the Former Yugoslav Republic of Macedonia, *var.* Macedonia, Mac. Makedonija, *abbrev.* FYR Macedonia, FYROM. ◆ *republic* SE Europe
Macedonia West *see* Dytikí Makedonía
59 Q16 **Maceió** *state capital* Alagoas, E Brazil
76 K15 **Macenta** Guinée-Forestière, SE Guinea
106 J12 **Macerata** Marche, C Italy
11 S11 **MacFarlane** ≈ Saskatchewan, C Canada
182 H7 **Macfarlane, Lake** *var.* Lake Mcfarlane. ◎ South Australia
Macgillicuddy's Reeks Mountains *see* Macgillycuddy's Reeks
97 B21 **Macgillycuddy's Reeks** *var.* Macgillicuddy's Reeks Mountains, *Ir.* Na Cruacha Dubha. ▲▲ SW Ireland
11 X16 **MacGregor** Manitoba, S Canada
149 O10 **Mach** Baluchistān, SW Pakistan
56 C6 **Machachi** Pichincha, C Ecuador
83 M19 **Machaila** Gaza, S Mozambique
Machaire Fíolta *see* Magherafelt
Machaire Rátha *see* Maghera
81 I19 **Machakos** Eastern, S Kenya
56 B8 **Machala** El Oro, SW Ecuador
83 J19 **Machaneng** Central, SE Botswana
83 M18 **Machanga** Sofala, E Mozambique
80 G13 **Machar Marshes** *wetland* SE Sudan
102 I8 **Machecoul** Loire-Atlantique, NW France
161 O8 **Macheng** Hubei, C China
155 J16 **Mācherla** Andhra Pradesh, C India
153 O11 **Machhapuchhre** ▲ C Nepal
19 T6 **Machias** Maine, NE USA
19 R3 **Machias River** ≈ Maine, NE USA
19 T6 **Machias River** ≈ Maine, NE USA
64 P5 **Machico** Madeira, Portugal, NE Atlantic Ocean
155 K16 **Machilīpatnam** *var.* Bandar Masulipatnam. Andhra Pradesh, E India
54 G5 **Machiques** Zulia, NW Venezuela
57 G15 **Machupicchu** Cusco, C Peru
83 M20 **Macia** *var.* Vila de Macia. Gaza, S Mozambique
Macías Nguema Biyogo *see* Bioco, Isla de
116 M13 **Măcin** Tulcea, SE Romania
183 T4 **Macintyre River** ≈ New South Wales/Queensland, SE Australia
181 Y7 **Mackay** Queensland, NE Australia
181 O7 **Mackay, Lake** *salt lake* Northern Territory/Western Australia
10 M13 **Mackenzie** British Columbia, W Canada
8 I9 **Mackenzie** ≈ Northwest Territories, NW Canada
195 Y6 **Mackenzie Bay** *bay* Antarctica
10 J1 **Mackenzie Bay** *bay* NW Canada
2 D9 **Mackenzie Delta** *delta* Northwest Territories, NW Canada
8 K3 **Mackenzie King Island** *island* Queen Elizabeth Islands, Northwest Territories, N Canada
8 H8 **Mackenzie Mountains** ▲▲ Northwest Territories, NW Canada
31 Q5 **Mackinac, Straits of** ◎ Michigan, N USA
194 K5 **Mackintosh, Cape** *headland* Antarctica
11 R15 **Macklin** Saskatchewan, S Canada
183 V6 **Macksville** New South Wales, SE Australia
183 V5 **Maclean** New South Wales, SE Australia
83 J24 **Maclear** Eastern Cape, SE South Africa
183 U6 **Macleay River** ≈ New South Wales, SE Australia
MacLeod *see* Fort Macleod
180 G9 **Macleod, Lake** ◎ Western Australia
10 I6 **Macmillan** ≈ Yukon Territory, NW Canada
30 J12 **Macomb** Illinois, N USA
107 B18 **Macomer** Sardegna, Italy, C Mediterranean Sea
82 Q13 **Macomia** Cabo Delgado, NE Mozambique
23 T5 **Macon** Georgia, SE USA
23 N4 **Macon** Mississippi, S USA
27 U3 **Macon** Missouri, C USA
103 R10 **Mâcon** *anc.* Matisco, Matisco Ædourum. Saône-et-Loire, C France
22 J6 **Macon, Bayou** ≈ Arkansas/Louisiana, S USA
82 G13 **Macondo** Moxico, E Angola
83 M16 **Macossa** Manica, C Mozambique
11 T12 **Macoun Lake** ◎ Saskatchewan, C Canada
30 K14 **Macoupin Creek** ≈ Illinois, N USA
Macouria *see* Tonate
83 N18 **Macovane** Inhambane, SE Mozambique
183 N17 **Macquarie Harbour** *inlet* Tasmania, SE Australia
192 J13 **Macquarie Island** *island* NZ, SW Pacific Ocean
183 T8 **Macquarie, Lake** *lagoon* New South Wales, SE Australia
183 Q6 **Macquarie Marshes** *wetland* New South Wales, SE Australia
175 O13 **Macquarie Ridge** *undersea feature* SW Pacific Ocean
183 Q6 **Macquarie River** ≈ New South Wales, SE Australia
183 P17 **Macquarie River** ≈ Tasmania, SE Australia
195 V5 **Mac. Robertson Land** *physical region* Antarctica
97 C21 **Macroom** *Ir.* Maigh Chromtha. SW Ireland
42 G5 **Macuelizo** Santa Bárbara, NW Honduras
182 G2 **Macumba River** ≈ South Australia
57 I16 **Macusani** Puno, S Peru
56 E8 **Macusari, Río** ≈ N Peru
41 U15 **Macuspana** Tabasco, SE Mexico
138 G10 **Ma'dabā** *var.* Mādabā, Madeba; *anc.* Medeba. 'Ammān, NW Jordan
172 G2 **Madagascar** *off.* Democratic Republic of Madagascar, *Malg.* Madagasikara; *prev.* Malagasy Republic. ◆ *republic* W Indian Ocean
172 I5 **Madagascar** *island* W Indian Ocean
130 L17 **Madagascar Basin** *undersea feature* W Indian Ocean
130 L16 **Madagascar Plain** *undersea feature* W Indian Ocean
67 Y14 **Madagascar Plateau** *var.* Madagascar Ridge, Madagascar Rise, *Rus.* Madagaskarskiy Khrebet. *undersea feature* W Indian Ocean
Madagascar Ridge/Madagascar Rise *see* Madagascar Plateau
Madagasikara *see* Madagascar
Madagaskarskiy Khrebet *see* Madagascar Plateau
64 N2 **Madalena** Pico, Azores, Portugal, NE Atlantic Ocean
77 Y6 **Madama** Agadez, NE Niger
114 J12 **Madan** Smolyan, S Bulgaria
155 I19 **Madanapalle** Andhra Pradesh, E India
186 D7 **Madang** Madang, N PNG
186 C6 **Madang** ◈ *province* N PNG
146 G7 **Madaniyat** *Rus.* Madeniyet. Qoraqalpoghiston Respublikasi, W Uzbekistan
Madanīyīn *see* Médenine
77 U11 **Madaoua** Tahoua, SW Niger
Madaras *see* Vtáčnik
153 U15 **Madaripur** Dhaka, C Bangladesh
77 U12 **Madarounfa** Maradi, S Niger
Madarska *see* Hungary
146 B13 **Madau** *Turkm.* Madaw. Balkanskiy Velayat, W Turkmenistan
186 H9 **Madau Island** *island* SE PNG
Madaw *see* Madau
19 S1 **Madawaska** Maine, NE USA
14 J13 **Madawaska** ≈ Ontario, SE Canada
Madawaska Highlands *see* Haliburton Highlands
166 M4 **Madaya** Mandalay, C Myanmar
107 K17 **Maddaloni** Campania, S Italy
29 O3 **Maddock** North Dakota, N USA
99 I14 **Made** Noord-Brabant, S Netherlands
Madeba *see* Ma'dabā
64 L9 **Madeira** *var.* Ilha de Madeira. *island* Madeira, Portugal, NE Atlantic Ocean
Madeira, Ilha de *see* Madeira
64 O5 **Madeira Islands** *Port.* Região Autoónoma da Madeira. ◈ *autonomous region* Madeira, Portugal, NE Atlantic Ocean
64 L9 **Madeira Plain** *undersea feature* E Atlantic Ocean
64 L9 **Madeira Ridge** *undersea feature* E Atlantic Ocean
59 F14 **Madeira, Rio** *Sp.* Río Madera. ≈ Bolivia/Brazil *see also* Madera, Río
101 J25 **Mädelegabel** ▲ Austria/Germany
15 X6 **Madeleine** ≈ Quebec, SE Canada
15 X5 **Madeleine, Cap de la** *headland* Quebec, SE Canada
13 Q13 **Madeleine, Îles de la** *Eng.* Magdalen Islands. *island group* Quebec, E Canada
29 U10 **Madelia** Minnesota, N USA
35 P3 **Madeline** California, W USA
30 K3 **Madeline Island** *island* Apostle Islands, Wisconsin, N USA
137 O15 **Maden** Elâzığ, SE Turkey
145 V12 **Madeniyet** Vostochnyy Kazakhstan, E Kazakhstan
Madeniyet *see* Madaniyat
40 H5 **Madera** Chihuahua, N Mexico
35 Q10 **Madera** California, W USA
56 L13 **Madera, Río** *Port.* Rio Madeira. ≈ Bolivia/Brazil *see also* Madeira, Rio
106 D6 **Madesimo** Lombardia, N Italy
141 O14 **Madhāb, Wādī** *dry watercourse* NW Yemen
153 R13 **Madhepura** *prev.* Madhipure. Bihār, NE India
Madhipure *see* Madhepura
153 Q13 **Madhubani** Bihār, N India
153 Q15 **Madhupur** Bihār, NE India
152 K15 **Madhya Pradesh** *prev.* Central Provinces and Berar. ◈ *state* C India
57 K15 **Madidi, Río** ≈ W Bolivia
155 F20 **Madikeri** *prev.* Mercara. Karnātaka, W India
27 O13 **Madill** Oklahoma, C USA
79 G21 **Madimba** Bas-Congo, SW Dem. Rep. Congo (Zaire)
138 M4 **Ma'dīn** Ar Raqqah, C Syria
Madīnah, Minṭaqat al *see* Al Madīnah
76 M14 **Madinani** NW Ivory Coast
141 O17 **Madīnat ash Sha'b** *prev.* Al Ittiḥād. SW Yemen
138 K3 **Madīnat ath Thawrah** *var.* Ath Thawrah. Ar Raqqah, N Syria Asia
173 O6 **Madingley Rise** *undersea feature* W Indian Ocean
79 E21 **Madingo-Kayes** Le Kouilou, S Congo
79 F21 **Madingou** La Bouenza, S Congo
Madioen *see* Madiun
23 U8 **Madison** Florida, SE USA
23 T3 **Madison** Georgia, SE USA
31 P15 **Madison** Indiana, N USA
27 P6 **Madison** Kansas, C USA
19 Q6 **Madison** Maine, NE USA
29 S9 **Madison** Minnesota, N USA
22 K5 **Madison** Mississippi, S USA
29 Q14 **Madison** Nebraska, C USA
29 R10 **Madison** South Dakota, N USA
21 V5 **Madison** Virginia, NE USA
21 Q5 **Madison** West Virginia, NE USA
30 L9 **Madison** *state capital* Wisconsin, N USA
21 T6 **Madison Heights** Virginia, NE USA
20 I6 **Madisonville** Kentucky, S USA
20 M10 **Madisonville** Tennessee, S USA
25 V9 **Madisonville** Texas, SW USA
169 R16 **Madiun** *prev.* Madioen. Jawa, C Indonesia
Madjene *see* Majene
14 J14 **Madoc** Ontario, SE Canada
Madoera *see* Madura, Pulau
81 J18 **Mado Gashi** North Eastern, E Kenya
159 R11 **Madoi** Qinghai, C China
189 O13 **Madolenihmw** Pohnpei, E Micronesia
118 I9 **Madona** *Ger.* Modohn. Madona, E Latvia
107 J23 **Madonie** ▲▲ Sicilia, Italy, C Mediterranean Sea
141 Y11 **Madrakah, Ra's** *headland* E Oman
32 I12 **Madras** Oregon, NW USA
Madras *see* Chennai
57 H14 **Madre de Dios** *off.* Departamento de Madre de Dios. ◈ *department* E Peru
63 F22 **Madre de Dios, Isla** *island* S Chile
57 J14 **Madre de Dios, Río** ≈ Bolivia/Peru
25 T16 **Madre, Laguna** ◎ Texas, SW USA
41 Q9 **Madre, Laguna** *lagoon* NE Mexico
37 Q12 **Madre Mount** ▲ New Mexico, SW USA
105 N8 **Madrid** ● (Spain) Madrid, C Spain
29 V14 **Madrid** Iowa, C USA
105 N7 **Madrid** ◈ *autonomous community* C Spain
105 N10 **Madridejos** Castilla-La Mancha, C Spain
104 L7 **Madrigal de las Altas Torres** Castilla-León, N Spain
104 K10 **Madrigalejo** Extremadura, W Spain
34 L3 **Mad River** ≈ California, W USA
42 J8 **Madriz** ◈ *department* NW Nicaragua
104 K10 **Madroñera** Extremadura, W Spain
181 N12 **Madura** Western Australia
Madura *see* Madurai
155 H22 **Madurai** *prev.* Madura, Mathurai. Tamil Nādu, S India
169 S16 **Madura, Pulau** *prev.* Madoera. *island* C Indonesia
169 S16 **Madura, Selat** *strait* C Indonesia
129 Q17 **Madzhalis** Respublika Dagestan, SW Russian Federation
114 K12 **Madzharovo** Khaskovo, S Bulgaria
83 M14 **Madzimoyo** Eastern, E Zambia
165 O12 **Maebashi** *var.* Maebasi, Mayebashi. Gunma, Honshū, S Japan
Maebasi *see* Maebashi
167 O6 **Mae Chan** Chiang Rai, NW Thailand
167 N7 **Mae Hong Son** *var.* Maehongson, Muai To. Mae Hong Son, NW Thailand
Mae Nam Khong *see* Mekong
167 Q7 **Mae Nam Nan** ≈ NW Thailand
167 O10 **Mae Nam Tha Chin** ≈ W Thailand
167 P7 **Mae Nam Yom** ≈ W Thailand
37 O3 **Maeser** Utah, W USA
Maeseyck *see* Maaseik
167 N9 **Mae Sot** *var.* Ban Mae Sot. Tak, W Thailand
Maestricht *see* Maastricht
167 O7 **Mae Suai** *var.* Ban Mae Suai. Chiang Rai, NW Thailand
167 O7 **Mae Tho, Doi** ▲ NW Thailand
172 I4 **Maevatanana** Mahajanga, C Madagascar
187 R13 **Maéwo** *prev.* Aurora. *island* C Vanuatu
171 S11 **Mafa** Pulau Halmahera, E Indonesia
83 I23 **Mafeteng** W Lesotho
99 J21 **Maffe** Namur, SE Belgium
183 P12 **Maffra** Victoria, SE Australia
81 K23 **Mafia** *island* E Tanzania
81 J23 **Mafia Channel** *sea waterway* E Tanzania
83 I21 **Mafikeng** North-West, N South Africa
60 J12 **Mafra** Santa Catarina, S Brazil
104 F10 **Mafra** Lisboa, C Portugal
143 Q17 **Mafraq** Abū Ẓaby, C UAE
Mafraq/Mafraq, Muḥāfaẓat al *see* Al Mafraq
123 T10 **Magadan** Magadanskaya Oblast', E Russian Federation
123 T9 **Magadanskaya Oblast'** ◈ *province* E Russian Federation
108 G11 **Magadino** Ticino, S Switzerland
63 G23 **Magallanes** *off.* Región de Magallanes y de la Antártica Chilena. ◈ *region* S Chile
Magallanes *see* Punta Arenas
Magallanes, Estrecho de *see* Magellan, Strait of
14 I10 **Maganasipi, Lac** ◎ Quebec, SE Canada
54 F6 **Magangué** Bolívar, N Colombia
Magareva *see* Mangareva
77 V12 **Magaria** Zinder, S Niger
186 F10 **Magarida** Central, SW PNG
171 O2 **Magat** ≈ Luzon, N Philippines
27 T11 **Magazine Mountain** ▲ Arkansas, C USA
76 I15 **Magburaka** C Sierra Leone
123 Q13 **Magdagachi** Amurskaya Oblast', SE Russian Federation
62 O12 **Magdalena** Buenos Aires, E Argentina
57 M15 **Magdalena** Beni, N Bolivia
40 F4 **Magdalena** Sonora, NW Mexico
37 Q13 **Magdalena** New Mexico, SW USA
54 F5 **Magdalena** *off.* Departamento del Magdalena. ◈ *province* N Colombia
40 E9 **Magdalena, Bahía** *bay* W Mexico
63 G19 **Magdalena, Isla** *island* Archipiélago de los Chonos, S Chile
40 D8 **Magdalena, Isla** *island* W Mexico
47 P6 **Magdalena, Río** ≈ C Colombia
40 F4 **Magdalena, Río** ≈ NW Mexico
Magdalen Islands *see* Madeleine, Îles de la
100 L13 **Magdeburg** Sachsen-Anhalt, C Germany
22 L6 **Magee** Mississippi, S USA
169 Q16 **Magelang** Jawa, C Indonesia
192 K7 **Magellan Rise** *undersea feature* C Pacific Ocean
63 H24 **Magellan, Strait of** *Sp.* Estrecho de Magallanes. *strait* Argentina/Chile
106 D7 **Magenta** Lombardia, NW Italy
Magerøy *see* Magerøya
92 K7 **Magerøya** *var.* Magerøy. *island* N Norway
164 C17 **Mage-shima** *island* Nansei-shotō, SW Japan
108 G11 **Maggia** Ticino, S Switzerland
108 G10 **Maggia** ≈ SW Switzerland
Maggiore, Lago *see* Maggiore, Lake
106 C6 **Maggiore, Lake** *It.* Lago Maggiore. ◎ Italy/Switzerland
44 I12 **Maggotty** W Jamaica
76 I10 **Maghama** Gorgol, S Mauritania
97 F14 **Maghera** *Ir.* Machaire Rátha. C Northern Ireland, UK
97 F15 **Magherafelt** *Ir.* Machaire Fíolta. C Northern Ireland, UK
188 H6 **Magicienne Bay** *bay* Saipan, S Northern Mariana Islands
105 O13 **Magina** ▲ S Spain
81 H24 **Magingo** Ruvuma, S Tanzania
112 H11 **Maglaj** Federacija Bosna I Hercegovina, N Bosnia and Herzegovina
107 Q19 **Maglie** Puglia, SE Italy
36 L2 **Magna** Utah, W USA
Magnesia *see* Manisa
14 G12 **Magnetawan** ≈ Ontario, S Canada
27 T14 **Magnolia** Arkansas, C USA
22 K7 **Magnolia** Mississippi, S USA
25 V10 **Magnolia** Texas, SW USA
Magnolia State *see* Mississippi
95 J15 **Magnor** Hedmark, S Norway
187 Y14 **Mago** *prev.* Mango. *island* Lau Group, E Fiji
83 L15 **Màgoé** Tete, NW Mozambique
15 Q13 **Magog** Quebec, SE Canada
83 J15 **Magoye** Southern, S Zambia
41 Q12 **Magozal** Veracruz-Llave, C Mexico
14 B7 **Magpie** ≈ Ontario, S Canada
11 Q17 **Magrath** Alberta, SW Canada
105 R10 **Magro** ≈ E Spain
76 I9 **Magta' Lahjar** *var.* Magta Lahjar, Magta' Lahjar, Magtá Lahjar. Brakna, SW Mauritania
83 L20 **Magude** Maputo, S Mozambique
77 Y12 **Magumeri** Borno, NE Nigeria
189 O14 **Magur Islands** *island group* Caroline Islands, C Micronesia
Magway *see* Magwe
166 L6 **Magwe** *var.* Magway. Magwe, W Myanmar
166 L6 **Magwe** *var.* Magway. ◈ *division* C Myanmar
Magyar-Becse *see* Bečej
Magyarkanizsa *see* Kanjiža
Magyarország *see* Hungary
Magyarzsombor *see* Zimbor
142 J4 **Mahābād** *var.* Mehabad; *prev.* Sāūjbulāgh. Āzarbāyjān-e Bākhtarī, NW Iran
172 H5 **Mahabo** Toliara, W Madagascar
Maha Chai *see* Samut Sakhon
155 D14 **Mahād** Mahārāshtra, W India
81 N17 **Mahadday Weyne** Shabeellaha Dhexe, C Somalia
79 Q17 **Mahagi** Orientale, NE Dem. Rep. Congo (Zaire)
Mahāil *see* Muhāyil
172 I4 **Mahajamba** *seasonal river* NW Madagascar
152 G10 **Mahājan** Rājasthān, NW India
172 I3 **Mahajanga** *var.* Majunga. Mahajanga, NW Madagascar
172 I3 **Mahajanga** ◈ *province* W Madagascar
172 I3 **Mahajanga** × Mahajanga, NW Madagascar
169 U10 **Mahakam, Sungai** *var.* Koetai, Kutai. ≈ Borneo, C Indonesia
83 I19 **Mahalapye** *var.* Mahalatswe. Central, SE Botswana
Mahalatswe *see* Mahalapye
Mahalla el Kubra *see* El Maḥalla el Kubra
171 O13 **Mahalona** Sulawesi, C Indonesia
Mahameru *see* Semeru, Gunung
143 S11 **Mahān** Kermān, E Iran
154 N12 **Mahānadi** ≈ E India
172 J5 **Mahanoro** Toamasina, E Madagascar
153 P13 **Mahārājganj** Bihār, N India
154 G13 **Mahārāshtra** ◈ *state* W India
172 I4 **Mahavavy** *seasonal river* N Madagascar
155 K24 **Mahaweli Ganga** ≈ C Sri Lanka
Mahbés *see* El Mahbas
155 J15 **Mahbūbābād** Andhra Pradesh, E India
155 H16 **Mahbūbnagar** Andhra Pradesh, C India
140 M8 **Mahd adh Dhahab** Al Madīnah, W Saudi Arabia
55 S9 **Mahdia** C Guyana
75 N6 **Mahdia** *var.* Al Mahdīyah, Mehdia. NE Tunisia
155 F20 **Mahe** *Fr.* Mahé; *prev.* Mayyali. Pondicherry, SW India
172 I16 **Mahé** × Mahé, NE Seychelles
172 H16 **Mahé** *island* Inner Islands, NE Seychelles
173 Y17 **Mahebourg** SE Mauritius
152 L10 **Mahendranagar** Far Western, W Nepal
81 I23 **Mahenge** Morogoro, SE Tanzania
185 F22 **Maheno** Otago, South Island, NZ
154 D9 **Mahesāna** Gujarāt, W India
154 F11 **Maheshwar** Madhya Pradesh, C India
151 F14 **Mahi** ≈ N India
184 Q10 **Mahia Peninsula** *peninsula* North Island, NZ
119 O16 **Mahilyow** *Rus.* Mogilëv. Mahilyowskaya Voblasts', E Belarus
119 M16 **Mahilyowskaya Voblasts'** *prev. Rus.* Mogilëvskaya Oblast'. ◈ *province* E Belarus
191 P7 **Mahina** Tahiti, W French Polynesia
185 E23 **Mahinerangi, Lake** ◎ South Island, NZ
83 L22 **Mahlabatini** KwaZulu/Natal, E South Africa
166 L5 **Mahlaing** Mandalay, C Myanmar
109 X8 **Mahldorf** Steiermark, SE Austria
Mahmūd-e 'Erāqī *see* Maḥmūd-e Rāqī
149 R4 **Maḥmūd-e Rāqī** *var.* Mahmūd-e 'Erāqī. Kāpīsā, NE Afghanistan
Mahmudiya *see* Al Maḥmūdīyah
29 S5 **Mahnomen** Minnesota, N USA
152 K14 **Mahoba** Uttar Pradesh, N India
105 Z9 **Mahón** *Cat.* Maó, *Eng.* Port Mahon; *anc.* Portus Magonis. Menorca, Spain, W Mediterranean Sea
18 D14 **Mahoning Creek Lake** ⊠ Pennsylvania, NE USA
105 Q10 **Mahora** Castilla-La Mancha, C Spain
Mähren *see* Moravia
Mährisch-Budwitz *see* Moravské Budějovice
Mährisch-Kromau *see* Moravský Krumlov
Mährisch-Neustadt *see* Uničov
Mährisch-Schönberg *see* Šumperk
Mährisch-Trübau *see* Moravská Třebová
Mährisch-Weisskirchen *see* Hranice
Māh-Shahr *see* Bandar-e Māhshahr
79 N19 **Mahulu** Maniema, E Dem. Rep. Congo (Zaire)
154 C12 **Mahuva** Gujarāt, W India
114 N11 **Mahya Dağı** ▲ NW Turkey
105 T6 **Maials** *var.* Mayals. Cataluña, NE Spain
191 O2 **Maiana** *prev.* Hall Island. *atoll* Tungaru, W Kiribati
191 S11 **Maiao** *var.* Tapuaemanu, Tubuai-Manu. *island* Îles du Vent, W French Polynesia
54 H4 **Maicao** La Guajira, N Colombia
Mai Ceu/Mai Chio *see* Maych'ew
103 U8 **Maîche** Doubs, E France
97 N22 **Maidenhead** S England, UK
11 S15 **Maidstone** Saskatchewan, S Canada
97 P22 **Maidstone** SE England, UK
77 Y13 **Maiduguri** Borno, NE Nigeria
108 I8 **Maienfeld** Sankt Gallen, NE Switzerland
116 J12 **Măieruş** *Hung.* Szászmagyarós. Braşov, C Romania
Maigh Chromtha *see* Macroom
Maigh Eo *see* Mayo
55 N9 **Maigualida, Sierra** ▲▲ S Venezuela
154 K9 **Maihar** Madhya Pradesh, C India
154 K11 **Maikala Range** ▲▲ C India
67 T10 **Maiko** ≈ W Dem. Rep. Congo (Zaire)
Mailand *see* Milano
152 L11 **Mailāni** Uttar Pradesh, N India
149 U10 **Māilsi** Punjab, E Pakistan
147 R8 **Maimak** Talasskaya Oblast', NW Kyrgyzstan
Maimāna *see* Meymaneh
Maimansingh *see* Mymensingh
171 V13 **Maimawa** Irian Jaya, E Indonesia
Maimuna *see* Al Maymūnah
101 G18 **Main** ≈ C Germany
115 F22 **Maïna** *ancient monument* Pelopónnisos, S Greece
115 E20 **Maínalo** ▲ S Greece
101 L22 **Mainburg** Bayern, SE Germany
Main Camp *see* Banana
14 E12 **Main Channel** *lake channel* Ontario, S Canada
79 I20 **Mai-Ndombe, Lac** *prev.* Lac Léopold II. ◎ W Dem. Rep. Congo (Zaire)
101 K20 **Main-Donau-Kanal** *canal* SE Germany
19 R6 **Maine** *off.* State of Maine; also known as Lumber State, Pine Tree State. ◈ *state* NE USA
102 K6 **Maine** *cultural region* NW France
102 J7 **Maine-et-Loire** ◈ *department* NW France
19 Q9 **Maine, Gulf of** *gulf* NE USA
77 X12 **Maïné-Soroa** Diffa, SE Niger
167 N2 **Maingkwan** *var.* Mungkawn. Kachin State, N Myanmar
Main Island *see* Bermuda
Mainistir Fhear Maí *see* Fermoy
Mainistirna Búille *see* Boyle
Mainistir na Corann *see* Midleton
Mainistir na Féile *see* Abbeyfeale
96 J5 **Mainland** *island* Orkney, N Scotland, UK
96 L2 **Mainland** *island* Shetland, NE Scotland, UK
159 P16 **Mainling** Xizang Zizhiqu, W China

◆ Country ● Country Capital ◇ Dependent Territory ○ Dependent Territory Capital ◈ Administrative Region × International Airport ▲ Mountain ▲▲ Mountain Range Volcano ≈ River ◎ Lake ⊠ Reservoir

152 K12 **Mainpuri** Uttar Pradesh, N India
103 N5 **Maintenon** Eure-et-Loir, C France
172 H4 **Maintirano** Mahajanga, W Madagascar
93 M15 **Mainua** Oulu, C Finland
101 G18 **Mainz** *Fr.* Mayence. Rheinland-Pfalz, SW Germany
76 I9 **Maio** *var.* Vila do Maio. Maio, S Cape Verde
76 E10 **Maio** *var.* Mayo. *island* Ilhas de Sotavento, SE Cape Verde
62 G12 **Maipo, Río** ≈ C Chile
62 H12 **Maipo, Volcán** ▲ W Argentina
61 E22 **Maipú** Buenos Aires, E Argentina
62 I11 **Maipú** Mendoza, E Argentina
62 H11 **Maipú** Santiago, C Chile
54 L5 **Maiquetía** Distrito Federal, N Venezuela
108 I10 **Maira** *It.* Mera. ≈ Italy/Switzerland
106 A9 **Maira** ≈ NW Italy
153 V12 **Mairābāri** Assam, NE India
44 K7 **Maisí** Guantánamo, E Cuba
118 H13 **Maišiagala** Vilnius, SE Lithuania
153 V17 **Maiskhal Island** *island* SE Bangladesh
167 N13 **Mai Sombun** Chumphon, SW Thailand
Maisur *see* Karnātaka, India
Maisur *see* Mysore, India
183 T8 **Maitland** New South Wales, SE Australia
182 I9 **Maitland** South Australia
14 F15 **Maitland** ≈ Ontario, S Canada
195 R1 **Maitri** *Indian research station* Antarctica
159 N15 **Maizhokunggar** Xizang Zizhiqu, W China
43 O10 **Maíz, Islas del** *var.* Corn Islands. *island group* SE Nicaragua
164 J12 **Maizuru** Kyōto, Honshū, SW Japan
54 F6 **Majagual** Sucre, N Colombia
41 Z13 **Majahual** Quintana Roo, E Mexico
Majardah, Wādī *see* Medjerda, Oued/Mejerda
Mājeej *see* Mejit Island
171 N13 **Majene** *prev.* Madjene. Sulawesi, C Indonesia
43 V15 **Majé, Serranía de** ⛰ E Panama
112 I11 **Majevica** ⛰ NE Bosnia and Herzegovina
81 H15 **Majī** Southern, S Ethiopia
141 X7 **Majīs** NW Oman
Majorca *see* Mallorca
Mājro *see* Majuro Atoll
Majunga *see* Mahajanga
189 Y3 **Majuro** ✕ Majuro Atoll, SE Marshall Islands
189 Y2 **Majuro Atoll** *var.* Mājro. *atoll* Ratak Chain, SE Marshall Islands
189 X2 **Majuro Lagoon** *lagoon* Majuro Atoll, SE Marshall Islands
76 H11 **Maka** C Senegal
79 F20 **Makabana** Le Niari, SW Congo
38 D9 **Makaha** *Haw.* Mākaha. Oahu, Hawaii, USA, C Pacific Ocean
38 B8 **Makahuena Point** *headland* Kauai, Hawaii, USA, C Pacific Ocean
38 D9 **Makakilo City** Oahu, Hawaii, USA, C Pacific Ocean
83 H18 **Makalamabedi** Central, C Botswana
Makale *see* Mek'elē
158 K17 **Makalu** *Chin.* Makaru Shan. ▲ China/Nepal
81 G23 **Makampi** Mbeya, S Tanzania
145 X12 **Makanchi** *Kaz.* Maqanshy. Vostochnyy Kazakhstan, E Kazakhstan
42 M8 **Makantaka** Región Autónoma Atlántico Norte, NE Nicaragua
190 B16 **Makapu Point** *headland* W Niue
185 C24 **Makarewa** Southland, South Island, NZ
117 O4 **Makariv** Kyyivs'ka Oblast', N Ukraine
185 D20 **Makarora** ≈ South Island, NZ
123 T13 **Makarov** Ostrov Sakhalin, Sakhalinskaya Oblast', SE Russian Federation
197 R9 **Makarov Basin** *undersea feature* Arctic Ocean
192 I5 **Makarov Seamount** *undersea feature* W Pacific Ocean
113 F15 **Makarska** *It.* Macarsca. Split-Dalmacija, SE Croatia
Makaru Shan *see* Makalu
127 O15 **Makar'yev** Kostromskaya Oblast', NW Russian Federation
82 L11 **Makasa** Northern, NE Zambia
Makasar *see* Ujungpandang
Makasar, Selat *see* Makassar Straits
Makassar *see* Ujungpandang
192 F7 **Makassar Straits** *Ind.* Selat Makasar. *strait* C Indonesia
144 G12 **Makat** *Kaz.* Maqat. Atyrau, SW Kazakhstan
191 T10 **Makatea** *island* Îles Tuamotu, C French Polynesia
139 U7 **Makātū** E Iraq
172 H6 **Makay** *var.* Massif du Makay. ⛰ SW Madagascar
114 J12 **Makaza** *pass* Bulgaria/Greece
Makedonija *see* Macedonia, FYR
190 B16 **Makefu** W Niue
191 V10 **Makemo** *atoll* Îles Tuamotu, C French Polynesia
76 I15 **Makeni** C Sierra Leone
Makenzen *see* Orlyak
Makeyevka *see* Makiyivka
129 Q16 **Makhachkala** *prev.* Petrovsk-Port. Respublika Dagestan, SW Russian Federation
144 F11 **Makhambet** Atyrau, W Kazakhstan
Makharadze *see* Ozurget'i
139 W13 **Makhfar Al Buşayyah** S Iraq
139 R4 **Makhmūr** N Iraq
138 I11 **Makhrūq, Wadi al** *dry watercourse* E Jordan
139 R4 **Makḩūl, Jabal** ⛰ C Iraq
141 R13 **Makhyah, Wādī** *dry watercourse* N Yemen
171 V13 **Maki** Irian Jaya, E Indonesia
185 G21 **Makikihi** Canterbury, South Island, NZ
191 O2 **Makin** *prev.* Pitt Island. *atoll* Tungaru, W Kiribati
81 I20 **Makindu** Eastern, S Kenya
145 Q8 **Makinsk** Akmola, N Kazakhstan
187 N10 **Makira** *off.* Makira Province. ◈ *province* SE Solomon Islands
Makira *see* San Cristobal
117 X8 **Makiyivka** *Rus.* Makeyevka; *prev.* Dmitriyevsk. Donets'ka Oblast', E Ukraine
140 L10 **Makkah** *Eng.* Mecca. Makkah, W Saudi Arabia
140 M10 **Makkah** *var.* Minţaqat Makkah. ◈ *province* W Saudi Arabia
13 R7 **Makkovik** Newfoundland, NE Canada
98 K6 **Makkum** Friesland, N Netherlands
Mako *see* Makung
111 M25 **Makó** *Rom.* Macău. Csongrád, SE Hungary
14 G9 **Makobe Lake** ◎ Ontario, S Canada
79 F18 **Makokou** Ogooué-Ivindo, NE Gabon
81 G23 **Makongolosi** Mbeya, S Tanzania
81 E19 **Makota** SW Uganda
79 G18 **Makoua** Cuvette, C Congo
110 M10 **Maków Mazowiecki** Mazowieckie, C Poland
111 K17 **Maków Podhalański** Małopolskie, S Poland
143 V14 **Makran** *cultural region* Iran/Pakistan
152 G12 **Makrāna** Rājasthān, N India
143 U15 **Makran Coast** *coastal region* SE Iran
119 F20 **Makrany** *Rus.* Mokrany. Brestskaya Voblasts', SW Belarus
Makrinoros *see* Makrynóros
115 H20 **Makrónisosi** *island* Kykládes, Greece, Aegean Sea
115 D17 **Makrynóros** *var.* Makrinoros. ⛰ C Greece
115 G19 **Makryplági** ▲ C Greece
Maksamaa *see* Maxmo
126 J15 **Maksatikha** *var.* Maksatha, Maksaticha. Tverskaya Oblast', W Russian Federation
154 G10 **Maksi** Madhya Pradesh, C India
142 I1 **Mākū** Āżarbāyjān-e Bākhtarī, NW Iran
153 Y11 **Mākum** Assam, NE India
Makun *see* Makung
161 R14 **Makung** *prev.* Mako, Makun. W Taiwan
164 B16 **Makurazaki** Kagoshima, Kyūshū, SW Japan
77 V15 **Makurdi** Benue, C Nigeria
38 L17 **Makushin Volcano** ※ Unalaska Island, Alaska, USA
83 K16 **Makwiro** Mashonaland West, N Zimbabwe
57 D15 **Mala** Lima, W Peru
Mala *see* Mallow, Ireland
Mala *see* Malaita, Solomon Islands
93 I14 **Malå** Västerbotten, N Sweden
190 G12 **Mala'atoli** Île Uvea, E Wallis and Futuna
171 P8 **Malabang** Mindanao, S Phippines
155 E21 **Malabār Coast** *coast* SW India
79 C16 **Malabo** *prev.* Santa Isabel. ● (Equatorial Guinea) Isla de Bioco, NW Equatorial Guinea
79 C16 **Malabo** ✕ Isla de Bioco, N Equatorial Guinea
Malaca *see* Málaga
Malacca *see* Melaka
168 I7 **Malacca, Strait of** *Ind.* Selat Malaka. *strait* Indonesia/Malaysia
Malacka *see* Malacky
111 G20 **Malacky** *Hung.* Malacka. Bratislavský Kraj, W Slovakia
33 R16 **Malad City** Idaho, NW USA
117 Q4 **Mala Divytsya** Chernihivs'ka Oblast', N Ukraine
119 J15 **Maladzyechna** *Pol.* Molodeczno, *Rus.* Molodechno. Minskaya Voblasts', C Belarus
190 D12 **Malaee** Île Futuna, N Wallis and Futuna
37 V15 **Malaga** New Mexico, SW USA
54 G8 **Málaga** Santander, C Colombia
104 M15 **Málaga** *anc.* Malaca. Andalucía, S Spain
104 L15 **Málaga** ◈ *province* Andalucía, S Spain
104 M15 **Málaga** ✕ Andalucía, S Spain
Malagasy Republic *see* Madagascar
105 N10 **Malagón** Castilla-La Mancha, C Spain
97 G18 **Malahide** *Ir.* Mullach Íde. E Ireland
187 N9 **Malaita** *off.* Malaita Province. ◈ *province* N Solomon Islands
187 N8 **Malaita** *var.* Mala. *island* N Solomon Islands
80 F13 **Malakal** Upper Nile, S Sudan
112 C10 **Mala Kapela** ⛰ NW Croatia
25 V7 **Malakoff** Texas, SW USA
Malakula *see* Malekula
149 V7 **Malakwāl** *var.* Mālikwāla. Punjab, E Pakistan
186 E7 **Malalamai** Madang, W PNG
GG Q11 **Malamala** Sulawesi, C Indonesia
169 S17 **Malang** Jawa, C Indonesia
83 O14 **Malanga** Niassa, N Mozambique
Malange *see* Malanje
92 I9 **Malangen** *sound* N Norway
82 C11 **Malanje** *var.* Malange. Malanje, NW Angola
82 C11 **Malanje** *var.* Malange. ◈ *province* N Angola
148 M16 **Malān, Rās** *headland* SW Pakistan
77 S13 **Malanville** NE Benin
Malapane *see* Ozimek
155 F21 **Malappuram** Kerala, SW India
43 T17 **Mala, Punta** *headland* S Panama
95 N16 **Mälaren** ◎ C Sweden
62 H13 **Malargüe** Mendoza, W Argentina
14 J8 **Malartic** Quebec, SE Canada
119 F20 **Malaryta** *Pol.* Maloryta, *Rus.* Malorita. Brestskaya Voblasts', SW Belarus
63 J19 **Malaspina** Chubut, SE Argentina
39 U12 **Malaspina Glacier** *glacier* Alaska, USA
137 N15 **Malatya** *anc.* Melitene. Malatya, SE Turkey
136 M14 **Malatya** ◈ *province* C Turkey
117 Q7 **Mala Vyska** *Rus.* Malaya Viska. Kirovohrads'ka Oblast', S Ukraine
83 M14 **Malawi** *off.* Republic of Malaŵi; *prev.* Nyasaland, Nyasaland Protectorate. ◆ *republic* S Africa
Malawi, Lake *see* Nyasa, Lake
93 J17 **Malax** *Fin.* Maalahti. Länsi-Suomi, W Finland
126 H14 **Malaya Vishera** Novgorodskaya Oblast', W Russian Federation
Malaya Viska *see* Mala Vyska
171 Q7 **Malaybalay** Mindanao, S Philippines
142 L6 **Malāyer** *prev.* Daulatabad. Hamadān, W Iran
168 L7 **Malay Peninsula** *peninsula* Malaysia/Thailand
192 D7 **Malaysia** *var.* Federation of Malaysia; *prev.* the separate territories of Federation of Malaya, Sarawak and Sabah (North Borneo) and Singapore. ◆ *monarchy* SE Asia
137 R14 **Malazgirt** Muş, E Turkey
15 R8 **Malbaie** ≈ Quebec, SE Canada
77 T12 **Malbaza** Tahoua, S Niger
110 J7 **Malbork** *Ger.* Marienburg, Marienburg in Westpreussen. Pomorskie, N Poland
100 N9 **Malchin** Mecklenburg-Vorpommern, N Germany
100 M9 **Malchiner See** ◎ NE Germany
99 D16 **Maldegem** Oost-Vlaanderen, NW Belgium
98 L13 **Malden** Gelderland, SE Netherlands
19 O11 **Malden** Massachusetts, NE USA
27 Y8 **Malden** Missouri, C USA
191 X4 **Malden Island** *prev.* Independence Island. *atoll* E Kiribati
173 Q6 **Maldives** *off.* Maldivian Divehi, Republic of Maldives. ◆ *republic* N Indian Ocean
Maldivian Divehi *see* Maldives
97 P21 **Maldon** E England, UK
61 G20 **Maldonado** Maldonado, S Uruguay
61 G20 **Maldonado** ◈ *department* S Uruguay
41 P17 **Maldonado, Punta** *headland* S Mexico
151 K19 **Male'** *Div.* Maale ● (Maldives) Male' Atoll, C Maldives
106 G6 **Malè** Trentino-Alto Adige, N Italy
76 K13 **Maléa** *var.* Maléya. Haute-Guinée, NE Guinea
115 G22 **Maléas, Akrotírio** *headland* S Greece
115 L17 **Maléas, Akrotírio** *headland* Lésvos, E Greece
151 K19 **Male' Atoll** *var.* Kaafu Atoll. *atoll* C Maldives
Malebo, Pool *see* Stanley Pool
154 E12 **Mālegaon** Mahārāshtra, W India
81 F15 **Malek** Jonglei, S Sudan
187 Q13 **Malekula** *var.* Malakula; *prev.* Mallicolo. *island* W Vanuatu
189 Y15 **Malem** Kosrae, E Micronesia
83 O15 **Malema** Nampula, N Mozambique
79 N23 **Malemba-Nkulu** Katanga, SE Dem. Rep. Congo (Zaire)
126 K9 **Malen'ga** Respublika Kareliya, NW Russian Federation
95 M20 **Målerås** Kalmar, S Sweden
103 O6 **Malesherbes** Loiret, C France
115 G18 **Malesína** Stereá Ellás, E Greece
Maléya *see* Maléa
129 O15 **Malgobek** Chechenskaya Respublika, SW Russian Federation
105 X5 **Malgrat de Mar** Cataluña, NE Spain
80 C9 **Malha** Northern Darfur, W Sudan
139 Q5 **Malḩāt** C Iraq
32 K14 **Malheur Lake** ◎ Oregon, NW USA
32 L14 **Malheur River** ≈ Oregon, NW USA
76 I13 **Mali** Moyenne-Guinée, NW Guinea
77 O9 **Mali** *off.* Republic of Mali, *Fr.* République du Mali; *prev.* French Sudan, Sudanese Republic. ◆ *republic* W Africa
171 Q16 **Maliana** W East Timor
167 O2 **Mali Hka** ≈ N Myanmar
Mali Idjoš *see* Mali Iđoš
112 K8 **Mali Iđoš** *var.* Mali Idjoš, *Hung.* Kishegyes; *prev.* Krivaja. Serbia, N Yugoslavia
112 K9 **Mali Kanal** *canal* N Yugoslavia
171 P12 **Maliku** Sulawesi, N Indonesia
Malik, Wadi al *see* Milk, Wadi el
Mālikwāla *see* Malakwāl
167 N11 **Mali Kyun** *var.* Tavoy Island. *island* Mergui Archipelago, S Myanmar
95 M19 **Målilla** Kalmar, S Sweden
112 B11 **Mali Lošinj** *It.* Lussinpiccolo. Primorje-Gorski Kotar, W Croatia
Malin *see* Malyn
171 P7 **Malindang, Mount** ▲ Mindanao, S Philippines
81 K20 **Malindi** Coast, SE Kenya
Malines *see* Mechelen
96 E13 **Malin Head** *Ir.* Cionn Mhálanna. *headland* NW Ireland
171 O11 **Malino, Gunung** ▲ Sulawesi, N Indonesia
113 M21 **Maliq** *var.* Maliqi. Korçë, SE Albania
Maliqi *see* Maliq
171 Q8 **Malita** Mindanao, S Philippines
154 G12 **Malkāpur** Mahārāshtra, C India
136 B10 **Malkara** Tekirdağ, NW Turkey
119 J19 **Mal'kavichy** *Rus.* Mal'kovichi. Brestskaya Voblasts', SW Belarus
Malkiye *see* Al Mālikīyah
114 L11 **Malko Sharkovo, Yazovir** ⊠ SE Bulgaria
114 N11 **Malko Tŭrnovo** Burgas, E Bulgaria
Mal'kovichi *see* Mal'kavichy
183 R12 **Mallacoota** Victoria, SE Australia
96 G10 **Mallaig** N Scotland, UK
182 I9 **Mallala** South Australia
75 W9 **Mallawi** C Egypt
105 R5 **Mallén** Aragón, NE Spain
106 F5 **Malles Venosta** Trentino-Alto Adige, N Italy
Mallicolo *see* Malekula
109 Q8 **Mallnitz** Salzburg, S Austria
105 W9 **Mallorca** *Eng.* Majorca; *anc.* Baleares Major. *island* Islas Baleares, Spain, W Mediterranean Sea
97 C20 **Mallow** *Ir.* Mala. SW Ireland
93 E15 **Malm** Nord-Trøndelag, C Norway
95 L19 **Malmbäck** Jönköping, S Sweden
92 J12 **Malmberget** Norrbotten, N Sweden
99 M20 **Malmédy** Liège, E Belgium
83 E25 **Malmesbury** Western Cape, SW South Africa
95 N16 **Malmköping** Södermanland, C Sweden
95 K23 **Malmö** Skåne, S Sweden
95 K23 **Malmo** ✕ Skåne, S Sweden
45 Q16 **Malmok** *headland* Bonaire, S Netherlands Antilles
95 M18 **Malmslätt** Östergötland, S Sweden
127 R16 **Malmyzh** Kirovskaya Oblast', NW Russian Federation
187 Q13 **Malo** *island* W Vanuatu
128 J7 **Maloarkhangel'sk** Orlovskaya Oblast', W Russian Federation
Maloelap *see* Maloelap Atoll
189 V6 **Maloelap Atoll** *var.* Maloelap. *atoll* E Marshall Islands
Maloenda *see* Malunda
108 I10 **Maloja** Graubünden, S Switzerland
82 L12 **Malole** Northern, NE Zambia
171 O3 **Malolos** Luzon, N Philippines
18 K6 **Malone** New York, NE USA
79 K25 **Malonga** Katanga, S Dem. Rep. Congo (Zaire)
111 L15 **Małopolska** *plateau* S Poland
111 K17 **Małopolskie** ◈ *province* S Poland
Malorita/Maloryta *see* Malaryta
126 K9 **Maloshuyka** Arkhangel'skaya Oblast', NW Russian Federation
114 G10 **Mal'ovitsa** ▲ W Bulgaria
145 V15 **Malovodnoye** Almaty, SE Kazakhstan
94 C10 **Måløy** Sogn og Fjordane, S Norway
128 K4 **Maloyaroslavets** Kaluzhskaya Oblast', W Russian Federation
122 G7 **Malozemel'skaya Tundra** *physical region* NW Russian Federation
104 J10 **Malpartida de Cáceres** Extremadura, W Spain
104 K9 **Malpartida de Plasencia** Extremadura, W Spain
106 C7 **Malpensa** ✕ (Milano) Lombardia, N Italy
76 J6 **Malqteïr** *desert* N Mauritania
118 J10 **Malta** Rēzekne, SE Latvia
33 V7 **Malta** Montana, NW USA
120 M11 **Malta** *off.* Republic of Malta. ◆ *republic* C Mediterranean Sea
109 R8 **Malta** *var.* Maltabach. ≈ S Austria
120 M11 **Malta** *island* Malta, C Mediterranean Sea
Maltabach *see* Malta
Malta, Canale di *see* Malta Channel
120 M11 **Malta Channel** *It.* Canale di Malta. *strait* Italy/Malta
83 D20 **Maltahöhe** Hardap, SW Namibia
97 N16 **Malton** N England, UK
171 R13 **Maluku** *off.* Propinsi Maluku, *Dut.* Molukken, *Eng.* Moluccas. ◈ *province* E Indonesia
171 R13 **Maluku** *Dut.* Molukken, *Eng.* Moluccas; *prev.* Spice Islands. *island group* E Indonesia
Maluku, Laut *see* Molucca Sea
77 V13 **Malumfashi** Katsina, N Nigeria
171 N13 **Malunda** *prev.* Maloenda. Sulawesi, C Indonesia
94 K13 **Malung** Dalarna, C Sweden
94 K13 **Malungsfors** Dalarna, C Sweden
186 M8 **Maluu** *var.* Malu'u. Malaita, N Solomon Islands
155 D16 **Mālvan** Mahārāshtra, W India
Malventum *see* Benevento
27 U12 **Malvern** Arkansas, C USA
29 S15 **Malvern** Iowa, C USA
44 I13 **Malvern** ▲ W Jamaica
Malvinas, Islas *see* Falkland Islands
117 N4 **Malyn** *Rus.* Malin. Zhytomyrs'ka Oblast', N Ukraine
129 O11 **Malyye Derbety** Respublika Kalmykiya, SW Russian Federation
Malyy Kavkaz *see* Lesser Caucasus
123 Q6 **Malyy Lyakhovskiy, Ostrov** *island* NE Russian Federation
Malyy Pamir *see* Little Pamir
122 N5 **Malyy Taymyr, Ostrov** *island* Severnaya Zemlya, N Russian Federation
144 E10 **Malyy Uzen'** *Kaz.* Kishiözen. ≈ Kazakhstan/Russian Federation
122 L14 **Malyy Yenisey** *var.* Ka-Krem. ≈ S Russian Federation
129 S3 **Mamadysh** Respublika Tatarstan, W Russian Federation
117 N14 **Mamaia** Constanța, E Romania
187 W14 **Mamanuca Group** *island group* Yasawa Group, W Fiji
146 L13 **Mamash** Lebapskiy Velayat, E Turkmenistan
79 O17 **Mambasa** Orientale, NE Dem. Rep. Congo (Zaire)
171 X13 **Mamberamo, Sungai** ≈ Irian Jaya, E Indonesia
79 G15 **Mambéré** ≈ SW Central African Republic
79 G15 **Mambéré-Kadéï** ◈ *prefecture* SW Central African Republic
Mambij *see* Manbij
79 H18 **Mambili** ≈ W Congo
83 N18 **Mambone** *var.* Nova Mambone. Inhambane, E Mozambique
171 O4 **Mamburao** Mindoro, N Philippines
172 I16 **Mamelles** *island* Inner Islands, NE Seychelles
99 M25 **Mamer** Luxembourg, SW Luxembourg
102 L6 **Mamers** Sarthe, NW France
79 D15 **Mamfe** Sud-Ouest, W Cameroon
145 P6 **Mamlyutka** Severnyy Kazakhstan, N Kazakhstan
36 M15 **Mammoth** Arizona, SW USA
33 S12 **Mammoth Hot Springs** Wyoming, C USA
Mamoedjoe *see* Mamuju
119 A14 **Mamonovo** *Ger.* Heiligenbeil. Kaliningradskaya Oblast', W Russian Federation
57 L14 **Mamoré, Rio** ≈ Bolivia/Brazil
76 I14 **Mamou** Moyenne-Guinée, W Guinea
22 H8 **Mamou** Louisiana, S USA
172 I14 **Mamoudzou** ○ (Mayotte) C Mayotte
172 I3 **Mampikony** Mahajanga, N Madagascar
77 P16 **Mampong** C Ghana
110 M7 **Mamry, Jezioro** *Ger.* Mauersee. ◎ NE Poland
171 N13 **Mamuju** *prev.* Mamoedjoe. Sulawesi, S Indonesia
83 F19 **Mamuno** Ghanzi, W Botswana
113 K19 **Mamuras** *var.* Mamurasi, Mamurras. Lezhë, C Albania
Mamurasi/Mamurras *see* Mamuras
76 L16 **Man** W Ivory Coast
55 X9 **Mana** NW French Guiana
56 A6 **Manabí** ◈ *province* W Ecuador
42 G4 **Manabique, Punta** *var.* Cabo Tres Puntas. *headland* E Guatemala
54 G11 **Manacacías, Río** ≈ C Colombia
58 F13 **Manacapuru** Amazonas, N Brazil
171 Q11 **Manado** *prev.* Menado. Sulawesi, C Indonesia
188 H5 **Managaha** *island* S Northern Mariana Islands
99 G20 **Manage** Hainaut, S Belgium
42 J10 **Managua** ● (Nicaragua) Managua, W Nicaragua
42 J10 **Managua** ◈ *department* W Nicaragua
42 J10 **Managua** ✕ Managua, W Nicaragua
42 J10 **Managua, Lago de** *var.* Xolotlán. ◎ W Nicaragua
Manah *see* Bilād Manaḩ
18 K16 **Manahawkin** New Jersey, NE USA
184 K11 **Manaia** Taranaki, North Island, NZ
172 J6 **Manakara** Fianarantsoa, SE Madagascar
152 J7 **Manāli** Himāchal Pradesh, NW India
131 U12 **Ma, Nam** *Vtn.* Sông Mã. ≈ Laos/Vietnam
Manama *see* Al Manāmah
186 D6 **Manam Island** *island* N PNG
67 Y13 **Mananara** ≈ SE Madagascar
182 M9 **Manangatang** Victoria, SE Australia
172 I6 **Mananjary** Fianarantsoa, SE Madagascar
76 L14 **Manankoro** Sikasso, SW Mali
76 J12 **Manantali, Lac de** ⊠ W Mali
Manáos *see* Manaus
185 B23 **Manapouri** Southland, South Island, NZ
185 B23 **Manapouri, Lake** ◎ South Island, NZ
58 F13 **Manaquiri** Amazonas, NW Brazil
Manar *see* Mannar
158 K5 **Manas** Xinjiang Uygur Zizhiqu, NW China
153 U12 **Manās** *var.* Dangme Chu. ≈ Bhutan/India
147 R8 **Manas, Gora** ▲ Kyrgyzstan/Uzbekistan
158 K3 **Manas Hu** ◎ NW China
153 P10 **Manaslu** ▲ C Nepal
37 S8 **Manassa** Colorado, C USA
21 W4 **Manassas** Virginia, NE USA
45 T5 **Manatí** C Puerto Rico
171 R16 **Manatuto** N East Timor
186 E8 **Manau** Northern, S PNG
54 H4 **Manaure** La Guajira, N Colombia
58 F12 **Manaus** *prev.* Manáos. *state capital* Amazonas, NW Brazil
136 G17 **Manavgat** Antalya, SW Turkey
184 M13 **Manawatu** ≈ North Island, NZ
184 L11 **Manawatu-Wanganui** *off.* Manawatu-Wanganui Region. ◈ *region* North Island, NZ
171 R7 **Manay** Mindanao, S Philippines
138 K2 **Manbij** *var.* Mambij, *Fr.* Membidj. Ḩalab, N Syria
105 N13 **Mancha Real** Andalucía, S Spain
102 I4 **Manche** ◈ *department* N France
97 L17 **Manchester** *Lat.* Mancunium. NW England, UK
23 S5 **Manchester** Georgia, SE USA
29 Y13 **Manchester** Iowa, C USA
21 N7 **Manchester** Kentucky, S USA
19 O10 **Manchester** New Hampshire, NE USA
20 K10 **Manchester** Tennessee, S USA
18 M9 **Manchester** Vermont, NE USA
97 L18 **Manchester** ✕ NW England, UK
149 P15 **Manchhar Lake** ◎ SE Pakistan
Man-chou-li *see* Manzhouli
131 X7 **Manchurian Plain** *plain* NE China
Máncio Lima *see* Japiim
Mancunium *see* Manchester
148 J15 **Mand** Baluchistān, SW Pakistan
Mand *see* Mand, Rūd-e
81 H25 **Manda** Iringa, SW Tanzania
172 H6 **Mandabe** Toliara, W Madagascar
162 I5 **Mandal** Hövsgöl, N Mongolia
162 L7 **Mandal** Töv, C Mongolia
95 E18 **Mandal** Vest-Agder, S Norway
166 L5 **Mandalay** Mandalay, C Myanmar
166 M6 **Mandalay** ◈ *division* C Myanmar
162 L9 **Mandalgovĭ** Dundgovĭ, C Mongolia
139 V7 **Mandalī** E Iraq
95 E18 **Mandalselva** ≈ S Norway
28 M5 **Mandan** North Dakota, N USA
Mandargiri Hill *see* Mandār Hill
153 R14 **Mandār Hill** *prev.* Mandargiri Hill. Bihār, NE India
170 M13 **Mandar, Teluk** *bay* Sulawesi, C Indonesia
107 C19 **Mandas** Sardegna, Italy, C Mediterranean Sea
Mandasor *see* Mandsaur
81 L16 **Mandera** North Eastern, NE Kenya
33 V13 **Manderson** Wyoming, C USA
44 J12 **Mandeville** C Jamaica
22 K9 **Mandeville** Louisiana, S USA
152 I7 **Mandi** Himāchal Pradesh, NW India
76 K14 **Mandiana** Haute-Guinée, E Guinea
149 U10 **Mandi Būrewāla** *var.* Būrewāla. Punjab, E Pakistan
152 G9 **Mandi Dabwāli** Haryāna, NW India
Mandidzudzure *see* Chimanimani
83 M15 **Mandié** Manica, NW Mozambique
83 N14 **Mandimba** Niassa, N Mozambique
57 Q19 **Mandioré, Laguna** ◎ E Bolivia
154 J10 **Mandla** Madhya Pradesh, C India
83 M20 **Mandlakazi** *var.* Manjacaze. Gaza, S Mozambique
95 E24 **Mandø** *var.* Manø. *island* W Denmark
Mandoúdhion/Mandoudi *see* Mantoúdi
115 G19 **Mándra** Attikí, C Greece
172 I7 **Mandrare** ≈ S Madagascar
114 M10 **Mandra, Yazovir** *salt lake* SE Bulgaria
107 L23 **Mandrazzi, Portella** *pass* Sicilia, Italy, C Mediterranean Sea
172 J3 **Mandritsara** Mahajanga, N Madagascar
143 O13 **Mand, Rūd-e** *var.* Mand. ≈ S Iran
154 F9 **Mandsaur** *prev.* Mandasor. Madhya Pradesh, C India
154 F11 **Māndu** Madhya Pradesh, C India
169 W8 **Mandul, Pulau** *island* N Indonesia
83 G15 **Mandundu** Western, W Zambia
180 I13 **Mandurah** Western Australia
107 P18 **Manduria** Puglia, SE Italy
155 G20 **Mandya** Karnātaka, C India
77 P12 **Mané** C Burkina
106 E8 **Manerbio** Lombardia, NW Italy
Manevichi *see* Manevychi
116 K3 **Manevychi** *Pol.* Maniewicze, *Rus.* Manevichi. Volyns'ka Oblast', NW Ukraine
107 N16 **Manfredonia** Puglia, SE Italy
107 N16 **Manfredonia, Golfo di** *gulf* Adriatic Sea, N Mediterranean Sea
77 P13 **Manga** C Burkina
59 L16 **Mangabeiras, Chapada das** ⛰ E Brazil

◆ Country ● Country Capital ◇ Dependent Territory ○ Dependent Territory Capital ◈ Administrative Region ✕ International Airport ▲ Mountain ⛰ Mountain Range ※ Volcano ≈ River ◎ Lake ⊠ Reservoir

79 J20 **Mangai** Bandundu, W Dem. Rep. Congo (Zaire)
190 L17 **Mangaia** island group S Cook Islands
184 M9 **Mangakino** Waikato, North Island, NZ
116 M15 **Mangalia** anc. Callatis. Constanța, SE Romania
78 J11 **Mangalmé** Guéra, SE Chad
155 E19 **Mangalore** Karnātaka, W India
191 Y13 **Mangareva** var. Magareva. island Îles Tuamotu, SE French Polynesia
83 I23 **Mangaung** Free State, C South Africa
Mangaung see Bloemfontein
154 K9 **Mangawān** Madhya Pradesh, C India
184 M11 **Mangaweka** Manawatu-Wanganui, North Island, NZ
184 N11 **Mangaweka** ▲ North Island, NZ
79 P17 **Mangbwalu** Orientale, NE Dem. Rep. Congo (Zaire)
101 L24 **Mangfall** ≈ SE Germany
169 P13 **Manggar** Pulau Belitung, W Indonesia
146 H8 **Manghit** Rus. Mangit. Qoraqalpoghiston Respublikasi, W Uzbekistan
166 M2 **Mangin Range** ▲▲ N Myanmar
139 R1 **Mangish** N Iraq
144 F15 **Mangistau** Kaz. Mangqystaū Oblysy; prev. Mangyshlaskaya. ◈ province SW Kazakhstan
Mangit see Manghit
54 A13 **Manglares, Cabo** headland SW Colombia
149 V6 **Mangla Reservoir** ⊟ NE Pakistan
159 N9 **Mangnai** var. Lao Mangnai. Qinghai, C China
Mango see Mago, Fiji
Mango see Sansanné-Mango, Togo
Mangoche see Mangochi
83 N14 **Mangochi** var. Mangoche; prev. Fort Johnston. Southern, SE Malawi
77 N14 **Mangodara** SW Burkina
172 H6 **Mangoky** ≈ W Madagascar
171 Q12 **Mangole, Pulau** island Kepulauan Sula, E Indonesia
184 J2 **Mangonui** Northland, North Island, NZ
Mangqystaū Oblysy see Mangistau
Mangqystaū Shyghanaghy see Mangyshlakskiy Zaliv
104 H7 **Mangualde** Viseu, N Portugal
61 H18 **Mangueira, Lagoa** ◎ S Brazil
77 X6 **Manguéni, Plateau du** ▲ NE Niger
26 K11 **Mangum** Oklahoma, C USA
79 O18 **Manguredjipa** Nord Kivu, E Dem. Rep. Congo (Zaire)
83 L16 **Mangwendi** Mashonaland East, E Zimbabwe
144 F15 **Mangyshlak, Plato** plateau SW Kazakhstan
144 E14 **Mangyshlakskiy Zaliv** Kaz. Mangqystaū Shyghanaghy. gulf SW Kazakhstan
Mangyshlaskaya see Mangistau
162 I5 **Manhan** Hövsgöl, N Mongolia
27 O4 **Manhattan** Kansas, C USA
99 L21 **Manhay** Luxembourg, SE Belgium
83 L21 **Manhiça** prev. Vila de Manhiça. Maputo, S Mozambique
83 L21 **Manhoca** Maputo, S Mozambique
59 N20 **Manhuaçu** Minas Gerais, SE Brazil
143 R11 **Mānī** Kermān, C Iran
54 H10 **Maní** Casanare, C Colombia
56 A6 **Manía, Bahía de** bay W Ecuador
83 M17 **Manica** var. Vila de Manica. Manica, W Mozambique
83 M17 **Manica** off. Província de Manica. ◈ province W Mozambique
83 L17 **Manicaland** ◈ province E Zimbabwe
15 U5 **Manic Deux, Réservoir** ⊟ Quebec, SE Canada
Manich see Manych
59 F14 **Manicoré** Amazonas, N Brazil
13 N11 **Manicouagan** Quebec, SE Canada
13 N11 **Manicouagan** ≈ Quebec, SE Canada
15 U6 **Manicouagan, Péninsule de** peninsula Quebec, SE Canada
13 N11 **Manicouagan, Réservoir** ◎ Quebec, E Canada
15 T4 **Manic Trois, Réservoir** ⊟ Quebec, SE Canada
79 M20 **Maniema** off. Région du Maniema. ◈ region E Dem. Rep. Congo (Zaire)
Maniewicze see Manevychi
160 F8 **Maniganggo** Sichuan, C China
11 Y15 **Manigotagan** Manitoba, S Canada
153 R13 **Manihāri** Bihār, N India
191 U9 **Manihi** island Îles Tuamotu, C French Polynesia
190 L13 **Manihiki** atoll N Cook Islands
175 U8 **Manihiki Plateau** undersea feature C Pacific Ocean
196 M14 **Maniitsoq** var. Manitsoq, Dan. Sukkertoppen. Kita, S Greenland
153 T15 **Manikganj** Dhaka, C Bangladesh
152 M14 **Mānikpur** Uttar Pradesh, N India
171 N4 **Manila** off. City of Manila. ● (Philippines) Luzon, N Philippines
27 Y9 **Manila** Arkansas, C USA
189 N16 **Manila Reef** reef W Micronesia
183 T6 **Manilla** New South Wales, SE Australia
192 F6 **Maniloa** island Tongatapu Group, S Tonga
123 U8 **Manily** Koryakskiy Avtonomnyy Okrug, E Russian Federation
171 V12 **Manim, Pulau** island E Indonesia
168 I11 **Maninjau, Danau** ◎ Sumatera, W Indonesia
153 W13 **Manipur** ◈ state NE India
153 X14 **Manipur Hills** hill range E India
136 C14 **Manisa** var. Manissa; prev. Saruhan, anc. Magnesia. Manisa, W Turkey
136 C13 **Manisa** var. Manissa. ◈ province W Turkey
Manissa see Manisa
31 O7 **Manistee** Michigan, N USA
31 P7 **Manistee River** ≈ Michigan, N USA
31 O4 **Manistique** Michigan, N USA
31 P4 **Manistique Lake** ◎ Michigan, N USA
11 W13 **Manitoba** ◈ province S Canada
11 X16 **Manitoba, Lake** ◎ Manitoba, S Canada
11 X17 **Manitou** Manitoba, S Canada
31 N2 **Manitou Island** island Michigan, N USA
14 H11 **Manitou Lake** ◎ Ontario, SE Canada
12 G15 **Manitoulin Island** island Ontario, S Canada
37 T5 **Manitou Springs** Colorado, C USA
14 G12 **Manitouwabing Lake** ◎ Ontario, S Canada
12 E12 **Manitouwadge** Ontario, S Canada
12 G15 **Manitowaning** Manitoulin Island, Ontario, S Canada
14 B7 **Manitowik Lake** ◎ Ontario, S Canada
31 N7 **Manitowoc** Wisconsin, N USA
Manîtsoq see Maniitsoq
139 O7 **Mānī', Wādī al** dry watercourse W Iraq
12 J14 **Maniwaki** Quebec, SE Canada
171 W13 **Maniwori** Irian Jaya, E Indonesia
54 E10 **Manizales** Caldas, W Colombia
112 F11 **Manjača** ▲ NW Bosnia and Herzegovina
Manjacaze see Mandlakazi
180 J14 **Manjimup** Western Australia
109 V4 **Mank** Niederösterreich, C Austria
79 I17 **Mankanza** Equateur, NW Dem. Rep. Congo (Zaire)
153 N12 **Mankāpur** Uttar Pradesh, N India
26 M3 **Mankato** Kansas, C USA
29 U10 **Mankato** Minnesota, N USA
117 O7 **Man'kivka** Cherkas'ka Oblast', C Ukraine
76 M15 **Mankono** C Ivory Coast
11 T17 **Mankota** Saskatchewan, S Canada
155 K23 **Mankulam** Northern Province, N Sri Lanka
39 Q9 **Manley Hot Springs** Alaska, USA
18 H10 **Manlius** New York, NE USA
105 W5 **Manlleu** Cataluña, NE Spain
29 V11 **Manly** Iowa, C USA
154 E13 **Manmād** Mahārāshtra, W India
182 J7 **Mannahill** South Australia
155 J23 **Mannar** var. Manar. Northern Province, NW Sri Lanka
155 I24 **Mannar, Gulf of** gulf India/Sri Lanka
155 J23 **Mannar Island** island N Sri Lanka
Mannersdorf see Mannersdorf am Leithagebirge
109 Y5 **Mannersdorf am Leithagebirge** var. Mannersdorf. Niederösterreich, E Austria
109 Y6 **Mannersdorf an der Rabnitz** Burgenland, E Austria
101 G20 **Mannheim** Baden-Württemberg, SW Germany
11 O12 **Manning** Alberta, W Canada
29 T14 **Manning** Iowa, C USA
28 K5 **Manning** North Dakota, N USA
21 S13 **Manning** South Carolina, SE USA
191 Y2 **Manning, Cape** headland Kiritimati, NE Kiribati
21 S3 **Mannington** West Virginia, NE USA
182 A1 **Mann Ranges** ▲▲ South Australia
107 C19 **Mannu** ≈ Sardegna, Italy, C Mediterranean Sea
11 R14 **Mannville** Alberta, SW Canada
76 J15 **Mano** ≈ Liberia/Sierra Leone
Manø see Mandø
39 O13 **Manokotak** Alaska, USA
171 V12 **Manokwari** Irian Jaya, E Indonesia
79 N22 **Manono** Shabo, SE Dem. Rep. Congo (Zaire)
25 T10 **Manor** Texas, SW USA
97 D16 **Manorhamilton** Ir. Cluainín. NW Ireland
103 S15 **Manosque** Alpes-de-Haute-Provence, SE France
12 L11 **Manouane, Lac** ◎ Quebec, SE Canada
163 W12 **Manp'o** var. Manp'ojin. NW North Korea
Manp'ojin see Manp'o
191 T4 **Manra** prev. Sydney Island. atoll Phoenix Islands, C Kiribati
105 V5 **Manresa** Cataluña, NE Spain
152 H9 **Mānsa** Punjab, NW India
82 J12 **Mansa** prev. Fort Rosebery. Luapula, N Zambia
76 G12 **Mansa Konko** C Gambia
15 Q11 **Manseau** Quebec, SE Canada
149 U5 **Mānsehra** North-West Frontier Province, NW Pakistan
9 Q9 **Mansel Island** island Nunavut, NE Canada
183 O12 **Mansfield** Victoria, SE Australia
97 M18 **Mansfield** C England, UK
27 S11 **Mansfield** Arkansas, C USA
22 G6 **Mansfield** Louisiana, S USA
19 O12 **Mansfield** Massachusetts, NE USA
31 T12 **Mansfield** Ohio, N USA
18 G12 **Mansfield** Pennsylvania, NE USA
18 M7 **Mansfield, Mount** ▲ Vermont, NE USA
59 M16 **Mansidão** Bahia, E Brazil
102 L11 **Mansle** Charente, W France
76 G12 **Mansôa** C Guinea-Bissau
47 V8 **Manso, Rio** ≈ C Brazil
Manṣūra see El Manṣūra
Mansurabad see Mehrān, Rūd-e
56 A6 **Manta** Manabí, W Ecuador
57 F14 **Mantaro, Río** ≈ C Peru
35 O8 **Manteca** California, W USA
54 J7 **Mantecal** Apure, C Venezuela
31 N11 **Manteno** Illinois, N USA
21 Y9 **Manteo** Roanoke Island, North Carolina, SE USA
Mantes-Gassicourt see Mantes-la-Jolie
103 N5 **Mantes-la-Jolie** prev. Mantes-Gassicourt, Mantes-sur-Seine, anc. Medunta. Yvelines, N France
Mantes-sur-Seine see Mantes-la-Jolie
36 L5 **Manti** Utah, W USA
Mantinea see Mantíneia
115 F20 **Mantíneia** anc. Mantinea. site of ancient city Pelopónnisos, S Greece
59 M21 **Mantiqueira, Serra da** ▲▲ S Brazil
29 W10 **Mantorville** Minnesota, N USA
115 G17 **Mantoúdi** var. Mandoudi; prev. Mandoúdhion. Évvoia, C Greece
Mantoue see Mantova
106 F8 **Mantova** Eng. Mantua, Fr. Mantoue. Lombardia, NW Italy
93 M19 **Mäntsälä** Etelä-Suomi, S Finland
93 L17 **Mänttä** Länsi-Suomi, W Finland
Mantua see Mantova
127 O14 **Manturovo** Kostromskaya Oblast', NW Russian Federation
93 M18 **Mäntyharju** Ita-Suomi, SE Finland
92 M13 **Mäntyjärvi** Lappi, N Finland
190 L16 **Manuae** island S Cook Islands
191 Q10 **Manuae** atoll Îles Sous le Vent, W French Polynesia
192 L16 **Manua Islands** island group E American Samoa
40 L5 **Manuel Benavides** Chihuahua, N Mexico
61 D21 **Manuel J.Cobo** Buenos Aires, E Argentina
58 M12 **Manuel Luís, Recife** reef E Brazil
61 F15 **Manuel Viana** Rio Grande do Sul, S Brazil
59 I14 **Manuel Zinho** Pará, N Brazil
191 V11 **Manuhangi** atoll Îles Tuamotu, C French Polynesia
185 E22 **Manuherikia** ≈ South Island, NZ
171 P13 **Manui, Pulau** island N Indonesia
Manukau see Manurewa
184 L6 **Manukau Harbour** harbor North Island, NZ
191 Z2 **Manulu Lagoon** ◎ Kiritimati, E Kiribati
182 J7 **Manunda Creek** seasonal river South Australia
57 K15 **Manupari, Río** ≈ N Bolivia
184 L6 **Manurewa** var. Manukau. Auckland, North Island, NZ
57 K15 **Manurimi, Río** ≈ NW Bolivia
186 D5 **Manus** ◈ province N PNG
186 D5 **Manus Island** var. Great Admiralty Island. island N PNG
171 T16 **Manuwui** Pulau Babar, E Indonesia
29 Q3 **Manvel** North Dakota, N USA
33 Z14 **Manville** Wyoming, C USA
22 G6 **Many** Louisiana, S USA
81 H21 **Manyara, Lake** ◎ NE Tanzania
128 L12 **Manych** var. Manich. ≈ SW Russian Federation
129 N13 **Manych-Gudilo, Ozero** salt lake SW Russian Federation
83 H14 **Manyinga** North Western, NW Zambia
105 O11 **Manzanares** Castilla-La Mancha, C Spain
44 H7 **Manzanillo** Granma, E Cuba
40 K14 **Manzanillo** Colima, SW Mexico
40 K14 **Manzanillo, Bahía** bay SW Mexico
37 S11 **Manzano Mountains** ▲▲ New Mexico, SW USA
37 R12 **Manzano Peak** ▲ New Mexico, SW USA
163 R6 **Manzhouli** var. Man-chou-li. Nei Mongol Zizhiqu, N China
Manzil Bū Ruqaybah see Menzel Bourguiba
139 X9 **Manzilīyah** E Iraq
83 L21 **Manzini** prev. Bremersdorp. C Swaziland
83 L21 **Manzini** ✈ (Mbabane) C Swaziland
78 G10 **Mao** Kanem, W Chad
45 N8 **Mao** NW Dominican Republic
Maó see Mahón
Maoemere see Maumere
159 W9 **Maojing** Gansu, N China
171 Y14 **Maoke, Pegunungan** Dut. Sneeuw-gebergte, Eng. Snow Mountains. ▲▲ Irian Jaya, E Indonesia
Maol Réidh, Caoc see Mweelrea
160 M15 **Maoming** Guangdong, S China
160 H8 **Maoxian** var. Mao Xian; prev. Fengyizhen. Sichuan, C China
83 L19 **Mapai** Gaza, SW Mozambique
158 H15 **Mapam Yumco** ◎ W China
83 I15 **Mapanza** Southern, S Zambia
54 J4 **Mapararí** Falcón, N Venezuela
41 U17 **Mapastepec** Chiapas, SE Mexico
169 V9 **Mapat, Pulau** island N Indonesia
171 Y15 **Mapi** Irian Jaya, E Indonesia
171 V11 **Mapia, Kepulauan** island group E Indonesia
40 L8 **Mapimí** Durango, C Mexico
83 N19 **Mapinhane** Inhambane, SE Mozambique
55 N7 **Mapire** Monagas, NE Venezuela
11 S17 **Maple Creek** Saskatchewan, S Canada
31 Q9 **Maple River** ≈ Michigan, N USA
29 P7 **Maple River** ≈ North Dakota/South Dakota, N USA
29 S13 **Mapleton** Iowa, C USA
29 U10 **Mapleton** Minnesota, N USA
29 R5 **Mapleton** North Dakota, N USA
32 F13 **Mapleton** Oregon, NW USA
36 L3 **Mapleton** Utah, W USA
192 K5 **Mapmaker Seamounts** undersea feature N Pacific Ocean
186 B6 **Maprik** East Sepik, NW PNG
83 L21 **Maputo** prev. Lourenço Marques. ● (Mozambique) Maputo, S Mozambique
83 L21 **Maputo** ◈ province S Mozambique
83 L21 **Maputo** ✈ Maputo, S Mozambique
67 V14 **Maputo** ≈ S Mozambique
Maqanshy see Makanchi
Maqat see Makat
113 K19 **Maqē** ≈ NW Albania
113 M19 **Maqellarë** Dibër, C Albania
159 S12 **Maqên** var. Dawu. Qinghai, C China
159 S11 **Maqên Gangri** ▲ C China
159 U12 **Maqu** Gansu, C China
104 M9 **Maqueda** Castilla-La Mancha, C Spain
82 B9 **Maquela do Zombo** Uíge, NW Angola
63 I16 **Maquinchao** Río Negro, C Argentina
29 Z13 **Maquoketa** Iowa, C USA
29 Y13 **Maquoketa River** ≈ Iowa, C USA
14 F13 **Mar** Ontario, S Canada
95 F14 **Mår** ◎ S Norway
81 G19 **Mara** ◈ region N Tanzania
191 P8 **Maraa** Tahiti, W French Polynesia
58 D12 **Maraã** Amazonas, NW Brazil
191 O8 **Maraa, Pointe** headland Tahiti, W French Polynesia
59 K14 **Marabá** Pará, NE Brazil
54 H5 **Maracaibo** Zulia, NW Venezuela
Maracaibo, Gulf of see Venezuela, Golfo de
54 H5 **Maracaibo, Lago de** var. Lake Maracaibo. inlet NW Venezuela
Maracaibo, Lake see Maracaibo, Lago de
58 K10 **Maracá, Ilha de** island NE Brazil
59 H20 **Maracaju, Serra de** ▲▲ S Brazil
58 I11 **Maracanaquará, Planalto** ▲▲ NE Brazil
54 L5 **Maracay** Aragua, N Venezuela
Marada see Marādah
75 R9 **Marādah** var. Marada. N Libya
77 U12 **Maradi** Maradi, S Niger
77 U11 **Maradi** ◈ department S Niger
81 E21 **Maragarazi** var. Muragarazi. ≈ Burundi/Tanzania
Maragha see Marāgheh
142 J3 **Marāgheh** var. Maragha. Āzarbāyjān-e Khāvarī, NW Iran
141 P7 **Marāh** var. Marrāt. Ar Riyāḍ, C Saudi Arabia
55 N11 **Marahuaca, Cerro** ▲ S Venezuela
27 R5 **Marais des Cygnes River** ≈ Kansas/Missouri, C USA
58 L11 **Marajó, Baía de** bay N Brazil
59 K12 **Marajó, Ilha de** island N Brazil
191 O2 **Marakei** atoll Tungaru, W Kiribati
Marakesh see Marrakech
81 I18 **Maralal** Rift Valley, C Kenya
83 G21 **Maralaleng** Kgalagadi, S Botswana
145 U8 **Maraldy, Ozero** ◎ NE Kazakhstan
182 C5 **Maralinga** South Australia
Máramarossziget see Sighetu Marmaţiei
187 N9 **Maramasike** var. Small Malaita. island N Solomon Islands
Maramba see Livingstone
194 H3 **Marambio** Argentinian research station Antarctica
116 H9 **Maramureș** ◈ county NW Romania
36 L15 **Marana** Arizona, SW USA
105 P7 **Maranchón** Castilla-La Mancha, C Spain
142 J2 **Marand** var. Merend. Āzarbāyjān-e Khāvarī, NW Iran
Marandellas see Marondera
58 L13 **Maranhão** off. Estado do Maranhão. ◈ state E Brazil
104 H10 **Maranhão, Barragem do** ⊟ C Portugal
149 O11 **Mārān, Koh-i** ▲ SW Pakistan
106 J7 **Marano, Laguna di** lagoon NE Italy
56 E9 **Marañón, Río** ≈ N Peru
102 J10 **Marans** Charente-Maritime, W France
83 M20 **Marão** Inhambane, S Mozambique
185 B23 **Mararoa** ≈ South Island, NZ
Maraş/Marash see Kahramanmaraş
107 M19 **Maratea** Basilicata, S Italy
104 G11 **Marateca** Setúbal, S Portugal
115 B20 **Marathiá, Akrotírio** headland Zákynthos, Iónioi Nísoi, Greece, C Mediterranean Sea
12 E12 **Marathon** Ontario, S Canada
23 Y17 **Marathon** Florida Keys, Florida, SE USA
24 L10 **Marathon** Texas, SW USA
Marathón see Marathónas
115 H19 **Marathónas** prev. Marathón. Attikí, C Greece
169 W9 **Maratua, Pulau** island N Indonesia
59 O18 **Maraú** Bahia, SE Brazil
143 R3 **Marāveh Tappeh** Golestān, N Iran
24 L11 **Maravillas Creek** ≈ Texas, SW USA
186 D8 **Marawaka** Eastern Highlands, C PNG
171 Q7 **Marawi** Mindanao, S Philippines
Marbat see Mirbāṭ
104 L16 **Marbella** Andalucía, S Spain
180 J7 **Marble Bar** Western Australia
36 L9 **Marble Canyon** canyon Arizona, SW USA
25 S10 **Marble Falls** Texas, SW USA
27 Y7 **Marble Hill** Missouri, C USA
33 T15 **Marbleton** Wyoming, C USA
Marburg see Maribor
Marburg see Marburg an der Lahn, Germany
101 H16 **Marburg an der Lahn** hist. Marburg. Hessen, W Germany
111 H23 **Marcal** ≈ W Hungary
42 G7 **Marcala** La Paz, SW Honduras
111 H24 **Marcali** Somogy, SW Hungary
83 A16 **Marca, Ponta da** headland SW Angola
59 I16 **Marcelândia** Mato Grosso, W Brazil
27 T3 **Marceline** Missouri, C USA
60 I13 **Marcelino Ramos** Rio Grande do Sul, S Brazil
55 Y12 **Marcel, Mont** ▲ S French Guiana
97 O19 **March** E England, UK
109 Z3 **March** var. Morava. ≈ C Europe see also Morava
106 I12 **Marche** Eng. Marches. ◈ region C Italy
103 N11 **Marche** cultural region C France
99 J21 **Marche-en-Famenne** Luxembourg, SE Belgium
104 K14 **Marchena** Andalucía, S Spain
57 B17 **Marchena, Isla** var. Bindloe Island. island Galapagos Islands, Ecuador, E Pacific Ocean
Marches see Marche
99 J20 **Marchin** Liège, E Belgium
181 S1 **Marchinbar Island** island Wessel Islands, Northern Territory, N Australia
62 L9 **Mar Chiquita, Laguna** ◎ C Argentina
103 Q10 **Marcigny** Saône-et-Loire, C France
23 W16 **Marco** Florida, SE USA
Marcodurum see Düren
59 O15 **Marcolândia** Pernambuco, E Brazil
106 I8 **Marco Polo** ✈ (Venezia) Veneto, NE Italy
Marcq see Mark
116 M8 **Mărculeşti** Rus. Markuleshty. N Moldova
29 S12 **Marcus** Iowa, C USA
39 S11 **Marcus Baker, Mount** ▲ Alaska, USA
192 I5 **Marcus Island** var. Minami Tori Shima. island E Japan
18 K8 **Marcy, Mount** ▲ New York, NE USA
149 T5 **Mardān** North-West Frontier Province, N Pakistan
63 N14 **Mar del Plata** Buenos Aires, E Argentina
137 Q16 **Mardin** Mardin, SE Turkey
137 Q16 **Mardin** ◈ province SE Turkey
137 Q16 **Mardin Dağları** ▲▲ SE Turkey
162 J9 **Mardzad** Övörhangay, C Mongolia
187 R17 **Maré** island Îles Loyauté, E New Caledonia
Marea Neagră see Black Sea
105 Z8 **Mare de Déu del Toro** ▲ Menorca, Spain, W Mediterranean Sea
181 W4 **Mareeba** Queensland, NE Australia
96 G8 **Maree, Loch** ◎ N Scotland, UK
Mareeq see Mereeg
Marek see Dupnitsa
76 J11 **Maréna** Kayes, W Mali
190 I2 **Marenanuka** atoll Tungaru, W Kiribati
29 X14 **Marengo** Iowa, C USA
102 J11 **Marennes** Charente-Maritime, W France
107 G23 **Marettimo, Isola** island Isole Egadi, S Italy
24 K10 **Marfa** Texas, SW USA
57 P17 **Marfil, Laguna** ◎ E Bolivia
Marganets see Marhanets'
25 Q4 **Margaret** Texas, SW USA
180 I14 **Margaret River** Western Australia
186 C7 **Margarima** Southern Highlands, W PNG
55 N4 **Margarita, Isla de** island N Venezuela
115 I25 **Margarítes** Kríti, Greece, E Mediterranean Sea
97 Q22 **Margate** prev. Mergate. SE England, UK
23 Z15 **Margate** Florida, SE USA
Margelan see Marghilon
103 P13 **Margeride, Montagnes de la** ▲▲ C France
Margherita see Jamaame
107 N16 **Margherita di Savoia** Puglia, SE Italy
Margherita, Lake see Ābaya Hāyk'
81 E18 **Margherita Peak** Fr. Pic Marguerite. ▲ Uganda/Dem. Rep. Congo (Zaire)
149 O4 **Marghī** Bāmīān, N Afghanistan
147 S10 **Marghilon** var. Margelan, Rus. Margilan. Farghona Wiloyati, E Uzbekistan
116 G9 **Marghita** Hung. Margitta. Bihor, NW Romania
Margilan see Marghilon
116 K8 **Marginea** Suceava, NE Romania
Margitta see Marghita
148 K9 **Mārgow, Dasht-e** desert SW Afghanistan
99 L18 **Margraten** Limburg, SE Netherlands
10 M15 **Marguerite** British Columbia, SW Canada
194 I6 **Marguerite Bay** bay Antarctica
Marguerite, Pic see Margherita Peak
117 T9 **Marhanets'** Rus. Marganets. Dnipropetrovs'ka Oblast', E Ukraine
186 B9 **Mari** Western, SW PNG
191 R12 **Maria** island Îles Australes, SW French Polynesia
191 Y12 **Maria** atoll Groupe Actéon, SE French Polynesia
40 I12 **María Cleofas, Isla** island C Mexico
62 H4 **María Elena** var. Oficina María Elena. Antofagasta, N Chile
95 G21 **Mariager** Århus, C Denmark
61 C22 **María Ignacia** Buenos Aires, E Argentina
183 P17 **Maria Island** island Tasmania, SE Australia
40 H12 **María Madre, Isla** island C Mexico
40 I12 **María Magdalena, Isla** island C Mexico
192 H6 **Mariana Islands** island group Guam/Northern Mariana Islands
175 N3 **Mariana Trench** var. Challenger Deep. undersea feature W Pacific Ocean
153 X12 **Mariāni** Assam, NE India
27 X11 **Marianna** Arkansas, C USA
23 R8 **Marianna** Florida, SE USA
172 J16 **Marianne** island Inner Islands, NE Seychelles
95 M19 **Mariannelund** Jönköping, S Sweden
61 D15 **Mariano I.Loza** Corrientes, NE Argentina
Mariano Machado see Ganda
111 A16 **Mariánské Lázně** Ger. Marienbad. Karlovarský Kraj, W Czech Republic
Máriaradna see Radna
33 S7 **Marias River** ≈ Montana, NW USA
Maria-Theresiopel see Subotica
Máriatölgyes see Dubnica nad Váhom
184 H1 **Maria van Diemen, Cape** headland North Island, NZ
109 V5 **Mariazell** Steiermark, E Austria
141 P15 **Mar'ib** W Yemen
95 I25 **Maribo** Storstrøm, S Denmark
109 W9 **Maribor** Ger. Marburg. NE Slovenia
Marica see Maritsa
35 R13 **Maricopa** California, W USA
Maricourt see Kangiqsujuaq
81 D15 **Maridi** Western Equatoria, SW Sudan
194 M11 **Marie Byrd Land** physical region Antarctica
193 P14 **Marie Byrd Seamount** undersea feature N Amundsen Sea
45 X11 **Marie-Galante** var. Ceyre to the Caribs. island SE Guadeloupe
45 Y6 **Marie-Galante, Canal de** channel S Guadeloupe
93 J20 **Mariehamn** Fin. Maarianhamina. Åland, SW Finland
44 C4 **Mariel** La Habana, W Cuba
99 H22 **Mariembourg** Namur, S Belgium
Marienbad see Mariánské Lázně
Marienburg see Alūksne, Latvia
Marienburg see Malbork, Poland
Marienburg see Feldioara, Romania
Marienburg in Westpreussen see Malbork
Marienhausen see Viļaka
83 D20 **Mariental** Hardap, SW Namibia
18 D13 **Marienville** Pennsylvania, NE USA
Marienwerder see Kwidzyń
58 C12 **Marié, Rio** ≈ NW Brazil
95 K17 **Mariestad** Västra Götaland, S Sweden
23 S3 **Marietta** Georgia, SE USA
31 U14 **Marietta** Ohio, N USA
27 N13 **Marietta** Oklahoma, C USA
81 H18 **Marigat** Rift Valley, W Kenya
103 S16 **Marignane** Bouches-du-Rhône, SE France
Marignano see Melegnano
45 O11 **Marigot** NE Dominica
122 K12 **Mariinsk** Kemerovskaya Oblast', S Russian Federation
129 Q3 **Mariinskiy Posad** Respublika Mariy El, W Russian Federation
119 E14 **Marijampolė** prev. Kapsukas. Marijampolė, S Lithuania
114 G12 **Marikostenovo** Blagoevgrad, SW Bulgaria
60 J9 **Marília** São Paulo, S Brazil
82 D11 **Marimba** Malanje, NW Angola
139 T1 **Marī Mīlā** E Iraq
104 G4 **Marín** Galicia, NW Spain
35 N10 **Marina** California, W USA
Marina di Catanzaro see Catanzaro Marina
Mar'ina Gorka see Mar"ina Horka
119 L17 **Mar"ina Horka** Rus. Mar'ina Gorka. Minskaya Voblasts', C Belarus
171 O4 **Marinduque** island C Philippines
31 S9 **Marine City** Michigan, N USA
31 N6 **Marinette** Wisconsin, N USA

◆ COUNTRY ● COUNTRY CAPITAL ◇ DEPENDENT TERRITORY ○ DEPENDENT TERRITORY CAPITAL ◈ ADMINISTRATIVE REGION ✈ INTERNATIONAL AIRPORT ▲ MOUNTAIN ▲▲ MOUNTAIN RANGE VOLCANO ≈ RIVER ◎ LAKE ⊟ RESERVOIR

60 I10 **Maringá** Paraná, S Brazil
83 N16 **Maringuè** Sofala, C Mozambique
104 F9 **Marinha Grande** Leiria, C Portugal
107 I15 **Marino** Lazio, C Italy
59 A15 **Mário Lobão** Acre, W Brazil
23 O5 **Marion** Alabama, S USA
27 Y11 **Marion** Arkansas, C USA
30 L17 **Marion** Illinois, N USA
31 P13 **Marion** Indiana, N USA
29 X13 **Marion** Iowa, C USA
27 O5 **Marion** Kansas, C USA
20 H6 **Marion** Kentucky, S USA
21 P9 **Marion** North Carolina, SE USA
31 S12 **Marion** Ohio, N USA
21 T12 **Marion** South Carolina, SE USA
21 Q7 **Marion** Virginia, NE USA
27 O5 **Marion Lake** ⊡ Kansas, C USA
21 S13 **Marion, Lake** ⊡ South Carolina, SE USA
27 S8 **Marionville** Missouri, C USA
55 N7 **Maripa** Bolívar, E Venezuela
55 X11 **Maripasoula** W French Guiana
35 Q9 **Mariposa** California, W USA
61 G19 **Mariscala** Lavalleja, S Uruguay
62 M4 **Mariscal Estigarribia** Boquerón, NW Paraguay
56 C6 **Mariscal Sucre** *var.* Quito. ✈ (Quito) Pichincha, C Ecuador
30 K16 **Marissa** Illinois, N USA
103 U14 **Maritime Alps** *Fr.* Alpes Maritimes, *It.* Alpi Marittime. ▲ France/Italy
Maritimes, Alpes *see* Maritime Alps
Maritime Territory *see* Primorskiy Kray
114 K11 **Maritsa** *var.* Marica, *Gk.* Évros, *Turk.* Meriç; *anc.* Hebrus. ≈ SW Europe *see also* Évros/Meriç
Maritsa *see* Simeonovgrad
Marittime, Alpi *see* Maritime Alps
Maritzburg *see* Pietermaritzburg
117 X9 **Mariupol'** *prev.* Zhdanov. Donets'ka Oblast', SE Ukraine
55 Q6 **Mariusa, Caño** ≈ NE Venezuela
142 J5 **Marīvān** *prev.* Dezh Shāhpūr. Kordestān, W Iran
129 R3 **Mariyets** Respublika Mariy El, W Russian Federation
Mariyskaya ASSR *see* Mariy El, Respublika
118 G4 **Märjamaa** *Ger.* Merjama. Raplamaa, NW Estonia
99 I15 **Mark** *Fr.* Marcq. ≈ Belgium/Netherlands
81 N17 **Marka** *var.* Merca. Shabeellaha Hoose, S Somalia
145 Z10 **Markakol', Ozero** *Kaz.* Marqaköl. ◎ E Kazakhstan
76 M12 **Markala** Ségou, W Mali
159 S15 **Markam** *var.* Gartog. Xizang Zizhiqu, W China
95 K21 **Markaryd** Kronoberg, S Sweden
142 L7 **Markazī** *off.* Ostān-e Markazī. ◈ *province* W Iran
14 F14 **Markdale** Ontario, S Canada
27 X10 **Marked Tree** Arkansas, C USA
98 N11 **Markelo** Overijssel, E Netherlands
98 J9 **Markermeer** ◎ C Netherlands
97 N20 **Market Harborough** C England, UK
97 N18 **Market Rasen** E England, UK
123 O10 **Markha** ≈ NE Russian Federation
12 H16 **Markham** Ontario, S Canada
25 V12 **Markham** Texas, SW USA
186 E7 **Markham** ≈ C PNG
195 Q11 **Markham, Mount** ▲ Antarctica
110 M11 **Marki** Mazowieckie, C Poland
158 F8 **Markit** Xinjiang Uygur Zizhiqu, NW China
117 Y5 **Markivka** *Rus.* Markovka. Luhans'ka Oblast', E Ukraine
35 Q7 **Markleeville** California, W USA
98 L8 **Marknesse** Flevoland, N Netherlands
79 H14 **Markounda** *var.* Marcounda. Ouham, NW Central African Republic
Markovka *see* Markivka
123 U7 **Markovo** Chukotskiy Avtonomnyy Okrug, NE Russian Federation
129 P8 **Marks** Saratovskaya Oblast', W Russian Federation
22 K2 **Marks** Mississippi, S USA
22 I7 **Marksville** Louisiana, S USA
101 I19 **Marktheidenfeld** Bayern, C Germany
101 J24 **Marktoberdorf** Bayern, S Germany
101 M18 **Marktredwitz** Bayern, E Germany
Markt-Übelbach *see* Übelbach
27 V3 **Mark Twain Lake** ⊡ Missouri, C USA
Markuleshty *see* Mărculeşti
101 E14 **Marl** Nordrhein-Westfalen, W Germany
182 E2 **Marla** South Australia
181 Y8 **Marlborough** Queensland, E Australia
97 M22 **Marlborough** S England, UK
185 I15 **Marlborough** *off.* Marlborough District. ◈ *unitary authority* South Island, NZ
103 P3 **Marle** Aisne, N France
31 S8 **Marlette** Michigan, N USA
25 T9 **Marlin** Texas, SW USA
21 S5 **Marlinton** West Virginia, NE USA
26 M12 **Marlow** Oklahoma, C USA
155 E17 **Marmagao** Goa, W India
Marmanda *see* Marmande
102 L13 **Marmande** *anc.* Marmanda. Lot-et-Garonne, SW France
136 C11 **Marmara** Balıkesir, NW Turkey
136 D11 **Marmara Denizi** *Eng.* Sea of Marmara. *sea* NW Turkey
114 N13 **Marmaraereğlisi** Tekirdağ, NW Turkey
Marmara, Sea of *see* Marmara Denizi
136 C16 **Marmaris** Muğla, SW Turkey
28 J6 **Marmarth** North Dakota, N USA
21 Q5 **Marmet** West Virginia, NE USA
106 H5 **Marmolada, Monte** ▲ N Italy
104 M13 **Marmolejo** Andalucía, S Spain
14 J14 **Marmora** Ontario, SE Canada
39 Q14 **Marmot Bay** *bay* Alaska, USA
103 Q4 **Marne** ◈ *department* N France
103 Q4 **Marne** ≈ N France
137 U10 **Marneuli** *prev.* Borchalo, Sarvani. S Georgia
78 I13 **Maro** Moyen-Chari, S Chad
54 L12 **Maroa** Amazonas, S Venezuela
172 J3 **Maroantsetra** Toamasina, NE Madagascar
191 W11 **Marokau** *atoll* Îles Tuamotu, C French Polynesia
172 J5 **Marolambo** Toamasina, E Madagascar
172 J2 **Maromokotro** ▲ N Madagascar
83 L16 **Marondera** *prev.* Marandellas. Mashonaland East, NE Zimbabwe
55 X9 **Maroni** *Dut.* Marowijne. ≈ French Guiana/Surinam
183 V2 **Maroochydore-Mooloolaba** Queensland, E Australia
171 N14 **Maros** Sulawesi, C Indonesia
116 H11 **Maros** *var.* Mureş, Mureşul, *Ger.* Marosch, Mieresch. ≈ Hungary/Romania *see also* Mureş
Marosch *see* Maros/Mureş
Maroshévíz *see* Toplița
Marosillye *see* Ilia
Marosludas *see* Luduş
Marosújvár/Marosújvárakna *see* Ocna Mureş
Marosvásárhely *see* Târgu Mureş
191 V14 **Marotiri** *var.* Îlots de Bass, Morotiri. *island group* Îles Australes, SW French Polynesia
78 G12 **Maroua** Extrême-Nord, N Cameroon
55 X12 **Marouini Rivier** ≈ SE Surinam
172 I3 **Marovoay** Mahajanga, NW Madagascar
55 W9 **Marowijne** ◈ *district* NE Surinam
Marowijne *see* Maroni
Marqaköl *see* Markakol', Ozero
193 P8 **Marquesas Fracture Zone** *tectonic feature* E Pacific Ocean
Marquesas Islands *see* Marquises, Îles
23 W17 **Marquesas Keys** *island group* Florida, SE USA
29 Y12 **Marquette** Iowa, C USA
31 N3 **Marquette** Michigan, N USA
103 N1 **Marquise** Pas-de-Calais, N France
191 X7 **Marquises, Îles** *Eng.* Marquesas Islands. *island group* N French Polynesia
183 Q6 **Marra Creek** ≈ New South Wales, SE Australia
80 B10 **Marra Hills** *plateau* W Sudan
80 B11 **Marra, Jebel** ▲ W Sudan
74 E7 **Marrakech** *var.* Marakesh, *Eng.* Marrakesh; *prev.* Morocco. W Morocco
Marrakesh *see* Marrakech
Marrāt *see* Marāh
183 N15 **Marrawah** Tasmania, SE Australia
182 I4 **Marree** South Australia
81 L17 **Marrehan** ▲ SW Somalia
83 N17 **Marromeu** Sofala, C Mozambique
104 J17 **Marroquí, Punta** *headland* SW Spain
183 N8 **Marrowie Creek** *seasonal river* New South Wales, SE Australia
83 O14 **Marrupa** Niassa, N Mozambique
182 D1 **Marryat** South Australia
75 Y10 **Marsa 'Alam** SE Egypt
75 R8 **Marsá al Burayqah** *var.* Al Burayqah. N Libya
81 J17 **Marsabit** Eastern, N Kenya
107 H23 **Marsala** *anc.* Lilybaeum. Sicilia, Italy, C Mediterranean Sea
121 P16 **Marsaxlokk Bay** *bay* SE Malta
65 G15 **Mars Bay** *bay* Ascension Island, C Atlantic Ocean
101 H15 **Marsberg** Nordrhein-Westfalen, W Germany
11 R15 **Marsden** Saskatchewan, S Canada
98 H7 **Marsdiep** *strait* NW Netherlands
103 R16 **Marseille** *Eng.* Marseilles; *anc.* Massilia. Bouches-du-Rhône, SE France
Marseille-Marignane *see* Provence
30 M11 **Marseilles** Illinois, N USA
Marseilles *see* Marseille
76 J16 **Marshall** W Liberia
39 N11 **Marshall** Alaska, USA
27 U9 **Marshall** Arkansas, C USA
31 N14 **Marshall** Illinois, N USA
31 Q10 **Marshall** Michigan, N USA
29 S9 **Marshall** Minnesota, N USA
27 T4 **Marshall** Missouri, C USA
21 O9 **Marshall** North Carolina, SE USA
25 X6 **Marshall** Texas, SW USA
189 S4 **Marshall Islands** *off.* Republic of the Marshall Islands. ◆ *republic* W Pacific Ocean
175 Q3 **Marshall Islands** *island group* W Pacific Ocean
192 K6 **Marshall Seamounts** *undersea feature* SW Pacific Ocean
29 W13 **Marshalltown** Iowa, C USA
19 P12 **Marshfield** Massachusetts, NE USA
27 T7 **Marshfield** Missouri, C USA
30 K6 **Marshfield** Wisconsin, N USA
44 H1 **Marsh Harbour** Great Abaco, W Bahamas
19 S3 **Mars Hill** Maine, NE USA
21 P9 **Mars Hill** North Carolina, SE USA
22 H10 **Marsh Island** *island* Louisiana, S USA
21 S11 **Marshville** North Carolina, SE USA
15 W5 **Marsoui** Quebec, SE Canada
15 R8 **Mars, Rivière à** ≈ Quebec, SE Canada
95 O15 **Märsta** Stockholm, C Sweden
95 H24 **Marstal** Fyn, C Denmark
95 I19 **Marstrand** Västra Götaland, S Sweden
25 U8 **Mart** Texas, SW USA
166 M9 **Martaban** *var.* Moktama. Mon State, S Myanmar
166 L9 **Martaban, Gulf of** *gulf* S Myanmar
107 Q19 **Martano** Puglia, SE Italy
Martapoera *see* Martapura
169 T13 **Martapura** *prev.* Martapoera. Borneo, C Indonesia
99 L23 **Martelange** Luxembourg, SE Belgium
114 L7 **Marten** Ruse, N Bulgaria
14 H10 **Marten River** Ontario, S Canada
11 T15 **Martensville** Saskatchewan, S Canada
Marteskirch *see* Târnăveni
Martes Tolosane *see* Martres-Tolosane
115 K25 **Mártha** Kríti, Greece, E Mediterranean Sea
183 Q6 **Marthaguy Creek** ≈ New South Wales, SE Australia
19 P13 **Martha's Vineyard** *island* Massachusetts, NE USA
108 C11 **Martigny** Valais, SW Switzerland
103 R16 **Martigues** Bouches-du-Rhône, SE France
111 J19 **Martin** *Ger.* Sankt Martin, *Hung.* Turócszentmárton; *prev.* Turčianský Svätý Martin. Žilinský Kraj, N Slovakia
28 L11 **Martin** South Dakota, N USA
20 G8 **Martin** Tennessee, S USA
105 S7 **Martín** ≈ E Spain
107 P18 **Martina Franca** Puglia, SE Italy
185 M14 **Martinborough** Wellington, North Island, NZ
25 S11 **Martindale** Texas, SW USA
35 N8 **Martinez** California, W USA
23 V3 **Martinez** Georgia, SE USA
41 Q13 **Martínez de La Torre** Veracruz-Llave, E Mexico
45 Y12 **Martinique** ◇ *French overseas department* E West Indies
1 O15 **Martinique** *island* E West Indies
Martinique Channel *see* Martinique Passage
45 X12 **Martinique Passage** *var.* Dominica Channel, Martinique Channel. *channel* Dominica/Martinique
23 Q5 **Martin Lake** ⊡ Alabama, S USA
115 G18 **Martíno** *prev.* Martínon. Stereá Ellás, C Greece
Martínon *see* Martíno
194 J11 **Martin Peninsula** *peninsula* Antarctica
39 S5 **Martin Point** *headland* Alaska, USA
109 V3 **Martinsberg** Niederösterreich, NE Austria
21 V3 **Martinsburg** West Virginia, NE USA
31 V13 **Martins Ferry** Ohio, N USA
Martinskirch *see* Târnăveni
31 O14 **Martinsville** Indiana, N USA
21 S8 **Martinsville** Virginia, NE USA
65 K16 **Martin Vaz, Ilhas** *island group* E Brazil
Martök *see* Martuk
184 M12 **Marton** Manawatu-Wanganui, North Island, NZ
105 N13 **Martos** Andalucía, S Spain
102 M16 **Martres-Tolosane** *var.* Martes Tolosane. Haute-Garonne, S France
92 M11 **Martti** Lappi, NE Finland
144 I9 **Martuk** *Kaz.* Martök. Aktyubinsk, NW Kazakhstan
137 U12 **Martuni** E Armenia
58 L11 **Marudá** Pará, E Brazil
169 V6 **Marudu, Teluk** *bay* East Malaysia
149 O8 **Ma'rūf** Kandahār, SE Afghanistan
164 H13 **Marugame** Kagawa, Shikoku, SW Japan
185 H16 **Maruia** ≈ South Island, NZ
98 M6 **Marum** Groningen, NE Netherlands
187 R13 **Marum, Mount** ▲ Ambrym, C Vanuatu
79 P23 **Marungu** ▲ SE Dem. Rep. Congo (Zaire)
191 Y12 **Marutea** *atoll* Groupe Actéon, C French Polynesia
143 O11 **Marv Dasht** *var.* Mervdasht. Fārs, S Iran
103 P13 **Marvejols** Lozère, S France
27 X12 **Marvell** Arkansas, C USA
36 L6 **Marvine, Mount** ▲ Utah, W USA
139 Q7 **Marwānīyah** C Iraq
152 F13 **Mārwār** *var.* Marwar Junction. Rājasthān, N India
Marwar Junction *see* Mārwār
11 R14 **Marwayne** Alberta, SW Canada
146 I14 **Mary** *prev.* Merv. Maryyskiy Velayat, S Turkmenistan
Mary *see* Maryyskiy Velayat
181 Z9 **Maryborough** Queensland, E Australia
182 M11 **Maryborough** Victoria, SE Australia
Maryborough *see* Port Laoise
83 G23 **Marydale** Northern Cape, W South Africa
117 W8 **Mar"yinka** Donets'ka Oblast', E Ukraine
Mary Island *see* Kanton
21 W4 **Maryland** *off.* State of Maryland; also known as America in Miniature, Cockade State, Free State, Old Line State. ◈ *state* NE USA
25 P7 **Maryneal** Texas, SW USA
97 J15 **Maryport** NW England, UK
13 U13 **Marystown** Newfoundland, SE Canada
36 K6 **Marysvale** Utah, W USA
35 O6 **Marysville** California, W USA
27 O3 **Marysville** Kansas, C USA
31 S13 **Marysville** Michigan, N USA
31 S9 **Marysville** Ohio, NE USA
32 H7 **Marysville** Washington, NW USA
27 R2 **Maryville** Missouri, C USA
21 N9 **Maryville** Tennessee, S USA
Mary Welayaty *see* Maryyskiy Velayat
146 I15 **Maryyskiy Velayat** *var.* Mary, *Turkm.* Mary Welayaty. ◈ *province* S Turkmenistan
Marzūq *see* Murzuq
42 J11 **Masachapa** *var.* Puerto Masachapa. Managua, W Nicaragua
81 G19 **Masai Mara National Reserve** *reserve* C Kenya
81 I21 **Masai Steppe** *grassland* NW Tanzania
81 F19 **Masaka** SW Uganda
169 T15 **Masalembo Besar, Pulau** *island* S Indonesia
137 Y13 **Masallı** *Rus.* Masally. S Azerbaijan
Masally *see* Masallı
171 N13 **Masamba** Sulawesi, C Indonesia
Masampo *see* Masan
163 Y16 **Masan** *prev.* Masampo. S South Korea
Masandam Peninsula *see* Musandam Peninsula
81 J25 **Masasi** Mtwara, SE Tanzania
Masawa *see* Massawa
42 J10 **Masaya** Masaya, W Nicaragua
42 J10 **Masaya** ◈ *department* W Nicaragua
171 P5 **Masbate** Masbate, N Philippines
171 P5 **Masbate** *island* C Philippines
74 I6 **Mascara** *var.* Mouaskar. NW Algeria
173 O7 **Mascarene Basin** *undersea feature* W Indian Ocean
173 O9 **Mascarene Islands** *island group* W Indian Ocean
173 N9 **Mascarene Plain** *undersea feature* W Indian Ocean
173 O7 **Mascarene Plateau** *undersea feature* W Indian Ocean
194 H5 **Mascart, Cape** *headland* Adelaide Island, Antarctica
62 J10 **Mascasín, Salinas de** *salt lake* C Argentina
40 K13 **Mascota** Jalisco, C Mexico
15 O12 **Mascouche** Quebec, SE Canada
126 J9 **Masel'gskaya** Respublika Kareliya, NW Russian Federation
83 J23 **Maseru** ● (Lesotho) W Lesotho
83 J23 **Maseru** ✈ W Lesotho
Mashaba *see* Mashava
160 K14 **Mashan** Guangxi Zhuangzu Zizhiqu, S China
83 K17 **Mashava** *prev.* Mashaba. Masvingo, SE Zimbabwe
143 U4 **Mashhad** *var.* Meshed. Khorāsān, NE Iran
165 S3 **Mashike** Hokkaidō, NE Japan
Mashīz *see* Bardsīr
149 N14 **Mashkai** ≈ SW Pakistan
143 X13 **Māshkel** *var.* Rūd-i Māshkel, Rūd-e Māshkīd. ≈ Iran/Pakistan
148 K12 **Māshkel, Hāmūn-i** *salt marsh* SW Pakistan
Māshkel, Rūd-i/Māshkīd, Rūd-e *see* Māshkel
83 K15 **Mashonaland Central** ◈ *province* N Zimbabwe
83 K16 **Mashonaland East** ◈ *province* NE Zimbabwe
83 J16 **Mashonaland West** ◈ *province* NW Zimbabwe
Mashtagi *see* Maştağa
141 S14 **Masīlah, Wādī al** *dry watercourse* SE Yemen
79 I21 **Masi-Manimba** Bandundu, SW Dem. Rep. Congo (Zaire)
81 F17 **Masindi** W Uganda
81 I19 **Masinga Reservoir** ⊡ S Kenya
Masīra *see* Maşīrah, Jazīrat
Masira, Gulf of *see* Maşīrah, Khalīj
141 Y10 **Maşīrah, Jazīrat** *var.* Masīra. *island* E Oman
141 Y10 **Maşīrah, Khalīj** *var.* Gulf of Masira. *bay* E Oman
Masis *see* Büyükağrı Dağı
79 O19 **Masisi** Nord Kivu, E Dem. Rep. Congo (Zaire)
Masjed-e Soleymān *see* Masjed Soleymān
142 L9 **Masjed Soleymān** *var.* Masjed-e Soleymān, Masjid-i Sulaiman. Khūzestān, SW Iran
Masjid-i Sulaiman *see* Masjed Soleymān
Maskat *see* Masqaţ
139 Q7 **Maskhān** C Iraq
141 X8 **Maskin** *var.* Miskin. NW Oman
97 B17 **Mask, Lough** *Ir.* Loch Measca. ◎ W Ireland
114 N10 **Maslen Nos** *headland* E Bulgaria
172 K3 **Masoala, Tanjona** *headland* NE Madagascar
Masohi *see* Amahai
31 Q9 **Mason** Michigan, N USA
31 R14 **Mason** Ohio, N USA
25 Q10 **Mason** Texas, SW USA
21 P4 **Mason** West Virginia, NE USA
185 B25 **Mason Bay** *bay* Stewart Island, NZ
30 K13 **Mason City** Illinois, N USA
29 V12 **Mason City** Iowa, C USA
Ma, Sông *see* Ma, Nam
18 B16 **Masontown** Pennsylvania, NE USA
141 Y8 **Masqaţ** *var.* Maskat, *Eng.* Muscat. ● (Oman) NE Oman
106 E10 **Massa** Toscana, C Italy
18 M11 **Massachusetts** *off.* Commonwealth of Massachusetts; also known as Bay State, Old Bay State, Old Colony State. ◈ *state* NE USA
19 P11 **Massachusetts Bay** *bay* Massachusetts, NE USA
35 R2 **Massacre Lake** ◎ Nevada, W USA
107 O18 **Massafra** Puglia, SE Italy
108 G11 **Massagno** Ticino, S Switzerland
78 G11 **Massaguet** Chari-Baguirmi, W Chad
Massakori *see* Massakory
78 G10 **Massakory** *var.* Massakori; *prev.* Dagana. Chari-Baguirmi, W Chad
78 H11 **Massalassef** Chari-Baguirmi, SW Chad
106 F13 **Massa Marittima** Toscana, C Italy
82 B11 **Massangano** Cuanza Norte, NW Angola
83 M18 **Massangena** Gaza, S Mozambique
80 J9 **Massawa** *var.* Masawa, *Amh.* Mits'iwa. E Eritrea
80 K9 **Massawa Channel** *channel* E Eritrea
18 J6 **Massena** New York, NE USA
78 H11 **Massenya** Chari-Baguirmi, SW Chad
10 I13 **Masset** Graham Island, British Columbia, SW Canada
102 L16 **Masseube** Gers, S France
14 E11 **Massey** Ontario, S Canada
103 P12 **Massiac** Cantal, C France
103 P12 **Massif Central** *plateau* C France
Massilia *see* Marseille
31 U12 **Massillon** Ohio, N USA
77 N12 **Massina** Ségou, W Mali
83 N19 **Massinga** Inhambane, SE Mozambique
83 L20 **Massingir** Gaza, SW Mozambique
195 Z10 **Masson Island** *island* Antarctica
Massoukou *see* Franceville
137 Z11 **Maştağa** *Rus.* Mashtagi, Mastaga. E Azerbaijan
Mastanli *see* Momchilgrad
184 M13 **Masterton** Wellington, North Island, NZ
18 M14 **Mastic** Long Island, New York, NE USA
149 O10 **Mastung** Baluchistān, SW Pakistan
119 J20 **Mastva** *Rus.* Mostva. ≈ SW Belarus
119 G17 **Masty** *Rus.* Mosty. Hrodzyenskaya Voblasts', W Belarus
164 F12 **Masuda** Shimane, Honshū, SW Japan
92 J11 **Masugnsbyn** Norrbotten, N Sweden
Masuku *see* Franceville
83 K17 **Masvingo** *prev.* Fort Victoria, Nyanda, Victoria. Masvingo, SE Zimbabwe
83 K18 **Masvingo** *prev.* Victoria. ◈ *province* SE Zimbabwe
138 H5 **Maşyāf** *Fr.* Misiaf. Ḩamāh, C Syria
Masyû Ko *see* Mashū-ko
110 E9 **Maszewo** Zachodniopomorskie, NW Poland
83 I17 **Matabeleland North** ◈ *province* W Zimbabwe
83 J18 **Matabeleland South** ◈ *province* S Zimbabwe
82 O13 **Mataca** Niassa, N Mozambique
14 G8 **Matachewan** Ontario, S Canada
79 F22 **Matadi** Bas-Congo, W Dem. Rep. Congo (Zaire)
25 O4 **Matador** Texas, SW USA
42 J9 **Matagalpa** Matagalpa, C Nicaragua
42 K9 **Matagalpa** ◈ *department* W Nicaragua
12 I12 **Matagami** Quebec, S Canada
25 U13 **Matagorda** Texas, SW USA
25 U13 **Matagorda Bay** *inlet* Texas, SW USA
25 U14 **Matagorda Island** *island* Texas, SW USA
25 U13 **Matagorda Peninsula** *headland* Texas, SW USA
191 Q8 **Mataiea** Tahiti, W French Polynesia
191 T9 **Mataiva** *atoll* Îles Tuamotu, C French Polynesia
183 O7 **Matakana** New South Wales, SE Australia
184 N7 **Matakana Island** *island* NE NZ
83 C15 **Matala** Huíla, SW Angola
190 G12 **Matala'a Pointe** *headland* Île Uvea, N Wallis and Futuna
155 K25 **Matale** Central Province, C Sri Lanka
190 E12 **Matalesina, Pointe** *headland* Île Alofi, W Wallis and Futuna
76 I10 **Matam** NE Senegal
184 M8 **Matamata** Waikato, North Island, NZ
77 V12 **Matamey** Zinder, S Niger
40 L8 **Matamoros** Coahuila de Zaragoza, NE Mexico
41 P15 **Matamoros** *var.* Izúcar de Matamoros. Puebla, S Mexico
41 Q8 **Matamoros** Tamaulipas, C Mexico
75 S13 **Ma'ţan as Sārah** SE Libya
82 J12 **Matanda** Luapula, N Zambia
81 J24 **Matandu** ≈ S Tanzania
15 V6 **Matane** Quebec, SE Canada
15 V6 **Matane** ≈ Quebec, SE Canada
77 S12 **Matankari** Dosso, SW Niger
39 R11 **Matanuska River** ≈ Alaska, USA
54 G7 **Matanza** Santander, N Colombia
44 D4 **Matanzas** Matanzas, NW Cuba
15 V7 **Matapédia** ≈ Quebec, SE Canada
15 V6 **Matapédia, Lac** ◎ Quebec, SE Canada
190 B17 **Mata Point** *headland* SE Niue
190 D12 **Matapu, Pointe** *headland* Île Futuna, W Wallis and Futuna
62 G12 **Mataquito, Río** ≈ C Chile
155 K26 **Matara** Southern Province, S Sri Lanka
115 D18 **Matarágka** *var.* Mataránga. Dytikí Ellás, C Greece
170 K16 **Mataram** Pulau Lombok, C Indonesia
Mataránga *see* Matarágka
181 Q3 **Mataranka** Northern Territory, N Australia
105 W6 **Mataró** *anc.* Illuro. Cataluña, E Spain
184 O8 **Matata** Bay of Plenty, North Island, NZ
192 K16 **Matātula, Cape** *headland* Tutuila, W American Samoa
185 D24 **Mataura** Southland, South Island, NZ
185 D24 **Mataura** ≈ South Island, NZ
Mata Uta *see* Matā'utu
190 G11 **Matā'utu** *var.* Mata Uta. ○ (Wallis and Futuna) Île Uvea, Wallis and Futuna
192 H16 **Matāutu** Upolu, C Samoa
190 G12 **Matā'utu, Baie de** *bay* Île Uvea, Wallis and Futuna
191 P7 **Matavai, Baie de** *bay* Tahiti, W French Polynesia
190 I16 **Matavera** Rarotonga, S Cook Islands
191 V16 **Mataveri** Easter Island, Chile, E Pacific Ocean
191 V17 **Mataveri** ✈ (Easter Island) Easter Island, Chile, E Pacific Ocean
184 P9 **Matawai** Gisborne, North Island, NZ
15 O10 **Matawin** ≈ Quebec, SE Canada
145 V13 **Matay** Almaty, SE Kazakhstan
14 K8 **Matchi-Manitou, Lac** ◎ Quebec, SE Canada
41 O10 **Matehuala** San Luis Potosí, C Mexico
45 V13 **Matelot** Trinidad, Trinidad and Tobago
83 M15 **Matenge** Tete, NW Mozambique
107 O18 **Matera** Basilicata, S Italy
111 O21 **Mátészalka** Szabolcs-Szatmár-Bereg, E Hungary
93 H17 **Matfors** Västernorrland, C Sweden
102 K11 **Matha** Charente-Maritime, W France
(0) F15 **Mathematicians Seamounts** *undersea feature* E Pacific Ocean
21 X6 **Mathews** Virginia, NE USA
25 S14 **Mathis** Texas, SW USA
152 J11 **Mathura** *prev.* Muttra. Uttar Pradesh, N India
Mathurai *see* Madurai
171 R7 **Mati** Mindanao, S Philippines
Matianus *see* Orūmīyeh, Daryācheh-ye
Matiara *see* Matiāri
149 Q15 **Matiāri** *var.* Matiara. Sind, SE Pakistan
41 S16 **Matías Romero** Oaxaca, SE Mexico
43 O13 **Matina** Limón, E Costa Rica
14 D10 **Matinenda Lake** ◎ Ontario, S Canada
19 R8 **Matinicus Island** *island* Maine, NE USA
Matisco/Matisco Ædourum *see* Mâcon
149 Q16 **Mātli** Sind, SE Pakistan
97 M18 **Matlock** C England, UK
59 F18 **Mato Grosso** *prev.* Vila Bela da Santissima Trindade. Mato Grosso, W Brazil
59 G17 **Mato Grosso** *off.* Estado de Mato Grosso; *prev.* Matto Grosso. ◈ *state* W Brazil
60 H8 **Mato Grosso do Sul** *off.* Estado de Mato Grosso do Sul. ◈ *state* S Brazil
59 I18 **Mato Grosso, Planalto de** *plateau* C Brazil
104 G6 **Matosinhos** *prev.* Matozinhos. Porto, NW Portugal
55 Z10 **Matoury** NE French Guiana
Matozinhos *see* Matosinhos
111 L21 **Mátra** ▲ N Hungary
141 Y8 **Maţraḩ** *var.* Mutrah. NE Oman
116 L12 **Mătrăşeşti** Vrancea, E Romania
108 M8 **Matrei Am Brenner** Tirol, W Austria
109 P8 **Matrei in Osttirol** Tirol, W Austria
76 I15 **Matru** SW Sierra Leone
75 U7 **Maţrūḩ** *var.* Mersa Maţrūḩ; *anc.* Paraetonium. NW Egypt
165 U16 **Matsubara** *var.* Matubara. Kagoshima, Tokuno-shima, SW Japan
164 G12 **Matsue** *var.* Matsuye, Matue. Shimane, Honshū, SW Japan
165 Q6 **Matsumae** Hokkaidō, NE Japan
164 M12 **Matsumoto** *var.* Matumoto. Nagano, Honshū, S Japan
164 K14 **Matsusaka** *var.* Matsuzaka, Matusaka. Mie, Honshū, SW Japan
161 S12 **Matsu Tao** *Chin.* Mazu Dao. *island* NW Taiwan
Matsutō *see* Mattō
164 F14 **Matsuyama** *var.* Matuyama. Ehime, Shikoku, SW Japan
Matsuye *see* Matsue
Matsuzaka *see* Matsusaka
164 M14 **Matsuzaki** Shizuoka, Honshū, S Japan
14 F8 **Mattagami** ≈ Ontario, S Canada
14 F8 **Mattagami Lake** ◎ Ontario, S Canada
62 K12 **Mattaldi** Córdoba, C Argentina
21 Y9 **Mattamuskeet, Lake** ◎ North Carolina, SE USA
21 W6 **Mattaponi River** ≈ Virginia, NE USA
14 I11 **Mattawa** Ontario, SE Canada
14 I11 **Mattawa** ≈ Ontario, SE Canada
19 S5 **Mattawamkeag** Maine, NE USA
19 S4 **Mattawamkeag Lake** ◎ Maine, NE USA

◆ Country ● Country Capital ◇ Dependent Territory ○ Dependent Territory Capital ◈ Administrative Region ✈ International Airport ▲ Mountain ▲ Mountain Range ⛰ Volcano ≈ River ◎ Lake ⊡ Reservoir

108 D11 **Matterhorn** *It.* Monte Cervino. ▲ Italy/Switzerland *see also* Cervino, Monte
35 W1 **Matterhorn** ▲ Nevada, W USA
32 L12 **Matterhorn** *var.* Sacajawea Peak. ▲ Oregon, NW USA
35 R8 **Matterhorn Peak** ▲ California, W USA
109 Y5 **Mattersburg** Burgenland, E Austria
108 E11 **Matter Vispa** ≈ S Switzerland
55 R7 **Matthews Ridge** N Guyana
44 K7 **Matthew Town** Great Inagua, S Bahamas
109 Q4 **Mattighofen** Oberösterreich, NW Austria
107 N16 **Mattinata** Puglia, SE Italy
141 T9 **Maṭṭī, Sabkhat** *salt flat* Saudi Arabia/UAE
18 M14 **Mattituck** Long Island, New York, NE USA
164 L11 **Mattō** *var.* Matsutō. Ishikawa, Honshū, SW Japan
Matto Grosso *see* Mato Grosso
30 M14 **Mattoon** Illinois, N USA
57 L16 **Mattos, Río** ≈ C Bolivia
Mattu *see* Metu
169 R9 **Matu** Sarawak, East Malaysia
57 E14 **Matucana** Lima, W Peru
Matudo *see* Matsudo
Matue *see* Matsue
187 Y15 **Matuku** *island* S Fiji
112 B9 **Matulji** Primorje-Gorski Kotar, NW Croatia
Matumoto *see* Matsumoto
55 P5 **Maturín** Monagas, NE Venezuela
Matusaka *see* Matsusaka
Matuura *see* Matsuura
Matuyama *see* Matsuyama
128 K11 **Matveyev Kurgan** Rostovskaya Oblast', SW Russian Federation
129 O8 **Matyshevo** Volgogradskaya Oblast', SW Russian Federation
153 O13 **Mau** *var.* Maunāth Bhanjan. Uttar Pradesh, N India
83 O14 **Maúa** Niassa, N Mozambique
102 M17 **Maubermé, Pic de** *var.* Tuc de Moubermé, *Sp.* Pico Mauberme; *prev.* Tuc de Mauberme. ▲ France/Spain *see also* Moubermé, Tuc de
Mauberme, Pico *see* Maubermé, Pic de/Moubermé, Tuc de
Mauberme, Tuc de *see* Maubermé, Pic de/Moubermé, Tuc de
103 Q2 **Maubeuge** Nord, N France
166 L8 **Maubin** Irrawaddy, SW Myanmar
152 L13 **Maudaha** Uttar Pradesh, N India
183 N9 **Maude** New South Wales, SE Australia
195 P3 **Maudheimvidda** *physical region* Antarctica
65 N22 **Maud Rise** *undersea feature* S Atlantic Ocean
109 Q4 **Mauerkirchen** Oberösterreich, NW Austria
Mauersee *see* Mamry, Jezioro
188 K2 **Maug Islands** *island group* N Northern Mariana Islands
103 Q15 **Mauguio** Hérault, S France
193 N5 **Maui** *island* Hawaii, USA, C Pacific Ocean
190 M16 **Mauke** *atoll* S Cook Islands
62 G13 **Maule** *off.* Región del Maule. ◐ *region* C Chile
102 J9 **Mauléon** Deux-Sèvres, W France
102 J16 **Mauléon-Licharre** Pyrénées-Atlantiques, SW France
62 G13 **Maule, Río** ≈ C Chile
63 G17 **Maullín** Los Lagos, S Chile
Maulmain *see* Moulmein
31 R11 **Maumee** Ohio, N USA
31 Q12 **Maumee River** ≈ Indiana/Ohio, N USA
27 U11 **Maumelle** Arkansas, C USA
27 T11 **Maumelle, Lake** ▣ Arkansas, C USA
171 O16 **Maumere** *prev.* Maoemere. Flores, S Indonesia
83 G17 **Maun** Ngamiland, C Botswana
Maunāth Bhanjan *see* Mau
Maunawai *see* Waimea
190 H16 **Maungaroa** ▲ Rarotonga, S Cook Islands
184 K3 **Maungatapere** Northland, North Island, NZ
184 K4 **Maungaturoto** Northland, North Island, NZ
191 R10 **Maupiti** *var.* Maurua. *island* Îles Sous le Vent, W French Polynesia
152 K14 **Mau Rānīpur** Uttar Pradesh, N India
22 K9 **Maurepas, Lake** ◎ Louisiana, S USA
103 T16 **Maures** ▲▲ SE France
103 O12 **Mauriac** Cantal, C France
Maurice *see* Mauritius
65 J20 **Maurice Ewing Bank** *undersea feature* SW Atlantic Ocean
182 C4 **Maurice, Lake** *salt lake* South Australia
18 I17 **Maurice River** ≈ New Jersey, NE USA
25 Y10 **Mauriceville** Texas, SW USA
98 K12 **Maurik** Gelderland, C Netherlands
76 H8 **Mauritania** *off.* Islamic Republic of Mauritania, *Ar.* Mūrītānīyah. ◆ *republic* W Africa
173 W15 **Mauritius** *off.* Republic of Mauritius, *Fr.* Maurice. ◆ *republic* W Indian Ocean
130 M17 **Mauritius** *island* W Indian Ocean
173 N9 **Mauritius Trench** *undersea feature* W Indian Ocean
102 H6 **Mauron** Morbihan, NW France
103 N13 **Maurs** Cantal, C France
Maurua *see* Maupiti
Maury Mid-Ocean Channel *see* Maury Seachannel
64 L6 **Maury Seachannel** *var.* Maury Mid-Ocean Channel. *undersea feature* N Atlantic Ocean
30 K8 **Mauston** Wisconsin, N USA
109 R8 **Mauterndorf** Salzburg, NW Austria
109 T4 **Mauthausen** Oberösterreich, N Austria
109 Q9 **Mauthen** Kärnten, S Austria
83 F15 **Mavinga** Cuando Cubango, SE Angola
83 M17 **Mavita** Manica, W Mozambique
115 K22 **Mavrópetra, Akrotírio** *headland* Thíra, Kykládes, Greece, Aegean Sea
115 F16 **Mavrovoúni** ▲ C Greece
184 Q8 **Mawhai Point** *headland* North Island, NZ
166 L3 **Mawlaik** Sagaing, C Myanmar
Mawlamyine *see* Moulmein
141 N14 **Mawr, Wādī** *dry watercourse* NW Yemen
195 X5 **Mawson** *Australian research station* Antarctica
195 X5 **Mawson Coast** *physical region* Antarctica
28 M4 **Max** North Dakota, N USA
41 W12 **Maxcanú** Yucatán, SE Mexico
Maxesibebi *see* Mount Ayliff
109 Q5 **Maxglan** ✕ (Salzburg) Salzburg, W Austria
93 K16 **Maxmo** *Fin.* Maksamaa. Länsi-Suomi, W Finland
21 T11 **Maxton** North Carolina, SE USA
25 R8 **May** Texas, SW USA
186 B6 **May** ≈ NW PNG
123 R10 **Maya** ≈ E Russian Federation
151 Q19 **Māyābandar** Andaman and Nicobar Islands, India, E Indian Ocean
Mayadin *see* Al Mayādīn
44 L5 **Mayaguana** *island* SE Bahamas
44 L5 **Mayaguana Passage** *passage* SE Bahamas
45 S6 **Mayagüez** W Puerto Rico
45 R6 **Mayagüez, Bahía de** *bay* W Puerto Rico
Mayals *see* Maials
79 G20 **Mayama** Le Pool, SE Congo
37 V8 **Maya, Mesa De** ▲ Colorado, C USA
143 R4 **Mayamey** Semnān, N Iran
42 F3 **Maya Mountains** *Sp.* Montañas Mayas. ▲▲ Belize/Guatemala
44 I7 **Mayarí** Holguín, E Cuba
Mayas, Montañas *see* Maya Mountains
18 I17 **May, Cape** *headland* New Jersey, NE USA
80 J11 **Maych'ew** *var.* Mai Chio, *It.* Mai Ceu. Tigray, N Ethiopia
138 I2 **Maydān Ikbiz** Ḥalab, N Syria
149 Q5 **Maydān Shahr** Wardag, E Afghanistan
80 O12 **Maydh** Sanaag, N Somalia
Maydī *see* Mīdī
Mayebashi *see* Maebashi
Mayence *see* Mainz
102 K6 **Mayenne** Mayenne, NW France
102 J6 **Mayenne** ◐ *department* NW France
102 J7 **Mayenne** ≈ N France
36 K12 **Mayer** Arizona, SW USA
22 J4 **Mayersville** Mississippi, S USA
11 P14 **Mayerthorpe** Alberta, SW Canada
21 S12 **Mayesville** South Carolina, SE USA
185 G19 **Mayfield** Canterbury, South Island, NZ
33 N14 **Mayfield** Idaho, NW USA
20 G7 **Mayfield** Kentucky, S USA
36 L5 **Mayfield** Utah, W USA
162 K9 **Mayhan** Övörhangay, C Mongolia
37 T14 **Mayhill** New Mexico, SW USA
145 T9 **Maykain** *Kaz.* Mayqayyng. Pavlodar, NE Kazakhstan
128 L14 **Maykop** Respublika Adygeya, SW Russian Federation
Maylibash *see* Maylybas
Mayli-Say *see* Mayluu-Suu
147 T9 **Mayluu-Suu** *prev.* Mayli-Say, *Kir.* Mayly-Say. Dzhalal-Abadskaya Oblast', W Kyrgyzstan
144 L14 **Maylybas** *prev.* Maylibash. Kyzylorda, S Kazakhstan
Mayly-Say *see* Mayluu-Suu
Maymana *see* Meymaneh
166 M5 **Maymyo** Mandalay, C Myanmar
123 V7 **Mayn** ≈ NE Russian Federation
129 Q5 **Mayna** Ul'yanovskaya Oblast', W Russian Federation
21 N8 **Maynardville** Tennessee, S USA
14 J13 **Maynooth** Ontario, SE Canada
10 I6 **Mayo** Yukon Territory, NW Canada
23 U9 **Mayo** Florida, SE USA
97 B16 **Mayo** *Ir.* Maigh Eo. *cultural region* W Ireland
Mayo *see* Maio
78 G12 **Mayo-Kébbi** *off.* Préfecture du Mayo-Kébbu, *var.* Mayo-Kébi. ◐ *prefecture* SW Chad
Mayo-Kébi *see* Mayo-Kébbi
79 F19 **Mayoko** Le Niari, SW Congo
171 P4 **Mayon Volcano** ※ Luzon, N Philippines
61 A24 **Mayor Buratovich** Buenos Aires, E Argentina
104 L4 **Mayorga** Castilla-León, N Spain
184 N6 **Mayor Island** *island* NE NZ
Mayor Pablo Lagerenza *see* Capitán Pablo Lagerenza
173 I14 **Mayotte** ◇ *French territorial collectivity* E Africa
Mayoumba *see* Mayumba
44 J13 **May Pen** C Jamaica
Mayqayyng *see* Maykain
171 O1 **Mayraira Point** *headland* Luzon, N Philippines
109 N8 **Mayrhofen** Tirol, W Austria
186 A6 **May River** East Sepik, NW PNG
123 R13 **Mayskiy** Amurskaya Oblast', SE Russian Federation
129 O15 **Mayskiy** Kabardino-Balkarskaya Respublika, SW Russian Federation
145 U9 **Mayskoye** Pavlodar, NE Kazakhstan
18 J17 **Mays Landing** New Jersey, NE USA
21 N4 **Maysville** Kentucky, S USA
27 R2 **Maysville** Missouri, C USA
79 D20 **Mayumba** *var.* Mayoumba. Nyanga, S Gabon
31 S8 **Mayville** Michigan, N USA
18 C11 **Mayville** New York, NE USA
29 Q4 **Mayville** North Dakota, N USA
Mayyali *see* Mahe
Mayyit, Al Baḥr al *see* Dead Sea
83 J15 **Mazabuka** Southern, S Zambia
Mazaca *see* Kayseri
Mazagan *see* El-Jadida
32 J7 **Mazama** Washington, NW USA
103 O15 **Mazamet** Tarn, S France
143 O4 **Māzandarān** *off.* Ostān-e Māzandarān. ◐ *province* N Iran
156 F7 **Mazar** Xinjiang Uygur Zizhiqu, NW China
107 H24 **Mazara del Vallo** Sicilia, Italy, C Mediterranean Sea
149 O2 **Mazār-e Sharīf** *var.* Mazār-i Sharif. Balkh, N Afghanistan
Mazār-i Sharif *see* Mazār-e Sharif
105 R13 **Mazarrón** Murcia, SE Spain
105 R14 **Mazarrón, Golfo de** *gulf* SE Spain
55 S9 **Mazaruni River** ≈ N Guyana
42 B6 **Mazatenango** Suchitepéquez, SW Guatemala
40 I10 **Mazatlán** Sinaloa, C Mexico
36 L12 **Mazatzal Mountains** ▲▲ Arizona, SW USA
118 D10 **Mažeikiai** Mažeikiai, NW Lithuania
118 D7 **Mazirbe** Talsi, NW Latvia
40 G5 **Mazocahui** Sonora, NW Mexico
57 I18 **Mazocruz** Puno, S Peru
Mazoe, Rio *see* Mazowe
79 N21 **Mazomeno** Maniema, E Dem. Rep. Congo (Zaire)
159 Q6 **Mazong Shan** ▲ N China
83 L16 **Mazowe** *var.* Rio Mazoe. ≈ Mozambique/Zimbabwe
110 L11 **Mazowieckie** ◐ *province* C Poland
Mazra'a *see* Al Mazra'ah
138 G6 **Mazraat Kfar Debiâne** C Lebanon
118 H7 **Mazsalaca** *Est.* Väike-Salatsi, *Ger.* Salisburg. Valmiera, N Latvia
110 L9 **Mazury** *physical region* NE Poland
119 M20 **Mazyr** *Rus.* Mozyr'. Homyel'skaya Voblasts', SE Belarus
107 K25 **Mazzarino** Sicilia, Italy, C Mediterranean Sea
Mba *see* Ba
83 L21 **Mbabane** ● (Swaziland) NW Swaziland
Mbacké *see* Mbaké
77 N16 **Mbahiakro** E Ivory Coast
79 I16 **Mbaïki** *var.* M'Baiki. Lobaye, SW Central African Republic
79 F14 **Mbakaou, Lac de** ◎ C Cameroon
76 G11 **Mbaké** *var.* Mbacké. W Senegal
82 L11 **Mbala** *prev.* Abercorn. Northern, NE Zambia
83 J18 **Mbalabala** *prev.* Balla Balla. Matabeleland South, SW Zimbabwe
81 G18 **Mbale** E Uganda
79 E16 **Mbalmayo** *var.* M'Balmayo. Centre, S Cameroon
81 H25 **Mbamba Bay** Ruvuma, S Tanzania
79 I18 **Mbandaka** *prev.* Coquilhatville. Equateur, NW Dem. Rep. Congo (Zaire)
82 B9 **M'Banza Congo** *var.* Mbanza Congo; *prev.* São Salvador, São Salvador do Congo. Zaire, NW Angola
79 G21 **Mbanza-Ngungu** Bas-Congo, W Dem. Rep. Congo (Zaire)
67 V11 **Mbarangandu** ≈ E Tanzania
81 E19 **Mbarara** SW Uganda
79 L15 **Mbari** ≈ SE Central African Republic
81 I24 **Mbarika Mountains** ▲▲ S Tanzania
83 J24 **Mbashe** ≈ S South Africa
Mbatiki *see* Batiki
79 F15 **Mbé** Nord, N Cameroon
81 J24 **Mbemkuru** *var.* Mbwemkuru. ≈ S Tanzania
Mbengga *see* Beqa
172 H13 **Mbéni** Grande Comore, NW Comoros
83 K18 **Mberengwa** Midlands, S Zimbabwe
81 G24 **Mbeya** Mbeya, SW Tanzania
81 G23 **Mbeya** ◐ *region* S Tanzania
79 E19 **Mbigou** Ngounié, C Gabon
Mbilua *see* Vella Lavella
79 F19 **Mbinda** Le Niari, SW Congo
79 D17 **Mbini** W Equatorial Guinea
Mbini *see* Uolo, Río
83 L18 **Mbizi** Masvingo, SE Zimbabwe
81 G23 **Mbogo** Mbeya, W Tanzania
79 N15 **Mboki** Haut-Mbomou, SE Central African Republic
79 G18 **Mbomo** Cuvette, NW Congo
79 L15 **Mbomou** ◐ *prefecture* SE Central African Republic
Mbomou/M'Bomu/Mbomu *see* Bomu
76 F11 **Mbour** W Senegal
76 I10 **Mbout** Gorgol, S Mauritania
79 J14 **Mbrès** *var.* Mbrés. Nana-Grébizi, C Central African Republic
79 L22 **Mbuji-Mayi** *prev.* Bakwanga. Kasai Oriental, S Dem. Rep. Congo (Zaire)
81 H21 **Mbulu** Arusha, N Tanzania
186 E5 **M'bunai** *var.* Bunai. Manus Island, N PNG
62 N8 **Mburucuyá** Corrientes, NE Argentina
Mbutha *see* Buca
Mbwemkuru *see* Mbemkuru
81 G21 **Mbwikwe** Singida, C Tanzania
13 O15 **McAdam** New Brunswick, SE Canada
25 O5 **McAdoo** Texas, SW USA
35 V2 **McAfee Peak** ▲ Nevada, W USA
27 P11 **McAlester** Oklahoma, C USA
25 S17 **McAllen** Texas, SW USA
21 S11 **McBee** South Carolina, SE USA
11 N14 **McBride** British Columbia, SW Canada
24 M9 **McCamey** Texas, SW USA
33 R15 **McCammon** Idaho, NW USA
35 X11 **McCarran** ✕ (Las Vegas) Nevada, W USA
39 T11 **McCarthy** Alaska, USA
30 M5 **McCaslin Mountain** *hill* Wisconsin, N USA
25 O2 **McClellan Creek** ≈ Texas, SW USA
21 T14 **McClellanville** South Carolina, SE USA
8 L6 **McClintock Channel** *channel* Nunavut, N Canada
195 R12 **McClintock, Mount** ▲ Antarctica
35 N2 **McCloud** California, W USA
35 N3 **McCloud River** ≈ California, W USA
35 Q9 **McClure, Lake** ▣ California, W USA
197 O8 **McClure Strait** *strait* Northwest Territories, N Canada
29 N4 **McClusky** North Dakota, N USA
21 T11 **McColl** South Carolina, SE USA
22 K7 **McComb** Mississippi, S USA
18 E16 **McConnellsburg** Pennsylvania, NE USA
31 T14 **McConnelsville** Ohio, N USA
28 M17 **McCook** Nebraska, C USA
21 P13 **McCormick** South Carolina, SE USA
11 W16 **McCreary** Manitoba, S Canada
27 W11 **McCrory** Arkansas, C USA
25 T10 **McDade** Texas, SW USA
23 O8 **McDavid** Florida, SE USA
35 T1 **McDermitt** Nevada, W USA
23 S4 **McDonough** Georgia, SE USA
36 L12 **McDowell Mountains** ▲▲ Arizona, SW USA
20 H8 **McEwen** Tennessee, S USA
35 R12 **McFarland** California, W USA
Mcfarlane, Lake *see* Macfarlane, Lake
27 P12 **McGee Creek Lake** ▣ Oklahoma, C USA
27 W13 **McGehee** Arkansas, C USA
35 X5 **McGill** Nevada, W USA
14 K11 **McGillivray, Lac** ◎ Quebec, SE Canada
39 P10 **Mcgrath** Alaska, USA
25 T8 **McGregor** Texas, SW USA
33 O12 **McGuire, Mount** ▲ Idaho, NW USA
83 M14 **Mchinji** *prev.* Fort Manning. Central, W Malawi
28 M7 **McIntosh** South Dakota, N USA
9 S7 **McKeand** ≈ Baffin Island, Nunavut, NE Canada
191 R4 **McKean Island** *island* Phoenix Islands, C Kiribati
30 J13 **McKee Creek** ≈ Illinois, N USA
18 C15 **Mckeesport** Pennsylvania, NE USA
21 V7 **McKenney** Virginia, NE USA
20 G8 **McKenzie** Tennessee, S USA
185 B20 **McKerrow, Lake** ◎ South Island, NZ
39 Q10 **McKinley, Mount** *var.* Denali. ▲ Alaska, USA
39 R10 **McKinley Park** Alaska, USA
34 K3 **McKinleyville** California, W USA
25 U6 **McKinney** Texas, SW USA
26 I5 **McKinney, Lake** ◎ Kansas, C USA
28 M7 **McLaughlin** South Dakota, N USA
25 O2 **McLean** Texas, SW USA
30 M16 **Mcleansboro** Illinois, N USA
11 O13 **McLennan** Alberta, W Canada
14 L9 **McLennan, Lac** ◎ Quebec, SE Canada
10 M13 **McLeod Lake** British Columbia, W Canada
27 N10 **McLoud** Oklahoma, C USA
32 G15 **McLoughlin, Mount** ▲ Oregon, NW USA
8 J4 **M'Clure Strait** *strait* NW Canada
37 U15 **McMillan, Lake** ▣ New Mexico, SW USA
32 G11 **McMinnville** Oregon, NW USA
20 K9 **McMinnville** Tennessee, S USA
195 R13 **McMurdo** *US research station* Antarctica
24 H9 **McNary** Texas, SW USA
37 N13 **Mcnary** Arizona, SW USA
27 N5 **McPherson** Kansas, C USA
McPherson *see* Fort McPherson
23 U6 **McRae** Georgia, SE USA
29 P4 **McVille** North Dakota, N USA
83 J25 **Mdantsane** Eastern Cape, SE South Africa
167 T6 **Me** Ninh Binh, N Vietnam
26 J7 **Meade** Kansas, C USA
39 O5 **Meade River** ≈ Alaska, USA
35 Y11 **Mead, Lake** ▣ Arizona/Nevada, W USA
24 M5 **Meadow** Texas, SW USA
11 S14 **Meadow Lake** Saskatchewan, C Canada
35 Y10 **Meadow Valley Wash** ≈ Nevada, W USA
22 J7 **Meadville** Mississippi, S USA
18 B12 **Meadville** Pennsylvania, NE USA
14 F14 **Meaford** Ontario, S Canada
Meáin, Inis *see* Inishmaan
104 G8 **Mealhada** Aveiro, N Portugal
13 R8 **Mealy Mountains** ▲▲ Newfoundland, E Canada
11 O10 **Meander River** Alberta, W Canada
32 E11 **Meares, Cape** *headland* Oregon, NW USA
47 V6 **Mearim, Rio** ≈ NE Brazil
Measca, Loch *see* Mask, Lough
97 F17 **Meath** *Ir.* An Mhí. *cultural region* E Ireland
11 T14 **Meath Park** Saskatchewan, S Canada
103 O5 **Meaux** Seine-et-Marne, N France
21 T9 **Mebane** North Carolina, SE USA
171 U12 **Mebo, Gunung** ▲ Irian Jaya, E Indonesia
94 I8 **Mebonden** Sør-Trøndelag, S Norway
82 A10 **Mebridege** ≈ NW Angola
35 W16 **Mecca** California, W USA
Mecca *see* Makkah
29 Y14 **Mechanicsville** Iowa, C USA
18 L10 **Mechanicville** New York, NE USA
99 H17 **Mechelen** *Eng.* Mechlin, *Fr.* Malines. Antwerpen, C Belgium
188 C8 **Mecherchar** *var.* Eil Malk. *island* Palau Islands, Palau
101 D17 **Mechernich** Nordrhein-Westfalen, W Germany
128 L12 **Mechetinskaya** Rostovskaya Oblast', SW Russian Federation
114 J11 **Mechka** ≈ S Bulgaria
Mechlin *see* Mechelen
61 D23 **Mechongué** Buenos Aires, E Argentina
115 L14 **Mecidiye** Edirne, NW Turkey
101 I24 **Meckenbeuren** Baden-Württemberg, S Germany
100 L8 **Mecklenburger Bucht** *bay* N Germany
100 M10 **Mecklenburgische Seenplatte** *wetland* NE Germany
100 L9 **Mecklenburg-Vorpommern** ◐ *state* NE Germany
83 Q15 **Meconta** Nampula, NE Mozambique
111 I25 **Mecsek** ▲▲ SW Hungary
83 P14 **Mecubúri** ≈ N Mozambique
83 Q14 **Mecúfi** Cabo Delgado, NE Mozambique
82 O13 **Mecula** Niassa, N Mozambique
168 I8 **Medan** Sumatera, E Indonesia
61 A24 **Médanos** *var.* Medanos. Buenos Aires, E Argentina
61 C19 **Médanos** Entre Ríos, E Argentina
155 K24 **Medawachchiya** North Central Province, N Sri Lanka
106 C8 **Mede** Lombardia, N Italy
74 J5 **Médéa** *var.* El Mediyya, Lemdiyya. N Algeria
Medeba *see* Ma'dabā
54 E8 **Medellín** Antioquia, NW Colombia
100 H9 **Medem** ≈ NW Germany
98 J8 **Medemblik** Noord-Holland, NW Netherlands
75 N7 **Médenine** *var.* Madanīyīn. SE Tunisia
76 G9 **Mederdra** Trarza, SW Mauritania
Medeshamstede *see* Peterborough
42 F4 **Medesto Mendez** Izabal, NE Guatemala
19 O11 **Medford** Massachusetts, NE USA
27 N8 **Medford** Oklahoma, C USA
32 G15 **Medford** Oregon, NW USA
30 K6 **Medford** Wisconsin, N USA
39 P10 **Medfra** Alaska, USA
116 M14 **Medgidia** Constanța, SE Romania
Medgyes *see* Mediaş
43 O5 **Media Luna, Arrecifes de la** *reef* E Honduras
60 G11 **Medianeira** Paraná, S Brazil
29 Y15 **Mediapolis** Iowa, C USA
116 I11 **Mediaş** *Ger.* Mediasch, *Hung.* Medgyes. Sibiu, C Romania
41 S15 **Medias Aguas** Veracruz-Llave, SE Mexico
Mediasch *see* Mediaş
106 G10 **Medicina** Emilia-Romagna, C Italy
33 X16 **Medicine Bow** Wyoming, C USA
37 S2 **Medicine Bow Mountains** ▲▲ Colorado/Wyoming, C USA
33 X16 **Medicine Bow River** ≈ Wyoming, C USA
11 R17 **Medicine Hat** Alberta, SW Canada
26 L7 **Medicine Lodge** Kansas, C USA
26 L7 **Medicine Lodge River** ≈ Kansas/Oklahoma, C USA
112 E7 **Međimurje** *off.* Međimurska Županija. ◐ *province* N Croatia
Međimurska Županija *see* Međimurje
54 G10 **Medina** Cundinamarca, C Colombia
18 E9 **Medina** New York, NE USA
29 O5 **Medina** North Dakota, N USA
31 T11 **Medina** Ohio, N USA
25 Q11 **Medina** Texas, SW USA
Medina *see* Al Madīnah
105 P6 **Medinaceli** Castilla-León, N Spain
104 L6 **Medina del Campo** Castilla-León, N Spain
104 L5 **Medina de Ríoseco** Castilla-León, N Spain
Médina Gonassé *see* Médina Gounas
76 H12 **Médina Gounas** *var.* Médina Gonassé. S Senegal
25 S12 **Medina River** ≈ Texas, SW USA
104 K16 **Medina Sidonia** Andalucía, S Spain
Medinat Israel *see* Israel
119 H14 **Medininkai** Vilnius, SE Lithuania
153 R16 **Medinīpur** West Bengal, NE India
Mediolanum *see* Saintes, France
Mediolanum *see* Milano, Italy
Mediomatrica *see* Metz
121 Q11 **Mediterranean Ridge** *undersea feature* C Mediterranean Sea
121 O16 **Mediterranean Sea** *Fr.* Mer Méditerranée. *sea* Africa/Asia/Europe
Méditerranée, Mer *see* Mediterranean Sea
79 N17 **Medje** Orientale, NE Dem. Rep. Congo (Zaire)
114 G7 **Medkovets** Montana, NW Bulgaria
93 J15 **Medle** Västerbotten, N Sweden
129 W7 **Mednogorsk** Orenburgskaya Oblast', W Russian Federation
123 W9 **Mednyy, Ostrov** *island* E Russian Federation
102 J12 **Médoc** *cultural region* SW France
159 Q16 **Mêdog** Xizang Zizhiqu, W China
28 J5 **Medora** North Dakota, N USA
79 E17 **Médouneu** Woleu-Ntem, N Gabon
106 I7 **Meduna** ≈ NE Italy
Medunta *see* Mantes-la-Jolie
Medvedica *see* Medveditsa
126 J16 **Medveditsa** *var.* Medvedica. ≈ W Russian Federation
129 O9 **Medveditsa** ≈ SW Russian Federation
112 E8 **Medvednica** ▲▲ NE Croatia
127 R15 **Medvedok** Kirovskaya Oblast', NW Russian Federation
123 S6 **Medvezh'i, Ostrova** *island group* NE Russian Federation
126 J9 **Medvezh'yegorsk** Respublika Kareliya, NW Russian Federation
109 T11 **Medvode** *Ger.* Zwischenwässern. NW Slovenia
128 J4 **Medyn'** Kaluzhskaya Oblast', W Russian Federation
180 J10 **Meekatharra** Western Australia
37 Q4 **Meeker** Colorado, C USA
13 T12 **Meelpaeg Lake** ◎ Newfoundland, E Canada
Meenen *see* Menen
101 M16 **Meerane** Sachsen, E Germany
101 D15 **Meerbusch** Nordrhein-Westfalen, W Germany
98 I12 **Meerkerk** Zuid-Holland, C Netherlands
99 L18 **Meerssen** *var.* Mersen. Limburg, SE Netherlands
152 J10 **Meerut** Uttar Pradesh, N India
33 U13 **Meeteetse** Wyoming, C USA
99 K17 **Meeuwen** Limburg, NE Belgium
81 J16 **Mēga** Oromo, C Ethiopia
81 J16 **Mēga Escarpment** *escarpment* S Ethiopia
Megála Kalívia *see* Megála Kalývia
115 E16 **Megála Kalývia** *var.* Megála Kalívia. Thessalía, C Greece
115 H14 **Megáli Panagiá** *var.* Megáli Panayía. Kentrikí Makedonía, N Greece
Megáli Panayía *see* Megáli Panagiá
Megáli Préspa, Límni *see* Prespa, Lake
114 K12 **Megálo Livádi** ▲ Bulgaria/Greece
115 E20 **Megalópoli** *prev.* Megalópolis. Pelopónnisos, S Greece
Megalópolis *see* Megalópoli
171 U12 **Megamo** Irian Jaya, E Indonesia
115 C18 **Meganísi** *island* Iónioi Nísoi, Greece, C Mediterranean Sea
Meganom, Mys *see* Mehanom, Mys
Mégantic *see* Lac-Mégantic
15 R12 **Mégantic, Mont** ▲ Quebec, SE Canada
115 G19 **Mégara** Attikí, C Greece
25 R5 **Megargel** Texas, SW USA
98 K13 **Megen** Noord-Brabant, S Netherlands
153 U13 **Meghālaya** ◐ *state* NE India
153 U16 **Meghna** ≈ S Bangladesh
137 V14 **Meghri** *Rus.* Megri. SE Armenia
115 Q23 **Megísti** *var.* Kastellórizon. *island* SE Greece
Megri *see* Meghri
Mehabad *see* Mahābād
116 F13 **Mehadia** *Hung.* Mehádia. Caraş-Severin, SW Romania
92 L7 **Mehamn** Finnmark, N Norway
117 U13 **Mehanom, Mys** *Rus.* Mys Meganom. *headland* S Ukraine
149 P14 **Mehar** Sind, SE Pakistan
180 J8 **Meharry, Mount** ▲ Western Australia
Mehdia *see* Mahdia
116 G14 **Mehedinți** ◐ *county* SW Romania
153 S15 **Meherpur** Khulna, W Bangladesh
21 W8 **Meherrin River** ≈ North Carolina/Virginia, SE USA
Meheso *see* Mī'ēso
191 T11 **Mehetia** *island* Îles du Vent, W French Polynesia
118 K6 **Mehikoorma** Tartumaa, E Estonia
Me Hka *see* Nmai Hka
143 N5 **Mehrabad** ✕ (Tehrān) Tehrān, N Iran
142 J7 **Mehrān** Īlām, W Iran
143 Q14 **Mehrān, Rūd-e** *prev.* Mansurabad. ≈ W Iran
143 Q9 **Mehrīz** Yazd, C Iran
149 R5 **Mehtarlām** *var.* Mehtar Lām, Meterlam, Methariam, Metharlam. Laghmān, E Afghanistan
103 N8 **Mehun-sur-Yèvre** Cher, C France
79 G14 **Meiganga** Adamaoua, NE Cameroon
160 H10 **Meigu** Sichuan, C China
163 W11 **Meihekou** *var.* Hailong. Jilin, NE China
99 L15 **Meijel** Limburg, SE Netherlands

◆ Country ● Country Capital ◇ Dependent Territory ○ Dependent Territory Capital ◐ Administrative Region ✕ International Airport ▲ Mountain ▲▲ Mountain Range ※ Volcano ≈ River ◎ Lake ▣ Reservoir

166 M5 **Meiktila** Mandalay, C Myanmar
Meilbhe, Loch see Melvin, Lough
108 G7 **Meilen** Zürich, N Switzerland
Meilu see Wuchuan
161 T12 **Meinhua Yu** island N Taiwan
101 J17 **Meiningen** Thüringen, C Germany
108 F9 **Meiringen** Bern, S Switzerland
101 O15 **Meissen** var. Meißen. Sachsen, E Germany
101 I15 **Meissner** ▲ C Germany
99 K25 **Meix-devant-Virton** Luxembourg, SE Belgium
Mei Xian see Meizhou
161 P13 **Meizhou** var. Meixian, Mei Xian. Guangdong, S China
67 P2 **Mejerda** var. Oued Medjerda, Wādī Majardah. ≈ Algeria/Tunisia see also Medjerda, Oued
42 F7 **Mejicanos** San Salvador, C El Salvador
Méjico see Mexico
62 G5 **Mejillones** Antofagasta, N Chile
189 V5 **Mejit Island** var. Mājeej. island Ratak Chain, NE Marshall Islands
79 F17 **Mékambo** Ogooué-Ivindo, NE Gabon
80 J10 **Mek'elē** var. Makale. Tigray, N Ethiopia
74 I10 **Mekerrhane, Sebkha** var. Sebkha Meqerghane, Sebkra Mekerrhane. salt flat C Algeria
Mekerrhane, Sebkra see Mekerrhane, Sebkha
76 G10 **Mékhé** NW Senegal
146 G14 **Mekhinli** Akhalskiy Velayat, C Turkmenistan
15 P9 **Mékinac, Lac** ◎ Quebec, SE Canada
Meklong see Samut Songhram
74 G6 **Meknès** N Morocco
131 U12 **Mekong** var. Lan-ts'ang Chiang, Cam. Mékôngk, Chin. Lancang Jiang, Lao. Mènam Khong, Th. Mae Nam Khong, Tib. Dza Chu, Vtn. Sông Tiên Giang. ≈ SE Asia
Mékôngk see Mekong
167 T15 **Mekong, Mouths of the** delta S Vietnam
38 L12 **Mekoryuk** Nunivak Island, Alaska, USA
77 R14 **Mékrou** ≈ N Benin
168 K9 **Melaka** var. Malacca. Melaka, Peninsular Malaysia
168 L9 **Melaka** var. Malacca. ◆ state Peninsular Malaysia
Melaka, Selat see Malacca, Strait of
175 O6 **Melanesia** island group W Pacific Ocean
175 P5 **Melanesian Basin** undersea feature W Pacific Ocean
171 R9 **Melanguane** Pulau Karakelang, N Indonesia
169 R11 **Melawi, Sungai** ≈ Borneo, N Indonesia
183 N12 **Melbourne** state capital Victoria, SE Australia
27 V9 **Melbourne** Arkansas, C USA
23 Y12 **Melbourne** Florida, SE USA
29 W14 **Melbourne** Iowa, C USA
92 G10 **Melbu** Nordland, C Norway
Melchor de Mencos see Ciudad Melchor de Mencos
63 F19 **Melchor, Isla** island Archipiélago de los Chonos, S Chile
40 M9 **Melchor Ocampo** Zacatecas, C Mexico
14 C11 **Meldrum Bay** Manitoulin Island, Ontario, S Canada
Meleda see Mljet
106 D8 **Melegnano** prev. Marignano. Lombardia, N Italy
188 F9 **Melekeok** var. Melekeiok. Babeldaob, N Palau
112 L9 **Melenci** Hung. Melencze. Serbia, N Yugoslavia
Melencze see Melenci
129 N4 **Melenki** Vladimirskaya Oblast', W Russian Federation
129 V6 **Meleuz** Respublika Bashkortostan, W Russian Federation
12 L6 **Mélèzes, Rivière aux** ≈ Quebec, C Canada
78 I11 **Melfi** Guéra, S Chad
107 M17 **Melfi** Basilicata, S Italy
11 U14 **Melfort** Saskatchewan, S Canada
104 H4 **Melgaço** Viana do Castelo, N Portugal
105 N4 **Melgar de Fernamental** Castilla-León, N Spain
74 L6 **Melghir, Chott** var. Chott Melrhir. salt lake E Algeria
94 H8 **Melhus** Sør-Trøndelag, S Norway
104 H3 **Melide** Galicia, NW Spain
Meligalá see Meligalás
115 E21 **Meligalás** prev. Meligalá. Pelopónnisos, S Greece
60 L12 **Mel, Ilha do** island S Brazil
120 E10 **Melilla** anc. Rusaddir, Russadir. Melilla, Spain, N Africa
71 N1 **Melilla** enclave Spain, N Africa
63 G18 **Melimoyu, Monte** ▲ S Chile
169 V11 **Melintang, Danau** ◎ Borneo, N Indonesia
117 U7 **Melioratyvne** Dnipropetrovs'ka Oblast', E Ukraine
62 G11 **Melipilla** Santiago, C Chile
115 I25 **Mélissa, Akrotírio** headland Kríti, Greece, E Mediterranean Sea
9 N15 **Melita** Manitoba, S Canada
Melita see Mljet
Melitene see Malatya
107 M23 **Melito di Porto Salvo** Calabria, SW Italy
117 U10 **Melitopol'** Zaporiz'ka Oblast', SE Ukraine
109 V4 **Melk** Niederösterreich, NE Austria
95 K15 **Mellan-Fryken** ◎ C Sweden
99 E17 **Melle** Oost-Vlaanderen, NW Belgium
100 G13 **Melle** Niedersachsen, NW Germany
95 J17 **Mellerud** Västra Götaland, S Sweden
102 K10 **Melle-sur-Bretonne** Deux-Sèvres, W France
29 P8 **Mellette** South Dakota, N USA
121 O15 **Mellieha** E Malta
80 B10 **Mellit** Northern Darfur, W Sudan
75 N7 **Mellita** × SE Tunisia
63 G21 **Mellizo Sur, Cerro** ▲ S Chile
100 G9 **Mellum** island NW Germany
83 L22 **Melmoth** KwaZulu/Natal, E South Africa
111 D16 **Mělník** Ger. Melnik. Středočeský Kraj, NW Czech Republic
122 J12 **Mel'nikovo** Tomskaya Oblast', C Russian Federation
61 G18 **Melo** Cerro Largo, NE Uruguay
Melodunum see Melun
Melrhir, Chott see Melghir, Chott
183 P7 **Melrose** New South Wales, SE Australia
182 I7 **Melrose** South Australia
29 T7 **Melrose** Minnesota, N USA
33 Q11 **Melrose** Montana, NW USA
37 V12 **Melrose** New Mexico, SW USA
108 I8 **Mels** Sankt Gallen, NE Switzerland
Melsetter see Chimanimani
33 V9 **Melstone** Montana, NW USA
101 I16 **Melsungen** Hessen, C Germany
92 L12 **Meltaus** Lappi, NW Finland
97 N19 **Melton Mowbray** C England, UK
82 Q13 **Meluco** Cabo Delgado, NE Mozambique
103 O5 **Melun** anc. Melodunum. Seine-et-Marne, N France
80 F12 **Melut** Upper Nile, SE Sudan
27 P5 **Melvern Lake** ⊡ Kansas, C USA
11 V16 **Melville** Saskatchewan, S Canada
Melville Bay/Melville Bugt see Qimusseriarsuaq
45 O11 **Melville Hall** × (Dominica) NE Dominica
181 O1 **Melville Island** island Northern Territory, N Australia
8 K5 **Melville Island** island Parry Islands, Northwest Territories, NW Canada
9 W9 **Melville, Lake** ◎ Newfoundland, E Canada
9 O7 **Melville Peninsula** peninsula Nunavut, NE Canada
Melville Sound see Viscount Melville Sound
25 Q9 **Melvin** Texas, SW USA
97 D15 **Melvin, Lough** Ir. Loch Meilbhe. ◎ S Northern Ireland, UK/Ireland
169 S12 **Memala** Borneo, C Indonesia
113 L22 **Memaliaj** Gjirokastër, S Albania
83 Q14 **Memba** Nampula, NE Mozambique
83 Q14 **Memba, Baia de** inlet NE Mozambique
Membidj see Manbij
Memel see Neman, NE Europe
Memel see Klaipėda, Lithuania
101 J23 **Memmingen** Bayern, S Germany
27 U1 **Memphis** Missouri, C USA
20 E10 **Memphis** Tennessee, S USA
25 P3 **Memphis** Texas, SW USA
20 E10 **Memphis** × Tennessee, S USA
15 Q13 **Memphrémagog, Lac** var. Lake Memphremagog. ◎ Canada/USA see also Memphremagog, Lake
19 N6 **Memphremagog, Lake** var. Lac Memphrémagog. ◎ Canada/USA see also Memphrémagog, Lac
117 Q2 **Mena** Chernihivs'ka Oblast', NE Ukraine
27 S12 **Mena** Arkansas, C USA
Menaam see Menaldum
Menado see Manado
106 D6 **Menaggio** Lombardia, N Italy
29 T6 **Menahga** Minnesota, N USA
77 R10 **Ménaka** Goa, E Mali
98 K5 **Menaldum** Fris. Menaam. Friesland, N Netherlands
Mènam Khong see Mekong
74 E7 **Menara** × (Marrakech) C Morocco
25 Q9 **Menard** Texas, SW USA
193 Q12 **Menard Fracture Zone** tectonic feature E Pacific Ocean
30 M7 **Menasha** Wisconsin, N USA
Mencezi Garagum see Tsentral'nyye Nizmennyye Garagumy
193 U9 **Mendaña Fracture Zone** tectonic feature E Pacific Ocean
169 S13 **Mendawai, Sungai** ≈ Borneo, C Indonesia
103 P13 **Mende** anc. Mimatum. Lozère, S France
81 J14 **Mendebo** ▲ C Ethiopia
80 J9 **Mendefera** prev. Adi Ugri. S Eritrea
197 S7 **Mendeleyev Ridge** undersea feature Arctic Ocean
129 T3 **Mendeleyevsk** Respublika Tatarstan, W Russian Federation
101 F15 **Menden** Nordrhein-Westfalen, W Germany
22 L6 **Mendenhall** Mississippi, S USA
38 L13 **Mendenhall, Cape** headland Nunivak Island, Alaska, USA
41 P9 **Méndez** var. Villa de Méndez. Tamaulipas, C Mexico
80 H13 **Mendī** Oromo, C Ethiopia
186 C7 **Mendi** Southern Highlands, W PNG
97 K22 **Mendip Hills** var. Mendips. hill range S England, UK
Mendips see Mendip Hills
34 L6 **Mendocino** California, W USA
34 J3 **Mendocino, Cape** headland California, W USA
(0) B8 **Mendocino Fracture Zone** tectonic feature NE Pacific Ocean
35 P10 **Mendota** California, W USA
30 L11 **Mendota** Illinois, N USA
30 K8 **Mendota, Lake** ◎ Wisconsin, N USA
62 I11 **Mendoza** Mendoza, W Argentina
62 I12 **Mendoza** off. Provincia de Mendoza. ◆ province W Argentina
108 H12 **Mendrisio** Ticino, S Switzerland
168 L10 **Mendung** Pulau Mendol, W Indonesia
54 I5 **Mene de Mauroa** Falcón, NW Venezuela
54 I5 **Mene Grande** Zulia, NW Venezuela
136 B14 **Menemen** İzmir, W Turkey
99 C18 **Menen** var. Meenen, Fr. Menin. West-Vlaanderen, W Belgium
163 Q8 **Menengiyn Tal** plain E Mongolia
189 R9 **Meneng Point** headland SW Nauru
92 L10 **Menesjärvi** Lapp. Menešjávri. Lappi, N Finland
Menešjávri see Menesjärvi
107 I24 **Menfi** Sicilia, Italy, C Mediterranean Sea
161 P7 **Mengcheng** Anhui, E China
160 F15 **Menghai** Yunnan, SW China
160 F15 **Mengla** Yunnan, SW China
65 F24 **Menguera Point** headland East Falkland, Falkland Islands
160 M13 **Mengzhu Ling** ▲ S China
160 H14 **Mengzi** Yunnan, SW China
Menin see Menen
182 L7 **Menindee** New South Wales, SE Australia
182 L7 **Menindee Lake** ◎ New South Wales, SE Australia
182 J10 **Meningie** South Australia
103 O5 **Mennecy** Essonne, N France
29 Q12 **Menno** South Dakota, N USA
114 H13 **Menoïkio** ▲ NE Greece
31 N5 **Menominee** Michigan, N USA
30 M5 **Menominee River** ≈ Michigan/Wisconsin, N USA
30 M8 **Menomonee Falls** Wisconsin, N USA
30 I6 **Menomonie** Wisconsin, N USA
83 D14 **Menongue** var. Vila Serpa Pinto, Port. Serpa Pinto. Cuando Cubango, C Angola
120 H8 **Menorca** Eng. Minorca; anc. Balearis Minor. island Islas Baleares, Spain, W Mediterranean Sea
105 S13 **Menor, Mar** lagoon SE Spain
39 S10 **Mentasta Lake** ◎ Alaska, USA
39 S10 **Mentasta Mountains** ▲ Alaska, USA
168 I13 **Mentawai, Kepulauan** island group W Indonesia
168 I12 **Mentawai, Selat** strait W Indonesia
168 M12 **Mentok** Pulau Bangka, W Indonesia
103 V15 **Menton** It. Mentone. Alpes-Maritimes, SE France
24 K8 **Mentone** Texas, SW USA
Mentone see Menton
31 U11 **Mentor** Ohio, N USA
169 U10 **Menyapa, Gunung** ▲ Borneo, N Indonesia
159 T9 **Menyuan** var. Menyuan Huizu Zizhixian. Qinghai, C China
Menyuan Huizu Zizhixian see Menyuan
74 M5 **Menzel Bourguiba** var. Manzil Bū Ruqaybah; prev. Ferryville. N Tunisia
136 M15 **Menzelet Barajı** ⊡ C Turkey
129 T4 **Menzelinsk** Respublika Tatarstan, W Russian Federation
180 K11 **Menzies** Western Australia
195 V6 **Menzies, Mount** ▲ Antarctica
40 J6 **Meoqui** Chihuahua, N Mexico
83 N14 **Meponda** Niassa, NE Mozambique
98 M8 **Meppel** Drenthe, NE Netherlands
100 E12 **Meppen** Niedersachsen, NW Germany
Meqerghane, Sebkha see Mekerrhane, Sebkha
105 T6 **Mequinenza, Embalse de** ⊡ NE Spain
30 M8 **Mequon** Wisconsin, N USA
Mera see Maira
182 D3 **Meramangye, Lake** salt lake South Australia
27 W5 **Meramec River** ≈ Missouri, C USA
Meran see Merano
168 K13 **Merangin** ≈ Sumatera, W Indonesia
106 G5 **Merano** Ger. Meran. Trentino-Alto Adige, N Italy
168 K8 **Merapuh Lama** Pahang, Peninsular Malaysia
106 D7 **Merate** Lombardia, N Italy
169 U13 **Meratus, Pegunungan** ▲ Borneo, N Indonesia
171 Y16 **Merauke, Sungai** ≈ Irian Jaya, E Indonesia
182 L9 **Merbein** Victoria, SE Australia
99 F21 **Merbes-le-Château** Hainaut, S Belgium
Merca see Marka
54 C13 **Mercaderes** Cauca, SW Colombia
Mercara see Madikeri
35 P9 **Merced** California, W USA
61 C20 **Mercedes** Buenos Aires, E Argentina
61 D15 **Mercedes** Corrientes, NE Argentina
62 J11 **Mercedes** prev. Villa Mercedes. San Luis, C Argentina
61 D19 **Mercedes** Soriano, SW Uruguay
25 S17 **Mercedes** Texas, SW USA
35 R9 **Merced Peak** ▲ California, W USA
35 P9 **Merced River** ≈ California, W USA
18 B13 **Mercer** Pennsylvania, NE USA
99 G18 **Merchtem** Vlaams Brabant, C Belgium
15 O13 **Mercier** Quebec, SE Canada
25 Q9 **Mercury** Texas, SW USA
184 M5 **Mercury Islands** island group N NZ
19 O9 **Meredith** New Hampshire, NE USA
65 B25 **Meredith, Cape** var. Cabo Belgrano headland West Falkland, Falkland Islands
37 V6 **Meredith, Lake** ◎ Colorado, C USA
25 N2 **Meredith, Lake** ⊡ Texas, SW USA
81 O16 **Mereeg** var. Mareeq, It. Meregh. Galguduud, E Somalia
117 V5 **Merefa** Kharkivs'ka Oblast', E Ukraine
Meregh see Mereeg
99 E17 **Merelbeke** Oost-Vlaanderen, NW Belgium
Merend see Marand
167 T12 **Mereuch** Môndól Kiri, E Cambodia
Mergate see Margate
144 F9 **Mergenevo** Zapadnyy Kazakhstan, NW Kazakhstan
167 N12 **Mergui** Tenasserim, S Myanmar
166 M12 **Mergui Archipelago** island group S Myanmar
114 L12 **Meriç** Edirne, NW Turkey
114 L12 **Meriç** Bul. Maritsa, Gk. Évros; anc. Hebrus. ≈ SE Europe see also Évros/Maritsa
41 X12 **Mérida** Yucatán, SW Mexico
104 J11 **Mérida** anc. Augusta Emerita. Extremadura, W Spain
54 I6 **Mérida** Mérida, W Venezuela
54 H7 **Mérida** off. Estado Mérida. ◆ state W Venezuela
18 M13 **Meriden** Connecticut, NE USA
22 M5 **Meridian** Mississippi, S USA
25 S8 **Meridian** Texas, SW USA
102 J13 **Mérignac** Gironde, SW France
102 J13 **Mérignac** × (Bordeaux) Gironde, SW France
93 J18 **Merikarvia** Länsi-Suomi, W Finland
183 R12 **Merimbula** New South Wales, SE Australia
182 L9 **Meringur** Victoria, SE Australia
Merín, Laguna see Mirim Lagoon
97 I19 **Merioneth** cultural region W Wales, UK
188 A11 **Merir** island Palau Islands, N Palau
188 B17 **Merizo** SW Guam
Merjama see Märjamaa
145 S16 **Merke** Zhambyl, S Kazakhstan
25 P7 **Merkel** Texas, SW USA
119 F15 **Merkinė** Varėna, S Lithuania
99 G16 **Merksem** Antwerpen, N Belgium
99 I15 **Merksplas** Antwerpen, N Belgium
Merkulovichi see Myerkulavichy
119 G15 **Merkys** ≈ S Lithuania
32 F15 **Merlin** Oregon, NW USA
61 C20 **Merlo** Buenos Aires, E Argentina
138 G8 **Meron, Haré** ▲ N Israel
74 K6 **Merouane, Chott** salt lake NE Algeria
80 F7 **Merowe** Northern, N Sudan
180 J12 **Merredin** Western Australia
97 I14 **Merrick** ▲ S Scotland, UK
32 H16 **Merrill** Oregon, NW USA
30 L5 **Merrill** Wisconsin, N USA
31 N11 **Merrillville** Indiana, N USA
19 O10 **Merrimack River** ≈ Massachusetts/New Hampshire, NE USA
28 L12 **Merriman** Nebraska, C USA
11 N17 **Merritt** British Columbia, SW Canada
23 Y12 **Merritt Island** Florida, SE USA
23 Y11 **Merritt Island** island Florida, SE USA
28 M12 **Merritt Reservoir** ⊡ Nebraska, C USA
183 S7 **Merriwa** New South Wales, SE Australia
183 O8 **Merriwagga** New South Wales, SE Australia
22 G8 **Merryville** Louisiana, S USA
80 K9 **Mersa Fatma** E Eritrea
102 M7 **Mer St-Aubin** Loir-et-Cher, C France
Mersa Maṭrûḥ see Maṭrûḥ
99 M24 **Mersch** Luxembourg, C Luxembourg
101 M15 **Merseburg** Sachsen-Anhalt, C Germany
Mersen see Meerssen
97 K18 **Mersey** ≈ NW England, UK
136 J17 **Mersin** İçel, S Turkey
168 L9 **Mersing** Johor, Peninsular Malaysia
118 E8 **Mērsrags** Talsi, NW Latvia
152 G12 **Merta** var. Merta City. Rājasthān, N India
Merta City see Merta
152 F12 **Merta Road** Rājasthān, N India
97 J21 **Merthyr Tydfil** S Wales, UK
104 H13 **Mértola** Beja, S Portugal
195 V16 **Mertz Glacier** glacier Antarctica
99 M24 **Mertzig** Diekirch, C Luxembourg
25 O9 **Mertzon** Texas, SW USA
81 I18 **Meru** Eastern, C Kenya
103 N4 **Méru** Oise, N France
81 I20 **Meru, Mount** ▲ NE Tanzania
Merv see Mary
Mervdasht see Marv Dasht
136 K11 **Merzifon** Amasya, N Turkey
101 D20 **Merzig** Saarland, SW Germany
36 L14 **Mesa** Arizona, SW USA
29 V4 **Mesabi Range** ▲ Minnesota, N USA
54 H6 **Mesa Bolívar** Mérida, NW Venezuela
107 Q18 **Mesagne** Puglia, SE Italy
39 P12 **Mesa Mountain** ▲ Alaska, USA
115 J25 **Mesará** lowland Kríti, Greece, E Mediterranean Sea
37 S14 **Mescalero** New Mexico, SW USA
101 G15 **Meschede** Nordrhein-Westfalen, W Germany
137 Q12 **Mescit Dağları** ▲ NE Turkey
189 V13 **Mesegon** island Chuuk, C Micronesia
Meseritz see Międzyrzecz
54 F11 **Mesetas** Meta, C Colombia
Meshchera Lowland see Meshcherskaya Nizina
128 M4 **Meshcherskaya Nizina** Eng. Meshchera Lowland. basin W Russian Federation
128 J5 **Meshchovsk** Kaluzhskaya Oblast', W Russian Federation
127 R9 **Meshchura** Respublika Komi, NW Russian Federation
Meshed see Mashhad
Meshed-i-Sar see Bābolsar
80 E13 **Meshra'er Req** Warab, S Sudan
37 R15 **Mesilla** New Mexico, SW USA
108 H10 **Mesocco** Ger. Misox. Ticino, S Switzerland
115 D18 **Mesolóngi** prev. Mesolóngion. Dytikí Ellás, W Greece
Mesolóngion see Mesolóngi
14 E8 **Mesomikenda Lake** ◎ Ontario, S Canada
61 D15 **Mesopotamia** var. Mesopotamia Argentina. physical region NE Argentina
Mesopotamia Argentina see Mesopotamia
35 Y10 **Mesquite** Nevada, W USA
82 Q13 **Messalo, Rio** var. Mualo. ≈ NE Mozambique
Messana/Messene see Messina
99 L25 **Messancy** Luxembourg, SE Belgium
107 M23 **Messina** var. Messana, Messene; anc. Zancle. Sicilia, Italy, C Mediterranean Sea
83 K19 **Messina** Northern, NE South Africa
Messina, Strait of see Messina, Stretto di
107 M23 **Messina, Stretto di** Eng. Strait of Messina. strait SW Italy
115 E21 **Messíni** Pelopónnisos, S Greece
115 E21 **Messinía** peninsula S Greece
115 E22 **Messiniakós Kólpos** gulf S Greece
122 J8 **Messoyakha** ≈ N Russian Federation
114 H11 **Mesta** Gk. Néstos, Turk. Kara Su. ≈ Bulgaria/Greece see also Néstos
Mestghanem see Mostaganem
137 R8 **Mestia** var. Mestiya. N Georgia
Mestiya see Mestia
115 K18 **Mestón, Akrotírio** headland Chíos, E Greece
106 H8 **Mestre** Veneto, NE Italy
59 M16 **Mestre, Espigão** ▲ E Brazil
169 N14 **Mesuji** ≈ Sumatera, W Indonesia
Mesule see Grosser Möseler
10 J10 **Meszah Peak** ▲ British Columbia, W Canada
54 G11 **Meta** off. Departamento del Meta. ◆ province C Colombia
15 Q8 **Metabetchouane** ≈ Quebec, SE Canada
9 S7 **Meta Incognita Peninsula** peninsula Baffin Island, Nunavut, NE Canada
22 K9 **Metairie** Louisiana, S USA
32 M6 **Metaline Falls** Washington, NW USA
62 K6 **Metán** Salta, N Argentina
82 N13 **Metangula** Niassa, N Mozambique
42 E7 **Metapán** Santa Ana, NW El Salvador
54 K9 **Meta, Río** ≈ Colombia/Venezuela
106 I11 **Metauro** ≈ C Italy
80 H11 **Metema** Amhara, N Ethiopia
115 D15 **Metéora** religious building Thessalía, C Greece
65 O20 **Meteor Rise** undersea feature SW Indian Ocean
186 G5 **Meteran** New Hanover, NE PNG
Meterlam/Methariam/Metharlam see Mehtarlām
115 G20 **Methanon** peninsula S Greece
32 J6 **Methow River** ≈ Washington, NW USA
19 O10 **Methuen** Massachusetts, NE USA
185 G19 **Methven** Canterbury, South Island, NZ
Metis see Metz
113 G15 **Metković** Dubrovnik-Neretva, SE Croatia
39 Y14 **Metlakatla** Annette Island, Alaska, USA
109 V13 **Metlika** Ger. Möttling. SE Slovenia
109 T8 **Metnitz** Kärnten, S Austria
27 W12 **Meto, Bayou** ≈ Arkansas, C USA
168 M15 **Metro** Sumatera, W Indonesia
30 M17 **Metropolis** Illinois, N USA
Metropolitan see Santiago
35 N8 **Metropolitan Oakland** × California, W USA
115 D15 **Métsovo** prev. Métsovon. Ípeiros, C Greece
Métsovon see Métsovo
23 V5 **Metter** Georgia, SE USA
99 H21 **Mettet** Namur, S Belgium
101 D20 **Mettlach** Saarland, SW Germany
Mettu see Metu
80 H13 **Metu** var. Mattu, Mettu. Oromo, C Ethiopia
169 T10 **Metulang** Borneo, N Indonesia
138 G8 **Metulla** Northern, N Israel
144 G14 **Metvyy Kultuk, Sor** salt flat SW Kazakhstan
103 T4 **Metz** anc. Divodurum Mediomatricum, Mediomatrica, Metis. Moselle, NE France
101 H22 **Metzingen** Baden-Württemberg, S Germany
168 G8 **Meulaboh** Sumatera, W Indonesia
99 D18 **Meulebeke** West-Vlaanderen, W Belgium
103 U6 **Meurthe** ≈ NE France
103 S5 **Meurthe-et-Moselle** ◆ department NE France
103 S4 **Meuse** ◆ department NE France
84 F10 **Meuse** Dut. Maas. ≈ W Europe see also Maas
Mexcala, Río see Balsas, Río
25 U8 **Mexia** Texas, SW USA
58 K11 **Mexiana, Ilha** island NE Brazil
40 C1 **Mexicali** Baja California, NW Mexico
27 V4 **Mexico** Missouri, C USA
18 H9 **Mexico** New York, NE USA
40 L7 **Mexico** off. United Mexican States, var. Méjico, México, Sp. Estados Unidos Mexicanos. ◆ federal republic N Central America
41 O14 **México** var. Ciudad de México, Eng. Mexico City. ● (Mexico) México, C Mexico
41 O13 **México** ◆ state S Mexico
(0) J13 **Mexico Basin** var. Sigsbee Deep. undersea feature C Gulf of Mexico
Mexico City see México
México, Golfo de see Mexico, Gulf of
44 B4 **Mexico, Gulf of** Sp. Golfo de México. gulf W Atlantic Ocean
Meyadine see Al Mayādīn
39 Y14 **Meyers Chuck** Etolin Island, Alaska, USA
148 M3 **Meymaneh** var. Maimāna, Maymana. Fāryāb, NW Afghanistan
143 N7 **Meymeh** Eşfahān, C Iran
123 V7 **Meynypil'gyno** Chukotskiy Avtonomnyy Okrug, NE Russian Federation
108 A10 **Meyrin** Genève, SW Switzerland
166 L7 **Mezaligon** Irrawaddy, SW Myanmar
41 O15 **Mezcala** Guerrero, S Mexico
114 H8 **Mezdra** Vratsa, NW Bulgaria
103 P16 **Mèze** Hérault, S France
127 O6 **Mezen'** Arkhangel'skaya Oblast', NW Russian Federation
127 P8 **Mezen'** ≈ NW Russian Federation
Mezen, Bay of see Mezenskaya Guba
103 Q13 **Mézenc, Mont** ▲ C France
127 O8 **Mezenskaya Guba** var. Bay of Mezen. bay NW Russian Federation
Mezha see Myazha
122 H6 **Mezhdusharskiy, Ostrov** island Novaya Zemlya, N Russian Federation
Mezhëvo see Myezhava
Mezhgor'ye see Mizhhir"ya
117 V8 **Mezhova** Dnipropetrovs'ka Oblast', E Ukraine
10 J12 **Meziadin Junction** British Columbia, W Canada
111 G16 **Mezileské Sedlo** var. Przełęcz Międzyleska. pass Czech Republic/Poland
102 L14 **Mézin** Lot-et-Garonne, SW France
111 M24 **Mezőberény** Békés, SE Hungary
111 M25 **Mezőhegyes** Békés, SE Hungary
111 M25 **Mezőkovácsháza** Békés, SE Hungary
111 M21 **Mezőkövesd** Borsod-Abaúj-Zemplén, NE Hungary
Mezőtelegd see Tileagd
111 M23 **Mezőtúr** Jász-Nagykun-Szolnok, E Hungary
40 K10 **Mezquital** Durango, C Mexico
106 G6 **Mezzolombardo** Trentino-Alto Adige, N Italy
82 L13 **Mfuwe** Northern, N Zambia
121 O15 **Mġarr** Gozo, N Malta
128 H6 **Mglin** Bryanskaya Oblast', W Russian Federation
Mhálanna, Cionn see Malin Head
154 G10 **Mhow** Madhya Pradesh, C India
Miadzioł Nowy see Myadzyel
171 O6 **Miagao** Panay Island, C Philippines
41 R17 **Miahuatlán** var. Miahuatlán de Porfirio Díaz. Oaxaca, SE Mexico
Miahuatlán de Porfirio Díaz see Miahuatlán
104 K10 **Miajadas** Extremadura, W Spain
Miajlar see Myājlār
36 M14 **Miami** Arizona, SW USA
23 Z16 **Miami** Florida, SE USA
27 R8 **Miami** Oklahoma, C USA
25 O2 **Miami** Texas, SW USA
23 Z16 **Miami** × Florida, SE USA
23 Z16 **Miami Beach** Florida, SE USA
23 Y15 **Miami Canal** canal Florida, SE USA
31 R14 **Miamisburg** Ohio, N USA
149 U10 **Miān Channūn** Punjab, E Pakistan
142 J4 **Miāndowāb** var. Mianduab, Miyāndoāb. Āžarbāyjān-e Bākhtarī, NW Iran
172 H5 **Miandrivazo** Toliara, C Madagascar
Mianduab see Miāndowāb
142 K3 **Mīāneh** var. Miyāneh. Āžarbāyjān-e Khāvarī, NW Iran
149 O16 **Miāni Hōr** lagoon S Pakistan
160 G10 **Mianning** Sichuan, C China
149 T7 **Miānwāli** Punjab, NE Pakistan
160 J7 **Mianxian** var. Mian Xian. Shaanxi, C China
160 I8 **Mianyang** Sichuan, C China
Mianyang see Xiantao
161 R3 **Miaodao Qundao** island group E China
161 S13 **Miaoli** N Taiwan
122 F11 **Miass** Chelyabinskaya Oblast', C Russian Federation
110 G8 **Miastko** Ger. Rummelsburg in Pommern. Pomorskie, N Poland

◆ Country ● Country Capital ◇ Dependent Territory ○ Dependent Territory Capital ◆ Administrative Region × International Airport ▲ Mountain ▲ Mountain Range 𝕏 Volcano ≈ River ◎ Lake ⊡ Reservoir

Miava see Myjava
11 O15 Mica Creek British Columbia, SW Canada
160 J7 Micang Shan ▲ C China
Mi Chai see Nong Khai
111 O19 Michalovce Ger. Grossmichel, Hung. Nagymihály. Košický Kraj, E Slovakia
99 M20 Michel, Baraque hill E Belgium
39 S5 Michelson, Mount ▲ Alaska, USA
45 P9 Miches E Dominican Republic
30 M4 Michigamme, Lake ◎ Michigan, N USA
30 M4 Michigamme Reservoir ⊟ Michigan, N USA
31 N4 Michigamme River ≈ Michigan, N USA
31 O7 Michigan off. State of Michigan; also known as Great Lakes State, Lake State, Wolverine State. ◈ state N USA
31 O11 Michigan City Indiana, N USA
31 O8 Michigan, Lake ◎ N USA
31 P2 Michipicoten Bay lake bay Ontario, N Canada
14 A8 Michipicoten Island island Ontario, S Canada
14 B7 Michipicoten River Ontario, S Canada
Michurin see Tsarevo
128 M6 Michurinsk Tambovskaya Oblast', W Russian Federation
Mico, Punta/Mico, Punto see Monkey Point
42 L10 Mico, Río ≈ SE Nicaragua
45 T12 Micoud SE Saint Lucia
189 N16 Micronesia off. Federated States of Micronesia. ◆ federation W Pacific Ocean
175 P4 Micronesia island group W Pacific Ocean
169 O9 Midai, Pulau island Kepulauan Natuna, W Indonesia
Mid-Atlantic Cordillera see Mid-Atlantic Ridge
65 M17 Mid-Atlantic Ridge var. Mid-Atlantic Cordillera, Mid-Atlantic Rise, Mid-Atlantic Swell. undersea feature Atlantic Ocean
Mid-Atlantic Rise/Mid-Atlantic Swell see Mid-Atlantic Ridge
99 E15 Middelburg Zeeland, SW Netherlands
83 H24 Middelburg Eastern Cape, S South Africa
83 K21 Middelburg Mpumalanga, NE South Africa
95 G23 Middelfart Fyn, C Denmark
98 G13 Middelharnis Zuid-Holland, SW Netherlands
99 B16 Middelkerke West-Vlaanderen, W Belgium
98 I9 Middenbeemster Noord-Holland, C Netherlands
98 I8 Middenmeer Noord-Holland, NW Netherlands
35 Q2 Middle Alkali Lake ◎ California, W USA
193 S6 Middle America Trench undersea feature E Pacific Ocean
151 P19 Middle Andaman island Andaman Islands, India, NE Indian Ocean
Middle Atlas see Moyen Atlas
21 R3 Middlebourne West Virginia, NE USA
23 W9 Middleburg Florida, SE USA
Middleburg Island see 'Eua
Middle Caicos see Grand Caicos
25 N8 Middle Concho River ≈ Texas, SW USA
Middle Congo see Congo (Republic of)
39 R6 Middle Fork Chandalar River ≈ Alaska, USA
39 Q7 Middle Fork Koyukuk River ≈ Alaska, USA
33 O12 Middle Fork Salmon River ≈ Idaho, NW USA
11 T15 Middle Lake Saskatchewan, S Canada
28 L13 Middle Loup River ≈ Nebraska, C USA
185 E22 Middlemarch Otago, South Island, NZ
31 T15 Middleport Ohio, N USA
29 U14 Middle Raccoon River ≈ Iowa, C USA
29 R3 Middle River ≈ Minnesota, N USA
21 N8 Middlesboro Kentucky, S USA
97 M15 Middlesbrough N England, UK
42 G3 Middlesex Stann Creek, C Belize
97 N22 Middlesex cultural region SE England, UK
13 P15 Middleton Nova Scotia, SE Canada
20 F10 Middleton Tennessee, S USA
30 L9 Middleton Wisconsin, N USA
39 S13 Middleton Island island Alaska, USA
34 M7 Middletown California, W USA
21 Y2 Middletown Delaware, NE USA
18 K15 Middletown New Jersey, NE USA
18 K13 Middletown New York, NE USA
31 R14 Middletown Ohio, N USA
18 G15 Middletown Pennsylvania, NE USA
141 N14 Mīdī var. Maydī. NW Yemen
103 O16 Midi, Canal du canal S France
102 K17 Midi de Bigorre, Pic du ▲ S France
102 K17 Midi d'Ossau, Pic du ▲ SW France
173 R7 Mid-Indian Basin undersea feature N Indian Ocean
173 P7 Mid-Indian Ridge var. Central Indian Ridge. undersea feature C Indian Ocean
103 N14 Midi-Pyrénées ◈ region S France
25 N8 Midkiff Texas, SW USA
14 G13 Midland Ontario, S Canada
31 R8 Midland Michigan, N USA
28 M10 Midland South Dakota, N USA
24 M8 Midland Texas, SW USA
83 K17 Midlands ◈ province C Zimbabwe
97 D21 Midleton Ir. Mainistir na Corann. SW Ireland
25 T7 Midlothian Texas, SW USA
96 K12 Midlothian cultural region S Scotland, UK
172 I7 Midongy Fianarantsoa, S Madagascar
102 K15 Midou ≈ SW France
192 J6 Mid-Pacific Mountains var. Mid-Pacific Seamounts. undersea feature NW Pacific Ocean
Mid-Pacific Seamounts see Mid-Pacific Mountains
171 Q7 Midsayap Mindanao, S Philippines
36 L3 Midway Utah, W USA
192 L5 Midway Islands ◇ US territory C Pacific Ocean
33 X14 Midwest Wyoming, C USA
27 N10 Midwest City Oklahoma, C USA
152 M10 Mid Western ◈ zone W Nepal
98 P5 Midwolda Groningen, NE Netherlands
137 Q16 Midyat Mardin, SE Turkey
114 F8 Midžhur SCr. Midžor. ▲ Bulgaria/Yugoslavia see also Midžor
113 Q14 Midžor Bul. Midzhur. ▲ Bulgaria/Yugoslavia see also Midzhur
164 K14 Mie off. Mie-ken. ◈ prefecture Honshū, SW Japan
111 L16 Miechów Małopolskie, S Poland
110 F11 Międzychód Ger. Mitteldorf. Wielkopolskie, C Poland
Międzyleska, Przełęcz see Mezileské Sedlo
110 O12 Międzyrzec Podlaski Lubelskie, E Poland
110 E11 Międzyrzecz Ger. Meseritz. Lubelskie, W Poland
Mie-ken see Mie
102 L16 Miélan Gers, S France
111 N16 Mielec Podkarpackie, SE Poland
95 L21 Mien ◎ S Sweden
41 O8 Mier Tamaulipas, C Mexico
116 J11 Miercurea-Ciuc Ger. Szeklerburg, Hung. Csíkszereda. Harghita, C Romania
Mieresch see Maros/Mureș
Mieres del Camín see Mieres del Camino
104 K2 Mieres del Camino var. Mieres del Camín. Asturias, NW Spain
99 K15 Mierlo Noord-Brabant, SE Netherlands
41 O10 Mier y Noriega Nuevo León, NE Mexico
Mies see Stříbro
80 K13 Mī'ēso var. Meheso, Miesso. Oromo, C Ethiopia
Miesso see Mī'ēso
110 D10 Mieszkowice Ger. Bärwalde Neumark. Zachodniopomorskie, W Poland
18 G14 Mifflinburg Pennsylvania, NE USA
18 F14 Mifflintown Pennsylvania, NE USA
41 R15 Miguel Alemán, Presa ⊟ SE Mexico
40 L9 Miguel Asua var. Miguel Auza. Zacatecas, C Mexico
Miguel Auza see Miguel Asua
43 S15 Miguel de la Borda var. Donoso. Colón, C Panama
41 N13 Miguel Hidalgo × (Guadalajara) Jalisco, SW Mexico
40 H7 Miguel Hidalgo, Presa ⊟ W Mexico
116 J14 Mihăileşti Giurgiu, S Romania
116 M14 Mihail Kogălniceanu var. Kogălniceanu; prev. Caramurat, Ferdinand. Constanța, SE Romania
117 N14 Mihai Viteazu Constanța, SE Romania
136 G12 Mihalıççık Eskişehir, NW Turkey
164 G13 Mihara Hiroshima, Honshū, SW Japan
165 N14 Mihara-yama ⩘ Miyako-jima, SE Japan
105 S8 Mijares ≈ E Spain
98 I11 Mijdrecht Utrecht, C Netherlands
165 S4 Mikasa Hokkaidō, NE Japan
Mikashevichi see Mikashevichy
119 K19 Mikashevichy Pol. Mikaszewicze, Rus. Mikashevichi. Brestskaya Voblasts', SW Belarus
Mikaszewicze see Mikashevichy
128 L5 Mikhaylov Ryazanskaya Oblast', W Russian Federation
Mikhaylovgrad see Montana
195 Z8 Mikhaylov Island island Antarctica
145 T6 Mikhaylovka Pavlodar, N Kazakhstan
129 N9 Mikhaylovka Volgogradskaya Oblast', SW Russian Federation
Mikhaylovka see Mykhaylivka
81 K24 Mikindani Mtwara, SE Tanzania
93 N18 Mikkeli Swe. Sankt Michel. Itä-Suomi, E Finland
110 M8 Mikołajki Ger. Nikolaiken. Warmińsko-Mazurskie, NE Poland
Míkonos see Mýkonos
114 I9 Mikre Lovech, N Bulgaria
114 C13 Mikrí Préspa, Límni ◎ N Greece
127 P4 Mikulkin, Mys headland NW Russian Federation
81 I23 Mikumi Morogoro, SE Tanzania
127 R10 Mikun' Respublika Komi, NW Russian Federation
164 K13 Mikuni Fukui, Honshū, SW Japan
165 X13 Mikura-jima island E Japan
29 V7 Milaca Minnesota, N USA
62 J10 Milagro La Rioja, C Argentina
56 B7 Milagro Guayas, SW Ecuador
31 P4 Milakokia Lake ◎ Michigan, N USA
30 J1 Milan Illinois, N USA
31 R10 Milan Michigan, N USA
27 T2 Milan Missouri, C USA
37 Q11 Milan New Mexico, SW USA
20 G9 Milan Tennessee, S USA
Milan see Milano
95 F15 Miland Telemark, S Norway
83 N15 Milange Zambézia, NE Mozambique
106 D8 Milano Eng. Milan, Ger. Mailand; anc. Mediolanum. Lombardia, N Italy
25 U10 Milano Texas, SW USA
136 C15 Milas Muğla, SW Turkey
119 K21 Milashavichy Rus. Milashevichi. Homyel'skaya Voblasts', SE Belarus
Milashevichi see Milashavichy
119 I18 Milavidy Rus. Milovidy. Brestskaya Voblasts', SW Belarus
107 L23 Milazzo anc. Mylae. Sicilia, Italy, C Mediterranean Sea
29 R8 Milbank South Dakota, N USA
19 T7 Milbridge Maine, NE USA
100 L11 Milde ≈ C Germany
14 F14 Mildmay Ontario, S Canada
182 L9 Mildura Victoria, SE Australia
137 X12 Mil Düzü Rus. Mil'skaya Ravnina, Mil'skaya Step'. physical region C Azerbaijan
160 H13 Mile Yunnan, SW China
Mile see Mili Atoll
181 Y10 Miles Queensland, E Australia
25 P8 Miles Texas, SW USA
33 X9 Miles City Montana, NW USA
11 U17 Milestone Saskatchewan, S Canada
107 N22 Mileto Calabria, SW Italy
107 K16 Miletto, Monte ▲ C Italy
18 M13 Milford Connecticut, NE USA
21 Y3 Milford var. Milford City. Delaware, NE USA
29 T11 Milford Iowa, C USA
19 S6 Milford Maine, NE USA
29 R16 Milford Nebraska, C USA
19 O10 Milford New Hampshire, NE USA
18 J13 Milford Pennsylvania, NE USA
25 T7 Milford Texas, SW USA
36 K6 Milford Utah, W USA
Milford see Milford Haven
Milford City see Milford
97 H21 Milford Haven prev. Milford. SW Wales, UK
27 O4 Milford Lake ⊟ Kansas, C USA
185 B21 Milford Sound Southland, South Island, NZ
185 B21 Milford Sound inlet South Island, NZ
Milhau see Millau
Milh, Bahr al see Razāzah, Buḩayrat ar
139 T10 Milh, Wādī al dry watercourse S Iraq
189 W8 Mili Atoll var. Mile. atoll Ratak Chain, SE Marshall Islands
110 H13 Milicz Dolnośląskie, SW Poland
107 L25 Militello in Val di Catania Sicilia, Italy, C Mediterranean Sea
123 V10 Mil'kovo Kamchatskaya Oblast', E Russian Federation
11 R17 Milk River Alberta, SW Canada
44 J13 Milk River ≈ C Jamaica
33 W7 Milk River ≈ Montana, NW USA
80 D9 Milk, Wadi el var. Wadi al Malik. ≈ C Sudan
99 L14 Mill Noord-Brabant, SE Netherlands
103 P14 Millau var. Milhau; anc. Æmilianum. Aveyron, S France
14 I14 Millbrook Ontario, SE Canada
23 U4 Milledgeville Georgia, SE USA
12 C12 Mille Lacs, Lac des ◎ Ontario, S Canada
29 V6 Mille Lacs Lake ◎ Minnesota, N USA
23 V4 Millen Georgia, SE USA
191 Y5 Millennium Island prev. Caroline Island, Thornton Island. atoll Line Islands, E Kiribati
29 O9 Miller South Dakota, N USA
30 K5 Miller Dam Flowage ◎ Wisconsin, N USA
39 U12 Miller, Mount ▲ Alaska, USA
128 L10 Millerovo Rostovskaya Oblast', SW Russian Federation
37 N17 Miller Peak ▲ Arizona, SW USA
31 T12 Millersburg Ohio, N USA
18 G15 Millersburg Pennsylvania, NE USA
185 D23 Millers Flat Otago, South Island, NZ
25 Q8 Millersview Texas, SW USA
106 B10 Millesimo Piemonte, NW Italy
17 N6 Milles Lacs, Lac des ◎ Ontario, SW Canada
25 Q13 Millett Texas, SW USA
103 N11 Millevaches, Plateau de plateau C France
182 K12 Millicent South Australia
98 M13 Millingen aan den Rijn Gelderland, SE Netherlands
20 E10 Millington Tennessee, S USA
19 R4 Millinocket Maine, NE USA
19 R4 Millinocket Lake ◎ Maine, NE USA
195 Z11 Mill Island island Antarctica
183 T3 Millmerran Queensland, E Australia
109 R9 Millstatt Kärnten, S Austria
97 B19 Milltown Malbay Ir. Sráid na Cathrach. W Ireland
18 J17 Millville New Jersey, NE USA
27 S13 Millwood Lake ⊟ Arkansas, C USA
Milne Bank see Milne Seamounts
186 G10 Milne Bay ◈ province SE PNG
64 J8 Milne Seamounts var. Milne Bank. undersea feature N Atlantic Ocean
29 Q6 Milnor North Dakota, N USA
19 R5 Milo Maine, NE USA
115 I22 Mílos Mílos, Kykládes, Greece, Aegean Sea
115 I22 Mílos island Kykládes, Greece, Aegean Sea
110 H11 Miłosław Wielkopolskie, C Poland
113 K19 Milot var. Miloti. Lezhë, C Albania
Miloti see Milot
117 Z5 Milove Luhans'ka Oblast', E Ukraine
Milovidy see Milavidy
182 L4 Milparinka New South Wales, SE Australia
35 N9 Milpitas California, W USA
Mil'skaya Ravnina/Mil'skaya Step' see Mil Düzü
14 G15 Milton Ontario, S Canada
185 E24 Milton Otago, South Island, NZ
21 Y4 Milton Delaware, NE USA
23 P8 Milton Florida, SE USA
18 G14 Milton Pennsylvania, NE USA
18 L7 Milton Vermont, NE USA
32 K11 Milton-Freewater Oregon, NW USA
97 N21 Milton Keynes SE England, UK
27 N3 Miltonvale Kansas, C USA
161 N10 Miluo Hunan, S China
30 M9 Milwaukee Wisconsin, N USA
Milyang see Miryang
Mimatum see Mende
37 Q15 Mimbres Mountains ▲ New Mexico, SW USA
182 D2 Mimili South Australia
102 J14 Mimizan Landes, SW France
Mimmaya see Minmaya
79 E19 Mimongo Ngounié, C Gabon
Min see Fujian
35 T7 Mina Nevada, W USA
143 S14 Mīnāb Hormozgān, SE Iran
Mina Baranis see Berenice
149 R9 Mīna Bāzār Baluchistān, SW Pakistan
165 X17 Minami-Iō-jima Eng. San Augustine. island SE Japan
165 R5 Minami-Kayabe Hokkaidō, NE Japan
164 C17 Minamitane Kagoshima, Tanega-shima, SW Japan
Minami Tori Shima see Marcus Island
62 J4 Mina Pirquitas Jujuy, NW Argentina
173 O3 Mīnā' Qābūs NE Oman
61 F19 Minas Lavalleja, S Uruguay
13 P15 Minas Basin bay Nova Scotia, SE Canada
61 F17 Minas de Corrales Rivera, NE Uruguay
44 A5 Minas de Matahambre Pinar del Río, W Cuba
104 J13 Minas de Ríotinto Andalucía, S Spain
60 K7 Minas Gerais off. Estado de Minas Gerais. ◈ state E Brazil
42 E5 Minas, Sierra de las ▲ E Guatemala
41 T15 Minatitlán Veracruz-Llave, E Mexico
166 L6 Minbu Magwe, W Myanmar
149 V10 Minchinābād Punjab, E Pakistan
63 G17 Minchinmávida, Volcán ▲ S Chile
96 G7 Minch, The var. North Minch. strait NW Scotland, UK
106 F8 Mincio anc. Mincius. ≈ N Italy
Mincius see Mincio
26 M11 Minco Oklahoma, C USA
171 Q7 Mindanao island S Philippines
Mindanao Sea see Bohol Sea
101 J23 Mindel ≈ S Germany
101 J23 Mindelheim Bayern, S Germany
Mindello see Mindelo
76 C9 Mindelo var. Mindello; prev. Porto Grande. São Vicente, N Cape Verde
14 I13 Minden Ontario, SE Canada
100 H13 Minden anc. Minthun. Nordrhein-Westfalen, NW Germany
22 G5 Minden Louisiana, S USA
29 O16 Minden Nebraska, C USA
35 Q6 Minden Nevada, W USA
182 L8 Mindona Lake seasonal lake New South Wales, SE Australia
171 O4 Mindoro island N Philippines
171 N5 Mindoro Strait strait W Philippines
159 S9 Mine Gansu, N China
97 E21 Mine Head Ir. Mionn Ard. headland S Ireland
97 J23 Minehead SW England, UK
59 J19 Mineiros Goiás, C Brazil
25 V6 Mineola Texas, SW USA
25 S13 Mineral Texas, SW USA
129 N15 Mineral'nyye Vody Stavropol'skiy Kray, SW Russian Federation
30 K9 Mineral Point Wisconsin, N USA
25 S6 Mineral Wells Texas, SW USA
36 K6 Minersville Utah, W USA
31 U12 Minerva Ohio, N USA
107 N17 Minervino Murge Puglia, SE Italy
103 O16 Minervois physical region S France
158 I10 Minfeng var. Niya. Xinjiang Uygur Zizhiqu, NW China
79 O25 Minga Katanga, SE Dem. Rep. Congo (Zaire)
137 W11 Mingäçevir Rus. Mingechaur, Mingechevir. C Azerbaijan
137 W11 Mingäçevir Su Anbarı Rus. Mingechaurskoye Vodokhranilishche, Mingechevirskoye Vodokhranilishche. ⊟ NW Azerbaijan
166 L8 Mingaladon × (Yangon) Yangon, SW Myanmar
13 P11 Mingan Quebec, E Canada
149 U5 Mingāora var. Mingora, Mongora. North-West Frontier Province, N Pakistan
146 K8 Mingbuloq Rus. Mynbulak. Nawoiy Wiloyati, N Uzbekistan
146 K9 Mingbuloq Botighi Rus. Vpadina Mynbulak. depression N Uzbekistan
Mingechaur/Mingechevir see Mingäçevir
Mingechaurskoye Vodokhranilishche/Mingechevirskoye Vodokhranilishche see Mingäçevir Su Anbarı
161 Q7 Mingguang prev. Jiashan. Anhui, S China
166 L4 Mingin Sagaing, C Myanmar
105 Q10 Minglanilla Castilla-La Mancha, C Spain
31 V13 Mingo Junction Ohio, N USA
Mingora see Mingāora
163 V7 Mingshui Heilongjiang, NE China
Mingteke Daban see Mintaka Pass
83 Q14 Minguri Nampula, NE Mozambique
159 U10 Minhe var. Shangchuankou. Qinghai, C China
166 L6 Minhla Magwe, W Myanmar
167 S14 Minh Lương Kiên Giang, S Vietnam
104 G5 Minho, Rio Sp. Miño. ≈ Portugal/Spain see also Miño
104 G5 Minho former province N Portugal
155 C24 Minicoy Island island SW India
33 P15 Minidoka Idaho, NW USA
118 C11 Minija ≈ W Lithuania
180 G9 Minilya Western Australia
14 E8 Minisinakwa Lake ◎ Ontario, S Canada
45 T12 Ministre Point headland S Saint Lucia
11 V15 Minitonas Manitoba, S Canada
Minius see Miño
161 R12 Min Jiang ≈ SE China
160 H10 Min Jiang ≈ C China
182 H9 Minlaton South Australia
165 Q6 Minmaya var. Mimmaya. Aomori, Honshū, C Japan
77 U14 Minna Niger, C Nigeria
165 P16 Minna-jima island Sakishima-shotō, SW Japan
27 N4 Minneapolis Kansas, C USA
29 U9 Minneapolis Minnesota, N USA
29 V8 Minneapolis-Saint Paul × Minnesota, N USA
9 N15 Minnedosa Manitoba, S Canada
26 J7 Minneola Kansas, C USA
29 S7 Minnesota off. State of Minnesota; also known as Gopher State, New England of the West, North Star State. ◈ state N USA
29 S9 Minnesota River ≈ Minnesota/South Dakota, N USA
29 V9 Minnetonka Minnesota, N USA
29 O3 Minnewaukan North Dakota, N USA
182 F7 Minnipa South Australia
104 H2 Miño Galicia, NW Spain
104 G5 Miño var. Mino, Minius, Port. Rio Minho. ≈ Portugal/Spain see also Minho, Rio
30 L4 Minocqua Wisconsin, N USA
30 L12 Minonk Illinois, N USA
Minorca see Menorca
28 M3 Minot North Dakota, N USA
159 U8 Minqin Gansu, N China
119 J16 Minsk ● (Belarus) Minskaya Voblasts', C Belarus
119 L16 Minsk × Minskaya Voblasts', C Belarus
Minskaya Oblast' see Minskaya Voblasts'
119 K16 Minskaya Voblasts' prev. Rus. Minskaya Oblast'. ◈ province C Belarus
119 J16 Minskaya Wzvyshsha ▲ C Belarus
110 N12 Mińsk Mazowiecki var. Nowo-Minsk. Mazowieckie, C Poland
31 Q13 Minster Ohio, N USA
79 F15 Minta Centre, C Cameroon
149 W2 Mintaka Pass Chin. Mingteke Daban. pass China/Pakistan
115 D20 Mínthi ▲ S Greece
Minthun see Minden
13 O14 Minto New Brunswick, SE Canada
10 H6 Minto Yukon Territory, W Canada
39 R9 Minto Alaska, USA
29 Q3 Minto North Dakota, N USA
12 K6 Minto, Lac ◎ Quebec, C Canada
195 R16 Minto, Mount ▲ Antarctica
11 U17 Minton Saskatchewan, S Canada
189 R15 Minto Reef atoll Caroline Islands, C Micronesia
37 R4 Minturn Colorado, C USA
107 J16 Minturno Lazio, C Italy
122 K13 Minusinsk Krasnoyarskiy Kray, S Russian Federation
108 G11 Minusio Ticino, S Switzerland
79 E17 Minvoul Woleu-Ntem, N Gabon
141 R13 Minwakh N Yemen
159 V11 Minxian var. Min Xian. Gansu, C China
Minya see El Minya
31 R6 Mio Michigan, N USA
Mionn Ard see Mine Head
158 L5 Miquan Xinjiang Uygur Zizhiqu, NW China
119 I17 Mir Hrodzyenskaya Voblasts', W Belarus
106 H8 Mira Veneto, NE Italy
104 G13 Mira, Rio ≈ S Portugal
12 K15 Mirabel var. Montreal. × (Montréal) Quebec, SE Canada
60 Q8 Miracema Rio de Janeiro, SE Brazil
54 G9 Miraflores Boyacá, C Colombia
40 G10 Miraflores Baja California Sur, W Mexico
44 L9 Miragoâne S Haiti
155 E16 Miraj Mahārāshtra, W India
61 E23 Miramar Buenos Aires, E Argentina
103 R15 Miramas Bouches-du-Rhône, SE France
102 K12 Mirambeau Charente-Maritime, W France
102 L13 Miramont-de-Guyenne Lot-et-Garonne, SW France
115 L25 Mirampéllou Kólpos gulf Kríti, Greece, E Mediterranean Sea
158 L8 Miran Xinjiang Uygur Zizhiqu, NW China
54 M5 Miranda off. Estado Miranda. ◈ state N Venezuela
Miranda de Corvo see Miranda do Corvo
105 O3 Miranda de Ebro La Rioja, N Spain
104 G8 Miranda do Corvo var. Miranda de Corvo. Coimbra, N Portugal
104 J6 Miranda do Douro Bragança, N Portugal
102 L15 Mirande Gers, S France
104 I6 Mirandela Bragança, N Portugal
25 R15 Mirando City Texas, SW USA
106 G9 Mirandola Emilia-Romagna, N Italy
60 I8 Mirandópolis São Paulo, S Brazil
60 K8 Mirassol São Paulo, S Brazil
104 J3 Miravalles ▲ NW Spain
42 L12 Miravalles, Volcán ⩘ NW Costa Rica
141 W13 Mirbāṭ var. Marbat. S Oman
44 M9 Mirebalais C Haiti
103 T6 Mirecourt Vosges, NE France
103 N16 Mirepoix Ariège, S France
Mirgorod see Myrhorod
139 W10 Mīr Ḩājī Khalīl E Iraq
169 T8 Miri Sarawak, East Malaysia
77 W12 Miria Zinder, S Niger
182 F5 Mirikata South Australia
54 K4 Mirimire Falcón, N Venezuela
61 H18 Mirim Lagoon var. Lake Mirim, Sp. Laguna Merín. lagoon Brazil/Uruguay
Mirim, Lake see Mirim Lagoon
Mírina see Mýrina
172 H14 Miringoni Mohéli, S Comoros
143 W11 Mīrjāveh Sīstān va Balūchestān, SE Iran
195 Z9 Mirny Russian research station Antarctica
123 O10 Mirnyy Respublika Sakha (Yakutiya), NE Russian Federation
Mironovka see Myronivka
110 F9 Mirosławiec Zachodniopomorskie, NW Poland
Mirovo see Vrattsa
100 N10 Mirow Mecklenburg-Vorpommern, N Germany
152 G6 Mirpur Jammu and Kashmir, NW India
Mirpur see New Mīrpur
149 P17 Mīrpur Batoro Sind, SE Pakistan
149 Q16 Mīrpur Khās Sind, SE Pakistan
149 P17 Mīrpur Sakro Sind, SE Pakistan
143 T14 Mīr Shahdād Hormozgān, S Iran
Mirtoan Sea see Mirtóo Pélagos
115 G21 Mirtóo Pélagos Eng. Mirtoan Sea; anc. Myrtoum Mare. sea S Greece
163 Z16 Miryang var. Milyang, Jap. Mitsuō. SE South Korea
Mirzachirla see Murzechirla
164 E14 Misaki Ehime, Shikoku, SW Japan
41 Q13 Misantla Veracruz-Llave, E Mexico
165 R7 Misawa Aomori, Honshū, C Japan
57 G14 Mishagua, Río ≈ C Peru
163 Z8 Mishan Heilongjiang, NE China
31 O11 Mishawaka Indiana, N USA
39 N6 Misheguk Mountain ▲ Alaska, USA
165 N14 Mishima var. Misima. Shizuoka, Honshū, S Japan
164 E12 Mi-shima island SW Japan
129 V4 Mishkino Respublika Bashkortostan, W Russian Federation
153 Y10 Mishmi Hills hill range NE India
161 N11 Mi Shui ≈ S China
Misiaf see Maṣyāf
107 J23 Misilmeri Sicilia, Italy, C Mediterranean Sea
Misima see Mishima
Misión de Guana see Guana
60 F13 Misiones off. Provincia de Misiones. ◈ province NE Argentina
62 P8 Misiones off. Departamento de las Misiones. ◈ department S Paraguay
Misión San Fernando see San Fernando
Miskin see Maskin
Miskito Coast see La Mosquitia
43 O7 Miskitos, Cayos island group NE Nicaragua
111 M21 Miskolc Borsod-Abaúj-Zemplén, NE Hungary
171 T12 Misool, Pulau island Maluku, E Indonesia
Misox see Mesocco
29 Y3 Misquah Hills hill range Minnesota, N USA
75 P7 Mişrātah var. Misurata. NW Libya
14 C7 Missanabie Ontario, S Canada

58 E10 **Missão Catrimani** Roraima, N Brazil
14 D6 **Missinaibi** ≈ Ontario, S Canada
14 C7 **Missinaibi Lake** ◎ Ontario, S Canada
11 T13 **Missinipe** Saskatchewan, C Canada
28 M11 **Mission** South Dakota, N USA
25 S17 **Mission** Texas, SW USA
12 F10 **Missisa Lake** ◎ Ontario, C Canada
18 M6 **Missisquoi Bay** *lake bay* Canada/USA
14 C10 **Mississagi** ≈ Ontario, S Canada
14 G15 **Mississauga** Ontario, S Canada
31 P12 **Mississinewa Lake** ⊟ Indiana, N USA
31 P12 **Mississinewa River** ≈ Indiana/Ohio, N USA
22 K4 **Mississippi** *off.* State of Mississippi; also known as Bayou State, Magnolia State. ◈ *state* SE USA
14 K13 **Mississippi** ≈ Ontario, SE Canada
22 M10 **Mississippi Delta** *delta* Louisiana, S USA
47 N1 **Mississippi Fan** *undersea feature* N Gulf of Mexico
14 L13 **Mississippi Lake** ◎ Ontario, SE Canada
(0) J11 **Mississippi River** ≈ C USA
22 M9 **Mississippi Sound** *sound* Alabama/Mississippi, S USA
33 P9 **Missoula** Montana, NW USA
27 T5 **Missouri** *off.* State of Missouri; also known as Bullion State, Show Me State. ◈ *state* C USA
25 V11 **Missouri City** Texas, SW USA
(0) J10 **Missouri River** ≈ C USA
15 Q6 **Mistassibi** ≈ Quebec, SE Canada
15 P6 **Mistassini** Quebec, SE Canada
15 P6 **Mistassini** ≈ Quebec, SE Canada
12 J11 **Mistassini, Lac** ◎ Quebec, SE Canada
109 Y3 **Mistelbach an der Zaya** Niederösterreich, NE Austria
107 L24 **Misterbianco** Sicilia, Italy, C Mediterranean Sea
95 N19 **Misterhult** Kalmar, S Sweden
57 H17 **Misti, Volcán** ▲ S Peru
Mistras *see* Mystrás
107 K23 **Mistretta** *anc.* Amestratus. Sicilia, Italy, C Mediterranean Sea
164 F12 **Misumi** Shimane, Honshū, SW Japan
Misurata *see* Mişrātah
83 O14 **Mitande** Niassa, N Mozambique
40 J13 **Mita, Punta de** *headland* C Mexico
55 W12 **Mitaraka, Massif du** ▲ NE South America
Mitau *see* Jelgava
181 X9 **Mitchell** Queensland, E Australia
14 E15 **Mitchell** Ontario, S Canada
28 I13 **Mitchell** Nebraska, C USA
32 J12 **Mitchell** Oregon, NW USA
29 P11 **Mitchell** South Dakota, N USA
23 P5 **Mitchell Lake** ⊟ Alabama, S USA
31 P7 **Mitchell, Lake** ◎ Michigan, N USA
21 P9 **Mitchell, Mount** ▲ North Carolina, SE USA
181 V3 **Mitchell River** ≈ Queensland, NE Australia
97 D20 **Mitchelstown** *Ir.* Baile Mhistéala. SW Ireland
14 M9 **Mitchinamécus, Lac** ◎ Quebec, SE Canada
Mitèmboni *see* Mitemele, Río
79 D17 **Mitemele, Río** *var.* Mitèmboni, Temboni, Utamboni. ≈ S Equatorial Guinea
149 S12 **Mithānkot** Punjab, E Pakistan
149 T7 **Mitha Tiwāna** Punjab, E Pakistan
149 R17 **Mithi** Sind, SE Pakistan
Míthimna *see* Míthymna
Mi Tho *see* My Tho
115 L16 **Míthymna** *var.* Míthimna. Lésvos, E Greece
190 L16 **Mitiaro** *island* S Cook Islands
Mitilíni *see* Mytilíni
15 U7 **Mitis** ≈ Quebec, SE Canada
41 R16 **Mitla** Oaxaca, SE Mexico
165 P13 **Mito** Ibaraki, Honshū, S Japan
92 N2 **Mitra, Kapp** *headland* W Svalbard
184 M13 **Mitre** ▲ North Island, NZ
185 B21 **Mitre Peak** ▲ South Island, NZ
39 O15 **Mitrofania Island** *island* Alaska, USA
Mitrovica/Mitrowitz *see* Sremska Mitrovica, Serbia, Yugoslavia
Mitrovica/Mitrovicë *see* Kosovska Mitrovica, Serbia, Yugoslavia
172 H12 **Mitsamiouli** Grande Comore, NW Comoros
172 I3 **Mitsinjo** Mahajanga, NW Madagascar
Mits'iwa *see* Massawa
172 H13 **Mitsoudjé** Grande Comore, NW Comoros
Mitspe Ramon *see* Mizpé Ramon
165 T5 **Mitsuishi** Hokkaidō, NE Japan
165 O11 **Mitsuke** *var.* Mituke. Niigata, Honshū, C Japan
Mitsuō *see* Miryang
164 C12 **Mitsushima** Nagasaki, Tsushima, SW Japan
100 G12 **Mittellandkanal** *canal* NW Germany
108 J7 **Mittelberg** Vorarlberg, NW Austria
Mitteldorf *see* Międzychód
Mittelstadt *see* Baia Sprie
Mitterburg *see* Pazin
109 P7 **Mittersill** Salzburg, NW Austria
101 N16 **Mittweida** Sachsen, E Germany
54 J13 **Mitú** Vaupés, SE Colombia
Mituke *see* Mitsuke
Mitumba, Chaîne des/Mitumba Range *see* Mitumba, Monts
79 O22 **Mitumba, Monts** *var.* Chaîne des Mitumba, Mitumba Range. ▲ E Dem. Rep. Congo (Zaire)
79 N23 **Mitwaba** Katanga, SE Dem. Rep. Congo (Zaire)
79 E18 **Mitzic** Woleu-Ntem, N Gabon
82 K11 **Miueru Wantipa, Lake** ◎ N Zambia
165 N14 **Miura** Kanagawa, Honshū, S Japan
165 Q10 **Miyagi** *off.* Miyagi-ken. ◈ *prefecture* Honshū, C Japan
138 M7 **Miyāh, Wādī al** *dry watercourse* E Syria
165 X13 **Miyake** Tōkyō, Miyako-jima, SE Japan
165 R8 **Miyako** Iwate, Honshū, C Japan
165 Q16 **Miyako-jima** *island* Sakishima-shotō, SW Japan
164 D16 **Miyakonojō** *var.* Miyakonzyô. Miyazaki, Kyūshū, SW Japan
Miyakonzyô *see* Miyakonojō
165 Q16 **Miyako-shotō** *island group* SW Japan
144 G11 **Miyaly** Atyrau, W Kazakhstan
Miyāndoāb *see* Miāndowāb
Miyāneh *see* Miāneh
164 D16 **Miyazaki** Miyazaki, Kyūshū, SW Japan
164 D16 **Miyazaki** *off.* Miyazaki-ken. ◈ *prefecture* Kyūshū, SW Japan
164 J12 **Miyazu** Kyōto, Honshū, SW Japan
Miyory *see* Myory
164 G12 **Miyoshi** *var.* Miyosi. Hiroshima, Honshū, SW Japan
Miyosi *see* Miyoshi
Miza *see* Mizë
81 H14 **Mīzan Teferī** Southern, S Ethiopia
Mizda *see* Mizdah
75 O8 **Mizdah** *var.* Mizda. NW Libya
113 K20 **Mizë** *var.* Miza. Fier, W Albania
97 A22 **Mizen Head** *Ir.* Carn Uí Néid. *headland* SW Ireland
116 H7 **Mizhhir"ya** *Rus.* Mezhgor'ye. Zakarpats'ka Oblast', W Ukraine
160 L4 **Mizhi** Shaanxi, C China
116 K13 **Mizil** Prahova, SE Romania
114 H7 **Miziya** Vratsa, NW Bulgaria
153 W15 **Mizo Hills** *hill range* E India
153 W15 **Mizoram** ◈ *state* NE India
138 F12 **Mizpé Ramon** *var.* Mitspe Ramon. Southern, S Israel
57 L19 **Mizque** Cochabamba, C Bolivia
57 M19 **Mizque, Río** ≈ C Bolivia
165 Q9 **Mizusawa** Iwate, Honshū, C Japan
95 M18 **Mjölby** Östergötland, S Sweden
95 G15 **Mjøndalen** Buskerud, S Norway
95 J19 **Mjörn** ◎ S Sweden
94 I13 **Mjøsa** *var.* Mjøsen. ◎ S Norway
Mjøsen *see* Mjøsa
81 G21 **Mkalama** Singida, C Tanzania
80 K13 **Mkata** ≈ C Tanzania
83 K14 **Mkushi** Central, C Zambia
83 L22 **Mkuze** KwaZulu/Natal, E South Africa
81 J22 **Mkwaja** Tanga, E Tanzania
111 D16 **Mladá Boleslav** *Ger.* Jungbunzlau. Středočeský Kraj, N Czech Republic
112 M12 **Mladenovac** Serbia, C Yugoslavia
114 L11 **Mladinovo** Khaskovo, S Bulgaria
113 O17 **Mlado Nagoričane** N FYR Macedonia
Mlanje *see* Mulanje
112 N12 **Mlava** ≈ E Yugoslavia
110 L9 **Mława** Mazowieckie, C Poland
113 G16 **Mljet** *It.* Meleda; *anc.* Melita. *island* S Croatia
116 K4 **Mlyniv** Rivnens'ka Oblast', NW Ukraine
83 I21 **Mmabatho** North-West, N South Africa
83 I19 **Mmashoro** Central, E Botswana
44 J7 **Moa** Holguín, E Cuba
76 J15 **Moa** ≈ Guinea/Sierra Leone
37 O6 **Moab** Utah, W USA
181 V1 **Moa Island** *island* Queensland, NE Australia
187 Y15 **Moala** *island* S Fiji
83 L21 **Moamba** Maputo, SW Mozambique
79 F19 **Moanda** *var.* Mouanda. Haut-Ogooué, SE Gabon
83 M15 **Moatize** Tete, NW Mozambique
79 P22 **Moba** Katanga, E Dem. Rep. Congo (Zaire)
Mobay *see* Montego Bay
79 K15 **Mobaye** Basse-Kotto, S Central African Republic
79 K15 **Mobayi-Mbongo** Equateur, NW Dem. Rep. Congo (Zaire)
25 P2 **Mobeetie** Texas, SW USA
27 U3 **Moberly** Missouri, C USA
23 N8 **Mobile** Alabama, S USA
23 N9 **Mobile Bay** *bay* Alabama, S USA
23 N8 **Mobile River** ≈ Alabama, S USA
29 N8 **Mobridge** South Dakota, N USA
Mobutu Sese Seko, Lac *see* Albert, Lake
45 N8 **Moca** N Dominican Republic
Moçamedes *see* Namibe
167 S6 **Môc Châu** Sơn La, N Vietnam
187 Z15 **Moce** *island* Lau Group, E Fiji
83 Q15 **Moçambique** Nampula, NE Mozambique
Mocha *see* Al Mukhā
193 T11 **Mocha Fracture Zone** *tectonic feature* SE Pacific Ocean
63 F14 **Mocha, Isla** *island* C Chile
56 C12 **Moche, Río** ≈ W Peru
167 S14 **Môc Hoa** Long An, S Vietnam
83 I20 **Mochudi** Kgatleng, SE Botswana
82 Q13 **Mocímboa da Praia** *var.* Vila de Mocímboa da Praia. Cabo Delgado, N Mozambique
94 L13 **Mockfjärd** Dalarna, C Sweden
21 R9 **Mocksville** North Carolina, SE USA
32 F8 **Moclips** Washington, NW USA
82 C13 **Môco** *var.* Morro de Môco. ▲ W Angola
54 D13 **Mocoa** Putumayo, SW Colombia
60 M8 **Mococa** São Paulo, S Brazil
Môco, Morro de *see* Môco
40 H8 **Mocorito** Sinaloa, C Mexico
40 J4 **Moctezuma** Chihuahua, N Mexico
41 N11 **Moctezuma** San Luis Potosí, C Mexico
40 G4 **Moctezuma** Sonora, NW Mexico
41 P12 **Moctezuma, Río** ≈ C Mexico
Mó, Cuan *see* Clew Bay
83 O16 **Mocuba** Zambézia, NE Mozambique
103 U12 **Modane** Savoie, E France
106 F9 **Modena** *anc.* Mutina. Emilia-Romagna, N Italy
36 I7 **Modena** Utah, W USA
35 O9 **Modesto** California, W USA
107 L25 **Modica** *anc.* Motyca. Sicilia, Italy, C Mediterranean Sea
79 K17 **Modjamboli** Equateur, N Dem. Rep. Congo (Zaire)
109 X4 **Mödling** Niederösterreich, NE Austria
Modohn *see* Madona
163 N8 **Modot** Hentiy, C Mongolia
171 V14 **Modowi** Irian Jaya, E Indonesia
112 I12 **Modračko Jezero** ⊟ NE Bosnia and Herzegovina
112 I10 **Modriča** Republika Srpska, N Bosnia and Herzegovina
183 O13 **Moe** Victoria, SE Australia
Moearatewe *see* Muaratewe
Moei, Mae Nam *see* Thaungyin
94 H13 **Moelv** Hedmark, S Norway
92 I10 **Moen** Troms, N Norway
Moen *see* Weno, Micronesia
Möen *see* Møn, Denmark
Moena *see* Muna, Pulau
36 M10 **Moenkopi Wash** ≈ Arizona, SW USA
185 F22 **Moeraki Point** *headland* South Island, NZ
99 F16 **Moerbeke** Oost-Vlaanderen, NW Belgium
99 H14 **Moerdijk** Noord-Brabant, S Netherlands
Moero, Lac *see* Mweru, Lake
101 D15 **Moers** *var.* Mörs. Nordrhein-Westfalen, W Germany
Moesi *see* Musi, Air
Moeskroen *see* Mouscron
96 J13 **Moffat** S Scotland, UK
185 C22 **Moffat Peak** ▲ South Island, NZ
152 H8 **Moga** Punjab, N India
79 N19 **Moga** Sud Kivu, E Dem. Rep. Congo (Zaire)
Mogadiscio/Mogadishu *see* Muqdisho
Mogador *see* Essaouira
104 J6 **Mogadouro** Bragança, N Portugal
167 N2 **Mogaung** Kachin State, N Myanmar
110 L13 **Mogielnica** Mazowieckie, C Poland
Mogilëv *see* Mahilyow
Mogilev-Podol'skiy *see* Mohyliv-Podil's'kyy
Mogilëvskaya Oblast' *see* Mahilyowskaya Voblasts'
110 I11 **Mogilno** Kujawsko-pomorskie, C Poland
60 L9 **Mogi-Mirim** *var.* Moji-Mirim. São Paulo, S Brazil
83 Q15 **Mogincual** Nampula, NE Mozambique
114 E13 **Moglenítsas** ≈ N Greece
106 H8 **Mogliano Veneto** Veneto, NE Italy
113 M21 **Moglicë** Korçë, SE Albania
123 O13 **Mogocha** Chitinskaya Oblast', S Russian Federation
122 J11 **Mogochin** Tomskaya Oblast', C Russian Federation
80 F13 **Mogogh** Jonglei, SE Sudan
171 U12 **Mogoi** Irian Jaya, E Indonesia
166 M4 **Mogok** Mandalay, C Myanmar
37 P14 **Mogollon Mountains** ▲ New Mexico, SW USA
36 M12 **Mogollon Rim** *cliff* Arizona, SW USA
61 E23 **Mogotes, Punta** *headland* E Argentina
42 J8 **Mogotón** ▲ NW Nicaragua
104 I14 **Moguer** Andalucía, S Spain
111 J26 **Mohács** Baranya, SW Hungary
185 C20 **Mohaka** ≈ North Island, NZ
28 M2 **Mohall** North Dakota, N USA
Moḥammadābād *see* Dargaz
74 F6 **Mohammedia** *prev.* Fédala. NW Morocco
74 F6 **Mohammed V** ✕ (Casablanca) W Morocco
Mohammerah *see* Khorramshahr
36 H10 **Mohave, Lake** ⊟ Arizona/Nevada, W USA
36 I12 **Mohave Mountains** ▲ Arizona, SW USA
36 I15 **Mohawk Mountains** ▲ Arizona, SW USA
18 J10 **Mohawk River** ≈ New York, NE USA
163 T3 **Mohe** Heilongjiang, NE China
95 L20 **Moheda** Kronoberg, S Sweden
172 H13 **Mohéli** *var.* Mwali, Mohilla, Mohila, *Fr.* Moili. *island* S Comoros
152 I11 **Mohendergarh** Haryāna, N India
38 K12 **Mohican, Cape** *headland* Nunivak Island, Alaska, USA
Mohn *see* Muhu
101 G15 **Möhne** ≈ W Germany
101 G15 **Möhne-Stausee** ⊟ W Germany
92 P2 **Mohn, Kapp** *headland* NW Svalbard
197 S14 **Mohns Ridge** *undersea feature* Greenland Sea/Norwegian Sea
57 I17 **Moho** Puno, SW Peru
Mohokare *see* Caledon
95 L17 **Moholm** Västra Götaland, S Sweden
36 J11 **Mohon Peak** ▲ Arizona, SW USA
81 J23 **Mohoro** Pwani, E Tanzania
Mohra *see* Moravice
Mohrungen *see* Morąg
116 M7 **Mohyliv-Podil's'kyy** *Rus.* Mogilev-Podol'skiy. Vinnyts'ka Oblast', C Ukraine
95 D17 **Moi** Rogaland, S Norway
116 K11 **Moinești** *Hung.* Mojnest. Bacău, E Romania
Móinteach Mílic *see* Mountmellick
14 J14 **Moira** ≈ Ontario, SE Canada
92 G13 **Mo i Rana** Nordland, C Norway
153 X14 **Moirāng** Manipur, NE India
115 J25 **Moíres** Kríti, Greece, E Mediterranean Sea
118 H6 **Mõisaküla** *Ger.* Moiseküll. Viljandimaa, S Estonia
Moiseküll *see* Mõisaküla
15 W4 **Moisie** Quebec, E Canada
15 W3 **Moisie** ≈ Quebec, SE Canada
102 M14 **Moissac** Tarn-et-Garonne, S France
78 I13 **Moïssala** Moyen-Chari, S Chad
55 O7 **Moitaco** Bolívar, E Venezuela
95 P15 **Möja** Stockholm, C Sweden
105 Q14 **Mojácar** Andalucía, S Spain
35 T13 **Mojave** California, W USA
35 V13 **Mojave Desert** *plain* California, W USA
35 V13 **Mojave River** ≈ California, W USA
Moji-Mirim *see* Mogi-Mirim
113 K15 **Mojkovac** Montenegro, SW Yugoslavia
Mojnest *see* Moinești
Móka *see* Mooka
153 Q13 **Mokāma** *prev.* Mokameh, Mukama. Bihār, N India
79 O25 **Mokambo** Katanga, SE Dem. Rep. Congo (Zaire)
Mokameh *see* Mokāma
38 D9 **Mokapu Point** *headland* Oahu, Hawaii, USA, C Pacific Ocean
184 L9 **Mokau** Waikato, North Island, NZ
184 L9 **Mokau** ≈ North Island, NZ
35 P7 **Mokelumne River** ≈ California, W USA
83 J23 **Mokhotlong** NE Lesotho
Mokil Atoll *see* Mwokil Atoll
95 N14 **Möklinta** Västmanland, C Sweden
184 L4 **Mokohinau Islands** *island group* N NZ
153 X12 **Mokokchūng** Nāgāland, NE India
78 F12 **Mokolo** Extrême-Nord, N Cameroon
185 D24 **Mokoreta** ≈ South Island, NZ
163 X17 **Mokp'o** *Jap.* Moppo. SW South Korea
113 L16 **Mokra Gora** ▲ S Yugoslavia
Mokrany *see* Makrany
129 O5 **Moksha** ≈ W Russian Federation
Moktama *see* Martaban
77 T14 **Mokwa** Niger, W Nigeria
99 J16 **Mol** *prev.* Moll. Antwerpen, N Belgium
107 O17 **Mola di Bari** Puglia, SE Italy
Molai *see* Moláoi
41 P13 **Molango** Hidalgo, C Mexico
115 F22 **Moláoi** *var.* Molai. Pelopónnisos, S Greece
41 Z12 **Molas del Norte, Punta** *var.* Punta Molas. *headland* SE Mexico
Molas, Punta *see* Molas del Norte, Punta
105 R11 **Molatón** ▲ C Spain
97 K18 **Mold** NE Wales, UK
Moldau *see* Moldova
Moldau *see* Vltava, Czech Republic
Moldavia *see* Moldova
Moldavian SSR/Moldavskaya SSR *see* Moldova
94 E9 **Molde** Møre og Romsdal, S Norway
Moldotau, Khrebet *see* Moldo-Too, Khrebet
147 V9 **Moldo-Too, Khrebet** *prev.* Khrebet Moldotau. ▲ C Kyrgyzstan
116 K9 **Moldova** ≈ N Romania
116 K9 **Moldova** *Eng.* Moldavia, *Ger.* Moldau. *former province* NE Romania
116 L9 **Moldova** *off.* Republic of Moldova, *var.* Moldavia; *prev.* Moldavian SSR, *Rus.* Moldavskaya SSR. ◆ *republic* SE Europe
116 F13 **Moldova Nouă** *Ger.* Neumoldowa, *Hung.* Újmoldova. Caraş-Severin, SW Romania
116 F13 **Moldova Veche** *Ger.* Altmoldowa, *Hung.* Ómoldova. Caraş-Severin, SW Romania
Moldoveanul *see* Vârful Moldoveanu
83 I20 **Molepolole** Kweneng, SE Botswana
44 L8 **Môle-St-Nicolas** NW Haiti
118 H13 **Molėtai** Molėtai, E Lithuania
107 O17 **Molfetta** Puglia, SE Italy
171 P11 **Molibagu** Sulawesi, N Indonesia
62 G12 **Molina** Maule, C Chile
105 Q7 **Molina de Aragón** Castilla-La Mancha, C Spain
105 R13 **Molina de Segura** Murcia, SE Spain
30 J11 **Moline** Illinois, N USA
27 P7 **Moline** Kansas, C USA
79 P23 **Moliro** Katanga, SE Dem. Rep. Congo (Zaire)
107 K16 **Molise** ◈ *region* S Italy
95 K15 **Molkom** Värmland, C Sweden
Moll *see* Mol
109 Q9 **Möll** ≈ S Austria
95 J22 **Mölle** Skåne, S Sweden
57 H18 **Mollendo** Arequipa, SW Peru
105 U5 **Mollerussa** Cataluña, NE Spain
108 H8 **Mollis** Glarus, NE Switzerland
95 J19 **Mölndal** Västra Götaland, S Sweden
95 J19 **Mölnlycke** Västra Götaland, S Sweden
117 U9 **Molochans'k** *Rus.* Molochansk. Zaporiz'ka Oblast', SE Ukraine
117 U10 **Molochna** *Rus.* Molochnaya. ≈ S Ukraine
Molochnaya *see* Molochna
117 U10 **Molochnyy Lyman** *bay* N Black Sea
Molodechno/Molodeczno *see* Maladzyechna
195 V3 **Molodezhnaya** *Russian research station* Antarctica
126 J14 **Mologa** ≈ NW Russian Federation
38 E9 **Molokai** *Haw.* Moloka'i. *island* Hawaii, USA, C Pacific Ocean
175 X3 **Molokai Fracture Zone** *tectonic feature* NE Pacific Ocean
126 K15 **Molokovo** Tverskaya Oblast', W Russian Federation
127 Q14 **Moloma** ≈ NW Russian Federation
183 R8 **Molong** New South Wales, SE Australia
83 H21 **Molopo** *seasonal river* Botswana/South Africa
115 F17 **Mólos** Stereá Ellás, C Greece
171 O11 **Molosipat** Sulawesi, N Indonesia
Molotov *see* Severodvinsk, Arkhangel'skaya Oblast', Russian Federation
Molotov *see* Perm', Permskaya Oblast', Russian Federation
79 G17 **Moloundou** Est, SE Cameroon
103 U5 **Molsheim** Bas-Rhin, NE France
9 O13 **Molson Lake** ◎ Manitoba, C Canada
Moluccas *see* Maluku
171 Q12 **Molucca Sea** *Ind.* Laut Maluku. *sea* E Indonesia
Molukken *see* Maluku
83 O15 **Molumbo** Zambézia, N Mozambique
171 T15 **Molu, Pulau** *island* Maluku, E Indonesia
83 P16 **Moma** Nampula, NE Mozambique
171 X14 **Momats** ≈ Irian Jaya, E Indonesia
42 J11 **Mombacho, Volcán** ⊼ SW Nicaragua
81 K21 **Mombasa** Coast, SE Kenya
81 J21 **Mombasa** ✕ Coast, SE Kenya
Mombetsu *see* Monbetsu
114 J12 **Momchilgrad** *prev.* Mastanli. Kŭrdzhali, S Bulgaria
99 F23 **Momignies** Hainaut, S Belgium
54 E6 **Momil** Córdoba, NW Colombia
42 I10 **Momotombo, Volcán** ⊼ W Nicaragua
56 B5 **Mompiche, Ensenada de** *bay* NW Ecuador
79 K18 **Mompono** Equateur, NW Dem. Rep. Congo (Zaire)
54 F6 **Mompós** Bolívar, NW Colombia
95 J24 **Møn** *prev.* Möen. *island* SE Denmark
36 L4 **Mona** Utah, W USA
Mona, Canal de la *see* Mona Passage
96 E8 **Monach Islands** *island group* NW Scotland, UK
103 V14 **Monaco** *var.* Monaco-Ville; *anc.* Monoecus. ● (Monaco) S Monaco
103 V14 **Monaco** *off.* Principality of Monaco. ◆ *monarchy* W Europe
Monaco *see* München
Monaco Basin *see* Canary Basin
Monaco-Ville *see* Monaco
96 I9 **Monadhliath Mountains** ▲ N Scotland, UK
55 O6 **Monagas** *off.* Estado Monagas. ◈ *state* NE Venezuela
97 F16 **Monaghan** *Ir.* Muineachán. N Ireland
97 E16 **Monaghan** *Ir.* Muineachán. *cultural region* N Ireland
43 S16 **Monagrillo** Herrera, S Panama
24 L8 **Monahans** Texas, SW USA
45 Q9 **Mona, Isla** *island* W Puerto Rico
45 Q9 **Mona Passage** *Sp.* Canal de la Mona. *channel* Dominican Republic/Puerto Rico
43 O14 **Mona, Punta** *headland* E Costa Rica
155 K25 **Monaragala** Uva Province, SE Sri Lanka
33 S9 **Monarch** Montana, NW USA
8 H14 **Monarch Mountain** ▲ British Columbia, SW Canada
Monasterio *see* Monesterio
Monasterzyska *see* Monastyrys'ka
Monastir *see* Bitola
Monastyriska *see* Monastyrys'ka
117 O7 **Monastyryshche** Cherkas'ka Oblast', C Ukraine
116 J6 **Monastyrys'ka** *Pol.* Monasterzyska, *Rus.* Monastyriska. Ternopil's'ka Oblast', W Ukraine
79 E15 **Monatélé** Centre, SW Cameroon
165 U2 **Monbetsu** *var.* Mombetsu, Monbetu. Hokkaidō, NE Japan
Monbetu *see* Monbetsu
106 B8 **Moncalieri** Piemonte, NW Italy
104 G4 **Monção** Viana do Castelo, N Portugal
105 Q5 **Moncayo** ▲ N Spain
105 Q5 **Moncayo, Sierra del** ▲ N Spain
126 J4 **Monchegorsk** Murmanskaya Oblast', NW Russian Federation
101 D15 **Mönchengladbach** *prev.* München-Gladbach. Nordrhein-Westfalen, W Germany
104 F14 **Monchique** Faro, S Portugal
104 G14 **Monchique, Serra de** ▲ S Portugal
21 S14 **Moncks Corner** South Carolina, SE USA
41 N7 **Monclova** Coahuila de Zaragoza, NE Mexico
Moncorvo *see* Torre de Moncorvo
13 P14 **Moncton** New Brunswick, SE Canada
104 F8 **Mondego, Cabo** *headland* N Portugal
104 G8 **Mondego, Rio** ≈ N Portugal
104 I2 **Mondoñedo** Galicia, NW Spain
99 N25 **Mondorf-les-Bains** Grevenmacher, SE Luxembourg
102 M7 **Mondoubleau** Loir-et-Cher, C France
30 J6 **Mondovi** Wisconsin, N USA
106 B9 **Mondovì** Piemonte, NW Italy
105 P3 **Mondragón** *var.* Arrasate. País Vasco, N Spain
107 J17 **Mondragone** Campania, S Italy
109 R5 **Mondsee** ◎ N Austria
115 G22 **Monemvasía** Pelopónnisos, S Greece
18 B15 **Monessen** Pennsylvania, NE USA
104 J12 **Monesterio** *var.* Monasterio. Extremadura, W Spain
14 L8 **Monet** Quebec, SE Canada
27 S8 **Monett** Missouri, C USA
27 X9 **Monette** Arkansas, C USA
14 G11 **Monetville** Ontario, S Canada
106 J7 **Monfalcone** Friuli-Venezia Giulia, NE Italy
104 H10 **Monforte** Portalegre, C Portugal
104 I4 **Monforte** Galicia, NW Spain
81 I24 **Monga** Lindi, SE Tanzania
79 L16 **Monga** Orientale, N Dem. Rep. Congo (Zaire)
81 F15 **Mongalla** Bahr el Gabel, S Sudan
153 U11 **Mongar** E Bhutan
167 U6 **Mong Cai** Quang Ninh, N Vietnam
180 I11 **Mongers Lake** *salt lake* Western Australia
186 K8 **Mongga** Kolombangara, NW Solomon Islands
167 O6 **Möng Hpayak** Shan State, E Myanmar
Monghyr *see* Munger
106 B10 **Mongioie** ▲ NW Italy
167 N5 **Möng Küng** Shan State, E Myanmar
Mongla *see* Mungla
188 C15 **Mongmong** C Guam
167 N6 **Möng Nai** Shan State, E Myanmar
78 I11 **Mongo** Guéra, C Chad
76 I14 **Mongo** ≈ N Sierra Leone
163 I8 **Mongolia** *Mong.* Mongol Uls. ◆ *republic* E Asia
131 V8 **Mongolia, Plateau of** *plateau* E Mongolia
Mongolküre *see* Zhaosu
Mongol Uls *see* Mongolia
79 E17 **Mongomo** E Equatorial Guinea
77 Y12 **Mongonu** *var.* Monguno. Borno, NE Nigeria
Mongora *see* Mingāora
78 K11 **Mongororo** Ouaddaï, SE Chad
Mongos, Chaîne des *see* Bongo, Massif des
79 I16 **Mongoumba** Lobaye, SW Central African Republic
Mongrove, Punta *see* Cayacal, Punta
83 G15 **Mongu** Western, W Zambia
76 I10 **Mônguel** Gorgol, SW Mauritania
Monguno *see* Mongonu
167 N4 **Möng Yai** Shan State, E Myanmar
167 O5 **Möng Yang** Shan State, E Myanmar
167 N3 **Möng Yu** Shan State, E Myanmar
162 K8 **Mönhbulag** Övörhangay, C Mongolia
Mönh Sarĭdag *see* Munku-Sardyk, Gora
186 F9 **Moni** ≈ S Papau New Guinea
115 I15 **Moní Megístis Lávras** *monastery* Kentrikí Makedonía, N Greece
115 F18 **Moní Osíou Loúkas** *monastery* Stereá Ellás, C Greece
54 F9 **Moniquirá** Boyacá, C Colombia
103 Q12 **Monistrol-sur-Loire** Haute-Loire, C France
35 V7 **Monitor Range** ▲ Nevada, W USA
115 I14 **Moní Vatopedíou** *monastery* Kentrikí Makedonía, N Greece
Monkchester *see* Newcastle upon Tyne
83 N14 **Monkey Bay** Southern, SE Malawi
43 N11 **Monkey Point** *var.* Punta Mico, Punte Mono, Punto Mico. *headland* SE Nicaragua
Monkey River *see* Monkey River Town
42 G3 **Monkey River Town** *var.* Monkey River. Toledo, SE Belize
14 M13 **Monkland** Ontario, SE Canada
79 J19 **Monkoto** Equateur, NW Dem. Rep. Congo (Zaire)
97 K21 **Monmouth** *Wel.* Trefynwy. SE Wales, UK
30 J12 **Monmouth** Illinois, N USA
32 F12 **Monmouth** Oregon, NW USA

◆ Country ● Country Capital ◇ Dependent Territory ○ Dependent Territory Capital ◈ Administrative Region ✕ International Airport ▲ Mountain ▲ Mountain Range ⊼ Volcano ≈ River ◎ Lake ⊟ Reservoir

97 K21 **Monmouth** *cultural region* SE Wales, UK
98 I10 **Monnickendam** Noord-Holland, C Netherlands
77 R15 **Mono** ≈ C Togo
Monoecus *see* Monaco
35 R8 **Mono Lake** ◎ California, W USA
115 O23 **Monólithos** Ródos, Dodekánisos, Greece, Aegean Sea
19 Q12 **Monomoy Island** *island* Massachusetts, NE USA
31 O12 **Monon** Indiana, N USA
29 Y12 **Monona** Iowa, C USA
30 L9 **Monona** Wisconsin, N USA
18 B15 **Monongahela** Pennsylvania, NE USA
18 B16 **Monongahela River** ≈ NE USA
107 P17 **Monopoli** Puglia, SE Italy
Mono, Punte *see* Monkey Point
111 K23 **Monor** Pest, C Hungary
Monostor *see* Beli Manastir
78 K8 **Monou** Borkou-Ennedi-Tibesti, NE Chad
105 S12 **Monóvar** País Valenciano, E Spain
105 R7 **Monreal del Campo** Aragón, NE Spain
107 I23 **Monreale** Sicilia, Italy, C Mediterranean Sea
23 T3 **Monroe** Georgia, SE USA
29 W14 **Monroe** Iowa, C USA
22 I5 **Monroe** Louisiana, S USA
31 S10 **Monroe** Michigan, N USA
18 K13 **Monroe** New York, NE USA
21 S11 **Monroe** North Carolina, SE USA
36 L6 **Monroe** Utah, W USA
32 H7 **Monroe** Washington, NW USA
30 L9 **Monroe** Wisconsin, N USA
27 V3 **Monroe City** Missouri, C USA
31 O15 **Monroe Lake** ⊡ Indiana, N USA
23 O7 **Monroeville** Alabama, S USA
18 C15 **Monroeville** Pennsylvania, NE USA
76 J16 **Monrovia** ● (Liberia) W Liberia
76 J16 **Monrovia** ✕ W Liberia
105 T7 **Monroyo** Aragón, NE Spain
99 F20 **Mons** *Dut.* Bergen. Hainaut, S Belgium
104 I8 **Monsanto** Castelo Branco, C Portugal
106 H8 **Monselice** Veneto, NE Italy
166 M9 **Mon State** ◈ *state* S Myanmar
98 G12 **Monster** Zuid-Holland, W Netherlands
95 N20 **Mönsterås** Kalmar, S Sweden
101 F17 **Montabaur** Rheinland-Pfalz, W Germany
106 G8 **Montagnana** Veneto, NE Italy
35 N1 **Montague** California, W USA
25 S5 **Montague** Texas, SW USA
183 S11 **Montague Island** *island* New South Wales, SE Australia
39 S12 **Montague Island** *island* Alaska, USA
39 S13 **Montague Strait** *strait* N Gulf of Alaska
102 J8 **Montaigu** Vendée, NW France
Montaigu *see* Scherpenheuvel
105 S7 **Montalbán** Aragón, NE Spain
106 G13 **Montalcino** Toscana, C Italy
104 H5 **Montalegre** Vila Real, N Portugal
114 G8 **Montana** *prev.* Ferdinand, Mikhaylovgrad. Montana, NW Bulgaria
108 D10 **Montana** Valais, SW Switzerland
39 R11 **Montana** Alaska, USA
114 G8 **Montana** ◈ *province* NW Bulgaria
33 T9 **Montana** *off.* State of Montana; *also known as* Mountain State, Treasure State. ◈ *state* NW USA
104 J10 **Montánchez** Extremadura, W Spain
Montañita *see* La Montañita
15 Q8 **Mont-Apica** Quebec, SE Canada
104 G10 **Montargil** Portalegre, C Portugal
104 G10 **Montargil, Barragem de** ⊡ C Portugal
103 O7 **Montargis** Loiret, C France
103 O4 **Montataire** Oise, N France
102 M14 **Montauban** Tarn-et-Garonne, S France
19 N14 **Montauk** Long Island, New York, NE USA
19 N14 **Montauk Point** *headland* Long Island, New York, NE USA
103 Q7 **Montbard** Côte d'Or, C France
103 U7 **Montbéliard** Doubs, E France
25 W11 **Mont Belvieu** Texas, SW USA
105 U6 **Montblanc** *var.* Montblanch. Cataluña, NE Spain
Montblanch *see* Montblanc
103 Q11 **Montbrison** Loire, E France
Montcalm, Lake *see* Dogai Coring
103 Q9 **Montceau-les-Mines** Saône-et-Loire, C France
103 U12 **Mont Cenis, Col du** *pass* E France
102 K15 **Mont-de-Marsan** Landes, SW France
103 O3 **Montdidier** Somme, N France
187 Q17 **Mont-Dore** Province Sud, S New Caledonia
20 K10 **Monteagle** Tennessee, S USA
57 M20 **Monteagudo** Chuquisaca, S Bolivia
41 R16 **Monte Albán** *ruins* Oaxaca, S Mexico
105 R11 **Montealegre del Castillo** Castilla-La Mancha, C Spain
59 N18 **Monte Azul** Minas Gerais, SE Brazil
14 M12 **Montebello** Quebec, SE Canada
106 H7 **Montebelluna** Veneto, NE Italy
60 G13 **Montecarlo** Misiones, NE Argentina
61 D16 **Monte Caseros** Corrientes, NE Argentina
60 J13 **Monte Castelo** Santa Catarina, S Brazil
106 F11 **Montecatini Terme** Toscana, C Italy
42 H7 **Montecillos, Cordillera de** ▲ W Honduras
62 I12 **Monte Comén** Mendoza, W Argentina
44 M8 **Monte Cristi** *var.* San Fernando de Monte Cristi. NW Dominican Republic
58 C13 **Monte Cristo** Amazonas, W Brazil
107 E14 **Montecristo, Isola di** *island* Archipelago Toscano, C Italy
Monte Croce Carnico, Passo di *see* Plöcken Pass
58 J12 **Monte Dourado** Pará, NE Brazil
40 L11 **Monte Escobedo** Zacatecas, C Mexico
106 I13 **Montefalco** Umbria, C Italy
107 H14 **Montefiascone** Lazio, C Italy
105 N14 **Montefrío** Andalucía, S Spain
44 I11 **Montego Bay** *var.* Mobay. W Jamaica
Montego Bay *see* Sangster
104 J8 **Montehermoso** Extremadura, W Spain
104 F10 **Montejunto, Serra de** ▲ C Portugal
Monteleone di Calabria *see* Vibo Valentia
54 E7 **Montelíbano** Córdoba, NW Colombia
103 R13 **Montélimar** *anc.* Acunum Acusio, Montilium Adhemari. Drôme, E France
104 K15 **Montellano** Andalucía, S Spain
35 Y2 **Montello** Nevada, W USA
30 L8 **Montello** Wisconsin, N USA
63 J18 **Montemayor, Meseta de** *plain* SE Argentina
41 O9 **Montemorelos** Nuevo León, NE Mexico
104 G11 **Montemor-o-Novo** Évora, S Portugal
104 G8 **Montemor-o-Velho** *var.* Montemor-o-Vélho. Coimbra, N Portugal
104 H7 **Montemuro, Serra de** ▲ N Portugal
102 K12 **Montendre** Charente-Maritime, W France
61 I15 **Montenegro** Rio Grande do Sul, S Brazil
113 J16 **Montenegro** *Serb.* Crna Gora. ◈ *republic* SW Yugoslavia
62 G10 **Monte Patria** Coquimbo, N Chile
45 O9 **Monte Plata** E Dominican Republic
83 P14 **Montepuez** Cabo Delgado, N Mozambique
83 P14 **Montepuez** ≈ N Mozambique
106 G13 **Montepulciano** Toscana, C Italy
62 L6 **Monte Quemado** Santiago del Estero, N Argentina
103 O6 **Montereau-Faut-Yonne** *anc.* Condate. Seine-St-Denis, N France
35 N11 **Monterey** California, W USA
20 L9 **Monterey** Tennessee, S USA
21 T5 **Monterey** Virginia, NE USA
Monterey *see* Monterrey
35 N10 **Monterey Bay** *bay* California, W USA
54 D6 **Montería** Córdoba, NW Colombia
57 N18 **Montero** Santa Cruz, C Bolivia
62 J7 **Monteros** Tucumán, C Argentina
104 I5 **Monterrei** Galicia, NW Spain
41 O8 **Monterrey** *var.* Monterey. Nuevo León, NE Mexico
32 F9 **Montesano** Washington, NW USA
107 M19 **Montesano sulla Marcellana** Campania, S Italy
107 N16 **Monte Sant' Angelo** Puglia, SE Italy
59 O16 **Monte Santo** Bahia, E Brazil
107 D18 **Monte Santu, Capo di** *headland* Sardegna, Italy, C Mediterranean Sea
59 M19 **Montes Claros** Minas Gerais, SE Brazil
107 K14 **Montesilvano Marina** Abruzzo, C Italy
23 P4 **Montevallo** Alabama, S USA
106 G12 **Montevarchi** Toscana, C Italy
29 S9 **Montevideo** Minnesota, N USA
61 F20 **Montevideo** ● (Uruguay) Montevideo, S Uruguay
37 S7 **Monte Vista** Colorado, C USA
23 T5 **Montezuma** Georgia, SE USA
29 W14 **Montezuma** Iowa, C USA
26 J6 **Montezuma** Kansas, C USA
103 U12 **Montgenèvre, Col de** *pass* France/Italy
97 K20 **Montgomery** E Wales, UK
23 Q5 **Montgomery** *state capital* Alabama, S USA
29 V9 **Montgomery** Minnesota, N USA
18 G13 **Montgomery** Pennsylvania, NE USA
21 Q5 **Montgomery** West Virginia, NE USA
97 K19 **Montgomery** *cultural region* E Wales, UK
Montgomery *see* Sāhīwāl
27 V4 **Montgomery City** Missouri, C USA
35 S8 **Montgomery Pass** *pass* Nevada, W USA
102 K12 **Montguyon** Charente-Maritime, W France
108 C10 **Monthey** Valais, SW Switzerland
27 V13 **Monticello** Arkansas, C USA
23 T4 **Monticello** Florida, SE USA
23 T8 **Monticello** Georgia, SE USA
30 M13 **Monticello** Illinois, N USA
31 O12 **Monticello** Indiana, N USA
29 Y13 **Monticello** Iowa, C USA
20 L7 **Monticello** Kentucky, S USA
29 V8 **Monticello** Minnesota, N USA
22 K7 **Monticello** Mississippi, S USA
27 V2 **Monticello** Missouri, C USA
18 J12 **Monticello** New York, NE USA
37 O7 **Monticello** Utah, W USA
106 F8 **Montichiari** Lombardia, N Italy
102 M12 **Montignac** Dordogne, SW France
99 G21 **Montignies-le-Tilleul** *var.* Montigny-le-Tilleul. Hainaut, S Belgium
14 J8 **Montigny, Lac de** ◎ Quebec, SE Canada
103 S6 **Montigny-le-Roi** Haute-Marne, N France
Montigny-le-Tilleul *see* Montignies-le-Tilleul
43 R16 **Montijo** Veraguas, S Panama
104 F11 **Montijo** Setúbal, W Portugal
104 J11 **Montijo** Extremadura, W Spain
Montilium Adhemari *see* Montélimar
104 M13 **Montilla** Andalucía, S Spain
102 L3 **Montivilliers** Seine-Maritime, N France
15 U7 **Mont-Joli** Quebec, SE Canada
14 M10 **Mont-Laurier** Quebec, SE Canada
15 X5 **Mont-Louis** Quebec, SE Canada
103 N17 **Mont-Louis** *var.* Mont Louis. Pyrénées-Orientales, S France
103 O10 **Montluçon** Allier, C France
15 R10 **Montmagny** Quebec, SE Canada
103 S3 **Montmédy** Meuse, NE France
103 P5 **Montmirail** Marne, N France
15 R9 **Montmorency** ≈ Quebec, SE Canada
102 M10 **Montmorillon** Vienne, W France
107 J14 **Montorio al Vomano** Abruzzo, C Italy
104 M13 **Montoro** Andalucía, S Spain
33 S16 **Montpelier** Idaho, NW USA
29 P6 **Montpelier** North Dakota, N USA
18 M7 **Montpelier** *state capital* Vermont, NE USA
103 Q15 **Montpellier** Hérault, S France
102 L12 **Montpon-Ménestérol** Dordogne, SW France
14 G8 **Montreal** ≈ Ontario, S Canada
14 C8 **Montreal** ≈ Ontario, S Canada
Montreal *see* Mirabel
12 K15 **Montréal** *Eng.* Montreal. Quebec, SE Canada
11 T14 **Montreal Lake** ◎ Saskatchewan, C Canada
14 B9 **Montreal River** Ontario, S Canada
103 N2 **Montreuil** Pas-de-Calais, N France
102 K8 **Montreuil-Bellay** Maine-et-Loire, NW France
108 C10 **Montreux** Vaud, SW Switzerland
108 B9 **Montricher** Vaud, W Switzerland
96 K10 **Montrose** E Scotland, UK
27 W14 **Montrose** Arkansas, C USA
37 Q6 **Montrose** Colorado, C USA
29 Y16 **Montrose** Iowa, C USA
18 H12 **Montrose** Pennsylvania, NE USA
21 X5 **Montross** Virginia, NE USA
15 O12 **Mont-St-Hilaire** Quebec, SE Canada
103 S3 **Mont-St-Martin** Meurthe-et-Moselle, NE France
45 V10 **Montserrat** *var.* Emerald Isle. ◇ *UK dependent territory* E West Indies
105 V5 **Montserrat** ▲ NE Spain
104 M7 **Montuenga** Castilla-León, N Spain
99 M19 **Montzen** Liège, E Belgium
37 N8 **Monument Valley** *valley* Arizona/Utah, SW USA
166 L4 **Monywa** Sagaing, C Myanmar
106 D7 **Monza** Lombardia, N Italy
83 J15 **Monze** Southern, S Zambia
105 T5 **Monzón** Aragón, NE Spain
25 T9 **Moody** Texas, SW USA
98 L13 **Mook** Limburg, SE Netherlands
165 O12 **Mooka** *var.* Mōka. Tochigi, Honshū, S Japan
182 K3 **Moomba** South Australia
14 G13 **Moon** ≈ Ontario, S Canada
Moon *see* Muhu
181 Y10 **Moonie** Queensland, E Australia
193 O5 **Moonless Mountains** *undersea feature* E Pacific Ocean
182 L13 **Moonlight Head** *headland* Victoria, SE Australia
Moon-Sund *see* Väinameri
182 H8 **Moonta** South Australia
Moor *see* Mór
180 I12 **Moora** Western Australia
98 H12 **Moordrecht** Zuid-Holland, C Netherlands
33 T9 **Moore** Montana, NW USA
27 N11 **Moore** Oklahoma, C USA
25 R12 **Moore** Texas, SW USA
191 S10 **Moorea** *island* Îles du Vent, W French Polynesia
21 U3 **Moorefield** West Virginia, NE USA
23 X14 **Moore Haven** Florida, SE USA
180 J11 **Moore, Lake** ◎ Western Australia
19 N7 **Moore Reservoir** ⊡ New Hampshire/Vermont, NE USA
44 G1 **Moores Island** *island* N Bahamas
21 R10 **Mooresville** North Carolina, SE USA
29 R5 **Moorhead** Minnesota, N USA
22 K4 **Moorhead** Mississippi, S USA
99 F18 **Moorsel** Oost-Vlaanderen, C Belgium
99 C18 **Moorslede** West-Vlaanderen, W Belgium
18 L8 **Moosalamoo, Mount** ▲ Vermont, NE USA
101 M22 **Moosburg** Bayern, SE Germany
33 S14 **Moose** Wyoming, C USA
12 H11 **Moose** ≈ Ontario, S Canada
12 H10 **Moose Factory** Ontario, S Canada
19 Q4 **Moosehead Lake** ◎ Maine, NE USA
11 U16 **Moose Jaw** Saskatchewan, S Canada
11 V14 **Moose Lake** Manitoba, C Canada
29 W6 **Moose Lake** Minnesota, N USA
19 P6 **Mooselookmeguntic Lake** ◎ Maine, NE USA
39 R12 **Moose Pass** Alaska, USA
19 P5 **Moose River** ≈ Maine, NE USA
18 J9 **Moose River** ≈ New York, NE USA
11 V16 **Moosomin** Saskatchewan, S Canada
12 H10 **Moosonee** Ontario, SE Canada
19 N12 **Moosup** Connecticut, NE USA
83 N16 **Mopeia** Zambézia, NE Mozambique
83 H18 **Mopipi** Central, C Botswana
Moppo *see* Mokp'o
77 N11 **Mopti** Mopti, C Mali
77 O11 **Mopti** ◈ *region* S Mali
57 H18 **Moquegua** Moquegua, SE Peru
57 H18 **Moquegua** *off.* Departamento de Moquegua. ◈ *department* S Peru
111 I23 **Mór** *Ger.* Moor. Fejér, C Hungary
78 G11 **Mora** Extrême-Nord, N Cameroon
104 G11 **Mora** Évora, S Portugal
105 N9 **Mora** Castilla-La Mancha, C Spain
94 L12 **Mora** Dalarna, C Sweden
29 V7 **Mora** Minnesota, N USA
37 T10 **Mora** New Mexico, SW USA
113 J17 **Morača** ≈ SW Yugoslavia
152 K10 **Morādābād** Uttar Pradesh, N India
105 U6 **Móra d'Ebre** *var.* Mora de Ebro. Cataluña, NE Spain
Mora de Ebro *see* Móra d'Ebre
105 S8 **Mora de Rubielos** Aragón, NE Spain
172 H4 **Morafenobe** Mahajanga, W Madagascar
110 K8 **Morąg** *Ger.* Mohrungen. Warmińsko-Mazurskie, NE Poland
111 L25 **Mórahalom** Csongrád, S Hungary
105 N11 **Moral de Calatrava** Castilla-La Mancha, C Spain
63 G19 **Moraleda, Canal** *strait* SE Pacific Ocean
54 J3 **Morales** Bolívar, N Colombia
54 D12 **Morales** Cauca, SW Colombia
42 F5 **Morales** Izabal, E Guatemala
172 J5 **Moramanga** Toamasina, E Madagascar
27 Q6 **Moran** Kansas, C USA
25 Q7 **Moran** Texas, SW USA
181 X7 **Moranbah** Queensland, NE Australia
44 L13 **Morant Bay** E Jamaica
96 G10 **Morar, Loch** ◎ N Scotland, UK
Morata *see* Goodenough Island
105 Q12 **Moratalla** Murcia, SE Spain
108 C8 **Morat, Lac de** *Ger.* Murtensee. ◎ W Switzerland
84 I11 **Morava** *var.* March. ≈ C Europe *see also* March
Morava *see* Moravia, Czech Republic
Morava *see* Velika Morava, Yugoslavia
29 W15 **Moravia** Iowa, C USA
111 F18 **Moravia** *Cz.* Morava, *Ger.* Mähren. *cultural region* E Czech Republic
111 H17 **Moravice** *Ger.* Mohra. ≈ NE Czech Republic
118 E12 **Moraviţa** Timiş, SW Romania
111 G17 **Moravská Třebová** *Ger.* Mährisch-Trübau. Pardubický Kraj, C Czech Republic
111 E19 **Moravské Budějovice** *Ger.* Mährisch-Budwitz. Jihlavský Kraj, C Czech Republic
111 F19 **Moravský Krumlov** *Ger.* Mährisch-Kromau. Brněnský Kraj, SE Czech Republic
96 J8 **Moray** *cultural region* N Scotland, UK
96 J8 **Moray Firth** *inlet* N Scotland, UK
42 B10 **Morazán** ◈ *department* NE El Salvador
154 C10 **Morbi** Gujarāt, W India
102 G7 **Morbihan** ◈ *department* NW France
Mörbisch *see* Mörbisch am See
109 Y5 **Mörbisch am See** *var.* Mörbisch. Burgenland, E Austria
95 N21 **Mörbylånga** Kalmar, S Sweden
102 J14 **Morcenx** Landes, SW France
Morcheh Khort *see* Mürcheh Khvort
11 X17 **Morden** Manitoba, S Canada
Mordovskaya ASSR/Mordvinia *see* Mordoviya, Respublika
129 N5 **Mordoviya, Respublika** *prev.* Mordovskaya ASSR, *Eng.* Mordovia, Mordvinia. ◈ *autonomous republic* W Russian Federation
128 M7 **Mordovo** Tambovskaya Oblast', W Russian Federation
Morea *see* Pelopónnisos
28 K8 **Moreau River** ≈ South Dakota, N USA
97 K16 **Morecambe** NW England, UK
97 K16 **Morecambe Bay** *inlet* NW England, UK
183 S4 **Moree** New South Wales, SE Australia
21 N5 **Morehead** Kentucky, S USA
21 X11 **Morehead City** North Carolina, SE USA
27 Y8 **Morehouse** Missouri, C USA
108 E10 **Mörel** Valais, SW Switzerland
54 D13 **Morelia** Caquetá, S Colombia
41 N14 **Morelia** Michoacán de Ocampo, S Mexico
105 T7 **Morella** País Valenciano, E Spain
40 I7 **Morelos** Chihuahua, N Mexico
41 O15 **Morelos** ◈ *state* S Mexico
154 H7 **Morena** Madhya Pradesh, C India
104 L12 **Morena, Sierra** ▲ S Spain
37 O14 **Morenci** Arizona, SW USA
31 R11 **Morenci** Michigan, N USA
116 J13 **Moreni** Dâmboviţa, S Romania
94 D9 **Møre og Romsdal** ◈ *county* S Norway
8 E13 **Moresby Island** *island* Queen Charlotte Islands, British Columbia, SW Canada
183 W2 **Moreton Island** *island* Queensland, E Australia
103 O3 **Moreuil** Somme, N France
35 V7 **Morey Peak** ▲ Nevada, W USA
127 U4 **More-Yu** ≈ NW Russian Federation
103 T9 **Morez** Jura, E France
Mórfou *see* Güzelyurt
Morfou Bay/Mórfou, Kólpos *see* Güzelyurt Körfezi
182 J8 **Morgan** South Australia
23 S7 **Morgan** Georgia, SE USA
25 S8 **Morgan** Texas, SW USA
22 J10 **Morgan City** Louisiana, S USA
20 H6 **Morganfield** Kentucky, S USA
35 O10 **Morgan Hill** California, W USA
21 Q9 **Morganton** North Carolina, SE USA
20 J7 **Morgantown** Kentucky, S USA
21 S2 **Morgantown** West Virginia, NE USA
108 B10 **Morges** Vaud, SW Switzerland
148 M4 **Morghāb, Daryā-ye** *var.* Murgab, Murghab, *Turkm.* Murgap Deryasy. ≈ Afghanistan/ Turkmenistan *see also* Murgab
Morghāb, Daryā-ye *see* Murgab
96 I9 **Mor, Glen** *var.* Glen Albyn, Great Glen. *valley* N Scotland, UK
103 T5 **Morhange** Moselle, NE France
158 M5 **Mori** *var.* Mori Kazak Zizhixian. Xinjiang Uygur Zizhiqu, NW China
165 R5 **Mori** Hokkaidō, NE Japan
35 Y6 **Moriah, Mount** ▲ Nevada, W USA
37 S11 **Moriarty** New Mexico, SW USA
54 J12 **Morichal** Guainía, E Colombia
Mori Kazak Zizhixian *see* Mori
163 U7 **Morin Dawa** *var.* Morin Dawa Daurzu Zizhiqi. Nei Mongol Zizhiqu, N China
Morin Dawa Daurzu Zizhiqi *see* Morin Dawa
8 J13 **Morinville** Alberta, SW Canada
165 R8 **Morioka** Iwate, Honshū, C Japan
183 T8 **Morisset** New South Wales, SE Australia
165 Q8 **Moriyoshi-yama** ▲ Honshū, C Japan
92 K13 **Morjärv** Norrbotten, N Sweden
129 R3 **Morki** Respublika Mariy El, W Russian Federation
123 N10 **Morkoka** ≈ NE Russian Federation
102 F5 **Morlaix** Finistère, NW France
95 M20 **Mörlunda** Kalmar, S Sweden
107 N19 **Mormanno** Calabria, SW Italy
36 L11 **Mormon Lake** ◎ Arizona, SW USA
35 Y10 **Mormon Peak** ▲ Nevada, W USA
Mormon State *see* Utah
45 Y5 **Morne-à-l'Eau** Grande Terre, N Guadeloupe
29 Y15 **Morning Sun** Iowa, C USA
193 S12 **Mornington Abyssal Plain** *undersea feature* SE Pacific Ocean
63 F22 **Mornington, Isla** *island* S Chile
181 T4 **Mornington Island** *island* Wellesley Islands, Queensland, N Australia
115 E18 **Mórnos** ≈ C Greece
149 P14 **Moro** Sind, SE Pakistan
32 I11 **Moro** Oregon, NW USA
186 E8 **Morobe** Morobe, C PNG
186 E8 **Morobe** ◈ *province* C PNG
31 N12 **Morocco** Indiana, N USA
74 E8 **Morocco** *off.* Kingdom of Morocco, *Ar.* Al Mamlakah. ◆ *monarchy* N Africa
Morocco *see* Marrakech
81 I22 **Morogoro** Morogoro, E Tanzania
81 H24 **Morogoro** ◈ *region* SE Tanzania
171 Q7 **Moro Gulf** *gulf* S Philippines
41 N13 **Moroleón** Guanajuato, C Mexico
172 H6 **Morombe** Toliara, W Madagascar
44 G5 **Morón** Ciego de Ávila, C Cuba
54 K5 **Morón** Carabobo, N Venezuela
Morón *see* Morón de la Frontera
163 N8 **Mörön** Hentiy, C Mongolia
162 I6 **Mörön** Hövsgöl, N Mongolia
56 D8 **Morona, Río** ≈ N Peru
56 C8 **Morona Santiago** ◈ *province* E Ecuador
172 H5 **Morondava** Toliara, W Madagascar
104 K14 **Morón de la Frontera** *var.* Morón. Andalucía, S Spain
172 G13 **Moroni** ● (Comoros) Grande Comore, NW Comoros
171 S10 **Morotai, Pulau** *island* Maluku, E Indonesia
Morotiri *see* Marotiri
81 H17 **Moroto** NE Uganda
Morozov *see* Bratan
128 M11 **Morozovsk** Rostovskaya Oblast', SW Russian Federation
97 L14 **Morpeth** N England, UK
Morphou *see* Güzelyurt
Morphou Bay *see* Güzelyurt Körfezi
28 I13 **Morrill** Nebraska, C USA
27 U11 **Morrilton** Arkansas, C USA
11 Q16 **Morrin** Alberta, SW Canada
184 M7 **Morrinsville** Waikato, North Island, NZ
11 X16 **Morris** Manitoba, S Canada
30 M11 **Morris** Illinois, N USA
29 S8 **Morris** Minnesota, N USA
14 M13 **Morrisburg** Ontario, SE Canada
197 R11 **Morris Jesup, Kap** *headland* N Greenland
182 B1 **Morris, Mount** ▲ South Australia
30 K10 **Morrison** Illinois, N USA
36 K13 **Morristown** Arizona, SW USA
18 J14 **Morristown** New Jersey, NE USA
21 O8 **Morristown** Tennessee, S USA
42 L11 **Morrito** Río San Juan, SW Nicaragua
35 P13 **Morro Bay** California, W USA
95 L22 **Mörrum** Blekinge, S Sweden
83 N16 **Morrumbala** Zambézia, NE Mozambique
83 N20 **Morrumbene** Inhambane, SE Mozambique
95 F21 **Mors** *island* NW Denmark
Mörs *see* Moers
25 N1 **Morse** Texas, SW USA
129 N6 **Morshansk** Tambovskaya Oblast', W Russian Federation
102 L5 **Mortagne-au-Perche** Orne, N France
102 J8 **Mortagne-sur-Sèvre** Vendée, NW France
104 G8 **Mortágua** Viseu, N Portugal
102 J5 **Mortain** Manche, N France
106 C8 **Mortara** Lombardia, N Italy
59 J17 **Mortes, Rio das** ≈ C Brazil
182 M12 **Mortlake** Victoria, SE Australia
Mortlock Group *see* Takuu Islands
189 Q17 **Mortlock Islands** *prev.* Nomoi Islands. *island group* C Micronesia
29 T9 **Morton** Minnesota, N USA
22 L5 **Morton** Mississippi, S USA
24 M5 **Morton** Texas, SW USA
32 H9 **Morton** Washington, NW USA
(0) D7 **Morton Seamount** *undersea feature* NE Pacific Ocean
45 U15 **Moruga** Trinidad, Trinidad and Tobago
183 P9 **Morundah** New South Wales, SE Australia
Moruroa *see* Mururoa
183 S11 **Moruya** New South Wales, SE Australia
103 Q8 **Morvan** *physical region* C France
185 G21 **Morven** Canterbury, South Island, NZ
183 O13 **Morwell** Victoria, SE Australia
127 N6 **Morzhovets, Ostrov** *island* NW Russian Federation
104 G4 **Mos** Galicia, NW Spain
128 J4 **Mosal'sk** Kaluzhskaya Oblast', W Russian Federation
101 H20 **Mosbach** Baden-Württemberg, SW Germany
95 E18 **Mosby** Vest-Agder, S Norway
33 V9 **Mosby** Montana, NW USA
32 M9 **Moscow** Idaho, NW USA
20 F10 **Moscow** Tennessee, S USA
Moscow *see* Moskva
101 D19 **Mosel** *Fr.* Moselle. ≈ W Europe *see also* Moselle
103 T4 **Moselle** ◈ *department* NE France
103 T6 **Moselle** *Ger.* Mosel. ≈ W Europe *see also* Mosel
32 K9 **Moses Lake** ◎ Washington, NW USA
83 I18 **Mosetse** Central, E Botswana
92 H4 **Mosfellsbær** Sudhurland, SW Iceland
185 F23 **Mosgiel** Otago, South Island, NZ
126 M11 **Mosha** ≈ NW Russian Federation
81 I20 **Moshi** Kilimanjaro, NE Tanzania
110 G12 **Mosina** Wielkolpolskie, C Poland
30 L6 **Mosinee** Wisconsin, N USA
92 F13 **Mosjøen** Nordland, C Norway
123 S12 **Moskal'vo** Ostrov Sakhalin, Sakhalinskaya Oblast', SE Russian Federation
92 I13 **Moskosel** Norrbotten, N Sweden
128 K4 **Moskovskaya Oblast'** ◈ *province* W Russian Federation
Moskovskiy *see* Moskva
128 J3 **Moskva** *Eng.* Moscow. ● (Russian Federation) Gorod Moskva, W Russian Federation
147 Q14 **Moskva** *Rus.* Moskovskiy; *prev.* Chubek. SW Tajikistan
128 L4 **Moskva** ≈ W Russian Federation
83 I20 **Mosomane** Kgatleng, SE Botswana
Moson and Magyaróvár *see* Mosonmagyaróvár
111 H21 **Mosoni-Duna** *Ger.* Kleine Donau. ≈ NW Hungary
111 H21 **Mosonmagyaróvár** *Ger.* Wieselburg-Ungarisch-Altenburg; *prev.* Moson and Magyaróvár, *Ger.* Wieselburg and Ungarisch-Altenburg. Győr-Moson-Sopron, NW Hungary

◆ Country ● Country Capital ◇ Dependent Territory ○ Dependent Territory Capital ◈ Administrative Region ✕ International Airport ▲ Mountain ▲ Mountain Range Volcano ≈ River ◎ Lake ⊡ Reservoir

Mospino see Mospyne
117 X8 **Mospyne** Rus. Mospino. Donets'ka Oblast', E Ukraine
54 B12 **Mosquera** Nariño, SW Colombia
37 U10 **Mosquero** New Mexico, SW USA
Mosquito Coast see La Mosquitia
31 U11 **Mosquito Creek Lake** ⊟ Ohio, N USA
Mosquito Gulf see Mosquitos, Golfo de los
23 X11 **Mosquito Lagoon** wetland Florida, SE USA
43 N10 **Mosquito, Punta** headland E Nicaragua
43 W14 **Mosquito, Punta** headland NE Panama
43 Q15 **Mosquitos, Golfo de los** Eng. Mosquito Gulf. gulf N Panama
95 H16 **Moss** Østfold, S Norway
Mossâmedes see Namibe
22 G8 **Moss Bluff** Louisiana, S USA
185 C23 **Mossburn** Southland, South Island, NZ
83 G26 **Mosselbaai** var. Mosselbai, Eng. Mossel Bay. Western Cape, SW South Africa
Mosselbaai/Mossel Bay see Mosselbaai
79 F20 **Mossendjo** Le Niari, SW Congo
183 N8 **Mossgiel** New South Wales, SE Australia
101 H22 **Mössingen** Baden-Württemberg, S Germany
181 W4 **Mossman** Queensland, NE Australia
59 P14 **Mossoró** Rio Grande do Norte, NE Brazil
23 N9 **Moss Point** Mississippi, S USA
183 S9 **Moss Vale** New South Wales, SE Australia
32 G9 **Mossyrock** Washington, NW USA
111 B15 **Most** Ger. Brüx. Ústecký Kraj, NW Czech Republic
121 P16 **Mosta** var. Musta. C Malta
74 I5 **Mostaganem** var. Mestghanem. NW Algeria
113 H14 **Mostar** Federacija Bosna I Hercegovina, S Bosnia and Herzegovina
61 J17 **Mostardas** Rio Grande do Sul, S Brazil
116 K14 **Mostiştea** ≈ S Romania
Mostva see Mastva
Mosty see Masty
116 H5 **Mostys'ka** L'vivs'ka Oblast', W Ukraine
Mosul see Al Mawşil
95 F15 **Møsvatnet** ◎ S Norway
80 J12 **Mot'a** Amhara, N Ethiopia
79 H16 **Motaba** ≈ N Congo
105 O10 **Mota del Cuervo** Castilla-La Mancha, C Spain
104 L5 **Mota del Marqués** Castilla-León, N Spain
42 F5 **Motagua, Río** ≈ Guatemala/Honduras
119 H19 **Motal'** Brestskaya Voblasts', SW Belarus
95 L17 **Motala** Östergötland, S Sweden
191 X7 **Motane** var. Mohotani. island Îles Marquises, NE French Polynesia
152 K13 **Moth** Uttar Pradesh, N India
Mother of Presidents/Mother of States see Virginia
96 I12 **Motherwell** C Scotland, UK
153 P12 **Motīhāri** Bihār, N India
105 Q10 **Motilla del Palancar** Castilla-La Mancha, C Spain
184 N7 **Motiti Island** island NE NZ
65 E25 **Motley Island** island SE Falkland Islands
83 J19 **Motloutse** ≈ E Botswana
41 V17 **Motozintla de Mendoza** Chiapas, SE Mexico
105 N15 **Motril** Andalucía, S Spain
116 G13 **Motru** Gorj, SW Romania
165 Q3 **Motsuta-misaki** headland Hokkaidō, NE Japan
28 L6 **Mott** North Dakota, N USA
Möttling see Metlika
107 O18 **Mottola** Puglia, SE Italy
184 P8 **Motu** ≈ North Island, NZ
185 I14 **Motueka** Tasman, South Island, NZ
185 I14 **Motueka** ≈ South Island, NZ
Motu Iti see Tupai
41 X12 **Motul** var. Motul de Felipe Carrillo Puerto. Yucatán, SE Mexico
Motul de Felipe Carrillo Puerto see Motul
191 U17 **Motu Nui** island Easter Island, Chile, E Pacific Ocean
191 Q10 **Motu One** var. Bellingshausen. atoll Îles Sous le Vent, W French Polynesia
190 I16 **Motutapu** island E Cook Islands
193 V15 **Motu Tapu** island Tongatapu Group, S Tonga
184 L5 **Motutapu Island** island N NZ
Motyca see Modica
Mouanda see Moanda
Mouaskar see Mascara
105 U3 **Moubermé, Tuc de** Fr. Pic de Maubermé, Sp. Pico Mauberme; prev. Tuc de Maubermé. ▲ France/Spain **see also** Maubermé, Pic de
45 N7 **Mouchoir Passage** passage SE Turks and Caicos Islands
76 I9 **Moudjéria** Tagant, SW Mauritania
108 C9 **Moudon** Vaud, W Switzerland
Mouhoun see Black Volta
79 E19 **Mouila** Ngounié, C Gabon
79 K14 **Mouka** Haute-Kotto, C Central African Republic
Moukden see Shenyang
183 N10 **Moulamein** New South Wales, SE Australia
Moulamein Creek see Billabong Creek
74 F6 **Moulay-Bousselham** NW Morocco
Moule see le Moule
80 M11 **Moulhoulé** N Djibouti
103 P9 **Moulins** Allier, C France
166 M9 **Moulmein** var. Maulmain, Mawlamyine. Mon State, S Myanmar
166 L8 **Moulmeingyun** Irrawaddy, SW Myanmar
74 G6 **Moulouya** var. Mulucha, Muluya, Mulwiya. seasonal river NE Morocco
23 O2 **Moulton** Alabama, S USA
29 W16 **Moulton** Iowa, C USA
25 T11 **Moulton** Texas, SW USA
23 T7 **Moultrie** Georgia, SE USA
21 S14 **Moultrie, Lake** ⊟ South Carolina, SE USA
22 K3 **Mound Bayou** Mississippi, S USA
30 L17 **Mound City** Illinois, N USA
27 R6 **Mound City** Kansas, C USA
27 Q2 **Mound City** Missouri, C USA
29 N7 **Mound City** South Dakota, N USA
78 H13 **Moundou** Logone-Occidental, SW Chad
27 P10 **Mounds** Oklahoma, C USA
21 R2 **Moundsville** West Virginia, NE USA
167 Q12 **Moŭng Roessei** Bătdâmbâng, W Cambodia
Moun Hou see Black Volta
8 H8 **Mountain** ≈ Northwest Territories, NW Canada
37 S12 **Mountainair** New Mexico, SW USA
35 V1 **Mountain City** Nevada, W USA
21 Q8 **Mountain City** Tennessee, S USA
27 U7 **Mountain Grove** Missouri, C USA
27 U9 **Mountain Home** Arkansas, C USA
33 N15 **Mountain Home** Idaho, NW USA
25 Q11 **Mountain Home** Texas, SW USA
29 W4 **Mountain Iron** Minnesota, N USA
29 T10 **Mountain Lake** Minnesota, N USA
23 S3 **Mountain Park** Georgia, SE USA
35 W12 **Mountain Pass** pass California, W USA
27 T12 **Mountain Pine** Arkansas, C USA
39 Y14 **Mountain Point** Annette Island, Alaska, USA
Mountain State see Montana, USA
Mountain State see West Virginia, USA
27 V7 **Mountain View** Arkansas, C USA
38 H12 **Mountain View** Hawaii, USA, C Pacific Ocean
27 V10 **Mountain View** Missouri, C USA
38 M11 **Mountain Village** Alaska, USA
21 R8 **Mount Airy** North Carolina, SE USA
83 K24 **Mount Ayliff** Xh. Maxesibebi. Eastern Cape, SE South Africa
29 U16 **Mount Ayr** Iowa, C USA
182 J9 **Mount Barker** South Australia
180 J14 **Mount Barker** Western Australia
183 P11 **Mount Beauty** Victoria, SE Australia
14 E16 **Mount Brydges** Ontario, S Canada
31 N16 **Mount Carmel** Illinois, N USA
30 K10 **Mount Carroll** Illinois, N USA
31 S9 **Mount Clemens** Michigan, N USA
185 E19 **Mount Cook** Canterbury, South Island, NZ
83 L16 **Mount Darwin** Mashonaland Central, NE Zimbabwe
19 S7 **Mount Desert Island** island Maine, NE USA
23 W11 **Mount Dora** Florida, SE USA
182 G5 **Mount Eba** South Australia
25 W8 **Mount Enterprise** Texas, SW USA
182 J4 **Mount Fitton** South Australia
83 J24 **Mount Fletcher** Eastern Cape, SE South Africa
14 F15 **Mount Forest** Ontario, S Canada
182 K12 **Mount Gambier** South Australia
181 W5 **Mount Garnet** Queensland, NE Australia
21 P6 **Mount Gay** West Virginia, NE USA
31 S12 **Mount Gilead** Ohio, N USA
186 C7 **Mount Hagen** Western Highlands, C PNG
18 J16 **Mount Holly** New Jersey, NE USA
21 R10 **Mount Holly** North Carolina, SE USA
27 T12 **Mount Ida** Arkansas, C USA
181 T6 **Mount Isa** Queensland, C Australia
21 U4 **Mount Jackson** Virginia, NE USA
18 D12 **Mount Jewett** Pennsylvania, NE USA
18 L13 **Mount Kisco** New York, NE USA
18 B15 **Mount Lebanon** Pennsylvania, NE USA
182 J8 **Mount Lofty Ranges** ▲ South Australia
180 J10 **Mount Magnet** Western Australia
184 N7 **Mount Maunganui** Bay of Plenty, North Island, NZ
97 E18 **Mountmellick** Ir. Móinteach Mílic. C Ireland
30 L10 **Mount Morris** Illinois, N USA
31 R9 **Mount Morris** Michigan, N USA
18 F10 **Mount Morris** New York, NE USA
18 B16 **Mount Morris** Pennsylvania, NE USA
30 K15 **Mount Olive** Illinois, N USA
21 V10 **Mount Olive** North Carolina, SE USA
21 N4 **Mount Olivet** Kentucky, S USA
29 Y15 **Mount Pleasant** Iowa, C USA
31 Q8 **Mount Pleasant** Michigan, N USA
18 C15 **Mount Pleasant** Pennsylvania, NE USA
21 T14 **Mount Pleasant** South Carolina, SE USA
20 I9 **Mount Pleasant** Tennessee, S USA
25 W6 **Mount Pleasant** Texas, SW USA
36 L4 **Mount Pleasant** Utah, W USA
63 N23 **Mount Pleasant** ✕ (Stanley) East Falkland, Falkland Islands
97 G25 **Mount's Bay** inlet SW England, UK
35 N2 **Mount Shasta** California, W USA
30 J13 **Mount Sterling** Illinois, N USA
21 N5 **Mount Sterling** Kentucky, S USA
18 E15 **Mount Union** Pennsylvania, NE USA
23 V6 **Mount Vernon** Georgia, SE USA
30 L16 **Mount Vernon** Illinois, N USA
20 M6 **Mount Vernon** Kentucky, S USA
27 S7 **Mount Vernon** Missouri, C USA
31 T13 **Mount Vernon** Ohio, N USA
32 K13 **Mount Vernon** Oregon, NW USA
25 W6 **Mount Vernon** Texas, SW USA
32 H7 **Mount Vernon** Washington, NW USA
20 L5 **Mount Washington** Kentucky, S USA
182 F8 **Mount Wedge** South Australia
30 L14 **Mount Zion** Illinois, N USA
181 Y9 **Moura** Queensland, NE Australia
58 F12 **Moura** Amazonas, NW Brazil
104 H12 **Moura** Beja, S Portugal
104 I12 **Mourão** Évora, S Portugal
76 L11 **Mourdiah** Koulikoro, W Mali
78 K7 **Mourdi, Dépression du** desert lowland Chad/Sudan
102 J16 **Mourenx** Pyrénées-Atlantiques, SW France
Mourgana see Mourgkána
115 C15 **Mourgkána** var. Mourgana. ▲ Albania/Greece
97 G16 **Mourne Mountains** Ir. Beanna Boirche. ▲ SE Northern Ireland, UK
115 I15 **Moúrtzeflos, Akrotírio** headland Límnos, E Greece
99 C19 **Mouscron** Dut. Moeskroen. Hainaut, W Belgium
Mouse River see Souris River
78 H10 **Moussoro** Kanem, W Chad
103 T11 **Moûtiers** Savoie, E France
172 J14 **Moutsamoudou** var. Mutsamudu. Anjouan, SE Comoros
74 K11 **Mouydir, Monts de** ▲ S Algeria
79 F20 **Mouyondzi** La Bouenza, S Congo
115 E16 **Mouzáki** prev. Mouzákion. Thessalía, C Greece
Mouzákion see Mouzáki
29 S13 **Moville** Iowa, C USA
82 E13 **Moxico** ◈ province E Angola
172 I14 **Moya** Anjouan, SE Comoros
40 L12 **Moyahua** Zacatecas, C Mexico
81 J16 **Moyalē** Oromo, C Ethiopia
76 I15 **Moyamba** W Sierra Leone
74 G7 **Moyen Atlas** Eng. Middle Atlas. ▲ N Morocco
78 H13 **Moyen-Chari** off. Préfecture du Moyen-Chari. ◈ prefecture S Chad
Moyen-Congo see Congo (Republic of)
83 J24 **Moyeni** var. Quthing. SW Lesotho
76 H13 **Moyenne-Guinée** ◈ state NW Guinea
79 D18 **Moyen-Ogooué** off. Province du Moyen-Ogooué, var. Le Moyen-Ogooué. ◈ province C Gabon
103 S4 **Moyeuvre-Grande** Moselle, NE France
33 N7 **Moyie Springs** Idaho, NW USA
145 S15 **Moynkum** prev. Fumanovka, Kaz. Fūrmanov. Zhambyl, S Kazakhstan
81 F16 **Moyo** NW Uganda
56 D10 **Moyobamba** San Martín, NW Peru
78 H10 **Moyto** Chari-Baguirmi, W Chad
158 G9 **Moyu** var. Karakax. Xinjiang Uygur Zizhiqu, NW China
122 M9 **Moyyero** ≈ N Russian Federation
145 Q15 **Moyynkum, Peski** Kaz. Moyynqum. desert S Kazakhstan
Moyynqum see Moyynkum, Peski
145 S12 **Moyynty** Zhezkazgan, C Kazakhstan
145 S12 **Moyynty** ≈ C Kazakhstan
Mozambika, Lakandranon' i see Mozambique Channel
83 M18 **Mozambique** off. Republic of Mozambique; prev. People's Republic of Mozambique, Portuguese East Africa. ◆ republic S Africa
Mozambique Basin see Natal Basin
Mozambique, Canal de see Mozambique Channel
83 P17 **Mozambique Channel** Fr. Canal de Mozambique, Mal. Lakandranon' i Mozambika. strait W Indian Ocean
172 L11 **Mozambique Escarpment** var. Mozambique Scarp. undersea feature SW Indian Ocean
172 L10 **Mozambique Plateau** var. Mozambique Rise. undersea feature SW Indian Ocean
Mozambique Rise see Mozambique Plateau
Mozambique Scarp see Mozambique Escarpment
129 O15 **Mozdok** Respublika Severnaya Osetiya, SW Russian Federation
57 K17 **Mozetenes, Serranías de** ▲ C Bolivia
128 J4 **Mozhaysk** Moskovskaya Oblast', W Russian Federation
129 T3 **Mozhga** Udmurtskaya Respublika, NW Russian Federation
Mozyr' see Mazyr
79 P22 **Mpala** Katanga, E Dem. Rep. Congo (Zaire)
79 G19 **Mpama** ≈ C Congo
81 E22 **Mpanda** Rukwa, W Tanzania
82 L11 **Mpande** Northern, NE Zambia
83 J18 **Mphoengs** Matabeleland South, SW Zimbabwe
81 F18 **Mpigi** S Uganda
82 L13 **Mpika** Northern, NE Zambia
83 J14 **Mpima** Central, C Zambia
82 J13 **Mpongwe** Copperbelt, C Zambia
82 K11 **Mporokoso** Northern, N Zambia
79 H20 **Mpouya** Plateaux, SE Congo
77 P16 **Mpraeso** C Ghana
82 L11 **Mpulungu** Northern, N Zambia
83 K21 **Mpumalanga** prev. Eastern Transvaal, Afr. Oos-Transvaal. ◈ province NE South Africa
83 D16 **Mpungu** Okavango, N Namibia
81 I22 **Mpwapwa** Dodoma, C Tanzania
Mqinvartsveri see Kazbek
110 M8 **Mrągowo** Ger. Sensburg. Warmińsko-Mazurskie, NE Poland,
129 V6 **Mrakovo** Respublika Bashkortostan, W Russian Federation
172 I13 **Mramani** Anjouan, E Comoros
112 F12 **Mrkonjić Grad** Republika Srpska, W Bosnia and Herzegovina
110 H9 **Mrocza** Kujawsko-pomorskie, NW Poland
126 I14 **Msta** ≈ NW Russian Federation
Mtkvari see Kura
Mtoko see Mutoko
128 K6 **Mtsensk** Orlovskaya Oblast', W Russian Federation
81 K24 **Mtwara** Mtwara, SE Tanzania
81 J25 **Mtwara** ◈ region SE Tanzania
104 G14 **Mu** ▲ S Portugal
193 V15 **Mu'a** Tongatapu, S Tonga
Muai To see Mae Hong Son
83 P16 **Mualama** Zambézia, NE Mozambique
Mualo see Messalo, Rio
79 E22 **Muanda** Bas-Congo, SW Dem. Rep. Congo (Zaire)
Muang Chiang Rai see Chiang Rai
167 R6 **Muang Ham** Houaphan, N Laos
167 S8 **Muang Hinboun** Khammouan, C Laos
Muang Kalasin see Kalasin
Muang Khammouan see Thakhèk
167 S11 **Muang Không** Champasak, S Laos
167 S10 **Muang Khôngxédôn** var. Khong Sedone. Salavan, S Laos
Muang Khon Kaen see Khon Kaen
167 Q6 **Muang Khoua** Phôngsali, N Laos
Muang Krabi see Krabi
Muang Lampang see Lampang
Muang Lamphun see Lamphun
Muang Loei see Loei
Muang Lom Sak see Lom Sak
Muang Nakhon Sawan see Nakhon Sawan
167 Q6 **Muang Namo** Oudômxai, N Laos
Muang Nan see Nan
167 Q6 **Muang Ngoy** Louangphabang, N Laos
167 Q5 **Muang Ou Tai** Phôngsali, N Laos
Muang Pak Lay see Pak Lay
Muang Pakxan see Pakxan
167 T10 **Muang Pakxong** Champasak, S Laos
167 S9 **Muang Phalan** var. Muang Phalane. Savannakhét, S Laos
Muang Phalane see Muang Phalan
Muang Phan see Phan
Muang Phayao see Phayao
Muang Phichit see Phichit
167 T9 **Muang Phin** Savannakhét, S Laos
Muang Phitsanulok see Phitsanulok
Muang Phrae see Phrae
Muang Roi Et see Roi Et
Muang Sakon Nakhon see Sakon Nakhon
Muang Samut Prakan see Samut Prakan
167 P6 **Muang Sing** Louang Namtha, N Laos
Muang Ubon see Ubon Ratchathani
Muang Uthai Thani see Uthai Thani
167 P7 **Muang Vangviang** Viangchan, C Laos
Muang Xaignabouri see Xaignabouli
Muang Xay see Xai
167 S9 **Muang Xépôn** var. Sepone. Savannakhét, S Laos
168 K10 **Muar** var. Bandar Maharani. Johor, Peninsular Malaysia
168 I9 **Muara** Sumatera, W Indonesia
168 L13 **Muarabeliti** Sumatera, W Indonesia
168 K12 **Muarabungo** Sumatera, W Indonesia
168 L13 **Muaraenim** Sumatera, W Indonesia
169 T11 **Muarajuloi** Borneo, C Indonesia
169 U12 **Muarakaman** Borneo, C Indonesia
168 H12 **Muarasigep** Pulau Siberut, W Indonesia
168 L12 **Muaratembesi** Sumatera, W Indonesia
169 T12 **Muaratewe** var. Muarateweh; prev. Moearatewe. Borneo, C Indonesia
Muarateweh see Muaratewe
169 U10 **Muarawahau** Borneo, N Indonesia
138 G13 **Mubārak, Jabal** ▲ S Jordan
153 N13 **Mubārakpur** Uttar Pradesh, N India
Mubarek see Muborak
81 F18 **Mubende** SW Uganda
77 Y14 **Mubi** Adamawa, NE Nigeria
146 M12 **Muborak** Rus. Mubarek. Qashqadaryo Wiloyati, S Uzbekistan
171 U12 **Mubrani** Irian Jaya, E Indonesia
67 U12 **Muchinga Escarpment** escarpment NE Zambia
129 N7 **Muchkapskiy** Tambovskaya Oblast', W Russian Federation
96 G10 **Muck** island W Scotland, UK
82 Q13 **Mucojo** Cabo Delgado, N Mozambique
82 F12 **Muconda** Lunda Sul, NE Angola
54 I10 **Muco, Río** ≈ E Colombia
83 O16 **Mucubela** Zambézia, NE Mozambique
42 J5 **Mucupina, Monte** ▲ N Honduras
136 J14 **Mucur** Kirşehir, C Turkey
143 U8 **Mūd** Khorāsān, E Iran
163 Y9 **Mudanjiang** var. Mu-tan-chiang. Heilongjiang, NE China
163 Y9 **Mudan Jiang** ≈ NE China
136 D11 **Mudanya** Bursa, NW Turkey
28 K8 **Mud Butte** South Dakota, N USA
155 G16 **Muddebihāl** Karnātaka, C India
27 P12 **Muddy Boggy Creek** ≈ Oklahoma, C USA
36 M6 **Muddy Creek** ≈ Utah, W USA
37 V7 **Muddy Creek Reservoir** ⊟ Colorado, C USA
33 W15 **Muddy Gap** Wyoming, C USA
35 Y11 **Muddy Peak** ▲ Nevada, W USA
183 R7 **Mudgee** New South Wales, SE Australia
29 S3 **Mud Lake** ◎ Minnesota, N USA
29 P7 **Mud Lake Reservoir** ⊟ South Dakota, N USA
167 N9 **Mudon** Mon State, S Myanmar
81 O14 **Mudug** off. Gobolka Mudug. ◈ region NE Somalia
81 O14 **Mudug** var. Mudugh. plain N Somalia
Mudugh see Mudug
83 Q15 **Muecate** Nampula, NE Mozambique
82 Q13 **Mueda** Cabo Delgado, NE Mozambique
42 L10 **Muelle de los Bueyes** Región Autónoma Atlántico Sur, SE Nicaragua
Muenchen see München
83 M14 **Muende** Tete, NW Mozambique
25 T5 **Muenster** Texas, SW USA
Muenster see Münster
43 O6 **Muerto, Cayo** reef NE Nicaragua
41 T17 **Muerto, Mar** lagoon SE Mexico
64 F11 **Muertos Trough** undersea feature N Caribbean Sea
83 H14 **Mufaya Kuta** Western, NW Zambia
82 J13 **Mufulira** Copperbelt, C Zambia
161 O10 **Mufu Shan** ▲ C China
Mugalzhar Taūlary see Mugodzhary, Gory
137 Y12 **Muğan Düzü** Rus. Muganskaya Ravnina, Muganskaya Step'. physical region S Azerbaijan
Muganskaya Ravnina/Muganskaya Step' see Muğan Düzü
106 K8 **Múggia** Friuli-Venezia Giulia, NE Italy
153 N14 **Mughal Sarāi** Uttar Pradesh, N India
Mughla see Muğla
141 W11 **Mughshin** var. Muqshin. S Oman
147 S12 **Mughsu** Rus. Muksu. ≈ C Tajikistan
164 H14 **Mugi** Tokushima, Shikoku, SW Japan
136 C16 **Muğla** var. Mughla. Muğla, SW Turkey
136 C16 **Muğla** var. Mughla. ◈ province SW Turkey
144 J11 **Mugodzhary, Gory** Kaz. Mugalzhar Taūlary. ▲ W Kazakhstan
83 O15 **Mugulama** Zambézia, NE Mozambique
139 U9 **Muḩammad** E Iraq
139 R8 **Muḩammadīyah** C Iraq
80 I6 **Muhammad Qol** Red Sea, NE Sudan
75 Y9 **Muhammad, Râs** headland E Egypt
Muhammerah see Khorramshahr
140 M12 **Muhāyil** var. Mahāil. 'Asīr, SW Saudi Arabia
139 O7 **Muḩaywir** W Iraq
101 H21 **Mühlacker** Baden-Württemberg, SW Germany
Mühlbach see Sebeş
Mühldorf see Mühldorf am Inn
101 N23 **Mühldorf am Inn** var. Mühldorf. Bayern, SE Germany
101 J15 **Mühlhausen** var. Mühlhausen in Thüringen. Thüringen, C Germany
Mühlhausen in Thüringen see Mühlhausen
195 Q2 **Mühlig-Hofmann Mountains** ▲ Antarctica
93 L14 **Muhos** Oulu, C Finland
138 K6 **Muḩ, Sabkhat al** ◎ C Syria
118 E5 **Muhu** Ger. Mohn, Moon. island W Estonia
81 F19 **Muhutwe** Kagera, NW Tanzania
Muhu Väin see Väinameri
98 J10 **Muiden** Noord-Holland, C Netherlands
193 W15 **Mui Hopohoponga** headland Tongatapu, S Tonga
Muikamachi see Muika
Muinchille see Cootehill
Muineachán see Monaghan
97 F19 **Muine Bheag** Eng. Bagenalstown. SE Ireland
56 B5 **Muisne** Esmeraldas, NW Ecuador
83 P14 **Muite** Nampula, NE Mozambique
41 Z11 **Mujeres, Isla** island E Mexico
116 G7 **Mukacheve** Hung. Munkács, Rus. Mukachevo. Zakarpats'ka Oblast', W Ukraine
Mukachevo see Mukacheve
169 R9 **Mukah** Sarawak, East Malaysia
Mukalla see Al Mukallā
Mukama see Mokāma
Mukāshafa/Mukashshafah see Mukayshīfah
139 S6 **Mukayshīfah** var. Mukāshafa, Mukashshafah. N Iraq
167 R9 **Mukdahan** Mukdahan, E Thailand
Mukden see Shenyang
165 Y15 **Mukojima-rettō** Eng. Parry group. island group SE Japan
146 M14 **Mukry** Lebapskiy Velayat, E Turkmenistan
Muksu see Mughsu
153 U14 **Muktagacha** var. Muktagachha Dhaka, N Bangladesh
Muktagachha see Muktagacha
82 K13 **Mukuku** Central, C Zambia
82 K11 **Mukupa Kaoma** Northern, NE Zambia
81 I18 **Mukutan** Rift Valley, W Kenya
83 F16 **Mukwe** Caprivi, NE Namibia
105 R13 **Mula** Murcia, SE Spain
151 K20 **Mulaku Atoll** var. Meemu Atoll. atoll C Maldives
83 J15 **Mulalika** Lusaka, C Zambia
163 X8 **Mulan** Heilongjiang, NE China
83 N15 **Mulanje** var. Mlanje. Southern, S Malawi
40 H5 **Mulatos** Sonora, NW Mexico
23 P3 **Mulberry Fork** ≈ Alabama, S USA
39 P12 **Mulchatna River** ≈ Alaska, USA
127 W4 **Mul'da** Respublika Komi, NW Russian Federation
101 M14 **Mulde** ≈ E Germany
27 R10 **Muldrow** Oklahoma, C USA
40 E7 **Mulegé** Baja California Sur, W Mexico
108 I10 **Mulegns** Graubünden, S Switzerland
79 M21 **Mulenda** Kasai Oriental, C Dem. Rep. Congo (Zaire)
24 M4 **Muleshoe** Texas, SW USA
83 O15 **Mulevala** Zambézia, NE Mozambique
183 P5 **Mulgoa Creek** seasonal river New South Wales, SE Australia
105 O15 **Mulhacén** var. Cerro de Mulhacén. ▲ S Spain
Mulhacén, Cerro de see Mulhacén
Mülhausen see Mulhouse
101 E24 **Mülheim** Baden-Württemberg, SW Germany
101 E15 **Mülheim** var. Mulheim an der Ruhr. Nordrhein-Westfalen, W Germany
Mulheim an der Ruhr see Mülheim
103 U7 **Mulhouse** Ger. Mülhausen. Haut-Rhin, NE France
160 G11 **Muli** var. Bowa, Muli Zangzu Zizhixian. Sichuan, C China
171 X15 **Muli** channel Irian Jaya, E Indonesia
163 Y9 **Muling** Heilongjiang, NE China
Mullach Íde see Malahide
Mullaitivu see Mullaittivu
155 K23 **Mullaittivu** var. Mullaitivu. Northern Province, N Sri Lanka
33 N8 **Mullan** Idaho, NW USA
28 M13 **Mullen** Nebraska, C USA
183 Q6 **Mullengudgery** New South Wales, SE Australia
21 Q6 **Mullens** West Virginia, NE USA
Müller-gerbergte see Muller, Pegunungan
169 T10 **Muller, Pegunungan** Dut. Müller-gerbergte. ▲ Borneo, C Indonesia
31 Q5 **Mullett Lake** ◎ Michigan, N USA
18 J16 **Mullica River** ≈ New Jersey, NE USA
25 R8 **Mullin** Texas, SW USA
97 E17 **Mullingar** Ir. An Muileann gCearr. C Ireland
21 T12 **Mullins** South Carolina, SE USA
96 G11 **Mull, Isle of** island W Scotland, UK
129 R5 **Mullovka** Ul'yanovskaya Oblast', W Russian Federation
95 K19 **Mullsjö** Västra Götaland, S Sweden
183 V4 **Mullumbimby** New South Wales, SE Australia
83 H15 **Mulobezi** Western, SW Zambia
83 C15 **Mulondo** Huíla, SW Angola
83 G15 **Mulonga Plain** plain W Zambia
79 N23 **Mulongo** Katanga, SE Dem. Rep. Congo (Zaire)
149 T10 **Multān** Punjab, E Pakistan
93 L17 **Multia** Länsi-Suomi, W Finland
Mulucha see Moulouya
83 J14 **Mulungushi** Central, C Zambia
83 K14 **Mulungwe** Central, C Zambia
Muluya see Moulouya
27 N7 **Mulvane** Kansas, C USA
183 O10 **Mulwala** New South Wales, SE Australia
Mulwiya see Moulouya
182 K6 **Mulyungarie** South Australia
154 D13 **Mumbai** prev. Bombay. Mahārāshtra, W India
154 D13 **Mumbai** ✕ Mahārāshtra, W India

◆ Country ● Country Capital ◇ Dependent Territory ○ Dependent Territory Capital ◈ Administrative Region ✕ International Airport ▲ Mountain ▲ Mountain Range Volcano ≈ River ◎ Lake ⊟ Reservoir

83 D14 **Mumbué** Bié, C Angola
186 E8 **Mumeng** Morobe, C PNG
171 V12 **Mumi** Irian Jaya, E Indonesia
Muminabad/Mŭ'minobod see Leningrad
129 Q13 **Mumra** Astrakhanskaya Oblast', SW Russian Federation
41 X12 **Muna** Yucatán, SE Mexico
123 O9 **Muna** ≈ NE Russian Federation
152 C12 **Munābāo** Rājasthān, NW India
Munamägi see Suur Munamägi
171 O14 **Muna, Pulau** prev. Moena. island C Indonesia
101 L18 **Münchberg** Bayern, E Germany
101 L23 **München** var. Muenchen, Eng. Munich, It. Monaco. Bayern, SE Germany
München-Gladbach see Mönchengladbach
108 E6 **Münchenstein** Basel-Land, NW Switzerland
10 L10 **Muncho Lake** British Columbia, W Canada
31 P13 **Muncie** Indiana, N USA
18 G13 **Muncy** Pennsylvania, NE USA
11 Q14 **Mundare** Alberta, SW Canada
25 Q5 **Munday** Texas, SW USA
31 N10 **Mundelein** Illinois, N USA
101 I15 **Münden** Niedersachsen, C Germany
105 Q12 **Mundo** ≈ S Spain
82 B12 **Munenga** Cuanza Sul, NW Angola
105 P11 **Munera** Castilla-La Mancha, C Spain
20 E9 **Munford** Tennessee, S USA
20 K7 **Munfordville** Kentucky, S USA
182 D5 **Mungala** South Australia
83 M16 **Mungári** Manica, C Mozambique
79 O16 **Mungbere** Orientale, NE Dem. Rep. Congo (Zaire)
153 Q13 **Munger** prev. Monghyr. Bihār, NE India
182 I2 **Mungeranie** South Australia
Mu Nggava see Rennell
169 O10 **Mungguresak, Tanjung** headland Borneo, N Indonesia
Mungiki see Bellona
183 R4 **Mungindi** New South Wales, SE Australia
Mungkawn see Maingkwan
153 T16 **Mungla** var. Mongla. Khulna, S Bangladesh
82 C13 **Mungo** Huambo, W Angola
188 F16 **Munguuy Bay** bay Yap, W Micronesia
82 E13 **Munhango** Bié, C Angola
Munich see München
105 S7 **Muniesa** Aragón, NE Spain
31 O4 **Munising** Michigan, N USA
Munkács see Mukacheve
95 I17 **Munkedal** Västra Götaland, S Sweden
95 K15 **Munkfors** Värmland, C Sweden
122 M14 **Munku-Sardyk, Gora** var. Mönh Sarĭdag. ▲ Mongolia/Russian Federation
99 E18 **Munkzwalm** Oost-Vlaanderen, NW Belgium
167 R10 **Mun, Mae Nam** ≈ E Thailand
153 U15 **Munshiganj** Dhaka, C Bangladesh
108 D8 **Münsingen** Bern, W Switzerland
103 U6 **Munster** Haut-Rhin, NE France
100 J11 **Munster** Niedersachsen, NW Germany
97 B20 **Munster** Ir. Cúige Mumhan. cultural region S Ireland
100 F13 **Münster** var. Muenster, Münster in Westfalen. Nordrhein-Westfalen, W Germany
108 F10 **Münster** Valais, S Switzerland
Münsterberg in Schlesien see Ziębice
Münster in Westfalen see Münster
100 E13 **Münsterland** cultural region NW Germany
100 F13 **Münster-Osnabruck** ✕ Nordrhein-Westfalen, NW Germany
31 R4 **Munuscong Lake** ⊚ Michigan, N USA
83 K17 **Munyati** ≈ C Zimbabwe
109 R3 **Münzkirchen** Oberösterreich, N Austria
92 K11 **Muodoslompolo** Norrbotten, N Sweden
92 M13 **Muojärvi** ⊚ NE Finland
167 S6 **Mương Khên** Hoa Binh, N Vietnam
Muong Sai see Xai
167 Q7 **Muong Xiang Ngeun** var. Xieng Ngeun. Louangphabang, N Laos
92 K11 **Muonio** Lappi, N Finland
Muonioälv/Muoniojoki see Muonionjoki
92 K11 **Muonionjoki** var. Muoniojoki, Swe. Muonioälv. ≈ Finland/Sweden
83 N17 **Mupa** ≈ C Mozambique
83 E16 **Mupini** Okavango, NE Namibia
80 F8 **Muqaddam, Wadi** ≈ N Sudan
138 K9 **Muqāţ** Al Mafraq, E Jordan
141 X7 **Muqaz** N Oman
81 N17 **Muqdisho** Eng. Mogadishu, It. Mogadiscio. ● (Somalia) Banaadir, S Somalia
81 N17 **Muqdisho** ✕ Banaadir, E Somalia
Muqshin see Mughshin
109 T8 **Mur** SCr. Mura. ≈ C Europe
Mura see Mur
137 T14 **Muradiye** Van, E Turkey
Muragarazi see Maragarazi
165 O10 **Murakami** Niigata, Honshū, C Japan
63 G22 **Murallón, Cerro** ▲ S Argentina
81 E20 **Muramvya** C Burundi
81 I19 **Murang'a** prev. Fort Hall. Central, SW Kenya
81 H16 **Murangering** Rift Valley, NW Kenya
Murapara see Murupara
140 M5 **Murār, Bi'r al** well NW Saudi Arabia
127 Q13 **Murashi** Kirovskaya Oblast', NW Russian Federation
103 O12 **Murat** Cantal, C France
114 N12 **Muratlı** Tekirdağ, NW Turkey
137 R14 **Murat Nehri** var. Eastern Euphrates; anc. Arsanias. ≈ NE Turkey
107 D20 **Muravera** Sardegna, Italy, C Mediterranean Sea
165 P10 **Murayama** Yamagata, Honshū, C Japan
121 R13 **Muraysah, Ra's al** headland N Libya
104 I6 **Murça** Vila Real, N Portugal
80 Q11 **Murcanyo** Bari, NE Somalia
143 N8 **Mūrcheh Khvort** var. Morcheh Khort. Eşfahān, C Iran
185 H15 **Murchison** Tasman, South Island, NZ
185 B22 **Murchison Mountains** ▲ South Island, NZ
180 I10 **Murchison River** ≈ Western Australia
105 R13 **Murcia** Murcia, SE Spain
105 Q13 **Murcia** ◐ autonomous community SE Spain
103 O13 **Mur-de-Barrez** Aveyron, S France
182 G8 **Murdinga** South Australia
28 M10 **Murdo** South Dakota, N USA
15 X6 **Murdochville** Quebec, SE Canada
109 W9 **Mureck** Steiermark, SE Austria
114 M13 **Mürefte** Tekirdağ, NW Turkey
116 I10 **Mureş** ◐ county N Romania
84 J11 **Mureş** var. Maros, Mureşul, Ger. Marosch, Mieresch. ≈ Hungary/Romania see also Maros
Mureşul see Maros/Mureş
102 M16 **Muret** Haute-Garonne, S France
27 T13 **Murfreesboro** Arkansas, C USA
21 W8 **Murfreesboro** North Carolina, SE USA
20 J9 **Murfreesboro** Tennessee, S USA
146 I14 **Murgab** prev. Murgap see also Morghāb, Daryā-ye. Maryyskiy Velayat, S Turkmenistan
146 J16 **Murgab** var. Murghab, Pash. Daryā-ye Morghāb, Turkm. Murgap Deryasy. ≈ Afghanistan/Turkmenistan see also Morghāb, Daryā-ye
Murgab see Murghob
Murgap see Murgab
Murgap Deryasy see Morghāb, Daryā-ye/Murgab
114 H9 **Murgash** ▲ W Bulgaria
Murghab see Morghāb, Daryā-ye/Murgab
147 U13 **Murghob** Rus. Murgab. SE Tajikistan
147 U13 **Murghob** Rus. Murgab. ≈ SE Tajikistan
181 Z10 **Murgon** Queensland, E Australia
190 I16 **Muri** Rarotonga, S Cook Islands
108 F7 **Muri** Aargau, W Switzerland
108 D8 **Muri** var. Muri bei Bern. Bern, W Switzerland
104 K3 **Murias de Paredes** Castilla-León, N Spain
Muri bei Bern see Muri
82 F11 **Muriege** Lunda Sul, NE Angola
189 P14 **Murilo Atoll** atoll Hall Islands, C Micronesia
Mūrītānīyah see Mauritania
100 N10 **Müritz** var. Müritzee. ⊚ NE Germany
Müritzee see Müritz
100 L10 **Müritz-Elde-Kanal** canal N Germany
184 K6 **Muriwai Beach** Auckland, North Island, NZ
92 J13 **Murjek** Norrbotten, N Sweden
126 J3 **Murmansk** Murmanskaya Oblast', NW Russian Federation
126 I4 **Murmanskaya Oblast'** ◐ province NW Russian Federation
197 V14 **Murmansk Rise** undersea feature SW Barents Sea
126 J3 **Murmashi** Murmanskaya Oblast', NW Russian Federation
128 M5 **Murmino** Ryazanskaya Oblast', W Russian Federation
101 K24 **Murnau** Bayern, SE Germany
103 X16 **Muro, Capo di** headland Corse, France, C Mediterranean Sea
107 M18 **Muro Lucano** Basilicata, S Italy
129 N4 **Murom** Vladimirskaya Oblast', W Russian Federation
122 I11 **Muromtsevo** Omskaya Oblast', C Russian Federation
165 R5 **Muroran** Hokkaidō, NE Japan
104 G3 **Muros** Galicia, NW Spain
104 F3 **Muros e Noia, Ría de** estuary NW Spain
164 H15 **Muroto** Kōchi, Shikoku, SW Japan
164 H15 **Muroto-zaki** headland Shikoku, SW Japan
116 L7 **Murovani Kurylivtsi** Vinnyts'ka Oblast', C Ukraine
110 G11 **Murowana Goślina** Wielkolpolskie, C Poland
32 M14 **Murphy** Idaho, NW USA
21 N10 **Murphy** North Carolina, SE USA
35 P8 **Murphys** California, W USA
30 L17 **Murphysboro** Illinois, N USA
29 V15 **Murray** Iowa, C USA
20 H8 **Murray** Kentucky, S USA
182 J10 **Murray Bridge** South Australia
175 X2 **Murray Fracture Zone** tectonic feature NE Pacific Ocean
192 H11 **Murray, Lake** ⊚ SW PNG
21 P12 **Murray, Lake** ⊡ South Carolina, SE USA
10 K8 **Murray, Mount** ▲ Yukon Territory, NW Canada
Murray Range see Murray Ridge
173 O3 **Murray Ridge** var. Murray Range. undersea feature N Arabian Sea
183 N10 **Murray River** ≈ SE Australia
182 K10 **Murrayville** Victoria, SE Australia
149 U5 **Murree** Punjab, E Pakistan
101 I21 **Murrhardt** Baden-Württemberg, S Germany
183 O9 **Murrumbidgee River** ≈ New South Wales, SE Australia
83 P15 **Murrupula** Nampula, NE Mozambique
183 T7 **Murrurundi** New South Wales, SE Australia
109 X9 **Murska Sobota** Ger. Olsnitz. NE Slovenia
154 G12 **Murtajāpur** prev. Murtazapur. Mahārāshtra, C India
77 S16 **Murtala Muhammed** ✕ (Lagos) Ogun, SW Nigeria
Murtazapur see Murtajāpur
108 C8 **Murten** Neuchâtel, W Switzerland
Murtensee see Morat, Lac de
182 L11 **Murtoa** Victoria, SE Australia
92 N13 **Murtovaara** Oulu, E Finland
Murua Island see Woodlark Island
155 D14 **Murud** Mahārāshtra, W India
184 O9 **Murupara** var. Murapara. Bay of Plenty, North Island, NZ
191 X12 **Mururoa** var. Moruroa. atoll Îles Tuamotu, SE French Polynesia
Murviedro see Sagunto
154 J9 **Murwāra** Madhya Pradesh, N India
183 V4 **Murwillumbah** New South Wales, SE Australia
146 H11 **Murzechirla** prev. Mirzachirla. Akhalskiy Velayat, C Turkmenistan
Murzuk see Murzuq
75 O11 **Murzuq** var. Marzūq, Murzuk. SW Libya
Murzuq, Edeyin see Murzuq, Idhān
75 N11 **Murzuq, Ḩamādat** plateau W Libya
75 O11 **Murzuq, Idhān** var. Edeyin Murzuq. desert SW Libya
109 W6 **Mürzzuschlag** Steiermark, E Austria
137 Q14 **Muş** var. Mush. Muş, E Turkey
137 Q14 **Muş** var. Mush. ◐ province E Turkey
186 F9 **Musa** ≈ S PNG
118 G11 **Mūša** ≈ Latvia/Lithuania
75 X8 **Mûsa, Gebel** ▲ NE Egypt
Musaiyib see Al Musayyib
Musa Khel see Mūsā Khel Bazār
149 R9 **Mūsā Khel Bazār** var. Musa Khel. Baluchistān, SW Pakistan
114 H10 **Musala** ▲ W Bulgaria
168 H10 **Musala, Pulau** island W Indonesia
83 J15 **Musale** Southern, S Zambia
141 Y9 **Muşallā** NE Oman
141 W6 **Musandam Peninsula** Ar. Masandam Peninsula. peninsula N Oman
Musay'id see Umm Sa'id
Muscat see Masqaţ
Muscat and Oman see Oman
29 Y14 **Muscatine** Iowa, C USA
Muscat Sīb Airport see Seeb
31 O15 **Muscatuck River** ≈ Indiana, N USA
30 K8 **Muscoda** Wisconsin, N USA
185 F19 **Musgrave, Mount** ▲ South Island, NZ
181 P9 **Musgrave Ranges** ▲ South Australia
Mush see Muş
138 H12 **Mushayyish, Qaşr al** castle Ma'ān, C Jordan
79 H20 **Mushie** Bandundu, W Dem. Rep. Congo (Zaire)
168 M13 **Musi, Air** prev. Moesi. ≈ Sumatera, W Indonesia
192 M4 **Musicians Seamounts** undersea feature N Pacific Ocean
54 D8 **Musinga, Alto** ▲ NW Colombia
29 T2 **Muskeg Bay** lake bay Minnesota, N USA
31 O8 **Muskegon** Michigan, N USA
31 O8 **Muskegon Heights** Michigan, N USA
31 P8 **Muskegon River** ≈ Michigan, N USA
31 T14 **Muskingum River** ≈ Ohio, N USA
95 P16 **Muskö** Stockholm, C Sweden
Muskogean see Tallahassee
27 Q10 **Muskogee** Oklahoma, C USA
14 H13 **Muskoka, Lake** ⊚ Ontario, S Canada
80 H8 **Musmar** Red Sea, NE Sudan
83 K14 **Musofu** Central, C Zambia
81 G19 **Musoma** Mara, N Tanzania
82 L13 **Musoro** Central, C Zambia
186 F4 **Mussau Island** island NE PNG
98 P7 **Musselkanaal** Groningen, NE Netherlands
33 V9 **Musselshell River** ≈ Montana, NW USA
82 C12 **Mussende** Cuanza Sul, NW Angola
102 L12 **Mussidan** Dordogne, SW France
99 L25 **Musson** Luxembourg, SE Belgium
152 J9 **Mussoorie** Uttar Pradesh, N India
Musta see Mosta
152 M13 **Mustafābād** Uttar Pradesh, N India
136 D12 **Mustafakemalpaşa** Bursa, NW Turkey
Mustafa-Pasha see Svilengrad
81 M15 **Mustahīl** Somali, E Ethiopia
24 M7 **Mustang Draw** valley Texas, SW USA
25 T14 **Mustang Island** island Texas, SW USA
Mustasaari see Korsholm
Mustér see Disentis
63 I19 **Musters, Lago** ⊚ S Argentina
45 Y14 **Mustique** island C Saint Vincent and the Grenadines
118 I6 **Mustla** Viljandimaa, S Estonia
118 J4 **Mustvee** Ger. Tschorna. Jõgevamaa, E Estonia
42 L9 **Musún, Cerro** ▲ NE Nicaragua
183 T7 **Muswellbrook** New South Wales, SE Australia
111 M18 **Muszyna** Małopolskie, SE Poland
136 I17 **Mut** İçel, S Turkey
75 V10 **Mût** var. Mut. C Egypt
109 V9 **Muta** N Slovenia
190 B15 **Mutalau** N Niue
Mu-tan-chiang see Mudanjiang
82 I13 **Mutanda** North Western, NW Zambia
59 O17 **Mutá, Ponta do** headland E Brazil
83 L17 **Mutare** var. Mutari; prev. Umtali. Manicaland, E Zimbabwe
Mutari see Mutare
54 D8 **Mutatá** Antioquia, NW Colombia
Mutina see Modena
83 L16 **Mutoko** prev. Mtoko. Mashonaland East, NE Zimbabwe
81 J20 **Mutomo** Eastern, S Kenya
Mutrah see Maţraḩ
79 M24 **Mutshatsha** Katanga, S Dem. Rep. Congo (Zaire)
165 R6 **Mutsu** var. Mutu. Aomori, Honshū, N Japan
165 R6 **Mutsu-wan** bay N Japan
108 E6 **Muttenz** Basel-Land, NW Switzerland
185 A26 **Muttonbird Islands** island group SW NZ
Mutu see Mutsu
83 O15 **Mutuáli** Nampula, N Mozambique
82 D13 **Mutumbo** Bié, C Angola
189 Y14 **Mutunte, Mount** var. Mount Buache. ▲ Kosrae, E Micronesia
155 K24 **Mutur** Eastern Province, E Sri Lanka
92 L13 **Muurola** Lappi, NW Finland
162 M14 **Mu Us Shamo** var. Ordos Desert. desert N China
82 B11 **Muxima** Bengo, NW Angola
126 I8 **Muyezerskiy** Respublika Kareliya, NW Russian Federation
81 E20 **Muyinga** NE Burundi
42 K9 **Muy Muy** Matagalpa, C Nicaragua
Muynak see Mŭynoq
146 G6 **Mŭynoq** Rus. Muynak. Qoraqalpoghiston Respublikasi, NW Uzbekistan
79 N22 **Muyumba** Katanga, SE Dem. Rep. Congo (Zaire)
149 V5 **Muzaffarābād** Jammu and Kashmir, NE Pakistan
149 S10 **Muzaffargarh** Punjab, E Pakistan
152 J9 **Muzaffarnagar** Uttar Pradesh, N India
153 P13 **Muzaffarpur** Bihār, N India
158 H6 **Muzat He** ≈ W China
83 L15 **Muze** Tete, NW Mozambique
122 H8 **Muzhi** Yamalo-Nenetskiy Avtonomnyy Okrug, N Russian Federation
102 H7 **Muzillac** Morbihan, NW France
Muzkol, Khrebet see Muzqŭl, Qatorkŭhi
112 L9 **Mužlja** Hung. Felsőmuzslya; prev. Gornja Mužlja. Serbia, N Yugoslavia
54 F9 **Muzo** Boyacá, C Colombia
83 J15 **Muzoka** Southern, S Zambia
39 Y15 **Muzon, Cape** headland Dall Island, Alaska, USA
40 M6 **Múzquiz** Coahuila de Zaragoza, NE Mexico
147 U13 **Muzqŭl, Qatorkŭhi** Rus. Khrebet Muzkol. ▲ SE Tajikistan
158 G10 **Muztag** ▲ NW China
158 D8 **Muztagata** ▲ NW China
158 K10 **Muztag Feng** var. Ulugh Muztag. ▲ W China
83 K17 **Mvuma** prev. Umvuma. Midlands, C Zimbabwe
82 L13 **Mwanya** Eastern, E Zambia
81 G20 **Mwanza** Mwanza, NW Tanzania
79 N23 **Mwanza** Katanga, SE Dem. Rep. Congo (Zaire)
81 F20 **Mwanza** ◐ region N Tanzania
82 M13 **Mwase Lundazi** Eastern, E Zambia
97 B17 **Mweelrea** Ir. Caoc Maol Réidh. ▲ W Ireland
79 K21 **Mweka** Kasai Occidental, C Dem. Rep. Congo (Zaire)
82 K12 **Mwenda** Luapula, N Zambia
79 L22 **Mwene-Ditu** Kasai Oriental, S Dem. Rep. Congo (Zaire)
83 L18 **Mwenezi** ≈ S Zimbabwe
79 O20 **Mwenga** Sud Kivu, E Dem. Rep. Congo (Zaire)
82 K11 **Mweru, Lake** var. Lac Moero. ⊚ Dem. Rep. Congo (Zaire)/Zambia
82 H13 **Mwinilunga** North Western, NW Zambia
189 V16 **Mwokil Atoll** var. Mokil Atoll. atoll Caroline Islands, E Micronesia
Myadel' see Myadzyel
118 J13 **Myadzyel** Pol. Miadzioł Nowy, Rus. Myadel'. Minskaya Voblasts', N Belarus
152 C12 **Myājlār** var. Miajlar. Rājasthān, NW India
123 T9 **Myakit** Magadanskaya Oblast', E Russian Federation
23 W13 **Myakka River** ≈ Florida, SE USA
126 L14 **Myaksa** Vologodskaya Oblast', NW Russian Federation
183 U8 **Myall Lake** ⊚ New South Wales, SE Australia
166 L7 **Myanaung** Irrawaddy, SW Myanmar
166 M4 **Myanmar** off. Union of Myanmar, var. Burma ◆ military dictatorship SE Asia
166 K8 **Myaungmya** Irrawaddy, SW Myanmar
118 N11 **Myazha** Rus. Mezha. Vitsyebskaya Voblasts', NE Belarus
119 O18 **Myerkulavichy** Rus. Merkulovichi. Homyel'skaya Voblasts', SE Belarus
119 N14 **Myezhava** Rus. Mezhëvo. Vitsyebskaya Voblasts', NE Belarus
166 L5 **Myingyan** Mandalay, C Myanmar
167 N2 **Myitkyina** Kachin State, N Myanmar
166 M5 **Myittha** Mandalay, C Myanmar
111 H19 **Myjava** Hung. Miava. Trenčiansky Kraj, W Slovakia
Myjeldino see Myyëldino
117 U9 **Mykhaylivka** Rus. Mikhaylovka. Zaporiz'ka Oblast', SE Ukraine
95 A18 **Mykines** Dan. Myggenaes Island Faeroe Islands
116 I5 **Mykolayiv** L'vivs'ka Oblast', W Ukraine
117 Q10 **Mykolayiv** Rus. Nikolayev. Mykolayivs'ka Oblast', S Ukraine
117 Q10 **Mykolayiv** ✕ Mykolayivs'ka Oblast', S Ukraine
Mykolayiv see Mykolayivs'ka Oblast'
117 P9 **Mykolayivka** Odes'ka Oblast', SW Ukraine
117 S13 **Mykolayivka** Respublika Krym, S Ukraine
117 P9 **Mykolayivs'ka Oblast'** var. Mykolayiv, Rus. Nikolayevskaya Oblast'. ◐ province S Ukraine
115 J20 **Mýkonos** Mýkonos, Kykládes, Greece, Aegean Sea
115 K20 **Mýkonos** var. Míkonos. island Kykládes, Greece, Aegean Sea
127 R7 **Myla** Respublika Komi, NW Russian Federation
Mylae see Milazzo
93 M19 **Myllykoski** Etelä-Suomi, S Finland
Mymensing see Mymensingh
153 U14 **Mymensingh** var. Maimansingh, Mymensing; prev. Nasirābād. Dhaka, N Bangladesh
93 K19 **Mynämäki** Länsi-Suomi, W Finland
145 S14 **Mynaral** Kaz. Myngaral. Zhambyl, S Kazakhstan
Mynbulak see Mingbuloq
Mynbulak, Vpadina see Mingbuloq Botighi
Myngaral see Mynaral
166 K5 **Myohaung** Arakan State, W Myanmar
163 W13 **Myohyang-sanmaek** ▲ C North Korea
164 M11 **Myōkō-san** ▲ Honshū, S Japan
83 J15 **Myooye** Central, C Zambia
118 K12 **Myory** prev. Miyory. Vitsyebskaya Voblasts', N Belarus
92 J4 **Mýrdalsjökull** glacier S Iceland
92 G10 **Myre** Nordland, C Norway
117 S5 **Myrhorod** Rus. Mirgorod. Poltavs'ka Oblast', NE Ukraine
115 J15 **Mýrina** var. Mírina. Límnos, SE Greece
117 P5 **Myronivka** Rus. Mironovka. Kyyivs'ka Oblast', N Ukraine
21 U13 **Myrtle Beach** South Carolina, SE USA
32 F14 **Myrtle Creek** Oregon, NW USA
183 P11 **Myrtleford** Victoria, SE Australia
32 E14 **Myrtle Point** Oregon, NW USA
115 K25 **Mýrtos** Kríti, Greece, E Mediterranean Sea
Myrtoum Mare see Mirtóo Pélagos
93 G17 **Myrviken** Jämtland, C Sweden
95 I15 **Mysen** Østfold, S Norway
126 L15 **Myshkin** Yaroslavskaya Oblast', NW Russian Federation
111 K17 **Myślenice** Małopolskie, S Poland
110 D10 **Myślibórz** Zachodniopomorskie, NW Poland
155 G20 **Mysore** var. Maisur. Karnātaka, W India
Mysore see Karnātaka
115 F21 **Mystrás** var. Mistras. Pelopónnisos, S Greece
127 T12 **Mysy** Komi-Permyatskiy Avtonomnyy Okrug, NW Russian Federation
111 K15 **Myszków** Śląskie, S Poland
167 T14 **My Tho** var. Mi Tho. Tiên Giang, S Vietnam
Mytilene see Mytilíni
115 L17 **Mytilíni** var. Mitilíni; anc. Mytilene. Lésvos, E Greece
128 K3 **Mytishchi** Moskovskaya Oblast', W Russian Federation
37 N3 **Myton** Utah, W USA
92 K2 **Mývatn** ⊚ C Iceland
127 T11 **Myyëldino** var. Myjeldino. Respublika Komi, NW Russian Federation
82 M13 **Mzimba** Northern, NW Malawi
82 M12 **Mzuzu** Northern, N Malawi

N

101 M19 **Naab** ≈ SE Germany
98 G12 **Naaldwijk** Zuid-Holland, W Netherlands
38 G12 **Naalehu** var. Nā'ālehu. Hawaii, USA, C Pacific Ocean
93 K19 **Naantali** Swe. Nådendal. Länsi-Suomi, W Finland
98 J10 **Naarden** Noord-Holland, C Netherlands
109 U4 **Naarn** ≈ N Austria
97 F18 **Naas** Ir. An Nás, Nás na Ríogh. C Ireland
92 M9 **Näätämöjoki** Lapp. Njávdám. ≈ NE Finland
83 E23 **Nababeep** var. Nababiep. Northern Cape, W South Africa
Nababiep see Nababeep
Nabadwip see Navadwip
164 J14 **Nabari** Mie, Honshū, SW Japan
Nabatié see Nabatîyé
138 G8 **Nabatîyé** var. An Nabatîyah at Taḩtā, Nabatié, Nabatiyet et Tahta. SW Lebanon
Nabatiyet et Tahta see Nabatîyé
187 X14 **Nabavatu** Vanua Levu, N Fiji
190 I2 **Nabeina** island Tungaru, W Kiribati
129 T4 **Naberezhnyye Chelny** prev. Brezhnev. Respublika Tatarstan, W Russian Federation
39 T10 **Nabesna** Alaska, USA
39 T10 **Nabesna River** ≈ Alaska, USA
75 N5 **Nabeul** var. Nābul. NE Tunisia
152 I9 **Nābha** Punjab, NW India
171 W13 **Nabire** Irian Jaya, E Indonesia
141 O15 **Nabī Shu'ayb, Jabal an** ▲ W Yemen
138 F10 **Nablus** var. Nābulus, Heb. Shekhem; anc. Neapolis, Bibl. Shechem. N West Bank
187 X14 **Nabouwalu** Vanua Levu, N Fiji
Nābul see Nabeul
Nābulus see Nablus
187 Y13 **Nabuna** Vanua Levu, N Fiji
83 Q14 **Nacala** Nampula, NE Mozambique
42 H8 **Nacaome** Valle, S Honduras
Na Cealla Beaga see Killybegs
Na-ch'ii see Nagqu
164 J15 **Nachikatsuura** var. Nachi-Katsuura. Wakayama, Honshū, SE Japan
81 J24 **Nachingwea** Lindi, SE Tanzania
111 F16 **Náchod** Hradecký Kraj, N Czech Republic
Na Clocha Liatha see Greystones
40 G3 **Naco** Sonora, NW Mexico
25 X8 **Nacogdoches** Texas, SW USA
40 G4 **Nacozari de García** Sonora, NW Mexico
Nada see Danzhou
77 O14 **Nadawli** NW Ghana
104 I3 **Nadela** Galicia, NW Spain
Nådendal see Naantali
144 M7 **Nadezhdinka** prev. Nadezhdinskiy. Kostanay, N Kazakhstan
Nadezhdinskiy see Nadezhdinka
Nadgan see Nadqān, Qalamat
187 W14 **Nadi** prev. Nandi. Viti Levu, W Fiji
187 X14 **Nadi** prev. Nandi. ✕ Viti Levu, W Fiji
154 D10 **Nadiād** Gujarāt, W India
Nadikdik see Knox Atoll
116 E11 **Nădlac** Ger. Nadlak, Hung. Nagylak. Arad, W Romania
Nadlak see Nădlac
74 H6 **Nador** prev. Villa Nador. NE Morocco
141 S9 **Nadqān, Qalamat** var. Nadgan. well E Saudi Arabia
111 N22 **Nádudvar** Hajdú-Bihar, E Hungary
121 O15 **Nadur** Gozo, N Malta
187 X13 **Naduri** prev. Nanduri. Vanua Levu, N Fiji
116 I7 **Nadvirna** Pol. Nadwórna, Rus. Nadvornaya. Ivano-Frankivs'ka Oblast', W Ukraine
126 J8 **Nadvoitsy** Respublika Kareliya, NW Russian Federation
Nadvornaya/Nadwórna see Nadvirna
122 I9 **Nadym** Yamalo-Nenetskiy Avtonomnyy Okrug, N Russian Federation
122 I9 **Nadym** ≈ C Russian Federation
186 E7 **Nadzab** Morobe, C PNG
77 X13 **Nafada** Gombe, E Nigeria
108 H8 **Näfels** Glarus, NE Switzerland
115 E18 **Náfpaktos** var. Návpaktos. Dytikí Ellás, C Greece
115 F20 **Náfplio** prev. Návplion. Pelopónnisos, S Greece
139 U6 **Naft Khāneh** E Iraq
149 N13 **Nāg** Baluchistān, SW Pakistan
171 P4 **Naga** off. Naga City; prev. Nueva Caceres. Luzon, N Philippines
Nagaarzê see Nagarzê
12 F11 **Nagagami** ≈ Ontario, S Canada
164 F14 **Nagahama** Ehime, Shikoku, SW Japan
153 X12 **Nāga Hills** ▲ NE India
165 P10 **Nagai** Yamagata, Honshū, C Japan
Na Gaibhlte see Galty Mountains
39 N16 **Nagai Island** island Shumagin Islands, Alaska, USA
153 X12 **Nāgāland** ◐ state NE India
164 M11 **Nagano** Nagano, Honshū, S Japan
164 M12 **Nagano** off. Nagano-ken. ◐ prefecture Honshū, S Japan
165 N11 **Nagaoka** Niigata, Honshū, C Japan
153 W12 **Nagaon** prev. Nowgong. Assam, NE India
155 J21 **Nāgappattinam** var. Negapatam, Negapattinam. Tamil Nādu, SE India
Nagara Nayok see Nakhon Nayok
Nagara Panom see Nakhon Phanom
Nagara Pathom see Nakhon Pathom
Nagara Sridharmaraj see Nakhon Si Thammarat
Nagara Svarga see Nakhon Sawan
155 H16 **Nāgārjuna Sāgar** ⊡ E India
42 I10 **Nagarote** León, SW Nicaragua

◆ Country ● Country Capital ◇ Dependent Territory ○ Dependent Territory Capital ◐ Administrative Region ✕ International Airport ▲ Mountain ▲ Mountain Range Volcano ≈ River ⊚ Lake ⊡ Reservoir

158 *M16* **Nagarzê** ***var.*** Nagaarzê. Xizang Zizhiqu, W China
164 C14 **Nagasaki** Nagasaki, Kyūshū, SW Japan
164 C14 **Nagasaki** ***off.*** Nagasaki-ken. ❖ *prefecture* Kyūshū, SW Japan
Nagashima *see* Kii-Nagashima
164 E12 **Nagato** Yamaguchi, Honshū, SW Japan
152 *F11* **Nāgaur** Rājasthān, NW India
154 *F10* **Nāgda** Madhya Pradesh, C India
98 *L8* **Nagele** Flevoland, N Netherlands
155 *H24* **Nāgercoil** Tamil Nādu, SE India
153 *X12* **Nāginimāra** Nāgāland, NE India
Na Gleannta *see* Glenties
165 T16 **Nago** Okinawa, Okinawa, SW Japan
154 *K9* **Nāgod** Madhya Pradesh, C India
155 *J26* **Nagoda** Southern Province, S Sri Lanka
101 *G22* **Nagold** Baden-Württemberg, SW Germany
Nagorno-Karabakhskaya Avtonomnaya Oblast *see* Nagornyy Karabakh
123 Q12 **Nagornyy** Respublika Sakha (Yakutiya), NE Russian Federation
137 *V12* **Nagornyy Karabakh** ***var.*** Nagorno-Karabakhskaya Avtonomnaya Oblast , ***Arm.*** Lerrnayin Gharabakh, ***Az.*** Dağliq Qarabağ. *former autonomous region* SW Azerbaijan
127 *R13* **Nagorsk** Kirovskaya Oblast', NW Russian Federation
164 K13 **Nagoya** Aichi, Honshū, SW Japan
154 *I12* **Nāgpur** Mahārāshtra, C India
156 *K10* **Nagqu** ***Chin.*** Na-ch'ii; ***prev.*** Hei-ho. Xizang Zizhiqu, W China
152 *J8* **Nāg Tibba Range** ▲ N India
45 *O8* **Nagua** NE Dominican Republic
111 *H25* **Nagyatád** Somogy, SW Hungary
Nagybánya *see* Baia Mare
Nagybecskerek *see* Zrenjanin
Nagydisznód *see* Cisnădie
Nagyenyed *see* Aiud
111 *N21* **Nagykálló** Szabolcs-Szatmár-Bereg, E Hungary
111 *G25* **Nagykanizsa** ***Ger.*** Grosskanizsa. Zala, SW Hungary
Nagykároly *see* Carei
111 *K22* **Nagykáta** Pest, C Hungary
Nagykikinda *see* Kikinda
111 *K23* **Nagykőrös** Pest, C Hungary
Nagy-Küküllő *see* Târnava Mare
Nagylak *see* Nădlac
Nagymihály *see* Michalovce
Nagyrőce *see* Revúca
Nagysomkút *see* Şomcuta Mare
Nagysurány *see* Šurany
Nagyszalonta *see* Salonta
Nagyszeben *see* Sibiu
Nagyszentmiklós *see* Sânnicolau Mare
Nagyszöllös *see* Vynohradiv
Nagyszombat *see* Trnava
Nagytapolcsány *see* Topoľčany
Nagyvárad *see* Oradea
165 S17 **Naha** Okinawa, Okinawa, SW Japan
152 *J8* **Nāhan** Himāchal Pradesh, NW India
Nahang, Rūd-e *see* Nihing
Nahariya *see* Nahariyya
138 *F8* **Nahariyya** ***var.*** Nahariya. Northern, N Israel
142 *L6* **Nahāvand** ***var.*** Nehavend. Hamadān, W Iran
101 *F19* **Nahe** ≈ SW Germany
Na h-Iarmhidhe *see* Westmeath
189 *O13* **Nahnalaud** ▲ Pohnpei, E Micronesia
Nahoi, Cape *see* Cumberland, Cape
63 *H16* **Nahuel Huapi, Lago** ◎ W Argentina
23 *W7* **Nahunta** Georgia, SE USA
40 *J6* **Naica** Chihuahua, N Mexico
11 *U15* **Naicam** Saskatchewan, S Canada
163 *T11* **Naiman Qi** Nei Mongol Zizhiqu, N China
158 *M4* **Naimin Bulak** *spring* NW China
13 *P6* **Nain** Newfoundland, NE Canada
143 *P8* **Nā'īn** Eşfahān, C Iran
152 *K10* **Naini Tāl** Uttar Pradesh, N India
154 *J11* **Nainpur** Madhya Pradesh, C India
96 *J8* **Nairn** N Scotland, UK
96 *I8* **Nairn** *cultural region* NE Scotland, UK
81 *I19* **Nairobi** ● (Kenya) Nairobi Area, S Kenya
81 *I19* **Nairobi** ✕ Nairobi Area, S Kenya
82 *P13* **Nairoto** Cabo Delgado, NE Mozambique
118 *G3* **Naissaar** *island* N Estonia
Naissus *see* Niš
187 Z14 **Naitaba** ***var.*** Naitauba; ***prev.*** Naitamba. *island* Lau Group, E Fiji
Naitamba/Naitauba *see* Naitaba
81 *I19* **Naivasha** Rift Valley, SW Kenya
81 *H19* **Naivasha, Lake** ◎ SW Kenya
Najaf *see* An Najaf
143 *N8* **Najafābād** ***var.*** Nejafabad. Eşfahān, C Iran
141 *N7* **Najd** ***var.*** Nejd. *cultural region* C Saudi Arabia
105 *O4* **Nájera** La Rioja, N Spain
105 *P4* **Najerilla** ≈ N Spain
152 *J9* **Najībābād** Uttar Pradesh, N India
Najima *see* Fukuoka
163 *Y11* **Najin** NE North Korea
139 *T9* **Najm al Ḩassūn** C Iraq
141 *O13* **Najrān** ***var.*** Abā as Su'ūd. Najrān, S Saudi Arabia
141 *P12* **Najrān** ***off.*** Minţaqat al Najrān. ❖ *province* S Saudi Arabia
165 T2 **Nakagawa** Hokkaidō, NE Japan
38 *F9* **Nakalele Pont** *headland* Maui, Hawaii, USA, C Pacific Ocean
164 D13 **Nakama** Fukuoka, Kyūshū, SW Japan
Nakambé *see* White Volta
Nakamti *see* Nek'emtē
164 F15 **Nakamura** Kōchi, Shikoku, SW Japan
186 H7 **Nakanai Mountains** ▲ New Britain, E PNG
164 H11 **Nakano-shima** *island* Oki-shotō, SW Japan
165 Q6 **Nakasato** Aomori, Honshū, C Japan
165 T5 **Nakasatsunai** Hokkaidō, NE Japan
165 W4 **Nakashibetsu** Hokkaidō, NE Japan
81 *F18* **Nakasongola** C Uganda
165 T1 **Nakatonbetsu** Hokkaidō, NE Japan
164 L13 **Nakatsugawa** ***var.*** Nakatugawa. Gifu, Honshū, SW Japan
Nakatu *see* Nakatsu
Nakatugawa *see* Nakatsugawa
Naka-umi *see* Nakano-umi
Nakdong *see* Naktong-gang
Nakel *see* Nakło nad Notecią
80 *J8* **Nakfa** N Eritrea
Nakhichevan' *see* Naxçıvan
123 S15 **Nakhodka** Primorskiy Kray, SE Russian Federation
122 J8 **Nakhodka** Yamalo-Nenetskiy Avtonomnyy Okrug, N Russian Federation
Nakhon Navok *see* Nakhon Nayok
167 P11 **Nakhon Nayok** ***var.*** Nagara Nayok, Nakhon Navok. Nakhon Nayok, C Thailand
167 O11 **Nakhon Pathom** ***var.*** Nagara Pathom, Nakorn Pathom. Nakhon Pathom, W Thailand
167 R8 **Nakhon Phanom** ***var.*** Nagara Panom. Nakhon Phanom, E Thailand
167 Q10 **Nakhon Ratchasima** ***var.*** Khorat, Korat. Nakhon Ratchasima, E Thailand
167 O9 **Nakhon Sawan** ***var.*** Muang Nakhon Sawan, Nagara Svarga. Nakhon Sawan, W Thailand
167 N15 **Nakhon Si Thammarat** ***var.*** Nagara Sridharmaraj, Nakhon Sithamnaraj. Nakhon Si Thammarat, SW Thailand
Nakhon Sithamnaraj *see* Nakhon Si Thammarat
139 *Y11* **Nakhrash** SE Iraq
10 *I9* **Nakina** British Columbia, W Canada
110 *H9* **Nakło nad Notecią** ***Ger.*** Nakel. Kujawsko-pomorskie, C Poland
39 *P13* **Naknek** Alaska, USA
152 *H8* **Nakodar** Punjab, NW India
82 *M11* **Nakonde** Northern, NE Zambia
Nakorn Pathom *see* Nakhon Pathom
95 *H24* **Nakskov** Storstrøm, SE Denmark
163 *Y15* **Naktong-gang** ***var.*** Nakdong, ***Jap.*** Rakutō-kō. ≈ C South Korea
83 *H18* **Nakuru** Rift Valley, SW Kenya
81 *H19* **Nakuru, Lake** ◎ Rift Valley, C Kenya
11 *O17* **Nakusp** British Columbia, SW Canada
149 *N15* **Nāl** ≈ W Pakistan
162 *M7* **Nalayh** Töv, C Mongolia
153 *V12* **Nalbāri** Assam, NE India
63 *G19* **Nalcayec, Isla** *island* Archipiélago de los Chonos, S Chile
129 *N15* **Nal'chik** Kabardino-Balkarskaya Respublika, SW Russian Federation
155 *I16* **Nalgonda** Andhra Pradesh, C India
153 *S14* **Nalhāti** West Bengal, NE India
153 *U14* **Nalitabari** Dhaka, N Bangladesh
155 *I17* **Nallamala Hills** ▲ E India
136 *G12* **Nallıhan** Ankara, NW Turkey
104 *K2* **Nalón** ≈ NW Spain
167 *N3* **Nalong** Kachin State, N Myanmar
75 *N8* **Nālūt** NW Libya
171 *T14* **Nama** Pulau Manawoka, E Indonesia
189 *Q16* **Nama** *island* C Micronesia
83 *O16* **Namacurra** Zambézia, NE Mozambique
188 *F9* **Namai Bay** *bay* Babeldaob, N Palau
29 *W2* **Namakan Lake** ◎ Canada/USA
143 *O6* **Namak, Daryācheh-ye** *marsh* N Iran
143 *T6* **Namak, Kavīr-e** *salt pan* NE Iran
167 *O6* **Namaklwe** Shan State, E Myanmar
Namaksār, Kowl-e/Namakzār, Daryācheh-ye *see* Namakzar
148 *I5* **Namakzar** ***Pash.*** Daryācheh-ye Namakzār, Kowl-e Namaksār. *marsh* Afghanistan/Iran
171 *V15* **Namalau** Pulau Jursian, E Indonesia
81 *I20* **Namanga** Rift Valley, S Kenya
147 *S10* **Namangan** Namangan Wiloyati, E Uzbekistan
Namanganskaya Oblast' *see* Namangan Wiloyati
147 *R10* **Namangan Wiloyati** ***Rus.*** Namanganskaya Oblast'. ❖ *province* E Uzbekistan
83 *Q14* **Namapa** Nampula, NE Mozambique
83 *C21* **Namaqualand** *physical region* S Namibia
81 *G18* **Namasagali** C Uganda
186 *H6* **Namatanai** New Ireland, NE PNG
83 *I14* **Nambala** Central, C Zambia
81 *J23* **Nambanje** Lindi, SE Tanzania
83 *G16* **Nambiya** Ngamiland, N Botswana
183 *V2* **Nambour** Queensland, E Australia
183 *V6* **Nambucca Heads** New South Wales, SE Australia
159 *N15* **Nam Co** ◎ W China
167 *R5* **Nâm Cum** Lai Châu, N Vietnam
Namdik *see* Namorik Atoll
167 *T6* **Nam Định** Nam Ha, N Vietnam
99 *I20* **Namêche** Namur, SE Belgium
30 *J4* **Namekagon Lake** ◎ Wisconsin, N USA
188 *F10* **Namekakl Passage** *passage* Babeldaob, N Palau
Namen *see* Namur
83 *P15* **Nametil** Nampula, NE Mozambique
163 *X14* **Nam-gang** ≈ C North Korea
163 *Y16* **Nam-gang** ≈ S South Korea
163 *Y17* **Namhae-do** ***Jap.*** Nankai-tō. *island* S South Korea
Namhoi *see* Foshan
83 *C19* **Namib Desert** *desert* W Namibia
83 *A15* **Namibe** ***Port.*** Moçâmedes, Mossâmedes. Namibe, SW Angola
83 *A15* **Namibe** ❖ *province* SE Angola
83 *C18* **Namibia** ***off.*** Republic of Namibia, ***var.*** South West Africa, ***Afr.*** Suidwes-Afrika, ***Ger.*** Deutsch-Südwestafrika; ***prev.*** German Southwest Africa, South-West Africa. ◆ *republic* S Africa
65 *O17* **Namibia Plain** *undersea feature* S Atlantic Ocean
165 *Q11* **Namie** Fukushima, Honshū, C Japan
165 *Q7* **Namioka** Aomori, Honshū, C Japan
40 *I5* **Namiquipa** Chihuahua, N Mexico
159 *P15* **Namjagbarwa Feng** ▲ W China
171 *R13* **Namlea** Pulau Buru, E Indonesia
158 *L16* **Namling** Xizang Zizhiqu, W China
Namnetes *see* Nantes
167 *R8* **Nam Ngum** ≈ C Laos
Namo *see* Namu Atoll
183 *R5* **Namoi River** ≈ New South Wales, SE Australia
189 *Q17* **Namoluk Atoll** *atoll* Mortlock Islands, C Micronesia
189 *O15* **Namonuito Atoll** *atoll* Caroline Islands, C Micronesia
189 *T9* **Namorik Atoll** ***var.*** Namdik. *atoll* Ralik Chain, S Marshall Islands
167 *Q6* **Nam Ou** ≈ N Laos
32 *M14* **Nampa** Idaho, NW USA
76 *M11* **Nampala** Ségou, W Mali
163 *W14* **Namp'o** SW North Korea
83 *P15* **Nampula** Nampula, NE Mozambique
83 *P15* **Nampula** ***off.*** Província de Nampula. ❖ *province* NE Mozambique
163 *W13* **Namsan-ni** NW North Korea
Namslau *see* Namysłów
93 *E15* **Namsos** Nord-Trøndelag, C Norway
93 *F14* **Namsskogan** Nord-Trøndelag, C Norway
123 *Q10* **Namsty** Respublika Sakha (Yakutiya), NE Russian Federation
167 *O6* **Nam Teng** ≈ E Myanmar
167 *P6* **Nam Tha** ≈ N Laos
167 *N4* **Namtu** Shan State, E Myanmar
10 *J15* **Namu** British Columbia, SW Canada
189 *T7* **Namu Atoll** ***var.*** Namo. *atoll* Ralik Chain, C Marshall Islands
187 *Y15* **Namuka-i-lau** *island* Lau Group, E Fiji
83 *O15* **Namuli, Mont** ▲ NE Mozambique
83 *P14* **Namuno** Cabo Delgado, N Mozambique
99 *I20* **Namur** ***Dut.*** Namen. Namur, SE Belgium
99 *H21* **Namur** ***Dut.*** Namen. ❖ *province* S Belgium
83 *D17* **Namutoni** Kunene, N Namibia
163 *Y16* **Namwŏn** ***Jap.*** Nangen. S South Korea
111 *H14* **Namysłów** ***Ger.*** Namslau. Opolskie, S Poland
167 *P7* **Nan** ***var.*** Muang Nan. Nan, NW Thailand
79 *G15* **Nana** ≈ W Central African Republic
165 *R5* **Nanae** Hokkaidō, NE Japan
79 *I14* **Nana-Grébizi** ❖ *prefecture* N Central African Republic
10 *L17* **Nanaimo** Vancouver Island, British Columbia, SW Canada
38 *C9* **Nanakuli** ***Haw.*** Nānākuli. Oahu, Hawaii, USA, C Pacific Ocean
79 *G15* **Nana-Mambéré** ❖ *prefecture* W Central African Republic
161 *R13* **Nan'an** Fujian, SE China
183 *U2* **Nanango** Queensland, E Australia
164 *L11* **Nanao** Ishikawa, Honshū, SW Japan
161 *Q14* **Nan'ao Dao** *island* S China
164 *L10* **Nanatsu-shima** *island* SW Japan
56 *F8* **Nanay, Río** ≈ NE Peru
160 *J8* **Nanbu** Sichuan, C China
163 *X7* **Nancha** Heilongjiang, NE China
161 *P10* **Nanchang** ***var.*** Nan-ch'ang, Nanch'ang-hsien. Jiangxi, S China
Nanch'ang-hsien *see* Nanchang
161 *P11* **Nancheng** Jiangxi, S China
Nan-ching *see* Nanjing
160 *J9* **Nanchong** Sichuan, C China
160 *J10* **Nanchuan** Chongqing Shi, C China
103 *T5* **Nancy** Meurthe-et-Moselle, NE France
185 *A22* **Nancy Sound** *sound* South Island, NZ
152 *L9* **Nanda Devi** ▲ NW India
42 *J11* **Nandaime** Granada, SW Nicaragua
160 *K13* **Nandan** Guangxi Zhuangzu Zizhiqu, S China
155 *H14* **Nānded** Mahārāshtra, C India
183 *S5* **Nandewar Range** ▲ New South Wales, SE Australia
Nandi *see* Nadi
160 *E13* **Nanding He** ≈ China/Vietnam
Nándorhgy *see* Oţelu Roşu
154 *E11* **Nandurbār** Mahārāshtra, W India
Nanduri *see* Naduri
155 *I17* **Nandyāl** Andhra Pradesh, E India
161 *P11* **Nanfeng** Jiangxi, S China
Nang *see* Nang Xian
79 *E15* **Nanga Eboko** Centre, C Cameroon
149 *W4* **Nanga Parbat** ▲ India/Pakistan
169 *R11* **Nangapinoh** Borneo, C Indonesia
149 *R5* **Nangarhār** ❖ *province* E Afghanistan
169 *S11* **Nangaserawai** ***var.*** Nangah Serawai. Borneo, C Indonesia
169 *Q12* **Nangatayap** Borneo, C Indonesia
Nangen *see* Namwŏn
103 *P5* **Nangis** Seine-et-Marne, N France
163 *X13* **Nangnim-sanmaek** ▲ C North Korea
161 *O4* **Nangong** Hebei, E China
159 *Q14* **Nangqên** Qinghai, C China
167 *Q10* **Nang Rong** Buri Ram, E Thailand
159 *O16* **Nang Xian** ***var.*** Nang. Xizang Zizhiqu, W China
Nan Hai *see* South China Sea
160 *L8* **Nan He** ≈ C China
160 *F12* **Nanhua** Yunnan, SW China
Naniwa *see* Ōsaka
155 *G20* **Nanjangūd** Karnātaka, W India
161 *Q8* **Nanjing** ***var.*** Nan-ching, Nanking; ***prev.*** Chianning, Chian-ning, Kiang-ning. Jiangsu, E China
Nankai-tō *see* Namhae-do
161 *O12* **Nankang** Jiangxi, S China
Nanking *see* Nanjing
161 *N13* **Nan Ling** ▲ S China
160 *L15* **Nanliu Jiang** ≈ S China
189 *P13* **Nan Madol** *ruins* Temwen Island, E Micronesia
160 *K15* **Nanning** ***var.*** Nan-ning; ***prev.*** Yung-ning. Guangxi Zhuangzu Zizhiqu, S China
196 *M15* **Nanortalik** Kitaa, S Greenland
Nanouki *see* Aranuka
160 *H13* **Nanpan Jiang** ≈ S China
152 *M11* **Nānpāra** Uttar Pradesh, N India
161 *Q12* **Nanping** ***var.*** Nan-p'ing; ***prev.*** Yenping. Fujian, SE China
160 *I7* **Nanping** Sichuan, C China
161 *R12* **Nanri Dao** *island* SE China
165 *S16* **Nansei-shotō** ***Eng.*** Ryukyu Islands. *island group* SW Japan
Nansei Syotō Trench *see* Ryukyu Trench
197 *T10* **Nansen Basin** *undersea feature* Arctic Ocean
197 *T10* **Nansen Cordillera** ***var.*** Arctic-Mid Oceanic Ridge, Nansen Ridge. *undersea feature* Arctic Ocean
Nansen Ridge *see* Nansen Cordillera
131 *T9* **Nan Shan** ▲ C China
Nansha Qundao *see* Spratly Islands
12 *K3* **Nantais, Lac** ◎ Quebec, NE Canada
103 *N5* **Nanterre** Hauts-de-Seine, N France
102 *I8* **Nantes** ***Bret.*** Naoned; ***anc.*** Condivincum, Namnetes. Loire-Atlantique, NW France
14 *G17* **Nanticoke** Ontario, S Canada
18 *H13* **Nanticoke** Pennsylvania, NE USA
21 *Y4* **Nanticoke River** ≈ Delaware/Maryland, NE USA
11 *Q17* **Nanton** Alberta, SW Canada
161 *S8* **Nantong** Jiangsu, E China
161 *S13* **Nant'ou** W Taiwan
103 *S10* **Nantua** Ain, E France
19 *Q13* **Nantucket** Nantucket Island, Massachusetts, NE USA
19 *Q13* **Nantucket Island** *island* Massachusetts, NE USA
19 *Q13* **Nantucket Sound** *sound* Massachusetts, NE USA
82 *P13* **Nantulo** Cabo Delgado, N Mozambique
189 *O12* **Nanuh** Pohnpei, E Micronesia
190 *D6* **Nanumaga** ***var.*** Nanumanga. *atoll* NW Tuvalu
Nanumanga *see* Nanumaga
190 *D5* **Nanumea Atoll** *atoll* NW Tuvalu
59 *O19* **Nanuque** Minas Gerais, SE Brazil
171 *R10* **Nanusa, Kepulauan** *island group* N Indonesia
163 *U4* **Nanweng He** ≈ NE China
160 *I10* **Nanxi** Sichuan, C China
161 *N10* **Nanxian** ***var.*** Nan Xian. Hunan, S China
161 *N7* **Nanyang** ***var.*** Nan-yang. Henan, C China
161 *P6* **Nanyang Hu** ◎ E China
165 *P10* **Nan'yō** Yamagata, Honshū, C Japan
81 *I18* **Nanyuki** Central, C Kenya
160 *M8* **Nanzhang** Hubei, C China
105 *T11* **Nao, Cabo de La** *headland* E Spain
12 *M9* **Naococane, Lac** ◎ Quebec, E Canada
153 *S14* **Naogaon** Rajshahi, NW Bangladesh
Naokot *see* Naukot
187 *R13* **Naone** Maewo, C Vanuatu
Naoned *see* Nantes
115 *E14* **Náousa** Kentrikí Makedonía, N Greece
35 *N8* **Napa** California, W USA
39 *O11* **Napaimiut** Alaska, USA
39 *N12* **Napakiak** Alaska, USA
122 *J7* **Napalkovo** Yamalo-Nenetskiy Avtonomnyy Okrug, N Russian Federation
12 *I16* **Napanee** Ontario, SE Canada
39 *N12* **Napaskiak** Alaska, USA
167 *S5* **Na Phac** Cao Băng, N Vietnam
184 *O11* **Napier** Hawke's Bay, North Island, NZ
195 *X3* **Napier Mountains** ▲ Antarctica
15 *O13* **Napierville** Quebec, SE Canada
23 *W15* **Naples** Florida, SE USA
25 *W5* **Naples** Texas, SW USA
Naples *see* Napoli
160 *I14* **Napo** Guangxi Zhuangzu Zizhiqu, S China
56 *D6* **Napo** ❖ *province* NE Ecuador
29 *O6* **Napoleon** North Dakota, N USA
31 *R11* **Napoleon** Ohio, N USA
Napoléon-Vendée *see* la Roche-sur-Yon
22 *J9* **Napoleonville** Louisiana, S USA
107 *K17* **Napoli** ***Eng.*** Naples, ***Ger.*** Neapel; ***anc.*** Neapolis. Campania, S Italy
107 *J18* **Napoli, Golfo di** *gulf* S Italy
57 *F7* **Napo, Río** ≈ Ecuador/Peru
191 *W9* **Napuka** *island* Îles Tuamotu, C French Polynesia
142 *J3* **Naqadeh** Āžarbāyjān-e Bākhtarī, NW Iran
139 *U6* **Naqnah** E Iraq
Nar *see* Nera
164 *J14* **Nara** Nara, Honshū, SW Japan
76 *L11* **Nara** Koulikoro, W Mali
164 *J14* **Nara** ***off.*** Nara-ken. ❖ *prefecture* Honshū, SW Japan
149 *R14* **Nāra Canal** *irrigation canal* S Pakistan
182 *K11* **Naracoorte** South Australia
183 *P8* **Naradhan** New South Wales, SE Australia
Naradhivas *see* Narathiwat
56 *B8* **Naranjal** Guayas, W Ecuador
57 *Q19* **Naranjos** Santa Cruz, E Bolivia
41 *Q12* **Naranjos** Veracruz-Llave, E Mexico
159 *Q6* **Naran Sebstein Bulag** *spring* NW China
143 *X12* **Narānū** Sīstān va Balūchestān, SE Iran
164 *B14* **Narao** Nagasaki, Nakadōri-jima, SW Japan
155 *J16* **Narasaraopet** Andhra Pradesh, E India
158 *J5* **Narat** Xinjiang Uygur Zizhiqu, W China
167 *P17* **Narathiwat** ***var.*** Naradhivas. Narathiwat, SW Thailand
37 *V10* **Nara Visa** New Mexico, SW USA
Nārāyāni *see* Gandak
Narbada *see* Narmada
Narbo Martius *see* Narbonne
103 *P16* **Narbonne** ***anc.*** Narbo Martius. Aude, S France
Narborough Island *see* Fernandina, Isla
104 *J2* **Narcea** ≈ NW Spain
152 *J9* **Narendranagar** Uttar Pradesh, N India
Nares Abyssal Plain *see* Nares Plain
64 *G11* **Nares Plain** ***var.*** Nares Abyssal Plain. *undersea feature* NW Atlantic Ocean
197 *P10* **Nares Strait** ***Dan.*** Nares Stræde. *strait* Canada/Greenland
Nares Stræde *see* Nares Strait
110 *O9* **Narew** ≈ E Poland
155 *F17* **Nargund** Karnātaka, W India
83 *D20* **Narib** Hardap, S Namibia
Narikrik *see* Knox Atoll
54 *B13* **Nariño** ***off.*** Departamento de Nariño. ❖ *province* SW Colombia
165 *P13* **Narita** Chiba, Honshū, S Japan
165 *P13* **Narita** ✕ (Tōkyō) Chiba, Honshū, S Japan
Narıya *see* An Nu'ayrīyah
152 *J8* **Nārkanda** Himāchal Pradesh, NW India
92 *L13* **Narkaus** Lappi, NW Finland
154 *E11* **Narmada** ***var.*** Narbada. ≈ C India
152 *H11* **Narnaul** ***var.*** Nārnaul. Haryāna, N India
107 *I14* **Narni** Umbria, C Italy
107 *J24* **Naro** Sicilia, Italy, C Mediterranean Sea
Narodichi *see* Narodychi
127 *V7* **Narodnaya, Gora** ▲ NW Russian Federation
117 *N3* **Narodychi** ***Rus.*** Narodichi. Zhytomyrs'ka Oblast', N Ukraine
128 *J4* **Naro-Fominsk** Moskovskaya Oblast', W Russian Federation
81 *H19* **Narok** Rift Valley, SW Kenya
104 *H2* **Narón** Galicia, NW Spain
183 *S11* **Narooma** New South Wales, SE Australia
Narova *see* Narva
Narovlya *see* Narowlya
149 *W8* **Nārowāl** Punjab, E Pakistan
119 *N20* **Narowlya** ***Rus.*** Narovlya. Homyel'skaya Voblasts', SE Belarus
93 *J17* **Närpes** ***Fin.*** Närpiö. Länsi-Suomi, W Finland
Närpiö *see* Närpes
183 *S5* **Narrabri** New South Wales, SE Australia
183 *P9* **Narrandera** New South Wales, SE Australia
183 *Q4* **Narran Lake** ◎ New South Wales, SE Australia
183 *Q4* **Narran River** ≈ New South Wales/Queensland, SE Australia
180 *J13* **Narrogin** Western Australia
183 *Q7* **Narromine** New South Wales, SE Australia
21 *R6* **Narrows** Virginia, NE USA
196 *M15* **Narsarsuaq** ✕ Kitaa, S Greenland
154 *I10* **Narsimhapur** Madhya Pradesh, C India
Narsingdi *see* Narsinghdi
153 *U15* **Narsinghdi** ***var.*** Narsingdi. Dhaka, C Bangladesh
154 *H9* **Narsinghgarh** Madhya Pradesh, C India
163 *Q11* **Nart** Nei Mongol Zizhiqu, N China
Nartës, Gjol i/Nartës, Laguna e *see* Nartës, Liqeni i
113 *J22* **Nartës, Liqeni i** ***var.*** Gjol i Nartës, Laguna e Nartës. ◎ SW Albania
115 *F17* **Narthàki** ▲ C Greece
129 *O15* **Nartkala** Kabardino-Balkarskaya Respublika, SW Russian Federation
118 *K3* **Narva** Ida-Virumaa, NE Estonia
118 *K4* **Narva** ***prev.*** Narova. ≈ Estonia/Russian Federation
118 *J3* **Narva Bay** ***Est.*** Narva Laht, ***Ger.*** Narwa-Bucht, ***Rus.*** Narvskiy Zaliv. *bay* Estonia/Russian Federation
Narva Laht *see* Narva Bay
126 *F13* **Narva Reservoir** ***Est.*** Narva Veehoidla, ***Rus.*** Narvskoye Vodokhranilishche. ▣ Estonia/Russian Federation
Narva Veehoidla *see* Narva Reservoir
92 *H10* **Narvik** Nordland, C Norway
Narvskiy Zaliv *see* Narva Bay
Narvskoye Vodokhranilishche *see* Narva Reservoir
Narwa-Bucht *see* Narva Bay
152 *I9* **Narwāna** Haryāna, NW India
127 *R4* **Nar'yan-Mar** ***prev.*** Beloshchel'ye, Dzerzhinskiy. Nenetskiy Avtonomnyy Okrug, NW Russian Federation
122 *J12* **Narym** Tomskaya Oblast', C Russian Federation
145 *Y10* **Narymskiy Khrebet** ***Kaz.*** Naryn Zhotasy. ▲ E Kazakhstan
147 *W9* **Naryn** Narynskaya Oblast', C Kyrgyzstan
147 *U8* **Naryn** ≈ Kyrgyzstan/Uzbekistan
145 *W16* **Narynkol** ***Kaz.*** Narynqol. Almaty, SE Kazakhstan
Naryn Oblasty *see* Narynskaya Oblast'
Narynqol *see* Narynkol
147 *V9* **Narynskaya Oblast'** ***Kir.*** Naryn Oblasty. ❖ *province* C Kyrgyzstan
Naryn Zhotasy *see* Narymskiy Khrebet
128 *J6* **Naryshkino** Orlovskaya Oblast', W Russian Federation
95 *L14* **Nås** Dalarna, C Sweden
92 *G13* **Nasa** ▲ C Norway
93 *H16* **Näsåker** Västernorrland, C Sweden
187 *Y14* **Nasau** Koro, C Fiji
116 *I9* **Năsăud** ***Ger.*** Nussdorf, ***Hung.*** Naszód. Bistriţa-Năsăud, N Romania
103 *P13* **Nasbinals** Lozère, S France
Na Sceirí *see* Skerries
Nase *see* Naze
185 *E22* **Naseby** Otago, South Island, NZ
143 *R10* **Nāşerīyeh** Kermān, C Iran
25 *X5* **Nash** Texas, SW USA
154 *E13* **Nāshik** ***prev.*** Nāsik. Mahārāshtra, W India
56 *E7* **Nashiño, Río** ≈ Ecuador/Peru
29 *W12* **Nashua** Iowa, C USA
33 *W7* **Nashua** Montana, NW USA
19 *O10* **Nashua** New Hampshire, NE USA
27 *S13* **Nashville** Arkansas, C USA
23 *U7* **Nashville** Georgia, SE USA
30 *L16* **Nashville** Illinois, N USA
31 *O14* **Nashville** Indiana, N USA
21 *V9* **Nashville** North Carolina, SE USA
20 *J8* **Nashville** *state capital* Tennessee, S USA
20 *J9* **Nashville** ✕ Tennessee, S USA
64 *H10* **Nashville Seamount** *undersea feature* NW Atlantic Ocean
112 *H9* **Našice** Osijek-Baranja, E Croatia
110 *M11* **Nasielsk** Mazowieckie, C Poland
93 *K18* **Näsijärvi** ◎ SW Finland
Nāsik *see* Nāshik
80 *G13* **Nasir** Upper Nile, SE Sudan
149 *Q12* **Nasīrābād** Baluchistān, SW Pakistan
148 *K15* **Nasīrābād** Baluchistān, SW Pakistan
Nasirābād *see* Mymensingh
Nasir, Buhayrat/Nâşir, Buḩeiret *see* Nasser, Lake
Nāsiri *see* Ahvāz
Nasiriya *see* An Nāşirīyah
Nás na Ríogh *see* Naas
107 *L23* **Naso** Sicilia, Italy, C Mediterranean Sea
Nasratabad *see* Zābol
10 *J11* **Nass** ≈ British Columbia, SW Canada
77 *V15* **Nassarawa** Nassarawa, C Nigeria
44 *H2* **Nassau** ● (Bahamas) New Providence, N Bahamas
44 *H2* **Nassau** ✕ New Providence, C Bahamas
190 *J13* **Nassau** *island* N Cook Islands
23 *W8* **Nassau Sound** *sound* Florida, SE USA
108 *L7* **Nassereith** Tirol, W Austria
95 *L19* **Nässjö** Jönköping, S Sweden
99 *K22* **Nassogne** Luxembourg, SE Belgium
12 *J6* **Nastapoka Islands** *island group* Nunavut, C Canada
93 *M19* **Nastola** Etelä-Suomi, S Finland
171 *O4* **Nasugbu** Luzon, N Philippines
94 *N11* **Näsviken** Gävleborg, C Sweden
Naszód *see* Năsăud
83 *I17* **Nata** Central, NE Botswana
54 *E11* **Natagaima** Tolima, C Colombia
59 *Q14* **Natal** Rio Grande do Norte, E Brazil
168 *I11* **Natal** Sumatera, N Indonesia
Natal *see* KwaZulu/Natal
173 *L10* **Natal Basin** ***var.*** Mozambique Basin. *undersea feature* W Indian Ocean
25 *R12* **Natalia** Texas, SW USA
67 *W15* **Natal Valley** *undersea feature* SW Indian Ocean
Natanya *see* Netanya
143 *O7* **Naţanz** Eşfahān, C Iran
13 *Q11* **Natashquan** Quebec, E Canada

◆ Country
● Country Capital
◇ Dependent Territory
○ Dependent Territory Capital
❖ Administrative Region
✕ International Airport
▲ Mountain
▲ Mountain Range
Volcano
≈ River
◎ Lake
▣ Reservoir

13 Q10 **Natashquan** Newfoundland/Quebec, E Canada
22 J7 **Natchez** Mississippi, S USA
22 G6 **Natchitoches** Louisiana, S USA
108 E10 **Naters** Valais, S Switzerland
Nathanya *see* Netanya
92 O3 **Nathorst Land** *physical region* W Svalbard
Nathula *see* Nacula
186 E9 **National Capital District** *province* S PNG
35 U17 **National City** California, W USA
184 M10 **National Park** Manawatu-Wanganui, North Island, NZ
77 R14 **Natitingou** NW Benin
40 B5 **Natividad, Isla** *island* W Mexico
165 Q10 **Natori** Miyagi, Honshū, C Japan
18 C14 **Natrona Heights** Pennsylvania, NE USA
81 H20 **Natron, Lake** ◎ Kenya/Tanzania
Natsrat *see* Nazerat
166 L7 **Nattalin** Pegu, C Myanmar
92 J12 **Nattavaara** Norrbotten, N Sweden
109 S3 **Natternbach** Oberösterreich, N Austria
95 M22 **Nättraby** Blekinge, S Sweden
169 P10 **Natuna Besar, Pulau** *island* Kepulauan Natuna, W Indonesia
169 O9 **Natuna Islands** *see* Natuna, Kepulauan
169 O9 **Natuna, Kepulauan** *var.* Natuna Islands. *island group* W Indonesia
169 N9 **Natuna, Laut** *sea* W Indonesia
21 N6 **Natural Bridge** *tourist site* Kentucky, C USA
173 V11 **Naturaliste Fracture Zone** *tectonic feature* E Indian Ocean
174 J10 **Naturaliste Plateau** *undersea feature* E Indian Ocean
Nau *see* Nov
103 O14 **Naucelle** Aveyron, S France
83 D20 **Nauchas** Hardap, C Namibia
108 K9 **Nauders** Tirol, W Austria
Naugard *see* Nowogard
118 F12 **Naujamiestis** Panevėžys, C Lithuania
118 E10 **Naujoji Akmenė** Akmenė, NW Lithuania
149 R16 **Naukot** *var.* Naokot. Sind, SE Pakistan
101 L16 **Naumburg** *var.* Naumburg an der Saale. Sachsen-Anhalt, C Germany
Naumburg am Queis *see* Nowogrodziec
Naumburg an der Saale *see* Naumburg
191 W15 **Naunau** *ancient monument* Easter Island, Chile, E Pacific Ocean
138 G10 **Nā'ūr** 'Ammān, W Jordan
189 Q8 **Nauru** *off.* Republic of Nauru; *prev.* Pleasant Island. ◆ *republic* W Pacific Ocean
175 P5 **Nauru** *island* W Pacific Ocean
189 Q9 **Nauru International** ✕ S Nauru
Nausari *see* Navsāri
19 Q12 **Nauset Beach** *beach* Massachusetts, NE USA
Naushahra *see* Nowshera
149 P14 **Naushahro Fīroz** Sind, SE Pakistan
Naushara *see* Nowshera
187 X14 **Nausori** Viti Levu, W Fiji
56 F9 **Nauta** Loreto, N Peru
153 O12 **Nautanwa** Uttar Pradesh, N India
41 R13 **Nautla** Veracruz-Llave, E Mexico
Nauzad *see* Now Zād
41 N6 **Nava** Coahuila de Zaragoza, NE Mexico
Navabad *see* Navobod
104 L6 **Nava del Rey** Castilla-León, N Spain
153 S15 **Navadwīp** *prev.* Nabadwip. West Bengal, NE India
104 M9 **Navahermosa** Castilla-La Mancha, C Spain
119 I16 **Navahrudak** *Pol.* Nowogródek, *Rus.* Novogrudok. Hrodzyenskaya Voblasts', W Belarus
119 I16 **Navahrudskaye Wzvyshsha** ▲ W Belarus
36 M8 **Navajo Mount** ▲ Utah, W USA
37 Q9 **Navajo Reservoir** ⊡ New Mexico, SW USA
104 K9 **Navalmoral de la Mata** Extremadura, W Spain
104 K10 **Navalvillar de Pelea** Extremadura, W Spain
97 F17 **Navan** *Ir.* An Uaimh. E Ireland
Navanagar *see* Jāmnagar
118 L12 **Navapolatsk** *Rus.* Novopolotsk. Vitsyebskaya Voblasts', N Belarus
149 P6 **Nāvar, Dasht-e** *Pash.* Dasht-i-Nawar. *desert* C Afghanistan
123 W6 **Navarin, Mys** *headland* NE Russian Federation
63 I25 **Navarino, Isla** *island* S Chile
105 Q4 **Navarra** *Eng./Fr.* Navarre. *autonomous community* N Spain
Navarre *see* Navarra
105 P4 **Navarrete** La Rioja, N Spain
61 C20 **Navarro** Buenos Aires, E Argentina
105 O12 **Navas de San Juan** Andalucía, S Spain
25 V10 **Navasota** Texas, SW USA
25 U9 **Navasota River** Texas, SW USA
44 I9 **Navassa Island** ◇ *US unincorporated territory* C West Indies
119 L19 **Navasyolki** *Rus.* Novosëlki. Homyel'skaya Voblasts', SE Belarus
119 H17 **Navayel'nya** *Pol.* Nowojelnia, *Rus.* Novoyel'nya. Hrodzyenskaya Voblasts', W Belarus
171 Y13 **Naver** Irian Jaya, E Indonesia
118 H5 **Navesti** C Estonia
104 J2 **Navia** Asturias, N Spain
104 J2 **Navia** NW Spain
59 I21 **Naviraí** Mato Grosso do Sul, SW Brazil
128 I6 **Navlya** Bryanskaya Oblast', W Russian Federation
187 X13 **Navoalevu** Vanua Levu, N Fiji
147 R12 **Navobod** *Rus.* Navabad, Novabad. C Tajikistan
147 P13 **Navobod** *Rus.* Navabad. W Tajikistan
Navoi *see* Nawoiy
Navoiyskaya Oblast' *see* Nawoiy Wiloyati
40 G7 **Navojoa** Sonora, NW Mexico
Navolat *see* Navolato
42 H9 **Navolato** *var.* Navolat. Sinaloa, C Mexico
187 Q13 **Navonda** Ambae, C Vanuatu
Návpaktos *see* Náfpaktos
Návplion *see* Náfplio
77 P14 **Navrongo** N Ghana
154 D12 **Navsāri** *var.* Nausari. Gujarāt, W India
187 X15 **Navua** Viti Levu, W Fiji
138 H8 **Nawá** Dar'ā, S Syria
Nawabashah *see* Nawābshāh
153 S14 **Nawabganj** Rajshahi, NW Bangladesh
153 S14 **Nawābganj** Uttar Pradesh, N India
149 Q15 **Nawābshāh** *var.* Nawabashah. Sind, S Pakistan
153 P14 **Nawāda** Bihār, N India
152 H11 **Nawalgarh** Rājasthān, N India
Nawāl, Sabkhat an *see* Noual, Sebkhet en
Nawar, Dasht-i- *see* Nāvar, Dasht-e
167 N4 **Nawnghkio** *var.* Nawngkio. Shan State, C Myanmar
Nawngkio *see* Nawnghkio
146 M11 **Nawoiy** *Rus.* Navoi. Nawoiy Wiloyati, C Uzbekistan
146 K8 **Nawoiy Wiloyati** *Rus.* Navoiyskaya Oblast'. *province* N Uzbekistan
137 U13 **Naxçıvan** *Rus.* Nakhichevan'. SW Azerbaijan
160 I10 **Naxi** Sichuan, C China
115 K21 **Náxos** *var.* Naxos. Náxos, Kykládes, Greece, Aegean Sea
115 K21 **Náxos** *island* Kykládes, Greece, Aegean Sea
40 J11 **Nayarit** *state* C Mexico
187 Y14 **Nayau** *island* Lau Group, E Fiji
143 S8 **Nāy Band** Khorāsān, E Iran
165 T2 **Nayoro** Hokkaidō, NE Japan
104 F9 **Nazaré** *var.* Nazare. Leiria, C Portugal
24 M4 **Nazareth** Texas, SW USA
Nazareth *see* Nazerat
173 O8 **Nazareth Bank** *undersea feature* W Indian Ocean
40 K9 **Nazas** Durango, C Mexico
57 F16 **Nazca** Ica, S Peru
(0) L17 **Nazca Plate** *tectonic feature*
193 U9 **Nazca Ridge** *undersea feature* E Pacific Ocean
165 V15 **Naze** *var.* Nase. Kagoshima, Amami-ōshima, SW Japan
138 G9 **Nazerat** *var.* Natsrat, *Ar.* En Nazira, *Eng.* Nazareth. Northern, N Israel
137 R14 **Nazik Gölü** ◎ E Turkey
136 C15 **Nazilli** Aydın, SW Turkey
137 P14 **Nazimiye** Tunceli, E Turkey
Nazinon *see* Red Volta
10 L15 **Nazko** British Columbia, SW Canada
129 O16 **Nazran'** Ingushskaya Respublika, SW Russian Federation
80 J13 **Nazrēt** *var.* Adama, Hadama. Oromo, C Ethiopia
Nazwāh *see* Nizwá
82 J13 **Nchanga** Copperbelt, C Zambia
82 J11 **Nchelenge** Luapula, N Zambia
Ncheu *see* Ntcheu
Ndaghamcha, Sebkra de *see* Te-n-Dghâmcha, Sebkhet
81 G21 **Ndala** Tabora, C Tanzania
82 B11 **N'Dalatando** *Port.* Salazar, Vila Salazar. Cuanza Norte, NW Angola
77 S14 **Ndali** C Benin
81 E18 **Ndeke** SW Uganda
78 J13 **Ndélé** Bamingui-Bangoran, N Central African Republic
79 E19 **Ndendé** Ngounié, S Gabon
79 E20 **Ndindi** Nyanga, S Gabon
78 G11 **Ndjamena** *var.* N'Djamena; *prev.* Fort-Lamy. ● (Chad) Chari-Baguirmi, W Chad
78 G11 **Ndjamena** ✕ Chari-Baguirmi, W Chad
79 D18 **Ndjolé** Moyen-Ogooué, W Gabon
82 J13 **Ndola** Copperbelt, C Zambia
Ndrhamcha, Sebkha de *see* Te-n-Dghâmcha, Sebkhet
79 L15 **Ndu** Orientale, N Dem. Rep. Congo (Zaire)
81 H21 **Nduguti** Singida, C Tanzania
186 M9 **Nduindui** Guadalcanal, C Solomon Islands
Nduke *see* Kolombangara
115 F16 **Néa Anchíalos** *var.* Nea Anhialos, Néa Ankhíalos. Thessalía, C Greece
Nea Anhialos/Néa Ankhíalos *see* Néa Anchíalos
115 H18 **Néa Artáki** Évvoia, C Greece
97 F15 **Neagh, Lough** ◎ E Northern Ireland, UK
32 F7 **Neah Bay** Washington, NW USA
115 J22 **Nea Kaméni** *island* Kykládes, Greece, Aegean Sea
181 O8 **Neale, Lake** ◎ Northern Territory, C Australia
182 G2 **Neales River** *seasonal river* South Australia
115 G14 **Néa Moudanía** *var.* Néa Moudhaniá. Kentrikí Makedonía, N Greece
Néa Moudhaniá *see* Néa Moudanía
116 K10 **Neamț** *county* NE Romania
Neapel *see* Napoli
115 D14 **Neápoli** *prev.* Neápolis. Dytikí Makedonía, N Greece
115 K25 **Neápoli** Kríti, Greece, E Mediterranean Sea
115 G22 **Neápoli** Pelopónnisos, S Greece
Neapolis *see* Napoli, Italy
Neapolis *see* Nablus, West Bank
Neápolis *see* Neápoli, Greece
38 D16 **Near Islands** *island group* Aleutian Islands, Alaska, USA
97 J21 **Neath** S Wales, UK
114 H13 **Néa Zíchni** *var.* Néa Zíkhni; *prev.* Néa Zíkhna. Kentrikí Makedonía, NE Greece
Néa Zíkhna/Néa Zíkhni *see* Néa Zíchni
42 C5 **Nebaj** Quiché, W Guatemala
77 P13 **Nebbou** S Burkina
146 B11 **Nebitdag** Balkanskiy Velayat, W Turkmenistan
54 M13 **Neblina, Pico da** ▲ NW Brazil
126 I13 **Nebolchi** Novgorodskaya Oblast', W Russian Federation
36 L4 **Nebo, Mount** ▲ Utah, W USA
28 L14 **Nebraska** *off.* State of Nebraska; also known as Blackwater State, Cornhusker State, Tree Planters State. *state* C USA
29 S16 **Nebraska City** Nebraska, C USA
107 K23 **Nebrodi, Monti** *var.* Monti Caronie. ▲ Sicilia, Italy, C Mediterranean Sea
10 L14 **Nechako** British Columbia, SW Canada
29 Q2 **Neche** North Dakota, N USA
25 V8 **Neches** Texas, SW USA
25 W8 **Neches River** Texas, SW USA
101 H20 **Neckar** SW Germany
101 H20 **Neckarsulm** Baden-Württemberg, SW Germany
192 L5 **Necker Island** *island* C British Virgin Islands
175 U3 **Necker Ridge** *undersea feature* N Pacific Ocean
61 D23 **Necochea** Buenos Aires, E Argentina
104 H2 **Neda** Galicia, NW Spain
115 E20 **Nédas** S Greece
25 Y11 **Nederland** Texas, SW USA
Nederland *see* Netherlands
98 K12 **Neder Rijn** *Eng.* Lower Rhine. C Netherlands
99 L16 **Nederweert** Limburg, SE Netherlands
95 G16 **Nedre Tokke** ◎ S Norway
Nedrigaylov *see* Nedryhayliv
117 S3 **Nedryhayliv** *Rus.* Nedrigaylov. Sums'ka Oblast', NE Ukraine
98 O11 **Neede** Gelderland, E Netherlands
33 T13 **Needle Mountain** ▲ Wyoming, C USA
35 Y14 **Needles** California, W USA
97 M24 **Needles, The** *rocks* Isle of Wight, S England, UK
62 O7 **Ñeembucú** *off.* Departamento de Ñeembucú. *department* SW Paraguay
30 M7 **Neenah** Wisconsin, N USA
11 W16 **Neepawa** Manitoba, S Canada
99 K16 **Neerpelt** Limburg, NE Belgium
74 M6 **Nefta** Tunisia
128 L15 **Neftegorsk** Krasnodarskiy Kray, SW Russian Federation
129 U3 **Neftekamsk** Respublika Bashkortostan, W Russian Federation
129 O14 **Neftekumsk** Stavropol'skiy Kray, SW Russian Federation
Neftezavodsk *see* Seydi
82 C10 **Negage** *var.* N'Gage. Uíge, NW Angola
Negapatam/Negapattinam *see* Nāgappattinam
169 T17 **Negara** Bali, Indonesia
169 T13 **Negara** Borneo, C Indonesia
Negara Brunei Darussalam *see* Brunei
31 N4 **Negaunee** Michigan, N USA
81 J15 **Negēlē** *var.* Negelli, *It.* Neghelli. Oromo, C Ethiopia
Negelli *see* Negēlē
Negeri Pahang Darul Makmur *see* Pahang
Negeri Selangor Darul Ehsan *see* Selangor
168 K9 **Negeri Sembilan** *var.* Negri Sembilan. *state* Peninsular Malaysia
92 P3 **Negerpynten** *headland* S Svalbard
Negev *see* HaNegev
Neghelli *see* Negēlē
116 I12 **Negoiu** *var.* Negoiul. ▲ S Romania
Negoiul *see* Negoiu
82 P13 **Negomane** *var.* Negomano. Cabo Delgado, N Mozambique
Negomano *see* Negomane
155 J25 **Negombo** Western Province, SW Sri Lanka
Negoreloye *see* Nyeharelaye
112 P12 **Negotin** Serbia, E Yugoslavia
113 P19 **Negotino** C FYR Macedonia
56 A10 **Negra, Punta** *headland* NW Peru
104 G3 **Negreira** Galicia, NW Spain
116 L10 **Negrești** Vaslui, E Romania
Negrești *see* Negrești-Oaș
116 H8 **Negrești-Oaș** *Hung.* Avasfelsőfalu; *prev.* Negrești. Satu Mare, NE Romania
44 H12 **Negril** W Jamaica
Negri Sembilan *see* Negeri Sembilan
63 K15 **Negro, Río** E Argentina
62 N7 **Negro, Río** NE Argentina
57 N17 **Negro, Río** E Bolivia
62 O5 **Negro, Río** C Paraguay
48 F6 **Negro, Río** N South America
61 E18 **Negro, Río** Brazil/Uruguay
Negro, Río *see* Sico Tinto, Río, Honduras
Negro, Río *see* Chixoy, Río, Guatemala/Mexico
171 P6 **Negros** *island* C Philippines
116 M15 **Negru Vodă** Constanța, SE Romania
13 P13 **Neguac** New Brunswick, SE Canada
14 B7 **Negwazu, Lake** ◎ Ontario, S Canada
Négyfalu *see* Săcele
32 F10 **Nehalem** Oregon, NW USA
32 F10 **Nehalem River** Oregon, NW USA
Nehavend *see* Nahāvand
143 V9 **Nehbandān** Khorāsān, E Iran
163 V6 **Nehe** Heilongjiang, NE China
193 Y14 **Neiafu** 'Uta Vava'u, N Tonga
45 N9 **Neiba** *var.* Neyba. SW Dominican Republic
Néid, Carn Uí *see* Mizen Head
92 M9 **Neiden** Finnmark, N Norway
Neidín *see* Kenmare
Néifinn *see* Nephin
103 S10 **Neige, Crêt de la** ▲ E France
173 O16 **Neiges, Piton des** ▲ C Réunion
15 R9 **Neiges, Rivière des** Québec, SE Canada
160 I10 **Neijiang** Sichuan, C China
30 K6 **Neillsville** Wisconsin, N USA
Nei Monggol Zizhiqu/Nei Mongol *see* Nei Mongol Zizhiqu
163 Q10 **Nei Mongol Gaoyuan** *plateau* NE China
163 O12 **Nei Mongol Zizhiqu** *var.* Nei Mongol, *Eng.* Inner Mongolia, Inner Mongolian Autonomous Region; *prev.* Nei Monggol Zizhiqu. *autonomous region* N China
161 O4 **Neiqiu** Hebei, E China
Neiriz *see* Neyrīz
101 Q16 **Neisse** *Cz.* Lužická Nisa, *Ger.* Lausitzer Neisse, *Pol.* Nisa, Nysa Łużycka. C Europe
Neisse *see* Nysa
54 E11 **Neiva** Huila, S Colombia
160 M7 **Neixiang** Henan, C China
Nejafabad *see* Najafābād
11 V9 **Nejanilini Lake** ◎ Manitoba, C Canada
Nejd *see* Najd
80 I13 **Nek'emtē** *var.* Lakemti, Nakamti. Oromo, C Ethiopia
128 M9 **Nekhayevskiy** Volgogradskaya Oblast', SW Russian Federation
30 K7 **Nekoosa** Wisconsin, N USA
95 M24 **Neksø** Bornholm, E Denmark
115 C16 **Nekyomanteío** *ancient monument* Ípeiros, W Greece
104 H7 **Nelas** Viseu, N Portugal
126 H16 **Nelidovo** Tverskaya Oblast', W Russian Federation
29 P13 **Neligh** Nebraska, C USA
123 R11 **Nel'kan** Khabarovskiy Kray, E Russian Federation
92 M10 **Nellim** *var.* Nellimö, *Lapp.* Njellim. Lappi, N Finland
Nellimö *see* Nellim
155 J18 **Nellore** Andhra Pradesh, E India
123 T14 **Nel'ma** Khabarovskiy Kray, SE Russian Federation
61 B17 **Nelson** Santa Fe, C Argentina
11 O17 **Nelson** British Columbia, SW Canada
185 I14 **Nelson** Nelson, South Island, NZ
97 L17 **Nelson** NW England, UK
29 P17 **Nelson** Nebraska, C USA
185 J14 **Nelson** *unitary authority* South Island, NZ
11 X12 **Nelson** Manitoba, C Canada
183 U8 **Nelson Bay** New South Wales, SE Australia
182 K13 **Nelson, Cape** *headland* Victoria, SE Australia
63 G23 **Nelson, Estrecho** *strait* SE Pacific Ocean
11 W12 **Nelson House** Manitoba, C Canada
30 J4 **Nelson Lake** ◎ Wisconsin, N USA
31 T14 **Nelsonville** Ohio, N USA
27 S2 **Nelsoon River** Iowa/Missouri, C USA
83 K21 **Nelspruit** Mpumalanga, NE South Africa
76 L10 **Néma** Hodh ech Chargui, SE Mauritania
118 D13 **Neman** *Ger.* Ragnit. Kaliningradskaya Oblast', W Russian Federation
84 I9 **Neman** *Bel.* Nyoman, *Ger.* Memel, *Lith.* Nemunas, *Pol.* Niemen, *Rus.* Neman. NE Europe
Nemausus *see* Nîmes
115 F19 **Neméa** Pelopónnisos, S Greece
Německý Brod *see* Havlíčkův Brod
14 D7 **Nemegosenda** Ontario, S Canada
14 D8 **Nemegosenda Lake** ◎ Ontario, S Canada
119 H14 **Nemenčinė** Vilnius, SE Lithuania
Nemetocenna *see* Arras
Nemirov *see* Nemyriv
103 O6 **Nemours** Seine-et-Marne, N France
Nemunas *see* Neman
165 W4 **Nemuro** Hokkaidō, NE Japan
165 W4 **Nemuro-hantō** *peninsula* Hokkaidō, NE Japan
165 W3 **Nemuro-kaikyō** *strait* Japan/Russian Federation
165 W4 **Nemuro-wan** *bay* N Japan
116 H5 **Nemyriv** *Rus.* Nemirov. L'vivs'ka Oblast', NW Ukraine
117 N7 **Nemyriv** *Rus.* Nemirov. Vinnyts'ka Oblast', C Ukraine
97 D19 **Nenagh** *Ir.* An tAonach. C Ireland
39 R9 **Nenana** Alaska, USA
39 R9 **Nenana River** Alaska, USA
187 P10 **Nendö** *var.* Swallow Island. *island* Santa Cruz Islands, E Solomon Islands
97 O19 **Nene** E England, UK
127 R4 **Nenetskiy Avtonomnyy Okrug** *autonomous district* NW Russian Federation
191 W11 **Nengonengo** *atoll* Îles Tuamotu, C French Polynesia
163 U6 **Nen Jiang** *var.* Nonni. NE China
163 V6 **Nenjiang** Heilongjiang, NE China
189 P16 **Neoch** *atoll* Caroline Islands, C Micronesia
115 D18 **Neochóri** Dytikí Ellás, C Greece
27 Q7 **Neodesha** Kansas, C USA
29 S14 **Neola** Iowa, C USA
115 M19 **Néon Karlovásí** *var.* Néon Karlovásion. Sámos, Dodekánisos, Greece, Aegean Sea
Néon Karlovásion *see* Néon Karlovásí
115 E16 **Néon Monastíri** Thessalía, C Greece
27 R8 **Neosho** Missouri, C USA
27 Q7 **Neosho River** Kansas/Oklahoma, C USA
123 N12 **Nepa** C Russian Federation
153 N10 **Nepal** *off.* Kingdom of Nepal. ◆ *monarchy* S Asia
152 M11 **Nepalganj** Mid Western, SW Nepal
14 L13 **Nepean** Ontario, SE Canada
36 L4 **Nephi** Utah, W USA
97 B16 **Nephin** *Ir.* Néifinn. ▲ W Ireland
67 T9 **Nepoko** NE Dem. Rep. Congo (Zaire)
18 K15 **Neptune** New Jersey, NE USA
182 G10 **Neptune Islands** *island group* South Australia
107 I14 **Nera** *anc.* Nar. C Italy
102 L14 **Nérac** Lot-et-Garonne, SW France
111 D16 **Neratovice** *Ger.* Neratowitz. Středočeský Kraj, C Czech Republic
Neratowitz *see* Neratovice
123 O13 **Nercha** S Russian Federation
123 O13 **Nerchinsk** Chitinskaya Oblast', S Russian Federation
123 P14 **Nerchinskiy Zavod** Chitinskaya Oblast', S Russian Federation
126 M15 **Nerekhta** Kostromskaya Oblast', NW Russian Federation
118 H10 **Nereta** Aizkraukle, S Latvia
106 K13 **Nereto** Abruzzo, C Italy
113 H15 **Neretva** Bosnia and Herzegovina/Croatia
115 C17 **Nerikós** *ruins* Lefkáda, Iónioi Nísoi, Greece, C Mediterranean Sea
118 B12 **Neringa** *Ger.* Nidden; *prev.* Nida. Neringa, SW Lithuania
83 F15 **Neriquinha** Cuando Cubango, SE Angola
118 I13 **Neris** *Bel.* Viliya, *Pol.* Wilia; *prev. Pol.* Wilja. Belarus/Lithuania
Neris *see* Viliya
105 N15 **Nerja** Andalucía, S Spain
126 L16 **Nerl'** W Russian Federation
105 P12 **Nerpio** Castilla-La Mancha, C Spain
104 J13 **Nerva** Andalucía, S Spain
98 L4 **Nes** Friesland, N Netherlands
94 G13 **Nesbyen** Buskerud, S Norway
92 L2 **Neskaupstadhur** Austurland, E Iceland
92 F13 **Nesna** Nordland, C Norway
26 K5 **Ness City** Kansas, C USA
Nesselsdorf *see* Kopřivnice
108 H7 **Nesslau** Sankt Gallen, NE Switzerland
96 I9 **Ness, Loch** ◎ N Scotland, UK
Nesterov *see* Zhovkva
114 I12 **Néstos** *Bul.* Mesta, *Turk.* Kara Su. Bulgaria/Greece *see also* Mesta
95 C14 **Nesttun** Hordaland, S Norway
Nesvizh *see* Nyasvizh
138 F9 **Netanya** *var.* Natanya, Nathanya. Central, C Israel
98 I9 **Netherlands** *off.* Kingdom of the Netherlands, *var.* Holland, *Dut.* Koninkrijk der Nederlanden, Nederland. ◆ *monarchy* NW Europe
45 S9 **Netherlands Antilles** *prev.* Dutch West Indies. ◇ *Dutch autonomous region* S Caribbean Sea
Netherlands East Indies *see* Indonesia
Netherlands Guiana *see* Surinam
Netherlands New Guinea *see* Irian Jaya
116 L4 **Netishyn** Khmel'nyts'ka Oblast', W Ukraine
138 E11 **Netivot** Southern, S Israel
107 O21 **Neto** S Italy
9 Q6 **Nettilling Lake** ◎ Baffin Island, Nunavut, N Canada
29 V3 **Nett Lake** ◎ Minnesota, N USA
107 I16 **Nettuno** Lazio, C Italy
Netum *see* Noto
41 U16 **Netzahualcóyotl, Presa** ⊡ SE Mexico
Netze *see* Noteć
Neu Amerika *see* Puławy
Neubetsche *see* Novi Bečej
Neubidschow *see* Nový Bydžov
Neubistritz *see* Nová Bystřice
100 N9 **Neubrandenburg** Mecklenburg-Vorpommern, NE Germany
101 K22 **Neuburg an der Donau** Bayern, S Germany
108 C8 **Neuchâtel** *Ger.* Neuenburg. Neuchâtel, W Switzerland
108 C8 **Neuchâtel** *Ger.* Neuenburg. *canton* W Switzerland
108 C8 **Neuchâtel, Lac de** *Ger.* Neuenburger See. ◎ W Switzerland
Neudorf *see* Spišská Nová Ves
100 L10 **Neue Elde** *canal* N Germany
Neuenburg *see* Neuchâtel
Neuenburg an der Elbe *see* Nymburk
Neuenburger See *see* Neuchâtel, Lac de
108 F7 **Neuenhof** Aargau, N Switzerland
100 H11 **Neuenland** ✕ (Bremen) Bremen, NW Germany
Neuenstadt *see* La Neuveville
101 C18 **Neuerburg** Rheinland-Pfalz, W Germany
99 K24 **Neufchâteau** Luxembourg, SE Belgium
103 S6 **Neufchâteau** Vosges, NE France
102 M3 **Neufchâtel-en-Bray** Seine-Maritime, N France
109 S3 **Neufelden** Oberösterreich, N Austria
Neugradisk *see* Nova Gradiška
Neuhaus *see* Jindřichův Hradec
Neuhäusel *see* Nové Zámky
108 G6 **Neuhausen** *var.* Neuhausen am Rheinfall. Schaffhausen, N Switzerland
Neuhausen am Rheinfall *see* Neuhausen
101 I17 **Neuhof** Hessen, C Germany
Neuhof *see* Zgierz
Neukuhren *see* Pionerskiy
Neu-Langenburg *see* Tukuyu
109 W4 **Neulengbach** Niederösterreich, NE Austria
113 G15 **Neum** Federacija Bosna I Hercegovina, S Bosnia and Herzegovina
Neumark *see* Nowy Targ, Nowy Sącz, Poland
Neumark *see* Nowe Miasto Lubawskie, Toruń, Poland
Neumarkt *see* Neumarkt im Hausruckkreis, Oberösterreich, Austria
Neumarkt *see* Neumarkt am Wallersee, Salzburg, Austria
Neumarkt *see* Środa Śląska, Wrocław, Poland
Neumarkt *see* Târgu Secuiesc, Covasna, Romania
Neumarkt *see* Târgu Mureș, Mureș, Romania
109 Q5 **Neumarkt am Wallersee** *var.* Neumarkt. Salzburg, NW Austria
109 R4 **Neumarkt im Hausruckkreis** *var.* Neumarkt. Oberösterreich, N Austria
101 L20 **Neumarkt in der Oberpfalz** Bayern, SE Germany
Neumarktl *see* Tržič
Neumoldowa *see* Moldova Nouă
100 J8 **Neumünster** Schleswig-Holstein, N Germany
109 X5 **Neunkirchen** *var.* Neunkirchen am Steinfeld. Niederösterreich, E Austria
101 E20 **Neunkirchen** Saarland, SW Germany
Neunkirchen am Steinfeld *see* Neunkirchen
Neuoderberg *see* Bohumín
63 I15 **Neuquén** Neuquén, SE Argentina
63 H14 **Neuquén** *off.* Provincia de Neuquén. *province* W Argentina
63 H14 **Neuquén, Río** W Argentina
Neurode *see* Nowa Ruda
100 N11 **Neuruppin** Brandenburg, NE Germany
Neusalz an der Oder *see* Nowa Sól
Neu Sandec/Neusandez *see* Małopolskie
101 K22 **Neusäss** Bayern, S Germany
Neusatz *see* Novi Sad
Neuschliss *see* Gherla
21 N8 **Neuse River** North Carolina, SE USA
109 Z5 **Neusiedl am See** Burgenland, E Austria
111 G22 **Neusiedler See** *Hung.* Fertő. ◎ Austria/Hungary
Neusohl *see* Banská Bystrica
101 D15 **Neuss** *anc.* Novaesium, Novesium. Nordrhein-Westfalen, W Germany
Neuss *see* Nyon
Neustadt *see* Neustadt an der Aisch, Bayern, Germany
Neustadt *see* Neustadt bei Coburg, Bayern, Germany
Neustadt *see* Prudnik, Opole, Poland
Neustadt *see* Baia Mare, Maramureș, Romania
100 I12 **Neustadt am Rübenberge** Niedersachsen, N Germany
101 J19 **Neustadt an der Aisch** *var.* Neustadt. Bayern, C Germany
Neustadt an der Haardt *see* Neustadt an der Weinstrasse
101 F20 **Neustadt an der Weinstrasse** *prev.* Neustadt an der Haardt, *hist.* Niewenstat, *anc.* Nova Civitas. Rheinland-Pfalz, SW Germany
101 K18 **Neustadt bei Coburg** *var.* Neustadt. Bayern, C Germany
Neustadt bei Pinne *see* Lwówek
Neustadt in Oberschlesien *see* Prudnik
Neustadtl *see* Novo mesto
Neustadtl in Mähren *see* Nové Město na Moravě
Neustettin *see* Szczecinek
108 M8 **Neustift im Stubaital** *var.* Stubaital. Tirol, W Austria
100 N10 **Neustrelitz** Mecklenburg-Vorpommern, NE Germany
Neutitschein *see* Nový Jičín
Neutra *see* Nitra
101 J22 **Neu-Ulm** Bayern, S Germany
Neuveville *see* La Neuveville
103 N12 **Neuvic** Corrèze, C France
Neuwarp *see* Nowe Warpno
100 G9 **Neuwerk** *island* NW Germany
101 E17 **Neuwied** Rheinland-Pfalz, W Germany
Neuzen *see* Terneuzen
126 H12 **Neva** NW Russian Federation
29 V14 **Nevada** Iowa, C USA
27 R6 **Nevada** Missouri, C USA
35 R5 **Nevada** *off.* State of Nevada; also known as Battle Born State, Sagebrush State, Silver State. *state* W USA
35 P6 **Nevada City** California, W USA
126 G16 **Nevel'** Pskovskaya Oblast', W Russian Federation
123 T14 **Nevel'sk** Ostrov Sakhalin, Sakhalinskaya Oblast', SE Russian Federation

◆ Country ● Country Capital ◇ Dependent Territory ○ Dependent Territory Capital Administrative Region ✕ International Airport ▲ Mountain Mountain Range Volcano River ◎ Lake ⊡ Reservoir

123 Q13 **Never** Amurskaya Oblast', SE Russian Federation
129 Q6 **Neverkino** Penzenskaya Oblast', W Russian Federation
103 P9 **Nevers** *anc.* Noviodunum. Nièvre, C France
18 J12 **Neversink River** ≈ New York, NE USA
183 Q6 **Nevertire** New South Wales, SE Australia
113 H15 **Nevesinje** Republika Srpska, S Bosnia and Herzegovina
118 G12 **Nevėžis** ≈ C Lithuania
128 M14 **Nevinnomyssk** Stavropol'skiy Kray, SW Russian Federation
45 W10 **Nevis** *island* Saint Kitts and Nevis
Nevoso, Monte *see* Veliki Snežnik
Nevrokop *see* Gotse Delchev
136 J14 **Nevşehir** *var.* Nevshehr. Nevşehir, C Turkey
136 J14 **Nevşehir** *var.* Nevshehr. ❖ *province* C Turkey
Nevshehr *see* Nevşehir
122 G10 **Nev'yansk** Sverdlovskaya Oblast', C Russian Federation
81 J25 **Newala** Mtwara, SE Tanzania
31 P16 **New Albany** Indiana, N USA
22 M2 **New Albany** Mississippi, S USA
29 Y11 **New Albin** Iowa, C USA
55 U8 **New Amsterdam** E Guyana
183 Q4 **New Angledool** New South Wales, SE Australia
21 Y2 **Newark** Delaware, NE USA
18 K14 **Newark** New Jersey, NE USA
18 G10 **Newark** New York, NE USA
31 T13 **Newark** Ohio, N USA
Newark *see* Newark-on-Trent
35 W5 **Newark Lake** ◎ Nevada, W USA
97 N18 **Newark-on-Trent** *var.* Newark. C England, UK
22 M7 **New Augusta** Mississippi, S USA
19 P12 **New Bedford** Massachusetts, NE USA
32 G11 **Newberg** Oregon, NW USA
21 X10 **New Bern** North Carolina, SE USA
20 F8 **Newbern** Tennessee, S USA
31 P4 **Newberry** Michigan, N USA
21 Q12 **Newberry** South Carolina, SE USA
18 F15 **New Bloomfield** Pennsylvania, NE USA
25 X5 **New Boston** Texas, SW USA
25 S11 **New Braunfels** Texas, SW USA
31 Q13 **New Bremen** Ohio, N USA
97 F18 **Newbridge** *Ir.* An Droichead Nua. C Ireland
18 B14 **New Brighton** Pennsylvania, NE USA
18 M12 **New Britain** Connecticut, NE USA
186 G7 **New Britain** *island* E PNG
192 I8 **New Britain Trench** *undersea feature* W Pacific Ocean
18 J15 **New Brunswick** New Jersey, NE USA
15 V8 **New Brunswick** *Fr.* Nouveau-Brunswick. ❖ *province* SE Canada
18 K13 **Newburgh** New York, NE USA
97 M22 **Newbury** S England, UK
19 P10 **Newburyport** Massachusetts, NE USA
77 T14 **New Bussa** Niger, W Nigeria
187 O17 **New Caledonia** *var.* Kanaky, *Fr.* Nouvelle-Calédonie. ◇ *French overseas territory* SW Pacific Ocean
187 O15 **New Caledonia** *island* SW Pacific Ocean
175 O10 **New Caledonia Basin** *undersea feature* W Pacific Ocean
183 T8 **Newcastle** New South Wales, SE Australia
13 O14 **Newcastle** New Brunswick, SE Canada
14 I15 **Newcastle** Ontario, SE Canada
97 C20 **Newcastle** *Ir.* An Caisleán Nua. SW Ireland
83 K22 **Newcastle** KwaZulu/Natal, E South Africa
97 G16 **Newcastle** *Ir.* An Caisleán Nua. SE Northern Ireland, UK
31 P13 **New Castle** Indiana, N USA
20 L5 **New Castle** Kentucky, S USA
27 N11 **Newcastle** Oklahoma, C USA
18 B13 **New Castle** Pennsylvania, NE USA
25 R6 **Newcastle** Texas, SW USA
36 J7 **Newcastle** Utah, W USA
21 S6 **New Castle** Virginia, NE USA
33 Z13 **Newcastle** Wyoming, C USA
45 W10 **Newcastle** × Nevis, Saint Kitts and Nevis
97 L14 **Newcastle** × NE England, UK
Newcastle *see* Newcastle upon Tyne
97 L18 **Newcastle-under-Lyme** C England, UK
97 M14 **Newcastle upon Tyne** *var.* Newcastle; *hist.* Monkchester, *Lat.* Pons Aelii. NE England, UK
181 Q4 **Newcastle Waters** Northern Territory, N Australia
Newchwang *see* Yingkou
18 K13 **New City** New York, NE USA
31 U13 **Newcomerstown** Ohio, N USA
18 G15 **New Cumberland** Pennsylvania, NE USA
21 R1 **New Cumberland** West Virginia, NE USA
152 I10 **New Delhi** ● (India) Delhi, N India
11 O17 **New Denver** British Columbia, SW Canada
28 J9 **Newell** South Dakota, N USA
21 Q13 **New Ellenton** South Carolina, SE USA
22 J6 **Newellton** Louisiana, S USA
28 K6 **New England** North Dakota, N USA
19 P8 **New England** *cultural region* NE USA
New England of the West *see* Minnesota
183 U5 **New England Range** ▲ New South Wales, SE Australia
64 G9 **New England Seamounts** *var.* Bermuda-New England Seamount Arc. *undersea feature* W Atlantic Ocean
38 M14 **Newenham, Cape** *headland* Alaska, USA
138 F11 **Newé Zohar** Southern, E Israel
18 D9 **Newfane** New York, NE USA
97 M23 **New Forest** *physical region* S England, UK
9 W10 **Newfoundland** *Fr.* Terre-Neuve. *island* Newfoundland, SE Canada
13 R9 **Newfoundland** *Fr.* Terre Neuve. ❖ *province* E Canada
65 J8 **Newfoundland Basin** *undersea feature* NW Atlantic Ocean
64 I8 **Newfoundland Ridge** *undersea feature* NW Atlantic Ocean
64 J8 **Newfoundland Seamounts** *undersea feature* N Sargasso Sea
18 G16 **New Freedom** Pennsylvania, NE USA
186 K9 **New Georgia** *island* New Georgia Islands, NW Solomon Islands
186 K8 **New Georgia Islands** *island group* NW Solomon Islands
186 L8 **New Georgia Sound** *var.* The Slot. *sound* E Solomon Sea
30 L9 **New Glarus** Wisconsin, N USA
13 Q15 **New Glasgow** Nova Scotia, SE Canada
New Goa *see* Panaji
186 A6 **New Guinea** *Dut.* Nieuw Guinea, *Ind.* Irian. *island* Indonesia/PNG
192 H8 **New Guinea Trench** *undersea feature* SW Pacific Ocean
32 I6 **Newhalem** Washington, NW USA
39 P13 **Newhalen** Alaska, USA
29 X13 **Newhall** Iowa, C USA
14 F16 **New Hamburg** Ontario, S Canada
19 N9 **New Hampshire** *off.* State of New Hampshire; also known as The Granite State. ❖ *state* NE USA
29 W12 **New Hampton** Iowa, C USA
186 G5 **New Hanover** *island* NE PNG
18 M13 **New Haven** Connecticut, NE USA
31 Q12 **New Haven** Indiana, N USA
27 W5 **New Haven** Missouri, C USA
97 P23 **Newhaven** SE England, UK
10 K13 **New Hazelton** British Columbia, SW Canada
New Hebrides *see* Vanuatu
175 P9 **New Hebrides Trench** *undersea feature* N Coral Sea
18 H15 **New Holland** Pennsylvania, NE USA
22 I9 **New Iberia** Louisiana, S USA
186 G5 **New Ireland** ❖ *province* NE PNG
186 G5 **New Ireland** *island* NE PNG
65 A24 **New Island** *island* W Falkland Islands
18 J15 **New Jersey** *off.* State of New Jersey; also known as The Garden State. ❖ *state* NE USA
18 C14 **New Kensington** Pennsylvania, NE USA
21 W6 **New Kent** Virginia, NE USA
27 O8 **Newkirk** Oklahoma, C USA
21 Q9 **Newland** North Carolina, SE USA
28 L6 **New Leipzig** North Dakota, N USA
14 H9 **New Liskeard** Ontario, S Canada
22 G7 **Newllano** Louisiana, S USA
19 N13 **New London** Connecticut, NE USA
29 Y15 **New London** Iowa, C USA
29 T8 **New London** Minnesota, N USA
27 V3 **New London** Missouri, C USA
30 M7 **New London** Wisconsin, N USA
27 Y8 **New Madrid** Missouri, C USA
180 J8 **Newman** Western Australia
194 M13 **Newman Island** *island* Antarctica
14 H15 **Newmarket** Ontario, S Canada
97 P20 **Newmarket** E England, UK
19 P10 **Newmarket** New Hampshire, NE USA
21 U4 **New Market** Virginia, NE USA
21 R2 **New Martinsville** West Virginia, NE USA
31 U14 **New Matamoras** Ohio, N USA
32 M12 **New Meadows** Idaho, NW USA
26 R12 **New Mexico** *off.* State of New Mexico; also known as Land of Enchantment, Sunshine State. ❖ *state* SW USA
149 V6 **New Mīrpur** *var.* Mīrpur. Sind, SE Pakistan
151 T17 **New Moore Island** *island* E India
23 S4 **Newnan** Georgia, SE USA
183 P17 **New Norfolk** Tasmania, SE Australia
22 K9 **New Orleans** Louisiana, S USA
22 K9 **New Orleans** × Louisiana, S USA
18 K12 **New Paltz** New York, NE USA
31 U12 **New Philadelphia** Ohio, N USA
184 K10 **New Plymouth** Taranaki, North Island, NZ
97 M24 **Newport** S England, UK
97 K22 **Newport** SE Wales, UK
27 W10 **Newport** Arkansas, C USA
31 N13 **Newport** Indiana, N USA
22 M3 **Newport** Kentucky, S USA
31 W9 **Newport** Minnesota, N USA
34 F12 **Newport** Oregon, NW USA
21 O13 **Newport** Rhode Island, NE USA
23 O9 **Newport** Tennessee, S USA
21 N6 **Newport** Vermont, NE USA
34 M7 **Newport** Washington, NW USA
23 X7 **Newport News** Virginia, NE USA
99 N20 **Newport Pagnell** SE England, UK
25 U12 **New Port Richey** Florida, SE USA
31 V9 **New Prague** Minnesota, N USA
46 H3 **New Providence** *island* N Bahamas
99 H24 **Newquay** SW England, UK
99 I20 **New Quay** SW Wales, UK
31 V10 **New Richland** Minnesota, N USA
13 X7 **New-Richmond** Quebec, SE Canada
31 R15 **New Richmond** Ohio, N USA
32 I5 **New Richmond** Wisconsin, N USA
44 G1 **New River** ≈ N Belize
57 T12 **New River** ≈ SE Guyana
23 R6 **New River** ≈ West Virginia, NE USA
44 G1 **New River Lagoon** ◎ N Belize
24 J8 **New Roads** Louisiana, S USA
20 L14 **New Rochelle** New York, NE USA
31 O4 **New Rockford** North Dakota, N USA
97 P23 **New Romney** SE England, UK
97 F20 **New Ross** *Ir.* Ros Mhic Thriúin. SE Ireland
97 F16 **Newry** *Ir.* An tIúr. SE Northern Ireland, UK
28 M5 **New Salem** North Dakota, N USA
New Sarum *see* Salisbury
29 W14 **New Sharon** Iowa, C USA
New Siberian Islands *see* Novosibirskiye Ostrova
23 X11 **New Smyrna Beach** Florida, SE USA
183 O7 **New South Wales** ❖ *state* SE Australia
39 O13 **New Stuyahok** Alaska, USA
21 N8 **New Tazewell** Tennessee, S USA
38 M12 **Newtok** Alaska, USA
23 S7 **Newton** Georgia, SE USA
29 W14 **Newton** Iowa, C USA
27 N6 **Newton** Kansas, C USA
19 O11 **Newton** Massachusetts, NE USA
22 M5 **Newton** Mississippi, S USA
18 J14 **Newton** New Jersey, NE USA
21 R9 **Newton** North Carolina, SE USA
25 Y9 **Newton** Texas, SW USA
97 J24 **Newton Abbot** SW England, UK
96 K13 **Newton St Boswells** SE Scotland, UK
97 I14 **Newton Stewart** S Scotland, UK
92 O2 **Newtontoppen** ▲ C Svalbard
28 K3 **New Town** North Dakota, N USA
97 J20 **Newtown** E Wales, UK
97 G15 **Newtownabbey** *Ir.* Baile na Mainistreach. E Northern Ireland, UK
97 G15 **Newtownards** *Ir.* Baile Nua na hArda. SE Northern Ireland, UK
29 U10 **New Ulm** Minnesota, N USA
28 K10 **New Underwood** South Dakota, N USA
25 V10 **New Waverly** Texas, SW USA
18 K14 **New York** New York, NE USA
18 G10 **New York** ❖ *state* NE USA
35 X13 **New York Mountains** ▲ California, W USA
184 K12 **New Zealand** *abbrev.* NZ. ◆ *commonwealth republic* SW Pacific Ocean
127 O15 **Neya** Kostromskaya Oblast', NW Russian Federation
Neyba *see* Neiba
143 Q12 **Neyrīz** *var.* Neiriz, Niriz. Fārs, S Iran
143 T4 **Neyshābūr** *var.* Nishapur. Khorāsān, NE Iran
155 J21 **Neyveli** Tamil Nādu, SE India
Nezhin *see* Nizhyn
33 N10 **Nezperce** Idaho, NW USA
22 H8 **Nezpique, Bayou** ≈ Louisiana, S USA
77 Y13 **Ngadda** ≈ NE Nigeria
N'Gage *see* Negage
185 G16 **Ngahere** West Coast, South Island, NZ
77 Z12 **Ngala** Borno, NE Nigeria
83 G17 **Ngamiland** ❖ *district* N Botswana
158 K16 **Ngamring** Xizang Zizhiqu, W China
81 K19 **Ngangerabeli Plain** *plain* SE Kenya
158 I14 **Ngangla Ringco** ◎ W China
158 G13 **Nganglong Kangri** ▲ W China
158 K15 **Ngangzê Co** ◎ W China
79 F14 **Ngaoundéré** *var.* N'Gaoundéré. Adamaoua, N Cameroon
81 E20 **Ngara** Kagera, NW Tanzania
188 F8 **Ngardmau Bay** *bay* Babeldaob, N Palau
188 F7 **Ngaregur** *island* Palau Islands, N Palau
184 L7 **Ngaruawahia** Waikato, North Island, NZ
184 N11 **Ngaruroro** ≈ North Island, NZ
190 I16 **Ngatangiia** Rarotonga, S Cook Islands
184 M6 **Ngatea** Waikato, North Island, NZ
166 L8 **Ngathainggyaung** Irrawaddy, SW Myanmar
Ngatik *see* Ngetik Atoll
Ngau *see* Gau
188 C7 **Ngcheangel** *var.* Kayangel Islands. *island* Palau Islands, N Palau
188 E10 **Ngchemiangel** Babeldaob, N Palau
188 C8 **Ngeaur** *var.* Angaur. *island* Palau Islands, S Palau
188 E10 **Ngerkeai** Babeldaob, N Palau
188 F9 **Ngermechau** Babeldaob, N Palau
188 C8 **Ngeruktabel** *prev.* Urukthapel. *island* Palau Islands, S Palau
188 F8 **Ngetbong** Babeldaob, N Palau
189 T17 **Ngetik Atoll** *var.* Ngatik; *prev.* Los Jardines. *atoll* Caroline Islands, E Micronesia
188 E10 **Ngetkip** Babeldaob, N Palau
Nggamea *see* Qamea
83 C16 **N'Giva** *var.* Ondjiva, *Port.* Vila Pereira de Eça. Cunene, S Angola
79 G20 **Ngo** Plateaux, SE Congo
167 S7 **Ngoc Lac** Thanh Hoa, N Vietnam
79 G17 **Ngoko** ≈ Cameroon/Congo
81 H19 **Ngorengore** Rift Valley, SW Kenya
159 Q11 **Ngoring Hu** ◎ C China
Ngorolaka *see* Banifing
81 H20 **Ngorongoro Crater** *crater* N Tanzania
79 D19 **Ngounié** *off.* Province de la Ngounié, *var.* La Ngounié. ❖ *province* S Gabon
79 D19 **Ngounié** ≈ Congo/Gabon
78 H10 **Ngoura** *var.* NGoura. Chari-Baguirmi, W Chad
78 G10 **Ngouri** *var.* NGouri; *prev.* Fort-Millot. Lac, W Chad
77 Y10 **Ngourti** Diffa, E Niger
77 Y11 **Nguigmi** *var.* N'Guigmi. Diffa, SE Niger
Nguimbo *see* Lumbala N'Guimbo
188 F15 **Ngulu Atoll** *atoll* Caroline Islands, W Micronesia
187 R14 **Nguna** *island* C Vanuatu
N'Gunza *see* Sumbe
169 U17 **Ngurah Rai** × (Bali) Bali, S Indonesia
77 W12 **Nguru** Yobe, NE Nigeria
Ngwaketze *see* Southern
83 I16 **Ngweze** ≈ S Zambia
83 M17 **Nhamatanda** Sofala, C Mozambique
58 G12 **Nhamundá, Rio** *var.* Jamundá, Yamundá. ≈ N Brazil
60 J7 **Nhandeara** São Paulo, S Brazil
N'Harea *see* Nharêa
82 D12 **Nharêa** *var.* N'Harea, Nhareia. Bié, W Angola
Nhareia *see* Nharêa
167 V12 **Nha Trang** Khanh Hoa, S Vietnam
182 L11 **Nhill** Victoria, SE Australia
83 L22 **Nhlangano** *prev.* Goedgegun. SW Swaziland
181 S1 **Nhulunbuy** Northern Territory, N Australia
77 N10 **Niafounké** Tombouctou, W Mali
31 N5 **Niagara** Wisconsin, N USA
14 H16 **Niagara** ≈ Ontario, S Canada
14 G15 **Niagara Escarpment** *hill range* Ontario, S Canada
14 H16 **Niagara Falls** Ontario, S Canada
18 D9 **Niagara Falls** New York, NE USA
17 S7 **Niagara Falls** *waterfall* Canada/USA
76 K12 **Niagassola** *var.* Nyagassola. Haute-Guinée, NE Guinea
77 R12 **Niamey** ● (Niger) Niamey, SW Niger
77 R12 **Niamey** × Niamey, SW Niger
77 R14 **Niamtougou** N Togo
79 O16 **Niangara** Orientale, NE Dem. Rep. Congo (Zaire)
77 O10 **Niangay, Lac** ◎ E Mali
77 N14 **Niangoloko** SW Burkina
27 U6 **Niangua River** ≈ Missouri, C USA
79 O17 **Nia-Nia** Orientale, NE Dem. Rep. Congo (Zaire)
19 N13 **Niantic** Connecticut, NE USA
163 U7 **Nianzishan** Heilongjiang, NE China
168 H10 **Nias, Pulau** *island* W Indonesia
82 O13 **Niassa** *off.* Província do Niassa. ❖ *province* N Mozambique
191 U10 **Niau** *island* Îles Tuamotu, C French Polynesia
95 G20 **Nibe** Nordjylland, N Denmark
189 Q8 **Nibok** N Nauru
118 C10 **Nīca** Liepāja, W Latvia
Nicaea *see* Nice
42 J9 **Nicaragua** *off.* Republic of Nicaragua. ◆ *republic* Central America
42 K11 **Nicaragua, Lago de** *var.* Cocibolca, Gran Lago, *Eng.* Lake Nicaragua. ◎ S Nicaragua
Nicaragua, Lake *see* Nicaragua, Lago de
64 D11 **Nicaraguan Rise** *undersea feature* NW Caribbean Sea
Nicaria *see* Ikaría
107 N21 **Nicastro** Calabria, SW Italy
103 V15 **Nice** *It.* Nizza; *anc.* Nicaea. Alpes-Maritimes, SE France
Nice *see* Côte d'Azur
Nicephorium *see* Ar Raqqah
12 M9 **Nichicun, Lac** ◎ Quebec, E Canada
164 D16 **Nichinan** *var.* Nitinan. Miyazaki, Kyūshū, SW Japan
44 E4 **Nicholas Channel** *channel* N Cuba
Nicholas II Land *see* Severnaya Zemlya
149 U2 **Nicholas Range** *Pash.* Selseleh-ye Kūh-e Vākhān, *Taj.* Qatorkūhi Vakhon. ▲ Afghanistan/Tajikistan
20 M6 **Nicholasville** Kentucky, S USA
44 G2 **Nicholls Town** Andros Island, NW Bahamas
21 U12 **Nichols** South Carolina, SE USA
55 U9 **Nickerie** ❖ *district* NW Surinam
55 V9 **Nickerie Rivier** ≈ NW Surinam
151 P22 **Nicobar Islands** *island group* India, E Indian Ocean
116 L9 **Nicolae Bălcescu** Botoşani, NE Romania
15 P11 **Nicolet** Quebec, SE Canada
15 Q12 **Nicolet** ≈ Quebec, SE Canada
31 Q4 **Nicolet, Lake** ◎ Michigan, N USA
29 U10 **Nicollet** Minnesota, N USA
61 F19 **Nico Pérez** Florida, S Uruguay
Nicopolis *see* Nikopol, Bulgaria
Nicopolis *see* Nikópoli, Greece
121 P2 **Nicosia** *Gk.* Lefkosía, *Turk.* Lefkoşa. ● (Cyprus) C Cyprus
107 K24 **Nicosia** Sicilia, Italy, C Mediterranean Sea
107 N22 **Nicotera** Calabria, SW Italy
42 K13 **Nicoya** Guanacaste, W Costa Rica
42 L14 **Nicoya, Golfo de** *gulf* W Costa Rica
42 L14 **Nicoya, Península de** *peninsula* NW Costa Rica
Nictheroy *see* Niterói
111 L15 **Nida** ≈ S Poland
Nida *see* Neringa
Nidaros *see* Trondheim
108 D8 **Nidau** Bern, W Switzerland
101 H17 **Nidda** ≈ W Germany
Nidden *see* Neringa
95 F17 **Nidelva** ≈ S Norway
110 L9 **Nidzica** *Ger.* Niedenburg. Warmińsko-Mazurskie, NE Poland,
100 H6 **Niebüll** Schleswig-Holstein, N Germany
Niedenburg *see* Nidzica
99 N25 **Niederanven** Luxembourg, C Luxembourg
103 V4 **Niederbronn-les-Bains** Bas-Rhin, NE France
Niederdonau *see* Niederösterreich
109 S7 **Niedere Tauern** ▲ C Austria
101 P14 **Niederlausitz** *Eng.* Lower Lusatia. *physical region* E Germany
109 U5 **Niederösterreich** *off.* Land Niederösterreich, *Eng.* Lower Austria, *Ger.* Niederdonau; *prev.* Lower Danube. ❖ *state* NE Austria
100 G12 **Niedersachsen** *Eng.* Lower Saxony, *Fr.* Basse-Saxe. ❖ *state* NW Germany
79 D17 **Niefang** *var.* Sevilla de Niefang. NW Equatorial Guinea
83 G23 **Niekerkshoop** Northern Cape, W South Africa
99 G17 **Niel** Antwerpen, N Belgium
Niélé *see* Niellé
76 M14 **Niellé** *var.* Niélé. N Ivory Coast
79 O22 **Niemba** Katanga, E Dem. Rep. Congo (Zaire)
111 G15 **Niemcza** *Ger.* Nimptsch. Dolnośląskie, SW Poland
Niemen *see* Neman
92 J13 **Niemisel** Norrbotten, N Sweden
111 H15 **Niemodlin** *Ger.* Falkenberg. Opolskie, S Poland
76 M13 **Niéna** Sikasso, SW Mali
100 H12 **Nienburg** Niedersachsen, N Germany
100 N13 **Nieplitz** ≈ NE Germany
111 L16 **Niepołomice** Małopolskie, S Poland
101 D14 **Niers** ≈ Germany/Netherlands
101 Q15 **Niesky** *Lus.* Niska. Sachsen, E Germany
Nieświeź *see* Nyasvizh
Nieuport *see* Nieuwpoort
98 O8 **Nieuw-Amsterdam** Drenthe, NE Netherlands
55 W9 **Nieuw Amsterdam** Commewijne, NE Surinam
99 M14 **Nieuw-Bergen** Limburg, SE Netherlands
98 O7 **Nieuw-Buinen** Drenthe, NE Netherlands
98 J12 **Nieuwegein** Utrecht, C Netherlands
98 P6 **Nieuwe Pekela** Groningen, NE Netherlands
98 P5 **Nieuweschans** Groningen, NE Netherlands
Nieuw Guinea *see* New Guinea
98 I11 **Nieuwkoop** Zuid-Holland, C Netherlands
98 M9 **Nieuwleusen** Overijssel, S Netherlands
98 J11 **Nieuw-Loosdrecht** Utrecht, C Netherlands
55 U9 **Nieuw Nickerie** Nickerie, NW Surinam
98 P5 **Nieuwolda** Groningen, NE Netherlands
99 B17 **Nieuwpoort** *var.* Nieuport. West-Vlaanderen, W Belgium
99 G14 **Nieuw-Vossemeer** Noord-Brabant, S Netherlands
98 P7 **Nieuw-Weerdinge** Drenthe, NE Netherlands
40 L10 **Nieves** Zacatecas, C Mexico
64 O11 **Nieves, Pico de las** ▲ Gran Canaria, Islas Canarias, Spain, NE Atlantic Ocean
103 P8 **Nièvre** ❖ *department* C France
Niewenstat *see* Neustadt an der Weinstrasse
136 J15 **Niğde** Niğde, C Turkey
136 J15 **Niğde** ❖ *province* C Turkey
83 J21 **Nigel** Gauteng, NE South Africa
77 V10 **Niger** *off.* Republic of Niger. ◆ *republic* W Africa
77 T14 **Niger** ❖ *state* C Nigeria
67 P8 **Niger** ≈ W Africa
Niger Cone *see* Niger Fan
67 P9 **Niger Delta** *delta* S Nigeria
67 P9 **Niger Fan** *var.* Niger Cone. *undersea feature* E Atlantic Ocean
77 T13 **Nigeria** *off.* Federal Republic of Nigeria. ◆ *federal republic* W Africa
77 T17 **Niger, Mouths of the** *delta* S Nigeria
185 C24 **Nightcaps** Southland, South Island, NZ
14 F7 **Night Hawk Lake** ◎ Ontario, S Canada
65 M19 **Nightingale Island** *island* S Tristan da Cunha, S Atlantic Ocean
38 M12 **Nightmute** Alaska, USA
114 G13 **Nigrita** Kentrikí Makedonía, NE Greece
148 J15 **Nihing** *Per.* Rūd-e Nahang. ≈ Iran/Pakistan
191 V10 **Nihiru** *atoll* Îles Tuamotu, C French Polynesia
Nihommatsu *see* Nihonmatsu
Nihon *see* Japan
165 P11 **Nihonmatsu** *var.* Nihommatsu, Nihonmatu. Fukushima, Honshū, C Japan
Nihonmatu *see* Nihonmatsu
62 I12 **Nihuil, Embalse del** ◎ W Argentina
165 O10 **Niigata** Niigata, Honshū, C Japan
165 O11 **Niigata** *off.* Niigata-ken. ❖ *prefecture* Honshū, C Japan
165 G14 **Niihama** Ehime, Shikoku, SW Japan
38 A8 **Niihau** *island* Hawaii, USA, C Pacific Ocean
165 X12 **Nii-jima** *island* E Japan
165 H12 **Niimi** Okayama, Honshū, SW Japan
165 O10 **Niitsu** *var.* Niitu. Niigata, Honshū, C Japan
Niitu *see* Niitsu
105 P15 **Níjar** Andalucía, S Spain
98 K11 **Nijkerk** Gelderland, C Netherlands
99 H16 **Nijlen** Antwerpen, N Belgium
98 L13 **Nijmegen** *Ger.* Nimwegen; *anc.* Noviomagus. Gelderland, SE Netherlands
98 N10 **Nijverdal** Overijssel, E Netherlands
190 G16 **Nikao** Rarotonga, S Cook Islands
Nikaria *see* Ikaría
126 I2 **Nikel'** Murmanskaya Oblast', NW Russian Federation
171 Q17 **Nikiniki** Timor, S Indonesia
131 Q15 **Nikitin Seamount** *undersea feature* E Indian Ocean
77 S14 **Nikki** E Benin
Niklasmarkt *see* Gheorgheni
39 P10 **Nikolai** Alaska, USA
Nikolaiken *see* Mikołajki
Nikolainkaupunki *see* Länsi-Suomi
Nikolayev *see* Mykolayiv
145 U15 **Nikolayevka** Almaty, SE Kazakhstan
145 O6 **Nikolayevka** Severnyy Kazakhstan, N Kazakhstan
129 P9 **Nikolayevsk** Volgogradskaya Oblast', SW Russian Federation
Nikolayevskaya Oblast' *see* Mykolayivs'ka Oblast'
123 S12 **Nikolayevsk-na-Amure** Khabarovskiy Kray, SE Russian Federation
129 P6 **Nikol'sk** Penzenskaya Oblast', W Russian Federation
127 O13 **Nikol'sk** Vologodskaya Oblast', NW Russian Federation
Nikol'sk *see* Ussuriysk
38 K17 **Nikolski** Umnak Island, Alaska, USA
Nikol'skiy *see* Satpayev
129 V7 **Nikol'skoye** Orenburgskaya Oblast', W Russian Federation
Nikol'sk-Ussuriyskiy *see* Ussuriysk
114 J7 **Nikopol** *anc.* Nicopolis. Pleven, N Bulgaria
117 S9 **Nikopol'** Dnipropetrovs'ka Oblast', SE Ukraine
115 C17 **Nikópoli** *anc.* Nicopolis. *site of ancient city* Ípeiros, W Greece
136 M12 **Niksar** Tokat, N Turkey
143 V14 **Nīkshahr** Sīstān va Balūchestān, SE Iran
113 J16 **Nikšić** Montenegro, SW Yugoslavia
191 R4 **Nikumaroro** *prev.* Gardner Island, Kemins Island. *atoll* Phoenix Islands, C Kiribati
191 P3 **Nikunau** *var.* Nukunau; *prev.* Byron Island. *atoll* Tungaru, W Kiribati
155 G21 **Nilambūr** Kerala, SW India
35 X16 **Niland** California, W USA
67 T3 **Nile** *Ar.* Nahr an Nīl. ≈ N Africa
80 G8 **Nile** *former province* NW Uganda
75 W7 **Nile Delta** *delta* N Egypt
67 T3 **Nile Fan** *undersea feature* E Mediterranean Sea
31 O11 **Niles** Michigan, N USA
31 V11 **Niles** Ohio, N USA
155 F20 **Nīleswaram** Kerala, SW India
14 K10 **Nilgaut, Lac** ◎ Quebec, SE Canada
158 I5 **Nilka** Xinjiang Uygur Zizhiqu, NW China
Nil, Nahr an *see* Nile
93 N16 **Nilsiä** Itä-Suomi, C Finland
154 F9 **Nīmach** Madhya Pradesh, C India
152 G14 **Nīmbāhera** Rājasthān, N India
76 L15 **Nimba, Monts** *var.* Nimba Mountains. ▲ W Africa
Nimba Mountains *see* Nimba, Monts
Nimburg *see* Nymburk
103 Q15 **Nîmes** *anc.* Nemausus, Nismes. Gard, S France
152 H11 **Nīm ka Thāna** Rājasthān, N India
183 R11 **Nimmitabel** New South Wales, SE Australia
Nimptsch *see* Niemcza
195 R11 **Nimrod Glacier** *glacier* Antarctica
Nimroze *see* Nīmrūz
148 K8 **Nīmrūz** *var.* Nimroze; *prev.* Chakhānsūr. ❖ *province* SW Afghanistan
81 F16 **Nimule** Eastern Equatoria, S Sudan
Nimwegen *see* Nijmegen
155 C23 **Nine Degree Channel** *channel* India/Maldives
18 G9 **Ninemile Point** *headland* New York, NE USA
173 S8 **Ninetyeast Ridge** *undersea feature* E Indian Ocean

◆ Country ● Country Capital ◇ Dependent Territory ○ Dependent Territory Capital ❖ Administrative Region × International Airport ▲ Mountain ▲ Mountain Range Volcano ≈ River ◎ Lake Reservoir

183 P13 **Ninety Mile Beach** *beach* Victoria, SE Australia
184 I2 **Ninety Mile Beach** *beach* North Island, NZ
21 P12 **Ninety Six** South Carolina, SE USA
163 Y9 **Ning'an** Heilongjiang, NE China
161 S9 **Ningbo** *var.* Ning-po, Yin-hsien; *prev.* Ninghsien. Zhejiang, SE China
161 U12 **Ningde** Fujian, SE China
161 P12 **Ningdu** Jiangxi, S China
186 A7 **Ningerum** Western, SW PNG
161 R9 **Ningguo** Anhui, E China
161 S9 **Ninghai** Zhejiang, SE China
Ning-hsia *see* Ningxia
Ninghsien *see* Ningbo
160 J15 **Ningming** Guangxi Zhuangzu Zizhiqu, S China
160 H11 **Ningnan** Sichuan, C China
Ning-po *see* Ningbo
Ningsia/Ningsia Hui/Ningsia Hui Autonomous Region *see* Ningxia
160 J5 **Ningxia** *off.* Ningxia Huizu Zizhiqu, *var.* Ning-hsia, Ningsia, *Eng.* Ningsia Hui, Ningsia Hui Autonomous Region. ◈ *autonomous region* N China
159 X10 **Ningxian** Gansu, N China
167 T7 **Ninh Binh** Ninh Binh, N Vietnam
167 V12 **Ninh Hoa** Khanh Hoa, S Vietnam
186 C4 **Ninigo Group** *island group* N PNG
39 Q12 **Ninilchik** Alaska, USA
27 N7 **Ninnescah River** ≈ Kansas, C USA
195 U16 **Ninnis Glacier** *glacier* Antarctica
165 R8 **Ninohe** Iwate, Honshū, C Japan
99 F18 **Ninove** Oost-Vlaanderen, C Belgium
171 O4 **Ninoy Aquino** ✕ (Manila) Luzon, N Philippines
Nio *see* Íos
29 P12 **Niobrara** Nebraska, C USA
28 M12 **Niobrara River** ≈ Nebraska/Wyoming, C USA
79 I20 **Nioki** Bandundu, W Dem. Rep. Congo (Zaire)
76 M11 **Niono** Ségou, C Mali
76 K11 **Nioro** *var.* Nioro du Sahel. Kayes, W Mali
76 G11 **Nioro du Rip** SW Senegal
Nioro du Sahel *see* Nioro
102 K10 **Niort** Deux-Sèvres, W France
172 H14 **Nioumachoua** Mohéli, S Comoros
186 C7 **Nipa** Southern Highlands, W PNG
11 U14 **Nipawin** Saskatchewan, S Canada
12 D12 **Nipigon** Ontario, S Canada
12 D11 **Nipigon, Lake** ◎ Ontario, S Canada
11 S13 **Nipin** ≈ Saskatchewan, C Canada
14 G11 **Nipissing, Lake** ◎ Ontario, S Canada
35 P13 **Nipomo** California, W USA
Nippon *see* Japan
138 K6 **Niqniqīyah, Jabal an** ▲ C Syria
62 I9 **Niquivil** San Juan, W Argentina
171 Y13 **Nirabotong** Irian Jaya, E Indonesia
Nirīz *see* Neyrīz
155 I14 **Nirmal** Andhra Pradesh, C India
153 Q13 **Nirmāli** Bihār, NE India
113 O14 **Niš** *Eng.* Nish, *Ger.* Nisch; *anc.* Naissus. Serbia, SE Yugoslavia
104 H9 **Nisa** Portalegre, C Portugal
Nisa *see* Neisse
141 P4 **Niṣab** Al Ḥudūd ash Shamālīyah, N Saudi Arabia
141 Q15 **Niṣāb** *var.* Anṣāb. SW Yemen
113 P14 **Nišava** *Bul.* Nishava. ≈ Bulgaria/Yugoslavia *see also* Nishava
107 K25 **Niscemi** Sicilia, Italy, C Mediterranean Sea
Nisch/Nish *see* Niš
165 R4 **Niseko** Hokkaidō, NE Japan
Nishapur *see* Neyshābūr
114 G9 **Nishava** *var.* Nišava. ≈ Bulgaria/Yugoslavia *see also* Nišava
118 L11 **Nishcha** *Rus.* Nishcha. ≈ N Belarus
165 C17 **Nishinoomote** Kagoshima, Tanega-shima, SW Japan
165 X15 **Nishino-shima** *Eng.* Rosario. *island* Ogasawara-shotō, SE Japan
165 I13 **Nishiwaki** *var.* Nisiwaki. Hyōgo, Honshū, SW Japan
141 U14 **Nishtūn** SE Yemen
Nisiros *see* Nísyros
Nisiwaki *see* Nishiwaki
Niska *see* Niesky
113 O14 **Niška Banja** Serbia, SE Yugoslavia
12 D6 **Niskibi** ≈ Ontario, C Canada
111 O15 **Nisko** Podkarpackie, SE Poland
10 H7 **Nisling** ≈ Yukon Territory, W Canada
99 H22 **Nismes** Namur, S Belgium
Nismes *see* Nîmes
116 M10 **Nisporeni** *Rus.* Nisporeny. W Moldova
Nisporeny *see* Nisporeni
95 K20 **Nissan** ≈ S Sweden
Nissan Islands *see* Green Islands
95 F16 **Nisser** ◎ S Norway
95 E21 **Nissum Bredning** *inlet* NW Denmark
29 U6 **Nisswa** Minnesota, N USA
Nistru *see* Dniester
115 M22 **Nísyros** *var.* Nisiros. *island* Dodekánisos, Greece, Aegean Sea
118 H8 **Nītaure** Cēsis, C Latvia
60 P10 **Niterói** *prev.* Nictheroy. Rio de Janeiro, SE Brazil
14 F16 **Nith** ≈ Ontario, S Canada
96 J13 **Nith** ≈ S Scotland, UK
Nitinan *see* Nichinan
111 I21 **Nitra** *Ger.* Neutra, *Hung.* Nyitra. Nitriansky Kraj, SW Slovakia
111 I20 **Nitra** *Ger.* Neutra, *Hung.* Nyitra. ≈ W Slovakia
111 I21 **Nitriansky Kraj** ◈ *region* SW Slovakia
21 Q5 **Nitro** West Virginia, NE USA
95 H14 **Nittedal** Akershus, S Norway
Niuatobutabu *see* Niuatoputapu
193 X13 **Niuatoputapu** *var.* Niuatobutabu; *prev.* Keppel Island. *island* N Tonga
193 U15 **Niu'Aunofa** *headland* Tongatapu, S Tonga
Niuchwang *see* Yingkou
190 B16 **Niue** ◇ *self-governing territory in free association with NZ* S Pacific Ocean
190 F10 **Niulakita** *var.* Nurakita. *atoll* S Tuvalu
190 E6 **Niutao** *atoll* NW Tuvalu
93 L15 **Nivala** Oulu, C Finland
102 I15 **Nive** ≈ SW France
99 G19 **Nivelles** Wallon Brabant, C Belgium
103 P8 **Nivernais** *cultural region* C France
15 N8 **Niverville, Lac** ◎ Quebec, SE Canada
27 T7 **Nixa** Missouri, C USA
35 R5 **Nixon** Nevada, W USA
25 S12 **Nixon** Texas, SW USA
Niya *see* Minfeng
146 K12 **Niyazov** Lebapskiy Velayat, NE Turkmenistan
155 H14 **Nizāmābād** Andhra Pradesh, C India
155 H15 **Nizām Sāgar** ◎ C India
127 N16 **Nizhegorodskaya Oblast'** ◈ *province* W Russian Federation
Nizhnegorskiy *see* Nyzhn'ohirs'kyy
129 S4 **Nizhnekamsk** Respublika Tatarstan, W Russian Federation
129 U3 **Nizhnekamskoye Vodokhranilishche** ▣ W Russian Federation
123 S14 **Nizhne Leninskoye** Yevreyskaya Avtonomnaya Oblast', SE Russian Federation
122 L13 **Nizhneudinsk** Irkutskaya Oblast', S Russian Federation
122 I10 **Nizhnevartovsk** Khanty-Mansiyskiy Avtonomnyy Okrug, C Russian Federation
123 Q7 **Nizhneyansk** Respublika Sakha (Yakutiya), NE Russian Federation
129 Q11 **Nizhniy Baskunchak** Astrakhanskaya Oblast', SW Russian Federation
129 O6 **Nizhniy Lomov** Penzenskaya Oblast', W Russian Federation
129 P3 **Nizhniy Novgorod** *prev.* Gor'kiy. Nizhegorodskaya Oblast', W Russian Federation
127 T8 **Nizhniy Odes** Respublika Komi, NW Russian Federation
Nizhniy Pyandzh *see* Panji Poyon
122 G10 **Nizhniy Tagil** Sverdlovskaya Oblast', C Russian Federation
127 T9 **Nizhnyaya-Omra** Respublika Komi, NW Russian Federation
127 P5 **Nizhnyaya Pesha** Nenetskiy Avtonomnyy Okrug, NW Russian Federation
117 Q3 **Nizhyn** *Rus.* Nezhin. Chernihivs'ka Oblast', NE Ukraine
136 M17 **Nizip** Gaziantep, S Turkey
141 X8 **Nizwá** *var.* Nazwāh. NE Oman
Nizza *see* Nice
106 C9 **Nizza Monferrato** Piemonte, NE Italy
Njávdám *see* Näätämöjoki
Njellim *see* Nellim
81 H24 **Njombe** Iringa, S Tanzania
81 G23 **Njombe** ≈ C Tanzania
92 I10 **Njunis** ▲ N Norway
93 H17 **Njurunda** Västernorrland, C Sweden
94 N11 **Njutånger** Gävleborg, C Sweden
79 D14 **Nkambe** Nord-Ouest, NW Cameroon
Nkata Bay *see* Nkhata Bay
79 F21 **Nkayi** *prev.* Jacob. La Bouenza, S Congo
83 J17 **Nkayi** Matabeleland North, W Zimbabwe
82 N13 **Nkhata Bay** *var.* Nkata Bay. Northern, N Malawi
81 E22 **Nkonde** Kigoma, N Tanzania
79 D15 **Nkongsamba** *var.* N'Kongsamba. Littoral, W Cameroon
83 E16 **Nkurenkuru** Okavango, N Namibia
77 Q15 **Nkwanta** E Ghana
167 O2 **Nmai Hka** *var.* Me Hka. ≈ N Myanmar
Noardwâlde *see* Noordwolde
39 N7 **Noatak** Alaska, USA
39 N7 **Noatak River** ≈ Alaska, USA
Nobeji *see* Noheji
164 E15 **Nobeoka** Miyazaki, Kyūshū, SW Japan
27 N11 **Noble** Oklahoma, C USA
31 P13 **Noblesville** Indiana, N USA
165 R5 **Noboribetsu** *var.* Noboribetu. Hokkaidō, NE Japan
Noboribetu *see* Noboribetsu
59 H18 **Nobres** Mato Grosso, W Brazil
107 N21 **Nocera Terinese** Calabria, S Italy
41 Q16 **Nochixtlán** *var.* Asunción Nochixtlán. Oaxaca, SE Mexico
25 S5 **Nocona** Texas, SW USA
63 K21 **Nodales, Bahía de los** *bay* S Argentina
27 Q2 **Nodaway River** ≈ Iowa/Missouri, C USA
27 R8 **Noel** Missouri, C USA
95 C17 **Nærbø** Rogaland, S Norway
95 I24 **Næstved** Storstrøm, SE Denmark
40 H3 **Nogales** Chihuahua, NW Mexico
40 F3 **Nogales** Sonora, NW Mexico
36 M17 **Nogales** Arizona, SW USA
Nogal Valley *see* Dooxo Nugaaleed
102 K15 **Nogaro** Gers, S France
110 J7 **Nogat** ≈ N Poland
164 D12 **Nōgata** Fukuoka, Kyūshū, SW Japan
129 P15 **Nogayskaya Step'** *steppe* SW Russian Federation
102 M6 **Nogent-le-Rotrou** Eure-et-Loir, C France
103 O4 **Nogent-sur-Oise** Oise, N France
103 P6 **Nogent-sur-Seine** Aube, N France
122 L10 **Noginsk** Evenkiyskiy Avtonomnyy Okrug, N Russian Federation
128 L3 **Noginsk** Moskovskaya Oblast', W Russian Federation
123 T12 **Nogliki** Ostrov Sakhalin, Sakhalinskaya Oblast', SE Russian Federation
164 K12 **Nōgōhaku-san** ▲ Honshū, SW Japan
162 D5 **Nogoonnuur** Bayan-Ölgiy, NW Mongolia
61 C18 **Nogoyá** Entre Ríos, E Argentina
111 K21 **Nógrád** *off.* Nógrád Megye. ◈ *county* N Hungary
105 U5 **Noguera Pallaresa** ≈ NE Spain
105 U4 **Noguera Ribagorçana** ≈ NE Spain
101 E19 **Nohfelden** Saarland, SW Germany
38 A8 **Nohili Point** *headland* Kauai, Hawaii, USA, C Pacific Ocean
104 G3 **Noia** Galicia, NW Spain
103 N16 **Noire, Montagne** ▲ S France
15 P12 **Noire, Rivière** ≈ Quebec, SE Canada
14 J10 **Noire, Rivière** ≈ Quebec, SE Canada
Noire, Rivière *see* Black River
102 G6 **Noires, Montagnes** ▲ NW France
102 H8 **Noirmoutier-en-l'Île** Vendée, NW France
102 H8 **Noirmoutier, Île de** *island* NW France
187 Q10 **Noka** Nendö, E Solomon Islands
83 G17 **Nokaneng** Ngamiland, NW Botswana
93 L18 **Nokia** Länsi-Suomi, W Finland
148 K11 **Nok Kundi** Baluchistān, SW Pakistan
30 L14 **Nokomis** Illinois, N USA
30 K5 **Nokomis, Lake** ▣ Wisconsin, N USA
78 G9 **Nokou** Kanem, W Chad
187 Q12 **Nokuku** Espiritu Santo, W Vanuatu
95 J18 **Nol** Västra Götaland, S Sweden
79 H16 **Nola** Sangha-Mbaéré, SW Central African Republic
25 P7 **Nolan** Texas, SW USA
127 R15 **Nolinsk** Kirovskaya Oblast', NW Russian Federation
95 B19 **Nólsoy** *Dan.* Nolsø *Island* Faeroe Islands
186 B7 **Nomad** Western, SW Papau New Guinea
164 B16 **Noma-zaki** *headland* Kyūshū, SW Japan
40 K10 **Nombre de Dios** Durango, C Mexico
42 I5 **Nombre de Dios, Cordillera** ▲ N Honduras
38 M9 **Nome** Alaska, USA
29 Q6 **Nome** North Dakota, N USA
38 M9 **Nome, Cape** *headland* Alaska, USA
Nōmi-jima *see* Nishi-Nōmi-jima
14 M11 **Nominingue, Lac** ◎ Quebec, SE Canada
Nomoi Islands *see* Mortlock Islands
164 B16 **Nomo-zaki** *headland* Kyūshū, SW Japan
193 X15 **Nomuka** *island* Nomuka Group, C Tonga
193 X15 **Nomuka Group** *island group* W Tonga
189 Q15 **Nomwin Atoll** *atoll* Hall Islands, C Micronesia
8 L10 **Nonacho Lake** ◎ Northwest Territories, NW Canada
Nondaburi *see* Nonthaburi
39 P12 **Nondalton** Alaska, USA
163 V10 **Nong'an** Jilin, NE China
167 P10 **Nong Bua Khok** Nakhon Ratchasima, C Thailand
167 Q9 **Nong Bua Lamphu** Udon Thani, E Thailand
167 R7 **Nông Hèt** Xiangkhoang, N Laos
Nongkaya *see* Nong Khai
167 Q8 **Nong Khai** *var.* Mi Chai, Nongkaya. Nong Khai, E Thailand
167 N14 **Nong Met** Surat Thani, SW Thailand
83 L22 **Nongoma** KwaZulu/Natal, E South Africa
167 P9 **Nong Phai** Phetchabun, C Thailand
153 U13 **Nongstoin** Meghālaya, NE India
83 C19 **Nonidas** Erongo, N Namibia
Nonni *see* Nen Jiang
40 I7 **Nonoava** Chihuahua, N Mexico
191 O3 **Nonouti** *prev.* Sydenham Island. *atoll* Tungaru, W Kiribati
167 O11 **Nonthaburi** *var.* Nondaburi, Nontha Buri. Nonthaburi, C Thailand
102 L11 **Nontron** Dordogne, SW France
181 P1 **Noonamah** Northern Territory, N Australia
28 K2 **Noonan** North Dakota, N USA
99 E14 **Noord-Beveland** *var.* North Beveland. *island* SW Netherlands
99 J14 **Noord-Brabant** *Eng.* North Brabant. ◈ *province* S Netherlands
98 H7 **Noorder Haaks** *spit* NW Netherlands
98 H9 **Noord-Holland** *Eng.* North Holland. ◈ *province* NW Netherlands
Noordhollandsch Kanaal *see* Noordhollands Kanaal
98 H8 **Noordhollands Kanaal** *var.* Noordhollandsch Kanaal. *canal* NW Netherlands
Noord-Kaap *see* Northern Cape
98 L8 **Noordoostpolder** *island* N Netherlands
45 P16 **Noordpunt** *headland* Curaçao, C Netherlands Antilles
98 I8 **Noord-Scharwoude** Noord-Holland, NW Netherlands
Noordwes *see* North-West
98 G11 **Noordwijk aan Zee** Zuid-Holland, W Netherlands
98 H11 **Noordwijkerhout** Zuid-Holland, W Netherlands
98 M7 **Noordwolde** *Fris.* Noardwâlde. Friesland, N Netherlands
Noordzee *see* North Sea
98 H10 **Noordzee-Kanaal** *canal* NW Netherlands
93 K18 **Noormarkku** *Swe.* Norrmark. Länsi-Suomi, W Finland
39 N8 **Noorvik** Alaska, USA
10 J17 **Nootka Sound** *inlet* British Columbia, W Canada
82 A9 **Nóqui** Zaire, NW Angola
95 L15 **Nora** Örebro, C Sweden
147 Q13 **Norak** *Rus.* Nurek. W Tajikistan
9 T14 **Noranda** Quebec, SE Canada
29 W12 **Nora Springs** Iowa, C USA
95 M14 **Norberg** Västmanland, C Sweden
14 K13 **Norcan Lake** ◎ Ontario, SE Canada
197 R12 **Nord** Avannaarsua, N Greenland
78 F13 **Nord** *Eng.* North. ◈ *province* N Cameroon
103 P2 **Nord** ◈ *department* N France
92 P1 **Nordaustlandet** *island* NE Svalbard
95 G24 **Nordborg** *Ger.* Nordburg. Sønderjylland, SW Denmark
Nordburg *see* Nordborg
95 F23 **Nordby** Ribe, W Denmark
11 P15 **Nordegg** Alberta, SW Canada
100 E9 **Norden** Niedersachsen, NW Germany
100 G10 **Nordenham** Niedersachsen, NW Germany
122 M6 **Nordenshel'da, Arkhipelag** *island group* N Russian Federation
92 O3 **Nordenskiold Land** *physical region* W Svalbard
100 E9 **Norderney** *island* NW Germany
100 J9 **Norderstedt** Schleswig-Holstein, N Germany
94 C11 **Nordfjord** *physical region* S Norway
94 D11 **Nordfjord** *fjord* S Norway
94 D11 **Nordfjordeid** Sogn og Fjordane, S Norway
92 G11 **Nordfold** Nordland, C Norway
Nordfriesische Inseln *see* North Frisian Islands
100 H7 **Nordfriesland** *cultural region* N Germany
101 K15 **Nordhausen** Thüringen, C Germany
25 T13 **Nordheim** Texas, SW USA
94 C13 **Nordhordland** *physical region* S Norway
100 E12 **Nordhorn** Niedersachsen, NW Germany
92 I1 **Nordhurfjördhur** Vestfirdhir, NW Iceland
92 J1 **Nordhurland Eystra** ◈ *region* N Iceland
92 I2 **Nordhurland Vestra** ◈ *region* N Iceland
172 H16 **Nord, Île du** *island* Inner Islands, NE Seychelles
95 F20 **Nordjylland** *off.* Nordjyllands Amt. ◈ *county* N Denmark
92 K7 **Nordkapp** *Eng.* North Cape. *headland* N Norway
92 O1 **Nordkapp** *headland* N Svalbard
92 L7 **Nordkinn** *headland* N Norway
79 N19 **Nord Kivu** *off.* Région du Nord Kivu. ◈ *region* E Dem. Rep. Congo (Zaire)
92 G12 **Nordland** ◈ *county* C Norway
101 J21 **Nördlingen** Bayern, S Germany
93 I16 **Nordmaling** Västerbotten, N Sweden
95 K15 **Nordmark** Värmland, C Sweden
Nord, Mer du *see* North Sea
94 F8 **Nordmøre** *physical region* S Norway
100 I8 **Nord-Ostee-Kanal** *canal* N Germany
(0) J3 **Nordostrundingen** *headland* NE Greenland
79 D14 **Nord-Ouest** *Eng.* North-West. ◈ *province* NW Cameroon
Nord-Ouest, Territoires du *see* Northwest Territories
103 N2 **Nord-Pas-de-Calais** ◈ *region* N France
101 F19 **Nordpfälzer Bergland** ▲ W Germany
Nord, Pointe *see* Fatua, Pointe
187 P16 **Nord, Province** ◈ *province* C New Caledonia
101 D14 **Nordrhein-Westfalen** *Eng.* North Rhine-Westphalia, *Fr.* Rhénanie du Nord-Westphalie. ◈ *state* W Germany
Nordsee/Nordsjøen/Nordsøen *see* North Sea
100 H7 **Nordstrand** *island* N Germany
93 E15 **Nord-Trøndelag** ◈ *county* C Norway
97 E19 **Nore** *Ir.* An Fheoir. ≈ S Ireland
29 Q14 **Norfolk** Nebraska, C USA
21 X7 **Norfolk** Virginia, NE USA
97 P19 **Norfolk** *cultural region* E England, UK
192 K10 **Norfolk Island** ◇ *Australian external territory* SW Pacific Ocean
175 P9 **Norfolk Ridge** *undersea feature* W Pacific Ocean
27 U8 **Norfork Lake** ▣ Arkansas/Missouri, C USA
98 N6 **Norg** Drenthe, NE Netherlands
Norge *see* Norway
95 D14 **Norheimsund** Hordaland, S Norway
25 S16 **Norias** Texas, SW USA
164 L12 **Norikura-dake** ▲ Honshū, S Japan
122 K8 **Noril'sk** Taymyrskiy (Dolgano-Nenetskiy) Avtonomnyy Okrug, N Russian Federation
14 I13 **Norland** Ontario, SE Canada
21 V8 **Norlina** North Carolina, SE USA
30 L13 **Normal** Illinois, N USA
27 N11 **Norman** Oklahoma, C USA
Norman *see* Tulita
186 G9 **Normanby Island** *island* SE PNG
Normandes, Îles *see* Channel Islands
58 G9 **Normandia** Roraima, N Brazil
102 L5 **Normandie** *Eng.* Normandy. *cultural region* N France
102 J5 **Normandie, Collines de** *hill range* NW France
Normandy *see* Normandie
25 V9 **Normangee** Texas, SW USA
21 Q10 **Norman, Lake** ▣ North Carolina, SE USA
44 K13 **Norman Manley** ✕ (Kingston) E Jamaica
181 U5 **Norman River** ≈ Queensland, NE Australia
181 U4 **Normanton** Queensland, NE Australia
16 L12 **Norman Wells** Northwest Territories, NW Canada
12 H12 **Normétal** Quebec, S Canada
11 V15 **Norquay** Saskatchewan, S Canada
94 N11 **Norra Dellen** ◎ C Sweden
93 G15 **Norråker** Jämtland, C Sweden
94 N12 **Norrala** Gävleborg, C Sweden
Norra Ny *see* Stöllet
92 G13 **Norra Storjfjället** ▲ N Sweden
92 I13 **Norrbotten** ◈ *county* N Sweden
Nørre Aaby *see* Nørre Åby
95 G23 **Nørre Åby** *var.* Nørre Aaby. Fyn, C Denmark
95 I24 **Nørre Alslev** Storstrøm, SE Denmark
95 E23 **Nørre Nebel** Ribe, W Denmark
95 G20 **Nørresundby** Nordjylland, N Denmark
21 N8 **Norris Lake** ▣ Tennessee, S USA
18 I15 **Norristown** Pennsylvania, NE USA
95 N17 **Norrköping** Östergötland, S Sweden
Norrmark *see* Noormarkku
94 N13 **Norrsundet** Gävleborg, C Sweden
95 P15 **Norrtälje** Stockholm, C Sweden
180 L12 **Norseman** Western Australia
93 I14 **Norsjö** Västerbotten, N Sweden
95 G16 **Norsjø** ◎ S Norway
123 R13 **Norsk** Amurskaya Oblast', SE Russian Federation
Norske Havet *see* Norwegian Sea
187 Q13 **Norsup** Malekula, C Vanuatu
191 V15 **Norte, Cabo** *headland* Easter Island, Chile, E Pacific Ocean
54 F7 **Norte de Santander** *off.* Departamento de Norte de Santander. ◈ *province* N Colombia
61 E21 **Norte, Punta** *headland* E Argentina
21 R13 **North** South Carolina, SE USA
North *see* Nord
18 L10 **North Adams** Massachusetts, NE USA
113 L17 **North Albanian Alps** *Alb.* Bjeshkët e Namuna, *SCr.* Prokletije. ▲ Albania/Yugoslavia
97 M15 **Northallerton** N England, UK
180 J12 **Northam** Western Australia
83 J20 **Northam** Northern, N South Africa
1 **North America** *continent*
1 N12 **North American Basin** *undersea feature* W Sargasso Sea
(0) C5 **North American Plate** *tectonic feature*
18 M11 **North Amherst** Massachusetts, NE USA
97 N20 **Northampton** C England, UK
97 M20 **Northamptonshire** *cultural region* C England, UK
151 P18 **North Andaman** *island* Andaman Islands, India, NE Indian Ocean
65 D25 **North Arm** East Falkland, Falkland Islands
21 Q13 **North Augusta** South Carolina, SE USA
173 W8 **North Australian Basin** *Fr.* Bassin Nord de l' Australie. *undersea feature* E Indian Ocean
31 R11 **North Baltimore** Ohio, N USA
11 T15 **North Battleford** Saskatchewan, S Canada
14 H11 **North Bay** Ontario, S Canada
12 H6 **North Belcher Islands** *island group* Belcher Islands, Nunavut, C Canada
29 R15 **North Bend** Nebraska, C USA
32 E14 **North Bend** Oregon, NW USA
96 K12 **North Berwick** SE Scotland, UK
North Beveland *see* Noord-Beveland
North Borneo *see* Sabah
183 P5 **North Bourke** New South Wales, SE Australia
North Brabant *see* Noord-Brabant
182 F2 **North Branch Neales** *seasonal river* South Australia
44 M6 **North Caicos** *island* NW Turks and Caicos Islands
26 L10 **North Canadian River** ≈ Oklahoma, C USA
31 U12 **North Canton** Ohio, N USA
13 R13 **North, Cape** *headland* Cape Breton Island, Nova Scotia, SE Canada
184 I1 **North Cape** *headland* North Island, NZ
186 G5 **North Cape** *headland* New Ireland, NE PNG
North Cape *see* Nordkapp
18 J17 **North Cape May** New Jersey, NE USA
12 C9 **North Caribou Lake** ◎ Ontario, C Canada
21 U10 **North Carolina** *off.* State of North Carolina; also known as Old North State, Tar Heel State, Turpentine State. ◈ *state* SE USA
North Celebes *see* Sulawesi Utara
155 J24 **North Central Province** ◈ *province* N Sri Lanka
31 S4 **North Channel** *lake channel* Canada/USA
97 G14 **North Channel** *strait* Northern Ireland/Scotland, UK
21 S14 **North Charleston** South Carolina, SE USA
31 N10 **North Chicago** Illinois, N USA
195 Y10 **Northcliffe Glacier** *glacier* Antarctica
31 Q14 **North College Hill** Ohio, N USA
25 O8 **North Concho River** ≈ Texas, SW USA
19 O8 **North Conway** New Hampshire, NE USA
27 V14 **North Crossett** Arkansas, C USA
28 L4 **North Dakota** *off.* State of North Dakota; also known as Flickertail State, Peace Garden State, Sioux State. ◈ *state* N USA
North Devon Island *see* Devon Island
97 O22 **North Downs** *hill range* SE England, UK
18 C11 **North East** Pennsylvania, NE USA
83 I18 **North East** ◈ *district* NE Botswana
65 G15 **North East Bay** *bay* Ascension Island, C Atlantic Ocean
38 L10 **Northeast Cape** *headland* Saint Lawrence Island, Alaska, USA
81 J17 **North Eastern** ◈ *province* Kenya
North East Frontier Agency/North East Frontier Agency of Assam *see* Arunāchal Pradesh
65 E25 **North East Island** *island* E Falkland Islands
189 V11 **Northeast Island** *island* Chuuk, C Micronesia
44 L12 **North East Point** *headland* E Jamaica
44 L6 **Northeast Point** *headland* Great Inagua, S Bahamas
44 K5 **Northeast Point** *headland* Acklins Island, SE Bahamas
191 Z2 **Northeast Point** *headland* Kiritimati, E Kiribati
44 H2 **Northeast Providence Channel** *channel* N Bahamas
101 J14 **Northeim** Niedersachsen, C Germany
29 X14 **North English** Iowa, C USA
138 G8 **Northern** ◈ *district* N Israel
82 M12 **Northern** ◈ *region* N Malawi
186 F8 **Northern** ◈ *province* S PNG
83 J20 **Northern** *off.* Northern Province; *prev.* Northern Transvaal. ◈ *province* NE South Africa
80 D7 **Northern** ◈ *state* N Sudan
82 K12 **Northern** ◈ *province* NE Zambia
80 B13 **Northern Bahr el Ghazal** ◈ *state* SW Sudan
Northern Border Region *see* Al Ḥudūd ash Shamālīyah
83 F24 **Northern Cape** *off.* Northern Cape Province, *Afr.* Noord-Kaap. ◈ *province* W South Africa
190 K14 **Northern Cook Islands** *island group* N Cook Islands
80 B8 **Northern Darfur** ◈ *state* NW Sudan
Northern Dvina *see* Severnaya Dvina
97 F14 **Northern Ireland** *var.* The Six Counties. *political division* UK
80 D9 **Northern Kordofan** ◈ *state* C Sudan
187 Z14 **Northern Lau Group** *island group* Lau Group, NE Fiji
188 K3 **Northern Mariana Islands** ◇ *US commonwealth territory* W Pacific Ocean
155 J23 **Northern Province** ◈ *province* N Sri Lanka
Northern Rhodesia *see* Zambia
Northern Sporades *see* Vóreioi Sporádes
182 D1 **Northern Territory** ◈ *territory* N Australia
Northern Transvaal *see* Northern
Northern Ural Hills *see* Severnyye Uvaly
84 I9 **North European Plain** *plain* N Europe
27 V2 **North Fabius River** ≈ Missouri, C USA
65 D24 **North Falkland Sound** *sound* N Falkland Islands
29 V9 **Northfield** Minnesota, N USA
19 O9 **Northfield** New Hampshire, NE USA
175 Q8 **North Fiji Basin** *undersea feature* N Coral Sea
97 Q22 **North Foreland** *headland* SE England, UK
35 P6 **North Fork American River** ≈ California, W USA

◆ COUNTRY ● COUNTRY CAPITAL ◇ DEPENDENT TERRITORY ○ DEPENDENT TERRITORY CAPITAL ◈ ADMINISTRATIVE REGION ✕ INTERNATIONAL AIRPORT ▲ MOUNTAIN ▲ MOUNTAIN RANGE △ VOLCANO ≈ RIVER ◎ LAKE ▣ RESERVOIR

39 *R7* **North Fork Chandalar River** Alaska, USA
28 *K7* **North Fork Grand River** North Dakota/South Dakota, N USA
21 *O6* **North Fork Kentucky River** Kentucky, S USA
39 *Q7* **North Fork Koyukuk River** Alaska, USA
39 *Q10* **North Fork Kuskokwim River** Alaska, USA
26 *K11* **North Fork Red River** Oklahoma/Texas, SW USA
26 *K3* **North Fork Solomon River** Kansas, C USA
23 *W14* **North Fort Myers** Florida, SE USA
31 *P5* **North Fox Island** *island* Michigan, N USA
100 *G6* **North Frisian Islands** ***var.*** Nordfriesische Inseln. *island group* N Germany
197 *N9* **North Geomagnetic Pole** *pole* Arctic Ocean
18 *M13* **North Haven** Connecticut, NE USA
184 *J5* **North Head** *headland* North Island, NZ
18 *L6* **North Hero** Vermont, NE USA
35 *O7* **North Highlands** California, W USA
North Holland *see* Noord-Holland
81 *I16* **North Horr** Eastern, N Kenya
151 *K21* **North Huvadhu Atoll** ***var.*** Gaafu Alifu Atoll. *atoll* S Maldives
65 *A24* **North Island** *island* W Falkland Islands
184 *N9* **North Island** *island* N NZ
21 *U14* **North Island** *island* South Carolina, SE USA
31 *O11* **North Judson** Indiana, N USA
North Kazakhstan *see* Severnyy Kazakhstan
31 *V10* **North Kingsville** Ohio, N USA
163 *Y13* **North Korea** ***off.*** Democratic People's Republic of Korea, ***Kor.*** Chosŏn-minjujuŭi-inmin-kanghwaguk. ◆ *republic* E Asia
153 *X11* **North Lakhimpur** Assam, NE India
184 *J3* **Northland** ***off.*** Northland Region. ◇ *region* North Island, NZ
192 K11 **Northland Plateau** *undersea feature* S Pacific Ocean
35 *X11* **North Las Vegas** Nevada, W USA
31 *O11* **North Liberty** Indiana, N USA
29 *X14* **North Liberty** Iowa, C USA
27 *V12* **North Little Rock** Arkansas, C USA
28 *M13* **North Loup River** Nebraska, C USA
151 *K18* **North Maalhosmadulu Atoll** ***var.*** North Malosmadulu Atoll, Raa Atoll. *atoll* N Maldives
31 *U10* **North Madison** Ohio, N USA
31 *P12* **North Manchester** Indiana, N USA
31 *P6* **North Manitou Island** *island* Michigan, N USA
29 *U10* **North Mankato** Minnesota, N USA
23 *Z15* **North Miami** Florida, SE USA
151 *K18* **North Miladummadulu Atoll** *atoll* N Maldives
North Minch *see* Minch, The
23 *W15* **North Naples** Florida, SE USA
175 *P8* **North New Hebrides Trench** *undersea feature* N Coral Sea
23 *Y15* **North New River Canal** Florida, SE USA
151 *K20* **North Nilandhe Atoll** ***var.*** Faafu Atoll. *atoll* C Maldives
36 *L2* **North Ogden** Utah, W USA
North Ossetia *see* Severnaya Osetiya-Alaniya, Respublika
35 *S10* **North Palisade** ▲ California, W USA
189 *U11* **North Pass** *passage* Chuuk Islands, C Micronesia
28 *M15* **North Platte** Nebraska, C USA
33 *X17* **North Platte River** C USA
65 *G14* **North Point** *headland* Ascension Island, C Atlantic Ocean
172 *I16* **North Point** *headland* Mahé, NE Seychelles
31 *S6* **North Point** *headland* Michigan, N USA
31 *R5* **North Point** *headland* Michigan, N USA
39 *S9* **North Pole** Alaska, USA
197 *R9* **North Pole** *pole* Arctic Ocean
23 *O4* **Northport** Alabama, S USA
23 *W14* **North Port** Florida, SE USA
32 *L6* **Northport** Washington, NW USA
32 *L12* **North Powder** Oregon, NW USA
29 *U13* **North Raccoon River** Iowa, C USA
North Rhine-Westphalia *see* Nordrhein-Westfalen
97 *M16* **North Riding** *cultural region* N England, UK
96 *G5* **North Rona** *island* NW Scotland, UK
96 *K4* **North Ronaldsay** *island* NE Scotland, UK
36 *L2* **North Salt Lake** Utah, W USA
11 *P15* **North Saskatchewan** Alberta/Saskatchewan, S Canada
35 *X5* **North Schell Peak** ▲ Nevada, W USA
North Scotia Ridge *see* South Georgia Ridge
86 *D10* **North Sea** ***Dan.*** Nordsøen, ***Dut.*** Noordzee, ***Fr.*** Mer du Nord, ***Ger.*** Nordsee, ***Nor.*** Nordsjøen; ***prev.*** German Ocean, ***Lat.*** Mare Germanicum. *sea* NW Europe
35 *T6* **North Shoshone Peak** ▲ Nevada, W USA
North Siberian Lowland/North Siberian Plain *see* Severo-Sibirskaya Nizmennost'
29 *R13* **North Sioux City** South Dakota, N USA
96 *K4* **North Sound, The** *sound* N Scotland, UK
183 *T4* **North Star** New South Wales, SE Australia
North Star State *see* Minnesota
183 *V3* **North Stradbroke Island** *island* Queensland, E Australia
North Sulawesi *see* Sulawesi Utara
North Sumatra *see* Sumatera Utara
14 *D17* **North Sydenham** Ontario, S Canada
18 *H9* **North Syracuse** New York, NE USA
184 *K9* **North Taranaki Bight** *gulf* North Island, NZ
12 *H9* **North Twin Island** *island* Nunavut, C Canada
96 *E8* **North Uist** *island* NW Scotland, UK
97 *L14* **Northumberland** *cultural region* N England, UK
181 *Y7* **Northumberland Isles** *island group* Queensland, NE Australia
13 *Q14* **Northumberland Strait** *strait* SE Canada
32 *G14* **North Umpqua River** Oregon, NW USA
45 *Q13* **North Union** Saint Vincent, Saint Vincent and the Grenadines
10 *L17* **North Vancouver** British Columbia, SW Canada
18 *K9* **Northville** New York, NE USA
97 *Q19* **North Walsham** E England, UK
39 *T10* **Northway** Alaska, USA
83 *G21* **North-West** ***off.*** North-West Province, ***Afr.*** Noordwes. ◇ *province* N South Africa
North-West *see* Nord-Ouest
64 *I6* **Northwest Atlantic Mid-Ocean Canyon** *undersea feature* N Atlantic Ocean
180 *G8* **North West Cape** *headland* Western Australia
38 *J9* **Northwest Cape** *headland* Saint Lawrence Island, Alaska, USA
82 *H13* **North Western** ◇ *province* W Zambia
155 *J24* **North Western Province** ◇ *province* W Sri Lanka
149 *U4* **North-West Frontier Province** ◇ *province* NW Pakistan
96 *H8* **North West Highlands** ▲ N Scotland, UK
192 J4 **Northwest Pacific Basin** *undersea feature* NW Pacific Ocean
191 *Y2* **Northwest Point** *headland* Kiritimati, E Kiribati
44 *G1* **Northwest Providence Channel** *channel* N Bahamas
13 *Q8* **North West River** Newfoundland, E Canada
8 J9 **Northwest Territories** ***Fr.*** Territoires du Nord-Ouest. ◇ *territory* NW Canada
97 *K18* **Northwich** C England, UK
25 *Q5* **North Wichita River** Texas, SW USA
18 *J17* **North Wildwood** New Jersey, NE USA
21 *R9* **North Wilkesboro** North Carolina, SE USA
19 *P8* **North Windham** Maine, NE USA
197 *Q6* **Northwind Plain** *undersea feature* Arctic Ocean
29 *V11* **Northwood** Iowa, C USA
29 *Q4* **Northwood** North Dakota, N USA
97 *M15* **North York Moors** *moorland* N England, UK
25 *V9* **North Zulch** Texas, SW USA
26 *K2* **Norton** Kansas, C USA
31 *S13* **Norton** Ohio, N USA
21 *P7* **Norton** Virginia, NE USA
39 *N9* **Norton Bay** *bay* Alaska, USA
Norton de Matos *see* Balombo
31 *O9* **Norton Shores** Michigan, N USA
38 *M10* **Norton Sound** *inlet* Alaska, USA
27 *Q3* **Nortonville** Kansas, C USA
102 *I8* **Nort-sur-Erdre** Loire-Atlantique, NW France
195 *N2* **Norvegia, Cape** *headland* Antarctica
18 *L13* **Norwalk** Connecticut, NE USA
29 *V14* **Norwalk** Iowa, C USA
31 *S11* **Norwalk** Ohio, N USA
19 *P7* **Norway** Maine, NE USA
31 *N5* **Norway** Michigan, N USA
93 *E17* **Norway** ***off.*** Kingdom of Norway, ***Nor.*** Norge. ◆ *monarchy* N Europe
11 *X13* **Norway House** Manitoba, C Canada
197 *R16* **Norwegian Basin** *undersea feature* NW Norwegian Sea
84 *D6* **Norwegian Sea** ***Nor.*** Norske Havet. *sea* NE Atlantic Ocean
197 *S17* **Norwegian Trench** *undersea feature* NE North Sea
14 *F16* **Norwich** Ontario, S Canada
97 *Q19* **Norwich** E England, UK
19 *N13* **Norwich** Connecticut, NE USA
18 *I11* **Norwich** New York, NE USA
29 *U9* **Norwood** Minnesota, N USA
31 *Q15* **Norwood** Ohio, N USA
14 *H11* **Nosbonsing, Lake** ◎ Ontario, S Canada
Nösen *see* Bistrița
165 T1 **Noshappu-misaki** *headland* Hokkaidō, NE Japan
165 P7 **Noshiro** ***var.*** Nosiro; ***prev.*** Noshirominato. Akita, Honshū, C Japan
Noshirominato/Nosiro *see* Noshiro
117 *Q3* **Nosivka** ***Rus.*** Nosovka. Chernihivs'ka Oblast', NE Ukraine
67 *T14* **Nosop** ***var.*** Nossob, Nossop. Botswana/Namibia
127 *S4* **Nosovaya** Nenetskiy Avtonomnyy Okrug, NW Russian Federation
Nosovka *see* Nosivka
143 *V11* **Noṣratābād** Sīstān va Balūchestān, E Iran
95 *J18* **Nossebro** Västra Götaland, S Sweden
96 *K6* **Noss Head** *headland* N Scotland, UK
Nossi-Bé *see* Be, Nosy
83 *E20* **Nossob** E Namibia
Nossob/Nossop *see* Nosop
172 *J2* **Nosy Be** × Antsirañana, N Madagascar
172 *J6* **Nosy Varika** Fianarantsoa, SE Madagascar
14 *L10* **Notawassi** Quebec, SE Canada
14 *M9* **Notawassi, Lac** ◎ Quebec, SE Canada
36 *J5* **Notch Peak** ▲ Utah, W USA
110 *G10* **Noteć** ***Ger.*** Netze. NW Poland
Nóties Sporádes *see* Dodekánisos
115 *J22* **Nótion Aigaíon** ***Eng.*** Aegean South. ◇ *region* E Greece
115 *H18* **Nótios Evvoïkós Kólpos** *gulf* E Greece
115 *B16* **Nótio Stenó Kérkyras** *strait* W Greece
107 *L25* **Noto** ***anc.*** Netum. Sicilia, Italy, C Mediterranean Sea
164 M10 **Noto** Ishikawa, Honshū, SW Japan
95 *G15* **Notodden** Telemark, S Norway
107 *L25* **Noto, Golfo di** *gulf* Sicilia, Italy, C Mediterranean Sea
164 L10 **Noto-hantō** *peninsula* Honshū, SW Japan
164 L11 **Noto-jima** *island* SW Japan
13 *T11* **Notre Dame Bay** *bay* Newfoundland, E Canada
15 *P6* **Notre-Dame-de-Lorette** Quebec, SE Canada
14 *L11* **Notre-Dame-de-Pontmain** Quebec, SE Canada
15 *T8* **Notre-Dame-du-Lac** Quebec, SE Canada
15 *Q6* **Notre-Dame-du-Rosaire** Quebec, SE Canada
15 *U8* **Notre-Dame, Monts** ▲ Quebec, S Canada
77 *R16* **Notsé** S Togo
14 *G14* **Nottawasaga** Ontario, S Canada
14 *G14* **Nottawasaga Bay** *lake bay* Ontario, S Canada
12 *I11* **Nottaway** Quebec, SE Canada
23 *S1* **Nottely Lake** ▣ Georgia, SE USA
95 *H16* **Nøtterøy** *island* S Norway
97 *M19* **Nottingham** C England, UK
9 P8 **Nottingham Island** *island* Nunavut, NE Canada
97 *N18* **Nottinghamshire** *cultural region* C England, UK
21 *V7* **Nottoway** Virginia, NE USA
21 *V7* **Nottoway River** Virginia, NE USA
76 *G7* **Nouâdhibou** ***prev.*** Port-Étienne. Dakhlet Nouâdhibou, W Mauritania
76 *G7* **Nouâdhibou** × Dakhlet Nouâdhibou, W Mauritania
76 *F7* **Nouâdhibou, Dakhlet** ***prev.*** Baie du Lévrier. *bay* W Mauritania
76 *F7* **Nouâdhibou, Râs** ***prev.*** Cap Blanc. *headland* NW Mauritania
76 *G9* **Nouakchott** ● (Mauritania) Nouakchott District, SW Mauritania
76 *G9* **Nouakchott** × Trarza, SW Mauritania
120 J11 **Noual, Sebkhet en** ***var.*** Sabkhat an Nawāl. *salt flat* C Tunisia
76 *G8* **Nouâmghâr** ***var.*** Nouamrhar. Dakhlet Nouâdhibou, W Mauritania
Nouamrhar *see* Nouâmghâr
Nouă Sulița *see* Novoselytsya
187 Q17 **Nouméa** ○ (New Caledonia) Province Sud, S New Caledonia
79 *E15* **Noun** C Cameroon
77 *N12* **Nouna** W Burkina
83 *H24* **Noupoort** Northern Cape, C South Africa
Nouveau-Brunswick *see* New Brunswick
Nouveau-Comptoir *see* Wemindji
15 *T4* **Nouvel, Lacs** ◎ Quebec, SE Canada
15 *W7* **Nouvelle** Quebec, SE Canada
15 *W7* **Nouvelle** Quebec, SE Canada
Nouvelle-Calédonie *see* New Caledonia
Nouvelle Écosse *see* Nova Scotia
103 *R3* **Nouzonville** Ardennes, N France
147 *Q11* **Nov** ***Rus.*** Nau. NW Tajikistan
59 *I21* **Nova Alvorada** Mato Grosso do Sul, SW Brazil
Novabad *see* Navobod
111 *D19* **Nová Bystřice** ***Ger.*** Neubistritz. Budějovický Kraj, S Czech Republic
116 *H13* **Novaci** Gorj, SW Romania
Nova Civitas *see* Neustadt an der Weinstrasse
Novaesium *see* Neuss
60 *H10* **Nova Esperança** Paraná, S Brazil
106 *H11* **Novafeltria** Marche, C Italy
60 *Q9* **Nova Friburgo** Rio de Janeiro, SE Brazil
82 *D12* **Nova Gaia** ***var.*** Cambundi-Catembo. Malanje, NE Angola
109 *S12* **Nova Gorica** W Slovenia
112 *G10* **Nova Gradiška** ***Ger.*** Neugradisk, ***Hung.*** Újgradiska. Brod-Posavina, NE Croatia
60 *K7* **Nova Granada** São Paulo, S Brazil
60 *O10* **Nova Iguaçu** Rio de Janeiro, SE Brazil
117 *S10* **Nova Kakhovka** ***Rus.*** Novaya Kakhovka. Khersons'ka Oblast', SE Ukraine
Nová Karvinná *see* Karviná
Nova Lamego *see* Gabú
Nova Lisboa *see* Huambo
112 *C11* **Novalja** Lika-Senj, W Croatia
119 *M14* **Novalukoml'** ***Rus.*** Novolukoml'. Vitsyebskaya Voblasts', N Belarus
Nova Mambone *see* Mambone
83 *P16* **Nova Nabúri** Zambézia, NE Mozambique
117 *Q9* **Nova Odesa** ***var.*** Novaya Odessa. Mykolayivs'ka Oblast', S Ukraine
60 *H10* **Nova Olímpia** Paraná, S Brazil
61 *I15* **Nova Prata** Rio Grande do Sul, S Brazil
14 *H12* **Novar** Ontario, S Canada
106 *C7* **Novara** ***anc.*** Novaria. Piemonte, NW Italy
Novaria *see* Novara
117 *P7* **Novarkanels'k** Kirovohrads'ka Oblast', C Ukraine
13 *P15* **Nova Scotia** ***Fr.*** Nouvelle Écosse. ◇ *province* SE Canada
(0) *M9* **Nova Scotia** *physical region* SE Canada
34 *M8* **Novato** California, W USA
192 M7 **Nova Trough** *undersea feature* W Pacific Ocean
116 *L7* **Nova Ushtsya** Khmel'nyts'ka Oblast', W Ukraine
83 *M17* **Nova Vanduzi** Manica, C Mozambique
117 *U5* **Nova Vodolaha** ***Rus.*** Novaya Vodolaga. Kharkivs'ka Oblast', E Ukraine
123 O12 **Novaya Chara** Chitinskaya Oblast', S Russian Federation
122 M12 **Novaya Igirma** Irkutskaya Oblast', C Russian Federation
Novaya Kakhovka *see* Nova Kakhovka
144 *E10* **Novaya Kazanka** Zapadnyy Kazakhstan, W Kazakhstan
126 *I12* **Novaya Ladoga** Leningradskaya Oblast', NW Russian Federation
129 *R5* **Novaya Malykla** Ul'yanovskaya Oblast', W Russian Federation
Novaya Odessa *see* Nova Odesa
123 Q5 **Novaya Sibir', Ostrov** *island* Novosibirskiye Ostrova, NE Russian Federation
Novaya Vodolaga *see* Nova Vodolaha
119 *P17* **Novaya Yel'nya** ***Rus.*** Novaya Yel'nya. Mahilyowskaya Voblasts', E Belarus
122 I6 **Novaya Zemlya** *island group* N Russian Federation
Novaya Zemlya Trough *see* East Novaya Zemlya Trough
114 *K10* **Nova Zagora** Sliven, C Bulgaria
105 *S12* **Novelda** País Valenciano, E Spain
111 *H19* **Nové Mesto nad Váhom** ***Ger.*** Waagneustadtll, ***Hung.*** Vágújhely. Trenčiansky Kraj, W Slovakia
111 *F17* **Nové Město na Moravě** ***Ger.*** Neustadtl in Mähren. Jihlavský Kraj, C Czech Republic
Novesium *see* Neuss
111 *I21* **Nové Zámky** ***Ger.*** Neuhäusel, ***Hung.*** Érsekújvár. Nitriansky Kraj, SW Slovakia
122 C7 **Novgorod** Novgorodskaya Oblast', W Russian Federation
Novgorod-Severskiy *see* Novhorod-Sivers'kyy
122 C7 **Novgorodskaya Oblast'** ◇ *province* W Russian Federation
117 *R8* **Novhorodka** Kirovohrads'ka Oblast', C Ukraine
117 *R2* **Novhorod-Sivers'kyy** ***Rus.*** Novgorod-Severskiy. Chernihivs'ka Oblast', NE Ukraine
31 *R10* **Novi** Michigan, N USA
Novi *see* Novi Vinodolski
112 *L9* **Novi Bečej** ***prev.*** Új-Becse, Vološinovo, ***Ger.*** Neubetsche, ***Hung.*** Törökbecse. Serbia, N Yugoslavia
25 *Q8* **Novice** Texas, SW USA
112 *A9* **Novigrad** Istra, NW Croatia
Novi Grad *see* Bosanski Novi
114 *G9* **Novi Iskŭr** Sofiya-Grad, W Bulgaria
106 *C9* **Novi Ligure** Piemonte, NW Italy
99 *L22* **Noville** Luxembourg, SE Belgium
194 *I10* **Noville Peninsula** *peninsula* Thurston Island, Antarctica
Noviodunum *see* Soissons, Aisne, France
Noviodunum *see* Nevers, Nièvre, France
Noviodunum *see* Nyon, Vaud, Switzerland
Noviomagus *see* Lisieux, France
Noviomagus *see* Nijmegen, Netherlands
114 *M8* **Novi Pazar** Shumen, NE Bulgaria
113 *M15* **Novi Pazar** ***Turk.*** Yenipazar. Serbia, S Yugoslavia
112 *K10* **Novi Sad** ***Ger.*** Neusatz, ***Hung.*** Újvidék. Serbia, N Yugoslavia
117 *T6* **Novi Sanzhary** Poltavs'ka Oblast', C Ukraine
112 *H12* **Novi Travnik** ***prev.*** Pučarevo. Federacija Bosna I Hercegovina, C Bosnia and Herzegovina
112 *B10* **Novi Vinodolski** ***var.*** Novi. Primorje-Gorski Kotar, NW Croatia
58 *F12* **Novo Airão** Amazonas, N Brazil
129 *N14* **Novoaleksandrovsk** Stavropol'skiy Kray, SW Russian Federation
Novoalekseyevka *see* Zhobda
129 *N9* **Novoanninskiy** Volgogradskaya Oblast', SW Russian Federation
58 *F13* **Novo Aripuanã** Amazonas, N Brazil
117 *Y6* **Novoaydar** Luhans'ka Oblast', E Ukraine
117 *X9* **Novoazovs'k** ***Rus.*** Novoazovsk. Donets'ka Oblast', E Ukraine
123 R14 **Novobureyskiy** Amurskaya Oblast', SE Russian Federation
129 *Q3* **Novocheboksarsk** Chuvashskaya Respublika, W Russian Federation
129 *R5* **Novocheremshansk** Ul'yanovskaya Oblast', W Russian Federation
128 *L12* **Novocherkassk** Rostovskaya Oblast', SW Russian Federation
129 *R6* **Novodevich'ye** Samarskaya Oblast', W Russian Federation
126 *M8* **Novodvinsk** Arkhangel'skaya Oblast', NW Russian Federation
Novograd-Volynskiy *see* Novohrad-Volyns'kyy
Novogrudok *see* Navahrudak
61 *I15* **Novo Hamburgo** Rio Grande do Sul, S Brazil
59 *H16* **Novo Horizonte** Mato Grosso, W Brazil
60 *K8* **Novo Horizonte** São Paulo, S Brazil
116 *M4* **Novohrad-Volyns'kyy** ***Rus.*** Novograd-Volynskiy. Zhytomyrs'ka Oblast', N Ukraine
144 *L14* **Novokazalinsk** *see* Ayteke Bi
128 *M8* **Novokhopersk** Voronezhskaya Oblast', W Russian Federation
129 *R6* **Novokuybyshevsk** Samarskaya Oblast', W Russian Federation
122 J13 **Novokuznetsk** ***prev.*** Stalinsk. Kemerovskaya Oblast', S Russian Federation
195 *R1* **Novolazarevskaya** *Russian research station* Antarctica
Novolukoml' *see* Novalukoml'
109 *V12* **Novo mesto** ***Ger.*** Rudolfswert; ***prev. Ger.*** Neustadtl. SE Slovenia
128 *K15* **Novomikhaylovskiy** Krasnodarskiy Kray, SW Russian Federation
112 *L8* **Novo Miloševo** Serbia, N Yugoslavia
Novomirgorod *see* Novomyrhorod
128 *L5* **Novomoskovsk** Tul'skaya Oblast', W Russian Federation
117 *U7* **Novomoskovs'k** ***Rus.*** Novomoskovsk. Dnipropetrovs'ka Oblast', E Ukraine
117 *V8* **Novomykolayivka** Zaporiz'ka Oblast', SE Ukraine
117 *Q7* **Novomyrhorod** ***Rus.*** Novomirgorod. Kirovohrads'ka Oblast', S Ukraine
129 *N8* **Novonikolayevskiy** Volgogradskaya Oblast', SW Russian Federation
129 *P10* **Novonikol'skoye** Volgogradskaya Oblast', SW Russian Federation
129 *X7* **Novoorsk** Orenburgskaya Oblast', W Russian Federation
128 *M13* **Novopokrovskaya** Krasnodarskiy Kray, SW Russian Federation
Novopolotsk *see* Navapolatsk
117 *Y5* **Novopskov** Luhans'ka Oblast', E Ukraine
Novoradomsk *see* Radomsko
Novo Redondo *see* Sumbe
129 *R8* **Novorepnoye** Saratovskaya Oblast', W Russian Federation
128 *K14* **Novorossiysk** Krasnodarskiy Kray, SW Russian Federation
Novorossiyskiy *see* Novorossiyskoye
144 *J10* **Novorossiyskoye** ***prev.*** Novorossiyskiy. Aktyubinsk, NW Kazakhstan
126 *F15* **Novorzhev** Pskovskaya Oblast', W Russian Federation
Novoselitsa *see* Novoselytsya
117 *S12* **Novoselivs'ke** Respublika Krym, S Ukraine
Novosëlki *see* Navasyolki
114 *G6* **Novo Selo** Vidin, NW Bulgaria
113 *M14* **Novo Selo** Serbia, C Yugoslavia
116 *K8* **Novoselytsya** ***Rom.*** Nouă Sulița, ***Rus.*** Novoselitsa. Chernivets'ka Oblast', W Ukraine
129 *U7* **Novosergiyevka** Orenburgskaya Oblast', W Russian Federation
128 *L11* **Novoshakhtinsk** Rostovskaya Oblast', SW Russian Federation
122 J12 **Novosibirsk** Novosibirskaya Oblast', C Russian Federation
122 J12 **Novosibirskaya Oblast'** ◇ *province* C Russian Federation
122 M4 **Novosibirskiye Ostrova** ***Eng.*** New Siberian Islands. *island group* N Russian Federation
128 *K6* **Novosil'** Orlovskaya Oblast', W Russian Federation
126 *G16* **Novosokol'niki** Pskovskaya Oblast', W Russian Federation
129 *Q6* **Novospasskoye** Ul'yanovskaya Oblast', W Russian Federation
129 *X8* **Novotroitsk** Orenburgskaya Oblast', W Russian Federation
Novotroitskoye *see* Brlik, Kazakhstan
Novotroitskoye *see* Novotroyits'ke, Ukraine
117 *T11* **Novotroyits'ke** ***Rus.*** Novotroitskoye. Khersons'ka Oblast', S Ukraine
Novoukrainka *see* Novoukrayinka
117 *Q8* **Novoukrayinka** ***Rus.*** Novoukrainka. Kirovohrads'ka Oblast', C Ukraine
129 *Q5* **Novoul'yanovsk** Ul'yanovskaya Oblast', W Russian Federation
129 *W8* **Novouralets** Orenburgskaya Oblast', W Russian Federation
Novo-Urgench *see* Urganch
116 *I4* **Novovolyns'k** ***Rus.*** Novovolynsk. Volyns'ka Oblast', NW Ukraine
117 *S9* **Novovorontsovka** Khersons'ka Oblast', S Ukraine
147 *Y7* **Novovoznesenovka** Issyk-Kul'skaya Oblast', E Kyrgyzstan
127 *R14* **Novovyatsk** Kirovskaya Oblast', NW Russian Federation
Novoyel'nya *see* Navayel'nya
117 *O6* **Novozhyvotiv** Vinnyts'ka Oblast', C Ukraine
128 *H6* **Novozybkov** Bryanskaya Oblast', W Russian Federation
112 *F9* **Novska** Sisak-Moslavina, NE Croatia
Nový Bohumín *see* Bohumín
111 *D15* **Nový Bor** ***Ger.*** Haida; ***prev.*** Bor u České Lípy, Hajda. Liberecký Kraj, N Czech Republic
111 *E16* **Nový Bydžov** ***Ger.*** Neubidschow. Hradecký Kraj, N Czech Republic
119 *G18* **Novy Dvor** ***Rus.*** Novyy Dvor. Hrodzyenskaya Voblasts', W Belarus
111 *I17* **Nový Jičín** ***Ger.*** Neutitschein. Ostravský Kraj, E Czech Republic
118 *K12* **Novy Pahost** ***Rus.*** Novyy Pogost. Vitsyebskaya Voblasts', NW Belarus
Novyy Bug *see* Novyy Buh
117 *R9* **Novyy Buh** ***Rus.*** Novyy Bug. Mykolayivs'ka Oblast', S Ukraine
117 *Q4* **Novyy Bykiv** Chernihivs'ka Oblast', N Ukraine
Novyy Dvor *see* Novy Dvor
Novyye Aneny *see* Anenii Noi
129 *P7* **Novyye Burasy** Saratovskaya Oblast', W Russian Federation
Novyy Margilan *see* Farghona
128 *K8* **Novyy Oskol** Belgorodskaya Oblast', W Russian Federation
Novyy Pogost *see* Novy Pahost
129 *R2* **Novyy Tor"yal** Respublika Mariy El, W Russian Federation
123 N12 **Novyy Uoyan** Respublika Buryatiya, S Russian Federation
122 J9 **Novyy Urengoy** Yamalo-Nenetskiy Avtonomnyy Okrug, N Russian Federation
Novyy Uzen' *see* Zhanaozen
111 *N16* **Nowa Dęba** Podkarpackie, SE Poland
111 *G15* **Nowa Ruda** ***Ger.*** Neurode. Dolnośląskie, SW Poland
110 *F12* **Nowa Sól** ***var.*** Nowasól, ***Ger.*** Neusalz an der Oder. Lubuskie, W Poland
27 *Q8* **Nowata** Oklahoma, C USA
142 *M6* **Nowbarān** Markazī, W Iran
110 *J8* **Nowe** Kujawski-pomorskie, C Poland
110 *K9* **Nowe Miasto Lubawskie** ***Ger.*** Neumark. Warmińsko-Mazurskie, NE Poland
110 *L13* **Nowe Miasto nad Pilicą** Mazowieckie, C Poland
110 *D8* **Nowe Warpno** ***Ger.*** Neuwarp. Zachodniopomorskie, NW Poland
Nowgong *see* Nagaon
110 *E8* **Nowogard** ***var.*** Nowógard, ***Ger.*** Naugard. Zachodniopomorskie, NW Poland
110 *N9* **Nowogród** Podlaskie, NE Poland
Nowogródek *see* Navahrudak
111 *E14* **Nowogrodziec** ***Ger.*** Naumburg am Queis. Dolnośląskie, SW Poland
Nowojelnia *see* Navayel'nya
Nowo-Minsk *see* Mińsk Mazowiecki
33 *V13* **Nowood River** Wyoming, C USA
Nowo-Święciany *see* Švenčionėliai
183 *S10* **Nowra-Bomaderry** New South Wales, SE Australia
149 *T5* **Nowshera** ***var.*** Naushahra, Naushara. North-West Frontier Province, NE Pakistan
110 *J7* **Nowy Dwór Gdański** ***Ger.*** Tiegenhof. Pomorskie, N Poland
110 *L11* **Nowy Dwór Mazowiecki** Mazowieckie, C Poland
111 *M17* **Nowy Sącz** ***Ger.*** Neu Sandec. Małopolskie, S Poland
111 *L18* **Nowy Targ** ***Ger.*** Neumark. Małopolskie, S Poland
110 *F11* **Nowy Tomyśl** ***var.*** Nowy Tomysl. Wielkolpolskie, C Poland
148 *M7* **Now Zād** ***var.*** Nauzad. Helmand, S Afghanistan
23 *N4* **Noxubee River** Alabama/Mississippi, S USA
122 I10 **Noyabr'sk** Yamalo-Nenetskiy Avtonomnyy Okrug, N Russian Federation
102 *L8* **Noyant** Maine-et-Loire, NW France
39 *X14* **Noyes Island** *island* Alexander Archipelago, Alaska, USA
103 *O3* **Noyon** Oise, N France
102 *I7* **Nozay** Loire-Atlantique, NW France

◆ COUNTRY ● COUNTRY CAPITAL ◇ DEPENDENT TERRITORY ○ DEPENDENT TERRITORY CAPITAL ◇ ADMINISTRATIVE REGION × INTERNATIONAL AIRPORT ▲ MOUNTAIN ▲ MOUNTAIN RANGE VOLCANO RIVER ◎ LAKE ▣ RESERVOIR

82 L12 **Nsando** Northern, NE Zambia
83 N16 **Nsanje** Southern, S Malawi
77 Q17 **Nsawam** SE Ghana
79 E16 **Nsimalen** × Centre, C Cameroon
82 K12 **Nsombo** Northern, NE Zambia
82 H13 **Ntambu** North Western, NW Zambia
83 N14 **Ntcheu** var. Ncheu. Central, S Malawi
79 D17 **Ntem** prev. Campo, Kampo. ⁓ Cameroon/Equatorial Guinea
83 I14 **Ntemwa** North Western, NW Zambia
Ntlenyana, Mount see Thabana Ntlenyana
79 I19 **Ntomba, Lac** var. Lac Tumba. ◎ NW Dem. Rep. Congo (Zaire)
81 E19 **Ntungamo** SW Uganda
81 E18 **Ntusi** SW Uganda
83 H18 **Ntwetwe Pan** *salt lake* NE Botswana
93 M15 **Nuasjärvi** ◎ C Finland
80 F11 **Nuba Mountains** ▲ C Sudan
68 I9 **Nubian Desert** *desert* NE Sudan
116 G10 **Nucet** *Hung.* Diófás. Bihor, W Romania
Nu Chiang see Salween
145 U9 **Nuclear Testing Ground** *nuclear site* Pavlodar, E Kazakhstan
56 E9 **Nucuray, Río** ⁓ N Peru
25 R14 **Nueces River** ⁓ Texas, SW USA
11 V9 **Nueltin Lake** ◎ Manitoba/Nunavut, C Canada
99 K15 **Nuenen** Noord-Brabant, S Netherlands
62 G6 **Nuestra Señora, Bahía** *bay* N Chile
61 D14 **Nuestra Señora Rosario de Caa Catí** Corrientes, NE Argentina
54 J9 **Nueva Antioquia** Vichada, E Colombia
Nueva Caceres see Naga
41 O7 **Nueva Ciudad Guerrera** Tamaulipas, C Mexico
55 N4 **Nueva Esparta** off. Estado Nueva Esparta. ◈ state NE Venezuela
44 C5 **Nueva Gerona** Isla de la Juventud, S Cuba
42 H8 **Nueva Guadalupe** San Miguel, E El Salvador
42 M11 **Nueva Guinea** Región Autónoma Atlántico Sur, SE Nicaragua
61 D19 **Nueva Helvecia** Colonia, SW Uruguay
63 J25 **Nueva, Isla** *island* S Chile
40 M14 **Nueva Italia** Michoacán de Ocampo, SW Mexico
56 D6 **Nueva Loja** var. Lago Agrio. Sucumbíos, NE Ecuador
42 F6 **Nueva Ocotepeque** prev. Ocotepeque. Ocotepeque, W Honduras
61 D19 **Nueva Palmira** Colonia, SW Uruguay
41 N6 **Nueva Rosita** Coahuila de Zaragoza, NE Mexico
42 E7 **Nueva San Salvador** prev. Santa Tecla. La Libertad, SW El Salvador
42 J8 **Nueva Segovia** ◈ *department* NW Nicaragua
Nueva Tabarca see Plana, Isla
Nueva Villa de Padilla see Nuevo Padilla
61 B21 **Nueve de Julio** Buenos Aires, E Argentina
44 H6 **Nuevitas** Camagüey, E Cuba
61 D18 **Nuevo Berlin** Río Negro, W Uruguay
40 I4 **Nuevo Casas Grandes** Chihuahua, N Mexico
43 T14 **Nuevo Chagres** Colón, C Panama
41 W15 **Nuevo Coahuila** Campeche, E Mexico
63 K17 **Nuevo, Golfo** *gulf* S Argentina
41 O7 **Nuevo Laredo** Tamaulipas, NE Mexico
41 N8 **Nuevo León** ◈ *state* NE Mexico
41 P10 **Nuevo Padilla** var. Nueva Villa de Padilla. Tamaulipas, C Mexico
56 E6 **Nuevo Rocafuerte** Napo, E Ecuador
162 G6 **Nuga** Dzavhan, W Mongolia
80 O13 **Nugaal** off. Gobolka Nugaal. ◈ *region* N Somalia
185 E24 **Nugget Point** *headland* South Island, NZ
186 J5 **Nuguria Islands** *island group* E PNG
184 P10 **Nuhaka** Hawke's Bay, North Island, NZ
138 M10 **Nuhaydayn, Wādī an** *dry watercourse* W Iraq
190 E7 **Nui Atoll** *atoll* W Tuvalu
Nu Jiang see Salween
Nûk see Nuuk
182 G7 **Nukey Bluff** *hill* South Australia
Nukha see Şäki
123 T9 **Nukh Yablonevyy, Gora** ▲ E Russian Federation
186 K7 **Nukiki** Choiseul Island, NW Solomon Islands
186 B6 **Nuku** Sandaun, NW PNG
193 W15 **Nuku** *island* Tongatapu Group, NE Tonga
193 U15 **Nukuʻalofa** Tongatapu, S Tonga
193 Y16 **Nukuʻalofa** ● (Tonga) Tongatapu, S Tonga
190 G12 **Nukuatea** *island* N Wallis and Futuna
190 F7 **Nukufetau Atoll** *atoll* C Tuvalu
190 G12 **Nukuhifala** *island* E Wallis and Futuna
191 W7 **Nuku Hiva** *island* Îles Marquises, NE French Polynesia
193 O8 **Nuku Hiva Island** *island* Îles Marquises, N French Polynesia
190 F9 **Nukulaelae Atoll** var. Nukulailai. *atoll* E Tuvalu
Nukulailai see Nukulaelae Atoll
190 G11 **Nukuloa** *island* N Wallis and Futuna
186 L6 **Nukumanu Islands** prev. Tasman Group. *island group* NE PNG
Nukunau see Nikunau
190 J9 **Nukunonu Atoll** *island* C Tokelau
190 J9 **Nukunonu Village** Nukunonu Atoll, C Tokelau
189 S18 **Nukuoro Atoll** *atoll* Caroline Islands, S Micronesia
146 H8 **Nukus** Qoraqalpoghiston Respublikasi, W Uzbekistan
190 G11 **Nukutapu** *island* N Wallis and Futuna
39 O9 **Nulato** Alaska, USA
39 O10 **Nulato Hills** ▲ Alaska, USA
105 T9 **Nules** País Valenciano, E Spain
Nuling see Sultan Kudarat
182 C6 **Nullarbor** South Australia
180 M11 **Nullarbor Plain** *plateau* South Australia/Western Australia
163 S12 **Nuluʻerhu Shan** ▲ N China
77 X14 **Numan** Adamawa, E Nigeria
165 S3 **Numata** Hokkaidō, NE Japan
81 C15 **Numatinna** ⁓ W Sudan
95 F14 **Numedalen** *valley* S Norway
95 G14 **Numedalslågen** var. Laagen. ⁓ S Norway
93 L19 **Nummela** Etelä-Suomi, S Finland
183 O11 **Numurkah** Victoria, SE Australia
196 L16 **Nunap Isua** var. Uummannarsuaq, *Dan.* Kap Farvel, *Eng.* Cape Farewell. *headland* S Greenland
9 N8 **Nunavut** ◈ *Territory* N Canada
54 H9 **Nunchia** Casanare, C Colombia
97 M20 **Nuneaton** C England, UK
153 W14 **Nungba** Manipur, NE India
38 L12 **Nunivak Island** *island* Alaska, USA
152 I5 **Nun Kun** ▲ NW India
98 L10 **Nunspeet** Gelderland, E Netherlands
107 C18 **Nuoro** Sardegna, Italy, C Mediterranean Sea
75 R12 **Nuqayy, Jabal** *hill range* S Libya
54 C9 **Nuquí** Chocó, W Colombia
143 O4 **Nūr** Māzandarān, N Iran
145 Q9 **Nura** ⁓ N Kazakhstan
143 N11 **Nūrābād** Fārs, C Iran
Nurakita see Niulakita
Nurata see Nurota
Nuratau, Khrebet see Nurota Tizmasi
136 L17 **Nur Dağları** ▲ S Turkey
Nurek see Norak
Nuremberg see Nürnberg
136 M15 **Nurhak** Kahramanmaraş, S Turkey
182 J9 **Nuriootpa** South Australia
129 S5 **Nurlat** Respublika Tatarstan, W Russian Federation
93 N15 **Nurmes** Itä-Suomi, E Finland
101 K20 **Nürnberg** *Eng.* Nuremberg. Bayern, S Germany
101 K20 **Nürnberg** × Bayern, SE Germany
146 M10 **Nurota** *Rus.* Nurata. Nawoiy Wiloyati, C Uzbekistan
147 N10 **Nurota Tizmasi** *Rus.* Khrebet Nuratau. ▲ C Uzbekistan
149 T8 **Nūrpur** Punjab, E Pakistan
183 P6 **Nurri, Mount** *hill* New South Wales, SE Australia
25 T13 **Nursery** Texas, SW USA
171 O16 **Nusa Tenggara** *Eng.* Lesser Sunda Islands. *island group* East Timor/ Indonesia
169 V17 **Nusa Tenggara Barat** off. Propinsi Nusa Tenggara Barat, *Eng.* West Nusa Tenggara. ◈ *province* S Indonesia
171 O16 **Nusa Tenggara Timur** off. Propinsi Nusa Tenggara Timur, *Eng.* East Nusa Tenggara. ◈ *province* S Indonesia
171 U14 **Nusawulan** Irian Jaya, E Indonesia
137 Q16 **Nusaybin** var. Nisibin. Manisa, SE Turkey
39 O14 **Nushagak Bay** *bay* Alaska, USA
39 O13 **Nushagak Peninsula** *headland* Alaska, USA
39 O13 **Nushagak River** ⁓ Alaska, USA
160 E11 **Nu Shan** ▲ SW China
149 N11 **Nushki** Baluchistān, SW Pakistan
Nussdorf see Năsăud
112 J9 **Nuštar** Vukovar-Srijem, E Croatia
99 L18 **Nuth** Limburg, SE Netherlands
100 N13 **Nuthe** ⁓ NE Germany
Nutmeg State see Connecticut
39 T10 **Nutzotin Mountains** ▲ Alaska, USA
64 I5 **Nuuk** var. Nûk, *Dan.* Godthaab, Godthåb. ○ (Greenland). Kitaa, SW Greenland
92 L13 **Nuupas** Lappi, NW Finland
191 O7 **Nuupere, Pointe** *headland* Moorea, W French Polynesia
191 O7 **Nuuroa, Pointe** *headland* Tahiti, W French Polynesia
162 M8 **Nüürst** Töv, C Mongolia
Nuwara see Nuwara Eliya
155 K25 **Nuwara Eliya** var. Nuwara. Central Province, S Sri Lanka
182 E7 **Nuyts Archipelago** *island group* South Australia
83 F17 **Nxaunxau** Ngamiland, NW Botswana
39 N12 **Nyac** Alaska, USA
122 H9 **Nyagan'** Khanty-Mansiyskiy Avtonomnyy Okrug, N Russian Federation
Nyagassola see Niagassola
81 I18 **Nyahururu** Central, W Kenya
182 M10 **Nyah West** Victoria, SE Australia
158 M15 **Nyainqêntanglha Feng** ▲ W China
159 N15 **Nyainqêntanglha Shan** ▲ W China
80 B11 **Nyala** Southern Darfur, W Sudan
83 M16 **Nyamapanda** Mashonaland East, NE Zimbabwe
81 H25 **Nyamtumbo** Ruvuma, S Tanzania
Nyanda see Masvingo
126 M11 **Nyandoma** Arkhangel'skaya Oblast', NW Russian Federation
83 M16 **Nyanga** prev. Inyanga. Manicaland, E Zimbabwe
79 D20 **Nyanga** off. Province de la Nyanga, var. La Nyanga. ◈ *province* SW Gabon
79 E20 **Nyanga** ⁓ Congo/Gabon
81 F20 **Nyantakara** Kagera, NW Tanzania
81 G19 **Nyanza** ◈ *province* W Kenya
81 E21 **Nyanza-Lac** S Burundi
68 J14 **Nyasa, Lake** var. Lake Malawi; prev. Lago Nyassa. ◎ E Africa
Nyasaland/Nyasaland Protectorate see Malawi
Nyassa, Lago see Nyasa, Lake
119 J17 **Nyasvizh** *Pol.* Nieśwież, *Rus.* Nesvizh. Minskaya Voblasts', C Belarus
166 M8 **Nyaunglebin** Pegu, SW Myanmar
166 M5 **Nyaung-u** Magwe, C Myanmar
95 H24 **Nyborg** Fyn, C Denmark
95 N21 **Nybro** Kalmar, S Sweden
119 J16 **Nyeharelaye** *Rus.* Negoreloye. Minskaya Voblasts', C Belarus
195 W3 **Nye Mountains** ▲ Antarctica
81 I19 **Nyeri** Central, C Kenya
118 M11 **Nyeshcharda, Vozyera** ◎ N Belarus
92 O2 **Ny-Friesland** *physical region* N Svalbard
95 L14 **Nyhammar** Dalarna, C Sweden
160 F7 **Nyikog Qu** ⁓ C China
158 L14 **Nyima** Xizang Zizhiqu, W China
83 L14 **Nyimba** Eastern, E Zambia
159 P16 **Nyingchi** Xizang Zizhiqu, W China
111 O21 **Nyírbátor** Szabolcs-Szatmár-Bereg, E Hungary
111 N21 **Nyíregyháza** Szabolcs-Szatmár-Bereg, NE Hungary
Nyiro see Ewaso Ng'iro
Nyitra see Nitra
Nyitrabánya see Handlová
93 K16 **Nykarleby** *Fin.* Uusikaarlepyy. Länsi-Suomi, W Finland
95 I25 **Nykøbing** Storstrøm, SE Denmark
95 I22 **Nykøbing** Vestsjælland, C Denmark
95 F21 **Nykøbing** Viborg, NW Denmark
95 N17 **Nyköping** Södermanland, S Sweden
95 L15 **Nykroppa** Värmland, C Sweden
83 J20 **Nylstroom** Northern, NE South Africa
183 P7 **Nymagee** New South Wales, SE Australia
183 V5 **Nymboida** New South Wales, SE Australia
183 U5 **Nymboida River** ⁓ New South Wales, SE Australia
111 D16 **Nymburk** var. Neuenburg an der Elbe, *Ger.* Nimburg. Středočeský Kraj, C Czech Republic
95 O16 **Nynäshamn** Stockholm, C Sweden
183 Q6 **Nyngan** New South Wales, SE Australia
Nyoman see Neman
108 A10 **Nyon** *Ger.* Neuss; *anc.* Noviodunum. Vaud, SW Switzerland
79 D16 **Nyong** ⁓ SW Cameroon
103 S14 **Nyons** Drôme, E France
79 D14 **Nyos, Lac** *Eng.* Lake Nyos. ◎ NW Cameroon
Nyos, Lake see Nyos, Lac
127 U11 **Nyrob** var. Nyrov. Permskaya Oblast', NW Russian Federation
Nyrov see Nyrob
111 H15 **Nysa** *Ger.* Neisse. Opolskie, S Poland
Nysa Łużycka see Neisse
Nyslott see Savonlinna
32 M13 **Nyssa** Oregon, NW USA
Nystad see Uusikaupunki
95 I25 **Nysted** Storstrøm, SE Denmark
127 U14 **Nytva** Permskaya Oblast', NW Russian Federation
165 P8 **Nyūdō-zaki** *headland* Honshū, C Japan
127 P9 **Nyukhcha** Arkhangel'skaya Oblast', NW Russian Federation
126 H8 **Nyuk, Ozero** var. Ozero Njuk. ◎ NW Russian Federation
127 O12 **Nyuksenitsa** var. Njuksenica. Vologodskaya Oblast', NW Russian Federation
79 O22 **Nyunzu** Katanga, SE Dem. Rep. Congo (Zaire)
123 O10 **Nyurba** Respublika Sakha (Yakutiya), NE Russian Federation
123 O11 **Nyuya** Respublika Sakha (Yakutiya), NE Russian Federation
117 T10 **Nyzhni Sirohozy** Khersons'ka Oblast', S Ukraine
117 U12 **Nyzhn'ohirs'kyy** *Rus.* Nizhnegorskiy. Respublika Krym, S Ukraine
81 G21 **Nzega** Tabora, C Tanzania
76 K15 **Nzérékoré** Guinée-Forestière, SE Guinea
82 A10 **N'Zeto** prev. Ambrizete. Zaire, NW Angola
79 M24 **Nzilo, Lac** prev. Lac Delcommune. ◎ SE Dem. Rep. Congo (Zaire)

O

29 O11 **Oacoma** South Dakota, N USA
29 N9 **Oahe Dam** *dam* South Dakota, N USA
28 M9 **Oahe, Lake** ▣ North Dakota/ South Dakota, N USA
38 C9 **Oahu** *Haw.* Oʻahu. *island* Hawaii, USA, C Pacific Ocean
165 V4 **O-Akan-dake** ▲ Hokkaidō, NE Japan
182 K8 **Oakbank** South Australia
19 P13 **Oak Bluffs** Martha's Vineyard, New York, NE USA
36 K4 **Oak City** Utah, W USA
37 R3 **Oak Creek** Colorado, C USA
35 P8 **Oakdale** California, W USA
22 H8 **Oakdale** Louisiana, S USA
29 P7 **Oakes** North Dakota, N USA
22 J4 **Oak Grove** Louisiana, S USA
97 N19 **Oakham** C England, UK
32 H7 **Oak Harbor** Washington, NW USA
21 R5 **Oak Hill** West Virginia, NE USA
35 N8 **Oakland** California, W USA
29 T15 **Oakland** Iowa, C USA
19 Q7 **Oakland** Maine, NE USA
21 T3 **Oakland** Maryland, NE USA
29 R14 **Oakland** Nebraska, C USA
31 N11 **Oak Lawn** Illinois, N USA
33 P16 **Oakley** Idaho, NW USA
26 I4 **Oakley** Kansas, C USA
31 N10 **Oak Park** Illinois, N USA
11 X16 **Oak Point** Manitoba, S Canada
32 G13 **Oakridge** Oregon, NW USA
20 M9 **Oak Ridge** Tennessee, S USA
184 K10 **Oakura** Taranaki, North Island, NZ
22 L7 **Oak Vale** Mississippi, S USA
14 G16 **Oakville** Ontario, S Canada
25 V8 **Oakwood** Texas, SW USA
185 F22 **Oamaru** Otago, South Island, NZ
96 F13 **Oa, Mull of** *headland* W Scotland, UK
171 O11 **Oan** Sulawesi, N Indonesia
185 J17 **Oaro** Canterbury, South Island, NZ
35 X2 **Oasis** Nevada, W USA
195 S15 **Oates Land** *physical region* Antarctica
183 P17 **Oatlands** Tasmania, SE Australia
36 I11 **Oatman** Arizona, SW USA
41 R16 **Oaxaca** var. Oaxaca de Juárez; prev. Antequera. Oaxaca, SE Mexico
41 Q16 **Oaxaca** ◈ *state* SE Mexico
Oaxaca de Juárez see Oaxaca
122 H9 **Ob'** ⁓ C Russian Federation
14 G9 **Obabika Lake** ◎ Ontario, S Canada
Obagan see Ubagan
118 M12 **Obal'** *Rus.* Obol'. Vitsyebskaya Voblasts', N Belarus
79 E16 **Obala** Centre, SW Cameroon
14 C6 **Oba Lake** ◎ Ontario, S Canada
164 J12 **Obama** Fukui, Honshū, SW Japan
96 H11 **Oban** W Scotland, UK
Oban see Halfmoon Bay
Obando see Puerto Inírida
104 I4 **O Barco** var. El Barco, El Barco de Valdeorras, O Barco de Valdeorras. Galicia, NW Spain
O Barco de Valdeorras see O Barco
Obbia see Hobyo
93 J16 **Obbola** Västerbotten, N Sweden
Obbrovazzo see Obrovac
Obchuga see Abchuha
Obdorsk see Salekhard
Óbecse see Bečej
118 I11 **Obeliai** Rokiškis, NE Lithuania
60 F13 **Oberá** Misiones, NE Argentina
108 E8 **Oberburg** Bern, W Switzerland
109 Q9 **Oberdrauburg** Salzburg, S Austria
Oberglogau see Głogówek
109 W4 **Ober Grafendorf** Niederösterreich, NE Austria
101 E15 **Oberhausen** Nordrhein-Westfalen, W Germany
Oberhollabrunn see Tulln
Oberlaibach see Vrhnika
101 Q15 **Oberlausitz** *physical region* E Germany
26 J2 **Oberlin** Kansas, C USA
22 H8 **Oberlin** Louisiana, S USA
31 T11 **Oberlin** Ohio, N USA
103 U5 **Obernai** Bas-Rhin, NE France
109 R4 **Obernberg-am-Inn** Oberösterreich, N Austria
Oberndorf see Oberndorf am Neckar
101 G23 **Oberndorf am Neckar** var. Oberndorf. Baden-Württemberg, SW Germany
109 Q5 **Oberndorf bei Salzburg** Salzburg, W Austria
Oberneustadtl see Kysucké Nové Mesto
183 S8 **Oberon** New South Wales, SE Australia
109 Q4 **Oberösterreich** off. Land Oberösterreich, *Eng.* Upper Austria. ◈ *state* NW Austria
Oberpahlen see Põltsamaa
101 M19 **Oberpfälzer Wald** ▲ SE Germany
109 Y6 **Oberpullendorf** Burgenland, E Austria
Oberradkersburg see Gornja Radgona
101 G18 **Oberursel** Hessen, W Germany
109 Q8 **Obervellach** Salzburg, S Austria
109 X7 **Oberwart** Burgenland, SE Austria
Oberwischau see Vişeu de Sus
109 T7 **Oberwölz** var. Oberwölz-Stadt. Steiermark, SE Austria
Oberwölz-Stadt see Oberwölz
31 S13 **Obetz** Ohio, N USA
Ob', Gulf of see Obskaya Guba
54 G8 **Obia** Santander, C Colombia
58 H12 **Óbidos** Pará, NE Brazil
104 F10 **Óbidos** Leiria, C Portugal
Obidovichi see Abidavichy
147 Q13 **Obigarm** W Tajikistan
165 T2 **Obihiro** Hokkaidō, NE Japan
Obi-Khingou see Khingov
147 P13 **Obikiik** SW Tajikistan
113 N16 **Obilić** Serbia, S Yugoslavia
129 O12 **Obil'noye** Respublika Kalmykiya, SW Russian Federation
20 F8 **Obion** Tennessee, S USA
20 F8 **Obion River** ⁓ Tennessee, S USA
171 S12 **Obi, Pulau** *island* Maluku, E Indonesia
165 S2 **Obira** Hokkaidō, NE Japan
129 N11 **Oblivskaya** Rostovskaya Oblast', SW Russian Federation
123 R14 **Obluch'ye** Yevreyskaya Avtonomnaya Oblast', SE Russian Federation
128 K4 **Obninsk** Kaluzhskaya Oblast', W Russian Federation
114 J8 **Obnova** Pleven, N Bulgaria
79 N15 **Obo** Haut-Mbomou, E Central African Republic
80 M11 **Obock** E Djibouti
Obol' see Obal'
Obolyanka see Abalyanka
171 V13 **Obome** Irian Jaya, E Indonesia
110 G11 **Oborniki** Wielkolpolskie, C Poland
79 G19 **Obouya** Cuvette, C Congo
128 J8 **Oboyan'** Kurskaya Oblast', W Russian Federation
126 M9 **Obozerskiy** Arkhangel'skaya Oblast', NW Russian Federation
112 L11 **Obrenovac** Serbia, N Yugoslavia
112 D12 **Obrovac** *It.* Obbrovazzo. Zadar, SW Croatia
Obrovo see Abrova
35 Q3 **Observation Peak** ▲ California, W USA
122 J8 **Obskaya Guba** *Eng.* Gulf of Ob'. *gulf* N Russian Federation
173 N13 **Ob' Tablemount** undersea feature S Indian Ocean
173 T10 **Ob' Trench** undersea feature E Indian Ocean
77 P16 **Obuasi** S Ghana
117 P5 **Obukhiv** *Rus.* Obukhov. Kyyivs'ka Oblast', N Ukraine
Obukhov see Obukhiv
127 U14 **Obva** ⁓ NW Russian Federation
117 V10 **Obytichna Kosa** *spit* SE Ukraine
117 V10 **Obytichna Zatoka** *gulf* SE Ukraine
105 O3 **Oca** ⁓ N Spain
23 W10 **Ocala** Florida, SE USA
40 M7 **Ocampo** Coahuila de Zaragoza, NE Mexico
54 G7 **Ocaña** Norte de Santander, N Colombia
105 N9 **Ocaña** Castilla-La Mancha, C Spain
106 H4 **O Carballiño** *Cast.* Carballiño Galicia, NW Spain
37 T9 **Ocate** New Mexico, SW USA
Ocavango see Okavango
54 D14 **Occidental, Cordillera** ▲ W Colombia
57 D14 **Occidental, Cordillera** ▲ W S America
21 Q6 **Oceana** West Virginia, NE USA
21 Z4 **Ocean City** Maryland, NE USA
18 J17 **Ocean City** New Jersey, NE USA
10 K15 **Ocean Falls** British Columbia, SW Canada
Ocean Island see Kure Atoll
Ocean Island see Banaba
64 J9 **Oceanographer Fracture Zone** *tectonic feature* NW Atlantic Ocean
35 U17 **Oceanside** California, W USA
22 M9 **Ocean Springs** Mississippi, S USA
Ocean State see Rhode Island
25 O9 **O C Fisher Lake** ▣ Texas, SW USA
117 Q10 **Ochakiv** *Rus.* Ochakov. Mykolayivs'ka Oblast', S Ukraine
Ochakov see Ochakiv
Ochamchira see Och'amch'ire
137 Q9 **Och'amch'ire** *Rus.* Ochamchira. W Georgia
Ochansk see Okhansk
127 T15 **Ocher** Permskaya Oblast', NW Russian Federation
115 I19 **Óchi** ▲ Évvoia, C Greece
165 W4 **Ochiishi-misaki** *headland* Hokkaidō, NE Japan
23 S9 **Ochlockonee River** ⁓ Florida/Georgia, SE USA
44 K12 **Ocho Rios** C Jamaica
Ochrida see Ohrid
Ochrida, Lake see Ohrid, Lake
101 J19 **Ochsenfurt** Bayern, C Germany
23 U7 **Ocilla** Georgia, SE USA
94 N13 **Ockelbo** Gävleborg, C Sweden
Ocker see Oker
95 I19 **Öckerö** Västra Götaland, S Sweden
23 U6 **Ocmulgee River** ⁓ Georgia, SE USA
116 H11 **Ocna Mureş** *Hung.* Marosújvár; prev. Ocna Mureşului; prev. *Hung.* Marosújvárakna. Alba, C Romania
Ocna Mureşului see Ocna Mureş
116 H11 **Ocna Sibiului** *Ger.* Salzburg, *Hung.* Vizakna. Sibiu, C Romania
116 H13 **Ocnele Mari** prev. Vioara. Vâlcea, S Romania
116 L7 **Ocniţa** *Rus.* Oknitsa. N Moldova
23 U4 **Oconee, Lake** ▣ Georgia, SE USA
23 U5 **Oconee River** ⁓ Georgia, SE USA
30 M9 **Oconomowoc** Wisconsin, N USA
30 M6 **Oconto** Wisconsin, N USA
30 M6 **Oconto Falls** Wisconsin, N USA
30 M6 **Oconto River** ⁓ Wisconsin, N USA
104 I3 **O Corgo** Galicia, NW Spain
41 V16 **Ocosingo** Chiapas, SE Mexico
42 J8 **Ocotal** Nueva Segovia, NW Nicaragua
42 F6 **Ocotepeque** ◈ *department* W Honduras
Ocotepeque see Nueva Ocotepeque
40 L13 **Ocotlán** Jalisco, SW Mexico
41 R16 **Ocotlán** var. Ocotlán de Morelos. Oaxaca, SE Mexico
Ocotlán de Morelos see Ocotlán
41 U16 **Ocozocuautla** Chiapas, SE Mexico
21 Y10 **Ocracoke Island** *island* North Carolina, SE USA
102 I3 **Octeville** Manche, N France
October Revolution Island see Oktyabr'skoy Revolyutsii, Ostrov
43 R17 **Ocú** Herrera, S Panama
83 Q14 **Ocua** Cabo Delgado, NE Mozambique
Ocumare see Ocumare del Tuy
54 M5 **Ocumare del Tuy** var. Ocumare. Miranda, N Venezuela
77 P17 **Oda** SE Ghana
165 G12 **Ōda** var. Oda. Shimane, Honshū, SW Japan
92 K3 **Ódáðahraun** *lava flow* C Iceland
165 Q7 **Ōdate** Akita, Honshū, C Japan
165 N14 **Odawara** Kanagawa, Honshū, S Japan
95 D14 **Odda** Hordaland, S Norway
95 G22 **Odder** Århus, C Denmark
Oddur see Xuddur
29 T13 **Odebolt** Iowa, C USA
104 H14 **Odeleite** Faro, S Portugal
25 Q4 **Odell** Texas, SW USA
25 T14 **Odem** Texas, SW USA
104 F13 **Odemira** Beja, S Portugal
136 C14 **Ödemiş** İzmir, SW Turkey
Ödenburg see Sopron
83 I22 **Odendaalsrus** Free State, C South Africa
Odenpäh see Otepää
95 H23 **Odense** Fyn, C Denmark
101 H19 **Odenwald** ▲ W Germany
84 H10 **Oder** *Cz./Pol.* Odra. ⁓ C Europe
Oderberg see Bohumín
100 P11 **Oderbruch** *wetland* Germany/Poland
Oderhaff see Szczeciński, Zalew
100 O11 **Oder-Havel-Kanal** *canal* NE Germany
Oderhellen see Odorheiu Secuiesc
100 P13 **Oder-Spree-Kanal** *canal* NE Germany
Odertal see Zdzieszowice
106 I7 **Oderzo** Veneto, NE Italy
16 J14 **Odesa** *Rus.* Odessa. Odes'ka Oblast', SW Ukraine
Odesa see Odes'ka Oblast'
95 L18 **Ödeshög** Östergötland, S Sweden
117 O9 **Odes'ka Oblast'** var. Odesa, *Rus.* Odesskaya Oblast'. ◈ *province* SW Ukraine
24 M8 **Odessa** Texas, SW USA
32 K8 **Odessa** Washington, NW USA
Odessa see Odesa
Odesskaya Oblast' see Odes'ka Oblast'
122 H12 **Odesskoye** Omskaya Oblast', C Russian Federation
Odessus see Varna
102 F6 **Odet** ⁓ NW France
104 I14 **Odiel** ⁓ SW Spain
76 L14 **Odienné** NW Ivory Coast
171 O4 **Odiongan** Tablas Island, C Philippines
116 L12 **Odobeşti** Vrancea, E Romania
110 H13 **Odolanów** *Ger.* Adelnau. Wielkopolskie, C Poland
167 R13 **Ŏdôngk** Kâmpóng Spoe, S Cambodia
25 N6 **O'donnell** Texas, SW USA
98 O7 **Odoorn** Drenthe, NE Netherlands
Odorhei see Odorheiu Secuiesc
116 J11 **Odorheiu Secuiesc** *Ger.* Oderhellen, *Hung.* Vámosudvarhely; prev. Odorhei; *Ger.* Hofmarkt. Harghita, C Romania
Odra see Oder
112 J9 **Odžaci** *Ger.* Hodschag, *Hung.* Hodság. Serbia, NW Yugoslavia
59 N14 **Oeiras** Piauí, E Brazil
104 F11 **Oeiras** Lisboa, C Portugal
101 G14 **Oelde** Nordrhein-Westfalen, W Germany
28 J11 **Oelrichs** South Dakota, N USA
Oels/Oels in Schlesien see Oleśnica
101 M17 **Oelsnitz** Sachsen, E Germany
29 X12 **Oelwein** Iowa, C USA
Oeniadae see Oiniádes
191 N17 **Oeno Island** *atoll* Pitcairn Islands, C Pacific Ocean
Oesel see Saaremaa
108 L7 **Oetz** var. Ötz. Tirol, W Austria
137 P11 **Of** Trabzon, NE Turkey
30 K15 **O'Fallon** Illinois, N USA
27 W4 **O'Fallon** Missouri, C USA
107 N16 **Ofanto** ⁓ S Italy
97 D18 **Offaly** *Ir.* Ua Uíbh Fhailí; prev. King's County. *cultural region* C Ireland
101 H18 **Offenbach** var. Offenbach am Main. Hessen, W Germany
Offenbach am Main see Offenbach
101 F22 **Offenburg** Baden-Württemberg, SW Germany
182 C2 **Officer Creek** *seasonal river* South Australia
Oficina María Elena see María Elena
Oficina Pedro de Valdivia see Pedro de Valdivia
115 K22 **Ofidoússa** *island* Kykládes, Greece, Aegean Sea
Ofiral see Sharm el Sheikh
92 H10 **Ofotfjorden** *fjord* N Norway
192 L16 **Ofu** *island* Manua Islands, E American Samoa
165 R9 **Ōfunato** Iwate, Honshū, C Japan
165 P8 **Oga** Akita, Honshū, C Japan
Ogaadeen see Ogadēn
165 Q9 **Ogachi** Akita, Honshū, C Japan

◆ Country ● Country Capital ◇ Dependent Territory ○ Dependent Territory Capital ◈ Administrative Region × International Airport ▲ Mountain ▲ Mountain Range ⛰ Volcano ⁓ River ◎ Lake ▣ Reservoir

165 P9 **Ogachi-tōge** *pass* Honshū, C Japan
81 N14 **Ogadēn** *Som.* Ogaadeen. *plateau* Ethiopia/Somalia
165 P8 **Oga-hantō** *peninsula* Honshū, C Japan
165 K13 **Ōgaki** Gifu, Honshū, SW Japan
28 L15 **Ogallala** Nebraska, C USA
168 M14 **Ogan, Air** ≈ Sumatera, W Indonesia
165 Y15 **Ogasawara-shotō** *Eng.* Bonin Islands. *island group* SE Japan
14 I9 **Ogascanane, Lac** ◎ Quebec, SE Canada
165 R7 **Ogawara-ko** ◎ Honshū, C Japan
77 T15 **Ogbomosho** Oyo, W Nigeria
29 U13 **Ogden** Iowa, C USA
36 L2 **Ogden** Utah, W USA
18 I6 **Ogdensburg** New York, NE USA
23 W5 **Ogeechee River** ≈ Georgia, SE USA
Oger *see* Ogre
146 F6 **Oghiyon Shūrkhogi** *wetland* NW Uzbekistan
165 N10 **Ogi** Niigata, Sado, C Japan
10 H5 **Ogilvie** Yukon Territory, NW Canada
10 H4 **Ogilvie** ≈ Yukon Territory, NW Canada
10 H5 **Ogilvie Mountains** ▲ Yukon Territory, NW Canada
Oginskiy Kanal *see* Ahinski Kanal
146 B10 **Oglanly** Balkanskiy Velayat, W Turkmenistan
23 T5 **Oglethorpe** Georgia, SE USA
23 T2 **Oglethorpe, Mount** ▲ Georgia, SE USA
106 F7 **Oglio** *anc.* Ollius. ≈ N Italy
103 T8 **Ognon** ≈ E France
123 R13 **Ogodzha** Amurskaya Oblast', S Russian Federation
77 W16 **Ogoja** Cross River, S Nigeria
12 C10 **Ogoki** ≈ Ontario, S Canada
12 D11 **Ogoki Lake** ◎ Ontario, C Canada
162 K10 **Ögöömör** Ömnögovĭ, S Mongolia
79 F19 **Ogooué** ≈ Congo/Gabon
79 E18 **Ogooué-Ivindo** *off.* Province de l'Ogooué-Ivindo, *var.* L'Ogooué-Ivindo. ◈ *province* N Gabon
79 E19 **Ogooué-Lolo** *off.* Province de l'Ogooué-Lolo, *var.* L'Ogooué-Lolo. ◈ *province* C Gabon
79 C19 **Ogooué-Maritime** *off.* Province de l'Ogooué-Maritime, *var.* L'Ogooué-Maritime. ◈ *province* W Gabon
165 D14 **Ogōri** Fukuoka, Kyūshū, SW Japan
114 H7 **Ogosta** ≈ NW Bulgaria
112 Q9 **Ogražden** *Bul.* Ograzhden. ▲ Bulgaria/FYR Macedonia *see also* Ograzhden
114 G12 **Ograzhden** | *Mac.* Ogražden. ▲ Bulgaria/FYR Macedonia *see also* Ogražden
118 G9 **Ogre** *Ger.* Oger. Ogre, C Latvia
118 H9 **Ogre** ≈ C Latvia
112 C10 **Ogulin** Karlovac, NW Croatia
77 S16 **Ogun** ◈ *state* SW Nigeria
146 A12 **Ogurdzhaly, Ostrov** *Turkm.* Ogurjaly Adasy. *island* W Turkmenistan
Ogurjaly Adasy *see* Ogurdzhaly, Ostrov
77 U16 **Ogwashi-Uku** Delta, S Nigeria
185 B23 **Ohai** Southland, South Island, NZ
147 Q10 **Ohangaron** *Rus.* Akhangaran. Toshkent Wiloyati, E Uzbekistan
147 Q10 **Ohangaron** *Rus.* Akhangaran. ≈ E Uzbekistan
83 C16 **Ohangwena** ◈ *district* N Namibia
30 M10 **O'Hare** ✕ (Chicago) Illinois, N USA
165 R6 **Ōhata** Aomori, Honshū, C Japan
184 L13 **Ohau** Manawatu-Wanganui, North Island, NZ
185 E20 **Ohau, Lake** ◎ South Island, NZ
Ohcejohka *see* Utsjoki
99 J20 **Ohey** Namur, SE Belgium
191 X15 **O'Higgins, Cabo** *headland* Easter Island, Chile, E Pacific Ocean
O'Higgins, Lago *see* San Martín, Lago
31 S12 **Ohio** *off.* State of Ohio; also known as The Buckeye State. ◈ *state* N USA
(0) L10 **Ohio River** ≈ N USA
Ohlau *see* Oława
101 H16 **Ohm** ≈ C Germany
193 W16 **Ohonua** 'Eua, E Tonga
23 V5 **Ohoopee River** ≈ Georgia, SE USA
100 L12 **Ohre** *Ger.* Eger. ≈ Czech Republic/Germany
Ohri *see* Ohrid
113 M20 **Ohrid** *Turk.* Ochrida, Ohri. SW FYR Macedonia
113 M20 **Ohrid, Lake** *var.* Lake Ochrida, *Alb.* Liqeni i Ohrit, *Mac.* Ohridsko Ezero. ◎ Albania/FYR Macedonia
Ohridsko Ezero/Ohrit, Liqeni i *see* Ohrid, Lake
184 L9 **Ohura** Manawatu-Wanganui, North Island, NZ
58 J9 **Oiapoque** Amapá, E Brazil
58 J10 **Oiapoque, Rio** *var.* Fleuve l'Oyapok, Oyapock. ≈ Brazil/French Guiana *see also* Oyapok, Fleuve l'
15 O9 **Oies, Île aux** *island* Quebec, SE Canada
92 L13 **Oijärvi** Oulu, C Finland
92 L12 **Oikarainen** Lappi, N Finland
188 F10 **Oikuul** Babeldaob, N Palau
18 C13 **Oil City** Pennsylvania, NE USA
18 C12 **Oil Creek** ≈ Pennsylvania, NE USA
35 R13 **Oildale** California, W USA
Oileán Ciarral *see* Castleisland
Oil Islands *see* Chagos Archipelago
115 D18 **Oiniádes** *anc.* Oeniadae. *site of ancient city* Dytikí Ellás, W Greece
115 L18 **Oinoússes** *island* E Greece
Oírr, Inis *see* Inisheer
99 J15 **Oirschot** Noord-Brabant, S Netherlands
103 N4 **Oise** ◈ *department* N France
103 P3 **Oise** ≈ N France
99 J14 **Oisterwijk** Noord-Brabant, S Netherlands
45 O14 **Oistins** S Barbados
165 E4 **Ōita** Ōita, Kyūshū, SW Japan
165 D14 **Ōita** *off.* Ōita-ken. ◈ *prefecture* Kyūshū, SW Japan
115 E17 **Oíti** ▲ C Greece
165 S4 **Oiwake** Hokkaidō, NE Japan
35 R14 **Ojai** California, W USA
94 K13 **Öje** Dalarna, C Sweden
93 J14 **Öjebyn** Norrbotten, N Sweden
165 B13 **Ojika-jima** *island* SW Japan
40 K5 **Ojinaga** Chihuahua, N Mexico
40 M11 **Ojo Caliente** *var.* Ojocaliente. Zacatecas, C Mexico
40 D6 **Ojo de Liebre, Laguna** *var.* Laguna Scammon, Scammon Lagoon. *lagoon* W Mexico
62 I7 **Ojos del Salado, Cerro** ▲ W Argentina
105 R7 **Ojos Negros** Aragón, NE Spain
40 M12 **Ojuelos de Jalisco** Aguascalientes, C Mexico
129 N4 **Oka** ≈ W Russian Federation
83 D19 **Okahandja** Otjozondjupa, C Namibia
184 L9 **Okahukura** Manawatu-Wanganui, North Island, NZ
184 J3 **Okaihau** Northland, North Island, NZ
83 D18 **Okakarara** Otjozondjupa, N Namibia
13 P5 **Okak Islands** *island group* Newfoundland, E Canada
10 M17 **Okanagan** ≈ British Columbia, SW Canada
11 N17 **Okanagan Lake** ◎ British Columbia, SW Canada
Ókanizsa *see* Kanjiža
83 C16 **Okankolo** Otjikoto, N Namibia
32 K6 **Okanogan River** ≈ Washington, NW USA
83 D18 **Okaputa** Otjozondjupa, N Namibia
149 V9 **Okāra** Punjab, E Pakistan
26 M10 **Okarche** Oklahoma, C USA
146 B13 **Okarem** *Turkm.* Ekerem. Balkanskiy Velayat, W Turkmenistan
189 X14 **Okat Harbor** *harbor* Kosrae, E Micronesia
22 M5 **Okatibbee Creek** ≈ Mississippi, S USA
83 C17 **Okaukuejo** Kunene, N Namibia
Okavanggo *see* Cubango/Okavango
83 E17 **Okavango** ◈ *district* NW Namibia
83 G17 **Okavango** *var.* Cubango, Kavango, Kavengo, Kubango, Okavanggo, *Port.* Ocavango. ≈ S Africa *see also* Cubango
83 G17 **Okavango Delta** *wetland* N Botswana
164 M12 **Okaya** Nagano, Honshū, S Japan
164 H13 **Okayama** Okayama, Honshū, SW Japan
164 H13 **Okayama** *off.* Okayama-ken. ◈ *prefecture* Honshū, SW Japan
164 L14 **Okazaki** Aichi, Honshū, C Japan
110 M12 **Okęcie** ✕ (Warszawa) Mazowieckie, C Poland
23 Y13 **Okeechobee** Florida, SE USA
23 Y14 **Okeechobee, Lake** ◎ Florida, SE USA
26 M9 **Okeene** Oklahoma, C USA
23 V8 **Okefenokee Swamp** *wetland* Georgia, SE USA
97 J24 **Okehampton** SW England, UK
27 P10 **Okemah** Oklahoma, C USA
77 U16 **Okene** Kogi, S Nigeria
100 K13 **Oker** *var.* Ocker. ≈ NW Germany
101 J14 **Oker-Stausee** ◎ C Germany
123 T12 **Okha** Ostrov Sakhalin, Sakhalinskaya Oblast', SE Russian Federation
127 U15 **Okhansk** *var.* Ochansk. Permskaya Oblast', NW Russian Federation
123 S10 **Okhotsk** Khabarovskiy Kray, E Russian Federation
192 J2 **Okhotsk, Sea of** *sea* NW Pacific Ocean
117 T4 **Okhtyrka** *Rus.* Akhtyrka. Sums'ka Oblast', NE Ukraine
83 E23 **Okiep** Northern Cape, W South Africa
Oki-guntō *see* Oki-shotō
164 H11 **Oki-kaikyō** *strait* SW Japan
165 P16 **Okinawa** Okinawa, SW Japan
165 S16 **Okinawa** *off.* Okinawa-ken. ◈ *prefecture* Okinawa, SW Japan
165 S16 **Okinawa** *island* SW Japan
165 U16 **Okinoerabu-jima** *island* Nansei-shotō, SW Japan
164 F15 **Okino-shima** *island* SW Japan
164 H11 **Oki-shotō** *var.* Oki-guntō. *island group* SW Japan
77 T16 **Okitipupa** Ondo, SW Nigeria
166 L8 **Okkan** Pegu, SW Myanmar
27 N10 **Oklahoma** *off.* State of Oklahoma; also known as The Sooner State. ◈ *state* C USA
27 N11 **Oklahoma City** *state capital* Oklahoma, C USA
25 Q4 **Oklaunion** Texas, SW USA
23 W10 **Oklawaha River** ≈ Florida, SE USA
27 P10 **Okmulgee** Oklahoma, C USA
Oknitsa *see* Ocniţa
22 M3 **Okolona** Mississippi, S USA
165 U2 **Okoppe** Hokkaidō, NE Japan
11 Q16 **Okotoks** Alberta, SW Canada
80 H6 **Oko, Wadi** ≈ NE Sudan
79 G19 **Okoyo** Cuvette, W Congo
77 S15 **Okpara** ≈ Benin/Nigeria
92 J8 **Øksfjord** Finnmark, N Norway
127 R4 **Oksino** Nenetskiy Avtonomnyy Okrug, NW Russian Federation
92 G13 **Oksskolten** ▲ C Norway
Oksu *see* Oqsu
144 M8 **Oktaybr'skiy** Kostanay, N Kazakhstan
186 B7 **Ok Tedi** Western, W PNG
Oktemberyan *see* Hoktemberyan
166 M7 **Oktwin** Pegu, C Myanmar
129 R6 **Oktyabr'sk** Samarskaya Oblast', W Russian Federation
Oktyabr'sk *see* Kandyagash
127 N12 **Oktyabr'skiy** Arkhangel'skaya Oblast', NW Russian Federation
122 E10 **Oktyabr'skiy** Kamchatskaya Oblast', E Russian Federation
129 T5 **Oktyabr'skiy** Respublika Bashkortostan, W Russian Federation
129 O11 **Oktyabr'skiy** Volgogradskaya Oblast', SW Russian Federation
Oktyabr'skiy *see* Aktsyabrski
129 V7 **Oktyabr'skoye** Orenburgskaya Oblast', W Russian Federation
122 M5 **Oktyabr'skoy Revolyutsii, Ostrov** *Eng.* October Revolution Island. *island* Severnaya Zemlya, N Russian Federation
164 C15 **Ōkuchi** *var.* Ōkuti. Kagoshima, Kyūshū, SW Japan
Okulovka *see* Uglovka
165 Q4 **Okushiri-tō** *var.* Okusiri Tô. *island* NE Japan
Okusiri Tô *see* Okushiri-tō
77 S15 **Okuta** Kwara, W Nigeria
Ōkuti *see* Ōkuchi
83 F19 **Okwa** *var.* Chapman's. ≈ Botswana/Namibia
123 T10 **Ola** Magadanskaya Oblast', E Russian Federation
27 T11 **Ola** Arkansas, C USA
Ola *see* Ala
35 T11 **Olacha Peak** ▲ California, W USA
92 J1 **Ólafsfjördhur** Nordhurland Eystra, N Iceland
92 H3 **Ólafsvík** Vesturland, W Iceland
Oláhbrettye *see* Bretea-Română
Oláhszentgyörgy *see* Sângeorz-Băi
Oláh-Toplicza *see* Toplița
35 T11 **Olancha** California, W USA
42 J5 **Olanchito** Yoro, C Honduras
42 J6 **Olancho** ◈ *department* E Honduras
95 O20 **Öland** *island* S Sweden
95 O19 **Ölands norra udde** *headland* S Sweden
95 N22 **Ölands södra udde** *headland* S Sweden
182 K7 **Olary** South Australia
27 R4 **Olathe** Kansas, C USA
61 C22 **Olavarría** Buenos Aires, E Argentina
92 O2 **Olav V Land** *physical region* C Svalbard
111 H14 **Oława** *Ger.* Ohlau. Dolnośląskie, SW Poland
107 D17 **Olbia** *prev.* Terranova Pausania. Sardegna, Italy, C Mediterranean Sea
44 G5 **Old Bahama Channel** *channel* Bahamas/Cuba
Old Bay State/Old Colony State *see* Massachusetts
10 H2 **Old Crow** Yukon Territory, NW Canada
Old Dominion *see* Virginia
Oldeberkeap *see* Oldeberkoop
98 M7 **Oldeberkoop** *Fris.* Oldeberkeap. Friesland, N Netherlands
98 L10 **Oldebroek** Gelderland, E Netherlands
98 L8 **Oldemarkt** Overijssel, N Netherlands
94 E11 **Olden** Sogn og Fjordane, C Norway
100 G10 **Oldenburg** Niedersachsen, NW Germany
100 K8 **Oldenburg** Schleswig-Holstein, N Germany
98 P10 **Oldenzaal** Overijssel, E Netherlands
18 J8 **Old Forge** New York, NE USA
Old Goa *see* Goa
97 L17 **Oldham** NW England, UK
39 Q14 **Old Harbor** Kodiak Island, Alaska, USA
44 J13 **Old Harbour** C Jamaica
97 C22 **Old Head of Kinsale** *Ir.* An Seancheann. *headland* SW Ireland
20 J8 **Old Hickory Lake** ▣ Tennessee, S USA
Old Line State *see* Maryland
Old North State *see* North Carolina
81 I17 **Ol Doinyo Lengeyo** ▲ C Kenya
11 Q16 **Olds** Alberta, SW Canada
19 O7 **Old Speck Mountain** ▲ Maine, NE USA
19 S6 **Old Town** Maine, NE USA
11 T17 **Old Wives Lake** ◎ Saskatchewan, S Canada
162 J7 **Öldziyt** Arhangay, C Mongolia
163 N10 **Öldziyt** Dornogovĭ, SE Mongolia
188 H6 **Oleai** *var.* San Jose. Saipan, S Northern Mariana Islands
18 E11 **Olean** New York, NE USA
110 O7 **Olecko** *Ger.* Treuburg. Warmińsko-Mazurskie, NE Poland
106 C7 **Oleggio** Piemonte, NE Italy
123 P11 **Olëkma** Amurskaya Oblast', SE Russian Federation
123 P12 **Olëkma** ≈ C Russian Federation
123 P11 **Olëkminsk** Respublika Sakha (Yakutiya), NE Russian Federation
117 W7 **Oleksandrivka** Donets'ka Oblast', E Ukraine
117 R7 **Oleksandrivka** *Rus.* Aleksandrovka. Kirovohrads'ka Oblast', C Ukraine
117 Q9 **Oleksandrivka** Mykolayivs'ka Oblast', S Ukraine
117 S7 **Oleksandriya** *Rus.* Aleksandriya. Kirovohrads'ka Oblast', C Ukraine
93 B20 **Ølen** Hordaland, S Norway
126 J4 **Olenegorsk** Murmanskaya Oblast', NW Russian Federation
123 N9 **Olenëk** Respublika Sakha (Yakutiya), NE Russian Federation
123 N9 **Olenëk** ≈ NE Russian Federation
123 O7 **Olenëkskiy Zaliv** *bay* N Russian Federation
126 K6 **Olenitsa** Murmanskaya Oblast', NW Russian Federation
102 I11 **Oléron, Île d'** *island* W France
111 H14 **Oleśnica** *Ger.* Oels, Oels in Schlesien. Dolnośląskie, SW Poland
111 I15 **Olesno** *Ger.* Rosenberg. Opolskie, S Poland
116 M3 **Olevs'k** *Rus.* Olevsk. Zhytomyrs'ka Oblast', N Ukraine
123 S15 **Ol'ga** Primorskiy Kray, SE Russian Federation
Olga, Mount *see* Kata Tjuta
92 P2 **Olgastretet** *strait* E Svalbard
162 D5 **Ölgiy** Bayan-Ölgiy, W Mongolia
95 F23 **Ølgod** Ribe, W Denmark
104 H14 **Olhão** Faro, S Portugal
93 L14 **Olhava** Oulu, C Finland
112 B12 **Olib** *It.* Ulbo. *island* W Croatia
83 B16 **Olifa** Kunene, NW Namibia
83 E20 **Olifants** *var.* Elephant River. ≈ E Namibia
83 E25 **Olifants** *var.* Elefantes. ≈ SW South Africa
83 G22 **Olifantshoek** Northern Cape, N South Africa
188 L15 **Olimarao Atoll** *atoll* Caroline Islands, C Micronesia
Ólimbos *see* Ólympos
Olimpo *see* Fuerte Olimpo
59 Q15 **Olinda** Pernambuco, E Brazil
Olinthos *see* Ólynthos
83 I20 **Oliphants Drift** Kgatleng, SE Botswana
Olisipo *see* Lisboa
Olita *see* Alytus
105 Q4 **Olite** Navarra, N Spain
62 K10 **Oliva** Córdoba, C Argentina
105 T11 **Oliva** País Valenciano, E Spain
104 I12 **Oliva de la Frontera** Extremadura, W Spain
Olivares *see* Olivares de Júcar
62 H9 **Olivares, Cerro de** ▲ N Chile
105 P9 **Olivares de Júcar** *var.* Olivares. Castilla-La Mancha, C Spain
22 L1 **Olive Branch** Mississippi, S USA
21 O5 **Olive Hill** Kentucky, S USA
35 O6 **Olivehurst** California, W USA
104 G7 **Oliveira de Azeméis** Aveiro, N Portugal
104 I11 **Olivenza** Extremadura, W Spain
11 N17 **Oliver** British Columbia, SW Canada
103 N7 **Olivet** Loiret, C France
29 Q12 **Olivet** South Dakota, N USA
29 T9 **Olivia** Minnesota, N USA
185 C20 **Olivine Range** ▲ South Island, NZ
108 H10 **Olivone** Ticino, S Switzerland
Ölkeyek *see* Ul'kayak
129 O9 **Ol'khovka** Volgogradskaya Oblast', SW Russian Federation
111 K16 **Olkusz** Małopolskie, S Poland
22 I6 **Olla** Louisiana, S USA
62 I4 **Ollagüe, Volcán** *var.* Oyahue, Volcán Oyahue. ▲ N Chile
189 U13 **Ollan** *island* Chuuk, C Micronesia
188 F7 **Ollei** Babeldaob, N Palau
Ollius *see* Oglio
108 C10 **Ollon** Vaud, W Switzerland
147 Q10 **Olmaliq** *Rus.* Almalyk. Toshkent Wiloyati, E Uzbekistan
104 M6 **Olmedo** Castilla-León, N Spain
56 B10 **Olmos** Lambayeque, W Peru
Olmütz *see* Olomouc
30 M15 **Olney** Illinois, N USA
25 R5 **Olney** Texas, SW USA
95 L22 **Olofström** Blekinge, S Sweden
187 N9 **Olomburi** Malaita, N Solomon Islands
111 H17 **Olomouc** *Ger.* Olmütz, *Pol.* Ołomuniec. Olomoucký Kraj, E Czech Republic
111 H18 **Olomoucký Kraj** ◈ region E Czech Republic
Ołomuniec *see* Olomouc
122 D7 **Olonets** Respublika Kareliya, NW Russian Federation
171 N3 **Olongapo** *off.* Olongapo City. Luzon, N Philippines
102 J16 **Oloron-Ste-Marie** Pyrénées-Atlantiques, SW France
192 L16 **Olosega** *island* Manua Islands, E American Samoa
105 W4 **Olot** Cataluña, NE Spain
146 K12 **Olot** *Rus.* Alat. Bukhoro Wiloyati, C Uzbekistan
112 I12 **Olovo** Federacija Bosna I Hercegovina, E Bosnia and Herzegovina
123 O14 **Olovyannaya** Chitinskaya Oblast', S Russian Federation
123 T7 **Oloy** ≈ NE Russian Federation
101 F16 **Olpe** Nordrhein-Westfalen, W Germany
109 N8 **Olperer** ▲ SW Austria
Olshanka *see* Vil'shanka
Ol'shany *see* Al'shany
Olsnitz *see* Murska Sobota
98 M10 **Olst** Overijssel, E Netherlands
110 L8 **Olsztyn** *Ger.* Allenstein. Warmińsko-Mazurskie, NE Poland,
110 L8 **Olsztynek** *Ger.* Hohenstein in Ostpreussen. Warmińsko-Mazurskie, NE Poland,
116 I14 **Olt** ◈ *county* SW Romania
116 I14 **Olt** *var.* Oltul, *Ger.* Alt. ≈ S Romania
108 E7 **Olten** Solothurn, NW Switzerland
116 K14 **Oltenița** *prev. Eng.* Oltenitsa, *anc.* Constantiola. Călărași, SE Romania
Oltenitsa *see* Oltenița
116 H14 **Olteț** ≈ S Romania
24 M4 **Olton** Texas, SW USA
137 R12 **Oltu** Erzurum, NE Turkey
Oltul *see* Olt
146 G7 **Oltynkŭl** Qoraqalpoghiston Respublikasi, NW Uzbekistan
161 S15 **Oluan Pi** *Eng.* Cape Olwanpi. *headland* S Taiwan
Ólubló *see* Stará L'ubovňa
137 R11 **Olur** Erzurum, NE Turkey
104 L15 **Olvera** Andalucía, S Spain
Ol'viopol' *see* Pervomays'k
Olwanpi, Cape *see* Oluan Pi
16 D5 **Olympia** *state capital* Washington, NW USA
115 D20 **Olympía** Dytikí Ellás, S Greece
182 H5 **Olympic Dam** South Australia
32 F7 **Olympic Mountains** ▲ Washington, NW USA
121 O3 **Ólympos** *var.* Troodos, *Eng.* Mount Olympus. ▲ C Cyprus
115 F15 **Ólympos** *var.* Ólimbos, *Eng.* Mount Olympus. ▲ N Greece
115 L17 **Ólympos** ▲ Lésvos, E Greece
16 C5 **Olympus, Mount** ▲ Washington, NW USA
Olympus, Mount *see* Ólympos
115 G14 **Ólynthos** *var.* Olinthos; *anc.* Olynthus. *site of ancient city* Kentrikí Makedonía, N Greece
Olynthus *see* Ólynthos
117 Q3 **Olyshivka** Chernihivs'ka Oblast', N Ukraine
123 W8 **Olyutorskiy, Mys** *headland* E Russian Federation
123 V8 **Olyutorskiy Zaliv** *bay* E Russian Federation
186 M10 **Om** ≈ W PNG
131 S6 **Om'** ≈ N Russian Federation
158 I13 **Oma** Xizang Zizhiqu, W China
165 R6 **Ōma** Aomori, Honshū, C Japan
127 P6 **Oma** ≈ NW Russian Federation
164 M12 **Ōmachi** *var.* Ômati. Nagano, Honshū, S Japan
165 Q8 **Ōmagari** Akita, Honshū, C Japan
97 E15 **Omagh** *Ir.* An Ómaigh. W Northern Ireland, UK
29 S15 **Omaha** Nebraska, C USA
83 E19 **Omaheke** ◈ *district* W Namibia
141 W10 **Oman** *off.* Sultanate of Oman, *Ar.* Salṭanat 'Umān; *prev.* Muscat and Oman. ◆ *monarchy* SW Asia
131 O10 **Oman Basin** *var.* Bassin d'Oman. *undersea feature* N Indian Ocean
Oman, Bassin d' *see* Oman Basin
131 N10 **Oman, Gulf of** *Ar.* Khalīj 'Umān. *gulf* N Arabian Sea
184 J3 **Omapere** Northland, North Island, NZ
185 E20 **Omarama** Canterbury, South Island, NZ
112 F11 **Omarska** Republika Srpska, NW Bosnia and Herzegovina
83 C18 **Omaruru** Erongo, NW Namibia
83 C19 **Omaruru** ≈ W Namibia
83 E17 **Omatako** ≈ NE Namibia
Ômati *see* Ōmachi
83 E18 **Omawewozonyanda** Omaheke, E Namibia
165 R6 **Ōma-zaki** *headland* Honshū, C Japan
Ombai *see* Alor, Pulau
83 C16 **Ombalantu** Omusati, N Namibia
79 H15 **Ombella-Mpoko** ◈ *prefecture* S Central African Republic
Ombetsu *see* Onbetsu
83 B17 **Ombombo** Kunene, NW Namibia
79 D19 **Omboué** Ogooué-Maritime, W Gabon
106 G13 **Ombrone** ≈ C Italy
80 F9 **Omdurman** *var.* Umm Durmān. Khartoum, C Sudan
165 N13 **Ōme** Tōkyō, Honshū, S Japan
106 C6 **Omegna** Piemonte, NE Italy
183 P12 **Omeo** Victoria, SE Australia
138 F11 **'Omer** Southern, C Israel
41 P16 **Ometepec** Guerrero, S Mexico
42 K11 **Ometepe, Isla de** *island* S Nicaragua
Om Hager *see* Om Hajer
80 I10 **Om Hajer** *var.* Om Hager. SW Eritrea
165 J13 **Ōmi-Hachiman** *var.* Ōmihachiman. Shiga, Honshū, SW Japan
10 L12 **Omineca Mountains** ▲ British Columbia, W Canada
113 F14 **Omiš** *It.* Almissa. Split-Dalmacija, S Croatia
112 B10 **Omišalj** Primorje-Gorski Kotar, NW Croatia
83 D19 **Omitara** Khomas, C Namibia
41 O16 **Omitlán, Río** ≈ S Mexico
39 X14 **Ommaney, Cape** *headland* Baranof Island, Alaska, USA
98 N9 **Ommen** Overijssel, E Netherlands
162 K11 **Ömnögovĭ** ◈ *province* S Mongolia
191 X7 **Omoa** Fatu Hira, NE French Polynesia
Omo Botego *see* Omo Wenz
Ómoldova *see* Moldova Veche
123 T7 **Omolon** Chukotskiy Avtonomnyy Okrug, NE Russian Federation
123 T7 **Omolon** ≈ NE Russian Federation
123 Q8 **Omoloy** ≈ NE Russian Federation
165 P8 **Omono-gawa** ≈ Honshū, C Japan
81 I14 **Omo Wenz** *var.* Omo Botego. ≈ Ethiopia/Kenya
122 H12 **Omsk** Omskaya Oblast', C Russian Federation
122 H11 **Omskaya Oblast'** ◈ *province* C Russian Federation
165 U2 **Ōmu** Hokkaidō, NE Japan
110 M9 **Omulew** ≈ NE Poland
116 J12 **Omul, Vârful** *prev.* Virful Omu. ▲ C Romania
83 D16 **Omundaungilo** Ohangwena, N Namibia
164 C14 **Ōmura** Nagasaki, Kyūshū, SW Japan
83 B17 **Omusati** ◈ *district* N Namibia
164 C14 **Ōmuta** Fukuoka, Kyūshū, SW Japan
127 S14 **Omutninsk** Kirovskaya Oblast', NW Russian Federation
Omu, Vîrful *see* Omul, Vârful
29 V7 **Onamia** Minnesota, N USA
21 Y5 **Onancock** Virginia, NE USA
14 E10 **Onaping Lake** ◎ Ontario, S Canada
30 M12 **Onarga** Illinois, N USA
15 R6 **Onatchiway, Lac** ◎ Quebec, SE Canada
29 S14 **Onawa** Iowa, C USA
165 U5 **Onbetsu** *var.* Ombetsu. Hokkaidō, NE Japan
83 B16 **Oncócua** Cunene, SW Angola
105 S9 **Onda** País Valenciano, E Spain
111 N18 **Ondava** ≈ NE Slovakia
Ondjiva *see* N'Giva
77 T16 **Ondo** Ondo, SW Nigeria
77 T16 **Ondo** ◈ *state* SW Nigeria
163 N8 **Öndörhaan** Hentiy, E Mongolia
83 D18 **Ondundazongonda** Otjozondjupa, N Namibia
151 K21 **One and Half Degree Channel** *channel* S Maldives
187 Z15 **Oneata** *island* Lau Group, E Fiji
126 L9 **Onega** Arkhangel'skaya Oblast', NW Russian Federation
122 E7 **Onega** ≈ NW Russian Federation
Onega Bay *see* Onezhskaya Guba
Onega, Lake *see* Onezhskoye Ozero
18 I10 **Oneida** New York, NE USA
20 M8 **Oneida** Tennessee, S USA
18 H9 **Oneida Lake** ◎ New York, NE USA
29 P13 **O'Neill** Nebraska, C USA
123 V12 **Onekotan, Ostrov** *island* Kuril'skiye Ostrova, SE Russian Federation
23 P3 **Oneonta** Alabama, S USA
18 J11 **Oneonta** New York, NE USA
190 I16 **Oneroa** *island* S Cook Islands
116 K11 **Onești** *Hung.* Onyest; *prev.* Gheorghe Gheorghiu-Dej. Bacău, E Romania
193 V15 **Onevai** *island* Tongatapu Group, S Tonga
108 A11 **Onex** Genève, SW Switzerland
126 K8 **Onezhskaya Guba** *Eng.* Onega Bay. *bay* NW Russian Federation
122 D7 **Onezhskoye Ozero** *Eng.* Lake Onega. ◎ NW Russian Federation
83 C16 **Ongandjera** Omusati, N Namibia
184 N12 **Ongaonga** Hawke's Bay, North Island, NZ
162 K9 **Ongi** Dundgovĭ, C Mongolia
162 J8 **Ongi** Övörhangay, C Mongolia
163 W14 **Ongjin** SW North Korea
155 J17 **Ongole** Andhra Pradesh, E India
162 K8 **Ongon** Övörhangay, C Mongolia
Ongtüstik Qazaqstan Oblysy *see* Yuzhnyy Kazakhstan
99 I21 **Onhaye** Namur, S Belgium
166 M8 **Onhne** Pegu, SW Myanmar
137 S9 **Oni** N Georgia
29 N9 **Onida** South Dakota, N USA
164 F15 **Onigajō-yama** ▲ Shikoku, SW Japan
172 H7 **Onilahy** ≈ S Madagascar
77 U16 **Onitsha** Anambra, S Nigeria
164 I13 **Ono** Hyōgo, Honshū, SW Japan
187 X15 **Ono** *island* SW Fiji
164 K12 **Ōno** Fukui, Honshū, SW Japan
164 E13 **Onoda** Yamaguchi, Honshū, SW Japan
187 Z16 **Ono-i-lau** *island* SE Fiji
164 D13 **Onojō** *var.* Ônozyô. Fukuoka, Kyūshū, SW Japan
Onomiti *see* Onomichi
163 O7 **Onon Gol** ≈ N Mongolia
Ononte *see* Orontes
55 N6 **Onoto** Anzoátegui, NE Venezuela
191 O3 **Onotoa** *prev.* Clerk Island. *atoll* Tungaru, W Kiribati
Ônozyô *see* Ōnojō
95 I19 **Onsala** Halland, S Sweden
83 E23 **Onseepkans** Northern Cape, W South Africa
104 F4 **Ons, Illa de** *island* NW Spain
180 H7 **Onslow** Western Australia
21 W11 **Onslow Bay** *bay* North Carolina, E USA
98 P6 **Onstwedde** Groningen, NE Netherlands
164 C16 **On-take** ▲ Kyūshū, SW Japan
35 T15 **Ontario** California, W USA
32 M13 **Ontario** Oregon, NW USA
12 D10 **Ontario** ◈ *province* S Canada
9 P14 **Ontario, Lake** ◎ Canada/USA
(0) L9 **Ontario Peninsula** *peninsula* Canada/USA
Onteniente *see* Ontinyent
105 S11 **Ontinyent** *var.* Onteniente. País Valenciano, E Spain
93 N15 **Ontojärvi** ◎ E Finland
30 L3 **Ontonagon** Michigan, N USA

◆ Country ◇ Dependent Territory ◈ Administrative Region ▲ Mountain ⛰ Volcano ◎ Lake
◆ Country Capital ○ Dependent Territory Capital ✕ International Airport ▲ Mountain Range ≈ River ▣ Reservoir

30 L3 **Ontonagon River** ≈ Michigan, N USA
186 M7 **Ontong Java Atoll** *prev.* Lord Howe Island. *atoll* N Solomon Islands
175 N5 **Ontong Java Rise** *undersea feature* W Pacific Ocean
Onuba *see* Huelva
55 W9 **Onverwacht** Para, N Surinam
Onyest *see* Onești
182 J7 **Oodla Wirra** South Australia
182 F2 **Oodnadatta** South Australia
182 C5 **Ooldea** South Australia
27 Q8 **Oologah Lake** ⊟ Oklahoma, C USA
Oos-Kaap *see* Eastern Cape
Oos-Londen *see* East London
99 E17 **Oostakker** Oost-Vlaanderen, NW Belgium
99 D15 **Oostburg** Zeeland, SW Netherlands
98 K9 **Oostelijk-Flevoland** *polder* C Netherlands
99 B16 **Oostende** *Eng.* Ostend, *Fr.* Ostende. West-Vlaanderen, NW Belgium
99 B16 **Oostende** ✈ West-Vlaanderen, NW Belgium
98 L12 **Oosterbeek** Gelderland, SE Netherlands
99 I14 **Oosterhout** Noord-Brabant, S Netherlands
98 O6 **Oostermoers Vaart** *var.* Hunze. ≈ NE Netherlands
99 F14 **Oosterschelde** *Eng.* Eastern Scheldt. *inlet* SW Netherlands
99 E14 **Oosterscheldedam** *dam* SW Netherlands
98 M7 **Oosterwolde** *Fris.* Easterwâlde. Friesland, N Netherlands
98 I9 **Oosthuizen** Noord-Holland, NW Netherlands
99 H16 **Oostmalle** Antwerpen, N Belgium
Oos-Transvaal *see* Mpumalanga
99 E15 **Oost-Souburg** Zeeland, SW Netherlands
99 E17 **Oost-Vlaanderen** *Eng.* East Flanders. ◈ *province* NW Belgium
98 J5 **Oost-Vlieland** Friesland, N Netherlands
98 F12 **Oostvoorne** Zuid-Holland, SW Netherlands
Ootacamund *see* Udagamandalam
98 O10 **Ootmarsum** Overijssel, E Netherlands
10 K14 **Ootsa Lake** ⊟ British Columbia, SW Canada
114 L8 **Opaka** Tŭrgovishte, N Bulgaria
79 M18 **Opala** Orientale, C Dem. Rep. Congo (Zaire)
127 Q13 **Oparino** Kirovskaya Oblast', NW Russian Federation
14 H8 **Opasatica, Lac** ◎ Quebec, SE Canada
112 B9 **Opatija** *It.* Abbazia. Primorje-Gorski Kotar, NW Croatia
111 N15 **Opatów** Świętokrzyskie, C Poland
111 I17 **Opava** *Ger.* Troppau. Ostravský Kraj, E Czech Republic
111 H16 **Opava** *Ger.* Oppa. ≈ NE Czech Republic
Opazova *see* Stara Pazova
Ópécska *see* Pecica
14 E8 **Opeepeesway Lake** ◎ Ontario, S Canada
23 R5 **Opelika** Alabama, S USA
22 I8 **Opelousas** Louisiana, S USA
186 G6 **Open Bay** *bay* New Britain, E PNG
14 I12 **Opeongo Lake** ◎ Ontario, SE Canada
99 K17 **Opglabbeek** Limburg, NE Belgium
33 W6 **Opheim** Montana, NW USA
39 P10 **Ophir** Alaska, USA
Ophiusa *see* Formentera
79 N18 **Opienge** Orientale, E Dem. Rep. Congo (Zaire)
185 G20 **Opihi** ≈ South Island, NZ
12 J9 **Opinaca** ≈ Quebec, C Canada
12 J10 **Opinaca, Réservoir** ⊟ Quebec, E Canada
117 T5 **Opishnya** *Rus.* Oposhnya. Poltavs'ka Oblast', NE Ukraine
98 I8 **Opmeer** Noord-Holland, NW Netherlands
77 V17 **Opobo** Akwa Ibom, S Nigeria
126 F16 **Opochka** Pskovskaya Oblast', W Russian Federation
110 L13 **Opoczno** Łodzkie, C Poland
111 I15 **Opole** *Ger.* Oppeln. Opolskie, S Poland
111 H15 **Opolskie** ◈ *province* S Poland
144 G13 **Opornyy** Mangistau, SW Kazakhstan
Oporto *see* Porto
Oposhnya *see* Opishnya
184 P8 **Opotiki** Bay of Plenty, North Island, NZ
23 Q7 **Opp** Alabama, S USA
Oppa *see* Opava
94 G9 **Oppdal** Sør-Trøndelag, S Norway
Oppeln *see* Opole
107 N23 **Oppido Mamertina** Calabria, SW Italy
Oppidum Ubiorum *see* Köln
94 F12 **Oppland** ◈ *county* S Norway
118 J12 **Opsa** *Rus.* Opsa. Vitsyebskaya Voblasts', NW Belarus
26 I8 **Optima Lake** ⊟ Oklahoma, C USA
184 J11 **Opunake** Taranaki, North Island, NZ
191 N6 **Opunohu, Baie d'** *bay* Moorea, W French Polynesia
83 B17 **Opuwo** Kunene, NW Namibia
146 H6 **Oqqal'a** *var.* Akkala, *Rus.* Karakala. Qoraqalpoghiston Respublikasi, NW Uzbekistan
147 V13 **Oqsu** *Rus.* Oksu. ≈ SE Tajikistan
147 P14 **Oqtogh, Qatorkŭhi** *Rus.* Khrebet Aktau. ▲ SW Tajikistan
146 M11 **Oqtosh** *Rus.* Aktash. Samarqand Wiloyati, C Uzbekistan
147 N11 **Oqtow Tizmasi** *Rus.* Khrebet Aktau. ▲ C Uzbekistan
30 J12 **Oquawka** Illinois, N USA
144 J10 **Or'** *Kaz.* Or. ≈ Kazakhstan/Russian Federation
36 M15 **Oracle** Arizona, SW USA
116 F9 **Oradea** *prev.* Oradea Mare, *Ger.* Grosswardein, *Hung.* Nagyvárad. Bihor, NW Romania
Oradea Mare *see* Oradea
113 M17 **Orahovac** *Alb.* Rahovec. Serbia, S Yugoslavia
112 H9 **Orahovica** Virovitica-Podravina, NE Croatia
152 K13 **Orai** Uttar Pradesh, N India
92 K12 **Orajärvi** Lappi, NW Finland
Or Akiva *see* Or 'Aqiva
Oral *see* Ural'sk
74 I5 **Oran** *var.* Ouahran, Wahran. NW Algeria
183 R8 **Orange** New South Wales, SE Australia
103 R14 **Orange** *anc.* Arausio. Vaucluse, SE France
25 Y10 **Orange** Texas, SW USA
21 V5 **Orange** Virginia, NE USA
21 R13 **Orangeburg** South Carolina, SE USA
58 J9 **Orange, Cabo** *headland* NE Brazil
29 S12 **Orange City** Iowa, C USA
Orange Cone *see* Orange Fan
172 J10 **Orange Fan** *var.* Orange Cone. *undersea feature* SW Indian Ocean
Orange Free State *see* Free State
25 S14 **Orange Grove** Texas, SW USA
18 K13 **Orange Lake** New York, NE USA
23 V10 **Orange Lake** ◎ Florida, SE USA
Orange Mouth/Orangemund *see* Oranjemund
23 W9 **Orange Park** Florida, SE USA
83 E23 **Orange River** *Afr.* Oranjerivier. ≈ S Africa
14 G15 **Orangeville** Ontario, S Canada
36 M5 **Orangeville** Utah, W USA
42 G1 **Orange Walk** Orange Walk, N Belize
42 F1 **Orange Walk** ◈ *district* NW Belize
100 N11 **Oranienburg** Brandenburg, NE Germany
98 O7 **Oranjekanaal** *canal* NE Netherlands
83 D23 **Oranjemund** *var.* Orangemund; *prev.* Orange Mouth. Karas, SW Namibia
Oranjerivier *see* Orange River
45 N16 **Oranjestad** ○ (Aruba) W Aruba
Oranje Vrystaat *see* Free State
Orany *see* Varėna
83 H18 **Orapa** Central, C Botswana
138 F9 **Or 'Aqiva** *var.* Or Akiva. Haifa, W Israel
112 I10 **Orašje** Federacija Bosna I Hercegovina, N Bosnia and Herzegovina
116 G11 **Orăștie** *Ger.* Broos, *Hung.* Szászváros. Hunedoara, W Romania
Orașul Stalin *see* Brașov
111 K18 **Orava** *Hung.* Árva, *Pol.* Orawa. ≈ N Slovakia
Oravainen *see* Oravais
93 K16 **Oravais** *Fin.* Oravainen. Länsi-Suomi, W Finland
Oravicabánya *see* Oravița
116 F13 **Oravița** *Ger.* Orawitza, *Hung.* Oravicabánya. Caraș-Severin, SW Romania
Orawa *see* Orava
185 B24 **Orawia** Southland, South Island, NZ
Orawitza *see* Oravița
103 P16 **Orb** ≈ S France
106 C9 **Orba** ≈ NW Italy
158 H12 **Orba Co** ◎ W China
108 B9 **Orbe** Vaud, W Switzerland
107 G14 **Orbetello** Toscana, C Italy
104 K3 **Orbigo** ≈ NW Spain
183 Q12 **Orbost** Victoria, SE Australia
95 O14 **Örbyhus** Uppsala, C Sweden
194 I1 **Orcadas** *Argentinian research station* South Orkney Islands, Antarctica
105 P12 **Orcera** Andalucía, S Spain
33 P9 **Orchard Homes** Montana, NW USA
37 P5 **Orchard Mesa** Colorado, C USA
18 D10 **Orchard Park** New York, NE USA
Orchid Island *see* Lan Yü
115 G18 **Orchómenos** *var.* Orhomenos, Orkhómenos; *prev.* Skripón, *anc.* Orchomenus. Stereá Ellás, C Greece
Orchomenus *see* Orchómenos
106 B7 **Orco** ≈ NW Italy
103 R8 **Or, Côte d'** *physical region* C France
29 O14 **Ord** Nebraska, C USA
Ordat' *see* Ordats'
119 O15 **Ordats'** *Rus.* Ordat'. Mahilyowskaya Voblasts', E Belarus
36 K8 **Orderville** Utah, W USA
104 H2 **Ordes** Galicia, NW Spain
35 V14 **Ord Mountain** ▲ California, W USA
Ordos Desert *see* Mu Us Shamo
188 B16 **Ordot** C Guam
137 N11 **Ordu** *anc.* Cotyora. Ordu, N Turkey
136 M11 **Ordu** ◈ *province* N Turkey
137 V14 **Ordubad** SW Azerbaijan
105 O3 **Orduña** País Vasco, N Spain
37 U6 **Ordway** Colorado, C USA
144 L8 **Ordzhonikidze** Kostanay, N Kazakhstan
117 T9 **Ordzhonikidze** Dnipropetrovs'ka Oblast', E Ukraine
Ordzhonikidze *see* Vladikavkaz, Russian Federation
Ordzhonikidze *see* Yenakiyeve, Ukraine
Ordzhonikidzeabad *see* Kofarnihon
55 U9 **Orealla** E Guyana
113 G15 **Orebić** *It.* Sabbioncello. Dubrovnik-Neretva, S Croatia
95 M16 **Örebro** Örebro, C Sweden
95 L16 **Örebro** ◈ *county* C Sweden
25 W6 **Ore City** Texas, SW USA
30 L10 **Oregon** Illinois, N USA
27 Q2 **Oregon** Missouri, C USA
31 R11 **Oregon** Ohio, N USA
32 H13 **Oregon** *off.* State of Oregon; also known as Beaver State, Sunset State, Valentine State, Webfoot State. ◈ *state* NW USA
32 G11 **Oregon City** Oregon, NW USA
95 P14 **Öregrund** Uppsala, C Sweden
Orekhov *see* Orikhiv
128 L3 **Orekhovo-Zuyevo** Moskovskaya Oblast', W Russian Federation
Orekhovsk *see* Arekhawsk
Orel *see* Oril'
128 J6 **Orël** Orlovskaya Oblast', W Russian Federation
56 E11 **Orellana** Loreto, N Peru
104 L11 **Orellana, Embalse de** ⊟ W Spain
36 L3 **Orem** Utah, W USA
Ore Mountains *see* Erzgebirge/Krušné Hory
129 V7 **Orenburg** *prev.* Chkalov. Orenburgskaya Oblast', W Russian Federation
129 V7 **Orenburg** ✈ Orenburgskaya Oblast', W Russian Federation
129 T7 **Orenburgskaya Oblast'** ◈ *province* W Russian Federation
Orense *see* Ourense
188 C8 **Oreor** *var.* Koror. ● (Palau) Oreor, N Palau
188 C8 **Oreor** *var.* Koror. *island* N Palau
185 B24 **Orepuki** Southland, South Island, NZ
114 L12 **Orestiáda** *prev.* Orestiás. Anatolikí Makedonía kai Thráki, NE Greece
Orestiás *see* Orestiáda
Öresund/Øresund *see* Sound, The
185 C23 **Oreti** ≈ South Island, NZ
184 L5 **Orewa** Auckland, North Island, NZ
65 A25 **Orford, Cape** *headland* West Falkland, Falkland Islands
44 B5 **Órganos, Sierra de los** ▲ W Cuba
37 R15 **Organ Peak** ▲ New Mexico, SW USA
105 N9 **Orgaz** Castilla-La Mancha, C Spain
Orgeyev *see* Orhei
162 I6 **Orgil** Hövsgöl, C Mongolia
105 O15 **Orgiva** *var.* Orjiva. Andalucía, S Spain
162 I9 **Orgön** Bayanhongor, C Mongolia
117 N9 **Orhei** *var.* Orheiu, *Rus.* Orgeyev. N Moldova
Orheiu *see* Orhei
105 R3 **Orhi** *var.* Orhy, Pico de Orhy, Pic d'Orhy. ▲ France/Spain *see also* Orhy
Orhomenos *see* Orchómenos
162 L6 **Orhon Gol** ≈ N Mongolia
102 J16 **Orhy** *var.* Orhi, Pico de Orhy, Pic d'Orhy. ▲ France/Spain *see also* Orhi
Orhy, Pic d'/Orhy, Pico de *see* Orhi/Orhy
34 L2 **Orick** California, W USA
32 L6 **Orient** Washington, NW USA
48 D6 **Oriental, Cordillera** ▲ Bolivia/Peru
48 D6 **Oriental, Cordillera** ▲ C Colombia
57 H16 **Oriental, Cordillera** ▲ C Peru
63 M15 **Oriente** Buenos Aires, E Argentina
105 R12 **Orihuela** País Valenciano, E Spain
117 V9 **Orikhiv** *Rus.* Orekhov. Zaporiz'ka Oblast', SE Ukraine
113 K22 **Orikum** *var.* Orikumi. Vlorë, SW Albania
Orikumi *see* Orikum
117 V6 **Oril'** *Rus.* Orel. ≈ E Ukraine
14 H14 **Orillia** Ontario, S Canada
93 M19 **Orimattila** Etelä-Suomi, S Finland
33 Y15 **Orin** Wyoming, C USA
47 R4 **Orinoco, Río** ≈ Colombia/Venezuela
186 C9 **Oriomo** Western, SW PNG
30 K11 **Orion** Illinois, N USA
29 Q5 **Oriska** North Dakota, N USA
153 P17 **Orissa** ◈ *state* NE India
Orissaar *see* Orissaare
118 E5 **Orissaare** *Ger.* Orissaar. Saaremaa, W Estonia
107 B19 **Oristano** Sardegna, Italy, C Mediterranean Sea
107 A19 **Oristano, Golfo di** *gulf* Sardegna, Italy, C Mediterranean Sea
54 D13 **Orito** Putumayo, SW Colombia
93 L18 **Orivesi** Häme, SW Finland
93 N17 **Orivesi** ◎ Länsi-Suomi, SE Finland
58 H12 **Oriximiná** Pará, NE Brazil
41 Q14 **Orizaba** Veracruz-Llave, E Mexico
41 Q14 **Orizaba, Volcán Pico de** *var.* Citlaltépetl. ▲ S Mexico
95 I16 **Ørje** Østfold, S Norway
113 I16 **Orjen** ▲ Bosnia and Herzegovina/Yugoslavia
Orjiva *see* Orgiva
94 G8 **Orkanger** Sør-Trøndelag, S Norway
94 G8 **Orkdalen** *valley* S Norway
95 K22 **Örkelljunga** Skåne, S Sweden
Orkhaniye *see* Botevgrad
Orkhómenos *see* Orchómenos
94 H9 **Orkla** ≈ S Norway
Orkney *see* Orkney Islands
65 J22 **Orkney Deep** *undersea feature* Scotia Sea/Weddell Sea
96 J4 **Orkney Islands** *var.* Orkney, Orkneys. *island group* N Scotland, UK
Orkneys *see* Orkney Islands
24 K8 **Orla** Texas, SW USA
35 N5 **Orland** California, W USA
23 X11 **Orlando** Florida, SE USA
23 X12 **Orlando** ✈ Florida, SE USA
107 K23 **Orlando, Capo d'** *headland* Sicilia, Italy, C Mediterranean Sea
Orlau *see* Orlová
103 N6 **Orléanais** *cultural region* C France
34 L2 **Orleans** California, W USA
19 Q12 **Orleans** Massachusetts, NE USA
103 N7 **Orléans** *anc.* Aurelianum. Loiret, C France
15 R10 **Orléans, Île d'** *island* Quebec, SE Canada
Orléansville *see* Chlef
111 F16 **Orlice** *Ger.* Adler. ≈ NE Czech Republic
122 L13 **Orlik** Respublika Buryatiya, S Russian Federation
127 Q14 **Orlov** *prev.* Khalturin. Kirovskaya Oblast', NW Russian Federation
111 I17 **Orlová** *Ger.* Orlau, *Pol.* Orłowa. Ostravský Kraj, E Czech Republic
Orlov, Mys *see* Orlovskiy, Mys
128 I6 **Orlovskaya Oblast'** ◈ *province* W Russian Federation
126 M5 **Orlovskiy, Mys** *var.* Mys Orlov. *headland* NW Russian Federation
Orłowa *see* Orlová
103 O5 **Orly** ✈ (Paris) Essonne, N France
119 G16 **Orlya** *Rus.* Orlya. Hrodzyenskaya Voblasts', W Belarus
114 M7 **Orlyak** *prev.* Makenzen, Trubchular, *Rom.* Trupcilar. Dobrich, NE Bulgaria
148 L16 **Ormāra** Baluchistān, SW Pakistan
171 P5 **Ormoc** *off.* Ormoc City, *var.* MacArthur. Leyte, C Philippines
23 X10 **Ormond Beach** Florida, SE USA
109 X10 **Ormož** *Ger.* Friedau. NE Slovenia
14 J13 **Ormsby** Ontario, SE Canada
97 K17 **Ormskirk** NW England, UK
Ormsö *see* Vormsi
15 N13 **Ormstown** Quebec, SE Canada
Ormuz, Strait of *see* Hormuz, Strait of
103 T8 **Ornans** Doubs, E France
102 K5 **Orne** ◈ *department* N France
102 K5 **Orne** ≈ N France
92 G12 **Ørnes** Nordland, C Norway
110 L7 **Orneta** Warmińsko-Mazurskie, NE Poland
95 P16 **Ornö** Stockholm, C Sweden
37 Q3 **Orno Peak** ▲ Colorado, C USA
93 I16 **Örnsköldsvik** Västernorrland, C Sweden
163 X13 **Oro** E North Korea
45 T6 **Orocovis** C Puerto Rico
54 H10 **Orocué** Casanare, E Colombia
77 N13 **Orodara** SW Burkina
105 S4 **Oroel, Peña de** ▲ N Spain
33 N10 **Orofino** Idaho, NW USA
162 I9 **Orog Nuur** ◎ S Mongolia
35 U14 **Oro Grande** California, W USA
37 S15 **Orogrande** New Mexico, SW USA
191 Q7 **Orohena, Mont** △ Tahiti, W French Polynesia
Orolaunum *see* Arlon
Orol Dengizi *see* Aral Sea
189 S15 **Oroluk Atoll** *atoll* Caroline Islands, C Micronesia
80 J13 **Oromo** ◈ *region* C Ethiopia
13 O15 **Oromocto** New Brunswick, SE Canada
191 S4 **Orona** *prev.* Hull Island. *atoll* Phoenix Islands, C Kiribati
191 V17 **Orongo** *ancient monument* Easter Island, Chile, E Pacific Ocean
138 I3 **Orontes** *var.* Ononte, *Ar.* Nahr el Aassi, Nahr al 'Aṣī. ≈ SW Asia
104 L9 **Oropesa** Castilla-La Mancha, C Spain
105 T8 **Oropesa** País Valenciano, E Spain
Oropeza *see* Cochabamba
163 U5 **Oroqen Zizhiqi** Nei Mongol Zizhiqu, N China
171 P7 **Oroquieta** *var.* Oroquieta City. Mindanao, S Philippines
40 J8 **Oro, Río del** ≈ C Mexico
59 O14 **Orós, Açude** ⊟ E Brazil
107 D18 **Orosei, Golfo di** *gulf* Tyrrhenian Sea, C Mediterranean Sea
111 M24 **Orosháza** Békés, SE Hungary
Orosirá Rodhópis *see* Rhodope Mountains
111 I22 **Oroszlány** Komárom-Esztergom, W Hungary
188 B16 **Orote Peninsula** *peninsula* W Guam
123 T9 **Orotukan** Magadanskaya Oblast', E Russian Federation
35 O5 **Oroville** California, W USA
32 K6 **Oroville** Washington, NW USA
35 O5 **Oroville, Lake** ⊟ California, W USA
(0) G15 **Orozco Fracture Zone** *tectonic feature* E Pacific Ocean
64 I7 **Orphan Knoll** *undersea feature* NW Atlantic Ocean
29 V3 **Orr** Minnesota, N USA
95 M21 **Orrefors** Kalmar, S Sweden
182 I7 **Orroroo** South Australia
31 T12 **Orrville** Ohio, N USA
94 L12 **Orsa** Dalarna, C Sweden
Orschowa *see* Orșova
Orschütz *see* Orzyc
119 O14 **Orsha** *Rus.* Orsha. Vitsyebskaya Voblasts', NE Belarus
129 Q2 **Orshanka** Respublika Mariy El, W Russian Federation
108 C11 **Orsières** Valais, SW Switzerland
122 E12 **Orsk** Orenburgskaya Oblast', W Russian Federation
116 F13 **Orșova** *Ger.* Orschowa, *Hung.* Orsova. Mehedinți, SW Romania
94 D10 **Ørsta** Møre og Romsdal, S Norway
95 O15 **Örsundsbro** Uppsala, C Sweden
136 D16 **Ortaca** Muğla, SW Turkey
107 M16 **Orta Nova** Puglia, SE Italy
136 I17 **Orta Toroslar** ▲ S Turkey
54 E11 **Ortega** Tolima, W Colombia
104 H1 **Ortegal, Cabo** *headland* NW Spain
Ortelsburg *see* Szczytno
102 J15 **Orthez** Pyrénées-Atlantiques, SW France
57 K14 **Orthon, Río** ≈ N Bolivia
60 J10 **Ortigueira** Paraná, S Brazil
104 H1 **Ortigueira** Galicia, NW Spain
106 H5 **Ortisei** *Ger.* Sankt-Ulrich. Trentino-Alto Adige, N Italy
40 F6 **Ortiz** Sonora, NW Mexico
54 L5 **Ortiz** Guárico, N Venezuela
Ortler *see* Ortles
106 F5 **Ortles** *Ger.* Ortler. ▲ N Italy
107 K14 **Ortona** Abruzzo, C Italy
29 R8 **Ortonville** Minnesota, N USA
147 W8 **Orto-Tokoy** Issyk-Kul'skaya Oblast', NE Kyrgyzstan
93 I15 **Örträsk** Västerbotten, N Sweden
100 J12 **Örtze** ≈ NW Germany
Oruba *see* Aruba
142 I3 **Orūmīyeh** *var.* Rizaiyeh, Urmia, Urmiyeh; *prev.* Reẓā'īyeh. Āẕarbāyjān-e Bākhtarī, NW Iran
142 J3 **Orūmīyeh, Daryācheh-ye** *var.* Matianus, Sha Hi, Urumi Yeh, *Eng.* Lake Urmia; *prev.* Daryācheh-ye Reẓā'īyeh. ◎ NW Iran
57 K19 **Oruro** Oruro, W Bolivia
57 J19 **Oruro** ◈ *department* W Bolivia
95 I18 **Orust** *island* S Sweden
Oruzgān/Orūzgān *see* Ūrūzgān
106 H13 **Orvieto** *anc.* Velsuna. Umbria, C Italy
194 K7 **Orville Coast** *physical region* Antarctica
114 H7 **Oryakhovo** Vratsa, NW Bulgaria
Oryokko *see* Yalu
117 R5 **Orzhytsya** Poltavs'ka Oblast', C Ukraine
110 M9 **Orzyc** *Ger.* Orschütz. ≈ NE Poland
110 N8 **Orzysz** *Ger.* Arys. Warmińsko-Mazurskie, NE Poland
94 I10 **Os** Hedmark, S Norway
95 C14 **Os** Hordaland, S Norway
127 U15 **Osa** Permskaya Oblast', NW Russian Federation
29 W11 **Osage** Iowa, C USA
27 U5 **Osage Beach** Missouri, C USA
27 P5 **Osage City** Kansas, C USA
27 U7 **Osage Fork River** ≈ Missouri, C USA
27 U5 **Osage River** ≈ Missouri, C USA
164 J13 **Ōsaka** *hist.* Naniwa. Ōsaka, Honshū, SW Japan
164 I13 **Ōsaka** *off.* Ōsaka-fu, *var.* Ōsaka Hu. ◈ *urban prefecture* Honshū, SW Japan
Ōsaka-fu/Ōsaka Hu *see* Ōsaka
145 R10 **Osakarovka** Karaganda, C Kazakhstan
29 T7 **Osakis** Minnesota, N USA
43 N16 **Osa, Península de** *peninsula* S Costa Rica
60 M10 **Osasco** São Paulo, S Brazil
27 R5 **Osawatomie** Kansas, C USA
26 L3 **Osborne** Kansas, C USA
173 S8 **Osborn Plateau** *undersea feature* E Indian Ocean
95 L21 **Osby** Skåne, S Sweden
Osca *see* Huesca
92 N2 **Oscar II Land** *physical region* W Svalbard
27 Y10 **Osceola** Arkansas, C USA
29 V15 **Osceola** Iowa, C USA
27 S6 **Osceola** Missouri, C USA
29 Q15 **Osceola** Nebraska, C USA
101 N15 **Oschatz** Sachsen, E Germany
100 K13 **Oschersleben** Sachsen-Anhalt, C Germany
31 R7 **Oscoda** Michigan, N USA
Ösel *see* Saaremaa
94 H6 **Osen** Sør-Trøndelag, S Norway
164 A14 **Ōse-zaki** *headland* Fukue-jima, SW Japan
147 T10 **Osh** Oshskaya Oblast', SW Kyrgyzstan
83 C16 **Oshakati** Oshana, N Namibia
83 C16 **Oshana** ◈ *district* N Namibia
14 H15 **Oshawa** Ontario, SE Canada
165 R10 **Oshika-hantō** *peninsula* Honshū, C Japan
83 C16 **Oshikango** Ohangwena, N Namibia
Oshikoto *see* Otjikoto
165 P5 **Ō-shima** *island* NE Japan
165 N14 **Ō-shima** *island* S Japan
165 Q5 **Oshima-hantō** ▲ Hokkaidō, NE Japan
83 D17 **Oshivelo** Otjikoto, N Namibia
28 K14 **Oshkosh** Nebraska, C USA
30 M7 **Oshkosh** Wisconsin, N USA
Oshmyany *see* Ashmyany
Osh Oblasty *see* Oshskaya Oblast'
77 T16 **Oshogbo** Osun, W Nigeria
147 S11 **Oshskaya Oblast'** *Kir.* Osh Oblasty. ◈ *province* SW Kyrgyzstan
79 J20 **Oshwe** Bandundu, C Dem. Rep. Congo (Zaire)
Osiek *see* Osijek
112 I9 **Osijek** *prev.* Osiek, Osjek, *Ger.* Esseg, *Hung.* Eszék. Osijek-Baranja, E Croatia
112 I9 **Osijek-Baranja** *off.* Osječko-Baranjska Županija. ◈ *province* E Croatia
106 J12 **Osimo** Marche, C Italy
122 M12 **Osinovka** Irkutskaya Oblast', C Russian Federation
Osintorf *see* Asintorf
112 N11 **Osipaonica** Serbia, NE Yugoslavia
Osipenko *see* Berdyans'k
Osipovichi *see* Asipovichy
Osječko-Baranjska Županija *see* Osijek-Baranja
Osjek *see* Osijek
29 W15 **Oskaloosa** Iowa, C USA
27 Q4 **Oskaloosa** Kansas, C USA
95 N20 **Oskarshamn** Kalmar, S Sweden
95 J21 **Oskarström** Halland, S Sweden
14 M8 **Oskélanéo** Quebec, SE Canada
Öskemen *see* Ust'-Kamenogorsk
Oskil *see* Oskol
117 W5 **Oskol** *Ukr.* Oskil. ≈ Russian Federation/Ukraine
93 D20 **Oslo** *prev.* Christiania, Kristiania. ● (Norway) Oslo, S Norway
93 D20 **Oslo** ◈ *county* S Norway
93 D21 **Oslofjorden** *fjord* S Norway
155 G15 **Osmānābād** Mahārāshtra, C India
136 J11 **Osmancık** Çorum, N Turkey
136 L16 **Osmaniye** Osmaniye, S Turkey
136 L16 **Osmaniye** ◈ *province* S Turkey
95 O16 **Ösmo** Stockholm, C Sweden
118 E3 **Osmussaar** *island* W Estonia
100 G13 **Osnabrück** Niedersachsen, NW Germany
110 D11 **Ośno Lubuskie** *Ger.* Drossen. Lubuskie, W Poland
113 P19 **Osogov Mountains** *var.* Osogovske Planine, Osogovski Planina, *Mac.* Osogovski Planini. ▲ Bulgaria/FYR Macedonia
Osogovske Planine/Osogovski Planina/Osogovski Planini *see* Osogov Mountains
165 R6 **Osore-yama** ▲ Honshū, C Japan
Oșorhei *see* Târgu Mureș
61 J16 **Osório** Rio Grande do Sul, S Brazil
63 G16 **Osorno** Los Lagos, C Chile
104 M4 **Osorno** Castilla-León, N Spain
11 N17 **Osoyoos** British Columbia, SW Canada
54 J6 **Ospino** Portuguesa, N Venezuela
98 K13 **Oss** Noord-Brabant, S Netherlands
104 H11 **Ossa** ▲ S Portugal
115 F15 **Óssa** ▲ C Greece
23 X6 **Ossabaw Island** *island* Georgia, SE USA
23 X6 **Ossabaw Sound** *sound* Georgia, SE USA
183 O16 **Ossa, Mount** ▲ Tasmania, SE Australia
104 H11 **Ossa, Serra d'** ▲ SE Portugal
77 U16 **Osse** ≈ S Nigeria
30 J6 **Osseo** Wisconsin, N USA
109 S9 **Ossiacher See** ◎ S Austria
18 K13 **Ossining** New York, NE USA
94 I12 **Ossjøen** ◎ S Norway
123 V9 **Ossora** Koryakskiy Avtonomnyy Okrug, E Russian Federation
126 I15 **Ostashkov** Tverskaya Oblast', W Russian Federation
100 H9 **Oste** ≈ NW Germany
Ostee *see* Baltic Sea
Ostend/Ostende *see* Oostende
117 P3 **Oster** Chernihivs'ka Oblast', N Ukraine
95 O14 **Österbybruk** Uppsala, C Sweden
95 M19 **Österbymo** Östergotland, S Sweden
94 K12 **Österdalälven** ≈ C Sweden
94 I12 **Østerdalen** *valley* S Norway
95 L18 **Östergötland** ◈ *county* S Sweden
100 H10 **Osterholz-Scharmbeck** Niedersachsen, NW Germany
Östermark *see* Teuva
Östermyra *see* Seinäjoki
Osterode/Osterode in Ostpreussen *see* Ostróda
101 J14 **Osterode am Harz** Niedersachsen, C Germany
94 C13 **Osterøy** *island* S Norway
Österreich *see* Austria
93 G16 **Östersund** Jämtland, C Sweden
95 N14 **Östervåla** Västmanland, C Sweden
101 H22 **Ostfildern** Baden-Württemberg, SW Germany
95 H16 **Østfold** ◈ *county* S Norway
100 E9 **Ostfriesische Inseln** *Eng.* East Frisian Islands. *island group* NW Germany
100 F10 **Ostfriesland** *historical region* NW Germany
95 P14 **Östhammar** Uppsala, C Sweden
Ostia Aterni *see* Pescara
106 G8 **Ostiglia** Lombardia, N Italy
95 J14 **Östmark** Värmland, C Sweden
95 K22 **Östra Ringsjön** ◎ S Sweden
111 I17 **Ostrava** Ostravský Kraj, E Czech Republic
111 H17 **Ostravský Kraj** ◈ *region* E Czech Republic
110 K8 **Ostróda** *Ger.* Osterode, Osterode in Ostpreussen. Warmińsko-Mazurskie, NE Poland
Ostrog/Ostróg *see* Ostroh
128 L8 **Ostrogozhsk** Voronezhskaya Oblast', W Russian Federation
116 L4 **Ostroh** *Pol.* Ostróg, *Rus.* Ostrog. Rivnens'ka Oblast', NW Ukraine
110 N9 **Ostrołęka** *Ger.* Wiesenhof, *Rus.* Ostrolenka. Mazowieckie, C Poland
111 A16 **Ostrov** *Ger.* Schlackenwerth. Karlovarský Kraj, W Czech Republic
126 F15 **Ostrov** *Latv.* Austrava. Pskovskaya Oblast', W Russian Federation
Ostrovets *see* Ostrowiec Świętokrzyski
113 M21 **Ostrovicës, Mali i** ▲ SE Albania
165 Z2 **Ostrov Iturup** *island* NE Russian Federation
114 L7 **Ostrovo** *prev.* Golema Ada. Razgrad, N Bulgaria
127 N15 **Ostrovskoye** Kostromskaya Oblast', NW Russian Federation

◆ Country ● Country Capital ◇ Dependent Territory ○ Dependent Territory Capital ◈ Administrative Region ✈ International Airport ▲ Mountain ▲ Mountain Range △ Volcano ≈ River ◎ Lake ⊟ Reservoir

Ostrów see Ostrów Wielkopolski
Ostrowiec see Ostrowiec Świętokrzyski
111 M14 **Ostrowiec Świętokrzyski** var. Ostrowiec, Rus. Ostrovets. Świętokrzyskie, C Poland
110 P13 **Ostrów Lubelski** Lubelskie, E Poland
110 N10 **Ostrów Mazowiecka** var. Ostrów Mazowiecki. Mazowieckie, C Poland
Ostrów Mazowiecki see Ostrów Mazowiecka
Ostrowo see Ostrów Wielkopolski
110 H13 **Ostrów Wielkopolski** var. Ostrów, Ger. Ostrowo. Wielkopolskie, C Poland
Ostryna see Astryna
110 I13 **Ostrzeszów** Wielkopolskie, C Poland
107 P18 **Ostuni** Puglia, SE Italy
Ostyako-Voguls'k see Khanty-Mansiysk
Osum see Osumit, Lumi i
114 I9 **Osŭm** ≈ N Bulgaria
164 C17 **Ōsumi-hantō** ▲ Kyūshū, SW Japan
164 C17 **Ōsumi-kaikyō** strait SW Japan
113 L22 **Osumit, Lumi i** var. Osum. ≈ SE Albania
77 T16 **Osun** ◈ state SW Nigeria
104 L14 **Osuna** Andalucía, S Spain
60 J8 **Osvaldo Cruz** São Paulo, S Brazil
Osveya see Asvyeya
18 J7 **Oswegatchie River** ≈ New York, NE USA
27 Q7 **Oswego** Kansas, C USA
18 H9 **Oswego** New York, NE USA
97 K19 **Oswestry** W England, UK
111 J16 **Oświęcim** Ger. Auschwitz. Małopolskie, S Poland
185 E22 **Otago** off. Otago Region. ◈ region South Island, NZ
185 F23 **Otago Peninsula** peninsula South Island, NZ
165 F13 **Ōtake** Hiroshima, Honshū, SW Japan
184 L13 **Otaki** Wellington, North Island, NZ
93 M15 **Otanmäki** Oulu, C Finland
145 T15 **Otar** Zhambyl, SE Kazakhstan
165 R4 **Otaru** Hokkaidō, NE Japan
185 C24 **Otatara** Southland, South Island, NZ
185 C24 **Otautau** Southland, South Island, NZ
93 M18 **Otava** Itä-Suomi, E Finland
111 B18 **Otava** Ger. Wottawa. ≈ SW Czech Republic
56 C6 **Otavalo** Imbabura, N Ecuador
83 D17 **Otavi** Otjozondjupa, N Namibia
165 P12 **Ōtawara** Tochigi, Honshū, S Japan
83 B16 **Otchinjau** Cunene, SW Angola
116 F12 **Oţelu Roşu** Ger. Ferdinandsberg, Hung. Nándorhgy. Caras-Severin, SW Romania
185 E21 **Otematata** Canterbury, South Island, NZ
118 I6 **Otepää** Ger. Odenpäh. Valgamaa, SE Estonia
32 K9 **Othello** Washington, NW USA
115 A15 **Othonoí** island Iónioi Nísoi, Greece, C Mediterranean Sea
Othris see Óthrys
115 F17 **Óthrys** var. Othris. ▲ C Greece
77 Q14 **Oti** ≈ N Togo
40 K10 **Otinapa** Durango, C Mexico
185 G17 **Otira** West Coast, South Island, NZ
37 V3 **Otis** Colorado, C USA
12 L10 **Otish, Monts** ▲ Quebec, E Canada
83 C17 **Otjikondo** Kunene, N Namibia
83 C17 **Otjikoto** var. Oshikoto. ◈ district N Namibia
83 E18 **Otjinene** Omaheke, NE Namibia
83 D18 **Otjiwarongo** Otjozondjupa, N Namibia
83 D18 **Otjosondu** var. Otjosundu. Otjozondjupa, C Namibia
Otjosundu see Otjosondu
83 D18 **Otjozondjupa** ◈ district C Namibia
112 C11 **Otočac** Lika-Senj, W Croatia
162 M14 **Otog Qi** Nei Mongol Zizhiqu, N China
112 J10 **Otok** Vukovar-Srijem, E Croatia
116 K14 **Otopeni** ✕ (Bucureşti) Bucureşti, S Romania
184 L8 **Otorohanga** Waikato, North Island, NZ
12 D9 **Otoskwin** ≈ Ontario, C Canada
165 G14 **Ōtoyo** Kōchi, Shikoku, SW Japan
95 E16 **Otra** ≈ S Norway
107 R19 **Otranto** Puglia, SE Italy
Otranto, Canale d' see Otranto, Strait of
107 Q18 **Otranto, Strait of** It. Canale d'Otranto. strait Albania/Italy
111 H18 **Otrokovice** Ger. Otrokowitz. Zlínský Kraj, E Czech Republic
Otrokowitz see Otrokovice
31 P10 **Otsego** Michigan, N USA
31 Q6 **Otsego Lake** ◎ Michigan, N USA
18 I11 **Otselic River** ≈ New York, NE USA
164 J13 **Ōtsu** var. Ôtu. Shiga, Honshū, SW Japan
94 G11 **Otta** Oppland, S Norway
189 U13 **Otta** island Chuuk, C Micronesia
94 F11 **Otta** ≈ S Norway
189 U13 **Otta Pass** passage Chuuk Islands, C Micronesia
95 J22 **Ottarp** Skåne, S Sweden
14 L12 **Ottawa** ● (Canada) Ontario, SE Canada
30 L11 **Ottawa** Illinois, N USA
27 Q5 **Ottawa** Kansas, C USA
31 R12 **Ottawa** Ohio, N USA
14 L12 **Ottawa** var. Uplands. ✕ Ontario, SE Canada
14 M12 **Ottawa** Fr. Outaouais. ≈ Ontario/Quebec, SE Canada
12 I4 **Ottawa Islands** island group Nunavut, C Canada
18 L8 **Otter Creek** ≈ Vermont, NE USA
36 L6 **Otter Creek Reservoir** ⊠ Utah, W USA
98 L11 **Otterlo** Gelderland, E Netherlands
94 D9 **Otterøya** island S Norway
29 S6 **Otter Tail Lake** ◎ Minnesota, N USA
29 R7 **Otter Tail River** ≈ Minnesota, C USA
95 H23 **Otterup** Fyn, C Denmark
99 H19 **Ottignies** Wallon Brabant, C Belgium
101 L23 **Ottobrunn** Bayern, SE Germany
29 X15 **Ottumwa** Iowa, C USA
Ôtu see Ōtsu
83 B16 **Otuazuma** Kunene, NW Namibia
Otuki see Ōtsuki
77 V16 **Oturkpo** Benue, S Nigeria
193 Y15 **Otu Tolu Group** island group SE Tonga
182 M13 **Otway, Cape** headland Victoria, SE Australia
63 H24 **Otway, Seno** inlet S Chile
Ötz see Oetz
108 L8 **Ötztaler Ache** ≈ W Austria
108 L9 **Ötztaler Alpen** It. Alpi Venoste. ▲ SW Austria
27 T12 **Ouachita, Lake** ⊠ Arkansas, C USA
27 R11 **Ouachita Mountains** ▲ Arkansas/Oklahoma, C USA
27 U13 **Ouachita River** ≈ Arkansas/Louisiana, C USA
Ouadaï see Ouaddaï
76 J7 **Ouadâne** var. Ouadane. Adrar, C Mauritania
78 K13 **Ouadda** Haute-Kotto, N Central African Republic
78 J10 **Ouaddaï** off. Préfecture du Ouaddaï, var. Ouadaï, Wadai. ◈ prefecture SE Chad
77 P13 **Ouagadougou** var. Wagadugu. ● (Burkina) C Burkina
77 P13 **Ouagadougou** ✕ C Burkina
77 O12 **Ouahigouya** NW Burkina
Ouahran see Oran
79 J14 **Ouaka** ◈ prefecture C Central African Republic
79 J15 **Ouaka** ≈ S Central African Republic
Oualam see Ouallam
76 M9 **Oualâta** var. Oualata. Hodh ech Chargui, SE Mauritania
77 R11 **Ouallam** var. Oualam. Tillabéri, W Niger
172 H14 **Ouanani** Mohéli, S Comoros
55 Z10 **Ouanary** E French Guiana
78 L13 **Ouanda Djallé** Vakaga, NE Central African Republic
79 N14 **Ouando** Haut-Mbomou, SE Central African Republic
79 L15 **Ouango** Mbomou, S Central African Republic
77 N14 **Ouangolodougou** var. Wangolodougou. N Ivory Coast
172 I13 **Ouani** Anjouan, SE Comoros
79 M15 **Ouara** ≈ E Central African Republic
76 K7 **Ouarâne** desert C Mauritania
15 O11 **Ouareau** ≈ Quebec, SE Canada
74 K7 **Ouargla** var. Wargla. NE Algeria
74 F8 **Ouarzazate** S Morocco
77 Q11 **Ouatagouna** Gao, E Mali
74 G6 **Ouazzane** var. Ouezzane, Ar. Wazan, Wazzan. N Morocco
Oubangui see Ubangi
Oubangui-Chari see Central African Republic
Oubari, Edeyen d' see Awbāri, Idhān
98 G13 **Oud-Beijerland** Zuid-Holland, SW Netherlands
98 F13 **Ouddorp** Zuid-Holland, SW Netherlands
77 P9 **Oudeïka** oasis C Mali
98 G13 **Oude Maas** ≈ SW Netherlands
99 E18 **Oudenaarde** Fr. Audenarde. Oost-Vlaanderen, SW Belgium
99 H14 **Oudenbosch** Noord-Brabant, S Netherlands
98 P6 **Oude Pekela** Groningen, NE Netherlands
Ouderkerk see Ouderkerk aan den Amstel
98 I10 **Ouderkerk aan den Amstel** var. Ouderkerk. Noord-Holland, C Netherlands
98 I6 **Oudeschild** Noord-Holland, NW Netherlands
99 G14 **Oude-Tonge** Zuid-Holland, SW Netherlands
98 I12 **Oudewater** Utrecht, C Netherlands
Oudjda see Oujda
98 L5 **Oudkerk** Friesland, N Netherlands
102 J7 **Oudon** ≈ NW France
98 I9 **Oudorp** Noord-Holland, NW Netherlands
83 G25 **Oudtshoorn** Western Cape, SW South Africa
99 I16 **Oud-Turnhout** Antwerpen, N Belgium
74 F7 **Oued-Zem** C Morocco
187 P16 **Ouégoa** Province Nord, C New Caledonia
76 L13 **Ouéléssébougou** var. Ouolossébougou. Koulikoro, SW Mali
77 N16 **Ouellé** E Ivory Coast
77 R16 **Ouémé** ≈ C Benin
77 O13 **Ouessa** S Burkina
102 D5 **Ouessant, Île d'** Eng. Ushant. island NW France
79 H17 **Ouésso** La Sangha, NW Congo
79 D15 **Ouest** Eng. West. ◈ province W Cameroon
190 G11 **Ouest, Baie de l'** bay Îles Wallis, Wallis and Futuna
15 Y7 **Ouest, Pointe de l'** headland Quebec, SE Canada
Ouezzane see Ouazzane
99 K20 **Ouffet** Liège, E Belgium
79 H14 **Ouham** ◈ prefecture NW Central African Republic
78 I13 **Ouham** ≈ Central African Republic/Chad
79 G14 **Ouham-Pendé** ◈ prefecture W Central African Republic
77 R16 **Ouidah** Eng. Whydah, Wida. S Benin
74 H6 **Oujda** Ar. Oudjda, Ujda. NE Morocco
76 I7 **Oujeft** Adrar, C Mauritania
93 L15 **Oulainen** Oulu, C Finland
Ould Yanja see Ould Yenjé
76 J10 **Ould Yenjé** var. Ould Yanja. Guidimaka, S Mauritania
93 L14 **Oulu** Swe. Uleåborg. Oulu, C Finland
93 M14 **Oulu** Swe. Uleåborg. ◈ province N Finland
93 L15 **Oulujärvi** Swe. Uleträsk. ◎ C Finland
93 M14 **Oulujoki** Swe. Uleälv. ≈ C Finland
93 L14 **Oulunsalo** Oulu, C Finland
106 A8 **Oulx** Piemonte, NE Italy
78 J9 **Oum-Chalouba** Borkou-Ennedi-Tibesti, NE Chad
76 M16 **Oumé** C Ivory Coast
74 F7 **Oum er Rbia** ≈ C Morocco
78 J10 **Oum-Hadjer** Batha, E Chad
92 K10 **Ounasjoki** ≈ N Finland
78 J7 **Ounianga Kébir** Borkou-Ennedi-Tibesti, N Chad
Ouolossébougou see Ouéléssébougou
Oup see Auob
99 K19 **Oupeye** Liège, E Belgium
99 N21 **Our** ≈ NW Europe
37 Q7 **Ouray** Colorado, C USA
103 R7 **Ource** ≈ C France
104 G9 **Ourém** Santarém, C Portugal
104 H4 **Ourense** Cast. Orense; Lat. Aurium. Galicia, NW Spain
104 I4 **Ourense** Cast. Orense. ◈ province Galicia, NW Spain
59 O15 **Ouricuri** Pernambuco, E Brazil
60 J9 **Ourinhos** São Paulo, S Brazil
104 G13 **Ourique** Beja, S Portugal
59 M20 **Ouro Preto** Minas Gerais, NE Brazil
Ours, Grand Lac de l' see Great Bear Lake
99 K20 **Ourthe** ≈ E Belgium
165 Q9 **Ōu-sanmyaku** ▲ Honshū, C Japan
97 M17 **Ouse** ≈ N England, UK
Ouse see Great Ouse
102 H7 **Oust** ≈ NW France
Outaouais see Ottawa
15 T4 **Outardes Quatre, Réservoir** ⊠ Quebec, SE Canada
15 T5 **Outardes, Rivière aux** ≈ Quebec, SE Canada
96 E8 **Outer Hebrides** var. Western Isles. island group NW Scotland, UK
30 K3 **Outer Island** island Apostle Islands, Wisconsin, N USA
35 S16 **Outer Santa Barbara Passage** passage California, SW USA
104 G3 **Outes** Galicia, NW Spain
83 C18 **Outjo** Kunene, N Namibia
11 T16 **Outlook** Saskatchewan, S Canada
93 N16 **Outokumpu** Itä-Suomi, E Finland
96 M2 **Out Skerries** island group NE Scotland, UK
187 Q16 **Ouvéa** island Îles Loyauté, NE New Caledonia
103 S14 **Ouvèze** ≈ SE France
182 L9 **Ouyen** Victoria, SE Australia
39 Q14 **Ouzinkie** Kodiak Island, Alaska, USA
137 O13 **Ovacık** Tunceli, E Turkey
106 C9 **Ovada** Piemonte, NE Italy
187 X14 **Ovalau** island C Fiji
62 G9 **Ovalle** Coquimbo, N Chile
83 C17 **Ovamboland** physical region N Namibia
54 L10 **Ovana, Cerro** ▲ S Venezuela
104 G7 **Ovar** Aveiro, N Portugal
114 L10 **Ovcharitsa, Yazovir** ⊠ SE Bulgaria
54 E6 **Ovejas** Sucre, NW Colombia
101 E16 **Overath** Nordrhein-Westfalen, W Germany
98 F13 **Overflakkee** island SW Netherlands
99 H19 **Overijse** Vlaams Brabant, C Belgium
98 N10 **Overijssel** ◈ province E Netherlands
98 M9 **Overijssels Kanaal** canal E Netherlands
92 K13 **Överkalix** Norrbotten, N Sweden
27 R4 **Overland Park** Kansas, C USA
99 L14 **Overloon** Noord-Brabant, SE Netherlands
99 K16 **Overpelt** Limburg, NE Belgium
35 Y10 **Overton** Nevada, W USA
25 W7 **Overton** Texas, SW USA
92 K13 **Övertorneå** Norrbotten, N Sweden
95 N18 **Överum** Kalmar, S Sweden
92 G13 **Överuman** ◎ N Sweden
162 H6 **Övgödiy** Dzavhan, C Mongolia
117 P11 **Ovidiopol'** Odes'ka Oblast', SW Ukraine
116 M14 **Ovidiu** Constanța, SE Romania
45 N10 **Oviedo** SW Dominican Republic
104 K2 **Oviedo** anc. Asturias. Asturias, NW Spain
104 K2 **Oviedo** ✕ Asturias, N Spain
Ovilava see Wels
118 D7 **Oviši** Ventspils, W Latvia
163 P10 **Ovoot** Sühbaatar, SE Mongolia
157 O4 **Övörhangay** ◈ province C Mongolia
94 E12 **Øvre Årdal** Sogn og Fjordane, S Norway
95 J14 **Övre Fryken** ◎ C Sweden
92 J11 **Övre Soppero** Norrbotten, N Sweden
117 N3 **Ovruch** Zhytomyrs'ka Oblast', N Ukraine
162 J8 **Övt** Övörhangay, C Mongolia
185 E24 **Owaka** Otago, South Island, NZ
79 H18 **Owando** prev. Fort-Rousset. Cuvette, C Congo
164 J14 **Owase** Mie, Honshū, SW Japan
27 P9 **Owasso** Oklahoma, C USA
29 V10 **Owatonna** Minnesota, N USA
173 O4 **Owen Fracture Zone** tectonic feature W Arabian Sea
185 H15 **Owen, Mount** ▲ South Island, NZ
185 H15 **Owen River** Tasman, South Island, NZ
44 D8 **Owen Roberts** ✕ Grand Cayman, Cayman Islands
20 I6 **Owensboro** Kentucky, S USA
35 T11 **Owens Lake** salt flat California, W USA
14 F14 **Owen Sound** Ontario, S Canada
14 F13 **Owen Sound** ◎ Ontario, S Canada
35 T10 **Owens River** ≈ California, W USA
186 F9 **Owen Stanley Range** ▲ S PNG
27 V5 **Owensville** Missouri, C USA
20 M4 **Owenton** Kentucky, S USA
77 U17 **Owerri** Imo, S Nigeria
184 M10 **Owhango** Manawatu-Wanganui, North Island, NZ
21 N5 **Owingsville** Kentucky, S USA
146 K10 **Owminzatovo-Toshi** Rus. Gory Auminzatau. ▲ N Uzbekistan
77 T16 **Owo** Ondo, SW Nigeria
31 R9 **Owosso** Michigan, N USA
35 V1 **Owyhee** Nevada, W USA
32 L14 **Owyhee, Lake** ◎ Oregon, NW USA
32 L15 **Owyhee River** ≈ Idaho/Oregon, NW USA
92 K1 **Öxarfjördhur** var. Axarfjördhur. fjord N Iceland
94 K12 **Oxberg** Dalarna, C Sweden
11 V17 **Oxbow** Saskatchewan, S Canada
95 O17 **Oxelösund** Södermanland, S Sweden
185 H18 **Oxford** Canterbury, South Island, NZ
97 M21 **Oxford** Lat. Oxonia. S England, UK
23 Q3 **Oxford** Alabama, S USA
22 L2 **Oxford** Mississippi, S USA
29 N16 **Oxford** Nebraska, C USA
18 I11 **Oxford** New York, NE USA
21 U8 **Oxford** North Carolina, SE USA
31 Q14 **Oxford** Ohio, N USA
18 H16 **Oxford** Pennsylvania, NE USA
11 X12 **Oxford House** Manitoba, C Canada
29 Y13 **Oxford Junction** Iowa, C USA
11 X12 **Oxford Lake** ◎ Manitoba, C Canada
97 M21 **Oxfordshire** cultural region S England, UK
Oxia see Oxyá
41 X12 **Oxkutzcab** Yucatán, SE Mexico
35 R15 **Oxnard** California, W USA
Oxonia see Oxford
14 I12 **Oxtongue** ≈ Ontario, SE Canada
Oxus see Amu Darya
115 E15 **Oxyá** var. Oxia. ▲ C Greece
164 L11 **Oyabe** Toyama, Honshū, SW Japan
Oyahue/Oyahue, Volcán see Ollagüe, Volcán
165 O12 **Oyama** Tochigi, Honshū, S Japan
47 U5 **Oyapock** ≈ E French Guiana
Oyapock see Oiapoque, Rio
55 Z10 **Oyapok, Baie de L'** bay Brazil/French Guiana
55 Z11 **Oyapok, Fleuve l'** var. Oyapock, Rio Oiapoque. ≈ Brazil/French Guiana **see also** Oiapoque, Rio
79 E17 **Oyem** Woleu-Ntem, N Gabon
11 R16 **Oyen** Alberta, SW Canada
95 I15 **Øyeren** ◎ S Norway
162 G6 **Oygon** Dzavhan, N Mongolia
96 I7 **Oykel** ≈ N Scotland, UK
123 R9 **Oymyakon** Respublika Sakha (Yakutiya), NE Russian Federation
79 H19 **Oyo** Cuvette, C Congo
77 S15 **Oyo** Oyo, W Nigeria
77 S15 **Oyo** ◈ state SW Nigeria
56 D13 **Oyón** Lima, C Peru
103 S10 **Oyonnax** Ain, E France
146 L10 **Oyoqighitma** Rus. Ayakagytma. Bukhoro Wiloyati, C Uzbekistan
146 M9 **Oyoqquduq** Rus. Ayakkuduk. Nawoiy Wiloyati, N Uzbekistan
32 F9 **Oysterville** Washington, NW USA
95 D14 **Øystese** Hordaland, S Norway
147 U10 **Oy-Tal** Oshskaya Oblast', SW Kyrgyzstan
147 T10 **Oy-Tal** ≈ SW Kyrgyzstan
145 S16 **Oytal** Zhambyl, S Kazakhstan
Oyyl see Uil
Ozarichi see Azarychy
23 R7 **Ozark** Alabama, S USA
27 S10 **Ozark** Arkansas, C USA
27 T8 **Ozark** Missouri, C USA
27 T8 **Ozark Plateau** plain Arkansas/Missouri, C USA
27 T6 **Ozarks, Lake of the** ⊠ Missouri, C USA
192 L10 **Ozbourn Seamount** undersea feature W Pacific Ocean
111 L20 **Ózd** Borsod-Abaúj-Zemplén, NE Hungary
112 D11 **Ozeblin** ▲ C Croatia
123 V11 **Ozernovskiy** Kamchatskaya Oblast', E Russian Federation
144 M7 **Ozërnoye** var. Ozërnyy. Kostanay, N Kazakhstan
Ozërnyy see Ozërnoye
115 D18 **Ozerós, Límni** ◎ W Greece
119 D14 **Ozersk** prev. Darkehnen, Ger. Angerapp. Kaliningradskaya Oblast', W Russian Federation
128 L4 **Ozery** Moskovskaya Oblast', W Russian Federation
Özgön see Uzgen
107 C17 **Ozieri** Sardegna, Italy, C Mediterranean Sea
111 I15 **Ozimek** Ger. Malapane. Opolskie, S Poland
129 R8 **Ozinki** Saratovskaya Oblast', W Russian Federation
Oziya see Ojiya
25 O10 **Ozona** Texas, SW USA
Ozorkov see Ozorków
110 J12 **Ozorków** Rus. Ozorkov. Łódź, C Poland
164 F14 **Ōzu** Ehime, Shikoku, SW Japan
137 R10 **Ozurget'i** prev. Makharadze. W Georgia

P

99 J17 **Paal** Limburg, NE Belgium
196 M14 **Paamiut** var. Pâmiut, Dan. Frederikshåb. Kitaa, S Greenland
167 N8 **Pa-an** Karen State, S Myanmar
101 L22 **Paar** ≈ SE Germany
83 E26 **Paarl** Western Cape, SW South Africa
93 L15 **Paavola** Oulu, C Finland
96 E8 **Pabbay** island NW Scotland, UK
153 T15 **Pabna** Rajshahi, W Bangladesh
109 U4 **Pabneukirchen** Oberösterreich, N Austria
118 H13 **Pabradė** Pol. Podbrodzie. Švenčionys, SE Lithuania
56 L13 **Pacahuaras, Río** ≈ N Bolivia
Pacaraima, Sierra/Pacaraim, Serra see Pakaraima Mountains
56 B11 **Pacasmayo** La Libertad, W Peru
42 D6 **Pacaya, Volcán de** ※ S Guatemala
115 K23 **Pachía** island Kykládes, Greece, Aegean Sea
107 L26 **Pachino** Sicilia, Italy, C Mediterranean Sea
56 F12 **Pachitea, Río** ≈ C Peru
154 I11 **Pachmarhi** Madhya Pradesh, C India
121 P3 **Páchna** var. Pakhna. SW Cyprus
115 H25 **Páchnes** ▲ Kríti, Greece, E Mediterranean Sea
54 F9 **Pacho** Cundinamarca, C Colombia
154 F12 **Pāchora** Mahārāshtra, C India
41 P13 **Pachuca** var. Pachuca de Soto. Hidalgo, C Mexico
Pachuca de Soto see Pachuca
27 W5 **Pacific** Missouri, C USA
192 L14 **Pacific-Antarctic Ridge** undersea feature S Pacific Ocean
32 F8 **Pacific Beach** Washington, NW USA
35 N10 **Pacific Grove** California, W USA
29 S15 **Pacific Junction** Iowa, C USA
198-199 **Pacific Ocean** ocean
131 Z10 **Pacific Plate** tectonic feature
113 J15 **Pačir** ▲ SW Yugoslavia
182 L5 **Packsaddle** New South Wales, SE Australia
32 H9 **Packwood** Washington, NW USA
Padalung see Phatthalung
168 J12 **Padang** Sumatera, W Indonesia
168 L9 **Padang Endau** Pahang, Peninsular Malaysia
Padangpandjang see Padangpanjang
168 I11 **Padangpanjang** prev. Padangpandjang. Sumatera, W Indonesia
168 I10 **Padangsidempuan** prev. Padangsidimpoean. Sumatera, W Indonesia
Padangsidimpoean see Padangsidempuan
126 I9 **Padany** Respublika Kareliya, NW Russian Federation
93 M18 **Padasjoki** Etelä-Suomi, S Finland
57 M22 **Padcaya** Tarija, S Bolivia
101 H14 **Paderborn** Nordrhein-Westfalen, NW Germany
Padeşul/Padeş, Vîrful see Padeş, Vârful
116 F12 **Padeş, Vârful** var. Padeşul; prev. Vîrful Padeş. ▲ W Romania
112 L10 **Padinska Skela** Serbia, N Yugoslavia
Padma see Brahmaputra
153 S14 **Padma** var. Ganges. ≈ Bangladesh/India **see also** Ganges
106 H8 **Padova** Eng. Padua; anc. Patavium. Veneto, NE Italy
82 A10 **Padrão, Ponta do** headland NW Angola
25 T16 **Padre Island** island Texas, SW USA
104 G3 **Padrón** Galicia, NW Spain
118 K13 **Padsvillye** Rus. Podsvil'ye. Vitsyebskaya Voblasts', N Belarus
182 K11 **Padthaway** South Australia
Padua see Padova
20 G7 **Paducah** Kentucky, S USA
25 P4 **Paducah** Texas, SW USA
105 N15 **Padul** Andalucía, S Spain
191 P8 **Paea** Tahiti, W French Polynesia
185 L14 **Paekakariki** Wellington, North Island, NZ
163 X11 **Paektu-san** var. Baitou Shan. ▲ China/North Korea
163 V15 **Paengnyŏng-do** island NW South Korea
184 M7 **Paeroa** Waikato, North Island, NZ
54 D12 **Páez** Cauca, SW Colombia
121 O3 **Páfos** var. Paphos. W Cyprus
121 O3 **Páfos** ✕ SW Cyprus
83 L19 **Pafúri** Gaza, SW Mozambique
112 C12 **Pag** It. Pago. Lika-Senj, W Croatia
112 B11 **Pag** It. Pago. island Zadar, SW Croatia
171 P7 **Pagadian** Mindanao, S Philippines
168 J13 **Pagai Selatan, Pulau** island Kepulauan Mentawai, W Indonesia
168 J13 **Pagai Utara, Pulau** island Kepulauan Mentawai, W Indonesia
188 K4 **Pagan** island C Northern Mariana Islands
115 G16 **Pagasitikós Kólpos** gulf E Greece
36 L8 **Page** Arizona, SW USA
29 Q5 **Page** North Dakota, N USA
118 D13 **Pagėgiai** Ger. Pogegen. Šilutė, SW Lithuania
21 S11 **Pageland** South Carolina, SE USA
81 G16 **Pager** ≈ NE Uganda
149 Q5 **Paghmān** Kābul, E Afghanistan
Pago see Pag
188 C16 **Pago Bay** bay E Guam, W Pacific Ocean
115 M20 **Pagóndas** var. Pagóndhas. Sámos, Dodekánisos, Greece, Aegean Sea
Pagóndhas see Pagóndas
192 J16 **Pago Pago** ○ (American Samoa) Tutuila, W American Samoa
37 R8 **Pagosa Springs** Colorado, C USA
38 H12 **Pahala** var. Pāhala. Hawaii, USA, C Pacific Ocean
168 K8 **Pahang** off. Negeri Pahang Darul Makmur. ◈ state Peninsular Malaysia
Pahang see Pahang, Sungai
168 L8 **Pahang, Sungai** var. Pahang, Sungei Pahang. ≈ Peninsular Malaysia
149 S8 **Pahārpur** North-West Frontier Province, NW Pakistan
185 B24 **Pahia Point** headland South Island, NZ
184 M13 **Pahiatua** Manawatu-Wanganui, North Island, NZ
38 H12 **Pahoa** Haw. Pāhoa. Hawaii, USA, C Pacific Ocean
23 Y14 **Pahokee** Florida, SE USA
35 X9 **Pahranagat Range** ▲ Nevada, W USA
35 W11 **Pahrump** Nevada, W USA
Pahsien see Chongqing
35 V9 **Pahute Mesa** ▲ Nevada, W USA
167 N7 **Pai** Mae Hong Son, NW Thailand
38 F10 **Paia** Haw. Pā'ia. Maui, Hawaii, USA, C Pacific Ocean
Pai-ch'eng see Baicheng
118 H4 **Paide** Ger. Weissenstein. Järvamaa, N Estonia
97 J24 **Paignton** SW England, UK
184 K3 **Paihia** Northland, North Island, NZ
93 M18 **Päijänne** ◎ S Finland
114 F13 **Païko** ▲ N Greece
57 M17 **Paila, Río** ≈ C Bolivia
167 Q12 **Pailin** Bătdâmbâng, W Cambodia
54 F6 **Pailitas** Cesar, N Colombia
38 F9 **Pailolo Channel** channel Hawaii, USA, C Pacific Ocean
93 K19 **Paimio** Swe. Pemar. Länsi-Suomi, W Finland
165 O16 **Paimi-saki** var. Yaeme-saki. headland Iriomote-jima, SW Japan
102 G5 **Paimpol** Côtes d'Armor, NW France
168 J12 **Painan** Sumatera, W Indonesia
63 G23 **Paine, Cerro** ▲ S Chile
31 U11 **Painesville** Ohio, N USA
31 S14 **Paint Creek** ≈ Ohio, N USA
36 L10 **Painted Desert** desert Arizona, SW USA
Paint Hills see Wemindji
30 M4 **Paint River** ≈ Michigan, N USA
25 P8 **Paint Rock** Texas, SW USA
21 O6 **Paintsville** Kentucky, S USA
Paisance see Piacenza
96 I12 **Paisley** W Scotland, UK
32 I15 **Paisley** Oregon, NW USA
105 R10 **País Valenciano** var. Valencia, Cat. València; anc. Valentia. ◈ autonomous community NE Spain
105 O3 **País Vasco** Basq. Euskadi, Eng. The Basque Country, Sp. Provincias Vascongadas. ◈ autonomous community N Spain
56 A9 **Paita** Piura, NW Peru
169 V6 **Paitan, Teluk** bay Sabah, East Malaysia
104 H7 **Paiva, Rio** ≈ N Portugal
92 K12 **Pajala** Norrbotten, N Sweden
104 K3 **Pajares, Puerto de** pass NW Spain
54 G9 **Pajarito** Boyacá, C Colombia
54 G4 **Pajaro** La Guajira, S Colombia
Pakanbaru see Pekanbaru
55 Q10 **Pakaraima Mountains** var. Serra Pacaraim, Sierra Pacaraima. ▲ N South America
167 P10 **Pak Chong** Nakhon Ratchasima, C Thailand
123 V8 **Pakhachi** Koryakskiy Avtonomnyy Okrug, E Russian Federation
Pakhna see Páchna
147 O11 **Pakhtakor** Jizzakh Wiloyati, C Uzbekistan
189 U16 **Pakin Atoll** atoll Caroline Islands, E Micronesia
149 Q12 **Pakistan** off. Islamic Republic of Pakistan, var. Islami Jamhuriya e Pakistan. ◆ republic S Asia
Pakistan, Islami Jamhuriya e see Pakistan
167 P8 **Pak Lay** var. Muang Pak Lay. Xaignabouli, C Laos
Paknam see Samut Prakan
166 L5 **Pakokku** Magwe, C Myanmar
110 I10 **Pakość** Ger. Pakosch. Kujawski-pomorskie, C Poland
Pakosch see Pakość
149 V10 **Pākpattan** Punjab, E Pakistan
167 O15 **Pak Phanang** var. Ban Pak Phanang. Nakhon Si Thammarat, SW Thailand
112 G9 **Pakrac** Hung. Pakrácz. Požega-Slavonija, NE Croatia
Pakrácz see Pakrac
118 F11 **Pakruojis** Pakruojis, N Lithuania
111 J24 **Paks** Tolna, S Hungary
Pak Sane see Paksan
Paksé see Pakxé
167 Q10 **Pak Thong Chai** Nakhon Ratchasima, C Thailand
149 R6 **Paktīā** ◈ province SE Afghanistan

◆ Country ● Country Capital ◇ Dependent Territory ○ Dependent Territory Capital ◈ Administrative Region ✕ International Airport ▲ Mountain ▲ Mountain Range ※ Volcano ≈ River ◎ Lake ⊠ Reservoir

149 Q7 **Paktīkā** ◈ *province* SE Afghanistan
171 N12 **Pakuli** Sulawesi, C Indonesia
81 F17 **Pakwach** NW Uganda
167 R8 **Pakxan** *var.* Muang Pakxan, Pak Sane. Bolikhamxai, C Laos
167 S10 **Pakxé** *var.* Paksé. Champasak, S Laos
78 G12 **Pala** Mayo-Kébbi, SW Chad
41 V14 **Palacios** Santa Fe, C Argentina
25 V13 **Palacios** Texas, SW USA
105 X5 **Palafrugell** Cataluña, NE Spain
107 L24 **Palagonia** Sicilia, Italy, C Mediterranean Sea
113 E17 **Palagruža** *It.* Pelagosa. *island* SW Croatia
115 G20 **Palaiá Epídavros** Pelopónnisos, S Greece
121 P3 **Palaichóri** *var.* Palekhori. C Cyprus
115 H25 **Palaiochóra** Kríti, Greece, E Mediterranean Sea
115 A15 **Palaiolastrítsa** *religious building* Kérkyra, Iónioi Nísoi, Greece, C Mediterranean Sea
115 J19 **Palaiópoli** Ándros, Kykládes, Greece, Aegean Sea
103 N5 **Palaiseau** Essonne, N France
Palakkad *see* Pālghāt
154 N11 **Pāla Laharha** Orissa, E India
83 G19 **Palamakoloi** Ghanzi, C Botswana
115 E16 **Palamás** Thessalía, C Greece
105 X5 **Palamós** Cataluña, NE Spain
118 J5 **Palamuse** *Ger.* Sankt-Bartholomäi. Jõgevamaa, E Estonia
183 Q14 **Palana** Tasmania, SE Australia
123 U9 **Palana** Koryakskiy Avtonomnyy Okrug, E Russian Federation
118 C11 **Palanga** *Ger.* Polangen. Palanga, NW Lithuania
143 V10 **Palangān, Kūh-e** ▲ E Iran
Palangkaraja *see* Palangkaraya
169 T12 **Palangkaraya** *prev.* Palangkaraja. Borneo, C Indonesia
155 H22 **Palani** Tamil Nādu, SE India
Palanka *see* Bačka Palanka
154 D9 **Pālanpur** Gujarāt, W India
Palantia *see* Palencia
83 I19 **Palapye** Central, SE Botswana
155 J19 **Pālār** ≈ SE India
104 H3 **Palas de Rei** Galicia, NW Spain
123 T9 **Palatka** Magadanskaya Oblast', E Russian Federation
23 W10 **Palatka** Florida, SE USA
188 B9 **Palau** *var.* Belau. ◆ *republic* W Pacific Ocean
131 Y14 **Palau Islands** *var.* Palau. *island group* N Palau
192 G16 **Palauli Bay** *bay* Savai'i, Samoa, C Pacific Ocean
167 N11 **Palaw** Tenasserim, S Myanmar
170 M6 **Palawan** *island* W Philippines
171 N6 **Palawan Passage** *passage* W Philippines
192 E7 **Palawan Trough** *undersea feature* S South China Sea
155 H23 **Pālayankottai** Tamil Nādu, SE India
107 L25 **Palazzola Acreide** *anc.* Acrae. Sicilia, Italy, C Mediterranean Sea
118 G3 **Paldiski** *prev.* Baltiski, *Eng.* Baltic Port, *Ger.* Baltischport. Harjumaa, NW Estonia
112 I13 **Pale** Republika Srpska, E Bosnia and Herzegovina
Palekhori *see* Palaichóri
168 L13 **Palembang** Sumatera, W Indonesia
63 G18 **Palena** Los Lagos, S Chile
63 G18 **Palena, Río** ≈ S Chile
104 M5 **Palencia** *anc.* Palantia, Pallantia. Castilla-León, NW Spain
104 M3 **Palencia** ◈ *province* Castilla-León, N Spain
35 X15 **Palen Dry Lake** ◎ California, W USA
41 V15 **Palenque** Chiapas, SE Mexico
41 V15 **Palenque** *var.* Ruinas de Palenque. *ruins* Chiapas, SE Mexico
45 O9 **Palenque, Punta** *headland* S Dominican Republic
Palenque, Ruinas de *see* Palenque
Palerme *see* Palermo
107 I23 **Palermo** *Fr.* Palerme; *anc.* Panhormus, Panormus. Sicilia, Italy, C Mediterranean Sea
25 V8 **Palestine** Texas, SW USA
25 V7 **Palestine, Lake** ⊞ Texas, SW USA
107 I15 **Palestrina** Lazio, C Italy
166 K5 **Paletwa** Chin State, W Myanmar
155 G21 **Pālghāt** *var.* Palakkad; *prev.* Pulicat. Kerala, SW India
152 F13 **Pāli** Rājasthān, N India
167 N16 **Palian** Trang, SW Thailand
189 O12 **Palikir** ● (Micronesia) Pohnpei, E Micronesia
Palimé *see* Kpalimé
107 L19 **Palinuro, Capo** *headland* S Italy
115 H15 **Palioúri, Akrotírio** *var.* Akra Kanestron. *headland* N Greece
33 R14 **Palisades Reservoir** ⊞ Idaho, NW USA
99 J23 **Paliseul** Luxembourg, SE Belgium
154 C11 **Pālitāna** Gujarāt, W India
118 F4 **Palivere** Läänemaa, W Estonia
41 V14 **Palizada** Campeche, SE Mexico
93 L18 **Pälkäne** Länsi-Suomi, W Finland
155 J22 **Palk Strait** *strait* India/Sri Lanka
155 J23 **Pallai** Northern Province, NW Sri Lanka
Pallantia *see* Palencia
106 C6 **Pallanza** Piemonte, NE Italy
129 Q9 **Pallasovka** Volgogradskaya Oblast', SW Russian Federation
Pallene/Pallíni *see* Kassándra
185 L15 **Palliser Bay** *bay* North Island, NZ
185 L15 **Palliser, Cape** *headland* North Island, NZ
191 U9 **Palliser, Îles** *island group* Îles Tuamotu, C French Polynesia
105 X9 **Palma** *var.* Palma de Mallorca. Mallorca, Spain, W Mediterranean Sea
105 X9 **Palma** × Mallorca, Spain, W Mediterranean Sea
82 Q12 **Palma** Cabo Delgado, N Mozambique
105 X10 **Palma, Badia de** *bay* Mallorca, Spain, W Mediterranean Sea
104 L13 **Palma del Río** Andalucía, S Spain
Palma de Mallorca *see* Palma
107 J25 **Palma di Montechiaro** Sicilia, Italy, C Mediterranean Sea
106 J7 **Palmanova** Friuli-Venezia Giulia, NE Italy
54 J7 **Palmarito** Apure, C Venezuela
43 N15 **Palmar Sur** Puntarenas, SE Costa Rica
60 I12 **Palmas** Paraná, S Brazil
59 K16 **Palmas** *var.* Palmas do Tocantins, C Brazil
Palmas do Tocantins *see* Palmas
54 D11 **Palmaseca** × (Cali) Valle del Cauca, SW Colombia
107 B21 **Palmas, Golfo di** *gulf* Sardegna, Italy, C Mediterranean Sea
44 I7 **Palma Soriano** Santiago de Cuba, E Cuba
23 Y12 **Palm Bay** Florida, SE USA
35 T14 **Palmdale** California, W USA
61 H14 **Palmeira das Missões** Rio Grande do Sul, S Brazil
82 A11 **Palmeirinhas, Ponta das** *headland* NW Angola
39 R11 **Palmer** Alaska, USA
19 N11 **Palmer** Massachusetts, NE USA
25 U7 **Palmer** Texas, SW USA
194 H4 **Palmer** *US research station* Antarctica
15 R11 **Palmer** ≈ Quebec, SE Canada
37 T5 **Palmer Lake** Colorado, C USA
194 J6 **Palmer Land** *physical region* Antarctica
14 F15 **Palmerston** Ontario, SE Canada
185 F22 **Palmerston** Otago, South Island, NZ
190 K15 **Palmerston** *island* S Cook Islands
Palmerston *see* Darwin
184 M12 **Palmerston North** Manawatu-Wanganui, North Island, NZ
76 L18 **Palmés, Cap des** *headland* SW Ivory Coast
23 V13 **Palmetto** Florida, SE USA
Palmetto State *see* South Carolina
107 M22 **Palmi** Calabria, SW Italy
54 D11 **Palmira** Valle del Cauca, W Colombia
56 F8 **Palmira, Río** ≈ N Peru
61 D19 **Palmitas** Soriano, SW Uruguay
Palmnicken *see* Yantarnyy
35 V15 **Palm Springs** California, W USA
27 V2 **Palmyra** Missouri, C USA
18 G10 **Palmyra** New York, NE USA
18 G15 **Palmyra** Pennsylvania, NE USA
21 V5 **Palmyra** Virginia, NE USA
Palmyra *see* Tudmur
192 L7 **Palmyra Atoll** ◇ *US privately owned unincorporated territory* C Pacific Ocean
154 P12 **Palmyras Point** *headland* E India
35 N9 **Palo Alto** California, W USA
25 O1 **Palo Duro Creek** ≈ Texas, SW USA
Paloe *see* Palu
Paloe *see* Denpasar, Bali, C Indonesia
168 L9 **Paloh** Johor, Peninsular Malaysia
80 F12 **Paloich** Upper Nile, SE Sudan
40 I3 **Palomas** Chihuahua, N Mexico
107 I15 **Palombara Sabina** Lazio, C Italy
105 S13 **Palos, Cabo de** *headland* SE Spain
104 I14 **Palos de la Frontera** Andalucía, S Spain
60 G11 **Palotina** Paraná, S Brazil
32 M9 **Palouse** Washington, NW USA
32 L9 **Palouse River** ≈ Washington, NW USA
35 Y16 **Palo Verde** California, W USA
57 E16 **Palpa** Ica, W Peru
95 M16 **Pålsboda** Örebro, C Sweden
93 M15 **Paltamo** Oulu, C Finland
171 N12 **Palu** *prev.* Paloe. Sulawesi, C Indonesia
137 P14 **Palu** Elâzığ, E Turkey
152 I11 **Palwal** Haryāna, N India
123 U6 **Palyavaam** ≈ NE Russian Federation
77 Q13 **Pama** SE Burkina
172 J14 **Pamandzi** × (Mamoudzou) Petite-Terre, E Mayotte
Pamangkat *see* Pemangkat
143 R11 **Pā Mazār** Kermān, C Iran
83 N19 **Pambarra** Inhambane, SE Mozambique
171 X12 **Pamdai** Irian Jaya, E Indonesia
103 N16 **Pamiers** Ariège, S France
147 T14 **Pamir** *var.* Daryā-ye Pāmīr, *Taj.* Dar"yoi Pomir. ≈ Afghanistan/Tajikistan *see also* Pāmīr, Daryā-ye
Pamir/Pāmīr, Daryā-ye *see* Pamirs
149 U1 **Pāmīr, Daryā-ye** *var.* Pamir, *Taj.* Dar"yoi Pomir. ≈ Afghanistan/Tajikistan *see also* Pamir
Pāmīr-e Khord *see* Little Pamir
131 Q8 **Pamirs** *Pash.* Daryā-ye Pāmīr, *Rus.* Pamir. ▲ C Asia
Pâmiut *see* Paamiut
21 X10 **Pamlico River** ≈ North Carolina, SE USA
21 Y10 **Pamlico Sound** *sound* North Carolina, SE USA
25 O2 **Pampa** Texas, SW USA
Pampa Aullagas, Lago *see* Poopó, Lago
61 B21 **Pampa Húmeda** *grassland* E Argentina
56 A10 **Pampa Las Salinas** *salt lake* NW Peru
57 F15 **Pampas** Huancavelica, C Peru
62 K13 **Pampas** *plain* C Argentina
55 O4 **Pampatar** Nueva Esparta, NE Venezuela
Pampeluna *see* Pamplona
104 H8 **Pampilhosa da Serra** *var.* Pampilhosa de Serra. Coimbra, N Portugal
173 Y15 **Pamplemousses** N Mauritius
54 G7 **Pamplona** Norte de Santander, N Colombia
105 Q3 **Pamplona** *Basq.* Iruña; *prev.* Pampeluna, *anc.* Pompaelo. Navarra, N Spain
114 I11 **Pamporovo** *prev.* Vasil Kolarov. Smolyan, S Bulgaria
136 D15 **Pamukkale** Denizli, W Turkey
21 W5 **Pamunkey River** ≈ Virginia, NE USA
152 K5 **Pamzal** Jammu and Kashmir, NW India
30 L14 **Pana** Illinois, N USA
41 Y11 **Panabá** Yucatán, SE Mexico
35 Y8 **Panaca** Nevada, W USA
115 E19 **Panachaikó** ▲ S Greece
14 F11 **Panache Lake** ◎ Ontario, S Canada
114 I10 **Panagyurishte** Pazardzhik, C Bulgaria
168 M16 **Panaitan, Pulau** *island* S Indonesia
115 D18 **Panaitolikó** ▲ C Greece
155 E17 **Panaji** *var.* Pangim, Panjim, New Goa. Goa, W India
43 T14 **Panama** *off.* Republic of Panama. ◆ *republic* Central America
43 T15 **Panamá** *var.* Ciudad de Panamá, *Eng.* Panama City. ● (Panama) Panamá, C Panama
43 U14 **Panamá** *off.* Provincia de Panamá. ◈ *province* E Panama
43 U15 **Panamá, Bahía de** *bay* N Gulf of Panama
193 T7 **Panama Basin** *undersea feature* E Pacific Ocean
43 T15 **Panama Canal** *canal* E Panama
23 R9 **Panama City** Florida, SE USA
43 T14 **Panama City** × Panamá, C Panama
Panama City *see* Panamá
23 Q9 **Panama City Beach** Florida, SE USA
43 T17 **Panamá, Golfo de** *var.* Gulf of Panama. *gulf* S Panama
Panama, Gulf of *see* Panamá, Golfo de
Panama, Isthmus of *see* Panamá, Istmo de
43 T15 **Panamá, Istmo de** *Eng.* Isthmus of Panama; *prev.* Isthmus of Darien. *isthmus* E Panama
35 U11 **Panamint Range** ▲ California, W USA
107 L22 **Panarea, Isola** *island* Isole Eolie, S Italy
106 G9 **Panaro** ≈ N Italy
171 P6 **Panay Gulf** *gulf* C Philippines
171 P5 **Panay Island** *island* C Philippines
35 W7 **Pancake Range** ▲ Nevada, W USA
112 M11 **Pančevo** *Ger.* Pantschowa, *Hung.* Pancsova. Serbia, N Yugoslavia
113 M15 **Pančićev Vrh** ▲ SW Yugoslavia
116 L12 **Panciu** Vrancea, E Romania
116 F10 **Pâncota** *Hung.* Pankota; *prev.* Pîncota. Arad, W Romania
Pancsova *see* Pančevo
83 N20 **Panda** Inhambane, SE Mozambique
171 X12 **Pandaidori, Kepulauan** *island group* E Indonesia
25 N11 **Pandale** Texas, SW USA
169 P12 **Pandang Tikar, Pulau** *island* N Indonesia
61 F20 **Pan de Azúcar** Maldonado, S Uruguay
118 H11 **Pandėlys** Rokiškis, NE Lithuania
155 F15 **Pandharpur** Mahārāshtra, W India
182 J1 **Pandie Pandie** South Australia
171 O12 **Pandiri** Sulawesi, C Indonesia
61 F20 **Pando** Canelones, S Uruguay
57 J14 **Pando** ◈ *department* N Bolivia
192 K9 **Pandora Bank** *undersea feature* W Pacific Ocean
95 G20 **Pandrup** Nordjylland, N Denmark
153 V12 **Pandu** Assam, NE India
79 J15 **Pandu** Equateur, NW Dem. Rep. Congo (Zaire)
Paneas *see* Bāniyās
59 F15 **Panelas** Mato Grosso, W Brazil
118 G12 **Panevėžys** Panevėžys, C Lithuania
Panfilov *see* Zharkent
129 N9 **Panfilovo** Volgogradskaya Oblast', SW Russian Federation
79 N17 **Panga** Orientale, N Dem. Rep. Congo (Zaire)
193 Y15 **Pangai** Lifuka, C Tonga
114 H13 **Pangaío** ▲ N Greece
79 G20 **Pangala** Le Pool, S Congo
81 J22 **Pangani** Tanga, E Tanzania
81 I21 **Pangani** ≈ NE Tanzania
186 K8 **Panggoe** Choiseul Island, NW Solomon Islands
79 N20 **Pangi** Maniema, E Dem. Rep. Congo (Zaire)
Pangim *see* Panaji
168 H8 **Pangkalanbrandan** Sumatera, W Indonesia
Pangkalanbun *see* Pangkalanbuun
169 R13 **Pangkalanbuun** *var.* Pangkalanbun. Borneo, C Indonesia
169 N12 **Pangkalpinang** Pulau Bangka, W Indonesia
11 U17 **Pangman** Saskatchewan, S Canada
Pang-Nga *see* Phang-Nga
9 S6 **Pangnirtung** Baffin Island, Nunavut, NE Canada
152 K6 **Pangong Tso** *var.* Bangong Co. ◎ China/India *see also* Bangong Co
36 K7 **Panguitch** Utah, W USA
186 J7 **Panguna** Bougainville Island, NE PNG
171 N8 **Pangutaran Group** *island group* Sulu Archipelago, SW Philippines
25 N2 **Panhandle** Texas, SW USA
Panhormus *see* Palermo
171 W14 **Paniai, Danau** ◎ Irian Jaya, E Indonesia
79 L21 **Pania-Mutombo** Kasai Oriental, C Dem. Rep. Congo (Zaire)
Panicherevo *see* Dolno Panicherevo
187 P16 **Panié, Mont** ▲ C New Caledonia
152 I10 **Pānīpat** Haryāna, N India
147 Q14 **Panj** *Rus.* Pyandzh; *prev.* Kirovabad. SW Tajikistan
147 P15 **Panj** *Rus.* Pyandzh. ≈ Afghanistan/Tajikistan
149 O5 **Panjāb** Bāmīān, C Afghanistan
147 O12 **Panjakent** *Rus.* Pendzhikent. W Tajikistan
148 L14 **Panjgūr** Baluchistān, SW Pakistan
Panjim *see* Panaji
163 U12 **Panjin** Liaoning, NE China
147 P14 **Panji Poyon** *Rus.* Nizhniy Pyandzh. SW Tajikistan
149 Q4 **Panjshīr** ≈ E Afghanistan
Pankota *see* Pâncota
77 W14 **Pankshin** Plateau, C Nigeria
163 Y10 **Pan Ling** ▲ N China
Panlong Jiang *see* Lô, Sông
154 J9 **Panna** Madhya Pradesh, C India
99 M16 **Panningen** Limburg, SE Netherlands
149 R13 **Pāno Āqil** Sind, SE Pakistan
121 P3 **Páno Léfkara** S Cyprus
121 O3 **Páno Panagiá** *var.* Pano Panayia. W Cyprus
Pano Panayia *see* Páno Panagiá
Panopolis *see* Akhmīm
29 U14 **Panora** Iowa, C USA
60 I8 **Panorama** São Paulo, S Brazil
115 I24 **Pánormos** Kríti, Greece, E Mediterranean Sea
Panormus *see* Palermo
163 W11 **Panshi** Jilin, NE China
59 H19 **Pantanal** *var.* Pantanalmato-Grossense. *swamp* SW Brazil
Pantanalmato-Grossense *see* Pantanal
61 H16 **Pântano Grande** Rio Grande do Sul, S Brazil
171 Q16 **Pantar, Pulau** *island* Kepulauan Alor, S Indonesia
21 X9 **Pantego** North Carolina, SE USA
107 G25 **Pantelleria** *anc.* Cossyra, Cosyra. Sicilia, Italy, C Mediterranean Sea
107 G25 **Pantelleria, Isola di** *island* SW Italy
Pante Macassar/Pante Makassar *see* Pante Makasar
171 Q16 **Pante Makasar** *var.* Pante Macassar, Pante Makassar. W East Timor
152 K10 **Pantnagar** Uttar Pradesh, N India
115 A15 **Pantokrátoras** ▲ Kérkyra, Iónioi Nísoi, Greece, C Mediterranean Sea
Pantschowa *see* Pančevo
41 P11 **Pánuco** Veracruz-Llave, E Mexico
41 P11 **Pánuco, Río** ≈ C Mexico
160 I12 **Panxian** Guizhou, S China
168 I10 **Panyabungan** Sumatera, N Indonesia
77 W14 **Panyam** Plateau, C Nigeria
157 N13 **Panzhihua** *prev.* Dukou, Tu-k'ou. Sichuan, C China
79 I22 **Panzi** Bandundu, SW Dem. Rep. Congo (Zaire)
42 E5 **Panzós** Alta Verapaz, E Guatemala
Pao-chi/Paoki *see* Baoji
Pao-king *see* Shaoyang
107 N20 **Paola** Calabria, SW Italy
121 P16 **Paola** E Malta
27 R5 **Paola** Kansas, C USA
31 O15 **Paoli** Indiana, N USA
187 R14 **Paonangisu** Éfaté, C Vanuatu
171 S13 **Paoni** *var.* Pauni. Pulau Seram, E Indonesia
37 Q5 **Paonia** Colorado, C USA
191 O7 **Paopao** Moorea, W French Polynesia
Pao-shan *see* Baoshan
Pao-ting *see* Baoding
Pao-t'ou/Paotow *see* Baotou
79 H14 **Paoua** Ouham-Pendé, W Central African Republic
Pap *see* Pop
111 H23 **Pápa** Veszprém, W Hungary
42 J12 **Papagayo, Golfo de** *gulf* NW Costa Rica
38 H11 **Papaikou** *var.* Pāpa'ikou. Hawaii, USA, C Pacific Ocean
41 R15 **Papaloapan, Río** ≈ S Mexico
184 L6 **Papakura** Auckland, North Island, NZ
41 Q13 **Papantla** *var.* Papantla de Olarte. Veracruz-Llave, E Mexico
Papantla de Olarte *see* Papantla
191 P8 **Papara** Tahiti, W French Polynesia
184 K4 **Paparoa** Northland, North Island, NZ
185 G16 **Paparoa Range** ▲ South Island, NZ
115 K20 **Pápas, Akrotirio** *headland* Ikaría, Dodekánisos, Greece, Aegean Sea
96 L2 **Papa Stour** *island* NE Scotland, UK
184 L6 **Papatoetoe** Auckland, North Island, NZ
185 E25 **Papatowai** Otago, South Island, NZ
96 K4 **Papa Westray** *island* NE Scotland, UK
191 T10 **Papeete** ○ (French Polynesia) Tahiti, W French Polynesia
100 F11 **Papenburg** Niedersachsen, NW Germany
98 H13 **Papendrecht** Zuid-Holland, SW Netherlands
191 Q7 **Papenoo** Tahiti, W French Polynesia
191 Q7 **Papenoo Rivière** ≈ Tahiti, W French Polynesia
191 N7 **Papetoai** Moorea, W French Polynesia
92 L3 **Papey** *island* E Iceland
Paphos *see* Páfos
40 H5 **Papigochic, Río** ≈ NW Mexico
118 E10 **Papilė** Akmenė, NW Lithuania
29 S15 **Papillion** Nebraska, C USA
15 T5 **Papinachois** ≈ Quebec, SE Canada
186 C9 **Papua, Gulf of** *gulf* S PNG
192 H8 **Papua New Guinea** *off.* Independent State of Papua New Guinea; *prev.* Territory of Papua and New Guinea, *abbrev.* PNG. ◆ *commonwealth republic* NW Melanesia
192 H8 **Papua Plateau** *undersea feature* N Coral Sea
112 G9 **Papuk** ▲ NE Croatia
167 N8 **Papun** Karen State, S Myanmar
42 L14 **Paquera** Puntarenas, W Costa Rica
55 V9 **Para** ◈ *district* N Surinam
58 I13 **Pará** *off.* Estado do Pará. ◈ *state* NE Brazil
Pará *see* Belém
180 I8 **Paraburdoo** Western Australia
57 E16 **Paracas, Península de** *peninsula* W Peru
59 L19 **Paracatu** Minas Gerais, NE Brazil
192 E6 **Paracel Islands** ◇ *disputed territory* SE Asia
182 I6 **Parachilna** South Australia
149 R6 **Pārachinār** North-West Frontier Province, NW Pakistan
112 N13 **Paraćin** Serbia, C Yugoslavia
14 K8 **Paradis** Quebec, SE Canada
39 N11 **Paradise** *var.* Paradise Hill. Alaska, USA
35 O5 **Paradise** California, W USA
35 X11 **Paradise** Nevada, W USA
Paradise Hill *see* Paradise
37 R11 **Paradise Hills** New Mexico, SW USA
Paradise of the Pacific *see* Hawaii
36 L13 **Paradise Valley** Arizona, SW USA
35 T2 **Paradise Valley** Nevada, W USA
115 O22 **Paradisi** × (Ródos) Ródos, Dodekánisos, Greece, Aegean Sea
154 P12 **Pārādwīp** Orissa, E India
Paraetonium *see* Maṭrūḥ
117 R4 **Parafiyivka** Chernihivs'ka Oblast', N Ukraine
36 K7 **Paragonah** Utah, W USA
27 X9 **Paragould** Arkansas, C USA
47 X8 **Paraguaçu** *var.* Paraguassú. ≈ E Brazil
60 J9 **Paraguaçu Paulista** São Paulo, S Brazil
54 H4 **Paraguaipoa** Zulia, NW Venezuela
62 O6 **Paraguarí** Paraguarí, S Paraguay
62 O7 **Paraguarí** *off.* Departamento de Paraguarí. ◈ *department* S Paraguay
55 O8 **Paragua, Río** ≈ SE Venezuela
57 O16 **Paraguá, Río** ≈ NE Bolivia
Paraguassú *see* Paraguaçu
62 N5 **Paraguay** ◆ *republic* C South America
47 U10 **Paraguay** *var.* Río Paraguay. ≈ C South America
Parahiba/Parahyba *see* Paraíba
59 P15 **Paraíba** *off.* Estado da Paraíba; *prev.* Parahiba, Parahyba. ◈ *state* E Brazil
Paraíba *see* João Pessoa
60 P9 **Paraíba do Sul, Rio** ≈ SE Brazil
Parainen *see* Pargas
43 N14 **Paraíso** Cartago, C Costa Rica
41 U14 **Paraíso** Tabasco, SE Mexico
57 O17 **Paraíso, Río** ≈ E Bolivia
Parajd *see* Praid
77 S14 **Parakou** C Benin
121 Q2 **Paralimni** E Cyprus
115 G18 **Paralímni, Límni** ◎ C Greece
55 W8 **Paramaribo** ● (Surinam) Paramaribo, N Surinam
55 W9 **Paramaribo** ◈ *district* N Surinam
55 W9 **Paramaribo** × Paramaribo, N Surinam
Paramithiá *see* Paramythiá
56 C13 **Paramonga** Lima, W Peru
123 V12 **Paramushir, Ostrov** *island* SE Russian Federation
115 C16 **Paramythiá** *var.* Paramithiá. Ípeiros, W Greece
62 M10 **Paraná** Entre Ríos, E Argentina
60 H11 **Paraná** *off.* Estado do Paraná. ◈ *state* S Brazil
47 U11 **Paraná** *var.* Alto Paraná. ≈ C South America
60 K12 **Paranaguá** Paraná, S Brazil
59 J20 **Paranaíba, Rio** ≈ E Brazil
61 C19 **Paraná Ibicuy, Río** ≈ E Argentina
59 H15 **Paranaíta** Mato Grosso, W Brazil
60 H9 **Paranapanema, Rio** ≈ S Brazil
60 K11 **Paranapiacaba, Serra do** ▲ S Brazil
60 H9 **Paranavaí** Paraná, S Brazil
143 N5 **Parandak** Markazī, W Iran
114 I12 **Paranéstio** Anatolikí Makedonía kai Thrakí, NE Greece
191 W11 **Paraoa** *atoll* Îles Tuamotu, C French Polynesia
184 L13 **Paraparaumu** Wellington, North Island, NZ
57 N20 **Parapeti, Río** ≈ SE Bolivia
54 L10 **Paraque, Cerro** ▲ W Venezuela
154 I11 **Parasiya** Madhya Pradesh, C India
115 M23 **Paraspóri, Akrotírio** *headland* Kárpathos, SE Greece
60 O10 **Parati** Rio de Janeiro, SE Brazil
59 K14 **Parauapebas** Pará, N Brazil
103 Q10 **Paray-le-Monial** Saône-et-Loire, C France
Parbatsar *see* Parvatsar
154 G13 **Parbhani** Mahārāshtra, C India
100 L10 **Parchim** Mecklenburg-Vorpommern, N Germany
Parchwitz *see* Prochowice
110 P13 **Parczew** Lubelskie, E Poland
60 L8 **Pardo, Rio** ≈ S Brazil
111 E16 **Pardubice** *Ger.* Pardubitz. Pardubický Kraj, C Czech Republic
111 E17 **Pardubický Kraj** ◈ region C Czech Republic
Pardubitz *see* Pardubice
119 F16 **Parechcha** *Pol.* Porzecze, *Rus.* Porech'ye. Hrodzyenskaya Voblasts', W Belarus
59 F17 **Parecis, Chapada dos** *var.* Serra dos Parecis. ▲ W Brazil
Parecis, Serra dos *see* Parecis, Chapada dos
104 M4 **Paredes de Nava** Castilla-León, N Spain
189 U12 **Parem** *island* Chuuk, C Micronesia
189 O12 **Parem Island** *island* E Micronesia
184 I1 **Parengarenga Harbour** *inlet* North Island, NZ
15 N8 **Parent** Quebec, SE Canada
102 J14 **Parentis-en-Born** Landes, SW France
Parenzo *see* Poreč
185 G20 **Pareora** Canterbury, South Island, NZ
171 N14 **Parepare** Sulawesi, C Indonesia
115 B16 **Párga** Ípeiros, W Greece
93 K20 **Pargas** *Swe.* Parainen. Länsi-Suomi, W Finland
64 O5 **Pargo, Ponta do** *headland* Madeira, Portugal, NE Atlantic Ocean
Paria, Golfo de *see* Paria, Gulf of
55 N6 **Pariaguán** Anzoátegui, NE Venezuela
45 X17 **Paria, Gulf of** *var.* Golfo de Paria. *gulf* Trinidad and Tobago/Venezuela
57 I15 **Pariamanu, Río** ≈ E Peru
36 L8 **Paria River** ≈ Utah, W USA
Parichi *see* Parychy
40 M14 **Paricutín, Volcán** ⩚ C Mexico
43 P16 **Parida, Isla** *island* SW Panama
55 T8 **Parika** NE Guyana
93 O18 **Parikkala** Etelä-Suomi, S Finland
58 E10 **Parima, Serra** *var.* Sierra Parima. ▲ Brazil/Venezuela *see also* Parima, Sierra
55 N11 **Parima, Sierra** *var.* Serra Parima. ▲ Brazil/Venezuela *see also* Parima, Serra
57 F17 **Parinacochas, Laguna** ◎ SW Peru
56 A9 **Pariñas, Punta** *headland* NW Peru
58 H12 **Parintins** Amazonas, N Brazil
103 O5 **Paris** *anc.* Lutetia, Lutetia Parisiorum, Parisii. ● (France) Paris, N France
191 Y2 **Paris** Kiritimati, E Kiribati
27 S11 **Paris** Arkansas, C USA
33 S16 **Paris** Idaho, NW USA
31 N14 **Paris** Illinois, N USA
20 M5 **Paris** Kentucky, S USA
27 V3 **Paris** Missouri, C USA
20 H8 **Paris** Tennessee, S USA
25 V5 **Paris** Texas, SW USA
Parisii *see* Paris
43 S16 **Parita** Herrera, S Panama
43 S16 **Parita, Bahía de** *bay* S Panama
Parkan/Párkány *see* Štúrovo
93 K18 **Parkano** Länsi-Suomi, W Finland
27 N6 **Park City** Kansas, C USA
36 L3 **Park City** Utah, W USA
36 I12 **Parker** Arizona, SW USA
23 R9 **Parker** Florida, SE USA
29 R11 **Parker** South Dakota, N USA
35 Z14 **Parker Dam** California, W USA
29 W13 **Parkersburg** Iowa, C USA
21 Q3 **Parkersburg** West Virginia, NE USA
29 T7 **Parkers Prairie** Minnesota, N USA
171 P8 **Parker Volcano** ⩚ Mindanao, S Philippines
181 W13 **Parkes** New South Wales, SE Australia
30 K4 **Park Falls** Wisconsin, N USA
Parkhar *see* Farkhor
14 E16 **Parkhill** Ontario, S Canada
29 T5 **Park Rapids** Minnesota, N USA
29 Q3 **Park River** North Dakota, N USA
29 Q11 **Parkston** South Dakota, N USA
10 L17 **Parksville** Vancouver Island, British Columbia, SW Canada
37 S3 **Parkview Mountain** ▲ Colorado, C USA
105 N8 **Parla** Madrid, C Spain
29 S8 **Parle, Lac qui** ⊞ Minnesota, N USA
115 F20 **Parlía Tyroú** Pelopónnisos, S Greece
155 G14 **Parli Vaijnāth** Mahārāshtra, C India
106 F9 **Parma** Emilia-Romagna, N Italy
31 T11 **Parma** Ohio, N USA
Parnahyba *see* Parnaíba

58 N13 **Parnaíba** var. Parnahyba. Piauí, E Brazil
65 J14 **Parnaíba Ridge** undersea feature C Atlantic Ocean
58 N13 **Parnaíba, Rio** ∽ NE Brazil
115 F18 **Parnassós** ▲ C Greece
185 J17 **Parnassus** Canterbury, South Island, NZ
182 H10 **Parndana** South Australia
115 H19 **Párnitha** ▲ C Greece
115 F21 **Párnon** ▲ S Greece
118 G5 **Pärnu** Ger. Pernau, Latv. Pērnava; prev. Rus. Pernov. Pärnumaa, SW Estonia
118 G6 **Pärnu** var. Parnu Jõgi, Ger. Pernau. ∽ SW Estonia
118 G5 **Pärnu-Jaagupi** Ger. Sankt-Jakobi. Pärnumaa, SW Estonia
Parnu Jõgi see Pärnu
118 G5 **Pärnu Laht** Ger. Pernauer Bucht. bay SW Estonia
118 F5 **Pärnumaa** off. Pärnu Maakond. ◆ province SW Estonia
153 T11 **Paro** W Bhutan
153 T11 **Paro** ✕ (Thimphu) W Bhutan
185 G17 **Paroa** West Coast, South Island, NZ
163 X14 **P'aro-ho** var. Hwach'ŏn-chŏsuji. ⊞ N South Korea
183 N6 **Paroo River** seasonal river New South Wales/Queensland, SE Australia
Paropamisus Range see Sefidkūh, Selseleh-ye
115 J21 **Páros** Páros, Kykládes, Greece, Aegean Sea
115 J21 **Páros** island Kykládes, Greece, Aegean Sea
36 K7 **Parowan** Utah, W USA
103 U13 **Parpaillon** ▲ SE France
108 I9 **Parpan** Graubünden, S Switzerland
62 G13 **Parral** Maule, C Chile
Parral see Hidalgo del Parral
183 T9 **Parramatta** New South Wales, SE Australia
21 Y6 **Parramore Island** island Virginia, NE USA
40 M8 **Parras** var. Parras de la Fuente. Coahuila de Zaragoza, NE Mexico
Parras de la Fuente see Parras
42 M14 **Parrita** Puntarenas, S Costa Rica
8 L5 **Parry Channel** channel N Canada
14 G13 **Parry Island** island Ontario, S Canada
8 M4 **Parry Islands** island group Nunavut, NW Canada
14 G12 **Parry Sound** Ontario, S Canada
110 F7 **Parsęta** Ger. Persante. ∽ NW Poland
28 L3 **Parshall** North Dakota, N USA
27 Q7 **Parsons** Kansas, C USA
20 H9 **Parsons** Tennessee, S USA
21 T3 **Parsons** West Virginia, NE USA
Parsonstown see Birr
100 P11 **Parsteiner See** ◎ NE Germany
107 I24 **Partanna** Sicilia, Italy, C Mediterranean Sea
108 J8 **Partenen** Graubünden, E Switzerland
102 K9 **Parthenay** Deux-Sèvres, W France
95 J19 **Partille** Västra Götaland, S Sweden
107 I23 **Partinico** Sicilia, Italy, C Mediterranean Sea
111 I20 **Partizánske** prev. Šimonovany; Hung. Simony. Trenčiansky Kraj, W Slovakia
58 H11 **Paru de Oeste, Rio** ∽ N Brazil
182 K9 **Paruna** South Australia
58 I11 **Paru, Rio** ∽ N Brazil
Parvān see Parwān
155 M14 **Pārvatipuram** Andhra Pradesh, E India
152 G12 **Parvatsar** prev. Parbatsar. Rājasthān, N India
149 Q5 **Parwān** Per. Parvān. ◆ province E Afghanistan
158 I15 **Paryang** Xizang Zizhiqu, W China
119 M18 **Parychy** Rus. Parichi. Homyel'skaya Voblasts', SE Belarus
83 J21 **Parys** Free State, C South Africa
35 T15 **Pasadena** California, W USA
25 W11 **Pasadena** Texas, SW USA
56 B8 **Pasaje** El Oro, SW Ecuador
137 T9 **P'asanauri** N Georgia
168 I13 **Pasapuat** Pulau Pagai Utara, W Indonesia
167 N7 **Pasawng** Kayah State, C Myanmar
114 L13 **Paşayiğit** Edirne, NW Turkey
23 N9 **Pascagoula** Mississippi, S USA
22 M8 **Pascagoula River** ∽ Mississippi, S USA
116 F12 **Paşcani** Hung. Páskán. Iaşi, NE Romania
109 T4 **Pasching** Oberösterreich, N Austria
32 K10 **Pasco** Washington, NW USA
56 E13 **Pasco** off. Departamento de Pasco. ◆ department C Peru
191 N11 **Pascua, Isla de** var. Rapa Nui, Eng. Easter Island. island E Pacific Ocean
63 G21 **Pascua, Río** ∽ S Chile
103 N1 **Pas-de-Calais** ◆ department N France
100 P10 **Pasewalk** Mecklenburg-Vorpommern, NE Germany
11 T10 **Pasfield Lake** ◎ Saskatchewan, C Canada
Pa-shih Hai-hsia see Bashi Channel
Pashkeni see Bolyarovo
Pashmakli see Smolyan
153 X10 **Pāsighāt** Arunāchal Pradesh, NE India
137 Q12 **Pasinler** Erzurum, NE Turkey
Pasi Oloy, Qatorkŭhi see Zaalayskiy Khrebet
42 E3 **Pasión, Río de la** ∽ N Guatemala
168 J12 **Pasirganting** Sumatera, W Indonesia
Pasirpangarayan see Bagansiapiapi
168 K6 **Pasir Puteh** var. Pasir Putih. Kelantan, Peninsular Malaysia
169 R9 **Pasir, Tanjung** headland East Malaysia
95 N20 **Påskallavik** Kalmar, S Sweden
Páskán see Paşcani
110 K7 **Pasłęk** Ger. Preußisch Holland. Warmińsko-Mazurskie, NE Poland
110 K7 **Pasłęka** Ger. Passarge. ∽ N Poland
148 K16 **Pasni** Baluchistān, SW Pakistan
63 I18 **Paso de Indios** Chubut, S Argentina
54 L7 **Paso del Caballo** Guárico, N Venezuela
61 E15 **Paso de los Libres** Corrientes, NE Argentina
61 E18 **Paso de los Toros** Tacuarembó, C Uruguay
35 P12 **Paso Robles** California, W USA
15 Y7 **Paspébiac** Quebec, SE Canada
11 U14 **Pasquia Hills** ▲ Saskatchewan, S Canada
149 W7 **Pasrūr** Punjab, E Pakistan
30 M1 **Passage Island** island Michigan, N USA
65 B24 **Passage Islands** island group W Falkland Islands
8 K5 **Passage Point** headland Banks Island, Northwest Territories, NW Canada
Passarge see Pasłęka
115 C15 **Passarón** ancient monument Ípeiros, W Greece
Passarowitz see Požarevac
101 O22 **Passau** Bayern, SE Germany
22 M9 **Pass Christian** Mississippi, S USA
107 L26 **Passero, Capo** headland Sicilia, Italy, C Mediterranean Sea
171 P5 **Passi** Panay Island, C Philippines
61 H14 **Passo Fundo** Rio Grande do Sul, S Brazil
60 H13 **Passo Fundo, Barragem de** ⊞ S Brazil
61 H15 **Passo Real, Barragem de** ⊞ S Brazil
59 L20 **Passos** Minas Gerais, NE Brazil
167 X10 **Passu Keah** island S Paracel Islands
118 J13 **Pastavy** Pol. Postawy, Rus. Postavy. Vitsyebskaya Voblasts', NW Belarus
56 D7 **Pastaza** ◆ province E Ecuador
56 D9 **Pastaza, Río** ∽ Ecuador/Peru
61 A21 **Pasteur** Buenos Aires, E Argentina
15 V3 **Pasteur** ∽ Quebec, SE Canada
147 Q12 **Pastigav** Rus. Pastigov. W Tajikistan
Pastigov see Pastigav
54 C13 **Pasto** Nariño, SW Colombia
38 M10 **Pastol Bay** bay Alaska, USA
37 O8 **Pastora Peak** ▲ Arizona, SW USA
105 O8 **Pastrana** Castilla-La Mancha, C Spain
169 S16 **Pasuruan** prev. Pasoeroean. Jawa, C Indonesia
118 F11 **Pasvalys** Pasvalys, N Lithuania
111 K21 **Pásztó** Nógrád, N Hungary
189 U12 **Pata** var. Patta. atoll Chuuk Islands, C Micronesia
36 M16 **Patagonia** Arizona, SW USA
63 H20 **Patagonia** physical region Argentina/Chile
Patalung see Phatthalung
154 D9 **Pātan** Gujarāt, W India
154 J10 **Pātan** Madhya Pradesh, C India
171 S11 **Patani** Pulau Halmahera, E Indonesia
Patani see Pattani
15 V7 **Patapédia Est** ∽ Quebec, SE Canada
116 K13 **Pătâriagele** prev. Pătiriagele. Buzău, SE Romania
Patavium see Padova
182 I5 **Patawarta Hill** ▲ South Australia
182 L10 **Patchewollock** Victoria, SE Australia
184 K11 **Patea** Taranaki, North Island, NZ
184 K11 **Patea** ∽ North Island, NZ
77 U15 **Pategi** Kwara, C Nigeria
81 K20 **Pate Island** var. Patta Island. island SE Kenya
105 S10 **Paterna** País Valenciano, E Spain
109 R9 **Paternion** Slvn. Špatrjan. Kärnten, S Austria
107 L24 **Paternò** anc. Hybla, Hybla Major. Sicilia, Italy, C Mediterranean Sea
32 J7 **Pateros** Washington, NW USA
18 J14 **Paterson** New Jersey, NE USA
32 J10 **Paterson** Washington, NW USA
185 C25 **Paterson Inlet** inlet Stewart Island, NZ
98 N6 **Paterswolde** Drenthe, NE Netherlands
152 H7 **Pathānkot** Himāchal Pradesh, N India
Pathein see Bassein
33 W15 **Pathfinder Reservoir** ⊞ Wyoming, C USA
167 O11 **Pathum Thani** var. Patumdhani, Prathum Thani. Pathum Thani, C Thailand
54 C12 **Patía** var. El Bordo. Cauca, SW Colombia
152 I9 **Patiāla** var. Puttiala. Punjab, NW India
54 B12 **Patía, Río** ∽ SW Colombia
188 D15 **Pati Point** headland NE Guam
Pătiriagele see Pătâriagele
56 C13 **Pativilca** Lima, W Peru
166 M1 **Pātkai Bum** var. Patkai Range. ▲ Myanmar/India
Patkai Range see Pātkai Bum
115 L20 **Pátmos** Pátmos, Dodekánisos, Greece, Aegean Sea
115 L20 **Pátmos** island Dodekánisos, Greece, Aegean Sea
153 P13 **Patna** var. Azimabad. Bihār, N India
154 M12 **Patnāgarh** Orissa, E India
171 O5 **Patnongon** Panay Island, C Philippines
137 S13 **Patnos** Ağrı, E Turkey
60 H12 **Pato Branco** Paraná, S Brazil
31 O16 **Patoka Lake** ◎ Indiana, N USA
92 L9 **Patoniva** Lapp. Buoddobohki. Lappi, N Finland
113 K21 **Patos** var. Patosi. Fier, SW Albania
Patos see Patos de Minas
59 K19 **Patos de Minas** var. Patos. Minas Gerais, NE Brazil
Patosi see Patos
61 I17 **Patos, Lagoa dos** lagoon S Brazil
62 J9 **Patquía** La Rioja, C Argentina
115 E19 **Pátra** Eng. Patras; prev. Pátrai. Dytikí Ellás, S Greece
Pátrai/Patras see Pátra
115 D18 **Patraïkós Kólpos** gulf S Greece
92 G2 **Patreksfjördhur** Vestfirdhir, W Iceland
24 M7 **Patricia** Texas, SW USA
63 F21 **Patricio Lynch, Isla** island S Chile
Patta see Pata
Patta Island see Pate Island
167 O16 **Pattani** var. Patani. Pattani, SW Thailand
167 P12 **Pattaya** Chon Buri, S Thailand
19 S4 **Patten** Maine, NE USA
35 O9 **Patterson** California, W USA
22 J10 **Patterson** Louisiana, S USA
35 R7 **Patterson, Mount** ▲ California, W USA
31 P4 **Patterson, Point** headland Michigan, N USA
107 L23 **Patti** Sicilia, Italy, C Mediterranean Sea
107 L23 **Patti, Golfo di** gulf Sicilia, Italy, C Mediterranean Sea
93 L14 **Pattijoki** Oulu, W Finland
193 Q4 **Patton Escarpment** undersea feature E Pacific Ocean
27 S2 **Pattonsburg** Missouri, C USA
(0) D6 **Patton Seamount** undersea feature NE Pacific Ocean
10 J12 **Pattullo, Mount** ▲ British Columbia, W Canada
Patuakhali see Patukhali
42 M5 **Patuca, Río** ∽ E Honduras
153 U16 **Patukhali** var. Patuakhali. Khulna, S Bangladesh
Patumdhani see Pathum Thani
40 M14 **Pátzcuaro** Michoacán de Ocampo, SW Mexico
42 C6 **Patzicía** Chimaltenango, S Guatemala
102 K16 **Pau** Pyrénées-Atlantiques, SW France
102 J12 **Pauillac** Gironde, SW France
166 L5 **Pauk** Magwe, W Myanmar
8 I6 **Paulatuk** Northwest Territories, NW Canada
42 K5 **Paulayá, Río** ∽ NE Honduras
22 M6 **Paulding** Mississippi, S USA
31 Q12 **Paulding** Ohio, N USA
29 S12 **Paullina** Iowa, C USA
59 P15 **Paulo Afonso** Bahia, E Brazil
38 M16 **Pauloff Harbor** var. Pavlor Harbour. Sanak Island, Alaska, USA
27 N12 **Pauls Valley** Oklahoma, C USA
166 L7 **Paungde** Pegu, C Myanmar
Pauni see Paoni
152 K9 **Pauri** Uttar Pradesh, N India
Pautalia see Kyustendil
142 J5 **Pāveh** Kermānshāh, NW Iran
128 L5 **Pavelets** Ryazanskaya Oblast', W Russian Federation
106 D8 **Pavia** anc. Ticinum. Lombardia, N Italy
118 C9 **Pāvilosta** Liepāja, W Latvia
127 P14 **Pavino** Kostromskaya Oblast', NW Russian Federation
114 J8 **Pavlikeni** Veliko Tŭrnovo, N Bulgaria
145 T8 **Pavlodar** Pavlodar, NE Kazakhstan
145 S9 **Pavlodar** off. Pavlodarskaya Oblast', Kaz. Pavlodar Oblysy. ◆ province NE Kazakhstan
Pavlodar Oblysy/Pavlodarskaya Oblast' see Pavlodar
Pavlograd see Pavlohrad
117 U7 **Pavlohrad** Rus. Pavlograd. Dnipropetrovs'ka Oblast', E Ukraine
Pavlor Harbour see Pauloff Harbor
145 R9 **Pavlovka** Akmola, C Kazakhstan
129 V4 **Pavlovka** Respublika Bashkortostan, W Russian Federation
129 Q7 **Pavlovka** Ul'yanovskaya Oblast', W Russian Federation
129 N3 **Pavlovo** Nizhegorodskaya Oblast', W Russian Federation
128 L9 **Pavlovsk** Voronezhskaya Oblast', W Russian Federation
128 L13 **Pavlovskaya** Krasnodarskiy Kray, SW Russian Federation
117 S7 **Pavlysh** Kirovohrads'ka Oblast', C Ukraine
106 F10 **Pavullo nel Frignano** Emilia-Romagna, C Italy
27 P8 **Pawhuska** Oklahoma, C USA
21 U13 **Pawleys Island** South Carolina, SE USA
167 N6 **Pawn** ∽ C Myanmar
30 K14 **Pawnee** Illinois, N USA
27 O9 **Pawnee** Oklahoma, C USA
37 U2 **Pawnee Buttes** ▲ Colorado, C USA
29 S17 **Pawnee City** Nebraska, C USA
26 K5 **Pawnee River** ∽ Kansas, C USA
31 O10 **Paw Paw** Michigan, N USA
31 O10 **Paw Paw Lake** Michigan, N USA
19 O12 **Pawtucket** Rhode Island, NE USA
Pax Augusta see Badajoz
115 I25 **Paximádia** island SE Greece
Pax Julia see Beja
115 B16 **Paxoí** island Iónioi Nísoi, Greece, C Mediterranean Sea
39 S10 **Paxson** Alaska, USA
30 M13 **Paxton** Illinois, N USA
126 J11 **Pay** Respublika Kareliya, NW Russian Federation
166 M8 **Payagyi** Pegu, SW Myanmar
108 C9 **Payerne** Ger. Peterlingen. Vaud, W Switzerland
32 M13 **Payette** Idaho, NW USA
32 M13 **Payette River** ∽ Idaho, NW USA
127 V2 **Pay-Khoy, Khrebet** ▲ NW Russian Federation
Payne see Kangirsuk
12 K4 **Payne, Lac** ◎ Quebec, NE Canada
29 T8 **Paynesville** Minnesota, N USA
169 S8 **Payong, Tanjung** headland East Malaysia
Payo Obispo see Chetumal
61 D18 **Paysandú** Paysandú, W Uruguay
61 D17 **Paysandú** ◆ department W Uruguay
102 I7 **Pays de la Loire** ◆ region NW France
36 L12 **Payson** Arizona, SW USA
36 L4 **Payson** Utah, W USA
127 W4 **Payyer, Gora** ▲ NW Russian Federation
Payzawat see Jiashi
137 Q11 **Pazar** Rize, NE Turkey
136 F10 **Pazarbaşı Burnu** headland NW Turkey
136 M16 **Pazarcık** Kahramanmaraş, S Turkey
114 I10 **Pazardzhik** prev. Tatar Pazardzhik. Pazardzhik, C Bulgaria
114 H11 **Pazardzhik** ◆ province C Bulgaria
54 H9 **Paz de Ariporo** Casanare, E Colombia
112 A10 **Pazin** Ger. Mitterburg, It. Pisino. Istra, NW Croatia
42 D7 **Paz, Río** ∽ El Salvador/Guatemala
113 O18 **Pčinja** ∽ N FYR Macedonia
193 V15 **Pea** Tongatapu, S Tonga
27 O6 **Peabody** Kansas, C USA
11 O12 **Peace** ∽ Alberta/British Columbia, W Canada
Peace Garden State see North Dakota
11 Q10 **Peace Point** Alberta, C Canada
11 O12 **Peace River** Alberta, W Canada
23 W13 **Peace River** ∽ Florida, SE USA
11 N17 **Peachland** British Columbia, SW Canada
36 J10 **Peach Springs** Arizona, SW USA
Peach State see Georgia
23 S4 **Peachtree City** Georgia, SE USA
189 Y13 **Peacock Point** point SE Wake Island
97 M18 **Peak District** physical region C England, UK
183 Q7 **Peak Hill** New South Wales, SE Australia
65 G15 **Peak, The** ▲ C Ascension Island
105 O13 **Peal de Becerro** Andalucía, S Spain
189 X11 **Peale Island** island N Wake Island
37 O6 **Peale, Mount** ▲ Utah, W USA
39 O4 **Peard Bay** bay Alaska, USA
23 Q7 **Pea River** ∽ Alabama/Florida, S USA
25 W11 **Pearland** Texas, SW USA
38 D9 **Pearl City** Oahu, Hawaii, USA, C Pacific Ocean
38 D9 **Pearl Harbor** inlet Oahu, Hawaii, USA, C Pacific Ocean
Pearl Islands see Perlas, Archipiélago de las
Pearl Lagoon see Perlas, Laguna de
22 M5 **Pearl River** ∽ Louisiana/Mississippi, S USA
25 Q13 **Pearsall** Texas, SW USA
23 U7 **Pearson** Georgia, SE USA
25 P4 **Pease River** ∽ Texas, SW USA
12 F7 **Peawanuk** Ontario, C Canada
83 P16 **Pebane** Zambézia, NE Mozambique
65 C23 **Pebble Island** island N Falkland Islands
65 C23 **Pebble Island Settlement** Pebble Island, N Falkland Islands
113 L16 **Peć** Alb. Pejë, Turk. Ipek. Serbia, S Yugoslavia
25 R8 **Pecan Bayou** ∽ Texas, SW USA
22 H10 **Pecan Island** Louisiana, S USA
60 L12 **Peças, Ilha das** island S Brazil
30 L10 **Pecatonica River** ∽ Illinois/Wisconsin, N USA
108 G10 **Peccia** Ticino, S Switzerland
Pechenegi see Pechenihy
Pechenezhskoye Vodokhranilishche see Pecheniz'ke Vodoskhovyshche
126 I2 **Pechenga** Fin. Petsamo. Murmanskaya Oblast', NW Russian Federation
117 V5 **Pechenihy** Rus. Pechenegi. Kharkivs'ka Oblast', E Ukraine
117 V5 **Pecheniz'ke Vodoskhovyshche** Rus. Pechenezhskoye Vodokhranilishche. ⊞ E Ukraine
127 U7 **Pechora** Respublika Komi, NW Russian Federation
127 R6 **Pechora** ∽ NW Russian Federation
Pechora Bay see Pechorskaya Guba
Pechora Sea see Pechorskoye More
127 S3 **Pechorskaya Guba** Eng. Pechora Bay. bay NW Russian Federation
122 H7 **Pechorskoye More** Eng. Pechora Sea. sea NW Russian Federation
116 E11 **Pecica** Ger. Petschka, Hung. Ópécska. Arad, W Romania
24 K8 **Pecos** Texas, SW USA
25 N11 **Pecos River** ∽ New Mexico/Texas, SW USA
111 I25 **Pécs** Ger. Fünfkirchen; Lat. Sopianae. Baranya, SW Hungary
43 T17 **Pedasí** Los Santos, S Panama
Pedde see Pedja
183 O17 **Pedder, Lake** ◎ Tasmania, SE Australia
44 M10 **Pedernales** SW Dominican Republic
55 Q5 **Pedernales** Delta Amacuro, NE Venezuela
25 R10 **Pedernales River** ∽ Texas, SW USA
62 H6 **Pedernales, Salar de** salt lake N Chile
Pedhoulas see Pedoulás
55 X11 **Pédima** var. Malavate. SW French Guiana
182 F1 **Pedirka** South Australia
171 S11 **Pediwang** Pulau Halmahera, E Indonesia
118 I5 **Pedja** var. Pedja Jõgi, Ger. Pedde. ∽ E Estonia
Pedja Jõgi see Pedja
121 O3 **Pedoulás** var. Pedhoulas. W Cyprus
59 N18 **Pedra Azul** Minas Gerais, NE Brazil
104 I3 **Pedrafita, Porto de** var. Puerto de Piedrafita. pass NW Spain
76 E9 **Pedra Lume** Sal, NE Cape Verde
43 P16 **Pedregal** Chiriquí, W Panama
54 J4 **Pedregal** Falcón, N Venezuela
40 L9 **Pedriceña** Durango, C Mexico
60 L11 **Pedro Barros** São Paulo, S Brazil
39 Q13 **Pedro Bay** Alaska, USA
62 H4 **Pedro de Valdivia** var. Oficina Pedro de Valdivia. Antofagasta, N Chile
62 P4 **Pedro Juan Caballero** Amambay, E Paraguay
63 L15 **Pedro Luro** Buenos Aires, E Argentina
105 O10 **Pedro Muñoz** Castilla-La Mancha, C Spain
155 J22 **Pedro, Point** headland NW Sri Lanka
182 K9 **Peebinga** South Australia
96 J13 **Peebles** SE Scotland, UK
31 S15 **Peebles** Ohio, N USA
96 J12 **Peebles** cultural region SE Scotland, UK
18 K13 **Peekskill** New York, NE USA
97 I16 **Peel** W Isle of Man
8 G7 **Peel** ∽ Northwest Territories/Yukon Territory, NW Canada
8 K5 **Peel Point** headland Victoria Island, Northwest Territories, NW Canada
8 M5 **Peel Sound** passage Nunavut, N Canada
100 N9 **Peene** ∽ NE Germany
99 K17 **Peer** Limburg, NE Belgium
14 H14 **Pefferlaw** Ontario, S Canada
185 I18 **Pegasus Bay** bay South Island, NZ
121 O3 **Pégeia** var. Peyia. SW Cyprus
109 V7 **Peggau** Steiermark, SE Austria
101 L19 **Pegnitz** Bayern, SE Germany
101 L19 **Pegnitz** ∽ SE Germany
105 T11 **Pego** País Valenciano, E Spain
166 L8 **Pegu** var. Bago. Pegu, SW Myanmar
166 L7 **Pegu** ◆ division S Myanmar
189 N13 **Pehleng** Pohnpei, E Micronesia
114 M12 **Pehlivanköy** Kırklareli, NW Turkey
77 R14 **Péhonko** C Benin
61 B21 **Pehuajó** Buenos Aires, E Argentina
Pei-ching see Beijing/Beijing Shi
100 J13 **Peine** Niedersachsen, C Germany
Pei-p'ing see Beijing/Beijing Shi
Peipsi Järv/Peipus-See see Peipus, Lake
118 J5 **Peipus, Lake** Est. Peipsi Järv, Ger. Peipus-See, Rus. Chudskoye Ozero. ◎ Estonia/Russian Federation
115 H19 **Peiraías** prev. Piraiévs, Eng. Piraeus. Attikí, C Greece
Peisern see Pyzdry
60 I8 **Peixe, Rio do** ∽ S Brazil
59 I16 **Peixoto de Azevedo** Mato Grosso, W Brazil
168 O11 **Pejantan, Pulau** island W Indonesia
Pejë see Peć
112 N11 **Pek** ∽ E Yugoslavia
167 R7 **Pèk** var. Xieng Khouang; prev. Xiangkhoang. Xiangkhoang, N Laos
169 Q16 **Pekalongan** Jawa, C Indonesia
168 K11 **Pekanbaru** var. Pakanbaru. Sumatera, W Indonesia
30 L12 **Pekin** Illinois, N USA
Peking see Beijing/Beijing Shi
Pelabohan Kelang/Pelabuhan Kelang see Pelabuhan Klang
168 J9 **Pelabuhan Klang** var. Kuala Pelabohan Kelang, Pelabohan Kelang, Pelabuhan Kelang, Port Klang, Port Swettenham. Selangor, Peninsular Malaysia
120 L11 **Pelagie, Isole** island group SW Italy
Pelagosa see Palagruža
22 L5 **Pelahatchie** Mississippi, S USA
169 T14 **Pelaihari** var. Pleihari. Borneo, C Indonesia
103 U14 **Pelat, Mont** ▲ SE France
116 F12 **Peleaga, Vârful** prev. Vîrful Peleaga. ▲ W Romania
Peleaga, Vîrful see Peleaga, Vârful
123 O11 **Peleduy** Respublika Sakha (Yakutiya), NE Russian Federation
14 C18 **Pelee Island** island Ontario, S Canada
45 Q11 **Pelée, Montagne** 𝕽 N Martinique
14 D18 **Pelee, Point** headland Ontario, S Canada
171 P12 **Pelei** Pulau Peleng, N Indonesia
Peleliu see Beliliou
171 P12 **Peleng, Pulau** island Kepulauan Banggai, N Indonesia
23 T7 **Pelham** Georgia, SE USA
111 E18 **Pelhřimov** Ger. Pilgram. Jihlavský Kraj, C Czech Republic
39 W13 **Pelican** Chichagof Island, Alaska, USA
191 Z3 **Pelican Lagoon** ◎ Kiritimati, E Kiribati
29 U6 **Pelican Lake** ◎ Minnesota, N USA
29 V3 **Pelican Lake** ◎ Minnesota, N USA
30 L5 **Pelican Lake** ◎ Wisconsin, N USA
44 G1 **Pelican Point** Grand Bahama Island, N Bahamas
83 B19 **Pelican Point** headland W Namibia
29 S6 **Pelican Rapids** Minnesota, N USA
Pelican State see Louisiana
11 U13 **Pelikan Narrows** Saskatchewan, C Canada
115 L18 **Pelinaío** ▲ Chíos, E Greece
Pelinnaeum see Pelinnaío
115 E16 **Pelinnaío** anc. Pelinnaeum. ruins Thessalía, C Greece
113 N20 **Pelister** ▲ SW FYR Macedonia
113 G15 **Pelješac** peninsula S Croatia
92 M12 **Pelkosenniemi** Lappi, NE Finland
29 W15 **Pella** Iowa, C USA
114 F13 **Pélla** site of ancient city Kentrikí Makedonía, N Greece
23 Q3 **Pell City** Alabama, S USA
61 A22 **Pellegrini** Buenos Aires, E Argentina
92 K12 **Pello** Lappi, NW Finland
100 G7 **Pellworm** island N Germany
10 H6 **Pelly** ∽ Yukon Territory, NW Canada
9 N7 **Pelly Bay** Nunavut, N Canada
10 I8 **Pelly Mountains** ▲ Yukon Territory, W Canada
Pélmonostor see Beli Manastir
37 P13 **Pelona Mountain** ▲ New Mexico, SW USA
Peloponnese/Peloponnesus see Pelopónnisos
115 E20 **Pelopónnisos** Eng. Peloponnese. ◆ region S Greece
115 E20 **Pelopónnisos** var. Morea, Eng. Peloponnese; anc. Peloponnesus. peninsula S Greece
107 L23 **Peloritani, Monti** anc. Pelorus and Neptunius. ▲ Sicilia, Italy, C Mediterranean Sea
107 M22 **Peloro, Capo** var. Punta del Faro. headland S Italy
Pelorus and Neptunius see Peloritani, Monti
61 H17 **Pelotas** Rio Grande do Sul, S Brazil
61 I14 **Pelotas, Rio** ∽ S Brazil
92 K10 **Peltovuoma** Lapp. Bealdovuopmi. Lappi, N Finland
19 R4 **Pemadumcook Lake** ◎ Maine, NE USA
169 Q16 **Pemalang** Jawa, C Indonesia
169 P10 **Pemangkat** var. Pamangkat. Borneo, C Indonesia
Pemar see Paimio
168 I9 **Pematangsiantar** Sumatera, W Indonesia
83 Q14 **Pemba** prev. Port Amelia, Porto Amélia. Cabo Delgado, NE Mozambique
81 J22 **Pemba** ◆ region E Tanzania
81 K21 **Pemba** island E Tanzania
83 Q14 **Pemba, Baia de** inlet NE Mozambique
81 J21 **Pemba Channel** channel E Tanzania
180 J14 **Pemberton** Western Australia
10 M16 **Pemberton** British Columbia, SW Canada
29 Q2 **Pembina** North Dakota, N USA
29 Q2 **Pembina** ∽ Canada/USA
11 P15 **Pembina** ∽ Alberta, SW Canada
171 X16 **Pembre** Irian Jaya, E Indonesia
14 K12 **Pembroke** Ontario, SE Canada
97 H21 **Pembroke** SW Wales, UK
23 W6 **Pembroke** Georgia, SE USA
21 U11 **Pembroke** North Carolina, SE USA
21 R7 **Pembroke** Virginia, NE USA
97 H21 **Pembroke** cultural region SW Wales, UK
Pembuang, Sungai see Seruyan, Sungai
43 S15 **Peña Blanca, Cerro** ▲ C Panama
104 K8 **Peña de Francia, Sierra de la** ▲ W Spain
104 G6 **Penafiel** var. Peñafiel. Porto, N Portugal
105 N6 **Peñafiel** Castilla-León, N Spain
105 N8 **Peñagolosa** ▲ E Spain
105 N7 **Peñalara, Pico de** ▲ C Spain

◆ Country ◆ Country Capital ◇ Dependent Territory ○ Dependent Territory Capital ◆ Administrative Region ✕ International Airport ▲ Mountain ▲ Mountain Range 𝕽 Volcano ∽ River ◎ Lake ⊞ Reservoir

171 X16 **Penambo, Banjaran** *var.* Banjaran Tama Abu, Penambo Range. ⛰ Indonesia/Malaysia
Penambo Range *see* Penambo, Banjaran
41 O10 **Peña Nevada, Cerro** ▲ C Mexico
Penang *see* Pinang, Pulau, Peninsular Malaysia
Penang *see* Pinang
Penang *see* George Town
60 J8 **Penápolis** São Paulo, S Brazil
104 L7 **Peñaranda de Bracamonte** Castilla-León, N Spain
105 S8 **Peñarroya** ▲ E Spain
104 L12 **Peñarroya-Pueblonuevo** Andalucía, S Spain
97 K22 **Penarth** S Wales, UK
104 K1 **Peñas, Cabo de** *headland* N Spain
63 F20 **Penas, Golfo de** *gulf* S Chile
Pen-ch'i *see* Benxi
79 H14 **Pendé** *var.* Logone Oriental. ~ Central African Republic/Chad
76 I14 **Pendembu** E Sierra Leone
29 R13 **Pender** Nebraska, C USA
Penderma *see* Bandırma
32 K11 **Pendleton** Oregon, NW USA
32 M7 **Pend Oreille, Lake** ◎ Idaho, NW USA
32 M7 **Pend Oreille River** ~ Idaho/Washington, NW USA
Pendzhikent *see* Panjakent
Peneius *see* Pineiós
104 G8 **Penela** Coimbra, N Portugal
14 G13 **Penetanguishene** Ontario, S Canada
151 H15 **Penganga** ~ C India
161 T12 **P'engchia Yu** *island* N Taiwan
79 M21 **Penge** Kasai Oriental, C Dem. Rep. Congo (Zaire)
Penghu Archipelago/P'enghu Ch'üntao/Penghu Islands *see* P'enghu Liehtao
161 R14 **P'enghu Liehtao** *var.* P'enghu Ch'üntao, Penghu Islands, *Eng.* Penghu Archipelago, Pescadores, *Jap.* Hoko-guntō, Hoko-shotō. *island group* W Taiwan
Penghu Shuidao/P'enghu Shuitao *see* Pescadores Channel
161 R4 **Penglai** *var.* Dengzhou. Shandong, E China
Peng-pu *see* Bengbu
Penhsihu *see* Benxi
Penibético, Sistema *see* Béticos, Sistemas
104 F10 **Peniche** Leiria, W Portugal
169 U17 **Penida, Nusa** *island* S Indonesia
Peninsular State *see* Florida
105 T8 **Peñíscola** País Valenciano, E Spain
40 M13 **Pénjamo** Guanajuato, C Mexico
Penki *see* Benxi
102 F7 **Penmarch, Pointe de** *headland* NW France
107 L15 **Penna, Punta della** *headland* C Italy
107 K14 **Penne** Abruzzo, C Italy
Penner *see* Penneru
155 J18 **Penneru** *var.* Penner. ~ C India
182 I10 **Penneshaw** South Australia
18 C14 **Penn Hills** Pennsylvania, NE USA
Penninae, Alpes/Pennine, Alpi *see* Pennine Alps
108 D11 **Pennine Alps** *Fr.* Alpes Pennines, *It.* Alpi Pennine; *Lat.* Alpes Penninae. ⛰ Italy/Switzerland
Pennine Chain *see* Pennines
97 L15 **Pennines** *var.* Pennine Chain. ⛰ N England, UK
Pennines, Alpes *see* Pennine Alps
21 O8 **Pennington Gap** Virginia, NE USA
18 I16 **Penns Grove** New Jersey, NE USA
18 I16 **Pennsville** New Jersey, NE USA
18 E14 **Pennsylvania** *off.* Commonwealth of Pennsylvania; also known as The Keystone State. ◈ *state* NE USA
18 G10 **Penn Yan** New York, NE USA
126 H16 **Peno** Tverskaya Oblast', W Russian Federation
19 R7 **Penobscot Bay** *bay* Maine, NE USA
19 S5 **Penobscot River** ~ Maine, NE USA
182 K12 **Penola** South Australia
40 K9 **Peñón Blanco** Durango, C Mexico
182 E7 **Penong** South Australia
43 S16 **Penonomé** Coclé, C Panama
190 L13 **Penrhyn** *atoll* N Cook Islands
192 M9 **Penrhyn Basin** *undersea feature* C Pacific Ocean
183 S9 **Penrith** New South Wales, SE Australia
97 K15 **Penrith** NW England, UK
23 O9 **Pensacola** Florida, SE USA
23 O9 **Pensacola Bay** *bay* Florida, SE USA
195 N7 **Pensacola Mountains** ⛰ Antarctica
182 L12 **Penshurst** Victoria, SE Australia
187 R13 **Pentecost** *Fr.* Pentecôte. *island* C Vanuatu
15 V4 **Pentecôte** ~ Quebec, SE Canada
Pentecôte *see* Pentecost
15 V4 **Pentecôte, Lac** ◎ Quebec, SE Canada
8 H15 **Penticton** British Columbia, SW Canada
96 J6 **Pentland Firth** *strait* N Scotland, UK
96 J12 **Pentland Hills** *hill range* S Scotland, UK
171 Q12 **Penu** Pulau Taliabu, E Indonesia
155 H18 **Penukonda** Andhra Pradesh, E India
166 L7 **Penwegon** Pegu, C Myanmar
24 M8 **Penwell** Texas, SW USA
97 J21 **Pen y Fan** ▲ SE Wales, UK
97 L16 **Pen-y-ghent** ▲ N England, UK
129 O6 **Penza** Penzenskaya Oblast', W Russian Federation
97 G25 **Penzance** SW England, UK
129 N6 **Penzenskaya Oblast'** ◈ *province* W Russian Federation
123 U7 **Penzhina** ~ E Russian Federation
123 U9 **Penzhinskaya Guba** *bay* E Russian Federation
Penzig *see* Pieńsk
36 K13 **Peoria** Arizona, SW USA
30 L12 **Peoria** Illinois, N USA
30 L12 **Peoria Heights** Illinois, N USA
31 N11 **Peotone** Illinois, N USA
18 J11 **Pepacton Reservoir** ⊡ New York, NE USA
76 I15 **Pepel** W Sierra Leone
30 I6 **Pepin, Lake** ⊡ Minnesota/Wisconsin, N USA
99 L20 **Pepinster** Liège, E Belgium
113 L20 **Peqin** *var.* Peqini. Elbasan, C Albania
Peqini *see* Peqin
40 D7 **Pequeña, Punta** *headland* W Mexico
168 J8 **Perak** ◈ *state* Peninsular Malaysia
105 R7 **Perales del Alfambra** Aragón, NE Spain
115 C15 **Pérama** *var.* Perama. Ípeiros, W Greece
92 M13 **Perä-Posio** Lappi, NE Finland
15 Z6 **Percé** Quebec, SE Canada
15 Z6 **Percé, Rocher** *island* Quebec, S Canada
102 L5 **Perche, Collines de** ⛰ N France
109 X4 **Perchtoldsdorf** Niederösterreich, NE Austria
180 L6 **Percival Lakes** *lakes* Western Australia
105 T3 **Perdido, Monte** ▲ NE Spain
23 O8 **Perdido River** ~ Alabama/Florida, S USA
Perece Vela Basin *see* West Mariana Basin
116 G7 **Perechyn** Zakarpats'ka Oblast', W Ukraine
54 E10 **Pereira** Risaralda, W Colombia
60 I7 **Pereira Barreto** São Paulo, S Brazil
59 G15 **Pereirinha** Pará, N Brazil
129 N10 **Perelazovskiy** Volgogradskaya Oblast', SW Russian Federation
129 S7 **Perelyub** Saratovskaya Oblast', W Russian Federation
31 P7 **Pere Marquette River** ~ Michigan, N USA
Peremyshl *see* Podkarpackie
116 I5 **Peremyshlyany** L'vivs'ka Oblast', W Ukraine
Pereshchepino *see* Pereshchepyne
116 L9 **Pereshchepyne** *Rus.* Pereshchepino. Dnipropetrovs'ka Oblast', E Ukraine
126 L16 **Pereslavl'-Zalesskiy** Yaroslavskaya Oblast', W Russian Federation
117 Y7 **Pereval's'k** Luhans'ka Oblast', E Ukraine
129 U7 **Perevolotskiy** Orenburgskaya Oblast', W Russian Federation
Pereyaslav-Khmel'nitskiy *see* Pereyaslav-Khmel'nyts'kyy
117 Q5 **Pereyaslav-Khmel'nyts'kyy** *Rus.* Pereyaslav-Khmel'nitskiy. Kyyivs'ka Oblast', N Ukraine
109 U4 **Perg** Oberösterreich, N Austria
61 B19 **Pergamino** Buenos Aires, E Argentina
106 G6 **Pergine Valsugana** *Ger.* Persen. Trentino-Alto Adige, N Italy
29 S6 **Perham** Minnesota, N USA
93 L16 **Perho** Länsi-Suomi, W Finland
116 E11 **Periam** *Ger.* Perjamosch, *Hung.* Perjámos. Timiş, W Romania
15 Q6 **Péribonca** ~ Quebec, SE Canada
12 L11 **Péribonca, Lac** ◎ Quebec, SE Canada
15 Q6 **Péribonca, Petite Rivière** ~ Quebec, SE Canada
15 Q7 **Péribonka** Quebec, SE Canada
40 I9 **Pericos** Sinaloa, C Mexico
169 Q10 **Perigi** Borneo, C Indonesia
102 L12 **Périgueux** *anc.* Vesuna. Dordogne, SW France
54 G5 **Perijá, Serranía de** ⛰ Columbia/Venezuela
115 H17 **Peristéra** *island* Vóreioi Sporádes, Greece, Aegean Sea
63 H20 **Perito Moreno** Santa Cruz, S Argentina
155 G22 **Periyāl** *var.* Periyār. ~ SW India
Periyār *see* Periyāl
155 G23 **Periyār Lake** ◎ S India
Perjámos/Perjamosch *see* Periam
27 O9 **Perkins** Oklahoma, C USA
116 L7 **Perkivtsi** Chernivets'ka Oblast', W Ukraine
43 U15 **Perlas, Archipiélago de las** *Eng.* Pearl Islands. *island group* SE Panama
43 O10 **Perlas, Cayos de** *reef* SE Nicaragua
43 N9 **Perlas, Laguna de** *Eng.* Pearl Lagoon. *lagoon* E Nicaragua
43 N10 **Perlas, Punta de** *headland* E Nicaragua
100 L11 **Perleberg** Brandenburg, N Germany
Perlepe *see* Prilep
168 I6 **Perlis** ◈ *state* Peninsular Malaysia
127 U14 **Perm'** *prev.* Molotov. Permskaya Oblast', NW Russian Federation
113 M22 **Përmet** *var.* Përmeti, Prëmet. Gjirokastër, S Albania
Përmeti *see* Përmet
127 U15 **Permskaya Oblast'** ◈ *province* NW Russian Federation
59 P15 **Pernambuco** *off.* Estado de Pernambuco. ◈ *state* E Brazil
Pernambuco *see* Recife
Pernambuco Abyssal Plain *see* Pernambuco Plain
47 Y6 **Pernambuco Plain** *var.* Pernambuco Abyssal Plain. *undersea feature* E Atlantic Ocean
65 K15 **Pernambuco Seamounts** *undersea feature* C Atlantic Ocean
182 H6 **Pernatty Lagoon** *salt lake* South Australia
Pernau *see* Pärnu
Pernauer Bucht *see* Pärnu Laht
Pērnava *see* Pärnu
114 G9 **Pernik** *prev.* Dimitrovo. Pernik, W Bulgaria
114 G10 **Pernik** ◈ *province* W Bulgaria
93 K20 **Perniö** *Swe.* Bjärnå. Länsi-Suomi, W Finland
109 X5 **Pernitz** Niederösterreich, E Austria
Pernov *see* Pärnu
103 O3 **Péronne** Somme, N France
14 L8 **Péronne, Lac** ◎ Quebec, SE Canada
106 A8 **Perosa Argentina** Piemonte, NE Italy
41 Q14 **Perote** Veracruz-Llave, E Mexico
Pérouse *see* Perugia
191 W15 **Pérouse, Bahía de la** *bay* Easter Island, Chile, E Pacific Ocean
Perovsk *see* Kyzylorda
103 O17 **Perpignan** Pyrénées-Orientales, S France
113 M20 **Përrenjas** *var.* Përrenjasi, Prenjas, Prenjasi. Elbasan, E Albania
Përrenjasi *see* Përrenjas
92 O2 **Perriertoppen** ▲ C Svalbard
25 S6 **Perrin** Texas, SW USA
23 Y16 **Perrine** Florida, SE USA
37 S12 **Perro, Laguna del** ◎ New Mexico, SW USA
102 G5 **Perros-Guirec** Côtes d'Armor, NW France
23 T9 **Perry** Florida, SE USA
23 T5 **Perry** Georgia, SE USA
29 U14 **Perry** Iowa, C USA
18 E10 **Perry** New York, NE USA
27 N9 **Perry** Oklahoma, C USA
27 Q3 **Perry Lake** ⊡ Kansas, C USA
31 R11 **Perrysburg** Ohio, N USA
25 O1 **Perryton** Texas, SW USA
39 O15 **Perryville** Alaska, USA
27 U11 **Perryville** Arkansas, C USA
27 Y6 **Perryville** Missouri, C USA
Persante *see* Parsęta
Persen *see* Pergine Valsugana
Pershay *see* Pyarshai
117 V7 **Pershotravens'k** Dnipropetrovs'ka Oblast', E Ukraine
117 W9 **Pershotravneve** Donets'ka Oblast', E Ukraine
Persia *see* Iran
Persian Gulf *see* The Gulf
Persis *see* Fārs
95 K22 **Perstorp** Skåne, S Sweden
137 O14 **Pertek** Tunceli, C Turkey
183 P16 **Perth** Tasmania, SE Australia
180 I13 **Perth** *state capital* Western Australia
14 L13 **Perth** Ontario, SE Canada
96 J11 **Perth** C Scotland, UK
180 I12 **Perth** ✈ Western Australia
96 J10 **Perth** *cultural region* C Scotland, UK
173 V10 **Perth Basin** *undersea feature* SE Indian Ocean
103 S15 **Pertuis** Vaucluse, SE France
103 Y16 **Pertusato, Capo** *headland* Corse, France, C Mediterranean Sea
30 L11 **Peru** Illinois, N USA
31 P12 **Peru** Indiana, N USA
57 E13 **Peru** *off.* Republic of Peru. ◆ *republic* W South America
Peru *see* Beru
193 T9 **Peru Basin** *undersea feature* E Pacific Ocean
193 U8 **Peru-Chile Trench** *undersea feature* E Pacific Ocean
112 F13 **Perućko Jezero** ◎ S Croatia
106 H13 **Perugia** *Fr.* Pérouse; *anc.* Perusia. Umbria, C Italy
Perugia, Lake of *see* Trasimeno, Lago
61 D15 **Perugorría** Corrientes, NE Argentina
60 M11 **Peruíbe** São Paulo, S Brazil
155 B21 **Perumalpār** *reef* India, N Indian Ocean
Perusia *see* Perugia
99 D20 **Péruwelz** Hainaut, SW Belgium
137 R15 **Pervari** Siirt, SE Turkey
129 O4 **Pervomaysk** Nizhegorodskaya Oblast', W Russian Federation
117 X7 **Pervomays'k** Luhans'ka Oblast', E Ukraine
117 P8 **Pervomays'k** *prev.* Ol'viopol'. Mykolayivs'ka Oblast', S Ukraine
117 S12 **Pervomays'ke** Respublika Krym, S Ukraine
129 V7 **Pervomayskiy** Orenburgskaya Oblast', W Russian Federation
128 M6 **Pervomayskiy** Tambovskaya Oblast', W Russian Federation
117 V6 **Pervomays'kyy** Kharkivs'ka Oblast', E Ukraine
122 F10 **Pervoural'sk** Sverdlovskaya Oblast', C Russian Federation
123 V11 **Pervyy Kuril'skiy Proliv** *strait* E Russian Federation
99 I19 **Perwez** Wallon Brabant, C Belgium
106 I11 **Pesaro** *anc.* Pisaurum. Marche, C Italy
35 N9 **Pescadero** California, W USA
Pescadores *see* P'enghu Liehtao
161 S14 **Pescadores Channel** *var.* Penghu Shuidao, P'enghu Shuitao. *channel* W Taiwan
107 K14 **Pescara** *anc.* Aternum, Ostia Aterni. Abruzzo, C Italy
107 K15 **Pescara** ~ C Italy
106 F11 **Pescia** Toscana, C Italy
108 C8 **Peseux** Neuchâtel, W Switzerland
127 P6 **Pesha** ~ NW Russian Federation
149 T5 **Peshāwar** North-West Frontier Province, N Pakistan
149 T6 **Peshāwar** ✈ North-West Frontier Province, N Pakistan
113 M19 **Peshkopi** *var.* Peshkopia, Peshkopija. Dibër, NE Albania
Peshkopia/Peshkopija *see* Peshkopi
114 I11 **Peshtera** Pazardzhik, C Bulgaria
31 N6 **Peshtigo** Wisconsin, N USA
31 N6 **Peshtigo River** ~ Wisconsin, N USA
Peski *see* Pyeski
127 S13 **Peskovka** Kirovskaya Oblast', NW Russian Federation
103 S8 **Pesmes** Haute-Saône, E France
104 H6 **Peso da Régua** *var.* Pêso da Regua. Vila Real, N Portugal
40 F5 **Pesqueira** Sonora, NW Mexico
102 J13 **Pessac** Gironde, SW France
111 J23 **Pest** *off.* Pest Megye. ◈ *county* C Hungary
126 J14 **Pestovo** Novgorodskaya Oblast', W Russian Federation
40 M15 **Petacalco, Bahía** *bay* W Mexico
Petach-Tikva/Petah Tiqva *see* Petah Tiqwa
138 F10 **Petah Tiqwa** *var.* Petach-Tikva, Petah Tiqva, Petakh Tikva. Tel Aviv, C Israel
Petakh Tikva *see* Petah Tiqwa
93 L17 **Petäjävesi** Länsi-Suomi, W Finland
22 M7 **Petal** Mississippi, S USA
115 I19 **Petalioí** *island* C Greece
115 H19 **Petalión, Kólpos** *gulf* E Greece
115 J19 **Pétalo** ▲ Ándros, Kykládes, Greece, Aegean Sea
34 M8 **Petaluma** California, W USA
99 L25 **Pétange** Luxembourg, SW Luxembourg
54 M5 **Petare** Miranda, N Venezuela
41 N16 **Petatlán** Guerrero, S Mexico
83 L14 **Petauke** Eastern, E Zambia
14 J12 **Petawawa** Ontario, SE Canada
14 J11 **Petawawa** ~ Ontario, SE Canada
Petchaburi *see* Phetchaburi
42 D2 **Petén** *off.* Departamento del Petén. ◈ *department* N Guatemala
42 D2 **Petén Itzá, Lago** *var.* Lago de Flores. ◎ N Guatemala
30 K7 **Petenwell Lake** ⊡ Wisconsin, N USA
14 D6 **Peterbell** Ontario, S Canada
182 I7 **Peterborough** South Australia
14 I14 **Peterborough** Ontario, SE Canada
97 N20 **Peterborough** *prev.* Medeshamstede. E England, UK
19 N10 **Peterborough** New Hampshire, NE USA
96 L8 **Peterhead** NE Scotland, UK
Peterhof *see* Luboń
193 Q14 **Peter I Island** ◇ *Norwegian dependency* Antarctica
194 H9 **Peter I Island** *var.* Peter I øy. *island* Antarctica
Peter I øy *see* Peter I Island
97 M14 **Peterlee** N England, UK
Peterlingen *see* Payerne
197 P14 **Petermann Bjerg** ▲ C Greenland
11 S12 **Peter Pond Lake** ◎ Saskatchewan, C Canada
39 X13 **Petersburg** Mytkof Island, Alaska, USA
30 K13 **Petersburg** Illinois, N USA
31 N16 **Petersburg** Indiana, N USA
29 Q3 **Petersburg** North Dakota, N USA
25 N5 **Petersburg** Texas, SW USA
21 V7 **Petersburg** Virginia, NE USA
21 T4 **Petersburg** West Virginia, NE USA
100 H12 **Petershagen** Nordrhein-Westfalen, NW Germany
55 S9 **Peters Mine** *var.* Peter's Mine. N Guyana
107 O21 **Petilia Policastro** Calabria, SW Italy
44 M9 **Pétionville** S Haiti
45 X6 **Petit-Bourg** Basse Terre, C Guadeloupe
15 Y5 **Petit-Cap** Quebec, SE Canada
45 Y6 **Petit Cul-de-Sac Marin** *bay* C Guadeloupe
12 K7 **Petite Rivière de la Baleine** ~ Quebec, NE Canada
44 M9 **Petite-Rivière-de-l'Artibonite** C Haiti
173 X16 **Petite Rivière Noire, Piton de la** ▲ C Mauritius
15 R9 **Petite-Rivière-St-François** Quebec, SE Canada
44 L9 **Petit-Goâve** S Haiti
Petitjean *see* Sidi-Kacem
13 N10 **Petit Lac Manicouagan** ◎ Quebec, E Canada
19 T7 **Petit Manan Point** *headland* Maine, NE USA
Petit Mécatina, Rivière du *see* Little Mecatina
11 N10 **Petitot** ~ Alberta/British Columbia, W Canada
45 S12 **Petit Piton** ▲ SW Saint Lucia
Petit-Popo *see* Aného
Petit St-Bernard, Col du *see* Little Saint Bernard Pass
13 O8 **Petitsikapau Lake** ◎ Newfoundland, E Canada
92 L11 **Petkula** Lappi, N Finland
41 X12 **Peto** Yucatán, SE Mexico
62 G10 **Petorca** Valparaíso, C Chile
31 Q5 **Petoskey** Michigan, N USA
138 G14 **Petra** *archaeological site* Ma'ān, W Jordan
Petra *see* Wādī Mūsā
115 F14 **Pétras, Sténa** *pass* N Greece
123 S16 **Petra Velikogo, Zaliv** *bay* SE Russian Federation
Petrel *see* Petrer
14 K15 **Petre, Point** *headland* Ontario, SE Canada
105 S12 **Petrer** *var.* Petrel. País Valenciano, E Spain
127 U11 **Petretsovo** Permskaya Oblast', NW Russian Federation
114 G12 **Petrich** Blagoevgrad, SW Bulgaria
187 P15 **Petrie, Récif** *reef* N New Caledonia
37 N11 **Petrified Forest** *prehistoric site* Arizona, SW USA
Petrikau *see* Piotrków Trybunalski
Petrikov *see* Pyetrykaw
116 H12 **Petrila** *Hung.* Petrilla. Hunedoara, W Romania
Petrilla *see* Petrila
112 E9 **Petrinja** Sisak-Moslavina, C Croatia
Petroaleksandrovsk *see* Türtkŭl
Petrőcz *see* Bački Petrovac
126 G12 **Petrodvorets** *Fin.* Pietarhovi. Leningradskaya Oblast', NW Russian Federation
Petrograd *see* Sankt-Peterburg
Petrokov *see* Piotrków Trybunalski
54 G6 **Petrólea** Norte de Santander, NE Colombia
14 D16 **Petrolia** Ontario, S Canada
25 S4 **Petrolia** Texas, SW USA
59 O15 **Petrolina** Pernambuco, E Brazil
45 T6 **Petrona, Punta** *headland* C Puerto Rico
Petropavl *see* Petropavlovsk
117 V7 **Petropavlivka** Dnipropetrovs'ka Oblast', E Ukraine
145 P6 **Petropavlovsk** *Kaz.* Petropavl. Severnyy Kazakhstan, N Kazakhstan
123 V11 **Petropavlovsk-Kamchatskiy** Kamchatskaya Oblast', E Russian Federation
60 P9 **Petrópolis** Rio de Janeiro, SE Brazil
116 H12 **Petroşani** *var.* Petroşeni, *Ger.* Petroschen, *Hung.* Petrozsény. Hunedoara, W Romania
Petroschen/Petroşeni *see* Petroşani
Petroskoi *see* Petrozavodsk
Petrovac/Petrovácz *see* Bački Petrovac
113 J17 **Petrovac na Moru** Montenegro, SW Yugoslavia
117 S8 **Petrove** Kirovohrads'ka Oblast', C Ukraine
113 O18 **Petrovec** C FYR Macedonia
Petrovgrad *see* Zrenjanin
129 P7 **Petrovsk** Saratovskaya Oblast', W Russian Federation
126 J9 **Petrovskiy Yam** Respublika Kareliya, NW Russian Federation
Petrovsk-Port *see* Makhachkala
129 P9 **Petrov Val** Volgogradskaya Oblast', SW Russian Federation
126 J11 **Petrozavodsk** *Fin.* Petroskoi. Respublika Kareliya, NW Russian Federation
Petrozsény *see* Petroşani
83 D20 **Petrusdal** Hardap, C Namibia
117 T7 **Petrykivka** Dnipropetrovs'ka Oblast', E Ukraine
Petsamo *see* Pechenga
Petschka *see* Pecica
Pettau *see* Ptuj
109 S5 **Pettenbach** Oberösterreich, C Austria
25 S13 **Pettus** Texas, SW USA
122 G11 **Petukhovo** Kurganskaya Oblast', C Russian Federation
Petuna *see* Songyuan
109 R4 **Peuerbach** Oberösterreich, N Austria
62 G12 **Peumo** Libertador, C Chile
123 T6 **Pevek** Chukotskiy Avtonomnyy Okrug, NE Russian Federation
27 X5 **Pevely** Missouri, C USA
Peyia *see* Pégeia
102 J15 **Peyrehorade** Landes, SW France
126 J14 **Peza** ~ NW Russian Federation
103 P16 **Pézenas** Hérault, S France
111 H20 **Pezinok** *Ger.* Bösing, *Hung.* Bazin. Bratislavský Kraj, W Slovakia
101 L22 **Pfaffenhofen an der Ilm** Bayern, SE Germany
108 G7 **Pfäffikon** Schwyz, C Switzerland
101 F20 **Pfälzer Wald** *hill range* W Germany
101 N22 **Pfarrkirchen** Bayern, SE Germany
101 G21 **Pforzheim** Baden-Württemberg, SW Germany
101 H24 **Pfullendorf** Baden-Württemberg, S Germany
108 K8 **Pfunds** Tirol, W Austria
101 G19 **Pfungstadt** Hessen, W Germany
83 L20 **Phalaborwa** Northern, NE South Africa
152 E11 **Phalodi** Rājasthān, NW India
152 E12 **Phalsund** Rājasthān, NW India
155 E15 **Phaltan** Mahārāshtra, W India
167 O7 **Phan** *var.* Muang Phan. Chiang Rai, NW Thailand
167 O14 **Phangan, Ko** *island* SW Thailand
166 M15 **Phang-Nga** *var.* Pang-Nga, Phangnga. Phangnga, SW Thailand
Phan Rang/Phanrang *see* Phan Rang-Thap Cham
167 V13 **Phan Rang-Thap Cham** *var.* Phanrang, Phan Rang, Phan Rang Thap Cham. Ninh Thuận, S Vietnam
167 U13 **Phan Ri** Binh Thuận, S Vietnam
167 U13 **Phan Thiêt** Binh Thuận, S Vietnam
Pharnacia *see* Giresun
25 S17 **Pharr** Texas, SW USA
Pharus *see* Hvar
167 N16 **Phatthalung** *var.* Padalung, Patalung. Phatthalung, SW Thailand
167 O7 **Phayao** *var.* Muang Phayao. Phayao, NW Thailand
11 U10 **Phelps Lake** ◎ Saskatchewan, C Canada
21 X9 **Phelps Lake** ◎ North Carolina, SE USA
23 R5 **Phenix City** Alabama, S USA
167 T8 **Pheo** Quang Binh, C Vietnam
Phet Buri *see* Phetchaburi
167 O11 **Phetchaburi** *var.* Bejraburi, Petchaburi, Phet Buri. Phetchaburi, SW Thailand
167 O9 **Phichit** *var.* Bichitra, Muang Phichit, Pichit. Phichit, C Thailand
22 M5 **Philadelphia** Mississippi, S USA
18 I7 **Philadelphia** New York, NE USA
18 I16 **Philadelphia** Pennsylvania, NE USA
18 I16 **Philadelphia** ✈ Pennsylvania, NE USA
Philadelphia *see* 'Ammān
28 L10 **Philip** South Dakota, N USA
99 H22 **Philippeville** Namur, S Belgium
Philippeville *see* Skikda
21 S3 **Philippi** West Virginia, NE USA
Philippi *see* Filippoi
195 Y9 **Philippi Glacier** *glacier* Antarctica
192 G6 **Philippine Basin** *undersea feature* W Pacific Ocean
131 X12 **Philippine Plate** *tectonic feature*
169 W6 **Philippines** *off.* Republic of the Philippines. ◆ *republic* SE Asia
131 X13 **Philippines** *island group* W Pacific Ocean
171 P3 **Philippine Sea** *sea* W Pacific Ocean
192 F6 **Philippine Trench** *undersea feature* W Philippine Sea
83 H23 **Philippolis** Free State, C South Africa
Philippopolis *see* Plovdiv, Bulgaria
Philippopolis *see* Shahbā', Syria
45 V9 **Philipsburg** Sint Maarten, N Netherlands Antilles
33 P10 **Philipsburg** Montana, NW USA
39 R6 **Philip Smith Mountains** ⛰ Alaska, USA
152 H8 **Phillaur** Punjab, N India
183 N13 **Phillip Island** *island* Victoria, SE Australia
25 N2 **Phillips** Texas, SW USA
30 K5 **Phillips** Wisconsin, N USA
26 K3 **Phillipsburg** Kansas, C USA
18 I14 **Phillipsburg** New Jersey, NE USA
21 S7 **Philpott Lake** ⊡ Virginia, NE USA
Phintias *see* Licata
167 P9 **Phitsanulok** *var.* Bisnulok, Muang Phitsanulok, Pitsanulok. Phitsanulok, C Thailand
Phlórina *see* Flórina
Phnom Penh *see* Phnum Penh
167 S13 **Phnum Penh** *var.* Phnom Penh. • (Cambodia) Phnum Penh, S Cambodia
167 S11 **Phnum Tbêng Meanchey** Preăh Vihéar, N Cambodia
36 K13 **Phoenix** *state capital* Arizona, SW USA
Phoenix Island *see* Rawaki
191 R3 **Phoenix Islands** *island group* C Kiribati
18 I15 **Phoenixville** Pennsylvania, NE USA
83 K22 **Phofung** *var.* Mont-aux-Sources. ▲ N Lesotho
167 Q10 **Phon** Khon Kaen, E Thailand
167 Q5 **Phôngsali** *var.* Phong Saly. Phôngsali, N Laos
Phong Saly *see* Phôngsali
167 Q8 **Phônhông** C Laos
167 R5 **Phô Rang** Lao Cai, N Vietnam
Phort Láirge, Cuan *see* Waterford Harbour
167 N10 **Phra Chedi Sam Ong** Kanchanaburi, W Thailand
167 O8 **Phrae** *var.* Muang Phrae, Prae. Phrae, NW Thailand
Phra Nakhon Si Ayutthaya *see* Ayutthaya
167 M14 **Phra Thong, Ko** *island* SW Thailand
Phu Cương *see* Thu Dâu Môt
166 M15 **Phuket** *var.* Bhuket, Puket, *Mal.* Ujung Salang; *prev.* Junkseylon, Salang. Phuket, SW Thailand
166 M15 **Phuket** ✈ Phuket, SW Thailand
166 M15 **Phuket, Ko** *island* SW Thailand
154 N12 **Phulabāni** *prev.* Phulbani. Orissa, E India
Phulbani *see* Phulabāni
167 U9 **Phu Lôc** Th,a Thiên-Huê, C Vietnam
167 S13 **Phumĭ Banam** Prey Vêng, S Cambodia

◆ Country • Country Capital ◇ Dependent Territory ○ Dependent Territory Capital ◈ Administrative Region ✈ International Airport ▲ Mountain ⛰ Mountain Range ☒ Volcano ~ River ◎ Lake ⊡ Reservoir

167 R13 **Phumĭ Choăm** Kâmpóng Speu, SW Cambodia
167 T11 **Phumĭ Kalêng** Stœng Trêng, NE Cambodia
167 S12 **Phumĭ Kâmpóng Trâbêk** *prev.* Phum Kompong Trabek. Kâmpóng Thum, C Cambodia
167 Q11 **Phumĭ Koŭk Kduŏch** Bătdâmbâng, NW Cambodia
167 T11 **Phumĭ Labăng** Rôtânôkiri, NE Cambodia
167 S11 **Phumĭ Mlu Prey** Preăh Vihéar, N Cambodia
167 R11 **Phumĭ Moŭng** Siĕmréab, NW Cambodia
167 Q12 **Phumĭ Prâmaôy** Poŭthĭsăt, W Cambodia
167 Q13 **Phumĭ Samĭt** Kaôh Kông, SW Cambodia
167 R11 **Phumĭ Sâmraông** *prev.* Phum Samrong. Siĕmréab, NW Cambodia
167 S12 **Phumĭ Siĕmbok** Stœng Trêng, N Cambodia
167 S11 **Phumĭ Thalabârĭvăt** Stœng Trêng, N Cambodia
167 R13 **Phumĭ Veal Renh** Kâmpôt, SW Cambodia
167 P13 **Phumĭ Yeay Sên** Kaôh Kông, SW Cambodia
Phum Kompong Trabek *see* Phumĭ Kâmpóng Trâbêk
Phum Samrong *see* Phumĭ Sâmraông
167 V11 **Phu My** Binh Đinh, C Vietnam
167 S14 **Phung Hiêp** Cân Thơ, S Vietnam
153 T12 **Phuntsholing** SW Bhutan
167 R15 **Phươc Long** Minh Hai, S Vietnam
167 R14 **Phu Quôc, Đao** *var.* Phu Quoc Island. *island* S Vietnam
Phu Quoc Island *see* Phu Quôc, Đao
167 S6 **Phu Tho** Vinh Phu, N Vietnam
Phu Vinh *see* Tra Vinh
189 T13 **Piaanu Pass** *passage* Chuuk Islands, C Micronesia
106 E8 **Piacenza** *Fr.* Paisance; *anc.* Placentia. Emilia-Romagna, N Italy
107 K14 **Pianella** Abruzzo, C Italy
107 M15 **Pianosa, Isola** *island* Archipelago Toscano, C Italy
171 U13 **Piar** Irian Jaya, E Indonesia
45 U14 **Piarco** *var.* Port of Spain. ✕ (Port-of-Spain) Trinidad, Trinidad and Tobago
110 M12 **Piaseczno** Mazowieckie, C Poland
116 I15 **Piatra** Teleorman, S Romania
116 L10 **Piatra-Neamţ** *Hung.* Karácsonkő. Neamţ, NE Romania
Piauhy *see* Piauí
59 N15 **Piauí** *off.* Estado do Piauí; *prev.* Piauhy. ◆ *state* E Brazil
106 I7 **Piave** ≈ NE Italy
107 K24 **Piazza Armerina** *var.* Chiazza. Sicilia, Italy, C Mediterranean Sea
81 G14 **Pibor** *Amh.* Pībor Wenz. ≈ Ethiopia/Sudan
81 G14 **Pibor Post** Jonglei, SE Sudan
Pībor Wenz *see* Pibor
Pibrans *see* Příbram
36 K11 **Picacho Butte** ▲ Arizona, SW USA
40 D4 **Picachos, Cerro** ▲ NW Mexico
103 O4 **Picardie** *Eng.* Picardy. ◆ *region* N France
Picardy *see* Picardie
22 L8 **Picayune** Mississippi, S USA
Piccolo San Bernardo, Colle di *see* Little Saint Bernard Pass
62 K5 **Pichanal** Salta, N Argentina
147 P12 **Pichandar** W Tajikistan
27 R8 **Picher** Oklahoma, C USA
62 G12 **Pichilemu** Libertador, C Chile
40 F9 **Pichilingue** Baja California Sur, W Mexico
56 B6 **Pichincha** ◆ *province* N Ecuador
56 C6 **Pichincha** ▲ N Ecuador
Pichit *see* Phichit
41 U15 **Pichucalco** Chiapas, SE Mexico
22 L5 **Pickens** Mississippi, S USA
21 O11 **Pickens** South Carolina, SE USA
14 G11 **Pickerel** ≈ Ontario, S Canada
14 H15 **Pickering** Ontario, S Canada
97 N16 **Pickering** N England, UK
31 S13 **Pickerington** Ohio, N USA
12 C10 **Pickle Lake** Ontario, C Canada
29 P12 **Pickstown** South Dakota, N USA
25 V6 **Pickton** Texas, SW USA
23 N1 **Pickwick Lake** ⊠ S USA
64 N2 **Pico** *var.* Ilha do Pico. *island* Azores, Portugal, NE Atlantic Ocean
63 J19 **Pico de Salamanca** Chubut, SE Argentina
1 P9 **Pico Fracture Zone** *tectonic feature* NW Atlantic Ocean
Pico, Ilha do *see* Pico
59 O14 **Picos** Piauí, E Brazil
63 I20 **Pico Truncado** Santa Cruz, SE Argentina
183 S9 **Picton** New South Wales, SE Australia
14 K15 **Picton** Ontario, SE Canada
185 K14 **Picton** Marlborough, South Island, NZ
63 H15 **Piċun Leufú, Arroyo** ≈ SW Argentina
Pidálion *see* Gkréko, Akrotíri
155 K25 **Pidurutalagala** ▲ S Sri Lanka
116 K6 **Pidvolochys'k** Ternopil's'ka Oblast', W Ukraine
107 K16 **Piedimonte Matese** Campania, S Italy
27 X7 **Piedmont** Missouri, C USA
21 P11 **Piedmont** South Carolina, SE USA
17 S12 **Piedmont** *escarpment* E USA
Piedmont *see* Piemonte
31 U13 **Piedmont Lake** ⊠ Ohio, N USA
104 M11 **Piedrabuena** Castilla-La Mancha, C Spain
Piedrafita, Puerto de *see* Pedrafita, Porto de
104 L8 **Piedrahita** Castilla-León, N Spain
41 N6 **Piedras Negras** *var.* Ciudad Porfirio Díaz. Coahuila de Zaragoza, NE Mexico
61 E21 **Piedras, Punta** *headland* E Argentina
57 I14 **Piedras, Río de las** ≈ E Peru
111 J16 **Piekary Śląskie** Śląskie, S Poland
93 M17 **Pieksämäki** Isä-Suomi, E Finland
109 V5 **Pielach** ≈ NE Austria
93 M16 **Pielavesi** Itä-Suomi, C Finland
93 N16 **Pielinen** *var.* Pielisjärvi. ◎ E Finland
Pielisjärvi *see* Pielinen
106 A8 **Piemonte** *Eng.* Piedmont. ◆ *region* NW Italy
111 L18 **Pieniny** ▲ Poland/Slovakia
111 E14 **Pieńsk** *Ger.* Penzig. Dolnośląskie, SW Poland
29 Q13 **Pierce** Nebraska, C USA
11 R14 **Pierceland** Saskatchewan, C Canada
115 E14 **Piéria** ▲ N Greece
29 N10 **Pierre** *state capital* South Dakota, N USA
102 K16 **Pierrefitte-Nestalas** Hautes-Pyrénées, S France
103 R14 **Pierrelatte** Drôme, E France
15 P11 **Pierreville** Quebec, SE Canada
15 O7 **Pierriche** ≈ Quebec, SE Canada
111 H20 **Piešt'any** *Ger.* Pistyan, *Hung.* Pöstyén. Trnavský, W Slovakia
109 X5 **Piesting** ≈ E Austria
Pietarhovi *see* Petrodvorets
Pietari *see* Sankt-Peterburg
Pietarsaari *see* Jakobstad
83 K23 **Pietermaritzburg** *var.* Maritzburg. KwaZulu/Natal, E South Africa
83 K20 **Pietersburg** Northern, NE South Africa
107 K24 **Pietraperzia** Sicilia, Italy, C Mediterranean Sea
107 N22 **Pietra Spada, Passo della** *pass* SW Italy
83 K22 **Piet Retief** Mpumalanga, E South Africa
116 I9 **Pietrosul, Vârful** *prev.* Vîrful Pietrosu. ▲ N Romania
116 J10 **Pietrosul, Vârful** *prev.* Vîrful Pietrosu. ▲ N Romania
Pietrosu, Vîrful *see* Pietrosul, Vârful
106 I6 **Pieve di Cadore** Veneto, NE Italy
14 C18 **Pigeon Bay** *lake bay* Ontario, S Canada
27 X8 **Piggott** Arkansas, C USA
83 L21 **Piggs Peak** NW Swaziland
Pigs, Bay of *see* Cochinos, Bahía de
61 A23 **Pigüé** Buenos Aires, E Argentina
41 O12 **Piguícas** ▲ C Mexico
193 W15 **Piha Passage** *passage* S Tonga
Pihkva Järv *see* Pskov, Lake
93 N18 **Pihlajavesi** ◎ SE Finland
93 J18 **Pihlava** Länsi-Suomi, W Finland
93 L16 **Pihtipudas** Länsi-Suomi, W Finland
40 L14 **Pihuamo** Jalisco, SW Mexico
189 U11 **Piis Moen** *var.* Pis. *atoll* Chuuk Islands, C Micronesia
41 U17 **Pijijiapán** Chiapas, SE Mexico
98 G12 **Pijnacker** Zuid-Holland, W Netherlands
42 H5 **Pijol, Pico** ▲ NW Honduras
Pikaar *see* Bikar Atoll
126 I13 **Pikalevo** Leningradskaya Oblast', NW Russian Federation
188 M15 **Pikelot** *island* Caroline Islands, C Micronesia
30 M5 **Pike River** ≈ Wisconsin, N USA
37 T5 **Pikes Peak** ▲ Colorado, C USA
21 P6 **Pikeville** Kentucky, S USA
20 L9 **Pikeville** Tennessee, S USA
Pikinni *see* Bikini Atoll
79 H18 **Pikounda** La Sangha, C Congo
110 G9 **Piła** *Ger.* Schneidemühl. Wielkopolskie, C Poland
62 N6 **Pilagá, Riacho** ≈ NE Argentina
61 D20 **Pilar** Buenos Aires, E Argentina
62 N7 **Pilar** *var.* Villa del Pilar. Ñeembucú, S Paraguay
62 N6 **Pilcomayo, Río** ≈ C South America
147 R12 **Pildon** *Rus.* Pil'don. C Tajikistan
Piles *see* Pylés
Pilgram *see* Pelhřimov
152 L10 **Pīlībhīt** Uttar Pradesh, N India
110 M13 **Pilica** ≈ C Poland
115 G16 **Pílio** ▲ C Greece
111 J22 **Pilisvörösvár** Pest, N Hungary
65 G15 **Pillar Bay** *bay* Ascension Island, C Atlantic Ocean
183 P17 **Pillar, Cape** *headland* Tasmania, SE Australia
Pillau *see* Baltiysk
183 R5 **Pilliga** New South Wales, SE Australia
44 H8 **Pilón** Granma, E Cuba
Pilos *see* Pýlos
11 W17 **Pilot Mound** Manitoba, S Canada
21 S8 **Pilot Mountain** North Carolina, SE USA
39 O14 **Pilot Point** Alaska, USA
25 T5 **Pilot Point** Texas, SW USA
32 K11 **Pilot Rock** Oregon, NW USA
38 M11 **Pilot Station** Alaska, USA
Pilsen *see* Plzeň
111 K18 **Pilsko** ▲ N Slovakia
Pilten *see* Piltene
118 D8 **Piltene** *Ger.* Pilten. Ventspils, W Latvia
111 M16 **Pilzno** Podkarpackie, SE Poland
Pilzno *see* Plzeň
37 N14 **Pima** Arizona, SW USA
58 H13 **Pimenta** Pará, N Brazil
59 F16 **Pimenta Bueno** Rondônia, W Brazil
56 B11 **Pimentel** Lambayeque, W Peru
105 S6 **Pina** Aragón, NE Spain
119 I20 **Pina** *Rus.* Pina. ≈ SW Belarus
40 E2 **Pinacate, Sierra del** ▲ NW Mexico
63 H22 **Pináculo, Cerro** ▲ S Argentina
191 X11 **Pinaki** *atoll* Îles Tuamotu, E French Polynesia
37 N15 **Pinaleno Mountains** ▲ Arizona, SW USA
171 P4 **Pinamalayan** Mindoro, N Philippines
169 Q10 **Pinang** Borneo, C Indonesia
168 J7 **Pinang** *var.* Penang. ◆ *state* Peninsular Malaysia
Pinang *see* Pinang, Pulau, Peninsular Malaysia
Pinang *see* George Town
168 J7 **Pinang, Pulau** *var.* Penang, Pinang; *prev.* Prince of Wales Island. *island* Peninsular Malaysia
44 B5 **Pinar del Río** Pinar del Río, W Cuba
114 N11 **Pınarhisar** Kırklareli, NW Turkey
171 O3 **Pinatubo, Mount** ▲ Luzon, N Philippines
11 Y16 **Pinawa** Manitoba, S Canada
11 Q17 **Pincher Creek** Alberta, SW Canada
30 L16 **Pinckneyville** Illinois, N USA
Pincota *see* Pâncota
111 L15 **Pińczów** Świętokrzyskie, C Poland
149 U7 **Pind Dādan Khān** Punjab, E Pakistan
Píndhos/Píndhos Óros *see* Píndos
149 V8 **Pindi Bhattiān** Punjab, E Pakistan
149 U6 **Pindi Gheb** Punjab, E Pakistan
115 D15 **Píndos** *var.* Píndhos Óros, *Eng.* Pindus Mountains; *prev.* Píndhos. ▲ C Greece
Pindus Mountains *see* Píndos
18 J16 **Pine Barrens** *physical region* New Jersey, NE USA
27 V12 **Pine Bluff** Arkansas, C USA
23 X11 **Pine Castle** Florida, SE USA
29 V7 **Pine City** Minnesota, N USA
181 P2 **Pine Creek** Northern Territory, N Australia
35 V4 **Pine Creek** ≈ Nevada, W USA
18 F13 **Pine Creek** ≈ Pennsylvania, NE USA
27 Q13 **Pine Creek Lake** ⊠ Oklahoma, C USA
33 T15 **Pinedale** Wyoming, C USA
11 X15 **Pine Dock** Manitoba, S Canada
11 Y16 **Pine Falls** Manitoba, S Canada
35 R10 **Pine Flat Lake** ⊠ California, W USA
127 N8 **Pinega** Arkhangel'skaya Oblast', NW Russian Federation
127 N8 **Pinega** ≈ NW Russian Federation
15 N12 **Pine Hill** Quebec, SE Canada
11 T12 **Pinehouse Lake** ◎ Saskatchewan, C Canada
21 T10 **Pinehurst** North Carolina, SE USA
115 D19 **Pineiós** ≈ S Greece
115 E16 **Pineiós** *var.* Piniós; *anc.* Peneius. ≈ C Greece
29 W10 **Pine Island** Minnesota, N USA
23 V15 **Pine Island** *island* Florida, SE USA
194 K10 **Pine Island Glacier** *glacier* Antarctica
25 X9 **Pineland** Texas, SW USA
23 V13 **Pinellas Park** Florida, SE USA
10 M13 **Pine Pass** *pass* British Columbia, W Canada
8 J10 **Pine Point** Northwest Territories, W Canada
28 K12 **Pine Ridge** South Dakota, N USA
29 U6 **Pine River** Minnesota, N USA
31 Q8 **Pine River** ≈ Michigan, N USA
30 M4 **Pine River** ≈ Wisconsin, N USA
106 A8 **Pinerolo** Piemonte, NE Italy
25 W6 **Pines, Lake O' the** ⊠ Texas, SW USA
Pines, The Isle of the *see* Juventud, Isla de la
Pine Tree State *see* Maine
21 N7 **Pineville** Kentucky, S USA
22 H7 **Pineville** Louisiana, S USA
27 R8 **Pineville** Missouri, C USA
21 R10 **Pineville** North Carolina, SE USA
21 Q6 **Pineville** West Virginia, NE USA
33 V8 **Piney Buttes** *physical region* Montana, NW USA
163 W9 **Ping'an** Jilin, NE China
160 H14 **Pingbian** *var.* Pingbian Miaozu Zizhixian. Yunnan, SW China
157 S9 **Pingdingshan** Henan, C China
161 R4 **Pingdu** Shandong, E China
189 W16 **Pingelap Atoll** *atoll* Caroline Islands, E Micronesia
160 K14 **Pingguo** Guangxi Zhuangzu Zizhiqu, S China
161 Q13 **Pinghe** Fujian, SE China
P'ing-hsiang *see* Pingxiang
161 N10 **Pingjiang** Hunan, S China
Pingkiang *see* Harbin
160 L8 **Pingli** Shaanxi, C China
159 W10 **Pingliang** *var.* P'ing-liang. Gansu, C China
159 W8 **Pingluo** Ningxia, N China
Pingma *see* Tiandong
167 O7 **Ping, Mae Nam** ≈ W Thailand
161 Q1 **Pingquan** Hebei, E China
29 P5 **Pingree** North Dakota, N USA
Pingsiang *see* Pingxiang
161 S14 **P'ingtung** *Jap.* Heitō. S Taiwan
160 I8 **Pingwu** Sichuan, C China
160 J15 **Pingxiang** Guangxi Zhuangzu Zizhiqu, S China
161 O11 **Pingxiang** *var.* P'ing-hsiang; *prev.* Pingsiang. Jiangxi, S China
161 S10 **Pingyang** Zhejiang, SE China
161 P5 **Pingyi** Shandong, E China
161 P5 **Pingyin** Shandong, E China
60 H13 **Pinhalzinho** Santa Catarina, S Brazil
60 I12 **Pinhão** Paraná, S Brazil
61 H17 **Pinheiro Machado** Rio Grande do Sul, S Brazil
104 I7 **Pinhel** Guarda, N Portugal
Piniós *see* Pineiós
168 I11 **Pini, Pulau** *island* Kepulauan Batu, W Indonesia
109 Y7 **Pinka** ≈ SE Austria
109 X7 **Pinkafeld** Burgenland, SE Austria
Pinkiang *see* Harbin
10 M12 **Pink Mountain** British Columbia, W Canada
166 M3 **Pinlebu** Sagaing, N Myanmar
38 J12 **Pinnacle Island** *island* Alaska, USA
180 I12 **Pinnacles, The** *tourist site* Western Australia
182 K10 **Pinnaroo** South Australia
Pinne *see* Pniewy
100 I9 **Pinneberg** Schleswig-Holstein, N Germany
115 I15 **Pínnes, Akrotírio** *headland* N Greece
Pinos, Isla de *see* Juventud, Isla de la
35 R14 **Pinos, Mount** ▲ California, W USA
105 R12 **Pinoso** País Valenciano, E Spain
105 N14 **Pinos-Puente** Andalucía, S Spain
41 Q17 **Pinotepa Nacional** *var.* Santiago Pinotepa Nacional. Oaxaca, SE Mexico
114 F13 **Pínovo** ▲ N Greece
187 R17 **Pins, Île des** *var.* Kunyé. *island* E New Caledonia
119 I20 **Pinsk** *Pol.* Pińsk. Brestskaya Voblasts', SW Belarus
14 D18 **Pins, Pointe aux** *headland* Ontario, S Canada
57 B16 **Pinta, Isla** *var.* Abingdon. *island* Galapagos Islands, Ecuador, E Pacific Ocean
127 Q12 **Pinyug** Kirovskaya Oblast', NW Russian Federation
57 B17 **Pinzón, Isla** *var.* Duncan Island. *island* Galapagos Islands, Ecuador, E Pacific Ocean
35 Y8 **Pioche** Nevada, W USA
106 F13 **Piombino** Toscana, C Italy
(0) C9 **Pioneer Fracture Zone** *tectonic feature* NE Pacific Ocean
122 L5 **Pioner, Ostrov** *island* Severnaya Zemlya, N Russian Federation
118 A13 **Pionerskiy** *Ger.* Neukuhren. Kaliningradskaya Oblast', W Russian Federation
110 N13 **Pionki** Mazowieckie, C Poland
184 L9 **Piopio** Waikato, North Island, NZ
110 K13 **Piotrków Trybunalski** *Ger.* Petrikau, *Rus.* Petrokov. Łodzkie, C Poland
152 F12 **Pīpār Road** Rājasthān, N India
115 I16 **Pipéri** *island* Vóreioi Sporádes, Greece, Aegean Sea
29 S10 **Pipestone** Minnesota, N USA
12 C9 **Pipestone** ≈ Ontario, C Canada
61 E21 **Pipinas** Buenos Aires, E Argentina
149 T7 **Piplān** *prev.* Liaqatabad. Punjab, E Pakistan
15 R5 **Pipmuacan, Réservoir** ⊠ Quebec, SE Canada
Piqan *see* Shanshan
31 R13 **Piqua** Ohio, N USA
105 P5 **Piqueras, Puerto de** *pass* N Spain
60 H11 **Piquiri, Rio** ≈ S Brazil
60 L9 **Piracicaba** São Paulo, S Brazil
Piraeus/Piraiévs *see* Peiraías
60 K10 **Piraju** São Paulo, S Brazil
60 K9 **Pirajuí** São Paulo, S Brazil
63 G21 **Pirámide, Cerro** ▲ S Chile
Piramiva *see* Pyramíva
109 R13 **Piran** *It.* Pirano. SW Slovenia
62 N6 **Pirané** Formosa, N Argentina
59 J18 **Piranhas** Goiás, S Brazil
Pirano *see* Piran
142 I4 **Pīrānshahr** Āžarbāyjān-e Bākhtarī, NW Iran
59 M19 **Pirapora** Minas Gerais, NE Brazil
60 I9 **Pirapòzinho** São Paulo, S Brazil
61 G19 **Piraraja** Lavalleja, S Uruguay
60 L9 **Pirassununga** São Paulo, S Brazil
45 V6 **Pirata, Monte** ▲ E Puerto Rico
60 I13 **Piratuba** Santa Catarina, S Brazil
114 I9 **Pirdop** *prev.* Srednogorie. Sofiya, W Bulgaria
191 P7 **Pirea** Tahiti, W French Polynesia
59 K18 **Pirenópolis** Goiás, S Brazil
153 S13 **Pirganj** Rajshahi, NW Bangladesh
Pirgi *see* Pyrgí
Pírgos *see* Pýrgos
61 F20 **Piriápolis** Maldonado, S Uruguay
114 G11 **Pirin** ▲ SW Bulgaria
Pirineos *see* Pyrenees
58 N13 **Piripiri** Piauí, E Brazil
118 H4 **Pirita** *var.* Pirita Jõgi. ≈ NW Estonia
Pirita Jõgi *see* Pirita
54 J6 **Píritu** Portuguesa, N Venezuela
93 L18 **Pirkkala** Länsi-Suomi, W Finland
101 F20 **Pirmasens** Rheinland-Pfalz, SW Germany
101 P16 **Pirna** Sachsen, E Germany
Piroe *see* Piru
113 Q15 **Pirot** Serbia, SE Yugoslavia
152 H6 **Pīr Panjāl Range** ▲ NE India
43 W16 **Pirre, Cerro** ▲ SE Panama
137 Y11 **Pirsaat** *Rus.* Pirsagat. ≈ E Azerbaijan
Pirsagat *see* Pirsaat
143 V11 **Pīr Shūrān, Selseleh-ye** ▲ SE Iran
92 M12 **Pirttikoski** Lappi, N Finland
Pirttikylä *see* Pörtom
171 R13 **Piru** *prev.* Piroe. Pulau Seram, E Indonesia
Piryatin *see* Pyryatyn
Pis *see* Piis Moen
106 F11 **Pisa** *var.* Pisae. Toscana, C Italy
Pisae *see* Pisa
189 V12 **Pisar** *atoll* Chuuk Islands, C Micronesia
Pisaurum *see* Pesaro
14 M10 **Piscatosine, Lac** ◎ Quebec, SE Canada
109 W7 **Pischeldorf** Steiermark, SE Austria
Pischk *see* Simeria
107 L19 **Pisciotta** Campania, S Italy
57 E16 **Pisco** Ica, SW Peru
116 G9 **Pişcolt** *Hung.* Piskolt. Satu Mare, NW Romania
57 E16 **Pisco, Río** ≈ E Peru
111 C18 **Písek** Budějovický Kraj, S Czech Republic
31 R14 **Pisgah** Ohio, N USA
158 F9 **Pishan** *var.* Guma. Xinjiang Uygur Zizhiqu, NW China
117 N8 **Pishchanka** Vinnyts'ka Oblast', C Ukraine
113 K21 **Pishë** Fier, SW Albania
143 X14 **Pīshīn** Sīstān va Balūchestān, SE Iran
149 O9 **Pishīn** North-West Frontier Province, NW Pakistan
149 N11 **Pishin Lora** *var.* Psein Lora, *Pash.* Pseyn Bowr. ≈ SW Pakistan
Pishma *see* Pizhma
Pishpek *see* Bishkek
171 O14 **Pising** Pulau Kabaena, C Indonesia
Pisino *see* Pazin
Piski *see* Simeria
Piskolt *see* Pişcolt
147 Q9 **Piskom** *Rus.* Pskem. ≈ E Uzbekistan
Piskom Tizmasi *see* Pskemskiy Khrebet
35 P13 **Pismo Beach** California, W USA
77 P12 **Pissila** C Burkina
62 H8 **Pissis, Monte** ▲ N Argentina
41 X12 **Piste** Yucatán, E Mexico
107 O18 **Pisticci** Basilicata, S Italy
106 F11 **Pistoia** *anc.* Pistoria, Pistoriæ. Toscana, C Italy
32 E15 **Pistol River** Oregon, NW USA
Pistoria/Pistoriæ *see* Pistoia
15 U5 **Pistuacanis** ≈ Quebec, SE Canada
Pistyan *see* Piešt'any
104 M5 **Pisuerga** ≈ N Spain
110 N8 **Pisz** *Ger.* Johannisburg. Warmińsko-Mazurskie, NE Poland
76 I13 **Pita** Moyenne-Guinée, NW Guinea
54 D12 **Pitalito** Huila, S Colombia
60 I11 **Pitanga** Paraná, S Brazil
182 M9 **Pitarpunga Lake** *salt lake* New South Wales, SE Australia
193 P10 **Pitcairn Island** *island* S Pitcairn Islands
193 P10 **Pitcairn Islands** ◇ *UK dependent territory* C Pacific Ocean
93 J14 **Piteå** Norrbotten, N Sweden
92 I13 **Piteälven** ≈ N Sweden
116 I13 **Piteşti** Argeş, S Romania
Pithagorio *see* Pythagóreio
180 I12 **Pithara** Western Australia
103 N6 **Pithiviers** Loiret, C France
152 L9 **Pithorāgarh** Uttar Pradesh, N India
188 B16 **Piti** W Guam
106 G13 **Pitigliano** Toscana, C Italy
40 F3 **Pitiquito** Sonora, NW Mexico
Pitkäranta *see* Pitkyaranta
38 M11 **Pitkas Point** Alaska, USA
126 H11 **Pitkyaranta** *Fin.* Pitkäranta. Respublika Kareliya, NW Russian Federation
96 J10 **Pitlochry** C Scotland, UK
18 I16 **Pitman** New Jersey, NE USA
112 G8 **Pitomača** Virovitica-Podravina, NE Croatia
35 O2 **Pit River** ≈ California, W USA
63 G15 **Pitrufquén** Araucanía, S Chile
Pitsanulok *see* Phitsanulok
Pitschen *see* Byczyna
Pitsunda *see* Bichvint'a
109 X6 **Pitten** ≈ E Austria
10 J14 **Pitt Island** *island* British Columbia, W Canada
Pitt Island *see* Makin
22 M3 **Pittsboro** Mississippi, S USA
21 T9 **Pittsboro** North Carolina, SE USA
27 R7 **Pittsburg** Kansas, C USA
25 W6 **Pittsburg** Texas, SW USA
18 B14 **Pittsburgh** Pennsylvania, NE USA
30 J14 **Pittsfield** Illinois, N USA
19 R6 **Pittsfield** Maine, NE USA
18 L11 **Pittsfield** Massachusetts, NE USA
183 U3 **Pittsworth** Queensland, E Australia
62 I8 **Pituil** La Rioja, NW Argentina
56 A10 **Piura** Piura, NW Peru
56 A9 **Piura** *off.* Departamento de Piura. ◆ *department* NW Peru
35 S13 **Piute Peak** ▲ California, W USA
113 J15 **Piva** ≈ SW Yugoslavia
117 V5 **Pivdenne** Kharkivs'ka Oblast', E Ukraine
117 P8 **Pivdennyy Buh** *Rus.* Yuzhnyy Bug. ≈ S Ukraine
54 F5 **Pivijay** Magdalena, N Colombia
109 T13 **Pivka** *prev.* Šent Peter, *Ger.* Sankt Peter, *It.* San Pietro del Carso. SW Slovenia
117 U13 **Pivnichno-Kryms'kyy Kanal** *canal* S Ukraine
113 J15 **Pivsko Jezero** ◎ SW Yugoslavia
111 M18 **Piwniczna** Małopolskie, S Poland
35 R12 **Pixley** California, W USA
127 Q15 **Pizhma** *var.* Pishma. ≈ NW Russian Federation
13 U13 **Placentia** Newfoundland, SE Canada
Placentia *see* Piacenza
13 U13 **Placentia Bay** *inlet* Newfoundland, SE Canada
171 P5 **Placer** Masbate, N Philippines
35 P7 **Placerville** California, W USA
44 F5 **Placetas** Villa Clara, C Cuba
113 Q18 **Plačkovica** ▲ E FYR Macedonia
36 L2 **Plain City** Utah, W USA
22 G4 **Plain Dealing** Louisiana, S USA
31 O14 **Plainfield** Indiana, N USA
18 K14 **Plainfield** New Jersey, NE USA
33 O8 **Plains** Montana, NW USA
24 L6 **Plains** Texas, SW USA
29 X10 **Plainview** Minnesota, N USA
29 Q13 **Plainview** Nebraska, C USA
25 N4 **Plainview** Texas, SW USA
26 K4 **Plainville** Kansas, C USA
115 L25 **Pláka, Akrotírio** *headland* Kríti, Greece, E Mediterranean Sea
115 J15 **Pláka, Akrotírio** *headland* Límnos, E Greece
113 N19 **Plakenska Planina** ▲ SW FYR Macedonia
44 K5 **Plana Cays** *islets* SE Bahamas
105 S12 **Plana, Isla** *var.* Nueva Tabarca. *island* E Spain
59 L18 **Planaltina** Goiás, S Brazil
83 O14 **Planalto Moçambicano** *plateau* N Mozambique
112 N10 **Plandište** Serbia, NE Yugoslavia
100 N13 **Plane** ≈ NE Germany
54 E6 **Planeta Rica** Córdoba, NW Colombia
29 P11 **Plankinton** South Dakota, N USA
30 M11 **Plano** Illinois, N USA
25 U6 **Plano** Texas, SW USA
23 W12 **Plant City** Florida, SE USA
22 J9 **Plaquemine** Louisiana, S USA
104 K9 **Plasencia** Extremadura, W Spain
112 P7 **Plaska** Podlaskie, NE Poland
114 C10 **Plaški** Karlovac, C Croatia
113 N19 **Plasnica** SW FYR Macedonia
13 N14 **Plaster Rock** New Brunswick, SE Canada
107 J24 **Platani** *anc.* Halycus. ≈ Sicilia, Italy, C Mediterranean Sea
115 G17 **Plataniá** Thessalía, C Greece
115 G24 **Plátanos** Kríti, Greece, E Mediterranean Sea
65 H18 **Plata, Río de la** *var.* River Plate. *estuary* Argentina/Uruguay
77 V15 **Plateau** ◆ *state* C Nigeria
79 G19 **Plateaux** *var.* Région des Plateaux. ◆ *province* C Congo
92 P1 **Platen, Kapp** *headland* NE Svalbard
Plate, River *see* Plata, Río de la
99 G22 **Plate Taille, Lac de la** *var.* L'Eau d'Heure. ◎ SE Belgium
Plathe *see* Płoty
39 N13 **Platinum** Alaska, USA
54 F5 **Plato** Magdalena, N Colombia
29 O11 **Platte** South Dakota, N USA
27 R3 **Platte City** Missouri, C USA
Plattensee *see* Balaton
27 R3 **Platte River** ≈ Iowa/Missouri, USA
29 Q15 **Platte River** ≈ Nebraska, C USA
37 T3 **Platteville** Colorado, C USA
30 K9 **Platteville** Wisconsin, N USA
101 N21 **Plattling** Bayern, SE Germany
27 R3 **Plattsburg** Missouri, C USA
18 L6 **Plattsburgh** New York, NE USA
29 S15 **Plattsmouth** Nebraska, C USA
101 M17 **Plauen** *var.* Plauen im Vogtland. Sachsen, E Germany
Plauen im Vogtland *see* Plauen
100 M10 **Plauer See** ◎ NE Germany
113 L16 **Plav** Montenegro, SW Yugoslavia
118 I10 **Pļaviņas** *Ger.* Stockmannshof. Aizkraukle, S Latvia
128 K5 **Plavsk** Tul'skaya Oblast', W Russian Federation
41 Z12 **Playa del Carmen** Quintana Roo, E Mexico
40 J12 **Playa Los Corchos** Nayarit, SW Mexico
37 P16 **Playas Lake** ◎ New Mexico, SW USA
41 S15 **Playa Vicenté** Veracruz-Llave, SE Mexico
167 U11 **Plây Cu** *var.* Pleiku. Gia Lai, C Vietnam
28 L3 **Plaza** North Dakota, N USA
63 I15 **Plaza Huincul** Neuquén, C Argentina
36 L3 **Pleasant Grove** Utah, W USA
29 V14 **Pleasant Hill** Iowa, C USA
27 R4 **Pleasant Hill** Missouri, C USA
Pleasant Island *see* Nauru
36 K13 **Pleasant, Lake** ⊠ Arizona, SW USA
19 P8 **Pleasant Mountain** ▲ Maine, NE USA
27 R5 **Pleasanton** Kansas, C USA

◆ Country ● Country Capital ◇ Dependent Territory ○ Dependent Territory Capital ◆ Administrative Region ✕ International Airport ▲ Mountain ▲ Mountain Range ▲ Volcano ◎ Lake ≈ River ⊠ Reservoir

25 R12 **Pleasanton** Texas, SW USA
185 G20 **Pleasant Point** Canterbury, South Island, NZ
19 R5 **Pleasant River** ∽ Maine, NE USA
18 J17 **Pleasantville** New Jersey, NE USA
103 N12 **Pléaux** Cantal, C France
111 B19 **Plechý** Ger. Plöckenstein. ▲ Austria/Czech Republic
Pleebo see Plibo
Pleihari see Pelaihari
Pleiku see Plây Cu
101 M16 **Pleisse** ∽ E Germany
Plencia see Plentzia
184 O7 **Plenty, Bay of** bay North Island, NZ
33 Y6 **Plentywood** Montana, NW USA
105 O2 **Plentzia** var. Plencia. País Vasco, N Spain
102 H5 **Plérin** Côtes d'Armor, NW France
126 M10 **Plesetsk** Arkhangel'skaya Oblast', NW Russian Federation
Pleshchenitsy see Plyeshchanitsy
Pleskau see Pskov
Pleskauer See see Pskov, Lake
Pleskava see Pskov
112 E8 **Pleso International** ✕ (Zagreb) Zagreb, NW Croatia
Pless see Pszczyna
15 Q11 **Plessisville** Quebec, SE Canada
110 H12 **Pleszew** Wielkopolskie, C Poland
12 L10 **Plétipi, Lac** ◎ Quebec, SE Canada
101 F15 **Plettenberg** Nordrhein-Westfalen, W Germany
114 I8 **Pleven** prev. Plevna. Pleven, N Bulgaria
114 I8 **Pleven** ◈ province N Bulgaria
Plevlja/Plevlje see Pljevlja
Plevna see Pleven
Plezzo see Bovec
Pliberk see Bleiburg
76 L17 **Plibo** var. Pleebo. SE Liberia
121 R11 **Pliny Trench** undersea feature C Mediterranean Sea
118 K13 **Plisa** Rus. Plissa. Vitsyebskaya Voblasts', N Belarus
Plissa see Plisa
112 D11 **Plitvica Selo** Lika-Senj, W Croatia
112 D11 **Plješevica** ▲ C Croatia
113 K14 **Pljevlja** prev. Plevlja, Plevlje. Montenegro, N Yugoslavia
Ploça see Plloçë
Plocce see Ploče
113 G15 **Ploče** It. Plocce; prev. Kardeljevo. Dubrovnik-Neretva, SE Croatia
113 K22 **Plloçë** var. Ploça. Vlorë, SW Albania
110 K11 **Płock** Ger. Plozk. Mazowieckie, C Poland
109 Q10 **Plöcken Pass** Ger. Plöckenpass, It. Passo di Monte Croce Carnico. pass SW Austria
Plöckenstein see Plechý
99 B19 **Ploegsteert** Hainaut, W Belgium
102 H6 **Ploërmel** Morbihan, NW France
Ploești see Ploiești
116 K13 **Ploiești** prev. Ploești. Prahova, SE Romania
115 L17 **Plomári** prev. Plomárion. Lésvos, E Greece
Plomárion see Plomári
103 O12 **Plomb du Cantal** ▲ C France
183 V6 **Plomer, Point** headland New South Wales, SE Australia
100 J8 **Plön** Schleswig-Holstein, N Germany
110 L11 **Płońsk** Mazowieckie, C Poland
119 J20 **Plotnitsa** Rus. Plotnitsa. Brestskaya Voblasts', SW Belarus
110 E8 **Płoty** Ger. Plathe. Zachodniopomorskie, NW Poland
102 G7 **Plouay** Morbihan, NW France
111 D15 **Ploučnice** Ger. Polzen. ∽ NE Czech Republic
114 I10 **Plovdiv** prev. Eumolpias, anc. Evmolpia, Philippopolis, Lat. Trimontium. Plovdiv, C Bulgaria 24.47
116 J11 **Plovdiv** ◈ province C Bulgaria
30 L6 **Plover** Wisconsin, N USA
Plozk see Płock
27 U11 **Plumerville** Arkansas, C USA
19 P10 **Plum Island** island Massachusetts, NE USA
32 M9 **Plummer** Idaho, NW USA
83 J18 **Plumtree** Matabeleland South, SW Zimbabwe
118 D11 **Plungė** Plungė, W Lithuania
113 J15 **Plužine** Montenegro, SW Yugoslavia
119 K14 **Plyeshchanitsy** Rus. Pleshchenitsy. Minskaya Voblasts', N Belarus
45 V10 **Plymouth** ○ (Montserrat) SW Montserrat
97 I24 **Plymouth** SW England, UK
31 O11 **Plymouth** Indiana, N USA
19 P12 **Plymouth** Massachusetts, NE USA
19 N8 **Plymouth** New Hampshire, NE USA
21 X9 **Plymouth** North Carolina, SE USA
30 M8 **Plymouth** Wisconsin, N USA
97 J20 **Plynlimon** ▲ C Wales, UK
126 G14 **Plyussa** Pskovskaya Oblast', W Russian Federation
111 B17 **Plzeň** Ger. Pilsen, Pol. Pilzno. Plzeňský Kraj, W Czech Republic
111 B17 **Plzeňský Kraj** ◈ region W Czech Republic
110 F11 **Pniewy** Ger. Pinne. Wielkolpolskie, C Poland
106 D8 **Po** ∽ N Italy
77 P13 **Pô** S Burkina
42 M13 **Poás, Volcán** ⚹ NW Costa Rica
77 S16 **Pobè** S Benin
123 S8 **Pobeda, Gora** ▲ NE Russian Federation
Pobeda Peak see Pobedy, Pik/Tomur Feng
147 Z7 **Pobedy, Pik** var. Pobeda Peak, Chin. Tomur Feng. ▲ China/Kyrgyzstan see also Tomur Feng
110 H11 **Pobiedziska** Ger. Pudewitz. Wielkolpolskie, C Poland
Po, Bocche del see Po, Foci del
27 W9 **Pocahontas** Arkansas, C USA
29 U12 **Pocahontas** Iowa, C USA
33 Q15 **Pocatello** Idaho, NW USA
167 S13 **Pochentong** ✕ (Phnum Penh) Phnum Penh, S Cambodia
128 I6 **Pochep** Bryanskaya Oblast', W Russian Federation
128 H4 **Pochinok** Smolenskaya Oblast', W Russian Federation
41 R17 **Pochutla** var. San Pedro Pochutla. Oaxaca, SE Mexico
62 I6 **Pocitos, Salar** var. Salar Quiróm. salt lake NW Argentina
101 O22 **Pocking** Bayern, SE Germany
186 I10 **Pocklington Reef** reef SE PNG
27 R11 **Pocola** Oklahoma, C USA
21 Y5 **Pocomoke City** Maryland, NE USA
59 L21 **Poços de Caldas** Minas Gerais, NE Brazil
126 H14 **Podberez'ye** Novgorodskaya Oblast', NW Russian Federation
Podbrodzie see Pabradė
127 U8 **Podcher'ye** Respublika Komi, NW Russian Federation
111 E16 **Poděbrady** Ger. Podiebrad. Středočeský Kraj, C Czech Republic
128 L9 **Podgorenskiy** Voronezhskaya Oblast', W Russian Federation
113 J17 **Podgorica** prev. Titograd. Montenegro, SW Yugoslavia
113 K17 **Podgorica** ✕ Montenegro, SW Yugoslavia
109 T13 **Podgrad** SW Slovenia
Podiebrad see Poděbrady
116 M5 **Podil's'ka Vysochina** plateau W Ukraine
Podium Anicensis see le Puy
122 L11 **Podkamennaya Tunguska** Eng. Stony Tunguska. ∽ C Russian Federation
113 N17 **Podkarpackie** ◈ province SE Poland
Pod Klošter see Arnoldstein
110 O9 **Podlaskie** ◈ province NE Poland
129 Q8 **Podlesnoye** Saratovskaya Oblast', W Russian Federation
128 K4 **Podol'sk** Moskovskaya Oblast', W Russian Federation
76 H10 **Podor** N Senegal
127 P12 **Podosinovets** Kirovskaya Oblast', NW Russian Federation
126 I12 **Podporozh'ye** Leningradskaya Oblast', NW Russian Federation
Podravska Slatina see Slatina, Croatia
112 J13 **Podromanlja** Republika Srpska, SE Bosnia & Herzegovina
Podsvil'ye see Padsvillye
116 L9 **Podu Iloaiei** prev. Podul Iloaiei. Iași, NE Romania
113 N15 **Podujevo** Serbia, S Yugoslavia
Podul Iloaiei see Podu Iloaiei
Podunajská Rovina see Little Alföld
126 M12 **Podyuga** Arkhangel'skaya Oblast', NW Russian Federation
56 A9 **Poechos, Embalse** ⊡ NW Peru
55 W10 **Poeketi** Sipaliwini, E Surinam
100 L8 **Poel** island N Germany
83 M20 **Poelela, Lagoa** ◎ S Mozambique
Poerwodadi see Purwodadi
Poetovio see Ptuj
83 E23 **Pofadder** Northern Cape, W South Africa
106 I9 **Po, Foci del** var. Bocche del Po. ∽ NE Italy
116 E12 **Pogăniș** ∽ W Romania
Pogegen see Pagėgiai
106 G12 **Poggibonsi** Toscana, C Italy
107 I14 **Poggio Mirteto** Lazio, C Italy
109 V4 **Pöggstall** Niederösterreich, N Austria
116 L13 **Pogoanele** Buzău, SE Romania
Pogónion see Delvináki
113 M21 **Pogradec** var. Pogradeci. Korçë, SE Albania
Pogradeci see Pogradec
123 S15 **Pogranichnyy** Primorskiy Kray, SE Russian Federation
38 M16 **Pogromni Volcano** ▲ Unimak Island, Alaska, USA
163 Z15 **P'ohang** Jap. Hokō. E South Korea
15 T9 **Pohénégamook, Lac** ◎ Quebec, SE Canada
93 L20 **Pohja** Swe. Pojo. Etelä-Suomi, SW Finland
Pohjanlahti see Bothnia, Gulf of
189 U16 **Pohnpei** ◈ state E Micronesia
189 O12 **Pohnpei** ✕ Pohnpei, E Micronesia
189 O12 **Pohnpei** prev. Ponape Ascension Island. island E Micronesia
111 F19 **Pohořelice** Ger. Pohrlitz. Brněnský Kraj, SE Czech Republic
109 V10 **Pohorje** Ger. Bacher. ▲ N Slovenia
117 N6 **Pohrebyshche** Vinnyts'ka Oblast', C Ukraine
Pohrlitz see Pohořelice
161 P9 **Po Hu** ⊡ E China
116 G15 **Poiana Mare** Dolj, S Romania
Poictiers see Poitiers
129 N6 **Poim** Penzenskaya Oblast', W Russian Federation
Poindo see Lhünzhub
195 Y13 **Poinsett, Cape** headland Antarctica
29 R9 **Poinsett, Lake** ◎ South Dakota, N USA
22 I10 **Point Au Fer Island** island Louisiana, S USA
39 X14 **Point Baker** Prince of Wales Island, Alaska, USA
25 U13 **Point Comfort** Texas, SW USA
Point de Galle see Galle
44 K10 **Pointe à Gravois** headland SW Haiti
22 L10 **Pointe a la Hache** Louisiana, S USA
45 Y6 **Pointe-à-Pitre** Grande Terre, C Guadeloupe
15 U7 **Pointe-au-Père** Quebec, SE Canada
15 V5 **Pointe-aux-Anglais** Quebec, SE Canada
45 T10 **Pointe du Cap** headland N Saint Lucia
79 E21 **Pointe-Noire** Le Kouilou, S Congo
45 X6 **Pointe Noire** Basse Terre, W Guadeloupe
79 E21 **Pointe-Noire** ✕ Le Kouilou, S Congo
45 U15 **Point Fortin** Trinidad, Trinidad and Tobago
38 M6 **Point Hope** Alaska, USA
39 N5 **Point Lay** Alaska, USA
18 B16 **Point Marion** Pennsylvania, NE USA
18 K16 **Point Pleasant** New Jersey, NE USA
21 P4 **Point Pleasant** West Virginia, NE USA
45 R14 **Point Salines** ✕ (St.George's) SW Grenada
102 L9 **Poitiers** prev. Poictiers; anc. Limonum. Vienne, W France
102 K9 **Poitou** cultural region W France
102 K10 **Poitou-Charentes** ◈ region W France
103 N3 **Poix-de-Picardie** Somme, N France
Pojo see Pohja
37 S10 **Pojoaque** New Mexico, SW USA
152 E11 **Pokaran** Rājasthān, NW India
183 R4 **Pokataroo** New South Wales, SE Australia
119 P18 **Pokats'** Rus. Pokot'. ∽ SE Belarus
29 V5 **Pokegama Lake** ◎ Minnesota, N USA
184 L6 **Pokeno** Waikato, North Island, NZ
153 O11 **Pokhara** Western, C Nepal
129 T6 **Pokhvistnevo** Samarskaya Oblast', W Russian Federation
55 W10 **Pokigron** Sipaliwini, C Surinam
92 L10 **Pokka** Lapp. Bohkká. Lappi, N Finland
79 N16 **Poko** Orientale, NE Dem. Rep. Congo (Zaire)
Pokot' see Pokats'
Po-ko-to Shan see Bogda Shan
147 S7 **Pokrovka** Talasskaya Oblast', NW Kyrgyzstan
Pokrovka see Kyzyl-Suu
117 V8 **Pokrovs'ke** Rus. Pokrovskoye. Dnipropetrovs'ka Oblast', E Ukraine
Pokrovskoye see Pokrovs'ke
Pola see Pula
37 N10 **Polacca** Arizona, SW USA
104 L2 **Pola de Laviana** Asturias, N Spain
104 K2 **Pola de Lena** Asturias, N Spain
104 L2 **Pola de Siero** Asturias, N Spain
191 Y3 **Poland** Kiritimati, E Kiribati
110 H12 **Poland** off. Republic of Poland, var. Polish Republic, Pol. Polska, Rzeczpospolita Polska; prev. Pol. Polska Rzeczpospolita Ludowa, Polish People's Republic. ◆ republic C Europe
Polangen see Palanga
110 G7 **Polanów** Ger. Pollnow. Zachodniopomorskie, NW Poland
136 H13 **Polatlı** Ankara, C Turkey
118 L12 **Polatsk** Rus. Polotsk. Vitsyebskaya Voblasts', N Belarus
110 F8 **Połczyn-Zdrój** Ger. Bad Polzin. Zachodniopomorskie, NW Poland
146 I16 **Polekhatum** prev. Pul'-I-Khatum. Akhalskiy Velayat, S Turkmenistan
149 Q3 **Pol-e Khomrī** var. Pul-i-Khumri. Baghlān, NE Afghanistan
197 S10 **Pole Plain** undersea feature Arctic Ocean
143 P5 **Pol-e Safīd** var. Pol-e-Sefid, Pul-i-Sefid. Māzandarān, N Iran
Pol-e-Sefid see Pol-e Safīd
118 B13 **Polessk** Ger. Labiau. Kaliningradskaya Oblast', W Russian Federation
Polesskoye see Polis'ke
171 N13 **Polewali** Sulawesi, C Indonesia
114 G11 **Polezhan** ▲ SW Bulgaria
78 F13 **Poli** Nord, N Cameroon
Poli see Pólis
107 M19 **Policastro, Golfo di** gulf S Italy
110 D8 **Police** Ger. Politz. Zachodniopomorskie, NW Poland
172 I17 **Police, Pointe** headland Mahé, NE Seychelles
115 L17 **Polichnítos** var. Polihnitos, Políkhnitos. Lésvos, E Greece
Poligiros see Polýgyros
107 P17 **Polignano a Mare** Puglia, SE Italy
103 S9 **Poligny** Jura, E France
Polihnitos see Polichnítos
Polikastro/Políkastron see Polýkastro
Políkhnitos see Polichnítos
114 K8 **Polikrayshte** Veliko Tŭrnovo, N Bulgaria
171 O3 **Polillo Islands** island group N Philippines
109 Q9 **Polinik** ▲ SW Austria
121 O2 **Polis** var. Poli. W Cyprus
Polish People's Republic see Poland
Polish Republic see Poland
117 O3 **Polis'ke** Rus. Polesskoye. Kyyivs'ka Oblast', N Ukraine
107 N22 **Polistena** Calabria, SW Italy
Politz see Police
Políyiros see Polýgyros
29 V14 **Polk City** Iowa, C USA
110 F13 **Polkowice** Ger. Heerwegen. Dolnośląskie, SW Poland
155 G22 **Pollāchi** Tamil Nādu, SE India
109 W7 **Pöllau** Steiermark, SE Austria
189 T13 **Polle** atoll Chuuk Islands, C Micronesia
Pollnow see Polanów
29 N7 **Pollock** South Dakota, N USA
92 L8 **Polmak** Finnmark, N Norway
30 L10 **Polo** Illinois, N USA
193 V15 **Poloa** island Tongatapu Group, N Tonga
42 E5 **Polochic, Río** ∽ C Guatemala
Pologi see Polohy
117 V9 **Polohy** Rus. Pologi. Zaporiz'ka Oblast', SE Ukraine
14 M10 **Polonais, Lac des** ◎ Quebec, SE Canada
61 G20 **Polonio, Cabo** headland E Uruguay
155 K24 **Polonnaruwa** North Central Province, C Sri Lanka
116 L5 **Polonne** Rus. Polonnoye. Khmel'nyts'ka Oblast', NW Ukraine
Polonnoye see Polonne
Polotsk see Polatsk
109 T7 **Pöls** var. Pölsbach. ∽ E Austria
Pölsbach see Pöls
Polska/Polska, Rzeczpospolita/Polska Rzeczpospolita Ludowa see Poland
114 L10 **Polski Gradets** Stara Zagora, C Bulgaria
114 K8 **Polsko Kosovo** Ruse, N Bulgaria
33 P8 **Polson** Montana, NW USA
117 T6 **Poltava** Poltavs'ka Oblast', NE Ukraine
Poltava see Poltavs'ka Oblast'
117 R5 **Poltavs'ka Oblast'** var. Poltava, Rus. Poltavskaya Oblast'. ◈ province NE Ukraine
Poltavskaya Oblast' see Poltavs'ka Oblast'
Poltoratsk see Ashgabat
118 I5 **Põltsamaa** Ger. Oberpahlen. Jõgevamaa, E Estonia
118 I4 **Põltsamaa** var. Põltsamaa Jõgi. ∽ C Estonia
Põltsamaa Jõgi see Põltsamaa
122 I8 **Poluy** ∽ N Russian Federation
118 J6 **Põlva** Ger. Põlwe. Põlvamaa, SE Estonia
93 N16 **Polvijärvi** Itä-Suomi, E Finland
Põlwe see Põlva
115 I22 **Polýaigos** island Kykládes, Greece, Aegean Sea
115 I22 **Polyaígou Folégandrou, Stenó** strait Kykládes, Greece, Aegean Sea
126 J3 **Polyarnyy** Murmanskaya Oblast', NW Russian Federation
127 W5 **Polyarnyy Ural** ▲ NW Russian Federation
115 G14 **Polýgyros** var. Poligiros, Políyiros. Kentrikí Makedonía, N Greece
114 F13 **Polýkastro** var. Polikastro; prev. Políkastron. Kentrikí Makedonía, N Greece
193 O9 **Polynesia** island group C Pacific Ocean
115 J15 **Polýochni** site of ancient city Límnos, E Greece
41 Y13 **Polyuc** Quintana Roo, E Mexico
109 V10 **Polzela** C Slovenia
Polzen see Ploučnice
56 D12 **Pomabamba** Ancash, C Peru
185 D23 **Pomahaka** ∽ South Island, NZ
106 F12 **Pomarance** Toscana, C Italy
104 G9 **Pombal** Leiria, C Portugal
76 D9 **Pombas** Santo Antão, NW Cape Verde
83 N19 **Pomene** Inhambane, SE Mozambique
110 G8 **Pomerania** cultural region Germany/Poland
110 D7 **Pomeranian Bay** Ger. Pommersche Bucht, Pol. Zatoka Pomorska. bay Germany/Poland
31 T15 **Pomeroy** Ohio, N USA
32 L10 **Pomeroy** Washington, NW USA
117 Q8 **Pomichna** Kirovohrads'ka Oblast', C Ukraine
186 H7 **Pomio** New Britain, E PNG
Pomir, Dar"yoi see Pamir/Pāmīr, Daryā-ye
27 T6 **Pomme de Terre Lake** ⊡ Missouri, C USA
29 S8 **Pomme de Terre River** ∽ Minnesota, N USA
Pommersche Bucht see Pomeranian Bay
35 T15 **Pomona** California, W USA
114 N9 **Pomorie** Burgas, E Bulgaria
Pomorska, Zatoka see Pomeranian Bay
110 H8 **Pomorskie** ◈ province N Poland
127 Q4 **Pomorskiy Proliv** strait NW Russian Federation
127 T10 **Pomozdino** Respublika Komi, NW Russian Federation
Pompaelo see Pamplona
23 Z15 **Pompano Beach** Florida, SE USA
107 K18 **Pompei** Campania, S Italy
33 V10 **Pompeys Pillar** Montana, NW USA
Ponape Ascension Island see Pohnpei
29 R13 **Ponca** Nebraska, C USA
27 O8 **Ponca City** Oklahoma, C USA
45 T6 **Ponce** C Puerto Rico
23 X10 **Ponce de Leon Inlet** inlet Florida, SE USA
22 K8 **Ponchatoula** Louisiana, S USA
26 M8 **Pond Creek** Oklahoma, C USA
155 J20 **Pondicherry** var. Puduchcheri, Fr. Pondichéry. Pondicherry, SE India
151 I20 **Pondicherry** var. Puduchcheri, Fr. Pondichéry. ◈ union territory India
Pondichéry see Pondicherry
197 N11 **Pond Inlet** Baffin Island, Nunavut, NE Canada
187 P16 **Ponérihouen** Province Nord, C New Caledonia
104 J4 **Ponferrada** Castilla-León, NW Spain
184 N13 **Pongaroa** Manawatu-Wanganui, North Island, NZ
167 Q12 **Pong Nam Ron** Chantaburi, S Thailand
81 C14 **Pongo** ∽ S Sudan
152 I7 **Pong Reservoir** ⊡ N India
111 N14 **Poniatowa** Lubelskie, E Poland
167 R12 **Pônhea Krêk** prev. Kâmpóng Chhnăng, C Cambodia
155 I20 **Ponnaiyār** ∽ SE India
11 Q15 **Ponoka** Alberta, SW Canada
129 U6 **Ponomarevka** Orenburgskaya Oblast', W Russian Federation
169 Q17 **Ponorogo** Jawa, C Indonesia
126 M5 **Ponoy** Murmanskaya Oblast', NW Russian Federation
122 F6 **Ponoy** ∽ NW Russian Federation
102 K11 **Pons** Charente-Maritime, W France
Pons see Ponts
Pons Aelii see Newcastle upon Tyne
Pons Vetus see Pontevedra
99 G20 **Pont-à-Celles** Hainaut, S Belgium
102 K16 **Pontacq** Pyrénées-Atlantiques, SW France
64 P3 **Ponta Delgada** São Miguel, Azores, Portugal, NE Atlantic Ocean
64 P3 **Ponta Delgado** ✕ São Miguel, Azores, Portugal, NE Atlantic Ocean
64 N2 **Ponta do Pico** ▲ Pico, Azores, Portugal, NE Atlantic Ocean
60 J11 **Ponta Grossa** Paraná, S Brazil
103 S5 **Pont-à-Mousson** Meurthe-et-Moselle, NE France
103 T9 **Pontarlier** Doubs, E France
106 G11 **Pontassieve** Toscana, C Italy
102 L4 **Pont-Audemer** Eure, N France
22 K9 **Pontchartrain, Lake** ◎ Louisiana, S USA
102 I8 **Pontchâteau** Loire-Atlantique, NW France
103 R10 **Pont-de-Vaux** Ain, E France
104 G4 **Ponteareas** Galicia, NW Spain
106 J6 **Pontebba** Friuli-Venezia Giulia, NE Italy
104 G4 **Ponte Caldelas** Galicia, NW Spain
107 J16 **Pontecorvo** Lazio, C Italy
104 G5 **Ponte da Barca** Viana do Castelo, N Portugal
104 G5 **Ponte de Lima** Viana do Castelo, N Portugal
106 F11 **Pontedera** Toscana, C Italy
104 H10 **Ponte de Sor** Portalegre, C Portugal
104 H2 **Pontedeume** Galicia, NW Spain
106 F6 **Ponte di Legno** Lombardia, N Italy
11 T17 **Ponteix** Saskatchewan, S Canada
59 N20 **Ponte Nova** Minas Gerais, NE Brazil
59 G18 **Pontes e Lacerda** Mato Grosso, W Brazil
104 G4 **Pontevedra** anc. Pons Vetus. Galicia, NW Spain
104 G3 **Pontevedra** ◈ province Galicia, NW Spain
104 G4 **Pontevedra, Ría de** estuary NW Spain
30 M12 **Pontiac** Illinois, N USA
31 R9 **Pontiac** Michigan, N USA
169 P11 **Pontianak** Borneo, C Indonesia
107 I16 **Pontino, Agro** plain C Italy
Pontisarae see Pontoise
102 H6 **Pontivy** Morbihan, NW France
102 F6 **Pont-l'Abbé** Finistère, NW France
103 N4 **Pontoise** anc. Briva Isarae, Cergy-Pontoise, Pontisarae. Val-d'Oise, N France
11 W13 **Ponton** Manitoba, C Canada
102 J5 **Pontorson** Manche, N France
22 M2 **Pontotoc** Mississippi, S USA
25 R9 **Pontotoc** Texas, SW USA
106 E10 **Pontremoli** Toscana, C Italy
108 J10 **Pontresina** Graubünden, S Switzerland
105 U5 **Ponts** var. Pons. Cataluña, NE Spain
103 R14 **Pont-St-Esprit** Gard, S France
97 K21 **Pontypool** Wel. Pontypŵl. SE Wales, UK
97 J22 **Pontypridd** S Wales, UK
Pontypŵl see Pontypool
43 R17 **Ponuga** Veraguas, SE Panama
184 L6 **Ponui Island** island N NZ
119 K14 **Ponya** Rus. Ponya. ∽ N Belarus
107 I17 **Ponziane, Isole** island C Italy
182 F7 **Poochera** South Australia
97 L24 **Poole** S England, UK
25 S6 **Poolville** Texas, SW USA
Poona see Pune
182 M8 **Pooncarie** New South Wales, SE Australia
183 N6 **Poopelloe Lake** seasonal lake New South Wales, SE Australia
57 K19 **Poopó** Oruro, C Bolivia
57 K19 **Poopó, Lago** var. Lago Pampa Aullagas. ◎ W Bolivia
184 L3 **Poor Knights Islands** island N NZ
39 P10 **Poorman** Alaska, USA
182 E3 **Pootnoura** South Australia
147 R10 **Pop** Rus. Pap. Namangan Wiloyati, E Uzbekistan
117 X7 **Popasna** Rus. Popasnaya. Luhans'ka Oblast', E Ukraine
Popasnaya see Popasna
54 D12 **Popayán** Cauca, SW Colombia
99 B18 **Poperinge** West-Vlaanderen, W Belgium
123 N7 **Popigay** Taymyrskiy (Dolgano-Nenetskiy) Avtonomnyy Okrug, N Russian Federation
123 N7 **Popigay** ∽ N Russian Federation
117 O5 **Popil'nya** Zhytomyrs'ka Oblast', N Ukraine
182 K8 **Popiltah Lake** seasonal lake New South Wales, SE Australia
33 X7 **Poplar** Montana, NW USA
11 Y14 **Poplar** ∽ Manitoba, C Canada
27 X8 **Poplar Bluff** Missouri, C USA
33 X6 **Poplar River** ∽ Montana, NW USA
41 P14 **Popocatépetl** ⚹ S Mexico
79 H21 **Popokabaka** Bandundu, SW Dem. Rep. Congo (Zaire)
107 J15 **Popoli** Abruzzo, C Italy
186 F9 **Popondetta** Northern, S PNG
112 F9 **Popovača** Sisak-Moslavina, NE Croatia
114 J10 **Popovitsa** Tŭrgovishte, C Bulgaria
114 L8 **Popovo** Tŭrgovishte, N Bulgaria
Popovo see Iskra
Popper see Poprad
30 M5 **Popple River** ∽ Wisconsin, N USA
111 L19 **Poprad** Ger. Deutschendorf, Hung. Poprád. Prešovský Kraj, E Slovakia
111 L18 **Poprad** Ger. Popper, Hung. Poprád. ∽ Poland/Slovakia
111 L19 **Poprad-Tatry** ✕ (Poprad) Prešovský Kraj, E Slovakia
21 X7 **Poquoson** Virginia, NE USA
149 O15 **Porāli** ∽ SW Pakistan
184 N12 **Porangahau** Hawke's Bay, North Island, NZ
59 K17 **Porangatu** Goiás, C Brazil
119 G18 **Porazava** Pol. Porozow, Rus. Porozovo. Hrodzyenskaya Voblasts', W Belarus
154 A11 **Porbandar** Gujarāt, W India
10 I13 **Porcher Island** island British Columbia, SW Canada
104 M13 **Porcuna** Andalucía, S Spain
14 F7 **Porcupine** Ontario, S Canada
64 M6 **Porcupine Bank** undersea feature N Atlantic Ocean
11 V15 **Porcupine Hills** ▲ Manitoba/Saskatchewan, S Canada
30 L3 **Porcupine Mountains** hill range Michigan, N USA
64 M7 **Porcupine Plain** undersea feature E Atlantic Ocean
8 G7 **Porcupine River** ∽ Canada/USA
106 I7 **Pordenone** anc. Portenau. Friuli-Venezia Giulia, NE Italy
54 H9 **Pore** Casanare, E Colombia
112 A9 **Poreč** It. Parenzo. Istra, NW Croatia
60 I9 **Porecatu** Paraná, S Brazil
Porech'ye see Parechcha
129 P4 **Poretskoye** Chuvashskaya Respublika, W Russian Federation
77 Q13 **Porga** N Benin
186 B7 **Porgera** Enga, W PNG
93 K18 **Pori** Swe. Björneborg. Länsi-Suomi, W Finland
185 L14 **Porirua** Wellington, North Island, NZ
92 I12 **Porjus** Norrbotten, N Sweden
126 G14 **Porkhov** Pskovskaya Oblast', W Russian Federation
55 O4 **Porlamar** Nueva Esparta, NE Venezuela
102 I8 **Pornic** Loire-Atlantique, NW France
186 B7 **Poroma** Southern Highlands, W PNG
123 T13 **Poronaysk** Ostrov Sakhalin, Sakhalinskaya Oblast', SE Russian Federation
115 G20 **Póros** Póros, S Greece
115 C19 **Póros** Kefallinía, Iónioi Nísoi, Greece, C Mediterranean Sea
115 G20 **Póros** island S Greece
81 G24 **Poroto Mountains** ▲ SW Tanzania
112 B10 **Porozina** Primorje-Gorski Kotar, NW Croatia
Porozovo/Porozow see Porazava
195 X15 **Porpoise Bay** bay Antarctica
65 G15 **Porpoise Point** headland NE Ascension Island
65 C25 **Porpoise Point** headland East Falkland, Falkland Islands
108 C6 **Porrentruy** Jura, NW Switzerland
106 F10 **Porretta Terme** Emilia-Romagna, C Italy
104 G4 **Porriño** Galicia, NW Spain
92 L7 **Porsangen** fjord N Norway

◆ Country ● Country Capital ◇ Dependent Territory ○ Dependent Territory Capital ◈ Administrative Region ✕ International Airport ▲ Mountain ▲ Mountain Range ⚹ Volcano ∽ River ◎ Lake ⊡ Reservoir

92 *K8* **Porsangerhalvøya** *peninsula* N Norway
95 *G16* **Porsgrunn** Telemark, S Norway
136 *E13* **Porsuk Çayı** ↝ C Turkey
Porsy *see* Boldumsaz
57 *N18* **Portachuelo** Santa Cruz, C Bolivia
182 *I9* **Port Adelaide** South Australia
97 *F15* **Portadown** *Ir.* Port An Dúnáin. S Northern Ireland, UK
31 *P10* **Portage** Michigan, N USA
18 *D15* **Portage** Pennsylvania, NE USA
30 *K8* **Portage** Wisconsin, N USA
30 *M3* **Portage Lake** ◎ Michigan, N USA
11 *X16* **Portage la Prairie** Manitoba, S Canada
31 *R11* **Portage River** ↝ Ohio, N USA
27 *Y8* **Portageville** Missouri, C USA
28 *L2* **Portal** North Dakota, N USA
10 *L17* **Port Alberni** Vancouver Island, British Columbia, SW Canada
14 *E15* **Port Albert** Ontario, S Canada
104 *I10* **Portalegre** *anc.* Ammaia, Amoea. Portalegre, E Portugal
104 *H10* **Portalegre** ◆ *district* C Portugal
37 *V12* **Portales** New Mexico, SW USA
39 *X14* **Port Alexander** Baranof Island, Alaska, USA
83 *I25* **Port Alfred** Eastern Cape, S South Africa
10 *J16* **Port Alice** Vancouver Island, British Columbia, SW Canada
22 *J8* **Port Allen** Louisiana, S USA
Port Amelia *see* Pemba
Port An Dúnáin *see* Portadown
32 *G7* **Port Angeles** Washington, NW USA
44 *L12* **Port Antonio** NE Jamaica
115 *D16* **Pórta Panagiá** *religious building* Thessalía, C Greece
25 *T14* **Port Aransas** Texas, SW USA
97 *E18* **Portarlington** *Ir.* Cúil an tSúdaire. C Ireland
183 *P17* **Port Arthur** Tasmania, SE Australia
25 *Y11* **Port Arthur** Texas, SW USA
96 *G12* **Port Askaig** W Scotland, UK
182 *I7* **Port Augusta** South Australia
44 *M9* **Port-au-Prince** ● (Haiti) C Haiti
44 *M9* **Port-au-Prince** ✕ E Haiti
22 *I8* **Port Barre** Louisiana, S USA
151 *Q19* **Port Blair** Andaman and Nicobar Islands, SE India
25 *X12* **Port Bolivar** Texas, SW USA
105 *X4* **Portbou** Cataluña, NE Spain
77 *N17* **Port Bouet** ✕ (Abidjan) SE Ivory Coast
182 *I8* **Port Broughton** South Australia
14 *F17* **Port Burwell** Ontario, S Canada
12 *G17* **Port Burwell** Quebec, NE Canada
182 *M13* **Port Campbell** Victoria, SE Australia
15 *V4* **Port-Cartier** Quebec, SE Canada
185 *F23* **Port Chalmers** Otago, South Island, NZ
23 *W14* **Port Charlotte** Florida, SE USA
38 *L9* **Port Clarence** Alaska, USA
10 *I13* **Port Clements** Graham Island, British Columbia, SW Canada
31 *S11* **Port Clinton** Ohio, N USA
14 *H17* **Port Colborne** Ontario, S Canada
15 *Y7* **Port-Daniel** Quebec, SE Canada
Port Darwin *see* Darwin
183 *O17* **Port Davey** *headland* Tasmania, SE Australia
44 *K8* **Port-de-Paix** NW Haiti
181 *W4* **Port Douglas** Queensland, NE Australia
10 *J13* **Port Edward** British Columbia, SW Canada
83 *K24* **Port Edward** KwaZulu/Natal, SE South Africa
58 *J12* **Portel** Pará, NE Brazil
104 *H12* **Portel** Évora, S Portugal
14 *E14* **Port Elgin** Ontario, S Canada
45 *Y14* **Port Elizabeth** Bequia, Saint Vincent and the Grenadines
83 *I26* **Port Elizabeth** Eastern Cape, S South Africa
96 *G13* **Port Ellen** W Scotland, UK
Portenau *see* Pordenone
97 *H16* **Port Erin** SW Isle of Man
45 *Q13* **Porter Point** *headland* Saint Vincent, Saint Vincent and the Grenadines
185 *G18* **Porters Pass** *pass* South Island, NZ
83 *E25* **Porterville** Western Cape, SW South Africa
35 *R12* **Porterville** California, W USA
Port-Étienne *see* Nouâdhibou
182 *L13* **Port Fairy** Victoria, SE Australia
184 *M4* **Port Fitzroy** Great Barrier Island, Auckland, NE NZ
Port Florence *see* Kisumu
Port-Francqui *see* Ilebo
79 *C18* **Port-Gentil** Ogooué-Maritime, W Gabon
182 *I7* **Port Germein** South Australia
22 *J6* **Port Gibson** Mississippi, S USA
39 *Q13* **Port Graham** Alaska, USA
77 *U17* **Port Harcourt** Rivers, S Nigeria
10 *J16* **Port Hardy** Vancouver Island, British Columbia, SW Canada
Port Harrison *see* Inukjuak
13 *R14* **Port Hawkesbury** Cape Breton Island, Nova Scotia, SE Canada
180 *I6* **Port Hedland** Western Australia
39 *O15* **Port Heiden** Alaska, USA
97 *I19* **Porthmadog** *var.* Portmadoc. NW Wales, UK
14 *I15* **Port Hope** Ontario, SE Canada
13 *S9* **Port Hope Simpson** Newfoundland, E Canada
65 *C24* **Port Howard Settlement** West Falkland, Falkland Islands
31 *T9* **Port Huron** Michigan, N USA
107 *K17* **Portici** Campania, S Italy
137 *Y13* **Port-Il'ic** *Rus.* Port Il'ich. SE Azerbaijan
Port Il'ich *see* Port-Ilic
104 *G14* **Portimão** *var.* Vila Nova de Portimão. Faro, S Portugal
25 *T17* **Port Isabel** Texas, SW USA
18 *J13* **Port Jervis** New York, NE USA
55 *S7* **Port Kaituma** NW Guyana
128 *K12* **Port Katon** Rostovskaya Oblast', SW Russian Federation
183 *S9* **Port Kembla** New South Wales, SE Australia
182 *F8* **Port Kenny** South Australia
Port Klang *see* Pelabuhan Klang
Port Láirge *see* Waterford
183 *S8* **Portland** New South Wales, SE Australia
182 *L13* **Portland** Victoria, SE Australia
184 *K4* **Portland** Northland, North Island, NZ
31 *Q13* **Portland** Indiana, N USA
19 *P8* **Portland** Maine, NE USA
31 *Q9* **Portland** Michigan, N USA
29 *Q4* **Portland** North Dakota, N USA
32 *G11* **Portland** Oregon, NW USA
20 *J8* **Portland** Tennessee, S USA
25 *T14* **Portland** Texas, SW USA
32 *G11* **Portland** ✕ Oregon, NW USA
182 *L13* **Portland Bay** *bay* Victoria, SE Australia
44 *K13* **Portland Bight** *bay* S Jamaica
97 *L24* **Portland Bill** *var.* Bill of Portland. *headland* S England, UK
Portland, Bill of *see* Portland Bill
183 *P15* **Portland, Cape** *headland* Tasmania, SE Australia
10 *J12* **Portland Inlet** *inlet* British Columbia, W Canada
184 *P11* **Portland Island** *island* E NZ
65 *F15* **Portland Point** *headland* SW Ascension Island
44 *J13* **Portland Point** *headland* C Jamaica
103 *P16* **Port-la-Nouvelle** Aude, S France
Portlaoighise *see* Port Laoise
97 *E18* **Port Laoise** *var.* Portlaoise, *Ir.* Portlaoighise; *prev.* Maryborough. C Ireland
25 *U13* **Port Lavaca** Texas, SW USA
182 *G9* **Port Lincoln** South Australia
39 *Q14* **Port Lions** Kodiak Island, Alaska, USA
76 *I15* **Port Loko** W Sierra Leone
65 *E24* **Port Louis** East Falkland, Falkland Islands
45 *Y5* **Port-Louis** Grande Terre, N Guadeloupe
173 *X16* **Port Louis** ● (Mauritius) NW Mauritius
Port Louis *see* Scarborough
Port-Lyautey *see* Kénitra
182 *K12* **Port MacDonnell** South Australia
183 *U7* **Port Macquarie** New South Wales, SE Australia
Portmadoc *see* Porthmadog
Port Mahon *see* Mahón
44 *K12* **Port Maria** C Jamaica
10 *K16* **Port McNeill** Vancouver Island, British Columbia, SW Canada
13 *P11* **Port-Menier** Île d'Anticosti, Quebec, E Canada
39 *N15* **Port Moller** Alaska, USA
44 *L13* **Port Morant** E Jamaica
44 *K13* **Portmore** C Jamaica
186 *D9* **Port Moresby** ● (PNG) Central/National Capital District, SW PNG
Port Natal *see* Durban
25 *Y11* **Port Neches** Texas, SW USA
182 *G9* **Port Neill** South Australia
15 *S6* **Portneuf** ↝ Quebec, SE Canada
15 *R6* **Portneuf, Lac** ◎ Quebec, SE Canada
83 *D23* **Port Nolloth** Northern Cape, W South Africa
18 *J17* **Port Norris** New Jersey, NE USA
Port-Nouveau-Québec *see* Kangiqsualujjuaq
104 *G6* **Porto** *Eng.* Oporto; *anc.* Portus Cale. Porto, NW Portugal
104 *G6* **Porto** *var.* Pôrto. ◆ *district* N Portugal
104 *G6* **Porto** ✕ Porto, W Portugal
61 *I16* **Porto Alegre** *var.* Pôrto Alegre. *state capital* Rio Grande do Sul, S Brazil
Porto Alexandre *see* Tombua
82 *B12* **Porto Amboim** Cuanza Sul, NW Angola
Porto Amélia *see* Pemba
Porto Bello *see* Portobelo
43 *T14* **Portobelo** *var.* Porto Bello, Puerto Bello. Colón, N Panama
60 *G10* **Pôrto Camargo** Paraná, S Brazil
25 *U13* **Port O'Connor** Texas, SW USA
Pôrto de Mós *see* Porto de Moz
58 *J12* **Porto de Moz** *var.* Pôrto de Mós. Pará, NE Brazil
64 *O5* **Porto do Moniz** Madeira, Portugal, NE Atlantic Ocean
59 *H16* **Porto dos Gaúchos** Mato Grosso, W Brazil
Porto Edda *see* Sarandë
107 *J24* **Porto Empedocle** Sicilia, Italy, C Mediterranean Sea
59 *H20* **Porto Esperança** Mato Grosso do Sul, SW Brazil
106 *E13* **Portoferraio** Toscana, C Italy
96 *G6* **Port of Ness** NW Scotland, UK
45 *U14* **Port-of-Spain** ● (Trinidad and Tobago) Trinidad, Trinidad and Tobago
Port of Spain *see* Piarco
103 *X15* **Porto, Golfe de** *gulf* Corse, France, C Mediterranean Sea
Porto Grande *see* Mindelo
106 *I7* **Portogruaro** Veneto, NE Italy
35 *P5* **Portola** California, W USA
187 *Q13* **Port-Olry** Espiritu Santo, C Vanuatu
93 *J17* **Pörtom** *Fin.* Pirttikylä. Länsi-Suomi, W Finland
Port Omna *see* Portumna
59 *G21* **Porto Murtinho** Mato Grosso do Sul, SW Brazil
59 *K16* **Porto Nacional** Tocantins, C Brazil
77 *S16* **Porto-Novo** ● (Benin) S Benin
23 *X10* **Port Orange** Florida, SE USA
32 *G8* **Port Orchard** Washington, NW USA
Porto Re *see* Kraljevica
32 *E15* **Port Orford** Oregon, NW USA
Porto Rico *see* Puerto Rico
106 *J13* **Porto San Giorgio** Marche, C Italy
107 *F14* **Porto San Stefano** Toscana, C Italy
64 *P5* **Porto Santo** *var.* Vila Baleira. Porto Santo, Madeira, Portugal, NE Atlantic Ocean
64 *Q5* **Porto Santo** ✕ Porto Santo, Madeira, Portugal, NE Atlantic Ocean
64 *P5* **Porto Santo** *var.* Ilha do Porto Santo. *island* Madeira, Portugal, NE Atlantic Ocean
60 *H9* **Porto São José** Paraná, S Brazil
59 *O19* **Porto Seguro** Bahia, E Brazil
107 *B17* **Porto Torres** Sardegna, Italy, C Mediterranean Sea
59 *J23* **Porto União** Santa Catarina, S Brazil
103 *Y16* **Porto-Vecchio** Corse, France, C Mediterranean Sea
59 *E15* **Porto Velho** *var.* Velho. *state capital* Rondônia, W Brazil
56 *A6* **Portoviejo** *var.* Puertoviejo. Manabí, W Ecuador
185 *B26* **Port Pegasus** *bay* Stewart Island, NZ
14 *H15* **Port Perry** Ontario, SE Canada
183 *N12* **Port Phillip Bay** *harbour* Victoria, SE Australia
182 *I8* **Port Pirie** South Australia
96 *G9* **Portree** N Scotland, UK
Port Rex *see* East London
Port Rois *see* Portrush
44 *K13* **Port Royal** E Jamaica
21 *R15* **Port Royal** South Carolina, SE USA
21 *R15* **Port Royal Sound** *inlet* South Carolina, SE USA
97 *F14* **Portrush** *Ir.* Port Rois. N Northern Ireland, UK
75 *W7* **Port Said** *Ar.* Būr Sa'īd. N Egypt
23 *R9* **Port Saint Joe** Florida, SE USA
23 *Y11* **Port Saint John** Florida, SE USA
83 *K24* **Port St.Johns** Eastern Cape, SE South Africa
103 *R16* **Port-St-Louis-du-Rhône** Bouches-du-Rhône, SE France
44 *K10* **Port Salut** SW Haiti
65 *E24* **Port Salvador** *inlet* East Falkland, Falkland Islands
65 *D24* **Port San Carlos** East Falkland, Falkland Islands
13 *S10* **Port Saunders** Newfoundland, SE Canada
83 *K24* **Port Shepstone** KwaZulu/Natal, E South Africa
45 *O11* **Portsmouth** *var.* Grand-Anse. NW Dominica
97 *N24* **Portsmouth** S England, UK
19 *P10* **Portsmouth** New Hampshire, NE USA
31 *S15* **Portsmouth** Ohio, N USA
21 *X7* **Portsmouth** Virginia, NE USA
14 *E17* **Port Stanley** Ontario, S Canada
65 *B25* **Port Stephens** *inlet* West Falkland, Falkland Islands
65 *B25* **Port Stephens Settlement** West Falkland, Falkland Islands
97 *F14* **Portstewart** *Ir.* Port Stíobhaird. N Northern Ireland, UK
Port Stíobhaird *see* Portstewart
80 *I7* **Port Sudan** Red Sea, NE Sudan
22 *L10* **Port Sulphur** Louisiana, S USA
Port Swettenham *see* Klang/Pelabuhan Klang
97 *J22* **Port Talbot** S Wales, UK
92 *L11* **Porttipahdan Tekojärvi** ◎ N Finland
32 *G7* **Port Townsend** Washington, NW USA
104 *H9* **Portugal** *off.* Republic of Portugal. ◆ *republic* SW Europe
105 *O2* **Portugalete** País Vasco, N Spain
54 *J6* **Portuguesa** *off.* Estado Portuguesa. ◆ *state* N Venezuela
Portuguese East Africa *see* Mozambique
Portuguese Guinea *see* Guinea-Bissau
Portuguese Timor *see* East Timor
Portuguese West Africa *see* Angola
97 *D18* **Portumna** *Ir.* Port Omna. W Ireland
Portus Cale *see* Porto
Portus Magnus *see* Almería
Portus Magonis *see* Mahón
103 *P17* **Port-Vendres** *var.* Port Vendres. Pyrénées-Orientales, S France
182 *H9* **Port Victoria** South Australia
187 *Q14* **Port-Vila** *var.* Vila. ● (Vanuatu) Éfaté, C Vanuatu
182 *I9* **Port Wakefield** South Australia
31 *N8* **Port Washington** Wisconsin, N USA
57 *J14* **Porvenir** Pando, NW Bolivia
63 *I24* **Porvenir** Magallanes, S Chile
61 *D18* **Porvenir** Paysandú, W Uruguay
93 *M19* **Porvoo** *Swe.* Borgå. Etelä-Suomi, S Finland
Porzecze *see* Parechcha
104 *M10* **Porzuna** Castilla-La Mancha, C Spain
61 *E14* **Posadas** Misiones, NE Argentina
104 *L13* **Posadas** Andalucía, S Spain
Poschega *see* Požega
108 *J11* **Poschiavino** ↝ Italy/Switzerland
108 *J10* **Poschiavo** *Ger.* Puschlav. Graubünden, S Switzerland
112 *D12* **Posedarje** Zadar, SW Croatia
Posen *see* Poznań
126 *L14* **Poshekhon'ye** Yaroslavskaya Oblast', W Russian Federation
92 *M13* **Posio** Lappi, NE Finland
Poskam *see* Zepu
Posnania *see* Poznań
171 *O12* **Poso** Sulawesi, C Indonesia
59 *P15* **Poço da Cruz, Açude** ⊞ E Brazil
171 *O12* **Poso, Danau** ◎ Sulawesi, C Indonesia
137 *R10* **Posof** Ardahan, NE Turkey
25 *R6* **Possum Kingdom Lake** ⊞ Texas, SW USA
25 *N6* **Post** Texas, SW USA
Postavy/Postawy *see* Pastavy
12 *I7* **Poste-de-la-Baleine** Quebec, NE Canada
99 *M17* **Postel** *prev.* Postheholt Limburg, SE Netherlands
83 *G22* **Postmasburg** Northern Cape, N South Africa
Pôsto Diuarum *see* Campo de Diauarum
59 *I16* **Pôsto Jacaré** Mato Grosso, W Brazil
109 *T12* **Postojna** *Ger.* Adelsberg, *It.* Postumia. SW Slovenia
Postumia *see* Postojna
29 *X12* **Postville** Iowa, C USA
Pöstyén *see* Piešt'any
113 *G14* **Posušje** Federacija Bosna I Herzegovina, SE Bosnia & Herzegovina
171 *O16* **Pota** Flores, C Indonesia
115 *G23* **Potamós** Antikýthira, S Greece
55 *S9* **Potaru River** ↝ C Guyana
83 *I21* **Potchefstroom** North-West, N South Africa
27 *R11* **Poteau** Oklahoma, C USA
25 *R12* **Poteet** Texas, SW USA
115 *G14* **Poteídaia** *site of ancient city* Kentrikí Makedonía, N Greece
Potentia *see* Potenza
107 *M18* **Potenza** *anc.* Potentia. Basilicata, S Italy
185 *A24* **Poteriteri, Lake** ◎ South Island, NZ
104 *M2* **Potes** Cantabria, N Spain
83 *J20* **Potgietersrus** Northern, NE South Africa
25 *S12* **Poth** Texas, SW USA
32 *J9* **Potholes Reservoir** ⊞ Washington, NW USA
137 *Q9* **P'ot'i** W Georgia
77 *X13* **Potiskum** Yobe, NE Nigeria
Potkozarje *see* Ivanjska
32 *M9* **Potlatch** Idaho, NW USA
33 *N9* **Pot Mountain** ▲ Idaho, NW USA
113 *H14* **Potoci** Federacija Bosna I Hercegovina, SE Bosnia & Herzegovina
21 *V3* **Potomac River** ↝ NE USA
27 *W6* **Potosi** Missouri, C USA
57 *L20* **Potosí** Potosí, S Bolivia
42 *H9* **Potosí** Chinandega, NW Nicaragua
57 *K21* **Potosí** ◆ *department* SW Bolivia
62 *H7* **Potrerillos** Atacama, N Chile
42 *H5* **Potrerillos** Cortés, NW Honduras
62 *H8* **Potro, Cerro del** ▲ N Chile
100 *N12* **Potsdam** Brandenburg, NE Germany
18 *J7* **Potsdam** New York, NE USA
109 *X5* **Pottendorf** Niederösterreich, E Austria
109 *X5* **Pottenstein** Niederösterreich, E Austria
18 *I15* **Pottstown** Pennsylvania, NE USA
18 *H14* **Pottsville** Pennsylvania, NE USA
155 *L25* **Pottuvil** Eastern Province, SE Sri Lanka
149 *U6* **Potwar Plateau** *plateau* NE Pakistan
102 *J7* **Pouancé** Maine-et-Loire, W France
15 *R6* **Poulin de Courval, Lac** ◎ Quebec, SE Canada
18 *L9* **Poultney** Vermont, NE USA
187 *O16* **Poum** Province Nord, W New Caledonia
59 *L21* **Pouso Alegre** Minas Gerais, NE Brazil
192 *I16* **Poutasi** Upolu, SE Samoa
167 *R12* **Poŭthĭsăt** *prev.* Pursat. Poŭthĭsăt, W Cambodia
167 *R12* **Poŭthĭsăt, Stœng** *prev.* Pursat. ↝ W Cambodia
102 *J9* **Pouzauges** Vendée, NW France
Po, Valle del *see* Po Valley
106 *F8* **Po Valley** *It.* Valle del Po. *valley* N Italy
111 *I19* **Považská Bystrica** *Ger.* Waagbistritz, *Hung.* Vágbeszterce. Trenčiansky Kraj, W Slovakia
126 *J10* **Povenets** Respublika Kareliya, NW Russian Federation
184 *Q9* **Poverty Bay** *inlet* North Island, NZ
112 *K12* **Povlen** ▲ W Yugoslavia
104 *G6* **Póvoa de Varzim** Porto, NW Portugal
129 *N8* **Povorino** Voronezhskaya Oblast', W Russian Federation
Povungnituk *see* Puvirnituq
12 *J3* **Povungnituk, Rivière de** ↝ Quebec, NE Canada
14 *H11* **Powassan** Ontario, S Canada
35 *U17* **Poway** California, W USA
33 *W14* **Powder River** Wyoming, C USA
33 *Y10* **Powder River** ↝ Montana/Wyoming, NW USA
32 *L12* **Powder River** ↝ Oregon, NW USA
33 *W13* **Powder River Pass** *pass* Wyoming, C USA
33 *U12* **Powell** Wyoming, C USA
65 *I22* **Powell Basin** *undersea feature* NW Weddell Sea
36 *M8* **Powell, Lake** ◎ Utah, W USA
37 *R4* **Powell, Mount** ▲ Colorado, C USA
10 *L17* **Powell River** British Columbia, SW Canada
31 *N5* **Powers** Michigan, N USA
28 *K2* **Powers Lake** North Dakota, N USA
21 *V6* **Powhatan** Virginia, NE USA
31 *V13* **Powhatan Point** Ohio, N USA
97 *J20* **Powys** *cultural region* E Wales, UK
187 *P17* **Poya** Province Nord, C New Caledonia
161 *P10* **Poyang Hu** ◎ S China
30 *L7* **Poygan, Lake** ◎ Wisconsin, N USA
109 *Y2* **Poysdorf** Niederösterreich, NE Austria
112 *N11* **Požarevac** *Ger.* Passarowitz. Serbia, NE Yugoslavia
41 *Q13* **Poza Rica** *var.* Poza Rica de Hidalgo. Veracruz-Llave, E Mexico
Poza Rica de Hidalgo *see* Poza Rica
112 *L13* **Požega** *Prev.* Slavonska Požega; *Ger.* Poschega, *Hung.* Pozsega. Požega-Slavonija, NE Croatia
112 *H9* **Požega-Slavonija** *off.* Požeško-Slavonska Županija. ◆ *province* NE Croatia
127 *U13* **Pozhva** Komi-Permyatskiy Avtonomnyy Okrug, NW Russian Federation
110 *G11* **Poznań** *Ger.* Posen, Posnania. Wielkolpolskie, C Poland
105 *O13* **Pozo Alcón** Andalucía, S Spain
62 *H3* **Pozo Almonte** Tarapacá, N Chile
104 *L12* **Pozoblanco** Andalucía, S Spain
105 *Q11* **Pozo Cañada** Castilla-La Mancha, C Spain
62 *N5* **Pozo Colorado** Presidente Hayes, C Paraguay
63 *J20* **Pozos, Punta** *headland* S Argentina
Pozsega *see* Požega
Pozsony *see* Bratislava
55 *N5* **Pozuelos** Anzoátegui, NE Venezuela
107 *L26* **Pozzallo** Sicilia, Italy, C Mediterranean Sea
107 *K17* **Pozzuoli** *anc.* Puteoli. Campania, S Italy
77 *P17* **Pra** ↝ S Ghana
111 *C19* **Prachatice** *Ger.* Prachatitz. Budějovický Kraj, S Czech Republic
Prachatitz *see* Prachatice
167 *P11* **Prachin Buri** *var.* Prachinburi. Prachin Buri, C Thailand
Prachuab Girikhand *see* Prachuap Khiri Khan
167 *O12* **Prachuap Khiri Khan** *var.* Prachuab Girikhand. Prachuap Khiri Khan, SW Thailand
111 *H16* **Praděd** *Ger.* Altvater. ▲ NE Czech Republic
54 *D11* **Pradera** Valle del Cauca, SW Colombia
103 *O17* **Prades** Pyrénées-Orientales, S France
59 *O19* **Prado** Bahia, SE Brazil
54 *E11* **Prado** Tolima, C Colombia
Prado del Ganso *see* Goose Green
Prae *see* Phrae
Prag/Praga/Prague *see* Praha
27 *O10* **Prague** Oklahoma, C USA
111 *D16* **Praha** *Eng.* Prague, *Ger.* Prag, *Pol.* Praga. ● (Czech Republic) Středočeský Kraj, NW Czech Republic
116 *J13* **Prahova** ◆ *county* SE Romania
116 *J13* **Prahova** ↝ S Romania
76 *E10* **Praia** ● (Cape Verde) Santiago, S Cape Verde
83 *M21* **Praia do Bilene** Gaza, S Mozambique
83 *M20* **Praia do Xai-Xai** Gaza, S Mozambique
116 *J10* **Praid** *Hung.* Parajd. Harghita, C Romania
26 *J3* **Prairie Dog Creek** ↝ Kansas/Nebraska, C USA
30 *J9* **Prairie du Chien** Wisconsin, N USA
27 *S9* **Prairie Grove** Arkansas, C USA
31 *P10* **Prairie River** ↝ Michigan, N USA
Prairie State *see* Illinois
25 *V11* **Prairie View** Texas, SW USA
167 *Q10* **Prakhon Chai** Buri Ram, E Thailand
109 *R4* **Pram** ↝ N Austria
109 *S4* **Prambachkirchen** Oberösterreich, N Austria
118 *H2* **Prangli** *island* N Estonia
154 *J13* **Prānhita** ↝ C India
172 *I15* **Praslin** *island* Inner Islands, NE Seychelles
115 *O23* **Prasonísi, Akrotírio** *headland* Ródos, Dodekánisos, Greece, Aegean Sea
111 *I14* **Praszka** Opolskie, S Poland
119 *M18* **Pratasy** *Rus.* Protasy. Homyel'skaya Voblasts', SE Belarus
167 *Q10* **Prathai** Nakhon Ratchasima, E Thailand
Prathet Thai *see* Thailand
Prathum Thani *see* Pathum Thani
63 *F21* **Prat, Isla** *island* S Chile
106 *G11* **Prato** Toscana, C Italy
103 *O17* **Prats-de-Mollo-la-Preste** Pyrénées-Orientales, S France
26 *L6* **Pratt** Kansas, C USA
108 *E6* **Pratteln** Basel-Land, NW Switzerland
193 *O2* **Pratt Seamount** *undersea feature* N Pacific Ocean
23 *P5* **Prattville** Alabama, S USA
Praust *see* Pruszcz Gdański
114 *M7* **Pravda** *prev.* Dogrular. Silistra, NE Bulgaria
119 *B14* **Pravdinsk** *Ger.* Friedland. Kaliningradskaya Oblast', W Russian Federation
104 *K2* **Pravia** Asturias, N Spain
118 *L12* **Prazaroki** *Rus.* Prozoroki. Vitsyebskaya Voblasts', N Belarus
Prázsmár *see* Prejmer
167 *S11* **Preăh Vihéar** Preăh Vihéar, N Cambodia
116 *J12* **Predeal** *Hung.* Predeál. Brașov, C Romania
109 *S8* **Predlitz** Steiermark, SE Austria
11 *V15* **Preeceville** Saskatchewan, S Canada
Preenkuln *see* Priekule
102 *K6* **Pré-en-Pail** Mayenne, NW France
109 *T4* **Pregarten** Oberösterreich, N Austria
54 *H7* **Pregonero** Táchira, NW Venezuela
118 *J10* **Preiļi** *Ger.* Preli. Preiļi, SE Latvia
116 *J12* **Prejmer** *Ger.* Tartlau, *Hung.* Prázsmár. Brașov, S Romania
113 *J16* **Prekornica** ▲ SW Yugoslavia
Preli *see* Preiļi
Prëmet *see* Përmet
100 *M12* **Premnitz** Brandenburg, NE Germany
25 *S15* **Premont** Texas, SW USA
113 *H14* **Prenj** ▲ S Bosnia and Herzegovina
Prenjas/Prenjasi *see* Përrenjas
22 *L7* **Prentiss** Mississippi, S USA
Preny *see* Prienai
100 *O10* **Prenzlau** Brandenburg, NE Germany
123 *N11* **Preobrazhenka** Irkutskaya Oblast', C Russian Federation
166 *J9* **Preparis Island** *island* SW Myanmar
Prerau *see* Přerov
111 *H18* **Přerov** *Ger.* Prerau. Olomoucký Kraj, E Czech Republic
Preschau *see* Prešov
14 *M14* **Prescott** Ontario, SE Canada
36 *K12* **Prescott** Arizona, SW USA
27 *T13* **Prescott** Arkansas, C USA
32 *L10* **Prescott** Washington, NW USA
30 *H6* **Prescott** Wisconsin, N USA
185 *A24* **Preservation Inlet** *inlet* South Island, NZ
112 *O7* **Preševo** Serbia, SE Yugoslavia
29 *N10* **Presho** South Dakota, N USA
58 *M13* **Presidente Dutra** Maranhão, E Brazil
60 *I8* **Presidente Epitácio** São Paulo, S Brazil
62 *N5* **Presidente Hayes** *off.* Departamento de Presidente Hayes. ◆ *department* C Paraguay
60 *I9* **Presidente Prudente** São Paulo, S Brazil
Presidente Stroessner *see* Ciudad del Este
Presidente Vargas *see* Itabira
60 *I8* **Presidente Venceslau** São Paulo, S Brazil
193 *O10* **President Thiers Seamount** *undersea feature* C Pacific Ocean
24 *J11* **Presidio** Texas, SW USA
Preslav *see* Veliki Preslav
111 *M19* **Prešov** *var.* Preschau, *Ger.* Eperies, *Hung.* Eperjes. Prešovský Kraj, E Slovakia
111 *M19* **Prešovský Kraj** ◆ *region* E Slovakia
113 *N20* **Prespa, Lake** *Alb.* Liqen i Prespës, *Gk.* Límni Megáli Préspa, Límni Prespa, *Mac.* Prespansko Ezero, *Serb.* Prespansko Jezero. ◎ SE Europe
Prespa, Limni/Prespansko Ezero/Prespansko Jezero/Prespës, Liqen i *see* Prespa, Lake
19 *S2* **Presque Isle** Maine, NE USA
18 *B11* **Presque Isle** *headland* Pennsylvania, NE USA
Pressburg *see* Bratislava
77 *P17* **Prestea** SW Ghana
111 *B17* **Přeštice** *Ger.* Pschestitz. Plzeňský Kraj, W Czech Republic
97 *K17* **Preston** NW England, UK
23 *S6* **Preston** Georgia, SE USA
33 *R16* **Preston** Idaho, NW USA
29 *Z13* **Preston** Iowa, C USA
29 *X11* **Preston** Minnesota, N USA
21 *O6* **Prestonsburg** Kentucky, S USA
96 *I13* **Prestwick** W Scotland, UK
83 *J21* **Pretoria** *var.* Epitoli, Tshwane. ● (South Africa-administrative capital) Gauteng, NE South Africa
Pretoria-Witwatersrand-Vereeniging *see* Gauteng
Pretusha *see* Pretushë
113 *M21* **Pretushë** *var.* Pretusha. Korçë, SE Albania

◆ Country ● Country Capital ◇ Dependent Territory ○ Dependent Territory Capital ◆ Administrative Region ✕ International Airport ▲ Mountain ▲ Mountain Range ☒ Volcano ↝ River ◎ Lake ⊞ Reservoir

Preussisch Eylau *see* Bagrationovsk
Preussisch-Stargard *see* Starogard Gdański
Preußisch Holland *see* Pasłęk
115 *C17* **Préveza** Ípeiros, W Greece
37 *V3* **Prewitt Reservoir** ⊞ Colorado, C USA
167 *S13* **Prey Vêng** Prey Vêng, S Cambodia
144 *M12* **Priaral'skiye Karakumy, Peski** *desert* SW Kazakhstan
123 *P14* **Priargunsk** Chitinskaya Oblast', S Russian Federation
38 *K14* **Pribilof Islands** *island group* Alaska, USA
113 *K14* **Priboj** Serbia, W Yugoslavia
111 *C17* **Příbram** *Ger.* Pibrans. Středočeský Kraj, W Czech Republic
36 *M4* **Price** Utah, W USA
37 *N5* **Price River** ≈ Utah, W USA
23 *N8* **Prichard** Alabama, S USA
25 *R8* **Priddy** Texas, SW USA
105 *P8* **Priego** Castilla-La Mancha, C Spain
104 *M14* **Priego de Córdoba** Andalucía, S Spain
118 *C10* **Priekule** *Ger.* Preenkuln. Liepāja, SW Latvia
118 *C12* **Priekulė** *Ger.* Prökuls. Gargždai, W Lithuania
119 *F14* **Prienai** *Pol.* Preny. Prienai, S Lithuania
83 *G23* **Prieska** Northern Cape, C South Africa
32 *M7* **Priest Lake** ◎ Idaho, NW USA
32 *M7* **Priest River** Idaho, NW USA
104 *M3* **Prieta, Peña** ▲ N Spain
40 *J10* **Prieto, Cerro** ▲ C Mexico
111 *J19* **Prievidza** *var.* Priewitz, *Ger.* Priwitz, *Hung.* Privigye. Trenčiansky Kraj, C Slovakia
Priewitz *see* Prievidza
112 *F10* **Prijedor** Republika Srpska, NW Bosnia & Herzegovina
113 *K14* **Prijepolje** Serbia, W Yugoslavia
Prikaspiyskaya Nizmennost' *see* Caspian Depression
113 *O19* **Prilep** *Turk.* Perlepe. S FYR Macedonia
108 *B9* **Prilly** Vaud, SW Switzerland
Priluki *see* Pryluky
62 *L10* **Primero, Río** ≈ C Argentina
29 *S12* **Primghar** Iowa, C USA
112 *B9* **Primorje-Gorski Kotar** *off.* Primorsko-Goranska Županija. ◆ *province* NW Croatia
118 *A13* **Primorsk** *Ger.* Fischhausen. Kaliningradskaya Oblast', W Russian Federation
126 *G12* **Primorsk** *Fin.* Koivisto. Leningradskaya Oblast', NW Russian Federation
Primorsk/Primorskoye *see* Prymors'k
123 *S14* **Primorskiy Kray** *prev. Eng.* Maritime Territory. ◆ *territory* SE Russian Federation
114 *N10* **Primorsko** *prev.* Keupriya. Burgas, E Bulgaria
128 *K13* **Primorsko-Akhtarsk** Krasnodarskiy Kray, SW Russian Federation
117 *U13* **Primors'kyy** Respublika Krym, S Ukraine
113 *D14* **Primošten** Šibenik-Knin, S Croatia
11 *R13* **Primrose Lake** ◎ Saskatchewan, C Canada
11 *T14* **Prince Albert** Saskatchewan, S Canada
83 *G25* **Prince Albert** Western Cape, SW South Africa
8 *J5* **Prince Albert Peninsula** *peninsula* Victoria Island, Northwest Territories, NW Canada
8 *J6* **Prince Albert Sound** *inlet* Northwest Territories, N Canada
8 *J5* **Prince Alfred, Cape** *headland* Northwest Territories, NW Canada
9 *P6* **Prince Charles Island** *island* Nunavut, NE Canada
195 *W6* **Prince Charles Mountains** ▲ Antarctica
Prince-Édouard, Île-du *see* Prince Edward Island
172 *M13* **Prince Edward Fracture Zone** *tectonic feature* SW Indian Ocean
13 *P14* **Prince Edward Island** *Fr.* Île-du Prince-Édouard. ◆ *province* SE Canada
13 *Q14* **Prince Edward Island** *Fr.* Île-du Prince-Édouard. *island* SE Canada
173 *M12* **Prince Edward Islands** *island group* S South Africa
21 *X4* **Prince Frederick** Maryland, NE USA
10 *M14* **Prince George** British Columbia, SW Canada
21 *W6* **Prince George** Virginia, NE USA
8 *L3* **Prince Gustaf Adolf Sea** *sea* Nunavut, N Canada
197 *Q3* **Prince of Wales, Cape** *headland* Alaska, USA
9 *N3* **Prince of Wales Icefield** *ice feature* Nunavut, N Canada
181 *V1* **Prince of Wales Island** *island* Queensland, E Australia
8 *L5* **Prince of Wales Island** *island* Queen Elizabeth Islands, Nunavut, NW Canada
39 *Y14* **Prince of Wales Island** *island* Alexander Archipelago, Alaska, USA
Prince of Wales Island *see* Pinang, Pulau
8 *J5* **Prince of Wales Strait** *strait* Northwest Territories, N Canada
8 *K4* **Prince Patrick Island** *island* Parry Islands, Northwest Territories, NW Canada
9 *N5* **Prince Regent Inlet** *channel* Nunavut, N Canada
10 *J13* **Prince Rupert** British Columbia, SW Canada
Prince's Island *see* Príncipe
21 *Y5* **Princess Anne** Maryland, NE USA
195 *R1* **Princess Astrid Kyst** *physical region* Antarctica
181 *W2* **Princess Charlotte Bay** *bay* Queensland, NE Australia
195 *W7* **Princess Elizabeth Land** *physical region* Antarctica
10 *J14* **Princess Royal Island** *island* British Columbia, SW Canada
45 *U15* **Princes Town** Trinidad, Trinidad and Tobago
11 *N17* **Princeton** British Columbia, SW Canada
30 *L11* **Princeton** Illinois, N USA
31 *N16* **Princeton** Indiana, N USA
29 *Z14* **Princeton** Iowa, C USA
20 *H7* **Princeton** Kentucky, S USA
29 *V8* **Princeton** Minnesota, N USA
27 *S1* **Princeton** Missouri, C USA
18 *J15* **Princeton** New Jersey, NE USA
21 *R6* **Princeton** West Virginia, NE USA
39 *S12* **Prince William Sound** *inlet* Alaska, USA
67 *P9* **Príncipe** *var.* Príncipe Island, *Eng.* Prince's Island. *island* N Sao Tome and Principe
Príncipe Island *see* Príncipe
32 *I13* **Prineville** Oregon, NW USA
28 *J11* **Pringle** South Dakota, N USA
25 *N1* **Pringle** Texas, SW USA
99 *H14* **Prinsenbeek** Noord-Brabant, S Netherlands
98 *L6* **Prinses Margriet Kanaal** *canal* N Netherlands
195 *T2* **Prinsesse Ragnhild Kyst** *physical region* Antarctica
195 *U2* **Prins Harald Kyst** *physical region* Antarctica
92 *N2* **Prins Karls Forland** *island* W Svalbard
43 *N8* **Prinzapolka** Región Autónoma Atlántico Norte, NE Nicaragua
42 *L8* **Prinzapolka, Río** ≈ NE Nicaragua
122 *H9* **Priob'ye** Khanty-Mansiyskiy Avtonomnyy Okrug, N Russian Federation
104 *H1* **Prior, Cabo** *headland* NW Spain
29 *V9* **Prior Lake** Minnesota, N USA
126 *H11* **Priozersk** *Fin.* Käkisalmi. Leningradskaya Oblast', NW Russian Federation
119 *J20* **Pripet** *Bel.* Prypyats', *Ukr.* Pryp"yat'. ≈ Belarus/Ukraine
119 *J20* **Pripet Marshes** *wetland* Belarus/Ukraine
Prishtinë *see* Priština
128 *J8* **Pristen'** Kurskaya Oblast', W Russian Federation
113 *N16* **Priština** *Alb.* Prishtinë. Serbia, S Yugoslavia
100 *M10* **Pritzwalk** Brandenburg, NE Germany
103 *R13* **Privas** Ardèche, E France
107 *I16* **Priverno** Lazio, C Italy
Privigye *see* Prievidza
112 *C12* **Privlaka** Zadar, SW Croatia
126 *M15* **Privolzhsk** Ivanovskaya Oblast', NW Russian Federation
129 *P7* **Privolzhskaya Vozvyshennost'** *var.* Volga Uplands. ▲ W Russian Federation
129 *P8* **Privolzhskoye** Saratovskaya Oblast', W Russian Federation
Priwitz *see* Prievidza
129 *N13* **Priyutnoye** Respublika Kalmykiya, SW Russian Federation
113 *M17* **Prizren** *Alb.* Prizreni. Serbia, S Yugoslavia
Prizreni *see* Prizren
107 *I24* **Prizzi** Sicilia, Italy, C Mediterranean Sea
113 *P18* **Probištip** NE FYR Macedonia
169 *S16* **Probolinggo** Jawa, C Indonesia
Probstberg *see* Wyszków
111 *F14* **Prochowice** *Ger.* Parchwitz. Dolnośląskie, SW Poland
29 *W5* **Proctor** Minnesota, N USA
25 *R8* **Proctor** Texas, SW USA
25 *R8* **Proctor Lake** ⊞ Texas, SW USA
155 *I18* **Proddatūr** Andhra Pradesh, E India
104 *H9* **Proença-a-Nova** Castelo Branco, C Portugal
95 *I24* **Præstø** Storstrøm, SE Denmark
99 *I21* **Profondeville** Namur, SE Belgium
41 *W11* **Progreso** Yucatán, SE Mexico
123 *R14* **Progress** Amurskaya Oblast', SE Russian Federation
129 *O15* **Prokhladnyy** Kabardino-Balkarskaya Respublika, SW Russian Federation
Prokletije *see* North Albanian Alps
Prökuls *see* Priekulė
113 *O15* **Prokuplje** Serbia, SE Yugoslavia
126 *H14* **Proletariy** Novgorodskaya Oblast', W Russian Federation
128 *M12* **Proletarsk** Rostovskaya Oblast', SW Russian Federation
128 *J8* **Proletarskiy** Belgorodskaya Oblast', W Russian Federation
166 *L7* **Prome** *var.* Pyè. Pegu, C Myanmar
60 *J8* **Promissão** São Paulo, S Brazil
60 *J8* **Promissão, Represa de** ⊞ S Brazil
127 *V4* **Promyshlennyy** Respublika Komi, NW Russian Federation
119 *O16* **Pronya** *Rus.* Pronya. ≈ E Belarus
10 *M11* **Prophet River** British Columbia, W Canada
30 *K11* **Prophetstown** Illinois, N USA
59 *P16* **Propriá** Sergipe, E Brazil
103 *X16* **Propriano** Corse, France, C Mediterranean Sea
Prościejów *see* Prostějov
Proskurov *see* Khmel'nyts'kyy
114 *H12* **Prosotsáni** Anatolikí Makedonía kai Thráki, NE Greece
171 *Q7* **Prosperidad** Mindanao, S Philippines
32 *J10* **Prosser** Washington, NW USA
Prossnitz *see* Prostějov
111 *G18* **Prostějov** *Ger.* Prossnitz, *Pol.* Prościejów. Olomoucký Kraj, E Czech Republic
117 *V8* **Prosyana** Dnipropetrovs'ka Oblast', E Ukraine
111 *L16* **Proszowice** Małopolskie, S Poland
Protasy *see* Pratasy
172 *J11* **Protea Seamount** *undersea feature* SW Indian Ocean
115 *D21* **Próti** *island* S Greece
114 *N8* **Provadiya** Varna, E Bulgaria
103 *S15* **Provence** *prev.* Marseille-Marignane. ✖ (Marseille) Bouches-du-Rhône, SE France
103 *T14* **Provence** *cultural region* SE France
103 *T14* **Provence-Alpes-Côte d'Azur** ◆ *region* SE France
20 *H6* **Providence** Kentucky, S USA
19 *N12* **Providence** *state capital* Rhode Island, NE USA
36 *L1* **Providence** Utah, W USA
Providence *see* Fort Providence
67 *X10* **Providence Atoll** *var.* Providence. *atoll* S Seychelles
14 *D12* **Providence Bay** Manitoulin Island, Ontario, S Canada
23 *R6* **Providence Canyon** *valley* Alabama/Georgia, S USA
22 *I5* **Providence, Lake** ◎ Louisiana, S USA
35 *X13* **Providence Mountains** ▲ California, W USA
44 *L6* **Providenciales** *island* W Turks and Caicos Islands
19 *Q12* **Provincetown** Massachusetts, NE USA
103 *P5* **Provins** Seine-et-Marne, N France
36 *L3* **Provo** Utah, W USA
11 *R15* **Provost** Alberta, SW Canada
112 *G13* **Prozor** Federacija Bosna I Hercegovina, SW Bosnia & Herzegovina
Prozoroki *see* Prazaroki
60 *I11* **Prudentópolis** Paraná, S Brazil
39 *R5* **Prudhoe Bay** Alaska, USA
39 *R4* **Prudhoe Bay** *bay* Alaska, USA
111 *H16* **Prudnik** *Ger.* Neustadt, Neustadt in Oberschlesien. Opolskie, S Poland
119 *J16* **Prudy** *Rus.* Prudy. Minskaya Voblasts', C Belarus
101 *D18* **Prüm** Rheinland-Pfalz, W Germany
101 *D18* **Prüm** ≈ W Germany
Prusa *see* Bursa
110 *I7* **Pruszcz Gdański** *Ger.* Praust. Pomorskie, N Poland
110 *M12* **Pruszków** *Ger.* Kaltdorf. Mazowieckie, C Poland
116 *K8* **Prut** *Ger.* Pruth. ≈ E Europe
Pruth *see* Prut
108 *L8* **Prutz** Tirol, W Austria
Pružana *see* Pruzhany
119 *G19* **Pruzhany** *Pol.* Prużana. Brestskaya Voblasts', SW Belarus
126 *I11* **Pryazha** Respublika Kareliya, NW Russian Federation
117 *U10* **Pryazovs'ke** Zaporiz'ka Oblast', SE Ukraine
Prychornomors'ka Nyzovyna *see* Black Sea Lowland
Prydniprovs'ka Nyzovyna/Prydnyaprows kaya Nizina *see* Dnieper Lowland
195 *Y7* **Prydz Bay** *bay* Antarctica
117 *R4* **Pryluky** *Rus.* Priluki. Chernihivs'ka Oblast', NE Ukraine
117 *V10* **Prymors'k** *Rus.* Primorsk; *prev.* Primorskoye. Zaporiz'ka Oblast', SE Ukraine
27 *Q9* **Pryor** Oklahoma, C USA
33 *U11* **Pryor Creek** ≈ Montana, NW USA
Pryp"yat'/Prypyats' *see* Pripet
110 *M10* **Przasnysz** Mazowieckie, C Poland
111 *K14* **Przedbórz** Łodzkie, S Poland
111 *P17* **Przemyśl** *Rus.* Peremyshl. Podkarpackie, SE Poland
111 *O16* **Przeworsk** Podkarpackie, SE Poland
Przheval'sk *see* Karakol
110 *L13* **Przysucha** Mazowieckie, SE Poland
115 *H18* **Psachná** *var.* Psahna, Psakhná. Évvoia, C Greece
Psahna/Psakhná *see* Psachná
115 *K18* **Psará** *island* E Greece
115 *I16* **Psathoúra** *island* Vóreioi Sporádes, Greece, Aegean Sea
Pschestitz *see* Přeštice
Psein Lora *see* Pishin Lora
117 *S5* **Psël** ≈ Russian Federation/Ukraine
115 *M21* **Psérimos** *island* Dodekánisos, Greece, Aegean Sea
Pseyn Bowr *see* Pishin Lora
Pskem *see* Piskom
147 *R8* **Pskemskiy Khrebet** *Uzb.* Piskom Tizmasi. ▲ Kyrgyzstan/Uzbekistan
126 *F14* **Pskov** *Ger.* Pleskau, *Latv.* Pleskava. Pskovskaya Oblast', W Russian Federation
118 *K6* **Pskov, Lake** *Est.* Pihkva Järv, *Ger.* Pleskauer See, *Rus.* Pskovskoye Ozero. ◎ Estonia/Russian Federation
126 *F15* **Pskovskaya Oblast'** ◆ *province* W Russian Federation
Pskovskoye Ozero *see* Pskov, Lake
112 *G9* **Psunj** ▲ NE Croatia
111 *J17* **Pszczyna** *Ger.* Pless. Śląskie, S Poland
Ptačnik/Ptacsnik *see* Vtáčnik
115 *D17* **Ptéri** ▲ C Greece
Ptich' *see* Ptsich
115 *E14* **Ptolemaïda** *prev.* Ptolemaïs. Dytikí Makedonía, N Greece
Ptolemaïs *see* Ptolemaïda, Greece
Ptolemaïs *see* 'Akko, Israel
119 *M19* **Ptsich** *Rus.* Ptich'. Homyel'skaya Voblasts', SE Belarus
119 *M18* **Ptsich** *Rus.* Ptich'. ≈ SE Belarus
109 *X10* **Ptuj** *Ger.* Pettau; *anc.* Poetovio. NE Slovenia
61 *A23* **Puán** Buenos Aires, E Argentina
192 *H15* **Pu'apu'a** Savai'i, C Samoa
192 *G15* **Puava, Cape** *headland* Savai'i, NW Samoa
56 *F12* **Pucallpa** Ucayali, C Peru
57 *J17* **Pucarani** La Paz, NW Bolivia
Pučarevo *see* Novi Travnik
157 *U12* **Pucheng** Fujian, SE China
160 *L6* **Pucheng** Shaanxi, C China
127 *N16* **Puchezh** Ivanovskaya Oblast', W Russian Federation
111 *I19* **Púchov** *Hung.* Puhó. Trenčiansky Kraj, W Slovakia
116 *J13* **Pucioasa** Dâmbovița, S Romania
110 *I6* **Puck** Pomorskie, N Poland
30 *L8* **Puckaway Lake** ◎ Wisconsin, N USA
63 *G15* **Pucón** Araucanía, S Chile
93 *M14* **Pudasjärvi** Oulu, C Finland
148 *L8* **Pūdeh Tal, Shelleh-ye** ≈ SW Afghanistan
129 *S1* **Pudem** Udmurtskaya Respublika, NW Russian Federation
Pudewitz *see* Pobiedziska
126 *K11* **Pudozh** Respublika Kareliya, NW Russian Federation
97 *M17* **Pudsey** N England, UK
Puduchcheri *see* Pondicherry
151 *H21* **Pudukkottai** Tamil Nādu, SE India
171 *Z13* **Pue** Irian Jaya, E Indonesia
41 *P14* **Puebla** *var.* Puebla de Zaragoza. Puebla, S Mexico
41 *P15* **Puebla** ◆ *state* S Mexico
104 *L11* **Puebla de Alcocer** Extremadura, W Spain
Puebla de Don Fabrique *see* Puebla de Don Fadrique
105 *P13* **Puebla de Don Fadrique** *var.* Puebla de Don Fabrique. Andalucía, S Spain
104 *J11* **Puebla de la Calzada** Extremadura, W Spain
104 *J5* **Puebla de Sanabria** Castilla-León, N Spain
104 *I4* **Puebla de Trives** *see* A Pobla de Trives
Puebla de Zaragoza *see* Puebla
37 *T6* **Pueblo** Colorado, C USA
37 *N10* **Pueblo Colorado Wash** *valley* Arizona, SW USA
61 *C16* **Pueblo Libertador** Corrientes, NE Argentina
40 *J10* **Pueblo Nuevo** Durango, C Mexico
42 *J8* **Pueblo Nuevo** Estelí, NW Nicaragua
54 *J3* **Pueblo Nuevo** Falcón, N Venezuela
42 *B6* **Pueblo Nuevo Tiquisate** *var.* Tiquisate. Escuintla, SW Guatemala
41 *Q11* **Pueblo Viejo, Laguna de** *lagoon* E Mexico
63 *J14* **Puelches** La Pampa, C Argentina
104 *L14* **Puente-Genil** Andalucía, S Spain
105 *Q3* **Puente la Reina** Navarra, N Spain
104 *L12* **Puente Nuevo, Embalse de** ⊞ S Spain
57 *D14* **Puente Piedra** Lima, W Peru
160 *F14* **Pu'er** Yunnan, SW China
45 *V6* **Puerca, Punta** *headland* E Puerto Rico
37 *R12* **Puerco, Rio** ≈ New Mexico, SW USA
57 *J17* **Puerto Acosta** La Paz, W Bolivia
63 *G19* **Puerto Aisén** Aisén, S Chile
41 *R17* **Puerto Ángel** Oaxaca, SE Mexico
Puerto Argentino *see* Stanley
41 *T17* **Puerto Arista** Chiapas, SE Mexico
43 *O16* **Puerto Armuelles** Chiriquí, SW Panama
Puerto Arrecife *see* Arrecife
54 *D14* **Puerto Asís** Putumayo, SW Colombia
54 *L9* **Puerto Ayacucho** Amazonas, SW Venezuela
57 *C18* **Puerto Ayora** Galapagos Islands, Ecuador, E Pacific Ocean
57 *C18* **Puerto Baquerizo Moreno** *var.* Baquerizo Moreno. Galapagos Islands, Ecuador, E Pacific Ocean
42 *G4* **Puerto Barrios** Izabal, E Guatemala
Puerto Bello *see* Portobelo
54 *F8* **Puerto Berrío** Antioquia, C Colombia
54 *F9* **Puerto Boyaca** Boyacá, C Colombia
54 *K4* **Puerto Cabello** Carabobo, N Venezuela
43 *N7* **Puerto Cabezas** *var.* Bilwi. Región Autónoma Atlántico Norte, NE Nicaragua
54 *L9* **Puerto Carreño** Vichada, E Colombia
54 *E4* **Puerto Colombia** Atlántico, N Colombia
42 *H4* **Puerto Cortés** Cortés, NW Honduras
54 *J4* **Puerto Cumarebo** Falcón, N Venezuela
Puerto de Cabras *see* Puerto del Rosario
55 *Q5* **Puerto de Hierro** Sucre, NE Venezuela
64 *O11* **Puerto de la Cruz** Tenerife, Islas Canarias, Spain, NE Atlantic Ocean
64 *Q11* **Puerto del Rosario** *var.* Puerto de Cabras. Fuerteventura, Islas Canarias, Spain, NE Atlantic Ocean
63 *J20* **Puerto Deseado** Santa Cruz, SE Argentina
40 *F8* **Puerto Escondido** Baja California Sur, W Mexico
41 *R17* **Puerto Escondido** Oaxaca, SE Mexico
60 *G12* **Puerto Esperanza** Misiones, NE Argentina
56 *D6* **Puerto Francisco de Orellana** *var.* Coca. Napo, N Ecuador
54 *H10* **Puerto Gaitán** Meta, C Colombia
Puerto Gallegos *see* Río Gallegos
60 *G12* **Puerto Iguazú** Misiones, NE Argentina
56 *F12* **Puerto Inca** Huánuco, N Peru
54 *L11* **Puerto Inírida** *var.* Obando. Guainía, E Colombia
42 *K13* **Puerto Jesús** Guanacaste, NW Costa Rica
41 *Z11* **Puerto Juárez** Quintana Roo, SE Mexico
55 *N5* **Puerto La Cruz** Anzoátegui, NE Venezuela
54 *E14* **Puerto Leguízamo** Putumayo, S Colombia
43 *N5* **Puerto Lempira** Gracias a Dios, E Honduras
Puerto Libertad *see* La Libertad
54 *I11* **Puerto Limón** Meta, E Colombia
54 *D13* **Puerto Limón** Putumayo, SW Colombia
Puerto Limón *see* Limón
105 *N11* **Puertollano** Castilla-La Mancha, C Spain
63 *K17* **Puerto Lobos** Chubut, SE Argentina
54 *I3* **Puerto López** La Guajira, N Colombia
105 *Q14* **Puerto Lumbreras** Murcia, SE Spain
41 *V17* **Puerto Madero** Chiapas, SE Mexico
63 *K17* **Puerto Madryn** Chubut, S Argentina
Puerto Magdalena *see* Bahía Magdalena
57 *J15* **Puerto Maldonado** Madre de Dios, E Peru
Puerto Masachapa *see* Masachapa
Puerto México *see* Coatzacoalcos
63 *G17* **Puerto Montt** Los Lagos, C Chile
41 *Z12* **Puerto Morelos** Quintana Roo, SE Mexico
54 *L10* **Puerto Nariño** Vichada, E Colombia
63 *H23* **Puerto Natales** Magallanes, S Chile
43 *X15* **Puerto Obaldía** San Blas, NE Panama
44 *H6* **Puerto Padre** Las Tunas, E Cuba
54 *L9* **Puerto Páez** Apure, C Venezuela
40 *E3* **Puerto Peñasco** Sonora, NW Mexico
55 *N5* **Puerto Píritu** Anzoátegui, NE Venezuela
45 *N8* **Puerto Plata** *var.* San Felipe de Puerto Plata. N Dominican Republic
45 *N8* **Puerto Plata** ✖ N Dominican Republic
Puerto Presidente Stroessner *see* Ciudad del Este
171 *N6* **Puerto Princesa** *off.* Puerto Princesa City. Palawan, W Philippines
Puerto Princesa City *see* Puerto Princesa
Puerto Príncipe *see* Camagüey
Puerto Quellón *see* Quellón
60 *F13* **Puerto Rico** Misiones, NE Argentina
57 *K14* **Puerto Rico** Pando, N Bolivia
54 *E12* **Puerto Rico** Caquetá, S Colombia
45 *U5* **Puerto Rico** *off.* Commonwealth of Puerto Rico; *prev.* Porto Rico. ◇ *US commonwealth territory* C West Indies
64 *F11* **Puerto Rico** *island* C West Indies
64 *G11* **Puerto Rico Trench** *undersea feature* NE Caribbean Sea
54 *I8* **Puerto Rondón** Arauca, E Colombia
Puerto San José *see* San José
63 *J21* **Puerto San Julián** *var.* San Julián. Santa Cruz, SE Argentina
63 *I22* **Puerto Santa Cruz** *var.* Santa Cruz. Santa Cruz, SE Argentina
Puerto Sauce *see* Juan L.Lacaze
57 *Q20* **Puerto Suárez** Santa Cruz, E Bolivia
54 *D13* **Puerto Umbría** Putumayo, SW Colombia
40 *J13* **Puerto Vallarta** Jalisco, SW Mexico
63 *G16* **Puerto Varas** Los Lagos, C Chile
42 *M13* **Puerto Viejo** Heredia, NE Costa Rica
Puertoviejo *see* Portoviejo
57 *B18* **Puerto Villamil** *var.* Villamil. Galapagos Islands, Ecuador, E Pacific Ocean
54 *F8* **Puerto Wilches** Santander, N Colombia
63 *H20* **Pueyrredón, Lago** *var.* Lago Cochrane. ◎ S Argentina
129 *R7* **Pugachëv** Saratovskaya Oblast', W Russian Federation
129 *T3* **Pugachëvo** Udmurtskaya Respublika, NW Russian Federation
32 *H8* **Puget Sound** *sound* Washington, NW USA
107 *O17* **Puglia** *var.* Le Puglie, *Eng.* Apulia. ◆ *region* SE Italy
107 *N17* **Puglia, Canosa di** *anc.* Canusium. Puglia, SE Italy
118 *I6* **Puhja** *Ger.* Kawelecht. Tartumaa, SE Estonia
Puhó *see* Púchov
105 *V4* **Puigcerdà** Cataluña, NE Spain
Puigmal *see* Puigmal d'Err
103 *N17* **Puigmal d'Err** *var.* Puigmal. ▲ S France
76 *I16* **Pujehun** S Sierra Leone
Puka *see* Pukë
185 *E20* **Pukaki, Lake** ◎ South Island, NZ
38 *F10* **Pukalani** Maui, Hawaii, USA, C Pacific Ocean
190 *J13* **Pukapuka** *atoll* N Cook Islands
191 *X9* **Pukapuka** *atoll* Îles Tuamotu, E French Polynesia
Pukari Neem *see* Purekkari Neem
191 *X11* **Pukarua** *var.* Pukaruha. *atoll* Îles Tuamotu, E French Polynesia
Pukaruha *see* Pukarua
14 *A7* **Pukaskwa** ≈ Ontario, S Canada
11 *V12* **Pukatawagan** Manitoba, C Canada
191 *X16* **Pukatikei, Maunga** ✱ Easter Island, Chile, E Pacific Ocean
182 *C1* **Pukatja** *var.* Ernabella. South Australia
163 *Y12* **Pukch'ŏng** E North Korea
113 *L18* **Pukë** *var.* Puka. Shkodër, N Albania
184 *L6* **Pukekohe** Auckland, North Island, NZ
184 *L7* **Pukemiro** Waikato, North Island, NZ
190 *D12* **Puke, Mont** ▲ Île Futuna, W Wallis and Futuna
Puket *see* Phuket
185 *C20* **Puketeraki Range** ▲ South Island, NZ
184 *N13* **Puketoi Range** ▲ North Island, NZ
185 *F21* **Pukeuri Junction** Otago, South Island, NZ
119 *L16* **Pukhavichy** *Rus.* Pukhovichi. Minskaya Voblasts', C Belarus
Pukhovichi *see* Pukhavichy
126 *M10* **Puksoozero** Arkhangel'skaya Oblast', NW Russian Federation
112 *A10* **Pula** *It.* Pola; *prev.* Pulj. Istra, NW Croatia
163 *U14* **Pulandian** *var.* Xinjin. Liaoning, NE China
163 *T14* **Pulandian Wan** *bay* NE China
189 *O15* **Pulap Atoll** *atoll* Caroline Islands, C Micronesia
18 *H9* **Pulaski** New York, NE USA
20 *I10* **Pulaski** Tennessee, S USA
21 *R7* **Pulaski** Virginia, NE USA
171 *Y14* **Pulau, Sungai** ≈ Irian Jaya, E Indonesia
110 *N13* **Puławy** *Ger.* Neu Amerika. Lubelskie, E Poland
101 *E16* **Pulheim** Nordrhein-Westfalen, W Germany
Pulicat *see* Pālghāt
155 *J19* **Pulicat Lake** *lagoon* SE India
Pul'-I-Khatum *see* Polekhatum
Pul-i-Khumri *see* Pol-e Khomrī
Pul-i-Sefid *see* Pol-e Safīd
Pulj *see* Pula
109 *W2* **Pulkau** ≈ NE Austria
93 *L15* **Pulkkila** Oulu, C Finland
122 *C7* **Pul'kovo** ✖ (Sankt-Peterburg) Leningradskaya Oblast', NW Russian Federation
32 *M9* **Pullman** Washington, NW USA
108 *B10* **Pully** Vaud, SW Switzerland
40 *F7* **Púlpita, Punta** *headland* W Mexico
110 *M10* **Pułtusk** Mazowieckie, C Poland
158 *H10* **Pulu** Xinjiang Uygur Zizhiqu, W China
137 *P13* **Pülümür** Tunceli, E Turkey
189 *N16* **Pulusuk** *island* Caroline Islands, C Micronesia
189 *N16* **Puluwat Atoll** *atoll* Caroline Islands, C Micronesia
25 *N11* **Pumpville** Texas, SW USA
191 *P7* **Punaauia** *var.* Hakapehi. Tahiti, W French Polynesia
56 *B8* **Puná, Isla** *island* SW Ecuador
185 *G16* **Punakaiki** West Coast, South Island, NZ
153 *T11* **Punakha** C Bhutan
57 *L18* **Punata** Cochabamba, C Bolivia
155 *E14* **Pune** *prev.* Poona. Mahārāshtra, W India
83 *M17* **Pungoè, Rio** *var.* Púnguè, Pungwe. ≈ C Mozambique
21 *X10* **Pungo River** ≈ North Carolina, SE USA
Púnguè/Pungwe *see* Pungoè, Rio
79 *N19* **Punia** Maniema, E Dem. Rep. Congo (Zaire)
62 *H8* **Punilla, Sierra de la** ▲ W Argentina
161 *P14* **Puning** Guangdong, S China
62 *G10* **Punitaqui** Coquimbo, C Chile
152 *H8* **Punjab** ◆ *state* NW India
149 *T9* **Punjab** *prev.* West Punjab, Western Punjab. ◆ *province* E Pakistan
131 *Q9* **Punjab Plains** *plain* N India
93 *O17* **Punkaharju** *var.* Punkasalmi. Isä-Suomi, E Finland

Punkasalmi see Punkaharju
57 I17 **Puno** Puno, SE Peru
57 H17 **Puno** *off.* Departamento de Puno. ◆ *department* S Peru
61 B24 **Punta Alta** Buenos Aires, E Argentina
63 H24 **Punta Arenas** *prev.* Magallanes. Magallanes, S Chile
45 T6 **Punta, Cerro de** ▲ C Puerto Rico
43 T15 **Punta Chame** Panamá, C Panama
57 G17 **Punta Colorada** Arequipa, SW Peru
40 F9 **Punta Coyote** Baja California Sur, W Mexico
62 G8 **Punta de Díaz** Atacama, N Chile
61 G20 **Punta del Este** Maldonado, S Uruguay
63 K17 **Punta Delgada** Chubut, SE Argentina
55 O5 **Punta de Mata** Monagas, NE Venezuela
55 O4 **Punta de Piedras** Nueva Esparta, NE Venezuela
42 F4 **Punta Gorda** Toledo, SE Belize
43 N11 **Punta Gorda** Región Autónoma Atlántico Sur, SE Nicaragua
23 W14 **Punta Gorda** Florida, SE USA
42 M11 **Punta Gorda, Río** ~ SE Nicaragua
62 H6 **Punta Negra, Salar de** *salt lake* N Chile
40 D5 **Punta Prieta** Baja California, NW Mexico
42 L13 **Puntarenas** Puntarenas, W Costa Rica
42 L13 **Puntarenas** *off.* Provincia de Puntarenas. ◆ *province* W Costa Rica
54 J4 **Punto Fijo** Falcón, N Venezuela
105 S4 **Puntón de Guara** ▲ N Spain
18 D14 **Punxsutawney** Pennsylvania, NE USA
93 M14 **Puolanka** Oulu, C Finland
57 J17 **Pupuya, Nevado** ▲ W Bolivia
161 O10 **Puqi** Hubei, C China
57 F16 **Puquio** Ayacucho, S Peru
122 J9 **Pur** ~ N Russian Federation
186 D7 **Purari** ~ S PNG
27 N11 **Purcell** Oklahoma, C USA
11 O16 **Purcell Mountains** ▲ British Columbia, SW Canada
105 P14 **Purchena** Andalucía, S Spain
27 S8 **Purdy** Missouri, C USA
118 I2 **Purekkari Neem** *prev.* Pukari Neem. *headland* N Estonia
37 U7 **Purgatoire River** ~ Colorado, C USA
Purgstall see Purgstall an der Erlauf
109 V5 **Purgstall an der Erlauf** *var.* Purgstall. Niederösterreich, NE Austria
154 O13 **Puri** *var.* Jagannath. Orissa, E India
Puriramya see Buriram
109 X4 **Purkersdorf** Niederösterreich, NE Austria
98 I9 **Purmerend** Noord-Holland, C Netherlands
151 G16 **Pūrna** ~ C India
Purnea see Pūrnia
153 R13 **Pūrnia** *prev.* Purnea. Bihār, NE India
Pursat see Poŭthĭsăt, Poŭthĭsăt, W Cambodia
Pursat see Poŭthĭsăt, Stœ̆ng, W Cambodia
Purulia see Puruliya
150 L13 **Puruliya** *prev.* Purulia. West Bengal, NE India
47 G7 **Purus, Rio** *Sp.* Río Purús. ~ Brazil/Peru
186 C9 **Purutu Island** *island* SW PNG
93 N17 **Puruvesi** ◎ SE Finland
22 L7 **Purvis** Mississippi, S USA
114 J11 **Pŭrvomay** *prev.* Borisovgrad. Plovdiv, C Bulgaria
169 R16 **Purwodadi** *prev.* Poerwodadi. Jawa, C Indonesia
169 P16 **Purwokerto** *prev.* Poerwokerto. Jawa, C Indonesia
169 P16 **Purworejo** *prev.* Poerworedjo. Jawa, C Indonesia
20 H8 **Puryear** Tennessee, S USA
154 H13 **Pusad** Mahārāshtra, C India
163 Z16 **Pusan** *off.* Pusan-gwangyŏksi, *var.* Busan, *Jap.* Fusan. SE South Korea
168 H7 **Pusatgajo, Pegunungan** ▲ Sumatera, NW Indonesia
Puschlav see Poschiavo
Pushkin see Tsarskoye Selo
129 Q8 **Pushkino** Saratovskaya Oblast', W Russian Federation
Pushkino see Biläsuvar
111 M22 **Püspökladány** Hajdú-Bihar, E Hungary
118 J3 **Püssi** *Ger.* Isenhof. Ida-Virumaa, NE Estonia
116 I5 **Pustomyty** L'vivs'ka Oblast', W Ukraine
126 F16 **Pustoshka** Pskovskaya Oblast', W Russian Federation
Pusztakalán see Călan
167 N1 **Putao** *prev.* Fort Hertz. Kachin State, N Myanmar
184 M8 **Putaruru** Waikato, North Island, NZ
Puteoli see Pozzuoli
161 R12 **Putian** Fujian, SE China
107 O17 **Putignano** Puglia, SE Italy
Putivl' see Putyvl'
41 Q16 **Putla** *var.* Putla de Guerrero. Oaxaca, SE Mexico
Putla de Guerrero see Putla
19 N12 **Putnam** Connecticut, NE USA
25 Q7 **Putnam** Texas, SW USA
18 M10 **Putney** Vermont, NE USA
111 L20 **Putnok** Borsod-Abaúj-Zemplén, NE Hungary
Putorana, Gory/Putorana Mountains see Putorana, Plato
122 L8 **Putorana, Plato** *var.* Gory Putorana, *Eng.* Putorana Mountains. ▲ N Russian Federation
62 H2 **Putre** Tarapacá, N Chile
155 J24 **Puttalam** North Western Province, W Sri Lanka
155 J24 **Puttalam Lagoon** *lagoon* W Sri Lanka
99 H17 **Putte** Antwerpen, C Belgium
98 K11 **Putten** Gelderland, C Netherlands
100 K7 **Puttgarden** Schleswig-Holstein, N Germany
Puttiala see Patiāla
101 D20 **Püttlingen** Saarland, SW Germany
54 D14 **Putumayo** *off.* Intendencia del Putumayo. ◆ *province* S Colombia
48 E7 **Putumayo, Río** *var.* Rio Içá. ~ NW South America *see also* Içá, Rio
169 P11 **Putus, Tanjung** *headland* Borneo, N Indonesia
116 J8 **Putyla** Chernivets'ka Oblast', W Ukraine
117 S3 **Putyvl'** *Rus.* Putivl'. Sums'ka Oblast', NE Ukraine
93 M18 **Puula** ◎ SE Finland
93 N18 **Puumala** Isä-Suomi, E Finland
118 I5 **Puurmani** *Ger.* Talkhof. Jõgevamaa, E Estonia
99 G17 **Puurs** Antwerpen, N Belgium
Pu'uUla'ula see Red Hill
38 A8 **Puuwai** Niihau, Hawaii, USA, C Pacific Ocean
12 J4 **Puvirnituq** *prev.* Povungnituk. Quebec, NE Canada
32 H8 **Puyallup** Washington, NW USA
161 O5 **Puyang** Henan, C China
161 R9 **Puyang Jiang** *var.* Tsien Tang. ~ SE China
103 O11 **Puy-de-Dôme** ◆ *department* C France
103 N15 **Puylaurens** Tarn, S France
102 M13 **Puy-l'Evêque** Lot, S France
103 N17 **Puymorens, Col de** *pass* S France
56 C7 **Puyo** Pastaza, C Ecuador
185 A24 **Puysegur Point** *headland* South Island, NZ
148 J8 **Pūzak, Hāmūn-e** *Pash.* Hāmūn-i-Puzak. ◎ SW Afghanistan
Puzak, Hāmūn-i- see Pūzak, Hāmūn-e
81 J23 **Pwani** *Eng.* Coast. ◆ *region* E Tanzania
79 O23 **Pweto** Katanga, SE Dem. Rep. Congo (Zaire)
97 I19 **Pwllheli** NW Wales, UK
189 O14 **Pwok** Pohnpei, E Micronesia
122 I9 **Pyakupur** ~ N Russian Federation
126 M6 **Pyalitsa** Murmanskaya Oblast', NW Russian Federation
126 K10 **Pyal'ma** Respublika Kareliya, NW Russian Federation
Pyandzh see Panj
126 I6 **Pyaozero, Ozero** ◎ NW Russian Federation
166 L9 **Pyapon** Irrawaddy, SW Myanmar
119 J15 **Pyarshai** *Rus.* Pershay. Minskaya Voblasts', C Belarus
122 K8 **Pyasina** ~ N Russian Federation
114 I10 **Pyasŭchnik, Yazovir** ⊡ C Bulgaria
Pyatikhatki see P"yatykhatky
117 S7 **P"yatykhatky** *Rus.* Pyatikhatki. Dnipropetrovs'ka Oblast', E Ukraine
166 M6 **Pyawbwe** Mandalay, C Myanmar
129 T3 **Pychas** Udmurtskaya Respublika, NW Russian Federation
Pyè see Prome
166 K6 **Pyechin** Chin State, W Myanmar
119 G17 **Pyeski** *Rus.* Peski. Hrodzyenskaya Voblasts', W Belarus
119 L19 **Pyetrykaw** *Rus.* Petrikov. Homyel'skaya Voblasts', SE Belarus
93 M16 **Pyhäjärvi** ◎ C Finland
93 O17 **Pyhäjärvi** ◎ SE Finland
93 L15 **Pyhäjoki** Oulu, W Finland
93 L15 **Pyhäjoki** ~ W Finland
93 M15 **Pyhäntä** Oulu, C Finland
93 M16 **Pyhäsalmi** Oulu, C Finland
93 O17 **Pyhäselkä** ◎ SE Finland
93 M19 **Pyhtää** *Swe.* Pyttis. Etelä-Suomi, S Finland
166 M6 **Pyinmana** Mandalay, C Myanmar
115 N24 **Pylés** *var.* Piles. Kárpathos, SE Greece
115 D21 **Pýlos** *var.* Pilos. Pelopónnisos, S Greece
18 B12 **Pymatuning Reservoir** ⊡ Ohio/Pennsylvania, NE USA
163 X15 **P'yŏngt'aek** NW South Korea
163 V14 **P'yŏngyang** *var.* P'yŏngyang-si, *Eng.* Pyongyang. ● (North Korea) SW North Korea
P'yŏngyang-si see P'yŏngyang
35 Q4 **Pyramid Lake** ◎ Nevada, W USA
37 P15 **Pyramid Mountains** ▲ New Mexico, SW USA
37 R5 **Pyramid Peak** ▲ Colorado, C USA
115 D17 **Pyramíva** *var.* Piramiva. ▲ C Greece
Pyrenaei Montes see Pyrenees
86 B12 **Pyrenees** *Fr.* Pyrénées, *Sp.* Pirineos; *anc.* Pyrenaei Montes. ▲ SW Europe
102 J16 **Pyrénées-Atlantiques** ◆ *department* SW France
103 N17 **Pyrénées-Orientales** ◆ *department* S France
115 L19 **Pyrgí** *var.* Pirgi. Chíos, E Greece
115 D20 **Pýrgos** *var.* Pírgos. Dytikí Ellás, S Greece
Pyritz see Pyrzyce
115 E19 **Pýrros** ~ S Greece
117 R4 **Pyryatyn** *Rus.* Piryatin. Poltavs'ka Oblast', NE Ukraine
110 D9 **Pyrzyce** *Ger.* Pyritz. Zachodniopomorskie, NW Poland
126 F15 **Pytalovo** *Latv.* Abrene; *prev.* Jaunlatgale. Pskovskaya Oblast', W Russian Federation
115 M20 **Pythagóreio** *var.* Pithagorio. Sámos, Dodekánisos, Greece, Aegean Sea
14 L11 **Pythonga, Lac** ◎ Quebec, SE Canada
94 E10 **Pyttegga** ▲ S Norway
Pyttis see Pyhtää
166 M7 **Pyu** Pegu, C Myanmar
166 M8 **Pyuntaza** Pegu, SW Myanmar
153 N11 **Pyuthan** Mid Western, W Nepal
110 H12 **Pyzdry** *Ger.* Peisern. Wielkopolskie, C Poland

Q

138 H13 **Qā' al Jafr** ◎ S Jordan
197 O11 **Qaanaaq** *var.* Qânâq, *Dan.* Thule. Avannaarsua, N Greenland
138 G7 **Qabb Eliâs** E Lebanon
Qabil see Al Qābil
Qabırrı see Iori
Qābis see Gabès
Qābis, Khalīj see Gabès, Golfe de
141 S14 **Qabr Hūd** C Yemen
Qacentina see Constantine
148 L4 **Qādes** Bādghīs, NW Afghanistan
139 T11 **Qādisīyah** S Iraq
143 O4 **Qā'emshahr** *prev.* 'Alīābad, Shāhī. Māzandarān, N Iran
143 U7 **Qā'en** *var.* Qain, Qāyen. Khorāsān, E Iran
141 U13 **Qafa** *spring/well* SW Oman
Qafṣah see Gafsa
163 V9 **Qagan Nur** ◎ NE China
163 Q11 **Qagan Nur** ◎ N China
Qagan Us see Dulan
158 H13 **Qagcaka** Xizang Zizhiqu, W China
Qahremānshahr see Bākhtarān
159 Q10 **Qaidam He** ~ C China
156 L8 **Qaidam Pendi** *basin* C China
Qain see Qā'en
Qala Āhangarān see Chaghcharān
139 U3 **Qalā Diza** *var.* Qal 'at Dīzah. NE Iraq
Qal'ah Sālih see Qal'at Ṣāliḥ
147 R13 **Qal'aikhum** *Rus.* Kalaikhum. S Tajikistan
Qala Nau see Qal'eh-ye Now
141 V17 **Qalansīyah** Suquṭrā, W Yemen
Qala Panja see Qal'eh-ye Panjeh
Qala Shāhar see Qal'eh Shahr
Qalāt see Kalāt
139 W9 **Qal'at Aḥmad** E Iraq
141 N11 **Qal'at Bīshah** 'Asīr, SW Saudi Arabia
138 H4 **Qal'at Burzay** Ḥamāh, W Syria
Qal 'at Dīzah see Qalā Diza
139 W9 **Qal'at Ḥusayh** E Iraq
139 V10 **Qal'at Majnūnah** S Iraq
139 X11 **Qal'at Ṣāliḥ** *var.* Qal'ah Sālih. E Iraq
139 V10 **Qal'at Sukkar** SE Iraq
Qalba Zhotasy see Kalbinskiy Khrebet
143 Q12 **Qal'eh Biābān** Fārs, S Iran
149 N4 **Qal'eh Shahr** *Pash.* Qala Shāhar. Sar-e Pol, N Afghanistan
148 L4 **Qal'eh-ye Now** *var.* Qala Nau. Bādghīs, NW Afghanistan
149 T2 **Qal'eh-ye Panjeh** *var.* Qala Panja. Badakhshān, NE Afghanistan
Qamar Bay see Qamar, Ghubbat al
141 U14 **Qamar, Ghubbat al** *Eng.* Qamar Bay. *bay* Oman/Yemen
141 V13 **Qamar, Jabal al** ▲ SW Oman
Qambar see Kambar
159 R14 **Qamdo** Xizang Zizhiqu, W China
75 R7 **Qamīnis** NE Libya
Qamishly see Al Qāmishlī
Qânâq see Qaanaaq
Qandahār see Kandahār
80 Q11 **Qandala** Bari, NE Somalia
Qandyaghash see Kandyagash
138 L2 **Qanṭārī** Ar Raqqah, N Syria
137 V13 **Qapiciğ Dağı** *Rus.* Gora Kapydzhik. ▲ SW Azerbaijan
158 H5 **Qapqal** *var.* Qapqal Xibe Zizhixian. Xinjiang Uygur Zizhiqu, NW China
Qapqal Xibe Zizhixian see Qapqal
Qapshagay Böyeni see Kapchagayskoye Vodokhranilishche
196 M15 **Qaqortoq** *Dan.* Julianehåb. Kitaa, S Greenland
75 U8 **Qâra** *var.* Qārah. NW Egypt
139 T4 **Qara Anjīr** N Iraq
Qarabāgh see Qarah Bāgh
Qaraböget see Karaboget
Qarabulaq see Karabulak
Qarabutaq see Karabutak
Qaraghandy/Qaraghandy Oblysy see Karaganda
Qaraghayly see Karagayly
139 U4 **Qara Gol** NE Iraq
Qārah see Qâra
148 J4 **Qarah Bāgh** *var.* Qarabāgh. Herāt, NW Afghanistan
138 G7 **Qaraoun, Lac de** *var.* Buḥayrat al Qir'awn. ◎ S Lebanon
Qaraoy see Karaoy
Qaraqoyyn see Karakoyyn, Ozero
Qara Qum see Garagumy
Qarasū see Karasu
Qaratal see Karatal
Qarataū see Karatau, Khrebet, Kazakhstan
Qarataū see Karatau, Zhambyl, Kazakhstan
Qaraton see Karaton
80 P13 **Qardho** *var.* Kardh, *It.* Gardo. Bari, N Somalia
142 M6 **Qareh Chāy** ~ N Iran
142 K2 **Qareh Sū** ~ NW Iran
Qariateïne see Al Qaryatayn
Qarkilik see Ruoqiang
147 O13 **Qarluq** *Rus.* Karluk. Surkhondaryo Wiloyati, S Uzbekistan
147 U12 **Qarokŭl** *Rus.* Karakul'. E Tajikistan
147 T12 **Qarokŭl** *Rus.* Ozero Karakul'. ◎ E Tajikistan
Qarqan see Qiemo
158 K9 **Qarqan He** ~ NW China
Qarqannah, Juzur see Kerkenah, Îles de
Qarqaraly see Karkaralinsk
149 O1 **Qarqīn** Jowzjān, N Afghanistan
Qars see Kars
Qarsaqbay see Karsakpay
146 M12 **Qarshi** *Rus.* Karshi; *prev.* Bek-Budi. Qashqadaryo Wiloyati, S Uzbekistan
146 L12 **Qarshi Chŭli** *Rus.* Karshinskaya Step. *grassland* S Uzbekistan
146 M13 **Qarshi Kanali** *Rus.* Karshinskiy Kanal. *canal* Turkmenistan/Uzbekistan
Qaryatayn see Al Qaryatayn
146 M12 **Qashqadaryo Wiloyati** *Rus.* Kashkadar'inskaya Oblast'. ◆ *province* S Uzbekistan
Qasigianguit see Qasigiannguit
197 N13 **Qasigiannguit** *var.* Qasigianguit, *Dan.* Christianshåb. Kitaa, C Greenland
Qaşim, Minṭaqat see Al Qaşim
139 P8 **Qaşr 'Amij** C Iraq
139 R9 **Qaşr Darwīshāh** C Iraq
142 J6 **Qaşr-e Shīrīn** Kermānshāh, W Iran
75 V10 **Qasr Farâfra** W Egypt
Qassim see Al Qaşim
141 O16 **Qa'ṭabah** SW Yemen
138 H7 **Qaṭanā** *var.* Katana. Dimashq, S Syria
143 N15 **Qatar** *off.* State of Qatar, *Ar.* Dawlat Qaṭar. ◆ *monarchy* SW Asia
Qatrana see Al Qaṭrānah
143 Q12 **Qaṭrūyeh** Fārs, S Iran
Qattara Depression/Qaṭṭārah, Munkhafaḍ al see Qaṭṭâra, Monkhafad el
75 U8 **Qaṭṭâra, Monkhafad el** *var.* Munkhafaḍ al Qaṭṭārah, *Eng.* Qattara Depression. *desert* NW Egypt
Qaṭṭīnah, Buḥayrat see Ḥimṣ, Buḥayrat
Qaydār see Qeydār
Qāyen see Qā'en
147 Q11 **Qayroqqum** *Rus.* Kayrakkum. NW Tajikistan
147 Q10 **Qayroqqum, Obanbori** *Rus.* Kayrakkumskoye Vodokhranilishche. ⊡ NW Tajikistan
139 U7 **Qazānīyah** *var.* Dhū Shaykh. E Iraq
Qazaqstan/Qazaqstan Respublikasy see Kazakhstan
137 T9 **Qazbegi** *Rus.* Kazbegi. NE Georgia
149 P15 **Qāzi Ahmad** *var.* Kazi Ahmad. Sind, SE Pakistan
137 Y12 **Qazimämmäd** *Rus.* Kazi Magomed. SE Azerbaijan
Qazris see Cáceres
142 M4 **Qazvīn** *var.* Kazvin. Qazvīn, N Iran
142 M5 **Qazvīn** ◆ *province* N Iran
187 Z13 **Qelelevu Lagoon** *lagoon* NE Fiji
75 X10 **Qena** *var.* Qinā; *anc.* Caene, Caenepolis. E Egypt
113 L23 **Qeparo** Vlorë, S Albania
Qeqertarssuaq see Qeqertarsuaq
197 N13 **Qeqertarsuaq** *var.* Qeqertarssuaq, *Dan.* Godhavn. Kitaa, Greenland
196 M13 **Qeqertarsuaq** *island* W Greenland
197 N13 **Qeqertarsuup Tunua** *Dan.* Disko Bugt. *inlet* W Greenland
Qerveh see Qorveh
143 S14 **Qeshm** Hormozgān, S Iran
143 R14 **Qeshm** *var.* Jazīreh-ye Qeshm, Qeshm Island. *island* S Iran
Qeshm Island/Qeshm, Jazīreh-ye see Qeshm
142 L4 **Qeydār** *var.* Qaydār. Zanjān, NW Iran
142 K5 **Qezel Owzan** *var.* Ki Zil Uzen, Qi Zil Uzun. ~ NW Iran
142 L5 **Qezel Owzan, Rūd-e** ~ NW Iran
Qian see Guizhou
Qian Gorlo see Qian Gorlos
163 V9 **Qian Gorlos** *var.* Qian Gorlo, Qian Gorlos Mongolzu Zizhixian, Qianguozhen. Jilin, NE China
Qian Gorlos Mongolzu Zizhixian/Qianguozhen see Qian Gorlos
161 N9 **Qianjiang** Hubei, C China
160 K10 **Qianjiang** Sichuan, C China
160 L14 **Qian Jiang** ~ S China
160 G9 **Qianning** *var.* Gartar. Sichuan, C China
163 U13 **Qian Shan** ▲ NE China
160 H10 **Qianwei** Sichuan, C China
160 J11 **Qianxi** Guizhou, S China
159 Q7 **Qiaowan** Gansu, N China
Qibilī see Kebili
158 K9 **Qiemo** *var.* Qarqan. Xinjiang Uygur Zizhiqu, NW China
160 J10 **Qijiang** Chongqing Shi, C China
159 N5 **Qijiaojing** Xinjiang Uygur Zizhiqu, NW China
149 P9 **Qila Saifullāh** Baluchistān, SW Pakistan
159 S9 **Qilian** Qinghai, C China
159 N8 **Qilian Shan** *var.* Kilien Mountains. ▲ N China
197 O11 **Qimusseriarsuaq** *Dan.* Melville Bugt, *Eng.* Melville Bay. *bay* NW Greenland
Qinā see Qena
159 W11 **Qin'an** Gansu, C China
Qing see Qinghai
163 W7 **Qing'an** Heilongjiang, NE China
161 R5 **Qingdao** *var.* Ching-Tao, Ch'ing-tao, Tsingtao, Tsintao, *Ger.* Tsingtau. Shandong, E China
163 V8 **Qinggang** Heilongjiang, NE China
Qinggil see Qinghe
159 P11 **Qinghai** *var.* Chinghai, Koko Nor, Qing, Qinghai Sheng, Tsinghai. ◆ *province* C China
159 S10 **Qinghai Hu** *var.* Ch'ing Hai, Tsing Hai, *Mong.* Koko Nor. ◎ C China
Qinghai Sheng see Qinghai
158 M3 **Qinghe** *var.* Qinggil. Xinjiang Uygur Zizhiqu, NW China
160 L4 **Qingjian** Shaanxi, C China
160 L9 **Qing Jiang** ~ C China
Qingjiang see Huaiyin
Qingkou see Ganyu
160 I12 **Qinglong** *var.* Liancheng. Guizhou, S China
161 Q2 **Qinglong** Hebei, E China
Qingshan see Dedu
159 R12 **Qingshuihe** Qinghai, C China
Qingyang see Jinjiang
163 V11 **Qingyuan** Liaoning, NE China
158 L13 **Qingzang Gaoyuan** *var.* Xizang Gaoyuan, *Eng.* Plateau of Tibet. *plateau* W China
161 Q4 **Qingzhou** *prev.* Yidu. Shandong, E China
157 R9 **Qin He** ~ C China
161 Q2 **Qinhuangdao** Hebei, E China
160 K7 **Qin Ling** ▲ C China
Qin Xian see Qinxian
161 N5 **Qinxian** *var.* Qin Xian. Shanxi, C China
161 N6 **Qinyang** Henan, C China
160 K15 **Qinzhou** Guangxi Zhuangzu Zizhiqu, S China
Qiong see Hainan
160 L17 **Qionghai** *prev.* Jiaji. Hainan, S China
160 H9 **Qionglai** Sichuan, C China
160 H8 **Qionglai Shan** ▲ C China
160 L17 **Qiongzhou Haixia** *var.* Hainan Strait. *strait* S China
163 U7 **Qiqihar** *var.* Ch'i-ch'i-ha-erh, Tsitsihar; *prev.* Lungkiang. Heilongjiang, NE China
143 P12 **Qīr** Fārs, S Iran
158 H10 **Qira** Xinjiang Uygur Zizhiqu, NW China
Qir'awn, Buḥayrat al see Qaraoun, Lac de
138 F11 **Qiryat Gat** *var.* Kiryat Gat. Southern, C Israel
138 G8 **Qiryat Shemona** Northern, N Israel
Qishlaq see Garmsār
141 U14 **Qishn** SE Yemen
138 G9 **Qishon, Naḥal** ~ N Israel
Qita Ghazzah see Gaza Strip
156 K5 **Qitai** Xinjiang Uygur Zizhiqu, NW China
163 Y8 **Qitaihe** Heilongjiang, NE China
141 W12 **Qitbīt, Wādī** *dry watercourse* S Oman
161 O5 **Qixian** *var.* Qi Xian, Zhaoge. Henan, C China
Qīzān see Jīzān
Qizil Orda see Kyzylorda
Qizil Qum/Qizilqum see Kyzyl Kum
147 V14 **Qizilrabot** *Rus.* Kyzylrabot. SE Tajikistan
146 J10 **Qizilrawbe** *Rus.* Kyzylrabat. Bukhoro Wiloyati, C Uzbekistan
Qi Zil Uzun see Qezel Owzan
139 S4 **Qizil Yār** N Iraq
146 G7 **Qizqetkan** *Rus.* Kazanketken. Qoraqalpoghiston Respublikasi, W Uzbekistan
Qoghaly see Kugaly
Qogir Feng see K2
143 N6 **Qom** *var.* Kum, Qum. Qom, N Iran
143 N6 **Qom** ◆ *province* N Iran
Qomisheh see Shahreẓā
Qomolangma Feng see Everest, Mount
142 M7 **Qom, Rūd-e** ~ C Iran
Qomsheh see Shahreẓā
Qomul see Hami
Qondūz see Kunduz
Qongyrat see Konyrat
Qoqek see Tacheng
Qorabowur Kirlari see Karabaur', Uval
Qoradaryo see Karadar'ya
146 G6 **Qorajar** *Rus.* Karadzhar. Qoraqalpoghiston Respublikasi, NW Uzbekistan
146 K12 **Qorakŭl** *Rus.* Karakul'. Bukhoro Wiloyati, C Uzbekistan
146 E5 **Qoraqalpoghiston** *Rus.* Karakalpakya. Qoraqalpoghiston Respublikasi, NW Uzbekistan
146 G7 **Qoraqalpoghiston Respublikasi** *Rus.* Respublika Karakalpakstan. ◆ *autonomous republic* NW Uzbekistan
146 H7 **Qoraŭzak** *Rus.* Karauzyak. Qoraqalpoghiston Respublikasi, NW Uzbekistan
Qorghazhyn see Kurgal'dzhino
138 H6 **Qornet es Saouda** ▲ NE Lebanon
146 L12 **Qorowulbozor** *Rus.* Karaulbazar. Bukhoro Wiloyati, C Uzbekistan
142 K5 **Qorveh** *var.* Qerveh, Qurveh. Kordestān, W Iran
Qosshaghyl see Koschagyl
Qostanay/Qostanay Oblysy see Kostanay
143 P12 **Qoṭbābād** Fārs, S Iran
143 R13 **Qoṭbābād** Hormozgān, S Iran
138 H6 **Qoubaïyât** *var.* Al Qubayyāt. N Lebanon
Qoussantîna see Constantine
158 K16 **Qowowuyag** see Cho Oyu
146 H6 **Qozoqdaryo** *Rus.* Kazakdar'ya. Qoraqalpoghiston Respublikasi, NW Uzbekistan
19 N11 **Quabbin Reservoir** ⊡ Massachusetts, NE USA
100 F12 **Quakenbrück** Niedersachsen, NW Germany
18 I15 **Quakertown** Pennsylvania, NE USA
182 M10 **Quambatook** Victoria, SE Australia
25 Q4 **Quanah** Texas, SW USA
167 V10 **Quang Ngai** *var.* Quangngai, Quang Nghia. Quang Ngai, C Vietnam
Quang Nghia see Quang Ngai
167 T9 **Quang Tri** Quang Tri, C Vietnam
Quan Long see Ca Mau
152 L4 **Quanshuigou** China/India
161 R13 **Quanzhou** *var.* Ch'uan-chou, Tsinkiang; *prev.* Chin-chiang. Fujian, SE China
160 M12 **Quanzhou** Guangxi Zhuangzu Zizhiqu, S China
11 V16 **Qu'Appelle** ~ Saskatchewan, S Canada
12 M3 **Quaqtaq** *prev.* Koartac. Quebec, NE Canada
61 E16 **Quaraí** Rio Grande do Sul, S Brazil
59 H24 **Quaraí, Rio** *Sp.* Río Cuareim. ~ Brazil/Uruguay *see also* Cuareim, Río
171 N13 **Quarles, Pegunungan** ▲ Sulawesi, C Indonesia
Quarnero see Kvarner
107 C20 **Quartu Sant' Elena** Sardegna, Italy, C Mediterranean Sea
29 X13 **Quasqueton** Iowa, C USA
173 X16 **Quatre Bornes** W Mauritius
172 I17 **Quatre Bornes** Mahé, NE Seychelles
137 X10 **Quba** *Rus.* Kuba. N Azerbaijan
Qubba see Ba'qūbah
143 T3 **Qūchān** *var.* Kuchan. Khorāsān, NE Iran
183 R10 **Queanbeyan** New South Wales, SE Australia
15 Q10 **Québec** *var.* Quebec. Quebec, SE Canada
14 K10 **Quebec** *var.* Quebec. ◆ *province* SE Canada
61 D17 **Quebracho** Paysandú, W Uruguay
101 K14 **Quedlinburg** Sachsen-Anhalt, C Germany
138 H10 **Queen Alia** ✕ ('Ammān) 'Ammān, C Jordan
10 L16 **Queen Bess, Mount** ▲ British Columbia, SW Canada
10 I14 **Queen Charlotte** British Columbia, SW Canada
65 B24 **Queen Charlotte Bay** *bay* West Falkland, Falkland Islands
10 H14 **Queen Charlotte Islands** *Fr.* Îles de la Reine-Charlotte. *island group* British Columbia, SW Canada
10 I15 **Queen Charlotte Sound** *sea area* British Columbia, W Canada
10 J16 **Queen Charlotte Strait** *strait* British Columbia, W Canada
27 U1 **Queen City** Missouri, C USA
25 X5 **Queen City** Texas, SW USA
8 L3 **Queen Elizabeth Islands** *Fr.* Îles de la Reine-Élisabeth. *island group* Nunavut, N Canada
195 Y10 **Queen Mary Coast** *physical region* Antarctica
65 N24 **Queen Mary's Peak** ▲ C Tristan da Cunha
196 M8 **Queen Maud Gulf** *gulf* Arctic Ocean
195 P11 **Queen Maud Mountains** ▲ Antarctica
Queen's County see Laois
181 U7 **Queensland** ◆ *state* N Australia
192 I9 **Queensland Plateau** *undersea feature* N Coral Sea
183 O16 **Queenstown** Tasmania, SE Australia
185 C22 **Queenstown** Otago, South Island, NZ
83 I24 **Queenstown** Eastern Cape, S South Africa
Queenstown see Cobh
32 F8 **Queets** Washington, NW USA
61 D18 **Queguay Grande, Río** ~ W Uruguay
59 O16 **Queimadas** Bahia, E Brazil
82 D11 **Quela** Malanje, NW Angola
83 O16 **Quelimane** *var.* Kilimane, Kilmain, Quilimane. Zambézia, NE Mozambique
63 G18 **Quellón** *var.* Puerto Quellón. Los Lagos, S Chile
Quelpart see Cheju-do
37 P12 **Quemado** New Mexico, SW USA
25 O12 **Quemado** Texas, SW USA
44 K7 **Quemado, Punta de** *headland* E Cuba
Quemoy see Chinmen Tao
62 K13 **Quemú Quemú** La Pampa, E Argentina
155 E17 **Quepem** Goa, W India
42 M14 **Quepos** Puntarenas, S Costa Rica
Que Que see Kwekwe
61 D23 **Quequén** Buenos Aires, E Argentina
61 D23 **Quequén Grande, Río** ~ E Argentina
61 C23 **Quequén Salado, Río** ~ E Argentina

◆ Country ● Country Capital ◇ Dependent Territory ○ Dependent Territory Capital ◆ Administrative Region ✕ International Airport ▲ Mountain ▲ Mountain Range ⩓ Volcano ~ River ◎ Lake ⊡ Reservoir

Quera *see* Chur
41 *N13* **Querétaro** Querétaro de Arteaga, C Mexico
40 *F4* **Querobabi** Sonora, NW Mexico
42 *M13* **Quesada** *var.* Ciudad Quesada, San Carlos. Alajuela, N Costa Rica
105 *O13* **Quesada** Andalucía, S Spain
161 *O7* **Queshan** Henan, C China
10 *M15* **Quesnel** British Columbia, SW Canada
37 *S9* **Questa** New Mexico, SW USA
102 *H7* **Questembert** Morbihan, NW France
57 *K22* **Quetena, Río** ↝ SW Bolivia
149 *O10* **Quetta** Baluchistān, SW Pakistan
Quetzalcoalco *see* Coatzacoalcos
Quetzaltenango *see* Quezaltenango
56 *B6* **Quevedo** Los Ríos, C Ecuador
42 *B6* **Quezaltenango** *var.* Quetzaltenango. Quezaltenango, W Guatemala
42 *A2* **Quezaltenango** *off.* Departamento de Quezaltenango, *var.* Quetzaltenango. ◆ *department* SW Guatemala
42 *E6* **Quezaltepeque** Chiquimula, SE Guatemala
170 M6 **Quezon** Palawan, W Philippines
161 *P5* **Qufu** Shandong, E China
82 *B12* **Quibala** Cuanza Sul, NW Angola
82 *B11* **Quibaxe** *var.* Quibaxi. Cuanza Norte, NW Angola
Quibaxi *see* Quibaxe
54 *D9* **Quibdó** Chocó, W Colombia
102 *G7* **Quiberon** Morbihan, NW France
102 *G7* **Quiberon, Baie de** *bay* NW France
54 *J5* **Quíbor** Lara, N Venezuela
42 *C4* **Quiché** *off.* Departamento del Quiché. ◆ *department* W Guatemala
99 *E21* **Quiévrain** Hainaut, S Belgium
40 *I9* **Quila** Sinaloa, C Mexico
83 *B14* **Quilengues** Huíla, SW Angola
Quilimane *see* Quelimane
57 *G15* **Quillabamba** Cusco, C Peru
57 *L18* **Quillacollo** Cochabamba, C Bolivia
62 *H4* **Quillagua** Antofagasta, N Chile
103 *N17* **Quillan** Aude, S France
11 *U15* **Quill Lakes** ◎ Saskatchewan, S Canada
62 *G11* **Quillota** Valparaíso, C Chile
155 *G23* **Quilon** *var.* Kolam, Kollam. Kerala, SW India
181 *V9* **Quilpie** Queensland, C Australia
149 *O4* **Quil-Qala** Bāmīān, N Afghanistan
62 *L7* **Quimilí** Santiago del Estero, C Argentina
57 *O19* **Quimome** Santa Cruz, E Bolivia
102 *F6* **Quimper** *anc.* Quimper Corentin. Finistère, NW France
Quimper Corentin *see* Quimper
102 *G7* **Quimperlé** Finistère, NW France
32 *F8* **Quinault** Washington, NW USA
32 *F8* **Quinault River** ↝ Washington, NW USA
35 *P5* **Quincy** California, W USA
23 *S8* **Quincy** Florida, SE USA
30 *I13* **Quincy** Illinois, N USA
19 *O11* **Quincy** Massachusetts, NE USA
32 *J9* **Quincy** Washington, NW USA
54 *E10* **Quindío** *off.* Departamento del Quindío. ◆ *province* C Colombia
54 *E10* **Quindío, Nevado del** ▲ C Colombia
62 *J10* **Quines** San Luis, C Argentina
39 *N13* **Quinhagak** Alaska, USA
76 *G13* **Quinhámel** W Guinea-Bissau
Qui Nhon/Quinhon *see* Quy Nhơn
Quinindé *see* Rosa Zárate
25 *U6* **Quinlan** Texas, SW USA
61 *H17* **Quinta** Rio Grande do Sul, S Brazil
105 *O10* **Quintanar de la Orden** Castilla-La Mancha, C Spain
41 *X13* **Quintana Roo** ◆ *state* SE Mexico
105 *S6* **Quinto** Aragón, NE Spain
108 *G10* **Quinto** Ticino, S Switzerland
27 *Q11* **Quinton** Oklahoma, C USA
62 *K12* **Quinto, Río** ↝ C Argentina
82 *A10* **Quinzau** Zaire, NW Angola
14 *H8* **Quinze, Lac des** ◎ Quebec, SE Canada
83 *B15* **Quipungo** Huíla, C Angola
62 *G13* **Quirihue** Bío Bío, C Chile
82 *D12* **Quirima** Malanje, NW Angola
183 *T6* **Quirindi** New South Wales, SE Australia
55 *P5* **Quiriquire** Monagas, NE Venezuela
14 *D10* **Quirke Lake** ◎ Ontario, S Canada
61 *B21* **Quiroga** Buenos Aires, E Argentina
104 *I4* **Quiroga** Galicia, NW Spain
Quiróm, Salar *see* Pocitos, Salar
56 *B9* **Quiroz, Río** ↝ NW Peru
82 *Q13* **Quissanga** Cabo Delgado, NE Mozambique
83 *M20* **Quissico** Inhambane, S Mozambique
25 *O4* **Quitaque** Texas, SW USA
82 *Q13* **Quiterajo** Cabo Delgado, NE Mozambique
23 *T6* **Quitman** Georgia, SE USA
22 *M6* **Quitman** Mississippi, S USA
25 *V6* **Quitman** Texas, SW USA
56 *C6* **Quito** ● (Ecuador) Pichincha, N Ecuador
Quito *see* Mariscal Sucre
58 *P13* **Quixadá** Ceará, E Brazil
83 *Q15* **Quixaxe** Nampula, NE Mozambique
160 *J9* **Qu Jiang** ↝ C China
161 *R10* **Qu Jiang** ↝ SE China
161 *N13* **Qujiang** *prev.* Maba. Guangdong, S China
160 *H12* **Qujing** Yunnan, SW China
Qulan *see* Kulan
146 *L10* **Quljuqtov-Toghi** *Rus.* Gory Kul'dzhuktau. ▲ C Uzbekistan
Qulsary *see* Kul'sary
Qulyndy Zhazyghy *see* Kulunda Steppe
Qum *see* Qom
Qumälisch *see* Lubartów
159 *P11* **Qumar He** ↝ C China
159 *Q12* **Qumarlêb** Qinghai, C China
Qumisheh *see* Shahreẓā
147 *O14* **Qumqurghon** *Rus.* Kumkurgan. Surkhondaryo Wiloyati, S Uzbekistan
Qunaytirah/Qunayṭirah, Muḥāfaẓat al/Qunaytra *see* Al Qunayṭirah
146 *G7* **Qŭnghirot** *Rus.* Kungrad. Qoraqalpoghiston Respublikasi, NW Uzbekistan
189 *V12* **Quoi** *island* Chuuk, C Micronesia
9 N8 **Quoich** ↝ Nunavut, NE Canada
83 *E26* **Quoin Point** *headland* SW South Africa
182 *I7* **Quorn** South Australia
147 *R10* **Qŭqon** *var.* Khokand, *Rus.* Kokand. Farghona Wiloyati, E Uzbekistan
Qurein *see* Al Kuwayt
147 *P14* **Qŭrghonteppa** *Rus.* Kurgan-Tyube. SW Tajikistan
Qurlurtuuq *see* Kugluktuk
Qurveh *see* Qorveh
Qusair *see* Quseir
137 *X10* **Qusar** *Rus.* Kusary. NE Azerbaijan
Quṣayr *see* Al Quṣayr
75 *Y10* **Quseir** *var.* Al Quṣayr, Qusair. E Egypt
142 *I2* **Qūshchī** Āẕarbāyjān-e Bākhtarī, N Iran
147 *N11* **Qŭshrabot** *Rus.* Kushrabat. Samarqand Wiloyati, C Uzbekistan
Qusmuryn *see* Kushmurun, Kostanay, Kazakhstan
Qusmuryn *see* Kushmurun, Ozero, Kazakhstan
Quṭayfah/Qutayfe/Quteife *see* Al Quṭayfah
Quthing *see* Moyeni
Quwair *see* Guwēr
147 *S10* **Quwasoy** *Rus.* Kuvasay. Farghona Wiloyati, E Uzbekistan
Qu Xian *see* Quzhou
159 *N16* **Qüxü** Xizang Zizhiqu, W China
167 *V13* **Quy Chanh** Ninh Thuận, S Vietnam
167 *V11* **Quy Nhơn** *var.* Quinhon, Qui Nhon. Binh Đinh, C Vietnam
147 *O11* **Qŭytosh** *Rus.* Koytash. Jizzakh Wiloyati, C Uzbekistan
161 *R10* **Quzhou** *var.* Qu Xian. Zhejiang, SE China
Qyteti Stalin *see* Kuçovë
Qyzylorda/Qyzylorda *see* Kyzylorda
Qyzyltū *see* Kishkenekol'
Qyzylzhar *see* Kyzylzhar

R

109 *R4* **Raab** Oberösterreich, N Austria
109 *X8* **Raab** *Hung.* Rába. ↝ Austria/Hungary *see also* Rába
Raab *see* Győr
109 *V2* **Raabs an der Thaya** Niederösterreich, E Austria
93 *L14* **Raahe** *Swe.* Brahestad. Oulu, W Finland
98 *M10* **Raalte** Overijssel, E Netherlands
99 *I14* **Raamsdonksveer** Noord-Brabant, S Netherlands
92 *L12* **Raanujärvi** Lappi, NW Finland
96 *G9* **Raasay** *island* NW Scotland, UK
118 *H3* **Raasiku** *Ger.* Rasik. Harjumaa, NW Estonia
112 *B11* **Rab** *It.* Arbe. Primorje-Gorski Kotar, NW Croatia
112 *B11* **Rab** *It.* Arbe. *island* NW Croatia
171 N16 **Raba** Sumbawa, S Indonesia
111 *G22* **Rába** *Ger.* Raab. ↝ Austria/Hungary *see also* Raab
112 *A10* **Rabac** Istra, NW Croatia
104 *I2* **Rábade** Galicia, NW Spain
80 *F10* **Rabak** White Nile, C Sudan
186 G9 **Rabaraba** Milne Bay, SE PNG
102 *K16* **Rabastens-de-Bigorre** Hautes-Pyrénées, S France
121 O16 **Rabat** W Malta
74 *F6* **Rabat** *var.* al Dar al Baida. ● (Morocco) NW Morocco
Rabat *see* Victoria
186 H6 **Rabaul** New Britain, E PNG
Rabbah Ammon/Rabbath Ammon *see* 'Ammān
28 *K8* **Rabbit Creek** ↝ South Dakota, N USA
14 *H10* **Rabbit Lake** ◎ Ontario, S Canada
187 Y14 **Rabi** *prev.* Rambi. *island* N Fiji
140 *K9* **Rābigh** Makkah, W Saudi Arabia
42 *D5* **Rabinal** Baja Verapaz, C Guatemala
168 *G9* **Rabi, Pulau** *island* NW Indonesia, East Indies
111 *L17* **Rabka** Małopolskie, S Poland
155 *F16* **Rabkavi** Karnātaka, W India
Rābniṭa *see* Rîbniṭa
109 *Y6* **Rabnitz** ↝ E Austria
126 *J7* **Rabocheostrovsk** Respublika Kareliya, NW Russian Federation
23 *U1* **Rabun Bald** ▲ Georgia, SE USA
75 *S11* **Rabyānah** SE Libya
75 *S11* **Rabyānah, Ramlat** *var.* Rebiana Sand Sea, Ṣaḥrā' Rabyānah. *desert* SE Libya
Rabyānah, Ṣaḥrā' *see* Rabyānah, Ramlat
116 *L11* **Răcăciuni** Bacău, E Romania
107 *J24* **Racalmuto** Sicilia, Italy, C Mediterranean Sea
116 *J14* **Răcari** Dâmboviṭa, SE Romania
Răcari *see* Durankulak
116 *F13* **Răcășdia** *Hung.* Rakasd. Caraș-Severin, SW Romania
106 *B9* **Racconigi** Piemonte, NE Italy
31 *T15* **Raccoon Creek** ↝ Ohio, N USA
13 *V13* **Race, Cape** *headland* Newfoundland, E Canada
22 *K10* **Raceland** Louisiana, S USA
19 *Q12* **Race Point** *headland* Massachusetts, NE USA
167 S14 **Rach Gia** Kiên Giang, S Vietnam
167 *S14* **Rach Gia, Vinh** *bay* S Vietnam
76 *J8* **Rachid** Tagant, C Mauritania
110 *L10* **Raciąż** Mazowieckie, C Poland
111 *I16* **Racibórz** *Ger.* Ratibor. Śląskie, S Poland
31 *N9* **Racine** Wisconsin, N USA
14 *D7* **Racine Lake** ◎ Ontario, S Canada
111 *J23* **Ráckeve** Pest, C Hungary
Rácz-Becse *see* Bečej
141 *O15* **Radā'** *var.* Ridā'. W Yemen
113 *O15* **Radan** ▲ SE Yugoslavia
63 *J19* **Rada Tilly** Chubut, SE Argentina
116 *K8* **Rădăuṭi** *Ger.* Radautz, *Hung.* Rádóc. Suceava, N Romania
116 *L8* **Rădăuṭi-Prut** Botoșani, NE Romania
Radautz *see* Rădăuṭi
Radbusa *see* Radbuza
111 *A17* **Radbuza** *Ger.* Radbusa. ↝ SE Czech Republic
20 *K6* **Radcliff** Kentucky, S USA
139 *O2* **Radd, Wādī ar** *dry watercourse* N Syria
95 *H16* **Råde** Østfold, S Norway
109 *V11* **Radeče** *Ger.* Ratschach. C Slovenia
Radein *see* Radenci
116 *J4* **Radekhiv** *Pol.* Radziechów, *Rus.* Radekhov. L'vivs'ka Oblast', W Ukraine
Radekhov *see* Radekhiv
109 *X9* **Radenci** *Ger.* Radein; *prev.* Radinci. NE Slovenia
109 *S9* **Radenthein** Kärnten, S Austria
21 *R7* **Radford** Virginia, NE USA
154 *C9* **Rādhanpur** Gujarāt, W India
Radinci *see* Radenci
129 *Q6* **Radishchevo** Ul'yanovskaya Oblast', W Russian Federation
12 *I9* **Radisson** Quebec, E Canada
11 *P16* **Radium Hot Springs** British Columbia, SW Canada
116 *F11* **Radna** *Hung.* Máriaradna. Arad, W Romania
114 *K10* **Radnevo** Stara Zagora, C Bulgaria
97 *J20* **Radnor** *cultural region* E Wales, UK
Radnót *see* Iernut
Rádóc *see* Rădăuṭi
101 *H24* **Radolfzell am Bodensee** Baden-Württemberg, S Germany
110 *M13* **Radom** Mazowieckie, C Poland
116 *I14* **Radomirești** Olt, S Romania
111 *K14* **Radomsko** *Rus.* Novoradomsk. Łodzkie, C Poland
117 *N4* **Radomyshl'** Zhytomyrs'ka Oblast', N Ukraine
113 *P19* **Radoviš** *prev.* Radovište. E FYR Macedonia
Radovište *see* Radoviš
94 *B13* **Radøy** *island* S Norway
109 *R7* **Radstadt** Salzburg, NW Austria
182 *E8* **Radstock, Cape** *headland* South Australia
119 *G15* **Radun'** *Rus.* Radun'. Hrodzyenskaya Voblasts', W Belarus
118 *F11* **Radviliškis** Radviliškis, N Lithuania
11 *U17* **Radville** Saskatchewan, S Canada
140 *K7* **Raḍwá, Jabal** ▲ W Saudi Arabia
111 *P16* **Radymno** Podkarpackie, SE Poland
116 *J5* **Radyvyliv** Rivnens'ka Oblast', NW Ukraine
Radziechów *see* Radekhiv
110 *I11* **Radziejów** Kujawsko-pomorskie, C Poland
110 *O12* **Radzyń Podlaski** Lubelskie, E Poland
8 *J7* **Rae** ↝ Nunavut, NW Canada
152 *M13* **Rāe Bareli** Uttar Pradesh, N India
Rae-Edzo *see* Edzo
21 *T11* **Raeford** North Carolina, SE USA
99 *M19* **Raeren** Liège, E Belgium
9 N7 **Rae Strait** *strait* Nunavut, N Canada
184 *L11* **Raetihi** Manawatu-Wanganui, North Island, NZ
191 *U13* **Raevavae** *var.* Raivavae. *island* Îles Australes, SW French Polynesia
Rafa *see* Rafah
62 *M10* **Rafaela** Santa Fe, E Argentina
138 *E11* **Rafah** *var.* Rafa, Rafaḥ, *Heb.* Rafiaḥ, Raphiah. SW Gaza Strip
79 *L15* **Rafaï** Mbomou, SE Central African Republic
141 *O4* **Rafḥah** Al Ḥudūd ash Shamālīyah, N Saudi Arabia
Rafiaḥ *see* Rafah
143 *R10* **Rafsanjān** Kermān, C Iran
80 *B13* **Raga** Western Bahr el Ghazal, SW Sudan
19 *S8* **Ragged Island** *island* Maine, NE USA
44 *I5* **Ragged Island Range** *island group* S Bahamas
184 *L7* **Raglan** Waikato, North Island, NZ
22 *G8* **Ragley** Louisiana, S USA
Ragnit *see* Neman
107 *K25* **Ragusa** Sicilia, Italy, C Mediterranean Sea
Ragusa *see* Dubrovnik
Ragusavecchia *see* Cavtat
171 P14 **Raha** Pulau Muna, C Indonesia
119 *N17* **Rahachow** *Rus.* Rogachëv. Homyel'skaya Voblasts', SE Belarus
67 *U6* **Rahad** *var.* Nahr ar Rahad. ↝ W Sudan
Rahad, Nahr ar *see* Rahad
Rahaeng *see* Tak
138 *F11* **Rahat** Southern, C Israel
140 *L8* **Raḥaṭ, Ḥarrat** *lavaflow* W Saudi Arabia
149 *S12* **Rahīmyār Khān** Punjab, SE Pakistan
95 *I14* **Råholt** Akershus, S Norway
Rahovec *see* Orahovac
191 *S10* **Raiatea** *island* Îles Sous le Vent, W French Polynesia
155 *H16* **Rāichūr** Karnātaka, C India
Raidestos *see* Tekirdağ
153 *S13* **Rāiganj** West Bengal, NE India
154 *M11* **Raigarh** Madhya Pradesh, C India
183 *O16* **Railton** Tasmania, SE Australia
36 *L8* **Rainbow Bridge** *natural arch* Utah, W USA
23 *Q3* **Rainbow City** Alabama, S USA
11 *N11* **Rainbow Lake** Alberta, W Canada
21 *R5* **Rainelle** West Virginia, NE USA
32 *G10* **Rainier** Oregon, NW USA
32 *H9* **Rainier, Mount** ⩕ Washington, NW USA
23 *Q2* **Rainsville** Alabama, S USA
12 *B11* **Rainy Lake** ◎ Canada/USA
12 *A11* **Rainy River** Ontario, C Canada
Raippaluoto *see* Replot
154 *K12* **Raipur** Madhya Pradesh, C India
154 *H10* **Raisen** Madhya Pradesh, C India
15 *N13* **Raisin** ↝ Ontario, SE Canada
31 *R11* **Raisin, River** ↝ Michigan, N USA
Raivavae *see* Raevavae
149 *W9* **Rāiwind** Punjab, E Pakistan
171 T12 **Raja Ampat, Kepulauan** *island group* E Indonesia
155 *L16* **Rājahmundry** Andhra Pradesh, E India
155 *I18* **Rājampet** Andhra Pradesh, E India
Rajang *see* Rajang, Batang
169 *S9* **Rajang, Batang** *var.* Rajang. ↝ East Malaysia
149 *S11* **Rājanpur** Punjab, E Pakistan
155 *H23* **Rājapālaiyam** Tamil Nādu, SE India
152 *E12* **Rājasthān** ◆ *state* NW India
153 *T15* **Rajbari** Dhaka, C Bangladesh
153 *R12* **Rajbiraj** Eastern, E Nepal
154 *G9* **Rājgarh** Madhya Pradesh, C India
152 *H10* **Rājgarh** Rājasthān, NW India
153 *P14* **Rājgir** Bihār, N India
110 *O8* **Rajgród** Podlaskie, NE Poland
154 *L12* **Rājim** Madhya Pradesh, C India
112 *C11* **Rajinac, Mali** ▲ W Croatia
154 *B10* **Rājkot** Gujarāt, W India
153 *R14* **Rājmahal** Bihār, NE India
153 *Q14* **Rājmahāl Hills** *hill range* N India
154 *K12* **Rāj Nāndgaon** Madhya Pradesh, C India
152 *I8* **Rājpura** Punjab, NW India
153 *S14* **Rajshahi** *prev.* Rampur Boalia. Rajshahi, W Bangladesh
153 *S13* **Rajshahi** ◆ *division* NW Bangladesh
190 *K13* **Rakahanga** *atoll* N Cook Islands
185 *H19* **Rakaia** Canterbury, South Island, NZ
185 *G19* **Rakaia** ↝ South Island, NZ
152 *H3* **Rakaposhi** ▲ N India
Rakasd *see* Răcășdia
169 N15 **Rakata, Pulau** *var.* Pulau Krakatau. *island* S Indonesia
158 *K16* **Raka Zangbo** ↝ W China
141 *U10* **Rakbah, Qalamat ar** *well* SE Saudi Arabia
Rakhine State *see* Arakan State
116 *I8* **Rakhiv** Zakarpats'ka Oblast', W Ukraine
141 *V13* **Rakhyūt** SW Oman
192 K9 **Rakiraki** Viti Levu, W Fiji
Rakka *see* Ar Raqqah
118 *I4* **Rakke** Lääne-Virumaa, NE Estonia
95 *I16* **Rakkestad** Østfold, S Norway
110 *F12* **Rakoniewice** *Ger.* Rakwitz. Wielkolpolskie, C Poland
Rakonitz *see* Rakovník
83 *H18* **Rakops** Central, C Botswana
111 *C16* **Rakovník** *Ger.* Rakonitz. Středočeský Kraj, W Czech Republic
114 *J10* **Rakovski** Plovdiv, C Bulgaria
Rakutō-kō *see* Naktong-gang
118 *I3* **Rakvere** *Ger.* Wesenberg. Lääne-Virumaa, N Estonia
Rakwitz *see* Rakoniewice
22 *L6* **Raleigh** Mississippi, S USA
21 *U9* **Raleigh** *state capital* North Carolina, SE USA
21 *Y11* **Raleigh Bay** *bay* North Carolina, SE USA
21 *U9* **Raleigh-Durham** ✕ North Carolina, SE USA
189 *S6* **Ralik Chain** *island group* Ralik Chain, W Marshall Islands
25 *N5* **Ralls** Texas, SW USA
18 *G13* **Ralston** Pennsylvania, NE USA
141 *O16* **Ramādah** W Yemen
Ramadi *see* Ar Ramādī
105 *N2* **Ramales de la Victoria** Cantabria, N Spain
138 *F10* **Ramallah** C West Bank
61 *C19* **Ramallo** Buenos Aires, E Argentina
155 *H20* **Rāmanagaram** Karnātaka, E India
155 *I23* **Rāmanāthapuram** Tamil Nādu, SE India
154 *N12* **Rāmapur** Orissa, E India
155 *I14* **Rāmāreddi** *var.* Kāmāreddi, Kamareddy. Andhra Pradesh, C India
138 *F10* **Ramat Gan** Tel Aviv, W Israel
103 *T6* **Rambervillers** Vosges, NE France
Rambi *see* Rabi
103 *N5* **Rambouillet** Yvelines, N France
186 E5 **Rambutyo Island** *island* N PNG
153 *Q12* **Ramechhap** Central, C Nepal
183 *R12* **Rame Head** *headland* Victoria, SE Australia
128 *L4* **Ramenskoye** Moskovskaya Oblast', W Russian Federation
126 *J15* **Rameshki** Tverskaya Oblast', W Russian Federation
153 P14 **Rāmgarh** Bihār, N India
152 *D11* **Rāmgarh** Rājasthān, NW India
142 *M9* **Rāmhormoz** *var.* Ram Hormuz, Ramuz. Khūzestān, SW Iran
Ram Hormuz *see* Rāmhormoz
Ram, Jebel *see* Ramm, Jabal
138 *F10* **Ramla** *var.* Ramle, Ramleh, *Ar.* Er Ramle. Central, C Israel
Ramle/Ramleh *see* Ramla
138 *F14* **Ramm, Jabal** *var.* Jebel Ram. ▲ SW Jordan
152 *K10* **Rāmnagar** Uttar Pradesh, N India
95 *N15* **Ramnäs** Västmanland, C Sweden
Râmnicul-Sărat *see* Râmnicu Sărat
116 *L12* **Râmnicu Sărat** *prev.* Râmnicul-Sărat, Rîmnicu-Sărat. Buzău, E Romania
116 *I13* **Râmnicu Vâlcea** *prev.* Rîmnicu Vîlcea. Vâlcea, C Romania
Ramokgwebana *see* Ramokgwebane
83 *J18* **Ramokgwebane** *var.* Ramokgwebana. Central, NE Botswana
128 *L7* **Ramon'** Voronezhskaya Oblast', W Russian Federation
35 *V17* **Ramona** California, W USA
56 *A10* **Ramón, Laguna** ◎ NW Peru
14 *G7* **Ramore** Ontario, S Canada
40 *M11* **Ramos** San Luis Potosí, C Mexico
41 *N8* **Ramos Arizpe** Coahuila de Zaragoza, NE Mexico
40 *J9* **Ramos, Río de** ↝ C Mexico
39 *R8* **Rampart** Alaska, USA
8 H8 **Ramparts** ↝ Northwest Territories, NW Canada
152 *K10* **Rāmpur** Uttar Pradesh, N India
154 *F9* **Rāmpura** Madhya Pradesh, C India
Rampur Boalia *see* Rajshahi
166 K6 **Ramree Island** *island* W Myanmar
141 *W6* **Rams** *var.* Ar Rams. Ra's al Khaymah, NE UAE
143 *N4* **Rāmsar** *prev.* Sakhtsar. Māzandarān, N Iran
93 *H16* **Ramsele** Västernorrland, N Sweden
21 *T9* **Ramseur** North Carolina, SE USA
97 *I16* **Ramsey** NE Isle of Man
97 *I16* **Ramsey Bay** *bay* NE Isle of Man
14 *E9* **Ramsey Lake** ◎ Ontario, S Canada
97 *Q22* **Ramsgate** SE England, UK
94 *M10* **Ramsjö** Gävleborg, C Sweden
154 *I12* **Rāmtek** Mahārāshtra, C India
Ramtha *see* Ar Ramthā
Ramuz *see* Rāmhormoz
118 *G12* **Ramygala** Panevėžys, C Lithuania
92 *G12* **Rana** ↝ C Norway
152 *H14* **Rāna Pratāp Sāgar** ◎ N India
169 V7 **Ranau** Sabah, East Malaysia
168 L14 **Ranau, Danau** ◎ Sumatera, W Indonesia
62 *H12* **Rancagua** Libertador, C Chile
99 *G22* **Rance** Hainaut, S Belgium
102 *H6* **Rance** ↝ NW France
60 *J9* **Rancharia** São Paulo, S Brazil
153 *P15* **Rānchi** Bihār, N India
61 *D21* **Ranchos** Buenos Aires, E Argentina
37 *S9* **Ranchos De Taos** New Mexico, SW USA
63 *G16* **Ranco, Lago** ◎ C Chile
95 *C16* **Randaberg** Rogaland, S Norway
29 *U7* **Randall** Minnesota, N USA
107 *L23* **Randazzo** Sicilia, Italy, C Mediterranean Sea
95 *G21* **Randers** Århus, C Denmark
92 *I12* **Randijaure** ◎ N Sweden
21 *T9* **Randleman** North Carolina, SE USA
19 *O11* **Randolph** Massachusetts, NE USA
29 *Q13* **Randolph** Nebraska, C USA
36 *M1* **Randolph** Utah, W USA
100 *P9* **Randow** ↝ NE Germany
95 *H14* **Randsfjorden** ◎ S Norway
92 *K13* **Råneå** Norrbotten, N Sweden
93 *F15* **Ranemsletta** Nord-Trøndelag, C Norway
76 *H10* **Ranérou** C Senegal
185 *E22* **Ranfurly** Otago, South Island, NZ
167 P17 **Rangae** Narathiwat, SW Thailand
153 *V16* **Rangamati** Chittagong, SE Bangladesh
184 *I2* **Rangaunu Bay** *bay* North Island, NZ
19 *P6* **Rangeley** Maine, NE USA
37 *O4* **Rangely** Colorado, C USA
25 *R7* **Ranger** Texas, SW USA
14 *C9* **Ranger Lake** Ontario, S Canada
14 *C9* **Ranger Lake** ◎ Ontario, S Canada
153 *V12* **Rangia** Assam, NE India
185 *I18* **Rangiora** Canterbury, South Island, NZ
191 *T9* **Rangiroa** *atoll* Îles Tuamotu, W French Polynesia
184 *N9* **Rangitaiki** ↝ North Island, NZ
185 *F19* **Rangitata** ↝ South Island, NZ
184 *M12* **Rangitikei** ↝ North Island, NZ
184 *L6* **Rangitoto Island** *island* N NZ
Rangkasbitoeng *see* Rangkasbitung
169 N16 **Rangkasbitung** *prev.* Rangkasbitoeng. Jawa, SW Indonesia
167 P9 **Rang, Khao** ▲ C Thailand
147 *V13* **Rangkŭl** *Rus.* Rangkul'. SE Tajikistan
Rangkul' *see* Rangkŭl
Rangoon *see* Yangon
153 *T13* **Rangpur** Rajshahi, N Bangladesh
155 *F18* **Rānibennur** Karnātaka, W India
153 *R15* **Rāniganj** West Bengal, NE India
149 *Q13* **Rānīpur** Sind, SE Pakistan
Rāniyah *see* Ṛānya
25 *N9* **Rankin** Texas, SW USA
9 O9 **Rankin Inlet** Nunavut, C Canada
183 *P8* **Rankins Springs** New South Wales, SE Australia
Rankovićevo *see* Kraljevo
108 *I7* **Rankweil** Vorarlberg, W Austria
Rann *see* Brežice
129 *T8* **Ranneye** Orenburgskaya Oblast', W Russian Federation
96 *I10* **Rannoch, Loch** ◎ C Scotland, UK
191 *U17* **Rano Kau** *var.* Rano Kao. *crater* Easter Island, Chile, E Pacific Ocean
167 N14 **Ranong** Ranong, SW Thailand
186 J8 **Ranongga** *var.* Ghanongga. *island* NW Solomon Islands
191 *W16* **Rano Raraku** *ancient monument* Easter Island, Chile, E Pacific Ocean
171 V12 **Ransiki** Irian Jaya, E Indonesia
92 *K12* **Rantajärvi** Norrbotten, N Sweden
93 *N17* **Rantasalmi** Isä-Suomi, SE Finland
169 U13 **Rantau** Borneo, C Indonesia
168 L10 **Rantau, Pulau** *var.* Pulau Tebingtinggi. *island* W Indonesia
171 N13 **Rantepao** Sulawesi, C Indonesia
30 *M13* **Rantoul** Illinois, N USA
93 *L15* **Rantsila** Oulu, C Finland
92 *L13* **Ranua** Lappi, NW Finland
139 *T3* **Ṛānya** *var.* Rāniyah. NE Iraq
157 *X3* **Raohe** Heilongjiang, NE China
74 *H9* **Raoui, Erg er** *desert* W Algeria
193 O10 **Rapa** *island* Îles Australes, S French Polynesia
191 *V14* **Rapa Iti** *island* Îles Australes, SW French Polynesia
106 *D10* **Rapallo** Liguria, NW Italy
Rapa Nui *see* Pascua, Isla de
Raphiah *see* Rafah
21 *V5* **Rapidan River** ↝ Virginia, NE USA
28 *J10* **Rapid City** South Dakota, N USA
15 *P8* **Rapide-Blanc** Quebec, SE Canada
14 *I8* **Rapide-Deux** Quebec, SE Canada
118 *K6* **Räpina** *Ger.* Rappin. Põlvamaa, SE Estonia
118 *G4* **Rapla** *Ger.* Rappel. Raplamaa, NW Estonia
118 *G4* **Raplamaa** *off.* Rapla Maakond. ◆ *province* NW Estonia
21 *X6* **Rappahannock River** ↝ Virginia, NE USA
Rappel *see* Rapla
108 *G7* **Rapperswil** Sankt Gallen, NE Switzerland
Rappin *see* Räpina
153 *N12* **Rāpti** ↝ N India
57 *K16* **Rapulo, Río** ↝ E Bolivia
Raqqah/Raqqah, Muḥāfaẓat al *see* Ar Raqqah
18 *J8* **Raquette Lake** ◎ New York, NE USA
18 *J6* **Raquette River** ↝ New York, NE USA
191 *V10* **Raraka** *atoll* Îles Tuamotu, C French Polynesia
191 *V10* **Raroia** *atoll* Îles Tuamotu, C French Polynesia
190 *H15* **Rarotonga** ✕ Rarotonga, S Cook Islands, C Pacific Ocean
190 *H16* **Rarotonga** *island* S Cook Islands, C Pacific Ocean
147 *P12* **Rarz** W Tajikistan
Ras al 'Ain *see* Ra's al 'Ayn
139 *N2* **Ra's al 'Ayn** *var.* Ras al 'Ain. Al Ḥasakah, N Syria
138 *H3* **Ra's al Basīṭ** Al Lādhiqīyah, W Syria
Ra's al-Hafgī *see* Ra's al Khafjī
141 *R5* **Ra's al Khafjī** *var.* Ra's al-Hafgi. Ash Sharqīyah, NE Saudi Arabia
Ras al-Khaimah/Ras al Khaimah *see* Ra's al Khaymah
143 *R15* **Ra's al Khaymah** *var.* Ras al Khaimah. Ra's al Khaymah, NE UAE
143 *R15* **Ra's al Khaymah** *var.* Ras al-Khaimah. ✕ Ra's al Khaymah, NE UAE

◆ Country
● Country Capital
◇ Dependent Territory
○ Dependent Territory Capital
◆ Administrative Region
✕ International Airport
▲ Mountain
▲ Mountain Range
⩕ Volcano
↝ River
◎ Lake
⊠ Reservoir

138 G13 **Ra's an Naqb** Ma'ān, S Jordan
61 B26 **Rasa, Punta** headland E Argentina
171 V12 **Rasawi** Irian Jaya, E Indonesia
Râşcani see Rîşcani
80 J10 **Ras Dashen Terara** ▲ N Ethiopia
151 K19 **Rasdu Atoll** atoll C Maldives
118 E12 **Raseiniai** Raseiniai, C Lithuania
75 X8 **Râs Ghârib** E Egypt
162 D6 **Rashaant** Bayan-Ölgiy, W Mongolia
162 L10 **Rashaant** Dundgovĭ, C Mongolia
162 J6 **Rashaant** Hövsgöl, N Mongolia
139 Y11 **Rashīd** E Iraq
75 V7 **Rashîd** Eng. Rosetta. N Egypt
142 M3 **Rasht** var. Resht. Gīlān, NW Iran
139 S2 **Rashwān** N Iraq
Rasik see Raasiku
113 M15 **Raška** Serbia, C Yugoslavia
119 P15 **Rasna** Rus. Ryasna. Mahilyowskaya Voblasts', E Belarus
116 J12 **Râşnov** prev. Rîşno, Rozsnyó, Hung. Barcarozsnyó. Braşov, C Romania
118 L11 **Rasony** Rus. Rossony. Vitsyebskaya Voblasts', N Belarus
Ra's Shamrah see Ugarit
129 N7 **Rasskazovo** Tambovskaya Oblast', W Russian Federation
119 O16 **Rasta** ≈ E Belarus
Rastadt see Rastatt
Rastâne see Ar Rastān
141 S6 **Ra's Tannūrah** Eng. Ras Tanura. Ash Sharqīyah, NE Saudi Arabia
Ras Tanura see Ra's Tannūrah
101 G21 **Rastatt** var. Rastadt. Baden-Württemberg, SW Germany
Rastenburg see Kętrzyn
149 V7 **Rasūlnagar** Punjab, E Pakistan
189 U6 **Ratak Chain** island group Ratak Chain, E Marshall Islands
119 K15 **Ratamka** Rus. Ratomka. Minskaya Voblasts', C Belarus
93 G17 **Ratan** Jämtland, C Sweden
152 G11 **Ratangarh** Rājasthān, NW India
Rat Buri see Ratchaburi
167 O11 **Ratchaburi** var. Rat Buri. Ratchaburi, W Thailand
29 W15 **Rathbun Lake** ⊡ Iowa, C USA
Ráth Caola see Rathkeale
166 K5 **Rathedaung** Arakan State, W Myanmar
100 M12 **Rathenow** Brandenburg, NE Germany
97 C19 **Rathkeale** Ir. Ráth Caola. SW Ireland
96 F13 **Rathlin Island** Ir. Reachlainn. island N Northern Ireland, UK
97 C20 **Ráthluirc** Ir. An Ráth. SW Ireland
Ratibor see Racibórz
Ratisbon/Ratisbona/Ratisbonne see Regensburg
Rätische Alpen see Rhaetian Alps
38 E17 **Rat Island** island Aleutian Islands, Alaska, USA
38 E17 **Rat Islands** island group Aleutian Islands, Alaska, USA
154 F10 **Ratlām** prev. Rutlam. Madhya Pradesh, C India
155 D15 **Ratnāgiri** Mahārāshtra, W India
155 K26 **Ratnapura** Sabaragamuwa Province, S Sri Lanka
116 J2 **Ratne** Rus. Ratno. Volyns'ka Oblast', NW Ukraine
Ratno see Ratne
Ratomka see Ratamka
37 U8 **Raton** New Mexico, SW USA
139 O7 **Ratqah, Wādī ar** dry watercourse W Iraq
Ratschach see Radeče
167 O16 **Rattaphum** Songkhla, SW Thailand
26 L6 **Rattlesnake Creek** ≈ Kansas, C USA
94 L13 **Rättvik** Dalarna, C Sweden
100 K9 **Ratzeburg** Mecklenburg-Vorpommern, N Germany
100 K9 **Ratzeburger See** ⊚ N Germany
10 J10 **Ratz, Mount** ▲ British Columbia, SW Canada
61 D22 **Rauch** Buenos Aires, E Argentina
41 U16 **Raudales** Chiapas, SE Mexico
Raudhatain see Ar Rawdatayn
Raudnitz an der Elbe see Roudnice nad Labem
92 K1 **Raufarhöfn** Nordhurland Eystra, NE Iceland
94 H13 **Raufoss** Oppland, S Norway
Raukawa see Cook Strait
184 Q8 **Raukumara** ▲ North Island, NZ
192 K11 **Raukumara Plain** undersea feature N Coral Sea
184 P8 **Raukumara Range** ▲ North Island, NZ
154 N11 **Rāulakela** var. Raurkela; prev. Rourkela. Orissa, E. India
95 F15 **Rauland** Telemark, S Norway
93 J19 **Rauma** Swe. Raumo. Länsi-Suomi, W Finland
94 F10 **Rauma** ≈ S Norway
Raumo see Rauma
118 H8 **Rauna** Cēsis, C Latvia
169 T17 **Raung, Gunung** ▲ Jawa, S Indonesia
Raurkela see Rāulakela
95 J22 **Raus** Skåne, S Sweden
165 W3 **Rausu** Hokkaidō, NE Japan
165 W3 **Rausu-dake** ▲ Hokkaidō, NE Japan
93 M17 **Rautalampi** Itä-Suomi, C Finland
93 N16 **Rautavaara** Itä-Suomi, C Finland
116 M9 **Răutel** ≈ C Moldova
93 O18 **Rautjärvi** Etelä-Suomi, S Finland
Rautu see Sosnovo
191 V11 **Ravahere** atoll Îles Tuamotu, C French Polynesia
107 J25 **Ravanusa** Sicilia, Italy, C Mediterranean Sea
143 S9 **Rāvar** Kermān, C Iran
147 Q11 **Ravat** Oshskaya Oblast', SW Kyrgyzstan
18 K11 **Ravena** New York, NE USA
106 H10 **Ravenna** Emilia-Romagna, N Italy
29 O15 **Ravenna** Nebraska, C USA
31 U11 **Ravenna** Ohio, N USA
101 I24 **Ravensburg** Baden-Württemberg, S Germany
181 W4 **Ravenshoe** Queensland, NE Australia
180 K13 **Ravensthorpe** Western Australia
21 Q4 **Ravenswood** West Virginia, NE USA
149 U9 **Rāvi** ≈ India/Pakistan
112 C9 **Ravna Gora** Primorje-Gorski Kotar, NW Croatia
109 U10 **Ravne na Koroškem** Ger. Gutenstein. N Slovenia
139 P6 **Rāwah** W Iraq
191 T4 **Rawaki** prev. Phoenix Island. atoll Phoenix Islands, C Kiribati
149 U6 **Rāwalpindi** Punjab, NE Pakistan
110 L13 **Rawa Mazowiecka** Łódzkie, C Poland
139 T2 **Ṛawāndiz** var. Rawandoz, Rawāndūz. N Iraq
Rawandoz/Rawāndūz see Ṛawāndiz
171 U12 **Rawas** Irian Jaya, E Indonesia
139 O4 **Rawḍah** ⊚ E Syria
110 G13 **Rawicz** Ger. Rawitsch. Wielkopolskie, C Poland
Rawitsch see Rawicz
180 M11 **Rawlinna** Western Australia
33 W16 **Rawlins** Wyoming, C USA
63 K17 **Rawson** Chubut, SE Argentina
159 R16 **Rawu** Xizang Zizhiqu, W China
153 P12 **Raxaul** Bihār, N India
28 K3 **Ray** North Dakota, N USA
169 S11 **Raya, Bukit** ▲ Borneo, C Indonesia
155 I18 **Rāyachoti** Andhra Pradesh, E India
Rāyadrug see Rāyagarha
155 M14 **Rāyagarha** prev. Rāyadrug. Orissa, E India
138 H7 **Rayak** var. Rayaq, Riyāq. E Lebanon
Rayaq see Rayak
139 T2 **Ṛāyat** E Iraq
169 N12 **Raya, Tanjung** headland Pulau Bangka, W Indonesia
13 R13 **Ray, Cape** headland Newfoundland, E Canada
123 Q13 **Raychikhinsk** Amurskaya Oblast', SE Russian Federation
129 U5 **Rayevskiy** Respublika Bashkortostan, W Russian Federation
11 Q17 **Raymond** Alberta, SW Canada
22 K6 **Raymond** Mississippi, S USA
32 F9 **Raymond** Washington, NW USA
183 T8 **Raymond Terrace** New South Wales, SE Australia
25 T17 **Raymondville** Texas, SW USA
11 U16 **Raymore** Saskatchewan, S Canada
39 Q8 **Ray Mountains** ▲ Alaska, USA
22 H9 **Rayne** Louisiana, S USA
41 O12 **Rayón** San Luis Potosí, C Mexico
40 G4 **Rayón** Sonora, NW Mexico
167 P12 **Rayong** Rayong, S Thailand
25 T5 **Ray Roberts, Lake** ⊚ Texas, SW USA
18 E15 **Raystown Lake** ⊡ Pennsylvania, NE USA
141 V13 **Raysūt** SW Oman
27 R4 **Raytown** Missouri, C USA
22 I5 **Rayville** Louisiana, S USA
142 L5 **Razan** Hamadān, W Iran
139 S9 **Razāzah, Buḥayrat ar** var. Baḥr al Milḥ. ⊚ C Iraq
114 L9 **Razboyna** ▲ E Bulgaria
Razdan see Hrazdan
Razdolnoye see Rozdol'ne
Razelm, Lacul see Razim, Lacul
139 U2 **Ṛazga** E Iraq
114 L8 **Razgrad** Razgrad, N Bulgaria
114 L8 **Razgrad** ❖ province N Bulgaria
117 N13 **Razim, Lacul** prev. Lacul Razelm. lagoon NW Black Sea
114 G11 **Razlog** Blagoevgrad, SW Bulgaria
118 K10 **Rāznas Ezers** ⊚ SE Latvia
102 E6 **Raz, Pointe du** headland NW France
Reachlainn see Rathlin Island
Reachrainn see Lambay Island
97 N22 **Reading** S England, UK
18 H15 **Reading** Pennsylvania, NE USA
48 C7 **Real, Cordillera** ▲ C Ecuador
62 K12 **Realicó** La Pampa, C Argentina
25 R15 **Realitos** Texas, SW USA
108 G9 **Realp** Uri, C Switzerland
167 Q12 **Reăng Kesei** Bătdâmbâng, W Cambodia
191 Y11 **Reao** atoll Îles Tuamotu, E French Polynesia
Reate see Rieti
180 L11 **Rebecca, Lake** ⊚ Western Australia
Rebiana Sand Sea see Rabyānah, Ramlat
126 H8 **Reboly** Respublika Kareliya, NW Russian Federation
165 S1 **Rebun** Rebun-tō, NE Japan
165 S1 **Rebun-tō** island NE Japan
106 J12 **Recanati** Marche, C Italy
Rechitsa see Rechytsa
109 Y7 **Rechnitz** Burgenland, SE Austria
119 J20 **Rechytsa** Rus. Rechitsa. Brestskaya Voblasts', SW Belarus
119 O19 **Rechytsa** Rus. Rechitsa. Homyel'skaya Voblasts', SE Belarus
59 Q15 **Recife** prev. Pernambuco. state capital Pernambuco, E Brazil
83 I26 **Recife, Cape** Afr. Kaap Recife. headland S South Africa
Recife, Kaap see Recife, Cape
172 I16 **Récifs, Îles aux** island Inner Islands, NE Seychelles
101 E14 **Recklinghausen** Nordrhein-Westfalen, W Germany
100 M8 **Recknitz** ≈ NE Germany
99 K23 **Recogne** Luxembourg, SE Belgium
61 C15 **Reconquista** Santa Fe, C Argentina
195 O6 **Recovery Glacier** glacier Antarctica
59 G15 **Recreio** Mato Grosso, W Brazil
27 X9 **Rector** Arkansas, C USA
110 E9 **Recz** Ger. Reetz Neumark. Zachodniopomorskie, NW Poland
99 L24 **Redange** var. Redange-sur-Attert. Diekirch, W Luxembourg
Redange-sur-Attert see Redange
18 C13 **Redbank Creek** ≈ Pennsylvania, NE USA
13 S9 **Red Bay** Quebec, E Canada
23 N2 **Red Bay** Alabama, S USA
35 N4 **Red Bluff** California, W USA
24 J8 **Red Bluff Reservoir** ⊡ New Mexico/Texas, SW USA
30 K6 **Red Bud** Illinois, N USA
30 J5 **Red Cedar River** ≈ Wisconsin, N USA
11 R17 **Redcliff** Alberta, SW Canada
83 K17 **Redcliff** Midlands, C Zimbabwe
182 L9 **Red Cliffs** Victoria, SE Australia
29 P17 **Red Cloud** Nebraska, C USA
22 L8 **Red Creek** ≈ Mississippi, S USA
11 P15 **Red Deer** Alberta, SW Canada
11 Q16 **Red Deer** ≈ Alberta, SW Canada
39 O11 **Red Devil** Alaska, USA
35 N3 **Redding** California, W USA
97 L20 **Redditch** W England, UK
29 P9 **Redfield** South Dakota, N USA
24 J12 **Redford** Texas, SW USA
45 V13 **Redhead** Trinidad, Trinidad and Tobago
182 I8 **Red Hill** South Australia
38 F10 **Red Hill** Haw. Pu'uUla'ula. ▲ Maui, Hawaii, USA, C Pacific Ocean
26 K7 **Red Hills** hill range Kansas, C USA
13 T12 **Red Indian Lake** ⊚ Newfoundland, E Canada
126 J16 **Redkino** Tverskaya Oblast', W Russian Federation
12 A10 **Red Lake** Ontario, C Canada
36 I10 **Red Lake** salt flat Arizona, SW USA
29 S4 **Red Lake Falls** Minnesota, N USA
29 R4 **Red Lake River** ≈ Minnesota, N USA
35 U15 **Redlands** California, W USA
18 G16 **Red Lion** Pennsylvania, NE USA
33 U11 **Red Lodge** Montana, NW USA
32 H13 **Redmond** Oregon, NW USA
36 L5 **Redmond** Utah, W USA
32 H8 **Redmond** Washington, NW USA
Rednitz see Regnitz
29 T15 **Red Oak** Iowa, C USA
18 K12 **Red Oaks Mill** New York, NE USA
102 I7 **Redon** Ille-et-Vilaine, NW France
45 W10 **Redonda** island SW Antigua and Barbuda
104 G4 **Redondela** Galicia, NW Spain
104 H11 **Redondo** Évora, S Portugal
39 Q12 **Redoubt Volcano** Ж Alaska, USA
11 Y16 **Red River** ≈ Canada/USA
131 U12 **Red River** var. Yuan, Chin. Yuan Jiang, Vtn. Sông Hông Hà. ≈ China/Vietnam
25 W4 **Red River** ≈ S USA
22 H7 **Red River** ≈ Louisiana, S USA
30 M6 **Red River** ≈ Wisconsin, N USA
Red Rock, Lake see Red Rock Reservoir
29 W14 **Red Rock Reservoir** var. Lake Red Rock. ⊡ Iowa, C USA
80 H7 **Red Sea** ❖ state NE Sudan
75 Y9 **Red Sea** anc. Sinus Arabicus. sea Africa/Asia
21 T11 **Red Springs** North Carolina, SE USA
8 I9 **Redstone** ≈ Northwest Territories, NW Canada
11 V17 **Redvers** Saskatchewan, S Canada
77 P13 **Red Volta** var. Nazinon, Fr. Volta Rouge. ≈ Burkina/Ghana
11 Q14 **Redwater** Alberta, SW Canada
28 M16 **Red Willow Creek** ≈ Nebraska, C USA
29 W9 **Red Wing** Minnesota, N USA
35 N9 **Redwood City** California, W USA
29 T9 **Redwood Falls** Minnesota, N USA
31 P7 **Reed City** Michigan, N USA
28 K6 **Reeder** North Dakota, N USA
35 R11 **Reedley** California, W USA
33 T11 **Reedpoint** Montana, NW USA
30 K8 **Reedsburg** Wisconsin, N USA
32 E13 **Reedsport** Oregon, NW USA
187 Q9 **Reef Islands** island group Santa Cruz Islands, E Solomon Islands
185 H16 **Reefton** West Coast, South Island, NZ
20 F8 **Reelfoot Lake** ⊚ Tennessee, S USA
97 D17 **Ree, Lough** Ir. Loch Rí. ⊚ C Ireland
Reengus see Ringas
35 U4 **Reese River** ≈ Nevada, W USA
98 M8 **Reest** ≈ E Netherlands
Reetz Neumark see Recz
137 N13 **Refahiye** Erzincan, C Turkey
23 N4 **Reform** Alabama, S USA
95 K20 **Reftele** Jönköping, S Sweden
25 T14 **Refugio** Texas, SW USA
110 E8 **Rega** ≈ NW Poland
Regar see Tursunzoda
101 O21 **Regen** Bayern, SE Germany
101 M20 **Regen** ≈ SE Germany
101 M21 **Regensburg** Eng. Ratisbon, Fr. Ratisbonne; hist. Ratisbona, anc. Castra Regina, Reginum. Bayern, SE Germany
101 M21 **Regenstauf** Bayern, SE Germany
74 I10 **Reggane** C Algeria
98 N9 **Regge** ≈ E Netherlands
Reggio see Reggio nell' Emilia
Reggio Calabria see Reggio di Calabria
107 M23 **Reggio di Calabria** var. Reggio Calabria, Gk. Rhegion; anc. Regium, Rhegium. Calabria, SW Italy
Reggio Emilia see Reggio nell' Emilia
106 F9 **Reggio nell' Emilia** var. Reggio Emilia, abbrev. Reggio; anc. Regium Lepidum. Emilia-Romagna, N Italy
116 I10 **Reghin** Ger. Sächsisch-Reen, Hung. Szászrégen; prev. Reghinul Săsesc, Ger. Sächsisch-Regen. Mureş, C Romania
Reghinul Săsesc see Reghin
11 U16 **Regina** Saskatchewan, S Canada
11 U16 **Regina** × Saskatchewan, S Canada
55 Z10 **Régina** E French Guiana
11 U16 **Regina Beach** Saskatchewan, S Canada
Reginum see Regensburg
Registan see Rīgestān
60 L11 **Registro** São Paulo, S Brazil
Regium see Reggio di Calabria
Regium Lepidum see Reggio nell' Emilia
101 K19 **Regnitz** var. Rednitz. ≈ SE Germany
40 K10 **Regocijo** Durango, W Mexico
104 H12 **Reguengos de Monsaraz** Évora, S Portugal
101 M18 **Rehau** Bayern, E Germany
83 D19 **Rehoboth** Hardap, C Namibia
Rehoboth/Rehovoth see Reḥovot
21 Z4 **Rehoboth Beach** Delaware, NE USA
138 F10 **Reḥovot** var. Rehoboth, Rekhovot, Rehovoth. Central, C Israel
81 J20 **Rei** spring/well S Kenya
Reichenau see Rychnov nad Kněžnou, Czech Republic
Reichenau see Bogatynia, Poland
101 M17 **Reichenbach** var. Reichenbach im Vogtland. Sachsen, E Germany
Reichenbach see Dzierżoniów
Reichenbach im Vogtland see Reichenbach
Reichenberg see Liberec
181 O11 **Reid** Western Australia
23 V6 **Reidsville** Georgia, SE USA
21 T8 **Reidsville** North Carolina, SE USA
Reifnitz see Ribnica
97 O22 **Reigate** SE England, UK
Reikjavik see Reykjavík
102 I10 **Ré, Île de** island W France
37 N15 **Reiley Peak** ▲ Arizona, SW USA
103 Q4 **Reims** Eng. Rheims; anc. Durocortorum, Remi. Marne, N France
63 G23 **Reina Adelaida, Archipiélago** island group S Chile
45 O16 **Reina Beatrix** × (Oranjestad) C Aruba
108 F7 **Reinach** Aargau, W Switzerland
108 E6 **Reinach** Basel-Land, NW Switzerland
64 O11 **Reina Sofía** × (Tenerife) Tenerife, Islas Canarias, Spain, NE Atlantic Ocean
29 W13 **Reinbeck** Iowa, C USA
100 J10 **Reinbek** Schleswig-Holstein, N Germany
11 U12 **Reindeer** ≈ Saskatchewan, C Canada
11 U11 **Reindeer Lake** ⊚ Manitoba/Saskatchewan, C Canada
Reine-Charlotte, Îles de la see Queen Charlotte Islands
Reine-Élisabeth, Îles de la see Queen Elizabeth Islands
94 F13 **Reineskarvet** ▲ S Norway
184 H1 **Reinga, Cape** headland North Island, NZ
105 N3 **Reinosa** Cantabria, N Spain
109 R8 **Reisseck** ▲ S Austria
21 W3 **Reisterstown** Maryland, NE USA
Reisui see Yŏsu
98 N5 **Reitdiep** ≈ NE Netherlands
191 V10 **Reitoru** atoll Îles Tuamotu, C French Polynesia
95 M17 **Rejmyre** Östergötland, S Sweden
Reka see Rijeka
Reka Ili see Ili
95 N16 **Rekarne** Västmanland, C Sweden 16.04
Rekhovot see Reḥovot
8 K9 **Reliance** Northwest Territories, C Canada
33 U16 **Reliance** Wyoming, C USA
74 I5 **Relizane** var. Ghelîzâne, Ghilizane. NW Algeria
182 I7 **Remarkable, Mount** ▲ South Australia
54 E8 **Remedios** Antioquia, N Colombia
43 Q16 **Remedios** Veraguas, W Panama
42 D8 **Remedios, Punta** headland SW El Salvador
Remi see Reims
99 N25 **Remich** Grevenmacher, SE Luxembourg
99 J19 **Remicourt** Liège, E Belgium
14 H8 **Rémigny, Lac** ⊚ Quebec, SE Canada
55 Z10 **Rémire** NE French Guiana
129 N13 **Remontnoye** Rostovskaya Oblast', SW Russian Federation
171 U14 **Remoon** Pulau Kur, E Indonesia
99 L20 **Remouchamps** Liège, E Belgium
103 R15 **Remoulins** Gard, S France
173 X16 **Rempart, Mont du** var. Mount Rempart. hill W Mauritius
101 E15 **Remscheid** Nordrhein-Westfalen, W Germany
29 S12 **Remsen** Iowa, C USA
94 I12 **Rena** Hedmark, S Norway
94 I11 **Rena** ≈ S Norway
Renaix see Ronse
118 H7 **Rencēni** Valmiera, N Latvia
118 D9 **Renda** Kuldīga, W Latvia
107 N20 **Rende** Calabria, SW Italy
99 K21 **Rendeux** Luxembourg, SE Belgium
Rendina see Rentína
30 L16 **Rend Lake** ⊡ Illinois, N USA
186 K9 **Rendova** island New Georgia Islands, NW Solomon Islands
100 I8 **Rendsburg** Schleswig-Holstein, N Germany
108 B9 **Renens** Vaud, SW Switzerland
14 K12 **Renfrew** Ontario, SE Canada
96 I12 **Renfrew** cultural region SW Scotland, UK
168 L11 **Rengat** Sumatera, W Indonesia
153 W12 **Rengma Hills** ▲ NE India
62 H12 **Rengo** Libertador, C Chile
116 M12 **Reni** Odes'ka Oblast', SW Ukraine
80 F11 **Renk** Upper Nile, E Sudan
93 L19 **Renko** Etelä-Suomi, S Finland
98 L12 **Renkum** Gelderland, SE Netherlands
182 K9 **Renmark** South Australia
186 L10 **Rennell** var. Mu Nggava. island S Solomon Islands
181 Q4 **Renner Springs Roadhouse** Northern Territory, N Australia
102 I6 **Rennes** Bret. Roazon; anc. Condate. Ille-et-Vilaine, NW France
195 S16 **Rennick Glacier** glacier Antarctica
11 Y16 **Rennie** Manitoba, S Canada
35 Q5 **Reno** Nevada, W USA
106 H10 **Reno** ≈ N Italy
35 Q5 **Reno-Cannon** × Nevada, W USA
83 F24 **Renoster** ≈ SW South Africa
15 T5 **Renouard, Lac** ⊚ Quebec, SE Canada
18 F13 **Renovo** Pennsylvania, NE USA
161 O3 **Renqiu** Hebei, E China
160 I9 **Renshou** Sichuan, C China
31 N12 **Rensselaer** Indiana, N USA
18 L11 **Rensselaer** New York, NE USA
105 Q2 **Rentería** Basq. Errenteria. País Vasco, N Spain
115 E17 **Rentína** var. Rendina. Thessalía, C Greece
29 T9 **Renville** Minnesota, N USA
77 O13 **Réo** W Burkina
15 O12 **Repentigny** Quebec, SE Canada
146 K13 **Repetek** Lebapskiy Velayat, E Turkmenistan
93 J16 **Replot** Fin. Raippaluoto. island W Finland
Reppen see Rzepin
Reps see Rupea
27 T7 **Republic** Missouri, C USA
32 K7 **Republic** Washington, NW USA
27 N3 **Republican River** ≈ Kansas/Nebraska, C USA
9 O7 **Repulse Bay** Northwest Territories, N Canada
56 F9 **Requena** Loreto, NE Peru
105 R10 **Requena** País Valenciano, E Spain
103 O14 **Réquista** Aveyron, S France
136 M12 **Reşadiye** Tokat, N Turkey
Reschenpass see Resia, Passo di
Reschitza see Reşiţa
113 N20 **Resen** Turk. Resne. SW FYR Macedonia
60 J11 **Reserva** Paraná, S Brazil
11 V15 **Reserve** Saskatchewan, S Canada
37 P13 **Reserve** New Mexico, SW USA
Reshetilovka see Reshetylivka
117 S6 **Reshetylivka** Rus. Reshetilovka. Poltavs'ka Oblast', NE Ukraine
Resht see Rasht
106 F5 **Resia, Passo di** Ger. Reschenpass. pass Austria/Italy
Resicabánya see Reşiţa
62 N7 **Resistencia** Chaco, NE Argentina
116 F12 **Reşiţa** Ger. Reschitza, Hung. Resicabánya. Caraş-Severin, W Romania
Resne see Resen
8 K4 **Resolute** var.. Qausuittuq. Nunavut, N Canada
Resolution see Fort Resolution
9 T7 **Resolution Island** island Nunavut, NE Canada
185 A23 **Resolution Island** island SW NZ
15 W7 **Restigouche** Quebec, SE Canada
11 W17 **Reston** Manitoba, S Canada
14 H11 **Restoule Lake** ⊚ Ontario, S Canada
54 F10 **Restrepo** Meta, C Colombia
42 B6 **Retalhuleu** Retalhuleu, SW Guatemala
42 A1 **Retalhuleu** off. Departamento de Retalhuleu. ❖ department SW Guatemala
97 N18 **Retford** C England, UK
103 Q3 **Rethel** Ardennes, N France
Rethimno/Réthimnon see Réthymno
115 I25 **Réthymno** var. Rethimno; prev. Réthimnon. Kríti, Greece, E Mediterranean Sea
Retiche, Alpi see Rhaetian Alps
99 J16 **Retie** Antwerpen, N Belgium
111 J21 **Rétság** Nógrád, N Hungary
109 W2 **Retz** Niederösterreich, NE Austria
173 N15 **Réunion** off. La Réunion. ◇ French overseas department W Indian Ocean
130 L17 **Réunion** island W Indian Ocean
105 U6 **Reus** Cataluña, E Spain
99 J15 **Reusel** Noord-Brabant, S Netherlands
108 F7 **Reuss** ≈ NW Switzerland
Reuţel see Ciuhuru
101 H22 **Reutlingen** Baden-Württemberg, S Germany
108 L7 **Reutte** Tirol, W Austria
99 M16 **Reuver** Limburg, SE Netherlands
28 K7 **Reva** South Dakota, N USA
Reval/Revel' see Tallinn
126 J4 **Revda** Murmanskaya Oblast', NW Russian Federation
122 F6 **Revda** Sverdlovskaya Oblast', C Russian Federation
103 N16 **Revel** Haute-Garonne, S France
11 O16 **Revelstoke** British Columbia, SW Canada
43 N13 **Reventazón, Río** ≈ E Costa Rica
106 G9 **Revere** Lombardia, N Italy
39 Y14 **Revillagigedo Island** island Alexander Archipelago, Alaska, USA
193 Y14 **Revillagigedo Islands** island group NW Mexico
103 R3 **Revin** Ardennes, N France
92 O3 **Revnosa** headland C Svalbard
Revolyutsii, Pik see Revolyutsiya, Qullai
147 T13 **Revolyutsiya, Qullai** Rus. Pik Revolyutsii. ▲ SE Tajikistan
111 L19 **Revúca** Ger. Grossrauschenbach, Hung. Nagyrőce. Banskobystrický Kraj, C Slovakia
154 K9 **Rewa** Madhya Pradesh, C India
152 I11 **Rewāri** Haryāna, N India
33 R14 **Rexburg** Idaho, NW USA
78 G13 **Rey Bouba** Nord, NE Cameroon
92 L3 **Reydharfjördhur** Austurland, E Iceland
57 K16 **Reyes** Beni, NW Bolivia
34 L8 **Reyes, Point** headland California, W USA
54 B12 **Reyes, Punta** headland SW Colombia
136 L17 **Reyhanlı** Hatay, S Turkey
43 U16 **Rey, Isla del** island Archipiélago de las Perlas, SE Panama
92 H2 **Reykhólar** Vestfirdhir, W Iceland
92 K2 **Reykjahlídh** Nordhurland Eystra, NE Iceland
92 I4 **Reykjanes** ❖ region SW Iceland
197 O16 **Reykjanes Basin** var. Irminger Basin. undersea feature N Atlantic Ocean
197 N17 **Reykjanes Ridge** undersea feature N Atlantic Ocean
92 H4 **Reykjavík** var. Reikjavik. ● (Iceland) Höfudhborgarsvaedhi, W Iceland
18 D13 **Reynoldsville** Pennsylvania, NE USA
41 P8 **Reynosa** Tamaulipas, C Mexico
Reẓā'īyeh see Orūmīyeh
Reẓā'īyeh, Daryācheh-ye see Orūmīyeh, Daryācheh-ye
102 I8 **Rezé** Loire-Atlantique, NW France
118 K10 **Rēzekne** Ger. Rositten; prev. Rus. Rezhitsa. Rēzekne, SE Latvia
Rezhitsa see Rēzekne
117 N9 **Rezina** NE Moldova
114 N11 **Rezovo** Turk. Rezve. Burgas, E Bulgaria
114 N11 **Rezovska Reka** Turk. Rezve Deresi. ≈ Bulgaria/Turkey see also Rezve Deresi
Rezve see Rezovo
114 N11 **Rezve Deresi** Bul. Rezovska Reka. ≈ Bulgaria/Turkey see also Rezovska Reka
Rhadames see Ghadāmis
Rhaedestus see Tekirdağ
108 J10 **Rhaetian Alps** Fr. Alpes Rhétiques, Ger. Rätische Alpen, It. Alpi Retiche. ▲ C Europe
108 I8 **Rhätikon** ▲ C Europe
101 G14 **Rheda-Wiedenbrück** Nordrhein-Westfalen, W Germany
98 M12 **Rheden** Gelderland, E Netherlands
Rhegion/Rhegium see Reggio di Calabria
Rheims see Reims
Rhein see Rhine
101 E17 **Rheinbach** Nordrhein-Westfalen, W Germany
100 F13 **Rheine** var. Rheine in Westfalen. Nordrhein-Westfalen, NW Germany
Rheine in Westfalen see Rheine
Rheinfeld see Rheinfelden
101 F24 **Rheinfelden** Baden-Württemberg, S Germany

◆ Country
● Country Capital
◇ Dependent Territory
○ Dependent Territory Capital
❖ Administrative Region
× International Airport
▲ Mountain
▲ Mountain Range
Ж Volcano
≈ River
⊚ Lake
⊡ Reservoir

108 E6 **Rheinfelden** var. Rheinfeld. Aargau, N Switzerland
101 E17 **Rheinisches Schiefergebirge** var. Rhine State Uplands, Eng. Rhenish Slate Mountains. ▲ W Germany
101 D18 **Rheinland-Pfalz** Eng. Rhineland-Palatinate, Fr. Rhénanie-Palatinat. ◈ state W Germany
101 G18 **Rhein/Main** ✕ (Frankfurt am Main) Hessen, W Germany
Rhénanie du Nord-Westphalie see Nordrhein-Westfalen
Rhénanie-Palatinat see Rheinland-Pfalz
98 K12 **Rhenen** Utrecht, C Netherlands
Rhenish Slate Mountains see Rheinisches Schiefergebirge
Rhétiques, Alpes see Rhaetian Alps
100 N10 **Rhin** ≈ NE Germany
Rhin see Rhine
84 F10 **Rhine** Dut. Rijn, Fr. Rhin, Ger. Rhein. ≈ W Europe
30 L5 **Rhinelander** Wisconsin, N USA
Rhineland-Palatinate see Rheinland-Pfalz
Rhine State Uplands see Rheinisches Schiefergebirge
100 N11 **Rhinkanal** canal NE Germany
81 F17 **Rhino Camp** NW Uganda
74 D7 **Rhir, Cap** headland W Morocco
106 D7 **Rho** Lombardia, N Italy
19 N12 **Rhode Island** off. State of Rhode Island and Providence Plantations; also known as Little Rhody, Ocean State. ◈ state NE USA
19 O13 **Rhode Island** island Rhode Island, NE USA
19 O13 **Rhode Island Sound** sound Maine/Rhode Island, NE USA
Rhodes see Ródos
Rhode-Saint-Genèse see Sint-Genesius-Rode
84 L14 **Rhodes Basin** undersea feature E Mediterranean Sea
Rhodesia see Zimbabwe
114 I12 **Rhodope Mountains** var. Rodhópi Óri, Bul. Rhodope Planina, Rodopi, Gk. Orosirá Rodhópis, Turk. Dospad Dagh. ▲ Bulgaria/Greece
Rhodope Planina see Rhodope Mountains
Rhodos see Ródos
101 I18 **Rhön** ▲ C Germany
103 Q10 **Rhône** ◈ department E France
86 C12 **Rhône** ≈ France/Switzerland
103 R12 **Rhône-Alpes** ◈ region E France
98 G13 **Rhoon** Zuid-Holland, SW Netherlands
96 G9 **Rhum** var. Rum. island W Scotland, UK
Rhuthun see Ruthin
97 J18 **Rhyl** NE Wales, UK
59 K18 **Rialma** Goiás, S Brazil
104 L3 **Riaño** Castilla-León, N Spain
105 O9 **Riansáres** ≈ C Spain
152 H6 **Riāsi** Jammu and Kashmir, NW India
168 K10 **Riau** off. Propinsi Riau. ◈ province W Indonesia
Riau Archipelago see Riau, Kepulauan
168 M11 **Riau, Kepulauan** var. Riau Archipelago, Dut. Riouw-Archipel. island group W Indonesia
105 O6 **Riaza** Castilla-León, N Spain
105 N6 **Riaza** ≈ N Spain
81 K17 **Riba** spring/well NE Kenya
104 H4 **Ribadavia** Galicia, NW Spain
104 J2 **Ribadeo** Galicia, NW Spain
104 L2 **Ribadesella** Asturias, N Spain
104 G10 **Ribatejo** former province C Portugal
143 Q8 **Ribāṭ-e Rīzāb** Yazd, C Iran
83 P15 **Ribáuè** Nampula, N Mozambique
97 K17 **Ribble** ≈ NW England, UK
95 F23 **Ribe** Ribe, W Denmark
95 F23 **Ribe** off. Ribe Amt, var. Ripen. ◈ county W Denmark
104 G3 **Ribeira** Galicia, NW Spain
64 O5 **Ribeira Brava** Madeira, Portugal, NE Atlantic Ocean
64 P3 **Ribeira Grande** São Miguel, Azores, Portugal, NE Atlantic Ocean
60 L8 **Ribeirão Preto** São Paulo, S Brazil
60 L11 **Ribeira, Rio** ≈ S Brazil
107 I24 **Ribera** Sicilia, Italy, C Mediterranean Sea
57 L14 **Riberalta** Beni, N Bolivia
105 W4 **Ribes de Freser** Cataluña, NE Spain
30 L6 **Rib Mountain** ▲ Wisconsin, N USA
109 U12 **Ribnica** Ger. Reifnitz. S Slovenia
117 N9 **Rîbniţa** var. Râbniţa, Rus. Rybnitsa. NE Moldova
100 M8 **Ribnitz-Damgarten** Mecklenburg-Vorpommern, NE Germany
111 D16 **Říčany** Ger. Ritschan. Středočeský Kraj, W Czech Republic
29 U7 **Rice** Minnesota, N USA
30 J5 **Rice Lake** Wisconsin, N USA
14 I15 **Rice Lake** ◎ Ontario, SE Canada
14 E8 **Rice Lake** ◎ Ontario, S Canada
23 V3 **Richard B.Russell Lake** ⊟ Georgia, SE USA
25 U6 **Richardson** Texas, SW USA
11 R11 **Richardson** ≈ Alberta, C Canada
10 I3 **Richardson Mountains** ▲ Yukon Territory, NW Canada
185 C21 **Richardson Mountains** ▲ South Island, NZ
42 F3 **Richardson Peak** ▲ SE Belize
76 G10 **Richard Toll** N Senegal
28 L5 **Richardton** North Dakota, N USA
14 F13 **Rich, Cape** headland Ontario, S Canada
102 L8 **Richelieu** Indre-et-Loire, C France
33 P15 **Richfield** Idaho, NW USA
36 K5 **Richfield** Utah, W USA
18 J10 **Richfield Springs** New York, NE USA
18 M6 **Richford** Vermont, NE USA
27 R6 **Rich Hill** Missouri, C USA
13 P14 **Richibucto** New Brunswick, SE Canada
108 G8 **Richisau** Glarus, NE Switzerland
23 S6 **Richland** Georgia, SE USA
27 U6 **Richland** Missouri, C USA
25 U8 **Richland** Texas, SW USA
32 K10 **Richland** Washington, NW USA
30 K8 **Richland Center** Wisconsin, N USA
21 W11 **Richlands** North Carolina, SE USA
21 Q7 **Richlands** Virginia, NE USA
25 R9 **Richland Springs** Texas, SW USA
183 S8 **Richmond** New South Wales, SE Australia
10 L17 **Richmond** British Columbia, SW Canada
14 L13 **Richmond** Ontario, SE Canada
15 Q12 **Richmond** Quebec, SE Canada
185 I14 **Richmond** Tasman, South Island, NZ
35 N8 **Richmond** California, W USA
31 Q14 **Richmond** Indiana, N USA
20 M6 **Richmond** Kentucky, S USA
27 S4 **Richmond** Missouri, C USA
25 V11 **Richmond** Texas, SW USA
36 L1 **Richmond** Utah, W USA
21 W6 **Richmond** state capital Virginia, NE USA
14 H15 **Richmond Hill** Ontario, S Canada
185 J15 **Richmond Range** ▲ South Island, NZ
27 S12 **Rich Mountain** ▲ Arkansas, C USA
31 S13 **Richwood** Ohio, N USA
21 R5 **Richwood** West Virginia, NE USA
104 K5 **Ricobayo, Embalse de** ⊟ NW Spain
Ricomagus see Riom
Ridā' see Radā'
98 H13 **Ridderkerk** Zuid-Holland, SW Netherlands
33 N16 **Riddle** Idaho, NW USA
32 F14 **Riddle** Oregon, NW USA
14 L13 **Rideau** ≈ Ontario, SE Canada
35 T12 **Ridgecrest** California, W USA
18 L13 **Ridgefield** Connecticut, NE USA
22 K5 **Ridgeland** Mississippi, S USA
21 R15 **Ridgeland** South Carolina, SE USA
20 F8 **Ridgely** Tennessee, S USA
14 D17 **Ridgetown** Ontario, S Canada
Ridgeway see Ridgway
21 R12 **Ridgeway** South Carolina, SE USA
18 D13 **Ridgway** var. Ridgeway. Pennsylvania, NE USA
11 W16 **Riding Mountain** ▲ Manitoba, S Canada
Ried see Ried im Innkreis
109 R4 **Ried im Innkreis** var. Ried. Oberösterreich, NW Austria
109 X8 **Riegersburg** Steiermark, SE Austria
108 E6 **Riehen** Basel-Stadt, NW Switzerland
92 J9 **Riehppegáisá** var. Rieppe. ▲ N Norway
99 K18 **Riemst** Limburg, NE Belgium
Rieppe see Riehppegáisá
101 O15 **Riesa** Sachsen, E Germany
63 H24 **Riesco, Isla** island S Chile
107 K25 **Riesi** Sicilia, Italy, C Mediterranean Sea
83 F25 **Riet** ≈ SW South Africa
83 I23 **Riet** ≈ SW South Africa
118 D11 **Rietavas** Plungė, W Lithuania
83 F19 **Rietfontein** Omaheke, E Namibia
107 I14 **Rieti** anc. Reate. Lazio, C Italy
84 D14 **Rif** var. Er Rif, Er Riff, Riff. ▲ N Morocco
Riff see Rif
37 Q4 **Rifle** Colorado, C USA
31 R7 **Rifle River** ≈ Michigan, N USA
81 H18 **Rift Valley** ◈ province Kenya
Rift Valley see Great Rift Valley
118 F9 **Rīga** Eng. Riga. ● (Latvia) Rīga, C Latvia
Rigaer Bucht see Riga, Gulf of
118 F6 **Riga, Gulf of** Est. Liivi Laht, Ger. Rigaer Bucht, Latv. Rīgas Jūras Līcis, Rus. Rizhskiy Zaliv; prev. Est. Riia Laht. gulf Estonia/Latvia
143 U12 **Rīgān** Kermān, SE Iran
Rīgas Jūras Līcis see Riga, Gulf of
15 N12 **Rigaud** ≈ Ontario/Quebec, SE Canada
33 R14 **Rigby** Idaho, NW USA
148 M10 **Rīgestān** var. Registan. desert region S Afghanistan
32 M11 **Riggins** Idaho, NW USA
13 R8 **Rigolet** Newfoundland, NE Canada
78 G9 **Rig-Rig** Kanem, W Chad
118 F4 **Riguldi** Läänemaa, W Estonia
Riia Laht see Riga, Gulf of
93 L19 **Riihimäki** Etelä-Suomi, S Finland
195 O2 **Riiser-Larsen Ice Shelf** ice shelf Antarctica
195 U2 **Riiser-Larsen Peninsula** peninsula Antarctica
65 P22 **Riiser-Larsen Sea** sea Antarctica
40 D2 **Riíto** Sonora, NW Mexico
112 B9 **Rijeka** Ger. Sankt Veit am Flaum, It. Fiume, Slvn. Reka; anc. Tarsatica. Primorje-Gorski Kotar, NW Croatia
99 I14 **Rijen** Noord-Brabant, S Netherlands
99 H15 **Rijkevorsel** Antwerpen, N Belgium
Rijn see Rhine
98 G11 **Rijnsburg** Zuid-Holland, W Netherlands
Rijssel see Lille
98 N10 **Rijssen** Overijssel, E Netherlands
98 G12 **Rijswijk** Eng. Ryswick. Zuid-Holland, W Netherlands
92 I10 **Riksgränsen** Norrbotten, N Sweden
165 U4 **Rikubetsu** Hokkaidō, NE Japan
165 R9 **Rikuzen-Takata** Iwate, Honshū, C Japan
27 O4 **Riley** Kansas, C USA
99 I17 **Rillaar** Vlaams Brabant, C Belgium
Rí, Loch see Ree, Lough
114 G11 **Rilska Reka** ≈ W Bulgaria
77 T12 **Rima** ≈ N Nigeria
141 N7 **Rimah, Wādī ar** var. Wādī ar Rummah. dry watercourse C Saudi Arabia
Rimaszombat see Rimavská Sobota
191 R12 **Rimatara** island Îles Australes, SW French Polynesia
111 L20 **Rimavská Sobota** Ger. Gross-Steffelsdorf, Hung. Rimaszombat. Banskobystrický Kraj, C Slovakia
11 Q15 **Rimbey** Alberta, SW Canada
95 P15 **Rimbo** Stockholm, C Sweden
95 M18 **Rimforsa** Östergötland, S Sweden
106 I11 **Rimini** anc. Ariminum. Emilia-Romagna, N Italy
Rîmnicu-Sărat see Râmnicu Sărat
Rîmnicu Vîlcea see Râmnicu Vâlcea
149 Y3 **Rimo Muztāgh** ▲ India/Pakistan
15 U7 **Rimouski** Quebec, SE Canada
158 M16 **Rinbung** Xizang Zizhiqu, W China
162 I5 **Rinchinlhümbe** Hövsgöl, N Mongolia
62 I5 **Rincón, Cerro** ▲ N Chile
104 M15 **Rincón de la Victoria** Andalucía, S Spain
Rincón del Bonete, Lago Artificial de see Río Negro, Embalse del
105 Q4 **Rincón de Soto** La Rioja, N Spain
94 G8 **Rindal** Møre og Romsdal, S Norway
115 J20 **Ríneia** island Kykládes, Greece, Aegean Sea
152 H11 **Rīngas** prev. Reengus, Ringus. Rājasthān, N India
95 H24 **Ringe** Fyn, C Denmark
94 H11 **Ringebu** Oppland, S Norway
Ringen see Rõngu
186 K8 **Ringi** Kolombangara, NW Solomon Islands
23 R1 **Ringgold** Georgia, SE USA
22 G5 **Ringgold** Louisiana, S USA
25 S5 **Ringgold** Texas, SW USA
95 E22 **Ringkøbing** Ringkøbing, W Denmark
95 E21 **Ringkøbing** off. Ringkøbing Amt. ◈ county W Denmark
95 E22 **Ringkøbing Fjord** fjord W Denmark
33 S10 **Ringling** Montana, NW USA
27 N13 **Ringling** Oklahoma, C USA
94 H13 **Ringsaker** Hedmark, S Norway
95 I23 **Ringsted** Vestsjælland, E Denmark
Ringus see Rīngas
92 I9 **Ringvassøya** island N Norway
18 K13 **Ringwood** New Jersey, NE USA
Rinn Duáin see Hook Head
100 H13 **Rinteln** Niedersachsen, NW Germany
Rio see Rio de Janeiro
115 E18 **Río** Dytikí Ellás, S Greece
56 C7 **Riobamba** Chimborazo, C Ecuador
60 P9 **Rio Bonito** Rio de Janeiro, SE Brazil
59 C16 **Rio Branco** state capital Acre, W Brazil
61 H18 **Río Branco** Cerro Largo, NE Uruguay
Rio Branco, Território de see Roraima
41 P8 **Río Bravo** Tamaulipas, C Mexico
63 G16 **Río Bueno** Los Lagos, C Chile
55 P5 **Río Caribe** Sucre, NE Venezuela
54 M5 **Río Chico** Miranda, N Venezuela
63 H18 **Río Cisnes** Aisén, S Chile
60 L9 **Rio Claro** São Paulo, S Brazil
45 V14 **Rio Claro** Trinidad, Trinidad and Tobago
54 J5 **Río Claro** Lara, N Venezuela
63 K15 **Río Colorado** Río Negro, E Argentina
62 K11 **Río Cuarto** Córdoba, C Argentina
60 P10 **Rio de Janeiro** var. Rio. state capital Rio de Janeiro, SE Brazil
60 P9 **Rio de Janeiro** off. Estado do Rio de Janeiro. ◈ state SE Brazil
43 R17 **Río de Jesús** Veraguas, S Panama
34 K3 **Rio Dell** California, W USA
60 K13 **Rio do Sul** Santa Catarina, S Brazil
63 I23 **Río Gallegos** var. Gallegos, Puerto Gallegos. Santa Cruz, S Argentina
61 I18 **Rio Grande** var. São Pedro do Rio Grande do Sul. Rio Grande do Sul, S Brazil
24 I9 **Rio Grande** ≈ Texas, SW USA
63 J24 **Río Grande** Tierra del Fuego, S Argentina
40 L10 **Río Grande** Zacatecas, C Mexico
42 J9 **Río Grande** León, NW Nicaragua
45 V5 **Río Grande** E Puerto Rico
25 R17 **Rio Grande City** Texas, SW USA
59 P14 **Rio Grande do Norte** off. Estado do Rio Grande do Norte. ◈ state E Brazil
61 G15 **Rio Grande do Sul** off. Estado do Rio Grande do Sul. ◈ state S Brazil
65 M17 **Rio Grande Fracture Zone** tectonic feature C Atlantic Ocean
65 J18 **Rio Grande Gap** undersea feature S Atlantic Ocean
Rio Grande Plateau see Rio Grande Rise
65 J18 **Rio Grande Rise** var. Rio Grande Plateau. undersea feature SW Atlantic Ocean
54 G4 **Ríohacha** La Guajira, N Colombia
43 S16 **Río Hato** Coclé, C Panama
25 T17 **Río Hondo** Texas, SW USA
56 D10 **Rioja** San Martín, N Peru
41 Y11 **Río Lagartos** Yucatán, SE Mexico
103 P11 **Riom** anc. Ricomagus. Puy-de-Dôme, C France
104 F10 **Rio Maior** Santarém, C Portugal
103 O12 **Riom-ès-Montagnes** Cantal, C France
60 J12 **Rio Negro** Paraná, S Brazil
63 I15 **Río Negro** off. Provincia de Río Negro. ◈ province C Argentina
61 D18 **Río Negro** ◈ department W Uruguay
47 V12 **Río Negro, Embalse del** var. Lago Artificial de Rincón del Bonete. ⊟ C Uruguay
107 M17 **Rionero in Vulture** Basilicata, S Italy
137 S9 **Rioni** ≈ W Georgia
105 P12 **Riópar** Castilla-La Mancha, C Spain
61 H16 **Rio Pardo** Rio Grande do Sul, S Brazil
37 R11 **Rio Rancho Estates** New Mexico, SW USA
42 L11 **Río San Juan** ◈ department S Nicaragua
54 E9 **Riosucio** Caldas, W Colombia
54 C7 **Ríosucio** Chocó, NW Colombia
62 K10 **Río Tercero** Córdoba, C Argentina
54 J5 **Río Tocuyo** Lara, N Venezuela
Riouw-Archipel see Riau, Kepulauan
59 J19 **Rio Verde** Goiás, C Brazil
41 O12 **Río Verde** var. Rioverde. San Luis Potosí, C Mexico
35 O8 **Rio Vista** California, W USA
112 M11 **Ripanj** Serbia, N Yugoslavia
106 J13 **Ripatransone** Marche, C Italy
Ripen see Ribe
22 M2 **Ripley** Mississippi, S USA
31 R15 **Ripley** Ohio, N USA
20 F9 **Ripley** Tennessee, S USA
21 Q4 **Ripley** West Virginia, NE USA
105 W4 **Ripoll** Cataluña, NE Spain
97 M16 **Ripon** N England, UK
30 M7 **Ripon** Wisconsin, N USA
107 L24 **Riposto** Sicilia, Italy, C Mediterranean Sea
99 L14 **Rips** Noord-Brabant, SE Netherlands
54 D9 **Risaralda** off. Departamento de Risaralda. ◈ province C Colombia
116 L8 **Rîşcani** var. Râşcani, Rus. Ryshkany. NW Moldova
152 J9 **Rishikesh** Uttar Pradesh, N India
165 S1 **Rishiri-tō** var. Risiri Tô. island NE Japan
165 S1 **Rishiri-yama** ⩓ Rishiri-tō, NE Japan
25 R7 **Rising Star** Texas, SW USA
31 Q15 **Rising Sun** Indiana, N USA
Risiri Tô see Rishiri-tō
102 L4 **Risle** ≈ N France
Rîşno see Râşnov
27 V13 **Rison** Arkansas, C USA
95 G17 **Risør** Aust-Agder, S Norway
92 H10 **Risøyhamn** Nordland, C Norway
101 I23 **Riss** ≈ S Germany
118 G4 **Risti** Ger. Kreuz. Läänemaa, W Estonia
15 V8 **Ristigouche** ≈ Quebec, SE Canada
93 N18 **Ristiina** Isä-Suomi, E Finland
93 N14 **Ristijärvi** Oulu, C Finland
188 C14 **Ritidian Point** headland N Guam
Ritschan see Říčany
35 R9 **Ritter, Mount** ▲ California, W USA
31 T12 **Rittman** Ohio, N USA
32 L9 **Ritzville** Washington, NW USA
Riva see Riva del Garda
61 A21 **Rivadavia** Buenos Aires, E Argentina
108 F7 **Riva del Garda** var. Riva. Trentino-Alto Adige, N Italy
106 B8 **Rivarolo Canavese** Piemonte, W Italy
42 K11 **Rivas** Rivas, SW Nicaragua
42 J11 **Rivas** ◈ department SW Nicaragua
103 R11 **Rive-de-Gier** Loire, E France
61 A22 **Rivera** Buenos Aires, E Argentina
61 F16 **Rivera** Rivera, NE Uruguay
61 F17 **Rivera** ◈ department NE Uruguay
35 P9 **Riverbank** California, W USA
76 K17 **River Cess** SW Liberia
28 M4 **Riverdale** North Dakota, N USA
30 I6 **River Falls** Wisconsin, N USA
11 T16 **Riverhurst** Saskatchewan, S Canada
183 O10 **Riverina** physical region New South Wales, SE Australia
80 G8 **River Nile** ◈ state NE Sudan
63 F19 **Rivero, Isla** island Archipiélago de los Chonos, S Chile
11 W16 **Rivers** Manitoba, S Canada
77 U17 **Rivers** ◈ state S Nigeria
185 D23 **Riversdale** Southland, South Island, NZ
83 F26 **Riversdale** Western Cape, SW South Africa
35 U15 **Riverside** California, W USA
25 W9 **Riverside** Texas, SW USA
37 U3 **Riverside Reservoir** ⊟ Colorado, C USA
10 K15 **Rivers Inlet** British Columbia, SW Canada
10 K15 **Rivers Inlet** inlet British Columbia, SW Canada
11 X15 **Riverton** Manitoba, S Canada
185 C24 **Riverton** Southland, South Island, NZ
30 L13 **Riverton** Illinois, N USA
36 L3 **Riverton** Utah, W USA
33 V15 **Riverton** Wyoming, C USA
14 G10 **River Valley** Ontario, S Canada
13 P14 **Riverview** New Brunswick, SE Canada
103 O17 **Rivesaltes** Pyrénées-Orientales, S France
36 H11 **Riviera** Arizona, SW USA
25 S15 **Riviera** Texas, SW USA
23 Z14 **Riviera Beach** Florida, SE USA
15 Q10 **Rivière-à-Pierre** Quebec, SE Canada
15 T9 **Rivière-Bleue** Quebec, SE Canada
15 T8 **Rivière-du-Loup** Quebec, SE Canada
173 Y15 **Rivière du Rempart** NE Mauritius
45 R12 **Rivière-Pilote** S Martinique
173 O17 **Rivière St-Etienne, Point de la** headland SW Réunion
13 S10 **Rivière-St-Paul** Quebec, E Canada
Rivière Sèche see Bel Air
116 K4 **Rivne** Pol. Równe, Rus. Rovno. Rivnens'ka Oblast', NW Ukraine
Rivne see Rivnens'ka Oblast'
116 K3 **Rivnens'ka Oblast'** var. Rivne, Rus. Rovenskaya Oblast'. ◈ province NW Ukraine
106 B8 **Rivoli** Piemonte, NW Italy
159 Q14 **Riwoqê** Xizang Zizhiqu, W China
99 H19 **Rixensart** Wallon Brabant, C Belgium
Riyadh/Riyāḍ, Minṭaqat ar see Ar Riyāḍ
Riyāq see Rayak
Rizaiyeh see Orūmīyeh
137 P11 **Rize** Rize, NE Turkey
137 P11 **Rize** prev. Çoruh. ◈ province NE Turkey
161 R5 **Rizhao** Shandong, E China
Rizhskiy Zaliv see Riga, Gulf of
Rizokarpaso/Rizokárpason see Dipkarpaz
107 O21 **Rizzuto, Capo** headland S Italy
95 F15 **Rjukan** Telemark, S Norway
95 D16 **Rjuven** ▲ S Norway
76 H9 **Rkîz** Trarza, W Mauritania
95 H14 **Roa** Oppland, S Norway
105 N5 **Roa** Castilla-León, N Spain
45 T9 **Road Town** ○ (British Virgin Islands) Tortola, C British Virgin Islands
96 F6 **Roag, Loch** inlet NW Scotland, UK
37 O5 **Roan Cliffs** cliff Colorado/Utah, W USA
21 P9 **Roan High Knob** var. Roan Mountain. ▲ North Carolina/Tennessee, SE USA
Roan Mountain see Roan High Knob
103 Q10 **Roanne** anc. Rodunma. Loire, E France
23 R4 **Roanoke** Alabama, S USA
21 S7 **Roanoke** Virginia, NE USA
21 Z9 **Roanoke Island** island North Carolina, SE USA
21 W8 **Roanoke Rapids** North Carolina, SE USA
21 X9 **Roanoke River** ≈ North Carolina/Virginia, SE USA
37 O4 **Roan Plateau** plain Utah, W USA
37 R5 **Roaring Fork River** ≈ Colorado, C USA
25 O5 **Roaring Springs** Texas, SW USA
42 J4 **Roatán** var. Coxen Hole, Coxin Hole. Islas de la Bahía, N Honduras
42 I4 **Roatán, Isla de** island Islas de la Bahía, N Honduras
Roat Kampuchea see Cambodia
Roazon see Rennes
143 T7 **Robāţ-e Chāh Gonbad** Khorāsān, E Iran
143 R7 **Robāţ-e Khān** Khorāsān, C Iran
143 T7 **Robāţ-e Khvosh Āb** Khorāsān, E Iran
143 R8 **Robāţ-e Posht-e Bādām** Khorāsān, NE Iran
175 S8 **Robbie Ridge** undersea feature W Pacific Ocean
21 T10 **Robbins** North Carolina, SE USA
183 N15 **Robbins Island** island Tasmania, SE Australia
21 N10 **Robbinsville** North Carolina, SE USA
182 J12 **Robe** South Australia
21 W9 **Robersonville** North Carolina, SE USA
25 P8 **Robert Lee** Texas, SW USA
35 V5 **Roberts Creek Mountain** ▲ Nevada, W USA
93 J15 **Robertsfors** Västerbotten, N Sweden
27 R11 **Robert S.Kerr Reservoir** ⊟ Oklahoma, C USA
38 L12 **Roberts Mountain** ▲ Nunivak Island, Alaska, USA
83 F26 **Robertson** Western Cape, SW South Africa
194 H4 **Robertson Island** island Antarctica
76 J16 **Robertsport** W Liberia
182 J8 **Robertstown** South Australia
Robert Williams see Caála
15 P7 **Roberval** Quebec, SE Canada
31 N15 **Robinson** Illinois, N USA
193 U11 **Robinson Crusoe, Isla** island Islas Juan Fernández, Chile, E Pacific Ocean
180 J9 **Robinson Range** ▲ Western Austral
182 M9 **Robinvale** Victoria, SE Australia
105 P11 **Robledo** Castilla-La Mancha, C Spain
54 G5 **Robles** var. La Paz, Robles La Paz. Cesar, N Colombia
Robles La Paz see Robles
11 V15 **Roblin** Manitoba, S Canada
11 S17 **Robsart** Saskatchewan, S Canada
11 N15 **Robson, Mount** ▲ British Columbia, SW Canada
25 T14 **Robstown** Texas, SW USA
25 P6 **Roby** Texas, SW USA
104 E11 **Roca, Cabo da** headland C Portugal
Rocadas see Xangongo
41 S14 **Roca Partida, Punta** headland C Mexico
47 X6 **Rocas, Atol das** island E Brazil
107 L18 **Roccadaspide** var. Rocca d'Aspide. Campania, S Italy
107 K15 **Roccaraso** Abruzzo, C Italy
106 H10 **Rocca San Casciano** Emilia-Romagna, C Italy
106 G13 **Roccastrada** Toscana, C Italy
61 G20 **Rocha** Rocha, E Uruguay
61 G19 **Rocha** ◈ department E Uruguay
97 L17 **Rochdale** NW England, UK
102 L11 **Rochechouart** Haute-Vienne, C France
99 J22 **Rochefort** Namur, SE Belgium
102 J11 **Rochefort** var. Rochefort sur Mer. Charente-Maritime, W France
Rochefort sur Mer see Rochefort
127 N10 **Rochegda** Arkhangel'skaya Oblast', NW Russian Federation
30 L10 **Rochelle** Illinois, N USA
25 Q9 **Rochelle** Texas, SW USA
13 P13 **Rocher Percé** island Rocher Percé, Quebec, E Canada
15 V3 **Rochers Ouest, Rivière aux** ≈ Quebec, SE Canada
97 O22 **Rochester** anc. Durobrivae. SE England, UK
31 O12 **Rochester** Indiana, N USA
29 W10 **Rochester** Minnesota, N USA
19 O9 **Rochester** New Hampshire, NE USA
18 F9 **Rochester** New York, NE USA
25 P5 **Rochester** Texas, SW USA
31 S9 **Rochester Hills** Michigan, N USA
Rocheuses, Montagnes/Rockies see Rocky Mountains
64 M6 **Rockall** island UK, N Atlantic Ocean
64 L6 **Rockall Bank** undersea feature N Atlantic Ocean
84 B8 **Rockall Rise** undersea feature N Atlantic Ocean
84 C9 **Rockall Trough** undersea feature N Atlantic Ocean
35 U2 **Rock Creek** ≈ Nevada, W USA
25 T10 **Rockdale** Texas, SW USA
195 N12 **Rockefeller Plateau** plateau Antarctica
30 K11 **Rock Falls** Illinois, N USA
23 Q5 **Rockford** Alabama, S USA
30 L10 **Rockford** Illinois, N USA
15 Q12 **Rock Forest** Quebec, SE Canada
11 T17 **Rockglen** Saskatchewan, S Canada
181 Y8 **Rockhampton** Queensland, E Australia
21 R11 **Rock Hill** South Carolina, SE USA
180 I13 **Rockingham** Western Australia
21 T11 **Rockingham** North Carolina, SE USA
30 J11 **Rock Island** Illinois, N USA
25 U12 **Rock Island** Texas, SW USA
14 C10 **Rock Lake** Ontario, S Canada
29 O2 **Rock Lake** North Dakota, N USA
14 I12 **Rock Lake** ◎ Ontario, SE Canada
14 M12 **Rockland** Ontario, SE Canada
19 R7 **Rockland** Maine, NE USA
182 L11 **Rocklands Reservoir** ⊟ Victoria, SE Australia
35 O7 **Rocklin** California, W USA
23 R3 **Rockmart** Georgia, SE USA
31 N16 **Rockport** Indiana, N USA
27 Q1 **Rock Port** Missouri, C USA
25 T14 **Rockport** Texas, SW USA
32 I7 **Rockport** Washington, NW USA
29 S11 **Rock Rapids** Iowa, C USA
30 K11 **Rock River** ≈ Illinois/Wisconsin, N USA
44 I3 **Rock Sound** Eleuthera Island, C Bahamas
33 U17 **Rock Springs** Wyoming, C USA
25 P11 **Rocksprings** Texas, SW USA
55 T9 **Rockstone** C Guyana
29 S12 **Rock Valley** Iowa, C USA
31 N14 **Rockville** Indiana, N USA
21 W3 **Rockville** Maryland, NE USA
25 U6 **Rockwall** Texas, SW USA
29 U13 **Rockwell City** Iowa, C USA
31 S10 **Rockwood** Michigan, N USA
20 M9 **Rockwood** Tennessee, S USA
25 Q8 **Rockwood** Texas, SW USA
37 U6 **Rocky Ford** Colorado, C USA
14 D9 **Rocky Island Lake** ◎ Ontario, S Canada
21 V9 **Rocky Mount** North Carolina, SE USA

◆ Country ● Country Capital ◇ Dependent Territory ○ Dependent Territory Capital ◈ Administrative Region ✕ International Airport ▲ Mountain ▲ Mountain Range ⩓ Volcano ≈ River ◎ Lake ⊟ Reservoir

21 S7 **Rocky Mount** Virginia, NE USA
33 Q8 **Rocky Mountain** ▲ Montana, NW USA
11 P15 **Rocky Mountain House** Alberta, SW Canada
37 T3 **Rocky Mountain National Park** national park Colorado, C USA
2 E12 **Rocky Mountains** var. Rockies, Fr. Montagnes Rocheuses. ▲ Canada/USA
42 H1 **Rocky Point** headland NE Belize
83 A17 **Rocky Point** headland NW Namibia
95 F14 **Rødberg** Buskerud, S Norway
95 I25 **Rødby** Storstrøm, SE Denmark
95 I25 **Rødbyhavn** Storstrøm, SE Denmark
13 T10 **Roddickton** Newfoundland, SE Canada
95 F23 **Rødding** Sønderjylland, SW Denmark
95 M22 **Rödeby** Blekinge, S Sweden
98 N6 **Roden** Drenthe, NE Netherlands
62 H9 **Rodeo** San Juan, W Argentina
103 O14 **Rodez** anc. Segodunum. Aveyron, S France
Rodholívos see Rodolívos
Rodhópi Óri see Rhodope Mountains
Ródhos/Rodi see Ródos
107 N15 **Rodi Garganico** Puglia, SE Italy
101 N20 **Roding** Bayern, SE Germany
113 J19 **Rodinit, Kepi i** headland W Albania
116 I9 **Rodnei, Munţii** ▲ N Romania
184 L4 **Rodney, Cape** headland North Island, NZ
38 L9 **Rodney, Cape** headland Alaska, USA
126 M16 **Rodniki** Ivanovskaya Oblast', W Russian Federation
119 Q16 **Rodnya** Rus. Rodnya. Mahilyowskaya Voblasts', E Belarus
Rodó see José Enrique Rodó
114 H13 **Rodolívos** var. Rodholívos. Kentrikí Makedonía, NE Greece
Rodopi see Rhodope Mountains
115 O22 **Ródos** var. Ródhos, Eng. Rhodes, It. Rodi. Ródos, Dodekánisos, Greece, Aegean Sea
115 O22 **Ródos** var. Ródhos, Eng. Rhodes, It. Rodi; anc. Rhodos. island Dodekánisos, Greece, Aegean Sea
Rodosto see Tekirdağ
59 A14 **Rodrigues** Amazonas, W Brazil
173 P8 **Rodrigues** var. Rodriquez. island E Mauritius
Rodriquez see Rodrigues
Rodunma see Roanne
180 I7 **Roebourne** Western Australia
83 J20 **Roedtan** Northern, NE South Africa
98 H11 **Roelofarendsveen** Zuid-Holland, W Netherlands
Roepat see Rupat, Pulau
Roer see Rur
99 M16 **Roermond** Limburg, SE Netherlands
99 C18 **Roeselare** Fr. Roulers; prev. Rousselaere. West-Vlaanderen, W Belgium
9 P8 **Roes Welcome Sound** strait Nunavut, N Canada
Roeteng see Ruteng
Rofreit see Rovereto
Rogachëv see Rahachow
57 L15 **Rogagua, Laguna** ◎ NW Bolivia
95 C16 **Rogaland** ◆ county S Norway
25 Y9 **Roganville** Texas, SW USA
109 W11 **Rogaška Slatina** Ger. Rohitsch-Sauerbrunn; prev. Rogatec-Slatina. E Slovenia
Rogatec-Slatina see Rogaška Slatina
112 J13 **Rogatica** Republica Srpska, SE Bosnia & Herzegovina
Rogatin see Rohatyn
93 F17 **Rogen** ◎ C Sweden
27 S9 **Rogers** Arkansas, C USA
29 P5 **Rogers** North Dakota, N USA
25 T9 **Rogers** Texas, SW USA
31 R5 **Rogers City** Michigan, N USA
Roger Simpson Island see Abemama
35 T14 **Rogers Lake** salt flat California, W USA
21 Q8 **Rogers, Mount** ▲ Virginia, NE USA
33 O16 **Rogerson** Idaho, NW USA
11 O16 **Rogers Pass** pass British Columbia, SW Canada
21 O8 **Rogersville** Tennessee, S USA
99 L16 **Roggel** Limburg, SE Netherlands
Roggeveen see Roggewein, Cabo
193 R10 **Roggeveen Basin** undersea feature E Pacific Ocean
191 X16 **Roggewein, Cabo** var. Roggeveen. headland Easter Island, Chile, E Pacific Ocean
103 Y13 **Rogliano** Corse, France, C Mediterranean Sea
107 N21 **Rogliano** Calabria, SW Italy
92 G12 **Rognan** Nordland, C Norway
100 K10 **Rögnitz** ≈ N Germany
Rogozhina/Rogozhinë see Rrogozhinë
110 G10 **Rogoźno** Wielkopolskie, C Poland
32 E15 **Rogue River** ≈ Oregon, NW USA
116 I6 **Rohatyn** Rus. Rogatin. Ivano-Frankivs'ka Oblast', W Ukraine
189 O14 **Rohi** Pohnpei, E Micronesia
Rohitsch-Sauerbrunn see Rogaška Slatina
149 Q13 **Rohri** Sind, SE Pakistan
152 I10 **Rohtak** Haryāna, N India
167 R9 **Roi Et** var. Muang Roi Et, Roi Ed. Roi Et, E Thailand
191 U9 **Roi Georges, Îles du** island group Îles Tuamotu, C French Polynesia
153 Y10 **Roing** Arunāchal Pradesh, NE India
118 E7 **Roja** Talsi, NW Latvia
61 B20 **Rojas** Buenos Aires, E Argentina
149 R12 **Rojhān** Punjab, E Pakistan
41 Q12 **Rojo, Cabo** headland C Mexico
45 Q10 **Rojo, Cabo** headland W Puerto Rico
168 K10 **Rokan Kiri, Sungai** ≈ Sumatera, W Indonesia
Rokha see Rokhah
149 R4 **Rokhah** var. Rokha. Kāpīsā, E Afghanistan
118 I11 **Rokiškis** Rokiškis, NE Lithuania
165 R7 **Rokkasho** Aomori, Honshū, C Japan
111 B17 **Rokycany** Ger. Rokytzan. Plzeňský Kraj, NW Czech Republic
117 P6 **Rokytne** Kyyivs'ka Oblast', N Ukraine
116 L3 **Rokytne** Rivnens'ka Oblast', NW Ukraine
Rokytzan see Rokycany
158 L11 **Rola Co** ◎ W China
29 V13 **Roland** Iowa, C USA
95 D15 **Røldal** Hordaland, S Norway
98 O7 **Rolde** Drenthe, NE Netherlands
29 O2 **Rolette** North Dakota, N USA
27 V6 **Rolla** Missouri, C USA
29 O2 **Rolla** North Dakota, N USA
108 A10 **Rolle** Vaud, W Switzerland
181 X8 **Rolleston** Queensland, E Australia
185 H19 **Rolleston** Canterbury, South Island, NZ
185 G18 **Rolleston Range** ▲ South Island, NZ
14 H8 **Rollet** Quebec, SE Canada
22 J4 **Rolling Fork** Mississippi, S USA
20 L6 **Rolling Fork** ≈ Kentucky, S USA
14 J11 **Rolphton** Ontario, SE Canada
Röm see Rømø
181 X10 **Roma** Queensland, E Australia
107 I15 **Roma** Eng. Rome. ● (Italy) Lazio, C Italy
95 P19 **Roma** Gotland, SE Sweden
21 T14 **Romain, Cape** headland South Carolina, SE USA
13 P11 **Romaine** ≈ Newfoundland/Quebec, E Canada
25 R17 **Roma Los Saenz** Texas, SW USA
114 H8 **Roman** Vratsa, NW Bulgaria
116 L10 **Roman** Hung. Románvásár. Neamţ, NE Romania
64 M13 **Romanche Fracture Zone** tectonic feature E Atlantic Ocean
61 C15 **Romang** Santa Fe, C Argentina
171 R15 **Romang, Pulau** var. Pulau Roma. island Kepulauan Damar, E Indonesia
171 R15 **Romang, Selat** strait Nusa Tenggara, S Indonesia
116 J11 **Romania** Bul. Rumŭniya, Ger. Rumänien, Hung. Románia, Rom. România, SCr. Rumunjska, Ukr. Rumuniya; prev. Republica Socialistă România, Roumania, Rumania, Socialist Republic of Romania, Rom. Romînia. ◆ republic SE Europe
117 T14 **Roman-Kash** ▲ S Ukraine
23 W16 **Romano, Cape** headland Florida, SE USA
44 G5 **Romano, Cayo** island C Cuba
123 O13 **Romanovka** Respublika Buryatiya, S Russian Federation
129 N8 **Romanovka** Saratovskaya Oblast', W Russian Federation
108 I6 **Romanshorn** Thurgau, NE Switzerland
103 R12 **Romans-sur-Isère** Drôme, E France
189 U12 **Romanum** island Chuuk, C Micronesia
Románvásár see Roman
39 S5 **Romanzof Mountains** ▲ Alaska, USA
Roma, Pulau see Romang, Pulau
103 S4 **Rombas** Moselle, NE France
23 R2 **Rome** Georgia, SE USA
18 I9 **Rome** New York, NE USA
Rome see Roma
31 S9 **Romeo** Michigan, N USA
Römerstadt see Rýmařov
Rometan see Romitan
103 P5 **Romilly-sur-Seine** Aube, N France
Romînia see Romania
146 L11 **Romitan** Rus. Rometan. Bukhoro Wiloyati, C Uzbekistan
21 U3 **Romney** West Virginia, NE USA
117 S4 **Romny** Sums'ka Oblast', NE Ukraine
95 E24 **Rømø** Ger. Röm. island SW Denmark
117 S5 **Romodan** Poltavs'ka Oblast', NE Ukraine
129 P5 **Romodanovo** Respublika Mordoviya, W Russian Federation
Romorantin see Romorantin-Lanthenay
103 N8 **Romorantin-Lanthenay** var. Romorantin. Loir-et-Cher, C France
94 F9 **Romsdal** physical region S Norway
94 F10 **Romsdalen** valley S Norway
94 E9 **Romsdalsfjorden** fjord S Norway
33 P8 **Ronan** Montana, NW USA
59 M14 **Roncador** Maranhão, E Brazil
186 M7 **Roncador Reef** reef N Solomon Islands
59 J17 **Roncador, Serra do** ▲ C Brazil
21 S6 **Ronceverte** West Virginia, NE USA
107 H14 **Ronciglione** Lazio, C Italy
104 L15 **Ronda** Andalucía, S Spain
94 G11 **Rondane** ▲ S Norway
104 L15 **Ronda, Serranía de** ▲ S Spain
95 H22 **Rønde** Århus, C Denmark
Rōndik see Rongrik Atoll
59 E16 **Rondônia** off. Estado de Rondônia; prev. Território de Rondônia. ◆ state W Brazil
59 I18 **Rondonópolis** Mato Grosso, W Brazil
94 G11 **Rondslottet** ▲ S Norway
95 P20 **Ronehamn** Gotland, SE Sweden
160 L13 **Rong'an** var. Chang'an, Rongan. Guangxi Zhuangzu Zizhiqu, S China
189 R4 **Rongelap Atoll** var. Rōnļap. atoll Ralik Chain, NW Marshall Islands
Rongerik see Rongrik Atoll
160 L13 **Rong Jiang** ≈ S China
160 K12 **Rongjiang** prev. Guzhou. Guizhou, S China
Rong, Kas see Rŭng, Kaôh
167 P8 **Rong Kwang** Phrae, NW Thailand
189 T4 **Rongrik Atoll** var. Rōndik, Rongerik. atoll Ralik Chain, N Marshall Islands
189 X2 **Rongrong** island SE Marshall Islands
160 L13 **Rongshui** var. Rongshui Miaozu Zizhixian. Guangxi Zhuangzu Zizhiqu, S China
Rongshui Miaozu Zizhixian see Rongshui
118 I6 **Rõngu** Ger. Ringen. Tartumaa, SE Estonia
160 L15 **Rongxian** var. Rong Xian. Guangxi Zhuangzu Zizhiqu, S China
Roniu see Ronui, Mont
189 N13 **Ronkiti** Pohnpei, E Micronesia
Rōnļap see Rongelap Atoll
95 L24 **Rønne** Bornholm, E Denmark
95 M22 **Ronneby** Blekinge, S Sweden
194 J7 **Ronne Entrance** inlet Antarctica
194 L6 **Ronne Ice Shelf** ice shelf Antarctica
99 E19 **Ronse** Fr. Renaix. Oost-Vlaanderen, SW Belgium
191 R8 **Ronui, Mont** var. Roniu. ✱ Tahiti, W French Polynesia
30 K14 **Roodhouse** Illinois, N USA
83 C19 **Rooibank** Erongo, W Namibia
65 N24 **Rookery Point** headland NE Tristan da Cunha
171 V13 **Roon, Pulau** island E Indonesia
173 V7 **Roo Rise** undersea feature E Indian Ocean
152 J9 **Roorkee** Uttar Pradesh, N India
99 H15 **Roosendaal** Noord-Brabant, S Netherlands
25 P10 **Roosevelt** Texas, SW USA
37 N3 **Roosevelt** Utah, W USA
47 T8 **Roosevelt** ≈ W Brazil
195 O13 **Roosevelt Island** island Antarctica
10 L10 **Roosevelt, Mount** ▲ British Columbia, W Canada
11 P17 **Roosville** British Columbia, SW Canada
29 X10 **Root River** ≈ Minnesota, N USA
111 N16 **Ropczyce** Podkarpackie, SE Poland
181 Q3 **Roper Bar** Northern Territory, N Australia
24 M5 **Ropesville** Texas, SW USA
102 K14 **Roquefort** Landes, SW France
61 C21 **Roque Pérez** Buenos Aires, E Argentina
58 E10 **Roraima** off. Estado de Roraima; prev. Território de Rio Branco, Território de Roraima. ◆ state N Brazil
58 F9 **Roraima, Mount** ▲ N South America
Ro Ro Reef see Malolo Barrier Reef
94 I9 **Røros** Sør-Trøndelag, S Norway
108 I7 **Rorschach** Sankt Gallen, NE Switzerland
93 E14 **Rørvik** Nord-Trøndelag, C Norway
119 G17 **Ros'** Rus. Ross'. Hrodzyenskaya Voblasts', W Belarus
119 G17 **Ros'** Rus. Ross'. ≈ W Belarus
117 O6 **Ros'** ≈ N Ukraine
44 K7 **Rosa, Lake** ◎ Great Inagua, S Bahamas
32 M9 **Rosalia** Washington, NW USA
191 W15 **Rosalia, Punta** headland Easter Island, Chile, E Pacific Ocean
45 P12 **Rosalie** E Dominica
35 T14 **Rosamond** California, W USA
35 S14 **Rosamond Lake** salt flat California, W USA
61 B18 **Rosario** Santa Fe, C Argentina
40 J11 **Rosario** Sinaloa, C Mexico
40 G6 **Rosario** Sonora, NW Mexico
62 O6 **Rosario** San Pedro, C Paraguay
61 E20 **Rosario** Colonia, SW Uruguay
54 H5 **Rosario** Zulia, NW Venezuela
Rosario see Rosarito
40 B4 **Rosario, Bahía del** bay NW Mexico
62 K6 **Rosario de la Frontera** Salta, N Argentina
61 C18 **Rosario del Tala** Entre Ríos, E Argentina
61 F16 **Rosário do Sul** Rio Grande do Sul, S Brazil
59 H18 **Rosário Oeste** Mato Grosso, W Brazil
40 E7 **Rosarito** Baja California, NW Mexico
40 B1 **Rosarito** var. Rosario. Baja California, NW Mexico
40 E7 **Rosarito** Baja California Sur, W Mexico
104 L9 **Rosarito, Embalse del** ⊠ W Spain
107 N22 **Rosarno** Calabria, SW Italy
56 B5 **Rosa Zárate** var. Quinindé. Esmeraldas, SW Ecuador
Roscianum see Rossano
29 O8 **Roscoe** South Dakota, N USA
25 P7 **Roscoe** Texas, SW USA
102 F5 **Roscoff** Finistère, NW France
Ros Comáin see Roscommon
97 C17 **Roscommon** Ir. Ros Comáin. C Ireland
31 Q7 **Roscommon** Michigan, N USA
97 C17 **Roscommon** Ir. Ros Comáin. cultural region C Ireland
Ros. Cré see Roscrea
97 D19 **Roscrea** Ir. Ros. Cré. C Ireland
45 X12 **Roseau** prev. Charlotte Town. ● (Dominica) SW Dominica
29 S2 **Roseau** Minnesota, N USA
173 Y16 **Rose Belle** SE Mauritius
183 O16 **Rosebery** Tasmania, SE Australia
21 U11 **Roseboro** North Carolina, SE USA
25 T9 **Rosebud** Texas, SW USA
33 W10 **Rosebud Creek** ≈ Montana, NW USA
32 F14 **Roseburg** Oregon, NW USA
22 J3 **Rosedale** Mississippi, S USA
99 H21 **Rosée** Namur, S Belgium
55 U8 **Rose Hall** E Guyana
173 X16 **Rose Hill** W Mauritius
80 H12 **Roseires, Reservoir** var. Lake Rusayris. ⊠ E Sudan
Rosenau see Rožnov pod Radhoštěm, Czech Republic
Rosenau see Rožňava, Slovakia
25 V11 **Rosenberg** Texas, SW USA
Rosenberg see Olesno, Poland
Rosenberg see Ružomberok, Slovakia
100 I10 **Rosengarten** Niedersachsen, N Germany
101 M24 **Rosenheim** Bayern, S Germany
Rosenhof see Zilupe
105 X4 **Roses** Cataluña, NE Spain
105 X4 **Roses, Golf de** gulf NE Spain
107 K14 **Roseto degli Abruzzi** Abruzzo, C Italy
11 S16 **Rosetown** Saskatchewan, S Canada
Rosetta see Rashīd
35 O7 **Roseville** California, W USA
30 J12 **Roseville** Illinois, N USA
29 V8 **Roseville** Minnesota, N USA
29 R7 **Rosholt** South Dakota, N USA
106 F12 **Rosignano Marittimo** Toscana, C Italy
116 J14 **Roşiori de Vede** Teleorman, S Romania
114 K8 **Rositsa** ≈ N Bulgaria
Rositten see Rēzekne
95 J23 **Roskilde** Roskilde, E Denmark
95 I23 **Roskilde** off. Roskilde Amt. ◆ county E Denmark
Ros Láir see Rosslare
128 H5 **Roslavl'** Smolenskaya Oblast', W Russian Federation
32 I8 **Roslyn** Washington, NW USA
99 K14 **Rosmalen** Noord-Brabant, S Netherlands
Ros Mhic Thriúin see New Ross
113 P19 **Rosoman** C FYR Macedonia
102 F6 **Rosporden** Finistère, NW France
185 F17 **Ross** West Coast, South Island, NZ
10 J7 **Ross** ≈ Yukon Territory, W Canada
Ross' see Ros'
96 H8 **Ross and Cromarty** cultural region N Scotland, UK
107 O20 **Rossano** anc. Roscianum. Calabria, SW Italy
22 L5 **Ross Barnett Reservoir** ⊠ Mississippi, S USA
11 W16 **Rossburn** Manitoba, S Canada
14 H13 **Rosseau** Ontario, S Canada
14 H13 **Rosseau, Lake** ◎ Ontario, S Canada
186 I10 **Rossel Island** prev. Yela Island. island SE PNG
195 P12 **Ross Ice Shelf** ice shelf Antarctica
13 P16 **Rossignol, Lake** ◎ Nova Scotia, SE Canada
83 C19 **Rössing** Erongo, W Namibia
195 Q14 **Ross Island** island Antarctica
Rossitten see Rybachiy
Rossiyskaya Federatsiya see Russian Federation
11 N17 **Rossland** British Columbia, SW Canada
97 F20 **Rosslare** Ir. Ros Láir. SE Ireland
97 F20 **Rosslare Harbour** Wexford, SE Ireland
101 M14 **Rosslau** Sachsen-Anhalt, E Germany
76 G10 **Rosso** Trarza, SW Mauritania
103 X14 **Rosso, Cap** headland Corse, France, C Mediterranean Sea
93 H16 **Rosson** Jämtland, C Sweden
97 K21 **Ross-on-Wye** W England, UK
Rossony see Rasony
128 L9 **Rossosh'** Voronezhskaya Oblast', W Russian Federation
181 Q7 **Ross River** Northern Territory, N Australia
10 J7 **Ross River** Yukon Territory, W Canada
205 O15 **Ross Sea** sea Antarctica
92 G13 **Røssvatnet** ◎ C Norway
23 R1 **Rossville** Georgia, SE USA
Rostak see Ar Rustāq
143 P14 **Rostāq** Hormozgān, S Iran
117 N5 **Rostavytsya** ≈ N Ukraine
11 T15 **Rosthern** Saskatchewan, S Canada
100 M8 **Rostock** Mecklenburg-Vorpommern, NE Germany
126 L16 **Rostov** Yaroslavskaya Oblast', W Russian Federation
Rostov see Rostov-na-Donu
128 L12 **Rostov-na-Donu** var. Rostov, Eng. Rostov-on-Don. Rostovskaya Oblast', SW Russian Federation
Rostov-on-Don see Rostov-na-Donu
128 L10 **Rostovskaya Oblast'** ◆ province SW Russian Federation
93 J14 **Rosvik** Norrbotten, N Sweden
23 S3 **Roswell** Georgia, SE USA
37 U14 **Roswell** New Mexico, SW USA
94 K12 **Rot** Dalarna, C Sweden
101 I23 **Rot** ≈ S Germany
104 J15 **Rota** Andalucía, S Spain
188 K9 **Rota** island S Northern Mariana Islands
25 P6 **Rotan** Texas, SW USA
Rotcher Island see Tamana
100 I11 **Rotenburg** Niedersachsen, NW Germany
Rotenburg see Rotenburg an der Fulda
101 I16 **Rotenburg an der Fulda** var. Rotenburg. Thüringen, C Germany
101 L18 **Roter Main** ≈ E Germany
101 K20 **Roth** Bayern, SE Germany
101 G16 **Rothaargebirge** ▲ W Germany
Rothenburg see Rothenburg ob der Tauber
101 J20 **Rothenburg ob der Tauber** var. Rothenburg. Bayern, S Germany
194 H6 **Rothera** UK research station Antarctica
185 I17 **Rotherham** Canterbury, South Island, NZ
97 M17 **Rotherham** N England, UK
96 H12 **Rothesay** W Scotland, UK
108 E7 **Rothrist** Aargau, N Switzerland
194 H6 **Rothschild Island** island Antarctica
171 P17 **Roti, Pulau** island S Indonesia
183 O8 **Roto** New South Wales, SE Australia
184 N8 **Rotoiti, Lake** ◎ North Island, NZ
Rotomagus see Rouen
107 N19 **Rotondella** Basilicata, S Italy
103 X15 **Rotondo, Monte** ▲ Corse, France, C Mediterranean Sea
185 I15 **Rotoroa, Lake** ◎ South Island, NZ
184 N8 **Rotorua** Bay of Plenty, North Island, NZ
184 N8 **Rotorua, Lake** ◎ North Island, NZ
101 N22 **Rott** ≈ SE Germany
108 F10 **Rotten** ≈ S Switzerland
109 T6 **Rottenmann** Steiermark, E Austria
98 H12 **Rotterdam** Zuid-Holland, SW Netherlands
18 K10 **Rotterdam** New York, NE USA
95 M21 **Rottnen** ◎ S Sweden
98 N4 **Rottumeroog** island Waddeneilanden, NE Netherlands
98 N4 **Rottumerplaat** island Waddeneilanden, NE Netherlands
101 G23 **Rottweil** Baden-Württemberg, S Germany
191 O7 **Rotui, Mont** ✱ Moorea, W French Polynesia
103 P1 **Roubaix** Nord, N France
111 C15 **Roudnice nad Labem** Ger. Raudnitz an der Elbe. Ústecký Kraj, NW Czech Republic
102 M4 **Rouen** anc. Rotomagus. Seine-Maritime, N France
171 X13 **Rouffaer Reserves** reserve Irian Jaya, E Indonesia
15 N10 **Rouge, Rivière** ≈ Quebec, SE Canada
20 J6 **Rough River** ≈ Kentucky, S USA
20 J6 **Rough River Lake** ⊠ Kentucky, S USA
Rouhaïbé see Ar Ruḥaybah
102 K11 **Rouillac** Charente, W France
Roulers see Roeselare
Roumania see Romania
173 Y15 **Round Island** var. Île Ronde. island NE Mauritius
14 J12 **Round Lake** ◎ Ontario, SE Canada
35 U7 **Round Mountain** Nevada, W USA
25 R10 **Round Mountain** Texas, SW USA
183 U5 **Round Mountain** ▲ New South Wales, SE Australia
25 S10 **Round Rock** Texas, SW USA
33 U10 **Roundup** Montana, NW USA
55 Y10 **Roura** NE French Guiana
Rourkela see Rāulakela
96 J4 **Rousay** island N Scotland, UK
Rousselaere see Roeselare
103 O17 **Roussillon** cultural region S France
15 V7 **Routhierville** Quebec, SE Canada
99 K25 **Rouvroy** Luxembourg, SE Belgium
14 I7 **Rouyn-Noranda** Quebec, SE Canada
Rouyuanchengzi see Huachi
92 L12 **Rovaniemi** Lappi, N Finland
106 E7 **Rovato** Lombardia, N Italy
127 N11 **Rovdino** Arkhangel'skaya Oblast', NW Russian Federation
Roven'ki see Roven'ky
117 Y8 **Roven'ky** var. Roven'ki. Luhans'ka Oblast', E Ukraine
Rovenskaya Oblast' see Rivnens'ka Oblast'
Rovenskaya Sloboda see Rovyenskaya Slabada
106 G7 **Rovereto** Ger. Rofreit. Trentino-Alto Adige, N Italy
167 S12 **Rôviĕng Tbong** Preăh Vihéar, N Cambodia
Rovigno see Rovinj
106 H8 **Rovigo** Veneto, NE Italy
112 A10 **Rovinj** It. Rovigno. Istra, NW Croatia
54 E10 **Rovira** Tolima, C Colombia
Rovno see Rivne
129 P9 **Rovnoye** Saratovskaya Oblast', W Russian Federation
82 Q12 **Rovuma, Rio** var. Ruvuma. ≈ Mozambique/Tanzania see also Ruvuma
119 O19 **Rovyenskaya Slabada** Rus. Rovenskaya Sloboda. Homyel'skaya Voblasts', SE Belarus
183 R5 **Rowena** New South Wales, SE Australia
21 T11 **Rowland** North Carolina, SE USA
9 P5 **Rowley** ≈ Baffin Island, Nunavut, NE Canada
9 P6 **Rowley Island** island Nunavut, NE Canada
173 W8 **Rowley Shoals** reef NW Australia
171 O4 **Roxas** Mindoro, N Philippines
171 P5 **Roxas City** Panay Island, C Philippines
21 U8 **Roxboro** North Carolina, SE USA
185 D23 **Roxburgh** Otago, South Island, NZ
96 K13 **Roxburgh** cultural region SE Scotland, UK
182 H5 **Roxby Downs** South Australia
95 M17 **Roxen** ◎ S Sweden
25 V5 **Roxton** Texas, SW USA
15 P12 **Roxton-Sud** Quebec, SE Canada
33 U8 **Roy** Montana, NW USA
37 U10 **Roy** New Mexico, SW USA
97 E17 **Royal Canal** Ir. An Chanáil Ríoga. canal C Ireland
30 L1 **Royale, Isle** island Michigan, N USA
37 S6 **Royal Gorge** valley Colorado, C USA
97 M20 **Royal Leamington Spa** var. Leamington, Leamington Spa. C England, UK
97 O23 **Royal Tunbridge Wells** var. Tunbridge Wells. SE England, UK
24 L9 **Royalty** Texas, SW USA
102 J11 **Royan** Charente-Maritime, W France
65 B24 **Roy Cove Settlement** West Falkland, Falkland Islands
103 O3 **Roye** Somme, N France
95 H15 **Røyken** Buskerud, S Norway
93 F14 **Røyrvik** Nord-Trøndelag, C Norway
25 U6 **Royse City** Texas, SW USA
97 O21 **Royston** E England, UK
23 U2 **Royston** Georgia, SE USA
114 L10 **Roza** prev. Gyulovo. Yambol, E Bulgaria
113 L16 **Rožaje** Montenegro, SW Yugoslavia
110 M10 **Różan** Mazowieckie, C Poland
117 O10 **Rozdil'na** Odes'ka Oblast', SW Ukraine
117 S12 **Rozdol'ne** Rus. Razdolnoye. Respublika Krym, S Ukraine
145 Q9 **Rozhdestvenka** Akmola, C Kazakhstan
116 I6 **Rozhnyativ** Ivano-Frankivs'ka Oblast', W Ukraine
116 J3 **Rozhyshche** Volyns'ka Oblast', NW Ukraine
Roznau am Radhost see Rožnov pod Radhoštěm
111 L19 **Rožňava** Ger. Rosenau, Hung. Rozsnyó. Košický Kraj, E Slovakia
116 K10 **Roznov** Neamţ, NE Romania
111 I18 **Rožnov pod Radhoštěm** Ger. Rosenau, Roznau am Radhost. Zlínský Kraj, E Czech Republic
Rózsahegy see Ružomberok
Rozsnyó see Râşnov, Romania
Rozsnyó see Rožňava, Slovakia
113 K18 **Rranxë** Shkodër, NW Albania
113 L18 **Rrëshen** var. Rresheni, Rrshen. Lezhë, C Albania
Rresheni see Rrëshen
Rrogozhina see Rrogozhinë
113 K20 **Rrogozhinë** var. Rogozhina, Rogozhinë, Rrogozhina. Tiranë, W Albania
Rrshen see Rrëshen
112 O13 **Rtanj** ▲ E Yugoslavia
129 O7 **Rtishchevo** Saratovskaya Oblast', W Russian Federation
184 N12 **Ruahine Range** var. Ruarine. ▲ North Island, NZ
185 L14 **Ruamahanga** ≈ North Island, NZ
Ruanda see Rwanda
184 M10 **Ruapehu, Mount** ▲ North Island, NZ
185 C25 **Ruapuke Island** island SW NZ
Ruarine see Ruahine Range
184 O9 **Ruatahuna** Bay of Plenty, North Island, NZ
184 Q8 **Ruatoria** Gisborne, North Island, NZ
184 K4 **Ruawai** Northland, North Island, NZ
15 N8 **Ruban** ≈ Quebec, SE Canada
81 I22 **Rubeho Mountains** ▲ C Tanzania
165 U3 **Rubeshibe** Hokkaidō, NE Japan
Rubezhnoye see Rubizhne
113 L18 **Rubik** Lezhë, C Albania
54 H7 **Rubio** Táchira, W Venezuela
117 X6 **Rubizhne** Rus. Rubezhnoye. Luhans'ka Oblast', E Ukraine
81 F20 **Rubondo Island** island N Tanzania
122 I13 **Rubtsovsk** Altayskiy Kray, S Russian Federation
39 P9 **Ruby** Alaska, USA
35 W3 **Ruby Dome** ▲ Nevada, W USA
35 W4 **Ruby Lake** ◎ Nevada, W USA
35 W4 **Ruby Mountains** ▲ Nevada, W USA
33 Q12 **Ruby Range** ▲ Montana, NW USA

◆ Country ● Country Capital ◇ Dependent Territory ○ Dependent Territory Capital ◆ Administrative Region ✕ International Airport ▲ Mountain ▲ Mountain Range ✱ Volcano ≈ River ◎ Lake ⊠ Reservoir

118 C10 **Rucava** Liepāja, SW Latvia
Rūdān see Dehbārez
Rudelstadt see Ciechanowiec
Rudensk see Rudzyensk
119 G14 **Rūdiškės** Trakai, S Lithuania
95 H24 **Rudkøbing** Fyn, C Denmark
145 V14 **Rudnichnyy** Kaz. Rūdnīchnyy. Almaty, SE Kazakhstan
127 S13 **Rudnichnyy** Kirovskaya Oblast', NW Russian Federation
114 N9 **Rudnik** Varna, E Bulgaria
Rudny see Rudnyy
128 H4 **Rudnya** Smolenskaya Oblast', W Russian Federation
129 O8 **Rudnya** Volgogradskaya Oblast', SW Russian Federation
144 M7 **Rudnyy** var. Rudny. Kostanay, N Kazakhstan
122 K3 **Rudol'fa, Ostrov** island Zemlya Frantsa-Iosifa, NW Russian Federation
81 H16 **Rudolf, Lake** var. Lake Turkana. ◎ N Kenya
Rudolfswert see Novo mesto
101 L17 **Rudolstadt** Thüringen, C Germany
31 Q4 **Rudyard** Michigan, N USA
33 S7 **Rudyard** Montana, NW USA
119 K16 **Rudzyensk** Rus. Rudensk. Minskaya Voblasts', C Belarus
104 L6 **Rueda** Castilla-León, N Spain
114 F10 **Ruen** ▲ Bulgaria/FYR Macedonia
80 G10 **Rufa'a** Gezira, C Sudan
102 L10 **Ruffec** Charente, W France
21 R14 **Ruffin** South Carolina, SE USA
81 J23 **Rufiji** ≈ E Tanzania
61 A20 **Rufino** Santa Fe, C Argentina
76 F11 **Rufisque** W Senegal
83 K14 **Rufunsa** Lusaka, C Zambia
118 J9 **Rugāji** Balvi, E Latvia
161 R7 **Rugao** Jiangsu, E China
97 M20 **Rugby** C England, UK
29 N3 **Rugby** North Dakota, N USA
100 N7 **Rügen** headland NE Germany
Ruhaybeh see Ar Ruḩaybah
161 N7 **Ru He** ≈ C China
81 E19 **Ruhengeri** NW Rwanda
Ruhja see Rūjiena
100 M10 **Ruhner Berg** hill N Germany
118 F7 **Ruhnu** var. Ruhnu Saar, Swe. Runö. island SW Estonia
Ruhnu Saar see Ruhnu
101 G15 **Ruhr** ≈ W Germany
91 W6 **Ruhr Valley** industrial region W Germany
161 S11 **Rui'an** var. Rui an. Zhejiang, SE China
161 P10 **Ruichang** Jiangxi, S China
24 J11 **Ruidosa** Texas, SW USA
37 S14 **Ruidoso** New Mexico, SW USA
161 P12 **Ruijin** Jiangxi, S China
160 D13 **Ruili** Yunnan, SW China
98 N8 **Ruinen** Drenthe, NE Netherlands
99 D17 **Ruiselede** West-Vlaanderen, W Belgium
64 P5 **Ruivo de Santana, Pico** ▲ Madeira, Portugal, NE Atlantic Ocean
40 J12 **Ruiz** Nayarit, SW Mexico
54 E10 **Ruiz, Nevado del** ☼ W Colombia
138 J9 **Rujaylah, Ḩarrat ar** salt lake N Jordan
Rujen see Rūjiena
118 H7 **Rūjiena** Est. Ruhja, Ger. Rujen. Valmiera, N Latvia
79 I18 **Ruki** ≈ W Dem. Rep. Congo (Zaire)
81 E22 **Rukwa** ◈ region SW Tanzania
81 F23 **Rukwa, Lake** ◎ SE Tanzania
25 P6 **Rule** Texas, SW USA
22 K3 **Ruleville** Mississippi, S USA
Rum see Rhum
112 K10 **Ruma** Serbia, N Yugoslavia
Rumadiya see Ar Ramādī
141 Q7 **Rumāḩ** Ar Riyāḑ, C Saudi Arabia
Rumaitha see Ar Rumaythah
Rumania/Rumänien see Romania
Rumänisch-Sankt-Georgen see Sângeorz-Băi
139 Y13 **Rumaylah** SE Iraq
139 P2 **Rumaylah, Wādī** dry watercourse NE Syria
171 U13 **Rumbati** Irian Jaya, E Indonesia
81 E14 **Rumbek** El Buhayrat, S Sudan
Rumburg see Rumburk
111 D14 **Rumburk** Ger. Rumburg. Ústecký Kraj, NW Czech Republic
44 J4 **Rum Cay** island C Bahamas
99 M26 **Rumelange** Luxembourg, S Luxembourg
99 D20 **Rumes** Hainaut, SW Belgium
19 P7 **Rumford** Maine, NE USA
110 I6 **Rumia** Pomorskie, N Poland
113 J17 **Rumija** ▲▲ SW Yugoslavia
103 T11 **Rumilly** Haute-Savoie, E France
139 O6 **Rūmiyah** W Iraq
Rummah, Wādī ar see Rimah, Wādī ar
Rummelsburg in Pommern see Miastko
165 S3 **Rumoi** Hokkaidō, NE Japan
82 M12 **Rumphi** var. Rumpi. Northern, N Malawi
Rumpi see Rumphi
29 V7 **Rum River** ≈ Minnesota, N USA
188 F16 **Rumung** island Caroline Islands, W Micronesia
Rumuniya/Rumŭniya/Rumunjska see Romania
185 G16 **Runanga** West Coast, South Island, NZ
184 P7 **Runaway, Cape** headland North Island, NZ
97 K18 **Runcorn** C England, UK
118 K10 **Rundāni** Ludza, E Latvia
83 L18 **Runde** var. Lundi. ≈ SE Zimbabwe
83 E16 **Rundu** var. Runtu. Okavango, NE Namibia
93 I16 **Rundvik** Västerbotten, N Sweden
81 G20 **Runere** Mwanza, N Tanzania
25 S13 **Runge** Texas, SW USA
167 Q13 **Rŭng, Kaôh** prev. Kas Rong. island SW Cambodia
79 O16 **Rungu** Orientale, NE Dem. Rep. Congo (Zaire)
81 F23 **Rungwa** Rukwa, W Tanzania
81 G22 **Rungwa** Singida, C Tanzania
94 M13 **Runn** ◎ C Sweden
24 M4 **Running Water Draw** valley New Mexico/Texas, SW USA
Runö see Ruhnu
Runtu see Rundu
189 V12 **Ruo** island Caroline Islands, C Micronesia
158 L9 **Ruoqiang** var. Jo-ch'iang, Uigh. Charkhlik, Charkhliq, Qarkilik. Xinjiang Uygur Zizhiqu, NW China
159 S7 **Ruo Shui** ≈ N China
92 L8 **Ruostefjelbma** var. Rustefjelbma Finnmark, N Norway
93 L18 **Ruovesi** Länsi-Suomi, W Finland
112 B9 **Rupa** Primorje-Gorski Kotar, NW Croatia
182 M11 **Rupanyup** Victoria, SE Australia
168 K9 **Rupat, Pulau** prev. Roepat. island W Indonesia
168 K10 **Rupat, Selat** strait Sumatera, W Indonesia
116 J11 **Rupea** Ger. Reps, Hung. Kőhalom; prev. Cohalm. Braşov, C Romania
99 G17 **Rupel** ≈ N Belgium
Rupella see la Rochelle
33 P15 **Rupert** Idaho, NW USA
21 R5 **Rupert** West Virginia, NE USA
Rupert House see Fort Rupert
12 J10 **Rupert, Rivière de** ≈ Quebec, C Canada
194 M13 **Ruppert Coast** physical region Antarctica
100 N11 **Ruppiner Kanal** canal NE Germany
55 S11 **Rupununi River** ≈ S Guyana
101 D16 **Rur** Dut. Roer. ≈ Germany/Netherlands
58 H13 **Rurópolis Presidente Medici** Pará, N Brazil
191 S12 **Rurutu** island Îles Australes, SW French Polynesia
Rusaddir see Melilla
83 L17 **Rusape** Manicaland, E Zimbabwe
Rusayris, Lake see Roseires, Reservoir
Ruschuk/Rusçuk see Ruse
114 K7 **Ruse** var. Ruschuk, Rustchuk, Turk. Rusçuk. Ruse, N Bulgaria
114 L7 **Ruse** ◈ province N Bulgaria
109 W10 **Ruše** NE Slovenia
114 K7 **Rusenski Lom** ≈ N Bulgaria
97 G17 **Rush** Ir. An Ros. E Ireland
161 S4 **Rushan** var. Xiacun. Shandong, E China
Rushan see Rŭshon
Rushanskiy Khrebet see Rushon, Qatorkŭhi
29 V7 **Rush City** Minnesota, N USA
37 V5 **Rush Creek** ≈ Colorado, C USA
29 X10 **Rushford** Minnesota, N USA
154 N13 **Rushikulya** ≈ E India
14 D8 **Rush Lake** ◎ Ontario, S Canada
30 M7 **Rush Lake** ◎ Wisconsin, N USA
28 J10 **Rushmore, Mount** ▲ South Dakota, N USA
147 S13 **Rŭshon** Rus. Rushan. S Tajikistan
147 S14 **Rushon, Qatorkŭhi** Rus. Rushanskiy Khrebet. ▲▲ SE Tajikistan
26 M12 **Rush Springs** Oklahoma, C USA
45 V15 **Rushville** Trinidad, Trinidad and Tobago
30 J13 **Rushville** Illinois, N USA
28 K12 **Rushville** Nebraska, C USA
183 O11 **Rushworth** Victoria, SE Australia
25 W8 **Rusk** Texas, SW USA
93 I14 **Rusksele** Västerbotten, N Sweden
118 C12 **Rusnė** Šilutė, W Lithuania
114 M10 **Rusokastrenska Reka** ≈ E Bulgaria
Russadir see Melilla
109 X3 **Russbach** ≈ NE Austria
11 V16 **Russell** Manitoba, S Canada
184 K2 **Russell** Northland, North Island, NZ
26 L4 **Russell** Kansas, C USA
21 O4 **Russell** Kentucky, S USA
20 L7 **Russell Springs** Kentucky, S USA
23 O2 **Russellville** Alabama, S USA
27 T11 **Russellville** Arkansas, C USA
20 J7 **Russellville** Kentucky, S USA
101 G18 **Rüsselsheim** Hessen, W Germany
92 K8 **Russenes** Finnmark, N Norway
Russia see Russian Federation
Russian America see Alaska
122 J11 **Russian Federation** off. Russian Federation, var. Russia, Latv. Krievija, Rus. Rossiyskaya Federatsiya. ◆ republic Asia/Europe
39 N11 **Russian Mission** Alaska, USA
34 M7 **Russian River** ≈ California, W USA
194 L13 **Russkaya** Russian research station Antarctica
122 J5 **Russkaya Gavan'** Novaya Zemlya, Arkhangel'skaya Oblast', N Russian Federation
122 J5 **Russkiy, Ostrov** island N Russian Federation
109 Y5 **Rust** Burgenland, E Austria
Rustaq see Ar Rustāq
137 U10 **Rust'avi** SE Georgia
21 T7 **Rustburg** Virginia, NE USA
Rustchuk see Ruse
Rustefjelbma see Ruostefjelbma
83 I21 **Rustenburg** North-West, N South Africa
22 H5 **Ruston** Louisiana, S USA
81 E21 **Rutana** SE Burundi
62 I4 **Rutana, Volcán** ▲ N Chile
Rutanzige, Lake see Edward, Lake
Rutba see Ar Ruţbah
104 M14 **Rute** Andalucía, S Spain
171 N16 **Ruteng** prev. Roeteng. Flores, C Indonesia
194 L8 **Rutford Ice Stream** ice feature Antarctica
35 X6 **Ruth** Nevada, W USA
101 G15 **Rüthen** Nordrhein-Westfalen, W Germany
14 D17 **Rutherford** Ontario, S Canada
21 Q10 **Rutherfordton** North Carolina, SE USA
97 J18 **Ruthin** Wel. Rhuthun. NE Wales, UK
108 G7 **Rüti** Zürich, N Switzerland
Rutlam see Ratlām
18 M9 **Rutland** Vermont, NE USA
97 N19 **Rutland** cultural region C England, UK
21 N8 **Rutledge** Tennessee, S USA
158 G12 **Rutog** var. Rutok. Xizang Zizhiqu, W China
Rutok see Rutog
79 P19 **Rutshuru** Nord Kivu, E Dem. Rep. Congo (Zaire)
98 L8 **Rutten** Flevoland, N Netherlands
129 Q17 **Rutul** Respublika Dagestan, SW Russian Federation
93 L14 **Ruukki** Oulu, C Finland
98 N11 **Ruurlo** Gelderland, E Netherlands
143 S15 **Ru'ūs al Jibāl** headland Oman/UAE
138 I7 **Ru'ūs aţ Ţiwāl, Jabal** ▲▲ W Syria
81 H23 **Ruvuma** ◈ region SE Tanzania
81 I25 **Ruvuma** var. Rio Rovuma. ≈ Mozambique/Tanzania see also Rovuma, Rio
Ruwais see Ar Ruways
138 L9 **Ruwayshid, Wadi ar** dry watercourse NE Jordan
141 Z10 **Ruways, Ra's ar** headland E Oman
79 P18 **Ruwenzori** ▲▲ Uganda/Dem. Rep. Congo (Zaire)
141 Y8 **Ruwī** NE Oman
114 F9 **Ruy** ▲ Bulgaria/Yugoslavia
Ruya see Luia, Rio
81 E20 **Ruyigi** E Burundi
129 P5 **Ruzayevka** Respublika Mordoviya, W Russian Federation
119 G18 **Ruzhany** Rus. Ruzhany. Brestskaya Voblasts', SW Belarus
114 I10 **Rŭzhevo Konare** var. Rŭzhevo Konare. Plovdiv, C Bulgaria
Ruzhin see Ruzhyn
114 G7 **Ruzhintsi** Vidin, NW Bulgaria
117 N5 **Ruzhyn** Rus. Ruzhin. Zhytomyrs'ka Oblast', N Ukraine
111 K19 **Ružomberok** Ger. Rosenberg, Hung. Rózsahegy. Žilinský Kraj, N Slovakia
111 C16 **Ruzyně** ✕ (Praha) Praha, C Czech Republic
81 D19 **Rwanda** off. Rwandese Republic; prev. Ruanda. ◆ republic C Africa
Rwandese Republic see Rwanda
95 G22 **Ry** Århus, C Denmark
Ryasna see Rasna
128 L5 **Ryazan'** Ryazanskaya Oblast', W Russian Federation
128 L5 **Ryazanskaya Oblast'** ◈ province W Russian Federation
128 M6 **Ryazhsk** Ryazanskaya Oblast', W Russian Federation
118 B13 **Rybachiy** Ger. Rossitten. Kaliningradskaya Oblast', W Russian Federation
126 J2 **Rybachiy, Poluostrov** peninsula NW Russian Federation
Rybach'ye see Balykchy
126 L15 **Rybinsk** prev. Andropov. Yaroslavskaya Oblast', W Russian Federation
126 K14 **Rybinskoye Vodokhranilishche** Eng. Rybinsk Reservoir, Rybinsk Sea. ⊞ W Russian Federation
Rybinsk Reservoir/Rybinsk Sea see Rybinskoye Vodokhranilishche
111 I16 **Rybnik** Śląskie, S Poland
Rybnitsa see Rîbniţa
111 F16 **Rychnov nad Kněžnou** Ger. Reichenau. Hradecký Kraj, N Czech Republic
110 I12 **Rychwał** Wielkolpolskie, C Poland
11 O13 **Rycroft** Alberta, W Canada
95 L21 **Ryd** Kronoberg, S Sweden
95 L20 **Rydaholm** Jönköping, S Sweden
194 I8 **Rydberg Peninsula** peninsula Antarctica
97 P23 **Rye** SE England, UK
33 T10 **Ryegate** Montana, NW USA
35 S3 **Rye Patch Reservoir** ⊞ Nevada, W USA
95 D15 **Ryfylke** physical region S Norway
95 H16 **Rygge** Østfold, S Norway
110 N13 **Ryki** Lubelskie, E Poland
Rykovo see Yenakiyeve
128 I7 **Ryl'sk** Kurskaya Oblast', W Russian Federation
183 S8 **Rylstone** New South Wales, SE Australia
111 H17 **Rýmařov** Ger. Römerstadt. Ostravský Kraj, E Czech Republic
144 E11 **Ryn-Peski** desert W Kazakhstan
165 N10 **Ryōtsu** var. Ryôtu. Niigata, Sado, C Japan
Ryôtu see Ryōtsu
110 K10 **Rypin** Kujawsko-pomorskie, C Poland
Ryshkany see Rîşcani
Ryssel see Lille
Ryswick see Rijswijk
95 M24 **Rytterknægten** hill E Denmark
192 G5 **Ryukyu Trench** var. Nansei Syotō Trench. undersea feature S East China Sea
110 D11 **Rzepin** Ger. Reppen. Lubuskie, W Poland
111 N16 **Rzeszów** Podkarpackie, SE Poland
126 I16 **Rzhev** Tverskaya Oblast', W Russian Federation
Rzhishchev see Rzhyshchiv
117 P5 **Rzhyshchiv** Rus. Rzhishchev. Kyyivs'ka Oblast', N Ukraine

S

138 E11 **Sa'ad** Southern, W Israel
109 P7 **Saalach** ≈ W Austria
101 L14 **Saale** ≈ C Germany
101 L17 **Saalfeld** var. Saalfeld an der Saale. Thüringen, C Germany
Saalfeld see Zalewo
Saalfeld an der Saale see Saalfeld
108 C8 **Saane** ≈ W Switzerland
101 D19 **Saar** Fr. Sarre. ≈ France/Germany
101 E20 **Saarbrücken** Fr. Sarrebruck. Saarland, SW Germany
Saarburg see Sarrebourg
Saare see Saaremaa
118 D6 **Sääre** var. Sjar. Saaremaa, W Estonia
118 D5 **Saaremaa** off. Saare Maakond. ◈ province W Estonia
118 E6 **Saaremaa** Ger. Oesel, Ösel; prev. Saare. island W Estonia
92 L12 **Saarenkylä** Lappi, N Finland
Saargemund see Sarreguemines
93 L17 **Saarijärvi** Länsi-Suomi, W Finland
Saar in Mähren see Žďár nad Sázavou
92 M10 **Saariselkä** Lapp. Suoločielgi. Lappi, N Finland
92 L10 **Saariselkä** hill range NE Finland
101 D20 **Saarland** Fr. Sarre. ◈ state SW Germany
Saarlautern see Saarlouis
101 D20 **Saarlouis** prev. Saarlautern. Saarland, SW Germany
108 E11 **Saaser Vispa** ≈ S Switzerland
137 X12 **Saatlı** Rus. Saatly. C Azerbaijan
Saatly see Saatlı
Saaz see Žatec
45 V9 **Saba** island N Netherlands Antilles
138 J7 **Sab' Ābār** var. Sab'a Biyar, Sa'b Bi'ār. Ḩimş, C Syria
Sab'a Biyar see Sab' Ābār
112 K11 **Šabac** Serbia, W Yugoslavia
105 W5 **Sabadell** Cataluña, E Spain
164 K12 **Sabae** Fukui, Honshū, SW Japan
169 V7 **Sabah** prev. British North Borneo, North Borneo. ◈ state East Malaysia
168 J8 **Sabak** var. Sabak Bernam. Selangor, Peninsular Malaysia
Sabak Bernam see Sabak
38 D16 **Sabak, Cape** headland Agattu Island, Alaska, USA
81 J20 **Sabaki** ≈ S Kenya
142 L2 **Sabalān, Kuhhā-ye** ▲ NW Iran
154 H7 **Sabalgarh** Madhya Pradesh, C India
44 E4 **Sabana, Archipiélago de** island group C Cuba
42 H7 **Sabanagrande** var. Sabana Grande. Francisco Morazán, S Honduras
54 E5 **Sabanalarga** Atlántico, N Colombia
41 W14 **Sabancuy** Campeche, SE Mexico
45 N8 **Sabaneta** NW Dominican Republic
54 J4 **Sabaneta** Falcón, N Venezuela
188 H4 **Sabaneta, Puntan** prev. Ushi Point. headland Saipan, S Northern Mariana Islands
171 X14 **Sabang** Irian Jaya, E Indonesia
116 L10 **Săbăoani** Neamţ, NE Romania
155 J26 **Sabaragamuwa Province** ◈ province C Sri Lanka
Sabaria see Szombathely
154 D10 **Sābarmati** ≈ NW India
171 S10 **Sabatai** Pulau Morotai, E Indonesia
141 Q15 **Sab'atayn, Ramlat as** desert C Yemen
107 I16 **Sabaudia** Lazio, C Italy
57 J19 **Sabaya** Oruro, S Bolivia
Sa'b Bi'ār see Sab' Ābār
Sabbioncello see Orebić
148 I8 **Şāberī, Hāmūn-e** var. Daryācheh-ye Hāmūn, Daryācheh-ye Sīstān. ◎ Afghanistan/Iran see also Sīstān, Daryācheh-ye
27 P2 **Sabetha** Kansas, C USA
75 P10 **Sabhā** C Libya
67 V13 **Sabi** var. Rio Save. ≈ Mozambique/Zimbabwe see also Save, Rio
118 E8 **Sabile** Ger. Zabeln. Talsi, NW Latvia
31 R14 **Sabina** Ohio, N USA
40 I3 **Sabinal** Chihuahua, N Mexico
25 Q12 **Sabinal** Texas, SW USA
25 Q11 **Sabinal River** ≈ Texas, SW USA
105 S4 **Sabiñánigo** Aragón, NE Spain
41 N6 **Sabinas** Coahuila de Zaragoza, NE Mexico
41 O8 **Sabinas Hidalgo** Nuevo León, NE Mexico
41 N6 **Sabinas, Río** ≈ NE Mexico
22 F9 **Sabine Lake** ◎ Louisiana/Texas, S USA
92 O3 **Sabine Land** physical region C Svalbard
25 W7 **Sabine River** ≈ Louisiana/Texas, SW USA
137 X12 **Sabirabad** C Azerbaijan
Sabkha see As Sabkhah
171 O4 **Sablayan** Mindoro, N Philippines
13 P16 **Sable, Cape** headland Newfoundland, SE Canada
23 X17 **Sable, Cape** headland Florida, SE USA
13 R16 **Sable Island** island Nova Scotia, SE Canada
14 L11 **Sables, Lac des** ◎ Quebec, SE Canada
14 E10 **Sables, Rivière aux** ≈ Ontario, S Canada
102 K7 **Sablé-sur-Sarthe** Sarthe, NW France
127 U7 **Sablya, Gora** ▲ NW Russian Federation
77 U14 **Sabon Birnin Gwari** Kaduna, C Nigeria
77 V11 **Sabon Kafi** Zinder, C Niger
104 I6 **Sabor, Rio** ≈ N Portugal
14 J8 **Sabourin, Lac** ◎ Quebec, SE Canada
102 J14 **Sabres** Landes, SW France
195 X13 **Sabrina Coast** physical region Antarctica
140 M11 **Sabt al Ulayā** 'Asīr, SW Saudi Arabia
104 I8 **Sabugal** Guarda, N Portugal
29 Z13 **Sabula** Iowa, C USA
141 N13 **Şabyā** Jīzān, SW Saudi Arabia
Sabzawar see Sabzevār
Sabzawaran see Sabzvārān
143 S4 **Sabzevār** var. Sabzawar. Khorāsān, NE Iran
143 T12 **Sabzvārān** var. Sabzawaran; prev. Jiroft. Kermān, SE Iran
Sacajawea Peak see Matterhorn
82 C9 **Sacandica** Uíge, NW Angola
42 A2 **Sacatepéquez** off. Departamento de Sacatepéquez. ◈ department S Guatemala
104 F11 **Sacavém** Lisboa, W Portugal
29 T13 **Sac City** Iowa, C USA
105 P8 **Sacedón** Castilla-La Mancha, C Spain
116 J12 **Săcele** Ger. Vierdörfer, Hung. Négyfalu; prev. Ger. Sieben Dörfer, Hung. Hétfalu. Braşov, C Romania
12 C8 **Sachigo** Ontario, C Canada
12 C7 **Sachigo** ≈ Ontario, C Canada
12 C8 **Sachigo Lake** ◎ Ontario, C Canada
163 Y16 **Sach'ŏn** Jap. Sansenhō; prev. Samch'ŏnpŏ. S South Korea
101 O15 **Sachsen** Eng. Saxony, Fr. Saxe. ◈ state E Germany
101 K14 **Sachsen-Anhalt** Eng. Saxony-Anhalt. ◈ state C Germany
109 R9 **Sachsenburg** Salzburg, S Austria
Sachsenfeld see Žalec
8 I5 **Sachs Harbour** Banks Island, Northwest Territories, N Canada
Sächsisch-Reen/Sächsisch-Regen see Reghin
18 H8 **Sackets Harbor** New York, NE USA
13 P14 **Sackville** New Brunswick, SE Canada
19 P9 **Saco** Maine, NE USA
19 P8 **Saco River** ≈ Maine/New Hampshire, NE USA
35 O7 **Sacramento** state capital California, W USA
37 T14 **Sacramento Mountains** ▲▲ New Mexico, SW USA
35 N6 **Sacramento River** ≈ California, W USA
35 N5 **Sacramento Valley** valley California, W USA
36 I10 **Sacramento Wash** valley Arizona, SW USA
105 N15 **Sacratif, Cabo** headland S Spain
116 F9 **Săcueni** prev. Săcuieni, Hung. Székelyhid. Bihor, W Romania
Săcuieni see Săcueni
105 R4 **Sádaba** Aragón, NE Spain
Sa da Bandeira see Lubango
138 I6 **Şadad** Ḩimş, W Syria
141 O13 **Şa'dah** NW Yemen
167 O16 **Sadao** Songkhla, SW Thailand
142 L8 **Sadd-e Dez, Daryācheh-ye** ◎ W Iran
19 S3 **Saddleback Mountain** hill Maine, NE USA
19 P6 **Saddleback Mountain** ▲ Maine, NE USA
167 S14 **Sa Đec** Đông Thap, S Vietnam
141 W13 **Sadḩ** S Oman
76 J11 **Sadiola** Kayes, W Mali
149 R12 **Sādiqābād** Punjab, E Pakistan
153 Y10 **Sadiya** Assam, NE India
139 W9 **Sa'dīyah, Hawr as** ◎ E Iraq
165 N9 **Sado** var. Sadoga-shima. island C Japan
Sadoga-shima see Sado
104 F12 **Sado, Rio** ≈ S Portugal
114 I8 **Sadovets** Pleven, N Bulgaria
129 O11 **Sadovoye** Respublika Kalmykiya, SW Russian Federation
105 W9 **Sa Dragonera** var. Isla Dragonera. island Islas Baleares, Spain, W Mediterranean Sea
95 H20 **Sæby** Nordjylland, N Denmark
105 P9 **Saelices** Castilla-La Mancha, C Spain
Saena Julia see Siena
Saetabicula see Alzira
114 O12 **Safaalan** Tekirdağ, NW Turkey
Safad see Ẕefat
Şafāqis see Sfax
192 I16 **Safata Bay** bay Upolu, Samoa, C Pacific Ocean
Safed see Ẕefat
Safed, Āb-i- see Sefīd, Darya-ye
139 X11 **Şaffāf, Ḩawr aş** wetland S Iraq
95 J16 **Säffle** Värmland, C Sweden
37 N15 **Safford** Arizona, SW USA
74 E7 **Safi** W Morocco
143 V9 **Safīdābeh** Khorāsān, E Iran
142 M4 **Safīd, Rūd-e** ≈ NW Iran
128 I4 **Safonovo** Smolenskaya Oblast', W Russian Federation
136 H11 **Safranbolu** Karabük, N Turkey
139 Y13 **Safwān** SE Iraq
158 J16 **Saga** var. Gya'gya. Xizang Zizhiqu, W China
164 C14 **Saga** Saga, Kyūshū, SW Japan
164 C13 **Saga** off. Saga-ken. ◈ prefecture Kyūshū, SW Japan
165 P10 **Sagae** Yamagata, Honshū, C Japan
166 L3 **Sagaing** Sagaing, C Myanmar
166 L5 **Sagaing** ◈ division N Myanmar
165 N13 **Sagamihara** Kanagawa, Honshū, S Japan
165 N14 **Sagami-nada** inlet SW Japan
Sagan see Żagań
29 Y3 **Saganaga Lake** ◎ Minnesota, N USA
155 F18 **Sāgar** Karnātaka, W India
154 I9 **Sāgar** prev. Saugor. Madhya Pradesh, C India
15 S8 **Sagard** Quebec, SE Canada
Sagarmatha see Everest, Mount
Sagebrush State see Nevada
143 V11 **Sāghand** Yazd, C Iran
19 N14 **Sag Harbor** Long Island, New York, NE USA
Saghez see Saqqez
31 R8 **Saginaw** Michigan, N USA
31 R8 **Saginaw Bay** lake bay Michigan, N USA
144 H11 **Sagiz** Atyrau, W Kazakhstan
64 H6 **Saglek Bank** undersea feature W Labrador Sea
13 P5 **Saglek Bay** bay SW Labrador Sea
Saglouc/Sagluk see Salluit
103 X15 **Sagonne, Golfe de** gulf Corse, France, C Mediterranean Sea
105 P13 **Sagra** ▲ S Spain
104 F14 **Sagres** Faro, S Portugal
37 S7 **Saguache** Colorado, C USA
44 J7 **Sagua de Tánamo** Holguín, E Cuba
44 E5 **Sagua la Grande** Villa Clara, C Cuba
15 R7 **Saguenay** ≈ Quebec, SE Canada
74 C9 **Saguia al Hamra** var. As Saqia al Hamra. ≈ N Western Sahara
Sagunt/Saguntum see Sagunto
105 S9 **Sagunto** var. Sagunt, Ar. Murviedro; anc. Saguntum. País Valenciano, E Spain
138 H10 **Saḩāb** 'Ammān, NW Jordan
54 E6 **Sahagún** Córdoba, NW Colombia
104 L4 **Sahagún** Castilla-León, N Spain
141 X8 **Şaḩam** N Oman
68 F9 **Sahara** desert Libya/Algeria
75 U9 **Sahara el Gharbîya** var. Aş Şaḩrā' al Gharbīyah, Eng. Western Desert. desert C Egypt
75 X9 **Sahara el Sharqîya** var. Aş Şaḩrā' ash Sharqīyah, Eng. Arabian Desert, Eastern Desert. desert E Egypt
Saharan Atlas see Atlas Saharien
152 J9 **Sahāranpur** Uttar Pradesh, N India
64 L10 **Saharan Seamounts** var. Saharian Seamounts. undersea feature E Atlantic Ocean
153 Q13 **Saharsa** Bihār, NE India
67 O7 **Sahel** physical region C Africa
153 R14 **Sāhibganj** Bihār, NE India
139 Q7 **Sahīlīyah** C Iraq
138 H4 **Sāḩilīyah, Jibāl as** ▲▲ NW Syria
114 M13 **Şahin** Tekirdağ, NW Turkey
149 U8 **Sāhīwāl** Punjab, E Pakistan
149 U9 **Sāhīwāl** prev. Montgomery. Punjab, E Pakistan
141 W11 **Saḩmah, Ramlat as** desert C Oman
139 T13 **Şaḩrā' al Ḩijārah** desert S Iraq
40 H5 **Sahuaripa** Sonora, NW Mexico
36 M16 **Sahuarita** Arizona, SW USA
40 L13 **Sahuayo** var. Sahuayo de José Mariá Morelos; prev. Sahuayo de Díaz, Sahuayo de Porfirio Díaz. Michoacán de Ocampo, SW Mexico
Sahuayo de Díaz/Sahuayo de José Mariá Morelos/Sahuayo de Porfirio Díaz see Sahuayo
173 W8 **Sahul Shelf** undersea feature N Timor Sea
167 P17 **Sai Buri** Pattani, SW Thailand
74 I6 **Saïda** NE Algeria
138 G7 **Saïda** var. Şaydā, Sayida; anc. Sidon. W Lebanon
Sa'īdābād see Sīrjān
80 B13 **Sa'id Bundas** Western Bahr el Ghazal, SW Sudan
186 E7 **Saidor** Madang, N PNG
153 S13 **Saidpur** var. Syedpur. Rajshahi, NW Bangladesh
108 C7 **Saignelégier** Jura, NW Switzerland
164 H11 **Saigō** Shimane, Dōgo, SW Japan
Saigon see Hô Chi Minh
162 I12 **Saihan Toroi** Nei Mongol Zizhiqu, N China
Saihon Tal see Sonid Youqi
Sai Hun see Syr Darya
92 M11 **Saija** Lappi, NE Finland
164 G14 **Saijō** Ehime, Shikoku, SW Japan
164 E15 **Saiki** Ōita, Kyūshū, SW Japan
93 N18 **Saimaa** ◎ SE Finland
93 N18 **Saimaa Canal** Fin. Saimaan Kanava, Rus. Saymenskiy Kanal. canal Finland/Russian Federation
Saimaan Kanava see Saimaa Canal
40 L10 **Saín Alto** Zacatecas, C Mexico
96 L12 **St Abb's Head** headland SE Scotland, UK
11 Y16 **St.Adolphe** Manitoba, S Canada
103 O15 **St-Affrique** Aveyron, S France
15 Q10 **St-Agapit** Quebec, SE Canada
97 O21 **St Albans** anc. Verulamium. E England, UK
18 L6 **Saint Albans** Vermont, NE USA

◆ Country ● Country Capital ◇ Dependent Territory ○ Dependent Territory Capital ◈ Administrative Region ✕ International Airport ▲ Mountain ▲▲ Mountain Range ☼ Volcano ≈ River ◎ Lake ⊞ Reservoir

21 Q5 **Saint Albans** West Virginia, NE USA
St Alban's Head *see* St.Aldhelm's Head
11 Q14 **St.Albert** Alberta, SW Canada
99 M24 **St. Aldhelm's Head** *var.* St.Alban's Head. *headland* S England, UK
15 S8 **St-Alexandre** Quebec, SE Canada
15 O11 **St-Alexis-des-Monts** Quebec, SE Canada
103 P2 **St-Amand-les-Eaux** Nord, N France
103 O9 **St-Amand-Montrond** *var.* St-Amand-Mont-Rond. Cher, C France
15 Q7 **St-Ambroise** Quebec, SE Canada
173 P16 **St-André** NE Réunion
14 M12 **St-André-Avellin** Quebec, SE Canada
102 K12 **St-André-de-Cubzac** Gironde, SW France
96 K11 **St Andrews** E Scotland, UK
23 Q9 **Saint Andrews Bay** *bay* Florida, SE USA
23 W7 **Saint Andrew Sound** *sound* Georgia, SE USA
Saint Anna Trough *see* Svyataya Anna Trough
44 J11 **St.Ann's Bay** C Jamaica
13 T10 **St.Anthony** Newfoundland, SE Canada
33 R13 **Saint Anthony** Idaho, NW USA
182 M11 **Saint Arnaud** Victoria, SE Australia
185 I15 **St.Arnaud Range** ▲▲ South Island, NZ
15 T8 **St-Arsène** Quebec, SE Canada
13 R10 **St-Augustin** Quebec, E Canada
23 X9 **Saint Augustine** Florida, SE USA
97 H24 **St Austell** SW England, UK
103 T4 **St-Avold** Moselle, NE France
103 N17 **St-Barthélemy** ▲▲ S France
102 L17 **St-Béat** Haute-Garonne, S France
97 I15 **St Bees Head** *headland* NW England, UK
173 P16 **St-Benoit** E Réunion
103 T13 **St-Bonnet** Hautes-Alpes, SE France
St.Botolph's Town *see* Boston
97 G21 **St Brides Bay** *inlet* SW Wales, UK
102 H5 **St-Brieuc** Côtes d'Armor, NW France
102 H5 **St-Brieuc, Baie de** *bay* NW France
102 L7 **St-Calais** Sarthe, NW France
15 Q10 **St-Casimir** Quebec, SE Canada
14 H16 **St.Catharines** Ontario, S Canada
45 S14 **St.Catherine, Mount** ▲ N Grenada
64 C11 **St Catherine Point** *headland* E Bermuda
23 X6 **Saint Catherines Island** *island* Georgia, SE USA
97 M24 **St Catherine's Point** *headland* S England, UK
103 N13 **St-Céré** Lot, S France
108 A10 **St.Cergue** Vaud, W Switzerland
103 R11 **St-Chamond** Loire, E France
33 S16 **Saint Charles** Idaho, NW USA
27 X4 **Saint Charles** Missouri, C USA
103 P13 **St-Chély-d'Apcher** Lozère, S France
Saint Christopher-Nevis *see* Saint Kitts and Nevis
31 S9 **Saint Clair** Michigan, N USA
14 D17 **St.Clair** ≈ Canada/USA
183 O17 **St.Clair, Lake** ◎ Tasmania, SE Australia
14 C17 **St.Clair, Lake** *var.* Lac à L'eau Claire. ◎ Canada/USA
31 S10 **Saint Clair Shores** Michigan, N USA
103 S10 **St-Claude** *anc.* Condate. Jura, E France
45 X6 **St-Claude** Basse Terre, SW Guadeloupe
23 X12 **Saint Cloud** Florida, SE USA
29 U8 **Saint Cloud** Minnesota, N USA
45 T9 **Saint Croix** *island* S Virgin Islands (US)
30 J4 **Saint Croix Flowage** ⊞ Wisconsin, N USA
19 T5 **Saint Croix River** ≈ Canada/USA
29 W7 **Saint Croix River** ≈ Minnesota/Wisconsin, N USA
45 S14 **St.David's** SE Grenada
97 H21 **St David's** SW Wales, UK
97 G21 **St David's Head** *headland* SW Wales, UK
64 C12 **St David's Island** *island* E Bermuda
173 O16 **St-Denis** ○ (Réunion) NW Réunion
103 U6 **St-Dié** Vosges, NE France
103 R5 **St-Dizier** *anc.* Desiderii Fanum. Haute-Marne, N France
15 N11 **St-Donat** Quebec, SE Canada
15 N11 **Ste-Adèle** Quebec, SE Canada
15 N11 **Ste-Agathe-des-Monts** Quebec, SE Canada
172 I16 **Sainte Anne** *island* Inner Islands, NE Seychelles
11 Y16 **Ste.Anne** Manitoba, S Canada
45 R12 **Ste-Anne** Grande Terre, E Guadeloupe
45 Y6 **Ste-Anne** SE Martinique
15 Q10 **Ste-Anne** ≈ Quebec, SE Canada
15 W6 **Ste-Anne-des-Monts** Quebec, SE Canada
14 M10 **Ste-Anne-du-Lac** Quebec, SE Canada
15 U4 **Ste-Anne, Lac** ◎ Quebec, SE Canada
15 S10 **Ste-Apolline** Quebec, SE Canada
15 U7 **Ste-Blandine** Quebec, SE Canada
15 R10 **Ste-Claire** Quebec, SE Canada
15 Q10 **Ste-Croix** Quebec, SE Canada
108 B8 **Ste.Croix** Vaud, SW Switzerland
103 P14 **Ste-Énimie** Lozère, S France
27 Y6 **Sainte Genevieve** Missouri, C USA
103 S12 **St-Egrève** Isère, E France
39 T12 **Saint Elias, Cape** *headland* Kayak Island, Alaska, USA
39 U11 **Saint Elias, Mount** ▲ Alaska, USA
10 G8 **Saint Elias Mountains** ▲▲ Canada/USA
55 Y10 **St-Élie** N French Guiana
103 O10 **St-Eloy-les-Mines** Puy-de-Dôme, C France
15 S7 **Ste-Maguerite Nord-Est** ≈ Quebec, SE Canada
15 R7 **Ste-Marguerite** ≈ Quebec, SE Canada
15 V4 **Ste-Marguerite, Pointe** *headland* Quebec, SE Canada
15 V3 **Ste-Marguesite** ≈ Quebec, SE Canada
15 R10 **Ste-Marie** Quebec, SE Canada
45 Q11 **Ste-Marie** NE Martinique
173 P16 **Ste-Marie** NE Réunion
103 U6 **Ste-Marie-aux-Mines** Haut-Rhin, NE France
12 J14 **Ste-Marie, Lac** ⊞ Quebec, S Canada
172 K4 **Sainte Marie, Nosy** *island* E Madagascar
102 L8 **Ste-Maure-de-Touraine** Indre-et-Loire, C France
103 R4 **Ste-Menehould** Marne, NE France
Ste-Perpétue *see* Ste-Perpétue-de-l'Islet
15 S9 **Ste-Perpétue-de-l'Islet** *var.* Ste-Perpétue. Quebec, SE Canada
45 X11 **Ste-Rose** Basse Terre, N Guadeloupe
173 P16 **Ste-Rose** E Réunion
11 W15 **Ste.Rose du Lac** Manitoba, S Canada
102 J11 **Saintes** *anc.* Mediolanum. Charente-Maritime, W France
45 X7 **Saintes, Canal des** *channel* SW Guadeloupe
Saintes, Îles des *see* les Saintes
173 P16 **Ste-Suzanne** N Réunion
15 P10 **Ste-Thècle** Quebec, SE Canada
103 Q12 **St-Étienne** Loire, E France
102 M4 **St-Étienne-du-Rouvray** Seine-Maritime, N France
Saint Eustatius *see* Sint Eustatius
14 M11 **Ste-Véronique** Quebec, SE Canada
15 T7 **St-Fabien** Quebec, SE Canada
15 P7 **St-Félicien** Quebec, SE Canada
15 O11 **St-Félix-de-Valois** Quebec, SE Canada
103 Y14 **St-Florent** Corse, France, C Mediterranean Sea
103 Y14 **St-Florent, Golfe de** *gulf* Corse, France, C Mediterranean Sea
103 P6 **St-Florentin** Yonne, C France
103 N9 **St-Florent-sur-Cher** Cher, C France
103 P12 **St-Flour** Cantal, C France
26 H2 **Saint Francis** Kansas, C USA
83 H26 **St.Francis, Cape** *headland* S South Africa
27 X10 **Saint Francis River** ≈ Arkansas/Missouri, C USA
22 J8 **Saint Francisville** Louisiana, S USA
15 Q12 **St-François** ≈ Quebec, SE Canada
45 Y6 **St-François** Grande Terre, E Guadeloupe
15 R11 **St-François, Lac** ◎ Quebec, SE Canada
27 X7 **Saint Francois Mountains** ▲▲ Missouri, C USA
St-Gall/Saint Gall/St.Gallen *see* Sankt Gallen
102 L16 **St-Gaudens** Haute-Garonne, S France
15 R12 **St-Gédéon** Quebec, SE Canada
181 X10 **Saint George** Queensland, E Australia
64 B12 **St George** N Bermuda
38 K15 **Saint George** Saint George Island, Alaska, USA
21 S14 **Saint George** South Carolina, SE USA
36 J8 **Saint George** Utah, W USA
13 R12 **St.George, Cape** *headland* Newfoundland, E Canada
9 W13 **St.George, Cape** *headland* New Ireland, NE PNG
38 J15 **Saint George Island** *island* Pribilof Islands, Alaska, USA
23 S10 **Saint George Island** *island* Florida, SE USA
99 J19 **Saint-Georges** Liège, E Belgium
15 R11 **St-Georges** Quebec, SE Canada
55 Z11 **St-Georges** E French Guiana
45 R14 **St.George's** ● (Grenada) SW Grenada
13 R12 **St.George's Bay** *inlet* Newfoundland, E Canada
97 G21 **Saint George's Channel** *channel* Ireland/Wales, UK
186 H6 **St.George's Channel** *channel* NE PNG
64 B11 **St George's Island** *island* E Bermuda
99 I21 **Saint-Gérard** Namur, S Belgium
St-Germain *see* St-Germain-en-Laye
15 P12 **St-Germain-de-Grantham** Quebec, SE Canada
103 N5 **St-Germain-en-Laye** *var.* St-Germain. Yvelines, N France
102 H8 **St-Gildas, Pointe du** *headland* NW France
103 R15 **St-Gilles** Gard, S France
102 I9 **St-Gilles-Croix-de-Vie** Vendée, NW France
173 O16 **St-Gilles-les-Bains** W Réunion
102 M16 **St-Girons** Ariège, S France
Saint Gotthard *see* Szentgotthárd
108 G9 **St.Gotthard Tunnel** *tunnel* Ticino, S Switzerland
97 H22 **St Govan's Head** *headland* SW Wales, UK
34 M7 **Saint Helena** California, W USA
65 F24 **Saint Helena** ◇ *UK dependent territory* C Atlantic Ocean
67 O12 **Saint Helena** *island* C Atlantic Ocean
83 E25 **St.Helena Bay** *bay* SW South Africa
65 M16 **Saint Helena Fracture Zone** *tectonic feature* C Atlantic Ocean
34 M7 **Saint Helena, Mount** ▲ California, W USA
21 S15 **Saint Helena Sound** *inlet* South Carolina, SE USA
31 Q7 **Saint Helen, Lake** ◎ Michigan, N USA
183 Q16 **Saint Helens** Tasmania, SE Australia
97 K18 **St Helens** NW England, UK
32 G10 **Saint Helens** Oregon, NW USA
32 H10 **Saint Helens, Mount** ⛰ Washington, NW USA
97 L26 **St Helier** ○ (Jersey) S Jersey, Channel Islands
15 S9 **St-Hilarion** Quebec, SE Canada
99 K22 **Saint-Hubert** Luxembourg, SE Belgium
15 T8 **St-Hubert** Quebec, SE Canada
15 P12 **St-Hyacinthe** Quebec, SE Canada
St.Iago de la Vega *see* Spanish Town
31 Q4 **Saint Ignace** Michigan, N USA
15 O10 **St-Ignace-du-Lac** Quebec, SE Canada
12 D12 **St.Ignace Island** *island* Ontario, S Canada
108 C7 **St.Imier** Bern, W Switzerland
97 G25 **St Ives** SW England, UK
29 U10 **Saint James** Minnesota, N USA
10 I15 **St.James, Cape** *headland* Graham Island, British Columbia, SW Canada
15 O13 **St-Jean** *var.* St-Jean-sur-Richelieu. Quebec, SE Canada
55 X9 **St-Jean** NW French Guiana
15 R8 **St-Jean** ≈ Quebec, SE Canada
Saint-Jean-d'Acre *see* 'Akko
102 K11 **St-Jean-d'Angély** Charente-Maritime, W France
103 N7 **St-Jean-de-Braye** Loiret, C France
102 I16 **St-Jean-de-Luz** Pyrénées-Atlantiques, SW France
103 T12 **St-Jean-de-Maurienne** Savoie, E France
102 I9 **St-Jean-de-Monts** Vendée, NW France
103 Q14 **St-Jean-du-Gard** Gard, S France
15 Q7 **St-Jean, Lac** ◎ Quebec, SE Canada
102 I16 **St-Jean-Pied-de-Port** Pyrénées-Atlantiques, SW France
15 S9 **St-Jean-Port-Joli** Quebec, SE Canada
St-Jean-sur-Richelieu *see* St-Jean
15 N12 **St-Jérôme** Quebec, SE Canada
25 T5 **Saint Jo** Texas, SW USA
13 O15 **St.John** New Brunswick, SE Canada
26 L6 **Saint John** Kansas, C USA
76 K16 **Saint John** ≈ C Liberia
45 T9 **Saint John** *island* C Virgin Islands (US)
22 I6 **Saint John, Lake** ◎ Louisiana, S USA
19 Q2 **Saint John** *Fr.* Saint-John. ≈ Canada/USA
45 W10 **St John's** ● (Antigua and Barbuda) Antigua, Antigua and Barbuda
13 V12 **St.John's** Newfoundland, E Canada
37 O12 **Saint Johns** Arizona, SW USA
31 Q9 **Saint Johns** Michigan, N USA
13 V12 **St.John's** ✕ Newfoundland, E Canada
23 X11 **Saint Johns River** ≈ Florida, SE USA
45 N12 **St.Joseph** W Dominica
173 P17 **St-Joseph** S Réunion
22 J6 **Saint Joseph** Louisiana, S USA
31 O10 **Saint Joseph** Michigan, N USA
27 R3 **Saint Joseph** Missouri, C USA
20 I10 **Saint Joseph** Tennessee, S USA
22 R9 **Saint Joseph Bay** *bay* Florida, SE USA
15 R11 **St-Joseph-de-Beauce** Quebec, SE Canada
12 C10 **St.Joseph, Lake** ◎ Ontario, C Canada
31 Q11 **Saint Joseph River** ≈ N USA
14 C11 **Saint Joseph's Island** *island* Ontario, S Canada
15 N11 **St-Jovite** Quebec, SE Canada
121 P16 **St Julian's** N Malta
St-Julien *see* St-Julien-en-Genevois
103 T10 **St-Julien-en-Genevois** *var.* St-Julien. Haute-Savoie, E France
102 M11 **St-Junien** Haute-Vienne, C France
103 Q11 **St-Just-St-Rambert** Loire, E France
96 D8 **St Kilda** *island* NW Scotland, UK
45 V10 **Saint Kitts** *island* Saint Kitts and Nevis
45 U10 **Saint Kitts and Nevis** *off.* Federation of Saint Christopher and Nevis, *var.* Saint Christopher-Nevis. ◆ *commonwealth republic* E West Indies
11 X16 **St.Laurent** Manitoba, S Canada
St-Laurent *see* St-Laurent-du-Maroni
55 X9 **St-Laurent-du-Maroni** *var.* St-Laurent. NW French Guiana
St-Laurent, Fleuve *see* St.Lawrence
102 J12 **St-Laurent-Médoc** Gironde, SW France
13 N12 **St.Lawrence** *Fr.* Fleuve St-Laurent. ≈ Canada/USA
13 Q12 **St.Lawrence, Gulf of** *gulf* NW Atlantic Ocean
38 K10 **Saint Lawrence Island** *island* Alaska, USA
14 M14 **Saint Lawrence River** ≈ Canada/USA
99 L25 **Saint-Léger** Luxembourg, SE Belgium
13 N14 **St.Léonard** New Brunswick, SE Canada
15 P11 **St-Léonard** Quebec, SE Canada
173 O17 **St-Leu** W Réunion
102 J4 **St-Lô** *anc.* Briovera, Laudus. Manche, N France
11 T15 **St.Louis** Saskatchewan, S Canada
103 V7 **St-Louis** Haut-Rhin, NE France
173 O17 **St-Louis** S Réunion
76 G10 **Saint Louis** NW Senegal
27 X4 **Saint Louis** Missouri, C USA
29 W5 **Saint Louis River** ≈ Minnesota, N USA
103 T7 **St-Loup-sur-Semouse** Haute-Saône, E France
15 O12 **St-Luc** Quebec, SE Canada
83 L22 **St.Lucia** KwaZulu/Natal, E South Africa
45 X13 **Saint Lucia** ◆ *commonwealth republic* SE West Indies
47 S3 **Saint Lucia** *island* SE West Indies
83 L22 **St.Lucia, Cape** *headland* E South Africa
45 Y13 **Saint Lucia Channel** *channel* Martinique/Saint Lucia
23 Y14 **Saint Lucie Canal** *canal* Florida, SE USA
23 Z13 **Saint Lucie Inlet** *inlet* Florida, SE USA
96 L2 **St Magnus Bay** *bay* N Scotland, UK
102 K10 **St-Maixent-l'École** Deux-Sèvres, W France
11 Y16 **St.Malo** Manitoba, S Canada
102 I5 **St-Malo** Ille-et-Vilaine, NW France
102 H4 **St-Malo, Golfe de** *gulf* NW France
44 L9 **St-Marc** C Haiti
44 L9 **St-Marc, Canal de** *channel* W Haiti
55 Y12 **Saint-Marcel, Mont** ▲ S French Guiana
103 S12 **St-Marcellin-le-Mollard** Isère, E France
96 K5 **St Margaret's Hope** NE Scotland, UK
32 M9 **Saint Maries** Idaho, NW USA
23 T9 **Saint Marks** Florida, SE USA
108 D11 **St.Martin** Valais, SW Switzerland
Saint Martin *see* Sint Maarten
31 O5 **Saint Martin Island** *island* Michigan, N USA
22 I9 **Saint Martinville** Louisiana, S USA
185 E20 **St.Mary, Mount** ▲ South Island, NZ
186 E8 **St.Mary, Mount** ▲ S PNG
182 I6 **Saint Mary Peak** ▲ South Australia
183 Q16 **Saint Marys** Tasmania, SE Australia
14 E16 **St.Marys** Ontario, S Canada
38 M11 **Saint Marys** Alaska, USA
23 W8 **Saint Marys** Georgia, SE USA
27 P4 **Saint Marys** Kansas, C USA
31 Q4 **Saint Marys** Ohio, N USA
21 R3 **Saint Marys** West Virginia, NE USA
23 W8 **Saint Marys River** ≈ Florida/Georgia, SE USA
31 Q4 **Saint Marys River** ≈ Michigan, N USA
102 D6 **St-Mathieu, Pointe** *headland* NW France
38 J12 **Saint Matthew Island** *island* Alaska, USA
21 R13 **Saint Matthews** South Carolina, SE USA
St.Matthew's Island *see* Zadetkyi Kyun
186 G4 **St.Matthias Group** *island group* NE PNG
108 C11 **St.Maurice** Valais, SW Switzerland
15 P9 **St-Maurice** ≈ Quebec, SE Canada
102 J13 **St-Médard-en-Jalles** Gironde, SW France
39 N10 **Saint Michael** Alaska, USA
St.Michel *see* Mikkeli
15 N10 **St-Michel-des-Saints** Quebec, SE Canada
103 S5 **St-Mihiel** Meuse, NE France
108 J10 **St.Moritz** *Ger.* Sankt Moritz, *Rmsch.* San Murezzan. Graubünden, SE Switzerland
102 H8 **St-Nazaire** Loire-Atlantique, NW France
Saint Nicholas *see* São Nicolau
Saint-Nicolas *see* Sint-Niklaas
103 N1 **St-Omer** Pas-de-Calais, N France
102 J11 **Saintonge** *cultural region* W France
15 S9 **St-Pacôme** Quebec, SE Canada
15 S10 **St-Pamphile** Quebec, SE Canada
15 S9 **St-Pascal** Quebec, SE Canada
14 J11 **St-Patrice, Lac** ◎ Quebec, SE Canada
11 R14 **St.Paul** Alberta, SW Canada
173 O16 **St-Paul** NW Réunion
38 K14 **Saint Paul** Saint Paul Island, Alaska, USA
29 V8 **Saint Paul** *state capital* Minnesota, N USA
29 P15 **Saint Paul** Nebraska, C USA
21 P7 **Saint Paul** Virginia, NE USA
77 Q17 **Saint Paul, Cape** *headland* S Ghana
103 O17 **St-Paul-de-Fenouillet** Pyrénées-Orientales, S France
65 K14 **Saint Paul Fracture Zone** *tectonic feature* E Atlantic Ocean
38 J14 **Saint Paul Island** *island* Pribilof Islands, Alaska, USA
102 J15 **St-Paul-les-Dax** Landes, SW France
21 U11 **Saint Pauls** North Carolina, SE USA
Saint Paul's Bay *see* San Pawl il-Bahar
191 R16 **St Paul's Point** *headland* Pitcairn Island, Pitcairn Islands
29 U10 **Saint Peter** Minnesota, N USA
97 L26 **St Peter Port** ○ (Guernsey) C Guernsey, Channel Islands
23 V13 **Saint Petersburg** Florida, SE USA
Saint Petersburg *see* Sankt-Peterburg
23 V13 **Saint Petersburg Beach** Florida, SE USA
173 P17 **St-Philippe** SE Réunion
45 Q11 **St-Pierre** NW Martinique
173 O17 **St-Pierre** SW Réunion
13 S13 **St-Pierre and Miquelon** *Fr.* Îles St-Pierre et Miquelon. ◇ *French territorial collectivity* NE North America
15 P11 **St-Pierre, Lac** ◎ Quebec, SE Canada
102 F5 **St-Pol-de-Léon** Finistère, NW France
103 O2 **St-Pol-sur-Ternoise** Pas-de-Calais, N France
St. Pons *see* St-Pons-de-Thomières
103 O16 **St-Pons-de-Thomières** *var.* St.Pons. Hérault, S France
103 P10 **St-Pourçain-sur-Sioule** Allier, C France
15 S11 **St-Prosper** Quebec, SE Canada
103 P3 **St-Quentin** Aisne, N France
15 R10 **St-Raphaël** Quebec, SE Canada
103 U15 **St-Raphaël** Var, SE France
15 Q10 **St-Raymond** Quebec, SE Canada
33 O9 **Saint Regis** Montana, NW USA
18 J7 **Saint Regis River** ≈ New York, NE USA
103 R15 **St-Rémy-de-Provence** Bouches-du-Rhône, SE France
15 V6 **St-René-de-Matane** Quebec, SE Canada
102 M9 **St-Savin** Vienne, W France
15 S8 **St-Siméon** Quebec, SE Canada
23 X7 **Saint Simons Island** *island* Georgia, SE USA
191 Y2 **Saint Stanislas Bay** *bay* Kiritimati, E Kiribati
13 O15 **St.Stephen** New Brunswick, SE Canada
39 X12 **Saint Terese** Alaska, USA
14 E17 **St.Thomas** Ontario, S Canada
29 Q2 **Saint Thomas** North Dakota, N USA
45 T9 **Saint Thomas** *island* W Virgin Islands (US)
Saint Thomas *see* São Tomé, Sao Tome and Principe
Saint Thomas *see* Charlotte Amalie, Virgin Islands (US)
15 P10 **St-Tite** Quebec, SE Canada
Saint-Trond *see* Sint-Truiden
103 U16 **St-Tropez** Var, SE France
Saint Ubes *see* Setúbal
102 L3 **St-Valéry-en-Caux** Seine-Maritime, N France
103 Q9 **St-Vallier** Saône-et-Loire, C France
106 B7 **St-Vincent** Valle d'Aosta, NW Italy
45 Q14 **Saint Vincent** *island* N Saint Vincent and the Grenadines
Saint Vincent *see* São Vicente
45 W14 **Saint Vincent and the Grenadines** ◆ *commonwealth republic* SE West Indies
Saint Vincent, Cape *see* São Vicente, Cabo de
102 I15 **St-Vincent-de-Tyrosse** Landes, SW France
182 I9 **Saint Vincent, Gulf** *gulf* South Australia
23 R10 **Saint Vincent Island** *island* Florida, SE USA
45 T12 **Saint Vincent Passage** *passage* Saint Lucia/Saint Vincent and the Grenadines
183 N18 **Saint Vincent, Point** *headland* Tasmania, SE Australia
Saint-Vith *see* Sankt-Vith
11 S14 **St.Walburg** Saskatchewan, S Canada
St Wolfgangsee *see* Wolfgangsee
102 M11 **St-Yrieix-la-Perche** Haute-Vienne, C France
Saint Yves *see* Setúbal
15 Y5 **St-Yvon** Quebec, SE Canada
188 H5 **Saipan** *island* ● (Northern Mariana Islands) S Northern Mariana Islands
188 H6 **Saipan Channel** *channel* S Northern Mariana Islands
188 H6 **Saipan International Airport** ✕ Saipan, S Northern Mariana Islands
74 G6 **Sais** ✕ (Fès) C Morocco
Saishū *see* Cheju
Saishū *see* Cheju-do
102 J16 **Saison** ≈ SW France
169 R10 **Sai, Sungai** ≈ Borneo, N Indonesia
165 N13 **Saitama** *off.* Saitama-ken. ◈ *prefecture* Honshū, S Japan
Saiyid Abid *see* Sayyid 'Abīd
57 J19 **Sajama, Nevado** ▲ W Bolivia
141 V13 **Sājir, Ras** *headland* S Oman
111 M20 **Sajószentpéter** Borsod-Abaúj-Zemplén, NE Hungary
83 F24 **Sak** ≈ SW South Africa
81 J18 **Saka** Coast, E Kenya
167 P11 **Sa Kaeo** Prachin Buri, C Thailand
164 J14 **Sakai** Ōsaka, Honshū, SW Japan
164 H14 **Sakaide** Kagawa, Shikoku, SW Japan
164 H12 **Sakaiminato** Tottori, Honshū, SW Japan
140 M3 **Sakākah** Al Jawf, NW Saudi Arabia
28 L4 **Sakakawea, Lake** ⊞ North Dakota, N USA
12 J9 **Sakami, Lac** ◎ Quebec, C Canada
79 O26 **Sakania** Katanga, SE Dem. Rep. Congo (Zaire)
146 K12 **Sakar** Lebapskiy Velayat, E Turkmenistan
172 H7 **Sakaraha** Toliara, SW Madagascar
146 I14 **Sakar-Chaga** *Turkm.* Sakarchäge. Maryyskiy Velayat, C Turkmenistan
Sakarchäge *see* Sakar-Chaga
Sak'art'velo *see* Georgia
136 F11 **Sakarya** ◈ *province* NW Turkey
136 F12 **Sakarya Nehri** ≈ NW Turkey
150 K13 **Sakasaul'skiy** *var.* Saksaul'skoye *Kaz.* Sekseūil. Kyzylorda, S Kazakhstan
Saksaul'skoye *see* Sakasaul'skiy
165 P9 **Sakata** Yamagata, Honshū, C Japan
123 P9 **Sakha (Yakutiya), Respublika** *var.* Respublika Yakutiya, Yakutiya, *Eng.* Yakutia. ◈ *autonomous republic* NE Russian Federation
Sakhalin *see* Sakhalin, Ostrov
192 I3 **Sakhalin, Ostrov** *var.* Sakhalin. *island* SE Russian Federation
123 U12 **Sakhalinskaya Oblast'** ◈ *province* SE Russian Federation
123 T12 **Sakhalinskiy Zaliv** *gulf* E Russian Federation
Sakhnovshchina *see* Sakhnovshchyna
117 U6 **Sakhnovshchyna** *Rus.* Sakhnovshchina. Kharkivs'ka Oblast', E Ukraine
Sakhon Nakhon *see* Sakon Nakhon
Sakhtsar *see* Rāmsar
Saki *see* Saky
137 W10 **Şäki** *Rus.* Sheki; *prev.* Nukha. NW Azerbaijan
118 E13 **Šakiai** *Ger.* Schaken. Šakiai, S Lithuania
165 O16 **Sakishima-shotō** *var.* Sakisima Syotô. *island group* SW Japan
Sakiz *see* Saqqez
Sakiz-Adasi *see* Chíos
155 F19 **Sakleshpur** Karnātaka, E India
167 S9 **Sakon Nakhon** *var.* Muang Sakon Nakhon, Sakhon Nakhon. Sakon Nakhon, E Thailand
149 P15 **Sakrand** Sind, SE Pakistan
83 F24 **Sak River** *Afr.* Sakrivier. Northern Cape, W South Africa
Sakrivier *see* Sak River
Saksaul'skiy *see* Saksaul'skoye
144 K13 **Saksaul'skoye** *prev.* Saksaul'skiy, *Kaz.* Sekseūil. Kzylorda, S Kazakhstan
95 I25 **Sakskøbing** Storstrøm, SE Denmark
165 N12 **Saku** Nagano, Honshū, S Japan
117 S13 **Saky** *Rus.* Saki. Respublika Krym, S Ukraine
76 E9 **Sal** *island* Ilhas de Barlavento, NE Cape Verde
129 N12 **Sal** ≈ SW Russian Federation
111 I21 **Sal'a** *Hung.* Sellye, Vágsellye. Nitriansky Kraj, SW Slovakia
95 N15 **Sala** Västmanland, C Sweden
15 N13 **Salaberry-de-Valleyfield** *var.* Valleyfield. Quebec, SE Canada
118 G7 **Salacgrīva** *Est.* Salatsi. Limbaži, N Latvia
107 M18 **Sala Consilina** Campania, S Italy
40 C2 **Salada, Laguna** ◎ NW Mexico
61 D14 **Saladas** Corrientes, NE Argentina
61 C21 **Saladillo** Buenos Aires, E Argentina
61 B16 **Saladillo, Río** ≈ C Argentina
25 T9 **Salado** Texas, SW USA
63 J16 **Salado, Arroyo** ≈ SE Argentina
37 Q12 **Salado, Rio** ≈ New Mexico, SW USA
61 D21 **Salado, Río** ≈ E Argentina
62 J12 **Salado, Río** ≈ C Argentina
41 N7 **Salado, Río** ≈ NE Mexico
143 N6 **Salafchegān** *var.* Sarafjagān. Qom, N Iran
77 Q15 **Salaga** C Ghana
192 G5 **Sala'ilua** Savai'i, W Samoa
116 G9 **Sălaj** ◈ *county* NW Romania
83 H20 **Salajwe** Kweneng, SE Botswana
78 H9 **Salal** Kanem, W Chad
80 I6 **Salala** Red Sea, NE Sudan
141 V13 **Şalālah** SW Oman
42 D5 **Salamá** Baja Verapaz, C Guatemala
42 J6 **Salamá** Olancho, C Honduras
62 G10 **Salamanca** Coquimbo, C Chile
41 N13 **Salamanca** Guanajuato, C Mexico
104 K7 **Salamanca** *anc.* Helmantica, Salmantica. Castilla-León, NW Spain
18 D11 **Salamanca** New York, NE USA
104 J7 **Salamanca** ◈ *province* Castilla-León, W Spain
63 J19 **Salamanca, Pampa de** *plain* S Argentina
78 J12 **Salamat** *off.* Préfecture du Salamat. ◈ *prefecture* SE Chad
78 I12 **Salamat, Bahr** ≈ S Chad
54 F5 **Salamina** Magdalena, N Colombia
115 G19 **Salamína** *var.* Salamís. Salamína, C Greece
115 G19 **Salamína** *island* C Greece
Salamís *see* Salamína

◆ Country
● Country Capital
◇ Dependent Territory
○ Dependent Territory Capital
◈ Administrative Region
✕ International Airport
▲ Mountain
▲▲ Mountain Range
⛰ Volcano
≈ River
◎ Lake
⊞ Reservoir

138 I5 **Salamīyah** var. As Salamīyah. Ḥamāh, W Syria
31 P12 **Salamonie Lake** ⊡ Indiana, N USA
31 P12 **Salamonie River** ≈ Indiana, N USA
Salang see Phuket
192 I16 **Salani** Upolu, SE Samoa
118 C11 **Salantai** Kretinga, NW Lithuania
104 K2 **Salas** Asturias, N Spain
105 O5 **Salas de los Infantes** Castilla-León, N Spain
102 M16 **Salat** ≈ S France
189 V13 **Salat** island Chuuk, C Micronesia
169 Q16 **Salatiga** Jawa, C Indonesia
189 V13 **Salat Pass** passage W Pacific Ocean
Salatsi see Salacgrīva
167 T10 **Salavan** var. Saravan, Saravane. Salavan, S Laos
129 V6 **Salavat** Respublika Bashkortostan, W Russian Federation
56 C12 **Salaverry** La Libertad, N Peru
171 T12 **Salawati, Pulau** island E Indonesia
193 R10 **Sala y Gomez** island Chile, E Pacific Ocean
Sala y Gomez Fracture Zone see Sala y Gomez Ridge
193 S10 **Sala y Gomez Ridge** var. Sala y Gomez Fracture Zone. tectonic feature SE Pacific Ocean
61 A22 **Salazar** Buenos Aires, E Argentina
54 G7 **Salazar** Norte de Santander, N Colombia
Salazar see N'Dalatando
173 P16 **Salazie** C Réunion
103 N8 **Salbris** Loir-et-Cher, C France
57 G15 **Salcantay, Nevado** ▲ C Peru
45 O8 **Salcedo** N Dominican Republic
39 S9 **Salcha River** ≈ Alaska, USA
119 H15 **Šalčininkai** Šalčininkai, SE Lithuania
Saldae see Béjaïa
54 E11 **Saldaña** Tolima, C Colombia
104 M4 **Saldaña** Castilla-León, N Spain
83 E25 **Saldanha** Western Cape, SW South Africa
Salduba see Zaragoza
61 B23 **Saldungaray** Buenos Aires, E Argentina
118 D9 **Saldus** Ger. Frauenburg. Saldus, W Latvia
183 P13 **Sale** Victoria, SE Australia
74 F6 **Salé** NW Morocco
74 F6 **Salé** × (Rabat) W Morocco
Salehābād see Andīmeshk
170 M16 **Saleh, Teluk** bay Nusa Tenggara, S Indonesia
122 H8 **Salekhard** prev. Obdorsk. Yamalo-Nenetskiy Avtonomnyy Okrug, N Russian Federation
192 H16 **Sālelologa** Savai'i, C Samoa
155 H21 **Salem** Tamil Nādu, SE India
27 V9 **Salem** Arkansas, C USA
30 L15 **Salem** Illinois, N USA
31 P15 **Salem** Indiana, N USA
19 P11 **Salem** Massachusetts, NE USA
27 V6 **Salem** Missouri, C USA
18 I16 **Salem** New Jersey, NE USA
31 U12 **Salem** Ohio, N USA
32 G12 **Salem** state capital Oregon, NW USA
29 Q11 **Salem** South Dakota, N USA
36 L4 **Salem** Utah, W USA
21 S7 **Salem** Virginia, NE USA
21 R3 **Salem** West Virginia, NE USA
107 H23 **Salemi** Sicilia, Italy, C Mediterranean Sea
Salemy see As Sālimī
94 K12 **Sälen** Dalarna, C Sweden
107 Q18 **Salentina, Campi** Puglia, SE Italy
107 Q18 **Salentina, Penisola** peninsula SE Italy
107 L18 **Salerno** anc. Salernum. Campania, S Italy
107 L18 **Salerno, Golfo di** Eng. Gulf of Salerno. gulf S Italy
Salerno, Gulf of see Salerno, Golfo di
Salernum see Salerno
97 K17 **Salford** NW England, UK
Salgir see Salhyr
111 K21 **Salgótarján** Nógrád, N Hungary
59 O15 **Salgueiro** Pernambuco, E Brazil
94 C13 **Salhus** Hordaland, S Norway
117 T12 **Salhyr** Rus. Salgir. ≈ S Ukraine
171 Q9 **Salibabu, Pulau** island N Indonesia
37 S6 **Salida** Colorado, C USA
102 J15 **Salies-de-Béarn** Pyrénées-Atlantiques, SW France
136 C14 **Salihli** Manisa, W Turkey
119 K18 **Salihorsk** Rus. Soligorsk. Minskaya Voblasts', S Belarus
119 K18 **Salihorskaye Vodaskhovishcha** ⊡ C Belarus
83 N14 **Salima** Central, C Malawi
166 L5 **Salin** Magwe, W Myanmar
27 N4 **Salina** Kansas, C USA
36 L5 **Salina** Utah, W USA
41 S17 **Salina Cruz** Oaxaca, SE Mexico
107 L22 **Salina, Isola** island Isole Eolie, S Italy
44 J5 **Salina Point** headland Acklins Island, SE Bahamas
56 A7 **Salinas** Guayas, W Ecuador
40 M11 **Salinas** var. Salinas de Hidalgo. San Luis Potosí, C Mexico
45 T6 **Salinas** C Puerto Rico
35 O10 **Salinas** California, W USA
Salinas, Cabo de see Salines, Cap de ses
Salinas de Hidalgo see Salinas
82 A13 **Salinas, Ponta das** headland W Angola
45 O10 **Salinas, Punta** headland S Dominican Republic
Salinas, Río see Chixoy, Río
35 O11 **Salinas River** ≈ California, W USA
22 H6 **Saline Lake** ◎ Louisiana, S USA
25 R17 **Salineno** Texas, SW USA
27 V14 **Saline River** ≈ Arkansas, C USA
30 M17 **Saline River** ≈ Illinois, N USA
105 X10 **Salines, Cap de ses** var. Cabo de Salinas. headland Mallorca, Spain, W Mediterranean Sea
Salisburg see Mazsalaca
45 O12 **Salisbury** var. Baroui. W Dominica
97 M23 **Salisbury** var. New Sarum. S England, UK
21 Y4 **Salisbury** Maryland, NE USA
27 T3 **Salisbury** Missouri, C USA
21 S9 **Salisbury** North Carolina, SE USA
Salisbury see Harare
9 Q7 **Salisbury Island** island Nunavut, NE Canada
Salisbury, Lake see Bisina, Lake
97 L23 **Salisbury Plain** plain S England, UK
21 R14 **Salkehatchie River** ≈ South Carolina, SE USA
138 I9 **Şalkhad** As Suwaydā', SW Syria
92 M12 **Salla** Lappi, NE Finland
103 U11 **Sallanches** Haute-Savoie, E France
105 V5 **Sallent** Cataluña, NE Spain
61 A22 **Salliqueló** Buenos Aires, E Argentina
27 R10 **Sallisaw** Oklahoma, C USA
80 I7 **Sallom** Red Sea, NE Sudan
12 J2 **Salluit** prev. Saglouc, Sagluk. Quebec, NE Canada
Sallûm, Khalīj as see Salûm, Gulf of
13 S11 **Sally's Cove** Newfoundland, E Canada
139 W9 **Salmān Bin 'Arāzah** E Iraq
Salmantica see Salamanca
142 I2 **Salmās** prev. Dilman, Shāpūr. Āzarbāyjān-e Bākhtarī, NW Iran
126 I11 **Salmi** Respublika Kareliya, NW Russian Federation
33 P12 **Salmon** Idaho, NW USA
11 N16 **Salmon Arm** British Columbia, SW Canada
192 L5 **Salmon Bank** undersea feature N Pacific Ocean
Salmon Leap see Leixlip
34 L2 **Salmon Mountains** ▲▲ California, W USA
14 J15 **Salmon Point** headland Ontario, SE Canada
33 N11 **Salmon River** ≈ Idaho, NW USA
18 K6 **Salmon River** ≈ New York, NE USA
33 N12 **Salmon River Mountains** ▲▲ Idaho, NW USA
18 I9 **Salmon River Reservoir** ⊡ New York, NE USA
93 K19 **Salo** Länsi-Suomi, W Finland
106 F7 **Salò** Lombardia, N Italy
Salona/Salonae see Solin
103 S15 **Salon-de-Provence** Bouches-du-Rhône, SE France
Salonica/Salonika see Thessaloníki
115 I14 **Salonikós, Akrotírio** headland Thásos, E Greece
116 F10 **Salonta** Hung. Nagyszalonta. Bihor, W Romania
104 I9 **Salor** ≈ W Spain
105 U6 **Salou** Cataluña, NE Spain
76 H11 **Saloum** ≈ C Senegal
42 H4 **Sal, Punta** headland NW Honduras
92 N3 **Salpynten** headland W Svalbard
138 I3 **Salqīn** Idlib, W Syria
93 F14 **Salsbruket** Nord-Trøndelag, C Norway
128 M13 **Sal'sk** Rostovskaya Oblast', SW Russian Federation
107 K25 **Salso** ≈ Sicilia, Italy, C Mediterranean Sea
107 J25 **Salso** ≈ Sicilia, Italy, C Mediterranean Sea
106 E9 **Salsomaggiore Terme** Emilia-Romagna, N Italy
Salt see As Salṭ
62 J6 **Salta** Salta, NW Argentina
62 K6 **Salta** off. Provincia de Salta. ⬖ province N Argentina
97 I24 **Saltash** SW England, UK
24 I8 **Salt Basin** basin Texas, SW USA
11 V16 **Saltcoats** Saskatchewan, S Canada
30 L13 **Salt Creek** ≈ Illinois, N USA
24 J9 **Salt Draw** ≈ Texas, SW USA
97 F21 **Saltee Islands** island group SE Ireland
92 G12 **Saltfjorden** inlet C Norway
24 I8 **Salt Flat** Texas, SW USA
27 N8 **Salt Fork Arkansas River** ≈ Oklahoma, C USA
31 T13 **Salt Fork Lake** ⊡ Ohio, N USA
26 J11 **Salt Fork Red River** ≈ Oklahoma/Texas, C USA
95 J23 **Saltholm** island E Denmark
41 N8 **Saltillo** Coahuila de Zaragoza, NE Mexico
182 L5 **Salt Lake** salt lake New South Wales, SE Australia
37 V15 **Salt Lake** ◎ New Mexico, SW USA
36 K2 **Salt Lake City** state capital Utah, W USA
61 C20 **Salto** Buenos Aires, E Argentina
61 D17 **Salto** Salto, N Uruguay
61 E17 **Salto** ⬖ department N Uruguay
107 I14 **Salto** ≈ C Italy
62 Q6 **Salto del Guairá** Canindeyú, E Paraguay
61 D17 **Salto Grande, Embalse de** var. Lago de Salto Grande. ⊡ Argentina/Uruguay
Salto Grande, Lago de see Salto Grande, Embalse de
35 W16 **Salton Sea** ◎ California, W USA
60 I12 **Salto Santiago, Represa de** ⊡ S Brazil
149 U7 **Salt Range** ▲▲ E Pakistan
36 M13 **Salt River** ≈ Arizona, SW USA
20 L5 **Salt River** ≈ Kentucky, S USA
27 V3 **Salt River** ≈ Missouri, C USA
95 F17 **Saltrød** Aust-Agder, S Norway
95 P16 **Saltsjöbaden** Stockholm, C Sweden
92 G12 **Saltstraumen** Nordland, C Norway
21 Q7 **Saltville** Virginia, NE USA
Saluces/Saluciae see Saluzzo
21 Q12 **Saluda** South Carolina, SE USA
21 X6 **Saluda** Virginia, NE USA
21 Q12 **Saluda River** ≈ South Carolina, SE USA
75 T7 **Salûm** var. As Sallūm. NW Egypt
152 F14 **Sālumbar** Rājasthān, N India
75 T7 **Salûm, Gulf of** Ar. Khalīj as Sallūm. gulf Egypt/Libya
171 O11 **Salumpaga** Sulawesi, N Indonesia
155 M14 **Sālūr** Andhra Pradesh, E India
55 Y9 **Salut, Îles du** island group N French Guiana
106 A9 **Saluzzo** Fr. Saluces; anc. Saluciae. Piemonte, NW Italy
63 F23 **Salvación, Bahía** bay S Chile
59 P17 **Salvador** prev. São Salvador. Bahia, E Brazil
65 E24 **Salvador** East Falkland, Falkland Islands
22 K10 **Salvador, Lake** ◎ Louisiana, S USA
Salvaleón de Higüey see Higüey
104 F10 **Salvaterra de Magos** Santarém, C Portugal
41 N13 **Salvatierra** Guanajuato, C Mexico
105 P3 **Salvatierra** Basq. Agurain. País Vasco, N Spain
Salwa/Salwah see As Salwā
166 M7 **Salween** Bur. Thanlwin, Chin. Nu Chiang, Nu Jiang. ≈ SE Asia
137 Y12 **Salyan** Rus. Sal'yany. SE Azerbaijan
153 N11 **Salyan** var. Sallyana. Mid Western, W Nepal
Sal'yany see Salyan
21 O6 **Salyersville** Kentucky, S USA
109 V6 **Salza** ≈ E Austria
109 Q7 **Salzach** ≈ Austria/Germany
109 Q6 **Salzburg** anc. Juvavum. Salzburg, N Austria
109 O8 **Salzburg** off. Land Salzburg. ⬖ state C Austria
Salzburg see Ocna Sibiului
Salzburg Alps see Salzburger Kalkalpen
109 Q7 **Salzburger Kalkalpen** Eng. Salzburg Alps. ▲▲ C Austria
100 J13 **Salzgitter** prev. Watenstedt-Salzgitter. Niedersachsen, C Germany
101 G14 **Salzkotten** Nordrhein-Westfalen, W Germany
100 K11 **Salzwedel** Sachsen-Anhalt, N Germany
152 D11 **Sām** Rājasthān, NW India
Šamac see Bosanski Šamac
54 G9 **Samacá** Boyacá, C Colombia
40 I7 **Samachique** Chihuahua, N Mexico
141 Y8 **Şamad** NE Oman
Sama de Langreo see Sama
Samaden see Samedan
57 M19 **Samaipata** Santa Cruz, C Bolivia
167 T10 **Samakhixai** var. Attapu, Attopeu. Attapu, S Laos
Samakov see Samokov
42 B6 **Samalá, Río** ≈ SW Guatemala
40 J3 **Samalayuca** Chihuahua, N Mexico
155 L16 **Sāmalkot** Andhra Pradesh, E India
45 P8 **Samaná** var. Santa Bárbara de Samaná. E Dominican Republic
45 P8 **Samaná, Bahía de** bay E Dominican Republic
44 K4 **Samana Cay** island SE Bahamas
136 K17 **Samandağı** Hatay, S Turkey
149 P3 **Samangān** ⬖ province N Afghanistan
Samangān see Āybak
165 T5 **Samani** Hokkaidō, NE Japan
54 C13 **Samaniego** Nariño, SW Colombia
171 Q5 **Samar** island C Philippines
129 S6 **Samara** prev. Kuybyshev. Samarskaya Oblast', W Russian Federation
129 S6 **Samara** × Samarskaya Oblast', W Russian Federation
129 T7 **Samara** ≈ W Russian Federation
117 V7 **Samara** ≈ E Ukraine
186 G10 **Samarai** Milne Bay, SE PNG
Samarang see Semarang
138 G9 **Samarian Hills** hill range N Israel
54 L9 **Samariapo** Amazonas, C Venezuela
169 V11 **Samarinda** Borneo, C Indonesia
Samarkand see Samarqand
Samarkandskaya Oblast' see Samarqand Wiloyati
Samarkandski/Samarkandskoye see Temirtau
Samarobriva see Amiens
147 N11 **Samarqand** Rus. Samarkand. Samarqand Wiloyati, C Uzbekistan
146 M11 **Samarqand Wiloyati** Rus. Samarkandskaya Oblast'. ⬖ province C Uzbekistan
139 S6 **Sāmarrā'** C Iraq
129 R7 **Samarskaya Oblast'** prev. Kuybyshevskaya Oblast'. ⬖ province W Russian Federation
153 Q13 **Samastīpur** Bihār, N India
76 L14 **Samatiguila** NW Ivory Coast
119 Q17 **Samatsevichy** Rus. Samotevichi. Mahilyowskaya Voblasts', E Belarus
Samawa see As Samāwah
137 Y11 **Şamaxı** Rus. Shemakha. C Azerbaijan
152 H6 **Samba** Jammu and Kashmir, NW India
79 K18 **Samba** Equateur, NW Dem. Rep. Congo (Zaire)
79 N21 **Samba** Maniema, E Dem. Rep. Congo (Zaire)
169 W10 **Sambaliung, Pegunungan** ▲▲ Borneo, N Indonesia
154 M11 **Sambalpur** Orissa, E India
67 X12 **Sambao** ≈ W Madagascar
169 Q10 **Sambas, Sungai** ≈ Borneo, N Indonesia
172 K2 **Sambava** Antsirañana, NE Madagascar
152 J10 **Sambhal** Uttar Pradesh, N India
152 H12 **Sāmbhar Salt Lake** ◎ N India
107 N21 **Sambiase** Calabria, SW Italy
116 H5 **Sambir** Rus. Sambor. L'vivs'ka Oblast', NW Ukraine
82 C13 **Sambo** Huambo, C Angola
Sambor see Sambir
61 E21 **Samborombón, Bahía** bay NE Argentina
99 H20 **Sambre** ≈ Belgium/France
43 V16 **Sambú, Río** ≈ SE Panama
163 Z14 **Samch'ŏk** Jap. Sanchoku. NE South Korea
Samch'ŏnpŏ see Sach'ŏn
81 I21 **Same** Kilimanjaro, NE Tanzania
108 J10 **Samedan** Ger. Samaden. Graubünden, S Switzerland
82 K12 **Samfya** Luapula, N Zambia
141 W13 **Samḥān, Jabal** ▲▲ SW Oman
115 C18 **Sámi** Kefallinía, Iónioi Nísoi, Greece, C Mediterranean Sea
56 F10 **Samiria, Río** ≈ N Peru
Samirum see Semīrom
137 V11 **Şämkir** Rus. Shamkhor. NW Azerbaijan
167 S7 **Sam, Nam** Vtn. Sông Chu. ≈ Laos/Vietnam
Samnān see Semnān
Sam Neua see Xam Nua
75 P10 **Samnū** C Libya
192 H15 **Samoa** off. Independent State of Samoa, var. Sāmoa; prev. Western Samoa ◆ monarchy W Polynesia
192 L9 **Sāmoa** island group American /Samoa
175 T9 **Samoa Basin** undersea feature W Pacific Ocean
Sāmoa-i-Sisifo see Samoa
112 D8 **Samobor** Zagreb, N Croatia
114 H10 **Samokov** var. Samakov. Sofiya, W Bulgaria
111 H21 **Šamorín** Ger. Sommerein, Hung. Somorja. Trnavský Kraj, W Slovakia
115 M19 **Sámos** prev. Limín Vathéos. Sámos, Dodekánisos, Greece, Aegean Sea
115 M20 **Sámos** island Dodekánisos, Greece, Aegean Sea
Samosch see Szamos
168 I9 **Samosir, Pulau** island W Indonesia
Samotevichi see Samatsevichy
Samothrace see Samothráki
115 K14 **Samothráki** Samothráki, NE Greece
115 J14 **Samothráki** anc. Samothrace. island NE Greece
115 A15 **Samothráki** island Iónioi Nísoi, Greece, C Mediterranean Sea
Samotschin see Szamocin
169 S13 **Sampit** Borneo, C Indonesia
169 S12 **Sampit, Sungai** ≈ Borneo, N Indonesia
Sampoku see Sanpoku
186 H7 **Sampun** New Britain, E PNG
79 N24 **Sampwe** Katanga, SE Dem. Rep. Congo (Zaire)
25 X8 **Sam Rayburn Reservoir** ⊡ Texas, SW USA
167 Q6 **Sam Sao, Phou** ▲▲ Laos/Thailand
95 H22 **Samsø** island E Denmark
95 H23 **Samsø Bælt** channel E Denmark
167 T7 **Sâm Sơn** Thanh Hoa, N Vietnam
136 L11 **Samsun** anc. Amisus. Samsun, N Turkey
136 K11 **Samsun** ⬖ province N Turkey
137 R9 **Samtredia** W Georgia
59 E15 **Samuel, Represa de** ⊡ W Brazil
167 O14 **Samui, Ko** island SW Thailand
Samundari see Samundri
149 U9 **Samundri** var. Samundari. Punjab, E Pakistan
137 X10 **Samur** ≈ Azerbaijan/Russian Federation
137 Y11 **Samur-Abşeron Kanalı** Rus. Samur-Apsheronskiy Kanal. canal E Azerbaijan
Samur-Apsheronskiy Kanal see Samur-Abşeron Kanalı
167 O11 **Samut Prakan** var. Muang Samut Prakan, Paknam. Samut Prakan, C Thailand
167 O11 **Samut Sakhon** var. Maha Chai, Samut Sakorn, Tha Chin. Samut Sakhon, C Thailand
Samut Sakorn see Samut Sakhon
167 O11 **Samut Songhram** prev. Meklong. Samut Songkhram, SW Thailand
77 N12 **San** Ségou, C Mali
111 O15 **San** ≈ SE Poland
141 O15 **Şan'ā'** Eng. Sana. ● (Yemen) W Yemen
112 F11 **Sana** ≈ NW Bosnia and Herzegovina
80 O12 **Sanaag** off. Gobolka Sanaag. ⬖ region N Somalia
114 J8 **Sanadinovo** Pleven, N Bulgaria
195 P1 **Sanae** South African research station Antarctica
139 Y10 **Sanāf, Hawr as** ◎ S Iraq
79 E15 **Sanaga** ≈ C Cameroon
54 D12 **San Agustín** Huila, SW Colombia
171 R8 **San Agustin, Cape** headland Mindanao, S Philippines
37 Q13 **San Agustin, Plains of** plain New Mexico, SW USA
38 M16 **Sanak Islands** island group Aleutian Islands, Alaska, USA
193 U10 **San Ambrosio, Isla** Eng. San Ambrosio Island. island W Chile
San Ambrosio Island see San Ambrosio, Isla
171 Q12 **Sanana** Pulau Sanana, E Indonesia
171 Q12 **Sanana, Pulau** island Maluku, E Indonesia
142 K5 **Sanandaj** prev. Sinneh. Kordestān, W Iran
35 P8 **San Andreas** California, W USA
2 C13 **San Andreas Fault** fault W USA
54 G8 **San Andrés** Santander, C Colombia
61 C20 **San Andrés de Giles** Buenos Aires, E Argentina
37 R14 **San Andres Mountains** ▲▲ New Mexico, SW USA
41 S15 **San Andrés Tuxtla** var. Tuxtla. Veracruz-Llave, E Mexico
25 P8 **San Angelo** Texas, SW USA
107 A20 **San Antioco, Isola di** island W Italy
42 F4 **San Antonio** Toledo, S Belize
62 G11 **San Antonio** Valparaíso, C Chile
188 H6 **San Antonio** Saipan, S Northern Mariana Islands
37 R13 **San Antonio** New Mexico, SW USA
25 R12 **San Antonio** Texas, SW USA
54 M11 **San Antonio** Amazonas, S Venezuela
54 I7 **San Antonio** Barinas, C Venezuela
55 O5 **San Antonio** Monagas, NE Venezuela
25 S12 **San Antonio** × Texas, SW USA
San Antonio see San Antonio del Táchira
105 V11 **San Antonio Abad** Eivissa, Spain, W Mediterranean Sea
25 U13 **San Antonio Bay** inlet Texas, SW USA
61 E22 **San Antonio, Cabo** headland E Argentina
44 A5 **San Antonio, Cabo de** headland W Cuba
105 T11 **San Antonio, Cabo de** headland E Spain
54 H7 **San Antonio de Caparo** Táchira, W Venezuela
62 J5 **San Antonio de los Cobres** Salta, NE Argentina
54 H7 **San Antonio del Táchira** var. San Antonio. Táchira, W Venezuela
35 T15 **San Antonio, Mount** ▲ California, W USA
63 K16 **San Antonio Oeste** Río Negro, E Argentina
25 T13 **San Antonio River** ≈ Texas, SW USA
54 J5 **Sanare** Lara, N Venezuela
103 T16 **Sanary-sur-Mer** Var, SE France
25 X8 **San Augustine** Texas, SW USA
141 T13 **Sanāw** var. Sanaw. NE Yemen
41 O11 **San Bartolo** San Luis Potosí, C Mexico
107 L16 **San Bartolomeo in Galdo** Campania, S Italy
106 K13 **San Benedetto del Tronto** Marche, C Italy
42 E3 **San Benito** Petén, N Guatemala
25 T17 **San Benito** Texas, SW USA
54 E6 **San Benito Abad** Sucre, N Colombia
35 P11 **San Benito Mountain** ▲ California, W USA
35 O10 **San Benito River** ≈ California, W USA
108 H10 **San Bernardino** Graubünden, S Switzerland
35 U15 **San Bernardino** California, W USA
62 H11 **San Bernardo** Santiago, C Chile
40 J8 **San Bernardo** Durango, C Mexico
164 G12 **Sanbe-san** ▲ Kyūshū, SW Japan
40 J12 **San Blas** Nayarit, C Mexico
40 H8 **San Blas** Sinaloa, C Mexico
43 V14 **San Blas** off. Comarca de San Blas. ⬖ special territory NE Panama
43 U14 **San Blas, Archipiélago de** island group NE Panama
23 Q10 **San Blas, Cape** headland Florida, SE USA
43 V14 **San Blas, Cordillera de** ▲▲ NE Panama
62 J8 **San Blas de los Sauces** Catamarca, NW Argentina
106 G8 **San Bonifacio** Veneto, NE Italy
29 S12 **Sanborn** Iowa, C USA
40 M7 **San Buenaventura** Coahuila de Zaragoza, NE Mexico
105 S5 **San Caprasio** ▲ N Spain
62 G13 **San Carlos** Bío Bío, C Chile
40 E9 **San Carlos** Baja California Sur, W Mexico
41 N5 **San Carlos** Coahuila de Zaragoza, NE Mexico
San Carlos, Estrecho de see Falkland Sound
41 P9 **San Carlos** Tamaulipas, C Mexico
42 L12 **San Carlos** Río San Juan, S Nicaragua
43 T16 **San Carlos** Panamá, C Panama
171 N3 **San Carlos** off. San Carlos City. Luzon, N Philippines
36 M14 **San Carlos** Arizona, SW USA
61 G20 **San Carlos** Maldonado, S Uruguay
54 K5 **San Carlos** Cojedes, N Venezuela
San Carlos see Quesada, Costa Rica
San Carlos see Luba, Equatorial Guinea
61 B17 **San Carlos Centro** Santa Fe, C Argentina
171 P6 **San Carlos City** Negros, C Philippines
San Carlos de Ancud see Ancud
63 H16 **San Carlos de Bariloche** Río Negro, SW Argentina
61 B21 **San Carlos de Bolívar** Buenos Aires, E Argentina
54 H6 **San Carlos del Zulia** Zulia, W Venezuela
54 L12 **San Carlos de Río Negro** Amazonas, S Venezuela
San Carlos, Estrecho de see Falkland Sound
36 M14 **San Carlos Reservoir** ⊡ Arizona, SW USA
42 M12 **San Carlos, Río** ≈ N Costa Rica
65 D24 **San Carlos Settlement** East Falkland, Falkland Islands
61 C23 **San Cayetano** Buenos Aires, E Argentina
103 O8 **Sancerre** Cher, C France
158 G7 **Sanchakou** Xinjiang Uygur Zizhiqu, NW China
Sanchoku see Samch'ŏk
41 O12 **San Ciro** San Luis Potosí, C Mexico
105 P10 **San Clemente** Castilla-La Mancha, C Spain
35 T16 **San Clemente** California, W USA
61 E21 **San Clemente del Tuyú** Buenos Aires, E Argentina
35 S17 **San Clemente Island** island Channel Islands, California, W USA
103 O9 **Sancoins** Cher, C France
187 N10 **San Cristobal** var. Makira. island SE Solomon Islands
61 B16 **San Cristóbal** Santa Fe, C Argentina
44 B4 **San Cristóbal** Pinar del Río, W Cuba
45 O9 **San Cristóbal** var. Benemérita de San Cristóbal. S Dominican Republic
54 H7 **San Cristóbal** Táchira, W Venezuela
San Cristóbal see San Cristóbal de Las Casas
41 U16 **San Cristóbal de Las Casas** var. San Cristóbal. Chiapas, SE Mexico
187 N10 **San Cristóbal, Isla** var. Chatham Island. island Galapagos Islands, Ecuador, E Pacific Ocean
42 D5 **San Cristóbal Verapaz** Alta Verapaz, C Guatemala
44 F6 **Sancti Spíritus** Sancti Spíritus, C Cuba
103 O11 **Sancy, Puy de** ▲ C France
95 D15 **Sand** Rogaland, S Norway
169 W7 **Sandakan** Sabah, East Malaysia
182 K9 **Sandalwood** South Australia
Sandalwood Island see Sumba, Pulau
94 D11 **Sandane** Sogn og Fjordane, S Norway
114 G12 **Sandanski** prev. Sveti Vrach. Blagoevgrad, SW Bulgaria
76 J11 **Sandaré** Kayes, W Mali
95 J19 **Sandared** Västra Götaland, S Sweden
94 N12 **Sandarne** Gävleborg, C Sweden
186 B5 **Sandaun** prev. West Sepik. ⬖ province NW PNG
96 K4 **Sanday** island NE Scotland, UK
31 P15 **Sand Creek** ≈ Indiana, N USA
95 H15 **Sande** Vestfold, S Norway
95 H16 **Sandefjord** Vestfold, S Norway
77 O15 **Sandégué** E Ivory Coast
77 P14 **Sandema** N Ghana
37 O11 **Sanders** Arizona, SW USA
24 M11 **Sanderson** Texas, SW USA
23 U4 **Sandersville** Georgia, SE USA
92 H4 **Sandgerdhi** Sudhurland, SW Iceland
28 K14 **Sand Hills** ▲▲ Nebraska, C USA
25 S14 **Sandia** Texas, SW USA
35 T17 **San Diego** California, W USA
25 S14 **San Diego** Texas, SW USA
136 F14 **Sandıklı** Afyon, W Turkey
152 L12 **Sandīla** Uttar Pradesh, N India
121 N15 **San Dimitri, Ras** var. San Dimitri Point. headland Gozo, NW Malta
168 J13 **Sanding, Selat** strait W Indonesia
30 J3 **Sand Island** island Apostle Islands, Wisconsin, N USA
95 C16 **Sandnes** Rogaland, S Norway
92 F13 **Sandnessjøen** Nordland, C Norway
79 L24 **Sandoa** Katanga, S Dem. Rep. Congo (Zaire)
111 N15 **Sandomierz** Rus. Sandomir. Świętokrzyskie, C Poland
Sandomir see Sandomierz
54 C13 **Sandoná** Nariño, SW Colombia
106 I7 **San Donà di Piave** Veneto, NE Italy
126 K14 **Sandovo** Tverskaya Oblast', W Russian Federation
166 K7 **Sandoway** Arakan State, W Myanmar
97 M24 **Sandown** S England, UK
95 B19 **Sandoy** Dan. Sandø Island Faeroe Islands
39 N16 **Sand Point** Popof Island, Alaska, USA
65 N24 **Sand Point** headland E Tristan da Cunha
31 R7 **Sand Point** headland Michigan, N USA
32 M7 **Sandpoint** Idaho, NW USA
93 H14 **Sandsele** Västerbotten, N Sweden
10 I14 **Sandspit** Moresby Island, British Columbia, SW Canada
27 P9 **Sand Springs** Oklahoma, C USA
29 W7 **Sandstone** Minnesota, N USA
36 K15 **Sand Tank Mountains** ▲▲ Arizona, SW USA
31 S8 **Sandusky** Michigan, N USA
31 S11 **Sandusky** Ohio, N USA
31 S12 **Sandusky River** ≈ Ohio, N USA
83 D22 **Sandverhaar** Karas, S Namibia
95 L24 **Sandvig** Bornholm, E Denmark
95 H15 **Sandvika** Akershus, S Norway
94 N13 **Sandviken** Gävleborg, C Sweden

◆ COUNTRY • COUNTRY CAPITAL ◇ DEPENDENT TERRITORY ○ DEPENDENT TERRITORY CAPITAL ⬖ ADMINISTRATIVE REGION × INTERNATIONAL AIRPORT ▲ MOUNTAIN ▲▲ MOUNTAIN RANGE VOLCANO ≈ RIVER ◎ LAKE ⊡ RESERVOIR

30 M11 **Sandwich** Illinois, N USA
Sandwich Island *see* Éfaté
Sandwich Islands *see* Hawaiian Islands
153 V16 **Sandwip Island** *island* SE Bangladesh
11 U12 **Sandy Bay** Saskatchewan, C Canada
183 N16 **Sandy Cape** *headland* Tasmania, SE Australia
36 L3 **Sandy City** Utah, W USA
31 U12 **Sandy Creek** ≈ Ohio, N USA
21 O5 **Sandy Hook** Kentucky, S USA
18 K15 **Sandy Hook** *headland* New Jersey, NE USA
146 J15 **Sandykachi** *Turkm.* Sandykgachy. Maryyskiy Velayat, S Turkmenistan
Sandykgachy *see* Sandykachi
146 L13 **Sandykly, Peski** *desert* E Turkmenistan
11 Q13 **Sandy Lake** Alberta, W Canada
12 B8 **Sandy Lake** Ontario, C Canada
12 B8 **Sandy Lake** ◎ Ontario, C Canada
23 S3 **Sandy Springs** Georgia, SE USA
24 H8 **San Elizario** Texas, SW USA
99 L25 **Sanem** Luxembourg, SW Luxembourg
42 K5 **San Esteban** Olancho, C Honduras
105 O6 **San Esteban de Gormaz** Castilla-León, N Spain
40 E5 **San Esteban, Isla** *island* NW Mexico
San Eugenio/San Eugenio del Cuareim *see* Artigas
62 H11 **San Felipe** *var.* San Felipe de Aconcagua. Valparaíso, C Chile
40 D3 **San Felipe** Baja California, NW Mexico
40 N12 **San Felipe** Guanajuato, C Mexico
54 K5 **San Felipe** Yaracuy, NW Venezuela
44 B5 **San Felipe, Cayos de** *island group* W Cuba
San Felipe de Aconcagua *see* San Felipe
San Felipe de Puerto Plata *see* Puerto Plata
37 R11 **San Felipe Pueblo** New Mexico, SW USA
San Feliú de Guixols *see* Sant Feliu de Guíxols
193 T10 **San Félix, Isla** *Eng.* San Felix Island. *island* W Chile
San Felix Island *see* San Félix, Isla
54 L11 **San Fernanado de Atabapo** Amazonas, S Venezuela
40 C4 **San Fernando** *var.* Misión San Fernando. Baja California, NW Mexico
41 P9 **San Fernando** Tamaulipas, C Mexico
171 N2 **San Fernando** Luzon, N Philippines
171 O3 **San Fernando** Luzon, N Philippines
104 J16 **San Fernando** *prev.* Isla de León. Andalucía, S Spain
45 U14 **San Fernando** Trinidad, Trinidad and Tobago
35 S15 **San Fernando** California, W USA
54 L7 **San Fernando** *var.* San Fernando de Apure. Apure, C Venezuela
San Fernando de Apure *see* San Fernando
62 L8 **San Fernando del Valle de Catamarca** *var.* Catamarca. Catamarca, NW Argentina
San Fernando de Monte Cristi *see* Monte Cristi
41 P9 **San Fernando, Río** ≈ C Mexico
23 X11 **Sanford** Florida, SE USA
19 P9 **Sanford** Maine, NE USA
21 T10 **Sanford** North Carolina, SE USA
25 N2 **Sanford** Texas, SW USA
39 T10 **Sanford, Mount** ▲ Alaska, USA
42 G8 **San Francisco** *var.* Gotera, San Francisco Gotera. Morazán, E El Salvador
43 R16 **San Francisco** Veraguas, C Panama
171 N2 **San Francisco** *var.* Aurora. Luzon, N Philippines
35 L8 **San Francisco** California, W USA
54 H5 **San Francisco** Zulia, NW Venezuela
34 M8 **San Francisco** ✕ California, W USA
35 N9 **San Francisco Bay** *bay* California, W USA
61 C24 **San Francisco de Bellocq** Buenos Aires, E Argentina
40 I6 **San Francisco de Borja** Chihuahua, N Mexico
42 J6 **San Francisco de la Paz** Olancho, C Honduras
40 J7 **San Francisco del Oro** Chihuahua, N Mexico
40 M12 **San Francisco del Rincón** Jalisco, SW Mexico
45 O8 **San Francisco de Macorís** C Dominican Republic
San Francisco de Satipo *see* Satipo
San Francisco Gotera *see* San Francisco
San Francisco Telixtlahuaca *see* Telixtlahuaca
107 K23 **San Fratello** Sicilia, Italy, C Mediterranean Sea
San Fructuoso *see* Tacuarembó
82 C12 **Sanga** Cuanza Sul, NW Angola
56 C5 **San Gabriel** Carchi, N Ecuador
159 S15 **Sa'ngain** Xizang Zizhiqu, W China
154 E13 **Sangamner** Mahārāshtra, W India
152 H12 **Sāngāner** Rājasthān, N India
Sangan, Koh-i- *see* Sangān, Kūh-e
149 N6 **Sangān, Kūh-e** *Pash.* Koh-i-Sangan. ▲▲ C Afghanistan
123 P10 **Sangar** Respublika Sakha (Yakutiya), NE Russian Federation
169 V11 **Sangasanga** Borneo, C Indonesia
103 N1 **Sangatte** Pas-de-Calais, N France
107 B19 **San Gavino Monreale** Sardegna, Italy, C Mediterranean Sea
57 D16 **Sangayan, Isla** *island* W Peru
30 L14 **Sangchris Lake** ▣ Illinois, N USA
171 N16 **Sangeang, Pulau** *island* S Indonesia
116 I10 **Sângeorgiu de Pădure** *prev.* Erdăt-Sângeorz, Sîngeorgiu de Pădure, *Hung.* Erdőszentgyörgy. Mureș, C Romania
116 I9 **Sângeorz-Băi** *var.* Singeroz Băi, *Ger.* Rumänisch-Sankt-Georgen, *Hung.* Oláhszentgyörgy; *prev.* Sîngeorz-Băi. Bistrița-Năsăud, N Romania
35 R10 **Sanger** California, W USA
25 T5 **Sanger** Texas, SW USA
Sângerei *see* Sîngerei
101 L15 **Sangerhausen** Sachsen-Anhalt, C Germany
45 S6 **San Germán** W Puerto Rico
San Germano *see* Cassino
161 N2 **Sanggan He** ≈ E China
169 Q11 **Sanggau** Borneo, C Indonesia
79 H16 **Sangha** ≈ Central African Republic/Congo
79 G16 **Sangha-Mbaéré** ◈ *prefecture* SW Central African Republic
149 Q15 **Sānghar** Sind, SE Pakistan
115 F22 **Sangiás** ▲ S Greece
Sangihe, Kepulauan *see* Sangir, Kepulauan
171 Q9 **Sangihe, Pulau** *var.* Sangir. *island* N Indonesia
54 G8 **San Gil** Santander, C Colombia
106 F12 **San Gimignano** Toscana, C Italy
148 M8 **Sangīn** *var.* Sangin. Helmand, S Afghanistan
107 O21 **San Giovanni in Fiore** Calabria, SW Italy
107 M16 **San Giovanni Rotondo** Puglia, SE Italy
106 G12 **San Giovanni Valdarno** Toscana, C Italy
Sangir *see* Sangihe, Pulau
171 Q10 **Sangir, Kepulauan** *var.* Kepulauan Sangihe. *island group* N Indonesia
162 K9 **Sangiyn Dalay** Dundgovĭ, C Mongolia
162 H9 **Sangiyn Dalay** Govĭ-Altay, C Mongolia
162 K11 **Sangiyn Dalay** Ömnögovĭ, S Mongolia
162 K8 **Sangiyn Dalay** Övörhangay, C Mongolia
163 Y15 **Sangju** *Jap.* Shōshū. C South Korea
167 R11 **Sangkha** Surin, E Thailand
169 W10 **Sangkulirang** Borneo, N Indonesia
169 W10 **Sangkulirang, Teluk** *bay* Borneo, N Indonesia
155 E16 **Sāngli** Mahārāshtra, W India
79 E16 **Sangmélima** Sud, S Cameroon
35 V15 **San Gorgonio Mountain** ▲ California, W USA
37 T8 **Sangre de Cristo Mountains** ▲▲ Colorado/New Mexico, C USA
61 A20 **San Gregorio** Santa Fe, C Argentina
61 F18 **San Gregorio de Polanco** Tacuarembó, C Uruguay
45 V14 **Sangre Grande** Trinidad, Trinidad and Tobago
159 N16 **Sangri** Xizang Zizhiqu, W China
152 H9 **Sangrūr** Punjab, NW India
44 I11 **Sangster** *off.* Sir Donald Sangster International Airport, *var.* Montego Bay. ✕ (Montego Bay) W Jamaica
59 G17 **Sangue, Rio do** ≈ W Brazil
105 R4 **Sangüesa** Navarra, N Spain
61 C16 **San Gustavo** Entre Ríos, E Argentina
Sangyuan *see* Wuqiao
40 C6 **San Hipólito, Punta** *headland* W Mexico
23 W15 **Sanibel** Sanibel Island, Florida, SE USA
23 V15 **Sanibel Island** *island* Florida, SE USA
60 F13 **San Ignacio** Misiones, NE Argentina
42 F2 **San Ignacio** *prev.* Cayo, El Cayo. Cayo, W Belize
57 L16 **San Ignacio** Beni, N Bolivia
57 O18 **San Ignacio** Santa Cruz, E Bolivia
42 M14 **San Ignacio** *var.* San Ignacio de Acosta. San José, W Costa Rica
40 E6 **San Ignacio** Baja California Sur, W Mexico
40 J10 **San Ignacio** Sinaloa, W Mexico
56 B9 **San Ignacio** Cajamarca, N Peru
San Ignacio de Acosta *see* San Ignacio
40 D7 **San Ignacio, Laguna** *lagoon* W Mexico
12 I6 **Sanikiluaq** Belcher Islands, Nunavut, C Canada
171 O3 **San Ildefonso Peninsula** *peninsula* Luzon, N Philippines
Saniquillie *see* Sanniquellie
61 D20 **San Isidro** Buenos Aires, E Argentina
43 N14 **San Isidro** *var.* San Isidro de El General. San José, SE Costa Rica
San Isidro de El General *see* San Isidro
54 E5 **San Jacinto** Bolívar, N Colombia
35 U16 **San Jacinto** California, W USA
35 V15 **San Jacinto Peak** ▲ California, W USA
61 F14 **San Javier** Misiones, NE Argentina
61 C16 **San Javier** Santa Fe, C Argentina
105 S13 **San Javier** Murcia, SE Spain
61 D18 **San Javier** Río Negro, W Uruguay
61 C16 **San Javier, Río** ≈ C Argentina
Sanjiang *see* Jinping
160 L12 **Sanjiang** *var.* Guyi, Sanjiang Dongzu Zizhixian. Guangxi Zhuangzu Zizhiqu, S China
Sanjiang Dongzu Zizhixian *see* Sanjiang
165 N11 **Sanjō** *var.* Sanzyô. Niigata, Honshū, C Japan
57 M15 **San Joaquín** Beni, N Bolivia
55 O6 **San Joaquín** Anzoátegui, NE Venezuela
35 O9 **San Joaquin River** ≈ California, W USA
35 P10 **San Joaquin Valley** *valley* California, W USA
61 A18 **San Jorge** Santa Fe, C Argentina
40 D3 **San Jorge, Bahía de** *bay* NW Mexico
San Jorge, Isla de *see* Weddell Island
63 J19 **San Jorge, Golfo** *var.* Gulf of San Jorge. *gulf* S Argentina
San Jorge, Gulf of *see* San Jorge, Golfo
188 K8 **San Jose** Tinian, S Northern Mariana Islands
35 N9 **San Jose** California, W USA
61 F14 **San José** Misiones, NE Argentina
57 P19 **San José** *var.* San José de Chiquitos. Santa Cruz, E Bolivia
42 M14 **San José** ● (Costa Rica) San José, C Costa Rica
42 C7 **San José** *var.* Puerto San José. Escuintla, S Guatemala
40 G6 **San José** Sonora, NW Mexico
105 U11 **San José** Eivissa, Spain, W Mediterranean Sea
54 H5 **San José** Zulia, NW Venezuela
42 M14 **San José** *off.* Provincia de San José. ◈ *province* W Costa Rica
61 E19 **San José** ◈ *department* S Uruguay
42 M13 **San José** ✕ Alajuela, C Costa Rica
San José *see* San José del Guaviare, Colombia
San José *see* San José de Mayo, S Uruguay
171 O3 **San Jose City** Luzon, N Philippines
San José de Cúcuta *see* Cúcuta
61 D16 **San José de Feliciano** Entre Ríos, E Argentina
55 O6 **San José de Guanipa** *var.* El Tigrito. Anzoátegui, NE Venezuela
62 I9 **San José de Jáchal** San Juan, W Argentina
40 G10 **San José del Cabo** Baja California Sur, W Mexico
54 G12 **San José del Guaviare** *var.* San José. Guaviare, S Colombia
61 E20 **San José de Mayo** *var.* San José. San José, S Uruguay
54 I10 **San José de Ocuné** Vichada, E Colombia
41 O9 **San José de Raíces** Nuevo León, NE Mexico
63 K17 **San José, Golfo** *gulf* E Argentina
40 F9 **San José, Isla** *island* W Mexico
43 U16 **San José, Isla** *island* SE Panama
25 U14 **San Jose Island** *island* Texas, SW USA
62 I10 **San Juan** San Juan, W Argentina
45 N9 **San Juan** *var.* San Juan de la Maguana. C Dominican Republic
57 E17 **San Juan** Ica, S Peru
45 U5 **San Juan** ○ (Puerto Rico) NE Puerto Rico
62 H10 **San Juan** *off.* Provincia de San Juan. ◈ *province* W Argentina
45 U5 **San Juan** *var.* Luis Muñoz Marin. ✕ NE Puerto Rico
San Juan *see* San Juan de los Morros
62 O7 **San Juan Bautista** Misiones, S Paraguay
35 O10 **San Juan Bautista** California, W USA
San Juan Bautista *see* Villahermosa
San Juan Bautista Cuicatlán *see* Cuicatlán
San Juan Bautista Tuxtepec *see* Tuxtepec
79 C17 **San Juan, Cabo** *headland* S Equatorial Guinea
105 S12 **San Juan de Alicante** País Valenciano, E Spain
54 H7 **San Juan de Colón** Táchira, NW Venezuela
40 L9 **San Juan de Guadalupe** Durango, C Mexico
San Juan de la Maguana *see* San Juan
54 G4 **San Juan del Cesar** La Guajira, N Colombia
40 L15 **San Juan de Lima, Punta** *headland* SW Mexico
42 I8 **San Juan de Limay** Estelí, NW Nicaragua
43 N12 **San Juan del Norte** *var.* Greytown. Río San Juan, SE Nicaragua
54 K4 **San Juan de los Cayos** Falcón, N Venezuela
40 M12 **San Juan de los Lagos** Jalisco, C Mexico
54 L5 **San Juan de los Morros** *var.* San Juan. Guárico, N Venezuela
40 K9 **San Juan del Río** Durango, C Mexico
41 O13 **San Juan del Río** Querétaro de Arteaga, C Mexico
42 J11 **San Juan del Sur** Rivas, SW Nicaragua
54 M9 **San Juan de Manapiare** Amazonas, S Venezuela
40 E7 **San Juanico** Baja California Sur, W Mexico
40 D7 **San Juanico, Punta** *headland* W Mexico
32 G6 **San Juan Islands** *island group* Washington, NW USA
40 I6 **San Juanito** Chihuahua, N Mexico
40 I12 **San Juanito, Isla** *island* C Mexico
37 R8 **San Juan Mountains** ▲▲ Colorado, C USA
54 E5 **San Juan Nepomuceno** Bolívar, NW Colombia
44 E5 **San Juan, Pico** ▲ C Cuba
191 W15 **San Juan, Punta** *headland* Easter Island, Chile, E Pacific Ocean
42 M12 **San Juan, Río** ≈ Costa Rica/Nicaragua
41 S15 **San Juan, Río** ≈ SE Mexico
37 O8 **San Juan River** ≈ Colorado/Utah, W USA
San Julián *see* Puerto San Julián
61 B17 **San Justo** Santa Fe, C Argentina
109 W5 **Sankt Aegyd-am-Neuwalde** Niederösterreich, E Austria
109 U9 **Sankt Andrä** *Slvn.* Šent Andraž. Kärnten, S Austria
Sankt Andrä *see* Szentendre
Sankt Anna *see* Sântana
108 K8 **Sankt Anton-am-Arlberg** Vorarlberg, W Austria
101 E16 **Sankt Augustin** Nordrhein-Westfalen, W Germany
Sankt-Bartholomäi *see* Palamuse
101 F24 **Sankt Blasien** Baden-Württemberg, SW Germany
109 R3 **Sankt Florian am Inn** Oberösterreich, N Austria
108 I7 **Sankt Gallen** *var.* St.Gallen, *Eng.* Saint Gall, *Fr.* St-Gall. Sankt Gallen, NE Switzerland
108 H8 **Sankt Gallen** *var.* St.Gallen, Eng, Saint Gall, *Fr.* St-Gall. ◈ *canton* NE Switzerland
108 J8 **Sankt Gallenkirch** Vorarlberg, W Austria
109 Q5 **Sankt Georgen** Salzburg, N Austria
Sankt Georgen *see* Đurđevac, Croatia
Sankt-Georgen *see* Sfântu Gheorghe, Romania
109 R6 **Sankt Gilgen** Salzburg, NW Austria
Sankt Gotthard *see* Szentgotthárd
101 E20 **Sankt Ingbert** Saarland, SW Germany
Sankt-Jakobi *see* Viru-Jaagupi, Lääne-Virumaa, Estonia
Sankt-Jakobi *see* Pärnu-Jaagupi, Pärnumaa, Estonia
Sankt Johann *see* Sankt Johann in Tirol
109 T7 **Sankt Johann am Tauern** Steiermark, E Austria
109 Q7 **Sankt Johann im Pongau** Salzburg, NW Austria
109 P6 **Sankt Johann in Tirol** *var.* Sankt Johann. Tirol, W Austria
Sankt-Johannis *see* Järva-Jaani
108 L8 **Sankt Leonhard** Tirol, W Austria
Sankt Margarethen *see* Sankt Margarethen im Burgenland
109 Y5 **Sankt Margarethen im Burgenland** *var.* Sankt Margarethen. Burgenland, E Austria
Sankt Martin *see* Martin
109 X8 **Sankt Martin an der Raab** Burgenland, SE Austria
109 U7 **Sankt Michael in Obersteiermark** Steiermark, SE Austria
Sankt Michel *see* Mikkeli
Sankt Moritz *see* St.Moritz
108 E11 **Sankt Niklaus** Valais, S Switzerland
109 S7 **Sankt Nikolai** *var.* Sankt Nikolai im Sölktal. Steiermark, SE Austria
Sankt Nikolai im Sölktal *see* Sankt Nikolai
109 U9 **Sankt Paul** *var.* Sankt Paul im Lavanttal. Kärnten, S Austria
Sankt Paul im Lavanttal *see* Sankt Paul
Sankt Peter *see* Pivka
109 W9 **Sankt Peter am Ottersbach** Steiermark, SE Austria
126 J13 **Sankt-Peterburg** *prev.* Leningrad, Petrograd, *Eng.* Saint Petersburg, *Fin.* Pietari. Leningradskaya Oblast', NW Russian Federation
100 H8 **Sankt Peter-Ording** Schleswig-Holstein, N Germany
109 V4 **Sankt Pölten** Niederösterreich, N Austria
109 W7 **Sankt Ruprecht** *var.* Sankt Ruprecht an der Raab. Steiermark, SE Austria
Sankt Ruprecht an der Raab *see* Sankt Ruprecht
Sankt-Ulrich *see* Ortisei
109 T4 **Sankt Valentin** Niederösterreich, C Austria
Sankt Veit am Flaum *see* Rijeka
109 T9 **Sankt Veit an der Glan** *Slvn.* Šent Vid. Kärnten, S Austria
99 M21 **Sankt-Vith** *var.* Saint-Vith. Liège, E Belgium
101 E20 **Sankt Wendel** Saarland, SW Germany
109 R6 **Sankt Wolfgang** Salzburg, NW Austria
79 K21 **Sankuru** ≈ C Dem. Rep. Congo (Zaire)
40 D8 **San Lázaro, Cabo** *headland* W Mexico
137 O16 **Şanlıurfa** *prev.* Sanli Urfa, Urfa, *anc.* Edessa. Şanlıurfa, S Turkey
137 O16 **Şanlıurfa** *prev.* Urfa. ◈ *province* SE Turkey
137 O16 **Şanlıurfa Yaylası** *plateau* SE Turkey
61 B18 **San Lorenzo** Santa Fe, C Argentina
57 M21 **San Lorenzo** Tarija, S Bolivia
56 C5 **San Lorenzo** Esmeraldas, N Ecuador
42 H8 **San Lorenzo** Valle, S Honduras
105 N8 **San Lorenzo de El Escorial** *var.* El Escorial. Madrid, C Spain
40 E5 **San Lorenzo, Isla** *island* NW Mexico
57 C14 **San Lorenzo, Isla** *island* W Peru
63 G20 **San Lorenzo, Monte** ▲ S Argentina
40 I9 **San Lorenzo, Río** ≈ C Mexico
104 J15 **Sanlúcar de Barrameda** Andalucía, S Spain
104 J14 **Sanlúcar la Mayor** Andalucía, S Spain
40 F11 **San Lucas** Baja California Sur, NW Mexico
40 E6 **San Lucas** *var.* Cabo San Lucas. Baja California Sur, W Mexico
40 G11 **San Lucas, Cabo** *var.* San Lucas Cape. *headland* W Mexico
San Lucas Cape *see* San Lucas, Cabo
62 J11 **San Luis** San Luis, C Argentina
42 E4 **San Luis** Petén, NE Guatemala
40 D2 **San Luis** *var.* San Luis Río Colorado. Sonora, NW Mexico
42 M7 **San Luis** Región Autónoma Atlántico Norte, NE Nicaragua
36 H15 **San Luis** Arizona, SW USA
37 T8 **San Luis** Colorado, C USA
54 J4 **San Luis** Falcón, N Venezuela
62 J11 **San Luis** *off.* Provincia de San Luis. ◈ *province* C Argentina
41 N12 **San Luis de la Paz** Guanajuato, C Mexico
40 K8 **San Luis del Cordero** Durango, C Mexico
40 D4 **San Luis, Isla** *island* NW Mexico
42 E6 **San Luis Jilotepeque** Jalapa, SE Guatemala
57 M16 **San Luis, Laguna de** ◎ NW Bolivia
35 P13 **San Luis Obispo** California, W USA
37 R7 **San Luis Peak** ▲ Colorado, C USA
41 N11 **San Luis Potosí** San Luis Potosí, C Mexico
41 N11 **San Luis Potosí** ◈ *state* C Mexico
35 O10 **San Luis Reservoir** ▣ California, W USA
San Luis Río Colorado *see* San Luis
37 S8 **San Luis Valley** *basin* Colorado, C USA
107 C19 **Sanluri** Sardegna, Italy, C Mediterranean Sea
61 D23 **San Manuel** Buenos Aires, E Argentina
36 M15 **San Manuel** Arizona, SW USA
106 F11 **San Marcello Pistoiese** Toscana, C Italy
107 N20 **San Marco Argentano** Calabria, SW Italy
54 E6 **San Marcos** Sucre, N Colombia
42 M14 **San Marcos** San José, C Costa Rica
42 B5 **San Marcos** San Marcos, W Guatemala
42 F6 **San Marcos** Ocotepeque, SW Honduras
41 O16 **San Marcos** Guerrero, S Mexico
25 S11 **San Marcos** Texas, SW USA
42 A5 **San Marcos** *off.* Departamento de San Marcos. ◈ *department* W Guatemala
San Marcos de Arica *see* Arica
40 E6 **San Marcos, Isla** *island* W Mexico
106 H11 **San Marino** ● (San Marino) C San Marino
106 I11 **San Marino** *off.* Republic of San Marino. ◆ *republic* S Europe
62 I11 **San Martín** Mendoza, C Argentina
54 F11 **San Martín** Meta, C Colombia
56 D11 **San Martín** *off.* Departamento de San Martín. ◈ *department* C Peru
194 I5 **San Martín** *Argentinian research station* Antarctica
63 H16 **San Martín de los Andes** Neuquén, W Argentina
104 M8 **San Martín de Valdeiglesias** Madrid, C Spain
63 G21 **San Martín, Lago** *var.* Lago O'Higgins. ◎ S Argentina
106 H6 **San Martino di Castrozza** Trentino-Alto Adige, N Italy
57 N16 **San Martín, Río** ≈ N Bolivia
San Martín Texmelucan *see* Texmelucan
35 N9 **San Mateo** California, W USA
55 O6 **San Mateo** Anzoátegui, NE Venezuela
42 B4 **San Mateo Ixtatán** Huehuetenango, W Guatemala
57 Q18 **San Matías** Santa Cruz, E Bolivia
63 K16 **San Matías, Golfo** *var.* Gulf of San Matías. *gulf* E Argentina
San Matías, Gulf of *see* San Matías
15 O8 **Sanmaur** Quebec, SE Canada
161 T10 **Sanmen Wan** *bay* E China
160 M6 **Sanmenxia** *var.* Shan Xian. Henan, C China
Sânmiclăuş Mare *see* Sânnicolau Mare
61 D14 **San Miguel** Corrientes, NE Argentina
57 L16 **San Miguel** Beni, N Bolivia
42 G8 **San Miguel** San Miguel, SE El Salvador
40 L6 **San Miguel** Coahuila de Zaragoza, N Mexico
40 J9 **San Miguel** *var.* San Miguel de Cruces. Durango, C Mexico
43 U16 **San Miguel** Panamá, SE Panama
35 P12 **San Miguel** California, W USA
42 B9 **San Miguel** ◈ *department* E El Salvador
41 N13 **San Miguel de Allende** Guanajuato, C Mexico
San Miguel de Cruces *see* San Miguel
San Miguel de Ibarra *see* Ibarra
61 D21 **San Miguel del Monte** Buenos Aires, E Argentina
62 J7 **San Miguel de Tucumán** *var.* Tucumán. Tucumán, N Argentina
43 V16 **San Miguel, Golfo de** *gulf* S Panama
35 P15 **San Miguel Island** *island* California, W USA
42 L11 **San Miguelito** Río San Juan, S Nicaragua
43 T15 **San Miguelito** Panamá, C Panama
57 N18 **San Miguel, Río** ≈ E Bolivia
56 D6 **San Miguel, Río** ≈ Colombia/Ecuador
40 I7 **San Miguel, Río** ≈ N Mexico
42 G8 **San Miguel, Volcán de** ⁂ SE El Salvador
161 Q12 **Sanming** Fujian, SE China
106 F11 **San Miniato** Toscana, C Italy
San Murezzan *see* St.Moritz
Sannār *see* Sennar
107 M15 **Sannicandro Garganico** Puglia, SE Italy
40 H6 **San Nicolás** Sonora, NW Mexico
61 C19 **San Nicolás de los Arroyos** Buenos Aires, E Argentina
35 R16 **San Nicolas Island** *island* Channel Islands, California, W USA
Sânnicolaul-Mare *see* Sânnicolau Mare
116 E11 **Sânnicolau Mare** *var.* Sânnicolaul-Mare, *Hung.* Nagyszentmiklós; *prev.* Sânmiclăuş Mare, Sînnicolau Mare. Timiş, W Romania
123 Q6 **Sannikova, Proliv** *strait* NE Russian Federation
76 K16 **Sanniquellie** *var.* Saniquillie. NE Liberia
165 R7 **Sannohe** Aomori, Honshū, C Japan
Sanntaler Alpen *see* Kamniško-Savinjske Alpe
111 O17 **Sanok** Podkarpackie, SE Poland
54 E5 **San Onofre** Sucre, NW Colombia
57 K21 **San Pablo** Potosí, S Bolivia
171 O4 **San Pablo** *off.* San Pablo City. Luzon, N Philippines
San Pablo Balleza *see* Balleza
35 N8 **San Pablo Bay** *bay* California, W USA
40 C6 **San Pablo, Punta** *headland* W Mexico
43 R16 **San Pablo, Río** ≈ C Panama
171 P4 **San Pascual** Burias Island, C Philippines
121 Q16 **San Pawl il-Bahar** *Eng.* Saint Paul's Bay. E Malta
61 C19 **San Pedro** Buenos Aires, E Argentina
62 K5 **San Pedro** Jujuy, N Argentina
60 G13 **San Pedro** Misiones, NE Argentina
42 H1 **San Pedro** Corozal, NE Belize
40 L8 **San Pedro** *var.* San Pedro de las Colonias. Coahuila de Zaragoza, NE Mexico
62 O5 **San Pedro** San Pedro, SE Paraguay
62 O6 **San Pedro** *off.* Departamento de San Pedro. ◈ *department* C Paraguay
77 N16 **San Pedro** ✕ (Yamoussoukro) C Ivory Coast
44 G6 **San Pedro** ≈ C Cuba
San Pedro *see* San Pedro del Pinatar
76 M17 **San-Pédro** S Ivory Coast
42 D5 **San Pedro Carchá** Alta Verapaz, C Guatemala
35 S16 **San Pedro Channel** *channel* California, W USA
62 I5 **San Pedro de Atacama** Antofagasta, N Chile
San Pedro de Durazno *see* Durazno
40 G5 **San Pedro de la Cueva** Sonora, NW Mexico
San Pedro de las Colonias *see* San Pedro
56 B11 **San Pedro de Lloc** La Libertad, NW Peru
105 S13 **San Pedro del Pinatar** *var.* San Pedro. Murcia, SE Spain
45 P9 **San Pedro de Macorís** SE Dominican Republic
40 C3 **San Pedro Mártir, Sierra** ▲▲ NW Mexico
San Pedro Pochutla *see* Pochutla
42 D2 **San Pedro, Río** ≈ Guatemala/Mexico
40 K10 **San Pedro, Río** ≈ C Mexico
104 J10 **San Pedro, Sierra de** ▲▲ W Spain
42 G5 **San Pedro Sula** Cortés, NW Honduras
San Pedro Tapanatepec *see* Tapanatepec
62 I4 **San Pedro, Volcán** ▲ N Chile
106 E7 **San Pellegrino Terme** Lombardia, N Italy
25 T16 **San Perlita** Texas, SW USA
San Pietro *see* Supetar
San Pietro del Carso *see* Pivka
107 A20 **San Pietro, Isola di** *island* W Italy
32 K7 **Sanpoil River** ≈ Washington, NW USA
165 O9 **Sanpoku** *var.* Sampoku. Niigata, Honshū, C Japan
40 C3 **San Quintín** Baja California, NW Mexico
40 B3 **San Quintín, Bahía de** *bay* NW Mexico
40 B3 **San Quintín, Cabo** *headland* NW Mexico
62 I12 **San Rafael** Mendoza, W Argentina
41 N9 **San Rafael** Nuevo León, NE Mexico
34 M8 **San Rafael** California, W USA

◆ COUNTRY ● COUNTRY CAPITAL ◇ DEPENDENT TERRITORY ○ DEPENDENT TERRITORY CAPITAL ◈ ADMINISTRATIVE REGION ✕ INTERNATIONAL AIRPORT ▲ MOUNTAIN ▲▲ MOUNTAIN RANGE ⁂ VOLCANO ≈ RIVER ◎ LAKE ▣ RESERVOIR

37 Q11 **San Rafael** New Mexico, SW USA
54 H4 **San Rafael** *var.* El Moján. Zulia, NW Venezuela
42 J8 **San Rafael del Norte** Jinotega, NW Nicaragua
42 J10 **San Rafael del Sur** Managua, SW Nicaragua
36 M5 **San Rafael Knob** ▲ Utah, W USA
35 Q14 **San Rafael Mountains** ▲ California, W USA
42 M13 **San Ramón** Alajuela, C Costa Rica
57 E14 **San Ramón** Junín, C Peru
61 F19 **San Ramón** Canelones, S Uruguay
62 K5 **San Ramón de la Nueva Orán** Salta, N Argentina
57 O16 **San Ramón, Río** ≈ E Bolivia
106 B11 **San Remo** Liguria, NW Italy
54 J3 **San Román, Cabo** *headland* NW Venezuela
61 C15 **San Roque** Corrientes, NE Argentina
188 I4 **San Roque** Saipan, S Northern Mariana Islands
104 K16 **San Roque** Andalucía, S Spain
25 R9 **San Saba** Texas, SW USA
25 Q9 **San Saba River** ≈ Texas, SW USA
61 D17 **San Salvador** Entre Ríos, E Argentina
42 F7 **San Salvador** ● (El Salvador) San Salvador, SW El Salvador
42 A10 **San Salvador** ◈ *department* C El Salvador
42 F8 **San Salvador** ✕ La Paz, S El Salvador
44 K4 **San Salvador** *prev.* Watlings Island. *island* E Bahamas
62 J5 **San Salvador de Jujuy** *var.* Jujuy. Jujuy, N Argentina
42 F7 **San Salvador, Volcán de** ☒ C El Salvador
77 Q14 **Sansanné-Mango** *var.* Mango. N Togo
45 S5 **San Sebastián** W Puerto Rico
63 J24 **San Sebastián, Bahía** *bay* S Argentina
Sansenhō *see* Sach'ŏn
106 H12 **Sansepolcro** Toscana, C Italy
107 M16 **San Severo** Puglia, SE Italy
112 F11 **Sanski Most** Federacija Bosna I Hercegovina, NW Bosnia & Herzegovina
171 W12 **Sansundi** Irian Jaya, E Indonesia
104 K11 **Santa Amalia** Extremadura, W Spain
60 F13 **Santa Ana** Misiones, NE Argentina
57 L16 **Santa Ana** Beni, N Bolivia
42 E7 **Santa Ana** Santa Ana, NW El Salvador
40 F4 **Santa Ana** Sonora, NW Mexico
35 T16 **Santa Ana** California, W USA
55 N6 **Santa Ana** Nueva Esparta, NE Venezuela
42 A9 **Santa Ana** ◈ *department* NW El Salvador
Santa Ana de Coro *see* Coro
42 E7 **Santa Ana, Volcán de** *var.* La Matepec. ☒ W El Salvador
40 J7 **Santa Barbara** Chihuahua, N Mexico
35 Q14 **Santa Barbara** California, W USA
42 G6 **Santa Bárbara** Santa Bárbara, W Honduras
54 L11 **Santa Bárbara** Amazonas, S Venezuela
54 I7 **Santa Bárbara** Barinas, W Venezuela
42 F5 **Santa Bárbara** ◈ *department* NW Honduras
Santa Bárbara *see* Iscuandé
35 Q15 **Santa Barbara Channel** *channel* California, W USA
Santa Bárbara de Samaná *see* Samaná
35 R16 **Santa Barbara Island** *island* Channel Islands, California, W USA
54 E5 **Santa Catalina** Bolívar, N Colombia
43 R15 **Santa Catalina** Bocas del Toro, W Panama
35 T17 **Santa Catalina, Gulf of** *gulf* California, W USA
40 F8 **Santa Catalina, Isla** *island* W Mexico
35 S16 **Santa Catalina Island** *island* Channel Islands, California, W USA
41 N8 **Santa Catarina** Nuevo León, NE Mexico
60 H13 **Santa Catarina** *off.* Estado de Santa Catarina. ◈ *state* S Brazil
Santa Catarina de Tepehuanes *see* Tepehuanes
60 L13 **Santa Catarina, Ilha de** *island* S Brazil
45 Q16 **Santa Catherina** Curaçao, C Netherlands Antilles
44 E5 **Santa Clara** Villa Clara, C Cuba
35 N9 **Santa Clara** California, W USA
36 J8 **Santa Clara** Utah, W USA
Santa Clara *see* Santa Clara de Olimar
61 F18 **Santa Clara de Olimar** *var.* Santa Clara. Cerro Largo, NE Uruguay
61 A17 **Santa Clara de Saguier** Santa Fe, C Argentina
Santa Coloma *see* Santa Coloma de Gramanet
105 X5 **Santa Coloma de Farners** *var.* Santa Coloma de Farnés. Cataluña, NE Spain
Santa Coloma de Farnés *see* Santa Coloma de Farners
105 W6 **Santa Coloma de Gramanet** *var.* Santa Coloma. Cataluña, NE Spain
104 G2 **Santa Comba** Galicia, NW Spain
Santa Comba *see* Uaco Cungo
104 H8 **Santa Comba Dão** Viseu, N Portugal
82 C10 **Santa Cruz** Uíge, NW Angola
57 N19 **Santa Cruz** *var.* Santa Cruz de la Sierra. Santa Cruz, C Bolivia
62 G12 **Santa Cruz** Libertador, C Chile
42 K13 **Santa Cruz** Guanacaste, W Costa Rica
44 I12 **Santa Cruz** W Jamaica
64 P6 **Santa Cruz** Madeira, Portugal, NE Atlantic Ocean
35 N10 **Santa Cruz** California, W USA
63 H20 **Santa Cruz** *off.* Provincia de Santa Cruz. ◈ *province* S Argentina
57 O18 **Santa Cruz** ◈ *department* E Bolivia
Santa Cruz *see* Viru-Viru
Santa Cruz *see* Puerto Santa Cruz
Santa Cruz Barillas *see* Barillas
59 O18 **Santa Cruz Cabrália** Bahia, E Brazil
Santa Cruz de El Seibo *see* El Seibo
64 N11 **Santa Cruz de la Palma** La Palma, Islas Canarias, Spain, NE Atlantic Ocean
Santa Cruz de la Sierra *see* Santa Cruz
105 O9 **Santa Cruz de la Zarza** Castilla-La Mancha, C Spain
42 C5 **Santa Cruz del Quiché** Quiché, W Guatemala
105 N8 **Santa Cruz del Retamar** Castilla-La Mancha, C Spain
Santa Cruz del Seibo *see* El Seibo
44 G7 **Santa Cruz del Sur** Camagüey, C Cuba
105 O11 **Santa Cruz de Mudela** Castilla-La Mancha, C Spain
64 Q11 **Santa Cruz de Tenerife** Tenerife, Islas Canarias, Spain, NE Atlantic Ocean
64 P11 **Santa Cruz de Tenerife** ◈ *province* Islas Canarias, Spain, NE Atlantic Ocean
60 K9 **Santa Cruz do Rio Pardo** São Paulo, S Brazil
61 H15 **Santa Cruz do Sul** Rio Grande do Sul, S Brazil
57 C17 **Santa Cruz, Isla** *var.* Indefatigable Island, Isla Chávez. *island* Galapagos Islands, Ecuador, E Pacific Ocean
40 F8 **Santa Cruz, Isla** *island* W Mexico
35 Q15 **Santa Cruz Island** *island* California, W USA
187 Q10 **Santa Cruz Islands** *island group* E Solomon Islands
63 I22 **Santa Cruz, Río** ≈ S Argentina
36 L15 **Santa Cruz River** ≈ Arizona, SW USA
61 C17 **Santa Elena** Entre Ríos, E Argentina
42 F2 **Santa Elena** Cayo, W Belize
25 R16 **Santa Elena** Texas, SW USA
56 A7 **Santa Elena, Bahía de** *bay* W Ecuador
55 R10 **Santa Elena de Uairén** Bolívar, E Venezuela
42 K12 **Santa Elena, Península** *peninsula* NW Costa Rica
56 A7 **Santa Elena, Punta** *headland* W Ecuador
104 L11 **Santa Eufemia** Andalucía, S Spain
107 N21 **Santa Eufemia, Golfo di** *gulf* S Italy
107 N21 **Santa Eufemia Lamezia Terme** Calabria, SE Italy
105 S4 **Santa Eulalia de Gállego** Aragón, NE Spain
105 V11 **Santa Eulalia del Río** Eivissa, Spain, W Mediterranean Sea
61 B17 **Santa Fe** Santa Fe, C Argentina
105 N14 **Santa Fe** Andalucía, S Spain
37 S10 **Santa Fe** *state capital* New Mexico, SW USA
61 B15 **Santa Fe** *off.* Provincia de Santa Fe. ◈ *province* C Argentina
Santa Fe *see* Bogotá
44 C6 **Santa Fé** *var.* La Fe. Isla de la Juventud, W Cuba
43 R16 **Santa Fé** Veraguas, C Panama
Santa Fe de Bogotá *see* Bogotá
60 J7 **Santa Fé do Sul** São Paulo, S Brazil
57 B18 **Santa Fe, Isla** *var.* Barrington Island. *island* Galapagos Islands, Ecuador, E Pacific Ocean
23 V9 **Santa Fe River** ≈ Florida, SE USA
59 M15 **Santa Filomena** Piauí, E Brazil
40 G10 **Santa Genoveva** ▲ W Mexico
153 S14 **Santahar** Rajshahi, NW Bangladesh
60 G11 **Santa Helena** Paraná, S Brazil
54 J5 **Santa Inés** Lara, N Venezuela
63 G24 **Santa Inés, Isla** *island* S Chile
62 J13 **Santa Isabel** La Pampa, C Argentina
43 U14 **Santa Isabel** Colón, N Panama
186 L8 **Santa Isabel** *var.* Bughotu. *island* N Solomon Islands
Santa Isabel *see* Malabo
58 D11 **Santa Isabel do Rio Negro** Amazonas, NW Brazil
61 C15 **Santa Lucia** Corrientes, NE Argentina
57 I17 **Santa Lucía** Puno, S Peru
61 F20 **Santa Lucía** *var.* Santa Lucia. Canelones, S Uruguay
42 B6 **Santa Lucía Cotzumalguapa** Escuintla, SW Guatemala
107 L23 **Santa Lucia del Mela** Sicilia, Italy, C Mediterranean Sea
35 O11 **Santa Lucia Range** ▲ California, W USA
40 D9 **Santa Margarita, Isla** *island* W Mexico
61 G15 **Santa Maria** Rio Grande do Sul, S Brazil
35 P13 **Santa Maria** California, W USA
64 Q4 **Santa Maria** ✕ Santa Maria, Azores, Portugal, NE Atlantic Ocean
64 P3 **Santa Maria** *island* Azores, Portugal, NE Atlantic Ocean
Santa Maria *see* Gaua.
62 J7 **Santa María** Catamarca, N Argentina
Santa María Asunción Tlaxiaco *see* Tlaxiaco
40 G9 **Santa María, Bahía** *bay* W Mexico
83 L21 **Santa Maria, Cabo de** *headland* S Mozambique
104 G15 **Santa Maria, Cabo de** *headland* S Portugal
44 J4 **Santa Maria, Cape** *headland* Long Island, C Bahamas
107 J17 **Santa Maria Capua Vetere** Campania, S Italy
59 M17 **Santa Maria da Vitória** Bahia, E Brazil
55 N9 **Santa Maria de Erebato** Bolívar, SE Venezuela
104 G7 **Santa Maria da Feira** Aveiro, N Portugal
55 N6 **Santa María de Ipire** Guárico, C Venezuela
Santa Maria del Buen Aire *see* Buenos Aires
40 J8 **Santa María del Oro** Durango, C Mexico
41 N12 **Santa María del Río** San Luis Potosí, C Mexico
Santa Maria di Castellabate *see* Castellabate
107 Q20 **Santa Maria di Leuca, Capo** *headland* SE Italy
108 K10 **Santa Maria-im-Münstertal** Graubünden, SE Switzerland
57 B18 **Santa María, Isla** *var.* Isla Floreana, Charles Island. *island* Galapagos Islands, Ecuador, E Pacific Ocean
40 J3 **Santa María, Laguna de** ◎ N Mexico
61 G16 **Santa Maria, Rio** ≈ S Brazil
43 R16 **Santa María, Río** ≈ C Panama
36 J12 **Santa Maria River** ≈ Arizona, SW USA
107 G15 **Santa Marinella** Lazio, C Italy
54 F4 **Santa Marta** Magdalena, N Colombia
104 J11 **Santa Marta** Extremadura, W Spain
Santa Maura *see* Lefkáda
35 S15 **Santa Monica** California, W USA
116 F10 **Sântana** *Ger.* Sankt Anna, *Hung.* Újszentanna; *prev.* Sîntana. Arad, W Romania
61 F16 **Santana, Coxilha de** *hill range* S Brazil
61 H16 **Santana da Boa Vista** Rio Grande do Sul, S Brazil
61 F16 **Santana do Livramento** *prev.* Livramento. Rio Grande do Sul, S Brazil
105 N2 **Santander** Cantabria, N Spain
54 F8 **Santander** *off.* Departamento de Santander. ◈ *province* C Colombia
Santander Jiménez *see* Jiménez
Sant'Andrea *see* Svetac
107 B20 **Sant'Antioco** Sardegna, Italy, C Mediterranean Sea
104 J13 **Santa Olalla del Cala** Andalucía, S Spain
35 R15 **Santa Paula** California, W USA
36 L4 **Santaquin** Utah, W USA
58 I12 **Santarém** Pará, N Brazil
104 G10 **Santarém** *anc.* Scalabis. Santarém, W Portugal
104 G10 **Santarém** ◈ *district* C Portugal
44 F4 **Santaren Channel** *channel* W Bahamas
54 K10 **Santa Rita** Vichada, E Colombia
188 B16 **Santa Rita** SW Guam
42 H5 **Santa Rita** Cortés, NW Honduras
40 E9 **Santa Rita** Baja California Sur, W Mexico
54 H5 **Santa Rita** Zulia, NW Venezuela
59 I19 **Santa Rita de Araguaia** Goiás, S Brazil
Santa Rita de Cassia *see* Cássia
61 D14 **Santa Rosa** Corrientes, NE Argentina
62 K13 **Santa Rosa** La Pampa, C Argentina
61 G14 **Santa Rosa** Rio Grande do Sul, S Brazil
58 E10 **Santa Rosa** Roraima, N Brazil
56 B8 **Santa Rosa** El Oro, SW Ecuador
57 I16 **Santa Rosa** Puno, S Peru
34 M7 **Santa Rosa** California, W USA
37 U11 **Santa Rosa** New Mexico, SW USA
55 O6 **Santa Rosa** Anzoátegui, NE Venezuela
42 A3 **Santa Rosa** *off.* Departamento de Santa Rosa. ◈ *department* SE Guatemala
Santa Rosa *see* Santa Rosa de Copán
63 J15 **Santa Rosa, Bajo de** *basin* E Argentina
42 F6 **Santa Rosa de Copán** *var.* Santa Rosa. Copán, W Honduras
54 E8 **Santa Rosa de Osos** Antioquia, C Colombia
35 Q15 **Santa Rosa Island** *island* California, W USA
23 O9 **Santa Rosa Island** *island* Florida, SE USA
40 E6 **Santa Rosalía** Baja California Sur, W Mexico
54 K6 **Santa Rosalía** Portuguesa, NW Venezuela
188 C15 **Santa Rosa, Mount** ▲ NE Guam
35 V16 **Santa Rosa Mountains** ▲ California, W USA
35 T2 **Santa Rosa Range** ▲ Nevada, W USA
62 M8 **Santa Sylvina** Chaco, N Argentina
Santa Tecla *see* Nueva San Salvador
61 B19 **Santa Teresa** Santa Fe, C Argentina
59 O20 **Santa Teresa** Espírito Santo, SE Brazil
107 M23 **Santa Teresa di Riva** Sicilia, Italy, C Mediterranean Sea
61 E21 **Santa Teresita** Buenos Aires, E Argentina
61 H19 **Santa Vitória do Palmar** Rio Grande do Sul, S Brazil
35 Q14 **Santa Ynez River** ≈ California, W USA
Sant Carles de la Rápida *see* Sant Carles de la Ràpita
105 U7 **Sant Carles de la Ràpita** *var.* Sant Carles de la Rápida. Cataluña, NE Spain
105 W5 **Sant Celoni** Cataluña, NE Spain
35 U17 **Santee** California, W USA
21 T13 **Santee River** ≈ South Carolina, SE USA
40 K15 **San Telmo, Punta** *headland* SW Mexico
107 O17 **Santeramo in Colle** Puglia, SE Italy
105 X5 **Sant Feliu de Guíxols** *var.* San Feliú de Guixols. Cataluña, NE Spain
105 W6 **Sant Feliu de Llobregat** Cataluña, NE Spain
106 C7 **Santhià** Piemonte, NE Italy
61 F15 **Santiago** Rio Grande do Sul, S Brazil
62 H11 **Santiago** *var.* Gran Santiago. ● (Chile) Santiago, C Chile
45 N8 **Santiago** *var.* Santiago de los Caballeros. N Dominican Republic
40 G10 **Santiago** Baja California Sur, W Mexico
41 O8 **Santiago** Nuevo León, NE Mexico
43 R16 **Santiago** Veraguas, S Panama
57 E16 **Santiago** Ica, SW Peru
104 G3 **Santiago** *var.* Santiago de Compostela, *Eng.* Compostella; *anc.* Campus Stellae. Galicia, NW Spain
62 H11 **Santiago** *off.* Región Metropolitana de Santiago, *var.* Metropolitan. ◈ *region* C Chile
62 H11 **Santiago** ✕ Santiago, C Chile
104 G3 **Santiago** ✕ Galicia, NW Spain
76 D10 **Santiago** *var.* São Tiago. *island* Ilhas de Sotavento, S Cape Verde
Santiago *see* Santiago de Cuba, Cuba
Santiago *see* Grande de Santiago, Río, Mexico
42 B6 **Santiago Atitlán** Sololá, SW Guatemala
43 Q16 **Santiago, Cerro** ▲ W Panama
Santiago de Compostela *see* Santiago
44 I8 **Santiago de Cuba** *var.* Santiago. Santiago de Cuba, E Cuba
Santiago de Guayaquil *see* Guayaquil
62 K8 **Santiago del Estero** Santiago del Estero, C Argentina
61 A15 **Santiago del Estero** *off.* Provincia de Santiago del Estero. ◈ *province* N Argentina
40 I8 **Santiago de los Caballeros** Sinaloa, W Mexico
Santiago de los Caballeros *see* Santiago, Dominican Republic
Santiago de los Caballeros *see* Guatemala, Guatemala
42 F8 **Santiago de María** Usulután, SE El Salvador
104 F12 **Santiago do Cacém** Setúbal, S Portugal
40 J12 **Santiago Ixcuintla** Nayarit, C Mexico
Santiago Jamiltepec *see* Jamiltepec
24 L11 **Santiago Mountains** ▲ Texas, SW USA
40 J9 **Santiago Papasquiaro** Durango, C Mexico
Santiago Pinotepa Nacional *see* Pinotepa Nacional
56 C8 **Santiago, Río** ≈ N Peru
40 M10 **San Tiburcio** Zacatecas, C Mexico
105 N2 **Santillana** Cantabria, N Spain
54 I5 **San Timoteo** Zulia, NW Venezuela
Santi Quaranta *see* Sarandë
Santissima Trinidad *see* Chilung
105 O12 **Santisteban del Puerto** Andalucía, S Spain
105 U7 **Sant Jordi, Golf de** *gulf* NE Spain
105 T8 **Sant Mateu** País Valenciano, E Spain
25 S7 **Santo** Texas, SW USA
Santo *see* Espiritu Santo
60 M10 **Santo Amaro, Ilha de** *island* SE Brazil
61 G14 **Santo Ângelo** Rio Grande do Sul, S Brazil
76 C9 **Santo Antão** *island* Ilhas de Barlavento, N Cape Verde
60 J10 **Santo Antônio da Platina** Paraná, S Brazil
58 C13 **Santo Antônio do Içá** Amazonas, N Brazil
57 Q18 **Santo Corazón, Río** ≈ E Bolivia
44 E5 **Santo Domingo** Villa Clara, C Cuba
45 O9 **Santo Domingo** *prev.* Ciudad Trujillo. ● (Dominican Republic) SE Dominican Republic
40 E8 **Santo Domingo** Baja California Sur, W Mexico
40 M10 **Santo Domingo** San Luis Potosí, C Mexico
42 L10 **Santo Domingo** Chontales, S Nicaragua
105 P4 **Santo Domingo de la Calzada** La Rioja, N Spain
56 B6 **Santo Domingo de los Colorados** Pichincha, NW Ecuador
Santo Domingo Tehuantepec *see* Tehuantepec
55 O6 **San Tomé** Anzoátegui, NE Venezuela
San Tomé de Guayana *see* Ciudad Guayana
105 R13 **Santomera** Murcia, SE Spain
105 O2 **Santoña** Cantabria, N Spain
Santorin/Santoríni *see* Thíra
60 M10 **Santos** São Paulo, S Brazil
65 J17 **Santos Plateau** *undersea feature* SW Atlantic Ocean
104 G6 **Santo Tirso** Porto, N Portugal
40 B2 **Santo Tomás** Baja California, NW Mexico
42 L10 **Santo Tomás** Chontales, S Nicaragua
42 G5 **Santo Tomás de Castilla** Izabal, E Guatemala
40 B2 **Santo Tomás, Punta** *headland* NW Mexico
57 H16 **Santo Tomás, Río** ≈ C Peru
57 B18 **Santo Tomás, Volcán** ☒ Galapagos Islands, Ecuador, E Pacific Ocean
61 F14 **Santo Tomé** Corrientes, NE Argentina
Santo Tomé de Guayana *see* Ciudad Guayana
98 H10 **Santpoort** Noord-Holland, W Netherlands
Santurce *see* Santurtzi
105 O2 **Santurtzi** *var.* Santurce, Santurzi. País Vasco, N Spain
Santurzi *see* Santurtzi
63 G20 **San Valentín, Cerro** ▲ S Chile
42 F8 **San Vicente** San Vicente, C El Salvador
40 C2 **San Vicente** Baja California, NW Mexico
188 H6 **San Vicente** Saipan, S Northern Mariana Islands
42 B9 **San Vicente** ◈ *department* E El Salvador
104 I10 **San Vicente de Alcántara** Extremadura, W Spain
105 N2 **San Vicente de Barakaldo** *var.* Baracaldo. País Vasco, N Spain
57 E15 **San Vicente de Cañete** *var.* Cañete. Lima, W Peru
104 M2 **San Vicente de la Barquera** Cantabria, N Spain
54 E12 **San Vicente del Caguán** Caquetá, S Colombia
42 F8 **San Vicente, Volcán de** ☒ C El Salvador
43 O15 **San Vito** Puntarenas, SE Costa Rica
106 I7 **San Vito al Tagliamento** Friuli-Venezia Giulia, NE Italy
107 H23 **San Vito, Capo** *headland* Sicilia, Italy, C Mediterranean Sea
107 P18 **San Vito dei Normanni** Puglia, SE Italy
160 L17 **Sanya** *var.* Ya Xian. Hainan, S China
83 J16 **Sanyati** ≈ N Zimbabwe
25 Q16 **San Ygnacio** Texas, SW USA
160 L6 **Sanyuan** Shaanxi, C China
123 P11 **Sanyyakhtakh** Respublika Sakha (Yakutiya), NE Russian Federation
82 C10 **Sanza Pombo** Uíge, NW Angola
Sanzyô *see* Sanjō
104 G14 **São Bartolomeu de Messines** Faro, S Portugal
60 M10 **São Bernardo do Campo** São Paulo, S Brazil
61 F15 **São Borja** Rio Grande do Sul, S Brazil
104 H14 **São Brás de Alportel** Faro, S Portugal
60 M10 **São Caetano do Sul** São Paulo, S Brazil
60 L9 **São Carlos** São Paulo, S Brazil
59 P16 **São Cristóvão** Sergipe, E Brazil
61 F15 **São Francisco de Assis** Rio Grande do Sul, S Brazil
58 K13 **São Félix** Pará, NE Brazil
São Félix *see* São Félix do Araguaia
59 J16 **São Félix do Araguaia** *var.* São Félix. Mato Grosso, W Brazil
59 J14 **São Félix do Xingu** Pará, NE Brazil
60 Q9 **São Fidélis** Rio de Janeiro, SE Brazil
76 D10 **São Filipe** Fogo, S Cape Verde
60 K12 **São Francisco do Sul** Santa Catarina, S Brazil
60 K12 **São Francisco, Ilha de** *island* S Brazil
59 P16 **São Francisco, Rio** ≈ E Brazil
61 G16 **São Gabriel** Rio Grande do Sul, S Brazil
60 P10 **São Gonçalo** Rio de Janeiro, SE Brazil
81 H23 **Sao Hill** Iringa, S Tanzania
60 R9 **São João da Barra** Rio de Janeiro, SE Brazil
104 G7 **São João da Madeira** Aveiro, N Portugal
58 M12 **São João de Cortês** Maranhão, E Brazil
59 M21 **São João del Rei** Minas Gerais, NE Brazil
59 N15 **São João do Piauí** Piauí, E Brazil
59 N14 **São João dos Patos** Maranhão, E Brazil
58 C11 **São Joaquim** Amazonas, NW Brazil
61 J14 **São Joaquim** Santa Catarina, S Brazil
60 L7 **São Joaquim da Barra** São Paulo, S Brazil
64 N2 **São Jorge** *island* Azores, Portugal, NE Atlantic Ocean
61 K14 **São José** Santa Catarina, S Brazil
60 M8 **São José do Rio Pardo** São Paulo, S Brazil
60 K8 **São José do Rio Preto** São Paulo, S Brazil
60 N10 **São Jose dos Campos** São Paulo, S Brazil
61 I17 **São Lourenço do Sul** Rio Grande do Sul, S Brazil
58 F11 **São Luís** Roraima, N Brazil
58 M12 **São Luís** *state capital* Maranhão, NE Brazil
58 M12 **São Luís, Ilha de** *island* NE Brazil
61 F14 **São Luiz Gonzaga** Rio Grande do Sul, S Brazil
104 I10 **São Mamede** ▲ C Portugal
São Mandol *see* São Manuel, Rio
47 U8 **São Manuel** ≈ C Brazil
59 H15 **São Manuel, Rio** *var.* São Mandol, Teles Pirés. ≈ C Brazil
58 C11 **São Marcelino** Amazonas, NW Brazil
58 N12 **São Marcos, Baía de** *bay* N Brazil
59 O20 **São Mateus** Espírito Santo, SE Brazil
60 J12 **São Mateus do Sul** Paraná, S Brazil
64 P3 **São Miguel** *island* Azores, Portugal, NE Atlantic Ocean
60 G13 **São Miguel d'Oeste** Santa Catarina, S Brazil
45 P9 **Saona, Isla** *island* SE Dominican Republic
172 H12 **Saondzou** ▲ Grande Comore, NW Comoros
103 R10 **Saône** ≈ E France
103 Q9 **Saône-et-Loire** ◈ *department* C France
76 D9 **São Nicolau** *Eng.* Saint Nicholas. *island* Ilhas de Barlavento, N Cape Verde
60 M10 **São Paulo** *state capital* São Paulo, S Brazil
60 K9 **São Paulo** *off.* Estado de São Paulo. ◈ *state* S Brazil
São Paulo de Loanda *see* Luanda
São Pedro do Rio Grande do Sul *see* Rio Grande
104 H7 **São Pedro do Sul** Viseu, N Portugal
64 K13 **São Pedro e São Paulo** *undersea feature* C Atlantic Ocean
59 M14 **São Raimundo das Mangabeiras** Maranhão, E Brazil
59 Q14 **São Roque, Cabo de** *headland* E Brazil
São Salvador/São Salvador do Congo *see* M'Banza Congo, Angola
São Salvador *see* Salvador, Brazil
60 N10 **São Sebastião, Ilha de** *island* S Brazil
83 N19 **São Sebastião, Ponta** *headland* C Mozambique
104 F13 **São Teotónio** Beja, S Portugal
São Tiago *see* Santiago
79 B18 **São Tomé** ● (Sao Tome and Principe) São Tomé, S Sao Tome and Principe
79 B18 **São Tomé** ✕ São Tomé, S Sao Tome and Principe
79 B18 **São Tomé** *Eng.* Saint Thomas. *island* S Sao Tome and Principe
79 B17 **Sao Tome and Principe** *off.* Democratic Republic of Sao Tome and Principe. ◆ *republic* E Atlantic Ocean
74 H9 **Saoura, Oued** ≈ NW Algeria
60 M10 **São Vicente** *Eng.* Saint Vincent. São Paulo, S Brazil
64 O5 **São Vicente** Madeira, Portugal, NE Atlantic Ocean
76 C9 **São Vicente** *Eng.* Saint Vincent. *island* Ilhas de Barlavento, N Cape Verde
São Vicente, Cabo de *see* São Vicente, Cabo de
104 F14 **São Vicente, Cabo de** *Eng.* Cape Saint Vincent, *Port.* Cabo de São Vicente. *headland* S Portugal
Sápai *see* Sápes
Sapaleri, Cerro *see* Zapaleri, Cerro
Saparoea *see* Saparua
171 S13 **Saparua** *prev.* Saparoea. C Indonesia
168 L11 **Sapat** Sumatera, W Indonesia
77 U17 **Sapele** Delta, S Nigeria
23 X7 **Sapelo Island** *island* Georgia, SE USA
23 X7 **Sapelo Sound** *sound* Georgia, SE USA
114 K13 **Sápes** *var.* Sápai. Anatolikí Makedonía kai Thráki, NE Greece
115 D22 **Sapiéntza** *island* S Greece
Sapir *see* Sappir
61 I15 **Sapiranga** Rio Grande do Sul, S Brazil
114 K13 **Sápka** ▲ NE Greece
56 D11 **Saposoa** San Martín, N Peru
119 F16 **Sapotskino** *Pol.* Sopockinie, *Rus.* Sopotskin. Hrodzyenskaya Voblasts', W Belarus
77 P13 **Sapoui** *var.* Sapouy. S Burkina
Sapouy *see* Sapoui
138 F12 **Sappir** *var.* Sapir. Southern, S Israel
165 S4 **Sapporo** Hokkaidō, NE Japan
107 M19 **Sapri** Campania, S Italy
169 T16 **Sapudi, Pulau** *island* S Indonesia
27 P9 **Sapulpa** Oklahoma, C USA
142 J4 **Saqqez** *var.* Saghez, Sakiz, Saqqiz. Kordestān, NW Iran
Saqqiz *see* Saqqez
139 U8 **Sarābādī** E Iraq
167 P10 **Sara Buri** *var.* Saraburi. Saraburi, C Thailand
24 K9 **Saragosa** Texas, SW USA
Saragossa *see* Zaragoza
Saragt *see* Serakhs
56 B8 **Saraguro** Loja, S Ecuador
128 M6 **Sarai** Ryazanskaya Oblast', W Russian Federation
Sarāi *see* Sarāy
154 M12 **Saraipāli** Madhya Pradesh, C India
149 T9 **Sarāi Sidhu** Punjab, E Pakistan
93 M15 **Säräisniemi** Oulu, C Finland
113 I14 **Sarajevo** ● (Bosnia and Herzegovina) Federacija Bosna I Hercegovina, SE Bosnia and Herzegovina
112 I13 **Sarajevo** ✕ Federacija Bosna I Hercegovina, C Bosnia and Herzegovina
143 V4 **Sarakhs** Khorāsān, NE Iran
115 H17 **Sarakíniko, Akrotírio** *headland* Évvoia, C Greece
115 I18 **Sarakinó** *island* Vóreioi Sporádes, Greece, Aegean Sea

◆ Country ● Country Capital ◇ Dependent Territory ○ Dependent Territory Capital ◈ Administrative Region ✕ International Airport ▲ Mountain ▲ Mountain Range ☒ Volcano ≈ River ◎ Lake ▣ Reservoir

129 V7 **Saraktash** Orenburgskaya Oblast', W Russian Federation
30 L15 **Sara, Lake** ▣ Illinois, N USA
23 N8 **Saraland** Alabama, S USA
55 V9 **Saramacca** ◈ *district* N Surinam
55 V10 **Saramacca Rivier** ∼ C Surinam
166 M2 **Saramati** ▲ N Myanmar
145 R10 **Saran'** *Kaz.* Saran. Karaganda, C Kazakhstan
18 K7 **Saranac Lake** New York, NE USA
18 K7 **Saranac River** ∼ New York, NE USA
Saranda *see* Sarandë
113 L23 **Sarandë** *var.* Saranda, *It.* Porto Edda; *prev.* Santi Quaranta. Vlorë, S Albania
61 H14 **Sarandi** Rio Grande do Sul, S Brazil
61 F19 **Sarandí del Yí** Durazno, C Uruguay
61 F19 **Sarandí Grande** Florida, S Uruguay
171 Q8 **Sarangani Islands** *island group* S Philippines
129 P5 **Saransk** Respublika Mordoviya, W Russian Federation
115 C14 **Sarantáporos** ∼ N Greece
114 H9 **Sarantsi** Sofiya, W Bulgaria
129 T3 **Sarapul** Udmurtskaya Respublika, NW Russian Federation
Sarâqeb *see* Sarāqib
138 I3 **Sarāqib** *Fr.* Sarâqeb. Idlib, N Syria
54 J5 **Sarare** Lara, N Venezuela
55 O10 **Sarariña** Amazonas, S Venezuela
143 S10 **Sar Ashk** Kermān, C Iran
23 V13 **Sarasota** Florida, SE USA
117 O11 **Sarata** Odes'ka Oblast', SW Ukraine
116 I10 **Sărăţel** *Hung.* Szeretfalva. Bistriţa-Năsăud, N Romania
25 X10 **Saratoga** Texas, SW USA
18 K10 **Saratoga Springs** New York, NE USA
129 P8 **Saratov** Saratovskaya Oblast', W Russian Federation
129 P8 **Saratovskaya Oblast'** ◈ *province* W Russian Federation
129 Q7 **Saratovskoye Vodokhranilishche** ▣ W Russian Federation
Saravan/Saravane *see* Salavan
169 S9 **Sarawak** ◈ *state* East Malaysia
Sarawak *see* Kuching
139 U6 **Sarāy** *var.* Sarāi. E Iraq
136 D10 **Saray** Tekirdağ, NW Turkey
76 J12 **Saraya** SE Senegal
143 W14 **Sarbāz** Sīstān va Balūchestān, SE Iran
143 U8 **Sarbīsheh** Khorāsān, E Iran
111 J24 **Sárbogárd** Fejér, C Hungary
Şărcad *see* Sarkad
27 S7 **Sarcoxie** Missouri, C USA
152 L11 **Sārda** *Nep.* Kali. ∼ India/Nepal
152 G10 **Sardārshahr** Rājasthān, NW India
107 C18 **Sardegna** *Eng.* Sardinia. ◈ *region* Italy, C Mediterranean Sea
107 A18 **Sardegna** *Eng.* Sardinia. *island* Italy, C Mediterranean Sea
42 K13 **Sardinal** Guanacaste, NW Costa Rica
54 G7 **Sardinata** Norte de Santander, N Colombia
Sardinia *see* Sardegna
120 K8 **Sardinia-Corsica Trough** *undersea feature* Tyrrhenian Sea, C Mediterranean Sea
22 L2 **Sardis** Mississippi, S USA
22 L2 **Sardis Lake** ▣ Mississippi, S USA
27 P12 **Sardis Lake** ▣ Oklahoma, C USA
92 H12 **Sarek** ▲ N Sweden
149 N3 **Sar-e Pol** *var.* Sar-i-Pul. Sar-e Pol, N Afghanistan
149 O3 **Sar-e Pol** ◈ *province* N Afghanistan
Sar-e Pol *see* Sar-e Pol-e Žahāb
142 J6 **Sar-e Pol-e Žahāb** *var.* Sar-e Pol, Sar-i Pul. Kermānshāh, W Iran
147 T13 **Sarez, Kŭli** *Rus.* Sarezskoye Ozero. ◎ SE Tajikistan
Sarezskoye Ozero *see* Sarez, Kŭli
64 G10 **Sargasso Sea** *sea* W Atlantic Ocean
149 U8 **Sargodha** Punjab, NE Pakistan
78 I13 **Sarh** *prev.* Fort-Archambault. Moyen-Chari, S Chad
143 P4 **Sārī** *var.* Sari, Sāri. Māzandarān, N Iran
115 N23 **Saría** *island* SE Greece
Sariasiya *see* Sariosiyo
40 F3 **Saric** Sonora, NW Mexico
188 K6 **Sarigan** *island* C Northern Mariana Islands
136 D14 **Sarıgöl** Manisa, SW Turkey
139 T6 **Sārihah** E Iraq
137 R12 **Sarıkamış** Kars, NE Turkey
169 R9 **Sarikei** Sarawak, East Malaysia
147 U12 **Sarikol Range** *Rus.* Sarykol'skiy Khrebet. ▲ China/Tajikistan
181 Y7 **Sarina** Queensland, NE Australia
Sarine *see* La Sarine
105 S5 **Sariñena** Aragón, NE Spain
147 O13 **Sariosiyo** *Rus.* Sariasiya. Surkhondaryo Wiloyati, S Uzbekistan
Sar-i-Pul *see* Sar-e Pol, Afghanistan
Sar-i Pul *see* Sar-e Pol-e Žahāb, Iran
Sariqamish Kŭli *see* Sarykamyshkoye Ozero
149 V1 **Sarī Qūl** *Rus.* Ozero Zurkul', *Taj.* Zŭrkŭl. ◎ Afghanistan/Tajikistan *see also* Zūrkūl
75 Q12 **Sarīr Tibistī** *var.* Serir Tibesti. *desert* S Libya
25 S15 **Sarita** Texas, SW USA
163 W14 **Sariwŏn** SW North Korea
114 P12 **Sarıyer** İstanbul, NW Turkey
97 L26 **Sark** *Fr.* Sercq. *island* Channel Islands
111 N24 **Sarkad** *Rom.* Şărcad. Békés, SE Hungary
145 W14 **Sarkand** Almaty, SW Kazakhstan
Sarkaṇi *see* Krasnogorskoye
152 D11 **Sarkāri Tala** Rājasthān, NW India
136 G15 **Şarkîkaraağaç** *var.* Şarki Karaağaç. Isparta, SW Turkey
136 L13 **Şarkışla** Sivas, C Turkey
136 C11 **Şarköy** Tekirdağ, NW Turkey
Sárköz *see* Livada
Sarlat *see* Sarlat-la-Canéda
102 M13 **Sarlat-la-Canéda** *var.* Sarlat. Dordogne, SW France
109 S3 **Sarleinsbach** Oberösterreich, N Austria
171 Y12 **Sarmi** Irian Jaya, E Indonesia
63 I19 **Sarmiento** Chubut, S Argentina
63 H25 **Sarmiento, Monte** ▲ S Chile
94 J11 **Särna** Dalarna, C Sweden
108 F8 **Sarnen** Obwalden, C Switzerland
108 F9 **Sarner See** ◎ C Switzerland
14 D16 **Sarnia** Ontario, S Canada
116 L3 **Sarny** Rivnens'ka Oblast', NW Ukraine
171 O13 **Saroako** Sulawesi, C Indonesia
118 L13 **Sarochyna** *Rus.* Sorochino. Vitsyebskaya Voblasts', N Belarus
168 L12 **Sarolangun** Sumatera, W Indonesia
165 U3 **Saroma** Hokkaidō, NE Japan
165 V3 **Saroma-ko** ◎ Hokkaidō, NE Japan
Saronic Gulf *see* Saronikós Kólpos
115 H20 **Saronikós Kólpos** *Eng.* Saronic Gulf. *gulf* S Greece
106 D7 **Saronno** Lombardia, N Italy
136 B11 **Saros Körfezi** *gulf* NW Turkey
111 N20 **Sárospatak** Borsod-Abaúj-Zemplén, NE Hungary
129 P12 **Sarpa** Respublika Kalmykiya, SW Russian Federation
129 P12 **Sarpa, Ozero** ◎ SW Russian Federation
113 M18 **Šar Planina** ▲ FYR Macedonia/Yugoslavia
95 I16 **Sarpsborg** Østfold, S Norway
139 U5 **Sarqalā** N Iraq
103 U4 **Sarralbe** Moselle, NE France
Sarre *see* Saar, France/Germany
Sarre *see* Saarland, Germany
103 U5 **Sarrebourg** *Ger.* Saarburg. Moselle, NE France
Sarrebruck *see* Saarbrücken
103 U4 **Sarreguemines** *prev.* Saargemund. Moselle, NE France
104 I3 **Sarria** Galicia, NW Spain
105 S8 **Sarrión** Aragón, NE Spain
42 F4 **Sarstoon** *Sp.* Río Sarstún. ∼ Belize/Guatemala
Sarstún, Río *see* Sarstoon
123 Q9 **Sartang** ∼ NE Russian Federation
103 X16 **Sartène** Corse, France, C Mediterranean Sea
102 K7 **Sarthe** ◈ *department* NW France
102 K7 **Sarthe** ∼ N France
115 H15 **Sárti** Kentrikí Makedonía, N Greece
165 T1 **Sarufutsu** Hokkaidō, NE Japan
Saruhan *see* Manisa
152 G9 **Sarūpsar** Rājasthān, NW India
137 U13 **Şärur** *prev.* Il'ichevsk. SW Azerbaijan
Sarvani *see* Marneuli
111 G23 **Sárvár** Vas, W Hungary
143 P11 **Sarvestān** Fārs, S Iran
171 W12 **Sarwon** Irian Jaya, E Indonesia
145 P17 **Saryagach** *Kaz.* Saryaghash. Yuzhnyy Kazakhstan, S Kazakhstan
Saryaghash *see* Saryagach
Saryarqa *see* Kazakhskiy Melkosopochnik
147 W8 **Sary-Bulak** Narynskaya Oblast', C Kyrgyzstan
147 U10 **Sary-Bulak** Oshskaya Oblast', SW Kyrgyzstan
117 S14 **Sarych, Mys** *headland* S Ukraine
147 Z7 **Sary-Dzhaz** *var.* Aksu He. ∼ China/Kyrgyzstan *see also* Aksu He
145 T14 **Saryesik-Atyrau, Peski** *desert* E Kazakhstan
144 G13 **Sarykamys** *Kaz.* Saryqamys. Mangistau, SW Kazakhstan
146 F8 **Sarykamyshkoye Ozero** *Uzb.* Sariqamish Kŭli. *salt lake* Kazakhstan/Uzbekistan
Sarykol'skiy Khrebet *see* Sarikol Range
144 M10 **Sarykopa, Ozero** ◎ C Kazakhstan
145 V15 **Saryozek** *Kaz.* Saryözek. Almaty, SE Kazakhstan
Saryqamys *see* Sarykamys
145 S13 **Saryshagan** *Kaz.* Saryshahan. Zhezkazgan, SE Kazakhstan
Saryshahan *see* Saryshagan
145 O13 **Sarysu** ∼ S Kazakhstan
147 T11 **Sary-Tash** Oshskaya Oblast', SW Kyrgyzstan
146 J15 **Saryyazynskoye Vodokhranilishche** ▣ S Turkmenistan
106 E10 **Sarzana** Liguria, NW Italy
188 B17 **Sasalaguan, Mount** ▲ S Guam
153 O14 **Sasarām** Bihār, N India
186 M8 **Sasari, Mount** ▲ Santa Isabel, N Solomon Islands
164 C13 **Sasebo** Nagasaki, Kyūshū, SW Japan
14 I9 **Saseginaga, Lac** ◎ Quebec, SE Canada
Saseno *see* Sazan
11 R13 **Saskatchewan** ◈ *province* SW Canada
11 U14 **Saskatchewan** ∼ Manitoba/Saskatchewan, C Canada
11 T15 **Saskatoon** Saskatchewan, S Canada
11 T15 **Saskatoon** ✕ Saskatchewan, S Canada
123 N7 **Saskylakh** Respublika Sakha (Yakutiya), NE Russian Federation
42 L7 **Saslaya, Cerro** ▲ N Nicaragua
38 G17 **Sasmik, Cape** *headland* Tanaga Island, Alaska, USA
119 N19 **Sasnovy Bor** *Rus.* Sosnovyy Bor. Homyel'skaya Voblasts', SE Belarus
129 N5 **Sasovo** Ryazanskaya Oblast', W Russian Federation
25 S12 **Saspamco** Texas, SW USA
109 W9 **Sass** *var.* Sassbach. ∼ SE Austria
76 M17 **Sassandra** S Ivory Coast
76 M17 **Sassandra** *var.* Ibo, Sassandra Fleuve. ∼ S Ivory Coast
Sassandra Fleuve *see* Sassandra
107 B17 **Sassari** Sardegna, Italy, C Mediterranean Sea
Sassbach *see* Sass
98 H11 **Sassenheim** Zuid-Holland, W Netherlands
Sassmacken *see* Valdemārpils
100 O7 **Sassnitz** Mecklenburg-Vorpommern, NE Germany
99 E16 **Sas van Gent** Zeeland, SW Netherlands
145 W12 **Sasykkol', Ozero** ◎ E Kazakhstan
117 O12 **Sasyk Kunduk, Ozero** ◎ SW Ukraine
76 J12 **Satadougou** Kayes, SW Mali
105 V11 **Sa Talaiassa** ▲ Eivissa, Spain, W Mediterranean Sea
164 C17 **Sata-misaki** *headland* Kyūshū, SW Japan
26 I7 **Satanta** Kansas, C USA
155 E15 **Sātāra** Mahārāshtra, W India
192 G15 **Sātaua** Savai'i, NW Samoa
188 M16 **Satawal** *island* Caroline Islands, C Micronesia
189 R17 **Satawan Atoll** *atoll* Mortlock Islands, C Micronesia
23 Y12 **Satellite Beach** Florida, SE USA
95 M14 **Säter** Dalarna, C Sweden
Sathmar *see* Satu Mare
23 V7 **Satilla River** ∼ Georgia, SE USA
57 F14 **Satipo** *var.* San Francisco de Satipo. Junín, C Peru
122 F11 **Satka** Chelyabinskaya Oblast', C Russian Federation
153 T16 **Satkhira** Khulna, SW Bangladesh
154 K9 **Satna** *prev.* Sutna. Madhya Pradesh, C India
103 R11 **Satolas** ✕ (Lyon) Rhône, E France
111 N20 **Sátoraljaújhely** Borsod-Abaúj-Zemplén, NE Hungary
145 O12 **Satpayev** *prev.* Nikol'skiy. Zhezkazgan, C Kazakhstan
154 G11 **Sātpura Range** ▲ C India
167 P12 **Sattahip** *var.* Ban Sattahip, Ban Sattahipp. Chon Buri, S Thailand
92 L11 **Sattanen** Lappi, NE Finland
Satul *see* Satun
116 H9 **Satulung** *Hung.* Kővárhosszúfalu. Maramureş, N Romania
Satul-Vechi *see* Staro Selo
116 G8 **Satu Mare** *Ger.* Sathmar, *Hung.* Szatmárnémeti. Satu Mare, NW Romania
116 G8 **Satu Mare** ◈ *county* NW Romania
167 N16 **Satun** *var.* Satul, Setul. Satun, SW Thailand
192 G16 **Satupaiteau** Savai'i, W Samoa
Sau *see* Sava
14 F14 **Sauble** ∼ Ontario, S Canada
14 F13 **Sauble Beach** Ontario, S Canada
61 C16 **Sauce** Corrientes, NE Argentina
Sauce *see* Juan L.Lacaze
36 K15 **Sauceda Mountains** ▲ Arizona, SW USA
61 C17 **Sauce de Luna** Entre Ríos, E Argentina
63 L15 **Sauce Grande, Río** ∼ E Argentina
40 K6 **Saucillo** Chihuahua, N Mexico
95 D15 **Sauda** Rogaland, S Norway
145 Q16 **Saudakent** *Kaz.* Saūdakent; *prev.* Baykadam *Kaz.* Bayqadam. Zhambyl, S Kazakhstan
92 J2 **Saudhárkrókur** Nordhurland Vestra, N Iceland
141 P9 **Saudi Arabia** *off.* Kingdom of Saudi Arabia, *Ar.* Al 'Arabīyah as Su'ūdīyah, Al Mamlakah al 'Arabīyah as Su'ūdīyah. ◆ *monarchy* SW Asia
101 D19 **Sauer** *var.* Sûre. ∼ NW Europe *see also* Sûre
101 F15 **Sauerland** *forest* W Germany
14 F14 **Saugeen** ∼ Ontario, S Canada
18 K12 **Saugerties** New York, NE USA
Saugor *see* Sāgar
10 K15 **Saugstad, Mount** ▲ British Columbia, SW Canada
Sāūjbulāgh *see* Mahābād
102 J11 **Saujon** Charente-Maritime, W France
29 T7 **Sauk Centre** Minnesota, N USA
30 L8 **Sauk City** Wisconsin, N USA
29 U7 **Sauk Rapids** Minnesota, N USA
55 Y11 **Saül** C French Guiana
103 O7 **Sauldre** ∼ C France
101 I23 **Saulgau** Baden-Württemberg, SW Germany
103 Q8 **Saulieu** Côte d'Or, C France
118 G8 **Saulkrasti** Rīga, C Latvia
15 S6 **Sault-aux-Cochons, Rivière du** ∼ Quebec, SE Canada
31 Q4 **Sault Sainte Marie** Michigan, N USA
12 F14 **Sault Ste.Marie** Ontario, S Canada
145 P7 **Saumalkol'** *prev.* Volodarskoye. Severnyy Kazakhstan, N Kazakhstan
190 E13 **Sauma, Pointe** *headland* Île Alofi, W Wallis and Futuna
171 T16 **Saumlaki** *var.* Saumlakki. Pulau Yamdena, E Indonesia
Saumlakki *see* Saumlaki
15 R12 **Saumon, Rivière au** ∼ Quebec, SE Canada
102 K8 **Saumur** Maine-et-Loire, NW France
185 F23 **Saunders, Cape** *headland* South Island, NZ
195 N13 **Saunders Coast** *physical region* Antarctica
65 B23 **Saunders Island** *island* NW Falkland Islands
65 C24 **Saunders Island Settlement** Saunders Island, NW Falkland Islands
82 F11 **Saurimo** *Port.* Henrique de Carvalho, Vila Henrique de Carvalho. Lunda Sul, NE Angola
55 S11 **Sauriwaunawa** S Guyana
82 D11 **Sautar** Malanje, NW Angola
45 S13 **Sauteurs** N Grenada
102 K13 **Sauveterre-de-Guyenne** Gironde, SW France
119 O14 **Sava** *Rus.* Sava. Mahilyowskaya Voblasts', E Belarus
84 H11 **Sava** *Eng.* Save, *Ger.* Sau, *Hung.* Száva. ∼ SE Europe
42 J5 **Savá** Colón, N Honduras
33 Y8 **Savage** Montana, NW USA
183 N16 **Savage River** Tasmania, SE Australia
77 R15 **Savalou** S Benin
30 K10 **Savanna** Illinois, N USA
23 X6 **Savannah** Georgia, SE USA
27 R2 **Savannah** Missouri, C USA
20 H10 **Savannah** Tennessee, S USA
21 O12 **Savannah River** ∼ Georgia/South Carolina, SE USA
Savannakhét *see* Khanthabouli
44 H12 **Savanna-La-Mar** W Jamaica
12 B10 **Savant Lake** ◎ Ontario, S Canada
155 F17 **Savanūr** Karnātaka, W India
93 J16 **Sävar** Västerbotten, N Sweden
Savaria *see* Szombathely
154 C11 **Sāvarkundla** *var.* Kundla. Gujarāt, W India
116 F11 **Săvârşin** *Hung.* Soborsin; *prev.* Săvirşin. Arad, W Romania
136 C13 **Savaştepe** Balıkesir, W Turkey
Savat *see* Sawot
83 N18 **Save** Inhambane, E Mozambique
102 L16 **Save** ∼ S France
83 L17 **Save** *var.* Sabi. ∼ Mozambique/Zimbabwe *see also* Sabi
Save *see* Sava
77 R15 **Savè** SE Benin
142 M6 **Sāveh** Markazī, W Iran
116 L8 **Săveni** Botoşani, NE Romania
103 N16 **Saverdun** Ariège, S France
103 U5 **Saverne** *var.* Zabern; *anc.* Tres Tabernae. Bas-Rhin, NE France
Savichi *see* Savichy
119 O21 **Savichy** *Rus.* Savichi. Homyel'skaya Voblasts', SE Belarus
106 B9 **Savigliano** Piemonte, NW Italy
Savigsivik *see* Savissivik
Savinichi *see* Savinichy
119 Q16 **Savinichy** *Rus.* Savinichi. Mahilyowskaya Voblasts', E Belarus
Savinski *see* Savinskiy
106 H11 **Savio** ∼ C Italy
Săvirşin *see* Săvârşin
197 O11 **Savissivik** *var.* Savigsivik. Avannaarsua, S Greenland
93 N18 **Savitaipale** Etelä-Suomi, S Finland
113 J15 **Šavnik** Montenegro, SW Yugoslavia
108 I9 **Savognin** Graubünden, S Switzerland
103 T12 **Savoie** ◈ *department* E France
106 C10 **Savona** Liguria, NW Italy
93 N17 **Savonlinna** *Swe.* Nyslott. Itä-Suomi, SE Finland
93 N17 **Savonranta** Itä-Suomi, SE Finland
38 K10 **Savoonga** Saint Lawrence Island, Alaska, USA
30 M13 **Savoy** Illinois, N USA
117 O8 **Savran'** Odes'ka Oblast', SW Ukraine
137 R11 **Şavşat** Artvin, NE Turkey
95 L19 **Sävsjö** Jönköping, S Sweden
Savu, Kepulauan *see* Sawu, Kepulauan
92 M11 **Savukoski** Lappi, NE Finland
Savu, Pulau *see* Sawu, Pulau
187 Y14 **Savusavu** Vanua Levu, N Fiji
171 O17 **Savu Sea** *Ind.* Laut Sawu. *sea* S Indonesia
83 H17 **Savute** Chobe, N Botswana
139 N7 **Şawāb 'Uqlat** *well* W Iraq
138 M7 **Şawāb, Wādī aş** *dry watercourse* W Iraq
152 H13 **Sawāi Mādhopur** Rājasthān, N India**Sawakin** *see* Suakin
167 R8 **Sawang Daen Din** Sakon Nakhon, E Thailand
167 O8 **Sawankhalok** *var.* Swankalok. Sukhothai, NW Thailand
165 P13 **Sawara** Chiba, Honshū, S Japan
37 R5 **Sawatch Range** ▲ Colorado, C USA
141 N12 **Sawdā', Jabal** ▲ SW Saudi Arabia
75 P9 **Sawdā', Jabal as** ▲ C Libya
Sawdirī *see* Sodiri
97 F14 **Sawel Mountain** ▲ C Northern Ireland, UK
Sawhāj *see* Sohāg
77 O15 **Sawla** N Ghana
147 P11 **Sawot** *Rus.* Savat. Sirdaryo Wiloyati, E Uzbekistan
141 X12 **Şawqirah** *var.* Suqrah. S Oman
141 X12 **Şawqirah, Dawhat** *var.* Ghubbat Sawqirah, Sukra Bay, Suqrah Bay. *bay* S Oman
Sawqirah, Ghubbat *see* Şawqirah, Dawhat
183 V5 **Sawtell** New South Wales, SE Australia
138 K7 **Şawt, Wādī aş** *dry watercourse* S Syria
171 O17 **Sawu, Kepulauan** *var.* Kepulauan Savu. *island group* S Indonesia
Sawu, Laut *see* Savu Sea
171 O17 **Sawu, Pulau** *var.* Pulau Savu. *island* Kepulauan Sawu, S Indonesia
105 S12 **Sax** País Valenciano, E Spain
Saxe *see* Sachsen
108 C11 **Saxon** Valais, SW Switzerland
Saxony *see* Sachsen
Saxony-Anhalt *see* Sachsen-Anhalt
77 R12 **Say** Niamey, SW Niger
15 V7 **Sayabec** Quebec, SE Canada
Sayaboury *see* Xaignabouli
145 U12 **Sayak** *Kaz.* Sayaq. Zhezkazgan, E Kazakhstan
57 D14 **Sayán** Lima, W Peru
131 T6 **Sayanskiy Khrebet** ▲ S Russian Federation
Sayaq *see* Sayak
146 K13 **Sayat** Lebapskiy Velayat, E Turkmenistan
42 D3 **Sayaxché** Petén, N Guatemala
Şaydā/Sayida *see* Saïda
141 T15 **Sayḩūt** E Yemen
29 U14 **Saylorville Lake** ▣ Iowa, C USA
Saymenskiy Kanal *see* Saimaa Canal
163 N10 **Saynshand** Dornogovĭ, SE Mongolia
162 J11 **Saynshand** Ömnögovĭ, S Mongolia
162 F7 **Sayn-Ust** Govĭ-Altay, W Mongolia
Say-Ötesh *see* Say-Utës
138 J7 **Şayqal, Baḩr** ◎ S Syria
Sayrab *see* Sayrob
158 H4 **Sayram Hu** ◎ NW China
26 K11 **Sayre** Oklahoma, C USA
18 H12 **Sayre** Pennsylvania, NE USA
18 K15 **Sayreville** New Jersey, NE USA
147 N13 **Sayrob** *Rus.* Sayrab. Surkhondaryo Wiloyati, S Uzbekistan
40 L13 **Sayula** Jalisco, SW Mexico
141 R14 **Say 'ūn** *var.* Saywūn. C Yemen
144 G14 **Say-Utës** *Kaz.* Say-Ötesh. Mangistau, SW Kazakhstan
10 K16 **Sayward** Vancouver Island, British Columbia, SW Canada
Saywūn *see* Say 'ūn
Sayyāl *see* As Sayyāl
139 U8 **Sayyid 'Abīd** *var.* Saiyid Abid. E Iraq
113 J22 **Sazan** *var.* Ishulli i Sazanit, *It.* Saseno. *island* SW Albania
Sazanit, Ishulli i *see* Sazan
Sazau/Sazawa *see* Sázava
111 E17 **Sázava** *var.* Sazau, *Ger.* Sazawa. ∼ C Czech Republic
126 J14 **Sazonovo** Vologodskaya Oblast', NW Russian Federation
102 G6 **Scaër** Finistère, NW France
97 J15 **Scafell Pike** ▲ NW England, UK
Scalabis *see* Santarém
96 M2 **Scalloway** N Scotland, UK
38 M11 **Scammon Bay** Alaska, USA
Scammon Lagoon/Scammon, Laguna *see* Ojo de Liebre, Laguna
84 F7 **Scandinavia** *geophysical region* NW Europe
Scania *see* Skåne
96 K5 **Scapa Flow** *sea basin* N Scotland, UK
107 K26 **Scaramia, Capo** *headland* Sicilia, Italy, C Mediterranean Sea
14 H15 **Scarborough** Ontario, SE Canada
45 Z16 **Scarborough** *prev.* Port Louis. Tobago, Trinidad and Tobago
97 N16 **Scarborough** N England, UK
185 I17 **Scargill** Canterbury, South Island, NZ
96 E7 **Scarp** *island* NW Scotland, UK
Scarpanto *see* Kárpathos
Scarpanto Strait *see* Karpathou, Stenó
107 G25 **Scauri** Sicilia, Italy, C Mediterranean Sea
Scealg, Bá na *see* Ballinskelligs Bay
Scebeli *see* Shebeli
100 K10 **Schaale** ∼ N Germany
100 K9 **Schaalsee** ◎ N Germany
99 G18 **Schaerbeek** Brussels, C Belgium
108 G6 **Schaffhausen** *Fr.* Schaffhouse. Schaffhausen, N Switzerland
108 G6 **Schaffhausen** *Fr.* Schaffhouse. ◈ *canton* N Switzerland
Schaffhouse *see* Schaffhausen
98 I8 **Schagen** Noord-Holland, NW Netherlands
Schaken *see* Šakiai
98 M10 **Schalkhaar** Overijssel, E Netherlands
109 R3 **Schärding** Oberösterreich, N Austria
100 G9 **Scharhörn** *island* NW Germany
Schässburg *see* Sighişoara
Schaulen *see* Šiauliai
30 M10 **Schaumburg** Illinois, N USA
Schebschi Mountains *see* Shebshi Mountains
98 P6 **Scheemda** Groningen, NE Netherlands
100 I10 **Scheessel** Niedersachsen, NW Germany
13 N8 **Schefferville** Quebec, E Canada
Schelde *see* Scheldt
99 D18 **Scheldt** *Dut.* Schelde, *Fr.* Escaut. ∼ W Europe
35 X5 **Schell Creek Range** ▲ Nevada, W USA
18 K10 **Schenectady** New York, NE USA
99 I17 **Scherpenheuvel** *Fr.* Montaigu. Vlaams Brabant, C Belgium
98 K11 **Scherpenzeel** Gelderland, C Netherlands
25 S12 **Schertz** Texas, SW USA
98 G11 **Scheveningen** Zuid-Holland, W Netherlands
98 G12 **Schiedam** Zuid-Holland, SW Netherlands
99 M24 **Schieren** Diekirch, NE Luxembourg
98 M4 **Schiermonnikoog** *Fris.* Skiermûntseach. Friesland, N Netherlands
98 M4 **Schiermonnikoog** *Fris.* Skiermûntseach. *island* Waddeneilanden, N Netherlands
99 K14 **Schijndel** Noord-Brabant, S Netherlands
Schil *see* Jiu
99 H16 **Schilde** Antwerpen, N Belgium
Schillen *see* Zhilino
103 V5 **Schiltigheim** Bas-Rhin, NE France
106 G7 **Schio** Veneto, NE Italy
98 H10 **Schiphol** ✕ (Amsterdam) Noord-Holland, C Netherlands
Schippenbeil *see* Sępopol
Schiria *see* Şiria
Schivelbein *see* Świdwin
115 D22 **Schíza** *island* S Greece
175 U3 **Schjetman Reef** *reef* Antarctica
Schlackenwerth *see* Ostrov
109 R7 **Schladming** Steiermark, SE Austria
Schlan *see* Slaný
Schlanders *see* Silandro
100 I7 **Schlei** *inlet* N Germany
101 D17 **Schleiden** Nordrhein-Westfalen, W Germany
Schlelau *see* Szydłowiec
100 I7 **Schleswig** Schleswig-Holstein, N Germany
29 T13 **Schleswig** Iowa, C USA
100 H8 **Schleswig-Holstein** ◈ *state* N Germany
Schlettstadt *see* Sélestat
108 F7 **Schlieren** Zürich, N Switzerland
Schlochau *see* Człuchów
Schloppe *see* Człopa
101 I18 **Schlüchtern** Hessen, C Germany
101 J17 **Schmalkalden** Thüringen, C Germany
109 W2 **Schmida** ∼ NE Austria
65 P19 **Schmidt-Ott Seamount** *var.* Schmitt-Ott Seamount, Schmitt-Ott Tablemount. *undersea feature* SW Indian Ocean
Schmiegel *see* Śmigiel
Schmitt-Ott Seamount/Schmitt-Ott Tablemount *see* Schmidt-Ott Seamount
15 V3 **Schmon** ∼ Quebec, SE Canada
101 M18 **Schneeberg** ▲ W Germany
Schneeberg *see* Veliki Snežnik
Schnee-Eifel *see* Schneifel
Schneekoppe *see* Sněžka
Schneidemühl *see* Piła
101 D18 **Schneifel** *var.* Schnee-Eifel. *plateau* W Germany
Schnelle Körös/Schnelle Kreisch *see* Crişul Repede
100 I11 **Schneverdingen** *var.* Schneverdingen (Wümme). Niedersachsen, NW Germany
Schneverdingen (Wümme) *see* Schneverdingen
Schoden *see* Skuodas
18 K10 **Schoharie** New York, NE USA
18 K11 **Schoharie Creek** ∼ New York, NE USA
115 J21 **Schoinoússa** *island* Kykládes, Greece, Aegean Sea
100 L13 **Schönebeck** Sachsen-Anhalt, C Germany
Schöneck *see* Skarszewy
100 O12 **Schönefeld** ✕ (Berlin) Berlin, NE Germany
101 K24 **Schongau** Bayern, S Germany
100 K13 **Schöningen** Niedersachsen, C Germany
Schönlanke *see* Trzcianka
Schönsee *see* Kowalewo Pomorskie
31 P10 **Schoolcraft** Michigan, N USA
98 O8 **Schoonebeek** Drenthe, NE Netherlands
98 I12 **Schoonhoven** Zuid-Holland, C Netherlands
98 H8 **Schoorl** Noord-Holland, NW Netherlands
Schooten *see* Schoten
101 F24 **Schopfheim** Baden-Württemberg, SW Germany
101 I21 **Schorndorf** Baden-Württemberg, S Germany
100 F10 **Schortens** Niedersachsen, NW Germany
99 H16 **Schoten** *var.* Schooten. Antwerpen, N Belgium
183 Q17 **Schouten Island** *island* Tasmania, SE Australia
186 C5 **Schouten Islands** *island group* NW PNG
98 E13 **Schouwen** *island* SW Netherlands
45 Q12 **Schœlcher** W Martinique
Schreiberhau *see* Szklarska Poręba
109 U2 **Schrems** Niederösterreich, E Austria
101 L22 **Schrobenhausen** Bayern, SE Germany
18 L8 **Schroon Lake** ◎ New York, NE USA
108 J8 **Schruns** Vorarlberg, W Austria
Schubin *see* Szubin
25 U11 **Schulenburg** Texas, SW USA
Schuls *see* Scuol
108 E8 **Schüpfheim** Luzern, C Switzerland
35 S6 **Schurz** Nevada, W USA
101 I24 **Schussen** ∼ S Germany
Schüttenhofen *see* Sušice
29 R15 **Schuyler** Nebraska, C USA
18 L10 **Schuylerville** New York, NE USA

101 K20 **Schwabach** Bayern, SE Germany
Schwabenalb *see* Schwäbische Alb
101 I23 **Schwäbische Alb** *var.* Schwabenalb, *Eng.* Swabian Jura. ▲ S Germany
101 I22 **Schwäbisch Gmünd** *var.* Gmünd. Baden-Württemberg, SW Germany
101 I21 **Schwäbisch Hall** *var.* Hall. Baden-Württemberg, SW Germany
101 H16 **Schwalm** ≈ C Germany
109 V9 **Schwanberg** Steiermark, SE Austria
108 H8 **Schwanden** Glarus, E Switzerland
101 M20 **Schwandorf** Bayern, SE Germany
109 S5 **Schwanenstadt** Oberösterreich, NW Austria
169 S11 **Schwaner, Pegunungan** ▲ Borneo, N Indonesia
109 W5 **Schwarza** ≈ E Austria
109 P9 **Schwarzach** ≈ S Austria
101 M20 **Schwarzach** *Cz.* Černice. ≈ Czech Republic/Germany
Schwarzach *see* Schwarzach im Pongau, Austria
Schwarzach *see* Svratka, Czech Republic
109 Q7 **Schwarzach im Pongau** *var.* Schwarzach. Salzburg, NW Austria
Schwarzawa *see* Svratka
101 N14 **Schwarze Elster** ≈ E Germany
Schwarze Körös *see* Crişul Negru
108 D9 **Schwarzenburg** Bern, W Switzerland
83 D21 **Schwarzrand** ▲ S Namibia
101 G23 **Schwarzwald** *Eng.* Black Forest. ▲ SW Germany
Schwarzwasser *see* Wda
39 P7 **Schwatka Mountains** ▲ Alaska, USA
109 N7 **Schwaz** Tirol, W Austria
109 Y4 **Schwechat** Niederösterreich, NE Austria
109 Y4 **Schwechat** ✕ (Wien) Wien, E Austria
100 P11 **Schwedt** Brandenburg, NE Germany
101 D19 **Schweich** Rheinland-Pfalz, SW Germany
Schweidnitz *see* Świdnica
101 J18 **Schweinfurt** Bayern, SE Germany
Schweiz *see* Switzerland
100 L9 **Schwerin** Mecklenburg-Vorpommern, N Germany
Schwerin *see* Skwierzyna
100 L9 **Schweriner See** ◎ N Germany
Schwertberg *see* Świecie
101 F15 **Schwerte** Nordrhein-Westfalen, W Germany
Schwiebus *see* Świebodzin
100 P13 **Schwielochsee** ◎ NE Germany
Schwihau *see* Švihov
Schwiz *see* Schwyz
108 G8 **Schwyz** *var.* Schwiz. Schwyz, C Switzerland
108 G8 **Schwyz** *var.* Schwiz. ◈ *canton* C Switzerland
14 J11 **Schyan** ≈ Quebec, SE Canada
Schyl *see* Jiu
107 I24 **Sciacca** Sicilia, Italy, C Mediterranean Sea
Sciasciamana *see* Shashemenē
107 L26 **Scicli** Sicilia, Italy, C Mediterranean Sea
97 F25 **Scilly, Isles of** *island group* SW England, UK
111 H17 **Šcinawa** *Ger.* Steinau an der Elbe. Dolnośląskie, SW Poland
Scio *see* Chíos
31 S14 **Scioto River** ≈ Ohio, N USA
36 L5 **Scipio** Utah, W USA
33 X6 **Scobey** Montana, NW USA
183 T7 **Scone** New South Wales, SE Australia
Scoresby Sound/Scoresbysund *see* Ittoqqortoormiit
Scoresby Sund *see* Kangertittivaq
Scorno, Punta dello *see* Caprara, Punta
34 K3 **Scotia** California, W USA
47 Y14 **Scotia Plate** *tectonic feature*
47 V15 **Scotia Ridge** *undersea feature* S Atlantic Ocean
194 H2 **Scotia Sea** *sea* SW Atlantic Ocean
29 Q12 **Scotland** South Dakota, N USA
25 R5 **Scotland** Texas, SW USA
96 H11 **Scotland** *national region* UK
21 W8 **Scotland Neck** North Carolina, SE USA
195 R13 **Scott Base** *NZ research station* Antarctica
10 J16 **Scott, Cape** *headland* Vancouver Island, British Columbia, SW Canada
26 I5 **Scott City** Kansas, C USA
27 Y7 **Scott City** Missouri, C USA
195 R14 **Scott Coast** *physical region* Antarctica
18 C15 **Scottdale** Pennsylvania, NE USA
195 Y11 **Scott Glacier** *glacier* Antarctica
195 Q17 **Scott Island** *island* Antarctica
26 L11 **Scott, Mount** ▲ Oklahoma, USA
32 G15 **Scott, Mount** ▲ Oregon, NW USA
34 M1 **Scott River** ≈ California, W USA
28 I13 **Scottsbluff** Nebraska, C USA
23 Q2 **Scottsboro** Alabama, S USA
31 P15 **Scottsburg** Indiana, N USA
183 P16 **Scottsdale** Tasmania, SE Australia
36 L13 **Scottsdale** Arizona, SW USA
45 O12 **Scotts Head Village** *var.* Cachacrou. S Dominica
192 L14 **Scott Shoal** *undersea feature* S Pacific Ocean
20 K7 **Scottsville** Kentucky, S USA
29 U14 **Scranton** Iowa, C USA
18 I13 **Scranton** Pennsylvania, NE USA
186 B6 **Screw** ≈ NW PNG
29 R14 **Scribner** Nebraska, C USA
Scrobesbyrig' *see* Shrewsbury
14 I14 **Scugog** ≈ Ontario, SE Canada
14 I14 **Scugog, Lake** ◎ Ontario, SE Canada
97 N17 **Scunthorpe** E England, UK
108 K9 **Scuol** *Ger.* Schuls. Graubünden, E Switzerland
Scupi *see* Skopje
Scutari *see* Shkodër
113 K17 **Scutari, Lake** *Alb.* Liqeni i Shkodrës, *SCr.* Skadarsko Jezero. ◎ Albania/Yugoslavia
Scyros *see* Skýros
Scythopolis *see* Bet She'an
25 U13 **Seadrift** Texas, SW USA
21 Y4 **Seaford** *var.* Seaford City. Delaware, NE USA
Seaford City *see* Seaford
15 H16 **Seaforth** Ontario, S Canada
24 M6 **Seagraves** Texas, SW USA
11 X9 **Seal** ≈ Manitoba, C Canada
182 M10 **Sea Lake** Victoria, SE Australia
83 G26 **Seal, Cape** *headland* S South Africa
65 D26 **Sea Lion Islands** *island group* SE Falkland Islands
19 S8 **Seal Island** *island* Maine, NE USA
25 V11 **Sealy** Texas, SW USA
35 X12 **Searchlight** Nevada, W USA
27 V11 **Searcy** Arkansas, C USA
19 R7 **Searsport** Maine, NE USA
35 N10 **Seaside** California, W USA
32 F10 **Seaside** Oregon, NW USA
18 K16 **Seaside Heights** New Jersey, NE USA
32 H8 **Seattle** Washington, NW USA
32 H9 **Seattle-Tacoma** ✕ Washington, NW USA
185 J16 **Seaward Kaikoura Range** ▲ South Island, NZ
42 J9 **Sébaco** Matagalpa, W Nicaragua
19 P8 **Sebago Lake** ◎ Maine, NE USA
169 S13 **Sebangan, Teluk** *bay* Borneo, C Indonesia
169 S13 **Sebanganu, Teluk** *bay* Borneo, C Indonesia
Sebaste/Sebastia *see* Sivas
23 Y12 **Sebastian** Florida, SE USA
40 C5 **Sebastián Vizcaíno, Bahía** *bay* NW Mexico
19 R6 **Sebasticook Lake** ◎ Maine, NE USA
34 M7 **Sebastopol** California, W USA
Sebastopol *see* Sevastopol'
169 W8 **Sebatik, Pulau** *island* N Indonesia
19 R5 **Sebec Lake** ◎ Maine, NE USA
76 K12 **Sébékoro** Kayes, W Mali
Sebenico *see* Šibenik
40 G6 **Seberi, Cerro** ▲ NW Mexico
116 H11 **Sebeş** *Ger.* Mühlbach, *Hung.* Szászsebes; *prev.* Sebeşu Săsesc. Alba, W Romania
Sebes-Körös *see* Crişul Repede
Sebeşu Săsesc *see* Sebeş
31 R8 **Sebewaing** Michigan, N USA
126 F16 **Sebezh** Pskovskaya Oblast', W Russian Federation
137 N12 **Şebinkarahisar** Giresun, N Turkey
116 F11 **Sebiş** *Hung.* Borossebes. Arad, W Romania
Sebkra Azz el Matti *see* Azzel Matti, Sebkha
19 Q4 **Seboomook Lake** ◎ Maine, NE USA
74 G6 **Sebou** *var.* Sebu. ≈ N Morocco
20 I6 **Sebree** Kentucky, S USA
23 X13 **Sebring** Florida, SE USA
Sebta *see* Ceuta
Sebu *see* Sebou
169 U13 **Sebuku, Pulau** *island* N Indonesia
169 W8 **Sebuku, Teluk** *bay* Borneo, N Indonesia
106 F10 **Secchia** ≈ N Italy
10 L17 **Sechelt** British Columbia, SW Canada
56 C12 **Sechin, Río** ≈ W Peru
56 A10 **Sechura, Bahía de** *bay* NW Peru
185 A22 **Secretary Island** *island* SW NZ
155 I15 **Secunderābād** *var.* Sikandarabad. Andhra Pradesh, C India
57 L17 **Sécure, Río** ≈ C Bolivia
118 D10 **Seda** Mažeikiai, NW Lithuania
27 T5 **Sedalia** Missouri, C USA
103 R3 **Sedan** Ardennes, N France
27 P7 **Sedan** Kansas, C USA
105 N3 **Sedano** Castilla-León, N Spain
104 H10 **Seda, Ribeira de** *stream* C Portugal
185 K15 **Seddon** Marlborough, South Island, NZ
185 H15 **Seddonville** West Coast, South Island, NZ
143 U7 **Sedeh** Khorāsān, E Iran
138 E11 **Sederot** Southern, S Israel
65 B23 **Sedge Island** *island* NW Falkland Islands
76 G12 **Sédhiou** SW Senegal
11 U16 **Sedley** Saskatchewan, S Canada
Sedlez *see* Siedlce
122 I11 **Sedel'nikovo** Omskaya Oblast', C Russian Federation
117 Q2 **Sedniv** Chernihivs'ka Oblast', N Ukraine
36 L11 **Sedona** Arizona, SW USA
Sedunum *see* Sion
118 F12 **Šeduva** Radviliškis, N Lithuania
141 Y8 **Seeb** *var.* Muscat Sīb Airport. ✕ (Masqaṭ) NE Oman
Seeb *see* As Sīb
108 M7 **Seefeld-in-Tirol** Tirol, W Austria
83 E22 **Seeheim Noord** Karas, S Namibia
Seeland *see* Sjælland
195 N9 **Seelig, Mount** ▲ Antarctica
Seeonee *see* Seoni
162 E6 **Seer** Hovd, W Mongolia
102 L5 **Sées** Orne, N France
101 J14 **Seesen** Niedersachsen, C Germany
Seesker Höhe *see* Szeskie Wzgórza
100 J10 **Seevetal** Niedersachsen, N Germany
109 V6 **Seewiesen** Steiermark, E Austria
136 J13 **Şefaatli** *var.* Kızılkoca. Yozgat, C Turkey
149 N3 **Sefid, Darya-ye** *Pash.* Āb-i-Safed. ≈ N Afghanistan
148 K5 **Sefid Kūh, Selseleh-ye** *Eng.* Paropamisus Range. ▲ W Afghanistan
74 G6 **Sefrou** N Morocco
185 E19 **Sefton, Mount** ▲ South Island, NZ
171 S13 **Segaf, Kepulauan** *island group* E Indonesia
169 W7 **Segama, Sungai** ≈ East Malaysia
168 L9 **Segamat** Johor, Peninsular Malaysia
77 S13 **Ségbana** NE Benin
Segestica *see* Sisak
Segesvár *see* Sighişoara
171 T12 **Seget** Irian Jaya, E Indonesia
Segewold *see* Sigulda
126 J9 **Segezha** Respublika Kareliya, NW Russian Federation
Seghedin *see* Szeged
Segna *see* Senj
107 I16 **Segni** Lazio, C Italy
Segodunum *see* Rodez
105 S9 **Segorbe** País Valenciano, E Spain
76 M12 **Ségou** *var.* Segu. Ségou, C Mali
76 M12 **Ségou** ◈ *region* SW Mali
54 E8 **Segovia** Antioquia, N Colombia
105 N7 **Segovia** Castilla-León, C Spain
104 M6 **Segovia** ◈ *province* Castilla-León, N Spain
Segoviao Wangkí *see* Coco, Río
126 J9 **Segozero, Ozero** ◎ NW Russian Federation
105 U5 **Segre** ≈ NE Spain
102 J7 **Segré** Maine-et-Loire, NW France
Segu *see* Ségou
38 I17 **Seguam Island** *island* Aleutian Islands, Alaska, USA
38 I17 **Seguam Pass** *strait* Aleutian Islands, Alaska, USA
77 Y7 **Séguédine** Agadez, NE Niger
76 M15 **Séguéla** W Ivory Coast
25 S11 **Seguin** Texas, SW USA
38 E17 **Segula Island** *island* Aleutian Islands, Alaska, USA
62 K10 **Segundo, Río** ≈ C Argentina
105 Q12 **Segura** ≈ S Spain
105 P13 **Sierra de Segura** ▲ S Spain
83 G18 **Sehithwa** Ngamiland, N Botswana
154 H10 **Sehore** Madhya Pradesh, C India
186 G9 **Sehulea** Normanby Island, S PNG
149 P15 **Sehwān** Sind, SE Pakistan
109 V8 **Seiersberg** Steiermark, SE Austria
26 L9 **Seiling** Oklahoma, C USA
103 S9 **Seille** ≈ E France
99 J20 **Seilles** Namur, SE Belgium
93 K17 **Seinäjoki** *Swe.* Östermyra. Länsi-Suomi, W Finland
12 B12 **Seine** ≈ Ontario, S Canada
102 M4 **Seine** ≈ N France
102 K4 **Seine, Baie de la** *bay* N France
Seine, Banc de la *see* Seine Seamount
103 O5 **Seine-et-Marne** ◈ *department* N France
102 L3 **Seine-Maritime** ◈ *department* N France
84 B14 **Seine Plain** *undersea feature* E Atlantic Ocean
84 B15 **Seine Seamount** *var.* Banc de la Seine. *undersea feature* E Atlantic Ocean
102 E6 **Sein, Île de** *island* NW France
171 Y14 **Seinma** Irian Jaya, E Indonesia
Seisbierrum *see* Sexbierum
109 U5 **Seitenstetten Markt** Niederösterreich, C Austria
Seiyu *see* Chŏnju
95 H22 **Sejerø** *island* E Denmark
110 P7 **Sejny** Podlaskie, NE Poland
81 G20 **Seke** Shinyanga, N Tanzania
164 L13 **Seki** Gifu, Honshū, SW Japan
161 U12 **Sekibi-sho** *island* China/Japan/Taiwan
165 U3 **Sekihoku-tōge** *pass* Hokkaidō, NE Japan
Sekondi *see* Sekondi-Takoradi
77 P17 **Sekondi-Takoradi** *var.* Sekondi. S Ghana
80 J11 **Sek'ot'a** Amhara, N Ethiopia
Seksaul *see* Saksaul'skiy
32 I9 **Selah** Washington, NW USA
168 J8 **Selangor** *var.* Negeri Selangor Darul Ehsan. ◈ *state* Peninsular Malaysia
Selânik *see* Thessaloníki
168 K10 **Selapanjang** Pulau Rantau, W Indonesia
167 R10 **Selaphum** Roi Et, E Thailand
171 T16 **Selaru, Pulau** *island* Kepulauan Tanimbar, E Indonesia
171 U13 **Selassi** Irian Jaya, E Indonesia
168 J7 **Selatan, Selat** *strait* Peninsular Malaysia
39 N8 **Selawik** Alaska, USA
39 N8 **Selawik Lake** ◎ Alaska, USA
171 N14 **Selayar, Selat** *strait* Sulawesi, C Indonesia
95 C14 **Selbjørnsfjorden** *fjord* S Norway
94 H8 **Selbusjøen** ◎ S Norway
97 M17 **Selby** N England, UK
29 N8 **Selby** South Dakota, N USA
21 Z4 **Selbyville** Delaware, NE USA
136 B15 **Selçuk** *var.* Akıncılar. İzmir, SW Turkey
39 Q13 **Seldovia** Alaska, USA
107 M18 **Sele** *anc.* Silarius. ≈ S Italy
42 B5 **Selegua, Río** ≈ W Guatemala
131 X7 **Selemdzha** ≈ SE Russian Federation
131 U7 **Selenga** *Mong.* Selenge Mörön. ≈ Mongolia/Russian Federation
162 K6 **Selenge** Bulgan, N Mongolia
162 J6 **Selenge** Hövsgöl, N Mongolia
79 I19 **Selenge** Bandundu, W Dem. Rep. Congo (Zaire)
162 L6 **Selenge** ◈ *province* N Mongolia
Selenge Mörön *see* Selenga
123 N14 **Selenginsk** Respublika Buryatiya, S Russian Federation
Selenica *see* Selenicë
113 K22 **Selenicë** *var.* Selenica. Vlorë, SW Albania
123 Q8 **Selennyakh** ≈ NE Russian Federation
100 J8 **Selenter See** ◎ N Germany
Sele Sound *see* Soela Väin
103 U6 **Sélestat** *Ger.* Schlettstadt. Bas-Rhin, NE France
Selety *see* Sileti
Seleucia *see* Silifke
92 I4 **Selfoss** Sudhurland, SW Iceland
28 M7 **Selfridge** North Dakota, N USA
76 I15 **Seli** ≈ N Sierra Leone
76 I11 **Sélibabi** *var.* Sélibaby. Guidimaka, S Mauritania
Sélibaby *see* Sélibabi
Selidovka/Selidovo *see* Selydove
126 I15 **Seliger, Ozero** ◎ W Russian Federation
36 J11 **Seligman** Arizona, SW USA
27 S8 **Seligman** Missouri, C USA
80 E6 **Selima Oasis** *oasis* N Sudan
76 L13 **Sélingué, Lac de** ▣ S Mali
Selinoús *see* Kréstena
18 G14 **Selinsgrove** Pennsylvania, NE USA
Selishche *see* Syelishcha
126 I16 **Selizharovo** Tverskaya Oblast', W Russian Federation
94 C10 **Selje** Sogn og Fjordane, S Norway
11 X16 **Selkirk** Manitoba, S Canada
96 K13 **Selkirk** SE Scotland, UK
96 K13 **Selkirk** *cultural region* SE Scotland, UK
11 O16 **Selkirk Mountains** ▲ British Columbia, SW Canada
9 O15 **Selkirk Rise** *undersea feature* SE Pacific Ocean
115 F21 **Sellasía** Pelopónnisos, S Greece
44 M9 **Selle, Pic de la** *var.* La Selle. ▲ SE Haiti
102 M8 **Selles-sur-Cher** Loir-et-Cher, C France
36 K16 **Sells** Arizona, SW USA
Sellye *see* Sal'a
23 P5 **Selma** Alabama, S USA
35 Q11 **Selma** California, W USA
20 G10 **Selmer** Tennessee, S USA
173 N17 **Sel, Pointe au** *headland* W Réunion
Selseleh-ye Kūh-e Vākhān *see* Nicholas Range
129 S2 **Selty** Udmurtskaya Respublika, NW Russian Federation
Selukwe *see* Shurugwi
62 L9 **Selva** Santiago del Estero, N Argentina
11 T9 **Selwyn Lake** ◎ Northwest Territories/Saskatchewan, C Canada
10 K6 **Selwyn Mountains** ▲ Yukon Territory, NW Canada
181 T6 **Selwyn Range** ▲ Queensland, C Australia
117 W8 **Selydove** *var.* Selidovka, *Rus.* Selidovo. Donets'ka Oblast', SE Ukraine
Selzaete *see* Zelzate
Seman *see* Semanit, Lumi i
168 M15 **Semangka, Teluk** *bay* Sumatera, SW Indonesia
113 D22 **Semanit, Lumi i** *var.* Seman. ≈ W Albania
169 Q16 **Semarang** *var.* Samarang. Jawa, C Indonesia
169 Q10 **Sematan** Sarawak, East Malaysia
171 P17 **Semau, Pulau** *island* S Indonesia
169 V8 **Sembakung, Sungai** ≈ Borneo, N Indonesia
79 G17 **Sembé** La Sangha, NW Congo
169 S13 **Sembulu, Danau** ◎ Borneo, N Indonesia
Semendria *see* Smederevo
117 R1 **Semenivka** Chernihivs'ka Oblast', N Ukraine
117 S6 **Semenivka** *Rus.* Semenovka. Poltavs'ka Oblast', NE Ukraine
129 O3 **Semenov** Nizhegorodskaya Oblast', W Russian Federation
Semenovka *see* Semenivka
169 S17 **Semeru, Gunung** *var.* Mahameru. ▲ Jawa, S Indonesia
Semey *see* Semipalatinsk
Semezhevo *see* Syemyezhava
128 L7 **Semiluki** Voronezhskaya Oblast', W Russian Federation
33 W16 **Seminoe Reservoir** ▣ Wyoming, C USA
27 O11 **Seminole** Oklahoma, C USA
24 M6 **Seminole** Texas, SW USA
23 S8 **Seminole, Lake** ▣ Florida/Georgia, SE USA
144 M8 **Semiozernoye** Kostanay, N Kazakhstan
145 V9 **Semipalatinsk** *Kaz.* Semey. Vostochnyy Kazakhstan, E Kazakhstan
143 O9 **Semīrom** *var.* Samirum. Eşfahān, C Iran
38 F17 **Semisopochnoi Island** *island* Aleutian Islands, Alaska, USA
169 R11 **Semitau** Borneo, C Indonesia
81 E18 **Semliki** ≈ Uganda/Dem. Rep. Congo (Zaire)
143 P5 **Semnān** *var.* Samnān. Semnān, N Iran
143 Q5 **Semnān** *off.* Ostān-e Semnān. ◈ *province* N Iran
99 K24 **Semois** ≈ SE Belgium
108 E8 **Sempacher See** ◎ C Switzerland
Sena *see* Vila de Sena
30 L12 **Senachwine Lake** ◎ Illinois, N USA
59 O14 **Senador Pompeu** Ceará, E Brazil
Sena Gallica *see* Senigallia
59 C15 **Sena Madureira** Acre, W Brazil
155 L25 **Senanayake Samudra** ◎ E Sri Lanka
83 G15 **Senanga** Western, SW Zambia
27 Y9 **Senath** Missouri, C USA
22 L2 **Senatobia** Mississippi, S USA
164 C16 **Sendai** Kagoshima, Kyūshū, SW Japan
165 Q10 **Sendai** Miyagi, Honshū, C Japan
165 Q11 **Sendai-wan** *bay* E Japan
101 J23 **Senden** Bayern, S Germany
154 F11 **Sendhwa** Madhya Pradesh, C India
111 H21 **Senec** *Ger.* Wartberg, *Hung.* Szenc; *prev.* Szempcz. Bratislavský Kraj, W Slovakia
27 P3 **Seneca** Kansas, C USA
27 R8 **Seneca** Missouri, C USA
32 K13 **Seneca** Oregon, NW USA
21 O11 **Seneca** South Carolina, SE USA
18 G11 **Seneca Lake** ◎ New York, NE USA
31 U13 **Senecaville Lake** ▣ Ohio, N USA
76 G11 **Senegal** *off.* Republic of Senegal, *Fr.* Sénégal. ◆ *republic* W Africa
76 H9 **Senegal** *Fr.* Sénégal. ≈ W Africa
31 O4 **Seney Marsh** *wetland* Michigan, N USA
101 P14 **Senftenberg** Brandenburg, E Germany
82 L11 **Senga Hill** Northern, NE Zambia
158 G13 **Sênggê Zangbo** ≈ W China
171 Z13 **Senggi** Irian Jaya, E Indonesia
129 R5 **Sengiley** Ul'yanovskaya Oblast', W Russian Federation
63 I19 **Senguerr, Río** ≈ S Argentina
83 J16 **Sengwa** ≈ C Zimbabwe
Senia *see* Senj
111 H19 **Senica** *Ger.* Senitz, *Hung.* Szenice. Trnavský Kraj, W Slovakia
Seniça *see* Sjenica
106 J11 **Senigallia** *anc.* Sena Gallica. Marche, C Italy
136 F15 **Senirkent** Isparta, SW Turkey
Senitz *see* Senica
112 C10 **Senj** *Ger.* Zengg, *It.* Segna; *anc.* Senia. Lika-Senj, NW Croatia
163 O10 **Senj** Dornogovĭ, SE Mongolia
92 H9 **Senja** *prev.* Senjen. *island* N Norway
Senjen *see* Senja
161 U12 **Senkaku-shotō** *island group* SW Japan
137 R12 **Şenkaya** Erzurum, NE Turkey
83 I16 **Senkobo** Southern, S Zambia
103 O4 **Senlis** Oise, N France
167 T12 **Senmonorom** Môndól Kiri, E Cambodia
80 G10 **Sennar** *var.* Sannār. Sinnar, C Sudan
Senno *see* Syanno
Senones *see* Sens
109 W11 **Senovo** E Slovenia
103 P6 **Sens** *anc.* Agendicum, Senones. Yonne, C France
Sensburg *see* Mrągowo
167 S11 **Sên, Stœng** ≈ C Cambodia
42 F7 **Sensuntepeque** Cabañas, NE El Salvador
112 L8 **Senta** *Hung.* Zenta. Serbia, N Yugoslavia
Šent Andraž *see* Sankt Andrä
171 Y13 **Sentani, Danau** ◎ Irian Jaya, E Indonesia
28 J5 **Sentinel Butte** ▲ North Dakota, N USA
10 M13 **Sentinel Peak** ▲ British Columbia, W Canada
59 N16 **Sento Sé** Bahia, E Brazil
Šent Peter *see* Pivka
Šent Vid *see* Sankt Veit an der Glan
Seo de Urgel *see* La See d'Urgel
154 I7 **Seondha** Madhya Pradesh, C India
154 J11 **Seoni** *prev.* Seeonee. Madhya Pradesh, C India
Seoul *see* Sŏul
184 I13 **Separation Point** *headland* South Island, NZ
169 V10 **Sepasu** Borneo, N Indonesia
186 B6 **Sepik** ≈ Indonesia/PNG
Sepone *see* Muang Xépôn
110 M7 **Sępopol** *Ger.* Schippenbeil. Warmińsko-Mazurskie, NE Poland,
116 F10 **Şepreuş** *Hung.* Seprős. Arad, W Romania
Seprős *see* Şepreuş
Şepşi-Sângeorz/Sepsiszentgyőrgy *see* Sfântu Gheorghe
15 W4 **Sept-Îles** Quebec, SE Canada
105 N6 **Sepúlveda** Castilla-León, N Spain
104 K8 **Sequeros** Castilla-León, N Spain
104 L5 **Sequillo** ≈ NW Spain
32 G7 **Sequim** Washington, NW USA
35 S11 **Sequoia National Park** *national park* California, W USA
137 Q14 **Şerafettin Dağları** ▲ E Turkey
129 N10 **Serafimovich** Volgogradskaya Oblast', SW Russian Federation
171 Q10 **Serai** Sulawesi, N Indonesia
99 K19 **Seraing** Liège, E Belgium
Sêraitang *see* Baima
Serajgonj *see* Shirajganj Ghat
146 I15 **Serakhs** *var.* Saragt. Akhalskiy Velayat, S Turkmenistan
171 W13 **Serami** Irian Jaya, E Indonesia
Seram, Laut *see* Ceram Sea
Serampore/Serampur *see* Shrīrāmpur
171 S13 **Seram, Pulau** *var.* Serang, *Eng.* Ceram. *island* Maluku, E Indonesia
169 N15 **Serang** Jawa, C Indonesia
Serang *see* Seram, Pulau
169 P9 **Serasan, Pulau** *island* Kepulauan Natuna, W Indonesia
169 P9 **Serasan, Selat** *strait* Indonesia/Malaysia
112 M12 **Serbia** *Ger.* Serbien, *Serb.* Srbija. ◈ *republic* Yugoslavia
Serbien *see* Serbia
Sercq *see* Sark
Serdica *see* Sofiya
129 O7 **Serdobsk** Penzenskaya Oblast', W Russian Federation
145 X9 **Serebryansk** Vostochnyy Kazakhstan, E Kazakhstan
123 Q12 **Serebryanyy Bor** Respublika Sakha (Yakutiya), NE Russian Federation
111 H20 **Sered'** *Hung.* Szered. Trnavský Kraj, SW Slovakia
117 S1 **Seredyna-Buda** Sums'ka Oblast', NE Ukraine
118 E13 **Seredžius** Jurbarkas, C Lithuania
136 I14 **Şereflikoçhisar** Ankara, C Turkey
106 D7 **Seregno** Lombardia, N Italy
103 P7 **Serein** ≈ C France
168 K9 **Seremban** Negeri Sembilan, Peninsular Malaysia
81 H20 **Serengeti Plain** *plain* N Tanzania
82 K13 **Serenje** Central, E Zambia
Seres *see* Sérres
116 J5 **Seret** ≈ W Ukraine
Seret/Sereth *see* Siret
115 I21 **Serfopoúla** *island* Kykládes, Greece, Aegean Sea
129 P4 **Sergach** Nizhegorodskaya Oblast', W Russian Federation
29 S13 **Sergeant Bluff** Iowa, C USA
163 P7 **Sergelen** Dornod, NE Mongolia
163 O9 **Sergelen** Sühbaatar, E Mongolia
168 H8 **Sergeulangit, Pegunungan** ▲ Sumatera, NW Indonesia
122 L5 **Sergeya Kirova, Ostrova** *island* N Russian Federation
Sergeyevichi *see* Syarhyeyevichy
145 O7 **Sergeyevka** Severnyy Kazakhstan, N Kazakhstan
Sergiopol *see* Ayagoz
59 P16 **Sergipe** *off.* Estado de Sergipe. ◈ *state* E Brazil
128 L3 **Sergiyev Posad** Moskovskaya Oblast', W Russian Federation
126 K5 **Sergozero, Ozero** ◎ NW Russian Federation
169 Q10 **Serian** Sarawak, East Malaysia
169 O15 **Seribu, Kepulauan** *island group* S Indonesia
115 I21 **Sérifos** *anc.* Seriphos. *island* Kykládes, Greece, Aegean Sea
115 I21 **Sérifou, Stenó** *strait* SE Greece
136 F16 **Serik** Antalya, SW Turkey
106 E7 **Serio** ≈ N Italy
Seriphos *see* Sérifos
Serir Tibesti *see* Sarīr Tibistī
129 S5 **Sernovodsk** Samarskaya Oblast', W Russian Federation
129 R2 **Sernur** Respublika Mariy El, W Russian Federation
110 M11 **Serock** Mazowieckie, C Poland
61 B18 **Serodino** Santa Fe, C Argentina
Seroei *see* Serui
105 P14 **Serón** Andalucía, S Spain
99 E14 **Serooskerke** Zeeland, SW Netherlands
105 T6 **Seròs** Cataluña, NE Spain
122 G10 **Serov** Sverdlovskaya Oblast', C Russian Federation
83 I19 **Serowe** Central, SE Botswana
104 H13 **Serpa** Beja, S Portugal
Serpa Pinto *see* Menongue
182 A4 **Serpentine Lakes** *salt lake* South Australia
45 T15 **Serpent's Mouth, The** *Sp.* Boca de la Serpiente. *strait* Trinidad and Tobago/Venezuela
Serpiente, Boca de la *see* Serpent's Mouth, The
128 K4 **Serpukhov** Moskovskaya Oblast', W Russian Federation
60 K13 **Serra do Mar** ▲ S Brazil
Sérrai *see* Sérres
107 N22 **Serra San Bruno** Calabria, SW Italy
103 S14 **Serres** Hautes-Alpes, SE France
114 H13 **Sérres** *var.* Seres; *prev.* Sérrai. Kentrikí Makedonía, NE Greece
62 J9 **Serrezuela** Córdoba, C Argentina
59 O16 **Serrinha** Bahia, E Brazil
59 M19 **Serro** *var.* Sêrro. Minas Gerais, NE Brazil
Sêrro *see* Serro
Sert *see* Siirt
Sertá *see* Sertã
104 H9 **Sertã** *var.* Sertá. Castelo Branco, C Portugal
60 L8 **Sertãozinho** São Paulo, S Brazil
160 F7 **Sêrtar** Sichuan, C China
171 W13 **Serui** *prev.* Seroei. Irian Jaya, E Indonesia
83 I19 **Serule** Central, E Botswana
169 S12 **Seruyan, Sungai** *var.* Sungai Pembuang. ≈ Borneo, N Indonesia
115 E14 **Sérvia** Dytikí Makedonía, N Greece
160 E7 **Sêrxü** Sichuan, C China
123 R13 **Seryshevo** Amurskaya Oblast', SE Russian Federation
Sesana *see* Sežana
169 V8 **Sesayap, Sungai** ≈ Borneo, N Indonesia
Sesdlets *see* Siedlce
79 N17 **Sese** Orientale, N Dem. Rep. Congo (Zaire)

◆ Country ● Country Capital ◇ Dependent Territory ○ Dependent Territory Capital ◈ Administrative Region ✕ International Airport ▲ Mountain ▲ Mountain Range Volcano ◎ Lake ≈ River ▣ Reservoir

81 F18 **Sese Islands** island group S Uganda
83 H16 **Sesheke** var. Sesheko. Western, SE Zambia
Sesheko see Sesheke
106 C8 **Sesia** anc. Sessites. ≈ NW Italy
104 F11 **Sesimbra** Setúbal, S Portugal
115 N22 **Seskió** island Dodekánisos, Greece, Aegean Sea
30 L16 **Sesser** Illinois, N USA
Sessites see Sesia
106 G11 **Sesto Fiorentino** Toscana, C Italy
106 E7 **Sesto San Giovanni** Lombardia, N Italy
106 A8 **Sestriere** Piemonte, NE Italy
106 D10 **Sestri Levante** Liguria, NW Italy
107 C20 **Sestu** Sardegna, Italy, C Mediterranean Sea
112 E8 **Sesvete** Zagreb, N Croatia
118 G12 **Šeta** Kėdainiai, C Lithuania
Setabis see Xátiva
165 Q4 **Setana** Hokkaidō, NE Japan
103 Q16 **Sète** prev. Cette. Hérault, S France
58 J11 **Sete Ilhas** Amapá, NE Brazil
59 L20 **Sete Lagoas** Minas Gerais, NE Brazil
60 G10 **Sete Quedas, Ilha das** island S Brazil
92 I10 **Setermoen** Troms, N Norway
95 E17 **Setesdal** valley S Norway
43 W16 **Setetule, Cerro** ▲ SE Panama
21 Q5 **Seth** West Virginia, NE USA
Setia see Sezze
74 K5 **Sétif** var. Stif. N Algeria
164 L13 **Seto** Aichi, Honshū, SW Japan
164 G13 **Seto-naikai** Eng. Inland Sea. sea S Japan
165 V16 **Setouchi** var. Setoushi. Kagoshima, Amami-Ō-shima, SW Japan
74 F6 **Settat** W Morocco
79 D20 **Setté Cama** Ogooué-Maritime, SW Gabon
11 W13 **Setting Lake** ◎ Manitoba, C Canada
97 L16 **Settle** N England, UK
189 Y12 **Settlement** E Wake Island
104 F11 **Setúbal** Eng. Saint Ubes, Saint Yves. Setúbal, W Portugal
104 F11 **Setúbal** ◈ district S Portugal
104 F12 **Setúbal, Baía de** bay W Portugal
Setul see Satun
12 B10 **Seul, Lac** ◎ Ontario, S Canada
103 R8 **Seurre** Côte d'Or, C France
137 U11 **Sevan** C Armenia
137 V12 **Sevana Lich** Eng. Lake Sevan, Rus. Ozero Sevan. ◎ E Armenia
Sevan, Lake/Sevan, Ozero see Sevana Lich
77 N11 **Sévaré** Mopti, C Mali
117 S14 **Sevastopol'** Eng. Sebastopol. Respublika Krym, S Ukraine
25 R14 **Seven Sisters** Texas, SW USA
10 K13 **Seven Sisters Peaks** ▲ British Columbia, SW Canada
99 M15 **Sevenum** Limburg, SE Netherlands
103 P14 **Séverac-le-Château** Aveyron, S France
14 H13 **Severn** ≈ Ontario, S Canada
97 L21 **Severn** Wel. Hafren. ≈ England/Wales, UK
127 O11 **Severnaya Dvina** var. Northern Dvina. ≈ NW Russian Federation
129 N16 **Severnaya Osetiya-Alaniya, Respublika** Eng. North Ossetia; prev. Respublika Severnaya Osetiya, Severo-Osetinskaya SSR. ◈ autonomous republic SW Russian Federation
Severnaya Osetiya, Respublika see Severnaya Osetiya-Alaniya Respublika
122 M5 **Severnaya Zemlya** var. Nicholas II Land. island group N Russian Federation
129 T5 **Severnoye** Orenburgskaya Oblast', W Russian Federation
35 S3 **Severn Troughs Range** ⛰ Nevada, W USA
127 W3 **Severnyy** Respublika Komi, NW Russian Federation
144 I13 **Severnyy Chink Ustyurta** ⛰ W Kazakhstan
127 Q13 **Severnyye Uvaly** var. Northern Ural Hills. hill range NW Russian Federation
145 O6 **Severnyy Kazakhstan** off. Severo-Kazakhstanskaya Oblast', var. North Kazakhstan, Kaz. Soltüstik Qazaqstan Oblysy. ◈ province N Kazakhstan
127 V9 **Severnyy Ural** ⛰ NW Russian Federation
Severo-Alichurskiy Khrebet see Alichuri Shimolí, Qatorkŭhi
123 N12 **Severobaykal'sk** Respublika Buryatiya, S Russian Federation
Severodonetsk see Syeverodonets'k
126 M8 **Severodvinsk** prev. Molotov, Sudostroy. Arkhangel'skaya Oblast', NW Russian Federation
Severo-Kazakhstanskaya Oblast' see Severnyy Kazakhstan
123 U11 **Severo-Kuril'sk** Sakhalinskaya Oblast', SE Russian Federation
126 J3 **Severomorsk** Murmanskaya Oblast', NW Russian Federation
Severo-Osetinskaya SSR see Severnaya Osetiya-Alaniya, Respublika
122 M7 **Severo-Sibirskaya Nizmennost'** var. North Siberian Plain, Eng. North Siberian Lowland. lowlands N Russian Federation
122 G10 **Severoural'sk** Sverdlovskaya Oblast', C Russian Federation
122 L11 **Severo-Yeniseyskiy** Krasnoyarskiy Kray, C Russian Federation
128 M11 **Severskiy Donets** Ukr. Sivers'kyy Donets'. ≈ Russian Federation/Ukraine **see also** Sivers'kyy Donets'
92 M9 **Sevettijärvi** Lappi, N Finland
36 M5 **Sevier Bridge Reservoir** ⊞ Utah, W USA
36 J4 **Sevier Desert** plain Utah, W USA
36 J5 **Sevier Lake** ◎ Utah, W USA
21 N9 **Sevierville** Tennessee, S USA
104 J14 **Sevilla** Eng. Seville; anc. Hispalis. Andalucía, SW Spain
104 J13 **Sevilla** ◈ province Andalucía, SW Spain
Sevilla de Niefang see Niefang
43 O16 **Sevilla, Isla** island SW Panama
Seville see Sevilla
114 J9 **Sevlievo** Gabrovo, N Bulgaria
Sevluš/Sevlyush see Vynohradiv
109 V11 **Sevnica** Ger. Lichtenwald. E Slovenia
128 I7 **Sevsk** Bryanskaya Oblast', W Russian Federation
76 J15 **Sewa** ≈ E Sierra Leone
39 R12 **Seward** Alaska, USA
29 R15 **Seward** Nebraska, C USA
10 G8 **Seward Glacier** glacier Yukon Territory, W Canada
197 Q3 **Seward Peninsula** peninsula Alaska, USA
Seward's Folly see Alaska
62 H12 **Sewell** Libertador, C Chile
98 K5 **Sexbierum** Fris. Seisbierrum. Friesland, N Netherlands
11 O13 **Sexsmith** Alberta, W Canada
41 W13 **Seybaplaya** Campeche, SE Mexico
173 N6 **Seychelles** off. Republic of Seychelles. ◆ republic W Indian Ocean
67 Z9 **Seychelles** island group NE Seychelles
173 N6 **Seychelles Bank** var. Le Banc des Seychelles. undersea feature W Indian Ocean
Seychelles, Le Banc des see Seychelles Bank
172 H17 **Seychellois, Morne** ▲ Mahé, NE Seychelles
92 L2 **Seydhisfjördhur** Austurland, E Iceland
146 J12 **Seydi** prev. Neftezavodsk. Lebapskiy Velayat, E Turkmenistan
136 G16 **Seydişehir** Konya, SW Turkey
136 J13 **Seyfe Gölü** ◎ C Turkey
Seyhan see Adana
136 K16 **Seyhan Barajı** ⊞ S Turkey
136 K17 **Seyhan Nehri** ≈ S Turkey
136 F13 **Seyitgazi** Eskişehir, W Turkey
128 J7 **Seym** ≈ W Russian Federation
117 S3 **Seym** ≈ N Ukraine
123 T9 **Seymchan** Magadanskaya Oblast', E Russian Federation
114 N12 **Seymen** Tekirdağ, NW Turkey
183 O11 **Seymour** Victoria, SE Australia
83 I25 **Seymour** Eastern Cape, S South Africa
29 W16 **Seymour** Iowa, C USA
27 U7 **Seymour** Missouri, C USA
25 Q5 **Seymour** Texas, SW USA
114 M12 **Şeytan Deresi** ≈ NW Turkey
109 S12 **Sežana** It. Sesana. SW Slovenia
103 P5 **Sézanne** Marne, N France
107 I16 **Sezze** anc. Setia. Lazio, C Italy
115 H25 **Sfákia** Kríti, Greece, E Mediterranean Sea
115 D21 **Sfaktiria** island S Greece
116 J11 **Sfântu Gheorghe** Ger. Sankt-Georgen, Hung. Sepsiszentgyörgy; prev. Şepşi-Sângeorz, Sfintu Gheorghe. Covasna, C Romania
117 N13 **Sfântu Gheorghe, Braţul** var. Gheorghe Braţul. ≈ E Romania
75 N6 **Sfax** Ar. Şafāqis. E Tunisia
75 N6 **Sfax** ✕ E Tunisia
Sfintu Gheorghe see Sfântu Gheorghe
98 H13 **'s-Gravendeel** Zuid-Holland, SW Netherlands
98 F11 **'s-Gravenhage** var. Den Haag, Eng. The Hague, Fr. La Haye. ● (Netherlands-seat of government) Zuid-Holland, W Netherlands
98 G12 **'s-Gravenzande** Zuid-Holland, W Netherlands
Shaan/Shaanxi Sheng see Shaanxi
159 X11 **Shaanxi** var. Shaan, Shaanxi Sheng, Shan-hsi, Shenshi, Shensi. ◈ province C China
Shaartuz see Shahrtuz
Shabani see Zvishavane
81 N17 **Shabeellaha Dhexe** off. Gobolka Shabeellaha Dhexe. ◈ region E Somalia
81 L17 **Shabeellaha Hoose** off. Gobolka Shabeellaha Hoose. ◈ region S Somalia
Shabeelle, Webi see Shebeli
114 O7 **Shabla** Dobrich, NE Bulgaria
114 O7 **Shabla, Nos** headland NE Bulgaria
13 N9 **Shabogama Lake** ◎ Newfoundland, E Canada
79 N20 **Shabunda** Sud Kivu, E Dem. Rep. Congo (Zaire)
141 Q15 **Shabwah** C Yemen
158 F8 **Shache** var. Yarkant. Xinjiang Uygur Zizhiqu, NW China
Shacheng see Huailai
195 R12 **Shackleton Coast** physical region Antarctica
195 Z10 **Shackleton Ice Shelf** ice shelf Antarctica
Shaddādī see Ash Shadādah
28 K7 **Shadehill Reservoir** ⊞ South Dakota, N USA
122 G11 **Shadrinsk** Kurganskaya Oblast', C Russian Federation
31 O12 **Shafer, Lake** ⊞ Indiana, N USA
35 R13 **Shafter** California, W USA
24 J11 **Shafter** Texas, SW USA
97 L23 **Shaftesbury** S England, UK
185 F22 **Shag** ≈ South Island, NZ
145 V9 **Shagan** ≈ E Kazakhstan
39 O11 **Shageluk** Alaska, USA
122 K14 **Shagonar** Respublika Tyva, S Russian Federation
185 F22 **Shag Point** headland South Island, NZ
144 J12 **Shagyray, Plato** plain SW Kazakhstan
Shāhābād see Eslāmābād
168 K9 **Shah Alam** Selangor, Peninsular Malaysia
117 O12 **Shahany, Ozero** ◎ SW Ukraine
138 H9 **Shahbā'** anc. Philippopolis. As Suwaydā', S Syria
Shahbān see Ad Dayr
149 P17 **Shāhbandar** Sind, SE Pakistan
149 P13 **Shāhdād Kot** Sind, SW Pakistan
143 T10 **Shāhdād, Namakzār-e** salt pan E Iran
149 Q15 **Shāhdādpur** Sind, SE Pakistan
154 K10 **Shahdol** Madhya Pradesh, C India
161 N7 **Sha He** ≈ C China
Shahepu see Linze
153 N13 **Shāhganj** Uttar Pradesh, N India
152 C11 **Shāhgarh** Rājasthān, NW India
Sha Hi see Orūmīyeh, Daryācheh-ye, Iran
Shāhī see Qā'emshahr, Māzandarān, Iran
139 Q6 **Shāhimah** var. Shahma. C Iraq
Shāhjahanabad see Delhi
152 L11 **Shāhjahānpur** Uttar Pradesh, N India
Shahma see Shāhimah
149 U7 **Shāhpur** Punjab, E Pakistan
Shāhpur see Shāhpur Chākar
152 G13 **Shāhpura** Rājasthān, N India
149 Q15 **Shāhpur Chākar** var. Shāhpur. Sind, SE Pakistan
148 M5 **Shahrak** Ghowr, C Afghanistan
143 Q11 **Shahr-e Bābak** Kermān, C Iran
143 N8 **Shahr-e Kord** var. Shahr Kord. Chahār Maḩall va Bakhtīārī, C Iran
143 O9 **Shahreẓā** var. Qomisheh, Qumisheh, Shahriza; prev. Qomsheh. Eşfahān, C Iran
147 S10 **Shahrikhon** Rus. Shakhrikhan. Andijon Wiloyati, E Uzbekistan
147 N12 **Shahrisabz** Rus. Shakhrisabz. Qashqadaryo Wiloyati, S Uzbekistan
147 P11 **Shahriston** Rus. Shakhristan. NW Tajikistan
Shahriza see Shahreẓā
Shahr-i-Zabul see Zābol
Shahr Kord see Shahr-e Kord
147 P14 **Shahrtuz** Rus. Shaartuz. SW Tajikistan
143 Q4 **Shāhrūd** prev. Emāmrūd, Emāmshahr. Semnān, N Iran
Shahsavār/Shahsawar see Tonekābon
Shaidara see Step' Nardara
Shaikh Ābid see Shaykh 'Ābid
Shaikh Fāris see Shaykh Fāris
Shaikh Najm see Shaykh Najm
138 K5 **Shā'īr, Jabal** ▲ C Syria
154 G10 **Shājāpur** Madhya Pradesh, C India
80 J8 **Shakal, Ras** headland NE Sudan
Shakhdarinskiy Khrebet see Shokhdara, Qatorkŭhi
Shakhrikhan see Shahrikhon
Shakhrisabz see Shahrisabz
Shakhristan see Shahriston
117 X8 **Shakhtars'k** Rus. Shakhtërsk. Donets'ka Oblast', SE Ukraine
Shakhtërsk see Shakhtars'k
145 R10 **Shakhtinsk** Karaganda, C Kazakhstan
128 L11 **Shakhty** Rostovskaya Oblast', SW Russian Federation
129 P2 **Shakhun'ya** Nizhegorodskaya Oblast', W Russian Federation
77 S15 **Shaki** Oyo, W Nigeria
81 J15 **Shakīso** Oromo, C Ethiopia
117 X8 **Shakmars'k** Donets'ka Oblast', E Ukraine
29 V9 **Shakopee** Minnesota, N USA
165 R3 **Shakotan-misaki** headland Hokkaidō, NE Japan
39 N9 **Shaktoolik** Alaska, USA
81 J14 **Shala Hāyk'** ◎ C Ethiopia
126 M10 **Shalakusha** Arkhangel'skaya Oblast', NW Russian Federation
145 U8 **Shalday** Pavlodar, NE Kazakhstan
129 P16 **Shali** Chechenskaya Respublika, SW Russian Federation
141 W12 **Shalīm** var. Shelim. S Oman
Shaliuhe see Gangca
144 F9 **Shalkar, Ozero** prev. Chelkar, Ozero. ◎ W Kazakhstan
21 V12 **Shallotte** North Carolina, SE USA
25 N5 **Shallowater** Texas, SW USA
126 K11 **Shal'skiy** Respublika Kareliya, NW Russian Federation
160 F9 **Shaluli Shan** ⛰ C China
81 F22 **Shama** ≈ C Tanzania
11 Z11 **Shamattawa** Manitoba, C Canada
12 F8 **Shamattawa** ≈ Ontario, C Canada
Shām, Bādiyat ash see Syrian Desert
Shamiya see Ash Shāmīyah
141 X8 **Shām, Jabal ash** var. Jebel Sham. ▲ NW Oman
Sham, Jebel see Shām, Jabal ash
Shamkhor see Şämkir
18 G14 **Shamokin** Pennsylvania, NE USA
25 P2 **Shamrock** Texas, SW USA
Sha'nabī, Jabal ash see Chambi, Jebel
139 Y12 **Shanāwah** E Iraq
159 T8 **Shandan** Gansu, N China
Shandī see Shendi
161 Q5 **Shandong** var. Lu, Shandong Sheng, Shantung. ◈ province E China
161 R4 **Shandong Bandao** var. Shantung Peninsula. peninsula E China
Shandong Peninsula see Shandong Bandao
Shandong Sheng see Shandong
139 U8 **Shandrūkh** E Iraq
83 J17 **Shangani** ≈ W Zimbabwe
161 O15 **Shangchuan Dao** island S China
Shangchuankou see Minhe
163 P12 **Shangdu** Nei Mongol Zizhiqu, N China
161 O11 **Shanggao** Jiangxi, S China
161 S8 **Shanghai** var. Shang-hai. Shanghai Shi, E China
Shanghai see Shanghai Shi
161 S8 **Shanghai Shi** var. Hu, Shanghai. ◈ municipality E China
161 P13 **Shanghang** Fujian, SE China
160 K14 **Shanglin** Guangxi Zhuangzu Zizhiqu, S China
83 G15 **Shangombo** Western, W Zambia
161 O6 **Shangqiu** var. Zhuji. Henan, C China
161 Q10 **Shangrao** Jiangxi, S China
161 S9 **Shangyu** var. Baiguan. Zhejiang, SE China
163 X9 **Shangzhi** Heilongjiang, NE China
160 L7 **Shangzhou** var. Shang Xian. Shaanxi, C China
163 W9 **Shanhetun** Heilongjiang, NE China
Shan-hsi see Shaanxi, China
Shan-hsi see Shanxi, China
159 O6 **Shankou** Xinjiang Uygur Zizhiqu, W China
184 M13 **Shannon** Manawatu-Wanganui, North Island, NZ
97 B19 **Shannon** ✕ W Ireland
97 C17 **Shannon** Ir. An tSionainn. ≈ W Ireland
167 N6 **Shan Plateau** plateau E Myanmar
158 M6 **Shanshan** var. Piqan. Xinjiang Uygur Zizhiqu, NW China
Shansi see Shanxi
167 N5 **Shan State** ◈ state E Myanmar
Shantar Islands see Shantarskiye Ostrova
123 S12 **Shantarskiye Ostrova** Eng. Shantar Islands. island group E Russian Federation
161 Q14 **Shantou** var. Shan-t'ou, Swatow. Guangdong, S China
Shantung see Shandong
Shantung Peninsula see Shandong Bandao
163 O14 **Shanxi** var. Jin, Shan-hsi, Shansi, Shanxi Sheng. ◈ province C China
Shan Xian see Sanmenxia
161 P6 **Shanxian** var. Shan Xian. Shandong, E China
Shanxi Sheng see Shanxi
160 L7 **Shanyang** Shaanxi, C China
161 O13 **Shaoguan** var. Shao-kuan, Cant. Kukong; prev. Ch'u-chiang. Guangdong, S China
Shao-kuan see Shaoguan
161 Q11 **Shaowu** Fujian, SE China
161 S9 **Shaoxing** Zhejiang, SE China
160 M12 **Shaoyang** prev. Tangdukou. Hunan, S China
160 M11 **Shaoyang** var. Baoqing, Shao-yang; prev. Pao-king. Hunan, S China
96 K5 **Shapinsay** island NE Scotland, UK
127 S4 **Shapkina** ≈ NW Russian Federation
Shāpūr see Salmās
158 M4 **Shaqiuhe** Xinjiang Uygur Zizhiqu, W China
139 T2 **Shaqlāwa** var. Shaqlāwah. E Iraq
Shaqlāwah see Shaqlāwa
138 I8 **Shaqqā** As Suwaydā', S Syria
141 P7 **Shaqrā'** Ar Riyāḍ, C Saudi Arabia
Shaqrā see Shuqrah
145 W10 **Shar** var. Charsk. Vostochnyy Kazakhstan, E Kazakhstan
149 O6 **Sharan** Urūzgān, SE Afghanistan
Sharaqpur see Sharqpur
Sharbaqty see Shcherbakty
141 X12 **Sharbatāt** S Oman
141 X12 **Sharbithāt, Ras** var. Ra's Sharbatāt. headland S Oman
14 K14 **Sharbot Lake** Ontario, SE Canada
145 P17 **Shardara** var. Chardara. Yuzhnyy Kazakhstan, S Kazakhstan
Shardara Dalasy see Step' Nardara
162 F8 **Sharga** Govī-Altay, W Mongolia
162 H6 **Sharga** Hövsgöl, N Mongolia
116 M7 **Sharhorod** Vinnyts'ka Oblast', C Ukraine
162 K10 **Sharhulsan** Ömnögovĭ, S Mongolia
165 V3 **Shari** Hokkaidō, NE Japan
Shari see Chari
139 T6 **Shārī, Buḩayrat** ◎ C Iraq
Sharjah see Ash Shāriqah
118 K12 **Sharkawshchyna** var. Sharkowshchyna, Pol. Szarkowszczyzna, Rus. Sharkovshchina. Vitsyebskaya Voblasts', NW Belarus
180 G9 **Shark Bay** bay Western Australia
141 Y9 **Sharkh** E Oman
Sharkovshchina/Sharkowshchyna see Sharkawshchyna
129 U6 **Sharlyk** Orenburgskaya Oblast', W Russian Federation
Sharm ash Shaykh see Sharm el Sheikh
75 Y9 **Sharm el Sheikh** var. Ofiral, Sharm ash Shaykh. E Egypt
18 B13 **Sharon** Pennsylvania, NE USA
26 H4 **Sharon Springs** Kansas, C USA
31 Q14 **Sharonville** Ohio, N USA
Sharourah see Sharūrah
29 O10 **Sharpe, Lake** ⊞ South Dakota, N USA
Sharqi, Al Jabal ash/Sharqi, Jebel esh see Anti-Lebanon
Sharqīyah, Al Minṭaqah ash see Ash Sharqīyah
138 I6 **Sharqīyat an Nabk, Jabal** ▲ W Syria
149 W8 **Sharqpur** var. Sharaqpur. Punjab, E Pakistan
141 Q13 **Sharūrah** var. Sharourah. Najrān, S Saudi Arabia
127 O14 **Shar'ya** Kostromskaya Oblast', NW Russian Federation
145 V15 **Sharyn** var. Charyn. ≈ SE Kazakhstan
Sharyn see Charyn
83 J18 **Shashe** Central, NE Botswana
83 J18 **Shashe** var. Shashi. ≈ Botswana/Zimbabwe
81 J14 **Shashemenē** var. Shashemenne, Shashhamana, It. Sciasciamana. Oromo, C Ethiopia
Shashemenne/Shashhamana see Shashemenē
Shashi see Shashe
Shashi/Sha-shih/Shasi see Jingzhou, Hubei
35 N3 **Shasta Lake** ⊞ California, W USA
35 N2 **Shasta, Mount** ▲ California, W USA
129 O4 **Shatki** Nizhegorodskaya Oblast', W Russian Federation
146 J13 **Shatlyk** Maryyskiy Velayat, C Turkmenistan
Shatra see Ash Shaṭrah
119 K17 **Shatsk** Rus. Shatsk. Minskaya Voblasts', C Belarus
129 N5 **Shatsk** Ryazanskaya Oblast', W Russian Federation
26 J9 **Shattuck** Oklahoma, C USA
145 P16 **Shaul'der** Yuzhnyy Kazakhstan, S Kazakhstan
11 S17 **Shaunavon** Saskatchewan, S Canada
Shavat see Showot
158 K4 **Shawan** Xinjiang Uygur Zizhiqu, NW China
14 G12 **Shawanaga** Ontario, S Canada
30 M6 **Shawano** Wisconsin, N USA
30 M6 **Shawano Lake** ◎ Wisconsin, N USA
15 P10 **Shawinigan** prev. Shawinigan Falls. Quebec, SE Canada
Shawinigan Falls see Shawinigan
15 P10 **Shawinigan-Sud** Quebec, SE Canada
138 J5 **Shawmarīyah, Jabal ash** ⛰ C Syria
27 O11 **Shawnee** Oklahoma, C USA
14 K12 **Shawville** Quebec, SE Canada
Shaykh see Ash Shakk
139 W9 **Shaykh 'Ābid** var. Shaikh Ābid. E Iraq
139 Y10 **Shaykh Fāris** var. Shaikh Fāris. E Iraq
139 T7 **Shaykh Ḥātim** E Iraq
Shaykh, Jabal ash see Hermon, Mount
139 X10 **Shaykh Najm** var. Shaikh Najm. E Iraq
139 W9 **Shaykh Sa'd** E Iraq
147 T14 **Shazud** SE Tajikistan
119 N18 **Shchadryn** Rus. Shchedrin. Homyel'skaya Voblasts', SE Belarus
119 H18 **Shchara** ≈ SW Belarus
Shchedrin see Shchadryn
Shcheglovsk see Kemerovo
128 K5 **Shchëkino** Tul'skaya Oblast', W Russian Federation
127 S7 **Shchel'yayur** Respublika Komi, NW Russian Federation
145 U8 **Shcherbakty** Kaz. Sharbaqty. Pavlodar, E Kazakhstan
128 K7 **Shchigry** Kurskaya Oblast', W Russian Federation
Shchitkovichi see Shchytkavichy
117 Q2 **Shchors** Chernihivs'ka Oblast', N Ukraine
117 T8 **Shchors'k** Dnipropetrovs'ka Oblast', E Ukraine
Shchuchin see Shchuchyn
145 Q7 **Shchuchinsk** prev. Shchuchye. Severnyy Kazakhstan, N Kazakhstan
Shchuchye see Shchuchinsk
119 G16 **Shchuchyn** Pol. Szczuczyn Nowogródzki, Rus. Shchuchin. Hrodzyenskaya Voblasts', W Belarus
119 K17 **Shchytkavichy** Rus. Shchitkovichi. Minskaya Voblasts', C Belarus
122 J13 **Shebalino** Respublika Altay, S Russian Federation
128 J9 **Shebekino** Belgorodskaya Oblast', W Russian Federation
Shebelē Wenz, Wabē see Shebeli
81 L14 **Shebeli** Amh. Wabē Shebelē Wenz, It. Scebeli, Som. Webi Shabeelle. ≈ Ethiopia/Somalia
113 M20 **Shebenikut, Maja e** ▲ E Albania
149 N2 **Sheberghān** var. Shibarghān, Shiberghan, Shiberghān. Jowzjān, N Afghanistan
144 F14 **Shebir** Mangistau, SW Kazakhstan
31 N8 **Sheboygan** Wisconsin, N USA
77 X15 **Shebshi Mountains** var. Schebschi Mountains. ⛰ E Nigeria
Shechem see Nablus
Shedadi see Ash Shadādah
13 P14 **Shediac** New Brunswick, SE Canada
128 L15 **Shedok** Krasnodarskiy Kray, SW Russian Federation
80 N12 **Sheekh** Woqooyi Galbeed, N Somalia
38 M11 **Sheenjek River** ≈ Alaska, USA
96 D13 **Sheep Haven** Ir. Cuan na gCaorach. inlet N Ireland
35 X10 **Sheep Range** ⛰ Nevada, W USA
98 M13 **'s-Heerenberg** Gelderland, E Netherlands
97 P22 **Sheerness** SE England, UK
13 Q15 **Sheet Harbour** Nova Scotia, SE Canada
185 H18 **Sheffield** Canterbury, South Island, NZ
97 M18 **Sheffield** N England, UK
23 O2 **Sheffield** Alabama, S USA
29 V12 **Sheffield** Iowa, C USA
25 N10 **Sheffield** Texas, SW USA
63 H22 **Shehuen, Río** ≈ S Argentina
Shekhem see Nablus
149 V8 **Shekhūpura** Punjab, NE Pakistan
Sheki see Şäki
126 L14 **Sheksna** Vologodskaya Oblast', NW Russian Federation
123 T5 **Shelagskiy, Mys** headland NE Russian Federation
27 V3 **Shelbina** Missouri, C USA
13 P16 **Shelburne** Nova Scotia, SE Canada
14 G14 **Shelburne** Ontario, S Canada
33 R7 **Shelby** Montana, NW USA
21 Q10 **Shelby** North Carolina, SE USA
31 S12 **Shelby** Ohio, N USA
30 L14 **Shelbyville** Illinois, N USA
31 P14 **Shelbyville** Indiana, N USA
20 L5 **Shelbyville** Kentucky, S USA
27 V2 **Shelbyville** Missouri, C USA
20 J10 **Shelbyville** Tennessee, S USA
25 X8 **Shelbyville** Texas, SW USA
30 L14 **Shelbyville, Lake** ⊞ Illinois, N USA
29 S12 **Sheldon** Iowa, C USA
38 M11 **Sheldons Point** Alaska, USA
Shelekhov Gulf see Shelikhova, Zaliv
123 U9 **Shelikhova, Zaliv** Eng. Shelekhov Gulf. gulf E Russian Federation
39 P14 **Shelikof Strait** strait Alaska, USA
Shelim see Shalīm
11 T14 **Shellbrook** Saskatchewan, S Canada
28 L3 **Shell Creek** ≈ North Dakota, N USA
Shellif see Chelif, Oued
22 I10 **Shell Keys** island group Louisiana, S USA
30 J4 **Shell Lake** Wisconsin, N USA
29 W12 **Shell Rock** Iowa, C USA
185 C26 **Shelter Point** headland Stewart Island, NZ
18 L13 **Shelton** Connecticut, NE USA
32 G8 **Shelton** Washington, NW USA
Shemakha see Şamaxı
145 W9 **Shemonaikha** Vostochnyy Kazakhstan, E Kazakhstan
129 Q4 **Shemursha** Chuvashskaya Respublika, W Russian Federation
38 D16 **Shemya Island** island Aleutian Islands, Alaska, USA
29 T16 **Shenandoah** Iowa, C USA
21 U4 **Shenandoah** Virginia, NE USA
21 U4 **Shenandoah Mountains** ridge West Virginia, NE USA
21 V3 **Shenandoah River** ≈ West Virginia, NE USA
77 W15 **Shendam** Plateau, C Nigeria
80 G8 **Shendi** var. Shandī. River Nile, NE Sudan
76 I15 **Shenge** SW Sierra Leone
145 U15 **Shengel'dy** Almaty, SE Kazakhstan
113 K18 **Shëngjin** var. Shëngjini. Lezhë, NW Albania
Shëngjini see Shëngjin
Shengking see Liaoning
Sheng Xian/Shengxian see Shengzhou
161 S9 **Shengzhou** var. Shengxian, Sheng Xian. Zhejiang, SE China
Shenking see Liaoning
127 N11 **Shenkursk** Arkhangel'skaya Oblast', NW Russian Federation
160 L3 **Shenmu** Shaanxi, C China
113 L19 **Shën Noj i Madh** ▲ C Albania
Shenshi/Shensi see Shaanxi
163 V12 **Shenyang** Chin. Shen-yang, Eng. Moukden, Mukden; prev. Fengtien. Liaoning, NE China
161 O15 **Shenzhen** Guangdong, S China
154 G8 **Sheopur** Madhya Pradesh, C India
116 L5 **Shepetivka** Rus. Shepetovka. Khmel'nyts'ka Oblast', NW Ukraine
Shepetovka see Shepetivka
25 W10 **Shepherd** Texas, SW USA
187 R14 **Shepherd Islands** island group C Vanuatu
20 K5 **Shepherdsville** Kentucky, S USA
183 O11 **Shepparton** Victoria, SE Australia
97 P22 **Sheppey, Isle of** island SE England, UK
Sherabad see Sherobod
9 O4 **Sherard, Cape** headland Nunavut, N Canada
97 L23 **Sherborne** S England, UK
76 H16 **Sherbro Island** island SW Sierra Leone
15 Q12 **Sherbrooke** Quebec, SE Canada
29 T11 **Sherburn** Minnesota, N USA
78 H6 **Sherda** Borkou-Ennedi-Tibesti, N Chad
80 G7 **Shereik** River Nile, N Sudan

◆ Country ● Country Capital ◇ Dependent Territory ○ Dependent Territory Capital ◈ Administrative Region ✕ International Airport ▲ Mountain ⛰ Mountain Range ⩫ Volcano ≈ River ◎ Lake ⊞ Reservoir

128 K3 **Sheremet'yevo** × (Moskva) Moskovskaya Oblast', W Russian Federation
153 P14 **Shergāti** Bihār, N India
27 U12 **Sheridan** Arkansas, C USA
33 W12 **Sheridan** Wyoming, C USA
182 G8 **Sheringa** South Australia
25 U5 **Sherman** Texas, SW USA
194 J10 **Sherman Island** *island* Antarctica
19 S4 **Sherman Mills** Maine, NE USA
29 O15 **Sherman Reservoir** ▣ Nebraska, C USA
147 N14 **Sherobod** *Rus.* Sherabad. Surkhondaryo Wiloyati, S Uzbekistan
147 O13 **Sherobod** *Rus.* Sherabad. ≈ S Uzbekistan
153 T14 **Sherpur** Dhaka, N Bangladesh
37 T4 **Sherrelwood** Colorado, C USA
99 J14 **'s-Hertogenbosch** *Fr.* Bois-le-Duc, *Ger.* Herzogenbusch. Noord-Brabant, S Netherlands
28 M2 **Sherwood** North Dakota, N USA
11 Q14 **Sherwood Park** Alberta, SW Canada
56 F13 **Sheshea, Río** ≈ E Peru
143 T5 **Sheshtamad** Khorāsān, NE Iran
29 S10 **Shetek, Lake** ◎ Minnesota, N USA
96 M2 **Shetland Islands** *island group* NE Scotland, UK
144 F14 **Shetpe** Mangistau, SW Kazakhstan
154 C11 **Shetrunji** ≈ W India
Shevchenko *see* Aktau
117 W5 **Shevchenkove** Kharkivs'ka Oblast', E Ukraine
81 H14 **Shewa Gīmīra** Southern, S Ethiopia
161 Q9 **Shexian** *var.* Huicheng, She Xian. Anhui, E China
161 R6 **Sheyang** *prev.* Hede. Jiangsu, E China
29 O4 **Sheyenne** North Dakota, N USA
29 P4 **Sheyenne River** ≈ North Dakota, N USA
96 G7 **Shiant Islands** *island group* NW Scotland, UK
123 U12 **Shiashkotan, Ostrov** *island* Kuril'skiye Ostrova, SE Russian Federation
31 R9 **Shiawassee River** ≈ Michigan, N USA
141 R14 **Shibām** C Yemen
Shibarghān *see* Sheberghān
165 O10 **Shibata** *var.* Sibata. Niigata, Honshū, C Japan
Shiberghan/Shiberghān *see* Sheberghān
Shibh Jazīrat Sīnā' *see* Sinai
Shibīn al Kawm *see* Shibîn el Kôm
75 W8 **Shibîn el Kôm** *var.* Shibīn al Kawm. N Egypt
143 O13 **Shīb, Kūh-e** ▲ S Iran
12 D8 **Shibogama Lake** ◎ Ontario, C Canada
Shibotsu-jima *see* Zelënyy, Ostrov
164 B16 **Shibushi** Kagoshima, Kyūshū, SW Japan
189 U13 **Shichiyo Islands** *island group* Chuuk, C Micronesia
Shickshock Mountains *see* Chic-Chocs, Monts
145 S9 **Shiderti** ≈ N Kazakhstan
145 S8 **Shiderty** Pavlodar, NE Kazakhstan
96 G10 **Shiel, Loch** ◎ N Scotland, UK
164 J13 **Shiga** *off.* Shiga-ken, *var.* Siga. ◈ *prefecture* Honshū, SW Japan
Shigatse *see* Xigazê
141 U13 **Shiḥan** *oasis* NE Yemen
Shih-chia-chuang/Shihmen *see* Shijiazhuang
158 K4 **Shihezi** Xinjiang Uygur Zizhiqu, NW China
Shiichi *see* Shyichy
113 K19 **Shijak** *var.* Shijaku. Durrës, W Albania
Shijaku *see* Shijak
161 O4 **Shijiazhuang** *var.* Shih-chia-chuang; *prev.* Shihmen. Hebei, E China
165 R5 **Shikabe** Hokkaidō, NE Japan
149 Q13 **Shikārpur** Sind, S Pakistan
189 V12 **Shiki Islands** *island group* Chuuk, C Micronesia
164 G14 **Shikoku** *var.* Sikoku. *island* SW Japan
192 H5 **Shikoku Basin** *var.* Sikoku Basin. *undersea feature* N Philippine Sea
164 G14 **Shikoku-sanchi** ▲ Shikoku, SW Japan
165 X4 **Shikotan, Ostrov** *Jap.* Shikotan-tō. *island* NE Russian Federation
Shikotan-tō *see* Shikotan, Ostrov
165 R4 **Shikotsu-ko** *var.* Sikotu Ko. ◎ Hokkaidō, NE Japan
81 N15 **Shilabo** Somali, E Ethiopia
129 X7 **Shil'da** Orenburgskaya Oblast', W Russian Federation
139 V3 **Shilēr, Āw-e** ≈ E Iraq
153 S12 **Shiliguri** *prev.* Siliguri. West Bengal, NE India
131 V7 **Shilka** ≈ S Russian Federation
18 H15 **Shillington** Pennsylvania, NE USA
153 V13 **Shillong** Meghālaya, NE India
128 M5 **Shilovo** Ryazanskaya Oblast', W Russian Federation
164 C14 **Shimabara** *var.* Simabara. Nagasaki, Kyūshū, SW Japan
164 C14 **Shimabara-wan** *bay* SW Japan
164 F12 **Shimane** *off.* Shimane-ken, *var.* Simane. ◈ *prefecture* Honshū, SW Japan
164 G11 **Shimane-hantō** *peninsula* Honshū, SW Japan
123 Q13 **Shimanovsk** Amurskaya Oblast', SE Russian Federation
Shimbir Berris *see* Shimbiris
80 O12 **Shimbiris** *var.* Shimbir Berris. ▲ N Somalia
165 T4 **Shimizu** Hokkaidō, NE Japan
164 M14 **Shimizu** *var.* Simizu. Shizuoka, Honshū, S Japan
152 I8 **Shimla** *prev.* Simla. Himāchal Pradesh, N India
Shimminato *see* Shinminato
165 N14 **Shimoda** *var.* Simoda. Shizuoka, Honshū, S Japan
165 O13 **Shimodate** *var.* Simodate. Ibaraki, Honshū, S Japan
155 F18 **Shimoga** Karnātaka, W India
164 C15 **Shimo-jima** *island* SW Japan
164 B15 **Shimo-Koshiki-jima** *island* SW Japan
81 J21 **Shimoni** Coast, S Kenya
164 D13 **Shimonoseki** *var.* Simonoseki; *hist.* Akamagaseki, Bakan. Yamaguchi, Honshū, SW Japan
126 G14 **Shimsk** Novgorodskaya Oblast', NW Russian Federation
141 W7 **Shināṣ** N Oman
148 J6 **Shīndand** Farāh, W Afghanistan
Shinei *see* Hsinying
25 T12 **Shiner** Texas, SW USA
167 N1 **Shingbwiyang** Kachin State, N Myanmar
145 W11 **Shingozha** Vostochnyy Kazakhstan, E Kazakhstan
164 J15 **Shingū** *var.* Singû. Wakayama, Honshū, SW Japan
14 F8 **Shining Tree** Ontario, S Canada
165 P9 **Shinjō** *var.* Sinzyô. Yamagata, Honshū, C Japan
96 I7 **Shin, Loch** ◎ N Scotland, UK
21 S3 **Shinnston** West Virginia, NE USA
138 I6 **Shinshār** *Fr.* Chinnchâr. Ḥimṣ, W Syria
Shinshū *see* Chinju
165 T4 **Shintoku** Hokkaidō, NE Japan
81 G20 **Shinyanga** Shinyanga, NW Tanzania
81 G20 **Shinyanga** ◈ *region* N Tanzania
165 Q10 **Shiogama** *var.* Siogama. Miyagi, Honshū, C Japan
164 M12 **Shiojiri** *var.* Sioziri. Nagano, Honshū, S Japan
164 I15 **Shiono-misaki** *headland* Honshū, SW Japan
165 Q12 **Shioya-zaki** *headland* Honshū, C Japan
114 J9 **Shipchenski Prokhod** *pass* C Bulgaria
160 G14 **Shiping** Yunnan, SW China
13 P13 **Shippagan** *var.* Shippegan. New Brunswick, SE Canada
Shippegan *see* Shippagan
18 F15 **Shippensburg** Pennsylvania, NE USA
37 O9 **Ship Rock** ▲ New Mexico, SW USA
37 P9 **Shiprock** New Mexico, SW USA
15 R6 **Shipshaw** ≈ Quebec, SE Canada
123 V10 **Shipunskiy, Mys** *headland* E Russian Federation
160 K7 **Shiquan** Shaanxi, C China
122 K13 **Shira** Respublika Khakasiya, S Russian Federation
153 T14 **Shirajganj Ghat** *var.* Serajgonj, Sirajganj. Rajshahi, C Bangladesh
165 P12 **Shirakawa** *var.* Sirakawa. Fukushima, Honshū, C Japan
164 M13 **Shirane-san** ▲ Honshū, S Japan
165 U14 **Shiranuka** Hokkaidō, NE Japan
195 N12 **Shirase Coast** *physical region* Antarctica
165 U3 **Shirataki** Hokkaidō, NE Japan
143 O11 **Shīrāz** *var.* Shīrāz. Fārs, S Iran
83 N15 **Shire** *var.* Chire. ≈ Malawi/Mozambique
162 G7 **Shiree** Dzavhan, W Mongolia
163 O9 **Shireet** Sühbaatar, SE Mongolia
165 W3 **Shiretoko-hantō** *headland* Hokkaidō, NE Japan
165 W3 **Shiretoko-misaki** *headland* Hokkaidō, NE Japan
129 N5 **Shiringushi** Respublika Mordoviya, W Russian Federation
148 M3 **Shīrīn Tagāb** Fāryāb, N Afghanistan
149 N2 **Shīrīn Tagāb** ≈ N Afghanistan
165 R6 **Shiriya-zaki** *headland* Honshū, C Japan
144 I12 **Shirkala, Gryada** *plain* W Kazakhstan
165 P10 **Shiroishi** *var.* Siroisi. Miyagi, Honshū, C Japan
Shirokoye *see* Shyroke
165 O10 **Shirone** *var.* Sirone. Niigata, Honshū, C Japan
164 L12 **Shirotori** Gifu, Honshū, SW Japan
197 T1 **Shirshov Ridge** *undersea feature* W Bering Sea
Shirshütür *see* Shirshyutyur, Peski
146 K12 **Shirshyutyur, Peski** *Turkm.* Shirshütür. *desert* E Turkmenistan
143 T3 **Shīrvān** *var.* Shirwān. Khorāsān, NE Iran
Shirwa, Lake *see* Chilwa, Lake
Shirwān *see* Shīrvān
159 N5 **Shisanjianfang** Xinjiang Uygur Zizhiqu, W China
38 M16 **Shishaldin Volcano** ▲ Unimak Island, Alaska, USA
Shishchitsy *see* Shyshchytsy
38 M8 **Shishmaref** Alaska, USA
Shisur *see* Ash Shişar
164 L13 **Shitara** Aichi, Honshū, SW Japan
152 D12 **Shiv** Rājasthān, NW India
151 E15 **Shivāji Sāgar** *prev.* Konya Reservoir ▣ W India
154 H8 **Shivpuri** Madhya Pradesh, C India
36 J9 **Shivwits Plateau** *plain* Arizona, SW USA
Shiwālik Range *see* Siwalik Range
160 M8 **Shiyan** Hubei, C China
160 H13 **Shizong** Yunnan, SW China
165 R10 **Shizugawa** Miyagi, Honshū, NE Japan
159 W8 **Shizuishan** *var.* Dawukou. Ningxia, N China
165 T5 **Shizunai** Hokkaidō, NE Japan
165 M14 **Shizuoka** *var.* Sizuoka. Shizuoka, Honshū, S Japan
164 M13 **Shizuoka** *off.* Shizuoka-ken, *var.* Sizuoka. ◈ *prefecture* Honshū, S Japan
Shklov *see* Shklow
119 N15 **Shklow** *Rus.* Shklov. Mahilyowskaya Voblasts', E Belarus
113 K18 **Shkodër** *var.* Shkodra, *It.* Scutari, *SCr.* Skadar. Shkodër, NW Albania
113 K17 **Shkodër** ◈ *district* NW Albania
Shkodra *see* Shkodër
Shkodrës, Liqeni i *see* Scutari, Lake
Shkumbî/Shkumbin *see* Shkumbinit, Lumi i
113 L20 **Shkumbinit, Lumi i** *var.* Shkumbî, Shkumbin. ≈ C Albania
Shligigh, Cuan *see* Sligo Bay
122 L4 **Shmidta, Ostrov** *island* Severnaya Zemlya, N Russian Federation
183 S10 **Shoalhaven River** ≈ New South Wales, SE Australia
11 W16 **Shoal Lake** Manitoba, S Canada
31 O15 **Shoals** Indiana, N USA
164 I13 **Shōdo-shima** *island* SW Japan
Shōka *see* Changhua
122 M5 **Shokal'skogo, Proliv** *strait* N Russian Federation
147 T14 **Shokhdara, Qatorkŭhi** *Rus.* Shakhdarinskiy Khrebet. ▲ SE Tajikistan
145 N9 **Sholaksay** Kostanay, N Kazakhstan
Sholāpur *see* Solāpur
Sholdaneshty *see* Şoldăneşti
145 P17 **Sholakkorgan** *var.* Chulakkurgan. Yuzhnyy Kazakhstan, S Kazakhstan
Shoqpar *see* Chokpar
155 G21 **Shoranūr** Kerala, SW India
155 G16 **Shorāpur** Karnātaka, C India
30 M11 **Shorewood** Illinois, N USA
Shorkazakhly, Solonchak *see* Kazakhlyshor, Solonchak
145 Q9 **Shortandy** Akmola, C Kazakhstan
Shortepa/Shor Tepe *see* Shūr Tappeh
186 J7 **Shortland Island** *var.* Alu. *island* NW Solomon Islands
Shosambetsu *see* Shosanbetsu
165 S2 **Shosanbetsu** *var.* Shosambetsu. Hokkaidō, NE Japan
33 O15 **Shoshone** Idaho, NW USA
35 T6 **Shoshone Mountains** ▲ Nevada, W USA
33 U12 **Shoshone River** ≈ Wyoming, C USA
83 I19 **Shoshong** Central, SE Botswana
33 V14 **Shoshoni** Wyoming, C USA
Shōshū *see* Sangju
117 S2 **Shostka** Sums'ka Oblast', NE Ukraine
185 C21 **Shotover** ≈ South Island, NZ
37 N12 **Show Low** Arizona, SW USA
Show Me State *see* Missouri
146 H9 **Showot** *Rus.* Shavat. Khorazm Wiloyati, W Uzbekistan
127 O4 **Shoyna** Nenetskiy Avtonomnyy Okrug, NW Russian Federation
126 M11 **Shozhma** Arkhangel'skaya Oblast', NW Russian Federation
117 Q7 **Shpola** Cherkas'ka Oblast', N Ukraine
Shqipëria/Shqipërisë, Republika e *see* Albania
22 G5 **Shreveport** Louisiana, S USA
97 K19 **Shrewsbury** *hist.* Scrobesbyrig'. W England, UK
152 D11 **Shri Mohangarh** *prev.* Sri Mohangorh. Rājasthān, NW India
153 S16 **Shrīrāmpur** *prev.* Serampore, Serampur. West Bengal, NE India
97 K19 **Shropshire** *cultural region* W England, UK
145 S16 **Shu** *Kaz.* Shū. Zhambyl, SE Kazakhstan
Shū *see* Chu
160 G13 **Shuangbai** Yunnan, SW China
163 W9 **Shuangcheng** Heilongjiang, NE China
160 E14 **Shuangjiang** Yunnan, SW China
163 U10 **Shuangliao** *var.* Zhengjiatun. Jilin, NE China
Shuang-liao *see* Liaoyuan
163 Y7 **Shuangyashan** *var.* Shuang-ya-shan. Heilongjiang, NE China
Shu'aymiah *see* Shu'aymīyah
141 W12 **Shu'aymīyah** *var.* Shu'aymiah. S Oman
144 I10 **Shubarkuduk** *Kaz.* Shubarqudyq. Aktyubinsk, W Kazakhstan
Shubarqudyq *see* Shubarkuduk
145 N12 **Shubar-Tengiz, Ozero** ◎ C Kazakhstan
39 S5 **Shublik Mountains** ▲ Alaska, USA
Shubrā al Khaymah *see* Shubrâ el Kheima
121 U13 **Shubrâ el Kheima** *var.* Shubrā al Khaymah. N Egypt
158 E8 **Shufu** Xinjiang Uygur Zizhiqu, NW China
147 S14 **Shughnon, Qatorkŭhi** *Rus.* Shugnanskiy Khrebet. ▲ SE Tajikistan
Shugnanskiy Khrebet *see* Shughnon, Qatorkŭhi
161 Q6 **Shu He** ≈ E China
Shuiding *see* Huocheng
Shuiji *see* Laixi
Shū-Ile Taūlary *see* Chu-Iliyskiye Gory
149 T10 **Shujāābād** Punjab, E Pakistan
163 W9 **Shulan** Jilin, NE China
158 E8 **Shule** Xinjiang Uygur Zizhiqu, NW China
Shuleh *see* Shule He
159 Q8 **Shule He** *var.* Shuleh, Sulo. ≈ C China
30 K9 **Shullsburg** Wisconsin, N USA
39 N16 **Shumagin Islands** *island group* Alaska, USA
146 G7 **Shumanay** Qoraqalpoghiston Respublikasi, W Uzbekistan
114 M8 **Shumen** Shumen, NE Bulgaria
114 M8 **Shumen** ◈ *province* NE Bulgaria
129 P4 **Shumerlya** Chuvashskaya Respublika, W Russian Federation
122 G11 **Shumikha** Kurganskaya Oblast', C Russian Federation
118 M12 **Shumilina** *Rus.* Shumilino. Vitsyebskaya Voblasts', NE Belarus
Shumilino *see* Shumilina
123 V11 **Shumshu, Ostrov** *island* SE Russian Federation
116 K5 **Shums'k** Ternopil's'ka Oblast', W Ukraine
39 O7 **Shungnak** Alaska, USA
Shunsen *see* Ch'unch'ŏn
160 M3 **Shuo Xian** Shanxi, NE China
Shuo Xian/Shuoxian *see* Shuozhou
161 N3 **Shuozhou** *var.* Shuoxian; *prev.* Shuo Xian. Shanxi, C China
141 P16 **Shuqrah** *var.* Shaqrā. SW Yemen
Shurab *see* Shŭrob
147 O14 **Shŭrchi** *Rus.* Shurchi. Surkhondaryo Wiloyati, S Uzbekistan
147 R11 **Shŭrob** *Rus.* Shurab. NW Tajikistan
143 T10 **Shūr, Rūd-e** ≈ E Iran
149 O2 **Shūr Tappeh** *var.* Shortepa, Shor Tepe. Balkh, N Afghanistan
83 K17 **Shurugwi** *prev.* Selukwe. Midlands, C Zimbabwe
142 L8 **Shūsh** *anc.* Susa, *Bibl.* Shushan. Khūzestān, SW Iran
Shushan *see* Shūsh
142 L9 **Shūshtar** *var.* Shustar, Shushter. Khūzestān, SW Iran
Shushter/Shustar *see* Shūshtar
141 T9 **Shuṭfah, Qalamat** *well* E Saudi Arabia
139 V9 **Shuwayjah, Hawr ash** *var.* Hawr as Suwayqiyah. ◎ E Iraq
126 M16 **Shuya** Ivanovskaya Oblast', W Russian Federation
39 Q14 **Shuyak Island** *island* Alaska, USA
166 M4 **Shwebo** Sagaing, C Myanmar
166 L7 **Shwedaung** Pegu, W Myanmar
166 M7 **Shwegyin** Pegu, SW Myanmar
167 N4 **Shweli** *Chin.* Longchuan Jiang. ≈ Myanmar/China
166 M6 **Shwemyo** Mandalay, C Myanmar
Shyghys Qazagastan Oblysy *see* Vostochnyy Kazakhstan
Shyghys Qongyrat *see* Shygys Konyrat
145 T12 **Shygys Konyrat** *var.* Vostochno-Kounradskiy, *Kaz.* Shyghys Qongyrat. Karaganda, C Kazakhstan
119 M19 **Shyichy** *Rus.* Shiichi. Homyel'skaya Voblasts', SE Belarus
145 Q17 **Shymkent** *prev.* Chimkent. Yuzhnyy Kazakhstan, S Kazakhstan
Shyngghyrlaū *see* Chingirlau
152 J5 **Shyok** Jammu and Kashmir, NW India
117 S9 **Shyroke** *Rus.* Shirokoye. Dnipropetrovs'ka Oblast', E Ukraine
117 O9 **Shyryayeve** Odes'ka Oblast', SW Ukraine
117 S5 **Shyshaky** Poltavs'ka Oblast', C Ukraine
119 K17 **Shyshchytsy** *Rus.* Shishchitsy. Minskaya Voblasts', C Belarus
149 Y3 **Siachen Muztāgh** ▲ NE Pakistan
Siadehan *see* Tākestān
148 M13 **Siāhān Range** ▲ W Pakistan
142 I1 **Siāh Chashmeh** Āzarbāyjān-e Bākhtarī, N Iran
149 W7 **Siālkot** Punjab, NE Pakistan
186 E7 **Sialum** Morobe, C PNG
Siam *see* Thailand
Siam, Gulf of *see* Thailand, Gulf of
Sian *see* Xi'an
Siang *see* Brahmaputra
Siangtan *see* Xiangtan
169 N8 **Siantan, Pulau** *island* Kepulauan Anambas, W Indonesia
54 H11 **Siare, Río** ≈ C Colombia
171 R6 **Siargao Island** *island* S Philippines
186 F7 **Siassi** Umboi Island, C PNG
115 D14 **Siátista** Dytikí Makedonía, N Greece
166 K4 **Siatlai** Chin State, W Myanmar
171 P6 **Siaton** Negros, C Philippines
171 P6 **Siaton Point** *headland* Negros, C Philippines
118 F11 **Šiauliai** *Ger.* Schaulen. Šiauliai, N Lithuania
171 Q10 **Siau, Pulau** *island* N Indonesia
83 J15 **Siavonga** Southern, SE Zambia
Siazan' *see* Siyäzän
Sibah *see* As Sībah
107 N20 **Sibari** Calabria, S Italy
Sibata *see* Shibata
129 X6 **Sibay** Respublika Bashkortostan, W Russian Federation
93 M19 **Sibbo** *Fin.* Sipoo. Etelä-Suomi, S Finland
112 D13 **Šibenik** *It.* Sebenico. Šibenik-Knin, S Croatia
Šibenik *see* Šibenik-Knin
112 E13 **Šibenik-Knin** *off.* Šibenska Županija. *var.* Šibenik. ◈ *province* S Croatia
Šibenska Županija *see* Šibenik-Knin
Siberia *see* Sibir'
Siberoet *see* Siberut, Pulau
168 H12 **Siberut, Pulau** *prev.* Siberoet. *island* Kepulauan Mentawai, W Indonesia
168 I12 **Siberut, Selat** *strait* W Indonesia
Sibetu *see* Shibetsu
149 P11 **Sibi** Baluchistān, SW Pakistan
186 B9 **Sibidiri** Western, SW PNG
123 N10 **Sibir'** *var.* Siberia. *physical region* NE Russian Federation
79 F20 **Sibiti** La Lékoumou, S Congo
81 G21 **Sibiti** ≈ C Tanzania
116 I12 **Sibiu** *Ger.* Hermannstadt, *Hung.* Nagyszeben. Sibiu, C Romania
116 I11 **Sibiu** ◈ *county* C Romania
29 S11 **Sibley** Iowa, C USA
169 R9 **Sibu** Sarawak, East Malaysia
Sibukawa *see* Shibukawa
42 G2 **Sibun** ≈ E Belize
79 I15 **Sibut** *prev.* Fort-Sibut. Kémo, S Central African Republic
171 P4 **Sibuyan Island** *island* C Philippines
171 P4 **Sibuyan Sea** *sea* C Philippines
189 U1 **Sibylla Island** *island* N Marshall Islands
11 N16 **Sicamous** British Columbia, SW Canada
Sichelburger Gebirge *see* Gorjanci/Žumberačko Gorje
167 N14 **Sichon** *var.* Ban Sichon, Si Chon. Nakhon Si Thammarat, SW Thailand
160 H9 **Sichuan** *var.* Chuan, Sichuan Sheng, Ssu-ch'uan, Szechuan, Szechwan. ◈ *province* C China
160 I9 **Sichuan Pendi** *basin* C China
Sichuan Sheng *see* Sichuan
103 S16 **Sicie, Cap** *headland* SE France
107 J24 **Sicilia** *Eng.* Sicily; *anc.* Trinacria. ◈ *region* Italy, C Mediterranean Sea
107 M24 **Sicilia** *Eng.* Sicily; *anc.* Trinacria. *island* Italy, C Mediterranean Sea
Sicilian Channel *see* Sicily, Strait of
Sicily *see* Sicilia
107 H24 **Sicily, Strait of** *var.* Sicilian Channel. *strait* C Mediterranean Sea
42 K5 **Sico Tinto, Río** *var.* Río Negro. ≈ NE Honduras
57 H16 **Sicuani** Cusco, S Peru
112 J10 **Šid** Serbia, NW Yugoslavia
115 A15 **Sidári** Kérkyra, Iónioi Nísoi, Greece, C Mediterranean Sea
169 Q11 **Sidas** Borneo, C Indonesia
98 O5 **Siddeburen** Groningen, NE Netherlands
154 D9 **Siddhapur** *prev.* Siddhpur, Sidhpur. Gujarāt, W India
Siddhpur *see* Siddhapur
155 I15 **Siddipet** Andhra Pradesh, C India
77 N14 **Sidéradougou** SW Burkina
107 N23 **Siderno** Calabria, SW Italy
Siders *see* Sierre
154 L9 **Sidhi** Madhya Pradesh, C India
Sidhirókastron *see* Sidirókastro
Sidhpur *see* Siddhapur
Sîdi al Hānī', Sabkhat *see* Sidi el Hani, Sebkhet de
75 U7 **Sîdi Barrâni** NW Egypt
74 I6 **Sidi Bel Abbès** *var.* Sidi bel Abbès, Sidi-Bel-Abbès. NW Algeria
74 E7 **Sidi-Bennour** W Morocco
74 M6 **Sidi Bouzid** *var.* Gammouda, Sīdī Bu Zayd. C Tunisia
74 D8 **Sidi-Ifni** SW Morocco
74 G6 **Sidi-Kacem** *prev.* Petitjean. N Morocco
114 G12 **Sidirókastro** *prev.* Sidhirókastron. Kentrikí Makedonía, NE Greece
194 L12 **Sidley, Mount** ▲ Antarctica
29 S16 **Sidney** Iowa, C USA
33 Y7 **Sidney** Montana, NW USA
28 J15 **Sidney** Nebraska, C USA
18 I11 **Sidney** New York, NE USA
31 R13 **Sidney** Ohio, N USA
23 T2 **Sidney Lanier, Lake** ▣ Georgia, SE USA
Sidon *see* Saïda
122 J9 **Sidorovsk** Yamalo-Nenetskiy Avtonomnyy Okrug, N Russian Federation
Sidra/Sidra, Gulf of *see* Surt, Khalīj, N Libya
Sidra *see* Surt, N Libya
Sīdī Bu Zayd *see* Sidi Bouzid
Siebenbürgen *see* Transylvania
Sieben Dörfer *see* Săcele
110 O12 **Siedlce** *Ger.* Sedlez, *Rus.* Sesdlets. Mazowieckie, C Poland
101 E16 **Sieg** ≈ W Germany
101 F16 **Siegen** Nordrhein-Westfalen, W Germany
109 X4 **Sieghartskirchen** Niederösterreich, E Austria
110 O11 **Siemiatycze** Podlaskie, NE Poland
167 T11 **Siĕmpang** Stœ̆ng Trêng, NE Cambodia
167 R11 **Siĕmréab** *prev.* Siemreap. Siĕmréab, NW Cambodia
Siemreap *see* Siĕmréab
106 G12 **Siena** *Fr.* Sienne; *anc.* Saena Julia. Toscana, C Italy
Sienne *see* Siena
92 K12 **Sieppijärvi** Lappi, NW Finland
110 J13 **Sieradz** Sieradz, C Poland
110 K10 **Sierpc** Mazowieckie, C Poland
24 I9 **Sierra Blanca** Texas, SW USA
37 S14 **Sierra Blanca Peak** ▲ New Mexico, SW USA
35 P5 **Sierra City** California, W USA
63 I16 **Sierra Colorada** Río Negro, S Argentina
62 I13 **Sierra del Nevado** ▲ W Argentina
63 J16 **Sierra Grande** Río Negro, E Argentina
76 G15 **Sierra Leone** *off.* Republic of Sierra Leone. ◆ *republic* W Africa
64 M13 **Sierra Leone Basin** *undersea feature* E Atlantic Ocean
66 K8 **Sierra Leone Fracture Zone** *tectonic feature* E Atlantic Ocean
Sierra Leone Ridge *see* Sierra Leone Rise
64 L13 **Sierra Leone Rise** *var.* Sierra Leone Ridge, Sierra Leone Schwelle. *undersea feature* E Atlantic Ocean
Sierra Leone Schwelle *see* Sierra Leone Rise
41 U17 **Sierra Madre** *var.* Sierra de Soconusco. ▲ Guatemala/Mexico
37 R2 **Sierra Madre** ▲ Colorado/Wyoming, C USA
(0) H15 **Sierra Madre del Sur** ▲ S Mexico
(0) G13 **Sierra Madre Occidental** *var.* Western Sierra Madre. ▲ C Mexico
(0) H13 **Sierra Madre Oriental** *var.* Eastern Sierra Madre. ▲ C Mexico
44 H8 **Sierra Maestra** ▲ E Cuba
40 L7 **Sierra Mojada** Coahuila de Zaragoza, NE Mexico
105 O14 **Sierra Nevada** ▲ S Spain
35 P6 **Sierra Nevada** ▲ W USA
54 F4 **Sierra Nevada de Santa Marta** ▲ NE Colombia
42 K5 **Sierra Río Tinto** ▲ NE Honduras
24 J10 **Sierra Vieja** ▲ Texas, SW USA
37 N16 **Sierra Vista** Arizona, SW USA
108 D10 **Sierre** *Ger.* Siders. Valais, SW Switzerland
36 L16 **Sierrita Mountains** ▲ Arizona, SW USA
Siete Moai *see* Ahu Akivi
76 M15 **Sifié** W Ivory Coast
115 I21 **Sífnos** *anc.* Siphnos. *island* Kykládes, Greece, Aegean Sea
115 I21 **Sífnou, Stenó** *strait* SE Greece
Siga *see* Shiga
103 P16 **Sigean** Aude, S France
Sighet *see* Sighetu Marmației
Sighetul Marmației *see* Sighetu Marmației
116 I8 **Sighetu Marmației** *var.* Sighet, Sighetul Marmației, *Hung.* Máramarossziget. Maramureş, N Romania
116 I11 **Sighişoara** *Ger.* Schässburg, *Hung.* Segesvár. Mureş, C Romania
168 G7 **Sigli** Sumatera, W Indonesia
92 J1 **Siglufjördhur** Nordhurland Vestra, N Iceland
101 H23 **Sigmaringen** Baden-Württemberg, S Germany
101 N20 **Signalberg** ▲ SE Germany
36 I13 **Signal Peak** ▲ Arizona, SW USA
Signan *see* Xi'an
194 H1 **Signy** *UK research station* South Orkney Islands, Antarctica
29 X15 **Sigourney** Iowa, C USA
115 K17 **Sígri, Akrotírio** *headland* Lésvos, E Greece
Sigsbee Deep *see* Mexico Basin
47 N2 **Sigsbee Escarpment** *undersea feature* N Gulf of Mexico
56 C8 **Sigsig** Azuay, S Ecuador
95 O15 **Sigtuna** Stockholm, C Sweden
42 H6 **Siguatepeque** Comayagua, W Honduras
105 P7 **Sigüenza** Castilla-La Mancha, C Spain
105 R4 **Sigües** Aragón, NE Spain
76 K13 **Siguiri** Haute-Guinée, NE Guinea
118 G8 **Sigulda** *Ger.* Segewold. Rīga, C Latvia
Sihanoukville *see* Kâmpóng Saôm
108 G8 **Sihlsee** ◎ NW Switzerland
93 K18 **Siikainen** Länsi-Suomi, W Finland
93 M16 **Siilinjärvi** Itä-Suomi, C Finland
137 R15 **Siirt** *var.* Sert; *anc.* Tigranocerta. Siirt, SE Turkey
137 R15 **Siirt** *var.* Sert. ◈ *province* SE Turkey
187 N8 **Sikaiana** *var.* Stewart Islands. *island group* W Solomon Islands
Sikandarabad *see* Secunderābād
152 J11 **Sikandra Rao** Uttar Pradesh, N India
10 M11 **Sikanni Chief** British Columbia, W Canada
10 M11 **Sikanni Chief** ≈ British Columbia, W Canada
152 H11 **Sīkar** Rājasthān, N India
76 M13 **Sikasso** Sikasso, S Mali
76 L13 **Sikasso** ◈ *region* SW Mali
167 N3 **Sikaw** Kachin State, C Myanmar
83 H14 **Sikelenge** Western, W Zambia
27 Y7 **Sikeston** Missouri, C USA
93 J14 **Sikfors** Norrbotten, N Sweden
123 T14 **Sikhote-Alin', Khrebet** ▲ SE Russian Federation
Siking *see* Xi'an
115 J22 **Síkinos** *island* Kykládes, Greece, Aegean Sea
153 S11 **Sikkim** *Tib.* Denjong. ◈ *state* N India
111 I26 **Siklós** Baranya, SW Hungary
Sikoku *see* Shikoku
Sikoku Basin *see* Shikoku Basin
83 G14 **Sikongo** Western, W Zambia
Sikotu Ko *see* Shikotsu-ko

Sikouri/Sikoúrion see Sykoúri
123 P8 **Siktyakh** Respublika Sakha (Yakutiya), NE Russian Federation
118 D12 **Silale** Šilalė, W Lithuania
106 G5 **Silandro** Ger. Schlanders. Trentino-Alto Adige, N Italy
41 N12 **Silao** Guanajuato, C Mexico
Silarius see Sele
153 W14 **Silchar** Assam, NE India
108 G9 **Silenen** Uri, C Switzerland
21 T9 **Siler City** North Carolina, SE USA
33 U11 **Silesia** Montana, NW USA
110 F13 **Silesia** physical region SW Poland
74 K12 **Silet** S Algeria
145 R8 **Sileti** var. Selety. ≈ N Kazakhstan
Siletitengiz see Siletiteniz, Ozero
145 R7 **Siletiteniz, Ozero** Kaz. Siletitengiz. ◎ N Kazakhstan
172 H16 **Silhouette** island Inner Islands, SE Seychelles
136 I17 **Silifke** anc. Seleucia. Içel, S Turkey
Siliguri see Shiliguri
156 J10 **Siling Co** ◎ W China
Silinhot see Xilinhot
192 G15 **Silisili** ▲ Savai'i, C Samoa
114 M6 **Silistra** var. Silistria; anc. Durostorum. Silistra, NE Bulgaria
116 M7 **Silistra** ◈ province NE Bulgaria
Silistria see Silistra
136 D10 **Silivri** İstanbul, NW Turkey
94 L13 **Siljan** ◎ C Sweden
95 G22 **Silkeborg** Århus, C Denmark
108 M8 **Sill** ≈ W Austria
105 S10 **Silla** País Valenciano, E Spain
62 H3 **Sillajguay, Cordillera** ▲ N Chile
118 K3 **Sillamäe** Ger. Sillamäggi. Ida-Virumaa, NE Estonia
Sillamäggi see Sillamäe
Sillein see Žilina
109 P9 **Sillian** Tirol, W Austria
112 B10 **Šilo** Primorje-Gorski Kotar, NW Croatia
27 R9 **Siloam Springs** Arkansas, C USA
25 X10 **Silsbee** Texas, SW USA
143 W15 **Sīlūp, Rūd-e** ≈ SE Iran
118 C12 **Šilutė** Ger. Heydekrug. Šilutė, W Lithuania
137 Q15 **Silvan** Dıyarbakır, SE Turkey
108 J10 **Silvaplana** Graubünden, S Switzerland
Silva Porto see Kuito
58 M12 **Silva, Recife do** reef E Brazil
154 D12 **Silvassa** Dādra and Nagar Haveli, W India
29 X4 **Silver Bay** Minnesota, N USA
37 P15 **Silver City** New Mexico, SW USA
18 D10 **Silver Creek** New York, NE USA
37 N12 **Silver Creek** ≈ Arizona, SW USA
27 P4 **Silver Lake** Kansas, C USA
32 I14 **Silver Lake** Oregon, NW USA
35 T9 **Silver Peak Range** ▲ Nevada, W USA
21 W3 **Silver Spring** Maryland, NE USA
Silver State see Nevada
Silver State see Colorado
37 Q7 **Silverton** Colorado, C USA
18 K16 **Silverton** New Jersey, NE USA
32 G11 **Silverton** Oregon, NW USA
25 N4 **Silverton** Texas, SW USA
104 G14 **Silves** Faro, S Portugal
54 D12 **Silvia** Cauca, SW Colombia
108 J9 **Silvrettagruppe** ▲ Austria/Switzerland
Sily-Vajdej see Vulcan
108 L7 **Silz** Tirol, W Austria
172 I13 **Sima** Anjouan, SE Comoros
Simabara see Shimabara
Simada see Shimada
83 H15 **Simakando** Western, W Zambia
Simane see Shimane
119 L20 **Simanichy** Rus. Simonichi. Homyel'skaya Voblasts', SE Belarus
160 F14 **Simao** Yunnan, SW China
153 P12 **Simara** Central, C Nepal
14 I8 **Simard, Lac** ◎ Quebec, SE Canada
136 D13 **Simav** Kütahya, W Turkey
136 D13 **Simav Çayı** ≈ NW Turkey
79 L18 **Simba** Orientale, N Dem. Rep. Congo (Zaire)
186 C7 **Simbai** Madang, N PNG
Simbirsk see Ul'yanovsk
14 F17 **Simcoe** Ontario, S Canada
14 H14 **Simcoe, Lake** ◎ Ontario, S Canada
80 J11 **Simēn** ▲ N Ethiopia
114 K11 **Simeonovgrad** prev. Maritsa. Khaskovo, S Bulgaria
116 G11 **Simeria** Ger. Pischk, Hung. Piski. Hunedoara, W Romania
107 L24 **Simeto** ≈ Sicilia, Italy, C Mediterranean Sea
168 G9 **Simeulue, Pulau** island NW Indonesia
117 T13 **Simferopol'** Respublika Krym, S Ukraine
117 T13 **Simferopol'** × Respublika Krym, S Ukraine
Simi see Sými
152 M9 **Simikot** Far Western, NW Nepal
54 F7 **Simití** Bolívar, N Colombia
114 G11 **Simitla** Blagoevgrad, SW Bulgaria
35 S15 **Simi Valley** California, W USA
Simizu see Shimizu
Simla see Shimla
Şimlăul Silvaniei/Şimleul Silvaniei see Şimleu Silvaniei
116 G9 **Şimleu Silvaniei** Hung. Szilágysomlyó; prev. Şimlăul Silvaniei, Şimleul Silvaniei. Sălaj, NW Romania
Simmer see Simmerbach
101 E19 **Simmerbach** var. Simmer. ≈ W Germany
101 F18 **Simmern** Rheinland-Pfalz, W Germany
22 I7 **Simmesport** Louisiana, S USA
119 F14 **Simnas** Alytus, S Lithuania
92 L13 **Simo** Lappi, NW Finland
Simoda see Shimoda
Simodate see Shimodate
92 M13 **Simojärvi** ◎ N Finland
92 L13 **Simojoki** ≈ NW Finland
41 U15 **Simojovel** var. Simojovel de Allende. Chiapas, SE Mexico
Simojovel de Allende see Simojovel
56 B7 **Simon Bolívar** var. Guayaquil. × (Quayaquil) Guayas, W Ecuador
54 L5 **Simon Bolívar** × (Caracas) Distrito Federal, N Venezuela
Simonichi see Simanichy
14 M12 **Simon, Lac** ◎ Quebec, SE Canada
Simonoseki see Shimonoseki
Šimonovany see Partizánske
Simonstad see Simon's Town
83 E26 **Simon's Town** var. Simonstad. Western Cape, SW South Africa
Simony see Partizánske
Simotuma see Shimotsuma
Simpeln see Simplon
99 M18 **Simpelveld** Limburg, SE Netherlands
108 E11 **Simplon** var. Simpeln. Valais, SW Switzerland
108 E11 **Simplon Pass** pass S Switzerland
106 C6 **Simplon Tunnel** tunnel Italy/Switzerland
Simpson see Fort Simpson
182 G1 **Simpson Desert** desert Northern Territory/South Australia
10 J9 **Simpson Peak** ▲ British Columbia, W Canada
9 N7 **Simpson Peninsula** peninsula Nunavut, NE Canada
21 P11 **Simpsonville** South Carolina, SE USA
95 L23 **Simrishamn** Skåne, S Sweden
123 U13 **Simushir, Ostrov** island Kuril'skiye Ostrova, SE Russian Federation
Sinā'/Sinai Peninsula see Sinai
168 G9 **Sinabang** Sumatera, W Indonesia
81 N15 **Sina Dhaqa** Galguduud, C Somalia
75 X8 **Sinai** var. Sinai Peninsula, Ar. Shibh Jazīrat Sīnā', Sīnā'. physical region NE Egypt
116 J12 **Sinaia** Prahova, SE Romania
188 B16 **Sinajana** C Guam
40 H8 **Sinaloa** ◈ state C Mexico
54 H4 **Sinamaica** Zulia, NW Venezuela
163 X14 **Sinan-ni** SE North Korea
Sinano Gawa see Shinano-gawa
Sināwan see Sīnāwin
75 N8 **Sīnāwin** var. Sīnāwan. NW Libya
83 J16 **Sinazongwe** Southern, S Zambia
166 L6 **Sinbaungwe** Magwe, W Myanmar
166 L5 **Sinbyugyun** Magwe, W Myanmar
54 E6 **Since** Sucre, NW Colombia
54 E6 **Sincelejo** Sucre, NW Colombia
166 J5 **Sinchaingbyin** var. Zullapara. Arakan State, W Myanmar
23 U4 **Sinclair, Lake** ▣ Georgia, SE USA
10 M14 **Sinclair Mills** British Columbia, SW Canada
149 Q14 **Sind** var. Sindh. ◈ province SE Pakistan
154 I8 **Sind** ≈ N India
95 H19 **Sindal** Nordjylland, N Denmark
171 P7 **Sindañgan** Mindanao, S Philippines
79 D19 **Sindara** Ngounié, W Gabon
152 E13 **Sindari** prev. Sindri. Rājasthān, N India
114 N8 **Sindel** Varna, E Bulgaria
101 H22 **Sindelfingen** Baden-Württemberg, SW Germany
155 G16 **Sindgi** Karnātaka, C India
Sindh see Sind
118 G5 **Sindi** Ger. Zintenhof. Pärnumaa, SW Estonia
136 C13 **Sındırgı** Balıkesir, W Turkey
77 N14 **Sindou** SW Burkina
Sindri see Sindari
149 T9 **Sind Sāgar Doāb** desert E Pakistan
128 M11 **Sinegorskiy** Rostovskaya Oblast', SW Russian Federation
123 S9 **Sinegor'ye** Magadanskaya Oblast', E Russian Federation
114 O12 **Sinekli** İstanbul, NW Turkey
104 F12 **Sines** Setúbal, S Portugal
104 F12 **Sines, Cabo de** headland S Portugal
92 L12 **Sinettä** Lappi, NW Finland
186 H6 **Sinewit, Mount** ▲ New Britain, C PNG
80 G11 **Singa** var. Sinja, Sinjah. Sinnar, E Sudan
78 J12 **Singako** Moyen-Chari, S Chad
Singan see Xi'an
168 K10 **Singapore** ● (Singapore) S Singapore
168 L10 **Singapore** off. Republic of Singapore. ◆ republic SE Asia
168 L10 **Singapore Strait** var. Strait of Singapore, Mal. Selat Singapura. strait Indonesia/Singapore
Singapore, Strait of/Singapura, Selat see Singapore Strait
169 U17 **Singaraja** Bali, C Indonesia
Singatoka see Sigatoka
167 O10 **Sing Buri** var. Singhaburi. Sing Buri, C Thailand
101 H24 **Singen** Baden-Württemberg, S Germany
Singeorgiu de Pădure see Sângeorgiu de Pădure
Singeorz-Băi/Singeroz Băi see Sângeorz-Băi
116 M9 **Sîngerei** var. Sângerei; prev. Lazovsk. N Moldova
Singhaburi see Sing Buri
81 H21 **Singida** Singida, C Tanzania
81 G22 **Singida** ◈ region C Tanzania
Singidunum see Beograd
166 M2 **Singkaling Hkamti** Sagaing, N Myanmar
171 N14 **Singkang** Sulawesi, C Indonesia
168 J11 **Singkarak, Danau** ◎ Sumatera, W Indonesia
169 N10 **Singkawang** Borneo, C Indonesia
168 M11 **Singkep, Pulau** island Kepulauan Lingga, W Indonesia
168 H9 **Singkilbaru** Sumatera, W Indonesia
183 T7 **Singleton** New South Wales, SE Australia
Singora see Songkhla
Singû see Shingū
Sining see Xining
107 D17 **Siniscola** Sardegna, Italy, C Mediterranean Sea
113 F14 **Sinj** Split-Dalmacija, SE Croatia
Sinja/Sinjah see Singa
Sinjajevina see Sinjavina
139 P3 **Sinjār** NW Iraq
139 P2 **Sinjār, Jabal** ▲ N Iraq
113 K15 **Sinjavina** var. Sinjajevina. ▲ SW Yugoslavia
80 I7 **Sinkat** Red Sea, NE Sudan
Sinkiang/Sinkiang Uighur Autonomous Region see Xinjiang Uygur Zizhiqu
Sînmartin see Târnăveni
163 V13 **Sinmi-do** island NW North Korea
Sinminato see Shinminato
101 I18 **Sinn** ≈ C Germany
Sinnamarie see Sinnamary
55 Y9 **Sinnamary** var. Sinnamarie. N French Guiana
Sin'anyō see Shinnanyō
80 G11 **Sinnar** ◈ state E Sudan
Sinneh see Sanandaj
18 E13 **Sinnemahoning Creek** ≈ Pennsylvania, NE USA
Sînnicolau Mare see Sânnicolau Mare
Sino/Sinoe see Greenville
Sinoe, Lacul see Sinoie, Lacul
Sinoia see Chinhoyi
117 N14 **Sinoie, Lacul** prev. Lacul Sinoe. lagoon SE Romania
59 H16 **Sinop** Mato Grosso, W Brazil
136 K10 **Sinop** anc. Sinope. Sinop, N Turkey
136 J10 **Sinop** ◈ province N Turkey
136 K10 **Sinop Burnu** headland N Turkey
Sinope see Sinop
163 Y12 **Sinp'o** E North Korea
101 H20 **Sinsheim** Baden-Württemberg, SW Germany
Sinsiro see Shinshiro
Sintana see Sântana
169 R11 **Sintang** Borneo, C Indonesia
99 F14 **Sint Annaland** Zeeland, SW Netherlands
98 L5 **Sint Annaparochie** Friesland, N Netherlands
45 V9 **Sint Eustatius** Eng. Saint Eustatius. island N Netherlands Antilles
99 G19 **Sint-Genesius-Rode** Fr. Rhode-Saint-Genèse. Vlaams Brabant, C Belgium
99 F16 **Sint-Gillis-Waas** Oost-Vlaanderen, N Belgium
99 H17 **Sint-Katelijne-Waver** Antwerpen, C Belgium
99 E18 **Sint-Lievens-Houtem** Oost-Vlaanderen, NW Belgium
45 V9 **Sint Maarten** Eng. Saint Martin. island N Netherlands Antilles
99 F14 **Sint Maartensdijk** Zeeland, SW Netherlands
99 L19 **Sint-Martens-Voeren** Fr. Fouron-Saint-Martin. Limburg, NE Belgium
99 J14 **Sint-Michielsgestel** Noord-Brabant, S Netherlands
Sîn-Miclăuş see Gheorgheni
45 O16 **Sint Nicholaas** S Aruba
99 F16 **Sint-Niklaas** Fr. Saint-Nicolas. Oost-Vlaanderen, N Belgium
99 K14 **Sint-Oedenrode** Noord-Brabant, S Netherlands
25 T14 **Sinton** Texas, SW USA
99 G14 **Sint Philipsland** Zeeland, SW Netherlands
99 G19 **Sint-Pieters-Leeuw** Vlaams Brabant, C Belgium
104 E11 **Sintra** prev. Cintra. Lisboa, W Portugal
99 J18 **Sint-Truiden** Fr. Saint-Trond. Limburg, NE Belgium
99 H14 **Sint Willebrord** Noord-Brabant, S Netherlands
163 V13 **Sinŭiju** W North Korea
80 P13 **Sinujiif** Nugaal, NE Somalia
Sinus Aelaniticus see Aqaba, Gulf of
Sinus Gallicus see Lion, Golfe du
Sinyang see Xinyang
Sinyavka see Sinyawka
119 I18 **Sinyawka** Rus. Sinyavka. Minskaya Voblasts', SW Belarus
Sinying see Hsinying
Sinyukha see Synyukha
Sinzi-ko see Shinji-ko
Sinzyô see Shinjō
111 I24 **Sió** ≈ W Hungary
171 O7 **Siocon** Mindanao, S Philippines
111 I24 **Siófok** Somogy, C Hungary
Siogama see Shiogama
83 G15 **Sioma** Western, SW Zambia
108 D11 **Sion** Ger. Sitten; anc. Sedunum. Valais, SW Switzerland
103 O11 **Sioule** ≈ C France
29 S12 **Sioux Center** Iowa, C USA
29 R13 **Sioux City** Iowa, C USA
29 R11 **Sioux Falls** South Dakota, N USA
12 B11 **Sioux Lookout** Ontario, S Canada
29 T12 **Sioux Rapids** Iowa, C USA
Sioux State see North Dakota
Sioziri see Shiojiri
171 P6 **Sipalay** Negros, C Philippines
55 V11 **Sipaliwini** ◈ district S Surinam
45 U15 **Siparia** Trinidad, Trinidad and Tobago
Siphnos see Sífnos
163 V11 **Siping** var. Ssu-p'ing, Szeping; prev. Ssu-p'ing-chieh. Jilin, NE China
11 X12 **Sipiwesk** Manitoba, C Canada
11 W13 **Sipiwesk Lake** ◎ Manitoba, C Canada
195 O11 **Siple Coast** physical region Antarctica
194 K12 **Siple Island** island Antarctica
194 K13 **Siple, Mount** ▲ Siple Island, Antarctica
Sipoo see Sibbo
112 G12 **Šipovo** Republika Srpska, W Bosnia and Herzegovina
23 O4 **Sipsey River** ≈ Alabama, S USA
168 I13 **Sipura, Pulau** island W Indonesia
(0) G16 **Siqueiros Fracture Zone** tectonic feature E Pacific Ocean
42 L10 **Siquia, Río** ≈ SE Nicaragua
43 N13 **Siquirres** Limón, E Costa Rica
54 J5 **Siquisique** Lara, N Venezuela
155 G19 **Sīra** Karnātaka, W India
95 D16 **Sira** ≈ S Norway
167 P12 **Siracha** var. Ban Si Racha, Si Racha. Chon Buri, S Thailand
107 L25 **Siracusa** Eng. Syracuse. Sicilia, Italy, C Mediterranean Sea
Sirajganj see Shirajganj Ghat
Sirakawa see Shirakawa
11 N14 **Sir Alexander, Mount** ▲ British Columbia, W Canada
137 O12 **Şiran** Gümüşhane, NE Turkey
77 Q12 **Sirba** ≈ E Burkina
143 O17 **Şīr Banī Yās** island W UAE
95 D17 **Sirdalsvatnet** ◎ S Norway
Sir Darya/Sirdaryo see Syr Darya
147 O11 **Sirdaryo Wiloyati** Rus. Syrdar'inskaya Oblast'. ◈ province E Uzbekistan
Sir Donald Sangster International Airport see Sangster
181 S3 **Sir Edward Pellew Group** island group Northern Territory, NE Australia
116 K8 **Siret** Ger. Sereth, Hung. Szeret. Suceava, N Romania
116 K8 **Siret** var. Siretul, Ger. Sereth, Rus. Seret, Ukr. Siret. ≈ Romania/Ukraine
Siretul see Siret
140 K3 **Sirḩān, Wādī as** dry watercourse Jordan/Saudi Arabia
152 I8 **Sirhind** Punjab, N India
116 F11 **Şiria** Ger. Schiria. Arad, W Romania
Siria see Syria
143 S14 **Sīrīk** Hormozgān, SE Iran
167 P8 **Sirikit Reservoir** ◎ N Thailand
58 K12 **Sirituba, Ilha** island NE Brazil
143 R11 **Sīrjān** prev. Sa'īdābād. Kermān, S Iran
182 H9 **Sir Joseph Banks Group** island group South Australia
92 K11 **Sirkka** Lappi, N Finland
Sirna see Sýrna
137 R16 **Şırnak** Şırnak, SE Turkey
137 S16 **Şırnak** ◈ province SE Turkey
Siroisi see Shiroishi
155 J14 **Sironcha** Mahārāshtra, C India
Sirone see Shirone
Síros see Sýros
Sirotino see Sirotsina
118 M12 **Sirotsina** Rus. Sirotino. Vitsyebskaya Voblasts', N Belarus
152 H9 **Sirsa** Haryāna, NW India
173 Y17 **Sir Seewoosagur Ramgoolam** × (Port Louis) SE Mauritius
155 E18 **Sirsi** Karnātaka, W India
Sirte see Surt
182 A2 **Sir Thomas, Mount** ▲ South Australia
Sirti, Gulf of see Surt, Khalīj
142 J5 **Sīrvān, Rūdkhāneh-ye** var. Nahr Diyālá, Sirwan. ≈ Iran/Iraq see also Diyālá, Nahr
118 H13 **Širvintos** Širvintos, SE Lithuania
Sirwan see Diyālá, Nahr/Sīrvān, Rūdkhāneh-ye
11 N15 **Sir Wilfrid Laurier, Mount** ▲ British Columbia, SW Canada
14 M10 **Sir-Wilfrid, Mont** ▲ Quebec, SE Canada
Sisačko-Moslavačka Županija see Sisak-Moslavina
112 E9 **Sisak** var. Siscia, Ger. Sissek, Hung. Sziszek; anc. Segestica. Sisak-Moslavina, C Croatia
167 R10 **Si Sa Ket** var. Sisaket, Sri Saket. Si Sa Ket, E Thailand
112 E9 **Sisak-Moslavina** off. Sisačko-Moslavačka Županija. ◈ province C Croatia
167 O8 **Si Satchanala** Sukhothai, NW Thailand
Siscia see Sisak
83 G22 **Sishen** Northern Cape, NW South Africa
137 V13 **Sisian** SE Armenia
197 N13 **Sisimiut** var. Holsteinborg, Holsteinsborg, Holstenborg, Holstensborg. Kitaa, S Greenland
30 M1 **Siskiwit Bay** lake bay Michigan, N USA
34 L1 **Siskiyou Mountains** ▲ California/Oregon, W USA
167 Q11 **Sisŏphŏn** Bătdâmbâng, NW Cambodia
108 E7 **Sissach** Basel-Land, NW Switzerland
186 B5 **Sissano** Sandaun, NW PNG
Sissek see Sisak
29 R7 **Sisseton** South Dakota, N USA
143 W9 **Sīstān, Daryācheh-ye** var. Daryācheh-ye Hāmūn, Hāmūn-e Şāberī. ◎ Afghanistan/Iran see also Şāberī, Hāmūn-e
143 V12 **Sīstān va Balūchestān** off. Ostān-e Sīstān va Balūchestān, var. Balūchestān va Sīstān. ◈ province SE Iran
103 T14 **Sisteron** Alpes-de-Haute-Provence, SE France
32 H13 **Sisters** Oregon, NW USA
65 G15 **Sisters Peak** ▲ N Ascension Island
21 R3 **Sistersville** West Virginia, NE USA
Sistova see Svishtov
Sitakund see Sitakunda
153 V16 **Sitakunda** var. Sitakund. Chittagong, SE Bangladesh
153 P12 **Sītāmarhi** Bihār, N India
152 L11 **Sītāpur** Uttar Pradesh, N India
Sitaş Cristuru see Cristuru Secuiesc
115 L25 **Siteía** var. Sitía. Kríti, Greece, E Mediterranean Sea
105 V6 **Sitges** Cataluña, NE Spain
115 H15 **Sithoniá** peninsula NE Greece
Sitía see Siteía
54 F4 **Sitionuevo** Magdalena, N Colombia
39 X13 **Sitka** Baranof Island, Alaska, USA
39 Q15 **Sitkinak Island** island Trinity Islands, Alaska, USA
166 M7 **Sittang** var. Sittoung. ≈ S Myanmar
99 L17 **Sittard** Limburg, SE Netherlands
Sitten see Sion
108 H7 **Sitter** ≈ NW Switzerland
109 U10 **Sittersdorf** Kärnten, S Austria
Sittoung see Sittang
166 K6 **Sittwe** var. Akyab. Arakan State, W Myanmar
42 L8 **Siuna** Región Autónoma Atlántico Norte, NE Nicaragua
153 R15 **Siuri** West Bengal, NE India
Siut see Asyūt
123 Q13 **Sivaki** Amurskaya Oblast', SE Russian Federation
136 M13 **Sivas** anc. Sebastia, Sebaste. Sivas, C Turkey
136 M13 **Sivas** ◈ province C Turkey
137 O15 **Siverek** Şanlıurfa, S Turkey
117 X6 **Sivers'k** Donets'ka Oblast', E Ukraine
126 G13 **Siverskiy** Leningradskaya Oblast', NW Russian Federation
117 X6 **Sivers'kyy Donets'** Rus. Severskiy Donets. ≈ Russian Federation/Ukraine see also Severskiy Donets
127 W5 **Sivomaskinskiy** Respublika Komi, NW Russian Federation
136 G13 **Sivrihisar** Eskişehir, W Turkey
99 F22 **Sivry** Hainaut, S Belgium
123 V9 **Sivuchiy, Mys** headland E Russian Federation
75 U9 **Siwa** var. Sīwah. NW Egypt
Sīwah see Siwa
152 J9 **Siwalik Range** var. Shiwalik Range. ▲ India/Nepal
153 O13 **Siwān** Bihār, N India
43 O14 **Sixaola, Río** ≈ Costa Rica/Panama
Six Counties, The see Northern Ireland
103 T16 **Six-Fours-les-Plages** Var, SE France
161 Q7 **Sixian** var. Si Xian. Anhui, E China
22 J9 **Six Mile Lake** ◎ Louisiana, S USA
139 V3 **Siyāh Gūz** E Iraq
155 L25 **Siyambalanduwa** Uva Province, SE Sri Lanka
137 Y10 **Siyäzän** Rus. Siazan'. NE Azerbaijan
Sizebolu see Sozopol
Sizuoka see Shizuoka
Sjar see Sääre
113 L15 **Sjenica** Turk. Seniça. Serbia, SW Yugoslavia
94 G11 **Sjoa** ≈ S Norway
95 K23 **Sjöbo** Skåne, S Sweden
95 I24 **Sjælland** Eng. Zealand, Ger. Seeland. island E Denmark
94 E9 **Sjøholt** Møre og Romsdal, S Norway
92 O1 **Sjuøyane** island group N Svalbard
Skadar see Shkodër
Skadarsko Jezero see Scutari, Lake
117 R11 **Skadovs'k** Khersons'ka Oblast', S Ukraine
92 I2 **Skagaströnd** prev. Höfdhakaupstadhur. Nordhurland Vestra, N Iceland
95 H19 **Skagen** Nordjylland, N Denmark
Skagerak see Skagerrak
95 L16 **Skagern** ◎ C Sweden
197 T17 **Skagerrak** var. Skagerak. channel N Europe
94 G12 **Skaget** ▲ S Norway
32 H7 **Skagit River** ≈ Washington, NW USA
39 W12 **Skagway** Alaska, USA
92 K8 **Skaidi** Finnmark, N Norway
115 F21 **Skála** Pelopónnisos, S Greece
116 K6 **Skalat** Pol. Skałat. Ternopil's'ka Oblast', W Ukraine
95 J22 **Skälderviken** inlet Denmark/Sweden
92 I12 **Skalka** ◎ N Sweden
114 I12 **Skalotí** Anatolikí Makedonía kai Thráki, NE Greece
95 G22 **Skanderborg** Århus, C Denmark
95 K22 **Skåne** prev. Eng. Scania. ◈ county S Sweden
75 N6 **Skanès** × (Sousse) E Tunisia
95 C15 **Skånevik** Hordaland, S Norway
95 M18 **Skänninge** Östergötland, S Sweden
95 J23 **Skanör** Skåne, S Sweden
115 H17 **Skantzoúra** island Vóreioi Sporádes, Greece, Aegean Sea
95 K18 **Skara** Västra Götaland, S Sweden
95 M17 **Skärblacka** Östergötland, S Sweden
95 I18 **Skärhamn** Västra Götaland, S Sweden
95 I14 **Skarnes** Hedmark, S Norway
119 M21 **Skarodnaye** Rus. Skorodnoye. Homyel'skaya Voblasts', SE Belarus
110 I8 **Skarszewy** Ger. Schöneck. Pomorskie, NW Poland
111 M14 **Skarżysko-Kamienna** Świętokrzyskie, C Poland
95 K16 **Skattkärr** Värmland, C Sweden
118 D12 **Skaudvilė** Tauragė, SW Lithuania
92 J12 **Skaulo** Norrbotten, N Sweden
111 K17 **Skawina** Małopolskie, S Poland
10 K12 **Skeena** ≈ British Columbia, SW Canada
10 J11 **Skeena Mountains** ▲ British Columbia, W Canada
97 O18 **Skegness** E England, UK
92 J4 **Skeidharársandur** coast S Iceland
93 J15 **Skellefteå** Västerbotten, N Sweden
93 I14 **Skellefteälven** ≈ N Sweden
93 J15 **Skelleftehamn** Västerbotten, N Sweden
25 O2 **Skellytown** Texas, SW USA
95 J19 **Skene** Västra Götaland, S Sweden
97 G17 **Skerries** Ir. Na Sceirí. E Ireland
95 H15 **Ski** Akershus, S Norway
115 G17 **Skíathos** Skíathos, Vóreioi Sporádes, Greece, Aegean Sea
115 G17 **Skíathos** island Vóreioi Sporádes, Greece, Aegean Sea
27 P9 **Skiatook** Oklahoma, C USA
27 P9 **Skiatook Lake** ▣ Oklahoma, C USA
97 B22 **Skibbereen** Ir. An Sciobairín. SW Ireland
92 I9 **Skibotn** Troms, N Norway
119 F16 **Skidal'** Rus. Skidel'. Hrodzyenskaya Voblasts', W Belarus
97 K15 **Skiddaw** ▲ NW England, UK
Skidel' see Skidal'
25 T14 **Skidmore** Texas, SW USA
95 G16 **Skien** Telemark, S Norway
Skiermûntseach see Schiermonnikoog
110 L12 **Skierniewice** Łodzkie, C Poland
74 L5 **Skikda** prev. Philippeville. NE Algeria
30 M16 **Skillet Fork** ≈ Illinois, N USA
95 L19 **Skillingaryd** Jönköping, S Sweden
115 B19 **Skinári, Akrotírio** headland Zákynthos, Iónioi Nísoi, Greece, C Mediterranean Sea
95 M15 **Skinnskatteberg** Västmanland, C Sweden
182 M12 **Skipton** Victoria, SE Australia
97 L16 **Skipton** N England, UK
Skiropoula see Skyropoúla
Skíros see Skýros
95 F21 **Skive** Viborg, NW Denmark
94 F11 **Skjåk** Oppland, S Norway
92 K2 **Skjálfandafljót** ≈ C Iceland
95 F22 **Skjern** Ringkøbing, W Denmark
95 F22 **Skjern Å** var. Skjern Aa. ≈ W Denmark
Skjern Aa see Skjern Å
92 G12 **Skjerstad** Nordland, C Norway
92 J8 **Skjervøy** Troms, N Norway
92 I10 **Skjold** Troms, N Norway
111 I17 **Skoczów** Śląskie, S Poland
95 I24 **Skælskør** Vestsjælland, E Denmark
109 T11 **Škofja Loka** Ger. Bischoflack. NW Slovenia
94 N12 **Skog** Gävleborg, C Sweden
95 K16 **Skoghall** Värmland, C Sweden
31 N10 **Skokie** Illinois, N USA
116 H6 **Skole** L'vivs'ka Oblast', W Ukraine
115 D19 **Skóllis** ▲ S Greece
167 S13 **Skon** Kâmpóng Cham, C Cambodia
115 H17 **Skópelos** Skópelos, Vóreioi Sporádes, Greece, Aegean Sea
115 H17 **Skópelos** island Vóreioi Sporádes, Greece, Aegean Sea
128 L5 **Skopin** Ryazanskaya Oblast', W Russian Federation
113 N18 **Skopje** var. Üsküb, Turk. Üsküp; prev. Skoplje, anc. Scupi. ● (FYR Macedonia) N FYR Macedonia
113 O18 **Skopje** × N FYR Macedonia
Skoplje see Skopje
110 I8 **Skórcz** Ger. Skurz. Pomorskie, N Poland
Skorodnoye see Skarodnaye
93 H16 **Skorped** Västernorrland, C Sweden
95 G21 **Skørping** Nordjylland, N Denmark
95 K18 **Skövde** Västra Götaland, S Sweden
123 Q13 **Skovorodino** Amurskaya Oblast', SE Russian Federation
19 Q6 **Skowhegan** Maine, NE USA
11 W15 **Skownan** Manitoba, S Canada
94 H13 **Skreia** Oppland, S Norway
Skripón see Orchómenos
118 H9 **Skrīveri** Aizkraukle, S Latvia
118 J11 **Skrudaliena** Daugvapils, SE Latvia
118 D9 **Skrunda** Kuldīga, W Latvia
95 C16 **Skudeneshavn** Rogaland, S Norway
83 L20 **Skukuza** Mpumalanga, NE South Africa
97 B22 **Skull** Ir. An Scoil. SW Ireland
22 L3 **Skuna River** ≈ Mississippi, S USA
29 X15 **Skunk River** ≈ Iowa, C USA
118 C10 **Skuodas** Ger. Schoden, Pol. Szkudy. Skuodas, NW Lithuania
95 K23 **Skurup** Skåne, S Sweden
Skurz see Skórcz
114 H8 **Skŭt** ≈ NW Bulgaria
94 O13 **Skutskär** Uppsala, C Sweden
95 B19 **Skúvoy** Dan. Skuø Island Faeroe Islands
Skvira see Skvyra
117 O5 **Skvyra** Rus. Skvira. Kyyivs'ka Oblast', N Ukraine
39 Q11 **Skwentna** Alaska, USA
110 E11 **Skwierzyna** Ger. Schwerin. Lubuskie, W Poland

◆ Country ● Country Capital ◇ Dependent Territory ○ Dependent Territory Capital ◈ Administrative Region × International Airport ▲ Mountain ▲ Mountain Range ※ Volcano ≈ River ◎ Lake ▣ Reservoir

36 K13 **Sky Harbour** × (Phoenix) Arizona, SW USA
96 G9 **Skye, Isle of** *island* NW Scotland, UK
32 I8 **Skykomish** Washington, NW USA
Skylge *see* Terschelling
63 F19 **Skyring, Peninsula** *peninsula* S Chile
63 H24 **Skyring, Seno** *inlet* S Chile
115 H17 **Skyropoúla** *var.* Skiropoula. *island* Vóreioi Sporádes, Greece, Aegean Sea
115 I17 **Skýros** *var.* Skíros. Skýros, Vóreioi Sporádes, Greece, Aegean Sea
115 I17 **Skýros** *var.* Skíros; *anc.* Scyros. *island* Vóreioi Sporádes, Greece, Aegean Sea
118 J12 **Slabodka** *Rus.* Slobodka. Vitsyebskaya Voblasts', NW Belarus
95 I23 **Slagelse** Vestsjælland, E Denmark
93 I14 **Slagnäs** Norrbotten, N Sweden
39 T10 **Slana** Alaska, USA
97 F20 **Slaney** *Ir.* An tSláine. ≈ SE Ireland
116 J13 **Slănic** Prahova, SE Romania
116 K11 **Slănic Moldova** Bacău, E Romania
113 H16 **Slano** Dubrovnik-Neretva, SE Croatia
126 F13 **Slantsy** Leningradskaya Oblast', NW Russian Federation
111 C16 **Slaný** *Ger.* Schlan. Střední Čechy, NW Czech Republic
111 I16 **Śląskie** ◈ *province* S Poland
12 C10 **Slate Falls** Ontario, S Canada
27 T4 **Slater** Missouri, C USA
112 H9 **Slatina** *Hung.* Szlatina *prev.* Podravska Slatina. Virovitica-Podravina, NE Croatia
116 I14 **Slatina** Olt, S Romania
25 N5 **Slaton** Texas, SW USA
95 H14 **Slattum** Akershus, S Norway
11 R10 **Slave** ≈ Alberta/Northwest Territories, C Canada
68 E11 **Slave Coast** *coastal region* W Africa
11 P13 **Slave Lake** Alberta, SW Canada
122 I13 **Slavgorod** Altayskiy Kray, S Russian Federation
Slavgorod *see* Slawharad
Slavonia *see* Slavonija
112 G9 **Slavonija** *Eng.* Slavonia, *Ger.* Slawonien, *Hung.* Szlavonia, Szlavonország. *cultural region* NE Croatia
Slavonska Požega *see* Požega
112 H10 **Slavonski Brod** *Ger.* Brod, *Hung.* Bród; *prev.* Brod, Brod na Savi. Brod-Posavina, NE Croatia
116 L4 **Slavuta** Khmel'nyts'ka Oblast', NW Ukraine
117 P2 **Slavutych** Chernihivs'ka Oblast', N Ukraine
123 R15 **Slavyanka** Primorskiy Kray, SE Russian Federation
114 J8 **Slavyanovo** Pleven, N Bulgaria
Slavyansk *see* Slov"yans'k
128 K14 **Slavyansk-na-Kubani** Krasnodarskiy Kray, SW Russian Federation
119 N20 **Slavyechna** *Rus.* Slovechna. ≈ Belarus/Ukraine
119 O16 **Slawharad** *Rus.* Slavgorod. Mahilyowskaya Voblasts', E Belarus
110 G7 **Sławno** Zachodniopomorskie, NW Poland
Slawonien *see* Slavonija
29 S10 **Slayton** Minnesota, N USA
97 N18 **Sleaford** E England, UK
97 A20 **Slea Head** *Ir.* Ceann Sléibhe. *headland* SW Ireland
96 G9 **Sleat, Sound of** *strait* NW Scotland, UK
Sledyuki *see* Slyedzyuki
12 I5 **Sleeper Islands** *island group* Nunavut, C Canada
31 O6 **Sleeping Bear Point** *headland* Michigan, N USA
29 T10 **Sleepy Eye** Minnesota, N USA
39 O11 **Sleetmute** Alaska, USA
Sléibhe, Ceann *see* Slea Head
Slēmānī *see* As Sulaymānīyah
195 O5 **Slessor Glacier** *glacier* Antarctica
22 L9 **Slidell** Louisiana, S USA
18 K12 **Slide Mountain** ▲ New York, NE USA
98 I13 **Sliedrecht** Zuid-Holland, C Netherlands
121 P16 **Sliema** N Malta
97 G16 **Slieve Donard** ▲ SE Northern Ireland, UK
Sligeach *see* Sligo
97 D16 **Sligo** *Ir.* Sligeach. NW Ireland
97 C16 **Sligo** *Ir.* Sligeach. *cultural region* NW Ireland
97 C15 **Sligo Bay** *Ir.* Cuan Shligigh. *inlet* NW Ireland
18 B13 **Slippery Rock** Pennsylvania, NE USA
95 P19 **Slite** Gotland, SE Sweden
114 L9 **Sliven** *var.* Slivno. Sliven, C Bulgaria
114 L10 **Sliven** ◈ *province* C Bulgaria
114 G9 **Slivnitsa** Sofiya, W Bulgaria
Slivno *see* Sliven
114 L7 **Slivo Pole** Ruse, N Bulgaria
29 S13 **Sloan** Iowa, C USA
35 X12 **Sloan** Nevada, W USA
Slobodka *see* Slabodka
127 R14 **Slobodskoy** Kirovskaya Oblast', NW Russian Federation
Slobodzeya *see* Slobozia
117 O10 **Slobozia** *Rus.* Slobodzeya. E Moldova
116 L14 **Slobozia** Ialomiţa, SE Romania
98 O5 **Slochteren** Groningen, NE Netherlands
119 H17 **Slonim** *Pol.* Słonim, *Rus.* Slonim. Hrodzyenskaya Voblasts', W Belarus
98 K7 **Sloter Meer** ◎ N Netherlands
Slot, The *see* New Georgia Sound
97 N22 **Slough** S England, UK
111 J20 **Slovakia** *off.* Slovenská Republika, *Ger.* Slowakei, *Hung.* Szlovákia, *Slvk.* Slovensko. ◆ *republic* C Europe
Slovak Ore Mountains *see* Slovenské rudohorie
Slovechna *see* Slavyechna
109 S12 **Slovenia** *off.* Republic of Slovenia, *Ger.* Slowenien, *Slvn.* Slovenija. ◆ *republic* SE Europe
Slovenija *see* Slovenia
109 V10 **Slovenj Gradec** *Ger.* Windischgraz. N Slovenia
109 W10 **Slovenska Bistrica** *Ger.* Windischfeistritz. NE Slovenia
Slovenská Republika *see* Slovakia
109 W10 **Slovenske Konjice** E Slovenia
111 K20 **Slovenské rudohorie** *Eng.* Slovak Ore Mountains, *Ger.* Slowakisches Erzgebirge, Ungarisches Erzgebirge. ▲▲ C Slovakia
Slovensko *see* Slovakia
117 Y7 **Slov"yanoserbs'k** Luhans'ka Oblast', E Ukraine
117 W6 **Slov"yans'k** *Rus.* Slavyansk. Donets'ka Oblast', E Ukraine
Slowakei *see* Slovakia
Slowakisches Erzgebirge *see* Slovenské rudohorie
Slowenien *see* Slovenia
110 D11 **Słubice** *Ger.* Frankfurt. Lubuskie, W Poland
119 K19 **Sluch** *Rus.* Sluch'. ≈ C Belarus
116 L4 **Sluch** ≈ NW Ukraine
99 D16 **Sluis** Zeeland, SW Netherlands
112 D10 **Slunj** *Hung.* Szluin. Karlovac, C Croatia
110 I11 **Słupca** Wielkolpolskie, C Poland
110 G6 **Słupia** *Ger.* Stolpe. ≈ NW Poland
110 G6 **Słupsk** *Ger.* Stolp. Pomorskie, N Poland
119 K18 **Slutsk** *Rus.* Slutsk. Minskaya Voblasts', S Belarus
119 O16 **Slyedzyuki** *Rus.* Sledyuki. Mahilyowskaya Voblasts', E Belarus
97 A17 **Slyne Head** *Ir.* Ceann Léime. *headland* W Ireland
27 U14 **Smackover** Arkansas, C USA
95 L20 **Småland** *cultural region* S Sweden
95 K20 **Smålandsstenar** Jönköping, S Sweden
Small Malaita *see* Maramasike
13 O8 **Smallwood Reservoir** ⊠ Newfoundland, S Canada
119 N14 **Smalyany** *Rus.* Smolyany. Vitsyebskaya Voblasts', NE Belarus
119 L15 **Smalyavichy** *Rus.* Smolevichi. Minskaya Voblasts', C Belarus
74 C9 **Smara** *var.* Es Semara. N Western Sahara
119 I14 **Smarhon'** *Pol.* Smorgonie, *Rus.* Smorgon'. Hrodzyenskaya Voblasts', W Belarus
112 M11 **Smederevo** *Ger.* Semendria. Serbia, N Yugoslavia
112 M12 **Smederevska Palanka** Serbia, C Yugoslavia
95 M14 **Smedjebacken** Dalarna, C Sweden
116 L13 **Smeeni** Buzău, SE Romania
Smela *see* Smila
107 D16 **Smeralda, Costa** *cultural region* Sardegna, Italy, C Mediterranean Sea
111 J22 **Śmigiel** *Ger.* Schmiegel. Wielkolpolskie, C Poland
117 Q6 **Smila** *Rus.* Smela. Cherkas'ka Oblast', C Ukraine
98 N7 **Smilde** Drenthe, NE Netherlands
11 S16 **Smiley** Saskatchewan, S Canada
25 T12 **Smiley** Texas, SW USA
Smilten *see* Smiltene
118 I8 **Smiltene** *Ger.* Smilten. Valka, N Latvia
123 T13 **Smirnykh** Ostrov Sakhalin, Sakhalinskaya Oblast', SE Russian Federation
11 Q13 **Smith** Alberta, W Canada
39 P4 **Smith Bay** *bay* Alaska, USA
12 I3 **Smith, Cape** *headland* Quebec, NE Canada
26 L3 **Smith Center** Kansas, C USA
10 K13 **Smithers** British Columbia, SW Canada
21 V10 **Smithfield** North Carolina, SE USA
36 L1 **Smithfield** Utah, W USA
21 X7 **Smithfield** Virginia, NE USA
12 I3 **Smith Island** *island* Nunavut, C Canada
Smith Island *see* Sumisu-jima
20 H7 **Smithland** Kentucky, S USA
21 T7 **Smith Mountain Lake** *var.* Leesville Lake. ⊠ Virginia, NE USA
34 L1 **Smith River** California, W USA
33 R9 **Smith River** ≈ Montana, NW USA
14 L13 **Smiths Falls** Ontario, SE Canada
33 N13 **Smiths Ferry** Idaho, NW USA
20 K7 **Smiths Grove** Kentucky, S USA
183 N15 **Smithton** Tasmania, SE Australia
18 L14 **Smithtown** Long Island, New York, NE USA
20 K9 **Smithville** Tennessee, S USA
25 T11 **Smithville** Texas, SW USA
Šmohor *see* Hermagor
35 Q4 **Smoke Creek Desert** *desert* Nevada, W USA
11 O14 **Smoky** ≈ Alberta, W Canada
182 E7 **Smoky Bay** South Australia
183 V6 **Smoky Cape** *headland* New South Wales, SE Australia
26 L4 **Smoky Hill River** ≈ Kansas, C USA
26 L4 **Smoky Hills** *hill range* Kansas, C USA
11 Q14 **Smoky Lake** Alberta, SW Canada
94 E8 **Smøla** *island* W Norway
128 H4 **Smolensk** Smolenskaya Oblast', W Russian Federation
128 H4 **Smolenskaya Oblast'** ◈ *province* W Russian Federation
Smolensk-Moscow Upland *see* Smolensko-Moskovskaya Vozvyshennost'
128 J3 **Smolensko-Moskovskaya Vozvyshennost'** *var.* Smolensk-Moscow Upland. ▲▲ W Russian Federation
Smolevichi *see* Smalyavichy
115 C15 **Smolikás** ▲ W Greece
114 I12 **Smolyan** *prev.* Pashmakli. Smolyan, S Bulgaria
114 I12 **Smolyan** ◈ *province* S Bulgaria
Smolyany *see* Smalyany
33 S15 **Smoot** Wyoming, C USA
12 G12 **Smooth Rock Falls** Ontario, S Canada
Smorgon'/Smorgonie *see* Smarhon'
95 K23 **Smygehamn** Skåne, S Sweden
194 I7 **Smyley Island** *island* Antarctica
21 Y3 **Smyrna** Delaware, NE USA
23 S3 **Smyrna** Georgia, SE USA
20 J9 **Smyrna** Tennessee, S USA
Smyrna *see* İzmir
97 I16 **Snaefell** ▲ C Isle of Man
92 H3 **Snaefellsjökull** ▲ W Iceland
10 J4 **Snake** ≈ Yukon Territory, NW Canada
29 O8 **Snake Creek** ≈ South Dakota, N USA
183 P13 **Snake Island** *island* Victoria, SE Australia
35 Y6 **Snake Range** ▲▲ Nevada, W USA
32 K10 **Snake River** ≈ NW USA
29 V6 **Snake River** ≈ Minnesota, N USA
28 L12 **Snake River** ≈ Nebraska, C USA
33 Q14 **Snake River Plain** *plain* Idaho, NW USA
93 F15 **Snåsa** Nord-Trøndelag, C Norway
21 O8 **Sneedville** Tennessee, S USA
98 K6 **Sneek** Friesland, N Netherlands
Sneeuw-gebergte *see* Maoke, Pegunungan
95 F22 **Snejbjerg** Ringkøbing, C Denmark
122 K9 **Snezhnogorsk** Taymyrskiy (Dolgano-Nenetskiy) Avtonomnyy Okrug, N Russian Federation
Snezhnoye *see* Snizhne
111 G15 **Sněžka** *Ger.* Schneekoppe. ▲ N Czech Republic
110 N8 **Śniardwy, Jezioro** *Ger.* Spirdingsee. ◎ NE Poland
Sniečkus *see* Visaginas
117 R10 **Snihurivka** Mykolayivs'ka Oblast', S Ukraine
116 I5 **Snilov** × (L'viv) L'vivs'ka Oblast', W Ukraine
111 O19 **Snina** *Hung.* Szinna. Prešovský Kraj, E Slovakia
117 Y8 **Snizhne** *Rus.* Snezhnoye. Donets'ka Oblast', SE Ukraine
92 J3 **Snækollur** ▲ C Iceland
94 G10 **Snøhetta** *var.* Snohetta. ▲ S Norway
92 G12 **Snøtinden** ▲ C Norway
97 I18 **Snowdon** ▲ NW Wales, UK
97 I18 **Snowdonia** ▲▲ NW Wales, UK
8 K10 **Snowdrift** ≈ Northwest Territories, NW Canada
Snowdrift *see* Łutsel'k'e
37 N12 **Snowflake** Arizona, SW USA
21 Y5 **Snow Hill** Maryland, NE USA
21 W10 **Snow Hill** North Carolina, SE USA
194 H3 **Snowhill Island** *island* Antarctica
11 V13 **Snow Lake** Manitoba, C Canada
37 R5 **Snowmass Mountain** ▲ Colorado, C USA
18 M10 **Snow, Mount** ▲ Vermont, NE USA
34 M5 **Snow Mountain** ▲ California, W USA
Snow Mountains *see* Maoke, Pegunungan
33 N7 **Snowshoe Peak** ▲ Montana, NW USA
182 I8 **Snowtown** South Australia
36 K1 **Snowville** Utah, W USA
35 X3 **Snow Water Lake** ◎ Nevada, W USA
183 Q11 **Snowy Mountains** ▲▲ New South Wales/Victoria, SE Australia
183 Q12 **Snowy River** ≈ New South Wales/Victoria, SE Australia
44 K5 **Snug Corner** Acklins Island, SE Bahamas
167 T13 **Snuŏl** Krâchéh, E Cambodia
116 J7 **Snyatyn** *Rus.* Snyatyn. Ivano-Frankivs'ka Oblast', W Ukraine
26 L12 **Snyder** Oklahoma, C USA
25 O6 **Snyder** Texas, SW USA
172 H3 **Soalala** Mahajanga, W Madagascar
172 J4 **Soanierana-Ivongo** Toamasina, E Madagascar
171 R11 **Soasiu** *var.* Tidore. Pulau Tidore, E Indonesia
54 G8 **Soatá** Boyacá, C Colombia
172 I5 **Soavinandriana** Antananarivo, C Madagascar
77 V13 **Soba** Kaduna, C Nigeria
163 Y16 **Sobaek-sanmaek** ▲▲ S South Korea
80 F13 **Sobat** ≈ E Sudan
171 Z14 **Sobger, Sungai** ≈ Irian Jaya, E Indonesia
171 V13 **Sobiei** Irian Jaya, E Indonesia
128 M3 **Sobinka** Vladimirskaya Oblast', W Russian Federation
129 S7 **Sobolevo** Orenburgskaya Oblast', W Russian Federation
Soborsin *see* Săvârşin
164 D15 **Sobo-san** ▲ Kyūshū, SW Japan
111 G14 **Sobótka** Dolnośląskie, SW Poland
59 O15 **Sobradinho** Bahia, E Brazil
Sobradinho, Barragem de *see* Sobradinho, Represa de
59 O16 **Sobradinho, Represa de** *var.* Barragem de Sobradinho. ⊠ E Brazil
58 O13 **Sobral** Ceará, E Brazil
105 T4 **Sobrarbe** *physical region* NE Spain
109 R10 **Soča** *It.* Isonzo. ≈ Italy/Slovenia
110 L11 **Sochaczew** Mazowieckie, C Poland
128 L15 **Sochi** Krasnodarskiy Kray, SW Russian Federation
114 G13 **Sochós** *var.* Sohos, Sokhós. Kentrikí Makedonía, N Greece
191 R11 **Société, Archipel de la** *var.* Archipel de Tahiti, Îles de la Société, *Eng.* Society Islands. *island group* W French Polynesia
Société, Îles de la/Society Islands *see* Société, Archipel de la
21 T11 **Society Hill** South Carolina, SE USA
175 W9 **Society Ridge** *undersea feature* C Pacific Ocean
62 I5 **Socompa, Volcán** ▲ N Chile
Soconusco, Sierra de *see* Sierra Madre
54 G8 **Socorro** Santander, C Colombia
37 R13 **Socorro** New Mexico, SW USA
Socotra *see* Suquṭrā
167 S14 **Soc Trăng** *var.* Khanh Hung. Soc Trăng, S Vietnam
105 P10 **Socuéllamos** Castilla-La Mancha, C Spain
35 W13 **Soda Lake** *salt flat* California, W USA
92 L11 **Sodankylä** Lappi, N Finland
Sodari *see* Sodiri
33 R15 **Soda Springs** Idaho, NW USA
Soddo/Soddu *see* Sodo
20 L10 **Soddy Daisy** Tennessee, S USA
95 N14 **Söderfors** Uppsala, C Sweden
94 N12 **Söderhamn** Gävleborg, C Sweden
95 N17 **Söderköping** Östergötland, S Sweden
95 N17 **Södermanland** ◈ *county* C Sweden
95 O16 **Södertälje** Stockholm, C Sweden
80 D10 **Sodiri** *var.* Sawdirī, Sodari. Northern Kordofan, C Sudan
81 I14 **Sodo** *var.* Soddo, Soddu. Southern, S Ethiopia
94 N11 **Södra Dellen** ◎ C Sweden
95 M19 **Södra Vi** Kalmar, S Sweden
18 G9 **Sodus Point** *headland* New York, NE USA
171 Q17 **Soe** *prev.* Soë. Timor, C Indonesia
169 N15 **Soekarno-Hatta** × (Jakarta) Jawa, S Indonesia
Soëla-Sund *see* Soela Väin
118 E5 **Soela Väin** *prev. Eng.* Sele Sound, *Ger.* Dagden-Sund, Soëla-Sund. *strait* W Estonia
Soemba *see* Sumba, Pulau
Soembawa *see* Sumbawa
Soemenep *see* Sumenep
Soengaipenoeh *see* Sungaipenuh
Soerabaja *see* Surabaya
101 G14 **Soest** Nordrhein-Westfalen, W Germany
98 J11 **Soest** Utrecht, C Netherlands
100 F11 **Soeste** ≈ NW Germany
98 J11 **Soesterberg** Utrecht, C Netherlands
115 E16 **Sofádes** *var.* Sofádhes. Thessalía, C Greece
Sofádhes *see* Sofádes
83 N18 **Sofala** Sofala, C Mozambique
83 N17 **Sofala** ◈ *province* C Mozambique
83 N18 **Sofala, Baia de** *bay* E Mozambique
172 J3 **Sofia** *seasonal river* NW Madagascar
Sofia *see* Sofiya
115 G19 **Sofikó** Pelopónnisos, S Greece
Sofi-Kurgan *see* Sopu-Korgon
114 G10 **Sofiya** *var.* Sophia, *Eng.* Sofia; *Lat.* Serdica. ● (Bulgaria) Sofiya-Grad, W Bulgaria
114 G9 **Sofiya** × Sofiya-Grad, W Bulgaria
114 H9 **Sofiya** ◈ *province* W Bulgaria
114 G9 **Sofiya-Grad** ◈ *municipality* W Bulgaria
Sofiyevka *see* Sofiyivka
117 S8 **Sofiyivka** *Rus.* Sofiyevka. Dnipropetrovs'ka Oblast', E Ukraine
123 R13 **Sofiysk** Khabarovskiy Kray, SE Russian Federation
123 S12 **Sofiysk** Khabarovskiy Kray, SE Russian Federation
126 I6 **Sofporog** Respublika Kareliya, NW Russian Federation
165 Y14 **Sōfu-gan** *island* Izu-shotō, SE Japan
Sog *see* Sog Xian
54 G9 **Sogamoso** Boyacá, C Colombia
136 I11 **Soğanlı Çayı** ≈ N Turkey
94 E12 **Sogn** *physical region* S Norway
94 E12 **Sogndal** *var.* Sogndalsfjøra. Sogn og Fjordane, S Norway
Sogndalsfjøra *see* Sogndal
95 E18 **Søgne** Vest-Agder, S Norway
94 D12 **Sognefjorden** *fjord* NE North Sea
94 C12 **Sogn Og Fjordane** ◈ *county* S Norway
162 I11 **Sogo Nur** ◎ N China
159 T12 **Sogruma** Qinghai, W China
163 X17 **Sŏgwip'o** S South Korea
156 K10 **Sog Xian** *var.* Sog. Xizang Zizhiqu, W China
75 X10 **Sohâg** *var.* Sawhāj, Suliag. C Egypt
Sohar *see* Şuḩār
64 H9 **Sohm Plain** *undersea feature* NW Atlantic Ocean
100 H7 **Soholmer Au** ≈ N Germany
Sohos *see* Sochós
Sohrau *see* Żory
99 F20 **Soignies** Hainaut, SW Belgium
159 R15 **Soila** Xizang Zizhiqu, W China
103 P4 **Soissons** *anc.* Augusta Suessionum, Noviodunum. Aisne, N France
164 H13 **Sōja** Okayama, Honshū, SW Japan
152 F13 **Sojat** Rājasthān, N India
163 W13 **Sŏjosŏn-man** *inlet* W North Korea
116 I4 **Sokal'** *Rus.* Sokal. L'vivs'ka Oblast', NW Ukraine
163 Y14 **Sokch'o** N South Korea
136 B15 **Söke** Aydın, SW Turkey
189 N12 **Sokehs Island** *island* E Micronesia
79 M24 **Sokele** Katanga, SE Dem. Rep. Congo (Zaire)
147 R11 **Sokh** *Uzb.* Sŭkh. ≈ Kyrgyzstan/Uzbekistan
Sokh *see* Sŭkh
Sokhós *see* Sochós
137 Q8 **Sokhumi** *Rus.* Sukhumi. NW Georgia
113 O14 **Sokobanja** Serbia, E Yugoslavia
77 R15 **Sokodé** C Togo
123 T10 **Sokol** Magadanskaya Oblast', E Russian Federation
126 M13 **Sokol** Vologodskaya Oblast', NW Russian Federation
110 P9 **Sokółka** Podlaskie, NE Poland
76 M11 **Sokolo** Ségou, W Mali
111 A16 **Sokolov** *Ger.* Falkenau an der Eger; *prev.* Falknov nad Ohří. Karlovarský Kraj, W Czech Republic
111 O16 **Sokołów Małopolski** Podkarpackie, SE Poland
110 O11 **Sokołów Podlaski** Mazowieckie, E Poland
76 G11 **Sokone** W Senegal
77 T12 **Sokoto** Sokoto, NW Nigeria
77 T12 **Sokoto** ◈ *state* NW Nigeria
77 S12 **Sokoto** ≈ NW Nigeria
Sokotra *see* Suquṭrā
147 U7 **Sokuluk** Chuyskaya Oblast', N Kyrgyzstan
116 L7 **Sokyryany** Chernivets'ka Oblast', W Ukraine
95 C16 **Sola** Rogaland, S Norway
187 R12 **Sola** Vanua Lava, N Vanuatu
95 C17 **Sola** × (Stavanger) Rogaland, S Norway
81 H18 **Solai** Rift Valley, W Kenya
152 I8 **Solan** Himāchal Pradesh, N India
185 A25 **Solander Island** *island* SW NZ
Solano *see* Bahía Solano
155 F15 **Solāpur** *var.* Sholāpur. Mahārāshtra, W India
93 H16 **Solberg** Västernorrland, C Sweden
116 K9 **Solca** *Ger.* Solka. Suceava, N Romania
105 O16 **Sol, Costa del** *coastal region* S Spain
106 F5 **Solda** Trentino-Alto Adige, N Italy
117 N9 **Şoldăneşti** *Rus.* Sholdaneshty. N Moldova
Soldau *see* Wkra
108 L8 **Sölden** Tirol, W Austria
27 P3 **Soldier Creek** ≈ Kansas, C USA
39 R12 **Soldotna** Alaska, USA
110 I10 **Solec Kujawski** Kujawsko-pomorskie, C Poland
61 B16 **Soledad** Santa Fe, C Argentina
55 E4 **Soledad** Atlántico, N Colombia
35 O11 **Soledad** California, W USA
55 O7 **Soledad** Anzoátegui, NE Venezuela
Soledad *see* East Falkland
Soledad, Isla *see* East Falkland
61 H15 **Soledade** Rio Grande do Sul, S Brazil
103 Y15 **Solenzara** Corse, France, C Mediterranean Sea
Soleure *see* Solothurn
94 C12 **Solheim** Hordaland, S Norway
127 N14 **Soligalich** Kostromskaya Oblast', NW Russian Federation
Soligorsk *see* Salihorsk
97 L20 **Solihull** C England, UK
127 U13 **Solikamsk** Permskaya Oblast', NW Russian Federation
129 V8 **Sol'-Iletsk** Orenburgskaya Oblast', W Russian Federation
57 G17 **Solimana, Nevado** ▲ S Peru
58 E13 **Solimões, Rio** ≈ C Brazil
113 E14 **Solin** *It.* Salona; *anc.* Salonae. Split-Dalmacija, S Croatia
101 E15 **Solingen** Nordrhein-Westfalen, W Germany
Solka *see* Solca
93 H16 **Sollefteå** Västernorrland, C Sweden
95 O15 **Sollentuna** Stockholm, C Sweden
94 L13 **Sollerön** Dalarna, C Sweden
101 I14 **Solling** *hill range* C Germany
95 O16 **Solna** Stockholm, C Sweden
128 K3 **Solnechnogorsk** Moskovskaya Oblast', W Russian Federation
123 R10 **Solnechnyy** Khabarovskiy Kray, SE Russian Federation
123 S13 **Solnechnyy** Respublika Sakha (Yakutiya), NE Russian Federation
94 H11 **Sølnkletten** ▲ S Norway
107 L17 **Solofra** Campania, S Italy
168 J11 **Solok** Sumatera, W Indonesia
42 C6 **Sololá** Sololá, W Guatemala
42 A2 **Sololá** *off.* Departamento de Sololá. ◈ *department* SW Guatemala
81 J16 **Sololo** Eastern, N Kenya
42 C4 **Soloma** Huehuetenango, W Guatemala
38 M9 **Solomon** Alaska, USA
27 N4 **Solomon** Kansas, C USA
187 N9 **Solomon Islands** *prev.* British Solomon Islands Protectorate. ◆ *commonwealth republic* W Pacific Ocean
186 L7 **Solomon Islands** *island group* PNG/Solomon Islands
26 M3 **Solomon River** ≈ Kansas, C USA
186 H8 **Solomon Sea** *sea* W Pacific Ocean
31 U11 **Solon** Ohio, N USA
117 T8 **Solone** Dnipropetrovs'ka Oblast', E Ukraine
171 P16 **Solor, Kepulauan** *island group* S Indonesia
128 M4 **Solotcha** Ryazanskaya Oblast', W Russian Federation
108 D7 **Solothurn** *Fr.* Soleure. Solothurn, NW Switzerland
108 D7 **Solothurn** *Fr.* Soleure. ◈ *canton* NW Switzerland
126 J7 **Solovetskiye Ostrova** *island group* NW Russian Federation
105 V5 **Solsona** Cataluña, NE Spain
113 E14 **Šolta** *It.* Solta. *island* S Croatia
Soltānābād *see* Kāshmar
142 L4 **Soltānīyeh** Zanjān, NW Iran
100 I11 **Soltau** Niedersachsen, NW Germany
126 G14 **Sol'tsy** Novgorodskaya Oblast', W Russian Federation
Soltüstik Qazaqstan Oblysy *see* Severnyy Kazakhstan
Solun *see* Thessaloníki
113 O19 **Solunska Glava** ▲ C FYR Macedonia
95 L22 **Sölvesborg** Blekinge, S Sweden
97 J15 **Solway Firth** *inlet* England/Scotland, UK
82 I13 **Solwezi** North Western, NW Zambia
165 Q11 **Sōma** Fukushima, Honshū, C Japan
136 C13 **Soma** Manisa, W Turkey
81 M14 **Somali** ◈ *region* E Ethiopia
81 O15 **Somalia** *off.* Somali Democratic Republic, *Som.* Jamuuriyada Demuqraadiga Soomaaliyeed, Soomaaliya; *prev.* Italian Somaliland, Somaliland Protectorate. ◆ *republic* E Africa
173 N6 **Somali Basin** *undersea feature* W Indian Ocean
67 Y8 **Somali Plain** *undersea feature* W Indian Ocean
112 J8 **Sombor** *Hung.* Zombor. Serbia, NW Yugoslavia
99 H20 **Sombreffe** Namur, S Belgium
40 L10 **Sombrerete** Zacatecas, C Mexico
45 V8 **Sombrero** *island* N Anguilla
151 Q21 **Sombrero Channel** *channel* Nicobar Islands, India
116 H9 **Şomcuta Mare** *Hung.* Nagysomkút; *prev.* Somcuţa Mare. Maramureş, N Romania
167 R9 **Somdet** Kalasin, E Thailand
99 L15 **Someren** Noord-Brabant, SE Netherlands
93 L19 **Somero** Länsi-Suomi, W Finland
33 P7 **Somers** Montana, NW USA
64 A12 **Somerset** *var.* Somerset Village. W Bermuda
37 Q5 **Somerset** Colorado, C USA
20 M7 **Somerset** Kentucky, S USA
19 O12 **Somerset** Massachusetts, NE USA
97 K23 **Somerset** *cultural region* SW England, UK
Somerset East *see* Somerset-Oos
64 A12 **Somerset Island** *island* W Bermuda
197 N9 **Somerset Island** *island* Queen Elizabeth Islands, Nunavut, NW Canada
Somerset Nile *see* Victoria Nile
83 I25 **Somerset-Oos** *Eng.* Somerset East. Eastern Cape, S South Africa
83 E26 **Somerset-Wes** *Eng.* Somerset West. Western Cape, SW South Africa
Somerset West *see* Somerset-Wes
Somers Islands *see* Bermuda
18 J17 **Somers Point** New Jersey, NE USA
19 P9 **Somersworth** New Hampshire, NE USA
36 H15 **Somerton** Arizona, SW USA
18 J14 **Somerville** New Jersey, NE USA
20 F10 **Somerville** Tennessee, S USA
25 U10 **Somerville** Texas, SW USA
25 T10 **Somerville Lake** ⊠ Texas, SW USA
Someş/Somesch/Someşul *see* Szamos
103 N2 **Somme** ◈ *department* N France
103 N2 **Somme** ≈ N France
95 L18 **Sommen** Jönköping, S Sweden
95 M18 **Sommen** ◎ S Sweden
101 K16 **Sömmerda** Thüringen, C Germany
Sommerein *see* Šamorín
Sommerfeld *see* Lubsko
55 Y11 **Sommet Tabulaire** *var.* Mont Itoupé. ▲ S French Guiana
111 H25 **Somogy** *off.* Somogy Megye. ◈ *county* SW Hungary
Somorja *see* Šamorín
105 N7 **Somosierra, Puerto de** *pass* N Spain
187 Y14 **Somosomo** Taveuni, N Fiji
42 I9 **Somotillo** Chinandega, NW Nicaragua
42 I8 **Somoto** Madriz, NW Nicaragua
110 I11 **Sompolno** Wielkolpolskie, C Poland
105 S3 **Somport** *var.* Puerto de Somport, *Fr.* Col du Somport; *anc.* Summus Portus. *pass* France/Spain *see also* Somport, Col du
102 J17 **Somport, Col du** *var.* Puerto de Somport, *Sp.* Somport; *anc.* Summus Portus. *pass* France/Spain *see also* Somport
Somport, Puerto de *see* Somport/Somport, Col du
99 K15 **Son** Noord-Brabant, S Netherlands
95 H15 **Son** Akershus, S Norway

◆ Country ● Country Capital ◇ Dependent Territory ○ Dependent Territory Capital ◈ Administrative Region × International Airport ▲ Mountain ▲▲ Mountain Range ※ Volcano ≈ River ◎ Lake ⊠ Reservoir

154 L9 **Son** *var.* Sone. ∽ C India
43 R16 **Soná** Veraguas, W Panama
154 M12 **Sonapur** *prev.* Sonepur. Orissa, E India
95 G24 **Sønderborg** *Ger.* Sonderburg. Sønderjylland, SW Denmark
Sonderburg *see* Sønderborg
95 F24 **Sønderjylland** *off.* Sønderjyllands Amt. ♦ *county* SW Denmark
101 K15 **Sondershausen** Thüringen, C Germany
Søndre Strømfjord *see* Kangerlussuaq
106 E6 **Sondrio** Lombardia, N Italy
Sone *see* Son
Sonepur *see* Sonapur
57 K22 **Sonequera** ▲ S Bolivia
167 V12 **Sông Câu** Phu Yên, C Vietnam
167 R15 **Sông Đôc** Minh Hai, S Vietnam
81 H25 **Songea** Ruvuma, S Tanzania
163 X10 **Songhua Hu** ◎ NE China
163 Y7 **Songhua Jiang** *var.* Sungari. ∽ NE China
161 S8 **Songjiang** Shanghai Shi, E China
Sŏngjin *see* Kimch'aek
167 O16 **Songkhla** *var.* Songkla, *Mal.* Singora. Songkhla, SW Thailand
Songkla *see* Songkhla
163 T13 **Song Ling** ▲ NE China
163 W14 **Songnim** SW North Korea
82 B10 **Songo** Uíge, NW Angola
83 M15 **Songo** Tete, NW Mozambique
79 F21 **Songololo** Bas-Congo, SW Dem. Rep. Congo (Zaire)
160 H7 **Songpan** *prev.* Sungpu. Sichuan, C China
163 Y17 **Sŏngsan** S South Korea
161 R11 **Songxi** Fujian, SE China
160 M6 **Songxian** *var.* Song Xian. Henan, C China
161 R10 **Songyin** Zhejiang, SE China
163 V9 **Songyuan** *var.* Fu-yü, Petuna; *prev.* Fuyu. Jilin, NE China
163 P11 **Sonid Youqi** *var.* Saihon Tal. Nei Mongol Zizhiqu, N China
163 P11 **Sonid Zuoqi** Nei Mongol Zizhiqu, N China
152 I10 **Sonīpat** Haryāna, N India
93 M15 **Sonkajärvi** Itä-Suomi, C Finland
167 R6 **Sơn La** Sơn La, N Vietnam
149 O16 **Sonmiāni** Baluchistān, S Pakistan
149 O16 **Sonmiāni Bay** *bay* S Pakistan
101 K18 **Sonneberg** Thüringen, C Germany
101 N24 **Sonntagshorn** ▲ Austria/Germany
Sonoita *see* Sonoyta
40 E3 **Sonoita, Rio** *var.* Río Sonoyta. ∽ Mexico/USA
35 N7 **Sonoma** California, W USA
35 T3 **Sonoma Peak** ▲ Nevada, W USA
35 P8 **Sonora** California, W USA
25 O10 **Sonora** Texas, SW USA
40 F5 **Sonora** ♦ *state* NW Mexico
35 X17 **Sonoran Desert** *var.* Desierto de Altar. *desert* Mexico/USA *see also* Altar, Desierto de
40 G5 **Sonora, Río** ∽ NW Mexico
40 E2 **Sonoyta** *var.* Sonoita. Sonora, NW Mexico
Sonoyta, Río *see* Sonoita, Rio
142 K6 **Sonqor** *var.* Sunqur. Kermānshāh, W Iran
105 N9 **Sonseca** *var.* Sonseca con Casalgordo. Castilla-La Mancha, C Spain
Sonseca con Casalgordo *see* Sonseca
54 E9 **Sonsón** Antioquia, W Colombia
42 E7 **Sonsonate** Sonsonate, W El Salvador
42 A9 **Sonsonate** ♦ *department* SW El Salvador
188 A10 **Sonsorol Islands** *island group* S Palau
112 J9 **Sonta** *Hung.* Szond; *prev.* Szonta. Serbia, NW Yugoslavia
167 S6 **Sơn Tây** *var.* Sontay. Ha Tây, N Vietnam
101 J25 **Sonthofen** Bayern, S Germany
Soochow *see* Suzhou
Soomaaliya/Soomaaliyeed, Jamuuriyada Demuqraadiga *see* Somalia
Soome Laht *see* Finland, Gulf of
Sooner State *see* Oklahoma
23 V5 **Soperton** Georgia, SE USA
167 S6 **Sop Hao** Houaphan, N Laos
Sophia *see* Sofiya
171 S10 **Sopi** Pulau Morotai, E Indonesia
Sopianae *see* Pécs
171 U13 **Sopinusa** Irian Jaya, E Indonesia
81 B14 **Sopo** ∽ W Sudan
Sopockinie/Sopotskin *see* Sapotskino
114 I9 **Sopot** Plovdiv, C Bulgaria
110 I7 **Sopot** *Ger.* Zoppot. Pomorskie, N Poland
167 O8 **Sop Prap** *var.* Ban Sop Prap. Lampang, NW Thailand
111 G22 **Sopron** *Ger.* Ödenburg. Győr-Moson-Sopron, NW Hungary
147 U11 **Sopu-Korgon** *var.* Sofi-Kurgan. Oshskaya Oblast', SW Kyrgyzstan
152 H5 **Sopur** Jammu and Kashmir, NW India
107 J15 **Sora** Lazio, C Italy
154 N13 **Sorada** Orissa, E India
93 H17 **Söråker** Västernorrland, C Sweden
57 J17 **Sorata** La Paz, W Bolivia
Sorau/Sorau in der Niederlausitz *see* Żary
105 Q14 **Sorbas** Andalucía, S Spain
Sord/Sórd Choluim Chille *see* Swords
15 O11 **Sorel** Quebec, SE Canada
183 P17 **Sorell** Tasmania, SE Australia
183 O17 **Sorell, Lake** ◎ Tasmania, SE Australia
106 E8 **Soresina** Lombardia, N Italy
95 D14 **Sørfjorden** *fjord* S Norway
94 N11 **Sörforsa** Gävleborg, C Sweden
103 R14 **Sorgues** Vaucluse, SE France
136 K13 **Sorgun** Yozgat, C Turkey
105 P5 **Soria** Castilla-León, N Spain
105 P6 **Soria** ♦ *province* Castilla-León, N Spain
61 D19 **Soriano** Soriano, SW Uruguay
61 D19 **Soriano** ♦ *department* SW Uruguay
92 O4 **Sørkapp** *headland* SW Svalbard
143 T5 **Sorkh, Kūh-e** ▲ NE Iran
Soro *see* Ghazal, Bahr el
95 I23 **Sorø** Vestsjælland, E Denmark
116 M8 **Soroca** *Rus.* Soroki. N Moldova
60 L10 **Sorocaba** São Paulo, S Brazil
Sorochino *see* Sarochyna
129 T7 **Sorochinsk** Orenburgskaya Oblast', W Russian Federation
Soroki *see* Soroca
188 H15 **Sorol** *atoll* Caroline Islands, W Micronesia
171 T12 **Sorong** Irian Jaya, E Indonesia
81 G17 **Soroti** C Uganda
Sørøy *see* Sørøya
92 J8 **Sørøya** *var.* Sørøy. *island* N Norway
104 G11 **Sorraia, Rio** ∽ C Portugal
92 I10 **Sørreisa** Troms, N Norway
107 K18 **Sorrento** *anc.* Surrentum. Campania, S Italy
104 H10 **Sor, Ribeira de** *stream* C Portugal
195 T3 **Sør Rondane Mountains** ▲ Antarctica
93 H14 **Sorsele** Västerbotten, N Sweden
107 B17 **Sorso** Sardegna, Italy, C Mediterranean Sea
171 P4 **Sorsogon** Luzon, N Philippines
105 U4 **Sort** Cataluña, NE Spain
126 H11 **Sortavala** Respublika Kareliya, NW Russian Federation
107 L25 **Sortino** Sicilia, Italy, C Mediterranean Sea
92 G10 **Sortland** Nordland, C Norway
94 G9 **Sør-Trøndelag** ♦ *county* S Norway
95 I15 **Sørumsand** Akershus, S Norway
118 D6 **Sõrve Säär** *headland* SW Estonia
95 K22 **Sösdala** Skåne, S Sweden
105 R4 **Sos del Rey Católico** Aragón, NE Spain
93 F15 **Sösjöfjällen** ▲ C Sweden
128 K7 **Sosna** ∽ W Russian Federation
62 H12 **Sosneado, Cerro** ▲ W Argentina
127 S9 **Sosnogorsk** Respublika Komi, NW Russian Federation
126 J8 **Sosnovets** Respublika Kareliya, NW Russian Federation
Sosnovets *see* Sosnowiec
129 Q3 **Sosnovka** Chuvashskaya Respublika, W Russian Federation
127 S16 **Sosnovka** Kirovskaya Oblast', NW Russian Federation
126 M6 **Sosnovka** Murmanskaya Oblast', NW Russian Federation
128 M6 **Sosnovka** Tambovskaya Oblast', W Russian Federation
126 H12 **Sosnovo** *Fin.* Rautu. Leningradskaya Oblast', NW Russian Federation
Sosnovyy Bor *see* Sasnovy Bor
111 J16 **Sosnowiec** *Ger.* Sosnowitz, *Rus.* Sosnovets. Śląskie, S Poland
Sosnowitz *see* Sosnowiec
117 R2 **Sosnytsya** Chernihivs'ka Oblast', N Ukraine
109 V10 **Šoštanj** N Slovenia
122 G10 **Sos'va** Sverdlovskaya Oblast', C Russian Federation
54 D12 **Sotará, Volcán** ⩕ S Colombia
76 D10 **Sotavento, Ilhas de** *var.* Leeward Islands. *island group* S Cape Verde
93 N15 **Sotkamo** Oulu, C Finland
41 P10 **Soto la Marina** Tamaulipas, C Mexico
41 P10 **Soto la Marina, Río** ∽ C Mexico
41 X12 **Sotuta** Yucatán, SE Mexico
79 F17 **Souanké** La Sangha, NW Congo
76 M17 **Soubré** S Ivory Coast
115 H24 **Soúda** *var.* Soúdha, *Eng.* Suda. Kríti, Greece, E Mediterranean Sea
Soúdha *see* Soúda
Soueida *see* As Suwaydā'
114 L12 **Souflí** *prev.* Souflíon. Anatolikí Makedonía kai Thráki, NE Greece
Souflíon *see* Souflí
45 S11 **Soufrière** W Saint Lucia
45 X6 **Soufrière** ⩕ Basse Terre, S Guadeloupe
102 M13 **Souillac** Lot, S France
173 Y17 **Souillac** S Mauritius
74 M5 **Souk Ahras** NE Algeria
74 E6 **Souk-el-Arba-Rharb** *var.* Souk el Arba du Rharb, Souk-el-Arba-du-Rharb, Souk-el-Arba-el-Rhab. NW Morocco
Soukhné *see* As Sukhnah
163 X14 **Sŏul** *off.* Sŏul-t'ŭkpyŏlsi, *Eng.* Seoul, *Jap.* Keijō; *prev.* Kyŏngsŏng. ● (South Korea) NW South Korea
102 J11 **Soulac-sur-Mer** Gironde, SW France
99 L19 **Soumagne** Liège, E Belgium
18 M14 **Sound Beach** Long Island, New York, NE USA
95 J22 **Sound, The** *Dan.* Øresund, *Swe.* Öresund. *strait* Denmark/Sweden
115 H20 **Soúnio, Akrotírio** *headland* C Greece
138 F8 **Soûr** *var.* Şūr; *anc.* Tyre. SW Lebanon
Sources, Mont-aux- *see* Phofung
104 G8 **Soure** Coimbra, N Portugal
11 W17 **Souris** Manitoba, S Canada
13 Q14 **Souris** Prince Edward Island, SE Canada
28 L2 **Souris River** *var.* Mouse River. ∽ Canada/USA
25 X10 **Sour Lake** Texas, SW USA
115 F17 **Sourpi** Thessalía, C Greece
104 H11 **Sousel** Portalegre, C Portugal
75 N6 **Sousse** *var.* Sūsah. NE Tunisia
14 H11 **South** ∽ Ontario, S Canada
South *see* Sud
83 G23 **South Africa** *off.* Republic of South Africa, *Afr.* Suid-Afrika. ◆ *republic* S Africa
48-49 **South America** *continent*
2 J17 **South American Plate** *tectonic feature*
97 M23 **Southampton** *hist.* Hamwih, *Lat.* Clausentum. S England, UK
19 N14 **Southampton** Long Island, New York, NE USA
9 P8 **Southampton Island** *island* Nunavut, NE Canada
151 P20 **South Andaman** *island* Andaman Islands, India, NE Indian Ocean
13 Q6 **South Aulatsivik Island** *island* Newfoundland, E Canada
182 E4 **South Australia** ♦ *state* S Australia
South Australian Abyssal Plain *see* South Australian Plain
192 G11 **South Australian Basin** *undersea feature* SW Indian Ocean
173 X12 **South Australian Plain** *var.* South Australian Abyssal Plain. *undersea feature* SE Indian Ocean
37 R13 **South Baldy** ▲ New Mexico, SW USA
23 Y14 **South Bay** Florida, SE USA
14 E12 **South Baymouth** Manitoulin Island, Ontario, S Canada
30 L10 **South Beloit** Illinois, N USA
31 O11 **South Bend** Indiana, N USA
25 R6 **South Bend** Texas, SW USA
32 F9 **South Bend** Washington, NW USA
South Beveland *see* Zuid-Beveland
South Borneo *see* Kalimantan Selatan
21 U7 **South Boston** Virginia, NE USA
182 F2 **South Branch Neales** *seasonal river* South Australia
21 U3 **South Branch Potomac River** ∽ West Virginia, NE USA
185 H19 **Southbridge** Canterbury, South Island, NZ
19 N12 **Southbridge** Massachusetts, NE USA
183 P17 **South Bruny Island** *island* Tasmania, SE Australia
18 L7 **South Burlington** Vermont, NE USA
44 M6 **South Caicos** *island* S Turks and Caicos Islands
South Cape *see* Ka Lae
23 V3 **South Carolina** *off.* State of South Carolina; also known as The Palmetto State. ♦ *state* SE USA
South Carpathians *see* Carpații Meridionali
South Celebes *see* Sulawesi Selatan
21 Q5 **South Charleston** West Virginia, NE USA
192 D7 **South China Basin** *undersea feature* SE South China Sea
169 R8 **South China Sea** *Chin.* Nan Hai, *Ind.* Laut Cina Selatan, *Vtn.* Biên Đông. *sea* SE Asia
33 Z10 **South Dakota** *off.* State of South Dakota; also known as The Coyote State, Sunshine State. ♦ *state* N USA
23 X10 **South Daytona** Florida, SE USA
37 R10 **South Domingo Pueblo** New Mexico, SW USA
97 N23 **South Downs** *hill range* SE England, UK
83 I21 **South East** ♦ *district* SE Botswana
65 H15 **South East Bay** *bay* Ascension Island, C Atlantic Ocean
183 O17 **South East Cape** *headland* Tasmania, SE Australia
38 K10 **Southeast Cape** *headland* Saint Lawrence Island, Alaska, USA
South-East Celebes *see* Sulawesi Tenggara
192 G12 **Southeast Indian Ridge** *undersea feature* Indian Ocean/Pacific Ocean
Southeast Island *see* Tagula Island
193 P13 **Southeast Pacific Basin** *var.* Belling Hausen Mulde. *undersea feature* SE Pacific Ocean
65 H15 **South East Point** *headland* SE Ascension Island
183 O14 **South East Point** *headland* Victoria, S Australia
191 Z3 **South East Point** *headland* Kiritimati, NE Kiribati
44 L5 **Southeast Point** *headland* Mayaguana, SE Bahamas
South-East Sulawesi *see* Sulawesi Tenggara
11 U12 **Southend** Saskatchewan, C Canada
97 P22 **Southend-on-Sea** E England, UK
83 H20 **Southern** *var.* Bangwaketse, Ngwaketze. ♦ *district* SE Botswana
81 I15 **Southern** ♦ *region* S Ethiopia
138 E13 **Southern** ♦ *district* S Israel
83 N15 **Southern** ♦ *region* S Malawi
83 I15 **Southern** ♦ *province* S Zambia
185 E19 **Southern Alps** ▲ South Island, NZ
190 K15 **Southern Cook Islands** *island group* S Cook Islands
180 K12 **Southern Cross** Western Australia
80 A12 **Southern Darfur** ♦ *state* W Sudan
186 B7 **Southern Highlands** ♦ *province* W PNG
11 V11 **Southern Indian Lake** ◎ Manitoba, C Canada
80 E11 **Southern Kordofan** ♦ *state* C Sudan
187 Z15 **Southern Lau Group** *island group* Lau Group, SE Fiji
173 S13 **Southern Ocean** *ocean*
21 T10 **Southern Pines** North Carolina, SE USA
155 J26 **Southern Province** ♦ *province* S Sri Lanka
96 I13 **Southern Uplands** ▲ S Scotland, UK
Southern Urals *see* Yuzhnyy Ural
183 P16 **South Esk River** ∽ Tasmania, SE Australia
11 U16 **Southey** Saskatchewan, S Canada
27 V2 **South Fabius River** ∽ Missouri, C USA
31 S10 **Southfield** Michigan, N USA
192 K10 **South Fiji Basin** *undersea feature* S Pacific Ocean
97 Q22 **South Foreland** *headland* SE England, UK
35 P7 **South Fork American River** ∽ California, W USA
28 K7 **South Fork Grand River** ∽ South Dakota, N USA
35 T12 **South Fork Kern River** ∽ California, W USA
39 Q7 **South Fork Koyukuk River** ∽ Alaska, USA
39 Q11 **South Fork Kuskokwim River** ∽ Alaska, USA
26 H2 **South Fork Republican River** ∽ C USA
26 L3 **South Fork Solomon River** ∽ Kansas, C USA
31 P5 **South Fox Island** *island* Michigan, N USA
20 G8 **South Fulton** Tennessee, S USA
195 U10 **South Geomagnetic Pole** *pole* Antarctica
65 J20 **South Georgia** *island* South Georgia and the South Sandwich Islands, SW Atlantic Ocean
65 K21 **South Georgia and the South Sandwich Islands** ◇ *UK dependent territory* SW Atlantic Ocean
47 Y14 **South Georgia Ridge** *var.* North Scotia Ridge. *undersea feature* SW Atlantic Ocean
181 Q1 **South Goulburn Island** *island* Northern Territory, N Australia
153 U16 **South Hatia Island** *island* SE Bangladesh
31 O10 **South Haven** Michigan, N USA
21 V7 **South Hill** Virginia, NE USA
South Holland *see* Zuid-Holland
21 P8 **South Holston Lake** ⊡ Tennessee/Virginia, S USA
175 N1 **South Honshu Ridge** *undersea feature* W Pacific Ocean
26 M6 **South Hutchinson** Kansas, C USA
151 K21 **South Huvadhu Atoll** *var.* Gaafu Dhaalu Atoll. *atoll* S Maldives
173 U14 **South Indian Basin** *undersea feature* Indian Ocean/Pacific Ocean
11 W11 **South Indian Lake** Manitoba, C Canada
81 I17 **South Island** *island* NW Kenya
185 C20 **South Island** *island* S NZ
65 B23 **South Jason** *island* Jason Islands, NW Falkland Islands
South Kalimantan *see* Kalimantan Selatan
South Kazakhstan *see* Yuzhnyy Kazakhstan
163 X15 **South Korea** *off.* Republic of Korea, *Kor.* Taehan Min'guk. ◆ *republic* E Asia
35 Q6 **South Lake Tahoe** California, W USA
25 N6 **Southland** Texas, SW USA
185 B23 **Southland** *off.* Southland Region. ♦ *region* South Island, NZ
29 N15 **South Loup River** ∽ Nebraska, C USA
151 K19 **South Maalhosmadulu Atoll** *var.* Baa Atoll. *atoll* N Maldives
14 E15 **South Maitland** ∽ Ontario, S Canada
192 E8 **South Makassar Basin** *undersea feature* E Java Sea
31 O6 **South Manitou Island** *island* Michigan, N USA
151 K18 **South Miladummadulu Atoll** *atoll* N Maldives
21 X8 **South Mills** North Carolina, SE USA
8 H9 **South Nahanni** ∽ Northwest Territories, NW Canada
39 P13 **South Naknek** Alaska, USA
14 M13 **South Nation** ∽ Ontario, SE Canada
44 F9 **South Negril Point** *headland* W Jamaica
151 K20 **South Nilandhe Atoll** *var.* Dhaalu Atoll. *atoll* C Maldives
36 L2 **South Ogden** Utah, W USA
18 M14 **Southold** Long Island, New York, NE USA
194 H1 **South Orkney Islands** *island group* Antarctica
137 S9 **South Ossetia** *former autonomous region* SW Georgia
South Pacific Basin *see* Southwest Pacific Basin
19 P7 **South Paris** Maine, NE USA
33 U15 **South Pass** *pass* Wyoming, C USA
189 U13 **South Pass** *passage* Chuuk Islands, C Micronesia
20 K10 **South Pittsburg** Tennessee, S USA
28 K15 **South Platte River** ∽ Colorado/Nebraska, C USA
31 T16 **South Point** Ohio, N USA
65 G15 **South Point** *headland* S Ascension Island
31 R6 **South Point** *headland* Michigan, N USA
South Point *see* Ka Lae
195 P9 **South Pole** *pole* Antarctica
183 P17 **Southport** Tasmania, SE Australia
97 K17 **Southport** NW England, UK
21 V12 **Southport** North Carolina, SE USA
19 P8 **South Portland** Maine, NE USA
14 H12 **South River** Ontario, S Canada
21 U11 **South River** ∽ North Carolina, SE USA
96 K5 **South Ronaldsay** *island* NE Scotland, UK
36 L2 **South Salt Lake** Utah, W USA
65 L21 **South Sandwich Islands** *island group* SE South Georgia and South Sandwich Islands
65 K21 **South Sandwich Trench** *undersea feature* SW Atlantic Ocean
11 S16 **South Saskatchewan** ∽ Alberta/Saskatchewan, S Canada
65 I21 **South Scotia Ridge** *undersea feature* S Scotia Sea
11 V10 **South Seal** ∽ Manitoba, C Canada
194 G4 **South Shetland Islands** *island group* Antarctica
65 H22 **South Shetland Trough** *undersea feature* Atlantic Ocean/Pacific Ocean
97 M14 **South Shields** NE England, UK
29 R13 **South Sioux City** Nebraska, C USA
192 J9 **South Solomon Trench** *undersea feature* W Pacific Ocean
183 V3 **South Stradbroke Island** *island* Queensland, E Australia
South Sulawesi *see* Sulawesi Selatan
South Sumatra *see* Sumatera Selatan
184 K11 **South Taranaki Bight** *bight* SE Tasman Sea
South Tasmania Plateau *see* Tasman Plateau
36 M15 **South Tucson** Arizona, SW USA
12 H9 **South Twin Island** *island* Nunavut, C Canada
96 E9 **South Uist** *island* NW Scotland, UK
South-West *see* Sud-Ouest
South-West Africa/South West Africa *see* Namibia
65 F15 **South West Bay** *bay* Ascension Island, C Atlantic Ocean
183 N18 **South West Cape** *headland* Tasmania, SE Australia
185 B26 **South West Cape** *headland* Stewart Island, NZ
38 J10 **Southwest Cape** *headland* Saint Lawrence Island, Alaska, USA
Southwest Indian Ocean Ridge *see* Southwest Indian Ridge
173 N11 **Southwest Indian Ridge** *var.* Southwest Indian Ocean Ridge. *undersea feature* SW Indian Ocean
192 L10 **Southwest Pacific Basin** *var.* South Pacific Basin. *undersea feature* SE Pacific Ocean
44 H2 **Southwest Point** *headland* Great Abaco, N Bahamas
191 X3 **South West Point** *headland* Kiritimati, NE Kiribati
65 G25 **South West Point** *headland* SW Saint Helena
25 P5 **South Wichita River** ∽ Texas, SW USA
97 Q20 **Southwold** E England, UK
19 Q12 **South Yarmouth** Massachusetts, NE USA
116 J10 **Sovata** *Hung.* Szováta. Mureș, C Romania
107 N22 **Soverato** Calabria, SW Italy
Sovetabad *see* Ghafurov
128 C2 **Sovetsk** *Ger.* Tilsit. Kaliningradskaya Oblast', W Russian Federation
127 Q15 **Sovetsk** Kirovskaya Oblast', NW Russian Federation
129 N10 **Sovetskaya** Rostovskaya Oblast', SW Russian Federation
Sovetskoye *see* Ketchenery
146 I15 **Sovet"yab** *prev.* Sovet"yap. Akhalskiy Velayat, S Turkmenistan
Sovet"yap *see* Sovet"yab
117 U12 **Sovyets'kyy** Respublika Krym, S Ukraine
83 I18 **Sowa** *var.* Sua. Central, NE Botswana
83 I18 **Sowa Pan** *salt lake* NE Botswana
83 J21 **Soweto** Gauteng, NE South Africa
Sōya-kaikyō *see* La Perouse Strait
165 T1 **Sōya-misaki** *headland* Hokkaidō, NE Japan
127 N7 **Soyana** ∽ NW Russian Federation
146 A8 **Soye, Mys** *var.* Mys Suz. *headland* NW Turkmenistan
82 A10 **Soyo** Zaire, NW Angola
80 J10 **Soyra** ▲ C Eritrea
Sozaq *see* Suzak
119 P16 **Sozh** *Rus.* Sozh. ∽ NE Europe
114 N10 **Sozopol** *prev.* Sizebolu *anc.* Apollonia. Burgas, E Bulgaria
172 J15 **Sœurs, Les** *island group* Inner Islands, W Seychelles
99 L20 **Spa** Liège, E Belgium
194 I7 **Spaatz Island** *island* Antarctica
144 M14 **Space Launching Centre** *space station* Kzylorda, S Kazakhstan
105 O7 **Spain** *off.* Kingdom of Spain, *Sp.* España; *anc.* Hispania, Iberia, *Lat.* Hispana. ◆ *monarchy* SW Europe
Spalato *see* Split
97 O19 **Spalding** E England, UK
14 D11 **Spanish** Ontario, S Canada
36 L3 **Spanish Fork** Utah, W USA
64 B12 **Spanish Point** *headland* C Bermuda
14 E9 **Spanish River** ∽ Ontario, S Canada
44 K13 **Spanish Town** *hist.* St.Iago de la Vega. C Jamaica
115 H24 **Spánta, Akrotírio** *headland* Kríti, Greece, E Mediterranean Sea
35 Q5 **Sparks** Nevada, W USA
Sparnacum *see* Épernay
95 N16 **Sparreholm** Södermanland, C Sweden
23 U4 **Sparta** Georgia, SE USA
30 K16 **Sparta** Illinois, N USA
31 P9 **Sparta** Michigan, N USA
21 R8 **Sparta** North Carolina, SE USA
20 L9 **Sparta** Tennessee, S USA
30 I7 **Sparta** Wisconsin, N USA
Sparta *see* Spárti
21 Q11 **Spartanburg** South Carolina, SE USA
115 F21 **Spárti** *Eng.* Sparta. Pelopónnisos, S Greece
107 B21 **Spartivento, Capo** *headland* Sardegna, Italy, C Mediterranean Sea
11 P17 **Sparwood** British Columbia, SW Canada
128 I4 **Spas-Demensk** Kaluzhskaya Oblast', W Russian Federation
128 M4 **Spas-Klepiki** Ryazanskaya Oblast', W Russian Federation
Spasovo *see* Kulen Vakuf
123 R15 **Spassk-Dal'niy** Primorskiy Kray, SE Russian Federation
128 M5 **Spassk-Ryazanskiy** Ryazanskaya Oblast', 111
N20 **Trebišov** *Hung.* Tőketerebes. Košický Kraj, E Slovakia
Trebitsch *see* Třebíč
Trebizond *see* Trabzon
ZaporizhzhyaŚląskie, S Poland
31 P9 **Sparta** Michigan, N USA
21 R8 **Sparta** North Carolina, SE USA
20 L9 **Sparta** Tennessee, S USA
30 I7 **Sparta** Wisconsin, N USA
Sparta *see* Spárti
21 Q11 **Spartanburg** South Carolina, SE USA
115 F21 **Spárti** *Eng.* Sparta. Pelopónnisos, S Greece
107 B21 **Spartivento, Capo** *headland* Sardegna, Italy, C Mediterranean Sea
11 P17 **Sparwood** British Columbia, SW Canada
128 I4 **Spas-Demensk** Kaluzhskaya Oblast', W Russian Federation
128 M4 **Spas-Klepiki** Ryazanskaya Oblast', W Russian Federation
Spasovo *see* Kulen Vakuf
123 R15 **Spassk-Dal'niy** Primorskiy Kray, SE Russian Federation
128 M5 **Spassk-Ryazanskiy** Ryazanskaya Oblast', W Russian Federation
115 H19 **Spáta** Attikí, C Greece
121 Q11 **Spátha, Akrotírio** *headland* Kríti, Greece, E Mediterranean Sea
Špatrjan *see* Paternion
28 I9 **Spearfish** South Dakota, N USA
25 O1 **Spearman** Texas, SW USA
65 C25 **Speedwell Island** *island* S Falkland Islands
65 C25 **Speedwell Island Settlement** S Falkland Islands
65 G25 **Speery Island** *island* S Saint Helena
45 N14 **Speightstown** NW Barbados
106 I13 **Spello** Umbria, C Italy
39 R12 **Spenard** Alaska, USA
Spence Bay *see* Taloyoak
31 O14 **Spencer** Indiana, N USA
29 T12 **Spencer** Iowa, C USA
29 P12 **Spencer** Nebraska, C USA
21 S9 **Spencer** North Carolina, SE USA
20 L9 **Spencer** Tennessee, S USA
21 Q4 **Spencer** West Virginia, NE USA
30 K6 **Spencer** Wisconsin, N USA
182 G10 **Spencer, Cape** *headland* South Australia
39 V13 **Spencer, Cape** *headland* Alaska, USA
182 H9 **Spencer Gulf** *gulf* South Australia
18 F9 **Spencerport** New York, NE USA
31 Q12 **Spencerville** Ohio, N USA
115 E17 **Spercheiáda** *var.* Sperhiada, Sperkhiás. Stereá Ellás, C Greece
115 E17 **Spercheiós** ∽ C Greece
Sperhiada *see* Spercheiáda
95 G14 **Sperillen** ◎ S Norway
Sperkhiás *see* Spercheiáda
101 I18 **Spessart** *hill range* C Germany
Spétsai *see* Spétses
115 G21 **Spétses** *prev.* Spétsai. Spétses, S Greece
115 G21 **Spétses** *island* S Greece
96 J8 **Spey** ∽ NE Scotland, UK
101 G20 **Speyer** *Eng.* Spires; *anc.* Civitas Nemetum, Spira. Rheinland-Pfalz, SW Germany
101 G20 **Speyerbach** ∽ W Germany
107 N20 **Spezzano Albanese** Calabria, SW Italy
Spice Islands *see* Maluku
100 F9 **Spiekeroog** *island* NW Germany
109 W9 **Spielfeld** Steiermark, SE Austria
65 N21 **Spiess Seamount** *undersea feature* S Atlantic Ocean
108 E9 **Spiez** Bern, W Switzerland
98 G13 **Spijkenisse** Zuid-Holland, SW Netherlands
39 T6 **Spike Mountain** ▲ Alaska, USA
115 J25 **Spíli** Kríti, Greece, E Mediterranean Sea
108 D10 **Spillgerten** ▲ W Switzerland
118 F9 **Spilva** ✕ (Rīga) Rīga, C Latvia
107 N17 **Spinazzola** Puglia, SE Italy
149 O9 **Spīn Būldak** Kandahār, S Afghanistan
Spira *see* Speyer
Spirdingsee *see* Śniardwy, Jezioro
Spires *see* Speyer
29 T11 **Spirit Lake** Iowa, C USA
29 T11 **Spirit Lake** ◎ Iowa, C USA
11 N13 **Spirit River** Alberta, W Canada

11 S14 **Spiritwood** Saskatchewan, S Canada
27 R11 **Spiro** Oklahoma, C USA
111 L19 **Spišská Nová Ves** *Ger.* Neudorf, Zipser Neudorf, *Hung.* Igló. Košický Kraj, E Slovakia
137 T11 **Spitak** NW Armenia
92 O2 **Spitsbergen** *island* NW Svalbard
Spittal *see* Spittal an der Drau
109 R9 **Spittal an der Drau** *var.* Spittal. Kärnten, S Austria
109 V3 **Spitz** Niederösterreich, NE Austria
94 D9 **Spjelkavik** Møre og Romsdal, S Norway
25 W10 **Splendora** Texas, SW USA
113 E14 **Split** *It.* Spalato. Split-Dalmacija, S Croatia
113 E14 **Split** ✕ Split-Dalmacija, S Croatia
113 E14 **Split-Dalmacija** *off.* Splitsko-Dalmatinska Županija. ◈ *province* S Croatia
11 X12 **Split Lake** ◎ Manitoba, C Canada
Splitsko-Dalmatinska Županija *see* Split-Dalmacija
108 H10 **Splügen** Graubünden, S Switzerland
Spodnji Dravograd *see* Dravograd
25 P12 **Spofford** Texas, SW USA
118 J11 **Špoģi** Daugvapils, SE Latvia
32 L8 **Spokane** Washington, NW USA
32 L8 **Spokane River** ≈ Washington, NW USA
106 I13 **Spoleto** Umbria, C Italy
30 I4 **Spooner** Wisconsin, N USA
30 K12 **Spoon River** ≈ Illinois, N USA
21 W5 **Spotsylvania** Virginia, NE USA
32 L8 **Sprague** Washington, NW USA
170 J5 **Spratly Island** *island* SW Spratly Islands
192 E6 **Spratly Islands** *Chin.* Nansha Qundao. ◇ *disputed territory* SE Asia
32 J12 **Spray** Oregon, NW USA
112 I11 **Spreča** ≈ N Bosnia and Herzegovina
100 P13 **Spree** ≈ E Germany
100 P13 **Spreewald** *wetland* NE Germany
101 P14 **Spremberg** Brandenburg, E Germany
25 W11 **Spring** Texas, SW USA
31 Q10 **Spring Arbor** Michigan, N USA
83 E23 **Springbok** Northern Cape, W South Africa
18 I15 **Spring City** Pennsylvania, NE USA
20 L9 **Spring City** Tennessee, S USA
36 L4 **Spring City** Utah, W USA
35 W3 **Spring Creek** Nevada, W USA
27 S9 **Springdale** Arkansas, C USA
31 Q14 **Springdale** Ohio, N USA
100 I13 **Springe** Niedersachsen, N Germany
37 U9 **Springer** New Mexico, SW USA
37 W7 **Springfield** Colorado, C USA
23 W5 **Springfield** Georgia, SE USA
30 K14 **Springfield** *state capital* Illinois, N USA
20 L6 **Springfield** Kentucky, S USA
18 M12 **Springfield** Massachusetts, NE USA
29 T10 **Springfield** Minnesota, N USA
27 T7 **Springfield** Missouri, C USA
31 R13 **Springfield** Ohio, N USA
32 G13 **Springfield** Oregon, NW USA
29 Q12 **Springfield** South Dakota, N USA
20 J8 **Springfield** Tennessee, S USA
18 M9 **Springfield** Vermont, NE USA
30 K14 **Springfield, Lake** ⊟ Illinois, N USA
55 T8 **Spring Garden** NE Guyana
30 K8 **Spring Green** Wisconsin, N USA
29 X11 **Spring Grove** Minnesota, N USA
22 G4 **Springhill** Louisiana, S USA
23 V12 **Spring Hill** Florida, SE USA
27 R4 **Spring Hill** Kansas, C USA
13 P15 **Springhill** Nova Scotia, SE Canada
20 I9 **Spring Hill** Tennessee, S USA
21 U10 **Spring Lake** North Carolina, SE USA
24 M4 **Springlake** Texas, SW USA
35 W11 **Spring Mountains** ▲▲ Nevada, W USA
65 B24 **Spring Point** West Falkland, Falkland Islands
27 W9 **Spring River** ≈ Arkansas/Missouri, C USA
27 S7 **Spring River** ≈ Missouri/Oklahoma, C USA
83 J21 **Springs** Gauteng, NE South Africa
185 H16 **Springs Junction** West Coast, South Island, NZ
181 X8 **Springsure** Queensland, E Australia
29 W11 **Spring Valley** Minnesota, N USA
18 K13 **Spring Valley** New York, NE USA
29 N12 **Springview** Nebraska, C USA
18 D11 **Springville** New York, NE USA
36 L3 **Springville** Utah, W USA
Sprottau *see* Szprotawa
15 V4 **Sproule, Pointe** *headland* Quebec, SE Canada
11 Q14 **Spruce Grove** Alberta, SW Canada
21 T4 **Spruce Knob** ▲ West Virginia, NE USA
35 X3 **Spruce Mountain** ▲ Nevada, W USA
21 P9 **Spruce Pine** North Carolina, SE USA
98 G13 **Spui** ≈ SW Netherlands
107 O19 **Spulico, Capo** *headland* S Italy
25 O5 **Spur** Texas, SW USA
97 O17 **Spurn Head** *headland* E England, UK
99 H20 **Spy** Namur, S Belgium
95 I15 **Spydeberg** Østfold, S Norway
185 J17 **Spy Glass Point** *headland* South Island, NZ
10 L17 **Squamish** British Columbia, SW Canada
19 O8 **Squam Lake** ◎ New Hampshire, NE USA
19 S2 **Squa Pan Mountain** ▲ Maine, NE USA
39 N16 **Squaw Harbor** Unga Island, Alaska, USA
14 E11 **Squaw Island** *island* Ontario, S Canada
107 O22 **Squillace, Golfo di** *gulf* S Italy
107 Q18 **Squinzano** Puglia, SE Italy
Sráid na Cathrach *see* Milltown Malbay
167 S11 **Srâlau** Stœng Trêng, N Cambodia
Srath an Urláir *see* Stranorlar
112 G10 **Srbac** Republika Srpska, N Bosnia & Herzegovina
Srbinje *see* Foča
Srbija *see* Serbia
Srbobran *see* Donji Vakuf
112 K9 **Srbobran** *var.* Bácsszenttamás, *Hung.* Szenttamás. Serbia, N Yugoslavia
167 R13 **Srê Âmběl** Kaôh Kông, SW Cambodia
112 K13 **Srebrenica** Republika Srpska, E Bosnia & Herzegovina
112 I11 **Srebrenik** Federacija Bosna I Hercegovina, E Bosnia & Herzegovina
114 M10 **Sredets** *prev.* Grudovo. Burgas, E Bulgaria
114 K10 **Sredets** *prev.* Syulemeshlii. Stara Zagora, C Bulgaria
114 M10 **Sredetska Reka** ≈ SE Bulgaria
123 U9 **Sredinnyy Khrebet** ▲▲ E Russian Federation
114 N7 **Sredishte** *Rom.* Beibunar; *prev.* Knyazhevo. Dobrich, NE Bulgaria
114 I10 **Sredna Gora** ▲▲ C Bulgaria
123 R7 **Srednekolymsk** Respublika Sakha (Yakutiya), NE Russian Federation
128 K7 **Srednerusskaya Vozvyshennost'** *Eng.* Central Russian Upland. ▲▲ W Russian Federation
122 L9 **Srednesibirskoye Ploskogor'ye** *var.* Central Siberian Uplands, *Eng.* Central Siberian Plateau. ▲▲ N Russian Federation
127 V13 **Sredniy Ural** ▲▲ NW Russian Federation
167 T12 **Srê Khtŭm** Môndól Kiri, E Cambodia
111 G12 **Śrem** Wielkolpolskie, C Poland
112 K10 **Sremska Mitrovica** *prev.* Mitrovica, *Ger.* Mitrowitz. Serbia, NW Yugoslavia
167 R11 **Srêng, Stœng** ≈ NW Cambodia
167 R11 **Srê Noy** Siĕmréab, NW Cambodia
Srepok, Sông *see* Srêpôk, Tônle
167 T12 **Srêpôk, Tônle** *var.* Sông Srepok. ≈ Cambodia/Vietnam
123 P13 **Sretensk** Chitinskaya Oblast', S Russian Federation
169 R10 **Sri Aman** Sarawak, East Malaysia
117 R4 **Sribne** Chernihivs'ka Oblast', N Ukraine
155 I25 **Sri Jayawardanapura** *var.* Sri Jayawardenepura; *prev.* Kotte. Western Province, W Sri Lanka
155 M14 **Srīkākulam** Andhra Pradesh, E India
155 I25 **Sri Lanka** *off.* Democratic Socialist Republic of Sri Lanka; *prev.* Ceylon. ◆ *republic* S Asia
130 F14 **Sri Lanka** *island* S Asia
153 V14 **Srimangal** Chittagong, E Bangladesh
Sri Mohangorh *see* Shri Mohangarh
152 H5 **Srīnagar** Jammu and Kashmir, N India
167 N10 **Srinagarind Reservoir** ◎ W Thailand
155 F19 **Sringeri** Karnātaka, W India
155 K25 **Sri Pada** *Eng.* Adam's Peak. ▲ S Sri Lanka
Sri Saket *see* Si Sa Ket
111 G14 **Środa Śląska** *Ger.* Neumarkt. Dolnośląskie, SW Poland
110 H12 **Środa Wielkopolska** Wielkolpolskie, C Poland
Srpska Kostajnica *see* Bosanska Kostajnica
113 G14 **Srpska, Republika** ◈ *republic* Bosnia & Herzegovina
Srpski Brod *see* Bosanski Brod
Ssu-ch'uan *see* Sichuan
Ssu-p'ing/Ssu-p'ing-chieh *see* Siping
Stablo *see* Stavelot
99 G15 **Stabroek** Antwerpen, N Belgium
Stackeln *see* Strenči
96 I5 **Stack Skerry** *island* N Scotland, UK
94 C10 **Stad** *peninsula* S Norway
100 I9 **Stade** Niedersachsen, N Germany
109 R5 **Stadl-Paura** Oberösterreich, NW Austria
119 L20 **Stadolichy** *Rus.* Stodolichi. Homyel'skaya Voblasts', SE Belarus
98 P7 **Stadskanaal** Groningen, NE Netherlands
101 H16 **Stadtallendorf** Hessen, C Germany
101 K23 **Stadtbergen** Bayern, S Germany
108 G7 **Stäfa** Zürich, NE Switzerland
95 K23 **Staffanstorp** Skåne, S Sweden
101 K18 **Staffelstein** Bayern, C Germany
97 L19 **Stafford** C England, UK
26 L6 **Stafford** Kansas, C USA
21 W4 **Stafford** Virginia, NE USA
97 L19 **Staffordshire** *cultural region* C England, UK
19 N12 **Stafford Springs** Connecticut, NE USA
115 H14 **Stágira** Kentrikí Makedonía, N Greece
118 G7 **Staicele** Limbaži, N Latvia
Ştaierdorf-Anina *see* Anina
109 V8 **Stainz** Steiermark, SE Austria
Stájerlakanina *see* Anina
117 Y7 **Stakhanov** Luhans'ka Oblast', E Ukraine
108 E11 **Stalden** Valais, SW Switzerland
Stalin *see* Varna
Stalinabad *see* Dushanbe
Stalingrad *see* Volgograd
Staliniri *see* Ts'khinvali
Stalino *see* Donets'k
Stalinobod *see* Dushanbe
Stalinov Štít *see* Gerlachovský štít
Stalinsk *see* Novokuznetsk
Stalinskaya Oblast' *see* Donets'ka Oblast'
Stalinski Zaliv *see* Varnenski Zaliv
Stalin, Yazovir *see* Iskŭr, Yazovir
8 K2 **Stallworthy, Cape** *headland* Nunavut, N Canada
111 N15 **Stalowa Wola** Podkarpackie, SE Poland
114 I11 **Stamboliyski** Plovdiv, C Bulgaria
114 J8 **Stamboliyski, Yazovir** ⊟ N Bulgaria
97 N19 **Stamford** E England, UK
18 L14 **Stamford** Connecticut, NE USA
25 P6 **Stamford** Texas, SW USA
25 Q6 **Stamford, Lake** ⊟ Texas, SW USA
108 I10 **Stampa** Graubünden, SE Switzerland
Stampalia *see* Astypálaia
27 T14 **Stamps** Arkansas, C USA
92 G11 **Stamsund** Nordland, C Norway
27 R2 **Stanberry** Missouri, C USA
195 O3 **Stancomb-Wills Glacier** *glacier* Antarctica
83 K21 **Standerton** Mpumalanga, E South Africa
31 R7 **Standish** Michigan, N USA
20 M6 **Stanford** Kentucky, S USA
33 S9 **Stanford** Montana, NW USA
95 P19 **Stånga** Gotland, SE Sweden
94 I13 **Stange** Hedmark, S Norway
83 L23 **Stanger** KwaZulu/Natal, E South Africa
Stanimaka *see* Asenovgrad
Stanislau *see* Ivano-Frankivs'k
35 P8 **Stanislaus River** ≈ California, W USA
Stanislav *see* Ivano-Frankivs'k
Stanislavskaya Oblast' *see* Ivano-Frankivs'ka Oblast'
Stanisławów *see* Ivano-Frankivs'k
Stanke Dimitrov *see* Dupnitsa
183 O15 **Stanley** Tasmania, SE Australia
65 E24 **Stanley** *var.* Port Stanley, Puerto Argentino ○ (Falkland Islands) East Falkland, Falkland Islands
33 O13 **Stanley** Idaho, NW USA
28 L3 **Stanley** North Dakota, N USA
21 U4 **Stanley** Virginia, NE USA
30 J6 **Stanley** Wisconsin, N USA
79 G21 **Stanley Pool** *var.* Pool Malebo. ◎ Congo/Dem. Rep. Congo (Zaire)
155 H20 **Stanley Reservoir** ⊟ S India
Stanleyville *see* Kisangani
42 G3 **Stann Creek** ◈ *district* SE Belize
Stann Creek *see* Dangriga
123 Q12 **Stanovoy Khrebet** ▲▲ SE Russian Federation
108 F8 **Stans** Unterwalden, C Switzerland
97 O21 **Stansted** ✕ (London) Essex, E England, UK
183 U4 **Stanthorpe** Queensland, E Australia
21 N6 **Stanton** Kentucky, S USA
31 Q8 **Stanton** Michigan, N USA
29 Q14 **Stanton** Nebraska, C USA
28 L5 **Stanton** North Dakota, N USA
25 N7 **Stanton** Texas, SW USA
32 H7 **Stanwood** Washington, NW USA
117 Y7 **Stanychno-Luhans'ke** Luhans'ka Oblast', E Ukraine
108 K7 **Stanzach** Tirol, W Austria
98 M9 **Staphorst** Overijssel, E Netherlands
14 D18 **Staples** Ontario, S Canada
29 T6 **Staples** Minnesota, N USA
28 M14 **Stapleton** Nebraska, C USA
25 S8 **Star** Texas, SW USA
111 M18 **Starachowice** Świętokrzyskie, C Poland
Stara Kanjiža *see* Kanjiža
111 M18 **Stará Ľubovňa** *Ger.* Altlublau, *Hung.* Prešovský Kraj, E Slovakia
112 L10 **Stara Pazova** *Ger.* Altpasua, *Hung.* Ópazova. Serbia, N Yugoslavia
Stara Planina *see* Balkan Mountains
114 L9 **Stara Reka** ≈ C Bulgaria
116 M5 **Stara Synyava** Khmel'nyts'ka Oblast', W Ukraine
116 I2 **Stara Vyzhivka** Volyns'ka Oblast', NW Ukraine
Staraya Belitsa *see* Staraya Byelitsa
119 M14 **Staraya Byelitsa** *Rus.* Staraya Belitsa. Vitsyebskaya Voblasts', NE Belarus
129 R5 **Staraya Mayna** Ul'yanovskaya Oblast', W Russian Federation
119 O18 **Staraya Rudnya** *Rus.* Staraya Rudnya. Homyel'skaya Voblasts', SE Belarus
126 H14 **Staraya Russa** Novgorodskaya Oblast', W Russian Federation
114 K10 **Stara Zagora** *Lat.* Augusta Trajana. Stara Zagora, C Bulgaria
116 K10 **Stara Zagora** ◈ *province* C Bulgaria
29 S8 **Starbuck** Minnesota, N USA
191 W4 **Starbuck Island** *prev.* Volunteer Island. *island* E Kiribati
27 V13 **Star City** Arkansas, C USA
112 F13 **Staretina** ▲▲ W Bosnia and Herzegovina
Stargard in Pommern *see* Stargard Szczeciński
110 E9 **Stargard Szczeciński** *Ger.* Stargard in Pommern. Zachodniopomorskie, NW Poland
187 N10 **Star Harbour** *harbor* San Cristobal, SE Solomon Islands
Stari Bečej *see* Bečej
113 F15 **Stari Grad** *It.* Cittavecchia. Split-Dalmacija, S Croatia
126 J16 **Staritsa** Tverskaya Oblast', W Russian Federation
23 V9 **Starke** Florida, SE USA
22 M4 **Starkville** Mississippi, S USA
186 B7 **Star Mountains** *Ind.* Pegunungan Sterren. ▲▲ Indonesia/PNG
101 L23 **Starnberg** Bayern, SE Germany
101 L24 **Starnberger See** ◎ SE Germany
Starobel'sk *see* Starobil's'k
117 X8 **Starobesheve** Donets'ka Oblast', E Ukraine
117 Y6 **Starobil's'k** *Rus.* Starobel'sk. Luhans'ka Oblast', E Ukraine
Starobin *see* Starobyn
119 K18 **Starobyn** *Rus.* Starobin. Minskaya Voblasts', S Belarus
128 H6 **Starodub** Bryanskaya Oblast', W Russian Federation
110 I8 **Starogard Gdański** *Ger.* Preussisch-Stargard. Pomorskie, N Poland
145 P16 **Staroikan** Yuzhnyy Kazakhstan, S Kazakhstan
Starokonstantinov *see* Starokostyantyniv
116 L5 **Starokostyantyniv** *Rus.* Starokonstantinov. Khmel'nyts'ka Oblast', NW Ukraine
128 K12 **Starominskaya** Krasnodarskiy Kray, SW Russian Federation
114 L7 **Staro Selo** *Rom.* Satul-Vechi; *prev.* Star-Smil. Silistra, NE Bulgaria
128 K12 **Staroshcherbinovskaya** Krasnodarskiy Kray, SW Russian Federation
129 V6 **Starosubkhangulovo** Respublika Bashkortostan, W Russian Federation
35 S4 **Star Peak** ▲ Nevada, W USA
Star-Smil *see* Staro Selo
97 J25 **Start Point** *headland* SW England, UK
Startsy *see* Kirawsk
Starum *see* Stavoren
119 L18 **Staryya Darohi** *Rus.* Staryye Dorogi. Minskaya Voblasts', S Belarus
Staryye Dorogi *see* Staryya Darohi
129 T2 **Staryye Zyatsy** Udmurtskaya Respublika, NW Russian Federation
117 U13 **Staryy Krym** Respublika Krym, S Ukraine
128 K8 **Staryy Oskol** Belgorodskaya Oblast', W Russian Federation
116 H6 **Staryy Sambir** L'vivs'ka Oblast', W Ukraine
101 L14 **Stassfurt** *var.* Staßfurt. Sachsen-Anhalt, C Germany
111 M15 **Staszów** Świętokrzyskie, C Poland
29 W13 **State Center** Iowa, C USA
18 E14 **State College** Pennsylvania, NE USA
18 K15 **Staten Island** *island* New York, NE USA
Staten Island *see* Estados, Isla de los
23 U8 **Statenville** Georgia, SE USA
23 W5 **Statesboro** Georgia, SE USA
States, The *see* United States of America
21 R9 **Statesville** North Carolina, SE USA
95 G16 **Stathelle** Telemark, S Norway
30 K15 **Staunton** Illinois, N USA
21 T5 **Staunton** Virginia, NE USA
95 C16 **Stavanger** Rogaland, S Norway
99 L21 **Stavelot** *Dut.* Stablo. Liège, E Belgium
95 G16 **Stavern** Vestfold, S Norway
Stavers Island *see* Vostok Island
98 J7 **Stavoren** *Fris.* Starum. Friesland, N Netherlands
128 M14 **Stavropol'** *prev.* Voroshilovsk. Stavropol'skiy Kray, SW Russian Federation
Stavropol' *see* Tol'yatti
128 M14 **Stavropol'skaya Vozvyshennost'** ▲▲ SW Russian Federation
128 M14 **Stavropol'skiy Kray** ◈ *territory* SW Russian Federation
115 H14 **Stavrós** Kentrikí Makedonía, N Greece
115 J24 **Stavrós, Akrotírio** *headland* Kríti, Greece, E Mediterranean Sea
115 K21 **Stavrós, Akrotírio** *headland* Náxos, Kykládes, Greece, Aegean Sea
114 I12 **Stavroúpoli** *prev.* Stavroúpolis. Anatolikí Makedonía kai Thráki, NE Greece
Stavroúpolis *see* Stavroúpoli
117 O6 **Stavyshche** Kyyivs'ka Oblast', N Ukraine
182 M11 **Stawell** Victoria, SE Australia
110 N9 **Stawiski** Podlaskie, NE Poland
14 G14 **Stayner** Ontario, S Canada
37 R3 **Steamboat Springs** Colorado, C USA
20 M8 **Stearns** Kentucky, S USA
39 N10 **Stebbins** Alaska, USA
108 K7 **Steeg** Tirol, W Austria
27 Y9 **Steele** Missouri, C USA
29 N5 **Steele** North Dakota, N USA
194 J5 **Steele Island** *island* Antarctica
30 K16 **Steeleville** Illinois, N USA
27 W6 **Steelville** Missouri, C USA
99 G14 **Steenbergen** Noord-Brabant, S Netherlands
Steenkool *see* Bintuni
11 O10 **Steen River** Alberta, W Canada
98 M8 **Steenwijk** Overijssel, N Netherlands
65 A23 **Steeple Jason** *island* Jason Islands, NW Falkland Islands
174 J8 **Steep Point** *headland* Western Australia
116 L9 **Ştefăneşti** Botoşani, NE Romania
Stefanie, Lake *see* Ch'ew Bahir
8 L5 **Stefansson Island** *island* Nunavut, N Canada
117 O10 **Ştefan Vodă** *Rus.* Suvorovo. SE Moldova
63 H18 **Steffen, Cerro** ▲ S Chile
108 D9 **Steffisburg** Bern, C Switzerland
95 J24 **Stege** Storstrøm, SE Denmark
116 G10 **Ştei** *Hung.* Vaskohsziklás. Bihor, W Romania
Steier *see* Steyr
Steierdorf/Steierdorf-Anina *see* Anina
109 T7 **Steiermark** *off.* Land Steiermark, *Eng.* Styria. ◈ *state* C Austria
101 J19 **Steigerwald** *hill range* C Germany
99 L17 **Stein** Limburg, SE Netherlands
Stein *see* Stein an der Donau, Austria
Stein *see* Kamnik, Slovenia
108 M8 **Steinach** Tirol, W Austria
Steinamanger *see* Szombathely
109 W3 **Stein an der Donau** *var.* Stein. Niederösterreich, NE Austria
Steinau an der Elbe *see* Ścinawa
11 Y16 **Steinbach** Manitoba, S Canada
Steiner Alpen *see* Kamniško-Savinjske Alpe
99 L24 **Steinfort** Luxembourg, W Luxembourg
100 H12 **Steinhuder Meer** ◎ NW Germany
93 E15 **Steinkjer** Nord-Trøndelag, C Norway
Stejarul *see* Karapelit
99 F16 **Stekene** Oost-Vlaanderen, NW Belgium
83 E26 **Stellenbosch** Western Cape, SW South Africa
98 F13 **Stellendam** Zuid-Holland, SW Netherlands
39 T12 **Steller, Mount** ▲ Alaska, USA
103 Y14 **Stello, Monte** ▲ Corse, France, C Mediterranean Sea
106 F5 **Stelvio, Passo dello** *pass* Italy/Switzerland
103 R3 **Stenay** Meuse, NE France
100 L12 **Stendal** Sachsen-Anhalt, C Germany
118 E8 **Stende** Talsi, NW Latvia
182 H10 **Stenhouse Bay** South Australia
95 J23 **Stenløse** Frederiksborg, E Denmark
95 L19 **Stensjön** Jönköping, S Sweden
95 K18 **Stenstorp** Västra Götaland, S Sweden
95 I18 **Stenungsund** Västra Götaland, S Sweden
Stepanakert *see* Xankändi
137 T11 **Step'anavan** N Armenia
100 K9 **Stepenitz** ≈ N Germany
29 O10 **Stephan** South Dakota, N USA
29 R3 **Stephen** Minnesota, N USA
27 T14 **Stephens** Arkansas, C USA
184 J13 **Stephens, Cape** *headland* D'Urville Island, Marlborough, SW NZ
21 V3 **Stephens City** Virginia, NE USA
182 L6 **Stephens Creek** New South Wales, SE Australia
184 K13 **Stephens Island** *island* C NZ
31 N5 **Stephenson** Michigan, N USA
13 S12 **Stephenville** Newfoundland, SE Canada
25 S7 **Stephenville** Texas, SW USA
145 P17 **Step' Nardara** *Kaz.* Shardara Dalasy; *prev.* Shaidara. *grassland* S Kazakhstan
145 R8 **Stepnogorsk** Akmola, C Kazakhstan
129 O15 **Stepnoye** Stavropol'skiy Kray, SW Russian Federation
145 Q8 **Stepnyak** Severnyy Kazakhstan, N Kazakhstan
192 J17 **Steps Point** *headland* Tutuila, W American Samoa
115 F17 **Stereá Ellás** *Eng.* Greece Central. ◈ *region* C Greece
83 J24 **Sterkspruit** Eastern Cape, SE South Africa
129 U6 **Sterlibashevo** Respublika Bashkortostan, W Russian Federation
39 R12 **Sterling** Alaska, USA
37 V3 **Sterling** Colorado, C USA
30 K11 **Sterling** Illinois, N USA
26 M5 **Sterling** Kansas, C USA
25 O8 **Sterling City** Texas, SW USA
31 S9 **Sterling Heights** Michigan, N USA
21 W3 **Sterling Park** Virginia, NE USA
37 V2 **Sterling Reservoir** ⊟ Colorado, C USA
22 I5 **Sterlington** Louisiana, S USA
129 U6 **Sterlitamak** Respublika Bashkortostan, W Russian Federation
Sternberg *see* Šternberk
111 H17 **Šternberk** *Ger.* Sternberg. Olomoucký Kraj, E Czech Republic
141 V17 **Sterōh** Suquţrā, S Yemen
110 G11 **Stęszew** Wielkolpolskie, C Poland
Stettin *see* Szczecin
Stettiner Haff *see* Szczeciński, Zalew
11 Q15 **Stettler** Alberta, SW Canada
31 V13 **Steubenville** Ohio, N USA
97 O21 **Stevenage** E England, UK
23 Q1 **Stevenson** Alabama, S USA
32 H11 **Stevenson** Washington, NW USA
182 E1 **Stevenson Creek** *seasonal river* South Australia
39 Q13 **Stevenson Entrance** *strait* Alaska, USA
30 L6 **Stevens Point** Wisconsin, N USA
39 R8 **Stevens Village** Alaska, USA
33 P10 **Stevensville** Montana, NW USA
93 E25 **Stevns Klint** *headland* E Denmark
10 J12 **Stewart** British Columbia, W Canada
10 J6 **Stewart** ≈ Yukon Territory, NW Canada
10 I6 **Stewart Crossing** Yukon Territory, NW Canada
63 H25 **Stewart, Isla** *island* S Chile
185 B25 **Stewart Island** *island* S NZ
181 W6 **Stewart, Mount** ▲ Queensland, E Australia
10 H6 **Stewart River** Yukon Territory, NW Canada
27 R3 **Stewartsville** Missouri, C USA
11 S16 **Stewart Valley** Saskatchewan, S Canada
29 W10 **Stewartville** Minnesota, N USA
Steyerlak-Anina *see* Anina
109 T5 **Steyr** *var.* Steier. Oberösterreich, N Austria
109 T5 **Steyr** ≈ NW Austria
29 P11 **Stickney** South Dakota, N USA
98 L5 **Stiens** Friesland, N Netherlands
Stif *see* Sétif
27 Q11 **Stigler** Oklahoma, C USA
107 N18 **Stigliano** Basilicata, S Italy
95 N17 **Stigtomta** Södermanland, C Sweden
10 I11 **Stikine** ≈ British Columbia, W Canada
Stilida/Stilís *see* Stylída
95 G22 **Stilling** Århus, C Denmark
29 W8 **Stillwater** Minnesota, N USA
27 O9 **Stillwater** Oklahoma, C USA
35 S5 **Stillwater Range** ▲▲ Nevada, W USA
18 I8 **Stillwater Reservoir** ⊟ New York, NE USA
107 O22 **Stilo, Punta** *headland* S Italy
27 R10 **Stilwell** Oklahoma, C USA
113 N17 **Štimlje** Serbia, S Yugoslavia
25 N1 **Stinnett** Texas, SW USA
113 P18 **Štip** E FYR Macedonia
Stira *see* Stýra
96 J12 **Stirling** C Scotland, UK
96 I12 **Stirling** *cultural region* C Scotland, UK
180 J14 **Stirling Range** ▲▲ Western Australia
93 E16 **Stjørdal** Nord-Trøndelag, C Norway
Stochód *see* Stokhid
101 H24 **Stockach** Baden-Württemberg, S Germany
25 S12 **Stockdale** Texas, SW USA
109 X3 **Stockerau** Niederösterreich, NE Austria
93 H20 **Stockholm** ● (Sweden) Stockholm, C Sweden
95 O15 **Stockholm** ◈ *county* C Sweden
Stockmannshof *see* Pļaviņas
97 L18 **Stockport** NW England, UK
65 K15 **Stocks Seamount** *undersea feature* C Atlantic Ocean
35 O8 **Stockton** California, W USA
26 L3 **Stockton** Kansas, C USA
27 S6 **Stockton** Missouri, C USA
30 K3 **Stockton Island** *island* Apostle Islands, Wisconsin, N USA
27 S7 **Stockton Lake** ⊟ Missouri, C USA
97 M15 **Stockton-on-Tees** *var.* Stockton on Tees. N England, UK
24 M10 **Stockton Plateau** *plain* Texas, SW USA
28 M16 **Stockville** Nebraska, C USA
93 H17 **Stöde** Västernorrland, C Sweden
Stodolichi *see* Stadolichy
167 S11 **Stœng Trêng** *prev.* Stung Treng. Stœng Trêng, NE Cambodia
113 M19 **Stogovo Karaorman** ▲ W FYR Macedonia
Stoke *see* Stoke-on-Trent
97 L19 **Stoke-on-Trent** *var.* Stoke. C England, UK
182 M15 **Stokes Point** *headland* Tasmania, SE Australia
116 J2 **Stokhid** *Pol.* Stochód, *Rus.* Stokhod. ≈ NW Ukraine
Stokhod *see* Stokhid
92 I4 **Stokkseyri** Sudhurland, SW Iceland
92 G10 **Stokmarknes** Nordland, C Norway
Stol *see* Veliki Krš
113 H15 **Stolac** Federacija Bosna I Hercegovina, S Bosnia and Herzegovina
Stolbce *see* Stowbtsy
101 D16 **Stolberg** *var.* Stolberg im Rheinland. Nordrhein-Westfalen, W Germany
Stolberg im Rheinland *see* Stolberg
123 P6 **Stolbovoy, Ostrov** *island* NE Russian Federation
Stolbtsy *see* Stowbtsy
119 J20 **Stolin** *Rus.* Stolin. Brestskaya Voblasts', SW Belarus
95 K14 **Stöllet** *var.* Norra Ny. Värmland, C Sweden
Stolp *see* Słupsk
Stolpe *see* Słupia
Stolpmünde *see* Ustka
115 F15 **Stómio** Thessalía, C Greece
14 J11 **Stonecliffe** Ontario, SE Canada
96 L10 **Stonehaven** NE Scotland, UK
97 M23 **Stonehenge** *ancient monument* Wiltshire, S England, UK

◆ Country ● Country Capital ◇ Dependent Territory ○ Dependent Territory Capital ◈ Administrative Region ✕ International Airport ▲ Mountain ▲▲ Mountain Range ⛰ Volcano ≈ River ◎ Lake ⊟ Reservoir

23 T3 **Stone Mountain** ▲ Georgia, SE USA
11 X16 **Stonewall** Manitoba, S Canada
21 S3 **Stonewood** West Virginia, NE USA
14 D17 **Stoney Point** Ontario, S Canada
92 H10 **Stonglandseidet** Troms, N Norway
65 N25 **Stonybeach Bay** bay Tristan da Cunha, SE Atlantic Ocean
35 N5 **Stony Creek** ≈ California, W USA
65 N25 **Stonyhill Point** headland S Tristan da Cunha
14 I14 **Stony Lake** ◎ Ontario, SE Canada
11 Q14 **Stony Plain** Alberta, SW Canada
21 R9 **Stony Point** North Carolina, SE USA
18 G8 **Stony Point** headland New York, NE USA
11 T10 **Stony Rapids** Saskatchewan, C Canada
39 P11 **Stony River** Alaska, USA
Stony Tunguska see Podkamennaya Tunguska
12 G10 **Stooping** ≈ Ontario, C Canada
100 I9 **Stör** ≈ N Germany
95 M15 **Storå** Örebro, S Sweden
95 J16 **Stora Gla** ◎ C Sweden
95 I16 **Stora Le** Nor. Store Le. ◎ Norway/Sweden
92 I12 **Stora Lulevatten** ◎ N Sweden
92 H13 **Storavan** ◎ N Sweden
93 I20 **Storby** Åland, SW Finland
94 E10 **Stordalen** Møre og Romsdal, S Norway
Storebelt see Storebælt
95 H23 **Storebælt** var. Store Bælt, Eng. Great Belt, Storebelt. channel Baltic Sea/Kattegat
95 M19 **Storebro** Kalmar, S Sweden
95 J24 **Store Heddinge** Storstrøm, SE Denmark
Store Le see Stora Le
93 E16 **Støren** Sør-Trøndelag, S Norway
95 B14 **Store Sotra** island S Norway
92 O4 **Storfjorden** fjord S Norway
95 L15 **Storfors** Värmland, C Sweden
92 G13 **Storforshei** Nordland, C Norway
Storhammer see Hamar
100 L10 **Störkanal** canal N Germany
93 F16 **Storlien** Jämtland, C Sweden
183 P17 **Storm Bay** inlet Tasmania, SE Australia
29 T12 **Storm Lake** Iowa, C USA
29 S13 **Storm Lake** ◎ Iowa, C USA
96 G7 **Stornoway** NW Scotland, UK
Storojineț see Storozhynets'
92 P1 **Storøya** island NE Svalbard
127 S10 **Storozhevsk** Respublika Komi, NW Russian Federation
Storozhinets see Storozhynets'
116 K8 **Storozhynets'** Ger. Storozynetz, Rom. Storojineț, Rus. Storozhinets. Chernivets'ka Oblast', W Ukraine
Storozynetz see Storozhynets'
92 H11 **Storriten** ▲ C Norway
19 N12 **Storrs** Connecticut, NE USA
94 I11 **Storsjøen** ◎ S Norway
93 N13 **Storsjön** ◎ C Sweden
93 F16 **Storsjön** ◎ C Sweden
92 J9 **Storslett** Troms, N Norway
92 I9 **Storsteinnes** Troms, N Norway
95 I24 **Storstrøm** off. Storstrøms Amt. ◈ county SE Denmark
93 J14 **Storsund** Norrbotten, N Sweden
93 F16 **Storsylen** ▲ S Norway
92 H11 **Stortoppen** ▲ N Sweden
93 H14 **Storuman** Västerbotten, N Sweden
93 H14 **Storuman** ◎ N Sweden
94 N13 **Storvik** Gävleborg, C Sweden
95 O14 **Storvreta** Uppsala, C Sweden
29 V13 **Story City** Iowa, C USA
11 V17 **Stoughton** Saskatchewan, S Canada
19 O11 **Stoughton** Massachusetts, NE USA
30 L9 **Stoughton** Wisconsin, N USA
97 L23 **Stour** ≈ E England, UK
97 P21 **Stour** ≈ S England, UK
27 T5 **Stover** Missouri, C USA
95 G21 **Støvring** Nordjylland, N Denmark
119 J17 **Stowbtsy** Pol. Stołbce, Rus. Stolbtsy. Minskaya Voblasts', C Belarus
25 X11 **Stowell** Texas, SW USA
97 P20 **Stowmarket** E England, UK
114 N8 **Stozher** Dobrich, NE Bulgaria
97 E14 **Strabane** Ir. An Srath Bán. W Northern Ireland, UK
121 S11 **Strabo Trench** undersea feature C Mediterranean Sea
27 T7 **Strafford** Missouri, C USA
183 N17 **Strahan** Tasmania, SE Australia
111 C18 **Strakonice** Ger. Strakonitz. Budějovický Kraj, S Czech Republic
Strakonitz see Strakonice
100 N8 **Stralsund** Mecklenburg-Vorpommern, NE Germany
99 L16 **Stramproy** Limburg, SE Netherlands
83 E26 **Strand** Western Cape, SW South Africa
94 E10 **Stranda** Møre og Romsdal, S Norway
97 G15 **Strangford Lough** Ir. Loch Cuan. inlet E Northern Ireland, UK
95 N16 **Strängnäs** Södermanland, C Sweden
97 E14 **Stranorlar** Ir. Srath an Urláir. NW Ireland
97 H14 **Stranraer** S Scotland, UK
11 U16 **Strasbourg** Saskatchewan, S Canada
103 V5 **Strasbourg** Ger. Strassburg; anc. Argentoratum. Bas-Rhin, NE France
37 U4 **Strasburg** Colorado, C USA
29 N7 **Strasburg** North Dakota, N USA
31 U12 **Strasburg** Ohio, N USA
21 U3 **Strasburg** Virginia, NE USA
117 N10 **Strășeni** var. Strasheny. C Moldova
Strasheny see Strășeni
109 T8 **Strassburg** Kärnten, S Austria
Strassburg see Strasbourg, France
Strassburg see Aiud, Romania
99 M25 **Strassen** Luxembourg, S Luxembourg
109 R5 **Strasswalchen** Salzburg, C Austria
14 F16 **Stratford** Ontario, S Canada
184 K10 **Stratford** Taranaki, North Island, NZ
35 Q11 **Stratford** California, W USA
29 V13 **Stratford** Iowa, C USA
27 O12 **Stratford** Oklahoma, C USA
25 N1 **Stratford** Texas, SW USA
30 K6 **Stratford** Wisconsin, N USA
Stratford see Stratford-upon-Avon
97 M20 **Stratford-upon-Avon** var. Stratford. C England, UK
183 O17 **Strathgordon** Tasmania, SE Australia
11 Q16 **Strathmore** Alberta, SW Canada
35 R11 **Strathmore** California, W USA
14 E16 **Strathroy** Ontario, S Canada
96 I6 **Strathy Point** headland N Scotland, UK
37 W4 **Stratton** Colorado, C USA
19 P6 **Stratton** Maine, NE USA
18 M10 **Stratton Mountain** ▲ Vermont, NE USA
101 N21 **Straubing** Bayern, SE Germany
100 O12 **Strausberg** Brandenburg, E Germany
32 K13 **Strawberry Mountain** ▲ Oregon, NW USA
29 X12 **Strawberry Point** Iowa, C USA
36 M3 **Strawberry Reservoir** ⊟ Utah, W USA
36 M4 **Strawberry River** ≈ Utah, W USA
25 R7 **Strawn** Texas, SW USA
113 P17 **Straža** ▲ Bulgaria/FYR Macedonia
111 I19 **Strážov** Hung. Sztrazsó. ▲ NW Slovakia
182 F7 **Streaky Bay** South Australia
182 E7 **Streaky Bay** bay South Australia
30 L12 **Streator** Illinois, N USA
Streckenbach see Świdnik
111 C17 **Středočeský Kraj** ◈ region C Czech Republic
Strednogorie see Pirdop
29 O6 **Streeter** North Dakota, N USA
25 U8 **Streetman** Texas, SW USA
116 G13 **Strehaia** Mehedinți, SW Romania
Strehlen see Strzelin
114 I10 **Strelcha** Pazardzhik, C Bulgaria
122 L12 **Strelka** Krasnoyarskiy Kray, C Russian Federation
126 L6 **Strel'na** ≈ NW Russian Federation
118 H7 **Strenči** Ger. Stackeln. Valka, N Latvia
108 K8 **Strengen** Tirol, W Austria
106 C6 **Stresa** Piemonte, NE Italy
Streshin see Streshyn
119 N18 **Streshyn** Rus. Streshin. Homyel'skaya Voblasts', SE Belarus
95 B18 **Streymoy** Dan. Strømø Island Faeroe Islands
95 G23 **Strib** Fyn, C Denmark
111 A17 **Stříbro** Ger. Mies. Plzeňský Kraj, W Czech Republic
186 B7 **Strickland** ≈ SW PNG
Striegau see Strzegom
Strigonium see Esztergom
98 H13 **Strijen** Zuid-Holland, SW Netherlands
63 H21 **Strobel, Lago** ◎ S Argentina
61 B25 **Stroeder** Buenos Aires, E Argentina
115 C20 **Strofádes** island Iónioi Nísoi, Greece, C Mediterranean Sea
Strofilia see Strofyliá
115 G17 **Strofyliá** var. Strofilia. Évvoia, C Greece
100 O10 **Strom** ≈ NE Germany
107 L22 **Stromboli** 🌋 Isola Stromboli, SW Italy
107 L22 **Stromboli, Isola** island Isole Eolie, S Italy
96 H9 **Stromeferry** N Scotland, UK
96 J5 **Stromness** N Scotland, UK
94 N11 **Strömsbruk** Gävleborg, C Sweden
29 Q15 **Stromsburg** Nebraska, C USA
95 K21 **Strömsnäsbruk** Kronoberg, S Sweden
95 I17 **Strömstad** Västra Götaland, S Sweden
93 G16 **Strömsund** Jämtland, C Sweden
93 G15 **Ströms Vattudal** valley N Sweden
27 V14 **Strong** Arkansas, C USA
Strongilí see Strongylí
107 O21 **Strongoli** Calabria, SW Italy
31 T11 **Strongsville** Ohio, N USA
115 Q23 **Strongylí** var. Strongilí. island SE Greece
96 K5 **Stronsay** island NE Scotland, UK
97 L21 **Stroud** C England, UK
27 O10 **Stroud** Oklahoma, C USA
18 I14 **Stroudsburg** Pennsylvania, NE USA
95 F21 **Struer** Ringkøbing, W Denmark
113 M20 **Struga** SW FYR Macedonia
Strugi-Kranyse see Strugi-Krasnyye
126 G14 **Strugi-Krasnyye** var. Strugi-Kranyse. Pskovskaya Oblast', W Russian Federation
114 G11 **Struma** Gk. Strymónas. ≈ Bulgaria/Greece see also Strymónas
97 G21 **Strumble Head** headland SW Wales, UK
113 Q19 **Strumeshnitsa** | Mac. Strumica. ≈ Bulgaria/FYR Macedonia
113 Q19 **Strumica** E FYR Macedonia
Strumica see Strumeshnitsa
114 G11 **Strumyani** Blagoevgrad, SW Bulgaria
31 V12 **Struthers** Ohio, N USA
114 I10 **Stryama** ≈ C Bulgaria
114 G13 **Strymónas** Bul. Struma. ≈ Bulgaria/Greece see also Struma
115 H14 **Strymonikós Kólpos** gulf N Greece
116 I6 **Stryy** L'vivs'ka Oblast', NW Ukraine
116 H6 **Stryy** ≈ W Ukraine
111 F14 **Strzegom** Ger. Striegau. Wałbrzych, SW Poland
110 E10 **Strzelce Krajeńskie** Ger. Friedeberg Neumark. Lubuskie, W Poland
111 I15 **Strzelce Opolskie** Ger. Gross Strehlitz. Opolskie, S Poland
182 K3 **Strzelecki Creek** seasonal river South Australia
182 J3 **Strzelecki Desert** desert South Australia
111 G15 **Strzelin** Ger. Strehlen. Dolnośląskie, SW Poland
110 I11 **Strzelno** Kujawsko-pomorskie, C Poland
111 N17 **Strzyżów** Podkarpackie, SE Poland
Stua Laighean see Leinster, Mount
23 Y13 **Stuart** Florida, SE USA
29 U14 **Stuart** Iowa, C USA
29 O13 **Stuart** Nebraska, C USA
21 S8 **Stuart** Virginia, NE USA
10 L13 **Stuart** ≈ British Columbia, SW Canada
39 N10 **Stuart Island** island Alaska, USA
10 L13 **Stuart Lake** ◎ British Columbia, SW Canada
185 B22 **Stuart Mountains** ⛰ South Island, NZ
182 F3 **Stuart Range** hill range South Australia
Stubaital see Neustift im Stubaital
95 I24 **Stubbekøbing** Storstrøm, SE Denmark
45 P14 **Stubbs** Saint Vincent, Saint Vincent and the Grenadines
109 V6 **Stübming** ≈ E Austria
114 J11 **Studen Kladenets, Yazovir** ⊟ S Bulgaria
185 G21 **Studholme** Canterbury, South Island, NZ
Stuhlweissenberg see Székesfehérvár
Stuhm see Sztum
12 C7 **Stull Lake** ◎ Ontario, C Canada
Stung Treng see Stœng Trêng
128 L4 **Stupino** Moskovskaya Oblast', W Russian Federation
27 U4 **Sturgeon** Missouri, C USA
14 G10 **Sturgeon** ≈ Ontario, S Canada
31 N6 **Sturgeon Bay** Wisconsin, N USA
14 G11 **Sturgeon Falls** Ontario, S Canada
12 C11 **Sturgeon Lake** ◎ Ontario, S Canada
30 M3 **Sturgeon River** ≈ Michigan, N USA
20 H6 **Sturgis** Kentucky, S USA
31 P11 **Sturgis** Michigan, N USA
28 J9 **Sturgis** South Dakota, N USA
112 D10 **Šturlić** Federacija Bosna I Hercegovina, NW Bosnia and Herzegovina
111 J22 **Štúrovo** Hung. Párkány; prev. Parkan. Nitriansky Kraj, W Slovakia
182 L4 **Sturt, Mount** hill New South Wales, SE Australia
181 P4 **Sturt Plain** plain Northern Territory, N Australia
181 T9 **Sturt Stony Desert** desert South Australia
83 J25 **Stutterheim** Eastern Cape, S South Africa
101 H21 **Stuttgart** Baden-Württemberg, SW Germany
27 W12 **Stuttgart** Arkansas, C USA
92 H2 **Stykkishólmur** Vesturland, W Iceland
115 F17 **Stylída** var. Stilida, Stilís. Stereá Ellás, C Greece
116 K2 **Styr** Rus. Styr'. ≈ Belarus/Ukraine
115 I19 **Stýra** var. Stira. Évvoia, C Greece
Styria see Steiermark
Su see Jiangsu
171 Q17 **Suai** W East Timor
54 G9 **Suaita** Santander, C Colombia
80 I7 **Suakin** var. Sawakin. Red Sea, NE Sudan
161 T13 **Suao** Jap. Suō. N Taiwan
Suao see Suau
40 G6 **Suaqui Grande** Sonora, NW Mexico
61 A16 **Suardi** Santa Fe, C Argentina
54 D11 **Suárez** Cauca, SW Colombia
186 G10 **Suau** var. Suao. Suaul Island, SE PNG
118 G12 **Subačius** Kupiškis, NE Lithuania
168 K9 **Subang** prev. Soebang. Jawa, C Indonesia
169 O16 **Subang** ✕ (Kuala Lumpur) Pahang, Peninsular Malaysia
153 V12 **Subansiri** ≈ NE India
118 I11 **Subate** Daugvapils, SE Latvia
139 N5 **Subaykhān** Dayr az Zawr, E Syria
159 P8 **Subei** var. Dangchengwan, Subei Mongolzu Zizhixian. Gansu, N China
Subei Mongolzu Zizhixian see Subei
169 P9 **Subi Besar, Pulau** island Kepulauan Natuna, W Indonesia
Subiyah see Aş Şubayhīyah
26 I7 **Sublette** Kansas, C USA
112 K8 **Subotica** Ger. Maria-Theresiopel, Hung. Szabadka. Serbia, N Yugoslavia
116 K9 **Suceava** Ger. Suczawa, Hung. Szucsava. Suceava, NE Romania
116 J9 **Suceava** ◈ county NE Romania
116 K9 **Suceava** Ger. Suczawa. ≈ N Romania
112 E12 **Sučevići** Zadar, SW Croatia
111 K17 **Sucha Beskidzka** Małopolskie, S Poland
111 M14 **Suchedniów** Świętokrzyskie, C Poland
42 A2 **Suchitepéquez** off. Departamento de Suchitepéquez. ◈ department SW Guatemala
Su-chou see Suzhou
Suchow see Suzhou, Jiangsu, China
Suchow see Xuzhou, Jiangsu, China
97 D17 **Suck** ≈ C Ireland
Sucker State see Illinois
186 F9 **Suckling, Mount** ▲ S PNG
57 L19 **Sucre** hist. Chuquisaca, La Plata. ● (Bolivia-legal capital) Chuquisaca, S Bolivia
54 E6 **Sucre** Santander, N Colombia
56 A7 **Sucre** Manabí, W Ecuador
54 E6 **Sucre** off. Departamento de Sucre. ◈ province N Colombia
55 O5 **Sucre** off. Estado Sucre. ◈ state NE Venezuela
56 D6 **Sucumbíos** ◈ province NE Ecuador
113 G15 **Sućuraj** Split-Dalmacija, S Croatia
58 K10 **Sucuriju** Amapá, NE Brazil
Suczawa see Suceava
79 E16 **Sud** Eng. South. ◈ province S Cameroon
126 K13 **Suda** ≈ NW Russian Federation
Suda see Soúda
117 U13 **Sudak** Respublika Krym, S Ukraine
24 M4 **Sudan** Texas, SW USA
80 C10 **Sudan** off. Republic of Sudan, Ar. Jumhuriyat as-Sudan; prev. Anglo-Egyptian Sudan. ◆ republic N Africa
Sudanese Republic see Mali
Sudan, Jumhuriyat as- see Sudan
14 F10 **Sudbury** Ontario, S Canada
97 P20 **Sudbury** E England, UK
Sud, Canal de see Gonâve, Canal de la
80 E13 **Sudd** swamp region S Sudan
100 K10 **Sude** ≈ N Germany
Sudest Island see Tagula Island
111 E15 **Sudeten** var. Sudetes, Sudetic Mountains, Cz./Pol. Sudety. ⛰ Czech Republic/Poland
Sudetes/Sudetic Mountains/Sudety see Sudeten
92 G1 **Sudhureyri** Vestfirdhir, NW Iceland
92 J4 **Sudhurland** ◈ region S Iceland
95 B19 **Sudhuroy** Dan. Suderø Island Faeroe Islands
126 M15 **Sudislavl'** Kostromskaya Oblast', NW Russian Federation
Südkarpaten see Carpații Meridionali
79 N20 **Sud Kivu** off. Région Sud Kivu. ◈ region E Dem. Rep. Congo (Zaire)
Südliche Morava see Južna Morava
100 E12 **Süd-Nord-Kanal** canal NW Germany
128 M3 **Sudogda** Vladimirskaya Oblast', W Russian Federation
Sudostroy see Severodvinsk
79 C15 **Sud-Ouest** Eng. South-West. ◈ province W Cameroon
173 X17 **Sud Ouest, Pointe** headland SW Mauritius
187 P17 **Sud, Province** ◈ province S New Caledonia
128 J8 **Sudzha** Kurskaya Oblast', W Russian Federation
81 D15 **Sue** ≈ S Sudan
105 S10 **Sueca** País Valenciano, E Spain
114 I10 **Sŭedinenie** Plovdiv, C Bulgaria
Suero see Alzira
75 X8 **Suez** Ar. As Suways, El Suweis. NE Egypt
75 W7 **Suez Canal** Ar. Qanāt as Suways. canal NE Egypt
75 X8 **Suez, Gulf of** Ar. Khalīj as Suways. gulf NE Egypt
11 R17 **Suffield** Alberta, SW Canada
21 X7 **Suffolk** Virginia, NE USA
97 P20 **Suffolk** cultural region E England, UK
142 J2 **Şūfiān** Āẕarbāyjān-e Khāvarī, N Iran
31 N12 **Sugar Creek** ≈ Illinois, N USA
30 L13 **Sugar Creek** ≈ Illinois, N USA
31 R3 **Sugar Island** island Michigan, N USA
25 V11 **Sugar Land** Texas, SW USA
19 P6 **Sugarloaf Mountain** ▲ Maine, NE USA
65 G24 **Sugar Loaf Point** headland N Saint Helena
136 G16 **Suğla Gölü** ◎ SW Turkey
123 T8 **Sugoy** ≈ E Russian Federation
158 F7 **Sugun** Xinjiang Uygur Zizhiqu, W China
147 U11 **Sugut, Gora** ▲ SW Kyrgyzstan
169 V6 **Sugut, Sungai** ≈ East Malaysia
159 O9 **Suhai Hu** ◎ C China
162 K14 **Suhait** Nei Mongol Zizhiqu, N China
141 X7 **Şuḩār** var. Sohar. N Oman
162 L6 **Sühbaatar** Selenge, N Mongolia
163 P9 **Sühbaatar** ◈ province E Mongolia
101 K17 **Suhl** Thüringen, C Germany
108 F7 **Suhr** Aargau, N Switzerland
161 O12 **Suichuan** Jiangxi, S China
Suid-Afrika see South Africa
160 L4 **Suide** Shaanxi, C China
Suidwes-Afrika see Namibia
163 Y9 **Suifenhe** Heilongjiang, NE China
Suigen see Suwŏn
163 W8 **Suihua** Heilongjiang, NE China
Súilí, Loch see Swilly, Lough
161 Q6 **Suining** Jiangsu, E China
160 I9 **Suining** Sichuan, C China
103 Q4 **Suippes** Marne, N France
97 E20 **Suir** Ir. An tSiúir. ≈ S Ireland
165 J13 **Suita** Ōsaka, Honshū, SW Japan
160 L16 **Suixi** Guangdong, S China
Sui Xian see Suizhou
163 T13 **Suizhong** Liaoning, NE China
161 N8 **Suizhou** prev. Sui Xian. Hubei, C China
149 P17 **Sujāwal** Sind, SE Pakistan
169 O16 **Sukabumi** prev. Soekaboemi. Jawa, C Indonesia
169 Q12 **Sukadana, Teluk** bay Borneo, W Indonesia
165 P11 **Sukagawa** Fukushima, Honshū, C Japan
Sukarnapura see Jayapura
Sukarno, Puntjak see Jaya, Puncak
147 R11 **Sŭkh** Rus. Sokh. Farghona Wiloyati, E Uzbekistan
Sŭkh see Sokh
114 N8 **Sukha Reka** ≈ NE Bulgaria
128 J5 **Sukhinichi** Kaluzhskaya Oblast', W Russian Federation
Sukhne see As Sukhnah
131 Q4 **Sukhona** var. Tot'ma. ≈ NW Russian Federation
167 O8 **Sukhothai** var. Sukotai. Sukhothai, W Thailand
Sukhumi see Sokhumi
Sukkertoppen see Maniitsoq
149 Q13 **Sukkur** Sind, SE Pakistan
Sukotai see Sukhothai
Sukra Bay see Şawqirah, Dawḩat
127 V15 **Suksun** Permskaya Oblast', NW Russian Federation
165 F15 **Sukumo** Kōchi, Shikoku, SW Japan
94 B12 **Sula** island S Norway
127 Q5 **Sula** ≈ NW Russian Federation
117 R5 **Sula** ≈ N Ukraine
42 H6 **Sulaco, Río** ≈ NW Honduras
Sulaimaniya see As Sulaymānīyah
149 S10 **Sulaimān Range** ⛰ C Pakistan
129 Q16 **Sulak** Respublika Dagestan, SW Russian Federation
129 Q16 **Sulak** ≈ SW Russian Federation
171 Q13 **Sula, Kepulauan** island group C Indonesia
136 I12 **Sulakyurt** var. Konur. Kırıkkale, N Turkey
171 P17 **Sulamu** Timor, S Indonesia
96 F5 **Sula Sgeir** island NW Scotland, UK
171 N13 **Sulawesi** Eng. Celebes. island C Indonesia
Sulawesi, Laut see Celebes Sea
171 N14 **Sulawesi Selatan** off. Propinsi Sulawesi Selatan, Eng. South Celebes, South Sulawesi. ◈ province C Indonesia
171 P12 **Sulawesi Tengah** off. Propinsi Sulawesi Tengah, Eng. Central Celebes, Central Sulawesi. ◈ province N Indonesia
171 O14 **Sulawesi Tenggara** off. Propinsi Sulawesi Tenggara, Eng. South-East Celebes, South-East Sulawesi. ◈ province C Indonesia
171 P11 **Sulawesi Utara** off. Propinsi Sulawesi Utara, Eng. North Celebes, North Sulawesi. ◈ province N Indonesia
139 T5 **Sulaymān Beg** N Iraq
95 D15 **Suldalsvatnet** ◎ S Norway
110 E12 **Sulechów** Ger. Züllichau. Lubuskie, W Poland
110 E11 **Sulęcin** Lubuskie, W Poland
77 U14 **Suleja** Niger, C Nigeria
111 K14 **Sulejów** Łodzkie, S Poland
96 I5 **Sule Skerry** island N Scotland, UK
Suliag see Sohâg
76 J16 **Sulima** S Sierra Leone
117 O13 **Sulina** Tulcea, SE Romania
117 N13 **Sulina Braţul** ≈ SE Romania
100 H12 **Sulingen** Niedersachsen, NW Germany
92 H12 **Suliskongen** ▲ C Norway
92 H12 **Sulitjelma** Nordland, C Norway
56 A9 **Sullana** Piura, NW Peru
23 N3 **Sulligent** Alabama, S USA
30 M14 **Sullivan** Illinois, N USA
31 N15 **Sullivan** Indiana, N USA
27 W5 **Sullivan** Missouri, C USA
Sullivan Island see Lanbi Kyun
96 M1 **Sullom Voe** NE Scotland, UK
103 O7 **Sully-sur-Loire** Loiret, C France
Sulmo see Sulmona
107 K15 **Sulmona** anc. Sulmo. Abruzzo, C Italy
Sulo see Shule He
114 M11 **Sülöğlu** Edirne, NW Turkey
22 G9 **Sulphur** Louisiana, S USA
27 O12 **Sulphur** Oklahoma, C USA
28 K9 **Sulphur Creek** ≈ South Dakota, N USA
24 M5 **Sulphur Draw** ≈ Texas, SW USA
25 W5 **Sulphur River** ≈ Arkansas/Texas, SW USA
25 V6 **Sulphur Springs** Texas, SW USA
24 M6 **Sulphur Springs Draw** ≈ Texas, SW USA
14 D8 **Sultan** Ontario, S Canada
Sultānābād see Arāk
Sultan Alonto, Lake see Lanao, Lake
136 G15 **Sultan Dağları** ⛰ C Turkey
114 N13 **Sultanköy** Tekirdağ, NW Turkey
171 Q7 **Sultan Kudarat** var. Nuling. Mindanao, S Philippines
152 M13 **Sultānpur** Uttar Pradesh, N India
171 O9 **Sulu Archipelago** island group SW Philippines
192 F7 **Sulu Basin** undersea feature SE South China Sea
Sülüktü see Sulyukta
Sulu, Laut see Sulu Sea
169 X6 **Sulu Sea** Ind. Laut Sulu. sea SW Philippines
145 O15 **Sulutobe** Kaz. Sulütöbe. Kzylorda, S Kazakhstan
147 Q11 **Sulyukta** Kir. Sülüktü. Oshskaya Oblast', SW Kyrgyzstan
Sulz see Sulz am Neckar
101 G22 **Sulz am Neckar** var. Sulz. Baden-Württemberg, SW Germany
101 L20 **Sulzbach-Rosenberg** Bayern, SE Germany
195 N13 **Sulzberger Bay** bay Antarctica
Sumail see Summēl
113 F15 **Sumartin** Split-Dalmacija, S Croatia
32 H6 **Sumas** Washington, NW USA
168 J10 **Sumatera** Eng. Sumatra. island W Indonesia
168 J12 **Sumatera Barat** off. Propinsi Sumatera Barat, Eng. West Sumatra. ◈ province W Indonesia
168 L13 **Sumatera Selatan** off. Propinsi Sumatera Selatan, Eng. South Sumatra. ◈ province W Indonesia
168 H10 **Sumatera Utara** off. Propinsi Sumatera Utara, Eng. North Sumatra. ◈ province W Indonesia
Sumatra see Sumatera
Šumava see Bohemian Forest
Sumayl see Summēl
139 U7 **Sumayr al Muḩammad** E Iraq
171 N17 **Sumba, Pulau** Eng. Sandalwood Island; prev. Soemba. island Nusa Tenggara, C Indonesia
146 D12 **Sumbar** ≈ W Turkmenistan
192 E9 **Sumbawa** prev. Soembawa. island Nusa Tenggara, C Indonesia
170 L16 **Sumbawabesar** Sumbawa, S Indonesia
81 F23 **Sumbawanga** Rukwa, W Tanzania
82 B12 **Sumbe** prev. N'Gunza, Port. Novo Redondo. Cuanza Sul, W Angola
96 M3 **Sumburgh Head** headland NE Scotland, UK
111 H23 **Sümeg** Veszprém, W Hungary
80 C12 **Sumeih** Southern Darfur, S Sudan
169 T16 **Sumenep** prev. Soemenep. Pulau Madura, C Indonesia
Sumgait see Sumqayıt, Azerbaijan
Sumgait see Sumqayıtçay, Azerbaijan
165 Y14 **Sumisu-jima** Eng. Smith Island. island SE Japan
139 Q2 **Summēl** var. Sumail, Sumayl. N Iraq
31 O5 **Summer Island** island Michigan, N USA
32 H15 **Summer Lake** ◎ Oregon, NW USA
11 N17 **Summerland** British Columbia, SW Canada
13 P14 **Summerside** Prince Edward Island, SE Canada
21 R5 **Summersville** West Virginia, NE USA
21 R5 **Summersville Lake** ⊟ West Virginia, NE USA
21 S13 **Summerton** South Carolina, SE USA
23 R2 **Summerville** Georgia, SE USA
21 S14 **Summerville** South Carolina, SE USA
39 R10 **Summit** Alaska, USA
35 V6 **Summit Mountain** ▲ Nevada, W USA
37 R8 **Summit Peak** ▲ Colorado, C USA
Summus Portus see Somport, Col du
29 X12 **Sumner** Iowa, C USA
22 K3 **Sumner** Mississippi, S USA
185 H17 **Sumner, Lake** ◎ South Island, NZ
37 U12 **Sumner, Lake** ⊟ New Mexico, SW USA
111 G17 **Šumperk** Ger. Mährisch-Schönberg. Olomoucký Kraj, E Czech Republic
42 F7 **Sumpul, Río** ≈ El Salvador/Honduras
137 Z11 **Sumqayıt** Rus. Sumgait. E Azerbaijan
137 Y11 **Sumqayıtçay** Rus. Sumgait. ≈ E Azerbaijan
147 R9 **Sumsar** Dzhalal-Abadskaya Oblast', W Kyrgyzstan
117 S3 **Sums'ka Oblast'** var. Sumy, Rus. Sumskaya Oblast'. ◈ province NE Ukraine
Sumskaya Oblast' see Sums'ka Oblast'
126 J8 **Sumskiy Posad** Respublika Kareliya, NW Russian Federation
21 S12 **Sumter** South Carolina, SE USA
117 T3 **Sumy** Sums'ka Oblast', NE Ukraine
Sumy see Sums'ka Oblast'
159 Q15 **Sumzom** Xizang Zizhiqu, W China
127 R15 **Suna** Kirovskaya Oblast', NW Russian Federation
126 I10 **Suna** ≈ NW Russian Federation
165 S3 **Sunagawa** Hokkaidō, NE Japan
153 V13 **Sunamganj** Chittagong, NE Bangladesh
159 S8 **Sunan** var. Hongwan, Sunan Yugurzu Zizhixian. Gansu, N China
163 W14 **Sunan** ✕ (P'yŏngyang) SW North Korea
Sunan Yugurzu Zizhixian see Sunan
19 N9 **Sunapee Lake** ◎ New Hampshire, NE USA
139 P4 **Sunaysilah** salt marsh N Iraq
20 M8 **Sunbright** Tennessee, S USA
33 R6 **Sunburst** Montana, NW USA
183 N12 **Sunbury** Victoria, SE Australia
21 X8 **Sunbury** North Carolina, SE USA
18 G14 **Sunbury** Pennsylvania, NE USA
61 A17 **Sunchales** Santa Fe, C Argentina
163 W13 **Sunch'ŏn** SW North Korea
163 Y16 **Sunch'ŏn** Jap. Junten. S South Korea

◆ Country
● Country Capital
◇ Dependent Territory
○ Dependent Territory Capital
◈ Administrative Region
✕ International Airport
▲ Mountain
⛰ Mountain Range
🌋 Volcano
≈ River
◎ Lake
⊟ Reservoir

36 K13 **Sun City** Arizona, SW USA
19 O9 **Suncook** New Hampshire, NE USA
Sunda Islands see Greater Sunda Islands
33 Z12 **Sundance** Wyoming, C USA
153 T17 **Sundarbans** wetland Bangladesh/India
154 M11 **Sundargarh** Orissa, E India
131 U15 **Sunda Shelf** undersea feature S South China Sea
Sunda Trench see Java Trench
131 U17 **Sunda Trough** undersea feature E Indian Ocean
95 O16 **Sundbyberg** Stockholm, C Sweden
97 M14 **Sunderland** var. Wearmouth. NE England, UK
101 F15 **Sundern** Nordrhein-Westfalen, W Germany
136 F12 **Sündiken Dağları** ⛰ C Turkey
24 M5 **Sundown** Texas, SW USA
11 P16 **Sundre** Alberta, SW Canada
14 H12 **Sundridge** Ontario, S Canada
93 H17 **Sundsvall** Västernorrland, C Sweden
26 H4 **Sunflower, Mount** ▲ Kansas, C USA
Sunflower State see Kansas
169 N14 **Sungaibuntu** Sumatera, SW Indonesia
168 K12 **Sungaidareh** Sumatera, W Indonesia
167 P17 **Sungai Kolok** var. Sungai Ko-Lok. Narathiwat, SW Thailand
168 K12 **Sungaipenuh** prev. Soengaipenoeh. Sumatera, W Indonesia
169 P11 **Sungaipinyuh** Borneo, C Indonesia
Sungari see Songhua Jiang
Sungaria see Dzungaria
Sungei Pahang see Pahang, Sungai
167 O8 **Sung Men** Phrae, NW Thailand
83 M15 **Sungo** Tete, NW Mozambique
168 M13 **Sungsang** Sumatera, W Indonesia
114 M9 **Sungurlare** Burgas, E Bulgaria
136 J12 **Sungurlu** Çorum, N Turkey
112 F9 **Sunja** Sisak-Moslavina, C Croatia
153 Q12 **Sun Koshi** ∼ E Nepal
94 F9 **Sunndalen** valley S Norway
94 F9 **Sunndalsøra** Møre og Romsdal, S Norway
95 K15 **Sunne** Värmland, C Sweden
95 O15 **Sunnersta** Uppsala, C Sweden
94 C11 **Sunnfjord** physical region S Norway
95 C15 **Sunnhordland** physical region S Norway
94 D10 **Sunnmøre** physical region S Norway
37 N4 **Sunnyside** Utah, W USA
32 J10 **Sunnyside** Washington, NW USA
35 N9 **Sunnyvale** California, W USA
30 L8 **Sun Prairie** Wisconsin, N USA
Sunqur see Sonqor
25 N1 **Sunray** Texas, SW USA
22 I8 **Sunset** Louisiana, S USA
25 S5 **Sunset** Texas, SW USA
Sunset State see Oregon
181 Z10 **Sunshine Coast** cultural region Queensland, E Australia
Sunshine State see Florida, USA
Sunshine State see New Mexico, USA
Sunshine State see South Dakota, USA
123 O10 **Suntar** Respublika Sakha (Yakutiya), NE Russian Federation
39 R10 **Suntrana** Alaska, USA
148 J15 **Suntsar** Baluchistān, SW Pakistan
163 W15 **Sunwi-do** island SW North Korea
163 W6 **Sunwu** Heilongjiang, NE China
77 O16 **Sunyani** W Ghana
Suō see Suao
93 M17 **Suolahti** Länsi-Suomi, W Finland
Suoločielgi see Saariselkä
Suomenlahti see Finland, Gulf of
Suomen Tasavalta/Suomi see Finland
93 N14 **Suomussalmi** Oulu, E Finland
165 E13 **Suō-nada** sea SW Japan
93 M17 **Suonenjoki** Itä-Suomi, C Finland
167 S13 **Suŏng** Kâmpóng Cham, C Cambodia
126 I10 **Suoyarvi** Respublika Kareliya, NW Russian Federation
Supanburi see Suphan Buri
57 D14 **Supe** Lima, W Peru
15 V7 **Supérieur, Lac** ◎ Quebec, SE Canada
Supérieur, Lac see Superior, Lake
36 M14 **Superior** Arizona, SW USA
33 O9 **Superior** Montana, NW USA
29 P17 **Superior** Nebraska, C USA
30 I3 **Superior** Wisconsin, N USA
41 S17 **Superior, Laguna** lagoon S Mexico
31 N2 **Superior, Lake** Fr. Lac Supérieur. ◎ Canada/USA
36 L13 **Superstition Mountains** ⛰ Arizona, SW USA
113 F14 **Supetar** It. San Pietro. Split-Dalmacija, S Croatia
167 O10 **Suphan Buri** var. Supanburi. Suphan Buri, W Thailand
171 V12 **Supiori, Pulau** island E Indonesia
188 K2 **Supply Reef** reef N Northern Mariana Islands
195 O7 **Support Force Glacier** glacier Antarctica
137 R10 **Sup'sa** var. Supsa. ∼ W Georgia
Sūq 'Abs see 'Abs
139 W12 **Sūq ash Shuyūkh** SE Iraq
138 H4 **Şuqaylibīyah** Ḩamāh, W Syria
161 Q6 **Suqian** Jiangsu, E China
Suqrah see Şawqirah
Suqrah Bay see Şawqirah, Dawḩat
141 V16 **Suquṭrā** var. Sokotra, Eng. Socotra. island SE Yemen
141 Z8 **Şūr** NE Oman
Şūr see Soûr
129 P5 **Sura** Penzenskaya Oblast', W Russian Federation
129 P4 **Sura** ∼ W Russian Federation
149 N12 **Sūrāb** Baluchistān, SW Pakistan
Surabaja see Surabaya
192 E8 **Surabaya** prev. Soerabaja, Surabaja. Jawa, C Indonesia
95 N15 **Surahammar** Västmanland, C Sweden
169 Q16 **Surakarta** Eng. Solo; prev. Soerakarta. Jawa, S Indonesia
Surakhany see Suraxanı
137 S10 **Surami** C Georgia
143 X13 **Sūrān** Sīstān va Balūchestān, SE Iran
111 I21 **Šurany** Hung. Nagysurány. Nitriansky Kraj, SW Slovakia
154 D12 **Sūrat** Gujarāt, W India
Suratdhani see Surat Thani
152 G9 **Sūratgarh** Rājasthān, NW India
167 N14 **Surat Thani** var. Suratdhani. Surat Thani, SW Thailand
119 Q16 **Suraw** Rus. Surov. ∼ E Belarus
137 Z11 **Suraxanı** Rus. Surakhany. E Azerbaijan
141 Y11 **Surayr** E Oman
138 K2 **Suraysāt** Ḩalab, N Syria
118 O12 **Surazh** Rus. Surazh. Vitsyebskaya Voblasts', NE Belarus
128 H6 **Surazh** Bryanskaya Oblast', W Russian Federation
191 V17 **Sur, Cabo** headland Easter Island, Chile, E Pacific Ocean
112 L11 **Surčin** Serbia, N Yugoslavia
116 H9 **Surduc** Hung. Szurduk. Sălaj, NW Romania
113 P16 **Surdulica** Serbia, SE Yugoslavia
99 L24 **Sûre** var. Sauer. ∼ W Europe see also Sauer
154 C10 **Surendranagar** Gujarāt, W India
18 K16 **Surf City** New Jersey, NE USA
183 V3 **Surfers Paradise** Queensland, E Australia
21 U13 **Surfside Beach** South Carolina, SE USA
102 J10 **Surgères** Charente-Maritime, W France
122 H10 **Surgut** Khanty-Mansiyskiy Avtonomnyy Okrug, C Russian Federation
122 K10 **Surgutikha** Krasnoyarskiy Kray, N Russian Federation
98 M6 **Surhuisterveen** Friesland, N Netherlands
105 V5 **Súria** Cataluña, NE Spain
143 P10 **Sūrīān** Fārs, S Iran
155 J15 **Suriāpet** Andhra Pradesh, C India
171 Q6 **Surigao** Mindanao, S Philippines
167 R10 **Surin** Surin, E Thailand
55 U11 **Suriname** off. Republic of Suriname, var. Surinam; prev. Dutch Guiana, Netherlands Guiana. ◆ republic N South America
Sūrīya/Sūrīyah, Al-Jumhūrīyah al-'Arabīyah as - see Syria
Surkhab, Darya-i- see Kahmard, Daryā-ye
Surkhandar'inskaya Oblast' see Surkhondaryo Wiloyati
Surkhandar'ya see Surkhondaryo
Surkhet see Birendranagar
147 R12 **Surkhob** ∼ C Tajikistan
147 P13 **Surkhondaryo** Rus. Surkhandar'ya. ∼ Tajikistan/Uzbekistan
147 N13 **Surkhondaryo Wiloyati** Rus. Surkhandar'inskaya Oblast'. ◐ province S Uzbekistan
137 P11 **Sürmene** Trabzon, NE Turkey
Surov see Suraw
129 N11 **Surovikino** Volgogradskaya Oblast', SW Russian Federation
35 N11 **Sur, Point** headland California, W USA
187 N15 **Surprise, Île** island N New Caledonia
61 E22 **Sur, Punta** headland E Argentina
Surrentum see Sorrento
28 M3 **Surrey** North Dakota, N USA
97 O22 **Surrey** cultural region SE England, UK
21 X7 **Surry** Virginia, NE USA
108 F8 **Sursee** Luzern, W Switzerland
129 P6 **Sursk** Penzenskaya Oblast', W Russian Federation
129 P5 **Surskoye** Ul'yanovskaya Oblast', W Russian Federation
75 P8 **Surt** var. Sidra, Sirte. N Libya
95 I19 **Surte** Västra Götaland, S Sweden
75 Q8 **Surt, Khalīj** Eng. Gulf of Sidra, Gulf of Sirti, Sidra. gulf N Libya
92 I5 **Surtsey** island S Iceland
137 N17 **Suruç** Şanlıurfa, S Turkey
168 L13 **Surulangun** Sumatera, W Indonesia
Süs see Susch
106 A8 **Susa** Piemonte, NE Italy
165 E12 **Susa** Yamaguchi, Honshū, SW Japan
Susa see Shūsh
113 E16 **Sušac** It. Cazza. island SW Croatia
Sūsah see Sousse
165 G14 **Susaki** Kōchi, Shikoku, SW Japan
165 I15 **Susami** Wakayama, Honshū, SW Japan
142 K9 **Sūsangerd** var. Susangird. Khūzestān, SW Iran
Susangird see Sūsangerd
35 P4 **Susanville** California, W USA
108 J9 **Susch** var. Süs. Graubünden, SE Switzerland
137 N12 **Suşehri** Sivas, N Turkey
Susiana see Khūzestān
111 B18 **Sušice** Ger. Schüttenhofen. Plzeňský Kraj, W Czech Republic
39 R11 **Susitna** Alaska, USA
39 R11 **Susitna River** ∼ Alaska, USA
129 Q3 **Suslonger** Respublika Mariy El, W Russian Federation
105 N14 **Suspiro del Moro, Puerto del** pass S Spain
18 H16 **Susquehanna River** ∼ New York/Pennsylvania, NE USA
13 O15 **Sussex** New Brunswick, SE Canada
18 J13 **Sussex** New Jersey, NE USA
21 W7 **Sussex** Virginia, NE USA
97 O23 **Sussex** cultural region S England, UK
183 S10 **Sussex Inlet** New South Wales, SE Australia
99 L17 **Susteren** Limburg, SE Netherlands
10 K12 **Sustut Peak** ▲ British Columbia, W Canada
123 S9 **Susuman** Magadanskaya Oblast', E Russian Federation
188 H6 **Susupe** Saipan, S Northern Mariana Islands
136 D12 **Susurluk** Balıkesir, NW Turkey
114 M13 **Susuzmüsellim** Tekirdağ, NW Turkey
136 F15 **Sütçüler** Isparta, SW Turkey
116 L13 **Suţeşti** Brăila, SE Romania
83 F25 **Sutherland** Western Cape, SW South Africa
28 L15 **Sutherland** Nebraska, C USA
96 I7 **Sutherland** cultural region N Scotland, UK
185 B21 **Sutherland Falls** waterfall South Island, NZ
32 F14 **Sutherlin** Oregon, NW USA
149 V10 **Sutlej** ∼ India/Pakistan
Sutna see Satna
35 P7 **Sutter Creek** California, W USA
39 R11 **Sutton** Alaska, USA
29 Q16 **Sutton** Nebraska, C USA
21 R4 **Sutton** West Virginia, NE USA
12 F8 **Sutton** ∼ Ontario, C Canada
97 M19 **Sutton Coldfield** C England, UK
21 R4 **Sutton Lake** ⊟ West Virginia, NE USA
15 P13 **Sutton, Monts** hill range Quebec, SE Canada
12 F8 **Sutton Ridges** ⛰ Ontario, C Canada
165 Q4 **Suttsu** Hokkaidō, NE Japan
39 P15 **Sutwik Island** island Alaska, USA
162 K7 **Süüj** Bulgan, C Mongolia
118 H5 **Suure-Jaani** Ger. Gross-Sankt-Johannis. Viljandimaa, S Estonia
118 J7 **Suur Munamägi** var. Munamägi, Ger. Eier-Berg. ▲ SE Estonia
118 F5 **Suur Väin** Ger. Grosser Sund. strait W Estonia
147 U8 **Suusamyr** Chuyskaya Oblast', C Kyrgyzstan
187 X14 **Suva** ● (Fiji) Viti Levu, W Fiji
187 X15 **Suva** ✕ Viti Levu, C Fiji
113 N18 **Suva Gora** ⛰ W FYR Macedonia
118 H11 **Suvainiškis** Rokiškis, NE Lithuania
Suvalkai/Suvalki see Suwałki
113 P15 **Suva Planina** ⛰ SE Yugoslavia
113 M17 **Suva Reka** Serbia, S Yugoslavia
128 K5 **Suvorov** Tul'skaya Oblast', W Russian Federation
117 N12 **Suvorove** Odes'ka Oblast', SW Ukraine
Suvorovo see Ştefan Vodă
Suwaik see As Suwayq
Suwaira see Aş Şuwayrah
110 O7 **Suwałki** Lith. Suvalkai, Rus. Suvalki. Podlaskie, NE Poland
167 R10 **Suwannaphum** Roi Et, E Thailand
23 V8 **Suwannee River** ∼ Florida/Georgia, SE USA
Şuwār see Aş Şuwār
190 K14 **Suwarrow** atoll N Cook Islands
Suwaydá/Suwaydā', Muḩāfaẓat as see As Suwaydā'
143 R16 **Suwaydān** var. Sweiham. Abū Ẓaby, E UAE
Suwayqiyah, Hawr as see Shuwayjah, Hawr ash
Suways, Khalīj as see Suez, Gulf of
Suways, Qanāt as see Suez Canal
Suweida see As Suwaydā'
Suweon see Suwŏn
163 X15 **Suwŏn** var. Suweon, Jap. Suigen. NW South Korea
Su Xian see Suzhou
143 R14 **Sūzā** Hormozgān, S Iran
145 P15 **Suzak** Kaz. Sozaq. Yuzhnyy Kazakhstan, S Kazakhstan
Suzaka see Suzuka
128 M3 **Suzdal'** Vladimirskaya Oblast', W Russian Federation
161 P7 **Suzhou** var. Su Xian. Anhui, E China
161 R8 **Suzhou** var. Soochow, Suchou, Suchow; prev. Wuhsien. Jiangsu, E China
Suz, Mys see Soye, Mys
165 M10 **Suzu** Ishikawa, Honshū, SW Japan
165 K14 **Suzuka** Mie, Honshū, SW Japan
165 N12 **Suzuka** var. Suzaka. Nagano, Honshū, S Japan
165 M10 **Suzu-misaki** headland Honshū, SW Japan
Svågälv see Svågan
94 M10 **Svågan** var. Svågälv. ∼ C Sweden
Svalava/Svaljava see Svalyava
92 O2 **Svalbard** ◇ Norwegian dependency Arctic Ocean
92 J2 **Svalbardhseyri** Nordhurland Eystra, N Iceland
95 K22 **Svalöv** Skåne, S Sweden
116 H7 **Svalyava** Cz. Svalava, Svaljava, Hung. Szolyva. Zakarpats'ka Oblast', W Ukraine
92 O2 **Svanbergfjellet** ▲ C Svalbard
95 M24 **Svaneke** Bornholm, E Denmark
95 L22 **Svängsta** Blekinge, S Sweden
95 J16 **Svanskog** Värmland, C Sweden
95 L16 **Svartå** Örebro, C Sweden
95 L15 **Svartälven** ∼ C Sweden
92 G12 **Svartisen** glacier C Norway
117 X6 **Svatove** Rus. Svatovo. Luhans'ka Oblast', E Ukraine
Svatovo see Svatove
Sväty Kríž nad Hronom see Žiar nad Hronom
167 Q11 **Svay Chék, Stœng** ∼ Cambodia/Thailand
167 S13 **Svay Riĕng** Svay Riĕng, S Cambodia
92 O3 **Sveagruva** Spitsbergen, W Svalbard
95 K23 **Svedala** Skåne, S Sweden
118 H12 **Svėdasai** Anykščiai, NE Lithuania
93 G18 **Sveg** Jämtland, C Sweden
118 C12 **Švėkšna** Šilutė, W Lithuania
94 C11 **Svelgen** Sogn og Fjordane, S Norway
95 H15 **Svelvik** Vestfold, S Norway
118 I13 **Švenčionėliai** Pol. Nowo-Święciany. Švenčionys, SE Lithuania
118 I13 **Švenčionys** Pol. Swięciany. Švenčionys, SE Lithuania
95 H24 **Svendborg** Fyn, C Denmark
95 K19 **Svenljunga** Västra Götaland, S Sweden
92 P2 **Svenskøya** island E Svalbard
93 G17 **Svenstavik** Jämtland, C Sweden
95 G20 **Svenstrup** Nordjylland, N Denmark
118 H12 **Šventoji** ∼ C Lithuania
117 Z8 **Sverdlovs'k** Rus. Sverdlovsk; prev. Imeni Sverdlova Rudnik. Luhans'ka Oblast', E Ukraine
Sverdlovsk see Yekaterinburg
129 W2 **Sverdlovskaya Oblast'** ◐ province C Russian Federation
8 M3 **Sverdrup Islands** island group Nunavut, N Canada
8 L3 **Sverdrup, Ostrov** island N Russian Federation
Sverige see Sweden
113 D15 **Svetac** prev. Sveti Andrea, It. Sant'Andrea. island SW Croatia
Sveti Andrea see Svetac
Sveti Nikola see Sveti Nikole
113 O18 **Sveti Nikole** prev. Sveti Nikola. C FYR Macedonia
Sveti Vrach see Sandanski
123 T14 **Svetlaya** Primorskiy Kray, SE Russian Federation
128 B2 **Svetlogorsk** Kaliningradskaya Oblast', W Russian Federation
122 K9 **Svetlogorsk** Krasnoyarskiy Kray, N Russian Federation
Svetlogorsk see Svyetlahorsk
129 N14 **Svetlograd** Stavropol'skiy Kray, SW Russian Federation
Svetlovodsk see Svitlovods'k
119 A14 **Svetlyy** Ger. Zimmerbude. Kaliningradskaya Oblast', W Russian Federation
129 Y8 **Svetlyy** Orenburgskaya Oblast', W Russian Federation
126 G11 **Svetogorsk** Fin. Enso. Leningradskaya Oblast', NW Russian Federation
Svetozarevo see Jagodina
111 B18 **Švihov** Ger. Schwihau. Plzeňský Kraj, W Czech Republic
112 E13 **Svilaja** ⛰ SE Croatia
112 N12 **Svilajnac** Serbia, C Yugoslavia
114 L11 **Svilengrad** prev. Mustafa-Pasha. Khaskovo, S Bulgaria
Svinecea Mare, Munte see Svinecea Mare, Vârful
116 F13 **Svinecea Mare, Vârful** var. Munte Svinecea Mare. ▲ SW Romania
95 B18 **Svínoy** Dan. Svinø. island Faeroe Islands
147 N14 **Svintsovyy Rudnik** Turkm. Swintsowyy Rudnik. Lebapskiy Velayat, E Turkmenistan
118 I13 **Svir** Rus. Svir'. Minskaya Voblasts', NW Belarus
126 I12 **Svir'** canal NW Russian Federation
Svir', Ozero see Svir, Vozyera
119 I14 **Svir, Vozyera** Rus. Ozero Svir'. ◎ C Belarus
114 J7 **Svishtov** prev. Sistova. Veliko Tŭrnovo, N Bulgaria
119 F18 **Svislach** Pol. Świsłocz, Rus. Svisloch'. Hrodzyenskaya Voblasts', W Belarus
119 M17 **Svislach** Rus. Svisloch'. Mahilyowskaya Voblasts', E Belarus
119 L17 **Svislach** Rus. Svisloch'. ∼ E Belarus
Svisloch' see Svislach
111 F17 **Svitavy** Ger. Zwittau. Pardubický Kraj, C Czech Republic
117 S6 **Svitlovods'k** Rus. Svetlovodsk. Kirovohrads'ka Oblast', C Ukraine
Svizzera see Switzerland
123 Q13 **Svobodnyy** Amurskaya Oblast', SE Russian Federation
114 G9 **Svoge** Sofiya, W Bulgaria
92 G11 **Svolvær** Nordland, C Norway
111 F18 **Svratka** Ger. Schwarzach, Schwarzawa. ∼ SE Czech Republic
113 P14 **Svrljig** Serbia, E Yugoslavia
197 U10 **Svyataya Anna Trough** var. Saint Anna Trough. undersea feature N Kara Sea
126 M4 **Svyatoy Nos, Mys** headland NW Russian Federation
119 N18 **Svyetlahorsk** Rus. Svetlogorsk. Homyel'skaya Voblasts', SE Belarus
Swabian Jura see Schwäbische Alb
97 P19 **Swaffham** E England, UK
23 V5 **Swainsboro** Georgia, SE USA
83 C19 **Swakop** ∼ W Namibia
83 C19 **Swakopmund** Erongo, W Namibia
97 M15 **Swale** ∼ N England, UK
Swallow Island see Nendö
99 M16 **Swalmen** Limburg, SE Netherlands
12 G8 **Swan** ∼ Ontario, C Canada
97 L24 **Swanage** S England, UK
182 M10 **Swan Hill** Victoria, SE Australia
11 P13 **Swan Hills** Alberta, W Canada
65 D24 **Swan Island** island C Falkland Islands
Swankalok see Sawankhalok
29 U10 **Swan Lake** ◎ Minnesota, N USA
21 Y10 **Swanquarter** North Carolina, SE USA
182 J9 **Swan Reach** South Australia
11 V15 **Swan River** Manitoba, S Canada
183 P17 **Swansea** Tasmania, SE Australia
97 J22 **Swansea** Wel. Abertawe. S Wales, UK
21 R13 **Swansea** South Carolina, SE USA
19 S7 **Swans Island** island Maine, NE USA
28 L17 **Swanson Lake** ⊟ Nebraska, C USA
31 R11 **Swanton** Ohio, N USA
110 G11 **Swarzędz** Poznań, C Poland
Swatow see Shantou
83 L22 **Swaziland** off. Kingdom of Swaziland. ◆ monarchy S Africa
93 G18 **Sweden** off. Kingdom of Sweden, Swe. Sverige. ◆ monarchy N Europe
Swedru see Agona Swedru
25 V12 **Sweeny** Texas, SW USA
33 R6 **Sweetgrass** Montana, NW USA
32 G12 **Sweet Home** Oregon, NW USA
25 T12 **Sweet Home** Texas, SW USA
27 T4 **Sweet Springs** Missouri, C USA
20 M10 **Sweetwater** Tennessee, S USA
25 P7 **Sweetwater** Texas, SW USA
33 V15 **Sweetwater River** ∼ Wyoming, C USA
Sweiham see Suwaydān
83 F26 **Swellendam** Western Cape, SW South Africa
111 G15 **Świdnica** Ger. Schweidnitz. Wałbrzych, SW Poland
111 O14 **Świdnik** Ger. Streckenbach. Lubelskie, E Poland
110 F8 **Świdwin** Ger. Schivelbein. Zachodniopomorskie, NW Poland
111 F15 **Świebodzice** Ger. Freiburg in Schlesien, Swiebodzice. Wałbrzych, SW Poland
110 E11 **Świebodzin** Ger. Schwiebus. Lubuskie, W Poland
Święciany see Švenčionys
110 I9 **Świecie** Ger. Schwertberg. Kujawsko-pomorskie, N Poland
111 L15 **Świętokrzyskie** ◐ province C Poland
11 T16 **Swift Current** Saskatchewan, S Canada
98 K9 **Swifterbant** Flevoland, C Netherlands
183 Q12 **Swifts Creek** Victoria, SE Australia
96 E13 **Swilly, Lough** Ir. Loch Súilí. inlet N Ireland
97 M22 **Swindon** S England, UK
Swinemünde see Świnoujście
110 D8 **Świnoujście** Ger. Swinemünde. Zachodniopomorskie, NW Poland
Swintsowyy Rudnik see Svintsovyy Rudnik
Świsłocz see Svislach
Swiss Confederation see Switzerland
108 E9 **Switzerland** off. Swiss Confederation, Fr. La Suisse, Ger. Schweiz, It. Svizzera; anc. Helvetia. ◆ federal republic C Europe
97 F17 **Swords** Ir. Sord, Sórd Choluim Chille. E Ireland
18 H13 **Swoyersville** Pennsylvania, NE USA
126 I10 **Syamozera, Ozero** ◎ NW Russian Federation
126 M13 **Syamzha** Vologodskaya Oblast', NW Russian Federation
118 N13 **Syanno** Rus. Senno. Vitsyebskaya Voblasts', NE Belarus
119 K16 **Syarhyeyevichy** Rus. Sergeyevichi. Minskaya Voblasts', C Belarus
126 I12 **Syas'stroy** Leningradskaya Oblast', NW Russian Federation
Sycaminum see Hefa
30 M10 **Sycamore** Illinois, N USA
128 J3 **Sychëvka** Smolenskaya Oblast', W Russian Federation
111 H14 **Syców** Ger. Gross Wartenberg. Dolnośląskie, SW Poland
14 E17 **Sydenham** ∼ Ontario, S Canada
Sydenham Island see Nonouti
183 T9 **Sydney** state capital New South Wales, SE Australia
13 R14 **Sydney** Cape Breton Island, Nova Scotia, SE Canada
Sydney Island see Manra
13 R14 **Sydney Mines** Cape Breton Island, Nova Scotia, SE Canada
Syedpur see Saidpur
119 K18 **Syelishcha** Rus. Selishche. Minskaya Voblasts', C Belarus
119 J18 **Syemyezhava** Rus. Semezhevo. Minskaya Voblasts', C Belarus
Syene see Aswân
117 X6 **Syeverodonets'k** Rus. Severodonetsk. Luhans'ka Oblast', E Ukraine
161 T6 **Sÿiao Shan** island SE China
100 H11 **Syke** Niedersachsen, NW Germany
94 D10 **Sykkylven** Møre og Romsdal, S Norway
115 F15 **Sykoúri** var. Sikouri; prev. Sikoúrion. Thessalía, C Greece
127 R11 **Syktyvkar** prev. Ust'-Sysol'sk. Respublika Komi, NW Russian Federation
23 Q4 **Sylacauga** Alabama, S USA
Sylarna see Sylene
94 J9 **Sylene** Swe. Sylarna. ▲ Norway/Sweden
153 V14 **Sylhet** Chittagong, NE Bangladesh
100 G6 **Sylt** island NW Germany
21 O10 **Sylva** North Carolina, SE USA
127 V15 **Sylva** ∼ NW Russian Federation
23 W5 **Sylvania** Georgia, SE USA
31 R11 **Sylvania** Ohio, N USA
11 Q15 **Sylvan Lake** Alberta, SW Canada
33 T13 **Sylvan Pass** pass Wyoming, C USA
23 T7 **Sylvester** Georgia, SE USA
25 P6 **Sylvester** Texas, SW USA
10 L11 **Sylvia, Mount** ▲ British Columbia, W Canada
122 K11 **Sym** ∼ C Russian Federation
115 N22 **Sými** var. Simi. island Dodekánisos, Greece, Aegean Sea
117 U8 **Synel'nykove** Dnipropetrovs'ka Oblast', E Ukraine
127 U6 **Synya** Respublika Komi, NW Russian Federation
117 P7 **Synyukha** Rus. Sinyukha. ∼ S Ukraine
Syōbara see Shōbara
195 V2 **Syowa** Japanese research station Antarctica
26 H6 **Syracuse** Kansas, C USA
29 S16 **Syracuse** Nebraska, C USA
18 H10 **Syracuse** New York, NE USA
Syracuse see Siracusa
Syrdar'inskaya Oblast' see Sirdaryo Wiloyati
Syrdariya see Syr Darya
144 L14 **Syr Darya** var. Sai Hun, Sir Darya, Syrdarya, Kaz. Syrdariya, Rus. Syrdar'ya, Uzb. Sirdaryo; anc. Jaxartes. ∼ C Asia
147 P10 **Syrdar'ya** Sirdaryo Wiloyati, E Uzbekistan
138 J6 **Syria** off. Syrian Arab Republic, var. Siria, Syrie, Ar. Al-Jumhūrīyah al-'Arabīyah as-Sūrīyah, Sūrīya. ◆ republic SW Asia
138 L9 **Syrian Desert** Ar. Al Hamad, Bādiyat ash Shām. desert SW Asia
Syrie see Syria
115 L22 **Sýrna** var. Sirna. island Kykládes, Greece, Aegean Sea
115 I20 **Sýros** var. Síros. island Kykládes, Greece, Aegean Sea
93 M18 **Sysmä** Etelä-Suomi, S Finland
127 R12 **Sysola** ∼ NW Russian Federation
Syulemeshlii see Sredets
129 S2 **Syumsi** Udmurtskaya Respublika, NW Russian Federation
114 K10 **Syuyutliyka** ∼ C Bulgaria
Syvash, Zaliv see Syvash, Zatoka
117 U12 **Syvash, Zatoka** Rus. Zaliv Syvash. inlet S Ukraine
129 Q6 **Syzran'** Samarskaya Oblast', W Russian Federation
Szabadka see Subotica
111 N21 **Szabolcs-Szatmár-Bereg** off. Szabolcs-Szatmár-Bereg Megye. ◐ county E Hungary
110 G10 **Szamocin** Ger. Samotschin. Wielkolpolskie, C Poland
116 H8 **Szamos** var. Someş, Someşul, Ger. Samosch, Somesch. ∼ Hungary/Romania
Szamosújvár see Gherla
110 G11 **Szamotuły** Poznań, C Poland
Szarkowszczyzna see Sharkawshchyna
111 M24 **Szarvas** Békés, SE Hungary
Szászmagyarós see Măieruş
Szászrégen see Reghin
Szászsebes see Sebeş
Szászváros see Orăştie
Szatmárrnémeti see Satu Mare
Száva see Sava
111 P15 **Szczebrzeszyn** Lubelskie, E Poland
110 D9 **Szczecin** Eng./Ger. Stettin. Zachodniopomorskie, NW Poland
110 G8 **Szczecinek** Ger. Neustettin. Zachodniopomorskie, NW Poland
110 D8 **Szczeciński, Zalew** var. Stettiner Haff, Ger. Oderhaff. bay Germany/Poland
111 K15 **Szczekociny** Śląskie, S Poland
110 N8 **Szczuczyn** Podlaskie, NE Poland
Szczuczyn Nowogródzki see Shchuchyn
110 M8 **Szczytno** Ger. Ortelsburg. Warmińsko-Mazurskie, NE Poland,
Szechuan/Szechwan see Sichuan
111 K21 **Szécsény** Nógrád, N Hungary
111 L25 **Szeged** Ger. Szegedin, Rom. Seghedin. Csongrád, SE Hungary
Szegedin see Szeged
111 N23 **Szeghalom** Békés, SE Hungary
Székelyhid see Săcueni
Székelykeresztúr see Cristuru Secuiesc

◆ Country ● Country Capital ◇ Dependent Territory ○ Dependent Territory Capital ◐ Administrative Region ✕ International Airport ▲ Mountain ⛰ Mountain Range ⩕ Volcano ∼ River ◎ Lake ⊟ Reservoir

111 I23 **Székesfehérvár** *Ger.* Stuhlweissenberg; *anc.* Alba Regia. Fejér, W Hungary
Szeklerburg *see* Miercurea-Ciuc
Szekler Neumarkt *see* Târgu Secuiesc
111 J25 **Szekszárd** Tolna, S Hungary
Szempcz/Szencz *see* Senec
Szenice *see* Senica
Szentágota *see* Agnita
111 J22 **Szentendre** *Ger.* Sankt Andrä. Pest, N Hungary
111 L24 **Szentes** Csongrád, SE Hungary
111 F23 **Szentgotthárd** *Eng.* Saint Gotthard, *Ger.* Sankt Gotthard. Vas, W Hungary
Szentgyörgy *see* Đurđevac
Szenttamás *see* Srbobran
Széphely *see* Jebel
Szeping *see* Siping
Szered *see* Sereď
111 N21 **Szerencs** Borsod-Abaúj-Zemplén, NE Hungary
Szeret *see* Siret
Szeretfalva *see* Sărăţel
110 N7 **Szeskie Wzgórza** *Ger.* Seesker Höhe. *hill* NE Poland
111 H25 **Szigetvár** Baranya, SW Hungary
Szilágysomlyó *see* Şimleu Silvaniei
Szinna *see* Snina
Sziszek *see* Sisak
Szitás-Keresztúr *see* Cristuru Secuiesc
111 E15 **Szklarska Poręba** *Ger.* Schreiberhau. Dolnośląskie, SW Poland
Szkudy *see* Skuodas
Szlatina *see* Slatina, Croatia
Szlavonia/Szlavonország *see* Slavonija
Szlovákia *see* Slovakia
Szluin *see* Slunj
111 L23 **Szolnok** Jász-Nagykun-Szolnok, C Hungary
Szolyva *see* Svalyava
111 G23 **Szombathely** *Ger.* Steinamanger; *anc.* Sabaria, Savaria. Vas, W Hungary
Szond/Szonta *see* Sonta
Szováta *see* Sovata
110 F13 **Szprotawa** *Ger.* Sprottau. Lubuskie, W Poland
Sztálinváros *see* Dunaújváros
Sztrazsó *see* Strážov
110 J8 **Sztum** *Ger.* Stuhm. Pomorskie, N Poland
110 H10 **Szubin** *Ger.* Schubin. Kujawsko-pomorskie, W Poland
Szucsava *see* Suceava
Szurduk *see* Surduc
111 M14 **Szydłowiec** *Ger.* Schlelau. Mazowieckie, C Poland

T

Taalintehdas *see* Dalsbruk
171 O4 **Taal, Lake** ◎ Luzon, NW Philippines
Taastrup *see* Tåstrup
111 I24 **Tab** Somogy, W Hungary
171 P4 **Tabaco** Luzon, N Philippines
186 G4 **Tabalo** Mussau Island, NE PNG
104 K5 **Tábara** Castilla-León, N Spain
186 H5 **Tabar Islands** *island group* NE PNG
Tabariya, Bahrat *see* Tiberias, Lake
143 S7 **Ţabas** *var.* Golshan. Khorāsān, C Iran
43 P15 **Tabasará, Serranía de** ▲ W Panama
41 U15 **Tabasco** ◈ *state* SE Mexico
Tabasco *see* Grijalva, Río
129 Q2 **Tabashino** Respublika Mariy El, W Russian Federation
58 B13 **Tabatinga** Amazonas, N Brazil
74 G9 **Tabelbala** W Algeria
11 Q17 **Taber** Alberta, SW Canada
171 V15 **Taberfane** Pulau Trangan, E Indonesia
95 L19 **Taberg** Jönköping, S Sweden
191 O3 **Tabiteuea** *prev.* Drummond Island. *atoll* Tungaru, W Kiribati
171 O5 **Tablas Island** *island* C Philippines
184 Q10 **Table Cape** *headland* North Island, NZ
13 S13 **Table Mountain** ▲ Newfoundland, E Canada
173 P17 **Table, Pointe de la** *headland* SE Réunion
27 S8 **Table Rock Lake** ▣ Arkansas/Missouri, C USA
36 K14 **Table Top** ▲ Arizona, SW USA
186 D8 **Tabletop, Mount** ▲ C PNG
123 R7 **Tabor** Respublika Sakha (Yakutiya), NE Russian Federation
29 S15 **Tabor** Iowa, C USA
111 D18 **Tábor** Budějovický Kraj, S Czech Republic
81 F21 **Tabora** Tabora, W Tanzania
81 F21 **Tabora** ◈ *region* C Tanzania
21 U12 **Tabor City** North Carolina, SE USA
147 Q10 **Taboshar** NW Tajikistan
76 L18 **Tabou** *var.* Tabu. S Ivory Coast
142 J2 **Tabrīz** *var.* Tebriz; *anc.* Tauris. Āžarbāyjān-e Khāvarī, NW Iran
Tabu *see* Tabou
191 W1 **Tabuaeran** *prev.* Fanning Island. *atoll* Line Islands, E Kiribati
171 O2 **Tabuk** Luzon, N Philippines
140 J4 **Tabūk** Tabūk, NW Saudi Arabia
140 J5 **Tabūk** *off.* Minţaqat Tabūk. ◈ *province* NW Saudi Arabia
187 Q13 **Tabwemasana, Mount** ▲ Espiritu Santo, W Vanuatu
95 O15 **Täby** Stockholm, C Sweden
41 N14 **Tacámbaro** Michoacán de Ocampo, SW Mexico
42 A5 **Tacaná, Volcán** ☒ Guatemala/Mexico
43 X16 **Tacarcuna, Cerro** ▲ SE Panama
Tachau *see* Tachov
158 J3 **Tacheng** *var.* Qoqek. Xinjiang Uygur Zizhiqu, NW China
54 H7 **Táchira** *off.* Estado Táchira. ◈ *state* W Venezuela
161 T13 **Tachoshui** N Taiwan
111 A17 **Tachov** *Ger.* Tachau. Plzeňský Kraj, W Czech Republic
171 Q5 **Tacloban** *off.* Tacloban City. Leyte, C Philippines
57 I19 **Tacna** Tacna, SE Peru
57 H18 **Tacna** *off.* Departamento de Tacna. ◈ *department* S Peru
32 H8 **Tacoma** Washington, NW USA
18 L11 **Taconic Range** ▲ NE USA
62 L6 **Taco Pozo** Formosa, N Argentina
57 M20 **Tacsara, Cordillera de** ▲ S Bolivia
61 F17 **Tacuarembó** *prev.* San Fructuoso. Tacuarembó, C Uruguay
61 E18 **Tacuarembó** ◈ *department* C Uruguay
61 F17 **Tacuarembó, Río** ≈ C Uruguay
83 I14 **Taculi** North Western, NW Zambia
171 Q8 **Tacurong** Mindanao, S Philippines
77 V8 **Tadek** ≈ NW Niger
74 J9 **Tademaït, Plateau du** *plateau* C Algeria
187 R17 **Tadine** Province des Îles Loyauté, E New Caledonia
80 L11 **Tadjoura** E Djibouti
80 M11 **Tadjoura, Golfe de** *Eng.* Gulf of Tajura. *inlet* E Djibouti
Tadmor/Tadmur *see* Tudmur
11 W10 **Tadoule Lake** ◎ Manitoba, C Canada
15 S8 **Tadoussac** Quebec, SE Canada
155 H18 **Tādpatri** Andhra Pradesh, E India
Tadzhikabad *see* Tojikobod
Tadzhikistan *see* Tajikistan
163 Y14 **T'aebaek-sanmaek** ▲ E South Korea
163 V15 **Taechŏng-do** *island* NW South Korea
163 X13 **Taedong-gang** ≈ C North Korea
163 Y16 **Taegu** *off.* Taegu-gwangyŏksi, *var.* Daegu, *Jap.* Taikyū. SE South Korea
Taehan-haehyŏp *see* Korea Strait
Taehan Min'guk *see* South Korea
163 Y15 **Taejŏn** *off.* Taejŏn-gwangyŏksi, *Jap.* Taiden. C South Korea
193 Z13 **Tafahi** *island* N Tonga
105 Q4 **Tafalla** Navarra, N Spain
75 M12 **Tafassâsset, Oued** ≈ SE Algeria
77 W7 **Tafassâsset, Ténéré du** *desert* N Niger
55 U11 **Tafelberg** ▲ S Suriname
97 J21 **Taff** ≈ SE Wales, UK
Tafila/Ţafilah, Muḩāfaẓat aţ *see* Aţ Ţafilah
77 N15 **Tafiré** N Ivory Coast
142 M6 **Tafresh** Markazī, W Iran
143 Q9 **Taft** Yazd, C Iran
35 R13 **Taft** California, W USA
25 T14 **Taft** Texas, SW USA
143 W12 **Taftān, Kūh-e** ▲ SE Iran
35 R13 **Taft Heights** California, W USA
189 Y14 **Tafunsak** Kosrae, E Micronesia
192 G16 **Tāga** Savai'i, SW Samoa
149 O6 **Tagāb** Kāpīsā, E Afghanistan
39 O8 **Tagagawik River** ≈ Alaska, USA
165 Q10 **Tagajō** *var.* Tagazyô. Miyagi, Honshū, C Japan
128 K12 **Taganrog** Rostovskaya Oblast', SW Russian Federation
128 K12 **Taganrog, Gulf of** *Rus.* Taganrogskiy Zaliv, *Ukr.* Tahanroz'ka Zatoka. *gulf* Russian Federation/Ukraine
Taganrogskiy Zaliv *see* Taganrog, Gulf of
76 J8 **Tagant** ◈ *region* C Mauritania
148 M14 **Tagas** Baluchistān, SW Pakistan
171 O4 **Tagaytay** Luzon, N Philippines
Tagazyô *see* Tagajō
171 P6 **Tagbilaran** *var.* Tagbilaran City. Bohol, C Philippines
106 B10 **Taggia** Liguria, NW Italy
77 V9 **Taghouaji, Massif de** ▲ C Niger
107 J15 **Tagliacozzo** Lazio, C Italy
106 J7 **Tagliamento** ≈ NE Italy
149 N3 **Tagow Bāy** *var.* Bai. Sar-e Pol, N Afghanistan
Tagtabazar *see* Takhtabazar
59 L17 **Taguatinga** Tocantins, C Brazil
186 I10 **Tagula** Tagula Island, SE PNG
186 I11 **Tagula Island** *prev.* Southeast Island, Sudest Island. *island* SE PNG
171 Q7 **Tagum** Mindanao, S Philippines
54 C7 **Tagún, Cerro** *elevation* Colombia/Panama
105 P7 **Tagus** *Port.* Rio Tejo, *Sp.* Río Tajo. ≈ Portugal/Spain
64 M9 **Tagus Plain** *undersea feature* E Atlantic Ocean
191 S10 **Tahaa** *island* Îles Sous le Vent, W French Polynesia
191 U10 **Tahanea** *atoll* Îles Tuamotu, C French Polynesia
Tahanroz'ka Zatoka *see* Taganrog, Gulf of
74 K12 **Tahat** ▲ SE Algeria
163 V12 **Ta He** ≈ NE China
163 U4 **Tahe** Heilongjiang, NE China
162 G9 **Tahilt** Govĭ-Altay, W Mongolia
191 T10 **Tahiti** *island* Îles du Vent, W French Polynesia
Tahiti, Archipel de *see* Société, Archipel de la
118 E4 **Tahkuna nina** *headland* W Estonia
148 K12 **Tāhlāb** ≈ W Pakistan
148 K12 **Tāhlāb, Dasht-i** *desert* SW Pakistan
27 R10 **Tahlequah** Oklahoma, C USA
35 Q6 **Tahoe City** California, W USA
35 P6 **Tahoe, Lake** ◎ California/Nevada, W USA
Tahoena *see* Tahuna
25 N6 **Tahoka** Texas, SW USA
32 F8 **Taholah** Washington, NW USA
77 T11 **Tahoua** Tahoua, W Niger
77 T11 **Tahoua** ◈ *department* W Niger
31 P3 **Tahquamenon Falls** *waterfall* Michigan, N USA
31 P4 **Tahquamenon River** ≈ Michigan, N USA
139 V10 **Taḩrīr** S Iraq
10 K17 **Tahsis** Vancouver Island, British Columbia, SW Canada
Tahta *see* Takhta
75 W9 **Ţahţa** C Egypt
136 L15 **Tahtalı Dağları** ▲ C Turkey
57 I14 **Tahuamanu, Río** ≈ Bolivia/Peru
56 F13 **Tahuanía, Río** ≈ E Peru
191 X7 **Tahuata** *island* Îles Marquises, NE French Polynesia
171 Q10 **Tahuna** *prev.* Tahoena. Pulau Sangihe, N Indonesia
76 L17 **Taï** SW Ivory Coast
161 P5 **Tai'an** Shandong, E China
191 R8 **Taiarapu, Presqu'île de** *peninsula* Tahiti, W French Polynesia
Taibad *see* Tāybād
160 K7 **Taibai Shan** ▲ C China
105 Q12 **Taibilla, Sierra de** ▲ S Spain
163 Q12 **Taibus Qi** *var.* Baochang. Nei Mongol Zizhiqu, N China
Taichū *see* T'aichung
161 S13 **T'aichung** *Jap.* Taichū; *prev.* Taiwan. C Taiwan
Taiden *see* Taejŏn
185 E23 **Taieri** ≈ South Island, NZ
115 E21 **Taïgetos** ▲ S Greece
161 N4 **Taihang Shan** ▲ C China
184 M11 **Taihape** Manawatu-Wanganui, North Island, NZ
161 O7 **Taihe** Anhui, E China
161 O12 **Taihe** Jiangxi, S China
Taihoku *see* T'aipei
161 R8 **Tai Hu** ◎ E China
161 P9 **Taihu** Anhui, E China
161 O6 **Taikang** Henan, C China
165 T5 **Taiki** Hokkaidō, NE Japan
166 L8 **Taikkyi** Yangon, SW Burma
Taikyū *see* Taegu
163 U8 **Tailai** Heilongjiang, NE China
168 I12 **Taileleo** Pulau Siberut, W Indonesia
182 J10 **Tailem Bend** South Australia
96 I8 **Tain** N Scotland, UK
161 S14 **T'ainan** *Jap.* Tainan; *prev.* Dainan. S Taiwan
115 E22 **Taínaro, Akrotírio** *headland* S Greece
161 Q11 **Taining** Fujian, SE China
191 W7 **Taiohae** *prev.* Madisonville. Nuku Hiva, NE French Polynesia
161 T13 **T'aipei** *Jap.* Taihoku; *prev.* Daihoku. ● (Taiwan) N Taiwan
168 J7 **Taiping** Perak, Peninsular Malaysia
163 S8 **Taiping Ling** ▲ NE China
165 Q4 **Taisei** Hokkaidō, NE Japan
165 G12 **Taisha** Shimane, Honshū, SW Japan
109 R4 **Taiskirchen** Oberösterreich, NW Austria
63 F20 **Taitao, Peninsula de** *peninsula* S Chile
Taitō *see* T'aitung
161 T14 **T'aitung** *Jap.* Taitō. S Taiwan
92 M13 **Taivalkoski** Oulu, E Finland
93 K19 **Taivassalo** Länsi-Suomi, W Finland
161 T14 **Taiwan** *off.* Republic of China, *var.* Formosa, Formo'sa. ◆ *republic* E Asia
192 F5 **Taiwan** *var.* Formosa. *island* E Asia
Taiwan *see* T'aichung
T'aiwan Haihsia/Taiwan Haixia *see* Taiwan Strait
Taiwan Shan *see* Chungyang Shanmo
161 R13 **Taiwan Strait** *var.* Formosa Strait, *Chin.* T'aiwan Haihsia, Taiwan Haixia. *strait* China/Taiwan
161 N4 **Taiyuan** *prev.* T'ai-yuan, T'ai-yüan, Yangku. Shanxi, C China
161 R7 **Taizhou** Jiangsu, E China
161 S10 **Taizhou** *prev.* Haimen, Jiaojiang. Zhejiang, SE China
Taizhou *see* Linhai
141 O16 **Ta'izz** SW Yemen
141 O16 **Ta'izz** × SW Yemen
75 P12 **Tajarhī** SW Libya
147 P13 **Tajikistan** *off.* Republic of Tajikistan, *Rus.* Tadzhikistan, *Taj.* Jumhurii Tojikiston; *prev.* Tajik S.S.R. ◆ *republic* C Asia
Tajik S.S.R *see* Tajikistan
165 O11 **Tajima** Fukushima, Honshū, C Japan
Tajoe *see* Tayu
Tajo, Río *see* Tagus
42 B5 **Tajumulco, Volcán** ▲ W Guatemala
105 P7 **Tajuña** ≈ C Spain
Tajura, Gulf of *see* Tadjoura, Golfe de
167 O9 **Tak** *var.* Rahaeng. Tak, W Thailand
189 U4 **Taka Atoll** *var.* Tōke. *atoll* Ratak Chain, N Marshall Islands
165 P12 **Takahagi** Ibaraki, Honshū, S Japan
165 H13 **Takahashi** *var.* Takahasi. Okayama, Honshū, SW Japan
Takahasi *see* Takahashi
189 P12 **Takaieu Island** *island* E Micronesia
184 I13 **Takaka** Tasman, South Island, NZ
170 M14 **Takalar** Sulawesi, C Indonesia
165 H13 **Takamatsu** *var.* Takamatu. Kagawa, Shikoku, SW Japan
Takamatu *see* Takamatsu
165 D14 **Takamori** Kumamoto, Kyūshū, SW Japan
165 D16 **Takanabe** Miyazaki, Kyūshū, SW Japan
170 M16 **Takan, Gunung** ▲ Pulau Sumba, S Indonesia
165 Q7 **Takanosu** Akita, Honshū, C Japan
Takao *see* Kaohsiung
165 L11 **Takaoka** Toyama, Honshū, SW Japan
184 N12 **Takapau** Hawke's Bay, North Island, NZ
191 U9 **Takapoto** *atoll* Îles Tuamotu, C French Polynesia
184 L5 **Takapuna** Auckland, North Island, NZ
165 J3 **Takarazuka** Hyōgo, Honshū, SW Japan
191 U9 **Takaroa** *atoll* Îles Tuamotu, C French Polynesia
165 N12 **Takasaki** Gunma, Honshū, S Japan
164 L12 **Takayama** Gifu, Honshū, SW Japan
164 K12 **Takefu** *var.* Takehu. Fukui, Honshū, SW Japan
Takehu *see* Takefu
164 C14 **Takeo** Saga, Kyūshū, SW Japan
Takeo *see* Takêv
164 C17 **Take-shima** *island* Nansei-shotō, SW Japan
142 M5 **Tākestān** *var.* Takistan; *prev.* Siadehan. Qazvin, N Iran
164 D14 **Taketa** Ōita, Kyūshū, SW Japan
167 R13 **Takêv** *prev.* Takeo. Takêv, S Cambodia
167 O10 **Tak Fah** Nakhon Sawan, C Thailand
139 T13 **Takhādīd** *well* S Iraq
149 R3 **Takhār** ◈ *province* NE Afghanistan
Takhiatash *see* Takhiatosh
146 H8 **Takhiatosh** *Rus.* Takhiatash. Qoraqalpoghiston Respublikasi, W Uzbekistan
167 S13 **Ta Khmau** Kândal, S Cambodia
146 H9 **Takhta** *Turkm.* Tahta. Dashkhovuzskiy Velayat, N Turkmenistan
146 J16 **Takhtabazar** *var.* Tagtabazar. Maryyskiy Velayat, S Turkmenistan
145 O8 **Takhtabrod** Severnyy Kazakhstan, N Kazakhstan
146 H7 **Takhtakūpir** *Rus.* Takhtakupyr. Qoraqalpoghiston Respublikasi, NW Uzbekistan
Takhtakupyr *see* Takhtakūpir
142 M8 **Takht-e Shāh, Kūh-e** ▲ C Iran
77 V12 **Takiéta** Zinder, S Niger
8 J8 **Takijuq Lake** ◎ Nunavut, NW Canada
165 S3 **Takikawa** Hokkaidō, NE Japan
165 U3 **Takinoue** Hokkaidō, NE Japan
Takistan *see* Tākestān
185 B23 **Takitimu Mountains** ▲ South Island, NZ
Takkaze *see* Tekezē
165 R7 **Takko** Aomori, Honshū, C Japan
10 L13 **Takla Lake** ◎ British Columbia, SW Canada
Takla Makan Desert *see* Taklimakan Shamo
158 H9 **Taklimakan Shamo** *Eng.* Takla Makan Desert. *desert* NW China
167 T12 **Takôk** Môndól Kiri, E Cambodia
39 P10 **Takotna** Alaska, USA
Takow *see* Kaohsiung
123 O12 **Taksimo** Respublika Buryatiya, S Russian Federation
164 C13 **Taku** Saga, Kyūshū, SW Japan
10 I10 **Taku** ≈ British Columbia, W Canada
166 M15 **Takua Pa** *var.* Ban Takua Pa. Phangnga, SW Thailand
77 W16 **Takum** Taraba, E Nigeria
191 V10 **Takume** *atoll* Îles Tuamotu, C French Polynesia
190 L16 **Takutea** *island* S Cook Islands
186 K6 **Takuu Islands** *prev.* Mortlock Group. *island group* NE PNG
119 L18 **Tal'** *Rus.* Tal'. Minskaya Voblasts', S Belarus
40 L13 **Tala** Jalisco, C Mexico
61 F19 **Tala** Canelones, S Uruguay
Talabriga *see* Aveiro, Portugal
Talabriga *see* Talavera de la Reina, Spain
119 N14 **Talachyn** *Rus.* Tolochin. Vitsyebskaya Voblasts', NE Belarus
149 U7 **Talagang** Punjab, E Pakistan
155 J23 **Talaimannar** Northern Province, NW Sri Lanka
117 R3 **Talalayivka** Chernihivs'ka Oblast', N Ukraine
43 O15 **Talamanca, Cordillera de** ▲ S Costa Rica
56 A9 **Talara** Piura, NW Peru
104 L11 **Talarrubias** Extremadura, W Spain
147 S8 **Talas** Talasskaya Oblast', NW Kyrgyzstan
147 S8 **Talas** ≈ NW Kyrgyzstan
186 G7 **Talasea** New Britain, E PNG
Talas Oblasty *see* Talasskaya Oblast'
147 S8 **Talasskaya Oblast'** *Kir.* Talas Oblasty. ◈ *province* NW Kyrgyzstan
147 S8 **Talasskiy Alatau, Khrebet** ▲ Kazakhstan/Kyrgyzstan
77 U12 **Talata Mafara** Zamfara, NW Nigeria
171 R9 **Talaud, Kepulauan** *island group* E Indonesia
104 M9 **Talavera de la Reina** *anc.* Caesarobriga, Talabriga. Castilla-La Mancha, C Spain
104 J11 **Talavera la Real** Extremadura, W Spain
186 F7 **Talawe, Mount** ▲ New Britain, C PNG
23 S5 **Talbotton** Georgia, SE USA
183 R7 **Talbragar River** ≈ New South Wales, SE Australia
62 G13 **Talca** Maule, C Chile
62 F13 **Talcahuano** Bío Bío, C Chile
154 N12 **Tālcher** Orissa, E India
25 W5 **Talco** Texas, SW USA
145 V14 **Taldykorgan** *Kaz.* Taldyqorghan; *prev.* Taldy-Kurgan. Almaty, SE Kazakhstan
Taldy-Kurgan/Taldyqorghan *see* Taldykorgan
147 Y7 **Taldy-Suu** Issyk-Kul'skaya Oblast', E Kyrgyzstan
147 U10 **Taldy-Suu** Oshskaya Oblast', SW Kyrgyzstan
Tal-e Khosravī *see* Yāsūj
193 Y15 **Taleki Tonga** *island* Otu Tolu Group, C Tonga
193 Y15 **Taleki Vavu'u** *island* Otu Tolu Group, C Tonga
102 J13 **Talence** Gironde, SW France
145 U16 **Talgar** *Kaz.* Talghar. Almaty, SE Kazakhstan
Talghar *see* Talgar
171 Q12 **Taliabu, Pulau** *island* Kepulauan Sula, C Indonesia
115 L22 **Taliarós, Akrotírio** *headland* Astypálaia, Kykládes, Greece, Aegean Sea
Ta-lien *see* Dalian
27 Q12 **Talihina** Oklahoma, C USA
Talimardzhan *see* Tollimarjon
Talin *see* T'alin
137 T12 **T'alin** *Rus.* Talin; *prev.* Verin T'alin. W Armenia
81 E15 **Tali Post** Bahr el Gabel, S Sudan
Taliq-an *see* Tāloqān
Talış Dağları *see* Talish Mountains
142 L2 **Talish Mountains** *Az.* Talış Dağları, *Per.* Kūhhā-ye Ţavālesh, *Rus.* Talyshskiye Gory. ▲ Azerbaijan/Iran
170 M16 **Taliwang** Sumbawa, C Indonesia
119 L17 **Tal'ka** *Rus.* Tal'ka. Minskaya Voblasts', C Belarus
Talkang *see* Dorbod
39 R11 **Talkeetna** Alaska, USA
39 R11 **Talkeetna Mountains** ▲ Alaska, USA
Talkhof *see* Puurmani
92 H2 **Tálknafjördhur** Vestfirdhir, W Iceland
139 Q3 **Tall 'Abţah** N Iraq
138 M2 **Tall Abyaḑ** *var.* Tell Abiad. Ar Raqqah, N Syria
23 Q4 **Talladega** Alabama, S USA
139 Q2 **Tall 'Afar** N Iraq
23 S8 **Tallahassee** *prev.* Muskogean. *state capital* Florida, SE USA
22 L2 **Tallahatchie River** ≈ Mississippi, S USA
Tall al Abyaḑ *see* At Tall al Abyaḑ
139 W12 **Tall al Laḩm** S Iraq
183 P11 **Tallangatta** Victoria, SE Australia
23 R4 **Tallapoosa River** ≈ Alabama/Georgia, S USA
103 T13 **Tallard** Hautes-Alpes, SE France
139 Q3 **Tall ash Sha'īr** N Iraq
23 Q5 **Tallassee** Alabama, S USA
139 R4 **Tall 'Azbah** NW Iraq
138 I5 **Tall Bīsah** Ḩimş, W Syria
139 R3 **Tall Ḩassūnah** N Iraq
139 Q2 **Tall Ḩuqnah** *var.* Tell Huqnah. N Iraq
Tallin *see* Tallinn
118 G3 **Tallinn** *Ger.* Reval, *Rus.* Tallin; *prev.* Revel. ● (Estonia) Harjumaa, NW Estonia
118 H3 **Tallinn** × Harjumaa, NW Estonia
138 H5 **Tall Kalakh** *var.* Tell Kalakh. Ḩimş, C Syria
139 R2 **Tall Kayf** NW Iraq
Tall Kūchak *see* Tall Kūshik
139 P2 **Tall Kūshik** *var.* Tall Kūchak. Al Ḩasakah, E Syria
31 U12 **Tallmadge** Ohio, N USA
22 J5 **Tallulah** Louisiana, S USA
139 Q2 **Tall 'Uwaynāt** NW Iraq
139 Q2 **Tall Zāhir** N Iraq
122 J13 **Tal'menka** Altayskiy Kray, S Russian Federation
122 K8 **Talnakh** Taymyrskiy (Dolgano-Nenetskiy) Avtonomnyy Okrug, N Russian Federation
117 P7 **Tal'ne** *Rus.* Tal'noye. Cherkas'ka Oblast', C Ukraine
Tal'noye *see* Tal'ne
80 E12 **Talodi** Southern Kordofan, C Sudan
188 B16 **Talofofo** SE Guam
188 B16 **Talofofo Bay** *bay* SE Guam
26 L9 **Taloga** Oklahoma, C USA
123 T10 **Talon** Magadanskaya Oblast', E Russian Federation
14 H11 **Talon, Lake** ◎ Ontario, S Canada
149 R2 **Tāloqān** *var.* Taliq-an. Takhār, NE Afghanistan
128 M8 **Talovaya** Voronezhskaya Oblast', W Russian Federation
9 N6 **Taloyoak** *prev.* Spence Bay. Nunavut, N Canada
25 Q8 **Talpa** Texas, SW USA
40 K13 **Talpa de Allende** Jalisco, C Mexico
23 S9 **Talquin, Lake** ▣ Florida, SE USA
Talsen *see* Talsi
162 H9 **Talshand** Govĭ-Altay, C Mongolia
118 E8 **Talsi** *Ger.* Talsen. Talsi, NW Latvia
143 V11 **Tal Sīāh** Sīstān va Balūchestān, SE Iran
62 G6 **Taltal** Antofagasta, N Chile
8 K10 **Taltson** ≈ Northwest Territories, NW Canada
168 K11 **Taluk** Sumatera, W Indonesia
92 J8 **Talvik** Finnmark, N Norway
182 M7 **Talyawalka Creek** ≈ New South Wales, SE Australia
Talyshskiye Gory *see* Talish Mountains
29 W14 **Tama** Iowa, C USA
Tama Abu, Banjaran *see* Penambo, Banjaran
169 U9 **Tamabo, Banjaran** ▲ East Malaysia
190 B16 **Tamakautoga** SW Niue
129 N7 **Tamala** Penzenskaya Oblast', W Russian Federation
77 P15 **Tamale** C Ghana
191 P3 **Tamana** *prev.* Rotcher Island. *atoll* Tungaru, W Kiribati
74 K12 **Tamanrasset** *var.* Tamenghest. S Algeria
74 J13 **Tamanrasset** *wadi* Algeria/Mali
166 M2 **Tamanthi** Sagaing, N Burma
97 I24 **Tamar** ≈ SW England, UK
Tamar *see* Tudmur
54 H9 **Támara** Casanare, C Colombia
54 F7 **Tamar, Alto de** ▲ C Colombia
173 X16 **Tamarin** E Mauritius
105 T5 **Tamarite de Litera** *var.* Tararite de Llitera. Aragón, NE Spain
111 I24 **Tamási** Tolna, S Hungary
Tamatave *see* Toamasina
41 O9 **Tamaulipas** ◈ *state* C Mexico
41 P10 **Tamaulipas, Sierra de** ▲ C Mexico
56 F12 **Tamaya, Río** ≈ E Peru
40 I9 **Tamazula** Durango, C Mexico
40 L14 **Tamazula** Jalisco, C Mexico
Tamazulápam *see* Tamazulapán
41 Q15 **Tamazulapán** *var.* Tamazulápam. Oaxaca, SE Mexico
41 P12 **Tamazunchale** San Luis Potosí, C Mexico
76 H11 **Tambacounda** SE Senegal
83 M16 **Tambara** Manica, C Mozambique
77 T13 **Tambawel** Sokoto, NW Nigeria
186 M9 **Tambea** Guadalcanal, C Solomon Islands
169 N10 **Tambelan, Kepulauan** *island group* W Indonesia
57 E15 **Tambo de Mora** Ica, W Peru
170 L16 **Tambora, Gunung** ☒ Sumbawa, S Indonesia
61 E17 **Tambores** Paysandú, W Uruguay
57 F14 **Tambo, Río** ≈ C Peru
56 F7 **Tamboryacu, Río** ≈ N Peru
128 M7 **Tambov** Tambovskaya Oblast', W Russian Federation
128 L6 **Tambovskaya Oblast'** ◈ *province* W Russian Federation
104 H3 **Tambre** ≈ NW Spain
169 V7 **Tambunan** Sabah, East Malaysia
81 C15 **Tambura** Western Equatoria, SW Sudan
Tamchaket *see* Tâmchekket
76 J9 **Tâmchekket** *var.* Tamchaket. Hodh el Gharbi, S Mauritania
167 T7 **Tam Điệp** Ninh Bình, N Vietnam
Tamdybulak *see* Tomdibuloq
54 H8 **Tame** Arauca, C Colombia
104 H6 **Tâmega, Rio** *Sp.* Río Támega. ≈ Portugal/Spain
115 H20 **Tamélos, Akrotírio** *headland* Kéa, Kykládes, Greece, Aegean Sea
Tamenghest *see* Tamanrasset
77 V8 **Tamgak, Adrar** ▲ C Niger
76 I13 **Tamgue** ▲ NW Guinea
41 Q12 **Tamiahua** Veracruz-Llave, E Mexico
41 Q12 **Tamiahua, Laguna de** *lagoon* E Mexico
23 Y16 **Tamiami Canal** *canal* Florida, SE USA
188 F17 **Tamil Harbor** *harbor* Yap, W Micronesia
155 H21 **Tamil Nādu** *prev.* Madras. ◈ *state* SE India
99 H20 **Tamines** Namur, S Belgium
116 E12 **Tamiš** *Ger.* Temesch, *Hung.* Temes, *SCr.* Tamiš. ≈ Romania/Yugoslavia
167 U10 **Tam Ky** Quang Nam-Đa Năng, C Vietnam
Tammerfors *see* Tampere
Tammisaari *see* Ekenäs
95 N14 **Tämnaren** ◎ C Sweden
191 Q7 **Tamotoe, Passe** *passage* Tahiti, W French Polynesia
23 V12 **Tampa** Florida, SE USA
23 V12 **Tampa** × Florida, SE USA
23 V13 **Tampa Bay** *bay* Florida, SE USA
93 L18 **Tampere** *Swe.* Tammerfors. Länsi-Suomi, W Finland
41 Q11 **Tampico** Tamaulipas, C Mexico
171 P14 **Tampo** Pulau Muna, C Indonesia
167 V11 **Tam Quan** Bình Định, C Vietnam
162 J13 **Tamsag Muchang** Nei Mongol Zizhiqu, N China
Tamsal *see* Tamsalu
118 I4 **Tamsalu** *Ger.* Tamsal. Lääne-Virumaa, NE Estonia
109 S8 **Tamsweg** Salzburg, SW Austria
166 L3 **Tamu** Sagaing, N Burma
41 P12 **Tamuín** San Luis Potosí, C Mexico
188 C15 **Tamuning** NW Guam
183 T6 **Tamworth** New South Wales, SE Australia
97 M19 **Tamworth** C England, UK
92 L8 **Tana** Finnmark, N Norway
92 M8 **Tana** *var.* Tenojoki, *Fin.* Teno, *Lapp.* Deatnu. ≈ Finland/Norway **see also** Teno
81 K19 **Tana** ≈ SE Kenya
164 I15 **Tanabe** Wakayama, Honshū, SW Japan
39 T10 **Tanacross** Alaska, USA
92 L7 **Tanafjorden** *fjord* N Norway
38 G17 **Tanaga Island** *island* Aleutian Islands, Alaska, USA
38 G17 **Tanaga Volcano** ▲ Tanaga Island, Alaska, USA
107 M18 **Tanagro** ≈ S Italy
80 H11 **T'ana Hāyk'** *Eng.* Lake Tana. ◎ NW Ethiopia
168 H11 **Tanahbela, Pulau** *island* Kepulauan Batu, W Indonesia
171 H15 **Tanahjampea, Pulau** *island* W Indonesia
168 H11 **Tanahmasa, Pulau** *island* Kepulauan Batu, W Indonesia
Tanais *see* Don
152 L10 **Tanakpur** Uttar Pradesh, N India
Tana, Lake *see* T'ana Hāyk'

◆ COUNTRY ● COUNTRY CAPITAL ◇ DEPENDENT TERRITORY ○ DEPENDENT TERRITORY CAPITAL ◈ ADMINISTRATIVE REGION × INTERNATIONAL AIRPORT ▲ MOUNTAIN ▲ MOUNTAIN RANGE ☒ VOLCANO ≈ RIVER ◎ LAKE ▣ RESERVOIR

181 P5 **Tanami Desert** *desert* Northern Territory, N Australia
167 T14 **Tân An** Long An, S Vietnam
39 Q9 **Tanana** Alaska, USA
Tananarive *see* Antananarivo
39 Q9 **Tanana River** ≈ Alaska, USA
95 C16 **Tananger** Rogaland, S Norway
188 H5 **Tanapag** Saipan, S Northern Mariana Islands
188 H5 **Tanapag, Puetton** *bay* Saipan, S Northern Mariana Islands
106 C9 **Tanaro** ≈ N Italy
163 Y12 **Tanch'ŏn** E North Korea
40 M14 **Tancitaro, Cerro** ※ C Mexico
153 N12 **Tānda** Uttar Pradesh, N India
77 O15 **Tanda** E Ivory Coast
116 L14 **Ţăndărei** Ialomiţa, SE Romania
63 N14 **Tandil** Buenos Aires, E Argentina
78 H12 **Tandjilé** *off.* Préfecture du Tandjilé. ◈ *prefecture* SW Chad
Tandjoeng *see* Tanjung
Tandjoengpandan *see* Tanjungpandan
Tandjoengpinang *see* Tanjungpinang
Tandjoengredeb *see* Tanjungredeb
149 Q16 **Tando Allāhyār** Sind, SE Pakistan
149 Q17 **Tando Bāgo** Sind, SE Pakistan
149 Q16 **Tando Muhammad Khān** Sind, SE Pakistan
182 L7 **Tandou Lake** *seasonal lake* New South Wales, SE Australia
94 L11 **Tandsjöborg** Gävleborg, C Sweden
155 H15 **Tāndūr** Andhra Pradesh, C India
164 C17 **Tanega-shima** *island* Nansei-shotō, SW Japan
165 R7 **Taneichi** Iwate, Honshū, C Japan
Tanen Taunggyi *see* Tane Range
167 N8 **Tane Range** *Bur.* Tanen Taunggyi. ▲▲ W Thailand
111 P15 **Tanew** ≈ SE Poland
21 W2 **Taneytown** Maryland, NE USA
74 H12 **Tanezrouft** *desert* Algeria/Mali
138 L7 **Ţanf, Jabal aţ** ▲ SE Syria
81 J21 **Tanga** Tanga, E Tanzania
81 I22 **Tanga** ◈ *region* E Tanzania
153 T14 **Tangail** Dhaka, C Bangladesh
186 I5 **Tanga Islands** *island group* NE PNG
155 K26 **Tangalla** Southern Province, S Sri Lanka
Tanganyika and Zanzibar *see* Tanzania
68 I13 **Tanganyika, Lake** ◎ E Africa
56 E7 **Tangarana, Río** ≈ N Peru
191 V16 **Tangaroa, Maunga** ※ Easter Island, Chile, E Pacific Ocean
74 G5 **Tanger** *var.* Tangiers, Tangier, *Fr./Ger.* Tangerk, *Sp.* Tánger; *anc.* Tingis. NW Morocco
169 N15 **Tangerang** Jawa, C Indonesia
Tangerk *see* Tanger
100 M12 **Tangermünde** Sachsen-Anhalt, C Germany
156 K10 **Tanggula Shan** *var.* Dangla, Tangla Range. ▲▲ W China
159 N13 **Tanggula Shan** ▲ W China
Tanggulashan *see* Tuotuoheyan
156 K10 **Tanggula Shankou** *pass* W China
161 N7 **Tanghe** Henan, C China
149 T5 **Tāngi** North-West Frontier Province, NW Pakistan
Tangier *see* Tanger
21 Y5 **Tangier Island** *island* Virginia, NE USA
Tangiers *see* Tanger
22 K8 **Tangipahoa River** ≈ Louisiana, S USA
Tangla Range *see* Tanggula Shan
164 J12 **Tango-hantō** *peninsula* Honshū, SW Japan
156 I10 **Tangra Yumco** *var.* Tangro Tso. ◎ W China
Tangro Tso *see* Tangra Yumco
157 T7 **Tangshan** *var.* T'ang-shan. Hebei, E China
77 R14 **Tanguiéta** NW Benin
163 X7 **Tangwang He** ≈ NE China
163 X7 **Tangyuan** Heilongjiang, NE China
92 M11 **Tanhua** Lappi, N Finland
171 U16 **Tanimbar, Kepulauan** *island group* Maluku, E Indonesia
Tanintharyi *see* Tenasserim
139 U4 **Tānjarō** ≈ E Iraq
131 T15 **Tanjong Piai** *headland* Peninsular Malaysia
Tanjore *see* Thanjāvūr
169 U12 **Tanjung** *prev.* Tandjoeng. Borneo, C Indonesia
169 W9 **Tanjungbatu** Borneo, N Indonesia
Tanjungkarang *see* Bandarlampung
169 N13 **Tanjungpandan** *prev.* Tandjoengpandan. Pulau Belitung, W Indonesia
168 M10 **Tanjungpinang** *prev.* Tandjoengpinang. Pulau Bintan, W Indonesia
169 V9 **Tanjungredeb** *var.* Tanjungredep; *prev.* Tandjoengredeb. Borneo, C Indonesia
Tanjungredep *see* Tanjungredeb
149 S8 **Tānk** North-West Frontier Province, NW Pakistan
187 S15 **Tanna** *island* S Vanuatu
93 F17 **Tännäs** Jämtland, C Sweden
Tannenhof *see* Krynica
108 K7 **Tannheim** Tirol, W Austria
Tannu-Tuva *see* Tyva, Respublika
171 Q12 **Tano** Pulau Taliabu, E Indonesia
77 O17 **Tano** ≈ S Ghana
152 D10 **Tanot** Rājasthān, NW India
77 V11 **Tanout** Zinder, C Niger
41 P12 **Tanquián** San Luis Potosí, C Mexico
77 R13 **Tansarga** E Burkina
167 T13 **Tan Son Nhat** × (Hô Chi Minh) Tây Ninh, S Vietnam
75 V8 **Tanta** *var.* Tantā, Tantâ. N Egypt
74 D9 **Tan-Tan** SW Morocco
41 P12 **Tantoyuca** Veracruz-Llave, E Mexico
152 J12 **Tāntpur** Uttar Pradesh, N India
Tan-tung *see* Dandong
38 M12 **Tanunak** Alaska, USA
166 L5 **Ta-nyaung** Magwe, W Burma
167 S5 **Tân Yên** Tuyên Quang, N Vietnam
81 F22 **Tanzania** *off.* United Republic of Tanzania, *Swa.* Jamhuri ya Muungano wa Tanzania; *prev.* German East Africa, Tanganyika and Zanzibar. ◆ *republic* E Africa
Tanzania, Jamhuri ya Muungano wa *see* Tanzania
163 U9 **Tao'an** *var.* Taoan, Taonan. Jilin, NE China
163 T8 **Tao'er He** ≈ NE China
159 U11 **Tao He** ≈ C China
T'aon-an *see* Baicheng
Taongi *see* Bokaak Atoll
107 M23 **Taormina** *anc.* Tauromenium. Sicilia, Italy, C Mediterranean Sea
37 S9 **Taos** New Mexico, SW USA
Taoudenit *see* Taoudenni
77 O6 **Taoudenni** *var.* Taoudenit. Tombouctou, N Mali
74 G6 **Taounate** N Morocco
161 S13 **T'aoyüan** *Jap.* Tōen. N Taiwan
118 I3 **Tapa** *Ger.* Taps. Lääne-Virumaa, NE Estonia
41 V17 **Tapachula** Chiapas, SE Mexico
Tapaiu *see* Gvardeysk
59 H14 **Tapajós, Rio** *var.* Tapajóz. ≈ NW Brazil
Tapajóz *see* Tapajós, Rio
61 C21 **Tapalqué** *var.* Tapalquén. Buenos Aires, E Argentina
Tapalquén *see* Tapalqué
Tapanahoni *see* Tapanahony Rivier
55 W11 **Tapanahony Rivier** *var.* Tapanahoni. ≈ E Suriname
41 T16 **Tapanatepec** *var.* San Pedro Tapanatepec. Oaxaca, SE Mexico
185 D23 **Tapanui** Otago, South Island, NZ
59 E14 **Tapauá** Amazonas, N Brazil
47 R7 **Tapauá, Rio** ≈ W Brazil
185 I14 **Tapawera** Tasman, South Island, NZ
61 I16 **Tapes** Rio Grande do Sul, S Brazil
76 K16 **Tapeta** C Liberia
154 H11 **Tāpi** *prev.* Tāpti. ≈ W India
104 J2 **Tapia de Casariego** Asturias, N Spain
56 F10 **Tapiche, Río** ≈ N Peru
167 N15 **Tapi, Mae Nam** *var.* Luang. ≈ SW Thailand
186 E8 **Tapini** Central, S PNG
Tapirapecó, Serra *see* Tapirapecó, Sierra
55 N13 **Tapirapecó, Sierra** *Port.* Serra Tapirapecó. ▲▲ Brazil/Venezuela
77 R13 **Tapoa** ≈ Benin/Niger
188 H5 **Tapochau, Mount** ▲ Saipan, S Northern Mariana Islands
111 H24 **Tapolca** Veszprém, W Hungary
21 X5 **Tappahannock** Virginia, NE USA
31 U13 **Tappan Lake** ▣ Ohio, N USA
165 Q6 **Tappi-zaki** *headland* Honshū, C Japan
Taps *see* Tapa
Tāpti *see* Tāpi
185 J16 **Tapuaenuku** ▲ South Island, NZ
171 N8 **Tapul Group** *island group* Sulu Archipelago, SW Philippines
58 E11 **Tapurmcuará** *var.* Tapuruquara. Amazonas, NW Brazil
Tapuruquara *see* Tapurmcuará
192 J17 **Taputapu, Cape** *headland* Tutuila, W American Samoa
141 W13 **Ţāqah** S Oman
139 T3 **Taqtaq** N Iraq
61 J15 **Taquara** Rio Grande do Sul, S Brazil
59 H19 **Taquari, Rio** ≈ C Brazil
60 L8 **Taquaritinga** São Paulo, S Brazil
122 I11 **Tara** Omskaya Oblast', C Russian Federation
83 I16 **Tara** Southern, S Zambia
113 J15 **Tara** ≈ SW Yugoslavia
112 K13 **Tara** ▲▲ W Yugoslavia
77 W15 **Taraba** ◈ *state* E Nigeria
77 X15 **Taraba** ≈ E Nigeria
75 O7 **Ţarābulus** *var.* Ţarābulus al Gharb, *Eng.* Tripoli. ● (Libya) NW Libya
75 O7 **Tarābulus** × NW Libya
Tarābulus/Ţarābulus ash Shām *see* Tripoli
Ţarābulus al Gharb *see* Ţarābulus
105 O7 **Taracena** Castilla-La Mancha, C Spain
117 N12 **Taraclia** *Rus.* Tarakilya. S Moldova
139 V10 **Tarād al Kahf** SE Iraq
183 R10 **Tarago** New South Wales, SE Australia
169 V8 **Tarakan** Borneo, C Indonesia
169 V9 **Tarakan, Pulau** *island* N Indonesia
Tarakilya *see* Taraclia
165 P16 **Tarama-jima** *island* Sakishima-shotō, SW Japan
184 K10 **Taranaki** *off.* Taranaki Region. ◈ *region* North Island, NZ
184 K10 **Taranaki, Mount** *var.* Egmont. ▲ North Island, NZ
105 O9 **Tarancón** Castilla-La Mancha, C Spain
188 M15 **Tarang Reef** *reef* C Micronesia
96 E7 **Taransay** *island* NW Scotland, UK
107 P18 **Taranto** *var.* Tarentum. Puglia, SE Italy
107 O19 **Taranto, Golfo di** *Eng.* Gulf of Taranto. *gulf* S Italy
Taranto, Gulf of *see* Taranto, Golfo di
62 G3 **Tarapacá** *off.* Región de Tarapacá. ◈ *region* N Chile
187 N9 **Tarapaina** Maramasike Island, N Solomon Islands
56 D10 **Tarapoto** San Martín, N Peru
138 M6 **Ţaraq an Na'jah** *hill range* E Syria
138 M6 **Ţaraq Sidāwī** *hill range* E Syria
103 Q11 **Tarare** Rhône, E France
Tararite de Llitera *see* Tamarite de Litera
184 M13 **Tararua Range** ▲▲ North Island, NZ
151 Q22 **Tarāsa Dwīp** *island* Nicobar Islands, India, NE Indian Ocean
103 Q15 **Tarascon** Bouches-du-Rhône, SE France
102 M17 **Tarascon-sur-Ariège** Ariège, S France
117 P6 **Tarashcha** Kyyivs'ka Oblast', N Ukraine
57 L18 **Tarata** Cochabamba, C Bolivia
57 I18 **Tarata** Tacna, SW Peru
190 H2 **Taratai** *atoll* Tungaru, W Kiribati
59 B15 **Tarauacá** Acre, W Brazil
59 B15 **Tarauacá, Rio** ≈ NW Brazil
191 Q8 **Taravao** Tahiti, W French Polynesia
191 R8 **Taravao, Baie de** *bay* Tahiti, W French Polynesia
191 Q8 **Taravao, Isthme de** *isthmus* Tahiti, W French Polynesia
103 X16 **Taravo** ≈ Corse, France, C Mediterranean Sea
190 J3 **Tarawa** × Tarawa, W Kiribati
190 H2 **Tarawa** *atoll* Tungaru, W Kiribati
184 N10 **Tarawera** Hawke's Bay, North Island, NZ
184 N8 **Tarawera, Lake** ◎ North Island, NZ
184 N8 **Tarawera, Mount** ▲ North Island, NZ
105 S8 **Tarayuela** ▲ N Spain
151 R16 **Taraz** *prev.* Aulie Ata, Auliye-Ata, Dzhambul, Zhambyl. Zhambyl, S Kazakhstan.
105 Q5 **Tarazona** Aragón, NE Spain
105 Q10 **Tarazona de la Mancha** Castilla-La Mancha, C Spain
145 X12 **Tarbagatay, Khrebet** ▲▲ China/Kazakhstan
96 J8 **Tarbat Ness** *headland* N Scotland, UK
149 U5 **Tarbela Reservoir** ▣ N Pakistan
96 H12 **Tarbert** W Scotland, UK
96 F7 **Tarbert** Western Isles, NW Scotland, UK
102 K16 **Tarbes** *anc.* Bigorra. Hautes-Pyrénées, S France
21 W9 **Tarboro** North Carolina, SE USA
Tarca *see* Torysa
106 J6 **Tarcento** Friuli-Venezia Giulia, NE Italy
182 F5 **Tarcoola** South Australia
105 S5 **Tardienta** Aragón, NE Spain
102 L11 **Tardoire** ≈ W France
183 U7 **Taree** New South Wales, SE Australia
92 K12 **Tärendö** Norrbotten, N Sweden
Tarentum *see* Taranto
74 C9 **Tarfaya** SW Morocco
116 J13 **Târgovişte** *prev.* Tîrgovişte. Dâmboviţa, S Romania
116 M12 **Târgu Bujor** *prev.* Tîrgu Bujor. Galaţi, E Romania
116 H13 **Târgu Cărbuneşti** *prev.* Tîrgu. Gorj, SW Romania
116 L9 **Târgu Frumos** *prev.* Tîrgu Frumos. Iaşi, NE Romania
116 H13 **Targu Jui** *prev.* Tîrgu Jiu. Gorj, W Romania
116 H9 **Târgu Lăpuş** *prev.* Tîrgu Lăpuş. Maramureş, N Romania
Târgul-Neamţ *see* Târgu-Neamţ
Târgul-Săcuiesc *see* Târgu Secuiesc
116 I10 **Târgu Mureş** *prev.* Oşorhei, Tîrgu Mures, *Ger.* Neumarkt, *Hung.* Marosvásárhely. Mureş, C Romania
116 K9 **Târgu-Neamţ** *var.* Târgul-Neamţ; *prev.* Tîrgu-Neamţ. Neamţ, NE Romania
116 K11 **Târgu Ocna** *Hung.* Aknavásár; *prev.* Tîrgu Ocna. Bacău, E Romania
116 K11 **Târgu Secuiesc** *Ger.* Neumarkt, Szekler Neumarkt, *Hung.* Kezdivásárhely; *prev.* Chezdi-Oşorheiu, Târgul-Săcuiesc, Tîrgu Secuiesc. Covasna, E Romania
145 X10 **Targyn** Vostochnyy Kazakhstan, E Kazakhstan
Tar Heel State *see* North Carolina
186 C7 **Tari** Southern Highlands, W PNG
143 P17 **Ţarīf** Abū Ẓaby, C UAE
104 K16 **Tarifa** Andalucía, S Spain
84 C14 **Tarifa, Punta de** *headland* SW Spain
57 M21 **Tarija** Tarija, S Bolivia
57 M21 **Tarija** ◈ *department* S Bolivia
141 R14 **Tarīm** C Yemen
Tarim Basin *see* Tarim Pendi
81 G19 **Tarime** Mara, N Tanzania
131 S8 **Tarim He** ≈ NW China
159 H8 **Tarim Pendi** *Eng.* Tarim Basin. *basin* NW China
149 N7 **Tarīn Kowt** *var.* Terinkot. Urūzgān, C Afghanistan
171 O12 **Taripa** Sulawesi, C Indonesia
117 Q12 **Tarkhankut, Mys** *headland* S Ukraine
27 Q1 **Tarkio** Missouri, C USA
122 J9 **Tarko-Sale** Yamalo-Nenetskiy Avtonomnyy Okrug, N Russian Federation
77 P17 **Tarkwa** S Ghana
171 O3 **Tarlac** Luzon, N Philippines
95 F22 **Tarm** Ringkøbing, W Denmark
57 E14 **Tarma** Junín, C Peru
103 N15 **Tarn** ◈ *department* S France
102 M15 **Tarn** ≈ S France
111 L22 **Tarna** ≈ C Hungary
92 G13 **Tärnaby** Västerbotten, N Sweden
149 P8 **Tarnak Rūd** ≈ SE Afghanistan
116 J11 **Târnava Mare** *Ger.* Grosse Kokel, *Hung.* Nagy-Küküllő; *prev.* Tîrnava Mare. ≈ S Romania
116 I11 **Târnava Mică** *Ger.* Kleine Kokel, *Hung.* Kis-Küküllo; *prev.* Tîrnava Mică. ≈ C Romania
116 I11 **Târnăveni** *Ger.* Marteskirch, Martinskirch, *Hung.* Dicsőszentmárton; *prev.* Sînmartin, Tîrnăveni. Mureş, C Romania
102 L14 **Tarn-et-Garonne** ◈ *department* S France
111 P18 **Tarnica** ▲ SE Poland
111 N15 **Tarnobrzeg** Podkarpackie, SE Poland
127 N12 **Tarnogskiy Gorodok** Vologodskaya Oblast', NW Russian Federation
Tarnopol *see* Ternopil'
111 M16 **Tarnów** Małopolskie, SE Poland
Tarnowice/Tarnowitz *see* Tarnowskie Góry
111 J16 **Tarnowskie Góry** *var.* Tarnowice, Tarnowskie Gory, *Ger.* Tarnowitz. Śląskie, S Poland
95 N14 **Tärnsjö** Västmanland, C Sweden
106 E9 **Taro** ≈ NW Italy
186 I6 **Taron** New Ireland, NE PNG
74 E8 **Taroudannt** *var.* Taroudant. SW Morocco
Taroudant *see* Taroudannt
23 V12 **Tarpon, Lake** ◎ Florida, SE USA
23 V12 **Tarpon Springs** Florida, SE USA
107 G14 **Tarquinia** *anc.* Tarquinii; *hist.* Corneto. Lazio, C Italy
Tarquinii *see* Tarquinia
Tarraco *see* Tarragona
76 D10 **Tarrafal** Santiago, S Cape Verde
105 V6 **Tarragona** *anc.* Tarraco. Cataluña, E Spain
105 T7 **Tarragona** ◈ *province* Cataluña, NE Spain
183 O17 **Tarraleah** Tasmania, SE Australia
23 P3 **Tarrant City** Alabama, S USA
185 D21 **Tarras** Otago, South Island, NZ
Tarrasa *see* Terrassa
105 U5 **Tàrrega** *var.* Tarrega. Cataluña, NE Spain
21 W9 **Tar River** ≈ North Carolina, SE USA
Tarsatica *see* Rijeka
136 J17 **Tarsus** İçel, S Turkey
62 K4 **Tartagal** Salta, N Argentina
137 V12 **Tärtär** *Rus.* Terter. ≈ SW Azerbaijan
102 J15 **Tartas** Landes, SW France
139 Q6 **Tārtasah** C Iraq
Tartlau *see* Prejmer
Tartous/Tartouss *see* Ţarţūs
118 J5 **Tartu** *Ger.* Dorpat; *prev. Rus.* Yurev, Yur'yev. Tartumaa, SE Estonia
118 I5 **Tartumaa** *off.* Tartu Maakond. ◈ *province* E Estonia
138 H5 **Ţarţūs** *Fr.* Tartouss; *anc.* Tortosa. Tarţūs, W Syria
138 H5 **Ţarţūs** *off.* Muḩāfaẓat Ţarţūs, *var.* Tartous, Tartus. ◈ *governorate* W Syria
164 C16 **Tarumizu** Kagoshima, Kyūshū, SW Japan
128 K4 **Tarusa** Kaluzhskaya Oblast', W Russian Federation
117 N11 **Tarutyne** Odes'ka Oblast', SW Ukraine
162 I7 **Tarvagatyn Nuruu** ▲▲ N Mongolia
106 J6 **Tarvisio** Friuli-Venezia Giulia, NE Italy
Tarvisium *see* Treviso
57 O16 **Tarvo, Río** ≈ E Bolivia
14 G8 **Tarzwell** Ontario, S Canada
40 K5 **Tasajera, Sierra de la** ▲▲ N Mexico
145 S13 **Tasaral** Zhezkazgan, C Kazakhstan
Tasböget *see* Tasbuget
145 N15 **Tasbuget** *Kaz.* Tasböget. Kzylorda, S Kazakhstan
108 E11 **Tasch** Valais, SW Switzerland
Tasek Kenyir *see* Kenyir, Tasik
122 J14 **Tashanta** Respublika Altay, S Russian Federation
Tashauz *see* Dashkhovuz
Tashi Chho Dzong *see* Thimphu
153 U11 **Tashigang** E Bhutan
137 T11 **Tashir** *prev.* Kalinino. N Armenia
143 Q11 **Ţashk, Daryācheh-ye** ◎ C Iran
Tashkent *see* Toshkent
Tashkentskaya Oblast' *see* Toshkent Wiloyati
146 J16 **Tashkepri** *Turkm.* Dashköpri. Maryyskiy Velayat, S Turkmenistan
Tash-Kömür *see* Tash-Kumyr
147 S9 **Tash-Kumyr** *Kir.* Tash-Kömür. Dzhalal-Abadskaya Oblast', W Kyrgyzstan
129 T7 **Tashla** Orenburgskaya Oblast', W Russian Federation
Tashqurghan *see* Kholm
122 J13 **Tashtagol** Kemerovskaya Oblast', S Russian Federation
95 H24 **Tåsinge** *island* C Denmark
12 M5 **Tasiujaq** Quebec, E Canada
77 W11 **Tasker** Zinder, C Niger
145 W12 **Taskesken** Vostochnyy Kazakhstan, E Kazakhstan
136 J10 **Taşköprü** Kastamonu, N Turkey
Taskuduk, Peski *see* Goshquduq Qum
186 G5 **Taskul** New Ireland, NE PNG
137 S13 **Taşlıçay** Ağrı, E Turkey
185 H14 **Tasman** *off.* Tasman District. ◈ *unitary authority* South Island, NZ
192 J12 **Tasman Basin** *var.* East Australian Basin. *undersea feature* S Tasman Sea
185 I14 **Tasman Bay** *inlet* South Island, NZ
192 I13 **Tasman Fracture Zone** *tectonic feature* S Indian Ocean
185 E19 **Tasman Glacier** *glacier* South Island, NZ
Tasman Group *see* Nukumanu Islands
183 N15 **Tasmania** *prev.* Van Diemen's Land. ◈ *state* SE Australia
183 Q16 **Tasmania** *island* SE Australia
185 H14 **Tasman Mountains** ▲▲ South Island, NZ
183 P17 **Tasman Peninsula** *peninsula* Tasmania, SE Australia
192 I11 **Tasman Plain** *undersea feature* W Tasman Sea
192 I12 **Tasman Plateau** *var.* South Tasmania Plateau. *undersea feature* SW Tasman Sea
192 I11 **Tasman Sea** *sea* SW Pacific Ocean
116 G9 **Tăşnad** *Ger.* Trestenberg, Trestendorf, *Hung.* Tasnád. Satu Mare, NW Romania
136 L11 **Taşova** Amasya, N Turkey
77 T10 **Tassara** Tahoua, W Niger
12 K4 **Tassialouc, Lac** ◎ Quebec, C Canada
Tassili du Hoggar *see* Tassili ta-n-Ahaggar
74 L11 **Tassili-n-Ajjer** *plateau* E Algeria
74 K14 **Tassili ta-n-Ahaggar** *var.* Tassili du Hoggar. *plateau* S Algeria
59 M15 **Tasso Fragoso** Maranhão, E Brazil
95 J23 **Tåstrup** *var.* Taastrup. København, E Denmark
145 O9 **Tasty-Taldy** Akmola, C Kazakhstan
143 W10 **Tāsūkī** Sīstān va Balūchestān, SE Iran
111 I22 **Tata** *Ger.* Totis. Komárom-Esztergom, NW Hungary
74 E8 **Tata** SW Morocco
Tataaihoa, Pointe *see* Vénus, Pointe
111 I22 **Tatabánya** Komárom-Esztergom, NW Hungary
191 X10 **Tatakoto** *atoll* Îles Tuamotu, E French Polynesia
75 N7 **Tataouine** *var.* Taţāwīn. SE Tunisia
55 O5 **Tataracual, Cerro** ▲ NE Venezuela
117 O12 **Tatarbunary** Odes'ka Oblast', SW Ukraine
119 M17 **Tatarka** *Rus.* Tatarka. Mahilyowskaya Voblasts', E Belarus
Tatar Pazardzhik *see* Pazardzhik
122 I12 **Tatarsk** Novosibirskaya Oblast', C Russian Federation
Tatarskaya ASSR *see* Tatarstan, Respublika
123 T13 **Tatarskiy Proliv** *Eng.* Tatar Strait. *strait* SE Russian Federation
129 R4 **Tatarstan, Respublika** *prev.* Tatarskaya ASSR. ◈ *autonomous republic* W Russian Federation
Tatar Strait *see* Tatarskiy Proliv
Taţāwīn *see* Tataouine
171 N12 **Tate** Sulawesi, N Indonesia
141 N11 **Tathlīth** 'Asīr, S Saudi Arabia
141 O11 **Tathlīth, Wādī** *dry watercourse* S Saudi Arabia
183 R11 **Tathra** New South Wales, SE Australia
129 P8 **Tatishchevo** Saratovskaya Oblast', W Russian Federation
39 S12 **Tatitlek** Alaska, USA
10 L15 **Tatla Lake** British Columbia, SW Canada
121 Q2 **Tatlısu** *Gk.* Akanthoú. N Cyprus
11 Z10 **Tatnam, Cape** *headland* Manitoba, C Canada
Tatra/Tátra *see* Tatra Mountains
111 K18 **Tatra Mountains** *Ger.* Tatra, *Hung.* Tátra, *Pol./Slvk.* Tatry. ▲▲ Poland/Slovakia
Tatry *see* Tatra Mountains
164 I13 **Tatsuno** *var.* Tatuno. Hyōgo, Honshū, SW Japan
145 S16 **Tatti** *var.* Tatty. Zhambyl, S Kazakhstan
Tatty *see* Tatti
60 L10 **Tatuí** São Paulo, S Brazil
37 V14 **Tatum** New Mexico, SW USA
25 X7 **Tatum** Texas, SW USA
Ta-t'ung/Tatung *see* Datong
Tatuno *see* Tatsuno
137 R14 **Tatvan** Bitlis, SE Turkey
95 C16 **Tau** Rogaland, S Norway
192 L17 **Ta'ū** *var.* Tau. *island* Manua Islands, E American Samoa
193 W15 **Tau** *island* Tongatapu Group, N Tonga
59 O14 **Tauá** Ceará, E Brazil
60 N10 **Taubaté** São Paulo, S Brazil
101 I19 **Tauber** ≈ SW Germany
101 I19 **Tauberbiscofsheim** Baden-Württemberg, C Germany
144 E14 **Tauchik** *Kaz.* Taūshyq. Mangistau, SW Kazakhstan
191 W10 **Tauere** *atoll* Îles Tuamotu, C French Polynesia
101 H17 **Taufstein** ▲ C Germany
190 I17 **Taukoka** *island* SE Cook Islands
145 T15 **Taukum, Peski** *desert* SE Kazakhstan
184 L10 **Taumarunui** Manawatu-Wanganui, North Island, NZ
59 A15 **Taumaturgo** Acre, W Brazil
27 X6 **Taum Sauk Mountain** ▲ Missouri, C USA
83 H22 **Taung** North-West, N South Africa
166 L6 **Taungdwingyi** Magwe, C Burma
166 M6 **Taunggyi** Shan State, C Burma
166 L5 **Taungtha** Mandalay, C Burma
166 K7 **Taungup** Arakan State, W Burma
149 S9 **Taunsa** Punjab, E Pakistan
97 K23 **Taunton** SW England, UK
19 O12 **Taunton** Massachusetts, NE USA
101 F18 **Taunus** ▲▲ W Germany
101 G18 **Taunusstein** Hessen, W Germany
184 N9 **Taupo** Waikato, North Island, NZ
184 M9 **Taupo, Lake** ◎ North Island, NZ
109 R8 **Taurach** *var.* Taurachbach. ≈ E Austria
Taurachbach *see* Taurach
118 D12 **Tauragė** *Ger.* Tauroggen. Tauragė, SW Lithuania
54 G10 **Tauramena** Casanare, C Colombia
184 N7 **Tauranga** Bay of Plenty, North Island, NZ
15 O10 **Taureau, Réservoir** ▣ Quebec, SE Canada
107 N22 **Taurianova** Calabria, SW Italy
Tauris *see* Tabrīz
184 I2 **Tauroa Point** *headland* North Island, NZ
Tauroggen *see* Tauragė
Tauromenium *see* Taormina
Taurus Mountains *see* Toros Dağları
Taus *see* Domažlice
Taūshyq *see* Tauchik
105 R5 **Tauste** Aragón, NE Spain
191 V16 **Tautara, Motu** *island* Easter Island, Chile, E Pacific Ocean
191 R8 **Tautira** Tahiti, W French Polynesia
Tauz *see* Tovuz
Ţavālesh, Kūhhā-ye *see* Talish Mountains
136 D15 **Tavas** Denizli, SW Turkey
Tavastehus *see* Hämeenlinna
Tavau *see* Davos
122 G10 **Tavda** Sverdlovskaya Oblast', C Russian Federation
122 G10 **Tavda** ≈ C Russian Federation
105 T11 **Tavernes de la Valldigna** País Valenciano, E Spain
81 I20 **Taveta** Coast, S Kenya
187 Y14 **Taveuni** *island* N Fiji
147 R13 **Tavildara** *Rus.* Tavil'dara, Tovil'-Dora. C Tajikistan
162 L8 **Tavin** Dundgovĭ, C Mongolia
104 H14 **Tavira** Faro, S Portugal
97 I24 **Tavistock** SW England, UK
167 N10 **Tavoy** *var.* Dawei. Tenasserim, S Burma
Tavoy Island *see* Mali Kyun
115 E16 **Tavropoú, Techníti Límni** ▣ C Greece
136 E13 **Tavşanlı** Kütahya, NW Turkey
187 X14 **Tavua** Viti Levu, W Fiji
97 J23 **Taw** ≈ SW England, UK
185 L14 **Tawa** Wellington, North Island, NZ
25 V6 **Tawakoni, Lake** ▣ Texas, SW USA
153 V11 **Tawang** Arunāchal Pradesh, NE India
169 R17 **Tawang, Teluk** *bay* Jawa, S Indonesia
31 R7 **Tawas Bay** ◎ Michigan, N USA
31 R7 **Tawas City** Michigan, N USA
169 V8 **Tawau** Sabah, East Malaysia
141 U10 **Ţawīl, Qalamat aţ** *well* SE Saudi Arabia
171 N9 **Tawitawi** *island* SW Philippines
Ţawkar *see* Tokar
Tāwūq *see* Dāqūq
Tawzar *see* Tozeur
41 O15 **Taxco** *var.* Taxco de Alarcón. Guerrero, S Mexico
Taxco de Alarcón *see* Taxco
158 D9 **Taxkorgan** *var.* Taxkorgan Tajik Zizhixian. Xinjiang Uygur Zizhiqu, NW China
Taxkorgan Tajik Zizhixian *see* Taxkorgan
96 J10 **Tay** ≈ C Scotland, UK
143 V6 **Tāybād** *var.* Taibad, Tāyybād, Tayyebāt. Khorāsān, NE Iran
Taybert at Turkz *see* Ţayyibat at Turkī
126 J3 **Taybola** Murmanskaya Oblast', NW Russian Federation
81 M16 **Tayeeglow** Bakool, C Somalia
96 K11 **Tay, Firth of** *inlet* E Scotland, UK
122 J12 **Tayga** Kemerovskaya Oblast', S Russian Federation
162 G8 **Taygan** Govĭ-Altay, C Mongolia
123 T9 **Taygonos, Mys** *headland* E Russian Federation
96 I11 **Tay, Loch** ◎ C Scotland, UK
11 N12 **Taylor** British Columbia, W Canada
29 O14 **Taylor** Nebraska, C USA
18 I13 **Taylor** Pennsylvania, NE USA
25 T10 **Taylor** Texas, SW USA
37 Q11 **Taylor, Mount** ▲ New Mexico, SW USA
37 R5 **Taylor Park Reservoir** ▣ Colorado, C USA
37 R6 **Taylor River** ≈ Colorado, C USA
21 P11 **Taylors** South Carolina, SE USA
20 L5 **Taylorsville** Kentucky, S USA
21 R6 **Taylorsville** North Carolina, SE USA
30 L14 **Taylorville** Illinois, N USA
140 K5 **Taymā'** Tabūk, NW Saudi Arabia
122 M10 **Taymura** ≈ C Russian Federation
123 O7 **Taymylyr** Respublika Sakha (Yakutiya), NE Russian Federation
122 L7 **Taymyr, Ozero** ◎ N Russian Federation
122 M6 **Taymyr, Poluostrov** *peninsula* N Russian Federation
122 L8 **Taymyrskiy (Dolgano-Nenetskiy) Avtonomnyy Okrug** *var.* Taymyrskiy Avtonomnyy Okrug. ◈ *autonomous district* N Russian Federation
167 S13 **Tây Ninh** Tây Ninh, S Vietnam

◆ Country
● Country Capital
◇ Dependent Territory
○ Dependent Territory Capital
◈ Administrative Region
× International Airport
▲ Mountain
▲▲ Mountain Range
※ Volcano
≈ River
◎ Lake
▣ Reservoir

122 L12 **Tayshet** Irkutskaya Oblast', S Russian Federation
171 N5 **Taytay** Palawan, W Philippines
169 Q16 **Tayu** prev. Tajoe. Jawa, C Indonesia
Tāyybād/Tayyebāt see Tāybād
138 L5 **Ţayyibah** var. At Taybé. Ḩimş, C Syria
138 I4 **Ţayyibat at Turkī** var. Taybert at Turkz. Ḩamāh, W Syria
145 P7 **Tayynsha** prev. Krasnoarmeysk. Severnyy Kazakhstan, N Kazakhstan
122 J10 **Taz** ≈ N Russian Federation
74 G6 **Taza** NE Morocco
139 T4 **Tāza Khurmātū** E Iraq
165 Q8 **Tazawa-ko** ◎ Honshū, C Japan
Taz, Bay of see Tazovskaya Guba
21 N8 **Tazewell** Tennessee, S USA
21 Q7 **Tazewell** Virginia, NE USA
75 S11 **Tāzirbū** SE Libya
39 S11 **Tazlina Lake** ◎ Alaska, USA
122 J8 **Tazovskiy** Yamalo-Nenetskiy Avtonomnyy Okrug, N Russian Federation
137 U10 **T'bilisi** Eng. Tiflis. ● (Georgia) SE Georgia
137 T10 **T'bilisi** ✕ S Georgia
79 E14 **Tchabal Mbabo** ▲ NW Cameroon
Tchad see Chad
Tchad, Lac see Chad, Lake
77 S15 **Tchaourou** E Benin
79 E20 **Tchibanga** Nyanga, S Gabon
Tchien see Zwedru
77 Z6 **Tchigaï, Plateau du** ▲ NE Niger
77 V9 **Tchighozérine** Agadez, C Niger
77 T10 **Tchin-Tabaradene** Tahoua, W Niger
78 G13 **Tcholliré** Nord, NE Cameroon
Tchongking see Chongqing
22 K4 **Tchula** Mississippi, S USA
110 I7 **Tczew** Ger. Dirschau. Pomorskie, N Poland
116 I10 **Teaca** Ger. Tekendorf, Hung. Teke; prev. Ger. Teckendorf. Bistriţa-Năsăud, N Romania
40 J11 **Teacapán** Sinaloa, C Mexico
190 A10 **Teafuafou** island Funafuti Atoll, C Tuvalu
25 U8 **Teague** Texas, SW USA
191 R9 **Teahupoo** Tahiti, W French Polynesia
190 H15 **Te Aiti Point** headland Rarotonga, S Cook Islands
65 D24 **Teal Inlet** East Falkland, Falkland Islands
185 B22 **Te Anau** Southland, South Island, NZ
185 B22 **Te Anau, Lake** ◎ South Island, NZ
41 U15 **Teapa** Tabasco, SE Mexico
184 Q7 **Te Araroa** Gisborne, North Island, NZ
184 M7 **Te Aroha** Waikato, North Island, NZ
Teate see Chieti
190 A9 **Te Ava Fuagea** channel Funafuti Atoll, SE Tuvalu
190 B8 **Te Ava I Te Lape** channel Funafuti Atoll, SE Tuvalu
190 B9 **Te Ava Pua Pua** channel Funafuti Atoll, SE Tuvalu
184 M8 **Te Awamutu** Waikato, North Island, NZ
171 X12 **Teba** Irian Jaya, E Indonesia
104 L15 **Teba** Andalucía, S Spain
128 M15 **Teberda** Karachayevo-Cherkesskaya Respublika, SW Russian Federation
74 M6 **Tébessa** NE Algeria
62 O7 **Tebicuary, Río** ≈ S Paraguay
168 L13 **Tebingtinggi** Sumatera, W Indonesia
168 I8 **Tebingtinggi** Sumatera, N Indonesia
Tebingtinggi, Pulau see Rantau, Pulau
Tebriz see Tabrīz
137 U9 **Tebulos Mt'a** Rus. Gora Tebulosmta. ▲ Georgia/Russian Federation
Tebulosmta, Gora see Tebulos Mt'a
41 Q14 **Tecamachalco** Puebla, S Mexico
40 B1 **Tecate** Baja California, NW Mexico
136 M13 **Tecer Dağları** ▲ C Turkey
103 O17 **Tech** ≈ S France
77 P16 **Techiman** W Ghana
117 N15 **Techirghiol** Constanţa, SE Romania
74 A12 **Techla** var. Techlé. SW Western Sahara
Techlé see Techla
63 H18 **Tecka, Sierra de** ▲ SW Argentina
Teckendorf see Teaca
40 K13 **Tecolotlán** Jalisco, SW Mexico
40 K14 **Tecomán** Colima, SW Mexico
35 V12 **Tecopa** California, W USA
40 G5 **Tecoripa** Sonora, NW Mexico
41 N16 **Tecpan** var. Tecpan de Galeana. Guerrero, S Mexico
Tecpan de Galeana see Tecpan
40 J11 **Tecuala** Nayarit, C Mexico
116 L12 **Tecuci** Galaţi, E Romania
31 R10 **Tecumseh** Michigan, N USA
29 S16 **Tecumseh** Nebraska, C USA
27 O11 **Tecumseh** Oklahoma, C USA
146 H14 **Tedzhen** Turkm. Tejen. Akhalskiy Velayat, S Turkmenistan
146 I15 **Tedzhen** Per. Harīrūd, Turkm. Tejen. ≈ Afghanistan/Iran see also Harīrūd
146 H15 **Tedzhenstroy** Turkm. Tejenstroy. Akhalskiy Velayat, S Turkmenistan
162 I7 **Teel** Arhangay, C Mongolia
97 L15 **Tees** ≈ N England, UK
14 E15 **Teeswater** Ontario, S Canada
190 A10 **Tefala** island Funafuti Atoll, C Tuvalu
58 D13 **Tefé** Amazonas, N Brazil
74 K11 **Tefedest** ▲ S Algeria
136 E16 **Tefenni** Burdur, SW Turkey
58 D13 **Tefé, Rio** ≈ NW Brazil
169 P16 **Tegal** Jawa, C Indonesia
100 O12 **Tegel** ✕ (Berlin) Berlin, NE Germany
99 M15 **Tegelen** Limburg, SE Netherlands
101 L24 **Tegernsee** ◎ SE Germany
107 M18 **Teggiano** Campania, S Italy
77 U14 **Tegina** Niger, C Nigeria
42 I7 **Tegucigalpa** ● (Honduras) Francisco Morazán, SW Honduras
42 H7 **Tegucigalpa** ✕ Central District, C Honduras
Tegucigalpa see Central District, Honduras
Tegucigalpa see Francisco Morazán, Honduras
77 U9 **Teguidda-n-Tessoumt** Agadez, C Niger
64 Q11 **Teguise** Lanzarote, Islas Canarias, Spain, NE Atlantic Ocean
122 K12 **Tegul'det** Tomskaya Oblast', C Russian Federation
35 S13 **Tehachapi** California, W USA
35 S13 **Tehachapi Mountains** ▲ California, W USA
Tehama see Tihāmah
Teheran see Tehrān
77 O14 **Téhini** NE Ivory Coast
143 N5 **Tehrān** var. Teheran. ● (Iran) Tehrān, N Iran
143 N6 **Tehrān** off. Ostān-e Tehrān, var. Tehran. ⬖ province N Iran
152 K9 **Tehri** Uttar Pradesh, N India
Tehri see Tikamgarh
41 Q15 **Tehuacán** Puebla, S Mexico
41 S17 **Tehuantepec** var. Santo Domingo Tehuantepec. Oaxaca, SE Mexico
41 S17 **Tehuantepec, Golfo de** var. Gulf of Tehuantepec. gulf S Mexico
Tehuantepec, Gulf of see Tehuantepec, Golfo de
Tehuantepec, Isthmus of see Tehuantepec, Istmo de
41 T16 **Tehuantepec, Istmo de** var. Isthmus of Tehuantepec. isthmus SE Mexico
(0) I16 **Tehuantepec Ridge** undersea feature E Pacific Ocean
41 S16 **Tehuantepec, Río** ≈ SE Mexico
191 W10 **Tehuata** atoll Îles Tuamotu, C French Polynesia
64 O11 **Teide, Pico de** ▲ Gran Canaria, Islas Canarias, Spain, NE Atlantic Ocean
97 I21 **Teifi** ≈ SW Wales, UK
80 B9 **Teiga Plateau** plateau W Sudan
97 J24 **Teignmouth** SW England, UK
Teisen see Chech'ŏn
116 H1 **Teiuş** Ger. Dreikirchen, Hung. Tövis. Alba, C Romania
169 U17 **Tejakula** Bali, C Indonesia
Tejen see Harīrūd/Tedzhen
Tejenstroy see Tedzhenstroy
35 S14 **Tejon Pass** pass California, W USA
Tejo, Rio see Tagus
41 O14 **Tejupilco** var. Tejupilco de Hidalgo. México, S Mexico
Tejupilco de Hidalgo see Tejupilco
184 P7 **Te Kaha** Bay of Plenty, North Island, NZ
29 S14 **Tekamah** Nebraska, C USA
184 I1 **Te Kao** Northland, North Island, NZ
185 F20 **Tekapo** ≈ South Island, NZ
185 F19 **Tekapo, Lake** ◎ South Island, NZ
184 P9 **Te Karaka** Gisborne, North Island, NZ
184 L7 **Te Kauwhata** Waikato, North Island, NZ
41 X12 **Tekax** var. Tekax de Álvaro Obregón. Yucatán, SE Mexico
Tekax de Álvaro Obregón see Tekax
Teke/Tekendorf see Teaca
136 A14 **Teke Burnu** headland W Turkey
114 M12 **Teke Deresi** ≈ NW Turkey
146 D10 **Tekedzhik, Gory** hill range NW Turkmenistan
145 V14 **Tekeli** Almaty, SE Kazakhstan
145 R7 **Teke, Ozero** ◎ N Kazakhstan
158 I5 **Tekes** Xinjiang Uygur Zizhiqu, NW China
145 W16 **Tekes** Almaty, SE Kazakhstan
Tekes see Tekes He
158 H5 **Tekes He** Rus. Tekes. ≈ China/Kazakhstan
80 I10 **Tekezē** var. Takkaze. ≈ Eritrea/Ethiopia
Tekhtin see Tsyakhtsin
136 C10 **Tekirdağ** It. Rodosto; anc. Bisanthe, Raidestos, Rhaedestus. Tekirdağ, NW Turkey
136 C10 **Tekirdağ** ⬖ province NW Turkey
155 N14 **Tekkali** Andhra Pradesh, E India
115 K15 **Tekke Burnu** Turk. İlyasbaba Burnu. headland NW Turkey
137 Q13 **Tekman** Erzurum, NE Turkey
32 M9 **Tekoa** Washington, NW USA
190 H16 **Te Kou** ▲ Rarotonga, S Cook Islands
Tekrit see Tikrīt
171 P12 **Teku** Sulawesi, N Indonesia
184 L9 **Te Kuiti** Waikato, North Island, NZ
42 H4 **Tela** Atlántida, NW Honduras
138 F12 **Telalim** Southern, S Israel
Telanaipura see Jambi
137 U10 **T'elavi** E Georgia
138 F10 **Tel Aviv** ⬖ district W Israel
Tel Aviv-Jaffa see Tel Aviv-Yafo
138 F10 **Tel Aviv-Yafo** var. Tel Aviv-Jaffa. Tel Aviv, C Israel
138 F10 **Tel Aviv-Yafo** ✕ Tel Aviv, C Israel
111 E18 **Telč** Ger. Teltsch. Jihlavský Kraj, C Czech Republic
186 B6 **Telefomin** Sandaun, NW Papua New Guinea
10 J10 **Telegraph Creek** British Columbia, W Canada
190 B10 **Telele** island Funafuti Atoll, C Tuvalu
60 J11 **Telêmaco Borba** Paraná, S Brazil
95 E15 **Telemark** ⬖ county S Norway
62 J13 **Telén** La Pampa, C Argentina
Teleneshty see Teleneşti
116 M9 **Teleneşti** Rus. Teleneshty. C Moldova
104 J4 **Teleno, El** ▲ NW Spain
116 I15 **Teleorman** ⬖ county S Romania
116 I14 **Teleorman** ≈ S Romania
25 V5 **Telephone** Texas, SW USA
35 U11 **Telescope Peak** ▲ California, W USA
Teles Pirés see São Manuel, Rio
97 L19 **Telford** C England, UK
108 L7 **Telfs** Tirol, W Austria
42 J8 **Telica** León, NW Nicaragua
42 J6 **Telica, Río** ≈ C Honduras
76 I13 **Télimélé** Guinée-Maritime, W Guinea
43 O14 **Telire, Río** ≈ Costa Rica/Panama
114 J8 **Telish** prev. Azizie. Pleven, N Bulgaria
41 R16 **Telixtlahuaca** var. San Francisco Telixtlahuaca. Oaxaca, SE Mexico
10 K13 **Telkwa** British Columbia, SW Canada
25 P4 **Tell** Texas, SW USA
Tell Abiad see Tall Abyaḑ
Tell Abiad/Tell Abyad see At Tall al Abyaḑ
31 O16 **Tell City** Indiana, N USA
38 M9 **Teller** Alaska, USA
Tell Huqnah see Tall Ḩuqnah
155 F20 **Tellicherry** var. Thalassery. Kerala, SW India
20 M10 **Tellico Plains** Tennessee, S USA
Tell Kalakh see Tall Kalakh
Tell Mardīkh see Ebla
54 E11 **Tello** Huila, C Colombia
Tell Shedadi see Ash Shadādah
37 Q7 **Telluride** Colorado, C USA
Tel'man/Tel'mansk see Gubadag
117 X9 **Tel'manove** Donets'ka Oblast', E Ukraine
162 H6 **Telmen Nuur** ◎ NW Mongolia
Teloekbetoeng see Bandarlampung
41 O15 **Teloloapán** Guerrero, S Mexico
Telo Martius see Toulon
127 V8 **Telposiz, Gora** ▲ NW Russian Federation
Telschen see Telšiai
63 J17 **Telsen** Chubut, S Argentina
118 D11 **Telšiai** Ger. Telschen. Telšiai, NW Lithuania
Teltsch see Telč
Telukbetung see Bandarlampung
168 H10 **Telukdalam** Pulau Nias, W Indonesia
14 H9 **Temagami** Ontario, S Canada
14 G9 **Temagami, Lake** ◎ Ontario, S Canada
190 H16 **Te Manga** ▲ Rarotonga, S Cook Islands
191 W12 **Tematangi** atoll Îles Tuamotu, S French Polynesia
41 X11 **Temax** Yucatán, SE Mexico
171 W14 **Tembagapura** Irian Jaya, E Indonesia
131 U5 **Tembenchi** ≈ N Russian Federation
55 P6 **Temblador** Monagas, NE Venezuela
105 N9 **Tembleque** Castilla-La Mancha, C Spain
Temboni see Mitemele, Río
35 U16 **Temecula** California, W USA
168 K7 **Temengor, Tasik** ⊠ Peninsular Malaysia
112 L9 **Temerin** Serbia, N Yugoslavia
Temes/Temesch see Tamiš
Temeschburg/Temeschwar see Timişoara
Temes-Kubin see Kovin
Temesvár/Temeswar see Timişoara
Teminaboean see Teminabuan
171 U12 **Teminabuan** prev. Teminaboean. Irian Jaya, E Indonesia
145 P17 **Temirlanovka** Yuzhnyy Kazakhstan, S Kazakhstan
145 R10 **Temirtau** prev. Samarkandski, Samarkandskoye. Karaganda, C Kazakhstan
14 H10 **Témiscaming** Quebec, SE Canada
Témiscamingue, Lac see Timiskaming, Lake
15 T8 **Témiscouata, Lac** ◎ Quebec, SE Canada
129 N5 **Temnikov** Respublika Mordoviya, W Russian Federation
191 Y13 **Temoe** island Îles Gambier, E French Polynesia
183 Q9 **Temora** New South Wales, SE Australia
40 H7 **Témoris** Chihuahua, W Mexico
40 I5 **Temósachic** Chihuahua, N Mexico
187 Q10 **Temotu** off. Temotu Province. ⬖ province E Solomon Islands
36 L14 **Tempe** Arizona, SW USA
Tempelburg see Czaplinek
107 C17 **Tempio Pausania** Sardegna, Italy, C Mediterranean Sea
42 K12 **Tempisque, Río** ≈ NW Costa Rica
25 T9 **Temple** Texas, SW USA
100 O12 **Tempelhof** ✕ (Berlin) Berlin, NE Germany
97 D19 **Templemore** Ir. An Teampall Mór. C Ireland
100 O11 **Templin** Brandenburg, NE Germany
41 P12 **Tempoal** var. Tempoal de Sánchez. Veracruz-Llave, E Mexico
Tempoal de Sánchez see Tempoal
41 P13 **Tempoal, Río** ≈ C Mexico
83 E14 **Tempué** Moxico, C Angola
128 J14 **Temryuk** Krasnodarskiy Kray, SW Russian Federation
99 G17 **Temse** Oost-Vlaanderen, N Belgium
63 F15 **Temuco** Araucanía, C Chile
185 G20 **Temuka** Canterbury, South Island, NZ
189 P13 **Temwen Island** island E Micronesia
56 C6 **Tena** Napo, C Ecuador
41 W13 **Tenabo** Campeche, E Mexico
Tenaghau see Aola
25 X7 **Tenaha** Texas, SW USA
39 X13 **Tenake** Chichagof Island, Alaska, USA
155 K16 **Tenāli** Andhra Pradesh, E India
Tenan see Ch'ŏnan
41 O14 **Tenancingo** var. Tenencingo de Degollado. México, S Mexico
191 X12 **Tenararo** island Groupe Actéon, SE French Polynesia
167 N12 **Tenasserim** Tenasserim, S Burma
167 N11 **Tenasserim** var. Tanintharyi. ⬖ division S Burma
98 O5 **Ten Boer** Groningen, NE Netherlands
97 I21 **Tenby** SW Wales, UK
80 K11 **Tendaho** Afar, NE Ethiopia
103 V14 **Tende** Alpes Maritimes, SE France
151 Q20 **Ten Degree Channel** strait Andaman and Nicobar Islands, India, E Indian Ocean
80 F11 **Tendelti** White Nile, E Sudan
76 G8 **Te-n-Dghâmcha, Sebkhet** var. Sebkha de Ndrhamcha, Sebkra de Ndaghamcha. salt lake W Mauritania
165 P10 **Tendō** Yamagata, Honshū, C Japan
74 H7 **Tendrara** NE Morocco
117 Q11 **Tendrivs'ka Kosa** spit S Ukraine
117 Q11 **Tendrivs'ka Zatoka** gulf S Ukraine
Tenencingo de Degollado see Tenancingo
77 N11 **Ténenkou** Mopti, C Mali
77 W9 **Ténéré** physical region C Niger
77 W9 **Ténére, Erg du** desert C Niger
64 O11 **Tenerife** island Islas Canarias, Spain, NE Atlantic Ocean
74 J5 **Ténès** NW Algeria
170 M15 **Tengah, Kepulauan** island group C Indonesia
169 V11 **Tenggarong** Borneo, C Indonesia
162 J15 **Tengger Shamo** desert N China
168 L8 **Tenggul, Pulau** island Peninsular Malaysia
Tengiz Köl see Tengiz, Ozero
145 P9 **Tengiz, Ozero** Kaz. Tengiz Köl. salt lake C Kazakhstan
76 M14 **Tengréla** var. Tingréla. N Ivory Coast
160 M14 **Tengxian** var. Teng Xian. Guangxi Zhuangzu Zizhiqu, S China
194 H2 **Teniente Rodolfo Marsh** Chilean research station South Shetland Islands, Antarctica
32 G9 **Tenino** Washington, NW USA
112 I9 **Tenja** Osijek-Baranja, E Croatia
188 B16 **Tenjo, Mount** ▲ W Guam
155 H23 **Tenkāsi** Tamil Nādu, SE India
79 N24 **Tenke** Katanga, SE Dem. Rep. Congo (Zaire)
Tenke see Tinca
123 Q7 **Tenkeli** Respublika Sakha (Yakutiya), NE Russian Federation
27 R10 **Tenkiller Ferry Lake** ⊠ Oklahoma, C USA
77 Q13 **Tenkodogo** S Burkina
181 Q5 **Tennant Creek** Northern Territory, C Australia
20 G9 **Tennessee** off. State of Tennessee; also known as The Volunteer State. ⬖ state SE USA
37 R5 **Tennessee Pass** pass Colorado, C USA
20 H10 **Tennessee River** ≈ S USA
23 N2 **Tennessee Tombigbee Waterway** canal Alabama/Mississippi, S USA
99 K22 **Tenneville** Luxembourg, SE Belgium
92 M11 **Tenniöjoki** ≈ NE Finland
92 L9 **Teno** var. Tenojoki, Lapp. Dealnu, Nor. Tana. ≈ Finland/Norway see also Tana
Tenojoki see Tana/Teno
169 U7 **Tenom** Sabah, East Malaysia
Tenos see Tínos
41 V15 **Tenosique** var. Tenosique de Pino Suárez. Tabasco, SE Mexico
Tenosique de Pino Suárez see Tenosique
22 I6 **Tensas River** ≈ Louisiana, S USA
23 O8 **Tensaw River** ≈ Alabama, S USA
74 E7 **Tensift** seasonal river W Morocco
171 O12 **Tentena** var. Tenteno. Sulawesi, C Indonesia
Tenteno see Tentena
183 U4 **Tenterfield** New South Wales, SE Australia
23 X16 **Ten Thousand Islands** island group Florida, SE USA
60 H9 **Teodoro Sampaio** São Paulo, S Brazil
59 N19 **Teófilo Otoni** var. Theophilo Ottoni. Minas Gerais, NE Brazil
116 K5 **Teofipol'** Khmel'nyts'ka Oblast', W Ukraine
191 Q8 **Teohatu** Tahiti, W French Polynesia
41 P14 **Teotihuacán** ruins México, S Mexico
Teotilán see Teotitlán del Camino
41 Q15 **Teotitlán del Camino** var. Teotilán. Oaxaca, S Mexico
190 G12 **Tepa** Île Uvea, E Wallis and Futuna
191 P8 **Tepaee, Récif** reef Tahiti, W French Polynesia
40 L14 **Tepalcatepec** Michoacán de Ocampo, SW Mexico
190 A16 **Tepa Point** headland SW Niue
40 L13 **Tepatitlán** var. Tepatitlán de Morelos. Jalisco, SW Mexico
Tepatitlán de Morelos see Tepatitlán
40 J9 **Tepehuanes** var. Santa Catarina de Tepehuanes. Durango, C Mexico
Tepelena see Tepelenë
113 L22 **Tepelenë** var. Tepelena, It. Tepeleni. Gjirokastër, S Albania
Tepeleni see Tepelenë
40 K12 **Tepic** Nayarit, C Mexico
111 C15 **Teplice** Ger. Teplitz; prev. Teplice-Šanov, Teplitz-Schönau. Ústecký Kraj, NW Czech Republic
Teplice-Šanov/Teplitz/Teplitz-Schönau see Teplice
117 O7 **Teplyk** Vinnyts'ka Oblast', C Ukraine
123 R10 **Teplyy Klyuch** Respublika Sakha (Yakutiya), NE Russian Federation
40 E5 **Tepoca, Cabo** headland NW Mexico
191 W9 **Tepoto** island Îles du Désappointement, C French Polynesia
92 L11 **Tepsa** Lappi, N Finland
190 B8 **Tepuka** atoll Funafuti Atoll, C Tuvalu
184 N7 **Te Puke** Bay of Plenty, North Island, NZ
40 L13 **Tequila** Jalisco, SW Mexico
41 O13 **Tequisquiapan** Querétaro de Arteaga, C Mexico
104 J5 **Tera** ≈ NW Spain
77 Q12 **Téra** Tillabéri, W Niger
191 V1 **Teraina** prev. Washington Island. atoll Line Islands, E Kiribati
81 F15 **Terakeka** Bahr el Gabel, S Sudan
107 J14 **Teramo** anc. Interamna. Abruzzo, C Italy
98 P7 **Ter Apel** Groningen, NE Netherlands
104 H11 **Tera, Ribeira de** ≈ S Portugal
185 K14 **Terawhiti, Cape** headland North Island, NZ
98 N12 **Terborg** Gelderland, E Netherlands
137 P13 **Tercan** Erzincan, NE Turkey
64 O2 **Terceira** ✕ Terceira, Azores, Portugal, NE Atlantic Ocean
64 O2 **Terceira** var. Ilha Terceira. island Azores, Portugal, NE Atlantic Ocean
Terceira, Ilha see Terceira
116 K6 **Terebovlya** Ternopil's'ka Oblast', W Ukraine
129 O15 **Terek** ≈ SW Russian Federation
Terekhovka see Tsyerakhowka
147 R9 **Terek-Say** Dzhalal-Abadskaya Oblast', W Kyrgyzstan
168 L7 **Terengganu** var. Trengganu. ⬖ state Peninsular Malaysia
129 X7 **Terensay** Orenburgskaya Oblast', W Russian Federation
58 N13 **Teresina** var. Therezina. state capital Piauí, NE Brazil
60 P9 **Teresópolis** Rio de Janeiro, SE Brazil
110 P12 **Terespol** Lubelskie, E Poland
191 V16 **Terevaka, Maunga** ⛰ Easter Island, Chile, E Pacific Ocean
103 P3 **Tergnier** Aisne, N France
43 O14 **Teribe, Río** ≈ NW Panama
126 K3 **Teriberka** Murmanskaya Oblast', NW Russian Federation
Terijoki see Zelenogorsk
Terinkot see Tarīn Kowt
Terisaqqan see Tersakkan
24 K12 **Terlingua** Texas, SW USA
24 K11 **Terlingua Creek** ≈ Texas, SW USA
62 K7 **Termas de Río Hondo** Santiago del Estero, N Argentina
136 M11 **Terme** Samsun, N Turkey
Termez see Termiz
Termia see Kýthnos
107 J23 **Termini Imerese** anc. Thermae Himerenses. Sicilia, Italy, C Mediterranean Sea
41 V14 **Términos, Laguna de** lagoon SE Mexico
77 X10 **Termit-Kaoboul** Zinder, C Niger
147 O14 **Termiz** Rus. Termez. Surkhondaryo Wiloyati, S Uzbekistan
107 L15 **Termoli** Molise, C Italy
Termonde see Dendermonde
98 P5 **Termunten** Groningen, NE Netherlands
171 R11 **Ternate** Pulau Ternate, E Indonesia
109 T5 **Ternberg** Oberösterreich, N Austria
99 E15 **Terneuzen** var. Neuzen. Zeeland, SW Netherlands
123 T14 **Terney** Primorskiy Kray, SE Russian Federation
107 I14 **Terni** anc. Interamna Nahars. Umbria, C Italy
109 X6 **Ternitz** Niederösterreich, E Austria
117 V7 **Ternivka** Dnipropetrovs'ka Oblast', E Ukraine
116 K6 **Ternopil'** Pol. Tarnopol, Rus. Ternopol'. Ternopil's'ka Oblast', W Ukraine
Ternopil' see Ternopil's'ka Oblast'
116 I6 **Ternopil's'ka Oblast'** var. Ternopil', Rus. Ternopol'skaya Oblast'. ⬖ province NW Ukraine
Ternopol' see Ternopil'
Ternopol'skaya Oblast' see Ternopil's'ka Oblast'
123 U13 **Terpeniya, Mys** headland Ostrov Sakhalin, SE Russian Federation
Térraba, Río see Grande de Térraba, Río
10 J13 **Terrace** British Columbia, W Canada
12 D12 **Terrace Bay** Ontario, S Canada
107 I16 **Terracina** Lazio, C Italy
93 F14 **Terråk** Troms, N Norway
26 M13 **Terral** Oklahoma, C USA
107 B19 **Terralba** Sardegna, Italy, C Mediterranean Sea
Terranova di Sicilia see Gela
Terranova Pausania see Olbia
105 W5 **Terrassa** Cast. Tarrasa. Cataluña, E Spain
15 O12 **Terrebonne** Quebec, SE Canada
22 J11 **Terrebonne Bay** bay Louisiana, SE USA
31 N14 **Terre Haute** Indiana, N USA
25 U6 **Terrell** Texas, SW USA
Terre Neuve see Newfoundland
33 Q14 **Terreton** Idaho, NW USA
103 T7 **Territoire-de-Belfort** ⬖ department E France
33 X9 **Terry** Montana, NW USA
28 I9 **Terry Peak** ▲ South Dakota, N USA
136 H14 **Tersakan Gölü** ◎ C Turkey
145 O10 **Tersakkan** Kaz. Terisaqqan. ≈ C Kazakhstan
98 J4 **Terschelling** Fris. Skylge. island Waddeneilanden, N Netherlands
78 H10 **Tersef** Chari-Baguirmi, C Chad
147 X8 **Terskey Ala-Too, Khrebet** ▲ Kazakhstan/Kyrgyzstan
Terter see Tärtär
105 R8 **Teruel** anc. Turba. Aragón, E Spain
105 R7 **Teruel** ⬖ province Aragón, E Spain
114 M7 **Tervel** prev. Kurtbunar, Rom. Curtbunar. Dobrich, NE Bulgaria
93 M16 **Tervo** Itä-Suomi, C Finland
92 L13 **Tervola** Lappi, NW Finland
Tervueren see Tervuren
99 H18 **Tervuren** var. Tervueren. Vlaams Brabant, C Belgium
112 H11 **Tešanj** Federacija Bosna I Hercegovina, N Bosnia and Herzegovina
Teschen see Cieszyn
83 M19 **Tesenane** Inhambane, S Mozambique
80 I9 **Teseney** var. Tessenei. W Eritrea
39 P5 **Teshekpuk Lake** ◎ Alaska, USA
162 K6 **Teshig** Bulgan, N Mongolia
165 T2 **Teshio** Hokkaidō, NE Japan
165 T2 **Teshio-sanchi** ▲ Hokkaidō, NE Japan
Těšín see Cieszyn
Tesio Gawa see Teshio-gawa
162 F5 **Tesiyn Gol** var. Tes-Khem. ≈ Mongolia/Russian Federation see also Tes-Khem
131 T7 **Tes-Khem** var. Tesiyn Gol. ≈ Mongolia/Russian Federation see also Tesiyn Gol
112 H11 **Teslić** Republika Srpska, N Bosnia and Herzegovina
10 I9 **Teslin** Yukon Territory, W Canada
10 I8 **Teslin** ≈ British Columbia/Yukon Territory, W Canada
77 Q8 **Tessalit** Kidal, NE Mali
77 V12 **Tessaoua** Maradi, S Niger
99 J17 **Tessenderlo** Limburg, NE Belgium
Tessenei see Teseney
14 L7 **Tessier, Lac** ◎ Quebec, SE Canada
Tessin see Ticino
97 M23 **Test** ≈ S England, UK
Testama see Tõstamaa
55 P4 **Testigos, Islas los** island group N Venezuela
37 S10 **Tesuque** New Mexico, SW USA
103 O17 **Têt** var. Tet. ≈ S France
54 G5 **Tetas, Cerro de las** ▲ NW Venezuela
83 M15 **Tete** Tete, NW Mozambique
83 M15 **Tete** off. Província de Tete. ⬖ province NW Mozambique
11 N15 **Tête Jaune Cache** British Columbia, SW Canada
184 O8 **Te Teko** Bay of Plenty, North Island, NZ
186 K9 **Tetepare** island New Georgia Islands, NW Solomon Islands
Teterev see Teteriv
116 M5 **Teteriv** Rus. Teterev. ≈ N Ukraine
100 M9 **Teterow** Mecklenburg-Vorpommern, NE Germany
114 I9 **Teteven** Lovech, N Bulgaria
191 T10 **Tetiaroa** atoll Îles du Vent, W French Polynesia
105 P14 **Tetica de Bacares** ▲ S Spain
Tetiyev see Tetiyiv
117 O6 **Tetiyiv** Rus. Tetiyev. Kyyivs'ka Oblast', N Ukraine
39 T10 **Tetlin** Alaska, USA
33 R8 **Teton River** ≈ Montana, NW USA
74 G5 **Tétouan** var. Tetouan, Tetuán. N Morocco
Tetova/Tetovë see Tetovo
114 L7 **Tetovo** Razgrad, N Bulgaria
113 N18 **Tetovo** Alb. Tetova, Tetovë, Turk. Kalkandelen. NW FYR Macedonia
115 E20 **Tetrázio** ▲ S Greece
Tetschen see Děčín
Tetuán see Tétouan
191 Q8 **Tetufera, Mont** ▲ Tahiti, W French Polynesia
129 R4 **Tetyushi** Respublika Tatarstan, W Russian Federation
108 I7 **Teufen** Sankt Gallen, NE Switzerland
40 L12 **Teul** var. Teul de Gonzáles Ortega. Zacatecas, C Mexico
107 B21 **Teulada** Sardegna, Italy, C Mediterranean Sea
Teul de Gonzáles Ortega see Teul
11 X16 **Teulon** Manitoba, S Canada
42 I7 **Teupasenti** El Paraíso, S Honduras
165 S2 **Teuri-tō** island NE Japan
100 G13 **Teutoburger Wald** Eng. Teutoburg Forest. hill range NW Germany

◆ Country ● Country Capital ◇ Dependent Territory ○ Dependent Territory Capital ⬖ Administrative Region ✕ International Airport ▲ Mountain ▲ Mountain Range ⛰ Volcano ≈ River ◎ Lake ⊠ Reservoir

Teutoburg Forest *see* Teutoburger Wald
93 K17 **Teuva** *Swe.* Östermark. Länsi-Suomi, W Finland
107 H15 **Tevere** *Eng.* Tiber. ≈ C Italy
138 G9 **Teverya** *var.* Tiberias, Tverya. Northern, N Israel
96 K13 **Teviot** ≈ SE Scotland, UK
Tevli *see* Tewli
122 H11 **Tevriz** Omskaya Oblast', C Russian Federation
185 B24 **Te Waewae Bay** *bay* South Island, NZ
97 L21 **Tewkesbury** C England, UK
119 F19 **Tewli** *Rus.* Tevli. Brestskaya Voblasts', SW Belarus
159 U12 **Têwo** *var.* Dêngkagoin. Gansu, C China
25 U12 **Texana, Lake** ◎ Texas, SW USA
27 S14 **Texarkana** Arkansas, C USA
25 X5 **Texarkana** Texas, SW USA
25 N9 **Texas** *off.* State of Texas; also known as The Lone Star State. ◈ *state* S USA
25 W12 **Texas City** Texas, SW USA
41 P14 **Texcoco** México, C Mexico
98 I6 **Texel** *island* Waddeneilanden, NW Netherlands
26 H8 **Texhoma** Oklahoma, C USA
25 N1 **Texhoma** Texas, SW USA
37 W12 **Texico** New Mexico, SW USA
24 L1 **Texline** Texas, SW USA
41 P14 **Texmelucan** *var.* San Martín Texmelucan. Puebla, S Mexico
27 O13 **Texoma, Lake** ⊠ Oklahoma/Texas, C USA
25 N9 **Texon** Texas, SW USA
83 J23 **Teyateyaneng** NW Lesotho
126 M16 **Teykovo** Ivanovskaya Oblast', W Russian Federation
126 M16 **Teza** ≈ W Russian Federation
41 Q13 **Teziutlán** Puebla, S Mexico
153 W12 **Tezpur** Assam, NE India
9 N10 **Tha-Anne** ≈ Nunavut, NE Canada
83 K23 **Thabana Ntlenyana** *var.* Thabantshonyana, Mount Ntlenyana. ▲ E Lesotho
Thabantshonyana *see* Thabana Ntlenyana
83 J23 **Thaba Putsoa** ▲ C Lesotho
167 Q8 **Tha Bo** Nong Khai, E Thailand
103 T12 **Thabor, Pic du** ▲ E France
Tha Chin *see* Samut Sakhon
166 M7 **Thagaya** Pegu, C Burma
Thai, Ao *see* Thailand, Gulf of
167 T6 **Thai Binh** Thai Binh, N Vietnam
167 S7 **Thai Hoa** Nghê An, N Vietnam
167 P9 **Thailand** *off.* Kingdom of Thailand, *Th.* Prathet Thai; *prev.* Siam. ◆ *monarchy* SE Asia
167 P13 **Thailand, Gulf of** *var.* Gulf of Siam, *Th.* Ao Thai, *Vtn.* Vinh Thai Lan. *gulf* SE Asia
Thai Lan, Vinh *see* Thailand, Gulf of
167 T6 **Thai Nguyên** Băc Thai, N Vietnam
167 S8 **Thakhèk** *prev.* Muang Khammouan. Khammouan, C Laos
153 S13 **Thakurgaon** Rajshahi, NW Bangladesh
149 S6 **Thal** North-West Frontier Province, NW Pakistan
166 M15 **Thalang** Phuket, SW Thailand
Thalassery *see* Tellicherry
167 Q10 **Thalat Khae** Nakhon Ratchasima, C Thailand
109 Q5 **Thalgau** Salzburg, NW Austria
108 G7 **Thalwil** Zürich, NW Switzerland
83 I20 **Thamaga** Kweneng, SE Botswana
Thamarīd *see* Thamarīt
141 V13 **Thamarīt** *var.* Thamarīd, Thumrayt. SW Oman
141 P16 **Thamar, Jabal** ▲ SW Yemen
184 M6 **Thames** Waikato, North Island, NZ
14 D17 **Thames** ≈ Ontario, S Canada
97 O22 **Thames** ≈ S England, UK
184 M6 **Thames, Firth of** *gulf* North Island, NZ
14 D17 **Thamesville** Ontario, S Canada
141 S13 **Thamūd** N Yemen
167 N9 **Thanbyuzayat** Mon State, S Burma
152 I9 **Thānesar** Haryāna, NW India
167 T7 **Thanh Hoa** Thanh Hoa, N Vietnam
Thanintari Taungdan *see* Bilauktaung Range
155 I21 **Thanjāvūr** *prev.* Tanjore. Tamil Nādu, SE India
Thanlwin *see* Salween
103 U7 **Thann** Haut-Rhin, NE France
167 O16 **Tha Nong Phrom** Phatthalung, SW Thailand
167 N13 **Thap Sakae** *var.* Thap Sakau. Prachuap Khiri Khan, SW Thailand
Thap Sakau *see* Thap Sakae
98 L10 **'t Harde** Gelderland, E Netherlands
152 D11 **Thar Desert** *var.* Great Indian Desert, Indian Desert. *desert* India/Pakistan
181 V10 **Thargomindah** Queensland, C Australia
150 D11 **Thar Pārkar** *desert* SE Pakistan
139 S7 **Tharthār al Furāt, Qanāt ath** *canal* C Iraq
139 R7 **Tharthār, Buḥayrat ath** ◎ C Iraq
139 R5 **Tharthār, Wādī ath** *dry watercourse* N Iraq
167 N13 **Tha Sae** Chumphon, SW Thailand
167 N15 **Tha Sala** Nakhon Si Thammarat, SW Thailand
114 I13 **Thásos** Thásos, E Greece
115 I14 **Thásos** *island* E Greece
37 N14 **Thatcher** Arizona, SW USA
167 T5 **Thât Khê** *var.* Tràng Dinh. Lang Sơn, N Vietnam
166 M8 **Thaton** Mon State, S Burma
167 S9 **That Phanom** Nakhon Phanom, E Thailand
167 R10 **Tha Tum** Surin, E Thailand
103 P16 **Thau, Bassin de** *var.* Étang de Thau. ◎ S France
Thau, Étang de *see* Thau, Bassin de
166 L3 **Thaungdut** Sagaing, N Burma
167 O8 **Thaungyin** *Th.* Mae Nam Moei. ≈ Burma/Thailand
167 R8 **Tha Uthen** Nakhon Phanom, E Thailand
109 W2 **Thaya** *var.* Dyje. ≈ Austria/Czech Republic *see also* Dyje
27 V8 **Thayer** Missouri, C USA
166 L6 **Thayetmyo** Magwe, C Burma
33 S15 **Thayne** Wyoming, C USA
166 M5 **Thazi** Mandalay, C Burma
Thebes *see* Thíva
44 L5 **The Carlton** *var.* Abraham Bay. Mayaguana, SE Bahamas
45 O14 **The Crane** *var.* Crane. S Barbados
32 I11 **The Dalles** Oregon, NW USA
28 M14 **Thedford** Nebraska, C USA
The Hague *see* 's-Gravenhage
Theiss *see* Tisa/Tisza
8 M9 **Thelon** ≈ Northwest Territories/Nunavut, N Canada
11 V15 **Theodore** Saskatchewan, S Canada
23 N8 **Theodore** Alabama, S USA
36 L13 **Theodore Roosevelt Lake** ⊠ Arizona, SW USA
Theodosia *see* Feodosiya
Theophilo Ottoni *see* Teófilo Otoni
9 N13 **The Pas** Manitoba, C Canada
31 T14 **The Plains** Ohio, N USA
Thera *see* Thíra
172 H17 **Thérèse, Île** *island* Inner Islands, NE Seychelles
Therezina *see* Teresina
115 L20 **Thérma** Ikaría, Dodekánisos, Greece, Aegean Sea
Thermae Himerenses *see* Termini Imerese
Thermae Pannonicae *see* Baden
Thermaic Gulf/Thermaicus Sinus *see* Thermaïkós Kólpos
121 Q8 **Thermaïkós Kólpos** *Eng.* Thermaic Gulf; *anc.* Thermaicus Sinus. *gulf* N Greece
Thermiá *see* Kýthnos
115 L17 **Thermís** Lésvos, E Greece
115 E18 **Thérmo** Dytikí Ellás, C Greece
33 V14 **Thermopolis** Wyoming, C USA
183 P10 **The Rock** New South Wales, SE Australia
195 O5 **Theron Mountains** ▲ Antarctica
115 G18 **Thespiés** Stereá Ellás, C Greece
115 E16 **Thessalía** *Eng.* Thessaly. ◈ *region* C Greece
14 C10 **Thessalon** Ontario, S Canada
115 G14 **Thessaloníki** *Eng.* Salonica, Salonika, *SCr.* Solun, *Turk.* Selânik. Kentrikí Makedonía, N Greece
115 G14 **Thessaloníki** ✕ Kentrikí Makedonía, N Greece
Thessaly *see* Thessalía
84 B12 **Theta Gap** *undersea feature* E Atlantic Ocean
97 P20 **Thetford** E England, UK
15 R11 **Thetford-Mines** Quebec, SE Canada
113 K17 **Theth** *var.* Thethi. Shkodër, N Albania
Thethi *see* Theth
99 L20 **Theux** Liège, E Belgium
45 V9 **The Valley** ○ (Anguilla) E Anguilla
27 N10 **The Village** Oklahoma, C USA
25 W10 **The Woodlands** Texas, SW USA
Thiamis *see* Thýamis
Thian Shan *see* Tien Shan
22 J9 **Thibodaux** Louisiana, S USA
29 S3 **Thief Lake** ◎ Minnesota, N USA
29 S3 **Thief River** ≈ Minnesota, C USA
29 S3 **Thief River Falls** Minnesota, N USA
Thièle *see* La Thielle
32 G14 **Thielsen, Mount** ▲ Oregon, NW USA
Thielt *see* Tielt
106 G7 **Thiene** Veneto, NE Italy
Thienen *see* Tienen
103 P11 **Thiers** Puy-de-Dôme, C France
76 F11 **Thiès** W Senegal
81 I19 **Thika** Central, S Kenya
Thikombia *see* Cikobia
151 K18 **Thiladhunmathi Atoll** *var.* Tiladummati Atoll. *atoll* N Maldives
Thimbu *see* Thimphu
153 T11 **Thimphu** *var.* Thimbu; *prev.* Tashi Chho Dzong. ● (Bhutan) W Bhutan
92 H2 **Thingeyri** Vestfirdhir, NW Iceland
92 I3 **Thingvellir** Sudhurland, SW Iceland
187 Q17 **Thio** Province Sud, C New Caledonia
103 T4 **Thionville** *Ger.* Diedenhofen. Moselle, NE France
115 K22 **Thíra** Thíra, Kykládes, Greece, Aegean Sea
115 K22 **Thíra** *prev.* Santorin, Santoríni, *anc.* Thera. *island* Kykládes, Greece, Aegean Sea
115 J22 **Thirasía** *island* Kykládes, Greece, Aegean Sea
97 M16 **Thirsk** N England, UK
14 F12 **Thirty Thousand Islands** *island group* Ontario, S Canada
Thiruvanathapuram *see* Trivandrum
95 F20 **Thisted** Viborg, NW Denmark
Thistil Fjord *see* Thistilfjördhur
92 L1 **Thistilfjördhur** *var.* Thistil Fjord. *fjord* NE Iceland
182 G9 **Thistle Island** *island* South Australia
Thithia *see* Cicia
Thiukhaoluang Phrahang *see* Luang Prabang Range
115 G18 **Thíva** *Eng.* Thebes; *prev.* Thívai. Stereá Ellás, C Greece
Thívai *see* Thíva
102 M12 **Thiviers** Dordogne, SW France
92 J4 **Thjórsá** ≈ C Iceland
9 N10 **Thlewiaza** ≈ Nunavut, NE Canada
8 L10 **Thoa** ≈ Northwest Territories, NW Canada
99 G14 **Tholen** Zeeland, SW Netherlands
99 F14 **Tholen** *island* SW Netherlands
26 L10 **Thomas** Oklahoma, C USA
21 T3 **Thomas** West Virginia, NE USA
27 U3 **Thomas Hill Reservoir** ⊠ Missouri, C USA
23 S5 **Thomaston** Georgia, SE USA
19 R7 **Thomaston** Maine, NE USA
25 T12 **Thomaston** Texas, SW USA
23 O6 **Thomasville** Alabama, S USA
23 T8 **Thomasville** Georgia, SE USA
21 S9 **Thomasville** North Carolina, SE USA
35 N5 **Thomes Creek** ≈ California, W USA
11 W12 **Thompson** Manitoba, C Canada
29 R4 **Thompson** North Dakota, N USA
(0) F8 **Thompson** ≈ Alberta/British Columbia, SW Canada
33 O8 **Thompson Falls** Montana, NW USA
29 Q10 **Thompson, Lake** ◎ South Dakota, N USA
34 M3 **Thompson Peak** ▲ California, W USA
27 S2 **Thompson River** ≈ Missouri, C USA
185 A22 **Thompson Sound** *sound* South Island, NZ
8 J5 **Thomsen** ≈ Banks Island, Northwest Territories, NW Canada
23 V4 **Thomson** Georgia, SE USA
103 T10 **Thonon-les-Bains** Haute-Savoie, E France
103 O15 **Thoré** *var.* Thore. ≈ S France
37 P11 **Thoreau** New Mexico, SW USA
Thorenburg *see* Turda
92 J3 **Thórisvatn** ◎ C Iceland
92 P4 **Thor, Kapp** *headland* S Svalbard
92 I4 **Thorlákshöfn** Sudhurland, SW Iceland
Thorn *see* Toruń
25 T10 **Thorndale** Texas, SW USA
14 H10 **Thorne** Ontario, S Canada
97 J14 **Thornhill** S Scotland, UK
25 U8 **Thornton** Texas, SW USA
Thornton Island *see* Millennium Island
14 H16 **Thorold** Ontario, S Canada
32 I9 **Thorp** Washington, NW USA
195 S3 **Thorshavnheiane** *physical region* Antarctica
92 L1 **Thórshöfn** Nordhurland Eystra, NE Iceland
Thospitis *see* Van Gölü
167 S14 **Thôt Nôt** Cân Thơ, S Vietnam
102 K8 **Thouars** Deux-Sèvres, W France
153 X14 **Thoubal** Manipur, NE India
102 K9 **Thouet** ≈ W France
Thoune *see* Thun
18 H7 **Thousand Islands** *island* Canada/USA
35 S15 **Thousand Oaks** California, W USA
114 L12 **Thrace** *cultural region* SE Europe
114 J13 **Thracian Sea** *Gk.* Thrakikó Pélagos; *anc.* Thracium Mare. *sea* Greece/Turkey
Thracium Mare/Thrakikó Pélagos *see* Thracian Sea
Thrá Lí, Bá *see* Tralee Bay
33 R11 **Three Forks** Montana, NW USA
11 Q16 **Three Hills** Alberta, SW Canada
183 N15 **Three Hummock Island** *island* Tasmania, SE Australia
184 H1 **Three Kings Islands** *island group* N NZ
175 P10 **Three Kings Rise** *undersea feature* W Pacific Ocean
77 O18 **Three Points, Cape** *headland* S Ghana
31 P10 **Three Rivers** Michigan, N USA
25 S13 **Three Rivers** Texas, SW USA
83 G24 **Three Sisters** Northern Cape, SW South Africa
32 H13 **Three Sisters** ▲ Oregon, NW USA
187 N10 **Three Sisters Islands** *island group* SE Solomon Islands
Thrissur *see* Trichūr
25 Q6 **Throckmorton** Texas, SW USA
180 M10 **Throssell, Lake** *salt lake* Western Australia
115 K25 **Thrýptis** ▲ Kríti, Greece, E Mediterranean Sea
167 T13 **Thu Dâu Môt** *var.* Phu Cuơng. Sông Be, S Vietnam
167 S6 **Thu Do** ✕ (Ha Nôi) Ha Nôi, N Vietnam
99 G21 **Thuin** Hainaut, S Belgium
149 Q12 **Thul** Sind, SE Pakistan
Thule *see* Qaanaaq
83 J18 **Thuli** *var.* Tuli. ≈ S Zimbabwe
Thumrayt *see* Thamarīt
108 D9 **Thun** *Fr.* Thoune. Bern, W Switzerland
12 C12 **Thunder Bay** Ontario, S Canada
30 M1 **Thunder Bay** *lake bay* S Canada
31 R6 **Thunder Bay** *lake bay* Michigan, N USA
31 R6 **Thunder Bay River** ≈ Michigan, N USA
27 N11 **Thunderbird, Lake** ⊠ Oklahoma, C USA
28 L8 **Thunder Butte Creek** ≈ South Dakota, N USA
108 E9 **Thuner See** ◎ C Switzerland
167 N15 **Thung Song** *var.* Cha Mai. Nakhon Si Thammarat, SW Thailand
108 H7 **Thur** ≈ N Switzerland
108 G6 **Thurgau** *Fr.* Thurgovie. ◈ *canton* NE Switzerland
Thurgovie *see* Thurgau
Thuringe *see* Thüringen
108 J7 **Thüringen** Vorarlberg, W Austria
101 J17 **Thüringen** *Eng.* Thuringia, *Fr.* Thuringe. ◈ *state* C Germany
101 J17 **Thüringer Wald** *Eng.* Thuringian Forest. ▲▲ C Germany
Thuringia *see* Thüringen
Thuringian Forest *see* Thüringer Wald
97 D19 **Thurles** *Ir.* Durlas. S Ireland
21 W2 **Thurmont** Maryland, NE USA
Thurø *see* Thurø By
95 H24 **Thurø By** *var.* Thurø. Fyn, C Denmark
14 M12 **Thurso** Quebec, SE Canada
96 J6 **Thurso** N Scotland, UK
194 I10 **Thurston Island** *island* Antarctica
108 I9 **Thusis** Graubünden, S Switzerland
115 C15 **Thýamis** *var.* Thiamis. ≈ W Greece
95 E21 **Thyborøn** *var.* Tyborøn. Ringkøbing, W Denmark
195 U3 **Thyer Glacier** *glacier* Antarctica
115 L20 **Thýmaina** *island* Dodekánisos, Greece, Aegean Sea
83 N15 **Thyolo** *var.* Cholo. Southern, S Malawi
183 U6 **Tia** New South Wales, SE Australia
54 H5 **Tía Juana** Zulia, NW Venezuela
160 J14 **Tiandong** *var.* Pingma. Guangxi Zhuangzu Zizhiqu, S China
161 O3 **Tianjin** *var.* Tientsin. Tianjin Shi, E China
Tianjin *see* Tianjin Shi
161 P3 **Tianjin Shi** *var.* Jin, Tianjin, T'ien-ching, Tientsin. ◈ *municipality* E China
159 S10 **Tianjun** *var.* Xinyuan. Qinghai, C China
160 J13 **Tianlin** *prev.* Leli. Guangxi Zhuangzu Zizhiqu, S China
Tian Shan *see* Tien Shan
159 W11 **Tianshui** Gansu, C China
150 I7 **Tianshuihai** Xinjiang Uygur Zizhiqu, W China
161 S10 **Tiantai** Zhejiang, SE China
160 J14 **Tianyang** Guangxi Zhuangzu Zizhiqu, S China
159 U9 **Tianzhu** *var.* Tianzhu Zangzu Zizhixian. Gansu, C China
Tianzhu Zangzu Zizhixian *see* Tianzhu
191 Q7 **Tiarei** Tahiti, W French Polynesia
74 J6 **Tiaret** *var.* Tihert. NW Algeria
77 N17 **Tiassalé** S Ivory Coast
192 I16 **Ti'avea** Upolu, SE Samoa
Tiba *see* Chiba
60 J11 **Tibagi** *var.* Tibaji. Paraná, S Brazil
60 J10 **Tibagi, Rio** *var.* Rio Tibají. ≈ S Brazil
Tibaji *see* Tibagi
Tibají, Rio *see* Tibagi, Rio
139 Q9 **Tibal, Wādī** *dry watercourse* S Iraq
54 G9 **Tibaná** Boyacá, C Colombia
79 F14 **Tibati** Adamaoua, N Cameroon
76 K15 **Tibé, Pic de** ▲ SE Guinea
Tiber *see* Tivoli, Italy
Tiber *see* Tevere, Italy
Tiberias *see* Teverya
138 G8 **Tiberias, Lake** *var.* Chinnereth, Sea of Bahr Tabariya, Sea of Galilee, *Ar.* Bahrat Tabariya, *Heb.* Yam Kinneret. ◎ N Israel
67 Q5 **Tibesti** *var.* Tibesti Massif, *Ar.* Tibistī. ▲▲ N Africa
Tibesti Massif *see* Tibesti
Tibetan Autonomous Region *see* Xizang Zizhiqu
Tibet, Plateau of *see* Qingzang Gaoyuan
Tibistī *see* Tibesti
14 K7 **Tiblemont, Lac** ◎ Quebec, SE Canada
139 X9 **Ţīb, Nahr aţ** ≈ S Iraq
Tibnī *see* At Tibnī
182 L4 **Tibooburra** New South Wales, SE Australia
95 L18 **Tibro** Västra Götaland, S Sweden
40 E5 **Tiburón, Isla** *var.* Isla del Tiburón. *island* NW Mexico
Tiburón, Isla del *see* Tiburón, Isla
23 W14 **Tice** Florida, SE USA
Tichau *see* Tychy
114 L8 **Ticha, Yazovir** ◎ NE Bulgaria
76 K9 **Tichît** *var.* Tichitt. Tagant, C Mauritania
Tichitt *see* Tichît
108 G11 **Ticino** *Fr./Ger.* Tessin. ◈ *canton* S Switzerland
106 D8 **Ticino** ≈ Italy/Switzerland
108 H11 **Ticino** *Ger.* Tessin. ≈ SW Switzerland
Ticinum *see* Pavia
41 X12 **Ticul** Yucatán, SE Mexico
95 K18 **Tidaholm** Västra Götaland, S Sweden
Tidjikdja *see* Tidjikja
76 J8 **Tidjikja** *var.* Tidjikdja; *prev.* Fort-Cappolani. Tagant, C Mauritania
Tidore *see* Soasiu
171 R11 **Tidore, Pulau** *island* E Indonesia
Tidra, Ile *see* Et Tîdra
77 N16 **Tiébissou** *var.* Tiebissou. C Ivory Coast
163 V11 **Tiefa** Liaoning, NE China
108 I9 **Tiefencastel** Graubünden, S Switzerland
Tiegenhof *see* Nowy Dwór Gdański
T'ieh-ling *see* Tieling
98 K13 **Tiel** Gelderland, C Netherlands
163 W7 **Tieli** Heilongjiang, NE China
163 V11 **Tieling** *var.* T'ieh-ling. Liaoning, NE China
152 L4 **Tielongtan** China/India
99 D17 **Tielt** *var.* Thielt. West-Vlaanderen, W Belgium
T'ien-ching *see* Tianjin Shi
99 I18 **Tienen** *var.* Thienen, *Fr.* Tirlemont. Vlaams Brabant, C Belgium
Tiên Giang, Sông *see* Mekong
147 X9 **Tien Shan** *Chin.* Thian Shan, Tian Shan, T'ien Shan, *Rus.* Tyan'-Shan'. ▲▲ C Asia
Tientsin *see* Tianjin
Tientsin *see* Tianjin Shi
167 U6 **Tiên Yên** Quang Ninh, N Vietnam
95 O14 **Tierp** Uppsala, C Sweden
62 H7 **Tierra Amarilla** Atacama, N Chile
37 R9 **Tierra Amarilla** New Mexico, SW USA
41 R15 **Tierra Blanca** Veracruz-Llave, E Mexico
41 O16 **Tierra Colorada** Guerrero, S Mexico
63 J17 **Tierra Colorada, Bajo de la** *basin* SE Argentina
63 I25 **Tierra del Fuego** *off.* Provincia de la Tierra del Fuego. ◈ *province* S Argentina
63 J24 **Tierra del Fuego** *island* Argentina/Chile
54 D7 **Tierralta** Córdoba, NW Colombia
104 K9 **Tiétar** ≈ W Spain
60 L10 **Tietê** São Paulo, S Brazil
60 J8 **Tietê, Rio** ≈ S Brazil
32 I9 **Tieton** Washington, NW USA
32 J6 **Tiffany Mountain** ▲ Washington, NW USA
31 S12 **Tiffin** Ohio, N USA
31 Q11 **Tiffin River** ≈ Ohio, N USA
Tiflis *see* T'bilisi
23 U7 **Tifton** Georgia, SE USA
171 R13 **Tifu** Pulau Buru, E Indonesia
38 L17 **Tigalda Island** *island* Aleutian Islands, Alaska, USA
115 I15 **Tigáni, Akrotírio** *headland* Límnos, E Greece
169 V6 **Tiga Tarok** Sabah, East Malaysia
117 O10 **Tighina** *Rus.* Bendery; *prev.* Bender. E Moldova
145 X9 **Tigiretskiy Khrebet** ▲ E Kazakhstan
79 F14 **Tignère** Adamaoua, N Cameroon
13 P14 **Tignish** Prince Edward Island, SE Canada
Tigranocerta *see* Siirt
80 I11 **Tigray** ◈ *province* N Ethiopia
41 O11 **Tigre, Cerro del** ▲ C Mexico
56 F8 **Tigre, Río** ≈ N Peru
139 X10 **Tigris** *Ar.* Dijlah, *Turk.* Dicle. ≈ Iraq/Turkey
76 G9 **Tiguent** Trarza, SW Mauritania
74 M10 **Tiguentourine** E Algeria
77 V10 **Tiguidit, Falaise de** *ridge* C Niger
141 N13 **Tihāmah** *var.* Tehama. *plain* Saudi Arabia/Yemen
Tihert *see* Tiaret
Ti-hua/Tihwa *see* Ürümqi
41 Q13 **Tihuatlán** Veracruz-Llave, E Mexico
40 B1 **Tijuana** Baja California, NW Mexico
42 E2 **Tikal** Petén, N Guatemala
154 I9 **Tīkamgarh** *prev.* Tehri. Madhya Pradesh, C India
158 L7 **Tikanlik** Xinjiang Uygur Zizhiqu, NW China
77 P12 **Tikaré** N Burkina
39 O12 **Tikchik Lakes** *lakes* Alaska, USA
191 T9 **Tikehau** *atoll* Îles Tuamotu, C French Polynesia
191 V9 **Tikei** *island* Îles Tuamotu, C French Polynesia
122 B11 **Tikhoretsk** Krasnodarskiy Kray, SW Russian Federation
126 I13 **Tikhvin** Leningradskaya Oblast', NW Russian Federation
193 P9 **Tiki Basin** *undersea feature* S Pacific Ocean
76 K13 **Tikinsso** ≈ NE Guinea
184 Q8 **Tikitiki** Gisborne, North Island, NZ
79 D16 **Tiko** Sud-Ouest, SW Cameroon
187 R11 **Tikopia** *island*, E Solomon Islands
139 S6 **Tikrīt** *var.* Tekrit. N Iraq
126 I8 **Tiksha** Respublika Kareliya, NW Russian Federation
126 I6 **Tikshozero, Ozero** ◎ NW Russian Federation
123 P7 **Tiksi** Respublika Sakha (Yakutiya), NE Russian Federation
42 A6 **Tilapa** San Marcos, SW Guatemala
42 L13 **Tilarán** Guanacaste, NW Costa Rica
99 J14 **Tilburg** Noord-Brabant, S Netherlands
14 D17 **Tilbury** Ontario, S Canada
182 K4 **Tilcha** South Australia
Tilcha Creek *see* Callabonna Creek
29 Q14 **Tilden** Nebraska, C USA
25 R13 **Tilden** Texas, SW USA
14 H10 **Tilden Lake** Ontario, S Canada
116 G9 **Tileagd** *Hung.* Mezőtelegd. Bihor, W Romania
77 Q8 **Tilemsi, Vallée de** ≈ C Mali
123 V8 **Tilichiki** Koryakskiy Avtonomnyy Okrug, E Russian Federation
Tiligul *see* Tilihul
Tiligul'skiy Liman *see* Tilihul's'kyy Lyman
117 P9 **Tilihul** *Rus.* Tiligul. ≈ SW Ukraine
117 P10 **Tilihul's'kyy Lyman** *Rus.* Tiligul'skiy Liman. ◎ S Ukraine
Tilimsen *see* Tlemcen
Tilio Martius *see* Toulon
77 R11 **Tillabéri** *var.* Tillabéry. Tillabéri, W Niger
77 R11 **Tillabéri** ◈ *department* SW Niger
Tillabéry *see* Tillabéri
32 F11 **Tillamook** Oregon, NW USA
32 E11 **Tillamook Bay** *inlet* Oregon, NW USA
151 Q22 **Tillanchāng Dwīp** *island* Nicobar Islands, India, NE Indian Ocean
95 N15 **Tillberga** Västmanland, C Sweden
Tillenberg *see* Dyleń
21 S10 **Tillery, Lake** ⊠ North Carolina, SE USA
77 T10 **Tillia** Tahoua, W Niger
23 N8 **Tillmans Corner** Alabama, S USA
14 F17 **Tillsonburg** Ontario, S Canada
115 N22 **Tílos** *island* Dodekánisos, Greece, Aegean Sea
183 N5 **Tilpa** New South Wales, SE Australia
Tilsit *see* Sovetsk
31 N13 **Tilton** Illinois, N USA
128 K7 **Tim** Kurskaya Oblast', W Russian Federation
54 D12 **Timaná** Huila, S Colombia
Timan Ridge *see* Timanskiy Kryazh
127 Q6 **Timanskiy Kryazh** *Eng.* Timan Ridge. *ridge* NW Russian Federation
185 G20 **Timaru** Canterbury, South Island, NZ
129 S6 **Timashevo** Samarskaya Oblast', W Russian Federation
128 K13 **Timashevsk** Krasnodarskiy Kray, SW Russian Federation
Timbaki/Timbákion *see* Tympáki
22 K10 **Timbalier Bay** *bay* Louisiana, S USA
22 K11 **Timbalier Island** *island* Louisiana, S USA
76 L10 **Timbedgha** *var.* Timbédra. Hodh ech Chargui, SE Mauritania
Timbédra *see* Timbedgha
32 G10 **Timber** Oregon, NW USA
181 O3 **Timber Creek** Northern Territory, N Australia
28 M8 **Timber Lake** South Dakota, N USA
54 D12 **Timbío** Cauca, SW Colombia
54 C12 **Timbiquí** Cauca, SW Colombia
83 O17 **Timbue, Ponta** *headland* C Mozambique
Timbuktu *see* Tombouctou
169 W8 **Timbun Mata, Pulau** *island* E Malaysia
77 P8 **Timétrine** *var.* Ti-n-Kâr. *oasis* C Mali
Timfi *see* Týmfi
Timfristos *see* Tymfristós
77 V9 **Timia** Agadez, C Niger
171 X14 **Timika** Irian Jaya, E Indonesia
74 I9 **Timimoun** C Algeria
Timiris, Cap *see* Timirist, Râs
76 F8 **Timirist, Râs** *var.* Cap Timiris. *headland* NW Mauritania
145 O7 **Timiryazevo** Severnyy Kazakhstan, N Kazakhstan
116 E11 **Timiş** ◈ *county* SW Romania
14 H9 **Timiskaming, Lake** *Fr.* Lac Témiscamingue. ◎ Ontario/Quebec, SE Canada
116 E11 **Timişoara** *Ger.* Temeschwar, Temeswar, *Hung.* Temesvár; *prev.* Temeschburg. Timiş, W Romania
116 E11 **Timişoara** ✕ Timiş, W Romania
Timkovichi *see* Tsimkavichy
77 U8 **Ti-m-Meghsoï** ≈ NW Niger
100 K8 **Timmerdorfer Strand** Schleswig-Holstein, N Germany
14 F7 **Timmins** Ontario, S Canada
21 S12 **Timmonsville** South Carolina, SE USA
30 K5 **Timms Hill** ▲ Wisconsin, N USA
112 P12 **Timok** ≈ E Yugoslavia
58 N13 **Timon** Maranhão, E Brazil
171 Q16 **Timor** *island* East Timor/Indonesia
171 Q17 **Timor Sea** *sea* E Indian Ocean
Timor Timur *see* East Timor
Timor Trench *see* Timor Trough
192 G8 **Timor Trough** *var.* Timor Trench. *undersea feature* NE Timor Sea
61 A21 **Timote** Buenos Aires, E Argentina
54 I6 **Timotes** Mérida, NW Venezuela
25 X8 **Timpson** Texas, SW USA
123 Q11 **Timpton** ≈ NE Russian Federation
93 H17 **Timrå** Västernorrland, C Sweden
20 J10 **Tims Ford Lake** ⊠ Tennessee, S USA
168 L7 **Timur, Banjaran** ▲ Peninsular Malaysia
171 Q8 **Tinaca Point** *headland* Mindanao, S Philippines
54 K5 **Tinaco** Cojedes, N Venezuela
64 Q11 **Tinajo** Lanzarote, Islas Canarias, Spain, NE Atlantic Ocean
187 P10 **Tinakula** *island* Santa Cruz Islands, E Solomon Islands
54 K5 **Tinaquillo** Cojedes, N Venezuela
116 F10 **Tinca** *Hung.* Tenke. Bihor, W Romania
155 J20 **Tindivanam** Tamil Nādu, SE India
74 E9 **Tindouf** W Algeria
74 E9 **Tindouf, Sebkha de** *salt lake* W Algeria
104 J2 **Tineo** Asturias, N Spain
77 R9 **Ti-n-Essako** Kidal, E Mali
183 T5 **Tingha** New South Wales, SE Australia
Tingis *see* Tanger
Tinglett *see* Tinglev
95 F24 **Tinglev** *Ger.* Tinglett. Sønderjylland, SW Denmark
56 E12 **Tingo María** Huánuco, C Peru

◆ Country ● Country Capital ◇ Dependent Territory ○ Dependent Territory Capital ◈ Administrative Region ✕ International Airport ▲ Mountain ▲▲ Mountain Range 𝔸 Volcano ≈ River ◎ Lake ⊠ Reservoir

Tingréla see Tengréla
158 K16 Tingri var. Xêgar. Xizang Zizhiqu, W China
95 M21 Tingsryd Kronoberg, S Sweden
95 P19 Tingstäde Gotland, SE Sweden
62 H12 Tinguiririca, Volcán ▲ C Chile
94 F9 Tingvoll Møre og Romsdal, S Norway
188 K8 Tinian island S Northern Mariana Islands
Ti-n-Kâr see Timétrine
Tinnevelly see Tirunelveli
95 G15 Tinnoset Telemark, S Norway
95 F15 Tinnsjø ◎ S Norway
Tino see Chino
115 J20 Tínos Tínos, Kykládes, Greece, Aegean Sea
115 J20 Tínos anc. Tenos. island Kykládes, Greece, Aegean Sea
153 R14 Tinpahar Bihār, NE India
153 X11 Tinsukia Assam, NE India
76 K10 Tintâne Hodh el Gharbi, S Mauritania
62 L7 Tintina Santiago del Estero, N Argentina
182 K10 Tintinara South Australia
104 I14 Tinto ~ SW Spain
77 S8 Ti-n-Zaouâtene Kidal, NE Mali
Tiobraid Árann see Tipperary
28 K3 Tioga North Dakota, N USA
18 G12 Tioga Pennsylvania, NE USA
25 T5 Tioga Texas, SW USA
35 Q8 Tioga Pass pass California, W USA
18 G12 Tioga River ~ New York/Pennsylvania, NE USA
Tioman Island see Tioman, Pulau
168 M9 Tioman, Pulau var. Tioman Island. island Peninsular Malaysia
18 C12 Tionesta Pennsylvania, NE USA
18 D12 Tionesta Creek ~ Pennsylvania, NE USA
168 J13 Tiop Pulau Pagai Selatan, W Indonesia
77 O12 Tiou NW Burkina
18 H11 Tioughnioga River ~ New York, NE USA
74 J5 Tipasa var. Tipaza. N Algeria
Tipaza see Tipasa
42 J10 Tipitapa Managua, W Nicaragua
31 R13 Tipp City Ohio, N USA
31 O12 Tippecanoe River ~ Indiana, N USA
97 D20 Tipperary Ir. Tiobraid Árann. S Ireland
97 D19 Tipperary Ir. Tiobraid Árann. cultural region S Ireland
35 R12 Tipton California, W USA
31 P13 Tipton Indiana, N USA
29 Y14 Tipton Iowa, C USA
27 U5 Tipton Missouri, C USA
36 I10 Tipton, Mount ▲ Arizona, SW USA
20 F8 Tiptonville Tennessee, S USA
12 E12 Tip Top Mountain ▲ Ontario, S Canada
155 G19 Tiptūr Karnātaka, W India
Tiquisate see Pueblo Nuevo Tiquisate
58 L13 Tiracambu, Serra do ▲ E Brazil
Tirana see Tiranë
113 K19 Tirana Rinas × Durrës, W Albania
113 L20 Tiranë var. Tirana. ● (Albania) Tiranë, C Albania
113 K20 Tiranë ◈ district W Albania
140 I5 Tirān, Jazīrat island Egypt/Saudi Arabia
106 F6 Tirano Lombardia, N Italy
182 I2 Tirari Desert desert South Australia
117 O10 Tiraspol Rus. Tiraspol'. E Moldova
184 M8 Tirau Waikato, North Island, NZ
136 C14 Tire İzmir, SW Turkey
137 O11 Tirebolu Giresun, N Turkey
96 F11 Tiree island W Scotland, UK
Tîrgovişte see Târgovişte
Tîrgu see Târgu Cărbuneşti
Tîrgu Bujor see Târgu Bujor
Tîrgu Frumos see Târgu Frumos
Tîrgu Jiu see Târgu Jiu
Tîrgu Lăpuş see Târgu Lăpuş
Tîrgu Mures see Târgu Mureş
Tîrgu-Neamţ see Târgu-Neamţ
Tîrgu Ocna see Târgu Ocna
Tîrgu Secuiesc see Târgu Secuiesc
149 T3 Tirich Mīr ▲ NW Pakistan
76 J5 Tiris Zemmour ◈ region N Mauritania
Tirlemont see Tienen
129 W5 Tirlyanskiy Respublika Bashkortostan, W Russian Federation
Tîrnava Mare see Târnava Mare
Tîrnava Mică see Târnava Mică
Tîrnăveni see Târnăveni
Tírnavos see Týrnavos
Tirnovo see Veliko Tŭrnovo
154 J11 Tirodi Madhya Pradesh, C India
108 K8 Tirol off. Land Tirol, var. Tyrol, It. Tirolo. ◈ state W Austria
Tirolo see Tirol
Tirreno, Mare see Tyrrhenian Sea
107 B19 Tirso ~ Sardegna, Italy, C Mediterranean Sea
95 H22 Tirstrup × (Århus) Århus, C Denmark
155 I21 Tiruchchirāppalli prev. Trichinopoly. Tamil Nādu, SE India
155 H23 Tirunelveli var. Tinnevelly. Tamil Nādu, SE India
155 J19 Tirupati Andhra Pradesh, E India
155 I20 Tiruppattūr Tamil Nādu, SE India
155 H21 Tiruppur Tamil Nādu, SW India
155 I20 Tiruvannāmalai Tamil Nādu, SE India
112 L10 Tisa Ger. Theiss, Hung. Tisza, Rus. Tissa, Ukr. Tysa. ~ SE Europe see also Tisza
Tischnowitz see Tišnov
11 U14 Tisdale Saskatchewan, S Canada
27 O13 Tishomingo Oklahoma, C USA
95 M17 Tisnaren ◎ S Sweden
111 F18 Tišnov Ger. Tischnowitz. Brnenský Kraj, SE Czech Republic
Tissa see Tisa/Tisza
74 J6 Tissemsilt N Algeria
153 S12 Tista ~ NE India
112 L8 Tisza Ger. Theiss, Rom./Slvn./SCr. Tisa, Rus. Tissa, Ukr. Tysa. ~ SE Europe see also Tisa
111 L23 Tiszaföldvár Jász-Nagykun-Szolnok, E Hungary
111 M22 Tiszafüred Jász-Nagykun-Szolnok, E Hungary
111 L23 Tiszakécske Bács-Kiskun, C Hungary
111 M21 Tiszaújváros prev. Leninváros. Borsod-Abaúj-Zemplén, NE Hungary
111 N21 Tiszavasvári Szabolcs-Szatmár-Bereg, NE Hungary
Titibu see Chichibu
57 I17 Titicaca, Lake ◎ Bolivia/Peru
190 H17 Titikaveka Rarotonga, S Cook Islands
154 M13 Titilāgarh Orissa, E India
168 K8 Titiwangsa, Banjaran ▲ Peninsular Malaysia
Titograd see Podgorica
Titose see Chitose
Titova Mitrovica see Kosovska Mitrovica
Titovo Užice see Užice
113 M18 Titov Vrv ▲ NW FYR Macedonia
94 F7 Titran Sør-Trøndelag, S Norway
31 Q8 Tittabawassee River ~ Michigan, N USA
116 J13 Titu Dâmboviţa, S Romania
79 M16 Titule Orientale, N Dem. Rep. Congo (Zaire)
23 X11 Titusville Florida, SE USA
18 C12 Titusville Pennsylvania, NE USA
76 G11 Tivaouane W Senegal
113 J17 Tivat Montenegro, SW Yugoslavia
14 E14 Tiverton Ontario, S Canada
97 J23 Tiverton SW England, UK
19 O12 Tiverton Rhode Island, NE USA
107 I15 Tivoli anc. Tiber. Lazio, C Italy
25 U13 Tivoli Texas, SW USA
141 Z8 Ţīwī NE Oman
Tiworo see Tioro, Selat
41 Y11 Tizimín Yucatán, SE Mexico
74 K5 Tizi Ouzou var. Tizi-Ouzou. N Algeria
74 D8 Tiznit SW Morocco
113 I14 Tjentište Republika Srpska, SE Bosnia and Herzegovina
Tjepoe/Tjepu see Cepu
98 L7 Tjeukemeer ◎ N Netherlands
Tjiamis see Ciamis
Tjiandjoer see Cianjur
Tjilatjap see Cilacap
Tjiledoeg see Ciledug
95 F23 Tjæreborg Ribe, W Denmark
95 I18 Tjörn island S Sweden
92 O3 Tjuvfjorden fjord S Svalbard
Tkvarcheli see Tqvarch'eli
40 L8 Tlahualilo Durango, N Mexico
41 P14 Tlalnepantla México, C Mexico
41 Q13 Tlapacoyán Veracruz-Llave, E Mexico
41 P16 Tlapa de Comonfort Guerrero, S Mexico
40 L13 Tlaquepaque Jalisco, C Mexico
Tlascala see Tlaxcala
41 P14 Tlaxcala var. Tlascala, Tlaxcala de Xicohténcatl. Tlaxcala, C Mexico
41 P14 Tlaxcala ◈ state S Mexico
Tlaxcala de Xicohténcatl see Tlaxcala
41 P14 Tlaxco var. Tlaxco de Morelos. Tlaxcala, S Mexico
Tlaxco de Morelos see Tlaxco
41 Q16 Tlaxiaco var. Santa María Asunción Tlaxiaco. Oaxaca, S Mexico
74 I6 Tlemcen var. Tilimsen, Tlemsen. NW Algeria
Tlemsen see Tlemcen
138 L4 Tlété Ouâte Rharbi, Jebel ▲ N Syria
116 J7 Tlumach Ivano-Frankivs'ka Oblast', W Ukraine
129 P17 Tlyarata Respublika Dagestan, SW Russian Federation
116 K10 Toaca, Vârful prev. Vîrful Toaca. ▲ NE Romania
Toaca, Vîrful see Toaca, Vârful
187 R13 Toak Ambrym, C Vanuatu
172 J4 Toamasina var. Tamatave. Toamasina, E Madagascar
172 J4 Toamasina ◈ province E Madagascar
172 J4 Toamasina × Toamasina, E Madagascar
21 X6 Toano Virginia, NE USA
191 U10 Toau atoll Îles Tuamotu, C French Polynesia
45 T6 Toa Vaca, Embalse ▣ C Puerto Rico
62 K13 Toay La Pampa, C Argentina
159 R14 Toba Xizang Zizhiqu, W China
164 K14 Toba Mie, Honshū, SW Japan
168 I9 Toba, Danau ◎ Sumatera, W Indonesia
45 Y16 Tobago island NE Trinidad and Tobago
149 Q9 Toba Kākar Range ▲ NW Pakistan
105 Q12 Tobarra Castilla-La Mancha, C Spain
149 U9 Toba Tek Singh Punjab, E Pakistan
171 R11 Tobelo Pulau Halmahera, E Indonesia
14 E12 Tobermory Ontario, S Canada
96 G10 Tobermory W Scotland, UK
165 S4 Tōbetsu Hokkaidō, NE Japan
180 M6 Tobin Lake ◎ Western Australia
11 U14 Tobin Lake ◎ Saskatchewan, C Canada
35 T4 Tobin, Mount ▲ Nevada, W USA
165 O9 Tobi-shima island C Japan
169 N13 Toboali Pulau Bangka, W Indonesia
144 M8 Tobol Kaz. Tobyl. Kostanay, N Kazakhstan
144 L8 Tobol Kaz. Tobyl. ~ Kazakhstan/Russian Federation
122 H11 Tobol'sk Tyumenskaya Oblast', C Russian Federation
Tobruch/Tobruk see Ţubruq
127 R3 Tobseda Nenetskiy Avtonomnyy Okrug, NW Russian Federation
Tobyl see Tobol
127 Q6 Tobysh ~ NW Russian Federation
54 F10 Tocaima Cundinamarca, C Colombia
59 K16 Tocantins off. Estado do Tocantins. ◈ state C Brazil
59 K15 Tocantins, Rio ~ N Brazil
23 T2 Toccoa Georgia, SE USA
165 O12 Tochigi off. Tochigi-ken, var. Totigi. ◈ prefecture Honshū, S Japan
165 O11 Tochio var. Totio. Niigata, Honshū, C Japan
95 I15 Töcksfors Värmland, C Sweden
42 J5 Tocoa Colón, N Honduras
62 H4 Tocopilla Antofagasta, N Chile
62 I4 Tocorpuri, Cerro de ▲ Bolivia/Chile
183 O10 Tocumwal New South Wales, SE Australia
54 K4 Tocuyo de La Costa Falcón, NW Venezuela
152 H13 Toda Rāisingh Rājasthān, N India
106 H13 Todi Umbria, C Italy
108 G9 Tödi ▲ NE Switzerland
171 T12 Todlo Irian Jaya, E Indonesia
165 S9 Todoga-saki headland Honshū, C Japan
59 P17 Todos os Santos, Baía de bay E Brazil
40 F10 Todos Santos Baja California Sur, W Mexico
40 B2 Todos Santos, Bahía de bay NW Mexico
Toeban see Tuban
Toekang Besi Eilanden see Tukangbesi, Kepulauan
Tōen see T'aoyüan
185 D25 Toetoes Bay bay South Island, NZ
11 Q14 Tofield Alberta, SW Canada
10 K17 Tofino Vancouver Island, British Columbia, SW Canada
189 X17 Tofol Kosrae, E Micronesia
95 J20 Tofta Halland, S Sweden
95 H15 Tofte Buskerud, S Norway
95 F24 Toftlund Sønderjylland, SW Denmark
193 X15 Tofua island Ha'apai Group, C Tonga
187 Q12 Toga island Torres Islands, N Vanuatu
80 N13 Togdheer off. Gobolka Togdheer. ◈ region NW Somalia
Toghyzaq see Toguzak
164 L11 Togi Ishikawa, Honshū, SW Japan
39 N13 Togiak Alaska, USA
171 O11 Togian, Kepulauan island group C Indonesia
77 Q15 Togo off. Togolese Republic; prev. French Togoland. ◆ republic W Africa
162 F8 Tögrög Govĭ-Altay, SW Mongolia
162 E7 Tögrög Hovd, W Mongolia
Togton-heyan see Tuotuoheyan
144 L7 Toguzak Kaz. Toghyzaq. ~ Kazakhstan/Russian Federation
37 P10 Tohatchi New Mexico, SW USA
191 O7 Tohiea, Mont ▲ Moorea, W French Polynesia
93 O17 Tohmajärvi Itä-Suomi, E Finland
137 N14 Tohma Çayı ~ C Turkey
93 L16 Toholampi Länsi-Suomi, W Finland
162 M10 Töhöm Dornogovĭ, SE Mongolia
23 X12 Tohopekaliga, Lake ◎ Florida, SE USA
164 M14 Toi Shizuoka, Honshū, S Japan
190 B15 Toi N Niue
93 L19 Toijala Länsi-Suomi, W Finland
171 P12 Toima Sulawesi, N Indonesia
164 D17 Toi-misaki headland Kyūshū, SW Japan
171 Q17 Toineke Timor, S Indonesia
Toirc, Inis see Inishturk
35 U6 Toiyabe Range ▲ Nevada, W USA
Tojikiston, Jumhurii see Tajikistan
147 R12 Tojikobod Rus. Tadzhikabad. C Tajikistan
164 G12 Tōjō Hiroshima, Honshū, SW Japan
39 T10 Tok Alaska, USA
164 K13 Tōkai Aichi, Honshū, SW Japan
111 N21 Tokaj Borsod-Abaúj-Zemplén, NE Hungary
165 N11 Tōkamachi Niigata, Honshū, C Japan
185 D25 Tokanui Southland, South Island, NZ
80 I7 Tokar var. Ţawkar. Red Sea, NE Sudan
136 L12 Tokat Tokat, N Turkey
136 L12 Tokat ◈ province N Turkey
Tokati Gawa see Tokachi-gawa
163 X15 Tŏkchŏk-gundo island group NW South Korea
Tōke see Taka Atoll
190 J9 Tokelau ◇ NZ overseas territory W Polynesia
Tőketerebes see Trebišov
Tokhtamyshbek see Tŭkhtamish
24 M6 Tokio Texas, SW USA
Tokio see Tōkyō
189 W11 Toki Point point NW Wake Island
Tokkuztara see Gongliu
147 V7 Tokmak Kir. Tokmok. Chuyskaya Oblast', N Kyrgyzstan
117 V9 Tokmak var. Velykyy Tokmak. Zaporiz'ka Oblast', SE Ukraine
Tokmok see Tokmak
184 Q8 Tokomaru Bay Gisborne, North Island, NZ
165 V3 Tokoro Hokkaidō, NE Japan
184 M8 Tokoroa Waikato, North Island, NZ
76 K14 Tokounou Haute-Guinée, C Guinea
38 M12 Toksook Bay Alaska, USA
Toksu see Xinhe
Toksum see Toksun
158 L6 Toksun var. Toksum. Xinjiang Uygur Zizhiqu, NW China
147 T8 Toktogul Talasskaya Oblast', NW Kyrgyzstan
147 T9 Toktogul'skoye Vodokhranilishche ▣ W Kyrgyzstan
Toktomush see Tŭkhtamish
193 Y14 Toku island Vava'u Group, N Tonga
165 U16 Tokunoshima Kagoshima, Tokuno-shima, SW Japan
165 U16 Tokuno-shima island Nansei-shotō, SW Japan
164 I14 Tokushima var. Tokusima. Tokushima, Shikoku, SW Japan
164 H14 Tokushima off. Tokushima-ken, var. Tokusima. ◈ prefecture Shikoku, SW Japan
Tokusima see Tokushima
164 E13 Tokuyama Yamaguchi, Honshū, SW Japan
165 N13 Tōkyō var. Tokio. ● (Japan) Tōkyō, Honshū, S Japan
165 O13 Tōkyō off. Tōkyō-to. ◈ capital district Honshū, S Japan
145 T12 Tokyrau ~ C Kazakhstan
149 O3 Tokzār Pash. Tukzār. Sar-e Pol, N Afghanistan
189 U12 Tol atoll Chuuk Islands, C Micronesia
184 Q9 Tolaga Bay Gisborne, North Island, NZ
172 I7 Tôlañaro prev. Faradofay, Fort-Dauphin. Toliara, SE Madagascar
162 D6 Tolbo Bayan-Ölgiy, W Mongolia
Tolbukhin see Dobrich
60 G11 Toledo Paraná, S Brazil
54 G8 Toledo Norte de Santander, N Colombia
105 N9 Toledo anc. Toletum. Castilla-La Mancha, C Spain
30 M14 Toledo Illinois, N USA
29 W13 Toledo Iowa, C USA
31 R11 Toledo Ohio, N USA
32 F12 Toledo Oregon, NW USA
32 G9 Toledo Washington, NW USA
42 F3 Toledo ◈ district S Belize
104 M9 Toledo ◈ province Castilla-La Mancha, C Spain
25 Y7 Toledo Bend Reservoir ▣ Louisiana/Texas, SW USA
104 M10 Toledo, Montes de ▲ C Spain
106 J12 Tolentino Marche, C Italy
Toletum see Toledo
94 H10 Tolga Hedmark, S Norway
158 J3 Toli Xinjiang Uygur Zizhiqu, NW China
172 H7 Toliara var. Toliary; prev. Tuléar. Toliara, SW Madagascar
172 H7 Toliara ◈ province SW Madagascar
Toliary see Toliara
54 D11 Tolima off. Departamento del Tolima. ◈ province C Colombia
171 N11 Tolitoli Sulawesi, C Indonesia
95 K22 Tollarp Skåne, S Sweden
100 N9 Tollense ~ NE Germany
100 N10 Tollensesee ◎ NE Germany
36 K13 Tolleson Arizona, SW USA
146 M13 Tollimarjon Rus. Talimardzhan. Qashqadaryo Wiloyati, S Uzbekistan
Tolmein see Tolmin
106 J6 Tolmezzo Friuli-Venezia Giulia, NE Italy
109 S11 Tolmin Ger. Tolmein, It. Tolmino. W Slovenia
Tolmino see Tolmin
111 J25 Tolna Ger. Tolnau. Tolna, S Hungary
111 I24 Tolna off. Tolna Megye. ◈ county SW Hungary
Tolnau see Tolna
79 I20 Tolo Bandundu, W Dem. Rep. Congo (Zaire)
Tolochin see Talachyn
190 D12 Toloke Île Futuna, W Wallis and Futuna
30 M13 Tolono Illinois, N USA
105 Q3 Tolosa País Vasco, N Spain
Tolosa see Toulouse
171 O13 Tolo, Teluk bay Sulawesi, C Indonesia
39 R9 Tolovana River ~ Alaska, USA
123 U10 Tolstoy, Mys headland E Russian Federation
63 G15 Toltén Araucanía, C Chile
63 G15 Toltén, Río ~ S Chile
54 E6 Tolú Sucre, NW Colombia
41 O14 Toluca var. Toluca de Lerdo. México, S Mexico
Toluca de Lerdo see Toluca
41 O14 Toluca, Nevado de ✱ C Mexico
129 R6 Tol'yatti prev. Stavropol'. Samarskaya Oblast', W Russian Federation
77 O12 Toma NW Burkina
30 K7 Tomah Wisconsin, N USA
30 L5 Tomahawk Wisconsin, N USA
117 T8 Tomakivka Dnipropetrovs'ka Oblast', E Ukraine
165 S4 Tomakomai Hokkaidō, NE Japan
165 S2 Tomamae Hokkaidō, NE Japan
104 G9 Tomar Santarém, W Portugal
123 T13 Tomari Ostrov Sakhalin, Sakhalinskaya Oblast', SE Russian Federation
115 C16 Tómaros ▲ W Greece
Tomaschow see Tomaszów Lubelski, Poland
Tomaschow see Tomaszów Mazowiecki, Poland
61 E16 Tomás Gomensoro Artigas, N Uruguay
117 N7 Tomashpil' Vinnyts'ka Oblast', C Ukraine
Tomaszów see Tomaszów Mazowiecki
111 P15 Tomaszów Lubelski Ger. Tomaschow. Lubelskie, E Poland
Tomaszów Mazowiecka see Tomaszów Mazowiecki
110 L13 Tomaszów Mazowiecki var. Tomaszów Mazowiecka; prev. Tomaszów, Ger. Tomaschow. Łodzkie, C Poland
40 J13 Tomatlán Jalisco, C Mexico
81 F15 Tombe Jonglei, S Sudan
23 N4 Tombigbee River ~ Alabama/Mississippi, S USA
82 A10 Tomboco Zaire, NW Angola
77 O10 Tombouctou Eng. Timbuktu. Tombouctou, N Mali
77 N9 Tombouctou ◈ region W Mali
37 N16 Tombstone Arizona, SW USA
83 A15 Tombua Port. Porto Alexandre. Namibe, SW Angola
83 J19 Tom Burke Northern, NE South Africa
146 L9 Tomdibuloq Rus. Tamdybulak. Nawoiy Wiloyati, N Uzbekistan
146 L9 Tomditow-Toghi ▲ N Uzbekistan
62 G13 Tomé Bío Bío, C Chile
58 L12 Tomé-Açu Pará, NE Brazil
95 L23 Tomelilla Skåne, S Sweden
105 O10 Tomelloso Castilla-La Mancha, C Spain
14 H10 Tomiko Lake ◎ Ontario, S Canada
77 N12 Tominian Ségou, C Mali
171 N12 Tomini, Gulf of var. Teluk Tomini; prev. Teluk Gorontalo. bay Sulawesi, C Indonesia
Tomini, Teluk see Tomini, Gulf of
165 Q11 Tomioka Fukushima, Honshū, C Japan
113 G14 Tomislavgrad Federacija Bosna I Hercegovina, SW Bosnia and Herzegovina
181 O9 Tomkinson Ranges ▲ South Australia/Western Australia
123 Q11 Tommot Respublika Sakha (Yakutiya), NE Russian Federation
171 Q11 Tomohon Sulawesi, N Indonesia
54 K9 Tomo, Río ~ E Colombia
113 L21 Tomorrit, Mali i ▲ S Albania
11 S17 Tompkins Saskatchewan, S Canada
20 K8 Tompkinsville Kentucky, S USA
171 N11 Tompo Sulawesi, N Indonesia
180 I8 Tom Price Western Australia
122 J12 Tomsk Tomskaya Oblast', C Russian Federation
122 I11 Tomskaya Oblast' ◈ province C Russian Federation
18 K16 Toms River New Jersey, NE USA
Tom Steed Lake see Tom Steed Reservoir
26 L12 Tom Steed Reservoir var. Tom Steed Lake. ▣ Oklahoma, C USA
171 U13 Tomu Irian Jaya, E Indonesia
158 H6 Tomur Feng var. Pik Pobedy, Pobeda Peak. ▲ China/Kyrgyzstan see also Pobedy, Pik
189 N13 Tomworoahlang Pohnpei, E Micronesia
41 U17 Tonalá Chiapas, SE Mexico
106 F6 Tonale, Passo del pass N Italy
164 I11 Tonami Toyama, Honshū, SW Japan
58 C12 Tonantins Amazonas, W Brazil
32 K6 Tonasket Washington, NW USA
55 Y9 Tonate var. Macouria. N French Guiana
18 D10 Tonawanda New York, NE USA
171 Q11 Tondano Sulawesi, C Indonesia
104 H7 Tondela Viseu, N Portugal
95 F24 Tønder Ger. Tondern. Sønderjylland, SW Denmark
Tondern see Tønder
143 N4 Tonekābon var. Shahsawar, Tonkābon; prev. Shahsavār. Māzandarān, N Iran
Tonezh see Tonyezh
193 Y14 Tonga off. Kingdom of Tonga, var. Friendly Islands. ◆ monarchy SW Pacific Ocean
175 R9 Tonga island group SW Pacific Ocean
83 K23 Tongaat KwaZulu/Natal, E South Africa
161 Q13 Tong'an var. Tong an. Fujian, SE China
27 Q4 Tonganoxie Kansas, C USA
39 Y13 Tongass National Forest reserve Alaska, USA
193 Y16 Tongatapu × Tongatapu, S Tonga
193 Y16 Tongatapu island Tongatapu Group, S Tonga
193 Y16 Tongatapu Group island group S Tonga
175 S9 Tonga Trench undersea feature S Pacific Ocean
161 N8 Tongbai Shan ▲ C China
161 P8 Tongcheng Anhui, E China
160 L6 Tongchuan Shaanxi, C China
160 L12 Tongdao var. Tongdao Dongzu Zizhixian; prev. Shuangjiang. Hunan, S China
159 T11 Tongde Qinghai, C China
99 K19 Tongeren Fr. Tongres. Limburg, NE Belgium
Tonggou see Tongyu
163 Y14 Tonghae NE South Korea
160 G13 Tonghai Yunnan, SW China
163 X8 Tonghe Heilongjiang, NE China
163 W11 Tonghua Jilin, NE China
163 Z6 Tongjiang Heilongjiang, NE China
163 Y13 Tongjosŏn-man prev. Broughton Bay. bay E North Korea
163 V7 Tongken He ~ NE China
167 T7 Tongking, Gulf of Chin. Beibu Wan, Vtn. Vinh Băc Bô. gulf China/Vietnam
163 U10 Tongliao Nei Mongol Zizhiqu, N China
161 Q9 Tongling Anhui, E China
161 R9 Tonglu Zhejiang, SE China
187 R14 Tongoa island Shepherd Islands, S Vanuatu
62 G9 Tongoy Coquimbo, C Chile
160 L11 Tongren Guizhou, S China
159 T11 Tongren Qinghai, C China
Tongres see Tongeren
153 U11 Tongsa var. Tongsa Dzong. C Bhutan
Tongsa Dzong see Tongsa
Tongshan see Xuzhou
160 L17 Tongshi Hainan, S China
159 P12 Tongtian He ~ C China
96 I6 Tongue N Scotland, UK
44 H3 Tongue of the Ocean strait C Bahamas
33 X10 Tongue River ~ Montana, NW USA
33 W11 Tongue River Resevoir ▣ Montana, NW USA
159 V11 Tongwei Gansu, C China
159 W9 Tongxin Ningxia, N China
163 U9 Tongyu var. Tonggou. Jilin, NE China
160 J11 Tongzi Guizhou, S China
40 G5 Tónichi Sonora, NW Mexico
81 D14 Tonj Warab, SW Sudan
152 H13 Tonk Rājasthān, N India
Tonkābon see Tonekābon
27 N8 Tonkawa Oklahoma, C USA
167 Q12 Tônlé Sap Eng. Great Lake. ◎ W Cambodia
102 L14 Tonneins Lot-et-Garonne, SW France
103 Q7 Tonnerre Yonne, C France
Tonoas see Dublon
35 U8 Tonopah Nevada, W USA
164 H13 Tonoshō Okayama, Shōdo-shima, SW Japan
43 S17 Tonosí Los Santos, S Panama
95 H16 Tønsberg Vestfold, S Norway
39 T11 Tonsina Alaska, USA
95 D17 Tonstad Vest-Agder, S Norway
193 X15 Tonumea island Nomuka Group, W Tonga
137 O11 Tonya Trabzon, NE Turkey
119 K20 Tonyezh Rus. Tonezh. Homyel'skaya Voblasts', SE Belarus
36 L3 Tooele Utah, W USA
122 L13 Toora-Khem Respublika Tyva, S Russian Federation
183 O5 Toorale East New South Wales, SE Australia
83 H25 Toorberg ▲ S South Africa
118 G5 Tootsi Pärnumaa, SW Estonia
183 U3 Toowoomba Queensland, E Australia
27 Q4 Topeka state capital Kansas, C USA
111 M18 Topla Hung. Toplya. ~ NE Slovakia
122 J12 Topki Kemerovskaya Oblast', S Russian Federation
Toplicza see Toplița
116 J10 Toplița Ger. Töplitz, Hung. Maroshévíz; prev. Toplița Română, Hung. Oláh-Toplicza, Toplicza. Harghita, C Romania
Toplița Română/Töplitz see Toplița
Toplya see Topla
111 I20 Topoľčany Hung. Nagytapolcsány. Nitriansky Kraj, SW Slovakia
40 G8 Topolobampo Sinaloa, C Mexico
116 I13 Topoloveni Argeş, S Romania
114 L11 Topolovgrad prev. Kavakli. Khaskovo, S Bulgaria
Topolya see Bačka Topola
126 I6 Topozero, Ozero ◎ NW Russian Federation
32 J10 Toppenish Washington, NW USA
181 P4 Top Springs Roadhouse Northern Territory, N Australia
189 U11 Tora island Chuuk, C Micronesia
Toraigh see Tory Island
189 U11 Tora Island Pass passage Chuuk Islands, C Micronesia
143 U5 Torbat-e Ḩeydarīyeh var. Turbat-i-Haidari. Khorāsān, NE Iran
143 V5 Torbat-e Jām var. Turbat-i-Jam. Khorāsān, NE Iran
39 Q11 Torbert, Mount ▲ Alaska, USA
31 P6 Torch Lake ◎ Michigan, N USA
Törcsvár see Bran
Torda see Turda
104 L6 Tordesillas Castilla-León, N Spain
92 K13 Töre Norrbotten, N Sweden
95 L17 Töreboda Västra Götaland, S Sweden
95 J21 Torekov Skåne, S Sweden
92 O3 Torell Land physical region SW Svalbard
117 Y8 Torez Donets'ka Oblast', SE Ukraine
101 N14 Torgau Sachsen, E Germany
Torgay Üstirti see Turgayskaya Stolovaya Strana
Torghay see Turgay
95 N22 Torhamn Blekinge, S Sweden
99 C17 Torhout West-Vlaanderen, W Belgium
106 B8 Torino Eng. Turin. Piemonte, NW Italy

◆ Country ● Country Capital ◇ Dependent Territory ○ Dependent Territory Capital ◈ Administrative Region × International Airport ▲ Mountain ▲ Mountain Range ✱ Volcano ~ River ◎ Lake ▣ Reservoir

165 U15 Tori-shima island Izu-shotō, SE Japan
81 F16 Torit Eastern Equatoria, S Sudan
186 H6 Toriu New Britain, E PNG
148 M4 Torkestān, Selseleh-ye Band-e var. Bandi-i Turkistan. ▲ NW Afghanistan
104 L7 Tormes ~ W Spain
Tornacum see Tournai
Torneå see Tornio
92 K12 Torneälven | var.Torniojoki, Fin. Tornionjoki. ~ Finland/Sweden
92 I11 Torneträsk ◎ N Sweden
13 O4 Torngat Mountains ▲ Newfoundland, NE Canada
24 H8 Tornillo Texas, SW USA
92 K13 Tornio Swe. Torneå. Lappi, NW Finland
Torniojoki/Tornionjoki see Torneälven
61 B23 Tornquist Buenos Aires, E Argentina
104 L6 Toro Castilla-León, N Spain
62 H9 Toro, Cerro del ▲ N Chile
77 R12 Torodi Tillabéri, SW Niger
Törökbecse see Novi Bečej
186 J7 Torokina Bougainville Island, NE PNG
111 L23 Törökszentmiklós Jász-Nagykun-Szolnok, E Hungary
42 G7 Torola, Río ~ El Salvador/Honduras
Toronaíos, Kólpos see Kassándras, Kólpos
14 H15 Toronto Ontario, S Canada
31 V12 Toronto Ohio, N USA
Toronto see Lester B.Pearson
27 P6 Toronto Lake ▣ Kansas, C USA
35 V16 Toro Peak ▲ California, W USA
126 H16 Toropets Tverskaya Oblast', W Russian Federation
81 G18 Tororo E Uganda
136 H16 Toros Dağları Eng. Taurus Mountains. ▲ S Turkey
183 N13 Torquay Victoria, SE Australia
97 J24 Torquay SW England, UK
104 M5 Torquemada Castilla-León, N Spain
35 S16 Torrance California, W USA
104 G12 Torrão Setúbal, S Portugal
104 H8 Torre, Alto da ▲ C Portugal
107 K18 Torre Annunziata Campania, S Italy
105 T8 Torreblanca País Valenciano, E Spain
104 L15 Torrecilla ▲ S Spain
105 P4 Torrecilla en Cameros La Rioja, N Spain
105 N13 Torredelcampo Andalucía, S Spain
107 K17 Torre del Greco Campania, S Italy
104 I6 Torre de Moncorvo var. Moncorvo, Tôrre de Moncorvo. Bragança, N Portugal
104 J9 Torrejoncillo Extremadura, W Spain
105 O8 Torrejón de Ardoz Madrid, C Spain
105 N7 Torrelaguna Madrid, C Spain
105 N2 Torrelavega Cantabria, N Spain
107 M16 Torremaggiore Puglia, SE Italy
104 M15 Torremolinos Andalucía, S Spain
182 I6 Torrens, Lake salt lake South Australia
Torrent/Torrent de l'Horta see Torrente
105 S10 Torrente var. Torrent, Torrent de l'Horta. País Valenciano, E Spain
40 L8 Torreón Coahuila de Zaragoza, NE Mexico
105 R13 Torre Pacheco Murcia, SE Spain
106 A8 Torre Pellice Piemonte, NE Italy
105 O13 Torreperogil Andalucía, S Spain
61 J15 Torres Rio Grande do Sul, S Brazil
Torrès, Îles see Torres Islands
187 Q11 Torres Islands Fr. Îles Torrès. island group N Vanuatu
104 G9 Torres Novas Santarém, C Portugal
181 V1 Torres Strait strait Australia/PNG
104 F10 Torres Vedras Lisboa, C Portugal
105 S13 Torrevieja País Valenciano, E Spain
186 B6 Torricelli Mountains ▲ NW PNG
96 G8 Torridon, Loch inlet NW Scotland, UK
106 D9 Torriglia Liguria, NW Italy
104 M9 Torrijos Castilla-La Mancha, C Spain
18 L12 Torrington Connecticut, NE USA
33 Z15 Torrington Wyoming, C USA
93 F16 Torröjen var. Torrön. ◎ C Sweden
Torrön see Torröjen
105 N15 Torrox Andalucía, S Spain
94 N13 Torsåker Gävleborg, C Sweden
95 N21 Torsås Kalmar, S Sweden
95 J14 Torsby Värmland, C Sweden
95 N16 Torshälla Södermanland, C Sweden
95 B19 Tórshavn Dan. Thorshavn Dependent territory capital Faeroe Islands
Torshiz see Kāshmar
45 T9 Tortola island C British Virgin Islands
106 D9 Tortona anc. Dertona. Piemonte, NW Italy
107 L23 Tortorici Sicilia, Italy, C Mediterranean Sea
105 U7 Tortosa anc. Dertosa. Cataluña, E Spain
Tortosa see Ţarţūs
105 U7 Tortosa, Cap headland E Spain
44 L8 Tortue, Île de la var. Tortuga Island. island N Haiti
55 Y10 Tortue, Montagne ▲ C French Guiana
Tortuga, Isla see La Tortuga, Isla
Tortuga Island see Tortue, Île de la
54 C11 Tortugas, Golfo gulf W Colombia
45 T5 Tortuguero, Laguna lagoon N Puerto Rico
137 Q12 Tortum Erzurum, NE Turkey
Torugart, Pereval see Turugart Shankou
137 O12 Torul Gümüşhane, NE Turkey
110 J10 Toruń Ger. Thorn. Toruń, Kujawsko-pomorskie, C Poland
95 K20 Torup Halland, S Sweden
118 I6 Tõrva Ger. Törwa. Valgamaa, S Estonia
Törwa see Tõrva
96 D13 Tory Island Ir. Toraigh. island NW Ireland
111 N19 Torysa Hung. Tarca. ~ NE Slovakia
Törzburg see Bran
126 J16 Torzhok Tverskaya Oblast', W Russian Federation
164 F15 Tosa-Shimizu var. Tosasimizu. Kōchi, Shikoku, SW Japan
Tosasimizu see Tosa-Shimizu
164 G15 Tosa-wan bay SW Japan
83 H21 Tosca North-West, N South Africa
106 F12 Toscana Eng. Tuscany. ◆ region C Italy
107 E14 Toscano, Archipelago Eng. Tuscan Archipelago. island group C Italy
106 G10 Tosco-Emiliano, Appennino Eng. Tuscan-Emilian Mountains. ▲ C Italy
Tōsei see Tungshih
165 N15 To-shima island Izu-shotō, SE Japan
147 Q9 Toshkent Eng./Rus. Tashkent. ● (Uzbekistan) Toshkent Wiloyati, E Uzbekistan
147 Q9 Toshkent × Toshkent Wiloyati, E Uzbekistan
147 P9 Toshkent Wiloyati Rus. Tashkentskaya Oblast'. ◆ province E Uzbekistan
126 H13 Tosno Leningradskaya Oblast', NW Russian Federation
159 Q10 Toson Hu ◎ C China
162 H6 Tosontsengel Dzavhan, NW Mongolia
Tosquduq Qumlari see Goshquduq Qum
105 U4 Tossal de l'Orri var. Llorri. ▲ NE Spain
61 A15 Tostado Santa Fe, C Argentina
118 F6 Tõstamaa Ger. Testama. Pärnumaa, SW Estonia
100 I10 Tostedt Niedersachsen, NW Germany
136 J11 Tosya Kastamonu, N Turkey
95 F15 Totak ◎ S Norway
105 R13 Totana Murcia, SE Spain
94 H13 Toten physical region S Norway
83 G18 Toteng Ngamiland, C Botswana
102 M3 Tôtes Seine-Maritime, N France
Totigi see Tochigi
Totio see Tochio
Totis see Tata
189 U13 Totiw island Chuuk, C Micronesia
127 N13 Tot'ma var. Totma. Vologodskaya Oblast', NW Russian Federation
Tot'ma see Sukhona
55 V9 Totness Coronie, N Suriname
42 C5 Totonicapán Totonicapán, W Guatemala
42 A2 Totonicapán off. Departamento de Totonicapán. ◆ department W Guatemala
61 B18 Totoras Santa Fe, C Argentina
187 Y15 Totoya island S Fiji
183 Q7 Tottenham New South Wales, SE Australia
164 I12 Tottori Tottori, Honshū, SW Japan
164 H12 Tottori off. Tottori-ken. ◆ prefecture Honshū, SW Japan
76 I6 Touâjîl Tiris Zemmour, N Mauritania
76 L15 Touba W Ivory Coast
76 G11 Touba W Senegal
74 E7 Toubkal, Jbel ▲ W Morocco
32 K10 Touchet Washington, NW USA
103 P7 Toucy Yonne, C France
77 O12 Tougan W Burkina
74 L7 Touggourt NE Algeria
77 Q12 Tougouri N Burkina
76 J13 Tougué Moyenne-Guinée, NW Guinea
76 K12 Toukoto Kayes, W Mali
103 S5 Toul Meurthe-et-Moselle, NE France
76 L16 Toulépleu var. Toulobli. W Ivory Coast
161 S14 Touliu C Taiwan
15 U3 Toulnustouc ~ Quebec, SE Canada
Toulobli see Toulépleu
103 T16 Toulon anc. Telo Martius, Tilio Martius. Var, SE France
30 K12 Toulon Illinois, N USA
102 M15 Toulouse anc. Tolosa. Haute-Garonne, S France
102 M15 Toulouse × Haute-Garonne, S France
77 N16 Toumodi C Ivory Coast
74 G9 Tounassine, Hamada hill range W Algeria
166 M7 Toungoo Pegu, C Burma
102 L8 Touraine cultural region C France
Tourane see Đă Nẵng
103 P1 Tourcoing Nord, N France
104 F2 Touriñán, Cabo headland NW Spain
76 J6 Tourine Tiris Zemmour, N Mauritania
102 J3 Tourlaville Manche, N France
99 D19 Tournai var. Tournay, Dut. Doornik; anc. Tornacum. Hainaut, SW Belgium
102 L16 Tournay Hautes-Pyrénées, S France
Tournay see Tournai
103 R12 Tournon Ardèche, E France
103 R9 Tournus Saône-et-Loire, C France
59 Q14 Touros Rio Grande do Norte, E Brazil
102 L8 Tours anc. Caesarodunum, Turoni. Indre-et-Loire, C France
183 Q17 Tourville, Cape headland Tasmania, SE Australia
162 L8 Töv ◆ province C Mongolia
54 H7 Tovar Mérida, NW Venezuela
128 L5 Tovarkovskiy Tul'skaya Oblast', W Russian Federation
Tovil'-Dora see Tavildara
Tövis see Teiuş
137 V11 Tovuz Rus. Tauz. W Azerbaijan
165 R7 Towada Aomori, Honshū, C Japan
184 K3 Towai Northland, North Island, NZ
18 H12 Towanda Pennsylvania, NE USA
29 W4 Tower Minnesota, N USA
171 N12 Towera Sulawesi, N Indonesia
Tower Island see Genovesa, Isla
180 M13 Tower Peak ▲ Western Australia
35 U11 Towne Pass pass California, W USA
29 N3 Towner North Dakota, N USA
33 R10 Townsend Montana, NW USA
181 X6 Townsville Queensland, NE Australia
Towoeti Meer see Towuti, Danau
148 K4 Towraghoudī Herāt, NW Afghanistan
21 X3 Towson Maryland, NE USA
171 O13 Towuti, Danau Dut. Towoeti Meer. ◎ Sulawesi, C Indonesia
Toxkan He see Ak-say
24 K9 Toyah Texas, SW USA
165 R4 Tōya-ko ◎ Hokkaidō, NE Japan
164 L11 Toyama Toyama, Honshū, SW Japan
164 L11 Toyama off. Toyama-ken. ◆ prefecture Honshū, SW Japan
164 L11 Toyama-wan bay W Japan
164 H15 Tōyo Kōchi, Shikoku, SW Japan
Toyohara see Yuzhno-Sakhalinsk
164 L14 Toyohashi var. Toyohasi. Aichi, Honshū, SW Japan
Toyohasi see Toyohashi
164 L14 Toyokawa Aichi, Honshū, SW Japan
164 I14 Toyooka Hyōgo, Honshū, SW Japan
164 L13 Toyota Aichi, Honshū, SW Japan
165 T1 Toyotomi Hokkaidō, NE Japan
Toytepa see Tuytepa
74 M6 Tozeur var. Tawzar. W Tunisia
39 Q8 Tozi, Mount ▲ Alaska, USA
137 Q9 Tqvarch'eli Rus. Tkvarcheli. NW Georgia
Trâblous see Tripoli
137 O11 Trabzon Eng. Trebizond; anc. Trapezus. Trabzon, NE Turkey
137 O11 Trabzon Eng. Trebizond. ◆ province NE Turkey
13 P13 Tracadie New Brunswick, SE Canada
Trachenberg see Żmigród
15 O11 Tracy Quebec, SE Canada
35 O8 Tracy California, W USA
29 S10 Tracy Minnesota, N USA
20 K10 Tracy City Tennessee, S USA
106 D7 Tradate Lombardia, N Italy
84 F6 Traena Bank undersea feature E Norwegian Sea
29 W13 Traer Iowa, C USA
104 J16 Trafalgar, Cabo de headland SW Spain
Traiectum ad Mosam/Traiectum Tungorum see Maastricht
Tráigh Mhór see Tramore
11 O17 Trail British Columbia, SW Canada
58 B11 Traíra, Serra do ▲ NW Brazil
109 V5 Traisen Niederösterreich, NE Austria
109 W4 Traisen ~ NE Austria
109 X4 Traiskirchen Niederösterreich, NE Austria
Trajani Portus see Civitavecchia
Trajectum ad Rhenum see Utrecht
119 H14 Trakai Ger. Traken, Pol. Troki. Trakai, SE Lithuania
Traken see Trakai
97 B20 Tralee Ir. Trá Lí. SW Ireland
97 A20 Tralee Bay Ir. Bá Thrá Lí. bay SW Ireland
Trá Lí see Tralee
Trälleborg see Trelleborg
Tralles see Aydın
61 J16 Tramandaí Rio Grande do Sul, S Brazil
108 C7 Tramelan Bern, W Switzerland
Trá Mhór see Tramore
97 E20 Tramore Ir. Tráigh Mhór, Trá Mhór. S Ireland
95 L18 Tranås Jönköping, S Sweden
62 J7 Trancas Tucumán, N Argentina
104 I7 Trancoso Guarda, N Portugal
95 H22 Tranebjerg Århus, C Denmark
95 K19 Tranemo Västra Götaland, S Sweden
167 N16 Trang Trang, S Thailand
171 V15 Trangan, Pulau island Kepulauan Aru, E Indonesia
Trâng Dinh see Thât Khê
183 Q7 Trangie New South Wales, SE Australia
94 K12 Trängslet Dalarna, C Sweden
107 N16 Trani Puglia, SE Italy
61 F17 Tranqueras Rivera, NE Uruguay
63 G17 Tranqui, Isla island S Chile
39 V6 Trans-Alaska pipeline oil pipeline Alaska, USA
195 Q10 Transantarctic Mountains ▲ Antarctica
Transcarpathian Oblast see Zakarpats'ka Oblast'
Transilvania see Transylvania
Transilvaniei, Alpi see Carpaţii Meridionali
Transjordan see Jordan
172 L11 Transkei Basin undersea feature SW Indian Ocean
122 E9 Trans-Siberian Railway Railroad Russian Federation
Transsylvanische Alpen/Transylvanian Alps see Carpaţii Meridionali
94 K12 Transtrand Dalarna, C Sweden
116 G10 Transylvania Eng. Ardeal, Transilvania, Ger. Siebenbürgen, Hung. Erdély. cultural region NW Romania
167 S14 Tra Ôn Vinh Long, S Vietnam
107 H23 Trapani anc. Drepanum. Sicilia, Italy, C Mediterranean Sea
167 S12 Trâpeăng Vêng Kâmpóng Thum, C Cambodia
Trapezus see Trabzon
114 L9 Trapoklovo Sliven, C Bulgaria
183 P13 Traralgon Victoria, SE Australia
76 H9 Trarza ◆ region SW Mauritania
Trasimenischersee see Trasimeno, Lago
106 H12 Trasimeno, Lago Eng. Lake of Perugia, Ger. Trasimenischersee. ◎ C Italy
95 J20 Träslövsläge Halland, S Sweden
Trás-os-Montes see Cucumbi
104 I6 Trás-os-Montes e Alto Douro former province N Portugal
167 Q12 Trat var. Bang Phra. Trat, S Thailand
Trá Tholl, Inis see Inishtrahull
Traù see Trogir
109 T4 Traun Oberösterreich, N Austria
109 S5 Traun ~ N Austria
Traun, Lake see Traunsee
101 N23 Traunreut Bayern, SE Germany
109 S5 Traunsee var. Traun. Gmundner See, Eng. Lake Traun. ◎ N Austria
Trautenau see Trutnov
21 P11 Travelers Rest South Carolina, SE USA
182 L8 Travellers Lake seasonal lake New South Wales, SE Australia
31 P6 Traverse City Michigan, N USA
29 R7 Traverse, Lake ◎ Minnesota/South Dakota, N USA
185 I16 Travers, Mount ▲ South Island, NZ
11 P17 Travers Reservoir ▣ Alberta, SW Canada
167 T14 Tra Vinh var. Phu Vinh. Tra Vinh, S Vietnam
25 S10 Travis, Lake ▣ Texas, SW USA
112 H12 Travnik Federacija Bosna I Hercegovina, C Bosnia and Herzegovina
109 V11 Trbovlje Ger. Trifail. C Slovenia
23 V13 Treasure Island Florida, SE USA
Treasure State see Montana
186 I8 Treasury Islands island group NW Solomon Islands
106 D9 Trebbia anc. Trebia. ~ NW Italy
100 N8 Trebel ~ NE Germany
103 O16 Trèbes Aude, S France
Trebia see Trebbia
111 F18 Třebíč Ger. Trebitsch. Jihlavský Kraj, S Czech Republic
113 I16 Trebinje Republika Srpska, S Bosnia and Herzegovina
Trebišnica see Trebišnjica
113 H16 Trebišnjica var. Trebišnica. ~ S Bosnia and Herzegovina
111 N20 Trebišov Hung. Tőketerebes. Košický Kraj, E Slovakia
Trebitsch see Třebíč
Trebizond see Trabzon
Trebnitz see Trzebnica
109 V12 Trebnje SE Slovenia
111 D19 Třeboň Ger. Wittingau. Budějovický Kraj, S Czech Republic
104 J15 Trebujena Andalucía, S Spain
100 I7 Treene ~ N Germany
Tree Planters State see Nebraska
109 S9 Treffen Kärnten, S Austria
Trefynwy see Monmouth
102 G5 Tréguier Côtes d'Armor, NW France
61 G18 Treinta y Tres Treinta y Tres, E Uruguay
61 F18 Treinta y Tres ◆ department E Uruguay
114 F9 Treklyanska Reka ~ W Bulgaria
102 K8 Trélazé Maine-et-Loire, NW France
63 K17 Trelew Chubut, SE Argentina
95 K23 Trelleborg var. Trälleborg. Skåne, S Sweden
113 P15 Trem ▲ SE Yugoslavia
15 N11 Tremblant, Mont ▲ Quebec, SE Canada
99 H17 Tremelo Vlaams Brabant, C Belgium
107 M15 Tremiti, Isole island group SE Italy
30 K12 Tremont Illinois, N USA
36 L1 Tremonton Utah, W USA
105 U4 Tremp Cataluña, NE Spain
30 J7 Trempealeau Wisconsin, N USA
15 P8 Trenche ~ Quebec, SE Canada
15 O7 Trenche, Lac ◎ Quebec, SE Canada
111 I20 Trenčiansky Kraj ◆ region W Slovakia
111 I19 Trenčín Ger. Trentschin, Hung. Trencsén. Trenčiansky Kraj, W Slovakia
Trencsén see Trenčín
Trengganu see Terengganu
61 A21 Trenque Lauquen Buenos Aires, E Argentina
14 J14 Trent ~ Ontario, SE Canada
97 N18 Trent ~ C England, UK
Trent see Trento
106 F5 Trentino-Alto Adige prev. Venezia Tridentina. ◆ region N Italy
106 G6 Trento Eng. Trent, Ger. Trient; anc. Tridentum. Trentino-Alto Adige, N Italy
14 J15 Trenton Ontario, SE Canada
23 V10 Trenton Florida, SE USA
23 R1 Trenton Georgia, SE USA
31 S10 Trenton Michigan, N USA
27 S2 Trenton Missouri, C USA
28 M17 Trenton Nebraska, C USA
18 J15 Trenton state capital New Jersey, NE USA
21 W10 Trenton North Carolina, SE USA
20 G9 Trenton Tennessee, S USA
36 L1 Trenton Utah, W USA
Trentschin see Trenčín
Treptow an der Rega see Trzebiatów
61 C23 Tres Arroyos Buenos Aires, E Argentina
61 J15 Três Cachoeiras Rio Grande do Sul, S Brazil
106 E7 Trescore Balneario Lombardia, N Italy
41 V17 Tres Cruces, Cerro ▲ SE Mexico
57 K18 Tres Cruces, Cordillera ▲ W Bolivia
113 N18 Treska ~ NW FYR Macedonia
113 I14 Treskavica ▲ SE Bosnia and Herzegovina
59 J20 Três Lagoas Mato Grosso do Sul, SW Brazil
40 H12 Tres Marías, Islas island group C Mexico
59 M19 Três Marias, Represa ▣ SE Brazil
63 F20 Tres Montes, Península headland S Chile
105 O3 Trespaderne Castilla-León, N Spain
60 G13 Três Passos Rio Grande do Sul, S Brazil
61 A23 Tres Picos, Cerro ▲ E Argentina
63 G17 Tres Picos, Cerro ▲ SW Argentina
60 I12 Três Pinheiros Paraná, S Brazil
59 M21 Três Pontas Minas Gerais, SE Brazil
Tres Puntas, Cabo see Manabique, Punta
60 P9 Três Rios Rio de Janeiro, SE Brazil
Tres Tabernae see Saverne
Trestenberg/Trestendorf see Tăşnad
41 R15 Tres Valles Veracruz-Llave, SE Mexico
94 H12 Tretten Oppland, S Norway
Treuburg see Olecko
101 K21 Treuchtlingen Bayern, S Germany
100 N13 Treuenbrietzen Brandenburg, E Germany
95 F16 Treungen Telemark, S Norway
63 H17 Trevelín Chubut, SW Argentina
Treves/Trèves see Trier
106 I13 Trevi Umbria, C Italy
106 E7 Treviglio Lombardia, N Italy
104 J4 Trevinca, Peña ▲ NW Spain
105 P3 Treviño Castilla-León, N Spain
106 I7 Treviso anc. Tarvisium. Veneto, NE Italy
97 G24 Trevose Head headland SW England, UK
Trg see Feldkirchen in Kärnten
183 P17 Triabunna Tasmania, SE Australia
21 W4 Triangle Virginia, NE USA
83 L18 Triangle Masvingo, SE Zimbabwe
115 L23 Tría Nisiá island Kykládes, Greece, Aegean Sea
Triberg see Triberg im Schwarzwald
101 G23 Triberg im Schwarzwald var. Triberg. Baden-Württemberg, SW Germany
153 P11 Tribhuvan × (Kathmandu) Central, C Nepal
54 C9 Tribugá, Golfo de gulf W Colombia
181 W4 Tribulation, Cape headland Queensland, NE Australia
108 M8 Tribulaun ▲ SW Austria
11 U17 Tribune Saskatchewan, S Canada
26 H5 Tribune Kansas, C USA
107 N18 Tricarico Basilicata, S Italy
107 Q19 Tricase Puglia, SE Italy
Trichinopoly see Tiruchchirāppalli
115 D18 Trichonída, Límni ◎ C Greece
155 G22 Trichūr var. Thrissur. Kerala, SW India
Tricorno see Triglav
183 O8 Trida New South Wales, SE Australia
35 S1 Trident Peak ▲ Nevada, W USA
Tridentum/Trient see Trento
109 T6 Trieben Steiermark, SE Austria
101 D19 Trier Eng. Treves, Fr. Trèves; anc. Augusta Treverorum. Rheinland-Pfalz, SW Germany
106 K7 Trieste Slvn. Trst. Friuli-Venezia Giulia, NE Italy
Trieste, Golfo di/Triest, Golf von see Trieste, Gulf of
106 J8 Trieste, Gulf of Cro. Tršćanski Zaljev, Ger. Golf von Triest, It. Golfo di Trieste, Slvn. Tržaški Zaliv. gulf S Europe
109 W4 Triesting ~ W Austria
Trifail see Trbovlje
116 L9 Trifeşti Iaşi, NE Romania
109 S10 Triglav It. Tricorno. ▲ NW Slovenia
104 I14 Trigueros Andalucía, S Spain
115 E16 Tríkala prev. Trikkala. Thessalía, C Greece
115 E17 Trikeriótis ~ C Greece
Trikkala see Tríkala
Trikomo/Tríkomon see İskele
97 F17 Trim Ir. Baile Átha Troim. E Ireland
108 E7 Trimbach Solothurn, NW Switzerland
109 Q5 Trimmelkam Oberösterreich, N Austria
29 U11 Trimont Minnesota, N USA
Trimontium see Plovdiv
Trinacria see Sicilia
155 K24 Trincomalee var. Trinkomali. Eastern Province, NE Sri Lanka
65 K16 Trindade, Ilha da island Brazil, W Atlantic Ocean
47 Y9 Trindade Spur undersea feature SW Atlantic Ocean
111 J17 Třinec Ger. Trzynietz. Ostravský Kraj, E Czech Republic
57 M16 Trinidad Beni, N Bolivia
54 H9 Trinidad Casanare, E Colombia
44 E6 Trinidad Sancti Spíritus, C Cuba
37 U8 Trinidad Colorado, C USA
61 E19 Trinidad Flores, S Uruguay
45 Y17 Trinidad island C Trinidad and Tobago
Trinidad see Jose Abad Santos
45 Y16 Trinidad and Tobago off. Republic of Trinidad and Tobago. ◆ republic SE West Indies
63 F22 Trinidad, Golfo gulf S Chile
61 B24 Trinidad, Isla island E Argentina
107 N16 Trinitapoli Puglia, SE Italy
55 X10 Trinité, Montagnes de la ▲ C French Guiana
25 W9 Trinity Texas, SW USA
13 U12 Trinity Bay inlet Newfoundland, E Canada
39 P15 Trinity Islands island group Alaska, USA
35 N2 Trinity Mountains ▲ California, W USA
35 S4 Trinity Peak ▲ Nevada, W USA
35 S5 Trinity Range ▲ Nevada, W USA
35 N2 Trinity River ~ California, W USA
25 V8 Trinity River ~ Texas, SW USA
Trinkomali see Trincomalee
173 Y15 Triolet NW Mauritius
107 O20 Trionto, Capo headland S Italy
115 J16 Tripití, Akrotírio headland Ágios Efstrátios, E Greece
138 G6 Tripoli var. Tarābulus, Ţarābulus ash Shām, Trâblous; anc. Tripolis. N Lebanon
29 X12 Tripoli Iowa, C USA
Tripoli see Ţarābulus
115 F20 Trípoli prev. Trípolis. Pelopónnisos, S Greece
Tripolis see Tripoli, Lebanon
Trípolis see Trípoli, Greece
29 Q12 Tripp South Dakota, N USA
153 V15 Tripura var. Hill Tippera. ◆ state NE India
108 K8 Trisanna ~ W Austria
100 H8 Trischen island NW Germany
65 M24 Tristan da Cunha ◇ dependency of Saint Helena SE Atlantic Ocean
67 P15 Tristan da Cunha island SE Atlantic Ocean
65 L18 Tristan da Cunha Fracture Zone tectonic feature S Atlantic Ocean
167 S14 Tri Tôn An Giang, S Vietnam
167 W10 Triton Island island S Paracel Islands
155 G24 Trivandrum var. Thiruvanathapuram. Kerala, SW India
111 H20 Trnava Ger. Tyrnau, Hung. Nagyszombat. Trnavský Kraj, W Slovakia
111 H20 Trnavský Kraj ◆ region W Slovakia
Trnovo see Veliko Tŭrnovo
Trobriand Island see Kiriwina Island
Trobriand Islands see Kiriwina Islands
11 Q16 Trochu Alberta, SW Canada
109 U7 Trofaiach Steiermark, SE Austria
93 F14 Trofors Troms, N Norway
113 E14 Trogir It. Traù. Split-Dalmacija, S Croatia
112 F13 Troglav ▲ Bosnia and Herzegovina/Croatia
107 M16 Troia Puglia, SE Italy
107 K24 Troina Sicilia, Italy, C Mediterranean Sea
173 O16 Trois-Bassins W Réunion
101 E17 Troisdorf Nordrhein-Westfalen, W Germany
74 H5 Trois Fourches, Cap des headland NE Morocco
15 T8 Trois-Pistoles Quebec, SE Canada
99 L21 Trois-Ponts Liège, E Belgium
15 P11 Trois-Rivières Quebec, SE Canada
55 Y12 Trois Sauts S French Guiana
99 M22 Troisvierges Diekirch, N Luxembourg
122 F11 Troitsk Chelyabinskaya Oblast', S Russian Federation
127 T9 Troitsko-Pechorsk Respublika Komi, NW Russian Federation
129 V7 Troitskoye Orenburgskaya Oblast', W Russian Federation
Troki see Trakai
94 F9 Trolla ▲ S Norway
95 J18 Trollhättan Västra Götaland, S Sweden
94 G9 Trollheimen ▲ S Norway
94 E9 Trolltindane ▲ S Norway
58 H11 Trombetas, Rio ~ NE Brazil
130 L16 Tromelin, Île island N Réunion
92 I9 Troms ◆ county N Norway
92 I9 Tromsø Fin. Tromssa. Troms, N Norway
84 F5 Tromsøflaket undersea feature W Barents Sea

◆ Country ● Country Capital ◇ Dependent Territory ○ Dependent Territory Capital ◆ Administrative Region × International Airport ▲ Mountain ▲ Mountain Range Volcano ~ River ◎ Lake ▣ Reservoir

Tromssa see Tromsø
94 H10 Tron ▲ S Norway
35 U12 Trona California, W USA
63 G16 Tronador, Cerro ▲ S Chile
94 H8 Trondheim Ger. Drontheim; prev. Nidaros, Trondhjem. Sør-Trøndelag, S Norway
94 H7 Trondheimsfjorden fjord S Norway
Trondhjem see Trondheim
107 J14 Tronto ≈ C Italy
Troodos see Ólympos
121 P3 Troódos var. Troodos Mountains. ▲ C Cyprus
Troodos Mountains see Troódos
96 I13 Troon W Scotland, UK
107 M22 Tropea Calabria, SW Italy
36 L7 Tropic Utah, W USA
64 L10 Tropic Seamount var. Banc du Tropique. undersea feature E Atlantic Ocean
Tropique, Banc du see Tropic Seamount
Tropoja see Tropojë
113 L17 Tropojë var. Tropoja. Kukës, N Albania
Troppau see Opava
95 O16 Trosa Södermanland, C Sweden
118 H12 Troškūnai Anykščiai, E Lithuania
101 G23 Trossingen Baden-Württemberg, SW Germany
117 T4 Trostyanets' Rus. Trostyanets. Sums'ka Oblast', NE Ukraine
117 N7 Trostyanets' Rus. Trostyanets. Vinnyts'ka Oblast', C Ukraine
116 L11 Trotuş ≈ E Romania
44 M8 Trou-du-Nord N Haiti
25 W7 Troup Texas, SW USA
8 I10 Trout ≈ Northwest Territories, NW Canada
33 N8 Trout Creek Montana, NW USA
32 H10 Trout Lake Washington, NW USA
12 B9 Trout Lake ⊚ Ontario, S Canada
33 T12 Trout Peak ▲ Wyoming, C USA
102 L4 Trouville Calvados, N France
97 L22 Trowbridge S England, UK
23 Q6 Troy Alabama, S USA
27 Q3 Troy Kansas, C USA
27 W4 Troy Missouri, C USA
18 L10 Troy New York, NE USA
21 S10 Troy North Carolina, SE USA
31 R13 Troy Ohio, N USA
25 T9 Troy Texas, SW USA
114 I9 Troyan Lovech, N Bulgaria
114 I9 Troyanski Prokhod pass N Bulgaria
145 N6 Troyebratskiy Severnyy Kazakhstan, N Kazakhstan
103 Q6 Troyes anc. Augustobona Tricassium. Aube, N France
117 X5 Troyits'ke Luhans'ka Oblast', E Ukraine
35 W7 Troy Peak ▲ Nevada, W USA
113 G15 Trpanj Dubrovnik-Neretva, S Croatia
Trščanski Zaljev see Trieste, Gulf of
Trst see Trieste
113 N14 Trstenik Serbia, C Yugoslavia
128 I6 Trubchevsk Bryanskaya Oblast', W Russian Federation
Trubchular see Orlyak
37 S10 Truchas Peak ▲ New Mexico, SW USA
143 P16 Trucial Coast physical region C UAE
Trucial States see United Arab Emirates
35 Q6 Truckee California, W USA
35 R5 Truckee River ≈ Nevada, W USA
129 Q13 Trudfront Astrakhanskaya Oblast', SW Russian Federation
14 I9 Truite, Lac à la ⊚ Quebec, SE Canada
42 K4 Trujillo Colón, NE Honduras
56 C12 Trujillo La Libertad, NW Peru
104 K10 Trujillo Extremadura, W Spain
54 I6 Trujillo Trujillo, NW Venezuela
54 I6 Trujillo off. Estado Trujillo. ◈ state W Venezuela
Truk see Chuuk
Truk Islands see Chuuk Islands
29 U10 Truman Minnesota, N USA
27 X10 Trumann Arkansas, C USA
36 J9 Trumbull, Mount ▲ Arizona, SW USA
114 F9 Trŭn Pernik, W Bulgaria
183 Q8 Trundle New South Wales, SE Australia
131 U13 Trung Phân physical region S Vietnam
Trupcilar see Orlyak
13 Q15 Truro Nova Scotia, SE Canada
97 H25 Truro SW England, UK
25 P5 Truscott Texas, SW USA
116 K9 Truşeşti Botoşani, NE Romania
116 H6 Truskavets' L'vivs'ka Oblast', W Ukraine
95 H22 Trustrup Århus, C Denmark
10 M11 Trutch British Columbia, W Canada
37 Q14 Truth Or Consequences New Mexico, SW USA
111 F15 Trutnov Ger. Trautenau. Hradecký Kraj, NE Czech Republic
103 P13 Truyère ≈ C France
114 K9 Tryavna Lovech, N Bulgaria
28 M14 Tryon Nebraska, C USA
94 I11 Trysilelva ≈ S Norway
112 D10 Tržac Federacija Bosna I Hercegovina, NW Bosnia and Herzegovina
Tržaški Zaliv see Trieste, Gulf of
110 G10 Trzcianka Ger. Schönlanke. Piła, Wielkopolskie, C Poland
110 E7 Trzebiatów Ger. Treptow an der Rega. Zachodniopomorskie, NW Poland
111 G14 Trzebnica Ger. Trebnitz. Dolnośląskie, SW Poland
109 T10 Tržič Ger. Neumarktl. NW Slovenia
Trzynietz see Třinec
Tsabong see Tshabong
162 G7 Tsagaanchuluut Dzavhan, C Mongolia
163 P7 Tsagaanders Dornod, NE Mongolia
163 S8 Tsagaannuur Dornod, E Mongolia
162 G8 Tsagaan-Olom Govĭ-Altay, C Mongolia
162 J8 Tsagaan-Ovoo Övörhangay, C Mongolia
162 D5 Tsagaantüngi Bayan-Ölgiy, NW Mongolia
129 P12 Tsagan Aman Respublika Kalmykiya, SW Russian Federation
23 V11 Tsala Apopka Lake ⊚ Florida, SE USA
Tsamkong see Zhanjiang
Tsangpo see Brahmaputra
162 L9 Tsant Dundgovĭ, C Mongolia
83 G17 Tsao Ngamiland, NW Botswana
172 I4 Tsaratanana Mahajanga, C Madagascar
114 N10 Tsarevo prev. Michurin. Burgas, E Bulgaria
Tsarigrad see İstanbul
Tsaritsyn see Volgograd
126 G13 Tsarskoye Selo prev. Pushkin. Leningradskaya Oblast', NW Russian Federation
117 T7 Tsarychanka Dnipropetrovs'ka Oblast', E Ukraine
83 H21 Tsatsu Southern, S Botswana
81 J20 Tsavo Coast, S Kenya
83 E21 Tsawisis Karas, S Namibia
Tschakathurn see Čakovec
Tschaslau see Čáslav
Tschenstochau see Częstochowa
Tschernembl see Črnomelj
28 K6 Tschida, Lake ⊞ North Dakota, N USA
Tschorna see Mustvee
83 I17 Tsebanana Central, NE Botswana
Tsefat see Ẕefat
162 G8 Tseel Govĭ-Altay, SW Mongolia
128 M13 Tselina Rostovskaya Oblast', SW Russian Federation
Tselinograd see Astana
Tselinogradskaya Oblast' see Akmola
162 J6 Tsengel Hövsgöl, N Mongolia
162 E7 Tsenher Hovd, W Mongolia
146 E12 Tsentral'nyye Garagumy Turkm. Merkezi Garagum. desert C Turkmenistan
83 E21 Tses Karas, S Namibia
Tseshevlya see Tsyeshawlya
162 E7 Tsetsegnuur Hovd, W Mongolia
162 J7 Tsetserleg Arhangay, C Mongolia
77 R16 Tsévié S Togo
83 G21 Tshabong var. Tsabong. Kgalagadi, SW Botswana
83 G20 Tshane Kgalagadi, SW Botswana
Tshangalele, Lac see Lufira, Lac de Retenue de la
83 H17 Tshauxaba Central, C Botswana
79 F21 Tshela Bas-Congo, W Dem. Rep. Congo (Zaire)
79 K22 Tshibala Kasai Occidental, S Dem. Rep. Congo (Zaire)
79 J22 Tshikapa Kasai Occidental, SW Dem. Rep. Congo (Zaire)
79 L22 Tshilenge Kasai Oriental, S Dem. Rep. Congo (Zaire)
79 L24 Tshimbalanga Katanga, S Dem. Rep. Congo (Zaire)
79 L22 Tshimbulu Kasai Occidental, S Dem. Rep. Congo (Zaire)
Tshiumbe see Chiumbe
79 M21 Tshofa Kasai Oriental, C Dem. Rep. Congo (Zaire)
79 K18 Tshuapa ≈ C Dem. Rep. Congo (Zaire)
Tshwane see Pretoria
114 G7 Tsibritsa ≈ NW Bulgaria
Tsien Tang see Puyang Jiang
114 I12 Tsigansko Gradishte ▲ Bulgaria/Greece
8 H7 Tsiigehtchic prev. Arctic Red River. Northwest Territories, NW Canada
127 Q7 Tsil'ma ≈ NW Russian Federation
119 J17 Tsimkavichy Rus. Timkovichi. Minskaya Voblasts', C Belarus
128 M11 Tsimlyansk Rostovskaya Oblast', SW Russian Federation
129 N11 Tsimlyanskoye Vodokhranilishche var. Tsimlyansk Vodoskhovshche, Eng. Tsimlyansk Reservoir ⊞ SW Russian Federation
Tsimlyansk Reservoir see Tsimlyanskoye Vodokhranilishche
Tsimlyansk Vodoskhovshche see Tsimlyanskoye Vodokhranilishche
Tsinan see Jinan
Tsing Hai see Qinghai Hu, China
Tsinghai see Qinghai, China
Tsingtao/Tsingtau see Qingdao
Tsingyuan see Baoding
Tsinkiang see Quanzhou
Tsintao see Qingdao
83 D17 Tsintsabis Otjikoto, N Namibia
172 H8 Tsiombe var. Tsihombe. Toliara, S Madagascar
123 O13 Tsipa ≈ S Russian Federation
172 H5 Tsiribihina ≈ W Madagascar
172 I5 Tsiroanomandidy Antananarivo, C Madagascar
189 U13 Tsis island Chuuk, C Micronesia
Tsitsihar see Qiqihar
129 Q3 Tsivil'sk Chuvashskaya Respublika, W Russian Federation
137 T9 Ts'khinvali prev. Staliniri. C Georgia
119 J19 Tsna ≈ SW Belarus
126 I15 Tsna var. Zna. ≈ W Russian Federation
162 K11 Tsoohor Ömnögovĭ, S Mongolia
164 K14 Tsu var. Tu. Mie, Honshū, SW Japan
165 O10 Tsubame var. Tubame. Niigata, Honshū, C Japan
165 V3 Tsubetsu Hokkaidō, NE Japan
165 O13 Tsuchiura var. Tutiura. Ibaraki, Honshū, S Japan
165 Q6 Tsugaru-kaikyō strait N Japan
164 E14 Tsukumi var. Tukumi. Ōita, Kyūshū, SW Japan
162 E5 Tsul-Ulaan Bayan-Ölgiy, W Mongolia
83 D17 Tsumeb Otjikoto, N Namibia
83 F17 Tsumkwe Otjozondjupa, NE Namibia
164 D15 Tsuno Miyazaki, Kyūshū, SW Japan
164 D12 Tsuno-shima island SW Japan
164 K12 Tsuruga var. Turuga. Fukui, Honshū, SW Japan
164 H12 Tsurugi-san ▲ Shikoku, SW Japan
165 P9 Tsuruoka var. Turuoka. Yamagata, Honshū, C Japan
164 C12 Tsushima var. Tsushima-tō, Tusima. island group SW Japan
Tsushima-tō see Tsushima
164 H12 Tsuyama var. Tuyama. Okayama, Honshū, SW Japan
83 G19 Tswaane Ghanzi, W Botswana
119 N16 Tsyakhtsin Rus. Tekhtin. Mahilyowskaya Voblasts', E Belarus
119 P19 Tsyerakhowka Rus. Terekhovka. Homyel'skaya Voblasts', SE Belarus
119 I17 Tsyeshawlya Rus. Cheshevlya, Tseshevlya. Brestskaya Voblasts', SW Belarus
Tsyurupinsk see Tsyurupyns'k
117 R10 Tsyurupyns'k Rus. Tsyurupinsk. Khersons'ka Oblast', S Ukraine
Tu see Tsu
186 C7 Tua ≈ C PNG
Tuaim see Tuam
184 L6 Tuakau Waikato, North Island, NZ
97 C17 Tuam Ir. Tuaim. W Ireland
185 K14 Tuamarina Marlborough, South Island, NZ
Tuamotu, Archipel des see Tuamotu, Îles
193 Q9 Tuamotu Fracture Zone tectonic feature E Pacific Ocean
191 W9 Tuamotu, Îles var. Archipel des Tuamotu, Dangerous Archipelago, Tuamotu Islands. island group N French Polynesia
Tuamotu Islands see Tuamotu, Îles
175 X10 Tuamotu Ridge undersea feature C Pacific Ocean
167 R5 Tuân Giao Lai Châu, N Vietnam
171 O2 Tuao Luzon, N Philippines
190 B15 Tuapa NW Niue
43 N7 Tuapi Región Autónoma Atlántico Norte, NE Nicaragua
128 K15 Tuapse Krasnodarskiy Kray, SW Russian Federation
169 U6 Tuaran Sabah, East Malaysia
104 I6 Tua, Rio ≈ N Portugal
192 H15 Tuasivi Savai'i, C Samoa
185 B24 Tuatapere Southland, South Island, NZ
36 M9 Tuba City Arizona, SW USA
138 H11 Ţubah, Qaşr aţ castle Ma'ān, C Jordan
Tubame see Tsubame
169 R16 Tuban prev. Toeban. Jawa, C Indonesia
141 O16 Tuban, Wādī dry watercourse SW Yemen
61 K14 Tubarão Santa Catarina, S Brazil
98 O10 Tubbergen Overijssel, E Netherlands
Tubeke see Tubize
101 H22 Tübingen var. Tuebingen. Baden-Württemberg, SW Germany
129 W6 Tubinskiy Respublika Bashkortostan, W Russian Federation
99 G19 Tubize Dut. Tubeke. Wallon Brabant, C Belgium
76 J16 Tubmanburg NW Liberia
75 T7 Ţubruq Eng. Tobruk, It. Tobruch. NE Libya
191 T13 Tubuai island Îles Australes, SW French Polynesia
Tubuai, Îles/Tubuai Islands see Australes, Îles
40 F3 Tubutama Sonora, NW Mexico
54 K4 Tucacas Falcón, N Venezuela
59 P16 Tucano Bahia, E Brazil
57 P19 Tucavaca, Río ≈ E Bolivia
110 H8 Tuchola Kujawsko-pomorskie, C Poland
111 M17 Tuchów Małopolskie, SE Poland
23 S3 Tucker Georgia, SE USA
27 W10 Tuckerman Arkansas, C USA
64 B12 Tucker's Town E Bermuda
Tuckum see Tukums
36 M15 Tucson Arizona, SW USA
62 J7 Tucumán off. Provincia de Tucumán. ◈ province N Argentina
Tucumán see San Miguel de Tucumán
37 V11 Tucumcari New Mexico, SW USA
58 H13 Tucunaré Pará, N Brazil
55 Q6 Tucupita Delta Amacuro, NE Venezuela
58 K13 Tucuruí, Represa de ⊞ NE Brazil
110 F9 Tuczno Zachodniopomorskie, NW Poland
Tuddo see Tudu
105 Q5 Tudela Basq. Tutera; anc. Tutela. Navarra, N Spain
104 M6 Tudela de Duero Castilla-León, N Spain
138 K6 Tudmur var. Tadmur, Tamar, Gk. Palmyra; Bibl. Tadmor. Ḩimş, C Syria
118 J4 Tudu Ger. Tuddo. Lääne-Virumaa, NE Estonia
Tuebingen see Tübingen
122 J14 Tuekta Respublika Altay, S Russian Federation
104 I5 Tuela, Rio ≈ N Portugal
153 X12 Tuensang Nāgāland, NE India
136 L15 Tufanbeyli Adana, C Turkey
Tüffer see Laško
186 F9 Tufi Northern, S PNG
193 O3 Tufts Plain undersea feature N Pacific Ocean
Tugalan see Kolkhozobod
67 V14 Tugela ≈ SE South Africa
21 P6 Tug Fork ≈ S USA
39 P15 Tugidak Island island Trinity Islands, Alaska, USA
171 O2 Tuguegarao Luzon, N Philippines
123 S12 Tugur Khabarovskiy Kray, SE Russian Federation
161 P4 Tuhai He ≈ E China
104 G4 Tui Galicia, NW Spain
77 O13 Tui var. Grand Balé. ≈ W Burkina
57 J16 Tuichi, Río ≈ W Bolivia
64 Q11 Tuineje Fuerteventura, Islas Canarias, Spain, NE Atlantic Ocean
43 X16 Tuira, Río ≈ SE Panama
Tuisarkan see Tūysarkān
Tujiabu see Yongxiu
129 W5 Tukan Respublika Bashkortostan, W Russian Federation
171 P14 Tukangbesi, Kepulauan Dut. Toekang Besi Eilanden. island group C Indonesia
147 V13 Tŭkhtamish Rus. Toktomush, prev. Tokhtamyshbek. SE Tajikistan
184 O12 Tukituki ≈ North Island, NZ
Tu-k'ou see Panzhihua
121 P12 Tūkrah NE Libya
8 H6 Tuktoyaktuk Northwest Territories, NW Canada
168 I9 Tuktuk Pulau Samosir, W Indonesia
Tukumi see Tsukumi
118 E9 Tukums Ger. Tuckum. Tukums, W Latvia
81 G24 Tukuyu prev. Neu-Langenburg. Mbeya, S Tanzania
Tukzār see Tokzār
41 O13 Tula var. Tula de Allende. Hidalgo, C Mexico
41 O11 Tula Tamaulipas, C Mexico
128 K5 Tula Tul'skaya Oblast', W Russian Federation
Tulach Mhór see Tullamore
Tula de Allende see Tula
159 N10 Tulage Ar Gol ≈ W China
186 M9 Tulaghi var. Tulagi. Florida Islands, C Solomon Islands
Tulagi see Tulaghi
41 P13 Tulancingo Hidalgo, C Mexico
35 R11 Tulare California, W USA
29 P9 Tulare South Dakota, N USA
35 Q12 Tulare Lake Bed salt flat California, W USA
37 S14 Tularosa New Mexico, SW USA
37 P13 Tularosa Mountains ▲ New Mexico, SW USA
37 S15 Tularosa Valley basin New Mexico, SW USA
83 E25 Tulbagh Western Cape, SW South Africa
56 C5 Tulcán Carchi, N Ecuador
117 N13 Tulcea Tulcea, E Romania
117 N13 Tulcea ◈ county SE Romania
Tul'chin see Tul'chyn
117 N7 Tul'chyn Rus. Tul'chin. Vinnyts'ka Oblast', C Ukraine
Tuléar see Toliara
35 O1 Tulelake California, W USA
116 J10 Tulgheş Hung. Gyergyótölgyes. Harghita, C Romania
Tul'govichi see Tul'havichy
119 N20 Tul'havichy Rus. Tul'govichi. Homyel'skaya Voblasts', SE Belarus
Tuli see Thuli
25 N4 Tulia Texas, SW USA
8 I9 Tulita prev. Fort Norman, Norman. Northwest Territories, NW Canada
20 J10 Tullahoma Tennessee, S USA
183 N12 Tullamarine × (Melbourne) Victoria, SE Australia
183 Q7 Tullamore New South Wales, SE Australia
97 E18 Tullamore Ir. Tulach Mhór. C Ireland
103 N12 Tulle anc. Tutela. Corrèze, C France
109 X3 Tulln var. Oberhollabrunn. Niederösterreich, NE Austria
109 W4 Tulln ≈ NE Austria
22 H6 Tullos Louisiana, S USA
97 F19 Tullow Ir. An Tullach. SE Ireland
181 W5 Tully Queensland, NE Australia
126 J3 Tuloma ≈ NW Russian Federation
114 K10 Tulovo Stara Zagora, C Bulgaria
27 P9 Tulsa Oklahoma, C USA
153 N11 Tulsipur Mid Western, W Nepal
128 K6 Tul'skaya Oblast' ◈ province W Russian Federation
128 L14 Tul'skiy Respublika Adygeya, SW Russian Federation
186 E5 Tulu Manus Island, N PNG
54 D10 Tuluá Valle del Cauca, W Colombia
116 M12 Tulucești Galați, E Romania
39 N12 Tuluksak Alaska, USA
41 Z12 Tulum, Ruinas de ruins Quintana Roo, SE Mexico
122 M13 Tulun Irkutskaya Oblast', S Russian Federation
169 R17 Tulungagung prev. Toeloengagoeng. Jawa, C Indonesia
186 J6 Tulun Islands var. Kilinailau Islands; prev. Carteret Islands. island group NE PNG
128 M4 Tuma Ryazanskaya Oblast', W Russian Federation
54 B12 Tumaco Nariño, SW Colombia
54 B12 Tumaco, Bahía de bay SW Colombia
Tuman-gang see Tumen
42 L8 Tuma, Río ≈ N Nicaragua
95 O16 Tumba Stockholm, C Sweden
Tumba, Lac see Ntomba, Lac
169 S12 Tumbangsenamang Borneo, C Indonesia
183 Q10 Tumbarumba New South Wales, SE Australia
56 A8 Tumbes Tumbes, NW Peru
56 A9 Tumbes off. Departamento de Tumbes. ◈ department NW Peru
19 P5 Tumbledown Mountain ▲ Maine, NE USA
11 N13 Tumbler Ridge British Columbia, W Canada
167 Q12 Tumbŏt, Phnum ▲ W Cambodia
182 G9 Tumby Bay South Australia
163 Y10 Tumen Jilin, NE China
163 Y11 Tumen Chin. Tumen Jiang, Kor. Tuman-gang, Rus. Tumyn'tszyan. ≈ E Asia
Tumen Jiang see Tumen
55 Q8 Tumeremo Bolívar, E Venezuela
155 G19 Tumkūr Karnātaka, W India
96 I10 Tummel ≈ C Scotland, UK
188 B15 Tumon Bay bay W Guam
77 P14 Tumu NW Ghana
58 I10 Tumuc Humac Mountains var. Serra Tumucumaque. ▲ N South America
Tumucumaque, Serra see Tumuc Humac Mountains
183 Q10 Tumut New South Wales, SE Australia
Tumyn'tszyan see Tumen
Tün see Ferdows
45 U14 Tunapuna Trinidad, Trinidad and Tobago
60 K11 Tunas Paraná, S Brazil
Tunbridge Wells see Royal Tunbridge Wells
114 L11 Tunca Nehri Bul. Tundzha. ≈ Bulgaria/Turkey see also Tundzha
137 O14 Tunceli var. Kalan. Tunceli, E Turkey
137 O14 Tunceli ◈ province C Turkey
152 J12 Tūndla Uttar Pradesh, N India
81 I25 Tunduru Ruvuma, S Tanzania
114 L10 Tundzha Turk. Tunca Nehri. ≈ Bulgaria/Turkey see also Tunca Nehri
155 H17 Tungabhadra ≈ S India
155 F17 Tungabhadra Reservoir ⊚ S India
191 P2 Tungaru prev. Gilbert Islands. island group W Kiribati
171 P7 Tungawan Mindanao, S Philippines
T'ung-shan see Xuzhou
161 Q16 Tungsha Tao Chin. Dongsha Qundao, Eng. Pratas Island. island S Taiwan
161 S13 Tungshih Jap. Tōsei. N Taiwan
8 H9 Tungsten Northwest Territories, W Canada
Tung-t'ing Hu see Dongting Hu
56 A13 Tungurahua ◈ province C Ecuador
95 F14 Tunhovdfjorden ⊚ S Norway
22 K2 Tunica Mississippi, S USA
75 N5 Tunis var. Tūnis. ● (Tunisia) NE Tunisia
75 N5 Tunis, Golfe de Ar. Khalīj Tūnis. gulf NE Tunisia
75 N6 Tunisia off. Republic of Tunisia, Ar. Al Jumhūrīyah at Tūnisīyah, Fr. République Tunisienne. ◆ republic N Africa
Tūnisīyah, Al Jumhūrīyah at see Tunisia
Tūnis, Khalīj see Tunis, Golfe de
54 G9 Tunja Boyacá, C Colombia
93 F14 Tunnsjøen ⊚ C Norway
39 N12 Tuntutuliak Alaska, USA
147 U8 Tunuk Chuyskaya Oblast', C Kyrgyzstan
13 Q6 Tunungayualok Island island Newfoundland, E Canada
62 H11 Tunuyán Mendoza, W Argentina
197 P14 Tunu ◈ province E Greenland
62 I11 Tunuyán, Río ≈ W Argentina
Tunxi see Huangshan
35 P9 Tuolumne River ≈ California, W USA
Tuong Buong see Tương Đương
167 R7 Tương Đương var. Tuong Buong. Nghê An, N Vietnam
160 I13 Tuoniang Jiang ≈ S China
159 N12 Tuotuo He ≈ C China
159 O12 Tuotuoheyan var. Tanggulashan, Togton-heyan. Qinghai, C China
Tüp see Tyup
60 J9 Tupã São Paulo, S Brazil
191 S10 Tupai var. Motu Iti. atoll Îles Sous le Vent, W French Polynesia
61 G15 Tupanciretã Rio Grande do Sul, S Brazil
22 M2 Tupelo Mississippi, S USA
59 K18 Tupiraçaba Goiás, S Brazil
57 L21 Tupiza Potosí, S Bolivia
11 N13 Tupper British Columbia, W Canada
18 J8 Tupper Lake ⊚ New York, NE USA
62 H11 Tupungato, Volcán ▲ W Argentina
163 T9 Tuquan Nei Mongol Zizhiqu, N China
54 C13 Túquerres Nariño, SW Colombia
153 U13 Tura Meghālaya, NE India
122 M10 Tura Evenkiyskiy Avtonomnyy Okrug, N Russian Federation
122 G10 Tura ≈ C Russian Federation
140 M10 Turabah Makkah, W Saudi Arabia
55 O8 Turagua, Cerro ▲ C Venezuela
184 L12 Turakina Manawatu-Wanganui, North Island, NZ
185 K15 Turakirae Head headland North Island, NZ
186 B8 Turama ≈ S PNG
122 K13 Turan Respublika Tyva, S Russian Federation
184 M10 Turangi Waikato, North Island, NZ
146 F11 Turan Lowland var. Turan Plain, Kaz. Turan Oypaty, Rus. Turanskaya Nizmennost', Turk. Turan Pesligi, Uzb. Turon Pasttekisligi. plain C Asia
Turan Oypaty/Turan Pesligi/Turan Plain/Turanskaya Nizmennost' see Turan Lowland
138 K7 Ţurāq al 'Ilab hill range S Syria
119 K20 Turaw Rus. Turov. Homyel'skaya Voblasts', SE Belarus
140 L2 Ţurayf Al Ḩudūd ash Shamālīyah, NW Saudi Arabia
Turba see Teruel
54 E5 Turbaco Bolívar, N Colombia
148 K15 Turbat Baluchistān, SW Pakistan
Turbat-i-Haidari see Torbat-e Ḩeydarīyeh
Turbat-i-Jam see Torbat-e Jām
54 D7 Turbo Antioquia, NW Colombia
Turčianský Svätý Martin see Martin
116 H10 Turda Ger. Thorenburg, Hung. Torda. Cluj, NW Romania
142 M7 Ţūreh Markazī, W Iran
191 X12 Tureia atoll Îles Tuamotu, SE French Polynesia
110 I12 Turek Wielkopolskie, C Poland
93 L19 Turenki Etelä-Suomi, S Finland
Turfan see Turpan
145 R8 Turgay Kaz. Torghay. Akmola, W Kazakhstan
145 N10 Turgay Kaz. Torgay. ≈ C Kazakhstan
144 M8 Turgayskaya Stolovaya Strana Kaz. Torgay Üstirti. plateau Kazakhstan/Russian Federation
Turgel see Türi
114 L8 Türgovishte prev. Eski Dzhumaya. Tŭrgovishte, N Bulgaria
114 L8 Türgovishte ◈ province N Bulgaria
136 C14 Turgutlu Manisa, W Turkey
136 L12 Turhal Tokat, N Turkey
118 H4 Türi Ger. Turgel. Järvamaa, N Estonia
105 S9 Turia ≈ E Spain
58 M12 Turiaçu Maranhão, E Brazil
Turin see Torino
116 I3 Turiys'k Volyns'ka Oblast', NW Ukraine
Turja see Tur"ya
116 H6 Turka L'vivs'ka Oblast', W Ukraine
Turkana, Lake see Rudolf, Lake
145 P16 Turkestan Kaz. Türkistan. Yuzhnyy Kazakhstan, S Kazakhstan
147 Q12 Turkestan Range Rus. Turkestanskiy Khrebet. ▲ C Asia
Turkestanskiy Khrebet see Turkestan Range
111 M23 Túrkeve Jász-Nagykun-Szolnok, E Hungary
25 O4 Turkey Texas, SW USA
136 H14 Turkey off. Republic of Turkey, Turk. Türkiye Cumhuriyeti. ◆ republic SW Asia
181 N4 Turkey Creek Western Australia
26 M9 Turkey Creek ≈ Oklahoma, C USA
37 T9 Turkey Mountains ▲ New Mexico, SW USA
29 X11 Turkey River ≈ Iowa, C USA
129 N7 Turki Saratovskaya Oblast', W Russian Federation
121 O1 Turkish Republic of Northern Cyprus ◇ disputed territory Cyprus
Türkistan see Turkestan
Turkistan, Bandi-i see Torkestān, Selseleh-ye Band-e
Türkiye Cumhuriyeti see Turkey
Türkmen Aylagy see Turkmenskiy Zaliv
146 A10 Turkmenbashi prev. Krasnovodsk. Balkanskiy Velayat, W Turkmenistan
Türkmengala see Turkmen-kala
146 G13 Turkmenistan off. Turkmenistan; prev. Turkmenskaya Soviet Socialist Republic. ◆ republic C Asia
146 J14 Turkmen-kala Turkm. Türkmengala; prev. Turkmen-Kala. Maryyskiy Velayat, S Turkmenistan
Turkmenskaya Soviet Socialist Republic see Turkmenistan
146 A11 Turkmenskiy Zaliv Turkm. Türkmen Aylagy. lake gulf W Turkmenistan
136 L16 Türkoğlu Kahramanmaraş, S Turkey
44 L6 Turks and Caicos Islands ◇ UK dependent territory N West Indies
64 G10 Turks and Caicos Islands island group N West Indies
45 N6 Turks Islands island group SE Turks and Caicos Islands
93 K19 Turku Swe. Åbo. Länsi-Suomi, W Finland
81 H17 Turkwel seasonal river NW Kenya
27 P9 Turley Oklahoma, C USA
35 P9 Turlock California, W USA
118 I12 Turmantas Zarasai, NE Lithuania
54 L5 Turmero Aragua, N Venezuela
Turmberg see Wieżyca

◆ Country ● Country Capital ◇ Dependent Territory ○ Dependent Territory Capital ◈ Administrative Region × International Airport ▲ Mountain ▲ Mountain Range Volcano ≈ River ⊚ Lake ⊞ Reservoir

184 N13 **Turnagain, Cape** *headland* North Island, NZ
Turnau *see* Turnov
42 H2 **Turneffe Islands** *island group* E Belize
18 M11 **Turners Falls** Massachusetts, NE USA
11 P16 **Turner Valley** Alberta, SW Canada
99 I16 **Turnhout** Antwerpen, N Belgium
109 V5 **Turnitz** Niederösterreich, E Austria
11 S12 **Turnor Lake** ⊚ Saskatchewan, C Canada
111 E15 **Turnov** *Ger.* Turnau. Liberecký Kraj, N Czech Republic
Tŭrnovo *see* Veliko Tŭrnovo
116 I15 **Turnu Măgurele** *var.* Turnu-Măgurele. Teleorman, S Romania
Turnu Severin *see* Drobeta-Turnu Severin
Turócszentmárton *see* Martin
Turoni *see* Tours
Turan Pasttekisligi *see* Turan Lowland
Turov *see* Turaw
Turpakkla *see* Turpoqqal'a
158 M6 **Turpan** *var.* Turfan. Xinjiang Uygur Zizhiqu, NW China
Turpan Depression *see* Turpan Pendi
158 M6 **Turpan Pendi** *Eng.* Turpan Depression. *depression* NW China
158 M5 **Turpan Zhan** Xinjiang Uygur Zizhiqu, W China
Turpentine State *see* North Carolina
146 J10 **Turpoqqal'a** *Rus.* Turpakkla. Khorazm Wiloyati, W Uzbekistan
44 H8 **Turquino, Pico** ▲ E Cuba
27 Y10 **Turrell** Arkansas, C USA
43 N14 **Turrialba** Cartago, E Costa Rica
96 K8 **Turriff** NE Scotland, UK
139 V7 **Tursāq** E Iraq
Turshiz *see* Kāshmar
Tursunzade *see* Tursunzoda
147 P13 **Tursunzoda** *Rus.* Tursunzade; *prev.* Regar. W Tajikistan
162 J4 **Turt** Hövsgöl, N Mongolia
146 I9 **Türtkŭl** *Rus.* Turtkul'; *prev.* Petroaleksandrovsk. Qoraqalpoghiston Respublikasi, W Uzbekistan
29 O9 **Turtle Creek** ↝ South Dakota, N USA
30 K4 **Turtle Flambeau Flowage** ⊠ Wisconsin, N USA
11 S14 **Turtleford** Saskatchewan, S Canada
28 M4 **Turtle Lake** North Dakota, N USA
92 K12 **Turtola** Lappi, NW Finland
122 M10 **Turu** ↝ N Russian Federation
Turuga *see* Tsuruga
147 V10 **Turugart Pass** *pass* China/Kyrgyzstan
158 E7 **Turugart Shankou** *var.* Pereval Torugart. *pass* China/Kyrgyzstan
122 K9 **Turukhan** ↝ N Russian Federation
122 K9 **Turukhansk** Krasnoyarskiy Kray, N Russian Federation
139 N3 **Ţurumbah** *well* NE Syria
Turuoka *see* Tsuruoka
144 H14 **Turush** Mangistau, SW Kazakhstan
60 K7 **Turvo, Rio** ↝ S Brazil
116 J2 **Tur"ya** *Pol.* Turja, *Rus.* Tur'ya. ↝ NW Ukraine
23 O4 **Tuscaloosa** Alabama, S USA
23 O4 **Tuscaloosa, Lake** ⊚ Alabama, S USA
Tuscan Archipelago *see* Toscano, Archipelago
Tuscan-Emilian Mountains *see* Tosco-Emiliano, Appennino
Tuscany *see* Toscana
35 V2 **Tuscarora** Nevada, W USA
18 F15 **Tuscarora Mountain** *ridge* Pennsylvania, NE USA
30 M14 **Tuscola** Illinois, N USA
25 P7 **Tuscola** Texas, SW USA
23 O2 **Tuscumbia** Alabama, S USA
92 O4 **Tusenøyane** *island group* S Svalbard
144 K13 **Tushybas, Zaliv** *prev.* Zaliv Paskevicha. *lake gulf* SW Kazakhstan
171 Y15 **Tusirah** Irian Jaya, E Indonesia
23 Q5 **Tuskegee** Alabama, S USA
94 E8 **Tustna** *island* S Norway
39 R12 **Tustumena Lake** ⊚ Alaska, USA
110 K13 **Tuszyn** Łodzkie, C Poland
137 S13 **Tutak** Ağrı, E Turkey
185 C20 **Tutamoe Range** ▲ North Island, NZ
Tutasev *see* Tutayev
126 L15 **Tutayev** *var.* Tutasev. Yaroslavskaya Oblast', W Russian Federation
Tutela *see* Tulle, France
Tutela *see* Tudela, Spain
Tutera *see* Tudela
155 H23 **Tuticorin** Tamil Nādu, SE India
113 L15 **Tutin** Serbia, S Yugoslavia
184 O10 **Tutira** Hawke's Bay, North Island, NZ
Tutiura *see* Tsuchiura
122 K10 **Tutonchany** Evenkiyskiy Avtonomnyy Okrug, N Russian Federation
114 L6 **Tutrakan** Silistra, NE Bulgaria
29 N5 **Tuttle** North Dakota, N USA
26 M11 **Tuttle** Oklahoma, C USA
27 O3 **Tuttle Creek Lake** ⊠ Kansas, C USA
101 H23 **Tuttlingen** Baden-Württemberg, S Germany
171 R16 **Tutuala** W East Timor
192 K17 **Tutuila** *island* W American Samoa
83 I18 **Tutume** Central, E Botswana
39 N7 **Tututalak Mountain** ▲ Alaska, USA
22 K3 **Tutwiler** Mississippi, S USA
162 L8 **Tuul Gol** ↝ N Mongolia
93 O16 **Tuupovaara** Itä-Suomi, E Finland
Tuva *see* Tyva, Respublika
190 E7 **Tuvalu** *prev.* Ellice Islands. ◆ *commonwealth republic* SW Pacific Ocean
Tuvana-i-Tholo *see* Tuvana-i-Colo
Tuvinskaya ASSR *see* Tyva, Respublika
Tuvutha *see* Tuvuca
141 P9 **Ţuwayq, Jabal** ▲ C Saudi Arabia
138 H13 **Ţuwayyil ash Shihāq** *desert* S Jordan
11 U16 **Tuxford** Saskatchewan, S Canada
167 U12 **Tu Xoay** Đăc Lăc, S Vietnam
40 L14 **Tuxpan** Jalisco, C Mexico
40 J12 **Tuxpan** Nayarit, C Mexico
41 Q12 **Tuxpán** *var.* Tuxpán de Rodríguez Cano. Veracruz-Llave, E Mexico
Tuxpán de Rodríguez Cano *see* Tuxpán
41 R15 **Tuxtepec** *var.* San Juan Bautista Tuxtepec. Oaxaca, S Mexico
41 U16 **Tuxtla** *var.* Tuxtla Gutiérrez. Chiapas, SE Mexico
Tuxtla *see* San Andrés Tuxtla
Tuxtla Gutiérrez *see* Tuxtla
Tuyama *see* Tsuyama
167 T5 **Tuyên Quang** Tuyên Quang, N Vietnam
167 U13 **Tuy Hoa** Binh Thuân, S Vietnam
167 V12 **Tuy Hoa** Phu Yên, S Vietnam
129 U5 **Tuymazy** Respublika Bashkortostan, W Russian Federation
142 L6 **Tūysarkān** *var.* Tuisarkan, Tuyserkān. Hamadān, W Iran
Tuyserkān *see* Tūysarkān
147 Q10 **Tuytepa** *Rus.* Toytepa. Toshkent Wiloyati, E Uzbekistan
145 W16 **Tuyuk** *Kaz.* Tuyyq. Almaty, SE Kazakhstan
Tuyyq *see* Tuyuk
136 I14 **Tuz Gölü** ⊚ C Turkey
127 Q15 **Tuzha** Kirovskaya Oblast', NW Russian Federation
113 K17 **Tuzi** Montenegro, SW Yugoslavia
139 T5 **Tūz Khurmātū** N Iraq
112 I11 **Tuzla** Federacija Bosna I Hercegovina, NE Bosnia and Herzegovina
117 N15 **Tuzla** Constanţa, SE Romania
137 T12 **Tuzluca** Igdır, NE Turkey
95 J20 **Tvååker** Halland, S Sweden
95 F17 **Tvedestrand** Aust-Agder, S Norway
126 J16 **Tver'** *prev.* Kalinin. Tverskaya Oblast', W Russian Federation
Tverya *see* Teverya
128 I15 **Tverskaya Oblast'** ◆ *province* W Russian Federation
126 I15 **Tvertsa** ↝ W Russian Federation
110 H13 **Twardogóra** *Ger.* Festenberg. Dolnośląskie, SW Poland
14 J14 **Tweed** Ontario, SE Canada
96 K13 **Tweed** ↝ England/Scotland, UK
98 O7 **Tweede-Exloërmond** Drenthe, NE Netherlands
183 V3 **Tweed Heads** New South Wales, SE Australia
98 M11 **Twello** Gelderland, E Netherlands
35 W15 **Twentynine Palms** California, W USA
25 P9 **Twin Buttes Reservoir** ⊠ Texas, SW USA
33 O15 **Twin Falls** Idaho, NW USA
39 N13 **Twin Hills** Alaska, USA
11 O11 **Twin Lakes** Alberta, W Canada
33 O12 **Twin Peaks** ▲ Idaho, NW USA
185 I14 **Twins, The** ▲ South Island, NZ
29 S5 **Twin Valley** Minnesota, N USA
100 G11 **Twistringen** Niedersachsen, NW Germany
185 E20 **Twizel** Canterbury, South Island, NZ
29 X5 **Two Harbors** Minnesota, N USA
11 R14 **Two Hills** Alberta, SW Canada
31 N7 **Two Rivers** Wisconsin, N USA
116 H8 **Tyachiv** Zakarpats'ka Oblast', W Ukraine
Tyan'-Shan' *see* Tien Shan
166 L3 **Tyao** ↝ Burma/India
117 R6 **Tyas'myn** ↝ N Ukraine
23 X6 **Tybee Island** Georgia, SE USA
Tyborøn *see* Thyborøn
111 J16 **Tychy** *Ger.* Tichau. Śląskie, S Poland
111 O16 **Tyczyn** Podkarpackie, SE Poland
94 I8 **Tydal** Sør-Trøndelag, S Norway
115 H24 **Tyflós** ↝ Kríti, Greece, E Mediterranean Sea
21 S3 **Tygart Lake** ⊠ West Virginia, NE USA
123 Q13 **Tygda** Amurskaya Oblast', SE Russian Federation
21 Q11 **Tyger River** ↝ South Carolina, SE USA
32 I11 **Tygh Valley** Oregon, NW USA
94 F12 **Tyin** ⊚ S Norway
29 S10 **Tyler** Minnesota, N USA
25 W7 **Tyler** Texas, SW USA
25 W7 **Tyler, Lake** ⊠ Texas, SW USA
22 K7 **Tylertown** Mississippi, S USA
22 K7 **Tylihuls'kyy Lyman** ⊚ SW Ukraine
Tylos *see* Bahrain
115 C15 **Týmfi** *var.* Timfi. ▲ W Greece
115 E17 **Tymfristós** *var.* Timfristos. ▲ C Greece
115 J25 **Tympáki** *var.* Timbaki; *prev.* Timbákion. Kríti, Greece, E Mediterranean Sea
123 Q12 **Tynda** Amurskaya Oblast', SE Russian Federation
29 Q12 **Tyndall** South Dakota, N USA
97 L14 **Tyne** ↝ N England, UK
97 M14 **Tynemouth** NE England, UK
97 L14 **Tyneside** *cultural region* NE England, UK
94 H10 **Tynset** Hedmark, S Norway
39 Q12 **Tyonek** Alaska, USA
Tyôsi *see* Chōshi
Tyras *see* Dniester, Moldova/Ukraine
Tyras *see* Bilhorod-Dnistrovs'kyy, Ukraine
Tyre *see* Soûr
95 G14 **Tyrifjorden** ⊚ S Norway
95 K22 **Tyringe** Skåne, S Sweden
123 R13 **Tyrma** Khabarovskiy Kray, SE Russian Federation
Tyrnau *see* Trnava
115 F15 **Týrnavos** *var.* Tírnavos. Thessalía, C Greece
129 N16 **Tyrnyauz** Kabardino-Balkarskaya Respublika, SW Russian Federation
Tyrol *see* Tirol
18 E14 **Tyrone** Pennsylvania, NE USA
97 E15 **Tyrone** *cultural region* W Northern Ireland, UK
182 M10 **Tyrrell, Lake** *salt lake* Victoria, SE Australia
84 H14 **Tyrrhenian Basin** *undersea feature* Tyrrhenian Sea, C Mediterranean Sea
120 L8 **Tyrrhenian Sea** *It.* Mare Tirreno. *sea* N Mediterranean Sea
Tysa *see* Tisa/Tisza
116 J7 **Tysmenytsya** Ivano-Frankivs'ka Oblast', W Ukraine
95 C14 **Tysnesøya** *island* S Norway
95 C14 **Tysse** Hordaland, S Norway
95 D14 **Tyssedal** Hordaland, S Norway
95 O17 **Tystberga** Södermanland, C Sweden
118 E12 **Tytuvėnai** Kelmė, C Lithuania
144 D14 **Tyub-Karagan, Mys** *headland* SW Kazakhstan
147 V8 **Tyugel'-Say** Narynskaya Oblast', C Kyrgyzstan
122 H11 **Tyukalinsk** Omskaya Oblast', C Russian Federation
129 V7 **Tyul'gan** Orenburgskaya Oblast', W Russian Federation
122 G11 **Tyumen'** Tyumenskaya Oblast', C Russian Federation
122 H11 **Tyumenskaya Oblast'** ◆ *province* C Russian Federation
147 Y7 **Tyup** *Kir.* Tüp. Issyk-Kul'skaya Oblast', NE Kyrgyzstan
122 L14 **Tyva, Respublika** *prev.* Tannu-Tuva, Tuva, Tuvinskaya ASSR. ◆ *autonomous republic* C Russian Federation
117 N7 **Tyvriv** Vinnyts'ka Oblast', C Ukraine
97 J21 **Tywi** ↝ S Wales, UK
97 I19 **Tywyn** W Wales, UK
83 K20 **Tzaneen** Northern, NE South Africa
Tzekung *see* Zigong
41 X12 **Tzucacab** Yucatán, SE Mexico

U

82 B12 **Uaco Cungo** *var.* Waku Kungo, *Port.* Santa Comba. Cuanza Sul, C Angola
UAE *see* United Arab Emirates
191 X7 **Ua Huka** *island* Îles Marquises, NE French Polynesia
58 E10 **Uaiacás** Roraima, N Brazil
Uamba *see* Wamba
Uanle Uen *see* Wanlaweyn
191 W7 **Ua Pu** *island* Îles Marquises, NE French Polynesia
81 L17 **Uar Garas** *spring/well* SW Somalia
58 G12 **Uatumã, Rio** ↝ C Brazil
Ua Uíbh Fhailí *see* Offaly
58 C11 **Uaupés, Rio** *var.* Río Vaupés. ↝ Brazil/Colombia *see also* Vaupés, Río
145 X9 **Uba** ↝ E Kazakhstan
145 N6 **Ubagan** *Kaz.* Obagan. ↝ Kazakhstan/Russian Federation
186 G7 **Ubai** New Britain, E PNG
79 J15 **Ubangi** *Fr.* Oubangui. ↝ C Africa
Ubangi-Shari *see* Central African Republic
116 M3 **Ubarts'** *Ukr.* Ubort'. ↝ Belarus/Ukraine *see also* Ubort'
54 F9 **Ubaté** Cundinamarca, C Colombia
60 N10 **Ubatuba** São Paulo, S Brazil
149 R12 **Ubauro** Sind, SE Pakistan
171 Q6 **Ubay** Bohol, C Philippines
103 U14 **Ubaye** ↝ SE France
Ubayid, Wadi al *see* Ubayyiḑ, Wādī al
139 N8 **Ubaylah** W Iraq
139 O10 **Ubayyiḑ, Wādī al** *var.* Wadi al Ubayid. *dry watercourse* SW Iraq
98 L13 **Ubbergen** Gelderland, E Netherlands
164 E13 **Ube** Yamaguchi, Honshū, SW Japan
105 O13 **Ubeda** Andalucía, S Spain
109 V7 **Ubelbach** *var.* Markt-Übelbach. Steiermark, SE Austria
59 L20 **Uberaba** Minas Gerais, SE Brazil
57 Q19 **Uberaba, Laguna** ⊚ E Bolivia
59 K19 **Uberlândia** Minas Gerais, SE Brazil
101 H24 **Überlingen** Baden-Württemberg, S Germany
77 U16 **Ubiaja** Edo, S Nigeria
104 K3 **Ubiña, Peña** ▲ NW Spain
57 H17 **Ubinas, Volcán** ※ S Peru
Ubol Rajadhani/Ubol Ratchathani *see* Ubon Ratchathani
167 P9 **Ubolratna Reservoir** ⊠ C Thailand
167 S10 **Ubon Ratchathani** *var.* Muang Ubon, Ubol Rajadhani, Ubol Ratchathani, Udon Ratchathani. Ubon Ratchathani, E Thailand
119 L20 **Ubort'** *Bel.* Ubarts'. ↝ Belarus/Ukraine *see also* Ubarts'
104 K15 **Ubrique** Andalucía, S Spain
Ubsu-Nur, Ozero *see* Uvs Nuur
79 M18 **Ubundu** Orientale, C Dem. Rep. Congo (Zaire)
137 X11 **Ucar** *Rus.* Udzhary. C Azerbaijan
56 G13 **Ucayali** *off.* Departamento de Ucayali. ◆ *department* E Peru
56 F10 **Ucayali, Río** ↝ C Peru
Uccle *see* Ukkel
146 J13 **Uch-Adzhi** *Turkm.* Üchajy. Maryyskiy Velayat, C Turkmenistan
Üchajy *see* Uch-Adzhi
129 X4 **Uchaly** Respublika Bashkortostan, W Russian Federation
145 W13 **Ucharal** *Kaz.* Üsharal. Almaty, E Kazakhstan
164 C17 **Uchinoura** Kagoshima, Kyūshū, SW Japan
165 R5 **Uchiura-wan** *bay* NW Pacific Ocean
Uchkuduk *see* Uchquduq
Uchkurghan *see* Uchqŭrgon
146 K8 **Uchquduq** *Rus.* Uchkuduk. Nawoiy Wiloyati, N Uzbekistan
147 S9 **Uchqŭrgon** *Rus.* Uchkurghan. Namangan Wiloyati, E Uzbekistan
Uchsay *see* Uchsoy
146 G6 **Uchsoy** *Rus.* Uchsay. Qoraqalpoghiston Respublikasi, NW Uzbekistan
Uchtagan Gumy *see* Uchtagan, Peski
146 D10 **Uchtagan, Peski** *Turkm.* Uchtagan Gumy. *desert* NW Turkmenistan
123 R11 **Uchur** ↝ E Russian Federation
100 O10 **Uckermark** *cultural region* E Germany
10 K17 **Ucluelet** Vancouver Island, British Columbia, SW Canada
122 M13 **Uda** ↝ S Russian Federation
123 R12 **Uda** ↝ E Russian Federation
123 N6 **Udachnyy** Respublika Sakha (Yakutiya), NE Russian Federation
155 G21 **Udagamandalam** *var.* Udhagamandalam; *prev.* Ootacamund. Tamil Nādu, SW India
152 F14 **Udaipur** *prev.* Oodeypore. Rājasthān, N India
Udayadhani *see* Uthai Thani
143 N16 **'Udayd, Khawr al** *var.* Khor al Udeid. *inlet* Qatar/Saudi Arabia
112 D11 **Udbina** Lika-Senj, W Croatia
95 I18 **Uddevalla** Västra Götaland, S Sweden
Uddjaur *see* Uddjaure
92 H13 **Uddjaure** *var.* Uddjaur. ⊚ N Sweden
Udeid, Khor al *see* 'Udayd, Khawr al
99 K14 **Uden** Noord-Brabant, SE Netherlands
Uden *see* Udenhout
99 J14 **Udenhout** *var.* Uden. Noord-Brabant, S Netherlands
155 H14 **Udgīr** Mahārāshtra, C India
Udhagamandalam *see* Udagamandalam
152 H6 **Udhampur** Jammu and Kashmir, NW India
139 X14 **'Udhaybah, 'Uqlat al** *well* S Iraq
106 J7 **Udine** *anc.* Utina. Friuli-Venezia Giulia, NE Italy
175 T14 **Udintsev Fracture Zone** *tectonic feature* S Pacific Ocean
Udipi *see* Udupi
Udmurtia *see* Udmurtskaya Respublika
129 S2 **Udmurtskaya Respublika** *Eng.* Udmurtia. ◆ *autonomous republic* NW Russian Federation
126 J15 **Udomlya** Tverskaya Oblast', W Russian Federation
Udon Ratchathani *see* Ubon Ratchathani
167 Q8 **Udon Thani** *var.* Ban Mak Khaeng, Udorndhani. Udon Thani, N Thailand
Udorndhani *see* Udon Thani
189 U12 **Udot** *atoll* Chuuk Islands, C Micronesia
123 S12 **Udskaya Guba** *bay* E Russian Federation
155 E19 **Udupi** *var.* Udipi. Karnātaka, SW India
Udzhary *see* Ucar
100 O9 **Uecker** ↝ NE Germany
100 P9 **Ueckermünde** Mecklenburg-Vorpommern, NE Germany
164 M12 **Ueda** *var.* Uyeda. Nagano, Honshū, S Japan
79 L16 **Uele** *var.* Welle. ↝ NE Dem. Rep. Congo (Zaire)
Uele (upper course) *see* Uolo, Río, Equatorial Guinea/Gabon
Uele (upper course) *see* Kibali, Dem. Rep. Congo (Zaire)
123 W5 **Uelen** Chukotskiy Avtonomnyy Okrug, NE Russian Federation
100 J11 **Uelzen** Niedersachsen, N Germany
164 J14 **Ueno** Mie, Honshū, SW Japan
129 V4 **Ufa** Respublika Bashkortostan, W Russian Federation
129 V4 **Ufa** ↝ W Russian Federation
146 A10 **Ufra** Balkanskiy Velayat, NW Turkmenistan
83 C18 **Ugab** ↝ C Namibia
118 D8 **Ugāle** Ventspils, NW Latvia
81 F17 **Uganda** *off.* Republic of Uganda. ◆ *republic* E Africa
138 G4 **Ugarit** *Ar.* Ra's Shamrah. *site of ancient city* Al Lādhiqīyah, NW Syria
39 O14 **Ugashik** Alaska, USA
107 Q19 **Ugento** Puglia, SE Italy
105 O15 **Ugíjar** Andalucía, S Spain
103 T11 **Ugine** Savoie, E France
127 V13 **Ugleural'skiy** Permskaya Oblast', NW Russian Federation
126 L15 **Uglich** Yaroslavskaya Oblast', W Russian Federation
126 I14 **Uglovka** *var.* Okulovka. Novgorodskaya Oblast', W Russian Federation
128 I4 **Ugra** ↝ W Russian Federation
147 V9 **Ugyut** Narynskaya Oblast', C Kyrgyzstan
111 H19 **Uherské Hradiště** *Ger.* Ungarisch-Hradisch. Zlínský kraj, E Czech Republic
111 H19 **Uherský Brod** *Ger.* Ungarisch-Brod. Zlínský kraj, E Czech Republic
111 B17 **Úhlava** *Ger.* Angel. ↝ W Czech Republic
Uhorshchyna *see* Hungary
31 T13 **Uhrichsville** Ohio, N USA
Uhuru Peak *see* Kilimanjaro
96 G8 **Uig** N Scotland, UK
82 B10 **Uíge** *Port.* Carmona, Vila Marechal Carmona. Uíge, NW Angola
82 B10 **Uíge** ◆ *province* N Angola
193 Y15 **Uiha** *island* Ha'apai Group, C Tonga
189 U13 **Uijec** *island* Chuuk, C Micronesia
163 X14 **Ŭijŏngbu** *Jap.* Giseifu. NW South Korea
144 H10 **Uil** *Kaz.* Oyyl. Aktyubinsk, W Kazakhstan
144 H10 **Uil** *Kaz.* Oyyl. ↝ W Kazakhstan
36 M3 **Uinta Mountains** ▲ Utah, W USA
83 C18 **Uis** Erongo, NW Namibia
83 I25 **Uitenhage** Eastern Cape, S South Africa
98 H9 **Uitgeest** Noord-Holland, W Netherlands
98 I11 **Uithoorn** Noord-Holland, C Netherlands
98 O4 **Uithuizen** Groningen, NE Netherlands
98 O4 **Uithuizermeeden** Groningen, NE Netherlands
189 R6 **Ujae Atoll** *var.* Wūjae. *atoll* Ralik Chain, W Marshall Islands
Ujain *see* Ujjain
111 I16 **Ujazd** Opolskie, S Poland
Új-Becse *see* Novi Bečej
Ujda *see* Oujda
189 N5 **Ujelang Atoll** *var.* Wujlān. *atoll* Ralik Chain, W Marshall Islands
111 N21 **Újfehértó** Szabolcs-Szatmár-Bereg, E Hungary
Újgradiska *see* Nova Gradiška
164 J13 **Uji** *var.* Udi. Kyōto, Honshū, SW Japan
81 E21 **Ujiji** Kigoma, W Tanzania
154 G10 **Ujjain** *prev.* Ujain. Madhya Pradesh, C India
Újlak *see* Ilok
'Ujmān *see* 'Ajmān
Újmoldova *see* Moldova Nouă
Újszentanna *see* Sântana
170 M14 **Ujungpandang** *var.* Macassar, Makassar; *prev.* Makasar. Sulawesi, C Indonesia
Ujung Salang *see* Phuket
Újvidék *see* Novi Sad
154 E11 **Ukāi Reservoir** ⊠ W India
81 G19 **Ukara Island** *island* N Tanzania
'Ukash, Wādī *see* 'Akāsh, Wādī
81 F19 **Ukerewe Island** *island* N Tanzania
139 S9 **Ukhaydhir** C Iraq
153 X13 **Ukhrul** Manipur, NE India
127 S9 **Ukhta** Respublika Komi, NW Russian Federation
34 L6 **Ukiah** California, W USA
32 K12 **Ukiah** Oregon, NW USA
99 G18 **Ukkel** *Fr.* Uccle. Brussels, C Belgium
118 G13 **Ukmergė** *Pol.* Wiłkomierz. Ukmergė, C Lithuania
Ukraina *see* Ukraine
116 L6 **Ukraine** *off.* Ukraine, *Rus.* Ukraina, *Ukr.* Ukrayina; *prev.* Ukrainian Soviet Socialist Republic, Ukrainskay S.S.R. ◆ *republic* SE Europe
Ukrainskay S.S.R./Ukrayina *see* Ukraine
82 B13 **Uku** Cuanza Sul, NW Angola
164 B13 **Uku-jima** *island* Gotō-rettō, SW Japan
83 F20 **Ukwi** Kgalagadi, SW Botswana
118 M13 **Ula** *Rus.* Ulla. Vitsyebskaya Voblasts', N Belarus
136 C16 **Ula** Muğla, SW Turkey
118 M13 **Ula** *Rus.* Ulla. ↝ N Belarus
162 L7 **Ulaanbaatar** *Eng.* Ulan Bator. ● (Mongolia) Töv, C Mongolia
163 N8 **Ulaan-Ereg** Hentiy, E Mongolia
162 E5 **Ulaangom** Uvs, NW Mongolia
162 E7 **Ulaantolgoy** Hovd, W Mongolia
162 I8 **Ulaan-Uul** Bayanhongor, C Mongolia
163 O10 **Ulaan-Uul** Dornogovĭ, SE Mongolia
159 R10 **Ulan** Qinghai, C China
Ulan Bator *see* Ulaanbaatar
162 L13 **Ulan Buh Shamo** *desert* N China
Ulanhad *see* Chifeng
163 T8 **Ulanhot** Nei Mongol Zizhiqu, N China
129 Q14 **Ulan Khol** Respublika Kalmykiya, SW Russian Federation
162 M13 **Ulansuhai Nur** ⊚ N China
123 N14 **Ulan-Ude** *prev.* Verkhneudinsk. Respublika Buryatiya, S Russian Federation
159 N12 **Ulan Ul Hu** ⊚ C China
187 N9 **Ulawa Island** *island* SE Solomon Islands
138 J7 **'Ulayyānīyah, Bi'r al** *var.* Al Hilbeh. *well* S Syria
123 S12 **Ul'banskiy Zaliv** *strait* E Russian Federation
Ulbo *see* Olib
113 J18 **Ulcinj** Montenegro, SW Yugoslavia
163 O7 **Uldz** Hentiy, NE Mongolia
Uleåborg *see* Oulu
Uleälv *see* Oulujoki
95 G16 **Ulefoss** Telemark, S Norway
Uleträsk *see* Oulujärvi
113 L19 **Ulëz** *var.* Ulëza. Dibër, C Albania
Ulëza *see* Ulëz
95 F22 **Ulfborg** Ringkøbing, W Denmark
98 N13 **Ulft** Gelderland, E Netherlands
162 G7 **Uliastay** Dzavhan, W Mongolia
188 F8 **Ulimang** Babeldaob, N Palau
67 T10 **Ulindi** ↝ W Dem. Rep. Congo (Zaire)
188 H14 **Ulithi Atoll** *atoll* Caroline Islands, W Micronesia
112 N10 **Uljma** Serbia, NE Yugoslavia
144 L11 **Ul'kayak** *Kaz.* Ölkeyek. ↝ C Kazakhstan
145 Q7 **Ul'ken-Karoy, Ozero** ⊚ N Kazakhstan
Ülkenözen *see* Bol'shoy Uzen'
Ülkenqobda *see* Bol'shaya Khobda
104 G3 **Ulla** ↝ NW Spain
Ulla *see* Ula
183 S10 **Ulladulla** New South Wales, SE Australia
153 T14 **Ullapara** Rajshahi, W Bangladesh
96 H7 **Ullapool** N Scotland, UK
95 J20 **Ullared** Halland, S Sweden
105 T7 **Ulldecona** Cataluña, NE Spain
92 I9 **Ullsfjorden** *fjord* N Norway
97 K15 **Ullswater** ⊚ NW England, UK
101 I22 **Ulm** Baden-Württemberg, S Germany
33 R8 **Ulm** Montana, NW USA
183 V5 **Ulmarra** New South Wales, SE Australia
116 K13 **Ulmeni** Buzău, C Romania
116 K14 **Ulmeni** Călăraşi, S Romania
42 L7 **Ulmukhuás** Región Autónoma Atlántico Norte, NE Nicaragua
188 C8 **Ulong** *var.* Aulong. *island* Palau Islands, N Palau
83 N14 **Ulonguè** *var.* Ulongwé. Tete, NW Mozambique
Ulongwé *see* Ulonguè
95 K19 **Ulricehamn** Västra Götaland, S Sweden
98 N5 **Ulrum** Groningen, NE Netherlands
163 Z16 **Ulsan** *Jap.* Urusan. SE South Korea
94 D10 **Ulsteinvik** Møre og Romsdal, S Norway
97 D15 **Ulster** ◆ *province* Northern Ireland, UK/Ireland
171 Q10 **Ulu** Pulau Siau, N Indonesia
123 Q11 **Ulu** Respublika Sakha (Yakutiya), NE Russian Federation
42 H5 **Ulúa, Río** ↝ NW Honduras
136 D12 **Ulubat Gölü** ⊚ NW Turkey
136 E12 **Uludağ** ▲ NW Turkey
Ulugh Muztag *see* Muztag Feng
158 D7 **Ulugqat** Xinjiang Uygur Zizhiqu, W China
136 J16 **Ulukışla** Niğde, S Turkey
189 O15 **Ulul** *island* Caroline Islands, C Micronesia
83 L22 **Ulundi** KwaZulu/Natal, E South Africa
158 M3 **Ulungur He** ↝ NW China
158 K2 **Ulungur Hu** ⊚ NW China
181 P8 **Uluru** *var.* Ayers Rock. *rocky outcrop* Northern Territory, C Australia
97 K16 **Ulverston** NW England, UK
183 O16 **Ulverstone** Tasmania, SE Australia
94 D13 **Ulvik** Hordaland, S Norway
93 J18 **Ulvila** Länsi-Suomi, W Finland
117 O8 **Ulyanivka** *Rus.* Ul'yanovka. Kirovohrads'ka Oblast', C Ukraine
Ul'yanovka *see* Ulyanivka
129 Q5 **Ul'yanovsk** *prev.* Simbirsk. Ul'yanovskaya Oblast', W Russian Federation
129 Q5 **Ul'yanovskaya Oblast'** ◆ *province* W Russian Federation
145 S10 **Ul'yanovskiy** Karaganda, C Kazakhstan
Ul'yanovskiy Kanal *see* Ul'yanow Kanali
146 M13 **Ul'yanow Kanali** *Rus.* Ul'yanovskiy Kanal. *canal* Turkmenistan/Uzbekistan
Ulyshylanshyq *see* Uly-Zhylanshyk
26 H6 **Ulysses** Kansas, C USA
145 O12 **Ulytau, Gory** ▲ C Kazakhstan
145 N11 **Uly-Zhylanshyk** *Kaz.* Ulyshylanshyq. ↝ C Kazakhstan
112 A9 **Umag** *It.* Umago. Istra, NW Croatia
Umago *see* Umag
189 V13 **Uman** *atoll* Chuuk Islands, C Micronesia
117 O7 **Uman'** *Rus.* Uman. Cherkas'ka Oblast', C Ukraine
41 W12 **Umán** Yucatán, SE Mexico
Umanak/Umanaq *see* Uummannaq
'Umān, Khalīj *see* Oman, Gulf of
'Umān, Salṭanat *see* Oman
154 K10 **Umaria** Madhya Pradesh, C India
149 R16 **Umar Kot** Sind, SE Pakistan
188 B17 **Umatac** SW Guam
188 A17 **Umatac Bay** *bay* SW Guam
139 S6 **Umayqah** C Iraq
126 J5 **Umba** Murmanskaya Oblast', NW Russian Federation
138 I8 **Umbāshī, Khirbat al** *ruins* As Suwaydā', S Syria
80 A12 **Umbelasha** ↝ W Sudan
106 H12 **Umbertide** Umbria, C Italy
61 B17 **Umberto** *var.* Humberto. Santa Fe, C Argentina
186 E7 **Umboi Island** *var.* Rooke Island. *island* C PNG
126 J4 **Umbozero, Ozero** ⊚ NW Russian Federation
106 H13 **Umbria** ◆ *region* C Italy
Umbrian-Machigian Mountains *see* Umbro-Marchigiano, Appennino

106 I12 **Umbro-Marchigiano, Appennino** *Eng.* Umbrian-Machigian Mountains. ▲ C Italy
93 J16 **Umeå** Västerbotten, N Sweden
93 H14 **Umeälven** ≈ N Sweden
39 Q5 **Umiat** Alaska, USA
83 K23 **Umlazi** KwaZulu/Natal, E South Africa
139 X10 **Umm al Baqar, Hawr** *var.* Birkat ad Dawaymah. *spring* S Iraq
141 U12 **Umm al Ḥayt, Wādī** *var.* Wādī Amilḥayt. *seasonal river* SW Oman
Umm al Qaiwain *see* Umm al Qaywayn
143 R15 **Umm al Qaywayn** *var.* Umm al Qaiwain. Umm al Qaywayn, NE UAE
139 Q5 **Umm al Ṭūz** C Iraq
138 J3 **Umm 'Āmūd** Ḥalab, N Syria
141 Y10 **Umm ar Ruṣāṣ** *var.* Umm Ruṣayṣ. W Oman
141 X9 **Ummas Samīn** *salt flat* C Oman
141 V9 **Umm az Zumūl** *oasis* E Saudi Arabia
80 A9 **Umm Buru** Western Darfur, W Sudan
80 A12 **Umm Dafag** Southern Darfur, W Sudan
Umm Durmān *see* Omdurman
138 F9 **Umm el Fahm** Haifa, N Israel
80 F9 **Umm Inderab** Northern Kordofan, C Sudan
80 C10 **Umm Keddada** Northern Darfur, W Sudan
140 J7 **Umm Lajj** Tabūk, W Saudi Arabia
138 L10 **Umm Maḥfur** ≈ N Jordan
139 Y13 **Umm Qaṣr** SE Iraq
Umm Ruṣayṣ *see* Umm ar Ruṣāṣ
80 F11 **Umm Ruwaba** *var.* Umm Ruwābah, Um Ruwāba. Northern Kordofan, C Sudan
Umm Ruwābah *see* Umm Ruwaba
143 N16 **Umm Sa'īd** *var.* Musay'īd. S Qatar
138 K10 **Umm Ṭuways, Wādī** *dry watercourse* N Jordan
38 J17 **Umnak Island** *island* Aleutian Islands, Alaska, USA
32 F13 **Umpqua River** ≈ Oregon, NW USA
82 D13 **Umpulo** Bié, C Angola
154 I12 **Umred** Mahārāshtra, C India
139 Y10 **Umr Sawān, Hawr** ◎ S Iraq
Um Ruwāba *see* Umm Ruwaba
Umtali *see* Mutare
83 J24 **Umtata** Eastern Cape, SE South Africa
77 V17 **Umuahia** Abia, SW Nigeria
60 H10 **Umuarama** Paraná, S Brazil
Umvuma *see* Mvuma
83 K18 **Umzingwani** ≈ S Zimbabwe
112 D11 **Una** ≈ Bosnia and Herzegovina/Croatia
112 E12 **Unac** ≈ W Bosnia and Herzegovina
23 T6 **Unadilla** Georgia, SE USA
18 I10 **Unadilla River** ≈ New York, NE USA
59 L18 **Unaí** Minas Gerais, SE Brazil
39 N10 **Unalakleet** Alaska, USA
38 K17 **Unalaska Island** *island* Aleutian Islands, Alaska, USA
185 I16 **Una, Mount** ▲ South Island, NZ
82 N13 **Unango** Niassa, N Mozambique
Unao *see* Unnāo
92 L12 **Unari** Lappi, N Finland
141 O6 **'Unayzah** *var.* Anaiza. Al Qaṣīm, C Saudi Arabia
138 L10 **'Unayzah, Jabal** ▲ Jordan/Saudi Arabia
Unci *see* Almería
57 K19 **Uncía** Potosí, C Bolivia
37 Q7 **Uncompahgre Peak** ▲ Colorado, C USA
37 P6 **Uncompahgre Plateau** *plain* Colorado, C USA
95 L17 **Unden** ◎ S Sweden
28 M4 **Underwood** North Dakota, N USA
171 T13 **Undur** Pulau Seram, E Indonesia
128 H6 **Unecha** Bryanskaya Oblast', W Russian Federation
39 N16 **Unga** Unga Island, Alaska, USA
Ungaria *see* Hungary
183 P8 **Ungarie** New South Wales, SE Australia
Ungarisch-Brod *see* Uherský Brod
Ungarisches Erzgebirge *see* Slovenské rudohorie
Ungarisch-Hradisch *see* Uherské Hradiště
Ungarn *see* Hungary
12 M4 **Ungava Bay** *bay* Quebec, E Canada
12 J2 **Ungava, Péninsule d'** *peninsula* Quebec, SE Canada
Ungeny *see* Ungheni
116 M9 **Ungheni** *Rus.* Ungeny. W Moldova
Unguja *see* Zanzibar
Üngüz Angyrsyndaky Garagum *see* Zaunguzskiye Garagumy
146 H11 **Unguz, Solonchakovyye Vpadiny** *salt marsh* C Turkmenistan
Ungvár *see* Uzhhorod
60 I12 **União da Vitória** Paraná, S Brazil
111 G17 **Uničov** *Ger.* Mährisch-Neustadt. Olomoucký Kraj, E Czech Republic
110 J12 **Uniejów** Łódzkie, C Poland
112 A11 **Unije** *island* W Croatia
38 L16 **Unimak Island** *island* Aleutian Islands, Alaska, USA
38 L16 **Unimak Pass** *strait* Aleutian Islands, Alaska, USA
27 W5 **Union** Missouri, C USA
32 L12 **Union** Oregon, NW USA
21 Q11 **Union** South Carolina, SE USA
21 R6 **Union** West Virginia, NE USA
62 J12 **Unión** San Luis, C Argentina
61 B25 **Unión, Bahía** *bay* E Argentina
31 Q13 **Union City** Indiana, N USA
31 Q10 **Union City** Michigan, N USA
18 C12 **Union City** Pennsylvania, NE USA
20 G8 **Union City** Tennessee, S USA
32 G14 **Union Creek** Oregon, NW USA
83 G25 **Uniondale** Western Cape, SW South Africa
40 K13 **Unión de Tula** Jalisco, SW Mexico
30 M9 **Union Grove** Wisconsin, N USA
45 Y15 **Union Island** *island* S Saint Vincent and the Grenadines
46 K5 **Union Reefs** *reef* SW Mexico
(0) D7 **Union Seamount** *undersea feature* NE Pacific Ocean
23 Q6 **Union Springs** Alabama, S USA
20 H6 **Uniontown** Kentucky, S USA
18 C16 **Uniontown** Pennsylvania, NE USA
27 T1 **Unionville** Missouri, C USA
141 V8 **United Arab Emirates** *Ar.* Al Imārāt al 'Arabīyah al Muttaḥidah, *abbrev.* UAE; *prev.* Trucial States. ◆ *federation* SW Asia
United Arab Republic *see* Egypt
97 H14 **United Kingdom** *off.* UK of Great Britain and Northern Ireland, *abbrev.* UK. ◆ *monarchy* NW Europe
United Mexican States *see* Mexico
United Provinces *see* Uttar Pradesh
16 L10 **United States of America** *off.* United States of America, *var.* America, The States, *abbrev.* U.S., USA. ◆ *federal republic*
126 J10 **Unitsa** Respublika Kareliya, NW Russian Federation
11 S15 **Unity** Saskatchewan, S Canada
Unity State *see* Wahda
105 Q8 **Universales, Montes** ▲ C Spain
27 X4 **University City** Missouri, C USA
187 Q13 **Unmet** Malekula, C Vanuatu
101 F15 **Unna** Nordrhein-Westfalen, W Germany
152 L12 **Unnão** *prev.* Unao. Uttar Pradesh, N India
187 R15 **Unpongkor** Erromango, S Vauautu
Unruhstadt *see* Kargowa
96 M1 **Unst** *island* NE Scotland, UK
101 K16 **Unstrut** ≈ C Germany
Unterdrauburg *see* Dravograd
Unterlimbach *see* Lendava
101 L23 **Unterschleissheim** Bayern, SE Germany
101 H24 **Untersee** ◎ Germany/Switzerland
100 O10 **Unterueckersee** ◎ NE Germany
108 F9 **Unterwalden** ⬖ *canton* C Switzerland
55 N12 **Unturán, Sierra de** ▲ Brazil/Venezuela
159 N11 **Unuli Horog** Qinghai, W China
136 M11 **Ünye** Ordu, W Turkey
Unza *see* Unzha
127 O14 **Unzha** *var.* Unza. ≈ NW Russian Federation
79 E17 **Uolo, Río** *var.* Eyo (lower course), Mbini, Uele (upper course), Woleu; *prev.* Benito. ≈ Equatorial Guinea/Gabon
55 Q10 **Uonán** Bolívar, SE Venezuela
161 T12 **Uotsuri-shima** *island* China/Japan/Taiwan
165 M11 **Uozu** Toyama, Honshū, SW Japan
42 L12 **Upala** Alajuela, NW Costa Rica
55 P7 **Upata** Bolívar, E Venezuela
79 M23 **Upemba, Lac** ◎ SE Dem. Rep. Congo (Zaire)
197 O12 **Upernavik** *var.* Upernivik. Kitaa, C Greenland
Upernivik *see* Upernavik
83 F22 **Upington** Northern Cape, W South Africa
Uplands *see* Ottawa
192 I16 **Upolu** *island* SE Samoa
38 G11 **Upolu Point** *headland* Hawaii, USA, C Pacific Ocean
Upper Austria *see* Oberösterreich
Upper Bann *see* Bann
14 M13 **Upper Canada Village** *tourist site* Ontario, SE Canada
18 I16 **Upper Darby** Pennsylvania, NE USA
28 L2 **Upper Des Lacs Lake** ⊠ North Dakota, N USA
185 L14 **Upper Hutt** Wellington, North Island, NZ
29 X11 **Upper Iowa River** ≈ Iowa, C USA
32 H15 **Upper Klamath Lake** ◎ Oregon, NW USA
34 M6 **Upper Lake** California, W USA
35 Q1 **Upper Lake** ◎ California, W USA
10 K9 **Upper Liard** Yukon Territory, W Canada
97 E16 **Upper Lough Erne** ◎ SW Northern Ireland, UK
80 F12 **Upper Nile** ⬖ *state* E Sudan
29 T3 **Upper Red Lake** ◎ Minnesota, N USA
31 S12 **Upper Sandusky** Ohio, N USA
Upper Volta *see* Burkina
95 O15 **Upplandsväsby** *var.* Upplands Väsby. Stockholm, C Sweden
95 O15 **Uppsala** Uppsala, C Sweden
95 O14 **Uppsala** ⬖ *county* C Sweden
38 J12 **Upright Cape** *headland* Saint Matthew Island, Alaska, USA
20 K6 **Upton** Kentucky, S USA
33 Y13 **Upton** Wyoming, C USA
141 N7 **'Uqlat aş Şuqūr** Al Qaşīm, W Saudi Arabia
Uqturpan *see* Wushi
54 C7 **Urabá, Golfo de** *gulf* NW Colombia
Uracas *see* Farallon de Pajaros
Uradar'ya *see* Ŭradaryo
147 N13 **Ŭradaryo** *Rus.* Uradar'ya. ≈ S Uzbekistan
162 M13 **Urad Qianqi** *var.* Xishanzui. Nei Mongol Zizhiqu, N China
165 U5 **Urahoro** Hokkaidō, NE Japan
165 T5 **Urakawa** Hokkaidō, NE Japan
129 X6 **Ural** *Kaz.* Zayyq. ≈ Kazakhstan/Russian Federation
183 T6 **Uralla** New South Wales, SE Australia
Ural Mountains *see* Ural'skiye Gory
144 F8 **Ural'sk** *Kaz.* Oral. Zapadnyy Kazakhstan, NW Kazakhstan
Ural'skaya Oblast' *see* Zapadnyy Kazakhstan
129 W5 **Ural'skiye Gory** *var.* Ural'skiy Khrebet, *Eng.* Ural Mountains. ▲ Kazakhstan/Russian Federation
Ural'skiy Khrebet *see* Ural'skiye Gory
138 I3 **Urām aş Şughrá** Ḥalab, N Syria
183 P10 **Urana** New South Wales, SE Australia
11 S10 **Uranium City** Saskatchewan, C Canada
58 F10 **Uraricoera** Roraima, N Brazil
47 S5 **Uraricoera, Rio** ≈ N Brazil
Ura-Tyube *see* Ŭroteppa
165 O13 **Urawa** Saitama, Honshū, S Japan
122 H10 **Uray** Khanty-Mansiyskiy Avtonomnyy Okrug, C Russian Federation
141 R7 **'Uray'irah** Ash Sharqīyah, E Saudi Arabia
30 M13 **Urbana** Illinois, N USA
31 R13 **Urbana** Ohio, N USA
29 V14 **Urbandale** Iowa, C USA
106 I11 **Urbania** Marche, C Italy
106 I11 **Urbino** Marche, C Italy
57 H16 **Urcos** Cusco, S Peru
144 D10 **Urda** Zapadnyy Kazakhstan, W Kazakhstan
105 N10 **Urda** Castilla-La Mancha, C Spain
162 E7 **Urdgol** Hovd, W Mongolia
Urdunn *see* Jordan
145 X12 **Urdzhar** *Kaz.* Ürzhar. Vostochnyy Kazakhstan, E Kazakhstan
97 L16 **Ure** ≈ N England, UK
119 K18 **Urechcha** *Rus.* Urech'ye. Minskaya Voblasts', S Belarus
Urech'ye *see* Urechcha
129 P2 **Uren'** Nizhegorodskaya Oblast', W Russian Federation
122 J9 **Urengoy** Yamalo-Nenetskiy Avtonomnyy Okrug, N Russian Federation
184 K10 **Urenui** Taranaki, North Island, NZ
187 Q12 **Ureparapara** *island* Banks Islands, N Vanuatu
40 G5 **Ures** Sonora, NW Mexico
Urfa *see* Şanlıurfa
146 H9 **Urganch** *Rus.* Urgench; *prev.* Novo-Urgench. Khorazm Wiloyati, W Uzbekistan
Urgench *see* Urganch
136 J14 **Ürgüp** Nevşehir, C Turkey
147 O12 **Urgut** Samarqand Wiloyati, C Uzbekistan
158 K3 **Urho** Xinjiang Uygur Zizhiqu, W China
152 G5 **Uri** Jammu and Kashmir, NW India
108 G9 **Uri** ⬖ *canton* C Switzerland
54 F11 **Uribe** Meta, C Colombia
54 H4 **Uribia** La Guajira, N Colombia
116 G12 **Uricani** *Hung.* Hobicaurikány. Hunedoara, SW Romania
57 M21 **Uriondo** Tarija, S Bolivia
40 I7 **Urique** Chihuahua, N Mexico
40 I7 **Urique, Río** ≈ N Mexico
56 E9 **Urituyacu, Río** ≈ N Peru
145 N7 **Uritskiy** Kostanay, N Kazakhstan
98 K8 **Urk** Flevoland, N Netherlands
136 B14 **Urla** İzmir, W Turkey
116 K13 **Urlaţi** Prahova, SE Romania
129 V4 **Urman** Respublika Bashkortostan, W Russian Federation
147 P12 **Urmetan** W Tajikistan
Urmia *see* Orūmīyeh
Urmia, Lake *see* Orūmīyeh, Daryācheh-ye
Urmiyeh *see* Orūmīyeh
113 N17 **Uroševac** *Alb.* Ferizaj. Serbia, S Yugoslavia
147 P11 **Ŭroteppa** *Rus.* Ura-Tyube. NW Tajikistan
54 D8 **Urrao** Antioquia, W Colombia
Ursat'yevskaya *see* Khowos
162 I11 **Urt** Ömnögovĭ, S Mongolia
129 X7 **Urtazym** Orenburgskaya Oblast', W Russian Federation
59 K18 **Uruaçu** Goiás, C Brazil
40 M14 **Uruapan** *var.* Uruapan del Progreso. Michoacán de Ocampo, SW Mexico
Uruapan del Progreso *see* Uruapan
57 G15 **Urubamba, Cordillera** ▲ C Peru
57 G14 **Urubamba, Río** ≈ C Peru
58 G12 **Urucará** Amazonas, N Brazil
61 E16 **Uruguaiana** Rio Grande do Sul, S Brazil
Uruguai, Rio *see* Uruguay
61 E18 **Uruguay** *off.* Oriental Republic of Uruguay; *prev.* La Banda Oriental. ◆ *republic* E South America
61 E15 **Uruguay** *var.* Rio Uruguai, Río Uruguay. ≈ E South America
Uruguay, Río *see* Uruguay
Urumchi *see* Ürümqi
158 L5 **Ürümqi** *var.* Tihwa, Urumchi, Urumqi, Urumtsi, Wu-lu-k'o-mu-shi, Wu-lu-mu-ch'i; *prev.* Ti-hua. *autonomous region capital* Xinjiang Uygur Zizhiqu, NW China
Urumtsi *see* Ürümqi
Urundi *see* Burundi
183 V6 **Urunga** New South Wales, SE Australia
188 C15 **Uruno Point** *headland* NW Guam
123 U13 **Urup, Ostrov** *island* Kuril'skiye Ostrova, SE Russian Federation
141 P11 **'Uruq al Mawārid** *desert* S Saudi Arabia
Urusan *see* Ulsan
129 T5 **Urussu** Respublika Tatarstan, W Russian Federation
184 K10 **Uruti** Taranaki, North Island, NZ
57 K19 **Uru Uru, Lago** ◎ W Bolivia
55 P9 **Uruyén** Bolívar, SE Venezuela
149 O7 **Ūrūzgān** *var.* Oruzgān, Orūzgān. Urūzgān, C Afghanistan
149 N6 **Ūrūzgān** *Per.* Orūzgān. ⬖ *province* C Afghanistan
165 T3 **Uryū-gawa** ≈ Hokkaidō, NE Japan
165 T2 **Uryū-ko** ◎ Hokkaidō, NE Japan
129 N8 **Uryupinsk** Volgogradskaya Oblast', SW Russian Federation
Ürzhar *see* Urdzhar
127 R16 **Urzhum** Kirovskaya Oblast', NW Russian Federation
116 K13 **Urziceni** Ialomiţa, SE Romania
U.S./USA *see* United States of America
164 E14 **Usa** Ōita, Kyūshū, SW Japan
119 L16 **Usa** *Rus.* Usa. ≈ C Belarus
127 T6 **Usa** ≈ NW Russian Federation
136 E14 **Uşak** *prev.* Ushak. Uşak, W Turkey
136 D14 **Uşak** *var.* Ushak. ⬖ *province* W Turkey
83 C19 **Usakos** Erongo, W Namibia
81 J21 **Usambara Mountains** ▲ NE Tanzania
81 G23 **Usangu Flats** *wetland* SW Tanzania
65 D24 **Usborne, Mount** ▲ East Falkland, Falkland Islands
100 O8 **Usedom** *island* NE Germany
99 M24 **Useldange** Diekirch, C Luxembourg
118 L12 **Ushacha** *Rus.* Ushacha. Vitsyebskaya Voblasts', N Belarus
Ushachi *see* Ushachy
118 L13 **Ushachy** *Rus.* Ushachi. Vitsyebskaya Voblasts', N Belarus
Ushak *see* Uşak
122 L4 **Ushakova, Ostrov** *island* Severnaya Zemlya, N Russian Federation
Ushant *see* Ouessant, Île d'
Üsharal *see* Ucharal
164 B15 **Ushibuka** *var.* Usibuka. Kumamoto, Shimo-jima, SW Japan
Ushi Point *see* Sabaneta, Puntan
145 V14 **Ushtobe** *Kaz.* Üshtöbe. Almaty, SE Kazakhstan
63 I25 **Ushuaia** Tierra del Fuego, S Argentina
39 R10 **Usibelli** Alaska, USA
Usibuka *see* Ushibuka
186 D7 **Usino** Madang, N PNG
127 U6 **Usinsk** Respublika Komi, NW Russian Federation
97 K22 **Usk** *Wel.* Wysg. ≈ SE Wales, UK
Uskočke Planine/Uskokengebirge *see* Gorjanci/Žumberačko Gorje
Uskoplje *see* Gornji Vakuf
Üsküb *see* Skopje
114 M11 **Üsküpdere** Kırklareli, NW Turkey
128 L7 **Usman'** Lipetskaya Oblast', W Russian Federation
118 D8 **Usmas Ezers** ◎ NW Latvia
127 U13 **Usol'ye** Permskaya Oblast', NW Russian Federation
41 T16 **Uspanapa, Río** ≈ SE Mexico
145 R11 **Uspenskiy** Zhezkazgan, C Kazakhstan
103 O11 **Ussel** Corrèze, C France
163 Z6 **Ussuri** *var.* Usuri, Wusuri, *Chin.* Wusuli Jiang. ≈ China/Russian Federation
123 S15 **Ussuriysk** *prev.* Nikol'sk, Nikol'sk-Ussuriyskiy, Voroshilov. Primorskiy Kray, SE Russian Federation
136 J10 **Usta Burnu** *headland* N Turkey
149 P13 **Usta Muhammad** Baluchistān, SW Pakistan
123 V11 **Ust'-Bol'sheretsk** Kamchatskaya Oblast', E Russian Federation
129 N9 **Ust'-Buzulukskaya** Volgogradskaya Oblast', SW Russian Federation
111 C16 **Ústecký Kraj** ⬖ *region* NW Czech Republic
108 G7 **Uster** Zürich, NE Switzerland
107 J22 **Ustica, Isola d'** *island* S Italy
122 M12 **Ust'-Ilimsk** Irkutskaya Oblast', C Russian Federation
111 C15 **Ústí nad Labem** *Ger.* Aussig. Ústecký Kraj, NW Czech Republic
111 F17 **Ústí nad Orlicí** *Ger.* Wildenschwert. Pardubický Kraj, E Czech Republic
Ustinov *see* Izhevsk
113 J14 **Ustiprača** Republika Srpska, SE Bosnia and Herzegovina
122 H11 **Ust'-Ishim** Omskaya Oblast', C Russian Federation
110 G6 **Ustka** *Ger.* Stolpmünde. Pomorskie, N Poland
123 V9 **Ust'-Kamchatsk** Kamchatskaya Oblast', E Russian Federation
145 X9 **Ust'-Kamenogorsk** *Kaz.* Öskemen. Vostochnyy Kazakhstan, E Kazakhstan
123 T10 **Ust'-Khayryuzovo** Koryakskiy Avtonomnyy Okrug, E Russian Federation
122 I14 **Ust'-Koksa** Respublika Altay, S Russian Federation
127 S11 **Ust'-Kulom** Respublika Komi, NW Russian Federation
123 Q8 **Ust'-Kuyga** Respublika Sakha (Yakutiya), NE Russian Federation
128 L14 **Ust'-Labinsk** Krasnodarskiy Kray, SW Russian Federation
123 R10 **Ust'-Maya** Respublika Sakha (Yakutiya), NE Russian Federation
123 R9 **Ust'-Nera** Respublika Sakha (Yakutiya), NE Russian Federation
123 P12 **Ust'-Nyukzha** Amurskaya Oblast', S Russian Federation
123 O7 **Ust'-Olenëk** Respublika Sakha (Yakutiya), NE Russian Federation
123 T9 **Ust'-Omchug** Magadanskaya Oblast', E Russian Federation
122 M13 **Ust'-Ordynskiy** Ust'-Ordynskiy Buryatskiy Avtonomnyy Okrug, S Russian Federation
122 M13 **Ust'-Ordynskiy Buryatskiy Avtonomnyy Okrug** ⬖ *autonomous district* S Russian Federation
127 N8 **Ust'-Pinega** Arkhangel'skaya Oblast', NW Russian Federation
122 K8 **Ust'-Port** Taymyrskiy (Dolgano-Nenetskiy) Avtonomnyy Okrug, N Russian Federation
114 L11 **Ustrem** *prev.* Vakav. Yambol, E Bulgaria
111 O18 **Ustrzyki Dolne** Podkarpackie, SE Poland
Ust'-Sysol'sk *see* Syktyvkar
127 R7 **Ust'-Tsil'ma** Respublika Komi, NW Russian Federation
Ust Urt *see* Ustyurt Plateau
127 O11 **Ust'ya** ≈ NW Russian Federation
117 R8 **Ustynivka** Kirovohrads'ka Oblast', C Ukraine
144 H15 **Ustyurt Plateau** *var.* Ust Urt, *Uzb.* Ustyurt Platosi. *plateau* Kazakhstan/Uzbekistan
Ustyurt Platosi *see* Ustyurt Plateau
126 K14 **Ustyuzhna** Vologodskaya Oblast', NW Russian Federation
158 J4 **Usu** Xinjiang Uygur Zizhiqu, NW China
171 O13 **Usu** Sulawesi, C Indonesia
164 E14 **Usuki** Ōita, Kyūshū, SW Japan
42 G8 **Usulután** Usulután, SE El Salvador
42 B9 **Usulután** ⬖ *department* SE El Salvador
41 W16 **Usumacinta, Río** ≈ Guatemala/Mexico
Usumbura *see* Bujumbura
Usuri *see* Ussuri
171 W14 **Uta** Irian Jaya, E Indonesia
36 K5 **Utah** *off.* State of Utah; also known as Beehive State, Mormon State. ⬖ *state* W USA
36 L3 **Utah Lake** ◎ Utah, W USA
Utaidhani *see* Uthai Thani
93 M14 **Utajärvi** Oulu, C Finland
Utamboni *see* Mitemele, Río
Utaradit *see* Uttaradit
165 T3 **Utashinai** *var.* Utasinai. Hokkaidō, NE Japan
Utasinai *see* Utashinai
193 Y14 **'Uta Vava'u** *island* Vava'u Group, N Tonga
37 V9 **Ute Creek** ≈ New Mexico, SW USA
118 H12 **Utena** Utena, E Lithuania
37 V10 **Ute Reservoir** ⊠ New Mexico, SW USA
167 O10 **Uthai Thani** *var.* Muang Uthai Thani, Udayadhani, Utaidhani. Uthai Thani, W Thailand
149 O15 **Uthal** Baluchistān, SW Pakistan
18 I10 **Utica** New York, NE USA
105 R10 **Utiel** País Valenciano, E Spain
11 O13 **Utikuma Lake** ◎ Alberta, W Canada
42 I4 **Utila, Isla de** *island* Islas de la Bahía, N Honduras
Utina *see* Udine
59 O17 **Utinga** Bahia, E Brazil
Utirik *see* Utrik Atoll
95 M22 **Utlängan** *island* S Sweden
117 U11 **Utlyuts'kyy Lyman** *bay* S Ukraine
95 P16 **Utö** Stockholm, C Sweden
25 Q12 **Utopia** Texas, SW USA
98 J11 **Utrecht** *Lat.* Trajectum ad Rhenum. Utrecht, C Netherlands
83 K22 **Utrecht** KwaZulu/Natal, E South Africa
98 I11 **Utrecht** ⬖ *province* C Netherlands
104 K14 **Utrera** Andalucía, S Spain
189 V4 **Utrik Atoll** *var.* Utirik, Utrōk, Utrōnk. *atoll* Ratak Chain, N Marshall Islands
Utrōk/Utrōnk *see* Utrik Atoll
95 B16 **Utsira** *island* SW Norway
92 L8 **Utsjoki** *var.* Ohcejohka. Lappi, N Finland
165 O12 **Utsunomiya** *var.* Utunomiya. Tochigi, Honshū, S Japan
129 P13 **Utta** Respublika Kalmykiya, SW Russian Federation
167 O8 **Uttaradit** *var.* Utaradit. Uttaradit, N Thailand
152 J8 **Uttarkāshi** Uttar Pradesh, N India
152 K11 **Uttar Pradesh** *prev.* United Provinces, United Provinces of Agra and Oudh. ⬖ *state* N India
45 T5 **Utuado** C Puerto Rico
158 K3 **Utubulak** Xinjiang Uygur Zizhiqu, W China
39 N5 **Utukok River** ≈ Alaska, USA
Utunomiya *see* Utsunomiya
187 P10 **Utupua** *island* Santa Cruz Islands, E Soloman Islands
144 G9 **Utva** ≈ NW Kazakhstan
189 Y15 **Utwe** Kosrae, E Micronesia
189 X15 **Utwe Harbor** *harbor* Kosrae, E Micronesia
162 J7 **Uubulan** Arhangay, C Mongolia
118 G6 **Uulu** Pärnumaa, SW Estonia
197 N13 **Uummannaq** *var.* Umanak, Umanaq. Kitaa, C Greenland
Uummannarsuaq *see* Nunap Isua
162 E4 **Üüreg Nuur** ◎ NW Mongolia
Uusikaarlepyy *see* Nykarleby
93 J19 **Uusikaupunki** *Swe.* Nystad. Länsi-Suomi, W Finland
129 S2 **Uva** Udmurtskaya Respublika, NW Russian Federation
113 L14 **Uvac** ≈ W Yugoslavia
25 Q12 **Uvalde** Texas, SW USA
155 K25 **Uva Province** ⬖ *province* SE Sri Lanka
119 O18 **Uvaravichy** *Rus.* Uvarovichi. Homyel'skaya Voblasts', SE Belarus
54 J11 **Uvá, Río** ≈ E Colombia
Uvarovichi *see* Uvaravichy
129 N7 **Uvarovo** Tambovskaya Oblast', W Russian Federation
122 H10 **Uvat** Tyumenskaya Oblast', C Russian Federation
190 G12 **Uvea, Île** *island* N Wallis and Futuna
81 E21 **Uvinza** Kigoma, W Tanzania
79 O20 **Uvira** Sud Kivu, E Dem. Rep. Congo (Zaire)
162 E5 **Uvs** ⬖ *province* NW Mongolia
162 F5 **Uvs Nuur** *var.* Ozero Ubsu-Nur. ◎ Mongolia/Russian Federation
164 F14 **Uwa** Ehime, Shikoku, SW Japan
164 F14 **Uwajima** *var.* Uwazima. Ehime, Shikoku, SW Japan
80 B5 **'Uwaynāt, Jabal al** *var.* Jebel Uweinat. ▲ Libya/Sudan
Uwazima *see* Uwajima
Uweinat, Jebel *see* 'Uwaynāt, Jabal al
14 H14 **Uxbridge** Ontario, S Canada
Uxellodunum *see* Issoudun
162 M15 **Uxin Qi** Nei Mongol Zizhiqu, N China
41 X12 **Uxmal, Ruinas** *ruins* Yucatán, SE Mexico
131 Q5 **Uy** ≈ Kazakhstan/Russian Federation
144 K15 **Uyaly** Kzylorda, S Kazakhstan
123 R8 **Uyandina** ≈ NE Russian Federation
122 L12 **Uyar** Krasnoyarskiy Kray, S Russian Federation
162 L10 **Üydzen** Ömnögovĭ, S Mongolia
Uyeda *see* Ueda
122 K5 **Uyedineniya, Ostrov** *island* N Russian Federation
77 V17 **Uyo** Akwa Ibom, S Nigeria
162 D8 **Üyönch** Hovd, W Mongolia
145 Q15 **Uyuk** Zhambyl, S Kazakhstan
141 V13 **'Uyūn** SW Oman
57 K20 **Uyuni** Potosí, W Bolivia
57 J20 **Uyuni, Salar de** *wetland* SW Bolivia
146 I9 **Uzbekistan** *off.* Republic of Uzbekistan. ◆ *republic* C Asia
158 D8 **Uzbel Shankou** *Rus.* Pereval Kyzyl-Dzhiik. *pass* China/Tajikistan
119 J17 **Uzda** *Rus.* Uzda. Minskaya Voblasts', C Belarus
103 N12 **Uzerche** Corrèze, C France
103 R14 **Uzès** Gard, S France
147 T10 **Uzgen** *Kir.* Özgön. Oshskaya Oblast', SW Kyrgyzstan
117 O3 **Uzh** ≈ N Ukraine
Uzhgorod *see* Uzhhorod
116 G7 **Uzhhorod** *Rus.* Uzhgorod; *prev.* Ungvár. Zakarpats'ka Oblast', W Ukraine
Uzi *see* Uji
112 K13 **Užice** *prev.* Titovo Užice. Serbia, W Yugoslavia
Uzin *see* Uzyn
128 L5 **Uzlovaya** Tul'skaya Oblast', W Russian Federation
108 H7 **Uznach** Sankt Gallen, NE Switzerland
145 U16 **Uzunagach** Almaty, SE Kazakhstan
136 B10 **Uzunköprü** Edirne, NW Turkey
118 D11 **Užventis** Kelmė, C Lithuania
117 P5 **Uzyn** *Rus.* Uzin. Kyyivs'ka Oblast', N Ukraine

V

Vääksy *see* Asikkala
83 H23 **Vaal** ≈ C South Africa
93 M14 **Vaala** Oulu, C Finland
93 N19 **Vaalimaa** Etelä-Suomi, SE Finland
99 M19 **Vaals** Limburg, SE Netherlands
93 J16 **Vaasa** *Swe.* Vasa; *prev.* Nikolainkaupunki. Vaasa, W Finland
98 L10 **Vaassen** Gelderland, E Netherlands
118 G11 **Vabalninkas** Biržai, NE Lithuania
Vabkent *see* Wobkent
111 J22 **Vác** *Ger.* Waitzen. Pest, N Hungary
61 I14 **Vacaria** Rio Grande do Sul, S Brazil
35 N7 **Vacaville** California, W USA
103 R15 **Vaccarès, Étang de** ◎ SE France
44 L10 **Vache, Île à** *island* SW Haiti
173 Y16 **Vacoas** W Mauritius
32 G10 **Vader** Washington, NW USA
94 D12 **Vadheim** Sogn og Fjordane, S Norway
154 D11 **Vadodara** *prev.* Baroda. Gujarāt, W India
92 M8 **Vadsø** *Fin.* Vesisaari. Finnmark, N Norway
95 L17 **Vadstena** Östergötland, S Sweden
108 I8 **Vaduz** ● (Liechtenstein) W Liechtenstein
Vág *see* Váh
127 N12 **Vaga** ≈ NW Russian Federation
94 G11 **Vågåmo** Oppland, S Norway
112 D12 **Vaganski Vrh** ▲ W Croatia

◆ COUNTRY ● COUNTRY CAPITAL ◇ DEPENDENT TERRITORY ○ DEPENDENT TERRITORY CAPITAL ⬖ ADMINISTRATIVE REGION ✈ INTERNATIONAL AIRPORT ▲ MOUNTAIN ▲ MOUNTAIN RANGE ⛰ VOLCANO ≈ RIVER ◎ LAKE ⊠ RESERVOIR

95 A19 **Vágar** *Dan.* Vágø *Island* Faeroe Islands
Vágbeszterce *see* Považská Bystrica
95 L19 **Vaggeryd** Jönköping, S Sweden
95 O16 **Vagnhärad** Södermanland, C Sweden
104 G7 **Vagos** Aveiro, N Portugal
Vágsellye *see* Sal'a
92 H10 **Vågsfjorden** *fjord* N Norway
94 C10 **Vågsøy** *island* S Norway
Vágújhely *see* Nové Mesto nad Váhom
111 I21 **Váh** *Ger.* Waag, *Hung.* Vág. ≈ W Slovakia
93 K16 **Vähäkyrö** Länsi-Suomi, W Finland
191 X11 **Vahitahi** *atoll* Îles Tuamotu, E French Polynesia
Vaidei *see* Vulcan
22 L4 **Vaiden** Mississippi, S USA
155 I23 **Vaigai** ≈ S India
191 V16 **Vaihu** Easter Island, Chile, E Pacific Ocean
118 I6 **Väike Emajõgi** ≈ S Estonia
118 I4 **Väike-Maarja** *Ger.* Klein-Marien. Lääne-Virumaa, NE Estonia
Väike-Salatsi *see* Mazsalaca
37 R4 **Vail** Colorado, C USA
193 V15 **Vaina** Tongatapu, S Tonga
118 E5 **Väinameri** *prev.* Muhu Väin, *Ger.* Moon-Sund. *sea* E Baltic Sea
93 N18 **Vainikkala** Etelä-Suomi, SE Finland
118 D10 **Vaiņode** Liepāja, SW Latvia
155 H23 **Vaippār** ≈ SE India
191 W11 **Vairaatea** *atoll* Îles Tuamotu, C French Polynesia
191 R8 **Vairao** Tahiti, W French Polynesia
103 R14 **Vaison-la-Romaine** Vaucluse, SE France
190 G11 **Vaitupu** Île Uvea, E Wallis and Futuna
190 F7 **Vaitupu** *atoll* C Tuvalu
Vajdahunyad *see* Hunedoara
Vajdej *see* Vulcan
78 K12 **Vakaga** ◆ *prefecture* NE Central African Republic
114 H10 **Vakarel** Sofiya, W Bulgaria
Vakav *see* Ustrem
137 O11 **Vakfıkebir** Trabzon, NE Turkey
122 J10 **Vakh** ≈ C Russian Federation
Vakhon, Qatorkŭhi *see* Nicholas Range
147 P14 **Vakhsh** SW Tajikistan
147 Q12 **Vakhsh** ≈ SW Tajikistan
129 P1 **Vakhtan** Nizhegorodskaya Oblast', W Russian Federation
94 C13 **Vaksdal** Hordaland, S Norway
127 O8 **Vashka** ≈ NW Russian Federation
Valachia *see* Wallachia
108 D11 **Valais** *Ger.* Wallis. ◆ *canton* SW Switzerland
113 M21 **Valamarës, Mali i** ▲ SE Albania
129 S2 **Valamaz** Udmurtskaya Respublika, NW Russian Federation
113 Q19 **Valandovo** SE FYR Macedonia
111 I18 **Valašské Meziříčí** *Ger.* Wallachisch-Meseritsch, *Pol.* Wałeckie Międzyrzecze. Zlínský Kraj, E Czech Republic
115 I17 **Valáxa** *island* Vóreioi Sporádes, Greece, Aegean Sea
95 K16 **Vålberg** Värmland, C Sweden
116 H12 **Vâlcea** *prev.* Vilcea. ◆ *county* SW Romania
63 J16 **Valcheta** Río Negro, E Argentina
15 P12 **Valcourt** Quebec, SE Canada
Valdai Hills *see* Valdayskaya Vozvyshennost'
104 M3 **Valdavia** ≈ N Spain
126 I15 **Valday** Novgorodskaya Oblast', W Russian Federation
126 I15 **Valdayskaya Vozvyshennost'** *var.* Valdai Hills. *hill range* W Russian Federation
104 L9 **Valdecañas, Embalse de** ⊠ W Spain
118 E8 **Valdemārpils** *Ger.* Sassmacken. Talsi, NW Latvia
95 N18 **Valdemarsvik** Östergötland, S Sweden
105 N8 **Valdemoro** Madrid, C Spain
105 O11 **Valdepeñas** Castilla-La Mancha, C Spain
104 L5 **Valderaduey** ≈ NE Spain
104 L5 **Valderas** Castilla-León, N Spain
105 T7 **Valderrobres** *var.* Vall-de-roures. Aragón, NE Spain
63 K17 **Valdés, Península** *peninsula* SE Argentina
39 S11 **Valdez** Alaska, USA
56 C5 **Valdéz** *var.* Limones. Esmeraldas, NW Ecuador
Valdia *see* Weldiya
103 U11 **Val d'Isère** Savoie, E France
63 G15 **Valdivia** Los Lagos, C Chile
Valdivia Bank *see* Valdivia Seamount
65 P17 **Valdivia Seamount** *var.* Valdivia Bank. *undersea feature* E Atlantic Ocean
103 N4 **Val-d'Oise** ◆ *department* N France
14 J8 **Val-d'Or** Quebec, SE Canada
23 U8 **Valdosta** Georgia, SE USA
94 G13 **Valdres** *physical region* S Norway
32 L13 **Vale** Oregon, NW USA
116 F9 **Valea lui Mihai** *Hung.* Érmihályfalva. Bihor, NW Romania
11 N15 **Valemount** British Columbia, SW Canada
59 O17 **Valença** Bahia, E Brazil
104 F4 **Valença do Minho** Viana do Castelo, N Portugal
59 N14 **Valença do Piauí** Piauí, E Brazil
103 N8 **Valençay** Indre, C France
103 R13 **Valence** *anc.* Valentia, Valentia Julia, Ventia. Drôme, E France
105 S10 **Valencia** País Valenciano, E Spain
54 K5 **Valencia** Carabobo, N Venezuela
105 R10 **Valencia** *Cat.* València. ◆ *province* País Valenciano, E Spain
105 S10 **Valencia** ✕ Valencia, E Spain
València/Valencia *see* País Valenciano
104 I10 **Valencia de Alcántara** Extremadura, W Spain
104 L4 **Valencia de Don Juan** Castilla-León, N Spain
105 U9 **Valencia, Golfo de** *var.* Gulf of Valencia. *gulf* E Spain
Valencia, Gulf of *see* Valencia, Golfo de
97 A21 **Valencia Island** *Ir.* Dairbhre. *island* SW Ireland
103 P2 **Valenciennes** Nord, N France
116 K13 **Vălenii de Munte** Prahova, SE Romania
Valentia *see* Valence, France
Valentia *see* País Valenciano
Valentia Julia *see* Valence
103 T8 **Valentigney** Doubs, E France
28 M12 **Valentine** Nebraska, C USA
24 J10 **Valentine** Texas, SW USA
Valentine State *see* Oregon
106 C8 **Valenza** Piemonte, NW Italy
94 I13 **Våler** Hedmark, S Norway
54 I6 **Valera** Trujillo, NW Venezuela
192 M11 **Valerie Guyot** *undersea feature* S Pacific Ocean
Valetta *see* Valletta
118 I7 **Valga** *Ger.* Walk, *Latv.* Valka. Valgamaa, S Estonia
118 I7 **Valgamaa** *off.* Valga Maakond. ◆ *province* S Estonia
43 Q15 **Valiente, Península** *peninsula* NW Panama
103 X16 **Valinco, Golfe de** *gulf* Corse, France, C Mediterranean Sea
112 L12 **Valjevo** Serbia, W Yugoslavia
Valjok *see* Válljohka
118 I7 **Valka** *Ger.* Walk. Valka, N Latvia
Valka *see* Valga
93 L18 **Valkeakoski** Länsi-Suomi, W Finland
93 M19 **Valkeala** Etelä-Suomi, S Finland
99 L18 **Valkenburg** Limburg, SE Netherlands
99 K15 **Valkenswaard** Noord-Brabant, S Netherlands
119 G15 **Valkininkai** Varėna, S Lithuania
117 U5 **Valky** Kharkivs'ka Oblast', E Ukraine
41 Y12 **Valladolid** Yucatán, SE Mexico
104 M5 **Valladolid** Castilla-León, NW Spain
104 L5 **Valladolid** ◆ *province* Castilla-León, N Spain
103 U15 **Vallauris** Alpes-Maritimes, SE France
Vall-de-roures *see* Valderrobres
105 S9 **Vall d'Uxó** País Valenciano, E Spain
95 E16 **Valle** Aust-Agder, S Norway
105 N2 **Valle** Cantabria, N Spain
42 H8 **Valle** ◆ *department* S Honduras
105 N8 **Vallecas** Madrid, C Spain
37 Q8 **Vallecito Reservoir** ⊠ Colorado, C USA
106 A7 **Valle d'Aosta** ◆ *region* NW Italy
41 O14 **Valle de Bravo** México, S Mexico
55 N5 **Valle de Guanape** Anzoátegui, N Venezuela
54 M6 **Valle de La Pascua** Guárico, N Venezuela
54 B11 **Valle del Cauca** *off.* Departamento del Valle del Cauca. ◆ *province* W Colombia
41 N13 **Valle de Santiago** Guanajuato, C Mexico
40 J7 **Valle de Zaragoza** Chihuahua, N Mexico
54 G5 **Valledupar** Cesar, N Colombia
76 G10 **Vallée de Ferlo** ≈ NW Senegal
57 M19 **Vallegrande** Santa Cruz, C Bolivia
41 P8 **Valle Hermoso** Tamaulipas, C Mexico
35 N8 **Vallejo** California, W USA
62 G8 **Vallenar** Atacama, N Chile
95 O15 **Vallentuna** Stockholm, C Sweden
121 P16 **Valletta** *prev.* Valetta. ● (Malta) E Malta
27 N6 **Valley Center** Kansas, C USA
29 Q5 **Valley City** North Dakota, N USA
32 I15 **Valley Falls** Oregon, NW USA
Valleyfield *see* Salaberry-de-Valleyfield
21 S4 **Valley Head** West Virginia, NE USA
25 T8 **Valley Mills** Texas, SW USA
75 W10 **Valley of the Kings** *ancient monument* E Egypt
29 R11 **Valley Springs** South Dakota, N USA
20 K5 **Valley Station** Kentucky, S USA
11 O13 **Valleyview** Alberta, W Canada
25 T5 **Valley View** Texas, SW USA
61 C21 **Vallimanca, Arroyo** ≈ E Argentina
92 L9 **Válljohka** *var.* Valjok. Finnmark, N Norway
107 M19 **Vallo della Lucania** Campania, S Italy
108 B9 **Vallorbe** Vaud, W Switzerland
105 V6 **Valls** Cataluña, NE Spain
94 N11 **Vallsta** Gävleborg, C Sweden
94 N12 **Vallvik** Gävleborg, C Sweden
11 T17 **Val Marie** Saskatchewan, S Canada
118 H7 **Valmiera** *Est.* Volmari, *Ger.* Wolmar. Valmiera, N Latvia
105 N3 **Valnera** ▲ N Spain
102 J3 **Valognes** Manche, N France
Valona *see* Vlorë
Valona Bay *see* Vlorës, Gjiri i
104 G6 **Valongo** *var.* Valongo de Gaia. Porto, N Portugal
Valongo de Gaia *see* Valongo
104 M5 **Valoria la Buena** Castilla-León, N Spain
119 J15 **Valozhyn** *Pol.* Wołożyn, *Rus.* Volozhin. Minskaya Voblasts', C Belarus
104 I5 **Valpaços** Vila Real, N Portugal
23 P8 **Valparaiso** Florida, SE USA
31 N11 **Valparaiso** Indiana, N USA
62 G11 **Valparaíso** Valparaíso, C Chile
40 L11 **Valparaíso** Zacatecas, C Mexico
62 G11 **Valparaíso** *off.* Región de Valparaíso. ◆ *region* C Chile
Valpo *see* Valpovo
112 I9 **Valpovo** *Hung.* Valpó. Osijek-Baranja, E Croatia
103 R14 **Valréas** Vaucluse, SE France
Vals *see* Vals-Platz
154 D12 **Valsād** *prev.* Bulsar. Gujarāt, W India
Valsbaai *see* False Bay
171 T12 **Valse Pisang, Kepulauan** *island group* E Indonesia
108 H9 **Vals-Platz** *var.* Vals. Graubünden, S Switzerland
171 X16 **Vals, Tanjung** *headland* Irian Jaya, SE Indonesia
93 N15 **Valtimo** Itä-Suomi, E Finland
115 D17 **Váltou** ▲▲ C Greece
129 O12 **Valuyevka** Rostovskaya Oblast', SW Russian Federation
128 K9 **Valuyki** Belgorodskaya Oblast', W Russian Federation
36 L2 **Val Verda** Utah, W USA
64 N12 **Valverde** Hierro, Islas Canarias, Spain, NE Atlantic Ocean
104 I13 **Valverde del Camino** Andalucía, S Spain
95 G23 **Vamdrup** Vejle, C Denmark
94 L12 **Våmhus** Dalarna, C Sweden
93 K18 **Vammala** Länsi-Suomi, W Finland
Vámosudvarhely *see* Odorheiu Secuiesc
137 S14 **Van** Van, E Turkey
25 V7 **Van** Texas, SW USA
137 T14 **Van** ◆ *province* E Turkey
137 T11 **Vanadzor** *prev.* Kirovakan. N Armenia
25 U5 **Van Alstyne** Texas, SW USA
33 W10 **Vananda** Montana, NW USA
116 I11 **Vânători** *Hung.* Héjjasfalva; *prev.* Vînători. Mureş, C Romania
191 W12 **Vanavana** *atoll* Îles Tuamotu, SE French Polynesia
Vana-Vändra *see* Vändra
122 M11 **Vanavara** Evenkiyskiy Avtonomnyy Okrug, C Russian Federation
15 Q8 **Van Bruyssel** Quebec, SE Canada
27 R10 **Van Buren** Arkansas, C USA
19 S1 **Van Buren** Maine, NE USA
27 W7 **Van Buren** Missouri, C USA
19 T5 **Vanceboro** Maine, NE USA
21 W10 **Vanceboro** North Carolina, SE USA
21 O4 **Vanceburg** Kentucky, S USA
Vanch *see* Vanj
10 L17 **Vancouver** British Columbia, SW Canada
32 G11 **Vancouver** Washington, NW USA
10 L17 **Vancouver** ✕ British Columbia, SW Canada
10 K16 **Vancouver Island** *island* British Columbia, SW Canada
Vanda *see* Vantaa
171 X13 **Van Daalen** ≈ Irian Jaya, E Indonesia
30 L15 **Vandalia** Illinois, N USA
27 V3 **Vandalia** Missouri, C USA
31 R13 **Vandalia** Ohio, N USA
25 U13 **Vanderbilt** Texas, SW USA
31 Q10 **Vandercook Lake** Michigan, N USA
10 L14 **Vanderhoof** British Columbia, SW Canada
18 K8 **Vanderwhacker Mountain** ▲ New York, NE USA
181 P1 **Van Diemen Gulf** *gulf* Northern Territory, N Australia
Van Diemen's Land *see* Tasmania
118 H5 **Vändra** *Ger.* Fennern; *prev.* Vana-Vändra. Pärnumaa, SW Estonia
Vandsburg *see* Więcbork
34 L4 **Van Duzen River** ≈ California, W USA
118 F13 **Vandžiogala** Kaunas, C Lithuania
41 N10 **Vanegas** San Luis Potosí, C Mexico
Vaner, Lake *see* Vänern
95 K17 **Vänern** *Eng.* Lake Vaner; *prev.* Lake Vener. ◎ S Sweden
95 J18 **Vänersborg** Västra Götaland, S Sweden
94 F12 **Vang** Oppland, S Norway
172 I7 **Vangaindrano** Fianarantsoa, SE Madagascar
137 S14 **Van Gölü** *Eng.* Lake Van; *anc.* Thospitis. *salt lake* E Turkey
186 L9 **Vangunu** *island* New Georgia Islands, NW Solomon Islands
24 J9 **Van Horn** Texas, SW USA
187 Q11 **Vanikolo** *var.* Vanikoro. *island* Santa Cruz Islands, E Solomon Islands
Vanikoro *see* Vanikolo
186 A5 **Vanimo** Sandaun, NW PNG
123 T13 **Vanino** Khabarovskiy Kray, SE Russian Federation
155 G19 **Vānīvilāsa Sāgara** ◎ SW India
147 S13 **Vanj** *Rus.* Vanch. S Tajikistan
116 G14 **Vânju Mare** *prev.* Vînju Mare. Mehedinţi, SW Romania
15 N12 **Vankleek Hill** Ontario, SE Canada
Van, Lake *see* Van Gölü
93 I16 **Vännäs** Västerbotten, N Sweden
93 I15 **Vännäsby** Västerbotten, N Sweden
102 H7 **Vannes** *anc.* Dariorigum. Morbihan, NW France
92 I8 **Vannøya** *island* N Norway
103 T12 **Vanoise, Massif de la** ▲▲ E France
83 E24 **Vanrhynsdorp** Western Cape, SW South Africa
21 P7 **Vansant** Virginia, NE USA
94 L13 **Vansbro** Dalarna, C Sweden
95 D18 **Vanse** Vest-Agder, S Norway
9 P7 **Vansittart Island** *island* Nunavut, NE Canada
93 M20 **Vantaa** *Swe.* Vanda. Etelä-Suomi, S Finland
93 L19 **Vantaa** ✕ (Helsinki) Etelä-Suomi, S Finland
32 J9 **Vantage** Washington, NW USA
187 Z14 **Vanua Balavu** *prev.* Vanua Mbalavu. *island* Lau Group, E Fiji
187 R12 **Vanua Lava** *island* Banks Islands, N Vanuatu
187 Y13 **Vanua Levu** *island* N Fiji
Vanua Mbalavu *see* Vanua Balavu
187 R12 **Vanuatu** *off.* Republic of Vanuatu; *prev.* New Hebrides. ◆ *republic* SW Pacific Ocean
175 P8 **Vanuatu** *island group* SW Pacific Ocean
31 Q12 **Van Wert** Ohio, N USA
187 Q17 **Vao** Province Sud, S New Caledonia
Vapincum *see* Gap
117 N7 **Vapnyarka** Vinnyts'ka Oblast', C Ukraine
103 T15 **Var** ◆ *department* SE France
103 U14 **Var** ≈ SE France
95 J18 **Vara** Västra Götaland, S Sweden
Varadinska Županija *see* Varaždin
118 J10 **Varakļani** Madona, C Latvia
106 C7 **Varallo** Piemonte, NE Italy
143 O5 **Varāmīn** *var.* Veramin. Tehrān, N Iran
153 N14 **Vārānasi** *prev.* Banaras, Benares, *hist.* Kasi. Uttar Pradesh, N India
127 T3 **Varandey** Nenetskiy Avtonomnyy Okrug, NW Russian Federation
92 M8 **Varangerbotn** Finnmark, N Norway
92 M8 **Varangerfjorden** *fjord* N Norway
92 M8 **Varangerhalvøya** *peninsula* N Norway
Varannó *see* Vranov nad Topl'ou
107 M15 **Varano, Lago di** ◎ SE Italy
118 J13 **Varapayeva** *Rus.* Voropayevo. Vitsyebskaya Voblasts', NW Belarus
Varasd *see* Varaždin
112 E7 **Varaždin** *Ger.* Warasdin, *Hung.* Varasd. Varaždin, N Croatia
112 E7 **Varaždin** *off.* Varadinska Županija. ◆ *province* N Croatia
106 C10 **Varazze** Liguria, NW Italy
95 J20 **Varberg** Halland, S Sweden
Vardak *see* Wardag
113 Q19 **Vardar** *Gk.* Axiós. ≈ FYR Macedonia/Greece *see also* Axiós
95 F23 **Varde** Ribe, W Denmark
137 V12 **Vardenis** E Armenia
92 N8 **Vardø** *Fin.* Vuoreija. Finnmark, N Norway
115 E18 **Vardoúsia** ▲▲ C Greece
Vareia *see* Logroño
100 G10 **Varel** Niedersachsen, NW Germany
119 G15 **Varėna** *Pol.* Orany. Varėna, S Lithuania
15 O12 **Varennes** Quebec, SE Canada
103 P10 **Varennes-sur-Allier** Allier, C France
112 I12 **Vareš** Federacija Bosna I Hercegovina, E Bosnia and Herzegovina
106 D7 **Varese** Lombardia, N Italy
116 J12 **Vârful Moldoveanu** *var.* Moldoveanul; *prev.* Vîrful Moldoveanu. ▲ C Romania
Varganzi *see* Warganza
95 J18 **Vårgårda** Västra Götaland, S Sweden
95 J18 **Vargön** Västra Götaland, S Sweden
95 C17 **Varhaug** Rogaland, S Norway
93 N17 **Varkaus** Itä-Suomi, C Finland
92 J2 **Varmahlidh** Nordhurland Vestra, N Iceland
95 J15 **Värmland** ◆ *county* C Sweden
95 K16 **Värmlandsnäs** *peninsula* S Sweden
114 N8 **Varna** *prev.* Stalin, *anc.* Odessus. Varna, E Bulgaria
114 N8 **Varna** ✕ Varna, E Bulgaria
114 N8 **Varna** ◆ *province* E Bulgaria
95 L20 **Värnamo** Jönköping, S Sweden
114 N8 **Varnenski Zaliv** *prev.* Stalinski Zaliv. *bay* E Bulgaria
114 N8 **Varnensko Ezero** *estuary* E Bulgaria
118 D11 **Varniai** Telšiai, W Lithuania
Varnoús *see* Baba
111 D14 **Varnsdorf** *Ger.* Warnsdorf. Ústecký Kraj, N Czech Republic
111 I23 **Várpalota** Veszprém, W Hungary
Varshava *see* Warszawa
118 K6 **Värska** Põlvamaa, SE Estonia
98 N12 **Varsseveld** Gelderland, E Netherlands
115 D19 **Vartholomió** *prev.* Vartholomión. Dytikí Ellás, S Greece
Vartholomión *see* Vartholomió
137 Q14 **Varto** Muş, E Turkey
95 K18 **Vartofta** Västra Götaland, S Sweden
93 O17 **Värtsilä** Itä-Suomi, E Finland
Värtsilä *see* Vyartsilya
117 R4 **Varva** Chernihivs'ka Oblast', NE Ukraine
59 H18 **Várzea Grande** Mato Grosso, SW Brazil
106 D9 **Varzi** Lombardia, N Italy
Varzimanor Ayni *see* Ayní
126 K5 **Varzuga** ≈ NW Russian Federation
103 P8 **Varzy** Nièvre, C France
111 G23 **Vas** *off.* Vas Megye. ◆ *county* W Hungary
Vasa *see* Vaasa
190 A9 **Vasafua** *island* Funafuti Atoll, C Tuvalu
111 O21 **Vásárosnamény** Szabolcs-Szatmár-Bereg, E Hungary
104 H13 **Vascão, Ribeira de** ≈ S Portugal
116 G10 **Vaşcău** *Hung.* Vaskoh. Bihor, NE Romania
Vascongadas, Provincias *see* País Vasco
Vashess Bay *see* Vaskess Bay
Vāsht *see* Khāsh
Vasilevichi *see* Vasilyevichy
115 G14 **Vasiliká** Kentrikí Makedonía, NE Greece
115 C18 **Vasilikí** Lefkáda, Iónioi Nísoi, Greece, C Mediterranean Sea
115 K25 **Vasilikí** Kríti, Greece, E Mediterranean Sea
119 G16 **Vasilishki** *Pol.* Wasiliszki, *Rus.* Vasilishki. Hrodzyenskaya Voblasts', W Belarus
Vasil Kolarov *see* Pamporovo
Vasil'kov *see* Vasyl'kiv
119 N19 **Vasilyevichy** *Rus.* Vasilevichi. Homyel'skaya Voblasts', SE Belarus
191 Y3 **Vaskess Bay** *var.* Vashess Bay. *bay* Kiritimati, E Kiribati
Vaskoh *see* Vaşcău
Vaskohsziklás *see* Ştei
116 M10 **Vaslui** Vaslui, C Romania
116 L11 **Vaslui** ◆ *county* NE Romania
31 R8 **Vassar** Michigan, N USA
95 E15 **Vassdalsegga** ▲ S Norway
60 P9 **Vassouras** Rio de Janeiro, SE Brazil
92 H11 **Vastenjaure** ◎ N Sweden
95 N15 **Västerås** Västmanland, C Sweden
93 G15 **Västerbotten** ◆ *county* N Sweden
94 K12 **Västerdalälven** ≈ C Sweden
95 O16 **Västerhaninge** Stockholm, C Sweden
94 M10 **Västernorrland** ◆ *county* C Sweden
95 N19 **Västervik** Kalmar, S Sweden
95 M15 **Västmanland** ◆ *county* C Sweden
107 L15 **Vasto** *anc.* Histonium. Abruzzo, C Italy
95 J19 **Västra Götaland** ◆ *county* S Sweden
95 J16 **Västra Silen** ◎ S Sweden
111 G23 **Vasvár** *Ger.* Eisenburg. Vas, W Hungary
117 U9 **Vasylivka** Zaporiz'ka Oblast', SE Ukraine
117 O5 **Vasyl'kiv** *Rus.* Vasil'kov. Kyyivs'ka Oblast', N Ukraine
122 I11 **Vasyugan** ≈ C Russian Federation
103 N8 **Vatan** Indre, C France
Vaté *see* Efate
107 G15 **Vatican City** *off.* Vatican City State. ◆ *papal state* S Europe
107 M22 **Vaticano, Capo** *headland* S Italy
92 K3 **Vatnajökull** *glacier* SE Iceland
95 P15 **Vätö** Stockholm, C Sweden
187 Z16 **Vatoa** *island* Lau Group, SE Fiji
172 J5 **Vatomandry** Toamasina, E Madagascar
116 J9 **Vatra Dornei** *Ger.* Dorna Watra. Suceava, NE Romania
116 J9 **Vatra Moldoviţei** Suceava, NE Romania
Vatter, Lake *see* Vättern
95 L18 **Vättern** *Eng.* Lake Vatter; *prev.* Lake Vetter. ◎ S Sweden
187 X5 **Vatulele** *island* SW Fiji
117 P7 **Vatutine** Cherkas'ka Oblast', C Ukraine
187 W15 **Vatu Vara** *island* Lau Group, E Fiji
103 R14 **Vaucluse** ◆ *department* SE France
103 S5 **Vaucouleurs** Meuse, NE France
108 B9 **Vaud** *Ger.* Waadt. ◆ *canton* SW Switzerland
15 N12 **Vaudreuil** Quebec, SE Canada
37 T12 **Vaughn** New Mexico, SW USA
54 I14 **Vaupés** *off.* Comisaría del Vaupés. ◆ *province* SE Colombia
54 J13 **Vaupés, Río** *var.* Rio Uaupés. ≈ Brazil/Colombia *see also* Uaupés, Rio
103 Q15 **Vauvert** Gard, S France
11 R17 **Vauxhall** Alberta, SW Canada
99 K23 **Vaux-sur-Sûre** Luxembourg, SE Belgium
172 J4 **Vavatenina** Toamasina, E Madagascar
193 Y14 **Vava'u Group** *island group* N Tonga
76 M16 **Vavoua** W Ivory Coast
129 S2 **Vavozh** Udmurtskaya Respublika, NW Russian Federation
155 K23 **Vavuniya** Northern Province, N Sri Lanka
119 G17 **Vawkavysk** *Pol.* Wołkowysk, *Rus.* Volkovysk. Hrodzyenskaya Voblasts', W Belarus
119 F17 **Vawkavyskaye Wzvyshsha** *Rus.* Volkovyskiye Vysoty. *hill range* W Belarus
95 P15 **Vaxholm** Stockholm, C Sweden
95 L21 **Växjö** *var.* Vexiö. Kronoberg, S Sweden
127 T1 **Vaygach, Ostrov** *island* NW Russian Federation
137 V13 **Vayk'** *prev.* Azizbekov. SE Armenia
127 P8 **Vazhgort** *prev.* Chasovo. Respublika Komi, NW Russian Federation
45 V10 **V.C.Bird** ✕ (St John's) Antigua, Antigua and Barbuda
95 C16 **Veavågen** Rogaland, S Norway
29 Q7 **Veblen** South Dakota, N USA
98 N9 **Vecht** *Ger.* Vechte. ≈ Germany/Netherlands *see also* Vechte
100 G12 **Vechta** Niedersachsen, NW Germany
100 E12 **Vechte** *Dut.* Vecht. ≈ Germany/Netherlands *see also* Vecht
118 I8 **Vecpiebalga** Cēsis, C Latvia
118 G9 **Vecumnieki** Bauska, C Latvia
Vedāvati *see* Hagari
95 J20 **Veddige** Halland, S Sweden
116 J15 **Vedea** ≈ S Romania
129 P16 **Vedeno** Chechenskaya Respublika, SW Russian Federation
98 O6 **Veendam** Groningen, NE Netherlands
98 K12 **Veenendaal** Utrecht, C Netherlands
99 E14 **Veere** Zeeland, SW Netherlands
24 M2 **Vega** Texas, SW USA
92 E13 **Vega** *island* C Norway
45 T5 **Vega Baja** C Puerto Rico
38 D17 **Vega Point** *headland* Kiska Island, Alaska, USA
95 F17 **Vegår** ◎ S Norway
99 K14 **Veghel** Noord-Brabant, S Netherlands
Veglia *see* Krk
114 E13 **Vegorítis, Límni** ◎ N Greece
11 Q14 **Vegreville** Alberta, SW Canada
95 K21 **Veinge** Halland, S Sweden
61 B21 **Veinticinco de Mayo** *var.* 25 de Mayo. Buenos Aires, E Argentina
63 I14 **Veinticinco de Mayo** La Pampa, C Argentina
119 F15 **Veisiejai** Lazdijai, S Lithuania
95 F23 **Vejen** Ribe, W Denmark
104 K16 **Vejer de la Frontera** Andalucía, S Spain
95 G23 **Vejle** Vejle, C Denmark
95 F23 **Vejle** *off.* Vejle Amt. ◆ *county* C Denmark
114 M7 **Vekilski** Shumen, NE Bulgaria
54 G3 **Vela, Cabo de la** *headland* NE Colombia
Vela Goa *see* Goa
113 F15 **Vela Luka** Dubrovnik-Neretva, S Croatia
61 G19 **Velázquez** Rocha, E Uruguay
101 E15 **Velbert** Nordrhein-Westfalen, W Germany
109 S9 **Velden** Kärnten, S Austria
Veldes *see* Bled
99 K15 **Veldhoven** Noord-Brabant, S Netherlands
112 C11 **Velebit** ▲▲ C Croatia
114 N11 **Veleka** ≈ SE Bulgaria
109 V10 **Velenje** *Ger.* Wöllan. N Slovenia
190 E12 **Vele, Pointe** *headland* Île Futuna, S Wallis and Futuna
113 O18 **Veles** *Turk.* Köprülü. C FYR Macedonia
113 M20 **Velešta** SW FYR Macedonia
115 F16 **Velestíno** *prev.* Velestínon. Thessalía, C Greece
Velestínon *see* Velestino
Velevshchina *see* Vyelyewshchyna
54 F9 **Vélez** Santander, C Colombia
105 Q13 **Vélez Blanco** Andalucía, S Spain
104 M17 **Vélez de la Gomera, Peñon de** *island group* S Spain
105 N15 **Vélez-Málaga** Andalucía, S Spain
105 Q13 **Vélez Rubio** Andalucía, S Spain
Velha Goa *see* Goa
Velho *see* Porto Velho
112 E8 **Velika Gorica** Zagreb, N Croatia
112 C9 **Velika Kapela** ▲▲ NW Croatia
Velika Kikinda *see* Kikinda
112 D10 **Velika Kladuša** Federacija Bosna I Hercegovina, NW Bosnia and Herzegovina
112 N11 **Velika Morava** *var.* Glavn'a Morava, Morava, *Ger.* Grosse Morava. ≈ C Yugoslavia
112 N12 **Velika Plana** Serbia, C Yugoslavia
109 U10 **Velika Raduha** ▲ N Slovenia
123 V7 **Velikaya** ≈ NE Russian Federation
126 F15 **Velikaya** ≈ W Russian Federation
Velikaya Berestovitsa *see* Vyalikaya Byerastavitsa
Velikaya Lepetikha *see* Velyka Lepetykha
Veliki Bečkerek *see* Zrenjanin
112 P12 **Veliki Krš** *var.* Stol. ▲ E Yugoslavia
114 L8 **Veliki Preslav** *prev.* Preslav. Shumen, NE Bulgaria
112 B9 **Veliki Risnjak** ▲ NW Croatia
109 T13 **Veliki Snežnik** *Ger.* Schneeberg, *It.* Monte Nevoso. ▲ SW Slovenia
112 J13 **Veliki Stolac** ▲ E Bosnia and Herzegovina
Velikiy Bor *see* Vyaliki Bor
126 G16 **Velikiye Luki** Pskovskaya Oblast', W Russian Federation
127 P12 **Velikiy Ustyug** Vologodskaya Oblast', NW Russian Federation
112 N11 **Veliko Gradište** Serbia, NE Yugoslavia
155 I18 **Velikonda Range** ▲▲ SE India
114 K9 **Veliko Tŭrnovo** *prev.* Tirnovo, Trnovo, Tŭrnovo. Veliko Tŭrnovo, N Bulgaria
114 K8 **Veliko Tŭrnovo** ◆ *province* N Bulgaria
Velikovec *see* Völkermarkt
127 R5 **Velikovisochnoye** Nenetskiy Avtonomnyy Okrug, NW Russian Federation
76 H12 **Vélingara** C Senegal
76 H11 **Vélingara** S Senegal
114 H11 **Velingrad** Pazardzhik, C Bulgaria
128 H3 **Velizh** Smolenskaya Oblast', W Russian Federation
111 F16 **Velká Deštná** *var.* Deštná, Grosskoppe, *Ger.* Deschnaer Koppe. ▲ NE Czech Republic

◆ Country ◇ Dependent Territory ◆ Administrative Region ▲ Mountain ⛰ Volcano ◎ Lake
● Country Capital ○ Dependent Territory Capital ✕ International Airport ▲▲ Mountain Range ≈ River ⊠ Reservoir

111 F18 **Velké Meziříčí** *Ger.* Grossmeseritsch. Jihlavský Kraj, C Czech Republic
92 N1 **Velkomstpynten** *headland* NW Svalbard
111 K21 **Veľký Krtíš** Banskobystrický Kraj, C Slovakia
186 J8 **Vella Lavella** *var.* Mbilua. *island* New Georgia Islands, NW Solomon Islands
107 I15 **Velletri** Lazio, C Italy
95 K23 **Vellinge** Skåne, S Sweden
155 I19 **Vellore** Tamil Nādu, SE India
Velobriga *see* Viana do Castelo
115 G21 **Velopoúla** *island* S Greece
98 M12 **Velp** Gelderland, SE Netherlands
Velsen *see* Velsen-Noord
98 H9 **Velsen-Noord** *var.* Velsen. Noord-Holland, W Netherlands
127 N12 **Vel'sk** *var.* Velsk. Arkhangel'skaya Oblast', NW Russian Federation
Velsuna *see* Orvieto
98 K10 **Veluwemeer** *lake channel* C Netherlands
28 M3 **Velva** North Dakota, N USA
115 E14 **Velvendós** *var.* Velvendos. Dytikí Makedonía, N Greece
117 S5 **Velyka Bahachka** Poltavs'ka Oblast', C Ukraine
117 S9 **Velyka Lepetykha** *Rus.* Velikaya Lepetikha. Khersons'ka Oblast', S Ukraine
117 O10 **Velyka Mykhaylivka** Odes'ka Oblast', SW Ukraine
117 W8 **Velyka Novosilka** Donets'ka Oblast', E Ukraine
117 S9 **Velyka Oleksandrivka** Khersons'ka Oblast', S Ukraine
117 T4 **Velyka Pysanivka** Sums'ka Oblast', NE Ukraine
116 G6 **Velykyy Bereznyy** Zakarpats'ka Oblast', W Ukraine
117 W4 **Velykyy Burluk** Kharkivs'ka Oblast', E Ukraine
Velykyy Tokmak *see* Tokmak
173 P7 **Vema Fracture Zone** *tectonic feature* W Indian Ocean
65 P18 **Vema Seamount** *undersea feature* SW Indian Ocean
93 F17 **Vemdalen** Jämtland, C Sweden
95 N19 **Vena** Kalmar, S Sweden
41 N11 **Venado** San Luis Potosí, C Mexico
62 L11 **Venado Tuerto** Entre Ríos, E Argentina
61 A19 **Venado Tuerto** Santa Fe, C Argentina
107 K16 **Venafro** Molise, C Italy
55 Q9 **Venamo, Cerro** ▲ E Venezuela
106 B8 **Venaria** Piemonte, NW Italy
103 U15 **Vence** Alpes-Maritimes, SE France
104 H5 **Venda Nova** Vila Real, N Portugal
104 G11 **Vendas Novas** Évora, S Portugal
102 J9 **Vendée** ◈ *department* NW France
103 Q6 **Vendeuvre-sur-Barse** Aube, NE France
102 M7 **Vendôme** Loir-et-Cher, C France
Venedig *see* Venezia
Vener, Lake *see* Vänern
106 I8 **Veneta, Laguna** *lagoon* NE Italy
Venetia *see* Venezia
39 S7 **Venetie** Alaska, USA
106 H8 **Veneto** *var.* Venezia Euganea. ◈ *region* NE Italy
114 M7 **Venets** Shumen, NE Bulgaria
128 L5 **Venev** Tul'skaya Oblast', W Russian Federation
106 I8 **Venezia** *Eng.* Venice, *Fr.* Venise, *Ger.* Venedig; *anc.* Venetia. Veneto, NE Italy
Venezia Euganea *see* Veneto
Venezia, Golfo di *see* Venice, Gulf of
Venezia Tridentina *see* Trentino-Alto Adige
54 K8 **Venezuela** *off.* Republic of Venezuela; *prev.* Estados Unidos de Venezuela, United States of Venezuela. ◆ *republic* N South America
Venezuela, Cordillera de *see* Costa, Cordillera de la
54 I4 **Venezuela, Golfo de** *Eng.* Gulf of Maracaibo, Gulf of Venezuela. *gulf* NW Venezuela
Venezuela, Gulf of *see* Venezuela, Golfo de
64 F11 **Venezuelan Basin** *undersea feature* E Caribbean Sea
155 D16 **Vengurla** Mahārāshtra, W India
39 O15 **Veniaminof, Mount** ▲ Alaska, USA
23 V14 **Venice** Florida, SE USA
22 L10 **Venice** Louisiana, S USA
Venice *see* Venezia
106 J8 **Venice, Gulf of** *It.* Golfo di Venezia, *Slvn.* Beneški Zaliv. *gulf* N Adriatic Sea
Venise *see* Venezia
94 K13 **Venjan** Dalarna, C Sweden
94 K13 **Venjansjön** ◎ C Sweden
155 J18 **Venkatagiri** Andhra Pradesh, E India
99 M15 **Venlo** *prev.* Venloo. Limburg, SE Netherlands
Venloo *see* Venlo
95 E18 **Vennesla** Vest-Agder, S Norway
107 M17 **Venosa** *anc.* Venusia. Basilicata, S Italy
Venoste, Alpi *see* Ötztaler Alpen
Venraij *see* Venray
99 M14 **Venray** *var.* Venraij. Limburg, SE Netherlands
118 C8 **Venta** *Ger.* Windau. ≈ Latvia/Lithuania
Venta Belgarum *see* Winchester
40 G9 **Ventana, Punta Arena de la** *var.* Punta de la Ventana. *headland* W Mexico
Ventana, Punta de la *see* Ventana, Punta Arena de la
61 B23 **Ventana, Sierra de la** *hill range* E Argentina
Ventia *see* Valence
191 S11 **Vent, Îles du** *var.* Windward Islands. *island group* Archipel de la Société, W French Polynesia
191 R10 **Vent, Îles Sous le** *var.* Leeward Islands. *island group* Archipel de la Société, W French Polynesia
106 B11 **Ventimiglia** Liguria, NW Italy
97 M24 **Ventnor** S England, UK
18 J17 **Ventnor City** New Jersey, NE USA
103 S14 **Ventoux, Mont** ▲ SE France
118 C8 **Ventspils** *Ger.* Windau. Ventspils, NW Latvia
54 M10 **Ventuari, Río** ≈ S Venezuela
35 R15 **Ventura** California, W USA
182 F8 **Venus Bay** South Australia
Venusia *see* Venosa
191 P7 **Vénus, Pointe** *var.* Pointe Tataaihoa. *headland* Tahiti, W French Polynesia
41 V16 **Venustiano Carranza** Chiapas, SE Mexico
41 N7 **Venustiano Carranza, Presa** ⊡ NE Mexico
61 B15 **Vera** Santa Fe, C Argentina
105 Q14 **Vera** Andalucía, S Spain
63 K18 **Vera, Bahía** *bay* E Argentina
41 R14 **Veracruz** *var.* Veracruz Llave. Veracruz-Llave, E Mexico
41 Q13 **Veracruz-Llave** *var.* Veracruz. ◈ *state* E Mexico
43 Q16 **Veraguas** *off.* Provincia de Veraguas. ◈ *province* W Panama
Veramin *see* Varāmīn
154 B12 **Verāval** Gujarāt, W India
106 C6 **Verbania** Piemonte, NW Italy
107 N20 **Verbicaro** Calabria, SW Italy
108 D11 **Verbier** Valais, SW Switzerland
Vercellae *see* Vercelli
106 C8 **Vercelli** *anc.* Vercellae. Piemonte, NW Italy
103 S13 **Vercors** *physical region* E France
93 E16 **Verdalsøra** Nord-Trøndelag, C Norway
Verde, Cabo *see* Cape Verde
44 J5 **Verde, Cape** *headland* Long Island, C Bahamas
104 M2 **Verde, Costa** *coastal region* N Spain
Verde Grande, Río/Verde Grande y de Belem, Río *see* Verde, Río
100 H11 **Verden** Niedersachsen, NW Germany
59 J19 **Verde, Rio** ≈ SE Brazil
57 P16 **Verde, Río** ≈ Bolivia/Brazil
40 M12 **Verde, Río** *var.* Río Verde Grande, Río Verde Grande y de Belem. ≈ C Mexico
41 Q16 **Verde, Río** ≈ SE Mexico
36 L13 **Verde River** ≈ Arizona, SW USA
Verdhikoúsa/Verdhikoússa *see* Verdikoússa
27 Q8 **Verdigris River** ≈ Kansas/Oklahoma, C USA
115 E15 **Verdikoússa** *var.* Verdhikoúsa, Verdhikoússa. Thessalía, C Greece
103 S15 **Verdon** ≈ SE France
15 O12 **Verdun** Québec, SE Canada
103 S4 **Verdun** *var.* Verdun-sur-Meuse; *anc.* Verodunum. Meuse, NE France
Verdun-sur-Meuse *see* Verdun
83 J21 **Vereeniging** Gauteng, NE South Africa
Veremeyki *see* Vyeramyeyki
127 T14 **Vereshchagino** Permskaya Oblast', NW Russian Federation
76 G14 **Verga, Cap** *headland* W Guinea
61 G18 **Vergara** Treinta y Tres, E Uruguay
108 G11 **Vergeletto** Ticino, S Switzerland
18 L8 **Vergennes** Vermont, NE USA
Veria *see* Véroia
104 I5 **Verín** Galicia, NW Spain
Verin T'alin *see* T'alin
118 K6 **Veriora** Põlvamaa, SE Estonia
117 T7 **Verkhivtseve** Dnipropetrovs'ka Oblast', E Ukraine
129 W3 **Verkhiye Kigi** Respublika Bashkortostan, W Russian Federation
Verkhnedvinsk *see* Vyerkhnyadzvinsk
122 L10 **Verkhneimbatsk** Krasnoyarskiy Kray, N Russian Federation
126 I3 **Verkhnetulomskiy** Murmanskaya Oblast', NW Russian Federation
126 I3 **Verkhnetulomskoye Vodokhranilishche** ⊡ NW Russian Federation
Verkhneudinsk *see* Ulan-Ude
123 P10 **Verkhnevilyuysk** Respublika Sakha (Yakutiya), NE Russian Federation
129 W5 **Verkhniy Avzyan** Respublika Bashkortostan, W Russian Federation
129 Q11 **Verkhniy Baskunchak** Astrakhanskaya Oblast', SW Russian Federation
117 T9 **Verkhniy Rohachyk** Khersons'ka Oblast', S Ukraine
123 Q11 **Verkhnyaya Amga** Respublika Sakha (Yakutiya), NE Russian Federation
127 V6 **Verkhnyaya Inta** Respublika Komi, NW Russian Federation
127 O10 **Verkhnyaya Toyma** Arkhangel'skaya Oblast', NW Russian Federation
128 K6 **Verkhov'ye** Orlovskaya Oblast', W Russian Federation
116 I8 **Verkhovyna** Ivano-Frankivs'ka Oblast', W Ukraine
123 P8 **Verkhoyanskiy Khrebet** ⛰ NE Russian Federation
117 T7 **Verkhn'odniprovs'k** Dnipropetrovs'ka Oblast', E Ukraine
101 G14 **Verl** Nordrhein-Westfalen, NW Germany
92 N1 **Verlegenhuken** *headland* N Svalbard
82 A9 **Vermelha, Ponta** *headland* NW Angola
103 P7 **Vermenton** Yonne, C France
11 R14 **Vermilion** Alberta, SW Canada
31 T11 **Vermilion** Ohio, N USA
22 I10 **Vermilion Bay** *bay* Louisiana, S USA
29 V4 **Vermilion Lake** ◎ Minnesota, N USA
14 F9 **Vermilion River** ≈ Ontario, S Canada
30 L12 **Vermilion River** ≈ Illinois, N USA
29 R12 **Vermillion** South Dakota, N USA
29 R12 **Vermillion River** ≈ South Dakota, N USA
15 O9 **Vermillon, Rivière** ≈ Québec, SE Canada
115 E14 **Vérmio** ⛰ N Greece
18 L8 **Vermont** *off.* State of Vermont; also known as The Green Mountain State. ◈ *state* NE USA
113 K16 **Vermosh** *var.* Vermoshi. Shkodër, N Albania
Vermoshi *see* Vermosh
37 O3 **Vernal** Utah, W USA
14 G11 **Verner** Ontario, S Canada
102 M5 **Verneuil-sur-Avre** Eure, N France
114 D13 **Vérno** ⛰ N Greece
11 N17 **Vernon** British Columbia, SW Canada
102 M4 **Vernon** Eure, N France
23 N3 **Vernon** Alabama, S USA
31 P15 **Vernon** Indiana, N USA
25 Q4 **Vernon** Texas, SW USA
32 G10 **Vernonia** Oregon, NW USA
14 G12 **Vernon, Lake** ◎ Ontario, S Canada
22 G7 **Vernon Lake** ⊡ Louisiana, S USA
23 Y13 **Vero Beach** Florida, SE USA
Verőcze *see* Virovitica
Verodunum *see* Verdun
115 E14 **Véroia** *var.* Veria, Vérroia, *Turk.* Karaferiye. Kentrikí Makedonía, N Greece
106 E8 **Verolanuova** Lombardia, N Italy
14 K14 **Verona** Ontario, SE Canada
106 G8 **Verona** Veneto, NE Italy
29 P6 **Verona** North Dakota, N USA
30 L9 **Verona** Wisconsin, N USA
61 E20 **Verónica** Buenos Aires, E Argentina
22 J9 **Verret, Lake** ◎ Louisiana, S USA
Vérroia *see* Véroia
103 N5 **Versailles** Yvelines, N France
31 P15 **Versailles** Indiana, N USA
20 M5 **Versailles** Kentucky, S USA
27 U5 **Versailles** Missouri, C USA
31 Q13 **Versailles** Ohio, N USA
Versecz *see* Vršac
108 A10 **Versoix** Genève, SW Switzerland
15 Z6 **Verte, Pointe** *headland* Quebec, SE Canada
111 I22 **Vértes** ⛰ NW Hungary
44 G6 **Vertientes** Camagüey, C Cuba
114 G13 **Vertískos** ⛰ N Greece
102 I8 **Vertou** Loire-Atlantique, NW France
Verulamium *see* St Albans
99 L19 **Verviers** Liège, E Belgium
103 Y14 **Vescovato** Corse, France, C Mediterranean Sea
99 L20 **Vesdre** ≈ E Belgium
117 U10 **Vesele** *Rus.* Veseloye. Zaporiz'ka Oblast', S Ukraine
111 D18 **Veselí nad Lužnicí** *var.* Weseli an der Lainsitz, *Ger.* Frohenbruck. Budějovický Kraj, S Czech Republic
114 M9 **Veselinovo** Shumen, E Bulgaria
128 L12 **Veselovskoye Vodokhranilishche** ⊡ SW Russian Federation
Veseloye *see* Vesele
117 Q9 **Veselynove** Mykolayivs'ka Oblast', S Ukraine
Veseya *see* Vyasyeya
128 M10 **Veshenskaya** Rostovskaya Oblast', SW Russian Federation
129 Q5 **Veshkayma** Ul'yanovskaya Oblast', W Russian Federation
Vesisaari *see* Vadsø
Vesontio *see* Besançon
103 T7 **Vesoul** *anc.* Vesulium, Vesulum. Haute-Saône, E France
95 J20 **Vessigebro** Halland, S Sweden
95 D17 **Vest-Agder** ◈ *county* S Norway
23 P4 **Vestavia Hills** Alabama, S USA
84 F6 **Vesterålen** *island* NW Norway
92 G10 **Vesterålen** *island group* N Norway
87 V3 **Vestervig** Viborg, NW Denmark
92 H2 **Vestfirdhir** ◈ *region* NW Iceland
92 G11 **Vestfjorden** *fjord* C Norway
95 G16 **Vestfold** ◈ *county* S Norway
95 B18 **Vestmanna** *Dan.* Vestmanhavn Faeroe Islands
92 I4 **Vestmannaeyjar** Sudhurland, S Iceland
94 E9 **Vestnes** Møre og Romsdal, S Norway
95 I23 **Vestsjælland** *off.* Vestsjællands Amt. ◈ *county* E Denmark
92 H3 **Vesturland** ◈ *region* W Iceland
92 G11 **Vestvågøya** *island* C Norway
Vesulium/Vesulum *see* Vesoul
Vesuna *see* Périgueux
107 K17 **Vesuvio** *Eng.* Vesuvius. ✻ S Italy
Vesuvius *see* Vesuvio
126 K14 **Ves'yegonsk** Tverskaya Oblast', W Russian Federation
111 I23 **Veszprém** *Ger.* Veszprim. Veszprém, W Hungary
111 H23 **Veszprém** *off.* Veszprém Megye. ◈ *county* W Hungary
Veszprim *see* Veszprém
Vetka *see* Vyetka
95 M19 **Vetlanda** Jönköping, S Sweden
129 P1 **Vetluga** Nizhegorodskaya Oblast', W Russian Federation
127 P14 **Vetluga** ≈ NW Russian Federation
127 O14 **Vetluzhskiy** Kostromskaya Oblast', NW Russian Federation
129 P2 **Vetluzhskiy** Nizhegorodskaya Oblast', W Russian Federation
107 H14 **Vetralla** Lazio, C Italy
114 M9 **Vetren** *prev.* Zhitarovo. Burgas, E Bulgaria
114 M8 **Vetrino** Varna, E Bulgaria
Vetrino *see* Vyetryna
122 L7 **Vetrovaya, Gora** ▲ N Russian Federation
Vetter, Lake *see* Vättern
106 J13 **Vettore, Monte** ▲ C Italy
99 A17 **Veurne** *var.* Furnes. West-Vlaanderen, W Belgium
31 Q15 **Vevay** Indiana, N USA
108 C10 **Vevey** *Ger.* Vivis; *anc.* Vibiscum. Vaud, SW Switzerland
Vexiö *see* Växjö
103 S13 **Veynes** Hautes-Alpes, SE France
103 N11 **Vézère** ≈ W France
114 I9 **Vezhen** ▲ C Bulgaria
136 K11 **Vezirköprü** Samsun, N Turkey
57 J18 **Viacha** La Paz, W Bolivia
27 R10 **Vian** Oklahoma, C USA
Viana de Castelo *see* Viana do Castelo
104 H12 **Viana do Alentejo** Évora, S Portugal
104 I4 **Viana do Bolo** Galicia, NW Spain
104 G5 **Viana do Castelo** *var.* Viana de Castelo; *anc.* Velobriga. Viana do Castelo, NW Portugal
104 G5 **Viana do Castelo** *var.* Viana de Castelo. ◈ *district* N Portugal
98 J12 **Vianen** Zuid-Holland, C Netherlands
167 Q8 **Viangchan** *Eng./Fr.* Vientiane. ● (Laos) C Laos
167 P6 **Viangphoukha** *var.* Vieng Pou Kha. Louang Namtha, N Laos
104 K13 **Viar** ≈ SW Spain
106 E11 **Viareggio** Toscana, C Italy
103 O14 **Viaur** ≈ S France
Vibiscum *see* Vevey
95 G21 **Viborg** Viborg, NW Denmark
29 R12 **Viborg** South Dakota, N USA
95 F21 **Viborg** *off.* Viborg Amt. ◈ *county* NW Denmark
107 N22 **Vibo Valentia** *prev.* Monteleone di Calabria; *anc.* Hipponium. Calabria, SW Italy
105 W5 **Vic** *var.* Vich; *anc.* Ausa, Vicus Ausonensis. Cataluña, NE Spain
102 K16 **Vic-en-Bigorre** Hautes-Pyrénées, S France
40 K10 **Vicente Guerrero** Durango, C Mexico
41 P10 **Vicente Guerrero, Presa** *var.* Presa de las Adjuntas. ⊡ NE Mexico
Vicentia *see* Vicenza
106 G8 **Vicenza** *anc.* Vicentia. Veneto, NE Italy
Vich *see* Vic
54 J10 **Vichada** *off.* Comisaría del Vichada. ◈ *province* E Colombia
54 K10 **Vichada, Río** ≈ E Colombia
61 G17 **Vichadero** Rivera, NE Uruguay
Vichegda *see* Vychegda
126 M16 **Vichuga** Ivanovskaya Oblast', W Russian Federation
103 P10 **Vichy** Allier, C France
26 K9 **Vici** Oklahoma, C USA
31 P10 **Vicksburg** Michigan, N USA
22 J5 **Vicksburg** Mississippi, S USA
103 O12 **Vic-sur-Cère** Cantal, C France
29 X14 **Victor** Iowa, C USA
59 I21 **Victor** Mato Grosso do Sul, SW Brazil
182 I10 **Victor Harbor** South Australia
61 C18 **Victoria** Entre Ríos, E Argentina
10 L17 **Victoria** Vancouver Island, British Columbia, SW Canada
45 R14 **Victoria** NW Grenada
42 H6 **Victoria** Yoro, NW Honduras
121 O15 **Victoria** *var.* Rabat. Gozo, NW Malta
116 I12 **Victoria** *Ger.* Viktoriastadt. Brașov, C Romania
172 H17 **Victoria** ● (Seychelles) Mahé, SW Seychelles
25 U13 **Victoria** Texas, SW USA
183 N12 **Victoria** ◈ *state* SE Australia
174 K7 **Victoria** ≈ Western Australia
Victoria *see* Labuan, East Malaysia
Victoria *see* Masvingo, Zimbabwe
Victoria Bank *see* Vitória Seamount
11 Y15 **Victoria Beach** Manitoba, S Canada
Victoria de Durango *see* Durango
Victoria de las Tunas *see* Las Tunas
83 I16 **Victoria Falls** Matabeleland North, W Zimbabwe
83 I16 **Victoria Falls** ✕ Matabeleland North, W Zimbabwe
83 I16 **Victoria Falls** *waterfall* Zambia/Zimbabwe
Victoria Falls *see* Iguaçu, Salto do
63 F19 **Victoria, Isla** *island* Archipiélago de los Chonos, S Chile
8 K6 **Victoria Island** *island* Northwest Territories/Nunavut, NW Canada
182 L8 **Victoria, Lake** ◎ New South Wales, SE Australia
68 I12 **Victoria, Lake** *var.* Victoria Nyanza. ◎ E Africa
195 S13 **Victoria Land** *physical region* Antarctica
166 L5 **Victoria, Mount** ▲ W Burma
187 X14 **Victoria, Mount** ▲ Viti Levu, W Fiji
186 E9 **Victoria, Mount** ▲ S PNG
81 F17 **Victoria Nile** *var.* Somerset Nile. ≈ C Uganda
Victoria Nyanza *see* Victoria, Lake
42 G3 **Victoria Peak** ▲ SE Belize
185 H16 **Victoria Range** ⛰ South Island, NZ
181 O3 **Victoria River** ≈ Northern Territory, N Australia
181 P3 **Victoria River Roadhouse** Northern Territory, N Australia
15 Q11 **Victoriaville** Quebec, SE Canada
Victoria-Wes *see* Victoria West
83 G24 **Victoria West** *Afr.* Victoria-Wes. Northern Cape, W South Africa
62 J13 **Victorica** La Pampa, C Argentina
195 T3 **Victor, Mount** ▲ Antarctica
35 U14 **Victorville** California, W USA
62 G9 **Vicuña** Coquimbo, N Chile
62 K11 **Vicuña Mackenna** Córdoba, C Argentina
Vicus Ausonensis *see* Vic
Vicus Elbii *see* Viterbo
33 X7 **Vida** Montana, NW USA
23 V6 **Vidalia** Georgia, SE USA
22 J7 **Vidalia** Louisiana, S USA
95 F22 **Videbæk** Ringkøbing, C Denmark
60 I13 **Videira** Santa Catarina, S Brazil
116 J14 **Videle** Teleorman, S Romania
Videm-Krško *see* Krško
Vídeň *see* Wien
104 H12 **Vidigueira** Beja, S Portugal
114 J9 **Vidima** ≈ N Bulgaria
114 G7 **Vidin** *anc.* Bononia. Vidin, NW Bulgaria
114 F8 **Vidin** ◈ *province* NW Bulgaria
154 H10 **Vidisha** Madhya Pradesh, C India
25 Y10 **Vidor** Texas, SW USA
95 L20 **Vidöstern** ◎ S Sweden
92 J13 **Vidsel** Norrbotten, N Sweden
118 H9 **Vidzemes Augstiene** ▲ C Latvia
118 J12 **Vidzy** *Rus.* Vidzy. Vitsyebskaya Voblasts', NW Belarus
63 L16 **Viedma** Río Negro, E Argentina
63 H22 **Viedma, Lago** ◎ S Argentina
45 O11 **Vieille Case** *var.* Itassi. N Dominica
104 M2 **Vieja, Peña** ▲ N Spain
40 E4 **Viejo, Cerro** ▲ NW Mexico
56 B9 **Viejo, Cerro** ▲ N Peru
118 E10 **Viekšniai** Akmenė, NW Lithuania
105 U3 **Vielha** *var.* Viella. Cataluña, NE Spain
Viella *see* Vielha
99 L21 **Vielsalm** Luxembourg, E Belgium
Vieng Pou Kha *see* Viangphoukha
23 T6 **Vienna** Georgia, SE USA
30 L17 **Vienna** Illinois, N USA
27 V5 **Vienna** Missouri, C USA
21 Q3 **Vienna** West Virginia, NE USA
Vienna *see* Wien, Austria
Vienna *see* Vienne, France
103 R11 **Vienne** *anc.* Vienna. Isère, E France
102 L10 **Vienne** ◈ *department* W France
102 L9 **Vienne** ≈ W France
Vientiane *see* Viangchan
Vientos, Paso de los *see* Windward Passage
45 V6 **Vieques** *var.* Isabel Segunda. E Puerto Rico
45 V6 **Vieques, Isla de** *island* E Puerto Rico
45 V6 **Vieques, Pasaje de** *passage* E Puerto Rico
45 V5 **Vieques, Sonda de** *sound* E Puerto Rico
Vierdörfer *see* Săcele
93 M15 **Vieremä** Itä-Suomi, C Finland
99 M14 **Vierlingsbeek** Noord-Brabant, SE Netherlands
101 G20 **Viernheim** Hessen, W Germany
101 D15 **Viersen** Nordrhein-Westfalen, W Germany
108 G8 **Vierwaldstätter See** *Eng.* Lake of Lucerne. ◎ C Switzerland
103 N8 **Vierzon** Cher, C France
40 L8 **Viesca** Coahuila de Zaragoza, NE Mexico
118 H10 **Viesīte** *Ger.* Eckengraf. Jēkabpils, S Latvia
107 N15 **Vieste** Puglia, SE Italy
167 T8 **Vietnam** *off.* Socialist Republic of Vietnam, *Vtn.* Công Hoa Xã Hôi Chu Nghia Việt Nam. ◆ *republic* SE Asia
167 S5 **Việt Quang** Ha Giang, N Vietnam
Vietri *see* Việt Tri
167 S6 **Việt Tri** *var.* Vietri. Vinh Phu, N Vietnam
30 L4 **Vieux Desert, Lac** ◎ Michigan/Wisconsin, N USA
45 Y13 **Vieux Fort** S Saint Lucia
45 X6 **Vieux-Habitants** Basse Terre, SW Guadeloupe
119 G14 **Vievis** Kaišiadorys, S Lithuania
171 N2 **Vigan** Luzon, N Philippines
106 D8 **Vigevano** Lombardia, N Italy
107 N18 **Viggiano** Basilicata, S Italy
58 L12 **Vigia** Pará, NE Brazil
41 Y12 **Vigía Chico** Quintana Roo, SE Mexico
45 T11 **Vigie** ✕ (Castries) NE Saint Lucia
102 K17 **Vignemale** *var.* Pic de Vignemale. ▲ France/Spain
Vignemale, Pic de *see* Vignemale
106 G10 **Vignola** Emilia-Romagna, C Italy
104 G4 **Vigo** Galicia, NW Spain
104 G4 **Vigo, Ría de** *estuary* NW Spain
94 D9 **Vigra** *island* S Norway
95 C17 **Vigrestad** Rogaland, S Norway
93 L15 **Vihanti** Oulu, C Finland
149 U10 **Vihāri** Punjab, E Pakistan
102 K8 **Vihiers** Maine-et-Loire, NW France
111 O19 **Vihorlat** ▲ E Slovakia
93 L19 **Vihti** Etelä-Suomi, S Finland
Viipuri *see* Vyborg
93 M16 **Viitasaari** Länsi-Suomi, W Finland
118 K3 **Viivikonna** Ida-Virumaa, NE Estonia
155 K16 **Vijayawāda** *prev.* Bezwada. Andhra Pradesh, SE India
Vijosa/Vijosë *see* Aóos, Albania/Greece
Vijosa/Vijosë *see* Vjosës, Lumi i, Albania/Greece
Vik *see* Vikøyri
92 J4 **Vík** Sudhurland, S Iceland
94 L13 **Vika** Dalarna, C Sweden
92 L12 **Vikajärvi** Lappi, N Finland
94 L13 **Vikarbyn** Dalarna, C Sweden
95 J22 **Viken** Skåne, S Sweden
95 L17 **Viken** ◎ C Sweden
95 G15 **Vikersund** Buskerud, S Norway
114 G11 **Vikhren** ▲ SW Bulgaria
11 R15 **Viking** Alberta, SW Canada
84 E7 **Viking Bank** *undersea feature* N North Sea
95 M14 **Vikmanshyttan** Dalarna, C Sweden
94 D12 **Vikøyri** *var.* Vik. Sogn og Fjordane, S Norway
93 H17 **Viksjö** Västernorrland, C Sweden
Viktoriastadt *see* Victoria
Vila *see* Port-Vila
Vila Arriaga *see* Bibala
Vila Artur de Paiva *see* Cubango
Vila Bela da Santissima Trindade *see* Mato Grosso
58 B12 **Vila Bittencourt** Amazonas, NW Brazil
Vila da Ponte *see* Cubango
64 O2 **Vila da Praia da Vitória** Terceira, Azores, Portugal, NE Atlantic Ocean
Vila de Aljustrel *see* Cangamba
Vila de Almoster *see* Chiange
Vila de João Belo *see* Xai-Xai
Vila de Macia *see* Macia
Vila de Manhiça *see* Manhiça
Vila de Manica *see* Manica
Vila de Mocímboa da Praia *see* Mocímboa da Praia
83 N16 **Vila de Sena** *var.* Sena. Sofala, C Mozambique
104 F14 **Vila do Bispo** Faro, S Portugal
104 G6 **Vila do Conde** Porto, NW Portugal
Vila do Maio *see* Maio
64 P3 **Vila do Porto** Santa Maria, Azores, Portugal, NE Atlantic Ocean
83 K15 **Vila do Zumbo** *prev.* Vila do Zumbu, Zumbo. Tete, NW Mozambique
Vila do Zumbu *see* Vila do Zumbo
104 I6 **Vila Flor** *var.* Vila Flôr. Bragança, N Portugal
105 V6 **Vilafranca del Penedès** *var.* Villafranca del Panadés. Cataluña, NE Spain
104 F10 **Vila Franca de Xira** *var.* Vilafranca de Xira. Lisboa, C Portugal
Vila Gago Coutinho *see* Lumbala N'Guimbo
104 G3 **Vilagarcía de Arousa** *var.* Villagarcía de Arosa. Galicia, NW Spain
Vila General Machado *see* Camacupa
Vila Henrique de Carvalho *see* Saurimo
102 I7 **Vilaine** ≈ NW France
Vila João de Almeida *see* Chibia
118 K8 **Viļaka** *Ger.* Marienhausen. Balvi, NE Latvia
104 I2 **Vilalba** Galicia, NW Spain
Vila Marechal Carmona *see* Uíge
Vila Mariano Machado *see* Ganda
172 G3 **Vilanandro, Tanjona** *headland* W Madagascar
Vilanculos *see* Vilankulo
118 J10 **Viļāni** Rēzekne, E Latvia
83 N19 **Vilankulo** *var.* Vilanculos. Inhambane, E Mozambique
Vila Norton de Matos *see* Balombo
104 G6 **Vila Nova de Famalicão** *var.* Vila Nova de Famalicao. Braga, N Portugal
104 I6 **Vila Nova de Foz Côa** *var.* Vila Nova de Fozcôa. Guarda, N Portugal
104 F6 **Vila Nova de Gaia** Porto, NW Portugal
Vila Nova de Portimão *see* Portimão
105 V6 **Vilanova i La Geltrú** Cataluña, NE Spain
Vila Pereira de Eça *see* N'Giva
104 H6 **Vila Pouca de Aguiar** Vila Real, N Portugal
104 H6 **Vila Real** *var.* Vila Rial. Vila Real, N Portugal
104 H6 **Vila Real** ◈ *district* N Portugal
105 T9 **Vila-real de los Infantes** *var.* Villarreal. País Valenciano, E Spain
104 H14 **Vila Real de Santo António** Faro, S Portugal
104 J7 **Vilar Formoso** Guarda, N Portugal
Vila Rial *see* Vila Real
59 J15 **Vila Rica** Mato Grosso, W Brazil

◆ Country ● Country Capital ◇ Dependent Territory ○ Dependent Territory Capital ◈ Administrative Region ✕ International Airport ▲ Mountain ⛰ Mountain Range ✻ Volcano ≈ River ◎ Lake ⊡ Reservoir

Vila Robert Williams see Caála
Vila Salazar see N'Dalatando
Vila Serpa Pinto see Menongue
Vila Teixeira da Silva see Bailundo
Vila Teixeira de Sousa see Luau
104 H9 **Vila Velha de Ródão** Castelo Branco, C Portugal
104 G5 **Vila Verde** Braga, N Portugal
104 H11 **Vila Viçosa** Évora, S Portugal
57 G15 **Vilcabamba, Cordillera de** ▲ C Peru
Vîlcea see Vâlcea
122 J4 **Vil'cheka, Zemlya** *Eng.* Wilczek Land. *island* Zemlya Frantsa-Iosifa, NW Russian Federation
95 F22 **Vildbjerg** Ringkøbing, C Denmark
Vileyka see Vilyeyka
93 H15 **Vilhelmina** Västerbotten, N Sweden
59 F17 **Vilhena** Rondônia, W Brazil
115 G19 **Vília** Attikí, C Greece
Viliya see Viliya
119 I14 **Viliya** *Lith.* Neris, *Rus.* Viliya. ≈ W Belarus
Viliya see Neris
118 H5 **Viljandi** *Ger.* Fellin. Viljandimaa, S Estonia
118 H5 **Viljandimaa** *off.* Viljandi Maakond. ◆ *province* SW Estonia
119 E14 **Vilkaviškis** *Pol.* Wyłkowyszki. Vilkaviškis, SW Lithuania
118 F13 **Vilkija** Kaunas, C Lithuania
197 V9 **Vil'kitskogo, Proliv** *strait* N Russian Federation
Vilkovo see Vylkove
57 L21 **Villa Abecia** Chuquisaca, S Bolivia
41 N5 **Villa Acuña** *var.* Ciudad Acuña. Coahuila de Zaragoza, NE Mexico
40 J4 **Villa Ahumada** Chihuahua, N Mexico
45 O9 **Villa Altagracia** C Dominican Republic
56 L13 **Villa Bella** Beni, N Bolivia
104 J3 **Villablino** Castilla-León, N Spain
54 K6 **Villa Bruzual** Portuguesa, N Venezuela
105 O9 **Villacañas** Castilla-La Mancha, C Spain
105 O12 **Villacarrillo** Andalucía, S Spain
104 M7 **Villacastín** Castilla-León, N Spain
Villa Cecilia see Ciudad Madero
109 S9 **Villach** *Slvn.* Beljak. Kärnten, S Austria
107 B20 **Villacidro** Sardegna, Italy, C Mediterranean Sea
Villa Concepción see Concepción
104 L4 **Villada** Castilla-León, N Spain
40 M10 **Villa de Cos** Zacatecas, C Mexico
54 L5 **Villa de Cura** *var.* Cura. Aragua, N Venezuela
Villa del Nevoso see Ilirska Bistrica
Villa del Pilar see Pilar
104 M13 **Villa del Río** Andalucía, S Spain
Villa de Méndez see Méndez
42 H6 **Villa de San Antonio** Comayagua, W Honduras
105 N4 **Villadiego** Castilla-León, N Spain
105 T8 **Villafames** País Valenciano, E Spain
41 U16 **Villa Flores** Chiapas, SE Mexico
104 J3 **Villafranca del Bierzo** Castilla-León, N Spain
105 S8 **Villafranca del Cid** País Valenciano, E Spain
104 J11 **Villafranca de los Barros** Extremadura, W Spain
105 N10 **Villafranca de los Caballeros** Castilla-La Mancha, C Spain
Villafranca del Panadés see Vilafranca del Penedès
106 F8 **Villafranca di Verona** Veneto, NE Italy
107 J23 **Villafrati** Sicilia, Italy, C Mediterranean Sea
Villagarcía de Arosa see Vilagarcía de Arousa
41 O9 **Villagrán** Tamaulipas, C Mexico
61 C17 **Villaguay** Entre Ríos, E Argentina
62 O6 **Villa Hayes** Presidente Hayes, S Paraguay
41 U15 **Villahermosa** *prev.* San Juan Bautista. Tabasco, SE Mexico
105 O11 **Villahermosa** Castilla-La Mancha, C Spain
64 O11 **Villahermoso** Gomera, Islas Canarias, Spain, NE Atlantic Ocean
Villa Hidalgo see Hidalgo
105 T12 **Villajoyosa** *var.* La Vila Jojosa. País Valenciano, E Spain
Villa Juárez see Juárez
Villalba see Collado Villalba
41 N8 **Villaldama** Nuevo León, NE Mexico
104 L5 **Villalón de Campos** Castilla-León, N Spain
61 A25 **Villalonga** Buenos Aires, E Argentina
104 L5 **Villalpando** Castilla-León, N Spain
40 K9 **Villa Madero** *var.* Francisco I.Madero. Durango, C Mexico
41 O9 **Villa Mainero** Tamaulipas, C Mexico
Villamaña see Villamañán
104 L4 **Villamañán** *var.* Villamaña. Castilla-León, N Spain
62 L10 **Villa María** Córdoba, C Argentina
61 C17 **Villa María Grande** Entre Ríos, E Argentina
57 K21 **Villa Martín** Potosí, SW Bolivia
104 K15 **Villamartin** Andalucía, S Spain
62 J8 **Villa Mazán** La Rioja, NW Argentina
Villa Mercedes see Mercedes
Villamil see Puerto Villamil
Villa Nador see Nador
54 G5 **Villanueva** La Guajira, N Colombia
42 H5 **Villanueva** Cortés, NW Honduras
40 L11 **Villanueva** Zacatecas, C Mexico
42 I9 **Villa Nueva** Chinandega, NW Nicaragua
37 T11 **Villanueva** New Mexico, SW USA
104 M12 **Villanueva de Córdoba** Andalucía, S Spain
105 O12 **Villanueva del Arzobispo** Andalucía, S Spain
104 K11 **Villanueva de la Serena** Extremadura, W Spain
104 L5 **Villanueva del Campo** Castilla-León, N Spain
105 O11 **Villanueva de los Infantes** Castilla-La Mancha, C Spain
61 C14 **Villa Ocampo** Santa Fe, C Argentina
40 J8 **Villa Ocampo** Durango, C Mexico
40 J7 **Villa Orestes Pereyra** Durango, C Mexico
105 N3 **Villarcayo** Castilla-León, N Spain
104 L5 **Villardefrades** Castilla-León, N Spain
105 S9 **Villar del Arzobispo** País Valenciano, E Spain
105 Q6 **Villaroya de la Sierra** Aragón, NE Spain
Villarreal see Vila-real de los Infantes
62 P6 **Villarrica** Guairá, SE Paraguay
63 G15 **Villarrica, Volcán** ☗ S Chile
105 P10 **Villarrobledo** Castilla-La Mancha, C Spain
105 N10 **Villarrubia de los Ojos** Castilla-La Mancha, C Spain
18 J17 **Villas** New Jersey, NE USA
105 O3 **Villasana de Mena** Castilla-León, N Spain
107 M23 **Villa San Giovanni** Calabria, S Italy
61 D18 **Villa San José** Entre Ríos, E Argentina
Villa Sanjurjo see Al-Hoceïma
105 P6 **Villasayas** Castilla-León, N Spain
107 C20 **Villasimius** Sardegna, Italy, C Mediterranean Sea
41 N6 **Villa Unión** Coahuila de Zaragoza, NE Mexico
40 K10 **Villa Unión** Durango, C Mexico
40 J10 **Villa Unión** Sinaloa, C Mexico
62 K12 **Villa Valeria** Córdoba, C Argentina
105 N8 **Villaverde** Madrid, C Spain
54 F10 **Villavicencio** Meta, C Colombia
104 L2 **Villaviciosa** Asturias, N Spain
104 L12 **Villaviciosa de Córdoba** Andalucía, S Spain
57 L22 **Villazón** Potosí, S Bolivia
14 J8 **Villebon, Lac** ⊚ Québec, SE Canada
Ville de Kinshasa see Kinshasa
102 J5 **Villedieu-les-Poêles** Manche, N France
Villefranche see Villefranche-sur-Saône
103 N16 **Villefranche-de-Lauragais** Haute-Garonne, S France
103 N14 **Villefranche-de-Rouergue** Aveyron, S France
103 R10 **Villefranche-sur-Saône** *var.* Villefranche. Rhône, E France
14 H9 **Ville-Marie** Quebec, SE Canada
102 M15 **Villemur-sur-Tarn** Haute-Garonne, S France
105 S11 **Villena** País Valenciano, E Spain
Villeneuve-d'Agen see Villeneuve-sur-Lot
102 L13 **Villeneuve-sur-Lot** *var.* Villeneuve-d'Agen; *hist.* Gajac. Lot-et-Garonne, SW France
103 P6 **Villeneuve-sur-Yonne** Yonne, C France
22 H8 **Ville Platte** Louisiana, S USA
103 R11 **Villeurbanne** Rhône, E France
101 G23 **Villingen-Schwenningen** Baden-Württemberg, S Germany
29 T15 **Villisca** Iowa, C USA
Villmanstrand see Lappeenranta
Vilna see Vilnius
119 H14 **Vilnius** *Pol.* Wilno, *Ger.* Wilna; *prev. Rus.* Vilna. ● (Lithuania) Vilnius, SE Lithuania
119 H14 **Vilnius** ✕ Vilnius, SE Lithuania
117 S7 **Vil'nohirs'k** Dnipropetrovs'ka Oblast', E Ukraine
117 U8 **Vil'nyans'k** Zaporiz'ka Oblast', SE Ukraine
93 L17 **Vilppula** Länsi-Suomi, W Finland
101 M20 **Vils** ≈ SE Germany
118 C5 **Vilsandi Saar** *island* W Estonia
117 P8 **Vil'shanka** *Rus.* Olshanka. Kirovohrads'ka Oblast', C Ukraine
101 O22 **Vilshofen** Bayern, SE Germany
155 J20 **Viluppuram** Tamil Nādu, SE India
113 I16 **Vilusi** Montenegro, SW Yugoslavia
99 G18 **Vilvoorde** *Fr.* Vilvorde. Vlaams Brabant, C Belgium
Vilvorde see Vilvoorde
119 J14 **Vilyeyka** *Pol.* Wilejka, *Rus.* Vileyka. Minskaya Voblasts', NW Belarus
123 P10 **Vilyuy** ≈ NE Russian Federation
123 P10 **Vilyuysk** Respublika Sakha (Yakutiya), NE Russian Federation
123 N10 **Vilyuyskoye Vodokhranilishche** ⊟ NE Russian Federation
104 G2 **Vimianzo** Galicia, NW Spain
95 M19 **Vimmerby** Kalmar, S Sweden
102 L5 **Vimoutiers** Orne, N France
93 L16 **Vimpeli** Länsi-Suomi, W Finland
79 G14 **Vina** ≈ Cameroon/Chad
62 G11 **Viña del Mar** Valparaíso, C Chile
19 R8 **Vinalhaven Island** *island* Maine, NE USA
105 T8 **Vinaròs** País Valenciano, E Spain
Vînători see Vânători
31 N15 **Vincennes** Indiana, N USA
195 Y12 **Vincennes Bay** *bay* Antarctica
25 O7 **Vincent** Texas, SW USA
95 H24 **Vindeby** Fyn, C Denmark
93 I15 **Vindeln** Västerbotten, N Sweden
95 F21 **Vinderup** Ringkøbing, C Denmark
Vindhya Mountains see Vindhya Range
153 N14 **Vindhya Range** *var.* Vindhya Mountains. ▲ N India
Vindobona see Wien
20 K6 **Vine Grove** Kentucky, S USA
18 J17 **Vineland** New Jersey, NE USA
116 E11 **Vinga** Arad, W Romania
95 M16 **Vingåker** Södermanland, C Sweden
167 S8 **Vinh** Nghê An, N Vietnam
104 I5 **Vinhais** Bragança, N Portugal
167 T9 **Vinh Linh** Quang Tri, C Vietnam
Vinh Loi see Bac Liêu
167 S14 **Vinh Long** *var.* Vinhlong. Vinh Long, S Vietnam
113 Q18 **Vinica** NE FYR Macedonia
109 V13 **Vinica** SE Slovenia
114 G8 **Vinishte** Montana, NW Bulgaria
27 Q8 **Vinita** Oklahoma, C USA
Vînju Mare see Vânju Mare
98 I11 **Vinkeveen** Utrecht, C Netherlands
116 L6 **Vin'kivtsi** Khmel'nyts'ka Oblast', W Ukraine
112 I10 **Vinkovci** *Ger.* Winkowitz, *Hung.* Vinkovcze. Vukovar-Srijem, E Croatia
Vinkovcze see Vinkovci
Vinnitsa see Vinnytsya
Vinnitskaya Oblast'/Vinnytsya see Vinnyts'ka Oblast'
116 M7 **Vinnyts'ka Oblast'** *var.* Vinnytsya, *Rus.* Vinnitskaya Oblast'. ◆ *province* C Ukraine
117 N6 **Vinnytsya** *Rus.* Vinnitsa. Vinnyts'ka Oblast', C Ukraine
117 N6 **Vinnytsya** ✕ Vinnyts'ka Oblast', N Ukraine
Vinogradov see Vynohradiv
194 L8 **Vinson Massif** ▲ Antarctica
94 G11 **Vinstra** Oppland, S Norway
116 K12 **Vintilă Vodă** Buzău, SE Romania
29 X13 **Vinton** Iowa, C USA
22 F9 **Vinton** Louisiana, S USA
155 J17 **Vinukonda** Andhra Pradesh, E India
Vioara see Ocnele Mari
83 E23 **Vioolsdrif** Northern Cape, SW South Africa
82 M13 **Viphya Mountains** ▲ C Malawi
171 Q4 **Virac** Catanduanes Island, N Philippines
126 K8 **Virandozero** Respublika Kareliya, NW Russian Federation
137 P16 **Viranşehir** Şanlıurfa, SE Turkey
154 D13 **Virār** Mahārāshtra, W India
11 W16 **Virden** Manitoba, S Canada
30 K14 **Virden** Illinois, N USA
Virdois see Virrat
102 J5 **Vire** Calvados, N France
102 J4 **Vire** ≈ N France
83 A15 **Virei** Namibe, SW Angola
Vîrful Moldoveanu see Vârful Moldoveanu
35 R5 **Virginia Peak** ▲ Nevada, W USA
45 U9 **Virgin Gorda** *island* C British Virgin Islands
83 I22 **Virginia** Free State, C South Africa
30 K13 **Virginia** Illinois, N USA
29 W4 **Virginia** Minnesota, N USA
21 T6 **Virginia** *off.* Commonwealth of Virginia; also known as Mother of Presidents, Mother of States, Old Dominion. ◆ *state* NE USA
21 Y7 **Virginia Beach** Virginia, NE USA
33 R11 **Virginia City** Montana, NW USA
35 Q6 **Virginia City** Nevada, W USA
14 H8 **Virginiatown** Ontario, S Canada
Virgin Islands see British Virgin Islands
45 T9 **Virgin Islands (US)** *var.* Virgin Islands of the United States; *prev.* Danish West Indies. ◇ *US unincorporated territory* E West Indies
45 T9 **Virgin Passage** *passage* Puerto Rico/Virgin Islands (US)
35 Y10 **Virgin River** ≈ Nevada/Utah, W USA
Virihaur see Virihaure
92 H12 **Virihaure** *var.* Virihaur. ⊚ N Sweden
167 T11 **Virôchey** Rôtânôkiri, NE Cambodia
93 N19 **Virolahti** Etelä-Suomi, S Finland
30 J8 **Viroqua** Wisconsin, N USA
112 G8 **Virovitica** *Ger.* Virovititz, *Hung.* Verőcze; *prev. Ger.* Werowitz. Virovitica-Podravina, NE Croatia
112 G8 **Virovitica-Podravina** *off.* Virovitičko-Podravska Županija. ◆ *province* NE Croatia
Virovititz see Virovitica
113 J17 **Virpazar** Montenegro, SW Yugoslavia
93 L17 **Virrat** *Swe.* Virdois. Länsi-Suomi, SW Finland
95 M20 **Virserum** Kalmar, S Sweden
99 K25 **Virton** Luxembourg, SE Belgium
118 F5 **Virtsu** *Ger.* Werder. Läänemaa, W Estonia
56 C12 **Virú** La Libertad, C Peru
Virudhunagar see Virudunagar
155 H23 **Virudunagar** *var.* Virudhunagar. Tamil Nādu, SE India
118 I3 **Viru-Jaagupi** *Ger.* Sankt-Jakobi. Lääne-Virumaa, NE Estonia
57 N19 **Viru-Viru** *var.* Santa Cruz. ✕ (Santa Cruz) Santa Cruz, C Bolivia
113 E15 **Vis** *It.* Lissa; *anc.* Issa. *island* S Croatia
Vis see Fish
118 I12 **Visaginas** *prev.* Sniečkus. Ignalina, E Lithuania
155 M15 **Visākhapatnam** Andhra Pradesh, SE India
35 R11 **Visalia** California, W USA
Višau see Vyškov
95 P19 **Visby** *Ger.* Wisby. Gotland, SE Sweden
197 N9 **Viscount Melville Sound** *prev.* Melville Sound. *sound* Northwest Territories/Nunavut, N Canada
99 L19 **Visé** Liège, E Belgium
112 K13 **Višegrad** Republika Srpska, E Bosnia and Herzegovina
58 L12 **Viseu** Pará, NE Brazil
104 H7 **Viseu** *prev.* Vizeu. Viseu, N Portugal
104 H7 **Viseu** *var.* Vizeu. ◆ *district* N Portugal
116 I8 **Vișeu** *Hung.* Visó; *prev.* Vișău. ≈ NW Romania
116 I8 **Vișeu de Sus** *var.* Vișeul de Sus, *Ger.* Oberwischau, *Hung.* Felsővisó. Maramureș, N Romania
Vișeul de Sus see Vișeu de Sus
127 R10 **Vishera** ≈ NW Russian Federation
95 J19 **Viskafors** Västra Götaland, S Sweden
95 J20 **Viskan** ≈ S Sweden
95 L21 **Vislanda** Kronoberg, S Sweden
Vislinskiy Zaliv see Vistula Lagoon
Visó see Vișeu
112 H13 **Visoko** Federacija Bosna I Hercegovina, C Bosnia and Herzegovina
106 A9 **Viso, Monte** ▲ NW Italy
108 E10 **Visp** Valais, SW Switzerland
108 E10 **Vispa** ≈ S Switzerland
95 M21 **Vissefjärda** Kalmar, S Sweden
100 I11 **Visselhövede** Niedersachsen, NW Germany
95 G23 **Vissenbjerg** Fyn, C Denmark
35 U17 **Vista** California, W USA
58 C11 **Vista Alegre** Amazonas, NW Brazil
114 J13 **Vistonída, Límni** ⊚ NE Greece
Vistula see Wisła
119 A14 **Vistula Lagoon** *Ger.* Frisches Haff, *Pol.* Zalew Wiślany, *Rus.* Vislinskiy Zaliv. *lagoon* Poland/Russian Federation
114 I8 **Vit** ≈ NW Bulgaria
Vitebsk see Vitsyebsk
Vitebskaya Oblast' see Vitsyebskaya Voblasts'
107 H14 **Viterbo** *anc.* Vicus Elbii. Lazio, C Italy
112 H12 **Vitez** Federacija Bosna I Hercegovina, C Bosnia and Herzegovina
167 S14 **Vi Thanh** Cân Thơ, S Vietnam
Viti see Fiji
186 E7 **Vitiaz Strait** *strait* NE PNG
104 J7 **Vitigudino** Castilla-León, N Spain
187 W15 **Viti Levu** *island* W Fiji
123 O11 **Vitim** ≈ C Russian Federation
123 O12 **Vitimskiy** Irkutskaya Oblast', C Russian Federation
109 V2 **Vitis** Niederösterreich, N Austria
Vitoria see Vitoria-Gasteiz
59 O20 **Vitória** Espírito Santo, SE Brazil
Vitoria Bank see Vitória Seamount
59 N18 **Vitória da Conquista** Bahia, E Brazil
105 P3 **Vitoria-Gasteiz** *var.* Vitoria, *Eng.* Vittoria. País Vasco, N Spain
65 J16 **Vitória Seamount** *var.* Victoria Bank, Vitoria Bank. *undersea feature* C Atlantic Ocean
112 F13 **Vitorog** ▲ SW Bosnia and Herzegovina
102 J6 **Vitré** Ille-et-Vilaine, NW France
103 R5 **Vitry-le-François** Marne, N France
114 D13 **Vítsoi** ▲ N Greece
118 N13 **Vitsyebsk** *Rus.* Vitebsk. Vitsyebskaya Voblasts', NE Belarus
118 K13 **Vitsyebskaya Voblasts'** *prev. Rus.* Vitebskaya Oblast'. ◆ *province* N Belarus
92 J11 **Vittangi** Norrbotten, N Sweden
103 R8 **Vitteaux** Côte d'Or, C France
103 S6 **Vittel** Vosges, NE France
95 N15 **Vittinge** Västmanland, C Sweden
107 K25 **Vittoria** Sicilia, Italy, C Mediterranean Sea
Vittoria see Vitoria-Gasteiz
106 I7 **Vittorio Veneto** Veneto, NE Italy
175 Q9 **Vitu Levu** *island* W Fiji
192 L6 **Vityaz Seamount** *undersea feature* C Pacific Ocean
175 Q7 **Vityaz Trench** *undersea feature* W Pacific Ocean
108 G8 **Vitznau** Luzern, W Switzerland
104 I1 **Viveiro** Galicia, NW Spain
105 S9 **Viver** País Valenciano, E Spain
103 Q13 **Viverais, Monts du** ▲ C France
122 L9 **Vivi** ≈ N Russian Federation
22 F4 **Vivian** Louisiana, S USA
29 N10 **Vivian** South Dakota, N USA
103 R13 **Viviers** Ardèche, E France
Vivis see Vevey
83 K19 **Vivo** Northern, NE South Africa
102 L10 **Vivonne** Vienne, W France
Vizakna see Ocna Sibiului
105 O2 **Vizcaya** *Basq.* Bizkaia. ◆ *province* País Vasco, N Spain
Vizcaya, Golfo de see Biscay, Bay of
136 C10 **Vize** Kırklareli, NW Turkey
122 K4 **Vize, Ostrov** *island* Severnaya Zemlya, N Russian Federation
Vizeu see Viseu
155 M15 **Vizianagaram** *var.* Vizianagram. Andhra Pradesh, E India
Vizianagram see Vizianagaram
103 S12 **Vizille** Isère, E France
127 R11 **Vizinga** Respublika Komi, NW Russian Federation
116 M13 **Viziru** Brăila, SE Romania
113 K21 **Vjosës, Lumi i** *var.* Vijosa, Vijosë, *Gk.* Aóos. ≈ Albania/Greece **see also** Aóos
99 H18 **Vlaams Brabant** ◆ *province* C Belgium
Vlaanderen see Flanders
98 G12 **Vlaardingen** Zuid-Holland, SW Netherlands
116 F10 **Vlădeasa, Vârful** *prev.* Vîrful Vlădeasa. ▲ NW Romania
Vlădeasa, Vîrful see Vlădeasa, Vârful
113 P16 **Vladičin Han** Serbia, SE Yugoslavia
129 O16 **Vladikavkaz** *prev.* Dzaudzhikau, Ordzhonikidze. Respublika Severnaya Osetiya, SW Russian Federation
128 M3 **Vladimir** Vladimirskaya Oblast', W Russian Federation
144 M7 **Vladimirovka** Kostanay, N Kazakhstan
Vladimirovka see Yuzhno-Sakhalinsk
128 L3 **Vladimirskaya Oblast'** ◆ *province* W Russian Federation
128 I3 **Vladimirskiy Tupik** Smolenskaya Oblast', W Russian Federation
Vladimir-Volynskiy see Volodymyr-Volyns'kyy
123 Q7 **Vladivostok** Primorskiy Kray, SE Russian Federation
117 U13 **Vladyslavivka** Respublika Krym, S Ukraine
98 P6 **Vlagtwedde** Groningen, NE Netherlands
Vlajna see Kukavica
112 J12 **Vlasenica** Republika Srpska, E Bosnia and Herzegovina
112 G12 **Vlašić** ▲ C Bosnia and Herzegovina
111 D17 **Vlašim** *Ger.* Wlaschim. Středočeský Kraj, C Czech Republic
113 P15 **Vlasotince** Serbia, SE Yugoslavia
123 Q7 **Vlasovo** Respublika Sakha (Yakutiya), NE Russian Federation
98 I11 **Vleuten** Utrecht, C Netherlands
98 I5 **Vlieland** *Fris.* Flylân. *island* Waddeneilanden, N Netherlands
98 I5 **Vliestroom** *strait* NW Netherlands
99 J14 **Vlijmen** Noord-Brabant, S Netherlands
99 E15 **Vlissingen** *Eng.* Flushing, *Fr.* Flessingue. Zeeland, SW Netherlands
Vlodava see Włodawa
Vlonë/Vlora see Vlorë
113 K22 **Vlorë** *prev.* Vlonë, *It.* Valona, Vlora. Vlorë, SW Albania
113 K22 **Vlorë** ◆ *district* SW Albania
113 K22 **Vlorës, Gjiri i** *var.* Valona Bay. *bay* SW Albania
Vlotslavsk see Włocławek
111 C16 **Vltava** *Ger.* Moldau. ≈ W Czech Republic
128 K3 **Vnukovo** ✕ (Moskva) Gorod Moskva, W Russian Federation
25 Q9 **Voca** Texas, SW USA
109 R5 **Vöcklabruck** Oberösterreich, NW Austria
112 D13 **Vodice** Šibenik-Knin, S Croatia
126 K10 **Vodlozero, Ozero** ⊚ NW Russian Federation
112 A10 **Vodnjan** *It.* Dignano d'Istria. Istra, NW Croatia
127 S9 **Vodnyy** Respublika Komi, NW Russian Federation
95 G20 **Vodskov** Nordjylland, N Denmark
92 H4 **Vogar** Sudhurland, SW Iceland
Vogelkop see Doberai, Jazirah
77 X15 **Vogel Peak** *prev.* Dim lang. ▲ E Nigeria
101 H17 **Vogelsberg** ▲ C Germany
106 D8 **Voghera** Lombardia, N Italy
112 I13 **Vogošća** Federacija Bosna I Hercegovina, SE Bosnia and Herzegovina
101 M17 **Vogtland** *historical region* E Germany
127 V12 **Vogul'skiy Kamen', Gora** ▲ NW Russian Federation
187 P16 **Voh** Province Nord, C New Caledonia
Vohémar see Iharaña
172 H8 **Vohimena, Tanjona** *Fr.* Cap Sainte Marie. *headland* S Madagascar
172 J6 **Vohipeno** Fianarantsoa, SE Madagascar
118 H5 **Võhma** *Ger.* Wöchma. Viljandimaa, S Estonia
81 J20 **Voi** Coast, S Kenya
76 K15 **Voinjama** N Liberia
103 S12 **Voiron** Isère, E France
109 V8 **Voitsberg** Steiermark, SE Austria
95 F24 **Vojens** *Ger.* Woyens. Sønderjylland, SW Denmark
112 K9 **Vojvodina** *Ger.* Wojwodina. *Region* N Yugoslavia
15 S6 **Volant** ≈ Quebec, SE Canada
Volaterrae see Volterra
43 P15 **Volcán** *var.* Hato del Volcán. Chiriquí, W Panama
Volchansk see Vovchans'k
Volchya see Vovcha
94 D10 **Volda** Møre og Romsdal, S Norway
98 J9 **Volendam** Noord-Holland, C Netherlands
126 L15 **Volga** Yaroslavskaya Oblast', W Russian Federation
29 R10 **Volga** South Dakota, N USA
122 C11 **Volga** ≈ NW Russian Federation
Volga-Baltic Waterway see Volgo-Baltiyskiy Kanal
Volga Hills/Volga Uplands see Privolzhskaya Vozvyshennost'
126 L13 **Volgo-Baltiyskiy Kanal** *Eng.* Volga-Baltic Waterway. *canal* NW Russian Federation
128 M12 **Volgodonsk** Rostovskaya Oblast', SW Russian Federation
129 O10 **Volgograd** *prev.* Stalingrad, Tsaritsyn. Volgogradskaya Oblast', SW Russian Federation
129 N9 **Volgogradskaya Oblast'** ◆ *province* SW Russian Federation
129 P10 **Volgogradskoye Vodokhranilishche** ⊟ SW Russian Federation
101 J19 **Volkach** Bayern, C Germany
109 U9 **Völkermarkt** *Slvn.* Velikovec. Kärnten, S Austria
126 I12 **Volkhov** Leningradskaya Oblast', NW Russian Federation
101 D20 **Völklingen** Saarland, SW Germany
Volkovysk see Vawkavysk
Volkovyskiye Vysoty see Vawkavyskaye Wzvyshsha
83 K22 **Volksrust** Mpumalanga, E South Africa
98 L8 **Vollenhove** Overijssel, N Netherlands
119 L16 **Vol'ma** *Rus.* Volma. ≈ C Belarus
Volmari see Valmiera
117 W9 **Volnovakha** Donets'ka Oblast', SE Ukraine
116 K6 **Volochys'k** Khmel'nyts'ka Oblast', W Ukraine
117 O6 **Volodarka** Kyyivs'ka Oblast', N Ukraine
117 W9 **Volodars'ke** Donets'ka Oblast', E Ukraine
129 R13 **Volodarskiy** Astrakhanskaya Oblast', SW Russian Federation
Volodarskoye see Saumalkol'
117 N8 **Volodars'k-Volyns'kyy** Zhytomyrs'ka Oblast', N Ukraine
116 K3 **Volodymerets'** Rivnens'ka Oblast', NW Ukraine
116 I3 **Volodymyr-Volyns'kyy** *Pol.* Włodzimierz, *Rus.* Vladimir-Volynskiy. Volyns'ka Oblast', NW Ukraine
126 L14 **Vologda** Vologodskaya Oblast', W Russian Federation
126 L12 **Vologodskaya Oblast'** ◆ *province* NW Russian Federation
128 K3 **Volokolamsk** Moskovskaya Oblast', W Russian Federation
128 K9 **Volokonovka** Belgorodskaya Oblast', W Russian Federation
115 G16 **Vólos** Thessalía, C Greece
126 M11 **Voloshka** Arkhangel'skaya Oblast', NW Russian Federation
Vološinovo see Novi Bečej
116 H7 **Volovets'** Zakarpats'ka Oblast', W Ukraine
114 K7 **Volovo** Ruse, N Bulgaria
Volozhin see Valozhyn
129 Q7 **Vol'sk** Saratovskaya Oblast', W Russian Federation
77 Q17 **Volta** ≈ SE Ghana
Volta Blanche see White Volta
77 P16 **Volta, Lake** ⊟ SE Ghana
Volta Noire see Black Volta
60 O9 **Volta Redonda** Rio de Janeiro, SE Brazil
Volta Rouge see Red Volta
106 F12 **Volterra** *anc.* Volaterrae. Toscana, C Italy
107 K17 **Volturno** ≈ S Italy
113 I15 **Volujak** ▲ SW Yugoslavia
Volunteer Island see Starbuck Island
65 F24 **Volunteer Point** *headland* East Falkland, Falkland Islands
Volunteer State see Tennessee
114 H13 **Vólvi, Límni** ⊚ N Greece
Volyn see Volyns'ka Oblast'
116 I3 **Volyns'ka Oblast'** *var.* Volyn, *Rus.* Volynskaya Oblast'. ◆ *province* NW Ukraine
Volynskaya Oblast' see Volyns'ka Oblast'
129 Q3 **Volzhsk** Respublika Mariy El, W Russian Federation
129 O10 **Volzhskiy** Volgogradskaya Oblast', SW Russian Federation
172 I7 **Vondrozo** Fianarantsoa, SE Madagascar
114 K9 **Voneshta Voda** Veliko Tŭrnovo, N Bulgaria
39 P10 **Von Frank Mountain** ▲ Alaska, USA
115 C17 **Vónitsa** Dytikí Ellás, W Greece
118 J6 **Võnnu** *Ger.* Wendau. Tartumaa, SE Estonia
98 G12 **Voorburg** Zuid-Holland, W Netherlands
98 H11 **Voorschoten** Zuid-Holland, W Netherlands
98 M11 **Voorst** Gelderland, E Netherlands
98 K11 **Voorthuizen** Gelderland, C Netherlands

◆ Country ● Country Capital ◇ Dependent Territory ○ Dependent Territory Capital ◆ Administrative Region ✕ International Airport ▲ Mountain ▲ Mountain Range ☗ Volcano ≈ River ⊚ Lake ⊟ Reservoir

92 L2 **Vopnafjördhur** Austurland, E Iceland
92 L2 **Vopnafjördhur** bay E Iceland
Vora see Vorë
119 H15 **Voranava** Pol. Werenów, Rus. Voronovo. Hrodzyenskaya Voblasts', W Belarus
108 I8 **Vorarlberg** off. Land Vorarlberg. ◆ state W Austria
109 X7 **Vorau** Steiermark, E Austria
98 N11 **Vorden** Gelderland, E Netherlands
108 H9 **Vorderrhein** ≈ SE Switzerland
92 J2 **Vordhufell** ▲ N Iceland
95 I24 **Vordingborg** Storstrøm, SE Denmark
113 K19 **Vorë** var. Vora. Tiranë, W Albania
115 H17 **Vóreioi Sporádes** var. Vórioi Sporádhes, Eng. Northern Sporades. island group E Greece
115 J17 **Vóreion Aigaíon** Eng. Aegean North. ◆ region SE Greece
115 G18 **Voreiós Evvoïkós Kólpos** gulf E Greece
197 S16 **Voring Plateau** undersea feature N Norwegian Sea
Vórioi Sporádhes see Vóreioi Sporádes
127 W4 **Vorkuta** Respublika Komi, NW Russian Federation
95 I14 **Vorma** ≈ S Norway
118 E4 **Vormsi** var. Vormsi Saar, Ger. Worms, Swed. Ormsö. island W Estonia
Vormsi Saar see Vormsi
129 N7 **Vorona** ≈ W Russian Federation
128 L7 **Voronezh** Voronezhskaya Oblast', W Russian Federation
128 L7 **Voronezh** ≈ W Russian Federation
128 K8 **Voronezhskaya Oblast'** ◆ province W Russian Federation
Voronovitsya see Voronovytsya
Voronovo see Voranava
117 N6 **Voronovytsya** Rus. Voronovitsya. Vinnyts'ka Oblast', C Ukraine
122 K7 **Vorontsovo** Taymyrskiy (Dolgano-Nenetskiy) Avtonomnyy Okrug, N Russian Federation
126 K3 **Voron'ya** ≈ NW Russian Federation
Voropayevo see Varapayeva
Voroshilov see Ussuriysk
Voroshilovgrad see Luhans'k, Ukraine
Voroshilovgrad see Luhans'ka Oblast', Ukraine
Voroshilovgradskaya Oblast' see Luhans'ka Oblast'
Voroshilovsk see Stavropol', Russian Federation
Voroshilovsk see Alchevs'k, Ukraine
137 V13 **Vorotan** Az. Bärgușad. ≈ Armenia/Azerbaijan
129 P3 **Vorotynets** Nizhegorodskaya Oblast', W Russian Federation
117 S3 **Vorozhba** Sums'ka Oblast', NE Ukraine
117 T5 **Vorskla** ≈ Russian Federation/Ukraine
99 I17 **Vorst** Antwerpen, N Belgium
83 G21 **Vorstershoop** North-West, N South Africa
118 H6 **Võrtsjärv** Ger. Wirz-See. ◎ SE Estonia
118 J7 **Võru** Ger. Werro. Võrumaa, SE Estonia
147 R11 **Vorukh** N Tajikistan
118 I7 **Võrumaa** off. Võru Maakond. ◆ province SE Estonia
83 G24 **Vosburg** Northern Cape, W South Africa
147 Q14 **Vose'** Rus. Vose; prev. Aral. SW Tajikistan
103 S6 **Vosges** ◆ department NE France
103 U6 **Vosges** ▲ NE France
126 K13 **Voskresenkoye** Vologodskaya Oblast', NW Russian Federation
128 L4 **Voskresensk** Moskovskaya Oblast', W Russian Federation
129 P2 **Voskresenskoye** Nizhegorodskaya Oblast', W Russian Federation
129 V6 **Voskresenskoye** Respublika Bashkortostan, W Russian Federation
94 D13 **Voss** Hordaland, S Norway
94 D13 **Voss** physical region S Norway
99 I16 **Vosselaar** Antwerpen, N Belgium
94 D13 **Vosso** ≈ S Norway
Vostochno-Kazakhstanskaya Oblast' see Shygys Konyrat
145 T12 **Vostochno-Kounradskiy** Kaz. Shyghys Qongyrat. Zhezkazgan, C Kazakhstan
123 S5 **Vostochno-Sibirskoye More** Eng. East Siberian Sea. sea Arctic Ocean
145 X10 **Vostochnyy Kazakhstan** off. Vostochno-Kazakhstanskaya Oblast', var. East Kazakhstan, Kaz. Shyghys Qazagastan Oblysy. ◆ province E Kazakhstan
Vostochnyy Sayan see Eastern Sayans
Vostock Island see Vostok Island
195 U10 **Vostok** Russian research station Antarctica
191 X5 **Vostok Island** var. Vostock Island; prev. Stavers Island. island Line Islands, SE Kiribati
129 T2 **Votkinsk** Udmurtskaya Respublika, NW Russian Federation
127 U15 **Votkinskoye Vodokhranilishche** var. Votkinsk Reservoir. ▣ NW Russian Federation
Votkinsk Reservoir see Votkinskoye Vodokhranilishche
60 J7 **Votuporanga** São Paulo, S Brazil
104 H7 **Vouga, Rio** ≈ N Portugal
115 E14 **Voúrinos** ▲ N Greece
115 G24 **Voúxa, Akrotírio** headland Kríti, Greece, E Mediterranean Sea
103 R4 **Vouziers** Ardennes, N France
117 V7 **Vovcha** Rus. Volchya. ≈ E Ukraine
117 V4 **Vovchans'k** Rus. Volchansk. Kharkivs'ka Oblast', E Ukraine
103 N6 **Voves** Eure-et-Loir, C France
79 M14 **Vovodo** ≈ S Central Africa Republic
94 M12 **Voxna** Gävleborg, C Sweden
94 L11 **Voxnan** ≈ C Sweden
114 F7 **Voynishka Reka** ≈ NW Bulgaria
127 T9 **Voyvozh** Respublika Komi, NW Russian Federation
126 M12 **Vozhega** Vologodskaya Oblast', NW Russian Federation
126 L12 **Vozhe, Ozero** ◎ NW Russian Federation
117 Q9 **Voznesens'k** Rus. Voznesensk. Mykolayivs'ka Oblast', S Ukraine
126 J12 **Voznesen'ye** Leningradskaya Oblast', NW Russian Federation
144 J14 **Vozrozhdeniya, Ostrov** Uzb. Wozrojdeniye Oroli. island Kazakhstan/Uzbekistan
95 G20 **Vrå** var. Vraa. Nordjylland, N Denmark
Vraa see Vrå
114 H9 **Vrachesh** Sofiya, NW Bulgaria
115 C19 **Vrachíonas** ▲ Zákynthos, Iónioi Nísoi, Greece, C Mediterranean Sea
117 P8 **Vradiyivka** Mykolayivs'ka Oblast', S Ukraine
113 G14 **Vran** ▲ SW Bosnia and Herzegovina
116 K12 **Vrancea** ◆ county E Romania
147 T14 **Vrang** SE Tajikistan
123 T4 **Vrangelya, Ostrov** Eng. Wrangel Island. island NE Russian Federation
112 H13 **Vranica** ▲ C Bosnia and Herzegovina
113 O16 **Vranje** Serbia, SE Yugoslavia
Vranov see Vranov nad Topl'ou
111 N19 **Vranov nad Topl'ou** var. Vranov, Hung. Varannó. Prešovský Kraj, E Slovakia
114 H8 **Vratsa** Vratsa, NW Bulgaria
114 H8 **Vratsa** ◆ province NW Bulgaria
114 F10 **Vrattsa** prev. Mirovo. Kyustendil, W Bulgaria
112 G11 **Vrbanja** ≈ NW Bosnia and Herzegovina
112 K9 **Vrbas** Serbia, NW Yugoslavia
112 G13 **Vrbas** ≈ N Bosnia and Herzegovina
112 E8 **Vrbovec** Zagreb, N Croatia
112 C9 **Vrbovsko** Primorje-Gorski Kotar, NW Croatia
111 E15 **Vrchlabí** Ger. Hohenelbe. Hradecký Kraj, NE Czech Republic
83 J22 **Vrede** Free State, E South Africa
100 E13 **Vreden** Nordrhein-Westfalen, NW Germany
83 E25 **Vredenburg** Western Cape, SW South Africa
99 I23 **Vresse-sur-Semois** Namur, SE Belgium
95 L16 **Vretstorp** Örebro, C Sweden
113 G15 **Vrgorac** prev. Vrhgorac. Split-Dalmacija, SE Croatia
Vrhgorac see Vrgorac
109 T12 **Vrhnika** Ger. Oberlaibach. W Slovenia
155 I21 **Vriddhāchalam** Tamil Nādu, SE India
98 N6 **Vries** Drenthe, NE Netherlands
98 O10 **Vriezenveen** Overijssel, E Netherlands
95 L20 **Vrigstad** Jönköping, S Sweden
108 H9 **Vrin** Graubünden, S Switzerland
112 E13 **Vrlika** Split-Dalmacija, S Croatia
113 M14 **Vrnjačka Banja** Serbia, C Yugoslavia
Vrondádhes/Vrondados see Vrontádos
115 L18 **Vrontádos** var. Vrondados; prev. Vrondádhes. Chíos, E Greece
98 N9 **Vroomshoop** Overijssel, E Netherlands
112 N10 **Vršac** Ger. Werschetz, Hung. Versecz. Serbia, NE Yugoslavia
112 M10 **Vršački Kanal** canal N Yugoslavia
83 H21 **Vryburg** North-West, N South Africa
83 K22 **Vryheid** KwaZulu/Natal, E South Africa
111 I18 **Vsetín** Ger. Wsetin. Zlínský Kraj, E Czech Republic
111 J20 **Vtáčnik** Hung. Madaras, Ptacsnik; prev. Ptačník. ▲ W Slovakia
Vuadil' see Wodil
Vuanggava see Vuaqava
114 I11 **Vúcha** ≈ SW Bulgaria
113 N16 **Vučitrn** Serbia, S Yugoslavia
99 J14 **Vught** Noord-Brabant, S Netherlands
117 W8 **Vuhledar** Donets'ka Oblast', E Ukraine
112 I9 **Vuka** ≈ E Croatia
113 K17 **Vukël** var. Vukli. Shkodër, N Albania
Vukli see Vukël
112 J9 **Vukovar** Hung. Vukovár. Vukovar-Srijem, E Croatia
112 I10 **Vukovar-Srijem** off. Vukovarsko-Srijemska Županija. ◆ province E Croatia
127 U8 **Vuktyl** Respublika Komi, NW Russian Federation
11 Q17 **Vulcan** Alberta, SW Canada
116 G12 **Vulcan** Ger. Wulkan, Hung. Zsilyvajdevulkán; prev. Crivadia Vulcanului, Vaidei, Hung. Sily-Vajdej, Vajdej. Hunedoara, W Romania
116 M12 **Vulcănești** Rus. Vulkaneshty. S Moldova
107 L22 **Vulcano, Isola** island Isole Eolie, S Italy
114 G7 **Vŭlchedrŭm** Montana, NW Bulgaria
114 N8 **Vŭlchidol** prev. Kurt-Dere. Varna, NE Bulgaria
Vulkaneshty see Vulcănești
36 J13 **Vulture Mountains** ▲ Arizona, SW USA
167 T14 **Vung Tau** prev. Fr. Cape Saint Jacques, Cap Saint-Jacques. Ba Ria-Vung Tau, S Vietnam
187 X15 **Vunisea** Kadavu, SE Fiji
Vuohčču see Vuotso
93 N15 **Vuokatti** Oulu, C Finland
93 M15 **Vuolijoki** Oulu, C Finland
92 J13 **Vuollerim** Norrbotten, N Sweden
Vuoreija see Vardø
92 L10 **Vuotso** Lapp. Vuohčču. Lappi, N Finland
114 J11 **Vŭrbitsa** prev. Filevo. Khaskovo, S Bulgaria
114 J12 **Vŭrbitsa** ≈ S Bulgaria
129 Q4 **Vurnary** Chuvashskaya Respublika, W Russian Federation
114 G8 **Vŭrshets** Montana, NW Bulgaria
119 F17 **Vyalikaya Byerastavitsa** Pol. Brzostowica Wielka, Rus. Bol'shaya Berëstovitsa; prev. Velikaya Berestovitsa. Hrodzyenskaya Voblasts', SW Belarus
119 N20 **Vyaliki Bor** Rus. Velikiy Bor. Homyel'skaya Voblasts', SE Belarus
119 J18 **Vyaliki Rozhan** Rus. Bol'shoy Rozhan. Minskaya Voblasts', S Belarus
126 H10 **Vyartsilya** Fin. Värtsilä. Respublika Kareliya, NW Russian Federation
119 K17 **Vyasyeya** Rus. Veseya. Minskaya Voblasts', C Belarus
127 R15 **Vyatka** ≈ NW Russian Federation
Vyatka see Kirov
127 S16 **Vyatskiye Polyany** Kirovskaya Oblast', NW Russian Federation
123 S14 **Vyazemskiy** Khabarovskiy Kray, SE Russian Federation
128 I4 **Vyaz'ma** Smolenskaya Oblast', W Russian Federation
129 N3 **Vyazniki** Vladimirskaya Oblast', W Russian Federation
129 O8 **Vyazovka** Volgogradskaya Oblast', SW Russian Federation
119 J14 **Vyazyn'** Rus. Vyazyn'. Minskaya Voblasts', NW Belarus
126 G11 **Vyborg** Fin. Viipuri. Leningradskaya Oblast', NW Russian Federation
127 P11 **Vychegda** var. Vichegda. ≈ NW Russian Federation
119 L14 **Vyelyewshchyna** Rus. Velevshchina. Vitsyebskaya Voblasts', N Belarus
119 P16 **Vyeramyeyki** Rus. Veremeyki. Mahilyowskaya Voblasts', E Belarus
118 K11 **Vyerkhnyadzvinsk** Rus. Verkhnedvinsk. Vitsyebskaya Voblasts', N Belarus
119 P18 **Vyetka** Rus. Vetka. Homyel'skaya Voblasts', SE Belarus
118 L12 **Vyetryna** Rus. Vetrino. Vitsyebskaya Voblasts', N Belarus
Vygonovskoye, Ozero see Vyhanawskaye, Vozyera
126 J9 **Vygozero, Ozero** ◎ NW Russian Federation
Vyhanashchanskaye Vozyera see Vyhanawskaye, Vozyera
119 I18 **Vyhanawskaye, Vozyera** var. Vyhanashchanskaye Vozyera, Rus. Ozero Vygonovskoye. ◎ SW Belarus
129 N4 **Vyksa** Nizhegorodskaya Oblast', W Russian Federation
117 O12 **Vylkove** Rus. Vilkovo. Odes'ka Oblast', SW Ukraine
127 R9 **Vym'** ≈ NW Russian Federation
116 H8 **Vynohradiv** Cz. Sevluš, Hung. Nagyszőllős, Rus. Vinogradov; prev. Sevlyush. Zakarpats'ka Oblast', W Ukraine
126 G13 **Vyritsa** Leningradskaya Oblast', NW Russian Federation
97 J19 **Vyrnwy** Wel. Afon Efyrnwy. ≈ E Wales, UK
145 X9 **Vyshe Ivanovskiy Belak, Gora** ▲ E Kazakhstan
117 P4 **Vyshhorod** Kyyivs'ka Oblast', N Ukraine
126 I15 **Vyshniy Volochek** Tverskaya Oblast', W Russian Federation
111 G18 **Vyškov** Ger. Wischau. Brněnský Kraz, SE Czech Republic
111 F17 **Vysoké Mýto** Ger. Hohenmauth. Pardubický Kraj, C Czech Republic
117 S9 **Vysokopillya** Khersons'ka Oblast', S Ukraine
128 K3 **Vysokovsk** Moskovskaya Oblast', W Russian Federation
126 K12 **Vytegra** Vologodskaya Oblast', NW Russian Federation
116 J8 **Vyzhnytsya** Chernivets'ka Oblast', W Ukraine

W

77 O14 **Wa** NW Ghana
Waadt see Vaud
Waag see Váh
Waagbistritz see Považská Bystrica
Waagneustadtl see Nové Mesto nad Váhom
81 M16 **Waajid** Gedo, SW Somalia
98 L13 **Waal** ≈ S Netherlands
187 O16 **Waala** Province Nord, W New Caledonia
99 I14 **Waalwijk** Noord-Brabant, S Netherlands
99 E16 **Waarschoot** Oost-Vlaanderen, NW Belgium
186 C7 **Wabag** Enga, W PNG
15 N7 **Wabano** ≈ Quebec, SE Canada
11 P11 **Wabasca** ≈ Alberta, SW Canada
31 P12 **Wabash** Indiana, N USA
29 X9 **Wabasha** Minnesota, N USA
31 N13 **Wabash River** ≈ N USA
14 C7 **Wabatongushi Lake** ◎ Ontario, S Canada
81 L15 **Wabē Gestro Wenz** ≈ SE Ethiopia
14 B9 **Wabos** Ontario, S Canada
11 W13 **Wabowden** Manitoba, C Canada
110 J9 **Wąbrzeźno** Kujawsko-pomorskie, N Poland
21 U12 **Waccamaw River** ≈ South Carolina, SE USA
23 U11 **Waccasassa Bay** bay Florida, SE USA
99 F16 **Wachtebeke** Oost-Vlaanderen, NW Belgium
25 T8 **Waco** Texas, SW USA
26 M3 **Waconda Lake** var. Great Elder Reservoir. ▣ Kansas, C USA
Wadai see Ouaddaï
Wad Al-Hajarah see Guadalajara
164 I12 **Wadayama** Hyōgo, Honshū, SW Japan
80 D10 **Wad Banda** Western Kordofan, C Sudan
75 P9 **Waddān** NW Libya
98 J4 **Waddeneilanden** Eng. West Frisian Islands. island group N Netherlands
98 J6 **Waddenzee** var. Wadden Zee. sea SE North Sea
10 L16 **Waddington, Mount** ▲ British Columbia, SW Canada
98 H12 **Waddinxveen** Zuid-Holland, C Netherlands
11 U15 **Wadena** Saskatchewan, S Canada
29 T6 **Wadena** Minnesota, N USA
108 G7 **Wädenswil** Zürich, N Switzerland
21 S11 **Wadesboro** North Carolina, SE USA
155 G16 **Wādi** Karnātaka, C India
138 G10 **Wādī as Sīr** var. Wadi es Sir. 'Ammān, NW Jordan
Wadi es Sir see Wādī as Sīr
80 F5 **Wadi Halfa** var. Wādī Ḥalfā'. Northern, N Sudan
138 G13 **Wādī Mūsā** var. Petra. Ma'ān, S Jordan
23 V4 **Wadley** Georgia, SE USA
Wad Madanī see Wad Medani
80 G10 **Wad Medani** var. Wad Madanī. Gezira, C Sudan
80 F10 **Wad Nimr** White Nile, C Sudan
165 U16 **Wadomari** Kagoshima, Okinoerabu-jima, SW Japan
111 K17 **Wadowice** Małopolskie, S Poland
35 R5 **Wadsworth** Nevada, W USA
31 T12 **Wadsworth** Ohio, N USA
25 T11 **Waelder** Texas, SW USA
Waereghem see Waregem
163 U13 **Wafangdian** var. Fuxian, Fu Xian. Liaoning, NE China
171 R13 **Waflia** Pulau Buru, E Indonesia
Wagadugu see Ouagadougou
98 K12 **Wageningen** Gelderland, SE Netherlands
55 V9 **Wageningen** Nickerie, NW Suriname
9 O8 **Wager Bay** inlet Nunavut, N Canada
183 P10 **Wagga Wagga** New South Wales, SE Australia
180 J13 **Wagin** Western Australia
108 H8 **Wägitaler See** ◎ SW Switzerland
29 P12 **Wagner** South Dakota, N USA
27 Q9 **Wagoner** Oklahoma, C USA
37 U10 **Wagon Mound** New Mexico, SW USA
32 J14 **Wagontire** Oregon, NW USA
110 H10 **Wągrowiec** Wielkopolskie, NW Poland
149 U6 **Wāh** Punjab, NE Pakistan
171 S13 **Wahai** Pulau Seram, E Indonesia
169 V10 **Wahau, Sungai** ≈ Borneo, C Indonesia
Wahaybah, Ramlat Al see Wahībah, Ramlat Āl
80 D13 **Wahda** var. Unity State. ◆ state S Sudan
38 D9 **Wahiawa** Haw. Wahiawā. Oahu, Hawaii, USA, C Pacific Ocean
Wahībah, Ramlat Ahl see Wahībah, Ramlat Āl
141 Y9 **Wahībah, Ramlat Āl** var. Ramlat Ahl Wahībah, Ramlat Al Wahaybah, Eng. Wahibah Sands. desert N Oman
Wahibah Sands see Wahībah, Ramlat Āl
101 E16 **Wahn** ✕ (Köln) Nordrhein-Westfalen, W Germany
29 R15 **Wahoo** Nebraska, C USA
29 R6 **Wahpeton** North Dakota, N USA
Wahran see Oran
36 J6 **Wah Wah Mountains** ▲ Utah, W USA
38 D9 **Waialua** Oahu, Hawaii, USA, C Pacific Ocean
38 D9 **Waianae** Haw. Wai'anae. Oahu, Hawaii, USA, C Pacific Ocean
184 Q8 **Waiapu** ≈ North Island, NZ
185 I17 **Waiau** Canterbury, South Island, NZ
185 I17 **Waiau** ≈ South Island, NZ
185 B23 **Waiau** ≈ South Island, NZ
101 H21 **Waiblingen** Baden-Württemberg, S Germany
Waidhofen see Waidhofen an der Ybbs, Niederösterreich, Austria
Waidhofen see Waidhofen an der Thaya, Niederösterreich, Austria
109 V2 **Waidhofen an der Thaya** var. Waidhofen. Niederösterreich, NE Austria
109 U5 **Waidhofen an der Ybbs** var. Waidhofen. Niederösterreich, E Austria
171 T11 **Waigeo, Pulau** island Maluku, E Indonesia
184 L5 **Waiheke Island** island N NZ
184 M7 **Waihi** Waikato, North Island, NZ
185 C20 **Waihou** ≈ North Island, NZ
Waikaboebak see Waikabubak
170 M17 **Waikabubak** prev. Waikaboebak. Pulau Sumba, C Indonesia
185 D23 **Waikaia** ≈ South Island, NZ
185 D23 **Waikaka** Southland, South Island, NZ
184 L13 **Waikanae** Wellington, North Island, NZ
184 M7 **Waikare, Lake** ◎ North Island, NZ
184 O9 **Waikaremoana, Lake** ◎ North Island, NZ
185 I17 **Waikari** Canterbury, South Island, NZ
184 L8 **Waikato** off. Waikato Region. ◆ region North Island, NZ
184 M8 **Waikato** ≈ North Island, NZ
182 J9 **Waikerie** South Australia
185 F23 **Waikouaiti** Otago, South Island, NZ
38 H11 **Wailea** Hawaii, USA, C Pacific Ocean
38 F10 **Wailuku** Maui, Hawaii, USA, C Pacific Ocean
185 H18 **Waimakariri** ≈ South Island, NZ
38 D9 **Waimanalo Beach** Oahu, Hawaii, USA, C Pacific Ocean
185 G15 **Waimangaroa** West Coast, South Island, NZ
185 G21 **Waimate** Canterbury, South Island, NZ
38 G11 **Waimea** var. Kamuela. Hawaii, USA, C Pacific Ocean
38 D9 **Waimea** var. Maunawai. Oahu, Hawaii, USA, C Pacific Ocean
38 B8 **Waimea** Kauai, Hawaii, USA, C Pacific Ocean
99 M20 **Waimes** Liège, E Belgium
154 J11 **Wainganga** var. Wain River. ≈ C India
Waingapoe see Waingapu
171 N17 **Waingapu** prev. Waingapoe. Pulau Sumba, C Indonesia
55 S7 **Waini** ≈ N Guyana
55 S7 **Waini Point** headland NW Guyana
Wain River see Wainganga
11 R15 **Wainwright** Alberta, SW Canada
39 O5 **Wainwright** Alaska, USA
184 K4 **Waiotira** Northland, North Island, NZ
184 M11 **Waiouru** Manawatu-Wanganui, North Island, NZ
171 W14 **Waipa** Irian Jaya, E Indonesia
184 L8 **Waipa** ≈ North Island, NZ
184 P9 **Waipaoa** ≈ North Island, NZ
185 D25 **Waipapa Point** headland South Island, NZ
185 I18 **Waipara** Canterbury, South Island, NZ
184 N12 **Waipawa** Hawke's Bay, North Island, NZ
184 K4 **Waipu** Northland, North Island, NZ
184 N12 **Waipukurau** Hawke's Bay, North Island, NZ
171 U14 **Wair** Pulau Kai Besar, E Indonesia
Wairakai see Wairakei
184 N9 **Wairakei** var. Wairakai. Waikato, North Island, NZ
185 M14 **Wairarapa, Lake** ◎ North Island, NZ
185 J15 **Wairau** ≈ South Island, NZ
184 P10 **Wairoa** Hawke's Bay, North Island, NZ
184 P10 **Wairoa** ≈ North Island, NZ
184 J4 **Wairoa** ≈ North Island, NZ
184 N9 **Waitahanui** Waikato, North Island, NZ
184 M6 **Waitakaruru** Waikato, North Island, NZ
185 F21 **Waitaki** ≈ South Island, NZ
184 K10 **Waitara** Taranaki, North Island, NZ
184 M7 **Waitoa** Waikato, North Island, NZ
184 L8 **Waitomo Caves** Waikato, North Island, NZ
184 L11 **Waitotara** Taranaki, North Island, NZ
184 L11 **Waitotara** ≈ North Island, NZ
32 L10 **Waitsburg** Washington, NW USA
Waitzen see Vác
184 L6 **Waiuku** Auckland, North Island, NZ
164 L10 **Wajima** var. Wazima. Ishikawa, Honshū, SW Japan
81 K17 **Wajir** North Eastern, NE Kenya
81 I14 **Waka** Southern, SW Ethiopia
79 J17 **Waka** Equateur, NW Dem. Rep. Congo (Zaire)
14 D9 **Wakami Lake** ◎ Ontario, S Canada
164 I12 **Wakasa** Tottori, Honshū, SW Japan
164 J12 **Wakasa-wan** bay C Japan
185 C22 **Wakatipu, Lake** ◎ South Island, NZ
11 T15 **Wakaw** Saskatchewan, S Canada
164 I14 **Wakayama** Wakayama, Honshū, SW Japan
164 I15 **Wakayama** off. Wakayama-ken. ◆ prefecture Honshū, SW Japan
26 K4 **Wa Keeney** Kansas, C USA
185 I14 **Wakefield** Tasman, South Island, NZ
97 M17 **Wakefield** N England, UK
27 O4 **Wakefield** Kansas, C USA
30 L4 **Wakefield** Michigan, N USA
21 U9 **Wake Forest** North Carolina, SE USA
Wakeham Bay see Kangiqsujuaq
189 Y11 **Wake Island** ◇ US unincorporated territory NW Pacific Ocean
189 Y12 **Wake Island** ✕ NW Pacific Ocean
189 Y12 **Wake Island** atoll NW Pacific Ocean
189 X12 **Wake Lagoon** lagoon Wake Island, NW Pacific Ocean
166 L8 **Wakema** Irrawaddy, SW Burma
Wakhan see Khandūd
164 H14 **Waki** Tokushima, Shikoku, SW Japan
165 T1 **Wakkanai** Hokkaidō, NE Japan
83 K22 **Wakkerstroom** Mpumalanga, E South Africa
14 C10 **Wakomata Lake** ◎ Ontario, S Canada
183 N10 **Wakool** New South Wales, SE Australia
Wakra see Al Wakrah
Waku Kungo see Uaco Cungo
186 J7 **Wakunai** Bougainville Island, NE PNG
Walachei/Walachia see Wallachia
155 K26 **Walawe Ganga** ≈ S Sri Lanka
111 F15 **Wałbrzych** Ger. Waldenburg, Waldenburg in Schlesien. Dolnośląskie, SW Poland
183 T6 **Walcha** New South Wales, SE Australia
101 K24 **Walchensee** ◎ SE Germany
99 D14 **Walcheren** island SW Netherlands
29 Z14 **Walcott** Iowa, C USA
33 W16 **Walcott** Wyoming, C USA
99 G21 **Walcourt** Namur, S Belgium
110 G9 **Wałcz** Ger. Deutsch Krone. Zachodniopomorskie, NW Poland
108 H7 **Wald** Zürich, N Switzerland
109 U3 **Waldaist** ≈ N Austria
180 I9 **Waldburg Range** ▲ Western Australia
37 R3 **Walden** Colorado, C USA
18 K13 **Walden** New York, NE USA
Waldenburg/Waldenburg in Schlesien see Wałbrzych
11 T15 **Waldheim** Saskatchewan, S Canada
Waldia see Weldiya
101 M23 **Waldkraiburg** Bayern, SE Germany
27 T14 **Waldo** Arkansas, C USA
23 V9 **Waldo** Florida, SE USA
19 R7 **Waldoboro** Maine, NE USA
21 W4 **Waldorf** Maryland, NE USA
32 F12 **Waldport** Oregon, NW USA
27 S11 **Waldron** Arkansas, C USA
195 Y13 **Waldron, Cape** headland Antarctica
101 F24 **Waldshut-Tiengen** Baden-Württemberg, S Germany
171 P12 **Walea, Selat** strait Sulawesi, C Indonesia
Wałeckie Międzyrzecze see Valašské Meziříčí
108 H8 **Walensee** ◎ NW Switzerland
38 L8 **Wales** Alaska, USA
97 J20 **Wales** Wel. Cymru. national region UK
9 O7 **Wales Island** island Nunavut, NE Canada
77 P14 **Walewale** N Ghana
99 M24 **Walferdange** Luxembourg, C Luxembourg
183 Q5 **Walgett** New South Wales, SE Australia
194 K10 **Walgreen Coast** physical region Antarctica
29 Q2 **Walhalla** North Dakota, N USA
21 O11 **Walhalla** South Carolina, SE USA
79 O19 **Walikale** Nord Kivu, E Dem. Rep. Congo (Zaire)
Walk see Valga, Estonia
Walk see Valka, Latvia
29 U5 **Walker** Minnesota, N USA
15 V4 **Walker, Lac** ◎ Quebec, SE Canada
35 S7 **Walker Lake** ◎ Nevada, W USA
35 R6 **Walker River** ≈ Nevada, W USA
28 K10 **Wall** South Dakota, N USA
173 U9 **Wallaby Plateau** undersea feature E Indian Ocean
33 N8 **Wallace** Idaho, NW USA
21 V11 **Wallace** North Carolina, SE USA
14 D17 **Wallaceburg** Ontario, S Canada
22 F5 **Wallace Lake** ▣ Louisiana, S USA
11 P13 **Wallace Mountain** ▲ Alberta, W Canada
116 J14 **Wallachia** var. Walachia, Ger. Walachei, Rom. Valachia. cultural region S Romania
Wallachisch-Meseritsch see Valašské Meziříčí
183 U4 **Wallangarra** New South Wales, SE Australia
182 I8 **Wallaroo** South Australia
32 L10 **Walla Walla** Washington, NW USA
45 V9 **Wallblake** ✕ (The Valley) C Anguilla
101 H19 **Walldürn** Baden-Württemberg, SW Germany
100 F12 **Wallenhorst** Niedersachsen, NW Germany
Wallenthal see Hațeg
109 S4 **Wallern** Oberösterreich, N Austria
Wallern see Wallern im Burgenland
109 Z5 **Wallern im Burgenland** var. Wallern. Burgenland, E Austria
18 M9 **Wallingford** Vermont, NE USA
25 V11 **Wallis** Texas, SW USA
Wallis see Valais
192 K9 **Wallis and Futuna** Fr. Territoire de Wallis et Futuna. ◇ French overseas territory C Pacific Ocean
108 G7 **Wallisellen** Zürich, N Switzerland

◆ Country ● Country Capital ◇ Dependent Territory ○ Dependent Territory Capital ◆ Administrative Region ✕ International Airport ▲ Mountain ▲ Mountain Range ▲ Volcano ≈ River ◎ Lake ▣ Reservoir

190 H11 **Wallis, Îles** *island group* N Wallis and Futuna
99 H19 **Wallon Brabant** ◈ *province* C Belgium
31 Q5 **Walloon Lake** ◎ Michigan, N USA
32 K10 **Wallula** Washington, NW USA
32 K10 **Wallula, Lake** ◎ Washington, NW USA
21 S8 **Walnut Cove** North Carolina, SE USA
35 N8 **Walnut Creek** California, W USA
26 K5 **Walnut Creek** ≈ Kansas, C USA
27 W9 **Walnut Ridge** Arkansas, C USA
25 S7 **Walnut Springs** Texas, SW USA
182 L10 **Walpeup** Victoria, SE Australia
187 R17 **Walpole, Île** *island* SE New Caledonia
39 N13 **Walrus Islands** *island group* Alaska, USA
97 L19 **Walsall** C England, UK
37 T7 **Walsenburg** Colorado, C USA
11 S17 **Walsh** Alberta, SW Canada
37 W7 **Walsh** Colorado, C USA
100 I11 **Walsrode** Niedersachsen, NW Germany
Waltenberg *see* Zalău
21 R14 **Walterboro** South Carolina, SE USA
Walter F. George Lake *see* Walter F. George Reservoir
23 R6 **Walter F. George Reservoir** *var.* Walter F. George Lake. ⊞ Alabama/Georgia, SE USA
26 M12 **Walters** Oklahoma, C USA
101 J16 **Waltershausen** Thüringen, C Germany
173 N10 **Walters Shoal** *var.* Walters Shoals. *reef* S Madagascar
Walters Shoals *see* Walters Shoal
22 M3 **Walthall** Mississippi, S USA
20 M4 **Walton** Kentucky, S USA
18 J11 **Walton** New York, NE USA
79 O20 **Walungu** Sud Kivu, E Dem. Rep. Congo (Zaire)
Walvisbaai *see* Walvis Bay
83 C19 **Walvis Bay** *Afr.* Walvisbaai. Erongo, NW Namibia
83 B19 **Walvis Bay** *bay* NW Namibia
Walvish Ridge *see* Walvis Ridge
65 O17 **Walvis Ridge** *var.* Walvish Ridge. *undersea feature* E Atlantic Ocean
171 X16 **Wamal** Irian Jaya, E Indonesia
171 U15 **Wamar, Pulau** *island* Kepulauan Aru, E Indonesia
77 V15 **Wamba** Nassarawa, C Nigeria
79 O17 **Wamba** Orientale, NE Dem. Rep. Congo (Zaire)
79 H22 **Wamba** *var.* Uamba. ≈ Angola/Dem. Rep. Congo (Zaire)
27 P4 **Wamego** Kansas, C USA
18 I10 **Wampsville** New York, NE USA
42 K6 **Wampú, Río** ≈ E Honduras
171 X16 **Wan** Irian Jaya, E Indonesia
Wan *see* Anhui
183 N4 **Wanaaring** New South Wales, SE Australia
185 D21 **Wanaka** Otago, South Island, NZ
185 D20 **Wanaka, Lake** ◎ South Island, NZ
171 W14 **Wanapiri** Irian Jaya, E Indonesia
14 F9 **Wanapitei** ≈ Ontario, S Canada
14 F10 **Wanapitei Lake** ◎ Ontario, S Canada
18 K14 **Wanaque** New Jersey, NE USA
171 U12 **Wanau** Irian Jaya, E Indonesia
185 F22 **Wanbrow, Cape** *headland* South Island, NZ
Wanchuan *see* Zhangjiakou
171 W13 **Wandai** *var.* Komeyo. Irian Jaya, E Indonesia
163 Z8 **Wanda Shan** ▲ NE China
197 R11 **Wandel Sea** *sea* Arctic Ocean
160 D13 **Wanding** *var.* Wandingzhen. Yunnan, SW China
Wandingzhen *see* Wanding
99 H20 **Wanfercée-Baulet** Hainaut, S Belgium
184 L12 **Wanganui** Manawatu-Wanganui, North Island, NZ
184 L11 **Wanganui** ≈ North Island, NZ
183 P11 **Wangaratta** Victoria, SE Australia
160 J8 **Wangcang** *prev.* Fengjiaba. Sichuan, C China
Wangda *see* Zogang
101 I24 **Wangen im Allgäu** Baden-Württemberg, S Germany
Wangerin *see* Węgorzyno
100 F9 **Wangerooge** *island* NW Germany
171 W13 **Wanggar** Irian Jaya, E Indonesia
160 J13 **Wangmo** *var.* Fuxing. Guizhou, S China
Wangolodougou *see* Ouangolodougou
161 S9 **Wangpan Yang** *sea* E China
163 Y10 **Wangqing** Jilin, NE China
167 P8 **Wang Saphung** Loei, C Thailand
167 O6 **Wan Hsa-la** Shan State, E Burma
55 W9 **Wanica** ◈ *district* N Suriname
79 M18 **Wanie-Rukula** Orientale, C Dem. Rep. Congo (Zaire)
Wankie *see* Hwange
Wanki, Río *see* Coco, Río
81 N17 **Wanlaweyn** *var.* Wanle Weyn, *It.* Uanle Uen. Shabeellaha Hoose, SW Somalia
Wanle Weyn *see* Wanlaweyn
180 I12 **Wanneroo** Western Australia
160 L17 **Wanning** Hainan, S China
167 Q8 **Wanon Niwat** Sakon Nakhon, E Thailand
155 H16 **Wanparti** Andhra Pradesh, C India
Wansen *see* Wiązów
160 L11 **Wanshan** Guizhou, S China
99 M14 **Wanssum** Limburg, SE Netherlands
184 N12 **Wanstead** Hawke's Bay, North Island, NZ
160 K9 **Wanxian** Chongqing Shi, C China
188 F16 **Wanyaan** Yap, Micronesia
160 K8 **Wanyuan** Sichuan, C China
161 O11 **Wanzai** Jiangxi, S China
99 J20 **Wanze** Liège, E Belgium
31 R12 **Wapakoneta** Ohio, N USA
12 D7 **Wapaseese** ≈ Ontario, C Canada
32 I10 **Wapato** Washington, NW USA
29 Y15 **Wapello** Iowa, C USA
11 N13 **Wapiti** ≈ Alberta/British Columbia, SW Canada
27 X7 **Wappapello Lake** ⊞ Missouri, C USA
18 K13 **Wappingers Falls** New York, NE USA
29 X13 **Wapsipinicon River** ≈ Iowa, C USA
14 L9 **Wapus** ≈ Quebec, SE Canada
160 H7 **Waqên** Sichuan, C China
21 Q7 **War** West Virginia, NE USA
80 D13 **Warab** Warab, SW Sudan
81 D14 **Warab** ◈ *state* SW Sudan
155 J15 **Warangal** Andhra Pradesh, C India
Warasdin *see* Varaždin
183 O16 **Waratah** Tasmania, SE Australia
183 O14 **Waratah Bay** *bay* Victoria, SE Australia
101 H15 **Warburg** Nordrhein-Westfalen, W Germany
182 I1 **Warburton Creek** *seasonal river* South Australia
180 M9 **Warburton** Western Australia
99 M20 **Warche** ≈ E Belgium
149 P5 **Wardag** *var.* Wardak, *Per.* Vardak. ◈ *province* E Afghanistan
Wardak *see* Wardag
32 K9 **Warden** Washington, NW USA
154 I12 **Wardha** Mahārāshtra, W India
121 N15 **Wardija, Ras il-** *var.* Wardija Point. *headland* Gozo, NW Malta
139 P3 **Wardīyah** N Iraq
185 E19 **Ward, Mount** ▲ South Island, NZ
10 L11 **Ware** British Columbia, W Canada
99 D18 **Waregem** *var.* Waereghem. West-Vlaanderen, W Belgium
99 J19 **Waremme** Liège, E Belgium
100 N10 **Waren** Mecklenburg-Vorpommern, NE Germany
171 W13 **Waren** Irian Jaya, E Indonesia
101 F14 **Warendorf** Nordrhein-Westfalen, W Germany
21 P12 **Ware Shoals** South Carolina, SE USA
98 N4 **Warffum** Groningen, NE Netherlands
81 O15 **Wargalo** Mudug, E Somalia
146 M12 **Warganza** *Rus.* Varganzi. Qashqadaryo Wiloyati, S Uzbekistan
Wargla *see* Ouargla
183 T4 **Warialda** New South Wales, SE Australia
154 F13 **Wāri Godri** Mahārāshtra, C India
167 R10 **Warin Chamrap** Ubon Ratchathani, E Thailand
25 R11 **Waring** Texas, SW USA
39 O8 **Waring Mountains** ▲ Alaska, USA
110 M12 **Warka** Mazowieckie, E Poland
184 L5 **Warkworth** Auckland, North Island, NZ
171 U12 **Warmandi** Irian Jaya, E Indonesia
83 E22 **Warmbad** Karas, S Namibia
98 H8 **Warmenhuizen** Noord-Holland, NW Netherlands
110 L8 **Warmińsko-Mazurskie** ◈ *province* NW Poland
97 L22 **Warminster** S England, UK
18 I15 **Warminster** Pennsylvania, NE USA
35 V8 **Warm Springs** Nevada, W USA
32 H12 **Warm Springs** Oregon, NW USA
21 S5 **Warm Springs** Virginia, NE USA
100 M8 **Warnemünde** Mecklenburg-Vorpommern, NE Germany
27 Q10 **Warner** Oklahoma, C USA
35 Q2 **Warner Mountains** ▲ California, W USA
23 T5 **Warner Robins** Georgia, SE USA
57 N18 **Warnes** Santa Cruz, C Bolivia
100 M9 **Warnow** ≈ NE Germany
Warnsdorf *see* Varnsdorf
98 M11 **Warnsveld** Gelderland, E Netherlands
154 I13 **Warora** Mahārāshtra, C India
182 L11 **Warracknabeal** Victoria, SE Australia
183 O13 **Warragul** Victoria, SE Australia
183 O4 **Warrego River** *seasonal river* New South Wales/Queensland, E Australia
183 Q6 **Warren** New South Wales, SE Australia
11 X16 **Warren** Manitoba, S Canada
27 V14 **Warren** Arkansas, C USA
31 S10 **Warren** Michigan, N USA
29 R3 **Warren** Minnesota, N USA
31 U11 **Warren** Ohio, N USA
18 D12 **Warren** Pennsylvania, NE USA
25 X10 **Warren** Texas, SW USA
97 G16 **Warrenpoint** *Ir.* An Pointe. SE Northern Ireland, UK
27 S4 **Warrensburg** Missouri, C USA
83 H22 **Warrenton** Northern Cape, N South Africa
23 U4 **Warrenton** Georgia, SE USA
27 W4 **Warrenton** Missouri, C USA
21 V8 **Warrenton** North Carolina, SE USA
21 V4 **Warrenton** Virginia, NE USA
77 U17 **Warri** Delta, S Nigeria
97 L18 **Warrington** C England, UK
23 O9 **Warrington** Florida, SE USA
23 P3 **Warrior** Alabama, S USA
182 L13 **Warrnambool** Victoria, SE Australia
29 T2 **Warroad** Minnesota, N USA
183 S6 **Warrumbungle Range** ▲ New South Wales, SE Australia
154 J12 **Wārsa** Mahārāshtra, C India
31 P11 **Warsaw** Indiana, N USA
20 L4 **Warsaw** Kentucky, S USA
27 T5 **Warsaw** Missouri, C USA
18 E10 **Warsaw** New York, NE USA
21 V10 **Warsaw** North Carolina, SE USA
21 X5 **Warsaw** Virginia, NE USA
Warsaw/Warschau *see* Warszawa
81 N17 **Warshiikh** Shabeellaha Dhexe, C Somalia
101 G15 **Warstein** Nordrhein-Westfalen, W Germany
110 M11 **Warszawa** *Eng.* Warsaw, *Ger.* Warschau, *Rus.* Varshava. ● (Poland) Mazowieckie, C Poland
110 J13 **Warta** Sieradz, C Poland
110 D11 **Warta** *Ger.* Warthe. ≈ W Poland
Wartberg *see* Senec
20 M9 **Wartburg** Tennessee, S USA
108 J7 **Warth** Vorarlberg, NW Austria
Warthe *see* Warta
169 U12 **Waru** Borneo, C Indonesia
171 T13 **Waru** Pulau Seram, E Indonesia
139 N6 **Wa'r, Wādī al** *dry watercourse* E Syria
183 U3 **Warwick** Queensland, E Australia
15 Q11 **Warwick** Quebec, SE Canada
97 M20 **Warwick** C England, UK
18 K13 **Warwick** New York, NE USA
29 P4 **Warwick** North Dakota, N USA
19 O12 **Warwick** Rhode Island, NE USA
97 L20 **Warwickshire** *cultural region* C England, UK
14 G14 **Wasaga Beach** Ontario, S Canada
77 U13 **Wasagu** Kebbi, NW Nigeria
36 M2 **Wasatch Range** ▲ W USA
35 R12 **Wasco** California, W USA
29 V10 **Waseca** Minnesota, N USA
14 H13 **Washago** Ontario, S Canada
19 S2 **Washburn** Maine, NE USA
28 M5 **Washburn** North Dakota, N USA
30 K3 **Washburn** Wisconsin, N USA
31 S14 **Washburn Hill** *hill* Ohio, N USA
154 H13 **Wāshīm** Mahārāshtra, C India
97 M14 **Washington** NE England, UK
23 U3 **Washington** Georgia, SE USA
30 L12 **Washington** Illinois, N USA
31 N15 **Washington** Indiana, N USA
29 X15 **Washington** Iowa, C USA
27 O3 **Washington** Kansas, C USA
27 W5 **Washington** Missouri, C USA
21 X9 **Washington** North Carolina, SE USA
18 B15 **Washington** Pennsylvania, NE USA
25 V10 **Washington** Texas, SW USA
36 J8 **Washington** Utah, W USA
21 V4 **Washington** Virginia, NE USA
32 I9 **Washington** *off.* State of Washington; also known as Chinook State, Evergreen State. ◈ *state* NW USA
Washington *see* Washington Court House
31 S14 **Washington Court House** *var.* Washington. Ohio, NE USA
21 W4 **Washington DC** ● (USA) District of Columbia, NE USA
31 O5 **Washington Island** *island* Wisconsin, N USA
Washington Island *see* Teraina
19 O7 **Washington, Mount** ▲ New Hampshire, NE USA
26 M11 **Washita River** ≈ Oklahoma/Texas, C USA
97 O18 **Wash, The** *inlet* E England, UK
32 L9 **Washtucna** Washington, NW USA
Wasiliszki *see* Vasilishki
110 P9 **Wasilków** Podlaskie, NE Poland
39 R11 **Wasilla** Alaska, USA
55 U9 **Wasjabo** Sipaliwini, NW Suriname
11 X11 **Waskaiowaka Lake** ◎ Manitoba, C Canada
11 T14 **Waskesiu Lake** Saskatchewan, C Canada
25 X7 **Waskom** Texas, SW USA
110 G13 **Wąsosz** Dolnośląskie, SW Poland
42 M6 **Waspam** *var.* Waspán. Región Autónoma Atlántico Norte, NE Nicaragua
Waspán *see* Waspam
165 T3 **Wassamu** Hokkaidō, NE Japan
108 G9 **Wassen** Uri, C Switzerland
98 G11 **Wassenaar** Zuid-Holland, W Netherlands
99 N24 **Wasserbillig** Grevenmacher, E Luxembourg
Wasserburg *see* Wasserburg am Inn
101 M23 **Wasserburg am Inn** *var.* Wasserburg. Bayern, SE Germany
101 I17 **Wasserkuppe** ▲ C Germany
103 R5 **Wassy** Haute-Marne, N France
171 N14 **Watampone** *var.* Bone. Sulawesi, C Indonesia
171 R13 **Watawa** Pulau Buru, E Indonesia
Watenstedt-Salzgitter *see* Salzgitter
18 M13 **Waterbury** Connecticut, NE USA
21 R11 **Wateree Lake** ⊞ South Carolina, SE USA
21 R12 **Wateree River** ≈ South Carolina, SE USA
97 E20 **Waterford** *Ir.* Port Láirge. S Ireland
31 S9 **Waterford** Michigan, N USA
97 E20 **Waterford** *Ir.* Port Láirge. *cultural region* S Ireland
97 E21 **Waterford Harbour** *Ir.* Cuan Phort Láirge. *inlet* S Ireland
98 G12 **Wateringen** Zuid-Holland, W Netherlands
99 G19 **Waterloo** Wallon Brabant, C Belgium
14 F16 **Waterloo** Ontario, S Canada
15 P12 **Waterloo** Quebec, SE Canada
30 K16 **Waterloo** Illinois, N USA
29 X13 **Waterloo** Iowa, C USA
18 G10 **Waterloo** New York, NE USA
30 L4 **Watersmeet** Michigan, N USA
23 V9 **Watertown** Florida, SE USA
18 I8 **Watertown** New York, NE USA
29 R9 **Watertown** South Dakota, N USA
30 M8 **Watertown** Wisconsin, N USA
22 L3 **Water Valley** Mississippi, S USA
27 O3 **Waterville** Kansas, C USA
17 V6 **Waterville** Maine, NE USA
29 V10 **Waterville** Minnesota, N USA
18 I10 **Waterville** New York, NE USA
14 E16 **Watford** Ontario, S Canada
97 N21 **Watford** SE England, UK
28 K4 **Watford City** North Dakota, N USA
141 X12 **Wāṭif** S Oman
18 G11 **Watkins Glen** New York, NE USA
Watlings Island *see* San Salvador
171 U15 **Watnil** Pulau Kai Kecil, E Indonesia
26 M10 **Watonga** Oklahoma, C USA
11 T16 **Watrous** Saskatchewan, S Canada
37 T10 **Watrous** New Mexico, SW USA
79 P16 **Watsa** Orientale, NE Dem. Rep. Congo (Zaire)
31 N12 **Watseka** Illinois, N USA
79 J19 **Watsikengo** Equateur, C Dem. Rep. Congo (Zaire)
182 C5 **Watson** South Australia
11 U15 **Watson** Saskatchewan, S Canada
195 O10 **Watson Escarpment** ▲ Antarctica
10 K9 **Watson Lake** Yukon Territory, W Canada
35 N10 **Watsonville** California, W USA
167 Q8 **Wattay** × (Viangchan) Viangchan, C Laos
109 N7 **Wattens** Tirol, W Austria
20 M9 **Watts Bar Lake** ⊞ Tennessee, S USA
108 H7 **Wattwil** Sankt Gallen, NE Switzerland
171 T14 **Watubela, Kepulauan** *island group* E Indonesia
101 N24 **Watzmann** ▲ SE Germany
186 E8 **Wau** Morobe, C PNG
81 D14 **Wau** *var.* Wāw. Western Bahr el Ghazal, S Sudan
29 Q8 **Waubay** South Dakota, N USA
29 Q8 **Waubay Lake** ◎ South Dakota, N USA
183 U7 **Wauchope** New South Wales, SE Australia
23 W13 **Wauchula** Florida, SE USA
30 M10 **Wauconda** Illinois, N USA
182 J7 **Waukaringa** South Australia
31 N10 **Waukegan** Illinois, N USA
30 M9 **Waukesha** Wisconsin, N USA
29 X11 **Waukon** Iowa, C USA
30 L8 **Waunakee** Wisconsin, N USA
30 L7 **Waupaca** Wisconsin, N USA
30 M8 **Waupun** Wisconsin, N USA
26 M13 **Waurika** Oklahoma, C USA
26 M12 **Waurika Lake** ⊞ Oklahoma, C USA
30 L6 **Wausau** Wisconsin, N USA
31 R11 **Wauseon** Ohio, N USA
30 L7 **Wautoma** Wisconsin, N USA
30 M9 **Wauwatosa** Wisconsin, N USA
22 L9 **Waveland** Mississippi, S USA
97 Q20 **Waveney** ≈ E England, UK
184 L11 **Waverley** Taranaki, North Island, NZ
29 W12 **Waverly** Iowa, C USA
27 T4 **Waverly** Missouri, C USA
29 R15 **Waverly** Nebraska, C USA
18 G12 **Waverly** New York, NE USA
20 H8 **Waverly** Tennessee, S USA
21 W7 **Waverly** Virginia, NE USA
99 H19 **Wavre** Wallon Brabant, C Belgium
166 M8 **Waw** Pegu, SW Burma
Wāw *see* Wau
14 B7 **Wawa** Ontario, S Canada
77 T14 **Wawa** Niger, W Nigeria
75 Q11 **Wāw al Kabīr** S Libya
43 N7 **Wawa, Río** *var.* Rio Huahua. ≈ NE Nicaragua
186 B8 **Wawoi** ≈ SW PNG
25 T7 **Waxahachie** Texas, SW USA
158 L9 **Waxxari** Xinjiang Uygur Zizhiqu, NW China
23 V7 **Waycross** Georgia, SE USA
180 K10 **Way, Lake** ◎ Western Australia
31 P9 **Wayland** Michigan, N USA
29 R13 **Wayne** Nebraska, C USA
18 K14 **Wayne** New Jersey, NE USA
21 P5 **Wayne** West Virginia, NE USA
23 V4 **Waynesboro** Georgia, SE USA
22 M7 **Waynesboro** Mississippi, S USA
20 H10 **Waynesboro** Tennessee, S USA
21 U5 **Waynesboro** Virginia, NE USA
18 B16 **Waynesburg** Pennsylvania, NE USA
27 U6 **Waynesville** Missouri, C USA
21 O10 **Waynesville** North Carolina, SE USA
26 L8 **Waynoka** Oklahoma, C USA
Wazan *see* Ouazzane
Wazima *see* Wajima
149 V7 **Wazīrābād** Punjab, NE Pakistan
Wazzan *see* Ouazzane
110 I8 **Wda** *var.* Czarna Woda, *Ger.* Schwarzwasser. ≈ N Poland
187 Q16 **Wé** Province des Îles Loyauté, E New Caledonia
97 O23 **Weald, The** *lowlands* SE England, UK
186 A9 **Weam** Western, SW PNG
97 L15 **Wear** ≈ N England, UK
Wearmouth *see* Sunderland
26 L10 **Weatherford** Oklahoma, C USA
25 S6 **Weatherford** Texas, SW USA
34 M3 **Weaverville** California, W USA
27 R7 **Webb City** Missouri, C USA
192 G8 **Weber Basin** *undersea feature* S Ceram Sea
Webfoot State *see* Oregon
18 F9 **Webster** New York, NE USA
29 Q8 **Webster** South Dakota, N USA
29 V13 **Webster City** Iowa, C USA
27 X5 **Webster Groves** Missouri, C USA
21 S4 **Webster Springs** *var.* Addison. West Virginia, NE USA
171 S11 **Weda, Teluk** *bay* Pulau Halmahera, E Indonesia
65 B25 **Weddell Island** *var.* Isla San Jose. *Island* W Falkland Islands
65 K22 **Weddell Plain** *undersea feature* SW Atlantic Ocean
65 K23 **Weddell Sea** *sea* SW Atlantic Ocean
65 B25 **Weddell Settlement** Weddell Island, W Falkland Islands
182 M11 **Wedderburn** Victoria, SE Australia
100 I9 **Wedel** Schleswig-Holstein, N Germany
92 N3 **Wedel Jarlsberg Land** *physical region* SW Svalbard
100 I12 **Wedemark** Niedersachsen, NW Germany
10 M17 **Wedge Mountain** ▲ British Columbia, SW Canada
23 R4 **Wedowee** Alabama, S USA
171 U15 **Weduar** Pulau Kai Besar, E Indonesia
35 N2 **Weed** California, W USA
15 Q12 **Weedon Centre** Quebec, SE Canada
18 E13 **Weedville** Pennsylvania, NE USA
100 F10 **Weener** Niedersachsen, NW Germany
29 S16 **Weeping Water** Nebraska, C USA
99 L16 **Weert** Limburg, SE Netherlands
98 I10 **Weesp** Noord-Holland, C Netherlands
183 S5 **Wee Waa** New South Wales, SE Australia
110 N7 **Węgorzewo** *Ger.* Angerburg. Warmińsko-Mazurskie, NE Poland
110 E9 **Węgorzyno** *Ger.* Wangerin. Zachodniopomorskie, NW Poland
110 N11 **Węgrów** *Ger.* Bingerau. Mazowieckie, E Poland
98 N5 **Wehe-Den Hoorn** Groningen, NE Netherlands
98 M12 **Wehl** Gelderland, E Netherlands
Wehlau *see* Znamensk
168 F7 **Weh, Pulau** *island* NW Indonesia
Wei *see* Weifang
161 P1 **Weichang** *prev.* Zhuizishan. Hebei, E China
Weichsel *see* Wisła
101 M16 **Weida** Thüringen, C Germany
Weiden *see* Weiden in der Oberpfalz
101 M19 **Weiden in der Oberpfalz** *var.* Weiden. Bayern, SE Germany
161 Q4 **Weifang** *var.* Wei, Wei-fang; *prev.* Weihsien. Shandong, E China
161 S4 **Weihai** Shandong, E China
160 K6 **Wei He** ≈ C China
Weihsien *see* Weifang
101 G17 **Weilburg** Hessen, W Germany
101 K24 **Weilheim** Bayern, SE Germany
183 P4 **Weilmoringle** New South Wales, SE Australia
101 L16 **Weimar** Thüringen, C Germany
25 U11 **Weimar** Texas, SW USA
160 L6 **Weinan** Shaanxi, C China
108 H6 **Weinfelden** Thurgau, NE Switzerland
101 I24 **Weingarten** Baden-Württemberg, S Germany
101 G20 **Weinheim** Baden-Württemberg, SW Germany
160 H11 **Weining** *var.* Weining Yizu Huizu Miaozu Zizhixian. Guizhou, S China
Weining Yizu Huizu Miaozu Zizhixian *see* Weining
181 V2 **Weipa** Queensland, NE Australia
11 Y11 **Weir River** Manitoba, C Canada
21 R1 **Weirton** West Virginia, NE USA
32 M13 **Weiser** Idaho, NW USA
160 F12 **Weishan** Yunnan, SW China
161 P6 **Weishan Hu** ◎ E China
101 M15 **Weisse Elster** *Eng.* White Elster. ≈ Czech Republic/Germany
Weisse Körös/Weisse Kreisch *see* Crişul Alb
108 L7 **Weissenbach am Lech** Tirol, W Austria
101 K21 **Weissenburg** Bayern, SE Germany
Weissenburg *see* Wissembourg, France
Weissenburg *see* Alba Iulia, Romania
101 M15 **Weissenfels** *var.* Weißenfels. Sachsen-Anhalt, C Germany
109 R9 **Weissensee** ◎ S Austria
Weissenstein *see* Paide
108 E11 **Weisshorn** *var.* Flüela Wisshorn. ▲ SW Switzerland
Weisskirchen *see* Bela Crkva
23 R3 **Weiss Lake** ⊞ Alabama, S USA
101 Q14 **Weisswasser** *Lus.* Běla Woda. Sachsen, E Germany
99 M22 **Weiswampach** Diekirch, N Luxembourg
109 U2 **Weitra** Niederösterreich, N Austria
161 O4 **Weixian** *var.* Wei Xian. Hebei, E China
159 V11 **Weiyuan** Gansu, C China
160 F14 **Weiyuan Jiang** ≈ SW China
109 W7 **Weiz** Steiermark, SE Austria
160 K16 **Weizhou Dao** *island* S China
110 I6 **Wejherowo** Pomorskie, NW Poland
27 Q8 **Welch** Oklahoma, C USA
24 M6 **Welch** Texas, SW USA
21 Q6 **Welch** West Virginia, NE USA
45 O14 **Welchman Hall** C Barbados
80 J11 **Weldiya** *var.* Waldia, *It.* Valdia. Amhara, N Ethiopia
21 W8 **Weldon** North Carolina, SE USA
25 V9 **Weldon** Texas, SW USA
99 M19 **Welkenraedt** Liège, E Belgium
193 O2 **Welker Seamount** *undersea feature* N Pacific Ocean
83 I22 **Welkom** Free State, C South Africa
14 H16 **Welland** Ontario, S Canada
14 G16 **Welland** ≈ Ontario, S Canada
97 O19 **Welland** ≈ C England, UK
14 H17 **Welland Canal** *canal* Ontario, S Canada
155 K25 **Wellawaya** Uva Province, SE Sri Lanka
Welle *see* Uele
181 T4 **Wellesley Islands** *island group* Queensland, N Australia
99 J22 **Wellin** Luxembourg, SE Belgium
97 N20 **Wellingborough** C England, UK
183 R7 **Wellington** New South Wales, SE Australia
14 J15 **Wellington** Ontario, SE Canada
185 L14 **Wellington** ● (NZ) Wellington, North Island, NZ
83 E26 **Wellington** Western Cape, SW South Africa
37 T2 **Wellington** Colorado, C USA
27 N7 **Wellington** Kansas, C USA
35 R7 **Wellington** Nevada, W USA
31 T11 **Wellington** Ohio, N USA
25 P3 **Wellington** Texas, SW USA
36 M4 **Wellington** Utah, W USA
185 M14 **Wellington** *off.* Wellington Region. ◈ *region* North Island, NZ
185 L14 **Wellington** × Wellington, North Island, NZ
Wellington *see* Wellington, Isla
63 F22 **Wellington, Isla** *var.* Wellington. *island* S Chile
183 P12 **Wellington, Lake** ◎ Victoria, SE Australia
29 X14 **Wellman** Iowa, C USA
24 M6 **Wellman** Texas, SW USA
97 K22 **Wells** SW England, UK
29 V11 **Wells** Minnesota, N USA
35 X2 **Wells** Nevada, W USA
25 W8 **Wells** Texas, SW USA
18 F12 **Wellsboro** Pennsylvania, NE USA
21 R1 **Wellsburg** West Virginia, NE USA
184 K4 **Wellsford** Auckland, North Island, NZ
180 L9 **Wells, Lake** ◎ Western Australia
181 N4 **Wells, Mount** ▲ Western Australia
97 P18 **Wells-next-the-Sea** E England, UK
31 T15 **Wellston** Ohio, N USA
27 O10 **Wellston** Oklahoma, C USA
18 E11 **Wellsville** New York, NE USA
31 V12 **Wellsville** Ohio, N USA
36 L1 **Wellsville** Utah, W USA
36 I14 **Wellton** Arizona, SW USA
109 S4 **Wels** *anc.* Ovilava. Oberösterreich, N Austria
99 K15 **Welschap** × (Eindhoven) Noord-Brabant, S Netherlands
100 P10 **Welse** ≈ NE Germany
22 H9 **Welsh** Louisiana, S USA
97 K19 **Welshpool** *Wel.* Y Trallwng. E Wales, UK
97 O21 **Welwyn Garden City** SE England, UK
79 K18 **Wema** Equateur, NW Dem. Rep. Congo (Zaire)
81 G21 **Wembere** ≈ C Tanzania
11 N13 **Wembley** Alberta, W Canada
12 I9 **Wemindji** *prev.* Nouveau-Comptoir, Paint Hills. Quebec, C Canada
99 G18 **Wemmel** Vlaams Brabant, C Belgium
32 J8 **Wenatchee** Washington, NW USA
160 M17 **Wenchang** Hainan, S China
161 R11 **Wencheng** *prev.* Daxue. Zhejiang, SE China
77 P16 **Wenchi** W Ghana
Wen-chou/Wenchow *see* Wenzhou
160 H8 **Wenchuan** *prev.* Weizhou. Sichuan, C China
Wendau *see* Võnnu
Wenden *see* Cēsis
161 S4 **Wendeng** Shandong, E China
81 J15 **Wendo** Southern, S Ethiopia
36 J2 **Wendover** Utah, W USA
14 D9 **Wenebegon** ≈ Ontario, S Canada
14 D8 **Wenebegon Lake** ◎ Ontario, S Canada
108 E9 **Wengen** Bern, W Switzerland

◆ Country ● Country Capital ◇ Dependent Territory ○ Dependent Territory Capital ◈ Administrative Region × International Airport ▲ Mountain ▲ Mountain Range ▲ Volcano ≈ River ◎ Lake ⊞ Reservoir

161 O13 **Wengyuan** prev. Longxian. Guangdong, S China
189 P15 **Weno** prev. Moen. Chuuk, C Micronesia
189 V12 **Weno** prev. Moen. atoll Chuuk Islands, C Micronesia
158 N13 **Wenquan** Qinghai, C China
159 H4 **Wenquan** var. Arixang. Xinjiang Uygur Zizhiqu, NW China
160 H14 **Wenshan** Yunnan, SW China
158 H6 **Wensu** Xinjiang Uygur Zizhiqu, W China
182 L8 **Wentworth** New South Wales, SE Australia
27 W4 **Wentzville** Missouri, C USA
159 V12 **Wenxian** var. Wen Xian. Gansu, C China
161 S10 **Wenzhou** var. Wen-chou, Wenchow. Zhejiang, SE China
34 L4 **Weott** California, W USA
99 I20 **Wépion** Namur, SE Belgium
100 O11 **Werbellinsee** ◎ NE Germany
99 L21 **Werbomont** Liège, E Belgium
83 G20 **Werda** Kgalagadi, S Botswana
Werder see Virtsu
81 N14 **Werder** Somalil, E Ethiopia
Werenów see Voranava
171 U13 **Weri** Irian Jaya, E Indonesia
98 I13 **Werkendam** Noord-Brabant, S Netherlands
101 M20 **Wernberg-Köblitz** Bayern, SE Germany
101 J18 **Werneck** Bayern, C Germany
101 K14 **Wernigerode** Sachsen-Anhalt, C Germany
Werowitz see Virovitica
101 J16 **Werra** ≈ C Germany
183 N12 **Werribee** Victoria, SE Australia
183 T6 **Werris Creek** New South Wales, SE Australia
Werro see Võru
Werschetz see Vršac
101 K23 **Wertach** ≈ S Germany
101 I19 **Wertheim** Baden-Württemberg, SW Germany
98 J8 **Wervershoof** Noord-Holland, NW Netherlands
Wervicq see Wervik
99 C18 **Wervik** var. Wervicq, Werwick. West-Vlaanderen, W Belgium
Werwick see Wervik
101 D14 **Wesel** Nordrhein-Westfalen, W Germany
Weseli an der Lainsitz see Veselí nad Lužnicí
Wesenberg see Rakvere
100 H12 **Weser** ≈ NW Germany
Wes-Kaap see Western Cape
25 S17 **Weslaco** Texas, SW USA
14 J13 **Weslemkoon Lake** ◎ Ontario, SE Canada
181 R1 **Wessel Islands** island group Northern Territory, N Australia
29 P9 **Wessington** South Dakota, N USA
29 P10 **Wessington Springs** South Dakota, N USA
25 T8 **West** Texas, SW USA
West see Ouest
30 M9 **West Allis** Wisconsin, N USA
182 E8 **Westall, Point** headland South Australia
West Antarctica see Lesser Antarctica
14 G11 **West Arm** Ontario, S Canada
West Azerbaijan see Āzarbāyjān-e Gharbī
138 F10 **West Bank** disputed region SW Asia
11 N17 **Westbank** British Columbia, SW Canada
14 E11 **West Bay** Manitoulin Island, Ontario, S Canada
22 L11 **West Bay** bay Louisiana, S USA
30 M8 **West Bend** Wisconsin, N USA
153 R16 **West Bengal** ◈ state NE India
West Borneo see Kalimantan Barat
29 Y14 **West Branch** Iowa, C USA
31 R7 **West Branch** Michigan, N USA
18 F13 **West Branch Susquehanna River** ≈ Pennsylvania, NE USA
97 L20 **West Bromwich** C England, UK
19 P8 **Westbrook** Maine, NE USA
29 T10 **Westbrook** Minnesota, N USA
29 Y15 **West Burlington** Iowa, C USA
96 L2 **West Burra** island NE Scotland, UK
30 J8 **Westby** Wisconsin, N USA
44 L6 **West Caicos** island W Turks and Caicos Islands
185 A24 **West Cape** headland South Island, NZ
174 L4 **West Caroline Basin** undersea feature SW Pacific Ocean
18 I16 **West Chester** Pennsylvania, NE USA
185 E18 **West Coast** off. West Coast Region. ◈ region South Island, NZ
25 V12 **West Columbia** Texas, SW USA
29 W10 **West Concord** Minnesota, N USA
29 V14 **West Des Moines** Iowa, C USA
37 Q6 **West Elk Peak** ▲ Colorado, C USA
44 F1 **West End** Grand Bahama Island, N Bahamas
44 F1 **West End Point** headland Grand Bahama Island, N Bahamas
98 O7 **Westerbork** Drenthe, NE Netherlands
98 N3 **Westereems** strait Germany/Netherlands
98 O9 **Westerhaar-Vriezenveensewijk** Overijssel, E Netherlands
100 G6 **Westerland** Schleswig-Holstein, N Germany
99 I17 **Westerlo** Antwerpen, N Belgium
19 N13 **Westerly** Rhode Island, NE USA
81 G18 **Western** ◈ province W Kenya
153 N11 **Western** ◈ zone C Nepal
186 A8 **Western** ◈ province SW PNG
186 J8 **Western** off. Western Province. ◈ province NW Solomon Islands
83 G15 **Western** ◈ province SW Zambia
180 K8 **Western Australia** ◈ state W Australia
80 A13 **Western Bahr el Ghazal** ◈ state SW Sudan
Western Bug see Bug
83 F25 **Western Cape** off. Western Cape Province, Afr. Wes-Kaap. ◈ province SW South Africa
80 A11 **Western Darfur** ◈ state W Sudan
Western Desert see Sahara el Gharbîya
118 G9 **Western Dvina** Bel. Dzvina, Ger. Düna, Latv. Daugava, Rus. Zapadnaya Dvina. ≈ W Europe
81 D15 **Western Equatoria** ◈ state SW Sudan
155 E16 **Western Ghats** ▲ SW India
186 C7 **Western Highlands** ◈ province C PNG
Western Isles see Outer Hebrides
80 C12 **Western Kordofan** ◈ state C Sudan
21 T3 **Westernport** Maryland, NE USA
155 J26 **Western Province** ◈ province SW Sri Lanka
74 B10 **Western Sahara** ◇ disputed territory N Africa
Western Samoa see Samoa
Western Sayans see Zapadnyy Sayan
Western Scheldt see Westerschelde
Western Sierra Madre see Madre Occidental, Sierra
99 E15 **Westerschelde** Eng. Western Scheldt; prev. Honte. inlet S North Sea
31 S13 **Westerville** Ohio, N USA
101 F17 **Westerwald** ▲ W Germany
65 C25 **West Falkland** var. Gran Malvina, Isla Gran Malvina. island W Falkland Islands
29 R5 **West Fargo** North Dakota, N USA
188 M15 **West Fayu Atoll** atoll Caroline Islands, C Micronesia
18 C11 **Westfield** New York, NE USA
30 L7 **Westfield** Wisconsin, N USA
West Flanders see West-Vlaanderen
27 S10 **West Fork** Arkansas, C USA
29 P16 **West Fork Big Blue River** ≈ Nebraska, C USA
29 U12 **West Fork Des Moines River** ≈ Iowa/Minnesota, C USA
25 S5 **West Fork Trinity River** ≈ Texas, SW USA
30 L16 **West Frankfort** Illinois, N USA
98 I8 **West-Friesland** physical region NW Netherlands
West Frisian Islands see Waddeneilanden
19 T5 **West Grand Lake** ◎ Maine, NE USA
18 M12 **West Hartford** Connecticut, NE USA
18 M13 **West Haven** Connecticut, NE USA
27 X12 **West Helena** Arkansas, C USA
28 M2 **Westhope** North Dakota, N USA
195 Y8 **West Ice Shelf** ice shelf Antarctica
47 R2 **West Indies** island group SE North America
West Irian see Irian Jaya
West Java see Jawa Barat
36 L3 **West Jordan** Utah, W USA
West Kalimantan see Kalimantan Barat
99 D14 **Westkapelle** Zeeland, SW Netherlands
31 O13 **West Lafayette** Indiana, N USA
31 T13 **West Lafayette** Ohio, N USA
West Lake see Kagera
29 Y14 **West Liberty** Iowa, C USA
21 O5 **West Liberty** Kentucky, S USA
Westliche Morava see Zapadna Morava
8 J13 **Westlock** Alberta, SW Canada
14 E17 **West Lorne** Ontario, S Canada
96 J12 **West Lothian** cultural region S Scotland, UK
99 H16 **Westmalle** Antwerpen, N Belgium
192 G6 **West Mariana Basin** var. Perece Vela Basin. undersea feature W Pacific Ocean
97 E17 **Westmeath** Ir. An Iarmhí, Na h-Iarmhidhe. cultural region C Ireland
27 Y11 **West Memphis** Arkansas, C USA
21 W2 **Westminster** Maryland, NE USA
21 O11 **Westminster** South Carolina, SE USA
22 I5 **West Monroe** Louisiana, S USA
18 D15 **Westmont** Pennsylvania, NE USA
27 O3 **Westmoreland** Kansas, C USA
35 W17 **Westmorland** California, W USA
186 E6 **West New Britain** ◈ province E PNG
West New Guinea see Irian Jaya
83 K18 **West Nicholson** Matabeleland South, S Zimbabwe
29 T14 **West Nishnabotna River** ≈ Iowa, C USA
175 P11 **West Norfolk Ridge** undersea feature W Pacific Ocean
25 P12 **West Nueces River** ≈ Texas, SW USA
West Nusa Tenggara see Nusa Tenggara Barat
29 T11 **West Okoboji Lake** ◎ Iowa, C USA
33 R16 **Weston** Idaho, NW USA
21 R4 **Weston** West Virginia, NE USA
97 J22 **Weston-super-Mare** SW England, UK
23 Z14 **West Palm Beach** Florida, SE USA
West Papua see Irian Jaya
188 E9 **West Passage** passage Babeldaob, N Palau
23 O9 **West Pensacola** Florida, SE USA
27 V8 **West Plains** Missouri, C USA
35 P7 **West Point** California, W USA
23 R5 **West Point** Georgia, SE USA
22 M3 **West Point** Mississippi, S USA
29 R14 **West Point** Nebraska, C USA
21 X6 **West Point** Virginia, NE USA
182 G10 **West Point** headland South Australia
65 B24 **Westpoint Island Settlement** Westpoint Island, NW Falkland Islands
23 R4 **West Point Lake** ⊡ Alabama/Georgia, SE USA
97 B16 **Westport** Ir. Cathair na Mart. W Ireland
185 G15 **Westport** West Coast, South Island, NZ
32 F10 **Westport** Oregon, NW USA
32 F9 **Westport** Washington, NW USA
31 S15 **West Portsmouth** Ohio, N USA
West Punjab see Punjab
11 V14 **Westray** Manitoba, C Canada
96 J4 **Westray** island NE Scotland, UK
14 F9 **Westree** Ontario, S Canada
97 L16 **West Riding** cultural region N England, UK
West River see Xi Jiang
30 J7 **West Salem** Wisconsin, N USA
65 H21 **West Scotia Ridge** undersea feature W Scotia Sea
West Sepik see Sandaun
173 N4 **West Sheba Ridge** undersea feature W Indian Ocean
West Siberian Plain see Zapadno-Sibirskaya Ravnina
31 S11 **West Sister Island** island Ohio, N USA
West-Skylge see West-Terschelling
West Sumatra see Sumatera Barat
98 J5 **West-Terschelling** Fris. West-Skylge. Friesland, N Netherlands
64 J7 **West Thulean Rise** undersea feature N Atlantic Ocean
29 X12 **West Union** Iowa, C USA
31 R15 **West Union** Ohio, N USA
21 R3 **West Union** West Virginia, NE USA
31 N13 **Westville** Illinois, N USA
21 R3 **West Virginia** off. State of West Virginia; also known as The Mountain State. ◈ state NE USA
99 A17 **West-Vlaanderen** Eng. West Flanders. ◈ province W Belgium
35 R7 **West Walker River** ≈ California/Nevada, W USA
35 P4 **Westwood** California, W USA
183 P9 **West Wyalong** New South Wales, SE Australia
171 Q16 **Wetar, Pulau** island Kepulauan Damar, E Indonesia
171 R16 **Wetar, Selat** var. Wetar Strait. strait Nusa Tenggara, S Indonesia
Wetar Strait see Wetar, Selat
11 Q15 **Wetaskiwin** Alberta, SW Canada
81 K21 **Wete** Pemba, E Tanzania
166 M4 **Wetlet** Sagaing, C Burma
37 T6 **Wet Mountains** ▲ Colorado, C USA
101 E15 **Wetter** Nordrhein-Westfalen, W Germany
101 H17 **Wetter** ≈ W Germany
99 F17 **Wetteren** Oost-Vlaanderen, NW Belgium
108 F7 **Wettingen** Aargau, N Switzerland
27 P11 **Wetumka** Oklahoma, C USA
23 Q5 **Wetumpka** Alabama, S USA
108 G7 **Wetzikon** Zürich, N Switzerland
101 G17 **Wetzlar** Hessen, W Germany
99 C18 **Wevelgem** West-Vlaanderen, W Belgium
38 M6 **Wevok** var. Wewuk. Alaska, USA
23 R9 **Wewahitchka** Florida, SE USA
186 C6 **Wewak** East Sepik, NW PNG
27 O11 **Wewoka** Oklahoma, C USA
Wewuk see Wevok
97 F20 **Wexford** Ir. Loch Garman. SE Ireland
97 F20 **Wexford** Ir. Loch Garman. cultural region SE Ireland
30 L7 **Weyauwega** Wisconsin, N USA
11 U17 **Weyburn** Saskatchewan, S Canada
Weyer see Weyer Markt
109 U5 **Weyer Markt** var. Weyer. Oberösterreich, N Austria
100 H11 **Weyhe** Niedersachsen, NW Germany
97 L24 **Weymouth** S England, UK
19 P11 **Weymouth** Massachusetts, NE USA
99 H18 **Wezembeek-Oppem** Vlaams Brabant, C Belgium
98 M9 **Wezep** Gelderland, E Netherlands
184 M9 **Whakamaru** Waikato, North Island, NZ
184 O8 **Whakatane** Bay of Plenty, North Island, NZ
184 O8 **Whakatane** ≈ North Island, NZ
9 O9 **Whale Cove** Nunavut, C Canada
96 M2 **Whalsay** island NE Scotland, UK
184 L11 **Whangaehu** ≈ North Island, NZ
184 M6 **Whangamata** Waikato, North Island, NZ
184 Q9 **Whangara** Gisborne, North Island, NZ
184 K3 **Whangarei** Northland, North Island, NZ
184 K3 **Whangaruru Harbour** inlet North Island, NZ
25 V12 **Wharton** Texas, SW USA
173 U8 **Wharton Basin** var. West Australian Basin. undersea feature E Indian Ocean
185 E18 **Whataroa** West Coast, South Island, NZ
8 K10 **Wha Ti** prev. Lac La Martre. Northwest Territories, W Canada
184 K6 **Whatipu** Auckland, North Island, NZ
33 Y16 **Wheatland** Wyoming, C USA
14 D18 **Wheatley** Ontario, S Canada
30 M10 **Wheaton** Illinois, N USA
29 R7 **Wheaton** Minnesota, N USA
37 T4 **Wheat Ridge** Colorado, C USA
25 P2 **Wheeler** Texas, SW USA
23 O2 **Wheeler Lake** ⊡ Alabama, S USA
35 Y6 **Wheeler Peak** ▲ Nevada, W USA
37 T9 **Wheeler Peak** ▲ New Mexico, SW USA
31 S15 **Wheelersburg** Ohio, N USA
21 R2 **Wheeling** West Virginia, NE USA
97 L16 **Whernside** ▲ N England, UK
182 F9 **Whidbey, Point** headland South Australia
180 I7 **Whim Creek** Western Australia
10 L17 **Whistler** British Columbia, SW Canada
21 W8 **Whitakers** North Carolina, SE USA
14 H15 **Whitby** Ontario, S Canada
97 N15 **Whitby** N England, UK
10 G6 **White** ≈ Yukon Territory, W Canada
13 T11 **White Bay** bay Newfoundland, E Canada
20 I8 **White Bluff** Tennessee, S USA
28 J6 **White Butte** ▲ North Dakota, N USA
19 R5 **White Cap Mountain** ▲ Maine, N USA
22 J9 **White Castle** Louisiana, S USA
182 M5 **White Cliffs** New South Wales, SE Australia
31 P8 **White Cloud** Michigan, N USA
11 P14 **Whitecourt** Alberta, SW Canada
25 O2 **White Deer** Texas, SW USA
White Elster see Weisse Elster
24 M5 **Whiteface** Texas, SW USA
18 K7 **Whiteface Mountain** ▲ New York, NE USA
29 W5 **Whiteface Reservoir** ⊡ Minnesota, N USA
33 O7 **Whitefish** Montana, NW USA
31 N9 **Whitefish Bay** Wisconsin, N USA
31 Q3 **Whitefish Bay** lake bay Canada/USA
14 E11 **Whitefish Falls** Ontario, S Canada
14 B7 **Whitefish Lake** ◎ Ontario, S Canada
29 U6 **Whitefish Lake** ◎ Minnesota, C USA
31 Q3 **Whitefish Point** headland Michigan, N USA
31 O4 **Whitefish River** ≈ Michigan, N USA
25 O4 **Whiteflat** Texas, SW USA
27 V12 **White Hall** Arkansas, C USA
30 K14 **White Hall** Illinois, N USA
31 O8 **Whitehall** Michigan, N USA
18 L9 **Whitehall** New York, NE USA
31 S13 **Whitehall** Ohio, N USA
30 J7 **Whitehall** Wisconsin, N USA
97 J15 **Whitehaven** NW England, UK
10 I8 **Whitehorse** territory capital Yukon Territory, W Canada
184 O7 **White Island** island NE NZ
14 K13 **White Lake** ◎ Ontario, SE Canada
22 H10 **White Lake** ◎ Louisiana, S USA
186 G7 **Whiteman Range** ▲ New Britain, E PNG
183 Q15 **Whitemark** Tasmania, SE Australia
35 S9 **White Mountains** ▲ California/Nevada, W USA
19 N7 **White Mountains** ▲ Maine/New Hampshire, NE USA
80 F11 **White Nile** ◈ state C Sudan
67 U7 **White Nile** var. Bahr el Jebel. ≈ S Sudan
81 E14 **White Nile** Ar. Al Baḥr al Abyaḍ, An Nīl al Abyaḍ, Bahr el Jebel. ≈ SE Sudan
25 W5 **White Oak Creek** ≈ Texas, SW USA
10 H9 **White Pass** pass Canada/USA
32 I9 **White Pass** pass Washington, NW USA
21 O9 **White Pine** Tennessee, S USA
18 K14 **White Plains** New York, NE USA
25 O5 **White River** ≈ Texas, SW USA
28 M11 **White River** South Dakota, N USA
27 W12 **White River** ≈ Arkansas, SE USA
37 P3 **White River** ≈ Colorado/Utah, C USA
31 N15 **White River** ≈ Indiana, N USA
31 O8 **White River** ≈ Michigan, N USA
28 K11 **White River** ≈ South Dakota, N USA
18 M8 **White River** ≈ Vermont, NE USA
37 N13 **Whiteriver** Arizona, SW USA
25 O5 **White River Lake** ⊡ Texas, SW USA
32 H11 **White Salmon** Washington, NW USA
18 I10 **Whitesboro** New York, NE USA
25 T5 **Whitesboro** Texas, SW USA
21 O7 **Whitesburg** Kentucky, S USA
White Sea see Beloye More
White Sea-Baltic Canal/White Sea Canal see Belomorsko-Baltiyskiy Kanal
63 I25 **Whiteside, Canal** channel S Chile
33 S10 **White Sulphur Springs** Montana, NW USA
21 R6 **White Sulphur Springs** West Virginia, NE USA
20 J6 **Whitesville** Kentucky, S USA
32 I10 **White Swan** Washington, NW USA
21 U12 **Whiteville** North Carolina, SE USA
20 F10 **Whiteville** Tennessee, S USA
77 Q13 **White Volta** var. Nakambé, Fr. Volta Blanche. ≈ Burkina/Ghana
30 M9 **Whitewater** Wisconsin, N USA
37 P14 **Whitewater Baldy** ▲ New Mexico, SW USA
23 X17 **Whitewater Bay** bay Florida, SE USA
31 Q14 **Whitewater River** ≈ Indiana/Ohio, N USA
11 V16 **Whitewood** Saskatchewan, S Canada
28 J9 **Whitewood** South Dakota, N USA
25 U5 **Whitewright** Texas, SW USA
97 I15 **Whithorn** S Scotland, UK
184 M6 **Whitianga** Waikato, North Island, NZ
19 N11 **Whitinsville** Massachusetts, NE USA
20 M8 **Whitley City** Kentucky, S USA
21 Q11 **Whitmire** South Carolina, SE USA
31 R10 **Whitmore Lake** Michigan, N USA
195 N9 **Whitmore Mountains** ▲ Antarctica
14 I12 **Whitney** Ontario, SE Canada
25 T8 **Whitney** Texas, SW USA
25 S8 **Whitney, Lake** ⊡ Texas, SW USA
35 S11 **Whitney, Mount** ▲ California, W USA
181 Y6 **Whitsunday Group** island group Queensland, E Australia
25 S6 **Whitt** Texas, SW USA
29 U12 **Whittemore** Iowa, C USA
39 R12 **Whittier** Alaska, USA
35 T15 **Whittier** California, W USA
83 I25 **Whittlesea** Eastern Cape, S South Africa
20 K10 **Whitwell** Tennessee, S USA
8 L10 **Wholdaia Lake** ◎ Northwest Territories, NW Canada
182 H7 **Whyalla** South Australia
Whydah see Ouidah
14 F13 **Wiarton** Ontario, S Canada
171 O13 **Wiau** Sulawesi, C Indonesia
111 H15 **Wiązów** Ger. Wansen. Dolnośląskie, SW Poland
33 Y8 **Wibaux** Montana, NW USA
27 N6 **Wichita** Kansas, C USA
25 R5 **Wichita Falls** Texas, SW USA
26 L11 **Wichita Mountains** ▲ Oklahoma, C USA
25 R5 **Wichita River** ≈ Texas, SW USA
96 K6 **Wick** N Scotland, UK
36 K13 **Wickenburg** Arizona, SW USA
24 L8 **Wickett** Texas, SW USA
180 I7 **Wickham** Western Australia
182 M14 **Wickham, Cape** headland Tasmania, SE Australia
20 G7 **Wickliffe** Kentucky, S USA
97 G19 **Wicklow** Ir. Cill Mhantáin. E Ireland
97 F19 **Wicklow** Ir. Cill Mhantáin. cultural region E Ireland
97 G19 **Wicklow Head** Ir. Ceann Chill Mhantáin. headland E Ireland
97 F18 **Wicklow Mountains** Ir. Sléibhte Chill Mhantáin. ▲ E Ireland
14 H10 **Wicksteed Lake** ◎ Ontario, S Canada
Wida see Ouidah
65 G15 **Wideawake Airfield** ✈ (Georgetown) SW Ascension Island
97 K18 **Widnes** C England, UK
110 H9 **Więcbork** Ger. Vandsburg. Kujawsko-pomorskie, C Poland
101 E17 **Wied** ≈ W Germany
101 F16 **Wiehl** Nordrhein-Westfalen, W Germany
111 L17 **Wieliczka** Małopolskie, S Poland
110 G12 **Wielkopolskie** ◈ province C Poland
111 J14 **Wieluń** Sieradz, C Poland
109 X4 **Wien** Eng. Vienna, Hung. Bécs, Slvk. Vídeň, Slvn. Dunaj; anc. Vindobona. ● (Austria) Wien, NE Austria
109 X4 **Wien** off. Land Wien, Eng. Vienna. ◈ state NE Austria
109 X5 **Wiener Neustadt** Niederösterreich, E Austria
110 G7 **Wieprza** Ger. Wipper. ≈ NW Poland
98 O10 **Wierden** Overijssel, E Netherlands
98 I7 **Wieringerwerf** Noord-Holland, NW Netherlands
Wieruschow see Wieruszów
111 I14 **Wieruszów** Ger. Wieruschow. Łódzkie, C Poland
109 V9 **Wies** Steiermark, SE Austria
Wiesbachhorn see Grosses Wiesbachhorn
101 G18 **Wiesbaden** Hessen, W Germany
Wieselburg and Ungarisch-Altenburg/Wieselburg-Ungarisch-Altenburg see Mosonmagyaróvár
Wiesenhof see Ostrołęka
101 G20 **Wiesloch** Baden-Württemberg, SW Germany
100 F10 **Wiesmoor** Niedersachsen, NW Germany
110 I7 **Wieżyca** Ger. Turmberg. hill Pomorskie, N Poland
97 L17 **Wigan** NW England, UK
37 U3 **Wiggins** Colorado, C USA
22 M8 **Wiggins** Mississippi, S USA
Wigorna Ceaster see Worcester
97 I14 **Wigtown** S Scotland, UK
97 H14 **Wigtown** cultural region SW Scotland, UK
97 I15 **Wigtown Bay** bay SW Scotland, UK
98 L13 **Wijchen** Gelderland, SE Netherlands
92 N1 **Wijdefjorden** fjord NW Svalbard
98 M10 **Wijhe** Overijssel, E Netherlands
98 J12 **Wijk bij Duurstede** Utrecht, C Netherlands
98 J13 **Wijk en Aalburg** Noord-Brabant, S Netherlands
99 H16 **Wijnegem** Antwerpen, N Belgium
14 E11 **Wikwemikong** Manitoulin Island, Ontario, S Canada
108 H7 **Wil** Sankt Gallen, NE Switzerland
29 R16 **Wilber** Nebraska, C USA
32 K8 **Wilbur** Washington, NW USA
27 Q11 **Wilburton** Oklahoma, C USA
182 M6 **Wilcannia** New South Wales, SE Australia
18 D12 **Wilcox** Pennsylvania, NE USA
Wilczek Land see Vil'cheka, Zemlya
109 U6 **Wildalpen** Steiermark, E Austria
31 O13 **Wildcat Creek** ≈ Indiana, N USA
108 L9 **Wilde Kreuzspitze** It. Picco di Croce. ▲ Austria/Italy
Wildenschwert see Ústí nad Orlicí
98 O6 **Wildervank** Groningen, NE Netherlands
100 G11 **Wildeshausen** Niedersachsen, NW Germany
108 D10 **Wildhorn** ▲ SW Switzerland
11 R17 **Wild Horse** Alberta, SW Canada
27 N12 **Wildhorse Creek** ≈ Oklahoma, C USA
28 L14 **Wild Horse Hill** ▲ Nebraska, C USA
109 W8 **Wildon** Steiermark, SE Austria
24 M2 **Wildorado** Texas, SW USA
29 R6 **Wild Rice River** ≈ Minnesota/North Dakota, N USA
Wilejka see Vilyeyka
195 Y9 **Wilhelm II Coast** physical region Antarctica
195 X9 **Wilhelm II Land** physical region Antarctica
55 U11 **Wilhelmina Gebergte** ▲ C Suriname
18 B13 **Wilhelm, Lake** ⊡ Pennsylvania, NE USA
92 O2 **Wilhelmøya** island C Svalbard
Wilhelm-Pieck-Stadt see Guben
109 W4 **Wilhelmsburg** Niederösterreich, E Austria
100 G10 **Wilhelmshaven** Niedersachsen, NW Germany
Wilia/Wilja see Neris
18 H13 **Wilkes Barre** Pennsylvania, NE USA
21 R9 **Wilkesboro** North Carolina, SE USA
195 W15 **Wilkes Coast** physical region Antarctica
189 W12 **Wilkes Island** island N Wake Island
195 X12 **Wilkes Land** physical region Antarctica
11 S15 **Wilkie** Saskatchewan, S Canada
194 I6 **Wilkins Ice Shelf** ice shelf Antarctica
182 D4 **Wilkinsons Lakes** salt lake South Australia
Wiłkomierz see Ukmergė
182 K11 **Willalooka** South Australia
32 G11 **Willamette River** ≈ Oregon, NW USA
183 O8 **Willandra Billabong Creek** seasonal river New South Wales, SE Australia
32 F9 **Willapa Bay** inlet Washington, NW USA
27 T7 **Willard** Missouri, C USA
37 S12 **Willard** New Mexico, SW USA
31 S12 **Willard** Ohio, N USA
36 L1 **Willard** Utah, W USA
186 G6 **Willaumez Peninsula** headland New Britain, E PNG
37 N15 **Willcox** Arizona, SW USA
37 N16 **Willcox Playa** salt flat Arizona, SW USA
99 G17 **Willebroek** Antwerpen, C Belgium
45 P16 **Willemstad** ○ (Netherlands Antilles) Curaçao, Netherlands Antilles
99 G14 **Willemstad** Noord-Brabant, S Netherlands
11 S11 **William** ≈ Saskatchewan, C Canada
23 O6 **William "Bill" Dannelly Reservoir** ⊡ Alabama, S USA
182 G3 **William Creek** South Australia
181 T15 **William, Mount** ▲ South Australia
36 K11 **Williams** Arizona, SW USA
29 X14 **Williamsburg** Iowa, C USA
20 M8 **Williamsburg** Kentucky, S USA

◆ Country ● Country Capital ◇ Dependent Territory ○ Dependent Territory Capital ◈ Administrative Region ✈ International Airport ▲ Mountain ▲ Mountain Range ※ Volcano ≈ River ◎ Lake ⊡ Reservoir

31 R15 **Williamsburg** Ohio, N USA
21 X6 **Williamsburg** Virginia, NE USA
10 M15 **Williams Lake** British Columbia, SW Canada
21 P6 **Williamson** West Virginia, NE USA
31 N13 **Williamsport** Indiana, N USA
18 G13 **Williamsport** Pennsylvania, NE USA
21 W9 **Williamston** North Carolina, SE USA
21 P11 **Williamston** South Carolina, SE USA
20 M4 **Williamstown** Kentucky, S USA
18 L10 **Williamstown** Massachusetts, NE USA
18 J16 **Willingboro** New Jersey, NE USA
11 Q14 **Willingdon** Alberta, SW Canada
25 W10 **Willis** Texas, SW USA
108 F8 **Willisau** Luzern, W Switzerland
83 F24 **Williston** Northern Cape, W South Africa
23 V10 **Williston** Florida, SE USA
28 J3 **Williston** North Dakota, N USA
21 Q13 **Williston** South Carolina, SE USA
10 L12 **Williston Lake** ⊠ British Columbia, W Canada
34 L5 **Willits** California, W USA
29 T8 **Willmar** Minnesota, N USA
10 K11 **Will, Mount** ▲ British Columbia, W Canada
31 T11 **Willoughby** Ohio, N USA
11 U17 **Willow Bunch** Saskatchewan, S Canada
32 J11 **Willow Creek** ~ Oregon, NW USA
39 R11 **Willow Lake** Alaska, USA
8 I9 **Willowlake** ~ Northwest Territories, NW Canada
83 H25 **Willowmore** Eastern Cape, S South Africa
30 L5 **Willow Reservoir** ⊠ Wisconsin, N USA
35 N5 **Willows** California, W USA
27 V7 **Willow Springs** Missouri, C USA
182 I7 **Wilmington** South Australia
21 Y2 **Wilmington** Delaware, NE USA
21 V12 **Wilmington** North Carolina, SE USA
31 R14 **Wilmington** Ohio, N USA
20 M6 **Wilmore** Kentucky, S USA
29 R8 **Wilmot** South Dakota, N USA
Wilna/Wilno *see* Vilnius
101 G16 **Wilnsdorf** Nordrhein-Westfalen, W Germany
99 G16 **Wilrijk** Antwerpen, N Belgium
100 I10 **Wilseder Berg** *hill* NW Germany
67 Z12 **Wilshaw Ridge** *undersea feature* W Indian Ocean
21 V9 **Wilson** North Carolina, SE USA
25 N5 **Wilson** Texas, SW USA
182 A7 **Wilson Bluff** *headland* South Australia/Western Australia
35 Y7 **Wilson Creek Range** ▲ Nevada, W USA
23 O1 **Wilson Lake** ⊠ Alabama, S USA
26 M4 **Wilson Lake** ⊠ Kansas, SE USA
37 P7 **Wilson, Mount** ▲ Colorado, C USA
183 P13 **Wilsons Promontory** *peninsula* Victoria, SE Australia
29 Y14 **Wilton** Iowa, C USA
19 P7 **Wilton** Maine, NE USA
28 M5 **Wilton** North Dakota, N USA
97 L22 **Wiltshire** *cultural region* S England, UK
99 M23 **Wiltz** Diekirch, NW Luxembourg
180 K9 **Wiluna** Western Australia
99 M23 **Wilwerwiltz** Diekirch, NE Luxembourg
29 P5 **Wimbledon** North Dakota, N USA
42 K7 **Wina** *var.* Güina. Jinotega, N Nicaragua
31 O12 **Winamac** Indiana, N USA
81 G19 **Winam Gulf** *var.* Kavirondo Gulf. *gulf* SW Kenya
83 I22 **Winburg** Free State, C South Africa
19 N10 **Winchendon** Massachusetts, NE USA
14 M13 **Winchester** Ontario, SE Canada
97 M23 **Winchester** *hist.* Wintanceaster, *Lat.* Venta Belgarum. S England, UK
32 M10 **Winchester** Idaho, NW USA
30 J14 **Winchester** Illinois, N USA
31 Q13 **Winchester** Indiana, N USA
20 M5 **Winchester** Kentucky, S USA
18 M10 **Winchester** New Hampshire, NE USA
20 K10 **Winchester** Tennessee, S USA
21 V3 **Winchester** Virginia, NE USA
99 L22 **Wincrange** Diekirch, NW Luxembourg
10 I5 **Wind** ~ Yukon Territory, NW Canada
183 S8 **Windamere, Lake** ◎ New South Wales, SE Australia
Windau *see* Ventspils, Latvia
Windau *see* Venta, Latvia/Lithuania
18 D15 **Windber** Pennsylvania, NE USA
23 T3 **Winder** Georgia, SE USA
97 K15 **Windermere** NW England, UK
14 C7 **Windermere Lake** ◎ Ontario, S Canada
31 U11 **Windham** Ohio, N USA
83 D19 **Windhoek** *Ger.* Windhuk. ● (Namibia) Khomas, C Namibia
83 D20 **Windhoek** × Khomas, C Namibia
Windhuk *see* Windhoek
15 O8 **Windigo** Quebec, SE Canada
15 O8 **Windigo** ~ Quebec, SE Canada
Windischfeistritz *see* Slovenska Bistrica
109 T6 **Windischgarsten** Oberösterreich, W Austria
Windischgraz *see* Slovenj Gradec
37 T16 **Wind Mountain** ▲ New Mexico, SW USA
29 T10 **Windom** Minnesota, N USA
37 Q7 **Windom Peak** ▲ Colorado, C USA
181 U9 **Windorah** Queensland, C Australia
37 O10 **Window Rock** Arizona, SW USA
31 N9 **Wind Point** *headland* Wisconsin, N USA
33 U14 **Wind River** ~ Wyoming, C USA
13 P15 **Windsor** Nova Scotia, SE Canada
14 C17 **Windsor** Ontario, S Canada
15 Q12 **Windsor** Quebec, SE Canada
97 N22 **Windsor** S England, UK
37 T3 **Windsor** Colorado, C USA
18 M12 **Windsor** Connecticut, NE USA
27 T5 **Windsor** Missouri, C USA
21 X9 **Windsor** North Carolina, SE USA
18 M12 **Windsor Locks** Connecticut, NE USA
25 R5 **Windthorst** Texas, SW USA
45 Z14 **Windward Islands** *island group* E West Indies
Windward Islands *see* Vent, Îles du, Archipel de la Société, French Polynesia
Windward Islands *see* Barlavento, Ilhas de, Cape Verde
44 K8 **Windward Passage** *Sp.* Paso de los Vientos. *channel* Cuba/Haiti
55 T9 **Wineperu** C Guyana
23 O3 **Winfield** Alabama, S USA
29 Y15 **Winfield** Iowa, C USA
27 O7 **Winfield** Kansas, C USA
25 W6 **Winfield** Texas, SW USA
21 Q4 **Winfield** West Virginia, NE USA
29 N5 **Wing** North Dakota, N USA
183 U7 **Wingham** New South Wales, SE Australia
12 G16 **Wingham** Ontario, S Canada
33 T8 **Winifred** Montana, NW USA
12 E8 **Winisk** ~ Ontario, S Canada
12 E9 **Winisk Lake** ◎ Ontario, C Canada
24 L8 **Wink** Texas, SW USA
36 M14 **Winkelman** Arizona, SW USA
11 X17 **Winkler** Manitoba, S Canada
109 Q9 **Winklern** Tirol, W Austria
Winkowitz *see* Vinkovci
32 G9 **Winlock** Washington, NW USA
77 P17 **Winneba** SE Ghana
29 U11 **Winnebago** Minnesota, N USA
29 R13 **Winnebago** Nebraska, C USA
30 M7 **Winnebago, Lake** ◎ Wisconsin, N USA
30 M7 **Winneconne** Wisconsin, N USA
35 T3 **Winnemucca** Nevada, W USA
35 R4 **Winnemucca Lake** ◎ Nevada, W USA
101 H21 **Winnenden** Baden-Württemberg, SW Germany
29 N11 **Winner** South Dakota, N USA
33 U9 **Winnett** Montana, NW USA
14 I9 **Winneway** Quebec, SE Canada
22 H6 **Winnfield** Louisiana, S USA
29 U4 **Winnibigoshish, Lake** ◎ Minnesota, N USA
25 X11 **Winnie** Texas, SW USA
11 Y16 **Winnipeg** Manitoba, S Canada
11 X16 **Winnipeg** × Manitoba, S Canada
(0) J8 **Winnipeg** ~ Manitoba, S Canada
11 X16 **Winnipeg Beach** Manitoba, S Canada
11 W14 **Winnipeg, Lake** ◎ Manitoba, C Canada
11 W15 **Winnipegosis** Manitoba, S Canada
11 W15 **Winnipegosis, Lake** ◎ Manitoba, C Canada
19 O8 **Winnipesaukee, Lake** ◎ New Hampshire, NE USA
22 J6 **Winnsboro** Louisiana, S USA
21 R12 **Winnsboro** South Carolina, SE USA
25 W6 **Winnsboro** Texas, SW USA
29 X10 **Winona** Minnesota, N USA
22 L4 **Winona** Mississippi, S USA
27 W7 **Winona** Missouri, C USA
25 W7 **Winona** Texas, SW USA
18 M7 **Winooski River** ~ Vermont, NE USA
98 P6 **Winschoten** Groningen, NE Netherlands
100 J10 **Winsen** Niedersachsen, N Germany
36 M11 **Winslow** Arizona, SW USA
19 Q7 **Winslow** Maine, NE USA
18 M12 **Winsted** Connecticut, NE USA
32 F14 **Winston** Oregon, NW USA
21 S9 **Winston Salem** North Carolina, SE USA
98 N5 **Winsum** Groningen, NE Netherlands
Wintanceaster *see* Winchester
23 W11 **Winter Garden** Florida, SE USA
10 J16 **Winter Harbour** Vancouver Island, British Columbia, SW Canada
23 W12 **Winter Haven** Florida, SE USA
23 X11 **Winter Park** Florida, SE USA
25 P8 **Winters** Texas, SW USA
29 U15 **Winterset** Iowa, C USA
98 O12 **Winterswijk** Gelderland, E Netherlands
108 G6 **Winterthur** Zürich, NE Switzerland
29 U9 **Winthrop** Minnesota, N USA
32 J7 **Winthrop** Washington, NW USA
181 V7 **Winton** Queensland, E Australia
185 C24 **Winton** Southland, South Island, NZ
21 X8 **Winton** North Carolina, SE USA
101 K15 **Wipper** ~ C Germany
101 K14 **Wipper** ~ C Germany
Wipper *see* Wieprza
182 G6 **Wirraminna** South Australia
182 F4 **Wirrida** South Australia
182 F7 **Wirrulla** South Australia
Wirsitz *see* Wyrzysk
Wirz-See *see* Võrtsjärv
97 O19 **Wisbech** E England, UK
Wisby *see* Visby
19 Q8 **Wiscasset** Maine, NE USA
Wischau *see* Vyškov
30 J5 **Wisconsin** *off.* State of Wisconsin; also known as The Badger State. ◆ *state* N USA
30 L8 **Wisconsin Dells** Wisconsin, N USA
30 L8 **Wisconsin, Lake** ⊠ Wisconsin, N USA
30 L7 **Wisconsin Rapids** Wisconsin, N USA
30 L7 **Wisconsin River** ~ Wisconsin, N USA
33 P11 **Wisdom** Montana, NW USA
21 P7 **Wise** Virginia, NE USA
39 Q7 **Wiseman** Alaska, USA
96 J12 **Wishaw** W Scotland, UK
29 O6 **Wishek** North Dakota, N USA
32 I11 **Wishram** Washington, NW USA
111 J17 **Wisła** Śląskie, S Poland
110 K11 **Wisła** *Eng.* Vistula, *Ger.* Weichsel. ~ C Poland
Wiślany, Zalew *see* Vistula Lagoon
111 M16 **Wisłoka** ~ SE Poland
100 L9 **Wismar** Mecklenburg-Vorpommern, N Germany
29 R14 **Wisner** Nebraska, C USA
103 V4 **Wissembourg** *var.* Weissenburg. Bas-Rhin, NE France
30 J6 **Wissota, Lake** ⊠ Wisconsin, N USA
97 O18 **Witham** ~ E England, UK
97 O17 **Withernsea** E England, UK
37 Q13 **Withington, Mount** ▲ New Mexico, SW USA
23 U8 **Withlacoochee River** ~ Florida/Georgia, SE USA
110 H11 **Witkowo** Wielkopolskie, C Poland
97 M21 **Witney** S England, UK
101 E15 **Witten** Nordrhein-Westfalen, W Germany
101 N14 **Wittenberg** Sachsen-Anhalt, E Germany
30 L6 **Wittenberg** Wisconsin, N USA
100 L11 **Wittenberge** Brandenburg, N Germany
103 U7 **Wittenheim** Haut-Rhin, NE France
180 I7 **Wittenoom** Western Australia
Wittingau *see* Třeboň
100 K12 **Wittingen** Niedersachsen, C Germany
101 E18 **Wittlich** Rheinland-Pfalz, SW Germany
100 F9 **Wittmund** Niedersachsen, NW Germany
100 M10 **Wittstock** Brandenburg, NE Germany
186 F6 **Witu Islands** *island group* E PNG
110 O7 **Wiżajny** Podlaskie, NE Poland
55 W10 **W.J. van Blommesteinmeer** ⊠ E Suriname
110 L11 **Wkra** *Ger.* Soldau. ~ C Poland
110 I6 **Władysławowo** Pomorskie, N Poland
Wlaschim *see* Vlašim
111 E14 **Wleń** *Ger.* Lähn. Dolnośląskie, SW Poland
110 J11 **Włocławek** *Ger./Rus.* Vlotslavsk. Kujawsko-pomorskie, C Poland
110 P13 **Włodawa** *Rus.* Vlodava. Lubelskie, SE Poland
Włodzimierz *see* Volodymyr-Volyns'kyy
111 K15 **Włoszczowa** Świętokrzyskie, C Poland
83 C19 **Wlotzkasbaken** Erongo, W Namibia
146 L11 **Wobkent** *Rus.* Vabkent. Bukhoro Wiloyati, C Uzbekistan
15 R12 **Woburn** Quebec, SE Canada
19 O11 **Woburn** Massachusetts, NE USA
Wocheiner Feistritz *see* Bohinjska Bistrica
Wöchma *see* Võhma
147 S11 **Wodil** *var.* Vuadil'. Farghona Wiloyati, E Uzbekistan
181 V14 **Wodonga** Victoria, SE Australia
111 I17 **Wodzisław Śląski** *Ger.* Loslau. Śląskie, S Poland
98 I11 **Woerden** Zuid-Holland, C Netherlands
98 I8 **Wognum** Noord-Holland, NW Netherlands
Wohlau *see* Wołów
108 F7 **Wohlen** Aargau, NW Switzerland
195 R2 **Wohlthat Mountains** ▲ Antarctica
Wōjjā *see* Wotje Atoll
Wojwodina *see* Vojvodina
171 V15 **Wokam, Pulau** *island* Kepulauan Aru, E Indonesia
97 N22 **Woking** SE England, UK
Woldenberg Neumark *see* Dobiegniew
188 K15 **Woleai Atoll** *atoll* Caroline Islands, W Micronesia
Woleu *see* Uolo, Río
79 E17 **Woleu-Ntem** *off.* Province du Woleu-Ntem, *var.* Le Woleu-Ntem. ◆ *province* W Gabon
32 F15 **Wolf Creek** Oregon, NW USA
26 K9 **Wolf Creek** ~ Oklahoma/Texas, SW USA
37 R7 **Wolf Creek Pass** *pass* Colorado, C USA
19 O9 **Wolfeboro** New Hampshire, NE USA
25 U5 **Wolfe City** Texas, SW USA
14 L15 **Wolfe Island** *island* Ontario, SE Canada
101 M14 **Wolfen** Sachsen-Anhalt, E Germany
100 J13 **Wolfenbüttel** Niedersachsen, C Germany
109 T4 **Wolfern** Oberösterreich, N Austria
109 Q6 **Wolfgangsee** *var.* Abersee, St Wolfgangsee. ◎ N Austria
39 P9 **Wolf Mountain** ▲ Alaska, USA
33 X7 **Wolf Point** Montana, NW USA
22 L8 **Wolf River** ~ Mississippi, S USA
30 M7 **Wolf River** ~ Wisconsin, N USA
109 U9 **Wolfsberg** Kärnten, SE Austria
100 K12 **Wolfsburg** Niedersachsen, N Germany
57 B17 **Wolf, Volcán** ✱ Galapagos Islands, Ecuador, E Pacific Ocean
100 O8 **Wolgast** Mecklenburg-Vorpommern, NE Germany
108 F8 **Wolhusen** Luzern, W Switzerland
110 D8 **Wolin** *Ger.* Wollin. Zachodniopomorskie, NW Poland
109 Y3 **Wolkersdorf** Niederösterreich, NE Austria
Wołkowysk *see* Vawkavysk
Wöllan *see* Velenje
8 J6 **Wollaston, Cape** *headland* Victoria Island, Northwest Territories, NW Canada
63 J25 **Wollaston, Isla** *island* S Chile
11 U11 **Wollaston Lake** Saskatchewan, C Canada
11 T10 **Wollaston Lake** ◎ Saskatchewan, C Canada
8 J6 **Wollaston Peninsula** *peninsula* Victoria Island, Northwest Territories/Nunavut, NW Canada
Wollin *see* Wolin
183 S9 **Wollongong** New South Wales, SE Australia
Wolmar *see* Valmiera
100 L13 **Wolmirstedt** Sachsen-Anhalt, C Germany
110 M11 **Wołomin** Mazowieckie, C Poland
110 G13 **Wołów** *Ger.* Wohlau. Dolnośląskie, SW Poland
Wołożyn *see* Valozhyn
14 G11 **Wolseley Bay** Ontario, S Canada
29 P10 **Wolsey** South Dakota, N USA
110 F12 **Wolsztyn** Wielkopolskie, W Poland
98 M7 **Wolvega** *Fris.* Wolvegea. Friesland, N Netherlands
Wolvegea *see* Wolvega
97 K19 **Wolverhampton** C England, UK
Wolverine State *see* Michigan
99 G18 **Wolvertem** Vlaams Brabant, C Belgium
99 H16 **Wommelgem** Antwerpen, N Belgium
186 D7 **Wonenara** *var.* Wonerara. Eastern Highlands, C PNG
Wonerara *see* Wonenara
Wongalara Lake *see* Wongalarroo Lake
183 N6 **Wongalarroo Lake** *var.* Wongalara Lake. *seasonal lake* New South Wales, SE Australia
163 Y15 **Wŏnju** *Jap.* Genshū. N South Korea
10 M12 **Wonowon** British Columbia, W Canada
163 X13 **Wŏnsan** SE North Korea
183 O13 **Wonthaggi** Victoria, SE Australia
23 N2 **Woodall Mountain** ▲ Mississippi, S USA
23 W7 **Woodbine** Georgia, SE USA
29 S14 **Woodbine** Iowa, C USA
18 J17 **Woodbine** New Jersey, NE USA
21 W4 **Woodbridge** Virginia, NE USA
183 V4 **Woodburn** New South Wales, SE Australia
32 G11 **Woodburn** Oregon, NW USA
20 K9 **Woodbury** Tennessee, S USA
183 V5 **Wooded Bluff** *headland* New South Wales, SE Australia
183 V3 **Woodenbong** New South Wales, SE Australia
35 R11 **Woodlake** California, W USA
35 N7 **Woodland** California, W USA
19 T5 **Woodland** Maine, NE USA
32 G10 **Woodland** Washington, NW USA
37 T5 **Woodland Park** Colorado, C USA
186 I9 **Woodlark Island** *var.* Murua Island. *island* SE PNG
Woodle Island *see* Kuria
11 T17 **Wood Mountain** ▲ Saskatchewan, S Canada
30 K15 **Wood River** Illinois, N USA
29 P16 **Wood River** Nebraska, C USA
39 R9 **Wood River** ~ Alaska, USA
39 O13 **Wood River Lakes** *lakes* Alaska, USA
182 C1 **Woodroffe, Mount** ▲ South Australia
21 P11 **Woodruff** South Carolina, SE USA
30 K4 **Woodruff** Wisconsin, N USA
25 T14 **Woodsboro** Texas, SW USA
31 U13 **Woodsfield** Ohio, N USA
181 P4 **Woods, Lake** ◎ Northern Territory, N Australia
11 Z16 **Woods, Lake of the** *Fr.* Lac des Bois. ◎ Canada/USA
25 Q6 **Woodson** Texas, SW USA
13 N14 **Woodstock** New Brunswick, SE Canada
14 F16 **Woodstock** Ontario, S Canada
30 M10 **Woodstock** Illinois, N USA
18 M9 **Woodstock** Vermont, NE USA
21 U4 **Woodstock** Virginia, NE USA
19 N8 **Woodsville** New Hampshire, NE USA
184 M12 **Woodville** Manawatu-Wanganui, North Island, NZ
22 J7 **Woodville** Mississippi, S USA
25 X9 **Woodville** Texas, SW USA
26 K9 **Woodward** Oklahoma, C USA
29 O5 **Woodworth** North Dakota, N USA
171 W12 **Wool** Irian Jaya, E Indonesia
183 V5 **Woolgoolga** New South Wales, E Australia
182 H6 **Woomera** South Australia
19 O12 **Woonsocket** Rhode Island, NE USA
29 P10 **Woonsocket** South Dakota, N USA
31 T12 **Wooster** Ohio, N USA
80 L12 **Woqooyi Galbeed** *off.* Gobolka Woqooyi Galbeed. ◆ *region* NW Somalia
108 E8 **Worb** Bern, C Switzerland
83 F26 **Worcester** Western Cape, SW South Africa
97 L20 **Worcester** *hist.* Wigorna Ceaster. W England, UK
19 N11 **Worcester** Massachusetts, NE USA
97 L20 **Worcestershire** *cultural region* C England, UK
32 H16 **Worden** Oregon, NW USA
109 O6 **Wörgl** Tirol, W Austria
171 V15 **Workai, Pulau** *island* Kepulauan Aru, E Indonesia
97 J15 **Workington** NW England, UK
98 K7 **Workum** Friesland, N Netherlands
33 V13 **Worland** Wyoming, C USA
Wormatia *see* Worms
99 N25 **Wormeldange** Grevenmacher, E Luxembourg
98 I9 **Wormer** Noord-Holland, C Netherlands
101 G19 **Worms** *anc.* Augusta Vangionum, Borbetomagus, Wormatia. Rheinland-Pfalz, SW Germany
Worms *see* Vormsi
101 K21 **Wörnitz** ~ S Germany
101 G21 **Wörth** Rheinland-Pfalz, SW Germany
25 U8 **Wortham** Texas, SW USA
109 S9 **Worther See** ◎ S Austria
97 O23 **Worthing** SE England, UK
29 S11 **Worthington** Minnesota, N USA
31 S13 **Worthington** Ohio, N USA
35 W8 **Worthington Peak** ▲ Nevada, W USA
171 Y13 **Wosi** Irian Jaya, E Indonesia
171 V13 **Wosimi** Irian Jaya, E Indonesia
189 R5 **Wotho Atoll** *var.* Wōtto. *atoll* Ralik Chain, W Marshall Islands
189 V5 **Wotje Atoll** *var.* Wōjjā. *atoll* Ratak Chain, E Marshall Islands
Wotoe *see* Wotu
Wottawa *see* Otava
Wōtto *see* Wotho Atoll
171 O13 **Wotu** *prev.* Wotoe. Sulawesi, C Indonesia
98 K11 **Woudenberg** Utrecht, C Netherlands
98 I13 **Woudrichem** Noord-Brabant, S Netherlands
43 N8 **Wounta** *var.* Huaunta. Región Autónoma Atlántico Norte, NE Nicaragua
171 P14 **Wowoni, Pulau** *island* C Indonesia
81 J17 **Woyamdero Plain** *plain* E Kenya
Woyens *see* Vojens
Wozrojdeniye Oroli *see* Vozrozhdeniya, Ostrov
Wrangel Island *see* Vrangelya, Ostrov
39 Y13 **Wrangell** Wrangell Island, Alaska, USA
38 C15 **Wrangell, Cape** *headland* Attu Island, Alaska, USA
39 S11 **Wrangell, Mount** ▲ Alaska, USA
39 T11 **Wrangell Mountains** ▲ Alaska, USA
197 S7 **Wrangel Plain** *undersea feature* Arctic Ocean
96 H6 **Wrath, Cape** *headland* N Scotland, UK
37 W3 **Wray** Colorado, C USA
44 K13 **Wreck Point** *headland* C Jamaica
83 C23 **Wreck Point** *headland* W South Africa
23 V4 **Wrens** Georgia, SE USA
97 K18 **Wrexham** NE Wales, UK
27 R13 **Wright City** Oklahoma, C USA
194 J12 **Wright Island** *island* Antarctica
13 N9 **Wright, Mont** ▲ Quebec, E Canada
25 X5 **Wright Patman Lake** ⊠ Texas, SW USA
36 M16 **Wrightson, Mount** ▲ Arizona, SW USA
23 U5 **Wrightsville** Georgia, SE USA
21 W12 **Wrightsville Beach** North Carolina, SE USA
35 T15 **Wrightwood** California, W USA
8 H9 **Wrigley** Northwest Territories, W Canada
111 G14 **Wrocław** *Eng./Ger.* Breslau. Dolnośląskie, SW Poland
110 F10 **Wronki** *Ger.* Fronicken. Wielkopolskie, NW Poland
110 H11 **Września** Wielkolpolskie, C Poland
110 F12 **Wschowa** Lubuskie, W Poland
Wsetin *see* Vsetín
180 I12 **Wubin** Western Australia
163 W9 **Wuchang** Heilongjiang, NE China
Wuchang *see* Wuhan
Wu-chou/Wuchow *see* Wuzhou
160 M16 **Wuchuan** *var.* Meilu. Guangdong, S China
160 K10 **Wuchuan** *prev.* Duru. Guizhou, S China
163 O13 **Wuchuan** Nei Mongol Zizhiqu, N China
163 V6 **Wudalianchi** Heilongjiang, NE China
159 O11 **Wudaoliang** Qinghai, C China
141 Q13 **Wuday'ah** *spring/well* S Saudi Arabia
77 V13 **Wudil** Kano, N Nigeria
160 G12 **Wuding** Yunnan, SW China
160 L4 **Wuding He** ~ C China
182 G8 **Wudinna** South Australia
157 P10 **Wudu** Gansu, C China
160 L9 **Wufeng** Hubei, C China
161 O11 **Wugong Shan** ▲ S China
157 P7 **Wuhai** Nei Mongol Zizhiqu, N China
161 O9 **Wuhan** *var.* Han-kou, Han-k'ou, Hanyang, Wuchang, Wu-han; *prev.* Hankow. Hubei, C China
161 Q7 **Wuhe** Anhui, E China
Wuhsi/Wu-hsi *see* Wuxi
Wuhsien *see* Suzhou
161 Q8 **Wuhu** *var.* Wu-na-mu. Anhui, E China
Wūjae *see* Ujae Atoll
160 K11 **Wu Jiang** ~ C China
Wujlān *see* Ujelang Atoll
77 W15 **Wukari** Taraba, E Nigeria
160 H11 **Wulian Feng** ▲ SW China
160 F13 **Wuliang Shan** ▲ SW China
160 K11 **Wuling Shan** ▲ S China
109 Y5 **Wulka** ~ E Austria
Wulkan *see* Vulcan
109 T3 **Wullowitz** Oberösterreich, N Austria
Wu-lu-k'o-mu-shi/Wu-lu-mu-ch'i *see* Ürümqi
79 D14 **Wum** Nord-Ouest, NE Cameroon
160 H12 **Wumeng Shan** ▲ SW China
160 K14 **Wuming** Guangxi Zhuangzu Zizhiqu, S China
100 I10 **Wümme** ~ NW Germany
Wu-na-mu *see* Wuhu
171 X13 **Wunen** Irian Jaya, E Indonesia
12 D9 **Wunnummin Lake** ◎ Ontario, C Canada
80 D13 **Wun Rog** Warab, S Sudan
101 M18 **Wunsiedel** Bayern, E Germany
100 I12 **Wunstorf** Niedersachsen, NW Germany
166 M3 **Wuntho** Sagaing, N Burma
101 F15 **Wupper** ~ W Germany
101 E15 **Wuppertal** *prev.* Barmen-Elberfeld. Nordrhein-Westfalen, W Germany
160 K5 **Wuqi** Shaanxi, C China
161 P4 **Wuqiao** *var.* Sangyuan. Hebei, E China
101 L23 **Würm** ~ SE Germany
77 T12 **Wurno** Sokoto, NW Nigeria
101 I19 **Würzburg** Bayern, SW Germany
101 N15 **Wurzen** Sachsen, E Germany
160 L9 **Wu Shan** ▲ C China
158 G7 **Wushi** *var.* Uqturpan. Xinjiang Uygur Zizhiqu, NW China
Wusih *see* Wuxi
65 N18 **Wüst Seamount** *undersea feature* S Atlantic Ocean
Wusuli Jiang/Wusuri *see* Ussuri
161 N3 **Wutai Shan** ▲ C China
160 H10 **Wutongqiao** Sichuan, C China
159 P6 **Wutongwozi Quan** *spring* NW China
99 H15 **Wuustwezel** Antwerpen, N Belgium
186 B4 **Wuvulu Island** *island* NW PNG
159 U9 **Wuwei** *var.* Liangzhou. Gansu, C China
161 R8 **Wuxi** *var.* Wuhsi, Wu-hsi, Wusih. Jiangsu, E China
Wuxing *see* Huzhou
160 L14 **Wuxuan** Guangxi Zhuangzu Zizhiqu, S China
160 K11 **Wuyang He** ~ S China
163 X6 **Wuyiling** Heilongjiang, NE China
157 T12 **Wuyi Shan** ▲ SE China
161 Q11 **Wuyishan** *prev.* Chong'an. Fujian, SE China
162 M13 **Wuyuan** Nei Mongol Zizhiqu, N China
160 L17 **Wuzhi Shan** ▲ S China
159 W8 **Wuzhong** Ningxia, N China
160 M14 **Wuzhou** *var.* Wu-chou, Wuchow. Guangxi Zhuangzu Zizhiqu, S China
18 H12 **Wyalusing** Pennsylvania, NE USA
182 M10 **Wycheproof** Victoria, SE Australia
97 K21 **Wye** *Wel.* Gwy. ~ England/Wales, UK
Wyłkowyszki *see* Vilkaviškis
97 P19 **Wymondham** E England, UK
29 R17 **Wymore** Nebraska, C USA
182 E5 **Wynbring** South Australia
181 N3 **Wyndham** Western Australia
29 R6 **Wyndmere** North Dakota, N USA
27 X11 **Wynne** Arkansas, C USA
27 N12 **Wynnewood** Oklahoma, C USA
183 O15 **Wynyard** Tasmania, SE Australia
11 U15 **Wynyard** Saskatchewan, S Canada
33 V11 **Wyola** Montana, NW USA
182 A4 **Wyola Lake** *salt lake* South Australia
31 P9 **Wyoming** Michigan, N USA
33 V14 **Wyoming** *off.* State of Wyoming; also known as The Equality State. ◆ *state* C USA
33 S15 **Wyoming Range** ▲ Wyoming, C USA
183 T8 **Wyong** New South Wales, SE Australia
110 G9 **Wyrzysk** *Ger.* Wirsitz. Wielkopolskie, C Poland
Wysg *see* Usk
110 O10 **Wysokie Mazowieckie** Łomża, E Poland
110 M11 **Wyszków** *Ger.* Probstberg. Mazowieckie, C Poland

◆ Country ● Country Capital ◇ Dependent Territory ○ Dependent Territory Capital ◆ Administrative Region × International Airport ▲ Mountain ▲ Mountain Range ✱ Volcano ~ River ◎ Lake ⊠ Reservoir

110 L11 **Wyszogród** Mazowieckie, C Poland
21 R7 **Wytheville** Virginia, NE USA

X

80 Q12 **Xaafuun** *It.* Hafun. Bari, NE Somalia
80 Q12 **Xaafuun, Raas** *var.* Ras Hafun. *headland* NE Somalia
Xábia *see* Jávea
42 C4 **Xaclbal, Río** *var.* Xalbal. ≈ Guatemala/Mexico
137 Y10 **Xaçmaz** *Rus.* Khachmas. N Azerbaijan
80 O12 **Xadeed** *var.* Haded. *physical region* N Somalia
159 O14 **Xagquka** Xizang Zizhiqu, W China
167 Q6 **Xai** *var.* Muang Xay, Muong Sai. Oudômxai, N Laos
158 F10 **Xaidulla** Xinjiang Uygur Zizhiqu, W China
167 Q7 **Xaignabouli** *prev.* Muang Xaignabouri, *Fr.* Sayaboury. Xaignabouli, N Laos
167 R7 **Xai Lai Leng, Phou** ▲ Laos/Vietnam
158 L15 **Xainza** Xizang Zizhiqu, W China
158 L16 **Xaitongmoin** Xizang Zizhiqu, W China
83 M20 **Xai-Xai** *prev.* João Belo, Vila de João Bel. Gaza, S Mozambique
Xalbal *see* Xaclbal, Río
80 P13 **Xalin** Nugaal, N Somalia
167 R6 **Xam Nua** *var.* Sam Neua. Houaphan, N Laos
82 D11 **Xá-Muteba** *Port.* Cinco de Outubro. Lunda Norte, NE Angola
83 C16 **Xangongo** *Port.* Rocadas. Cunene, SW Angola
137 W12 **Xankändi** *Rus.* Khankendi; *prev.* Stepanakert. SW Azerbaijan
137 V11 **Xanlar** *Rus.* Khanlar. NW Azerbaijan
114 J13 **Xánthi** Anatolikí Makedonía kai Thráki, NE Greece
60 H13 **Xanxerê** Santa Catarina, S Brazil
81 O15 **Xarardheere** Mudug, E Somalia
131 W8 **Xar Moron** ≈ NE China
Xarra *see* Xarrë
113 L23 **Xarrë** *var.* Xarra. Vlorë, S Albania
82 D12 **Xassengue** Lunda Sul, NW Angola
105 S11 **Xátiva** *var.* Jativa; *anc.* Setabis. País Valenciano, E Spain
Xauen *see* Chefchaouen
60 K10 **Xavantes, Represa de** *var.* Represa de Chavantes. ⊞ S Brazil
158 I7 **Xayar** Xinjiang Uygur Zizhiqu, W China
Xäzär Dänizi *see* Caspian Sea
167 S8 **Xé Bangfai** ≈ C Laos
167 T9 **Xé Banghiang** *var.* Bang Hieng. ≈ S Laos
Xégar *see* Tingri
31 R14 **Xenia** Ohio, N USA
Xeres *see* Jeréz de la Frontera
115 E15 **Xeriás** ≈ C Greece
115 G17 **Xeró** ▲ Évvoia, C Greece
83 H18 **Xhumo** Central, C Botswana
161 N15 **Xiachuan Dao** *island* S China
Xiacun *see* Rushan
Xiaguan *see* Dali
159 U11 **Xiahe** *var.* Labrang. Gansu, C China
161 Q13 **Xiamen** *var.* Hsia-men; *prev.* Amoy. Fujian, SE China
160 L6 **Xi'an** *var.* Changan, Sian, Signan, Siking, Singan, Xian. Shaanxi, C China
160 L10 **Xianfeng** Hubei, C China
Xiang *see* Hunan
161 N7 **Xiangcheng** Henan, C China
160 F10 **Xiangcheng** *prev.* Qagchêng. Sichuan, C China
160 M8 **Xiangfan** *var.* Xiangyang. Hubei, C China
161 N10 **Xiang Jiang** ≈ S China
Xiangkhoang *see* Pèk
167 Q7 **Xiangkhoang, Plateau de** *var.* Plain of Jars. *plateau* N Laos
161 N11 **Xiangtan** *var.* Hsiang-t'an, Siangtan. Hunan, S China
161 N11 **Xiangxiang** Hunan, S China
Xiangyang *see* Xiangfan
161 S10 **Xianju** Zhejiang, SE China
160 F8 **Xianshui He** ≈ C China
161 N9 **Xiantao** *var.* Mianyang. Hubei, C China
161 R10 **Xianxia Ling** ▲▲ SE China
160 K6 **Xianyang** Shaanxi, C China
158 L5 **Xiaocaohu** Xinjiang Uygur Zizhiqu, W China
163 W6 **Xiao Hinggan Ling** *Eng.* Lesser Khingan Range. ▲▲ NE China
160 M6 **Xiao Shan** ▲▲ C China
160 M12 **Xiao Shui** ≈ S China
161 P6 **Xiaoxian** *var.* Xiao Xian. Anhui, E China
160 I10 **Xichang** Sichuan, C China
41 P11 **Xicoténcatl** Tamaulipas, C Mexico
Xieng Khouang *see* Pèk
Xieng Ngeun *see* Muong Xiang Ngeun
159 X10 **Xifeng** Gansu, C China
160 J11 **Xifeng** Guizhou, S China
Xigang *see* Helan
158 L16 **Xigazê** *var.* Jih-k'a-tse, Shigatse, Xigaze. Xizang Zizhiqu, W China
160 I8 **Xi He** ≈ C China
159 W11 **Xihe** Gansu, C China
Xihuachi *see* Heshui
159 Q7 **Xijian Quan** *spring* NW China
159 W10 **Xiji** Ningxia, N China
160 M14 **Xi Jiang** *var.* Hsi Chiang, *Eng.* West River. ≈ S China
160 K15 **Xijin Shuiku** ⊞ S China
Xilaganí *see* Xylaganí
160 I13 **Xilin** *prev.* Bada. Guangxi Zhuangzu Zizhiqu, S China
163 Q10 **Xilinhot** *var.* Silinhot. Nei Mongol Zizhiqu, N China
Xilokastro *see* Xylókastro
Xin *see* Xinjiang Uygur Zizhiqu
161 R10 **Xin'anjiang Shuiku** ⊞ SE China
Xin'anzhen *see* Xinyi
163 Q7 **Xin Barag Youqi** *var.* Altan Emel. Nei Mongol Zizhiqu, N China
163 R7 **Xin Barag Zuoqi** *var.* Amgalang. Nei Mongol Zizhiqu, N China
163 W12 **Xinbin** Liaoning, NE China
161 O7 **Xincai** Henan, C China
159 V8 **Xincheng** *var.* Yinchuanzhan. Ningxia, N China
161 O13 **Xinfeng** Jiangxi, S China
161 O14 **Xinfengjiang Shuiku** ⊞ S China
163 T13 **Xingcheng** Liaoning, NE China
82 E11 **Xinge** Lunda Norte, NE Angola
161 P12 **Xingguo** Jiangxi, S China
159 S11 **Xinghai** Qinghai, C China
161 R7 **Xinghua** Jiangsu, E China
Xingkai Hu *see* Khanka, Lake
161 P13 **Xingning** Guangdong, S China
160 I13 **Xingren** Guizhou, S China
161 O4 **Xingtai** Hebei, E China
59 J14 **Xingu, Rio** ≈ C Brazil
159 P6 **Xingxingxia** Xinjiang Uygur Zizhiqu, NW China
160 I13 **Xingyi** Guizhou, S China
158 I6 **Xinhe** *var.* Toksu. Xinjiang Uygur Zizhiqu, NW China
Xin Hot *see* Abag Qi
159 T10 **Xining** *var.* Hsining, Hsi-ning, Sining. *province capital* Qinghai, C China
161 O4 **Xinji** *prev.* Shulu. Hebei, E China
161 P10 **Xinjian** Jiangxi, S China
Xinjiang *see* Xinjiang Uygur Zizhiqu
162 D8 **Xinjiang Uygur Zizhiqu** *var.* Sinkiang, Sinkiang Uighur Autonomous Region, Xin, Xinjiang. ◈ *autonomous region* NW China
160 H9 **Xinjin** Sichuan, C China
Xinjin *see* Pulandian
163 U12 **Xinmin** Liaoning, NE China
160 M12 **Xinning** Hunan, S China
Xinpu *see* Lianyungang
161 P5 **Xinwen** *prev.* Suncun. Shandong, E China
Xin Xian *see* Xinzhou
161 N6 **Xinxiang** Henan, C China
161 O8 **Xinyang** *var.* Hsin-yang, Sinyang. Henan, C China
161 Q6 **Xinyi** *var.* Xin'anzhen. Jiangsu, E China
161 Q6 **Xinyi He** ≈ E China
161 O11 **Xinyu** Jiangxi, S China
158 I5 **Xinyuan** *var.* Künes. Xinjiang Uygur Zizhiqu, NW China
Xinyuan *see* Tianjun
162 M14 **Xinzhao Shan** ▲ N China
161 N3 **Xinzhou** *var.* Xin Xian. Shanxi, C China
104 H4 **Xinzo de Limia** Galicia, NW Spain
Xions *see* Książ Wielkopolski
161 O7 **Xiping** Henan, C China
159 T11 **Xiqing Shan** ▲▲ C China
59 N16 **Xique-Xique** Bahia, E Brazil
115 E14 **Xirovoúni** ▲ N Greece
Xishanzui *see* Urad Qianqi
160 J11 **Xishui** Guizhou, S China
161 O9 **Xishui** Hubei, C China
163 R10 **Xi Ujimqin Qi** *var.* Bayan Ul Hot. Nei Mongol Zizhiqu, N China
160 K11 **Xiushan** Sichuan, C China
161 O10 **Xiu Shui** ≈ S China
158 J16 **Xixabangma Feng** ▲ W China
160 M7 **Xixia** Henan, C China
Xixón *see* Gijón
Xixona *see* Jijona
Xizang *see* Xizang Zizhiqu
Xizang Gaoyuan *see* Qingzang Gaoyuan
160 E9 **Xizang Zizhiqu** *var.* Thibet, Tibetan Autonomous Region, Xizang, *Eng.* Tibet. ◈ *autonomous region* W China
163 U14 **Xizhong Dao** *island* N China
Xolotlán *see* Managua, Lago de
159 N9 **Xorkol** Xinjiang Uygur Zizhiqu, NW China
41 X14 **Xpujil** Quintana Roo, E Mexico
Xuancheng *see* Xuanzhou
167 T9 **Xuân Đuc** Quang Binh, C Vietnam
160 L9 **Xuan'en** Hubei, C China
160 K8 **Xuanhan** Sichuan, C China
161 O2 **Xuanhua** Hebei, E China
161 P4 **Xuanhui He** ≈ E China
161 Q8 **Xuanzhou** *var.* Xuancheng. Anhui, E China
161 N7 **Xuchang** Henan, C China
137 X10 **Xudat** *Rus.* Khudat. NE Azerbaijan
81 M16 **Xuddur** *var.* Hudur, *It.* Oddur. Bakool, SW Somalia
80 O13 **Xudun** Nugaal, N Somalia
160 L11 **Xuefeng Shan** ▲▲ S China
42 F2 **Xunantunich** *ruins* Cayo, W Belize
163 W6 **Xun He** ≈ NE China
160 L7 **Xun He** ≈ C China
160 L14 **Xun Jiang** ≈ S China
163 W5 **Xunke** Heilongjiang, NE China
161 P13 **Xunwu** Jiangxi, S China
161 O3 **Xushui** Hebei, E China
160 L16 **Xuwen** Guangdong, S China
160 I11 **Xuyong** *var.* Yongning. Sichuan, C China
161 P6 **Xuzhou** *var.* Hsu-chou, Suchow, Tongshan; *prev.* T'ung-shan. Jiangsu, E China
114 K13 **Xylaganí** *var.* Xilaganí. Anatolikí Makedonía kai Thráki, NE Greece
115 F19 **Xylókastro** *var.* Xilokastro. Pelopónnisos, S Greece

Y

160 H9 **Ya'an** *var.* Yaan. Sichuan, C China
182 L10 **Yaapeet** Victoria, SE Australia
79 D15 **Yabassi** Littoral, W Cameroon
81 J15 **Yabēlo** Oromo, C Ethiopia
114 H9 **Yablanitsa** Lovech Oblast, W Bulgaria
43 N7 **Yablis** Región Autónoma Atlántico Norte, NE Nicaragua
123 O14 **Yablonovyy Khrebet** ▲▲ S Russian Federation
162 J14 **Yabrai Shan** ▲▲ NE China
45 U6 **Yabucoa** E Puerto Rico
160 J11 **Yachi He** ≈ S China
32 H10 **Yacolt** Washington, NW USA
54 M10 **Yacuaray** Amazonas, S Venezuela
57 M22 **Yacuiba** Tarija, S Bolivia
57 K16 **Yacuma, Río** ≈ C Bolivia
155 H16 **Yādgir** Karnātaka, C India
21 R8 **Yadkin River** ≈ North Carolina, SE USA
21 R9 **Yadkinville** North Carolina, SE USA
129 P3 **Yadrin** Chuvashskaya Respublika, W Russian Federation
165 O16 **Yaeyama-shotō** *var.* Yaegama-shotō. *island group* SW Japan
75 O8 **Yafran** NW Libya
165 S2 **Yagashiri-tō** *island* NE Japan
65 H21 **Yaghan Basin** *undersea feature* SE Pacific Ocean
123 S9 **Yagodnoye** Magadanskaya Oblast', E Russian Federation
Yagotin *see* Yahotyn
78 G12 **Yagoua** Extrême-Nord, NE Cameroon
159 Q11 **Yagradagzê Shan** ▲ C China
Yaguachi *see* Yaguachi Nuevo
56 B7 **Yaguachi Nuevo** *var.* Yaguachi. Guayas, W Ecuador
Yaguarón, Río *see* Jaguarão, Rio
117 Q11 **Yahorlyts'kyy Lyman** *bay* S Ukraine
117 Q5 **Yahotyn** *Rus.* Yagotin. Kyyivs'ka Oblast', N Ukraine
40 L12 **Yahualica** Jalisco, SW Mexico
79 L17 **Yahuma** Orientale, N Dem. Rep. Congo (Zaire)
136 K15 **Yahyalı** Kayseri, C Turkey
167 N15 **Yai, Khao** ▲ SW Thailand
164 M14 **Yaizu** Shizuoka, Honshū, S Japan
160 G9 **Yajiang** Sichuan, C China
119 O14 **Yakawlyevichi** *Rus.* Yakovlevichi. Vitsyebskaya Voblasts', NE Belarus
163 S6 **Yakeshi** Nei Mongol Zizhiqu, N China
32 I9 **Yakima** Washington, NW USA
32 J10 **Yakima River** ≈ Washington, NW USA
114 G7 **Yakimovo** Montana, NW Bulgaria
Yakkabag *see* Yakkabogh
147 N12 **Yakkabogh** *Rus.* Yakkabag. Qashqadaryo Wiloyati, S Uzbekistan
148 L12 **Yakmach** Baluchistān, SW Pakistan
77 O12 **Yako** W Burkina
39 W13 **Yakobi Island** *island* Alexander Archipelago, Alaska, USA
79 K16 **Yakoma** Equateur, N Dem. Rep. Congo (Zaire)
114 H11 **Yakoruda** Blagoevgrad, SW Bulgaria
Yakovlevichi *see* Yakawlyevichi
129 T2 **Yakshur-Bod'ya** Udmurtskaya Respublika, NW Russian Federation
165 Q5 **Yakumo** Hokkaidō, NE Japan
164 B17 **Yaku-shima** *island* Nansei-shotō, SW Japan
39 V12 **Yakutat** Alaska, USA
39 U12 **Yakutat Bay** *inlet* Alaska, USA
Yakutia/Yakutiya/Yakutiya, Respublika *see* Sakha (Yakutiya), Respublika
123 Q10 **Yakutsk** Respublika Sakha (Yakutiya), NE Russian Federation
167 O17 **Yala** Yala, SW Thailand
182 D6 **Yalata** South Australia
31 S9 **Yale** Michigan, N USA
180 I11 **Yalgoo** Western Australia
114 O12 **Yalıköy** İstanbul, NW Turkey
79 L14 **Yalinga** Haute-Kotto, C Central African Republic
119 M17 **Yalizava** *Rus.* Yelizovo. Mahilyowskaya Voblasts', E Belarus
44 L13 **Yallahs Hill** ▲ E Jamaica
22 L3 **Yalobusha River** ≈ Mississippi, S USA
79 H15 **Yaloké** Ombella-Mpoko, W Central African Republic
160 E7 **Yalong Jiang** ≈ C China
136 E11 **Yalova** Yalova, NW Turkey
136 E11 **Yalova** ◈ *province* NW Turkey
Yaloveny *see* Ialoveni
Yalpug *see* Ialpug
Yalpug, Ozero *see* Yalpuh, Ozero
117 N12 **Yalpuh, Ozero** *Rus.* Ozero Yalpug. ◎ SW Ukraine
117 T14 **Yalta** Respublika Krym, S Ukraine
163 W12 **Yalu** *Chin.* Yalu Jiang, *Jap.* Oryokko, *Kor.* Amnok-kang. ≈ China/North Korea
Yalu Jiang *see* Yalu
136 F14 **Yalvaç** Isparta, SW Turkey
165 R9 **Yamada** Iwate, Honshū, C Japan
165 D14 **Yamaga** Kumamoto, Kyūshū, SW Japan
165 P10 **Yamagata** Yamagata, Honshū, C Japan
165 P9 **Yamagata** *off.* Yamagata-ken. ◈ *prefecture* Honshū, C Japan
164 C16 **Yamagawa** Kagoshima, Kyūshū, SW Japan
164 E13 **Yamaguchi** *var.* Yamaguti. Yamaguchi, Honshū, SW Japan
164 E13 **Yamaguchi** *off.* Yamaguchi-ken, *var.* Yamaguti. ◈ *prefecture* Honshū, SW Japan
Yamaguti *see* Yamaguchi
127 X5 **Yamalo-Nenetskiy Avtonomnyy Okrug** ◈ *autonomous district* N Russian Federation
122 J7 **Yamal, Poluostrov** *peninsula* N Russian Federation
165 N13 **Yamanashi** *off.* Yamanashi-ken, *var.* Yamanasi. ◈ *prefecture* Honshū, S Japan
Yamanasi *see* Yamanashi
Yamanīyah, Al Jumhūrīyah al *see* Yemen
129 W5 **Yamantau** ▲ W Russian Federation
Yamasaki *see* Yamazaki
15 P12 **Yamaska** ≈ Quebec, SE Canada
192 G4 **Yamato Ridge** *undersea feature* S Sea of Japan
164 I13 **Yamazaki** *var.* Yamasaki. Hyōgo, Honshū, SW Japan
183 V5 **Yamba** New South Wales, SE Australia
81 D16 **Yambio** *var.* Yambiyo. Western Equatoria, S Sudan
Yambiyo *see* Yambio
114 L10 **Yambol** *Turk.* Yanboli. Yambol, E Bulgaria
114 M11 **Yambol** ◈ *province* E Bulgaria
79 M17 **Yambuya** Orientale, N Dem. Rep. Congo (Zaire)
171 T15 **Yamdena, Pulau** *prev.* Jamdena. *island* Kepulauan Tanimbar, E Indonesia
165 O14 **Yame** Fukuoka, Kyūshū, SW Japan
166 M6 **Yamethin** Mandalay, C Burma
186 C6 **Yaminbot** East Sepik, NW PNG
181 U9 **Yamma Yamma, Lake** ◎ Queensland, C Australia
76 M16 **Yamoussoukro** ● (Ivory Coast) C Ivory Coast
37 P3 **Yampa River** ≈ Colorado, C USA
117 S2 **Yampil'** Sums'ka Oblast', NE Ukraine
116 M8 **Yampil'** Vinnyts'ka Oblast', C Ukraine
123 T9 **Yamsk** Magadanskaya Oblast', E Russian Federation
152 J8 **Yamuna** *prev.* Jumna. ≈ N India
152 I9 **Yamunānagar** Haryāna, N India
Yamundá *see* Nhamundá, Rio
145 U8 **Yamyshevo** Pavlodar, NE Kazakhstan
159 N16 **Yamzho Yumco** ◎ W China
123 Q8 **Yana** ≈ NE Russian Federation
186 H9 **Yanaba Island** *island* SE PNG
155 L16 **Yanam** *var.* Yanaon. Pondicherry, E India
160 L5 **Yan'an** *var.* Yanan. Shaanxi, C China
Yanaon *see* Yanam
129 U3 **Yanaul** Respublika Bashkortostan, W Russian Federation
118 O12 **Yanavichy** *Rus.* Yanovichi. Vitsyebskaya Voblasts', NE Belarus
Yanboli *see* Yambol
140 K8 **Yanbu' al Baḥr** Al Madīnah, W Saudi Arabia
21 T8 **Yanceyville** North Carolina, SE USA
161 R7 **Yancheng** Jiangsu, E China
159 W8 **Yanchi** Ningxia, N China
160 L5 **Yanchuan** Shaanxi, C China
183 O10 **Yanco Creek** *seasonal river* New South Wales, SE Australia
183 O6 **Yanda Creek** *seasonal river* New South Wales, SE Australia
182 K4 **Yandama Creek** *seasonal river* New South Wales/South Australia
161 S11 **Yandang Shan** ▲▲ SE China
Yandua *see* Yadua
159 O6 **Yandun** Xinjiang Uygur Zizhiqu, W China
76 L13 **Yanfolila** Sikasso, SW Mali
79 M18 **Yangambi** Orientale, N Dem. Rep. Congo (Zaire)
158 M15 **Yangbajain** Xizang Zizhiqu, W China
Yangchow *see* Yangzhou
160 M15 **Yangchun** Guangdong, S China
161 N2 **Yanggao** Shanxi, C China
Yanggeta *see* Yaqeta
Yangiabad *see* Yangiobod
Yangibazar *see* Dzhany-Bazar, Kyrgyzstan
Yangi-Bazar *see* Kofarnihon, Tajikistan
Yangiklshak *see* Yangiqishloq
146 M13 **Yangi-Nishon** *Rus.* Yang-Nishan. Qashqadaryo Wiloyati, S Uzbekistan
147 Q9 **Yangiobod** *Rus.* Yangiabad. Toshkent Wiloyati, E Uzbekistan
147 O10 **Yangiqishloq** *Rus.* Yangiklshak. Jizzakh Wiloyati, C Uzbekistan
147 P11 **Yangiyer** Sirdaryo Wiloyati, E Uzbekistan
147 P9 **Yangiyŭl** *Rus.* Yangiyul'. Toshkent Wiloyati, E Uzbekistan
160 M15 **Yangjiang** Guangdong, S China
Yangku *see* Taiyuan
Yang-Nishan *see* Yangi-Nishon
166 L8 **Yangon** *Eng.* Rangoon. ● (Burma) Yangon, S Burma
166 M8 **Yangon** *Eng.* Rangoon. ◈ *division* S Burma
160 K17 **Yangpu Gang** *harbor* Hainan, S China
161 N4 **Yangquan** Shanxi, C China
161 N13 **Yangshan** Guangdong, S China
167 U12 **Yang Sin, Chu** ▲ S Vietnam
Yangtze *see* Chang Jiang, C China
Yangtze Kiang *see* Chang Jiang
161 R7 **Yangzhou** *var.* Yangchow. Jiangsu, E China
160 L5 **Yan He** ≈ C China
163 Y10 **Yanji** Jilin, NE China
Yanji *see* Longjing
29 Q12 **Yankton** South Dakota, N USA
Yannina *see* Ioánnina
123 Q7 **Yano-Indigirskaya Nizmennost'** *plain* NE Russian Federation
Yanovichi *see* Yanavichy
155 K24 **Yan Oya** ≈ N Sri Lanka
158 K6 **Yanqi** *var.* Yanqi Huizu Zizhixian. Xinjiang Uygur Zizhiqu, NW China
Yanqi Huizu Zizhixian *see* Yanqi
161 P2 **Yan Shan** ▲▲ E China
161 Q10 **Yanshan** Jiangxi, S China
160 H14 **Yanshan** *prev.* Hekou. Yunnan, SW China
163 X8 **Yanshou** Heilongjiang, NE China
123 Q7 **Yanskiy Zaliv** *bay* N Russian Federation
183 O4 **Yantabulla** New South Wales, SE Australia
161 R4 **Yantai** *var.* Yan-t'ai; *prev.* Chefoo, Chih-fu. Shandong, E China
118 A13 **Yantarnyy** *Ger.* Palmnicken. Kaliningradskaya Oblast', W Russian Federation
114 J9 **Yantra** Gabrovo, N Bulgaria
114 K9 **Yantra** ≈ N Bulgaria
160 G11 **Yanyuan** Sichuan, C China
161 P5 **Yanzhou** Shandong, E China
79 E16 **Yaoundé** *var.* Yaunde. ● (Cameroon) Centre, S Cameroon
188 I14 **Yap** ◈ *state* W Micronesia
188 F16 **Yap** *island* Caroline Islands, W Micronesia
57 M18 **Yapacani, Río** ≈ C Bolivia
171 W14 **Yapa Kopra** Irian Jaya, E Indonesia
Yapan *see* Yapen, Selat
Yapanskoye More *see* Japan, Sea of
77 P15 **Yapei** N Ghana
12 M10 **Yapeitso, Mont** ▲ Quebec, E Canada
171 W12 **Yapen, Pulau** *prev.* Japen. *island* E Indonesia
171 W12 **Yapen, Selat** *var.* Yapan. *strait* Irian Jaya, E Indonesia
61 E15 **Yapeyú** Corrientes, NE Argentina
136 I11 **Yapraklı** Çankırı, N Turkey
174 M3 **Yap Trench** *var.* Yap Trough. *undersea feature* SE Philippine Sea
Yap Trough *see* Yap Trench
Yapurá *see* Caquetá, Río, Brazil/Colombia
Yapurá *see* Japurá, Rio, Brazil/Colombia
197 I12 **Yaqaga** *island* N Fiji
197 H12 **Yaqeta** *prev.* Yanggeta. *island* Yasawa Group, NW Fiji
40 G6 **Yaqui** Sonora, NW Mexico
32 E12 **Yaquina Bay** *bay* Oregon, NW USA
40 G6 **Yaqui, Río** ≈ NW Mexico
54 K5 **Yaracuy** *off.* Estado Yaracuy. ◈ *state* NW Venezuela
146 E13 **Yaradzhi** *Turkm.* Yarajy. Akhalskiy Velayat, C Turkmenistan
Yarajy *see* Yaradzhi
127 Q15 **Yaransk** Kirovskaya Oblast', NW Russian Federation
136 F17 **Yardımcı Burnu** *headland* SW Turkey
97 Q19 **Yare** ≈ E England, UK
127 S9 **Yarega** Respublika Komi, NW Russian Federation
116 I7 **Yaremcha** Ivano-Frankivs'ka Oblast', W Ukraine
189 Q9 **Yaren** SW Nauru
127 Q10 **Yarensk** Arkhangel'skaya Oblast', NW Russian Federation
155 F16 **Yargatti** Karnātaka, W India
164 M12 **Yariga-take** ▲ Honshū, S Japan
141 O15 **Yarīm** W Yemen
54 F14 **Yarí, Río** ≈ SW Colombia
54 K5 **Yaritagua** Yaracuy, N Venezuela
Yarkand *see* Yarkant He
Yarkant *see* Shache
158 E9 **Yarkant He** *var.* Yarkand. ≈ NW China
149 U3 **Yarkhūn** ≈ NW Pakistan
Yarlung Zangbo Jiang *see* Brahmaputra
116 L6 **Yarmolyntsi** Khmel'nyts'ka Oblast', W Ukraine
163 T11 **Yar Moron** ≈ N China
13 O16 **Yarmouth** Nova Scotia, SE Canada
Yarmouth *see* Great Yarmouth
Yaroslav *see* Jarosław
126 L15 **Yaroslavl'** Yaroslavskaya Oblast', W Russian Federation
126 K14 **Yaroslavskaya Oblast'** ◈ *province* W Russian Federation
123 N11 **Yaroslavskiy** Respublika Sakha (Yakutiya), NE Russian Federation
183 P13 **Yarram** Victoria, SE Australia
183 O11 **Yarrawonga** Victoria, SE Australia
182 L4 **Yarriarraburra Swamp** *wetland* New South Wales, SE Australia
122 I8 **Yar-Sale** Yamalo-Nenetskiy Avtonomnyy Okrug, N Russian Federation
122 K11 **Yartsevo** Krasnoyarskiy Kray, C Russian Federation
128 I4 **Yartsevo** Smolenskaya Oblast', W Russian Federation
54 E8 **Yarumal** Antioquia, NW Colombia
187 W14 **Yasawa Group** *island group* NW Fiji
77 V12 **Yashi** Katsina, N Nigeria
77 S14 **Yashikera** Kwara, W Nigeria
147 T14 **Yashilkŭl** *Rus.* Ozero Yashil'kul'. ◎ SE Tajikistan
Yashil'kul', Ozero *see* Yashilkŭl
165 P9 **Yashima** Akita, Honshū, C Japan
129 P13 **Yashkul'** Respublika Kalmykiya, SW Russian Federation
146 F13 **Yashlyk** Akhalskiy Velayat, C Turkmenistan
Yasinovataya *see* Yasynuvata
114 N10 **Yasna Polyana** Burgas, SE Bulgaria
167 R10 **Yasothon** Yasothon, E Thailand
183 R10 **Yass** New South Wales, SE Australia
Yassy *see* Iaşi
164 H12 **Yasugi** Shimane, Honshū, SW Japan
143 N10 **Yāsūj** *var.* Yesuj; *prev.* Tal-e Khosravī. Kohkīlūyeh va Būyer Aḥmadī, C Iran
136 M11 **Yasun Burnu** *headland* N Turkey
117 X8 **Yasynuvata** *Rus.* Yasinovataya. Donets'ka Oblast', SE Ukraine
136 C15 **Yatağan** Muğla, SW Turkey
165 Q7 **Yatate-tōge** *pass* Honshū, C Japan
187 Q17 **Yaté** Province Sud, S New Caledonia
27 P6 **Yates Center** Kansas, C USA
185 B21 **Yates Point** *headland* South Island, NZ
9 N9 **Yathkyed Lake** ◎ Nunavut, NE Canada
171 T16 **Yatoke** Pulau Babar, E Indonesia
79 M18 **Yatolema** Orientale, N Dem. Rep. Congo (Zaire)
164 C15 **Yatsushiro** *var.* Yatusiro. Kumamoto, Kyūshū, SW Japan
164 C15 **Yatsushiro-kai** *bay* SW Japan
138 F11 **Yatta** *var.* Yuta. S West Bank
81 J20 **Yatta Plateau** *plateau* SE Kenya
Yatusiro *see* Yatsushiro
57 F17 **Yauca, Río** ≈ SW Peru
45 S6 **Yauco** W Puerto Rico
Yaunde *see* Yaoundé
Yavan *see* Yovon
Yavarí *see* Javari, Rio
56 G9 **Yavari Mirim, Río** ≈ NE Peru
40 G7 **Yavaros** Sonora, NW Mexico
154 I13 **Yavatmāl** Mahārāshtra, C India
54 M9 **Yaví, Cerro** ▲ C Venezuela
43 W16 **Yaviza** Darién, SE Panama
138 F10 **Yavne** Central, W Israel
116 H5 **Yavoriv** *Pol.* Jaworów, *Rus.* Yavorov. L'vivs'ka Oblast', NW Ukraine
Yavorov *see* Yavoriv
164 F14 **Yawatahama** Ehime, Shikoku, SW Japan
Ya Xian *see* Sanya
136 L17 **Yayladaği** Hatay, S Turkey
127 V13 **Yayva** Permskaya Oblast', NW Russian Federation
127 V12 **Yayva** ≈ NW Russian Federation
143 Q9 **Yazd** *var.* Yezd. Yazd, C Iran
143 Q8 **Yazd** *off.* Ostān-e Yazd, *var.* Yezd. ◈ *province* C Iran
Yazgulemskiy Khrebet *see* Yazgulom, Qatorkŭhi
147 S13 **Yazgulom, Qatorkŭhi** *Rus.* Yazgulemskiy Khrebet. ▲▲ S Tajikistan
22 K5 **Yazoo City** Mississippi, S USA
22 K5 **Yazoo River** ≈ Mississippi, S USA
129 Q5 **Yazykovo** Ul'yanovskaya Oblast', W Russian Federation
109 U4 **Ybbs** Niederösterreich, NE Austria
109 U4 **Ybbs** ≈ C Austria
95 G22 **Yding Skovhøj** *hill* C Denmark
115 G20 **Ýdra** *var.* Ídhra, Idra. Ýdra, S Greece
115 G21 **Ýdra** *var.* Ídhra. *island* S Greece
115 G20 **Ýdras, Kólpos** *strait* S Greece
167 N10 **Ye** Mon State, S Myanmar
183 O12 **Yea** Victoria, SE Australia
78 I5 **Yebbi-Bou** Borkou-Ennedi-Tibesti, N Chad
158 F9 **Yecheng** *var.* Kargilik. Xinjiang Uygur Zizhiqu, NW China
105 R11 **Yecla** Murcia, SE Spain
40 H6 **Yécora** Sonora, NW Mexico
Yedintsy *see* Edineţ
126 J13 **Yefimovskiy** Leningradskaya Oblast', NW Russian Federation
128 K6 **Yefremov** Tul'skaya Oblast', W Russian Federation
Yêgainnyin *see* Henan
137 U12 **Yeghegis** *Rus.* Yekhegis. ≈ C Armenia
145 T10 **Yegindybulak** *Kaz.* Egindibulaq. Karaganda, C Kazakhstan
128 L4 **Yegor'yevsk** Moskovskaya Oblast', W Russian Federation
Yehuda, Haré *see* Judaean Hills
81 E15 **Yei** ≈ S Sudan
161 P8 **Yeji** *var.* Yejiaji. Anhui, E China
Yejiaji *see* Yeji
122 G10 **Yekaterinburg** *prev.* Sverdlovsk. Sverdlovskaya Oblast', C Russian Federation
Yekaterinodar *see* Krasnodar
Yekaterinoslav *see* Dnipropetrovs'k
123 R13 **Yekaterinoslavka** Amurskaya Oblast', SE Russian Federation
129 O7 **Yekaterinovka** Saratovskaya Oblast', W Russian Federation
76 K16 **Yekepa** NE Liberia
129 T3 **Yelabuga** Respublika Tatarstan, W Russian Federation
Yela Island *see* Rossel Island
129 O8 **Yelan'** Volgogradskaya Oblast', SW Russian Federation
117 Q9 **Yelanets'** *Rus.* Yelanets. Mykolayivs'ka Oblast', S Ukraine
123 S13 **Yel'ban'** Khabarovskiy Kray, E Russian Federation
128 L7 **Yelets** Lipetskaya Oblast', W Russian Federation
127 W4 **Yeletskiy** Respublika Komi, NW Russian Federation
76 J11 **Yélimané** Kayes, W Mali
Yelisavetpol *see* Gäncä
Yelizavetgrad *see* Kirovohrad

◆ Country ● Country Capital ◇ Dependent Territory ○ Dependent Territory Capital ◈ Administrative Region ✕ International Airport ▲ Mountain ▲▲ Mountain Range ⩓ Volcano ≈ River ◎ Lake ⊞ Reservoir

123 T12 **Yelizavety, Mys** *headland* SE Russian Federation
Yelizovo *see* Yalizava
129 S5 **Yelkhovka** Samarskaya Oblast', W Russian Federation
96 M1 **Yell** *island* NE Scotland, UK
155 E17 **Yellāpur** Karnātaka, W India
11 U17 **Yellow Grass** Saskatchewan, S Canada
Yellowhammer State *see* Alabama
11 O15 **Yellowhead Pass** *pass* Alberta/British Columbia, SW Canada
8 K10 **Yellowknife** *territory capital* Northwest Territories, W Canada
8 K9 **Yellowknife** ⁓ Northwest Territories, NW Canada
23 P8 **Yellow River** ⁓ Alabama/Florida, S USA
30 I4 **Yellow River** ⁓ Wisconsin, N USA
30 J6 **Yellow River** ⁓ Wisconsin, N USA
30 K7 **Yellow River** ⁓ Wisconsin, N USA
Yellow River *see* Huang He
157 V8 **Yellow Sea** *Chin.* Huang Hai, *Kor.* Hwang-Hae. *sea* E Asia
33 S13 **Yellowstone Lake** ⊚ Wyoming, C USA
33 T13 **Yellowstone National Park** *national park* Wyoming, NW USA
33 Y8 **Yellowstone River** ⁓ Montana/Wyoming, NW USA
96 L1 **Yell Sound** *strait* N Scotland, UK
27 U9 **Yellville** Arkansas, C USA
122 K10 **Yeloguy** ⁓ C Russian Federation
146 J14 **Yëloten** *prev.* Iolotan', *Turkm.* Yolöten. Maryyskiy Velayat, S Turkmenistan
119 M20 **Yel'sk** *Rus.* Yel'sk. Homyel'skaya Voblasts', SE Belarus
77 T13 **Yelwa** Kebbi, W Nigeria
21 R15 **Yemassee** South Carolina, SE USA
141 O15 **Yemen** *off.* Republic of Yemen, *Ar.* Al Jumhūrīyah al Yamanīyah, Al Yaman. ◆ *republic* SW Asia
116 M4 **Yemil'chyne** Zhytomyrs'ka Oblast', N Ukraine
126 M10 **Yemtsa** Arkhangel'skaya Oblast', NW Russian Federation
126 M10 **Yemtsa** ⁓ NW Russian Federation
127 R10 **Yemva** *prev.* Zheleznodorozhnyy. Respublika Komi, NW Russian Federation
77 U17 **Yenagoa** Bayelsa, S Nigeria
117 X7 **Yenakiyeve** *Rus.* Yenakiyevo; *prev.* Ordzhonikidze, Rykovo. Donets'ka Oblast', E Ukraine
Yenakiyevo *see* Yenakiyeve
166 L6 **Yenangyaung** Magwe, W Myanmar
167 S5 **Yên Bai** Yên Bai, N Vietnam
183 P9 **Yenda** New South Wales, SE Australia
77 Q14 **Yendi** NE Ghana
158 E8 **Yengisar** Xinjiang Uygur Zizhiqu, NW China
121 R1 **Yenierenköy** *var.* Yialousa, *Gk.* Agialoúsa. NE Cyprus
Yenipazar *see* Novi Pazar
136 E12 **Yenişehir** Bursa, NW Turkey
Yenisei Bay *see* Yeniseyskiy Zaliv
122 K12 **Yeniseysk** Krasnoyarskiy Kray, C Russian Federation
197 W10 **Yeniseyskiy Zaliv** *var.* Yenisei Bay. *bay* N Russian Federation
129 Q12 **Yenotayevka** Astrakhanskaya Oblast', SW Russian Federation
126 L4 **Yenozero, Ozero** ⊚ NW Russian Federation
Yenping *see* Nanping
39 Q11 **Yentna River** ⁓ Alaska, USA
180 M10 **Yeo, Lake** *salt lake* Western Australia
183 R7 **Yeoval** New South Wales, SE Australia
97 K23 **Yeovil** SW England, UK
40 H6 **Yepachic** Chihuahua, N Mexico
181 Y8 **Yeppoon** Queensland, E Australia
128 M5 **Yerakhtur** Ryazanskaya Oblast', W Russian Federation
Yeraliyev *see* Kuryk
146 F12 **Yerbent** Akhalskiy Velayat, C Turkmenistan
123 N11 **Yerbogachen** Irkutskaya Oblast', C Russian Federation
137 T12 **Yerevan** *Eng.* Erivan. ● (Armenia) C Armenia
137 U12 **Yerevan** ✕ C Armenia
145 R9 **Yereymentau** *var.* Jermentau, Yermentau, *Kaz.* Ereymentaū. Akmola, C Kazakhstan
129 O12 **Yergeni** *hill range* SW Russian Federation
Yeriho *see* Jericho
35 R6 **Yerington** Nevada, W USA
136 J13 **Yerköy** Yozgat, C Turkey
114 L13 **Yerlisu** Edirne, NW Turkey
Yermak *see* Aksu
145 R9 **Yermentau** *Kaz.* Ereymentaū, *prev.* Jermentau. Akmola, C Kazakhstan
145 R9 **Yermentau, Gory** ▲ C Kazakhstan
127 R5 **Yermitsa** Respublika Komi, NW Russian Federation
35 V14 **Yermo** California, W USA
123 P13 **Yerofey Pavlovich** Amurskaya Oblast', SE Russian Federation
99 F15 **Yerseke** Zeeland, SW Netherlands
129 Q8 **Yershov** Saratovskaya Oblast', W Russian Federation
127 P9 **Yërtom** Respublika Komi, NW Russian Federation
56 D13 **Yerupaja, Nevado** ▲ C Peru
Yerushalayim *see* Jerusalem
105 R4 **Yesa, Embalse de** ⊟ NE Spain
145 V15 **Yesik** *Kaz.* Esik; *prev.* Issyk. Almaty, SE Kazakhstan
145 O8 **Yesil'** *Kaz.* Esil. Akmola, C Kazakhstan
136 K15 **Yeşilhisar** Kayseri, C Turkey
136 L11 **Yeşilırmak** *anc.* Iris. ⁓ N Turkey
37 U12 **Yeso** New Mexico, SW USA
Yeso *see* Hokkaidō
129 N15 **Yessentuki** Stavropol'skiy Kray, SW Russian Federation
122 M9 **Yessey** Evenkiyskiy Avtonomnyy Okrug, N Russian Federation
105 P12 **Yeste** Castilla-La Mancha, C Spain
Yesuj *see* Yāsūj
183 T4 **Yetman** New South Wales, SE Australia
76 L4 **Yetti** *physical region* N Mauritania
166 M4 **Ye-u** Sagaing, C Myanmar
102 H9 **Yeu, Île d'** *island* NW France
Yevlakh *see* Yevlax
137 W11 **Yevlax** *Rus.* Yevlakh. C Azerbaijan
117 S13 **Yevpatoriya** Respublika Krym, S Ukraine
128 K12 **Yeya** ⁓ SW Russian Federation
158 I10 **Yeyik** Xinjiang Uygur Zizhiqu, W China
128 K12 **Yeysk** Krasnodarskiy Kray, SW Russian Federation
Yezd *see* Yazd
Yezerishche *see* Yezyaryshcha
Yezo *see* Hokkaidō
118 N11 **Yezyaryshcha** *Rus.* Yezerishche. Vitsyebskaya Voblasts', NE Belarus
Yialí *see* Gyalí
Yialousa *see* Yenierenköy
163 V7 **Yi'an** Heilongjiang, NE China
Yiannitsá *see* Giannitsá
160 I10 **Yibin** Sichuan, C China
158 K13 **Yibug Caka** ⊚ W China
160 M9 **Yichang** Hubei, C China
160 L5 **Yichuan** Shaanxi, C China
157 W3 **Yichun** Heilongjiang, NE China
163 X6 **Yichun** *var.* I-ch'un. Heilongjiang, NE China
161 O11 **Yichun** Jiangxi, S China
Yidu *see* Qingzhou
188 C15 **Yigo** NE Guam
161 Q5 **Yi He** ⁓ E China
163 X8 **Yilan** Heilongjiang, NE China
136 C9 **Yıldız Dağları** ▲ NW Turkey
136 L13 **Yıldızeli** Sivas, N Turkey
163 U4 **Yilehuli Shan** ▲ NE China
163 S7 **Yimin He** ⁓ NE China
159 W8 **Yinchuan** *var.* Yinch'uan, Yin-ch'uan, Yinchwan. Ningxia, N China
Yinchuanzhan *see* Xincheng
Yinchwan *see* Yinchuan
Yindu He *see* Indus
161 N14 **Yingde** Guangdong, S China
161 O7 **Ying He** ⁓ C China
163 U13 **Yingkou** *var.* Ying-k'ou, Yingkow; *prev.* Newchwang, Niuchwang. Liaoning, NE China
Yingkow *see* Yingkou
161 P9 **Yingshan** Hubei, C China
Yingshan *see* Guangshui
161 Q10 **Yingtan** Jiangxi, S China
Yin-hsien *see* Ningbo
158 H5 **Yining** *var.* I-ning, *Uigh.* Gulja, Kuldja. Xinjiang Uygur Zizhiqu, NW China
160 K11 **Yinjiang** Guizhou, S China
166 L4 **Yinmabin** Sagaing, C Myanmar
163 N13 **Yin Shan** ▲ N China
Yin-tu Ho *see* Indus
159 P15 **Yi'ong Zangbo** ⁓ W China
Yioúra *see* Gyáros
81 J14 **Yirga 'Alem** *It.* Irgalem. Southern, S Ethiopia
61 E19 **Yí, Río** ⁓ C Uruguay
81 E14 **Yirol** El Buhayrat, S Sudan
Yirshi *see* Yirxie
163 S8 **Yirxie** *prev.* Yirshi. Nei Mongol Zizhiqu, N China
161 Q5 **Yishui** Shandong, E China
Yisrael/Yisra'el *see* Israel
Yíthion *see* Gýtheio
Yitiaoshan *see* Jingtai
163 W10 **Yitong** Jilin, NE China
159 P5 **Yiwu** *var.* Aratürük. Xinjiang Uygur Zizhiqu, NW China
163 U12 **Yiwulü Shan** ▲ N China
163 T12 **Yi Xian** Liaoning, NE China
161 N10 **Yiyang** Hunan, S China
161 Q10 **Yiyang** Jiangxi, S China
161 N13 **Yizhang** Hunan, S China
93 K19 **Yläne** Länsi-Suomi, W Finland
93 L14 **Yli-Ii** Oulu, C Finland
93 L14 **Ylikiiminki** Oulu, C Finland
92 N13 **Yli-Kitka** ⊚ NE Finland
93 K17 **Ylistaro** Länsi-Suomi, W Finland
92 K13 **Ylitornio** Lappi, NW Finland
93 L15 **Ylivieska** Oulu, W Finland
93 L18 **Ylöjärvi** Länsi-Suomi, W Finland
95 N17 **Yngaren** ⊚ C Sweden
25 T12 **Yoakum** Texas, SW USA
77 X13 **Yobe** ◈ *state* NE Nigeria
165 R3 **Yobetsu-dake** ✳ Hokkaidō, NE Japan
80 L11 **Yoboki** C Djibouti
22 M4 **Yockanookany River** ⁓ Mississippi, S USA
22 L2 **Yocona River** ⁓ Mississippi, S USA
171 Y15 **Yodom** Irian Jaya, E Indonesia
169 Q16 **Yogyakarta** *prev.* Djokjakarta, Jogjakarta, Jokyakarta. Jawa, C Indonesia
169 P17 **Yogyakarta** *off.* Daerah Istimewa Yogyakarta, *var.* Djokjakarta, Jogjakarta, Jokyakarta. ◈ *autonomous district* S Indonesia
165 Q3 **Yoichi** Hokkaidō, NE Japan
42 G6 **Yojoa, Lago de** ⊚ NW Honduras
79 G16 **Yokadouma** Est, SE Cameroon
Yōkaiti *see* Yōkaichi
164 K13 **Yokkaichi** *var.* Yokkaiti. Mie, Honshū, SW Japan
Yokkaiti *see* Yokkaichi
79 E15 **Yoko** Centre, C Cameroon
165 V15 **Yokoate-jima** *island* Nansei-shotō, SW Japan
165 R6 **Yokohama** Aomori, Honshū, C Japan
165 O14 **Yokosuka** Kanagawa, Honshū, S Japan
164 G12 **Yokota** Shimane, Honshū, SW Japan
165 Q9 **Yokote** Akita, Honshū, C Japan
77 Y14 **Yola** Adamawa, E Nigeria
79 L19 **Yolombo** Equateur, C Dem. Rep. Congo (Zaire)
Yolöten *see* Yëloten
165 Y15 **Yome-jima** *island* Ogasawara-shotō, SE Japan
76 K16 **Yomou** Guinée-Forestière, SE Guinea
171 Y15 **Yomuka** Irian Jaya, E Indonesia
188 C16 **Yona** E Guam
164 H12 **Yonago** Tottori, Honshū, SW Japan
165 N16 **Yonaguni** Okinawa, SW Japan
165 N16 **Yonaguni-jima** *island* Nansei-shotō, SW Japan
165 T16 **Yonaha-dake** ▲ Okinawa, SW Japan
163 X14 **Yonan** SW North Korea
165 P10 **Yonezawa** Yamagata, Honshū, C Japan
161 Q12 **Yong'an** *var.* Yongan. Fujian, SE China
159 T9 **Yongchang** Gansu, N China
161 P7 **Yongcheng** Henan, C China
163 Z15 **Yŏngch'ŏn** *Jap.* Eisen. SE South Korea
160 I10 **Yongchuan** Chongqing Shi, C China
159 U10 **Yongdeng** Gansu, C China
131 W9 **Yongding He** ⁓ E China
161 P11 **Yongfeng** Jiangxi, S China
158 L5 **Yongfengqu** Xinjiang Uygur Zizhiqu, W China
160 L13 **Yongfu** Guangxi Zhuangzu Zizhiqu, S China 24.57
163 X13 **Yŏnghŭng** E North Korea
159 U10 **Yongjing** Gansu, C China
163 Y15 **Yŏngju** *Jap.* Eishū. C South Korea
Yongning *see* Xuyong
160 E12 **Yongping** Yunnan, SW China
160 G12 **Yongren** Yunnan, SW China
160 L10 **Yongshun** *var.* Lingxi. Hunan, S China
161 P10 **Yongxiu** *var.* Tujiabu. Jiangxi, S China
160 M12 **Yongzhou** Hunan, S China
18 K14 **Yonkers** New York, NE USA
103 Q7 **Yonne** ◈ *department* C France
103 P6 **Yonne** ⁓ C France
54 H9 **Yopal** *var.* El Yopal. Casanare, C Colombia
158 E8 **Yopurga** *var.* Yukuriawat. Xinjiang Uygur Zizhiqu, NW China
180 J12 **York** Western Australia
97 M16 **York** *anc.* Eboracum, Eburacum. N England, UK
23 N5 **York** Alabama, S USA
29 Q15 **York** Nebraska, C USA
18 G16 **York** Pennsylvania, NE USA
21 R11 **York** South Carolina, SE USA
14 J13 **York** ⁓ Ontario, SE Canada
15 X6 **York** ⁓ Quebec, SE Canada
181 V1 **York, Cape** *headland* Queensland, NE Australia
182 I9 **Yorke Peninsula** *peninsula* South Australia
182 I9 **Yorketown** South Australia
19 P9 **York Harbor** Maine, NE USA
21 X6 **York River** ⁓ Virginia, NE USA
97 M16 **Yorkshire** *cultural region* N England, UK
97 L16 **Yorkshire Dales** *physical region* N England, UK
11 V16 **Yorkton** Saskatchewan, S Canada
25 T12 **Yorktown** Texas, SW USA
21 X6 **Yorktown** Virginia, NE USA
30 M11 **Yorkville** Illinois, N USA
42 I5 **Yoro** Yoro, C Honduras
42 H5 **Yoro** ◈ *department* N Honduras
165 T16 **Yoron-jima** *island* Nansei-shotō, SW Japan
77 N13 **Yorosso** Sikasso, S Mali
35 R8 **Yosemite National Park** *national park* California, W USA
129 Q3 **Yoshkar-Ola** Respublika Mariy El, W Russian Federation
Yosino Gawa *see* Yoshino-gawa
171 Y16 **Yos Sudarso, Pulau** *var.* Pulau Dolak, Pulau Kolepom; *prev.* Jos Sudarso. *island* E Indonesia
163 Y17 **Yŏsu** *Jap.* Reisui. S South Korea
165 R4 **Yotei-zan** ▲ Hokkaidō, NE Japan
97 D21 **Youghal** *Ir.* Eochaill. S Ireland
97 D21 **Youghal Bay** *Ir.* Cuan Eochaille. *inlet* S Ireland
18 C15 **Youghiogheny River** ⁓ Pennsylvania, NE USA
160 K14 **You Jiang** ⁓ S China
183 Q9 **Young** New South Wales, SE Australia
11 T15 **Young** Saskatchewan, S Canada
61 E18 **Young** Río Negro, W Uruguay
182 G5 **Younghusband, Lake** *salt lake* South Australia
182 J10 **Younghusband Peninsula** *peninsula* South Australia
184 Q10 **Young Nicks Head** *headland* North Island, NZ
185 D20 **Young Range** ▲ South Island, NZ
191 Q15 **Young's Rock** *island* Pitcairn Island, Pitcairn Islands
11 R16 **Youngstown** Alberta, SW Canada
31 V12 **Youngstown** Ohio, N USA
159 N9 **Youshashan** Qinghai, C China
Youth, Isle of *see* Juventud, Isla de la
77 N11 **Youvarou** Mopti, C Mali
160 K10 **Youyang** Sichuan, C China
163 Y7 **Youyi** Heilongjiang, NE China
147 P13 **Yovon** *Rus.* Yavan. SW Tajikistan
136 J13 **Yozgat** Yozgat, C Turkey
136 K13 **Yozgat** ◈ *province* C Turkey
62 O6 **Ypacaraí** *var.* Ypacaray. Central, S Paraguay
Ypacaray *see* Ypacaraí
62 P5 **Ypané, Río** ⁓ C Paraguay
Ypres *see* Ieper
114 I13 **Ypsário** *var.* Ipsario. ▲ Thásos, E Greece
31 R10 **Ypsilanti** Michigan, N USA
34 M1 **Yreka** California, W USA
Yrendagüé *see* General Eugenio A. Garay
186 G5 **Ysabel Channel** *channel* N PNG
14 K8 **Yser, Lac** ⊚ Quebec, SE Canada
147 Y8 **Yshtyk** Issyk-Kul'skaya Oblast', E Kyrgyzstan
Yssel *see* IJssel
103 Q12 **Yssingeaux** Haute-Loire, C France
95 K23 **Ystad** Skåne, S Sweden
Ysyk-Köl *see* Balykchy, Kyrgyzstan
Ysyk-Köl *see* Issyk-Kul', Ozero, Kyrgyzstan
Ysyk-Köl Oblasty *see* Issyk-Kul'skaya Oblast'
96 L8 **Ythan** ⁓ NE Scotland, UK
Y Trallwng *see* Welshpool
94 C13 **Ytre Arna** Hordaland, S Norway
94 B12 **Ytre Sula** *island* S Norway
93 G17 **Ytterhogdal** Jämtland, C Sweden
Yu *see* Henan
Yuan Jiang *see* Red River
161 S13 **Yüanlin** *Jap.* Inrin. C Taiwan
161 N3 **Yuanping** Shanxi, C China
161 O11 **Yuan Shui** ⁓ S China
35 O6 **Yuba City** California, W USA
35 O6 **Yuba River** ⁓ California, W USA
80 H13 **Yubdo** Oromo, C Ethiopia
165 U3 **Yūbetsu** Hokkaidō, NE Japan
Yūbetsu-gawa *see* Yabetsu-gawa
41 X12 **Yucatán** ◈ *state* SE Mexico
47 O3 **Yucatan Basin** *var.* Yucatan Deep. *undersea feature* N Caribbean Sea
Yucatán, Canal de *see* Yucatan Channel
41 Y10 **Yucatan Channel** *Sp.* Canal de Yucatán. *channel* Cuba/Mexico
Yucatan Deep *see* Yucatan Basin
Yucatan Peninsula *see* Yucatán, Península de
41 X13 **Yucatán, Península de** *Eng.* Yucatan Peninsula. *peninsula* Guatemala/Mexico
36 I11 **Yucca** Arizona, SW USA
35 V15 **Yucca Valley** California, W USA
161 P4 **Yucheng** Shandong, E China
161 N4 **Yuci** Shanxi, C China
131 X5 **Yudoma** ⁓ E Russian Federation
161 P12 **Yudu** Jiangxi, C China
Yue *see* Guangdong
160 M12 **Yuecheng Ling** ▲ S China
181 P7 **Yuendumu** Northern Territory, N Australia
160 H10 **Yuexi** Sichuan, C China
161 N10 **Yueyang** Hunan, S China
127 U14 **Yug** Permskaya Oblast', NW Russian Federation
127 P13 **Yug** ⁓ NW Russian Federation
123 R10 **Yugorenok** Respublika Sakha (Yakutiya), NE Russian Federation
122 H9 **Yugorsk** Khanty-Mansiyskiy Avtonomnyy Okrug, C Russian Federation
122 H7 **Yugorskiy Poluostrov** *peninsula* NW Russian Federation
112 M13 **Yugoslavia** *off.* Federal Republic of Yugoslavia, *SCr.* Jugoslavija, Savezna Republika Jugoslavija. ◆ *federal republic* SE Europe
146 K14 **Yugo-Vostochnyye Garagumy** *prev.* Yugo-Vostochnyye Karakumy. *desert* E Turkmenistan
Yugo-Vostochnyye Karakumy *see* Yugo-Vostochnyye Garagumy
161 S10 **Yuhuan Dao** *island* SE China
160 L14 **Yu Jiang** ⁓ S China
123 S7 **Yukagirskoye Ploskogor'ye** *plateau* NE Russian Federation
118 L11 **Yukhavichy** *Rus.* Yukhovichi. Vitsyebskaya Voblasts', N Belarus
128 J4 **Yukhnov** Kaluzhskaya Oblast', W Russian Federation
Yukhovichi *see* Yukhavichy
79 J20 **Yuki** *var.* Yuki Kengunda. Bandundu, W Dem. Rep. Congo (Zaire)
Yuki Kengunda *see* Yuki
26 M10 **Yukon** Oklahoma, C USA
(0) F4 **Yukon** ⁓ Canada/USA
Yukon *see* Yukon Territory
39 S7 **Yukon Flats** *salt flat* Alaska, USA
8 F8 **Yukon Territory** *var.* Yukon, *Fr.* Territoire du Yukon. ◈ *territory* NW Canada
137 T16 **Yüksekova** Hakkâri, SE Turkey
123 N10 **Yukta** Evenkiyskiy Avtonomnyy Okrug, C Russian Federation
165 O13 **Yukuhashi** *var.* Yukuhasi. Fukuoka, Kyūshū, SW Japan
Yukuhasi *see* Yukuhashi
Yukuriawat *see* Yopurga
127 O9 **Yula** ⁓ NW Russian Federation
181 P8 **Yulara** Northern Territory, N Australia
129 W6 **Yuldybayevo** Respublika Bashkortostan, W Russian Federation
23 W8 **Yulee** Florida, SE USA
158 K7 **Yuli** *var.* Lopnur. Xinjiang Uygur Zizhiqu, NW China
161 T14 **Yüli** C Taiwan
160 L15 **Yulin** Guangxi Zhuangzu Zizhiqu, S China
160 L4 **Yulin** Shaanxi, C China
161 T14 **Yüli Shan** ▲ E Taiwan
160 F11 **Yulongxue Shan** ▲ SW China
36 H14 **Yuma** Arizona, SW USA
37 W3 **Yuma** Colorado, C USA
54 K5 **Yumare** Yaracuy, N Venezuela
63 G14 **Yumbel** Bío Bío, C Chile
79 N19 **Yumbi** Maniema, E Dem. Rep. Congo (Zaire)
159 R8 **Yumen** *var.* Laojunmiao, Yümen. Gansu, N China
159 Q7 **Yumenzhen** Gansu, N China
158 J3 **Yumin** Xinjiang Uygur Zizhiqu, NW China
Yun *see* Yunnan
136 G14 **Yunak** Konya, W Turkey
45 O8 **Yuna, Río** ⁓ E Dominican Republic
38 I17 **Yunaska Island** *island* Aleutian Islands, Alaska, USA
160 M6 **Yuncheng** Shanxi, C China
57 L18 **Yungas** *physical region* E Bolivia
Yungki *see* Jilin
Yung-ning *see* Nanning
160 I12 **Yun Gui Gaoyuan** *plateau* SW China
Yunjinghong *see* Jinghong
160 M15 **Yunkai Dashan** ▲ S China
Yunki *see* Jilin
160 E11 **Yun Ling** ▲ SW China
161 N9 **Yunmeng** Hubei, C China
157 N14 **Yunnan** *var.* Yun, Yunnan Sheng, Yünnan, Yun-nan. ◈ *province* SW China
Yunnan *see* Kunming
Yunnan Sheng *see* Yunnan
165 P15 **Yunomae** Kumamoto, Kyūshū, SW Japan
161 N8 **Yun Shui** ⁓ C China
182 J7 **Yunta** South Australia
161 Q14 **Yunxiao** Fujian, SE China
160 K9 **Yunyang** Sichuan, C China
193 S9 **Yupanqui Basin** *undersea feature* E Pacific Ocean
Yuratishki *see* Yuratsishki
119 I15 **Yuratsishki** *Pol.* Juraciszki, *Rus.* Yuratishki. Hrodzyenskaya Voblasts', W Belarus
Yurev *see* Tartu
122 J12 **Yurga** Kemerovskaya Oblast', S Russian Federation
56 E10 **Yurimaguas** Loreto, N Peru
129 P3 **Yurino** Respublika Mariy El, W Russian Federation
41 N13 **Yuriria** Guanajuato, C Mexico
127 T13 **Yurla** Komi-Permyatskiy Avtonomnyy Okrug, NW Russian Federation
Yuruá, Río *see* Juruá, Rio
114 M13 **Yürük** Tekirdağ, NW Turkey
158 G10 **Yurungkax He** ⁓ W China
127 Q14 **Yur'ya** *var.* Jarja. Kirovskaya Oblast', NW Russian Federation
Yur'yev *see* Tartu
127 N16 **Yur'yevets** Ivanovskaya Oblast', W Russian Federation
128 M3 **Yur'yev-Pol'skiy** Vladimirskaya Oblast', W Russian Federation
117 V7 **Yur"yivka** Dnipropetrovs'ka Oblast', E Ukraine
42 I7 **Yuscarán** El Paraíso, S Honduras
161 P12 **Yu Shan** ▲ S China
126 I7 **Yushkozero** Respublika Kareliya, NW Russian Federation
159 R13 **Yushu** Qinghai, C China
129 P12 **Yusta** Respublika Kalmykiya, SW Russian Federation
126 I10 **Yustozero** Respublika Kareliya, NW Russian Federation
137 Q11 **Yusufeli** Artvin, NE Turkey
164 F14 **Yusuhara** Kōchi, Shikoku, SW Japan
127 T14 **Yus'va** Permskaya Oblast', NW Russian Federation
Yuta *see* Yatta
161 P2 **Yutian** Hebei, E China
158 H10 **Yutian** *var.* Keriya. Xinjiang Uygur Zizhiqu, NW China
62 K5 **Yuto** Jujuy, NW Argentina
62 P7 **Yuty** Caazapá, S Paraguay
160 G13 **Yuxi** Yunnan, SW China
161 O2 **Yuxian** *prev.* Yu Xian. Hebei, E China
165 Q9 **Yuzawa** Akita, Honshū, C Japan
127 N16 **Yuzha** Ivanovskaya Oblast', W Russian Federation
Yuzhno-Alichurskiy Khrebet *see* Alichuri Janubí, Qatorkŭhi
Yuzhno-Kazakhstanskaya Oblast' *see* Yuzhnyy Kazakhstan
123 T13 **Yuzhno-Sakhalinsk** *Jap.* Toyohara; *prev.* Vladimirovka. Ostrov Sakhalin, Sakhalinskaya Oblast', SE Russian Federation
129 P14 **Yuzhno-Sukhokumsk** Respublika Dagestan, SW Russian Federation
145 Z10 **Yuzhnyy Altay, Khrebet** ▲ E Kazakhstan
Yuzhnyy Bug *see* Pivdennyy Buh
145 O15 **Yuzhnyy Kazakhstan** *off.* Yuzhno-Kazakhstanskaya Oblast', *Eng.* South Kazakhstan, *Kaz.* Ongtüstik Qazaqstan Oblysy; *prev.* Chimkentskaya Oblast'. ◈ *province* S Kazakhstan
123 U10 **Yuzhnyy, Mys** *headland* E Russian Federation
129 W6 **Yuzhnyy Ural** *var.* Southern Urals. ▲ W Russian Federation
159 V10 **Yuzhong** Gansu, C China
Yuzhou *see* Chongqing
103 N5 **Yvelines** ◈ *department* N France
108 B9 **Yverdon** *var.* Yverdon-les-Bains, *Ger.* Iferten; *anc.* Eborodunum. Vaud, W Switzerland
Yverdon-les-Bains *see* Yverdon
102 M3 **Yvetot** Seine-Maritime, N France
Yylanly *see* Il'yaly

Z

147 T12 **Zaalayskiy Khrebet** *Taj.* Qatorkŭhi Pasi Oloy. ▲ Kyrgyzstan/Tajikistan
Zaamin *see* Zomin
Zaandam *see* Zaanstad
98 I10 **Zaanstad** *prev.* Zaandam. Noord-Holland, C Netherlands
Zabadani *see* Az Zabdānī
119 L18 **Zabalatstsye** *Rus.* Zabolot'ye. Homyel'skaya Voblasts', SE Belarus
112 L9 **Žabalj** *Ger.* Josefsdorf, *Hung.* Zsablya; *prev.* Józseffalva;. Serbia, N Yugoslavia
Zāb aş Şaghīr, Nahraz *see* Little Zab
123 P14 **Zabaykal'sk** Chitinskaya Oblast', S Russian Federation
Zāb-e Kūchek, Rūdkhāneh-ye *see* Little Zab
Zabeln *see* Sabile
Zabéré *see* Zabré
Zabern *see* Saverne
141 N16 **Zabīd** W Yemen
141 O16 **Zabīd, Wādī** *dry watercourse* SW Yemen
Żabinka *see* Zhabinka
Ząbkowice *see* Ząbkowice Śląskie
111 G15 **Ząbkowice Śląskie** *var.* Ząbkowice, *Ger.* Frankenstein, Frankenstein in Schlesien. Dolnośląskie, SW Poland
110 P10 **Zabłudów** Podlaskie, NE Poland
112 D8 **Zabok** Krapina-Zagorje, N Croatia
143 W9 **Zābol** *var.* Shahr-i-Zabul, Zabul; *prev.* Nasratabad. Sīstān va Balūchestān, E Iran
Zābol *see* Zābul
143 W13 **Zābolī** Sīstān va Balūchestān, SE Iran
Zabolot'ye *see* Zabalatstsye
77 Q13 **Zabré** *var.* Zabéré. S Burkina
111 G17 **Zábřeh** *Ger.* Hohenstadt. Olomoucký Kraj, E Czech Republic
111 J16 **Zabrze** *Ger.* Hindenburg, Hindenburg in Oberschlesien. Śląskie, S Poland
149 O7 **Zābul** *Per.* Zābol. ◈ *province* SE Afghanistan
Zabul *see* Zābol
42 E6 **Zacapa** Zacapa, E Guatemala
42 A3 **Zacapa** *off.* Departamento de Zacapa. ◈ *department* E Guatemala
40 M14 **Zacapú** Michoacán de Ocampo, SW Mexico
41 V14 **Zacatal** Campeche, SE Mexico
40 M11 **Zacatecas** Zacatecas, C Mexico
40 L10 **Zacatecas** ◈ *state* C Mexico
42 F8 **Zacatecoluca** La Paz, S El Salvador
41 P15 **Zacatepec** Morelos, S Mexico
41 Q13 **Zacatlán** Puebla, S Mexico
144 F8 **Zachagansk** Zapadnyy Kazakhstan, NW Kazakhstan
115 D20 **Zacháro** *var.* Zaharo, Zakháro. Dytikí Ellás, S Greece
22 J8 **Zachary** Louisiana, S USA
117 U6 **Zachepylivka** Kharkivs'ka Oblast', E Ukraine
Zachist'ye *see* Zachystsye
110 E9 **Zachodniopomorskie** ◈ NW Poland
119 L14 **Zachystsye** *Rus.* Zachist'ye. Minskaya Voblasts', NW Belarus
40 L13 **Zacoalco** *var.* Zacoalco de Torres. Jalisco, SW Mexico
Zacoalco de Torres *see* Zacoalco
41 P13 **Zacualtipán** Hidalgo, C Mexico
112 C12 **Zadar** *It.* Zara; *anc.* Iader. Zadar, W Croatia
112 C12 **Zadar** *off.* Zadarsko-Kninska Županija *prev.* Zadar-Knin. ◈ *province* SW Croatia
Zadar-Knin *see* Zadar
166 M14 **Zadetkyi Kyun** *var.* St. Matthew's Island. *island* Mergui Archipelago, S Myanmar
67 Q9 **Zadié** *var.* Djadié. ⁓ NE Gabon
159 Q13 **Zadoi** Qinghai, C China
128 L7 **Zadonsk** Lipetskaya Oblast', W Russian Federation
75 X8 **Za'farāna** E Egypt
149 W7 **Zafarwāl** Punjab, E Pakistan
121 Q1 **Zafer Burnu** *var.* Cape Andreas, Cape Apostolas Andreas, *Gk.* Akrotíri Apostólou Andréa. *headland* NE Cyprus
107 J23 **Zafferano, Capo** *headland* Sicilia, Italy, C Mediterranean Sea
114 M7 **Zafirovo** Silistra, NE Bulgaria
115 L23 **Zaforá** *island* Kykládes, Greece, Aegean Sea
104 J12 **Zafra** Extremadura, W Spain
110 E13 **Żagań** *var.* Zagań, Żegań, *Ger.* Sagan. Lubuskie, W Poland
118 F10 **Žagarė** *Pol.* Žagory. Joniškis, N Lithuania
75 W7 **Zagazig** *var.* Az Zaqāzīq. N Egypt
74 M5 **Zaghouan** *var.* Zaghwān. NE Tunisia
Zaghwān *see* Zaghouan
115 G16 **Zagorá** Thessalía, C Greece
Zagorod'ye *see* Zaharoddzye
Žagory *see* Žagarė
Zágráb *see* Zagreb
112 E8 **Zagreb** *Ger.* Agram, *Hung.* Zágráb. ● (Croatia) Zagreb, N Croatia
112 E8 **Zagreb** *prev.* Grad Zagreb. ◈ *province* NC Croatia
142 L7 **Zāgros, Kūhhā-ye** *Eng.* Zagros Mountains. ▲ W Iran
Zagros Mountains *see* Zāgros, Kūhhā-ye
112 O12 **Žagubica** Serbia, E Yugoslavia
111 L22 **Zagyva** ⁓ N Hungary
Zaharo *see* Zacháro

◆ Country
● Country Capital
◇ Dependent Territory
○ Dependent Territory Capital
◈ Administrative Region
✕ International Airport
▲ Mountain
▲ Mountain Range
✳ Volcano
⁓ River
⊚ Lake
⊟ Reservoir

119 G19 **Zaharoddzye** *Rus.* Zagorod'ye. *physical region* SW Belarus
143 W11 **Zāhedān** *var.* Zahidan; *prev.* Duzdab. Sīstān va Balūchestān, SE Iran
Zahidan *see* Zāhedān
Zaḩlah *see* Zahlé
138 H7 **Zahlé** *var.* Zaḩlah. C Lebanon
Zähmet *see* Zakhmet
111 O20 **Záhony** Szabolcs-Szatmár-Bereg, NE Hungary
141 N13 **Zahrān** 'Asīr, S Saudi Arabia
139 R12 **Zahrat al Baṭn** *hill range* S Iraq
120 H11 **Zahrez Chergui** *var.* Zahrez Chergúi. *marsh* N Algeria
129 S4 **Zainsk** Respublika Tatarstan, W Russian Federation
82 A10 **Zaire** *prev.* Congo. ◈ *province* NW Angola
Zaire *see* Congo (Democratic Republic of)
Zaire *see* Congo (river)
112 P13 **Zaječar** Serbia, E Yugoslavia
83 L18 **Zaka** Masvingo, E Zimbabwe
122 M14 **Zakamensk** Respublika Buryatiya, S Russian Federation
116 G7 **Zakarpats'ka Oblast'** *Eng.* Transcarpathian Oblast, *Rus.* Zakarpatskaya Oblast'. ◈ *province* W Ukraine
Zakarpatskaya Oblast' *see* Zakarpats'ka Oblast'
Zakataly *see* Zaqatala
Zakháro *see* Zacháro
Zakhidnyy Buh/Zakhodni Buh *see* Bug
146 J14 **Zakhmet** *Turkm.* Zähmet. Maryyskiy Velayat, C Turkmenistan
139 Q1 **Zākhō** *var.* Zākhū. N Iraq
Zākhū *see* Zākhō
Zákinthos *see* Zákynthos
111 L18 **Zakopane** Małopolskie, S Poland
78 J12 **Zakouma** Salamat, S Chad
115 L25 **Zákros** Kríti, Greece, E Mediterranean Sea
115 C19 **Zákynthos** *var.* Zákinthos. Zákynthos, W Greece
115 C20 **Zákynthos** *var.* Zákinthos, *It.* Zante. *island* Iónioi Nísoi, Greece, C Mediterranean Sea
115 C19 **Zakýnthou, Porthmós** *strait* SW Greece
111 G24 **Zala** *off.* Zala Megye. ◈ *county* W Hungary
111 G24 **Zala** ≈ W Hungary
138 M4 **Zalābiyah** Dayr az Zawr, C Syria
111 G24 **Zalaegerszeg** Zala, W Hungary
104 K11 **Zalamea de la Serena** Extremadura, W Spain
104 J13 **Zalamea la Real** Andalucía, S Spain
163 U7 **Zalantun** *var.* Butha Qi. Nei Mongol Zizhiqu, N China
111 G23 **Zalaszentgrót** Zala, SW Hungary
Zalatna *see* Zlatna
116 G9 **Zalău** *Ger.* Waltenberg, *Hung.* Zilah; *prev. Ger.* Zillenmarkt. Sălaj, NW Romania
109 V10 **Žalec** *Ger.* Sachsenfeld. C Slovenia
117 S9 **Zalenodol's'k** Dnipropetrovs'ka Oblast', E Ukraine
110 K8 **Zalewo** *Ger.* Saalfeld. Warmińsko-Mazurskie, NE Poland
141 N9 **Zalim** Makkah, W Saudi Arabia
80 A11 **Zalingei** *var.* Zalinje. Western Darfur, W Sudan
Zalinje *see* Zalingei
116 K7 **Zalishchyky** Ternopil's'ka Oblast', W Ukraine
Zallah *see* Zillah
98 J13 **Zaltbommel** Gelderland, C Netherlands
126 H15 **Zaluch'ye** Novgorodskaya Oblast', NW Russian Federation
Zamak *see* Zamakh
141 Q14 **Zamakh** *var.* Zamak. N Yemen
136 K15 **Zamantı Irmağı** ≈ C Turkey
Zambesi/Zambeze *see* Zambezi
83 G14 **Zambezi** North Western, W Zambia
83 K15 **Zambezi** *var.* Zambesi, *Port.* Zambeze. ≈ S Africa
83 O15 **Zambézia** *off.* Província da Zambézia. ◈ *province* C Mozambique
83 I14 **Zambia** *off.* Republic of Zambia; *prev.* Northern Rhodesia. ◆ *republic* S Africa
171 O8 **Zamboanga** *off.* Zamboanga City. Mindanao, S Philippines
54 E5 **Zambrano** Bolívar, N Colombia
110 N10 **Zambrów** Łomża, E Poland
83 L14 **Zambué** Tete, NW Mozambique
77 T13 **Zamfara** ≈ NW Nigeria
56 C9 **Zamora** Zamora Chinchipe, S Ecuador
104 K6 **Zamora** Castilla-León, NW Spain
104 K5 **Zamora** ◈ *province* Castilla-León, NW Spain
Zamora *see* Barinas
56 A13 **Zamora Chinchipe** ◈ *province* S Ecuador
40 M13 **Zamora de Hidalgo** Michoacán de Ocampo, SW Mexico
111 P15 **Zamość** *Rus.* Zamoste. Lubelskie, E Poland
Zamoste *see* Zamość
160 G7 **Zamtang** *prev.* Gamda. Sichuan, C China
75 O8 **Zamzam, Wādī** *dry watercourse* NW Libya
79 F20 **Zanaga** La Lékoumou, S Congo
41 T16 **Zanatepec** Oaxaca, SE Mexico
105 P9 **Záncara** ≈ C Spain
Zancle *see* Messina
158 G14 **Zanda** Xizang Zizhiqu, W China
98 H10 **Zandvoort** Noord-Holland, W Netherlands
39 P8 **Zane Hills** *hill range* Alaska, USA
31 T13 **Zanesville** Ohio, N USA
Zanga *see* Hrazdan
142 L4 **Zanjān** *var.* Zenjan, Zinjan. Zanjān, NW Iran
142 L4 **Zanjān** *off.* Ostān-e Zanjān, *var.* Zenjan, Zinjan. ◈ *province* NW Iran
Zante *see* Zákynthos
81 J22 **Zanzibar** Zanzibar, E Tanzania
81 J22 **Zanzibar** ◈ *region* E Tanzania
81 J22 **Zanzibar** *Swa.* Unguja. *island* E Tanzania
81 J22 **Zanzibar Channel** *channel* E Tanzania
165 P10 **Zaō-san** ▲ Honshū, C Japan
161 N8 **Zaoyang** Hubei, C China
161 Q6 **Zaozhuang** Shandong, E China
28 L4 **Zap** North Dakota, N USA
112 L13 **Zapadna Morava** *Ger.* Westliche Morava. ≈ C Yugoslavia
126 H16 **Zapadnaya Dvina** Tverskaya Oblast', W Russian Federation
Zapadnaya Dvina *see* Western Dvina
122 I9 **Zapadno-Sibirskaya Ravnina** *Eng.* West Siberian Plain. *plain* C Russian Federation
Zapadnyy Bug *see* Bug
144 E9 **Zapadnyy Kazakhstan** *off.* Zapadno-Kazakhstanskaya Oblast', *Eng.* West Kazakhstan, *Kaz.* Batys Qazaqstan Oblysy; *prev.* Ural'skaya Oblast'. ◈ *province* NW Kazakhstan
122 K13 **Zapadnyy Sayan** *Eng.* Western Sayans. ▲ S Russian Federation
63 H15 **Zapala** Neuquén, W Argentina
62 I4 **Zapaleri, Cerro** *var.* Cerro Sapaleri. ▲ N Chile
25 Q16 **Zapata** Texas, SW USA
44 D5 **Zapata, Península de** *peninsula* W Cuba
61 G19 **Zapicán** Lavalleja, S Uruguay
65 J19 **Zapiola Ridge** *undersea feature* SW Atlantic Ocean
65 L19 **Zapiola Seamount** *undersea feature* S Atlantic Ocean
126 I2 **Zapolyarnyy** Murmanskaya Oblast', NW Russian Federation
117 U8 **Zaporizhzhya** *Rus.* Zaporozh'ye; *prev.* Aleksandrovsk. Zaporiz'ka Oblast', SE Ukraine
Zaporizhzhya *see* Zaporiz'ka Oblast'
117 U9 **Zaporiz'ka Oblast'** *var.* Zaporizhzhya, *Rus.* Zaporozhskaya Oblast'. ◈ *province* SE Ukraine
Zaporozhskaya Oblast' *see* Zaporiz'ka Oblast'
Zaporozh'ye *see* Zaporizhzhya
40 L14 **Zapotiltic** Jalisco, SW Mexico
158 G13 **Zapug** Xizang Zizhiqu, W China
137 V10 **Zaqatala** *Rus.* Zakataly. NW Azerbaijan
159 P13 **Zaqên** Qinghai, W China
159 Q13 **Za Qu** ≈ C China
136 M13 **Zara** Sivas, C Turkey
Zara *see* Zadar
Zarafshan *see* Zarafshon
147 P12 **Zarafshon** *Rus.* Zeravshan. W Tajikistan
146 L9 **Zarafshon** *Rus.* Zarafshan. Nawoiy Wiloyati, N Uzbekistan
Zarafshon *see* Zeravshan
147 O12 **Zarafshon, Qatorkŭhi** *Rus.* Zeravshanskiy Khrebet, *Uzb.* Zarafshon Tizmasi. ▲ Tajikistan/Uzbekistan
Zarafshon Tizmasi *see* Zarafshon, Qatorkŭhi
54 E7 **Zaragoza** Antioquia, N Colombia
40 I5 **Zaragoza** Chihuahua, N Mexico
41 N6 **Zaragoza** Coahuila de Zaragoza, NE Mexico
41 O10 **Zaragoza** Nuevo León, NE Mexico
105 R5 **Zaragoza** *Eng.* Saragossa; *anc.* Caesaraugusta, Salduba. Aragón, NE Spain
105 R6 **Zaragoza** ◈ *province* Aragón, NE Spain
105 R5 **Zaragoza** ✕ Aragón, NE Spain
143 S10 **Zarand** Kermān, C Iran
148 J9 **Zaranj** Nimrūz, SW Afghanistan
118 I11 **Zarasai** Zarasai, E Lithuania
62 N12 **Zárate** *prev.* General José F.Uriburu. Buenos Aires, E Argentina
105 Q2 **Zarautz** *var.* Zarauz. País Vasco, N Spain
Zarauz *see* Zarautz
Zaravecchia *see* Biograd na Moru
Zarāyīn *see* Zarēn
128 L4 **Zaraysk** Moskovskaya Oblast', W Russian Federation
55 N6 **Zaraza** Guárico, N Venezuela
Zarbdar *see* Zarbdor
147 P11 **Zarbdor** *Rus.* Zarbdar. Jizzakh Wiloyati, C Uzbekistan
142 M8 **Zard Kūh** ▲ SW Iran
126 I5 **Zarechensk** Murmanskaya Oblast', NW Russian Federation
149 Q7 **Zareh Sharan** Paktīkā, E Afghanistan
39 Y14 **Zarembo Island** *island* Alexander Archipelago, Alaska, USA
139 V4 **Zarēn** *var.* Zarāyīn. E Iraq
149 Q7 **Zarghūn Shahr** *var.* Katawaz. Paktīkā, SE Afghanistan
77 V13 **Zaria** Kaduna, C Nigeria
116 K2 **Zarichne** Rivnens'ka Oblast', NW Ukraine
122 J13 **Zarinsk** Altayskiy Kray, S Russian Federation
116 J12 **Zărnești** *Hung.* Zernest. Brașov, C Romania
115 J25 **Zarós** Kríti, Greece, E Mediterranean Sea
100 O9 **Zarow** ≈ NE Germany
Zarqa/Zarqā', Muḩāfaẓat az *see* Az Zarqā'
111 G20 **Záruby** ▲ W Slovakia
56 B8 **Zaruma** El Oro, SW Ecuador
110 E13 **Żary** *Ger.* Sorau, Sorau in der Niederlausitz. Lubuskie, W Poland
54 D10 **Zarzal** Valle del Cauca, W Colombia
42 I7 **Zarzalar, Cerro** ▲ S Honduras
152 I5 **Zāskār** ≈ NE India
152 I5 **Zāskār Range** ▲ NE India
119 K15 **Zaslawye** Minskaya Voblasts', C Belarus
116 K7 **Zastavna** Chernivets'ka Oblast', W Ukraine
111 B16 **Žatec** *Ger.* Saaz. Ústecký Kraj, NW Czech Republic
Zaumgarten *see* Chrzanów
146 G10 **Zaunguzskiye Garagumy** *Turkm.* Üngüz Angyrsyndaky Garagum. *desert* N Turkmenistan
25 X9 **Zavalla** Texas, SW USA
99 H18 **Zaventem** Vlaams Brabant, C Belgium
99 H18 **Zaventem** ✕ (Brussel/Bruxelles) Vlaams Brabant, C Belgium
Zavertse *see* Zawiercie
114 L7 **Zavet** Razgrad, NE Bulgaria
129 O12 **Zavetnoye** Rostovskaya Oblast', SW Russian Federation
156 M3 **Zavhan Gol** ≈ W Mongolia
112 H12 **Zavidovići** Federacija Bosna I Hercegovina, N Bosnia and Herzegovina
123 R13 **Zavitinsk** Amurskaya Oblast', SE Russian Federation
Zawia *see* Az Zāwiyah
111 K15 **Zawiercie** *Rus.* Zavertse. Śląskie, S Poland
75 P11 **Zawīlah** *var.* Zuwaylah, *It.* Zueila. C Libya
138 I4 **Zāwiyah, Jabal az** ▲ NW Syria
109 Y3 **Zaya** ≈ NE Austria
166 M8 **Zayatkyi** Pegu, C Myanmar
145 Y11 **Zaysan** Vostochnyy Kazakhstan, E Kazakhstan
Zaysan Köl *see* Zaysan, Ozero
145 Y11 **Zaysan, Ozero** *Kaz.* Zaysan Köl. ◎ E Kazakhstan
159 R16 **Zayü** *var.* Gyigang. Xizang Zizhiqu, W China
Zayyq *see* Ural
44 F6 **Zaza** ≈ C Cuba
116 K5 **Zbarazh** Ternopil's'ka Oblast', W Ukraine
116 J5 **Zboriv** Ternopil's'ka Oblast', W Ukraine
111 F18 **Zbraslav** Brněnský Kraj, SE Czech Republic
116 K6 **Zbruch** ≈ W Ukraine
Žďár *see* Žďár nad Sázavou
111 F17 **Žďár nad Sázavou** *Ger.* Saar in Mähren; *prev.* Žďár. Jihlavský Kraj, C Czech Republic
116 K4 **Zdolbuniv** *Pol.* Zdolbunów, *Rus.* Zdolbunov. Rivnens'ka Oblast', NW Ukraine
Zdolbunov/Zdolbunów *see* Zdolbuniv
110 J13 **Zduńska Wola** Sieradz, C Poland
117 O4 **Zdvizh** ≈ N Ukraine
Zdzięciół *see* Dzyatlava
111 I16 **Zdzieszowice** *Ger.* Odertal. Opolskie, S Poland
Zealand *see* Sjælland
188 K6 **Zealandia Bank** *undersea feature* C Pacific Ocean
63 H20 **Zeballos, Monte** ▲ S Argentina
83 K20 **Zebediela** Northern, NE South Africa
113 L18 **Zebë, Mal** *var.* Mali i Zebës. ▲ NE Albania
Zebës, Mali i *see* Zebë, Mal
21 V9 **Zebulon** North Carolina, SE USA
112 K8 **Žednik** *Hung.* Bácsjózseffalva. Serbia, N Yugoslavia
99 C15 **Zeebrugge** West-Vlaanderen, NW Belgium
183 N16 **Zeehan** Tasmania, SE Australia
99 L14 **Zeeland** Noord-Brabant, SE Netherlands
29 N7 **Zeeland** North Dakota, N USA
99 E14 **Zeeland** ◈ *province* SW Netherlands
83 I21 **Zeerust** North-West, N South Africa
98 K10 **Zeewolde** Flevoland, C Netherlands
138 G8 **Ẕefat** *var.* Safed, Tsefat, *Ar.* Safad. Northern, N Israel
Zegań *see* Żagań
Zehden *see* Cedynia
100 O11 **Zehdenick** Brandenburg, NE Germany
Zē-i Bādīnān *see* Great Zab
Zeiden *see* Codlea
146 M14 **Zeidskoye Vodokhranilishche** ⊡ E Turkmenistan
Zē-i Kōya *see* Little Zab
181 P7 **Zeil, Mount** ▲ Northern Territory, C Australia
98 J12 **Zeist** Utrecht, C Netherlands
101 M16 **Zeitz** Sachsen-Anhalt, E Germany
159 T11 **Zêkog** Qinghai, C China
Zelaya Norte *see* Atlántico Norte, Región Autónoma
Zelaya Sur *see* Atlántico Sur, Región Autónoma
99 F17 **Zele** Oost-Vlaanderen, NW Belgium
110 N12 **Żelechów** Lubelskie, E Poland
113 H14 **Zelena Glava** ▲ SE Bosnia and Herzegovina
113 I14 **Zelengora** ▲ S Bosnia and Herzegovina
126 I5 **Zelenoborskiy** Murmanskaya Oblast', NW Russian Federation
129 R3 **Zelenodol'sk** Respublika Tatarstan, W Russian Federation
126 G12 **Zelenogorsk** *Fin.* Terijoki. Leningradskaya Oblast', NW Russian Federation
128 K3 **Zelenograd** Moskovskaya Oblast', W Russian Federation
118 B13 **Zelenogradsk** *Ger.* Cranz, Kranz. Kaliningradskaya Oblast', W Russian Federation
129 O15 **Zelenokumsk** Stavropol'skiy Kray, SW Russian Federation
165 X4 **Zelënyy, Ostrov** *var.* Shibotsu-jima. *island* NE Russian Federation
Železna Kapela *see* Eisenkappel
Železna Vrata *see* Demir Kapija
112 L11 **Železniki** Serbia, N Yugoslavia
98 N12 **Zelhem** Gelderland, E Netherlands
113 N18 **Želino** NW FYR Macedonia
113 M14 **Željin** ▲ C Yugoslavia
101 K17 **Zella-Mehlis** Thüringen, C Germany
109 P7 **Zell am See** *var.* Zell-am-See. Salzburg, S Austria
109 N7 **Zell am Ziller** Tirol, W Austria
Zelle *see* Celle
109 W2 **Zellerndorf** Niederösterreich, NE Austria
109 U7 **Zeltweg** Steiermark, S Austria
119 G17 **Zel'va** *Pol.* Zelwa. Hrodzyenskaya Voblasts', W Belarus
118 H13 **Zelva** Ukmergė, C Lithuania
Zelwa *see* Zel'va
99 E16 **Zelzate** *var.* Selzaete. Oost-Vlaanderen, NW Belgium
118 E11 **Žemaičių Aukštumas** *physical region* W Lithuania
118 C12 **Žemaičių Naumiestis** Šilutė, SW Lithuania
Zembin *see* Zyembin
129 N6 **Zemetchino** Penzenskaya Oblast', W Russian Federation
79 M15 **Zémio** Haut-Mbomou, E Central African Republic
41 R16 **Zempoaltepec, Cerro** ▲ SE Mexico
99 G17 **Zemst** Vlaams Brabant, C Belgium
112 L11 **Zemun** Serbia, N Yugoslavia
Zendajan *see* Zendeh Jan
148 J5 **Zendeh Jan** *var.* Zendajan, Zindajān. Herāt, NW Afghanistan
Zengg *see* Senj
112 H12 **Zenica** Federacija Bosna I Hercegovina, C Bosnia and Herzegovina
Zenjan *see* Zanjān
Zen'kov *see* Zin'kiv
Zenshū *see* Chŏnju
Zenta *see* Senta
Zentûzi *see* Zentsūji
82 B11 **Zenza do Itombe** Cuanza Norte, NW Angola
112 H12 **Žepče** Federacija Bosna I Hercegovina, N Bosnia and Herzegovina
23 W12 **Zephyrhills** Florida, SE USA
192 L9 **Zephyr Reef** *reef* Pacific Ocean
158 F9 **Zepu** *var.* Poskam. Xinjiang Uygur Zizhiqu, NW China
147 Q12 **Zeravshan** *Taj./Uzb.* Zarafshon. ≈ Tajikistan/Uzbekistan
Zeravshan *see* Zarafshon
Zeravshanskiy Khrebet *see* Zarafshon, Qatorkŭhi
101 M14 **Zerbst** Sachsen-Anhalt, E Germany
145 P8 **Zerenda** Severnyy Kazakhstan, N Kazakhstan
110 H12 **Żerków** Wielkopolskie, C Poland
108 E11 **Zermatt** Valais, SW Switzerland
Zernest *see* Zărnești
108 J9 **Zernez** Graubünden, SE Switzerland
128 L12 **Zernograd** Rostovskaya Oblast', SW Russian Federation
Zestafoni *see* Zestap'oni
137 S9 **Zestap'oni** *Rus.* Zestafoni. C Georgia
98 H12 **Zestienhoven** ✕ (Rotterdam) Zuid-Holland, SW Netherlands
113 J16 **Zeta** ≈ SW Yugoslavia
8 L6 **Zeta Lake** ◎ Victoria Island, Nunavut, N Canada
98 L12 **Zetten** Gelderland, SE Netherlands
101 M17 **Zeulenroda** Thüringen, C Germany
100 H10 **Zeven** Niedersachsen, NW Germany
98 M12 **Zevenaar** Gelderland, SE Netherlands
99 H14 **Zevenbergen** Noord-Brabant, S Netherlands
131 X6 **Zeya** ≈ SE Russian Federation
Zeya Reservoir *see* Zeyskoye Vodokhranilishche
143 T11 **Zeynalābād** Kermān, C Iran
123 R12 **Zeyskoye Vodokhranilishche** *Eng.* Zeya Reservoir. ⊡ SE Russian Federation
104 H8 **Zêzere, Rio** ≈ C Portugal
Zgerzh *see* Zgierz
138 H6 **Zgharta** N Lebanon
110 K12 **Zgierz** *Ger.* Neuhof, *Rus.* Zgerzh. Łódź, C Poland
111 E14 **Zgorzelec** *Ger.* Görlitz. Dolnośląskie, SW Poland
Zhabdün *see* Zhongba
119 F19 **Zhabinka** *Pol.* Żabinka, *Rus.* Zhabinka. Brestskaya Voblasts', SW Belarus
Zhaggo *see* Luhuo
159 R15 **Zhag'yab** Xizang Zizhiqu, W China
144 L9 **Zhailma** *Kaz.* Zhayylma. Kostanay, N Kazakhstan
145 V16 **Zhalanash** Almaty, SE Kazakhstan
Zhalashash *see* Dzhalagash
145 S7 **Zhalauly, Ozero** ◎ NE Kazakhstan
144 E9 **Zhalpaktal** *prev.* Furmanovo. Zapadnyy Kazakhstan, W Kazakhstan
119 G16 **Zhaludok** *Rus.* Zheludok. Hrodzyenskaya Voblasts', W Belarus
Zhaman-Akkol', Ozero *see* Akkol', Ozero
Zhambyl *see* Taraz
145 Q14 **Zhambyl** *off.* Zhambylskaya Oblast', *Kaz.* Zhambyl Oblysy; *prev.* Dzhambulskaya Oblast'. ◈ *province* S Kazakhstan
Zhambyl Oblysy/Zhambylskaya Oblast' *see* Zhambyl
Zhamo *see* Bomi
145 S12 **Zhamshy** ≈ C Kazakhstan
144 M15 **Zhanadar'ya** Kzylorda, S Kazakhstan
145 O15 **Zhanakorgan** *Kaz.* Zhangaqorghan. Kzylorda, S Kazakhstan
159 N16 **Zhanang** Xizang Zizhiqu, W China
145 T12 **Zhanaortalyk** Zhezkazgan, C Kazakhstan
144 F15 **Zhanaozen** *Kaz.* Zhangaözen, *prev.* Novyy Uzen'. Mangistau, W Kazakhstan
145 Q16 **Zhanatas** Zhambyl, S Kazakhstan
Zhangaözen *see* Zhanaozen
Zhangaqazaly *see* Ayteke Bi
Zhangaqorghan *see* Zhanakorgan
161 O2 **Zhangbei** Hebei, E China
Zhangdian *see* Zibo
163 X9 **Zhangguangcai Ling** ▲ NE China
145 W10 **Zhangiztobe** Vostochnyy Kazakhstan, E Kazakhstan
159 W11 **Zhangjiachuan** Gansu, N China
160 L10 **Zhangjiajie** *var.* Dayong. Hunan, S China
161 O2 **Zhangjiakou** *var.* Changkiakow, Zhang-chia-k'ou, *Eng.* Kalgan; *prev.* Wanchuan. Hebei, E China
161 Q13 **Zhangping** Fujian, SE China
161 Q13 **Zhangpu** Fujian, SE China
163 U11 **Zhangwu** Liaoning, NE China
159 S8 **Zhangye** Gansu, N China
161 Q13 **Zhangzhou** Fujian, SE China
163 W6 **Zhan He** ≈ NE China
Zhänibek *see* Dzhanybek
160 L16 **Zhanjiang** *var.* Chanchiang, Chan-chiang, *Cant.* Tsamkong, *Fr.* Fort-Bayard. Guangdong, S China
Zhansügirov *see* Dzhansugurov
163 V8 **Zhaodong** Heilongjiang, NE China
Zhaoge *see* Qixian
160 H11 **Zhaojue** Sichuan, C China
161 N14 **Zhaoqing** Guangdong, S China
158 H5 **Zhaosu** *var.* Mongolküre. Xinjiang Uygur Zizhiqu, NW China
160 H11 **Zhaotong** Yunnan, SW China
163 V9 **Zhaoyuan** Heilongjiang, NE China
163 V9 **Zhaozhou** Heilongjiang, NE China
145 X13 **Zharbulak** Vostochnyy Kazakhstan, E Kazakhstan
158 J15 **Zhari Namco** ◎ W China
144 I12 **Zharkamys** *Kaz.* Zharqamys. Aktyubinsk, W Kazakhstan
145 W15 **Zharkent** *prev.* Panfilov. Almaty, SE Kazakhstan
126 H17 **Zharkovskiy** Tverskaya Oblast', W Russian Federation
145 W11 **Zharma** Vostochnyy Kazakhstan, E Kazakhstan
144 F14 **Zharmysh** Mangistau, SW Kazakhstan
Zharqamys *see* Zharkamys
118 L13 **Zhary** *Rus.* Zhary. Vitsyebskaya Voblasts', N Belarus
Zhaslyk *see* Jasliq
158 J14 **Zhaxi Co** ◎ W China
Zhayylma *see* Zhailma
Zhdanov *see* Beylăqan, Azerbaijan
Zhdanov *see* Mariupol', Ukraine
Zhe *see* Zhejiang
161 R10 **Zhejiang** *var.* Che-chiang, Chekiang, Zhe, Zhejiang Sheng. ◈ *province* SE China
Zhejiang Sheng *see* Zhejiang
145 S7 **Zhelezinka** Pavlodar, N Kazakhstan
119 C14 **Zheleznodorozhnyy** *Ger.* Gerdauen. Kaliningradskaya Oblast', W Russian Federation
Zheleznodorozhnyy *see* Yemva
128 J7 **Zheleznogorsk** Kurskaya Oblast', W Russian Federation
129 N15 **Zheleznovodsk** Stavropol'skiy Kray, SW Russian Federation
Zhëltyye Vody *see* Zhovti Vody
Zheludok *see* Zhaludok
Zhem *see* Emba
160 K7 **Zhenba** Shaanxi, C China
160 I13 **Zhenfeng** Guizhou, S China
Zhengjiatun *see* Shuangliao
159 X10 **Zhengning** Gansu, N China
163 Q12 **Zhengxiangbai Qi** Nei Mongol Zizhiqu, N China
161 N6 **Zhengzhou** *var.* Ch'eng-chou, Chengchow; *prev.* Chenghsien. Henan, C China
161 R8 **Zhenjiang** *var.* Chenkiang. Jiangsu, E China
163 U9 **Zhenlai** Jilin, NE China
160 I11 **Zhenxiong** Yunnan, SW China
160 K11 **Zhenyuan** *prev.* Wuyang. Guizhou, S China
161 R11 **Zherong** Fujian, SE China
Zhetiqara *see* Dzhetygara
144 F15 **Zhetybay** Mangistau, SW Kazakhstan
145 P17 **Zhetysay** *var.* Dzhetysay. Yuzhnyy Kazakhstan
160 M11 **Zhexi Shuiku** ⊡ C China
145 O12 **Zhezdy** Zhezkazgan, C Kazakhstan
145 O12 **Zhezkazgan** *Kaz.* Zhezqazghan; *prev.* Dzhezkazgan. Zhezkazgan, C Kazakhstan
Zhezqazghan *see* Zhezkazgan
160 M9 **Zhicheng** Hubei, C China
Zhidachov *see* Zhydachiv
159 Q12 **Zhidoi** Qinghai, C China
122 M13 **Zhigalovo** Irkutskaya Oblast', S Russian Federation
129 R6 **Zhigulevsk** Samarskaya Oblast', W Russian Federation
118 D13 **Zhilino** *Ger.* Schillen. Kaliningradskaya Oblast', W Russian Federation
129 O8 **Zhirnovsk** Volgogradskaya Oblast', SW Russian Federation
Zhitarovo *see* Vetren
Zhitkovichi *see* Zhytkavichy
129 P10 **Zhitkur** Volgogradskaya Oblast', SW Russian Federation
Zhitomir *see* Zhytomyr
Zhitomirskaya Oblast' *see* Zhytomyrs'ka Oblast'
128 J5 **Zhizdra** Kaluzhskaya Oblast', W Russian Federation
119 N18 **Zhlobin** Homyel'skaya Voblasts', SE Belarus
Zhmerinka *see* Zhmerynka
116 M7 **Zhmerynka** *Rus.* Zhmerinka. Vinnyts'ka Oblast', C Ukraine
149 R9 **Zhob** *var.* Fort Sandeman. Baluchistān, SW Pakistan
149 R8 **Zhob** ≈ C Pakistan
144 I10 **Zhobda** *prev.* Novoalekseyevka. Aktyubinsk, W Kazakhstan
Zhodino *see* Zhodzina
119 L15 **Zhodzina** *Rus.* Zhodino. Minskaya Voblasts', C Belarus
123 Q5 **Zhokhova, Ostrov** *island* Novosibirskiye Ostrova, NE Russian Federation
Zholkev/Zholkva *see* Zhovkva
Zholsaly *see* Dzhusaly
Zhondor *see* Jondor
158 I15 **Zhongba** *var.* Zhabdün. Xizang Zizhiqu, W China
160 F11 **Zhongdian** Yunnan, SW China
Zhonghua Renmin Gongheguo *see* China
159 V9 **Zhongning** Ningxia, N China
161 N15 **Zhongshan** Guangdong, S China
195 X7 **Zhongshan** *Chinese research station* Antarctica
160 M6 **Zhongtiao Shan** ▲ C China
159 V9 **Zhongwei** Ningxia, N China
160 K9 **Zhongxian** *var.* Zhong Xian. Chongqing Shi, C China
161 N9 **Zhongxiang** Hubei, C China
161 O7 **Zhoukou** *var.* Zhoukouzhen. Henan, C China
Zhoukouzhen *see* Zhoukou
161 S9 **Zhoushan** Zhejiang, S China
161 S9 **Zhoushan Qundao** *Eng.* Zhoushan Islands. *island group* SE China
116 I5 **Zhovkva** *Pol.* Żółkiew, *Rus.* Zholkev, Zholkva; *prev.* Nesterov. L'vivs'ka Oblast', NW Ukraine
117 S7 **Zhovti Vody** *Rus.* Zhëltyye Vody. Dnipropetrovs'ka Oblast', E Ukraine
117 Q10 **Zhovtneve** *Rus.* Zhovtnevoye. Mykolayivs'ka Oblast', S Ukraine
Zhovtnevoye *see* Zhovtneve
114 K9 **Zhrebchevo, Yazovir** ⊡ C Bulgaria
163 V13 **Zhuanghe** Liaoning, NE China
159 W11 **Zhuanglang** Gansu, C China
145 P15 **Zhuantobe** *Kaz.* Zhūantöbe. Yuzhnyy Kazakhstan, S Kazakhstan
161 Q5 **Zhucheng** Shandong, E China
159 V12 **Zhugqu** Gansu, C China
161 N15 **Zhuhai** Guangdong, S China
Zhuizishan *see* Weichang
Zhuji *see* Shangqiu
128 I5 **Zhukovka** Bryanskaya Oblast', W Russian Federation
161 O3 **Zhuozhou** *prev.* Zhuo Xian. Hebei, E China
162 L14 **Zhuozi Shan** ▲ N China
Zhuravichi *see* Zhuravichy
119 O17 **Zhuravichy** *Rus.* Zhuravichi. Homyel'skaya Voblasts', SE Belarus
145 Q8 **Zhuravlevka** Akmola, N Kazakhstan
117 Q4 **Zhurivka** Kyyivs'ka Oblast', N Ukraine
144 J11 **Zhuryn** Aktyubinsk, W Kazakhstan
145 T15 **Zhusandala, Step'** *grassland* SE Kazakhstan
160 L8 **Zhushan** Hubei, C China
161 N11 **Zhuzhou** Hunan, S China
116 I6 **Zhydachiv** *Pol.* Żydaczów, *Rus.* Zhidachov. L'vivs'ka Oblast', NW Ukraine
Zhympity *see* Dzhambeyty
119 K19 **Zhytkavichy** *Rus.* Zhitkovichi. Homyel'skaya Voblasts', SE Belarus
117 N4 **Zhytomyr** *Rus.* Zhitomir. Zhytomyrs'ka Oblast', NW Ukraine
Zhytomyr *see* Zhytomyrs'ka Oblast'
116 M4 **Zhytomyrs'ka Oblast'** *var.* Zhytomyr, *Rus.* Zhitomirskaya Oblast'. ◈ *province* N Ukraine
153 U15 **Zia** ✕ (Dhaka) Dhaka, C Bangladesh
111 J20 **Žiar nad Hronom** *var.* Svätý Kríž nad Hronom, *Ger.* Heiligenkreuz, *Hung.* Garamszentkereszt. Banskobystrický Kraj, C Slovakia
161 Q4 **Zibo** *var.* Zhangdian. Shandong, E China

◆ COUNTRY ● COUNTRY CAPITAL ◇ DEPENDENT TERRITORY ○ DEPENDENT TERRITORY CAPITAL ◈ ADMINISTRATIVE REGION ✕ INTERNATIONAL AIRPORT ▲ MOUNTAIN ▲ MOUNTAIN RANGE VOLCANO ≈ RIVER ◎ LAKE ⊡ RESERVOIR

160 *L4* **Zichang** *prev.* Wayaobu. Shaanxi, C China
Zichenau *see* Ciechanów
111 *G15* **Ziębice** *Ger.* Münsterberg in Schlesien. Dolnośląskie, SW Poland
Ziebingen *see* Cybinka
Ziegenhais *see* Głuchołazy
110 *E12* **Zielona Góra** *Ger.* Grünberg, Grünberg in Schlesien, Grüneberg. Lubuskie, W Poland
99 *F14* **Zierikzee** Zeeland, SW Netherlands
160 *I10* **Zigong** *var.* Tzekung. Sichuan, C China
76 *G12* **Ziguinchor** SW Senegal
41 *N16* **Zihuatanejo** Guerrero, S Mexico
Zilah *see* Zalău
129 *W7* **Zilair** Respublika Bashkortostan, W Russian Federation
136 *L12* **Zile** Tokat, N Turkey
111 *J18* **Žilina** *Ger.* Sillein, ***Hung.*** Zsolna. Žilinský Kraj, N Slovakia
111 *J19* **Žilinský Kraj** ◈ *region* N Slovakia
75 *Q9* **Zillah** *var.* Zallah. C Libya
Zillenmarkt *see* Zalău
109 *N7* **Ziller** ≈ W Austria
Zillertal Alps *see* Zillertaler Alpen
109 *N8* **Zillertaler Alpen** ***Eng.*** Zillertal Alps, ***It.*** Alpi Aurine. ▲ Austria/Italy
118 *K10* **Zilupe** *Ger.* Rosenhof. Ludza, E Latvia
41 *O13* **Zimapán** Hidalgo, C Mexico
83 *I16* **Zimba** Southern, S Zambia
83 *J17* **Zimbabwe** *off.* Republic of Zimbabwe; *prev.* Rhodesia. ◆ *republic* S Africa
116 *H10* **Zimbor** ***Hung.*** Magyarzsombor. Sălaj, NW Romania
Zimmerbude *see* Svetlyy
116 *J15* **Zimnicea** Teleorman, S Romania
114 *L9* **Zimnitsa** Yambol, E Bulgaria
129 *N12* **Zimovniki** Rostovskaya Oblast', SW Russian Federation
Zindajān *see* Zendeh Jan
77 *V12* **Zinder** Zinder, S Niger
77 *W11* **Zinder** ◈ *department* S Niger
77 *P12* **Ziniaré** C Burkina
Zinjan *see* Zanjān
141 *P16* **Zinjibār** SW Yemen
117 *T4* **Zin'kiv** *var.* Zen'kov. Poltavs'ka Oblast', NE Ukraine
Zinov'yevsk *see* Kirovohrad
Zintenhof *see* Sindi
31 *N10* **Zion** Illinois, N USA
54 *F10* **Zipaquirá** Cundinamarca, C Colombia
Zipser Neudorf *see* Spišská Nová Ves
111 *H23* **Zirc** Veszprém, W Hungary
113 *D14* **Žirje** ***It.*** Zuri. *island* S Croatia
Zirknitz *see* Cerknica
108 *M7* **Zirl** Tirol, W Austria
101 *K20* **Zirndorf** Bayern, SE Germany
160 *M11* **Zi Shui** ≈ C China
109 *Y3* **Zistersdorf** Niederösterreich, NE Austria
41 *O14* **Zitácuaro** Michoacán de Ocampo, SW Mexico
101 *Q16* **Zittau** Sachsen, E Germany
112 *I12* **Živinice** Federacija Bosna I Hercegovina, E Bosnia and Herzegovina
Ziwa Magharibi *see* Kagera
81 *J14* **Ziway Hāyk'** ◎ C Ethiopia
161 *N12* **Zixing** Hunan, S China
129 *W7* **Ziyanchurino** Orenburgskaya Oblast', W Russian Federation
160 *K8* **Ziyang** Shaanxi, C China
111 *I20* **Zlaté Moravce** ***Hung.*** Aranyosmarót. Nitriansky Kraj, SW Slovakia
112 *K13* **Zlatibor** ▲ W Yugoslavia
114 *L9* **Zlati Voyvoda** Sliven, E Bulgaria
116 *G11* **Zlatna** *Ger.* Kleinschlatten, *Hung.* Zalatna; *prev. Ger.* Goldmarkt. Alba, C Romania
114 *I8* **Zlatna Panega** Lovech, N Bulgaria
114 *N8* **Zlatni Pyasŭtsi** Dobrich, NE Bulgaria
122 F11 **Zlatoust** Chelyabinskaya Oblast', C Russian Federation
111 *M19* **Zlatý Stôl** *Ger.* Goldener Tisch, ***Hung.*** Aranyosasztal. ▲ C Slovakia
113 *P18* **Zletovo** NE FYR Macedonia
111 *H18* **Zlín** *prev.* Gottwaldov. Zlínský Kraj, SE Czech Republic
113 H19 **Zlinský Kraj** ◈ *region* E Czech Republic
75 *O7* **Zlīṭan** W Libya
110 *F9* **Złocieniec** *Ger.* Falkenburg in Pommern. Zachodniopomorskie, NW Poland
110 *J13* **Złoczew** Sieradz, S Poland
Złoczów *see* Zolochiv
111 *F14* **Złotoryja** *Ger.* Goldberg. Dolnośląskie, W Poland
110 *G9* **Złotów** Wielkopolskie, NW Poland
110 *G13* **Żmigród** *Ger.* Trachenberg. Dolnośląskie, SW Poland
128 *J6* **Zmiyevka** Orlovskaya Oblast', W Russian Federation
117 *V5* **Zmiyiv** Kharkivs'ka Oblast', E Ukraine
Zna *see* Tsna
Znaim *see* Znojmo
128 *M7* **Znamenka** Tambovskaya Oblast', W Russian Federation
Znamenka *see* Znam"yanka
119 *C14* **Znamensk** *Ger.* Wehlau. Kaliningradskaya Oblast', W Russian Federation
117 *R7* **Znam"yanka** ***Rus.*** Znamenka. Kirovohrads'ka Oblast', C Ukraine
110 *H10* **Żnin** Kujawsko-pomorskie, C Poland
111 *F19* **Znojmo** *Ger.* Znaim. Brněnský Kraj, S Czech Republic
79 *N16* **Zobia** Orientale, N Dem. Rep. Congo (Zaire)
83 *N15* **Zóbuè** Tete, NW Mozambique
98 *G12* **Zoetermeer** Zuid-Holland, W Netherlands
108 *E7* **Zofingen** Aargau, N Switzerland
159 *R15* **Zogang** *var.* Wangda. Xizang Zizhiqu, W China
106 *E7* **Zogno** Lombardia, N Italy
142 *M10* **Zohreh, Rūd-e** ≈ SW Iran
160 *H7* **Zoigê** Sichuan, C China
Zółkiew *see* Zhovkva
108 *D8* **Zollikofen** Bern, W Switzerland
Zolochev *see* Zolochiv
117 *U4* **Zolochiv** ***Rus.*** Zolochev. Kharkivs'ka Oblast', E Ukraine
116 *J5* **Zolochiv** ***Pol.*** Złoczów, ***Rus.*** Zolochev. L'vivs'ka Oblast', W Ukraine
117 *X7* **Zolote** ***Rus.*** Zolotoye. Luhans'ka Oblast', E Ukraine
117 *Q6* **Zolotonosha** Cherkas'ka Oblast', C Ukraine
Zolotoye *see* Zolote
Zólyom *see* Zvolen
83 *N15* **Zomba** Southern, S Malawi
Zombor *see* Sombor
99 *D17* **Zomergem** Oost-Vlaanderen, NW Belgium
147 *P11* **Zomin** ***Rus.*** Zaamin. Jizzakh Wiloyati, C Uzbekistan
79 *I15* **Zongo** Equateur, N Dem. Rep. Congo (Zaire)
136 *G10* **Zonguldak** Zonguldak, NW Turkey
136 *H10* **Zonguldak** ◈ *province* NW Turkey
99 *K17* **Zonhoven** Limburg, NE Belgium
142 *J2* **Zonūz** Āẕarbāyjān-e Khāvarī, NW Iran
103 *Y16* **Zonza** Corse, France, C Mediterranean Sea
Zoppot *see* Sopot
Zorgho *see* Zorgo
77 *Q13* **Zorgo** *var.* Zorgho. C Burkina
104 *K10* **Zorita** Extremadura, W Spain
147 *U14* **Zorkŭl** ***Rus.*** Ozero Zorkul'. ◎ SE Tajikistan
Zorkul', Ozero *see* Zorkŭl
56 *A8* **Zorritos** Tumbes, N Peru
111 *J16* **Żory** *var.* Zory, *Ger.* Sohrau. Śląskie, S Poland
76 *K15* **Zorzor** N Liberia
99 *E18* **Zottegem** Oost-Vlaanderen, NW Belgium
77 *R15* **Zou** ≈ S Benin
78 *H6* **Zouar** Borkou-Ennedi-Tibesti, N Chad
76 *J6* **Zouérat** *var.* Zouérate, Zouîrât. Tiris Zemmour, N Mauritania
Zouérate *see* Zouérat
Zoug *see* Zug
Zouîrât *see* Zouérat
76 *M16* **Zoukougbeu** C Ivory Coast
98 *M5* **Zoutkamp** Groningen, NE Netherlands
99 *J18* **Zoutleeuw** *Fr.* Leau. Vlaams Brabant, C Belgium
112 *L9* **Zrenjanin** *prev.* Petrovgrad, Veliki Bečkerek, *Ger.* Grossbetschkerek, ***Hung.*** Nagybecskerek. Serbia, N Yugoslavia
112 *E10* **Zrinska Gora** ▲ C Croatia
Zsablya *see* Žabalj
101 *N16* **Zschopau** ≈ E Germany
Zsebely *see* Jebel
Zsibó *see* Jibou
Zsil/Zsily *see* Jiu
Zsilyvajdevulkán *see* Vulcan
Zsolna *see* Žilina
Zsombolya *see* Jimbolia
Zsupanya *see* Županja
55 *N7* **Zuata** Anzoátegui, NE Venezuela
105 *N14* **Zubia** Andalucía, S Spain
65 *P16* **Zubov Seamount** *undersea feature* E Atlantic Ocean
126 *I16* **Zubtsov** Tverskaya Oblast', W Russian Federation
108 *M8* **Zuckerhütl** ▲ SW Austria
Zueila *see* Zawīlah
76 *M16* **Zuénoula** C Ivory Coast
105 *S5* **Zuera** Aragón, NE Spain
141 *V13* **Ẓufār** *Eng.* Dhofar. *physical region* SW Oman
108 *G8* **Zug** *Fr.* Zoug. Zug, C Switzerland
108 *G8* **Zug** *Fr.* Zoug. ◈ *canton* C Switzerland
137 *R9* **Zugdidi** W Georgia
108 *G8* **Zuger See** ◎ NW Switzerland
101 *K25* **Zugspitze** ▲ S Germany
99 *E15* **Zuid-Beveland** *var.* South Beveland. *island* SW Netherlands
98 *K10* **Zuidelijk-Flevoland** *polder* C Netherlands
Zuider Zee *see* IJsselmeer
98 *G12* **Zuid-Holland** *Eng.* South Holland. ◈ *province* W Netherlands
98 *N5* **Zuidhorn** Groningen, NE Netherlands
98 *O6* **Zuidlaardermeer** ◎ NE Netherlands
98 *O6* **Zuidlaren** Drenthe, NE Netherlands
99 *K14* **Zuid-Willemsvaart Kanaal** *canal* S Netherlands
98 *N8* **Zuidwolde** Drenthe, NE Netherlands
Zuitaizi *see* Kangxian
105 *O14* **Zújar** Andalucía, S Spain
104 *L11* **Zújar** ≈ W Spain
104 *L11* **Zújar, Embalse del** ▣ W Spain
80 *J9* **Zula** E Eritrea
54 *G6* **Zulia** *off.* Estado Zulia. ◈ *state* NW Venezuela
Zullapara *see* Sinchaingbyin
Züllichau *see* Sulechów
105 *P3* **Zumárraga** País Vasco, N Spain
112 *D8* **Žumberačko Gorje** *var.* Gorjanči, Uskocke Planine, Žumberak, *Ger.* Uskokengebirge; ***prev.*** Sichelbuger Gebirge. ▲ Croatia/Slovenia *see also* Gorjanci
Žumberak *see* Gorjanci/Žumberačko Gorje
194 *K7* **Zumberge Coast** *coastal feature* Antarctica
Zumbo *see* Vila do Zumbo
29 *W10* **Zumbro Falls** Minnesota, N USA
29 *W10* **Zumbro River** ≈ Minnesota, N USA
29 *W10* **Zumbrota** Minnesota, N USA
99 *H15* **Zundert** Noord-Brabant, S Netherlands
Zungaria *see* Dzungaria
77 *U14* **Zungeru** Niger, C Nigeria
37 *O11* **Zuni** New Mexico, SW USA
37 *P11* **Zuni Mountains** ▲ New Mexico, SW USA
160 *J11* **Zunyi** Guizhou, S China
160 *J15* **Zuo Jiang** ≈ China/Vietnam
108 *J9* **Zuoz** Graubünden, SE Switzerland
112 *I10* **Županja** ***Hung.*** Zsupanya. Vukovar-Srijem, E Croatia
113 *M17* **Žur** Serbia, S Yugoslavia
129 *T2* **Zura** Udmurtskaya Respublika, NW Russian Federation
139 *V8* **Zurbāṭīyah** E Iraq
Zuri *see* Žirje
108 *F7* **Zürich** ***Eng./Fr.*** Zurich, ***It.*** Zurigo. Zürich, N Switzerland
108 *G6* **Zürich** ***Eng./Fr.*** Zurich. ◈ *canton* N Switzerland
Zurich, Lake *see* Zürichsee
108 *G7* **Zürichsee** ***Eng.*** Lake Zurich. ◎ NE Switzerland
Zurigo *see* Zürich
149 *V1* **Zŭrkŭl** ***Pash.*** Sarī Qūl, ***Rus.*** Ozero Zurkul'. ◎ Afghanistan/Tajikistan ***see also*** Sarī Qūl
Zurkul', Ozero *see* Sarī Qūl/Zŭrkŭl
110 *K10* **Żuromin** Mazowieckie, N Poland
108 *J8* **Zürs** Vorarlberg, W Austria
77 *T13* **Zuru** Kebbi, W Nigeria
108 *F6* **Zurzach** Aargau, N Switzerland
101 *J22* **Zusam** ≈ S Germany
98 *M11* **Zutphen** Gelderland, E Netherlands
75 *N7* **Zuwārah** NW Libya
Zuwaylah *see* Zawīlah
127 *R14* **Zuyevka** Kirovskaya Oblast', NW Russian Federation
161 *N10* **Zuzhou** Hunan, S China
Zvenigorodka *see* Zvenyhorodka
117 *P6* **Zvenyhorodka** ***Rus.*** Zvenigorodka. Cherkas'ka Oblast', C Ukraine
123 *N12* **Zvezdnyy** Irkutskaya Oblast', C Russian Federation
83 *K18* **Zvishavane** ***prev.*** Shabani. Matabeleland South, S Zimbabwe
111 *J20* **Zvolen** *Ger.* Altsohl, ***Hung.*** Zólyom. Banskobystrický Kraj, C Slovakia
112 *J12* **Zvornik** E Bosnia and Herzegovina
98 *M5* **Zwaagwesteinde** ***Fris.*** De Westerein. Friesland, N Netherlands
98 *H10* **Zwanenburg** Noord-Holland, C Netherlands
98 *L8* **Zwarte Meer** ◎ N Netherlands
98 *M9* **Zwarte Water** ≈ N Netherlands
98 *M8* **Zwartsluis** Overijssel, E Netherlands
76 *L17* **Zwedru** *var.* Tchien. E Liberia
98 *O8* **Zweeloo** Drenthe, NE Netherlands
101 *E20* **Zweibrücken** *Fr.* Deux-Ponts; ***Lat.*** Bipontium. Rheinland-Pfalz, SW Germany
108 *D9* **Zweisimmen** Fribourg, W Switzerland
101 *M15* **Zwenkau** Sachsen, E Germany
109 *V3* **Zwettl** Wien, NE Austria
109 *T3* **Zwettl an der Rodl** Oberösterreich, N Austria
99 *D18* **Zwevegem** West-Vlaanderen, W Belgium
101 *M17* **Zwickau** Sachsen, E Germany
101 *O21* **Zwiesel** Bayern, SE Germany
98 *H13* **Zwijndrecht** Zuid-Holland, SW Netherlands
101 *N16* **Zwikauer Mulde** ≈ E Germany
Zwischenwässern *see* Medvode
Zwittau *see* Svitavy
110 *N13* **Zwoleń** Mazowieckie, SE Poland
98 *M9* **Zwolle** Overijssel, E Netherlands
22 *G6* **Zwolle** Louisiana, S USA
110 *K12* **Żychlin** Łodzkie, C Poland
Żydaczów *see* Zhydachiv
119 *L14* **Zyembin** ***Rus.*** Zembin. Minskaya Voblasts', C Belarus
Zyôetu *see* Jōetsu
110 *L12* **Żyrardów** Mazowieckie, C Poland
123 S8 **Zyryanka** Respublika Sakha (Yakutiya), NE Russian Federation
145 *Y9* **Zyryanovsk** Vostochnyy Kazakhstan, E Kazakhstan
111 *J17* **Żywiec** *Ger.* Bäckermühle Schulzenmühle. Śląskie, S Poland

◆ Country ● Country Capital ◇ Dependent Territory ○ Dependent Territory Capital ◈ Administrative Region ✕ International Airport ▲ Mountain ▲ Mountain Range ⩕ Volcano ≈ River ◎ Lake ▣ Reservoir

PICTURE CREDITS

DORLING KINDERSLEY *would like to express their thanks to the following individuals, companies, and institutions for their help in preparing this atlas.*

Earth Resource Mapping Ltd., Egham, Surrey
Brian Groombridge, World Conservation Monitoring Centre, Cambridge
The British Library, London
British Library of Political and Economic Science, London
The British Museum, London
The City Business Library, London
King's College, London
National Meteorological Library and Archive, Bracknell
The Printed Word, London
The Royal Geographical Society, London
University of London Library
Paul Beardmore
Philip Boyes
Hayley Crockford
Alistair Dougal
Reg Grant
Louise Keane
Zoe Livesley
Laura Porter
Jeff Eidenshink
Chris Hornby
Rachelle Smith
Ray Pinchard
Robert Meisner
Fiona Strawbridge

Every effort has been made to trace the copyright holders and we apologize in advance for any unintentional omissions. We would be pleased to insert the appropriate acknowledgment in any subsequent edition of this publication.

Adams Picture Library: 86CLA; **G Andrews:** 186CR; **Ardea London Ltd:** K Ghana 150C; M Iljima 132TC; R Waller 148TR; Art Directors **Aspect Picture Library:** P Carmichael 160TR; 131CR(below); G Tompkinson 190TRB; **Axiom:** C Bradley 148CA, 158CA; J Holmes xivCRA, xxivBCR, xxviiCRB, 150TCR, 165C(below), 166TL, J Morris 75TL, 77CRB, J Spaull 134BL; **Bridgeman Art Library, London / New York:** Collection of the Earl of Pembroke, Wilton House xxBC; **The J. Allan Cash Photolibrary:** xlBR, xliiCLA, xlivCL, 10BC, 60CL, 69CLB, 70CL, 72CLB, 75BR, 76BC, 87BL, 109BR, 138BCL, 141TL, 154CR, 178BR, 181TR; **Bruce Coleman Ltd:** 86BC, 98CL, 100TC; S Alden 192BC(below); Atlantide xxviTCR, 138BR; E Bjurstrom 141BR; S Bond 96CRB; T Buchholz xvCL, 92TR, 123TCL; J Burton xxiiiC; J Cancalosi 181TRB; B J Coates xxvBL, 192CL; B Coleman 63TL; B & C Colhoun 2TR, 36CB; A Compost xxiiiCBR; Dr S Coyne 45TL; G Cubitt xviTCL, 169BR, 178TR, 184TR; P Davey xxviiCLB, 121TL(below); N Devore 189CBL; S J Doylee xxiiCRR; H Flygare xviiCRA; M P L Fogden 17C(above) ; Jeff Foott Productions xxiiiCRB, 11CRA; M Freeman 91BRA; P van Gaalen 86TR; G Gualco 140C; B Henderson 194CR; Dr C Henneghien 69C; HPH Photography, H Van den Berg 69CR; C Hughes 69BCL; C James xxxixTC; J Johnson 39CR, 197TR; J Jurka 91CA; S C Kaufman 28C; S J Krasemann 33TR; H Lange 10TRB, 68CA; C Lockwood 32BC; L C Marigo xxiiBC, xxviiCLA, 49CRA, 59BR; M McCoy 187TR; D Meredith 3CR; J Murray xvCR, 179BR; Orion Press 165CR(above); Orion Services & Trading Co. Inc. 164CR; C Ott 17BL; Dr E Pott 9TR, 40CL, 87C, 93TL, 194CLB; F Prenzel 186BC, 193BC; M Read 42BR, 43CRB; H Reinhard xxiiCR, xxviiTR, 194BR; L Lee Rue III 151BCL; J Shaw xixTL; K N Swenson 194BC; P Terry 115CR; N Tomalin 54BCL; P Ward 78TC; S Widstrand 57TR; K Wothe 91C, 173TCL; J T Wright 127BR; **Colorific:** Black Star / L Mulvehil 156CL; Black Star / R Rogers 57BR; Black Star / J Rupp 161BCR; Camera Tres / C. Meyer 59BRA; R Caputo / Matrix 78CL; J. Hill 117CLB; M Koene 55TR; G Satterley xliiCLAR; M Yamashita 156BL, 167CR(above); **Comstock:** 108CRB; Corbis UK Ltd: 170TR, 170BL; **D Cousens:** 147 CRA; **Sue Cunningham Photographic:** 51CR; S Alden 192BC(below) **James Davis Travel Photography:** xxxviTCB, xxxviTR, xxxviCL, 13CA, 19BC, 49TLB, 56BCR, 57CLA, 61BCL, 93BC, 94TC, 102TR, 120CB, 158BC, 179CRA, 191BR; **G Dunnet:** 124CA; **Environmental Picture Library:** Chris Westwood 126C; **Eye Ubiquitous:** xlCA; L. Fordyce 12CLA; L Johnstone 6CRA, 28BLA, 30CB; S. Miller xxiCA; M Southern 73BLA; **Chris Fairclough Colour Library:** xliBR; **Ffotograff:** N. Tapsell 158CL **FLPA -Images of nature:** 123TR; **Geoscience Features:** xviBCR, xviBR, 102CL, 108BC, 122BR; Solar Film 64TC; **gettyone stone**: 131BC, 133BR, 164CR(above); G Johnson 130BL; R Passmore 120TR; D Austen 187CL; G Allison 186CL; L Ulrich 17TL; M Vines 17BL; R Wells 193BL; **Robert Harding Picture Library:** xviiTC, xxivCR, xxxC, xxxvTC, 2TLB, 3CA, 15CRB, 15CR, 37BC, 38CRA, 50BL, 95BR, 99CR, 114CR, 122BL, 131CLA, 142CB, 143TL, 147TR, 168TR, 168CA, 166BR; P G. Adam 13TCB; D Atchison-Jones 70BLA; J Bayne 72BCL; B Schuster 80CR; C Bowman 50BR, 53CA, 62CL, 70CRL; C Campbell xxiBC; G Corrigan 159CRB, 161CRB; P Craven xxxvBL; R Cundy 69BR; Delu 79BC; A Durand 111BR; Financial Times 142BR; R Frerck 51BL; T Gervis 3BCL, 7CR; I Griffiths xxxCL, 77TL; T Hall 166CRA; D Harney 142CA; S Harris xliiiBCL; G Hellier xvCRB, 135BL; F Jackson 137BCR; Jacobs xxxviiTL; P Koch 139TR; F Joseph Land 122TR; Y Marcoux 9BR; S Massif xvBC; A Mills 88CLB; L Murray 114TR; R Rainford xlivBL; G Renner 74CB, 194C; C Rennie 48CL, 116BR; R Richardson 118CL; P Van Riel 48BR; E Rooney 124TR; Sassoon xxivCL, 148CLB; P Scholey 176TR; M Short 137TL; E Simanor xxviiCR; V Southwell 139CR; J Strachan 42TR, 111BL, 132BCR; C Tokeley 131CLA; A C Waltham 161C; T Waltham xviiBL, xxiiCLLL, 138CRB; Westlight 37CR; N Wheeler 139BL; A Williams xxxviiiBR, xlTR; A Woolfitt 95BRA; Paul Harris: 168TC; **Hutchison Library:** 131CR (above) 6BL; P. Collomb 137CR; C. Dodwell 130TR; S Errington 70BCL; P. Hellyer 142BC; J. Horner xxxiTC; R. Ian Lloyd 134CRA; N. Durrell McKenna xxviBCR; J.Nowell 135CLB, 143TC; A Zvoznikov xxiiCL; **Image Bank:** 87BR; J Banagan 190BCA; A Becker xxivBCL; M Khansa 121CR, M Isy-Schwart 193CR(above), 191CL; Khansa K Forest 163TR; Lomeo xxivTCR; T Madison 170TL(below); C Molyneux xxiiCRRR; C Navajas xviiiTR; Ocean Images Inc. 192CLB; J van Os xviiTCR; S Proehl 6CL; T Rakke xixTC, 64CL; M Reitz 196CA; M Romanelli 166CL(below); G A Rossi 151BCR, 176BLA; B Roussel 109TL; S Satushek xviiBCR; Stock Photos / J M Spielman xxivTRL; **Images Colour Library:** xxiiCLL, xxxixTR, xliCR, xliiiBL, 3BR, 19BR, 37TL, 44TL, 62TC, 91BR, 102CLB, 103CR, 150CL, 180CA; 164BC, 165TL; **Impact Photos:** J & G Andrews 186BL; C. Bluntzer 156BR; Cosmos / G. Buthaud 65BC; S Franklin 126BL; A. le Garsmeur 131C; A Indge xxviiTC; C Jones xxxiCB, 70BL; V. Nemirousky 137BR; J Nicholl 76TCR; C. Penn 187C(below); G Sweeney xviiBR, 196CB, 196TR, J & G Andrews 186TR; **JVZ Picture Library:** T Nilson 135TC; **Frank Lane Picture Agency:** xxiTCR, xxiiiBL, 93TR; A Christiansen 58CRA; J Holmes xivBL; S. McCutcheon 3C; Silvestris 173TCR; D Smith xxiiBCL; W Wisniewsli 195BR; **Leeds Castle Foundation:** xxxviiBC; **Magnum:** Abbas 83CR, 136CA; S Franklin 134CRB; D Hurn 4BCL; P. Jones-Griffiths 191BL; H Kubota xviBCL, 156CLB; F Maver xviBL; S McCurry 73CL, 133BCR; G. Rodger 74TR; C Steele Perkins 72BL; **Mountain Camera / John Cleare:** 153TR; C Monteath 153CR; **Nature Photographers:** E.A. Janes 112CL; **Natural Science Photos:** M Andera 110C; **Network Photographers Ltd.:** C Sappa / Rapho 119BL; **N.H.P.A.:** N. J. Dennis xxiiiCL; D Heuchlin xxiiiCLA; S Krasemann 15BL, 25BR, 38TC; K Schafer 49CB; R Tidman 160CLB; D Tomlinson 145CR; M Wendler 48TR; **Nottingham Trent University:** T Waltham xivCL, xvBR; **Novosti:** 144BLA; **Oxford Scientific Films:** D Allan xxiiTR; H R Bardarson xviiiBC; D Bown xxiiiCBLL; M Brown 140BL; M Colbeck 147CAR; W Faidley 3TL; L Gould xxiiiTRB; D Guravich xxiiiTR; P Hammerschmidy / Okapia 87CLA; M Hill 57TL, 195TR; C Menteath ; J Netherton 2CRB; S Osolinski 82CA; R Packwood 72CA; M Pitts 179TC; N Rosing xxiiiCBL, 9TR, 197BR; D Simonson 57C; Survival Anglia / C Catton 137TR; R Toms xxiiiBR; K Wothe xxiBL, xviiCLA; **Panos Pictures:** B Aris 133C; P Barker xxivBR; T Bolstao 153BR; N Cooper 82CB, 153TC; J-L Dugast 166C(below), 167BR; J Hartley 73CA, 90CL; J Holmes 149BC; J Morris 76CLB; M Rose 146TR; D Sansoni 155CL; C Stowers 163TL; **Edward Parker:** 49TL, 49CLB; **Pictor International:** xivBR, xvBRA, xixTCL, xxCL, 3CLA, 17BR, 20TR, 20CRB, 23BCA, 23CL, 26CB, 27BC, 30CA, 33TRB, 34BC, 34BR, 34CR, 38CB, 38CL, 43CL, 63BR, 65TC, 82CL, 83CLB, 99BR, 107CLA, 166TR, 171CL(above), 180CLB, 185TL; **Pictures Colour Library:** xxiBCL, xxiiBR, xxviBCL, 6BR, 15TR, 8TR, 16CL(above), 19TL, 20BL, 24C, 24CLA, 27TR, 32TRB, 36BC, 41CA, 43CRA, 68BL, 90TCB, 94BL, 99BL, 106CA, 107CLB, 107CR, 107BR, 117BL, 164BC, 192BL, K Forest 165TL(below); **Planet Earth Pictures:** 193CR(below); D Barrett 148CB, 184CA; R Coomber 16BL; G Douwma 172BR; E Edmonds 173BR; J Lythgoe 196BL; A Mounter 172CR; M Potts 6CA; P Scoones xxTR; J Walencik 110TR; J Waters 53BCL; **Popperfoto:** Reuters / J Drake xxxiiCLA; **Rex Features:** 165CR; Antelope xxxiiCLB; M Friedel xxiCR; I McIlgorm xxxCBR; J Shelley xxxCR; Sipa Press xxxCR; Sipa Press / Alix xxxCBL; Sipa Press / Chamussy 176BL; **Robert Harding Picture Library:** C. Tokeley 131TL; J Strachan 132BL; Franz Joseph Land 122TR; Franz Joseph Land 364/7088 123BL, 169C(above), 170C(above), 168CL, Tony Waltham 186CR(below), Y Marcoux 9BR; **Russia & Republics Photolibrary:** M Wadlow 118CR, 119CL, 124BC, 124CL, 125TL, 125BR, 126TCR; **Science Photo Library:** Earth Satellite Corporation xixTRB, xxxiCR, 49BCL; F Gohier xiCR; J Heseltine xviTCB; K Kent xvBLA; P Menzell xvBL; N.A.S.A. xBC; D Parker xivBC; University of Cambridge Collection Air Pictures 87CLB; RJ Wainscoat / P Arnold, Inc. xiBC; D Weintraub xiBL; **South American Pictures:** 57BL, 62TR; R Francis 52BL; Guyana Space Centre 50TR; T Morrison 49CRB, 49BL, 50CR, 52TR, 54TR, 60BL, 61C; **Southampton Oceanography:** xviiiBL; **Sovofoto / Eastfoto:** xxxiiCBR; **Spectrum Colour Library:** 50BC, 160BC; J King 145BR; **Frank Spooner Pictures:** Gamma-Liason/Vogel 131CL(above); 26CRB; E. Baitel xxxiiBC; Bernstein xxxiCL; Contrast 112CR; Diard / Photo News 113CL; Liaison / C. Hires xxxiiTCB; Liaison / Nickelsberg xxxiiTR; Marleen 113TL; Novosti 116CA; P. Piel xxxCA; N Quidu 135CL; H Stucke 188CLB, 190CA; Torrengo / Figaro 78BR; A Zamur 113BL; **Still Pictures:** C Caldicott 77TC; A Crump 189CL; M & C Denis-Huot xxiiBL, 78CR, 81BL; M Edwards xxiCRL, 53BL, 64CR, 69BLA, 155BR; J Frebet 53CLB; H Giradet 53TC; E Parker 52CL; M Gunther 121BC; **Tony Stone Images:** xxviTR, 4CA, 7BL, 7CL, 13CRB, 39BR, 58C, 97BC, 101BR, 106TR, 109CL, 109CRB, 164CLB, 165C,180CB, 181BR, 188BC, 192TR; G Allison 18TR, 31CRB, 187CRB; D Armand 14TCB; D Austen 180TR, 186CL, 187CL; J Beatty 74CL; O Benn xxviBR; K Biggs xxiTL; R Bradbury 44BR; R A Butcher xxviTL; J Callahan xxviiCRA; P Chesley 185BCL, 188C; W Clay 30BL, 31CRA; J Cornish 96BL, 107TL; C Condina 41CB; T Craddock xxivTR; P Degginger 36CLB; Demetrio 5BR; N DeVore xxivBC; A Diesendruck 60BR; S Egan 87CRA, 96BR; R Elliot xxiiBCR; S Elmore 19C; J Garrett 73CR; S Grandadam 14BR; R Grosskopf 28BL; D Hanson 104BC; C Harvey 69TL; G Hellier 110BL, 165CR; S Huber 103CRB; D Hughs xxxiBR; A Husmo 91TR; G Irvine 31BC; J Jangoux 58CL; D Johnston xviiTR; A Kehr 113C; R Koskas xviTR; J Lamb 96CRA; J Lawrence 75CRA; L Lefkowitz 7CA; M Lewis 45CLA; S Mayman 55BR; Murray & Associates 45CR; G Norways 104CA; N Parfitt xxviiCL, 68TCR, 81TL; R Passmore 121TR; N Press xviBCA; E Pritchard 88CA, 90CLR; T Raymond 21BL, 29TR; L Resnick 74BR; M Rogers 80BR; A Sacks 28TCB; C Saule 90CR; S Schulhof xxivTC; P Seaward 34CL; M Segal 32BL; V Shenai 152CL; R Sherman 26CL; H Sitton 136CR; R Smith xxvBLA, 56C; S Studd 108CLA; H Strand 49BR, 63TR; P Tweedie 177CR; L Ulrich 17BL; M Vines 17TC; A B Wadham 60CR; J Warden 63CLB; R Wells 23CRA, 193BL; G Yeowell 34BL; **Telegraph Colour Library:** 61CRB, 61TCR, 157TL; R Antrobus xxxixBR; J Sims 26BR; **Topham Picturepoint:** xxxiCBL, 162BR, 168TR, 168BC; **Travel Ink:** A Cowin 88TR; **Trip:** 140BR, 144CA, 155CRA; B Ashe 159TR; D Cole 190BCL, 190CR; D Davis 89BL; I Deineko xxxiTR; J Dennis 22BL; Dinodia 154CL; Eye Ubiquitous / L Fordyce 2CLB; A Gasson 149CR; W Jacobs 43TL, 54BL, 177BC, 178CLA, 185BCR, 186BL; P Kingsbury 112C; K Knight 177BR; V Kolpakov 147BL; T Noorits 87TL, 119BR, 146CL; R Power 41TR; N Ray 166BL, 168TC; C Rennie 116CLB; V Sidoropolev 145TR; E Smith 183BC, 183TL; **Woodfin Camp & Associates:** 92BLR; **World Pictures:** xvCRA, xviiCRA, 9CRB, 22CL, 23BC, 24BL, 35BL, 40TR, 51TR, 71BR, 80TCR, 82TR, 83BL, 86BCR, 96TC, 98BL, 100CR, 101CR, 103BC, 105TC, 157BL, 161BCL, 162CLB, 172CLB, 172BC, 179BL, 182CB, 183C, 184CL, 185CR; 121BR, 121TT; **Zefa Picture Library:** xviBLR, xviiBCL, xviiiCL, 3CL, 8BC, 8CT, 9CR, 13BC, 14TC, 16TR, 21TL, 22CRB, 25BL, 32TCR, 36BCR, 59BCL, 65TCL, 69CLA, 79TL, 81BR, 87CRB, 92C, 98C, 99TL, 100BL, 107TR, 118CRB, 120BL; 122C(below), 124CLA, 164BR, 183TR; Anatol 113BR; Barone 114BL; Brandenburg 5C; A J Brown 44TR; H J Clauss 55CLB; Damm 71BC; Evert 92BL; W Felger 3BL; J Fields 189CRA; R Frerck 4BL; G Heil 56BR; K Heibig 115BR; Heilman 28BC; Hunter 8C; Kitchen 10TR, 8CL, 8BL, 9TR; Dr H Kramarz 7BLA, 123CR(below); Mehlio 155BL; J F Raga 24TR; Rossenbach 105BR; Streichan 89TL; T Stewart 13TR, 19CR; Sunak 54BR, 162TR; D H Teuffen 95TL; B Zaunders 40BC. **Additional Photography:** Geoff Dann; Rob Reichenfeld; H Taylor; Jerry Young.